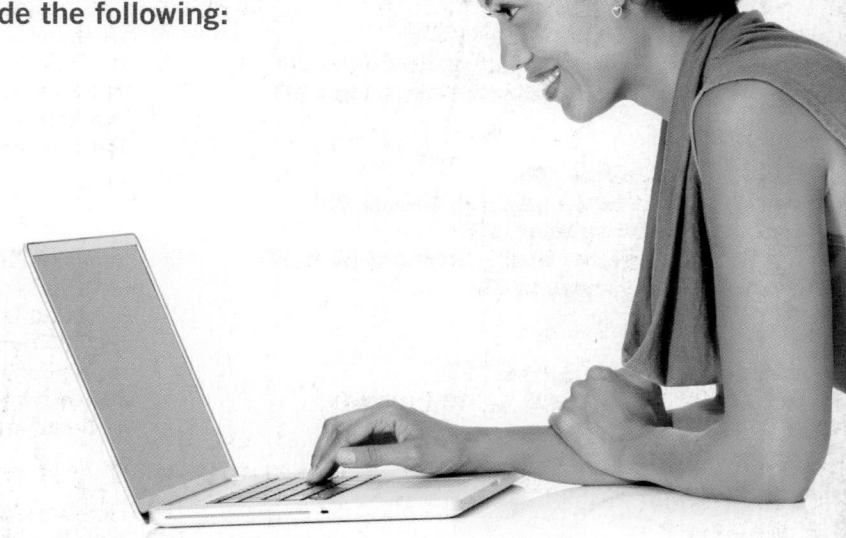

Maternal Child Nursing Care

SIXTH EDITION

MATERNITY

Shannon E. Perry, RN, PhD, FAAN
Professor Emerita, School of Nursing
San Francisco State University
San Francisco, California

Deitra Leonard Lowdermilk, RNC, PhD, FAAN
Clinical Professor Emerita, School of Nursing
University of North Carolina at Chapel Hill
Chapel Hill, North Carolina

Kitty Cashion, RN-BC, MSN
Clinical Nurse Specialist, College of Medicine,
    Department of Obstetrics and Gynecology, Division
    of Maternal-Fetal Medicine
University of Tennessee Health Science Center
Memphis, Tennessee

Kathryn Rhodes Alden, EdD, MSN, RN, IBCLC
Associate Professor, School of Nursing
University of North Carolina at Chapel Hill
Chapel Hill, North Carolina

Associate Editor

Ellen F. Olshansky, PhD, RN, WHNP-BC, NC-BC, FAAN
Professor and Chair, Department of Nursing
Suzanne Dworak-Peck School of Social Work
University of Southern California
Los Angeles, California

PEDIATRIC

Marilyn J. Hockenberry, PhD, RN, PPCNP-BC, FAAN
Bessie Baker Professor of Nursing and Professor of
    Pediatrics
Associate Dean of Research Affairs, School of Nursing
Chair, Duke Institutional Review Board
Duke University
Durham, North Carolina

David Wilson, MS, RNC-NIC (deceased)
Staff
Children's Hospital at Saint Francis
Tulsa, Oklahoma

Cheryl C. Rodgers, PhD, RN, CPNP, CPON
Assistant Professor
Duke University School of Nursing
Durham, North Carolina

ELSEVIER

ELSEVIER

3251 Riverport Lane
St. Louis, Missouri 63043

MATERNAL CHILD NURSING CARE, SIXTH EDITION

ISBN: 978-0-323-54938-7

Notices

Practitioners and researchers must always rely on their own experience and knowledge in evaluating and using any information, methods, compounds or experiments described herein. Because of rapid advances in the medical sciences, in particular, independent verification of diagnoses and drug dosages should be made. To the fullest extent of the law, no responsibility is assumed by Elsevier, authors, editors or contributors for any injury and/or damage to persons or property as a matter of products liability, negligence or otherwise, or from any use or operation of any methods, products, instructions, or ideas contained in the material herein.

Previous editions copyrighted 2014, 2010, 2006, 2002, and 1998.

Library of Congress Cataloging-in-Publication Data

Names: Perry, Shannon E., author. | Olshansky, Ellen Frances, 1949- editor.
Title: Maternal child nursing care : maternity pediatrics / Shannon E. Perry, Marilyn J. Hockenberry, Deitra Leonard Lowdermilk, David Wilson, Kitty Cashion, Cheryl C. Rodgers, Kathryn Rhodes Alden ; associate editor, Ellen Olshansky.
Description: Sixth edition. | St. Louis, Missouri : Elsevier, [2018] | Includes bibliographical references and index.
Identifiers: LCCN 2017036656 | ISBN 9780323549387 (hardcover : alk. paper)
Subjects: | MESH: Maternal-Child Nursing–methods | Pediatric Nursing–methods | Maternal Health | Infant Health | Child Health
Classification: LCC RG951 | NLM WY 157.3 | DDC 618.92/00231–dc23 LC record available at https://lccn.loc.gov/2017036656

Senior Content Strategist: Sandra Clark
Senior Content Development Specialist: Heather Bays
Publishing Services Manager: Julie Eddy
Book Production Specialist: Clay S. Broeker
Design Direction: Brian Salisbury

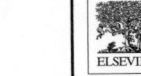
Printed in Canada

Last digit is the print number: 9 8 7 6 5 4 3 2

Debbie Fraser, MN, RNC-NIC
Associate Professor
Director
Nurse Practitioner Program
Faculty of Health Disciplines
Athabasca University
Advanced Practice Nurse
NICU St. Boniface Hospital
Winnipeg, Canada

Pat Mahaffee Gingrich, MSN, RN, WHNP-BC
Assistant Professor
School of Nursing
University of North Carolina at Chapel Hill
Chapel Hill, North Carolina

Evolve Contributors

Key Points
Joanna Cain, BSN, BA, RN
President and Founder
Auctorial Pursuits, Inc.
Austin, Texas

Review Questions
Daryle Wane, PhD, ARNP, FNP-BC
Baccalaureate Degree Nursing Program Director
Professor of Nursing
BSN Faculty
Pasco-Hernando State College
New Port Richey, Florida

Test Bank
Linda Turchin, RNH, MSN, CNE
Assistant Professor, Nursing
Fairmont State University
Fairmont, West Virginia

REVIEWERS

Michael D. Aldridge, PhD, RN, CNE
Assistant Professor of Nursing
Pediatric Nursing
Concordia University Texas
Austin, Texas

Sandy Barker, RN, MSN
Master Nursing Instructor
Nursing
Tennessee College of Applied Technology
Elizabethton, Tennessee

Judy Carlyle, MSN, RN
Faculty
Arkansas Rural Nursing Education Consortium
Nashville, Arkansas

Brigit Carter, PhD, RN, CCRN
Assistant Professor
School of Nursing
Duke University
Durham, North Carolina

Janie Corbitt, RN, MLS
Instructor of Nursing (retired)
Milledgeville, Georgia

Stephanie Evans, PhD, APRN, PNP-PC
Assistant Professor
Harris College of Nursing and Health Sciences
Texas Christian University
Fort Worth, Texas

Vanessa Lynn Flannery, MSN, PHCNS-BC, CNE
Associate Professor
Morehead State University
Morehead, Kentucky

Kari Gali, DNP, RN, CPNP
Post-Doctoral Fellow
Case Western Reserve University
Cleveland, Ohio

Terry Hadler, MSN, RN
Assistant Professor
Dakota Wesleyan University
Mitchell, South Dakota

Teresa Howell, DNP, RN, CNE
Department of Nursing
Morehead State University
Morehead, Kentucky

Kathleen S. Jordon, DNP, MS, FNP-BC, ENP-BC, SANE-P
Clinical Assistant Professor
School of Nursing
University of North Carolina at Charlotte
Nurse Practitioner
Emergency Department
Mid-Atlantic Emergency Medicine Associates
Charlotte, North Carolina

Christina D. Keller, MSN, RN, CHS
Instructor
Nursing
Radford University Clinical Simulation Center
Radford, Virginia

Rebecca M. Padgett, MSN, RN
Nursing Faculty
Jefferson Davis Community College
Brewton, Alabama

Latoya Rawlins, DNP, RN-BC, CNE
Assistant Professor
School of Nursing
Rutgers, The State University of New Jersey
New Brunswick, New Jersey

Debra Lee Stayer, RN, PhD, CCRN-K
Assistant Professor
Nursing
Bloomsburg University
Bloomsburg, Pennsylvania

Michelle Van Wyhe, DNP, ARNP-BC
Professor of Nursing
Northwestern College
Nurse Practitioner
Orange City Area Health System
Orange City, Iowa

Donna Wilsker, RN, BSN, MSN
Assistant Professor
Nursing
Lamar University
Beaumont, Texas

MATERNITY

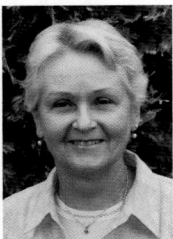

Shannon E. Perry is Professor Emerita, School of Nursing, San Francisco State University, San Francisco, California. She received her diploma in nursing from St. Joseph Hospital School of Nursing, Bloomington, Illinois; a BSN from Marquette University; an MSN from the University of Colorado Medical Center; and a PhD in Educational Psychology from Arizona State University. She completed a 2-year postdoctoral fellowship in perinatal nursing at the University of California, San Francisco, as a Robert Wood Johnson Clinical Nurse Scholar.

Dr. Perry has had clinical experience in obstetrics, pediatrics, gynecology, and neonatal nursing. She has taught in schools of nursing in several states for over 30 years and was director of the School of Nursing at San Francisco State University. She is a Fellow in the American Academy of Nursing. Dr. Perry's experience in international nursing includes teaching in the United Kingdom, Ireland, Italy, Thailand, Ghana, and China, as well as participating in health missions in Ghana, Kenya, and Honduras.

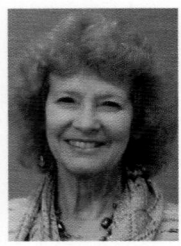

Deitra Leonard Lowdermilk is Clinical Professor Emerita, School of Nursing, University of North Carolina at Chapel Hill. She received her BSN from East Carolina University and her MEd and PhD in Education from the University of North Carolina at Chapel Hill. She is certified in in-patient obstetrics by the National Certification Corporation. She is a Fellow in the American Academy of Nursing. In addition to being a nurse educator for more than 34 years, Dr. Lowdermilk has clinical experience in maternity and women's health care.

Dr. Lowdermilk has been recognized for her expertise in nursing education and women's health by state and national nursing organizations and by her alma mater, East Carolina University. A few examples include Educator of the Year by the Association of Women's Health, Obstetric and Neonatal Nurses and by the North Carolina Nurses Association. Dr. Lowdermilk also is co-author of *Maternity and Women's Health Care* (eleventh edition), *Maternity Nursing* (eighth edition), and *Maternal and Child Health* (fifth edition). In Fall 2010, the East Carolina University College of Nursing named the Neonatal Intensive Care and Midwifery Laboratory in honor of Dr. Lowdermilk. In 2011, she was named as one of the first 40 nurses inducted into the College of Nursing Hall of Fame.

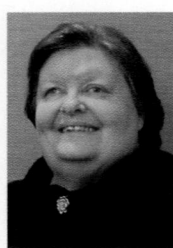

Kitty Cashion is a Clinical Nurse Specialist in the Maternal-Fetal Medicine Division, College of Medicine, Department of Obstetrics and Gynecology at The University of Tennessee Health Science Center in Memphis. She received her BSN from the University of Tennessee College of Nursing in Memphis and her MSN in parent-child nursing from the Vanderbilt University School of Nursing in Nashville, Tennessee. Ms. Cashion is certified as a high risk perinatal nurse through the American Nurses Credentialing Center.

Ms. Cashion's job responsibilities at the University of Tennessee include providing education regarding low- and high-risk obstetrics to staff nurses in West Tennessee community hospitals. For over 20 years, Ms. Cashion has been an adjunct clinical instructor in maternal-child nursing at Northwest Mississippi Community College in Senatobia, Mississippi, and Union University in Germantown, Tennessee. Ms. Cashion has contributed many chapters to maternity nursing textbooks over the years and also co-authored several major maternity nursing textbooks.

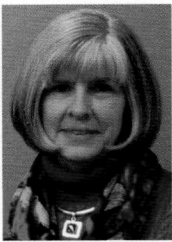

Kathryn Rhodes Alden is Associate Professor at the University of North Carolina at Chapel Hill School of Nursing, where she has taught clinical and didactic in maternal/newborn nursing for 29 years. She has received numerous awards for excellence in nursing education at the University of North Carolina, being recognized for clinical and classroom teaching expertise as well as for academic counseling. Dr. Alden was instrumental in the adoption of simulation-based learning for nursing education as well as for interprofessional education.

Dr. Alden earned a BSN from University of North Carolina at Charlotte, an MSN from the University of North Carolina at Chapel Hill, and a doctorate in adult education from North Carolina State University. She has clinical experience as a staff nurse in pediatrics, pediatric intensive care, and neonatal intensive care, as well as in postpartum home care of mothers, newborns, and families. She has served as a nursing administrator and coordinator of quality improvement. Dr. Alden has been an international board certified lactation consultant for more than 20 years and has extensive experience working as an inpatient lactation consultant and a lactation educator.

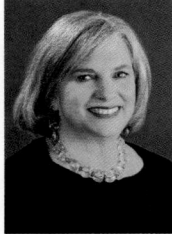

Ellen F. Olshansky is Professor and Founding Chair of the Department of Nursing in the Suzanne Dworak-Peck School of Social Work at the University of Southern California. She earned a BA in Social Work from the University of California, Berkeley, and a BS, MS, and PhD from the University of California, San Francisco School of Nursing. She is a Fellow in the American Academy of Nursing and the Western Academy of Nursing through the Western Institute of Nursing.

Dr. Olshansky is a women's health nurse practitioner, certified through the National Certification Corporation, and her research focuses on women's health across the lifespan, with an emphasis on reproductive health. She is one of the founders of the Orange County Women's Health Project, which promotes women's health and wellness in Orange County, California. She recently completed a 10-year term as editor of the *Journal of Professional Nursing*, the official journal of the American Association of Colleges of Nursing. She has published extensively in numerous nursing and other health-related journals as well as authoring many book chapters and editorials.

PEDIATRIC

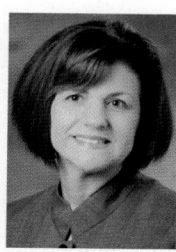

Marilyn J. Hockenberry is the Bessie Baker Distinguished Professor of Nursing and Professor of Pediatrics at Duke University. She is the Associate Dean of Research Affairs in the Duke School of Nursing. Her research focuses on symptom management and treatment-related side effects experienced by children who have cancer. Dr. Hockenberry's current National Institutes of Health–funded research studies are evaluating the treatment-related symptoms and neurocognitive deficits of leukemia treatment.

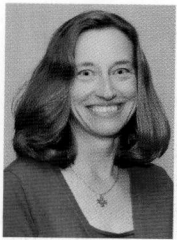

Cheryl C. Rodgers is an Assistant Professor at Duke University School of Nursing in Durham. Her research focuses on symptom assessment and symptom management among children undergoing cancer treatment or stem cell transplant. Dr. Rodgers is certified as a primary care pediatric nurse practitioner and a pediatric oncology nurse. She has over 25 years of clinical experience caring for children with hematologic and oncologic diseases.

This sixth edition of *Maternal Child Nursing Care* combines essential maternity and pediatric nursing information into one text. The text focuses on the care of women during their reproductive years and the care of children from birth through adolescence. The issues and concerns of childbearing women and the health care of children are the primary concentrations. The promotion of wellness and the management of common women's health problems and child development in the context of the family are also addressed. As we move further into the twenty-first century, this edition of *Maternal Child Nursing Care* is designed to address the changing needs of women during their childbearing years and children during their developing years.

Maternal Child Nursing Care was developed to provide students with the knowledge and skills they need to become competent critical thinkers and to attain the sensitivity needed to become caring nurses. This sixth edition has been revised and refined in response to comments and suggestions from educators, clinicians, and students. It includes the most accurate, current, and clinically relevant information available.

APPROACH

Professional nursing practice continues to evolve and adapt to society's changing health priorities. The rapidly changing health care delivery system offers new opportunities for nurses to alter the practice of maternity and pediatric nursing and to improve the way care is given. Increasingly, nursing practice must be evidence based. It is incumbent on nurses to use the most up-to-date and scientifically supported information on which to base their care. To assist nurses in providing this type of care, Evidence-Based Practice boxes with implications for practice are included throughout the text.

Consumers of maternity and pediatric care vary in age, ethnicity, culture, language, social status, marital status, and sexual orientation. They seek care from a variety of health care providers in numerous health care settings, including the home. To meet the needs of these consumers, clinical education must offer students a variety of health care experiences in settings that include hospitals and birth centers, homes, clinics, private physicians' offices, shelters for the homeless or for women and children in need of protection, and other community-based settings.

Care management has been used as an organizing framework for discussion in the nursing care chapters. Interprofessional care is emphasized because this approach demonstrates how nursing must collaborate with other health care disciplines to provide the most comprehensive care possible to women and children. Nursing Care Plans reinforce the problem-solving approach to patient care. In chapters that focus on complications of childbearing, reproductive conditions, and childhood illnesses, medical interventions are included along with nursing care management. Throughout the discussion of assessment and care, we alert the nurse to signs of potential problems and provide informational boxes that highlight warning signs and emergency situations.

Patient education is an essential component of the nursing care of women and children. The chapter on women's health promotion and screening emphasizes teaching for self-care to promote wellness and to encourage preventive care. The chapter on transition to parenthood focuses on teaching for new parents and infants at home. Special boxes highlight community care throughout the text. Family-Centered Care boxes incorporate family considerations important to the care of women

and children. Issues concerning grandparents, siblings, and different family constellations are addressed. In the pediatric chapters, these boxes focus on the special learning needs of families. Legal Tips are integrated into the maternity section to emphasize issues related to the care of women and infants. Alerts are located throughout the text to draw attention to important information on medications, nursing care, and safety.

This sixth edition features a contemporary design with logical, easy-to-follow headings and an attractive four-color design that highlights important content and increases visual appeal. Hundreds of color photographs and drawings throughout the text, many of them new, illustrate important concepts and techniques to further enhance comprehension. To help students learn essential information quickly and efficiently, we have included numerous features that prioritize, condense, simplify, and emphasize important aspects of nursing care. In addition, the text encourages students to think critically.

SPECIAL FEATURES

- **Atraumatic Care** boxes emphasize the importance of providing competent care without creating undue physical and psychologic distress. Although many of the boxes provide suggestions for managing pain, atraumatic care also considers approaches to promoting self-esteem and preventing embarrassment.

- **Clinical Reasoning Case Studies** present students with real-life situations and encourage them to make appropriate clinical judgments. A focus on interprofessional care encourages students to think beyond the nursing role to include collaboration with other health care professionals. Answer guidelines are provided in *TEACH for Nurses*.

- **Community Focus** boxes emphasize community issues, provide resources and guidance, and illustrate nursing care in a variety of settings.

- **Cultural Considerations** boxes describe beliefs and practices about pregnancy, labor and birth, parenting, and women's health concerns.

- **Emergency Treatment** boxes alert students to the signs and symptoms of various emergency situations and provide interventions for immediate implementation.

- **Evidence-Based Practice** is incorporated in new boxes that integrate findings from recent studies on selected clinical practices topics; relevant Quality and Safety Education for Nurses (QSEN) competencies are identified in these boxes.

- **Family-Centered Care** boxes highlight the needs and concerns of families that should be addressed when family-centered care is provided.

- **Guidelines** boxes provide students with examples of various approaches to implementing care.

- **Legal Tips** are integrated throughout Part 1 to provide students with relevant information to deal with important legal matters in the context of maternity nursing.

- **Medication Guide** boxes and **Medication Alerts** include key information about medications used in maternity and newborn care, including their indications, adverse effects, and nursing considerations.

- **Nursing Alerts** call the reader's attention to critical information that could lead to deteriorating or emergency situations.

- **Nursing Care Plans** are provided for many commonly encountered situations and disorders. Rationales are included for nursing interventions that might not be immediately evident to students. The care plans present a brief case study to help students conceptualize how to individualize patient care.

- **Patient Teaching** boxes assist students to help patients and families become involved in their own care with optimal outcomes.

- **Resources,** including websites and contact information for organizations and educational resources available for the topics discussed, are listed throughout.

- **Safety Alerts** call the reader's attention to potentially dangerous situations that should be addressed by the nurse.

- During assessment, the nurse must be alert for **Signs of Potential Complications;** these are included in chapters that cover uncomplicated pregnancy and childbirth.

- A highly detailed, cross-referenced **Index** allows readers to quickly access needed information.

TEACHING AND LEARNING PACKAGE

Several ancillaries for this text have been developed for instructors and students to use in classroom and clinical settings.

For Students

Evolve: Evolve is an innovative website that provides a wealth of content, resources, and state-of-the-art information on maternity and pediatric nursing. Learning resources for students include Animations, Case Studies, Content Updates, Glossary, Printable Key Points, Nursing Skills, and NCLEX-Style Review Questions.

Simulation Learning System (SLS): The Simulation Learning System (SLS) is an online toolkit that helps instructors and facilitators effectively incorporate medium- to high-fidelity simulation into their nursing curriculum. Detailed patient scenarios promote and enhance the clinical decision-making skills of students at all levels. The SLS provides detailed instructions for preparation and implementation of the simulation experience, debriefing questions that encourage critical thinking, and learning resources to reinforce student comprehension. Each scenario in the SLS complements the textbook content and helps bridge the gap between lectures and clinical practice. The SLS provides the perfect environment for students to practice what they are learning in the text for a true-to-life, hands-on learning experience.

Study Guide: This comprehensive and challenging study aid presents a variety of questions to enhance learning of key concepts and content from the text. Multiple-choice and matching questions and Critical Thinking Case Studies are included. Answers for all questions are included at the back of the study guide.

Virtual Clinical Excursions: Virtual Hospital and Workbook Companion: A virtual hospital and workbook package has been developed as a virtual clinical experience to expand student opportunities for critical thinking. This package guides students through a virtual clinical environment and helps users apply textbook content to virtual patients in that environment. Case studies are presented that allow students to use this textbook as a reference to assess, diagnose, plan, implement, and evaluate "real" patients using clinical scenarios. The state-of-the-art technologies reflected in this virtual hospital demonstrate cutting-edge learning opportunities for students and facilitate knowledge retention of the information found in the textbook. The clinical simulations and workbook represent the next generation of research-based learning tools that promote critical thinking and meaningful learning.

For Instructors

Evolve includes these teaching resources for instructors:

Image Collection, containing more than 700 full-color illustrations and photographs from the text, helps instructors develop presentations and explain key concepts.

PowerPoint Slides, with lecture notes for each chapter of the text, assist in presenting materials in the classroom. *Case Studies* and *Audience Response Questions* for i-clicker are included.

TEACH for Nurses includes teaching strategies; in-class case studies; and links to animations, nursing skills, and nursing curriculum standards such as QSEN, concepts, and BSN Essentials.

Test Bank in ExamView format contains more than 1850 NCLEX-style test items, including alternate-format questions. An answer key with page references to the text, rationales, and NCLEX-style coding is included.

ACKNOWLEDGMENTS

Thanks to Pat Gingrich for preparing the Evidence-Based Practice boxes in Part 1 and to those parents who permitted us to use photos of their infants and families. Very special thanks to Heather Bays, Clay Broeker, and Laurie Gower, whose support was crucial for the completion of this project. Thanks also to those faculty and students who provided reports and offered suggestions to ensure accuracy.

Shannon E. Perry
Deitra Leonard Lowdermilk
Kitty Cashion
Kathryn Rhodes Alden
Ellen F. Olshansky

We are fortunate to have worked for many years with David Wilson, who served as a co-editor on numerous editions. We miss him greatly with this edition. We are grateful to the many nursing faculty members, practitioners, and students who have offered their comments, recommendations, and suggestions. This edition could not have been completed without the dedication of these special people. We are also grateful to the editorial staff at Elsevier, especially Sandra Clark, Heather Bays, and Clay Broeker, for their support and commitment to excellence.

Marilyn J. Hockenberry
Cheryl C. Rodgers

The authors would like to acknowledge the following individuals for contributions to the ninth edition of *Wong's Essentials of Pediatric Nursing*: Rose A.U. Baker, PhD, PMHCNS-BC; Annette L. Baker, RN, BSN, MSN, CPNP; Raymond Barfield, MD, PhD; Amy Barry, RN, MSN, PNP-BC; Heather Bastardi, MSN, BSN, PNP; Debra Brandon, PhD, RN, CNS, FAAN; Terri L. Brown, MSN, RN, CPN; Meg Bruening, PhD,MPH, RD; Rosalind Bryant, PhD, RN, PPCNP-BC; Cynthia J. Camille, MSN, RN, CPNP, FNP-BC; Patricia M. Conlon, MS, APRN, CNS, CNP; Erin Connelly, APRN, CPNP; Martha R. Curry, MS, RN, CPNP; Amy Delaney, RN, MSN, CPNP-AC/P; Sharron L. Docherty, PhD, PNP-BC, FAAN; Angela Drummond, MS, APRN, CPNP; Jan M. Foote, DNP, ARNP, CPNP, FAANP; Quinn Franklin, MS; Debbie Fraser, MN, RNC-NIC; Teri A. Huddleston Lavenbarg, MSN, APRN, PPCNP-BC, FNP-BC, CDE; Patricia Barry McElfresh, MN, RN, PNP-BC; Tara Taneski Merck, CPNP; Mary A. Mondozzi, MSN, BSN, RN; Rebecca A. Monroe, MSN, RN, CPNP; Kim Mooney-Doyle, PhD, RN, CPNP-AC; Patricia O'Brien, MSN, RN, CPNP-AC; Cynthia A. Prows, MSN, CNS, FAAN; Patricia Ring, MSN, RN, CPNP; Maureen Sheehan, MS, CPNP; Anne Feierabend Stanton, MSN, APRN, PCNS-BC; Barbara J. Wheeler, RN, BN, MN, IBCLC; and Kristina Wilson, PhD, CCC-SLP.

CONTENTS

1

21st Century Maternity Nursing

Ellen F. Olshansky

ℯ http://evolve.elsevier.com/Perry/maternal

Maternity nursing encompasses care of childbearing women and their families through all stages of pregnancy and childbirth and the first 6 weeks after birth. Some practitioners also include preconception as part of maternity nursing because of the importance of counseling related to planning for pregnancy. Throughout the prenatal period, nurses, nurse practitioners, and nurse-midwives provide care for women in clinics and physicians' offices and teach classes to help families prepare for childbirth. Nurses and nurse-midwives care for childbearing families during labor and birth in hospitals, and nurse-midwives also care for childbearing families in birthing centers (e.g., www.birthcenters.org), and in the home. Nurses with special training may provide intensive care for high-risk neonates in special care units and high-risk mothers in antepartum units, in critical care obstetric units, or in the home. Maternity nurses teach about pregnancy; the process of labor, birth, and recovery; newborn care, and parenting skills. They provide continuity of care throughout the childbearing cycle. This chapter presents a general overview of issues and trends related to the health and health care of women and infants.

Nurses caring for women have helped make the health care system more responsive to women's needs. They have been critically important in developing strategies to improve the well-being of women, their families, and their infants and have led the efforts to implement clinical practice guidelines and to practice using an evidence-based approach. Through professional associations, nurses have a voice in setting standards and influencing health policy by actively participating in the education of the public and state and federal legislators (e.g., www.nursingworld.org; www.can-nurses.ca; www.awhonn.org; www.capwhn.ca). Some nurses hold elective office and influence policy directly. For example, Mary Wakefield, a nurse, served for a time as Acting Deputy Secretary of the Health Resources and Services Administration (HRSA), the agency that oversees approximately 7000 community clinics that serve low-income and uninsured people.

ADVANCES IN THE CARE OF MOTHERS AND INFANTS

Although tremendous advances have taken place in the care of mothers and their infants during the past 150 years (Box 1.1), serious problems exist in the United States related to the health and health care of mothers and infants. Lack of access to prepregnancy and pregnancy-related care for all women and the lack of reproductive health services for adolescents are major concerns. Sexually transmitted infections, including acquired immunodeficiency syndrome (AIDS), continue to adversely affect reproduction.

EFFORTS TO REDUCE HEALTH DISPARITIES

Racial and ethnic diversity is increasing within the United States. It is estimated that by 2060, 43% of the population will be composed of non-Hispanic Whites, resulting in this previous "majority" group no longer being in the majority. Predicted distribution of other ethnic groups is: 14% African-American, 28% Hispanic, 11% Asian-American, 2% American Indians and Alaska Natives, and 0.7% Native Hawaiian and other Pacific Islanders (Colby & Ortman, 2015). These percentages are estimates and therefore do not add up to 100% exactly; the intent here is to show trends.

These trends reflect a slight decrease in non-Hispanic whites and a slight increase in the other ethnic groups: African-Americans, Hispanics, Asian-Americans, Alaskan Natives, Native Hawaiians, and other Pacific Islanders.

African-Americans, Native Americans, Hispanics, Alaska Natives, and Asian/Pacific Islanders experience significant disparities in morbidity and mortality rates compared to Caucasians. Shorter life expectancy, higher infant and maternal mortality rates, more birth defects, and more sexually transmitted infections are found among these ethnic and racial minority groups. The disparities are thought to result from a complex interaction among biologic factors, environment, socioeconomic factors, and health behaviors. Social determinants of health are those nonbiologic factors that have profound influences on health. Disparities in education and income are associated with differences in morbidity and mortality.

The HRSA Health Disparities Collaboratives are part of a national effort to eliminate disparities and improve delivery systems of health care for all people in the United States who are cared for in HRSA-supported health centers. The National Partnership for Action to End Health Disparities (NPA), sponsored by the Office of Minority Health, has developed priorities to address and end health disparities (NPA, 2016). The Institute for Healthcare Improvement (IHI, 2016) has implemented virtual training sessions on Advancing Safer Maternal and Newborn Care (www.ihi.org/education/WebTraining/Expeditions/AdvancingSaferMaternalandNewbornCare/Pages/default.aspx). The National Institutes of Health (NIH) have a commitment to improve

1

BOX 1.1   Historic Overview of Milestones in the Care of Mothers and Infants

1847—James Young Simpson in Edinburgh, Scotland, used ether for an internal podalic version and birth; the first reported use of obstetric anesthesia

1861—Ignaz Semmelweis wrote *The Cause, Concept and Prophylaxis of Childbed Fever*

1906—First US program for prenatal nursing care established

1908—Childbirth classes started by the American Red Cross

1909—First White House Conference on Children convened

1911—First milk bank in the United States established in Boston

1912—US Children's Bureau established

1915—Radical mastectomy determined to be effective treatment for breast cancer

1916—Margaret Sanger established first American birth control clinic in Brooklyn, New York

1918—Condoms became legal in the United States

1923—First US hospital center for premature infant care established at Sarah Morris Hospital in Chicago, Illinois

1929—The modern tampon (with an applicator) invented and patented

1933—Sodium pentothal used as anesthesia for childbirth; *Natural Childbirth* published by Grantly Dick-Read

1934—Dionne quintuplets born in Ontario, Canada, and survive partly due to donated breast milk

1935—Sulfonamides introduced as cure for puerperal fever

1941—Penicillin used as a treatment for infection

1941—Papanicolaou (Pap) test introduced

1942—Premarin approved by the Food and Drug Administration (FDA) as treatment for menopausal symptoms

1953—Virginia Apgar, an anesthesiologist, published Apgar scoring system of neonatal assessment

1956—Oxygen determined to cause retrolental fibroplasia (now known as retinopathy of prematurity)

1958—Edward Hon reported on the recording of the fetal electrocardiogram (ECG) from the maternal abdomen (first commercial electronic fetal monitor produced in the late 1960s)

1958—Ian Donald, a Glasgow physician, was first to report clinical use of ultrasound to examine the fetus

1959—*Thank You, Dr. Lamaze* published by Marjorie Karmel

1959—Cytologic studies demonstrated that Down syndrome is associated with a particular form of nondisjunction now known as trisomy 21

1960—American Society for Psychoprophylaxis in Obstetrics (ASPO/Lamaze) formed

1960—International Childbirth Education Association founded

1960—Birth control pill introduced in the United States

1962—Thalidomide found to cause birth defects

1963—Title V of the Social Security Act amended to include comprehensive maternity and infant care for women who were low income and high risk

1963—Testing for PKU begun

1965—Supreme Court ruled that married people have the right to use birth control

1967—Rh₀(D) immune globulin produced for treatment of Rh incompatibility

1967—Reva Rubin published article on maternal role attainment

1968—Rubella vaccine became available

1969—Nurses Association of the American College of Obstetricians and Gynecologists (NAACOG) founded; renamed Association of Women's Health, Obstetric and Neonatal Nurses (AWHONN) and incorporated as a 501(c)(3) organization in 1993

1969—Mammogram became available

1972—Special Supplemental Food Program for Women, Infants, and Children (WIC) started

1973—Abortion legalized in United States

1974—First standards for obstetric, gynecologic, and neonatal nursing published by NAACOG

1975—The Pregnant Patient's Bill of Rights published by the International Childbirth Education Association

1976—First home pregnancy kits approved by FDA

1978—Louise Brown, first test-tube baby, born

1987—Safe Motherhood initiative launched by World Health Organization and other international agencies

1991—Society for Advancement of Women's Health Research founded

1992—Office of Research on Women's Health authorized by US Congress

1993—Female condom approved by FDA

1993—Human embryos cloned at George Washington University

1993—Family and Medical Leave Act enacted

1994—DNA sequences of *BRCA1* and *BRCA2* identified

1994—Zidovudine guidelines to reduce mother-to-fetus transmission of HIV published

1996—FDA mandated folic acid fortification in all breads and grains sold in United States

1998—Newborns' and Mothers' Health Act went into effect

1998—Canadian Obstetric, Gynecologic, and Neonatal Nurses (COGNN) becomes AWHONN Canada

1999—First emergency contraceptive pill for pregnancy prevention (Plan B) approved by FDA

2000—Working draft of sequence and analysis of human genome completed

2006—Human papilloma virus (HPV) vaccine available

2010—Centenary of the death of Florence Nightingale

2010—Patient Protection and Affordable Care Act signed into law by President Obama

2011—AWHONN Canada becomes the Canadian Association of Perinatal and Women's Health Nurses (CAPWHN)

2012—US Supreme Court upheld individual mandate but not the Medicaid expansion provisions of the Patient Protection and Affordable Care Act

2012—Scientists reported findings of the ENCODE (**Enc**yclopedia **of D**NA **E**lements) project showing that 80% of the human genome is active

2016—Zika virus discovered, spread by mosquitos, and sexually transmitted by sperm if a male is infected, affects the fetus/neonate (microcephaly)

---

the health of minorities and provide funding for research and training of minority researchers (www.nih.gov). The National Institute of Nursing Research includes in its strategic plan support of research that promotes health equity and eliminates health disparities.

The Centers for Disease Control and Prevention (CDC) publishes reports of recent trends and variation in health disparities and inequalities in some social and health indicators and provides data against which to measure progress in eliminating disparities. Topics specific to perinatal nursing that are addressed are infant deaths, preterm births, and adolescent pregnancy and childbirth. In 2015, the US Department of Health and Human Services (USDHHS) released a progress report on

its HHS Disparities Action Plan that provides a vision of "a nation free of disparities in health and health care" (USDHHS, 2015). Through this plan, HHS will promote evidence-based programs, integrated approaches, and best practices to reduce disparities. The Action Plan complements the 2011 National Stakeholder Strategy for Achieving Health Equity prepared by the NPA. Since this strategy was developed, much progress has been made in addressing disparities and health equity through a comprehensive, community-driven approach to achieve health equity through collaboration and synergy (NPA, 2016). Through these initiatives, the United States is making a concerted effort to eliminate health disparities.

CONTEMPORARY ISSUES AND TRENDS

HEALTHY PEOPLE 2020 GOALS

Healthy People provides science-based 10-year national objectives for improving the health of all Americans. It has four overarching goals: (1) attaining high-quality, longer lives free of preventable disease, disability, injury, and premature death; (2) achieving health equity, eliminating disparities, and improving the health of all groups; (3) creating social and physical environments that promote good health for all; and (4) promoting quality of life, healthy development, and healthy behaviors across all life stages (www.healthypeople.gov/2020/about/default.aspx). The goals of *Healthy People 2020* are based on assessments of major risks to health and wellness, changes in public health priorities, and issues related to the health preparedness and prevention of our nation. Of the objectives of *Healthy People 2020*, 33 are related to maternal, infant, and child health (Box 1.2).

MILLENNIUM DEVELOPMENT GOALS

The United Nations Millennium Development Goals (MDGs) are eight goals that were to be achieved by 2015, responding to the main development challenges in the world (www.un.org/millenniumgoals). Goals three through five of the MDGs relate specifically to women and children.

In September 2015, the United Nations site in New York City hosted a conference of world leaders, where they adopted the 2030 Agenda for Sustainable Development. This 2030 agenda consists of 17 Sustainable Development Goals (SDGs), also referred to as Global Goals, which are now replacing the MDGs (United Nations Development Programme, 2016). The majority of these SDGs are related to the environment and eliminating poverty, in many ways collectively encompassing social determinants of health, all of which are relevant to childbearing and childrearing. They are listed in Box 1.3.

INTEGRATIVE HEALTH CARE

Integrative health care encompasses complementary and alternative therapies in combination with conventional Western modalities of treatment. Many popular alternative healing modalities offer human-centered care based on philosophies that recognize the value of the patient's input and honor the individual's beliefs, values, and desires. The focus of these modalities is on the whole person, not just on a disease complex. Patients often find that alternative modalities are more

---

BOX 1.2   *Healthy People 2020* Maternal, Infant, and Child Health Objectives

- Reduce the rate of fetal and infant deaths.
- Reduce the 1-year mortality rate for infants with Down syndrome.
- Reduce the rate of child deaths.
- Reduce the rate of adolescent and young adult deaths.
- Reduce the rate of maternal mortality.
- Reduce maternal illness and complications caused by pregnancy (complications during hospitalized labor and delivery).
- Reduce the incidence of cesarean births among low-risk (full-term, singleton, vertex presentation) women.
- Reduce the incidence of low birth weight (LBW) and very low birth weight (VLBW). births.
- Reduce the incidence of preterm births.
- Increase the proportion of pregnant women who receive early and adequate prenatal care.
- Increase abstinence from alcohol, cigarettes, and illicit drugs in pregnant women.
- Increase the proportion of pregnant women who attend a series of prepared childbirth classes.
- Increase the proportion of mothers who achieve a recommended weight gain during their pregnancies.
- Increase the proportion of women of childbearing potential who have an intake of at least 400 mcg of folic acid from fortified foods or dietary supplements.
- Reduce the proportion of women of childbearing potential who have low red blood cell folate concentrations.
- Increase the proportion of women delivering a live birth; increase the number of those who receive preconception care services and practice key recommended preconception health behaviors.
- Reduce the proportion of people 18 to 44 years of age who have impaired fecundity (i.e., a physical barrier preventing pregnancy or carrying a pregnancy to term).
- Decrease postpartum relapse of smoking in women who quit smoking during pregnancy.
- Increase the proportion of women giving birth who attend a postpartum care visit with a health worker.
- Increase the proportion of infants who are placed on their backs to sleep.
- Increase the proportion of infants who are breastfed.
- Increase the proportion of employers who have worksite lactation programs.
- Reduce the proportion of breastfed newborns who receive formula supplementation within the first 2 days of life.
- Increase the proportion of live births that occur in facilities that provide recommended care for lactating mothers and their babies.
- Reduce the occurrence of fetal alcohol syndrome (FAS).
- Reduce the proportion of children diagnosed with a disorder through newborn blood spot screening who experience developmental delay requiring special education services.
- Reduce the proportion of children with cerebral palsy born as LBW infants (less than 2500 g).
- Reduce the occurrence of neural tube defects.
- Increase the proportion of young children with an autism spectrum disorder (ASD) and other developmental delays who are screened, evaluated, and enrolled in early intervention services in a timely manner.
- Increase the proportion of children, including those with special health care needs, who have access to a medical home.
- Increase the proportion of children with special health care needs who receive their care in family-centered, comprehensive, coordinated systems.
- Increase appropriate newborn blood-spot screening and follow-up testing.
- Increase the number of states, including the District of Columbia, that verify through linkage with vital records that all newborns are screened shortly after birth for conditions mandated by their state-sponsored screening program.
- Increase the proportion of screen-positive children who receive follow-up testing within the recommended time period.
- Increase the proportion of children with a diagnosed condition identified through newborn screening who have an annual assessment of services needed and received.
- Increase the proportion of VLBW infants born at level III hospitals or subspecialty perinatal centers.

Adapted from HealthyPeople.gov. (2012). *Maternal, infant, and child health.* Retrieved from www.healthypeople.gov/2020/topicsobjectives2020/objectiveslist.aspx?topicId=26.

BOX 1.3 United Nations Sustainable Development Goals

1. No poverty
2. Zero hunger
3. Good health and well-being
4. Quality education
5. Gender equality
6. Clean water and sanitation
7. Affordable and clean energy
8. Decent work and economic growth
9. Industry, innovation, and infrastructure
10. Reduced inequalities
11. Sustainable cities and communities
12. Responsible consumption and production
13. Climate action
14. Life below water
15. Life on land
16. Peace, justice and strong institutions
17. Partnerships for the goals

From United Nations Development Programme. (2016). Sustainable Development Goals. Retrieved from http://www.un.org/sustainabledevelopment/sustainable-development-goals/.

---

consistent with their own belief systems and also allow for more patient autonomy in health care decisions (Fig. 1.1). Examples of alternative modalities include acupuncture, macrobiotics, herbal medicines, massage therapy, biofeedback, meditation, yoga, chelation therapy, and guided imagery (See Fig 1.1). Chelation therapy is an alternative therapy that consists of infusing intravenous substances to remove calcium and heavy metals from hardened arteries.

The National Center for Complementary and Integrative Health (NCCIH) (https://nccih.nih.gov) is a US government agency that supports research and evaluation of various alternative and complementary modalities and provides information to health care consumers about such modalities. It is one of the 27 institutes and centers included in the NIH.

INTERPROFESSIONAL EDUCATION

Interprofessional education (IPE) consists of faculty and students from two or more health professions who create and foster a collaborative learning environment. The underlying premise of interprofessional collaboration is that patient care will improve when health professionals work together. Numerous organizations, including the World Health

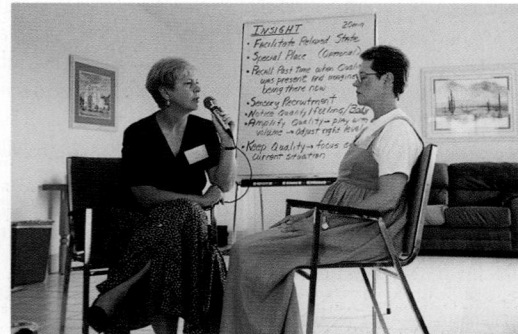

FIG 1.1 Nurse and patient during guided imagery session. (Courtesy of Nurses Certificate Program in Interactive Imagery, Foster City, CA.)

BOX 1.4 Interprofessional Education and Collaboration

The Interprofessional Education Collaborative builds on earlier work, in which practice competencies were identified to include the following:
1. Values/ethics for interprofessional practice
2. Roles/responsibilities
3. Interprofessional communication
4. Teams and teamwork

In 2013, The Interprofessional Education Collaborative developed a new collaborative that expands the number of health professionals involved (https://ipecollaborative.org/uploads/IPEC-2016-Updated-Core-Competencies-Report__final_release_.PDF).

Organization (WHO), the National Academy of Medicine, the National Academies of Practice, and the American Public Health Association, have expressed support of interprofessional education. See Box 1.4 for a description of the practice competencies related to IPE.

Teamwork and communication are key aspects of IPE. Failure to communicate is a major cause of errors in health care. The Situation-Background-Assessment-Recommendation (SBAR) technique provides a specific framework for communication among health care providers about a patient's condition, reducing the potential for errors. SBAR is an easy to remember, useful, concrete mechanism for communicating important information that requires a clinician's immediate attention (Kaiser Permanente of Colorado, 2014) (Table 1.1). A specific program to enhance teamwork and collaboration is TeamSTEPPS, which was developed by the Department of Defense Patient Safety Program in collaboration with the Agency for Healthcare Research and Quality (AHRQ) as a teamwork system for health professionals to provide higher-quality, safer patient care (www.teamstepps.ahrq.gov/about-2cl_3.htm). It provides an evidence base to improve communication and teamwork skills. Through this system, health care teams use information, people, and resources to achieve the best possible clinical outcomes, increase team awareness and clarify roles and responsibilities of team members, resolve conflicts and improve sharing of information, and eliminate barriers to quality and safety.

PROBLEMS WITH THE US HEALTH CARE SYSTEM

Structure of the Health Care Delivery System

The US health care delivery system is often fragmented and expensive and is inaccessible to many. Opportunities exist for nurses to alter nursing practice and improve the way care is delivered through managed care, integrated delivery systems, and redefined roles. Information about health and health care is readily available on the Internet (e-health). Consumers use this information to participate in their own care and consult health care providers with a knowledge base that was previously difficult to access.

Reducing Medical Errors

Medical errors are the third leading cause of death in the United States (Leapfrog Group, 2015; Makary & Daniel, 2016). Since the Institute of Medicine (IOM) released its report, *To Err Is Human: Building a Safer Health System* (IOM, 2000), a concerted effort has been under way to analyze causes of errors and develop strategies to prevent them. Hayes, Jackson, Davidson, and Power and colleagues (2015) explored how nurses can decrease interruptions and distractions that contribute to medical errors. Recognizing the multifaceted causes of medical errors, the Agency for Healthcare Research and Quality (AHRQ) prepared a fact sheet in 2000, *20 Tips to Help Prevent Medical Errors*, which was

TABLE 1.1 Sample SBAR Report to Physician or Nurse-Midwife*

S	**Situation** Hello, I am Ellen Olshansky on the mother/baby unit, and I'm calling about Mary Smith, who just gave birth 12 hours ago. I have just assessed her, and she saturated a peripad in the last hour. Her blood pressure is 112/62, pulse 86, and respirations 18. I think she is bleeding excessively.
B	**Background** Mrs. Smith is 12 hours' postpartum after giving birth vaginally to a 9-lb, 12-oz term infant after an uncomplicated pregnancy. She had a rapid labor, just over 4 hours, and had no analgesia. She plans to bottle-feed this baby. She had an IV with 10 units of oxytocin (Pitocin), but it was completed and discontinued about 2 hours ago. This is her sixth birth. All were uncomplicated, and she had an uneventful recovery from them.
A	**Assessment** Her fundus becomes firm after massage but relaxes again. She has a slightly malodorous vaginal discharge. She has voided, and her bladder feels empty. I think she might have retained placenta and she needs to be examined.
R	**Recommendation** I would like you to come and examine her immediately. Do you want her IV restarted? Do you want her to have a hemoglobin and hematocrit?

IV, Intravenous infusion; *SBAR*, Situation-Background-Assessment-Recommendation.
*The SBAR tool was developed by Kaiser Permanente, and the example was prepared by Shannon E. Perry.

TABLE 1.2 Selected Safe Practices for Better Health Care

Safe Practice	Practice Statement
Safe Practice 2: Culture Measurement, Feedback, and Intervention	Health care organizations must measure their culture, provide feedback to leadership and staff, and undertake interventions that reduce patient safety risk.
Safe Practice 5: Informed Consent	Ask each patient or legal surrogate to "teach back" in his or her own words key information about the proposed treatments or procedures for which he or she is being asked to provide informed consent.
Safe Practice 12: Patient Care Information	Ensure that care information is transmitted and appropriately documented in a timely manner and a clearly understandable form to patients and all of the patients' health care providers/professionals, within and between care settings, who need that information to provide continued care.
Safe Practice 19: Hand Hygiene	Comply with current Centers for Disease Control and Prevention (CDC) hand hygiene guidelines.

CT, Computed tomography.
From National Quality Forum. (2013). *Safe practices for better healthcare—2013 update: A consensus report.* Washington, DC: NQF. In Health Care Facilities Accreditation Program. Retrieved from http://www.hfap.org/pdf/patient_safety.pdf.

BOX 1.5 National Quality Forum Serious Reportable Events Pertaining to Maternal and Child Health

- Maternal death or serious injury associated with labor or birth in a low-risk pregnancy while being cared for in a health care facility
- Death or serious injury of a neonate associated with labor or delivery in a low-risk pregnancy
- Artificial insemination with the wrong donor sperm or wrong egg

From National Quality Forum. (2011). Serious reportable events in healthcare—2011 update: A consensus report. Washington, DC: NQF.

updated in 2014, for patients and the public. Patients are encouraged to be knowledgeable consumers of health care and ask questions of providers, including physicians, midwives, nurses, and pharmacists.

In 2002, the National Quality Forum (NQF) published a list of Serious Reportable Events in Healthcare. The list was most recently updated in 2011 (NQF, 2011), resulting in a total of 29 events. Of these 29 events, three pertain directly to maternity and newborn care (Box 1.5).

The NQF published *Safe Practices for Better Healthcare* in 2003 and updated it most recently in 2013 (http://www.hfap.org/pdf/patient_safety.pdf). The 34 safe practices included should be used in all applicable health care settings to reduce the risk for harm that results from processes, systems, and environments of care. Table 1.2 contains a selection of practices from that document.

High Cost of Health Care

Health care is one of the fastest-growing sectors of the US economy. Currently 17.5% of the gross domestic product is spent on health care (Centers for Medicare & Medicaid, 2015). These high costs are related to higher prices, readily accessible technology, and greater obesity. Most researchers agree that caring for the increased number of low–birth weight (LBW) infants in neonatal intensive care units contributes significantly to overall health care costs.

Nurse-midwifery and advanced practice nursing care have helped contain some health care costs. However, not all insurance carriers reimburse nurse practitioners and clinical nurse specialists as direct care providers, nor do they reimburse for all services provided by nurse-midwives, a situation that continues to be a problem. Nurses must become involved in the politics of cost containment because they, as knowledgeable experts, can provide solutions to many health care problems at a relatively low cost. Nurse practitioners are among the health care providers included in the Affordable Care Act (ACA). Despite this, only 21 states and the District of Columbia allow nurse practitioners to practice to their fullest potential without physician involvement (American Academy of Nurse Practitioners, 2015).

Limited Access to Care

Barriers to access must be removed so pregnancy outcomes and care of children can be improved. The most significant barrier to access is the inability to pay. Some improvement in ability to pay has been seen due to the ACA. The uninsured rate in 2014 was 10.4%, or 33 million people, which was lower than the rate of 13.3%, or 41.8 million people, in 2013 (Smith & Medalia, 2015). Lack of transportation and dependent child care are other barriers. In addition to a lack of insurance and high costs, a lack of providers for low-income women exists because many physicians either refuse to take Medicaid patients or take only a few such patients. This presents a serious problem because a significant proportion of births are to mothers who receive Medicaid.

Health Care Reform

In early 2010, President Barack Obama signed into law the Patient Protection and Affordable Care Act, commonly referred to as *Obamacare*. The Act aims to make insurance affordable, contain costs, strengthen and improve Medicare and Medicaid, and reform the insurance market. There are provisions to promote prevention and improve public health; improve the quality of care for all Americans; reduce waste, fraud, and abuse; and reform the health delivery system. There are some immediate benefits, but the fate of the ACA is uncertain in the current political climate.

In 2012, 26 states, several individuals, and the National Federation of Independent Business brought suit challenging the constitutionality of the individual mandate (requirement for most Americans to have minimum essential health insurance) and the Medicaid expansion (expand the scope of coverage and increase the number of individuals the states must cover). The Supreme Court upheld the individual mandate but not the Medicaid expansion. The debate continues on how the plan will be implemented and there is much uncertainty regarding health care reform.

The Association of Women's Health, Obstetric and Neonatal Nurses (AWHONN) advocated successfully for the inclusion in the ACA of contraceptive methods, services, and counseling, without any out-of-pocket costs to women; preventive services such as mammograms, well-woman visits, and screening for gestational diabetes; and providing breastfeeding equipment and counseling for pregnant and nursing women in new insurance plans. Work continues on implementation.

ACCOUNTABLE CARE ORGANIZATIONS

In 2011, the Center for Medicaid and Medicare Services (CMS) finalized new rules under the ACA to help health care providers and hospitals better coordinate care for Medicare patients through Accountable Care Organizations (ACOs). An ACO is a group of health care providers and health care agencies that are accountable for improving the health of populations while containing costs. These groups of health care providers and hospitals voluntarily come together to coordinate high-quality care, eliminate duplication of services, and prevent medical errors, which results in savings of health care dollars.

HEALTH LITERACY

Health literacy involves a spectrum of abilities, ranging from reading an appointment slip to interpreting medication instructions. These skills must be assessed routinely to recognize a problem and accommodate patients with limited literacy skills. Most education materials are written at too high a level for the average adult; e-health literacy has emerged as a concept. Individuals use the Internet for diagnosis, but more than half of these individuals seek the opinion of a medical professional rather than trying to care for themselves based on the information accessed (Dickens & Piano, 2013).

The CDC (2016a) has a health literacy website (www.cdc.gov/healthliteracy) that highlights implementation of goals and strategies of the National Action Plan to Improve Health Literacy. Health literacy is part of the Patient Protection and Affordable Care Act.

As a result of the increasingly multicultural US population, there is a more urgent need to address health literacy as a component of culturally and linguistically competent care. Older adults, racial or ethnic minorities, and those whose income is at or below the poverty level are most

---

BOX 1.6   Maternal-Infant Biostatistical Terminology

Abortus: An embryo or fetus that is removed or expelled from the uterus at 20 weeks of gestation or less, weighs 500 g or less, or measures 25 cm or less

Birth rate: Number of live births in 1 year per 1000 population

Fertility rate: Number of births per 1000 women between 15 and 44 years of age (inclusive), calculated on an annual basis

Infant mortality rate: Number of deaths of infants younger than 1 year of age per 1000 live births

Maternal mortality rate: Number of maternal deaths from births and complications of pregnancy, childbirth, and puerperium (the first 42 days after termination of the pregnancy) per 100,000 live births

Pregnancy-associated deaths: All deaths during pregnancy and within the 1 year following the end of pregnancy

Pregnancy-related deaths (subset of pregnancy-associated): Deaths that are a complication of pregnancy, an aggravation of an unrelated condition by the physiology of pregnancy, or a chain of events initiated by the pregnancy

Neonatal mortality rate: Number of deaths of infants younger than 28 days of age per 1000 live births

Perinatal mortality rate: Number of stillbirths and number of neonatal deaths per 1000 live births

Stillbirth: An infant who at birth demonstrates no signs of life such as breathing, heartbeat, or voluntary muscle movements

---

vulnerable. Lower health literacy is associated with adverse health outcomes (Dickens & Piano, 2013).

Health care providers contribute to health literacy by using simple, common words; avoiding jargon; and assessing whether the patient understands the discussion. Speaking slowly and clearly and focusing on what is important increase understanding.

TRENDS IN FERTILITY AND BIRTH RATE

Fertility trends and birth rates reflect women's needs for health care. Box 1.6 defines biostatistical terminology useful in analyzing maternal health care. In 2015, the fertility rate in the United States declined by 1% as compared with 2014 (down from 62.9 to 62.5 births per 1000 women ages 15-44). There was a decline in births among Hispanic and non-Hispanic white women, and the rate was unchanged for non-Hispanic black women. Among women in their early 20s, there was a record low birth rate in 2015. There was a lesser decline for women in their late 20s, with an increase for women in their 30s and early 40s. The birth rate also fell among unmarried women, which is notable as this was the seventh year in a row in which this group experienced a decline in birth rate. The teenage birth rate (ages 15-19) decreased by 8% (down to 22.3 births per 1000 young women ages 15 to 19. Fertility rates declined among teenagers in all racial groups (Martin, Hamilton, Osterman, et al., 2017).

LOW–BIRTH WEIGHT AND PRETERM BIRTH

The risks of morbidity and mortality increase for newborns weighing less than 2500 g (5 lb, 8 oz)—low–birth weight (LBW) infants. Multiple births contribute to the incidence of LBW. There has been a 9% decline in triplet and higher order multiple births from 2014 to 2015 and a decline in the twin birth rate during this same year. This is particularly significant because the rate of twin births in 2014 had been at an all-time high (Martin et al., 2017).

Non-Hispanic black infants are almost twice as likely as non-Hispanic white infants to be of LBW and to die in the first year of life. Cigarette smoking is associated with LBW, prematurity, and intrauterine growth restriction, with a higher rate among non-Hispanic white women and non-Hispanic black women (Tong, Dietz, Morrow, et al., 2013).

The percentage of infants born preterm (i.e., born before 37 weeks of gestation) was 9.63% in 2015, which is slightly higher than the 2014 rate of 9.57%. Non-Hispanic black and Hispanic black women experienced increased rates of preterm births (Martin et al., 2017).

INTERNATIONAL INFANT MORTALITY TRENDS

In 2010, the infant mortality rate in the United States (6.1/1000) ranked twenty-sixth, when compared with those of other industrialized countries (MacDorman, Mathew, Mohangoo, et al., 2014). Decreases in the infant mortality rate in the United States do not keep pace with the rates of other industrialized countries. One reason for this is the high rate of LBW infants in the United States in contrast with the rates in other countries.

MATERNAL MORTALITY

Worldwide approximately 800 women die each day of problems related to pregnancy or childbirth. In the United States in 2011, the annual maternal mortality rate (number of deaths per 100,000 live births) was 17.8; the rate decreased to 15.9 in 2012, and then increased again to 17.3 in 2013 (CDC, 2016b). Although the overall number of maternal deaths is small, maternal mortality remains a significant problem because a high proportion of deaths are preventable, primarily through improving the access to and use of prenatal care services. In the United States, there is significant racial disparity in the rates of maternal death, which are highest in non-Hispanic black women, followed by non-Hispanic white women (CDC, 2016b).

The leading causes of maternal death attributable to pregnancy differ over the world. In the United States, the three major causes are cardiovascular diseases, non-cardiovascular diseases, and infection (CDC, 2016b). Unsafe abortion is an additional cause. Factors that are strongly related to maternal death include age (younger than 20 years and 35 years or older), lack of prenatal care, low educational attainment, unmarried status, and non-Caucasian race. Worldwide strategies to reduce maternal mortality rates include improving access to skilled attendants at birth, providing postabortion care, improving family planning services, and providing adolescents with better reproductive health services.

MATERNAL MORBIDITY

Although mortality is the traditional measure of maternal health and maternal health is often measured by neonatal outcomes, pregnancy complications are important. Currently no surveillance method is available to measure the incidence of maternal morbidity (Firoz, Chou, von Dadelszen, et al., 2013).

Maternal morbidity includes such conditions as acute renal failure, amniotic fluid embolism, cerebrovascular accident, eclampsia, pulmonary embolism, liver failure, obstetric shock, respiratory failure, septicemia, and complications of anesthesia (pulmonary, cardiac, central nervous system). Maternal morbidity results in high-risk pregnancy. The diagnosis of high risk imposes a situational crisis on the family. The combined efforts of interprofessional health care teams that includes nurses, physicians, and others are required to care for these patients, who often need the expertise of health care providers trained in both critical care obstetrics and intensive care medicine or nursing.

Obesity

Approximately 25% of women who were pregnant in 2014 in the United States were obese (Branum, Kirmeyer, Gregory, 2016). The two most frequently reported maternal medical risk factors are hypertension associated with pregnancy and diabetes, both of which are associated with obesity. Decreased fertility, congenital anomalies, miscarriage, and fetal death are also associated with obesity. Obesity in pregnancy is associated with higher risks, and there are significant disparities in obesity associated with race and ethnicity (Marshall, Guild, Cheng, et al., 2014).

REGIONALIZATION OF PERINATAL HEALTH CARE SERVICES

Not all facilities can develop and maintain the full spectrum of services required for high-risk perinatal patients. A regionalized system focusing on integrated delivery of graded levels of hospital-based perinatal health care services is effective and results in improved outcomes for mothers and their newborns. This system of coordinated care can be extended to preconception and ambulatory prenatal care services. In 2015, ACOG and the Society for Maternal-Fetal Medicine (SMFM) published a consensus statement on levels of maternal care (ACOG & SMFM, 2015).

Ambulatory Prenatal Care

Guidelines have been established regarding the level of care that can be expected at any given facility. In ambulatory settings, providers must distinguish themselves by the level of care they provide. Basic care is provided by obstetricians, family physicians, certified nurse-midwives, and other advanced practice clinicians approved by local governance. Routine risk-oriented prenatal care, education, and support are provided. Providers offering specialty care are obstetricians who must provide fetal diagnostic testing and management of obstetric and medical complications in addition to basic care. Subspecialty care is provided by maternal-fetal medicine specialists and reproductive geneticists and includes the aforementioned in addition to genetic testing, advanced fetal therapies, and management of severe maternal and fetal complications. Collaboration among providers to meet the woman's needs is the key to reducing perinatal morbidity and mortality.

HIGH-TECHNOLOGY CARE

Advances in scientific knowledge and the large number of high-risk pregnancies have contributed to a health care system that emphasizes high-technology care. Maternity care has extended to preconception counseling, more and better scientific techniques to monitor the mother and fetus, more definitive tests for hypoxia and acidosis, and neonatal intensive care units. The labors of virtually all women who give birth in hospitals in the United States are monitored electronically despite the lack of evidence of efficacy of such monitoring. The numbers of assisted labors and births are increasing. Internet-based information is available to the public that enhances interactions among health care providers, families, and community providers. Point-of-care testing is available. Personal data assistants are used to enhance comprehensive care; the medical record is increasingly in electronic form.

Strides are being made in identifying genetic codes, and genetic engineering is taking place. Women's health has expanded to emphasize care of older women, new cancer-screening techniques, advances in the diagnosis and treatment of breast cancer, and work on an AIDS vaccine. In general, high-technology care has flourished, whereas "health" care has become relatively neglected. Nurses must use caution and prospective planning and assess the effect of the emerging technology.

BOX 1.7   American Nurses Association's Principles for Social Networking and the Nurse

- Nurses must not transmit or place online individually identifiable patient information.
- Nurses must observe ethically prescribed professional patient-nurse boundaries.
- Nurses should understand that patients, colleagues, institutions, and employers may view postings.
- Nurses should take advantage of privacy settings and seek to separate personal and professional information online.
- Nurses should bring content that could harm a patient's privacy, rights, or welfare to the attention of appropriate authorities.
- Nurses should participate in developing institutional policies governing online contact.

From American Nurses Association. (2011). *Fact sheet: Navigating the world of social media.* Washington, DC: Author.

Telehealth is an umbrella term for the use of communication technologies and electronic information to provide or support health care when the participants are separated by distance. It permits specialists, including nurses, to provide health care and consultation when distance separates them from those needing care. This technology has the potential to save billions of dollars annually for health care, but these technologic advances have also contributed to higher health care costs..

Social Media

Social media uses Internet-based technologies to allow users to create their own content and participate in dialog. The most common social media platforms are Facebook, Twitter, and LinkedIn, with others also gaining in popularity. Social media can be integrated into nursing practice, facilitating communication among nurses and between nurses and other health care providers and patients (Casella, Mills, Usher, et al., 2014). However, there are pitfalls for nurses using this technology. Patient privacy and confidentiality can be violated, and institutions and colleagues can be cast in unfavorable lights with negative consequences for those posting the information. Nursing students have been expelled from school, and nurses have been fired or reprimanded by a Board of Nursing for injudicious posts. To help make nurses aware of their responsibilities when using social media, the American Nurses Association (ANA) published six principles for social networking and the nurse (Box 1.7). Brous (2013) referred to the *White Paper: A Nurse's Guide to the Use of Social Media* that was published by the National Council of State Boards of Nursing (NCSBN, 2011; https://www.ncsbn.org/Social_Media.pdf), detailing issues of confidentiality and privacy, possible consequences of inappropriate use of social media, common myths and misunderstandings of social media, and tips on how to avoid problems.

COMMUNITY-BASED CARE

A shift in settings from acute care institutions to ambulatory settings, including the home, has occurred. Even childbearing women at high risk are cared for on an outpatient basis or in the home. Technology previously available only in the hospital is now found in the home. This has affected the organizational structure of care, the skills required in providing such care, and the costs to consumers.

Home health care also has a community focus. Nurses are involved in providing care for women and infants in homeless shelters and adolescents in school-based clinics and in promoting health at community sites, churches, and shopping malls. Nursing education curricula are increasingly community based.

CHILDBIRTH PRACTICES

Prenatal care can promote better pregnancy outcomes by providing early risk assessment and promoting healthy behaviors such as improved nutrition and smoking cessation. Preconception care ideally begins before pregnancy because early decisions lay the foundation for the entire perinatal year. If at all possible, education continues in each trimester of pregnancy and extends through the early postpartum weeks. Some health care providers today promote preconception care as an important component of perinatal services. Preconception or early-pregnancy classes also emphasize health-promoting behavior and choices of care.

In the United States, most women received care in the first trimester. There is disparity, however, in receiving prenatal care by race and ethnicity, with non-Hispanic black women and Hispanic women receiving significantly later prenatal care as compared to non-Hispanic whites. In spite of these statistics, substantial gains have been made in the use of prenatal care since the early 1990s, which are attributed to the expansion in the 1980s of Medicaid coverage for pregnant women.

Women can choose physicians or nurse-midwives as primary care providers. In 2015, doctors of medicine attended 84% of births in hospitals, certified nurse-midwives attended 8.1%, and doctors of osteopathy attended 7.1% (Martin et al., 2017). Women who choose nurse-midwives as their primary care providers participate more actively in childbirth decisions, receive fewer interventions during labor, and are less likely to give birth prematurely (Sandall, Soltani, Gates, et al., 2013). From 2014 to 2015, there was a decline in the rate of cesarean births from 32.2% to 32.0% (Martin et al.), although Thielking (2015) reported that the approximately 1/3 rate for cesarean births is too high for resulting benefits, as benefits usually plateau at about a 19% cesarean birth rate.

INVOLVING CONSUMERS AND PROMOTING SELF-MANAGEMENT

Self-management of health care is appealing to both patients and the health care system because of its potential to reduce health care costs. Maternity care is especially suited to self-management because childbearing is primarily health focused, women are usually well when they enter the system, and visits to health care providers can present the opportunity for health and illness interventions. Measures to improve health and reduce risks associated with poor pregnancy outcomes and illness can be addressed. Topics such as nutrition education, stress management, smoking cessation, alcohol and drug treatment, prevention of violence, improvement of social supports, and parenting education are appropriate for such encounters.

INTERNATIONAL CONCERNS

Access to prenatal care and family planning education, care for women experiencing postpartum hemorrhage, obstructed labors with no access to hospital care or operative birth, fistulas due to obstructed labors, and HIV-positive parents are major international concerns. The high maternal and infant mortality in developing countries is a serious problem with limited resources to address the contributing factors. Two concerns that nurses in the United States and Canada might encounter are female genital mutilation and human trafficking.

Female genital mutilation, infibulation, and *circumcision* are terms used to describe procedures in which part or all of the female external

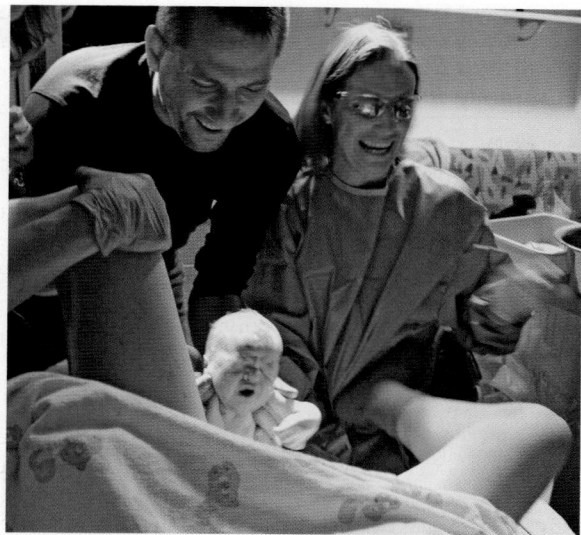

FIG 1.2 Father "catching" newborn daughter who cried before her lower body had emerged. (Courtesy of Darren and Julie Nelson, Loveland, CO.)

genitalia is removed for cultural or nontherapeutic reasons (WHO, 2016). Worldwide, many women undergo such procedures. The International Council of Nurses and other health professionals have spoken out against procedures that result in mutilation as harmful to women's health. Although it is illegal in the United States to perform female genital mutilation on a person younger than 18 years of age, it is estimated that 513,000 women and girls in the United States have experienced or are at risk for female genital mutilation (Office of Women's Health, 2015).

Human trafficking is a serious crime, an illegal business that exists in the United States and internationally, in which mostly women and children are "trafficked," or forced into hard labor, sex work, and even organ donation (Budiani-Saberi, Raja, Findley, et al., 2014; United Nations Office on Drugs & Crime, 2016). Health care professionals may interact with victims who are in captivity. This provides an opportunity to identify victims, intervene to help them obtain necessary health services, and provide information about ways to escape from their situation (Fig. 1.2) (see Chapter 3). The National Human Trafficking Resource Center (1-888-373-7888) can provide assistance.

THE FUTURE OF NURSING

In 2008, the Robert Wood Johnson Foundation and the IOM initiated a 2-year process to meet the need to assess and transform the nursing profession. The IOM appointed a committee that developed four key messages: (1) nurses should practice to the full extent of their education and training; (2) nurses should achieve higher levels of education and training through an improved education system that promotes seamless academic progression; (3) nurses should be full partners with physicians and other health care professionals in redesigning health care in the United States; and (4) effective workforce planning and policy-making require better data collection and an improved information infrastructure (IOM, 2010). Throughout the United States individual states and nursing organizations are making concerted efforts to implement the recommendations of the report. In 2015, a meeting was convened to assess the progress toward the goals outlined in the original report (National Academy of Sciences, 2015). Efforts continue toward meeting the recommendations of the original IOM report.

TRENDS IN NURSING PRACTICE

The increasing complexity of care for maternity and women's health patients has contributed to specialization of nurses working with these patients. This specialized knowledge is gained through experience, advanced degrees, and certification programs. Nurses in advanced practice (e.g., nurse practitioners and nurse-midwives) may provide primary care throughout a woman's life, including during the pregnancy cycle. In some settings, the clinical nurse specialist and nurse practitioner roles are blended, and nurses deliver high-quality, comprehensive, and cost-effective care in a variety of settings. In other settings, nurses educated in both critical care and high-risk obstetrics provide care in obstetric critical care units. Lactation consultants provide services in the hospital setting, in clinics and physician offices, and during home visits.

NURSING INTERVENTIONS CLASSIFICATION

When the National IOM proposed that all patient records be computerized by 2000, a need for a common language to describe the contributions of nurses to patient care became evident. Nurses from the University of Iowa developed a comprehensive standardized language that describes interventions that are performed by generalist or specialist nurses. This language is included in the Nursing Interventions Classification (NIC) (Bulechek, Buthcer, Dochterman, et al., 2013). Interventions commonly used by maternal-child nurses include those in Box 1.8.

EVIDENCE-BASED PRACTICE

Evidence-based practice—providing care based on evidence gained through research and clinical trials—is increasingly emphasized. Although not all practice can be evidence-based, practitioners must use the best available information on which to base their interventions. In 2013, AWHONN developed a draft document of quality measures for women's health and perinatal nursing, comparing NQF measures with AWHONN Nursing Care Quality measures (AWHONN, 2013). Discussion of nursing care and evidence-based practice boxes throughout this text provide examples of evidence-based practice in perinatal and women's health nursing (see Evidence-Based Practice box).

Cochrane Pregnancy and Childbirth Database

The Cochrane Pregnancy and Childbirth Database was first planned in 1976 with a small grant from the World Health Organization to Dr. Iain Chalmers and colleagues at Oxford. In 1993, the Cochrane Collaboration was formed, and the Oxford Database of Perinatal Trials became known as the Cochrane Pregnancy and Childbirth Database. The Cochrane Collaboration oversees up-to-date, systematic reviews of randomized controlled trials of health care and disseminates these reviews. The premise of the project is that these types of studies provide the most reliable evidence about the effects of care.

The evidence from these studies should encourage practitioners to implement useful measures and abandon those that are useless or harmful. Studies are ranked in the following six categories:
1. Beneficial forms of care
2. Forms of care that are likely to be beneficial
3. Forms of care with a trade-off between beneficial and adverse effects
4. Forms of care with unknown effectiveness
5. Forms of care that are unlikely to be beneficial
6. Forms of care that are likely to be ineffective or harmful

Joanna Briggs Institute

Established in 1996 as an initiative of the Royal Adelaide Hospital and the University of Adelaide in Australia, the Joanna Briggs Institute (JBI)

BOX 1.8   Childbearing Care Interventions

Level 1 Domain: Family
- Care that supports the family

Level 2 Class: Childbearing Care
- Interventions to assist in the preparation for childbirth and management of the psychologic and physiologic changes before, during, and immediately after childbirth

Level 3: Interventions
- Amnioinfusion
- Birthing
- Bleeding reduction: antepartum uterus
- Bleeding reduction: postpartum uterus
- Cesarean birth care
- Childbirth preparation
- Circumcision care
- Electronic fetal monitoring: antepartum
- Electronic fetal monitoring: intrapartum
- Environmental management: attachment process
- Family integrity promotion: childbearing family
- Family planning: contraception
- Family planning: infertility
- Family planning: unplanned pregnancy
- Fertility preservation
- Genetic counseling
- Grief work facilitation: perinatal death
- High-risk pregnancy care
- Infant care: newborn
- Infant care: preterm
- Intrapartal care
- Intrapartal care: high-risk delivery
- Kangaroo care
- Labor induction
- Labor suppression
- Lactation support
- Lactation suppression
- Newborn care
- Nonnutritive sucking
- Phototherapy: neonate
- Postpartal care
- Preconception counseling
- Pregnancy termination care
- Prenatal care
- Reproductive technology management
- Resuscitation: fetus
- Resuscitation: neonate
- Risk identification: childbearing family
- Surveillance: late pregnancy
- Tube care: umbilical line
- Ultrasonography: limited obstetric

From Bulechek, G. M., Butcher, H. K., Dochterman, J. M., et al. (2013). *Nursing interventions classification (NIC)* (6th ed.). St. Louis, MO: Mosby.

EVIDENCE-BASED PRACTICE

Seeking and Evaluating Evidence: A Necessary Competency for Quality and Safety

Throughout this text you will see Evidence-Based Practice boxes. These boxes provide examples of how a nurse might conduct an inquiry into an identified practice question. Curiosity and access to a virtual or real library are all the nurse needs to be confident that his or her practice has a sound foundation of evidence.

A literature search may reveal up to three levels of evidence. The first layer consists of primary studies. The strongest of these are randomized controlled trials. Well-designed studies, even small ones, add another piece to the puzzle.

These primary studies may be combined into the second level of evidence. In systematic analyses such as those in the Cochrane Database, the researcher uses a methodology to identify all studies relevant to a particular question. If the data are similar enough, they can be pooled into a meta-analysis. If the evidence is strong, some analyses will form the basis for recommendations for practice and guide further inquiry.

At the tertiary level, professional organizations such as the Agency for Healthcare Research and Quality (AHRQ) (www.ahrq.gov) or the National Guidelines Clearinghouse (NGC) (guideline.gov) may decide to address a broad practice question by sorting through all the available primary and secondary evidence and consulting experienced clinicians. After thoughtful review, the committee of experts in the organization crafts its consensus statement. These recommendations for best practice stand on the shoulders of the systematic analysts, who stand on the many shoulders of the primary researchers.

Provided that the professional organization is well-respected and the process is rigorous, these guidelines in the consensus statement carry enormous authority. Individuals and institutions may choose to adopt them with confidence. An example of this is the Association of Women's Health, Obstetric and Neonatal Nurses (AWHONN) (www.awhonn.org) Late Preterm Infant Initiative. This initiative began in 2005 in response to the confusion that surrounded the care of infants who do not qualify for NICU admission yet require extra vigilance. Nurseries can adapt these recommendations to their specific institutions, enabling nurses to become more effective at caring for the unique problems of this population of neonates. Like AWHONN, most of the professional organizations make their guidelines available free of charge on their websites.

To develop common language and goals for nursing education, the Quality and Safety Education for Nurses (QSEN) (www.qsen.org) Project expert panel identified six competencies necessary to enable the new nurse to continuously improve the health care system: patient-centered care, teamwork and collaboration, evidence-based practice, quality improvement, safety, and informatics. Most nursing challenges require a combination of these competencies. Each competency is further defined as having targets for knowledge, skills, and attitude. The Evidence-Based Practice boxes in this textbook include examples that illustrate each of these targets specific to that competency. A mastery of QSEN competencies greatly enriches the nurse's ability to identify and improve patient and health care–system problems and communicate within the interdisciplinary team.

Pat Mahaffee Gingrich

NICU, Neonatal intensive care unit.

uses a collaborative approach for evaluating evidence from a range of sources (www.joannabriggs.edu.au). The JBI has formed collaborations with a variety of universities and hospitals around the world including in the United States and Canada. The JBI uses the following grades of recommendation for evidence of feasibility, appropriateness, meaningfulness, and effectiveness: *A,* strong support that merits application; *B,* moderate support that warrants consideration of application; and *C,* not supported (JBI, 2013). The JBI provides another source for perinatal nurses to access information to support evidence-based practice.

OUTCOMES-ORIENTED PRACTICE

Outcomes of care (i.e., the effectiveness of interventions and quality of care) are receiving increased emphasis. Outcomes-oriented care measures effectiveness of care against benchmarks or standards. It is a measure of the value of nursing using quality indicators and assesses whether or not the patient benefitted from the care provided (Moorhead, Johnson, Maas, et al., 2013). The Outcome and Assessment Information Set (OASIS) is an example of an outcome system important for nursing. Its use is required by the CMS in all home health organizations that are Medicare accredited. The Nursing Outcomes Classification (NOC) is an effort to identify outcomes and related measures that can be used for evaluation of care of individuals, families, and communities across the care continuum (Moorhead et al.).

A GLOBAL PERSPECTIVE

Advances in medicine and nursing have resulted in increased knowledge and understanding in the care of mothers and infants and reduced perinatal morbidity and mortality rates. However, these advances have affected predominantly the industrialized nations. With more knowledge and implementation of interventions in other countries (e.g., antiretroviral treatment for mother during pregnancy and for baby as well, more education about prevention of transmission), the rates of HIV have the potential to decrease worldwide. Without intervention, rates of HIV transmission to infants range from 15% to 45%, but with interventions it is possible to decrease the rate to 5% (WHO, 2017).

The Zika virus is a recently discovered concern (CDC, 2016c). This is a virus that is spread via bites from infected mosquitos and may be spread through sexual intercourse with an infected partner. The virus can also be spread to a fetus, leading to microcephaly. Currently there is no vaccine for this virus, and much more research is needed to better understand and treat this infectious disease. More discussion about the Zika virus is included in Chapter 4.

As the world becomes smaller because of travel and communication technologies, nurses and other health care providers are gaining a global perspective and participating in activities to improve the health and health care of people worldwide. Nurses participate in medical outreach, providing obstetric, surgical, ophthalmologic, orthopedic, or other services (Fig. 1.3); attend international meetings; conduct research; and provide international consultation. International student and faculty exchanges occur. More articles about health and health care in various countries are appearing in nursing journals. Several schools of nursing in the United States are World Health Organization Collaborating Centers.

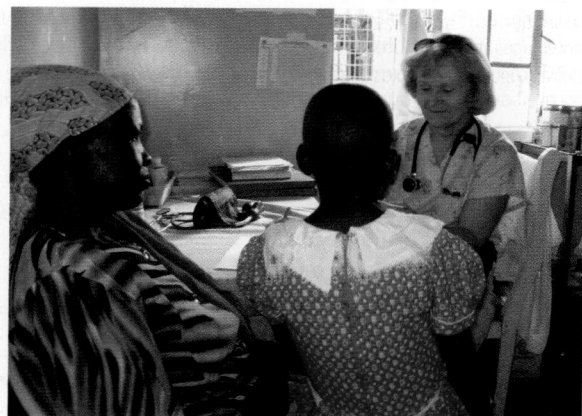

FIG 1.3 Nurse interviewing a young girl accompanied by her mother in a clinic in rural Kenya. (Courtesy of Shannon Perry, Phoenix, AZ.)

STANDARDS OF PRACTICE AND LEGAL ISSUES IN DELIVERY OF CARE

Several organizations have described standards of practice in perinatal and women's health nursing. These organizations include the ANA, which publishes standards for maternal-child health nursing; the AWHONN, which publishes standards of practice and education for perinatal nurses (Box 1.9); the American College of Nurse-Midwives (ACNM), which publishes standards of practice for midwives; and the National Association of Neonatal Nurses (NANN), which publishes standards of practice for neonatal nurses. These standards reflect current knowledge, represent levels of practice agreed on by leaders in the specialty, and can be used for clinical benchmarking.

In addition to these more formalized standards, agencies have their own policies, procedures, and protocols that outline standards to be followed in that setting. In legal terms, the standard of care is that level of practice that a reasonably prudent nurse would provide in the same or similar circumstances. In determining legal negligence, the care given is compared with the standard of care. If the standard was not met and harm resulted, negligence occurred. The number of legal suits in the perinatal area typically has been high. As a consequence, malpractice insurance costs are high for physicians, nurse-midwives, and nurses who work in labor and birth settings.

> **LEGAL TIP Standard of Care**   When a nurse is uncertain about how to perform a procedure, he or she should consult the agency's policies and procedures documents. These guidelines are the standard of care for that agency.

PREVENTION OF ERRORS IN NURSING CARE

Medical errors are now the third leading cause of death (Makary & Daniel, 2016). To decrease the risk for errors in the administration of medications, in 2009 The Joint Commission (TJC) developed an official list of abbreviations, acronyms, and symbols *not* to use, which was updated in 2013 (Glassman, 2013) (Table 1.3). In addition, each agency must develop its own list.

SENTINEL EVENTS

TJC (2015) revised its definition of a sentinel event as any event that is not due to underlying conditions or natural courses of a patient's condition that affects a patient, resulting in death, permanent harm, or severe temporary harm. This refers to perinatal events, specifically the need for receiving 4 or more units of blood products and/or admission to the ICU.

FAILURE TO RESCUE

Failure to rescue is the failure to recognize or act on early signs of distress. Key components of failure to rescue are (1) careful surveillance and identification of complications, and (2) quick action to initiate appropriate interventions and activate a team response. For the perinatal nurse, this involves careful surveillance, timely identification of complications, appropriate interventions, and activation of a team response to minimize patient harm. Maternal complications that are appropriate for process measurement are placental abruption, postpartum hemorrhage, uterine rupture, eclampsia, and amniotic fluid embolism (Simpson, Knox, Martin, et al., 2011). Fetal complications include nonreassuring

BOX 1.9 Standards of Care for Women and Newborns

Standards That Define the Nurse's Responsibility to the Patient

Assessment
- Collection of health data of the woman or newborn

Diagnosis
- Analysis of data to determine nursing diagnosis

Outcome Identification
- Identification of expected outcomes that are individualized

Planning
- Development of a plan of care

Implementation
- Performance of interventions for the plan of care

Evaluation
- Evaluation of the effectiveness of interventions in relation to expected outcomes

Standards of Professional Performance That Delineate Roles and Behaviors for Which the Professional Nurse Is Accountable

Quality of Care
- Systematic evaluation of nursing practice

Performance Appraisal
- Self-evaluation in relation to professional practice standards and other regulations

Education
- Participation in ongoing educational activities to maintain knowledge for practice

Collegiality
- Contribution to the development of peers, students, and others

Ethics
- Use of American Nurses Association (ANA) Code of Ethics for Nurses with Interpretive Statements (ANA, 2015) to guide practice collaboration
- Involvement of patient, significant others, and other health care providers in the provision of patient care

Research
- Use of research findings in practice

Resource Utilization
- Consideration of factors related to safety, effectiveness, and costs in planning and delivering patient care

Practice Environment
- Contribution to the environment of care delivery

Accountability
- Legal and professional responsibility for practice

From Association of Women's Health, Obstetric and Neonatal Nurses. (2009). *Standards and guidelines for professional practice in the care of women and newborns* (7th ed.). Washington, DC: Author.

TABLE 1.3 The Joint Commission "Do Not Use" List

Do Not Use	Potential Problem	Use Instead
IU (International Unit)	Mistaken for IV (intravenous) or the number 10 (ten)	Write "International Unit"
Lack of leading zero (.X mg)	Decimal point is missed	Write "0.X mg"
MS	Can mean morphine sulfate or magnesium sulfate	Write "morphine sulfate"
MSO₄ and MgSO₄	Confused for one another	Write "magnesium sulfate"
Q.D., QD, q.d., qd (daily)	Mistaken for each other	Write "daily"
Q.O.D., QOD, q.o.d, qod (every other day)	Period after the Q mistaken for "I" and the "O" mistaken for "I"	Write "every other day"
Trailing zero (X.0 mg)*	Decimal point is missed	Write "X mg"
U, u (unit)	Mistaken for "0" (zero), the number "4" (four), or "cc"	Write "unit"
Additional Abbreviations, Acronyms, and Symbols*		
> (greater than) < (less than)	Misinterpreted as the number "7" (seven) or the letter "L"; confused for one another	Write "greater than" Write "less than"
Abbreviations for drug names	Misinterpreted because of similar abbreviations for multiple drugs	Write drug names in full
Apothecary units	Unfamiliar to many practitioners Confused with metric units	Use metric units
@	Mistaken for the number "2" (two)	Write "at"
cc	Mistaken for U (units) when poorly written	Write "mL" or "ml" or "milliliters" ("mL" is preferred)
μg	Mistaken for mg (milligrams) resulting in one-thousandfold overdose	Write "mcg" or "micrograms"

*For possible future inclusion in the Official "Do Not Use" List. From The Joint Commission. The Joint Commission "Do Not Use" list, updated 2012. Retrieved from www.jointcommission.org/PatientSafety/DoNotUseList.
See "dnu_list.pdf" and "Facts about the Official Do Not Use List of Abbreviations." Cited in *Pharmacy Technician*. (2015). Retrieved from http://pharmacytechniciantoday.com/joint-commission-do-not-use-list/.

fetal heart rate and pattern, prolapsed umbilical cord, shoulder dystocia, and uterine hyperstimulation (Simpson et al.).

ETHICAL ISSUES IN PERINATAL NURSING AND WOMEN'S HEALTH CARE

Ethical concerns and debates have multiplied with the increased use of technology and scientific advances. For example, with reproductive technology pregnancy is now possible in women who thought they would never bear children, including some who are menopausal or postmenopausal. Should scarce resources be devoted to achieving pregnancies in older women? Is giving birth to a child at an older age worth the risks involved? Should older parents be encouraged to conceive a baby when they may not live to see the child reach adulthood? Should a woman who is HIV positive have access to assisted reproduction services? Should third-party payers assume the costs of reproductive technology such as the use of induced ovulation and in vitro fertilization? With induced ovulation and in vitro fertilization, multiple pregnancies occur, and multifetal pregnancy reduction (selectively terminating one or more fetuses) may be considered. Questions about informed consent and allocation of resources must be addressed with innovations such as intrauterine fetal surgery, fetoscopy, therapeutic insemination, genetic engineering, stem cell research, surrogate childbearing, surgery for infertility, "test tube" babies, fetal research, and treatment of very low–birth weight (VLBW) babies. The introduction of long-acting contraceptives has created moral choices and policy dilemmas for health care providers and legislators (i.e., should some women [substance abusers, women with low incomes, or women who are HIV positive] be required to take the contraceptives?). With the potential benefits from fetal tissue transplantation, what research is ethical? What are the rights of the embryo? Should cloning of humans be permitted? Discussion and debate about these issues will continue for many years. Nurses and patients, together with scientists, physicians, attorneys, lawmakers, ethicists, and clergy, must be involved in the discussions.

REFERENCES

Agency for Healthcare Research and Quality. (2014). *20 Tips to Help Prevent Medical Errors: Patient Fact Sheet*, December 2014, Rockville, MD. Retrieved from http://archive.ahrq.gov/patients-consumers/care-planning/errors/20tips/index.html.

American Academy of Nurse Practitioners. (2015). *AANP Voices Support for Senate Bill Empowering Nurse Practitioners in the Veterans Health Administration*. Retrieved from https://www.aanp.org/press-room/press-releases/166-press-room/2015-press-releases/1730-aanp-voices-support-for-senate-bill-empowering-nurse-practitioners-in-the-veterans-health-administration.

American College of Obstetricians and Gynecologists. (2015). Levels of maternal care. Obstetric Care Consensus No. 2. *Obstetrics and Gynecology*, *1225*, 502–515. Retrieved from http://www.acog.org/Resources-And-Publications/Obstetric-Care-Consensus-Series/Levels-of-Maternal-Care.

American Nurses Association. (2015). *Code of ethics for nurses with interpretive statements*. Silver Spring, MD: Author.

Association of Women's Health, Obstetric and Neonatal Nurses. (2013). *Women's health and perinatal nursing quality draft measures specifications*. Retrieved from https://c.ymcdn.com/sites/www.awhonn.org/resource/resmgr/Downloadables/perinatalqualitymeasures.pdf.

Branum, A. M., Kirmeyer, S. E., & Gregory, E. C. S. (2016). Prepregnancy body mass index by maternal characteristics and state: Data from the birth certificate, 2014. *National Vital Statistics Reports*, *65*(6), 1–11.

Brous, E. (2013). How to avoid pitfalls in social media. *American Nurse Today*, *8*(5), Retrieved from https://americannursetoday.com/how-to-avoid-the-pitfalls-of-social-media/.

Budiani-Saberi, D. A., Raja, K. R., Findley, K. C., et al. (2014). Human trafficking for organ removal in India: A victim-centered, evidence-based report. *Transplantation*, *97*(4), 380–384.

Bulechek, G. M., Butcher, H. K., Dochterman, J. M., et al. (2013). *Nursing interventions classification (NIC)* (6th ed.). St. Louis, MO: Mosby.

Casella, E., Mills, J., & Usher, K. (2014). Social media and nursing practice: Changing the balance between the social and technical aspects of work. *Collegian*, *21*, 121–126.

Centers for Disease Control and Prevention. (2013a). CDC Health disparities & inequalities report—United States, 2013. *Morbidity and Mortality Weekly Report*, *62*(3 suppl), 1–187.

Centers for Disease Control and Prevention. (2016a). *Health literacy*. Retrieved from www.cdc.gov/healthliteracy.

Centers for Disease Control and Prevention. (2016b). *Pregnancy mortality surveillance system*, 2016. Retrieved from https://www.cdc.gov/reproductivehealth/maternalinfanthealth/pmss.html.

Centers for Disease Control and Prevention. (2016c). *Zika and pregnancy*. Retrieved from http://www.cdc.gov/zika/pregnancy/question-answers.html.

Centers for Medicare and Medicaid. (2015). *NHE fact sheet*. Retrieved from https://www.cms.gov/research-statistics-data-and-systems/statistics-trends-and-reports/nationalhealthexpenddata/nhe-fact-sheet.html.

Colby, S. L., & Ortman, J. (2015). *Projections of the size and composition of the US population: 2014-2016*. US Census Bureau. Retrieved from https://www.census.gov/library/publications/2015/demo/p25-1143.html.

Dickens, C., & Piano, M. R. (2013). Health literacy and nursing: An update. *American Journal of Nursing*, *113*(6), 52–57.

Firoz, T., Chou, D., von Dadelszen, P., et al. for the Maternal Morbidity Working Group. (2013). Measuring maternal health: Focus on maternal morbidity. *Bulletin of the World Health Organization*, *91*, 794–796. Retrieved from http://www.who.int/bulletin/volumes/91/10/13-117564/en/.

Glassman, P. (2013). *The Joint Commission's "Do Not Use" list: Brief review (NEW)*. In Making Health Care Safer II: An Updated Critical Analysis of the Evidence for Patient Safety Practices. Evidence Reports/Technology Assessments, No. 211. Rockville, MD: Agency for Healthcare Research and Quality.

Hayes, C., Jackson, D., Davidson, P. M., & Power, T. (2015). Medication errors in hospitals: A literature review of disruptions to nursing practice during medication administration. *Journal of Clinical Nursing*, *24*(21–22), 3063–3076. (epub Aug 9, 2015).

Institute for Healthcare Improvement. (2016). Retrieved from http://www.ihi.org/education/WebTraining/Expeditions/AdvancingSaferMaternalandNewbornCare/Pages/default.aspx.

Institute of Medicine. (2000). *To err is human: Building a safer health system*. L. T. Kohn, J. M. Corrigan, & M. S. Donaldson (Eds.). Washington, DC: National Academy Press.

Institute of Medicine. (2010). *The future of nursing: Leading change, advancing health*. Washington, DC: National Academy of Sciences.

Interprofessional Education Collaborative. (2016). Retrieved from https://ipecollaborative.org/About_IPEC.html.

The Joanna Briggs Institute. (2013). *JBI grading recommendations*. Retrieved from http://joannabriggs.org/jbi-approach.html#tabbed-nav-Grades-of-Recommendation.

The Joint Commission. (2009). *Official "do not use" list*, Retrieved from http://www.jointcommission.org/assets/1/18/dnu_list.pdf. 2009.

The Joint Commission. (2015). *Comprehensive accreditation manual for hospitals*, Update 2. Sentinel events. Retrieved from http://www.jointcommission.org/assets/1/6/CAMH_24_SE_all_CURRENT.pdf.

Kaiser Permanente of Colorado. (2014). *SBAR technique for communication: A situational briefing model*. Retrieved from http://www.ihi.org/resources/Pages/Tools/SBARTechniqueforCommunicationASituationalBriefingModel.aspx.

Leapfrog Group. (2015). *Hospital errors are the third leading cause of death in the U.S., and new hospital safety scores show improvements are slow*. Washington, DC: Author. Retrieved from http://www.hospitalsafetygrade.org/newsroom/display/hospitalerrors-thirdleading-causeofdeathinus-improvementstooslow.

MacDorman, M. F., Mathews, T. J., Mohangoo, A. D., et al. (2014). International comparisons of infant mortality and related factors: United States and Europe, 2010. *National Vital Statistics Reports*, *63*(5), Retrieved from http://www.cdc.gov/nchs/data/nvsr/nvsr63/nvsr63_05.pdf.

Makary, M. A., & Daniel, M. (2016). Medical error—The third leading cause of death in the United States. *British Medical Journal*, *353*, i2139,

Marshall, N. E., Guild, C., Cheng, Y. W., et al. (2014). Racial disparities in pregnancy outcomes in obese women. *Journal of Maternal Fetal Neonatal Medicine*, *27*(2), 122–126.

Martin, J. A., Hamilton, B. E., Osterman, M. J. K., et al. (2017). Births: Final data for 2015. *National Vital Statistics Report*, *66*(1). Retrieved from https://www.cdc.gov/nchs/data/nvsr/nvsr66/nvsr66_01.pdf.

Moorhead, S., Johnson, M., Maas, M., et al. (Eds.), (2013). *Nursing outcomes classification (NOC)* (5th ed.). St. Louis, MO: Elsevier.

National Academy of Sciences. (2015). *Assessing progress on the Institute of Medicine report on the Future of Nursing*. Retrieved from http://www.nationalacademies.org/hmd/~/media/Files/Report%20Files/2015/AssessingFON_releaseslides/Nursing-Report-in-brief.pdf.

National Partnership for Action to End Health Disparities. (2016). *NPA background*. Rockville, MD: US Department of Health & Human Services, Office of Minority Health. Retrieved from http://minorityhealth.hhs.gov/npa/templates/browse.aspx?1v1=1&1v1id=45.

National Quality Forum. (2011). *Serious reportable events in healthcare—2011 update: a consensus report*. Washington, DC: NQF.

National Quality Forum. (2013). *Safe Practices for Better Healthcare—2013 update: a consensus report*. Washington, DC: NQF. In Health Care Facilities Accreditation Program. Retrieved from http://www.hfap.org/pdf/patient_safety.pdf.

Office of Women's Health. (2015). *Female genital cutting*. Retrieved from http://womenshealth.gov/publications/our-publications/fact-sheet/female-genital-cutting.html.

Sandall, J., Soltani, H., Gates, S., et al. (2013). Midwife-led continuity models of care for childbearing women. *The Cochrane Library*, issue 8. John Wiley & Sons.

Simpson, K. R., Knox, E., Martin, M., et al. (2011). Michigan Health & Hospital Association Keystone Obstetrics: A statewide collaborative for perinatal patient safety in Michigan. *Joint Commission Journal on Quality and Patient Safety, 37*(12), 544–552.

Smith, J. C., & Medalia, C. (2015). *Health insurance coverage in the United States: 2014*. Current Population Report. US Census Bureau. P60-253.

Washington, DC: US Government Printing Office. Retrieved from https://www.census.gov/content/dam/Census/library/publications/2015/demo/p60-253.pdf.

Thielking, M. (2015). *Sky-high C-section rates in the US don't translate to better birth outcomes. Stat*. Retrieved from https://www.statnews.com/2015/12/01/cesarean-section-childbirth/.

Tong, V. T., Dietz, P. M., Morrow, B., et al. (2013). Trends in smoking before, during, and after pregnancy—Pregnancy risk assessment monitoring system, United States, 40 sites, 2000-2010. *Morbidity and Mortality Weekly Report, 62*(6), 1–19.

United Nations Development Programme. (2016). *Sustainable Development Goals*. Retrieved from http://www.un.org/sustainabledevelopment/sustainable-development-goals/.

United Nations Office on Drugs and Crime. (2016). *Human trafficking*. Retrieved from https://www.unodc.org/unodc/en/human-trafficking/what-is-human-trafficking.html.

US Department of Health and Human Services, Office of Disease Prevention and Health Promotion. (2015). *National action plan to improve health literacy*. Washington, DC: Author. Retrieved from http://minorityhealth.hhs.gov/omh/browse.aspx?lvl=2&lvlid=10.

World Health Organization. (2016). *WHO guidelines on the management of health complications from female genital mutilation*. Geneva, Switzerland: World Health Organization. Retrieved from http://www.who.int/mediacentre/news/releases/2016/female-genital-mutilation-guidelines/en/.

World Health Organization. (2017). *Mother-to-child transmission of HIV*. Geneva, Switzerland: World Health Organization. Retrieved from http://www.who.int/hiv/topics/mtct/about/en/.

2

The Family, Culture, Spirituality, and Home Care

Shannon E. Perry

http://evolve.elsevier.com/Perry/maternal

The composition, structure, and function of the American family have changed dramatically in recent years, largely in response to economic, demographic, sociocultural, and technologic trends that influence family life and health. Despite current efforts to improve the overall health of the nation, there is widespread concern about family health and well-being as a reflection of individual, community, and national health status. Recent economic changes have further reduced the ability to access health care. In addition to facing significant barriers in accessing needed services, women and families are faced with the challenge of overcoming discrimination in health care practices. It is critical to consider racial and ethnic differences and sexual orientation when addressing the health status of women. American women with a minority racial or ethnic affiliation share poorer outcomes in a wide variety of conditions. Lesbian women may conceal sexual orientation for fear of discrimination. As cultural diversity increases and demographics change, nurses must become culturally competent in order to recognize and reduce or eliminate health disparities (Freund, 2012).

As perinatal health trends emerge, nurses are assuming greater roles in assessing family health status and providing care across the perinatal continuum. This continuum begins with family planning and continues with the following categories of care: preconception, prenatal, intrapartum, postpartum, newborn, and interconception (between pregnancies). Depending on the needs of the individual family unit, independent self-management, outpatient care, home care, low-risk hospitalization, or specialized intensive care may be appropriate at different points along this continuum.

THE FAMILY IN CULTURAL AND SPIRITUAL CONTEXT

The family and its cultural and spiritual context play an important role in defining the work of maternity nurses. Despite modern stresses and strains, the family forms a social network that acts as a potent support system for its members. Family health-seeking behavior and relationships with health care professionals are influenced by culturally related health beliefs and spiritual values. Ultimately, all of these factors have the power to affect maternal and child health outcomes. The current emphasis in working with families is on wellness and empowerment for families to achieve control over their lives. It is essential that nurses become culturally competent and cognizant of spirituality in its various meanings and interpretations in order to provide appropriate care.

DEFINING FAMILY

The family has traditionally been viewed as the primary unit of socialization. The family plays a pivotal role in health care, representing the

primary target of health care delivery for maternal and newborn nurses. As one of society's most important institutions, the family represents a primary social group that influences and is influenced by other people and institutions. A variety of family configurations exist. Each of these is characterized by certain structural features.

FAMILY ORGANIZATION AND STRUCTURE

The *nuclear family* has long represented the traditional American family in which husband, wife, and their children (either biologic or adopted) live as an independent unit, sharing roles, responsibilities, and economic resources (Fig. 2.1). Today the number of families living in a nuclear family structure is steadily decreasing in response to societal changes. By race and Hispanic origin, this family structure is represented as follows (Lofquist, Lugaila, O'Connell, et al., 2012):

- Caucasian: 51.1%
- Hispanic: 50.1%
- African-American: 28.5%
- Asian: 59.7%
- American Indian and Alaska Native: 40.1%
- Native Hawaiian and Pacific Islander: 51.3%

Many nuclear families have other relatives living in the same household. These extended family members include grandparents, aunts, uncles, or other people related by blood. Members of extended families can also live in close proximity to the nuclear family. Due to societal changes, Internet access, and increased mobility, these families may also be a long-distance unit (Fig. 2.2). The *extended family* is becoming more common as American society ages. The extended family provides social, emotional, and financial support to one another. It is therefore important for nurses to recognize the desire for people of many cultures to include their family in making important decisions even if extended family members are not physically close. This has implications for privacy and sharing individual health information under the Health Insurance Portability and Accountability Act (HIPAA) rules.

Multigenerational families, consisting of three or more generations of relatives (grandparents, children, grandchildren) are becoming increasingly common. In 2015, they made up 5.9% of all households (US Census Bureau, 2015). This type of arrangement can create stress for some as children must care for their parents as well as their own children. Other types of multigenerational families consist of grandparents supporting children and grandchildren or as sole caregivers for the grandchildren.

No-biologic-parent families are those in which children live independently in foster or kinship care such as living with a grandparent. In 2012, an estimated 7 million children in the United States live with grandparents (Ellis & Simmons, 2014). Of these grandparents, 2.7 million

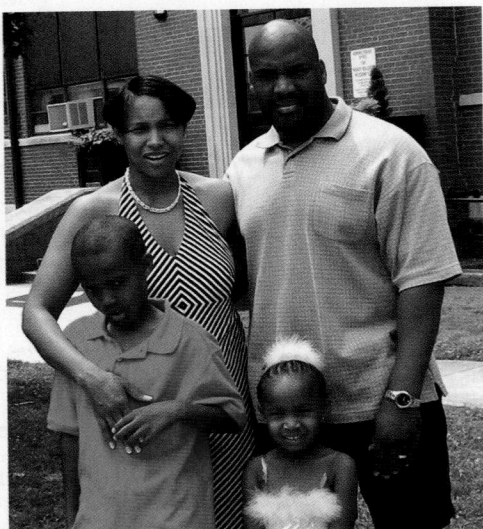

FIG 2.1 Nuclear family. (Courtesy of Makeba Felton, Wake Forest, NC.)

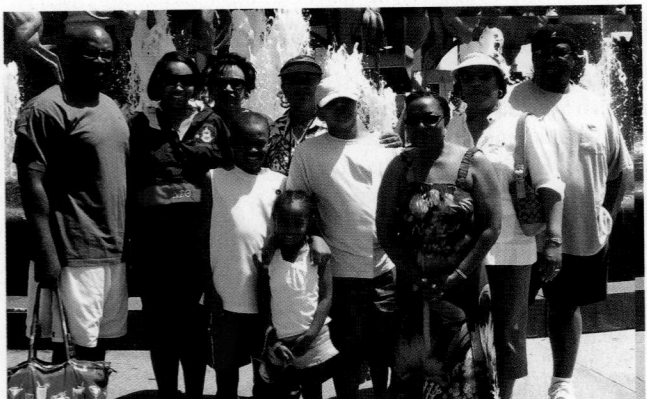

FIG 2.2 Extended family. (Courtesy of Makeba Felton, Wake Forest, NC.)

are responsible for most of the basic needs (i.e., food, shelter, and clothing) of one or more grandchildren (US Census Bureau, 2011).

Married-blended families, those formed as a result of divorce and remarriage, consist of unrelated family members (stepparents, stepchildren, stepsiblings) who join to create a new household. These family groups frequently involve a biologic or adoptive parent whose spouse may or may not have adopted the child.

Cohabiting-parent families are those in which children live with two unmarried biologic parents or two adoptive parents. Hispanic children are almost twice as likely as African-American children to live in cohabiting-parent families and about four times as likely as Caucasian children to live in this kind of family arrangement (Lofquist et al., 2012).

Single-parent families comprise an unmarried biologic or adoptive parent who may or may not be living with other adults. The single-parent family may result from the loss of a spouse by death, divorce, separation, or desertion; from either an unplanned or planned pregnancy, including those achieved through reproductive technology; or from the adoption of a child by an unmarried woman or man. This family structure is continually on the rise. In 2012, 24% of children lived with only their mothers, 4% lived with only their fathers, and 4% lived with neither of their biologic parents (America's Children, 2013). The single-parent family tends to be vulnerable economically and socially, creating an

unstable and deprived environment for the growth of children. This in turn affects health status, school achievement, and high-risk behaviors for these children (Scharte & Bolte, 2012). Some families become more stable with the absence of drugs, alcohol, and/or physical/emotional abuse.

Homosexual families (lesbian, gay, bisexual, transgender [LGBT]) may live together with or without children. Usually formed by same-sex couples, they can also consist of single LGBT parents or multiple parenting figures. Children in LGBT families may be the offspring of previous heterosexual unions, conceived by one member of a lesbian couple through natural or therapeutic insemination, conceived by a gay couple using a surrogate, or adopted. Approximately 594,000 same-sex couple households lived in the United States in 2010, raising about 115,000 children younger than 18 years of age. When these children are combined with LGBT parents who are raising children, almost 2 million children are being raised by LGBT parents in the United States (Siegel & Perrin, 2013).

THE FAMILY IN SOCIETY

The social context for the family can be viewed in relation to social and demographic trends that define the population as a whole. Racial and ethnic diversity of the population has grown dramatically, necessitating consideration of such diversity in provision of health care. According to the 2010 census, approximately 36% of the population belongs to a racial or ethnic minority group (Centers for Disease Control and Prevention [CDC], 2016).

THEORETIC APPROACHES TO UNDERSTANDING FAMILIES

FAMILY NURSING

Family plays a pivotal role in health care, representing the primary target of health care delivery for maternal and newborn nurses. It is crucial that nurses assist families as they incorporate new additions into their family (see Nursing Care Plan). When treating the woman and family with respect and dignity, health care professionals listen to and honor perspectives and choices of the woman and family. They share information with families in ways that are positive, useful, timely, complete, and accurate. The family is supported in participating in the care and decision making at the level of their choice.

Families are viewed as part of the interprofessional health care team and as the unit of care. Because so many variables affect ways of relating, the nurse must be aware that family members may interact and communicate with each other in ways that are distinct from those of the nurse's own family of origin. Most families will hold some beliefs about health that are different from those of the nurse. Their beliefs can conflict with principles of health care management predominant in the Western health care system.

Family nursing interventions occur within nurse-family relationships through therapeutic conversation (Bell, 2013; Wright & Bell, 2009). This necessitates interacting with family members present during caregiving, asking about those who may be absent, and actively listening to words and noting expressions to facilitate understanding. To do this within time constraints, Wright and Leahey (1999, 2013) developed a format for a brief therapeutic interview (Table 2.1).

FAMILY THEORIES

A **family theory** can be used to describe families and how the family unit responds to events both within and outside the family. Each family theory makes certain assumptions about the family and has inherent

◎ NURSING CARE PLAN

Incorporating the Infant Into the Family

Case Study

Corita, who is Mexican-American and 23 years of age, gave birth to her first baby at term, a healthy male infant weighing 3600 grams. Her husband, Juan, also Mexican-American, was present at the birth and is very excited to have a son whom he named Jesus. Soon after birth, the infant latched readily and sucked strongly for 5 minutes before falling asleep. The nurse assisted Juan to hold Jesus in an appropriate position. Juan asked several questions of the nurse: how often should Jesus be fed, what are the red spots on the back of his neck, why is he bundled so tightly in his blanket.

Assessment

What are signs that Corita and Juan have prepared for incorporating the baby into the family?

Defining Characteristics

Corita demonstrates appropriate baby feeding techniques and Juan demonstrates basic baby care techniques
The couple provide safe a environment for the baby
Corita and Juan use support systems appropriately

Nursing Diagnosis

Readiness for Enhanced Childbearing Process

Expected Outcomes

Corita and Juan will convey confidence in their knowledge of newborn care.
Corita and Juan will demonstrate attachment behaviors toward Jesus.
Jesus' physical, nutritional, and social needs will be met.

Nursing Interventions	Rationales
Assess baseline knowledge of newborn care.	To identify knowledge deficits
Provide written literature on newborn care.	To allow time to understand new information
Teach Corita and Juan newborn care.	Demonstrating proper care improves confidence and reduces anxiety

Case Study (Continued)

Corita and Jesus were discharged 2 days after his birth. Corita's lochia was diminishing, her perineum was healing, she was breastfeeding successfully, and both Corita and Juan were comfortable holding Jesus and changing diapers. Corita's mother is planning to stay with them to cook and help as needed for 1 week. Corita and Juan welcome her input about caring for Jesus and interpreting his behavioral cues.

Assessment

What are the signs of enhanced parenting?

Defining Characteristics

Willingness of Juan and Corita to enhance parenting
Bonding and attachment
Fulfillment of emotional and physical needs of Jesus
Realistic expectations of Jesus

Nursing Diagnosis

Readiness for Enhanced Parenting

Expected Outcomes

Corita and Juan express satisfaction in role of parent
Corita and Juan will express confidence in their ability to parent

Baby care routines are adequate
Family will enjoy spending time together

Nursing Interventions	Rationales
Discuss with Corita and Juan their perceptions and philosophy of parenting.	To provide an opportunity to clarify the parent's perceptions
Support Corita and Juan as they adapt to the changing family needs.	Recogning and appreciating the efforts of Corita and Juan enhances their motivation to continue to improve
Explore Juan's and Corita's value system and their spiritual beliefs and practices	Values and spirituality provide a basis for moral and ethical reasoning and enhance the meaning of life

Case Study (Continued)

Corita and Juan have increasing confidence in their infant caregiving skills, and breastfeeding is going well. Jesus is gaining weight and sleeping several hours at a time. Juan is ready to resume their sexual relationship, while Corita is somewhat hesitant, fearing that penile penetration will be painful.

Assessment

What was their usual pattern of sexual relations prior and during pregnancy? Does Corita still have lochia? How comfortable are Corita and Juan discussing their sexual relations?

Defining Characteristics

Demonstrate mutual respect between partners
Demonstrate understanding of partner's hesitance in resuming sexual relations
Understand physiologic changes due to pregnancy and childbirth
Express desire to enhance communication between partners

Nursing Diagnosis

Readiness for Enhanced Relationship

Expected Outcomes

Corita and Juan will communicate effectively.
Corita will articulate ways to mutually meet physical and emotional needs of herself and Juan.
Corita and Juan will understand the changes in sexuality related to pregnancy and childbirth.
Corita and Juan will express satisfaction with sharing of information and ideas between partners.
Corita and Juan's sexual relationship will resume when both partners are ready.

Nursing Interventions	Rationales
Assess communication techniques and effectiveness of couple and family.	To be able to counsel and/or refer appropriately as needed
Encourage Corita and Juan to share information and ideas.	To enhance communication
Teach Corita and Juan normal changes in sexuality due to pregnancy and postpartum status.	So they can better understand what is normal and resume sexual relations when they are both comfortable
Refer as needed to colleagues in other disciplines.	To facilitate enhanced communication

TABLE 2.1   Key Ingredients of a 15-Minute (or Shorter) Family Interview

Ingredient	Exemplars
Manners	Introduce yourself to patients and families, preferably by your full name (i.e., Ms., Mrs., Mr. Jones).
	Make eye contact with all members of the family.
	Inquire about relationship of persons with the patient.
	Always call your patients by name.
Therapeutic Conversations	Interview is purposeful and time-limited
	Provide opportunity for patient and family to be acknowledged.
	Involve patients in information giving and decision making.
	Routinely invite families to accompany the patient to the unit/clinic.
	Invite families to ask questions during patient orientation.
	Routinely consult families and patients about their ideas for treatment and discharge.
Family Genograms and Ecomaps	Draw a quick genogram (and if indicated, an ecomap) for all families (see Figs. 2.4 and 2.5).
	Acknowledge that illness is a family affair.
	Include essential information such as ages, occupation, school grade, religion, ethnic background, and current health status of all family members.
Therapeutic Questions	Think of at least three questions to routinely ask all families.
	Basic themes include sharing of information, expectations of hospitalization, clinic, or home care visit, challenges, sufferings, and most pressing concerns/problems.
Commending Family and Individual Strengths	Offer at least two commendations to family on strengths, resources, or competencies that were observed or reported to the nurse. These are observations of behavior patterns rather than one-time occurrences.
	Evaluate usefulness of the interview and conclude.

From Wright, L. M., & Leahey, M. (1999). Maximizing time, minimizing suffering: The 15-minute (or less) family interview. *Journal of Family Nursing, 5*(3), 259-273.

strengths and limitations. Most nurses use a combination of theories in their work with families. For more in depth information about family theories, a textbook describing various family theories can be consulted. Use of a family theory can guide assessment and interventions for the family.

FAMILY ASSESSMENT

When selecting a family assessment framework, an appropriate model for a perinatal nurse is one that is a health-promotion rather than an illness-care model. The low-risk family can be assisted in promoting a healthy pregnancy, childbirth, and integration of the newborn into the family. The high-risk perinatal family has illness-care needs, and the nurse can help meet those needs while also promoting the health of the childbearing family.

BOX 2.1   Calgary Family Assessment Model

There are three major categories of the Calgary Family Assessment Model (CFAM)—structural, developmental, and functional. Each category has several subcategories. In this box, only the major categories are included. A few sample questions are included.

Structural Assessment
- Determine the members of the family, relationship among family members, and context of family.
- Genograms and ecomaps (see Figs. 2.4; 2.5) are useful in outlining the internal and external structures of a family.

Sample Questions
- Who are the members of your family?
- Has anyone moved in or out lately?
- Are there any family members who do not live with you?

Developmental Assessment
- Describe the life cycle—that is, the typical trajectory most families experience.

Sample Questions
- When you think back, what do you most enjoy about your life?
- What do you regret about your life?
- Have you made plans for your care as your health declines?

Functional Assessment
- Evaluate the way in which individuals behave in relation to each other in instrumental and expressive aspects. (Instrumental aspects are activities of daily living; expressive aspects include communication, problem solving, roles, etc.)

Sample Questions
- Who in the family is responsible for making sure Grandma takes her medicine?
- Whose turn is it to make dinner for Grandma?
- How can we get Martin to help with Grandma's care?

Data from Wright, L. M., & Leahey, M. (2013). *Nurses and families: A guide to family assessment and intervention* (6th ed.). Philadelphia, PA: FA Davis.

A family assessment tool such as the Calgary Family Assessment Model (CFAM) (Box 2.1) can be used as a guide for assessing aspects of the family. Such an assessment is based on "the nurse's personal and professional life experiences, beliefs, and relationships with those being interviewed" (Wright & Leahy, 2013) and is not "the truth" about the family but, rather, one perspective at one point in time.

The CFAM comprises three major categories: structural, developmental, and functional. Several subcategories are within each category. The three assessment categories and the many subcategories can be conceptualized as a branching diagram (Fig. 2.3). These categories and subcategories can be used to guide the assessment that will provide data to help the nurse better understand the family and formulate a nursing care plan. The nurse asks questions of family members about themselves to gain understanding of the structure, development, and function of the family at this point in time. Not all questions within the subcategories should be asked at the first interview, and some questions may not be appropriate for all families. Although individuals are the ones interviewed, the focus of the assessment is on interaction of individuals within the family.

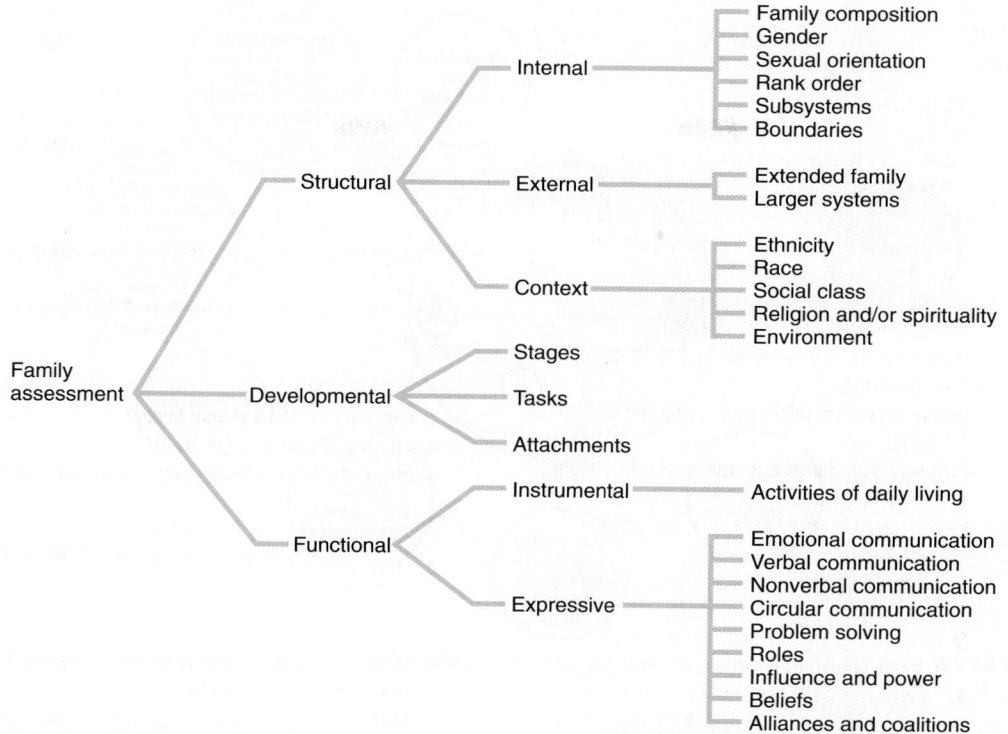

FIG 2.3 Branching diagram of Calgary Family Assessment Model (CFAM). (From Wright, L. M., & Leahy, M. [2013]. *Nurses and families: A guide to family assessment and intervention* (6th ed.) Philadelphia, PA: FA Davis.)

GRAPHIC REPRESENTATIONS OF FAMILIES

A family **genogram** (family tree format depicting relationships of family members over at least three generations) (Fig. 2.4) provides valuable information about a family and can be placed in the nursing care plan for easy access by care providers. An **ecomap**, a graphic portrayal of social relationships of the woman and family, may also help the nurse understand the social environment of the family and identify support systems available to them (Fig. 2.5). Software is available to generate genograms and ecomaps (www.interpersonaluniverse.net).

THE FAMILY IN A CULTURAL CONTEXT

CULTURAL FACTORS RELATED TO FAMILY HEALTH

The **culture** of an individual and a group is influenced by religion, environment, and historic events and plays a powerful role in the individual's and group's behaviors and patterns of human interaction. Culture is not static; it is an ongoing process that influences a woman throughout her entire life, from birth to death. Culture is an essential element of what defines us as people.

Cultural knowledge includes beliefs and values about each facet of life and is passed from one generation to the next. Cultural beliefs and traditions relate to food, language, religion, spirituality, art, health and healing practices, kinship relationships, and all other aspects of community, family, and individual life. Culture has also been shown to have a direct effect on health behaviors. Values, attitudes, and beliefs that are culturally acquired may influence perceptions of illness, as well as health care–seeking behavior and response to treatment. The political, social, and economic context of people's lives is also part of the cultural experience.

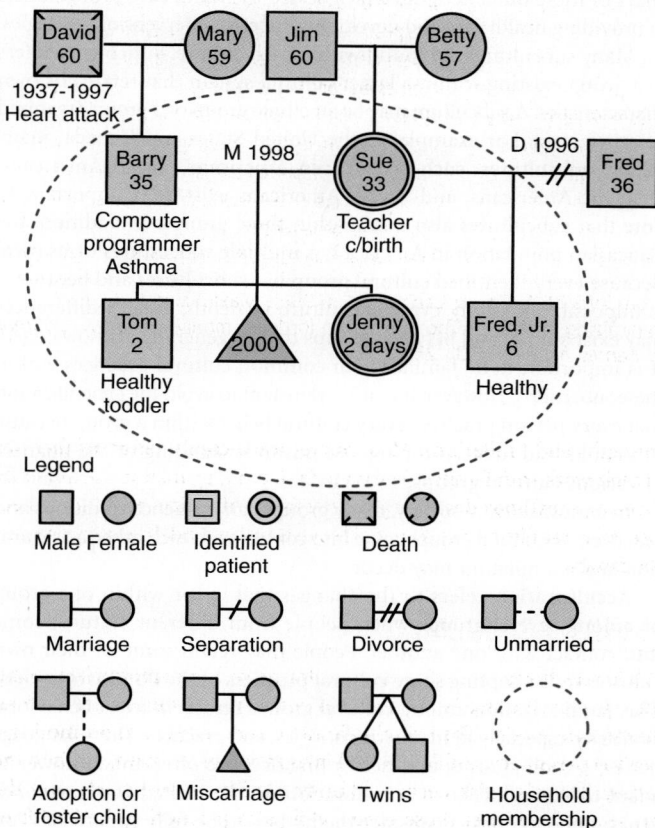

FIG 2.4 Example of a family genogram.

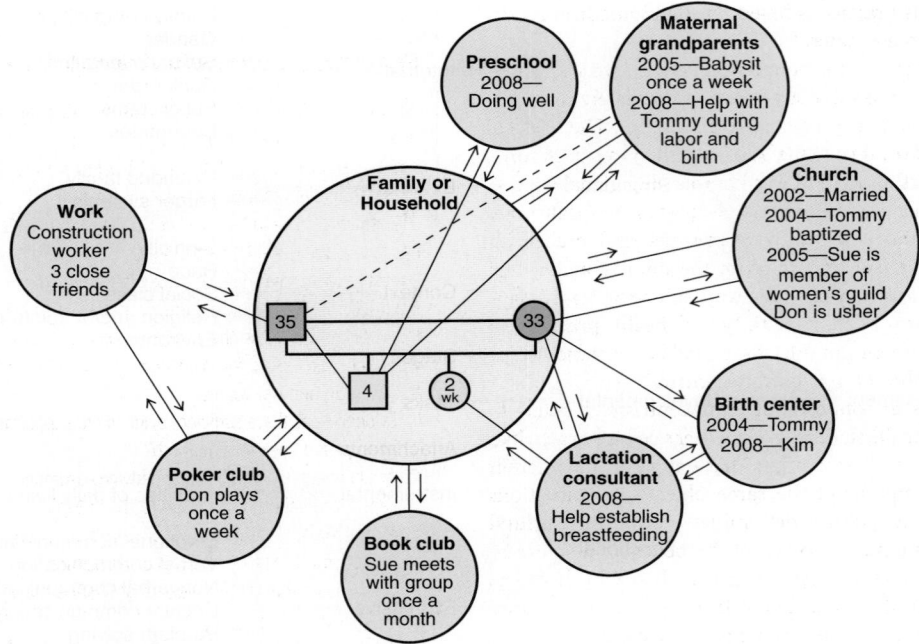

FIG 2.5 Example of an ecomap. An ecomap describes social relationships and depicts available supports.

Culture, shared beliefs, and values of a group play a powerful role in an individual's behavior, particularly when the individual is faced with health care issues. Understanding a culture can provide insight into how a person reacts to illness, pain, and invasive medical procedures, as well as patterns of human interaction and expressions of emotion. The effect of these influences must be assessed by health care professionals in providing health care and developing effective intervention strategies.

Many subcultures are found within each culture. Subculture refers to a group existing within a larger cultural system that retains its own characteristics. A subculture may be an ethnic group or a group organized in other ways. For example, in the United States and Canada, many ethnic subcultures such as African-Americans, Asian-Americans, Hispanic-Americans, and Native Americans exist. It is important to note that subcultures also exist within these groups. In addition, the Caucasian population in America has multiple subcultures of its own. Because every identified cultural group has subcultures and because it is impossible to study every subculture in depth, greater differences may exist among and between groups than is generally acknowledged. It is important to be familiar with common cultural practices within these subgroups. However, it is also important to avoid the generalization that every person practices every cultural belief within a group because this could lead to stereotyping and misunderstanding of the nuances of various cultural groups.

In a multicultural society, many groups can influence traditions and practices. As cultural groups come into contact with each other, acculturation and assimilation may occur.

Acculturation refers to the changes that occur within one group or among several groups when people from different cultures come into contact with one another. People may retain some of their own culture while adopting some cultural practices of the dominant society. This familiarization among cultural groups results in overt behavioral similarity, especially in mannerisms, styles, and practices. Dress, language patterns, food choices, and health practices are often much slower to adapt to the influence of acculturation. In the United States, second-generation Americans consider themselves to be fully American (Pew Research Center, 2013).

During times of family transitions such as childbearing or during crisis or illness, a woman may rely on old cultural patterns even after she has become acculturated in many ways. This is consistent with the family developmental theory that states that during times of stress, people revert to practices and behaviors that are most comfortable and familiar (Carter & McGoldrick, 1999).

Assimilation occurs when a cultural group loses its cultural identity and becomes part of the dominant culture. Assimilation is the process by which groups "melt" into the mainstream, thus accounting for the notion of a "melting pot," a phenomenon that has been said to occur in the United States. This is illustrated by individuals who identify themselves as being of Irish or German descent without having any remaining cultural practices or values linked specifically to that culture such as food preparation techniques, style of dress, or proficiency in the language associated with their reported cultural heritage. Spector (2013) asserts that in the United States, the melting pot, with its dream of a common culture, is a myth. Instead, a mosaic phenomenon exists in which we must accept and appreciate the differences among people.

IMPLICATIONS FOR NURSING

As our society becomes more culturally diverse, it is essential that nurses become culturally competent. Nurses must examine their own beliefs so that they have a better appreciation and understanding of the beliefs of their patients. To promote culturally congruent practice, a new standard has been added to *Nursing: Scope and Standards of Practice,* 3rd edition (American Nurses Association, 2015b). Standard 8 directs nurses to practice "in a manner that is congruent with cultural diversity and inclusion principles" (Cipriano, 2016, p. 15). Understanding the concepts of ethnocentrism and cultural relativism may help nurses care for families in a multicultural society.

Ethnocentrism is the view that one's own way of doing things is best (Giger, 2013). Although the United States is a culturally diverse nation, the prevailing practice of health care is based on the beliefs and practices held by members of the dominant culture, primarily Caucasians of European descent. This practice is based on the biomedical model that focuses on curing disease states.

Pregnancy and childbirth in this biomedical perspective are viewed as processes with inherent risks that are most appropriately managed by using scientific knowledge and advanced technology. The medical perspective stands in direct contrast to the belief systems of many cultures. Among many women, birth is viewed as a completely normal process that can be managed with a minimum of involvement from health care practitioners. When encountering behavior in women unfamiliar with the biomedical model or those who reject it, the nurse may become frustrated and impatient and may label the women's behavior as inappropriate and believe that it conflicts with "good" health practices. If the Western health care system provides the nurse's only standard for judgment, the behavior of the nurse is ethnocentric.

Cultural relativism is the opposite of ethnocentrism. It refers to learning about and applying the standards of another's culture to activities within that culture. The nurse recognizes that people from different cultural backgrounds comprehend the same objects and situations differently. In other words, culture determines viewpoint. Cultural relativism does not require nurses to accept the beliefs and values of another culture. Instead, nurses recognize that the behavior of others can be based on a system of logic different from their own. Cultural relativism affirms the uniqueness and value of every culture.

CHILDBEARING BELIEFS AND PRACTICES

Nurses working with childbearing families care for families from many different cultures and ethnic groups. To provide culturally competent care, the nurse must assess the beliefs and practices of patients. When working with childbearing families, a nurse considers all aspects of culture including communication, space, time orientation, and family roles.

Communication often creates the most challenging obstacle for nurses working with patients from diverse cultural groups. Communication is not merely the exchange of words. Instead, it involves (1) understanding the individual's language, including subtle variations in meaning and distinctive dialects; (2) appreciating individual differences in interpersonal style; and (3) accurately interpreting the volume of speech as well as the meanings of touch and gestures. For example, members of some cultural groups tend to speak loudly when they are excited, with great emotion and with vigorous and animated gestures; this is true whether their excitement is related to positive or negative events or emotions. It is important, therefore, for the nurse to avoid rushing to judgment regarding a person's intent when he or she is speaking, especially in a language not understood by the nurse. Instead, the nurse should withhold an interpretation of what has been expressed until it is possible to clarify the patient's intent. The nurse needs to enlist the assistance of a person who can help verify with the patient the true intent and meaning of the communication (see Clinical Reasoning Case Study).

Inconsistencies between the language of patients and the language of providers present a significant barrier to effective health care. For example, there are many dialects of Spanish that vary by geographic location. Because of the diversity of cultures and languages within the US and Canadian populations, health care agencies are increasingly seeking the services of interpreters (of oral communication from one language to another) or translators (of written words from one language to another) to bridge these gaps and fulfill their obligation for culturally and linguistically appropriate health care (Box 2.2). Finding the best possible interpreter in the circumstance is critically important as well. Ideally, interpreters should have the same native language and be of the same religion or have the same country of origin as the patient.

CLINICAL REASONING CASE STUDY
Providing Culturally Appropriate Care

Elisabeth, a 22-year-old first-generation Mexican-American, comes into your office for her initial prenatal visit. You are concerned because Elisabeth's fundal height is consistent with 32 weeks of gestation and this is her first prenatal visit. Elisabeth, who lives with her husband, four children (ages 6, 4, 3 years, and 15 months), her mother, her aunt, and her uncle, states that she has been doing well this pregnancy and did not start prenatal care in her previous pregnancies until she was almost ready to give birth. She also comments that all the babies were full term with uneventful labors and births. In obtaining the history, you note the presence of a safety pin in Elisabeth's shirt and wonder what this is for. You want to provide culturally appropriate care to this woman and her family.

1. Evidence—Is there sufficient evidence to support the components of culturally appropriate care for Elisabeth?
2. Assumptions—Describe an underlying assumption about culturally appropriate care for Elisabeth in relation to these topics:
   a. The view of pregnancy in Elisabeth's culture
   b. The role of family in Elisabeth's culture
   c. The acceptability for women of Elisabeth's age to begin having children at such young ages
   d. The religious or spiritual beliefs that Elisabeth may have that affect contraception
3. What implications and priorities for nursing care can be made at this time?
4. Does the evidence objectively support your conclusion?

Interpreters should have specific health-related language skills and experience and help bridge the language and cultural barriers between the patient and the health care provider. The person interpreting also should be mature enough to be trusted with private information. However, because the nature of nursing care is not always predictable and because nursing care that is provided in a home or community setting does not always allow expert, experienced, or mature adult interpreters, ideal interpretive services sometimes are impossible to find when they are needed. In crisis or emergency situations or when family members are having extreme stress or emotional upset, it may be necessary to use relatives, neighbors, or children as interpreters. If this situation occurs, the nurse must ensure that the patient is in agreement and comfortable with using the available interpreter to assist. Having a man or a child interpret for a woman can create embarrassment and interfere with obtaining an accurate history or detail of symptoms.

When using an interpreter, the nurse respects the family by creating an atmosphere of respect and privacy. Questions should be addressed to the woman and not to the interpreter. Even though an interpreter will of necessity be exposed to sensitive and privileged information about the family, the nurse should take care to ensure that confidentiality is maintained. A quiet location free from interruptions is ideal for interpretive services to take place. Culturally and linguistically appropriate educational materials that are easy to read, with appropriate text and graphics, should be available to assist the woman and her family in understanding health care information. To ensure understanding and avoid liability issues, it is important to make certain that the material has been translated by someone who is trained appropriately.

PERSONAL SPACE

Cultural traditions define the appropriate personal space for various social interactions. Although the need for personal space varies from person to person and with the situation, the actual physical dimensions of comfort zones differ from culture to culture. Actions such as touching,

BOX 2.2   Working With an Interpreter

Step 1: Before the Interview
- Outline your statements and questions. List the key pieces of information you want/need to know.
- Learn something about the culture so that you can converse informally with the interpreter.

Step 2: Meeting with the Interpreter
- Introduce yourself to the interpreter and converse informally. This is the time to find out how well he or she speaks English. No matter how proficient or what age the interpreter is, be respectful. Some ways to show respect are to ask a cultural question to acknowledge that you can learn from the interpreter, or you could learn one word or phrase from the interpreter.
- Emphasize that you do want the patient to ask questions, because some cultures consider this inappropriate behavior.
- Make sure the interpreter is comfortable with the technical terms you need to use. If not, take some time to explain them.

Step 3: During the Interview
- Ask your questions and explain your statements (see Step 1).
- Make sure that the interpreter understands which parts of the interview are most important. You usually have limited time with the interpreter, and you want to have adequate time at the end for patient questions.
- Try to get a "feel" for how much is "getting through." No matter what the language is, if in relating information to the patient, the interpreter uses far fewer or far more words than you do, something else is going on.
- Stop now and then and ask the interpreter, "How is it going?" You may not get a totally accurate answer, but you will have emphasized to the interpreter your strong desire to focus on the task at hand. If there are language problems, (1) speak slowly; (2) use gestures (e.g., fingers to count or point to body parts); and (3) use pictures.
- Ask the interpreter to elicit questions. This may be difficult, but it is worth the effort.
- Identify cultural issues that may conflict with your requests or instructions.
- Use the interpreter to help problem solve or at least give insight into possibilities for solutions.

Step 4: After the Interview
- Speak to the interpreter and try to get an idea of what went well and what could be improved. This will help you be more effective in the future with this or another interpreter.
- Make notes on what you learned for your future reference or to help a colleague.

Remember
- Your interview is a *collaboration* between you and the interpreter. *Listen* as well as speak.

Notes
- The interpreter may be a child, grandchild, or sibling of the patient. Be sensitive to the fact that the child is playing an adult role.
- Be sensitive to cultural and situational differences (e.g., an interview with someone from urban Germany will likely be different from an interview with someone from a transitional refugee camp).
- Younger females telling older males what to do may be a problem for both a female nurse and a female interpreter. This is not the time to pioneer new gender relations. Be aware that in some cultures it is difficult for a woman to talk about some topics with a husband or a father present.

Courtesy of Elizabeth Whalley, PhD, San Francisco State University.

placing the woman in proximity to others, taking away personal possessions, and making decisions for the woman can decrease personal security and heighten anxiety. Conversely, respecting the need for distance allows the woman to maintain control over personal space and supports personal autonomy, thereby increasing her sense of security. Nurses must touch patients. However, they frequently do so without any awareness of the emotional distress they may be causing.

TIME ORIENTATION

Time orientation is a fundamental way in which culture affects health behaviors. People in cultural groups may be relatively more oriented to past, present, or future. Those who focus on the past strive to maintain tradition or the status quo and have little motivation for formulating goals. In contrast, individuals who focus primarily on the present neither plan for the future nor consider the experiences of the past. These individuals do not necessarily adhere to strict schedules and are often described as "living for the moment" or "marching to their own drummer." Individuals oriented to the future maintain a focus on achieving long-term goals.

The time orientation of the childbearing family may affect nursing care. For example, talking to a family about bringing the infant to the clinic for follow-up examinations (events in the future) may be difficult for the family who is focused on the present concerns of day-to-day survival. Because a family with a future-oriented sense of time plans far in advance, thinking about the long-term consequences of present actions, they may be more likely to return as scheduled for follow-up visits. Despite the differences in time orientation, each family can be equally concerned for the well-being of its newborn.

FAMILY ROLES

Family roles involve the expectations and behaviors associated with a member's position in the larger family system (e.g., mother, father, grandparent). Social class and cultural norms also affect these roles, with distinct expectations for men and women clearly determined by social norms. For example, culture may influence whether a man actively participates in pregnancy and childbirth, yet maternity care providers working in the Western health care system expect fathers to be involved. This can create a significant conflict between the nurse and the role expectations of very traditional Mexican or Arabic families, who usually view the birthing experience as a female affair (see Cultural Considerations box). The way that health care practitioners manage such a family's care molds its experience and perception of the Western health care system.

🌐 CULTURAL CONSIDERATIONS

Questions to Ask to Elicit Cultural Expectations About Childbearing

1. What do you and your family think you should do to remain healthy during pregnancy?
2. What can you do to improve your health and the health of your baby?
3. What foods will help make a healthy baby?
4. Who do you want with you during your labor?
5. What can your labor support person do to help you be most comfortable during labor?
6. What actions are important for you and your family after the baby's birth?
7. What do you and your family expect from the nurse(s) caring for you?
8. How will family members participate in your pregnancy, childbirth, and parenting?

In maternity nursing, the nurse supports and nurtures the beliefs that promote physical or emotional adaptation to childbearing. However, if certain beliefs might be harmful, the nurse should carefully explore them with the woman and use them in the reeducation and modification process. Table 2.2 provides examples of some cultural beliefs and practices surrounding childbearing. The cultural beliefs and customs in the table are categorized on the basis of distinct cultural traditions and are not practiced by all members of the cultural group in every part of the country. Women from these cultural and ethnic groups may adhere to a few, all, or none of the practices listed. In using this table as a guide, the nurse should take care to avoid making stereotypic assumptions about any person based on sociocultural-spiritual affiliations. Nurses should exercise sensitivity in working with every family, being careful to assess the ways in which they apply their own mixture of cultural traditions.

TABLE 2.2   Traditional* Cultural Beliefs and Practices: Childbearing and Parenting

Pregnancy	Childbirth	Parenting

Hispanic-American

(Based primarily on knowledge of Mexican-Americans; members of the Hispanic community have their origins in Spain, Cuba, Central and South America, Mexico, Puerto Rico, and other Spanish-speaking countries.)

Pregnancy	Childbirth	Parenting
Pregnancy • Pregnancy desired soon after marriage • Late prenatal care • Expectant mother influenced strongly by mother or mother-in-law • Cool air in motion considered dangerous during pregnancy • Unsatisfied food cravings thought to cause a birthmark • Some pica observed in the eating of ashes or dirt (not common) • Milk avoided because it causes large babies and difficult births • Many predictions about sex of baby • May be unacceptable and frightening to have pelvic examination by male health care provider • Use of herbs to treat common complaints of pregnancy • Drinking chamomile tea thought to ensure effective labor • May wear ribbon or band around pregnant belly in belief that baby will be born healthy • Need a balance of hot and cold	*Labor* • Use of *partera* or lay midwife preferred in some places; expectant mother may prefer presence of mother rather than husband • After birth of baby, mother's legs brought together to prevent air from entering uterus • Loud behavior in labor *Postpartum* • Diet may be restricted after birth; for first 2 days only boiled milk and toasted tortillas permitted (special foods to restore warmth to body) • Avoid cold foods • Bed rest for 3 days after birth • Mother's head and feet protected from cold air; bathing permitted after 14 days • Mother often cared for by her own mother • Forty-day restriction on sexual intercourse • Mother may want baby's first wet diaper to wipe her face in belief that it aids in making "mask of pregnancy" go away	*Newborn* • Breastfeeding begun after third day; colostrum may be considered "filthy" or "spoiled" or just not enough nourishment • Need a balance of heat and cold to promote milk flow • Olive oil or castor oil given to stimulate passage of meconium • Male infant not circumcised • Female infant's ears pierced • Belly band used to prevent umbilical hernia • Religious medal worn by mother during pregnancy; placed around infant's neck • Infant protected from *mal de ojo* ("evil eye") • Various remedies used to treat *mal de ojo* and fallen fontanel (depressed fontanel)

African-American

(Members of the African-American community, many of whom are descendants of slaves, have different origins. Today a number of black Americans have emigrated from Africa, the West Indies, the Dominican Republic, Haiti, and Jamaica.)

Pregnancy	Childbirth	Parenting

Pregnancy
 • Acceptance of pregnancy depends on economic status
 • Pregnancy thought to be state of "wellness," which is often the reason for delay in seeking prenatal care, especially by lower-income African-Americans
 • Old wives' tales include beliefs that having a picture taken during pregnancy will cause stillbirth and reaching up will cause cord to strangle baby
 • Craving for certain foods, including chicken and greens, and nonfood substances such as clay, starch, and dirt (pica)
 • Pregnancy may be viewed by African-American men as a sign of their virility
 • Self-treatment for various discomforts of pregnancy, including constipation, nausea, vomiting, headache, and heartburn
	Labor
	 • Use of "Granny midwife" in certain parts of United States
	 • Varied emotional responses: some cry out, some display stoic behavior to avoid calling attention to selves
	 • Woman may arrive at hospital in far-advanced labor
	 • Emotional support often provided by other women, especially the woman's own mother
	
	 Postpartum
	 • Vaginal bleeding seen as sign of sickness; tub baths and shampooing of hair prohibited
	 • Sassafras tea thought to have healing power
	 • Eating liver thought to cause heavier vaginal bleeding because of its high "blood" content
		Newborn
		 • Feeding very important:
		   • "Good" baby thought to eat well
		   • Early introduction of solid foods
		   • May breastfeed or bottle-feed; breastfeeding may be considered embarrassing
		 • Parents fearful of spoiling baby
		 • Commonly call baby by nicknames
		 • May use excessive clothing to keep baby warm
		 • Belly band used to prevent umbilical hernia
		 • Abundant use of oil on baby's scalp and skin
		 • Strong feeling of family, community, and religion
		 • African-American minister and church important in recovery

Continued

TABLE 2.2 Traditional* Cultural Beliefs and Practices: Childbearing and Parenting—cont'd

Pregnancy	Childbirth	Parenting

Asian-American
(Typically refers to groups from China, Korea, the Philippines, Japan, Southeast Asia [particularly Thailand], Indochina, and Vietnam.)

Pregnancy
- Pregnancy considered time when mother "has happiness in her body"
- Pregnancy seen as natural process
- Strong preference for female health care provider
- Belief in theory of hot and cold
- May omit soy sauce in diet to prevent dark-skinned baby
- Prefer soup made with ginseng root as general strength tonic
- Milk usually excluded from diet because it causes stomach distress
- Inactivity or sleeping late may cause difficult birth
- Korean women practice Tae-kyo (think about good things and maintain a calm attitude)
- Many diagnostic tests such as amniocentesis, ultrasonography, or drawing blood considered unnecessary and dangerous
- Sexual intercourse in last 2 months of pregnancy may be restricted

Labor
- Mother attended by other women, especially her own mother
- Father does not actively participate
- May moan or grunt
- Cesarean birth not desired

Postpartum
- Must protect self from *yin* (cold forces) for 30 days
- Ambulation limited
- Shower and bathing prohibited for about 10 days
- Warm room
- Diet:
  - Warm fluids
  - Some women are vegetarians
  - Korean mother served seaweed soup with rice
  - Chinese diet high in hot foods
  - Chinese mother avoids fruits and vegetables

Newborn
- Concept of family important and valued
- Father is head of household; wife plays a subordinate role
- Birth of boy preferred
- May delay naming child
- Some groups (e.g., Vietnamese) believe colostrum is dirty; therefore they may delay breastfeeding until milk comes in
- Traditionally Filipino babies are not circumcised at birth

European-American
(Members of the European-American [Caucasian] community have their origins in countries such as Ireland, Great Britain, Germany, Italy, and France.)

Pregnancy
- Pregnancy viewed as a condition that requires medical attention to ensure health
- Emphasis on early prenatal care
- Variety of childbirth education programs available, and participation encouraged
- Technology driven
- Emphasis on nutritional science
- Involvement of the father valued
- Written sources of information valued

Labor
- Birth is a public concern
- Technology dominated
- Birthing process in institutional setting valued
- Involvement of father expected
- Physician seen as head of team

Postpartum
- Emphasis or focus on early bonding
- Medical interventions for dealing with discomfort
- Early ambulation and activity emphasized
- Self-management valued

Newborn
- More women breastfeeding
- Breastfeeding begins as soon as possible after childbirth

Parenting
- Motherhood and transition to parenting seen as stressful time
- Nuclear family valued, although single parenting and other forms of parenting more acceptable than in the past
- Women often deal with multiple roles
- Early return to prenatal activities

Native American
(Many different tribes exist within the Native-American culture; viewpoints vary according to tribal customs and beliefs.)

Pregnancy
- Pregnancy considered a normal, natural process
- Late prenatal care
- Avoid heavy lifting
- Herb teas encouraged

Labor
- Prefers female attendant, although husband, mother, or father may assist with birth
- Birth may be attended by whole family
- Herbs may be used to promote uterine activity
- Birth may occur in squatting position

Postpartum
- Herbal teas to stop bleeding

Newborn
- Infant not fed colostrum
- Use of herbs to increase flow of milk
- Use of cradle boards for infant
- Babies not handled often

Note: Most of these cultural beliefs and customs reflect the traditional culture and are not universally practiced. These lists are not intended to stereotype patients but, rather, to serve as guidelines while discussing meaningful cultural beliefs with a woman and her family. Examples of other cultural beliefs and practices are found throughout this text.

*Variations in some beliefs and practices exist within subcultures of each group.

Data from Amaro, H. (1994). Women in the Mexican-American community: religion, culture, and reproductive attitudes and experiences, *Journal of Comparative Psychology 16*(1):6–19; D'Avanzo, C. (2008). *Mosby's pocket guide to cultural health assessment* (4th ed.). St. Louis, MO: Mosby; Giger, J. N. (2013). *Transcultural nursing: Assessment and intervention* (6th ed.). St. Louis, MO: Mosby; Mattson, S. (1995). Culturally sensitive prenatal care for Southeastern Asians, *Journal of Obstetric, Gynecologic, and Neonatal Nursing 24*(4):335–341; Spector, R. (2013). *Cultural diversity in health and illness* (8th ed.). Upper Saddle River, NJ: Prentice-Hall

DEVELOPING CULTURAL COMPETENCE

Cultural competence has many names and definitions, all of which have subtle shades of difference but which are essentially the same: multiculturalism, cultural sensitivity, and intercultural effectiveness. Cultural competence involves acknowledging, respecting, and appreciating ethnic, cultural, and linguistic diversity. Culturally competent professionals act in ways that meet the needs of the patient and are respectful of ways and traditions that may be very different from their own. In today's society, it is critically important that nurses develop more than technical skills. At every level of preparation and throughout their professional lives, nurses must engage in a continual process of developing and refining attitudes and behaviors that will promote culturally competent care (Giger, 2013).

Key components of culturally competent care include the following:

- Recognizing that differences exist between one's own culture and that of the patient
- Educating and promoting healthy behaviors in a cultural context that has meaning for patients
- Taking abstract knowledge about other cultures and applying it in a practical way so that the quality of service improves and policies are enacted that meet the needs of all patients
- Communicating respect for a wide range of differences, including patient use of nontraditional healing practices and alternative therapies
- Recognizing the importance of culturally different communication styles, problem-solving techniques, concepts of space and time, and desires to be involved with care decisions
- Anticipating the need to address varying degrees of language ability and literacy, as well as barriers to care and compliance with treatment

In addition to issues of preserving and promoting human dignity, the development of cultural competence is of equal importance in terms of health outcomes. Nurses who relate effectively with patients are able to motivate them in the direction of health-promoting behaviors. Provider competence to address language barriers facilitates appropriate tailoring of health messages and preventive health teaching. Cross-cultural experiences also present an opportunity for the health care professional to expand cultural sensitivity, awareness, and skills (Fig. 2.6).

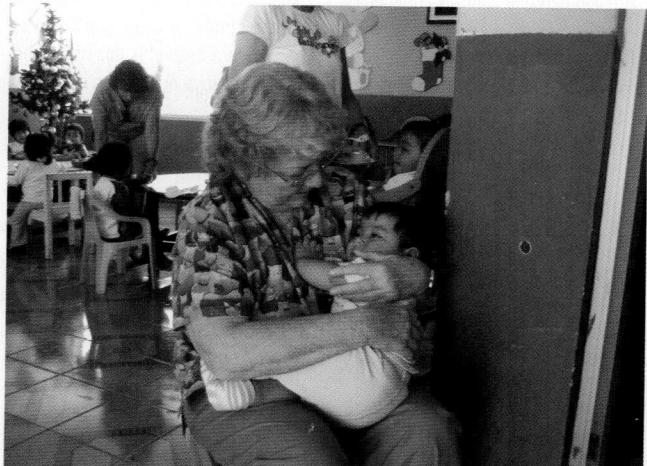

FIG 2.6 Nurse volunteering in a day care center in Ecuador. (Courtesy of CoraLee Thompson, RN, BA, CNP [ret].)

SPIRITUALITY AND THE FAMILY

Spirituality is an aspect of humans that is above and beyond the mind and body. It "speaks to what gives ultimate meaning and purpose to one's life. It is that part of people that seeks healing and reconciliation with self or others" (Puchalski, 2006). Spirituality is important in all phases of life; it relates to deep and important things and will affect how patients face health issues (Giske & Cone, 2015). While religion is a more organized or rule-driven form of spirituality, one can be spiritual without being a member of an organized religion.

Many studies of religion and health suggest that religious people are healthier and generally live longer than nonreligious people. Those who attend church once a week are less likely to become ill than those who do not. The studies did not control for rates of smoking and alcohol use, so no inference can be made as to whether the improved health status was from better habits or religion. In general, it is known that religious people do tend to have healthier lifestyles overall than people who are not religious (Condon, 2004). Spiritual wellness can be estimated by answering questions such as those suggested in Box 2.3

Spirituality is a component of holistic nursing and thus a professional responsibility. The International Council of Nurses Code of Ethics for Nurses (2012) states that: "In providing care, the nurse promotes an environment in which the human rights, values, customs and spiritual beliefs of the individual, family, and community are respected" (p. 2). The American Nurses Association Code of Ethics for Nurses With Interpretive Statements states that: "Factors such as culture, value systems, religious or spiritual beliefs, lifestyle, social support system, sexual orientation or gender expression and primary language are to be considered when planning individual, family and population-centered care" (American Nurses Association, 2015, p. 1). NANDA-I includes two nursing diagnoses

BOX 2.3   Spiritual Wellness Self-Assessment

1. How do you describe your purpose in life?
2. What activities do you do regularly that bring you joy?
3. What goals do you have for 6 months from now?
4. What goals do you have for 2 years from now?
5. What activities make you feel nourished?
6. What kinds of things do you do for yourself every day?
7. What do you hope for in the future?
8. Are there people to whom you can reach out?
9. On whom can you count for encouragement and/or support?
10. Are there others to whom you give encouragement and/or support?
11. Who loves you?
12. Whom do you love or care about?
13. In what areas are you growing?
14. How do you go about forgiving yourself?
15. How do you go about forgiving others?
16. To whom do you confide your hopes, dreams, and pain?
17. Do you believe in some kind of higher power?
18. What do you hope for in the future?
19. When do you reach out to people?
20. Do you look forward to getting up in the morning?
21. Would you like to live to be 100?

The more questions you answer in the positive, the higher the level of spiritual wellness.

Adapted from Condon, M. (2004). *Women's health: Body, mind, spirit: An integrated approach to wellness and illness.* Upper Saddle River, NJ: Prentice-Hall.

related to spirituality: Readiness for Enhanced Spiritual Well-Being and Spiritual Distress (Ackley, Ladwig, & Makic, 2017).

Spirituality is a component of basic professional nursing education; graduates are to include spirituality in assessments and provide spiritually and culturally appropriate health promotion (American Association of Colleges of Nursing, 2008). The Joint Commission (2016) includes among patient rights the right to religious and other spiritual services; religion, spiritual beliefs, values, and preferences are to be taken into account in the provision of care. Thus, many health care and nursing organizations and associations recognize the importance of spiritual care and incorporate the provision of such care into their standards.

Spiritual care encompasses those "interventions, individual or communal, that facilitate the ability to experience the integration of the body, mind, and spirit to achieve wholeness, health, and a sense of connection to self, others, and a higher power" (American Nurses Association and Health Ministries Association, 2005, p. 38). Spirituality is of relevance for all of nursing, not just for those in palliative care or for dying patients (Giske & Cone, 2015).

Religious preference is usually included with demographic information on initial contact with health care organizations. Hospital chaplains and other clergy use the information to arrange visits with parishioners or others who desire their services. Nurses can use the information to pose questions about preferences or requests for prayers, blessings, counseling, or visits from clergy. Taylor (2012) provided a guide for nurses by describing a number of religions and the rituals and relation to health important to those denominations.

Baptisms, b'nai mitzvah, salat, anointings, blessings, communion services, sacrament of the sick, and other religious observances and practices may occur. Memorial services may be held in the hospital chapel or prayer room. Occasionally weddings are performed within a hospital. Nurses may be requested to provide the space and opportunity for such events to occur. At times they may be invited or requested to participate. Depending on preferences, the nurse may choose to remain for the service or decline respectfully. The nurse need not be of the same religion, or any religion, to provide support by his or her presence.

The Pause, which originated in an emergency room after the death of a patient, is a minute or two of taking time to acknowledge a lost human life, and is an example of the recognition of the individual in this sad time as well as giving support to those health care providers who worked to save the life (Bartels, 2014). After a death, the staff are asked to remain and bear witness, to be together and present in this time of grief and loss. The staff is able to be together and achieve some type of closure or resolution surrounding the unsuccessful efforts to resuscitate the individual. Use of the Pause is growing and winning advocates.

Spiritual Assessment

As part of patient assessments, questions related to spirituality and religion should be included. Questions can be directed to patients as well as the family. Examples of such questions are in Box 2.4.

The FICA Spiritual Assessment Tool (Box 2.5) is a short and simple guide for spiritual assessment. Small cards are available to assist health care professionals to guide assessments.

Brussat and Brussat (1996) described characteristics of the spiritually literate person as being present, having compassion, being connected, having hope, being kind and listening, having meaning and openness, and using silence. All of these are characteristics of a nurse who is interested in providing spiritual care.

To provide spiritual care, the nurse must understand the meaning of spirituality to the person for whom care is provided (Gordon, Kelly, & Mitchell, 2011). The nurse must listen attentively to learn what is

---

BOX 2.4   Spiritual Assessment Questions

- Who or what provides the patient with strength and hope?
- Does the patient use prayer in his or her life?
- How does the patient express his or her spirituality?
- How would the patient describe his or her philosophy of life?
- What type of spiritual/religious support does the patient desire?
- What is the name of the patient's clergy, ministers, chaplains, pastor, rabbi?
- What does suffering mean to the patient?
- What does dying mean to the patient?
- What are the patient's spiritual goals?
- Is there a role of church/synagogue in the patient's life?
- How does faith help the patient cope with illness?
- How does the patient keep going day after day?
- What helps the patient get through this health care experience?
- How has illness affected the patient and his or her family?

Adapted from The Joint Commission, *Standards FAQ details, medical record—Spiritual assessment*. Retrieved from https://www.jointcommission.org/standards_information/jcfaqdetails.aspx?StandardsFAQId=765&StandardsFAQChapterId=29&ProgramId=0&ChapterId=0&IsFeatured=False&IsNew=False&Keyword=spiritual.

BOX 2.5   FICA Spiritual Assessment Tool*

F - Faith and Belief
"Do you consider yourself spiritual or religious?" or "Is spirituality something important to you" or "Do you have spiritual beliefs that help you cope with stress/difficult times?" (Contextualize to reason for visit if it is not the routine history).
  If the patient responds "No," the health care provider might ask, "What gives your life meaning?" Sometimes patients respond with answers such as family, career, or nature.
  (The question of meaning should also be asked even if people answer yes to spirituality.)

I - Importance
"What importance does your spirituality have in your life? Has your spirituality influenced how you take care of yourself, your health? Does your spirituality influence you in your healthcare decision making? (e.g., advance directives, treatment, etc.)

C - Community
"Are you part of a spiritual community? Communities such as churches, temples, and mosques, or a group of like-minded friends, family, or yoga, can serve as strong support systems for some patients. Can explore further: Is this of support to you and how? Is there a group of people you really love or who are important to you?"

A - Address in Care
"How would you like me, your healthcare provider, to address these issues in your healthcare?" (With the newer models including diagnosis of spiritual distress A also refers to the Assessment and Plan of patient spiritual distress or issues within a treatment or care plan.)

From Puchalski, C. (2006). Spiritual assessment in clinical practice. *Psychiatric Annals, 36*(3), 150-155. Used with permission from George Washington Institute for Spirituality and Health (GWish), Washington, DC.
*Copyright 1996 by C. Pulchalski.

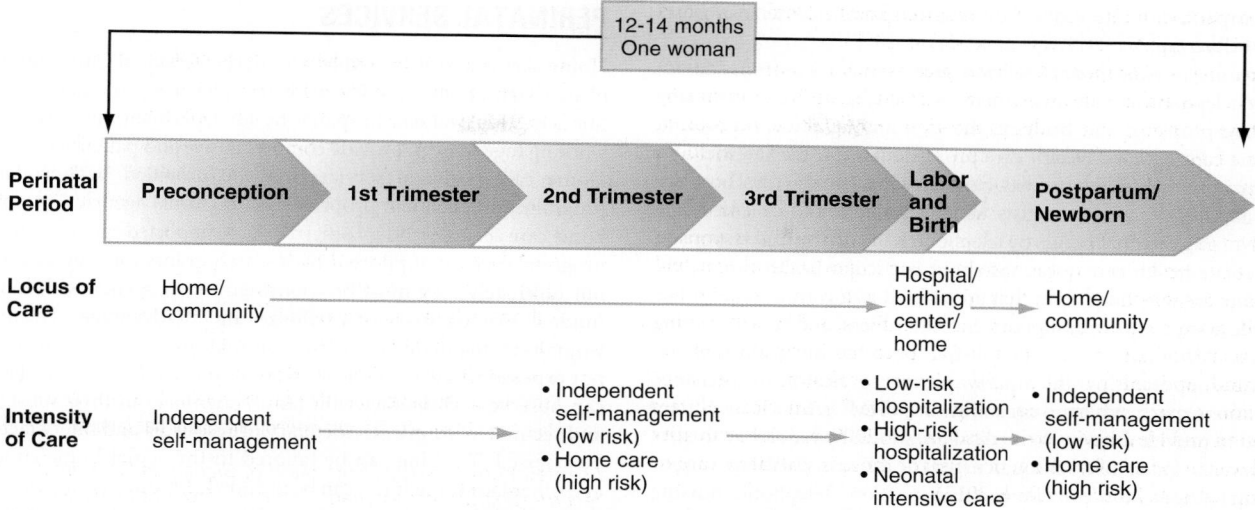

FIG 2.7 Perinatal continuum of care.

important to the patient, what gives meaning to her life, what gives hope and strength, and what are her fears and concerns (Burkhardt & Nagai-Jacobson, 2015). Only then can the nurse respond appropriately and provide spiritual care that is healing.

Parish nursing or faith community nursing is another opportunity to provide spiritual care. Parish nurses work through their church, synagogue, mosque, or faith community to promote health, manage disease, coordinate care, and assist with access to health care through classes, home visits, and other types of outreach (Wordsworth, Moore, & Woodhouse, 2016). These visits do not replace community health visits but supplement them.

HOME CARE IN THE COMMUNITY

Modern home care nursing has its foundation in public health nursing, which provided comprehensive care to sick and well patients in their own homes. Specialized maternity home care nursing services began in the 1980s when public health maternity nursing services were limited and services had not kept pace with the changing practices of high-risk obstetrics and emerging technology. Lengthy antepartum hospitalizations for such conditions as preterm labor and gestational hypertension created nursing care challenges for staff members of inpatient units.

Many women expressed their concerns about the negative effect of antepartum hospitalizations on the family as well as the costs and burdens of lengthy hospitalization. Although clinical indications showed that a new nursing care approach was needed, home health care did not become a viable alternative until third-party payers (i.e., public or private organizations or employer groups that pay for health care) pushed for cost containment in maternity services.

In the current health care system, home care is an important component of health care delivery along the perinatal continuum of care (Fig. 2.7). The growing demand for home care is based on several factors:

- Interest in family birthing alternatives
- Shortened hospital stays
- New technologies that facilitate home-based assessments and treatments
- Reimbursement by third-party payers

As health care costs continue to rise and because millions of American families lack health insurance, there is greater demand for innovative,

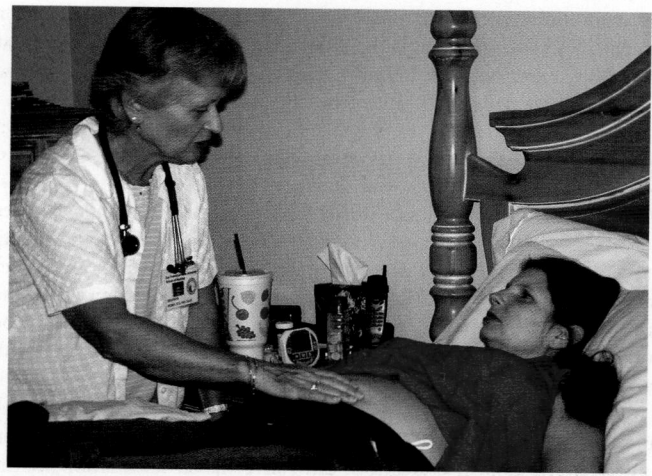

FIG 2.8 Home care nurse visits with a woman in preterm labor at home on bedrest. (Courtesy of Shannon Perry, Phoenix, AZ.)

cost-effective methods of health care delivery in the community. Large health care systems are developing clinically integrated health care delivery networks whose goals are: (1) improved coordination of care and care outcomes; (2) better communication among health care providers; (3) increased patient, payer, and provider satisfaction; and (4) reduced cost. The integration of clinical services changes the focus of care to a continuum of services that are increasingly community based.

COMMUNICATION AND TECHNOLOGY APPLICATIONS

As maternity care continues to consist of frequent and brief contacts with health care providers throughout the prenatal and postpartum periods, services that link maternity patients throughout the perinatal continuum of care have assumed increasing importance. These services include critical pathways, telephonic nursing assessments, discharge planning, specialized education programs, parent support groups, home visiting programs, nurse advice lines, and perinatal home care (Fig. 2.8). Hospitals may provide cross-training for hospital-based nurses to make postpartum home visits or to staff outpatient centers for post-partum follow-up.

Telephonic nursing through services such as warm lines, nurse advice lines, and telephonic nursing assessments is a valuable means of managing health care problems and bridging the gaps among acute, outpatient, and home care services. Health care professionals use the Internet and Skype to communicate with patients. Newborns in distress in rural hospitals can be assessed by neonatologists using high-definition telemedicine robots. Nursing care that occurs by telephone is interactive and responsive to immediate health care questions about particular health care needs. *Warm lines* are telephone lines that are offered as a community service to provide new parents with support, encouragement, and basic parenting education. *Nurse advice lines*, or toll-free nurse consultation services, often are supported by third-party payers or health maintenance organizations/managed care organizations (HMOs/MCOs) and are designed to provide answers to medical questions. Nurse care managers are prepared to guide callers through urgent health care situations, suggest treatment options, and provide health education. Telephonic nursing assessments or nurse consultation, assessment, and health education that take place during a telephone conversation can be added to the nursing care plan in conjunction with skilled nursing visits, or they may comprise a separate nursing contact for the woman. Telephonic nursing assessments are commonly used after a postpartum home care visit to reassess a woman's knowledge about the signs and symptoms of adequate hydration in breastfeeding or, after initiating home phototherapy, to assess the caregiver's knowledge regarding problems with equipment.

GUIDELINES FOR NURSING PRACTICE

The Association of Women's Health, Obstetric, and Neonatal Nurses (AWHONN, 2009) defines home care as the provision of technical, psychologic, and other therapeutic support in the woman's home rather than in an institution. The scope of nursing care delivered in the home is necessarily limited to practices deemed safe and appropriate to be carried out in an environment that is physically separated from a health care institution and its resources. Nursing practice at home is consistent with federal and state regulations that direct home care practice. The nurse demonstrates practice competence through formalized orientation and ongoing clinical education and performance evaluation in the respective home care agency. Standards for practice from key specialty organizations such as AWHONN, the National Association of Neonatal Nurses (NANN), ACOG, the American Academy of Pediatrics (AAP), and the Intravenous Nursing Society (INS) provide the basis for clinical protocols and pathways and organizational programs in home care practice. The Joint Commission (www.jointcommission.org) provides criteria for home care procedures based on Centers for Medicare & Medicaid Services (CMS) regulations (www.cms.gov).

A wide range of professional health care services and products can be delivered or used in the home by means of technology and telecommunication. For example, telehealth and telemedicine make it possible for patients in the home to be interviewed and assessed by a specialist located hundreds of miles away. Home health care can be viewed as an extension of in-hospital care.

Essentially, the primary difference between health care in a hospital and home care is the absence of the continuous presence of professional health care providers in a patient's home. Generally, but not always, home health care entails intermittent care by a professional who visits the patient's home for a particular reason and/or provides care onsite for fewer than 4 hours at a time. The home health care agency maintains on-call professional staff to assist home care patients who have questions about their care and for emergencies, such as equipment failure.

PERINATAL SERVICES

Home care is best delivered by an interprofessional care team. Nurses, obstetricians, maternal-fetal medicine, pharmacy, mental health practitioners, social workers, the public health department, and case managers working together can provide comprehensive and patient-centered care. Home care perinatal services may be provided by hospital-based programs, independent proprietary (for-profit) agencies, or nonprofit home care agencies and by official or tax-supported agencies. Innovative programs may be supported by research grants for a period of years, but ultimately they must be sponsored by an agency with long-term funding. Home visits have advantages and disadvantages. The pregnant woman can maintain bed rest if indicated, and vulnerable neonates are not exposed to the weather or external sources of infection. The nurse can observe and interact with family members in their most natural and secure environment. Adequacy of resources and safety factors can be assessed. Teaching can be tailored to the actual home conditions, and other family members can be included. A home visit is less expensive than a day's hospitalization, but a 60- to 90-minute visit requires 2.5 to 3 hours of nursing time, including travel and documentation. Areas of challenge include limited availability of nurses with expertise in maternity care and concerns about the nurse's physical safety in the community. One alternative that is less expensive is contacting women via telephone or the Internet.

Visits for outreach and health promotion are an integral part of community (or public) health nursing. In countries with national health systems, a nurse or midwife may see all women during pregnancy and after birth. In the United States, visits of this sort have been provided mainly to low-income families without health insurance and Medicaid recipients who use the clinics provided by local health departments. Until recently, private insurers did not reimburse for health promotion visits. MCOs now recognize that anticipatory guidance can be cost-effective, but home visitation programs for the most part still target specific, high-risk populations, such as adolescents and women at risk for preterm labor.

Home care agencies are subject to regulation by governmental and professional organizations and provide interdisciplinary services including social work, nutrition, and occupational and physical therapy. Increasingly, their caseloads are made up of women who require high-technology care, such as infusions or home monitoring. Although the home health nurse develops the care plan, all care must be ordered by a physician. In addition, interventions must meet the insurer's criteria for reimbursement, and services are limited to registered patients. Preconception care and low-risk antepartum care can usually be provided more efficiently in offices and clinics. High-risk antepartum care can be provided by home care agencies; for example, women with hyperemesis gravidarum who require parenteral nutrition may be treated at home. Conditions requiring bed rest, such as preterm labor and hypertension, are other common indications for home care. Other conditions often managed with home care include cardiac disease, substance abuse, and diabetes in pregnancy.

Insurers may reimburse for at least one postpartum visit to families after early discharge or in the presence of high-risk factors. Many neonates who require long-term high-technology care are also managed with home care.

PATIENT SELECTION AND REFERRAL

The office- or hospital-based nurse is often the key person in making effective referrals to home care. When considering a referral to home care, the following factors are evaluated:

- Health status of mother and fetus or infant: Is the condition serious enough to warrant home care, and is it stable enough for intermittent observation to be sufficient?
- Availability of professionals to provide the needed services within the woman's community.
- Family resources, including psychosocial, social, and economic resources: Will the family be able to provide care between nursing visits? Are relationships supportive? Is third-party reimbursement available, or can it be negotiated with the insurer? Could a voluntary or tax-supported community agency provide needed care without payment?
- Cost-effectiveness: Is it more reasonable for the woman to receive these services at home or to go to a local outpatient facility to receive them?

Community referrals should not be limited to women with physiologic complications of pregnancy that require medical treatment. Women at risk (e.g., young adolescents, families with a history of abuse, members of vulnerable population groups, developmentally disabled individuals) may need follow-up care at home. As we move more and more into an interdisciplinary health care society, it is crucial that nurses communicate with social workers to tap into valuable community resources that women can use in their own communities after being discharged.

Standardized forms simplify the referral process and ensure that all needed information will be forwarded to the home health agency. The nursing assessment should include the woman's physical and psychologic status, her level of knowledge about self-management activities, her willingness to learn, the availability of caregivers and social support in the home, and her level of comfort with home care. If the referral is for a mother-and-infant home care visit, the nursing assessment should include newborn data.

High-technology home care requires additional information to be collected from the chart and consultation with the referring physician and other members of the health care team before a home care referral is made. These additional data include the medical diagnosis, medical prognosis, prescribed therapies, medication history, drug-dosing information, potential ancillary supplies, type of infusion and access device, and the available systems of social support for the woman and family. The nursing assessment and therapy data provide baseline information for the home care nurse and other health care providers involved in the care plan.

Whenever a referral is called in to a home health care agency, a member of the nursing or admissions staff determines the agency's ability to accept the woman for service. The use of telecommunication modalities such as fax machines, cellular phones, electronic files, and the Internet to transmit information has eliminated delays in initiating home care services, even in more remote rural areas.

CARE MANAGEMENT

PREPARING FOR THE HOME VISIT

Home care is an excellent example of the benefits of interprofessional care. The home care nurse reviews the available clinical data, demographic information, and completed care plan form and consults with the home care pharmacist or other health care team members who have previously contacted the woman to determine the goals of the visit. At this point, the nurse uses the medical diagnosis and the location of the case on the perinatal continuum as a starting point to organize the woman's care. The nurse reviews agency policies and procedures, professional literature about diagnosis, and community resources as part of the previsit preparation work (Box 2.6).

FIRST HOME CARE VISIT

Making the first home care visit can be stressful for the nurse and the woman. The home care nurse is faced with an unknown environment controlled by the woman and her family. The woman and her family also experience feelings about the unknown, such as anxiety about the way the nurse will treat them or what the nurse will do during the visit. The challenge for the home care nurse is to establish a positive nurse-patient relationship that includes the family and provide the prescribed home care services within the time provided for the initial home visit. One of the most important roles of the home care nurse is modeling health-related behaviors for the woman and others who are in the home during the visit.

ASSESSMENT AND NURSING DIAGNOSES

The major areas of the assessment are demographics, medical history, general health history, medication history, physical assessment, psychosocial assessment (Box 2.7), and the home and community environment. Information can be obtained from patient records sent to the home care agency at the time of referral or from the previsit interview. These data will be used to develop and complete the nursing care plan, which is required for many licensed home health care agencies.

The nursing care plan is developed in collaboration with the woman, based on her health care needs. Home care nurses working in home health care agencies regulated by the CMS use a nursing care plan that includes patient demographics, the health care provider's orders, home care goals, and the woman's level of functioning. This document is initiated at the time of referral to the home care agency and must be updated every 60 days or as specified by state regulations. The frequency of the skilled nursing visit may vary with the individual plan of care and reimbursement criteria established by the third-party payers.

NURSING CONSIDERATIONS

There are several areas of concern when caring for a woman in the home. In home care, the woman or family members are responsible for administration of medications in the absence of the nurse. A careful medication history should be obtained to see if the woman is taking her medications correctly and understands their desired action and potential side effects. It is important that women and caretakers have a clear understanding of medication regimens and are notified when medications change in any way.

Nurses have to be skilled at performing various procedures such as venipuncture and administration of intravenous medications or fluids. Nurses must be sure that women know how to respond in emergency situations. Women need to be able to have 24-hour access to resources in the community in emergency situations. Women and family members are also encouraged to learn how to perform cardiopulmonary resuscitation (CPR), especially for infants.

⚡ **SAFETY ALERT**

The homes of women using electronic home health care equipment, such as phototherapy equipment or infusion pumps, require physical inspection of any electrical outlets, electrical cords, and extension cords that will be used. Homes with faulty electrical wiring may place the woman at risk for being involved in an electrical fire; faulty wiring may require inspection and repair by a professional electrician before electronic devices are used. Findings from the assessment are incorporated into the nursing care plan.

BOX 2.6   Protocol for Perinatal Home Visits

Previsit Interventions
- Contact the family to arrange details for home visit.
  - Identify self, credentials, and agency role.
  - Review purpose of home visit follow-up.
  - Schedule convenient time for visit.
  - Confirm address and route to family home.
- Review and clarify appropriate data.
  - Review all available assessment data for mother and fetus or infant (i.e., referral forms, hospital discharge summaries, identified learning needs of the family).
  - Review records of any previous nursing contacts.
  - Contact other professional caregivers as necessary to clarify data (e.g., obstetrician, nurse-midwife, pediatrician, referring nurse).
- Identify community resources and teaching materials appropriate to meet those needs already identified.
- Plan the visit, and prepare a bag with equipment, supplies, and materials necessary for assessments of mother and fetus or infant, actual care anticipated, and teaching.

In-Home Interventions: Establishing a Relationship
- Reintroduce yourself, and establish the purpose of the visit for mother, infant, and family; offer the family the opportunity to clarify their expectations of the contact.
- Spend a brief time socially interacting with the family to become acquainted and establish a trusting relationship.

In-Home Interventions: Working With the Family
- Conduct a systematic assessment of the mother and the fetus or newborn to determine their physiologic adjustment and any existing complications (see Fig. 2.8).
- Throughout the visit, collect data to assess the emotional adjustment of individual family members to the pregnancy or birth and lifestyle changes. Note any evidence of family-newborn bonding and sibling rivalry; note relationships among mother, father, children, and grandparents.
- Determine the adequacy of the support system.
  - To what extent does someone help with cooking, cleaning, and other home-management tasks?
  - To what extent is help being provided in caring for the newborn and any other children?
  - Are support persons encouraging the new mother to care for herself and get adequate rest?
  - Who is providing helpful information? Emotional support?
- Throughout the visit, observe the home environment for adequacy of resources.
  - Space: privacy, safe play of children, sleeping

- Overall cleanliness and state of repair
- Number of steps pregnant woman/new mother must climb
- Adequacy of cooking arrangements
- Adequacy of refrigeration and other food storage areas
- Adequacy of bathing, toilet, and laundry facilities
- Arrangements in home for newborn: sleeping, bathing, formula preparation (if needed), layette items, and diapers
- Throughout the visit, observe the home environment for overall state of repair and existence of safety hazards.
  - Storage of medications, household cleaners, and other substances hazardous to children
  - Presence of peeling paint on furniture, walls, or pipes
  - Factors that contribute to falls, such as dim lighting, broken steps, scatter rugs
  - Presence of vermin
  - Use of crib or playpen that fails to meet safety guidelines
  - Existence of emergency plan in case of fire; fire alarm or extinguisher
- Provide care to the mother, the newborn, or both as prescribed by their respective primary care provider or in accord with agency protocol.
- Provide teaching on the basis of previously identified needs.
- Refer the family to appropriate community agencies or resources, such as warm lines and support groups.
- Ensure that the woman knows potential problems to watch for and who to call if they occur.
- Ensure that used disposable items have been handled appropriately and that reusable items are cleaned and repacked appropriately in the nurse's bag.

In-Home Interventions: Ending the Visit
- Summarize the activities and main points of the visit.
- Clarify future expectations, including the schedule of the next visit.
- Review the teaching plan, and provide major points in writing.
- Provide information about reaching the nurse or agency if needed before the next scheduled visit.

Postvisit Interventions
- Document the visit thoroughly, using the necessary agency forms to serve as a legal record of the visit and to allow third-party reimbursement, as possible.
- Initiate the plan of care on which the next encounter with the woman and/or family will be based.
- Communicate appropriately (e.g., by telephone, letter, progress notes, or referral form) with the primary care provider, other health care professionals, or referral agencies on behalf of the woman and family.

Oral explanations should be supplemented with clearly written instructions. General information to promote well-being includes nutrition and common discomforts of pregnancy. The need for childbirth education and preparation can be addressed by using books or videos and supplemented by individual teaching at home. Coping with bed rest or other limitation of activity is a problem for many women with high-risk pregnancies. The nurse can share strategies that others have used, such as support groups for women on bed rest using Facebook or Skype, help with time management, and provide information about support services. Teaching about infant care or the special needs of the preterm infant may be appropriate during the prenatal period.

⚡ SAFETY ALERT

In caring for the home care patient, Occupational Safety and Health Administration (OSHA) guidelines should be followed. The use of strict handwashing techniques, sharps containers, gloves, personal protective equipment (PPE), and proper equipment is essential in preventing the spread of disease to the care provider, the woman, and her family.

The home care nurses should adhere to personal safety measures such as parking the car for access to a quick departure and should never enter a home where guns are visible.

BOX 2.7 Psychosocial Assessment

Language
- Identify the primary language spoken in the home.
- Assess whether there are any language barriers to receiving support.

Community Resources/Access to Care
- Identify primary and secondary means of transportation.
- Identify community agencies family uses for health care and support.
- Assess cultural and psychosocial barriers to receiving care.

Social Support
- Determine the people living with the pregnant woman.
- Identify who assists with household chores.
- Identify who assists with child care and parenting activities.
- Identify who the pregnant woman turns to for problems or during a crisis.

Interpersonal Relationships
- Identify the way decisions are made in the family.
- Identify the family's perception of the need for home care.
- Identify roles of adults in caring for family members.

Caregiver
- Identify the primary caregiver for home care treatments.
- Identify other caregivers and their roles.
- Assess the caregiver's knowledge of treatments and the care process.
- Identify potential strain from the caregiver role.
- Identify the level of satisfaction with the caregiver role.

Stress and Coping
- Identify what the woman perceives as lifestyle changes and their effect on her and her family.
- Identify the changes she and her family have made to adjust to her health condition and home health care treatments.

Clear documentation of assessments, problems identified, treatments and interventions performed, and the woman's response is essential. Third-party payers base reimbursement on the nurse's written record of providing skilled nursing care and assessments that support the woman's continuing need for those services. The nurse must promptly inform the health care provider by telephone, fax, or electronic file of any significant changes. When new orders are transmitted by telephone, a written copy must be sent for the physician's signature.

REFERENCES

Ackley, B. J., Ladwig, G. B., & Makic, M. B. F. (2017). *Nursing diagnosis handbook. An evidence-based guide to planning care.* St. Louis , MO: Elsevier.

American Association of Colleges of Nursing. (2008). *The essentials of baccalaureate education for professional nursing practice.* Washington, DC: Author.

American Nurses Association. (2015). *Code of ethics for nurses with interpretive statements.* Silver Spring, MD: Author.

American Nurses Association. (2015). *Nursing: Scope and standards of practice.* Silver Spring, MD: Author.

American Nurses Association and Health Ministries Association. (2005). *Faith community nursing: Scope & standards of practice.* Silver Spring, MD: American Nurses Association.

America's Children. (2013). *Key national indicators of well-being.* Retrieved from www.childstats.gov/pdf/ac2013/ac_13.pdf.

Association of Women's Health, Obstetric, and Neonatal Nurses. (2009). *Standards for professional nursing practice in the care of women and newborns* (7th ed.). Washington, DC: Author.

Bartels, J. B. (2014). The pause. *Critical Care Nurse, 34*(1), 74–75.

Bell, J. M. (2013). Family nursing is more than family centered care. *Journal of Family Nursing, 19*(4), 411–417.

Brussat, F., & Brussat, M. (1996). *Spiritual literacy: Reading the sacred in everyday life.* New York, NY: Scribner.

Burkhardt, P., & Nagai-Jacobson, M. G. (2015). Tips for spiritual care-giving. *Beginnings (American Holistic Nurses' Association), 35*(5), 6–7.

Carter, B., & McGoldrick, M. (1999). *The expanded family life cycle: Individual, family, and social perspectives* (3rd ed.). Boston: Allyn & Bacon.

Centers for Disease Control and Prevention. (2016). *Minority Health.* Retrieved from www.cdc.gov/MinorityHealth/index.html.

Cipriano, P. F. (2016). Attaining a culturally congruent practice. *American Nurse Today, 11*(5), 15.

Condon, M. (2004). *Women's health: Body, mind, spirit. An integrated approach to wellness and illness.* Upper Saddle River, NJ: Prentice-Hall.

Ellis, R. R., & Simmons, T. (2014). *Coresident grandparents and their grandchildren: 2012. Population characteristics.* US Census Bureau, 2012 American Community Survey. Retrieved from census.gov/content/dam/Census/library/publications/2014/demo/p.20-576.pdf.

Freund, K. (2012). Health disparities among women. In L. Goldman & A. Schafer (Eds.), *Goldman's Cecil medicine* (24th ed.). Philadelphia, PA: Elsevier.

Giger, J. N. (2013). *Transcultural nursing: Assessment and intervention* (6th ed.). St. Louis, MO: Mosby.

Giske, T., & Cone, P. H. (2015). Discerning the healing path—how nurses assist patient spirituality in diverse health care settings. *Journal of Clinical Nursing, 24*, 2926–2935.

Gordon, T., Kelly, E., & Mitchell, D. (2011). *Spiritual care for healthcare professionals: Reflecting on clinical practice.* London, UK: Radcliffe Publishing.

International Council of Nurses. (2012). *ICN code of ethics for nurses.* Geneva, Switzerland: Author.

Joint Commission. (2016). *Comprehensive accreditation manual for hospitals (CAMH).* Oak Brook, IL: Joint Commission Resources.

Lofquist, D., Lugaila, T., O'Connell, M., & Feliz, S. (2012). *Households and families: 2010.* Retrieved from www.census.gov/prod/cen2010/briefs/c2010br-14.pdf.

Pew Research Center. (2013). *Second-generation Americans. A portrait of the adult children of immigrants.* Washington, DC: Pew Research Center. Retrieved from www.pewsocialtrends.org/files/2013/02/FINAL_immigrant_generations_report_2-7-13.pdf.

Puchalski, C. (2006). Spiritual assessment in clinical practice. *Psychiatric Annals, 36*(3), 150–155.

Scharte, M., & Bolte, G. (2012). Increased health risks of children with single mothers: The impact of socio-economic and environmental factors. *Journal of Public Health, 23*(3), 469–475.

Siegel, B. S., & Perrin, E. C. (2013). Policy statement: Promoting the well-being of children whose parents are gay or lesbian. *Pediatrics, 13*(4), 827–830.

Spector, R. (2013). *Cultural diversity in health and illness* (8th ed.). Upper Saddle River, NJ: Prentice-Hall.

Taylor, E. J. (2012). *Religion: A clinical guide for nurses.* New York: Springer.

US Census Bureau. (2015). *Children characteristics: American community survey 1-year estimates.* Retrieved from https://factfinder.census.gov/faces/tableservices/jsf/pages/productview.xhtml?src=bkmk.

US Census Bureau. (2011). *Population estimates.* Retrieved from www.census.gov/popest/data/national/asrh/2011/index.html.

Wordsworth, H., Moore, R., & Woodhouse, D. (2016). Parish nursing: A unique resource for community and district nurses. *British Journal of Community Nursing, 21*(2), 66–74.

Wright, L. M., & Bell, J. M. (2009). *Beliefs and illness: A model for healing.* Calgary, Canada: 4th Floor Press.

Wright, L. M., & Leahey, M. (1999). Maximizing time, minimizing suffering: The 15-minute (or less) family interview. *Journal of Family Nursing, 5*(3), 259–271.

Wright, L. M., & Leahy, M. (2013). *Nurses and families: A guide to family assessment and intervention* (6th ed.). Philadelphia, PA: FA Davis.

3

Assessment and Health Promotion

Ellen F. Olshansky

e http://evolve.elsevier.com/Perry/maternal

Care of the well woman is focused on health promotion and illness prevention, recognizing that a woman is a bio-psycho-social-spiritual being, requiring a holistic approach to nursing care. To encourage appropriate health-promotion activities, it is important to conduct systematic health assessments and screenings. This chapter presents an overview of the nurse's role in encouraging health promotion and illness prevention in women. It provides guidelines for how to conduct a complete history and physical examination. This chapter also includes a schedule of screening tests recommended for women at different stages of their lives. As a background to understanding assessment, a review of female anatomy and physiology as well as the menstrual cycle is presented. Facilitators and barriers to women entering the health care system and risk factors for women's health across the life cycle are described. Anticipatory guidance suggestions, including nutrition and stress management, are included. Violence against women, particularly intimate partner violence (IPV) and battering of women, is discussed because it is often in the health care setting that the woman is able to acknowledge being in an abusive relationship. Examples of health-promotion efforts in the community are presented in an effort to emphasize community health approaches to care, especially since much of well woman care occurs in the community.

FEMALE REPRODUCTIVE SYSTEM

The female reproductive system consists of external structures visible from the pubis to the perineum and internal structures located in the pelvic cavity. The external and internal female reproductive structures develop and mature in response to estrogen and progesterone. This process starts in fetal life and continues through puberty and the childbearing years. Reproductive structures atrophy with age or in response to a decrease in ovarian hormone production. A complex nerve and blood supply supports the functions of these structures. The appearance of the external genitalia varies greatly among women. Heredity, age, race, and the number of children a woman has borne influence the size, shape, and color of her external organs.

EXTERNAL STRUCTURES

The external genital organs, or vulva, include all structures visible externally from the pubis to the perineum. These include the mons

pubis, labia majora, labia minora, clitoris, vestibular glands, vaginal vestibule, vaginal orifice, and urethral opening. The external genital organs are illustrated in Fig. 3.1.

The mons pubis is a fatty pad that lies over the anterior surface of the symphysis pubis. In the postpubertal female, the mons is covered with coarse, curly hair. The labia majora are two rounded folds of fatty tissue covered with skin that extend downward and backward from the mons pubis. The labia are highly vascular structures that develop hair on the outer surfaces after puberty. They protect the inner vulvar structures. The labia minora are two flat, reddish folds of tissue visible when the labia majora are separated. There are no hair follicles on the labia minora, but many sebaceous follicles and a few sweat glands are present. The interior of the labia minora is comprised of connective tissue and smooth muscle and is supplied with extremely sensitive nerve endings. Anteriorly, the labia minora fuse to form the prepuce (the hoodlike covering of the clitoris) and the frenulum (the fold of tissue under the clitoris). The labia minora join to form a thin, flat tissue called the *fourchette* underneath the vaginal opening at midline. The clitoris is located underneath the prepuce. It is a small structure composed of erectile tissue with numerous sensory nerve endings. During sexual arousal, the clitoris increases in size.

The vaginal vestibule is an almond-shaped area enclosed by the labia minora that contains openings to the urethra, Skene glands, vagina, and Bartholin glands. The urethra is not a reproductive organ but is discussed here because of its location. It usually is found about 2.5 cm below the clitoris. Skene glands are located on each side of the urethra and produce mucus, which aids in lubrication of the vagina. The vaginal opening is in the lower portion of the vestibule and varies in shape and size. The hymen, a connective tissue membrane that surrounds the vaginal opening, can be perforated during strenuous exercise, insertion of tampons, masturbation, and vaginal intercourse. Bartholin glands lie under the constrictor muscles of the vagina and are located posteriorly on the sides of the vaginal opening, although the ductal opening usually is not visible. During sexual arousal, the glands secrete clear mucus to lubricate the vaginal introitus.

The area between the fourchette and the anus is the perineum, a skin-covered muscular area that covers the pelvic structures. The perineum forms the base of the perineal body, a wedge-shaped mass that serves as an anchor for the muscles, fascia, and ligaments of the pelvis. The muscles and ligaments form a sling that supports the pelvic organs.

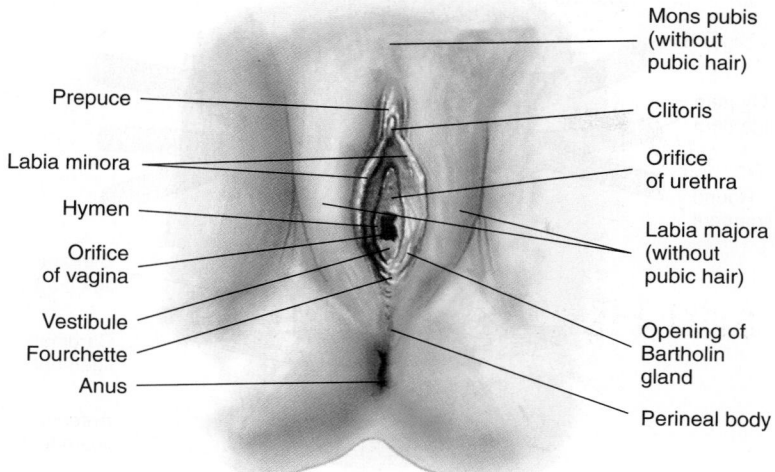

FIG 3.1 External female genitalia.

Labels: Prepuce, Labia minora, Hymen, Orifice of vagina, Vestibule, Fourchette, Anus, Mons pubis (without pubic hair), Clitoris, Orifice of urethra, Labia majora (without pubic hair), Opening of Bartholin gland, Perineal body

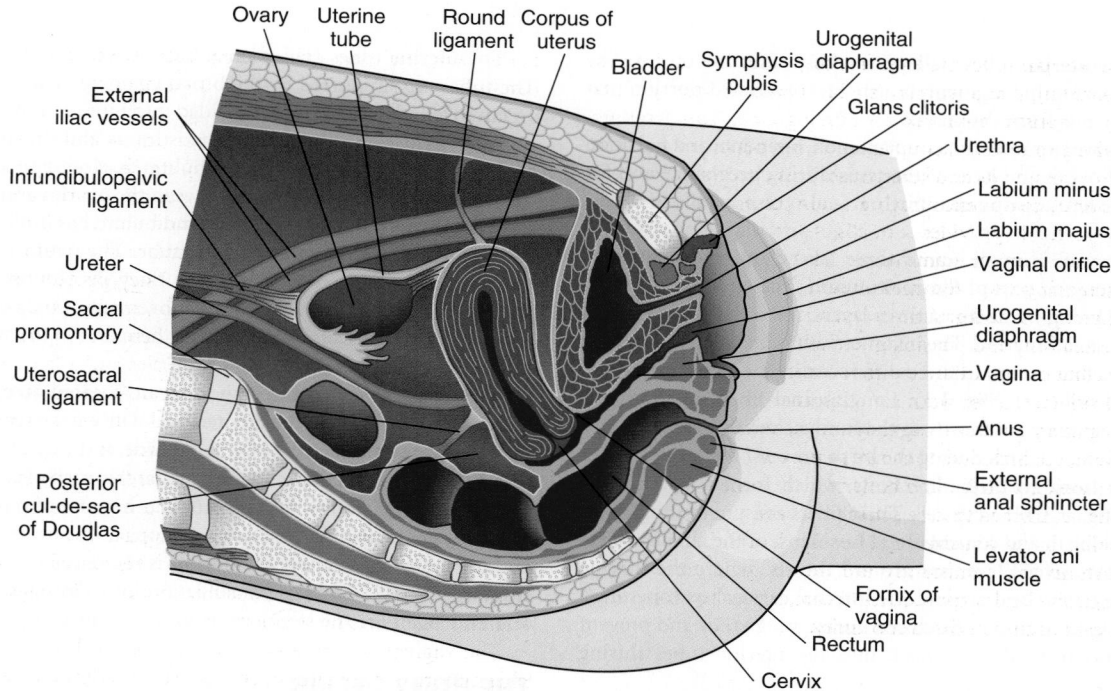

FIG 3.2 Midsagittal view of female pelvic organs with woman lying supine.

Labels: Ovary, Uterine tube, Round ligament, Corpus of uterus, Bladder, Symphysis pubis, Urogenital diaphragm, Glans clitoris, Urethra, Labium minus, Labium majus, Vaginal orifice, Urogenital diaphragm, Vagina, Anus, External anal sphincter, Levator ani muscle, Fornix of vagina, Rectum, Cervix, Posterior cul-de-sac of Douglas, Uterosacral ligament, Sacral promontory, Ureter, Infundibulopelvic ligament, External iliac vessels

INTERNAL STRUCTURES

The internal structures include the vagina, uterus, uterine tubes (fallopian tubes), and ovaries. The description of these structures follows.

The vagina is a fibromuscular, collapsible, tubular structure that lies between the bladder and rectum and extends from the vulva to the uterus. During the reproductive years, the mucosal lining is arranged in transverse folds called *rugae*. These rugae allow the vagina to expand during childbirth. Estrogen deprivation that occurs after childbirth, during lactation, and at menopause causes dryness and thinning of the vaginal walls and smoothing of the rugae. The vagina, particularly the lower segment, has few sensory nerve endings. Vaginal secretions are slightly acidic (pH 4 to 5) so that vaginal susceptibility to infections is limited. The vagina serves as a passageway for menstrual flow, as a female organ of copulation, and as a part of the birth canal for vaginal childbirth. The uterine cervix projects into a blind vault at the upper end of the vagina. Anterior, posterior, and lateral pockets called *fornices* (singular: *fornix*) surround the cervix. The internal pelvic organs can be palpated through the thin walls of these fornices.

The uterus is a muscular organ shaped like an upside-down pear that sits midline in the pelvic cavity between the bladder and rectum and above the vagina. Four pairs of ligaments support the uterus: cardinal, uterosacral, round, and broad. Single anterior and posterior ligaments also support the uterus. The *cul-de-sac of Douglas* is a deep pouch, or recess, posterior to the cervix formed by the posterior ligament.

The uterus is divided into two major parts: an upper triangular portion called the *corpus* and a lower cylindric portion called the *cervix* (Fig. 3.2). The fundus is the dome-shaped top of the uterus and is the

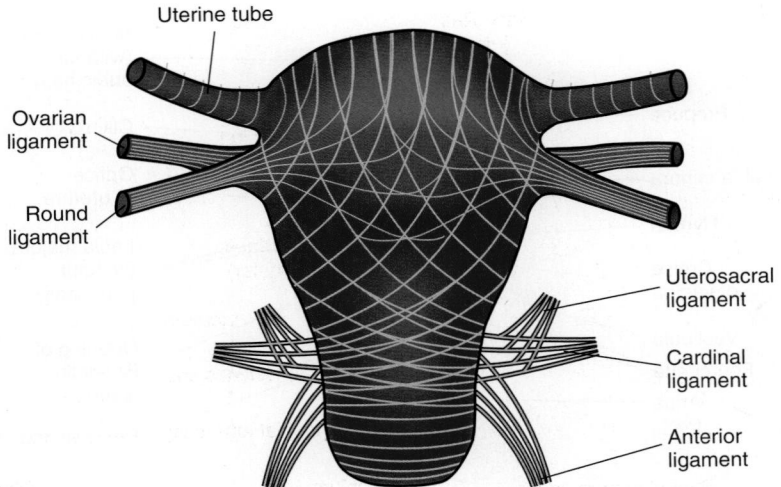

FIG 3.3 Schematic arrangement of directions of muscle fibers. Note that uterine muscle fibers are continuous with supportive ligaments of the uterus.

site at which the uterine tubes (fallopian tubes) enter the uterus. The isthmus, or lower uterine segment, is a short, constricted portion that separates the corpus from the cervix.

The uterus serves for reception, implantation, retention, and nutrition of the fertilized ovum and later of the fetus during pregnancy and for expulsion of the fetus during childbirth. It is also responsible for cyclic menstruation.

The uterine wall is made up of three layers: the endometrium, the myometrium, and part of the peritoneum. The endometrium is a highly vascular lining made up of three layers, the outer two of which are shed during menstruation. The myometrium is made up of layers of smooth muscles that extend in three different directions (longitudinal, transverse, and oblique) (Fig. 3.3). Longitudinal fibers of the outer myometrial layer are found mostly in the fundus, and this arrangement assists in expelling the fetus during the birth process. The middle layer contains fibers from all three directions, which form a figure-eight pattern encircling large blood vessels. These fibers assist in ligating blood vessels after childbirth and control blood loss. Most of the circular fibers of the inner myometrial layer are around the site where the uterine tubes enter the uterus and around the internal cervical os (opening). These fibers help keep the cervix closed during pregnancy and prevent menstrual blood from flowing back into the uterine tubes during menstruation.

The cervix is made up of mostly fibrous connective tissue and elastic tissue, making it possible for the cervix to stretch during vaginal childbirth. The opening between the uterine cavity and the canal that connects the uterine cavity to the vagina (endocervical canal) is the internal os. The narrowed opening between the endocervix and the vagina is the external os, a small circular opening in women who have never been pregnant. The cervix feels firm (like the end of a nose) with a dimple in the center that marks the external os.

The outer portion of the cervix is covered with a layer of squamous epithelium. The mucosa of the cervical canal is covered with columnar epithelium and contains numerous glands that secrete mucus in response to ovarian hormones. The squamo-columnar junction, where the two types of cells meet, is usually located just inside the external cervical os. This junction is also called the *transformation zone* and is the most common site for neoplastic changes. Cells from this site are scraped for the Papanicolaou (Pap) test (see discussion later in this chapter).

The uterine tubes (fallopian tubes) attach to the uterine fundus. The tubes are supported by the broad ligaments and range from 8 to 14 cm in length. The tubes are divided into four sections: the interstitial portion is closest to the uterus; the isthmus and the ampulla are the middle portions; and the infundibulum is closest to the ovary. The uterine tubes provide a passage between the ovaries and the uterus for the movement of the ovum. The infundibulum has fimbriated (fringed) ends, which pull the ovum into the tube. The ovum is pushed along the tubes to the uterus by rhythmic contractions of muscles of the tubes and by the current produced by the movement of the cilia that line the tubes. The ovum is usually fertilized by the sperm in the ampulla portion of one of the tubes.

The ovaries are almond-shaped organs located on each side of the uterus below and behind the uterine tubes. During the reproductive years, they are approximately 3 cm long, 2 cm wide, and 1 cm thick; they diminish in size after menopause. Before menarche, each ovary has a smooth surface; after menarche, they are nodular because of repeated ruptures of follicles at ovulation. The two functions of the ovaries are ovulation and hormone production. Ovulation is the release of a mature ovum from the ovary at intervals (usually monthly). Estrogen, progesterone, and androgen are the steroid hormones produced by the ovaries.

THE BONY PELVIS

The bony pelvis serves three primary purposes: protection of the pelvic structures, accommodation of the growing fetus during pregnancy, and anchorage of the pelvic support structures. The two innominate (hip) bones (consisting of ilium, ischium, and pubis), the sacrum, and the coccyx make up the four bones of the pelvis (Fig. 3.4). Cartilage and ligaments form the symphysis pubis, sacrococcygeal joint, and two sacroiliac joints that separate the pelvic bones.

The pelvis is divided into two parts: the false pelvis and the true pelvis (Fig. 3.5). The false pelvis is the upper portion above the pelvic brim or inlet. The true pelvis is the lower, curved, bony canal, which includes the inlet, the cavity, and the outlet through which the fetus passes during vaginal birth. The upper portion of the outlet is at the level of the ischial spines, and the lower portion is at the level of the ischial tuberosities and the pubic arch. Variations that occur in the size and shape of the pelvis are usually related to age, race, and sex. Pelvic ossification is complete at about 20 years of age.

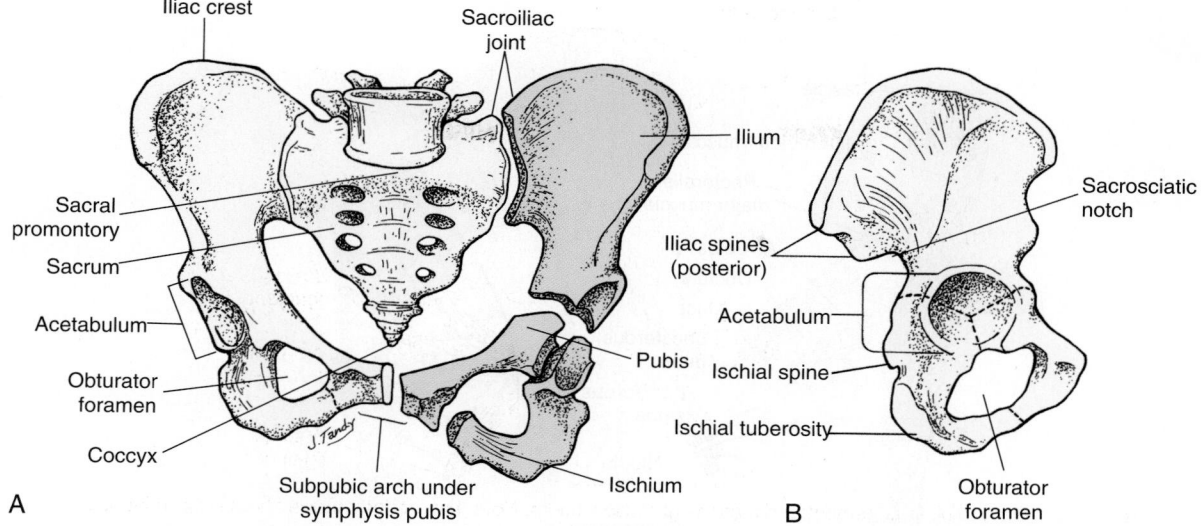

FIG 3.4 Adult female bony pelvis. **A,** Anterior view. **B,** External view of innominate bone (fused).

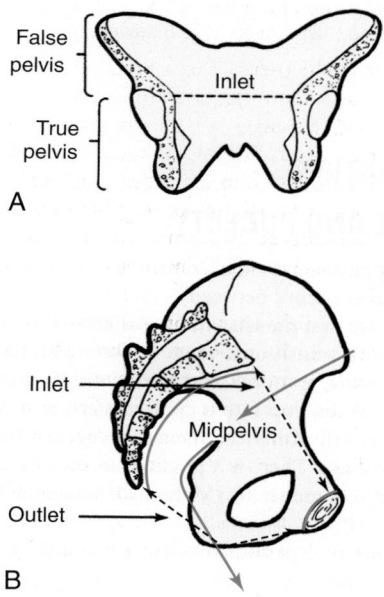

FIG 3.5 Female pelvis. **A,** Cavity of false pelvis is shallow. **B,** Cavity of true pelvis is irregularly curved canal *(arrows)*.

BREASTS

The breasts are paired mammary glands located between the second and sixth ribs (Fig. 3.6). About two thirds of the breast overlies the pectoralis muscle, between the sternum and midaxillary line, with an extension to the *tail of Spence*. The lower one third of the breast overlies the serratus anterior muscle. The breasts are attached to the muscles by connective tissue or fascia. Besides their function of lactation, breasts function as organs for sexual arousal in the mature adult female.

The breasts of the healthy, mature woman are approximately equal in size and shape but often are not absolutely symmetric. The size and shape vary with the woman's age, heredity, and nutrition. However, the contour should be smooth with no retractions, dimpling, or masses. Estrogen stimulates growth of the breasts by inducing fat deposition

in the breasts, development of stromal tissue (i.e., increase in its amount and elasticity), and growth of the extensive ductile system. Estrogen also increases the vascularity of breast tissue.

Once ovulation begins in puberty, progesterone levels increase. The increase in progesterone causes maturation of mammary gland tissue, specifically the lobules and acinar structures. During adolescence, fat deposition and growth of fibrous tissue contribute to the increase in the size of the glands. Full development of the breasts is not achieved until after the end of the first pregnancy or in the early period of lactation.

Each mammary gland is composed of a number of lobes that are divided into lobules. Lobules are clusters of acini. An acinus is a saclike terminal part of a compound gland emptying through a narrow lumen or duct. The acini are lined with epithelial cells that secrete colostrum and milk. Just below the epithelium is the myoepithelium (*myo*, or muscle), which contracts to expel milk from the acini. Mammary glands are modified sweat glands.

The ducts from the clusters of acini that form the lobules merge to form larger ducts draining the lobes. Ducts from the lobes converge in a single nipple (mammary papilla) surrounded by an areola. The anatomy of the ducts is similar for each breast but varies among women. Protective fatty tissue surrounds the glandular structures and ducts. *Cooper's ligaments*, or fibrous suspensory ligaments, separate and support the glandular structures and ducts. Cooper's ligaments provide support to the mammary glands while permitting their mobility on the chest wall (see Fig. 3.6). The round nipple is usually slightly elevated above the breast. On each breast the nipple projects slightly upward and laterally. It contains multiple openings from the milk ducts. The nipple is surrounded by fibromuscular tissue and covered by wrinkled skin (the areola). Except during pregnancy and lactation, there is usually no discharge from the nipple.

The nipple and surrounding areola are usually more deeply pigmented than the skin of the breast. The rough appearance of the areola is caused by sebaceous glands, known as Montgomery tubercles, directly beneath the skin. These glands secrete a fatty substance thought to lubricate the nipple. Smooth muscle fibers in the areola contract to cause the nipple to become erect, making it easier for the breastfeeding infant to grasp.

The vascular supply to the mammary gland is abundant. In the nonpregnant state, there is no obvious vascular pattern in the skin. The

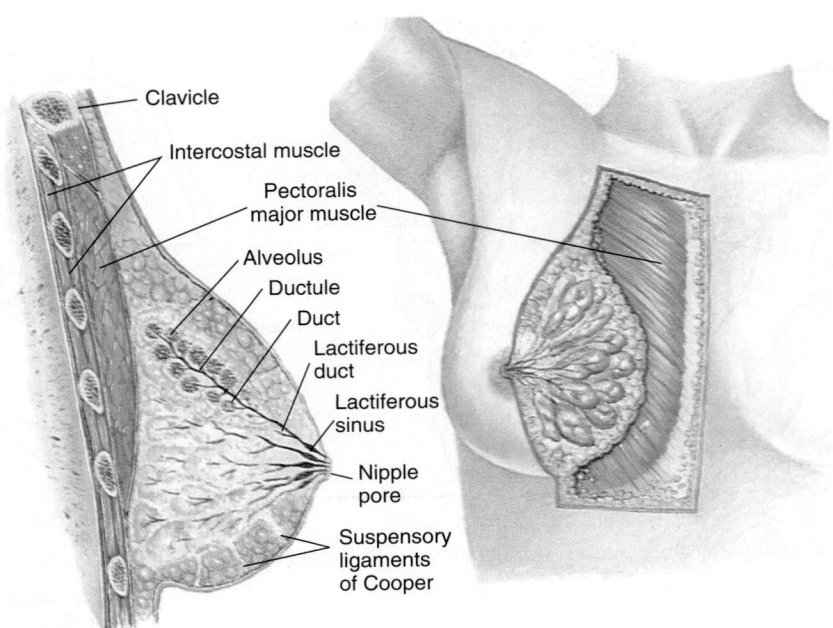

FIG 3.6 Anatomy of the breast showing position and major structures. (Adapted from Ball, J. W., Dains, J. E., Flynn, J. A., et al. [2016]. *Seidel's guide to physical examination* (8th ed.). St. Louis, MO: Elsevier.)

Labels in figure:
- Clavicle
- Intercostal muscle
- Pectoralis major muscle
- Alveolus
- Ductule
- Duct
- Lactiferous duct
- Lactiferous sinus
- Nipple pore
- Suspensory ligaments of Cooper

normal skin is smooth without tightness or shininess. The skin covering the breasts contains an extensive superficial lymphatic network that serves the entire chest wall and is continuous with the superficial lymphatics of the neck and abdomen. The lymphatics form a rich network in the deeper portions of the breasts. The primary deep lymphatic pathway drains laterally toward the axillae.

The breasts change in size and nodularity in response to cyclic ovarian changes throughout reproductive life. Increasing levels of both estrogen and progesterone in the 3 to 4 days before menstruation increase the vascularity of the breasts, induce growth of the ducts and acini, and promote water retention. The epithelial cells lining the ducts proliferate in number, the ducts dilate, and the lobules distend. The acini become enlarged and secretory, and lipid (fat) is deposited within their epithelial cell lining. As a result, breast swelling, tenderness, and discomfort are common symptoms just before the onset of menstruation. After menstruation, cellular proliferation begins to regress, acini begin to decrease in size, and retained water is lost. After breasts have undergone changes numerous times in response to the ovarian cycle, the proliferation and involution (regression) are not uniform throughout the breast. In time, after repeated hormonal stimulation, small, persistent areas of nodulations may develop. This normal physiologic change must be remembered when breast tissue is examined. Nodules may develop just before and during menstruation, when the breast is most active. The physiologic alternations in breast size and activity reach their minimum level about 5 to 7 days after menstruation stops. Therefore breast self-examination (BSE) (systematic palpation of breasts to detect signs of breast cancer or other changes) is best carried out during this phase of the menstrual cycle. Although monthly BSE used to be recommended to all women, there is very little evidence that BSE or a clinical breast exam by a health care provider helps to detect breast cancer early when a woman also gets a screening mammogram (United States Preventive Task Force [USPTF], 2016). However, all women should be familiar with how their breats normally appear and feel, and report any changes to a health care provider immediately.

MENSTRUATION

MENARCHE AND PUBERTY

Although young girls secrete small, rather constant amounts of estrogen, a marked increase occurs between 8 and 11 years of age. The term menarche denotes first menstruation. Puberty is a broader term that denotes the entire transitional stage between childhood and sexual maturity. Increasing amounts and variations in gonadotropin and estrogen secretion develop into a cyclic pattern at least 1 year before menarche. In North America, menarche occurs in most girls at about 13 years of age. There is a possible correlation between obesity and decreased age of menarche (Mohamad, Jamshidi, & Nouri-Jelyani, 2013).

Initially, menstrual periods are irregular, unpredictable, painless, and anovulatory (no ovum is released from the ovary). After 1 or more years, a hypothalamic-pituitary rhythm develops and the ovary produces adequate cyclic estrogen to make a mature ovum. Ovulatory (ovum released from the ovary) periods tend to be regular, with estrogen dominating the first half of the cycle and progesterone dominating the second half of the cycle.

Although pregnancy can occur in exceptional cases of true precocious puberty, most pregnancies in young girls occur after the normally timed menarche. All young adolescents of both sexes would benefit from knowing that pregnancy can occur at any time after the onset of menses.

MENSTRUAL CYCLE

Menstruation is the periodic uterine bleeding that begins approximately 14 days after ovulation. It is controlled by a feedback system of three cycles: endometrial, hypothalamic-pituitary, and ovarian. The average length of a menstrual cycle is 28 days, but variations are normal. The first day of bleeding is designated as day 1 of the menstrual cycle, or menses (Fig. 3.7). The average duration of menstrual flow is 5 days

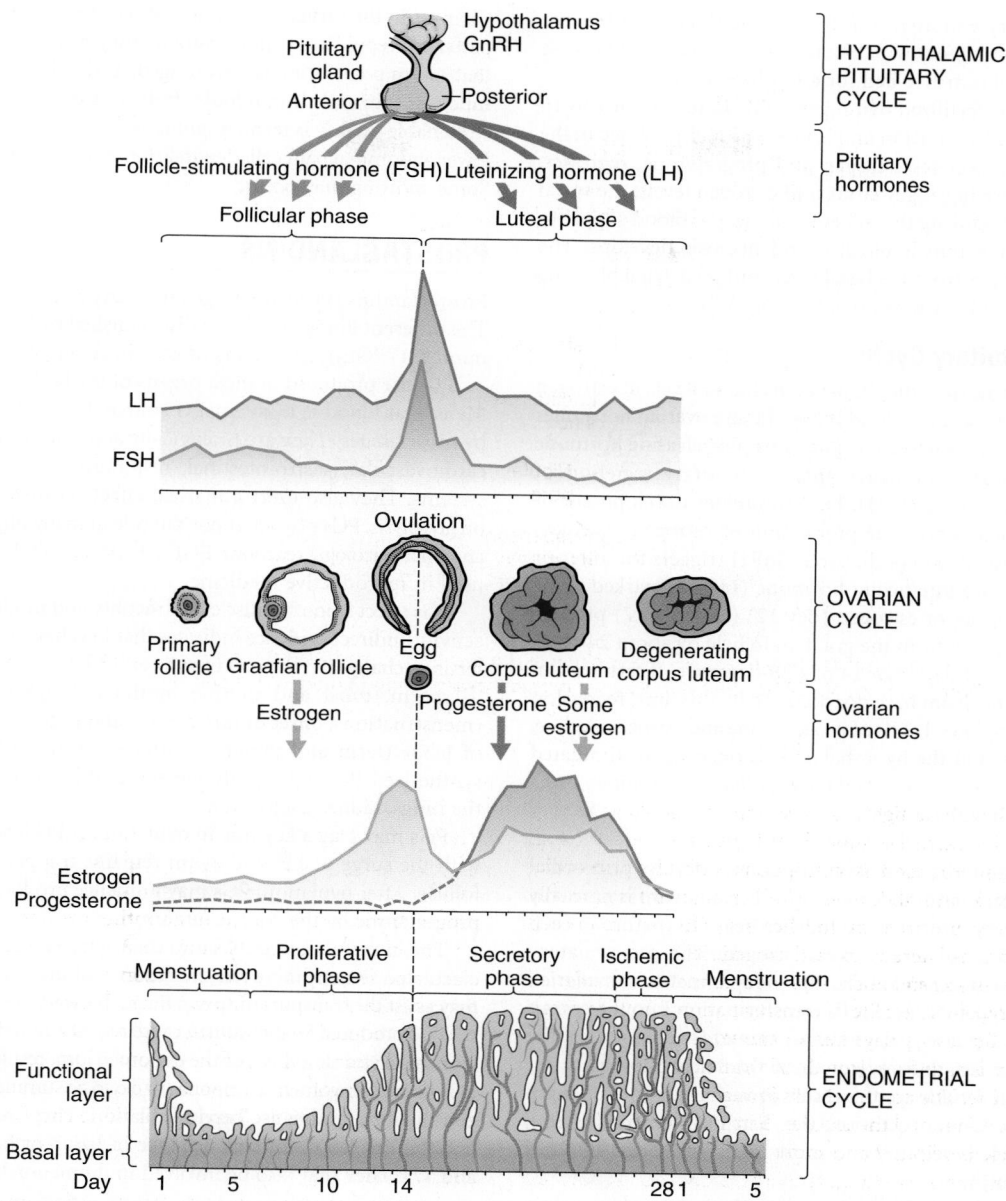

FIG 3.7 Menstrual cycle: hypothalamic-pituitary, ovarian, and endometrial. *GnRH,* Gonadotropin-releasing hormone.

(with a range of 3 to 6 days) and the average blood loss is 50 mL (with a range of 20 to 80 mL), but these vary greatly.

For about 50% of women, menstrual blood does not appear to clot. The menstrual blood clots within the uterus, but the clot usually liquefies before being discharged from the uterus. Uterine discharge includes mucus and epithelial cells in addition to blood.

The menstrual cycle is a complex interplay of events that occur simultaneously in the endometrium, the hypothalamus, the pituitary glands, and the ovaries. The menstrual cycle prepares the uterus for pregnancy. When pregnancy does not occur, menstruation follows. A woman's age, physical and emotional status, and environment influence the regularity of her menstrual cycles.

Endometrial Cycle

The four phases of the endometrial cycle are (1) the menstrual phase, (2) the proliferative phase, (3) the secretory phase, and (4) the ischemic phase (see Fig. 3.7). During the menstrual phase, shedding of the functional two thirds of the endometrium (the compact and spongy layers) is initiated by periodic vasoconstriction in the upper layers of the endometrium. The basal layer is always retained, and regeneration begins near the end of the cycle from cells derived from the remaining glandular remnants or stromal cells in this layer.

The proliferative phase is a period of rapid growth lasting from about the fifth day to the time of ovulation. The endometrial surface is completely restored in approximately 4 days, or slightly before bleeding ceases. From this point on, an eightfold to tenfold thickening occurs, with a leveling off of growth at ovulation. The proliferative phase depends on estrogen stimulation derived from ovarian follicles.

The secretory phase extends from the day of ovulation to about 3 days before the next menstrual period. After ovulation, large amounts of progesterone are produced. An edematous, vascular, functional endometrium is now apparent. At the end of the secretory phase, the fully matured secretory endometrium reaches the thickness of heavy, soft velvet. It becomes luxuriant with blood and glandular secretions—a suitable protective and nutritive bed for a fertilized ovum.

Implantation of the fertilized ovum generally occurs about 7 to 10 days after ovulation. If fertilization and implantation do not occur, the corpus luteum, which secretes estrogen and progesterone, regresses. With the rapid decrease in progesterone and estrogen levels, the spiral arteries go into spasm. During the ischemic phase, the blood supply to the functional endometrium is blocked and necrosis develops. The functional layer separates from the basal layer, and menstrual bleeding begins, marking day 1 of the next cycle (see Fig. 3.7).

Hypothalamic-Pituitary Cycle

Toward the end of the normal menstrual cycle, blood levels of estrogen and progesterone decrease. Low blood levels of these ovarian hormones stimulate the hypothalamus to secrete gonadotropin-releasing hormone (GnRH). In turn, GnRH stimulates anterior pituitary secretion of follicle-stimulating hormone (FSH). FSH stimulates development of ovarian graafian follicles and their production of estrogen. Estrogen levels begin to decrease, and hypothalamic GnRH triggers the anterior pituitary gland to release luteinizing hormone (LH). A marked surge of LH and a smaller peak of estrogen (day 12) (see Fig. 3.7) precede the expulsion of the ovum from the graafian follicle by about 24 to 36 hours. LH peaks at about day 13 or 14 of a 28-day cycle. If fertilization and implantation of the ovum have not occurred by this time, regression of the corpus luteum follows. Levels of progesterone and estrogen decline, menstruation occurs, and the hypothalamus is once again stimulated to secrete GnRH. This process is called the *hypothalamic-pituitary cycle*.

Ovarian Cycle

The primitive graafian follicles contain immature oocytes (primordial ova). Before ovulation, a monthly process in which an ovum is normally released from the ovary, from 1 to 30 follicles begin to mature in each ovary under the influence of FSH and estrogen. The pre-ovulatory surge of LH affects a selected follicle. The oocyte matures, *ovulation* occurs, and the empty follicle begins its transformation into the corpus luteum. This follicular phase (pre-ovulatory phase) (see Fig. 3.7) of the ovarian cycle varies in length from woman to woman. Almost all variations in ovarian cycle length are the result of variations in the length of the follicular phase. On rare occasions (i.e., 1 in 100 menstrual cycles), more than one follicle is selected and more than one oocyte matures and undergoes ovulation.

After ovulation, estrogen levels drop. For 90% of women, only a small amount of withdrawal bleeding occurs, and it goes unnoticed. In 10% of women, there is sufficient bleeding for it to be visible, resulting in what is termed *midcycle bleeding*.

The luteal phase begins immediately after ovulation and ends with the start of menstruation. This postovulatory phase of the ovarian cycle usually requires 14 days (range 13 to 15 days). The corpus luteum reaches its peak of functional activity 8 days after ovulation, secreting the steroids *estrogen* and *progesterone*. Coincident with this time of peak luteal functioning, the fertilized ovum is implanted in the endometrium. If no implantation occurs, the corpus luteum regresses and steroid levels drop. Two weeks after ovulation, if fertilization and implantation do not occur, the functional layer of the uterine endometrium is shed through menstruation.

Other Cyclic Changes

When the hypothalamic-pituitary-ovarian axis functions properly, other tissues undergo predictable responses. Before ovulation, the woman's basal body temperature is often less than 37° C (98.6° F); after ovulation, with increasing progesterone levels, her basal body temperature rises.

Changes in the cervix and cervical mucus follow a generally predictable pattern. Preovulatory and postovulatory mucus is viscous (thick) so that sperm penetration is discouraged. At the time of ovulation, cervical mucus is thin and clear. It looks, feels, and stretches like egg white. This stretchable quality is termed *spinnbarkeit*. Some women have localized lower abdominal pain called *mittelschmerz* that coincides with ovulation. Some spotting may occur.

PROSTAGLANDINS

Prostaglandins (PGs) are oxygenated fatty acids classified as hormones. The different kinds of PGs are distinguished by letters (PGE and PGF), numbers (PGE$_2$), and letters of the Greek alphabet (PGF$_{2\alpha}$).

PGs are produced in most organs of the body, including the uterus. Menstrual blood is a potent PG source. PGs are metabolized quickly by most tissues. They are biologically active in minute amounts in the cardiovascular, gastrointestinal, respiratory, urogenital, and nervous systems. They also exert a marked effect on metabolism, particularly on glycolysis. PGs play an important role in many physiologic, pathologic, and pharmacologic reactions. PGF$_{2\alpha}$, PGE$_4$, and PGE$_2$ are most commonly used in reproductive medicine.

PGs affect smooth muscle contractility and modulation of hormonal activity. Indirect evidence indicates that PGs have an effect on ovulation, fertility, changes in the cervix and cervical mucus that affect receptivity to sperm, tubal and uterine motility, sloughing of endometrium (menstruation), onset of miscarriage and induced abortion, and onset of labor (term and preterm). After exerting biologic actions, newly synthesized PGs are rapidly metabolized by tissues in such organs as the lungs, kidneys, and liver.

PGs may play a key role in ovulation. If PG levels do not rise along with the surge of LH, the ovum remains trapped within the graafian follicle. After ovulation, PGs may influence production of estrogen and progesterone by the corpus luteum.

The introduction of PGs into the vagina or the uterine cavity (from ejaculated semen) increases the motility of uterine musculature, which may assist the transport of sperm through the uterus and into the oviduct.

PGs produced by the woman cause regression of the corpus luteum and regression and sloughing of the endometrium, resulting in menstruation. PGs increase myometrial response to oxytocic stimulation, enhance uterine contractions, and cause cervical dilation. They may be a factor in the initiation of labor, the maintenance of labor, or both (see Chapters 13 and 17). They may also be involved in dysmenorrhea (see Chapter 4).

CLIMACTERIC AND MENOPAUSE

The climacteric is a transitional phase during which ovarian function and hormone production decline. This phase spans the years from the onset of premenopausal ovarian decline to the postmenopausal time when symptoms stop. Menopause (from Latin *mensis*, month, and Greek *pauses*, to cease) refers only to the last menstrual period. However, unlike menarche, menopause can be dated with certainty only 1 year after menstruation ceases. The average age at natural menopause is 51.4 years, with an age range of 35 to 60 years. *Perimenopause* is a period preceding menopause that lasts about 4 years. During this time, ovarian function declines. Ova slowly diminish, and menstrual cycles may be anovulatory, resulting in irregular bleeding. The ovary stops producing estrogen, and eventually menses no longer occur.

SEXUAL RESPONSE

The hypothalamus and anterior pituitary glands in females regulate the production of FSH and LH. The target tissue for these hormones is the ovary, which produces ova and secretes estrogen and progesterone. A feedback mechanism between hormone secretion from the ovaries, the hypothalamus, and the anterior pituitary gland aids in the control of the production of sex cells and sex steroid hormone secretion.

Although the first outward appearance of maturing sexual development occurs at an earlier age in females, both females and males achieve physical maturity at approximately 17 years of age; however, individual development varies greatly. Anatomic and reproductive differences notwithstanding, women and men are more alike than different in their physiologic response to sexual excitement and orgasm. For example, the glans clitoris and the glans penis are embryonic homologs. Little difference exists between female and male sexual response; the physical response is essentially the same whether stimulated by coitus, fantasy, or masturbation. Physiologic sexual response can be analyzed in terms of two processes: vasocongestion and myotonia (increased muscular tension).

Sexual stimulation results in increased circulation to circum-vaginal blood vessels (lubrication in the female), causing engorgement and distention of the genitals. Venous congestion is localized primarily in the genitalia, but it also occurs to a lesser degree in the breasts and other parts of the body. Arousal is characterized by myotonia, resulting in voluntary and involuntary rhythmic contractions. Examples of sexually stimulated myotonia are pelvic thrusting, facial grimacing, and spasms of the hands and feet (carpopedal spasms).

Although other sex researchers have noted various sexual response cycles, the sexual response cycle is classically divided into four phases: excitement, plateau, orgasm, and resolution, according to the seminal work of Masters and Johnson (1966). The four phases occur progressively, with no sharp dividing line between any two phases. The time, intensity, and duration for cyclic completion also vary for individuals and situations, and there are other models to explain sexual response, though less prevalent than the Masters and Johnson model. Sexuality and sexual response may change during pregnancy and postpartum, emphasizing the need to discuss with women possible sexual changes during this time. Specific issues related to this period (and prior procedures such as episiotomy) must be considered in counseling to promote healthy sexuality during the postpartum period. Despite these alternate models of sexual response, it is still common to describe the classic four stages in which specific body changes take place in sequence, and this description is useful in educating and talking with women who may have concerns about possible sexual dysfunction.

BARRIERS TO ENTERING THE HEALTH CARE SYSTEM

FINANCIAL ISSUES

Access to care varies greatly, depending on type and size of the system, source of payment for services, private versus public programs, availability of and accessibility to providers, individual preferences, and insurance coverage or ability to pay. The existing system continues to be oriented to treatment of acute or episodic conditions rather than to the promotion of health and comprehensive care, despite the fact that people are discharged earlier from hospitals, requiring more care in homes and community settings.

In the United States, disparity among races and socioeconomic classes affects many facets of life including health. Limited finances is associated with lack of access to care, delay in seeking care, few prevention activities, and little accurate information about health and the health care system. Women use health care services more often than men but are more likely than men to have difficulty in financing the services. Many poor women have traditionally been underinsured or uninsured, but rules about health insurance and who and what are covered are undergoing a transition with the Affordable Care Act (ACA) (USDHHS, 2015). With the new presidential administration, the future of the ACA is uncertain; insurance coverage of preexisting conditions and various preventive health services is not assured. With a greater focus on preventive health care services, nurses, advanced practice nurses, including nurse practitioners, nurse-midwives, and clinical nurse specialists, are critical to the provision of high quality, safe, effective, and accessible health care.

CULTURAL ISSUES

We live in a multicultural society with constantly changing demographics, and for nursing care of women to be optimal, cultural differences must be addressed with great sensitivity and competency. Nurses are in excellent positions to be responsible for providing culturally sensitive and competent health care (Douglas, Rosenkoetter, Pacquiao, et al., 2016). A variety of reasons are given to explain some of the differences in accessing care when financial barriers are adjusted. Some women experience racial discrimination or disrespectful, disillusioning, or discouraging encounters with community service providers such as social services and health care providers. Many women do not seek care from the health care system because of lack of trust. A lack of cross-cultural communication also presents problems. Desired health outcomes are best achieved when the health care provider has knowledge of and understanding about the culture, language, values, priorities, and health beliefs of those in various ethnic groups. Conversely, members of these various groups should understand the health goals to be achieved and the methods proposed to do so. Language differences can produce profound barriers between patients and providers. Even with an interpreter, misinformation can occur on both sides of the communication.

Providers must consider culturally based differences that could affect the treatment of diverse groups of women, and the women themselves must share practices and beliefs that could influence their responses to treatment or willingness to adhere to treatment. For example, women in some cultures value privacy to such an extent that they are reluctant to disrobe and, as a result, avoid physical examination unless absolutely necessary. Other women rely on their husbands to make major decisions, including those affecting the woman's health. Religious beliefs may dictate a plan of care, as with birth control measures or blood transfusions. Some cultural groups prefer folk medicine, homeopathy, or prayer to traditional Western medicine; others attempt combinations of some or all practices. Nurses can integrate into their own practice various holistic approaches to care, in accordance with Dossey's (2013) Theory of Integral Nursing. It is critically important to be sensitive to cultural differences and at the same time not stereotype and assume that a woman has certain beliefs because of her ethnic background. Although the amount of health information on the Internet is increasing, information in languages other than English is limited and not all information on the Internet is accurate, making health literacy an important issue in culturally competent care.

GENDER ISSUES

Gender influences communications between health care professionals and patients and may influence access to health care in general. Researchers have reported significant male-female differences in receipt of major diagnostic and therapeutic interventions, especially with cardiac and kidney problems. Women tend to use primary care services more often than do men and, some believe, more effectively. The gender of the provider plays a role. The concept of "gender concordance," in which the patient's gender matches the health care provider's gender, was found to be important for women seeking Pap tests (Lin & Chen, 2014).

Sexual orientation may produce another barrier. Nurses and other health care professionals need to understand the specific health care needs and issues related to sexual orientation, particularly since many lesbian, gay, bisexual, and transgender (LGBT) individuals feel stigmatized and are reluctant to seek health care (Olshansky & Zender, 2015). Some lesbians may not disclose their sexual orientation to health care professionals because they feel they may be at risk for hostility, inadequate health care, or breach of confidentiality. In many health care settings, heterosexuality is assumed, and the setting may be one in which the woman does not feel welcome (magazines, brochures, and environment reflect heterosexual couples, or the health care provider shows discomfort interacting with the woman). Lesbians themselves may hold beliefs that are incorrect (e.g., that they have immunity to human immunodeficiency virus [HIV], sexually transmitted infections [STIs], and certain cancers [e.g., cervical]). The perceived lack of risk can result in lesbians avoiding health care, as well as in health care providers giving incorrect advice or not providing appropriate screening for these women. Not all gynecologic cancers are related to sexual activity; lesbians who have never had children may be more at risk for breast, ovarian, and endometrial cancers. Their risk for heart disease, cancer of the lung, and colon cancer is not different from that of the heterosexual woman. To offset stereotypes, it is necessary for providers to develop an approach that does not assume that all patients are heterosexual. More content related to this issue needs to be included in nursing curricula.

CARING FOR THE WELL WOMAN ACROSS THE LIFE SPAN: THE NEED FOR HEALTH PROMOTION AND DISEASE PREVENTION

Maintaining optimal health is a goal for all women. Essential components of health maintenance are the identification of unrecognized problems and potential risks and the education and health promotion needed to reduce them. Current trends in the health care of women have expanded beyond a reproductive focus. A holistic approach to women's health care goes beyond only reproductive needs and includes a woman's health needs throughout her lifetime, with attention to physical, mental, emotional, social, and spiritual health. Women's health is considered to be part of the primary health care delivery system with assessment and screening focusing on a multisystem evaluation that emphasizes the maintenance and enhancement of wellness. Prevention of cardiovascular disease, promotion of mental health, and prevention of cancers beyond just reproductive-related cancers are all components of well-woman care. It is important to consider all aspects of women's health, particularly in light of the fact that the leading causes of death in women in the United States include more than just reproductive health conditions (Box 3.1).

Even when focusing on reproductive health, it is critical to take a holistic approach to the health of women. This is especially important for women in their childbearing years because conditions that increase a woman's health risks are related not only to her well-being but also to the well-being of both mother and baby in the event of a pregnancy. Prenatal care is an example of prevention that is practiced after conception. However, prevention and health maintenance are needed before conception because many of the mother's risks can be identified and eliminated, or at least modified.

As a female progresses through developmental ages and stages, she is faced with conditions that are age related. An overview of conditions and circumstances that increase health risks in women across the life span is presented in the next section.

> ### BOX 3.1 Top 10 Leading Causes of Death in Women in the United States
>
> 1. Heart disease
> 2. Malignant neoplasm (cancer)
> 3. Chronic lower respiratory disease
> 4. Stroke
> 5. Alzheimer's disease
> 6. Unintentional injury
> 7. Diabetes mellitus
> 8. Influenza and pneumonia
> 9. Nephritis
> 10. Septicemia

Data from Centers for Disease Control and Prevention (2015). *Leading causes of death in females United States, 2013.* Retrieved from http://www.cdc.gov/women/lcod/2013/index.htm.

ADOLESCENTS

All teenagers undergo progressive development of sex characteristics. They experience the developmental tasks of adolescence such as establishing identity and sexual orientation, emancipating from family, and establishing career goals. Some of these processes can produce great stress for the adolescent, and the health care provider should treat her very carefully. Female teenagers who enter the health care system usually do so for screening or because of a problem such as episodic illness or accidents. Previous guidelines recommended that young women should be screened with Pap tests at 18 years of age or when they become sexually active. Current guidelines suggest that Pap tests begin at 21 years of age (Sammarco, 2016), but controversy exists about the evidence to support these new guidelines, with some health care providers advising earlier testing, especially if a woman is sexually active at a younger age. Gynecologic problems are often associated with menses (either bleeding irregularities or dysmenorrhea), vaginitis or leukorrhea, STIs, contraception, or pregnancy. The adolescent is also at risk for use of street drugs, for eating disorders, and for stress, depression, and anxiety.

Many women first enter the health care delivery system for a Pap test or for contraception. Visits to the nurse may be their only contact with the system unless they become ill. Some women postpone examination until a specific need arises such as pregnancy, infertility, pain, abnormal bleeding, or vaginal discharge. Recently the availability of the human papillomavirus (HPV) vaccine has created another reason for young women to enter the health care system (Berg, Taylor, & Woods, 2015).

Teenage Pregnancy

Most young women begin having sex in the mid- to late teens. The average age at first intercourse is 18 (Guttmacher Institute, 2016), meaning that many begin sexual activity at an earlier age. A sexually active teenager who does not use contraception has a 90% chance of pregnancy within 1 year. The unintended pregnancy rate increased from 48% to 51% between 2001 and 2008, but it has since decreased to 45% based on 2011 data (Guttmacher Institute). The teen pregnancy rate has also decreased, but 77% of teen pregnancies are unplanned (USDHHS, 2016a).

Effective educational programs about sex and family life are imperative to control the rate of teen pregnancy and STIs. The nurse can provide information regarding the need for child spacing, methods of family planning that are consistent with religious and personal preferences, non-contraceptive benefits of certain methods, the appropriate use of methods selected, and the protection of future fertility when so desired.

Pregnancy in the teenager who is 16 years of age or younger often introduces additional stress into an already stressful developmental period. The emotional level of such teenagers is commonly characterized by impulsiveness and self-centered behavior, and they often place primary importance on the beliefs and actions of their peers. In attempts to establish a personal and independent identity, many teenagers do not realize the consequence of their behavior; their thinking processes do not include planning for the future.

Teenagers usually lack the financial resources to support a pregnancy and may not have the maturity to avoid teratogens or seek prenatal care and instruction or follow-up care. Children of teen mothers may be at risk for abuse or neglect because of the teenager's inadequate knowledge of growth, development, and parenting. Implementation of specialized adolescent programs in schools, communities, and health care systems is demonstrating continued success in reducing the birth rate in teenagers.

YOUNG AND MIDDLE ADULTHOOD

Because women 20 to 40 years of age have a need for contraception, pelvic and breast screening, and pregnancy care, they may prefer to use their gynecologic or obstetric provider as their primary care provider. During these years the woman may be "juggling" family, home, and career responsibilities, with resulting increases in stress-related conditions. Health maintenance includes not only pelvic and breast screening but also promotion of a healthy lifestyle (i.e., good nutrition, regular exercise, no smoking, moderate or no alcohol consumption, sufficient rest, stress reduction, and referral for medical conditions and other specific problems). Common conditions requiring well-woman care include vaginitis, urinary tract infections, menstrual variations, obesity, sexual and relationship issues, and pregnancy.

Parenthood After 35 Years of Age

The woman older than 35 years of age does not have a different physical response to a pregnancy per se but, rather, has had health status changes as a result of time and the aging process. These changes may be responsible for age-related pregnancy conditions. For example, a woman with type 2 diabetes may not have had expression of her diabetes at 22 years of age but may have full-blown disease at 38 years of age. Other chronic or debilitating diseases or conditions increase in severity with time, and these in turn may predispose to increased risks during pregnancy. Of significance to women in this age group is the risk for certain genetic anomalies (e.g., Down syndrome). The opportunity for genetic counseling should be available to all women (see Chapter 6).

LATE REPRODUCTIVE AGE

Women of later reproductive age are often experiencing change and reordering personal priorities. In general, the goals of education, career, marriage, and family have been achieved and now the woman has increased time and opportunity for new interests and activities. Divorce rates are high at this age, and children leaving home may produce an "empty nest syndrome," resulting in increased levels of depression. Chronic diseases also become more apparent. Most problems for the well woman are associated with perimenopause (e.g., bleeding irregularities and vasomotor symptoms). Health maintenance screening continues to be of importance because some conditions such as breast disease or ovarian cancer occur more often during this stage.

APPROACHES TO CARE AT SPECIFIC STAGES OF A WOMAN'S LIFE

There are certain specific approaches to care of women at different stages of their lives. Several of these approaches are described in the next section.

PRECONCEPTION COUNSELING AND CARE

Preconception health promotion provides women and their partners with information that is needed to make decisions about their reproductive future. Preconception care guides couples on how to avoid unintended pregnancies, identify and manage risk factors in their lives and their environment, and identify healthy behaviors that promote the well-being of the woman and her potential fetus. It has been estimated that 32% of pregnant women experience some complications of pregnancy, including mental health issues (mostly depression) and factors that lead to the need for cesarean birth (CDC, 2016a). In addition, 9.63% of births result in preterm infants, and 8.07% result in low–birth weight (LBW) infants (Martin, Hamilton, Osterman, et al., 2017).

Activities that promote healthy mothers and babies must be initiated before the period of critical fetal organ development, which is between 17 and 56 days after fertilization. By the end of the eighth week after conception and certainly by the end of the first trimester, any major structural anomalies in the fetus are already present. Because many women do not realize that they are pregnant and do not seek prenatal care until well into the first trimester, the rapidly growing fetus may be exposed to many types of intrauterine environmental hazards during this most vulnerable developmental phase. These hazards include drugs, viruses, and chemicals. In many instances, counseling can promote behavior modification before damage is done, or the woman can make an informed decision about her willingness to accept potential hazards.

Preconception care is important for women who have had a problem with a previous pregnancy (e.g., miscarriage or preterm birth). Although causes are not always identifiable, in many cases problems can be discovered and treated and do not recur in subsequent pregnancies. Preconception care is also important to minimize fetal malformations. For example, the offspring of women who have pre-existing diabetes mellitus have significantly more congenital anomalies than do children of mothers without diabetes. The rate of malformation is greatly reduced when the woman with pre-existing diabetes has excellent blood glucose control at the time she becomes pregnant and maintains euglycemia (normal blood glucose level) throughout the period of organ development in the fetus. The incidence of neural tube defects such as spina bifida and anencephaly is decreased significantly with the daily intake of 400 mcg of supplemental folic acid.

The components of preconception care such as health promotion, risk assessment, and interventions are outlined in Box 3.2.

PREGNANCY

A woman's entry into health care is often associated with pregnancy, for either diagnosis or actual prenatal care. Early entry into prenatal care (i.e., within the first 12 weeks of pregnancy) allows for identification of the woman at risk for complications and initiation of measures to prevent problems or treat them if they arise. The US Department of Health and Human Services and the National Institute of Child Health and Human Development (2013) emphasized the importance of early and consistent prenatal care to improve outcomes for both mother and infant. Major goals of prenatal care are listed in Box 3.3 and should be addressed in the first visit. Extensive discussion of pregnancy is found in Unit 3.

FERTILITY CONTROL AND INFERTILITY

Although the unintended pregnancy rate is slowly decreasing, the problem of unintended pregnancies remains significant (Guttmacher Institute, 2016). The majority of these occur in women who either do not use contraception or who experienced a contraceptive failure. Education

BOX 3.2   Components of Preconception Care

Health Promotion: General Teaching
- Nutrition
  - Healthy diet, including folic acid
  - Optimal weight
- Exercise and rest
- Avoidance of substance abuse (tobacco, alcohol, "recreational" drugs)
- Use of risk-reducing sex practices
- Attending to family and social needs

Risk Factor Assessment
- Chronic diseases
  - Diabetes, heart disease, hypertension, asthma, thyroid disease, kidney disease, anemia, mental illness
- Infectious diseases
  - HIV/AIDS, other sexually transmitted infections, vaccine-preventable diseases (e.g., rubella, hepatitis B, HPV)
- Reproductive history
  - Contraception
  - Pregnancies—unplanned pregnancy, pregnancy outcomes
  - Infertility
- Genetic or inherited conditions (e.g., sickle cell anemia, Down syndrome, cystic fibrosis)
- Medications and medical treatment
  - Prescription medication use (especially those contraindicated in pregnancy), over-the-counter medication use, radiation exposure
- Personal behaviors and exposures
  - Smoking, alcohol consumption, illicit drug use
  - Overweight or underweight; eating disorders
  - Folic acid supplement use
  - Spouse or partner and family situation, including intimate partner violence
  - Availability of family or other support systems
  - Readiness for pregnancy (e.g., age, life goals, stress)
- Environmental (home, workplace) conditions
  - Safety hazards
  - Toxic chemicals
  - Radiation

Interventions
- Anticipatory guidance or teaching
  - Treatment of medical conditions and results
  - Medications
  - Cessation or reduction in substance use and abuse
  - Immunizations (e.g., rubella, hepatitis)
- Nutrition, diet, weight management
- Exercise
- Referral for genetic counseling
- Referral to and use of:
  - Family planning services
  - Family and social needs management

BOX 3.3   Major Goals of Prenatal Care

- Define health status of mother and fetus.
- Determine the gestational age of the fetus, and monitor fetal development.
- Identify the woman at risk for complications, and minimize the risk whenever possible.
- Provide appropriate education and counseling.

starting their families until they are in their 30s or 40s, which allows more time to be exposed to factors that affect fertility negatively (including age-related infertility for the woman). In addition, STIs, which can predispose to decreased fertility, are becoming more common, and many women and men are in workplaces and home settings where they may be exposed to reproductive environmental hazards.

Infertility can cause emotional pain for many couples, and the inability to produce offspring sometimes results in feelings of failure and places inordinate stress on the couple's relationship. Much time, money, and emotional investment can be used for testing and treatment in efforts to build a family.

Steps toward prevention of infertility should be undertaken as part of ongoing routine health care, and information about how women may prevent some causes of infertility is especially appropriate in preconception counseling. Primary care providers can undertake initial evaluation and counseling before couples are referred to specialists. For additional information about infertility, see Chapter 5.

MENSTRUAL PROBLEMS

Irregularities or problems with the menstrual period are among the most common concerns of women and often cause them to seek help from the health care system. Common menstrual disorders include amenorrhea, dysmenorrhea, premenstrual syndrome, endometriosis, and menorrhagia or metrorrhagia. Simple explanation and counseling may handle the concern; however, history and examination must be completed, as well as laboratory or diagnostic tests, if indicated. Questions should never be considered inconsequential, and age-specific reading materials are recommended, especially for teenagers. See Chapter 4 for an in-depth discussion of menstrual problems.

PERIMENOPAUSE

The body responds to this natural transition in a number of ways, most of which are caused by the decrease in estrogen. Most women seeking health care during the perimenopausal period do so because of irregular bleeding. Others are concerned about vasomotor symptoms (hot flashes and flushes). Although fertility is greatly reduced during this period, women are urged to maintain some method of birth control because pregnancies still can occur. All women need to have factual information, the dispelling of myths, a thorough examination, and periodic health screenings thereafter.

IDENTIFICATION OF RISK FACTORS TO WOMEN'S HEALTH

In caring for women at all stages of life, it is important to understand the various and complex risk factors that can affect a woman's health. This section describes these risk factors. A thorough and systematic health history can elicit information about risk factors that exist for each woman.

is the key to encouraging women to make family planning choices based on preference and actual benefit-to-risk ratios. Providers can influence the user's motivation and ability to use the method correctly (see Chapter 5).

Women also enter the health care system because of their desire to become pregnant. Approximately 12.3% of women in the United States have some degree of infertility (CDC, 2016b). Many couples have delayed

SOCIAL, CULTURAL, AND GENETIC FACTORS

Differences exist among people from different socioeconomic levels and ethnic groups with respect to risk for illness and distribution of disease and death. Some diseases are more common among people of selected ethnicity (e.g., sickle cell anemia in African-Americans, Tay-Sachs disease in Ashkenazi Jews, adult lactase deficiency in Chinese individuals, β-thalassemia in Mediterranean individuals, and cystic fibrosis in northern Europeans). Cultural and religious influences also increase health risks because the woman and her family may have life and societal values and a view of health and illness that dictate practices different from those expected in the Judeo-Christian Western model. These may include food taboos or frequencies, methods of hygiene, effects of climate, care-seeking behaviors, willingness to undergo screening and diagnostic procedures, and conflicts in values.

Socioeconomic status affects birth outcomes. The rates of perinatal and maternal deaths, preterm births, and LBW infants are considerably higher in disadvantaged populations. Social consequences for poor women as single parents are great because many mothers with few skills are caught in the bind of insufficient income to afford child care. These families generate fewer and fewer resources and increase their risks for health problems. Multiple roles for women in general produce overload, conflict, and stress, resulting in higher risks for mental health problems.

SUBSTANCE USE AND ABUSE

Use of illicit drugs and inappropriate use of prescription drugs continue to increase and are found in all ages, races, ethnic groups, and socio-economic levels. Addiction to substances is seen as a biopsychosocial disease, with several factors leading to risk. These include biogenetic predisposition, lack of resilience to stressful life experiences, and poor social support. Women are less likely than men to abuse drugs, but the rate in women is increasing significantly. See Chapter 11 for more details about substance use and abuse during pregnancy.

Prescription Drug Use

Psychotherapeutic medications such as stimulants, sleeping pills, tran-quilizers, and pain relievers are used by an estimated 2.3% of American women (Substance Abuse and Mental Health Services Administration, 2015). Such medications can bring relief from undesirable conditions such as insomnia, anxiety, and pain. Because the medications have mind-altering capacity, misuse can produce psychologic and physical dependency in the same manner as illicit drugs. Risk-to-benefit ratios should be considered when such medications are used for more than a very short period. Depression and anxiety are the most common mental health problems in women (depression used to be considered the most common, but recently it is noted that depression occurs comorbidly with anxiety). Many kinds of medications are used to treat depression and anxiety. All of these psychotherapeutic drugs can have some effect on the fetus and must be monitored very carefully.

Illicit Drug Use
Marijuana

Marijuana is a substance derived from the cannabis plant. It is usually rolled into a cigarette and smoked, but it also may be mixed into food and eaten. Marijuana produces distorted perceptions, difficulty with problem solving as well as with thinking and memory, altered state of awareness, relaxation, mild euphoria, reduced inhibition, and mood changes (National Institute on Drug Abuse, 2016a). Marijuana is the most frequently used illicit drug, although a number of states have legalized it for recreational use.

Cocaine

Cocaine is a powerful central nervous system stimulant that is addictive because of the tremendous sense of euphoria that it creates. It can be snorted, smoked, or injected (National Institute on Drug Abuse, 2016b). Crack or rock cocaine is a form of the drug that is exceedingly potent and even more highly addictive. (Some say that an individual is "hooked" after the first use or at least after two or three "hits.") After ingestion of cocaine, an intensely pleasurable high results that is followed by an uncomfortable low; this increases the urge to continue taking the drug.

Predisposing factors and problems associated with cocaine use are polydrug use; poor nutrition; poverty; STIs; hepatitis B infection; dysfunctional family systems; employment difficulties; stress; anger; poor self-esteem; and previous or present physical, emotional, and sexual abuse. Cocaine use is especially concentrated among poor women of color.

Cocaine affects all major body systems. Among other complications, it produces cardiovascular stress (including tachycardia and hypertension) that can lead to heart attack or stroke, liver disease, central nervous system simulation that can cause seizures, and even perforation of the nasal septum. Needle-borne diseases such as hepatitis B and acquired immunodeficiency syndrome (AIDS) are common among cocaine users.

Opiates

The opiates include opium, heroin, meperidine, morphine, codeine, and methadone. Heroin is one of the most commonly abused drugs of this class. It is usually taken by intravenous injection but can be smoked or "snorted." The signs and symptoms of heroin use are euphoria, relaxation, relief from pain, "nodding out" (apathy, detachment from reality, impaired judgment, and drowsiness), constricted pupils, nausea, constipation, slurred speech, and respiratory depression.

Opiate use has become a priority problem area for the US Department of Health and Human Services with the recognition that prescription drugs, of which some opiates are a part, contribute to this serious abuse of opiates. Drug overdose, much of which occurs due to opiate abuse, is the leading cause of death due to injury (USDHHS, 2016b).

Methamphetamine

Methamphetamine is a relatively cheap and highly addictive stimulant. Over the past few years, use of this dangerous drug has decreased. Methamphetamine makes many users feel hypersexual and uninhibited, leading to more sex and less protection from pregnancy and STIs.

The active metabolite of methamphetamine is amphetamine, a central nervous system stimulant known as both "speed" and "meth." The crystalline form, which is smoked, is known as "ice." Methamphetamine causes a person to experience an elevated mood state as well as increased energy and creates addiction within a short period (Medline Plus, 2016). It can lead to cardiac problems, including irregular heartbeat and hypertension and, over time, can create cognitive and mental as well as dental problems (National Institute on Drug Abuse, 2014). Most of the effects of amphetamines are similar to those of cocaine.

Phencyclidine

Phencyclidine (PCP) is a synthetic drug known by various names ("peace pill," "elephant," "angel dust," "hog"). PCP causes a person to experience dissociative symptoms that include distorted perceptions and detached feelings, memory loss, depression, delusions, hallucinations, anxiety, panic, and disordered thinking, and high doses can cause seizures, coma, and possibly death (National Institute on Drug Abuse, 2016c). Because some effects mimic the signs and symptoms of schizophrenia, a user may be admitted to a psychiatric unit.

Other Illicit Drugs

A number of street drugs pose risks to users. A few are derived from organic materials, but more and more are produced synthetically in laboratories. Sedatives such as "downers," "yellow jackets," or "red devils" are used to come off of "highs." Hallucinogens alter perceptions and body function. Lysergic acid diethylamide (LSD) produces vivid changes in sensation, often with agitation, euphoria, paranoia, and a tendency toward antisocial behavior. Its use may lead to flashbacks, chronic psychosis, and violent behavior.

Alcohol Consumption

Current data estimates that 5.3 million women drink to such an extent that it endangers their health (National Institute on Alcohol Abuse and Alcoholism, 2016). About one-third of alcoholics are women, and many relate the onset of their drinking problem to stressful events. Women who are problem drinkers are often depressed, have more motor vehicle injuries, and have a higher incidence of attempted suicide than do women in the general population. They are also at risk for alcohol-related liver damage. Early case finding and treatment are important in alcoholism for both the ill individual and family members.

Cigarette Smoking

Tobacco use is the leading cause of preventable death and illness. Smoking is linked to cardiovascular disease, various types of cancers (especially lung and cervical), chronic lung disease, and negative pregnancy outcomes. Premature death is estimated to occur in 480,000 people annually because of either smoking or being exposed to secondhand smoke, with cigarette smoking being the leading cause of preventable deaths. However, it is also estimated that 46.6 million adults in the United States smoke; 14.8% of women are smokers (CDC, 2016c). Women who smoke decrease their life span by 14.5 years compared with nonsmokers, but recent data indicate that the sooner a person quits smoking, the sooner he or she can decrease the risk for early death (American Cancer Society [ACS], 2015). Box 3.4 includes guidelines for smoking cessation.

Tobacco contains nicotine, which is an addictive substance that creates physical and psychologic dependence. Recently, alternatives to cigarettes have been used, including electronic cigarettes (e-cigarettes), smokeless tobacco, and water pipes. These alternative methods, however, may cause serious side effects due to the chemicals used in them and may have deleterious effects on the developing fetus (England, Bunnell, Pechacek, et al., 2015).

Cigarette smoking impairs fertility in both women and men, may reduce the age for menopause, and increases the risk for osteoporosis after menopause. Passive, or secondhand, smoke (environmental tobacco smoke) contains similar hazards and presents additional problems for the smoker and harm for the nonsmoker. Smoking during pregnancy may have adverse consequences for the infant, such as low-birth weight.

Caffeine

Caffeine is found in society's most popular drinks: coffee, tea, and soft drinks. It is a stimulant that can affect mood and interrupt body functions by producing anxiety and sleep interruptions. Heart dysrhythmias may be made worse by caffeine, and there can be interactions with certain medications such as lithium. Birth defects have not been related to caffeine consumption; however, high intake has been related to a slight decrease in birth weight and may also increase the risk for miscarriage. The March of Dimes (2013) recommends that pregnant women, or women who are trying to conceive, limit their caffeine intake to no more than 200 mg/day, which is the equivalent of one 12-ounce cup of coffee.

BOX 3.4 Interventions for Smoking Cessation: The Five *A's*

Ask
- What was her age when she started smoking?
- How many cigarettes does she smoke a day? When was her last cigarette?
- Has she tried to quit?
- Does she want to quit?

Advise
- Give her information about the effects of smoking on pregnancy and her fetus, on her own future health, and on the members of her household.

Assess
- What were her reasons for not being able to quit before, or what made her start again?
- Does she have anyone who can help her?
- Does anyone else smoke at home?
- Does she have friends or family who have quit successfully?

Assist
- Provide support; give self-help materials.
- Encourage her to set a quit date.
- Refer to a smoking-cessation program, or provide information about nicotine replacement products (not recommended during pregnancy) if she is interested.
- Teach and encourage the use of stress-reduction activities.
- Provide for follow-up with a phone call, letter, or clinic visit.

Arrange Follow-up
- Arrange to follow the woman to find out about smoking-cessation status.
- Make a phone call around the time of her quit date. Assess her status at every prenatal visit.
- Congratulate her on her success, or provide support for her if she relapses.
- Referral to intensive treatment may be necessary.

Adapted from Fiore, C. (2012). *Tobacco use and dependence: A 2011 update of treatments.* Retrieved from http://www.medscape.org/viewarticle/757167 (reviewed May 15, 2016).

NUTRITION PROBLEMS AND EATING DISORDERS

Good nutrition is essential for optimal health. A well-balanced diet helps prevent illness and also is used to treat certain health problems. Conversely, poor eating habits, eating disorders, and obesity are linked to disease and debility. *Dietary Guidelines for Americans* (Office of Disease Prevention and Health Promotion [ODPHP], 2015) provides evidence-based recommendations to promote health and reduce risks for chronic diseases through diet and physical activity. This guide contains resources for health professionals and consumers on dietary guidelines. Previously, the US government advocated the Food Pyramid, followed by MyPlate. The 2015 recommendations include five guidelines: (1) follow a healthy eating pattern across the life span, (2) focus on variety, nutrient density, and amount, (3) limit calories from added sugars and saturated fats, and reduce sodium intake, (4) shift to healthier food and beverage choices, and (5) support healthy eating patterns for all.

In addition to specific guidelines for healthy eating, environmental factors play an important role in nutrition. Environmental factors are part of what is referred to as social determinants of health, in which the availability of resources is a critical factor in nutrition and health.

Nutritional Deficiencies

Overt disease caused by a lack of certain nutrients is rarely seen in the United States. However, insufficient amounts or imbalances of nutrients do pose problems for individuals and families. Overweight or underweight status, malabsorption, listlessness, fatigue, frequent colds and other minor infections, constipation, dull hair and nails, and dental caries are examples of problems that can be related to nutrition and indicate the need for further nutritional assessment. Poor nutrition, especially related to obesity and high fat and cholesterol intake, may lead to more serious conditions such as heart diseases, malignant neoplasms, cerebrovascular diseases, and diabetes.

Other dietary extremes also produce risk. For example, insufficient amounts of calcium can lead to osteoporosis, too much sodium can aggravate hypertension, and megadoses of vitamins can cause adverse effects in several body systems. Fad weight-loss programs and yo-yo dieting (repeated and cyclic weight gain and weight loss) result in nutritional imbalances and, in some instances, medical problems. Such diets and programs are not appropriate for weight maintenance. Adolescent pregnancy produces special nutritional requirements because the metabolic needs of pregnancy are superimposed on the teenager's own needs for growth and maturation at a time when eating habits are not ideal. Neural tube defects are more common in infants born to women with a diet poor in folate. In their childbearing years, women should ingest at least 0.4 mg (400 mcg) of folic acid daily in addition to consuming a diet rich in folate-containing foods (CDC, 2016d).

Obesity

During the past 20 years, obesity has increased dramatically in the United States. More than one third of women in the United States are obese (body mass index [BMI] of 30 or greater), with adults 40 to 59 years of age having the highest prevalence. The BMI is defined as a measure of an adult's weight in relation to his or her height, specifically the adult's weight in kilograms divided by the square of his or her height in meters (Box 3.5). It is estimated that one-third of adults (CDC, 2015a) and one-sixth of children and adolescents are in the obese range (CDC, 2015b). Overweight and obesity are known risk factors for premature death, diabetes, heart disease, stroke, hypertension, type 2 diabetes, gallbladder disease, diverticular disease, some anemias, oral disease, constipation, osteoarthritis, gout, osteoporosis, respiratory dysfunction, sleep apnea, and some types of cancer (uterine, breast, esophageal, colorectal, kidney, and pancreatic) (ACS, 2016a). In addition, obesity is associated with high cholesterol, menstrual irregularities, hirsutism (excess body/facial hair), stress incontinence, depression, complications of pregnancy, increased surgical risk, and shortened life span. Pregnant women who are morbidly obese are at increased risk for hypertension, diabetes, gallbladder disease, postterm pregnancy, and musculoskeletal problems.

BOX 3.5 Ideal Body Weight With Body Mass Index

BMI 18.5 or less—Underweight
BMI 18.5 to 24.9—Normal weight
BMI 25.0 to 29.9—Overweight
BMI 30.0 to 34.5—Obese
BMI 35.0 to 40—Very obese

Source: Centers for Disease Control and Prevention (2015). *About adult BMI.* https://www.cdc.gov/healthyweight/assessing/bmi/adult_bmi/.

Eating Disorders

Eating disorders are estimated to have a prevalence of 20 million women and 10 million men in the United States. Eating disorders are considered a mental illness, and the mortality rate is the highest of all mental illnesses (Sammarco, 2016).

Anorexia nervosa and bulimia are two forms of eating disorders, although there are additional forms, such as binge eating disorders or other specified feeding or eating disorders. Some women, especially adolescents, do not have symptoms that lend themselves to a diagnosis of anorexia nervosa or bulimia, but they do fall under an unspecified category and require accurate diagnosis and prompt treatment (Sammarco, 2016). Eating disorders can affect not only the woman, but her family as well. Treatment must be personalized, including nutritional and behavioral/psychotherapeutic approaches.

It is important to assess for and treat women with eating disorders early because they are at increased risk for serious physical problems as well as diminished quality of life (Sammarco, 2016). Eating disorders during pregnancy are also associated with increased risk to the pregnant woman and her fetus.

Anorexia Nervosa

Some women have a distorted view of their bodies and, no matter what their weight, perceive themselves to be much too heavy. As a result, they undertake strict and severe diets and rigorous extreme exercise. This chronic eating disorder is known as *anorexia nervosa*. Women can carry this condition to the point of starvation, with resulting endocrine and metabolic abnormalities. If not corrected, significant complications of dysrhythmias, amenorrhea, cardiomyopathy, and heart failure occur and, in the extreme, can lead to death. The condition commonly begins during adolescence in young women who have some degree of personality disorder. They gradually lose weight over several months, have amenorrhea, and are abnormally concerned with body image. A coexisting depression usually accompanies anorexia.

There are no specific tests to diagnose anorexia nervosa. A medical history, physical examination, and screening tests help identify women at risk for eating disorders. Several tools are available to use in primary care settings. The SCOFF questionnaire, developed by Morgan, Reid, & Lacey (1999) is still in use and is easy to administer and can help the nurse decide whether an eating disorder is likely and whether the woman needs further assessment and possibly psychiatric and medical intervention (Hautala, Junnila, Alin, et al., 2009). See Box 3.6 for a description of the SCOFF.

Bulimia Nervosa

Bulimia refers to secret, uncontrolled binge eating alternating with methods to prevent weight gain: self-induced vomiting, laxatives or

---

BOX 3.6 Screening for Eating Disorders: SCOFF Questions

Each question scores 1 point. A score of 2 or more indicates the person may have anorexia nervosa or bulimia.

1. Do you make yourself Sick (i.e., induce vomiting) because you feel too full?
2. Do you worry about loss of Control over the amount you eat?
3. Have you recently lost more than One stone (6.4 kg [14 lbs]) in a 3-month period?
4. Do you think you are too Fat even if others think you are too thin?
5. Does Food dominate your life?

From Morgan, J., Reid, F., & Lacey, J. (1999). The SCOFF questionnaire: Assessment of a new screening tool for eating disorders, *British Medical Journal, 319*(7223), 1467–1468.

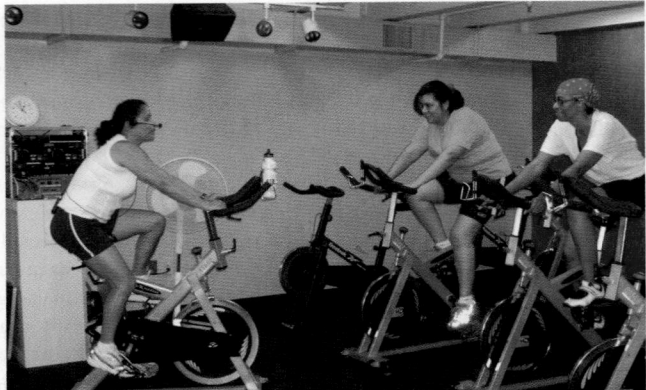

FIG 3.8 Exercise should be part of one's regular health routine. A cycle class is fun and provides moderate to vigorous exercise. (Courtesy of Shari Rivera Sharpe, Chapel Hill, NC.)

 GUIDELINES

Kegel Exercise

Description and Rationale

Kegel exercise, or pelvic muscle exercise, is a technique used to strengthen the muscles that support the pelvic floor. This exercise involves regularly tightening (contracting) and relaxing the muscles that support the bladder and urethra. By strengthening these pelvic muscles, a woman can prevent or reduce accidental urine loss.

Specific Instructions

1. Each contraction should be as intense as possible without contracting the abdomen, thighs, or buttocks.
2. Contractions should be held for at least 10 seconds. The woman may have to start with as little as 2 seconds per contraction until her muscles get stronger.
3. The woman should rest for 10 seconds or more between contractions so that the muscles have time to recover and each contraction can be as strong as the woman can make it.
4. The woman should feel the pulling up over the three muscle layers so that the contraction reaches the highest level of her pelvis.

Data from Sampselle, C. (2003). Behavior interventions in young and middle-aged women: Simple interventions to combat a complex problem, *American Journal of Nursing, 103*(suppl), 9–19; Sampselle, C. (2000). Behavioral interventions for urinary incontinence in women: Evidence for practice, *Journal of Midwifery Women's Health, 45*(2), 94–103; Sampselle, C., Wyman, J., Thomas, K., et al. (2000). Continence for women: A test of AWHONN's evidence-based protocol, *Journal of Obstetric, Gynecologic, and Neonatal Nursing, 29*(1), 312–317.

diuretics, strict diets, fasting, and rigorous exercise. During a binge episode, a large number of calories are consumed, usually consisting of sweets and "junk foods." Binges occur at least twice per week. Bulimia usually begins in early adulthood (18 to 25 years of age) and is found primarily in females. Complications can include dehydration and electrolyte imbalance, gastrointestinal abnormalities, and cardiac dysrhythmias. Unlike those with anorexia, individuals with bulimia may feel shame or disgust about their disorder and tend to seek help earlier. The SCOFF screening assessment also can be used to assess patients with bulimia (see Box 3.6).

LACK OF EXERCISE

Exercise contributes to good health by lowering risks for a variety of conditions that are influenced by obesity and a sedentary lifestyle. It is effective in the prevention of cardiovascular disease and in the management of chronic conditions such as hypertension, arthritis, diabetes, respiratory disorders, and osteoporosis (Fig. 3.8). Exercise also contributes to stress reduction and weight maintenance. Women report that engaging in regular exercise improves their body image and self-esteem and acts as a mood enhancer. Aerobic exercise produces cardiovascular involvement because an increased amount of oxygen is delivered to working muscles. Anaerobic exercise such as weight training improves individual muscle mass without stress on the cardiovascular system. Because women are concerned about both cardiovascular and bone health, weight-bearing aerobic exercises such as walking, running, racket sport, and dancing are preferred. However, excessive or strenuous exercise can lead to hormone imbalances, resulting in amenorrhea and its consequences. Physical injury is also a potential risk.

One particular exercise that is important for women is Kegel exercise, or pelvic muscle exercise. This exercise is used to strengthen the muscles that support the pelvic floor and should be practiced regularly. Instructions for this exercise are in presented in the Guidelines box.

Physical activity and exercise counseling for persons of all ages should be undertaken at schools, work sites, and primary care settings. Specific recommendations include 20 to 30 minutes of moderate activity at least 3 times per week. Few Americans exercise this often, and physical inactivity increases with age, especially during adolescence and early adulthood. Even small increases in activity can be beneficial. During pregnancy, an ongoing exercise regimen can be continued but intensity and duration should be decreased. Sedentary women should obtain medical clearance to initiate exercise during pregnancy and should begin with low-intensity and low-impact workouts.

STRESS

The modern woman faces increasing levels of stress and, as a result, is prone to a variety of stress-induced complaints and illnesses. Stress often occurs because of multiple roles in which coping with job and financial responsibilities conflicts with parenting and duties at home. To add to this burden, women are socialized to be caregivers, which is emotionally draining, creating additional stress. They also may find themselves in positions of minimal power that do not allow them control over their everyday environments. Some stress is normal and contributes to positive outcomes. Many women thrive in busy surroundings. However, excessive or high levels of ongoing stress trigger physical reactions such as rapid heart rate, elevated blood pressure, slowed digestion, release of additional neurotransmitters and hormones, muscle tenseness, and a weakened immune system. Consequently, constant stress can contribute to clinical illnesses such as flare-ups of arthritis or asthma, frequent colds or infections, gastrointestinal upsets, cardiovascular problems, and infertility. Box 3.7 lists symptoms that may be related to chronic or extreme stress. Psychologic symptoms such as anxiety, irritability, eating disorders, depression, insomnia, and substance abuse have also been associated with stress.

Because it is neither possible nor desirable to avoid all stress, women must learn how to manage it. The nurse should assess each woman for signs of stress, using therapeutic communication skills to determine risk factors and the woman's ability to function. Some women must be referred for counseling or other mental health therapy. Women experiencing major life changes such as separation and divorce, bereavement, serious illness, and unemployment also need special attention.

Many centers offer support groups to help women prevent or manage stress. Social support and good coping skills can improve a woman's self-esteem and give her a sense of mastery. Anticipatory guidance for developmental or expected situational crises can help her plan strategies

BOX 3.7 Stress Symptoms

Physical

- Perspiration/sweaty hands
- Increased heart rate
- Trembling
- Nervous tics
- Dryness of throat and mouth
- Tiring easily
- Urinating frequently
- Sleeping problems
- Diarrhea, indigestion, vomiting
- Butterflies in stomach
- Headaches
- Premenstrual tension
- Pain in neck and lower back
- Loss of appetite or overeating
- Susceptibility to illness

Behavioral

- Stuttering and other speech difficulties
- Crying for no apparent reason
- Acting impulsively
- Startling easily
- Laughing in a high-pitched and nervous tone of voice
- Grinding teeth
- Increasing smoking
- Increasing use of drugs and alcohol
- Being accident prone

Psychologic

- Feeling anxious
- Feeling scared
- Feeling irritable
- Feeling moody
- Having low self-esteem
- Being afraid of failure
- Being unable to concentrate
- Embarrassing easily
- Worrying about the future
- Being preoccupied with thoughts or tasks
- Forgetful

Adapted from State University of New York Counseling Center (2002). *Stress management.* Buffalo, NY: University of Buffalo, State University of New York.

for dealing with potentially stressful events. Role playing, relaxation techniques, biofeedback, meditation, desensitization, imagery, assertiveness training, yoga, diet, exercise, and weight control are all techniques nurses can include in their repertoire of helping skills.

DEPRESSION, ANXIETY, AND OTHER MENTAL HEALTH CONDITIONS

Women experience depression and/or anxiety frequently. Women are twice as likely as men to suffer from anxiety panic attacks and suffer more major depression than men (Anxiety and Depression Association of America, 2016). Nurses must be alert to the symptoms of serious mental disorders such as depression and anxiety and make referrals to mental health practitioners when necessary. In addition, depression is sometimes described as a cotraveler because it is exists comorbidly with

other physical conditions. Depression and/or anxiety create difficulties for quality of life and, at the extreme, a risk for suicide. Recent research (Cohen, Edmundson, & Kronish, 2014) indicates that persons with comorbid anxiety and depression are at greater risk for developing cardiac disease. In addition to depression and anxiety, women experience other mental health disorders, such as bipolar disease.

SLEEP DISORDERS

Many women suffer from sleep disorders, including difficulty initiating sleep or staying asleep and experiencing nonrestorative sleep. During pregnancy and postpartum, many factors can negatively affect sleep, and restless leg syndrome may result. Sleep disorders are correlated with physical and mental health problems, including depression, pain, and fibromyalgia. Women experience sleep and sleep problems at various stages across the life span (Shaver, 2015). It is important that the nurse talk with the woman about her sleep patterns and discuss ways to improve sleep, such as avoiding alcohol before going to sleep and sleeping in a regular pattern.

ENVIRONMENTAL AND WORKPLACE HAZARDS

Environmental hazards in the home, the workplace, and the community can contribute to poor health at all ages. Categories and examples of health-damaging hazards include the following: (1) pathogenic agents, including viruses, bacteria, fungi, parasites; (2) natural and synthetic chemicals, including natural toxins from animals, insects, and plants, consumer and industrial products such as pesticides and hydrocarbon gases, medical and diagnostic devices, tobacco, fuels, and drug and alcohol abuse; (3) radiation, including radon, heat waves, sound waves; (4) food substances, including added components that are not necessary for nutrition; and (5) physical objects, including moving vehicles, machinery, weapons, water, and building materials.

Environmental hazards can affect fertility, fetal development, live birth, and the child's future mental and physical development. Children are at special risk for poisoning from lead found in paint and soil. Everyone is at risk from air pollutants such as tobacco smoke, carbon monoxide, smog, suspended particles (dust, ash, and asbestos), and cleaning solvents; noise pollution; pesticides; chemical additives; and poor preparation of food. Workers also face safety and health risks caused by ergonomically poor work stations and stress. It is important that risk assessments continue to be in effect to identify and understand environmental problems in public health. The March of Dimes (http://www.marchofdimes.org) provides information about various risks posed in the environment to pregnant women and their fetuses.

RISKY SEXUAL PRACTICES

Potential risks related to sexual activity include undesired pregnancy and STIs. The risks are particularly high for adolescents and young adults who engage in sexual intercourse at earlier and earlier ages. Adolescents report many reasons for wanting to be sexually active: peer pressure, desire to love and be loved, experimentation, to enhance self-esteem, and to have fun. However, many teenagers do not have the decision-making or values-clarification skills needed to take this important step. They may also lack knowledge about contraception and STIs. Many do not believe that becoming pregnant or getting an STI will happen to them.

Although some STIs can be cured with antibiotics, many cause significant problems. Possible sequelae include infertility, ectopic pregnancy, neonatal morbidity and mortality, genital cancers, AIDS, and even death.

Choice of contraceptive method has an impact on the risk for contracting an STI. No method of contraception offers complete protection, unless it is abstinence that is consistently used. (See Chapter 4 for a discussion of STIs and Chapter 5 for a discussion of contraception.)

Prevention of STIs is predicated on the reduction of high-risk behaviors by educating toward a behavioral change. Behaviors of concern include multiple and casual sexual partners and unsafe sexual practices. Specific self-management measures to prevent STIs are listed in Box 3.8. The abuse of alcohol and drugs is a high-risk behavior, resulting in impaired judgment and thoughtless acts. Behavioral changes must come from within; therefore the nurse must provide sufficient information for the individual or group to "buy into" the need for change. Education is a powerful tool in health promotion and prevention of STIs and pregnancy. However, it works best when delivered in a way that considers the language, culture, and lifestyle of the intended listener.

RISK FOR CERTAIN MEDICAL CONDITIONS

Most women of reproductive age are relatively healthy. Heart disease; lung, breast, colon, and other nongynecologic cancers; chronic lung disease; and diabetes are all concerns for adult women because they are among the leading causes of death in women. Certain medical conditions present during pregnancy can have deleterious effects on both the woman and the fetus. Of particular concern are risks from all forms of diabetes, urinary tract disorders, thyroid disease, hypertensive disorders of pregnancy, cardiac disease, and seizure disorders. Effects on the fetus vary and include intrauterine growth restriction, macrosomia, anemia, prematurity, immaturity, and stillbirth. Effects on the woman also can be severe. These conditions are discussed in later chapters.

RISK FOR CERTAIN GYNECOLOGIC CONDITIONS

Women are at risk throughout their reproductive years for pelvic inflammatory disease, endometriosis, STIs and other vaginal infections (see Chapter 4), uterine fibroids, uterine deformities such as bicornuate uterus, ovarian cysts, interstitial cystitis, and urinary incontinence related to pelvic relaxation. Uterine deformities, in fact, are conditions that are congenital and are therefore present in some women at times other than the reproductive years. These gynecologic conditions may contribute negatively to pregnancy by causing infertility, miscarriage, preterm labor,

and fetal and neonatal problems. Gynecologic cancers also affect women's health, although the risk for most cancers is low in pregnancy. Risk factors depend on the type of cancer. The impact of developing a gynecologic problem or cancer on women and their families is shaped by a number of factors, including the specific type of problem or cancer, the implications of the diagnosis for the woman and her family, and the timing of the occurrence in the woman's and the family's lives.

FEMALE GENITAL MUTILATION

Female genital mutilation (FGM), *infibulation (surgical closure of the labia majora)*, and *circumcision* are terms used to describe procedures in which part or all of the female external genitalia is removed for cultural or nontherapeutic reasons (WHO, 2016). These procedures are attempts to control women through controlling their sexuality. FGM is supposed to remove sexual desire so that the girl will not become sexually active until married. FGM is practiced in more than 45 countries, with the majority of these countries being in Africa. As emigrants from these countries arrive in North America, nurses in the United States and Canada will see patients who have had such procedures performed. Although it is illegal in the United States to perform FGM on a person younger than 18 years of age, it is estimated that 513,000 women and girls in the United States have experienced or are at risk for FGM (Office of Women's Health, 2015).

Female circumcision occurs in women of many different ethnic, cultural, and religious backgrounds. Although circumcision is usually performed during childhood, some communities circumcise infants or older females. The procedure involves the removal of a portion of the clitoris but may extend to the removal of the entire clitoris and labia minora. In addition, the labia majora, which are often stitched together over the urethral and vaginal openings, may be affected.

The extent of the circumcision site affects the seriousness of complications. Common complications include bleeding, pain, local scarring, keloid or cyst formation, and infection. Impaired drainage of urine and menstrual blood may lead to chronic pelvic infections, pelvic and back pain, and chronic urinary tract infections. Some women may require surgery before vaginal examination, intercourse, or childbirth if the vaginal opening is obstructed.

FGM in the United States is punishable by fines, imprisonment, and deportation. An obstetric care provider may incise the closed labia to deliver a baby or remove cysts but may not sew the labia back to its previous state, reinfibulation. If performed on a minor, FGM is considered child abuse in the United States. FGM is recognized internationally as a violation of the human rights of girls and women. It reflects deep-rooted inequality between the sexes, and constitutes an extreme form of discrimination against women. FGM is nearly always carried out on minors and it is a violation of the rights of children. The practice also violates a person's rights to health, security, and physical integrity; the right to be free from torture and cruel, inhuman, or degrading treatment; and the right to life when the procedure results in death (WHO, 2016).

Nurses are providing care to a growing number of women who have emigrated from the Middle East, Asia, and Africa, where female circumcision is more common. Nurses must be sensitive to the unique needs of these patients, especially if these women have concerns about maintaining or restoring the intactness of the circumcision after childbirth.

HUMAN TRAFFICKING

Human trafficking is actually a form of slavery in which people are forced into the United States in order to become part of the unpaid labor force, usually in sweatshops or in domestic work, or in order to

BOX 3.9 Screening for Victims of Human Trafficking

If human trafficking is suspected, the nurse should ask simple questions that are not threatening and that mostly require a "yes" or "no" response, as follows:

- Is the place where you sleep clean?
- Do you have enough food?
- Have you been threatened or harmed physically? Has your family been threatened?
- Are you free to talk to people outside of your home or job?
- Are you free to come and go as you please?
- Are you ever forced to have sex?
- Are you ever forced to work?
- Where are you from?
- How did you get here?
- Do you know where you are now?
- Do you have money? If you earn money, do you keep it? Or are you forced to give it to someone?
- Do you have identification papers?

Adapted from Green, C. (2016). Human trafficking: Preparing for a unique patient population. *American Nurse Today*, 11(1), 9–12.

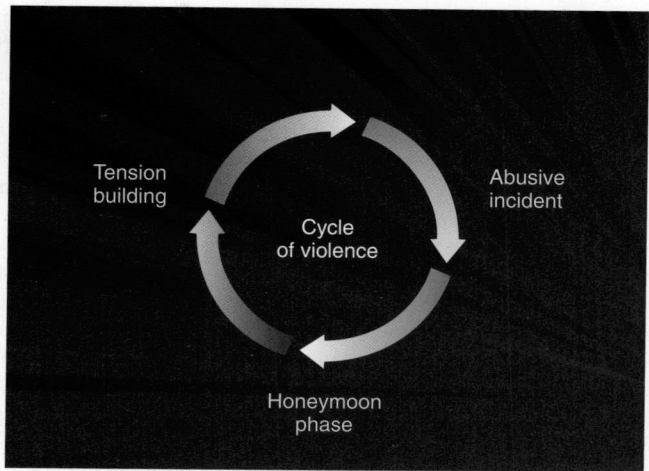

FIG 3.9 Cycle of violence.

serve as sex slaves (Green, 2016). The majority of these trafficking slaves are women and children, and many women have some interaction with health care providers. Thus, the implications for nursing are that it is imperative that signs of trafficking are recognized so that appropriate care can be delivered. In fact, it is mandatory that nurses report any suspected minor (younger than 18 years of age) human trafficking victims. Green (2016) recommended asking simple "yes" or "no" questions in order to screen for suspected trafficking (Box 3.9). Certain findings on history are also indicative of possible trafficking (see "History" section later in this chapter).

INTIMATE PARTNER VIOLENCE

Intimate partner violence (IPV) is the most common form of violence experienced by women worldwide, with a reported incidence of one of every six women having been a victim of domestic violence. In the United States, IPV is a significant social problem and a major health care problem that affects millions of women and men each year and costs millions of dollars. The US Department of Justice, Office on Violence Against Women (2015) describes violence and abuse as including one or more of the following: physical, sexual, emotional, economic, and psychologic factors. One in four women in the United States has experienced severe physical violence by a current or former intimate partner. In addition, 5.2 million women were victimized by stalkers. It is estimated that 18.3% of women in the United States are raped at some point in their lives. It is also important to note that sometimes IPV is committed by women against men. Statistics are not clear, as there is much inconsistency in reporting of IPV (Sammarco, 2016).

Although *IPV* is the preferred term, *wife battering, spousal abuse,* and *domestic* or *family violence* are also terms that may be applied to a pattern of assaultive and coercive behaviors inflicted by a male partner in a marriage or other heterosexual, significant, intimate relationship. Because IPV is common, with women being abused frequently, routine assessment of violence against women should be included in primary care histories. Common elements of IPV are physical abuse; psychologic or emotional abuse; sexual assault; isolation; and controlling all aspects of the victim's life, including money, shelter, time, and food.

Battering is neither random nor constant; rather, it occurs in repeated cycles. Health care providers often refer to the "cycle of violence" (Fig. 3.9). A three-phase cycle includes a period of increasing tension leading to the battery. The battery consists of slaps, punches to the face and head, kicking, stomping, choking, pushing, breaking of bones, burns from irons, and mutilations from knives and guns. The honeymoon phase is characterized by a period of calm and remorse in which the male partner displays kind, loving behavior and pleas for forgiveness. This honeymoon phase lasts until stress or other factors cause conflict and tension to mount again toward another episode of battering. Over time, the tension and battering phases last longer and the calm phase becomes shorter until there is no honeymoon phase.

Because violence against women crosses all ethnic, educational, religious, and socioeconomic backgrounds and there are often misconceptions regarding who is at risk for being abused, it is important to differentiate myths from facts about this serious and often devastating condition.

Battering During Pregnancy

Estimates of prevalence of battering in pregnancy vary, but it is estimated that 300,000 pregnant women annually are affected by intimate partner violence (Domestic Shelters, 2017). Most women abused before pregnancy will be abused during pregnancy, and the incidence may escalate. Abuse also may happen for the first time during pregnancy. Pregnant adolescents are abused at higher rates than are adult women; thus they should be considered at high risk. Battering during pregnancy in teenagers constitutes a particularly difficult situation. Adolescents may be more trapped in the abusive relationship than adult women because of their inexperience. They may ignore the violence because the jealous and controlling behavior is interpreted as love and devotion. Because pregnancy in young adolescent girls is frequently the result of sexual abuse, feelings about the pregnancy should be assessed.

During pregnancy, the nurse should assess for abuse at each prenatal visit and for labor and birth. Battering episodes initiate or increase in pregnancy for a variety of reasons: (1) the biopsychosocial stresses of pregnancy may strain the relationship beyond the couple's ability to cope, and frustration is followed by violence; (2) the man may be jealous of the fetus, resenting the intrusion into the couple's relationship and the woman's displacement of attention; (3) the man may be angry at the unborn child or the woman; and (4) the beating may be the man's conscious or subconscious attempt to end the pregnancy. After birth, the mother may be so physically and emotionally drained that she may have difficulty bonding with her infant. She may be at risk for becoming an abusive mother whether or not she remains in the abusive relationship.

A pregnant woman is often accompanied by a male partner to the prenatal appointment, especially if the woman does not speak English and the partner does. Unless an interpreter is available, it is difficult to interview the woman alone; in addition, asking questions about abuse through an interpreter is more difficult unless the interpreter is a woman and can communicate the nurse's sensitivity and concern accurately.

It is imperative that the woman has knowledge of resources available to her and a plan of action if she stays with the battering partner. First, the nurse should provide services and telephone numbers of a hotline and the battered women's shelter or other safe haven. The woman can be offered use of a telephone to call the shelter if this is an option she chooses. If she chooses to go back to the abuser, a safety plan includes necessities for a quick escape: a bag packed with personal items for an overnight stay (can be hidden or left with a neighbor), money or a checkbook, an extra set of car keys, and any legal documents for identification. Legal options such as those for restraining orders or arrest of the perpetrator also are important aspects of the safety plan. A restraining order can be obtained from the county court or police department 24 hours a day. Shelters also can be helpful with assistance in obtaining orders of protection. If the woman chooses not to act in the middle of a violent episode, she may use the hotline or shelter for some counseling when the threat of harm is no longer present.

LEGAL TIP Reporting Requirements for Domestic Violence

Domestic violence is considered a crime in all states, but it varies by state between being a misdemeanor or a felony offense; in the majority of states, domestic violence is a misdemeanor. Forty states and the District of Columbia have laws that mandate reporting by health care providers in situations in which the woman has an injury that may be caused by a deadly weapon. Some states also require reports when there is a reason to believe that the woman's injury may have resulted from an illegal act or act of violence. Because of the wide variation from state to state in mandatory reporting, nurses must be knowledgeable about the reporting requirements of the state in which they practice.

SPIRITUAL APPROACHES TO WOMEN'S HEALTH PROMOTION

Many women find that spirituality is helpful in maintaining wellness as well as coping with illness. *Spirituality* refers to the essence of our being and humanity, reflected in a connection to a Sacred Source (Burkhardt & Nagai-Jacobson, 2013). The concept of Sacred Source is experienced in different ways, with some experiencing it as a person, some as a presence, and some as a nondescribable mystery (Burkhardt & Nagai-Jacobson). The idea of connection is important, and experiencing this connection in a sacred space is central to spirituality. Spirituality may be experienced within a context of organized religion. Nurses, taking a holistic approach to women's wellness, must be sensitive and nonjudgmental to the spiritual aspect of their patients. In an optimal healing approach to care, nurses can facilitate and encourage the patient to express her spirituality in a way that is comfortable for the patient.

ASSESSMENT OF THE WOMAN: HISTORY AND PHYSICAL EXAMINATION

Trends in women's health have expanded beyond a reproductive focus to include a holistic approach to health care across the life span and place women's health within the scope of primary care. Women's health assessment and screening focus on a systems evaluation that begins with a careful history and physical examination. During assessment and evaluation, the responsibility for self-management, health promotion, and enhancement of wellness is emphasized.

In a market-driven system such as managed care, specific guidelines may be provided for health screening by the insurer or the managed care organization. A nurse often takes the history, orders diagnostic tests, interprets test results, makes referrals, coordinates care, and directs attention to problems requiring medical intervention. Advanced practice nurses who have specialized in women's health such as nurse practitioners, clinical nurse specialists, and nurse-midwives perform complete physical examinations, including gynecologic examinations.

HISTORY

Contact with the woman usually begins with an interview, which is an integral part of the history. This interview should be conducted in a private, relaxed setting (Fig. 3.10). The nurse is seated and makes sure that the woman is comfortable. The woman is addressed by her title and name (e.g., Mrs. Martinez), and the nurse introduces herself or himself using name and title. It is important to phrase questions in a sensitive and nonjudgmental manner. Body language should match oral communication. The nurse is aware of a woman's vulnerability and assures her of strict confidentiality. For many women, fear, anxiety, and modesty make the physical examination a dreaded and stressful experience. Many women are uninformed, misguided by myths, or afraid they will appear ignorant by asking questions about sexual or reproductive functioning. The woman is assured that no question is irrelevant.

The history begins with an open-ended question such as "What brings you to the office/clinic/hospital today?" and is furthered by other questions such as "Is there anything else?" and "Tell me about it." Additional ways to encourage women to share information include the following:

Facilitation: Using a word or posture that communicates interest such as leaning forward, making eye contact, or saying "Mm-hmmm" or "Go on"

Reflection: Repeating a word or phrase that a woman has used

Clarification: Asking the woman what is meant by a stated word or phrase

Empathic responses: Acknowledging the feelings of a woman by statements such as "That must have been frightening"

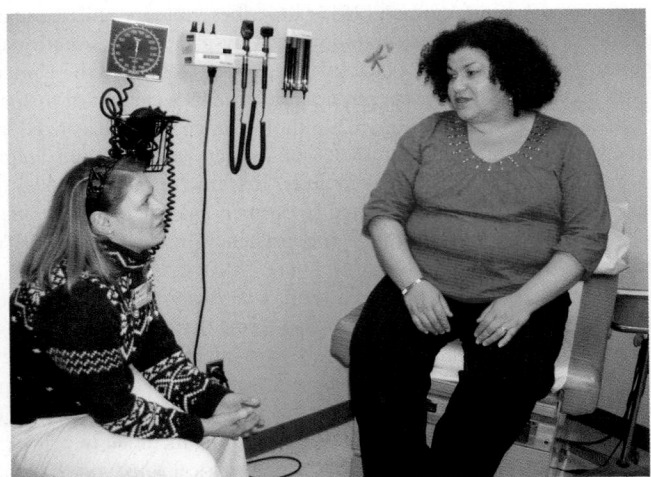

FIG 3.10 Nurse interviews a woman as part of routine history and physical examination. (Courtesy of Ed Lowdermilk, Chapel Hill, NC.)

Confrontation: Identifying something about the woman's behavior or feelings not expressed verbally or apparently inconsistent with her history

Interpretation: Putting into words what you infer about the woman's feelings or about the meaning of her symptoms, events, or other matters

Nurses need to develop rapport and trust with their patients as they take a history. Because communication within a caring context is core to nursing practice, nurses are well suited to taking a comprehensive patient history. Nurses should ask questions incrementally to build a comprehensive understanding. They should also share insights with the woman by eliciting her concerns or thoughts as well as offering clarification to her. Trust is a key aspect of the nurse-patient relationship, and it is critical that nursing approaches to establishing trust are developed and respected by the entire team (Rortveit, Hansen, Leiknes, et al., 2015).

At a woman's first visit, she is often expected to fill out a form with biographic and historical data before meeting with the examiner. This form aids the health care provider in completing the history during the interview. Most forms include information about the following categories:

- Biographic data
- Reason for seeking care
- Present health or history of present illness
- Past health
- Family history
- Screening for abuse (Fig. 3.11)
- Review of systems
- Functional assessment (activities of daily living)

Box 3.10 describes a complete health history based on the categories just mentioned.

Nurses should screen all women entering the health care system for abuse. Abuse is a life-threatening public health problem that affects millions of women and their children. The risk for intimate partner violence increases during pregnancy and after separation or divorce. Help for the woman may depend on the sensitivity with which the nurse screens for abuse, the discovery of abuse, and subsequent intervention. The nurse must be familiar with the laws governing abuse in the state in which she or he practices.

It also is important that the nurse is alert to any indication from the woman that she is being abused, despite the fact that she may not have specifically stated that she is in an abusive relationship. Box 3.11 provides a list of signs of IPV. If a male partner is present, he should be asked to leave the room because the woman may not disclose experiences of abuse in his presence, or he may try to answer questions for her to protect himself. The same procedure applies to partners of lesbians or the adult children of older women.

There is no universally accepted screening tool for all populations regarding IPV. The Guidelines Box presents a suggested list of questions to screen for IPV.

A therapeutic relationship and skillful interviewing help women disclose and describe their abuse. Language is important when talking with women. For example, using the term *victim* connotes powerlessness and hopelessness; a more empowering term is *survivor*. Women who have identified their abuse may appear passive, hostile, anxious, depressed, or hysterical because they may think they are at the mercy of the man's temper or that he is "out of control." In addition, they may be embarrassed, afraid, angry, sad, and shocked.

Pocket cards listing emergency numbers (abuse counseling, legal protection, and emergency shelter) can be obtained from local police departments, women's shelters, or emergency departments. It is helpful to have these on hand in the setting where screening is done.

Human trafficking is another important situation to which the nurse should be alert in the history. Signs that a woman may be a victim of human trafficking include demonstrating an exaggerated startle response,

ABUSE ASSESSMENT SCREEN

- Are you with a spouse or partner who threatens or physically hurts you?
  - Yes ______ No ______
- Are you with a spouse or partner who emotionally hurts you?
  - Yes ______ No ______
- Within the past year or in this pregnancy (if the woman is pregnant) has anyone hit, slapped, kicked, or otherwise hurt you?
  - Yes ______ No ______
  - If yes, by whom ________________
  - Number of times ________________
  - Mark the area of injury on the body map.
- Has anyone forced you to have sexual activities that made you uncomfortable?
  - Yes ______ No ______
  - If yes, by whom ________________
  - Number of times ________________
- Are you afraid of your partner or anyone you listed above?
  - Yes ______ No ______

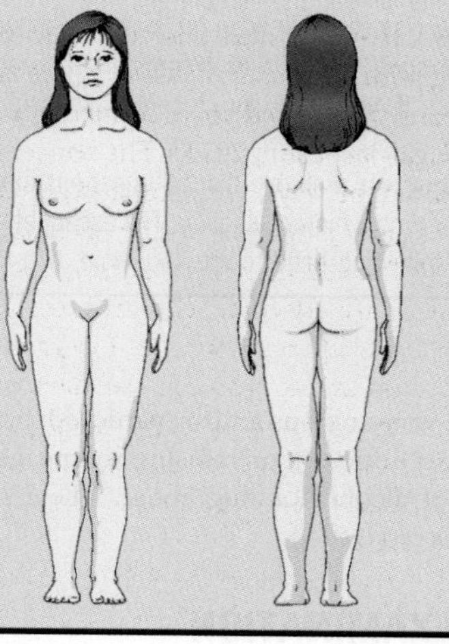

FIG 3.11 Screening for intimate partner violence. (Adapted from American College of Obstetricians and Gynecologists [ACOG] [2012]. *Are you being abused? Screening tool for domestic violence.* Retrieved from www.acog.org/About_ACOG/ACOG_Departments/Violence_Against_Women/Are_you_being_abused; Nursing Research Consortium on Violence and Abuse [1991].)

BOX 3.10   Health History and Review of Systems

Identifying data: Name, age, race, sex, marital status, occupation, religion, and ethnicity

Reason for seeking care: A response to the question, "What problem or symptom brought you here today?" More than one reason? Focus on the one she thinks is most important.

Present health: Current health status is described with attention to the following:

- *Use of safety measures:* seat belts, bicycle helmets, designated driver
- *Exercise and leisure activities:* regularity
- *Sleep patterns:* length and quality
- *Sexuality:* Is she sexually active? With men, women, or both? Risk-reducing sex practices?
- *Diet, including beverages:* 24-hour dietary recall
- *Nicotine, alcohol, illicit or recreational drug use:* type, amount, frequency, duration, and reactions
- *Environmental and chemical hazards:* home, school, work, and leisure setting; exposure to extreme heat or cold, noise, industrial toxins such as asbestos or lead, pesticides, radiation, cat feces, or cigarette smoke

History of present illness: A chronologic narrative of the problem that includes a description of the following: location, quality or character, quantity or severity, timing (onset, duration, frequency), setting, factors that aggravate or relieve, associated factors, and woman's perception of the meaning of the symptom

Past health:

- *Infectious diseases:* e.g., measles, mumps, rubella, tuberculosis (TB), hepatitis, sexually transmitted infections (STIs)
- *Chronic disease and system disorders:* e.g., arthritis, cancer, diabetes, heart, lung, kidney
- *Adult injuries, accidents*
- *Hospitalizations, operations, blood transfusions*
- *Obstetric history*
- *Allergies:* medications, previous transfusion reactions, environmental allergies
- *Immunizations:* e.g., diphtheria, pertussis, tetanus, mumps, rubella, influenza hepatitis A, hepatitis B, HPV
- *Last date of screening tests:* e.g., Pap test, mammogram, cholesterol test
- *Current medications:* name, dose, frequency, duration, reason for taking, and compliance with prescription medications; home remedies, over-the-counter drugs, vitamin and mineral or herbal supplements used

Family history: Information about the ages and health of family members. Check for history of diabetes, heart disease, or other chronic disorders.

Screen for abuse: Has she ever been hit, kicked, slapped, or forced to have sex against her wishes? Verbally or emotionally abused? History of childhood sexual abuse? If yes, has she received counseling or does she need referral?

Review of systems: It is probable that all questions in each system will not be included every time a history is taken. The essential areas to be explored are listed in the following head-to-toe sequence. If a woman gives a positive response to a question about an essential area, more detailed questions should be asked.

- *General:* weight change, fatigue, weakness, fever, chills, or night sweats
- *Skin:* skin, hair, and nail changes; itching, bruising, bleeding, rashes, sores, lumps, or moles
- *Lymph nodes:* enlargement, inflammation, pain, or drainage
- *Head:* trauma, vertigo (dizziness), convulsive disorder, syncope (fainting); headache: location, frequency, pain type, nausea and vomiting, or visual symptoms present
- *Eyes:* glasses, contact lenses, blurriness, tearing, itching, photophobia, diplopia, inflammation, trauma, cataracts, glaucoma, or acute visual loss
- *Ears:* hearing loss, tinnitus (ringing), vertigo, discharge, pain, fullness, recurrent infections, or mastoiditis
- *Nose and sinuses:* trauma, rhinitis, nasal discharge, epistaxis, obstruction, sneezing, itching, allergy, or smelling impairment
- *Mouth, throat, and neck:* hoarseness, voice changes, soreness, ulcers, bleeding gums, goiter, swelling, or enlarged nodes
- *Breasts:* masses, pain, lumps, dimpling, nipple discharge, fibrocystic changes, or implants; breast self-examination practice
- *Respiratory:* shortness of breath, wheezing, cough, sputum, hemoptysis
- *Cardiovascular:* hypertension, rheumatic fever, murmurs, angina, palpitations, dyspnea, tachycardia, orthopnea, edema, chest pain, cough, cyanosis, cold extremities, ascites, phlebitis, or skin color changes
- *Gastrointestinal:* appetite, nausea, vomiting, indigestion, dysphagia, abdominal pain, ulcers, bleeding with stools or black, tarry stools, diarrhea, constipation, bowel movement frequency, food intolerance, hemorrhoids, jaundice, or hepatitis
- *Genitourinary:* frequency, hesitancy, urgency, polyuria, dysuria, hematuria, nocturia, incontinence, stones, infection, or urethral discharge; menstrual history, dyspareunia, discharge, sores, itching
- *Sexual health and sexual activity:* with men, women, or both; contraceptive use; sexually transmitted infections
- *Peripheral vascular:* coldness, numbness and tingling, leg edema, varicose veins, thromboses, or emboli
- *Endocrine:* heat and cold intolerance, dry skin, excessive sweating, polyuria, polydipsia, polyphagia, thyroid problems, diabetes, or secondary sex characteristic changes
- *Hematologic:* anemia, easy bruising, bleeding, petechiae, purpura, or transfusions
- *Musculoskeletal:* muscle weakness, pain, joint stiffness, scoliosis, lordosis, kyphosis, range-of-motion, instability, redness, swelling, arthritis, or gout
- *Neurologic:* loss of sensation, numbness, tingling, tremors, weakness, vertigo, paralysis, fainting, twitching, blackouts, seizures, convulsions, loss of consciousness or memory
- *Mental status:* moodiness, depression, anxiety, obsessions, delusions, illusions, or hallucinations
- *Functional assessment:* ability to care for self

---

appearing to be very anxious and/or panicked, having a flat affect and social withdrawal/difficulty or refusing to engage in conversation, or showing signs of alcohol or dug abuse. These signs require further investigation (Green, 2016).

PHYSICAL EXAMINATION

In preparation for the physical examination, the woman is instructed to undress and she is given a gown to wear during the examination. She is usually given the opportunity to undress privately. Objective data are recorded by system or location. A general statement of overall health status is a good way to start. Findings are described in detail.

- **General appearance:** age, race, sex, state of health, posture, height, weight, development, dress, hygiene, affect, alertness, orientation, cooperativeness, and communication skills
- **Vital signs:** temperature, pulse, respirations, blood pressure
- **Skin:** color; integrity; texture; hydration; temperature; edema; excessive perspiration; unusual odor; presence and description of lesions; hair texture and distribution; nail configuration, color, texture, and condition; presence of nail clubbing

BOX 3.11   Signs of Intimate Partner Violence

- Overuse of health services
- Vague, nonspecific complaints
- Chronic pain
- Depression, anxiety
- Missed appointments
- Unexplainable injuries or bruising
- Nonadherence to treatment
- Untreated serious injuries
- Injuries not matching the description
- Intimate partner never leaving the patient's side
- Intimate partner insisting on telling the story of the injury

From American College of Physicians (2016). *Asking right questions key to detecting abuse.* From Berthold, J. (2009). Posted on ACP website in 2016. Retrieved from http://www.acpinternist.org/archives/2009/03/abuse.htm

 GUIDELINES

Communicating With Abused Women

What Not to Say
1. Do not ask "why." This question "revictimizes" and blames the victim.
2. Do not talk negatively about the abuser to the victim. She may become defensive and stop talking.
3. Do not talk directly to the abuser about your suspicions of abuse. The abuser will assume the victim told you, and the victim risks retaliation.

What to Say
1. "I'm afraid for your safety (and the safety of your children)."
2. "I believe you."
3. "It is progressive and will only get worse."
4. "You deserve better than this. You deserve to be treated with respect."
5. "You are not alone."
6. "It is a crime."
7. "I'm here for you."

What to Do
1. Empower the victim.
2. Sit down with her.
3. Assure her of total privacy and confidentiality (but only if you can).
4. Use your best listening skills.
5. Call 911 and report any incident of imminent danger.
6. Give the woman the telephone number of the nearest battered women's shelter.

Questions adapted from American College of Obstetricians and Gynecologists (2012). Committee option No. 518. Intimate partner violence. *Obstetrics and Gynecology, 119*, 412–417.

- **Head:** size, shape, trauma, masses, scars, rashes, or scaling; facial symmetry; presence of edema or puffiness
- **Eyes:** pupil size, shape, reactivity, conjunctival injection, scleral icterus, fundal papilledema, hemorrhage, lids, extraocular movements, visual fields and acuity
- **Ears:** shape and symmetry, tenderness, discharge, external canal, and tympanic membranes; hearing—Weber should be midline (loudness of sound equal in both ears) and Rinne negative (no conductive or sensorineural hearing loss); should be able to hear whisper at 3 feet
- **Nose:** symmetry, tenderness, discharge, mucosa, turbinate inflammation, frontal or maxillary sinus tenderness; discrimination of odors

- **Mouth and throat:** hygiene; condition of teeth; dentures; appearance of lips, tongue, buccal and oral mucosa; erythema; edema; exudate; tonsillar enlargement; palate; uvula; gag reflex; ulcers
- **Neck:** mobility, masses, range of motion, tracheal deviation, thyroid size, carotid bruits
- **Lymphatic:** cervical, intraclavicular, axillary, trochlear, or inguinal adenopathy; size, shape, tenderness, and consistency
- **Breasts:** skin changes, dimpling, symmetry, scars, tenderness, discharge, masses; characteristics of nipples and areolae
- **Heart:** rate, rhythm, murmurs, rubs, gallops, clicks, heaves, or precordial movements
- **Peripheral vascular:** jugular vein distention, bruits, edema, swelling, vein distention, Homans' sign, or tenderness of extremities
- **Lungs:** chest symmetry with respirations, wheezes, crackles, rhonchi, vocal fremitus, whispered pectoriloquy, percussion, and diaphragmatic excursion; breath sounds equal and clear bilaterally
- **Abdomen:** shape, scars, bowel sounds, consistency, tenderness, rebound, masses, guarding, organomegaly, liver span, percussion (tympany, shifting, dullness), or costovertebral angle tenderness
- **Extremities:** edema, ulceration, tenderness, varicosities, erythema, tremor, or deformity
- **Genitourinary:** external genitalia, perineum, vaginal mucosa, cervix; inflammation, tenderness, discharge, bleeding, ulcers, nodules, or masses; internal vaginal support, bimanual and rectovaginal palpation of cervix, uterus, and adnexa
- **Rectal:** sphincter tone, masses, hemorrhoids, rectal wall contour, tenderness, and stool for occult blood
- **Musculoskeletal:** posture, symmetry of muscle mass, muscle atrophy, weakness, appearance of joints, tenderness or crepitus, joint range of motion, instability, redness, swelling, or spinal deviation
- **Neurologic:** mental status, orientation, memory, mood, speech clarity and comprehension, cranial nerves II to XII, sensation, strength, deep tendon and superficial reflexes, gait, balance, and coordination with rapid alternating motions

CULTURAL CONSIDERATIONS AND COMMUNICATION VARIATIONS IN THE HISTORY AND PHYSICAL

Recognizing signs and symptoms of disease and deciding to seek treatment are influenced by cultural perceptions. Culture evolves over time and is a system of symbols that are learned, shared, and passed on through generations of a social group. In recognizing the value of these differences, the nurse can modify the plan of care to meet the needs of each woman. Modifications may be necessary for the physical examination. In many cultures, a woman examiner is preferred. In some cultures, it may be considered inappropriate for the woman to disrobe completely for the physical examination. Communication may be hindered by cultural beliefs, even when the nurse and woman speak the same language.

HISTORY AND PHYSICAL EXAMINATION IN WOMEN WITH DISABILITIES

Women with emotional or physical disorders have special needs. Women who have vision, hearing, emotional, or physical disabilities should be respected and involved in the assessment and physical examination to the full extent of their capabilities. The nurse should communicate openly, directly, and with sensitivity. It is often helpful to learn about the disability directly from the woman while maintaining eye contact. Family and significant others should be relied on only when necessary.

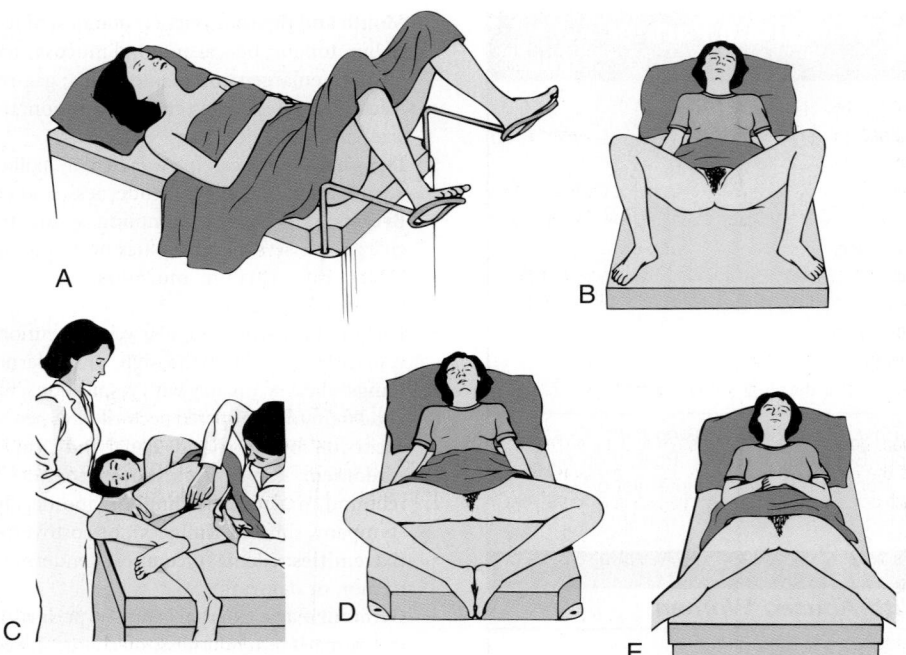

FIG 3.12 Lithotomy and variable positions for women who have a disability. **A,** Lithotomy position. **B,** *M*-shaped position. **C,** Side-lying position. **D,** Diamond-shaped position. **E,** V-shaped position.

The assessment and physical examination can be adapted to each woman's individual needs.

Communication with a woman who is hearing-impaired can be accomplished without difficulty. Many of these women can read lips, write, or both. The interviewer who speaks and enunciates each word slowly and in full view may be easily understood. If a woman is not comfortable with lip reading, she may use an interpreter. In this case, it is important to continue to address the woman directly, avoiding the temptation to speak directly with the interpreter.

The visually impaired woman needs to be oriented to the examination room and may have her guide dog with her. As with all patients, the visually impaired woman needs a full explanation of what the examination entails before proceeding. Before touching her, the nurse explains, "Now I am going to take your blood pressure. I am going to place the cuff on your right arm." The woman can be asked if she would like to touch each of the items that will be used in the examination to reduce her anxiety.

Many women with physical disabilities cannot comfortably lie in the lithotomy position for the pelvic examination. Several alternative positions may be used, including a lateral (side-lying) position, a *V*-shaped position, a diamond-shaped position, and an *M*-shaped position (Fig. 3.12). The woman can be asked what has worked best for her previously. If she has never had a pelvic examination or has never had a comfortable pelvic examination, the nurse proceeds slowly by showing her a picture of various positions and asking her which one she prefers. The nurse's support and reassurance can help the woman relax, which will make the examination go more smoothly.

HISTORY AND PHYSICAL EXAMINATION IN ADOLESCENT GIRLS (13 TO 19 YEARS OF AGE)

As a young woman matures, she should be asked the same questions that are included in any history. Particular attention should be paid to hints about risky behaviors, eating disorders, and depression. Sexual activity is addressed after rapport has been established. It is best to talk to a teenager with the parent (or partner or friend) out of the room. The nurse should engage with the patient in a sensitive manner, using active listening and conveying a nonjudgmental stance.

Injury prevention should be a part of the counseling at routine health examinations, with special attention to seat belts, helmets, firearms, recreational hazards, and sports involvement. The use of drugs and alcohol and the nonuse of seat belts contribute to motor vehicle injuries, accounting for a significant proportion of accidental deaths in women. Contraceptives/STI prevention information may be needed for teenagers who are sexually active.

To provide developmentally appropriate care, it is important to review the major tasks for women in this stage of life. Major tasks for teenagers include values assessment; education and work goal setting; formation of peer relationships that focus on love, commitment, and becoming comfortable with sexuality; and separation from parents. The teenager is egocentric as she progresses rapidly through emotional and physical change. Her feelings of invulnerability may lead to misconceptions such as the belief that unprotected sexual intercourse will not lead to pregnancy.

PELVIC EXAMINATION

Many women fear the gynecologic portion of the physical examination. The nurse can be instrumental in allaying these fears by providing information and assisting the woman to express her feelings to the examiner.

The woman is assisted into the lithotomy position (see Fig. 3.12, *A*) for the pelvic examination. When she is in the lithotomy position, the woman's hips and knees are flexed, with buttocks at the edge of the table, and her feet are supported by heel or knee stirrups.

Some women prefer to keep their shoes or socks on, especially if the stirrups are not padded. Many women express feelings of vulnerability and strangeness when in the lithotomy position. During the procedure, the nurse assists the woman with relaxation techniques (Box 3.12).

1. Wash hands. Assemble equipment (see illustration below).
2. Ask woman to empty her bladder before the examination (obtain clean-catch urine specimen as needed).
3. Assist with relaxation techniques. Have the woman place her hands on her chest at about the level of the diaphragm and breathe deeply and slowly.
4. Encourage the woman to become involved with the examination if she shows interest. For example, a mirror can be placed so that she can see the area being examined.
5. Assess for and treat signs of problems such as supine hypotension.
6. Warm the speculum in warm water if a prewarmed one is not available.
7. Instruct the woman to bear down when the speculum is being inserted.
8. Apply gloves and assist the examiner with collection of specimens for cytologic examination, such as a Pap test. After handling specimens, remove gloves and wash hands.
9. Lubricate the examiner's fingers with water or water-soluble lubricant before bimanual examination.
10. Assist the woman at completion of the examination to a sitting position and then a standing position.
11. Provide tissues to wipe lubricant from perineum.
12. Provide privacy for the woman while she is dressing.

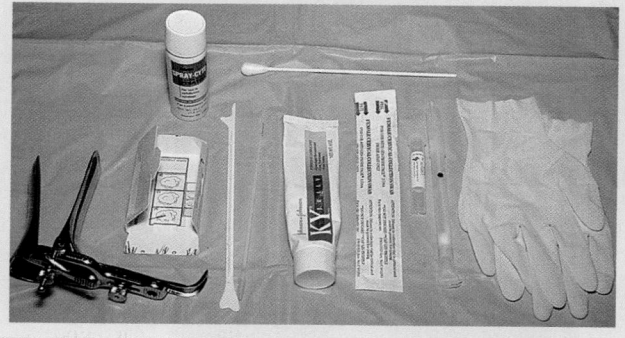

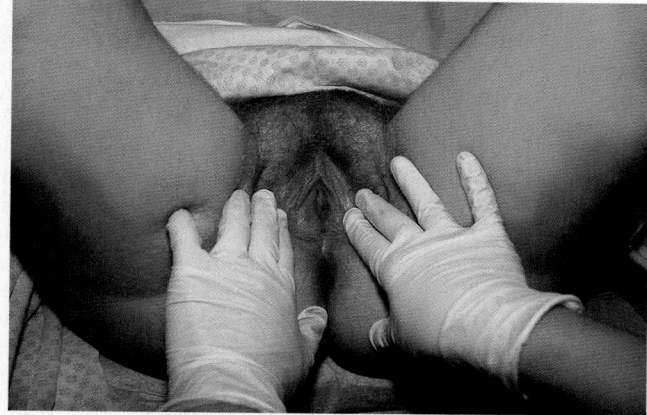

FIG 3.13 External examination: separation of the labia. (From Wilson, S. F., & Giddens, J. F. [2013]. *Health assessment for nursing practice* (5th ed.). St. Louis, MO: Mosby.)

Many women find it distressing to attempt to converse in the lithotomy position. Most women appreciate an explanation of the procedure as it unfolds, as well as coaching for the type of sensations they may expect. Generally, however, women prefer not to have to respond to questions until they are again upright and at eye level with the examiner. Being asked questions during the procedure, especially if they cannot see their questioner's eyes, may make women tense.

A teenager's first speculum examination is the most important because she will develop perceptions that will remain with her for future examinations. What the examination entails should be discussed with the teenager while she is dressed. Models or illustrations can be used to show exactly what will happen. All of the necessary equipment should be assembled so there are no interruptions. Pediatric specula that are 1 to 1.5 cm wide can be inserted with minimal discomfort. If the teenager is sexually active, a small adult speculum may be used.

External Inspection

The examiner wears gloves and sits at the foot of the table for the inspection of the external genitalia and the speculum examination. In good lighting, external genitalia are inspected for sexual maturity, clitoris, labia, perineum, and lesions indicative of STIs. After childbirth or other trauma, healed scars may be present.

External Palpation

Before touching the woman, the examiner explains what is going to be done and what the woman should expect to feel (e.g., pressure). The examiner may touch the woman in a less sensitive area such as the inner thigh to alert her that the genitalia examination is beginning. This gesture may put the woman more at ease. The labia are spread apart to expose the structures in the vestibule: urinary meatus, Skene glands, vaginal orifice, and Bartholin glands (Fig. 3.13). To assess Skene glands, the examiner inserts one finger into the vagina and "milks" the area of the urethra. Any exudate from the urethra or the Skene glands is cultured. Masses and erythema of either structure are assessed further. Ordinarily the openings to the Skene glands are not visible; prominent openings may be seen if the glands are infected (e.g., with gonorrhea). During the examination, the examiner keeps in mind the data from the review of systems such as history of burning on urination.

The vaginal orifice is examined. Hymenal tags are normal findings. With one finger still in the vagina, the examiner repositions the index finger near the posterior part of the orifice. With the thumb outside the posterior part of the labia majora, the examiner compresses the area of Bartholin glands located at the 8 o'clock and 4 o'clock positions and looks for swelling, discharge, and pain.

The support of the anterior and posterior vaginal wall is assessed. The examiner spreads the labia with the index and middle finger and asks the woman to strain down. Any bulge from the anterior wall (urethrocele or cystocele) or posterior wall (rectocele) is noted and compared with the history, such as difficulty starting the stream of urine or constipation.

The perineum (area between the vagina and anus) is assessed for scars from old lacerations or episiotomies, thinning, fistulas, masses, lesions, and inflammation. The anus is assessed for hemorrhoids, hemorrhoidal tags, and integrity of the anal sphincter. The anal area is also assessed for lesions, masses, abscesses, and tumors. If there is a history of STI, the examiner may want to obtain a culture specimen from the anal canal at this time. Throughout the genital examination, the examiner notes any odor, which may indicate infection or poor hygiene.

Vulvar Self-Examination

The pelvic examination provides a good opportunity for the practitioner to emphasize the need for regular *vulvar self-examination (VSE)* and to teach this procedure. Because there has been a dramatic increase in cancerous and precancerous conditions of the vulva in recent years, VSE should be an integral part of preventive health care for all women

(ACS, 2016b). VSE should be performed monthly between menses or more often if there are symptoms or a history of serious vulvar disease. Most lesions, including malignancy, condyloma acuminatum (wart-like growth), and Bartholin cysts, can be seen or palpated and are easily treated if diagnosed early.

The VSE can be performed by the practitioner and woman together by using a mirror. A simple diagram of the anatomy of the vulva can be given to the woman, with instructions to perform the examination herself that evening to reinforce what she has learned. She does the examination in a sitting position with adequate lighting, holding a mirror in one hand and using the other hand to expose the tissues surrounding the vaginal introitus. She then systematically examines the mons pubis, clitoris, urethra, labia majora, perineum, and perianal area and palpates the vulva, noting any changes in appearance or abnormalities such as ulcers, lumps, warts, and changes in pigmentation.

Internal Examination

A vaginal speculum consists of two blades and a handle. Specula come in a variety of types and styles. A vaginal speculum is used to view the vaginal vault and cervix. The speculum is gently placed into the vagina and inserted to the back of the vaginal vault. The blades are opened to reveal the cervix and are locked into the open position. The cervix is inspected for position and appearance of the os: color, lesions, bleeding, and discharge (Fig. 3.14, A–D). Cervical findings that are not within normal limits include ulcerations, masses, inflammation, and excessive protrusion into the vaginal vault. Anomalies such as a cockscomb (a protrusion over the cervix that looks like a rooster's comb), a hooded or collared cervix (seen in diethylstilbestrol [DES] daughters), or polyps are noted.

Collection of Specimens

The collection of specimens for cytologic examination is an important part of the gynecologic examination. Infection can be diagnosed by examination of specimens collected during the pelvic examination. These infections include candidiasis, trichomoniasis, bacterial vaginosis, group B streptococcus, gonorrhea, chlamydia, and herpes simplex virus. Once the diagnoses have been made, treatment can be instituted.

Papanicolaou Test

Carcinogenic conditions, whether potential or actual, can be determined by examination of cells from the cervix collected during the pelvic examination (i.e., a Pap test) (Box 3.13).

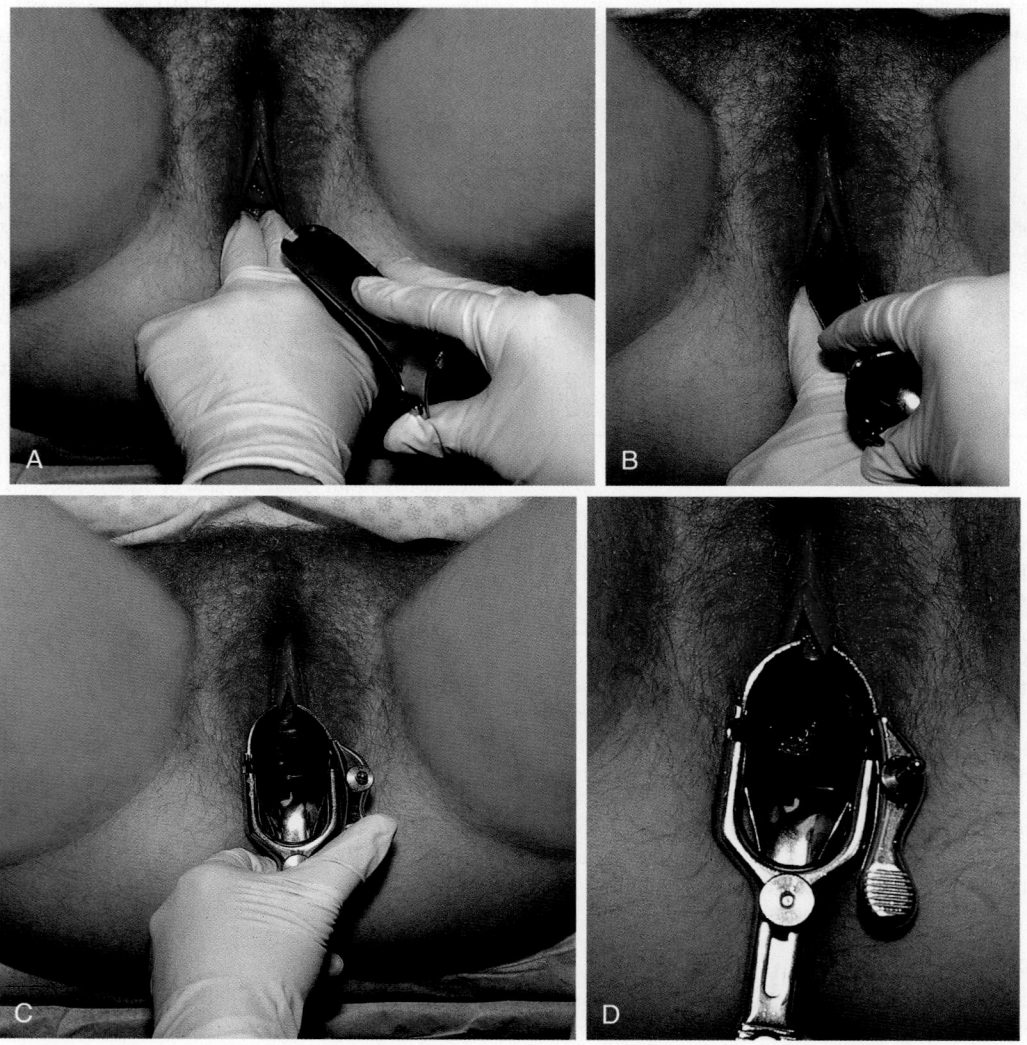

FIG 3.14 Insertion of speculum for vaginal examination. **A,** Opening of the introitus. **B,** Oblique insertion of the speculum. **C,** Final insertion of the speculum. **D,** Opening of the speculum blades. (From Wilson, S. F., & Giddens, J. F. [2013]. *Health assessment for nursing practice* (5th ed.). St. Louis, MO: Mosby.)

BOX 3.13 Papanicolaou Test

- In preparation, make sure the woman has not douched, used vaginal medications, or had sexual intercourse for 24 to 48 hours before the procedure. Reschedule the test if the woman is menstruating. Midcycle is the best time for the test.
- Explain to the woman the purpose of the test and the sensations she will feel as the specimen is obtained (e.g., pressure but not pain).
- The woman is assisted into a lithotomy position. A speculum is inserted into the vagina.
- The cytologic specimen is obtained before any digital examination of the vagina is made or endocervical bacteriologic specimens are taken. A cotton swab may be used to remove excess cervical discharge before the specimen is collected.
- The specimen is obtained by using an endocervical sampling device (Cytobrush, Cervex-brush, spatula, or broom) (see Figs. *A* and *B*). If the two-sample method of obtaining cells is used, the Cytobrush is inserted into the canal and rotated 90 to 180 degrees, followed by a gentle smear of the entire transformation zone by using a spatula. Broom devices are inserted and rotated 360 degrees 5 times. They obtain endocervical and ectocervical samples at the same time. If the patient has had a hysterectomy, the vaginal cuff is sampled. Areas that appear abnormal on visualization will require colposcopy and biopsy. If using a one-slide technique, the spatula sample is smeared first. This is followed by applying the Cytobrush sample (rolling the brush in the opposite direction from which it was obtained), which is less subject to drying artifact; then the slide is sprayed with preservative within 5 seconds. The ThinPrep or SurePath Pap Test is a liquid-based method of preserving cells that reduces blood, mucus, and inflammation. The Pap specimen is obtained in the manner described above except that the cervix is not swabbed before collection of the sample. The collection device (brush, spatula, or broom) is rinsed in a vial of preserving solution that is provided by the laboratory. The sealed vial with solution is sent off to the appropriate laboratory. A special processing device filters the contents, and a thin layer of cervical cells is deposited on a slide, which is then examined microscopically. The AutoPap and Papnet tests are similar to the ThinPrep test. If cytology is abnormal, liquid-based methods allow follow-up testing for human papillomavirus (HPV) DNA with the same sample.

- Label the slides or vial with the woman's name and site. Include on the form to accompany the specimens the woman's name, age, parity, and chief complaint or reason for taking the cytologic specimens.
- Send specimens to the pathology laboratory promptly for staining, evaluation, and a written report, with special reference to abnormal elements, including cancer cells.
- Advise the woman that repeated tests may be necessary if the specimen is not adequate.
- Instruct the woman concerning routine checkups for cervical and vaginal cancer. Women vaccinated against HPV should follow the same screening guidelines as unvaccinated women. Current recommendations of the US Preventive Services Task Force (USPSTF, 2014) and the American Cancer Society (ACS) (2015) for Pap tests are that women 21 to 65 years of age be screened every 3 years, or for women 30 to 65 years of age every 5 years (if they had a Pap test plus HPV test that were both negative). These guidelines recommend no screening in women younger than 21 years of age, although if a girl becomes sexually active, the guidelines recommend that she get a Pap test within 3 years of initiating sexual activity or at 21 years of age, whichever comes first. Women with high-risk factors such as exposure to diethylstilbestrol (DES) in utero, those treated for cervical intraepithelial neoplasia (CIN) 2, CIN 3, cervical cancer, or human immunodeficiency virus (HIV) may need more frequent screening.
- Young women who have been treated with excisional procedures for dysplasia have had an increase in premature births. A large majority of the cervical dysplasias in adolescents caused by HPV resolve on their own without treatment. It is important to avoid unnecessary instrumentation and procedures that negatively affect the cervix. Women who have had a complete hysterectomy for noncancerous reasons who have no history of high-grade CIN may have routine cervical cytology testing discontinued. Women who are older than 65 years of age who have not had serious cervical precancer or cancer in the past 20 years may discontinue cervical cancer screening (ACS, 2015).
- Record the examination date on the woman's record.
- Communicate findings to the woman per agency protocol.

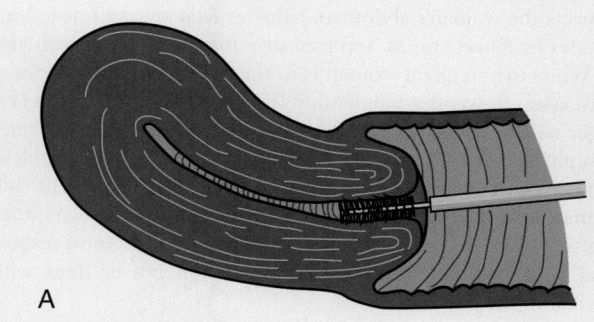

A

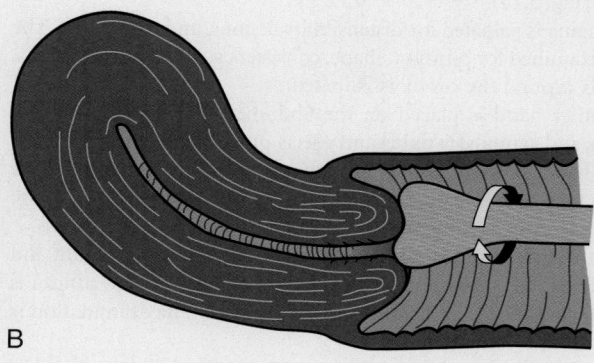

B

Adapted from American Cancer Society. (2015). *Cancer prevention and early detection facts and figures, 2015-2016*. Atlanta, GA: Author. Retrieved from https://www.cancer.org/content/dam/cancer-org/research/cancer-facts-and-statistics/cancer-prevention-and-early-detection-facts-and-figures/cancer-prevention-and-early-detection-facts-and-figures-2015-2016.pdf; US Preventive Services Task Force. (2014). *US preventive services task force issues new cervical cancer screening recommendations*. Retrieved from https://www.uspreventiveservicestaskforce.org/Page/Name/us-preventive-services-task-force-issues-new-cervical-cancer-screening-recommendations.

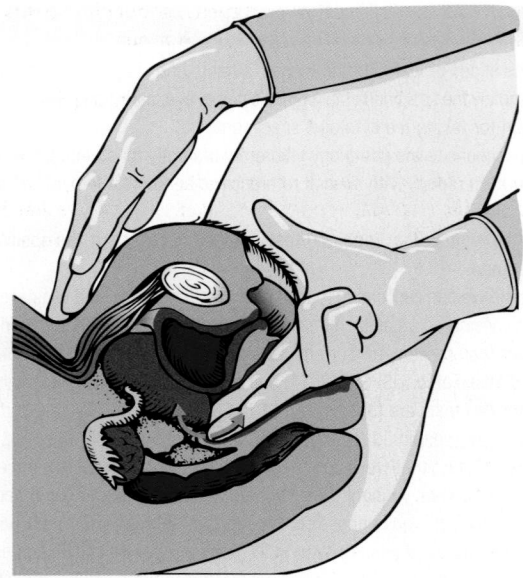

FIG 3.15 Bimanual palpation of the uterus. (From Ball, J., Dains, J., Flynn, J., et al. [2015]. *Seidel's guide to physical examination* [8th ed.]. St. Louis: Elsevier.)

Vaginal Wall Examination

After the specimens are obtained, the vagina is viewed when the speculum is rotated. The speculum blades are unlocked and partially closed. As the speculum is withdrawn, it is rotated; the vaginal walls are inspected for color, lesions, rugae, fistulas, and bulging.

Bimanual Palpation

The examiner stands for this part of the examination. A small amount of lubricant is placed on the first and second fingers of the gloved hand for the internal examination. To avoid tissue trauma and contamination, the thumb is abducted, and the ring and little fingers are flexed into the palm (Fig. 3.15).

The vagina is palpated for distensibility, lesions, and tenderness. The cervix is examined for position, shape, consistency, motility, and lesions. The fornix around the cervix is palpated.

The other hand is placed on the abdomen halfway between the umbilicus and symphysis pubis and exerts pressure downward toward the pelvic hand. Upward pressure from the pelvic hand traps reproductive structures for assessment by palpation. The uterus is assessed for position, size, shape, consistency, regularity, motility, masses, and tenderness.

With the abdominal hand moving to the right lower quadrant and the fingers of the pelvic hand in the right lateral fornix, the adnexa is assessed for position, size, tenderness, and masses. The examination is repeated on the woman's left side.

Just before the intravaginal fingers are withdrawn, the woman is asked to tighten her vagina around the fingers as much as she can. If the muscle response is weak, the woman is assessed for her knowledge about Kegel exercise.

Rectovaginal Palpation

To prevent contamination of the rectum from organisms in the vagina (e.g., *Neisseria gonorrhoeae*), it is necessary to change gloves, add fresh lubricant, and then reinsert the index finger into the vagina and the middle finger into the rectum (Fig. 3.16). Insertion is facilitated if the woman strains down. The maneuvers of the abdominovaginal examination are repeated. The rectovaginal examination permits assessment of the rectovaginal septum, the posterior surface of the uterus, and the

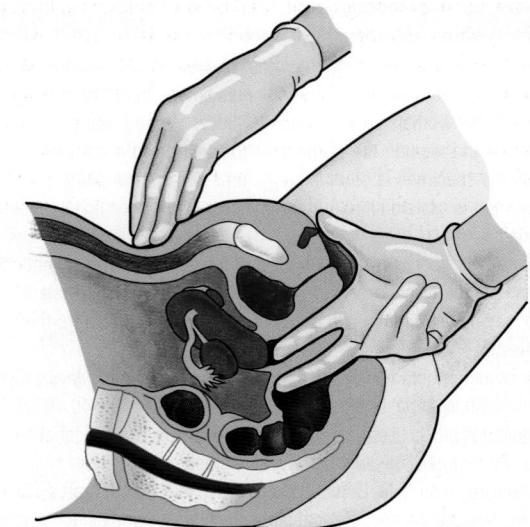

FIG 3.16 Rectovaginal examination. (From Ball, J., Dains, J., Flynn, J., et al. [2015]. *Seidel's guide to physical examination* [8th ed.]. St. Louis: Elsevier.)

region behind the cervix and the adnexa. The vaginal finger is removed and folded into the palm, leaving the middle finger free to rotate 360 degrees. The rectum is palpated for rectal tenderness and masses.

After the rectal examination, the woman is assisted into a sitting position, given tissues or wipes to cleanse herself, and afforded privacy to dress. The examiner returns after the woman is dressed to discuss findings and the plan of care.

Pelvic Examination During Pregnancy

The pelvic examination during pregnancy is done in the same way as it is during a routine examination on a nonpregnant woman. Pelvic measurements are completed, and uterine size is estimated. A Pap test may be done initially and cytologic specimens collected to test for gonorrhea, chlamydia, human papillomavirus, herpes simplex virus, and group B streptococcus. As the pregnancy progresses, the nurse inspects the woman's abdomen, palpates fetal size and position, auscultates fetal heart tones, and measures fundal height at each visit.

While the pregnant woman is in the lithotomy position, the nurse must assess for supine hypotension (decrease in blood pressure) caused by the weight of the uterus pressing on the vena cava and aorta. Symptoms of supine hypotension include pallor, dizziness, faintness, breathlessness, tachycardia, nausea, clammy skin, and sweating. To prevent this, the woman who is lying supine should have a pillow or wedge under one hip. She should be positioned on her side until symptoms resolve and vital signs stabilize. The vaginal examination can be done with the woman in the lateral position.

Pelvic Examination After Hysterectomy

The pelvic examination after hysterectomy is done much as it is done on a woman with a uterus. Vaginal screening using the Pap test is not recommended in women who have had a total hysterectomy with removal of the cervix for benign disease. Because of the epidemic of human papillomavirus, which causes vaginal intraepithelial neoplasia, sampling of the vaginal walls after hysterectomy may still be practiced, with schedules varying from every year to every 2 to 3 years.

Laboratory and Diagnostic Procedures

The following laboratory and diagnostic procedures are ordered at the discretion of the clinician, considering the patient and family history:

hemoglobin, fasting blood glucose, total blood cholesterol, lipid profile, urinalysis, syphilis serology (Venereal Disease Research Laboratories [VDRL] or rapid plasma reagent [RPR]) and other screening tests for STIs, mammogram, tuberculosis skin testing, hearing, visual acuity, electrocardiogram, chest x-ray, pulmonary function, fecal occult blood, flexible sigmoidoscopy, and bone mineral density (dual energy x-ray absorptiometry [DEXA] scan). Results of these tests may be reported in person, by phone call, or by letter. Tests hepatitis B, and drug screening may be offered with informed consent in high-risk populations. These test results are usually reported in person. HIV testing is recommended as routine for all adults (women and men), although patients should be told that they will be tested unless they opt out.

HEALTH SCREENING FOR WOMEN ACROSS THE LIFE SPAN

To promote wellness and prevent illness, it is imperative that women adhere to specific screening guidelines to detect conditions that, if found early, are amenable to treatment and/or cure. Table 3.1 summarizes the screening procedures for women across the life span.

TABLE 3.1   Health Screening Guidelines and Immunization Recommendations for Women 18 Years of Age and Older

Intervention	Recommendation*
Physical Examination	
Blood pressure	Every visit, but at least every 2 years
Height and weight	Every visit, but at least every 2 years
Pelvic examination	Annually until age 70; recommended for any woman who has ever been sexually active
Breast Examination	
Clinical examination	Every 3 years, 20 to 39 years of age; after 40 years of age with periodic examination, preferably annually
High risk	Annually after 18 years of age with history of premenopausal breast cancer in first-degree relative
Risk Groups	
Skin examination	Family history of skin cancer or increased exposure to sunlight every 3 years between 20 and 40 years of age; annually after 40 years of age; monthly mole self-examinations also recommended
Oral cavity examination	History of mouth lesions or exposure to tobacco or excessive alcohol at least annually
Laboratory and Diagnostic Tests	
Blood cholesterol (fasting lipoprotein analysis)	Beginning at 45 years of age if level is within normal limits, every 5 years; more often if abnormal levels or have risk factors for coronary artery disease
Papanicolaou (Pap) test	Between 21 and 65 years of age—every 3 years with Pap test done
	Between 30 and 65 years of age—every 5 years if Pap test plus human papillomavirus (HPV) test done
	After 65 years of age and three negative tests and no risks and after total hysterectomy for benign disease—women may choose to stop screening
Mammography†	Every 1 to 2 years between 40 and 49 years of age or earlier if at high risk
	Annually after 40 years of age
	Annually after 50 years of age
	Biennially, 50 to 74 years of age
	After 75 years of age, discuss with your health care provider
Colon cancer screening	Use one of these three methods:
	Fecal occult blood test annually 50 to 74 years of age
	Flexible sigmoidoscopy every 5 years 50 to 74 years of age
	Colonoscopy every 10 years 50 to 74 years of age
	After 75 years of age, discuss with your health care provider
Hearing screen	Starting at 18 years of age, then every 10 years until 49 years of age
	Every 3 years after 50 years of age
	Annually with exposure to excessive noise or when loss is suspected
Vision screen	At least once between 20 and 29 years of age; at least twice between 30 and 39 years of age;
	Every 2 to 4 years between 40 and 64 years of age; every 1 to 2 years after 65 years of age
Risk Groups	
Fasting blood sugar	Annually with family history of diabetes or gestational diabetes or if significantly obese; every 3 to 5 years for all women older than 45 years of age
Thyroid-stimulating hormone (TSH) test	As determined by the health care provider
Sexually transmitted infection test (e.g., gonorrhea, syphilis, herpes)	As needed if sexually active with multiple partners and engaging in risky sexual behaviors; be aware of sensitive issues with transgender persons
Chlamydia test	If sexually active, yearly until 25 years of age; after 25 years of age, test as needed when sexually active with new or multiple partners

Continued

TABLE 3.1   Health Screening Guidelines and Immunization Recommendations for Women 18 Years of Age and Older—cont'd

Intervention	Recommendation*
Cholesterol screening	Starting at 20 years of age if at increased risk for heart disease; discuss with health care provider
Colorectal cancer screening	Starting at 50 years of age, unless at higher risk; use of fecal occult blood screening, sigmoidoscopy, or colonoscopy
Diabetes screening	Routine testing, and especially if blood pressure is over 135/80
Human immunodeficiency virus (HIV) test	At least once between 18 and 64 years of age to determine HIV status; test if there is a high risk for HIV infection
Hepatitis C test	Recommended for all persons born between 1945 and 1964, and others based on risk.
Tuberculin skin test	Annually with exposure to persons with tuberculosis or in risk categories for close contact with the disease
Endometrial biopsy	At menopause for women at risk for endometrial cancer; repeat as needed
Bone mineral density testing	All women 65 years of age and older at least once; repeat testing as needed; younger women with risk for osteoporosis may need periodic screenings
Immunizations	
Tetanus-diphtheria-pertussis (Td/Tdap)	Tdap vaccine once; then booster is given every 10 years
Measles, mumps, rubella	Once if born after 1956 and no evidence of immunity
Hepatitis A	Primary series of two injections for all who are in risk categories
Hepatitis B	Primary series of three injections for all who are in risk categories
Influenza	Annually
Pneumococcal	1–2 doses between 19 and 64 years of age; 1 dose after 65 years of age
Herpes zoster (shingles)	One dose at 65 years of age
Human papillomavirus (HPV) vaccine	Primary series of three injections for girls 9 years of age to women 26 years of age; intended for those not previously exposed to HPV

*The information in this table is only a guide; health care providers will individualize the timing of tests and immunizations for each woman.
†Note: No consensus has been reached regarding mammograms for women between 40 and 49 years of age; therefore various recommendations are listed. Women are urged to discuss circumstances with their health care providers.
Data from American Cancer Society. (2015): Cancer prevention and early detection facts and figures, 2015–2016. Atlanta, GA: Author. Retrieved from http://old.cancer.org/acs/groups/content/@editorial/documents/document/acspc-044552.pdf; Centers for Disease Control and Prevention. *Cancer prevention & early detection facts and figures.* Retrieved from http://www.cancer.org/acs/groups/content/@research/documents/webcontent/acspc-045101.pdf; Advisory Committee on Immunization Practices. (2016). *Recommended adult immunization schedule, United States.* Retrieved from http://www.cdc.gov/vaccines/acip/recs/index.html; Workowski, K. A., Bolan, G. A. (2015). Sexually transmitted diseases treatment guidelines 2010, *Morbidity and Mortality Weekly Report, 64*(RR3), 1–127; Retrieved from http://www.cdc.gov/mmwr/preview/mmwrhtml/rr6403a1.htm; National Women's Health Information Center. (2013). *Screening tests for women.* Retrieved from http://www.womenshealth.gov/screening-tests-and-vaccines/screening-tests-for-women/; US Preventive Services Task Force. (2014). *US preventive services task force issues new cervical cancer screening recommendations.* Retrieved from https://www.uspreventiveservicestaskforce.org/Page/Name/us-preventive-services-task-force-issues-new-cervical-cancer-screening-recommendations.

REFERENCES

American Cancer Society. (2015). *Cancer prevention and early detection facts and figures, 2015-2016.* Atlanta, GA: Author. Retrieved from https://www.cancer.org/content/dam/cancer-org/research/cancer-facts-and-statistics/cancer-prevention-and-early-detection-facts-and-figures/cancer-prevention-and-early-detection-facts-and-figures-2015-2016.pdf.

American Cancer Society. (2016a). *Does body weight affect cancer risk?* Retrieved from http://www.cancer.org/cancer/cancercauses/dietandphysicalactivity/bodyweightandcancerrisk/body-weight-and-cancer-risk-effects.

American Cancer Society. (2016b). *Can vulvar cancer be prevented?* Retrieved from https://www.cancer.org/cancer/vulvar-cancer/causes-risks-prevention/prevention.html.

Anxiety and Depression Association of America. (2016). *Facts and statistics.* Retrieved from https://www.adaa.org/about-adaa/press-room/facts-statistic.

Berg, J. A., Taylor, D., & Woods, N. F. (2015). Women at midlife. In E. F. Olshansky (Ed.), *Women's health and wellness across the lifespan.* Philadelphia, PA: Wolters Kluwer.

Burkhardt, M. A., & Nagai-Jacobson, M. G. (2013). Spirituality and health. In B. M. Dossey & L. Keegan (Eds.), *Holistic nursing: A handbook for practice* (ed. 6, pp. 721–749). Burlington, MA: Jones & Bartlett.

Centers for Disease Control and Prevention. (2015a). *Adult obesity facts.* Atlanta, GA: Author. Retrieved from http://www.cdc.gov/obesity/data/adult.html.

Centers for Disease Control and Prevention. (2015b). *Childhood overweight and obesity.* Atlanta, GA: Author. Retrieved from http://www.cdc.gov/obesity/childhood/index.html.

Centers for Disease Control and Prevention. (2016a). *Birthweight and gestation.* Atlanta, GA: CDC. http://www.cdc.gov/nchs/fastats/birthweight.htm.

Centers for Disease Control and Prevention. (2016b). *Current cigarette smoking among adults in the United States.* Atlanta, GA: Author. Retrieved from http://www.cdc.gov/tobacco/data_statistics/fact_sheets/adult_data/cig_smoking/.

Centers for Disease Control and Prevention. (2016c). *Infertility.* Retrieved from https://www.cdc.gov/nchs/fastats/infertility.htm.

Centers for Disease Control and Prevention. (2016d). *Folic acid.* Atlanta, GA: Author. Retrieved from https://www.cdc.gov/ncbddd/folicacid/recommendations.html.

Cohen, B. E., Edmundson, D., & Kronish, I. M. (2014). State of the art review: Depression, stress, anxiety, and cardiovascular disease. *American Journal of Hypertension, 28*(11), 1295–1302.

Domestic Shelters. (2017). *When pregnancy triggers violence: Facts to know about the danger of abuse during pregnancy.* Retrieved from https://

www.domesticshelters.org/domestic-violence-articles-information/when-pregnancy-triggers-violence#.WI6x4hsrKqE.

Douglas, M. K., Rosenkoetter, M., Pacquiao, D. F., & Centers for Disease Control and Prevention. (2016). *Births: Method of delivery*. Atlanta, GA: CDC. Retrieved from http://www.cdc.gov/nchs/fastats/delivery.htm.

Dossey, B. M. (2013). Integral and holistic nursing; Local to global. In B. M. Dossey & L. Keegan (Eds.), *Holistic nursing: A handbook for practice* (ed. 6). Burlington, MA: Jones & Bartlett.

England, L. C., Bunnell, R. E., Pechacek, T. F., et al. (2015). Nicotine and the developing human: A neglected element in the electronic cigarette debate. *American Journal of Preventive Medicine, 49*(2), 286–293.

Green, C. (2016). Human trafficking: Preparing for a unique patient population. *American Nurse Today, 11*(1), 9–12.

Guttmacher Institute. (2016). *Unintended pregnancy in the United States*. New York, NY. Retrieved from https://www.guttmacher.org/fact-sheet/unintended-pregnancy-united-states.

Hautala, L., Junnila, J., Alin, J., et al. (2009). Uncovering hidden eating disorders using the SCOFF questionnaire: Cross-sectional survey of adolescents and comparison with nurse assessments. *International Journal of Nursing Studies, 46*(11), 1439–1447.

Lin, T.-F., & Chen, J. (2014). Effect of physician gender on demand for Pap tests. *Economics Research International, 2014*, 647169, doi:10.1155/2014/647169.

March of Dimes. (2013). *Eating and nutrition*. Retrieved from www.marchofdimes.com/pregnancy/caffeine-in-pregnancy.aspx.

Martin, J. A., Hamilton, B. E., Osterman, M. J. K., et al. (2017). Births: Final data for 2015. *National Vital Statistics Reports, 66*(1), Division of Vital Statistics. Retrieved from https://www.cdc.gov/nchs/data/nvsr/nvsr66/nvsr66_01.pdf.

Masters, W., & Johnson, V. (1966). *Human sexual response*. New York: Bantam Books.

Mohamad, K., Jamshidi, L., & Nouri-Jelyani, K. (2013). Is age of menarche related with body mass index? *Iranian Journal of Public Health, 42*(9), 1043–1048.

Morgan, J., Reid, F., & Lacey, J. (1999). The SCOFF questionnaire: Assessment of a new screening tool for eating disorders. *BMJ (Clinical Research Ed.), 319*(7223), 1467–1468.

National Institute on Alcohol Abuse and Alcoholism. (2016). *Alcohol: A women's health issue*. Retrieved from https://pubs.niaaa.nih.gov/publications/brochurewomen/women.htm.

National Institute on Drug Abuse. (2014). *Drug facts: Methamphetamine*. Retrieved from https://www.drugabuse.gov/publications/drugfacts/methamphetamine.

National Institute on Drug Abuse. (2016a). *Drug facts: Marijuana*. Retrieved from https://www.drugabuse.gov/publications/drugfacts/marijuana.

National Institute on Drug Abuse. (2016b). *What is cocaine?* Retrieved from https://www.drugabuse.gov/publications/drugfacts/cocaine.

National Institute on Drug Abuse. (2016c). *What are hallucinogens?* Retrieved from https://www.drugabuse.gov/publications/drugfacts/hallucinogens.

Office of Disease Prevention and Health Promotion. (2015). *2015-2020 Dietary guidelines for Americans*. Retrieved from https://health.gov/dietaryguidelines/.

Office of Women's Health. (2015). *Female genital cutting*. Retrieved from http://womenshealth.gov/publications/our-publications/fact-sheet/female-genital-cutting.html.

Olshansky, E. F., & Zender, R. (2015). Wellness for special populations of women. In E. Olshansky (Ed.), *Women's health and wellness across the lifespan*. Philadelphia, PA: Wolters Kluwer.

Rørtveit, K., Hansen, B. S., Leiknes, I., et al. (2015). Patients' experiences of trust in the patient-nurse relationship: A systematic review of qualitative studies. *Open Journal of Nursing, 5*(3), 195–209.

Sammarco, A. (2016). *Women's health issues across the life cycle: A quality of life perspective*. Burlington, MA: Jones & Bartlett.

Shaver, J. L. F. (2015). Promoting healthy sleep. In E. F. Olshansky (Ed.), *Women's health and wellness across the lifespan*. Philadelphia, PA: Wolters Kluwer.

Substance Abuse and Mental Health Services Administration (SAMHSA). (2015). *Specific populations and prescription drug misuse and abuse*. Retrieved from https://www.samhsa.gov/prescription-drug-misuse-abuse/specific-populations.

US Department of Health & Human Services/National Institute of Child Health & Human Development. (2013). *What is prenatal care and why is it important?* Retrieved from https://www.nichd.nih.gov/health/topics/pregnancy/conditioninfo/Pages/prenatal-care.aspx.

US Department of Health & Human Services. (2015). *About the law*. Retrieved from http://www.hhs.gov/healthcare/about-the-law/.

US Department of Health & Human Services. (2016a). *Trends in teen pregnancy and childbearing*. Office of Adolescent Health. Rockville, MD. Retrieved from http://www.hhs.gov/ash/oah/adolescent-health-topics/reproductive-health/teen-pregnancy/trends.html.

US Department of Health & Human Services. (2016b). *The U.S. opioid epidemic*. Washington, DC. Retrieved from http://www.hhs.gov/opioids/about-the-epidemic/.

US Department of Justice, Office on violence against women. (2015). *Domestic violence*. Washington, DC: Dept. of Justice. Retrieved from https://www.justice.gov/ovw/domestic-violence.

US National Library of Medicine, & National Institutes of Health. (2016). Methamphetamines. *Medline Plus*. Retrieved from https://www.nlm.nih.gov/medlineplus/methamphetamine.html.

US Preventive Services Task Force. (2016). *Breast cancer screening*. Retrieved from https://www.uspreventiveservicestaskforce.org/Page/Document/UpdateSummaryFinal/breast-cancer-screening.

World Health Organization. (2016). *Female genital mutilation*. New York, NY: UNICEF. Retrieved from http://www.who.int/mediacentre/factsheets/fs241/en/.

4

Reproductive System Concerns

Ellen F. Olshansky

http://evolve.elsevier.com/Perry/maternal

The reproductive system consists of many components. Problems may occur at any point in the menstrual cycle. Many factors, including anatomic abnormalities, physiologic imbalances, and lifestyle, can affect the menstrual cycle. The average woman is likely to have some concerns related to her menstrual and gynecologic health at some point in her life and will experience bleeding, pain, discharge, or infections associated with her reproductive organs or functions. This chapter provides information on common menstrual problems; sexually transmitted infections, and selected other infections that can affect reproductive functions; abnormal bleeding problems; and problems associated with perimenopause and postmenopause. Benign breast conditions are also discussed. Breast cancer is included because it is the most common reproductive cancer occurring in women.

MENSTRUAL DISORDERS

Knowledge of the normal parameters of menstruation is essential to the assessment of menstrual cycle experiences and disorders. Chapter 3 provides additional information on the menstrual cycle and endocrine physiology.

Once the irregular nature of menses in the first 1 to 2 years after menarche subsides and a cyclic, predictable pattern of monthly bleeding is established, women may worry about any deviation from that pattern or from what they have been told is normal for all menstruating women. A woman may be concerned about her ability to conceive and bear children without this monthly evidence. Amenorrhea or excess menstrual bleeding can be a source of severe distress and concern for a woman.

AMENORRHEA

Amenorrhea, the absence of menstrual flow, is a clinical sign of a variety of disorders. Generally, the following circumstances should be evaluated: (1) the absence of both menarche and secondary sexual characteristics by 13 years of age; (2) the absence of menses by 15 years of age, regardless of normal growth and development (primary amenorrhea); (3) the absence of menstruation within 5 years of breast development, or (4) a 6-month or more cessation of menses after a period of menstruation (secondary amenorrhea) (Lobo, 2017).

A moderately obese girl (20% to 30% above ideal weight) may have early-onset menstruation, whereas delay of onset is known to be related to malnutrition (starvation such as that with anorexia). Girls who exercise strenuously before menarche can have delayed onset of menstruation until about 18 years of age (Lobo, 2017).

Although amenorrhea is not a disease, it is often a sign of one. Still, most commonly and most benignly, amenorrhea is a result of pregnancy.

It also can result from anatomic abnormalities such as outflow tract obstruction, anterior pituitary disorders, other endocrine disorders such as polycystic ovary syndrome, hypothyroidism or hyperthyroidism, chronic diseases such as type 1 diabetes, medications such as phenytoin (Dilantin), drug abuse (alcohol, tranquilizers, opiates, marijuana, cocaine), or oral contraceptive use.

Hypogonadotropic Amenorrhea

Hypogonadotropic amenorrhea reflects a problem in the central hypothalamic-pituitary axis. In rare instances, a pituitary lesion or genetic inability to produce follicle-stimulating hormone (FSH) and luteinizing hormone (LH) is at fault. However, Lobo (2017) has noted that women without a lesion who had a low level of gonadotropins were believed to have primary pituitary failure, which was referred to as *hypogonadotropic hypogonadism,* but it has been noted that gonadotropin-releasing hormone (GnRH) stimulation results in increased FSH and LH levels. This suggests a hypothalamic defect with lack of adequate GnRH synthesis or a defect in a CNS neurotransmitter.

Hypogonadotropic amenorrhea often results from hypothalamic suppression as a result of stress (in the home, school, or workplace) or a sudden and severe weight loss, eating disorders, strenuous exercise, or mental illness (Wambach & Alexander, 2012). Research on the interaction between nervous system or neurotransmitter functions and hormone regulation throughout the body has demonstrated a biologic basis for the relation of stress to physiologic processes. Women who are more than 20% underweight for height or who have had rapid weight loss and women with eating disorders such as anorexia nervosa may report amenorrhea. Amenorrhea is one of the classic signs of anorexia nervosa; and the interrelation of disordered eating, amenorrhea, and premature osteoporosis has been described as the female athlete triad (Mielke, Parsons, & Greenberg, 2015; Thein-Nissenbaum, 2013). A loss of calcium from the bone, comparable to that seen in postmenopausal women, may occur with this type of amenorrhea.

Exercise-associated amenorrhea can occur in women undergoing vigorous physical and athletic training and is thought to be associated with many factors, including body composition (height, weight, and percentage of body fat); type, intensity, and frequency of exercise; nutritional status; and presence of emotional or physical stressors. Women who participate in sports emphasizing low body weight are at greatest risk, including the following (Lobo, 2017):

- Sports in which performance is subjectively scored (e.g., dance, gymnastics)
- Endurance sports favoring participants with low body weight (e.g., distance running, cycling)

- Sports in which body contour–revealing clothing is worn (e.g., swimming, diving, volleyball)
- Sports with weight categories for participation (e.g., rowing, martial arts)
- Sports in which prepubertal body shape favors success (e.g., gymnastics, figure skating)

Assessment of amenorrhea begins with a thorough history and physical examination. Specific components of the assessment process depend on the patient's age—adolescent, young adult, or perimenopausal—and whether she has menstruated previously.

An important initial step, often overlooked, is to be sure that the woman is not pregnant. Once pregnancy has been ruled out by a β-human chorionic gonadotropin (hCG) pregnancy test, diagnostic tests may include a complete blood count (CBC), urinalysis, and serum chemistries in order to rule out any systemic conditions. FSH level, thyroid-stimulating hormone (TSH) and prolactin levels, radiographic or computed tomography (CT) scan of the sellaturcica, a progestational challenge, and possible pelvic sonogram are performed (Lobo, 2017).

Management

When amenorrhea is caused by hypothalamic disturbances, the nurse is an ideal health professional to assist women because many of the causes are potentially reversible (e.g., stress, weight loss for nonorganic reasons). Counseling and education are primary interventions and appropriate nursing roles. When a stressor known to predispose a woman to hypothalamic amenorrhea is identified, initial management involves addressing the stressor. Together the woman and nurse plan how the woman can decrease or discontinue medications known to affect menstruation, correct weight loss, deal more effectively with psychologic stress, address emotional distress, and alter exercise routine.

The nurse works with the woman to help her identify, cope with, and eliminate sources of stress in her life. Deep-breathing exercises and relaxation techniques are simple yet effective stress-reduction measures. Referral for biofeedback or massage therapy also may be useful. In some instances, referrals for psychotherapy may be indicated.

If a woman's exercise program is thought to contribute to her amenorrhea, several options exist for management. She may decide to decrease the intensity, frequency, or duration of her training or modify her diet to include the appropriate nutrition for her age. Accepting the former alternative may be difficult for one who is committed to a strenuous exercise regimen. The woman and nurse may have several sessions before the woman elects to try exercise reduction. Many young female athletes may not understand the consequences of low bone density or osteoporosis; nurses can point out the connection between low bone density and stress fractures. The nurse and woman should also investigate other factors that may be contributing to the amenorrhea and develop plans for altering lifestyle and decreasing stress.

Research on recommended dosages of calcium, vitamin D, and potassium is inconclusive for women experiencing amenorrhea associated with the female athlete triad. Oral contraceptives may be helpful in amenorrheic women but are usually not used in young women with amenorrhea associated with the female athlete triad unless there are specific issues that warrant such treatment, which are best discussed with the woman's health care provider (Drakh, 2016).

CYCLIC PERIMENSTRUAL PAIN AND DISCOMFORT

Cyclic perimenstrual pain and discomfort (CPPD) is a useful concept to describe women's experiences of discomfort during the menstrual cycle (Sharp, Taylor, Thomas, et al., 2002; Taylor, 2005). This concept includes dysmenorrhea, premenstrual syndrome (PMS), and premenstrual dysphoric disorder (PMDD) as well as symptom clusters that occur before and after the menstrual flow starts. Symptoms occur cyclically and can include mood swings as well as pelvic pain and physical discomforts. These symptoms can range from mild to severe and can last 1 or 2 days or up to 2 weeks. CPPD is a health problem that can have a significant effect on a woman's quality of life. The following discussion focuses on the three main conditions of CPPD.

Dysmenorrhea

Dysmenorrhea, pain during or shortly before menstruation, is one of the most common gynecologic problems in women of all ages. Many adolescents have dysmenorrhea in the first 3 years after menarche. Young adult women 17 to 24 years of age are most likely to report painful menses. Approximately 75% of women report some level of discomfort associated with menses, and approximately 15% report severe dysmenorrhea (Mendiratta, 2017). However, the amount of disruption in women's lives is difficult to determine. Researchers have estimated that as many as 10% of women with dysmenorrhea have severe enough pain to interfere with their functioning for 1 to 3 days a month. Menstrual problems, including dysmenorrhea, are relatively more common in women who smoke and are obese. Severe dysmenorrhea is also associated with early menarche, nulliparity, and lack of physical exercise (Mendiratta). Traditionally dysmenorrhea is differentiated as primary or secondary. Symptoms usually begin with menstruation, although some women have discomfort several hours before onset of flow. The range and severity of symptoms are different from woman to woman and from cycle to cycle in the same woman. Symptoms of dysmenorrhea may last several hours or several days.

Pain is usually located in the suprapubic area or lower abdomen. Women describe the pain as sharp, cramping, or gripping, or as a steady dull ache. For some women pain radiates to the lower back or upper thighs.

Primary Dysmenorrhea

Primary dysmenorrhea is a condition associated with ovulatory cycles. Research has shown that primary dysmenorrhea has a biochemical basis and arises from the release of prostaglandins with menses. During the luteal phase and subsequent menstrual flow, prostaglandin F_2-alpha ($PGF_{2\alpha}$) is secreted. Excessive release of $PGF_{2\alpha}$ increases the amplitude and frequency of uterine contractions and causes vasospasm of the uterine arterioles, resulting in ischemia and cyclic lower abdominal cramps. Systemic responses to $PGF_{2\alpha}$ include backache, weakness, sweats, gastrointestinal symptoms (anorexia, nausea, vomiting, and diarrhea), and central nervous system symptoms (dizziness, syncope, headache, and poor concentration). Pain usually begins at the onset of menstruation and lasts 12 to 72 hours (Mendiratta, 2017).

Primary dysmenorrhea usually appears 6 to 12 months after menarche when ovulation is established. Anovulatory bleeding, common in the first few months or years after menarche, is painless. Because both estrogen and progesterone are necessary for primary dysmenorrhea to occur, it is experienced only with ovulatory cycles. This problem is more common among women in their late teens and early twenties than in women in older age-groups; the incidence declines with age. Psychogenic factors may influence symptoms, but symptoms are definitely related to ovulation and do not occur when ovulation is suppressed.

Management. Management of primary dysmenorrhea depends on the severity of the problem and the individual woman's response to various treatments. Important components of nursing care are information and support. Because menstruation is so closely linked to reproduction and sexuality, menstrual problems such as dysmenorrhea can have a negative influence on sexuality and self-worth. Nurses can correct myths and misinformation about menstruation and dysmenorrhea by providing facts about what is normal. Women need support to foster their feelings of positive sexuality and self-worth.

Often, nurses can offer more than one alternative for alleviating menstrual discomfort and dysmenorrhea, which gives women options to try to decide which works best for them. Several of these alternatives are discussed in the following paragraphs.

Heat (a patch or wrap) that is applied to the lower abdomen minimizes cramping by increasing vasodilation and muscle relaxation and minimizing uterine ischemia. Aerobic exercise has also been found to help alleviate pain (Mendiratta, 2017). Relaxation training, biofeedback, transcutaneous electrical nerve stimulation (TENS), Lamaze (notably a childbirth method, but also a breathing technique that can help with pain reduction), hypnotherapy, imagery, and desensitization are also used to decrease menstrual discomfort, although evidence is insufficient to determine their effectiveness (Mendiratta). Research findings from Chien and colleagues (2013) concluded that an 8-week yoga intervention decreased serum homocysteine levels, alleviating dysmenorrhea in women with primary dysmenorrhea (Fig. 4.1).

Exercise helps relieve menstrual discomfort through increased vasodilation and subsequent decreased ischemia. It also releases endogenous opiates (specifically beta-endorphins), suppresses prostaglandins, and shunts blood flow away from the viscera, resulting in reduced pelvic congestion. One specific exercise that nurses can suggest is pelvic rocking. Pelvic rocking is done by putting one's hands and feet on the floor, with a hand directly under the shoulders. Then breathe in and hollow the back and push out the abdomen, and breathe out and arch the back and contract the abdomen (Healthwise Staff, 2015).

In addition to maintaining good nutrition at all times, specific dietary changes are helpful in decreasing some of the systemic symptoms associated with dysmenorrhea. Decreased intake of salt and refined sugar intake 7 to 10 days before expected menses may reduce fluid retention. Natural diuretics such as asparagus, cranberry juice, peaches, parsley, or watermelon may help reduce edema and related discomforts. A low-fat vegetarian diet and vitamin E intake may also help minimize dysmenorrheal symptoms (Mendiratta, 2017).

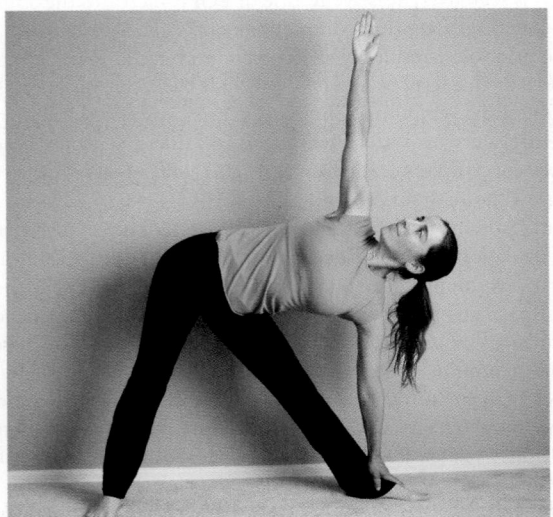

FIG 4.1 Yoga asana: triangle pose. Helpful for assisting digestion and stretching and strengthening the spine; also used for dysmenorrheal and pelvic congestion. (Courtesy of Julie Perry Nelson, Loveland, CO.)

Medications used to treat primary dysmenorrhea include prostaglandin synthesis inhibitors, primarily nonsteroidal antiinflammatory drugs (NSAIDs) (Mendiratta, 2017) (Table 4.1). NSAIDs are most effective if started several days before menses or at least by the onset of bleeding. All NSAIDs have potential gastrointestinal side effects, including nausea, vomiting, and indigestion. Women taking NSAIDs should be instructed to report dark-colored stool because this may be an indication of gastrointestinal bleeding.

> **! NURSING ALERT**
>
> If one NSAID is ineffective, often a different one may be effective. If the second drug is unsuccessful after a 6-month trial, combined oral contraceptive pills (OCPs) may be used. Women with a history of aspirin sensitivity or allergy should avoid all NSAIDs.

OCPs are a reasonable choice for women who want to use a contraceptive agent. The benefits of their use are attributed to decreased prostaglandin synthesis associated with an atrophic decidualized endometrium. Combined OCPs, which contain both estrogen and progesterone, are effective in relieving symptoms of primary dysmenorrhea for approximately 90% of women. No single OCP, including low-dose and extended-cycle OCPs, has been shown to be superior to another for the relief of primary dysmenorrhea (Mendiratta, 2017). OCPs are a particularly good choice for therapy because they combine contraception with a positive effect on dysmenorrhea, menstrual flow, and menstrual irregularities. Adolescents may benefit from use of the long-acting injectable contraceptive (depot medroxyprogesterone), but more research is needed. Since OCPs have side effects, women may not wish to use them for dysmenorrhea. They may be contraindicated for some women. (See Chapter 5 for a complete discussion of OCPs.)

Over-the-counter (OTC) preparations that are indicated for primary dysmenorrhea contain the same active ingredients (e.g., ibuprofen or naproxen sodium) as prescription preparations. However, the labeled recommended dose may be subtherapeutic. Preparations containing acetaminophen are even less effective because acetaminophen does not have the antiprostaglandin properties of NSAIDs.

Alternative and complementary therapies are increasingly popular and used in developed countries. Therapies such as acupuncture, acupressure, biofeedback, desensitization, hypnosis, massage, reiki, relaxation exercises, and therapeutic touch have been used to treat pelvic pain. Herbal preparations have long been used for managing menstrual problems, including dysmenorrhea (Table 4.2). Herbal medicines may be valuable in treating dysmenorrhea. However, it is essential that women understand that these therapies are not without potential toxicity and may cause drug interactions.

> **! NURSING ALERT**
>
> Nurses must routinely ask women about use of herbal and other alternative therapies and document their use.

Secondary Dysmenorrhea

Secondary dysmenorrhea is menstrual pain that develops later in life than primary dysmenorrhea, typically after 25 years of age. It is associated with pelvic pathology such as adenomyosis, endometriosis, pelvic inflammatory disease, endometrial polyps, or submucous or interstitial myomas (fibroids). Women with secondary dysmenorrhea often have other symptoms that may suggest the underlying cause. For example, heavy menstrual flow with dysmenorrhea suggests a diagnosis of leiomyomata, adenomyosis, or endometrial polyps. Pain associated with endometriosis often begins a few days before menses but can be present

TABLE 4.1		**Nonsteroidal Antiinflammatory Agents Used to Treat Dysmenorrhea**			
Drug	**Brand Name and Status**	**Recommended Dosage (Oral)***	**Common Side Effects†**	**Comments**	**Contraindications**
Diclofenac	Cataflam Rx	100 mg initially, then 50 mg q 8 hours	Nausea, diarrhea, constipation, abdominal distress, dyspepsia, heartburn, flatulence, dizziness, tinnitus, itching, rash	Enteric coated; immediate release	**For all NSAIDs:** Do not give if woman has hemophilia or bleeding ulcers; do not give if woman has had an allergic or anaphylactic reaction to aspirin or another NSAID; do not give if woman is taking anticoagulant medication
Ibuprofen	Motrin Rx, Advil OTC, Nuprin OTC, Motrin IB OTC	400 mg q6–8h, 200 mg q4–6h up to 1200 mg/day	See diclofenac	If GI upset occurs, take with food, milk, or antacids; avoid alcoholic beverages; do not take with aspirin; stop taking and call care provider if rash occurs	
Ketoprofen	Orudis Rx	25–50 mg q6–8h up to 300 mg/day	See diclofenac	See ibuprofen	
	Orudis KT OTC, Actron OTC	12.5 mg q6–8h up to 75 mg/day			
Meclofenamate	Meclomen Rx	100 mg tid up to 300 mg	See diclofenac	See ibuprofen	
Mefenamic acid	Ponstel Rx	500 mg initially, then 250 mg q6h/day	See diclofenac	Very potent and effective prostaglandin-synthesis inhibitor; antagonizes already formed prostaglandins; increased incidence of adverse GI side effects	
Naproxen	Naprosyn Rx	500 mg initially, then 250 mg q6–8h or 500 mg q hr (long-acting formula) not to exceed 1250 mg/day on first day; subsequent doses not to exceeed 100 mg/day	See diclofenac	See ibuprofen	
Naproxen sodium	Anaprox Rx	550 mg initially, then 275 mg q6–8h *or* 550 mg q12h up to 1375 mg/day	See diclofenac	See ibuprofen	
	Aleve OTC	440 mg initially, then 220 mg q6–8h up to 660 mg/day			
Celecoxib	Celebrex	400 mg initially, then 200 mg bid	See diclofenac	See ibuprofen	

*Dosages are current recommendations and should be verified before use. Recommended doses for over-the-counter preparations are generally less than recommendations for therapeutic doses. As-needed dosing is recommended by manufacturer; scheduled dosing may be more effective.
†Risk with all NSAIDs is gastrointestinal ulceration, possible bleeding, and prolonged bleeding time. Incidence of side effects is dose related. Reported incidence is 1% to 10%.
Data from Calis, K. A. (2016). Dysmenorrhea medication. *Medscape.* Retrieved from http://emedicine.medscape.com/article/253812-medication#2; Mendiratta, V. (2017). Primary and secondary dysmenorrhea, premenstrual syndrome, and premenstrual dysphoric disorder. In R. A. Lobo, D. M. Gershenson, G. M. Lentz, et al. (Eds.), *Comprehensive gynecology* (7th ed.). Philadelphia, PA: Elsevier.

at ovulation and continue through the first days of menses or start after menstrual flow has begun. In contrast to primary dysmenorrhea, the pain of secondary dysmenorrhea is often characterized by dull lower-abdominal aching that radiates to the back or thighs. Often women experience feelings of bloating or pelvic fullness. In addition to a physical examination with a careful pelvic examination, diagnosis may be assisted by ultrasound examination, dilation and curettage (D&C), endometrial biopsy, or laparoscopy. Treatment is directed toward removal of the underlying pathology. Many of the measures described for pain relief of primary dysmenorrhea are also helpful for women with secondary dysmenorrhea.

Premenstrual Syndrome

Approximately 75% of women experience premenstrual symptoms at some time in their reproductive lives (Mendiratta, 2017). Establishing a universal definition of premenstrual syndrome (PMS) is difficult, given that so many symptoms have been associated with the condition and at least two different syndromes have been recognized: PMS and premenstrual dysphoric disorder (PMDD).

PMS is a complex, poorly understood condition that includes one or more of a large number (more than 150) of physical and psychologic symptoms beginning in the luteal phase of the menstrual cycle, occurring to such a degree that lifestyle or work is affected, and followed by a

TABLE 4.2 Herbal Medicinals Taken Orally for Menstrual Disorders

Symptoms or Indications	Herbal Therapy*	Action
Menstrual cramping, dysmenorrhea	Black haw	Uterine antispasmodic
	Fennel	Uterotonic
	Catnip	Uterine antispasmodic
	Dong quai	Uterotonic; antiinflammatory
	Ginger	Antiinflammatory
	Motherwort	Uterotonic
	Wild yam	Uterine antispasmodic
	Valerian	Uterine antispasmodic
Premenstrual discomfort, tension	Black cohosh root	Estrogen-like luteinizing hormone suppressant; binds to estrogen receptors
	Chamomile	Antispasmodic
Breast pain	Chaste tree fruit	Decreases prolactin levels
	Bugleweed	Antigonadotropic; decreases prolactin levels
Menorrhea, metrorrhagia	Lady's mantle	Uterotonic
	Raspberry	Uterotonic
	Shepherd's purse	Uterotonic

*Many women's herbs do not have rigorous scientific studies backing their use; most uses and properties of herbs have not been validated by the US Food and Drug Administration.
Data from Annie's Remedy. (2012). *Herbal remedies for dysmenorrhea.* Retrieved from www.anniesremedy.com; National Center for Complementary and Alternative Medicine. (2010). *Herbs at a glance.* Retrieved from https://nccih.nih.gov/health/herbsataglance.htm.

symptom-free period. Symptoms include fluid retention (abdominal bloating, pelvic fullness, edema of the lower extremities, breast tenderness, and weight gain), behavioral or emotional changes (depression, crying spells, irritability, panic attacks, and impaired ability to concentrate), premenstrual cravings (sweets, salt, increased appetite, and food binges), headache, fatigue, and backache.

All age-groups are affected, with women in their twenties and thirties most frequently reporting symptoms. Ovarian function is necessary for the condition to occur because it does not occur before puberty, after menopause, or during pregnancy. The condition is not dependent on the presence of monthly menses: women who have had a hysterectomy without bilateral salpingo-oophorectomy (BSO) still can have cyclic symptoms.

PMDD is a more severe variant of PMS in which women have marked irritability, dysphoria, mood lability, anxiety, fatigue, appetite changes, and a sense of feeling overwhelmed (Mendiratta, 2017). The most common symptoms are those associated with mood disturbances, and PMDD is listed as a condition in the *Diagnostic and Statistical Manual of Mental Disorders,* fifth edition *(DSM-5)* (American Psychiatric Association [APA], 2014).

A diagnosis of PMS is made when a specific group of symptoms consistent with PMS occur in the luteal phase and resolve within a few days of menses onset. These symptoms can be physical and/or behavioral, including breast tenderness, bloating, and headache; irritability, anxiety, and depression (Mendiratta, 2017).

For a diagnosis of PMDD, the following criteria must be met (APA, 2014):

- Five or more affective and physical symptoms are present in the week before menses and begin to improve in the follicular phase of the menstrual cycle.

- At least one of the symptoms is marked affective lability, marked irritability or anger, depressed mood or feelings of hopelessness or self-deprecating thoughts, or anxiety.
- One or more of the following additional symptoms, reaching a total of 5 symptoms when combined with the above symptoms: decreased interest in usual activities, subjective difficulty concentrating, lethargy, marked change in appetite (overeating, food cravings), hypersomnia or insomnia, feeling overwhelmed, physical symptoms of breast tenderness, muscle pain, bloating, weight gain
- Symptoms interfere markedly with work or interpersonal relationships.
- Symptoms are not caused by an exacerbation of another condition or disorder.
- Must confirm that symptoms are occurring, evidenced through daily ratings
- Symptoms are not caused by physiologic effects of a substance or a specific medical treatment.

These criteria must be confirmed by prospective daily ratings for at least two menstrual cycles.

The causes of PMS and PMDD continue to be investigated, but there is general agreement that they are distinct psychiatric and medical syndromes rather than an exacerbation of an underlying psychiatric disorder. They do not occur if there is no ovarian function. A number of biologic and neuroendocrine etiologies have been suggested; however, none have been conclusively substantiated as the causative factor. It is likely that biologic, psychosocial, and sociocultural factors contribute to PMS and PMDD.

Management

There is little agreement on management. A careful, detailed history and daily log of symptoms and mood fluctuations spanning several cycles may give direction to a plan of management. Any changes that help a woman with PMS exert control over her life have a positive effect. For this reason, lifestyle changes are often effective in its treatment.

Education is an important component of the management of PMS. Nurses can advise women that self-help modalities often result in significant symptom improvement. Women have found a number of complementary and alternative therapies to be useful in managing the symptoms of PMS. Diet and exercise changes can provide symptom relief for some women. Nurses can suggest that women do not smoke and limit their consumption of refined sugar, salt, red meat, alcohol, and caffeinated beverages. Women can be encouraged to include whole grains, legumes, seeds, nuts, vegetables, fruits, and vegetable oils in their diets; reduce the amount of salt, sugar, and caffeine in their diets; and incorporate 60 minutes or more of physical exercise daily (a monthly program that varies in intensity and type of exercise according to PMS symptoms is best). Women who exercise regularly seem to have less premenstrual anxiety than do nonathletic women. Researchers believe aerobic exercise increases beta-endorphin levels to offset symptoms of depression and elevate mood.

Use of natural diuretics may also help reduce fluid retention (see the "Management" section on dysmenorrhea earlier in the chapter for more information). Nutritional supplements may assist in symptom relief. Calcium and vitamin B_6 have been shown to be moderately effective in relieving symptoms, to have few side effects, and to be safe. Daily supplements of evening primrose oil are reportedly useful in relieving breast symptoms with minimal side effects, but research reports are conflicting. Chasteberry has been found to alleviate symptoms of PMS (Jafari & Orenstein, 2015). Other herbal therapies have long been used to treat PMS; however, research on effectiveness is lacking, or studies are flawed.

Nurses can explain the relation between cyclic estrogen fluctuation and changes in serotonin levels, which can lead to mood changes. Serotonin is one of the brain chemicals that assists in coping with normal life stresses. Different management strategies recommended for PMS help to produce a more stable mood by maintaining serotonin levels. Support groups or individual or couples counseling may be helpful. Stress-reduction techniques also may help with symptom management.

If these strategies do not provide significant symptom relief in 1 to 2 months, medication is often added. Many medications have been used in treatment of PMS, but no single medication alleviates all PMS symptoms. Medications often used in the treatment of PMS include diuretics, prostaglandin inhibitors (NSAIDs), progesterone, and OCPs. These have been used mainly for the physical symptoms. Studies of progesterone have not shown that it is an effective treatment (Mendiratta, 2017). Serotonergic-activating agents, including the selective serotonin reuptake inhibitors (SSRIs) such as fluoxetine (Prozac or Sarafem), sertraline (Zoloft), citalopram (Celexa), escitalopram (Lexapro), and paroxetine (Paxil CR) are approved by the US Food and Drug Administration (FDA) as agents for PMS and are the first-line pharmacologic therapy (Mendiratta). Use of these medications during the luteal phase of the menstrual cycle is less expensive and has fewer side effects than drugs used before the development of these serotonergic activating agents. (Mendiratta). Common side effects are headaches, sleep disturbances, dizziness, weight gain, dry mouth, and decreased libido.

ENDOMETRIOSIS

Endometriosis is characterized by the presence and growth of endometrial tissue outside of the uterus. The tissue may be implanted on the ovaries; anterior and posterior cul-de-sac; broad, uterosacral, and round ligaments; rectovaginal septum; sigmoid colon; appendix; pelvic peritoneum; cervix; and inguinal area (Fig. 4.2). Endometrial lesions have been found in the vagina and surgical scars and on the vulva, perineum, and bladder. They have also been found on sites far from the pelvic area such as the thoracic cavity, gallbladder, and heart. A cystic lesion of endometriosis found in the ovary is sometimes described as a chocolate cyst because of the dark coloring of the contents of the cyst caused by the presence of old blood.

Endometrial tissue contains uterine glands and stroma (connective tissue) and responds to cyclic hormone stimulation in the same way that the uterine endometrium does but often out of phase with it. The tissue grows during the proliferative and secretory phases of the cycle. During or immediately after menstruation the tissue bleeds, resulting in an inflammatory response with subsequent fibrosis and adhesions to adjacent organs.

The overall incidence of endometriosis is 5% to 15% in reproductive-age women, 30% to 45% in infertile women, and 33% in women with chronic pelvic pain (Advincula, Troung, & Lobo, 2017). Although the condition usually develops in the third or fourth decade of life, endometriosis has been found in adolescents with disabling pelvic pain or abnormal vaginal bleeding. Endometriosis may worsen with repeated cycles, or it may remain asymptomatic and undiagnosed, eventually disappearing after menopause. However, it has been reported to occur in about 5% of postmenopausal women receiving menopausal hormone therapy. Endometriosis has been thought to be a rare occurrence in adolescents, but currently it is estimated that approximately 50% of teens with pelvic pain are found to have endometriosis (Advincula et al., 2017).

Several theories concerning the cause of endometriosis have been suggested. However, the etiology and pathology of this condition continue to be poorly understood. One of the most widely accepted theories is transplantation or retrograde menstruation. According to this theory, endometrial tissue is refluxed through the uterine tubes (also referred to as fallopian tubes) during menstruation into the peritoneal cavity, where it implants on the ovaries and other organs. Retrograde menstruation has been documented in a number of menstruating women. For most women endometrial tissue outside the uterus is destroyed before it can implant or seed in the peritoneal cavity or elsewhere. A recent theory is that there is an interaction between the amount of retrograde menstruation and an individual woman's immunologic response, which may be influenced by ethnic and genetic variability (Advincula et al., 2017).

There is a wide variation of symptoms among among women with endometriosis. It is interesting that often the extent of pain is not correlated with severity of endometriosis (Advincula et al., 2017). The major symptoms of endometriosis are pelvic pain, dysmenorrhea, and dyspareunia (painful intercourse). Women may also have chronic noncyclic pelvic pain, pelvic heaviness, or pain radiating into the thighs. Many women report bowel symptoms such as diarrhea, pain with defecation, and constipation caused by avoiding defecation because of the pain. Other symptoms include abnormal bleeding (hypermenorrhea, menorrhagia, or premenstrual staining) and pain during exercise as a result of adhesions (Advincula et al.).

Impaired fertility may result from adhesions around the uterus that pull the uterus into a fixed, retroverted position. Adhesions around the uterine tubes may block the fimbriated ends or prevent the spontaneous movement that carries the ovum to the uterus.

Management

Treatment is based on the severity of symptoms and the goals of the woman or couple. Women without pain who do not want to become pregnant need no treatment. In women with mild pain who may desire a future pregnancy, treatment may be limited to use of NSAIDs during menstruation (see earlier discussion of these medications).

Suppression of endogenous estrogen production and subsequent endometrial lesion growth is the cornerstone of management of the disease. Two main classes of medications are used to suppress endogenous

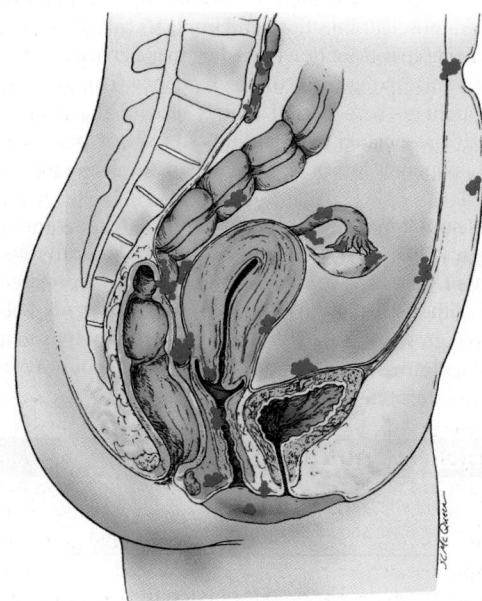

FIG 4.2 Common sites of endometriosis. (From Lobo, R.A., Gershenson, D.M., Lentz, G.M., et al. [2017]. *Comprehensive gynecology* [7th ed.]. Philadelphia, PA: Elsevier.)

estrogen levels: GnRH agonists and androgen derivatives. GnRH agonist therapy (leuprolide [Lupron], nafarelin acetate [Synarel], goserelin acetate [Zoladex]) acts by suppressing pituitary gonadotropin secretion. FSH and LH stimulation of the ovary declines markedly, and ovarian function decreases significantly. A medically induced menopause develops, resulting in anovulation and amenorrhea. Shrinkage of already established endometrial tissue, significant pain relief, and interruption in further lesion development follow. The hypoestrogenism results in hot flashes in almost all women. Trabecular bone loss is common, although most loss is reversible within 12 to 24 months after the medication is stopped (Advincula et al., 2017).

Leuprolide (3.75 mg intramuscular injection given once a month) (Medscape, 2017), nafarelin (200 mg administered twice daily by nasal spray) (MedicineNet.com, 2017), and goserelin (3.6 mg every 28 days by subcutaneous implant) (Drugs.com, 2017) are effective and well tolerated. These medications reduce endometrial lesions and pelvic pain associated with endometriosis and have posttreatment pregnancy rates similar to that of danazol (Danocrine) therapy. Common side effects of these drugs are those of natural menopause—hot flashes and vaginal dryness. Occasionally women report headaches and muscle aches. Treatment is usually limited to 6 months to minimize bone loss. Although unlikely, it is possible for a woman to become pregnant while taking a GnRH agonist. Because the potential teratogenicity of this drug is unclear, women should use a barrier contraceptive during treatment.

Danazol, a mildly androgenic synthetic steroid, suppresses FSH and LH secretion, thus producing anovulation and hypogonadotropism. This results in decreased secretion of estrogen and progesterone and regression of endometrial tissue. Danazol can produce side effects severe enough to cause a woman to discontinue the drug, including masculinizing traits (weight gain, edema, decreased breast size, oily skin, hirsutism, and deepening of the voice), all of which often disappear when treatment is discontinued. Other side effects are amenorrhea, hot flashes, vaginal dryness, insomnia, and decreased libido. Migraine headaches, dizziness, fatigue, and depression are also reported. Danazol treatment has been reported to adversely affect lipids, with a decrease in high-density lipoprotein levels and an increase in low-density lipoprotein levels. Danazol should never be prescribed when pregnancy is suspected, and barrier contraception should be used with it because ovulation may not be suppressed. Danazol can produce pseudohermaphroditism in female fetuses. The medication is contraindicated in women with liver disease and should be used with caution in women with cardiac and renal disease. Danazol is less frequently used to treat endometriosis than other medical therapies (Advincula et al., 2017).

Women who have early symptomatic disease and who can postpone pregnancy may be treated with continuous OCPs that have a low estrogen-to-progestin ratio to shrink endometrial tissue. The OCPs are taken continuously for 6 to 12 months, without any withdrawal time of the OCP. This approach is believed to lead to a more complete suppression, thus decreasing the endometriosis (Advincula et al., 2017). There can be some breakthrough bleeding, however. Any low-dose OCPs can be used if taken for 15 weeks, followed by 1 week of withdrawal. This therapy is associated with minimal side effects and can be taken for extended periods. Limited data exist on the effectiveness of progestogen-only medications for treating pain related to endometriosis.

Continuous combined hormone therapy (OCPs, estrogen/progestin patch, estrogen/progestin vaginal ring) for menstrual suppression and administration of NSAIDs are the usual treatment for adolescents younger than 16 years of age who have endometriosis. GnRH agonist therapy for severe symptoms may have possible adverse effects on bone mineralization in adolescents, and bone mineral density should be carefully monitored.

Surgical intervention is often needed for severe, acute, or incapacitating symptoms. Decisions regarding the extent and type of surgery are influenced by a woman's age, desire for children, and location of the disease. For women who do not want to preserve their ability to have children, the only definite cure is total abdominal hysterectomy (TAH) with bilateral salpingectomy and oophorectomy (BSO). In women who want children and in whom the disease does not prevent bearing children, reproductive capacity should be retained through careful removal by laparoscopic surgery or laser therapy (coagulation, vaporization, or resection) of all endometrial tissue possible with retention of ovarian function (Advincula et al., 2017).

Regardless of the type of treatment (short of TAH with BSO), endometriosis recurs in approximately 40% of women. Thus for many women, endometriosis is a chronic disease with conditions such as chronic pain or infertility. Counseling and education are critical components of nursing care for women with endometriosis. Women need an honest discussion of treatment options, with review of the potential risks and benefits of each option. Because pelvic pain is a subjective, personal experience that can be frightening, support is important. Sexual dysfunction resulting from dyspareunia is common and may necessitate referral for counseling. Support groups for women with endometriosis may be found in some locations. Resolve (www.resolve.org), an organization for infertile couples, or the Endometriosis Association (www.ivf.com/endohtml.html) may also be helpful. The nursing care discussed in the previous section on dysmenorrhea is appropriate for managing chronic pelvic pain and dysmenorrhea experienced by women with endometriosis (see Nursing Care Plan).

ALTERATIONS IN CYCLIC BLEEDING

Women often experience changes in amount, duration, interval, or regularity of menstrual cycle bleeding. Commonly women worry about menstruation that is infrequent (**oligomenorrhea**), is scanty at normal intervals (**hypomenorrhea**), is excessive (**menorrhagia**), or occurs between periods (**metrorrhagia**).

Treatment depends on the cause and may include education and reassurance. For example, the nurse or health care provider informs women that OCPs can cause scanty menstrual flow and midcycle spotting. Progestin intramuscular injections and implants can also cause midcycle bleeding. A single episode of heavy bleeding may signal an early pregnancy loss such as a miscarriage or ectopic pregnancy. This type of bleeding is often thought to be a period that is heavier than usual, perhaps delayed, and is associated with abdominal pain or pelvic discomfort. When early pregnancy loss is suspected, hematocrit and pregnancy tests are indicated.

Uterine leiomyomas (fibroids or myomas) are a common cause of menorrhagia. Fibroids are benign tumors of the smooth muscle of the uterus with an unknown cause. Fibroids occur in approximately 70% of women, with about 50% having symptoms (Ryntz & Lobo, 2017). Other uterine growths ranging from endometrial polyps to adenocarcinoma and endometrial cancer are common causes of heavy menstrual bleeding and intermenstrual bleeding.

> ### ❗ NURSING ALERT
>
> If the woman herself considers the amount or duration of bleeding to be excessive, the problem should be investigated.

Treatment for menorrhagia depends on the cause of the bleeding. If the bleeding is related to the contraceptive method (e.g., an intrauterine device [IUD]), the health care professional provides factual information and reassurance and discusses other contraceptive options.

NURSING CARE PLAN
The Woman With Endometriosis

Case Study
Terri is a 28-year-old married woman who has come to the Well Women's Clinic. She complains of having heavy menstrual periods that are accompanied by severe pelvic and abdominal pain (pain scale rating 7–8) that sometimes radiates down her thighs and that the pain has worsened over the last year or so. She has tried over-the-counter ibuprofen for the pain with some relief. She confides that sexual intercourse is often painful and that she no longer enjoys sexual relations. She says this has caused stress for her and tension between her and her husband. She added that they would like to have a child but she has not been able to conceive, although they have been trying to achieve a pregnancy for about 1 year. She states tearfully, "I feel like a failure. I hope that you can find out why I have such bad pain and bleeding and why I can't get pregnant. I am really afraid of what you are going to find and that there is nothing that can be done."

After further assessment and diagnostic testing, endometriosis is diagnosed. The treatment plan is to suppress endogenous estrogen production and subsequent endometrial lesion growth using GnRH agonist therapy for 6 months.

Assessment
What are the common signs of acute and chronic pain associated with endometriosis?

Defining Characteristics
Self-report of pain characteristics and intensity
Alteration in ability to continue previous activities
Self-focusing
Protective behavior
Alteration in sleep pattern

Nursing Diagnosis
Acute and Chronic Pain related to menstruation secondary to endometriosis

Expected Outcome
Terri will verbalize a decrease in intensity and frequency of pain during each menstrual cycle.

Nursing Interventions	Rationales
Assess location, type, and duration of pain and history of discomfort.	To determine severity of dysmenorrhea
Administer nonsteroidal antiinflammatory drugs as indicated.	To assist with pain relief
Administer hormone-altering medications as ordered.	To suppress ovulation and subsequently suppress endometrial tissue lesion growth
Provide information about use of nonpharmacologic methods such as heat.	To increase blood flow to the pelvic region

Assessment
What factors interfere with Terri's understanding of endometriosis and its treatment?

Defining Characteristics
Insufficient information about endometriosis
Verbalization of problem
Inappropriate or exaggerated behavior

Nursing Diagnosis
Deficient Knowledge related to insufficient understanding about disease process and prescribed therapy and the effects on self-care

Expected Outcome
Terri will verbalize correct understanding of endometriosis and the use of self-care methods and prescribed therapies.

Nursing Interventions	Rationales
Assess woman's current understanding of the disorder and related therapies.	To validate the accuracy of knowledge base
Give information to woman regarding the disorder and treatment regimen.	To empower the woman to become a partner in her own care

Assessment
What characteristics of low self-esteem are manifested by Terri?

Defining Characteristics
Self-negating statements of feeling like a failure
Situational challenge to self-worth
Underestimates ability to deal with situation

Nursing Diagnosis
Situational Low Self-Esteem related to inability to get pregnant

Expected Outcome
Terri will verbalize positive feelings of self-worth.

Nursing Interventions	Rationales
Provide therapeutic communication. Include husband as appropriate.	To validate feelings and provide support
Refer to support group.	To enhance feelings of self-worth through group communication

Assessment
What are common signs of anxiety for women who have endometriosis?

Defining Characteristics
Fear of what is wrong with her
Feeling of inadequacy
Helplessness
Awareness of physiologic symptoms

Nursing Diagnosis
Anxiety related to stressors, unmet needs, current health status, and unknown outcomes of diagnosis and treatment

Expected Outcome
Terri will report a decreased number of anxious feelings.

Nursing Interventions	Rationales
Provide opportunity to discuss feelings.	To identify source of anxiety.
Provide and reinforce information about endometriosis and the prescribed therapy.	To keep expectations realistic and dispel myths or inaccuracies.
Provide emotional support.	To encourage verbalization of feelings.

Continued

The Woman With Endometriosis—cont'd

Assessment
What types of stressors does Terri exhibit?

Defining Characteristics
Negative impact from stress
Tension
Impaired functioning

Nursing Diagnosis
Stress Overload related to emotional and physiologic effects of having endometriosis and infertility

Expected Outcome
Terri will verbalize understanding and accept the emotional and physiologic responses to 1 disorder.

Nursing Interventions	Rationales
Provide therapeutic communication.	To validate feelings of the effects of pain and stress on her life.

If there is no known cause for the bleeding and anatomic causes have been ruled out, therapy is aimed at reducing the amount of heavy bleeding using medical rather than surgical approaches. Current options for treatment include estrogens, progestogen, NSAIDS, antifibrinolytic agents, and GnRH (Ryntz & Lobo, 2017). Nurses focus on the correct administration of these treatments and reducing potential adverse side effects, such as gastrointestinal distress with NSAIDS.

If bleeding is related to the presence of fibroids, the degree of disability and discomfort associated with the fibroids and the woman's plans for childbearing influence treatment decisions. Treatment options include medical and surgical management. Most fibroids can be monitored by frequent examinations to judge growth, if any, and correction of anemia if present. It is important to warn women with metrorrhagia to avoid using aspirin because of its tendency to increase bleeding. Medical treatment is directed toward temporarily reducing symptoms, shrinking the myoma, and reducing its blood supply. This reduction is often accomplished with the use of a GnRH agonist. There is evidence that following cessation of treatment, blood loss may return to levels that existed prior to treatment (Ryntz & Lobo, 2017). If the woman wishes to retain childbearing potential, a myomectomy may be performed. Myomectomy, or removal of the tumors only by laparoscopic or hysteroscopic resection or laser surgery, is particularly difficult if multiple myomas must be removed. One in four women will have a hysterectomy performed within 20 years of having a myomectomy. If the woman does not want to preserve her childbearing function or if she has severe symptoms (severe anemia, severe pain, considerable disruption of lifestyle), uterine artery embolization (UAE) (procedure that blocks blood supply to fibroid), or hysterectomy (removal of uterus) may be performed. Neither procedure is considered to be very effective unless the cause of the excessive bleeding is fibroids (Ryntz & Lobo). Important nursing roles include reassurance, counseling, education, and support.

Dysfunctional Uterine Bleeding

Abnormal uterine bleeding (AUB) is any form of uterine bleeding that is irregular in amount, duration, or timing and is not related to regular menstrual bleeding. Box 4.1 lists possible causes of AUB. Although often used interchangeably, the terms *AUB* and *dysfunctional uterine bleeding (DUB)* are not synonymous. AUB can have organic causes such as systemic diseases, reproductive tract disease, as well as hormonal causes, while DUB occurs in the absence of organic, systemic causes.

DUB can be anovulatory or ovulatory but is most commonly caused by anovulation. When no surge of LH occurs or if insufficient progesterone is produced by the corpus luteum to support the endometrium, it will begin to involute and shed. This process most often occurs at the extremes of a woman's reproductive years, when the menstrual cycle is just becoming established at menarche or when it draws to a close at menopause. DUB also occurs with any condition that gives rise to

chronic anovulation associated with continuous estrogen production. Such conditions include obesity, hyperthyroidism and hypothyroidism, polycystic ovary syndrome, and any of the endocrine conditions discussed in the sections on amenorrhea and oligomenorrhea. A diagnosis of DUB is made only after ruling out all other organic causes of abnormal menstrual bleeding.

Management

The most effective medical treatment of acute bleeding episodes of DUB is administration of oral or intravenous estrogen. Dilation and curettage (D&C) may be done if the bleeding has not stopped in 12 to 24 hours. An oral conjugated estrogen and progestin regimen is usually given for at least 3 months after the acute phase has passed. Such long-term treatment will help prevent recurrence of the pattern of DUB and hemorrhage. If the woman wants contraception, she should continue to take OCPs. If she has no need for contraception, the treatment may be stopped to assess the woman's bleeding pattern. If her menses does not resume, a progestin regimen (e.g., medroxyprogesterone, 10 mg each day for 10 days before the expected date of her menstrual period) may be prescribed after ruling out pregnancy. This is done to prevent persistent anovulation with chronic unopposed endogenous estrogen hyperstimulation of the endometrium, which can result in eventual atypical tissue changes. This approach usually successfully leads to regular withdrawal bleeding (Ryntz & Lobo, 2017).

If the recurrent, heavy bleeding is not controlled by hormone therapy or D&C, ablation of the endometrium through laser treatment may be performed. Nursing roles include informing patients of their options, counseling and education as indicated, and referring to the appropriate specialists and health care services.

Nursing assessments for women who have a menstrual disorder include the following:
- Taking a thorough menstrual, obstetric, sexual, and contraceptive history.
- Exploring the woman's perceptions of her condition, cultural or ethnic influences, lifestyle, and patterns of coping.
- Evaluating the amount of pain or bleeding experienced and its effect on daily activities.
- Noting any home remedies and prescriptions to relieve discomfort. A symptom diary, in which the woman records emotions, behaviors, physical symptoms, diet, and exercise and rest patterns, is a useful diagnostic tool.

In addition to the medical, surgical, and nursing interventions discussed with each problem, additional nursing interventions may include the following:
- Accepting the woman's symptoms as valid.
- Correlating data from the daily diary of emotional status, subjective feelings, and physical state with physiologic changes.

BOX 4.1   Possible Causes of Abnormal Uterine Bleeding

Pregnancy-Related Conditions
- Threatened or spontaneous miscarriage
- Retained products of conception after elective abortion
- Ectopic pregnancy
- Placenta previa/placental abruption
- Trophoblastic disease

Lower Reproductive Tract Infections
- Cervicitis
- Endometritis
- Myometritis
- Salpingitis

Benign Anatomic Abnormalities
- Adenomyosis
- Leiomyomata
- Polyps of the cervix or endometrium

Neoplasms
- Endometrial hyperplasia
- Cancer of cervix and endometrium
- Hormonally active tumors (rare)
- Vaginal tumors (rare)

Malignant Lesions
- Cervical squamous cell carcinoma
- Endometrial adenocarcinoma
- Estrogen-producing ovarian tumors
- Testosterone-producing ovarian tumors
- Leiomyosarcoma

Trauma
- Genital injury (accidental, coital trauma, sexual abuse)
- Foreign body
- Lacerations

Systemic Conditions
- Adrenal hyperplasia and Cushing's disease
- Blood dyscrasias
- Coagulopathies
- Hypothalamic suppression (from stress, weight loss, excessive exercise)
- Polycystic ovary disease
- Thyroid disease
- Pituitary adenoma or hyperprolactinemia
- Severe organ disease (renal or liver failure)

Iatrogenic Causes
- Medications with estrogenic activity
- Anticoagulants
- Exogenous hormone use (oral contraceptives, menopausal hormone therapy)
- Selective serotonin reuptake inhibitors
- Tamoxifen
- Intrauterine devices
- Herbal preparation (ginseng)

Modified from Albers, J. R., Hull, S. K., Wesley, R. M. (2004). Abnormal uterine bleeding, *American Family Physician, 69*, 1915–1926, 1931–1932; Ryntz, T., & Lobo, R. A. (2017). Abnormal uterine bleeding: Etiology and management of acute and chronic excessive bleeding. In R. A. Lobo, D. M. Gershenson, G. M. Lentz, et al. (Eds.), *Comprehensive gynecology* (7th ed.). Philadelphia, PA: Elsevier.

BOX 4.2   Sexually Transmitted Infections

Bacteria
- Chlamydia
- Gonorrhea
- Syphilis
- Group B streptococci

Protozoa
- Trichomoniasis

Viruses
- Human immunodeficiency virus
- Herpes simplex virus, types 1 and 2
- Viral hepatitis A and B
- Human papillomavirus

- Encouraging the woman to express her feelings about her symptoms.
- Providing information about therapeutic options (pharmacologic and nonpharmacologic) so the woman (couple) makes (make) choices considered best for her (them).
- Providing information about local support groups.

INFECTIONS

Infections of the reproductive tract can occur throughout a woman's life and are often the cause of significant reproductive morbidity, including ectopic pregnancy and tubal factor infertility. The direct economic costs of these infections can be substantial, and the indirect cost is equally overwhelming. Some consequences of maternal infection such as infertility last a lifetime. The emotional costs may include damaged relationships and lowered self-esteem. Nurses and other health care personnel must be aware of universal precautions to prevent transmission of infections.

SEXUALLY TRANSMITTED INFECTIONS

Sexually transmitted infections (STIs) are infections or infectious disease syndromes transmitted primarily by sexual contact. The term sexually transmitted infection includes more than 25 infectious organisms that are transmitted through sexual activity and the dozens of clinical syndromes that they cause (Box 4.2). STIs are among the most common health problems in the United States today, with increases seen in 2014 in the three nationally reportable STIs (chlamydia, gonorrhea, and syphilis) (CDC, 2017b). The following discussion focuses on the most common STIs in women. Chapter 25 discusses neonatal effects.

Prevention

Preventing infection (primary prevention) is the most effective way of reducing the adverse consequences of STIs for women. Prompt diagnosis and treatment of current infections (secondary prevention) also can prevent complications and transmission to others. Preventing the spread of STIs requires that women at risk for transmitting or acquiring infections change their behavior. A critical first step is to include questions about a woman's sexual history, sexual risk behaviors, and drug-related risky behaviors as a part of her assessment. The CDC (2017a) has created the "five Ps" as a guide to questions that help to assess risky behaviors: partners, practices, prevention of pregnancy, protection from STIs, and past history of STIs (Box 4.3). Identification of risk factors

BOX 4.3   Assessing Sexually Transmitted Infection and Human Immunodeficiency Virus Risk Behaviors: The Five Ps

Partners
- Have your partners been men, women, both?
- Ever thought that a sex partner put you at risk for AIDS or an STI (IV drug user, bisexual)?

Practices
- Are you sexually active now?
- If no, have you had sex in the past?
- Ever had an oral, vaginal, or anal sexual experience with another person?
- With how many different people? 1? 2 or 3? 4 to 10? More than 10?

Prevention of Pregnancy
- Do you use male condoms? Female condoms? Other barriers?

Protection From STIs
- Ever injected drugs using shared equipment, including street drugs, steroids?
- Ever had sex with a person who uses and shares?
- Ever had sex while so stoned, high, or drunk that you can't remember the details?
- Ever exchanged sex for drugs, money, shelter?
- Ever had sex against your will?
- What do you do to protect yourself from HIV and STIs?
- Ever had a blood transfusion?
- Ever had sex with a person who had a blood transfusion?
- Ever had sex with a person with hemophilia?
- Ever received donor semen, egg, transplanted organ or tissue?
- Ever shared equipment for tattoo, body piercing?

Past History of STIs
- Ever had an STI (herpes, gonorrhea, genital warts, chlamydia)?
- Ever had a test for HIV?
- Ever worried about AIDS and would like to talk with someone about it?

From Centers for Disease Control and Prevention. (2017). *Sexually transmitted disease treatment guidelines.* Retrieved from https://www.cdc.gov/std/tg2015/clinical.htm.

or risky behaviors is followed by prevention counseling. Techniques that are effective in providing prevention counseling include using open-ended questions, using understandable language, and reassuring the woman that treatment will be provided regardless of considerations such as ability to pay, language spoken, or lifestyle. Prevention messages should include descriptions of specific actions to prevent contracting or transmitting STIs (e.g., refraining from sexual activity when STI-related symptoms are present) and should be individualized for each woman, giving attention to her specific risk factors.

To be motivated to take preventive actions, a woman must believe that acquiring a disease will be serious for her and that she is at risk for infection. Most individuals tend to underestimate their personal risk for infection in a given situation. Thus many women may not perceive themselves as being at risk for contracting an STI, and telling them that they should carry condoms may not be well received. Although levels of awareness of STIs are generally high, widespread misconceptions or specific gaps in knowledge also exist. Therefore nurses have a responsibility to provide their patients with accurate, comprehensive information about transmission and symptoms of STIs and the behaviors that place them at risk for contracting an infection.

Primary preventive measures are individual activities aimed at avoiding infection. Risk-free options include complete abstinence from sexual activities that transmit semen, blood, or other body fluids or that allow for skin-to-skin contact (CDC, 2017b). Involvement in a mutually monogamous relationship with an uninfected partner also eliminates the risk for contracting STIs.

Sexually Transmitted Infections/Human Immunodeficiency Virus Prevention Strategies

An essential component of primary prevention is counseling the woman regarding sexual practices so she can avoid acquiring or transmitting STIs, including attaining knowledge of her partner, reducing her number of partners, practicing low-risk sex, avoiding the exchange of body fluids, and vaccination.

Reducing the number of partners and avoiding partners who have had many previous sexual partners decrease a woman's chances of contracting an STI. Discussing each new partner's previous sexual history and exposure to STIs augments other efforts to reduce risk; however, sexual partners are not always truthful about their sexual history.

Women should be taught low-risk sexual practices and which sexual practices to avoid. Sexual fantasizing is safe, as are caressing, hugging, body rubbing, and massage. Mutual masturbation is low risk as long as there is no contact with a partner's semen or vaginal secretions. All sexual activities are safe when both partners are monogamous, trustworthy, and known (by testing) to be free of disease. Anal-genital intercourse, anal-oral contact, and anal-digital activity are high-risk sexual behaviors and should be avoided.

The physical barrier promoted for the prevention of sexual transmission of human immunodeficiency virus (HIV) and other STIs is the latex male condom. The nurse should remind women to use a condom with every sexual encounter; to use latex or plastic male condoms rather than natural skin condoms for STI protection; to use a condom with a current expiration date; to use each one only once; and to handle it carefully to avoid damaging it with fingernails, teeth, or other sharp objects. Condoms should be stored away from high heat. Although it is not ideal, women may choose to safely carry condoms in wallets, shoes, or inside a bra. They can be taught the differences among condoms: price ranges, sizes, and where they can be purchased. Explicit instructions for how to apply a male condom are included in Chapter 5.

The female condom (i.e., a lubricated polyurethane sheath with a ring on each end that is inserted into the vagina) has been shown in laboratory studies to be an effective mechanical barrier to viruses, including HIV. Studies suggest that, while more costly than the male condom, the female condom is managed by the woman, adding to its effectiveness in preventing transmission of STIs (CDC, 2017b). What is important and should be stressed by nurses is the consistent use of condoms for every act of sexual intimacy when there is the possibility of transmission of disease.

Evidence has shown that vaginal spermicides do not protect against certain STIs (e.g., chlamydia, cervical gonorrhea) and that frequent use of spermicides containing nonoxynol-9 has been associated with genital lesions and may increase HIV transmission. Condoms lubricated with nonoxynol-9 are not recommended (CDC, 2017b).

Vaccination is an effective method for the prevention of some STIs such as hepatitis B and human papillomavirus (HPV). Hepatitis B vaccine is recommended for women at high risk for STIs. A vaccine is available for HPV types 6, 11, 16, and 18 for girls and women 9 to 26 years of age and for boys 9 to 21 years of age (CDC, 2017b) (see later discussion).

It is important to counsel women to be alert for situations that make it hard to talk about and practice risk reduction. These situations include romantic times when condoms are not available and when alcohol or drugs make it difficult to make wise decisions.

SEXUALLY TRANSMITTED BACTERIAL INFECTIONS

Chlamydia

Chlamydia trachomatis is the most frequently reported infectious disease in the United States, yet many cases are asymptomatic (CDC, 2017a). These infections are often silent and highly destructive; their sequelae and complications are very serious. In women, chlamydial infections are difficult to diagnose; the symptoms, if present, are nonspecific, and the organism is expensive to culture.

Acute salpingitis, or pelvic inflammatory disease, is the most serious complication of chlamydial infections. Past chlamydial infections are associated with an increased risk for ectopic pregnancy and tubal factor infertility. Furthermore, chlamydial infection of the cervix causes inflammation, resulting in microscopic cervical ulcerations that may increase the risk for acquiring HIV infection. More than one-half of infants born to mothers with chlamydia will develop conjunctivitis or pneumonia after perinatal exposure to the mother's infected cervix. *C. trachomatis* is the most common infectious cause of ophthalmia neonatorum.

Sexually active women younger than 25 years of age are the ones most likely to become infected with chlamydia (CDC, 2017b). Women older than 30 years of age have the lowest rate of infection. Risky behaviors, including multiple partners and not using barrier methods of birth control, increase a woman's risk for chlamydial infection.

Screening and Diagnosis

In addition to obtaining information regarding the presence of risk factors (e.g., women younger than 25 years of age, older women who do not use barrier contraceptives, women with new or multiple partners), the nurse inquires about the presence of any symptoms. Although infection is usually asymptomatic, some women may experience spotting or postcoital bleeding, mucoid or purulent cervical discharge, or dysuria. Bleeding results from inflammation and erosion of the cervical columnar epithelium.

Laboratory diagnosis of chlamydia is by culture (expensive and labor-intensive), DNA probe (relatively less expensive but less sensitive), enzyme immunoassay (also relatively less expensive but less sensitive), and nucleic acid amplification tests (NAATs) (expensive but have relatively higher sensitivity) of urine specimens or specimens from the endocervix/vagina (CDC, 2017a). All pregnant women should have cervical cultures for chlamydia at the first prenatal visit. Screening late in the third trimester (36 weeks) may be carried out if the woman was positive previously or if she is younger than 25 years of age, has a new sex partner, or has multiple sex partners.

Management

The CDC (2015b) recommendations for the treatment of chlamydial infections include doxycycline or azithromycin (Table 4.3). Azithromycin is often prescribed when compliance is a problem because only one dose is needed. Because chlamydia is often asymptomatic, women must take all prescribed medication. All exposed sexual partners should be treated. Women treated with doxycycline or azithromycin do not need to be retested unless symptoms continue (CDC, 2017b).

Gonorrhea

Gonorrhea is probably the oldest communicable disease in the United States. An estimated 820,000 American men and women contract gonorrhea each year (CDC, 2017a). The incidence of drug-resistant cases of gonorrhea, in particular penicillinase-producing *Neisseria gonorrhoeae,* is increasing dramatically in the United States.

Gonorrhea is caused by the aerobic, gram-negative diplococci *N. gonorrhoeae.* It is almost exclusively transmitted by sexual contact. The principal means of transmission is genital-to-genital contact during sexual activity; however, it is also spread by oral-genital and anal-genital contact. There is also evidence that infection may spread in females from vagina to rectum. Although the organism has been recovered from inanimate objects artificially inoculated with the bacteria, there is no evidence that natural transmission occurs this way.

Age is probably the most important risk factor associated with gonorrhea. In the United States, the highest reported rates of infection are among sexually active teenagers and young adults. The majority of those contracting gonorrhea are younger than 20 years of age and engage in sexual activities with multiple partners. Routine screening is advised for all sexually active women younger than 25 years of age and older women who are at risk due to multiple sex partners or a new sex partner.

Women are often asymptomatic; but, when they are symptomatic, they may have a greenish-yellow purulent endocervical discharge or may experience menstrual irregularities. Women may complain of pain (i.e., chronic or acute severe pelvic or lower abdominal pain) or menses that last longer or are more painful than normal. Gonococcal rectal infection may occur in women after anal intercourse. Individuals with rectal gonorrhea may be completely asymptomatic or may experience severe symptoms with profuse purulent anal discharge, rectal pain, and blood in the stool. Rectal itching, fullness, pressure, and pain are also common symptoms, as is diarrhea. A diffuse vaginitis with vulvitis is the most common form of gonococcal infection in prepubertal girls. Signs of infection may include vaginal discharge, dysuria, or swollen, reddened labia.

Gonococcal infections in pregnancy potentially affect both mother and infant. Women with cervical gonorrhea may develop salpingitis in the first trimester. Perinatal complications of gonococcal infection include premature rupture of the membranes, preterm birth, chorioamnionitis, neonatal sepsis, intrauterine growth restriction, and maternal postpartum sepsis. Amniotic infection syndrome—manifested by placental, fetal, and umbilical cord inflammation following premature rupture of the membranes—may result from gonorrheal infection during pregnancy.

Screening and Diagnosis

All pregnant women should be screened at the first prenatal visit, and infected women and those identified with risky behaviors rescreened at 36 weeks of gestation. Gonococcal infection cannot be diagnosed reliably by clinical signs and symptoms alone. Individuals may have "classic" symptoms, vague symptoms that may be attributed to a number of conditions, or no symptoms at all. Cultures should be obtained from the endocervix, the rectum, and when indicated, the pharynx. Thayer-Martin cultures are recommended to diagnose gonorrhea in women. Because coinfection is common, any woman suspected of having gonorrhea should have a chlamydial culture and serologic test for syphilis unless one has been done within the past 2 months.

Management

Management of gonorrhea is becoming more challenging as drug-resistant strains are increasing. The treatment of choice for uncomplicated urethral, endocervical, and rectal infections in pregnant and nonpregnant women is ceftriaxone given intramuscularly once. The CDC also recommends concomitant treatment for chlamydia because coinfection is common (CDC, 2017b) (see Table 4.3). All women with both gonorrhea and syphilis should also be treated for syphilis according to CDC guidelines (see discussion of syphilis in the "Syphilis" section later in this chapter).

Gonorrhea is highly communicable. Recent (past 30 days) sexual partners should be examined, cultured, and treated with appropriate regimens. Most treatment failures result from reinfection. The woman needs to be informed of this and of the consequences of reinfection in

TABLE 4.3 Sexually Transmitted Infections and Drug Therapies for Women*

Disease	Nonpregnant Women (13–17 Years)	Nonpregnant Women (>18 Years)	Pregnant Women	Lactating Women[†]
Chlamydia	*Recommended:* Azithromycin, 1 g orally once or Doxycycline, 100 mg orally bid for 7 days *Alternatives:* Erythromycin base 500 mg orally qid for 7 days or Erythromycin ethylsuccinate 800 mg orally qid for 7 days or Levofloxacin 500 mg orally once a day for 7 days or Ofloxacin 300 mg orally bid for 7 days	*Recommended:* Azithromycin, 1 g orally once or Doxycycline, 100 mg orally bid for 7 days *Alternatives:* Erythromycin base 500 mg orally qid for 7 days or Erythromycin ethylsuccinate 800 mg orally qid for 7 days or Levofloxacin 500 mg orally once a day for 7 days or Ofloxacin 300 mg orally bid for 7 days	*Recommended:* Azithromycin, 1 g orally once *Alternatives:* Amoxicillin, 500 mg orally tid for 7 days or Erythromycin base 500 mg orally qid for 7 days or Erythromycin base 250 mg orally qid for 14 days or Erythromycin ethylsuccinate 800 mg orally qid for 7 days or Erythromycin ethylsuccinate 400 mg orally qid for 14 days	*Recommended:* Azithromycin, 1 g orally once *Alternatives:* Amoxicillin, 500 mg orally tid for 7 days or Erythromycin base 500 mg orally qid for 7 days or Erythromycin base 250 mg orally qid for 14 days or Erythromycin ethylsuccinate 800 mg orally qid for 7 days or Erythromycin ethylsuccinate 400 mg orally qid for 14 days
Gonorrhea	*Recommended:* Ceftriaxone, 125 mg IM once (adolescents who weigh >45 kg can be treated with any regimen recommended for adults) Plus treatment for chlamydia as above	*Recommended:* Ceftriaxone, 250 mg IM once Plus Azithromycin 1 gm orally in a single dose	*Recommended:* Ceftriaxone, 250 mg IM once Plus Azithroymycin 1 gm orally in a single dose	*Recommended:* Ceftriaxone, 250 mg IM once Plus Azithromycin 1 gm orally in a single dose
Syphilis	**Primary, secondary, early-latent disease:** *Recommended:* Benzathine penicillin G, 2.4 million units IM once **Late-latent or unknown-duration disease:** *Recommended:* Benzathine penicillin G, 7.2 million units total, administered as three doses, 2.4 million units each, at 1-week intervals **Penicillin allergy:** Doxycycline, 100 mg orally qid for 14 days or Tetracycline, 500 mg orally qid for 14 days	**Primary, secondary, early-latent disease:** *Recommended:* Benzathine penicillin G, 2.4 million units IM once **Late-latent or unknown-duration disease:** *Recommended:* Benzathine penicillin G, 7.2 million units total, administered as three doses, 2.4 million units each, at 1-week intervals **Penicillin allergy:** Doxycycline, 100 mg orally qid for 14 days or Tetracycline, 500 mg orally qid for 14 days	**Primary, secondary, early-latent disease:** *Recommended:* Benzathine penicillin G, 2.4 million units IM once (some experts recommend a second dose of benzathine penicillin, 2.4 million units, 1 week later) **Late-latent or unknown-duration disease:** *Recommended:* Benzathine penicillin G, 7.2 million units total, administered as three doses, 2.4 million units each, at 1-week intervals No proven alternatives to penicillin in pregnancy Pregnant women who have a history of allergy to penicillin should be desensitized and treated with penicillin	**Primary, secondary, early-latent disease:** *Recommended:* Benzathine penicillin G, 2.4 million units IM once
Human papillomavirus	*Recommended for external genital warts:* **Patient-applied:** Podofilox, 0.5% solution, or gel to wart bid for 3 days followed by 4-day rest for ≤4 cycles or Imiquimod, 5% cream, hs 3 times a week for ≤16 weeks or Sinecatechins 15% ointment tid for ≤16 weeks	*Recommended for external genital warts:* **Patient-applied:** Podofilox, 0.5% solution, or gel to wart bid for 3 days followed by 4-day rest for ≤4 cycles or Imiquimod, 5% cream, hs 3 times a week for ≤16 wk or Sinecatechins 15% ointment tid for ≤16 wk	*Recommended for external genital warts:* **Provider applied:** Cryotherapy with liquid nitrogen or cryoprobe or TCA or BCA 80%–90% weekly Imiquimod, podophyllin (Podocon-25), sinecatechins, and podofilox should not be used in pregnancy	*Recommended for external genital warts:* **Provider applied:** Cryotherapy with liquid nitrogen or cryoprobe or TCA or BCA 80%–90% weekly Imiquimod, podophyllin, sinecatechins, and podofilox should not be used during lactation

Disease	Nonpregnant Women (13–17 Years)	Nonpregnant Women (>18 Years)	Pregnant Women	Lactating Women†
	Provider-applied: Cryotherapy with liquid nitrogen or cryoprobe _or_ Podophyllin resin, 10%–25% in tincture of benzoin compound weekly (wash off in 1–4 hours). Repeat weekly as necessary _or_ Trichloracetic acid (TCA) or bichloracetic acid (BCA) 80%–90% weekly	**Provider-applied:** Cryotherapy with liquid nitrogen or cryoprobe _or_ Podophyllin resin, 10%–25% in tincture of benzoin compound weekly (wash off in 1–4 hours). Repeat weekly as necessary _or_ TCA or BCA 80%–90% weekly		
Genital herpes simplex virus (HSV-1 or HSV-2)	**Primary infection:** Acyclovir, 400 mg orally tid for 7–10 days _or_ Acyclovir, 200 mg orally 5 times a day for 7–10 days _or_ Valacyclovir, 1 g orally bid for 7–10 days _or_ Famciclovir, 250 mg orally tid for 7–10 days **Recurrent infection:** Acyclovir, 400 mg orally tid for 5 days _or_ Acyclovir, 800 mg orally bid for 5 days _or_ Acyclovir, 800 mg orally tid for 2 days _or_ Valacyclovir, 500 mg orally bid for 3 days _or_ Valacyclovir, 1 g orally once a day for 5 days Famciclovir, 125 mg orally bid for 5 days _or_ Famciclovir 1000 mg orally bid for 1 day _or_ Famciclovir, 500 mg once, then 250 mg bid for 2 days **Suppression therapy:** _Take daily for 1 year or more:_ Acyclovir, 400 mg orally bid _or_ Famciclovir, 250 mg orally bid _or_ Valacyclovir, 500 mg orally once a day _or_ Valacyclovir, 1 g orally once a day	**Primary infection:** Acyclovir, 400 mg orally tid for 7–10 days _or_ Acyclovir, 200 mg orally 5 times a day for 7-10 days _or_ Valacyclovir, 1 g orally bid for 7–10 days _or_ Famciclovir, 250 mg orally tid for 7–10 days **Recurrent infection:** Acyclovir, 400 mg orally tid for 5 days _or_ Acyclovir, 800 mg orally bid for 5 days _or_ Acyclovir, 800 mg orally tid for 2 days _or_ Valacyclovir, 500 mg orally bid for 3 days _or_ Valacyclovir, 1 g orally once a day for 5 days Famciclovir, 125 mg orally bid for 5 days or Famciclovir, 1000 mg orally bid for 1 day _or_ Famciclovir 500 mg once, then 250 mg bid for 2 days **Suppression therapy:** _Take daily for 1 year or more:_ Acyclovir, 400 mg orally bid _or_ Famciclovir, 250 mg orally bid _or_ Valacyclovir, 500 mg orally once a day _or_ Valacyclovir, 1 g orally once a day	No increase in birth defects beyond the general population has been found with acyclovir use in pregnancy Acyclovir, 400 mg orally tid for 7 days for first episode or severe recurrent infection; may be given IV if infection is severe Suppression therapy with acyclovir 400 ms orally tid or valacyclovir 500 mg orally bid; if taken 4 weeks before the birth, women with recurrent infections can reduce the need for a cesarean birth	Acyclovir usually is considered compatible with breastfeeding Acyclovir, 400 mg tid for 7 days

bid, Twice daily; _hs,_ at bedtime; _HSV,_ herpes simplex virus; _IM,_ intramuscularly; _IV,_ intravenously; _qid,_ four times daily; _tid,_ three times daily.
*List is not inclusive of all drugs that may be used as alternatives.
†These medications are usually compatible with breastfeeding.
Data from Centers for Disease Control and Prevention. (2017). _Sexually transmitted diseases treatment guidelines._ Retrieved from http://www.cdc.gov/std/tg2015/clinical.htm.

terms of chronicity, complications, and potential infertility. Women are counseled to use condoms. All women with gonorrhea should be offered confidential counseling and testing for HIV infection.

Syphilis

Syphilis, one of the earliest described STIs, is caused by *Treponema pallidum,* a motile spirochete. Transmission is thought to be by entry through microscopic abrasions in the subcutaneous tissue, which can occur during sexual intercourse. The disease can also be transmitted through kissing, biting, or oral-genital sex. Transplacental transmission may occur at any time during pregnancy; the degree of risk is related to the quantity of spirochetes in the maternal bloodstream. Syphilis rates increased in women and men in 2014-2015, with an increase of 18.1% in men and 27.3% in women. This increase in syphilis rates in women raises concerns about congenital syphilis (CDC, 2017b). In 2013–2014, the rate rose for men by 14.5% and for women by 22.7% (CDC, 2017b).

Syphilis is a complex disease that can lead to serious systemic disease and even death when untreated. Infection manifests itself in distinct stages with different symptoms and clinical manifestations. Primary syphilis is characterized by a primary lesion, the chancre, which appears 5 to 90 days after infection (Fig. 4.3, *A*). This lesion often begins as a painless papule at the site of inoculation and erodes to form a nontender, shallow, indurated, clean ulcer several millimeters to centimeters in size. Secondary syphilis occurs 6 weeks to 6 months after the appearance of the chancre. It is characterized by a widespread, symmetric, maculopapular rash on the palms and soles and generalized lymphadenopathy.

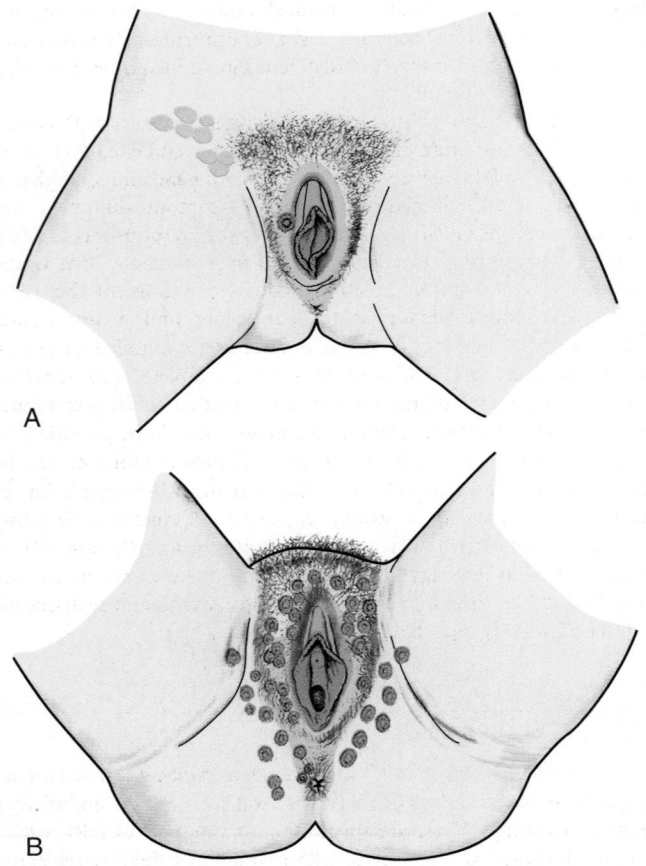

FIG 4.3 Syphilis. **A,** Primary stage: chancre with inguinal adenopathy. **B,** Secondary stage: condylomata lata.

The infected individual also may experience fever, headache, and malaise. Condylomata lata (broad, painless, pink-gray, wartlike infectious lesions) may develop on the vulva, perineum, or anus (see Fig. 4.3, *B*). If the woman is untreated, she enters a latent phase that is asymptomatic for the majority of individuals. Left untreated, about one-third of these women will develop tertiary syphilis. Neurologic, cardiovascular, musculoskeletal, or multiorgan system complications can develop in the third stage.

Screening and Diagnosis

All women who are diagnosed with another STI or with HIV should be screened for syphilis. All high-risk pregnant women should be screened for syphilis at the first prenatal visit, again in the late third trimester, and at the time of giving birth if high risk. Diagnosis depends on microscopic examination of primary and secondary lesion tissue and serology during latency and late infection. A test for antibodies may not be reactive in the presence of active infection because it takes time for the immune system of the body to develop antibodies to any antigens. Up to one-third of people with early primary syphilis may have nonreactive serologic tests. Two types of serologic tests are used: nontreponemal and treponemal. Nontreponemal antibody tests such as Venereal Disease Research Laboratory (VDRL) and rapid plasma reagin (RPR) are used as screening tests. False-positive results are not unusual, particularly when conditions such as acute infection, autoimmune disorders, malignancy, pregnancy, and drug addiction exist and after immunization or vaccination. The treponemal tests, fluorescent treponemal antibody absorbed, and microhemagglutination assays for antibody to *T. pallidum* are used to confirm positive results. Test results in patients with early primary or incubating syphilis may be negative. Seroconversion usually takes place 6 to 8 weeks after exposure; thus testing should be repeated in 1 to 2 months when a suggestive genital lesion exists.

Tests (e.g., wet preparations and cultures) for concomitant STIs (e.g., chlamydia, gonorrhea) should be done. HIV testing is also offered if indicated.

Management

Penicillin G is the preferred drug for treating patients with all stages of syphilis, including pregnant women (see Table 4.3). Although doxycycline, tetracycline, and erythromycin are alternative treatments for penicillin-allergic patients, both tetracycline and doxycycline are contraindicated in pregnancy, and erythromycin is unlikely to cure a fetal infection. Therefore if necessary, pregnant women should receive skin testing and be treated with penicillin or be desensitized. Specific protocols are recommended by the CDC (2017b).

> **⚠ NURSING ALERT**
>
> Patients treated for syphilis may experience a Jarisch-Herxheimer reaction. This is an acute febrile reaction often accompanied by headache, myalgias, and arthralgias that develop within the first 24 hours of treatment. The reaction may be treated symptomatically with analgesics and antipyretics. If treatment precipitates this reaction in the second half of pregnancy, women are at risk for preterm labor and birth. They should be advised to contact their health care provider if they notice any change in fetal movement or have any contractions.

Monthly follow-up is mandatory, so repeated treatment may be given if needed. The nurse should emphasize the necessity of long-term serologic testing even in the absence of symptoms. The woman should be advised to practice sexual abstinence until treatment is completed, all evidence of primary and secondary syphilis is gone, and serologic evidence of a cure is demonstrated. Women should be told to notify all partners who may have been exposed. They should be informed that the disease is reportable. Preventive measures should be discussed.

> **LEGAL TIP Reporting a Communicable Disease** Both gonorrhea and syphilis are reportable communicable diseases (CDC, 2015). Health care providers are legally responsible for reporting all cases of gonorrhea and syphilis to health authorities, usually the local health department in the patient's county of residence. Women should be informed that the case will be reported, told why, and informed of the possibility of being contacted by a health department epidemiologist.

Pelvic Inflammatory Disease

Pelvic inflammatory disease (PID) is an infectious process that most commonly involves the uterine tubes, causing salpingitis; the uterus, causing endometritis; and, more rarely, the ovaries and peritoneal surfaces. Multiple organisms have been found to cause PID. In the past, the most common causative organisms were *N. gonorrhoeae* and *C. trachomatis*, as well as a wide variety of anaerobic and aerobic bacteria. PID encompasses a wide variety of pathologic processes; the infection can be acute, subacute, or chronic and can have a wide range of symptoms.

Most PID results from the ascending spread of microorganisms from the vagina and endocervix to the upper genital tract. This spread most commonly occurs at the end of or just after menses following reception of an infectious agent. During the menstrual period, several factors facilitate the development of an infection: the cervical os is slightly open, the cervical mucus barrier is absent, and menstrual blood is an excellent medium for growth. PID also may develop after a miscarriage or an induced abortion, pelvic surgery, or childbirth.

Risk factors for acquiring PID are those associated with the risk for contracting an STI, including young age, multiple partners, high rate of new partners, and a history of STIs. Women who use IUDs may be at increased risk for PID if they have more than one sexual partner or if the partner has other sexual partners because they are at higher risk for acquiring an STI. Most of this risk occurs at the time of placement and in the 3 weeks after IUD insertion (Gardella et al., 2017). PID tends to recur.

Women who have had PID are at increased risk for ectopic pregnancy, infertility, and chronic pelvic pain. After a single episode of PID, a woman's risk for ectopic pregnancy increases sevenfold compared with the risk for women who have never had it. Other problems associated with PID include dyspareunia, pyosalpinx (pus in the uterine tubes), tubo-ovarian abscess, and pelvic adhesions.

The symptoms of PID vary, depending on whether the infection is acute, subacute, or chronic; however, pain is common to all types of infection. It may be dull, cramping, intermittent (subacute) or severe, persistent, and incapacitating (acute). Women may also report one or more of the following: fever, chills, nausea and vomiting, increased vaginal discharge, symptoms of a urinary tract infection, and irregular bleeding. Abdominal pain is usually present.

Screening and Diagnosis

PID is difficult to diagnose because of the accompanying wide variety of symptoms. The CDC (2017b) recommends treatment for PID in all sexually active young women and others at risk for STIs if the following criteria are present and no other cause or causes of the illness are found: lower abdominal tenderness, bilateral adnexal tenderness, and cervical motion tenderness. Other criteria for diagnosing PID include an oral temperature of 38.3° C (100.9° F) or above, abnormal cervical or vaginal discharge, elevated erythrocyte sedimentation rate, elevated C-reactive protein, and laboratory documentation of cervical infection with *N. gonorrhoeae* or *C. trachomatis*. Elevated C-reactive protein is not considered to be reliable in guiding treatment (Gardella, Eckert, & Lentz, 2017).

Management

Perhaps the most important nursing intervention is prevention counseling. Primary prevention includes education in avoiding contracting STIs; secondary prevention involves preventing a lower genital tract infection from ascending to the upper genital tract. Instructing women in self-protective behaviors such as practices to avoid contracting STIs and using barrier methods is critical. Women using hormonal contraception or an IUD and those who have chosen tubal ligation must be reminded to use a condom with intercourse when indicated. Also important is the detection of asymptomatic gonorrheal and chlamydial infections through routine screening of women who practice risky behaviors or have specific risk factors such as age.

Although treatment regimens vary with the infecting organism, generally a broad-spectrum antibiotic is used (Gardella et al., 2017). Treatment for mild-to–moderately severe PID may be oral (e.g., ceftriaxone plus doxycycline with or without metronidazole) or parenteral (e.g., cefotetan or cefoxitin plus doxycycline [oral]), and regimens can be administered in inpatient or outpatient settings. It was previously recommended that pregnant women be hospitalized and given parenteral antibiotics, but current guidelines do not support this practice (Gardella et al.).

The woman with acute PID should be on bed rest in a semi-Fowler's position. Comfort measures include analgesics for pain and all other nursing measures applicable to a patient confined to bed. Few pelvic examinations should be done during the acute phase of the disease. During the recovery phase, the woman should restrict her activity and make every effort to get adequate rest and a nutritionally sound diet. Follow-up laboratory work after treatment should include endocervical cultures for a test of cure.

Health education is central to effective management of PID. Nurses should explain the nature of the disease to women and encourage them to comply with all therapy and prevention recommendations, emphasizing the need to take all medication, even if symptoms disappear. Any potential problems (such as a lack of money for prescriptions or a lack of transportation to return for follow-up appointments) that would prevent a woman from completing a course of treatment should be identified, referrals made for assistance as needed, and the importance of follow-up visits stressed. Women should be counseled to refrain from sexual intercourse until their treatment is completed. Contraceptive counseling, including information on barrier methods such as condoms, the contraceptive sponge, and the diaphragm, should be provided.

The potential or actual loss of reproductive capabilities can be devastating and can adversely affect the woman's self-concept. Part of the nurse's role is to help the woman adjust her self-concept to fit reality and accept alterations in a way that promotes health. Because PID is so closely tied to sexuality, body image, and self-concept, the woman diagnosed with it needs supportive care. Her feelings should be discussed, and her partner(s) included when appropriate.

SEXUALLY TRANSMITTED VIRAL INFECTIONS

Human Papillomavirus

Human papillomavirus (HPV), also known as *condylomata acuminata* or *genital warts,* is the most common viral STI seen in ambulatory health care settings. There are approximately 100 types of HPV, which is a double-stranded DNA virus, with about 40 of these types found to be causes of anogenital infections. There are several that can cause genital cancers, with two specific types (16 and 18) that are highly

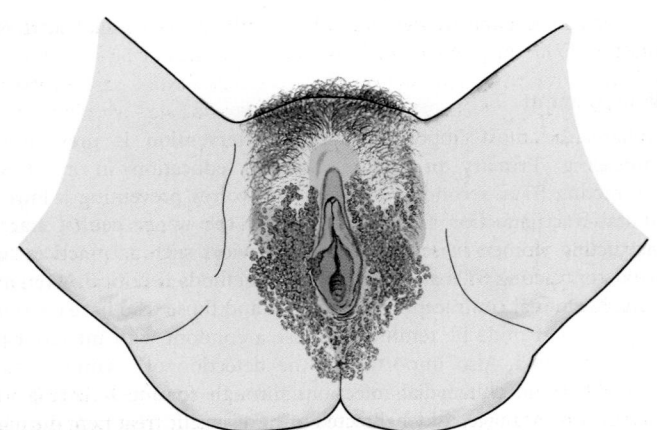

FIG 4.4 Human papillomavirus infection. Genital warts or condylomataacuminata.

oncogenic, meaning they are highest risk for causing cancers of the cervix, vagina, vulva, penis, and oropharyngeal area (CDC, 2017b). HPV is the primary cause of cervical neoplasia.

In women, HPV lesions are most commonly seen in the posterior part of the introitus. Lesions also are found on the buttocks, vulva, vagina, anus, and cervix (Fig. 4.4). Typically the lesions are small (2 to 3 mm in diameter and 10 to 15 mm in height), soft, papillary swellings occurring singly or in clusters on the genital and anal-rectal region. Infections of long duration may appear as a cauliflower-like mass. In moist areas such as the vaginal introitus, the lesions may appear to have multiple fine, fingerlike projections. Vaginal lesions are often multiple. Flat-topped papules, 1 to 4 mm in diameter, are seen most often on the cervix. Often these lesions are visualized only under magnification. Warts are usually flesh colored or slightly darker on Caucasian women, black on African-American women, and brownish on Asian women. The lesions are usually painless; but they may be uncomfortable, particularly when very large, inflamed, or ulcerated. Chronic vaginal discharge, pruritus, or dyspareunia can occur.

HPV infections are thought to be more common in pregnant than in nonpregnant women, with an increase in incidence from the first trimester to the third trimester. Furthermore, a significant proportion of preexisting HPV lesions enlarge greatly during pregnancy, a proliferation presumably resulting from the relative state of immunosuppression present during this period. Lesions may become so large during pregnancy that they affect urination, defecation, mobility, and fetal descent, although birth by cesarean is rarely necessary. Cesarean birth may be performed when extensive growths are present. Initial observation of large growths can be misleading, suggesting that the entire vagina is involved. However, all of the growth may derive from one stalk; and in such cases it may be possible to push the large mass to the side, allowing the baby to pass through.

Screening and Diagnosis

A woman with HPV lesions may complain of symptoms such as a profuse, irritating vaginal discharge; itching; dyspareunia; or postcoital bleeding. She also may report "bumps" on her vulva or labia. History of a known exposure is important; however, because of the potentially long latency period and the possibility of subclinical infections in men, the lack of a history of known exposure cannot be used to exclude a diagnosis of HPV infection.

Physical inspection of the vulva, the perineum, the anus, the vagina, and the cervix is essential whenever HPV lesions are suspected or seen in one area. Because speculum examination of the vagina may block some lesions, it is important to rotate the speculum blades until all areas are visualized. When lesions are visible, the characteristic appearance previously described is considered diagnostic. However, in many instances cervical lesions are not visible, and some vaginal or vulvar lesions also may be unobservable to the naked eye. Because of the potential spread of vulvar or vaginal lesions to the anus, gloves should be changed between vaginal and rectal examinations.

Viral screening and typing for HPV are available but not standard practice. History, evaluation of signs and symptoms, Papanicolaou (Pap) test, and physical examination are used in making a diagnosis. The HPV-DNA test can be used in women older than 30 years of age in combination with the Pap test to screen for types of HPV that are likely to cause cancer or in women with abnormal Pap test results American Cancer Society (ACS, 2016). (ACS, 2016b). The only definitive diagnostic test for presence of HPV is histologic evaluation of a biopsy specimen.

Management

Untreated warts may resolve on their own in young women since their immune systems may be strong enough to fight the HPV infection. Treatment of genital warts, if needed, is often difficult. No therapy has been shown to eradicate HPV. Therefore the goal of treatment is removal of warts and relief of signs and symptoms. The patient often must make multiple office visits; frequently many different treatment modalities will be used.

Treatment of genital warts should be guided by preference of the woman, available resources, and experience of the health care provider. No one of the treatments is superior to all other treatments, and no one treatment is ideal for all warts (CDC, 2017b). Imiquimod, podophyllin, and podofilox are common treatments but should not be used during pregnancy because there is limited data on the safety of such treatments (see Table 4.3). Because the lesions can proliferate and become friable during pregnancy, many experts recommend their removal using cryotherapy or various surgical techniques, and providers must be specifically trained in such techniques (CDC).

Women who have discomfort associated with genital warts may find that bathing with an oatmeal solution and drying the area with cool air from a hair dryer provides some relief. Keeping the area clean and dry also decreases the growth of the warts. Cotton underwear and loose-fitting clothes that decrease friction and irritation may lessen discomfort. Women should be advised to maintain a healthy lifestyle to aid the immune system and be counseled regarding diet, rest, stress reduction, and exercise.

Patient counseling is essential. Women must understand the virus, how it is transmitted, that no immunity is conferred with infection, and that reinfection is likely with repeated contact (CDC, 2017b). Counseling includes all sexually active women with multiple partners or a history of HPV to use latex condoms for intercourse to decrease acquisition or transmission of the infection. Semiannual or annual health examinations are recommended to assess disease recurrence and screening for cervical cancer. Women who have been treated for HPV infections should have at least annual Pap tests.

Prevention

Preventive strategies that have been suggested include abstinence from all sexual activity, staying in a long-term monogamous relationship, and prophylactic vaccination. Two vaccines, Cervarix and Gardasil, are available; other vaccines continue to be investigated. Cervarix prevents infection from HPV viruses 16 and 18, whereas Gardasil prevents infection from viruses 6, 11, 16, and 18. Both can be administered to girls and women 9 to 26 years of age. The CDC recommends 2 doses for girls ages 9 to 14, and 3 doses for girls and young women ages 15 to 26 (Meites, Kempe, & Markowitz, 2016). Boys, too, can be vaccinated, beginning at 9 to 21 years of age (CDC, 2017b). Practitioners should stay current with results of these clinical trials and make recommendations about vaccination based on the outcomes of the research.

Herpes Simplex Virus

Unknown until the middle of the twentieth century, herpes simplex virus (HSV) infection is now widespread in the United States, especially in women. It results in painful, recurrent ulcers. It is caused by two different antigen subtypes of HSV: HSV type 1 (HSV-1) and HSV type 2 (HSV-2). HSV-2 is usually transmitted sexually, and HSV-1 nonsexually. Although HSV-1 is more commonly associated with gingivostomatitis and oral labial ulcers (fever blisters) and HSV-2 with genital lesions, neither type is exclusively associated with the respective sites.

Although HSV infection is not a reportable disease, it is estimated that approximately 75% of people who have sex with an infected partner will become infected themselves with this incurable virus (Gardella et al., 2017). Women between 15 and 34 years of age are most likely to become infected, especially if they have multiple partners. Recurrent HSV infections are much more common. Most persons infected with HSV-2 have not been diagnosed, and most infections are transmitted by persons who are unaware that they are infected.

An initial HSV genital infection is characterized by multiple painful lesions, fever, chills, malaise, and severe dysuria and may last 2 to 3 weeks. Women generally have a more severe clinical course than do men. Women with primary genital herpes have many lesions that progress from macules to papules; they then progress to form vesicles, pustules, and ulcers that crust and heal without scarring (Fig. 4.5). These ulcers are extremely tender, and primary infections may be bilateral. Women also may have itching, inguinal tenderness, and lymphadenopathy. Severe vulvar edema may develop, and women may have difficulty sitting. HSV cervicitis is common with initial HSV-2 infections. The cervix may appear normal or be friable, reddened, ulcerated, or necrotic. A heavy, watery-to-purulent vaginal discharge is common. Extragenital lesions may be present because of autoinoculation. Urinary retention and dysuria may occur secondary to autonomic involvement of the sacral nerve root.

Women with recurrent episodes of HSV infections commonly have only local symptoms that are usually less severe than those associated with the initial infection. Systemic symptoms are usually absent, although the characteristic prodromal genital tingling is common. Recurrent lesions are unilateral, are less severe, and usually last 5 to 7 days. Lesions begin as vesicles and progress rapidly to ulcers. Few women with recurrent disease have cervicitis.

During pregnancy, maternal infection with HSV-2 can have adverse effects on both the mother and fetus. Viremia occurs during the primary infection, and congenital infection is possible although rare. Primary infections during the first trimester have been associated with increased miscarriage rates (CDC, 2017b).

Screening and Diagnosis

Although a diagnosis of herpes infection may be suspected from the history and physical examination, it is confirmed by laboratory studies. A viral culture is obtained by swabbing exudate during the vesicular stage of the disease.

Management

Genital herpes is a chronic and recurring disease for which there is no known cure. Management is directed toward specific treatment during primary and recurrent infections, prevention, self-help measures, and psychologic support.

Oral medications used for treating the first clinical HSV infection include acyclovir, famciclovir, and valacyclovir. These medications are considered for episodic or suppressive therapy for recurrent HSV. Intravenous acyclovir may be used for women with severe disease . The safety of acyclovir, valacyclovir, and famciclovir therapy during pregnancy has not been established; however, acyclovir may be used to reduce the symptoms of HSV if the benefits to the woman outweigh the potential harm to the fetus, and this decision to treat must be discussed with the woman's health care provider . Continued investigation of HSV therapy with these medications during pregnancy is needed.

Cleaning lesions twice a day with saline helps prevent secondary infection. Bacterial infection must be treated with appropriate antibiotics. Measures that may increase comfort for women when lesions are active include warm sitz baths with baking soda; keeping lesions dry by using cool air from a hair dryer or patting dry with a soft towel; wearing cotton underwear and loose clothing; using drying aids such as hydrogen peroxide, Burow's solution, or oatmeal baths; and applying cool, wet, black tea bags to lesions. Women can also apply compresses with an infusion of cloves or peppermint oil and clove oil to lesions.

Oral analgesics such as aspirin or ibuprofen may be used to relieve pain and systemic symptoms associated with initial infections. Because the mucous membranes affected by herpes are extremely sensitive, any topical agents should be used with caution. Nonantiviral ointments, especially those containing cortisone, should be avoided. A thin layer of lidocaine ointment or an antiseptic spray may be applied to decrease discomfort, especially if walking is difficult.

Counseling and education are critical components of the nursing care of women with herpes infections. Information regarding the etiology, signs and symptoms, transmission, and treatment should be provided. The nurse should explain that each woman is unique in her response to herpes and emphasize the variability of symptoms. Women should be helped to understand when viral shedding and thus transmission to a partner are most likely. They should be counseled to refrain from sexual contact from the onset of prodrome until complete healing of lesions.

Some authorities recommend consistent use of condoms for all persons with genital herpes. Condoms may not prevent transmission, particularly male-to-female transmission; however, this does not mean that the partners should avoid all intimacy. Women can be encouraged to maintain close contact with their partners while avoiding contact with lesions. They should be taught how to look for herpetic lesions using a mirror and good light source and a wet cloth or finger covered with a finger cot to rub lightly over the labia. The nurse should ensure that women understand that, when lesions are active, sharing intimate articles (e.g., washcloths or wet towels) that come into contact with the

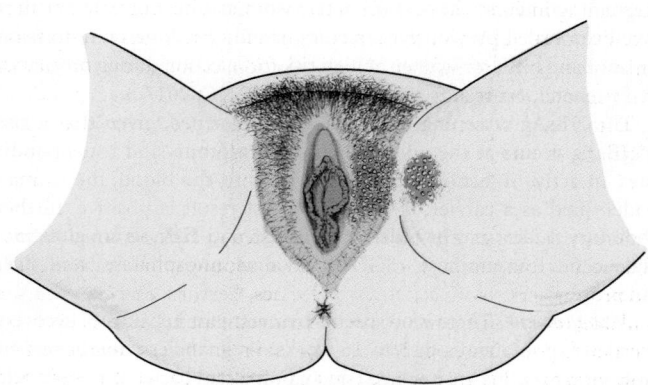

FIG 4.5 Herpes genitalis.

lesions should be avoided. Only plain soap and water are needed to clean hands that have come in contact with herpetic lesions; isolation is neither necessary nor appropriate.

Stress, menstruation, trauma, febrile illnesses, chronic illness, and ultraviolet light have all been found to trigger genital herpes. Women may wish to keep a diary to identify stressors that seem to be associated with recurrent herpes attacks so they can avoid these stressors when possible. The role of exercise in reducing stress can be discussed. Referral for stress-reduction therapy, yoga, or meditation classes may be indicated. Avoiding excessive heat, sun, and hot baths and using a lubricant during sexual intercourse to reduce friction also may be helpful. Women in their childbearing years should be counseled regarding the risk for herpes infection during pregnancy. They should be instructed to use condoms if there is any risk for contracting an STI from a sexual partner. If they become pregnant while taking acyclovir, the risk for birth defects does not appear to be higher than for the general population; however, continued use should be based on whether the benefits for the woman outweigh the possible risks to the fetus. Acyclovir does enter breast milk, but the amount of medication ingested during breastfeeding is very low and usually not a health concern (CDC, 2017c).

Because neonatal HSV infection is such a devastating disease, prevention is critical. Women with a history of HSV are often placed on acyclovir for suppression during the last few weeks of pregnancy to try to prevent an outbreak at the time of labor and birth. This could prevent the need for cesarean birth and also decrease the risk of neonatal infection. Current recommendations include carefully examining and questioning all women about symptoms at onset of labor (CDC, 2017c). If visible lesions or prodromal symptoms are not present at onset of labor, vaginal birth is acceptable. Cesarean birth within 4 hours after labor begins or membranes rupture is recommended if visible lesions are present. Infants who are born through an infected vagina should be observed carefully and cultured. Some experts recommend presumptive treatment of infants who were exposed to HSV during birth. Because HSV infection may be associated with cervical dysplasia, women must be encouraged to have annual Pap tests and gynecologic examinations.

The emotional effect of contracting an incurable STI such as herpes is considerable. At diagnosis, many emotions may surface—helplessness, anger, denial, guilt, anxiety, shame, or inadequacy. Women need the opportunity to discuss their feelings and help in learning to live with the disease. Herpes can affect a woman's sexuality, her sexual practices, and her current and future relationships. She may need help in raising the issue with her partner or future partners.

Hepatitis

Five different viruses (hepatitis viruses A, B, C, D, and E) account for almost all cases of viral hepatitis in humans. Hepatitis viruses A, B, and C are discussed here. Hepatitis D and E viruses, common among users of intravenous drugs and recipients of multiple blood transfusions, are not included in this discussion.

Hepatitis A

Hepatitis A virus (HAV) infection is acquired primarily through the fecal-oral route by ingestion of contaminated food, particularly milk, shellfish, or polluted water, or via person-to-person contact. Influenza-like symptoms with malaise, fatigue, anorexia, nausea, pruritus, fever, and upper–right-quadrant pain characterize HAV infection. Serologic testing to detect the immunoglobulin M (IgM) antibody confirms acute infections. Because HAV infection is self-limited and does not result in chronic infection or chronic liver disease, treatment is usually supportive. Women who become dehydrated from nausea and vomiting or who have fulminating hepatitis A may need to be hospitalized. Medications that might cause liver damage or that are metabolized in the liver should be used with caution. No specific diet or activity restrictions are necessary. Hepatitis A vaccine and immunoglobulin (IG) for intramuscular administration are effective in preventing most hepatitis A infections (CDC, 2017c).

Hepatitis B

Hepatitis B virus (HBV) infection is an STI and is the virus most threatening to the fetus and neonate. It is caused by a large DNA virus and is associated with three antigens and their antibodies: hepatitis B surface antigen (HBsAg), HBV antigen (HBeAg), HBV core antigen (HBcAg), antibody to HBsAg (anti-HBs), antibody to HBeAg (anti-HBe), and antibody to HBcAg (anti-HBc). Screening for active or chronic disease or disease immunity is based on testing for these antigens and their antibodies.

Populations at risk include women of Asian, Pacific Island (Polynesian, Micronesian, Melanesian), or Alaskan-Eskimo descent and those born in Haiti or sub-Saharan Africa. Women who have a history of acute or chronic liver disease, who work or receive treatment in a dialysis unit, or who have household or sexual contact with a hemodialysis patient are at greater risk. Women who work or live in institutions for the mentally handicapped are considered to be at risk, as are those with a history of multiple blood transfusions. Health care workers and public safety workers exposed to blood in the workplace are at risk. Behaviors such as multiple sexual partners and a history of intravenous drug use increase the risk for contracting HBV infections.

HBsAg has been found in blood, saliva, sweat, tears, vaginal secretions, and semen. Drug abusers who share needles are at risk. Perinatal transmission most often occurs in infants of mothers who have acute hepatitis infection late in the third trimester or during the intrapartum or postpartum periods from exposure to HBsAg-positive vaginal secretions, blood, amniotic fluid, saliva, and breast milk. HBsAg has also been transmitted by artificial insemination. Although it can be transmitted by blood transfusion, the incidence of such infections has decreased significantly since testing of blood for HBsAg became routine.

HBV infection is a disease of the liver and is often a silent infection. In the adult, its course can be fulminating and the outcome fatal. Symptoms of HBV infection are similar to those of hepatitis A: arthralgias, arthritis, lassitude, anorexia, nausea, vomiting, headache, fever, and mild abdominal pain. Later the woman may have clay-colored stools, dark urine, increased abdominal pain, and jaundice. Between 5% and 10% of individuals with HBV have persistent HBsAg and become chronic hepatitis B carriers.

Screening and diagnosis. All women at high risk for contracting HBV should be screened on a regular basis. However, screening only individuals at high risk may not identify up to 50% of HBsAg-positive women. Screening for the presence of HBsAg is recommended on all pregnant women at the first prenatal visit, regardless of whether they have been tested previously; screening should be done on admission for labor and birth for women at high risk for infection during pregnancy or if prenatal test results are not available (CDC, 2017c).

The HBsAg screening test is usually performed, given that a rise in HBsAg occurs at the onset of clinical symptoms and usually indicates an active infection. If HBsAg persists in the blood, the woman is identified as a carrier. If the HBsAg test result is positive, further laboratory studies may be ordered: anti-HBe, anti-HBc, serum glutamic-oxaloacetic transaminase (SGOT), alkaline phosphatase, and liver panel.

Management. There is no specific treatment for hepatitis B. Recovery is usually spontaneous in 3 to 16 weeks. Pregnancies complicated by acute viral hepatitis are managed on an outpatient basis. Women should be advised to increase bed rest; eat a high-protein, low-fat diet; and increase their fluid intake. They should avoid medications metabolized in the liver and alcohol. Pregnant women with a definite exposure to HBV should be given HBIG and begin the hepatitis B vaccine series within 14 days of the most recent contact to prevent infection (CDC, 2017c). Vaccination during pregnancy is not thought to pose risks to the fetus.

All nonimmune women at high or moderate risk for hepatitis should be informed of the availability of hepatitis B vaccine. Vaccination is recommended for all individuals who have had multiple sex partners within the past 6 months (CDC, 2017b). In addition, intravenous drug users, residents of correctional or long-term care facilities, persons seeking care for an STI, prostitutes, women whose partners are intravenous drug users or bisexual, and women whose occupation exposes them to high risk should be vaccinated. The vaccine is given in a series of three (four if rapid protection is needed) doses over a 6-month period, with the first two doses given at least 1 month apart. The vaccine is given in the deltoid muscle.

Patient education includes explaining the meaning of hepatitis B infection, including transmission, state of infectivity, and sequelae. The nurse also should explain the need for immunoprophylaxis for household members and sexual contacts. To decrease transmission of the virus, women with hepatitis B or those who test positive for HBV should be advised to maintain a high level of personal hygiene (e.g., wash hands after using the toilet; carefully dispose of tampons, pads, and bandages in plastic bags; avoid sharing razor blades, toothbrushes, needles, or manicure implements; have male partner use a condom if unvaccinated and without hepatitis; avoid sharing saliva through kissing or sharing silverware or dishes; and wipe up blood spills immediately with soap and water). They should inform all health care providers of their carrier state. Postpartum women should be reassured that breastfeeding is not contraindicated if their infants received prophylaxis at birth and are currently on the immunization schedule.

Hepatitis C

Hepatitis C virus (HCV) infection is the most common chronic bloodborne infection in the United States and is responsible for nearly 50% of the cases of chronic viral hepatitis. It is estimated that 6% of infants born to HCV-infected pregnant women will actually become infected with HCV, with transmission occurring during the birth process. However, there is no known way to prevent such transmission (CDC, 2017b). The most common risk factor for pregnant women is a history of intravenous drug use. Other risk factors include STIs such as HBV and HIV, multiple sex partners, and a history of blood transfusions. HCV is readily transmitted through exposure to blood.

Currently there is no vaccine to prevent HCV. Its transmission through breastfeeding has not been reported. The CDC (2017b) does not recommend routine testing for HCV in pregnant women unless they are considered to be at high risk.

The Food and Drug Administration (US FDA, 2017) has approved several drugs for the treatment of hepatitis C, although more study is needed to determine the safety of these drugs during pregnancy.

Human Immunodeficiency Virus

Approximately 25% of people currently living with HIV are women, but over the past 10 years, there has been an estimated decrease of 40% of newly diagnosed cases of HIV in women (CDC, 2017c). The largest proportion of HIV is found in African-American women, followed by Caucasian and Hispanic/Latinas (CDC). There is also a high prevalence rate of HIV in transgender women (CDC).

Severe depression of the cellular immune system associated with HIV infection characterizes acquired immunodeficiency syndrome (AIDS). Although behaviors that place women at risk have been well documented, all women should be assessed for the possibility of HIV exposure. The most commonly reported opportunistic diseases are *Pneumocystis (jirovecii)* pneumonia (PCP), *Candida* esophagitis, and wasting syndrome. Other viral infections such as HSV and cytomegalovirus infections seem to be more prevalent in women than in men. There is a higher incidence of adnexal masses in women with PID who are also HIV positive, but antibiotics are often as effective in HIV-positive women with PID as they are in HIV-negative women with PID (Gardella et al., 2017). The clinical course of HPV infection in women with HIV infection is accelerated, and recurrence is more frequent in non–HIV-infected women.

Once HIV enters the body, seroconversion to HIV positivity usually occurs within 6 to 12 weeks. Although HIV seroconversion may be totally asymptomatic, it usually is accompanied by a viremic, influenza-like response. Symptoms include fever, headache, night sweats, malaise, generalized lymphadenopathy, myalgias, nausea, diarrhea, weight loss, sore throat, and rash.

Laboratory studies may reveal leukopenia, thrombocytopenia, anemia, and an elevated erythrocyte sedimentation rate. HIV has a strong affinity for surface-marker proteins on T lymphocytes. This affinity leads to significant T-cell destruction. Both clinical and epidemiologic studies have shown that declining CD4 levels are strongly associated with increased incidence of AIDS-related diseases and death in many different groups of HIV-infected persons.

Screening and Diagnosis

Screening, teaching, and counseling regarding HIV risk factors; indications for being tested; and testing are major roles for nurses caring for women today. A number of behaviors place women at risk for HIV infection, including intravenous drug use, high-risk sex partners, multiple sex partners, and a previous history of multiple STIs. HIV infection is usually diagnosed by using HIV-1 and HIV-2 antibody tests. Antibody testing is done first with a sensitive screening test such as the enzyme immunoassay. Reactive screening tests must be confirmed by an additional test such as the Western blot or an immunofluorescence assay. If a positive antibody test is confirmed by a supplemental test, it means that a woman is infected with HIV and is capable of infecting others. HIV antibodies are detectable in at least 95% of patients within 3 months after infection. Although a negative antibody test usually indicates that a person is not infected, antibody tests cannot exclude recent infection.

The FDA has approved six methods of rapid testing for HIV, variously using a blood sample obtained by fingerstick or venipuncture, serum, or plasma or an oral fluid sample. The tests have accuracy rates of 98% to 99%. If the results are reactive, further testing is done. Quick results mean that patients do not have to make extra visits for follow-up standard tests, and the oral test provides an option for patients who do not want to have a blood test.

The CDC (2016b) recommends offering HIV testing to all women whose behavior places them at risk for HIV infection. It may be useful to allow women to self-select for HIV testing. On entry to the health care system, a woman can be handed written information about the risk factors for the AIDS virus and asked to inform the nurse if she believes she is at risk. She should be told that she does not have to say why she may be at risk, only that she thinks she might be.

Counseling for HIV Testing

All pregnant women should receive HIV risk-reduction counseling and be notified that they will be tested for antibody to HIV as part of the routine prenatal testing unless the test is declined (American Academy of Pediatrics [AAP] & ACOG, 2012) (Box 4.4). Counseling before and after HIV testing is standard nursing practice today. It is a nursing responsibility to assess a woman's understanding of the information

BOX 4.4 Human Immunodeficiency Virus Screening

- Pregnant women are ethically obligated to seek reasonable care during pregnancy and to avoid causing harm to the fetus. Women's health nurses should be advocates for the fetus while also showing acceptance of the pregnant woman's decision regarding testing and/or treatment for HIV.
- Without treatment, the incidence of perinatal transmission from an HIV-positive mother to her fetus is approximately 25%. Triple-drug antiviral or highly active antiretroviral therapy (HAART) during pregnancy decreases perinatal transmission to less than 1% (CDC, 2014).
- The Centers for Disease Control and Prevention (CDC, 2014) recommend testing for HIV infections for all pregnant women as early as possible in pregnancy and a second test in the third trimester for women in certain geographic areas and those who are at high risk for HIV infection.
- Testing has the potential to identify HIV-positive women who can then be treated. Health care providers have an obligation to ensure that pregnant women are well informed about HIV symptoms, testing, and methods of decreasing maternal-fetal transmission. The CDC and the American College of Obstetricians and Gynecologists (ACOG) recommend universal opt-out screening, which means that all pregnant women are offered HIV screening but have the opportunity to opt-out if desired (ACOG, 2011; CDC, 2014). The Association of Women's Health, Obstetric and Neonatal Nurses (AWHONN, 2008) supports this system of HIV screening that allows all pregnant women to be offered screening.

From American College of Obstetricians and Gynecologists. (2011). Committee opinion no. 418. Prenatal and perinatal human immunodeficiency virus testing—Expanded recommendations. *Obstetrics & Gynecology, 104*(5 Part 1), 1119–1124; AWHONN. (2008). *HIV screening procedures for pregnant women and newborns—Policy position statement.* Washington, DC: Author; Centers for Disease Control and Prevention. (2014). Reducing HIV transmission from mother-to-child: An opt-out approach to HIV screening. Retrieved from www.cdc.gov/hiv/group/gender/pregnantwomen/opt-out.html.

such a test would provide and to be sure the woman thoroughly understands the emotional, legal, and medical implications of a positive or negative test before the test is performed.

! NURSING ALERT

Counseling associated with HIV testing has two components: pretest and posttest. During pretest counseling, a personalized risk assessment is conducted, the meaning of positive and negative test results is explained, informed consent for HIV testing is obtained, and women are helped to develop a realistic plan for reducing risk and preventing infection. Posttest counseling includes informing the patient of the test results, reviewing the meaning of the results, and reinforcing prevention messages. All pretest and posttest counseling should be documented.

Given the strong social stigma attached to HIV infection, nurses must consider the issue of confidentiality and documentation before providing counseling and offering HIV testing to patients.

LEGAL TIP HIV Testing If HIV test results are placed in the patient's medical record, the appropriate place for all health information, they are available to all who have access to the medical record. The woman is informed of this availability before testing. Informed consent must be obtained before an HIV test is performed. In some states, written consent is mandated. In many sites, HIV testing is performed unless a patient declines to be tested (i.e., opt-out testing). Nurses must know which procedures are being used for informed consent in their facility.

Unless rapid testing is done, there is generally a 1- to 3-week waiting period after testing for HIV before test results become available; this can be a very anxious time for the woman. It is helpful if the nurse informs her that this time period between blood drawing and test results is routine. Test results must always be communicated in person, and the woman should be informed in advance that this is the procedure. Whenever possible, the person who provided the pretest counseling should also tell the woman her test results.

When some women are informed of negative results, they may escalate risk behaviors because they equate negativity with immunity. Others may believe that negative means "bad" and positive means "good." The woman's reaction to a negative test should be explored by asking, "How do you feel?" Counseling sessions for women with an HIV-negative result are another opportunity to provide education. Emphasis can be placed on ways in which a woman can remain HIV free. She should be reminded that, if she has been exposed to HIV in the past 6 months, she should be retested, and that she should have ongoing testing if she continues high-risk behaviors.

In posttest counseling of an HIV-positive woman, privacy with no interruptions is essential. Adequate time for the counseling sessions also should be provided. The nurse should make sure that the woman understands what a positive test means and review the reliability of the test results. Risk-reduction practices should be reemphasized. Referral for appropriate medical evaluation and follow-up should be made, and the need or desire for psychosocial or psychiatric referrals should be assessed.

The importance of early medical evaluation so a baseline assessment can be made and prophylactic medication begun should be stressed. If possible, the nurse should make a referral or appointment for the woman at the posttest counseling session.

Management

During the initial contact with an HIV-infected woman, the nurse should establish what the woman knows about HIV infection and that she is being cared for by a health care provider or facility with expertise in caring for persons with HIV infections, including AIDS. Psychologic referral also may be indicated. Resources such as counseling for financial assistance, legal advocacy, suicide prevention, and death and dying may be appropriate. All women who are drug users should be referred to a substance-abuse program. A major focus of counseling is prevention of transmission of HIV to partners.

Nurses counseling seropositive women wishing contraceptive information can recommend oral contraceptives and latex condoms or tubal sterilization or vasectomy and latex condoms. The nurse can suggest female condoms or abstinence to women whose male partners refuse to use condoms.

No cure is available for HIV infections at this time. Rare and unusual diseases are characteristic of HIV infections. Opportunistic infections and concurrent diseases are managed vigorously with treatment specific to the infection or disease. Routine gynecologic care for HIV-positive women should include a pelvic examination every 6 months. Thorough Pap screening is essential because of the greatly increased incidence of abnormal findings on examination. In addition, HIV-positive women should be screened for syphilis, gonorrhea, chlamydia, and other vaginal infections and treated if infections are present. General prevention strategies are an important part of care (e.g., smoking cessation, sound nutrition) as is antiretroviral therapy. Discussion of the medical care of HIV-positive women or women with AIDS is beyond the scope of this chapter because of the rapidly changing recommendations. The reader is referred to the CDC (www.cdc.gov), AIDS hotline (800-342-2437), and Internet websites such as HIV/AIDS Treatment Information Service (www.hivatis.org) for current information and recommendations.

Pregnancy and Human Immunodeficiency Virus

Transmission of the virus from mother to infant can occur throughout the perinatal period. Exposure may occur to the fetus through the maternal circulation as early as the first trimester of pregnancy, to the infant during labor and birth by inoculation or ingestion of maternal blood and other infected fluids, or to the infant through breast milk. Because the HIV antibody crosses the placenta, definite diagnosis of HIV in children younger than 18 months of age is based on laboratory evidence of HIV in blood or tissues by culture, nucleic acid, or antigen detection. With proper treatment and adherence to prescribed medication for both the pregnant women and, later, for her neonate, HIV-positive women can have a less than 1% chance of transmitting HIV to their babies (CDC, 2017c).

HIV counseling and testing should be offered to all women at their initial entry into prenatal care as part of routine prenatal testing unless the woman opts out of the screening. Universal testing versus selective testing for maternal HIV is recommended because it results in a greater number of women being screened and treated and can reduce the likelihood of perinatal transmission and maintain the health of the woman. The CDC (2017b) also recommends retesting in the third trimester for women known to be at high risk for HIV and rapid HIV testing in labor for women with unknown HIV status.

Perinatal transmission of HIV has decreased significantly in the past decade because of the administration of antiretroviral prophylaxis (e.g., zidovudine) to pregnant women in the prenatal and the perinatal periods. Treatment of HIV-infected women with the triple-drug antiviral therapy or highly active antiretroviral therapy (HAART) during pregnancy should be used for all HIV-infected women regardless of their CD4 cell counts (Hughes & Cu-Uvin, 2016). Women who are infected with HIV and need treatment for their own health should start the therapy as soon as possible, even in the first trimester, and continue throughout the pregnancy. Women who are taking the therapy as prophylaxis usually start therapy after the first trimester.

Antiviral therapy is administered orally and continued throughout pregnancy. The major side effect of this therapy is bone marrow suppression. Periodic hematocrit, white blood cell count, and platelet count assessments should be performed. Women who are HIV positive should also be vaccinated against hepatitis B, pneumococcal infection, *Haemophilus influenzae* type B, and viral influenza. To support any pregnant woman's immune system, appropriate counseling is provided about optimal nutrition, sleep, rest, exercise, and stress reduction. Use of condoms is encouraged to minimize further exposure to HIV if her partner is the source.

In the intrapartum period, antiretroviral therapy is recommended and the decision to have a cesarean birth versus a vaginal birth is dependent on the amount of viral load (Hughes & Cu-Uvin, 2016). The US Department of Health and Human Services Clinical Guidelines Portal (2015) recommends a scheduled cesarean birth at 38 weeks of gestation for women with a viral load of more than 1000 copies/mL. A vaginal birth may be an option for HIV-infected women who have a viral load of less than 1000 copies/mL at 36 weeks, if a woman has ruptured membranes and labor is progressing rapidly, or if she declines a cesarean birth. Intravenous zidovudine is recommended for all HIV-infected pregnant women during the intrapartum period, except for those with a low viral load (<1000 copies) who have been on highly active anti-retroviral therapy (HAART) during pregnancy (Choudhary, 2015). The drug is administered 3 hours before a scheduled cesarean birth and continued until the baby is born. It should be given during labor if the woman is having a vaginal birth, and to the infant for 6 weeks after birth (Hughes & Cu-Uvin). Fetal scalp electrode and scalp pH sampling should be avoided because these procedures may result in inoculation of the virus into the fetus. Similarly, the use of forceps or a vacuum extractor should be avoided when possible. Avoidance of breastfeeding is recommended in the United States and most developed countries (Hughes & Cu-Uvin).

Women who have HIV but who are without symptoms may have an unremarkable postpartum course. Immunosuppressed women with symptoms may be at increased risk for postpartum urinary tract infections (UTIs), vaginitis, postpartum endometritis, and poor wound healing. Good perineal hygiene should be stressed. Women who are HIV positive but who were not on antiretroviral drugs before pregnancy should be tested in the postpartum period to determine whether therapy that was initiated in pregnancy should be continued. After the initial bath, the newborn can be with the mother. In planning for discharge, comprehensive care and support services need to be arranged. After discharge, the woman and her infant are referred to health care providers who are experienced in the treatment of HIV and AIDS and associated conditions for intensive monitoring and follow-up.

Zika Virus

The Zika virus is spread by bites from the Aedes mosquito. It is also spread via sexual contact through semen. Women who become pregnant and are infected by the Zika virus have an increased risk for giving birth to an infant with microcephaly. Zika virus has also been associated with risk for Guillain-Barré syndrome, a neurologic condition that can lead to muscle weakness and possibly paralysis. The Aedes mosquito has been found predominantly in Africa, Southeast Asia, the Caribbean, Central America, South America, and the Pacific Islands, with a few recent cases found in the southeastern United States (CDC, 2016a). Pregnant women and women considering becoming pregnant should avoid traveling to areas that are known to have the Aedes mosquito. Women should use condoms with male partners who may have been exposed to the Zika virus (CDC, 2016a).

VAGINAL INFECTIONS

Vaginal discharge and itching of the vulva and vagina are among the most common reasons a woman seeks help from a health care provider. More women complain of vaginal discharge than any other gynecologic symptom. Women who have adequate endogenous or exogenous estrogen have vaginal secretions. Vaginal discharge resulting from infection must be distinguished from normal secretions. Normal vaginal secretions (or leukorrhea) are clear to cloudy in appearance. The discharge may turn yellow after drying; is slightly slimy; is nonirritating; and has a mild, inoffensive odor. Normal vaginal secretions are acidic, with a pH range of 4 to 5. The amount of leukorrhea differs with phases of the menstrual cycle, with greater amounts occurring at ovulation and just before menses. Leukorrhea is also increased during pregnancy. Normal vaginal secretions contain lactobacilli and epithelial cells.

Vaginitis, or abnormal vaginal discharge, is an infection caused by a microorganism. The most common vaginal infections are bacterial vaginosis (BV), candidiasis, and trichomoniasis. Although streptococcus B is considered normal vaginal flora, it may also cause infection. Vulvovaginitis (i.e., inflammation of the vulva and vagina) may be caused by vaginal infection; copious leukorrhea, which can cause maceration of tissues; and chemical irritants, allergens, and foreign bodies, which may produce inflammatory reactions.

Bacterial Vaginosis

Bacterial vaginosis (BV), formerly called *nonspecific vaginitis, Haemophilus vaginitis,* or *Gardnerella,* is the most common type of symptomatic vaginitis today (Gardella et al., 2017). It is associated with preterm labor and birth. The exact cause of BV is unknown. It is a syndrome in which

TABLE 4.4 Wet Smear Tests for Vaginal Infections

Infection	Test	Positive Findings
Trichomoniasis	Saline wet smear (vaginal secretions mixed with normal saline on a glass slide)	Presence of many white blood cell protozoa
Candidiasis	Potassium hydroxide (KOH) preparation (vaginal secretions mixed with KOH on a glass slide)	Presence of hyphae and pseudohyphae (buds and branches of yeast cells)
Bacterial vaginosis	Normal saline smear	Presence of clue cells (vaginal epithelial cells coated with bacteria)
	Whiff test (vaginal secretions mixed with KOH)	Release of fishy odor

normal, hydrogen peroxide–producing lactobacilli are replaced with high concentrations of anaerobic bacteria (e.g., *Gardnerella*, *Mobiluncus*). With the increase of anaerobes, the level of vaginal amines is raised, and the normal acidic pH of the vagina is altered. Epithelial cells slough, and numerous bacteria attach to their surfaces (clue cells). When the amines are volatilized, the characteristic odor of BV occurs.

Many women with BV complain of a characteristic "fishy odor." The odor may be noticed by the woman or her partner after heterosexual intercourse because semen releases the vaginal amines. When present, the BV discharge is usually profuse; thin; and white, gray, or milky in appearance. Some women also may experience mild irritation or pruritus.

Screening and Diagnosis

A focused history may help distinguish BV from other vaginal infections if the woman is symptomatic. Reports of fishy odor and increased thin vaginal discharge are most significant, and a report of increased odor after intercourse is also suggestive of BV. The nurse should question women with previous occurrence of similar symptoms, diagnosis, and treatment because women with BV often have been treated incorrectly because of misdiagnosis.

Microscopic examination of vaginal secretions is always performed (Table 4.4). Both normal saline and 10% potassium hydroxide (KOH) smears are made. The presence of clue cells (vaginal epithelial cells coated with bacteria) on wet saline smear is highly diagnostic because the phenomenon is specific to BV. Vaginal secretions are tested for pH and amine odor. Nitrazine paper is sensitive enough to detect a pH of 4.5 or greater. The fishy odor of BV will be released when KOH is added to vaginal secretions on the lip of the withdrawn speculum.

Management

Treatment of BV with oral metronidazole (Flagyl) or trinidazole or intravaginal metronidazole gel (Metrogel) or clindamycin cream (Cleocin) are comparable, and the decision regarding which to use is based on the preference of the woman (Gardella et al., 2017).

Several adverse outcomes are associated with BV during pregnancy: preterm labor and birth, premature rupture of the membranes, intraamniotic infection, and postpartum endometritis. Therefore, pregnant women should be treated to relieve vaginal symptoms and the signs of infection. Metronidazole is not recommended if the woman is breastfeeding. If it is necessary to prescribe it, she can suspend breastfeeding

temporarily (pump and discard milk to maintain supply) and resume breastfeeding 12 to 24 hours after taking the last dose.

Candidiasis

Vulvovaginal candidiasis, or yeast infection, is the second most common type of vaginal infection in the United States (Up-to-Date, 2017). Although vaginal candidiasis infections are common in healthy women, those seen in women with HIV infection are often more severe and persistent. Genital candidiasis lesions may be painful, and coalescing ulcerations necessitate continuous prophylactic therapy.

The most common organism is *Candida albicans*. It is estimated that 90% of yeast infections in women are caused by this organism. However, in the past 10 years the incidence of non–*C. albicans* infections has increased steadily. It is common for as many as 80% of women to experience chronic or recurrent infections; those with recurrent vulvovaginal infections are those women with four or more infections per year (Gardella et al., 2017). Numerous factors have been identified as predisposing a woman to yeast infections. These include antibiotic therapy, particularly broad-spectrum antibiotics such as ampicillin, tetracycline, cephalosporins, and metronidazole; diabetes, especially when uncontrolled; pregnancy; obesity; diets high in refined sugars or artificial sweeteners; use of corticosteroids and exogenous hormones; and immunosuppressed states. Clinical observations and research have suggested that tight-fitting clothing and underwear or pantyhose made of nonabsorbent materials create an environment in which a vaginal fungus can grow.

The most common symptom of yeast infection is vulvar and possibly vaginal pruritus. The itching may be mild or intense, interfere with rest and activities, and occur during or after intercourse. Some women report a feeling of dryness. Others may have painful urination as the urine flows over the vulva. The latter usually occurs in women who have **excoriations** resulting from scratching. Most often the discharge is thick, white, lumpy, and cottage cheese–like. The discharge may be found in patches on the vaginal walls, cervix, and labia. Commonly the vulva is red and swollen, as are the labial folds, vagina, and cervix. Although there is no odor characteristic of yeast infections, sometimes a yeasty or musty smell is noted.

Screening and Diagnosis

In addition to noting the onset and course of the woman's symptoms, the history is a valuable screening tool for identifying predisposing risk factors. Physical examination should include a thorough inspection of the vulva and vagina. A speculum examination is always done. Commonly saline and KOH wet smear and vaginal pH are obtained (see Table 4.4). Vaginal pH is normal (less than 4.5) with a yeast infection. The characteristic pseudohypha (bud or branching of a fungus) may be seen on a wet smear done with normal saline; however, they may be confused with other cells and artifacts.

Management

A number of antifungal preparations are available for the treatment of *C. albicans*. Many of these medications (e.g., miconazole [Monistat] and clotrimazole [Gyne-Lotrimin]) are available as over-the-counter (OTC) agents. Exogenous lactobacillus (in the form of dairy products [yogurt] or powder, tablet, capsule, or suppository supplements) and garlic have been suggested for prevention and treatment of vulvovaginal candidiasis, but have not been found to be effective (Gardella et al., 2017). The first time a woman suspects that she may have a yeast infection, she should see a health care provider for confirmation of the diagnosis and treatment recommendation. If she has another infection, she may wish to purchase an OTC preparation and self-treat. If she elects to do this, she should always be counseled to seek care for numerous recurrent

BOX 4.5   Patient Teaching Prevention of Genital Tract Infections in Women

- Practice genital hygiene (e.g. avoid douching and hard soaps, wash using singular front-to-back motion).
- Choose underwear or hosiery with a cotton crotch.
- Avoid tight-fitting clothing (especially tight jeans).
- Select cloth car seat covers instead of vinyl.
- Limit the time spent in damp exercise clothes (especially swimsuits, leotards, and tights).
- Limit exposure to bath salts or bubble bath.
- Avoid colored or scented toilet tissue.
- If sensitive, discontinue use of feminine hygiene deodorant sprays.
- Use condoms.
- Void before and after intercourse.
- Decrease dietary sugar.
- Drink yeast-active milk and eat yogurt (with lactobacilli).
- Do not douche.

or chronic yeast infections. If vaginal discharge is extremely thick and copious, vaginal debridement with a cotton swab followed by application of vaginal medication may be effective.

Women who have extensive irritation, swelling, and discomfort of the labia and vulva may find sitz baths helpful in decreasing inflammation and increasing comfort. Adding colloidal oatmeal powder to the bath may also increase the woman's comfort. Not wearing underpants to bed may help decrease symptoms and prevent recurrences. Completing the full course of treatment prescribed is essential to removing the pathogen. Medication should be continued even during menstruation. Women should be counseled not to use tampons during menses because the medication will be absorbed by the tampon. If possible, intercourse is avoided during treatment; if this is not feasible, the woman's partner should use a condom to prevent introduction of more organisms. Suggested measures to prevent genital tract infections are listed in Box 4.5.

Trichomoniasis

Trichomonas vaginalis is almost always an STI and is also a common cause of vaginal infection (5% to 50% of all vaginitis) and discharge (Gardella et al., 2017).

Trichomoniasis is caused by *T. vaginalis,* an anaerobic, one-celled protozoan with characteristic flagella. Although trichomoniasis may be asymptomatic, women commonly experience characteristically yellowish-to-greenish, frothy, mucopurulent, copious, malodorous discharge. Inflammation of the vulva, vagina, or both may be present, and the woman may complain of irritation and pruritus. Dysuria and dyspareunia are often present. Typically the discharge worsens during and after menstruation. The cervix and vaginal walls may demonstrate characteristic "strawberry spots" or tiny petechiae, although this does not occur in the majority of women with trichomoniasis, and the cervix may bleed on contact. In severe infections, the vaginal walls, the cervix, and occasionally the vulva are acutely inflamed.

Screening and Diagnosis

In addition to obtaining a history of current symptoms, it is important to obtain a history of similar symptoms and previous treatment. A thorough sexual history includes information about the treatment of her partner or partners and if she has had subsequent sexual contact with new partners.

A speculum examination is always performed, even though it may be uncomfortable for the woman. Any of the classic signs may or may not be seen on physical examination. The typical one-celled flagellate trichomonads are easily distinguished on a normal saline wet preparation (see Table 4.4). The pH of the discharge is greater than 5.0. Because trichomoniasis is an STI, once diagnosis is confirmed, the appropriate laboratory studies for other STIs should be carried out.

Management

The recommended treatment is a class of drugs called nitroimidazoles, including metronidazole or tinidazole orally in a single dose. For pregnant women, metronidazole is considered safe, but tinidazole is a category C drug (Gardella et al., 2017). Although the male partner is usually asymptomatic, he should receive treatment also because he often harbors the trichomonads in the urethra or prostate. Nurses need to discuss the importance of partner treatment with their patients. If partners are not treated, the infection will likely recur.

Women with trichomoniasis need to understand the sexual transmission of this disease. The woman should know that the organism can be present without symptoms, perhaps for several months, and that determining when she became infected is impossible.

Group B Streptococcus

Group B streptococcus (GBS) may be considered a normal vaginal flora in a woman who is not pregnant. It is estimated to be present in 25% of healthy pregnant women (CDC, 2016b). However, GBS infection is associated with poor pregnancy outcomes. These infections are an important factor in perinatal and neonatal morbidity and mortality, usually resulting from vertical transmission from the birth canal of the infected mother to the infant during birth (CDC, 2016b).

Risk factors for neonatal GBS infection include positive prenatal culture for GBS in the current pregnancy; preterm birth of less than 37 weeks of gestation; premature rupture of membranes for longer than 18 hours; intrapartum maternal fever higher than 38° C (100.4° F); and a positive history for early-onset neonatal GBS (CDC, 2016b). To decrease the risk for neonatal GBS infection, it is recommended that all women be screened at 35 to 37 weeks of gestation for GBS using a rectovaginal culture and that intravenous antibiotic prophylaxis (IAP) be offered to all who test positive. If a culture is not available at onset of labor or if risk factors are present, IAP is also offered. A rapid polymerase chain reaction (PCR) test for GBS is available for use in laboring women when GBS culture results are not available. This possibly avoids unnecessary IAP. It is not recommended before a cesarean birth if labor or rupture of membranes has not occurred. The recommended treatment is penicillin G, 5 million units in an intravenous loading dose and then 2.5 million units intravenously every 4 hours during labor. Ampicillin, 2 g intravenous loading dose, followed by 1 g intravenously every 4 hours, is an alternative therapy (CDC, 2016b).

CONCERNS OF LESBIAN, GAY, BISEXUAL, TRANSSEXUAL, QUEER (LGBT) COMMUNITY

It is important to note that persons in the LGBT community are at risk for STIs. In women's health, it is particularly important to understand the specific issues related to women who have sex with women (WSW). The CDC (2017c) has issued guidelines that are specific to WSW as well as other populations. WSW are at risk for acquiring bacterial, viral, and protozoal infections from current and prior partners, both male and female. They should not be presumed to be at low or no risk for STIs because of their sexual orientation. It is critical for effective screening that health care providers discuss sexual orientation with their patients in an open, accepting manner.

TABLE 4.5 Pregnancy and Fetal Effects of Common Sexually Transmitted Infections

Infection	Maternal Effects	Fetal Effects
Chlamydia	Premature rupture of membranes Preterm labor Postpartum endometritis	Low birth weight
Gonorrhea	Miscarriage Preterm labor Amniotic infection syndrome Chorioamnionitis Postpartum endometritis Postpartum sepsis Premature rupture of membranes	Preterm birth IUGR
Group B streptococci	Urinary tract infection Chorioamnionitis Postpartum endometritis Sepsis Meningitis (rare)	Preterm birth
Herpes simplex virus	Intrauterine infection (rare)	Congenital infection (rare)
Human papillomavirus (HPV)	Dystocia from large lesions Excessive bleeding from lesions after birth trauma	
Syphilis	Miscarriage Preterm labor	IUGR Preterm birth Stillbirth Congenital infection
Zika virus		Microcephaly

IUGR, Intrauterine growth restriction.
Data from Gilbert, E. (2011). *Manual of high risk pregnancy and delivery* (5th ed.). St. Louis, MO: Mosby; Duff, P., Sweet, R., & Edwards, R. (2013). Maternal and fetal infections. In R. K. Creasy, R. Resnik, J. D. Iams, et al. (Eds), *Creasy and Resnik's maternal-fetal medicine: Principles and practice* (7th ed.). Philadelphia, PA: Saunders; Gardella, C., Eckert, L.O., & Lentz G. M. (2017). Genital tract infections: Vulva, vagina, cervix, toxic shock syndrome, endometritis, and salpingitis. In R. A. Lobo, D. M. Gershenson, G. M. Lentz, et al. *Comprehensive gynecology* (7th ed.). Philadelphia, PA: Elsevier.

EFFECTS OF SEXUALLY TRANSMITTED INFECTIONS ON PREGNANCY AND THE FETUS

STIs in pregnancy are discussed in Chapter 12. Table 4.5 describes the effects of several common STIs on pregnancy and the fetus. It is difficult to predict these effects with certainty. Factors such as co-infection with other STIs and at what point in pregnancy the infection was treated can affect outcomes.

INFECTION CONTROL

Infection-control measures are essential to protect care providers and prevent health care–associated infection of patients, regardless of the infectious agent. The risk for occupational transmission varies with the disease. Even when the risk is low as with HIV, the existence of any risk warrants reasonable precautions. Precautions against airborne disease transmission are available in all health care agencies. **Standard Precautions** (precautions to use in care of all persons for infection control) are listed in Box 4.6.

BENIGN PROBLEMS

Fibrocystic Changes

Women often experience a benign breast problem at some point in adulthood, with fibrocystic changes being very common (Sandadi, Rock, Orr, et al., 2017). Fibrocystic changes occur in varying degrees in breasts of healthy women. The etiologic agent responsible for these changes has not been found. One theory is that estrogen excess and progesterone deficiency in the luteal phase of the menstrual cycle may cause changes in breast tissue.

Fibrocystic changes are characterized by lumpiness, with or without tenderness, in both breasts. Single simple cysts can also occur. Symptoms are often cyclical, usually developing approximately 1 week before menstruation begins and subsiding approximately 1 week after menstruation ends. Symptoms include dull heavy pain and a sense of fullness and tenderness often in the upper outer quadrants of the breasts. Physical examination may reveal excessive nodularity that often feels like peas (Sandadi et al., 2017). Larger cysts are often described as feeling like water-filled balloons. Women in their twenties report the most severe pain. Women in their thirties have premenstrual pain and tenderness; small multiple nodules are usually present. Women in their forties usually do not report severe pain, but cysts are tender and often regress in size (Sandadi et al.).

Steps in the workup of a breast lump may begin with ultrasonography to determine whether it is fluid filled or solid. Fluid-filled cysts are aspirated, and the woman is monitored on a routine basis for the development of other cysts. If the lump is solid, a mammogram is obtained. A fine-needle aspiration (FNA) is performed, regardless of the woman's age, to determine the nature of the lump (Sandadi et al., 2017).

Management depends on the severity of the symptoms. A low-fat, nutrient-dense diet with decreased saturated fat is advised, and sometimes, despite lack of clear evidence, eliminating methylxanthines (colas, coffee, tea, chocolate) is also advised. Some practitioners suggest that women take mild diuretics shortly before menses, as well as decreasing alcohol intake (Sandadi et al., 2017). Other pain-relief measures include taking analgesics or NSAIDs, wearing a supportive bra, and applying heat or cold to the breasts.

Evening primrose oil and vitamin E supplements may be effective for some women, although more research is needed. Oral contraceptives, danazol, bromocriptine, and tamoxifen have also been used with varying degrees of success.

Fibroadenoma

The next most common benign neoplasm of the breast is a fibroadenoma. It is the single most common type of tumor seen in the adolescent population, although it can also occur in women in their thirties. Fibroadenomas are discrete, usually solitary lumps averaging 2.5 cm in diameter (Sandadi et al., 2017). Occasionally the woman with a fibroadenoma experiences tenderness in the tumor during the menstrual cycle. Fibroadenomas do not increase in size in response to the menstrual cycle as cysts do. They increase in size during pregnancy and decrease in size as the woman ages. The cause of fibroadenomas is unknown.

Diagnosis is made by reviewing patient history and physical examination. Mammography, ultrasound, or magnetic resonance imaging (MRI) helps determine the type of lesion. Fine needle aspiration (FNA) may be used to determine underlying pathologic conditions. Surgical excision may be necessary if the lump is suspicious or if the symptoms are severe. Periodic observation of masses by professional physical examination or mammography may be all that is necessary for masses not

BOX 4.6 Standard Precautions

Medical history and examination cannot reliably identify all persons infected with human immunodeficiency virus (HIV) or other bloodborne pathogens. Therefore Standard Precautions should be used consistently in the care of all persons. These precautions apply to blood; body fluids; and all secretions and excretions, except sweat, nonintact skin, and mucous membranes. The following infection-control practices should be applied during the delivery of health care to reduce the risk for transmission of microorganisms from known and unknown sources of infection:

1. *Hand hygiene.* During the delivery of health care, avoid unnecessary touching of surfaces in close proximity to the patient to prevent both contamination of clean hands from environmental surfaces and transmission of pathogens from contaminated hands to surfaces. Wash dirty or contaminated hands with either a nonantimicrobial or an antimicrobial soap and water. If hands are not visibly soiled, decontaminate them with an alcohol-based hand rub, or they may be washed with an antimicrobial soap and water. Perform hand hygiene (1) before having direct contact with patients; (2) after contact with blood, body fluids, excretions, mucous membranes, nonintact skin, or wound dressings; (3) after contact with a patient's intact skin (e.g., when taking a pulse or blood pressure or lifting a patient); (4) if hands will be moving from a contaminated to a clean body site during patient care; (5) after contact with inanimate objects (including medical equipment) in the immediate vicinity of the patient; and (6) after removing gloves. Wash hands with nonantimicrobial soap and water or with antimicrobial soap and water if contact with spores (e.g., *Clostridium difficile* or *Bacillus anthracis*) is likely to have occurred. The physical action of washing and rinsing hands under such circumstances is recommended because alcohols, chlorhexidine, iodophors, and other antiseptic agents have poor activity against spores. Do not wear artificial fingernails or extenders if duties include direct contact with patients at high risk for infection and associated adverse outcomes.

2. *Personal protective equipment (PPE).* Observe the following principles of use:
   - *Gloves.* Wear gloves when a reasonably anticipated possibility exists that contact with blood or other potentially infectious materials, mucous membranes, nonintact skin, or potentially contaminated intact skin (e.g., of a patient incontinent of stool or urine) might occur. Gloves should be worn during infant eye prophylaxis, care of the umbilical cord, care of the circumcision site, parenteral procedures, diaper changes, contact with colostrum, and postpartum assessments. Wear gloves with fit and durability appropriate to the task. Remove gloves after contact with a patient or the surrounding environment (including medical equipment), using proper technique to prevent hand contamination. Do not wear the same pair of gloves for the care of more than one patient. Change gloves during patient care if the hands will move from a contaminated (e.g., perineal area) to a clean (e.g., face) body site.

   - *Gowns.* Wear a gown that is appropriate to the task to protect the skin and prevent soiling or contamination of clothing during procedures and patient-care activities when contact with blood, body fluids, secretions, or excretions is anticipated. Remove the gown and perform hand hygiene before leaving the patient's environment. Do not reuse gowns, even for repeated contacts with the same patient. Routine donning of gowns on entrance into a high-risk unit (e.g., intensive care unit [ICU], neonatal intensive care unit [NICU]) is not indicated.

   - *Mouth, nose, eye protection.* Use PPE to protect the mucous membranes of the eyes, nose, and mouth during procedures and patient-care activities that are likely to generate splashes or sprays of blood, body fluids, secretions, and excretions. Select masks, goggles, face shields, and combinations of each according to the need anticipated by the task performed.

   - *Respiratory hygiene and cough etiquette.* Post signs at entrances and in strategic places (e.g., elevators, cafeterias) within ambulatory and inpatient settings with instructions to patients and other persons with symptoms of a respiratory infection to cover their mouth and nose when coughing or sneezing, use and dispose of tissues, and perform hand hygiene after hands have been in contact with respiratory secretions. Provide tissues and no-touch receptacles (e.g., foot pedal–operated lid or open, plastic-lined wastebasket) for disposal of tissues. Provide resources and instructions for performing hand hygiene in or near waiting areas in ambulatory and inpatient settings; provide conveniently located dispensers of alcohol-based hand rubs and, where sinks are available, supplies for handwashing. During periods of increased prevalence of respiratory infections in the community, offer masks to coughing patients and other symptomatic persons (e.g., persons who accompany ill patients) on entry into the facility, and encourage them to maintain special separation, ideally a distance of at least 3 feet, from others in common waiting areas.

3. *Safe injection practices.* The following recommendations apply to the use of needles, cannulas that replace needles, and, where applicable, intravenous delivery systems:
   - Use aseptic technique to prevent contamination of sterile injection equipment. Needles, cannulas, and syringes are sterile, single-use items; they should not be reused for another patient. Use fluid infusion and administration sets (i.e., intravenous bags, tubing, and connectors) for one patient only, and dispose of appropriately after use. Use single-dose vials for parenteral medications whenever possible. If multidose vials must be used, both the needle (or cannula) and the syringe used to access the multidose vial must be sterile. Do not keep multidose vials in the immediate patient treatment area, and store in accordance with manufacturer recommendations; discard if sterility is compromised or questionable.

Modified from Wisconsin Department of Health Services. (2016). *Infection control and prevention: Standard precautions.* Retrieved from https://www.dhs.wisconsin.gov/ic/precautions.htm.

needing surgical intervention (Sandadi et al., 2017). Women need to recognize changes in their breasts and seek further evaluation from a clinician.

Nipple Discharge

Nipple discharge is a common occurrence that concerns many women. Although most nipple discharge is physiologic, it is important to evaluate each woman who has this problem thoroughly because some women will be found to have a serious endocrine disorder or malignancy. Most nipple discharge is elicited (i.e., discharge is a result of the breast being compressed or stimulated) and is usually not a concern unless the woman is postmenopausal or a mass is present in the breast (Sandadi et al., 2017).

Another form of breast discharge not related to malignancy is galactorrhea, a bilaterally spontaneous, milky, sticky discharge. It is a normal finding in pregnancy. It can also occur as the result of elevated prolactin levels caused by a thyroid disorder, pituitary tumor, or chest wall surgery or trauma. Obtaining a complete medication history on each woman is essential, as some medications can precipitate galactorrhea in some women (Sandadi et al., 2017).

Diagnostic tests that may be indicated include a physical examination, mammography, ultrasound or magnetic resonance imaging (MRI), as well as ductoscopy to microscopically evaluate the discharge (Sandadi et al., 2017).

Mammary Duct Ectasia

Mammary duct ectasia is a benign inflammation of the ducts behind the nipple. It occurs most often in perimenopausal women. In mammary duct ectasia, nipple discharge is thick; sticky; and colored white, brown, green, or purple. The woman frequently experiences a burning pain, an itching, or a palpable mass behind the nipple (American Cancer Society, 2016a).

The workup includes a mammogram and aspiration and culture of fluid. Treatment is usually symptomatic; mild pain relievers, warm compresses applied to the breast, or wearing a supportive bra may provide relief. If a mass is present or an abscess occurs, treatment may include a local excision of the affected duct or ducts (Sandadi et al., 2017).

Intraductal Papilloma

Intraductal papilloma is a rare benign condition that develops within the terminal nipple ducts. The cause is unknown. It usually occurs in women between 30 and 50 years of age. The papilloma is usually too small to be palpated, and the characteristic sign is spontaneous unilateral nipple discharge that is serous, serosanguineous, or bloody. After eliminating the possibility of malignancy, the affected segments of the ducts and breasts are surgically excised (Sandadi et al., 2017). Table 4.6 compares manifestations of benign breast diseases.

Nursing Care

The history should focus on risk factors for breast diseases, events related to the breast mass, and health maintenance practices. Risk factors for breast cancer are discussed later in this chapter. Information related to the breast mass should include how, when, and by whom the mass was discovered. The following patient information is documented: presence of pain, whether symptoms increase with menses, dietary habits, smoking habits, and use of oral contraceptives. The woman's emotional status, including her stress level, fears, and concerns and her ability to cope, also should be assessed.

Physical examination may include assessment of the breasts for symmetry, masses (size, number, consistency, mobility), and nipple discharge.

Nursing actions might include the following:

- Discuss the intervals for and facets of breast screening, including professional examination and mammography (see Table 3.3). Women with breast implants may need special views of the breast, and precautions might have to be taken to prevent rupturing the implant during mammography.
- Provide written educational materials.

- Encourage the verbalization of fears and concerns about treatment and prognosis.
- Provide specific information regarding the woman's condition and treatment, including dietary changes, drug therapy, comfort measures, stress management, and surgery.
- Demonstrate correct breast self-examination technique if the woman desires to practice.
- Describe pain-relieving strategies in detail, and collaborate with the primary health care provider to ensure effective pain control.
- Encourage discussion of feelings about body image.
- Refer to a support group or stress-management resource if needed to cope with long-term consequences of benign breast conditions.

CANCER OF THE BREAST

The United States has one of the highest rates of carcinoma in the world. After skin cancer, breast cancer is the most frequently diagnosed cancer and the leading cause of cancer deaths in Hispanic women, and the second-leading cause of cancer deaths in white, black, Asian/Pacific Islander, and American Indian/Alaskan Native women (CDC, 2016c). One in eight American women will develop breast cancer in her lifetime (Sandadi et al., 2017). No clear method for prevention has been formulated. The prognosis for and survival of the woman are improved with early detection. Therefore, women must be educated about risk factors, early detection, and screening.

Although the exact cause of breast cancer is still unknown, researchers have identified certain factors that increase a woman's risk for developing a malignancy. Box 4.7 lists these factors. The most important predictor for breast cancer is age; the risk increases as the woman ages.

Much discussion has taken place about possible links between breast cancer and hormone therapy; several large research studies, including the Women's Health Initiative, have found that the risk for breast cancer increases when a woman is taking combined estrogen and progesterone but declines quickly once therapy is stopped. No consensus about possible links has been reached (Sandadi et al., 2017).

Although studies have shown no correlation between breast implants and the development of breast cancer, recently the Food and Drug Administration has found a small correlation between breast implants and anaplastic large cell lymphoma (ALCL), which can occur in other parts of the body, but also very rarely in the breast (Pruthi, 2015). The incidence of ALCL is very small, but is something for a woman to consider when deciding to have breast implants.

Although most breast cancers are not related to genetic factors, the identification of the *BRCA1* and *BRCA2* genes has demonstrated the role of heredity and genetic mutations in this disease. Only approximately 5% to 10% of all breast cancers are attributed to heredity. Women who have abnormalities in the *BRCA1* and *BRCA2* genes and develop cancer,

TABLE 4.6 Comparison of Common Manifestations of Benign Breast Masses

Fibrocystic Changes	Fibroadenoma	Lipoma	Intraductal Papilloma	Mammary Duct Ectasia
Multiple lumps	Single lump	Single lump	Single or multiple	Mass behind nipple
Nodular	Well delineated	Well delineated	Not well delineated	Not well delineated
Palpable	Palpable	Palpable	Nonpalpable	Palpable
Movable	Movable	Movable	Nonmobile	Nonmobile
Round, smooth	Round, lobular	Round, lobular	Small, ball-like	Irregular
Firm or soft	Firm	Soft	Firm or soft	Firm
Tenderness influenced by menstrual cycle	Usually asymptomatic	Nontender	Usually nontender	Painful, burning, itching
Bilateral	Unilateral	Unilateral	Unilateral	Unilateral
May or may not have nipple discharge	No nipple discharge	No nipple discharge	Serous or bloody nipple discharge	Thick, sticky nipple discharge

BOX 4.7 Risk Factors for Breast Cancer*

Risks That Are Not Modifiable

- Age—risk increases with age
- Previous history of breast cancer
- Family history of breast cancer, especially a mother or sister (particularly significant if premenopausal)
- Inherited genetic mutations in *BRCA1* and *BRCA2* genes
- Previous history of ovarian, endometrial, colon, or thyroid cancer
- High breast tissue density
- Early menarche (before 12 years of age)
- Late menopause (after 55 years of age)
- Previous history of benign breast disease with epithelial hyperplasia
- Race (Caucasian women have highest incidence)

Lifestyle and Modifiable Risks

- Nulliparity or first pregnancy after 30 years of age
- Not breastfeeding
- Postmenopausal use of combined estrogen-progestin replacement therapy
- Obesity after menopause
- Alcohol consumption of more than one drink per day
- Sedentary lifestyle
- Vitamin D—low levels increase risk

Risk factors are cumulative (i.e., the more risk factors that are present, the greater is the likelihood of breast cancer occurring).

Data from American Cancer Society. (2011). *Breast cancer*. Retrieved from www.cancer.org; American Cancer Society. (2012). *Cancer facts and figures*. Atlanta, GA: Author.

BOX 4.8 Risk Factors Included in the Breast Cancer Risk Assessment Tool

- Woman's age
- Number of first-degree relatives affected
- Age of woman at menarche
- Age of woman at first live birth
- Number of breast biopsies
- History of atypical hyperplasia in biopsy specimens

tend to develop it earlier in life and in a usually more aggressive, bilateral form (Sandadi et al., 2017). Other genetic mutations that can cause breast cancer include Li-Fraumeni syndrome, which is related to the *p53* gene, and Cowden syndrome, which is related to the *PTEN* gene (Sandadi et al.).

Information about breast cancer risks can be confusing, and women can overestimate or underestimate their risks. Women and health professionals can use the Breast Cancer Risk Assessment Tool to calculate risk. This tool was developed and verified by the National Cancer Institute (NCI) to predict the risk for breast cancer in 5 years and over the lifetime (to 90 years of age) of a woman. The risk factors used are listed in Box 4.8. The tool is available at https://www.cancer.gov/bcrisktool/. Although the clinical applicability of risk factors has limits, it is important to screen women more frequently if they are at higher risk and help them to change risks that are modifiable, such as losing weight and limiting alcohol intake.

Prevention

Chemoprevention is the use of medications to reduce cancer risk. Tamoxifen and raloxifene block the effect of estrogen on breast tissue. Studies have shown that these two drugs can reduce the risk for breast cancer, and the FDA has approved them for such use (Sandadi et al., 2017) (see Medication Guides for tamoxifen and raloxifene). The role of aromatase inhibitors (e.g., anastrozole) also is being examined to see if these drugs are effective for prevention.

MEDICATION GUIDE

Tamoxifen (Nolvadex)

Action

Antiestrogenic effects; attaches to hormone receptors on cancer cells and prevents natural hormones from attaching to the receptors

Indications

For treatment of advanced-stage or metastatic breast cancer; for treatment of early-stage breast cancer after breast cancer surgery and radiation therapy; to reduce the incidence of breast cancer in women at high risk

Dosage

20 mg orally daily for 5 years

Adverse Reactions

Common side effects include hot flashes, night sweats, nausea, vaginal bleeding or discharge, and mood swings. Hair loss is an uncommon effect. Serious side effects include deep vein thrombosis, increased risk for endometrial cancer, and stroke.

Nursing Considerations

The medication may be taken on an empty stomach or with food. Missed doses should be taken as soon as possible, but taking two doses at once is not recommended. A barrier or nonhormonal form of contraception is recommended in premenopausal women because tamoxifen may be harmful to the fetus if pregnancy should occur.

Data from Medscape (2017). *Tamoxifen*. Retrieved from http://reference.medscape.com/drug/nolvadex-soltamox-tamoxifen-342183.

Surgical prophylaxis (bilateral mastectomy, oophorectomy) can reduce the risk for breast cancer, but it should be considered only for people who are at very high risk (Sandadi et al., 2017).

Screening and Diagnosis

Breast cancer in its earliest form can be detected by a mammogram before it is felt by a woman. More than half of all lumps are discovered in the upper outer quadrant of the breast. The most common presenting symptom is a lump or thickening of the breast. The lump may feel hard and fixed or soft and spongy. It may have well-defined or irregular borders. It may be fixed to the skin, thereby causing dimpling to occur. A nipple discharge that is bloody or clear also may be present.

Early detection and diagnosis reduce the risk for mortality because cancer is found when it is smaller, lesions are more localized, and the tendency is to have a lower percentage of positive nodes. However, cultural factors may influence a woman's decision to participate in breast cancer screening. Knowledge of these factors and use of culturally sensitive messages and materials that appeal to the unique concerns, beliefs, and reading abilities of target groups assist the nurse in helping women overcome barriers to seeking care. It is important to understand the perspectives of women from various ethnic groups in terms of how they view the health care system and why they choose or do not choose to seek health screening, such as mammograms. Other barriers to breast cancer screening include older age, expense, lack of health insurance, fear, lack of knowledge, and organizational barriers such as scheduling problems and lack of available services.

Raloxifene Hydrochloride (Evista)

Action
A selective estrogen receptor modulator, serving as an agonist and antagonist to estrogen receptor sites

Indications
Treatment and prevention of osteoporosis; reduction in the risk for invasive breast cancer in postmenopausal women with osteoporosis; and reduction of risk for invasive breast cancer in postmenopausal women at high risk for invasive breast cancer

Dosage
60 mg orally daily for 5 years

Adverse Reactions
Common side effects include hot flashes, nausea, peripheral edema, joint pain, leg cramps, flulike symptoms, and sweating. Serious and life-threatening side effects can occur from existing condition. Women who have had or are at risk for a heart attack have increased risk for dying from a stroke. Risk for blood clots in the legs and lungs is increased. Raloxifene is contraindicated in women with an active or past history of venous thromboembolism.

Nursing Considerations
The medication may be taken on an empty stomach or with food. Missed doses should be taken as soon as possible, but taking two doses at once is not recommended. The woman should contact her health care provider if leg pain or feeling of warmth in lower legs, swelling of hands and feet, sudden chest pain or shortness of breath, or sudden changes in vision occur. Calcium 1500 mg plus vitamin D 400 to 800 International Units daily are recommended.

Data from Medscape (2017). *Raloxifene.* Retrieved from http://reference.medscape.com/drug/evista-raloxifene-342794.

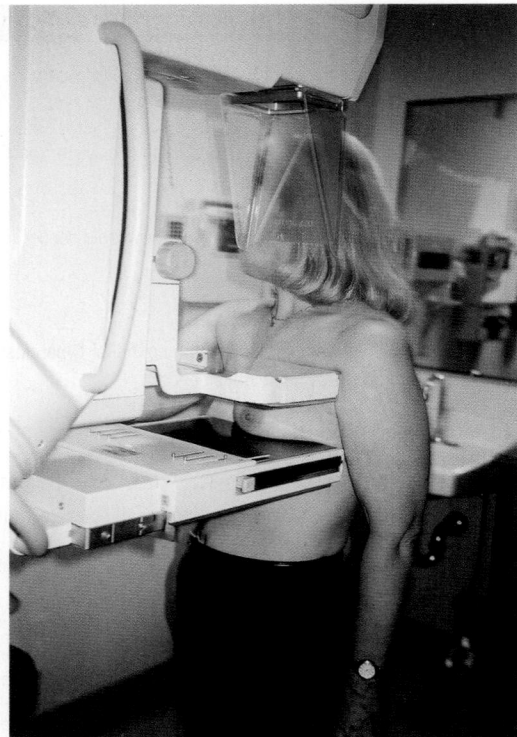

FIG 4.6 Patient undergoing mammography. (Courtesy of Shannon Perry, Phoenix, AZ.)

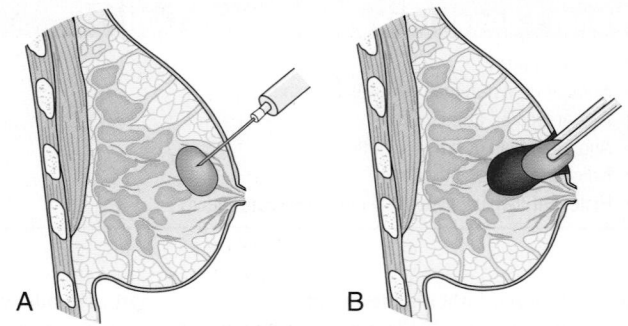

FIG 4.7 Diagnosis. **A,** Needle aspiration. **B,** Open biopsy. (Redrawn from National Women's Health Resource Center. [1995]. Breast health. *National Women's Health Report, 13*[5], 3.)

Clinical examination by a qualified health care provider and screening mammography (X-ray film examination of the breast) (Fig. 4.6) may aid in the early detection of breast cancers. A diagnostic mammogram is performed when a screening mammogram identifies something that needs further inspection or when the woman or examiner finds a breast symptom that is new.

When a suspicious finding on a mammogram is noted or a lump is detected, the diagnosis is confirmed by needle aspiration, a core needle biopsy, or surgical excision (Fig. 4.7). Ultrasound may also be used to assess a specific area of abnormality found during a mammogram procedure (Sandadi et al., 2017). Women need specific information regarding advantages and disadvantages of these procedures in making a decision about which one is most appropriate for them.

Laboratory examination of breast tissue determines if cancer is present and, if so, the extent. Other tests performed to determine the spread of the cancer include digital mammography, CT, MRI, and three-dimensional mammography (tomosynthesis), among other tests (Sandadi et al., 2017).

An important step in evaluating a breast cancer is to test for the presence of estrogen and progesterone receptors in the biopsied tissue. Cancer cells may contain one, both, or neither of these receptors. Breast cancers that contain estrogen receptors are often called *ER-positive* cancers, whereas those containing progesterone receptors are called *PR-positive* cancers. Women with hormone-positive tumors tend to respond better to treatment and have higher survival rates than the general population (Sandadi et al., 2017).

An HER2/neu test also may be performed on the biopsied breast tissue. HER2/neu is a growth-promoting hormone. In approximately 18% to 20% of breast cancers, excessive amounts of the hormone are present, causing the cancer to be more aggressive in spreading than other types of breast cancer (Sandadi et al., 2017).

Medical Management
Controversy continues regarding the best treatment for breast cancer. Nodal involvement, tumor size, receptor status, and aggressiveness are important variables for treatment selection. Medical management of breast cancer includes surgery, breast reconstruction, radiation therapy, adjuvant hormone therapy, biologic targeted therapy, and chemotherapy. Many women face difficult decisions about the various treatment options. Box 4.9 lists questions that must be addressed in decision making.

Most health care providers recommend that the malignant mass and the axillary nodes, specifically the sentinel node, be removed for staging purposes (Sandadi et al., 2017). The treatment can be conservative or more radical. The most frequently recommended surgical approaches for the treatment of breast cancer are lumpectomy and total simple mastectomy. Breast-conserving surgery such as a **lumpectomy**

BOX 4.9   Decision-Making Questions to Ask

1. What kind of breast cancer is it (invasive or noninvasive)?
2. What stage is cancer (i.e., how extensive is the spread)?
3. Did the cancer test positive for hormone (estrogen) (may be slower growing)?
4. Which further tests are recommended?
5. What are the treatment options? (pros and cons of each, including side effects)
6. If surgery is recommended, what will the scar look like?
7. If a mastectomy is done, can breast reconstruction be done (at the time of surgery or later)?
8. How long will the woman be in the hospital? What kind of postoperative care will she need?
9. How long will treatment last if radiation or chemotherapy is recommended? What effects can the woman expect from these treatments?
10. What community resources are available for support?

(Fig. 4.8, *A*) or partial mastectomy (e.g., quadrantectomy, wide excision) (see Fig. 4.8, *B*) is the removal of the breast tumor and a small amount of surrounding tissue. Sampling of axillary lymph nodes usually occurs through a separate incision at the time of these procedures, and the surgery is usually followed by radiation therapy to the remaining breast tissue (Sandadi et al.). These procedures are for the primary treatment of women with early-stage (I or II) breast cancer. Lumpectomy offers survival equivalent to that with modified radical mastectomy.

A total **simple mastectomy** (see Fig. 4.8, *C*) is the removal of the breast containing the tumor. A **modified radical mastectomy** is the removal of the breast tissue, skin, and fascia of the pectoralis muscle and dissection of the axillary nodes. A **radical mastectomy** (see Fig. 4.8, *D*), although rarely performed, is the removal of the breast and underlying pectoralis muscles and complete axillary node dissection. After surgery, follow-up treatment may include radiation, chemotherapy, or hormone therapy (Sandadi et al., 2017). The decision to include follow-up therapy is based on the stage of disease, age and menopausal status of the woman, the woman's preference, and her hormone receptor status. Follow-up treatment is usually initiated to decrease the risk for recurrence in women who have no evidence of metastasis.

Radiation is usually recommended as follow-up therapy for women who have stage I or II cancer. Radiation can be external for 5 to 6 weeks or as short as 3 weeks. Internal radiation is in the form of needles, seeds, wires, or catheters filled with a radioactive substance that is inserted into the breast near the tumor. Hormone therapy with tamoxifen, an estrogen agonist, is recommended for women older than 50 years of age for at least 5 years (see Medication Guide for tamoxifen).

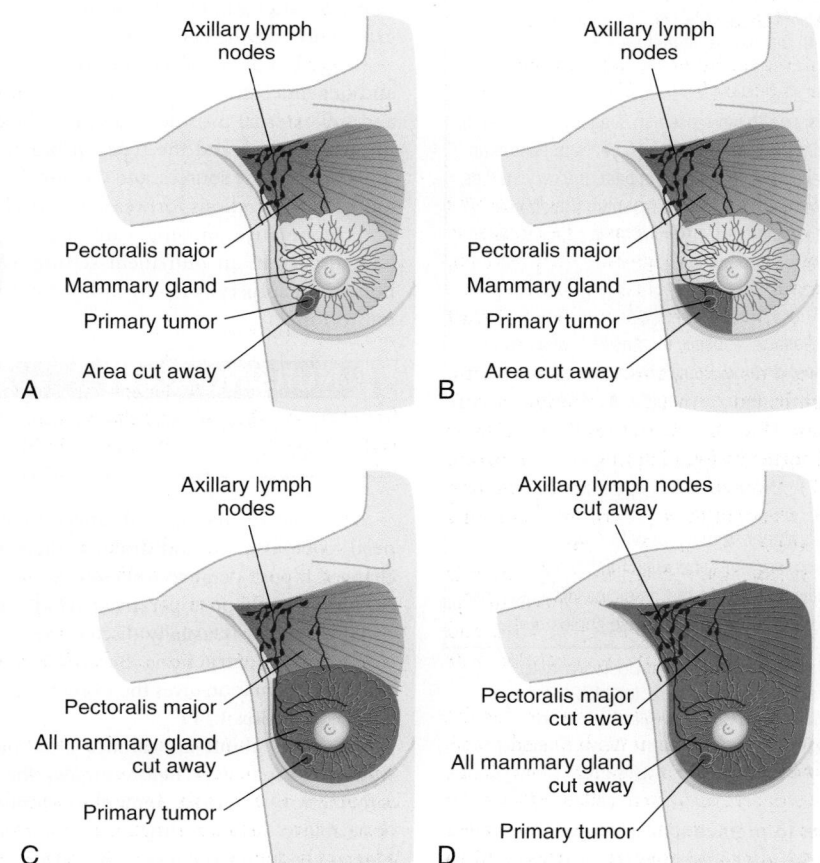

FIG 4.8 Surgical alternatives for breast cancer. **A,** Lumpectomy. **B,** Partial mastectomy (quadrantectomy, wide excision). **C,** Total (simple) mastectomy. **D,** Radical mastectomy.

Aromatase inhibitors markedly suppress plasma estrogen levels in postmenopausal women by inhibiting or inactivating aromatase, the enzyme responsible for synthesizing estrogens from androgenic substrates. Aromatase inhibitors such as anastrozole, letrozole, and exemestane have been shown to be effective agents in hormone therapy for breast cancer. In early-stage breast cancer, adjuvant therapy with anastrozole appears to be superior to adjuvant therapy with tamoxifen in reducing recurrence in postmenopausal women (see Medication Guide for anastrozole). The aromatase inhibitors appear to be well tolerated, with a lower incidence of adverse effects compared to tamoxifen in post-menopausal women (Sandadi et al., 2017). More research is needed to determine how long a woman should take an aromatase inhibitor. Chlebowski and Budoff (2016) have suggested possibly continued use of an aromatase inhibitor for 10 years in postmenopausal women who are hormone receptor–positive, In the past, the only studies conducted looked at 5 years of treatment.

💊 MEDICATION GUIDE

Anastrozole (Arimidex)

Action
An aromatase inhibitor; inhibits the conversion of androgens to estrogen

Indication
For adjuvant treatment of early breast cancer in postmenopausal women who have received 5 years of tamoxifen therapy, or instead of tamoxifen if a woman cannot tolerate it (e.g., develops deep vein thrombosis); first-line treatment of postmenopausal women with hormone receptor–positive or hormone recep-tor–unknown locally advanced or metastatic cancer; adjuvant treatment of postmenopausal women with hormone receptor–positive early breast cancer. There is a risk for osteoporosis with aromatase inhibitors.

Dosage and Route
1 mg once a day by mouth for 5 years (with new research suggesting 10 years)
   Possibly continued use of an aromatase inhibitor for 10 years in postmeno-pausal women who are hormone receptor–positiveIn the past, the only studies conducted looked at 5 years of treatment, but recent research (Chlebowski & Gudoff, 2016) suggests a possible benefit of 10 years of treatment. More research is needed as these are very new findings.

Adverse Reactions
Common side effects include hot flashes, nausea, increased sweating, joint or muscle pain, fluid retention, vaginal dryness, constipation, dizziness, fatigue, headache; severe side effects include severe allergic reactions (e.g., rash, hives, difficulty breathing), vomiting, chest pain, severe bone pain, calf pain or tenderness

Nursing Considerations
The medication may be taken on an empty stomach or with food. The woman should use caution if driving or using machinery because this medication may cause drowsiness or dizziness. Advise her that the medicine may decrease bone strength, increase her risk for fractures, and increase cholesterol.

Data from Medscape (2017). *Anastrozole.* Retrieved from http://reference.medscape.com/drug/arimidex-anastrozole-342208; Chlebowski, R. T., & Budoff, M. J. (2016). Changing adjuvant breast-cancer therapy with a signal for prevention. *New England Journal of Medicine, 375*(3), 274-275.

Chemotherapy is often given to premenopausal women who have positive nodes. Therapy for more advanced tumors usually includes surgery followed by chemotherapy, radiation, or both (Sandadi et al., 2017).

The goals of surgical breast reconstruction are achievement of symmetry and preservation of body image. Surgical reconstruction can be done immediately or at a later date. Immediate reconstruction at the time of mastectomy does not change survival rates or interfere with therapy or the treatment of recurrent disease.

Surgical options for breast reconstruction include implants and flap procedures. Implants are made of silicone or saline or a combination of both and can be inserted at the same time as a mastectomy or later. They are placed underneath the chest muscle versus on top of it, as in the case of breast augmentation. Silicone implants have been deemed safe and are options for women having breast reconstruction following mastectomy.

Flap procedures are done by plastic and reconstructive surgeons who specialize in microsurgery. During flap reconstruction a breast is created using tissue taken from other parts of the body such as the abdomen, back, or buttocks, or thighs, which is then transplanted to the chest by reconnecting the blood vessels to new ones in the chest region.

After a woman has recovered from initial reconstructive surgery, she may choose to have nipple and areolar reconstruction. Nipple reconstruction is achieved by using an autologous skin graft to construct a nipple, either from tissue from the remaining nipple or from a donor site (Sandadi et al., 2017).

Nursing Care

Surgery may be performed in an outpatient surgical setting or as an inpatient procedure, depending on which type of surgery is being performed. Nursing care and teaching are focused on the perioperative period. Before surgery, the nurse assesses the woman's psychologic readiness, specific teaching needs related to the procedure, and what to expect after surgery. A visit from a woman who has had a similar experience may be beneficial before and after surgery.

There is a discussion of reconstruction surgery, including the risks and benefits before the surgery if appropriate. A discussion of partial and full external prostheses also may be appropriate, including where to purchase one and the types of bras that may be worn. Local ACS units can provide sources, and volunteers of Reach to Recovery can offer hints and suggestions for wearing apparel and coping with prostheses.

Postoperative nursing care focuses on recovery. Women who had surgery in an outpatient setting usually go home within a few hours after surgery. A 24- to 48-hour stay is usual after modified radical mastectomy.

⚠ NURSING ALERT

Avoid taking blood pressure, giving injections, or taking blood from the arm on the affected side.

The woman may have drainage tubes from the incision site that need to be assessed and drained. Incision care may include dressing changes. If postoperative arm exercises are appropriate, these are initiated during the early postoperative period (Box 4.10).

The woman is usually discharged to home after being given self-management instructions. Because teaching time is short, providing printed information gives the woman and her family something to refer to at home (Box 4.11).

Concerns about appearance after breast surgery may affect the woman's self-concept. Before surgery, the woman and her partner need information about the woman's postoperative appearance. They need to be able to discuss feelings and concerns about accepting the changes. Nurses can help the couple communicate these feelings and concerns. Information about community resources and support groups such as Reach to Recovery are often beneficial.

BOX 4.10   Exercises After Breast Surgery

It is important to talk to your health care provider before starting any exercises. A physical or occupational therapist can help design an exercise program for you.

Exercises in Lying Position

These exercises should be performed on a bed or the floor while lying on your back with your knees and hips bent, feet flat.

Wand Exercise

This exercise helps increase the forward motion of the shoulders. You will need a broom handle, yardstick, or other similar object to perform it.

- Hold the wand in both hands with palms facing up.
- Lift the wand up over your head (as far as you can), using your unaffected arm to help lift it until you feel a stretch in your affected arm.
- Hold for 5 seconds.
- Lower arms and repeat 5 to 7 times.

Elbow Winging

This exercise helps increase the mobility of the front of your chest and shoulder. It may take several weeks of regular exercise before your elbows will get close to the bed (or floor).

- Clasp your hands behind your neck with your elbows pointing toward the ceiling.
- Move your elbows apart and down toward the bed (or floor).
- Repeat 5 to 7 times

Exercises in Sitting Position

Shoulder Blade Stretch

This exercise helps increase the mobility of the shoulder blades.

- Sit in a chair very close to a table with your back against the chair back.
- Place the unaffected arm on the table with your elbow bent and palm down. Do not move this arm during the exercise.
- Place the affected arm on the table, palm down with your elbow straight.
- Without moving your trunk, slide the affected arm toward the opposite side of the table. You should feel your shoulder blade move as you do this.
- Relax your arm and repeat 5 to 7 times.

Shoulder Blade Squeeze

This exercise also helps increase the mobility of the shoulder blade.

- Facing straight ahead, sit in a chair in front of a mirror without resting on the back of the chair.
- Arms should be at your sides with elbows bent.
- Squeeze shoulder blades together, bringing your elbows behind you. Keep your shoulders level as you do this exercise. Do not lift them up toward your ears.
- Return to the starting position and repeat 5 to 7 times.

Side Bending

This exercise helps increase the mobility of the trunk/body.

- Clasp your hands together in front of you and lift your arms slowly over your head, straightening your arms.
- When your arms are over your head, bend your trunk to the right while bending at the waist and keeping your arms overhead.
- Return to the starting position and bend to the left.
- Repeat 5 to 7 times.

Exercises in Standing Position

Chest Wall Stretch

This exercise helps stretch the chest wall.

- Stand facing a corner with toes approximately 8 to 10 inches from the corner.
- Bend your elbows and place forearms on the wall, one on each side of the corner. Your elbows should be as close to shoulder height as possible.
- Keep your arms and feet in position and move your chest toward the corner. You will feel a stretch across your chest and shoulders.
- Return to starting position and repeat 5 to 7 times.
- Be sure you keep your shoulders dropped far away from your ears as you do this stretch.

Shoulder Stretch

This exercise helps increase the mobility in the shoulder.

- Stand facing the wall with your toes approximately 8 to 10 inches from it.
- Place your hands on the wall. Use your fingers to "climb the wall," reaching as high as you can until you feel a stretch.
- Return to starting position and repeat 5 to 7 times.
- Be sure you keep your shoulders dropped far away from your ears as you raise your arms.

Modified from American Cancer Society (2016). *Exercises after breast surgery*. Retrieved from http://www.cancer.org/cancer/breastcancer/moreinformation/exercises-after-breast-surgery.

BOX 4.11   Patient Teaching After a Mastectomy Without and With Reconstruction

- Wash hands well before and after touching incision area or drains.
- Empty surgical drains twice a day and as needed, recording the date, time, drain sites (if more than one drain is present), and amount of drainage in milliliters in the diary that you will take to each surgical checkup until your drains are removed. (Before discharge you may receive a graduated container for emptying drains and measuring drainage.)
- Avoid driving, lifting more than 10 pounds, or reaching above your head until given permission by the surgeon.
- Take medications for pain as soon as pain begins.
- Perform arm exercises as directed.
- Call health care provider if inflammation of incision or swelling of the incision or the arm occurs.
- Avoid tight clothing, tight jewelry, and other causes of decreased circulation in the affected arm.

- Until drains are removed, wear loose-fitting underwear (camisole or half-slip) and clothes, pinning surgical drains inside of clothing. (You will be taught how to do this safely.)
- After drains are removed and surgical sites are healing and still tender, wear a mastectomy bra or camisole with a cotton-filled, muslin temporary prosthesis. Temporary prostheses of this type are often available from Reach to Recovery.
- Avoid depilatory creams; strong deodorants; and shaving of affected chest area, axilla, and arm.
- Sponge bathe for the first 48 hours; then you may shower. Thoroughly dry yourself afterward and reapply fresh dressings.
- Return to the surgeon's office for incision check, drain inspection, and possible drain removal as directed.

Continued

BOX 4.11 Patient Teaching After a Mastectomy Without and With Reconstruction—cont'd

- Contact Reach to Recovery or a breast center nursing staff member for assistance in obtaining external prosthesis and lingerie when dressings, drains, and staples are removed and wound is healing and nontender.
- Contact insurance company for information about coverage of prosthesis and wig if needed. Obtain prescriptions for prosthesis and wig to submit with receipts of purchase for these items to the insurance company. If insurance does not pay for these items, contact hospital or agency social worker or local American Cancer Society for assistance.
- Practice breast self-exam (BSE) of unaffected side and affected surgical site and axilla.
- Keep follow-up visits for professional examination, mammography, and testing to detect recurrent breast cancer.
- Expect decreased sensation and tingling at incision sites and in the affected arm for weeks to months after surgery.
- Resume sexual activities as desired.

- Participate in breast cancer survivor support group if desired.
- Encourage mother, sisters, and daughters (if applicable) to learn and practice BSE and have annual professional breast examinations and mammography (if appropriate).

Additional Nursing Care for Women Undergoing Mastectomy With Reconstruction
- Apply no tight compression of the reconstructed breasts until approved by the plastic surgeon.
- Wear loosely fitting garments for first 3 to 4 weeks.
- Know that surgery is still a work in progress and that final cosmetic result of reconstruction takes many weeks.
- Assess skin for potential of poor peripheral circulation that may cause skin necrosis, and report any skin changes immediately.
- See drain care instructions under axillary dissection section.

REFERENCES

Advincula, A., Troung, M., & Lobo, R. A. (2017). Endometriosis: Etiology, pathology, diagnosis, management. In R. A. Lobo, D. M. Gershenson, G. M. Lentz, et al. (Eds.), *Comprehensive gynecology* (7th ed.). Philadelphia, PA: Mosby.

American Academy of Pediatrics & American College of Obstetricians and Gynecologists. (2012). *Guidelines for perinatal care* (7th ed.). Washington, DC: Author.

American Cancer Society. (2016a). *Non-cancerous breast conditions: Duct ectasia.* Retrieved from http://www.cancer.org/healthy/findcancerearly/womenshealth/non-cancerousbreastconditions/non-cancerous-breast-conditions-duct-ectasia.

American Cancer Society. (2016b). *The American Cancer Society guidelines for the prevention and early detection of cervical cancer.* Retrieved from http://www.cancer.org/ccervical-cancer/prevention-and-early-detection/cervical-cancer-screening-guidelines.html.

American Psychiatric Association. (2014). *Diagnostic and statistical manual of mental disorders* (5th ed.) Washington, DC: Author. Arlington.

Centers for Disease Control and Prevention. (2015). *National notifiable diseases surveillance system (NNDSS).* Retrieved from https://wwwn.cdc.gov/nndss/conditions/notifiable/2015/infectious-diseases/.

Centers for Disease Control and Prevention. (2016a). *Areas with Zika.* Retrieved from http://www.cdc.gov/zika/about/index.html.

Centers for Disease Control and Prevention. (2016b). *Prevention in newborns: Preventing early-onset group B strep disease (GBS).* Retrieved from http://www.cdc.gov/groupbstrep/about/prevention.html.

Centers for Disease Control and Prevention. (2016c). *Breast cancer statistics.* Retrieved from http://www.cdc.gov/cancer/breast/statistics/.

Centers for Disease Control and Prevention. (2017a). *Sexually transmitted diseases.* Retrieved from https://www.cdc.gov/std/treatment/.

Centers for Disease Control and Prevention. (2017b). *Sexually transmitted diseases treatment guidelines.* Retrieved from https://www.cdc.gov/std/tg2015/clinical.htm.

Centers for Disease Control and Prevention. (2017c). *Sexually transmitted diseases treatment guidelines: Special populations.* Retrieved from https://www.cdc.gov/std/tg2015/specialpops.htm.

Chien, L. W., Chang, H. C., & Liu, C. F. (2013). Effect of yoga on serum homocysteine and nitric oxide levels in adolescent women with and without dysmenorrhea. *Journal of Complementary and Alternative Medicine, 19*(1), 20–23.

Chlebowski, R. T., & Budoff, M. J. (2016). Changing adjuvant breast cancer therapy with a signal for prevention. *New England Journal of Medicine, 375*(3), 274–275.

Choudhary, M. C. (2015). *Antiretroviral therapy for pregnant HIV-infected patients. Medscape.* Retrieved from http://emedicine.medscape.com/article/2042311-overview#a2.

Department of Health and Human Services. (2015). *Clinical guidelines portal—AIDS info.* Retrieved from https://aidsinfo.nih.gov/guidelines/html/3/perinatal-guidelines/182/transmission-and-mode-of-delivery.

Drakh, A. (2016). Low energy availability in female athletes: Oral contraceptives in athletes. *Medscape News and Perspective.* Retrieved from http://emedicine.medscape.com/article/312312-overview#a10.

Drugs.com. (2017). *Goserelin dosage.* Retrieved from https://www.drugs.com/dosage/goserelin.html.

Gardella, C., Eckert, L. O., & Lentz, G. M. (2017). Genital tract infections: vulva, vagina, cervix, toxic shock syndrome, endometritis, and salpingitis. In R. A. Lobo, D. M. Gershenson, G. M. Lentz, et al. (Eds.), *Comprehensive gynecology* (7th ed.). Philadelphia, PA: Mosby.

Healthwise Staff. (2015). *Pelvic rocking. WebMD.* Retrieved from http://www.webmd.com/fitness-exercise/pelvic-rocking.

Hughes, B., & Cu-Uvin, S. (2016). *Use of antiretroviral medications in pregnant HIV-infected patients and their infants in resource-rich settings.* Retrieved from www.uptodate.com/contents/antiretroviral-treatment-of-pregnant-hiv-infected-women-and-antiretroviral-prophylaxis-of-their-infants-in-resource-rich-settings.

Jafari, M., & Orenstein, G. (2015). Women and herbal medicine. In E. F. Olshansky (Ed.), *Women's health and wellness across the lifespan.* Philadelphia, PA: Wolters Kluwer.

Lobo, R. A. (2017). Primary and secondary amenorrhea and precocious puberty. In R. A. Lobo, D. M. Gershenson, G. M. Lentz, et al. (Eds.), *Comprehensive gynecology* (7th ed.). Philadelphia, PA: Mosby.

MedicineNet.com. (2017). *Nafarelin, Synarel.* Retrieved from http://www.medicinenet.com/nafarelin/page3.htm.

Medscape. (2017). *Leuprolide.* Retrieved from http://reference.medscape.com/drug/lupron-leuprolide-342221.

Meites, E., Kempe, A., & Markowitz, L. E. (2016). Use of a 2-dose schedule for human papillomavirus vaccination—Updated recommendations of the Advisory Committee on Immunization Practices. *Morbidity and Mortality Weekly Report, 65,* 1405–1408.

Mendiratta, V. (2017). Primary and secondary dysmenorrhea, premenstrual syndrome, and premenstrual dysphoric disorder. In R. A. Lobo, D. M. Gershenson, G. M. Lentz, et al. (Eds.), *Comprehensive gynecology* (7th ed.). Philadelphia, PA: Mosby.

Mielke, R., Parsons, K., & Greenberg, C. S. (2015). Puberty through early adulthood. In E. F. Olshansky (Ed.), *Women's health and wellness across the lifespan.* Philadelphia, PA: Wolters Kluwer.

Pruthi, S. (2015). *Is there a correlation between breast implants and cancer? And if so, how serious is the risk? Mayo Clinic.* Retrieved from http://

www.mayoclinic.org/healthy-lifestyle/womens-health/expert-answers/breast-implants-and-cancer/faq-20057774.

Ryntz, T., & Lobo, R. A. (2017). Abnormal uterine bleeding: etiology and management of acute and chronic excessive bleeding. In R. A. Lobo, D. M. Gershenson, G. M. Lentz, et al. (Eds.), *Comprehensive gynecology* (7th ed.). Philadelphia, PA: Mosby.

Sandadi, S., Rock, D. T., Orr, J. W., & Valea, F. A. (2017). Breast diseases: Detection, management, and surveillance of breast disease. In R. A. Lobo, D. M. Gershenson, G. M. Lentz, et al. (Eds.), *Comprehensive gynecology* (7th ed.). Philadelphia, PA: Mosby.

Sharp, B. A. C., Taylor, D. L., Thomas, K. K., Killeen, M. B., & Dawood, M. Y. (2002). Cyclic premenstrual pain and discomfort: the scientific basis for practice. *Journal of Obstetrics, Gynecologic, and Neonatal Nursing, 31*(6), 637–649.

Taylor, D. L. (2005). Premenstrual symptoms and syndromes: guidelines for management and self care. *Advanced Studies in Medicine, 5*(5), 228–241.

Thein-Nissenbaum, J. (2013). Long term consequences of the female athlete triad. *Maturitas, 75*(2), 107–112.

UpToDate. (2017). *Candida vulvovaginitis*. Retrieved from http://www.uptodate.com/contents/candida-vulvovaginitis.

Wambach, C. M., & Alexander, C. J. (2012). Menstrual disorders. In P. J. DiSaia, G. Chaudhuri, L. C. Giudice, et al. (Eds.), *Women's health review: A clinical update in obstetrics-gynecology*. Philadelphia, PA: Saunders.

5

Infertility, Contraception, and Abortion

Ellen F. Olshansky

http://evolve.elsevier.com/Perry/maternal

INFERTILITY

INCIDENCE

Infertility is a serious concern that affects 1 in 4 couples of reproductive age, with increasing incidence correlated with increased age (Crawford & Steiner, 2015; Lobo, 2017). Commonly infertility is considered to be a diagnosis for couples who have not achieved pregnancy after 1 year of regular, unprotected intercourse when the woman is less than 35 years of age or after 6 months when the woman is older than 35 years of age. *Fecundity* is the term used to describe the chance of achieving pregnancy and subsequent live birth within one menstrual cycle. Fecundity averages 20% in couples who are not experiencing reproductive problems (American Society of Reproductive Medicine [ASRM], 2012).

Probable causes of infertility include the trend toward delaying pregnancy until later in life, a time when fertility decreases naturally and the prevalence of diseases such as endometriosis and ovulatory dysfunction increases. Questions exist regarding whether there has been an increase in male infertility or whether male infertility is more readily identified because of improvements in diagnosis.

For the couple experiencing infertility, diagnosis and treatment strategies require considerable physical, emotional, and financial investment over an extended period of time. Feelings connected with infertility are many and complex, often interfering with quality of life. It is common for infertile couples to experience anxiety from the need to undergo many tests and examinations and from a perception of feeling "different" from their fertile friends and relatives. The following four goals provide a framework for nurses who care for infertile persons:

- Provide the couple with accurate information about human reproduction, infertility treatments, and prognosis for pregnancy. Dispel any myths or inaccuracies from friends or the mass media that the couple may believe to be true.
- Help the couple and the health care team accurately identify and treat possible causes of infertility.
- Provide emotional support. The couple may benefit from anticipatory guidance, counseling, and support group meetings, either face-to-face or online. The organization RESOLVE (www.resolve.org) provides online support, advocacy, and education about infertility for both the infertility community and health care providers.
- Guide and educate those who fail to conceive biologically about other forms of treatment such as in vitro fertilization (IVF), donor eggs or semen, surrogate motherhood, and adoption. Support the couple in their decisions regarding their future family.

It is important for nurses to encourage all healthy women and men to maintain a normal body mass index (BMI) and avoid sexually transmitted infections (STIs) and exposures to substances or habits (such as smoking) that impair reproductive ability. While these health-promoting activities will not ensure fertility, they will enhance overall health as the individual or couple is coping with the stresses of infertility.

FACTORS ASSOCIATED WITH INFERTILITY

Although exact percentages vary somewhat with populations, approximately 85% to 90% of couples seeking infertility care are treated with medication or surgery, with 3% being treated with in vitro fertilization or other assisted reproductive methods (ASRM, 2016). About 40% of infertility is related to a male factor or a combined male and female factor (ASRM, 2016). About 20% of infertility is unexplained (Lobo, 2017). For those couples and individuals for whom a specific cause of infertility is not detected, the focus of infertility treatment has shifted from attempting to correct a specific pathology to recommending and initiating the treatment that is most effective in achieving pregnancy for this unique couple at this time in their reproductive life span. Assisted reproductive technologies (ARTs) have proven to be effective, even in couples who experience unexplained infertility.

Unassisted human conception requires a normally developed reproductive tract in both the male and female partners. For simplification, each live birth necessitates synchronization of the following:

- The male must deposit semen with sperm that has the capacity to fertilize an egg close to the cervix at the time of ovulation. The sperm must be able to ascend through the uterus and uterine tubes (male factor). The cervix must be sufficiently open to allow semen to enter the uterus and provide a nurturing environment for sperm (cervical factor).
- The uterine tubes must be able to capture the ovum, transport semen to the ovum, and transport the fertilized embryo to the uterus (tubal factor).
- Ovulation of a healthy oocyte must occur, ideally within the parameters of a regular, predictable menstrual cycle (ovarian factor).
- The uterus must be receptive to implantation of the embryo and capable of nourishing the growth and development of the fetus throughout the normal duration of pregnancy (uterine factor).

An alteration in one or more of these structures, functions, or processes results in some degree of impaired fertility. Boxes 5.1 and 5.2 list factors affecting female and male infertility.

For conception to occur, both partners must have normal, intact hypothalamic-pituitary-gonadal hormonal axes that support the formation of sperm in the male and ova in the female. Sperm can remain viable within a woman's reproductive tract for at least 3 days and for as long as 5 days. The oocyte can only be successfully fertilized for 12 to 24 hours after ovulation. The couple seeking pregnancy should be taught about the menstrual cycle and ways to detect ovulation (see Chapter 3). They should be counseled to have intercourse 2 to 3 times

BOX 5.1 Factors Affecting Female Fertility

Ovarian Factors
- Developmental anomalies
- Anovulation—primary
  - Pituitary or hypothalamic hormone disorders
  - Adrenal gland disorders (rare)
  - Congenital adrenal hyperplasia (rare)
- Anovulation—secondary
  - Disruption of hypothalamic-pituitary-ovarian axis
  - Anorexia
  - Insufficient body fat in athletic women
  - Increased prolactin levels
  - Thyroid disorders
  - Premature ovarian failure
  - Polycystic ovary syndrome
- Medications
  - Oral contraceptives
  - Progestins
  - Antidepressant and antipsychotic drugs
  - Corticosteroids
  - Chemotherapy

Tubal/Peritoneal Factors
- Developmental anomalies of the tubes (see Fig. 5.1)
- Reduced tubal motility
- Inflammation within the tube
- Tubal adhesions
- Disruption caused by tubal pregnancy
- Endometriosis

Uterine Factors
- Developmental anomalies of the uterus (see Fig. 5.1)
- Endometrial and myometrial fibroid tumors
- Asherman's syndrome (uterine adhesions or scar tissue)

Vaginal-Cervical Factors
- Vaginal-cervical infections
- Cervical mucus inadequate
- Isoimmunization (development of sperm antibodies)

Other Factors
- Nutritional deficiencies
- Obesity
- Thyroid dysfunction (hyperthyroidism and hypothyroidism)
- Idiopathic conditions

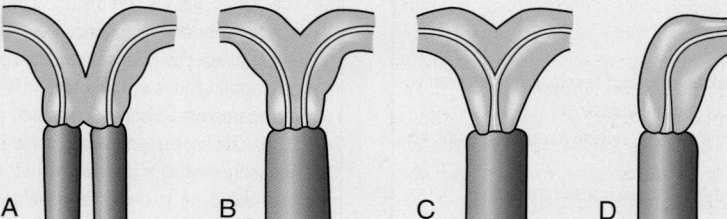

FIG 5.1 Abnormal uterus. **A,** Complete bicornuate uterus with vagina divided by a septum. **B,** Complete bicornuate uterus with normal vagina. **C,** Partial bicornuate uterus with normal vagina. **D,** Unicornuate uterus.

a week; or, if timed intercourse does not increase anxiety, they should be encouraged to engage in intercourse the day before and the day of ovulation. Fertility decreases markedly 24 hours after ovulation.

CARE MANAGEMENT

Infertility care management includes a team of health care providers, including an obstetric care provider, fertility specialist, embryologist, genetic counselor, and mental health provider or counselor. The nurse is a key member of the care management team and assists in the assessment and education of the infertile couple. As part of the assessment process, he or she obtains information from the couple through interview and physical examination, including if this couple's situation is one of primary (never experienced pregnancy) or secondary (previous pregnancy) infertility. Religious, cultural, and ethnic data may place restrictions on use of available treatments.

In addition, the nurse obtains and monitors results of diagnostic testing. Some of the information and data needed to investigate impaired fertility are of a sensitive, personal nature. The couple may experience feelings of invasion of privacy, and the nurse must exercise tact and express concern for their well-being throughout the interview. The tests and examinations associated with infertility diagnosis and treatment are occasionally painful and often intrusive. The couple's intimacy and feelings of romantic attachment are often impaired as they engage in

this process. A high level of motivation is needed to endure the investigation and subsequent treatment. Because multiple factors involving both partners are common, the investigation of impaired fertility is conducted systematically and simultaneously for both male and female partners. Both partners must be interested in the solution to the problem. The medical investigation requires time (3 to 4 months) and considerable financial expense. Box 5.3 describes the status of insurance coverage for infertility treatment.

Assessment of Female Infertility

Evaluation for infertility should be offered to couples who have failed to become pregnant after 1 year of regular intercourse or after 6 months if the woman is older than 35 years of age. Investigation of impaired fertility begins for the woman with a complete history and physical examination. A complete general physical examination should include height and weight and estimation of BMI. Both obesity and being underweight are associated with anovulation disorders. Signs and symptoms of androgen excess such as excess body hair or pigmentation changes should be noted. The general physical examination is followed by a specific assessment of the reproductive tract. A history of infections of the genitourinary tract and any signs of infections, especially STIs that could impair tubal patency, should be assessed. Bimanual examination of internal organs may reveal lack of mobility of the uterus or abnormal contours of the uterus and tubes. A woman may have an

BOX 5.2   Factors Affecting Male Fertility

Hormonal Disorders
- Congenital disorders
- Tumors of the pituitary gland or hypothalamus
- Trauma to the pituitary gland or hypothalamus
- Hyperprolactinemia
- Excess of androgens, estrogen, or cortisol
- Drugs and substance abuse (recreational and prescribed drugs)
- Chronic illnesses
- Nutritional deficiencies
- Obesity
- Endocrine disorders (e.g., diabetes)

Testicular Factors
- Congenital disorders
- Undescended testes
- Hypospadias
- Varicocele
- Viral infections (e.g., mumps)
- Sexually transmitted infections (e.g. gonorrhea, chlamydial infection)
- Obstructive lesions of the epididymis and vas deferens
- Environmental toxins
- Trauma
- Torsion
- Castration
- Systemic illnesses
- Antisperm antibodies
- Changes in sperm from cigarette smoking or use of heroin, marijuana, amyl nitrate, butyl nitrate, ethyl chloride, or methaqualone
- Decrease in libido from use of heroin, methadone, selective serotonin reuptake inhibitors, or barbiturates
- Impotence from use of alcohol or antihypertensive medications

Factors Associated With Sperm Transport
- Drugs
- Sexually transmitted infections of the epididymis
- Ejaculatory dysfunction
- Premature ejaculation

Idiopathic Male Infertility

BOX 5.4   Summary of Findings Favorable to Fertility

1. Follicular development, ovulation, and luteal development are supportive of pregnancy:
   a. Basal body temperature (presumptive evidence of ovulatory cycles) is biphasic, with temperature elevation that persists for 12 to 14 days before menstruation.
   b. Cervical mucus characteristics change appropriately during phases of the menstrual cycle.
   c. Days 3 to 10 follicle-stimulating hormone (FSH) levels are low enough to verify the presence of adequate ovarian follicles.
   d. Day 3 estradiol levels are low enough to verify the presence of adequate ovarian follicles.
   e. Woman reports a history of regular, predictable menses with consistent premenstrual and menstrual symptoms.
2. The luteal phase is supportive of pregnancy:
   a. Levels of plasma progesterone are adequate to indicate ovulation.
   b. Luteal phase of menstrual cycle is of sufficient duration to support pregnancy.
3. Cervical factors are receptive to sperm during expected time of ovulation:
   a. Cervical os is open.
   b. Cervical mucus is clear, watery, abundant, and slippery and demonstrates good spinnbarkeit and arborization (fern pattern) at time of ovulation.
   c. Cervical examination reveals no lesions or infections.
4. The uterus and uterine tubes support pregnancy:
   a. Uterine and tubal patency are documented by (1) spillage of dye into the peritoneal cavity, and (2) outlines of uterine and tubal cavities of adequate size and shape with no abnormalities.
   b. Laparoscopic examination verifies normal development of internal genitals and absence of adhesions, infections, endometriosis, and other lesions.
5. The male partner's reproductive structures are normal:
   a. There is no evidence of developmental anomalies of penis, testicular atrophy, or varicocele (varicose veins on the spermatic vein in the groin).
   b. There is no evidence of infection in prostate, seminal vesicles, and urethra.
   c. Testes are more than 4 cm in largest diameter.
6. Semen is supportive of pregnancy:
   a. Sperm (number per milliliter) are adequate in ejaculate.
   b. Most sperm show normal morphology.
   c. Most sperm are motile, forward moving.
   d. No autoimmunity exists.
   e. Seminal fluid is normal.

BOX 5.3   Insurance Coverage for Infertility

As of October 2016, only 15 states had mandated some form of insurance coverage for infertility. These mandates included in vitro fertilization in some states, whereas others only covered some diagnostic tests. Some states require health maintenance organizations (HMOs) to cover some costs, whereas in others HMOs are exempt. Patients need information about what they can expect from their insurers. The state Insurance Commissioner's office can provide information about an individual state. The website for the American Society for Reproductive Medicine (www.asrm.org) has more complete information.

abnormal uterus and tubes as a result of congenital abnormalities during fetal development). These uterine abnormalities increase risk for early pregnancy loss.

Laboratory data, including routine urine and blood tests, are collected. The initial clinic visit serves as a preconceptional visit and as initial assessment of possible causes of infertility. The woman should be taking folic acid supplements, and all immunizations should be current to prepare for possible pregnancy.

Diagnostic Testing

The basic infertility survey of the female involves evaluation of the cervix, uterus, tubes, and peritoneum; detection of ovulation; and hormone analysis. Timing and descriptions of common tests are presented in Table 5.1.

Previous status regarding ovulation can be evaluated through menstrual history, serum hormone studies, and use of an ovulation predictor kit. If the woman is older than 35 years of age, the clinician may choose to assess "ovarian reserve" or how many potential ova remain within the ovaries. A common evaluation of ovarian reserve is measurement of follicle-stimulating hormone (FSH) levels on the third day of the menstrual cycle. The uterus and fallopian/uterine tubes can be visualized for abnormalities and tubal patency through hysterosalpingogram (x-ray film examination of the uterine cavity and tubes after

TABLE 5.1 General Tests for Impaired Fertility

Test or Examination	Timing (Menstrual Cycle Days)	Rationale
Hysterosalpingogram (HSG) (uterine abnormalities, tubal patency)	7–10	Late follicular, early proliferative phase; will not disrupt a fertilized ovum; may open uterine tubes before time of ovulation
Chlamydia immunoglobulin G antibodies (tubal patency)	Variable	Negative antibody test may indicate tubal patency assessment (HSG); not needed in low-risk women
Hysterosalpingo-contrast sonography (uterine abnormalities, tubal patency)	7–10	Late follicular, early proliferative phase; will not disrupt a fertilized ovum; evaluates tubal patency, uterine cavity, and myometrium
Serum progesterone (ovulation)	7 days before expected menses	Midluteal-phase progesterone levels; check adequacy of corpus luteum progesterone production
Assessment of cervical mucus (ovulation)	Variable, ovulation	Cervical mucus should have low viscosity, spinnbarkeit (ability to stretch) during ovulation
Basal body temperature (ovulation)	Chart entire cycle	Elevation occurs in response to progesterone; documents ovulation
Urinary ovulation predictor kit (ovulation)	Variable, ovulation	Detects timing of lutein hormone surge before ovulation
Semen analysis (male factor)	2–7 days after abstinence	Detects ability of sperm to fertilize egg
Sperm penetration assay (male factor)	After 2 days but ≤1 week of abstinence	Evaluates ability of sperm to penetrate egg
Follicle-stimulating hormone (FSH) level (ovarian reserve)	Day 3	High FSH levels (>20) indicate that pregnancy will not occur with woman's own eggs; value <10 indicates adequate ovarian reserve
Clomiphene citrate challenge test (CCCT) (ovarian reserve)	Administer clomiphene 100 mg days 5 through 9	Assess FSH on days 3 and 10 in presence of clomiphene stimulation; high FSH levels (>20) indicate that pregnancy will not occur with woman's own eggs; FSH <15 suggestive of adequate ovarian reserve

From Genetics & IVF Institute. (2013). *Fertility: Clomiphene citrate test.* Retrieved from http://www.givf.com/fertility/clomidchallengetest.shtml.

instillation of radiopaque contrast material through the cervix). If the woman is at risk for endometriosis (implants of endometrial tissue outside of the uterus) or adhesions, diagnostic laparoscopy may be indicated. Test findings favorable for fertility are summarized in Box 5.4.

Assessment of Male Infertility

The systematic investigation of infertility in the male patient begins with a thorough history and physical examination. Assessment of the male patient proceeds in a manner similar to that of the female patient, starting with noninvasive tests.

Diagnostic Testing and Semen Analysis

The basic test for male infertility is semen analysis. A complete semen analysis, study of the effects of cervical mucus on sperm forward motility and survival, and evaluation of the ability of the sperm to penetrate an ovum provide basic information. Sperm counts vary from day to day and depend on emotional and physical status and sexual activity. Therefore, a single analysis may be inconclusive. A minimum of two analyses must be performed several weeks apart to assess male fertility.

Semen is collected by ejaculation into a clean container or a plastic sheath that does not contain a spermicidal agent. The specimen is usually collected by masturbation following 2 to 7 days of abstinence from ejaculation. The semen is examined at the collection site or taken to the laboratory in a sealed container within 2 hours of ejaculation. Exposure to excessive heat or cold is avoided. Commonly accepted values for semen characteristics are given in Box 5.5. If results are in the fertile range, no further sperm evaluation is necessary. If results are not within this range, the test is repeated. If subsequent results are still in the subfertile range, further evaluation is needed to identify the problem.

Hormone analyses are done for testosterone, gonadotropin, FSH, and luteinizing hormone (LH). The sperm penetration assay and other alternative tests may be used to evaluate the ability of sperm to penetrate an egg. Testicular biopsy may be warranted. Scrotal ultrasound may be used to examine the testes for presence of varicoceles and identify abnormalities

in the scrotum and spermatic cord. Transrectal ultrasound is used to evaluate the ejaculatory ducts, seminal vesicles, and vas deferens.

BOX 5.5 Semen Analysis: Normal Values

- Semen volume at least 1.5 mL
- Semen pH 7.2 or higher
- Sperm density greater than 15 million/mL
- Total sperm count greater than 39 million per ejaculate
- Normal morphologic features greater than 4% (normal oval)
- Motility (important consideration in sperm evaluation)—percentage of forward-moving sperm estimated with respect to abnormally motile and nonmotile sperm, 40%
- Liquification—usually within 15 minutes but no longer than 60 minutes

Note: These values are not absolute but are only relative to final evaluation of the couple as a single reproductive unit. Values also differ according to source used as a reference.

Data from World Health Organization. (2010). *Laboratory manual for the examination of human semen* (5th ed.). Geneva, Switzerland: Author.

Psychosocial Considerations

Infertility is recognized as a major life stressor that can affect self-esteem; relations with the spouse or partner, family, and friends; and careers. Psychologic responses to the diagnosis of infertility may tax a couple's capacity for giving and receiving physical and sexual closeness. The prescriptions and taboos for achieving conception may add tension to a couple's sexual functioning. They may report decreased desire for intercourse, orgasmic dysfunction, or midcycle erectile disorders.

To be able to deal comfortably with a couple's sexuality, nurses must be comfortable with their own sexuality so they can better help couples understand why aspects of sexual intimacy need to be shared with health care professionals. Nurses need current factual knowledge about human sexual practices and must be accepting of the preferences and activities of others without being judgmental. They must be skilled in

CLINICAL REASONING CASE STUDY
Infertility

Diane is a 39-year-old accountant who has recently married for the first time. Charles is 41 years of age and has two children from a previous marriage. Diane has a history of amenorrhea dating back to when she was in college and a member of the track team. Currently her menstrual periods are irregular. She wants to have a baby "before it's too late," and she and Charles have been having unprotected sex for almost 1 year. They have come to the fertility clinic today for an evaluation. Diane tells the nurse that she has heard about the success of in vitro fertilization (IVF) and wants to know if she will be able to have it performed. How should the nurse respond to Diane's comments and questions?

1. Evidence—Is evidence sufficient to draw conclusions about what response the nurse should give?
2. Assumptions—Describe underlying assumptions about the following issues:
   a. Age and fertility: Is Diane's age a factor in her concern regarding infertility?
   b. Infertility as a major life stressor: To what extent can infertility or the fear of being infertile cause stress?
   c. Success rates for IVF pregnancy and birth: Is IVF a reasonable treatment to consider (after having a thorough workup)?
   d. Causes of female infertility: What are some of the reasons that Diane may be infertile?
3. What implications and priorities for nursing care can be drawn at this time?
4. Describe the roles and responsibilities of members of the interprofessional health care team who may be caring for Diana and Charles.

interviewing and therapeutic use of self, sensitive to the nonverbal cues of others, and knowledgeable regarding each couple's sociocultural and religious beliefs (see Clinical Reasoning Case Study).

The couple facing infertility exhibits behaviors of the grieving process such as those associated with other types of loss. The loss of one's genetic continuity with the generations to come can provoke decreased self-esteem, a sense of inadequacy as a woman or a man, and feelings of loss of control over personal destiny. Infertile individuals can perceive dissatisfaction with their marriages or partner relationships. Not all people have all the reactions described, nor can it be predicted how long any reaction will last for an individual. Often a mental health counselor with experience and expertise dealing with infertility can be very helpful to an individual or couple.

If the couple does not conceive, they should be assessed regarding their desire to be referred for help with adoption, donor eggs or semen, surrogacy, or other reproductive alternatives. The couple may choose to continue in a child-free state. Both health care providers and patients should have a list of agencies, support groups, and other resources within their community such as the ASRM (www.asrm.org) and RESOLVE (www.resolve.org).

Nonmedical Treatments

Both men and women can benefit from healthy lifestyle changes that result in a BMI within the normal range; moderate daily exercise; and abstinence from alcohol, nicotine, and recreational drugs. For the woman with a BMI >27 and polycystic ovary syndrome, losing just 5% to 10% of body weight can restore ovulation within 6 months. Anovulatory women with a BMI <17 who have eating disorders or intense exercise regimens benefit from weight gain. Nevertheless, this population sometimes is reluctant to alter their behaviors, and counseling should be advised.

Simple changes in lifestyle may be effective in the treatment of subfertile men. Only water-soluble lubricants should be used during intercourse because many commonly used lubricants contain spermicides or have spermicidal properties. Instead of wearing briefs, the male should wear boxer shorts and loose pants because these tend to decrease scrotal temperature and may prevent a decrease in sperm count. High scrotal temperatures can be caused by daily hot tub baths or saunas that keep the testes at temperatures too high for efficient spermatogenesis. These conditions lead to only lessened fertility and should not be used as a means of contraception.

Most herbal remedies have not been proven clinically to promote fertility or to be safe in early pregnancy and should be taken by the woman only as prescribed by a physician or nurse-midwife who has expertise in herbology. Relaxation, osteopathy, stress management (e.g., aromatherapy, yoga), and nutritional and exercise counseling have been reported to increase pregnancy rates in some women. Herbs to avoid while trying to conceive include licorice root, yarrow, wormwood, ephedra, fennel, goldenseal, lavender, juniper, flaxseed, pennyroyal, passionflower, wild cherry, cascara, sage, thyme, and periwinkle. All supplements or herbs should be purchased from trusted sources to ensure that they do not contain contaminants.

Medical Therapy

One goal of infertility assessment and treatment is to determine which couples are likely to respond to conventional therapies in a timely manner. Another goal is early referral of couples who will need ARTs to conceive. In general, any fertility treatment is more likely to result in a live birth in women who are younger than 35 years of age, with successful outcomes decreasing for women older than 40 years of age.

Pharmacologic therapy for female infertility is often directed at treating ovulatory dysfunction by either stimulating or enhancing ovulation so more oocytes mature. These medications include (1) clomiphene citrate as initial therapy for many women with intermittent anovulation; (2) a combination of clomiphene and metformin for women with anovulation and insulin resistance; (3) human menopausal gonadotropin (HMG), FSH, and recombinant FSH (rFSH) to stimulate follicle formation in women who do not respond to clomiphene therapies; (4) human chorionic gonadotropin to induce ovulation when follicles are ripe; (5) gonadotropin-releasing hormone (GnRH) agonists at the beginning of a cycle to sequence HMG therapies; (6) progesterone to support the luteal phase of the cycle; and (7) bromocriptine (Parlodel) for women who have excess prolactin (Lobo, 2017).

Treatment of certain medical conditions may result in improved fertility. The woman who is hypothyroid benefits from thyroid hormone supplementation. Treatment of endometriosis could include trials of danazol, progesterone, continuous combined oral contraceptives, or GnRH agonists to suppress menstruation and shrink endometrial implants. This regimen would be followed by ovulation induction. Adrenal hyperplasia is treated with prednisone. Any infections present in the infertile couple should be treated with appropriate antimicrobial therapy.

Clomiphene citrate (with the possible addition of metformin) is often the initial pharmacologic treatment of the infertile woman because it is inexpensive and the side-effect profile is less than other medications that induce ovulation. There is an increased risk for giving birth to twins or higher order multiples with clomiphene therapy.

The more powerful medications used to induce ovulation include GnRH agonists followed by gonadotropin therapy. These medications are extremely potent and require daily ovarian ultrasonography and monitoring of estradiol levels to prevent hyperstimulation of the ovaries. Combinations of these medications are used with ART to stimulate ovulation before harvesting eggs.

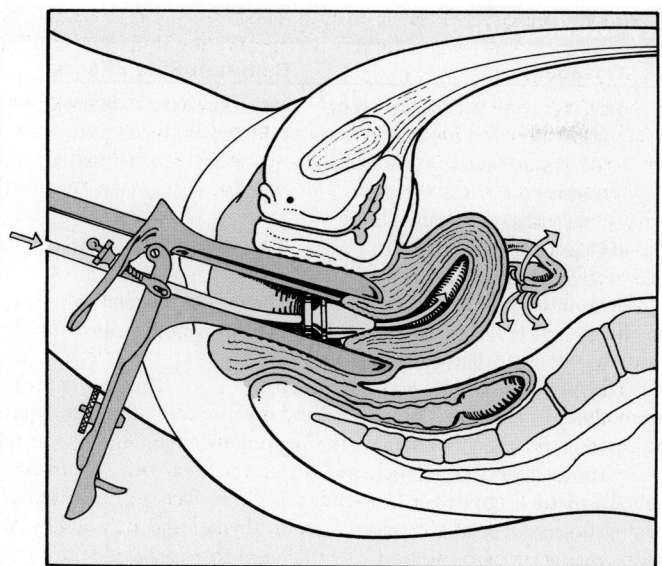

FIG 5.2 Hysterosalpingography. Note that the contrast medium flows through the intrauterine cannula and out through the uterine tubes.

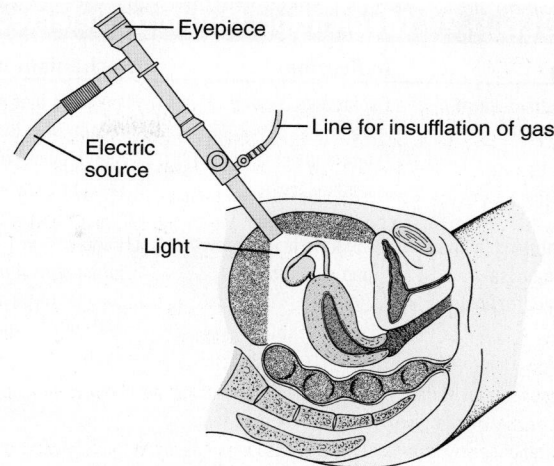

FIG 5.3 Laparoscopy.

Drug therapy may be indicated for male infertility. As with women, problems with the thyroid or adrenal glands are corrected with appropriate medications. Infections are identified and treated with antimicrobials. FSH, HMG, and clomiphene may be used to stimulate spermatogenesis in men with hypogonadism. Men who do not respond to these therapies are candidates for intracytoplasmic sperm injection (ICSI), which is a procedure that injects sperm directly into the egg as part of IVF. ICSI has enabled men with very low sperm counts to achieve biologic reproduction.

The infertility specialist is responsible for fully informing patients about the prescribed medications. The nurse must be ready to answer patients' questions and confirm their understanding of the drug, its administration, potential side effects, and expected outcomes. Because information varies with each drug, the nurse must consult the medication package inserts, pharmacology references, health care provider, and pharmacist as necessary. The nurse should also provide anticipatory guidance regarding the time given for a medication trial before referral to a specialist in ART would be indicated if the couple wants to continue to attempt to become pregnant.

Table 5.2 includes information on selected medications for infertility treatment.

Surgical Therapies

A number of surgical procedures may be used for problems causing female infertility. Ovarian tumors must be excised. Whenever possible, functional ovarian tissue is left intact. Scar tissue adhesions caused by chronic infections may cover much of the ovary. These adhesions usually necessitate surgery to free and expose the ovary so ovulation can occur.

Hysterosalpingography is useful for identification of tubal obstruction and also for the release of blockage as demonstrated in Fig. 5.2. During laparoscopy, delicate adhesions may be divided and removed, and endometrial implants may be destroyed by electrocoagulation or laser, as illustrated in Fig. 5.3. Laparotomy and microsurgery may be required for extensive repair of the damaged tube. Prognosis depends on the degree to which tubal patency and function can be restored. In general, laparoscopic surgery for tubal patency is most effective in younger women with distal tubal damage. Older women or those with significant proximal disease should be referred for ARTs that bypass the uterine tube.

In women with uterine abnormalities, reconstructive surgery (e.g., the unification operation for bicornuate uterus) can improve the ability to conceive and carry a fetus to term. Surgical removal of tumors or fibroids involving the endometrium or muscular walls of the uterus may also improve the woman's chance of conceiving and maintaining a pregnancy to viability, depending on the location and size of the fibroid or tumor. Surgical treatment of uterine tumors or maldevelopment that results in successful pregnancy usually necessitates birth by cesarean surgery near term gestation because the enlarging uterus can rupture as a result of weakness in the area of reconstructive surgery.

Chronic inflammation and infection can be eliminated by radial chemocautery (destruction of tissue with chemicals) or thermocautery (destruction of tissue with heat, usually electrical) of the cervix, cryosurgery (destruction of tissue by application of extreme cold, usually liquid nitrogen), or conization (excision of a cone-shaped piece of tissue from the endocervix). When the cervix has been deeply cauterized or frozen or when extensive conization has been performed, the cervix may produce less mucus. Therefore, the absence of a mucus bridge from the vagina to the uterus can make sperm migration difficult or impossible. Therapeutic intrauterine insemination may be necessary to carry the sperm directly through the internal os of the cervix.

Surgical procedures may also be used for problems causing male infertility. Surgical repair of varicocele has been relatively successful in increasing sperm count but not fertility rates. Microsurgery to reanastomose (restore tubal continuity) the sperm ducts after vasectomy may restore fertility.

Assisted Reproductive Therapies

The Centers for Disease Control and Prevention (CDC) (2014) defines *ART* as fertility treatments in which both eggs and sperm are handled. In general, these treatments involve removing the eggs from the woman, fertilizing the eggs in the laboratory, and returning the embryo or embryos to the woman or surrogate carrier. Births that were conceived through ART comprise over 1.5% of all infants born in the United States each year since 2013 (Kaplan, 2015).

Some of the ARTs for treatment of infertility include in vitro fertilization–embryo transfer (IVF-ET), gamete intrafallopian transfer (GIFT) (Fig. 5.4), zygote intrafallopian transfer (ZIFT), ovum transfer (oocyte donation), embryo adoption, embryo hosting and surrogate motherhood, therapeutic donor insemination (TDI), ICSI, assisted embryo hatching, and preimplantation genetic diagnosis (PGD).

TABLE 5.2   Medication Guide to Selected Infertility Medications

Drug	Indication	Mechanism of Action	Dosage	Common Side Effects
Clomiphene citrate	Ovulation induction, treatment of luteal-phase inadequacy	Thought to bind to estrogen receptors in the pituitary gland, blocking them from detecting estrogen	Tablets, starting with 50 mg/day by mouth for 5 days beginning on fifth day of menses; if ovulation does not occur, may increase dose next cycle; variable dosage	Vasomotor flushes, abdominal discomfort, nausea and vomiting, breast tenderness, ovarian enlargement
Menotropins (human menopausal gonadotropins)	Ovarian follicular growth and maturation	LH and FSH in 1:1 ratio, direct stimulation of ovarian follicle; given sequentially with hCG to induce ovulation	IM injections; dosage regimen variable based on ovarian response Initial dose is 75 International Units of FSH and 75 International Units of LH (1 ampule) daily for 7–12 days (not to exceed 12 days) followed by 5000 to 10,000 International Units hCG (if serum estradiol <2000 pg/mL	Ovarian enlargement, ovarian hyperstimulation, local irritation at injection site, multifetal gestations
Follitropins (purified FSH)	Treatment of polycystic ovary syndrome; follicle stimulation for assisted reproductive techniques	Direct action on ovarian follicle	Subcutaneous or IM injections; dosage regimen variable	Ovarian enlargement, ovarian hyperstimulation, local irritation at injection site, multifetal gestations
Human chorionic gonadotropin (hCG)	Ovulation induction	Direct action on ovarian follicle to stimulate meiosis and rupture of the follicle	5000–10,000 International Units IM 1 day after last dose of menotropins; dosage regimen variable	Local irritation at injection site; headaches, irritability, edema, depression, fatigue
GnRH agonists (nafarelin acetate, leuprolide acetate)	Treatment of endometriosis, uterine fibroids	Desensitization and downward regulation of GnRH receptors of pituitary gland, resulting in suppression of LH, FSH, and ovarian function	Nafarelin, 200 mcg (1 spray) intranasally twice daily for 6 months; leuprolide acetate 3.75 mg IM every month for 3–6 months	Nafarelin—irritation, nosebleeds Both nafarelin and leuprolide—hot flashes, vaginal dryness, myalgia and arthralgia, headaches, mild bone loss (usually reversible within 12–18 months after treatment)
Progesterone	Treatment of luteal-phase inadequacy	Direct stimulation of endometrium	Vaginal gel 8%, 1 prefilled applicator per day; after ovulation induction, continue through 10–12 weeks of pregnancy	Breast tenderness, local irritation, headaches
GnRH antagonists (ganirelix acetate, cetrorelix acetate)	Controlled ovarian stimulation for infertility treatment	Suppress gonadotropin secretion, inhibit premature LH surges in women undergoing ovarian hyperstimulation	250 mcg daily subcutaneously, usually in the early to midfollicular phase of the menstrual cycle; usually followed by hCG administration	Abdominal pain, headache, vaginal bleeding, irritation at the injection site
Metformin	Restores cyclic ovulation and menses in many women with polycystic ovary syndrome	Induces ovulation through reducing insulin resistance, thus affecting gonadotropins and androgens; simulates the ovary	Initial dose is 500 mg daily and titrated up over several weeks to 1500 mg/day; administered orally	Nausea, vomiting, diarrhea, lactic acidosis, liver dysfunction
Letrozole	Ovulation induction	Aromatase inhibitor that inhibits E_2 production, which causes an increase in LH:FHS ratio	2.5- to 5-mg tablets administered orally for 5 days beginning on cycle day 3 to 7	Hot flashes, headaches, breast tenderness; may increase risk for congenital anomalies

Data from American Society for Reproductive Medicine. (2013). *Medications for inducing ovulation: A patient guide*. Retrieved from www.asrm. org/Factsheetsandbooklets; Facts and Comparisons. (2013). *A to Z drug facts*. Retrieved from www.factsandcomparisons.com; Casper, R.F., & Mitwally, M.F.M. (2016). Ovulation induction with letrozole. *UpToDate*. Retrieved from https://www.uptodate.com/contents/ovulation-induction-with-letrozole; Medscape. (2017). *Menotropins*. Retrieved from http://reference.medscape.com/drug/menopur-repronex-menotropins-342877; Lobo R. (2017). Infertility: Etiology, diagnostic evaluation, management, prognosis. In R. A. Lobo, D. M. Gershenson, G. M. Lentz, et al. (Eds.), *Comprehensive gynecology* (7th ed.). Philadelphia, PA: Elsevier.

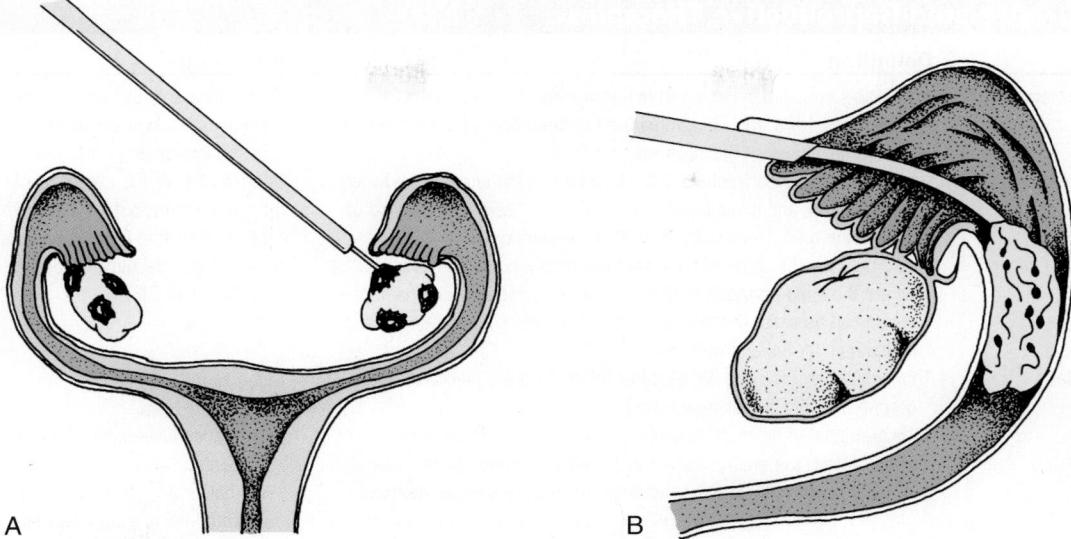

FIG 5.4 Gamete intrafallopian transfer (GIFT). **A,** Through laparoscopy a ripe follicle is located, and fluid containing the egg is removed. **B,** The sperm and egg are placed separately in the uterine tube, where fertilization occurs.

BOX 5.6   Issues to Be Addressed by Infertile Couples Before Treatment

- Risk for multiple gestation
- Possible need for multifetal reduction
- Possible need for donor oocytes, sperm, or embryos or for gestational carrier (surrogate mother)
- Whether or how to disclose facts of conception to offspring
- Freezing embryos for later use and what to do with extra embryos
- Possible risk for long-term effects of medications and treatment on women, children, and families
- Potential mental health effects (anxiety, depression) related to infertility treatment

---

Table 5.3 describes these procedures and the possible indications for ARTs. Donor sperm and donor eggs can be used with ARTs. In addition, surrogates may carry the couple's biologic child. ARTs are associated with many ethical and legal issues (Box 5.6).

The lack of or misleading information about success rates and the risks and benefits of treatment alternatives prevent couples from making informed decisions. Nurses can provide information so couples have an accurate understanding of their chances for a successful pregnancy and live birth. Nurses also can provide anticipatory guidance about the moral and ethical dilemmas regarding the use of ARTs. If a couple is fortunate enough to have multiple embryos available, they may choose to preserve these for later implantation, which has potential legal implications.

LEGAL TIP Cryopreservation of Human Embryos Couples who have extra embryos frozen for possible transfer must be fully informed before consenting to the procedure. They must make decisions regarding the disposal of embryos in the event of death or divorce. If they no longer want the embryos, they may consider donating them to other couples, contributing them to research, or disposing of them.

Complications

Other than the established risks associated with laparoscopy and general anesthesia, few risks are associated with IVF-ET, GIFT, and ZIFT. The more common transvaginal needle aspiration for egg retrieval requires only local or intravenous analgesia. Congenital anomalies occur no more frequently than among naturally conceived embryos. Multiple gestations are more likely and are associated with increased risks for both the mother and fetuses. Nevertheless, ectopic pregnancies do occur more often and pose significant maternal risk (Lobo, 2017).

PREIMPLANTATION GENETIC DIAGNOSIS

PGD is a form of early genetic testing designed to allow identification of embryos with serious genetic abnormalities. Those embryos would not be used in ART. Genetic testing improves the likelihood of successful pregnancy. Micromanipulation allows removal of a single cell from a multicellular embryo for genetic study (i.e., embryo biopsy) (ASRM, 2014). PGD is used clinically in numerous centers around the world. Couples must be counseled about their options and choices and the implications of their choices when genetic analysis is considered.

ADOPTION

Couples may choose to build their family by adopting children who are not their own biologically. With increased availability of birth control and abortion and an increase in single mothers who choose to keep their babies, the availability of healthy newborn infants in the United States is limited (Greenblatt, 2011). Infants with diverse ethnic and racial heritages, infants with special needs, older children, and foreign adoptions are other options (Fig. 5.5).

CONTRACEPTION

The CDC noted that the capability of Americans to engage in effective family planning as a result of the modern era of contraception was one of the 10 greatest public health achievements of the 20th century (CDC, 2013). Nevertheless, nearly half of all pregnancies in the United States are

TABLE 5.3   Assisted Reproductive Therapies

Procedure	Definition	Indications
In vitro fertilization–embryo transfer (IVF-ET)	A woman's eggs are collected from her ovaries, fertilized in the laboratory with sperm, and transferred to her uterus after normal embryo development has occurred.	Tubal disease or blockage; severe male infertility; endometriosis; unexplained infertility; cervical factor; immunologic infertility
Gamete intrafallopian transfer (GIFT)	Oocytes are retrieved from the ovary, placed in a catheter with washed motile sperm, and immediately transferred into the fimbriated end of the uterine tube. Fertilization occurs in the uterine tube.	Same as for IVF-ET, except there must be normal tubal anatomy, patency, and absence of previous tubal disease in at least one uterine tube
IVF-ET and GIFT with donor sperm	This process is the same as described previously except in cases where the male partner's fertility is severely compromised and donor sperm can be used; if donor sperm are used, the woman must have indications for IVF and GIFT.	Severe male infertility; azoospermia; indications for IVF-ET or GIFT
Zygote intrafallopian transfer (ZIFT)	This process is similar to IVF-ET; after IVF the ova are placed in one uterine tube during the zygote stage.	Same as for GIFT
Donor oocyte	Eggs are donated by an IVF procedure, and the donated eggs are inseminated. The embryos are transferred into the recipient's uterus, which is hormonally prepared with estrogen/progesterone therapy.	Early menopause; surgical removal of ovaries; congenitally absent ovaries; autosomal or sex-linked disorders; lack of fertilization in repeated IVF attempts because of subtle oocyte abnormalities or defects in oocyte-spermatozoa interaction
Donor embryo (embryo adoption)	A donated embryo is transferred to the uterus of an infertile woman at the appropriate time (normal or induced) of the menstrual cycle.	Infertility not resolved by less aggressive forms of therapy; absence of ovaries; male partner azoospermic or severely compromised
Gestational carrier (embryo host); surrogate mother	A couple undertakes an IVF cycle, and the embryo(s) is/are transferred to another woman's uterus (the carrier), who has contracted with the couple to carry the baby to term. The carrier has no genetic investment in the child. Surrogate motherhood is a process by which a woman is inseminated with semen from the infertile woman's partner and then carries the baby to term.	Congenital absence or surgical removal of uterus; reproductively impaired uterus, myomas, uterine adhesions, or other congenital abnormalities; medical condition that might be life-threatening during pregnancy (e.g., diabetes; immunologic problems; or severe heart, kidney, or liver disease)
Therapeutic donor insemination (TDI)	Donor sperm are used to inseminate the female partner.	Male partner is azoospermic or has very low sperm count; couple has genetic defect; male partner has antisperm antibodies
Intracytoplasmic sperm injection	One sperm cell is selected to be injected directly into the egg to achieve fertilization. It is used with IVF.	Same as TDI
Assisted hatching	The zona pellucida is penetrated chemically or manually to create an opening for the dividing embryo to hatch and implant into the uterine wall.	Recurrent miscarriages; to improve implantation rate in women with previously unsuccessful IVF attempts; advanced age

Data from American Society for Reproductive Medicine. (2016). *Assisted reproductive technologies: A guide for patients*. Retrieved from https://www.asrm.org/BOOKLET_Assisted_Reproductive_Technologies/.

not planned (Rivlin & Westhoff, 2017). Among adolescent women who were 19 years of age or younger, more than 80% of those who became pregnant did not intend to do so (CDC, 2015). The nurse can play a vital role in preventing unplanned and/or unwanted pregnancy through counseling and education regarding family planning, contraception, and effective birth control. Family planning is the conscious decision about when to conceive or to avoid pregnancy throughout the reproductive years. Contraception is defined as the intentional prevention of pregnancy during sexual intercourse. Birth control is the device and/or practice used to decrease the risk for conceiving or bearing offspring.

With the wide assortment of birth control options available, it is possible for a woman to use several different contraceptive methods at various stages throughout her fertile years. Nurses provide information about the various methods and help couples compare and contrast available contraceptive options. Providing adequate instruction about how to use a contraceptive method, when to use a backup method, and when to use emergency contraception (EC) can decrease the risk for unintended pregnancy. The Community Focus box presents information about contraceptive education.

🏠 COMMUNITY FOCUS

Education for Contraceptive Use: Student Activity

A suggested activity to learn more about contraceptive use is to observe a nurse doing contraceptive counseling in a family planning clinic. An alternative suggestion is to prepare information on several common contraceptive methods to present to adolescents at a health course in school or at a group meeting, such as for the Girl Scouts, Girls Inc., or a church youth group.

CARE MANAGEMENT

An interprofessional approach may help a woman choose and correctly use an appropriate contraceptive method. Nurses, nurse-midwives, nurse practitioners, other advanced practice nurses, and physicians have the knowledge and expertise to help a woman make decisions about contraception that will satisfy her personal, social, cultural, and interpersonal needs.

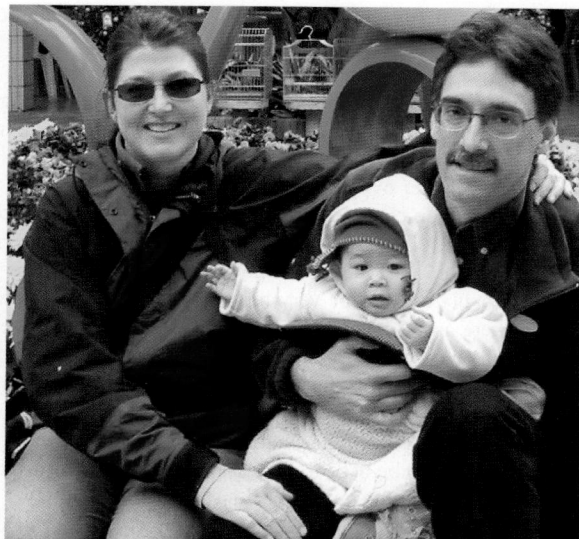

FIG 5.5 After two miscarriages, this couple chose foreign adoption. (Courtesy of Shannon Perry, Phoenix, AZ.)

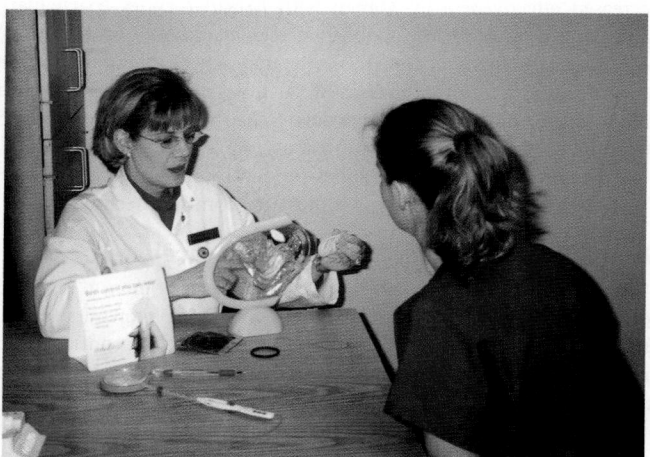

FIG 5.6 Nurse counseling a woman about contraceptive methods. (Courtesy of Dee Lowdermilk, Chapel Hill, NC.)

Assessment for the couple desiring contraception involves assessment of the woman's medical and reproductive history (menstrual, obstetric, gynecologic, contraceptive), physical examination, and sometimes current laboratory tests. The nurse must determine the woman's knowledge about reproduction, contraception, and STIs and her sexual partner's commitment to any particular method. Fig. 5.6 illustrates contraceptive counseling. The nurse obtains information about the frequency of coitus, number of sexual partners (present and past), and any objections that she or her partner might have about specific birth control methods. In addition, the nurse must determine a woman's willingness to touch her genitals. Religious and cultural factors may influence a couple's choice regarding a particular contraceptive method. The couple may believe in certain reproductive myths. Unbiased patient teaching is fundamental to initiating and maintaining any form of contraception. The nurse counters myths with facts, clarifies misinformation, and fills in gaps in knowledge. The ideal contraceptive should be safe, effective, easily available, economical, acceptable, simple to use, and promptly reversible. Although no method may ever achieve all of these objectives, significant

advances in the development of new contraceptive technologies have occurred over the past 30 years.

Contraceptive failure rate refers to the percentage of contraceptive users expected to have an unplanned pregnancy during the first year even when they use a method consistently and correctly. Contraceptive effectiveness varies from couple to couple and depends on both the properties of the method and the characteristics of the user (Box 5.7). Effectiveness of a method can be expressed as theoretic (i.e., how effective the method is with perfect use) and typical (i.e., how effective the method is with typical use). Failure rates decrease over time, either because a user gains experience with and uses a method more appropriately or because the less effective users stop using the method. Safety of a method may be affected by a woman's medical history (e.g., thromboembolic problems and contraceptive methods containing estrogen). Nevertheless, in most instances pregnancy would be more dangerous to the woman with medical problems than a particular contraceptive method. In addition, many contraceptive methods have health promotion effects. Barrier methods such as the male condom offer some protection from acquiring STIs, and oral contraceptives lower the incidence of ovarian and endometrial cancer.

Following assessment and analysis, the couple determines possible contraceptive methods that are appropriate for their unique situation. Factors to consider when determining a contraceptive method are effectiveness, convenience, affordability, duration of action of method, reversibility of method, time of return to fertility, effects on uterine bleeding patterns, side effects, adverse events, health promotion effects of methods, effect of method on transmission of STIs, and medical contraindications for use.

The most effective reversible contraceptive methods at preventing pregnancy are the long-acting, reversible contraceptive (LARC) methods (e.g., contraceptive implants, intrauterine contraception). With these methods, theoretic and typical pregnancy rates are the same because the method requires no user intervention after correct insertion. Effective methods include those that prevent pregnancy through exogenous hormones (estrogen and/or progestins) such as contraceptive injections, oral contraceptive pills, contraceptive patches, and vaginal rings. Each of these methods involves user interventions; thus typical-use pregnancy rates are higher than pregnancy rates with perfect use. The least effective contraceptive methods include the barrier methods and natural family planning. Examples include condoms, diaphragms, cervical caps, spermicides, withdrawal, and periodic abstinence during perceived ovulation. Effectiveness rates for these methods vary from user to user, depending on correct application of the method and consistency of use.

Expected outcomes related to contraceptive counseling are that the couple will verbalize understanding about appropriate contraceptive methods, state they are satisfied with the method chosen, use the method correctly and consistently, experience no adverse sequelae as a result of the chosen contraceptive method, and prevent unplanned pregnancy. The nurse assists with obtaining appropriate informed consent concerning contraception or sterilization, provides appropriate education to the couple, and documents the couple's understanding of the contraceptive method chosen. Evaluation involves achievement of patient-centered outcomes when the couple engage in effective use of the chosen contraceptive device, experience no adverse sequelae, and achieve pregnancy only when they desire to do so.

METHODS OF CONTRACEPTION

The following discussion of contraceptive methods provides the nurse with information needed for patient teaching. After implementing the appropriate teaching for contraceptive use, the nurse supervises return demonstrations and practice to assess patient understanding (see Clinical Reasoning Case Study). The couple is given written instructions, telephone numbers, and/or email contact information for questions. If the woman has difficulty understanding written instructions, she and her partner, if available, are offered graphic material, a telephone number to call as necessary, and an opportunity to return for further instruction.

Coitus Interruptus

Coitus interruptus (withdrawal) involves the male partner withdrawing his penis from the woman's vagina before he ejaculates. Although coitus interruptus has been criticized as being an ineffective method of contraception, it is a good choice for couples who do not have another contraceptive available. Effectiveness is similar to barrier methods and depends on the man's ability to withdraw his penis before ejaculation. The percentage of women who experience an unintended pregnancy within the first year of typical use (failure rate) of withdrawal ranges from 4% when used consistently and correctly to 22% as a typical failure rate (Rivlin & Westhoff, 2017). Coitus interruptus does not protect against STIs or human immunodeficiency virus (HIV) infection.

Fertility Awareness Methods

Fertility awareness methods (FAMs) of contraception depend on identifying the beginning and end of the fertile period of the menstrual cycle. When women who want to use FAMs are educated about the menstrual cycle, the following three phases are identified:

1. Infertile phase: Before ovulation
2. Fertile phase: About 5 to 7 days around the middle of the cycle, including several days before and during ovulation and the day after ovulation
3. Infertile phase: After ovulation

Although ovulation can be unpredictable in many women, teaching the woman about how she can directly observe her fertility patterns is an empowering tool. In addition, knowledge about the signs and symptoms of ovulation can be very helpful when the couple desires pregnancy. There are nearly a dozen categories of FAMs. To prevent pregnancy, each one uses a combination of charts, records, calculations, tools, observations, and either abstinence (natural family planning [NFP]) or barrier methods of birth control during the fertile period of the menstrual cycle. The charts and calculations associated with these methods can also be used to increase the likelihood of detecting the optimal timing of intercourse to achieve conception.

Advantages of these methods include low-to-no cost, absence of chemicals and hormones, and lack of alteration in the menstrual flow pattern. Disadvantages of FAMs include adherence needed for strict record keeping, unintentional interference from external influences that may alter the woman's core body temperature and vaginal secretions, decreased effectiveness in women with irregular cycles (particularly adolescents who have not established regular patterns of ovulation), decreased spontaneity of coitus, and the necessity of attending possibly time-consuming training sessions by qualified instructors. The typical failure rate for most FAMs is 24% during the first year of use (Rivlin & Westhoff, 2017). FAMs do not protect against STIs or HIV infection.

FAMs involve several techniques to identify high-risk, fertile days. The following discussion includes the most common techniques.

Natural Family Planning (Periodic Abstinence)

Natural family planning (NFP), or periodic abstinence, provides contraception by using methods that rely on avoiding intercourse during fertile days. NFP methods are the only methods of contraception acceptable to the Roman Catholic Church. Signs and symptoms of fertility awareness most commonly used with abstinence are menstrual bleeding, cervical mucus, and basal body temperature. Development and marketing of ovulation predictor kits have also been very helpful for couples who choose NFP. Several application products have been developed for smart phones, which make FAM record tracking convenient and portable.

The human ovum can be fertilized no later than 16 to 24 hours after ovulation. Motile sperm have been recovered from the uterus and uterine tubes as long as 7 days after coitus. However, their ability to fertilize the ovum probably lasts no longer than 24 hours. Pregnancy is unlikely to occur if a couple abstains from intercourse for 4 days before and 3 or 4 days after ovulation (fertile period). Unprotected intercourse on the other days of the cycle (safe period) should not result in pregnancy. Nevertheless, the exact time of ovulation cannot be predicted accurately, and couples may find it difficult to abstain from sexual intercourse for several days before and after ovulation. Women with irregular menstrual periods have the greatest risk for failure with this form of contraception.

Calendar Rhythm Method

Practice of the calendar rhythm method is based on the number of days in each cycle, counting from the first day of the menstrual cycle (first day of menstrual vaginal bleeding). The fertile period is determined after accurately recording the lengths of menstrual cycles for 6 months. The beginning of the fertile period is estimated by subtracting 18 days

---

CLINICAL REASONING CASE STUDY

Contraception for Adolescents

Maria is a 16-year-old Hispanic female who comes to the family planning clinic seeking contraception. She has recently become sexually active and tells the nurse that she is concerned that her mother will find out. She also has many questions about the type of contraception to use. She seeks the nurse's advice to help in her decision making.

1. Evidence—Is there sufficient evidence to draw conclusions about advice to give Maria?
2. Assumptions—What assumptions can be made about contraception for adolescents:
   a. Types of contraception: What methods are appropriate (safe and effective) for an adolescent young woman?
   b. Legal issues: With whom is this young woman engaging in sexual intercourse? Is it consensual? Does she need parental consent to obtain contraception?
   c. Implications of culture on choice: Are there any cultural issues?
3. What implications and priorities for nursing care can be drawn at this time?
4. Describe the roles and responsibilities of members of the interprofessional health care team who may be involved in caring for Maria.

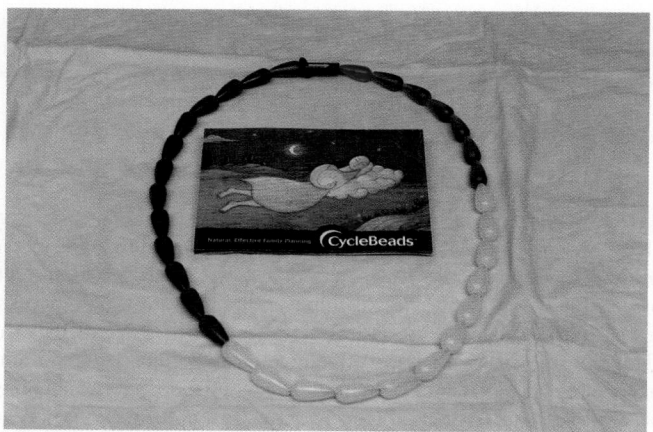

FIG 5.7 CycleBeads. *Red bead* marks the first day of the menstrual cycle. *White beads* mark days that are likely to be fertile days; therefore unprotected intercourse should be avoided. *Brown beads* are days when pregnancy is unlikely and unprotected intercourse is permitted. (Courtesy of Dee Lowdermilk, Chapel Hill, NC.)

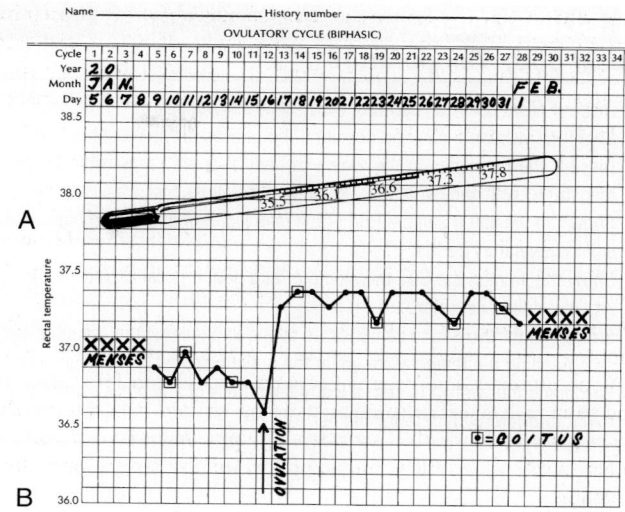

FIG 5.8 **A,** Special thermometer for recording basal body temperature, marked in tenths to enable the person to read it more easily. **B,** Basal temperature record shows decrease and sharp increase at time of ovulation. Biphasic curve indicates ovulatory cycle. A digital thermometer may also be used.

from the length of the shortest cycle. The end of the fertile period is determined by subtracting 11 days from the length of the longest cycle. If the shortest cycle is 24 days and the longest is 30 days, application of the formula to calculate the fertile period is as follows:

Shortest cycle, 24 − 18 = day 6

Longest cycle, 30 − 11 = day 19

To avoid conception the couple would abstain during the fertile period, days 6 through 19.

If the woman has very regular cycles of 28 days each, the formula indicates the fertile days to be as follows:

Longest cycle, 28 − 11 = day 17

To avoid conception, the couple would abstain from days 10 through 17 because ovulation occurs on day 14 ± 2 days. A major drawback of the calendar method is that the couple is attempting to predict future events with past data. The unpredictability of the menstrual cycle is also not taken into consideration. The calendar rhythm method is most useful as an adjunct to the basal body temperature or cervical mucus method.

Standard Days Method

The standard days method (SDM) is essentially a modified form of the calendar rhythm method that has a "fixed" number of days of fertility for each cycle (i.e., days 8 to 19). A CycleBeads necklace (i.e., a color-coded string of beads) can be purchased as a concrete tool to track fertility (Fig. 5.7) or as a smart phone application. Day 1 of the menstrual flow is counted as the first day to begin counting. Women who use this device are taught to avoid unprotected intercourse on days 8 to 19 (white beads on CycleBeads necklace). Although this method is useful to women whose cycles are 26 to 32 days long, it is unreliable for those who have longer or shorter cycles (Contracept.org, 2016a).

Basal Body Temperature Method

The basal body temperature (BBT) is the lowest body temperature of a healthy person, taken immediately after waking and before getting out of bed. The BBT usually varies from 36.2°C (97.16°F) to 36.3°C (97.34°F) during menses and for approximately 5 to 7 days afterward (Fig. 5.8).

About the time of ovulation a slight drop in temperature (approximately 0.5°C [35.8°F]) may occur in some women, but others may have no decrease at all. After ovulation, in concert with the increasing progesterone levels of the early luteal phase of the cycle, the BBT increases slightly (approximately 0.4°C [36.2°F] to 0.8°C [36.6°F]). The temperature remains on an elevated plateau until 2 to 4 days before menstruation. Then BBT decreases to the low levels recorded during the previous cycle unless pregnancy has occurred. In pregnant women, the temperature remains elevated. If ovulation fails to occur, the pattern of lower body temperature continues throughout the cycle.

To use this method the fertile period is defined as the day of first temperature drop, or first elevation, through 3 consecutive days of elevated temperature. Abstinence begins the first day of menstrual bleeding and lasts through 3 consecutive days of sustained temperature rise. The decrease and subsequent increase in temperature are referred to as the *thermal shift*. When the temperatures of the entire month are recorded on a graph, the pattern described is more apparent. It is more difficult to perceive day-to-day variations without the entire picture (see Guidelines box). Either a glass mercury thermometer or a digital thermometer may be used for BBT, but the thermometer must measure the temperature within one-tenth of a degree. The glass mercury thermometer needs no batteries but is fragile and can break. If a mercury thermometer does break, it is important to put on rubber, nitrile, or latex gloves and pick up all broken pieces and place on a paper towel. Put the folded paper towel with the contents in it securely into a zip-lock bag, label it, and contact the local health department regarding disposal. A digital thermometer requires batteries but may have a history recall function and an audible beep when the temperature assessment is finished. Digital thermometers that monitor temperature throughout the day combined with an accelerometer to monitor movement have been cleared for use by the Food and Drug Administration (FDA). These devices can be wirelessly uploaded to a computer through a companion device. Their use in FAM needs further research. Guidelines for BBT recording is included in the Guidelines box, and Fig. 5.8 depicts a graph of what a BBT recording looks like.

Infection, fatigue, less than 3 hours of sleep per night, awakening late, and anxiety may cause temperature fluctuations and alter the

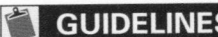

GUIDELINES
Basal Body Temperature

- Discuss basal body temperature (BBT) with the woman.
- Show the woman a diagram depicting the phases of the menstrual cycle.
- Discuss the hormones in the woman's body that are responsible for her menstrual cycle and ovulation. Leave time for questions.
- Show the woman a sample BBT graph (see Fig. 5.8) and the biphasic line seen in ovulatory cycles.
- Show the woman the BBT thermometer and how it is calibrated.
- Provide a demonstration.
- Encourage the woman to demonstrate taking and reading the thermometer and graphing the temperature while the nurse watches.
- Encourage the woman to start a log to keep track of any other activity that might interfere with determining her true BBT.

expected pattern. If a new BBT thermometer is purchased, this fact is noted on the chart because the readings may vary slightly. Jet lag, alcohol taken the evening before, or sleeping in a heated waterbed must also be noted on the chart because each affects the BBT. Therefore the BBT alone is not a reliable method of predicting ovulation.

Cervical Mucus Ovulation-Detection Method

The cervical mucus ovulation-detection method (i.e., Billings method or Creighton model ovulation method) requires that the woman recognize and interpret the cyclic changes in the amount and consistency of cervical mucus that characterize her own unique pattern of changes at the time of ovulation. Cervical mucus changes before and during ovulation to facilitate and promote the viability and motility of sperm. Without adequate cervical mucus, coitus does not result in conception. This method requires that a woman check the quantity and character of mucus on the vulva or introitus with her fingers or tissue paper each day for several months. This way she can learn how her cervical mucus responds to ovulation during her menstrual cycles. To ensure an accurate assessment of changes, the cervical mucus should be free from semen, contraceptive gels or foams, and blood or discharge from vaginal infections for at least one full cycle. Other factors that create difficulty in identifying mucus changes include douches and vaginal deodorants, being in the sexually aroused state (which thins the mucus), and taking medications such as antihistamines (which dry the mucus). Intercourse is considered safe without restriction beginning the fourth day after the last day of wet, clear, slippery mucus, which would indicate that ovulation has occurred 2 to 3 days previously.

Some women find this method unacceptable if they are uncomfortable touching their genitals. Whether or not a woman wants to use this method for contraception, it is to her advantage to learn to recognize mucus characteristics at ovulation (see Guidelines box).

Symptothermal Method

The symptothermal method combines the BBT and cervical mucus methods with awareness of secondary phase–related symptoms of the menstrual cycle. The woman gains fertility awareness as she learns the psychologic and physiologic symptoms that mark the phases of her cycle. Secondary symptoms include increased libido, midcycle spotting, mittelschmerz (cramplike pain before ovulation), pelvic fullness or tenderness, and vulvar fullness.

The woman is taught to palpate her cervix to assess for changes indicating ovulation: the cervical os dilates slightly, the cervix softens and rises in the vagina, and cervical mucus is copious and slippery. The

woman notes days on which coitus, changes in routine, illness, and other changes that might affect BBT have occurred (Fig. 5.9). Calendar calculations and cervical mucus changes are used to estimate the onset of the fertile period; changes in cervical mucus or the BBT are used to estimate the end of the fertile period.

TwoDay Method of Family Planning

Based on monitoring and the recording of cervical secretions, an algorithm for identifying the fertile window has been developed by the Institute for Reproductive Health at Georgetown University (Contracept. org, 2016b). The TwoDay algorithm appears to be simpler to teach, learn, and use than other natural methods. Results suggest that the algorithm can be an effective alternative for low-literacy populations or for programs that find current NFP methods too time-consuming or otherwise not feasible to incorporate within their services. Two questions are posed. Each day the woman is to ask herself, (1) "Did I note secretions today?" and (2) "Did I note secretions yesterday?" If the answer to either question is yes, she should avoid coitus or use a backup method of birth control. If the answer to both questions is no, her probability of getting pregnant is low. Further studies are needed to determine the efficacy of the TwoDay algorithm in avoiding pregnancy and to assess its acceptability to users and providers.

Home Predictor Test Kits for Ovulation

Although the methods previously discussed are characteristic of ovulation, they do not prove that ovulation actually occurred or indicate the exact timing. The urine predictor test for ovulation is a major addition to the NFP and fertility-awareness methods to help women who want to plan the time of their pregnancies and for those who are trying to conceive (Fig. 5.10). The urine predictor test for ovulation detects the sudden surge of LH that occurs approximately 12 to 24 hours before ovulation. Unlike BBT, this test is not affected by illness, emotions, or physical activity. For home use, a test kit contains sufficient material for several days' testing during each cycle. A positive response indicating an LH surge is noted by a color change that is easy to interpret. Directions for use of urine predictor test kits vary with the manufacturer.

The Marquette Model

The Marquette Model (MM) is a natural family planning method that was developed through the Marquette University College of Nursing Institute for Natural Family Planning. The MM uses cervical monitoring along with the ClearPlan Easy Fertility Monitor. The ClearPlan monitor is a handheld device that uses test strips to measure urinary metabolites of estrogen and LH. The monitor provides the user with "low," "high," and "peak" fertility readings. The MM incorporates the use of the monitor as an aid to learning NFP and fertility awareness.

Research continues on the efficacy of available home test kits and devices for the prevention of pregnancy (Leiva et al., 2014). With more research and development, women and men will have greater access to pregnancy prevention methods.

Breastfeeding: Lactational Amenorrhea Method

The lactational amenorrhea method (LAM) can be a highly effective, *temporary* method of birth control. The LAM is more popular in underdeveloped countries and traditional societies in which breastfeeding is used to prolong birth intervals. The method has seen limited use in the United States because most American women do not establish breastfeeding patterns that provide maximum protection against pregnancy, and therefore it is recommended that breastfeeding mothers consider another form of reliable contraception (Rivlin & Westhoff, 2017).

When the infant suckles at the mother's breast, a surge of prolactin is released. Prolactin inhibits estrogen production and suppresses

GUIDELINES
Cervical Mucus Characteristics

Setting the Stage

- Show charts of the menstrual cycle along with changes in the cervical mucus.
- Have the woman practice assessing mucus using raw egg white.
- Supply her with a basal body temperature (BBT) log and graph if she does not already have one.
- Explain that the assessment of cervical mucus characteristics is best when mucus is not mixed with semen, contraceptive jellies or foams, or discharge from infections.

Benefits of Noting Cervical Mucus Characteristics

- To alert the couple to the reestablishment of ovulation while breastfeeding and after discontinuation of oral contraception
- To note anovulatory cycles at any time and at the beginning of menopause
- To help couples plan a pregnancy

Content Related to Cervical Mucus

- Explain to the woman (or couple) how cervical mucus changes throughout the menstrual cycle.

- Right before ovulation the watery, thin, clear mucus becomes more abundant and thick. It feels like a lubricant and can be stretched approximately 5 cm between the thumb and forefinger; this is called *spinnbarkeit*. This characteristic indicates the period of maximum fertility. Sperm deposited in this type of mucus can survive until ovulation occurs.

Assessment Technique

- Stress that good hand washing is imperative to begin and end all self-assessment.
- Start observation from the last day of menstrual flow.
- Assess cervical mucus several times a day for several cycles. Mucus can be obtained from vaginal introitus; there is no need to reach into vagina to cervix.
- Record findings on the same record on which her BBT is entered.

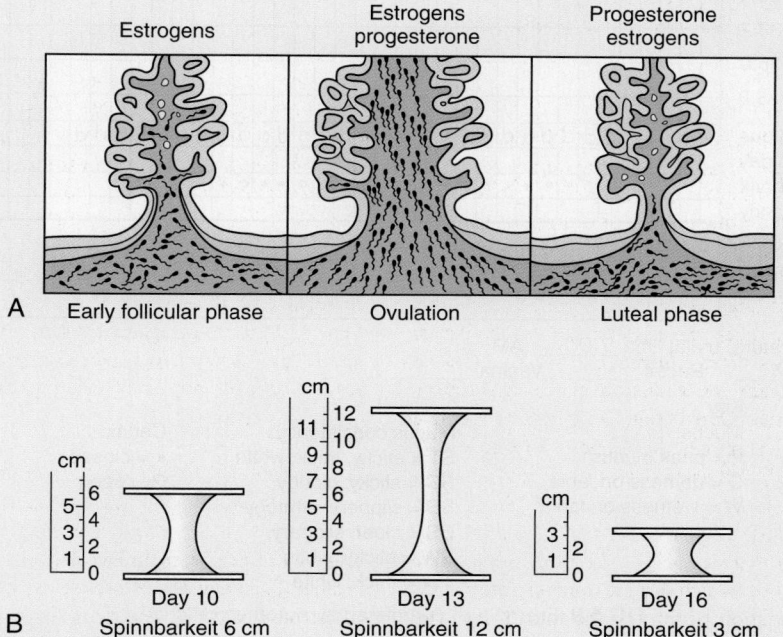

ovulation and the return of menses. LAM works best if the mother is exclusively breastfeeding, if she has not had a menstrual flow since birth, and if the infant is younger than 6 months of age. Effectiveness is enhanced by frequent feedings at intervals of less than 4 hours during the day and no more than 6 hours during the night, long duration of each feeding, and no bottle supplementation. The woman should be counseled that disruption of the breastfeeding pattern or formula supplementation can increase the risk for pregnancy. The typical failure rate is 2% if used correctly, which means exclusive breastfeeding for up to 6 months after birth (Rivlin & Westhoff, 2017).

Barrier Methods

Barrier contraceptives have gained in popularity not only as a contraceptive method but also as protection against the spread of STIs such as human papilloma virus and herpes simplex virus (HSV). Some male condoms and female vaginal methods provide a physical barrier to several STIs, and some male condoms provide protection against HIV. Spermicides serve as chemical barriers against semen and inhibit the ability of sperm to fertilize the ovum.

The nurse should remember that any user of a barrier method of contraception must also be aware of emergency contraception (EC) options in case there is a failure of the method. An example of a barrier method failure would be if a condom broke during intercourse. In this instance, EC would be indicated to prevent unplanned pregnancy.

Spermicides

Spermicides such as nonoxynol-9 (N-9) work by reducing the mobility of the sperm. The chemicals attack the sperm flagella and body, thereby preventing the sperm from reaching the cervical os. N-9, the most commonly used spermicidal chemical in the United States, is a surfactant

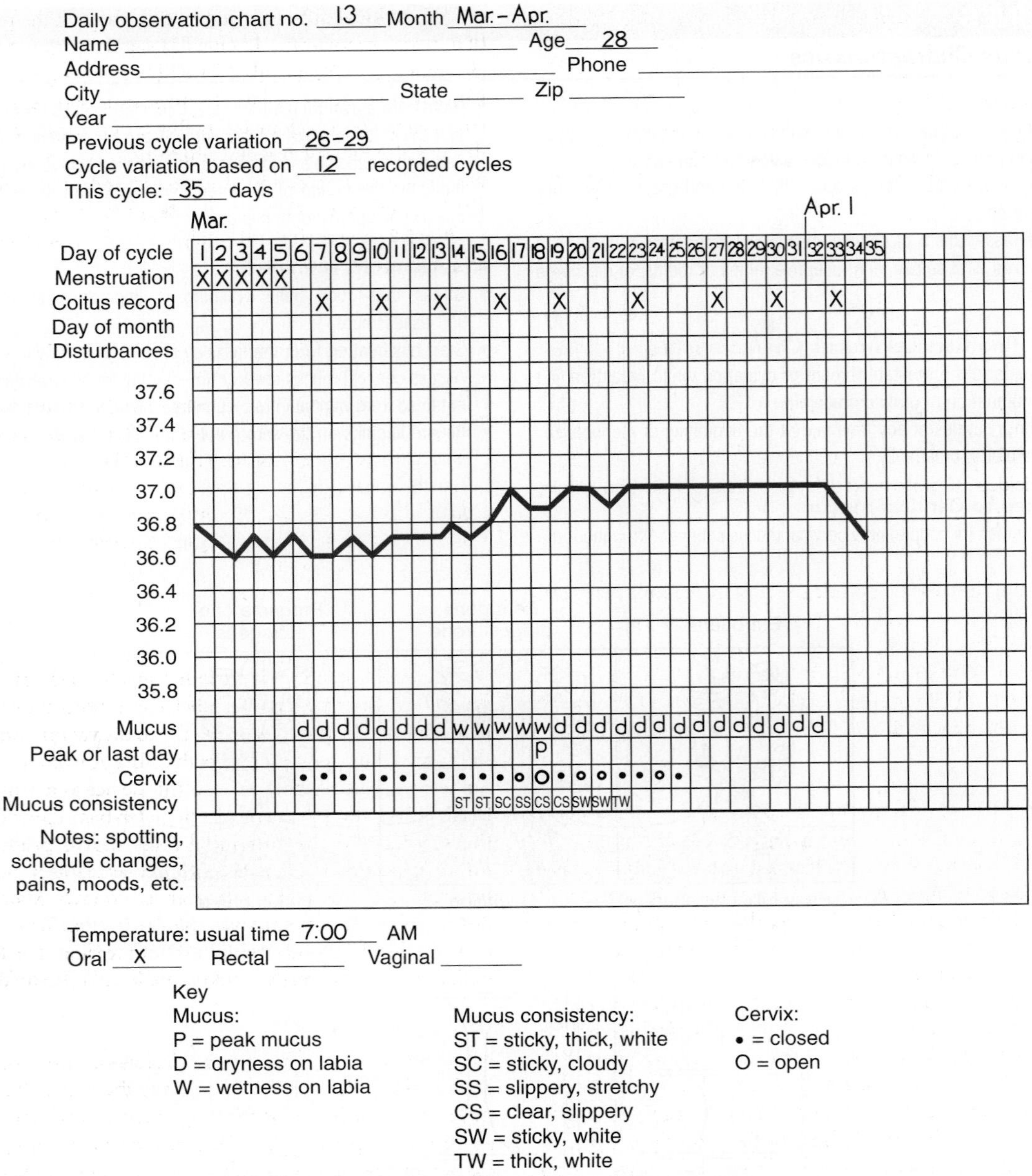

Daily observation chart no. ___13___ Month _Mar. – Apr.___
Name _____ Age ___28___
Address _____ Phone _____
City _____ State _____ Zip _____
Year _____
Previous cycle variation __26–29_____
Cycle variation based on __12__ recorded cycles
This cycle: __35__ days

	Mar.																														Apr. 1					
Day of cycle	1	2	3	4	5	6	7	8	9	10	11	12	13	14	15	16	17	18	19	20	21	22	23	24	25	26	27	28	29	30	31	32	33	34	35
Menstruation	X	X	X	X	X																														
Coitus record							X			X			X			X			X				X			X			X			X			

Day of month
Disturbances

Temperature scale (°C):
37.6
37.4
37.2
37.0
36.8
36.6
36.4
36.2
36.0
35.8

Mucus					d	d	d	d	d	d	d	d	w	w	w	w	w	d	d	d	d	d	d	d	d	d	d	d	d	d	d				
Peak or last day																	P																		
Cervix			•	•	•	•	•	•	•	•	•	•	•	•	○	O	•	○	•	○	•	•	•	○	•										
Mucus consistency													ST	ST	SC	SS	CS	CS	SW	SW	TW														

Notes: spotting, schedule changes, pains, moods, etc.

Temperature: usual time __7:00__ AM
Oral __X___ Rectal _____ Vaginal _____

Key
Mucus:
P = peak mucus
D = dryness on labia
W = wetness on labia

Mucus consistency:
ST = sticky, thick, white
SC = sticky, cloudy
SS = slippery, stretchy
CS = clear, slippery
SW = sticky, white
TW = thick, white

Cervix:
• = closed
O = open

FIG 5.9 Example of completed symptothermal chart.

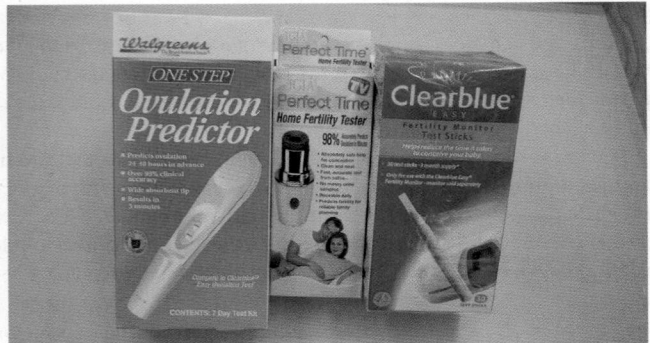

FIG 5.10 Examples of ovulation predictor tests.

that destroys the sperm cell membrane. Results from data analyses now suggest that frequent use (more than 2 times a day) of N-9 or the use of N-9 as a lubricant during intercourse may increase the transmission of HIV and can cause lesions (World Health Organization, 2016). There is no evidence that the addition of spermicides to male condoms decreases the risk for subsequent pregnancy. Women with high-risk behaviors that increase their likelihood of contracting HIV and other STIs are advised to avoid the use of spermicidal products containing N-9, including lubricated condoms, diaphragms, and cervical caps to which N-9 is added.

Intravaginal spermicides are marketed and sold without prescriptions as aerosol foams, tablets, suppositories, creams, films, and gels (Fig. 5.11). Preloaded, single-dose applicators small enough to be carried in a small purse are available. Effectiveness of spermicides depends on consistent and accurate use. Not more than 1 hour before sexual intercourse, the spermicide should be inserted high into the vagina so

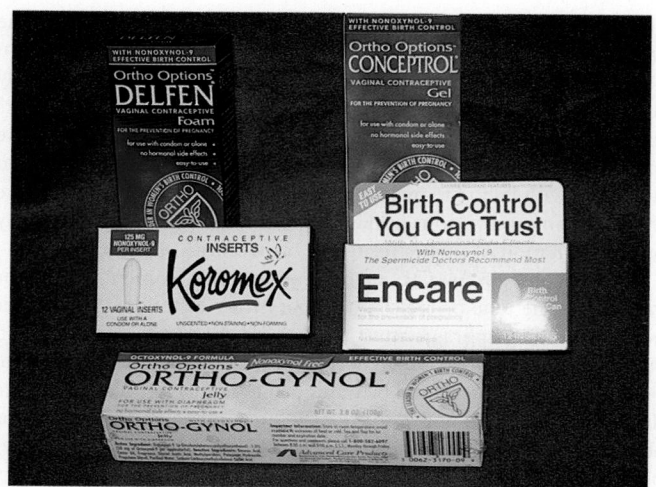

FIG 5.11 Spermicides. (Courtesy of Marjorie Pyle, RNC, Life Circle, Costa Mesa, CA.)

it makes contact with the cervix. Spermicide must be reapplied for each additional act of intercourse, even if a barrier method is used. Studies have shown varying effectiveness rates for spermicidal use alone. The typical failure rate is 15% to 29% (Rivlin & Westhoff, 2017). Some female barrier methods (e.g., diaphragm, cervical caps) offer more effective protection against pregnancy with the addition of spermicides.

Condoms

The male condom is a thin, stretchable sheath that covers the penis before genital, oral, or anal contact and is removed when the penis is withdrawn from the partner's orifice after ejaculation. Condoms are made of latex rubber, which, if intact, provides a barrier to sperm and STIs (including HIV); polyurethane (strong, thin plastic); or natural membranes (animal tissue). In addition to providing a physical barrier for sperm, nonspermicidal latex condoms also provide a barrier for STIs (particularly gonorrhea, chlamydia, and trichomonas) and HIV transmission. Condoms lubricated with N-9 are not recommended for preventing STIs or HIV and do not increase protection against pregnancy, as noted earlier. Latex condoms break down with oil-based lubricants (e.g., petroleum jelly and suntan oil) and should be used only with water-based or silicone lubricants. Because of the growing number of people with latex allergies, condom manufacturers have begun using polyurethane, which is thinner and stronger than latex.

> ❗ **NURSING ALERT**
>
> All patients should be questioned about the potential for latex allergy. Latex condom use is contraindicated for patients with latex sensitivity.

Although polyurethane condoms are as effective for STI prevention as latex condoms, they are more likely to slip or lose contour when compared to latex condoms. Therefore, with perfect use latex condoms offer better protection against pregnancy as compared with polyurethane condoms. Polyurethane condoms do offer pregnancy protection equivalent to that of most barrier products. A small percentage of condoms are made from lamb cecum (natural skin). Natural skin condoms do not provide the same protection against STIs and HIV infection as latex condoms. Natural skin condoms contain small pores that may allow passage of viruses such as hepatitis B, HSV, and HIV and are not generally recommended.

A functional difference in condom shape is the presence or absence of a sperm reservoir tip. To enhance vaginal stimulation, some condoms are contoured and rippled or have ribbed or roughened surfaces. Thinner construction increases heat transmission and sensitivity; a variety of colors increases condom acceptability and attractiveness. A wet jelly or dry powder lubricates some condoms. The typical failure rate for the use of the male condom is approximately 15% (Rivlin & Westhoff, 2017). Effective condom use is a skill that must be taught.

Box 5.8 summarizes advantages and disadvantages of male condoms and nursing considerations.

> ❗ **NURSING ALERT**
>
> It is a false assumption that everyone knows how to use condoms. To prevent unintended pregnancy and the spread of STIs, it is essential that condoms be used correctly. Proper instruction in use must be provided. The sheath is applied over the erect penis before insertion and before the loss of preejaculatory drops of semen. All types of condoms must be discarded after each single use. Condoms are available without prescription from a variety of sources, including vending machines.

The female condom is a vaginal sheath made of nitrile, a nonlatex, synthetic rubber and has flexible rings at both ends (Fig. 5.12, A). The closed end of the pouch is inserted into the vagina and anchored around the cervix; the open ring covers the labia. A woman whose partner will not wear a male condom can use this device as a protective mechanical barrier. Rewetting drops or oil- or water-based lubricants may be used to help decrease the distracting noise that is produced while penile thrusting occurs. The female condom is available in one size, is intended for single use only, and is sold over the counter. Male condoms should not be used concurrently because the friction from both sheaths can increase the likelihood of either or both tearing. The typical failure rate in the first year of female condom use is 21% (Rivlin & Westhoff, 2017).

Diaphragm

The contraceptive diaphragm is a shallow, dome-shaped, latex or silicone device with a flexible rim that covers the cervix. The diaphragm is a mechanical barrier to the meeting of sperm with the ovum. By holding spermicide in place against the cervix for the 6 hours it takes to destroy the sperm, the diaphragm also provides a chemical barrier to pregnancy. Diaphragms are available in a wide range of diameters (50 to 95 mm) and differ in the inner construction of the circular rim. The types of rims are coil spring, arcing spring, and wide-seal rim. The diaphragm should be the largest size the woman can wear without being aware of its presence. The typical failure rate of the diaphragm combined with spermicide ranges from 13% to 17%, but it is possible that the failure rate can be reduced to 4% to 8% with correct and consistent use (Rivlin & Westhoff, 2017).

The woman using a diaphragm needs an annual gynecologic examination to assess its fit, seeking the largest size that does not cause discomfort. Rivlin & Westhoff (2017) note that no data exist that support a correlation between fit and effectiveness, despite the fact that it has commonly been believed that weight change (gain or loss), birth, miscarriage, or abdominal and pelvic surgery may change the appropriate fit. Because various types of diaphragms are on the market, the nurse uses the package insert when teaching the woman how to use and care for the diaphragm (see Patient Teaching box). A newer diaphragm, called Caya, that is sold over-the-counter and comes in only one size, has been approved by the FDA (Rivlin & Westhoff, 2017).

BOX 5.8 Male Condoms

Mechanism of Action

Sheath is applied over the erect penis before insertion or loss of preejaculatory drops of semen. If used correctly, condoms prevent sperm from entering the cervix. Spermicide-coated condoms cause ejaculated sperm to be immobilized rapidly, thus increasing contraceptive effectiveness.

Advantages

- Safe
- No side effects
- Readily available
- Premalignant changes in cervix can be prevented or ameliorated in women whose partners use condoms
- Method of male nonsurgical contraception

Disadvantages

- Sexual activity must be interrupted to apply sheath.
- Sensation may be altered.
- If used improperly, spillage of sperm can result in pregnancy.
- Condoms occasionally may tear during intercourse.

Sexually Transmitted Infection Protection

If a condom is used throughout the act of intercourse and there is no unprotected contact with female genitals, a latex rubber condom, which is impermeable to viruses, can act as a protective measure against sexually transmitted infections.

Nursing Considerations

Teach the male patient to do the following:

- Use a new condom (check expiration date) for each act of sexual intercourse or other acts between partners that involve contact with the penis.
- Place the condom after the penis is erect and before intimate contact.
- Place the condom on the head of the penis (A) and unroll it all the way to the base (B).
- Leave an empty space at the tip (A); remove any air remaining in the tip by gently pressing air out toward the base of the penis.
- If a lubricant is desired, use water-based products such as K-Y lubricating jelly. Do not use petroleum-based products because they can cause the condom to break.
- After ejaculation, carefully withdraw the still-erect penis from the vagina, holding onto the condom rim; remove and discard the condom.
- Store unused condoms in a cool, dry place.
- Do not use condoms that are sticky, brittle, or obviously damaged.

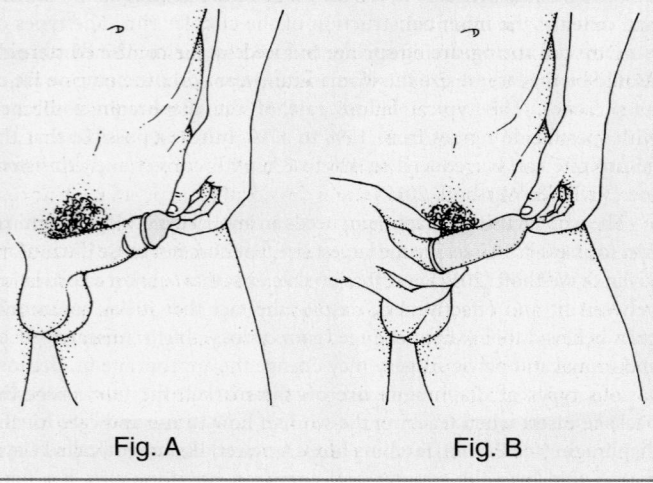

Fig. A   Fig. B

Disadvantages of diaphragm use include the reluctance of some women to insert and remove it. Although it can be inserted up to 6 hours before intercourse, a cold diaphragm and a cold gel temporarily reduce vaginal response to sexual stimulation if insertion occurs immediately before intercourse. Some women or couples object to the messiness of the spermicide. These annoyances associated with diaphragm use, along with failure to insert the device once foreplay has begun, are the most common reasons for failures of this method. Side effects may include irritation of tissues related to contact with spermicides.

The diaphragm is not a good option for women with poor vaginal muscle tone or recurrent urinary tract infections. For proper placement, the diaphragm must rest behind the pubic symphysis and completely cover the cervix. To decrease the chance of exerting urethral pressure, the woman should be reminded to empty her bladder before diaphragm insertion and immediately after intercourse. Diaphragms are contraindicated for women with pelvic relaxation (uterine prolapse) or a large cystocele. Women with a latex allergy should not use latex diaphragms.

Cervical Cap

The FemCap is the only type of cervical cap available in the United States (see Fig. 5.12, *B*). It comes in three sizes and is made of silicone rubber. The cap fits snugly around the base of the cervix close to the junction of the cervix and vaginal fornices. It is recommended that the cap remain in place no less than 6 hours and no more than 48 hours at a time. It is left in place at least 6 hours after the last act of intercourse. The seal provides a physical barrier to sperm; spermicide inside the cap adds a chemical barrier. The extended period of wear may be an added convenience for women.

Instructions for the actual insertion and use of the cervical cap closely resemble the instructions for use of the contraceptive diaphragm. Some of the differences are that the cervical cap can be inserted hours before sexual intercourse without a later need for additional spermicide, the cervical cap requires less spermicide than the diaphragm when initially inserted, and no additional spermicide is required for repeated acts of intercourse. Effectiveness of the first-generation FemCap has been found to be comparable to that of the diaphragm (Rivlin & Westhoff, 2017).

Although reported in very small numbers, **toxic shock syndrome (TSS)** can occur in association with the use of the contraceptive diaphragm and cervical caps. The nurse should instruct the woman about ways to reduce her risk for TSS. These measures include prompt removal 6 to 8 hours after intercourse, not using the diaphragm or cervical caps during menses, and learning and watching for danger signs of TSS.

! NURSING ALERT

The nurse should alert the woman who uses a diaphragm or cervical cap as a contraceptive method for signs of TSS. The most common signs include a sunburn type of rash, diarrhea, dizziness, faintness, weakness, sore throat, aching muscles and joints, sudden high fever, and vomiting.

The angle of the uterus, the vaginal muscle tone, and the shape of the cervix may interfere with the ease of fitting and use of the cervical cap. Correct fitting requires time, effort, and skill of both the woman and the clinician, although the FemCap may be easier to fit than previous types of cervical caps.

Because of the potential risk for TSS associated with the use of the cervical cap, another form of birth control is recommended for use during menstrual bleeding and up to at least 6 weeks after birth. The cap should be refitted after any gynecologic surgery or birth and after

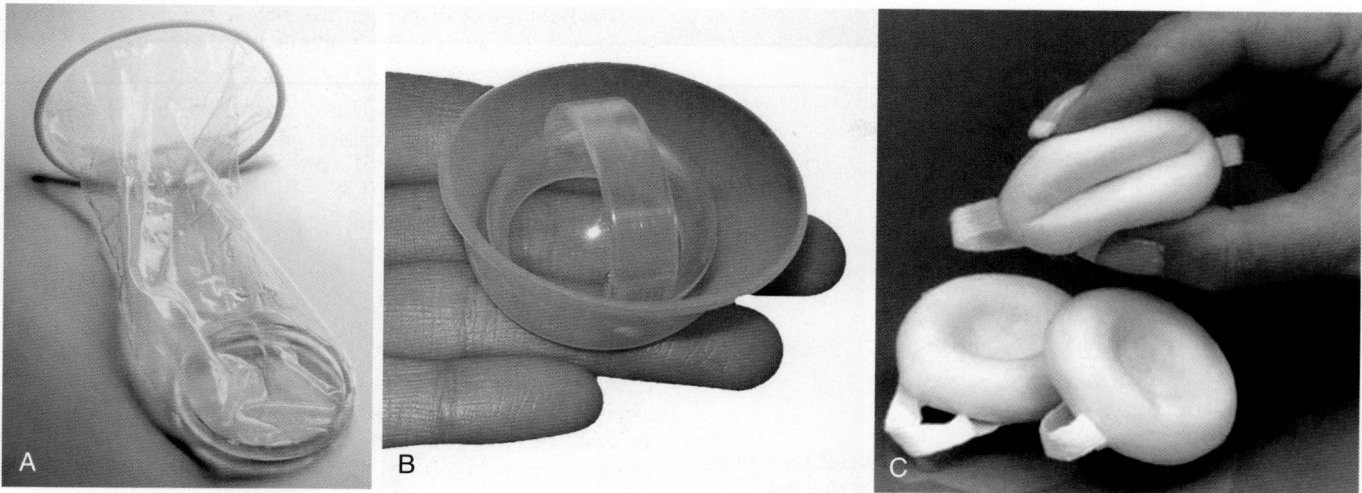

FIG 5.12 Barrier methods. **A,** Female condom (FC2). **B,** FemCap. **C,** Contraceptive sponge. (A, Courtesy of The Female Health Company, Chicago, IL. B, Courtesy of FemCap, Del Mar, CA. C, Courtesy of Allendale Pharmaceuticals, Allendale, NJ.)

major weight losses or gains. Otherwise the size should be checked at least once a year.

Women who are not good candidates for wearing the cervical cap include those with abnormal Papanicolaou (Pap) test results, those who cannot be fitted properly with the existing cap sizes or who find the insertion and removal of the device too difficult, those with a history of TSS or with vaginal or cervical infections, and those who experience allergic responses to the cap or to spermicide.

Contraceptive Sponge

The vaginal sponge is a small, round, polyurethane sponge that contains N-9 spermicide (see Fig. 5.12, *C*). It is designed to fit over the cervix (one size fits all). The side that is placed next to the cervix is concave for better fit. The opposite side has a woven polyester loop to be used for removal of the sponge.

The sponge must be moistened with water before it is inserted into the vagina to cover the cervix. It provides protection for up to 24 hours and for repeated instances of sexual intercourse. It should be left in place for at least 6 hours after the last act of intercourse and no more than 24 to 30 hours. Wearing it longer than 24 to 30 hours may put the woman at risk for TSS. The typical failure rate of the vaginal sponge is greater than that of the diaphragm (Center for Young Women's Health, 2016).

Hormonal Methods

Many different hormonal contraception therapies using different delivery methods are available in the United States today. General classes are described in Table 5.4. Because of the wide variety of preparations available, the woman and nurse must read the package insert for information about specific products prescribed. Formulations include combined estrogen-progestin steroidal medications or progestational agents. The formulations are administered orally, transdermally, vaginally, by implantation, or by injection.

Combined Estrogen-Progestin Contraceptives

Oral contraceptives. The normal menstrual cycle is maintained through hormonal feedback mechanisms. FSH and LH are secreted in response to fluctuating levels of ovarian estrogen and progesterone. Regular ingestion of combined oral contraceptive pills (COCs) suppresses the action of the hypothalamus and anterior pituitary gland, leading

TABLE 5.4	Hormonal Contraception	
Composition	**Route of Administration**	**Duration of Effect**
Combination Estrogen and Progestin		
Synthetic estrogens and progestins in varying doses and formulations	Oral	24 hours (extended cycle possible with daily pill for 12 weeks)
	Transdermal patch	7 days
	Vaginal ring insertion	3 weeks
Progestin Only		
• Norethindrone, norgestrel	Oral	24 hours
• Medroxyprogesterone acetate	Intramuscular or subcutaneous injection	3 months
• Etonogestrel	Subdermal implant	Up to 3 years
• Levonorgestrel	Intrauterine device	1 year

to insufficient secretion of FSH and LH; therefore follicles do not mature, and ovulation is inhibited.

Other contraceptive effects are induced by the combined steroids. Maturation of the endometrium is altered, making the uterine lining a less favorable site for implantation. COCs also have a direct effect on the endometrium; thus from 1 to 4 days after the last COC is taken the endometrium sloughs and bleeds as a result of hormone withdrawal. The withdrawal bleeding is usually less profuse than that of normal menstruation and may last only 2 to 3 days. Some women have no bleeding at all. The cervical mucus remains thick from the effect of the progestin. Cervical mucus under the effect of progesterone does not provide as suitable an environment for sperm penetration as does the thin, watery mucus that the healthy reproductive woman produces before and during ovulation.

Monophasic pills provide fixed dosages of estrogen and progestin. They alter the amount of progestin and sometimes estrogen within each cycle. These preparations reduce the total dosage of hormones in a single cycle without sacrificing contraceptive efficacy. To maintain adequate hormone levels for contraception and enhance compliance,

PATIENT TEACHING
Use and Care of the Diaphragm

Positions for Insertion of Diaphragm

Squatting

- Squatting is the most commonly used position, and most women find it satisfactory.

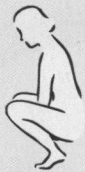

Leg-Up Method

- Another position is to raise the left foot (if right hand is used for insertion) on a low stool and, while in a bending position, insert the diaphragm.

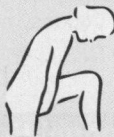

Chair Method

- Another practical method for diaphragm insertion is to sit far forward on the edge of a chair.

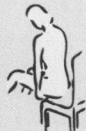

Reclining

- You may prefer to insert the diaphragm while in a semireclining position in bed.

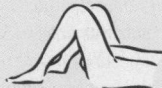

Inspection of Diaphragm

Your diaphragm must be inspected carefully before each use. The best way to do this is:

- Hold the diaphragm up to a light source. Carefully stretch it at the area of the rim, on all sides, to make sure that there are no holes. Remember, it is possible to puncture the diaphragm with sharp fingernails.
- Another way to check for pinholes is to carefully fill the diaphragm with water. If there is any problem, it will be seen immediately.
- If your diaphragm is puckered, especially near the rim, this could mean thin spots.
- The diaphragm should not be used if you see any of these; consult your health care provider.

Preparation of Diaphragm

- Rinse off cornstarch (see section, below, on care of diaphragm, noting that it should be dusted with cornstarch when stored). Your diaphragm must always be used with a spermicidal lubricant to be effective. Pregnancy cannot be prevented effectively by the diaphragm alone.

- Always empty your bladder before inserting the diaphragm. Place about 2 tsp of contraceptive jelly or contraceptive cream on the side of the diaphragm that will rest against the cervix (or whichever way you have been instructed). Spread it around to coat the surface and the rim. This aids in insertion and offers a more complete seal. Many women also spread some jelly or cream on the other side of the diaphragm (Fig. A).

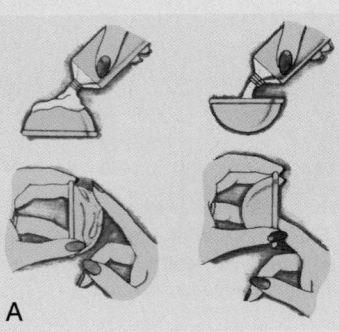

A

Insertion of Diaphragm

- The diaphragm can be inserted as long as 6 hours before intercourse. Hold it between your thumb and fingers. The dome can be either up or down, as directed by your health care provider. Place your index finger on the outer rim of the compressed diaphragm (Fig. B).

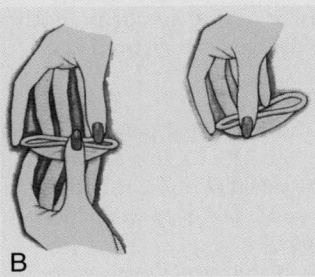

B

- Use the fingers of the other hand to spread the labia (lips of the vagina). This will aid in guiding the diaphragm into place.
- Insert the diaphragm into the vagina. Direct it inward and downward as far as it will go to the space behind and below the cervix (Fig. C).

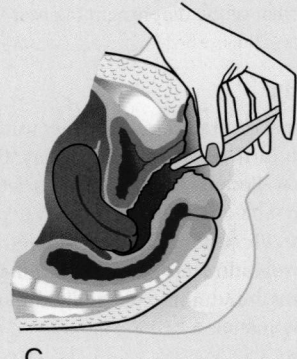

C

PATIENT TEACHING

Use and Care of the Diaphragm—cont'd

- Tuck the front of the rim of the diaphragm behind the pubic bone so the rubber hugs the front wall of the vagina (Fig. D).

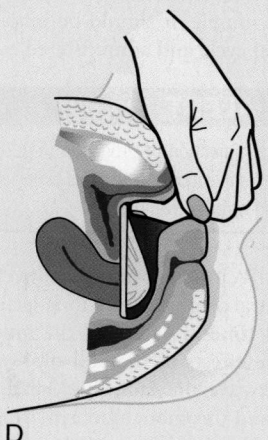

D

- Feel for your cervix through the diaphragm to be certain that it is placed properly and covered securely by the rubber dome (Fig. E).

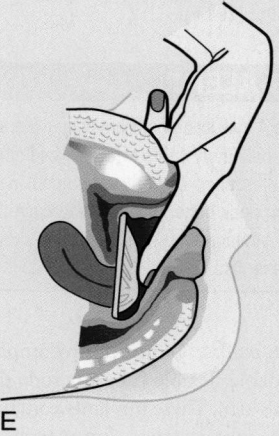

E

General Information

- Regardless of the time of the month, you must use your diaphragm every time intercourse takes place. It must be left in place for at least 6 hours after the last intercourse. If you remove it before the 6-hour period, your chance of becoming pregnant could be greatly increased. If you have repeated acts of intercourse, you must add more spermicide for each act.

Removal of Diaphragm

- The only proper way to remove the diaphragm is to insert your forefinger up and over the top side of the diaphragm and slightly to the side.
- Next turn the palm of your hand downward and backward, hooking the forefinger firmly on top of the inside of the upper rim of the diaphragm, breaking the suction.
- Pull the diaphragm down and out. This avoids the possibility of tearing it with the fingernails. You should not remove it by trying to catch the rim from below the dome (Fig. F).

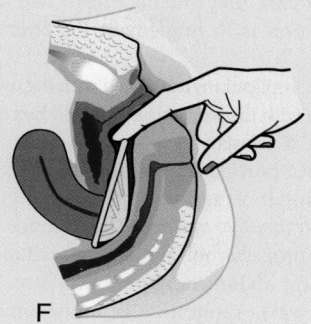

F

Care of Diaphragm

- When using a vaginal diaphragm, avoid using oil-based products such as certain body lubricants, mineral oil, baby oil, vaginal lubricants, or vaginitis preparations. These products can weaken the rubber.
- A little care means longer wear for your diaphragm. After each use, wash it in warm water and mild soap. Do not use detergent soaps, cold-cream soaps, deodorant soaps, and soaps containing oil products because they can weaken the rubber.
- After washing, dry the diaphragm thoroughly. All water and moisture should be removed with a towel. Dust the diaphragm with cornstarch. Scented talc, body powder, baby powder, and the like should not be used because they can weaken the rubber.
- To clean the introducer (if one is used), wash with mild soap and warm water, rinse, and dry thoroughly.
- Place the diaphragm back in the plastic case for storage. Do not store it near a radiator or heat source or exposed to light for an extended period.

COCs should be taken at the same time each day. Taken exactly as directed, COCs prevent ovulation, and pregnancy cannot occur. The overall user effectiveness rate of COCs is 91% (CDC, 2011).

Because taking the pill does not relate directly to the sexual act, COC acceptability may be increased. Improvement in sexual response may occur once the possibility of pregnancy is not an issue. For many women, it is convenient to know when to expect the next menstrual flow.

Contraindications for COC use include a history of thromboembolic disorders, cerebrovascular or coronary artery disease, breast cancer, estrogen-dependent tumors, pregnancy, impaired liver function, liver tumor, lactation less than 6 weeks postpartum, smoking if older than 35 years of age, migraine with aura, surgery with prolonged immobilization or any surgery on the legs, hypertension ($\geq$160/100), and diabetes mellitus (of more than 20 years' duration) with vascular disease.

The effectiveness of oral contraceptives is decreased when the following medications are taken simultaneously:
- Anticonvulsants such as barbiturates, oxcarbazepine, phenytoin, phenobarbital, carbamazepine, primidone, and topiramate
- Systemic antifungals such as griseofulvin
- Antituberculosis drugs such as rifampicin and rifabutin
- Anti-HIV protease inhibitors such as nelfinavir and amprenavir

After discontinuing oral contraception, fertility usually returns quickly, but fertility rates may be slightly lower the first 3 to 12 months after discontinuation.

Nursing considerations. Many different preparations of oral hormonal contraceptives are available. Because of these wide variations in pills, each woman must be clear about the unique dosage regimen for the preparation prescribed for her and follow directions on the package

BOX 5.9   Signs of Potential Complications: Oral Contraceptives

Before oral contraceptives are prescribed and periodically throughout hormone therapy, the woman is alerted to stop taking the pill and report immediately any of the following symptoms to the health care provider. The mnemonic ACHES helps in remembering this list:

A—Abdominal pain: may indicate a problem with the liver or gallbladder

C—Chest pain or shortness of breath: may indicate a possible clot problem within the lungs or heart

H—Headaches (sudden or persistent): may be caused by cerebrovascular accident or hypertension

E—Eye problems: may indicate vascular accident or hypertension

S—Severe leg pain: may indicate a thromboembolic process

insert. Directions for care after missing one or two tablets also vary. A simple recommendation is to implement EC after two missed pills, regardless of dose.

Signs of potential complications associated with the use of oral contraceptives must be reviewed with the woman, as noted in Box 5.9. Oral contraceptives do not protect a woman against STIs. Male condoms used in combination with COCs provide protection against STIs, and this combination gives excellent protection against unplanned pregnancy.

Transdermal contraceptive system. The contraceptive patch delivers continuous levels of progesterone and ethynyl estradiol. The patch can be applied to the lower abdomen, upper outer arm, buttock, or upper torso (except the breasts). Application is on the same day once a week for 3 weeks but not at the same site, followed by a week without the patch. Withdrawal bleeding occurs during the "no patch" week. Mechanisms of action, contraindications, and side effects are similar to those of COCs. The typical failure rate during the first year of use is less than 9% (CDC, 2011).

Vaginal contraceptive ring. The vaginal ring (made of ethylene vinyl acetate co-polymer) delivers continuous levels of progesterone and ethynyl estradiol. Mechanisms of action, contraindications, and side effects are similar to those of COCs. One vaginal ring is worn for 3 weeks, followed by 1 week without the ring. Withdrawal bleeding occurs during the "no ring" week. The ring can be inserted by the woman and does not have to be fitted. Some wearers may experience vaginal discomfort, usually related to increased vaginal discharge; but other wearers report that the ring alleviates symptoms of vaginitis. Some couples say that the ring can be felt during intercourse. Although it is not recommended that the ring be removed for intercourse, contraceptive effectiveness would not decrease if it were replaced within 3 hours. The typical failure rate of the vaginal contraceptive ring is less than 9% during the first year of use (CDC, 2011).

Progestin-Only Contraception

Progestin-only methods impair fertility by inhibiting ovulation, thickening and decreasing the amount of cervical mucus, thinning the endometrium, and altering cilia in the uterine tubes. Because progestin-only methods do not contain estrogen, they may be used in certain instances such as lactation, when estrogen would not be recommended.

Oral progestins (minipill). Progestin-only pills are less effective than COCs. Because minipills contain such a low dose of progestin, they must be taken at the same time every day. If the pill is taken more than 3 hours late (27 hours after the last pill), a backup contraceptive method must be initiated. Much of the contraceptive effectiveness of the minipill depends on progestin-induced changes in cervical mucus, and this effect lasts about 24 hours after oral ingestion of the pill. Users often complain of irregular vaginal bleeding. Effectiveness is increased if minipills are

taken correctly. There are two instances in which the minipill is quite effective: in lactating women and women older than 40 years of age. The reduced fecundity of lactation and the perimenopause period enhance the contraceptive effects of the minipill.

Injectable progestins. Depot medroxyprogesterone acetate (DMPA; Depo-Provera) is given subcutaneously or intramuscularly in the deltoid or gluteus maximus muscle. It should be initiated during the first 5 days of the menstrual cycle and administered every 11 to 13 weeks.

! NURSING ALERT

When administering an injection of progestin (e.g., DMPA), the site should not be massaged after the injection because this action can hasten the absorption and shorten the period of effectiveness.

Advantages of DMPA include a contraceptive effectiveness comparable to that of combined oral contraceptives, long-lasting effects, requirement of injections only 4 times a year, and the unlikelihood of lactation being impaired. Side effects at the end of 1 year include decreased bone mineral density, weight gain, lipid changes, increased risk for venous thrombosis and thromboembolism, irregular vaginal spotting, decreased libido, and breast changes. Other disadvantages include no protection against STIs (including HIV). Return to fertility may be delayed as long as up to 18 months after discontinuing DMPA, with the median time being 10 months. The typical failure rate is 6% in the first year of use (CDC, 2011).

! NURSING ALERT

Women who use DMPA may lose significant bone mineral density with increasing duration of use. It is unknown if this effect is reversible. It is unknown if use of DMPA during adolescence or early adulthood, a critical period of bone accretion, will reduce peak bone mass and increase the risk for osteoporotic fracture in later life. Women who receive DMPA should be counseled about calcium intake and exercise.

Implantable progestins. Contraceptive implants consist of one or more nonbiodegradable flexible tubes or rods that are inserted under the skin of a woman's arm. These implants contain a progestin hormone and are effective for contraception for at least 3 years. They must be removed at the end of the recommended time. The only available implant in the United States is a single-rod etonogestrel implant (Implanon, Nexplanon), which is FDA approved. Three other devices are also used globally, but they are unavailable in the United States. One of these implants is Norplant, which used to be commonly used in the United States, but due to difficulties in insertion and removal (because it contains 6 rods), it is no longer used (Rivlin & Westhoff, 2017).

Insertion and removal of the single-rod etonogestrel capsule are minor surgical procedures involving a local anesthetic, a small incision, and no sutures. The capsule is placed subdermally in the inner aspect of the nondominant upper arm. The progestin prevents some, but not all, ovulatory cycles and thickens cervical mucus. Other advantages of the single-rod implant are that it provides long-term continuous contraception that is not related to frequency of coitus and is quickly reversible. The single-rod implant can be inserted immediately after the birth in breastfeeding women without affecting lactation. Irregular menstrual bleeding is the most common side effect. Less common side effects include headache, nervousness, nausea, skin changes, and vertigo. The implant does not protect against STIs. As in other hormonal contraception methods, condoms should be used for protection against STIs. Implants are considered to be as effective or even more effective than sterilization and IUDs, making them some of the most effective contraceptive methods (Rivlin & Westhoff, 2017).

Emergency Contraception

Emergency contraception (EC) offers protection against pregnancy after intercourse occurs in instances such as broken condoms, sexual assault, dislodged cervical cap, disruption of use of any other method, or any other case of unprotected intercourse. Methods that are available in the United States that could provide postcoital contraception include the following:

- Ella (Ulipristal): single 30-mg pill containing an antiprogestin
- Plan B One-Step: single progestin-only pill containing 1.5 mg levonorgestrel
- Next Choice: two levonorgestrel 0.75-mg tablets taken orally 12 hours apart or both together
- Combined oral: estrogen-progestin contraceptive pills (e.g., 100-mcg ethinyl estradiol plus 0.5 mg levonorgestrel); two doses given 12 hours apart (Yuzpe regimen)
- Copper intrauterine device (IUD) insertion within 120 hours of intercourse

Plan B One-Step and Next Choice are approved by the FDA for over-the-counter sale to women 17 years of age and older with proof of age. Adolescents 16 years of age and younger require a prescription. Ella is available only with a prescription. States vary in the ability of pharmacists to dispense EC, and some states have implemented refusal legislation (Guttmacher Institute, 2016a).

In general, for the most effectiveness, EC should be taken by a woman as soon as possible but within 72 hours of unprotected intercourse or a birth control mishap (e.g., broken condom, dislodged ring or cervical cap, missed oral contraceptive pills, late for injection) to prevent unintended pregnancy. Research has shown a moderate amount of effectiveness between 72 and 120 hours, but no data are available for effectiveness after 120 hours (Rivlin & Westhoff, 2017).

If taken before ovulation, EC prevents ovulation by inhibiting follicular development. If taken after ovulation occurs, there is little effect on ovarian hormone production or the endometrium. To minimize the side effect of nausea that occurs with high doses of estrogen and progestin (Yuzpe regimen), the woman can be advised to take an over-the-counter antiemetic 1 hour before each dose. Nausea is not as common with the Plan B (One-Step regimen). Women with contraindications for estrogen use should use progestin-only EC. No medical contraindications for EC exist, except pregnancy and undiagnosed abnormal vaginal bleeding. If the woman does not begin menstruation within 21 days after taking the pills, she should be evaluated for pregnancy. EC is ineffective if the woman is pregnant since the pills do not disturb an implanted pregnancy. Risk for pregnancy is reduced by approximately 75% with EC (Rivlin & Westhoff, 2017).

> **! NURSING ALERT**
>
> EC will not protect the woman against pregnancy if she engages in unprotected intercourse in the days or weeks that follow treatment. Because ingestion of EC pills may delay ovulation, the woman should be cautioned that she needs to establish a reliable form of birth control to prevent unintended pregnancy. Information about EC method options and access to providers is available on the Internet at www.NOT-2-LATE.com or by calling 888-NOT-2-LATE.

IUDs containing copper (see later discussion) provide another EC option. The IUD should be inserted within 5 days of unprotected intercourse, resulting in an estimated 99% effectiveness in preventing pregnancy (Rivlin & Westhoff, 2017). This method is suggested only for women who wish to have the benefit of long-term contraception.

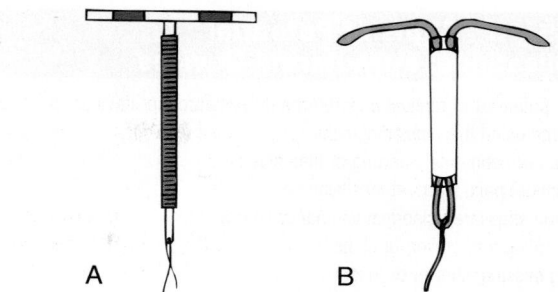

FIG 5.13 Intrauterine devices. **A,** Copper T380A. **B,** Levonorgestrel-releasing intrauterine device.

The risk for pregnancy is reduced by as much as 99% with emergency insertion of the copper-releasing IUD.

Contraceptive counseling should be provided to all women requesting EC, including a discussion of modification of risky sexual behaviors to prevent STIs and unwanted pregnancy.

Intrauterine Devices

An intrauterine device (IUD) is a small T-shaped device with bendable arms for insertion through the cervix into the uterine cavity. Two strings hang from the base of the stem through the cervix and protrude into the vagina for the woman to feel for assurance that the device has not been dislodged (Fig. 5.13). There is one FDA-approved copper-bearing IUD in the United States. This is the Copper T380A (ParaGard, Frazier, Pennsylvania) IUD, which is made of radiopaque polyethylene and fine solid copper and is approved for 10 years of use. The copper primarily serves as a spermicide and inflames the endometrium, preventing fertilization. Sometimes women experience an increase in bleeding and cramping within the first year after insertion, but nonsteroidal antiinflammatory drugs (NSAIDs) can provide pain relief. The cumulative failure rate over 12 years of use of the copper IUD is 1.7% (Rivlin & Westhoff, 2017).

Another type of IUD releases levonorgestrel from its vertical reservoir. This is the levonorgestrel intrauterine system (IUS) (Mirena, Bayer, New Jersey), which is effective for up to 5 years. It works by impairing sperm motility, irritating the lining of the uterus, and exerting some anovulatory effects. Uterine cramping and uterine bleeding are usually decreased with this device, although irregular spotting is common in the first few months following insertion. The cumulative failure rate over 5 years of use is 1.1% (Rivlin & Westhoff, 2017). IUDs offer constant contraception without the need to remember to take pills each day or engage in other manipulation before or between coital acts. If pregnancy can be excluded, either device (the Copper T380A or the levonorgestrel intrauterine system) can be placed at any time during the menstrual cycle. These devices may be inserted immediately after childbirth or following a first-trimester abortion. The contraceptive effects are reversible. When pregnancy is desired, the health care provider removes the device.

Disadvantages of IUD use include increased risk for pelvic inflammatory disease within the first 20 days after insertion, especially if infection is present at the time of insertion. There is also a slight risk for uterine perforation. Neither the Copper T380A nor the levonorgestrel intrauterine system offers protection against STIs or HIV. The Copper T380A is more likely to be associated with regular menses that may have heavier flow. Women who have the levonorgestrel intrauterine system are more likely to experience scant, irregular episodes of vaginal bleeding or amenorrhea.

Nursing Considerations

The woman should be taught to check for the presence of the IUD thread after menstruation to rule out expulsion of the device. If pregnancy

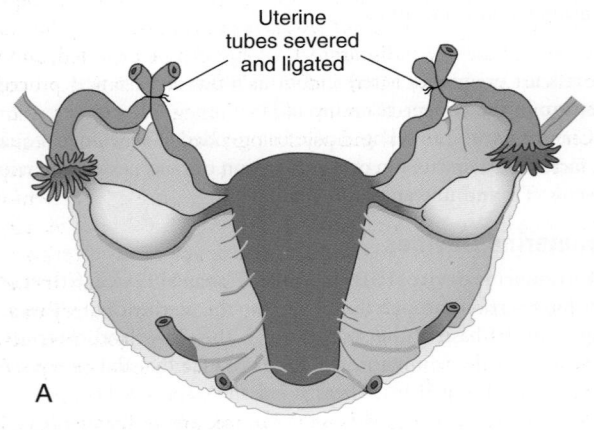

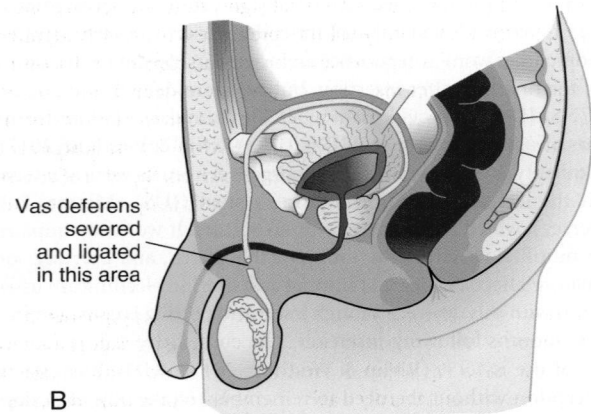

FIG 5.14 Sterilization. **A,** Uterine tubes ligated and severed (tubal ligation). **B,** Sperm duct ligated and severed (vasectomy).

occurs with the IUD in place, the IUD should be removed immediately in the first trimester if the strings are visible. Later in pregnancy ultrasound examination should be used to localize the IUD and rule out placenta previa. Retention of the IUD during pregnancy increases the risk for septic miscarriage and ectopic pregnancy. Some women allergic to copper develop a rash, necessitating removal of the copper-bearing IUD. Signs of potential complications of intrauterine contraception are listed in Box 5.10.

Sterilization

Sterilization refers to surgical procedures intended to render the person infertile. Most procedures involve the occlusion of the passageways for the ova and sperm (Fig. 5.14). For the woman the uterine tubes are occluded; for the man the sperm ducts (vas deferens) are occluded. Only surgical removal of the ovaries (oophorectomy) or uterus (hysterectomy) or both results in absolute **sterility** for the woman. All other

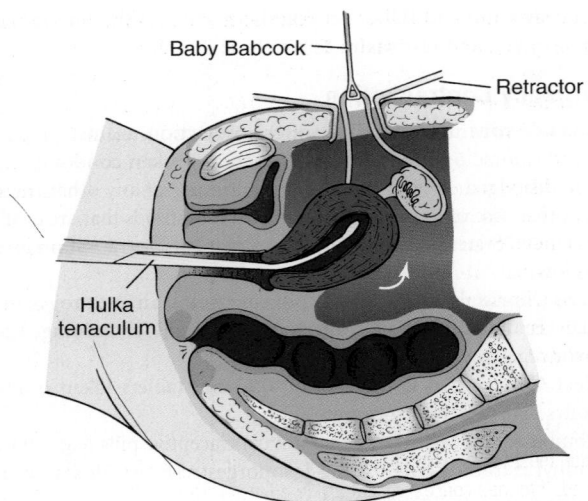

FIG 5.15 Use of minilaparotomy to gain access to uterine tubes for occlusion procedures. Tenaculum is used to lift uterus upward *(arrow)* toward incision.

PATIENT TEACHING
What to Expect After Tubal Ligation

- You should expect no change in hormones and their influence.
- Your menstrual period will be about the same as before the sterilization.
- You may feel pain at ovulation.
- It is highly unlikely that you will become pregnant.
- You should not have a change in sexual functioning; you may enjoy sexual relations more because you will not be concerned about becoming pregnant.
- Sterilization offers no protection against sexually transmitted infections; therefore, you may need to use condoms.

sterilization procedures have a small but definite failure rate (i.e., pregnancy may result).

Female Sterilization

Female sterilization (bilateral **tubal ligation**) may be done immediately after giving birth (within 24 to 48 hours), concomitantly with abortion, or as an interval procedure (during any phase of the menstrual cycle). Half of all female sterilization procedures are performed immediately after a pregnancy. Sterilization procedures can be done safely on an outpatient basis. The failure rate for methods of female sterilization vary by the method and the woman's age, but this is a very effective and safe method, with one study demonstrating a failure rate of 57 out of 1000 in the first year. However, it is important to emphasize that this form of birth control is considered to be permanent (Rivlin & Westhoff, 2017).

Tubal occlusion. A laparoscopic approach or a minilaparotomy may be used for tubal ligation (Fig. 5.15), tubal electrocoagulation, or the application of bands or clips. Electrocoagulation and ligation are considered to be permanent methods. Essure is another permanent method in which a soft insert is placed into each fallopian tube, forming a barrier that grows around the inserts. The couple is told to use a backup contraceptive method for the first 3 months. Another method, the bands or clips, has the theoretic advantage of possible removal and return of tubal patency (see Patient Teaching box).

Tubal reconstruction. Restoration of tubal continuity (reanastomosis) and function is technically feasible except after laparoscopic tubal electrocoagulation. Sterilization reversal is costly, difficult (requiring microsurgery), and uncertain. The success rate varies with the extent of tubal destruction and removal. The risk for ectopic pregnancy after tubal reanastomosis is approximately 10%, significantly higher than the risk of 3% in the general population (Tubal Reversal, 2017).

Laws and regulations. All states have strict regulations for informed consent. Many states permit voluntary sterilization of any mature, rational woman without reference to her marital or pregnancy status. Although the partner's consent is not required by law, the woman is encouraged to discuss the situation with her partner, and health care providers may request the partner's consent. Sterilization of minors or mentally incompetent individuals is restricted by most states and often requires the approval of a board of eugenicists or other court-appointed individuals.

LEGAL TIP Sterilization If federal funds are used for sterilization, the person must be at least 21 years of age on the day the consent form is signed. Informed consent must include an explanation of the risks, benefits, and alternatives; a statement that describes sterilization as a permanent, irreversible method of birth control; and a statement that mandates a 30-day waiting period between giving consent and the sterilization. Informed consent must be in the person's native language, or an interpreter must be provided to read the consent form to the person. Signed consent forms expire after 180 days, so they must be re-signed if the sterilization procedure is still desired but has not yet been performed.

Male Sterilization

Vasectomy is the sealing, tying, or cutting of a man's vas deferens so the sperm cannot travel from the testes to the penis. Vasectomy is the easiest and most commonly used operation for male sterilization. The surgery can be performed with local anesthesia on an outpatient basis. Pain, bleeding, infection, and other postsurgical complications are considered to be possible disadvantages to the surgical procedure.

Two methods are used for scrotal entry: conventional and no-scalpel vasectomy. The surgeon identifies and immobilizes the vas deferens through the scrotum. Then the vas is ligated or cauterized (see Fig. 5.14, *B*). Surgeons vary in their techniques to occlude the vas deferens: ligation with sutures, division, cautery, application of clips, excision of a segment of the vas, fascial interposition, or some combination of these methods.

Vasectomy has no effect on potency (ability to achieve and maintain erection) or volume of ejaculate. Endocrine production of testosterone continues, so secondary sex characteristics are not affected. Sperm production continues, but sperm are unable to leave the epididymis and are lysed by the immune system. Vasectomy does not change the man's transmission of the HIV virus if he is infected. He will need to be instructed to engage in a number of ejaculations until there are no viable sperm remaining above the area of the surgery. Until this occurs, as documented by semen analysis, the couple should use backup contraception.

Complications after bilateral vasectomy are uncommon and usually not serious. They include bleeding (usually external), suture reaction, and reaction to the anesthetic agent. Men occasionally develop a hematoma, infection, or epididymitis. Less common are painful granulomas from accumulation of sperm. Vasectomy is highly effective and safe. It is estimated that 5% to 7% of men in the United States request reversal of vasectomy (Rivlin & Westhoff, 2017), and although reanastomosis is possible, it is important to emphasize that men should view the decision to have vasectomy as permanent.

Tubal reconstruction. Microsurgery to reanastomose (restore tubal continuity) the sperm ducts can be accomplished successfully (i.e., sperm in the ejaculate) in 86% of cases; however, the fertility rate following reanastomosis is only about 50% (Baker & Sabanegh, 2013). The rate of success decreases as the time since the procedure was initially performed increases. The vasectomy may result in permanent changes in the testes that leave men unable to father children. The changes are those ordinarily seen only in older adults (e.g., interstitial fibrosis [scar tissue between the seminiferous tubules]). In addition, some men develop antibodies against their own sperm (autoimmunization).

Nursing Considerations

The nurse plays an important role in helping people make decisions so all requirements for informed consent are met. The nurse also provides information about alternatives to sterilization such as contraception.

Information must be given about what is entailed in the various procedures, how much discomfort or pain can be expected, and what type of care is needed. Many individuals fear sterilization procedures because of imagined effects on sexual functioning. They need reassurance concerning the hormonal and psychologic basis of sexual functioning. The fact that uterine tube occlusion or vasectomy has no biologic sequelae in terms of sexual adequacy needs to be communicated and reinforced. If sex drive is affected, it can be a sign of emotional or other physical issues and should discussed with a physician or nurse practitioner.

Preoperative care includes health assessment, which includes a psychologic assessment, physical examination, and laboratory tests. The nurse confirms that the individual understands printed instructions. Ambivalence and extreme fear of the procedure should be reported to the health care provider.

Postoperative care depends on the procedure performed (e.g., laparoscopy, laparotomy for tubal occlusion, or vasectomy). General care includes recovery after anesthesia, vital signs, fluid-electrolyte balance (intake and output, laboratory values), prevention of or early identification and treatment of infection or hemorrhage, control of discomfort, and assessment of emotional response to the procedure and recovery.

Discharge planning depends on the type of procedure performed. In general, the patient is given written instructions about observing for and reporting symptoms and signs of complications, the type of recovery to be expected, and the date and time for a follow-up appointment.

ABORTION

Induced abortion is the purposeful interruption of a pregnancy before 20 weeks of gestation. (Spontaneous abortion or miscarriage is discussed in Chapter 12.) If the abortion is performed at the woman's request, the term elective abortion is usually used; if performed for reasons of maternal or fetal health or disease, the term therapeutic abortion applies. Many factors contribute to a woman's decision to have an abortion. Indications include (1) preservation of the life or health of the mother, (2) genetic disorders of the fetus, (3) rape or incest, and (4) the pregnant woman's request. The control of birth, dealing as it does with human sexuality and the question of life and death, is one of the most emotional components of health care. It has been the most controversial social issue in the last half of the twentieth century and continues to be so today. Regulations exist to protect the mother from the complications of abortion.

Abortion is regulated in most countries, including the United States. Before 1970 legal abortion was not widely available in the United States. However, in January 1973 the US Supreme Court set aside previous antiabortion laws and legalized it. This decision established a trimester approach to abortion, but controversy remains, and there are continuing attempts to change this law.

Following the US Supreme Court ruling in 1973 in the case of *Roe versus Wade,* the decision of first-trimester abortion was deemed to be between the pregnant woman and her health care provider, and state laws determining abortion to be illegal were struck down. During the second trimester, abortion is left to the discretion of the individual states to regulate procedures as long as these regulations are reasonably related to the woman's health. In the third trimester, abortions may be limited or even prohibited by state regulation unless the restriction interferes with the life or health of the pregnant woman (*Roe v. Wade*, 1973). Hospitals maintained by Roman Catholics and some of those maintained by strict fundamentalists forbid abortion (and often sterilization) despite legal challenges.

Currently 38 states legislate that abortion be performed by a licensed physician. Nurse practitioners can perform aspiration abortions in six states: California, Montana, New Hampshire, New York, Rhode Island, and Vermont. In these states plus six additional states, nurse practitioners can prescribe medication abortions (Guttmacher Institute, 2016b; Levi et al., 2015). Congress has legislated that Medicaid funds can only be used to pay for abortion when a woman's life is endangered. States vary on the financing of abortions, with 17 states using their own funds to pay for them, depending on the circumstances surrounding the procedure. States also vary regarding parental notification and/or consent regarding abortion, with 37 states providing legislation for some type of parental involvement in the abortion of a pregnant daughter who is a minor. Individual health care providers may refuse to participate in abortion in 45 states (Guttmacher Institute).

In the United States it is estimated that 50% of pregnancies are unintended, with about 40% of those unintended pregnancies ending in elective abortion (Rivlin & Westhoff, 2017). The number of abortions in the United States has decreased by 13% since 2008 (Rivlin & Westhoff). Most abortions occur in women who already have children, and abortion rates tend to be higher in women whose income is below the poverty level.

The Association of Women's Health, Obstetric and Neonatal Nurses (AWHONN, 2016) supports a nurse's right to choose whether to participate in abortion procedures in keeping with her or his "personal, moral, ethical, or religious beliefs." AWHONN also advocates that "nurses have a professional obligation to inform their employers, at the time of employment, of any attitudes and beliefs that may interfere with essential job functions." Levi and colleagues (2015) describe why they choose to provide abortion services and why this is an important role for nursing.

Rates of biologic complications after abortions such as ectopic pregnancy, infection, or hemorrhage tend to be low if the woman aborts during the first trimester. Psychologic sequelae of induced abortion are uncommon and may be related to circumstances and support systems surrounding the pregnant woman such as the attitudes reflected by friends, family, and health care workers. The woman facing an abortion is pregnant and exhibits the emotional responses shared by all pregnant women, including the possibility of depression.

Nurses and other health care providers often struggle with the same values and moral convictions as those of the pregnant woman. The conflicts and doubts of the nurse can be readily communicated to women who are already anxious. Regardless of personal views on abortion, nurses who provide care to women seeking abortion have an ethical responsibility to counsel women about their options and make appropriate referrals.

LEGAL TIP **Institutional Policies for Nurses' Rights and Responsibilities Related to Abortion** Nurses' rights and responsibilities related to caring for abortion patients should be protected through policies that describe how the institution accommodates the nurse's ethical or moral beliefs and what the nurse should do to avoid patient abandonment in such situations. Nurses should know what policies are in place in their institutions and encourage such policies to be written. Nurses and nurse practitioners play an important role in the care of a woman choosing to have an elective abortion.

BOX 5.11 **Selected Nursing Diagnoses for Women Having Elective Abortion**

- Decisional conflict related to
  - Value system
- Fear related to
  - Abortion procedure
  - Potential complications
  - Implications for future pregnancies
  - What others might think
- Grieving related to
  - Distress at loss or feelings of guilt
- Risk for infection related to
  - Effects of the procedure
  - Lack of understanding of preoperative and postoperative self-care
- Acute pain related to
  - Effects of the procedure or postoperative events

CARE MANAGEMENT

A thorough assessment is conducted through history, physical examination, and laboratory tests. The length of pregnancy and the condition of the woman must be determined to select the appropriate type of abortion procedure. An ultrasound examination should be performed before a second-trimester abortion is done. If the woman is Rh-negative, she is a candidate for prophylaxis against Rh isoimmunization. She should receive $Rh_o(D)$ immune globulin within 72 hours after the abortion if she is D-negative and if Coombs' test results are negative (if the woman is unsensitized or isoimmunization has not developed).

The woman's understanding of alternatives, the types of abortions, and expected recovery is assessed. Misinformation and gaps in knowledge are identified and corrected. The record is reviewed for the signed informed consent, and the woman's understanding is verified. General preoperative, operative, and postoperative assessments are performed.

Analysis of data leads to identification of the appropriate nursing diagnoses for the woman undergoing elective abortion. Potential nursing diagnoses are listed in Box 5.11. Counseling about abortion includes helping the woman identify how she perceives the pregnancy, providing information about the choices available (i.e., having an abortion or carrying the pregnancy to term and then either keeping the infant or placing the baby for adoption), and informing about the types of abortion procedures and risks.

First-Trimester Abortion

Methods for performing early elective abortion (up to 10 weeks of gestation) include surgical (aspiration) and medical methods (mifepristone with prostaglandin and methotrexate with misoprostol). The earlier an abortion is performed, the safer it is, reducing the need for later-term abortions.

Surgical (Aspiration) Abortion

Aspiration (vacuum or suction curettage) is the most common procedure in the first trimester. Aspiration abortion is usually performed under local anesthesia in a health care provider's office, a clinic, or a hospital. The ideal time for performing this procedure is 8 to 12 weeks after the last menstrual period (gestational age of 10 weeks) (Rivlin & Westhoff, 2017). The suction procedure for performing an early elective abortion usually requires less than 5 minutes.

A bimanual examination is done before the procedure to assess uterine size and position. A speculum is inserted, and the cervix is anesthetized with a local anesthetic agent. The cervix is dilated if necessary, and a cannula connected to suction is inserted into the uterine cavity. The products of conception are evacuated from the uterus.

During the procedure, the woman is kept informed about what to expect next (e.g., menstrual-like cramping and sounds of the suction machine). The nurse assesses the woman's vital signs. The aspirated uterine contents must be inspected carefully to ascertain whether all fetal parts and adequate placental tissue have been evacuated. After the abortion, the woman rests on the table until she is ready to stand. She remains in the recovery area or waiting room for 1 to 3 hours for detection of excessive cramping or bleeding; then she is discharged.

Bleeding after the operation is normally about the equivalent of a heavy menstrual period, and cramps are rarely severe. Excessive vaginal bleeding and infection such as endometritis or salpingitis are the most common complications of induced abortion. Retained products of conception are the primary cause of vaginal bleeding. Evacuation of the uterus, uterine massage, and administration of oxytocin or methylergonovine (Methergine) may be necessary to decrease vaginal bleeding. Prophylactic antibiotics to decrease the risk for infection are commonly prescribed. Generally, postabortion pain can be relieved with NSAIDs such as ibuprofen.

Nursing considerations. Instructions following a surgical abortion differ among health care providers. For example, there is disagreement as to whether tampons should not be used for at least 3 days or should be avoided for up to 3 weeks, or whether resumption of sexual intercourse may be permitted within 1 week or discouraged for 2 weeks. The woman may shower daily. Instruction is given to watch for excessive bleeding and other signs of complications and to avoid douches of any type. The woman can expect her menstrual period to resume 4 to 6 weeks after the day of the procedure. The nurse offers information about the birth control method the woman prefers if contraceptive counseling has not been done during the counseling interview that usually precedes the decision to have an abortion. The woman must be strongly encouraged to return for her follow-up visit so complications can be detected and an acceptable contraceptive method prescribed. A pregnancy test may also be performed to determine if the pregnancy has been terminated successfully.

⚡ SAFETY ALERT

The woman who has an induced abortion should be given clear instructions to return immediately to the health care facility or emergency department for any of the following symptoms:
- Fever greater than 38° C (100.4° F)
- Chills
- Bleeding greater than two saturated pads in 2 hours or heavy bleeding lasting a few days
- Foul-smelling vaginal discharge
- Severe abdominal pain, cramping, or backache
- Abdominal tenderness (when pressure applied)

Data from Paul, M., & Stein, T. (2011). Abortion. In R. A. Hatcher, J. Trussell, & A. L. Nelson (Eds.), *Contraceptive technology*. Atlanta, GA: Ardent Media.

Medical Abortion

Early abortion using medication rather than surgery has been popular in Canada and Europe for more than 15 years, but medical abortion is a relatively new procedure in the United States. Medical abortions are available for use in the United States for up to 9 weeks after the last menstrual period. Methotrexate, misoprostol, and mifepristone are the drugs used in the current regimens to induce early abortion. Medication abortions increased from 6% in 2011 to 31% in 2014. However, the overall abortion rate has declined (Guttmacher Institute, 2017).

Misoprostol and Mifepristone

Misoprostol (Cytotec) is a prostaglandin analog that acts directly on the cervix to soften and dilate and on the uterine muscle to stimulate contractions. Mifepristone, formerly known as RU 486, was approved by the FDA in 2000. It works by preventing progesterone from binding to receptors, thereby blocking the action of progesterone, which is necessary for maintaining pregnancy (Rivlin & Westhoff, 2017).

Mifepristone may be taken up to 7 weeks after the last menstrual period. The FDA-approved regimen is that the woman takes 600 mg of mifepristone orally; 48 hours later she returns to the office and takes 400 mcg of misoprostol orally (unless abortion has already occurred and been confirmed) (Rivlin & Westhoff, 2017). Two weeks after the administration of mifepristone, the woman must return to the office for a clinical examination or ultrasound to confirm that the pregnancy has been terminated.

With any medical abortion regimen, the woman usually experiences bleeding and cramping. Side effects of the medications include nausea, vomiting, diarrhea, headache, dizziness, fever, and chills. These are attributed to misoprostol and usually subside in a few hours after administration.

Second-Trimester Abortion

Because the great majority of induced abortions in the United States occur in the first trimester, only about 10% are performed in the second trimester. Second-trimester abortion is associated with more complications and costs than first-trimester abortions. Dilation and evacuation (D&E) accounts for almost all procedures performed in the United States. This term is also often referred to as *dilation and curettage (D&C)*.

In general, medical administration of second-trimester abortions involves the same drugs (misoprostol and mifepristone) used in medical termination of pregnancy during the first trimester. The D&E procedure is often chosen by patients because it has a lower risk for retained products of conception and a decreased hospitalization time (Rivlin & Westhoff, 2017).

Dilation and Evacuation

D&E can be performed at any point up to 20 weeks of gestation, although it is more often performed between 13 and 16 weeks. After 16 weeks, the cervix requires more dilation because the products of conception are larger. Often laminaria are inserted several hours or several days before the procedure, or misoprostol can be applied to the cervix to soften the tissue. The procedure is similar to that of vaginal aspiration, except that a larger cannula is used and other instruments may be needed to remove the fetus and placenta. Nursing care includes monitoring vital signs, providing emotional support, administering analgesics, and postoperative monitoring. Disadvantages of D&E include possible long-term harmful effects on the cervix.

Nursing Considerations

The woman considering an abortion will need help to explore the meaning of the various alternatives for elective abortion and consequences to herself and her significant others. It is often difficult for a woman to express her true feelings (e.g., what abortion means to her now and in the future and what support or regret her friends and peers may demonstrate). A calm, matter-of-fact approach on the part of the nurse can be helpful. Clarifying, restating, and reflecting statements; open-ended questions; and feedback are communication techniques that can be used to maintain a realistic focus on the situation and bring the woman's problems into the open. Sometimes the partner or family are involved and may also need support as there may be conflicting feelings among family members of the partner. The woman may have been a victim of human trafficking (see Chapter 3). If family or friends cannot be involved, scheduling time for nursing personnel to give the necessary support is an essential component of the care plan.

Information about alternatives to abortion such as referral to adoption agencies or support services if the woman chooses to keep her baby is provided. If a decision is made to have an abortion, the woman must be assured of continued support. Information about what is entailed in various procedures, how much discomfort or pain can be expected, and what type of care is needed must be given. A discussion of the various feelings, including depression, guilt, regret, and relief, that the woman might experience after the abortion is needed. Information about community resources for postabortion counseling may be needed.

Evidence of long-term depression after elective abortion has been inconclusive. Guilt and anxiety may occur more with young women, women with poor social support, multiparous women, and women with a history of psychiatric illness. Women having second-trimester abortions may have more emotional distress than women having abortions in the first trimester. Because symptoms can vary among women who have had abortions, nurses must assess women for grief reactions and facilitate the grieving process through active listening and nonjudgmental support and care.

REFERENCES

American Society for Reproductive Medicine. (2012). *Age and fertility*. Retrieved from https://www.asrm.org/uploadedFiles/ASRM _Content/Resources/Patient_Resources/Fact_Sheets_and_Info_Booklets/ agefertility.pdf.

American Society for Reproductive Medicine. (2014). *Preimplantation genetic testing*. Retrieved from http://www.asrm.org/uploadedFiles/ASRM_ Content/Resources/Patient_Resources/Fact_Sheets_and_Info_Booklets/ PGT_2014.pdf.

American Society for Reproductive Medicine. (2016). *Quick facts about infertility*. Retrieved from https://www.asrm.org/detail.aspx?id=2322.

Association of Women's Health, Obstetric and Neonatal Nurses. (2016). Position statement: Midwifery. *Journal of Obstetric, Gynecologic, & Neonatal Nursing, 45*(3), 454–457.

Baker, K., & Sabanegh, E. (2013). Obstructive azoospermia: Reconstructive techniques and results. *Clinics (Sao Paulo), 68*(1 suppl), 61–73. Retrieved from https://www.ncbi.nlm.nih.gov/pmc/articles/PMC3583161/.

Center for Young Women's Health. (2016). *Contraceptive sponge*. Division of Adolescent and Young Adult Medicine, Division of Gynecology, Boston Children's Hospital. Retrieved from http://youngwomenshealth.org/ 2013/08/22/contraceptive-sponge/.

Centers for Disease Control and Prevention. (2011). *Effectiveness of family planning methods*. Retrieved from https://www.asrm.org/uploadedFiles/ ASRM_Content/Resources/Patient_Resources/Fact_Sheets _and_Info_Booklets/agefertility.pdf.

Centers for Disease Control and Prevention. (2013). *Ten great public health achievements in the 20th century*. Retrieved from https://www.cdc.gov/ about/history/tengpha.htm.

Centers for Disease Control and Prevention. (2014). *What is assisted reproductive technology?* Retrieved from https://www.cdc.gov/art/ whatis.html.

Centers for Disease Control and Prevention. (2015). *Unintended pregnancy prevention*. Retrieved from https://www.cdc.gov/reproductivehealth/ unintendedpregnancy/.

Contracept.org. (2016a). *Fertility awareness methods: Standard days method*. Retrieved from http://www.contracept.org/calendar.php.

Contracept.org. (2016b). *Fertility awareness methods: The TwoDay method*. Retrieved from http://www.contracept.org/twoday-method.php.

Crawford, N. M., Steiner, A. Z. (2015). Age-related infertility. *Obstetrics and Gynecology Clinics of North America, 42*(1), 15–25.

Greenblatt, A. (2011). *Fewer babies available for adoption by US parents. National Public Radio*. Retrieved from http://www.npr.org/2011/ 11/17/142344354/fewer-babies-available-for-adoption-by-u-s -parents.

Guttmacher Institute. (2016a). *Emergency contraception*. Retrieved from https://www.guttmacher.org/sites/default/files/pdfs/spibs/spib_EC.pdf.

Guttmacher Institute. (2016b). *An overview of abortion laws, as of August 1, 2016*. Retrieved from https://www.guttmacher.org/state-policy/explore/ overview-abortion-laws.

Guttmacher Institute. (2017). *Induced abortion in the US*. Retrieved from https://www.guttmacher.org/fact-sheet/induced-abortion-united-states.

Kaplan, K. (2015). *More than 1.5% of American babies owe their births to IVF, report says. Los Angeles Times*. Retrieved from http://www.latimes.com/ science/sciencenow/la-sci-sn-ivf-live-birth s-success-rate-20150303-story.html.

Leiva, R., Burhan, U., Kyrillos, E., Fehring, R., McLaren, R., Dalzell, C., et al. (2014). Use of ovulation predictor kits as adjuncts when using fertility awareness methods (FAMs): A pilot study. *Journal of the American Board of Family Medicine, 27*(3), 427–429.

Levi, A. J., Banks, E., Dieseldorff, J., & Tueros, V. S. (2015). *The clinician speaks: Why I am an abortion provider. Women's Healthcare, May*, 46-49. Retrieved from http://npwomenshealthcare.com/wp-content/ uploads/2015/05/Comm_M15.pdf.

Lobo, R. A. (2017). Infertility: Etiology, diagnostic evaluation, management, prognosis. In R. A. Lobo, D. M. Gershenson, G. M. Lentz, & F. A. Valea (Eds.), *Comprehensive gynecology* (7th ed.). Philadelphia, PA: Mosby.

Rivlin, K., & Westhoff, C. (2017). Family planning. In R. A. Lobo, D. M. Gershenson, G. M. Lentz, & F. A. Valea (Eds.), *Comprehensive gynecology* (7th ed.). Philadelphia, PA: Mosby.

Roe v. Wade, 410 US 113, 154 (1973).

Tubal Reversal. (2017). *Risks of tubal reversal surgery*. Retrieved from https:// www.tubal-reversal.net/tubal-reversal/risks-of-tubal-reversal-surgery/.

World Health Organization. (2016). *Nonoxynol-9 ineffective in preventing HIV infection*. Retrieved from http://www.who.int/mediacentre/news/notes/ release55/en/.

6

Genetics, Conception, and Fetal Development

Ellen F. Olshansky

ⓔ http://evolve.elsevier.com/Perry/maternal

This chapter presents a brief discussion of genetics and the role of the nurse in genetics. It also provides an overview of the process of fertilization and of the development of the normal embryo and fetus.

GENETICS

Recent advances in molecular biology and genomics have revolutionized the field of health care by providing the tools needed to determine the hereditary component of many diseases as well as improve our ability to predict susceptibility to disease, onset and progression of disease, and response to medications (Calzone, Jenkins, Nicoli, et al., 2013; McCarthy, McLeod, & Ginsburg, 2013).

Since the human genome was sequenced, there has been a gradual shift from genetics to genomics. Genetics refers to the study of a particular gene, whereas genomics refers to the study of the entire genome. Genes are the basic physical units of inheritance that are passed from parents to offspring and contain the information needed to specify traits. The genome is the entire set of genetic instructions found in a cell. For these and other definitions of genetic terms, check out the *Talking Glossary of Genetic Terms* (www.genome.gov/Glossary).

With growing public interest in *personalized genomic information* (information about much or all of an individual's genome), increasing development of practice guidelines, mounting commercial pressures, and ever-increasing opportunities for individuals, families, and communities to participate in the direction and design of their genomic health care, genetic services are rapidly becoming an integral part of routine health care (Manolio, Chisholm, Ozenberger, et al., 2013). Moreover, many individuals and families have participated in *direct-to-consumer genetic testing* (testing marketed directly to consumers through television, print advertisements, and websites). Although much of the information provided by direct-to-consumer testing companies is recreational (ancestry information, information about types of ear wax, and bitter taste perception), some of the information provided is health related and could be interpreted as diagnostic. Because of this, direct-to-consumer testing that is provided without the involvement of competent health care professionals may be not only unhelpful, but also harmful (Beery, 2013). However, recently it has been reported that more negotiation is occurring between direct-to-consumer testing and the FDA to create regulations (Gever, 2015).

More recently, attention has turned toward "precision medicine" or "personalized medicine," which emphasizes a focus away from the notion that "one size fits all" and toward the understanding that each individual's uniqueness influences how best to determine medical treatment (US Food and Drug Administration [FDA], 2016). Personalized medicine holds promise for tailored treatments for individuals based on their own personal makeup.

Epigenetics is another more recent concept. Epigenetics refers to the variations in phenotype that occur due to the influence of the environment and our lifestyle on genetics. Moore (2015) has written eloquently on this new concept that he believes is key to understanding an individual's development as a unique human being.

Genetic disorders affect people of all ages, from all socioeconomic levels, and from all racial and ethnic backgrounds. Genetic disorders affect not only individuals but also families, communities, and society. Advances in genetic testing and genetically based treatments have altered the care provided to affected individuals. Improvements in diagnostic capability have resulted in earlier diagnosis and enabled individuals who previously would have died in childhood to survive into adulthood. However, for most genetic conditions, therapeutic or preventive measures do not exist or are very limited. Consequently, the most useful means of reducing the incidence of these disorders is by preventing their transmission. It is standard practice to assess all pregnant women for heritable disorders to identify potential problems.

NURSING EXPERTISE IN GENETICS AND GENOMICS

Because of their front-line position in the health care system and their long-standing history of providing holistic family-centered care, nurses are likely to be one of the first health care professionals to whom individuals and families turn with questions about genetic risk and susceptibility and to seek guidance regarding the complexities of genetic testing and interpretation. Nowhere is this more apparent than in maternity and women's health care. A growing number of maternity and women's health nurses provide information about the availability of genetic tests, answer questions about them, and order and interpret genetic tests. Although most of these tests are used to determine a patient's risk for having a child affected by a genetic condition such as Down syndrome

(DS), cystic fibrosis (CF), or sickle cell disease, the number of genetic tests used to determine the presence of, or susceptibility to, adult-onset disorders (e.g., hereditary colorectal cancer, hereditary breast and ovarian cancer, and Huntington's disease [HD]) continues to rise. Additionally, nurses working in maternity and women's health are caring for an increasing number of individuals and families who are dealing with complex ethical, legal, and social issues associated with genetic testing and the experience of living with someone who has a genetic condition (Wilke, Gallo, Yao, et al., 2013).

Essential Competencies in Genetics and Genomics for All Nurses

Nearly 50 organizations, including the Association of Women's Health, Obstetric and Neonatal Nurses (AWHONN) and the National Association of Neonatal Nurses (NANN), have endorsed the *Essential Nursing Competencies and Curricula Guidelines for Genetics and Genomics* (www.genome.gov/17517146). According to these guidelines, which were developed by an independent panel of nurse leaders (consensus panel) from clinical, research, and academic settings and published by the American Nurses Association and the National Human Genome Research Institute (NHGRI) of the National Institutes of Health (NIH) (Greco, Tinley, & Seibert, 2011), all nurses need to have minimal competencies in genetics and genomics regardless of their academic preparation, practice setting, or specialty. Some of the competencies most relevant to nurses in the area of maternity and women's health include the following:

- Construct a pedigree from collected family history information using standardized symbols and terminology
- Develop a plan of care that incorporates genetic and genomic assessment information
- Recognize when one's own attitudes and values related to genetics and genomic science may affect care provided to patients
- Provide patients with credible, accurate, appropriate, and current genetic and genomic information, resources, services, and/or technologies that facilitate decision making
- Demonstrate in practice the importance of tailoring genetic and genomic information and services to patients based on their culture, religion, knowledge level, literacy, and preferred language
- Assess patients' knowledge, perceptions, and responses to genetic and genomic information
- Facilitate referrals for specialized genetic and genomic services for patients as needed

Expanded Roles for Maternity and Women's Health Nurses

Expanded roles for nurses with expertise in genetics and genomics are developing in many areas of maternity and women's health nursing. These areas include but are not limited to prenatal screening and testing; carrier testing during pregnancy; newborn screening; palliative care for infants with life-threatening genetic conditions and their families; the identification and care of individuals with genetic conditions and their families; and the care of women with genetic conditions who require specialized care during pregnancy, such as women with neuromuscular disease, CF, and factor V Leiden deficiency (DeLuca, Zanni, Bonhomme, et al., 2013; Frazer, Porter, & Gross, 2013; Johnson, Giarelli, Lewis, et al., 2013; Prows, Hopkin, Barnoy, et al., 2013; Wilke et al., 2013). As an example, the Oncology Nursing Society (ONS) (www.ons.org) has taken an active role in providing oncology nurses with the education and resources they need to integrate genetics and genomics into all phases of care for individuals and families affected by cancer, including information specifically related to cancers affecting women.

HUMAN GENOME PROJECT AND IMPLICATIONS FOR CLINICAL PRACTICE

The Human Genome Project was a publicly funded international effort coordinated by the NIH and the US Department of Energy (www.doegenomes.org). When the Human Genome Project was initiated in 1990, the ultimate goal of the project was to map the human genome (the complete set of genetic instructions in the nucleus of each human cell) by 2005. Considering that the human genome consists of approximately 3 billion base pairs of DNA, many people regarded this as an impossible task. However, by 2003 a substantially complete version of the human genome was announced.

The Human Genome Project found that all human beings are 99.9% identical at the DNA level (NHGRI, 2016). This finding that human beings are 99.9% identical at the DNA level should help discourage the use of science as a justification for drawing precise racial boundaries around certain groups of people. A more recent effort by the NHGRI called the **Enc**yclopedia **o**f **D**NA **E**lements, or the ENCODE Project, was organized to identify the genome's functional elements (ENCODE, 2016). Researchers found that more than 80% of the human genome is linked to a specific biologic function, and that proteins interact with DNA in more than 4 million regulatory regions. This finding made clearer the active genome in which genes are turned on and off by proteins using sites that may be at a great distance from the genes. Identification of regulatory regions will help explain varied functions of different types of cells. (www.genome.gov/pfv.cfm?pageID=27549810).

IMPORTANCE OF FAMILY HISTORY

Completion of the Human Genome Project and the resultant identification of the inherited causes for many diseases has resulted in renewed interest in family history. Although it is easy to be impressed by the more than 3600 genetic tests currently available through the Genetic Testing Registry (GTR), which can be accessed at its website (www.ncbi.nlm.nih.gov/gtr), family history will most likely continue to be the single most cost-effective piece of genetic information. In 2008, Solomon, Jack, and Feero described a complete three-generation family history that includes ancestry information concerning both sides of family as the best genetic "test" applicable to preconception care. When nurses and other clinicians conduct a family history, they can gain not only valuable information about the structure of the family and diseases that affect various individuals in the family, but also a rich understanding of family relationships, social context, occupations, lifestyle, and health habits (American College of Obstetricians and Gynecologists [ACOG], 2011a). The process of collecting this information often facilitates the development of a relationship between the patient/family and the clinician. In 2004, the US Department of Health and Human Services launched the Family History Initiative by designating Thanksgiving Day as National Family History Day. The US Surgeon General encouraged families to use their family gatherings as a time to talk about and collect important family health history. A number of family history tools are available free of charge online. One of the most widely used family history tools is the My Family Health Portrait (https://familyhistory.hhs.gov). Another helpful tool is the family health history tool, *Does it run in the family?* that was developed by the Genetic Alliance (www.doesitruninthefamily.org). The Centers for Disease Control and Prevention (CDC) also provides links to family history resources (https://www.cdc.gov/genomics/famhistory/index.htm).

The preconception period is an ideal time to review family history and provide personalized recommendations based on family history

(ACOG, 2011a). It is also one of the best times to counsel couples about carrier testing options that are based on known population-specific risks (Bodurtha & Strauss, 2012). Finally, the preconception period is an optimal time to refer couples, when appropriate, to specialists in high-risk pregnancy and genetics.

GENE IDENTIFICATION AND TESTING

Initial efforts to sequence and analyze the human genome have proven invaluable in the identification of genes involved in disease and in the development of genetic tests. In an effort to bridge the transition from discovery to diagnostics and treatments, the NIH launched the Genetic Testing Registry (GTR) in 2012. The GTR (www.ncbi.nlm.nih.gov/gtr) is a free online tool that can be used to obtain a list of available genetic tests. The GTR website also includes links to other resources such as *GeneReviews* and Online Mendelian Inheritance in Man (OMIM). *GeneReviews* is a collection of expert-authored, peer-reviewed disease descriptions presented in a standardized format and focused on clinically relevant and medically actionable information on the diagnosis, management, and genetic counseling of individuals and families with specific inherited conditions. OMIM is an online catalog of human genes and genetic disorders.

Genetic testing involves the analysis of human DNA, **ribonucleic acid (RNA)**, which has a major role in protein synthesis, chromosomes (threadlike packages of genes and other DNA in the nucleus of a cell), or proteins to detect abnormalities related to an inherited condition. Genetic tests can be used to directly examine the DNA and RNA that make up a gene (direct or molecular testing), look at markers that are coinherited with a gene that causes a genetic condition (linkage analysis), examine the protein products of genes (biochemical testing), or examine chromosomes (cytogenetic testing). Cytogenetic analysis of malignant tissue has become a mainstay of oncology.

Most of the genetic tests now offered in clinical practice are tests for single-gene disorders in patients with clinical symptoms or who have a family history of a genetic disease (http://iml.dartmouth.edu/education/cme/Genetics). Some of these genetic tests are prenatal tests or tests used to identify the genetic status of a pregnancy at risk for a genetic condition. Current prenatal testing options include maternal serum screening (a blood test used to see if a pregnant woman is at increased risk for carrying a fetus with a neural tube defect or a chromosomal abnormality such as DS, trisomy 18, or trisomy 13), fetal ultrasound or sonogram (an imaging technique using high-frequency sound waves to produce images of the fetus inside the uterus), invasive procedures (chorionic villus sampling and amniocentesis), and noninvasive prenatal testing for fetal aneuploidy (a blood test that uses cell-free DNA from the plasma of pregnant women to screen for DS and, in some cases, trisomy 13 and trisomy 18 (see Chapter 10 for more in-depth information).

Another type of genetic test is the **carrier** screening test used to identify individuals who have a gene mutation for a genetic condition but do not show symptoms of the condition because it is an autosomal recessive condition (e.g., CF, sickle cell disease, and Tay-Sachs disease). A third type of genetic testing is **predictive testing**, which is used to clarify the genetic status of asymptomatic family members. The two types of predictive testing are presymptomatic and predispositional. Mutation analysis for Huntington disease (HD), a neurodegenerative disorder, is an example of **presymptomatic testing**. If the gene mutation for HD is present, symptoms of HD are certain to appear if the individual lives long enough. Testing for a *BRCA1* gene mutation to determine breast cancer susceptibility is an example of predispositional testing. **Predispositional testing** differs from presymptomatic testing in that a positive result (indicating that a *BRCA1* mutation is present) does not indicate a 100% risk for developing the condition (breast cancer).

In addition to using genetic tests to test for single-gene disorders in patients with clinical symptoms or who have a family history of a genetic disease, genetic tests are used for population-based screening. For example, each year in the United States, approximately 4 million infants undergo newborn screening (Bodurtha & Strauss, 2012). Newborn screening is a mandatory, state-supported public health program. Initially, newborn screening in the United States was only concerned with a few conditions such as phenylketonuria (PKU). However, with the advent of tandem mass spectrometry, the number of conditions included in newborn screening grew rapidly (DeLuca et al., 2013). Currently, most states test newborns for 31 core disorders and 26 secondary disorders (McCarthy et al., 2013). A complete list of conditions tested for in each state is available on the National Newborn Screening and Genetics Resource website (http://genes-r-us.uthscsa.edu). (See Chapter 23.)

Another type of population-based screening is carrier screening for single-gene disorders such as CF, sickle cell disease, and Tay-Sachs disease either preconceptionally or prenatally. In 2001, ACOG and the American College of Medical Genetics (ACMG) recommended that clinicians offer carrier screening for CF to individuals with a family history of CF, reproductive partners of individuals who have CF, and couples in whom one or both partners are Caucasian and are planning a pregnancy or seeking prenatal care. Ten years later, in 2011, ACOG updated its recommendations and emphasized that it is not a straightforward or easy task to assign an ethnicity to a person and, therefore, the recommendation was updated to offer to screen all women of reproductive age to determine if they are carriers of CF (ACOG, 2011b). Recommendations for newborn screening for CF appeared in 2004, and soon after this many newborn screening programs in the United States began offering newborn screening for CF. One outcome of this broader carrier and newborn screening for CF is that more and more individuals are being informed they have a CF mutation. However, the correlation between genotype (an individual's collection of genes) and phenotype (an individual's observable traits) is poor for many of the more than 1900 CF mutations identified to date. That is, whereas some CF mutations are associated with significant health problems (poor growth, greasy stools, and chronic respiratory problems), others are not. Because of this, the significance of many CF mutations is uncertain. As a result, nurses and other health care professionals are increasingly being asked to communicate results with uncertain significance to individuals and families during the preconception, prenatal, and newborn periods. A coherent and systematic approach is needed for the introduction of new tests into population-based screening programs.

The use of genome sequencing (e.g., whole-genome sequencing and next-generation sequencing) has entered the clinical setting (Conley, Biesecker, Gonsalves, et al., 2013; McCarthy et al., 2013; Wade, Tarini, & Wilfond, 2013). It is difficult to determine the cost for sequencing a particular genome as there are many factors to consider (National Human Genome Research Institute, 2016).

PHARMACOGENOMICS

One of the most promising clinical applications of the Human Genome Project has been pharmacogenomic testing (the use of genetic information to guide a patient's drug therapy). Associations between genetic variation and drug effect have been observed for a number of commonly used drugs, including warfarin, an anticoagulant commonly used to reduce the risk for thromboembolic events in patients with a history of deep vein thrombosis, pulmonary embolism, myocardial infarction, or atrial fibrillation (McCarthy et al., 2013). Warfarin is a drug with a narrow therapeutic index; it can result in serious bleeding with supratherapeutic doses and thromboembolic events with subtherapeutic doses. Because of this and the fact that there is a great deal of interpatient and intrapatient dose variation, warfarin is one of the most common causes of serious adverse drug reactions. There is mounting evidence that genotype-guided warfarin dosing may not only help reduce the serious adverse drug reactions commonly associated with its use, but also increase dosing accuracy, shorten the time to dose stabilization, and help identify individuals who may require more frequent monitoring. In August 2007, the FDA approved updated labeling for warfarin. The updated labeling acknowledges that individuals with variations in their *CYP2C9* and *VKORC1* genes may require a lower initial dose of warfarin. However, there are not enough clinical data yet to recommend that this type of testing be mandatory, but there are some FDA-approved drugs with pharmacogenomic labeling (US Department of Health and Human Services, 2016).

Pharmacogenomic testing can also be used to target therapies. Trastuzumab (Herceptin), a monoclonal antibody that specifically targets HER2/neu overexpressing breast tumors, is an example of a drug for which an obligatory genetic test has been developed (McCarthy et al., 2013). The purpose of this obligatory genetic test is to identify the subset of women with breast cancer who overexpress HER2/neu. Women who overexpress HER2/neu are most likely the only breast cancer patients who will benefit from taking trastuzumab (www.herceptin .com/index.jsp).

GENE THERAPY

The aim of gene therapy is to correct defective genes that are responsible for disease development. Generally, gene therapy involves inserting a healthy copy of the defective gene into the somatic cells (any cell of the body except sperm and egg cells) of the affected individual. Although the early optimism about gene therapy was probably never fully justified, gene therapy has now moved from preclinical to clinical studies for many diseases. These diseases range from hemophilia and other single-gene disorders to complex disorders such as cancer, HIV, and cardiovascular disorders. Major challenges to gene therapy include determining how to target the right gene to the right location in the right cells, expressing the transferred gene at the right time, and minimizing adverse reactions.

ETHICAL, LEGAL, AND SOCIAL IMPLICATIONS

Because of widespread concern about misuse of the information gained through genetics research, a percentage of the Human Genome Project budget was designated for the study of the ethical, legal, and social implications (ELSI) of human genome research (Genetics Home Reference, 2017a). Two large ELSI programs were created to identify, analyze, and address the ELSIs of human genome research at the same time that the basic science issues were being studied. During the past decade, issues of high priority for these programs were as follows:

- Privacy and fairness in the use and interpretation of genetic information
- Clinical integration of new genetics technologies
- Issues surrounding genetics research, such as possible discrimination and stigmatization
- Education for professionals and the general public about genetics, genetics health care, and ELSI of human genome research

Both ELSI programs have excellent websites that include much educational information, as well as links to other informative sites (www.genome.gov/10001618; www.ornl.gov/sci/techresources/Human _Genome/elsi/elsi.shtml; https://www.genome.gov/elsi/). The major risk associated with genetic testing concerns what happens with the information gained through testing. It may result in increased anxiety and altered family relationships; it may be difficult to keep confidential; and it may result in discrimination and stigmatization. More important, there is a large gap between the ability to test for a genetic condition and the ability to treat that same condition. Informed consent is difficult to ensure when some of the outcomes, benefits, and risks of genetic testing remain unknown.

FACTORS INFLUENCING THE DECISION TO UNDERGO GENETIC TESTING

The decision to undergo genetic testing is seldom autonomous and based solely on the needs and preferences of the individual being tested. Instead, it is often a decision based on feelings of responsibility and commitment to others. For example, a woman who is receiving treatment for breast cancer may undergo *BRCA1/BRCA2* mutation testing not because she wants to find out if she carries a *BRCA1* or *BRCA2* mutation but, instead, because her two unaffected sisters have asked her to be tested and she feels a sense of responsibility and commitment to them. A female airline pilot with a family history of HD, who has no desire to find out if she has the gene mutation associated with HD, may undergo mutation analysis for HD because she feels she has an obligation to her family, her employer, and the people who fly with her.

Decisions about genetic testing are shaped and, in many instances, constrained by factors such as social norms where care is received and socioeconomic status. Most pregnant women in the United States now have at least one ultrasound examination, many undergo some type of multiple-marker screening, and a growing number undergo other types of prenatal testing (see Chapter 8). The range of prenatal testing options available to a pregnant woman and her family may vary, based on where the pregnant woman receives prenatal care and her socioeconomic status. Certain types of prenatal testing may not be available in smaller communities and rural settings (e.g., chorionic villus sampling and fluorescent in situ hybridization [FISH] analysis). In addition, certain types of genetic testing may not be offered in conservative medical communities (e.g., preimplantation diagnosis). Some types of genetic testing are expensive and typically not covered by health insurance. Because of this, these tests may be available only to a relatively small number of individuals and families—those who can afford to pay for them (Badzek, Henaghan, Turner, et al., 2013). (See Chapter 10 for more information on prenatal testing).

Cultural and ethnic differences also have a significant impact on decisions about genetic testing. When prenatal diagnosis was first introduced, the principal constituency was a self-selected group of Caucasian, well-informed, middle- to upper-class women. Today the widespread use of genetic testing has introduced prenatal testing to new groups of women, women who had not previously considered genetic services. The fact that many of the women currently undergoing prenatal testing may not share mainstream US views about the role of medicine and prenatal care, the meaning of *disability*, or how to respond to scientific risks and uncertainties, further amplifies the complexity of ethical issues associated with prenatal testing.

CLINICAL GENETICS

Genetic Transmission

Human development is a complicated process that depends on the systematic unraveling of instructions found in the genetic material of the egg and the sperm. Development from conception to birth of a normal, healthy baby occurs without incident in most cases; occasionally, however, some anomaly in the genetic code of the embryo creates a birth defect or disorder.

Genes and Chromosomes

The hereditary material carried in the nucleus of each of the somatic cells determines an individual's characteristics. This material, called *DNA* (deoxyribonucleic acid), forms threadlike strands known as *chromosomes*. Each chromosome is composed of many smaller segments of DNA referred to as *genes*. Genes or combinations of genes contain coded information that determines an individual's unique characteristics. The code is found in the specific linear order of the molecules that combine to form the strands of DNA. Genes control both the types of proteins that are made and the rate at which they are produced. Genes never act in isolation; they always interact with other genes and the environment.

All normal human somatic cells contain 46 chromosomes arranged as 23 pairs of homologous (matched) chromosomes; one chromosome of each pair is inherited from each parent. There are 22 pairs of *autosomes,* which control most traits in the body, and one pair of sex chromosomes. The larger female chromosome is called the *X;* the smaller male chromosome is the *Y.* Whereas the Y chromosome is primarily concerned with sex determination, the X chromosome contains genes that are involved in much more than sex determination. Generally, the presence of a Y chromosome causes an embryo to develop as a male; in the absence of a Y chromosome, the individual develops as a female. Thus in a normal female, the homologous pair of sex chromosomes are XX, and in a normal male, the homologous pair are XY.

Homologous chromosomes (except the X and Y chromosomes in males) have the same number and arrangement of genes. In other words, if one chromosome has a gene for hair color, its partner chromosome also will have a gene for hair color and these hair-color genes will have the same loci or be located in the same place on the two chromosomes. Although both genes code for hair color, they may not code for the same hair color. Genes at corresponding loci on homologous chromosomes that code for different forms or variations of the same trait are called alleles. An individual having two copies of the same allele for a given trait is said to be homozygous for that trait. With two different alleles, the individual is heterozygous for the trait.

The term genotype typically is used to refer to the genetic makeup of an individual when discussing a specific gene pair, but at times, genotype is used to refer to an individual's entire genetic makeup or all the genes that the individual can pass on to future generations. Phenotype refers to the observable expression of an individual's genotype, such as physical features, a biochemical or molecular trait, and even a psychologic trait. A trait or disorder is considered *dominant* if it is expressed or phenotypically apparent when only one copy of the gene is present. It is considered *recessive* if it is expressed only when two copies of the alleles associated with the trait are present.

As more is learned about genetics and genomics, the concepts of dominance and recessivity have become more complex, especially in X-linked disorders. For example, traits considered to be recessive may be expressed even when only one copy of a gene located on the X chromosome is present. This occurs frequently in males because males have only one X chromosome; thus they have only one copy of the genes located on the X chromosome. Whichever gene is present on the one X chromosome determines which trait is expressed. Females, conversely, have two X chromosomes, so they have two copies of the genes located on the X chromosome. However, in any female somatic cell, only one X chromosome is functioning (otherwise there would be inequality in gene dosage between males and females). This process, known as *X-inactivation* or the *Lyon hypothesis,* is generally a random occurrence. That is, there is a 50-50 chance as to whether the maternal X or the paternal X is inactivated. Occasionally the percentage of cells that have the X with an abnormal or mutant gene is very high. This helps explain why hemophilia, an X-linked recessive disorder, can clinically manifest itself in a female known to be a heterozygous carrier (a female who has only one copy of the gene mutation). It also helps explain why traditional methods of carrier detection are less effective for X-linked recessive disorders; the possible range for enzyme activity values can vary greatly, depending on which X chromosome is inactivated.

CHROMOSOMAL ABNORMALITIES

Chromosomal abnormalities are a major cause of reproductive loss, congenital problems, and gynecologic disorders. Errors resulting in chromosomal abnormalities can occur in mitosis (cell division occurring in somatic cells that results in two identical daughter cells containing a diploid number of chromosomes) or meiosis (division of a sex cell into two and four haploid cells). These errors can occur in either the autosomes or the sex chromosomes. Even without the presence of obvious structural malformations, small deviations in chromosomes can cause problems in fetal development.

The pictorial analysis of the number, form, and size of an individual's chromosomes is known as a karyotype. Cells from any nucleated, replicating body tissue (not red blood cells, nerves, or muscles) can be used. The most commonly used tissues are white blood cells and fetal cells in amniotic fluid. The cells are grown in a culture and arrested when they are in metaphase (during metaphase, the chromosomes are condensed and visible with a light microscope), and then the cells are dropped onto a slide. This breaks the cell membranes and spreads the chromosomes, making them easier to visualize. Next, the cells are stained with special stains (e.g., Giemsa stain) that create striping or "banding" patterns. These patterns aid in the analysis because they are consistent from person to person. Once the chromosome spreads are photographed or scanned by a computer, they are cut out and arranged in a specific numeric order according to their length and shape. The chromosomes are numbered from largest to smallest, 1 to 22, and the sex chromosomes are designated by the letter *X* or *Y.* Each chromosome is divided into two "arms" designated by *p* (short arm) and *q* (long arm). A female karyotype is designated as 46,XX, and a male karyotype is designated as 46,XY. Fig. 6.1 illustrates the chromosomes in a body cell and a karyotype.

Autosomal Abnormalities

Autosomal abnormalities involve differences in the number or structure of autosome chromosomes (pairs 1 to 22). They result from unequal distribution of the genetic material during gamete (egg and sperm) formation.

Abnormalities of Chromosome Number

A euploid cell is a cell with the correct or normal number of chromosomes within the cell. Because most gametes are haploid (1N, 23 chromosomes) and most somatic cells are diploid (2N, 46 chromosomes), they are both considered euploid cells. Deviations from the correct number of chromosomes per cell can be one of two types: (1) polyploidy, in which the deviation is an exact multiple of the haploid number of chromosomes or one chromosome set (23 chromosomes); or (2) aneuploidy, in which the numeric deviation is not an exact multiple of the haploid set. A triploid (3N) cell is an example of a polyploidy. It has 69 chromosomes. A tetraploid (4N) cell, also an example of a polyploidy, has 92 chromosomes.

Aneuploidy is the most commonly identified chromosome abnormality in humans and the leading genetic cause of intellectual disability.

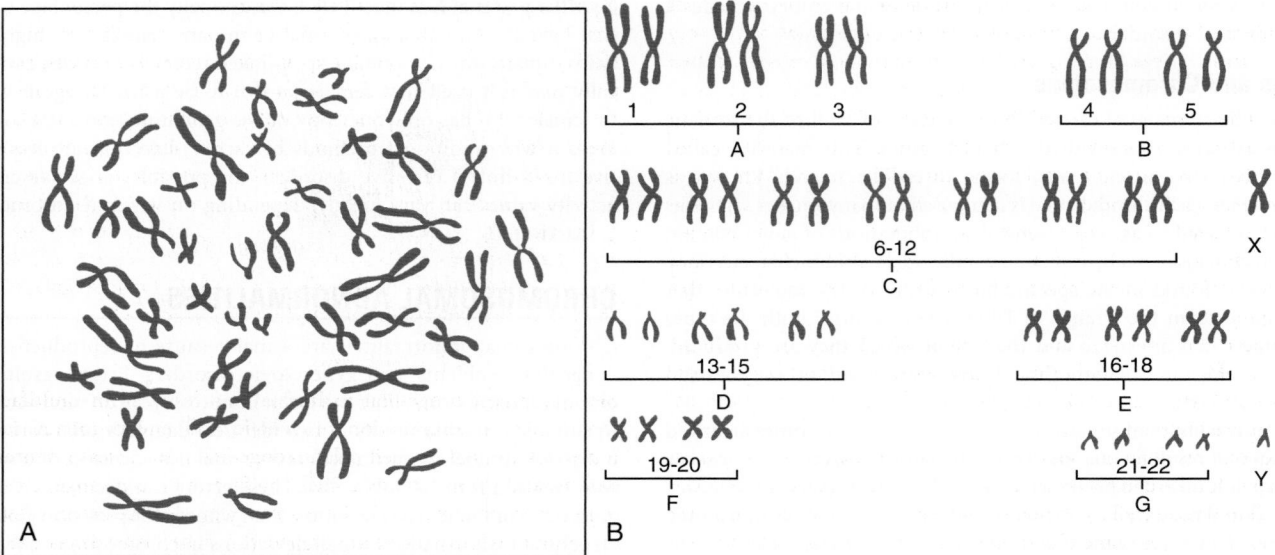

FIG 6.1 Chromosomes during cell division. **A,** Example of a photomicrograph. **B,** Chromosomes arranged in karyotype; female and male sex-determining chromosomes.

A monosomy is the product of the union between a normal gamete and a gamete that is missing a chromosome. Monosomic individuals have only 45 chromosomes in each of their cells. The product of the union of a normal gamete with a gamete containing an extra chromosome is a trisomy. The most common autosomal aneuploid conditions involve trisomies. Trisomic individuals have 47 chromosomes in most or all of their cells.

The vast majority of trisomies occur during oogenesis (the process by which a premeiotic female germ cell divides into a mature egg); the incidence of these types of chromosomal errors increases exponentially with advancing maternal age. Although variation exists among trisomies with regard to the parent and stage of origin of the extra chromosome, most trisomies are maternal meiosis I (MI) errors. This means that most trisomies are caused by nondisjunction during the first meiotic division. The first meiotic division involves the segregation of homologous or similar chromosomes. One pair of chromosomes fails to separate. One resulting cell contains both chromosomes, and the other contains none. The fact that most trisomies are maternal MI errors is not that surprising, because maternal MI occurs over a long time span. It is initiated in precursor cells during fetal development, but it is not completed until the time those cells undergo ovulation after menarche.

The most common trisomy abnormality is DS. Approximately 1 in every 691 newborns has DS; there are over 400,000 individuals with DS living in the United States (Prows et al., 2013; CDC, 2016; www.cdc .gov/ncbddd/birthdefects/DownSyndrome.html; http://ndsccenter.org; www.ndss.org). Ninety-five percent of individuals with DS have trisomy 21 (nondisjunction) or an extra chromosome 21 (47,XX+21, female with DS; or 47,XY+21, male with DS) (CDC, 2016). Another type of DS, translocation, occurs when extra chromosome 21 material is present in every cell of the individual but it is attached to another chromosome. In the third type of DS, mosaicism, extra chromosome 21 material is found in some but not all of the cells.

Although the risk for having a child with DS increases with maternal age (incidence is approximately 1 in 1200 for a 25-year-old woman; 1 in 350 for a 35-year-old woman; and 1 in 10 for a 49-year-old woman), children with DS can be born to mothers of any age. The risk for a mother over age 40 of having a second child with DS is about 1% (Sole-Smith, 2014).

Other autosomal trisomies that maternity nurses might see are trisomy 18 (Edwards syndrome) and trisomy 13 (Patau syndrome). Trisomy 18 is more common than trisomy 13; it occurs in about 1 of 5000 live births versus 1 of 16,000 live births for trisomy 13 (Genetics Home Reference, 2017b). Infants with trisomy 18 and trisomy 13 usually have severe to profound intellectual disabilities. Although both conditions have a poor prognosis, with the vast majority of affected infants dying before they reach their first birthday, a growing number of infants with these trisomies are living longer, and a small number are actually living into their 40s and 50s.

Nondisjunction can also occur during mitosis. If this occurs early in development, when cell lines are forming, the individual has a mixture of cells, some with a normal number of chromosomes and others either missing a chromosome or containing an extra chromosome. This condition is known as *mosaicism*. The most common form of mosaicism in autosomes is mosaic DS.

Abnormalities of Chromosome Structure

Structural abnormalities can occur in any chromosome. Types of structural abnormalities include translocation, duplication, deletion, microdeletion, and inversion. Translocation results when there is an exchange of chromosomal material between two chromosomes. Exposure to certain drugs, viruses, and radiation can cause translocations, but often they arise for no apparent reason.

The two major types of translocation are reciprocal and robertsonian. Reciprocal translocations are the most common. In a reciprocal translocation, either the parts of the two chromosomes are exchanged equally (balanced translocation) or a part of a chromosome is transferred to a different chromosome, creating an unbalanced translocation because there is extra chromosomal material—extra of one chromosome but correct amount or deficient amount of the other chromosome. In a balanced translocation, the individual is phenotypically normal because there is no extra chromosome material; it is just rearranged. In an unbalanced translocation, the individual will be both genotypically and phenotypically abnormal.

In a robertsonian translocation, the short arms (p arms) of two different acrocentric chromosomes (chromosomes with very short p arms) break, leaving sticky ends that then cause the two long arms (q arms) to stick together. This forms a new, large chromosome that is made of the two long arms. The individual with a balanced robertsonian translocation has 45 chromosomes. Because the short arm of acrocentric chromosomes contains genes for ribosomal RNA and these genes are represented elsewhere, the individual usually does not show any symptoms. The individual may produce an unbalanced gamete (sperm or egg with too many or two few genes). This can lead to reproductive difficulties such as miscarriages or birth defects.

In duplication, there is an extra chromosomal segment within the same homologous or another nonhomologous chromosome. Clinical findings are highly variable and depend on which of the chromosomal segments are involved.

Deletions result in the loss of chromosomal material and partial monosomy for the chromosome involved. Microdeletions are deletions too small to be detected by standard cytogenetic techniques. Whenever a portion of a chromosome is deleted from one chromosome and added to another, the gamete produced may have either extra copies of genes or too few copies. The clinical effects produced may be mild or severe depending on the amount of genetic material involved. Two of the more common conditions are the deletion of the short arm of chromosome 5 (cri du chat syndrome) and the deletion of the long arm of chromosome 18.

Inversions are deviations in which a portion of the chromosome has been rearranged in reverse order. Few birth defects have been attributed to the presence of inversions, but it is suspected that inversions may be responsible for problems with infertility and miscarriages.

Sex Chromosome Abnormalities

Several sex chromosome abnormalities are caused by nondisjunction during gametogenesis in either parent. The most common deviation in females is *Turner syndrome,* or monosomy X (45,X). The affected female exhibits juvenile external genitalia with undeveloped ovaries. She is short in stature and often has webbing of the neck, a low hairline in the back, low-set ears, and lymphedema of her hands and feet. Intelligence may be impaired. Most affected embryos miscarry spontaneously. In most cases of Turner syndrome, it is the paternal X or Y that is lost. Turner syndrome is a common cause of infertility (Genetics Home Reference, 2017c).

The most common deviation in males is *Klinefelter syndrome,* or trisomy XXY. The affected male has poorly developed secondary sexual characteristics and small testes. He is infertile, usually tall, and effeminate and may be slow to learn. Males who have mosaic Klinefelter syndrome may be fertile.

PATTERNS OF GENETIC TRANSMISSION

Heritable characteristics are those that can be passed on to offspring. The patterns by which genetic material is transmitted to the next generation are affected by the number of genes involved in the expression of the trait. Many phenotypic characteristics result from two or more genes on different chromosomes acting together (referred to as *multifactorial inheritance*); others are controlled by a single gene (*unifactorial inheritance*). Specialists in genetics (e.g., geneticists, genetic counselors, and nurses with advanced expertise in genetics) predict the probability of the presence of an abnormal gene from the known occurrence of the trait in the individual's family and the known patterns by which the trait is inherited.

Multifactorial Inheritance

Most common congenital malformations result from multifactorial inheritance, a combination of genetic and environmental factors. Examples are cleft lip, cleft palate, congenital heart disease, neural tube defects, and pyloric stenosis. Each malformation can range from mild to severe, depending on the number of genes for the defect present or the amount of environmental influence. A neural tube defect can range from spina bifida (a bony defect in the lumbar region of the vertebrae with little or no neurologic impairment) to anencephaly (absence of brain development, which is always fatal). Some malformations occur more often in one sex. For example, pyloric stenosis and cleft lip are more common in males, and cleft palate is more common in females.

Unifactorial Inheritance

If a single gene controls a particular trait or disorder, its pattern of inheritance is referred to as *unifactorial mendelian* or *single-gene inheritance*. The number of single-gene disorders far exceeds the number of chromosomal abnormalities. Potential patterns of inheritance for single-gene disorders include autosomal dominant, autosomal recessive, and X-linked dominant and recessive modes of inheritance (Fig. 6.2).

Autosomal Dominant Inheritance

Autosomal dominant inheritance disorders are those in which only one copy of a variant allele is needed for phenotypic expression. The variant allele may be a result of a mutation—a spontaneous and permanent change in the normal gene structure in which case the disorder occurs for the first time in the family. Usually an affected individual comes from multiple generations having the disorder. An affected parent who is heterozygous for the trait has a 50% chance of passing the variant allele to each offspring (see Fig. 6.2, *B* and *C*). There is a vertical pattern of inheritance (i.e., there is no skipping of generations; if an individual has an autosomal dominant disorder such as HD, so must one of his or her parents). Males and females are equally affected.

Autosomal dominant disorders are not always expressed with the same severity of symptoms. For example, a woman who has an autosomal

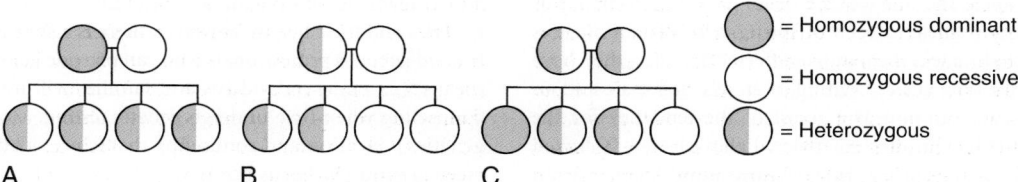

FIG 6.2 Possible offspring in three types of matings. **A,** Homozygous-dominant parent and homozygous-recessive parent. Children: all heterozygous, displaying dominant trait. **B,** Heterozygous parent and homozygous-recessive parent. Children: 50% heterozygous, displaying dominant trait; 50% homozygous, displaying recessive trait. **C,** Both parents heterozygous. Children: 25% homozygous, displaying dominant trait; 25% homozygous, displaying recessive trait; 50% heterozygous, displaying dominant trait.

dominant disorder may show few symptoms and may not become aware of her diagnosis until after she gives birth to a severely affected child. Predicting whether an offspring will have a minor or severe abnormality is not possible. Sometimes an individual can acquire a de novo mutation (new mutation that spontaneously occurred in a gene carried by an individual germ cell) that can result in an autosomal dominant disorder (Prows et al., 2013). Examples of autosomal dominant disorders are HD, Marfan syndrome, neurofibromatosis, myotonic dystrophy, Stickler syndrome, Treacher Collins syndrome, and achondroplasia (dwarfism).

Autosomal Recessive Inheritance

Autosomal recessive inheritance disorders are those in which both genes of a pair associated with the disorder must be abnormal for the disorder to be expressed. Heterozygous individuals have only one variant allele and are unaffected clinically because their normal gene overshadows the variant allele. They are known as *carriers* of the recessive trait. Because these recessive traits are inherited by generations of the same family, an increased incidence of the disorder occurs in consanguineous matings (closely related parents). For the trait to be expressed, two carriers must each contribute a variant allele to the offspring (see Fig. 6.2, *C*). The chance of the trait occurring in each child is 25%. A clinically normal offspring may be a carrier of the gene. Autosomal recessive disorders have a horizontal pattern of inheritance rather than the vertical pattern seen with autosomal dominant disorders. That is, autosomal recessive disorders are usually observed in one or more siblings but not in earlier generations. Males and females are equally affected.

Inborn Errors of Metabolism

More than 350 *inborn errors of metabolism* have been recognized. Most inborn errors of metabolism (IEMs), such as phenylketonuria, galactosemia, maple syrup urine disease, Tay-Sachs disease, sickle cell anemia, and CF, are autosomal recessive inherited disorders. IEMs occur when a gene mutation reduces the efficiency of encoded enzymes to a level at which normal metabolism cannot occur. Defective enzyme action interrupts the normal series of chemical reactions from the affected point onward. The result may be an accumulation of a damaging product, such as phenylalanine in PKU, or the absence of a necessary product, such as the lack of melanin in albinism caused by lack of tyrosinase. Diagnostic and carrier testing is available for a growing number of IEMs. In addition, many states in the United States have started screening for specific IEMs as part of their expanded newborn screening programs using tandem mass spectrometry. However, many of the deaths caused by IEMs are the result of enzyme variants not currently screened for in many of the newborn screening programs. (See discussion of IEMs in Chapter 25.)

X-Linked Dominant Inheritance

X-linked dominant inheritance disorders occur in males and heterozygous females, but because of X inactivation, affected females are usually less severely affected than affected males and they are more likely to transmit the variant allele to their offspring. Heterozygous females (females who have one wild-type allele and one variant allele) have a 50% chance of transmitting the variant allele to each offspring. The variant allele is often lethal in affected males since, unlike affected females, they have no normal gene (wild-type allele). Mating of an affected male and an unaffected female is uncommon as a result of the tendency for the variant allele to be lethal in affected males. Relatively few X-linked dominant disorders have been identified. Two examples are vitamin D–resistant rickets and Rett syndrome.

X-Linked Recessive Inheritance

Abnormal genes for X-linked recessive inheritance disorders are carried on the X chromosome. Females may be heterozygous or homozygous for traits carried on the X chromosome because they have two X chromosomes. Males are hemizygous because they have only one X chromosome, which carries genes with no alleles on the Y chromosome. Therefore X-linked recessive disorders are most commonly manifested in the male with the abnormal gene on his single X chromosome. Hemophilia, color blindness, and Duchenne muscular dystrophy are X-linked recessive disorders.

The male with an X-linked recessive disorder receives the disease-associated allele from his carrier mother on her affected X chromosome. Female carriers (those heterozygous for the trait) have a 50% probability of transmitting the disease-associated allele to each offspring. An affected male can pass the disease-associated allele to his daughters but not to his sons. The daughters will be carriers of the trait if they receive a normal gene on the X chromosome from their mother. They will be affected only if they receive a disease-associated allele on the X chromosome from both their mother and their father.

GENETIC COUNSELING

It is standard practice in obstetrics to determine whether a heritable disorder exists in a couple or in anyone in either of their families. The goal of screening is to detect or define risk for disease in low-risk populations and identify those for whom diagnostic testing may be appropriate. A nurse can obtain a genetics history using a questionnaire or checklist such as the one in Fig. 6.3.

Genetic counseling is a professional service that provides genetics information, education, and support to individuals and families with ongoing or potential genetic health concerns. It is typically provided by a team of genetics specialists that includes clinical geneticists (physicians), medical geneticists, genetics fellows, genetics counselors, and, advanced practice genetics nurse specialists. Cytogeneticists, biochemical geneticists, and molecular geneticists support the clinical genetics team by providing laboratory expertise that helps with the diagnosis and management of individuals and families affected by genetic conditions.

Genetic counseling occurs in regional genetics centers, major medical centers, outreach or satellite genetics clinics, public health clinics, some community hospitals, and now that genetics has entered the mainstream of health care, in a wide variety of other settings. These include but are not limited to managed health care organizations, commercial facilities, and private practices. A number of specialized groups provide genetics education and counseling for individuals and families affected by specific genetic disorders, such as DS, CF, diabetes, muscular dystrophy, HD, and cancer. Genetic counseling also is offered over the Internet.

Individuals and families seek out or are referred for genetic counseling for a wide variety of reasons and at all stages of their lives. Some seek preconception or prenatal information; others are referred after the birth of a child with a birth defect or a suspected genetic condition or after a pregnancy loss. Still others seek information because they have a family history of a genetic condition. Regardless of the setting or the individual's and family's stage of life, genetic counseling should be offered and available to all individuals and families who have questions about genetics and their health. However, there is a shortage of appropriately trained genetics professionals who can provide genetic counseling. This means that many individuals and families will not be offered genetic counseling when they undergo genetic testing. Moreover, some of the genetics education and counseling that is provided will be inadequate (see Community Focus box).

ESTIMATION OF RISK

Most families with a history of genetic disease want an answer to the following question: What is the chance that our future children will

Risk Factors for Genetic Disorders

Answer the following questions about risk factors. If you answer "yes" to any of them, you may be at increased risk for having a baby with a genetic disorder.

_____Will you be age 35 years or older when your baby is due?

_____Will the baby's father be age 50 years or older when your baby is due?

_____If you or the baby's father are of Mediterranean or Asian descent, do either of you or does anyone in your families have thalassemia?

_____Is there a family history of neural tube defects?

_____Have you or the baby's father ever had a child with a neural tube defect?

_____Is there a family history of congenital heart defects?

_____Is there a family history of Down syndrome?

_____Have you or the baby's father ever had a child with Down syndrome?

_____If you or the baby's father are of Eastern European Jewish, French Canadian, or Cajun descent, is there a family history of Tay-Sachs disease?

_____If you or your partner are of Eastern European Jewish descent, is there a family history of Canavan disease or any other genetic disorders?

_____If you or your partner are African-American, is there a family history of sickle cell disease or sickle cell trait?

_____Is there a family history of hemophilia?

_____Is there a family history of muscular dystrophy?

_____Is there a family history of cystic fibrosis?

_____Is there a family history of Huntington's disease?

_____Does anyone in your family or the family of the baby's father have cystic fibrosis?

_____Is anyone in your family or the family of the baby's father's mentally retarded?

_____If so, was that person tested for fragile X syndrome?

_____Do you, the baby's father, anyone in your families, or any of your children have any other genetic diseases, chromosomal disorders, or birth defects?

_____Do you have a metabolic disorder such as diabetes or phenylketonuria?

_____Do you have a history of pregnancy issues (miscarriage or stillbirth)?

FIG 6.3 Questionnaire for identifying couples having increased risk for offspring with genetic disorders. (Courtesy of American College of Obstetricians and Gynecologists. [2010]. *Your pregnancy and childbirth month to month* [5th ed.]. Washington, DC: Author.)

have this disease? Because the answer to this question may have profound implications for individual family members and the family as a whole, health care professionals must be able to answer this question as accurately as they can in a timely manner. In some cases, estimation of risk is rather straightforward; in other cases, it is complicated.

If a couple has not yet had children but they are known to be at risk for having children with a genetic disease, they will be given an occurrence risk. Once the mating of a couple has produced one or more children with a genetic disease, the couple will be given a recurrence risk. Both occurrence and recurrence risks are determined by the mode of inheritance for the genetic disease in question. For genetic diseases caused by a factor that segregates during cell division (genes and chromosomes), risk can be estimated with a high degree of accuracy by application of mendelian principles.

In an autosomal dominant disorder, both the occurrence and recurrence risk is 50%, or one in two, that a subsequent offspring will be affected when one parent is affected and the other is not. The recurrence risk for autosomal recessive disorders is 25%, or 1 in 4, if both parents are carriers (they each have one recessive disease gene and one normal gene). Occasionally an individual homozygous for a recessive disease gene mates with an individual who is a carrier of the same recessive gene. In this case, the recurrence risk is 50%, or 1 in 2. If two individuals affected by an autosomal recessive disorder mate, all of their children will be affected. For X-linked disorders, recurrence risk is related to the sex of the child. Translocation chromosomes have a high risk for recurrence.

A number of autosomal disorders display fairly complex patterns of inheritance, making estimation of risk somewhat difficult. For example,

COMMUNITY FOCUS

Resources for Genetic Disorders

- Select a hereditary disorder such as CF, muscular dystrophy, hemophilia, Tay-Sachs disease, or sickle cell anemia. Visit the website of the national organization. Locate accredited care centers that are in your community. Do the centers offer preconception counseling?
- Visit the Genetic Alliance website at www.geneticalliance.org. Select a disorder, and go to the disease information search link. Review the patient information sections about clinical description, insurance issues, research, and treatment.
- Share your findings with your classmates in a clinical conference.
- Existing genetics resources include the following:
  - Centers for Disease Control and Prevention (www.cdc.gov/genetics/activities/ogdp.htm)
  - Genetic Alliance (www.geneticalliance.org/)
  - National Coalition for Health Professional Education in Genetics (www.nchpeg.org/)
  - Genetics Education Program for Nurses at Cincinnati Children's Hospital Medical Center (www.cincinnatichildrens.org/ed/clinical/gpnf/default.htm)
  - NHGRI Education (www.genome.gov/Education/)
  - National Center for Biotechnology Information (www.ncbi.nlm.nih.gov/)
  - Other websites, such as www.hsl.unc.edu/Services/Guides/focusonclingen.cfm

Some of these resources may be in health care professionals' own communities, but others are regional, national, and international resources.

if a child is born with a genetic disease and there has been no history of the disease in the family, the disease may have been caused by a new mutation (this is more likely if the disease in question is an autosomal dominant disorder, such as achondroplasia). If the child's genetic disease has been caused by a new mutation, the recurrence risk for the parents' subsequent children is low (1% to 2%), but it is not as low as that for the general population. Offspring of the affected child may have a substantially elevated occurrence risk.

The risk for recurrence for multifactorial conditions can be estimated empirically. An empiric risk is based not on genetics theory but, rather, on experience and observation of the disorder in other families. Recurrence risks are determined by applying the frequency of a similar disorder in other families to the case under consideration.

An important concept to be emphasized to individuals and families during a genetic counseling session is that *each pregnancy is an independent event.* For example, in monogenic disorders in which the risk factor is 1 in 4 that the child will be affected, the risk remains the same no matter how many affected children are already in the family. Families may maintain the erroneous assumption that the presence of one affected child ensures that the next three will be free of the disorder. However, "chance has no memory." The risk is 1 in 4 for each pregnancy. Conversely, in a family with a child who has a disorder with multifactorial causes, the risk increases with each subsequent child born with the disorder.

INTERPRETATION OF RISK

The guiding principle for genetics counselors has traditionally been nondirectiveness. According to the principle of nondirectiveness, the individual who is providing genetic counseling respects the right of the individual or family being counseled to make autonomous decisions. Counselors using a nondirective approach avoid making recommendations, and they try to communicate genetics information in an unbiased

manner. The first step in providing nondirective counseling is becoming aware of one's own values and beliefs. Another important step is recognizing how one's values and beliefs can influence or interfere with the communication of genetics information.

If the individual who is providing genetic counseling has difficulty being nonjudgmental and objective, he or she may either intentionally or unintentionally influence the decision-making process. Individuals and families also may pressure the counselor to make decisions for them with questions such as "What would you do if you were me?" Families and individuals need education, guidance, and support throughout the counseling process. They should be given the facts and possible consequences as well as all of the assistance they need in problem solving, but the final decision regarding a course of action must be their own.

MULTIPLE ROLES FOR NURSES IN GENETICS

Nurses play many roles in genetics. Some nurses play a key role in the identification of families in need of genetic counseling, and they collaborate with other health care professionals as part of interprofessional teams to make referrals to specialists in genetics. Other nurses take a more active role in genetic counseling.

Probably the most important of all nursing functions is to provide emotional support during all aspects of the counseling process. Feelings that are generated under the real or imagined threat posed by a genetic disorder are as varied as the individuals being counseled. Responses may include a variety of stress reactions, such as apathy, denial, anger, hostility, fear, embarrassment, grief, and loss of self-esteem. Guilt and self-blame are universal reactions. Many look on the disorder as a stigma, especially if the disorder is visible to others. Old wives' tales, superstitions, and long-held misconceptions may influence a family's reaction to a genetic disorder.

Nurses are ideally positioned to help individuals and families maximize the benefits of the genetics revolution, but first, nurses need (1) a working knowledge of human genetics, (2) an awareness of recent advances in genetics and genomics, and (3) an understanding of the potential effects of genomic discoveries on individual and family well-being. More research is needed concerning the family experience of genetic testing. Nurses must understand why individuals and families decide to undergo or to forgo genetic testing. Nurses also need to be aware of how individuals and families define and manage ethical, legal, and social issues that emerge during the genetic testing experience.

CELL DIVISION AND CONCEPTION

CELL DIVISION

Cells are reproduced by two different methods: mitosis and meiosis. In mitosis, the body cells replicate to yield two cells with the same genetic makeup as the parent cell. First the cell makes a copy of its DNA, and then it divides. Each daughter cell receives one copy of the genetic material. Mitotic division facilitates growth and development or cell replacement.

Meiosis, the process by which germ cells divide and decrease their chromosomal number by half, produces gametes (eggs and sperm). Each homologous pair of chromosomes contains one chromosome received from the mother and one from the father; thus meiosis results in cells that contain one of each of the 23 pairs of chromosomes. Because these germ cells contain 23 single chromosomes, half of the genetic material of a normal somatic cell, they are called *haploid.* This halving of the genetic material is accomplished by replicating the DNA once and then dividing twice. When the female gamete (egg or ovum) and

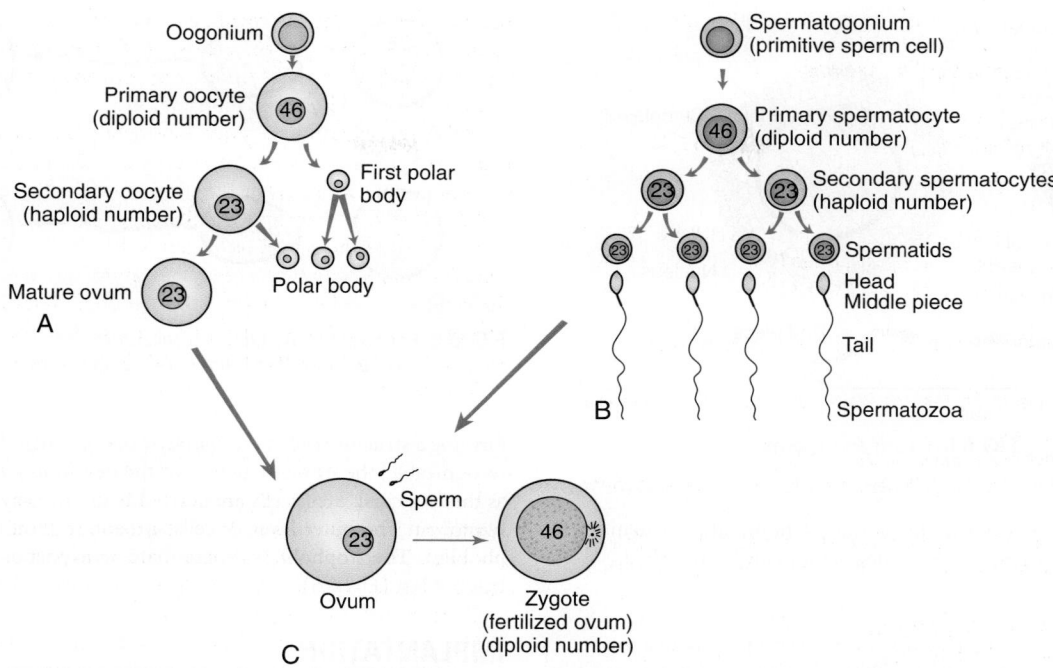

FIG 6.4 Gametogenesis and fertilization. **A,** Oogenesis. Gametogenesis in the female produces one mature ovum and three polar bodies. Note relative difference in overall size between ovum and sperm. **B,** Spermatogenesis. Gametogenesis in the male produces four mature gametes, the sperm. **C,** Fertilization results in the single-cell zygote and restoration of the diploid number of chromosomes.

the male gamete (spermatozoon) unite to form the zygote, the diploid number of human chromosomes (46, or 23 pairs) is restored.

The process of DNA replication and cell division in meiosis allows different alleles (genes on corresponding loci that code for variations of the same trait) for genes to be distributed at random by each parent and then rearranged on the paired chromosomes. The chromosomes then separate and proceed to different gametes. Because the two parents have genotypes derived from four different grandparents, many combinations of genes on each chromosome are possible. This random mixing of alleles accounts for the variation of traits seen in the offspring of the same two parents.

GAMETOGENESIS

Oogenesis, the process of egg (ovum) formation, begins during fetal life of the female. All the cells that may undergo meiosis in a woman's lifetime are contained in her ovaries at birth. The majority of the estimated 2 million primary oocytes (the cells that undergo the first meiotic division) degenerate spontaneously. Only 400 to 500 ova will mature during the approximately 35 years of a woman's reproductive life. The primary oocytes begin the first meiotic division (i.e., they replicate their DNA) during fetal life, but they remain suspended at this stage until puberty (Fig. 6.4, *A*). Then, usually monthly, one primary oocyte matures and completes the first meiotic division, yielding two unequal cells: the secondary oocyte and a small polar body. Both contain 22 autosomes and one X sex chromosome.

At ovulation, the second meiotic division begins. However, the ovum does not complete the second meiotic division unless fertilization occurs. At fertilization, when the sperm is united with the mature ovum, a second polar body and the **zygote** (the united egg and sperm) are produced (see Fig. 6.4, *C*). The three polar bodies degenerate.

When a male reaches puberty, his testes begin the process of **spermatogenesis**. The cells that undergo meiosis in the male are called

spermatocytes. The primary spermatocyte, which undergoes the first meiotic division, contains the diploid number of chromosomes. The cell has already copied its DNA before division, so four alleles for each gene are present. The cell is still considered diploid because the copies are bound together (i.e., one allele plus its copy on each chromosome).

During the first meiotic division, two haploid secondary spermatocytes are formed. Each secondary spermatocyte contains 22 autosomes and one sex chromosome; one contains the X chromosome (plus its copy) and the other, the Y chromosome (plus its copy). During the second meiotic division, the male produces two gametes with an X chromosome and two gametes with a Y chromosome, all of which will develop into viable sperm (see Fig. 6.4, *B*).

CONCEPTION

Conception, defined as the union of a single egg and sperm, marks the beginning of a pregnancy. Conception occurs not as an isolated event but as part of a sequential process. This sequential process includes gamete (egg and sperm) formation, ovulation (release of the egg), union of the gametes (which results in an embryo), and implantation in the uterus.

Ovum

Meiosis occurs in the female in the ovarian follicles and produces an egg, or ovum. Each month one ovum matures with a host of surrounding supportive cells. At ovulation, the ovum is released from the ruptured ovarian follicle. High estrogen levels increase the motility of the uterine tubes so that their cilia can capture the ovum and propel it through the tube toward the uterine cavity. An ovum cannot move by itself.

Two protective layers surround the ovum (Fig. 6.5). The inner layer is a thick, acellular layer called the *zona pellucida*. The outer layer, called the *corona radiata,* is composed of elongated cells.

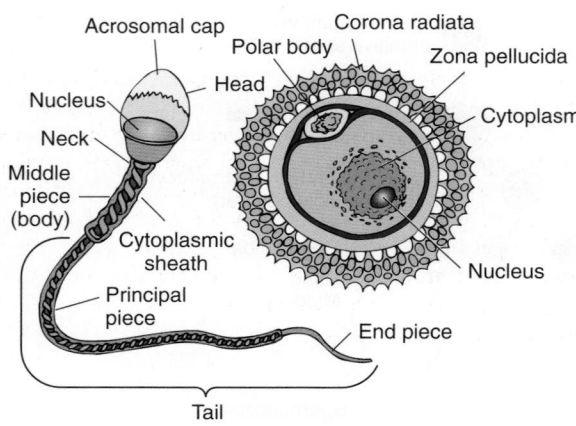

FIG 6.5 Ovum and sperm.

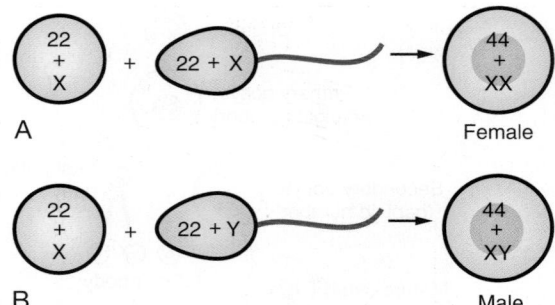

FIG 6.6 Fertilization. **A,** Ovum fertilized by X-bearing sperm to form female zygote. **B,** Ovum fertilized by Y-bearing sperm to form male zygote.

Ova are considered fertile for about 24 hours after ovulation. If unfertilized by a sperm, the ovum degenerates and is resorbed.

Sperm

Ejaculation during sexual intercourse normally propels about a teaspoon of semen containing as many as 200 to 500 million sperm into the vagina. The sperm swim by means of the flagellar movement of their tails. Some sperm can reach the site of fertilization within 5 minutes, but average transit time is 4 to 6 hours. Sperm remain viable within the woman's reproductive system for an average of 2 to 3 days. Most sperm are lost in the vagina, within the cervical mucus, or in the endometrium; or they enter the tube that contains no ovum.

As sperm travel through the female reproductive tract, enzymes are produced to aid in their capacitation. *Capacitation* is a physiologic change that removes the protective coating from the heads of the sperm. Small perforations then form in the acrosome (a cap on the sperm) and allow enzymes (e.g., hyaluronidase) to escape (see Fig. 6.5). These enzymes are necessary for the sperm to penetrate the protective layers of the ovum before fertilization.

FERTILIZATION

Fertilization takes place in the ampulla (the outer third) of the uterine tube. When a sperm successfully penetrates the membrane surrounding the ovum, both sperm and ovum are enclosed within the membrane and the membrane becomes impenetrable to other sperm; this process is termed the *zona reaction*. The second meiotic division of the secondary oocyte is then completed, and the nucleus of the ovum becomes the female pronucleus. The head of the sperm enlarges to become the male pronucleus, and the tail degenerates. The nuclei fuse and the chromosomes combine, restoring the diploid number (46) (Fig. 6.6). Conception, the formation of the zygote (the first cell of the new individual), has been achieved.

Mitotic cellular replication, called *cleavage*, begins as the zygote travels the length of the uterine tube into the uterus. This voyage takes 3 to 4 days. Because the fertilized egg divides rapidly with no increase in size, successively smaller cells, called *blastomeres*, are formed with each division. A 16-cell morula, a solid ball of cells, is produced within 3 days and is still surrounded by the protective zona pellucida (Fig. 6.7, *A*). Further development occurs as the morula floats freely within the uterus. Fluid passes through the zona pellucida into the intercellular spaces between the blastomeres, separating them into two parts: the trophoblast (which gives rise to the placenta) and the embryoblast (which gives rise to the embryo). A cavity forms within the cell mass as the spaces come together,

forming a structure called the *blastocyst cavity.* When the cavity becomes recognizable, the whole structure of the developing embryo is known as the *blastocyst.* Stem cells are derived from the inner cell mass of the blastocyst. The outer layer of cells surrounding the cavity is the trophoblast. The trophoblast differentiates into villous and extravillous trophoblast (Fig. 6.8).

IMPLANTATION

The zona pellucida degenerates, the trophoblast cells displace endometrial cells at the implantation site, and the blastocyst embeds in the endometrium, usually in the anterior or posterior fundal region. Between 6 and 10 days after conception, the trophoblast secretes enzymes that enable it to burrow into the endometrium until the entire blastocyst is covered. This is known as *implantation.* Endometrial blood vessels erode, and some women have implantation bleeding (slight spotting and bleeding at the time of the first missed menstrual period). Chorionic villi, fingerlike projections, develop out of the trophoblast and extend into the blood-filled spaces of the endometrium. These villi are vascular processes that obtain oxygen and nutrients from the maternal bloodstream and dispose of carbon dioxide and waste products into the maternal blood.

After implantation, the endometrium is called the *decidua.* The portion directly under the blastocyst, where the chorionic villi tap into the maternal blood vessels, is the *decidua basalis.* The portion covering the blastocyst is the *decidua capsularis,* and the portion lining the rest of the uterus is the *decidua vera* (Fig. 6.9).

THE EMBRYO AND FETUS

Pregnancy lasts approximately 10 lunar months, 9 calendar months, 40 weeks, or 280 days. Length of pregnancy is computed from the first day of the last menstrual period (LMP) until the day of birth. However, conception occurs approximately 2 weeks after the first day of the LMP. Thus the postconception age of the fetus is 2 weeks less, for a total of 266 days or 38 weeks. *Postconception age* is used in the discussion of fetal development.

Intrauterine development is divided into three stages: ovum or preembryonic, embryo, and fetus (see Fig. 6.19). The stage of the ovum lasts from conception until day 14. This period covers cellular replication, blastocyst formation, initial development of the embryonic membranes, and establishment of the primary germ layers.

PRIMARY GERM LAYERS

During the third week after conception, the embryonic disk differentiates into three primary germ layers: the ectoderm, the mesoderm, and the

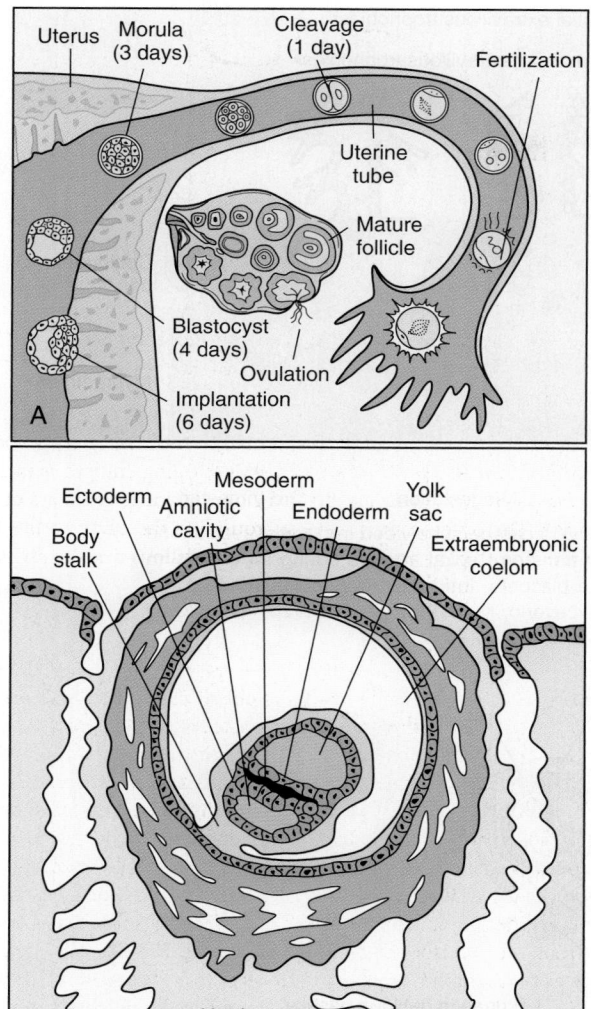

FIG 6.7 First weeks of human development. **A,** Follicular development in ovary, ovulation, fertilization, and transport of early embryo down uterine tube and into uterus, where implantation occurs. **B,** Blastocyst embedded in endometrium. Germ layers forming. (A, From Carlson, B.M. [2013]. *Human embryology and developmental biology* [5th ed.]. St. Louis, MO: Mosby; B, Adapted from Langley, L.L., Telford, I.R., Christensen, J.B. [1980]. *Dynamic human anatomy and physiology* [5th ed.]. New York, NY: McGraw-Hill.)

endoderm (or entoderm) (see Fig. 6.7, *B*). All tissues and organs of the embryo develop from these three layers.

The ectoderm, the upper layer of the embryonic disk, gives rise to the epidermis, glands (anterior pituitary, cutaneous, and mammary), nails and hair, central and peripheral nervous systems, lens of the eyes, tooth enamel, and floor of the amniotic cavity.

The mesoderm, the middle layer, develops into the bones and teeth, muscles (skeletal, smooth, and cardiac), dermis and connective tissue, cardiovascular system and spleen, and urogenital system.

The endoderm, the lower layer, gives rise to the epithelium lining the respiratory tract and digestive tract, including the oropharynx, liver and pancreas, urethra, bladder, and vagina. The endoderm forms the roof of the yolk sac.

DEVELOPMENT OF THE EMBRYO

The stage of the embryo lasts from day 15 until approximately 8 weeks after conception, when the embryo measures approximately 3 cm from crown to rump. The embryonic stage is the most critical time in the development of the organ systems and the main external features. Developing areas with rapid cell division are the most vulnerable to malformation caused by environmental teratogens (substances or exposure that causes abnormal development). At the end of the eighth week, all organ systems and external structures are present and the embryo is unmistakably human. (See Fig. 6.19 and Visible Embryo, www.visembryo.com, for a pictorial view of normal and abnormal development.)

MEMBRANES

At the time of implantation, two fetal membranes that will surround the developing embryo begin to form. The chorion develops from the trophoblast and contains the chorionic villi on its surface. The villi burrow into the decidua basalis and increase in size and complexity as the vascular processes develop into the placenta. The chorion becomes the covering of the fetal side of the placenta. It contains the major umbilical blood vessels that branch out over the surface of the placenta. As the embryo grows, the decidua capsularis stretches. The chorionic villi on this side atrophy and degenerate, leaving a smooth chorionic membrane.

The inner cell membrane, the amnion, develops from the interior cells of the blastocyst. The cavity that develops between this inner cell mass and the outer layer of cells (trophoblast) is the amniotic cavity (see Fig. 6.7, *B*). As it grows larger, the amnion forms on the side opposite the developing blastocyst (see Fig. 6.7, *B*, and Fig. 6.9). The developing embryo draws the amnion around itself to form a fluid-filled sac. The amnion becomes the covering of the umbilical cord and covers the chorion on the fetal surface of the placenta. As the embryo grows larger, the amnion enlarges to accommodate the embryo/fetus and the surrounding amniotic fluid. The amnion eventually comes in contact with the chorion surrounding the fetus (see the Critical Reasoning Case Study).

CLINICAL REASONING CASE STUDY
Ingestion of Alcohol During Pregnancy

Sandra is 12 weeks pregnant, confirmed by ultrasound, and has just come for her first prenatal visit. She stated that she drinks wine with dinner almost every night. Now that she has a confirmed pregnancy, she is worried about her alcohol and medication intake during the first trimester of pregnancy. What information should the nurse provide Sandra?

1. Evidence—Is there sufficient evidence to draw conclusions about what information the nurse should provide Sandra?
2. Assumptions—Describe an underlying assumption about the following factors:
   a. Sandra's motivation to learn about fetal development
   b. Sandra's understanding of fetal development
   c. Sandra's knowledge about alcohol intake and medication use during pregnancy
   d. Why dating the pregnancy is important
   e. Sandra being worried about possible negative effects on the fetus of alcohol intake and medications
3. What implications and priorities for nursing care can be drawn at this time?
4. What are the opportunities for interprofessional practice? Which members of the interprofessional health care team might be involved in providing care for Sandra?

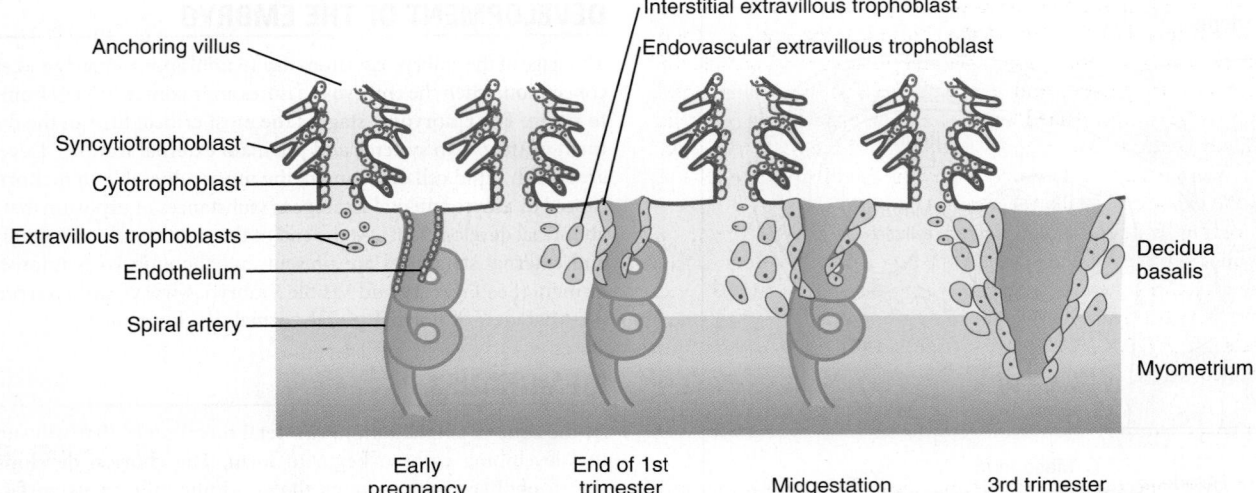

FIG 6.8 Extravillous trophoblasts are found outside the villus and can be subdivided into endovascular and interstitial categories. Endovascular trophoblasts invade and transform spiral arteries during pregnancy to create low-resistance blood flow that is characteristic of the placenta. Interstitial trophoblasts invade the decidua and surround spiral arteries. (From Cunningham, F., Leveno, K., Bloom, S., et al. [2014]. *Williams obstetrics* [24th ed.]. New York, NY: McGraw-Hill.)

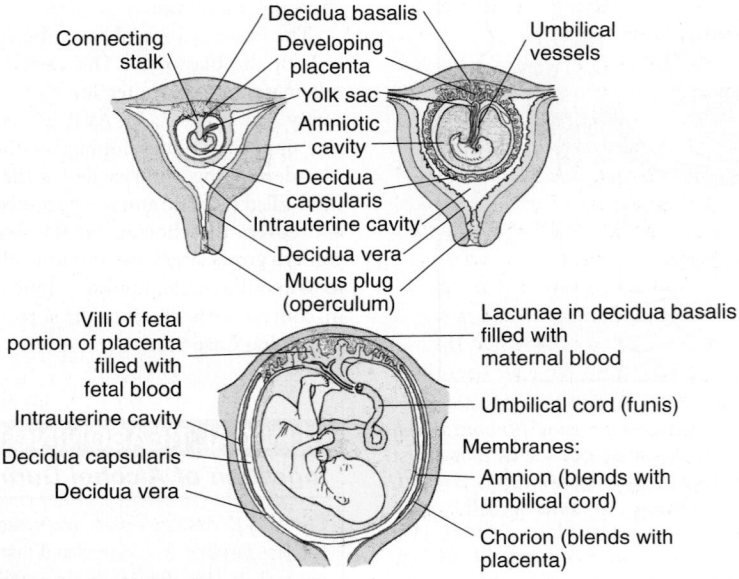

FIG 6.9 Development of fetal membranes. Note gradual obliteration of intrauterine cavity as decidua capsularis and decidua vera meet. Also note thinning of uterine wall. Chorionic and amnionic membranes are in apposition to each other but may be peeled apart.

AMNIOTIC FLUID

The amniotic cavity initially derives its fluid by diffusion from the maternal blood. Fluid secreted by the respiratory and gastrointestinal tracts of the fetus also enters the amniotic cavity (Moore, Persaud, & Torchia, 2013). The amount of fluid increases weekly, and 700 to 1000 mL of transparent liquid is normally present at term. The volume of amniotic fluid changes constantly. The fetus swallows fluid, and fluid flows into and out of the fetal lungs. Beginning in week 11, the fetus urinates into the fluid, increasing its volume.

Amniotic fluid serves many functions. It helps maintain a constant body temperature. It serves as a source of oral fluid and as a repository for waste and assists in maintenance of fluid and electrolyte homeostasis.

It cushions the fetus from trauma by blunting and dispersing outside forces. It allows freedom of movement for musculoskeletal development. It acts as a barrier to infection and allows fetal lung development (Moore et al., 2013). The fluid keeps the embryo from tangling with the membranes, facilitating symmetric growth. If the embryo does become tangled with the membranes, amputations of extremities or other deformities can occur from constricting amniotic bands.

YOLK SAC

When the amniotic cavity and amnion are forming, another blastocyst cavity forms on the other side of the developing embryonic disk (see Fig. 6.7, *B*). This cavity becomes surrounded by a membrane, forming the yolk sac. The yolk sac aids in transferring maternal nutrients and oxygen, which have diffused through the chorion, to the embryo. Blood vessels form to aid transport. Blood cells and plasma are manufactured in the yolk sac during the second and third weeks while uteroplacental circulation is being established and is forming primitive blood cells until hematopoietic activity begins. At the end of the third week, the primitive heart begins to beat and circulate the blood through the embryo, the connecting stalk, the chorion, and the yolk sac.

The folding in of the embryo during the fourth week results in incorporation of part of the yolk sac into the embryo's body as the primitive digestive system. Primordial germ cells arise in the yolk sac and move into the embryo. The shrinking remains of the yolk sac degenerate (see Fig. 6.7, *B*), and by the fifth or sixth week, the remnant has separated from the embryo.

UMBILICAL CORD

By day 14 after conception, the embryonic disk, the amniotic sac, and the yolk sac are attached to the chorionic villi by the connecting stalk. During the third week, the blood vessels develop to supply the embryo with maternal nutrients and oxygen. During the fifth week, the embryo has curved inward on itself from both ends, bringing the connecting stalk to the ventral side of the embryo. The connecting stalk becomes compressed from both sides by the amnion and forms the narrower umbilical cord (see Fig. 6.7). Two arteries carry blood from the embryo to the chorionic villi, and one vein returns blood to the embryo. Approximately 1% of umbilical cords contain only two vessels: one artery and one vein. This occurrence is sometimes associated with congenital malformations (Kaiser Permanente, 2017).

The cord rapidly increases in length. At term, the cord is 2 cm in diameter and ranges from 30 to 90 cm in length (with an average of 55 cm). It twists spirally on itself and loops around the embryo/fetus. A true knot is rare, but false knots occur as folds or kinks in the cord and may jeopardize circulation to the fetus. Connective tissue called *Wharton's jelly* prevents compression of the blood vessels and ensures continued nourishment of the embryo/fetus. Compression can occur if the cord lies between the fetal head and the pelvis or is twisted around the fetal body. When the cord is wrapped around the fetal neck, it is called a nuchal cord.

Because the placenta develops from the chorionic villi, the umbilical cord is usually located centrally. A peripheral location is less common and is known as a *battledore placenta* (see Chapter 12 for more information). The blood vessels are arrayed out from the center to all parts of the placenta (Fig. 6.10).

PLACENTA

Structure

The placenta begins to form at implantation. During the third week after conception, the trophoblast cells of the chorionic villi continue to invade the decidua basalis. As the uterine capillaries are tapped, the endometrial spiral arteries fill with maternal blood. The chorionic villi grow into the spaces with two layers of cells: the outer syncytium and the inner cytotrophoblast. A third layer develops into anchoring septa, dividing the projecting decidua into separate areas called *cotyledons*. In each of the 15 to 20 cotyledons, the chorionic villi branch out and a complex system of fetal blood vessels forms. Each cotyledon is a functional unit. The whole structure is the placenta (see Fig. 6.10).

The maternal-placental-embryonic circulation is in place by day 17, when the embryonic heart starts beating. By the end of the third week, embryonic blood is circulating between the embryo and the chorionic villi. In the intervillous spaces, maternal blood supplies oxygen and

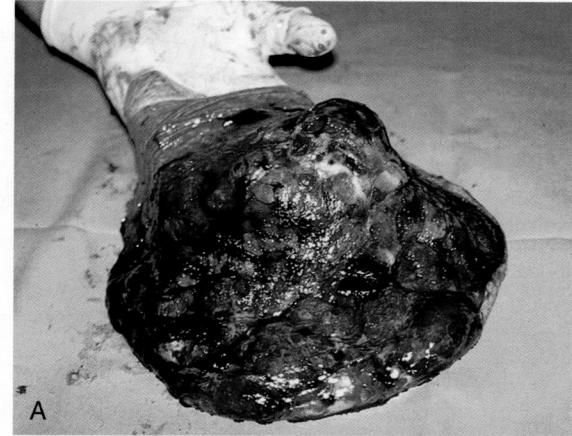

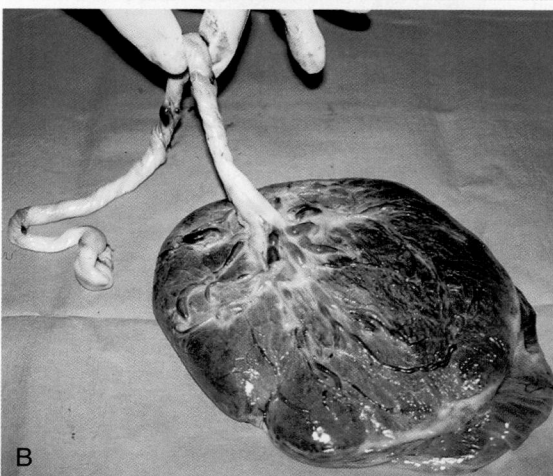

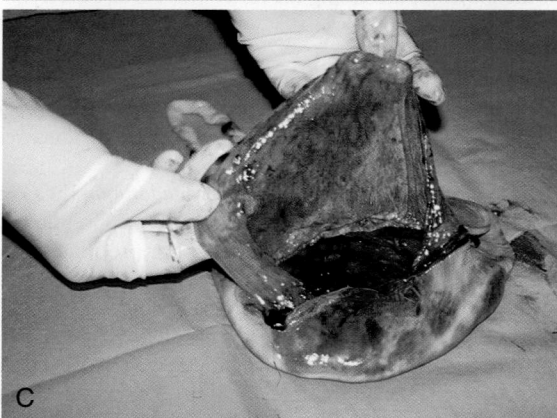

FIG 6.10 Term placenta. **A,** Maternal (or uterine) surface, showing cotyledons and grooves. **B,** Fetal (or amniotic) surface, showing blood vessels running under amnion and converging to form umbilical vessels at attachment of umbilical cord. **C,** Amnion and smooth chorion are arranged to show that they are (1) fused and (2) continuous with margins of placenta. (Courtesy of Marjorie Pyle, RNC, Lifecircle, Costa Mesa, CA.)

nutrients to the embryonic capillaries in the villi (Fig. 6.11). Waste products and carbon dioxide diffuse into the maternal blood.

The placenta functions as a means of metabolic exchange. Exchange is minimal at this time because the two cell layers of the villous membrane are too thick. Permeability increases as the cytotrophoblast thins and disappears; by the fifth month, only the single layer of syncytium is left

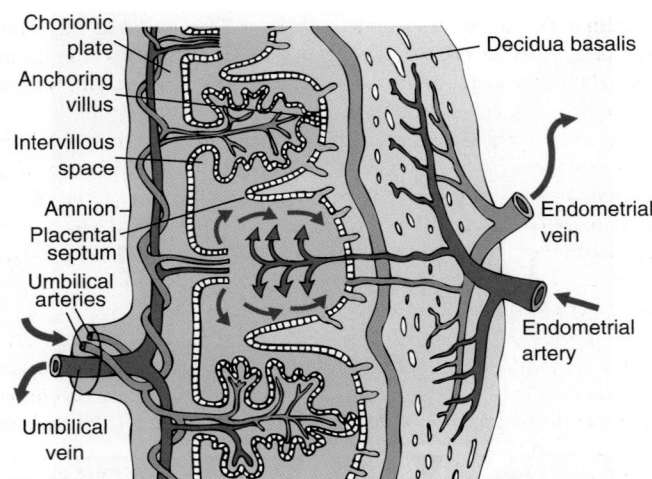

FIG 6.11 Schematic drawing of placenta illustrating how it supplies oxygen and nutrition to embryo and removes its waste products. Deoxygenated blood leaves fetus through the umbilical arteries and enters placenta, where it is oxygenated. Oxygenated blood leaves placenta through the umbilical vein, which enters the fetus via the umbilical cord.

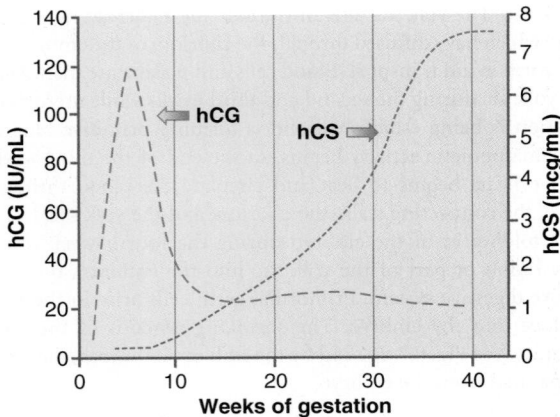

FIG 6.12 Distinct profile for the concentrations of human chorionic gonadotropin (hCG) and human chorionic somatomammotropin (hCS) in serum of women through normal pregnancy. *IU*, International units. (Adapted from Cunningham, F., Leveno, K., Bloom, S., et al. [2014]. *Williams obstetrics* [24th ed.]. New York, NY: McGraw-Hill.)

between the maternal blood and the fetal capillaries. The syncytium is the functional layer of the placenta. By the eighth week, genetic testing may be done on a sample of chorionic villi obtained by aspiration biopsy; however, limb defects have been associated with chorionic villi sampling done before 10 weeks. The structure of the placenta is complete by the twelfth week. The placenta continues to grow wider until 20 weeks, when it covers about half of the uterine surface. It then continues to grow thicker. The branching villi continue to develop within the body of the placenta, increasing the functional surface area.

Functions

One of the early functions of the placenta is as an endocrine gland that produces four hormones necessary to maintain the pregnancy and support the embryo/fetus. The hormones are produced in the syncytium.

The protein hormone *human chorionic gonadotropin* (hCG) can be detected in the maternal serum by 8 to 10 days after conception, shortly after implantation. This hormone is the basis for pregnancy tests. The hCG preserves the function of the ovarian corpus luteum, ensuring a continued supply of estrogen and progesterone needed to maintain the pregnancy. Miscarriage occurs if the corpus luteum stops functioning before the placenta can produce sufficient estrogen and progesterone. The hCG reaches its maximum level at 50 to 70 days and then begins to decrease.

The other protein hormone produced by the placenta is *human chorionic somatomammotropin* (hCS) or *human placental lactogen* (hPL). This substance is similar to a growth hormone and stimulates maternal metabolism to supply needed nutrients for fetal growth. hCS increases the resistance to insulin, facilitates glucose transport across the placental membrane, and stimulates breast development to prepare for lactation (Fig. 6.12).

The placenta eventually produces more of the steroid hormone *progesterone* than the corpus luteum does during the first few months of pregnancy. Progesterone maintains the endometrium, decreases the contractility of the uterus, and stimulates maternal metabolism and development of breast alveoli.

By 7 weeks after fertilization, the placenta is producing most of the maternal estrogens, which are steroid hormones. The major estrogen

secreted by the placenta is estriol, whereas the ovaries produce mostly estradiol. Estriol levels may be measured to determine placental functioning. Estrogen stimulates uterine growth and uteroplacental blood flow. It causes a proliferation of the breast glandular tissue and stimulates myometrial contractility. Placental estrogen production increases greatly toward the end of pregnancy. One theory for the cause of the onset of labor is the decrease in circulating levels of progesterone and the increased levels of estrogen (Fig. 6.13).

The metabolic functions of the placenta are respiration, nutrition, excretion, and storage. Oxygen diffuses from the maternal blood across the placental membrane into the fetal blood, and carbon dioxide diffuses in the opposite direction. In this way, the placenta functions as lungs for the fetus.

Carbohydrates, proteins, calcium, and iron are stored in the placenta for ready access to meet fetal needs. Water, inorganic salts, carbohydrates, proteins, fats, and vitamins pass from the maternal blood supply across the placental membrane into the fetal blood, supplying nutrition. Water and most electrolytes with a molecular weight less than 500 readily diffuse through the membrane. Hydrostatic and osmotic pressures aid in the flow of water and some solutions. Facilitated and active transport assist in the transfer of glucose, amino acids, calcium, iron, and substances with higher molecular weights. Amino acids and calcium are transported against the concentration gradient between the maternal blood and fetal blood.

The fetal concentration of glucose is lower than the glucose level in the maternal blood because of its rapid metabolism by the fetus. This fetal requirement demands larger concentrations of glucose than simple diffusion can provide. Therefore maternal glucose moves into the fetal circulation by active transport.

Pinocytosis is a mechanism used for transferring large molecules, such as albumin and gamma globulins, across the placental membrane. This mechanism conveys the maternal immunoglobulins that provide early passive immunity to the fetus.

Metabolic waste products of the fetus cross the placental membrane from the fetal blood into the maternal blood. The maternal kidneys then excrete them. Many viruses can cross the placental membrane and infect the fetus. Some bacteria and protozoa first infect the placenta and then infect the fetus. Drugs can also cross the placental membrane and may harm the fetus. Caffeine, alcohol, nicotine, carbon monoxide and other toxic substances in cigarette smoke, and prescription

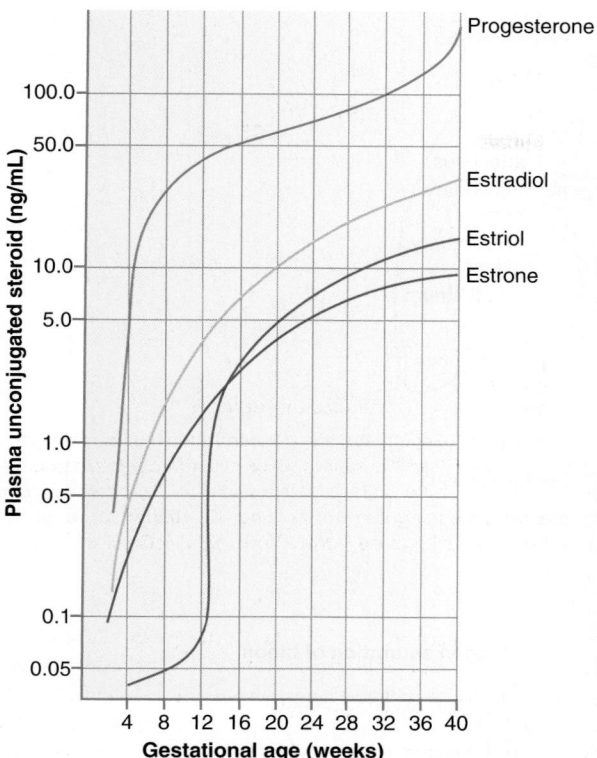

FIG 6.13 Plasma levels of progesterone, estradiol, estrone, and estriol in women during the course of gestation. (From Cunningham, F., Leveno, K., Bloom, S., et al. [2014]. *Williams obstetrics* [24th ed.]. New York, NY: McGraw-Hill.)

BOX 6.1 Developmentally Toxic Exposures in Humans

- Aminopterin
- Androgens
- Angiotensin-converting enzyme inhibitors
- Carbamazepine
- Cigarette smoking
- Cocaine
- Coumarin anticoagulants
- Cytomegalovirus
- Diethylstilbestrol
- Ethanol (>1 drink/day)
- Etretinate
- Hyperthermia
- Iodides
- Ionizing radiation (>10 rads)
- Isotretinoin
- Lead
- Lithium
- Methimazole
- Methyl mercury
- Parvovirus B19
- Penicillamine
- Phenytoin
- Radioiodine
- Rubella
- Syphilis
- Tetracycline
- Thalidomide
- Toxoplasmosis
- Trimethadione
- Valproic acid
- Varicella

---

and recreational drugs (e.g., marijuana, cocaine) readily cross the placenta (Box 6.1).

Although no direct link exists between the fetal blood in the vessels of the chorionic villi and the maternal blood in the intervillous spaces, only one cell layer separates them. Breaks occasionally occur in the placental membrane. Fetal erythrocytes then leak into the maternal circulation, and the mother may develop antibodies to the fetal red blood cells. This is often the way the Rh-negative mother becomes sensitized to the erythrocytes of her Rh-positive fetus (see the discussion of isoimmunization in Chapter 19).

Although the placenta and fetus are analogous to living tissue transplants, they are not destroyed by the host mother (Mor & Abrahams, 2014). Either the placental hormones suppress the immunologic response, or the tissue evokes no response.

Placental function depends on the maternal blood pressure supplying the circulation. Maternal arterial blood, under pressure in the small uterine spiral arteries, spurts into the intervillous spaces (see Fig. 6.11). As long as rich arterial blood continues to be supplied, pressure is exerted on the blood already in the intervillous spaces, pushing it toward drainage by the low-pressure uterine veins. At term gestation, 10% of the maternal cardiac output goes to the uterus.

If there is interference with the circulation to the placenta, the placenta cannot supply the embryo or fetus. Vasoconstriction, such as that caused by hypertension or cocaine use, diminishes uterine blood flow. Decreased maternal blood pressure or decreased cardiac output also diminishes uterine blood flow.

When a woman lies on her back with the pressure of the uterus compressing the vena cava, blood return to the right atrium is diminished (see Fig. 16.5 and the discussion of supine hypotension in Chapter 16). Excessive maternal exercise that diverts blood to the muscles away from the uterus compromises placental circulation. Optimum circulation is achieved when the woman is lying at rest on her side. Decreased uterine circulation may lead to intrauterine growth restriction of the fetus and infants who are small for gestational age.

Braxton Hicks contractions seem to enhance the movement of blood through the intervillous spaces, aiding placental circulation. However, prolonged contractions or intervals that are too short between contractions during labor can reduce the blood flow to the placenta.

FETAL MATURATION

This stage of the fetus lasts from 9 weeks (when the fetus becomes recognizable as a human being) until the pregnancy ends. Changes during the fetal period are not as dramatic, because refinement of structure and function is taking place. The fetus is less vulnerable to teratogens except for those that affect central nervous system functioning.

Viability refers to the capability of the fetus to survive outside the uterus. With modern technology and advances in maternal and neonatal care, infants who are 22 to 25 weeks of gestation are now considered to be on the threshold of viability (Cunningham, Leveno, Bloom, et al., 2014). The limitations on survival outside the uterus when an infant is born at this early stage are based on central nervous system function and oxygenation capability of the lungs.

FETAL CIRCULATORY SYSTEM

The cardiovascular system is the first organ system to function in the developing human. Blood vessel and blood cell formation begins in the third week and supplies the embryo with oxygen and nutrients from the mother. By the end of the third week, the tubular heart begins to beat and the primitive cardiovascular system links the embryo, connecting stalk, chorion, and yolk sac. During the fourth and fifth weeks, the heart develops into a four-chambered organ. By the end of the embryonic stage, the heart is developmentally complete.

The fetal lungs do not function for respiratory gas exchange, so a special circulatory pathway, the ductus arteriosus, bypasses the lungs. Oxygen-rich blood from the placenta flows rapidly through the umbilical vein into the fetal abdomen (Fig. 6.14). When the umbilical vein reaches the liver, it divides into two branches; one branch circulates some oxygenated blood through the liver. Most of the blood passes through the ductus venosus into the inferior vena cava. There it mixes with the deoxygenated blood from the fetal legs and abdomen on its way to the

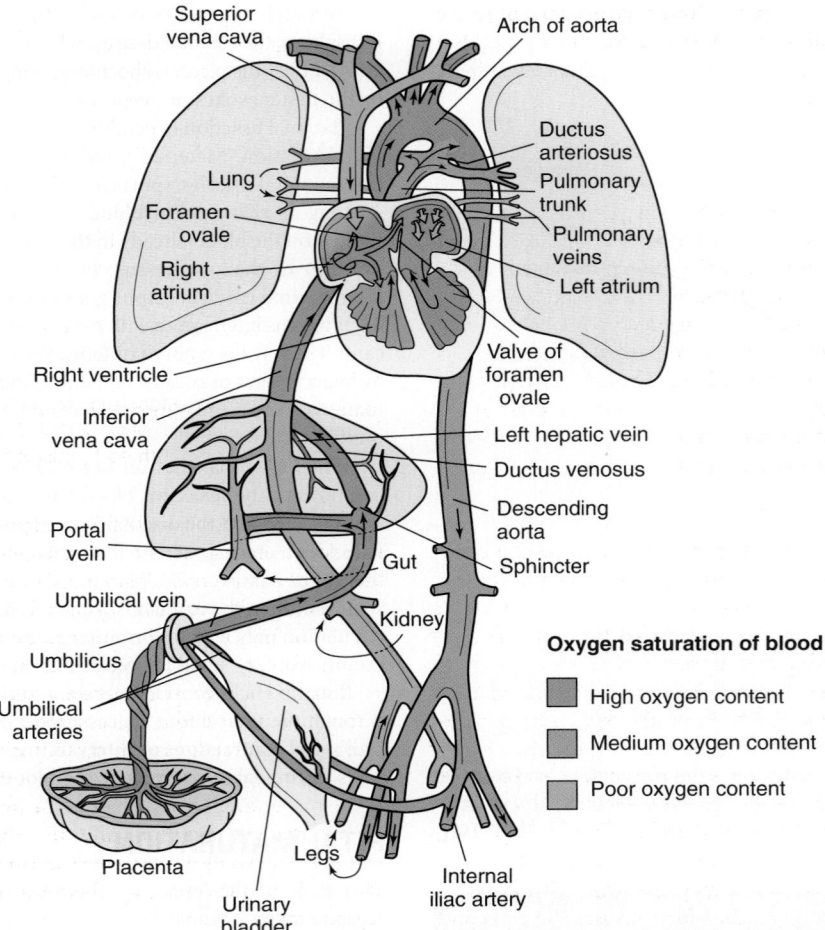

FIG 6.14 Schematic illustration of fetal circulation. The *colors* indicate the oxygen saturation of the blood, and the *arrows* show the course of the blood from the placenta to the heart. The organs are not drawn to scale. Observe that three shunts permit most of the blood to bypass the liver and lungs: (1) ductus venosus, (2) foramen ovale, and (3) ductus arteriosus. A small amount of highly oxygenated blood from the inferior vena cava remains in the right atrium and mixes with poorly oxygenated blood from the superior vena cava. This medium oxygenated blood then passes into the right ventricle. The poorly oxygenated blood returns to the placenta for oxygen and nutrients through the umbilical arteries. (From Moore, K.L., Persaud, T.V.N., Torchia, M.G. [2016]. *The developing human: Clinically oriented embryology* [10th ed.]. Philadelphia, PA: Elsevier.)

right atrium. Most of this blood passes straight through the right atrium and through the foramen ovale, an opening into the left atrium. There it mixes with the small amount of deoxygenated blood returning from the fetal lungs through the pulmonary veins.

The blood flows into the left ventricle and is squeezed out into the aorta, where the arteries supplying the heart, head, neck, and arms receive most of the oxygen-rich blood. This pattern of supplying the highest levels of oxygen and nutrients to the head, neck, and arms enhances the cephalocaudal (head-to-rump) development of the embryo/fetus.

Deoxygenated blood returning from the head and arms enters the right atrium through the superior vena cava. This blood is directed downward into the right ventricle, where it is squeezed into the pulmonary artery. A small amount of blood circulates through the resistant lung tissue, but the majority follows the path with less resistance through the ductus arteriosus into the aorta, distal to the point of exit of the arteries supplying the head and arms with oxygenated blood. The oxygen-poor blood flows through the abdominal aorta into the internal iliac arteries, where the umbilical arteries direct most of it back through the umbilical cord to the placenta. There the blood gives up its wastes and carbon dioxide in exchange for nutrients and oxygen. The blood

remaining in the iliac arteries flows through the fetal abdomen and legs, ultimately returning through the inferior vena cava to the heart.

The following three special characteristics enable the fetus to obtain sufficient oxygen from the maternal blood:
- Fetal hemoglobin carries 20% to 30% more oxygen than maternal hemoglobin.
- The hemoglobin concentration of the fetus is about 50% greater than that of the mother.
- The fetal heart rate (FHR) is 110 to 160 beats/min, making the cardiac output per unit of body weight higher than that of an adult.

HEMATOPOIETIC SYSTEM

Hematopoiesis, the formation of blood, occurs in the yolk sac (see Fig. 6.7, *B*) beginning in the third week. Hematopoietic stem cells seed the fetal liver during the fifth week, and hematopoiesis begins there during the sixth week. This accounts for the relatively large size of the liver between the seventh and ninth weeks. Stem cells seed the fetal bone marrow, spleen and thymus, and lymph nodes between weeks 8 and 11. (For more information about stem cells, see https://stemcells.nih.gov.)

The antigenic factors that determine blood type are present in the erythrocytes soon after the sixth week. For this reason, the Rh-negative woman is at risk for isoimmunization in any pregnancy that lasts longer than 6 weeks after fertilization.

RESPIRATORY SYSTEM

The respiratory system begins development during embryonic life and continues through fetal life and into childhood. The development of the respiratory tract begins in week 4 and continues through week 17 with formation of the larynx, trachea, bronchi, and lung buds. Between 16 and 24 weeks, the bronchi and terminal bronchioles enlarge and vascular structures and primitive alveoli are formed. Between 24 weeks and term birth, more alveoli form. Specialized alveolar cells, type I and type II cells, secrete pulmonary surfactants to line the interior of the alveoli. After 32 weeks, sufficient surfactant is present in developed alveoli to provide infants with a good chance of survival.

Pulmonary Surfactants

The detection of the presence of pulmonary surfactants, surface-active phospholipids, in amniotic fluid has been used to determine the degree of fetal lung maturity, or the ability of the lungs to function after birth. Lecithin (L) is the most critical alveolar surfactant required for postnatal lung expansion. It is detectable at approximately 21 weeks and increases in amount after week 24. Another pulmonary phospholipid, sphingomyelin (S), remains constant in amount. Thus the measure of lecithin in relation to sphingomyelin, or the L/S ratio, is used to determine fetal lung maturity. When the L/S ratio reaches 2:1, the infant's lungs are considered to be mature. This occurs at approximately 35 weeks of gestation (Mercer, 2014).

Certain maternal conditions that cause decreased maternal placental blood flow, such as maternal hypertension, placental dysfunction, infection, or corticosteroid use, accelerate lung maturity. This apparently is caused by the resulting fetal hypoxia, which stresses the fetus and increases the blood levels of corticosteroids that accelerate alveolar and surfactant development.

Conditions such as gestational diabetes and chronic glomerulonephritis can slow fetal lung maturity. The use of intrabronchial synthetic surfactant in the treatment of respiratory distress syndrome in the newborn has greatly improved the chances of survival for preterm infants (see Chapter 25).

Fetal respiratory movements have been seen on ultrasound as early as week 11. These fetal respiratory movements may aid in development of the chest wall muscles and regulate lung fluid volume. The fetal lungs produce fluid that expands the air spaces in the lungs. The fluid drains into the amniotic fluid or is swallowed by the fetus.

Shortly before birth, secretion of lung fluid decreases. Absorption of lung fluid begins during labor as fetal catecholamines and endogenous steroids are released in response to labor. The normal birth process squeezes out approximately one third of the fluid. Infants born by cesarean do not benefit from this squeezing process; thus they may have more respiratory difficulty at birth. The fluid remaining in the lungs at birth is usually resorbed into the infant's bloodstream within 2 hours of birth.

GASTROINTESTINAL SYSTEM

During the fourth week, the shape of the embryo changes from being almost straight to a C shape as both ends fold in toward the ventral surface. A portion of the yolk sac is incorporated into the body from head to tail as the primitive gut (digestive system).

The foregut produces the pharynx, part of the lower respiratory tract, the esophagus, the stomach, the first half of the duodenum, the liver, the pancreas, and the gallbladder. These structures evolve during

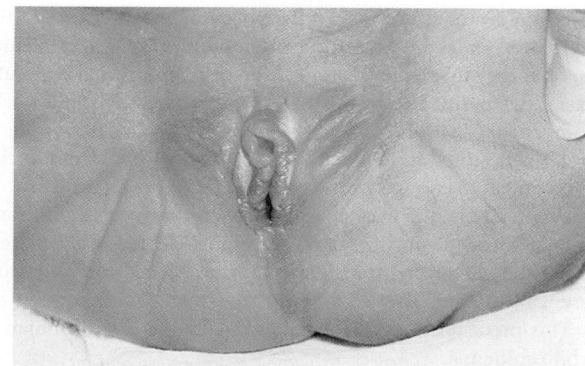

FIG 6.15 Anorectal malformation (imperforate anus). (From Moore, K.L., Persaud, T.V.N., Torchia, M.G. [2016]. *The developing human: Clinically oriented embryology* [10th ed.]. Philadelphia, PA: Elsevier.)

the fifth and sixth weeks. Malformations that can occur in these areas include esophageal atresia, hypertrophic pyloric stenosis, duodenal stenosis or atresia, and biliary atresia (see Chapter 41).

The midgut becomes the distal half of the duodenum, the jejunum and ileum, the cecum and appendix, and the proximal half of the colon. The midgut loop projects into the umbilical cord between weeks 5 and 10. A malformation, omphalocele, results if the midgut fails to return to the abdominal cavity, causing the intestines to protrude from the umbilicus. Meckel diverticulum is the most common malformation of the midgut. It occurs when a remnant of the yolk stalk that failed to degenerate attaches to the ileum, leaving a blind sac.

The hindgut develops into the distal half of the colon, the rectum and parts of the anal canal, the urinary bladder, and the urethra. Anorectal malformations are the most common abnormalities of the digestive system.

The fetus swallows amniotic fluid beginning in the fifth month. Gastric emptying and intestinal peristalsis occur. Fetal nutrition and elimination needs are taken care of by the placenta. As the fetus nears term, fetal waste products accumulate in the intestines as dark-green to black, tarry meconium. Normally this substance is passed through the rectum within 24 hours of birth. Sometimes with a breech presentation or fetal hypoxia, meconium is passed in utero into the amniotic fluid. The failure to pass meconium after birth may indicate atresia somewhere in the digestive tract; an imperforate anus (Fig. 6.15); or meconium ileus, in which a firm meconium plug blocks passage (seen in infants with CF).

The metabolic rate of the fetus is relatively low, but the infant has great growth and development needs. Beginning in week 9, the fetus synthesizes glycogen for storage in the liver. Between 26 and 30 weeks, the fetus begins to lay down stores of brown fat in preparation for extrauterine cold stress. Thermoregulation in the neonate requires increased metabolism and adequate oxygenation (see Chapter 22).

The gastrointestinal system is mature by 36 weeks. Digestive enzymes (except pancreatic amylase and lipase) are present in sufficient quantity to facilitate digestion. The neonate cannot digest starches or fats efficiently. Little saliva is produced.

HEPATIC SYSTEM

The liver and biliary tract develop from the foregut during the fourth week of gestation. Hematopoiesis begins during the sixth week and requires that the liver is large. The embryonic liver is prominent, occupying most of the abdominal cavity. Bile, a constituent of meconium, begins to form in the twelfth week.

Glycogen is stored in the fetal liver beginning at week 9 or 10. At term, glycogen stores are twice those of the adult. Glycogen is the major source of energy for the fetus and for the neonate stressed by in utero hypoxia, extrauterine loss of the maternal glucose supply, the work of breathing, or cold stress.

Iron is also stored in the fetal liver. If maternal intake is sufficient, the fetus can store enough iron to last for 5 months after birth.

During fetal life, the liver does not have to conjugate bilirubin for excretion because the unconjugated bilirubin is cleared by the placenta. Therefore the glucuronyl transferase enzyme needed for conjugation is present in the fetal liver in amounts less than those required after birth. This predisposes the neonate, especially the preterm infant, to hyperbilirubinemia.

Coagulation factors II, VII, IX, and X cannot be synthesized in the fetal liver because of the lack of vitamin K synthesis in the sterile fetal gut. This coagulation deficiency persists after birth for several days and is the rationale for the prophylactic administration of vitamin K to the newborn (see Chapter 23).

RENAL SYSTEM

The kidneys form during the fifth week and begin to function approximately 4 weeks later. Urine is excreted into the amniotic fluid and forms a major part of the amniotic fluid volume. Oligohydramnios is indicative of renal dysfunction. Because the placenta acts as the organ of excretion and maintains fetal water and electrolyte balance, the fetus does not need functioning kidneys while in utero. At birth, however, the kidneys are required immediately for excretory and acid-base regulatory functions.

A fetal renal malformation can be diagnosed in utero. Corrective or palliative fetal surgery may treat the malformation successfully, or plans can be made for treatment immediately after birth.

At term, the fetus has fully developed kidneys. However, the glomerular filtration rate (GFR) is low, and the kidneys lack the ability to concentrate urine. This makes the newborn more susceptible to both overhydration and dehydration.

NEUROLOGIC SYSTEM

The nervous system originates from the ectoderm during the third week after fertilization. The open neural tube forms during the fourth week. It initially closes at what will be the junction of the brain and spinal cord, leaving both ends open. The embryo folds in on itself lengthwise at this time, forming a head fold in the neural tube at this junction. The cranial end of the neural tube closes, and then the caudal end closes. During week 5, different growth rates cause more flexures in the neural tube, delineating three brain areas: the forebrain, the midbrain, and the hindbrain.

The forebrain develops into the eyes (cranial nerve II) and cerebral hemispheres. The development of all areas of the cerebral cortex continues throughout fetal life and into childhood. The olfactory system (cranial nerve I) and thalamus also develop from the forebrain. Cranial nerves III and IV (oculomotor and trochlear) form from the midbrain. The hindbrain forms the medulla, the pons, the cerebellum, and the remainder of the cranial nerves. Brain waves can be recorded on an electroencephalogram by week 8.

The spinal cord develops from the long end of the neural tube. Another ectodermal structure, the neural crest, develops into the peripheral nervous system. By the eighth week, nerve fibers traverse throughout the body. By week 11 or 12, the fetus makes respiratory movements, moves all extremities, and changes position in utero. The fetus can suck his or her thumb, swim in the amniotic fluid pool, and turn somersaults and can occasionally tie a knot in the umbilical cord.

At term, the fetal brain is approximately one-fourth the size of an adult brain. Neurologic development continues. Stressors on the fetus and neonate (e.g., chronic poor nutrition or hypoxia, drugs, environmental toxins, trauma, disease) damage the central nervous system long after the vulnerable embryonic time for malformations in other organ systems. Neurologic insult can result in cerebral palsy, neuromuscular impairment, intellectual disability, and learning disabilities.

Sensory Awareness

Purposeful movements of the fetus have been demonstrated in response to a firm touch transmitted through the mother's abdomen. Because it can feel, the fetus requires anesthesia when invasive procedures are done.

Fetuses respond to sound by 24 weeks. Different types of music evoke different movements. The fetus can be soothed by the sound of the mother's voice. Acoustic stimulation can be used to evoke a fetal heart rate response. The fetus becomes accustomed (habituates) to noises heard repeatedly. Hearing is fully developed at birth.

The fetus is able to distinguish taste. By the fifth month, when the fetus is swallowing amniotic fluid, a sweetener added to the fluid causes the fetus to swallow faster. The fetus also reacts to temperature changes. A cold solution placed into the amniotic fluid can cause fetal hiccups.

The fetus can see. Eyes have both rods and cones in the retina by the seventh month. A bright light shone on the mother's abdomen in late pregnancy causes abrupt fetal movements. During sleep time, rapid eye movements (REMs) have been observed similar to those occurring in children and adults while dreaming.

ENDOCRINE SYSTEM

The thyroid gland develops along with structures in the head and neck during the third and fourth weeks. The secretion of thyroxine begins during the eighth week. Maternal thyroxine does not readily cross the placenta; therefore the fetus that does not produce thyroid hormones will be born with congenital hypothyroidism. If untreated, hypothyroidism can result in severe intellectual disability. Screening for hypothyroidism is typically included in newborn screening after birth.

The adrenal cortex is formed during the sixth week and produces hormones by the eighth or ninth week. As term approaches, the fetus produces more cortisol. This is believed to aid in initiation of labor by decreasing the maternal progesterone and stimulating production of prostaglandins.

The pancreas forms from the foregut during the fifth through eighth weeks. The islets of Langerhans develop during the twelfth week. Insulin is produced by week 20. In fetuses of mothers with uncontrolled diabetes, maternal hyperglycemia produces fetal hyperglycemia, stimulating hyperinsulinemia and islet cell hyperplasia. This results in a macrosomic (large) fetus. The hyperinsulinemia also blocks lung maturation, placing the neonate at risk for respiratory distress and hypoglycemia when the maternal glucose source is lost at birth. Control of the maternal glucose level before and during pregnancy minimizes problems for the fetus and infant.

REPRODUCTIVE SYSTEM

Sex differentiation begins in the embryo during the seventh week. Female and male external genitalia are indistinguishable until after the ninth week. Distinguishing characteristics appear around the ninth week and are fully differentiated by the twelfth week. When a Y chromosome is present, testes are formed. By the end of the embryonic period, testosterone is being secreted and causes formation of the male genitalia. By week 28, the testes begin descending into the scrotum. After birth, low levels of testosterone continue to be secreted until the pubertal surge.

The female, with two X chromosomes, forms ovaries and female external genitalia. By the sixteenth week, oogenesis has been established. At birth, the ovaries contain the female's lifetime supply of ova. Most female hormone production is delayed until puberty. However, the fetal endometrium responds to maternal hormones, and withdrawal bleeding or vaginal discharge (pseudomenstruation) may occur at birth when these hormones are lost. The high level of maternal estrogen also stimulates mammary engorgement and secretion of fluid ("witch's milk") in newborn infants of both sexes.

MUSCULOSKELETAL SYSTEM

Bones and muscles develop from the mesoderm by the fourth week of embryonic development. At that time, the cardiac muscle is already beating. The mesoderm next to the neural tube forms the vertebral column and ribs. The parts of the vertebral column grow toward each other to enclose the developing spinal cord. Ossification, or bone formation, begins. If there is a defect in the bony fusion, various forms of spina bifida can occur. A large defect affecting several vertebrae may allow the membranes and spinal cord to pouch out from the back, producing neurologic deficits and skeletal deformity.

The flat bones of the skull develop during the embryonic period, and ossification continues throughout childhood. At birth, connective tissue sutures exist where the bones of the skull meet. The areas where more than two bones meet (called *fontanels*) are especially prominent. The sutures and fontanels allow the bones of the skull to mold, or move during birth, enabling the head to pass through the birth canal.

The bones of the shoulders, arms, hips, and legs appear in the sixth week as a continuous skeleton with no joints. Differentiation occurs, producing separate bones and joints. Ossification will continue through childhood to allow growth. Beginning in the seventh week, muscles contract spontaneously. Arm and leg movements are visible on ultrasound examination, although the mother does not perceive them until sometime between 16 and 20 weeks.

INTEGUMENTARY SYSTEM

The epidermis begins as a single layer of cells derived from the ectoderm at 4 weeks. By the seventh week, there are two layers of cells. The cells of the superficial layer are sloughed and become mixed with the sebaceous gland secretions to form the white, cheesy vernix caseosa, the material that protects the skin of the fetus. The vernix is thick at 24 weeks but becomes scant by term.

The basal layer of the epidermis is the germinal layer, which replaces lost cells. Until 17 weeks, the skin is thin and wrinkled, with blood vessels visible underneath. The skin thickens, and all layers are present at term. After 32 weeks, as subcutaneous fat is deposited under the dermis, the skin becomes less wrinkled and red in appearance.

By 16 weeks, the epidermal ridges are present on the palms of the hands, the fingers, the bottoms of the feet, and the toes. These handprints and footprints are unique to that infant.

Hairs form from hair bulbs in the epidermis that project into the dermis. Cells in the hair bulb keratinize to form the hair shaft. As the cells at the base of the hair shaft proliferate, the hair grows to the surface of the epithelium. Very fine hairs, called lanugo, appear first at 12 weeks on the eyebrows and upper lip. By 20 weeks, they cover the entire body. At this time, the eyelashes, eyebrows, and scalp hair are beginning to grow. By 28 weeks, the scalp hair is longer than the lanugo, which thins and may disappear by term gestation.

Fingernails and toenails develop from thickened epidermis at the tips of the digits beginning during the tenth week. They grow slowly. Fingernails usually reach the fingertips by 32 weeks, and toenails reach toe tips by 36 weeks.

IMMUNOLOGIC SYSTEM

During the third trimester, albumin and globulin are present in the fetus. The only immunoglobulin (Ig) that crosses the placenta, IgG, provides passive acquired immunity to specific bacterial toxins. The fetus produces IgM by the end of the first trimester. This is produced in response to blood group antigens, gram-negative enteric organisms, and some viruses. IgA is not produced by the fetus; however, colostrum, the precursor to breast milk, contains large amounts of IgA and can provide passive immunity to the neonate who is breastfed.

The normal term neonate can fight infection, but not as effectively as an older child. The preterm infant is at much greater risk for infection.

Table 6.1 summarizes embryonic and fetal development.

TABLE 6.1 Milestones in Human Development Before Birth Since Last Menstrual Period (LMP)		
4 Weeks	**8 Weeks**	**12 Weeks**
External Appearance		
Body flexed, C shaped; arm and leg buds present; head at right angles to body	Body fairly well formed; nose flat, eyes far apart; digits well formed; head elevating; tail almost disappeared; eyes, ears, nose, and mouth recognizable	Nails appearing; resembles a human; head erect but disproportionately large; skin pink, delicate
Crown-to-Rump Measurement; Weight		
0.4–0.5 cm; 0.4 g	2.5–3 cm; 2 g	6–9 cm; 19 g

Continued

TABLE 6.1   Milestones in Human Development Before Birth Since Last Menstrual Period (LMP)—cont'd

4 Weeks	8 Weeks	12 Weeks
Gastrointestinal System Stomach at midline and fusiform; conspicuous liver; esophagus short; intestine a short tube	Intestinal villi developing; small intestines coil within umbilical cord; palatal folds present; liver very large	Bile secreted; palatal fusion complete; intestines have withdrawn from cord and assume characteristic positions
Musculoskeletal System All somites present	First indication of ossification—occiput, mandible, and humerus; fetus capable of some movement; definitive muscles of trunk, limbs, and head well represented	Some bones well outlined, ossification spreading; upper cervical to lower sacral arches and bodies ossify; smooth muscle layers indicated in hollow viscera
Circulatory System Heart develops, double chambers visible, begins to beat; aortic arch and major veins completed	Main blood vessels assume final plan; enucleated red cells predominate in blood	Blood forming in marrow
Respiratory System Primary lung buds appear	Pleural and pericardial cavities forming; branching bronchioles; nostrils closed by epithelial plugs	Lungs acquire definite shape; vocal cords appear
Renal System Rudimentary ureteral buds appear	Earliest secretory tubules differentiating; bladder-urethra separates from rectum	Kidneys able to secrete urine; bladder expands as a sac
Nervous System Well-marked midbrain flexure; no hindbrain or cervical flexures; neural groove closed	Cerebral cortex begins to acquire typical cells; differentiation of cerebral cortex, meninges, ventricular foramina, cerebrospinal fluid circulation; spinal cord extends entire length of spine	Brain structural configuration almost complete; cord shows cervical and lumbar enlargements; fourth ventricle foramina are developed; sucking present
Sensory Organs Eye and ear appearing as optic vessel and otocyst	Primordial choroid plexuses develop; ventricles large relative to cortex; development progressing; eyes converging rapidly; internal ears developing	Earliest taste buds indicated; characteristic organization of eyes attained
Genital System Genital ridge appears (fifth week)	Testes and ovaries distinguishable; external genitalia sexless but begin to differentiate	Sex recognizable; internal and external sex organs specific

16 Weeks	20 Weeks	24 Weeks
External Appearance Head still dominant; face looks human; eyes, ears, and nose approach typical appearance on gross examination; arm/leg ratio proportionate; scalp hair appears	Vernix caseosa appears; lanugo appears; legs lengthen considerably; sebaceous glands appear	Body lean but fairly well proportioned; skin red and wrinkled; vernix caseosa present; sweat glands forming

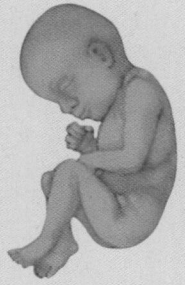

Crown-to-Rump Measurement; Weight 11.5–13.5 cm; 100 g	16–18.5 cm; 300 g	23 cm; 600 g
Gastrointestinal System Meconium in bowel; some enzyme secretion; anus open	Enamel and dentine depositing; ascending colon recognizable	

TABLE 6.1 Milestones in Human Development Before Birth Since Last Menstrual Period (LMP)—cont'd

16 Weeks	20 Weeks	24 Weeks
Musculoskeletal System Most bones distinctly indicated throughout body; joint cavities appear; muscular movements can be detected	Sternum ossifies; fetal movements strong enough for mother to feel	
Circulatory System Heart muscle well developed; blood formation active in spleen		Blood formation increases in bone marrow and decreases in liver
Respiratory System Elastic fibers appear in lungs; terminal and respiratory bronchioles appear	Nostrils reopen; primitive respiratory-like movements begin	Alveolar ducts and sacs present; lecithin begins to appear in amniotic fluid (weeks 26–27)
Renal System Kidneys in position; attain typical shape		
Nervous System Cerebral lobes delineated; cerebellum assumes some prominence	Brain grossly formed; cord myelination begins; spinal cord ends at level of first sacral vertebra (S-1)	Cerebral cortex layered typically; neuronal proliferation in cerebral cortex ends
Sensory Organs General sense organs differentiated	Nose and ears ossify	Can hear
Genital System Testes in position for descent into scrotum; vagina open		Testes at inguinal ring in descent to scrotum

28 Weeks	30–31 Weeks	36 and 40 Weeks
External Appearance Lean body, less wrinkled and red; nails appear	Subcutaneous fat beginning to collect; more rounded appearance; skin pink and smooth; has assumed birth position	**36 Weeks** Skin pink, body rounded; general lanugo disappearing; body usually plump **40 Weeks** Skin smooth and pink; scant vernix caseosa; moderate to profuse hair; lanugo on shoulders and upper body only; nasal and alar cartilage apparent
Crown-to-Rump Measurement; Weight 27 cm; 1100 g	31 cm; 1800–2100 g	**36 Weeks** 35 cm; 2200–2900 g **40 Weeks** 40 cm; 3200+ g
Musculoskeletal System Astragalus (talus, ankle bone) ossifies; weak, fleeting movements, minimum tone	Middle fourth phalanxes ossify; permanent teeth primordia seen; can turn head to side	**36 Weeks** Distal femoral ossification centers present; sustained, definite movements; fair tone; can turn and elevate head **40 Weeks** Active, sustained movement; good tone; may lift head
Respiratory System Lecithin forming on alveolar surfaces	L/S ratio = 1.2:1	**36 Weeks** L/S ratio ≥2:1 **40 Weeks** Pulmonary branching only two-thirds complete

Continued

TABLE 6.1   Milestones in Human Development Before Birth Since Last Menstrual Period (LMP)—cont'd

28 Weeks	30–31 Weeks	36 and 40 Weeks
Renal System		**36 Weeks** Formation of new nephrons ceases
Nervous System Appearance of cerebral fissures, convolutions rapidly appearing; indefinite sleep-wake cycle; cry weak or absent; weak suck reflex		**36 Weeks** End of spinal cord at level of third lumbar vertebra (L-3); definite sleep-wake cycle **40 Weeks** Myelination of brain begins; patterned sleep-wake cycle with alert periods; cries when hungry or uncomfortable; strong suck reflex
Sensory Organs Eyelids reopen; retinal layers completed, light receptive; pupils capable of reacting to light	Sense of taste present; aware of sounds outside mother's body	
Genital System	Testes descending to scrotum	**40 Weeks** Testes in scrotum; labia majora well developed

MULTIFETAL PREGNANCY

TWINS

The incidence of twinning is 1 in 43 pregnancies. There has been a steady rise in multiple births since 1973, partly attributed to the availability of assisted reproductive technologies and the increasing age at which women give birth (Benirschke, 2014). The twin rate was at its highest incidence in 2014 but then declined in 2015 (Martin, Hamilton, Osterman, et al., 2017) . This is partly attributed to the availability of assisted reproductive technologies and the increasing age at which women give birth as well as use of ovulation-enhancing drugs (Benirschke, 2014).

Dizygotic Twins

When two mature ova are produced in one ovarian cycle, both have the potential to be fertilized by separate sperm. This results in two zygotes, or dizygotic twins (Fig. 6.16). There are always two amnions, two chorions, and two placentas that may be fused (Fig. 6.17). These dizygotic or fraternal twins may be the same sex or different sexes and are genetically no more alike than siblings born at different times. Dizygotic twinning occurs in families with a history of twinning, more often among African-American women than Caucasian women, and least often among Asian-American women. Dizygotic twinning increases in frequency with maternal age up to 35 years, with parity, and with the use of fertility drugs.

Monozygotic Twins

Identical or monozygotic twins develop from one fertilized ovum, which then divides (Fig. 6.18). They are the same sex and have the same genotype. If division occurs soon after fertilization, two embryos, two amnions, two chorions, and two placentas that may be fused will develop. Most often, division occurs between 4 and 8 days after fertilization, and there are two embryos, two amnions, one chorion, and one placenta. Rarely, division occurs after the eighth day after fertilization. In this case, there are two embryos within a common amnion and a common chorion with one placenta. This often causes circulatory problems because the umbilical cords may tangle together and one or both fetuses may die. If division occurs very late, cleavage may not be complete and

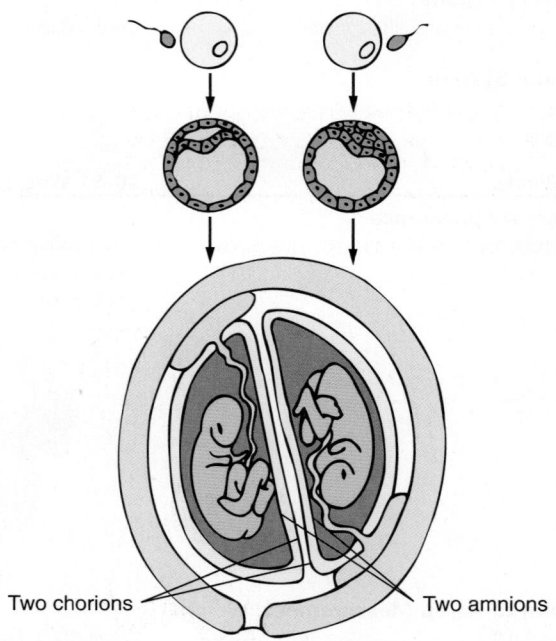

Two chorions   Two amnions

FIG 6.16 Formation of dizygotic twins. There is fertilization of two ova, two implantations, two placentas, two chorions, and two amnions.

conjoined or "Siamese" twins may result. Monozygotic twinning occurs in approximately 3.5 to 4 per 1000 births (Benirschke, 2014). There is no association with race, heredity, maternal age, or parity. Fertility drugs increase the incidence of monozygotic twinning.

Conjoined Twins

Conjoined twins are a type of monozygotic twins in which there is incomplete embryonic division at 13 to 15 days postconception (see Fig. 6.18). The estimated frequency is 1.5 in 100,000 births (Malone & D'Alton, 2014). Prenatal diagnosis is possible with three-dimensional ultrasonography. Cesarean birth minimizes trauma to mother and fetuses.

OTHER MULTIFETAL PREGNANCIES

The occurrence of multifetal pregnancies with three or more fetuses has increased with the use of fertility drugs and in vitro fertilization, but in 2015 it decreased by 9% from the previous year to 103.6 triplets per 100,000 births (Martin et al., 2017). They can occur from the division of one zygote into two, with one of the two dividing again, producing identical triplets. Triplets can also be produced (1) from two zygotes, one dividing into a set of identical twins and the second zygote a single fraternal sibling or (2) from three zygotes. Quadruplets, quintuplets, sextuplets, and so on have similar possible derivations.

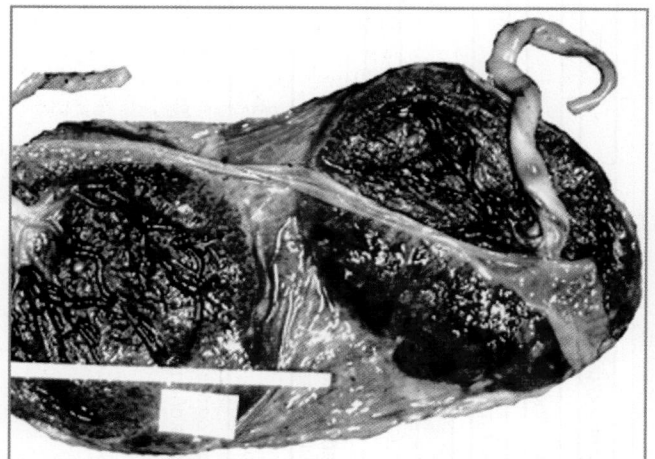

FIG 6.17 Diamniotic dichorionic (separate) twin placentas. (From Benirschke, K. [2014]. Multiple gestation: The biology of twinning. In Creasy, R., Resnik, R., Iams, J., et al. [eds.]. *Creasy & Resnik's maternal-fetal medicine: Principles and practice* [7th ed.] Philadelphia, PA: Saunders.)

NONGENETIC FACTORS INFLUENCING DEVELOPMENT

Congenital disorders may be inherited or may be caused by environmental factors or by inadequate maternal nutrition. *Congenital* means that the condition was present at birth. Some congenital malformations may be the result of teratogens, that is, environmental substances or exposures that result in functional or structural disability. In contrast to other forms of developmental disabilities, disabilities caused by teratogens are theoretically totally preventable. Known human teratogens are drugs and chemicals, infections, exposure to radiation, and certain maternal conditions such as diabetes and PKU (Box 6.2). A teratogen has the greatest effect on the organs and parts of an embryo during its periods of rapid growth and differentiation. This occurs during the embryonic period, specifically from days 15 to 60. During the first 2 weeks of development, teratogens either have no effect on the embryo or have effects so severe that they cause miscarriage. Brain growth and development continue during the fetal period, and teratogens can severely affect mental development throughout gestation (Fig. 6.19).

In addition to genetic makeup and the influence of teratogens, the adequacy of maternal nutrition influences development. The embryo and fetus must obtain the nutrients they need from the mother's diet; they cannot tap the maternal reserves. Malnutrition during pregnancy produces low–birth-weight (LBW) newborns who are susceptible to infection. Malnutrition also affects brain development during the latter half of gestation and can result in learning disabilities in the child. Inadequate folic acid is associated with neural tube defects.

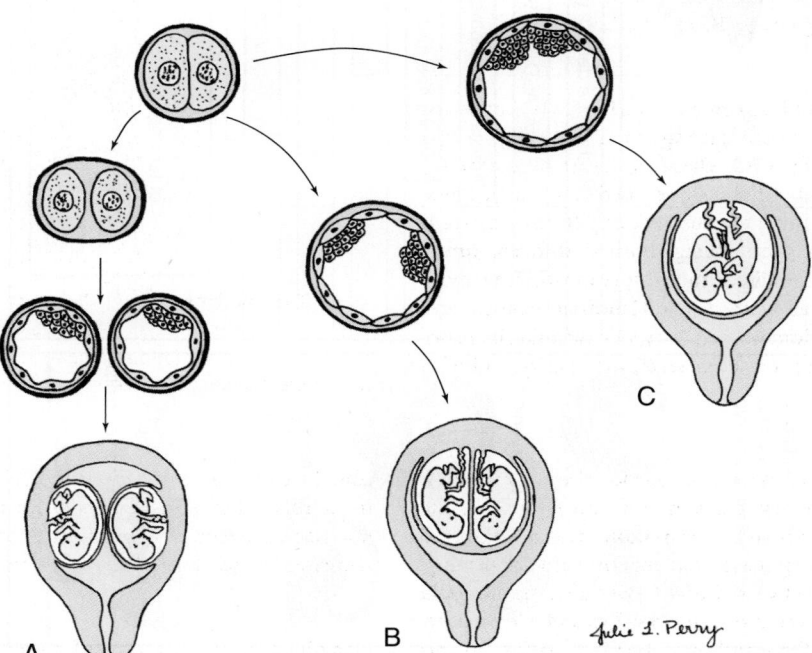

FIG 6.18 Formation of monozygotic twins. **A,** One fertilization: blastomeres separate, resulting in two implantations, two placentas, and two sets of membranes. **B,** One blastomere with two inner cell masses, one fused placenta, one chorion, and separate amnions. **C,** One blastomere with incomplete separation of cell mass resulting in conjoined twins.

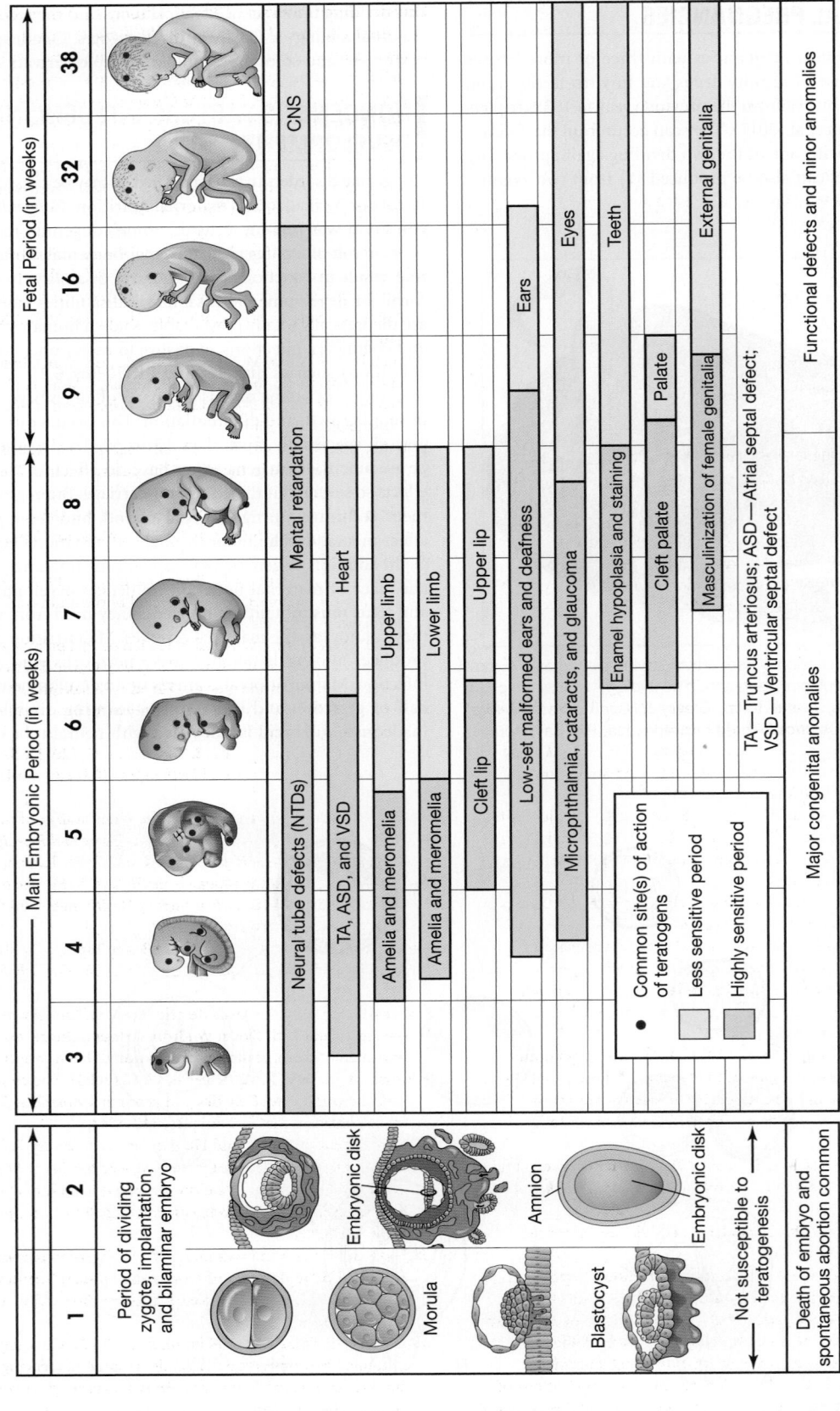

FIG 6.19 Critical periods in human development. *Dark color* denotes highly sensitive periods; *light color* indicates stages that are less sensitive to teratogens. *CNS,* Central nervous system. (From Moore, K.L., Persaud, T.V.N., Torchia, M.G. [2013]. *Before we are born: Essentials of embryology and birth defects* [8th ed.]. Philadelphia, PA: Saunders.)

BOX 6.2   Etiology of Human Malformations

Environmental
- Maternal conditions
  - Alcoholism, diabetes, endocrinopathies, phenylketonuria, smoking, nutritional problems
- Infectious agents
  - Rubella, toxoplasmosis, syphilis, herpes simplex, cytomegalic inclusion disease, varicella, Venezuelan equine encephalitis
- Mechanical problems (deformations)
  - Amniotic band constrictions, umbilical cord constraint, disparity in uterine size and uterine contents
- Chemicals, drugs, radiation, hyperthermia

Genetic
- Single-gene disorders
- Chromosomal abnormalities

Unknown
- Polygenic/multifactorial (gene-environment interactions)
- "Spontaneous" errors of development
- Other unknowns

Modified from Parikh, A.S., Mitchell, A.L. (2015). Congenital anomalies. In Martin, R.J., Fanaroff, A.A., Walsh, M.C. (Eds.), *Fanaroff and Martin's neonatal-perinatal medicine: Diseases of the fetus and infant* (10th ed.). Philadelphia, PA: Saunders.

REFERENCES

American College of Obstetricians and Gynecologists. (2011a). Family history as a risk assessment tool. *Obstetrics and Gynecology, 117*(3), 747–750.

American College of Obstetricians and Gynecologists. (2011b). *Update on carrier screening for cystic fibrosis.* Retrieved from http://www.acog.org/Resources-And-Publications/Committee-Opinions/Committee-on-Genetics/Update-on-Carrier-Screening-for-Cystic-Fibrosis.

Badzek, L., Henaghan, M., Turner, M., & Monsen, R. (2013). Ethical, legal, and social issues in the translation of genomics into health care. *Journal of Nursing Scholarship, 45*(1), 15–24.

Beery, T. (2013). Genetic and genomic testing in clinical practice: What you need to know. *Rehabilitation Nursing, 39*(2), 1–6.

Benirschke, K. (2014). Multiple gestation: The biology of twinning. In R. Creasy, R. Resnik, J. Iams, et al. (Eds.), *Creasy and Resnik's maternal-fetal medicine: Principles and practice* (7th ed.). Philadelphia, PA: Saunders.

Bodurtha, J., & Strauss, J. F. (2012). Genomics and perinatal care. *New England Journal of Medicine, 366*(1), 64–73.

Calzone, K. A., Jenkins, J., Nicoli, N., et al. (2013). Relevance of genomics to healthcare and nursing practice. *Journal of Nursing Scholarship, 45*(1), 1–2.

Centers for Disease Control and Prevention. (2016). *Facts about Down syndrome.* Retrieved from www.cdc.gov/ncbddd/birthdefects/DownSyndrome.html.

Conley, Y., Biesecker, L. G., Gonsalves, S., et al. (2013). Current and emerging technology approaches in genomics. *Journal of Nursing Scholarship, 45*(1), 5–14.

Cunningham, F., Leveno, K., Bloom, S., et al. (2014). *Williams' obstetrics* (24th ed.). New York: McGraw-Hill.

DeLuca, J., Zanni, K. L., Bonhomme, N., & Kemper, A. R. (2013). Implications of newborn screening for nurses. *Journal of Nursing Scholarship, 45*(1), 25–33.

ENCODE Project. (2016). *ENcyclopedia Of DNA Elements.* National Human Genome Research Institute, National Institutes of Health, Bethesda, MD. Retrieved from https://www.genome.gov/10005107/encode-project/.

Frazer, K. L., Porter, S., & Goss, C. (2013). The genetics and implications of neuromuscular diseases in pregnancy. *The Journal of Perinatal & Neonatal Nursing, 27*(3), 205–214, quiz 215–216.

Genetics Home Reference. (2017a). What were some of the ethical, legal, and social implications addressed by the Human Genome Project? *National Library of Medicine.* https://ghr.nlm.nih.gov/primer/hgp/elsi.

Genetics Home Reference. (2017b). Trisomy 13. *National Library of Medicine.* https://ghr.nlm.nih.gov/condition/trisomy-13#statistics.

Genetics Home Reference. (2017c). Turner syndrome. *National Library of Medicine.* https://ghr.nlm.nih.gov/condition/turner-syndrome#genes.

Gever, J. (2015). *Update: Direct-to-Consumer genetic testing. Medpage Today.* Retrieved from http://www.medpagetoday.com/genetics/genetictesting/55439.

Greco, K. E., Tinley, S., & Seibert, D. (2011). *Essential genetic and genomic competencies for nurses with graduate degrees.* Consensus Panel, Silver Springs, MD: American Nurses Association.

Johnson, N. L., Giarelli, E., Lewis, C., & Rice, C. E. (2013). Genomics and autism spectrum disorder. *Journal of Nursing Scholarship, 45*(1), 69–78.

Kaiser Permanente. (2017). Prenatal ultrasound findings: What is a single umbilical artery? *Kaiser Genetics Department.* https://mydoctor.kaiserpermanente.org/ncal/Images/GEN_US%20SUA%20handout_tcm63-10027.pdf.

Malone, F., & D'Alton, M. (2014). Multiple gestation: Clinical characteristics and management. In R. Creasy, R. Resnik, J. Iams, et al. (Eds.), *Creasy and Resnik's maternal-fetal medicine: Principles and practice* (7th ed.). Philadelphia, PA: Saunders.

Manolio, T. A., Chisholm, R. L., Ozenberger, B., et al. (2013). Implementing genomic medicine in the clinic: The future is here. *Genetics in Medicine, 15*(4), 258–267.

Martin, J. A., Hamilton, B. E., Osterman, M. J. K., Driscoll, A. K., & Mathews, T. J. (2017). Births: Final data for 2015. *National Vital Statistics Reports, 66*(1), 1–69.

McCarthy, J. J., McLeod, H. L., & Ginsburg, G. S. (2013). Genomic medicine: A decade of successes, challenges, and opportunities. *Science Translational Medicine, 5*(189), 1–17.

Mercer, B. (2014). Assessment and induction of fetal pulmonary maturity. In R. Creasy, R. Resnik, J. Iams, et al. (Eds.), *Creasy and Resnik's maternal-fetal medicine: Principles and practice* (7th ed.). Philadelphia, PA: Saunders.

Moore, D. S. (2015). *The developing genome: An introduction to behavioral epigenetics.* Oxford University Press.

Moore, K. L., Persaud, T. V. N., & Torchia, M. G. (2013). *Before we are born. Essentials of embryology and birth defects* (8th ed.). Philadelphia, PA: Saunders.

Mor, G., Abrahams, V., et al. (2014). The immunology of pregnancy. In R. Creasy, R. Resnik, & J. Iams (Eds.), *Creasy and Resnik's maternal-fetal medicine: Principles and practice* (7th ed.). Philadelphia, PA: Saunders.

National Human Genome Research Institute. (2016). *The cost of sequencing a human genome. National Institutes of Health.* Retrieved from https://www.genome.gov/sequencingcosts/.

Prows, C. A., Hopkin, R. J., Barnoy, S., & Van Riper, M. (2013). An update of childhood genetic disorders. *Journal of Nursing Scholarship, 45*(1), 34–42.

Sole-Smith, V. (2014). Doctors describe some of the known risk factors for having a child with Down syndrome. *Parents.* Retrieved from http://www.parents.com/health/down-syndrome/down-syndrome-risks/.

Solomon, B. D., Jack, B. W., & Feero, W. G. (2008). The clinical content of preconception care: Genetics and genomics. *American Journal of Obstetrics and Gynecology, 199*(6; 2 suppl), S340–S344.

US Department of Health and Human Services. (2016). *Table of pharmacogenomics biomarkers in drug labeling.* Silver Springs, MD: Food and Drug Administration. Retrieved from http://www.fda.gov/Drugs/ScienceResearch/ResearchAreas/Pharmacogenetics/ucm083378.htm.

US Food and Drug Administration. (2016). *Precision medicine. Science and research.* US Department of Health and Human Services. Retrieved from http://www.fda.gov/ScienceResearch/SpecialTopics/PrecisionMedicine/default.htm.

Wade, C. H., Tarini, B. A., & Wilfond, B. S. (2013). Growing up in the genomic era: Implications of whole-genome sequencing for children, families, and pediatric practice. *Annual Review of Genomics and Human Genetics, 14*, 535–555.

Wilke, D. J., Gallo, A. M., Yao, Y., et al. (2013). Reproductive health choices for young adults with sickle cell disease or trait: Randomized controlled trial immediate posttest effects. *Nursing Research, 62*(5), 352–361.

7

Anatomy and Physiology of Pregnancy

Kathryn R. Alden

http://evolve.elsevier.com/Perry/maternal

The goal of maternity care is a healthy pregnancy with a physically safe and emotionally satisfying outcome for mother, infant, and family. Consistent health supervision and surveillance are of utmost importance. Moreover, many maternal adaptations are unfamiliar to pregnant women and their families. Helping the pregnant woman recognize the relationship between her physical status and the plan for her care can enhance her ability to be an active participant in care management along with members of the interprofessional health care team.

GRAVIDITY AND PARITY

An understanding of the following terms used to describe pregnancy and the pregnant woman is essential to the study of maternity care:

Gravida: A woman who is pregnant
Gravidity: Pregnancy
Nulligravida: A woman who has never been pregnant and is not currently pregnant
Primigravida: A woman who is pregnant for the first time
Multigravida: A woman who has had two or more pregnancies
Parity: The number of pregnancies in which the fetus or fetuses have reached 20 weeks of gestation, not the number of fetuses (e.g., twins) born. Parity is not affected by whether the fetus is born alive or is stillborn (i.e., showing no signs of life at birth).
Nullipara: A woman who has not completed a pregnancy with a fetus or fetuses who have reached at least 20 weeks of gestation
Primipara: A woman who has completed one pregnancy with a fetus or fetuses who have reached 20 weeks of gestation or more
Multipara: A woman who has completed two or more pregnancies to 20 weeks of gestation or more
Preterm: A pregnancy that has reached 20 weeks of gestation but ends before 37 weeks 0 days of gestation
Late preterm: A pregnancy that has reached between 34 weeks 0 days and 36 weeks 6 days of gestation
Early term: A pregnancy that has reached between 37 weeks 0 days and 38 weeks 6 days of gestation
Full term: A pregnancy that has reached between 39 weeks 0 days and 40 weeks 6 days of gestation
Late term: A pregnancy that has reached between 41 weeks 0 days and 41 weeks 6 days of gestation
Postterm: A pregnancy that has reached 42 weeks 0 days and beyond of gestation
Viability: The capacity to live outside the uterus; there are no clear limits of gestational age or weight. Infants born at 22 to 25 weeks of gestation are considered to be on the threshold of viability and are especially vulnerable to brain injury if they survive.

Gravidity and parity information is obtained during history-taking interviews. Obtaining and documenting this information accurately is important in planning care for a pregnant woman.

Information may be recorded in medical records in a variety of ways because no one standardized system exists. It is important that the nurse understand the documentation system used by the health care facility.

Two commonly used systems of summarizing the obstetric history are discussed here. Gravidity and parity may be described with only two digits: the first digit indicates the number of pregnancies the woman has had, including the present one, and parity the number of pregnancies that have reached 20 weeks or more of gestation. For example, the abbreviation gravida 1, para 0 (1/0) means that a woman is pregnant for the first time (primigravida) and has not carried a pregnancy to 20 weeks or more (nullipara). If a woman had twins at 36 weeks with her first pregnancy, she would be gravida 1, para 1.

Another system consisting of five digits is commonly used. The first digit represents gravidity (the number of pregnancies), the second digit represents the number of pregnancies that ended in term births (including early, full, late term, or postterm births) at 37 weeks 0 days and beyond, the third indicates the number of pregnancies that ended in preterm birth (between 20 weeks 0 days and 36 weeks 6 days gestation), the fourth identifies the number of pregnancies that ended in miscarriage (spontaneous abortion) or elective termination (therapeutic abortion) before 20 weeks, and the fifth is the number of children currently living. The acronym GTPAL (gravidity, term, preterm, abortions, living children) can be helpful in remembering this system of notation. For example, if a woman pregnant only once gives birth at week 35 and the infant survives, the abbreviation that represents this information is 1-0-1-0-1. During her next pregnancy the abbreviation is 2-0-1-0-1. Additional examples are in Table 7.1.

PREGNANCY TESTS

Early detection of pregnancy allows for early initiation of prenatal care. Human chorionic gonadotropin (hCG) is the earliest biologic marker for pregnancy. Pregnancy tests are based on the recognition of hCG or a beta (β) subunit of hCG. Production of β-hCG begins as early as the day of implantation and can be detected in maternal serum or urine as soon as 7 to 8 days before the expected menses. hCG levels usually double approximately every 2 days for the first 4 weeks of pregnancy. The hCG level rises until it peaks at 60 to 70 days and then declines to lowest levels at about 100 to 130 days as the placenta becomes the primary source of estrogen and progesterone. Plasma levels of hCG remain at this lower level for the remainder of the pregnancy. Higher

TABLE 7.1   Obstetric History Using Five-Digit and Two-Digit System

	FIVE-DIGIT SYSTEM					TWO-DIGIT SYSTEM
	G	T	P	A	L	G/P
Condition	Gravidity	Term Birth	Preterm Births	Abortions and Miscarriages	Living Children	Gravidity/Parity
Olivia is pregnant for the first time.	1	0	0	0	0	1/0
She carries the pregnancy to term, and the neonate survives.	1	1	0	0	1	1/1
She is pregnant again.	2	1	0	0	1	2/1
Her second pregnancy ends in miscarriage at 10 weeks.	2	1	0	1	1	2/1
During her third pregnancy, she gives birth at 36 weeks to twins.	3	1	1	1	3	3/2

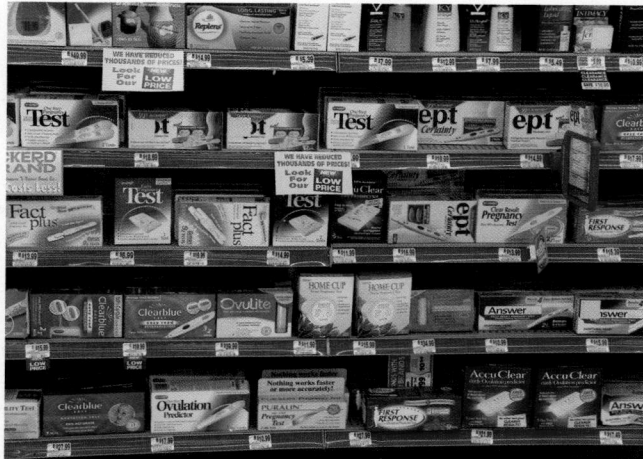

FIG 7.1 Many pregnancy test products are available over the counter. (Courtesy of Dee Lowdermilk, Chapel Hill, NC.)

than normal levels of hCG are associated with abnormal gestation (e.g., fetus with Down syndrome, gestational trophoblastic disease) or multiple gestation. An abnormally slow increase in hCG or lower levels can indicate impending miscarriage or ectopic pregnancy (Liu, 2014).

Serum and urine pregnancy tests are performed in clinics, offices, women's health centers, and laboratory settings. Urine tests can also be done at home. Both serum and urine tests can provide accurate results.

Quantitative serum testing—the β-hCG test—has a high level of accuracy because it measures the exact amount of hCG in the blood and can detect even small amounts. hCG levels greater than 25 International Units/L are diagnostic for pregnancy. For serum testing, a 7- to 10-mL sample of venous blood is collected (Pagana, Pagana, & Pagana, 2017).

Sandwich-type immunoassay testing is the most popular method of testing for pregnancy and is the basis for most home pregnancy tests. It uses a specific monoclonal antibody (anti-hCG) with enzymes that bond with hCG in urine. Many different pregnancy tests are available (Fig. 7.1). With these one-step tests, the woman usually applies urine to a strip or absorbent-tipped applicator and reads the results. The test kits come with directions for collection of the specimen, the testing procedure, and reading of results.

The accuracy of the results is related to following the instructions correctly (see Community Focus box). However, instructions for some home pregnancy tests do not comply with the recommended guidelines for use of plain language, and many instructions are written at a seventh-grade reading level or above, which limits understanding by some users. A positive test result is indicated by a simple color change reaction or a digital reading. Most manufacturers of the kits provide a toll-free telephone number to call if users have concerns or questions about test

CLINICAL REASONING CASE STUDY

Pregnancy Testing

When her menstrual period was 10 days late, Regine purchased a home pregnancy test on her way home from work and performed the test that evening. The result was negative. Regine and her partner have been trying to get pregnant so that the baby will be born when she is on summer break from her teaching job at the elementary school. She is disappointed that the test was negative and she calls the clinic to ask the nurse if she should come in for a blood test to see if she is pregnant.

1. Evidence—Is there sufficient evidence to draw conclusions about the advice the nurse should provide to Regine?
2. Assumptions—What assumptions can be made about the following issues?
   a. Proper use of home pregnancy tests
   b. Factors that can affect results of home pregnancy tests
   c. Human chorionic gonadotropin (hCG) levels in pregnancy
3. What are the implications and priorities for providing information to Regine?
4. Does the evidence objectively support your conclusion?

procedures or results. A common error in performing home pregnancy tests is doing the test too early in pregnancy before a significant rise in hCG level; this can cause a false-negative result (Pagana et al., 2017) (see Clinical Reasoning Case Study).

Interpreting the results of pregnancy tests requires some judgment. The type of pregnancy test and its degree of sensitivity (the ability to detect low levels of a substance) and specificity (the ability to discern the absence of a substance) must be considered in conjunction with the woman's history. This includes the date of her last normal menstrual period, her usual cycle length, and results of previous pregnancy tests. It is important to know about any medications or other substances she is taking. Medications such as anticonvulsants and tranquilizers can cause false-positive results, whereas diuretics and promethazine can

TABLE 7.2   Signs of Pregnancy

Time of Occurrence (Gestational Age)	Sign	Other Possible Cause
Presumptive		
3–4 weeks	Breast changes	Premenstrual changes, oral contraceptives
4 weeks	Amenorrhea	Stress, vigorous exercise, early menopause, endocrine problems, malnutrition
4–14 weeks	Nausea, vomiting	Gastrointestinal virus, food poisoning
6–12 weeks	Urinary frequency	Infection, pelvic tumors
12 weeks	Fatigue	Stress, illness
16–20 weeks	Quickening	Gas, peristalsis
Probable		
5 weeks	Goodell sign	Pelvic congestion
6–8 weeks	Chadwick sign	Pelvic congestion
6–12 weeks	Hegar sign	Pelvic congestion
4–12 weeks	Positive pregnancy test (serum)	Hydatidiform mole, choriocarcinoma
6–12 weeks	Positive pregnancy test (urine)	False-positive result may be caused by pelvic infection, tumors
16 weeks	Braxton Hicks contractions	Myomas, other tumors
16–28 weeks	Ballottement	Tumors, cervical polyps
Positive		
5–6 weeks	Visualization of fetus by real-time ultrasound examination	No other causes
6 weeks	Fetal heart tones detected by ultrasound	No other causes
16 weeks	Visualization of fetus by radiographic study	No other causes
8–17 weeks	Fetal heart tones detected by Doppler ultrasound stethoscope	No other causes
17–19 weeks	Fetal heart tones detected by fetal stethoscope	No other causes
19–22 weeks	Fetal movements palpated by examiner	No other causes
Late pregnancy	Fetal movements visible to examiner	No other causes

PATIENT TEACHING

Home Pregnancy Testing

1. Follow the manufacturer's instructions carefully. Do not omit steps.
2. Review the manufacturer's list of foods, medications, and other substances that can affect the test results.
3. Use a first-voided morning urine specimen.
4. If the test done at the time of your missed period is negative, repeat the test in 1 week if you still have not had a period.
5. If you have questions about the test, contact the manufacturer.
6. Contact your health care provider for follow-up if the test result is positive or if the test result is negative and you still have not had a period.

cause false-negative results (Pagana et al. 2017). Improper collection of the specimen, hormone-producing tumors, and laboratory errors can also cause inaccurate results.

Women who use a home pregnancy test should be advised about the variations in accuracy and to use caution when interpreting results. Whenever there is any question, further evaluation or retesting may be appropriate (see Patient Teaching box).

ADAPTATIONS TO PREGNANCY

Maternal physiologic adaptations are attributed to the hormones of pregnancy and to mechanical pressures arising from the enlarging uterus and other tissues. These adaptations protect the woman's normal physiologic functioning, meet the metabolic demands that pregnancy imposes on her body, and provide a nurturing environment for fetal development and growth. Although pregnancy is a normal phenomenon, problems can occur.

SIGNS OF PREGNANCY

Some physiologic adaptations are recognized as the signs and symptoms of pregnancy. Three commonly used categories of these signs and symptoms are as follows:

- **Presumptive**—Subjective changes reported by the woman (e.g., amenorrhea, fatigue, breast changes). These can be caused by conditions other than pregnancy.
- **Probable**—Objective changes assessed by an examiner (e.g., Hegar sign, ballottement, pregnancy tests). When combined with the presumptive signs and symptoms, these changes strongly suggest pregnancy.
- **Positive**—Objective signs assessed by an examiner that can be attributed only to the presence of the fetus (e.g., hearing fetal heart tones, visualizing the fetus, palpating fetal movements). These are definitive signs that confirm pregnancy.

Table 7.2 summarizes these signs of pregnancy in relation to when they might occur and gives other possible causes for their occurrence.

REPRODUCTIVE SYSTEM AND BREASTS

Uterus

Changes in Size, Shape, and Position

High levels of estrogen and progesterone stimulate phenomenal uterine growth in the first trimester. Early uterine enlargement results from increased vascularity and dilation of blood vessels, hyperplasia (production of new muscle fibers and fibroelastic tissue) and hypertrophy

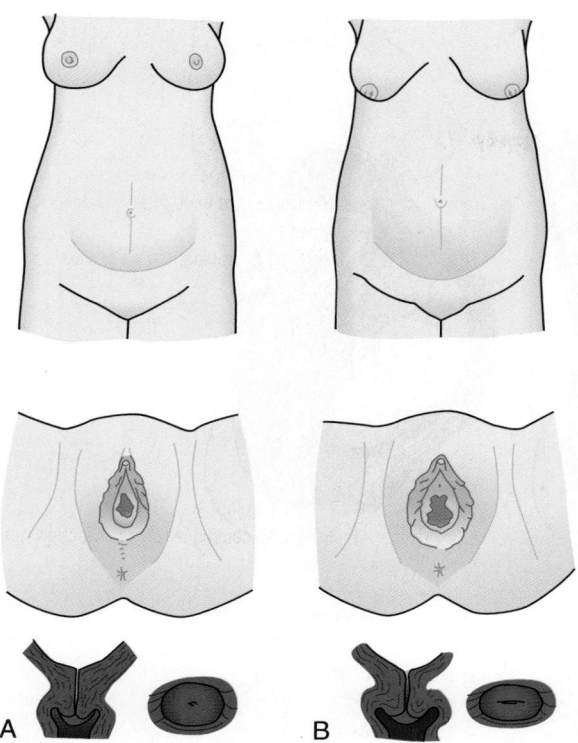

FIG 7.2 Comparison of abdomen, vulva, and cervix in **A,** nullipara, and **B,** multipara, at the same stage of pregnancy.

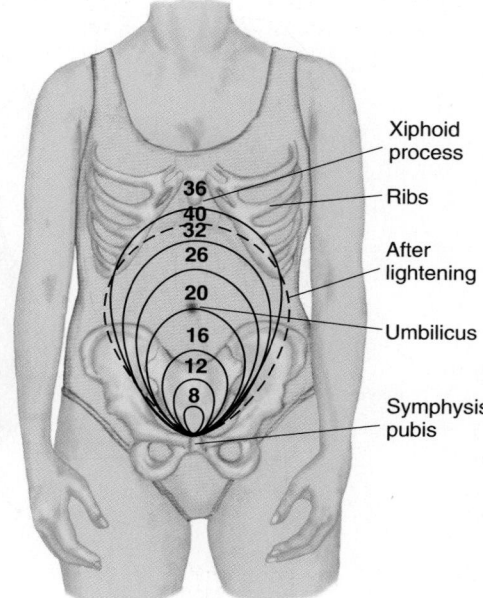

FIG 7.3 Height of fundus by weeks of normal gestation with a single fetus. *Dashed line,* Height after lightening. (From Leifer, G. [2012]. *Maternity nursing: An introductory text* [11th ed.]. St. Louis, MO: Saunders.)

(enlargement of preexisting muscle fibers and fibroelastic tissue), and development of the decidua. Uterine weight increases dramatically from 4 g to 70 g in the nonpregnant state to 1200 g at term gestation. Volume increases from 10 mL before pregnancy to 5 L at term. By 7 weeks of gestation, the uterus is the size of a large hen's egg; by 10 weeks, it is the size of an orange (twice its nonpregnant size); and by 12 weeks, it is the size of a grapefruit. After the third month, uterine enlargement is primarily the result of mechanical pressure of the growing fetus.

As the uterus enlarges, it also changes in shape and position. At conception the uterus is shaped like an upside-down pear. During the second trimester, as the muscular walls strengthen and become more elastic, the uterus becomes spherical or globular. Later, as the fetus lengthens, the uterus becomes larger and more ovoid and rises out of the pelvis into the abdominal cavity.

The pregnancy may "show" after the fourteenth week, although this depends to some degree on the woman's height and weight. Abdominal enlargement may be less apparent in the nullipara with good abdominal muscle tone (Fig. 7.2). Posture also influences the type and degree of abdominal enlargement that occurs. In normal pregnancies, the uterus enlarges at a predictable rate.

As the uterus grows, it can be palpated above the symphysis pubis sometime between the twelfth and fourteenth weeks of pregnancy (Fig. 7.3). The uterus rises gradually to the level of the umbilicus by 20 weeks of gestation and nearly reaches the xiphoid process at term. Between weeks 38 and 40, fundal height decreases as the fetus begins to descend into the pelvis (lightening) in preparation for birth (see Fig. 7.3, *dashed line*). Generally lightening occurs in the nullipara about 2 weeks before the onset of labor and in the multipara at the start of labor.

Uterine enlargement is determined by measuring fundal height (see Fig. 8.8). This measurement is commonly used to estimate the weeks of gestation. However, variations in the position of the fundus or the fetus, variations in the amount of amniotic fluid present, the presence

of more than one fetus, maternal obesity, and differences in examiner technique can reduce the accuracy of this estimation.

Generally the uterus rotates to the right as it enlarges and rises in the abdomen, probably because of the presence of the rectosigmoid colon on the left side. However, the extensive hypertrophy (enlargement) of the round ligaments keeps the uterus in the midline. Eventually the growing uterus touches the anterior abdominal wall and displaces the intestines to either side of the abdomen (Fig. 7.4). When a pregnant woman is standing, most of her uterus rests against the anterior abdominal wall and contributes to altering her center of gravity.

At approximately 6 weeks of gestation, softening and compressibility of the lower uterine segment (uterine isthmus) occurs (Hegar sign) (Fig. 7.5). This results in exaggerated uterine anteflexion during the first 3 months of pregnancy. In this position, the uterine fundus presses on the urinary bladder, causing the woman to have urinary frequency.

Changes in Contractility

Soon after the fourth month of pregnancy, uterine contractions may be felt through the abdominal wall. These are referred to as Braxton Hicks contractions. Braxton Hicks contractions are irregular and painless contractions that occur intermittently throughout pregnancy. Although Braxton Hicks contractions are not painful, some women complain that they are annoying. After the twenty-eighth week, these contractions become more definite, but they usually cease with walking or exercise. Braxton Hicks contractions can be mistaken for true labor; however, they do not increase in intensity or duration or cause cervical dilation. Conversely, premature labor contractions can be mistaken for Braxton Hicks contractions, which can lead to a delay in seeking treatment.

Uteroplacental Blood Flow

Placental perfusion depends on the maternal blood flow to the uterus. Uterine blood flow increases 10-fold over the course of pregnancy as the uterus increases in size. In a normal-term pregnancy, one sixth of the total maternal blood volume is within the uterine vascular system. The rate of blood flow through the uterus averages 450 to 650 mL/

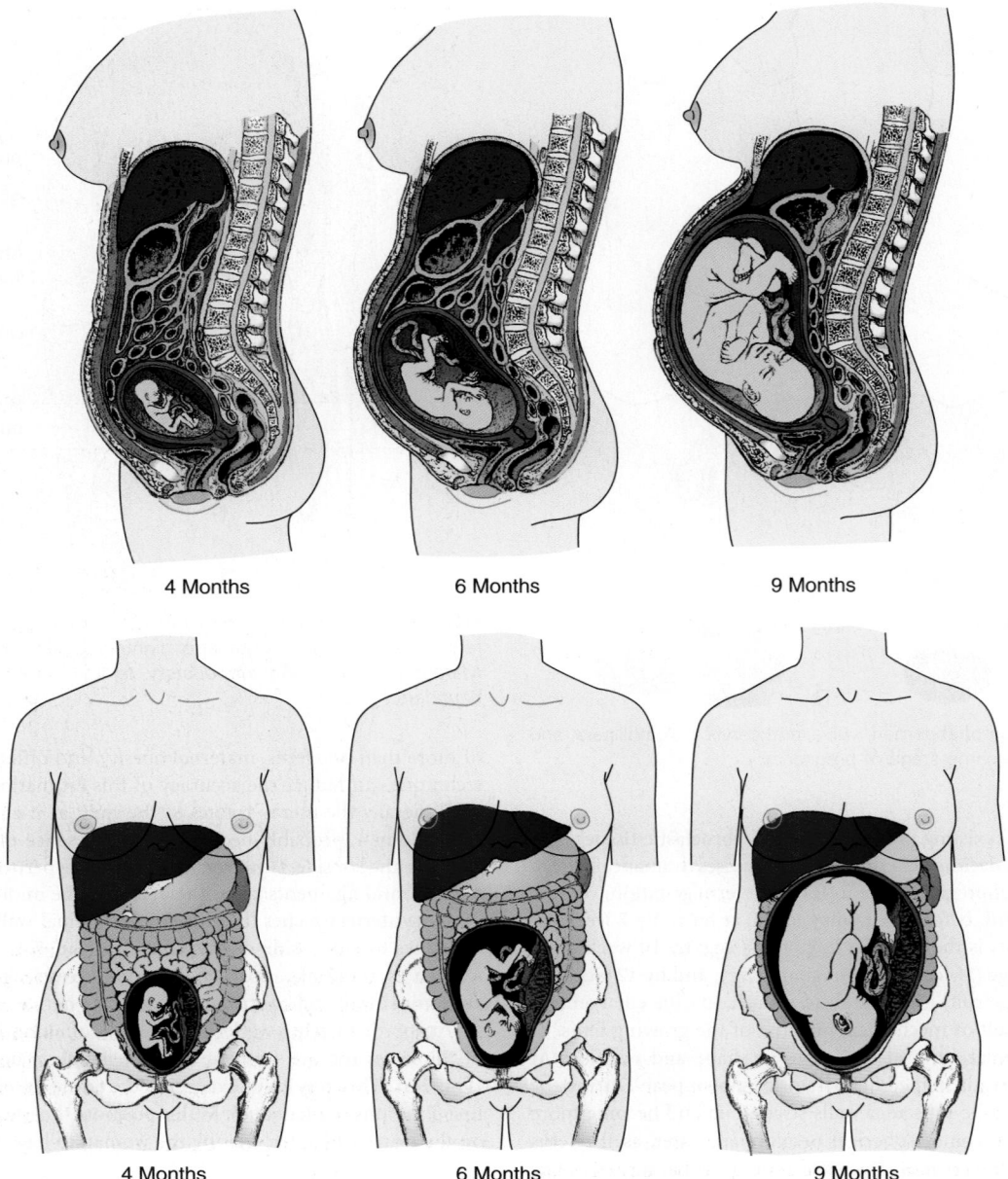

FIG 7.4 Displacement of internal abdominal structures and diaphragm by the enlarging uterus at 4, 6, and 9 months of gestation.

minute at term, and oxygen consumption of the gravid uterus increases to meet fetal needs, with the greatest consumption occurring during the last trimester when fetal growth is accelerated. Three factors known to decrease uterine blood flow are low maternal arterial pressure, uterine contractions, and maternal supine position. Estrogen stimulation can increase uterine blood flow. Doppler ultrasound examination may be used to measure uterine blood flow velocity, especially in pregnancies at risk because of conditions associated with decreased placental perfusion (e.g., hypertension, intrauterine growth restriction, diabetes mellitus, multiple gestation) (Blackburn, 2013).

By using an ultrasound device or a fetal stethoscope to auscultate fetal heart tones, the examiner may also hear the uterine souffle or bruit, a rushing or blowing sound of maternal blood flowing through uterine arteries to the placenta that is synchronous with the maternal pulse. The funic souffle, which is synchronous with the fetal heart rate

and is caused by fetal blood coursing through the umbilical cord, may also be heard, as well as the fetus's actual heartbeat (see Fig. 8.7).

Cervical Changes

The cervix consists primarily of collagen-rich connective tissue and is responsive to hormonal changes of pregnancy. This results in the cervix being a firm, nondistensible, closed structure that maintains the pregnancy and changing to a soft, highly elastic tissue that dilates and becomes almost indistinguishable during labor in preparation for birth.

In a normal, unscarred cervix, softening of the cervical tip can be observed about the beginning of the sixth week. This probable sign of pregnancy, Goodell sign, is due to increased vascularity, slight hypertrophy, and hyperplasia (increase in number of cells).

The glands near the external os proliferate beneath the stratified squamous epithelium, giving the cervix the velvety appearance

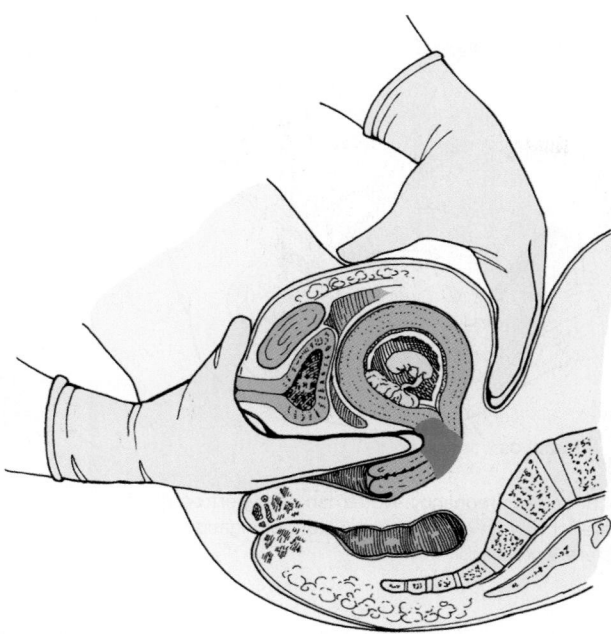

FIG 7.5 Hegar sign. Bimanual examination for assessing compressibility and softening of isthmus (lower uterine segment) while the cervix is still firm.

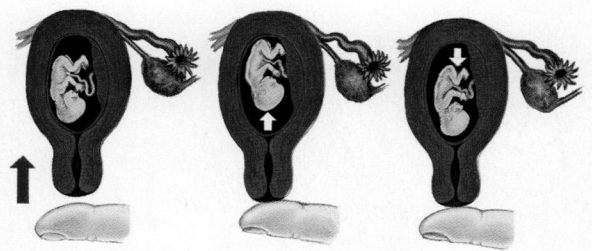

FIG 7.6 Internal ballottement (18 weeks).

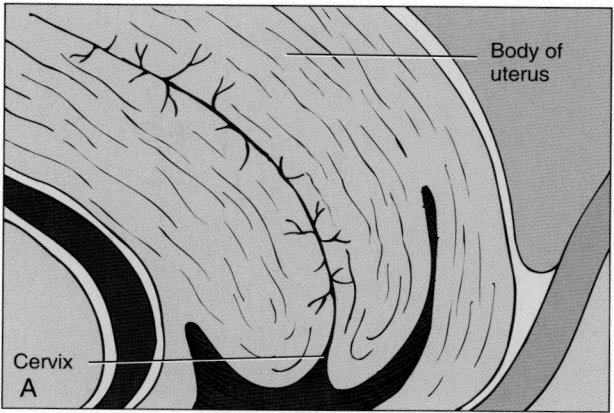

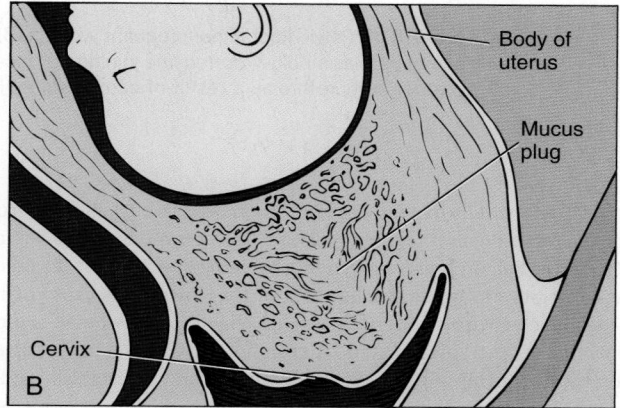

FIG 7.7 A, Cervix in nonpregnant woman. **B,** Cervix during pregnancy.

characteristic of pregnancy. Friability (tissue is easily damaged) is increased and can result in slight bleeding after vaginal examination or after coitus with deep penetration.

Pregnancy can also cause the squamocolumnar junction, the site for obtaining cells for cervical cancer screening, to be located away from the cervix. Because of these changes, evaluation of abnormal Papanicolaou (Pap) tests during pregnancy can be complicated. However, careful assessment of all pregnant women is important because cervical cancer is the most common gynecologic malignancy occurring during pregnancy. Approximately 3% of all invasive cervical cancers occur during pregnancy (Salani, Billingsley, & Crafton, 2014).

The cervix of the nullipara is rounded. Lacerations of the cervix can occur during the birth process. After birth, with or without lacerations, the cervix becomes more oval in the horizontal plane and the external os appears as a transverse slit (see Fig. 7.2).

Changes Related to the Presence of the Fetus

Passive movement of the unengaged fetus is called ballottement and can be identified by the examiner generally between the sixteenth and eighteenth weeks. Ballottement is a technique of palpating a floating structure by bouncing it gently and feeling it rebound. To palpate the fetus, the examiner places a finger within the vagina and taps gently upward on the cervix, causing the fetus to rise. The fetus then sinks, and a gentle tap is felt on the finger (Fig. 7.6).

Quickening is the first recognition of fetal movements, or "feeling life." It can be detected by the multiparous woman as early as 14 to 16 weeks of gestation. The nulliparous woman may not notice these sensations until the eighteenth week or later. Quickening is commonly described as a flutter and is difficult to distinguish from peristalsis. Fetal movements gradually increase in intensity and frequency as pregnancy progresses. The week in which quickening occurs provides a tentative clue in dating the duration of gestation.

Vagina and Vulva

Pregnancy hormones prepare the vagina for stretching during labor and birth by causing the vaginal mucosa to thicken, the connective tissue to loosen, the smooth muscle to hypertrophy, and the vaginal vault to lengthen. Increased vascularity results in a violet-blue vaginal mucosa and cervix. This is known as the Chadwick sign and can be evident as early as the sixth week but is easily noted by the eighth week of pregnancy.

Leukorrhea is a white or slightly gray mucoid vaginal discharge with a faint musty odor. This copious mucoid fluid occurs in response to cervical stimulation by estrogen and progesterone. The fluid is whitish because of the presence of many exfoliated vaginal epithelial cells caused by the hyperplasia of normal pregnancy. This normal vaginal discharge is never pruritic or blood stained. The mucus fills the endocervical canal, resulting in the formation of the mucus plug (operculum) (Fig. 7.7). The operculum acts as a barrier against bacterial invasion of the uterus during pregnancy.

The vaginal microbiome changes during pregnancy with an increase in at least four species of *Lactobacillus* and a decrease in anaerobic

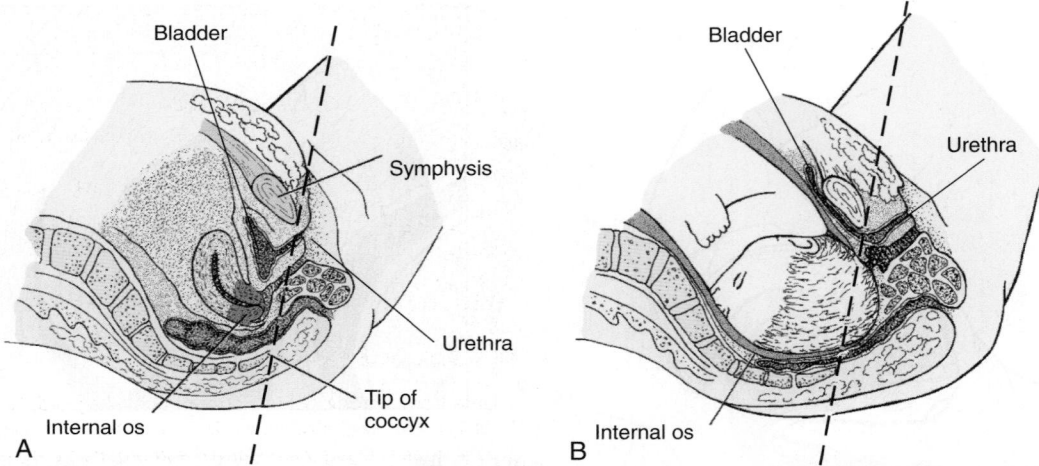

FIG 7.8 A, Pelvic floor in nonpregnant woman. **B,** Pelvic floor at end of pregnancy. Note marked hypertrophy and hyperplasia below *dotted line* joining tip of coccyx and inferior margin of symphysis. Note elongation of bladder and urethra as a result of compression. Fat deposits are increased.

bacteria. This results in a lower pH of vaginal secretions, ranging from about 3.5 to 6.0 (nonpregnant, 4.0 to 5.0). Alterations in the vaginal microbiome help to prevent ascending bacterial infections of the uterus that contribute to preterm labor and birth. However, because of the glycogen-rich environment of the vagina, the pregnant woman is more vulnerable to other infections such as candidiasis. Changes in the vaginal microbiome during pregnancy may be important in establishing the upper gastrointestinal microbiota of the neonate (Prince, Antony, Ma, et al., 2014; Romero, Hassan, Gajer, et al., 2014).

The increased vascularity of the vagina and other pelvic viscera results in heightened sensitivity that can lead to a high degree of sexual interest and arousal, especially during the second trimester of pregnancy. The increased congestion, plus the relaxed walls of the blood vessels and the heavy uterus, can result in edema and varicosities of the vulva. The edema and varicosities usually resolve during the postpartum period.

External structures of the perineum are enlarged during pregnancy because of increased vascularity, hypertrophy of the perineal body, and deposition of fat (Fig. 7.8). The labia majora of nulliparous women approximate (come together) and obscure the vaginal introitus; those of the parous woman separate and gape after childbirth and perineal or vaginal injury. See Fig. 7.2 for a comparison of the nullipara and the multipara in relation to the pregnant abdomen, vulva, and cervix.

Breasts

Fullness, heightened sensitivity, tingling, and heaviness of the breasts begin in the early weeks of gestation in response to increased levels of estrogen and progesterone. Breast sensitivity varies from mild tingling to sharp pain. Nipples and areolae become more pigmented; secondary pinkish areolae develop, extending beyond the primary areolae; and nipples become more erectile. Hypertrophy of Montgomery tubercles may be seen around the nipples. These sebaceous (oil) glands embedded in the primary areolae secrete lubricating and antiinfective substances to help protect the nipples and areolae during breastfeeding.

The richer blood supply to the breasts causes the vessels beneath the skin to dilate. Once barely noticeable, the blood vessels become visible, often appearing in an intertwining bluish network beneath the surface of the skin. Venous congestion in the breasts is more obvious in primigravidas. Striae gravidarum, or stretch marks, can appear at the outer aspects of the breasts.

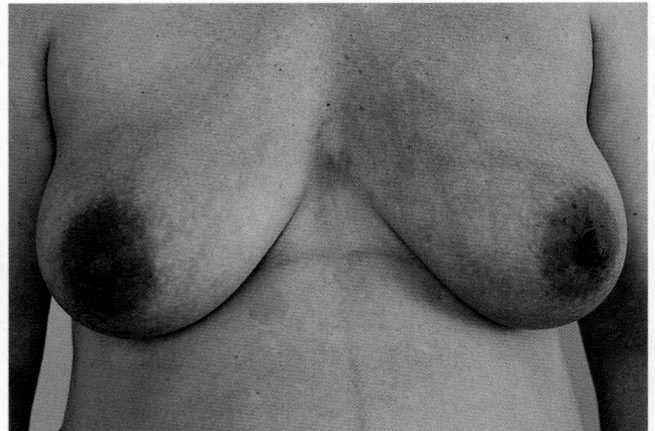

FIG 7.9 Enlarged breasts in pregnancy with venous network and darkened areolae and nipples. (From Ball, J.W., Dains, J.E, Flynn, J.A., et al. [2015]. *Mosby's guide to physical examination* [8th ed.]. St. Louis, MO: Mosby.)

During the second and third trimesters, growth of the mammary glands accounts for the progressive breast enlargement (Fig. 7.9). The high levels of luteal and placental hormones in pregnancy promote proliferation of the lactiferous ducts and lobule-alveolar tissue so that palpation of the breasts reveals a generalized coarse nodularity. Glandular tissue displaces connective tissue, resulting in the tissue becoming softer and looser.

Prolactin, produced by the anterior pituitary gland, stimulates production of colostrum by the end of the first trimester. During the second trimester, human placental lactogen stimulates secretion of colostrum. This is lactogenesis stage I. By the sixteenth week, the breasts are prepared for full lactation; as such, if a woman has a spontaneous or therapeutic abortion after this time, she will produce colostrum. Although development of the mammary glands is functionally complete by midpregnancy, lactation is inhibited until the progesterone level decreases after birth (Lawrence & Lawrence, 2016). See Chapter 24 for a discussion of lactation.

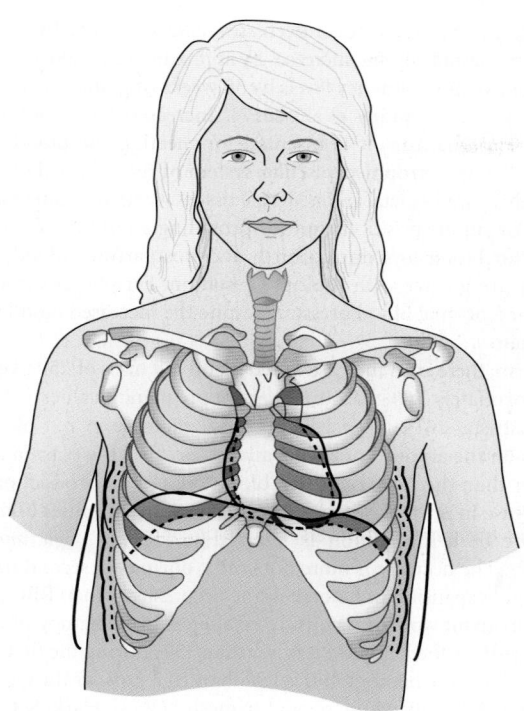

FIG 7.10 Changes in position of heart in pregnancy. *Broken line,* nonpregnant state; *solid line,* change that occurs in pregnancy.

TABLE 7.3 Cardiovascular Changes in Pregnancy	
Parameter	**Change**
Heart rate	Increases 15 to 20 beats/min
Blood pressure	
Systolic	Slight or no decrease from prepregnancy levels
Diastolic	Slight decrease to midpregnancy (24–32 weeks) and gradual return to prepregnancy levels by end of pregnancy
Blood volume	Increases by 1200–1500 mL or 40%–45% above prepregnancy level
Cardiac output	Increases 30%–50%

Data from Antony, K.M., Racusin, D.A., Aagaard, K., & Dildy, G.A. (2017). Maternal physiology. In S.G. Gabbe, J.R. Niebyl, J.L. Simpson, et al. (Eds.), *Obstetrics: Normal and problem pregnancies* (7th ed.), Philadelphia, PA: Elsevier.

GENERAL BODY SYSTEMS

Cardiovascular System

Maternal adjustments to pregnancy involve extensive anatomic and physiologic changes in the cardiovascular system. Cardiovascular adaptations protect the woman's normal physiologic functioning, meet the metabolic demands pregnancy imposes on her body, and provide for fetal developmental and growth needs.

Slight cardiac hypertrophy (enlargement) is probably secondary to increased blood volume and cardiac output that occur in pregnancy. The heart returns to its normal size within 6 months after birth (Antony, Racusin, Aagaard, et al., 2017). As the diaphragm is displaced upward by the enlarging uterus, the heart is elevated upward and rotated forward to the left (Fig. 7.10). The apical impulse, or point of maximal intensity (PMI), is shifted upward and laterally about 1 to 1.5 cm. The degree of shift depends on the duration of pregnancy and the size and position of the uterus.

The changes in heart size and position and the increases in blood volume and cardiac output contribute to common auscultatory changes. By the end of the first trimester, there is audible splitting of S_1 and S_2. The majority of pregnant women also have a third heart sound (S_3) after midpregnancy due to rapid diastolic filling. Approximately 96% of women develop systolic ejection murmurs which are most audible over the left sternal border. These auscultatory changes are transient and usually disappear shortly after birth (Antony et al., 2017).

Maternal heart rate begins to increase at about 5 weeks of gestation, reaching a peak of 15 to 20 beats/minute over the prepregnancy baseline by 32 weeks and persisting until term. This represents an increase of approximately 17% over the prepregnancy heart rate (Antony et al., 2017).

Pregnancy has limited effects on cardiac rhythm. Pregnant women may experience sinus dysrhythmia or premature atrial or ventricular contractions. Women with preexisting heart disease need close medical and obstetric supervision throughout pregnancy and may be at increased risk for arrhythmias during labor (Antony et al., 2017) (see Chapter 11).

Cardiac Output

Cardiac output increases 30% to 50% during pregnancy, reaching a peak by 25 to 30 weeks and declining to about a 20% increase at 40 weeks of gestation. This elevated cardiac output is largely a result of increased stroke volume and heart rate and occurs in response to increased tissue demands for oxygen (Monga & Mastrobattista, 2014). Cardiac output increases with any exertion such as labor and birth. Table 7.3 summarizes cardiovascular changes in pregnancy.

Blood Pressure

Blood pressure is influenced by two major factors: cardiac output (CO) and systemic vascular resistance (SVR). Although cardiac output increases significantly during pregnancy, maternal blood pressure remains the same or decreases slightly. This is due to reduced SVR caused primarily by the vasodilatory effects of progesterone, prostaglandins, and relaxin. The uteroplacental vascular system holds a large percentage of the maternal blood volume, which also contributes to decreased SVR (Monga & Mastrobattista, 2014). Systemic vascular resistance is lowest at 16 to 34 weeks and increases gradually, approximating nonpregnant values by term. During the first trimester, systolic blood pressure usually remains the same as the prepregnancy level but can decrease slightly as pregnancy advances. Diastolic blood pressure begins to decrease in the first trimester, continues to drop until 24 to 32 weeks, and gradually increases, returning to prepregnancy levels by term (Blackburn, 2013).

Various factors influence maternal blood pressure. These include age, activity level, presence of health problems, circadian rhythm, alcohol consumption, smoking, anxiety, and pain. Maternal position also affects blood pressure readings. Brachial blood pressure is highest when the woman is sitting; lowest when she is lying in the lateral recumbent position; and intermediate when she is supine, except for some women who experience hypotensive syndrome (see later discussion). At each prenatal visit, blood pressure should be measured in the same arm and with the woman in a seated position with her back and arm supported and her upper arm at the level of the right atrium. The position and arm used should be recorded along with the reading. If an elevated reading is found, the woman is given time to rest and the reading is repeated.

The type of equipment influences blood pressure readings. The proper-size cuff is essential for accuracy. A cuff that is too small yields

BOX 7.1   Procedure for Blood Pressure Measurement

- Measure BP with the woman seated or in the lateral recumbent position with the arm at heart level. If the woman is seated for BP measurement, both of her feet should be planted on a firm surface (she should *not* cross her legs) and her back should be supported.
- Allow a period of quiet rest before measuring the BP.
- Use the right arm each time. Measure BP over the brachial artery whenever possible.
- Support the weight of the woman's arm in a horizontal position roughly at heart level. BP will be higher when the woman holds up her arm.
- Use the proper-size cuff. The ideal cuff has a bladder length that is 80% and a width that is 40% of the arm circumference.
- Use both Korotkoff phase IV (muffling of sound) and phase V (disappearance of sound) for recording the diastolic value.
- Use measurement devices that have been validated and calibrated according to manufacturer guidelines.

BP, Blood pressure
Data from Sibai, B. (2017). Preeclampsia and hypertensive disorders. In S.G. Gabbe, J.R. Niebyl, J.L. Simpson, et al. (Eds.), *Obstetrics: Normal and problem pregnancies* (7th ed.), Philadelphia, PA: Elsevier; Witcher, P.M. (2017). Caring for the laboring woman with hypertensive disorders complicating pregnancy. In B. B. Kennedy, & S. M. Baird (Eds.), *Intrapartum management modules: A perinatal education program* (5th ed.). Philadelphia, PA: Wolters Kluwer.

a falsely high reading; a cuff that is too large yields a falsely low reading (Box 7.1).

Caution should be used when comparing auscultatory and oscillatory blood pressure readings because discrepancies can occur. Automated monitors can give inaccurate readings in women with hypertensive conditions.

Assessment of the *mean arterial pressure* (MAP) (mean of the blood pressure in the arterial circulation) can increase the diagnostic value of the findings. Automated blood pressure monitors display the MAP. MAP is one of several biomarkers that has been examined as a predictor of preeclampsia (Gallo, Wright, Casanova, et al., 2016; O'Gorman, Wright, Syngelaki, et al., 2016).

Some degree of compression of the vena cava occurs in any woman who lies on her back during the second half of pregnancy. Cardiac output is reduced by as much as 25% to 30% when a pregnant woman is turned from left lateral recumbent to supine position. Some women experience a fall of more than 30 mm Hg in their systolic pressure. After 4 to 5 minutes, a reflex bradycardia is noted, cardiac output is reduced by half, and the woman feels faint. This condition is called *supine hypotensive syndrome* or *vena caval syndrome* (Monga & Mastrobattista, 2014) (see Fig. 16.5).

Compression of the iliac veins and inferior vena cava by the uterus causes increased venous pressure and reduced blood flow in the legs, except when the woman is in the lateral position. These alterations contribute to the dependent edema, varicose veins in the legs and vulva, and hemorrhoids that can develop in the latter part of term pregnancy and contributes to the increased risk for venous thromboembolism (VTE).

Blood Volume and Composition

Total blood volume (TBV), consisting of plasma and red blood cell volume, increases significantly during pregnancy by 40% to 50%. During the first half of pregnancy, TBV increases rapidly, peaks around 28 to 34 weeks, and then stabilizes or decreases slightly by term. In a singleton pregnancy, plasma volume increases by approximately 1200 to 1500 mL, or 50% above prepregnancy levels by 30 weeks of gestation, decreasing slightly by term (Antony et al., 2017). Increased blood volume is a protective mechanism. It is essential for meeting the blood volume needs of the hypertrophied vascular system of the enlarged uterus, for adequately hydrating fetal and maternal tissues when the woman assumes an erect or supine position, and for providing a fluid reserve to compensate for blood loss during birth and postpartum. Blood volume increases are greater with multiple gestation. Peripheral vasodilation allows for a normal blood pressure despite the increased blood volume in pregnancy.

By term, there is an increase in red blood cell mass of 250 to 450 mL, or approximately 20% to 30% over prepregnancy values (Monga & Mastrobattista, 2014). The percentage of increase in red blood cells depends on the amount of iron available. Because the plasma increase is greater than the increase in red blood cell (RBC) production, there is a decrease in normal hemoglobin and hematocrit values (Table 7.4). This state of hemodilution is referred to as *physiologic anemia of pregnancy*. The decrease is more noticeable during the second trimester, when rapid expansion of blood volume occurs faster than RBC production. A pregnant woman is considered anemic if the hemoglobin is less than 11 g/dL or the hematocrit is less than 33% during the first or third trimester, or if the hemoglobin is less than 10.5 g/dL or the hematocrit is less than 32% during the second trimester (West, Hark, & Catalano, 2017).

The total white blood cell count increases during the second trimester and peaks during the third trimester. This increase is primarily in the granulocytes; the lymphocyte count stays about the same throughout pregnancy (see Table 7.4).

Circulation and Coagulation Times

Pregnancy is considered a hypercoagulable state in which women are at a five- to six-fold increased risk for thromboembolic disease (Antony et al., 2017). The circulation time decreases slightly by week 32 and returns to near normal by term. There is a greater tendency for blood to coagulate during pregnancy because of increases in various clotting factors (i.e., factors VII, VIII, IX, X, and fibrinogen) and decreases in factors that inhibit coagulation (e.g., protein S). This tendency, combined with the fact that fibrinolytic activity (the splitting up or dissolving of a clot) is depressed during pregnancy and the postpartum period, provides a protective function to decrease the chance of bleeding but also makes the woman more vulnerable to thrombosis, especially after cesarean birth.

Respiratory System

Upper Respiratory Tract

The upper respiratory tract becomes more vascular in response to elevated levels of estrogen. As the capillaries become engorged, edema and hyperemia develop within the nose, pharynx, larynx, trachea, and bronchi. This congestion within the tissues of the respiratory tract gives rise to several conditions commonly seen during pregnancy, including nasal and sinus stuffiness, epistaxis (nosebleed), changes in the voice, and marked inflammatory response to even a mild upper respiratory infection (Antony et al., 2017). Increased vascularity of the upper respiratory tract also can cause the tympanic membranes and eustachian tubes to swell, giving rise to symptoms of impaired hearing, earache, or a sense of fullness in the ears.

Structural Adaptations

Structural and ventilatory adaptations occur during pregnancy to provide for maternal and fetal needs. Maternal oxygen consumption increases

TABLE 7.4 Laboratory Values for Pregnant and Nonpregnant Women

Values	Nonpregnant	Pregnant
Hematologic		
Complete Blood Count		
Hemoglobin, g/dL	12–16*	>11*
Hematocrit, packed cell volume, %	37–47	>33*
RBC volume, per mL	1400	1650
Plasma volume, per mL	2400	40%–45% increase
RBC count, million/mm^3	4.2–5.4	5–6.25; 20%–30% increase
White blood cells, total per mm^3	5000–10,000	5000–15,000
Neutrophils, %	55–70	60–85
Lymphocytes, %	20–40	15–40
Erythrocyte sedimentation rate, mm/hr	20	Elevated in second and third trimesters
Mean corpuscular hemoglobin concentration (MCHC) (g/dL packed RBCs) g/dL packed RBCs	32–36	No change
Mean corpuscular hemoglobin (MCH) (pg), pg	27–31	No change
Mean corpuscular volume (MCV), per mm^3	80–95	No change
Blood Coagulation and Fibrinolytic Activity†		
Factor VII	65–140	Increases in pregnancy, returns to normal in early puerperium
Factor VIII	55–145	Increases during pregnancy and immediately after birth
Factor IX	60–140	Same as factor VII
Factor X	45–155	Same as factor VII
Factor XI	65–135	Decreases in pregnancy
Factor XII	50–150	Same as factor VII
Prothrombin time (PT), sec	11–12.5	Decreases slightly in pregnancy
Partial thromboplastin time (PTT), sec	60–70	Decreases slightly in pregnancy and decreases during second and third stages of labor (indicates clotting at placental site)
Bleeding time, min	1–9 (Ivy method)	No appreciable change
Coagulation time, min	6–10 (Lee-White method)	No appreciable change
Platelets, per mm^3	150,000–400,000	No significant change until 3–5 days after birth and then increases rapidly (may predispose woman to thrombosis) and gradually returns to normal
Fibrinolytic activity		Decreases in pregnancy and then abruptly returns to normal (protection against thromboembolism)
Fibrinogen, mg/dL	200–400	Levels increase late in pregnancy
Mineral/Vitamin Concentrations		
Vitamin B$_{12}$, folic acid, ascorbic acid	Normal	Moderate decrease
Blood Glucose		
Fasting, mg/dL	70–105	60–90 before breakfast; 60–105 before lunch, dinner, bedtime snack
2-hr postprandial, mg/dL	<140	<120
Acid-Base Values in Arterial Blood		
Po$_2$, mm Hg	80–100	104–108 (increased)
Pco$_2$, mm Hg	35–45	27–32 (decreased)
Sodium bicarbonate (HCO$_3$), mEq/L	21–28	18–31 (decreased)
Blood pH	7.35–7.45	7.40–7.45 (slightly increased, more alkaline)
Hepatic		
Bilirubin, total, mg/dL	≤1	Unchanged
Serum cholesterol, mg/dL	120–200	Increases from 16–32 weeks of pregnancy; remains at this level until after birth
Serum alkaline phosphatase, units/L	30–120	Increases from week 12 of pregnancy to 6 weeks after birth
Serum albumin, g/dL	3.5–5	Increases 25% by term
Renal		
Bladder capacity, mL	1300	1500
Renal plasma flow, mL/min	490–700	Increases by 25%–30%
Glomerular filtration rate, mL/min	88–128	Increases by 30%–50%
Nonprotein nitrogen, mg/dL	25–40	Decreases
Blood urea nitrogen, mg/dL	10–20	Decreases
Serum creatinine, mg/dL	0.5–1.1	Decreases

Continued

TABLE 7.4   Laboratory Values for Pregnant and Nonpregnant Women—cont'd

Values	Nonpregnant	Pregnant
Serum uric acid, mg/dL	2.7–7.3	Decreases but returns to prepregnancy level by end of pregnancy
Urine glucose	Negative	Present in 20% of pregnant women
Intravenous pyelogram	Normal	Slight to moderate hydroureter and hydronephrosis; right kidney larger than left kidney

pg, Picogram; *RBC*, red blood cell.

*At sea level. Permanent residents of higher levels (e.g., Denver) require higher levels of hemoglobin.

†Pregnancy represents a hypercoagulable state.

Data from Blackburn, S. (2013). *Maternal, fetal, and neonatal physiology: A clinical perspective* (4th ed.). Maryland Heights, MO: Saunders; Antony, K.M., Racusin, D.A., Aagaard, K., et al. (2017). Maternal physiology. In S.G. Gabbe, J.R. Niebyl, J.L. Simpson, et al. (Eds.), *Obstetrics: Normal and problem pregnancies* (7th ed.). Philadelphia, PA: Elsevier; Landon, M.B., Catalano, P.J., & Gabbe, S.G. (2017). Diabetes mellitus complicating pregnancy. In S.G. Gabbe, J.R. Niebyl, J.L. Simpson, et al. (Eds.), *Obstetrics: Normal and problem pregnancies* (7th ed.). Philadelphia, PA: Elsevier; Pagana, K.D., Pagana, T.J., & Pagana, T.N. (2017). *Mosby's diagnostic and laboratory test reference* (13th ed.). St. Louis, MO: Mosby; Samuels, P. (2017). Hematologic complications of pregnancy. In S.G. Gabbe, J.R. Niebyl, J.L. Simpson, et al. (Eds.), *Obstetrics: Normal and problem pregnancies* (7th ed.). Philadelphia, PA: Elsevier.

during pregnancy by 20% to 40% above nonpregnant levels. This increase is necessary to support the needs of the fetus, placenta, and changes in maternal organs (Antony et al., 2017). As pregnancy progresses, the enlarging uterus places upward pressure on the diaphragm causing the level of the diaphragm to rise by as much as 4 cm. The costal angle increases, and the lower rib cage appears to flare out. Ligaments of the rib cage relax due to the effects of progesterone, permitting increased chest expansion. The transverse diameter of the thoracic cage increases by about 2 cm and the circumference by 5 to 7 cm. Consequently there is little change in total lung capacity.

With advancing pregnancy, chest breathing replaces abdominal breathing, and it becomes less possible for the diaphragm to descend with inspiration. Thoracic breathing is accomplished primarily by the diaphragm rather than by the costal muscles (Blackburn, 2013).

Pulmonary Function

Tidal volume (the amount of air exchanged during normal inspiration and expiration) increases by 40% during pregnancy. Respiratory rate does not change during pregnancy, although minute ventilation (volume of gas expelled from the lungs per minute) increases by 30% to 50%. This is likely related to increased progesterone and increased basal metabolic rate (Monga & Mastrobattista, 2014).

Pregnancy is a state of chronic mild hyperventilation with reduced arterial carbon dioxide ($PaCO_2$) and increased oxygen (PaO_2) over nonpregnant levels. Respiratory changes in pregnancy are shown in Table 7.5. Progesterone may be responsible for increasing the sensitivity of the respiratory center receptors so that $PaCO_2$ decreases, the base excess (HCO_3, or bicarbonate) decreases, and pH increases slightly. These alterations in acid-base balance create a state of respiratory alkalosis (see Table 7.4). These changes also facilitate the transport of CO_2 from the fetus to the mother and O_2 release from the mother to the fetus.

Renal System

The kidneys are responsible for maintaining electrolyte and acid-base balance, regulating extracellular fluid volume, excreting waste products, and conserving essential nutrients.

Anatomic Changes

Changes in renal structure result from hormonal activity (estrogen and progesterone), pressure from an enlarging uterus, and an increase in blood volume. As early as the tenth week of pregnancy, the renal pelves and the ureters dilate. Dilation of the ureters is more pronounced above the pelvic brim, in part because they are compressed between the uterus

TABLE 7.5   Respiratory Changes in Pregnancy

Parameter	Change
Respiratory rate	Unchanged or slightly increased
Tidal volume	Increased 40%
Vital capacity	Unchanged
Inspiratory capacity	Increased 6%
Expiratory reserve volume	Decreased 20%
Total lung capacity	Unchanged to slightly decreased
Minute ventilation	Increased 30%–50%
Oxygen consumption	Increased 20%–40%

Data from Monga, M., Mastrobattista, J.M. (2014). Maternal cardiovascular, respiratory, and renal adaptation to pregnancy. In R.K. Creasy, R. Resnik, J.D. Iams, et al. (Eds.). *Creasy & Resnik's maternal-fetal medicine: Principles and practice*, (7th ed.). Philadelphia, PA: Saunders.

and the pelvic brim. In most women, the ureters below the pelvic brim are normal size. The smooth-muscle walls of the ureters undergo hyperplasia and hypertrophy and muscle tone relaxation. The ureters elongate, become tortuous, and form single or double curves. In the latter part of pregnancy, the renal pelvis and ureter dilate more on the right side than on the left because the heavy uterus is displaced to the right by the sigmoid colon (Monga & Mastrobattista, 2014).

Because of these changes, a larger volume of urine is held in the pelves and ureters and urine flow rate is slowed. Urinary stasis or stagnation has several consequences:

- A lag occurs between the time urine is formed and when it reaches the bladder. Therefore, clearance test results may reflect substances contained in glomerular filtrate several hours before.
- Stagnated urine is an excellent medium for the growth of microorganisms. In addition, the urine of pregnant women contains more nutrients, including glucose, that increase the pH (making the urine more alkaline). This makes pregnant women more susceptible to urinary tract infection (Cheung & Lafayette, 2013).

Bladder irritability, nocturia, and urinary frequency and urgency (without dysuria) are commonly reported in early pregnancy. These bladder symptoms may return near term, especially after lightening occurs.

Urinary frequency results initially from increased bladder sensitivity and later from compression of the bladder (see Fig. 7.8). In the second trimester, the bladder is pulled up out of the true pelvis into the abdomen. The urethra lengthens to 7.5 cm as the bladder is displaced upward. The pelvic congestion that occurs in pregnancy is reflected in hyperemia of the bladder and urethra. This increased vascularity causes the bladder mucosa to be easily traumatized. Bladder tone may decrease, which increases the bladder capacity to 1500 mL. At the same time, the bladder is compressed by the enlarging uterus, resulting in the urge to void even if the bladder contains only a small amount of urine.

Functional Changes

In normal pregnancy renal function is altered considerably. Renal plasma flow (RPF) rises significantly from early in pregnancy, peaking by the end of the first trimester. RPF remains elevated above nonpregnant levels throughout pregnancy, although it begins to decrease after 34 weeks of gestation. The glomerular filtration rate (GFR) increases by 50% during the first trimester and remains elevated throughout pregnancy. These changes are caused by pregnancy hormones; an increase in blood volume; and the woman's posture, physical activity, and nutritional intake. The woman's kidneys must manage the increased metabolic and circulatory demands of the maternal body as well as the excretion of fetal waste products. The increase in GFR results in increased creatinine clearance and a reduction in serum creatinine, blood urea nitrogen (BUN), and uric acid levels (Antony et al., 2017).

Renal function is most efficient when the woman lies in the lateral recumbent position and least efficient when the woman assumes a supine position. A side-lying position increases renal perfusion, which increases urine output and decreases edema. When the pregnant woman is lying supine, the heavy uterus compresses the vena cava and the aorta, and cardiac output decreases. As a result, blood flow to the brain and heart is continued at the expense of other organs, including the kidneys and uterus.

Fluid and Electrolyte Balance

By term gestation, there is an increase in total body water of 6.5 to 8.5 L. This additional water content can be attributed to expansion of maternal blood volume; water content of the fetus, placenta, and amniotic fluid; intracellular fluid in the uterus and breasts; extravascular fluid; and increase in adipose tissue (Antony et al., 2017).

Selective renal tubular reabsorption maintains sodium and water balance, regardless of changes in dietary intake and losses through sweat, vomitus, or diarrhea. To prevent excessive sodium depletion, the maternal kidneys undergo a significant adaptation by increasing tubular reabsorption. Because of the need for increased maternal intravascular and extracellular fluid volume, additional sodium is needed to expand fluid volume and maintain an isotonic state. About 900 mEq of sodium is cumulatively retained during pregnancy, although maternal serum levels of sodium decrease by 3 to 4 mmol/L (Antony et al., 2017).

> #### ⚡ SAFETY ALERT
>
> As efficient as the renal system is, it can be overstressed by excessive dietary sodium intake or restriction or by use of diuretics. Severe hypovolemia and reduced placental perfusion are two consequences of using diuretics during pregnancy.

The capacity of the kidneys to excrete water is more efficient during the early weeks than later in pregnancy. As a result, some women feel thirsty in early pregnancy because of the greater amount of water loss. The pooling of fluid in the legs in the latter part of pregnancy decreases renal blood flow and GFR. This pooling is sometimes referred to as *physiologic* or *dependent edema* and requires no treatment. The normal diuretic response to the water load is triggered when the woman lies down, preferably on her side, and the pooled fluid reenters general circulation.

Normally the kidney reabsorbs almost all the glucose and other nutrients from the plasma filtrate. However, in pregnant women tubular reabsorption of glucose is impaired, causing glucosuria to occur at varying times and to varying degrees (Cheung & Lafayette, 2013). Nonpregnant women excrete less than 100 mg/day, whereas pregnant women with normal blood glucose levels excrete 1 to 10 g of glucose each day (Antony et al., 2017). The mechanism by which this occurs is unclear, although it may be related to the increased GFR and tubular flow rate that exceeds the capacity for tubular reabsorption of glucose (Blackburn, 2013). Although glucosuria can be found in normal pregnancies (2+ levels can be seen with increased anxiety states), the possibility of diabetes mellitus and gestational diabetes must be considered.

During normal pregnancy, there is an increase in urinary excretion of protein and albumin, most notable after 20 weeks of gestation (Cheung & Lafayette, 2013). This is due to increased GFR and impaired proximal tubular function. It is considered abnormal when proteinuria exceeds 300 mg/24 hours or albuminuria is greater than 30 mg/24 hours. The amount of protein excreted is not an indication of the severity of renal disease, nor does an increase in protein excretion in a pregnant woman with known renal disease necessarily indicate a progression in her disease. However, a pregnant woman with hypertension and proteinuria must be evaluated carefully because she may be at greater risk for adverse pregnancy outcomes (Antony et al., 2017).

Integumentary System

Alterations in hormone balance and mechanical stretching are responsible for several changes in the integumentary system during pregnancy. Hyperpigmentation is stimulated by the anterior pituitary hormone *melanotropin,* which is increased during pregnancy. Darkening of the nipples, areolae, axillae, and vulva occurs at about the sixteenth week of gestation. Melasma (also called *chloasma* or *mask of pregnancy*) is a blotchy, brownish hyperpigmentation of the skin over the cheeks, nose, and forehead, especially in pregnant women with dark complexions. Melasma appears in 50% to 70% of pregnant women, beginning after the sixteenth week and increasing gradually until term. The sun intensifies this pigmentation in susceptible women. Melasma caused by normal pregnancy usually fades after birth but often recurs with oral contraceptive use or subsequent pregnancies (Wang & Kroumpouzos, 2017).

The linea nigra (Fig. 7.11) is a pigmented line extending from the symphysis pubis to the top of the fundus in the midline. This line is known as the *linea alba* before hormone-induced pigmentation. In

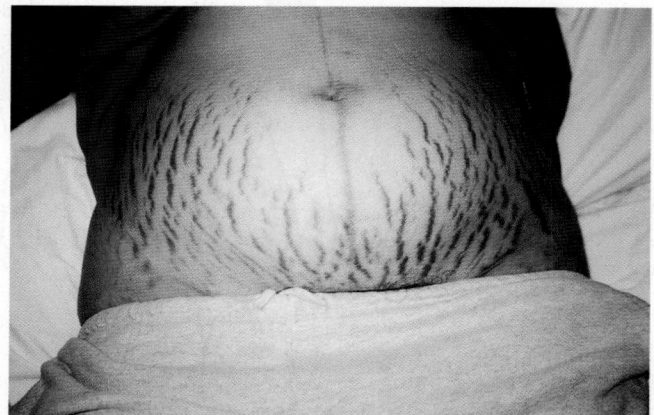

FIG 7.11 Striae gravidarum and linea nigra in a dark-skinned person. (Courtesy of Shannon Perry, Phoenix, AZ.)

primigravidas, the extension of the linea nigra, beginning in the third month, keeps pace with the rising height of the fundus; in multigravidas, the entire line often appears earlier than the third month. Not all pregnant women develop linea nigra, and some women notice hair growth along the line with or without the change in pigmentation.

Striae gravidarum or stretch marks (see Fig. 7.11) appear in 50% to 80% of pregnant women during the second half of pregnancy. Striae reflect separation within the underlying connective (collagen) tissue of the skin. These slightly depressed streaks tend to occur over areas of maximum stretch (the abdomen, thighs, and breasts). The stretching sometimes causes a sensation that resembles itching. The tendency to develop striae may be familial. After birth they usually fade, although they never disappear completely. No topical therapy has been shown to affect the course of striae, although pulsed laser therapy can reduce redness of early lesions (Rapini, 2014).

Angiomatas, commonly known as vascular spiders, are tiny star-shaped or branched, slightly raised, and pulsating end-arterioles usually found on the neck, thorax, face, and arms. Angiomatas appear during the second to fifth months of pregnancy as a result of increased blood flow to the skin due to rising estrogen levels during pregnancy and usually disappear within the first three months postpartum (Wang & Kroumpouzos, 2017).

Pinkish red, diffusely mottled, or well-defined blotches are seen over the palmar surfaces of the hands in about 70% of Caucasian women and 30% of African-American women during pregnancy (Wang & Kroumpouzos, 2017). These color changes, called palmar erythema, are related to increased estrogen levels.

Some dermatologic conditions have been identified as unique to pregnancy or as having an increased incidence during pregnancy. The most common dermatologic symptom during pregnancy is itching (pruritis). Mild pruritus, also known as pruritus gravidarum, usually occurs over the abdomen. Less than 2% of women have significant pruritus that requires further evaluation (Wang & Kroumpouzos, 2017). The problem usually resolves during the postpartum period.

The most common specific dermatosis during pregnancy is polymorphic eruption of pregnancy (PEP), also known as pruritic urticarial papules and plaques of pregnancy (PUPPP). PEP occurs in approximately 1 in 130 to 1 in 300 pregnancies and is more common in multiple gestations. Although it can cause significant maternal discomfort, it is not associated with adverse outcomes for the mother or fetus. Mild PEP is usually treated with oral antihistamines and topical antipruritic and corticosteroid creams. Oral steroids may be needed in more severe cases (Wang & Kroumpouzos, 2017). See Chapter 11 and Fig. 11.7.

The effect of pregnancy on acne is variable. In some women, the skin clears and looks radiant. Acne can worsen or occur for the first time during pregnancy or postpartum. Commonly used topical treatments for acne (e.g., benzoyl peroxide, topical antibiotics) are considered safe during pregnancy; topical retinoids should be avoided in the first trimester (Tyler & Zirwas, 2013).

Nail and hair growth may be accelerated. Some women notice thinning and softening of the nails. Hirsutism, the excessive growth of hair or growth of hair in unusual places, is commonly reported. An increase in fine hair growth can occur but tends to disappear after pregnancy. However, growth of coarse or bristly hair does not usually disappear after pregnancy. The rate of scalp hair loss slows during pregnancy; increased hair loss may be noted in the postpartum period (Rapini, 2014).

Musculoskeletal System

The gradually changing body and increasing weight of pregnancy usually cause noticeable changes in a woman's posture (Fig. 7.12). Abdominal distention causes the pelvis to tilt forward, abdominal muscle tone decreases, and weight bearing increases; these changes require a realignment of the spinal curvatures. The woman's center of gravity shifts forward. An increase in the normal lumbosacral curve (lordosis) develops, and a compensatory curvature in the cervicodorsal region (exaggerated anterior flexion of the head) develops to help her maintain balance. Aching, numbness, and weakness of the upper extremities can result. Large breasts and a stoop-shouldered stance further accentuate the lumbar and dorsal curves. The ligamentous and muscular structures of the middle and lower spine can be severely stressed. These and related changes often cause musculoskeletal discomfort such as back pain, especially in older women or those with a back disorder or a faulty sense of balance.

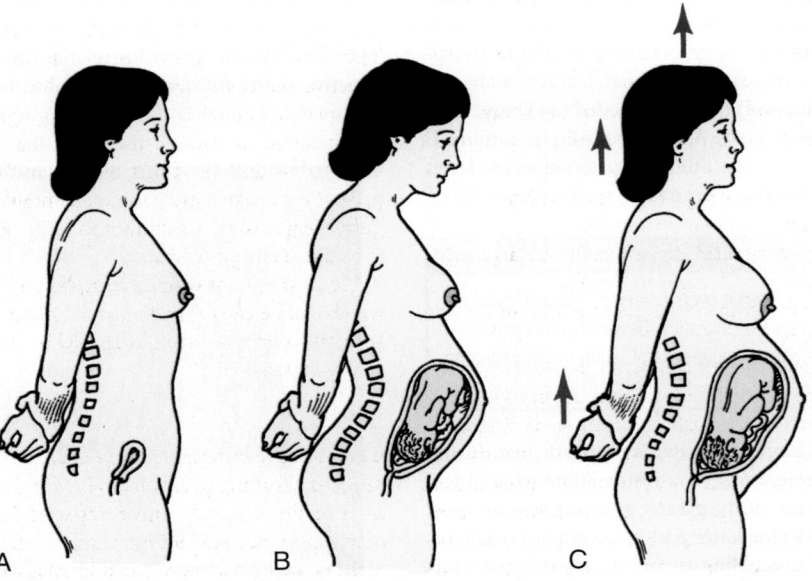

FIG 7.12 Postural changes during pregnancy. **A,** Nonpregnant. **B,** Incorrect posture during pregnancy. **C,** Correct posture during pregnancy.

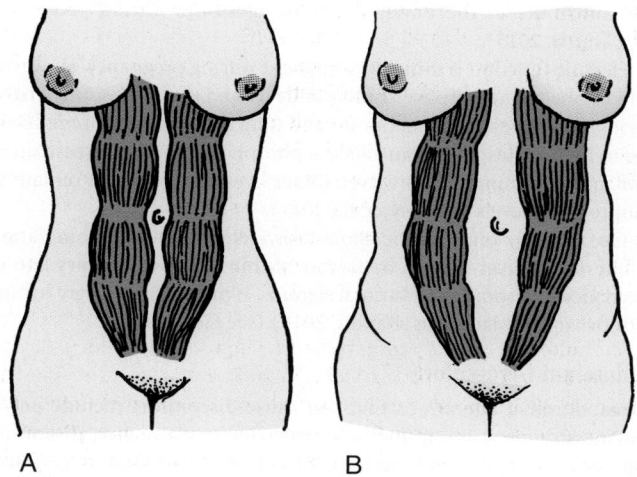

FIG 7.13 Possible change in rectus abdominis muscles during pregnancy. **A,** Normal position in nonpregnant woman. **B,** Diastasis recti abdominis in pregnant woman.

The hormones relaxin and progesterone cause loosening of ligaments of the pubic symphysis and sacroiliac joints to facilitate labor and birth. By 28 to 32 weeks of gestation, the symphysis widens from approximately 3 to 4 mm to 7.7 to 7.9 mm. Separation of the symphysis pubis and the instability of the sacroiliac joints can cause pain and difficulty in walking. A waddling gait is common. Obesity or multifetal pregnancy tends to increase pelvic instability (Antony et al., 2017).

> ⚡ **SAFETY ALERT**
>
> Pregnant women are at increased risk for falling due to the shifting center of gravity, impaired balance, and joint laxity.

The muscles of the abdominal wall stretch and ultimately lose some tone. During the third trimester, the rectus abdominis muscles can separate (**diastasis recti abdominis**) (Fig. 7.13), allowing abdominal contents to protrude at the midline. The umbilicus flattens or protrudes. After birth, the muscles gradually regain tone. However, separation of the muscles can persist.

Neurologic System

Little is known about specific alterations in function of the neurologic system during pregnancy aside from hypothalamic-pituitary neurohormonal changes.

Specific physiologic alterations resulting from pregnancy can cause the following neurologic or neuromuscular symptoms:

- Compression of pelvic nerves or vascular stasis caused by enlargement of the uterus can result in sensory changes in the legs.
- Dorsolumbar lordosis can cause pain because of traction on nerves or compression of nerve roots.
- Edema involving the peripheral nerves can result in **carpal tunnel syndrome** during the last trimester. The syndrome is characterized by paresthesia (abnormal sensation such as burning or tingling) and pain in the hand, radiating to the elbow. The sensations are caused by edema that compresses the median nerve beneath the carpal ligament of the wrist. Smoking and alcohol consumption can impair the microcirculation and worsen the symptoms. The dominant hand is usually affected most, although many women report symptoms in both hands. Symptoms usually regress after pregnancy. In some cases, surgical treatment is necessary.

- Acroesthesia (numbness and tingling of the hands) is caused by the stoop-shouldered stance (see Fig. 7.12, *B*) assumed by some women during pregnancy. The condition is associated with traction on segments of the brachial plexus.
- Tension headache is common when anxiety or uncertainty complicates pregnancy. However, vision problems unrelated to pregnancy such as refractive errors, sinusitis, or migraine may also be responsible for headaches.
- Lightheadedness, faintness, and even syncope (fainting) are common during early pregnancy. Vasomotor instability, postural hypotension, or hypoglycemia may be responsible.
- Hypocalcemia can cause neuromuscular problems such as muscle cramps or tetany.
- Corneal thickening and decreased intraocular pressure occur during pregnancy, and resolve within a few weeks after birth (Antony et al., 2017).

Gastrointestinal System
Appetite

During pregnancy, a woman's appetite and food intake fluctuate. Up to 70% of pregnant women experience nausea with or without vomiting ("morning sickness"), possibly in response to increasing levels of hCG and altered carbohydrate metabolism (Antony et al., 2017). Nausea and vomiting of pregnancy (NVP) appears at about 4 to 6 weeks of gestation and usually subsides by the end of the third month (first trimester) of pregnancy (see Chapter 9). Severity varies from mild distaste for certain foods to more severe vomiting. The condition can be triggered by the sight or odor of various foods. By the end of the second trimester, the appetite increases in response to increasing metabolic needs. Rarely does NVP have harmful effects on the embryo, the fetus, or the woman. Whenever the vomiting is severe or persists beyond the first trimester or when it is accompanied by fever, pain, or weight loss, further evaluation is necessary and medical intervention is likely (see Chapter 12).

Women can have changes in their sense of taste, leading to cravings and changes in dietary intake. Some women have nonfood cravings (**pica**) such as for ice, clay, and laundry starch. Pica should be considered as a potential factor in cases of iron deficiency anemia or poor weight gain (Antony et al., 2017) (see Chapter 9 for a discussion of nutrition in pregnancy).

Mouth

The gums can become hyperemic, spongy, and swollen during pregnancy. They tend to bleed easily because the increasing levels of estrogen cause selective increased vascularity and connective tissue proliferation (a nonspecific gingivitis). An **epulis** (gingival granuloma gravidarum) is a red, raised nodule on the gums that bleeds easily. This lesion may develop around the third month and often continues to enlarge as pregnancy progresses. It is usually managed by avoiding trauma to the gums (e.g., using a soft toothbrush). An epulis commonly regresses spontaneously after birth.

Some pregnant women complain of **ptyalism** (excessive salivation), which can be caused by the unconscious decrease in swallowing by the woman when nauseated or caused by stimulation of salivary glands by eating starch.

Esophagus, Stomach, and Intestines

Increased progesterone causes decreased tone and motility of smooth muscles, resulting in esophageal regurgitation (reflux), slower emptying time of the stomach, and reverse peristalsis. As a result, the woman may experience acid indigestion, or heartburn (**pyrosis**), beginning as early as the first trimester and intensifying through the third trimester.

The incidence of hiatal hernia is increased during pregnancy as a result of the upward displacement of the stomach by the enlarging uterus, which causes a widening of the hiatus of the diaphragm. Hiatal hernia occurs more often in multiparas and older or obese women.

In response to increased needs during pregnancy, iron is absorbed more readily in the small intestine. Even when the woman is deficient in iron, it continues to be absorbed in sufficient amounts for the fetus to have a normal hemoglobin level.

Smooth muscle relaxation and reduced peristalsis caused by increased progesterone and estrogen result in an increase in water absorption from the colon and can cause constipation. Constipation can also result from food choices, lack of fluids, iron supplementation, decreased activity level, abdominal distention by the pregnant uterus, and displacement and compression of the intestines. If the pregnant woman has hemorrhoids and is constipated, the hemorrhoids can evert or bleed during straining at stool.

The maternal gut microbiome changes during pregnancy. The bacterial diversity within the gut seems to decrease as pregnancy progresses. By the third trimester, there is an overall increase in *Proteobacteria* and a decrease in *Faecalibacterium,* which creates a gut microbiome that is similar to proinflammatory and prodiabetogenic states (Koren et al., 2012). Gestational changes in maternal vaginal and gut microbiomes seem to be adaptive responses that protect the fetus and contribute to establishing the neonatal microbiome (Mueller, Bakacs, Combellick, et al., 2015).

Gallbladder and Liver

The gallbladder is often distended because of its decreased muscle tone during pregnancy. Increased emptying time and thickening of bile caused by prolonged retention are typical changes. These features, together with slight hypercholesterolemia from increased progesterone levels,

can contribute to the development of gallstones during pregnancy (Blackburn, 2013).

Hepatic function is difficult to appraise during pregnancy. However, only minor changes in liver function develop. Liver size is unchanged during pregnancy. Serum albumin and total protein levels are reduced due to hemodilution. Serum alkaline phosphatase levels increase up to four times the nonpregnant level. Other liver function tests remain at nonpregnant levels (Antony et al., 2017).

Occasionally intrahepatic cholestasis (retention and accumulation of bile in the liver caused by factors within the liver) occurs late in pregnancy in response to placental steroids. It can result in severe itching with or without jaundice (Rapini, 2014) (see Chapter 11).

Abdominal Discomfort

Intraabdominal alterations that can cause discomfort include pelvic heaviness or pressure, round ligament tension, flatulence, distention and bowel cramping, and uterine contractions. In addition to displacement of intestines, pressure from the expanding uterus causes an increase in venous pressure in the pelvic organs. Although most abdominal discomfort is a consequence of normal maternal alterations, the health care provider must be constantly alert to the possibility of disorders such as bowel obstruction or an inflammatory process.

Appendicitis can be difficult to diagnose in pregnancy because the appendix is displaced upward and laterally, high and to the right, away from McBurney's point (Fig. 7.14). See Chapter 12 for more information.

Endocrine System

Profound endocrine changes are essential for pregnancy maintenance, normal fetal growth, and postpartum recovery. Hormones, their sources, and their effects on the pregnancy are presented in Table 7.6.

TABLE 7.6	Hormones and Effects of Changes During Pregnancy	
Hormone	**Source**	**Effects of Changes During Pregnancy**
Human chorionic gonadotropin (hCG)	Fertilized ovum and chorionic villi	Maintains corpus luteum production of estrogen and progesterone until placenta takes over the function
Progesterone	Corpus luteum until 14 weeks of gestation, then the placenta	Suppresses secretion of FSH and LH by the anterior pituitary gland; maintains pregnancy by relaxing smooth muscles, decreasing uterine contractility; causes fat to deposit in subcutaneous tissues over the maternal abdomen, back, and upper thighs; decreases mother's ability to use insulin
Estrogen	Corpus luteum until 14 weeks of gestation, then the placenta	Suppresses secretion of FSH and LH by the anterior pituitary gland; causes fat to deposit in subcutaneous tissues over the maternal abdomen, back, and upper thighs; promotes enlargement of genitals, uterus, and breasts; increases vascularity; relaxes pelvic ligaments and joints; interferes with folic acid metabolism; increases the level of total body proteins; promotes retention of sodium and water; decreases secretion of hydrochloric acid and pepsin; decreases mother's ability to use insulin
Serum prolactin	Anterior pituitary gland	Prepares breasts for lactation
Oxytocin	Posterior pituitary gland	Stimulates uterine contractions; stimulates milk ejection from breasts
Human chorionic somatomammotropin (previously called *human placental lactogen*)	Placenta	Acts as a growth hormone; contributes to breast development; decreases maternal metabolism of glucose; increases the amount of fatty acids for metabolic needs
Thyroxine-binding globulin, thyroxine, triiodothyronine	Thyroid gland	With adequate iodine intake, little or no enlargement of thyroid gland. Total T_3 and T_4 levels are slightly increased, peak by midpregnancy; by term are 10% to 15% lower than nonpregnant
Parathyroid	Parathyroid glands	Controls calcium and magnesium metabolism
Insulin	Pancreas	Increases production of insulin to compensate for insulin antagonism caused by placental hormones; effect of insulin antagonists is to decrease tissue sensitivity to insulin or ability to use insulin
Cortisol	Adrenal glands	Stimulates production of insulin; increases peripheral resistance to insulin
Aldosterone	Adrenal glands	Stimulates reabsorption of excess sodium from the renal tubules

FSH, Follicle-stimulating hormone; *LH,* luteinizing hormone.

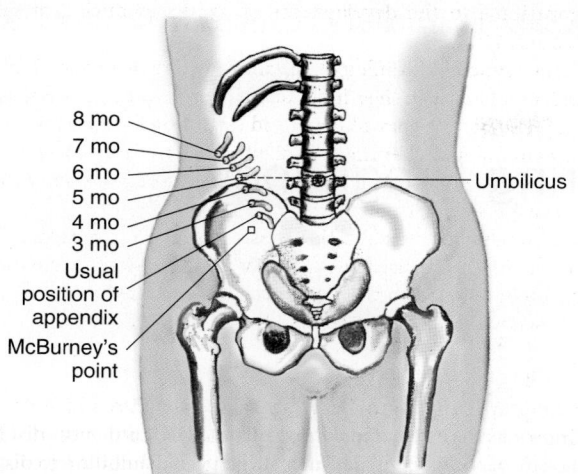

8 mo
7 mo
6 mo
5 mo
4 mo
3 mo
Usual position of appendix
McBurney's point

Umbilicus

FIG 7.14 Change in position of appendix in pregnancy. Note McBurney's point.

REFERENCES

Antony, K. M., Racusin, D. A., Aagaard, K., & Dildy, G. A. (2017). Maternal physiology. In S. G. Gabbe, J. R. Niebyl, J. L. Simpson, et al. (Eds.), *Obstetrics: Normal and problem pregnancies* (7th ed.). Philadelphia, PA: Elsevier.

Blackburn, S. (2013). *Maternal, fetal, & neonatal physiology: A clinical perspective* (4th ed.). Maryland Heights, MO: Saunders.

Cheung, K. L., & Lafayette, R. A. (2013). Renal physiology of pregnancy. *Advances in Chronic Kidney Disease, 20*(3), 209–214.

Gallo, D. M., Wright, D., Casanova, C., et al. (2016). Competing risks model in screening for preeclampsia by maternal factors and biomarkers at 19-24 weeks gestation. *American Journal of Obstetrics and Gynecology, 214*(5), 619.e1–619.e17.

Koren, O., Goodrich, J. K., Cullender, T. C., et al. (2012). Host remodeling of the gut microbiome and metabolic changes during pregnancy. *Cell, 150*(3), 470–480.

Lawrence, R. A., & Lawrence, R. M. (2016). *Breastfeeding: A guide for the medical profession* (8th ed.). Philadelphia, PA: Elsevier.

Liu, J. H. (2014). Endocrinology of pregnancy. In R. K. Creasy, R. Resnik, J. D. Iams, et al. (Eds.), *Creasy & Resnik's maternal-fetal medicine: Principles and practice* (7th ed.). Philadelphia, PA: Saunders.

Monga, M., & Mastrobattista, J. M. (2014). Maternal cardiovascular, respiratory, and renal adaptation to pregnancy. In R. K. Creasy, R. Resnik, J. D. Iams, et al. (Eds.), *Creasy & Resnik's maternal-fetal medicine: Principles and practice* (7th ed.). Philadelphia, PA: Saunders.

Mueller, N. T., Bakacs, E., Combellick, J., et al. (2015). The infant microbiome development: Mom matters. *Trends in Molecular Medicine, 21*(2), 109–117.

O'Gorman, N., Wright, D., Syngelaki, A., et al. (2016). Competing risks model in screening for preeclampsia by maternal factors and biomarkers at 11-13 weeks gestation. *American Journal of Obstetrics and Gynecology, 214*(1), e1–e103.

Pagana, K. D., Pagana, T. J., & Pagana, T. N. (2017). *Mosby's diagnostic and laboratory test reference* (13th ed.). St. Louis, MO: Elsevier.

Prince, A. L., Antony, K. M., Ma, J., & Aagaard, K. M. (2014). The microbiome and development: A mother's perspective. *Seminars in Reproductive Medicine, 32*(1), 14–22.

Rapini, R. P. (2014). The skin and pregnancy. In R. K. Creasy, R. Resnik, J. D. Iams, et al. (Eds.), *Creasy & Resnik's maternal-fetal medicine: Principles and practice* (7th ed.). Philadelphia, PA: Saunders.

Romero, R., Hassan, S., Gajer, P., et al. (2014). The vaginal microbiota of pregnant women who subsequently have spontaneous pre-term labor and delivery and those with a normal delivery at term. *Microbiome, 2*(18), 1–19.

Salani, R., Billingsley, C. C., & Crafton, S. M. (2014). Cancer and pregnancy: An overview. *American Journal of Obstetrics and Gynecology, 211*(1), 7–14.

Tyler, K. H., & Zirwas, M. J. (2013). Pregnancy and dermatologic therapy. *Journal of the American Academy of Dermatology, 68*(4), 663–671.

Wang, A. R., & Kroumpouzos, G. (2017). Skin disease and pregnancy. In S. G. Gabbe, J. R. Niebyl, J. L. Simpson, et al. (Eds.), *Obstetrics: Normal and problem pregnancies* (7th ed.). Philadelphia, PA: Elsevier.

West, E. H., Hark, L., & Catalano, P. M. (2017). Nutrition during pregnancy. In S. G. Gabbe, J. R. Niebyl, J. L. Simpson, et al. (Eds.), *Obstetrics: Normal and problem pregnancies* (7th ed.). Philadelphia, PA: Elsevier.

8

Nursing Care of the Family During Pregnancy

Kathryn R. Alden

e http://evolve.elsevier.com/Perry/maternal

The prenatal period is a time of physical and psychologic preparation for birth and parenthood. Becoming a parent is considered one of the maturational milestones of adult life. It is a time of intense learning for parents and those close to them. The prenatal period provides a unique opportunity for nurses and other members of the interprofessional health care team to influence pregnancy outcome and family health. Health promotion interventions can affect the well-being of the woman, her unborn child, and the rest of her family for many years.

Regular prenatal visits, ideally beginning soon after the first missed menstrual period, offer opportunities to safeguard the health of the expectant mother and her fetus. Prenatal health care enables discovery, diagnosis, and treatment of preexisting maternal disorders and any disorders that develop during the pregnancy. Prenatal care is designed to monitor the growth and development of the fetus and to identify abnormalities that will interfere with the course of normal labor. Prenatal care also provides education and support for maternal self-care and parenting and includes the spouse or partner or significant other.

Pregnancy, or gestation, lasts about 40 weeks or 280 days. It is often described in terms of **trimesters**. The first trimester lasts from weeks 1 through 13; the second, from weeks 14 through 26; and the third, from weeks 27 to 40. A pregnancy is considered to be at term if it advances to a gestational age of 37 weeks 0 days or more. The focus of this chapter is on the health care needs of the expectant family over the course of pregnancy, which is known as the *prenatal period*.

DIAGNOSIS OF PREGNANCY

Women suspect pregnancy when they miss a menstrual period. Many women come to the first prenatal visit after a positive home pregnancy test; however, in some women the clinical diagnosis of pregnancy before the second missed period is difficult. Physical variations, obesity, or tumors, for example, confound even the experienced examiner. Accuracy is important, however, because emotional, social, health, or legal consequences of an inaccurate diagnosis, either positive or negative, can be extremely serious.

SIGNS AND SYMPTOMS

The physical cues of pregnancy vary greatly; therefore, the diagnosis of pregnancy is uncertain for a time. Many of the indicators of pregnancy are clinically useful in the diagnosis of pregnancy and are classified as presumptive, probable, or positive (see Table 7.2).

ESTIMATING DATE OF BIRTH

After the diagnosis of pregnancy, the woman's first question usually concerns when she will give birth. The *estimated date of delivery* (EDD), also known as the estimated date of birth (EDB), is determined based on the date of the woman's last menstrual period and the first accurate ultrasound examination. Accurate dating of pregnancy is vital to promoting healthy outcomes for the woman and the fetus. The EDB is important for planning prenatal care, scheduling specific prenatal screening tests, assessing fetal growth, and making critical decisions for managing pregnancy complications. The most accurate assessment of the EDB is based on ultrasound measurement of the embryo or fetus during the first trimester of pregnancy (American College of Obstetricians and Gynecologists [ACOG], American Institute of Ultrasound in Medicine, & Society for Maternal-Fetal Medicine, 2014).

Naegele's rule is a common method for calculating the EDB. It is based on the woman's accurate recall of her last menstrual period (LMP). It assumes that the woman has a 28-day cycle and that fertilization occurred on the 14th day. According to Naegele's rule, after determining the first day of the LMP, subtract 3 calendar months and add 7 days (Box 8.1). Only about 5% of women give birth spontaneously on the EDB as determined by Naegele's rule. Most women give birth during the period extending from 7 days before to 7 days after the EDB.

ADAPTATION TO PREGNANCY

Pregnancy affects all family members, and each family member must adapt to the pregnancy and interpret its meaning in light of his or her own needs. This process of family adaptation to pregnancy takes place within a cultural environment influenced by societal trends. Dramatic changes have occurred in Western society in recent years, and the nurse must be prepared to support not only traditional families in the childbearing experience but also nontraditional families including single-parent families, same-sex couples, adoptive families, reconstituted families, and dual-career families.

The nurse must remember that the family, traditional or nontraditional, is the best source of information about their beliefs, needs, and concerns. Through effective communication with every family, the nurse can assess their specific needs and use this information as the basis for the plan of care.

MATERNAL ADAPTATION

Women of all ages use the months of pregnancy to adapt to the maternal role, a complex process of social and cognitive learning. Early in pregnancy nothing seems to be happening, and a woman may spend much time sleeping secondary to the increased fatigue of this stage. With the perception of fetal movement in the second trimester, the woman turns her attention inward to her pregnancy and to relationships with her mother and other women who have been or who are pregnant.

BOX 8.1   Use of Naegele's Rule

December 10, 2016, is the first day of the last menstrual period (LMP).

	Month	Day	Year
LMP	12	10	2016
	−3	+7	
Estimated date of birth:	9	17	2017

The estimated date of birth (EDB) is September 17, 2017.

Pregnancy is a maturational milestone that can be stressful but also rewarding as the woman prepares for a new level of caring and responsibility. Her self-concept changes in readiness for parenthood as she prepares for her new role. She moves gradually from being self-contained and independent to being committed to a lifelong concern for another human being. This growth requires mastery of certain developmental tasks: accepting the pregnancy, identifying with the role of mother, reordering the relationships between herself and her mother and between herself and her partner, establishing a relationship with the unborn child, and preparing for the birth experience. The partner's emotional support is an important factor in successfully accomplishing these developmental tasks. Single women with limited support can have difficulty making this adaptation.

Accepting the Pregnancy

The first step in adapting to the maternal role is accepting the idea of pregnancy and assimilating the pregnant state into the woman's way of life. Mercer (1995) described this process as cognitive restructuring and credited Rubin (1975, 1984) as the nurse theorist who pioneered our understanding of maternal role attainment. The degree of acceptance is reflected in the woman's emotional responses. Many women are upset initially when they discover they are pregnant, especially if the pregnancy is unintended. Eventual acceptance of pregnancy parallels the growing acceptance of the reality of a child. However, nonacceptance of the pregnancy does not equate with rejection of the child, because a woman can dislike being pregnant but feel love for the child to be born.

Women who are happy and pleased about their pregnancy often view it as biologic fulfillment and part of their life plan. They have high self-esteem and tend to be confident about outcomes for themselves, their babies, and other family members. Despite a general feeling of well-being, many women are surprised to experience *emotional lability,* that is, rapid and unpredictable changes in mood. These swings in emotions and increased sensitivity to others are disconcerting to the expectant mother and those around her. Increased irritability and explosions of tears and anger can alternate with feelings of great joy and cheerfulness apparently with little or no provocation.

Profound hormonal changes that are part of the maternal response to pregnancy can be responsible for mood changes. Other reasons such as concerns about finances and changes in lifestyle contribute to this seemingly erratic behavior.

Most women have ambivalent feelings during pregnancy whether the pregnancy was intended or not. Ambivalence—having conflicting feelings simultaneously—is considered a normal response for people preparing for a new role. For example, during pregnancy some women feel great pleasure that they are fulfilling a lifelong dream, but they also feel great regret that life as they know it is ending.

Even women who are pleased to be pregnant can experience feelings of hostility toward the pregnancy or unborn child from time to time. Such incidents as a partner's chance remark about the attractiveness of a slim, nonpregnant woman or news of a colleague's promotion can give rise to ambivalent feelings. Body sensations, feelings of dependence, or the realization of the responsibilities of child care also can generate such feelings.

Intense feelings of ambivalence that persist through the third trimester can indicate an unresolved conflict with the motherhood role (Mercer, 1995). After the birth of a healthy child, memories of these ambivalent feelings usually are dismissed. If the child is born with a defect, however, a woman may look back at the times when she did not want the pregnancy and feel intense guilt. She may believe that her ambivalence caused the birth defect. She then will need assurance that her feelings were not responsible for the problem.

Identifying With the Mother Role

The process of identifying with the mother role begins early in each woman's life when she is being mothered as a child. Her social group's perception of what constitutes the feminine role can subsequently influence her choosing between motherhood or a career, being married or single, being independent rather than interdependent, or being able to manage multiple roles. Practice roles, such as playing with dolls, babysitting, and taking care of siblings can increase her understanding of what being a mother involves.

Many women have always wanted a baby, liked children, and looked forward to motherhood. Their high motivation to become a parent promotes acceptance of pregnancy and eventual prenatal and parental adaptation. Other women have not considered in any detail what motherhood means to them. During pregnancy, these women must resolve conflicts such as not wanting the pregnancy and child-related or career-related decisions.

Reordering Personal Relationships

Close relationships of a pregnant woman undergo change during pregnancy as she prepares emotionally for the new role of mother. As family members learn their new roles, periods of tension and conflict can occur. An understanding of the typical patterns of adjustment can help the nurse reassure the pregnant woman and explore issues related to social support. Promoting effective communication patterns between the expectant mother and her own mother and between the expectant mother and her partner are common nursing interventions provided during the prenatal visits.

The woman's relationship with her mother is significant in adaptation to pregnancy and motherhood. Important components in the pregnant woman's relationship with her mother are the mother's availability (past and present), her reactions to the daughter's pregnancy, respect for her daughter's autonomy, and the willingness to reminisce (Mercer, 1995).

The mother's reaction to the daughter's pregnancy signifies her acceptance of the grandchild and of her daughter. If the mother is supportive, the daughter has an opportunity to discuss pregnancy and labor with a knowledgeable and accepting woman (Fig. 8.1). Reminiscing about the pregnant woman's early childhood and sharing the prospective grandmother's account of her childbirth experience help the daughter anticipate and prepare for labor and birth.

Although the woman's relationship with her mother is significant in considering her adaptation to pregnancy, the most important person to the pregnant woman is usually the father of her child (Fig. 8.2). With same-sex couples, the most important person is the partner. Women express two major needs within this relationship during pregnancy: feeling loved and valued and having the child accepted by the partner.

The marital or committed partner relationship is not static but evolves over time. The addition of a child changes forever the nature of the bond between partners. This can be a time when couples grow closer, and the pregnancy has a maturing effect on the partners' relationship as they assume new roles and discover new aspects of each other.

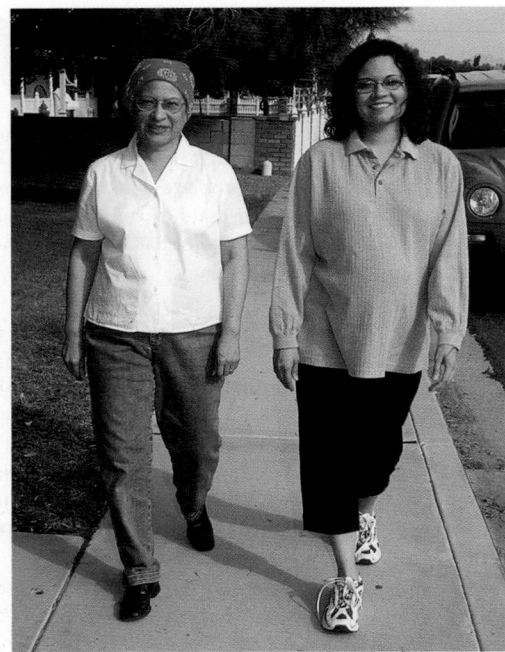

FIG 8.1 A pregnant woman and her mother enjoying a walk together. (Courtesy of Michael S. Clement, MD, Mesa, AZ.)

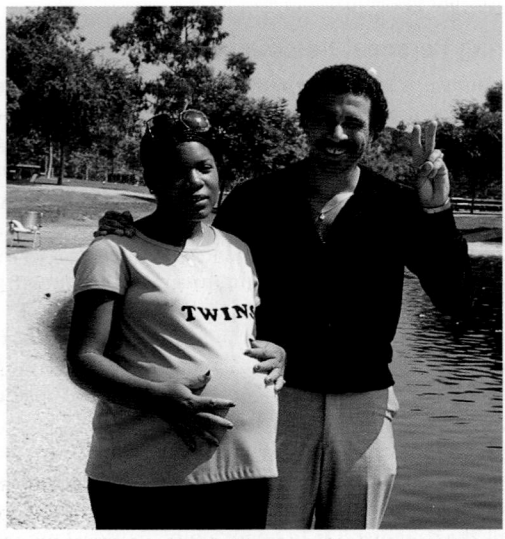

FIG 8.2 A prospective mother and father walk together. Women respond positively to their partner's interest and concern. (Courtesy of Marjorie Pyle, RNC, Lifecircle, Costa Mesa, CA.)

Partners who trust and support each other are able to share mutual-dependency needs (Mercer, 1995).

Sexual expression during pregnancy is highly individual. The sexual relationship is affected by physical, emotional, and interactional factors, as well as the couple's knowledge about sexual activity during pregnancy. As pregnancy progresses, changes in body shape, body image, and levels of discomfort influence both partners' desire for sexual expression. During the first trimester, the woman's sexual desire usually decreases, especially if she has breast tenderness, nausea, or fatigue. As she progresses into the second trimester, however, her sense of well-being combined with the increased pelvic congestion that occurs at this time often increases her desire for sexual release. In the third trimester, somatic

complaints and physical bulkiness can increase her physical discomfort and again diminish her interest in sex.

Partners need to feel free to discuss their sexual responses during pregnancy with each other, their health care provider, and nurses involved in their care (see later discussion).

Establishing a Relationship With the Fetus

Emotional attachment—feelings of being tied by affection or love—begins during the prenatal period as women use fantasizing and daydreaming to prepare themselves for motherhood (Rubin, 1975, 1984). They think of themselves as mothers and imagine maternal qualities they would like to possess. Expectant parents desire to be warm, loving, and close to their child. They try to anticipate changes that the child will bring into their lives and wonder how they will react to noise, disorder, reduced freedom, and caregiving activities. The mother-child relationship progresses through pregnancy as a developmental process that unfolds in three phases.

In phase 1, the woman accepts the biologic fact of pregnancy. She needs to be able to state, "I am pregnant," and incorporate the idea of a child into her body and self-image. The woman's thoughts center on herself and the reality of her pregnancy. The child is viewed as part of herself, not a separate and unique person.

In phase 2, the woman accepts the growing fetus as distinct from herself. This is usually accomplished by the fifth month. She can now say, "I am going to have a baby." This differentiation of the child from the woman's self permits the beginning of the mother-child relationship that involves not only caring but also responsibility. Attachment of a mother to her child is enhanced by experiencing a planned or desired pregnancy, and it increases when ultrasound examination and quickening confirm the reality of the fetus. With acceptance of the reality of the child (hearing the heartbeat and feeling the fetus move) and an overall feeling of well-being, the woman enters a quiet period and becomes more introspective. A fantasy child becomes precious to her. As she seems to withdraw and concentrate her interest on the unborn child, her partner sometimes feels left out. If there are children in the family, they can become more demanding in their efforts to redirect the mother's attention to themselves.

During phase 3 of the attachment process, the woman prepares realistically for the birth and parenting of the child. She expresses the thought, "I am going to be a mother," and defines the nature and characteristics of the child. She may, for example, speculate about the child's sex (if unknown) and personality traits based on patterns of fetal activity.

Although the mother alone experiences the child within, both parents and siblings believe the unborn child responds in a very individualized, personal manner. Family members may interact a great deal with the unborn child by talking to the fetus and stroking the mother's abdomen, especially when the fetus shifts position (Fig. 8.3). The fetus may have a nickname used by family members.

Preparing for Birth

Many women actively prepare for birth by reading books and information on various websites, watching videos, attending parenting classes, and talking to other women. They seek the best caregiver possible for advice, monitoring, and caring. The multiparous woman has her own history of labor and birth that influences her approach to preparation for this birth experience.

Anxiety can arise from concern about a safe passage for herself and her child during the birth process (Mercer, 1995; Rubin, 1975, 1984). Some women do not express this concern overtly, but they give cues to the nurse by making plans for care of the new baby and other children in case "anything should happen." Many women fear the pain of labor

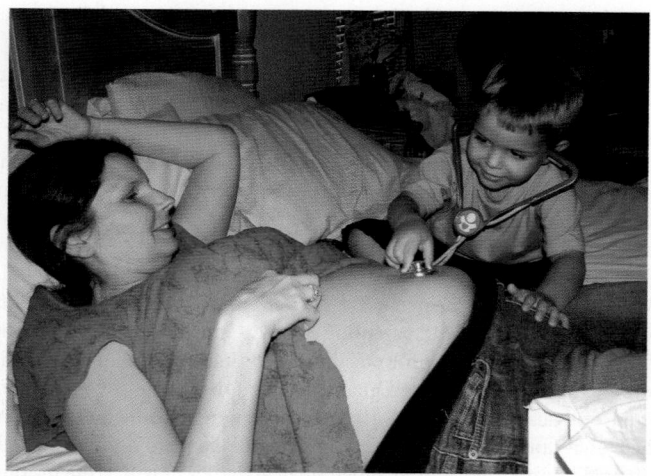

FIG 8.3 A 4-year-old likes to examine his pregnant mother's abdomen. (Courtesy of Kara George, Phoenix, AZ.)

and birth because they do not understand anatomy and the birth process. Education by the nurse can alleviate many of these fears.

Toward the end of the third trimester, breathing is difficult, and fetal movements become vigorous enough to disturb the woman's sleep. Backaches, frequency and urgency of urination, constipation, and varicose veins can become troublesome. The bulkiness and awkwardness of her body interfere with the woman's ability to care for other children, perform routine work-related duties, and assume a comfortable position for sleep and rest. By this time most women become impatient for labor to begin, whether the birth is anticipated with joy, dread, or a mixture of both. A strong desire to see the end of pregnancy, to be over and done with it, makes women at this stage ready to move on to birth.

PATERNAL ADAPTATION

The father's beliefs and feelings about the ideal mother and father and his cultural expectations of appropriate behavior during pregnancy affect his response to his partner's need for him. One man may engage in nurturing behavior. Another may feel lonely and alienated as the woman becomes physically and emotionally engrossed in the unborn child. He may seek friends and relationships outside the home or become interested in a new hobby or involved with his work. Some men view pregnancy as proof of their masculinity and their dominant role. To others, pregnancy has no meaning in terms of responsibility to either mother or child. However, for most men, pregnancy is a time of preparation for the parental role with intense learning.

Accepting the Pregnancy

The ways fathers adjust to the parental role has been the subject of considerable research. In older societies, the man enacted the ritual couvade; that is, he behaved in specific ways and respected taboos associated with pregnancy and giving birth so his new status was recognized and endorsed. Some men experience pregnancy-like symptoms, such as nausea, weight gain, and other physical symptoms. This phenomenon is known as the couvade syndrome. Changing cultural and professional attitudes have encouraged fathers' participation in the birth experience.

The man's emotional response to becoming a father, his concerns, and his informational needs change during the course of pregnancy. Phases of the developmental pattern become apparent. May (1982) described the following three phases characterizing the developmental tasks experienced by the expectant father:

- The *announcement phase* lasts from a few hours to a few weeks. The developmental task is to accept the biologic fact of pregnancy. Men react to the confirmation of pregnancy with joy or dismay, depending on whether the pregnancy is desired, unplanned, or unwanted. Ambivalence in the early stages of pregnancy is common. If pregnancy is unplanned or unwanted, some men find the alterations in life plans and lifestyles difficult to accept. Some men engage in extramarital affairs for the first time during their partner's pregnancy. Others batter their wives for the first time or escalate the frequency of battering episodes (See Chapter 3 and later discussion in this chapter).
- The second phase, the *moratorium phase*, is the period when he adjusts to the reality of pregnancy. The developmental task is to accept the pregnancy. Men appear to put conscious thought of the pregnancy aside for a time. They become more introspective and engage in many discussions about their philosophy of life, religion, childbearing, and childrearing practices and their relationships with family members, particularly with their father. Depending on the man's readiness for the pregnancy, this phase can be relatively short or persist until the last trimester.
- The third phase, the *focusing phase*, begins in the last trimester and is characterized by the father's active involvement in both the pregnancy and his relationship with his child. The developmental task is to negotiate with his partner the role he is to play in labor and to prepare for parenthood. In this phase, the man concentrates on his experience of the pregnancy and begins to think of himself as a father.

Identifying With the Father Role

Each man brings to pregnancy attitudes that affect the way in which he adjusts to the pregnancy and the parental role. His memories of the fathering he received from his own father, the experiences he has had with child care, and the perceptions of the male and father roles within his social group will guide his selection of the tasks and responsibilities he will assume. Some men are highly motivated to nurture and love a child. They are excited and pleased about the anticipated role of father. Others are more detached or even hostile to the idea of fatherhood.

Reordering Personal Relationships

The partner's main role in pregnancy is to nurture and respond to the pregnant woman's feelings of vulnerability. The partner also must deal with the reality of the pregnancy. The partner's support indicates involvement in the pregnancy and preparation for attachment to the child.

Some aspects of a partner's behavior can indicate rivalry, and it can be especially evident during sexual activity. For example, some men protest that fetal movements prevent sexual gratification or feel that they are being watched by the fetus during sexual activity. However, feelings of rivalry are often unconscious and not verbalized, but expressed in subtle behaviors.

The woman's increased introspection can cause her partner to feel uneasy as she becomes preoccupied with thoughts of the child and of her motherhood, with her growing dependence on her health care provider, and with her reevaluation of the couple's relationship.

Establishing a Relationship With the Fetus

The father-child attachment can be as strong as the mother-child relationship, and fathers can be as competent as mothers in nurturing their infants. The father-child attachment also begins during pregnancy. A father may rub or kiss the maternal abdomen; try to listen, talk, or sing to the fetus; or play with the fetus as he notes movement. Calling the unborn child by name or nickname helps confirm the reality of pregnancy and promotes attachment.

Men prepare for fatherhood in many of the same ways as women do for motherhood—by reading and fantasizing about the baby. Daydreaming about their role as father is common in the last weeks before the birth; however, men rarely describe their thoughts unless they are reassured that such daydreams are normal.

Nurses can help fathers identify concerns and prepare for the reality of a baby by asking questions such as the following:

- How do you expect the baby to look and act?
- How do you envision life as a father?
- How will you be involved in helping to care for the baby?
- How will having a baby affect your relationship with your partner?

Some fathers do not wish to answer such questions when they are asked but need time to think them through or discuss them with their partners.

As the birth date approaches, men have more questions about fetal and newborn behaviors. Some men are shocked or amazed at the smallness of clothes and furniture for the baby. If an expectant father can imagine only an older child and has difficulty visualizing or talking about an infant, this situation must be explored. The nurse can tell the father about the unborn child's ability to respond to light, sound, and touch and encourage him to feel and talk to the fetus. Discussions with new fathers, as in childbirth classes, may be welcomed.

Some men become involved by choosing the child's name and anticipating the child's sex, if it is not already known. Some couples select the name of the child as early as the first month of pregnancy. Family tradition, religious customs, and the continuation of the parent's name or names of relatives or friends are important in the selection process.

Preparing for Birth

The days and weeks immediately before the expected day of birth are characterized by anticipation and anxiety. Boredom and restlessness are common as the couple focuses on the birth process; however, during the last 2 months of pregnancy, many expectant fathers experience a surge of creative energy at home and on the job. They become dissatisfied with their present living space. If possible, they tend to act on the need to alter the environment (e.g., remodeling, painting). This activity is their way of sharing in the childbearing experience. They are able to channel the anxiety and other feelings experienced during the final weeks before birth into productive activities. This behavior earns recognition and compliments from friends, relatives, and their partners.

Major concerns for the man are getting the woman to a health care facility in time for the birth and not appearing ignorant. Many men want to be able to recognize labor and determine when it is appropriate to leave for the hospital or call the obstetric care provider. They fantasize different situations and plan what they will do in response to them or rehearse taking various routes to the hospital, timing each route at different times of the day.

Some prospective fathers have questions about the labor suite's furniture and equipment, nursing staff, and location, as well as the availability of the obstetric and anesthesia care providers. Others want to know what is expected of them when their partners are in labor. The man also may have fears concerning safe passage of his child and partner and the possible death or complications of his partner and child. It is important he verbalize these fears; otherwise he cannot help his mate deal with her spoken or unspoken apprehension.

With the exception of childbirth preparation classes, a man has few opportunities to learn ways to be an involved and active partner in this rite of passage into parenthood. Mothers often sense the tensions and apprehensions of the unprepared, unsupportive father, and it can increase their fears.

ADAPTATION TO PARENTHOOD FOR THE NONPREGNANT PARTNER

The same fears, questions, and concerns can affect birth partners who are not the biologic fathers or who are the nonpregnant partner in a same-sex couple. Much attention is paid to the needs of the pregnant woman, but the nonpregnant partner's needs receive less attention. Nonpregnant female partners, also referred to as co-mothers, can feel excluded by heterocentric maternity care service structures, but are likely to feel included by nursing staff (Cherguit, Burns, Pettle, et al., 2012). Nonpregnant partners will be better prepared for the changes that come with pregnancy and parenting if they are included and considered in the process. In addition to dealing with their own feelings and the care of their partner, nonpregnant partners in a same-sex couple are often not acknowledged or accepted as a parent-to-be from within their own families and in society in general. Partners need to be kept informed, supported, and included in all activities in which the mother desires their participation. Nurses can do much to promote pregnancy and birth as a family experience by providing information about resources for same-sex parents such as community and on-line support groups.

SIBLING ADAPTATION

Sharing the spotlight with a new brother or sister can be the first major crisis for a child. The older child often experiences a sense of loss or feels jealous at being "replaced" by the new sibling. Some of the factors that influence the child's response are age, the parents' attitudes, the role of the father, the length of separation from the mother, the facility visitation policy, and the way the child has been prepared for the change.

A mother with other children must devote time and effort to reorganizing her relationships with them. She needs to prepare siblings for the baby's birth (Fig. 8.4) and begin the process of role transition in the family by including the children in the pregnancy and being sympathetic to older children's concerns about losing their places in the family hierarchy. No child willingly gives up a familiar position.

Siblings' responses to pregnancy vary with their age and dependency needs. The 1-year-old infant seems largely unaware of the process, but the 2-year-old child notices the change in his or her mother's appearance

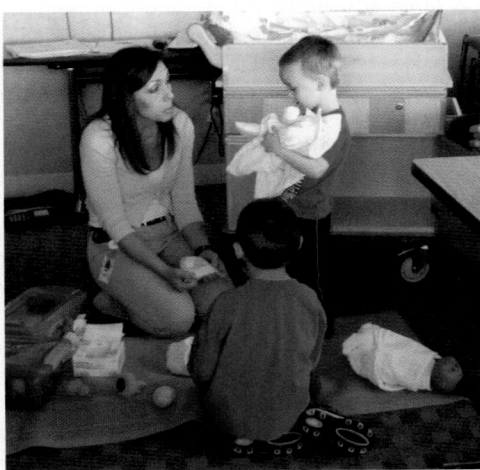

FIG 8.4 A preschooler in a sibling class learns about childbirth and infant care using dolls and a bunny. (Courtesy of Julie and Darren Nelson, Loveland, CO.)

and may comment that "Mommy's fat." Toddlers' need for sameness in the environment makes children aware of any change. They can exhibit more clinging behavior and sometimes regress in toilet training or eating.

By 3 or 4 years of age, children like to be told the story of their own beginning and accept a comparison of their own development with that of the present pregnancy. They like to listen to the fetal heartbeat and feel the baby moving in utero (see Fig. 8.3). Sometimes they worry about how the baby is being fed and clothed.

School-age children take a more clinical interest in their mother's pregnancy. They may want to know in more detail, "How did the baby get in there?" and "How will it get out?" Children in this age-group notice pregnant women in stores, churches, and schools and sometimes seem shy if they need to approach a pregnant woman directly. On the whole, they look forward to the new baby, see themselves as "mothers" or "fathers," and enjoy buying baby supplies and readying a place for the baby. Because they still think in concrete terms and base judgments on the here and now, they respond positively to their mother's current good health.

Early and middle adolescents preoccupied with the establishment of their own sexual identity can have difficulty accepting the overwhelming evidence of the sexual activity of their parents. They reason that if they are too young for such activity, certainly their parents are too old. They seem to take on a critical parental role and may ask, "What will people think?" or "How can you let yourself get so fat?" or "How can you let yourself get pregnant?" Many pregnant women with teenage children will confess that the attitudes of their teenagers are the most difficult aspect of their current pregnancy.

Late adolescents do not appear to be unduly disturbed. They are busy making plans for their own lives and realize that they soon will be gone from home. Parents usually report they are comforting and act more as other adults than as children.

GRANDPARENT ADAPTATION

Most grandparents are delighted at the prospect of a new baby in the family. It reawakens the feelings of their own youth, the excitement of giving birth, and their delight in the behavior of the parents-to-be when they were infants. They set up a memory store of the child's first smiles, first words, and first steps that they can use later for "claiming" the newborn as a member of the family. These behaviors provide a link between the past and present for the parents and grandparents-to-be.

In addition, the grandparent is the historian who transmits the family history, a resource person who shares knowledge based on experience; a role model; and a support person. The grandparent's presence and support can strengthen family systems by widening the circle of support and nurturance (Fig. 8.5). Other sources of information cannot replace the unique contribution that grandparents make (www.grandparents.com; www.grandparenting.org).

For some expectant grandparents, a first pregnancy in a child is undeniable evidence that they are growing older. Many think of a grandparent as old, white-haired, and becoming feeble of mind and body; however, some people face grandparenthood while still in their 30s or 40s. Some individuals react negatively to the news that they will be grandparents, indicating that they are not ready for the new role.

In some family units, expectant grandparents are nonsupportive and can inadvertently decrease the self-esteem of the parents-to-be. Mothers may talk about their terrible pregnancies; fathers may discuss the endless cost of rearing children; and mothers-in-law may complain that their sons are neglecting them because their concern is now directed toward the pregnant daughters-in-law.

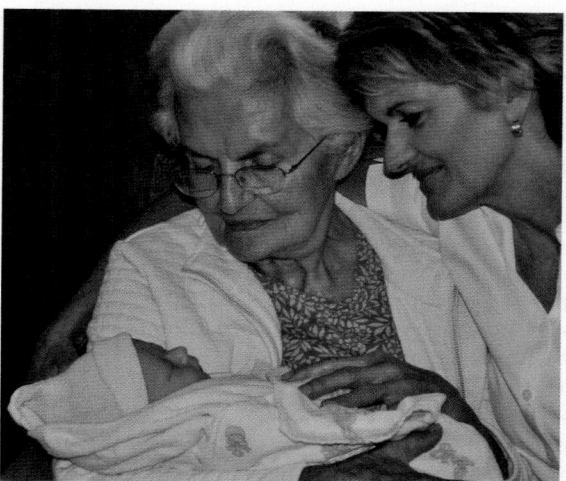

FIG 8.5 A great-grandmother and grandmother admiring the new baby. (Courtesy of Barbara Wilson, West Jordan, UT.)

CARE MANAGEMENT

Prenatal care occurs in physician or midwifery offices, public health or hospital clinics, or in the patient's home. Optimal care is provided by an interprofessional team that includes the obstetric care provider, nurses, and other health care professionals and support groups (Gregory, Ramos, & Jauniaux, 2017). Family physicians, nurse practitioners, physician assistants, public health nurses, registered dieticians, childbirth educators, maternal-fetal medicine specialists, and other health care professionals may be part of the care team, based on the individual needs of the woman. Psychiatric care providers and social workers may be involved if the woman has mental health issues such as a history of depression. The team works collaboratively to provide care that optimizes pregnancy outcomes.

The goal of prenatal care is to promote the health and well-being of the pregnant woman, her fetus, the newborn, and the family. It includes education about healthy lifestyle behaviors such as nutrition and physical activity, self-care for the common pregnancy discomforts, and information about changes in the mother and growth of the developing fetus. Routine screening is offered during pregnancy to help identify existing risk factors and potential problems so that efforts to reduce risk for harm to mother or baby and management of identified conditions can be initiated at the earliest opportunity. Major emphasis is placed on preventive aspects of care, primarily to support the pregnant woman in self-management between visits with health care professionals and to help her to recognize and report changes that can signal problems early so that adverse effects for her or her unborn child can be prevented or minimized. If health behaviors must be modified in early pregnancy, nurses need to understand psychosocial factors that can influence the woman. In holistic care, nurses provide information and guidance about the physical changes and the psychosocial impact of pregnancy on the woman and members of her family. The goals of prenatal nursing care, therefore, are to foster a safe birth for the mother and infant and to promote satisfaction of the mother and family with the pregnancy and birth experience.

According to the National Center for Health Statistics (NCHS), more than 75% of women in the United States receive pregnancy care in the first trimester. Women who are least likely to begin early prenatal care are non-Hispanic African-American, non-Hispanic Native Hawaiian/ Other Pacific Islander, and non-Hispanic American Indian/Alaska Native mothers (Martin, Hamilton, Sutton, et al., 2012). Although women of middle or high socioeconomic status routinely seek prenatal care, women's reasons for delaying prenatal care include cost, lack of insurance, child care, transportation barriers, or inability to take time off from work. Lack of culturally sensitive care providers, discrimination based on sexual orientation, and barriers to communication resulting from differences in language also interfere with access to care. Likewise, immigrant women who come from cultures in which prenatal care is not emphasized may not know to seek routine prenatal care. Birth outcomes in these populations are less positive, with higher rates of maternal and fetal or newborn complications. In particular, problems with preterm birth, low birth weight (LBW; less than 2500 g), and infant mortality are associated with lack of adequate prenatal care.

The availability of advanced practice nurses (nurse practitioners and certified nurse-midwives [CNM]) as independent providers of care or in collaborative practice with physicians improves the availability and accessibility of prenatal care (American College of Nurse-Midwives [ACNM], 2012). A regular schedule of home visits by nurses aids in reducing barriers to care and contributes to improved maternal and infant outcomes (Meghea, You, Raffo, et al., 2015; Olds, Kitzman, Knudtson, et al., 2014; Roman, Raffo, Zhu, et al., 2014).

The traditional model for provision of prenatal care has been used for more than a century. The initial visit usually occurs in the first trimester, with monthly visits through week 28 of pregnancy. Thereafter, visits are scheduled every 2 weeks until week 36 and then every week until birth. Today the trend is toward individualizing the schedule of care. Women with low-risk pregnancies may have fewer routine prenatal visits, whereas those at risk for complications may be seen more frequently than the traditional schedule (American Academy of Pediatrics [AAP] & ACOG, 2012).

Group prenatal care is an alternative model to traditional care during pregnancy. In group prenatal care, authority is shifted from the provider to the woman and other women who have similar due dates. The model creates an atmosphere that facilitates learning, encourages discussion, and develops mutual support. CenteringPregnancy (Centering Healthcare Institute, 2016) is a well-known model of group prenatal care that involves three components: health care assessment, education, and peer support. Groups consist of 8 to 12 women at similar gestational ages who participate in 10 sessions lasting about 90 minutes each. At each meeting, the first 30 to 40 minutes consist of assessments (by the woman herself and by the health care provider), and the remaining 60 to 75 minutes are spent in guided education and group discussion of specific issues such as discomforts of pregnancy and preparation for labor and birth. Families and partners are encouraged to participate. Benefits associated with group prenatal care include improved birth outcomes such as lower rates of preterm birth, increased knowledge, improved satisfaction, increased psychosocial well-being, and higher breastfeeding initiation rates (Fiset, Hoffman, & Ehrenthal, et al., 2016; Heberlein, Picklesimer, Billings, et al., 2016; Herrman, Rogers, & Ehrenthal, 2012; Picklesimer, Billings, Hale, et al., 2012).

Prenatal care is ideally a multidisciplinary activity in which nurses work collaboratively with health care providers (physicians and certified nurse-midwives), nutritionists, social workers, and others to provide holistic care. The case management model, which makes use of care maps and critical pathways, is one system that promotes comprehensive care with limited overlap in services. To emphasize the nursing role, care management for the initial visit and follow-up visits is organized around the central elements of the nursing process: assessment, nursing diagnoses, expected outcomes, plan of care and interventions, and evaluation.

In recent years, the concept of preconception care has been recognized as an important contributor to positive pregnancy outcomes (see Chapter 3). If women can be taught healthy lifestyle behaviors and then practice them before conception—specifically good nutrition, entering pregnancy with as healthy a weight as possible, adequate intake of folic acid, avoidance of alcohol and tobacco use, and prevention of sexually transmitted infections (STIs) and other health hazards—a healthier pregnancy will result. Likewise, women who have health problems related to chronic diseases such as diabetes mellitus can be counseled regarding their special needs with the intent to minimize maternal and fetal complications.

INITIAL VISIT

Once the presence of pregnancy has been confirmed and the woman's desire to continue the pregnancy has been validated, prenatal care is begun. The assessment process begins at the initial prenatal visit and is continued throughout the pregnancy. Assessment techniques include the interview, physical examination, and laboratory tests. Because the initial visit and follow-up visits are distinctly different in content and process, they are described separately.

Prenatal Interview

The therapeutic relationship between the nurse and the woman is established during the initial assessment interview. During this interview, the nurse has the opportunity to gain the woman's trust.

The pregnant woman and family members who are present should be told that the first prenatal visit is longer and more detailed than future visits. The initial evaluation includes a comprehensive health history emphasizing the current pregnancy, previous pregnancies, the family, a psychosocial profile, a physical assessment, diagnostic testing, and an overall risk assessment.

One or more family members often accompany the pregnant woman. With the woman's permission, the nurse includes those accompanying the woman in the initial prenatal interview. Observations and information about the woman's family are then included in the database. For example, if the woman has small children with her, the nurse can ask about her plans for child care during the time of labor and birth. The nurse notes any special needs that are identified during this first interview (e.g., wheelchair access, assistance in getting on and off the examining table, difficulty speaking and/or understanding English, and cognitive deficits).

Reason for Seeking Care

Although pregnant women are scheduled for routine prenatal visits, they often come to the health care provider seeking information or reassurance about a particular concern. When the woman is asked a broad, open-ended question such as, "How have you been feeling?," she may reveal problems that could otherwise be overlooked. The woman's chief concerns should be recorded in her own words to alert other personnel to the priority of needs as identified by her. At the initial visit, the desire for information about what is normal in the course of pregnancy is typical.

Current Pregnancy

The presumptive signs of pregnancy, such as nausea and vomiting, can be of great concern to the woman. A review of symptoms she is experiencing and how she is coping with them helps establish a database to develop a plan of care. Some early teaching may be provided at this time.

Obstetric and Gynecologic History

Data are gathered on the woman's age at menarche, menstrual history, and contraceptive history; any infertility or reproductive system conditions; history of STIs; sexual history; and detailed history of all pregnancies, including the present pregnancy, and their outcomes. The date of the last Papanicolaou (Pap) test and the result are noted. The date of her LMP is obtained to calculate the EDB.

Health History

The health history includes physical conditions or surgical procedures that can affect the pregnancy or that can be affected by the pregnancy. For example, a pregnant woman who has diabetes, hypertension, or epilepsy requires special care. A careful history of any allergies and the type of reaction, medication use, and immunizations must be included. Because most women are anxious during the initial interview, the nurse's attention to cues, such as a MedicAlert bracelet, can prompt the woman to recall allergies, chronic diseases, or medications being taken such as cortisone, insulin, or anticonvulsants.

The woman is asked to list any previous surgical procedures. If she has had uterine surgery or extensive repair of the pelvic floor, a cesarean birth may be necessary; appendectomy rules out appendicitis as a cause of right lower quadrant pain in pregnancy; and spinal surgery may contraindicate the use of spinal or epidural anesthesia. The nurse notes any injury involving the pelvis as from a motor vehicle accident or childhood nutritional deficit.

Women who have chronic or handicapping conditions often forget to mention them during the initial assessment because they have become so adapted to them. Special shoes or a limp can indicate the existence of a pelvic structural defect, which is an important consideration in pregnant women. The nurse who observes these special characteristics and inquires about them with sensitivity can obtain individualized data that will provide the basis for a comprehensive nursing care plan. Observations are vital components of the interview process because they prompt the nurse and woman to focus on the specific needs of the woman and her family.

Nutritional History

The woman's nutritional history is an important component of the prenatal history because her nutritional status has a direct effect on the growth and development of the fetus. A dietary assessment can reveal special dietary practices, food allergies, eating behaviors, the practice of *pica* (the consumption of nonfood substances), and other factors related to her nutritional status (see Box 9.6). Body mass index should be calculated on all women at the first prenatal visit to provide the basis for counseling about weight gain, physical activity, and healthy food choices. Significant maternal, fetal, and neonatal risks are associated with obesity and pregnancy; these include miscarriage, congenital anomalies, gestational diabetes, preeclampsia, preterm birth, dysfunctional labor, shoulder dystocia, postpartum hemorrhage, wound infection, stillbirth, and neonatal death (ACOG, 2013a; Lim & Mahmood, 2015; West, Hark, & Catalano, 2017). Referral to a nutritionist is recommended for women with specific nutritional issues including obesity, multiple gestation, inadequate weight gain, adolescent pregnancy, food allergies or intolerances, diabetes, eating disorders, history of low birth weight infants, and social factors such as poverty that limit nutritional intake (West et al).

Pregnant women are usually motivated to learn about healthy lifestyle behaviors and respond well to advice generated by this assessment. Women with a history of bariatric surgery are nutritionally at risk and should be followed closely throughout pregnancy to ensure adequate caloric and micronutrient intake. Maternal weight gain and fetal growth should be closely monitored (Magdaleno, Pereira, Chaim, et al., 2012; Stotland, Bodnar, & Abrams, 2014) (see Chapter 9).

History of Drug and Herbal Preparation Use

The prenatal history includes past and present use of drugs (legal over-the-counter [OTC] and prescription medications; vitamin supplements

such as A, C, D, and E; herbal preparations; caffeine; alcohol; nicotine, and street drugs (e.g., marijuana, cocaine, heroin). This is because many substances cross the placenta and can therefore pose a risk to the developing fetus. See Chapter 11 for discussion of substance abuse during pregnancy. Increasing numbers of individuals are using herbal preparations, and this includes pregnant women. Therefore, it is important for health care providers to question prenatal women regarding the use of herbal preparations and document their responses. Information about allergies to medications and the type of reaction should also be obtained and recorded in the health record.

The immunization record should be reviewed for vaccinations against diseases such as rubella (German measles), varicella (chickenpox), seasonal influenza, hepatitis B, and pertussis (whooping cough) that can pose a particular risk to pregnant women or their infants during pregnancy and immediately following birth. Recommendations for vaccinations during the perinatal period are discussed later in this chapter.

Family History

The family history provides information about the woman's immediate family, including parents, siblings, and children. These data help identify familial or genetic disorders or conditions that could affect the health status of the woman or her fetus.

Social, Experiential, and Occupational History

Situational factors such as the family's ethnic and cultural background and socioeconomic status are assessed while the history is obtained. The following information may be obtained in several encounters. The nurse explores the woman's perception of this pregnancy by asking questions that focus on the following issues:

- Was this pregnancy planned or unintended? Is it desired or wanted?
- Is the woman pleased, displeased, accepting, or nonaccepting?
- Will any changes related to finances, career, or living accommodations occur as a result of the pregnancy?

The nurses assesses the family and social support system by questioning the woman about the following areas:

- What primary support is available to her?
- Are changes needed to promote adequate support?
- What are the existing relationships among the mother, father or partner, siblings, and expectant grandparents?
- What preparations are being made for her care and that of dependent family members during labor and for the care of the infant after birth?
- Is financial, educational, or other support needed from the community?
- What are the woman's ideas about childbearing, her expectations of the infant's behavior, and her outlook on life and the maternal role?

Other questions can provide perspective on the woman's perceptions about becoming a mother. Examples of issues to explore include the following:

- What does the woman think it will be like to have a baby in the home?
- How is her life going to change by having a baby?
- How prepared does she feel for becoming a mother?

During interviews throughout the pregnancy, nurses should remain alert to the appearance of potential parenting problems, such as depression, lack of family support, and inadequate living conditions. Nurses assess the woman's attitude toward health care, particularly during childbearing, her expectations of health care providers, and her view of the relationship between herself and the nurse.

Coping mechanisms and patterns of interacting are identified through observation and conversation with the mother. Early in the pregnancy the nurse should determine the woman's knowledge in various areas: pregnancy, maternal changes, fetal growth, self-care, and care of the newborn, including feeding. Asking about attitudes toward unmedicated or medicated labor and birth and about her knowledge of the availability of parenting skills classes is important. Before planning for nursing care, the nurse obtains information about the woman's decision-making abilities and living habits (i.e., exercise, sleep, diet, recreational interests, personal hygiene, clothing). Common concerns that can be sources of stress during childbearing include the baby's welfare, labor and birth process, behaviors of the newborn, the woman's relationship with her partner and her family, changes in body image, and physical symptoms.

The nurse explores attitudes concerning the range of acceptable sexual behavior during pregnancy by asking questions such as the following: What has your family (partner, friends) told you about sex during pregnancy? To gain insight into the woman's sexual self-concept, the nurse can ask questions such as the following: How do you feel about the changes in your appearance? How does your partner feel about your body now? How do you feel about wearing maternity clothes?

Women are questioned regarding their occupation—past and present—because this can adversely affect maternal and fetal health. For some women, heavy lifting and exposure to chemicals and radiation are part of their daily work, and these activities can negatively affect the pregnancy. Standing for long periods at a retail checkout line or in front of a classroom is associated with orthostatic hypotension. For others, long hours of sitting at a desk working on a computer can contribute to carpal tunnel syndrome or circulatory stasis in the legs.

Mental Health Screening

As part of routine prenatal care, all women should be assessed and screened for mental health issues. Perinatal depression is the most common complication of pregnancy and, if untreated, can have serious adverse effects on the mother, her newborn, and her family. ACOG recommends screening for depression and anxiety symptoms at least once during the perinatal period using a standardized, validated instrument such as the Edinburgh Postnatal Depression Scale (ACOG, 2015b). Appropriate follow-up and treatment, including referral to mental health care providers, is essential whenever there is a positive screen. Women are usually unlikely to initiate discussions with health care professionals related to mental health concerns, but they may be more willing to disclose issues and concerns when they are informed that the screening is part of routine prenatal care, when health care professionals are interested and sensitive, and when they are informed about the prevalence of mental health issues during the perinatal period (Byatt, Biebel, & Friedman, 2013; Kingston, Austin, & Heaman, 2015). When mental health issues are identified, appropriate referral and follow-up are needed. Risk factors for depression or anxiety during pregnancy include lack of support from partner, indadequate social support, history of intimate partner violence, personal history of mental illness, unintended pregnancy, pregnancy complications or loss, and stressful life events (Biaggi, Conroy, Pawlby, et al., 2016).

Intimate Partner Violence

Intimate partner violence (IPV), also known as battering, domestic abuse, or domestic violence, occurs in as many as 20% of pregnancies (AAP & ACOG, 2012). Rates of IPV during pregnancy are higher in developing countries than in the United States (James, Brody, & Hamilton, 2013). Estimates of IPV are low primarily because many women are afraid to disclose the abuse for fear of retaliation and escalation of violence (World Health Organization, 2013). In some cases, women do not recognize that they are being abused; they may not realize that psychologic aggression exhibited as public humiliation, coercive control,

threats of harm, or damage to personal property are forms of IPV (Breiding, Basile, Smith, et al., 2015).

The greatest predictor of violence during pregnancy is IPV prior to pregnancy; violence tends to worsen during pregnancy (James et al., 2013). Risk factors for IPV during pregnancy include younger age (especially adolescents), unintended pregnancy, lower income, and lower level of education (James et al; Martin-de-las-Heras, Velasco, Luna Jde, et al., 2015).

Reproductive coercion, defined as contraceptive sabotage and pregnancy coercion, is common in abusive relationships. This increases the risk for unintended pregnancy, which, in turn, increases the risk for IPV during pregnancy (Clark, Allen, Goyal, et al., 2014; Han & Stewart, 2014).

IPV begins or escalates during pregnancy for a variety of reasons. Pregnancy tends to be a time of increased autonomy and self-awareness for women. A woman's focus on her body, preoccupation with the fetus, and reduced physical and emotional availability can trigger jealous and possessive responses by the partner, especially if the pregnancy was unintended. After birth, the mother may be so physically and emotionally drained that she may have difficulty bonding with her infant; she has little time or energy to focus on the partner, which can trigger more violence. She may be at risk for becoming an abusive mother whether or not she remains in the abusive relationship (Campo, 2015).

Physical assault, especially to the abdomen, and sexual trauma increase the risk for spontaneous abortion (miscarriage), antepartum hemorrhage, abruptio placentae, preterm birth, low birth weight, maternal death, and neonatal death (Donovan, Spracklen, Schweizer, et al., 2016; Liu, McFarlane, Maddoux, et al., 2016). Trauma to the genital tract (e.g., vaginal and anal tears), urinary tract infections, and STIs are increased among victims of IPV (Martin, Acara, & Pollock, 2012). Psychologic effects of IPV include greater tendency to engage in risk-taking behaviors such as use of illicit drugs; lower self-esteem, posttraumatic stress disorder, and depression that can extend into the postpartum period (Udo, Lewis, Tobin, et al., 2016). Victims of IPV lack autonomy and are more likely to enter prenatal care later in pregnancy (Martin et al).

IPV occurs more frequently in pregnant adolescents than in adult women (Alhusen, Ray, Sharps, et al., 2015; Stöckl, March, Pallitto, et al., 2014). Battering during pregnancy in teenagers constitutes a particularly difficult situation. Adolescents may be more trapped in the abusive relationship than adult women because of their inexperience. They may ignore the violence because the jealous and controlling behavior is interpreted as love and devotion. Because pregnancy in young adolescent girls is frequently the result of sexual abuse, feelings about the pregnancy should be assessed.

Women are unlikely to initiate conversation with health care professionals about IPV, therefore it is critical that routine screening is done. ACOG recommends screening for IPV at the first prenatal visit, at least once every trimester, and at the postpartum visit (ACOG, 2012). It is essential that the screening is done in a safe, private setting with the woman alone (Association of Women's Health, Obstetric, and Neonatal Nurses [AWHONN], 2015).

There are a variety of screening tools for IPV. A simple and widely used tool is the Abuse Assessment Screen consisting of 5 items with a diagram for the abused woman to mark areas where she has been injured (McFarlane, Parker & Bullock, 1992).

Nurses can ask the woman screening questions with routine assessments during pregnancy. Examples of questions that might be asked include the following:

- Are you with a spouse or partner who threatens or physically hurts you? If yes, who?
- Within the past year or in this pregnancy, has anyone hit, slapped, kicked, or otherwise hurt you? If yes, who? Are you currently with that person?

• Has anyone forced you to have sexual activities that made you uncomfortable? If yes, who? Are you currently with that person?

A pregnant woman is often accompanied by her partner to the prenatal appointment, especially if the woman does not speak English and the partner does. Unless an interpreter is available, it is difficult to interview the woman alone; in addition, asking questions about abuse through an interpreter is more difficult unless the interpreter is a woman and can effectively communicate the nurse's sensitivity and concern.

If a woman discloses IPV, the first step is to assess for immediate danger and to take action to protect the woman and her children, if needed. A complete physical examination is needed to assess for injuries and to observe the woman's behaviors and verbal responses when asked about the various injuries (Bianchi, Cesario, & McFarlane, 2016). The next step is to help the woman formulate a safety plan. It is imperative that the woman is aware of resources available to her and has a plan of action if she stays with the battering partner. The nurse should provide telephone numbers of a hotline and the battered women's shelter or other safe haven. The woman can be offered use of a telephone to call the shelter if this is an option she chooses. If she chooses to remain with the abuser, a safety plan includes necessities for a quick escape: a bag packed with personal items for an overnight stay (can be hidden or left with a neighbor), money or a checkbook, an extra set of car keys, and any legal documents for identification. Legal options such as those for restraining orders or arrest of the perpetrator also are important aspects of the safety plan. A restraining order can be obtained from the county court or police department 24 hours a day. Shelters also can be helpful with assistance in obtaining orders of protection. If the woman chooses not to act in the middle of a violent episode, she may use the hotline or shelter for some counseling when the threat of harm is no longer present.

Nurses should be aware that victims of human trafficking can be seen in prenatal settings because of unintended pregnancy. Similar to victims of IPV, these women are likely to exhibit signs of physical abuse or neglect such as scars, bruises, burns, unusual bald patches, or tattoos that can be a sign of branding. They are likely to be accompanied by someone who never leaves them alone and speaks for them. They may not speak English and may lack identification documents. If the woman is alone, she may have her cell phone on and in speaker mode so that the person on the other end can hear everything that is said during the visit. Nurses and other health care providers must be creative in getting the woman alone for questioning. Strategies might include sending the other person to the front desk to fill out paperwork, interviewing the woman in the restroom, or telling her she needs to go for testing and cannot take her cell phone. With the consent of suspected or confirmed victims of human trafficking, intervention plans can be developed. An excellent resource is the National Human Trafficking Resource Center (www.polarisproject.org/what-we-do/national-human-trafficking-hotline/the-nhtrc/overview) (1-888-373-7888) (Tracy & Konstantopoulos, 2012).

Review of Systems

During this portion of the interview, the woman is asked to identify and describe preexisting or concurrent problems in any of the body systems, and her mental status is assessed. The nurse questions the woman about physical symptoms she has experienced, such as shortness of breath or pain. Pregnancy affects and is affected by all body systems; therefore, information on the current status of the body systems is important in planning care. For each sign or symptom described, the following additional data should be obtained: location, quality, quantity, chronology, aggravating or alleviating factors, and associated manifestations (signs or symptoms that occur with the primary symptom).

Physical Examination

The initial physical examination provides the baseline for assessing subsequent changes. The nurse should determine the woman's needs for basic information regarding reproductive anatomy and provide this information, along with a demonstration of the equipment that may be used and an explanation of the procedure itself. The interaction requires an unhurried, sensitive, and gentle approach with a matter-of-fact attitude.

The physical examination begins with assessment of vital signs and height and weight (for calculation of body mass index [BMI] see Chapter 9). The bladder should be empty before pelvic examination; the woman may be asked to provide a urine specimen at this time if not already provided.

Each examiner develops a routine for proceeding with the physical examination; most choose the head-to-toe progression. Heart and lung sounds are evaluated, and extremities are examined. Distribution, amount, and quality of body hair are of particular importance because the findings reflect nutritional status, endocrine function, and attention to hygiene. The thyroid gland is assessed carefully. The height of the fundus is noted if the first examination is done after the first trimester of pregnancy. During the examination, the nurse must remain alert to the woman's cues that give direction to the remainder of the assessment and that indicate a potential threatening condition such as supine hypotension—low blood pressure (BP) that occurs while the woman is lying on her back, causing feelings of faintness (see Emergency Treatment box). See Chapter 3 for a detailed description of the physical examination.

Whenever a pelvic examination is performed, the tone of the pelvic musculature and the woman's knowledge of Kegel exercises are assessed (see Chapter 3). Particular attention is paid to the size of the uterus because this is an indication of the duration of gestation. During the examination, the nurse can coach the woman in breathing and relaxation techniques, as needed. One vaginal examination during early pregnancy is recommended; another is usually not performed until late in the third trimester unless indicated by the woman's health status.

Laboratory Tests

The laboratory data yielded by the analysis of the specimens obtained during the examination provide important information concerning the symptoms of pregnancy and the woman's health status.

Urine, cervical, and blood samples are obtained during the initial visit for a variety of recommended screening and diagnostic tests for infectious diseases and metabolic conditions that can affect the mother and/or developing fetus. (A list of the various tests is found in Table 8.1.) Women should receive information about the various tests and the purpose for each test and be provided an opportunity to opt-out of testing. All pregnant women should receive human immunodeficiency

---

✚ **EMERGENCY TREATMENT**

Supine Hypotension

Signs and Symptoms
- Pallor
- Dizziness, faintness, breathlessness
- Tachycardia
- Nausea
- Clammy (damp, cool) skin; sweating

Interventions
- Position woman on her side until her signs and symptoms subside and vital signs stabilize within normal limits.

TABLE 8.1   Laboratory Tests in the Prenatal Period

Laboratory Test	Purpose
Hemoglobin, hematocrit, WBC, differential	Detects anemia; detects infection
Hemoglobin electrophoresis	Identifies women with hemoglobinopathies (e.g., sickle cell anemia, thalassemia)
Blood type, Rh, and irregular antibody	Identifies women whose fetuses are at risk for developing erythroblastosis fetalis or hyperbilirubinemia in neonatal period due to Rh or ABO incompatibility
Rubella titer	Determines immunity to rubella
Tuberculin skin test; chest X-ray after 20 weeks of gestation in women with reactive tuberculin tests	Screens for exposure to tuberculosis
Urinalysis, including microscopic examination of urinary sediment; pH, specific gravity, color, glucose, albumin, protein, RBCs, WBCs, casts, acetone; hCG	Identifies women with glycosuria, renal disease, hypertensive disease of pregnancy; infection; occult hematuria; hCG for confirmation of pregnancy
Urine culture	Identifies women with asymptomatic bacteriuria
Renal function tests: BUN, creatinine, electrolytes, creatinine clearance, total protein excretion	Evaluates level of possible renal compromise in women with a history of diabetes, hypertension, or renal disease
Pap test	Screens for cervical intraepithelial neoplasia; if a liquid-based test is used, may also screen for HPV
Cervical cultures for *Neisseria gonorrhoeae, Chlamydia*	Screens for asymptomatic infection at first visit
Vaginal/anal culture	GBS test done at 35–37 weeks for infection
RPR, VDRL, or FTA-ABS	Identifies women with untreated syphilis, done at first visit
HIV antibody, hepatitis B surface antigen, toxoplasmosis	Screens for the specific infections
1-hour glucose tolerance	Screens for gestational diabetes; done at initial visit for women with risk factors; done at 24–28 weeks for pregnant women at risk whose initial screen was negative and for others who were not previously tested
3-hour glucose tolerance	Tests for gestational diabetes in women with elevated glucose level after 1-hour test; must have two elevated readings for diagnosis
Cardiac evaluation: ECG, chest X-ray, and echocardiogram	Evaluates cardiac function in women with a history of hypertension or cardiac disease

BUN, Blood urea nitrogen; *ECG,* electrocardiogram; *FTA-ABS,* fluorescent treponemal antibody absorption; *GBS,* group B streptococcus; *hCG,* human chorionic gonadotropin; *HIV,* human immunodeficiency virus; *HPV,* human papillomavirus; *RBCs,* red blood cells; *RPR,* rapid plasma reagin; *WBCs,* white blood cells; *VDRL,* Venereal Disease Research Laboratory.

virus (HIV) risk-reduction counseling and be notified that they will be tested for antibody to HIV as part of the routine prenatal testing unless they decline the test (AAP & ACOG, 2012). If the woman refuses testing for HIV, this should be documented. The Centers for Disease Control and Prevention (CDC) also recommend testing during the first prenatal visit for syphilis, chlamydia, and hepatitis B. Screening for *Neisseria gonorrhoeae* is done for women who are at risk (CDC, 2016b). Screening for HIV, syphilis, chlamydia, and gonorrhea is repeated in the third trimester for women who are at high risk for contracting these infections. A purified protein derivative (PPD) tuberculin test may be administered to assess exposure to tuberculosis in women who are at high risk. The urine is tested for protein, glucose, and leukocytes; urine culture may also be done. During the pelvic examination, Pap test and culture for chlamydia and gonorrhea are done. In addition, pregnant women and fathers with certain ancestry or a family history of various genetically linked disorders may choose to undergo genetic testing (see Chapter 3). Antenatal testing for risk factors in pregnancy is discussed in Chapter 10.

FOLLOW-UP VISITS

The timing of follow-up visits varies according to the model of care and the individual needs of the pregnant woman. The pattern of interviewing the woman first and then assessing physical changes and performing laboratory tests continues. Patient education is part of every prenatal visit.

Interview

Follow-up visits are briefer and less comprehensive than the initial prenatal visit. At each of these follow-up visits, the woman is asked to

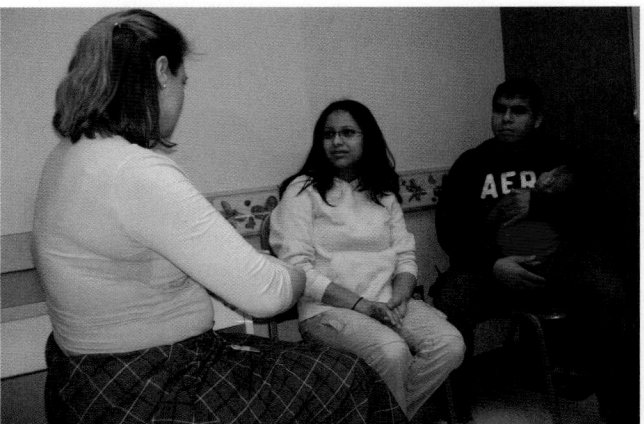

FIG 8.6 A prenatal interview. (Courtesy of Dee Lowdermilk, Chapel Hill, NC.)

summarize relevant events that have occurred since the previous visit. She is asked about her general emotional and physiologic well-being, and any complaints, problems, and questions she may have. Family needs also are identified and explored (Fig. 8.6).

Emotional changes are common during pregnancy, and therefore asking whether the woman has experienced any mood swings, reactions to changes in her body image, bad dreams, or worries is reasonable. The nurse documents the reactions of the partner and other family members to the pregnancy and the woman's emotional changes.

During the third trimester, it is important to assess current family situations and their effect on the woman as well as siblings' and grandparents' responses to the pregnancy and the coming child. This is a time to assess the woman and her family's knowledge of warning signs of emergencies, signs of preterm and term labor, the labor process and concerns about labor, and fetal development and methods to assess fetal well-being. The nurse should ask if the woman is planning to attend childbirth preparation classes and what she knows about management of discomfort during labor.

A review of the woman's physical systems is appropriate at each prenatal visit, and any suspicious signs or symptoms are assessed in depth. This review of systems includes identifying any discomforts reflecting adaptations to pregnancy. The nurse inquires about success with self-care measures as well as outcomes of prescribed therapy.

Physical Examination

Reevaluation is a constant aspect of a pregnant woman's care. Physiologic changes are documented as the pregnancy progresses and reviewed for possible deviations from normal progress.

At each visit, physical parameters are measured. BP is measured using the same arm at every visit. The woman's weight is assessed, and the appropriateness of the gestational weight gain is evaluated in relationship to her BMI. Urine may be checked by dipstick, and the presence and degree of edema are noted. For examination of the abdomen, the woman lies on her back with her arms by her side and head supported by a pillow. A small wedge is placed under her right hip to tilt her slightly to the left. The bladder should be empty. Abdominal inspection is followed by measurement of the height of the fundus (see Fig. 8.8). While the woman lies on her back, the nurse should be alert for the occurrence of supine hypotension (see the Emergency Treatment box).

The information provided through the interview and the physical examination reflects the status of maternal adaptations. When any of the findings are outside the expected range, an in-depth examination is performed. For example, careful interpretation of BP is important in the risk factor analysis of all pregnant women. Signs and symptoms other than hypertension also can be present that indicate potential complications (Table 8.2).

Fetal Assessment

Gestational Age

In an uncomplicated pregnancy, fetal gestational age is estimated after the duration of pregnancy and the EDB are determined. Fetal gestational age is determined from the menstrual history, contraceptive history, pregnancy test result, and the following findings obtained during the clinical evaluation:

- First uterine evaluation: date, size
- Fetal heart first heard: date, method (Doppler stethoscope, fetoscope)
- Date of quickening
- Current fundal height, estimated fetal weight (EFW)
- Current week of gestation by history of LMP and/or ultrasound examination
- Ultrasound examination: date, week of gestation, biparietal diameter (BPD)
- Reliability of dates

Quickening usually occurs between 16 and 20 weeks of gestation and is initially experienced as a fluttering sensation. The mother's report should be recorded. Multiparous women often perceive fetal movement earlier than primigravidas.

Ultrasonography (also called a *sonogram*) in early pregnancy is used to determine the estimated date of birth and to establish the duration of pregnancy. Ultrasound can detect a multiple gestation pregnancy and provide information about the well-being of the fetus or fetuses (see Chapter 10 for further discussion).

TABLE 8.2 Signs of Potential Complications: First, Second, and Third Trimesters

Signs and Symptoms	Possible Causes
First Trimester	
Severe vomiting	Hyperemesis gravidarum
Chills, fever	Infection
Burning on urination	Infection
Diarrhea	Infection
Abdominal cramping, vaginal bleeding	Miscarriage, ectopic pregnancy
Second and Third Trimesters	
Persistent, severe vomiting	Hyperemesis gravidarum, hypertension, preeclampsia
Sudden discharge of fluid from vagina before 37 weeks	Preterm premature rupture of membranes (PPROM)
Vaginal bleeding, severe abdominal pain	Miscarriage, placenta previa, abruptio placentae
Chills, fever, burning on urination, diarrhea	Infection
Severe backache or flank pain	Kidney infection or stones; preterm labor
Change in fetal movements: absence of fetal movements after quickening, any unusual change in pattern or amount	Fetal jeopardy or intrauterine fetal death
Uterine contractions, pelvic pressure, cramping before 37 weeks	Preterm labor
Visual disturbances: blurring, double vision, or spots	Hypertensive conditions, preeclampsia
Swelling of face or fingers and over sacrum	Hypertensive conditions, preeclampsia
Headaches: severe, frequent, or continuous	Hypertensive conditions, preeclampsia
Muscular irritability or seizures	Hypertensive conditions, preeclampsia
Epigastric or abdominal pain (perceived as heartburn or severe stomachache)	Hypertensive conditions, preeclampsia; abruptio placentae
Glycosuria, positive glucose tolerance test reaction	Gestational diabetes mellitus

Fetal Heart Tones

The fetal heart tones (FHTs) are assessed routinely at prenatal care visits. Early in pregnancy, the fetal heartbeat can be detected during ultrasound examination. Late in the first trimester, the heartbeat can be heard with a Doppler device that transmits fetal heart tones through a speaker or attached earpieces (Fig. 8.7, *B*). As the uterus grows and becomes an abdominal organ, the fetal heartbeat can also be auscultated with a fetoscope (see Fig. 8.7, *A*). Many practitioners use the Doppler device because it allows the mother and others who are present to easily hear the fetal heartbeat. Another tool for assessing fetal heart tones is the Pinard horn, which is a fetoscope commonly used by midwives and in much of Europe (see Fig. 8.7, *C*).

To detect the heartbeat before the fetal position can be palpated by Leopold maneuvers (see Chapter 16), the Doppler or fetoscope is moved around the abdomen until the heartbeat is heard. Each nurse develops a set pattern for searching the abdomen for the heartbeat—for example, starting first in the midline about 2 to 3 cm above the symphysis pubis,

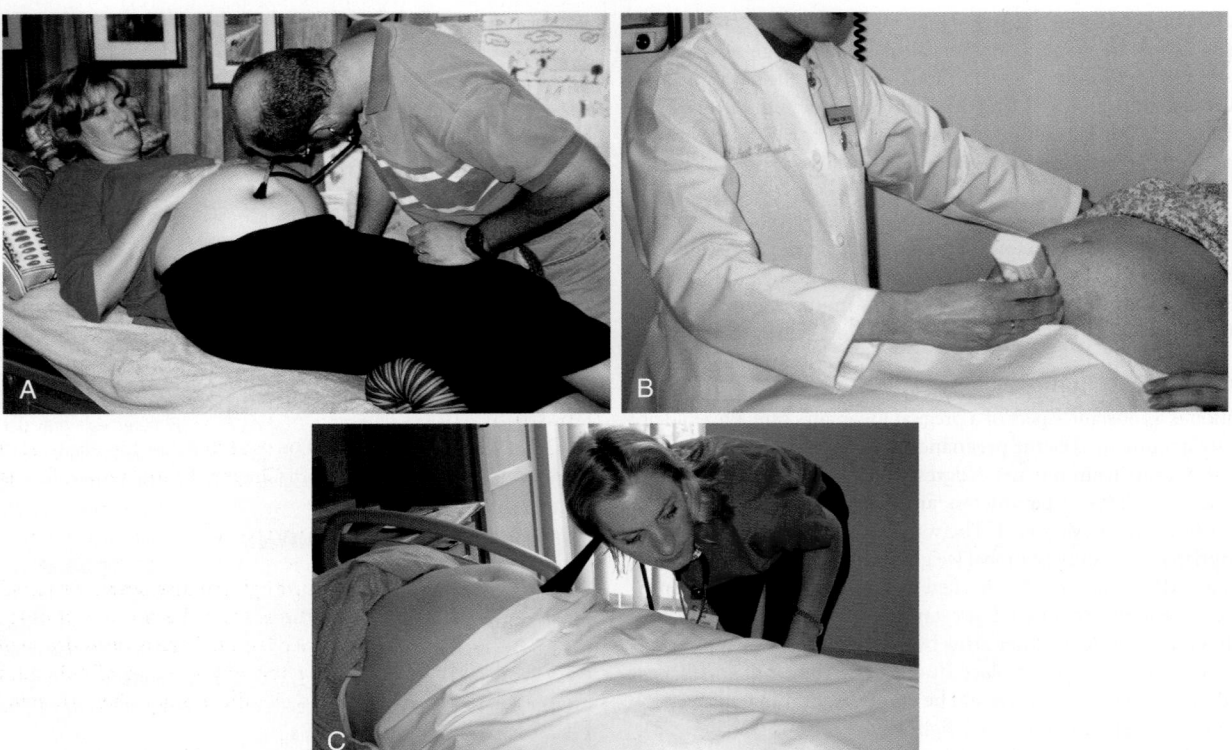

FIG 8.7 Detecting fetal heartbeat. **A,** Father can listen to the fetal heart with a fetoscope (first detectable at 18 to 20 weeks with a fetoscope). **B,** Doppler ultrasound stethoscope (fetal heartbeat detectable at 12 weeks). **C,** Pinard fetoscope. Note: Hands should not touch the fetoscope while listening. (A, Courtesy of Shannon Perry, Phoenix, AZ. B, Courtesy of Dee Lowdermilk, Chapel Hill, NC. C, Courtesy of Julie Perry Nelson, Loveland, CO.)

then moving to the left lower quadrant, and so on. The heartbeat is counted for 1 minute, and the quality and rhythm noted. A normal rate and rhythm are other good indicators of fetal health. Once the heartbeat is noted, its absence is cause for immediate investigation.

Health Status

The assessment of fetal health status often includes consideration of fetal movement. Absence of fetal movement is correlated with fetal death; women who report decreased fetal movement have an increased risk for adverse outcomes (AAP & ACOG, 2012). The mother is instructed to note the extent and timing of fetal movements and to report immediately if the pattern changes or if movement ceases. See Chapter 10 for more information on maternal assessment of fetal movement.

Fetal health status is investigated intensively if any maternal or fetal complications arise (e.g., gestational hypertension, intrauterine growth restriction (IUGR), premature rupture of membranes [PROM], irregular or absent FHR, or decreased or absent fetal movements after quickening). Careful, precise, and concise recording of the woman's responses and laboratory results contributes to the continuous supervision vital to promoting the well-being of the mother and fetus.

Fundal Height

During the second trimester, the uterus becomes an abdominal organ. The fundal height (measurement of the height of the uterus above the symphysis pubis) is one indicator of fetal growth. The measurement also provides a gross estimate of the duration of pregnancy. From gestational weeks (GW) 18 to 30, the height of the fundus in centimeters is approximately the same as the number of weeks of gestation (±2

GW), if the woman's bladder is empty at the time of measurement. As much as a 3 cm variation is possible if the bladder is full. For example, a woman of 28 weeks of gestation with an empty bladder would measure from 26 to 30 cm. The fundal height measurement can aid in identifying risk factors. A stable or decreased fundal height can indicate intrauterine growth restriction (IUGR); an excessive increase can indicate the presence of multifetal gestation (more than one fetus) or polyhydramnios.

A disposable paper metric tape measure is preferred for measuring fundal height; plastic retractable tape measures should be cleaned after use and prior to retraction. To increase the reliability of the measurement, the same person examines the pregnant woman at each of her prenatal visits, but often this is not possible. All clinicians who examine a particular pregnant woman should be consistent in their measurement technique. Ideally a protocol should be established for the health care setting in which the measurement technique is explicitly set forth, and the woman's position on the examining table, the measuring device, and method of measurement used are specified. Conditions under which the measurements are taken also can be described in the woman's records, including whether the bladder was empty and whether the uterus was relaxed or contracted at the time of measurement.

Various positions for measuring fundal height have been described. The woman can be supine with her head elevated and/or knees flexed. Measurements obtained with the woman in the various positions differ, making it even more important to standardize the fundal height measurement technique.

Placement of the tape measure also can vary. The tape can be placed in the middle of the woman's abdomen and the measurement made from the upper border of the symphysis pubis to the upper border of the

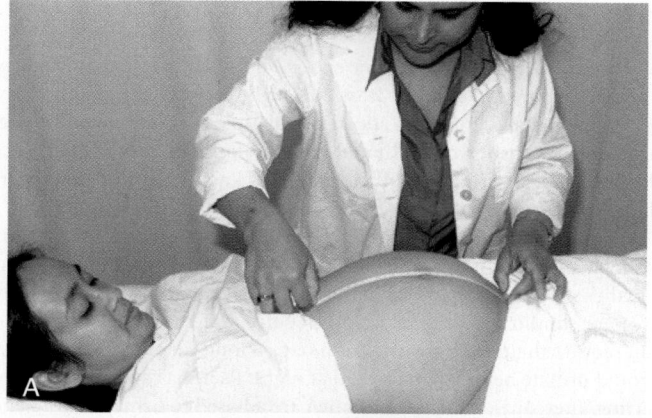

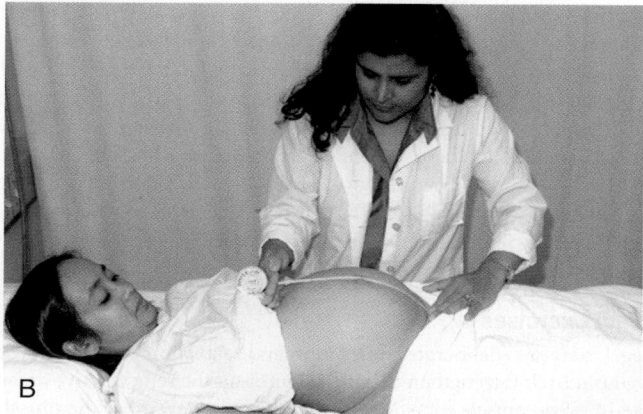

FIG 8.8 Measurement of fundal height from symphysis pubis that **A,** includes the upper curve of the fundus and **B,** does not include the upper curve of the fundus. Note position of the hands and measuring tape. (Courtesy of Chris Rozales, San Francisco, CA.)

fundus, with the tape measure held in contact with the skin for the entire length of the uterus (Fig. 8.8, *A*). In another measurement technique, the upper curve of the fundus is not included in the measurement. Instead, one end of the tape measure is held at the upper border of the symphysis pubis with one hand, and the other hand is placed at the upper border of the fundus. The tape is placed between the middle and index fingers of the other hand, and the point where these fingers intercept the tape measure is taken as the measurement (see Fig. 8.8, *B*).

Laboratory Tests

The number of routine laboratory tests done during follow-up visits in pregnancy is limited. A clean-catch urine specimen is obtained to test for glucose, protein, nitrites, and leukocytes at each visit. Urine specimens for culture and sensitivity are obtained, and cervical and vaginal smears and blood tests are repeated as necessary.

Sequential integrated screening (SIS) is an option for women who begin prenatal care before 14 weeks of gestation; it involves two blood tests and one ultrasound. This multiple marker screen can identify the following conditions: Down syndrome (trisomy 21), trisomy 18, neural tube defects (anencephaly and spina bifida), abdominal wall defects (gastroschisis and omphalocele), and Smith-Lemli-Opitz syndrome.

(ACOG, 2013c) recommends glucose screening for all pregnant women. Assessment for risk factors can be done through review of the medical history, screening for clinical risk factors, or measurement of blood glucose levels. Risk factors that warrant early screening include obesity, history of gestational diabetes mellitus (GDM), or known

impairment of glucose metabolism. If GDM is not diagnosed with early screening, blood glucose testing is repeated at 24 to 28 weeks. The standard screening test for GDM is a 1-hour, 50-g oral glucose tolerance test (GTT). If the glucose level is elevated, further testing is done using a 3-hour, 100-g GTT (see Chapter 11).

Group B streptococcus (GBS) testing is recommended between 35 and 37 weeks of gestation; cultures collected earlier will not accurately predict GBS status at time of birth. GBS culture results are only valid for 5 weeks. If birth has not occurred by the end of that time period, the test should be repeated. All pregnant women should have GBS testing, even those who are scheduled for a cesarean birth, because labor can begin or membranes can rupture prior to the routine administration of prophylactic antibiotics. Women with a history of GBS in a previous pregnancy should be retested with each pregnancy (ACOG, 2011/2015).

Other diagnostic tests may be used to assess the health status of the pregnant woman and fetus. See Chapter 10 for more information.

NURSING INTERVENTIONS

After obtaining information through the assessment process, the data are analyzed to identify deviations from the norm and unique needs of the pregnant woman and her family. Care is optimized with a collaborative approach involving the physician or CNM, nurse, other relevant health care professionals, the woman, her partner, and her family.

The nurse-patient relationship is critical in setting the tone for further interaction. The techniques of active listening with an attentive expression and using touch and eye contact (if culturally appropriate), have their place, as does recognizing the woman's feelings and her right to express these feelings. The interaction may occur in various formal or informal settings. A clinical setting, home visits, or telephone conversations all provide opportunities for contact and can be used effectively.

Education for Self-Management

The expectant mother needs information on many topics. The nurse who is observant, listens, and is familiar with typical concerns of expectant parents can anticipate the questions that will be asked and can encourage mothers and their partners to discuss what is on their minds. Printed literature can be given to supplement the individualized teaching the nurse provides. To be most effective, educational materials should be appropriate for the pregnant woman's or couple's ethnicity, culture, and literacy level and the agency's resources. Women often avidly read books, pamphlets, and web information related to their own pregnancy experience. Nurses should be familiar with the educational materials that are distributed to expectant parents as well as popular web-based resources related to pregnancy. Nurses can direct pregnant women and their families to reliable websites that contain accurate information.

Because family members are common sources for health information, it is also important to include them in health education endeavors during pregnancy (US Department of Health and Human Services Office of Disease Prevention and Promotion, 2013). This can enhance their ability to be supportive of the pregnant woman as she progresses through pregnancy.

Pregnant women who receive conflicting advice or instruction are likely to grow increasingly frustrated with members of the health care team and the care provided. Several topics that can cause concerns in pregnant women are discussed in the following sections.

Expected Maternal and Fetal Changes

Most expectant parents are curious about the growth and development of the fetus and the changes that occur in the mother's body during pregnancy. Mothers are often more tolerant of the discomforts related to the progressing pregnancy if they understand the underlying causes. Educational literature (printed, electronic, or web-based materials) that describes fetal and maternal changes can be used to explain changes as they occur. Couples can track the development of their growing fetus through websites such as www.babycenter.com/fetal-development or www.parents.com/pregnancy/stages/fetal-development/. There are also apps for smart phones that provide periodic updates on fetal development.

Nutrition

Good nutrition is important for the maintenance of maternal health during pregnancy and the provision of adequate nutrients for embryonic and fetal development. Assessing a woman's nutritional status and weight gain and providing ongoing education about nutrition are part of the nurse's responsibilities in providing prenatal care. Education for pregnant women includes recommendations about daily intake of nutrients, calories, vitamins, and minerals. Based on the woman's BMI, the recommended weight gain during pregnancy is discussed. Additional information regarding nutrition during pregnancy may include foods high in iron, the importance of taking prenatal vitamins, and recommendations to avoid alcohol and to limit caffeine intake. Pregnant women are instructed about how to avoid food-borne illnesses such as listeriosis. At each visit, the nurse assesses for practice of pica. In some settings, a nutritionist counsels women individually or conducts classes for pregnant women about nutrition during pregnancy. Nurses can refer women to a nutritionist if a need is identified during the nursing assessment. (For detailed information concerning maternal and fetal nutritional needs and related nursing care, see Chapter 9.)

Personal Hygiene

During pregnancy, the sebaceous (sweat) glands are highly active because of hormonal influences, and women often perspire freely. They can be informed that the increase is normal and that their previous patterns of perspiration will return after the postpartum period. Baths and warm showers can be therapeutic because they relax tense, tired muscles; help counter insomnia; and make the pregnant woman feel fresh. Tub bathing is not restricted even in late pregnancy because little water enters the vagina unless under pressure. However, late in pregnancy, when the woman's center of gravity lowers, she is at risk for falling. Tub bathing is contraindicated after rupture of the membranes.

Prevention of Urinary Tract Infections

Because of physiologic changes that occur in the renal system during pregnancy (see Chapter 7), infections of the lower urinary tract (acute urethritis, acute cystitis) are common. *Escherichia coli* (*E. coli*) is the most common causative organism for urinary tract infection (UTI) in pregnant women (Duff & Birsner, 2017). Although UTIs can be asymptomatic, typical symptoms include frequency, urgency, dysuria, dribbling, and hesitancy; gross hematuria can occur. Women should be instructed to inform their health care provider promptly if they experience these symptoms. Urinary tract infections pose a risk to the mother and fetus, and thus their prevention or early treatment is essential. Oral antibiotics are commonly prescribed.

The nurse can assess the woman's understanding and use of appropriate hand hygiene techniques before and after urinating and the importance of wiping the perineum from front to back. Soft, absorbent toilet tissue, preferably white and unscented, should be used; harsh, scented, or printed toilet paper can cause irritation. Bubble bath or other bath oils should be avoided because these can irritate the urethra. Women should wear all-cotton undergarments and avoid wearing tight-fitting slacks or jeans for long periods; anything that allows a buildup of heat and moisture in the genital area can foster the growth of bacteria.

Some women do not consume enough fluid. The nurse should advise pregnant women to drink at least 2 L (eight glasses) of liquid per day, preferably water, to maintain adequate fluid intake that ensures frequent urination. Pregnant women should not limit fluids in an effort to reduce the frequency of urination. Women need to know that if urine appears dark (concentrated), they must increase their fluid intake.

The nurse should review healthy urination practices with the woman. Women are told not to ignore the urge to urinate because holding urine lengthens the time bacteria are in the bladder and allows them to multiply. Women should plan ahead when they are faced with situations that can require them to delay urination (e.g., a long car ride). They always should urinate before going to bed at night. Bacteria can be introduced during intercourse; therefore, women are advised to urinate before and after intercourse, and then drink a large glass of water to promote additional urination. Consumption of cranberry juice has been considered preventive for UTI based on the acidity of the juice. There appears to be greater benefit from cranberry supplements compared with cranberry juice. Recent evidence indicates that the value of using cranberry supplements is related to the component proanthocyanidins (PAC), which prevent adhesion of bacteria to the bladder wall. Cranberry capsules are the best source of PAC, although it has been shown that there is high variability in the amount of PAC in commercially available products (Chughtai, Thomas, & Howell, 2016).

Kegel Exercises

Kegel exercises (deliberate contraction and relaxation of the pubococcygeus muscle) strengthen the muscles around the reproductive organs and improve muscle tone. Many women are not aware of the muscles of the pelvic floor until it is pointed out that these are the muscles used during urination and sexual intercourse that can be consciously controlled. The muscles of the pelvic floor encircle the vaginal outlet, and they need to be exercised because an exercised muscle can then stretch and contract readily at the time of birth. Practice of pelvic muscle exercises during pregnancy also results in fewer complaints of urinary incontinence in late pregnancy and postpartum (Kocaöz, Erogul, & Sivaslioglu, 2013).

Several ways of performing Kegel exercises have been described. The method described in the Patient Teaching box: Kegel Exercises in Chapter 3 demonstrates evidence-based nursing care. This method was developed by nurses involved in a research utilization project for continence in women. Teaching has been effective if the woman reports an increased ability to control urine flow and greater muscular control during sexual intercourse.

Preparation for Breastfeeding

During the first prenatal visit, the nurse asks if the woman is planning to breastfeed. A woman's decision about the method of infant feeding is usually made before pregnancy; thus it is essential to educate women of childbearing age about the benefits of breastfeeding. The woman and her partner are encouraged to decide which method of feeding is suitable for them; however, the benefits of breastfeeding should be emphasized. Once the couple has been given information about the advantages and disadvantages of breastfeeding and formula-feeding, they can make an informed choice. Most women who choose to breastfeed do so because they are aware of the numerous benefits (see Chapter 24). Lack of knowledge about the benefits of breastfeeding and perceived personal and social disadvantages to breastfeeding can influence a woman not to breastfeed. Modesty issues, effect on the mother's figure, lack of support by the partner and family, incompatibility with lifestyle, and lack of confidence are among the reasons cited by women

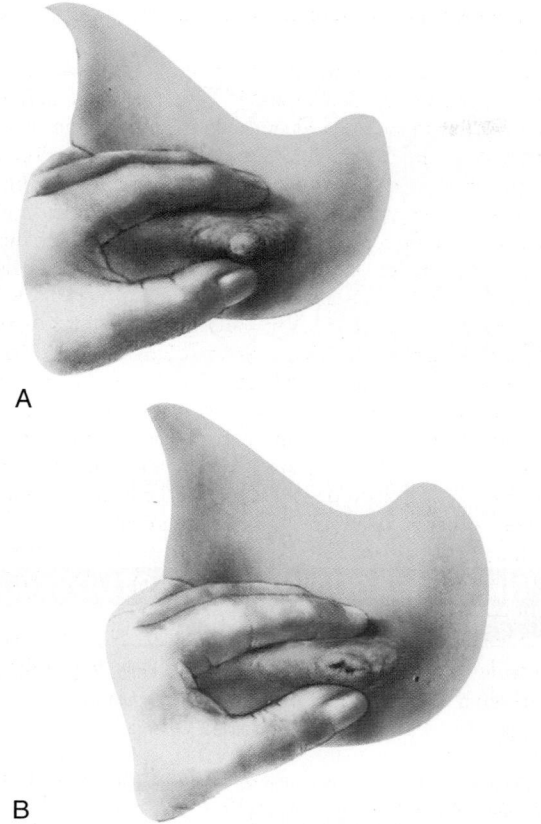

A

B

FIG 8.9 Test for inverted nipples **A,** Normal nipple everts with gentle pressure. **B,** Inverted nipple inverts with gentle pressure. (Adapted from Lawrence, R.A., & Lawrence, R.M. [2016]. *Breastfeeding: A guide for the medical profession* [8th ed.]. St. Louis, MO: Mosby.)

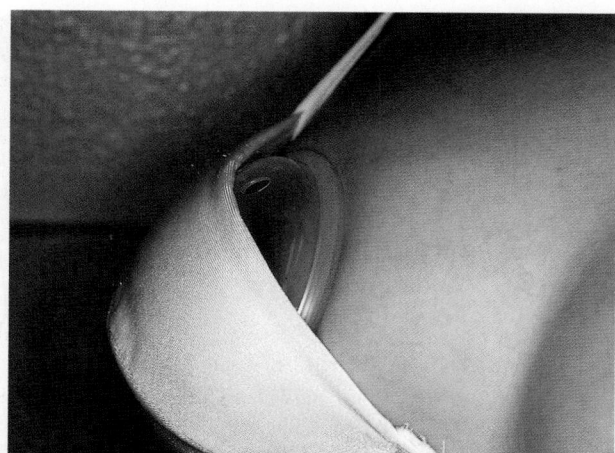

FIG 8.10 Breast shell in place inside bra; sometimes recommended for flat or inverted nipples. (Courtesy of Michael S. Clement, MD, Mesa, AZ.)

who decide to formula-feed their infants (Lawrence & Lawrence, 2016; Nelson, 2012).

Assessment of breasts during the prenatal period can reveal potential concerns related to breastfeeding. Scars on the breast can indicate previous breast reduction surgery, which can affect milk production. The woman may have breast implants; this may affect successful breastfeeding. Asymmetry of the breasts or tubular-shaped breasts suggest a lack of glandular tissue and potential problems with adequate milk production. Examination of the breasts can reveal flat or inverted nipples, which can affect the baby's ability to successfully latch on to the breast. To determine if nipples are inverted, a woman can perform a test on her nipples to determine freedom of protrusion (Fig. 8.9). The woman places her thumb and forefinger on her areola and presses inward gently. A normal nipple will evert or stand erect while an inverted nipple will appear to withdraw (Lawrence & Lawrence, 2016).

Exercises to break the adhesions that cause the nipple to invert do not work and can cause uterine contractions. Some clinicians recommend the prenatal use of breast shells (Fig. 8.10) during the last trimester for women with flat or inverted nipples, although evidence to support their effectiveness is lacking. They can be uncomfortable and cause irritation to the nipple or areola. Breast stimulation is contraindicated in women at risk for preterm labor; therefore, the decision to suggest the use of breast shells to women with flat or inverted nipples must be made judiciously (Lawrence & Lawrence, 2016).

There is no special preparation of the nipples or breasts for breastfeeding. The woman is taught to cleanse the nipples with warm water to keep the ducts from being blocked with dried colostrum. Soap, ointments, alcohol, and tinctures should not be applied because they remove protective oils that keep the nipples supple. Breast pads with plastic liners should be avoided. Women with nipple piercings should be instructed to remove the jewelry during pregnancy to allow the nipple to recover, which will help prevent infection (Lawrence & Lawrence, 2016).

A bra that fits well and provides support promotes comfort as breasts increase in size during pregnancy. The woman who plans to breastfeed may want to purchase a nursing bra that will accommodate her increased breast size during the last few months of pregnancy and during lactation.

The nurse explores the mother's questions and concerns related to breastfeeding and recommends sources of information including books and websites. The mother may appreciate a list of local breastfeeding resources that includes prenatal breastfeeding classes as well as lactation consultants and services they provide such as inpatient and outpatient consultations, home visits, and breast pump rentals.

Oral Health

Oral health during pregnancy is especially important because it can affect maternal health and pregnancy outcomes (Hartnett, Haber, Krainovich-Miller et al., 2016). There is an increased incidence of gingivitis (swelling and inflammation of the gums) and periodontitis (infection of gums that can cause damage to soft tissues and bone) during pregnancy. Studies have shown an association between periodontal disease and preterm birth, LBW, VLBW, preeclampsia, and gestational diabetes (Corbella, Taschieri, Del Fabbro, et al., 2016; Jared & Boggess, 2012; Parihar, Katoch, Rajguru, et al., 2015).

Health care providers should assess oral health at the initial prenatal visit and at intervals throughout pregnancy (ACOG, 2013/2015). It only takes 1 minute to complete an oral examination, so it can easily be incorporated into routine care. The provider or nurse should inquire about the woman's last dental visit. If it was more than 6 months earlier, she should schedule a dental examination soon (Oral Health Care During Pregnancy Expert Workgroup, 2012). A high percentage of women do not have regular dental care, primarily due to financial barriers; those with insurance are more likely to visit the dentist (Cigna Corporation, 2015).

Because calcium and phosphorus in the teeth are fixed in enamel, the old adage "for every child a tooth" is not true. There is no scientific evidence to support the belief that filling teeth or even dental extraction involving the administration of local or nitrous oxide–oxygen anesthesia

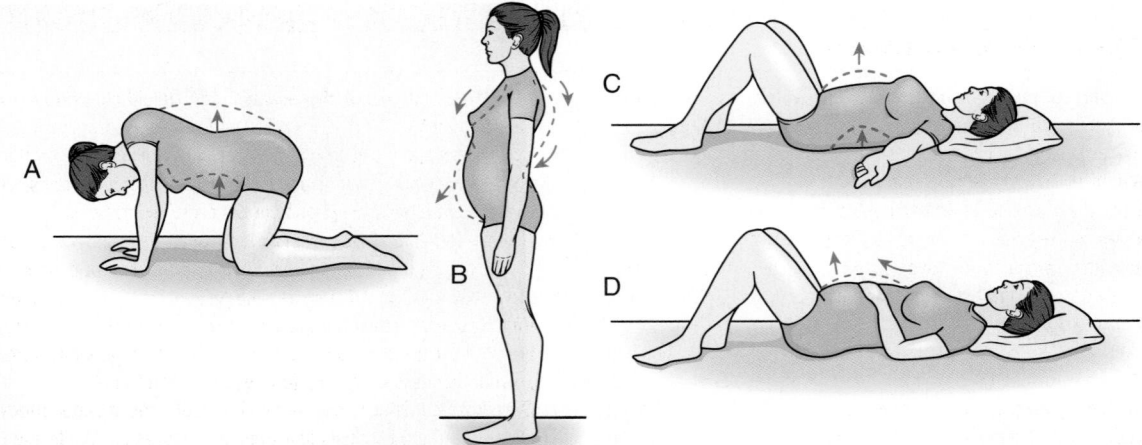

FIG 8.11 Exercises. **A, B,** and **C,** Pelvic rocking relieves low backache (excellent for relief of menstrual cramps as well). **D,** Abdominal breathing aids relaxation and lifts abdominal wall off uterus.

precipitates miscarriage or preterm labor. Antibacterial therapy should be considered for prevention of sepsis, especially in pregnant women who have had rheumatic heart disease or nephritis.

Diagnosis and treatment of oral health problems, including necessary dental X-rays and the use of local anesthetics or nitrous oxide–oxygen anesthesia, are considered safe during pregnancy. Dental care and nonemergent procedures are best scheduled during the second trimester when the woman is past the stage of feeling nauseated and can sit comfortably in the chair. To avoid supine hypotension during dental procedures, the pregnant woman in her second or third trimester is positioned in the dental chair with a small pillow under her right hip (Oral Health Care During Pregnancy Expert Workgroup, 2012).

Nurses can teach pregnant women about the importance of dental hygiene, including regular brushing and flossing. Women who experience nausea and vomiting episodes can prevent erosion of tooth enamel by rinsing with a solution of baking soda after vomiting.

Physical Activity

Physical activity during pregnancy has minimal risks and promotes a feeling of well-being in the pregnant woman. It improves physical fitness, enhances psychologic well-being, improves circulation, promotes relaxation and rest, and counteracts boredom (Price, Amini, & Kappeler, 2012). Regular exercise helps with weight management and can reduce the risk for gestational diabetes, cesarean birth, and giving birth to a large for gestational age infant (ACOG, 2015a; Domenjoz Kayser, Boulvain, 2014). Detailed exercise tips for pregnancy are presented in the Patient Teaching box: Exercise Tips for Pregnant Women. Exercises that help relieve the low back pain that often arises during the second trimester because of the increased weight of the fetus are demonstrated in Fig. 8.11 (see Clinical Reasoning Case Study). Some women enjoy prenatal exercise or yoga classes, where they receive physical benefits along with support of other pregnant women.

Posture and Body Mechanics

Skeletal and musculature changes and hormonal changes in pregnancy can predispose the woman to backache and possible injury. As pregnancy progresses, the woman's center of gravity changes, pelvic joints soften and relax, and stress is placed on abdominal musculature. Poor posture and body mechanics contribute to the discomfort and potential for injury. To minimize these problems, women can learn good body posture and body mechanics (Fig. 8.12). Strategies to prevent or relieve backache are presented in the Patient Teaching box: Posture and Body Mechanics.

CLINICAL REASONING CASE STUDY
Exercise in Pregnancy

Lourdes is 16 weeks pregnant with her second child. She wants to avoid gaining extra weight during this pregnancy and would like to continue her exercise habits: walking and Zumba classes. What guidance can you give to Lourdes?

1. Evidence—Is the evidence sufficient to make a recommendation for or against exercising during pregnancy?
2. Assumptions—Describe the underlying assumptions for each of the following issues:
   1. Physiologic changes in pregnancy that affect balance, movement, respiration, and cardiac function
   2. Maternal physiologic response during exercise
   3. Benefits of exercise
3. What implications and priorities for nursing care can be drawn at this time?
4. Does the evidence objectively support your conclusion?
5. Describe the roles/responsibilities of members of the interprofessional health care team who may be involved in caring for Lourdes.

Rest and Relaxation

Nurses encourage women to plan regular rest periods, particularly as pregnancy advances. The side-lying position is recommended because it promotes uterine perfusion and fetoplacental oxygenation by eliminating pressure on the ascending vena cava and descending aorta, which can lead to supine hypotension (Fig. 8.13). The woman should be shown how to rise slowly from a side-lying position to prevent placing strain on the back and to minimize the orthostatic hypotension caused by changes in position common in the later part of pregnancy. To stretch and rest back muscles at home or work, the nurse can show the woman the way to do the following exercises:

- Stand behind a chair. Support and balance self by using the back of the chair (Fig. 8.14). Squat for 30 seconds; stand for 15 seconds. Repeat 6 times, several times per day, as needed.
- While sitting in a chair, lower head to knees for 30 seconds. Raise head. Repeat 6 times, several times per day, as needed.

Conscious relaxation is the process of releasing tension from the mind and body through deliberate effort and practice. The techniques for conscious relaxation are numerous and varied. Box 8.2 gives some

PATIENT TEACHING

Exercise Tips for Pregnant Women

- *Consult your health care provider* when you know or suspect you are pregnant. Discuss your health and pregnancy history, your current exercise regimen, and the exercises you would like to continue throughout pregnancy.
- *Seek help* in determining an exercise routine that is well within your limit of tolerance, especially if you have not been exercising regularly.
- *Consider decreasing weight-bearing exercises* (jogging, running) and concentrating on non–weight-bearing activities such as swimming, cycling, or stretching. If you are a runner, starting in your seventh month, you may wish to walk instead.
- *Avoid risky activities* such as surfing, mountain climbing, skydiving, and racquetball because such activities, which require precise balance and coordination, can be dangerous. Avoid activities that require holding your breath and bearing down (Valsalva maneuver). Jerky, bouncy motions also should be avoided.
- *Exercise regularly* every day if possible, as long as you are healthy, to improve muscle tone and increase or maintain your stamina. Exercising sporadically can place undue strain on your muscles. Thirty minutes of moderate physical exercise is recommended. This activity can be broken up into shorter segments with rest in between. For example, exercise for 10 to 15 minutes, rest for 2 to 3 minutes, and then exercise for another 10 to 15 minutes.
- *Consider decreasing your exercise level* as your pregnancy progresses. The normal alterations of advancing pregnancy, such as decreased cardiac reserve and increased respiratory effort, can produce physiologic stress if you exercise strenuously for a long time.
- *Take your pulse* every 10 to 15 minutes while you are exercising. If it is more than 140 beats/min, slow down until it returns to a maximum of 90 beats/min. You should be able to converse easily while exercising. If you cannot, you need to slow down.
- *Avoid becoming overheated* for extended periods. It is best not to exercise for more than 35 minutes, especially in hot, humid weather. As your body temperature rises, the heat is transmitted to your fetus. Prolonged or repeated elevation of fetal temperature can result in birth defects, especially during the first 3 months of pregnancy. Your temperature should not exceed 38° C.
- *Do not use hot tubs and saunas.*
- *Perform warm-up and stretching exercises* to prepare your joints for more strenuous exercise and lessen the likelihood of strain or injury to your joints.

After the fourth month of pregnancy, you should not perform exercises flat on your back.
- *Include a cool-down period* of mild activity involving your legs after an exercise period to help bring your respiration, heart, and metabolic rates back to normal and prevent blood from pooling in the exercised muscles.
- *Rest for 10 minutes after exercising,* lying on your side. As the uterus grows, it puts pressure on a major vein in your abdomen that carries blood to your heart. Lying on your side removes the pressure and promotes return circulation from your extremities and muscles to your heart, thereby increasing blood flow to your placenta and fetus. You should rise gradually from the floor to prevent dizziness or fainting (orthostatic hypotension).
- *Stay hydrated.* Drink two or three 8-ounce glasses of water after you exercise to replace the body fluids lost through perspiration. While exercising, drink water whenever you feel the need.
- *Increase your caloric intake* to replace the calories burned during exercise and provide the extra energy needs of pregnancy. Choose high-protein foods such as fish, milk, cheese, eggs, and meat.
- *Take your time.* This is not the time to be competitive or train for activities requiring speed or long endurance.
- *Wear a supportive bra.* Your increased breast weight can cause changes in posture and put pressure on the ulnar nerve.
- *Wear supportive shoes.* As your uterus grows, your center of gravity shifts and you compensate for this by arching your back. These natural changes can make you feel off balance and more likely to fall.
- *Stop exercising immediately* if you experience shortness of breath, dizziness, numbness, tingling, pain of any kind, more than four uterine contractions per hour, decreased fetal activity, or vaginal bleeding, and consult your health care provider.
- *Recognize signs of danger,* including vaginal bleeding; blurred vision; nausea; dizziness; fainting; breathlessness; heart palpitations; increased swelling in your hands, feet, and ankles; sharp pain in the abdomen and chest; and sudden change in body temperature.
- *Avoid the following exercises* during pregnancy: downhill snow skiing because the center of gravity changes and there is a risk for falls; contact sports such as ice hockey, soccer, and basketball; and scuba diving because the pressure from the water could put the fetus at risk for decompression sickness.

PATIENT TEACHING

Posture and Body Mechanics

To Prevent or Relieve Backache
Do pelvic tilt:
- Pelvic tilt (rock) on hands and knees (see Fig. 8.11, *A*) and while sitting in straight-back chair
- Pelvic tilt (rock) in standing position against a wall, or lying on floor (see Fig. 8.11, *B* and *C*)
- Perform abdominal muscle contractions during pelvic tilt while standing, lying, or sitting to help strengthen rectus abdominis muscle (see Fig. 8.11, *D*). Use good body mechanics.
- Use leg muscles to reach objects on or near floor. Bend at the knees, not from the back. Bend knees to lower body to squatting position. Keep feet 12 to 18 inches apart to provide a solid base to maintain balance (see Fig. 8.12, *A*).
- Lift with the legs. To lift a heavy object (e.g., young child) place one foot slightly in front of the other and keep it flat while lowering onto one knee.

Lift the weight, holding it close to the body and never higher than the chest. To stand up or sit down, place one leg slightly behind the other while rising or lowering the body (see Fig. 8.12, *B*).

To Restrict the Lumbar Curve
- For prolonged standing (e.g., ironing, employment), place one foot on low footstool or box; change positions often.
- Move car seat forward so that knees are bent and higher than hips. If needed, use a small pillow to support the low back area.
- Sit in chairs low enough to allow both feet to be placed on the floor, preferably with knees higher than hips.

To Prevent Round Ligament Pain and Strain on Abdominal Muscles
- Implement the suggestions given in Table 8.2.

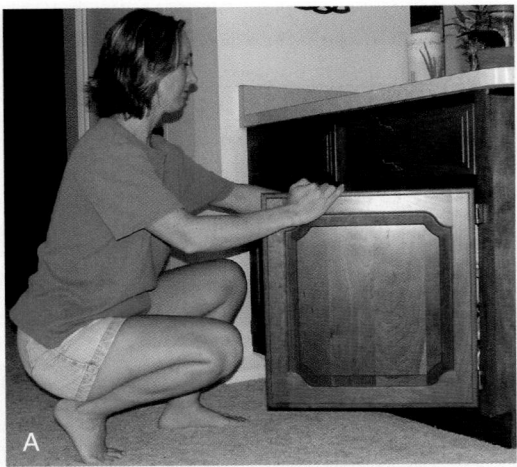

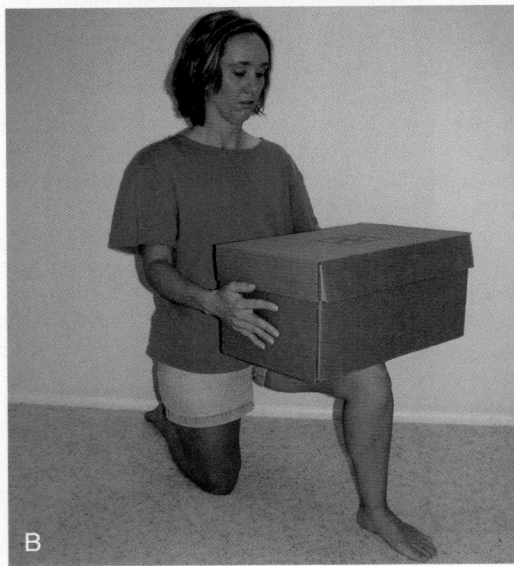

FIG 8.12 Correct body mechanics. **A,** Squatting. **B,** Lifting. (Courtesy of Julie Perry Nelson, Loveland, CO.)

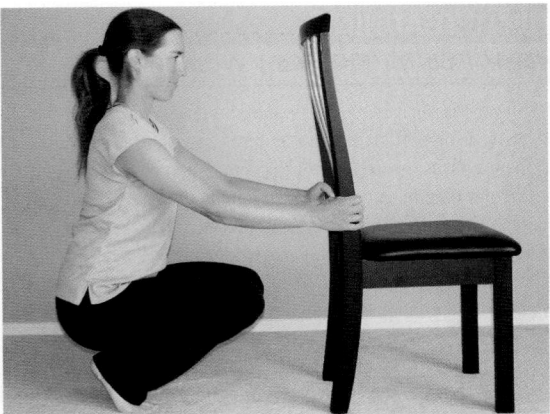

FIG 8.14 Squatting for muscle relaxation and strengthening and for keeping leg and hip joints flexible. (Courtesy of Julie Perry Nelson, Loveland, CO.)

BOX 8.2 Conscious Relaxation Tips

Preparation—Loosen clothing; assume a comfortable sitting or side-lying position with all parts of your body well supported with pillows. The use of soothing music is optional.

Beginning—Allow yourself to feel warm and comfortable. Inhale and exhale slowly and imagine peaceful relaxation coming over each part of your body, starting with the neck and working down to the toes. People who learn conscious relaxation often speak of feeling relaxed even if some discomfort is present.

Maintenance—Use imagery (fantasy or daydream) to maintain the state of relaxation. Using *active imagery*, imagine yourself moving or doing some activity and experiencing its sensations. Using *passive imagery*, imagine yourself watching a scene such as a lovely sunset.

Awakening—Return to the wakeful state gradually. Slowly begin to take in stimuli from the surrounding environment.

Further retention and development of the skill—Practice regularly for some periods each day (e.g., at the same hour for 10 to 15 minutes each day to feel refreshed, revitalized, and invigorated).

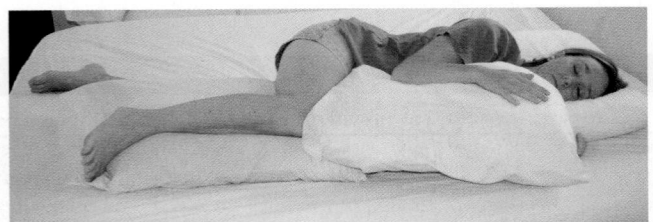

FIG 8.13 Side-lying position for rest and relaxation. (Courtesy of Julie Perry Nelson, Loveland, CO.)

guidelines. The ability to relax consciously and intentionally is beneficial for the following reasons:
- To relieve the normal discomforts related to pregnancy
- To reduce stress and therefore diminish pain perception during the childbearing cycle
- To heighten self-awareness and trust in one's own ability to control responses and functions
- To help cope with stress in everyday life situations

Employment

Employment of pregnant women usually has no adverse effects on pregnancy outcomes. Job discrimination that is based strictly on pregnancy is illegal. However, some job environments pose potential risk to the fetus (e.g., dry-cleaning plants, chemistry laboratories, parking garages). Excessive fatigue is usually the deciding factor in the termination of employment. Strategies to improve safety during pregnancy are described in the Patient Teaching box: Safety During Pregnancy.

Women with sedentary jobs need to walk around at intervals to counter the usual sluggish circulation in the legs. They also should neither sit nor stand in one position for long periods, and they should avoid crossing their legs at the knees, because all of these activities can increase the risk for varices and thrombophlebitis. Standing for long periods also increases the risk for preterm labor. The pregnant woman's chair should provide adequate back support. Use of a footstool can prevent pressure on veins, relieve strain on varicosities, minimize edema of the feet, and prevent backache.

Clothing

Some women continue to wear their usual clothes during pregnancy as long as they fit and feel comfortable. If maternity clothing is needed,

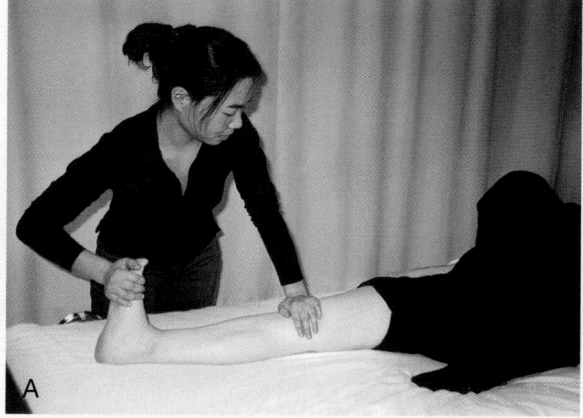

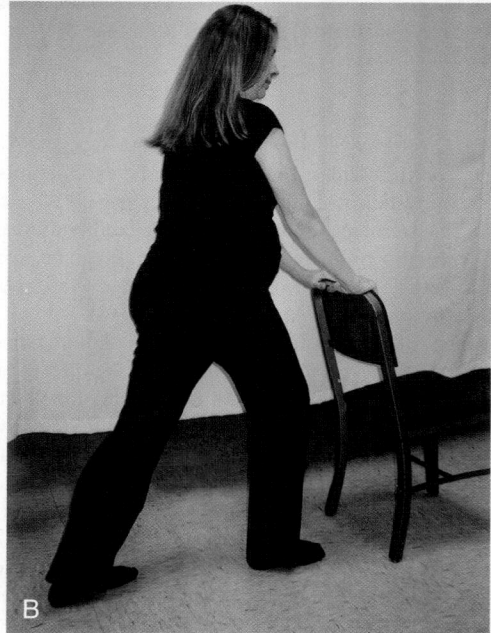

FIG 8.16 Relief of muscle spasm (leg cramps). **A,** Another person dorsiflexes foot with knee extended. **B,** Woman stands and leans forward, thereby dorsiflexing foot of the affected leg. (Courtesy of Shannon Perry, Phoenix, AZ.)

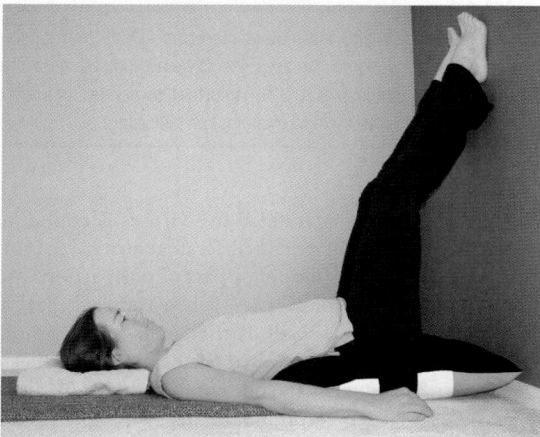

FIG 8.15 Position for resting legs and reducing edema and varicosities. Encourage the woman with vulvar varicosities to include a pillow under her hips. (Courtesy of Julie Perry Nelson, Loveland, CO.)

outfits can be purchased new or found at thrift shops or garage sales in good condition. Comfortable, loose clothing is recommended. Tight bras and belts, stretch pants, garters, tight-top knee socks, panty girdles, and other constrictive clothing should be avoided because tight clothing over the perineum increases the risk for vaginitis and miliaria (heat rash), and impaired circulation in the legs can cause varicosities.

Maternity bras are constructed to accommodate the increased breast weight, chest circumference, and size of breast tail tissue (under the arm). A well-fitting support bra can help prevent neckache and backache.

Maternal support hose give considerable comfort and promote greater venous emptying in women with large varicose veins. Ideally, support stockings should be put on before the woman gets out of bed in the morning. Fig. 8.15 demonstrates a position for resting the legs and reducing swelling and varicosities.

Comfortable shoes that provide firm support and promote good posture and balance are advisable. Very high heels and platform shoes are not recommended because of the changes in the pregnant woman's center of gravity and softening of the pelvic joints in later pregnancy, which can cause her to lose her balance. In addition, in the third trimester, the woman's pelvis tilts forward, and her lumbar curve increases. The resulting leg aches and cramps are aggravated by nonsupportive shoes. Exercises to relieve leg cramps are shown in Fig. 8.16.

Travel

Travel is not contraindicated in low-risk pregnant women; women with high-risk pregnancies are advised to avoid long-distance travel after fetal viability has been reached to avert possible economic and psychologic consequences of giving birth to a preterm infant far from home. Pregnant women should not travel to areas in which medical care is poor, water is untreated, or diseases such as malaria or Zika are prevalent. Women who contemplate foreign travel should be aware that many health

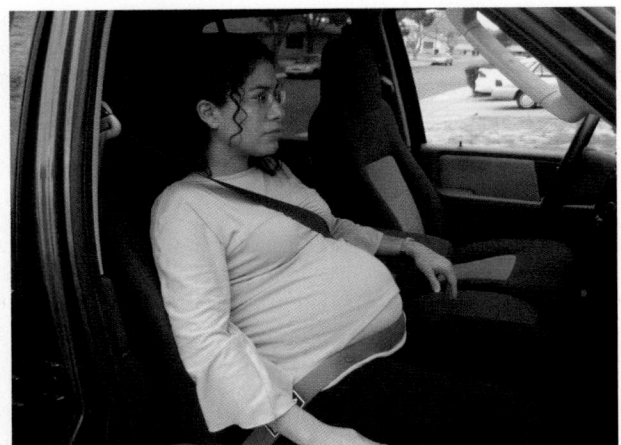

FIG 8.17 Proper use of seatbelt and headrest. (Courtesy of Brian and Mayannyn Sallee, Minot, ND.)

insurance carriers do not cover a birth in a foreign setting or even hospitalization for preterm labor. In addition, some vaccinations for foreign travel are contraindicated during pregnancy (e.g., BCG vaccine for tuberculosis). The woman should assess the availability of medical care if she experiences any problems while traveling. Pregnant women who are accustomed to living and working abroad need to seek advice from their health care provider (Morof & Carroll, 2016).

Pregnant women who travel for long distances should schedule periods of activity and rest. Prolonged periods of sitting during car or air travel increase the risk for venous stasis and thromboembolism. Six hours per day of sitting is the maximum amount of time for driving; the woman should stop at least every 2 hours to walk around for 10 minutes (Gregory et al., 2017). While sitting, the woman can practice deep breathing, foot circling, and alternately contracting and relaxing different muscle groups. She should avoid becoming fatigued.

A combination lap belt and shoulder harness is the most effective automobile restraint, and both should be used whether the mother is a driver or passenger seated in the front or back seats. The lap belt should be worn low across the pelvic bones as snugly as is comfortable. The shoulder harness should be worn above the gravid uterus and below the neck to prevent chafing (Fig. 8.17). The pregnant woman should sit upright. The headrest should be used to prevent whiplash injury. Airbags if present should remain engaged, but the steering wheel should be tilted upward, away from the abdomen and the seat moved back away from the steering wheel as much as possible.

Airline travel in large commercial jets poses little risk to a healthy pregnant woman. She is advised to inquire about restrictions or recommendations from her carrier. Most health care providers allow air travel up to 36 weeks of gestation for domestic travel and 32 to 35 weeks for international destinations in women without health- or pregnancy-related complications. Metal detectors used at airport security checkpoints emit low levels of radiation and should not pose an increased risk for harm to the fetus (Morof & Carroll, 2016). Exposure to cosmic radiation while in flight is below the dose that can cause harm at any stage of gestation (Health Physics Society, 2016). Women who fly frequently (e.g., flight attendants) should be aware of the increased exposure. The 8% humidity at which the cabins of commercial airlines are maintained can result in some water loss; hydration (with water) should therefore be maintained. The lower oxygen tension on commercial airliners does not create problems for women with uncomplicated pregnancies; however, those with severe anemia, sickle cell disease, or preexisting cardiovascular problems may experience issues. Sitting in the cramped seat of an airliner

for prolonged periods can increase the risk for superficial and deep vein thrombosis, therefore the woman is encouraged to take a walk around the aircraft during each hour of travel and to wear graduated compression stockings to minimize this risk (Morof & Carroll).

Medications and Herbal Preparations

Although much has been learned in recent years about fetal drug toxicity, the possible teratogenicity of many medications, both prescription and OTC, is still unknown. This is especially true for new medications and combinations of drugs. Moreover, certain subclinical errors or deficiencies in intermediate metabolism in the fetus may cause an otherwise harmless drug to be converted into a hazardous one. The greatest danger of drug-caused developmental defects in the fetus extends from the time of fertilization through the first trimester, a time when the woman may not realize she is pregnant. Self-treatment must be discouraged. The use of all drugs, including OTC medications, herbs, and vitamins, should be limited and a careful record kept of all therapeutic and nontherapeutic agents used.

The use of complementary and alternative medicine by pregnant women is widespread (Frawley, Adams, Sibbritt, et al., 2013). There is limited research evidence about the safety of herbal preparations, especially during pregnancy. Although the use of complementary and alternative therapies is consistent with the holistic, woman-centered approach to care, caution is warranted in their use because of the lack of evidence related to their safety and efficacy.

> **! NURSING ALERT**
>
> Although complementary and alternative medicine (CAM) may benefit the woman during pregnancy, some practices should be avoided because they can increase the risk for complications. It is important to ask the woman about OTC products (including herbals and vitamins) she is using.

Immunizations

Immunization with live or attenuated live viruses is contraindicated during pregnancy because of potential teratogenicity; recommended vaccination with these agents should be part of postpartum care. Live-virus vaccines include those for measles (rubeola and rubella), varicella (chickenpox), and mumps, as well as the Sabin (oral) poliomyelitis vaccine (no longer used in the United States). Vaccines that can be administered during pregnancy include combined tetanus-diphtheria-acellular pertussis (Tdap), recombinant hepatitis B, and influenza (inactivated) vaccines (CDC, 2016a).

Reported cases of pertussis (whooping cough) have increased significantly in the United States and Canada in recent years. Pertussis can cause serious and life-threatening complications in mothers and infants. To provide maximal maternal antibody response and transfer passive immunity to the infant, Tdap should be administered between 27 and 36 weeks of gestation. Maternal antipertussis antibodies are short lived, and antibody levels drop significantly during the first year after vaccination. As a result, it is unlikely that a Tdap vaccination in one pregnancy will transfer passive immunity from mother to infant in a subsequent pregnancy. Therefore, the recommendation is to administer Tdap to a pregnant woman during every pregnancy regardless of her prior vaccination history. If Tdap is not administered during pregnancy, it should be given immediately postpartum. Adolescents and adults (parents, grandparents, siblings, child care workers, and health care personnel) who will have close contact with an infant less than 12 months of age should receive a single dose of Tdap if not vaccinated previously (CDC, 2013; 2016a).

All women who are pregnant during the influenza season (November to March) should be offered an influenza vaccination. The injectable inactivated influenza vaccine is safe throughout pregnancy. The intranasal influenza vaccine is contraindicated during pregnancy because it contains a live virus (ACOG, 2014).

Rh Immune Globulin

Testing to determine the pregnant woman's blood type is done at the first prenatal visit. Rh-negative women will also have an antibody screen in the first and third trimester. Women with Rh-negative (D-negative) blood type who are carrying an Rh-positive (D-positive) fetus can develop antibodies against the D antigen on the fetal red blood cell, causing lysis of the fetal red blood cells. This can lead to life-threatening hemolytic disease of the fetus and newborn (Aitken & Tichy, 2015).

Prophylactic Rh immune globulin can be administered to the Rh-negative (D-negative) pregnant woman to prevent formation of antibodies (alloimmunization) by destroying any fetal red blood cells in the maternal circulation before her immune system recognizes the D-positive antigen and begins to produce antibodies (Blackburn, 2013). A dose of 300 micrograms of Rh immune globulin is routinely administered at 26 to 30 weeks to all Rh-negative women without evidence of anti-D alloimmunization. If she gives birth to an Rh-positive infant, the dose of Rh

immune globulin is repeated within 72 hours after birth (see Medication Guide in Chapter 19). Other indications for administration of Rh immune globulin to Rh-negative women during pregnancy include chorionic villus sampling, amniocentesis, spontaneous or therapeutic abortion, ectopic pregnancy, external cephalic version, and abdominal trauma (Moise, 2017).

Substance Use

Any drug or environmental agent that enters the pregnant woman's bloodstream has the potential to cross the placenta and harm the fetus. The nurse inquires about the use of any substances at the initial prenatal visit and at all subsequent visits. See Chapter 11 for information on substance use during pregnancy.

Normal Discomforts

Pregnant women have physical symptoms that would be considered abnormal in the nonpregnant state. They need explanations of the causes of the discomforts and advice on ways to relieve them. Information about the physiology, prevention, and self-management of discomforts experienced during the three trimesters is given in Table 8.3. Nurses can do much to allay a first-time mother's anxiety about such symptoms

TABLE 8.3 Discomforts Related to Pregnancy

Discomfort	Physiology	Education for Self-Management
First Trimester		
Breast changes: pain, tingling, tenderness, enlargement	Hypertrophy of mammary glandular tissue and increased vascularization, pigmentation, and size and prominence of nipples and areolae caused by hormonal stimulation	Wear supportive maternity bras with pads to absorb discharge, may be worn at night; wash with warm water and keep dry; breast tenderness may interfere with sexual expression or foreplay but is temporary
Urgency and frequency of urination	Vascular engorgement and altered bladder function caused by hormones; bladder capacity reduced by enlarging uterus and fetal presenting part	Empty bladder regularly; perform Kegel exercises; limit fluid intake before bedtime; wear perineal pad; report pain or burning sensation to primary health care provider
Languor and malaise; fatigue (early pregnancy, most common)	Unexplained; may be caused by increasing levels of estrogen, progesterone, and hCG or by elevated basal body temperature; psychologic response to pregnancy and its required physical and psychologic adaptations	Rest as needed; eat well-balanced diet to prevent anemia
Nausea and vomiting, also known as morning sickness, occurs in 50%–75% of pregnant women; starts between first and second missed periods and lasts until about fourth missed period; can occur any time during day; fathers also may have symptoms	Cause unknown; may result from hormonal changes, possibly hCG; may be partly emotional, reflecting pride in, ambivalence about, or rejection of pregnant state	Avoid empty or overloaded stomach; maintain good posture—give stomach ample room; stop smoking; eat dry carbohydrate on awakening; remain in bed until feeling subsides, or alternate dry carbohydrate every other hour with fluids such as hot herbal decaffeinated tea, milk, or clear coffee until feeling subsides; eat five or six small meals per day; avoid fried, odorous, spicy, greasy, or gas-forming foods; wear acupressure bands used to treat motion sickness; ginger or acupuncture may be helpful; vitamin B$_6$ + doxylamine (Diclegis) may be ordered; consult primary health care provider if intractable vomiting occurs
Ptyalism (excessive salivation) can occur starting 2–3 weeks after first missed period	Possibly caused by elevated estrogen levels; may be related to reluctance to swallow because of nausea	Use astringent mouthwash, chew gum, eat hard candy as comfort measures
Gingivitis and epulis (hyperemia, hypertrophy, bleeding, tenderness of the gums); condition disappears spontaneously 1–2 months after birth	Increased vascularity and proliferation of connective tissue from estrogen stimulation	Eat well-balanced diet with adequate protein and fresh fruits and vegetables; brush teeth gently with soft toothbrush, and observe good dental hygiene; avoid infection; see dentist

Continued

TABLE 8.3   Discomforts Related to Pregnancy—cont'd

Discomfort	Physiology	Education for Self-Management
Nasal stuffiness; epistaxis (nosebleed)	Hyperemia of mucous membranes related to increased estrogen levels	Use humidifier; avoid trauma; normal saline nose drops or spray may be used
Leukorrhea: often noted throughout pregnancy	Hormonally stimulated cervix becomes hypertrophic and hyperactive, producing abundant amount of mucus	Not preventable; do not douche; wear perineal pads; perform hygienic practices such as wiping front to back; report to primary health care provider if accompanied by pruritus, foul odor, or change in character or color
Psychosocial dynamics, mood swings, mixed feelings	Hormonal and metabolic adaptations; feelings about female role, sexuality, timing of pregnancy, and resultant changes in life and lifestyle	Participate in pregnancy support group; communicate concerns to partner, family, and health care provider; request referral for supportive services if needed (financial assistance)

Second Trimester

Discomfort	Physiology	Education for Self-Management
Pigmentation deepens: darkening of areola and vulva; linea nigra; melasma (mask of pregnancy), acne, oily skin	Melanocyte-stimulating hormone (from anterior pituitary gland)	Not preventable; usually resolves during puerperium
Spider nevi (angiomas) appear over neck, thorax, face, and arms during second or third trimester	Focal networks of dilated arterioles (end arteries) from increased concentration of estrogens	Not preventable; they fade slowly during late puerperium; rarely disappear completely
Pruritus (noninflammatory)	Unknown cause; various types: nonpapular; closely aggregated pruritic papules	Keep fingernails short and clean; contact primary health care provider for diagnosis of cause
	Increased excretory function of skin and stretching of skin possible factors	Not preventable; use comfort measures for symptoms; distraction; tepid baths with sodium bicarbonate or oatmeal added to water; lotions and oils; change of soaps or reduction in use of soap; loose clothing; oral or topical antihistamines or topical steroid cream if recommended by health care provider
Palpitations	Unknown; should not be accompanied by persistent cardiac irregularity	Not preventable; contact primary health care provider if accompanied by symptoms of cardiac decompensation
Supine hypotension (vena cava syndrome) and bradycardia	Caused by pressure of gravid uterus on ascending vena cava when woman is supine; reduces uteroplacental and renal perfusion	Side-lying position or semi-sitting posture, with knees slightly flexed (see Emergency Treatment box: Supine Hypotension)
Faintness and, rarely, syncope (orthostatic hypotension) may persist throughout pregnancy	Vasomotor lability or postural hypotension from hormones; in late pregnancy may be caused by venous stasis in lower extremities	Moderate exercise, deep breathing, vigorous leg movement; avoid sudden changes in position and warm, crowded areas; move slowly and deliberately; keep environment cool; avoid hypoglycemia by eating five or six small meals per day; wear elastic hose; sit as necessary; if symptoms are serious, contact primary health care provider
Food cravings	Cause unknown; craving influenced by culture or geographic area	Not preventable; satisfy craving unless it interferes with well-balanced diet; report unusual cravings to primary health care provider
Heartburn (pyrosis or acid indigestion): burning sensation, occasionally with burping and regurgitation of a little sour-tasting fluid	Progesterone slows gastrointestinal (GI) tract motility and digestion, reverses peristalsis, relaxes cardiac sphincter, and delays emptying time of stomach; stomach displaced upward and compressed by enlarging uterus	Limit or avoid gas-producing or fatty foods and large meals; maintain good posture; sip milk for temporary relief; drink hot herbal tea; primary health care provider may prescribe antacid between meals; contact primary health care provider for persistent symptoms
Constipation	GI tract motility slowed because of progesterone, resulting in increased resorption of water and drying of stool; intestines compressed by enlarging uterus; predisposition to constipation because of oral iron supplementation	Drink 2 L (8–10 glasses) of water per day; include fiber in diet; engage in moderate exercise; maintain regular schedule for bowel movements; use relaxation techniques and deep breathing; do not take stool softener, laxatives, mineral oil, other drugs, or enemas without first consulting primary health care provider
Flatulence with bloating and belching	Reduced GI motility because of progesterone, allowing time for bacterial action that produces gas; swallowing air	Chew foods slowly and thoroughly; avoid gas-producing foods, fatty foods, large meals; exercise; maintain regular bowel habits

TABLE 8.3 Discomforts Related to Pregnancy—cont'd

Discomfort	Physiology	Education for Self-Management
Varicose veins (varicosities): can be associated with aching legs and tenderness; can be present in legs and vulva; hemorrhoids are varicosities in perianal area	Hereditary predisposition; relaxation of smooth muscle walls of veins because of hormones causing tortuous dilated veins in legs and pelvic vasocongestion; condition aggravated by enlarging uterus, gravity, and bearing down for bowel movements; thrombi from leg varices rare but can occur in hemorrhoids	Avoid lengthy standing or sitting, constrictive clothing, and constipation and bearing down with bowel movements; moderate exercise; rest with legs and hips elevated (see Fig. 8.15); wear support stockings; thrombosed hemorrhoid may be evacuated; relieve swelling and pain with warm sitz baths, local application of astringent compresses
Headaches (through week 26)	Emotional tension (more common than vascular migraine headache); eye strain (refractory errors); vascular engorgement and congestion of sinuses resulting from hormone stimulation	Conscious relaxation; contact primary health care provider for constant "splitting" headache to assess for preeclampsia; OTC analgesics may be used if recommended by health care provider (e.g., acetaminophen)
Carpal tunnel syndrome (involves thumb, second, and third fingers, lateral side of little finger)	Compression of median nerve resulting from changes in surrounding tissues; pain, numbness, tingling, burning; loss of skilled movements (typing); dropping of objects	Not preventable; elevate affected arms; splinting of affected hand may help; regressive after pregnancy; surgery is curative
Periodic numbness, tingling of fingers (acrodysesthesia)	Brachial plexus traction syndrome resulting from drooping of shoulders during pregnancy (occurs especially at night and early morning)	Maintain good posture; wear supportive maternity bra; condition will disappear after birth if lifting and carrying baby do not aggravate it
Round ligament pain (tenderness)	Stretching of ligament caused by enlarging uterus	Not preventable; rest, maintain good body mechanics to avoid overstretching ligament; relieve cramping by squatting or bringing knees to chest; sometimes heat helps
Joint pain, backache, and pelvic pressure; hypermobility of joints	Relaxation of symphyseal and sacroiliac joints because of hormones, resulting in unstable pelvis; exaggerated lumbar and cervicothoracic curves caused by change in center of gravity resulting from enlarging abdomen	Maintain good posture and body mechanics; avoid fatigue; wear low-heeled shoes; abdominal support may be useful; conscious relaxation; sleep on firm mattress; apply local heat or ice; get back rubs; do pelvic tilt exercises; rest; condition will disappear 6–8 weeks after the birth
Third Trimester		
Shortness of breath and dyspnea occur in 60% of pregnant women	Expansion of diaphragm limited by enlarging uterus; diaphragm is elevated about 4 cm; some relief after lightening	Good posture; sleep with extra pillows; avoid overloading stomach; stop smoking; contact health care provider if symptoms worsen to rule out anemia, emphysema, and asthma
Insomnia (later weeks of pregnancy)	Fetal movements, muscle cramping, urinary frequency, shortness of breath, or other discomforts	Reassurance; conscious relaxation; back massage or effleurage; support of body parts with pillows; warm milk or warm shower or bath before bedtime
Psychosocial responses: mood swings, mixed feelings, increased anxiety	Hormonal and metabolic adaptations; feelings about impending labor, birth, and parenthood	Reassurance and support from significant other and health care providers; improved communication with partner, family, and others
Urinary frequency and urgency return	Vascular engorgement and altered bladder function caused by hormones; bladder capacity reduced by enlarging uterus and fetal presenting part	Empty bladder regularly; Kegel exercises; limit fluid intake before bedtime; reassurance; wear perineal pad; contact health care provider for pain or burning sensation
Perineal discomfort and pressure	Pressure from enlarging uterus, especially when standing or walking; worse with multifetal gestation	Rest, conscious relaxation, and good posture; contact health care provider for assessment and treatment if pain is present
Braxton Hicks contractions	Intensification of uterine contractions in preparation for work of labor	Reassurance; rest; change of position; practice breathing techniques when contractions are bothersome; effleurage; differentiate from preterm labor
Leg cramps (gastrocnemius spasm), especially when reclining	Compression of nerves supplying lower extremities because of enlarging uterus; reduced level of diffusible serum calcium or elevation of serum phosphorus; aggravating factors: fatigue, poor peripheral circulation, pointing toes when stretching legs or when walking, drinking more than 1 L (1 qt) of milk per day	Use massage and heat over affected muscle; dorsiflex foot until spasm relaxes (see Fig. 8.16); stand on cold surface; oral supplementation with calcium carbonate or calcium lactate tablets; aluminum hydroxide gel, 30 mL, with each meal removes phosphorus by absorbing it (consult primary health care provider before taking these remedies)
Ankle edema (nonpitting) to lower extremities	Edema aggravated by prolonged standing, sitting, poor posture, lack of exercise, constrictive clothing, or hot weather	Ample fluid intake for natural diuretic effect; put on support stockings before arising; rest periodically with legs and hips elevated (see Fig. 8.15); exercise moderately; contact health care provider if generalized edema develops; diuretics are contraindicated

by telling her about them in advance and using terminology that the woman (or couple) can understand. Understanding the rationale for treatment promotes their participation in their care. Interventions should be individualized, with attention given to the woman's lifestyle and culture (see Nursing Care Plan).

Recognizing Potential Complications

One of the most important responsibilities of care providers is to alert the pregnant woman to signs and symptoms that indicate a potential complication of pregnancy. The woman needs to know how and to whom to report such warning signs. She and her family should receive

NURSING CARE PLAN

Adolescent Pregnancy

Case Study

Monica, 16 years of age, is 6 weeks pregnant with her first child; this is her first prenatal visit to the OB clinic. She hopes to marry Rick, the father of her baby, but her parents say she is too young. She lives with her parents, and Rick lives nearby. Very few of her friends have children, and she admits she knows very little about pregnancy and childbirth. She wonders what to expect. Monica's parents are upset about her pregnancy but will try to support her. She has started experiencing nausea in the mornings and says she feels more tired than usual; she has also noticed that she needs to urinate more frequently.

Assessment

What are the normal discomforts of pregnancy that Monica might experience? What are signs of possible problems that she might notice?

Defining Characteristics

Verbalization of problem
Lack of personal experience with pregnancy
Lack of exposure to other pregnant women

Nursing Diagnosis

Deficient Knowledge related to lack of information about discomforts of pregnancy

Expected Outcomes

Monica will recognize that increased knowledge and skill will help her cope with the discomforts of pregnancy.
Monica will demonstrate understanding of normal pregnancy and common discomforts.
Monica will express satisfaction with her increase in knowledge.

Nursing Interventions	Rationales
Establish a trusting relationship with the patient; develop mutual goals for learning.	To enhance learning
Assess her knowledge about pregnancy.	To identify knowledge deficits and to establish a baseline for teaching
Select teaching strategies appropriate to the material, the patient's age, learning style, and learning preferences.	To better meet Monica's needs
List common discomforts of pregnancy, and provide information and skills needed for understanding discomforts of pregnancy and how to deal with them.	To decrease Monica's anxiety, to relieve her discomfort, and increase her sense of competence

Case Study (Continued)

Monica is now in her sixth month of pregnancy. Most of the discomforts of pregnancy have been resolved, and she is feeling well. She missed her last appointment with the midwife because she was "busy" and wasn't having any problems so did not see the need to keep the appointment. She has plans to go with her girlfriend to visit friends in the next state and will be gone at least 2 weeks. She said that she will call the midwife if she has any problems or

questions. She plans to keep her 9-month appointment, but she is afraid of needles and does not see the need to have any blood samples taken.

Assessment

What are signs of problems during the second trimester of pregnancy? What are the risks of not keeping prenatal appointments? Of not undergoing screening?

Defining Characteristics

Increasing blood pressure
Excessive weight gain
Proteinuria
Abnormal blood profile
Refusing prenatal screening
Lack of compliance with prenatal care

Nursing Diagnosis

Risk for Injury: Maternal or Fetal related to inadequate prenatal care and screening

Expected Outcomes

Monica will keep prenatal appointments; her parents will encourage visits to the midwife.
She will undergo appropriate prenatal screening.
Monica will experience an uncomplicated pregnancy and give birth to a healthy baby at term.

Nursing Interventions	Rationales
Provide information using therapeutic communication and confidentiality.	To establish relationship and build trust
Discuss importance of ongoing prenatal care and possible risks to adolescent patient and fetus.	To reinforce that ongoing assessment is crucial to the health and well-being of Monica and her fetus, even if she feels well. Adolescents are more at risk for some complications that may be avoided or managed early if prenatal visits are maintained.
Discuss risks of alcohol, tobacco, and recreational drug use during pregnancy.	To minimize risks to Monica and her fetus because adolescents have a higher abuse rate than the rest of the pregnant population
Assess for evidence of STI, and provide information regarding sexual practices.	To minimize risk to Monica and her fetus because adolescents are more at risk for STIs
Screen for preeclampsia on an ongoing basis.	To minimize risk because adolescents are more at risk for preeclampsia

Case Study (Continued)

When Monica was 8 months pregnant, she tearfully said that her girlfriends don't want a "fat, pregnant" person to go out with them and that her boyfriend spends more time with his friends than with her. She asked him to go to parenting classes with her, but he would rather go to football practice. Her mother is not

◉ NURSING CARE PLAN

Adolescent Pregnancy—cont'd

sympathetic; she told Monica that it is her own fault she is pregnant and that she will just have to deal with it.

Assessment

What are characteristics of social isolation? What measures can Monica take to establish satisfying relationships?

Defining Characteristics

Absence of supportive significant other
Expressed feelings of aloneness
Expressed feelings of difference from others
Sad, dull affect

Nursing Diagnosis

Social Isolation related to body image changes of pregnant adolescent as evidenced by patient statements and concerns

Expected Outcomes

Monica will identify support systems.
She will report decreased feelings of social isolation.
She will participate in childbirth and preparation for parenting classes.

Nursing Interventions	Rationales
Discuss with Monica changes in relationships that have occurred as a result of pregnancy.	To determine extent of isolation from family, peers, and father of baby
Provide referrals and resources appropriate for developmental stage of patient	To give information for patient support
Provide information regarding parenting classes, breastfeeding classes, and childbirth preparation classes.	To give further information and group support, which lessens social isolation

a printed list of warning signs, written at the appropriate literacy level and in their language, that warrant a call to the health care provider (HCP) or clinic; phone numbers for the HCP or clinic should be listed.

The nurse answers questions as they arise during pregnancy. Pregnant women often have difficulty deciding when to report signs and symptoms. The mother is encouraged to refer to the printed list of potential complications and to listen to her body. If she senses that something is wrong, she should call her care provider. Several signs and symptoms must be discussed moreextensively. These include vaginal bleeding, alteration in fetal movements, symptoms of preeclampsia, rupture of membranes, and preterm labor (see Table 8.2).

Sexual Counseling

Sexual counseling of expectant couples includes providing information, countering misinformation, providing reassurance of normality, and suggesting alternative behaviors. The uniqueness of each couple is considered within a biopsychosocial framework. Nurses can initiate discussion about sexual adaptations during pregnancy, based on sound knowledge about the physical, social, and emotional responses to sex during pregnancy. Not all maternity nurses are comfortable dealing with the sexual concerns of their patients. Nurses should be aware of their personal strengths and limitations in dealing with sexual content and be prepared to make referrals if necessary.

Some women merely need permission to be sexually active during pregnancy. Others, however, need to be given information about the physiologic changes that occur during pregnancy, have the myths that are associated with sex during pregnancy dispelled, and participate in open discussions of positions for intercourse that decrease pressure on the gravid abdomen (Fig. 8.18). Such tasks are within the purview of the nurse and should be an integral component of the health care rendered.

Some couples need to be referred for sex therapy or family therapy. Couples with long-standing problems with sexual dysfunction that are intensified by pregnancy are candidates for sex therapy. Whenever a sexual problem is a symptom of a more serious relationship problem, family therapy can be beneficial.

Sexual History

The couple's sexual history provides a basis for counseling, but history taking also is an ongoing process. The couple's receptivity to changes in attitudes, body image, partner relationships, and physical status are

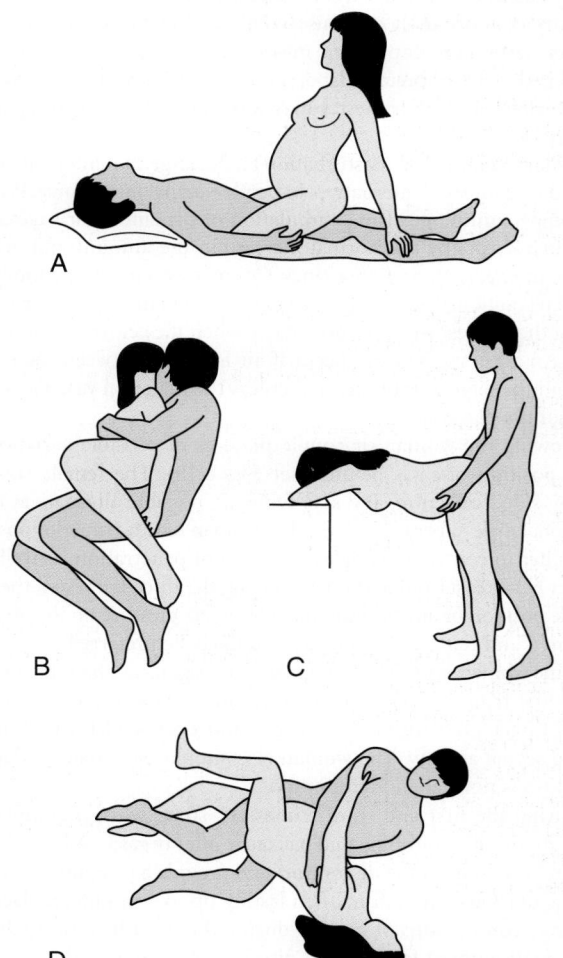

FIG 8.18 Positions for sexual intercourse during pregnancy. **A,** Female superior. **B,** Side by side. **C,** Rear entry. **D,** Facing each other.

relevant topics throughout pregnancy. The history reveals the woman's knowledge of female anatomy and physiology and her attitudes about sex during pregnancy, as well as her perceptions of the pregnancy, the health status of the couple, and the quality of their relationship.

Countering Misinformation

Many myths and much of the misinformation related to sex and pregnancy are masked by seemingly unrelated issues. For example, a discussion about the baby's ability to hear and see in utero can be prompted by questions about the baby being an "unseen observer" of the couple's sexual activities. The counselor must be extremely sensitive to the concerns behind such questions when counseling in this highly charged emotional area.

Safety and Comfort During Sexual Activity

For most women, there are no restrictions on sexual intercourse during pregnancy. However, pregnant women should be aware that they are likely to experience alternations in sexual desire and comfort during sexual activity. Uterine activity can increase with sexual intercourse; this can be related to breast stimulation, orgasm, or prostaglandins in male ejaculate. For the majority of women, this is not a problem. However, a history of more than one miscarriage; a threatened miscarriage in the first trimester; impending miscarriage in the second trimester; threatened or actual preterm labor; and PROM, bleeding, or abdominal pain during the third trimester may warrant caution regarding coitus and orgasm.

Solitary and mutual masturbation and oral-genital intercourse may be used by couples as alternatives to penile-vaginal intercourse. Partners who enjoy cunnilingus (oral stimulation of the clitoris or vagina) can feel "turned off" by the normal increase in the amount and odor of vaginal discharge during pregnancy. Couples who practice cunnilingus should be cautioned against the blowing of air into the vagina, particularly during the last few weeks of pregnancy when the cervix can be slightly open. An air embolism can occur if air is forced between the uterine wall and the fetal membranes and enters the maternal vascular system through the placenta.

Showing the woman or couple pictures of possible variations of coital position often is helpful (see Fig. 8.18). The female-superior, side-by-side, rear-entry, and side-lying are possible alternatives to the traditional male-superior position. The woman astride (superior position) allows her to control the angle and depth of penetration, as well as to protect her breasts and abdomen. During the third trimester, the side-by-side position or any position that places less pressure on the pregnant abdomen and requires less energy will likely be preferred.

Some women, especially multiparas, have significant breast tenderness in the first trimester. The nurse can recommend a coital position that avoids direct pressure on the breasts and decreased breast fondling during sexual activity. The woman also should be reassured that this condition is normal and temporary.

During the first and third trimesters, some women complain of lower abdominal cramping and backache after orgasm. A back rub can often relieve some of the discomfort and provide a pleasant experience. A tonic uterine contraction, often lasting up to 1 minute, replaces the rhythmic contractions of orgasm during the third trimester. Changes in the FHR without fetal distress also have been reported.

Risk-reduction measures against the acquisition and transmission of STIs (e.g., syphilis, gonorrhea, chlamydia, herpes simplex virus [HSV], HIV) are advised during sexual activity at all times, including during pregnancy. Because these diseases can be transmitted to the woman and her fetus, using condoms is recommended throughout pregnancy if the woman is at risk for acquiring an STI (e.g., adolescents) (AAP & ACOG, 2012).

Psychosocial Support

Esteem, affection, trust, concern, consideration of cultural and religious responses, and listening are all components of the emotional support given to the pregnant woman and her family. The woman's satisfaction with her relationships—partner and family—and their support, her feeling of competence, and her sense of being in control are important issues to be addressed in the third trimester. A discussion of fetal responses to stimuli, such as sound and light, as well as patterns of sleeping and waking, can be helpful. Other common concerns for the pregnant woman and her partner include fear of pain, loss of control, and possible birth of the infant before reaching the hospital; anxieties about parenthood; parental concerns about the safety of the mother and unborn child; siblings and their acceptance of the new baby; social and economic responsibilities; and issues arising from conflicts in cultural, religious, or personal value systems. In addition, the woman may have concerns about the father's or partner's commitment to the pregnancy and to the couple's relationship. Providing the prospective parents with an opportunity to discuss their concerns and validating the normality of their responses can meet their needs to varying degrees. Anticipatory guidance and health promotion strategies can help partners cope with their concerns. Nurses can facilitate and encourage open dialog between the expectant mother and her partner.

VARIATIONS IN PRENATAL CARE

The course of prenatal care described thus far may seem to suggest that the experiences of childbearing women are similar and that nursing interventions are uniformly consistent across all populations. Although typical patterns of response to pregnancy are easily recognized and many aspects of prenatal care indeed are consistent, pregnant women and their families enter the health care system with unique concerns and needs. The nurse's ability to assess unique needs and to tailor interventions to the woman and her family is the hallmark of expertise in providing care. Variations that influence prenatal care include culture, maternal age, medical and obstetric history, and number of fetuses.

CULTURAL INFLUENCES

All health care professionals are responsible for providing safe, evidence-based care that helps people to attain and maintain their optimal state of health. Services that are offered in a way that respects people's cultural and linguistic preferences have been demonstrated to improve the quality of health care and to reduce health disparities. The US Department of Health and Human Services Office of Minority Health (2013) has developed standards for the delivery of culturally and linguistically appropriate health care; the standards can be accessed at http://minorityhealth.hhs.gov.

Prenatal care as we know it is a phenomenon of Western health practices. In the US model of health care, women are encouraged to seek prenatal care as early as possible in pregnancy by visiting a physician or certified nurse-midwife. This recommendation not only is unfamiliar but also seems strange to women of other cultures.

Many cultural variations are found in prenatal care. Even if the prenatal care described is familiar to a woman, some practices can conflict with the beliefs and practices of a subculture group to which she belongs. Because of these and other factors, such as lack of money, lack of transportation, and language barriers, women from diverse cultures may not seek prenatal care until late in pregnancy or they may not participate in the prenatal care system at all. A concern for modesty can be a deterrent to seeking prenatal care. For some women, exposing body parts, especially to a male, is considered a serious violation of their modesty. For many women, an invasive procedure such as a vaginal

🏠 COMMUNITY FOCUS

Cultural Childbearing Needs

Select an immigrant or other minority group in your community, and identify childbearing-related beliefs and practices that are unique to that group. Are there stores in the area that sell items that meet that group's needs? Does the community center have activities or classes that are directed toward the group? Are perinatal education programs available in languages other than English; do they provide essential information while incorporating cultural patterns? What could you, as a nurse, contribute to the community that would help meet the needs of that group?

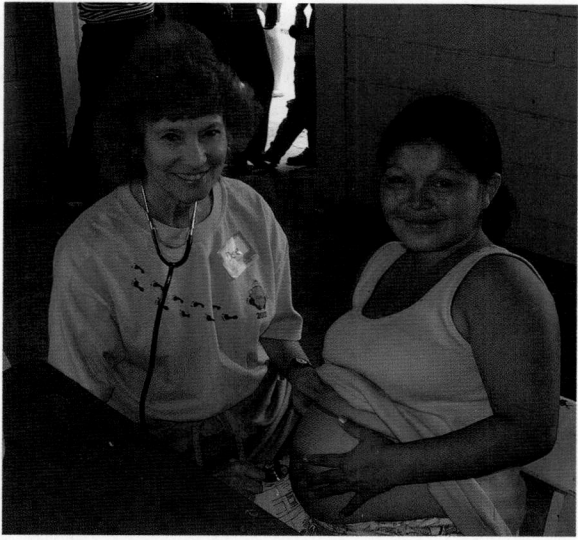

FIG 8.19 A young woman from Honduras wearing a red muñeco given to her by her mother to ensure a safe birth. (Courtesy of Dee Lowdermilk, Chapel Hill, NC.)

examination is so threatening that they cannot discuss it, even with their own husbands. Many women prefer a female health care provider. Too often, health care providers assume women lose this modesty during pregnancy and labor, but actually most women value and appreciate efforts to maintain their modesty.

Because pregnancy is considered a normal process and the woman is in a state of health, many cultural groups regard care from a health care professional to be necessary only in times of illness. Therefore, the services of a clinician are considered inappropriate during pregnancy. Western medicine's view of problems in pregnancy can differ from that of members of other cultural groups.

Although pregnancy is considered normal by many, certain practices are expected of women of all cultures to promote a good outcome. Cultural prescriptions tell women what to do, and cultural proscriptions establish taboos. The purposes of these practices are to prevent maternal illness resulting from a pregnancy-induced imbalanced state and to protect the vulnerable fetus. Prescriptions and proscriptions regulate the woman's emotional response, clothing, activity, rest, sexual activity, and dietary practices. Exploring her beliefs, perceptions of the meaning of childbearing, and health care practices can help health care professionals foster the woman's self-actualization, promote attainment of the maternal role, and positively influence her relationship with her partner.

To provide culturally responsive care, nurses must be knowledgeable about practices and customs, although it is not possible to know all there is to know about every culture and subculture or the many lifestyles that exist. It is important to learn about the varied cultures in the setting where each nurse practices. When exploring cultural beliefs and practices related to childbearing, the nurse can support and nurture those beliefs that promote physical or emotional adaptation. However, if potentially harmful beliefs or activities are identified, the nurse should sensitively provide education and propose modifications (see Community Focus box).

Emotional Response

Virtually all cultures emphasize the importance of maintaining a socially harmonious and agreeable environment for a pregnant woman. A lifestyle with minimal stress is important in promoting positive outcomes for the mother and baby. Harmony with other people must be fostered, and visits from extended family members may be required to demonstrate pleasant and noncontroversial relationships. If discord exists in a relationship, it is usually dealt with in culturally prescribed ways.

Some cultural proscriptions involve forms of magic. For example, some Mexicans believe pregnant women should not be allowed to witness an eclipse of the moon because it can cause a cleft palate in the infant. They also believe that exposure to an earthquake can precipitate preterm birth, miscarriage, or a breech presentation. In some cultures, a pregnant woman must not ridicule someone with an affliction for fear her child might be born with the same handicap. A mother should not hate a

person lest her child resemble that person. Dental work should not be done during pregnancy because it may cause a baby to have a cleft lip. A folk belief widely held in many cultures is that the pregnant woman should refrain from raising her arms above her head and from tying knots because such movements tie knots in the umbilical cord and can cause it to wrap around the baby's neck. Another belief is that placing a knife under the bed of a laboring woman will "cut" her pain.

Physical Activity and Rest

Norms that regulate the physical activity of mothers during pregnancy vary tremendously. Some cultural groups encourage women to be active, to walk, and to engage in normal, although not strenuous, activities to ensure that the baby is healthy and not too large. Conversely, some groups believe that any activity is dangerous, and family members willingly take over the work of the pregnant woman, believing that this inactivity protects the mother and child. The mother is encouraged simply to produce the succeeding generation. If health care professionals are unaware of this belief, they can misinterpret their behavior as laziness or nonadherence with the desired prenatal health care regimen. It is important for the nurse to find out how each pregnant woman views activity and rest.

Clothing

Although most cultural groups do not prescribe specific clothing to be worn during pregnancy, modesty is an expectation of many. Amulets, medals, and beads are worn by women from some cultures to promote health or protect the woman and fetus from danger. For example, some Mexican women of the US Southwest and women of Central America wear a cord beneath the breasts and knotted over the umbilicus. This cord, called a *muñeco*, is thought to prevent morning sickness and ensure a safe birth (Fig. 8.19).

Sexual Activity

In most cultures, sexual activity is not prohibited until the end of pregnancy. Some groups view sexual activity as necessary to keep the birth canal lubricated. Others may have definite proscriptions against sexual intercourse, requiring abstinence throughout the pregnancy because it is thought that sexual intercourse can harm the mother and fetus.

Diet

Nutritional information given by Western health care providers can be a source of conflict for some cultural groups. Such a conflict commonly is not known by health care providers unless they understand the dietary beliefs and practices of the people for whom they are caring. For example, some religious groups have strict regulations regarding preparation of food, and if meat cannot be prepared as prescribed, they omit meats from their diets. Many cultures permit pregnant women to eat only warm foods.

AGE DIFFERENCES

The age of the childbearing couple can have a significant influence on their physical and psychosocial adaptation to pregnancy. Normal developmental processes that occur in both very young and older mothers are interrupted by pregnancy and require a different type of adaptation to pregnancy than that of the woman of typical childbearing age. Although the individuality of each pregnant woman is recognized, special needs of expectant mothers 15 years of age or younger or those 35 years of age or older are summarized.

Adolescents

Teenage pregnancy is a worldwide problem. The United States has one of the highest teen birth rates among industrialized nations, although rates have steadily declined since the most recent peak in 1991. The birth rate for 2015 for teens 15 to 19 years of age decreased to the historic low of 22.3 births per 1000 women (Martin, Hamilton, Osterman, et al., 2017). Hispanic adolescents have the highest birth rate, although the rate for non-Hispanic black adolescents also is high (Martin et al). Most of these young women are unmarried, and many are not ready for the emotional, psychosocial, and financial responsibilities of parenthood.

Numerous adolescent pregnancy-prevention programs have had varying degrees of success. Characteristics of programs that make a difference are those that have sustained commitment to adolescents over a long time, involve the parents and other adults in the community, promote abstinence and personal responsibility, and assist adolescents to develop a clear strategy for reaching goals such as a college education or a career.

When adolescents become pregnant and decide to give birth, they are much less likely than older women to receive adequate prenatal care, often receiving no health care at all. These young women also are more likely to smoke and less likely to gain adequate weight during pregnancy. Neonates born to adolescents are at increased risk for LBW, VLBW, and infant death. Adolescents are at increased risk for maternal anemia, preterm birth, preeclampsia and/or HELLP syndrome, postpartum hemorrhage, and chorioamnionitis, but do not have an increased likelihood of cesarean birth (Kawakita, Wilson, Grantz, et al., 2016; Torvie, Callegari, Schiff, et al., 2015).

Delayed entry into prenatal care can be the result of late recognition of pregnancy, denial of pregnancy, or confusion about the available services. Such a delay in care can leave an inadequate time before birth to attend to correctable problems. The very young pregnant adolescent is at higher risk for each of the variables associated with poor pregnancy outcomes (e.g., socioeconomic factors) and for those conditions associated with a first pregnancy, regardless of age (e.g., gestational hypertension).

The role of the nurse in reducing the risks and consequences of adolescent pregnancy is to encourage early and continued prenatal care; to provide early and ongoing education about pregnancy, birth, and parenting (Fig. 8.20); and to refer the adolescent, if necessary, for appropriate social support services, which can help decrease the effects of a negative socioeconomic environment (see Nursing Care Plan).

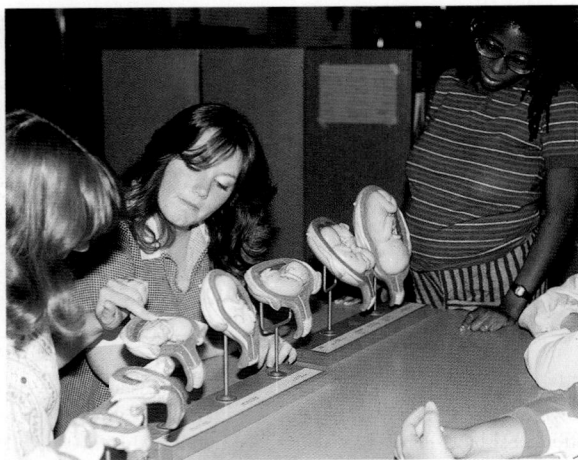

FIG 8.20 Pregnant adolescents review fetal development. (Courtesy of Marjorie Pyle, RNC, Lifecircle, Costa Mesa, CA.)

Adolescents often see the nurse as trustworthy and someone who will maintain confidentiality, as well as provide them with accurate information. Therefore, effective communication is essential in providing care to the pregnant adolescent (US Department of Health and Human Services Office of Adolescent Health, 2013) (see Nursing Care Plan).

Women Older Than 35 Years of Age

Two groups of older parents have emerged in the population of women having a child late in their childbearing years. One group consists of multiparous women who intentionally or unintentionally become pregnant in the peri-menopausal period. The other group consists of primigravidas: women who have deliberately delayed childbearing until their late 30s or early 40s and those who previously were unable to conceive due to fertility problems and became pregnant through assisted reproductive technology.

Birth rates for women from 35 to 39 years of age increased in 2015 to 51.8 births per 1000 women; this is the highest rate since 1962. Birth rates for women 40 to 44 years of age have risen steadily over the last 30 years to the 2015 rate of 11.0 births per 1000 women. Births to women over 44 years of age have increased since 1997 (Martin et al., 2017).

As maternal age advances, there is a greater chance of preexisting conditions such as hypertension and diabetes (Gregory et al., 2017). Pregnancy for women older than 35 years of age is associated with increased risk for miscarriage, stillbirth, diabetes, hypertension, placenta previa, placental abruption, cesarean birth, and pregnancy-related mortality. These women are more likely than younger primiparas to have infants with chromosomal abnormalities, LBW infants, preterm birth, and multiple gestation (Creanga, Berg, Syverson, et al., 2015; Johnson & Tough, 2012; Mills & Lavender, 2014).

Multiparous Women

For some multiparous women older than 35 years of age, pregnancy is desired, such as with a new marriage or partner. For others, it may be unplanned. Some multiparous women have never used contraceptives because of personal choice or lack of knowledge concerning contraceptives. Others may have used contraceptives successfully during the childbearing years, but as menopause approaches they cease menstruating regularly or stop using contraceptives and consequently become pregnant.

Pregnancy can bring feelings of joy as women consider continuing the maternal role and expanding the family. For some older multiparas, pregnancy can evoke feelings of isolation. She may feel that pregnancy separates her from her peer group and that her age is a hindrance to close associations with young mothers.

Primiparous Women

Reasons for delaying pregnancy include a desire to obtain advanced education, career priorities, and use of effective contraceptive measures. Women with infertility issues may not delay pregnancy deliberately but may become pregnant at a later age through the use of assisted reproductive technology. There is evidence of increased risk for preterm labor and preeclampsia for women older than 40 years of age who conceive through assisted reproductive technology and oocyte donation (Gregory et al., 2017).

Many primigravidas older than 35 years of age deliberately choose parenthood. They often are successfully established in a career and a lifestyle with a partner that includes time for self-attention, the establishment of a home with accumulated possessions, and freedom to travel. When asked the reason they chose pregnancy later in life, many reply, "Because time is running out."

The dilemma of choice includes the recognition that being a parent will have positive and negative consequences. Couples should discuss the joys, responsibilities, and challenges of childbearing and childrearing before committing themselves to this lifelong venture. Partners in this group seem to share the preparation for parenthood, planning for a family-centered birth, and desire to be loving and competent parents; however, the reality of child care can prove difficult for such parents.

First-time mothers older than 35 years of age select the "right time" for pregnancy; this time is influenced by their awareness of the increasing possibility of infertility or of genetic defects in infants of older women. Such women seek information about pregnancy from books, friends, and electronic resources. They actively try to prevent fetal disorders and are careful in searching for the best possible maternity care. They identify sources of stress in their lives. They have concerns about having enough energy and stamina to meet the demands of parenting and their new roles and relationships.

If older women with a history of infertility become pregnant through assisted reproductive technology, they can suddenly have negative or ambivalent feelings about the pregnancy. They can experience a multifetal pregnancy that can create emotional and physical problems. Adjusting to parenting two or more infants requires adaptability and additional resources.

During pregnancy, parents explore the possibilities and responsibilities of changing identities and new roles. They must prepare a safe and nurturing environment during pregnancy and after birth. They must integrate the child into an established family system and negotiate new roles (parent roles, sibling roles, grandparent roles) for family members.

Adverse perinatal outcomes are more common in older primiparas than in younger women, even when they receive adequate prenatal care. The occurrence of these complications is quite stressful for the new parents, and nursing interventions that provide information and psychosocial support are needed, as well as care for physical needs.

MULTIFETAL PREGNANCY

With the increased use of assistive reproductive technology and ovulation-induction agents, the incidence of multifetal pregnancy has risen. In the United States, the twin birth rate for 2015 was 33.5 per 1000 births; this was slightly lower than the all-time high of 33.9 in 2014. The birth rate for triplets and higher-order multiples in 2015 was 113.5 per 100,000 live births; this represents a 46% decline since 1998 (Martin et al., 2017).

A multifetal pregnancy, or pregnancy with more than one fetus, places the mother and fetuses at increased risk for adverse outcomes. Maternal physiologic adaptation to pregnancy is more dramatic with multiple fetuses. Levels of pregnancy hormones such as human chorionic gonadotropin are significantly increased over a singleton pregnancy; this increases the risk for hyperemesis gravidarum. The maternal blood volume is increased, resulting in an increased strain on the maternal cardiovascular system. Anemia often develops because of a greater demand for iron by the fetuses. Marked uterine distention, increased pressure on the adjacent viscera and pelvic vasculature, and diastasis of the rectus abdominis muscles can occur (see Fig. 7.13). Multifetal gestation increases the risk for many pregnancy complications including spontaneous abortion, gestational diabetes, hypertension, preeclampsia, placenta previa, and postpartum hemorrhage. Preterm birth is more likely with multifetal gestation; the risk rises as the number of fetuses increases. Intrauterine growth restriction or discordant growth, LBW, very low birth weight (VLBW), congenital abnormalities, neonatal death, and cerebral palsy are more common in multifetal gestation. There can be local shunting of blood between placentas (twin-to-twin transfusion); this causes the recipient twin to be larger and the donor twin to be small, pallid, dehydrated, malnourished, and hypovolemic. However, the larger twin can develop congestive heart failure during the first 24 hours after birth. The risk for death of one or more fetuses increases significantly with higher-order multiples (Newman & Unal, 2017).

If the presence of more than three fetuses is diagnosed, parents may receive counseling regarding selective reduction to reduce the incidence of premature birth and improve the opportunities for the remaining fetuses to grow to term gestation (ACOG, 2013b). This situation poses an ethical dilemma for many couples, especially those who have worked hard to overcome problems with infertility and have strong values regarding right to life. Nurses can initiate discussions with couples to help them identify resources (e.g., a minister, priest, rabbi, or mental health counselor) to aid in the decision-making process.

The likelihood of a multifetal pregnancy is increased if any or a combination of the following factors is noted during a careful assessment:
- History of dizygotic twins in the female lineage
- Use of fertility drugs
- More rapid uterine growth for the number of weeks of gestation
- Polyhydramnios
- Palpation of more than the expected number of small or large fetal parts
- Asynchronous fetal heartbeats or more than one fetal electrocardiographic tracing
- Ultrasound evidence of more than one fetus

The diagnosis of multifetal pregnancy comes as a shock to many expectant parents. They need additional support and education to help them cope with the changes they face.

The prenatal care for women with multifetal pregnancies includes changes in the pattern of care and modifications in other aspects. Prenatal visits are scheduled more frequently. Frequent ultrasound examinations, nonstress tests, and FHR monitoring will be performed. The pregnant woman needs information related to self-management of a multifetal pregnancy because guidelines differ in comparison with a singleton pregnancy. Specific instruction should be provided regarding nutrition so that she consumes a well-balanced diet with adequate caloric intake and gains weight appropriately. Other pertinent information includes maternal adaptations during pregnancy, management of discomforts, and the risk for preterm labor and birth, including warning signs and when to call the provider. The uterine distention associated with multifetal pregnancy can cause the backache commonly experienced by pregnant women to be even worse. Maternal support hose may be worn to control leg varicosities. If risk factors such as premature dilation of the cervix or bleeding are present, abstinence from orgasm and nipple stimulation during the last trimester is recommended to help avert preterm labor. Some practitioners recommend bed rest beginning at 20 weeks in women carrying multiple fetuses to prevent preterm labor. Other practitioners question the value of prolonged bed rest. If bed rest is recommended, the mother assumes a lateral position to promote increased placental perfusion. If birth is delayed until after the thirty-sixth week, the risk for morbidity and mortality decreases for the neonates.

Multiple newborns can place a strain on finances, space, workload, and the woman's and family's coping capabilities. Lifestyle changes can be necessary. Parents need assistance in making realistic plans for the care of the infants (e.g., whether to breastfeed and whether to raise them as "alike" or as separate people). Parents should be referred to national organizations such as Parents of Twins and Triplets (www.bigtent.com/groups/nashpotato), Mothers of Twins (www.nomotc.org), and the La Leche League (www.llli.org) for further support.

PERINATAL EDUCATION

The goal of perinatal education is to assist women and their family members to make informed, safe decisions about pregnancy, labor and birth, infant care, and early parenthood. It also is to assist them to comprehend the long-lasting potential that empowering birth experiences have in the lives of women and that early experiences have on the development of children and the family.

Pregnant women consider maternity care providers and childbirth education classes as the most valuable sources of information about pregnancy and birth. However, time with providers for education during prenatal visits is limited, and only about half of pregnant women report having ever attended a childbirth education class. Attendance at formal childbirth classes has declined in recent years. Women are turning to electronic media for information. A majority of women seek information from online resources such as pregnancy websites, blogs, emails, apps, and social media, as well as television shows about labor and birth (Declercq, Sakala, Corry, et al., 2013). Yet, women do not typically discuss information they have retrieved from these sources with their health care providers. Many women are unable to differentiate between commercially sponsored and not-for-profit websites; they cannot assess the accuracy of the information they are reading or hearing (Lima-Pereira, Bermúdez-Tamayo, & Jasienska, 2012). Nurses can help to fill the education gap by talking with pregnant women about the sources and types of information they are finding through the Internet and other technology-based resources, offering to answer questions and directing women to sites that present current, accurate information about pregnancy, birth, newborn care, breastfeeding, parenting, and other issues of interest (Demirci, Cohen, Parker, et al., 2016).

CLASSES FOR EXPECTANT PARENTS

The perinatal education program is an expansion of the earlier childbirth education movement that originally offered a set of classes in the third trimester of pregnancy to prepare parents for birth. Today perinatal education programs consist of a menu of class series and activities from preconception through the early months of parenting. In recent years, women have moved from enrolling in a series of classes that span several weeks to classes that are done in 1 or 2 days. The most common focus of classes is labor and birth (Declercq et al., 2013). Some classes are offered through distance education.

Expectant parents and their families have different interests and information needs as the pregnancy progresses. Parents may select a variety of classes such as the following:

- Early pregnancy ("early bird") classes provide fundamental information including (1) fetal development, (2) physiologic and emotional changes of pregnancy, (3) human sexuality, and (4) the nutritional needs of the mother and fetus. The classes often address environmental and workplace hazards. Exercises, nutrition, warning signs, drugs, and self-medication also are topics of interest and concern.
- Midpregnancy classes emphasize the woman's participation in self-management. Classes provide information on preparation for breastfeeding and formula feeding, infant care, basic hygiene, common discomforts and simple safe remedies, infant health, parenting, and planning for labor and birth.
- Late pregnancy classes emphasize different methods of coping with labor and birth, and these are often the basis for various prenatal classes. These include Lamaze, Bradley, and Dick-Read. These classes usually include a tour of the birthing facility. Because fear of pain in labor is a key issue for many women, childbirth preparation classes provide information on management of discomfort during labor and birth. Topics include nonpharmacologic methods to reduce discomfort such as relaxation and breathing techniques, imagery and visualization, and biofeedback. Pharmacologic interventions such as intravenous medications and epidural analgesia are also discussed. An emphasis on nonpharmacologic pain management strategies helps couples manage the labor and birth with dignity and increased comfort. Most instructors teach a flexible approach, which helps couples learn and master many techniques to use during labor.
- Perinatal education programs offer classes to meet specific learning needs. These include classes for adolescents, first-time mothers older than 35 years of age, single women, adoptive parents, parents of multiples, or women with special needs such as those with visual or hearing impairments. In some agencies, classes are also offered in languages other than English. Refresher classes for parents with children not only review coping techniques for labor and birth but also help couples prepare for sibling reactions and adjustments to a new baby. Cesarean birth classes are available for couples who have this kind of birth scheduled because of breech presentation or other risk factors. Other classes focus on vaginal birth after cesarean (VBAC) because many women can successfully give birth vaginally after previous cesarean birth.

For the most part, the pregnant woman and her partner attend perinatal education classes, although sometimes a friend or relative is the designated support person (Fig. 8.21). There are also classes for grandparents and siblings to prepare them for their attendance at birth or the arrival of the baby. Siblings often see a film about birth and learn ways they can help welcome the baby. They also learn to cope with

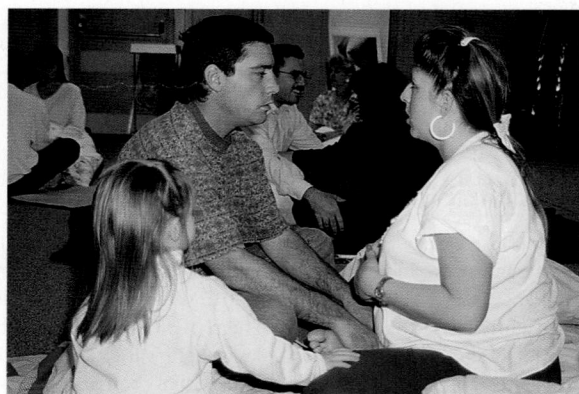

FIG 8.21 Learning relaxation exercises in a family-centered childbirth education class. (Courtesy of Marjorie Pyle, RNC, Lifecircle, Costa Mesa, CA.)

changes that include a reduction in parental time and attention. Grandparents learn about current child care practices and how to help their adult children adapt to parenting in a supportive way.

Perinatal classes include discussion of support systems that people can use during pregnancy, labor and birth, and in the postpartum period. Such support systems help parents function independently and effectively. During all the classes, the open expression of feelings and concerns about any aspect of pregnancy, birth, and parenting is welcomed. Perinatal education is focused on health promotion and emphasizes how a healthy body is best able to adapt to the changes that accompany pregnancy. Without this context of health, routine care and testing for risks can contribute to a mindset of families that pregnancy is a state of illness as opposed to a healthy mind-body-spirit event.

Some of the decisions the childbearing family must consider are the decision to have a baby, followed by choices of a health care provider and type of care (a midwifery model [natural oriented] versus a medical [intervention oriented] model); the place for birth (hospital, birthing center, home); the type of infant feeding (breast or formula); and infant care. If a woman has had a cesarean birth, she may consider having a vaginal birth. Perinatal education can provide information to help childbearing families make informed decisions about these issues.

Previous pregnancy and childbirth experiences are important influences on current learning needs. The woman's (and support person's) age, cultural background, personal philosophy with regard to labor and birth, socioeconomic status, spiritual beliefs, and learning styles are assessed to develop the best plan to help the woman meet her needs.

PERINATAL CARE CHOICES

Often the first decision the woman makes is to select her primary health care provider for the pregnancy and birth. This decision usually affects where the birth will take place. The nurse can provide information about the different types of obstetric health care providers and the kind of care to expect from each one. Women are encouraged to ask potential care providers a series of pertinent questions (Box 8.3). Women report that the primary reasons for choosing a particular care provider or

group are that they "accept my health insurance," they "are a good match for what I value/want," and they "attend births at a hospital I like" (Declercq et al., 2013).

PHYSICIANS

Physicians (obstetricians, family medicine physicians) attended 91% of hospital births in the United States in 2015 (Martin et al., 2017). In general, family practice physicians provide care for primarily low-risk pregnant women and refer high-risk women to obstetricians. Obstetricians provide care for low-risk and high-risk pregnant women. High-risk pregnant women are often referred to maternal-fetal medicine specialists for part or all of their care. Care often includes pharmacologic and medical management of problems as well as use of technologic procedures.

MIDWIVES

Increasing numbers of pregnant women are choosing certified nurse-midwives (CNM) and certified midwives (CM) as their obstetric care providers. In 2015, 8.1% of all hospital births and 32.3% of out-of-hospital births were attended by a CNM or other midwife (Hamilton, Martin, & Osterman, 2016).

The midwifery model of care emphasizes the natural ability of women to experience pregnancy, labor, and birth with minimal intervention. Compared with the medical model of care, midwifery care throughout pregnancy, labor, and birth is associated with benefits for mothers and babies. These include reduced use of epidurals and fewer episiotomies and instrument-assisted births. Midwifery care is associated with an increased likelihood of spontaneous vaginal birth (Sandall, Soltani, Gates, et al., 2013).

The services provided by midwives are dependent on their licensing and certification as well as the practice regulations in each state. Women who are interested in midwifery care should explore the various types of midwives, the care that is available, where they are allowed to practice and attend births, and reimbursement by insurance companies (see Evidence-Based Practice box.)

In the United States, there are three types of credentialed professional midwives: certified nurse midwives (CNM), certified midwives (CM), and certified professional midwives (CPM). CMs and CPMs are known as direct-entry midwives. Certified nurse midwives are registered nurses with education in the two disciplines of nursing and midwifery. CNMs are legally approved to practice in all 50 states and the District of Columbia. Fewer states allow CMs and CPMs to practice.

CERTIFIED NURSE-MIDWIVES

CNMs are certified by the American College of Nurse Midwives (ACNM). Nurse midwifery programs are graduate level; since 2010, ACNM has mandated that entry into practice requires at least a master's degree. CNMs are trained to provide women's health care throughout the lifespan, not just during pregnancy and birth. Nurse-midwives practice collaboratively with physicians or independently with an arrangement for physician backup. They usually see low-risk women. Care is often noninterventionist, and the woman and her family are encouraged to be active participants in the care. Certified nurse-midwives co-manage and/or refer pregnant women with complications to physicians.

DIRECT-ENTRY MIDWIVES

Certified midwives (CM) are trained in midwifery schools, colleges, or universities. A nursing degree is not required, although a bachelor's

---

BOX 8.3 Questions to Ask When Seeking a Maternity Care Provider

The Coalition for Improving Maternity Services, a group of more than 50 nursing and maternity care–oriented organizations, produced a document to assist women in selecting their perinatal care. After some explanation of choices, the nurse can encourage women to ask potential care providers the following questions:

- Who can be with me during labor and birth?
- What happens during a normal labor and birth in your setting?
- How do you allow for differences in culture and beliefs?
- May I walk and move around during labor? What position do you suggest for birth?
- How do you make sure everything goes smoothly when my nurse, doctor, nurse-midwife, or agency works with one another?
- What things do you normally do to a woman in labor?
- How do you help mothers stay as comfortable as they can be? Besides drugs, how do you help mothers relieve the pain of labor?
- What if my baby is born early or has special problems?
- Do you circumcise babies?
- How do you help mothers who want to breastfeed?

Modified from Coalition for Improving Maternity Services. (2000). *Having a baby? 10 questions to ask.* Retrieved from www.motherfriendly.org/Resources/Documents/Having_a_Baby-English.pdf.

EVIDENCE-BASED PRACTICE

Outcomes of Midwifery Care

Ask the Question

PICOT Question: For pregnant women contemplating birth options, especially in rural settings, what are the differences between outcomes for births attended by midwives and physicians? What is the relative safety of home births, compared with hospital births?

Search for the Evidence

Search Strategies: English research-based publications since 2013 on birth, midwife, home birth (or homebirth), and rural birth were included

Databases Used: Cochrane Collaborative Database, National Guideline Clearinghouse (AHRQ), CINAHL, PubMed, UpToDate, PLoS ONE, and the professional websites for ACOG and AWHONN

Critical Appraisal of the Evidence

Pregnant women who live in underserved rural areas or who desire alternatives to physician-attended hospital birth may choose midlevel health care providers, most commonly midwives. Midwives include masters-prepared Certified Nurse Midwives (CNMs), and non-nurse Certified Professional Midwives (CPMs) who have been prepared in programs that meet the International Confederation of Midwives (ICM) Global Standards of Midwife Education (ACOG, 2016).

- A systematic analysis of 15 randomized controlled trials noted that births led by midwives were associated with less preterm birth, greater maternal satisfaction, and fewer interventions including regional analgesia, instrumental birth, amniotomy, and episiotomy than physician-led births. Cesarean births, adverse events, and intact perineum were similar between groups. (Sandall, Soltani, Gates et al, 2016). Studies that took place in countries where health care systems are highly coordinated between hospitals and various levels of health care providers may limit generalizability to the less well-integrated system in the United States (ACOG, 2016).
- Rural childbirth has its own challenges, including distance, few local health options, limited insurance, poverty, and care for other children, that may increase the risk for mother and baby. CNMs attend about 1 in 3 rural births, and more in states that do not require the CNM to be supervised by an MD (Kozhimannil, Hennings-Smith, & Hung et al, 2016).
- Less than 1% of US births, or about 35,000 per year, occur at home, and about one-fourth of those are unplanned or unattended (ACOG, 2016). Pregnant women who inquire about home birth may seek to avoid interventions or prefer a noninstitutional setting. Although high-quality evidence is limited, observational studies suggest that home births are associated with fewer interventions, perineal lacerations, and infections (ACOG, 2016). However, in over 1 million home births from 2006 to 2009, the risk for neonatal mortality was two to three times that of hospital births, with no significant difference between certified and uncertified midwives (Grunebaum, et al, 2016). In addition, the risk for neonatal seizures or neurologic dysfunction was triple for home births, compared to medical settings (ACOG, 2016).

Apply the Evidence: Nursing Implications

- ACOG (2016) recommends the following to improve outcomes for home births: Attendance by physician, CNM, or midwife prepared to ICM standards; access

to consultation; and access to timely transport to the appropriate health care facility. In addition, fetal malpresentation, multiple gestation, and a history of cesarean birth are absolute contraindications to home birth.

- Interprofessional practice between physicians and CNMs improves health care coverage and options. State authority for CNMs to practice autonomously has been proven to increase access to care for rural pregnant women (Kozhimannil, et al., 2016).
- Nurses can educate women as to safe practices and reasonable expectations for their birth, and confidently recommend certified birth attendants in medical facilities for women examining their options.
- Medical facilities should smoothly coordinate the transfer in of an attempted home birth, and provide compassionate care and welcome to the transferring patient, family, and attendant, without judgment.
- Policy advocates can examine countries with highly coordinated and integrated birth systems, such as Canada and England, and seek to replicate their successful birth outcomes.

Quality and Safety Competencies: Evidence-Based Practice*
Knowledge

Describe EBP to include the components of research evidence, clinical expertise, and patient/family values.

Assess patient and family experiences and preferences for birth, and present options, including education about risks and benefits of each.

Skills

Question rationale for routine approaches to care that result in less-than-desired outcomes or adverse events.

Encourage the pregnant woman to have realistic goals and expectations within the context of safe birth settings. Coordinate with health care team for smooth transfers.

Attitudes

Value the need for continuous improvement in clinical practice based on new knowledge.

Advocate for a low-intervention, homelike atmosphere within the medical setting.

References

American College of Obstetrics and Gynecologists. (2016). Committee opinion #669: Planned home birth. *Obstetrics and Gynecology, 128*(2), e26–e31.

Grunebaum, A., McCullough, L. B., Arabin, B., et al. (2016). Neonatal mortality of planned home birth in the United States in relation to professional certification of birth attendants. *PLoS ONE, 11*(5), e0155721.

Kozhimannil, K. B., Henning-Smith, C., & Hung, P. (2016). The practice of midwifery in rural US hospitals. *The Journal of Midwifery and Women's Health, 61*(4), 411–418.

Sandall, J., Soltani, H., Gates, S., et al. (2016). Midwife-led continuity models versus other models of care for childbearing women (review). *Cochrane Database of Systematic Reviews, 2016*(4), CD004667.

Pat Mahaffee Gingrich

*Adapted from QSEN at www.qsen.org/.

degree and specific health and science courses are required prior to entering a CM training program. Certified midwives are credentialed by the ACNM based on a certification examination; a graduate degree is required for entry into practice.

Certified professional midwives (CPM) meet the standards of certification set by the North American Registry of Midwives (NARM) in collaboration with Midwives Alliance of North America (MANA). They

are educated in midwifery programs in colleges, universities, or midwifery schools, or through self-study and apprenticeship.

TRADITIONAL OR LAY MIDWIVES

Independent or *lay midwives* are also known as traditional or community-based midwives. These midwives are not certified. They are usually trained through self-study and apprenticeship. It is up to the woman seeking care from a lay midwife to assess the level of experience and expertise of a lay midwife. Lay midwives can legally practice and are licensed in some states, although there are specific requirements and guidelines that must be followed. Care by lay midwives is usually not covered by third-party payers.

DOULAS

There are primarily two types of doulas involved in the care of childbearing women. The most common is a labor doula who is trained to provide physical, emotional, and informational support to women and their partners during labor and birth. The doula does not become involved with clinical tasks. There are also postpartum doulas who provide support and care for women, newborns, and families during the first weeks after birth (Ahlemeyer & Mahon, 2015). Some doulas are certified by Doula International (DONA) or Childbirth and Postpartum Professional Association (CAPPA), while others provide care without having any certification.

Continuous labor support provided by a doula has been shown to decrease the use of pain medication, shorten labor, increase satisfaction with the birth experience, increase the likelihood of a spontaneous vaginal birth, and increase breastfeeding rates and duration (Gruber, Cupito, & Dobson, 2013; Hodnett, Gates, Hofmeyr, et al., 2013). There are no known risks associated with labor support by a doula.

A doula typically meets with the woman and her husband or partner during pregnancy. At this meeting, she ascertains the woman's expectations and desires for the birth experience. The doula focuses efforts on assisting the woman to achieve her goals. Doulas work collaboratively with nurses and other health care providers and the husband or other supportive individuals, but their primary goal is to assist the woman. Doulas who are also trained medical interpreters can enhance the care of women with limited English proficiency (Maher, Crawford-Carr, & Neidigh, 2012).

Doulas can be found through community contacts, health care providers, childbirth educators, or websites; a number of organizations offer information or referral services. It is important that the expectant mother is comfortable with the doula who will be attending her (see Box 8.4 for a list of questions to ask when arranging for a doula).

BIRTH PLANS

The birth plan is a natural evolution of a contemporary wellness-oriented lifestyle in which women assume a level of responsibility for their own health. The birth plan is a tool with which parents can explore their childbirth options and choose those that are most important to them. The plan must be viewed as tentative because the realities of what is feasible may change as the actual labor and birth unfold. It is understood to be a preference list based on a best-case scenario.

It is useful for the nurse in a prenatal practice setting to initiate a discussion of choices and birth planning. Some maternity practices provide printed material describing available options and giving answers to commonly asked questions, and tours of the birth setting are offered by almost all birthing facilities. The nurse can provide couples with pertinent information and make them aware of the various options for care and the advantages and consequences of each so they can begin making informed decisions. Early plans can be modified as the couple learns more details in their childbirth classes. Topics for the expectant parents to consider when creating a birth plan are listed in Box 8.5.

Nurses can direct women and their partners to websites with information about creating a birth plan (http://americanpregnancy.org/labor-and-birth/birth-plan/). The birth plan can serve as a means of open

---

BOX 8.4 Questions to Ask When Choosing a Labor Doula

To discover the specific training, experience, and services offered by anyone who provides labor support, potential patients, nursing supervisors, physicians, midwives, and others should ask the following questions of that person:
- What training have you had?
- Tell me about your experience with birth, both personally and as a doula.
- What is your philosophy about childbirth and supporting women and their partners through labor?
- May we meet to discuss our birth plans and the role you will play in supporting me through childbirth?
- May we call you with questions or concerns before and after the birth?
- When do you try to join women in labor? Do you come to our home or meet us at the hospital?
- Do you meet with us after the birth to review the labor and answer questions?
- Do you work with one or more backup doulas for times when you are not available? May we meet them?
- What is your fee?

Adapted from Doula International. (2016). *Position paper: The birth doula's role in maternity care.* Retrieved from http://www.dona.org/wp-content/uploads/2016/09/DONA-Birth-Position-Paper.pdf.

BOX 8.5 Creating a Birth Plan

Topics for birth plan discussion and decision-making may include any or all of the following:

Partner's participation: Attend prenatal visits? Childbirth and parent education classes? Present during labor? During birth? During cesarean birth?

Birth setting: Hospital delivery room or birthing room (if available)? A birthing center? Home?

Labor management: Walk around during labor? Use a rocking chair? Use a shower? Use a Jacuzzi, if available? Intermittent versus continuous use of an electronic fetal monitor? Have music or dimmed lighting? Have older children or other people present? Is telemetry monitoring available? Consider stimulation of labor? Consider medication—what kind?

Birth: Positions—Side-lying? On hands and knees, kneeling, or squatting? Use a birthing bed or delivery table? Will you be photographing, videotaping, or recording any of the labor or birth? Who would you like to be present—partner, older siblings, other family members, or friends? What do you know about the use of forceps? Episiotomy? Will your partner want to cut the umbilical cord? Emergency considerations/contingencies (e.g., cesarean)?

Immediately after birth: Do you want to hold the baby skin-to-skin right away? Breastfeed immediately?

Postpartum care: What kind of care do you anticipate—labor, delivery, recovery, postpartum room; mother-baby couplet care? How long does your insurance company provide coverage for you to stay? Would you like to attend self-management classes, or do you prefer to get such information from media sources? On which subjects?

---

communication between the pregnant woman and her partner and between the couple and health care providers. An early introduction to the idea of a birth plan allows the couple time to think about events or situations that could make their childbearing experience more meaningful and those they would prefer to avoid (Anderson & Kilpatrick, 2012).

Traditionally, birth plans are created prenatally and implemented on admission to the labor and birth unit. However, when women without predesigned birth plans are admitted, nurses can use a template with simple questions about preferences for care to help them develop a simple birth plan (Anderson & Kilpatrick, 2012). This is in accordance with the AWHONN position statement on nursing support of laboring women, specifically creating individualized care plans for laboring women based on their needs, desires, and expectations (AWHONN, 2011).

BIRTH SETTING CHOICES

The three primary options for birth settings are the hospital, free-standing birth center, and home. Women consider several factors in choosing a setting for birth, including the preference of their health care provider, characteristics of the birthing unit, and reimbursement by third-party payers.

While the majority of births occur in hospital settings, out-of-hospital births are gradually increasing. In 2015, 1.5% of births occurred outside the hospital setting. Of those births, 63.1% were at home and 30.9% occurred in free-standing birth centers; the remainder took place in a health care provider's office, clinic, or other location (Martin et al., 2017).

Hospital

The types of labor and birth services in hospital settings vary greatly, from the traditional labor and delivery rooms with separate postpartum and newborn units to in-hospital birthing centers where all or almost all care takes place in a single unit.

Labor, delivery, and recovery (LDR) and labor, delivery, recovery, and postpartum (LDRP) rooms offer families a comfortable, private space for labor and birth (Fig. 8.22). Women are admitted to LDR units, labor and give birth, and spend the first 1 to 2 hours postpartum there for immediate recovery and to have time with their families to bond with their newborns. After this period, the mothers and newborns move to a postpartum unit and nursery or mother-baby unit for the duration of their stay.

In LDRP units, the same nursing staff usually provides total care from admission through postpartum discharge. The woman and her family may stay in this unit for 6 to 48 hours after giving birth. The units are furnished to provide a homelike atmosphere, as LDR units are, but have accommodations for family members to stay overnight (see Fig. 8.22, *A*).

Both units have fetal monitors, emergency resuscitation equipment for mother and newborn, and heated cribs or warming units for the newborn. Often this equipment is out of sight in cabinets or closets when it is not being used (see Fig. 8.22, *B*).

Birth Centers

Free-standing birth centers are usually built in locations separate from the hospital but are often located nearby so that quick transfer of the woman or newborn can occur when needed. These birth centers offer families a safe and cost-effective alternative to hospital or home birth. The centers are usually staffed by certified nurse midwives or physicians who also have privileges at the local hospital. Only women at low risk for complications are included for care.

Birth centers typically have homelike accommodations, including a double bed for the couple and a crib for the newborn (Fig. 8.23, *A*). Emergency equipment and drugs are usually in cabinets, out of view but easily accessible. Private bathroom facilities are incorporated into each birth unit. There may be an early labor lounge or a living room and small kitchen (see Fig. 8.23, *B*). The family is admitted to the birth center for labor and birth and will remain there until discharge, which often takes place within 6 hours of the birth.

Services provided by the free-standing birth centers include those necessary for safe management of low-risk pregnant women during the childbearing cycle. Attendance at birthing and parenting classes is

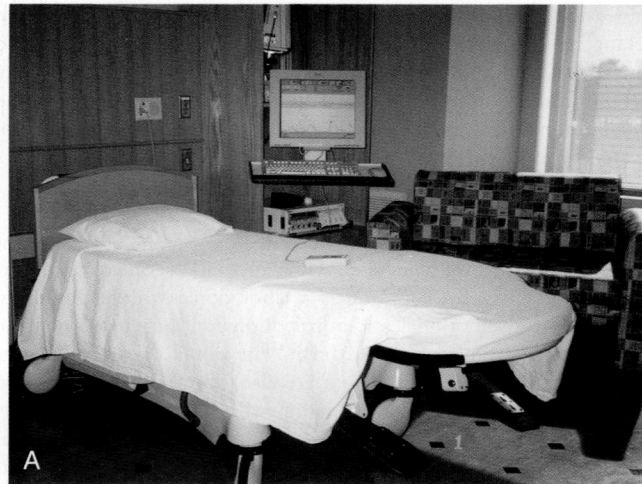

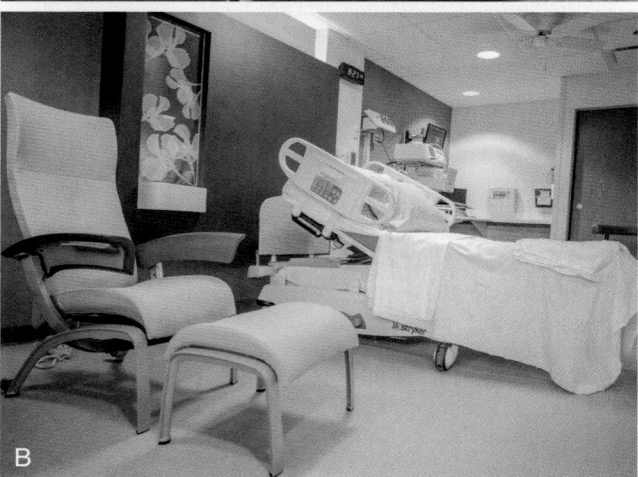

FIG 8.22 Labor, delivery, recovery, and postpartum (LDRP) units. (A, Courtesy of Dee Lowdermilk, Chapel Hill, NC. B, Courtesy of Mercy Hospital, St. Louis, MO.)

required of all patients. Expectant families develop birth plans. They must understand that some situations require transfer to a hospital, and they must agree to abide by those guidelines.

Birth centers and hospitals with comprehensive birthing programs usually provide resources for parents such as a lending library that includes books and DVDs, reference files on related topics, and supplies and reference materials for childbirth educators. The centers may also have referral files for community resources that offer services relating to birth and early parenting, including support groups (e.g., for single parents, for postbirth support, and for parents of twins), genetic counseling, women's issues, and consumer action.

Ambulance service and emergency procedures must be readily available. Fees vary with the services provided by birthing centers but typically are less than or equal to those charged by local hospitals. Some base fees on the ability of the family to pay (a reduced-fee sliding scale). Several third-party payers, as well as Medicaid and the Civilian Health and Medical Programs of the Uniformed Services (TRICARE/CHAMPVA) recognize and reimburse these centers.

Home Birth

Home birth has always been popular in certain countries, such as the Netherlands. In developing countries, hospitals or adequate lying-in

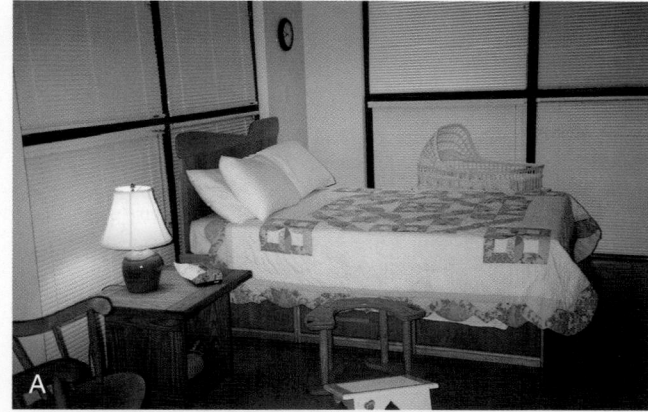

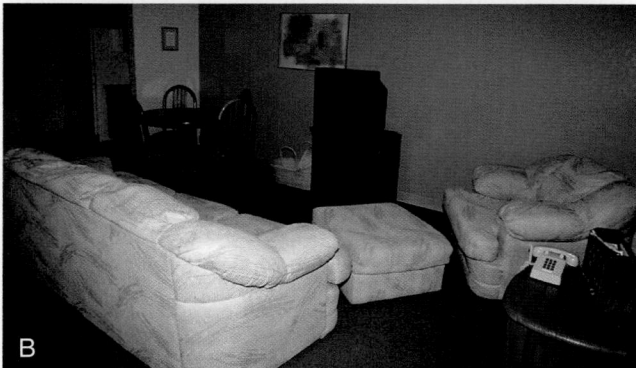

FIG 8.23 Birth center. **A,** Note the double bed, baby crib, and birthing stool. **B,** Lounge and kitchen. (**A,** Courtesy of Dee Lowdermilk, Chapel Hill, NC. **B,** Courtesy of Michael S. Clement, MD, Mesa, AZ. Photo location: Bethany Birth Center, Phoenix, AZ.)

facilities often are unavailable to most pregnant women, and home birth is a necessity. The number of planned home births in the United States is gradually increasing.

Home birth remains a controversial topic in American health care. According to ACOG (2016), while women have the option of making an informed decision about where they will give birth, the safest setting for birth is a hospital or an accredited birthing center. Women considering home birth need to be informed about risks and benefits; specifically, home birth is associated with fewer interventions, although it carries an increased risk for perinatal death and serious neurologic dysfunction in the infant. ACOG stresses the importance of appropriate selection of candidates for home birth (i.e., low-risk pregnancy) and identifies absolute contraindications to home birth: fetal malpresentation, multiple gestation, or prior cesarean birth. The woman should be attended by an obstetric physician, certified nurse-midwife, or other professional midwife with appropriate education and licensure. There should be availability for safe and timely transport to a hospital and ready access to consultation (ACOG, 2016).

Large-scale studies have documented the safety of planned home birth for healthy, low-risk women who are attended by CNMs and when there is a system in place for transfer to a hospital facility (Cheyney, Bovbjerg, Everson, et al., 2014; Cox, Schlegel, Payne, et al., 2013; McIntyre, 2012). The National Perinatal Association (2008) and the American College of Nurse-Midwives (ACNM, 2011) support planned home birth for carefully selected low-risk women within a system that provides hospitalization as needed. National groups supporting home birth are the Home Oriented Maternity Experience (HOME) and the National

Association of Parents for Safe Alternatives in Childbirth (NAPSAC). These groups work to foster more humane childbearing practices at all levels, integrating the alternatives for childbirth to meet the needs of the total population.

There are advantages of planned home birth. The family is in control of the experience. The birth may be more physiologically normal in familiar surroundings. The mother may be more relaxed than she would be in the hospital environment. Care providers who participate in home births tend to be more support oriented and less intervention oriented. The family can assist in and be a part of the happy event, and contact with the newborn is immediate and sustained. In addition, home birth may be less expensive than a hospital or birth center. Serious infection may be less likely, assuming strict aseptic principles are followed, because people generally are relatively immune to their own home bacteria.

REFERENCES

Ahlemeyer, J., & Mahon, S. (2015). Doulas for childbearing women. *American Journal of Maternal/Child Nursing, 40*(2), 122–127.

Aitken, S. L., & Tichy, E. M. (2015). Rh(O)D immune globulin products for prevention of alloimmunization during pregnancy. *American Journal of Health-System Pharmacists, 72*(4), 267–276.

Alhusen, J. L., Ray, E., Sharps, P., & Bullock, L. (2015). Intimate partner violence during pregnancy: Maternal and neonatal outcomes. *Journal of Women's Health, 24*(1), 100–106.

American Academy of Pediatrics and American College of Obstetricians and Gynecologists. (2012). *Guidelines for perinatal care* (7th ed.). Washington, DC: Author.

American College of Nurse-Midwives. (2011). *Position statement: Home birth*. Retrieved from http://www.midwife.org/ACNM/files/ACNMLibraryData/UPLOADFILENAME/000000000251/Home%20Birth%20Aug%202011.pdf.

American College of Nurse-Midwives. (2012). *Midwifery: Evidence-based practice*. Silver Spring, MD: Author. Retrieved from WWW.midwife.org/ACNM/files/ccLibraryFiles/Filename/000000002128/Midwifery%20Evidence-based%20Practice%20Issue%20Brief%20FINALMAY%202012.pdf.

American College of Obstetricians and Gynecologists. (2011 reaffirmed 2015). Committee opinion no. 485: Prevention of early-onset group B streptococcal disease in newborns. *Obstetrics and Gynecology, 117*(4), 1019–1027.

American College of Obstetricians and Gynecologists. (2012). Committee opinion no. 518: Intimate partner violence. *Obstetrics and Gynecology, 119*(2), 412–417.

American College of Obstetricians and Gynecologists. (2013 reaffirmed 2015). Committee opinion no. 569: Oral health care during pregnancy and through the lifespan. *Obstetrics and Gynecology, 122*(2 Pt. 1), 417–422.

American College of Obstetricians and Gynecologists. (2013a). Committee opinion no. 549: Obesity in pregnancy. *Obstetrics and Gynecology, 121*(1), 213–217.

American College of Obstetricians and Gynecologists. (2013b). Committee opinion no. 553: Multifetal pregnancy reduction. *Obstetrics and Gynecology, 121*(2), 405–410.

American College of Obstetricians and Gynecologists. (2013c). Practice bulletin no. 137: Gestational diabetes mellitus. *Obstetrics and Gynecology, 122*(2 Pt. 1), 406–416.

American College of Obstetricians and Gynecologists. (2014). Committee opinion no. 608: Influenza vaccination during pregnancy. *Obstetrics and Gynecology, 124*(3), 648–651.

American College of Obstetricians and Gynecologists. (2015a). Committee opinion no. 630: Screening for perinatal depression. *Obstetrics and Gynecology, 125*(5), 1268–1271.

American College of Obstetricians and Gynecologists. (2015b). Committee opinion no. 650: Physical activity and exercise during pregnancy and the postpartum period. *Obstetrics and Gynecology, 126*(6), e135–e142.

American College of Obstetricians and Gynecologists. (2016). Committee opinion no. 669: Planned home birth. *Obstetrics and Gynecology, 128*(2), e26–e31.

American College of Obstetricians and Gynecologists, American Institute of Ultrasound in Medicine, & Society for Maternal-Fetal Medicine. (2014). Committee opinion no. 611: Method for estimating due date. *Obstetrics and Gynecology, 124*(4), 863–866.

Anderson, C. J., & Kilpatrick, C. (2012). Patients' birth plans: Theories, strategies, and implications for nurses. *Nursing for Women's Health, 16*(3), 211–218.

Association of Women's Health, Obstetric and Neonatal Nurses. (2011). Nursing support for laboring women. *Journal of Obstetric, Gynecologic, and Neonatal Nursing, 40*(5), 665–666.

Association of Women's Health, Obstetric, and Neonatal Nurses (AWHONN). (2015). AWHONN position statement: Intimate partner violence. *Journal of Obstetric, Gynecologic, and Neonatal Nursing, 44*(3), 405–408.

Biaggi, A., Conroy, S., Pawlby, S., & Pariante, C. M. (2016). Identifying the women at risk of antenatal anxiety and depression: A systematic review. *Journal of Affective Disorders, 191*, 62–77.

Bianchi, A. L., Cesario, S. K., & McFarlane, J. (2016). Interrupting intimate partner violence during pregnancy with an effective screening and assessment program. *Journal of Obstetric, Gynecologic, and Neonatal Nursing, 45*(4), 579–591.

Blackburn, S. (2013). *Maternal, fetal, and neonatal physiology* (3rd ed.). Maryland Heights, MO: Saunders.

Breiding, M. J., Basile, K. C., Smith, S. G., et al. (2015). *Intimate partner surveillance: Uniform definitions and recommended data elements, Version 2.0*. Retrieved from http://www.cdc.gov/violenceprevention/pdf/intimatepartnerviolence.pdf.

Byatt, N., Biebel, K., & Friedman, L. (2013). Patient's views on depression care in obstetric settings: How do they compare to the views of health care professionals? *General Hospital Psychiatry, 35*(6), 598–604.

Campo, M. (2015). *Domestic and family violence in pregnancy and early parenthood: overview and emerging interventions*. Retrieved from https://aifs.gov.au/cfca/publications/domestic-and-family-violence-pregnancy-and-early-parenthood.

Centering Healthcare Institute (2016). *CenteringPregnancy*. Retrieved from https://www.centeringhealthcare.org/what-we-do/centering-pregnancy.

Centers for Disease Control and Prevention. (2013). *Intimate partner violence*. Retrieved from http://www.cdc.gov/violenceprevention/intimatepartnerviolence.

Centers for Disease Control and Prevention. (2013). Updated recommendations for use of tetanus toxoid, reduced diphtheria toxoid, and acellular pertussis vaccine (Tdap) in pregnant women—Advisory Committee on Immunization Practices (ACIP), 2012. *Morbidity and Mortality Weekly Report, 62*(7), 131–135.

Centers for Disease Control and Prevention. (2016a). *Information for adult patients: 2016 recommended immunizations for adults by health conditions*. Retrieved from http://www.cdc.gov/vaccines/schedules/downloads/adult/adult-schedule-easy-read.pdf.

Centers for Disease Control and Prevention. (2016b). *STDs and pregnancy—CDC fact sheet*. Retrieved from www.cdc.gov/std/pregnancy/stdfact-pregnancy.htm.

Cherguit, J., Burns, J., Pettle, S., & Tasker, F. (2012). Lesbian co-mothers' experiences of maternity healthcare services. *Journal of Advanced Nursing, 69*(6), 1269–1278.

Chervenak, F., McCullough, L., Brent, R., et al. (2013). Planned home birth: The professional responsibility response. *American Journal of Obstetrics and Gynecology, 208*(1), 31–38.

Cheyney, M., Bovbjerg, M., Everson, C., et al. (2014). Outcomes of care for 16,924 planned home births in the United States: The Midwives Alliance of North America Statistics Project, 2004-2009. *Journal of Midwifery and Women's Health, 59*(1), 17–27.

Chughtai, B., Thomas, D., & Howell, A. (2016). Variability of commercial cranberry products for the prevention of uropathogenic bacterial adhesion. *American Journal of Obstetrics and Gynecology, 215*(1), 122–123.

Cigna Corporation (2015). *Healthy smiles for mom and baby: Insights into expecting and new mothers' oral health habits*. Retrieved from http://www.cigna.com/assets/docs/newsroom/cigna-study-healthy-smiles-for-mom-and-baby-2015.pdf.

Clark, L. E., Allen, R. H., Goyal, V., et al. (2014). Reproductive coercion and co-occurring intimate partner violence in obstetrics and gynecology patients. *American Journal of Obstetrics and Gynecology, 210*(1), 42.e1–42.e8.

Corbella, S., Taschieri, S., Del Fabbro, M., et al. (2016). Adverse pregnancy outcomes and periodontitis: A systematic review and meta-analysis exploring potential association. *Quintessence International, 47*(3), 193–204.

Cox, K. J., Schlegel, R., Payne, P., et al. (2013). Outcomes of planned home births attended by certified nurse-midwives in southeastern Pennsylvania, 1983-2008. *Journal of Midwifery and Women's Health, 58*(2), 145–149.

Creanga, A. A., Berg, C. J., Syverson, C., et al. (2015). Pregnancy-related mortality in the United States, 2006-2010. *Obstetrics and Gynecology, 125*(1), 5–12.

Declercq, E. R., Sakala, C., Corry, M. P., et al. (2013). *Listening to mothers III: Pregnancy and birth*. New York, NY: Childbirth Connection.

Demirci, J. R., Cohen, S. M., Parker, M., et al. (2016). Access, use, and preferences for technology-based perinatal and breastfeeding support among childbearing women. *Journal of Perinatal Education, 25*(1), 29–36.

Domenjoz, I., Kayser, B., & Boulvain, M. (2014). Effect of physical activity during pregnancy on mode of delivery. *American Journal of Obstetrics and Gynecology, 211*(4), 401.e1–401.e11.

Donovan, B. M., Spracklen, C. N., Schweizer, M. L., et al. (2016). Intimate partner violence during pregnancy and the risk for adverse infant outcomes: A systematic review and meta-analysis. *BJOG: An International Journal of Obstetrics and Gynaecology, 123*(8), 1289–1299.

Duff, P., & Birsner, M. (2017). Maternal and perinatal infection-bacterial. In S. G. Gabbe, J. R. Niebyl, J. L. Simpson, et al. (Eds.), *Obstetrics: Normal and problem pregnancies* (7th ed.). Philadelphia, PA: Elsevier.

Fiset, K. L., Hoffman, M. K., & Ehrenthal, D. B. (2016). Centering prenatal care: Can a care model impact preterm birth rates? *Obstetrics and Gynecology, 127*(1 suppl), 1s–2s.

Frawley, J., Adams, J., Sibbritt, D., et al. (2013). Prevalence and determinants of complementary and alternative medicine use during pregnancy: Results from a nationally representative sample of Australian pregnant women. *Australian and New Zealand Journal of Obstetrics and Gynaecology, 53*(4), 347–352.

Gregory, K. D., Ramos, D. E., & Jauniaux, E. R. M. (2017). Preconception and prenatal care. In S. G. Gabbe, J. R. Niebyl, J. L. Simpson, et al. (Eds.), *Obstetrics: Normal and problem pregnancies* (7th ed.). Philadelphia, PA: Elsevier.

Gruber, K. J., Cupito, S. H., & Dobson, C. F. (2013). Impact of doulas on healthy birth outcomes. *Journal of Perinatal Education, 22*(1), 49–58.

Hamilton, B. E., Martin, J. A., & Osterman, M. J. K. (2016). Births: Preliminary data for 2015. *National Vital Statistics Reports, 65*(3), 1–63.

Han, A., & Stewart, D. E. (2014). Maternal and fetal outcomes of intimate partner violence associated with pregnancy in the Latin American and Caribbean regions. *International Journal of Gynaecology and Obstetrics, 124*(1), 6–11.

Hartnett, E., Haber, J., Krainovich-Miller, B., et al. (2016). Oral health in pregnancy. *Journal of Obstetric, Gynecologic, and Neonatal Nursing, 45*(4), 565–573.

Health Physics Society. (2016). *Pregnancy and flying*. Retrieved from http://hps.org/publicinformation/ate/faqs/pregnancyandflying.html.

Heberlein, E. C., Picklesimer, A. H., Billings, D. L., et al. (2016). The comparative effects of group prenatal care on psychosocial outcomes. *Archives of Women's Mental Health, 19*(2), 259–269.

Herrman, J. W., Rogers, S., & Ehrenthal, D. B. (2012). Women's perceptions of CenteringPregnancy: A focus group study. *American Journal of Maternal Child Nursing, 37*(1), 19–26.

Hodnett, E., Gates, S., Hofmeyr, G., & Sakala, C. (2013). Continuous support for women during childbirth. *Cochrane Database of Systematic Reviews, 2013*(7), CD003766.

James, L., Brody, D., & Hamilton, A. (2013). Risk factors for domestic violence during pregnancy: A meta-analysis review. *Violence and Victims*, *28*(3), 359–380.

Jared, H., & Boggess, K. (2012) *Periodontal diseases and adverse pregnancy outcomes: A review of the evidence and implications for practice. American Dental Hygienists' Association.* Retrieved from www.cdeworld.com/courses/20006.

Johnson, J. A., & Tough, S. (2012). Delayed childbearing. *Journal of Obstetrics and Gynaecology of Canada, 34*(1), 80–93.

Kawakita, T., Wilson, K., Grantz, K. L., et al. (2016). Adverse maternal and neonatal outcomes in adolescent pregnancy. *Journal of Pediatric and Adolescent Gynecology, 29*(2), 130–136.

Kingston, D., Austin, M., & Heaman, M. (2015). Barriers and facilitators of mental health screening in pregnancy. *Journal of Affective Disorders, 186*, 350–357.

Kocaöz, S., Erogul, K., & Sivaslioglu, A. (2013). Role of pelvic floor muscle exercises in the prevention of stress urinary incontinence during pregnancy and the postpartum period. *Gynecologic and Obstetric Investigation, 75*(1), 34–40.

Lawrence, R. A., & Lawrence, R. M. (2016). *Breastfeeding: A guide for the medical profession* (8th ed.). St. Louis, MO: Elsevier.

Lim, C. C., & Mahmood, T. (2015). Obesity in pregnancy. *Best Practice and Research Clinical Obstetrics and Gynecology, 29*(3), 309–319.

Lima-Pereira, P., Bermúdez-Tamayo, C., & Jasienska, G. (2012). Use of the Internet as a source of health information among participants of antenatal classes. *Journal of Clinical Nursing, 21*(3-4), 322–330.

Liu, F., McFarlane, J., Maddoux, J. A., et al. (2016). Perceived fertility control and pregnancy outcomes among abused women. *Journal of Obstetric, Gynecologic and Neonatal Nursing, 45*(4), 592–600.

Magdaleno, R., Pereira, B. G., Chaim, E. A., & Turato, E. R. (2012). Pregnancy after bariatric surgery: A current view of maternal, obstetrical, and perinatal challenges. *Archives of Gynecology and Obstetrics, 285*(3), 559–566.

Maher, S., Crawford-Carr, A., & Neidigh, K. (2012). The role of the interpreter/doula in the maternity setting. *Nursing for Women's Health, 16*(6), 472–481.

Martin, J. A., Hamilton, B. E., Osterman, M. J., et al. (2017). Births: Final data for 2015. *National Vital Statistics Reports, 66*(1), Hyattsville, MD: National Center for Health Statistics.

Martin, J. A., Hamilton, B. E., Osterman, M. J., et al. (2013). Births: Final data for 2012. *National Vital Statistics Reports, 62*(9), Hyattsville, MD: National Center for Health Statistics.

Martin, J. A., Hamilton, B. E., Sutton, P. D., et al. (2012). Births: Final data for 2010. *National Vital Statistics Reports, 61*(1), Hyattsville, MD: National Center for Health Statistics.

Martin, J. A., Osterman, M. J., & Thoma, M. E. (2016). *Declines in triplet and higher-order multiple births in the United States, 1998-2014. NCHS Data Brief no. 243.* Hyattsville, MD: National Center for Health Statistics.

Martin, S. L., Acara, J., & Pollock, M. D. (2012). *Violence against women during pregnancy and the postpartum period.* Harrisburg, PA: VAWnet.

Martin-de-las-Heras, S., Velasco, C., Luna Jde, D., & Martin, A. (2015). Unintended pregnancy and intimate partner violence around pregnancy in a population-based study. *Women and Birth, 28*(2), 101–105.

Mathews, T. J., & Hamilton, B. E. (2014). *First births to older women continue to rise. NCHS data brief no. 152.* Hyattsville, MD: National Center for Health Statistics.

May, K. (1982). Three phases of father involvement in pregnancy. *Nursing Research, 31*(6), 337–342.

McFarlane, J., Parker, B., & Bullock, L. (1992). Assessing for abuse during pregnancy: Severity and frequency of injuries and associated entry into prenatal care. *Journal of the American Medical Association, 267*(23), 3176–3178.

McIntyre, M. (2012). Safety of non-medically led primary maternity care models: A critical review of the international literature. *Australian Health Review, 36*(2), 140–147.

Meghea, C. I., You, Z., Raffo, J., et al. (2015). Statewide Medicaid enhanced prenatal care programs and infant mortality. *Pediatrics, 136*(2), 334–342.

Mercer, R. (1995). *Becoming a mother.* New York, NY: Springer.

Mills, T. A., & Lavender, T. (2014). Advanced maternal age. *Obstetrics, Gynaecology, and Reproductive Medicine, 24*(2), 85–90.

Moise, K. J. (2017). Red cell alloimmunization. In S. G. Gabbe, J. R. Niebyl, J. L. Simpson, et al. (Eds.), *Obstetrics: Normal and problem pregnancies* (7th ed.). Philadelphia, PA: Elsevier.

Morof, D. F., & Carroll, D. (2016). Advising travelers with specific needs. In Centers for Disease Control and Prevention. *CDC health information for international travel 2016.* New York, NY: Oxford University Press.

National Perinatal Association. (2008) *Position paper: Choice of birth setting.* Retrieved from www.nationalperinatal.org/advocacy/pdf/Choice-of-Birth-Setting.pdf.

Nelson, A. M. (2012). A meta-synthesis related to infant feeding decision making. *American Journal of Maternal Child Nursing, 37*(4), 247–252.

Newman, R., & Unal, E. R. (2017). Multiple gestations. In S. G. Gabbe, J. R. Niebyl, J. L. Simpson, et al. (Eds.), *Obstetrics: Normal and problem pregnancies* (7th ed.). Philadelphia, PA: Elsevier.

Olds, D. L., Kitzman, H., Knudtson, M. D., et al. (2014). Effect of home visiting by nurses on maternal and child mortality. *JAMA Pediatrics, 168*(9), 800–806.

Oral Health Care During Pregnancy Expert Workgroup (2012). *Oral health care during pregnancy: A national consensus statement—summary of an expert workgroup meeting.* Washington, DC: National Maternal and Child Oral Health Resource Center. Retrieved from http://www.mchoralhealth.org/PDFs/Oralhealthpregnancyconsensusmeetingsummary.pdf.

Parihar, A. S., Katoch, V., Rajguru, S. A., et al. (2015). Periodontal disease: A possible risk-factor for adverse pregnancy outcome. *Journal of International Oral Health, 7*(7), 137–142.

Picklesimer, A. H., Billings, D., Hale, N., et al. (2012). The effect of CenteringPregnancy group prenatal care on preterm birth in a low-income population. *American Journal of Obstetrics and Gynecology, 206*(5), 415.e1–415.e7.

Price, B., Amini, S., & Kappeler, K. (2012). Exercise in pregnancy: Effect on fitness and obstetric outcomes—a randomized trial. *Medicine and Science in Sports and Exercise, 44*(12), 2263–2269.

Roman, L., Raffo, J. E., Zhu, Q., & Meghea, C. I. (2014). A statewide Medicaid enhanced prenatal program: Impact on birth outcomes. *JAMA Pediatrics, 168*(3), 220–227.

Rubin, R. (1975). Maternal tasks in pregnancy. *Maternal and Child Nursing Journal, 4*(3), 143–153.

Rubin, R. (1984). *Maternal identity and the maternal experience.* New York, NY: Springer.

Salinsky, E. (2013). *Effect of provider payment reforms on maternal and child health services.* National Governor's Association, May, 2013: NGA paper.

Sandall, J., Soltani, H., Gates, S., et al. (2013). Midwife-led continuity models versus other models of care for childbearing women. *Cochrane Database of Systematic Reviews, 2013*(8), CD004667.

Stöckl, H., March, L., Pallitto, C., Garcia-Moreno, C., & WHO Multi-Country Study Team. (2014). Intimate partner violence among adolescents and young women: Prevalence and associated factors in nine countries: a cross-sectional study. *BMC Public Health, 14*, 751.

Stotland, N. E., Bodnar, L. M., & Abrams, B. (2014). Maternal nutrition. In R. K. Creasy, R. Resnik, J. D. Iams, C. J. Lockwood, T. R. Moore, & M. F. Greene (Eds.), *Creasy & Resnik's maternal-fetal medicine: Principles and practice* (7th ed.). Philadelphia, PA: Elsevier.

Torvie, A. J., Callegari, L. S., Schiff, M. A., & Debiec, K. E. (2015). Labor and delivery outcomes among young adolescents. *American Journal of Obstetrics and Gynecology, 213*(1), 95.e1–95.e8.

Tracy, E. E., & Konstantopoulos, W. M. (2012). Human trafficking: A call for heightened awareness and advocacy by obstetrician-gynecologists. *Obstetrics and Gynecology, 119*(5), 1045–1047.

Udo, I. E., Lewis, J. B., Tobin, J. N., & Ickovics, J. R. (2016). Intimate partner victimization and health risk behaviors among pregnant adolescents. *American Journal of Public Health, 106*(8), 1457–1459.

US Department of Health and Human Services Office of Adolescent Health. (2013). *Teen pregnancy and childbearing.* Retrieved from http://

www.hhs.gov/ash/oah/adolescent-health-topics/reproductive-health/teen-pregnancy.

US Department of Health and Human Services Office of Disease Prevention and Health Promotion. (2013). *Healthy People 2020: Maternal, infant, and child health*. Retrieved from http://healthypeople.gov/2020.

US Department of Health and Human Services Office of Minority Health. (2013). *National standards for culturally and linguistically appropriate services (CLAS) in health and health care*. Retrieved from http://www.thinkculturalhealth.hhs.gov.

West, E. H., Hark, L., & Catalano, P. M. (2017). Nutrition during pregnancy. In S. G. Gabbe, J. R. Niebyl, J. L. Simpson, M. B. Landon, & H. L. Calan (Eds.), *Obstetrics: Normal and problem pregnancies* (7th ed.). Philadelphia, PA: Elsevier.

World Health Organization. (2013). *Responding to partner violence and sexual violence against women: WHO clinical and policy guidelines*. Geneva, Switzerland: WHO. Retrieved from http://apps.who.int/iris/bitstream/10665/85240/1/9789241548595_eng.pdf.

9

Maternal and Fetal Nutrition

Ellen F. Olshansky

http://evolve.elsevier.com/Perry/maternal

Nutrition is one of the many factors that influence the outcome of pregnancy (Fig. 9.1). Indeed, maternal nutritional status is an especially significant factor, both because it is potentially alterable and because good nutrition before and during pregnancy is an important preventive measure for a variety of problems. These problems include birth of low–birth-weight (LBW) (birth weight of 2500 g or less) and preterm infants. Evidence is growing that a mother's nutrition and lifestyle affect the long-term health of her children. Thus the importance of good nutrition must be emphasized with all women of childbearing potential. Key components of nutrition care during the preconception period and pregnancy include the following:

- Nutrition assessment, including of weight and height, and adequacy and quality of dietary intake and habits
- Diagnosis of nutrition-related problems or risk factors such as diabetes, phenylketonuria (PKU), and obesity
- Interventions based on an individual's dietary goals to promote appropriate weight gain, including ingesting a variety of foods, appropriate use of dietary supplements, and physical activity
- Evaluation with referral to a nutritionist or dietitian as necessary

NUTRIENT NEEDS BEFORE CONCEPTION

The first trimester of pregnancy is crucial in terms of embryonic and fetal organ development. A healthy diet before conception and during pregnancy is the best way to ensure that adequate nutrients are available for the developing fetus. Folate or folic acid intake is of particular concern in the periconception period. Folate is the form in which this vitamin is found naturally in foods, and folic acid is the form used in fortification of grain products and other foods and in vitamin supplements. Neural tube defects (NTDs), or failures in closure of the neural tube, are more common in infants of women with poor folic acid intake. Proper closure of the neural tube is required for normal formation of the spinal cord, and the neural tube begins to close within the first month of gestation, often before the woman realizes that she is pregnant. Therefore, all adolescents and women who are capable of becoming pregnant should take 0.4 mg (400 mcg) of folic acid every day, in addition to consuming dietary sources of folate (Box 9.1). A woman who has had a pregnancy involving a child with NTD should take 0.4 mg of folic acid daily, even if she is not planning another pregnancy. If she does become pregnant, she should consult with her health care provider. Some health care providers will prescribe a 4 mg folic acid supplement daily through the first 3 months of pregnancy, and ideally for the month prior to conception, although some health care providers believe that the lower dose of 0.4 mg is adequate (Centers for Disease Control and Prevention [CDC], 2016).

Maternal and fetal risks in pregnancy are increased when the mother is significantly underweight or overweight when pregnancy begins.

Overweight and obese women who lose weight before pregnancy are likely to have healthier pregnancies. Counseling in regard to healthy diet and lifestyle practices, as well as behavioral modification techniques, should be available to women before they become pregnant (American College of Obstetricians and Gynecologist [ACOG], 2013a). Ideally, all women will achieve their desirable body weights before conception.

NUTRIENT NEEDS DURING PREGNANCY

Nutrient needs are determined, at least in part, by the stage of gestation. The amount of fetal growth varies during the different stages of pregnancy. During the first trimester, the synthesis of fetal tissues places relatively few demands on maternal nutrition. Therefore during the first trimester, when the embryo or fetus is very small, the needs are only slightly increased over those before pregnancy. In contrast, the last trimester is a period of accelerated fetal growth when most of the fetal stores of energy sources and minerals are deposited. Thus as fetal growth progresses during the second and third trimesters, the pregnant woman's need for some nutrients increases greatly. Factors that contribute to the increase in nutrient needs include the following:

- Development and growth of the uterine-placental-fetal unit
- Total blood volume (TBV), consisting of plasma and red blood cell volume, increases significantly during pregnancy by 40% to 50%. During the first half of pregnancy, TBV increases rapidly, peaks around 28 to 34 weeks, and then stabilizes or decreases slightly by term. In a singleton pregnancy, plasma volume increases by approximately 1200 to 1500 mL, or 50% above prepregnancy levels by 30 weeks of gestation, decreasing slightly by term (Antony, Racusin, Aagaard, et al., 2017). Increased blood volume is a protective mechanism. It is essential for meeting the blood volume needs of the hypertrophied vascular system of the enlarged uterus, for adequately hydrating fetal and maternal tissues when the woman assumes an erect or supine position, and for providing a fluid reserve to compensate for blood loss during birth and postpartum. Blood volume increases are greater with multiple gestation. Peripheral vasodilation allows for a normal blood pressure despite the increased blood volume in pregnancy.
- Maternal mammary development
- 20% increase in metabolic rate during pregnancy

Dietary Reference Intakes (DRIs) (US Department of Health and Human Services [USDHHS], 2017) have been established for the people of the United States and Canada and are updated regularly. The DRIs include recommendations for daily nutritional intakes that meet the needs of almost all of the healthy members of the population. They are different from the nutritional labeling on foods, which is based on Reference Daily Intakes (RDIs). The DRIs are divided into age, sex, and life-stage categories (e.g., infancy, pregnancy, and lactation), and they

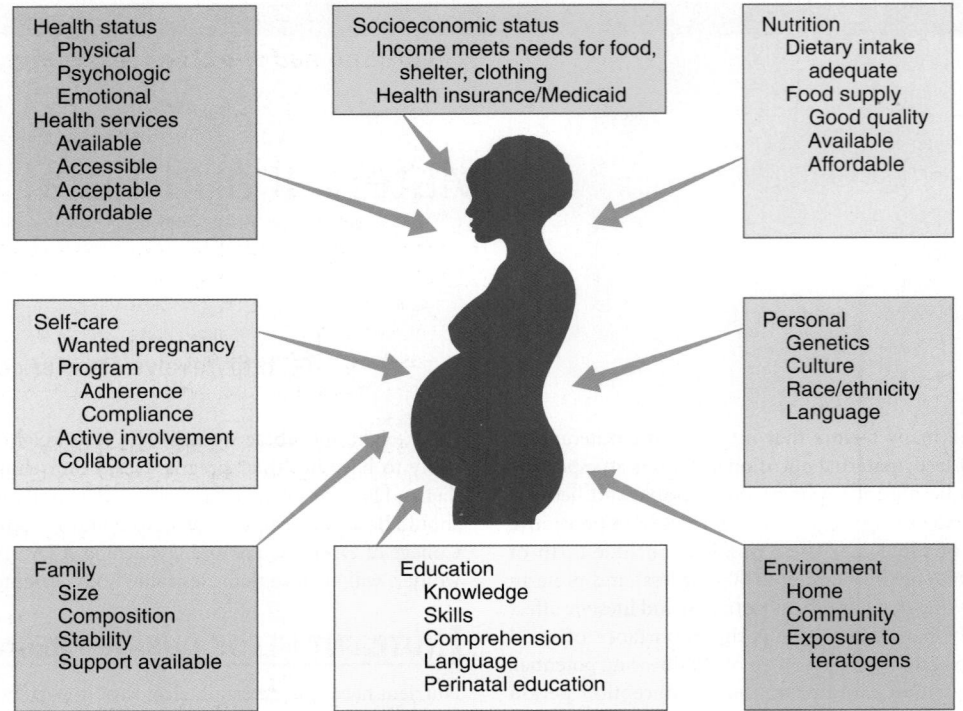

FIG 9.1 Factors that influence the outcome of pregnancy.

can be used as goals in planning the diets of individuals (Table 9.1). The USDHHS and the US Department of Agriculture (USDA) (2015) have also developed guidelines for nutrition, with the most recent guidelines covering 2015 to 2020.

ENERGY NEEDS

Energy (kilocalories) needs are met by carbohydrate, fat, and protein in the diet. No specific recommendations exist for the amount of carbohydrate and fat in the diet of the pregnant women, but the intake of these nutrients should be adequate to support the recommended weight gain. Longitudinal assessment of weight gain during pregnancy is the best way to determine whether the kilocalorie intake is adequate; very underweight or active women may require more than the recommended increase in kilocalories to sustain the desired rate of weight gain. Although protein can be used to supply energy, its primary role is to provide amino acids for the synthesis of new tissues (see discussion later in this chapter).

Weight Gain

The desirable weight gain during pregnancy varies among women. The primary factor to consider in making a weight-gain recommendation is the appropriateness of the prepregnancy weight for the woman's height—that is, whether the woman's weight was normal before pregnancy or whether she was underweight or overweight. Whenever possible, the woman should achieve a weight in the normal range for her height before pregnancy. Maternal and fetal risks in pregnancy are increased when the mother is significantly underweight or overweight before pregnancy and when weight gain during pregnancy is either too low or too high. Severely underweight women are more likely to have preterm labor and to give birth to LBW infants. Both normal-weight and underweight women with inadequate weight gain have an increased risk for giving birth to an infant with intrauterine growth restriction

(IUGR). Greater than expected weight gain during pregnancy may occur for many reasons. It may also lead to several risks, noted in the section under Excessive Weight Gain.

A commonly used method of evaluating the appropriateness of weight for height is the body mass index (BMI), which is calculated by the following formula:

$$BMI = Weight \div Height^2$$

in which the weight is in kilograms and height is in meters. Thus for a woman who weighed 51 kg before pregnancy and is 1.57 m tall:

$$BMI = 51 kg \div (1.57\, m)^2, or\ 20.7$$

Prepregnant BMI can be classified into the following categories: less than 18.5, underweight or low; 18.5 to 24.9, normal; 25 to 29.9, overweight or high; and 30 or greater, obese (CDC, 2015). The BMI can be calculated on this website: www.nhlbi.nih.gov/guidelines/obesity/BMI/bmicalc.htm

At the first prenatal visit, the pregnant woman should be helped to establish a weight-gain goal for pregnancy that is suited to her prepregnancy weight. Progress toward this goal should be monitored at each visit.

For women with single fetuses, current recommendations are that women with normal BMI should gain 11.5 to 16 kg (25 to 35 lbs) during pregnancy (ACOG, 2013a; Institute of Medicine, 2009).

Pattern of Weight Gain

The optimal rate of weight gain depends on the stage of pregnancy. During the first and second trimesters, growth takes place primarily in maternal tissues; during the third trimester, growth occurs primarily in fetal tissues. During the first trimester of singleton pregnancy, the average total weight gain is only 2 to 4 lbs. Thereafter the recommended weight gain increases to approximately 1 lb per week for an underweight woman and a woman of normal weight. The recommended weekly

BOX 9.1   Food Sources of Folate

Foods Providing 500 mcg or More per Serving
- Liver: chicken, turkey, goose (100 g [3.5 oz])

Foods Providing 200 mcg or More per Serving
- Liver: lamb, beef, veal (100 g [3.5 oz])

Foods Providing 100 mcg or More per Serving
- Legumes, cooked (½ cup)
- Peas: black-eyed, chickpea (garbanzo)
- Beans: black, kidney, pinto, red, navy
- Lentils
- Vegetables (½ cup)
  - Asparagus
  - Spinach, cooked
- Papaya (1 medium)
- Breakfast cereal, ready-to-eat ½ to 1 cup)
- Wheat germ (¼ cup)

Foods Providing 50 mcg or More per Serving
- Vegetables (½ cup)
  - Broccoli
  - Beans: lima beans, baked beans, or pork and beans
  - Greens: collards or mustard, cooked
  - Spinach, raw
- Fruits (½ cup)
  - Avocado
  - Orange or orange juice
- Pasta, cooked (1 cup)
- Rice, cooked (1 cup)

Foods Providing 20 mcg or More per Serving
- Bread (1 slice)
- Egg (1 large)
- Corn (½ cup)

CLINICAL REASONING CASE STUDY
Nutrition and the Overweight Pregnant Woman

Angela is a 28-year old Hispanic woman who has missed her period for 2 consecutive months and suspects that she is pregnant. She comes for her initial appointment for diagnosis and care. She is married and cooks for her husband and her brother, who lives with her. She emigrated to the United States 3 years ago and does not speak much English. She appears to be overweight for her height (5 ft 2 in. [1.57 meters] tall, 172 lbs [78 kg]). Angela tells you that this is the weight she has been for several years. When her pregnancy is confirmed, you are asked to plan a diet with Angela that meets the minimum daily requirements and allows for growth of the pregnancy. You know that it is important to include consideration of personal preferences and cultural factors in your plan. With Angela, identify barriers to implementing the plan.

1. Evidence—Is there sufficient evidence to draw conclusions about an appropriate nutrition plan, considering personal preferences and cultural factors?
2. Assumptions—What assumptions can be made about the following?
   a. The daily food guide that Angela should follow
   b. Indicators of nutritional risk in pregnancy, particularly the risk for obesity
   c. How cooking for others influences what Angela eats
   d. How Angela's prepregnancy obesity may affect her pregnancy (her growing fetus and herself)
3. What are the nursing priorities in this situation?
4. Describe the roles/responsibilities of other health care professionals who would potentially be involved in Angela's care.

weight gain during the second and third trimesters is 0.6 lb for overweight women and 0.5 lb for obese women. There is not enough information available to make firm recommendations about optimal weight gain for women with more than two fetuses, but provisional recommendations have been made for all prepregnancy BMI categories except the underweight category. The provisional recommendations for a gestation with more than two fetuses suggest that normal-weight women gain 17 to 25 kg, overweight women gain 14 to 23 kg, and obese women gain 11 to 19 kg (ACOG, 2013a).

The recommended energy (kcal) intake corresponds to the recommended pattern of gain (see Table 9.1). Recommendations include 1800 kcals/day during the first trimester, 2200 kcals/day during the second trimester, and 2400 kcals/day during the third trimester (Medline, 2016). These recommendations are most appropriate for singleton pregnancy and may need to be adjusted in multiple gestation. The amount of food providing the needed increase in energy is not large. The additional kcals needed during the second trimester can be provided by one additional serving from any one of the following groups: milk, yogurt, or cheese (all skim milk products); fruits; vegetables; and bread, cereal, rice, or pasta. In the third trimester, an additional one-third of a serving will provide the needed kcal.

The reasons for an inadequate weight gain (less than 1 kg per month for normal-weight women or less than 0.5 kg per month for obese women during the last two trimesters) or excessive weight gain (more than 3 kg per month) should be evaluated thoroughly. Possible reasons for deviations from the expected rate of weight gain, besides inadequate or excessive dietary intake, include measurement or recording errors or differences in weight of clothing or time of day. An exceptionally high gain is likely to be caused by an accumulation of fluids, and a gain of more than 3 kg in a month, especially after the twentieth week of gestation, often indicates the development of preeclampsia.

Hazards of Restricting Adequate Weight Gain

An obsession with thinness and dieting pervades the North American culture. Figure-conscious women may find it difficult to make the transition from guarding against weight gain before pregnancy to valuing weight gain during pregnancy. In counseling these women, the nurse can emphasize the positive effects of good nutrition as well as the adverse effects of maternal malnutrition (manifested by poor weight gain) on infant growth and development. This counseling includes information on the components of weight gain during pregnancy (Table 9.2) and the amount of this weight that will be lost at birth. Because lactation can help reduce maternal energy stores gradually, this also provides an opportunity to promote breastfeeding.

Pregnancy is not a time for a weight-reduction diet. Even overweight or obese pregnant women need to gain at least enough weight to equal the weight of the products of conception (fetus, placenta, and amniotic fluid). If they limit their energy intake to prevent weight gain, they may also excessively limit their intake of important nutrients. Moreover, dietary restriction results in catabolism of fat stores, which in turn augments the production of ketones. The long-term effects of mild ketonemia during pregnancy are not known, but ketonuria is associated with the occurrence of preterm labor. It should be stressed to obese women (and to all pregnant women) that the quality of the weight gain is important, with emphasis placed on the consumption of nutrient-dense foods and the avoidance of empty-calorie foods (see Clinical Reasoning Case Study).

TABLE 9.1   Recommendations for Daily Intakes of Selected Nutrients During Pregnancy and Lactation

Nutrient (Units)	Recommendation for Nonpregnant Woman*	Recommendation for Pregnancy*	Recommendation for Lactation*	Role in Relation to Pregnancy and Lactation	Food Sources
Energy (kilocalories [kcal] or kilojoules [kJ]†)	Variable	First trimester, same as nonpregnant; second trimester, nonpregnant needs + 340 kcal (1424 kJ); third trimester, nonpregnant needs + 452 kcal (1892 kJ)	First 6 months, nonpregnant needs + 330 kcal (1382 kJ); second 6 months, nonpregnant needs + 400 kcal (1675 kJ)	Growth of fetal and maternal tissues; milk production	Carbohydrate, fat, and protein
Protein (g)	46	First trimester, same as nonpregnant; second and third trimesters, nonpregnant needs + 25 g‡	Nonpregnant needs + 25 g	Synthesis of the products of conception; growth of maternal tissue and expansion of blood volume; secretion of milk protein during lactation	Meats, eggs, cheese, yogurt, legumes (dry beans and peas, peanuts), nuts, grains
Water (L) in food and beverages	2.7	3	3.8	Expansion of blood volume, excretion of wastes; milk secretion	Water and beverages made with water, milk, juices; all foods, especially frozen desserts, fruits, lettuce and other fresh vegetables
Fiber (g)	25	28	29	Promotes regular bowel elimination; reduces long-term risk for heart disease, diverticulosis, and diabetes	Whole grains, bran, vegetables, fruits, nuts and seeds
Minerals					
Calcium (mg)	1300/1000	1300/1000	1300/1000	Fetal skeleton and tooth formation; maintenance of maternal bone and tooth mineralization	Milk, cheese, yogurt, sardines or other fish eaten with bones left in, dark green leafy vegetables except spinach or Swiss chard, calcium-set tofu, baked beans, tortillas
Iron (mg)	15/18	30	10/9	Maternal hemoglobin formation, fetal liver iron storage	Liver, meats, whole grain or enriched breads and cereals, dark green leafy vegetables, legumes, dried fruits
Zinc (mg)	9/8	12/11	13/12	Component of numerous enzyme systems, possibly important in preventing congenital malformations	Liver, shellfish, meats, whole grains, milk
Iodine (mcg)	150	220	290	Increased maternal metabolic rate	Iodized salt, seafood, milk and milk products, commercial yeast breads, rolls, and donuts
Magnesium (mg)	360/310–320	400/350–360	360/310–320	Involved in energy and protein metabolism, tissue growth, muscle action	Nuts, legumes, cocoa, meats, whole grains

TABLE 9.1   Recommendations for Daily Intakes of Selected Nutrients During Pregnancy and Lactation—cont'd

Nutrient (Units)	Recommendation for Nonpregnant Woman*	Recommendation for Pregnancy*	Recommendation for Lactation*	Role in Relation to Pregnancy and Lactation	Food Sources
Fat-Soluble Vitamins					
A (mcg)	700	750/770	1200/1300	Essential for cell development, tooth bud formation, bone growth	Dark green leafy vegetables, dark yellow vegetables and fruits, liver, fortified margarine and butter
D (mcg)	5	5	5	Involved in absorption of calcium and phosphorus, improves mineralization	Fortified milk and breakfast cereals; salmon, tuna, and other oily fish; butter, liver
E (mg)	15	15	19	Antioxidant (protects cell membranes from damage), especially important for preventing breakdown of red blood cells (RBCs)	Vegetable oils, dark green leafy vegetables, whole grains, liver, nuts and seeds, cheese, fish
Water-Soluble Vitamins					
C (mg)	65/75	80/85	115/120	Tissue formation and integrity, formation of connective tissue, enhancement of iron absorption	Citrus fruits, strawberries, melons, broccoli, tomatoes, peppers, raw dark green leafy vegetables
Folate (mcg)	400	600	500	Prevention of neural tube defects, increased maternal RBC formation	Fortified ready-to-eat cereals and other grain products, dark green leafy vegetables, oranges, broccoli, asparagus, artichokes, liver
B₆ or pyridoxine (mg)	1.2/1.3	1.9	2	Involved in protein metabolism	Meats, liver, dark green leafy vegetables, whole grains
B₁₂ (mcg)	2.4	2.6	2.8	Production of nucleic acids and proteins, especially important in formation of RBCs and neural functioning	Milk and milk products, eggs, meats, liver, fortified soy milk

*When two values appear, separated by a diagonal slash, the first is for females younger than 19 years and the second is for those 19 to 50 years of age.
†The international metric unit of energy measurement is the joule (J). 1 kcal = 4.184 kJ.
‡Add an additional 25 g in twin pregnancies.
Data from Otten J.J., Helwig J.P., Meyers L.D. (Eds.). (2006). *Dietary reference intakes: The essential guide to nutrient requirements.* Washington, DC, 2006, National Academies Press.

TABLE 9.2   Tissues Contributing to Maternal Weight Gain at 40 Weeks of Gestation

Tissue	Kilograms	Pounds
Fetus	3.2–3.9	7–8.5
Placenta	0.9–1.1	2–2.5
Amniotic fluid	0.9	2
Increase in uterine tissue	0.9	2
Breast tissue	0.5–1.8	1–4
Increased blood volume	1.8–2.3	4–5
Increased tissue fluid	1.4–2.3	3–5
Increased stores (fat)	1.8–2.7	4–6

Excessive Weight Gain

In the United States, 60% of women who give birth are overweight or obese; only 30% follow the weight gain recommendations for pregnancy, with most women gaining excessive amounts (Centers for Disease Control and Prevention, 2014). Weight gain is important, but pregnancy is not an excuse for uncontrolled dietary indulgence. The woman should place an emphasis on the quality of her food intake as she considers her needs and those of her fetus. Obesity during pregnancy is associated with increased use of health care services and longer hospital stays. During pregnancy, an emphasis on regular physical activity and a healthy dietary intake can help avert excessive weight gain (see Clinical Reasoning Case Study). Excessive weight gained during pregnancy can be difficult to lose after pregnancy, thus contributing to chronic overweight or obesity—an etiologic factor in a host of chronic diseases, including hypertension, diabetes mellitus, and arteriosclerotic heart disease. The woman who gains 18 kg (22 lbs) or more is especially at risk. Food energy intake and particularly intake of fat is likely to be high among pregnant women, especially low-income women. When obesity is present (either preexisting obesity or obesity that develops during pregnancy), there is an increased likelihood of preeclampsia; gestational diabetes; macrosomia and cephalopelvic disproportion; operative vaginal birth; emergency cesarean birth; postpartum hemorrhage; wound, genital tract, or urinary tract infection; birth trauma; and late fetal death. Maternal obesity is also associated with increased risk for miscarriage, congenital anomalies, growth abnormalities, and stillbirth (March of Dimes, 2015; Mayo Clinic, 2016). In addition, the infant of a woman who is obese during pregnancy is more likely to be obese and to develop diabetes as an adult (see Evidence-Based Practice box).

PROTEIN

Protein, with its essential constituent *nitrogen*, is the nutritional element basic to growth. Adequate protein intake is essential to meet increasing demands in pregnancy.

These demands arise from the following:

- The rapid growth of the fetus
- The enlargement of the uterus and its supporting structures, the mammary glands, and the placenta
- The increase in the maternal circulating blood volume and the subsequent demand for increased amounts of plasma protein to maintain colloidal osmotic pressure
- The formation of amniotic fluid

Milk, meat, eggs, and cheese are complete protein foods with a high biologic value. Legumes (dried beans and peas), whole grains, and nuts

---

EVIDENCE-BASED PRACTICE

Weight Management in Pregnancy

Ask the Question

PICOT Question: For obese and overweight pregnant women, what weight management interventions are associated with improved outcomes?

Search for the Evidence

Search Strategies English research-based publications on pregnancy, obesity, weight gain, diet, exercise were included.

Databases Used Cochrane Collaborative Database, National Guideline Clearinghouse (AHRQ), CINAHL, PubMed, UpToDate, Joanna Briggs Institute, and the professional websites for AWHONN and ACOG.

Critical Appraisal of the Evidence

- Half of all reproductive age women are overweight or obese (Spencer et al., 2015) and are more likely to have gestational weight gain (GWG) in excess of recommendations (Jarman, Yuan, Pakseresht, et al., 2016). GWG in obese women tends to accelerate during the second trimester (Overcash, Hull, Moore, et al., 2015).
- Excessive GWG during pregnancy is associated with poor outcomes, due to gestational diabetes, gestational hypertension, fetal macrosomia (Stang & Huffman, 2016), stillbirth, and long-term maternal and childhood obesity (Spencer, Hauk, MacDonald-Wicks, et al., 2015).
- Interventions promoting diet, exercise, or both resulted in significantly less gestational hypertension, and may lower the risk for cesarean birth, fetal macrosomia, and neonatal respiratory distress. Dietary interventions were associated with the best outcomes. Obese and overweight pregnant women benefited the most from interventions (Muktabhant, Lawrie, Lumbiganon, et al., 2015).

Apply the Evidence: Nursing Implications

- Preconceptional counseling should include prevention of obesity, ideally from childhood. Prepregnancy weight loss improves fertility and decreases preterm birth, gestational diabetes, preeclampsia, assisted delivery, and fetal anomalies (Stang & Huffman, 2016).
- Nurses are frequently the main educators about nutrition and food choices. Successful interventions for pregnant women have utilized individual or group counseling, goal-setting, food diaries, supportive emails or text messages, with follow-up lasting weeks or months (Spencer et al., 2015). Messages may need to be tailored to body mass index categories (Jarman et al., 2016).
- Activity needs to be frequent, fun, and affordable. An excellent idea is encouraging the patient to walk with other pregnant women, which provides

social support and increased safety. Encourage this healthy habit in the postpartum period, to decrease weight retention and improve subsequent pregnancy outcomes. In addition, the nurse can advocate for low-cost indoor facilities in the community.

Quality and Safety Competencies: Evidence-Based Practice*
Knowledge

Explain the role of evidence in determining best clinical practice.

Both dietary and exercise counseling work best for weight management in pregnancy.

Skills

Locate evidence reports related to clinical practice topics and guidelines.

Tailoring dietary and exercise counseling to women before, during, and after pregnancy utilizing a variety of techniques can improve maternal and newborn outcomes.

Attitudes

Appreciate the importance of regularly reading relevant professional journals.

Systematic reviews and professional guidelines highlight interventions that have evidence of success, such as motivational goal setting for weight management.

References

Jarman, M., Yuan, Y., Pakseresht, M., et al. (2016). Patterns and trajectories of gestational weight gain, a prospective cohort study. *Canadian Medical Association Journal, 4*(2), e338–e345.

Muktabhant, B., Lawrie, T. A., Lumbiganon, P., et al. (2015). Diet and exercise, or both, for preventing excessive weight gain in pregnancy. *Cochrane Database of Systematic Reviews, 2015*(6), CD007145.

Overcash, R. T., Hull, A. D., Moore, T. R., ET AL. (2015). Early second trimester weight gain in obese women predicts excessive gestational weight gain in pregnancy. *Maternal Child Health, 19*(11), 2412–2418.

Spencer, L., Hauk, R. M., MacDonald-Wicks, L., et al. (2015). The effect of weight management interventions that include a diet component on weight-related outcomes in pregnant and postpartum women: a systematic review protocol. *JBI Database of Systematic Review and Implementation Reports, 13*(1), 88–98.

Stang, J., & Huffman, L. G. (2016). Position of the Academy of Nutrition and Dietetics: Obesity, reproduction, and pregnancy outcomes. *Journal of the Academy of Nutrition and Dietetics, 116*(4), 677–691.

Pat Mahaffee Gingrich

*Adapted from QSEN at www.qsen.org/.

TABLE 9.3 Daily Food Guide for Pregnancy and Lactation

Food Group	Daily Amount of Food Recommended for Women*	Serving Size
Grains	6- to 8-ounce equivalents At least half of grain servings should be whole grains. Whole grains are those that contain the entire grain kernel (bran, germ, endosperm) (e.g., whole wheat or cornmeal, oatmeal, and brown rice). Refined grains have been milled to remove the bran and germ (e.g., white flour, white bread, degermed cornmeal, white rice, and corn or flour tortillas).	1-ounce equivalent = 1 slice bread, 1 cup ready-to-eat cereal, or ½ cup cooked rice or pasta or cooked cereal
Vegetables Vary the vegetables consumed to take advantage of the different nutrients they offer	2½ to 3 cups Weekly intake should include at least the following: 3 cups dark green vegetables (e.g., spinach or greens, broccoli, bok choy, romaine lettuce); 2 cups orange vegetables (e.g., carrots; acorn, butternut, or Hubbard squash; sweet potatoes); 3 cups dry beans or peas (e.g., black, navy, or kidney beans; chickpeas; black-eyed peas; split peas; lentils; soybeans; tofu); 3 cups starchy vegetables (corn, green peas, potatoes); and 6½ cups of other vegetables (e.g., artichokes, asparagus, bean sprouts, green beans, cauliflower, cucumber, tomatoes, iceberg or head lettuce).	1 cup = 2 cups raw leafy greens; 1 cup of other vegetables, raw or cooked; or 1 cup of vegetable juice
Fruits	2 cups	1 cup = 1 cup raw, frozen, or canned fruit; 1 cup 100% juice; or ½ cup dried fruit
Milk, yogurt, and cheese (milk group)	3 cups Most milk group choices should be fat free or low fat.	1 cup = 1 cup milk or yogurt; 1½ ounces natural cheese; 2 ounces processed cheese (e.g., American); 2 cups cottage cheese; 1½ cups ice cream (choose fat-free or low-fat most often)
Meat, poultry, fish, dry beans, eggs, and nuts (meat and beans† groups)	5½- to 6½-ounce equivalents Most meat and poultry choices should be lean or low fat. Fish, nuts, and seeds contain healthy oils, so choose these foods frequently instead of meat or poultry. (Note: Avoid shark, swordfish, king mackerel, or tilefish because they have too much mercury; white albacore tuna must be limited to 6 ounces/week.)	1 ounce-equivalent = 1 ounce (30 g) meat, poultry, or fish; ¼ cup cooked dried beans†; 1 egg; 1 tablespoon (15 mL) peanut butter; ½ ounce nuts or seeds
Oils	6 teaspoons (30 mL) Choose oils rather than solid fats. Solid fats are fats that are solid at room temperature, such as butter, shortening, stick margarine, and pork, chicken, or beef fat. Read the label: choose products with no trans fats, limit intake of saturated fats, and choose oils high in monounsaturated and polyunsaturated fats.	1 teaspoon = 1 teaspoon liquid oil (e.g., olive, canola, sunflower, safflower, peanut, soybean, cottonseed) or soft margarine (tub or squeeze bottle); 1 tablespoon mayonnaise or Italian salad dressing; ¾ tablespoon Thousand Island salad dressing; 8 large olives; ⅙ medium avocado; ⅓ ounce dry roasted peanuts, mixed nuts, cashews, sunflower seeds†

*These are approximate amounts based on a relatively sedentary lifestyle and should be individualized. Intake may have to be increased for women with a more active lifestyle or multiple gestation, those who are underweight before pregnancy, or those exhibiting poor gestational weight gain. Needs during lactation may also be greater than these recommendations.
†Beans are also part of the vegetable group; avocados are also part of the fruit group, and nuts and seeds are part of the meat and beans group.
From US Department of Agriculture. (2017). *Making healthy choices in each food group.* Retrieved from https://www.choosemyplate.gov/moms-making-healthy-food-choices.

are also valuable sources of protein. In addition, these protein-rich foods are a source of other nutrients such as calcium, iron, and B vitamins. Plant sources of protein often provide needed dietary fiber. The recommended daily food plan (Table 9.3) is a guide to the amounts of these foods that would supply the quantities of protein needed. The recommendations provide for only a modest increase in protein intake (25 g daily) over the prepregnant levels in adult women.

Protein intake in many people in the United States is relatively high; thus many women may not need to increase their protein intake at all during pregnancy. Three servings of milk, yogurt, or cheese (four for adolescents) and two servings (5 to 6 oz [140 to 168 g]) of meat, poultry, or fish would supply most of the recommended protein for a pregnant woman. Additional protein is provided by vegetables and breads, cereals, rice, or pasta. Pregnant adolescents, women from impoverished backgrounds, and women adhering to unusual diets such as a macrobiotic (highly restricted vegetarian) diet are those whose protein intake is most likely to be inadequate. High-protein supplements are not recommended because of potentially harmful effects on the fetus.

OMEGA-3 FATTY ACIDS

The long-chain polyunsaturated fatty acids (LC-PUFAs) docosahexaenoic acid (DHA) and arachidonic acid (AA) are considered essential to fetal brain development and neurologic function. Supplementation of omega-3 (n-3) LC-PUFA during pregnancy has been associated with reduced risk for preterm birth and improved neurologic and visual development in the offspring. However, there is a lack of conclusive evidence on the specific beneficial effects of DHA supplementation (Gould, Smithers,

& Makrides, 2013). Many providers recommend at least 300 mg/day of DHA for pregnant women. Some prenatal vitamins contain DHA; fish oil supplements are another source of DHA. Women can get adequate amounts of DHA by eating 8 to 12 ounces of seafood per week. Because of the risk for fetal neurotoxicity of methylmercury, pregnant women are cautioned to select fish species known to have lower levels of methylmercury.

> ## ⚡ SAFETY ALERT
>
> High levels of mercury can harm the developing nervous system of the fetus or young child, and certain fish are especially high in mercury. Women who may become pregnant, women who are pregnant or nursing, and young children need to follow some precautions: (1) avoid eating shark, swordfish, king mackerel, and tilefish; (2) check local advisories about the safety of fish caught by family and friends in local bodies of water, but if no advisory is available, limit intake of these fish to 6 ounces and eat no other fish that week; and (3) eat as much as 12 ounces per week of a variety of commercially caught fish and shellfish low in mercury, such as shrimp, salmon, pollock, catfish, and canned light tuna (but limit intake of albacore or "white" tuna and tuna steaks, which contain more mercury, to 6 ounces per week) (US Food and Drug Administration [FDA], 2013).

FLUIDS

Water is the main substance of cells, blood, lymph, amniotic fluid, and other vital body fluids. It is essential during the exchange of nutrients and waste products across cell membranes. It also aids in maintaining body temperature. A good fluid intake promotes regular bowel function, which is sometimes a problem during pregnancy. The recommended daily intake is about 8 to 10 glasses (2.3 L) of fluid. Water, milk, and decaffeinated tea are good sources. Foods in the diet should supply an additional 700 mL or more of fluid. Dehydration may increase the risk for cramping, contractions, and preterm labor.

MINERALS AND VITAMINS

In general, the nutrient needs of pregnant women, with perhaps the exception of folate and iron, can be met through dietary sources. Counseling about the need for a varied diet rich in vitamins and minerals should be a part of early prenatal care of every pregnant woman and should be reinforced throughout pregnancy. It has been suggested that taking a micronutrient supplement (including vitamins and trace minerals) before and during pregnancy reduces the risk for congenital defects, LBW, and preterm birth, as well as preeclampsia. Although there is no conclusive evidence to support this suggestion and further research is needed on maternal and fetal benefits of micronutrient supplementation, prenatal vitamins are frequently recommended (Mayo Clinic, 2017). Supplements are especially advisable for women with known nutritional risk factors. Box 9.2 includes information about such nutritional risk factors. It is important that the pregnant woman understand that the use of a vitamin-mineral supplement does not lessen the need to consume a nutritious, well-balanced diet.

Iron

Iron is needed to allow transfer of adequate iron to the fetus and to permit expansion of the maternal red blood cell (RBC) mass. By term, there is an increase in red blood cell mass of 250 to 450 mL, or approximately 20% to 30% over prepregnancy values (Monga & Mastrobattista, 2014). The percentage of increase in RBCs depends on the amount of iron available. Because the plasma increase is greater than the increase in RBC production, there is a decrease in normal hemoglobin and

> ### BOX 9.2   Indicators of Nutritional Risk in Pregnancy
>
> - Adolescence or less than 2 years postmenarche
> - Frequent pregnancies: three within 2 years
> - Poor fetal outcome in a previous pregnancy
> - Poverty/food insecurity
> - Poor dietary habits with resistance to change
> - Use of tobacco, alcohol, or drugs
> - Weight at conception under or over normal weight
> - Problems with weight gain
> - Any weight loss
> - Weight gain of less than 1 kg/month after the first trimester
> - Weight gain of more than 3 kg/month after the first trimester
> - Multifetal pregnancy
> - Low hemoglobin and/or hematocrit values
> - Diabetes
> - Chronic illness, including an eating disorder, that affects intake, absorption, or metabolism of nutrients

hematocrit values (see Table 7.4). This state of hemodilution is referred to as physiologic anemia of pregnancy. The decrease is more noticeable during the second trimester, when rapid expansion of blood volume occurs faster than RBC production. A pregnant woman is considered anemic if the hemoglobin is less than 11 g/dL or the hematocrit is less than 33% during the first or third trimester, or if the hemoglobin is less than 10.5 g/dL or the hematocrit is less than 32% during the second trimester (West, Hark, & Catalano, 2017). This is a normal adaptation during pregnancy.

Poor iron status, which can result in iron deficiency anemia, is relatively common among women in the childbearing years. Anemic women are poorly prepared to tolerate hemorrhage at the time of birth. In addition, women who have iron deficiency anemia during early pregnancy are at increased risk for preterm birth. Iron deficiency during the third trimester apparently does not carry the same risk. In the United States, anemia is most common among adolescents, African-American women, and women of lower socioeconomic status.

A supplement of 30 mg of at least 30 mg ferrous iron daily (World Health Organization, 2017) starting by 12 weeks of gestation helps ensure an adequate iron intake. Iron supplements may be poorly tolerated during the nausea prevalent in the first trimester, and starting the supplement after this point may improve tolerance. If maternal iron deficiency anemia is present (preferably diagnosed by measurement of serum ferritin, a storage form of iron), increased dosages may be required and must be discussed with the woman's health care provider. Certain foods taken with an iron supplement can promote or inhibit absorption of iron from the supplement. See Patient Teaching box later in the chapter regarding iron supplementation. Even when a woman is taking an iron supplement, she should also include good food sources of iron in her daily diet (see Table 9.1).

Calcium

There is no increase in the DRI of calcium during pregnancy and lactation compared with the recommendation for the nonpregnant woman (see Table 9.1). The normal amount for the nonpregnant woman appears to provide sufficient calcium for fetal bone and tooth development to proceed while maintaining maternal bone mass. Milk and yogurt are especially rich sources of calcium. Nevertheless, many women do not consume these foods or do not consume adequate amounts to provide the recommended intakes of calcium. One problem that can interfere with milk consumption is lactose intolerance, the inability to digest

BOX 9.3   Calcium Sources for Women Who Do Not Drink Milk

Each of the following provides approximately the same amount of calcium as 1 cup of milk:

Fish
- 3-oz can of sardines
- 4½-oz can of salmon (if bones are eaten)

Beans and Legumes
- 3 cups of cooked dried beans
- 2½ cups of refried beans
- 2 cups of baked beans with molasses
- 1 cup of tofu (calcium added in processing)

Greens
- 1 cup of collards
- 1½ cups of kale or turnip greens

Baked Products
- 3 pieces of cornbread
- 3 English muffins
- 4 slices of French toast
- 2 (7-inch diameter) waffles

Fruits
- 11 dried figs
- 1⅛ cups of orange juice with calcium added

Sauces
- 3 oz of creamy pesto sauce
- 5 oz of cheese sauce

milk sugar (lactose) caused by the lack of the lactase enzyme in the small intestine. It is relatively common in adults, particularly African-Americans, Asians, Native Americans, and Inuits (Alaskan Natives). Milk consumption can cause abdominal cramping, bloating, and diarrhea in such people, although many lactose-intolerant individuals can tolerate small amounts of milk without symptoms. Yogurt, sweet acidophilus milk, buttermilk, cheese, chocolate milk, and cocoa may be tolerated even when fresh fluid milk is not. Commercial lactase supplements (e.g., Lactaid) are widely available to consume with milk, and many supermarkets stock lactase-treated milk. The lactase in these products hydrolyzes, or digests, the lactose in milk, making it possible for lactose-intolerant people to drink milk.

In some cultures it is uncommon for adults to drink milk. For example, Puerto Ricans and other Hispanic people may use milk only as an additive in coffee. Pregnant women from these cultures may need to consume nondairy sources of calcium (Box 9.3). If calcium intake appears low and the woman does not change her dietary habits despite counseling, a calcium supplement may be needed daily, to be determined by the woman and her health care provider. Calcium supplements may also be recommended when a pregnant woman experiences leg cramps caused by an imbalance in the calcium-to-phosphorus ratio.

⚡ SAFETY ALERT

Bone meal, which is sometimes used as a calcium source by pregnant women, is frequently contaminated with lead. Lead freely crosses the placenta; thus regular maternal intake of bone meal may result in high levels of lead in the fetus. Women should ask their provider about which calcium supplements are safe.

Other Minerals and Electrolytes

Magnesium

Diets of women in the childbearing years are likely to be low in magnesium. Adolescents and low-income women are especially at risk. Dairy products, nuts, whole grains, and green leafy vegetables are good sources of magnesium (US Department of Health and Human Services, 2016a).

Sodium

During pregnancy the need for sodium increases slightly, primarily because the body water is expanding (e.g., the expanding blood volume). Sodium is essential for maintaining body water balance. In the past, dietary sodium was routinely restricted in an effort to control the peripheral edema that commonly occurs during pregnancy. It is now recognized that moderate peripheral edema is normal in pregnancy, occurring as a response to the fluid-retaining effects of elevated levels of estrogen. Sodium is not routinely restricted in pregnancy, and restriction has not proved effective in reducing the rates of preeclampsia. Severe sodium restriction may make it difficult for pregnant women to achieve an adequate diet. Grain, milk, and meat products, which are good sources of nutrients needed during pregnancy, are significant sources of sodium. In addition, sodium restriction may stress the adrenal glands and the kidneys as they attempt to retain adequate sodium. In general, sodium restriction is necessary only if the woman has a medical condition such as renal or liver failure or hypertension that warrants such a restriction.

Excessive intake of sodium is discouraged during pregnancy because it may contribute to development of hypertension in salt-sensitive individuals. An adequate sodium intake for pregnant and lactating women, as well as for nonpregnant women in the childbearing years, is estimated to be 1.5 g/day (Fisk, 2015). Table salt (sodium chloride) is the richest source of sodium, with approximately 2.3 g of sodium contained in 1 teaspoon (5 g) of salt. Most canned foods contain added salt unless the label states otherwise. Large amounts of sodium are also found in many processed foods, including meats (e.g., smoked or cured meats, cold cuts, and corned beef), frozen entrees and meals, baked goods, mixes for casseroles or grain products, soups, and condiments. Products low in nutritive value and excessively high in sodium include pretzels, potato and other chips (except salt free), pickles, catsup, prepared mustard, steak and Worcestershire sauces, some soft drinks, and bouillon. A moderate sodium intake can usually be achieved by salting food lightly during cooking; adding no additional salt at the table; and avoiding low-nutrient, high-sodium foods.

Potassium

Diets including adequate intake of potassium are associated with reduced risk for hypertension. Potassium has been identified as one of the nutrients most likely to be lacking in the diets of women of childbearing years. A diet including 8 to 10 servings of unprocessed fruits and vegetables daily, along with moderate amounts of low-fat meats and dairy products, has been effective in reducing sodium intake while providing adequate amounts of potassium.

Zinc

Zinc is a constituent of numerous enzymes involved in major metabolic pathways. Zinc deficiency is associated with malformations of the central nervous system in infants. When large amounts of iron and folic acid are consumed, the absorption of zinc is inhibited and the serum zinc levels are reduced as a result. Because iron and folic acid supplements are commonly prescribed during pregnancy, pregnant women should be encouraged to consume good sources of zinc daily (see Table 9.1). Women with anemia who receive high-dose iron supplements also need supplements of zinc and copper.

Fluoride

There is no evidence that prenatal fluoride supplementation reduces the child's likelihood of tooth decay during the preschool years. No increase in fluoride intake over the nonpregnant DRI is recommended during pregnancy (Lee, 2015).

Fat-Soluble Vitamins

The fat-soluble vitamins include vitamins A, D, E, and K. These are of special concern during pregnancy because vitamin E intake is among the nutrients most likely to be lacking in the diets of women of childbearing age; intake of vitamins A and D is also low in the diets of some women. Fat-soluble vitamins are stored in the body tissues; in the event of prolonged overdoses, these vitamins can reach toxic levels. Because of the high potential for toxicity, pregnant women are advised to take fat-soluble vitamin supplements only as prescribed. However, toxicity from dietary sources is very unlikely.

Vitamin E is needed for protection against oxidative stress, and pregnancy is associated with increased oxidative stress. Oxidative stress above that usually associated with pregnancy has been proposed as an explanation for the etiology of preeclampsia, although supplementation with vitamin E has not been effective in reducing rates of preeclampsia. Vegetable oils and nuts are especially good sources of vitamin E, and whole grains and green leafy vegetables are moderately good sources.

Adequate intake of vitamin A is needed so that sufficient amounts of the vitamin can be stored in the fetus. A well-chosen diet, including adequate amounts of deep yellow and deep green vegetables and fruits such as leafy greens, broccoli, carrots, cantaloupe, and apricots, provides sufficient amounts of carotenes that can be converted in the body to vitamin A. Congenital malformations have occurred in infants of mothers who took excessive amounts of preformed vitamin A (from supplements) during pregnancy; thus supplements are not recommended routinely for pregnant women. Vitamin A analogs (e.g., isotretinoin [Accutane]), which are prescribed for the treatment of cystic acne, are a special concern. Isotretinoin use during early pregnancy has been associated with an increased incidence of heart malformations, facial abnormalities, cleft palate, hydrocephalus, and deafness and blindness in the infant, as well as an increased risk for miscarriage. Topical agents such as tretinoin (Retin-A) do not appear to enter the circulation in substantial amounts, but their safety in pregnancy has not been confirmed.

Vitamin D plays an important role in absorption and metabolism of calcium. The main food sources of this vitamin are enriched or fortified foods such as milk and ready-to-eat cereals. Vitamin D is also produced in the skin by the action of ultraviolet light (in sunlight). A severe deficiency may lead to neonatal hypocalcemia and tetany, as well as to hypoplasia of the tooth enamel. Women with lactose intolerance and those who do not include milk in their diet for any reason are at risk for vitamin D deficiency. Other risk factors for deficiency are dark skin, with African-American women being at high risk for deficiency; habitual use of clothing that covers most of the skin (e.g., Muslim women with extensive body covering); and living in northern latitudes where sunlight exposure is limited, especially during the winter. Use of recommended amounts of sunscreen with a sun protection factor (SPF) rating of 15 or greater reduces skin vitamin D production by as much as 99%, thus bringing about a need for regular intake of fortified foods or a supplement.

Water-Soluble Vitamins

Body stores of water-soluble vitamins are much smaller than those of fat-soluble vitamins, and the water-soluble vitamins, in contrast to fat-soluble vitamins, are readily excreted in the urine. Therefore good sources of these vitamins must be consumed frequently. Toxicity with overdose is less likely than it is in people taking fat-soluble vitamins.

Folate/Folic Acid

Because of the increase in RBC production during pregnancy, as well as the nutritional requirements of the rapidly growing cells in the fetus and placenta, pregnant women should consume 0.4 mg (400 mcg) of folic acid daily (CDC, 2016). All women of childbearing potential need careful counseling about including good sources of folate in their diets (see Box 9.1). Supplemental folic acid is usually prescribed to ensure that intake is adequate.

Pyridoxine (Vitamin B$_6$)

Pyridoxine, or vitamin B$_6$, is essential for carbohydrate, protein, and fat metabolism and is involved in the synthesis of red blood cells, antibodies, and neurotransmitters. Although the recommended intake during pregnancy is 1.9 mg/day (US Department of HHS, 2016b), there is evidence that larger doses are effective for some women in reducing nausea and vomiting (West, Hark, & Catalano, 2017).

Vitamin B$_{12}$

Vitamin B$_{12}$ is involved in production of nucleic acids and protein; it is especially important in formation of RBCs and neural functioning. It is found in milk and milk products, eggs, meats, liver, and fortified soy milk. The recommended dietary allowance of Vitamin B12 for pregnant women is 2.6 mcg and for lactating women it is 2.8 mcg (US Department of HHS, 2016c).

Vitamin C

Vitamin C, or ascorbic acid, plays an important role in tissue formation and enhances the absorption of iron. The vitamin C needs of most women are readily met by a diet that includes at least one or two daily servings of citrus fruit or juice or another good source of the vitamin (see Table 9.1), but women who smoke need more.

OTHER NUTRITIONAL ISSUES DURING PREGNANCY

Alcohol

Alcohol use is contraindicated throughout pregnancy. There is no safe amount or type of alcohol during pregnancy, and there is no time during pregnancy when alcohol consumption is without risk. Because alcohol is a teratogen, it can cause birth defects, impaired cognitive and psychomotor development, and emotional and behavioral problems. Fetal alcohol syndrome can result from maternal alcohol consumption; this severe disorder involves growth restriction, central nervous system abnormalities, and facial dysmorphia (ACOG, 2013b).

Caffeine

The safety of caffeine use in pregnancy is not yet clear. Data suggest that excess caffeine intake can contribute to IUGR (Sengpiel, Elind, Bacelis, et al., 2013). In their review, Jahanfar and Jaafara (2013) found that there is insufficient evidence to determine whether caffeine has any effect on pregnancy outcome. Although the evidence about caffeine is far from conclusive, ACOG and the March of Dimes recommend a daily intake of no more than 200 mg of caffeine (ACOG Committee on Obstetric Practice, 2013c). Caffeine is found not only in coffee but also in tea, some soft drinks, and chocolate.

Artificial Sweeteners

Aspartame (NutraSweet, Equal), acesulfame potassium (Sunett), and sucralose (Splenda) are artificial sweeteners commonly used in low- or no-calorie beverages and low-calorie food products. They have not been found to have adverse effects on the mother or fetus and therefore are approved by the US Food and Drug Administration (FDA) (2015) for use during pregnancy. However, Aspartame, which contains phenylalanine, should be avoided by pregnant women with PKU. Stevia (stevioside) is a sweetener sold as a dietary supplement; no acceptable daily intake has been established for Stevia. Agave is another dietary supplement sweetener, but little is known about its safety or effects in pregnancy.

Pica and Food Cravings

Pica, which is the practice of consuming nonfood substances (e.g., clay, dirt, and laundry starch) or excessive amounts of foodstuffs low in nutritional value (e.g., cornstarch, ice or freezer frost, baking powder, or baking soda), is often influenced by the woman's cultural background (Fig. 9.2). In the United States, it appears to be most common among African-American and Hispanic women, women from rural areas, and women with a family history of pica. One problem with pica is that regular and heavy consumption of low-nutrient products may cause more nutritious foods to be displaced from the diet. As an example, cornstarch ingestion is popular among African-American women. It is a source of "empty" kilocalories; half a cup (64 g) provides 240 kcal but almost no vitamins, minerals, or protein. In addition, the pica items consumed may interfere with the absorption of nutrients, especially minerals. Women with pica have been found to have lower hemoglobin levels than do those without pica. Craving and chewing ice may be associated with iron deficiency during pregnancy, although the cause is unclear.

Moreover, there is a risk that nonfood items are contaminated with heavy metals or other toxic substances. Among Mexican-American women, consumption of "tierra" includes both soil and pulverized Mexican pottery. Lead contamination of soils and soil-based products has caused high levels of lead in pregnant women and their newborns. Regular household use of Mexican pottery in cooking or serving food or ingestion of ground pottery must be included in interviews or questionnaires regarding nutrition intake of pregnant women. The possibility of pica must be considered when pregnant women are found to be anemic, and the nurse should provide counseling about the health risks associated with pica.

The practice of pica, as well as details of the types and amounts of products ingested, is likely to be discovered only by the sensitive interviewer who has developed a relationship of trust with the woman. It has been proposed that pica and food cravings (e.g., the urge to have ice cream, pickles, or pizza) during pregnancy are caused by an innate

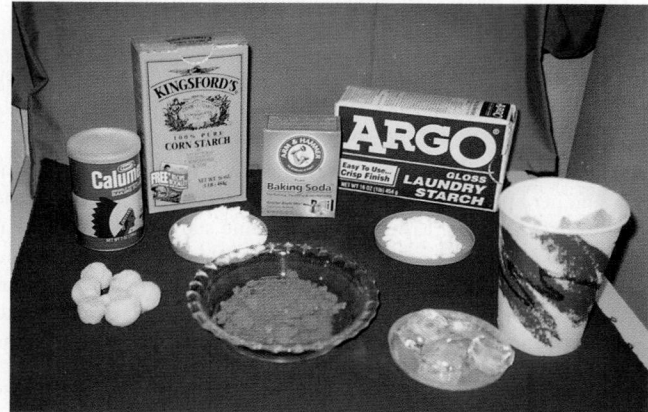

FIG 9.2 Nonfood substances consumed in pica: baking powder, cornstarch, baking soda, laundry starch, and ice. Some individuals practice poly-pica, consuming more than one of these or other nonfood substances. (Courtesy of Shannon Perry, Phoenix, AZ.)

drive to consume nutrients missing from the diet. However, research has not supported this hypothesis.

Many women experience food cravings during pregnancy. In general, consuming foods to satisfy the cravings is not harmful. However, there is some concern that it can lead to dietary imbalances, especially if the cravings involve pica. The nurse can suggest choosing healthy alternatives for cravings, eating small amounts of the craved foods (buying single servings), eating regularly and including healthy snacks to avoid drops in blood glucose levels, and using distraction to curb the craving (take a walk or make a call to a friend).

Adolescent Pregnancy Needs

Many adolescent females have diets that provide less than the recommended intakes of key nutrients, including calcium and iron. Pregnant adolescents and their infants are at increased risk for complications during pregnancy and parturition. Growth of the pelvis is delayed in comparison with growth in stature, and this helps explain why cephalopelvic disproportion and other mechanical problems associated with labor are common among young adolescents. Competition for nutrients between the growing adolescent and the fetus may also contribute to some of the poor outcomes apparent in teen pregnancies. Recommended weight-gain goals are not different from those of adult women. Pregnant adolescents are encouraged to choose a weight-gain goal at the upper end of the range for their BMI. BMI is calculated the same as for adult women rather than by using the adolescent BMI growth charts available from the Centers for Disease Control and Prevention (2015). Adolescent females who have given birth have greater percentages of total fat and visceral fat (associated with the metabolic syndrome and cardiovascular disease) than those who have never given birth (Chang, Choi, Richardson, et al., 2013); thus, the adolescent mother needs careful teaching regarding nutritional intake and physical activity to control body weight in the postpartum period.

Efforts to improve the nutritional health of pregnant adolescents focus on the following:

- Improving the nutrition knowledge, meal planning, and selection and food preparation skills of young women
- Promoting access to prenatal care
- Developing nutrition interventions and educational programs that are effective with adolescents
- Striving to understand the factors that create barriers to change in the adolescent population

Preeclampsia

There has been speculation that the poor intake of various nutrients might contribute to development of preeclampsia, but no definitive evidence exists. At present, a diet adequate in the recommended nutrients (see Table 9.1), along with use of a supplement that provides micronutrients both before and during pregnancy, appears to be the best means of reducing the risk for preeclampsia.

Physical Activity During Pregnancy

Moderate exercise during pregnancy yields numerous benefits, including improving muscle tone, potentially shortening the course of labor, and promoting a sense of well-being. If no medical or obstetric problems contraindicate physical activity, pregnant women should engage in 20 to 30 minutes of moderate physical exercise on most, if not all, days of the week (ACOG, 2015a). Two nutritional concepts are especially important for women who choose to exercise during pregnancy. First, a liberal amount of fluid should be consumed before, during, and after exercise because dehydration can trigger premature labor. Second, the kilocalorie intake should be sufficient to meet the increased needs of pregnancy and the demands of exercise.

NUTRIENT NEEDS DURING LACTATION

Nutritional needs during lactation are similar in many ways to those during pregnancy. Needs for energy (kilocalories), protein, calcium, iodine, zinc, the B vitamins (thiamine, riboflavin, niacin, pyridoxine, and vitamin B_{12}), and vitamin C remain greater than nonpregnant needs. The recommendations for some of these (e.g., vitamin C, zinc, and protein) are slightly to moderately higher than during pregnancy (Otten, Helwig, Meyers, et al., 2006) (see Table 9.1). This allowance covers the amount of the nutrients released in the milk, as well as the needs of the mother for tissue maintenance. In the case of iron and folic acid, the recommendation during lactation is lower than that during pregnancy. Both of these nutrients are essential for RBC formation and thus for maintaining the increase in the blood volume that occurs during pregnancy. With the decrease in maternal blood volume to nonpregnant levels after birth, maternal iron and folic acid needs also decrease. Many lactating women have a delay in the return of menses, which also conserves blood cells and reduces iron and folic acid needs. It is especially important that the calcium intake be adequate; if it is not, a supplement may be needed.

The recommended energy intake for the first 6 months is an increase of 400 to 500 kcal more than the woman's nonpregnant intake (Mayo Clinic, 2015). It becomes difficult to obtain adequate nutrients for maintenance of lactation if total caloric intake is less than 1800 kcal. Because of the deposition of energy stores, the woman who has gained the optimal amount of weight during pregnancy is heavier after birth than at the beginning of pregnancy. As a result of the caloric demands of lactation, the lactating mother usually experiences a gradual but steady weight loss. Most women rapidly lose several kilograms during the first month after birth, whether or not they breastfeed. After the first month, the average loss during lactation is 0.5 to 1 kg a month, and a woman who is overweight may be able to lose up to 2 kg without decreasing her milk supply.

Fluid intake must be adequate to maintain milk production, but the mother's level of thirst is the best guide to the right amount. There is no need to consume more fluids than those needed to satisfy thirst.

Smoking, alcohol intake, and excessive caffeine intake should be avoided during lactation. Smoking not only may impair milk production but also exposes the infant to the risk of passive smoking. It is speculated that the infant's psychomotor development may be affected by maternal alcohol use, and alcohol use may impair the milk-ejection reflex. Caffeine intake can lead to a reduced iron concentration in milk and consequently contribute to the development of anemia in the infant. The caffeine concentration in milk is only approximately 1% of the mother's plasma level, but caffeine levels build up in the infant. Breastfed infants of mothers who drink large amounts of coffee or caffeine-containing soft drinks may be unusually active and wakeful (La Leche League International, 2016).

CARE MANAGEMENT

During pregnancy, nutrition plays a key role in achieving an optimal outcome for the mother and her unborn baby. The motivation to learn about nutrition is usually greater during pregnancy because parents strive to "do what's right for the baby." Optimal nutrition cannot eliminate all problems that may arise during pregnancy, but it does establish a good foundation for supporting the needs of the mother and her Unborn baby.

ASSESSMENT

Ideally a nutritional assessment is performed before conception so that any recommended changes in diet, lifestyle, and weight can be undertaken before the woman becomes pregnant. Information on nutrition and diet is obtained from an interview and review of the woman's health records, physical examination, and laboratory results.

Obstetric and Gynecologic Effects on Nutrition

Nutrition reserves may be depleted in the multiparous woman or one who has had frequent pregnancies (especially three pregnancies within 2 years). A history of preterm birth or the birth of an LBW or small-for-gestational-age (SGA) infant may indicate inadequate dietary intake. Birth of a large-for-gestational-age (LGA) infant often indicates the existence of maternal diabetes mellitus. Contraceptive methods also may affect reproductive health. Increased menstrual blood loss often occurs during the first 3 to 6 months after placement of an intrauterine contraceptive device; consequently the user may have low iron stores or even iron deficiency anemia. Oral contraceptive agents are associated with decreased menstrual losses and increased iron stores; however, oral contraceptives may interfere with folic acid metabolism.

Health History

Chronic maternal illnesses such as diabetes mellitus, renal disease, liver disease, cystic fibrosis or other malabsorptive disorders, seizure disorders and the use of anticonvulsant agents, hypertension, and PKU may affect a woman's nutritional status and dietary needs. In women with illnesses that have resulted in nutrition deficits or that require dietary treatment (e.g., diabetes mellitus, PKU), it is extremely important for nutritional care to be started and for the condition to be optimally controlled before conception. A registered dietitian can provide in-depth counseling for the woman who requires medical nutrition therapy during pregnancy and lactation.

Usual Maternal Diet

The woman's usual food and beverage intake; the adequacy of her income and other resources to meet her nutritional needs; any dietary modifications, food allergies, and intolerances; all medications and nutrition supplements being taken; as well as pica and cultural dietary requirements should be ascertained. In addition, the presence and severity of nutrition-related discomforts of pregnancy such as nausea and vomiting, constipation, and pyrosis (heartburn) should be determined. The nurse should be alert to any evidence of eating disorders such as anorexia nervosa, bulimia, or frequent and rigorous dieting before or during pregnancy.

The effect of food allergies and intolerances on nutritional status varies. Lactose intolerance is of special concern in pregnant and lactating women because no other food group equals milk and milk products in terms of calcium content. If a woman has lactose intolerance, the interviewer should explore her intake of other calcium sources (see Box 9.3).

The assessment must include an evaluation of the woman's financial status and her knowledge of sound dietary practices. The quality of the diet improves with increasing socioeconomic status and educational level. Poor women may not have access to adequate refrigeration and cooking facilities and may find it difficult to obtain adequate nutritious food. Foodborne illnesses may cause adverse effects in pregnancy, and the woman's understanding of safe food-handling practices such as the following should be assessed:

- Cleansing hands, food preparation surfaces, and utensils frequently
- Avoiding contact between raw meat, fish, or poultry and other foods that will not be cooked before consumption
- Storing foods properly
- Cooking foods to a safe temperature

It is important to obtain a thorough diet history. Box 9.4 provides a simple tool for doing so. When potential problems are identified, they should be followed up with a careful interview.

PHYSICAL EXAMINATION

Anthropometric (body) measurements provide short-term and long-term information on a woman's nutritional status and are thus essential to the assessment. At a minimum, the woman's height and weight must be determined at the time of her first prenatal visit, and her weight should be measured at each subsequent visit (see earlier discussion of BMI).

A careful physical examination can reveal objective signs of malnutrition (Table 9.4). It is important to note, however, that some of these signs are nonspecific and that the physiologic changes of pregnancy may complicate the interpretation of physical findings. For example, lower-extremity edema often occurs when kilocalorie and protein deficiencies are present, but it may also be a normal finding in the third trimester of pregnancy. The interpretation of physical findings is made easier by a thorough health history and by laboratory testing if indicated.

LABORATORY TESTING

The only nutrition-related laboratory testing needed by most pregnant women is a hematocrit or hemoglobin measurement to screen for the presence of anemia. Because of the physiologic anemia of pregnancy, the reference values for hemoglobin and hematocrit must be adjusted during pregnancy. The lower limit of the normal range for hemoglobin during pregnancy is 11 g/dL in the first and third trimesters and

---

TABLE 9.4 Physical Assessment of Nutritional Status

Signs of Good Nutrition	Signs of Poor Nutrition
General Appearance	
Alert, responsive, energetic, good endurance	Listless, apathetic, cachectic, easily fatigued, looks tired
Muscles	
Well developed, firm, good tone, some fat under skin	Flaccid, poor tone, tender, "wasted" appearance
Gastrointestinal Function	
Good appetite and digestion, normal regular elimination, no palpable organs or masses	Anorexia, indigestion, constipation or diarrhea, liver or spleen enlargement
Cardiovascular Function	
Normal heart rate and rhythm, no murmurs, normal blood pressure for age	Rapid heart rate, enlarged heart, abnormal rhythm, elevated blood pressure
Hair	
Shiny, lustrous, firm, not easily plucked, healthy scalp	Stringy, dull, brittle, dry, thin and sparse, depigmented, can be easily plucked
Skin (General)	
Smooth, slightly moist, good color	Rough, dry, scaly, pale, pigmented, irritated, easily bruised, petechiae
Face and Neck	
Skin color uniform, smooth, pink, healthy appearance; no enlargement of thyroid gland; lips not chapped or swollen	Scaly, swollen, skin dark over cheeks and under eyes, lumpiness or flakiness of skin around nose and mouth; thyroid enlarged; lips swollen, angular lesions or fissures at corners of mouth
Oral Cavity	
Reddish pink mucous membranes and gums; no swelling or bleeding of gums; tongue healthy pink or deep reddish in appearance, not swollen or smooth, surface papillae present; teeth bright and clean, no cavities, no pain, no discoloration	Gums spongy, bleed easily, inflamed or receding; tongue swollen, scarlet and raw, magenta color, beefy, hyperemic and hypertrophic papillae, atrophic papillae; teeth with unfilled caries, absent teeth, worn surfaces, mottled
Eyes	
Bright, clear, shiny, no sores at corners of eyelids, membranes moist and healthy pink color, no prominent blood vessels or mound of tissue (Bitot spots) on sclera, no fatigue circles beneath	Eye membranes pale, redness of membrane, dryness, signs of infection, redness and fissuring of eyelid corners, dryness of eye membrane, dull appearance of cornea, blue sclerae
Extremities	
No tenderness, weakness, or swelling; nails firm and pink	Edema, tender calves, tingling, weakness; nails spoon-shaped, brittle
Skeleton	
No malformations	Bowlegs, knock-knees, chest deformity at diaphragm, beaded ribs, prominent scapulae

BOX 9.4   Food Intake Questionnaire

Which of the following did you eat or drink yesterday? If the way you ate yesterday wasn't the way you usually eat, choose a recent day that was typical for you.

Food or Drink	Number of Servings	Food or Drink	Number of Servings
Beer, wine, other alcoholic drinks	_____	Orange or grapefruit juice	_____
Tea	_____	Fruit juice other than orange or grapefruit	_____
Coffee		Soft drinks	_____
Caffeinated	_____	Milk	_____
Decaffeinated	_____	Cereal with milk	_____
Fruit drink	_____	Yogurt	_____
Water	_____	Pizza	_____
Cheese	_____	Melon (e.g., watermelon, cantaloupe,	_____
Macaroni and cheese	_____	honeydew)	
Other foods with cheese (e.g., lasagna,		Berries (kind)	_____
enchiladas, cheeseburgers)	_____	Apples	_____
Orange or grapefruit	_____	Other fruit	_____
Bananas	_____	Broccoli	_____
Peaches or apricots	_____	Green beans	_____
Green salad	_____	Potatoes (other than fried)	_____
Spinach or greens	_____	Corn	_____
Green peas	_____	Other vegetables	_____
Sweet potatoes	_____	Chicken or turkey	_____
Carrots	_____	Egg	_____
Meat	_____	Nuts	_____
Fish	_____	Hot dog	_____
Peanut butter	_____	Cold cuts (e.g., bologna)	_____
Dried beans or peas	_____	Roll/bagel	_____
Bacon or sausage	_____	Noodles	_____
Bread	_____	Chips	_____
Rice	_____	Cake	_____
Spaghetti or other pasta	_____	Donut or pastry	_____
Tortillas	_____	Cookie	_____
French fries	_____	Pie	_____

Are you often bothered by any of the following? (Circle all that apply.)
Nausea   Vomiting   Heartburn   Constipation

Are you on a special diet? No _____ Yes _____
  If yes, what kind?
_____

Do you try to limit the amount or kind of food you eat to control your weight? No _____ Yes _____

Do you avoid any foods for health or religious reasons? No _____ Yes _____
  If yes, what foods?
_____

Do you take any prescribed drugs or medications? No _____ Yes _____
  If yes, what are they?
_____

Do you take any over-the-counter medications (e.g., aspirin, cold medicines, acetaminophen [Tylenol])? No _____ Yes _____
  If yes, what are they?
_____

Do you take any herbal supplements? No _____ Yes _____
  If yes, what are they?
_____

Do you ever have trouble affording the food you need? No _____ Yes _____

Do you have any help getting the food you need? No _____ Yes _____
  If yes, what kind? SNAP (Food stamps) _____ WIC _____ School lunch or breakfast _____
  Food from a food pantry, soup kitchen, or food bank _____ Other _____

10.5 g/dL in the second trimester (compared with 12 g/dL in the nonpregnant state). The lower limit of the normal range for hematocrit is 33% during the first and third trimesters and 32% in the second trimester (compared with 36% in the nonpregnant state) (Rigby & Ramus, 2016). Cutoff values for anemia are higher in women who smoke or live at high altitudes because the decreased oxygen-carrying capacity of their RBCs causes them to produce more RBCs than other women produce.

A woman's history or physical findings may indicate the need for additional testing. These tests might include a complete blood cell count with a differential to identify megaloblastic or macrocytic anemia and measurement of levels of specific vitamins or minerals believed to be lacking in the diet.

⚡ SAFETY ALERT

Pregnant women who contract listeriosis, a disease resulting from infection with the bacteria *Listeria*, are at increased risk for miscarriage, premature birth, and stillbirth (US Food & Drug Administration, 2016). During pregnancy, women should not consume unpasteurized milk or products made with unpasteurized milk, including soft cheeses such as Brie, Camembert, and the soft Mexican cheeses queso blanco, queso fresco, panela, and asadero. Hot dogs, luncheon meats, bologna, and deli meats should be eaten only if they have been reheated to be steaming hot. Deli-made and other store-bought salads such as egg, chicken, ham, and seafood should not be eaten.

NUTRITION CARE AND TEACHING

For many women with uncomplicated pregnancies, the nurse can serve as the primary source of nutrition education. The registered dietitian, who has specialized training in diet evaluation and planning, nutritional needs during illness, ethnic and cultural food patterns, as well as translating nutrient needs into food patterns, frequently serves as a consultant. Pregnant women with serious nutritional problems, those with intervening illnesses such as diabetes (either preexisting or gestational), and any others requiring in-depth dietary counseling should be referred to the dietitian. Nutrition care involves an interprofessional team, including the nurse, dietitian, physician, nurse-midwife, and social worker, who collaborate in helping the woman achieve nutrition-related expected outcomes. Nutritional care and teaching generally involve the following:

- Educating the woman about nutritional needs during pregnancy and the components of an adequate diet, if necessary
- Helping her individualize her diet so that she achieves an adequate intake while conforming to her personal, family, cultural, financial, and health circumstances
- Discussing with her strategies for coping with the nutrition-related discomforts of pregnancy
- Helping her use nutrition supplements appropriately
- Consulting with and making referrals to other professionals or services as indicated

Two programs that provide nutrition services are the Supplemental Nutrition Assistance Program (SNAP or food stamps) and the Special Supplemental Nutrition Program for Women, Infants and Children (WIC), which provides vouchers for selected foods for pregnant and lactating women as well as for infants and children at nutritional risk. WIC foods include items such as eggs, milk (or cheese, soy milk, or tofu), juice, fortified cereals, legumes, and peanut butter. WIC participants receive nutrition counseling, and the program encourages breastfeeding (see Nursing Care Plan).

BOX 9.5 Dietary Guidelines 2015–2020

Follow a healthy eating pattern that accounts for all foods and beverages within an appropriate kilocalorie level. A healthy eating pattern includes the following:
- A variety of vegetables from all of the subgroups: dark green, red and orange, legumes (beans and peas), starchy, and other
- Fruits, especially whole fruits
- Grains, at least half of which are whole grains
- Fat-free or low-fat dairy, including milk, yogurt, cheese, and/or fortified soy beverages
- A variety of protein foods, including seafood, lean meats and poultry, eggs, legumes (beans and peas), and nuts, seeds, and soy products
- Oils

A healthy eating pattern limits the following:
- Saturated fats and trans fats, added sugars and sodium
- Less than 10% of kilocalories per day from added sugars
- Less than 10% of kilocalories per day from added fats
- Less than 2300 milligrams per day of sodium
- If alcohol is consumed, it should be limited to one drink/day for women and two drinks/day for men, and only by adults of drinking age

From US Department of Health and Human Services, & US Department of Agriculture. (2015). *Dietary guidelines for Americans 2015-2020.* Retrieved from http://health.gov/dietaryguidelines/2015/guidelines/.

Adequate Dietary Intake

Nutrition teaching can take place in a one-on-one interview or in a group setting. In either case, teaching should emphasize the importance of choosing a varied diet composed of readily available foods (rather than specialized diet supplements). Good nutrition practices (and avoidance of poor practices such as smoking and alcohol or drug use) are essential content for prenatal classes designed for women in early pregnancy.

The USDHHS and USDA (2015) collaboratively have developed the most recent dietary guidelines. (Box 9.5 summarizes these guidelines.)

Pregnancy

The pregnant woman must understand what adequate weight gain during pregnancy means, recognize the reasons for its importance, and be able to evaluate her own gain in terms of the desirable pattern. Many women, particularly those who have worked hard to control their weight before pregnancy, may find it difficult to understand why the weight-gain goal is so high when a newborn infant is so small. The nurse can explain that maternal weight gain consists of increases in the weight of many tissues, not just the growing fetus (see Table 9.2).

Dietary overindulgence, which may result in excessive fat stores that persist after giving birth, should be discouraged. Nevertheless, it is best not to focus unduly on weight gain because this could result in feelings of stress and guilt in the woman who does not follow the preferred pattern of gain. Teaching regarding weight gain during pregnancy is summarized in Box 9.2.

Postpartum

An important goal of postpartum nutrition is for the woman to lose the weight gained during pregnancy. Retention of this weight can contribute to overweight/obesity and the development of later health problems including the metabolic syndrome, cardiovascular disease, and diabetes.

NURSING CARE PLAN

Nutrition During Pregnancy

Case Study

Mercedes is a 27-year-old married woman who is pregnant with her first child. Mercedes and her wife planned this pregnancy, and it was achieved through artificial insemination using a friend as a sperm donor. Mercedes is an avid tennis player and plays competitive tennis. She is a vegetarian and strives to keep her weight down to enhance her playing ability. Mercedes is 5 ft 8 in. tall; her current weight is 122 lbs (body mass index [BMI] is 18.5 [normal is 18.5–24.9]). She has asked for help in planning a nutritional diet that supports the fetus but restricts her weight gain. She is in her first trimester and experiencing nausea in the early morning.

Assessment

What are the nutritional requirements of a mother and fetus during pregnancy? Can nutritional requirements be met on a vegetarian diet? What are signs of inadequate nutrition?

Defining Characteristics

Lack of knowledge of nutritional intake to support fetal growth
Inadequate food intake (less than recommended daily allowances)
Nausea and perceived inability to ingest food

Nursing Diagnosis

Deficient Knowledge related to nutritional requirements during pregnancy

Expected Outcomes

Mercedees will describe nutritional requirements and exhibit evidence of incorporating requirements into her diet.
Mercedes will eat a balanced, healthy diet and take prenatal vitamins and iron as prescribed.
Mercedes will exhibit an appropriate weight gain.
Mercedes will maintain normal hematocrit and hemoglobin.

Nursing Interventions	Rationales
Assess current diet history/intake.	To determine need for additions or changes in present dietary pattern
Review basic nutritional requirements for a healthy vegetarian diet by using recommended dietary guidelines.	To provide knowledge baseline for discussion
Discuss increased nutrient needs (kilocalories, protein, minerals, vitamins) that occur as a result of being pregnant.	To increase knowledge needed for altered dietary requirements
Discuss relation between weight gain and fetal growth.	To reinforce interdependence of fetus and mother
Calculate appropriate total weight gain range during pregnancy using Mercedes' BMI as a guide, and discuss recommended rates of weight gain during various trimesters of pregnancy.	To provide concrete measures of dietary success
Review food preferences, cultural eating patterns or beliefs, and prepregnancy eating patterns.	To enhance integration of new dietary needs
Discuss how to fit nutritional needs into usual dietary patterns and how to alter any identified nutritional deficits or excesses.	To increase chances of success with dietary alterations
Discuss what changes can be made in diet, activity, and lifestyle.	To ensure well-being of the fetus

Assessment

What are the signs of excessive nausea and vomiting?

Defining Characteristics

Reports of nausea or "feeling sick to stomach;" vomiting
Gagging sensation
Increased salivation
Increased swallowing
Decreased skin turgor
Concentrated urine

Nursing Diagnosis

Nausea related to physiologic alterations of first trimester of pregnancy

Expected Outcomes

Nausea will not be so severe that it interferes with adequate nutrient intake.
Nausea will not substantially reduce quality of life.
Mercedes will maintain adequate fluid intake.

Nursing Interventions	Rationales
Assess state of hydration, and assess pattern of weight gain during pregnancy.	To ensure that Mercedes does not have a deficient fluid volume; to ensure that nausea is not preventing adequate energy intake
Review nausea history (i.e., frequency of episodes of nausea, likelihood of nausea progressing to vomiting, factors precipitating or associated with nausea, and any relief measure that Mercedes has tried).	To determine severity of problem and to begin to identify effective and ineffective measures for coping with nausea
Review measures for prevention or relief of morning sickness.	To ensure that Mercedes is knowledgeable about measures that are often effective in alleviating morning sickness
Discuss with Mercedes what relief measures she will try.	To determine whether Mercedes understands how to implement measures

Case Study (Continued)

Mercedes in now in the middle of the second trimester. Her nausea has resolved, and she is able to eat and drink as she wishes. She has resumed playing tennis but has stopped playing competitively. She has gained 3 lbs over her prepregnancy weight and is pleased that she is not gaining "too much weight." She has set a goal of a 10-lb weight gain during pregnancy; she has heard that limiting her weight will ensure an easier labor and birth and she won't have to lose all that baby fat after birth.

Assessment

What are the hazards of gaining too little weight during pregnancy? How does an inadequate weight gain affect the fetus?

Defining Characteristics

Inadequate food intake (less than recommended daily allowances)
Inadequate weight gain
Lack of information or misinformation about nutrition
Lack of knowledge about the detrimental effects on fetal growth and development of an inadequate nutritional intake

NURSING CARE PLAN

Nutrition During Pregnancy—cont'd

Nursing Diagnosis	Nursing Interventions	Rationales
Imbalanced Nutrition: Less Than Body Requirements related to inadequate intake of needed nutrients	Review recent diet history (including food aversions) using food diary 24-hour recall, or food frequency approach.	To ascertain dietary inadequacies contributing to insufficient weight gain
Expected Outcomes	Review normal activity and exercise routines, and discuss eating patterns and reasons that lead to decreased food intake.	To determine level of energy expenditure and to identify habits that contribute to inadequate weight gain
Mercedes will verbalize minimum nutritional requirements to support fetal growth and development.	Review optimal weight gain guidelines and their rationale.	To ensure that Mercedes is knowledgeable about healthful weight gain rates
Mercedes will demonstrate ability to plan a vegetarian diet that meets minimum requirements.		
Mercedes' weekly weight gain will be increased to appropriate rate using her BMI and recommended weight gain ranges as guidelines.	Set target weight gains for remaining weeks of pregnancy.	To establish set, measureable goals

The need for a varied diet with food from all the food groups continues throughout lactation. The lactating woman should be advised to consume an additional 450 to 500 calories per day (American Academy of Pediatrics [AAP], 2012), and she should receive counseling if her diet appears to be inadequate in any nutrients. Special attention should be given to her zinc, vitamin B_6, and folic acid intake because the recommendations for these remain higher than for nonpregnant women (see Table 9.1). Sufficient calcium is needed to allow for both milk formation and maintenance of maternal bone mass. It may be difficult for lactating women to consume enough of these nutrients without careful meal planning.

Obese women and normal-weight women who gain more than the recommended amount of weight during pregnancy are less likely to breastfeed than normal-weight women with appropriate weight gain. Obese women who do choose to breastfeed have a statistically shorter period of lactation than normal-weight women (Leonard, Labiner-Wolfe, Geraghty, et al., 2011). The woman who does not breastfeed can lose weight gradually if she consumes a balanced diet that provides slightly less than her daily energy expenditure, although overweight and obese women with excessive weight gain during pregnancy have an increased likelihood of failing to return to their prepregnancy weights. A reasonable weight-loss goal for nonlactating women is 0.5 to 0.9 kg per week; a loss of 1 kg per month is recommended for most lactating women. Those at risk for obesity and overweight need follow-up to ensure that they know how to make wise food choices, primarily from fruits, vegetables, whole grains, lean meats, and low-fat dairy products. An hour of moderately vigorous physical activity (e.g., walking, jogging, swimming, cycling, aerobic dance) most days of the week will improve the ability of the woman to lose weight gradually and maintain the weight loss.

Daily Food Guide and Menu Planning

The daily food plan (see Table 9.3) can be used as a guide for educating women about nutritional needs during pregnancy and lactation. This food plan is general enough to be used by women from a wide variety of cultures, including those who follow a vegetarian diet. One of the more helpful teaching strategies is to help the woman plan daily menus that follow the food plan and are affordable, have realistic preparation times, and are compatible with personal preferences and cultural practices. Information regarding cultural food patterns is provided later in this chapter.

Medical Nutrition Therapy

During pregnancy and lactation, the food plan for women with special medical nutrition therapy may have to be modified. Members of the interprofessional health care team are often involved in nutrition therapy. These health care team members include the obstetric care provider; specialists such as endocrinologists; nurses; registered dietitians; and social workers.

The registered dietitian can instruct these women about their diets and assist them in meal planning. The nurse should understand the basic principles of the diet and be able to reinforce the teaching.

The nurse should be especially aware of the dietary modifications necessary for women with diabetes mellitus (either gestational or preexisting). This disease is relatively common, and fetal morbidity and mortality occur more often in pregnancies complicated by hyperglycemia or hypoglycemia (see discussion of diabetes in Chapter 11). Every effort should be made to maintain blood glucose levels in the recommended range throughout pregnancy. The food plan of the woman with diabetes usually includes four to six meals and snacks daily, with the daily carbohydrate intake distributed fairly evenly among the meals and snacks. The complex carbohydrates—fibers and starches—should be well represented in the diet. To maintain strict control of the blood glucose level, the pregnant woman with diabetes usually must monitor her own blood glucose several times daily.

Counseling About Iron Supplementation

The nutrition supplement most commonly needed during pregnancy is iron, but routine supplementation with iron during pregnancy is not recommended. If supplementation is indicated, this should be decided in consultation with the woman's health care provider. However, a variety of dietary factors can affect the completeness of absorption of an iron supplement. The Patient Teaching box summarizes important points regarding iron supplementation.

Coping With Nutrition-Related Discomforts of Pregnancy

The most common nutrition-related discomforts of pregnancy are nausea and vomiting (or "morning sickness"), constipation, and pyrosis.

Nausea and Vomiting

Nausea and vomiting of pregnancy (NVP) is most common during the first trimester. Usually, NVP causes only mild to moderate problems nutritionally, although it may be a source of substantial discomfort. Antiemetic medications, vitamin B_6, ginger, and P6 acupressure may be effective in reducing the severity of nausea, although the evidence supporting them is not strong (ACOG, 2015b). The pregnant woman may find the suggestions in Box 9.6 helpful in alleviating NVP.

PATIENT TEACHING
Iron Supplementation

- Iron supplementation should be taken upon the recommendation of the health care provider.
- A diet rich in vitamin C (in citrus fruits, tomatoes, melons, and strawberries) and heme iron (in meats) increases the absorption of the iron supplement; therefore include these in the diet often.
- Bran, tea, coffee, milk, oxalates (in spinach and Swiss chard), and egg yolk decrease iron absorption. Avoid consuming them at the same time as the supplement.
- Iron is absorbed best if it is taken when the stomach is empty; that is, take it between meals with a beverage other than tea, coffee, or milk.
- Iron can be taken at bedtime if abdominal discomfort occurs when it is taken between meals.
- If an iron dose is missed, take it as soon as it is remembered if that is within 13 hours of the scheduled dose. Do not double up on the dose.
- Keep the supplement in a childproof container and out of the reach of any children in the household.
- The iron may cause stools to be black or dark green.
- Constipation is common with iron supplementation. A diet high in fiber with adequate fluid intake is recommended.

BOX 9.6   Suggestions for Managing Nausea and Vomiting During Pregnancy

- Eat dry, starchy foods such as dry toast, melba toast, or crackers on awakening in the morning and at other times when nausea occurs.
- Avoid consuming excessive amounts of fluids early in the day or when nauseated (but compensate by drinking fluids at other times).
- Eat small amounts frequently (every 2 to 3 hours), and avoid large meals that distend the stomach.
- Avoid skipping meals and thus becoming extremely hungry, which may worsen nausea. Have a snack such as cereal with milk, a small sandwich, or yogurt before bedtime.
- Avoid sudden movements. Get out of bed slowly.
- Decrease intake of fried and other fatty foods. Try high-carbohydrate foods such as toast, rice, or potatoes. Some women find high-protein meals or snacks helpful.
- Breathe fresh air to help relieve nausea. Keep the environment well ventilated (e.g., open a window), go for a walk outside, or decrease cooking odors by using an exhaust fan.
- Eat foods served at cool temperatures and foods that give off little aroma. Avoid spicy foods.
- Avoid brushing teeth immediately after eating.
- Try salty and tart foods (e.g., potato chips and lemonade) during periods of nausea. Sucking a lemon slice may help.
- Try herbal teas such as those made with raspberry leaf or peppermint to decrease nausea.
- Vitamin B_6 or a medicine such as Diclegis (made of vitamin B_6 and doxylamine) may be recommended by the health care provider.

Hyperemesis gravidarum, or severe and persistent vomiting causing weight loss, dehydration, and electrolyte abnormalities, occurs in up to 1% of pregnant women. Intravenous fluid and electrolyte replacement, enteral tube feeding, and rarely total parenteral nutrition have been used to nourish women with hyperemesis gravidarum. There is very limited evidence that acupressure and ginger might provide some relief (see Chapter 12 for more information).

Constipation

Improved bowel function generally results from increasing the intake of fiber (e.g., bran and whole-wheat products, popcorn, and raw or lightly steamed vegetables) in the diet. Fiber helps create a bulky stool that stimulates intestinal peristalsis. The recommendation for pregnant women for fiber is 25 to 30 g daily. An adequate fluid intake (at least 8 to 10 cups [2.3 L]/day) helps hydrate the fiber and increase the bulk of the stool. Making a habit of regular physical activity that uses large muscle groups (walking, swimming, water aerobics) also helps stimulate bowel motility (American Pregnancy Association, 2015).

Pyrosis

Pyrosis, or heartburn, is usually caused by reflux of gastric contents into the esophagus. This condition can be minimized by eating small, frequent meals rather than two or three larger meals daily. Because fluids increase the distention of the stomach, they should not be consumed with foods. The woman needs to drink adequate amounts between meals. Avoiding spicy foods may help alleviate the problem. Reflux can be exacerbated by lying down immediately after eating and wearing clothing that is tight across the abdomen.

Cultural Influences

Consideration of a woman's cultural food preferences enhances communication and provides a greater opportunity for following the agreed-on pattern of intake. Women in most cultures are encouraged to eat a diet typical for them. The nurse needs to be aware of what constitutes a typical diet for each cultural or ethnic group present in her patient population. However, several variations may occur within one cultural group. Thus a careful exploration of individual preferences is needed. Although ethnic and cultural food beliefs may seem at first glance to conflict with the dietary instruction provided by physicians, nurses, and dietitians, it is often possible for the empathic health care provider to identify cultural beliefs that are congruent with the modern understanding of pregnancy and fetal development. Many cultural food practices have some merit or the culture would not have survived. Food cravings during pregnancy are considered normal by many cultures, but the kinds of cravings often are culturally specific. Cultural influences on food intake usually lessen if the woman and her family become more integrated into the dominant culture. Nutritional beliefs and the practices of selected cultural groups are summarized in Table 9.5.

Vegetarian Diets

Vegetarian diets represent another cultural effect on nutritional status. Foods basic to almost all vegetarian diets are vegetables, fruits, legumes, nuts, seeds, and grains, but with many variations. Lacto-vegetarians include milk products. Lacto-ovovegetarians consume eggs and dairy products in addition to plant products. Strict vegetarians, or vegans, consume only plant products. All of these types of vegetarian diets, if they are well planned, can be nutritionally adequate for pregnant and lactating women. Because vitamin B_{12} is found only in foods of animal origin, this diet is deficient in vitamin B_{12}. As a result, strict vegetarians should take a supplement or regularly consume vitamin B_{12}–fortified foods such as fortified soy milk two or three times a day or take a supplement. Vitamin B_{12} deficiency can result in megaloblastic anemia, glossitis (inflamed red tongue), and neurologic deficits in the mother. Infants born to affected mothers are likely to have megaloblastic anemia and exhibit neurodevelopmental delays. The diet should be carefully planned to include adequate minerals. Iron and zinc may not be as well absorbed from plant foods as they are from meats, and calcium intake can be low if milk products are avoided. Plant proteins tend to be "incomplete," in that they lack one or more amino acids required for growth and the maintenance of body tissues. However, the daily consumption of a variety of different plant proteins—grains, dried beans and peas, nuts, and seeds—can provide all of the essential amino acids.

TABLE 9.5   Popular Foods of Various Cultural and Ethnic Groups

Cultural or Ethnic Group or Eating Pattern	FOOD GROUPS				
	Grains	**Vegetable**	**Fruit**	**Dairy**	**Protein**
Mexican	Tortilla Taco shell Posole (corn soup) Rice Postres (pastries)*	*Other vegetables:* Chayote (Mexican squash) Jicama (root vegetable) Nopales (cactus leaves) Tomato Corn	Avocado Mango Papaya Plátano (cooking banana) Zapote (sweet, yellowish fruit)	Queso blanco (white Mexican cheese) Custard (1 cup = 1 cup milk serving) Leche (milk)	Chorizo (sausage)* Chicken, beef, goat, or pork Beans, dried, cooked
African-American soul food (Southern-style cooking)	Biscuit Cornbread Grits, rice, macaroni, or noodles Hominy Crackers Hush puppies	*Dark green:* Collard, kale, mustard, or turnip greens *Orange:* Sweet potatoes *Other:* Okra Snap, pole (green), lima, and butter beans Turnips Summer squash (yellow or zucchini) Coleslaw	Blackberries Melons Muscadines (grapes) Peaches	Buttermilk	Pork (cured ham and uncured cuts), chicken, beef, fish Peas or beans (black-eyed, crowder, purple-hull, or cream)
Vegetarian	Whole-grain bread Cereal, cooked or ready-to-eat Brown rice Whole-grain pasta Bagel	All	All	Milk and cheese (lacto-vegetarians) Soy milk, calcium-fortified Soy cheese	Cooked dried beans or peas Tofu (soybean curd) or tempeh (fermented soy) Nuts or seeds Peanut butter Egg (ovovegetarians)
Italian	Breadsticks, breads Gnocchi (dumplings) Polenta (cornmeal mush) Risotto (creamy rice dish) Pastas	*Dark green:* Spinach *Other:* Artichoke Eggplant Mushrooms Marinara sauce	Berries Figs Pomegranate	Cheeses (e.g., mozzarella, Parmesan, Romano, ricotta) Gelato (Italian ice cream)	Veal or beef Fish Sausage* Luncheon meats* Lentils Squid Almonds, pistachios
Chinese	Rice or millet Rice vermicelli (thin rice pasta) Cellophane noodles (bean thread) Steamed rolls Rice congee (soup) Rice sticks	*Other:* Pea pods Yard-long beans Baby corn Bamboo shoots Straw mushrooms Eggplant Bitter melon	Guava Lychee Persimmon Pummelo Kumquat Star fruit	Soy milk	Pork, fish, chicken Shrimp, crab, lobster Tofu or tempeh
Indian (south Asia)	Breads: roti (chapati), naan, paratha, batura, puris, dosa, idli Rice or rice pilau Pooha, upma, sabudana	*Dark green:* Saag (mixed greens and potatoes) Spinach *Other:* Green peppers Cabbage Eggplant Green beans Methi (fenugreek leaves) Cucumbers Chutney or vegetable pickles	Mango Dates Raisins Melons Figs Fruit juices and nectars	Yogurt	Dal (lentils, mung beans, other dried beans) Beef, chicken (some are vegetarian)

Continued

TABLE 9.5 Popular Foods of Various Cultural and Ethnic Groups—cont'd

Cultural or Ethnic Group or Eating Pattern	FOOD GROUPS				
	Grains	Vegetable	Fruit	Dairy	Protein
Native American[†]	Bread	*Orange:*	Berries		Wild game (deer, rabbit, elk, beaver)
	Fry bread	Winter squash (hard outer shell)	Cherries		Lamb
	Wild rice or oats	*Starchy:*	Plums		Salmon and other fish
	Popcorn	Potato	Apples		Clams, mussels
	Tortilla	Corn	Peaches		Crab
	Mush (cooked cereal)	*Other:*			Duck or quail
		Rhubarb			
Middle Eastern	Rice or bulgur (cracked wheat)	*Yellow:*	Apricots	Yogurt	Lamb, goat, fish
	Couscous	Pumpkin or winter squash (butternut)	Grapes		Almonds
	Bread	*Other:*	Melons		Pistachio nuts
	Pita	Peppers	Dried fruits: dates, raisins, apricots		Dried beans and peas, lentils
		Tomatoes			Eggs
		Grape leaves			
		Cucumbers			
		Fava beans			
		Eggplant			

*High fat, use sparingly.
[†]Varies widely depending on tribal grouping and locale.

REFERENCES

American Academy of Pediatrics. (2012). Breastfeeding and the use of human milk. *Pediatrics, 129*, e827–e841. Retrieved from http://pediatrics. aappublications.org/content/129/3/e827.full.pdf+html.

American College of Obstetricians and Gynecologists. (2015a). *Physical activity and exercise during pregnancy and the postpartum period.* Retrieved from http://www.acog.org/Resources-And-Publications/ Committee-Opinions/Committee-on-Obstetric-Practice/Physical-Activity -and-Exercise-During-Pregnancy-and-the-Postpartum-Period.

American College of Obstetricians and Gynecologists. (2015b). Practice bulletin no. 153: Nausea and vomiting of pregnancy. *Obstetrics and Gynecology, 126*(3), e12–e24.

American College of Obstetricians and Gynecologists. (2013a). Practice bulletin no. 548: Weight gain during pregnancy. *Obstetrics and Gynecology, 2013*, 121–122.

American College of Obstetricians and Gynecologists. (2013b). *Committee opinion no. 496: At-risk drinking and alcohol dependence: Obstetric and gynecologic implications.* Retrieved from www.acog.org/ Resources-And-Publications/Committee-Opinions/Committee-on-Health -Care-for-Underserved-Women/At-Risk-Drinking-and-Alcohol -Dependence-Obstetric-and-Gynecologic-Implications.

American College of Obstetricians and Gynecologists. (2013c). *Moderate caffeine consumption during pregnancy.* Retrieved from www.acog.org/ Resources-And-Publications/Committee-Opinions/ Committee-on-Obstetric-Practice/Moderate-Caffeine-Consumption -During-Pregnancy.

American Pregnancy Association. (2015). *Pregnancy and constipation.* Retrieved from http://americanpregnancy.org/pregnancy-health/ constipation-during-pregnancy/.

Antony, K. M., Racusin, D. A., Aagaard, K., et al. (2017). Maternal physiology. In S. G. Gabbe, J. R. Niebyl, J. L. Simpson, et al. (Eds.), *Obstetrics: Normal and problem pregnancies* (7th ed.). Philadelphia: Elsevier.

Centers for Disease Control and Prevention. (2015). *What is BMI?* Retrieved from https://www.cdc.gov/healthyweight/assessing/bmi/adult_bmi/.

Centers for Disease Control and Prevention. (2016). *Folic acid.* Retrieved from https://www.cdc.gov/ncbddd/folicacid/faqs.html.

Chang, T., Choi, H., Richardson, C. R., et al. (2013). Implications of teen birth for overweight and obesity in adulthood. *American Journal of Obstetrics and Gynecology, 209*(2), 110.e1–110.e7.

Drugs.com. (2017). *Ferrous sulfate dosage.* Retrieved from https:// www.drugs.com/dosage/ferrous-sulfate.html.

Fisk, M. (2015). *How much sodium is too much for pregnant women?* Retrieved from http://www.livestrong.com/article/493914-how-much-sodiu m-is-too-much-for-pregnant-women/.

Gould, J. F., Smithers, L. G., & Makrides, M. (2013). The effect of maternal omega-3 (n-3) LCPUFA supplementation on early childhood cognitive and visual development: A systematic review and meta-analysis of randomized controlled trials. *American Journal of Clinical Nutrition, 97*(3), 532–544.

Institute of Medicine. (2009). *Weight gain during pregnancy: Reexamining the guidelines.* Washington, DC: National Academies Press.

Jahanfar, S., & Jaafara, S. H. (2013). Effects of restricted caffeine intake by mother on fetal, neonatal and pregnancy outcome. *Cochrane Database of Systematic Review, 2013*(2), CD006965.

La Leche League International. (2016). *Wht effect does the mother's consumption of caffeine have on the breastfeeding infant?* Retrieved from http://www.llli.org/faq/caffeine.html.

Lee, S. (2015). *What are safe levels of fluoride for pregnant women and newborns?* Retrieved from http://www.livestrong.com/article/493681-what -are-safe-levels-of-flouride-for-pregnant-women-newborns/.

Leonard, S. A., Labiner-Wolfe, J., Geraghty, S. R., et al. (2011). Associations between high prepregnancy body mass index, breast-milk expression, and breast-milk production and feeding. *American Journal of Clinical Nutrition, 93*(3), 556–563.

March of Dimes. (2015). *Being overweight during pregnancy.* Retrieved from www.marchofdimes.org/pregnancy/being-overweight-during -pregnancy.aspx.

Mayo Clinic (2015). *Breast-feeding nutrtion: Tips for moms.* Retrieved from http://www.mayoclinic.org/healthy-lifestyle/infant-and-toddler-health/in -depth/breastfeeding-nutrition/art-20046912.

Mayo Clinic (2016). *Pregnancy and obesity: Know the risks.* Retrieved from http://www.mayoclinic.org/healthy-lifestyle/pregnancy-week-by-week/in -depth/pregnancy-and-obesity/art-20044409.

Mayo Clinic. (2017). *Pregnancy week by week: Prenatal vitamins: Why they matter/how to choose.* Retrieved from http://www.mayoclinic.org/healthy-lifestyle/pregnancy-week-by-week/in-depth/prenatal-vitamins/art-20046945.

Medline. (2016). *Eating right during pregnancy.* US National Library of Medicine. Retrieved from https://medlineplus.gov/ency/patientinstructions/000584.htm.

Monga, M., & Mastrobattista, J. M. (2014). Maternal cardiovascular, respiratory, and renal adaptation to pregnancy. In R. K. Creasy, R. Resnik, J. D. Iams, et al. (Eds.), *Creasy & Resnik's maternal-fetal medicine: Principles and practice* (7th ed.). Philadelphia: Saunders.

Otten, J. J., Helwig, J. P., & Meyers, L. D. (Eds.), (2006). *Dietary reference intakes: The essential guide to nutrient requirements.* Washington, DC: National Academies Press.

Rigby, F. B., & Ramus, R. M. (2016). Anemia and and thrombocytopenia in pregnancy. *Medscape.* Retrieved from http://emedicine.medscape.com/article/261586-overview.

Sengpiel, V., Elind, E., Bacelis, J., et al. (2013). Maternal caffeine intake during pregnancy is associated with birth weight but not with gestational length: Results from a large prospective observational cohort study. *British Medical Journal, 11*(42).

US Department of Health and Human Services. (2016a). *Magnesium: Fact sheet for health professionals.* Retrieved from https://ods.od.nih.gov/factsheets/Magnesium-HealthProfessional/.

US Department of Health and Human Services. (2016b). *Vitamin B6: Dietary supplement fact sheet.* Retrieved from https://ods.od.nih.gov/factsheets/VitaminB6-HealthProfessional/.

US Department of Health and Human Services. (2016c). *Vitamin B12: Dietary supplement fact sheet.* Retrieved from https://ods.od.nih.gov/factsheets/VitaminB12-HealthProfessional/.

US Department of Health and Human Services. (2017). *Dietary guidelines.* Retrieved from https://health.gov/dietaryguidelines/.

US Department of Health and Human Services and U.S. Department of Agriculture. (2015). *2015 – 2020 Dietary Guidelines for Americans. 8th ed.* Available at Retrieved from http://health.gov/dietaryguidelines/2015/guidelines/.

US Food and Drug Administration. (2013). *Food safety for moms-to-be: While you're pregnant—methylmercury.*

US Food and Drug Administration. (2015). *Additional information about high-intensity sweeteners permitted for use in food in the United States.* Retrieved from https://www.fda.gov/Food/IngredientsPackagingLabeling/FoodAdditivesIngredients/ucm397725.htm.

US Food and Drug Administration. (2016). *Food safety for moms-to-be: While you're pregnant—Listeria.* Retrieved from http://www.fda.gov/Food/ResourcesForYou/HealthEducators/ucm083320.htm.

West, E. H., Hark, L., & Catalano, P. M. (2017). Nutrition during pregnancy. In S. G. Gabbe, J. R. Niebyl, J. L. Simpson, et al. (Eds.), *Obstetrics: Normal and problem pregnancies* (7th ed.). Philadelphia: Elsevier.

World Health Organization. (2017). *Daily iron and folic acid supplementation during pregnancy.* Retrieved from http://www.who.int/elena/titles/guidance_summaries/daily_iron_pregnancy/en/.

10

Assessment of High-Risk Pregnancy

Kitty Cashion

ⓔ http://evolve.elsevier.com/Perry/maternal

In the most recent year for which data are available, nearly 4 million births occurred in the United States (Martin, Hamilton, Osterman, et al., 2017). Many of these were the result of pregnancies considered to be *high risk* because the life or health of the mother, fetus, or newborn was jeopardized by circumstances coincidental with or unique to the pregnancy. Care of these high-risk patients requires the combined efforts of an interprofessional health care team. Team members may include professionals such as obstetric providers, maternal/fetal medicine specialists, nurses, pharmacists, social workers, and nutritionists. Factors associated with a diagnosis of a high-risk pregnancy are identified in this chapter. Diagnostic techniques often used to monitor the maternal-fetal unit at risk are also described.

ASSESSMENT OF RISK FACTORS

Pregnancies can be designated as high risk for any of several undesirable outcomes. In the past, risk factors were evaluated only from a medical standpoint. Therefore, only adverse medical, obstetric, or physiologic conditions were considered to place the woman at risk. Today a more comprehensive approach to high-risk pregnancy is used, and the factors associated with high-risk childbearing are grouped into broad categories based on threats to health and pregnancy outcome. Categories of risk include biophysical, psychosocial, sociodemographic, and environmental (Box 10.1). Risk factors are interrelated and cumulative in their effects.

Biophysical risks include factors that originate within the mother or fetus and affect the development or functioning of either one or both. Examples include genetic disorders, problems related to nutritional and general health status, and medical or obstetric-related illnesses. Box 10.2 lists common risk factors for several pregnancy-related problems.

Psychosocial risks consist of maternal behaviors and adverse lifestyles that have a negative effect on the health of the mother or fetus. These risks may include emotional distress, history of depression or other mental health problems, disturbed interpersonal relationships such as intimate partner violence, substance use or abuse, inadequate social support, and unsafe cultural practices.

Sociodemographic risks arise from the mother and her family. These risks may place the mother and fetus at risk. Examples include lack of prenatal care, low income, single marital status, and being a member of a minority ethnic group (see Box 10.1).

Environmental factors include hazards in the workplace and the woman's general environment and may include environmental chemicals (e.g., lead, mercury), anesthetic gases, and radiation (Chambers & Scialli, 2014; Cunningham, Leveno, Bloom, et al., 2014).

ANTEPARTUM TESTING

Standard prenatal tests that are done for all pregnant women are discussed in Chapter 8 and listed in Table 8.1. This chapter concentrates on the testing that is done for high-risk pregnancies rather than for those considered routine. Antepartum testing has two major goals. The first is to identify fetuses at risk for injury due to interrupted oxygenation so that permanent injury or death may be prevented. The second goal is to identify appropriately oxygenated fetuses so that unnecessary intervention can be avoided (Miller, Miller, & Cypher, 2017). In most cases, monitoring begins by 32 to 34 weeks of gestation and continues regularly until birth. Assessment tests should be selected on the basis of their effectiveness, and the results must be interpreted in light of the complete clinical picture. Box 10.3 lists common maternal and fetal indications for antepartum testing that are supported by available evidence (Miller et al).

The remainder of this chapter describes maternal and fetal assessment tests that are often used to monitor high-risk pregnancies.

BIOPHYSICAL ASSESSMENT

DAILY FETAL MOVEMENT COUNT

Assessment of fetal activity by the mother is a simple yet valuable method for monitoring the condition of the fetus. The **daily fetal movement count (DFMC)** (also called *kick count*) can be assessed at home and is noninvasive, inexpensive, and simple to understand and usually does not interfere with a daily routine. It is frequently used to monitor the fetus in pregnancies complicated by conditions that may affect fetal oxygenation (see Box 10.2). The presence of movements is generally a reassuring sign of fetal health. During the third trimester, the fetus makes about 30 gross body movements each hour. The mother is able to recognize 70% to 80% of these movements (Greenberg & Druzin, 2017).

Several different protocols are used for counting. One recommendation is to count once a day for 60 minutes (Fig. 10.1). Fig. 10.1 is an example of a form used to record fetal kick counts. Other common recommendations are that mothers count fetal activity 2 or 3 times daily (e.g., after meals or before bedtime) for 2 hours or until 10 movements are counted or that they count all fetal movements in a 12-hour period each day until a minimum of 10 movements are counted. Except for establishing a very low number of daily fetal movements or a trend toward decreased motion, the clinical value of the absolute number of fetal movements has not been established, other than in the situation

BOX 10.1 Categories of High-Risk Factors

Biophysical Factors

- *Genetic considerations.* Genetic factors may interfere with normal fetal or neonatal development, result in congenital anomalies, or create difficulties for the mother. These factors include defective genes, transmissible inherited disorders and chromosomal anomalies, multiple gestation, large fetal size, and ABO incompatibility.
- *Nutritional status.* Adequate nutrition, without which fetal growth and development cannot proceed normally, is one of the most important determinants of pregnancy outcome. Conditions that influence nutritional status include the following: young age; three pregnancies in the previous 2 years; tobacco, alcohol, or drug use; inadequate dietary intake because of chronic illness or food fads; inadequate or excessive weight gain; and hematocrit value less than 33%.
- *Medical and obstetric disorders.* Complications of current and past pregnancies, obstetric-related illnesses, and pregnancy losses put the woman at risk (see Box 10.2).

Psychosocial Factors

- *Smoking.* A strong, consistent, causal relation has been established between maternal smoking and reduced birth weight. Risks include low–birth weight infants, higher neonatal mortality rates, increased rates of miscarriage, and increased incidence of premature rupture of membranes. These risks are aggravated by low socioeconomic status, poor nutritional status, and concurrent use of alcohol.
- *Caffeine.* Birth defects in humans have not been related to caffeine consumption. However, pregnant women who consume more than 200 mg of caffeine daily (equivalent to about 12 ounces of coffee per day) may be at increased risk for giving birth to infants with intrauterine growth restriction (IUGR).
- *Alcohol.* Although the exact effects of alcohol in pregnancy have not been quantified and its mode of action is largely unexplained, it exerts adverse effects on the fetus, resulting in fetal alcohol syndrome, fetal alcohol effects, learning disabilities, and hyperactivity.
- *Drugs.* The developing fetus may be affected adversely by drugs through several mechanisms. They can be teratogenic, cause metabolic disturbances, produce chemical effects, or cause depression or alteration of central nervous system function. This category includes medications prescribed by a health care provider or bought over the counter and commonly abused drugs such as heroin, cocaine, and marijuana (see Chapter 11 for more information about drug and alcohol abuse).
- *Psychologic status.* Childbearing triggers profound and complex physiologic, psychologic, and social changes, with evidence to suggest a relationship between emotional distress and birth complications. This risk factor includes conditions such as specific intrapsychic disturbances and addictive lifestyles; a history of child abuse or intimate partner violence; inadequate support systems; family disruption or dissolution; maternal role changes or conflicts; noncompliance with cultural norms; unsafe cultural, ethnic, or religious practices; and situational crises.

Sociodemographic Factors

- *Low income.* Poverty underlies many other risk factors and leads to inadequate financial resources for food and prenatal care, poor general health, increased risk for medical complications of pregnancy, and greater prevalence of adverse environmental influences.

- *Lack of prenatal care.* Failure to diagnose and treat complications early is a major risk factor arising from financial barriers or lack of access to care; depersonalization of the system resulting in long waits, routine visits, variability in health care personnel, and unpleasant physical surroundings; lack of understanding of the need for early and continued care or cultural beliefs that do not support the need; and fear of the health care system and its providers.
- *Age.* Women at both ends of the childbearing age spectrum have an increased incidence of poor outcomes; however, age may not be a risk factor in all cases. Physiologic and psychologic risks should be evaluated.
- *Adolescents.* Possible pregnancy and birth complications include anemia, preeclampsia, prolonged labor, and contracted pelvis and cephalopelvic disproportion. Long-term social implications of early motherhood are lower educational attainment, lower income, increased dependence on government support programs, higher divorce rates, and higher parity.
- *Mature mothers.* The risks to older mothers are not from age alone but from other considerations such as number and spacing of previous pregnancies, genetic disposition of the parents, medical history, lifestyle, nutrition, and prenatal care. The increased likelihood of chronic diseases and complications that arise from more invasive medical management of a pregnancy and labor combined with demographic characteristics put an older woman at risk. Conditions more likely to be experienced by mature women include chronic hypertension and preeclampsia, diabetes, prolonged labor, cesarean birth, placenta previa, placental abruption, and death. Her fetus is at greater risk for low birth weight and macrosomia, chromosomal abnormalities, congenital malformations, and neonatal death.
- *Parity.* The number of previous pregnancies is a risk factor associated with age and includes all first pregnancies, especially a first pregnancy at either end of the childbearing age continuum. The incidence of preeclampsia and dystocia is increased with a first birth.
- *Marital status.* The increased mortality and morbidity rates for unmarried women, including an increased risk for preeclampsia, are often related to inadequate prenatal care and a young childbearing age.
- *Residence.* The availability and quality of prenatal care vary widely with geographic residence. Women in metropolitan areas have more prenatal visits than those in rural areas who have fewer opportunities for specialized care and consequently a higher incidence of maternal mortality. Health care in the inner city, where residents are usually poorer and begin childbearing earlier and continue longer, may be of lower quality than in a more affluent neighborhood.
- *Ethnicity.* Although ethnicity by itself is not a major risk, race is associated with some poor pregnancy outcomes. In the United States, for example, African-American women have the highest rates of preterm birth, almost twice as high as those of other racial and ethnic groups (Simhan, Iams, & Romero, 2017).
- *Environmental factors.* Various environmental substances can affect fertility and fetal development, the chance of a live birth, and the child's subsequent mental and physical development. Environmental influences include infections, radiation, chemicals such as mercury and lead, therapeutic drugs, illicit drugs, industrial pollutants, cigarette smoke, stress, and diet. Paternal exposure to mutagenic agents in the workplace has been associated with an increased risk for miscarriage.

BOX 10.2   Specific Pregnancy Problems and Related Risk Factors

Polyhydramnios
Poorly controlled diabetes mellitus
Fetomaternal hemorrhage
Fetal congenital anomalies (e.g., gastrointestinal obstruction, CNS abnormalities)
Genetic disorders
Twin-twin transfusion syndrome

Intrauterine Growth Restriction
Maternal Causes
Hypertensive disorders
Pregestational diabetes
Cyanotic heart disease
Autoimmune disease
Restrictive pulmonary disease
Multifetal gestation
Malabsorptive disease/malnutrition
Living at a high altitude
Tobacco/substance abuse

Fetal Causes
Genetic disorders
Teratogenic exposure
Fetal infection

Oligohydramnios
Renal agenesis (Potter syndrome)
Premature rupture of membranes
Prolonged pregnancy
Uteroplacental insufficiency
Severe intrauterine growth restriction (IUGR)
Maternal hypertensive disorders
Maternal dehydration/hypovolemia

Chromosomal Abnormalities
Advanced maternal age
Parental chromosomal rearrangements
Previous pregnancy with autosomal trisomy
Abnormal ultrasound findings during the current pregnancy (e.g., fetal structural anomalies, IUGR, amniotic fluid volume abnormalities)
Increased risk, as calculated from noninvasive screening results (e.g., nuchal translucency and maternal serum analytes)

Data from Baschat, A.A, & Galan, H.L. (2017). Intrauterine growth restriction. In S.G. Gabbe, J.R. Niebyl, J.L. Simpson, et al. (Eds.), *Obstetrics: Normal and problem pregnancies* (7th ed.). Philadelphia, PA: Elsevier; Driscoll, D.A., Simpson, J.L., Holzgreve, W., et al. (2017). Genetic screening and prenatal genetic diagnosis. In S.G. Gabbe, J.R. Niebyl, J.L. Simpson, et al. (Eds.), *Obstetrics: Normal and problem pregnancies* (7th ed.). Philadelphia, PA: Elsevier; Gilbert, W.M. (2017). Amniotic fluid disorders. In S.G. Gabbe, J.R. Niebyl, J.L. Simpson, et al. (Eds.), *Obstetrics: Normal and problem pregnancies* (7th ed.). Philadelphia, PA: Elsevier.

BOX 10.3   Common Maternal and Fetal Indications for Antepartum Testing

- Diabetes
- Chronic hypertension
- Preeclampsia (with or without severe features)
- Suspected or confirmed fetal growth restriction
- Multiple gestation
- Oligohydramnios
- Preterm premature rupture of membranes
- Late-term or postterm gestation
- Previous stillbirth
- Decreased fetal movement
- Systemic lupus erythematosus
- Renal disease
- Cholestasis of pregnancy

From Miller, L., Miller, D., & Cypher, R. (2017). *Mosby's pocket guide to fetal monitoring: A multidisciplinary approach* (8th ed.). St. Louis, MO: Elsevier.

record findings on a daily fetal movement record, and when to notify the health care provider.

⚡ SAFETY ALERT

In assessing fetal movements, it is important to remember that they are usually not present during the fetal sleep cycle; they may be reduced temporarily if the woman is taking depressant medication, drinking alcohol, or smoking a cigarette. They do not decrease as the woman nears term. Obesity decreases perception of fetal movements and consequently the ability of the mother to count them.

ULTRASONOGRAPHY

Diagnostic ultrasonography is an important, safe technique in antepartum fetal surveillance. It is considered by many to be the most valuable diagnostic tool used in obstetrics (Richards, 2017). It provides critical information to health care providers regarding fetal activity and gestational age, normal versus abnormal fetal growth curves, fetal and placental anatomy, fetal well-being, and visual assistance with which invasive tests can be performed more safely (Driscoll, Simpson, Holzgreve, et al., 2017; Richards, 2017).

Sound is a form of wave energy that causes small particles in a medium to oscillate. The frequency of sound, which refers to the number of peaks or waves that move over a given point per unit of time, is expressed in hertz (Hz). Sound with a frequency of one cycle, or one peak per second, has a frequency of 1 Hz. When directional beams of sound strike an object, an echo is returned. The time delay between the emission of the sound and the return and direction of the echo is noted. From these data, the distance and location of an object can be calculated. Ultrasound is sound frequency higher than that detectable by humans (>20,000 Hz). Ultrasound images are a reflection of the strength of the sending beam, the strength of the returning echo, and the density of the medium (e.g., muscle [uterus], bone, tissue [placenta], fluid, or blood) through which the beam is sent and returned.

An ultrasound examination can be performed either abdominally or transvaginally during pregnancy. Ultrasound scans produce a two- or three-dimensional view of the area being examined and can be used to create pictorial images (Fig. 10.2, *A* and *B*). Box 10.4 explains the differences in these scans and the views they produce.

in which fetal movements cease entirely for 12 hours (the so-called *fetal alarm signal*). A count of fewer than three fetal movements within 1 hour warrants further evaluation by a nonstress test or a contraction stress test and a complete or modified biophysical profile (see later discussion). Women should be taught the significance of the presence or absence of fetal movements, the procedure for counting, how to

Fetal Movement Chart

This chart will help to keep track of your baby's well-being. Carefully count the number of movements your baby makes during the same hour every evening, when babies are typically most active. For example, between 9 and 10 p.m.

If your baby has not moved for 12 hours, please contact 602.406.3521. Be sure to bring this chart with you when visiting your doctor.

Daily Chart of Baby Kicks							
DAYS OF WEEK	MONDAY	TUESDAY	WEDNESDAY	THURSDAY	FRIDAY	SATURDAY	SUNDAY
DATE							
KICKS							
DATE							
KICKS							
DATE							
KICKS							
DATE							
KICKS							
DATE							
KICKS							
DATE							
KICKS							
DATE							
KICKS							
DATE							
KICKS							
DATE							
KICKS							

Fetal movement (kick count) chart. Courtesy of St. Joseph's Hospital and Medical Center, Phoenix, AZ.

FIG 10.1 Fetal movement (kick count) chart. (Courtesy of St Joseph Hospital and Medical Center, Phoenix, AZ.)

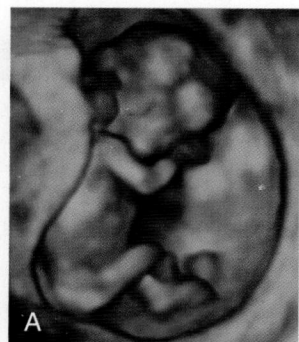 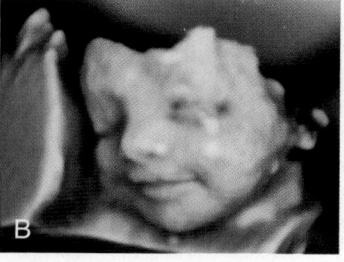

FIG 10.2 Fetus seen on three-dimensional ultrasound. **A,** View of fetus at 15 weeks and 3 days of gestation. **B,** Close-up view of fetal face at 28 weeks and 5 days of gestation. (A, Courtesy of Christina and Eva Gardner, Marion, AR; B, Courtesy of Constance Wheeler, Lakeland, TN.)

Abdominal ultrasonography is more useful after the first trimester when the pregnant uterus becomes an abdominal organ. During the procedure, the woman should have a full bladder to displace the uterus upward to provide a better image of the fetus. Transmission gel or paste is applied to the woman's abdomen to enhance the transmission and reception of the sound waves before a transducer is moved over the skin. She is positioned with small pillows under her head and knees. The display panel is positioned so the woman or her partner (or both) can observe the images on the screen if they desire.

Transvaginal ultrasonography, in which the probe is inserted into the vagina, allows pelvic anatomic features to be evaluated in greater detail and intrauterine pregnancy to be diagnosed earlier. A transvaginal ultrasound examination does not require that the woman have a full bladder. It is especially useful in obese women whose thick abdominal layers cannot be penetrated adequately with an abdominal approach. A transvaginal ultrasound may be performed with the woman in a lithotomy position or with her pelvis elevated by towels, cushions, or a folded pillow. This pelvic tilt is optimal to image the pelvic structures.

A protective cover such as a condom, the finger of a clean surgical glove, or a special probe cover provided by the manufacturer is used to cover the transducer probe. The probe is lubricated with a water-soluble gel and placed in the vagina either by the examiner or by the woman herself. During the examination, the position of the probe or the tilt of the examining table may be changed so the complete pelvis is in view. The procedure is not physically painful, although the woman feels pressure as the probe is moved. Transvaginal ultrasonography is optimally used in the first trimester to detect ectopic pregnancies, monitor the developing embryo, help identify abnormalities, and help establish gestational age. In some instances, it may be used along with abdominal scanning to evaluate for preterm labor in second- and third-trimester pregnancies.

Levels of Ultrasonography

The American College of Obstetricians and Gynecologists (ACOG) and several other organizations, including the American College of Radiology, the American Institute for Ultrasound in Medicine (AIUM), and the Society for Maternal Fetal Medicine (SMFM) describe three levels of ultrasonography (ACOG & AIUM, 2016c):

1. *Standard* (also called *basic*) examinations are done most frequently and can be performed by ultrasonographers or other health care professionals, including nurses, who have had special training. Indications for standard ultrasonography are described in detail in the next section. In the second and third trimesters, a standard ultrasound examination is used to evaluate fetal presentation, amniotic fluid volume (AFV), cardiac activity, placental position, fetal growth parameters, and number of fetuses. It is also used to perform an anatomic survey of the fetus.

2. *Limited* examinations are performed to determine a specific piece of information about the pregnancy, such as identifying fetal presentation during labor or estimating AFV. These examinations are usually performed by the woman's obstetric health care provider in the office or clinic or the labor and birth unit.

3. *Specialized* (also called *detailed*) or *targeted* examinations are performed if a woman is suspected of carrying an anatomically or physiologically abnormal fetus. Indications for this comprehensive examination include abnormal history or laboratory findings or the results of a previous standard or limited ultrasound examination. Specialized ultrasonography is performed by highly trained and experienced personnel.

Indications for Use

Major indications for obstetric sonography are listed by trimester in Table 10.1. During the first trimester, ultrasound examination is performed to obtain information regarding the number, size, and location of gestational sacs; the presence or absence of fetal cardiac and body movements; the presence or absence of uterine abnormalities (e.g., bicornuate uterus or fibroids) or adnexal masses (e.g., ovarian cysts or an ectopic pregnancy); and pregnancy dating.

During the second and third trimesters, ultrasonography is used to assess fetal viability, number, position, gestational age, growth pattern, and anomalies; amniotic fluid volume; placental location and condition; presence of uterine fibroids or anomalies; presence of adnexal masses; and cervical length.

Ultrasonography provides earlier diagnoses, allowing therapy to be instituted earlier in the pregnancy, thereby decreasing the severity and duration of morbidity, both physical and emotional, for the family. For instance, early diagnosis provides time for the family to make informed

---

BOX 10.4   Types of Ultrasound Scans

Two-Dimensional (2D)
- Sound waves are sent straight down from the ultrasound transducer.
- The image produced includes only two dimensions (length and width), so it appears flat.
- The image is viewed in black, white, or shades of gray.
- This is the standard medical scan used in pregnancy.

Three-Dimensional (3D)
- Sound waves are sent out at different angles. The returning echoes are processed by a computer program, which adds a third dimension (depth) to the 2D scan, producing a three-dimensional image.
- The image is usually displayed in sepia tones rather than in black and white.
- This scan can be used for diagnostic or management purposes. Viewing certain anomalies using a 3D scan provides further information that assists in planning for care at birth and for the neonate. These images are also often requested by pregnant women and families simply for their own enjoyment.

Four-Dimensional (4D)
- This scan adds a fourth dimension (time) to the 3D scan.
- The images produced are recorded and played back in succession. As the image is continuously updated, the fetus is viewed in real time.

TABLE 10.1   Major Uses of Ultrasonography During Pregnancy

First Trimester	Second Trimester	Third Trimester
Confirm pregnancy	Establish or confirm dates	Confirm gestational age
Confirm viability	Confirm viability	Confirm viability
Determine gestational age	Detect polyhydramnios, oligohydramnios	Detect macrosomia
Rule out ectopic pregnancy	Detect congenital anomalies	Detect congenital anomalies
Detect multiple gestation	Detect intrauterine growth restriction (IUGR)	Detect IUGR
Determine cause of vaginal bleeding	Assess placental location	Determine fetal position
Visualization during chorionic villus sampling	Visualization during amniocentesis	Detect placenta previa or placental abruption
Detect maternal abnormalities such as bicornuate uterus, ovarian cysts, fibroids	Evaluate for preterm labor	Visualization during amniocentesis, external version
		Biophysical profile
		Amniotic fluid volume assessment
		Doppler flow studies
		Detect placental maturity
		Evaluate for preterm labor

decisions regarding possible intrauterine surgery, termination of the pregnancy, or preparing to care for an infant with a disorder.

Fetal Heart Activity

Fetal heart activity can be demonstrated by about 6 weeks of gestation using transvaginal ultrasound. When the fetus is in a favorable position, good views of the fetal cardiac anatomy using transvaginal ultrasound are possible in most patients at 13 weeks of gestation (Richards, 2017). Fetal death can be confirmed by lack of heart motion along with the presence of fetal scalp edema and maceration and overlap of the cranial bones.

Gestational Age

Gestational dating by ultrasonography is indicated for conditions such as uncertainty regarding the date of the last normal menstrual period, recent discontinuation of oral contraceptives, a bleeding episode during the first trimester, uterine size that does not agree with dates, and other high-risk conditions. Gestational dating may best be done using ultrasound measurements and ignoring menstrual dates. However, all recent guidelines on establishing gestational age include references to menstrual dates. A standard set of measurements has been accepted as being the most useful for determining gestational age. These measurements include the crown-rump length in the first trimester and the biparietal diameter (BPD), head circumference, abdominal circumference, and femur length after the first trimester (Fig. 10.3). Gestational age calculation using a combination of these measurements is the most accepted method of ultrasound dating after the first trimester. An ultrasound examination performed for pregnancy dating before 22 weeks of gestation is comparable to one performed during the first trimester in terms of accuracy. However, after that time ultrasound dating is less reliable because of variability in fetal size (Richards, 2017).

Fetal Growth

Fetal growth is determined by both intrinsic growth potential and environmental factors. Conditions that require ultrasound assessment of fetal growth include poor maternal weight gain or pattern of weight gain, previous pregnancy with intrauterine growth restriction (IUGR), chronic infections, ingestion of drugs (tobacco, alcohol, and over-the-counter and street drugs), maternal diabetes, hypertension, multifetal pregnancy, and other medical or surgical complications.

Serial evaluations of BPD, limb length, and abdominal circumference can allow differentiation among size discrepancies resulting from inaccurate dates, true IUGR, and macrosomia. IUGR may be symmetric (the fetus is small in all parameters) or asymmetric (head and body growth do not match). Symmetric IUGR reflects a chronic or long-standing insult and may be caused by low genetic growth potential, intrauterine infection, chromosomal anomaly, maternal undernutrition, or heavy smoking. Asymmetric growth suggests an acute or late-occurring deprivation such as placental insufficiency resulting from hypertension, renal disease, or cardiovascular disease. Reduced fetal growth is still one of the most frequent conditions associated with stillbirth. Macrosomic infants (those weighing 4000 g or more) are at increased risk for traumatic injury and asphyxia during birth. Macrosomia may also be characterized as symmetric or asymmetric.

Fetal Anatomy

Anatomic structures that can be identified by ultrasonography (depending on the gestational age) include the following: head (including ventricles and blood vessels), neck, spine, heart, stomach, small bowel, liver, kidneys, bladder, and limbs. Ultrasonography permits the confirmation of normal anatomy and detection of major fetal malformations. The presence of an anomaly may influence the location of birth (e.g., a subspecialty center versus a basic care center) and the method of birth (vaginal versus cesarean) to optimize neonatal outcomes. For example, plans are often made for a fetus with a condition that will require immediate surgery to be born in or near a hospital able to provide that care rather than in a small community hospital that is totally unequipped to meet the newborn's needs.

Fetal Genetic Disorders and Physical Anomalies

A prenatal screening technique called *nuchal translucency* (NT) screening uses ultrasound measurement of fluid in the nape of the fetal neck between 10 and 14 weeks of gestation to identify possible fetal abnormalities (Fig. 10.4). Mandatory training and quality assurance for professionals who perform NT measurement is critical to ensure accurate results. A fluid collection greater than 3 mm is considered abnormal (ACOG, 2016b). When combined with abnormal maternal serum marker levels, elevated NT indicates a possible increased risk for certain chromosomal

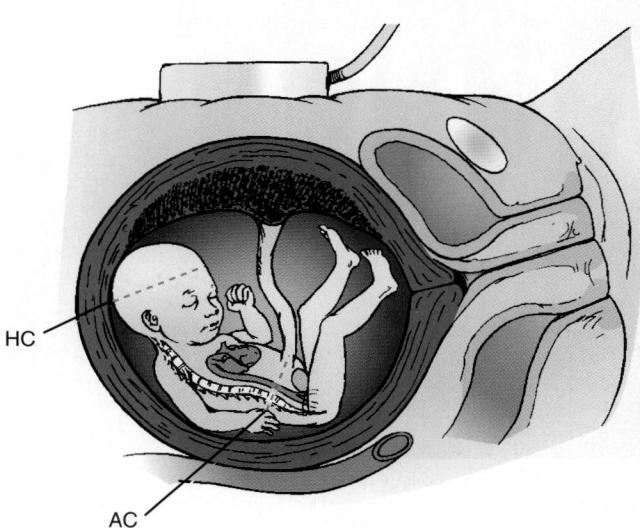

FIG 10.3 Appropriate planes of sections (*dotted lines*) for head circumference (HC) and abdominal circumference (AC).

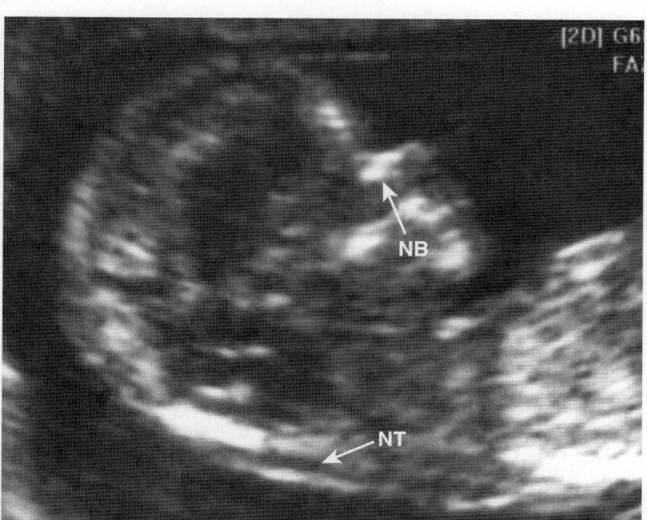

FIG 10.4 Midsagittal view of a 12-week fetus showing the nuchal translucency (NT) and nasal bone (NB). (From S.G. Gabbe, J.R. Niebyl, J.L. Simpson, et al. (Eds.). [2017]. *Obstetrics: Normal and problem pregnancies* [7th ed.]. Philadelphia, PA: Elsevier.)

abnormalities in the fetus, including trisomies 13, 18, and 21. An elevated NT alone indicates an increased risk for congenital heart defects. If the NT is abnormal, diagnostic genetic testing is recommended (ACOG & AIUM, 2016c; Driscoll et al., 2017).

Other ultrasound findings that predict trisomy 21 are an absent nasal bone, shortened femur or humerus, echogenic intracardiac focus, echogenic bowel, pyelectasis (enlargement of the renal pelvis, the part of the kidney that collects urine), and an abnormally fast or slow fetal heart rate (Driscoll et al., 2017; Richards, 2017). These findings are considered soft markers only; they are not diagnostic for the anomaly. Women with positive screening results for a chromosomal abnormality should be referred for genetic counseling and offered an invasive diagnostic test (Driscoll et al.).

Placental Position and Appearance

One of the major advantages of ultrasound is its ability to diagnose serious problems related to placental location in a timely manner. Between 18 and 23 weeks of gestation, the edge of the placenta extends to or covers the internal os of the cervix in about 2% of pregnancies. However, most cases of placenta previa diagnosed during the second trimester resolve by term, primarily because of the elongation of the lower uterine segment as pregnancy advances. Therefore, if placenta previa is diagnosed during the second trimester, repeated ultrasounds should be performed as pregnancy progresses until the placenta moves well away from the cervical os or it becomes clear that the previa will persist (Richards, 2017).

Another use for ultrasound is assessment of placental appearance. Many changes observed in the placenta are related to calcification, fibrosis, and infarction. These changes tend to become more apparent as pregnancy progresses, but their clinical significance is not clear. It has recently been recognized that a "globular" placenta, with a narrow

base in comparison to height, is associated with an increased rate of IUGR, fetal death, and other complications (Richards, 2017).

Adjunct to Other Invasive Tests

The safety of amniocentesis is increased when the positions of the fetus, placenta, umbilical cord, and pockets of amniotic fluid can be identified accurately. Ultrasound scanning has reduced risks previously associated with amniocentesis such as fetomaternal hemorrhage from a pierced placenta. Percutaneous umbilical blood sampling and chorionic villus sampling also are guided by ultrasonography to identify the cord and chorion frondosum accurately.

Fetal Well-Being

Physiologic parameters of the fetus that can be assessed with ultrasound scanning include AFV, vascular waveforms from the fetal circulation, heart motion, fetal breathing movements (FBMs), fetal urine production, and fetal limb and head movements. Assessment of these parameters, alone or in combination, yields a fairly reliable picture of fetal well-being. The significance of these findings is discussed in the following sections.

Doppler blood flow analysis. One of the major advances in perinatal medicine is the ability to study blood flow noninvasively in the woman, fetus, and placenta using ultrasound. Doppler blood flow analysis uses systolic/diastolic flow ratios and resistance indices to estimate blood flow in various arteries. Thus, it provides an indication of fetal adaptation and reserve. The vessels most often studied are the fetal umbilical and middle cerebral arteries and the maternal uterine arteries. Severe restriction of umbilical artery blood flow as indicated by absent or reversed flow during diastole has been associated with intrauterine growth restriction (Fig. 10.5) (Miller et al., 2017). Doppler ultrasound has been demonstrated to be of value in reducing perinatal mortality and unnecessary obstetric interventions in fetuses with IUGR (Greenberg & Druzin,

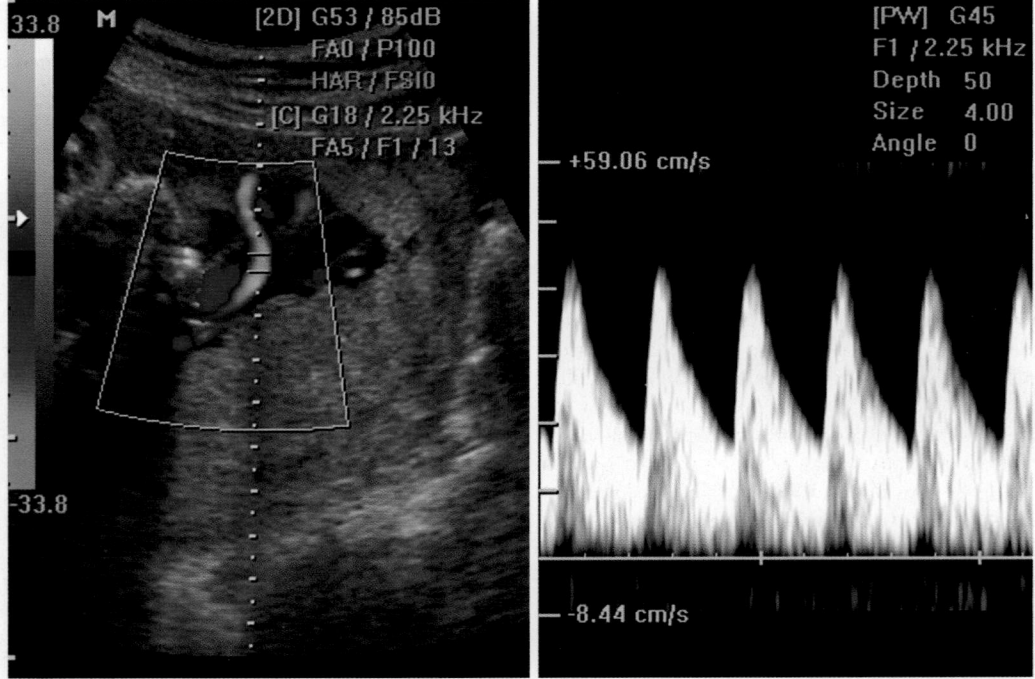

FIG 10.5 Color and spectral Doppler evaluation of the umbilical artery. The coiling arteries and vein are shown *(left panel)*. Red indicates flow toward the transducer, and blue indicates flow away. The sample gate for the pulse Doppler is superimposed. The result of the pulse Doppler is shown *(right panel)* depicting a normal flow velocity waveform. (From S.G. Gabbe, J.R. Niebyl, J.L. Simpson, et al. (Eds.). [2017]. *Obstetrics: Normal and problem pregnancies* [7th ed.]. Philadelphia, PA: Elsevier.)

2017). Significantly increased peak systolic velocity in the middle cerebral artery has been found to predict moderate to severe fetal anemia. Abnormal maternal uterine artery Doppler waveforms have been used to predict fetal growth restriction (Miller et al.).

Amniotic fluid volume. Accurate measurement of amniotic fluid volume (AFV) using ultrasound is difficult, and evidence indicates that the estimates produced poorly predict abnormal values. However, the measurement is still frequently performed in clinical practice. Differences in the amount of pressure placed on the ultrasound transducer by the sonographer can affect the accuracy of measurement. Use of greater pressure when placing the ultrasound transducer on the maternal abdomen can yield a lower measurement, while less pressure can result in a higher measurement (Gilbert, 2017).

Abnormalities in AFV are frequently associated with fetal disorders. Subjective determinants of oligohydramnios (decreased fluid) include a fundal height that is small for gestational age and a fetus that is easily palpated. An objective criterion of decreased AFV is met if the maximum vertical pocket of amniotic fluid is less than 1 to 2 cm (Gilbert, 2017). Increased amniotic fluid is called polyhydramnios or sometimes just *hydramnios*. Subjective criteria for polyhydramnios include a fundal height that is large for gestational age and a fetus that cannot easily be palpated or that is ballotable. Polyhydramnios is usually objectively defined as pockets of amniotic fluid measuring more than 8 cm (Gilbert).

The total AFV can be evaluated by a method in which the vertical depths (in centimeters) of the largest pocket of amniotic fluid in all four quadrants surrounding the maternal umbilicus are totaled, providing an amniotic fluid index (AFI). An AFI of less than 5 cm indicates oligohydramnios. With polyhydramnios, the AFI is 25 cm or more (Gilbert, 2017). Oligohydramnios is associated with congenital anomalies (e.g., renal agenesis [Potter syndrome]) and premature rupture of membranes. Polyhydramnios is associated with gastrointestinal and central nervous system abnormalities, multiple fetuses, and fetal hydrops (Gilbert).

Biophysical profile. Real-time ultrasound permits detailed assessment of the physical and physiologic characteristics of the developing fetus and cataloging of normal and abnormal biophysical responses to stimuli. The biophysical profile (BPP) is a noninvasive dynamic assessment of a fetus that is based on acute and chronic markers of fetal disease. The BPP includes AFV, FBMs, fetal movements, and fetal tone determined by ultrasound and fetal heart rate (FHR) reactivity determined by means of the nonstress test. Therefore the BPP can be considered a physical examination of the fetus, including determination of vital signs. FHR reactivity, FBMs, fetal movement, and fetal tone reflect current central nervous system (CNS) status, whereas the AFV demonstrates the adequacy of placental function over a longer period of time (Miller et al., 2017). BPP scoring and management are detailed in Tables 10.2 and 10.3.

The BPP is used frequently in the late second and the third trimester for antepartum fetal testing because it is a reliable predictor of fetal well-being. A BPP of 8 or 10 with a normal AFV is considered normal. Advantages of the test include excellent sensitivity and a low false-negative rate (Miller et al., 2017). One limitation of the test is that, if the fetus is in a quiet sleep state, the BPP can require a long period of observation. Also, unless the ultrasound examination is videotaped, it cannot be reviewed (Greenberg & Druzin, 2017).

Modified biophysical profile. The modified BPP (mBPP) is being used increasingly as a way to shorten the testing time required for the complete BPP by assessing the components that are most predictive of perinatal outcome. The mBPP combines the nonstress test, which assesses the current fetal condition, with measurement of the quantity of amniotic fluid, an indicator of placental function over a longer period of time.

TABLE 10.2   Scoring the Biophysical Profile

Biophysical Variable	Score 2	Score 0
Fetal breathing movements	At least one episode of fetal breathing movements of at least 30-second duration in a 30-minute observation	Absent fetal breathing movements or less than 30 seconds of sustained fetal breathing movements in 30 minutes
Fetal movements	At least three trunk/limb movements in 30 minutes	Fewer than three episodes of trunk/limb movements in 30 minutes
Fetal tone	At least one episode of active extension with return to flexion of fetal limb or trunk; opening and closing of hand considered normal tone	Absence of movement or slow extension/flexion
Amniotic fluid index (AFI)	Deepest vertical pocket >2 cm	Deepest vertical pocket ≤2 cm
Nonstress test	Reactive	Nonreactive

From Miller, L., Miller, D., & Cypher, R. (2017). *Mosby's pocket guide to fetal monitoring: A multidisciplinary approach* (8th ed.). St. Louis, MO: Elsevier.

TABLE 10.3   Biophysical Profile Management

Score	Interpretation	Management
10	Normal; low risk for chronic asphyxia	Repeat testing at weekly to twice-weekly intervals.
8	Normal; low risk for chronic asphyxia	Repeat testing at weekly to twice-weekly intervals.
6	Suspect chronic asphyxia	If ≥36–37 weeks of gestation or <36 weeks with positive testing for fetal pulmonary maturity, consider delivery; if <36 weeks and/or fetal pulmonary maturity testing negative, repeat biophysical profile in 4–6 hours; deliver if oligohydramnios is present.
4	Suspect chronic asphyxia	If ≥36 weeks of gestation, deliver; if <32 weeks of gestation, repeat score.
0–2	Strongly suspect chronic asphyxia	Extend testing time to 120 min; if persistent score ≤4, deliver, regardless of gestational age.

Modified from Manning, F.A., Harman, C.R., Morrison, I., et al. (1990). Fetal assessment based on fetal biophysical profile scoring. *American Journal of Obstetrics and Gynecology, 162*(3), 703-709; Manning, F.A. (1992). Biophysical profile scoring. In J. Nijhuis (Ed.), *Fetal behavior.* New York: Oxford University Press.

It is recommended that the amniotic fluid volume be determined by measuring a single deepest pocket of fluid instead of using the AFI. Desired test results are a reactive nonstress test and a single deepest vertical pocket of amniotic fluid that is more than 2 cm (Greenberg & Druzin, 2017; Miller et al., 2017).

Nursing Role

Although a growing number of nurses with additional training/education perform ultrasound scans and BPPs in certain centers, the main roles of nurses are counseling and educating women about the procedure. Ultrasound is widely used and in fact is considered a standard part of current prenatal care. Unlike many diagnostic tests, most women look forward to and enjoy their prenatal ultrasound. Exposure to diagnostic ultrasonography during pregnancy appears to be safe for the fetus. Nevertheless, because there is the possibility that unrecognized harm exists, ultrasound should be used only by qualified health professionals to provide medical benefit to patients (Richards, 2017).

Nonmedical Ultrasounds

Three- and four-dimensional ultrasonography for nonmedical purposes has become increasingly popular with pregnant women and their families. Although insurance does not cover the cost, women can have ultrasound images made of the fetus, just as professional photographs are often taken of infants and children. Both AIUM and ACOG have published statements that strongly discourage this practice. Although ultrasonography is considered safe, exposure of the fetus to high-frequency soundwaves without a clear medical indication for doing so should be avoided. In addition, casual ultrasonography performed by people who are not qualified health care professionals could give false reassurance to women or result in the discovery of abnormalities in settings that are not conducive to discussion and follow-up of findings (ACOG & AIUM, 2016c; AIUM, 2012; Richards, 2017). Helping the expectant family to understand the role of ultrasound beyond providing a picture of the fetus is a component of prenatal education.

MAGNETIC RESONANCE IMAGING

Magnetic resonance imaging (MRI) is a noninvasive radiologic technique used for obstetric and gynecologic diagnosis. Similar to computed tomography (CT), MRI provides excellent pictures of soft tissue. Unlike CT, ionizing radiation is not used. Therefore vascular structures within the body can be visualized and evaluated without injecting an iodinated contrast medium, thus eliminating any known biologic risk. Similar to sonography, MRI is noninvasive and can provide images in multiple planes, but no interference occurs from skeletal, fatty, or gas-filled structures, and imaging of deep pelvic structures does not require a full bladder.

With MRI, the examiner can evaluate fetal structure (CNS, thorax, abdomen, genitourinary tract, musculoskeletal system) and overall growth, the placenta (position, density, and presence of gestational trophoblastic disease), and the quantity of amniotic fluid. Maternal structures (uterus, cervix, adnexa, and pelvis), the biochemical status (pH, adenosine triphosphate content) of tissues and organs, and soft-tissue, metabolic, or functional anomalies can also be evaluated.

The woman is placed on a table in the supine position and moved into the bore of the main magnet, which is similar in appearance to a CT scanner. Depending on the reason for the study, the procedure may take from 20 to 60 minutes, during which time the woman must be perfectly still except for short breaks. Because of the long time needed to produce MRIs, the fetus will probably move, which will obscure anatomic details. The only way to ensure that this problem does not occur is to administer a sedative to the woman, but this approach should be reserved for selected cases in which visualization of fetal detail is critical.

MRI has little effect on the fetus. Concerns that the FHR or fetal movement would decrease have not been supported.

▌BIOCHEMICAL ASSESSMENT

Biochemical assessment involves biologic examination (e.g., of chromosomes in exfoliated cells) and chemical determinations (e.g., lecithin/

TABLE 10.4 Summary of Biochemical Monitoring Techniques

Test	Possible Findings	Clinical Significance
Maternal Blood		
Coombs test	Titer of 1:8 and increasing	Significant Rh incompatibility
Cell-free DNA screening	>Normal amount of DNA from specific chromosomes	Fetus with trisomy 13, 18, or 21
AFP	See AFP later in table	
Amniotic Fluid Analysis		
Lung profile:		Fetal lung maturity
L/S ratio	2:1	
Phosphatidylglycerol	Present	
LBC	≥50,000/μL	
Creatinine	>2 mg/dL	Gestational age >36 weeks
Lipid cells	>10%	Gestational age >35 weeks
AFP	High levels after 15 weeks of gestation	Open neural tube or other defect
Osmolality	Declines after 20 weeks of gestation	Advancing gestational age
Genetic disorders Sex-linked Chromosomal Metabolic	Dependent on cultured cells for karyotype and enzymatic activity	Counseling possibly required

AFP, Alpha-fetoprotein; *L/S*, lecithin/sphingomyelin; *LBC*, lamellar body count.

BOX 10.5 Fetal Rights

Amniocentesis, percutaneous umbilical blood sampling (PUBS), and chorionic villus sampling (CVS) are prenatal tests used for diagnosing fetal defects in pregnancy. They are invasive and carry risks to the mother and fetus. A consideration of induced abortion is linked to the performance of these tests because no treatment for genetically affected fetuses has been developed; therefore the issue of fetal rights is a key ethical concern in prenatal testing for fetal defects.

sphingomyelin [L/S] ratio, phosphatidylglycerol [PG]), or lamellar body count (LBC) (Table 10.4). Procedures used to obtain the needed specimens include amniocentesis, percutaneous umbilical blood sampling, chorionic villus sampling, and maternal blood sampling (Box 10.5).

AMNIOCENTESIS

Amniocentesis is performed to obtain amniotic fluid, which contains fetal cells. Under direct ultrasonographic visualization, a needle is inserted transabdominally into the uterus and amniotic fluid is withdrawn into a syringe. Then the various assessments are performed on the fluid sample (Fig. 10.6). Amniocentesis is possible after week 14 of pregnancy, when the uterus becomes an abdominal organ and sufficient amniotic fluid is available for testing. Indications for the procedure include prenatal diagnosis of genetic disorders or congenital anomalies (neural tube defects [NTDs] in particular), assessment of pulmonary maturity, and (rarely) diagnosis of fetal hemolytic disease.

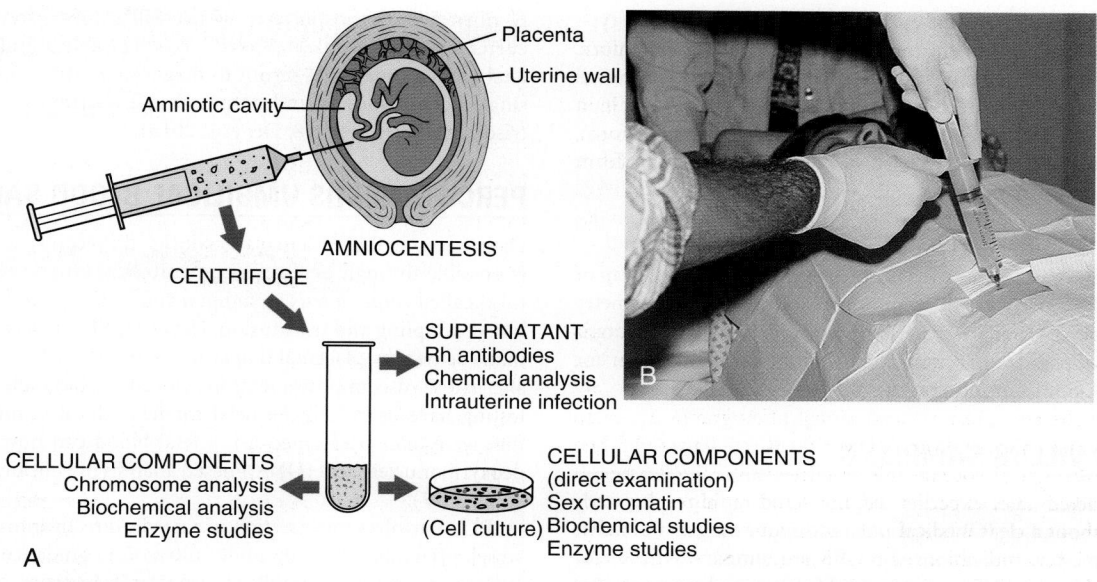

FIG 10.6 A, Amniocentesis and laboratory use of amniotic fluid aspirant. **B,** Transabdominal amniocentesis. (B, Courtesy of Marjorie Pyle, RNC, Lifecircle, Costa Mesa, CA.)

Complications in the mother and fetus occur only rarely and include the following:

- *Maternal:* Leakage of amniotic fluid, hemorrhage, fetomaternal hemorrhage with possible maternal Rh isoimmunization, infection, labor, placental abruption, inadvertent damage to the intestines or bladder, and amniotic fluid embolism (anaphylactoid syndrome of pregnancy)
- *Fetal:* Death, hemorrhage, infection (amnionitis), and direct injury from the needle

Many of the complications have been minimized or eliminated by using ultrasonography to direct the procedure.

⚡ SAFETY ALERT

Because of the possibility of fetomaternal hemorrhage, administering Rh_oD immunoglobulin to the woman who is Rh negative is standard practice after an amniocentesis.

Indications for Use
Genetic Concerns

Families in several different categories are considered to be at increased risk for having a child with a genetic disorder. These include the following (ACOG & SMFM, 2016a):

- Older maternal age (35 years of age or older)
- Older paternal age (there is no consensus, but usually considered to be 40 to 50 years of age)
- Parents who are affected by or are carriers of genetic disorders, including sickle cell anemia, Tay-Sachs disease, and cystic fibrosis
- Women with a prior child with a structural birth defect or with a structural fetal defect identified by ultrasound during their current pregnancy
- Women with a prior child with a chromosomal abnormality

In the past, prenatal assessment of genetic disorders focused on women and their partners who were included in one of these categories. Now, however, ACOG and SMFM (2016a) recommend that all pregnant women, regardless of age or other risk factors, be offered genetic screening or diagnostic testing (Box 10.6).

BOX 10.6 Prenatal Screening and Testing for Fetal Genetic Disorders

All pregnant women should be offered the option of screening or diagnostic testing for fetal genetic disorders, regardless of age or other risk factors. Genetic testing should be discussed as early as possible in pregnancy, ideally at the first prenatal visit. Health care providers must carefully explain the difference in screening tests, which assess whether a woman is at increased risk for having a fetus affected by a genetic disorder, and diagnostic tests, which determine with as much certainty as possible whether a specific genetic disorder or condition is present in the fetus. It is also important that women understand the benefits and limitations of all prenatal screening and diagnostic testing, including the conditions for which tests are available and the conditions that will not be detected by testing (ACOG & SMFM, 2016a).

Biochemical analysis of enzymes in amniotic fluid can detect inborn errors of metabolism or fetal structural anomalies. For example, alpha-fetoprotein (AFP) levels in amniotic fluid are assessed as a follow-up for elevated levels in maternal serum. High AFP levels in amniotic fluid help confirm the diagnosis of an NTD such as spina bifida or anencephaly or an abdominal wall defect such as omphalocele. The elevation results from the increased leakage of cerebrospinal or abdominal fluid into the amniotic fluid through the closure defect.

Fetal Lung Maturity

Late in pregnancy, accurate assessment of fetal lung maturity is possible by examining amniotic fluid to determine the L/S ratio or for the presence of PG. However, because both of these tests require considerable time, technical expertise, and cost to perform, they are generally used as primary tests only in special clinical circumstances. They may also be used as secondary tests if simpler and less expensive automated tests indicate lung immaturity (Mercer, 2014).

In the past, the TDx FLM assay and a subsequent modification, the TDx FLM II assay, were used as primary tests for fetal lung maturity. These assays determined the surfactant-to-albumin (S/A) ratio. However, they are no longer available for use in the United States. Instead, the LBC has become the primary test for determining fetal lung maturity.

Lamellar bodies are surfactant-containing particles secreted by type II pneumocytes. The number of lamellar bodies found in the amniotic fluid increases with the onset of functional fetal pulmonary maturity. The LBC compares favorably with the L/S ratio and the PG test in predicting fetal lung maturity. The automated test is simple to perform, and almost all hospital laboratories have the equipment used to perform it (Mercer, 2014) (see Table 10.4).

Fetal Hemolytic Disease

In the past, amniocentesis was used for identification and follow-up of fetal hemolytic disease in cases of isoimmunization. Doppler velocimetry of the fetal middle cerebral artery has now replaced serial amniocentesis as the method of choice to accurately and noninvasively monitor for fetal anemia in isoimmunized pregnancies (Moise, 2017).

CHORIONIC VILLUS SAMPLING

The combined advantages of earlier diagnosis and rapid results made chorionic villus sampling (CVS) a popular technique for genetic studies in the first trimester. Indications for CVS are similar to those for amniocentesis, although CVS cannot be used for maternal serum marker screening because no fluid is obtained. CVS performed in the second trimester carries no greater risk for pregnancy loss than amniocentesis and is considered equal to amniocentesis in diagnostic accuracy. When performed after the first trimester, the procedure is better known as *late CVS* or *placental biopsy* (Driscoll et al., 2017).

CVS can be performed in the first or second trimester, ideally between 10 and 13 weeks of gestation, and involves the removal of a small tissue specimen from the fetal portion of the placenta (Driscoll et al., 2017). Because chorionic villi originate in the zygote, this tissue reflects the genetic makeup of the fetus.

CVS procedures can be accomplished either transcervically or transabdominally. In transcervical sampling, a sterile catheter is introduced through the cervical canal toward the placenta under continuous ultrasonographic guidance, and a small portion of the chorionic villi is aspirated with a syringe) (Driscoll et al., 2017).

If the abdominal approach is used, an 18- or 20-gauge spinal needle with stylet is inserted under sterile conditions through the abdominal wall into the placenta under ultrasound guidance. The stylet is then withdrawn, and the chorionic tissue is aspirated into a syringe. The transabdominal approach is preferred if genital herpes, cervicitis, or a bicornuate uterus is present (Driscoll et al., 2017).

CVS is a relatively safe procedure. Pregnancy loss with CVS is similar to that of second-trimester amniocentesis. The incidence of IUGR, placental abruption, and preterm birth is no higher in women undergoing CVS than would be expected in the general population. In the early 1990s, there was controversy concerning an increased risk for fetal limb reduction defects associated with CVS. However, the consensus of further studies is that, when CVS is performed by experienced individuals after 9 completed weeks of gestation, the risk for limb reduction defects is no higher than it is in the general population (Driscoll et al., 2017).

> ## ⚡ SAFETY ALERT
>
> Because of the possibility of fetomaternal hemorrhage, women who are Rh negative should receive Rh₀D immunoglobulin after CVS to prevent isoimmunization, regardless of whether the procedure is performed transcervically or transabdominally, unless the fetus is known to be Rh negative (Driscoll et al., 2017).

Because amniocentesis and CVS are invasive tests, their use is associated with a small but concerning risk for pregnancy loss and infection.

Noninvasive diagnostic tests, which will someday replace them, are currently in development. These tests will be able to isolate and analyze fetal DNA in maternal serum to diagnose multiple disorders such as single gene disorders and chromosomal aberrations, in addition to trisomies (Latendresse & Deneris, 2015).

PERCUTANEOUS UMBILICAL BLOOD SAMPLING

Direct access to the fetal circulation during the second and third trimesters is possible through percutaneous umbilical blood sampling (PUBS) (also called *cordocentesis* or *funipuncture*). PUBS can be used for fetal blood sampling and transfusion. However, PUBS has been replaced in many centers by placental biopsy because it is a safer, easier, and faster alternative. Also, improvements in cytogenetic and molecular diagnostic testing have decreased the need for fetal blood samples. Many tests that were once performed using fetal blood can now be done using deoxyribonucleic acid (DNA)–based analysis of chorionic villi (Driscoll et al., 2017).

PUBS involves the insertion of a needle directly into a fetal umbilical vessel, preferably the vein, under ultrasound guidance (Figs. 10.7 and 10.8). Puncture of the umbilical cord near its insertion into the placenta is technically easier but is associated with a higher risk for contamination with maternal blood. Alternatively, free loops of umbilical cord or the intrahepatic vein may be used as puncture sites instead. Generally a small amount of blood is removed and tested immediately to ensure that it is fetal in origin (Driscoll et al., 2017). The most common genetic indication for the use of PUBS is evaluation of mosaic results found on amniocentesis or CVS, when a sample of fetal blood is required to determine the specific mutation. PUBS is also used to assess for fetal anemia, infection, and thrombocytopenia (Wapner, 2014). Bleeding from the cord puncture site is the most common complication of the procedure. Transient fetal bradycardia can also occur. Maternal complications are rare but include amnionitis and transplacental hemorrhage (Driscoll et al.).

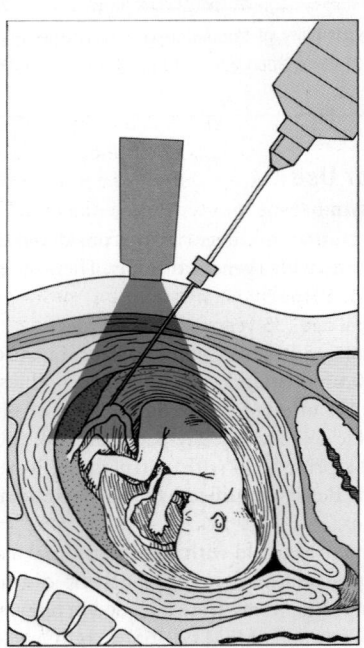

FIG 10.7 Technique for percutaneous umbilical blood sampling guided by ultrasound.

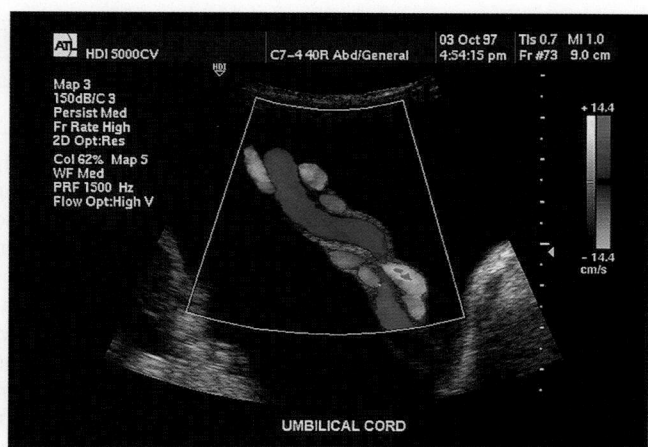

FIG 10.8 Umbilical cord as seen on ultrasound at 26 weeks of gestation. (Courtesy of Advanced Technology Laboratories, Bothell, WA.)

MATERNAL ASSAYS

Alpha-Fetoprotein

Maternal serum **alpha-fetoprotein (AFP)** levels are used as a screening tool for NTDs in pregnancy. Through this technique, approximately 80% to 85% of all open NTDs and open abdominal wall defects can be detected early. Screening is recommended for all pregnant women.

The cause of NTDs is not well understood, but 95% of all affected infants are born to women with no family history of similar anomalies (Wapner, 2014). The defect occurs in approximately 1 in 1000 live births. Risk factors for NTDs include a history of this disorder in a prior pregnancy, folic acid deficiency, pregestational diabetes, and teratogen exposure (e.g., valproic acid [Depakote], carbamazepine [Tegretol]) (Wolf, 2014).

AFP is produced in the fetal gastrointestinal tract and liver, and increasing levels are detectable in the serum of pregnant women from 14 to 34 weeks of gestation. Although amniotic fluid AFP measurement is diagnostic for NTD, maternal serum AFP is a screening tool only. Maternal serum AFP (MSAFP) screening can be performed with reasonable reliability any time between 15 and 20 weeks of gestation (16 to 18 weeks being ideal) (Wapner, 2014).

Once the maternal level of AFP is determined, it is compared with normal values for each week of gestation. Values also should be correlated with maternal age, weight, race, presence of a multifetal pregnancy, and whether the woman has insulin-dependent diabetes. Until recently, an amniocentesis to obtain fluid for determining amniotic fluid AFP and acetylcholinesterase levels was recommended as standard follow-up testing when the AFP level in maternal serum was found to be elevated. A targeted ultrasound performed by an experienced sonographer, however, has since been shown to be as sensitive and specific for identifying NTDs as the amniotic fluid AFP and acetylcholinesterase measurements, which require invasive testing via amniocentesis (Wapner, 2014).

Multiple Marker Screens

Screening to detect fetal chromosomal abnormalities, particularly trisomy 21 (Down syndrome) is available, beginning at 11 to 14 weeks of gestation (Cunningham et al., 2014). This first-trimester screen includes measurement of two maternal biochemical markers, pregnancy-associated placental protein A (PAPP-A) and human chorionic gonadotropin (hCG) or the free beta–human chorionic gonadotropin (β-hCG) subunit, and evaluation of fetal nuchal translucency (NT), or a combination of both. In the presence of a fetus with trisomy 21, hCG levels and the NT measurement are higher than normal in the first trimester, whereas PAPP-A levels are lower than normal. First-trimester screening using PAPP-A and hCG or β-hCG levels has been shown to be as accurate for detecting fetuses with trisomy 21 as triple screening in the second trimester (Cunningham et al., 2014; Driscoll et al., 2017; Wapner, 2014). Another biochemical marker that can be measured during the first trimester, at 8 to 10 weeks of gestation, is a disintegrin and metalloproteinase 12 (ADAM 12), a glycoprotein that is synthesized by the placenta and secreted throughout pregnancy. Decreased levels of ADAM 12 are found in women carrying a fetus with trisomy 21 (Wapner).

About one-third of all fetuses with an increased NT have a chromosomal abnormality; half of these have trisomy 21. Combining the serum marker and NT values results in the detection of Down syndrome in 79% to 87% of cases. These results are comparable to those obtained with quad screening (see discussion following) in the second trimester (Cunningham et al., 2014).

Assessment of the fetal nasal bone by ultrasound during the first trimester provides another way to predict trisomy 21. The nasal bone cannot be identified on ultrasound in about one-fourth to one-third of fetuses who have trisomy 21 (Wapner, 2014).

In the second trimester, triple screening and quad screening are available to screen for fetuses with trisomy 21 and trisomy 18. The triple-marker screen, performed at 16 to 18 weeks of gestation, measures the levels of three maternal serum markers: MSAFP, unconjugated estriol, and hCG. In the presence of a fetus with trisomy 21, the MSAFP and unconjugated estriol levels are low, whereas the hCG level is elevated. Low values in all three markers are associated with trisomy 18 (Cunningham et al., 2014).

The quad screen adds an additional marker, a placental hormone called inhibin A, to increase the accuracy of screening for Down syndrome in women younger than 35 years of age. Elevated inhibin A levels indicate the possibility of Down syndrome (Cunningham et al., 2014; Wapner, 2014). The addition of inhibin A to the other three markers increases the detection rate for Down syndrome to about 75% in women younger than 35 years of age and to more than 80% in women 35 years of age or older (Driscoll et al. 2017). Similar to triple marker screening, the optimal time to perform the quad screen is between 16 and 18 weeks of gestation (Wapner).

The ability of multiple marker tests to detect chromosomal abnormalities depends on the accuracy of gestational age assessment. These tests are screening procedures only and are not diagnostic. A positive screening test result indicates an increased risk but is not diagnostic of trisomy 21 or another chromosome abnormality. Women with positive screening results should be offered diagnostic testing by amniocentesis or CVS for fetal karyotyping (Cunningham et al., 2014) (see Box 10.6). In the future, noninvasive prenatal diagnosis will likely replace amniocentesis and CVS as diagnostic, or confirmatory, testing (Latendresse & Deneris, 2015).

Coombs Test

The indirect Coombs test is a screening tool for Rh incompatibility. If the maternal titer for Rh antibodies is greater than 1:8, amniocentesis for determination of bilirubin in amniotic fluid is indicated to establish the severity of fetal hemolytic anemia. However, middle cerebral artery Doppler studies to determine the degree of fetal hemolysis have now replaced serial amniocentesis (see earlier discussion) (Moise, 2017). The Coombs test can also detect other antibodies that may place the fetus at risk for incompatibility with maternal antigens.

Cell-Free (DNA) Screening

The newest screening test for aneuploidy, **cell-free DNA (cfDNA)**, is performed using a sample of maternal blood. The cfDNA screening test is an example of *noninvasive prenatal testing (NIPT)*. Aneuploidy is defined as having one or more extra or missing chromosomes in the 23 pairs each individual normally possesses (ACOG, 2016b). Common aneuploidies are trisomies 13, 18, and 21, each of which results from an extra chromosome. cfDNA also provides a definitive diagnosis noninvasively for fetal Rh status, fetal gender, and certain paternally transmitted single gene disorders (ACOG & SMFM, 2016b; Cunningham et al., 2014; Driscoll et al., 2017; Latendresse & Deneris, 2015).

Maternal plasma contains small fragments of cfDNA, resulting from the breakdown of both maternal and fetal cells (Driscoll et al., 2017; Latendresse & Deneris, 2015). Normal amounts of cfDNA, which vary throughout pregnancy, are known and compared with those obtained from the maternal sample. The test cannot actually distinguish fetal from maternal DNA, but it can accurately predict the fetal status by measuring the amount of cfDNA circulating in maternal blood and comparing it with known standards. If the fetus has a normal karyotype, the amount of DNA is consistent with the known standard for the normal amount. However, if more than the expected amount of chromosome 21 DNA, for example, is detected, it can then be assumed that the fetus is contributing the extra amount and therefore has trisomy 21. The same is true for trisomies 13 and 18. The test has a detection rate of more than 99% for trisomies 21 and 18, but a lower rate (approximately 80%) for trisomy 13 (Latendresse & Deneris, 2015). Women should understand that although the cfDNA screen results nearly match those of diagnostic tests, cfDNA is still a screening test. Therefore, women with positive cfDNA results are referred for amniocentesis or CVS to confirm the findings (ACOG & SMFM, 2016b; Latendresse & Deneris) (see Box 10.6).

The accuracy of the test depends on the proportion of fetal to maternal DNA in the maternal plasma, which must be at least 4%. As pregnancy progresses, the fetal contribution to the amount of cfDNA in maternal circulation increases. cfDNA screening for the detection of fetal chromosomal abnormalities is optimally performed at 10 to 12 weeks of gestation, by which time the average fetal DNA fraction should have reached approximately 10% of the maternal DNA (Driscoll et al., 2017; Latendresse & Deneris, 2015). The test is offered to women considered to be at risk for chromosomal abnormalities (i.e., aneuploidies), including those with advanced maternal age, screen-positive maternal serum screens, or ultrasound abnormalities. Women who have previously given birth to a child with a chromosomal abnormality are also candidates for the screen (Cunningham et al., 2014; Latendresse & Deneris). The cfDNA test is simple to perform; a sample of maternal blood is obtained by venipuncture and sent to a commercial laboratory. The test is less sensitive in women who are obese. Currently cfDNA testing is not recommended for use in multifetal pregnancies (Latendresse & Deneris).

FETAL CARE CENTERS

With developing technology, diagnosis and subsequent treatment options exist for some fetal anomalies. Fetal care centers have evolved in response to the need to provide diagnostic and therapeutic options as well as support services for families with a fetal anomaly diagnosis (ACOG, 2011). These families need access to an interprofessional team able to provide multiple services such as genetic counseling, support from social workers and chaplains, a palliative care team skilled in perinatal issues, and ethics consultation because of the complex emotional stressors they face. Care coordination is critical for the successful management of high-risk pregnancies. Many fetal care centers have a staff member, often a nurse, who coordinates care and assists the family in navigating multiple appointments with members of the interprofessional team.

ANTEPARTUM ASSESSMENT USING ELECTRONIC FETAL MONITORING

INDICATIONS

First- and second-trimester antepartum assessment is directed primarily at the diagnosis of fetal anomalies. The goal of third-trimester testing is to determine whether the intrauterine environment continues to support the fetus. The testing is often used to determine the timing of childbirth for women at risk for interrupted oxygenation to the fetus by any of several mechanisms (see Box 10.2). Evidence-based recommendations for condition-specific testing schemes in cases of identified risk factors have been difficult to develop and often do not exist. Condition-specific testing used as a strategy to prevent fetal death is unlikely to be effective, given the many fetal deaths that occur in pregnancies considered to be low risk or with no identifiable risk factors. In short, there is no ideal single test or testing strategy for all high-risk pregnancies (Greenberg & Druzin, 2017).

The ability to detect and prevent impending fetal death depends on the group of pregnant women selected for testing, the predictive value of the tests used, and the clinician's ability to respond to abnormal test results. Maternal assessment of fetal movement is suggested as a first-line screening test for fetal well-being (see earlier discussion of daily fetal movement count). When electronic fetal monitoring and ultrasound are used for antepartum fetal evaluation, the nonstress test and the mBPP are the primary tests performed. The complete BPP and the contraction stress test are used for follow-up evaluation in patients who have a persistently nonreactive nonstress test or abnormal mBPP score. Traditionally testing has begun at 32 to 34 weeks of gestation, with earlier initiation of testing recommended for women with multiple high-risk conditions. Testing is usually performed once or twice weekly (Greenberg & Druzin, 2017).

NONSTRESS TEST

The **nonstress test (NST)** is the most widely applied technique for antepartum evaluation of the fetus. The basis for the NST is that the normal fetus produces characteristic heart rate patterns in response to fetal movement, uterine contractions, or stimulation. In the term fetus, accelerations are associated with movement more than 85% of the time. The most common reason for the absence of FHR accelerations is the quiet fetal sleep state. However, CNS depressant medications, chronic smoking, and the presence of fetal malformations can also adversely affect the test (Greenberg & Druzin, 2017). The NST can be performed easily and quickly in an outpatient setting because it is noninvasive, easy to perform and interpret, relatively inexpensive, and has no known contraindications. Disadvantages include the requirement for twice-weekly testing, a high false-positive rate, and a higher false-negative rate than is achieved with most other methods. The test also is slightly less sensitive in detecting fetal compromise than the contraction stress test or the BPP (Greenberg & Druzin; Miller et al., 2017).

Procedure

The woman is seated in a reclining chair (or in the semi-Fowler's position) with a slight lateral tilt to optimize uterine perfusion and prevent supine hypotension. The FHR is recorded with a Doppler transducer, and a tocodynamometer is applied to detect uterine contractions or fetal movements. The tracing is observed for signs of fetal activity and a concurrent acceleration of FHR. If evidence of fetal movement is not apparent on the tracing, the woman may be asked to depress a button on a handheld event marker connected to the monitor when she feels fetal movement. The movement is then noted on the tracing. Because

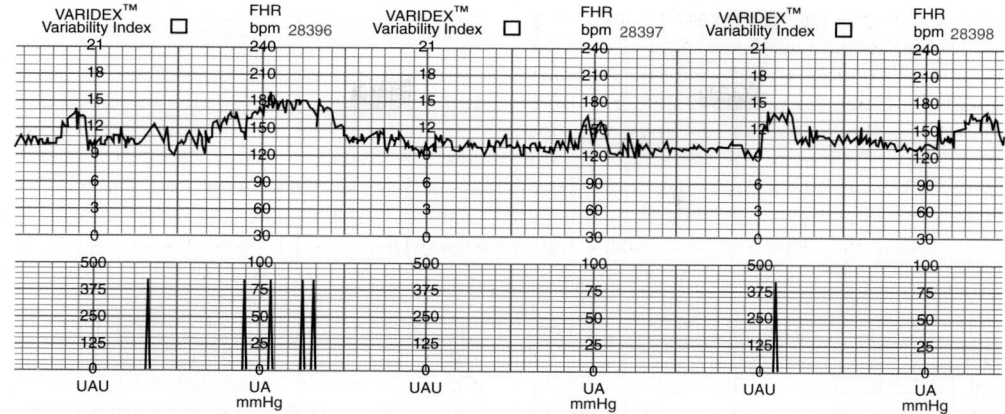

FIG 10.9 Reactive nonstress test. (From S.G. Gabbe, J.R. Niebyl, J.L. Simpson, et al. [Eds.]. [2017]. *Obstetrics: Normal and problem pregnancies* [7th ed.]. Philadelphia, PA: Elsevier.)

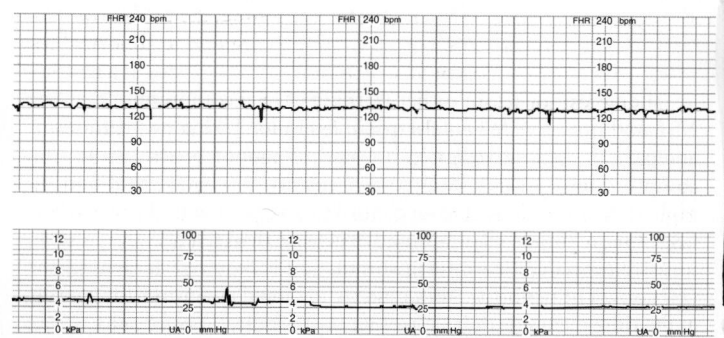

FIG 10.10 Segment of nonreactive nonstress test in term pregnancy. The lack of accelerations meeting minimum criteria continued for 40 minutes. (From Miller, L., Miller, D., & Cypher, R. [2017]. *Mosby's pocket guide to fetal monitoring: A multidisciplinary approach* [8th ed.]. St. Louis, MO: Elsevier.)

BOX 10.7   Interpretation of the Nonstress Test

Reactive test: Two accelerations in a 20-minute period, each lasting at least 15 seconds and peaking at least 15 beats/min above the baseline. (Before 32 weeks of gestation, an acceleration is defined as a rise of at least 10 beats/min lasting at least 10 seconds from onset to offset) (see Fig. 10.9).

Nonreactive test: A test that does not demonstrate at least two qualifying accelerations within a 20-minute window (see Fig. 10.10).

From Miller, L., Miller, D., & Cypher, R. (2017). *Mosby's pocket guide to fetal monitoring: A multidisciplinary approach* (8th ed.). St. Louis, MO: Elsevier.

almost all accelerations are accompanied by fetal movement, the movements need not be recorded for the test to be considered reactive. The test is usually completed within 20 to 30 minutes, but more time may be required if the fetus must be awakened from a sleep state.

Care providers sometimes attempt to increase fetal activity by manually stimulating the fetus or having the woman drink orange juice to increase her blood sugar level. Although these practices are common, there is no evidence that they increase fetal activity (Greenberg & Druzin, 2017).

Vibroacoustic stimulation (VAS; see later discussion) is often used to change the fetal state from quiet to active sleep if the initial NST result is nonreactive. After 26 weeks of gestation, VAS may significantly increase the number of reactive NSTs obtained, thus shortening the time required to complete the test (Greenberg & Druzin, 2017).

Interpretation

NST results are either reactive (Fig. 10.9) or nonreactive (Fig. 10.10). Box 10.7 lists criteria for both results. A reactive NST is considered normal, while a nonreactive test requires further evaluation. The testing period is often extended, usually for an additional 20 minutes, with the expectation that the fetal sleep state will change and the test will become reactive. During this time, VAS (see later discussion) may be used to stimulate fetal activity. If the test does not meet the criteria after 40 minutes, a contraction stress test or BPP should be performed. Once

the NST is initiated, it is usually repeated once or twice weekly for the remainder of the pregnancy (Greenberg & Druzin, 2017; Miller et al., 2017) (see Clinical Reasoning Case Study).

VIBROACOUSTIC STIMULATION

Vibroacoustic stimulation (VAS) (also called the *fetal acoustic stimulation test [FAST]*) is another method of testing antepartum FHR response. This test is generally performed in conjunction with the NST and uses a combination of sound and vibration to stimulate the fetus. Whether the acoustic or the vibratory component alters the fetal state is unclear. The fetus is monitored for 5 minutes before stimulation to obtain a baseline FHR. If the fetal baseline pattern is nonreactive, the sound source (usually a laryngeal stimulator) is then activated for 3 seconds on the maternal abdomen over the fetal head. The desired result is a reactive NST, which usually occurs within 3 minutes of stimulation. The accelerations produced may have a significant increase in duration (Fig. 10.11). The stimulus may be repeated at 1-minute intervals up to 3 times when no response is noted. Further evaluation is needed with BPP or contraction stress test if the pattern is still nonreactive. VAS is safe for use during pregnancy. No long-term evidence of hearing loss has been found in children followed up to 4 years of age who were exposed to VAS during pregnancy (Greenberg & Druzin, 2017).

CONTRACTION STRESS TEST

The contraction stress test (CST) or *oxytocin challenge test (OCT)* was the first widely used electronic fetal assessment test. It was devised

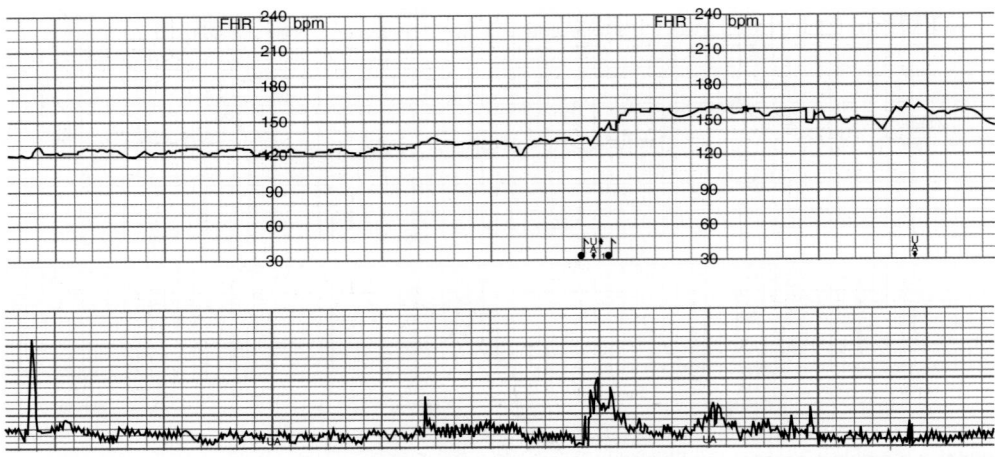

FIG 10.11 Reactive nonstress test after vibroacoustic stimulation. The stimulus was applied at the point marked by the musical notes. A sustained fetal heart rate acceleration was produced. (From S.G. Gabbe, J.R. Niebyl, J.L. Simpson, et al. (Eds.). [2017]. *Obstetrics: Normal and problem pregnancies* [7th ed.]. Philadelphia, PA: Elsevier.)

CLINICAL REASONING CASE STUDY

Fetal Assessment Using the Nonstress Test

LaTonya is a 30-year-old G5 T3 P0 A1 L3 who is now at 32 weeks of gestation. LaTonya was diagnosed with diabetes 4 years ago and also has chronic hypertension. Her physician has scheduled her for twice-weekly nonstress testing, and this appointment is her first. You are the nurse assigned to perform LaTonya's nonstress test (NST) today. As you help her get comfortable and attach the fetal heart rate and contraction monitors, LaTonya grumbles, "I don't see why I had to come get this test done. It was really hard to find a babysitter for my kids, and I live on the other side of town!"

1. Evidence—Is there sufficient evidence regarding the benefits of performing fetal assessment using the nonstress test during the third trimester of pregnancy in women who have preexisting diabetes and chronic hypertension?
2. Assumptions—Describe an underlying assumption about each of the following issues:
   a. The physiologic principle on which the NST is based
   b. Advantages of the NST
   c. The desired result of the NST
   d. LaTonya's understanding of why the test is necessary
3. What implications and priorities for nursing care can be drawn at this time?
4. Does the evidence objectively support your argument (conclusion)?
5. Interprofessional care—Describe the roles/responsibilities of health care professionals who might be involved in LaTonya's care.

as a graded stress test of the fetus, and its purpose was to identify the jeopardized fetus that was stable at rest but showed evidence of compromise after stress. Uterine contractions decrease uterine blood flow and placental perfusion. If this decrease is sufficient to produce hypoxia in the fetus, a deceleration in FHR results.

! NURSING ALERT

In a healthy fetoplacental unit, uterine contractions do not usually produce late decelerations, whereas if interrupted oxygenation is present, contractions produce late decelerations.

The CST provides an earlier warning of fetal compromise than the NST and produces fewer false-positive results. Like most methods of antepartum fetal surveillance, however, it cannot predict acute fetal compromise (e.g., umbilical cord accidents, placental abruption, or rapid deterioration of glucose control in a woman with diabetes). The CST is more time-consuming and expensive than the NST. It is also an invasive procedure if oxytocin stimulation is required. In general the CST cannot be performed on women who should not give birth vaginally at the time the test is done. Absolute contraindications for the CST are the following: preterm labor, placenta previa, vasa previa, cervical insufficiency, multiple gestation, and previous classic uterine incision for cesarean birth (Greenberg & Druzin, 2017; Miller et al., 2017). Because of these disadvantages, the CST is generally used as a backup, rather than a primary method of antepartum testing.

Procedure

The woman is placed in the semi-Fowler's position or sits in a reclining chair with a slight lateral tilt to optimize uterine perfusion and avoid supine hypotension. She is monitored electronically with a fetal ultrasound transducer and a uterine tocodynamometer. The tracing is observed for 10 to 20 minutes for baseline rate and variability and the possible occurrence of spontaneous contractions. The two methods of CST are the nipple-stimulated contraction test and the more commonly used oxytocin-stimulated contraction test.

Nipple-Stimulated Contraction Test

Several methods of nipple stimulation have been described. In one approach, the woman applies warm, moist washcloths to both breasts for several minutes. She is then asked to massage one nipple for 10 minutes. Massaging the nipple causes a release of oxytocin from the posterior pituitary gland. An alternative approach is for her to massage one nipple through her clothes for 2 minutes, rest for 5 minutes, and repeat the cycles of massage and rest as necessary to achieve adequate uterine activity. When adequate contractions or hyperstimulation (defined as uterine contractions lasting more than 90 seconds or five or more contractions in 10 minutes) occurs, stimulation should be stopped.

Oxytocin-Stimulated Contraction Test

Exogenous oxytocin can be used to stimulate uterine contractions. An intravenous (IV) infusion is begun, and a dilute solution of oxytocin

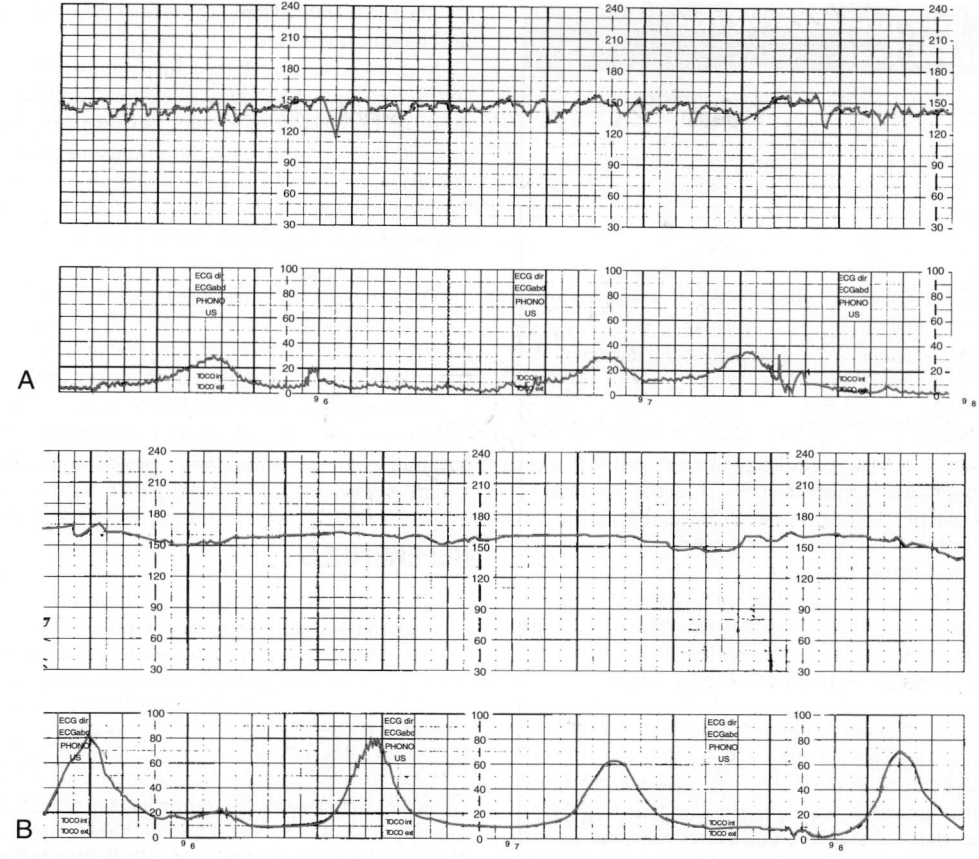

FIG 10.12 Contraction stress test (CST). **A,** Negative CST. **B,** Positive CST. (From Tucker, S. [2004]. *Pocket guide to fetal monitoring and assessment* [5th ed.]. St. Louis, MO: Mosby.)

(e.g., 30 units in 500 mL of fluid) is infused into the tubing of the main IV line through a piggyback port and delivered by an infusion pump to ensure an accurate dose. One method of oxytocin infusion is to begin at 0.5 milliunits/min and double the dose every 20 minutes until three uterine contractions of moderate intensity, each lasting 40 to 60 seconds, are observed within a 10-minute period. These criteria for contractions were selected to approximate the stress experienced by the fetus during the first stage of labor (Greenberg & Druzin, 2017).

Interpretation

CST results are negative, positive, equivocal, suspicious, or unsatisfactory. If no late decelerations are observed with the contractions, the findings are considered negative (Fig. 10.12, *A*). Repetitive late decelerations render the test results positive (see Fig. 10.12, *B*). Table 10.5 lists criteria for each possible test result and the clinical significance of each.

The desired CST result is negative because it has consistently been associated with good fetal outcomes. The likelihood of fetal death occurring within 1 week of a negative CST is less than 1 in 1000. Positive CST results have been associated with intrauterine fetal death, late FHR decelerations in labor, IUGR, and meconium-stained amniotic fluid (Greenberg & Druzin, 2017). A positive CST result usually leads to hospitalization for further close observation or birth. Unsatisfactory, suspicious, and equivocal tests require further evaluation, either by prolonged monitoring or repeat testing, often the following day (Miller et al., 2017).

PSYCHOLOGIC CONSIDERATIONS RELATED TO HIGH-RISK PREGNANCY

Once a pregnancy has been identified as high risk, the pregnant woman and her fetus are monitored carefully throughout the remainder of the pregnancy. All women who undergo antepartum assessments are at risk for real and potential problems and may feel anxious. In most instances, the tests are ordered because of suspected fetal compromise, deterioration of a maternal condition, or both. In the third trimester, pregnant women are most concerned about protecting themselves and their fetuses and consider themselves most vulnerable to outside influences. The label of *high risk* often increases this sense of vulnerability.

When a woman is diagnosed with a high-risk pregnancy, she and her family will likely experience stress related to the diagnosis. The woman may exhibit various psychologic responses, including anxiety, low self-esteem, guilt, frustration, and inability to function. A high-risk pregnancy can also affect parental attachment, accomplishment of the tasks of pregnancy, and family adaptation to the pregnancy. If the woman is fearful for her well-being, she may continue to feel ambivalent about the pregnancy or may not accept its reality. She may not be able to complete preparations for the baby or go to childbirth classes if she is placed on restricted activity at home or hospitalized. The family may become frustrated because they cannot engage in activities that prepare them for parenthood. The nurse can help the woman and her family regain control and balance in their lives by providing support and

TABLE 10.5 Interpretation of the Contraction Stress Test

Interpretation	Clinical Significance
Negative	
At least three uterine contractions in a 10-minute period, with no late or significant variable decelerations	Usually resume routine weekly testing schedule
Positive	
Late decelerations occur with 50% or more of contractions, even if there are fewer than three contractions in 10 minutes	Usually warrants hospital admission for further evaluation and/or delivery
Suspicious or Equivocal	
Prolonged, variable, or late decelerations occurring with less than 50% of the contractions	Further evaluation needed, either by prolonged monitoring or repeat testing the next day
Equivocal-Hyperstimulatory	
Decelerations that occur in the presence of contractions more frequent than every 2 minutes or lasting longer than 90 seconds	Further evaluation needed, either by prolonged monitoring or repeat testing the next day
Unsatisfactory	
Failure to produce three contractions within a 10-minute window or inability to trace the fetal heart rate	Further evaluation needed, either by prolonged monitoring or repeat testing the next day

From Miller, L., Miller, D., & Cypher, R. [2017]. *Mosby's pocket guide to fetal monitoring: A multidisciplinary approach* (8th ed.). St. Louis, MO: Elsevier.

encouragement, information about the pregnancy problem and its management, and opportunities to make as many choices as possible about the woman's care.

THE NURSE'S ROLE IN ASSESSMENT AND MANAGEMENT OF THE HIGH-RISK PREGNANCY

Nursing interventions for all pregnant women include education, anticipatory guidance, counseling for family adaptation, assessment, and planning of appropriate interventions. Providing care to women facing a high-risk pregnancy draws on the nurse's unique knowledge in understanding the physiologic and psychosocial needs when a pregnancy is complicated by a maternal or fetal issue. Along with receiving a diagnosis of a maternal or fetal health concern, mothers may experience loss and grief, increased stress, uncertainty, information needs, and decision-making dilemmas (Lalor, Begley, & Galavan, 2009).

High-risk pregnancies are often accompanied by additional testing and procedures. In these situations, the nurse's role is one of educator and supporter as women undergo procedures such as ultrasonography, MRI, CVS, PUBS, and amniocentesis. In some instances, the nurse may assist the health care provider with the test or procedure. When educating the woman and her family, the nurse must explain the purpose of each test, how it is performed, and the difference between screening and diagnostic tests. The nurse must also be aware of potential moral and ethical implications associated with certain tests. For example, women

and their families may need to make a decision about pregnancy termination based on test results.

In many settings, nurses actually perform tests such as NSTs, CSTs, and BPPs; conduct an initial assessment; and begin necessary interventions for nonreassuring results. Nurses who perform these tests have had additional education and training and function under guidance of established protocols and in collaboration with obstetric providers. Patient teaching, which is an integral component of this role, involves preparing the woman for the test, interpreting the findings, and providing psychosocial support when needed.

Women with high-risk pregnancies will likely receive many different services from multiple care providers. For all childbearing families, effective care management requires that members of the interprofessional health care team cooperate, communicate, and collaborate to provide care that promotes the best possible outcomes for mothers and babies. This coordination of care is even more essential in meeting the needs of families who are dealing with the additional stressors associated with a high-risk pregnancy (Barron, 2014).

REFERENCES

American College of Obstetricians and Gynecologists. (2011). Maternal-fetal intervention and fetal care centers. *Obstetrics & Gynecology, 118*(2 Pt. 1), 405–410.

American College of Obstetricians and Gynecologists, & Society for Maternal Fetal Medicine. (2016a). Practice bulletin no. 162. Prenatal diagnostic testing for genetic disorders. *Obstetrics & Gynecology, 127*(5), e108–e122.

American College of Obstetricians and Gynecologists, & Society for Maternal Fetal Medicine. (2016b). Practice bulletin no. 163. Screening for fetal aneuploidy. *Obstetrics & Gynecology, 127*(5), e123–e137.

American College of Obstetricians and Gynecologists, & American Institute of Ultrasound in Medicine. (2016c). Practice bulletin no. 175. Ultrasound in Pregnancy. *Obstetrics & Gynecology, 128*(6), e241–e256.

American Institute of Ultrasound in Medicine. (2012). *Official statement: Prudent use in pregnancy.* Laurel, MD: American Institute of Ultrasound in Medicine.

Barron, M. L. (2014). Antenatal care. In K. R. Simpson & P. Creehan (Eds.), *AWHONN's Perinatal Nursing* (4th ed.). Philadelphia, PA: Lippincott Williams & Wilkins.

Chambers, C., & Scialli, A. R. (2014). Teratogenesis and environmental exposure. In R. K. Creasy, R. Resnik, J. D. Iams, et al. (Eds.), *Creasy and Resnik's maternal-fetal medicine: Principles and practice* (7th ed.). Philadelphia, PA: Saunders.

Cunningham, F., Leveno, K., Bloom, S., et al. (2014). *Williams obstetrics* (24th ed.). New York, NY: McGraw-Hill Education.

Driscoll, D. A., Simpson, J. L., Holzgreve, W., et al. (2017). Genetic screening and prenatal genetic diagnosis. In S. G. Gabbe, J. R. Niebyl, J. L. Simpson, et al. (Eds.), *Obstetrics: Normal and problem pregnancies* (7th ed.). Philadelphia, PA: Elsevier.

Gilbert, W. M. (2017). Amniotic fluid disorders. In S. G. Gabbe, J. R. Niebyl, J. L. Simpson, et al. (Eds.), *Obstetrics: Normal and problem pregnancies* (7th ed.). Philadelphia, PA: Elsevier.

Greenberg, M. B., & Druzin, M. L. (2017). Antepartum fetal evaluation. In S. G. Gabbe, J. R. Niebyl, J. L. Simpson, et al. (Eds.), *Obstetrics: Normal and problem pregnancies* (7th ed.). Philadelphia, PA: Elsevier.

Lalor, J., Begley, C., & Galavan, E. (2009). Recasting hope: A process of adaptation following fetal anomaly diagnosis. *Social Science & Medicine, 68*, 462–472.

Latendresse, G., & Deneris, A. (2015). An update on current prenatal testing options: First trimester and noninvasive prenatal testing. *Journal of Midwifery & Women's Health, 60*(1), 24–36.

Martin, J. A., Hamilton, B. E., Osterman, M. J. K., et al. (2017). Births: Final data for 2015. *National Vital Statistics Reports, 66*(1), 1–70.

Mercer, B. M. (2014). Assessment and induction of fetal pulmonary maturity. In R. K. Creasy, R. Resnik, J. D. Iams, et al. (Eds.), *Creasy and Resnik's maternal-fetal medicine: Principles and practice* (7th ed.). Philadelphia, PA: Saunders.

Miller, L., Miller, D., & Cypher, R. (2017). *Mosby's pocket guide to fetal monitoring: A multidisciplinary approach* (8th ed.). St. Louis, MO: Elsevier.

Moise, K. (2017). Red cell alloimmunization. In S. G. Gabbe, J. R. Niebyl, J. L. Simpson, et al. (Eds.), *Obstetrics: Normal and problem pregnancies* (7th ed.). Philadelphia, PA: Elsevier.

Richards, D. S. (2017). Obstetrical ultrasound: Imaging, dating, growth, and anomaly. In S. G. Gabbe, J. R. Niebyl, J. L. Simpson, et al. (Eds.), *Obstetrics: Normal and problem pregnancies* (7th ed.). Philadelphia, PA: Elsevier.

Simhan, H. N., Iams, J. D., & Romero, R. (2017). Preterm labor and birth. In S. G. Gabbe, J. R. Niebyl, J. L. Simpson, et al. (Eds.), *Obstetrics: Normal and problem pregnancies* (7th ed.). Philadelphia, PA: Elsevier.

Wapner, R. J. (2014). Prenatal diagnosis of congenital disorders. In R. K. Creasy, R. Resnik, J. D. Iams, et al. (Eds.), *Creasy and Resnik's maternal-fetal medicine: Principles and practice* (7th ed.). Philadelphia, PA: Saunders.

Wolf, R. B. (2014). Skeletal imaging. In R. K. Creasy, R. Resnik, J. D. Iams, et al. (Eds.), *Creasy and Resnik's maternal-fetal medicine: Principles and practice* (7th ed.). Philadelphia, PA: Saunders.

11

High-Risk Perinatal Care: Preexisting Conditions

Kitty Cashion

http://evolve.elsevier.com/Perry/maternal

For most women, pregnancy represents a normal part of life. However, for some women it presents a significant risk because it is superimposed on a chronic illness. Providing safe and effective care for women experiencing high-risk pregnancy and their fetuses is a challenge. Although unique maternal and fetal needs prompted by the chronic illness exist, these women also experience the feelings, needs, and concerns associated with a normal pregnancy. The primary objective of nursing care is to achieve optimal outcomes for both the pregnant woman and the fetus. With the active participation of well-motivated women in the treatment plan and careful management from an interprofessional health care team, positive outcomes are often possible.

This chapter focuses on metabolic disorders, including diabetes mellitus and thyroid disorders; cardiovascular disorders; selected disorders of the respiratory, integumentary, and central nervous systems; and autoimmune disorders. Substance abuse is also discussed. For each disorder, management throughout the entire perinatal period (antepartum, intrapartum, and postpartum) is included in this chapter; thus all the information for each condition is located in one place in the text.

DIABETES MELLITUS

Worldwide, the incidence of diabetes mellitus has been steadily growing for the past 3 decades, especially in low- and middle-income countries. This growth is mostly because of increases in overweight, obesity, and physical inactivity. An estimated 422 million people now have diabetes (World Health Organization [WHO], 2016). In 2012, an estimated 29.1 million people in the United States (9.3% of the total population) had diabetes. Of these, 8.1 million were undiagnosed (Centers for Disease Control and Prevention [CDC], 2014). If this trend continues, it is predicted that by 2050 as many as 1 in 3 adults in the United States will have diabetes. The prevalence of diabetes among women of childbearing age is increasing in the United States, which will greatly affect the care of mothers and children for years to come (Moore, Hauguel de Mouzon, & Catalano, 2014).

It is estimated that diabetes complicates as many as 6% to 7% of pregnancies. While 90% of women with diabetes during pregnancy have gestational diabetes, the number of pregnant women who have type 1 or type 2 diabetes is growing (American Diabetes Association [ADA], 2016b; Landon, Catalano, & Gabbe, 2017; Moore et al., 2014). The perinatal mortality rate for well-managed diabetic pregnancies, excluding major congenital malformations, is approximately the same as for any other pregnancy. The key to an optimal pregnancy outcome is strict maternal glucose control before conception and

throughout the gestational period (Landon et al.). Consequently, for women with diabetes, much emphasis is placed on preconception counseling.

Pregnancy complicated by diabetes is considered high risk. It is most successfully managed by an interprofessional team approach involving the obstetrician, maternal fetal medicine specialist (perinatologist), internist or endocrinologist, ophthalmologist, nephrologist, neonatologist, nurse, nutritionist or dietitian, and social worker. A favorable outcome also requires commitment and active participation by the pregnant woman and her family.

PATHOGENESIS

Diabetes mellitus refers to a group of metabolic diseases characterized by hyperglycemia resulting from defects in insulin secretion, insulin action, or both (ADA, 2016a). Insulin, produced by the beta cells in the islets of Langerhans in the pancreas, regulates blood glucose levels by enabling glucose to enter adipose and muscle cells, where it is used for energy. When insulin is insufficient or ineffective in promoting glucose uptake by the muscle and adipose cells, glucose accumulates in the bloodstream, and hyperglycemia results. Hyperglycemia causes hyperosmolarity of the blood, which attracts intracellular fluid into the vascular system, resulting in cellular dehydration and expanded blood volume. Consequently, the kidneys function to excrete large volumes of urine (polyuria) in an attempt to regulate excess vascular volume and excrete the unusable glucose (glycosuria). Polyuria, along with cellular dehydration, causes excessive thirst (polydipsia).

The body compensates for its inability to convert carbohydrate (glucose) into energy by burning proteins (muscle) and fats. However, the end products of this metabolism are ketones and fatty acids, which in excess quantities produce ketoacidosis and acetonuria. Weight loss occurs as a result of the breakdown of fat and muscle tissue. This tissue breakdown causes a state of starvation that compels the individual to eat excessive amounts of food (polyphagia).

Over time, diabetes causes significant changes in the microvascular and macrovascular circulations. These structural changes affect a variety of organ systems, particularly the heart, the eyes, the kidneys, and the nerves. Complications resulting from diabetes include premature atherosclerosis, retinopathy, nephropathy, and neuropathy.

Diabetes may be caused either by impaired insulin secretion, when the beta cells of the pancreas are destroyed by an autoimmune process, or by inadequate insulin action in target tissues at one or more points along the metabolic pathway. Both of these conditions are commonly present in the same person; and determining which, if either, abnormality is the primary cause of the disease is difficult (ADA, 2016a). For additional information on diabetes, visit the ADA website at www.diabetes.org.

CLASSIFICATION

The current classification system includes four groups: type 1 diabetes, type 2 diabetes, other specific types (e.g., diabetes caused by genetic defects in beta cell function or insulin action, disease or injury of the pancreas, or drug-induced diabetes), and gestational diabetes mellitus (GDM) (ADA, 2016a; Moore et al., 2014). *Pregestational diabetes mellitus* is the label sometimes given to type 1 or type 2 diabetes that existed before pregnancy.

Type 1 accounts for 5% to 10% of all diabetes and includes cases that are caused primarily by pancreatic islet beta cell destruction and that are prone to ketoacidosis. People with type 1 diabetes usually have an abrupt onset of illness at a young age and an absolute insulin deficiency. Type 1 diabetes includes cases thought to be caused by an autoimmune process and those for which the cause is unknown (ADA, 2016a; Landon et al., 2017).

Type 2 is the most prevalent form of the disease, accounting for 90% to 95% of all diabetes. It includes individuals who have insulin resistance and usually relative (rather than absolute) insulin deficiency (ADA, 2016a). Although type 2 diabetes was once believed to affect mostly older individuals, increasing numbers of children and adolescents have been diagnosed with the disorder since the early 1990s (Moore et al., 2014). Specific causes of type 2 diabetes are unknown at this time. It often goes undiagnosed for years because hyperglycemia develops gradually and is often not severe enough for the person to recognize the classic signs of polyuria, polydipsia, and polyphagia. Most people who develop type 2 diabetes are obese or have an increased amount of body fat distributed primarily in the abdominal area. Other risk factors for the development of type 2 diabetes include aging, a sedentary lifestyle, family history and genetics, puberty, hypertension, and prior gestational diabetes. Type 2 diabetes often has a strong genetic predisposition (ADA, 2016a; Moore et al.).

The traditional definition of GDM is carbohydrate intolerance with the onset or first recognition occurring during pregnancy (American College of Obstetricians and Gynecologists [ACOG], 2013/2015). This definition is appropriate whether or not management includes medication in addition to dietary changes or the diabetes persists after pregnancy. It does not exclude the possibility that the glucose intolerance preceded the pregnancy or that medication might be required for optimal glucose control (Landon et al., 2017). The ADA has adopted a new definition for gestational diabetes that excludes women with preexisting diabetes (type 1 or type 2) that is diagnosed during pregnancy. This definition for GDM is simply diabetes diagnosed during the second or third trimester of pregnancy that is clearly not overt (preexisting) diabetes (ADA, 2016a).

Classification of Diabetes in Pregnancy

Dr. Priscilla White, a physician who worked with pregnant women with diabetes during the 1940s, developed a system specifically to further classify diabetes in this group of women (Table 11.1). White's system was based on age at diagnosis, duration of illness, and presence of end-organ, especially eye and kidney, involvement (Landon et al., 2017; Moore et al., 2014). Her classification system has been modified through the years, changing her original definitions and adding increasing complexity, which has resulted in confusion (Sacks & Metzger, 2013). It is still frequently used, however, to assess maternal and fetal risk.

A new system has since been developed by the ADA that further classifies type 1 and type 2 diabetes as (a) without vascular complications and (b) with vascular complications that are specified. This distinction

TABLE 11.1 White's Classification of Diabetes in Pregnancy

Gestational Diabetes

Class A₁	Woman has two or more abnormal values on OGTT but her fasting and postprandial glucose values are diet controlled.
Class A₂	Woman was not known to have diabetes before pregnancy but requires either insulin or oral hypoglycemic medication for blood glucose control.

Pregestational Diabetes

Class B	Onset of disease occurs after 20 years of age, and duration of illness is <10 years.
Class C	Onset of disease occurs between 10 and 19 years of age, or duration of illness is 10 to 19 years or both.
Class D	Onset of disease occurs before 10 years of age, or duration of illness is >20 years or both.
Class F	Woman has developed diabetic nephropathy.
Class R	Woman has developed retinitis proliferans.
Class T	Woman has had a renal transplant.

OGTT, Oral glucose tolerance test.
Data from Landon, M.B., Catalano, P.M., & Gabbe, S.G. (2017). Diabetes mellitus complicating pregnancy. In S.G. Gabbe, J.R. Niebyl, J.L. Simpson, et al. (Eds.), *Obstetrics: Normal and problem pregnancies* (7th ed.). Philadelphia, PA: Elsevier; Moore, T.R.H, Hauguel-deMouzon, S., & Catalano, P. (2014). Diabetes in pregnancy. In R. K. Creasy, R. Resnik, J. D. Iams, et al. (Eds.), *Creasy and Resnik's maternal-fetal medicine: Principles and practice* (7th ed.). Philadelphia, PA: Saunders.

is important, because perinatal risk increases with vascular complications regardless of the duration of illness. Only women whose glucose intolerance was diagnosed during pregnancy but who do not meet the criteria defining type 1 or type 2 diabetes are included in the gestational diabetes category. It has been suggested that White's modified classification system be replaced by the new ADA system in clinical practice (Sacks & Metzger, 2013).

METABOLIC CHANGES ASSOCIATED WITH PREGNANCY

Normal pregnancy is characterized by complex alterations in maternal glucose metabolism, insulin production, and metabolic homeostasis. During normal pregnancy, adjustments in maternal metabolism allow for adequate nutrition for the mother and the developing fetus. Glucose, the primary fuel used by the fetus, is transported across the placenta through the process of carrier-mediated facilitated diffusion, meaning that the glucose levels in the fetus are directly proportional to maternal levels. Although glucose crosses the placenta, insulin does not. Around the tenth week of gestation, the fetus begins to secrete its own insulin at levels adequate to use the glucose obtained from the mother. Therefore, as maternal glucose levels rise, fetal glucose levels are increased, resulting in increased fetal insulin secretion.

During the first trimester of pregnancy, the pregnant woman's metabolic status is significantly influenced by the rising levels of estrogen and progesterone. These hormones stimulate the beta cells in the pancreas to increase insulin production, which promotes increased peripheral use of glucose and decreased blood glucose, with fasting levels being reduced by approximately 10% (Fig. 11.1, *A*). At the same time, an increase in tissue glycogen stores and a decrease in hepatic glucose

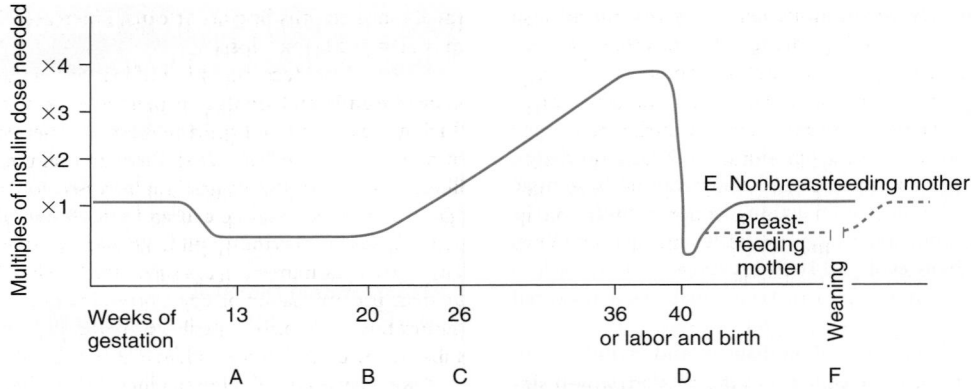

FIG 11.1 Changing insulin needs during pregnancy. A, First trimester: Insulin need is reduced because of increased insulin production by pancreas and increased peripheral sensitivity to insulin; nausea, vomiting, and decreased food intake by mother and glucose transfer to embryo or fetus contribute to hypoglycemia. B, Second trimester: Insulin needs begin to increase as placental hormones, cortisol, and insulinase act as insulin antagonists, decreasing effectiveness of insulin. C, Third trimester: Insulin needs may double or even quadruple but usually level off after 36 weeks of gestation. D, Day of birth: Maternal insulin requirements decrease drastically to approach prepregnancy levels. E, Breastfeeding mother maintains lower insulin requirements, as much as 25% less than those of prepregnancy; insulin needs of nonbreastfeeding mother return to prepregnancy levels in 7 to 10 days. F, Weaning of breastfeeding infant causes mother's insulin needs to return to prepregnancy levels.

production occur, which further encourage lower fasting glucose levels. As a result of these normal metabolic changes of pregnancy, women with insulin-dependent diabetes are prone to hypoglycemia during the first trimester.

During the second and third trimesters, pregnancy exerts a "diabetogenic" effect on the maternal metabolic status. Because of the major hormonal changes, decreased tolerance to glucose, increased insulin resistance, decreased hepatic glycogen stores, and increased hepatic production of glucose occur. Rising levels of human chorionic somatomammotropin, estrogen, progesterone, prolactin, cortisol, and insulinase increase insulin resistance through their actions as insulin antagonists. Insulin resistance is a glucose-sparing mechanism that ensures an abundant supply of glucose for the fetus. Maternal insulin requirements gradually increase from approximately 18 to 24 weeks of gestation to approximately 36 weeks of gestation. Maternal insulin requirements may double or quadruple by the end of the pregnancy (see Fig. 11.1, B and C).

At birth, expulsion of the placenta prompts an abrupt drop in levels of circulating placental hormones, cortisol, and insulinase (see Fig. 11.1, D). Maternal tissues quickly regain their prepregnancy sensitivity to insulin. For the nonbreastfeeding mother, the prepregnancy insulin-carbohydrate balance usually returns in approximately 7 to 10 days (see Fig. 11.1, E). Lactation uses maternal glucose; therefore the breastfeeding mother's insulin requirements remain lower during lactation. On completion of weaning, the mother's prepregnancy insulin requirement is reestablished (see Fig. 11.1, F).

PREGESTATIONAL DIABETES MELLITUS

Only about 10% of pregnancies complicated by diabetes occur in women who have preexisting disease (Landon et al., 2017). Women who have pregestational diabetes mellitus can have either type 1 or 2 diabetes, which may be complicated by vascular disease, retinopathy, nephropathy, or other diabetic complications. Type 2 is a more common diagnosis than type 1. Almost all women with pregestational diabetes are insulin dependent during pregnancy. According to White's classification system, these women fall into classes B through T (see Table 11.1).

The diabetogenic state of pregnancy imposed on the compromised metabolic system of the woman with pregestational diabetes has significant implications. The normal hormonal changes of pregnancy affect glycemic control, and pregnancy may accelerate the progress of vascular complications.

During the first trimester, when maternal blood glucose levels are normally reduced and the insulin response to glucose is enhanced, glycemic control is improved. The insulin dose for the woman with well-controlled diabetes may have to be reduced to prevent hypoglycemia. Nausea, vomiting, and cravings typical of early pregnancy result in dietary fluctuations that influence maternal glucose levels and may necessitate a reduction in the insulin dose.

Because insulin requirements steadily increase after the first trimester, the insulin dose must be adjusted accordingly to prevent hyperglycemia. Insulin resistance begins as early as 14 to 16 weeks of gestation and continues to rise until it stabilizes during the last few weeks of pregnancy.

PRECONCEPTION COUNSELING

Preconception counseling is recommended for all women of reproductive age who have diabetes because it is associated with less perinatal mortality and fewer congenital anomalies (Landon et al., 2017; Moore et al., 2014). Under ideal circumstances, women with pregestational diabetes are counseled before the time of conception to plan the optimal time for pregnancy, establish glycemic control before conception, and diagnose any vascular complications of diabetes. However, estimates indicate that less than 20% of women with diabetes in the United States participate in preconception counseling (Landon et al.).

The woman's partner should be included in the counseling to assess the couple's level of understanding related to the effects of pregnancy on the diabetic condition and the potential complications of pregnancy as a result of diabetes. The couple should also be informed of the anticipated alterations in management of diabetes during pregnancy and the need for an interprofessional team approach to health care. Financial implications of diabetic pregnancy and other demands related to frequent maternal and fetal surveillance should be discussed. In addition, medications the woman is currently taking must be assessed for safety during pregnancy. Medications that carry risk for adverse maternal or fetal outcomes should be changed to ones that are safer but equally effective. Preconception counseling should also include discussion of microvascular and macrovascular complications that carry significant risk for maternal morbidity and mortality during pregnancy such as coronary artery disease and renal insufficiency. Renal transplantation may be necessary prior to conception. Contraception is another important aspect of preconception counseling to assist the couple in planning effectively for pregnancy. They should be encouraged to use reliable contraception until glycemic control is optimal.

MATERNAL RISKS AND COMPLICATIONS

Although maternal morbidity and mortality rates have improved significantly, the pregnant woman with diabetes remains at risk for the development of complications during pregnancy. Poor glycemic control around the time of conception and in the early weeks of pregnancy is associated with an increased incidence of spontaneous abortion (miscarriage). Women with good glycemic control before conception and in the first trimester are no more likely to miscarry than women who do not have diabetes (Moore et al., 2014).

Poor glycemic control later in pregnancy, particularly in women without vascular disease, increases the rate of fetal macrosomia. Macrosomia has been defined as a birth weight more than 4000 to 4500 g or greater than the 90th percentile. It occurs in approximately 40% of pregestational diabetic pregnancies and up to 50% of pregnancies complicated by GDM (Landon et al., 2017). Infants born to women with diabetes tend to have a disproportionate increase in shoulder, trunk, and chest size. Because of this tendency, the risk for shoulder dystocia is greater in these babies than in other macrosomic infants. Therefore, women with diabetes face an increased likelihood of cesarean birth because of failure of fetal descent or labor progress or of operative vaginal birth (birth involving the use of episiotomy, forceps, or vacuum extractor) (Moore et al., 2014).

Women with preexisting diabetes are at risk for several obstetric and medical complications. In general, the risk for developing these complications increases with the duration and severity of the woman's diabetes. For example, more than one third of women who have had diabetes for more than 20 years develop preeclampsia. Women with nephropathy and hypertension in addition to diabetes are also increasingly likely to develop preeclampsia. Poor glycemic control at the beginning of pregnancy is also related to the development of preeclampsia. The rate of hypertensive disorders in all types of pregnancies complicated by diabetes is 15% to 30%. Chronic hypertension occurs in 10% to 20% of all pregnant women with diabetes and in up to 40% of women who have preexisting renal or retinal vascular disease (Moore et al., 2014).

Hydramnios (polyhydramnios) frequently develops during the third trimester of pregnancy in women with diabetes. Its cause is unknown. One theory is that hydramnios in women with diabetes is caused by an increased glucose concentration in amniotic fluid resulting from maternal and fetal hyperglycemia, which induces fetal polyuria. The complications most frequently associated with hydramnios (usually defined as an amniotic fluid index [AFI] greater than 24 to 25 cm) are placental abruption, uterine dysfunction, and postpartum hemorrhage (Cunningham, Leveno, Bloom, et al., 2014).

Infections are more common and more serious in pregnant women with diabetes than in those without the disease. Disorders of carbohydrate metabolism alter the normal resistance of the body to infection. The inflammatory response, leukocyte function, and vaginal pH are all affected. Vaginal infections, particularly monilial vaginitis, are more common. Urinary tract infections (UTIs) are also more prevalent.

Infection is serious because it causes increased insulin resistance and may result in ketoacidosis.

Ketoacidosis (accumulation of ketones in the blood resulting from hyperglycemia and leading to metabolic acidosis) occurs most often during the second and third trimesters, when the diabetogenic effect of pregnancy is greatest. When the maternal metabolism is stressed by illness or infection, the woman is at increased risk for diabetic ketoacidosis (DKA). DKA can also be caused by poor compliance with treatment or the onset of previously undiagnosed diabetes (Moore et al., 2014). The use of beta-mimetic drugs such as terbutaline (Brethine) for tocolysis to treat preterm labor or corticosteroids given to enhance fetal lung maturation may also contribute to the risk for hyperglycemia and subsequent DKA (Mercer, 2014; Simhan, Berghella, & Iams, 2014).

DKA may occur with blood glucose levels barely exceeding 200 mg/dL, compared with 300 to 350 mg/dL in the nonpregnant state. In response to stress factors such as infection or illness, hyperglycemia (a greater than normal amount of glucose in the blood) occurs as a result of increased hepatic glucose production and decreased peripheral glucose use. Stress hormones, which act to impair insulin action and further contribute to insulin deficiency, are released. Fatty acids are mobilized from fat stores to enter the circulation. As they are oxidized, ketone bodies are released into the peripheral circulation. The woman's buffering system is unable to compensate, and metabolic acidosis develops. The excessive blood glucose and ketone bodies result in osmotic diuresis with subsequent loss of fluid and electrolytes, volume depletion, and cellular dehydration. DKA is a medical emergency. Prompt treatment is necessary to prevent maternal coma or death. Ketoacidosis occurring at any time during pregnancy can lead to intrauterine fetal death. The incidence of DKA has decreased in recent years because of advances in clinical management and blood glucose monitoring (Inturrisi, Lintner, & Sorem, 2013). It affects only about 1% to 2% of pregnant women with diabetes. The rate of intrauterine fetal demise (IUFD) with DKA, formerly approximately 35%, is 10% or less (Moore et al., 2014) (Table 11.2).

The risk for hypoglycemia (a less than normal amount of glucose in the blood) is also increased during pregnancy. Early in pregnancy, when hepatic production of glucose is diminished and peripheral use of glucose is enhanced, hypoglycemia occurs frequently, often during sleep. Later in pregnancy, it may also result as insulin doses are adjusted to maintain euglycemia (a normal blood glucose level). Women with a prepregnancy history of severe hypoglycemia are at increased risk for severe hypoglycemia during gestation. Mild-to-moderate hypoglycemic episodes do not appear to have significant damaging effects on fetal well-being (see Table 11.2).

FETAL AND NEONATAL RISKS AND COMPLICATIONS

From the moment of conception, the infant of a woman with diabetes faces an increased risk for complications that may occur during the antepartum, intrapartum, or neonatal periods. Infant morbidity and mortality rates associated with diabetic pregnancy are significantly reduced with strict control of maternal glucose levels before and during pregnancy.

Despite improvements in the care of pregnant women with diabetes, the perinatal mortality rate is three times higher for women with diabetes than for women who do not have this disease. Miscarriage rates for women with preexisting diabetes are as high as 30%. Major causes of perinatal mortality are congenital malformations, respiratory distress syndrome, and extreme prematurity. IUFD (sometimes called *stillbirth*) remains a major concern. Approximately 4% of all stillbirths occur in women whose pregnancies are complicated by preexisting diabetes.

TABLE 11.2   Differentiation of Hypoglycemia (Insulin Shock) and Hyperglycemia (Diabetic Ketoacidosis)

Causes	Onset	Symptoms	Interventions
Hypoglycemia (Insulin Shock)			
Excess insulin	Rapid (regular insulin)	Irritability	Check blood glucose level when symptoms first appear.
Insufficient food (delayed or missed meals)	Gradual (modified insulin or oral hypoglycemic agents)	Hunger	If blood glucose is <70 mg/dL, eat 2–4 glucose tablets or gel (8–16 g carbohydrate) immediately.
Excessive exercise or work		Sweating	
Indigestion, diarrhea, vomiting		Nervousness	Recheck blood glucose level in 15 minutes. If glucose level is still <70 mg/dL, eat 2–4 additional glucose tablets.
		Personality change	
		Weakness	
		Fatigue	Recheck blood glucose level in 15 minutes. If glucose level is still <70 mg/dL, notify health care provider immediately.
		Blurred or double vision	
		Dizziness	
		Headache	If woman is unconscious, administer 50% dextrose IV push, 5%–10% dextrose in water IV drip, or 1 mg glucagon intramuscularly.
		Pallor; clammy skin	
		Shallow respirations	
		Rapid pulse	
		Laboratory values	Obtain blood and urine specimens for laboratory testing.
		Urine: Negative for sugar and acetone	
		Blood glucose: <70 mg/dL	
Hyperglycemia (DKA)			
Insufficient insulin	Slow (hours to days)	Thirst	Notify primary health care provider.
Excess or wrong kind of food		Nausea or vomiting	Administer insulin in accordance with blood glucose levels.
Infection, injuries, illness		Abdominal pain	
Emotional stress		Constipation	Give IV fluids such as normal saline solution or one-half normal saline solution; potassium when urinary output is adequate; bicarbonate for pH <7.
Insufficient exercise		Drowsiness	
		Dim vision	
		Increased urination	Monitor laboratory testing of blood and urine.
		Headache	
		Flushed, dry skin	
		Rapid breathing	
		Weak, rapid pulse	
		Acetone (fruity) breath odor	
		Laboratory values	
		Urine: Positive for sugar and acetone	
		Blood glucose: >200 mg/dL	

DKA, Diabetic ketoacidosis; *IV,* intravenous.

Poor glycemic control is the most consistent finding in women who had a stillbirth. In addition to hyperglycemia, other causes of stillbirth include congenital abnormalities, placental insufficiency or fetal growth restriction, macrosomia or polyhydramnios, or obstructed labor (intrapartum stillbirth) (Inturrisi, 2017; Reddy & Spong, 2014).

Hyperglycemia during the first trimester of pregnancy, when organs and organ systems are forming, is the main cause of diabetes-associated birth defects. Anomalies commonly seen in infants born to women with diabetes affect primarily the cardiovascular system and the central nervous system (CNS) (Inturrisi, 2017; Moore et al., 2014) (see Chapter 25).

Hypoglycemia that occurs in the first few hours after birth is also a risk for infants born to mothers with diabetes. For further discussion of neonatal complications related to maternal diabetes, see Chapter 25.

CARE MANAGEMENT

ASSESSMENT AND NURSING DIAGNOSES

When a pregnant woman with diabetes initiates prenatal care, a thorough evaluation of her health status is completed. At the initial visit, a complete physical examination is performed. In addition to the routine prenatal examination, specific efforts are made to assess for acute and chronic complications of diabetes (Daley, 2014), especially retinopathy, nephropathy, peripheral and autonomic neuropathy, peripheral vasculopathy, and cardiac involvement.

Routine prenatal laboratory tests are performed, and baseline renal function may be assessed with a 24-hour urine collection for total protein excretion and creatinine clearance. Urinalysis and culture are performed to assess for the presence of a UTI, which is common in diabetic pregnancy. Because of the risk for coexisting thyroid disease, thyroid function tests may also be performed (see later discussion of thyroid disorders). The glycosylated hemoglobin A1c level may be measured to assess recent glycemic control.

With prolonged hyperglycemia, some of the hemoglobin remains saturated with glucose for the life of the red blood cell (RBC). Therefore, a test for glycosylated hemoglobin provides a "diabetic report card," a prediction of past glycemic control. Because red blood cells turn over more rapidly during pregnancy, A1c levels are normally lower in pregnant women than in nonpregnant individuals. Therefore, the estimation of glycemic control provided by the test applies to a shorter period of

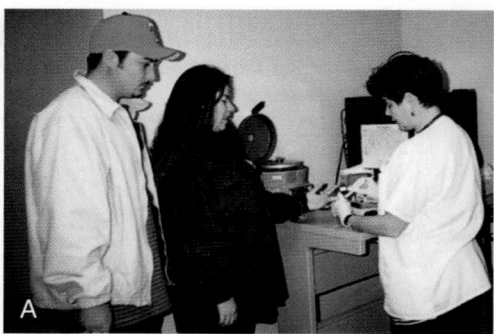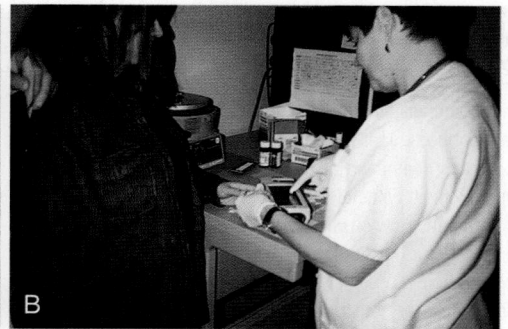

FIG 11.2 **A,** Clinic nurse collects blood to determine glucose level. **B,** Nurse interprets glucose value displayed by monitor. (Courtesy of Dee Lowdermilk, UNC Ambulatory Care Clinics, Chapel Hill, NC.)

time, only the previous 2 to 6 weeks. Hemoglobin A1c levels less than 6 to 6.5 in early pregnancy have been associated with the lowest rates of adverse fetal outcomes (ADA, 2016a; Inturrisi, 2017). Fasting blood glucose or random (1 to 2 hours after eating) glucose levels may be assessed during antepartum visits (Fig. 11.2).

> ### ❗ NURSING ALERT
>
> Iron deficiency anemia falsely increases the A1c level (Inturrisi, 2017). Self-monitoring blood glucose records should be reviewed at every prenatal visit. Accuracy of reporting should be reviewed periodically by accessing the meter memory and addressed if falsification of blood glucose results is detected. Most meters can be downloaded using manufacturer software, but this cannot replace logging, which affords more information for both the health care provider and the woman.

TABLE 11.3 Target Blood Glucose Levels During Pregnancy

Time of Day	Target Plasma Glucose Level (mg/dL)
Premeal or fasting	60–105
Postmeal (1 hour)	<140
Postmeal (2 hours)	≤120
2 AM to 6 AM	>60

Data from Landon, M.B., Catalano, P.M., & Gabbe, S.G. (2017). Diabetes mellitus complicating pregnancy. In S.G. Gabbe, J.R. Niebyl, J.L. Simpson, et al. (Eds.), *Obstetrics: Normal and problem pregnancies* (7th ed.). Philadelphia, PA: Elsevier.

Potential nursing diagnoses for the woman with pregestational diabetes include the following:
- *Deficient Knowledge* related to
  - diabetic pregnancy, management, and potential effects on pregnant woman and fetus
  - insulin administration and its effects
  - hypoglycemia and hyperglycemia
  - diabetic diet
- *Anxiety, Grieving, Powerlessness, Disturbed Body Image, Situational Low Self-Esteem, Spiritual Distress, Ineffective Role Performance, Interrupted Family Processes* related to
  - stigma of being labeled "diabetic"
  - effects of diabetes and its potential sequelae on the pregnant woman and the fetus
- *Risk for Injury* to fetus related to
  - disruption of oxygen transfer from environment to fetus
  - birth trauma
- *Risk for Injury* to mother related to
  - improper insulin administration
  - hypoglycemia and hyperglycemia
  - cesarean or operative vaginal birth
  - postpartum infection

INTERVENTIONS

Antepartum

Because of her high-risk status, a woman with pregestational diabetes is monitored much more frequently and thoroughly than other pregnant women. During the first and second trimesters of pregnancy, her routine prenatal care visits are scheduled every 1 to 2 weeks. In the last trimester, she will likely be seen 1 or 2 times each week. In the past, routine hospitalization for management of the diabetes, such as for insulin dose changes, was common. With the availability of improved home glucose monitoring and the growing reluctance of third-party payers to reimburse for hospitalization, pregnant women with diabetes generally now are managed as outpatients. Some patient and family education and maternal and fetal assessment may be performed in the home, depending on the woman's insurance coverage and care provider preference.

Achieving and maintaining constant euglycemia is the primary goal of medical therapy. Blood glucose levels should be in the range of 60 to 105 mg/dL before meals and 140 mg/dL or less when measured 1 hour after a meal. Postmeal glucose levels at 2 hours should be no higher than 120 mg/dL (Landon et al., 2017) (Table 11.3). Euglycemia is achieved through a combination of diet, insulin, and exercise. Providing the woman with the knowledge, skill, and motivation she needs to achieve and maintain excellent blood glucose control is the primary nursing goal.

Achieving euglycemia requires commitment on the part of the woman and her family to make the necessary lifestyle changes, which can sometimes seem overwhelming. Maintaining tight blood glucose control necessitates that the woman follow a consistent daily schedule. She must get up, go to bed, eat, exercise, and take insulin at the same time each day. Blood glucose measurements are done frequently (6 to 8 times each day) to determine how well the major components of therapy (diet, insulin, and exercise) are working together to control blood glucose levels. The pregnant woman with diabetes should wear a medical identification bracelet at all times and carry insulin, syringes or pens, a blood glucose meter, and glucose tablets with her whenever she is

COMMUNITY FOCUS

Accessibility of Diabetes Supplies

Visit your local pharmacy, and examine the diabetes equipment and supplies that are available. Locate glucose meters, urine test strips, insulin syringes, and insulin pens. How much does each of these items cost? Check to see which items are covered by most types of insurance and Medicaid. Read the instructions for use of each item. How easily could you follow the instructions? Could a woman with low literacy skills read and understand them? Do the instructions contain illustrations? Are the instructions written in more than one language (e.g., in Spanish or French) in addition to English? Does the pharmacy have someone who can teach women? How can you use the information you have obtained in this exercise in your patient teaching?

PATIENT TEACHING

Dietary Management for Pregnant Women With Diabetes

- Follow the prescribed diet plan.
- Eat a well-balanced diet, including daily food requirements for a normal pregnancy.
- Divide daily food intake among three meals and two or three snacks, depending on individual needs.
- Eat a substantial bedtime snack to prevent a severe drop in blood glucose level during the night.
- Take daily vitamins and iron as prescribed by your health care provider.
- Avoid foods high in refined sugar.
- Eat consistently each day; never skip meals or snacks.
- Eat foods high in dietary fiber.
- Avoid alcohol and nicotine; limit caffeine.
- Avoid excessive use of nonnutritive sweeteners.

away from home (see Community Focus box: Accessibility of Diabetes Supplies).

Because the woman with pregestational diabetes is at increased risk for infections and neurologic changes, foot and general skin care are important. A daily bath that includes thorough perineal and foot care is recommended. For dry skin, lotions, creams, or oils can be applied. Tight clothing should be avoided. Shoes or slippers that fit properly should be worn at all times and are best worn with socks or stockings. Feet should be inspected regularly; toenails should be cut straight across, and professional help should be sought for any foot problems. Extremes of temperature should be avoided.

Diet

The woman with pregestational diabetes has usually had nutrition counseling regarding management of her diabetes. However, because pregnancy produces special nutrition concerns and needs, the woman must be educated to incorporate these changes into dietary planning. The woman who has "controlled" her diabetes for several years may find it difficult to adjust to the changes in her insulin and dietary needs mandated by pregnancy. Nutrition counseling is usually provided by a registered dietitian. Counseling should address general nutrition principles appropriate for all pregnant women as well as diabetes-specific nutritional needs.

Dietary management during diabetic pregnancy must be based on blood (not urine) glucose levels. The diet is individualized to allow for increased fetal and metabolic requirements, with consideration of such factors as prepregnancy weight and dietary habits, overall health, ethnic background, lifestyle, stage of pregnancy, knowledge of nutrition, and insulin therapy. The dietary goals are to promote weight gain consistent with a normal pregnancy, prevent ketoacidosis, and minimize wide fluctuation of blood glucose levels.

For women with a body mass index (BMI) of 22 to 27, dietary counseling includes advice to consume about 35 kcal/kg of ideal body weight per day. In contrast, obese women with a BMI of 30 or greater may be managed with a caloric intake as low as 15 kcal/kg of actual weight per day (Landon et al., 2017). The average diet includes 2200 calories (first trimester) to 2500 calories (second and third trimesters). Total calories may be distributed among three meals and one evening snack or, more commonly, three meals and two or three snacks. Meals should be eaten on time and never skipped. Going more than 4 hours without food intake increases the risk for episodes of hypoglycemia. Snacks must be planned carefully in accordance with insulin therapy to prevent fluctuations in blood glucose levels. A large bedtime snack of at least 25 g of complex carbohydrate with some protein or fat is recommended to help prevent hypoglycemia and starvation ketosis during the night (Moore et al., 2014).

The ideal diet is composed of 40% to 60% complex high-fiber carbohydrates, 20% protein, and 30% to 40% fat, with less than 10% as saturated fat (Landon et al., 2017) (see Patient Teaching box: Dietary Management for Pregnant Women with Diabetes). Complex carbohydrates that are high in fiber content are recommended because the starch and protein in such foods help regulate the blood glucose level by more sustained glucose release (Moore et al., 2014).

Exercise

Being active for 30 to 60 minutes per day is encouraged. Daily activity has been shown to: increase insulin sensitivity, thus lowering blood glucose levels; increase utilization of glucose, especially after a meal; improve glucose control, perhaps eliminating the need for insulin therapy; reduce the risk for excessive weight gain; and reduce the weight of the newborn by approximately 150 g. Physical activity can be divided into 10 to 20 minute periods after each meal (Daley, 2014; Inturrisi, 2017).

Women with pregestational diabetes who are poorly controlled or have vascular disease should avoid vigorous exercise during pregnancy. Walking and swimming are two forms of exercise with minimal risk and may be the exercises of choice for previously sedentary women (Daley, 2014). Women should check their blood glucose levels before, during, and after exercising. If the blood glucose is less than 100 mg/dL, they should consume 15 to 30 g of carbohydrate to prevent hypoglycemia. Women should avoid exercise if they have positive urine ketones or a blood glucose greater than 200 mg/dL because hyperglycemia and ketosis can worsen with physical activity (Inturrisi, 2017). Exercising with another person is prudent for safety reasons.

! NURSING ALERT

Uterine contractions may occur during exercise. The woman should be advised to stop exercising immediately if they are detected.

Insulin Therapy

Adequate insulin is the primary factor in the maintenance of euglycemia during pregnancy, thus ensuring proper glucose metabolism of the woman and fetus. Insulin requirements during pregnancy change dramatically as the pregnancy progresses, necessitating frequent adjustments in the dose. In the first trimester, from weeks 3 to 7 of gestation, insulin requirements are increased, followed by a decrease between weeks 7 and 15 of gestation. The commonly prescribed insulin dose is

PATIENT TEACHING
Self-Administration of Insulin

Procedure for Mixing NPH (Intermediate-Acting) and Rapid-Acting Insulin

- Wash hands thoroughly, and gather supplies. Be sure that insulin syringe corresponds to concentration of insulin you are using.
- Check insulin bottle to be certain that it is the appropriate type, and check expiration date.
- Gently rotate (do not shake) the insulin vial to mix the insulin.
- Wipe off the rubber stopper of each vial with alcohol.
- Draw into syringe the amount of air equal to the total dose.
- Inject air equal to NPH dose into NPH vial. Remove syringe from vial.
- Inject air equal to rapid-acting insulin dose into vial, and leave syringe in vial.
- Invert rapid-acting vial, and withdraw insulin dose.
- Without adding more air to NPH vial, carefully withdraw NPH dose.

Procedure for Self-Injection of Insulin

- Select proper injection site.
- Injection site should be clean. No need to use alcohol. If alcohol is used, let it dry before injecting.
- Puncture the skin at a 90-degree angle.
- Slowly inject the insulin.
- As you withdraw the needle, cover the injection site with sterile gauze and apply gentle pressure to prevent bleeding.
- Record insulin dose and time of injection.

BOX 11.1 Helpful Hints for Using Insulin

- The most common type of insulin used during pregnancy is a biosynthetic human insulin (Humulin) made by programming *Escherichia coli* bacteria to produce insulin.
- Insulin is classified either as rapid acting, short acting, intermediate acting, or long acting (see Table 11.4).
- Unopened vials of insulin should be stored in the refrigerator until reaching their expiration date. Insulin should not be frozen. Vials currently in use can be stored at room temperature for up to 1 month. They should not be left in a car or exposed to extreme heat as in the sun.
- Regular insulin can be mixed with NPH insulin in the same syringe. Lispro insulin can also be mixed in a syringe with NPH insulin. Once mixed, the syringe can be used immediately or stored for future use. If it is used later, the syringe should be rotated 20 times before injection.
- Glargine insulin is usually administered at bedtime. It cannot be mixed with any other insulin in the same syringe. Prepared syringes are stable for 2 weeks in the refrigerator.
- Insulin may be administered by pen injector, jet injector, or insulin pump, in addition to syringe.
- The abdomen is the preferred injection site because insulin is best absorbed there. Other possible injection sites are the upper outer arm (not the deltoid area), the thighs, and the buttocks.
- Each injection should be given 2 inches from the previous injection in one quadrant before moving to another quadrant.

TABLE 11.4 Common Insulin Preparations

Type of Insulin	Examples Generic (Trade) Name	Onset of Action	Peak of Action	Duration of Action
Rapid-acting	Lispro (Humalog)	15 min	30–90 min	4–5 hr
	Aspart (NovoLog)	15 min	1–3 hr	3–5 hr
Short-acting	Humulin R	30 min	2–4 hr	5–7 hr
	Novolin R	30 min	2.5–5 hr	6–8 hr
Intermediate-acting	Humulin NPH	1–2 hr	6–12 hr	18–24 hr
	Novolin N	1.5 hr	4–20 hr	24 hr
	Humulin L	1–3 hr	6–12 hr	18–24 hr
	Novolin L	2.5 hr	7–15 hr	22 hr
Long-acting	Glargine (Lantus)	1 hr	None	24 hr
	Detemir (Levemir)	1–2 hr	None	24 hr

hr, Hour; *L*, lente; *min*, minutes; *NPH* (or *N*), neutral protamine Hagedorn; *R*, regular.
Data from Landon, M.B., Catalano, P.M., & Gabbe, S.G. (2017). Diabetes mellitus complicating pregnancy. In S.G. Gabbe, J.R. Niebyl, J.L. Simpson, et al. (Eds.), *Obstetrics: Normal and problem pregnancies* (7th ed.). Philadelphia, PA: Elsevier.

0.7 units/kg in the first trimester for women with type 1 diabetes. During the second and third trimesters, because of insulin resistance, the dose must be increased significantly to maintain target glucose levels. Insulin requirements normally peak at 36 weeks of gestation and drop significantly after that (Moore et al., 2014).

For the woman with type 1 pregestational diabetes who has typically been accustomed to one injection per day of intermediate-acting insulin, multiple daily injections of mixed insulin are a new experience. The woman with type 2 diabetes previously treated with an oral hypoglycemic agent is faced with the task of learning to self-administer injections of insulin. The nurse is instrumental in educating and supporting women with pregestational diabetes in regard to insulin administration and adjustment of the insulin dose to maintain euglycemia (see Patient Teaching box: Self-Administration of Insulin and Box 11.1).

Since 1982, most insulin preparations have been produced by inserting portions of deoxyribonucleic acid (DNA) ("recombinant DNA") into special laboratory-cultivated bacteria or yeast cells. The cells then produce synthetic human insulin (Humulin), which is less likely to cause antibody formation than animal-derived (beef or pork) insulin. More recently, insulin products called *insulin analogues*, in which the structure differs slightly from human insulin, have been produced. This small alteration in insulin structure results in changes in the onset and peak of action of the medication. The most commonly used insulin preparations include rapid-acting, short-acting, intermediate-acting, and long-acting (Landon et al., 2017) (Table 11.4). Mixtures of short- and intermediate-acting insulins in several proportions are also available but usually are not in the correct percentages to be effective in pregnancy. Therefore, they are rarely used.

Lispro (Humalog) and aspart (NovoLog) are commonly prescribed rapid-acting insulin analogues that have replaced regular insulin (Landon et al., 2017). Rapid-acting insulins have a faster onset of action and peak effect than regular insulin, so their use may help to prevent hypoglycemia between meals (Daley, 2014). Rapid-acting insulins are convenient to use because they are injected immediately before mealtime. Because their effects last only 3 to 5 hours, most patients require a longer-acting insulin in addition to the rapid-acting insulin to maintain optimal blood glucose levels (see Table 11.4).

Glargine (Lantus) and detemir (Levemir) are long-acting insulin analogues that have been designed to more accurately mimic basal insulin secretion. Small amounts of these insulins are released slowly, with no pronounced peak. Glargine insulin may be combined with rapid-acting insulin to prevent hypoglycemia. When it is administered with rapid-acting insulin, unpredictable spikes in insulin levels and resulting hypoglycemia appear to occur less often. Both glargine and detemir appear to be safe for use during pregnancy (Landon et al., 2017) (see Table 11.4).

Insulin is usually administered in three to five injections per day. Many women with insulin-dependent diabetes take a combination of intermediate-acting and rapid-acting insulin before breakfast and dinner. Usually two-thirds of the daily insulin dose, with intermediate-acting and rapid-acting insulin combined in a 2 : 1 ratio, is given before breakfast. The remaining one-third is administered in the evening. It may be given as a combination of rapid- and intermediate-acting insulin before dinner or split, with rapid-acting insulin at dinner and intermediate-acting insulin at bedtime (Landon et al., 2017).

Insulin is still usually administered by drawing up the correct dose from a vial into a syringe and injecting it subcutaneously. Some women, however, may have difficulty drawing up the dose correctly, especially if mixing insulins in a syringe is required. Using prefilled syringes that have been stored in a refrigerator is one solution to this problem. Prefilled insulin pens are also available for use (Fig. 11.3). In addition to ensuring that the correct dose of insulin is administered, the pen is convenient for use away from home because there is no need to carry vials and syringes. The woman simply turns a dial on the pen to select her correct dose and then injects it. Some individuals believe that pen injections, because of the needle's small length and gauge, are less painful than those administered using a traditional syringe and needle. A disadvantage of insulin pens, however, is that they are more expensive than syringes and needles.

The continuous subcutaneous insulin infusion (CSII) system, commonly referred to as *the insulin pump,* is used increasingly during pregnancy. The CSII system is designed to mimic more closely the function of the pancreas in secreting insulin (Fig. 11.4). The portable battery-powered insulin pump is worn similar to a pager during most daily activities. The pump infuses rapid-acting insulin (usually lispro) (Landon et al., 2017) at a set basal rate and has the capacity to deliver up to four different basal rates in 24 hours, although only three or four

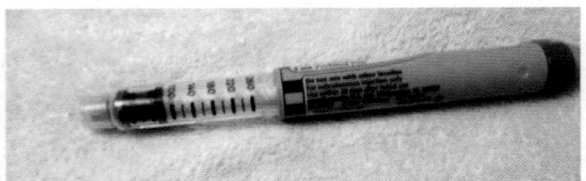

FIG 11.3 An insulin pen provides an accurate and convenient way to administer insulin. (Courtesy of Barbra Manning, RN, MSN, Senatobia, MS.)

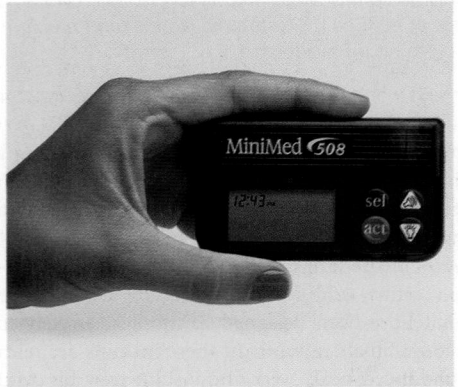

FIG 11.4 Insulin pump shows basal rate for pregnant women with diabetes. (Courtesy of MiniMed, Inc., Sylmar, CA.)

rates are necessary to provide individualized glycemic control. The pump also delivers bolus doses of insulin before meals to control postprandial blood glucose levels or to correct elevations in blood glucose. A fine-gauge plastic catheter is inserted into subcutaneous tissue, usually in the abdomen, and attached to the pump syringe by connecting tubing. The subcutaneous catheter and connecting tubing are changed every 2 to 3 days. Although the insulin pump is convenient and generally provides good glycemic control, complications such as pump failure, precipitation of insulin inside the pump mechanism, abscess formation, and poor uptake from the infusion site can still occur. To safely use the pump during pregnancy, the woman must monitor her blood glucose levels frequently. Therefore use of the insulin pump requires a knowledgeable, motivated woman and skilled health care providers (Daley, 2014).

Self-Monitoring of Blood Glucose

Blood glucose testing at home using a glucose meter is considered the standard of care for monitoring blood glucose levels during pregnancy. It provides the most important tool available to the woman to assess her degree of glycemic control. The newer meters are calibrated to provide plasma (rather than whole blood) glucose values. The nurse must be knowledgeable about the specific glucose meter that the woman uses in order to troubleshoot problems, assess accuracy of technique, and determine accuracy of reported results. To perform blood glucose monitoring, a drop of blood is obtained and placed on a test strip. Most glucose meters allow the user to obtain the blood sample from the forearm or palm rather than a finger. Fingersticks are recommended during pregnancy, however, because use of other sites can affect the accuracy of results. After a specified amount of time, the glucose level is displayed by the meter (see Patient Teaching box: Self-Monitoring of Blood Glucose Level). Blood glucose levels are routinely measured at various times throughout the day such as before breakfast, lunch, and dinner; 1 to 2 hours after each meal; at bedtime; and in the middle of the night if nighttime insulin is being adjusted. When any adjustment in the insulin dose or diet is made, more frequent measurement of blood glucose is warranted. If nausea, vomiting, or diarrhea occurs or if infection is present, the woman is asked to monitor her blood glucose levels more closely than usual.

PATIENT TEACHING
Self-Monitoring of Blood Glucose Level

- Gather supplies, check expiration date, and read instructions on testing materials. Prepare glucose meter for use according to manufacturer's instructions.
- Wash hands in warm water (warmth increases circulation).
- Select site on side of any finger (all fingers should be used in rotation).
- Pierce site with lancet (may use automatic spring-loaded, puncturing device). Cleaning the site with alcohol is not necessary.
- Drop hand down to side; with other hand, gently squeeze finger from hand to fingertip.
- Allow blood to be drawn into glucose test strip.
- Determine blood glucose value using glucose reflectance meter following manufacturer's instructions.
- Record results displayed.
- Repeat as instructed by health care provider and as needed for signs of hypoglycemia or hyperglycemia.

! NURSING ALERT

Hyperglycemia is most likely to be identified in 2-hour postmeal values because blood glucose levels peak approximately 2 hours after a meal.

PATIENT TEACHING
Treatment for Hypoglycemia

- Be familiar with signs and symptoms of hypoglycemia (nervousness, headache, fatigue, shaking, irritability, tachycardia, hunger, blurred vision, sweaty skin, tingling of mouth or extremities).
- Check blood glucose level immediately when hypoglycemic symptoms occur.
- If blood glucose is less than 70 mg/dL, immediately eat 2 to 4 glucose tablets or gel (8–16 g carbohydrate). If glucose tablets or gel are not available, then other simple carbohydrates (15 g) can be eaten or drunk instead. Examples are as follows:
  - ½ cup (4 oz) unsweetened orange juice
  - ½ cup (4 oz) regular (not diet) soda
  - 5 or 6 hard candies
  - 1 cup (8 oz) skim milk
- Rest for 15 minutes, and then recheck blood glucose.
- If glucose level is greater than 70 mg/dL, eat a meal to stabilize the sugar level.
- If glucose level is still less than 70 mg/dL, eat 2 to 4 additional glucose tablets.
- Wait 15 minutes, and then recheck blood glucose. If level is still less than 70 mg/dL, notify your health care provider immediately.
- If nausea related to hypoglycemia prevents ingestion of carbohydrates, inject 0.15 mg glucagon intramuscularly. This will elevate the blood glucose enough to allow eating.

PATIENT TEACHING
What to Do When Illness Occurs

- Be sure to take insulin even if unable to eat or appetite is less than normal. (Insulin needs are increased with illness or infection.)
- Call your health care provider, and relay the following information:
  - Symptoms of illness (e.g., nausea, vomiting, diarrhea)
  - Elevated temperature
  - Most recent blood glucose level
  - Urine ketones
  - Time and amount of last insulin dose
- Increase oral intake of fluids to prevent dehydration.
- Rest as much as possible.
- If you are unable to reach your health care provider and blood glucose exceeds 200 mg/dL with moderate urine ketones present, seek emergency treatment at the nearest health care facility. Do not attempt to self-treat for this condition.

Target levels of blood glucose during pregnancy are lower than nonpregnant values (see Table 11.3). Acceptable fasting levels are generally between 60 and 90 mg/dL, and 1-hour postmeal levels should be 140 mg/dL or less. Two-hour postmeal levels should be 120 mg/dL or less (Landon et al., 2017). The woman should be told to report recurrent episodes of hypoglycemia (less than 70 mg/dL) and hyperglycemia (more than 200 mg/dL) to her health care provider so adjustments in diet or insulin therapy can be made.

Pregnant women with diabetes are much more likely to develop hypoglycemia than hyperglycemia. Most episodes of mild or moderate hypoglycemia can be treated with oral intake of 15 g of carbohydrate, preferably in the form of commercial glucose tablets (see Patient Teaching box: Treatment for Hypoglycemia). If severe hypoglycemia occurs and the woman experiences a decrease in or loss of consciousness or an inability to swallow, she will require a parenteral injection of glucagon or intravenous (IV) glucose. Because hypoglycemia can develop rapidly and impaired judgment can be associated with even moderate episodes, family members, friends, and work colleagues must be able to recognize signs and symptoms quickly and initiate proper treatment if necessary.

Some women with long-term pregestational diabetes develop hypoglycemia unawareness, a condition in which early symptoms of hypoglycemia are not recognized. Women with hypoglycemia unawareness should test their blood glucose levels more frequently, especially during the night, in order to detect hypoglycemia earlier. Glycemic thresholds in women with hypoglycemia unawareness should be higher than for other women with diabetes in order to avoid dangerous hypoglycemia. The threshold for recognition of hypoglycemia should be determined at the first prenatal visit so that individual guidelines for hypoglycemia can be determined and the woman and her family educated.

Hyperglycemia is less likely to occur than hypoglycemia, although it can rapidly progress to DKA, which is associated with an increased risk for fetal death (Inturrisi, 2017; Landon et al., 2017). Women and family members should be particularly alert for signs and symptoms of hyperglycemia when infections or other illnesses occur (see Patient Teaching box: What to Do When Illness Occurs).

Urine Testing

Urine testing for glucose is not beneficial during pregnancy. Because of the lowered renal threshold for glucose, the degree of glycosuria does not accurately reflect the blood glucose level. However, urine testing for ketones continues to have a place in diabetic management. Monitoring for urine ketones may detect inadequate caloric or carbohydrate intake or skipped meals or snacks. Testing may also be performed when illness occurs or when the blood glucose level is 250 mg/dL or greater, because of the increased risk for ketoacidosis. The woman should be told to report moderate levels of urine ketones to her health care provider (Daley, 2014).

Complications Requiring Hospitalization

Occasionally hospitalization is necessary to regulate insulin therapy and stabilize glucose levels. Infection, which can lead to hyperglycemia and DKA, is an indication for hospitalization, regardless of gestational age. Hospitalization during the third trimester for close maternal and fetal observation may be indicated for women whose diabetes is poorly controlled. In addition, women with diabetes are more likely than women who do not have diabetes to also have preexisting hypertension or develop preeclampsia, which may necessitate hospitalization (Moore et al., 2014).

Fetal Surveillance

Diagnostic techniques for fetal surveillance are often performed to assess fetal growth and well-being. The goals of fetal surveillance are to detect fetal compromise as early as possible and prevent IUFD or unnecessary preterm birth.

The estimated date of birth is determined early in pregnancy. A baseline ultrasound is obtained during the first trimester to assess gestational age. Follow-up ultrasound examinations are usually performed during the pregnancy (as often as every 3 to 4 weeks) to monitor fetal growth; estimate fetal weight; and detect hydramnios, macrosomia, and congenital anomalies.

Because the fetus of a woman with diabetes is at increased risk for neural tube defects (e.g., spina bifida, anencephaly, microcephaly), measurement of maternal serum alpha-fetoprotein is performed between 15 and 20 weeks of gestation (ideally between 16 and 18 weeks of gestation) (Wapner, 2014). In addition, a detailed ultrasound study to examine the fetus for neural tube defects and other anomalies should be performed between 18 and 20 weeks of gestation (Moore et al., 2014).

Ultrasound measurement of the fetal nuchal translucency (NT) in conjunction with maternal serum screening between 11 and 14 weeks of gestation has been found to increase the detection of heart defects and other anomalies in women with pregestational diabetes (Miller, de Veciana, Turan, et al., 2013). Fetal echocardiography may be performed between 20 and 22 weeks of gestation to detect cardiac anomalies, especially in women who had less than desirable glucose control early in pregnancy, as demonstrated by a hemoglobin A1c level greater than 6% at the first prenatal visit (Moore et al., 2014). Some practitioners repeat this fetal surveillance test at 34 weeks of gestation. Doppler studies of the umbilical artery may be performed in women with vascular disease to detect placental compromise.

Most fetal surveillance measures are concentrated in the third trimester, when the risk for fetal compromise is greatest. The goals of antepartum testing during the third trimester are to monitor fetal growth and ensure fetal well-being. Pregnant women should be taught how to make daily fetal movement counts, beginning at 28 weeks of gestation (see Chapter 10) (Moore et al., 2014).

The nonstress test (NST) is the preferred primary method to evaluate fetal well-being. It is usually begun by 32 weeks of gestation and performed at least twice weekly. If the NST is nonreactive, a biophysical profile or contraction stress test will be performed. Testing often begins earlier, between 28 and 32 weeks of gestation, in women who have vascular disease, poor glucose control, or suspected fetal growth restriction (Landon et al., 2017) (see Chapter 10).

Determination of Birth Date and Mode of Birth

The optimal time for birth is between 39 and 40 weeks of gestation, as long as good metabolic control is maintained and parameters of antepartum fetal surveillance remain within normal limits. Induction of labor at 39 weeks of gestation is often planned for women with well-controlled diabetes who do not have vascular disease (Landon et al., 2017). Reasons to proceed with birth before full-term gestation include poor metabolic control, coexisting hypertension, and nonreassuring responses to fetal testing (Moore et al., 2014).

To confirm fetal lung maturity, an amniocentesis should be performed when birth will occur before 38 weeks of gestation. For the pregnancy complicated by diabetes, fetal lung maturation is best predicted by the amniotic fluid phosphatidylglycerol (greater than 3%). If the fetal lungs are still immature, birth should be postponed until 40 weeks of gestation as long as fetal assessment test results remain reassuring. After that time, however, the benefits of conservative management are outweighed by the increasing risk for fetal compromise if the pregnancy is allowed to continue. Birth, despite poor fetal lung maturity, may be necessary when testing suggests fetal compromise or worsening maternal condition, such as deteriorating renal function or preeclampsia with severe features (Moore et al., 2014).

Although vaginal birth is expected for most women with pregestational diabetes, the cesarean rate for these women is as high as 80% (Cunningham et al., 2014). ACOG (2016) states that although the diagnosis of fetal macrosomia is imprecise, prophylactic cesarean birth may be considered when the estimated fetal weight is at least 4500 g in women with diabetes. This recommendation may reduce the risk for shoulder dystocia to some degree for an individual woman, but the benefit to a larger group of women is unclear (Moore et al., 2014.).

Intrapartum

During the intrapartum period, the woman with pregestational diabetes must be monitored closely to prevent complications related to dehydration, hypoglycemia, and hyperglycemia. An IV line is inserted for infusion of a maintenance fluid. Initially this infusion will be either normal saline or lactated Ringer's solution. Once active labor begins or glucose levels fall below 70 mg/dL, a piggybacked pump-controlled infusion of a solution containing 5% dextrose should be added (Landon et al., 2017). The dextrose provides the energy (calories) necessary for the woman to accomplish the work and manage the stress of labor and birth. Most commonly, insulin is administered by continuous infusion, piggybacked into the main IV line. Only rapid- or short-acting insulin can be administered intravenously. Insulin may also be given intermittently by subcutaneous injection as needed to maintain glucose levels within the target range. Determinations of blood glucose levels are made every hour, and fluids and insulin are adjusted to maintain the blood glucose level between 90 and 110 mg/dL (Moore et al., 2014). Maintaining this target glucose level is essential because hyperglycemia during labor can cause metabolic problems in the neonate, particularly hypoglycemia (Daley, 2014).

During labor, continuous fetal heart monitoring is necessary. The woman should assume an upright or side-lying position during labor to prevent supine hypotension caused by a large fetus or polyhydramnios. Labor, whether spontaneous or induced, is allowed to progress as long as expected rates of cervical dilation and fetal descent are maintained and fetal well-being is evident. Failure to progress in labor may indicate a macrosomic infant and cephalopelvic disproportion, necessitating a cesarean birth. The woman is observed and treated during labor for complications of diabetes such as hyperglycemia, ketosis, and ketoacidosis. During second-stage labor, shoulder dystocia may occur with the birth of a macrosomic infant (see Chapter 17). A neonatologist, pediatrician, or neonatal nurse practitioner will likely be present at the birth to initiate neonatal assessment and care.

If a cesarean birth is planned, it should be scheduled in the early morning to facilitate glycemic control. Women should take their full dose of insulin the night before surgery. No morning insulin is given on the day of surgery, and the woman is given nothing by mouth (Daley, 2014; Landon et al., 2017). Regional (spinal or epidural) anesthesia is recommended because hypoglycemia can be detected earlier if the woman is awake. After surgery, glucose levels should be monitored carefully.

Postpartum

During the first 24 hours postpartum, insulin requirements decrease substantially because the major source of insulin resistance, the placenta, has been removed. Women with preexisting diabetes usually only require 50% of their most recent pregnancy insulin dose on the first postpartum day, provided they are eating a full diet (Daley, 2014). Women who give birth by cesarean may need an IV infusion of glucose and insulin until they resume a regular diet (Moore et al., 2014). A subcutaneous dose of insulin should be given at least 1 hour before discontinuing IV insulin.

After birth, several days may be required to reestablish carbohydrate homeostasis (see Fig. 11.1, *D* and *E*). Blood glucose levels are carefully monitored in the postpartum period, and the insulin dose is adjusted appropriately. The woman who has insulin-dependent diabetes must realize the importance of eating on time, even if the baby needs feeding or other pressing demands exist. Women with type 2 diabetes may resume taking their prepregnancy oral hypoglycemics if these medications are compatible with breastfeeding and provide adequate glycemic control.

Possible postpartum complications include preeclampsia or eclampsia, hemorrhage, and infection. Hemorrhage is a possibility if the mother's uterus was overdistended (hydramnios, macrosomic fetus) or overstimulated (oxytocin induction). Postpartum infections such as endometritis are more likely to occur in women with diabetes than in women who do not have diabetes.

Women with diabetes are encouraged to breastfeed. In addition to the benefits of breastfeeding for all mothers and infants, breastfeeding may offer longer-term benefits for both women with diabetes and their children. Weight control and glucose levels may both be improved in breastfeeding women in the first 3 months postpartum. Infants of women with diabetes have a decreased risk for childhood obesity, if they are breastfed for at least 6 months (ADA, 2016b; Inturrisi, 2017). Children who were exclusively breastfed also have a significantly lower risk for developing non–insulin-dependent diabetes (Moore et al., 2014).

Insulin requirements in breastfeeding women decrease because of the carbohydrate used in human milk production. Because glucose levels are lower than normal, breastfeeding women are at increased risk for hypoglycemia after breastfeeding, particularly after late-night nursing sessions (Moore et al., 2014). Women should check their blood glucose level just before breastfeeding. If it is less than 100 mg/dL, they should consume 15 g carbohydrate (see Patient Teaching box: Treatment for Hypoglycemia) without taking insulin. Women should also be aware that frequent hypoglycemia can reduce breast milk production. Breastfeeding mothers with hyperglycemia are at increased risk for mastitis (Inturrisi, 2017). Insulin, glyburide, and metformin are all considered safe for use while breastfeeding (Spencer, 2015). The insulin dose must be recalculated at weaning (see Fig. 11.1, *F*).

The mother may have early breastfeeding difficulties. Poor metabolic control may delay lactogenesis and contribute to decreased milk production (Moore et al., 2014). Initial contact with and opportunity to breastfeed the infant may be delayed for mothers who gave birth by cesarean or if infants are placed in neonatal intensive care units or special care nurseries for observation during the first few hours after birth. Support and assistance from nursing staff and lactation specialists can facilitate the mother's early experience with breastfeeding and encourage her to continue.

The new mother needs information about family planning and contraception. Although family planning is important for all women, it is essential for the woman with diabetes in order to safeguard her own health and promote optimal outcomes in future pregnancies. The risks and benefits of contraceptive methods should be discussed with the mother and her partner before discharge from the hospital. Barrier methods have become the preferred interim method of contraception for women with diabetes because they are safe, inexpensive options that do not affect carbohydrate metabolism or have no inherent risks. An intrauterine device (IUD) may also be used without concerns about an increased risk for infection (Landon et al., 2017).

Use of oral contraceptives by women with diabetes is controversial because of the possible increased risk for thromboembolic and vascular complications, myocardial infarction, and the effect on carbohydrate metabolism (Landon et al,, 2017). In nonsmoking women who are younger than 35 years of age and do not have vascular disease, combination low-dose oral contraceptives may be prescribed if they are not breastfeeding. Progestin-only oral contraceptives also may be used because they do not significantly affect glucose levels (Cunningham et al., 2014). Close monitoring of blood pressure and lipid levels is necessary to detect complications (Landon et al.).

Opinion is divided about the use of long-acting parenteral progestins, such as medroxyprogesterone (Depo-Provera). Some health care providers recommend their use, particularly in women who are noncompliant with daily-dosing oral contraceptives. In contrast, other health care providers believe this method may adversely affect glycemic control. In addition, although Depo-Provera may lower serum triglyceride and high-density lipoprotein (HDL) cholesterol levels, it does not lower total cholesterol or low-density lipoprotein (LDL) levels. For this reason, it is not recommended as a first-choice method for contraception for women with diabetes (Landon et al., 2017). Implants that contain only progesterone (e.g., Nexplanon) may be used by many women with diabetes because they do not significantly affect glucose levels (Cunningham et al., 2014).

Transdermal (patch) and transvaginal (vaginal ring) are also contraceptive options, particularly effective in women who prefer weekly or every-third-week dosing, respectively. For women who weigh more than 90 kg (198 lb), the contraceptive failure rate with transdermal administration is higher than in normal-weight women. Therefore, this method is contraindicated in obese women. In addition, women who choose the patch as their contraceptive method may be at risk for developing thromboembolic disease (Cunningham et al., 2014).

The risks associated with pregnancy increase with the duration and severity of diabetes. In addition, pregnancy may contribute to the vascular changes associated with diabetes. This information needs to be thoroughly discussed with the woman and her partner. Sterilization is often recommended for the woman who has completed her family, who has poor metabolic control, or who has significant vascular problems. Vasectomy for the partner is very effective and is safer than surgical sterilization in the woman with diabetes.

GESTATIONAL DIABETES MELLITUS

Gestational diabetes mellitus (GDM) complicates approximately 9.2% of all pregnancies (a range of 2% to 18%, depending on the race and ethnicity of the population and the method of diagnosis) in the United States (Inturrisi, 2017). It occurs more often now worldwide than in the past, probably because of increasing rates of overweight and obesity and the stricter criteria for diagnosis now being used by some health care practitioners (Landon et al., 2017). According to White's classification system, women with GDM fall into classes A_1 and A_2 (see Table 11.1). It is more likely to occur among Hispanic, African-American, Native-American, Asian, and Pacific Islander women than in Caucasians and is likely to recur in future pregnancies; the risk for development of overt diabetes later in life is also increased (Inturrisi; Landon et al.). This tendency is especially true of women whose GDM is diagnosed early in pregnancy and who have elevated fasting glucose levels (Landon et al.). Classic risk factors for GDM include a family history of diabetes and a previous pregnancy that resulted in an unexplained stillbirth or the birth of a malformed or macrosomic fetus. Other risk factors for GDM include obesity, hypertension, glycosuria, and maternal age older than 25 years. However, more than half of all women diagnosed with GDM do not have these risk factors (Landon et al.).

GDM is diagnosed during the second half of pregnancy. As fetal nutrient demands rise during the late second and the third trimesters, maternal nutrient ingestion induces greater and more sustained levels of blood glucose. At the same time, maternal insulin resistance is also increasing because of the insulin-antagonistic effects of the placental hormones, cortisol, and insulinase. Consequently, maternal insulin demands rise as much as threefold. Most pregnant women are capable of increasing insulin production to compensate for insulin resistance and maintain euglycemia. However, when the pancreas is unable to produce sufficient insulin or the insulin is not used effectively, GDM can result.

FETAL RISKS

No increase in the incidence of birth defects has been found among infants of women who develop GDM after the first trimester because the critical period of organ formation has already passed by that time (Moore, et al., 2014). Obesity (BMI >30) also contributes to congenital defects even in the absence of GDM. As with pregestational diabetes, infants born to women with GDM are at risk for macrosomia and associated risks for birth trauma and electrolyte imbalances including neonatal hypoglycemia.

CARE MANAGEMENT

SCREENING FOR GESTATIONAL DIABETES MELLITUS

Early Pregnancy Screening

All pregnant women not known to have pregestational diabetes should be screened for GDM by history, clinical risk factors, or laboratory screening of blood glucose levels (ACOG, 2013/2015). Based on history and clinical risk factors, some women are at low risk for developing GDM; therefore, glucose testing for this population may not be cost-effective. This group includes normal-weight women younger than 25 years of age who have no family history of diabetes, are not members of an ethnic or a racial group known to have a high prevalence of the disease, and have no history of abnormal glucose tolerance or adverse obstetric outcomes usually associated with GDM. However, only 10% of pregnant women meet all of these criteria (ACOG).

Increasing rates of obesity and diabetes have resulted in more women of childbearing age with type 2 diabetes, many of whom are undiagnosed when they become pregnant. Both the ADA and ACOG recommend that women with high-risk factors for type 2 diabetes (i.e., severe obesity, a strong family history of type 2 diabetes, and a history of GDM in a previous pregnancy) be tested for preexisting diabetes at their initial prenatal visit by one of the methods used to diagnose diabetes in the nonpregnant population (ADA, 2016a; Inturrisi, 2017; Landon et al., 2017). Screening early in pregnancy diagnoses women with preexisting diabetes so that appropriate treatment and postpartum follow-up are possible. If early screening indicates that these women do not have preexisting diabetes, they should be rescreened at 24 to 28 weeks of gestation for GDM (ADA, 2016a; Landon et al.; Inturrisi).

Screening at 24 to 28 Weeks of Gestation

Two different blood glucose screening methods for GDM are used in the United States. ACOG still recommends the two-step screening method that has been used for many years. The first step is a screen consisting of a 50-g oral glucose load followed by a plasma glucose measurement 1 hour later. The woman need not be fasting when the screen is done. A glucose value of 130 to 140 mg/dL is considered a positive screen. An initial positive screening result is followed by step 2, a 3-hour oral glucose tolerance test (OGTT) on another day. ACOG recommends use of the two-step screening procedure because there is no evidence that the one-step method (see later discussion) leads to clinically significant improvement in maternal or newborn outcomes. Use of the one-step method does, however, significantly increase health care costs because more women will be diagnosed with GDM and thus will require more visits, tests, and procedures than pregnant women who do not have this disease (ACOG, 2013/2015).

The OGTT is administered after an overnight fast and at least 3 days of unrestricted diet (at least 150 g of carbohydrate) and physical activity. The woman is instructed to avoid caffeine because it increases glucose levels and to abstain from smoking for 12 hours before the test. The 3-hour OGTT requires a fasting blood glucose level, which is drawn before giving a 100-g glucose load. Blood glucose levels are then drawn 1, 2, and 3 hours later. The woman is diagnosed with GDM if two or more values are met or exceeded (ACOG, 2013/2015). Two different sets of glucose values are commonly used to diagnose GDM following the 100-g OGTT (Fig. 11.5). At this time, use of one set of glucose values cannot be clearly recommended over the other. Therefore, providers are urged to select one set of blood glucose values and use it consistently in their practice (ACOG).

An international consensus group, the International Association of Diabetes and Pregnancy Study Groups (IADPSG), consisting of representatives from multiple obstetric and diabetic organizations including the ADA, recommends a different (one-step) method of screening and diagnosis. If the tests done early in pregnancy for preexisting diabetes are normal, a 75-g OGTT diagnostic test is administered between 24 and 28 weeks of gestation. The 75-g OGTT requires a fasting blood glucose level, which is drawn before giving the glucose load. Blood glucose levels are then drawn 1 and 2 hours later. A diagnosis of GDM is made if only one glucose value is exceeded (Fig. 11.6). The one-step method of screening and diagnosis significantly increases the incidence of GDM because the upper limit of normal for the blood glucose value at each sampling time is lower than in the two-step method. Therefore, more cases of GDM are diagnosed. Most practitioners in the United

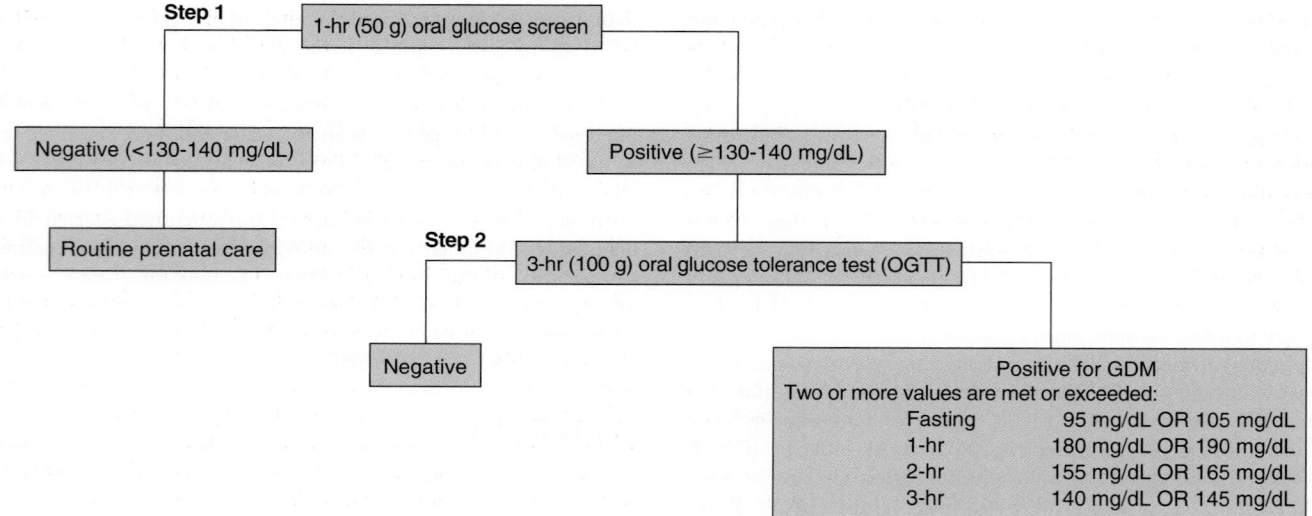

FIG 11.5 Two-step method for diagnosing gestational diabetes mellitus (GDM), recommended by the American College of Obstetricians and Gynecologists (ACOG). (Data from American College of Obstetricians and Gynecologists. [2013/2015]. *Practice bulletin no. 137: Gestational diabetes mellitus.* Washington, DC: American College of Obstetricians and Gynecologists.)

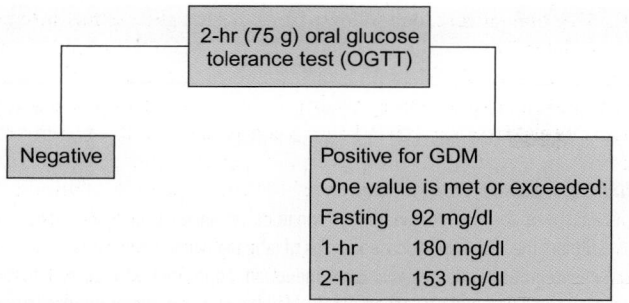

FIG 11.6 One-step method for diagnosing gestational diabetes mellitus (GDM), recommended by the International Association of Diabetes in Pregnancy Study Groups (IADPSG). (Data from American College of Obstetricians and Gynecologists. [2013/2015]. *Practice bulletin no. 137: Gestational diabetes mellitus*. Washington, DC: American College of Obstetricians and Gynecologists.)

States continue to use the two-step approach to screening for GDM. However, many countries in Europe and Asia, as well as some health care providers in the United States, have adopted the IADPSG recommendations for screening and diagnosing GDM (ADA, 2016a; Inturrisi, 2017; Landon et al., 2017) (see Evidence-Based Practice box).

Nursing diagnoses and expected outcomes of care for women with GDM are basically the same as those for women with pregestational diabetes. The time frame for planning may be shortened with GDM, however, because the diagnosis is made later in pregnancy (see Nursing Care Plan).

INTERVENTIONS

Antepartum

When the diagnosis of GDM is made, treatment begins immediately, allowing little or no time for the woman and her family to adjust to the diagnosis before they are expected to participate in the treatment plan. With each step of the treatment plan, the nurse and other health care providers should educate the woman and her family, providing detailed and comprehensive explanations to ensure understanding, participation, and adherence to the necessary interventions. Potential complications should be discussed, and the need for maintaining euglycemia throughout the remainder of the pregnancy reinforced. Knowing that GDM typically disappears when the pregnancy is over may be reassuring for the woman and her family.

As with pregestational diabetes, the aim of therapy in women with GDM is strict blood glucose control. Fasting blood glucose levels less than 95 mg/dL, 1-hour postmeal blood glucose levels less than 140 mg/dL, and 2-hour postmeal glucose levels less than 120 mg/dL are recommended (Landon et al., 2017). These levels are very similar to but not exactly the same as those recommended for women with preexisting diabetes (see Table 11.3).

Diet

Dietary modification is the mainstay of treatment for GDM. The woman with GDM is placed on a standard diabetic diet. The usual prescription is 2000 to 2500 kcal/day, which represents approximately 35 kcal/kg/day of present pregnancy weight. For overweight or obese women, a reduction to 25 kcal/kg/day and 15 kcal/kg/day (present pregnancy weight), respectively, may be advised. The usual carbohydrate intake is restricted to approximately 50% to 60% of caloric intake. However, some authorities believe that a diet containing this much carbohydrate will cause excessive weight gain and postmeal hyperglycemia, resulting

in a need for insulin therapy in 50% of women with GDM. Therefore, they recommend limiting carbohydrate intake to 33% to 40% of calories (Landon et al., 2017). Dietary counseling by a registered dietitian is recommended.

Exercise

There are few published studies on the benefits of exercise in women with GDM. In adults who are not pregnant, exercise increases lean muscle mass and improves sensitivity to insulin. Therefore, a moderate exercise program is recommended for overweight or obese women with GDM in order to improve blood sugar control and facilitate weight loss (ACOG, 2013/2015).

Monitoring of Blood Glucose

Blood glucose monitoring is necessary to determine whether euglycemia can be maintained by diet and exercise. The frequency and timing of blood glucose monitoring should be individualized for each woman. A typical schedule for monitoring blood glucose is on rising in the morning, 1 or 2 hours after breakfast, before and after lunch, before dinner, and at bedtime (Moore et al., 2014). Alternatively, women may be instructed to check a fasting blood glucose level and then continue to monitor their values 2 hours after each meal (Inturrisi, 2017; Landon et al., 2017). Women with GDM usually perform self-monitoring at home with a review of their results at prenatal visits to determine the effectiveness of diet and exercise. If glycemic thresholds are not met, then pharmacologic intervention is indicated.

Pharmacologic Therapy

Approximately 25% to 50% of women with GDM require insulin or oral medication during the pregnancy to maintain satisfactory blood glucose levels, despite compliance with the prescribed diet (Landon et al., 2017). If fasting plasma glucose levels are persistently greater than 95 mg/dL, 1-hour postmeal levels are persistently greater than 140 mg/dL, or 2-hour postmeal levels are persistently greater than 120 mg/dL, pharmacologic therapy is begun (ACOG, 2013/2015).

For over 1 decade, oral hypoglycemic therapy has been used as an alternative to insulin in women with GDM who require medication in addition to diet for blood glucose control. Women who are unable or unwilling to take insulin by injection or are cognitively impaired also may be candidates for oral hypoglycemic medication. Glyburide and metformin are both used for blood glucose control in women with GDM and both cross the placenta. While both appear to be safe for use during pregnancy, long-term studies are lacking, so the effects of glyburide and metformin over time on women with GDM and their children are unknown (ADA, 2016b; Daley, 2014).

Glyburide is the oral agent most frequently prescribed in the United States (Moore et al., 2014). Several studies have shown that glyburide controls blood glucose levels as well as insulin does in women with GDM. However, other studies found that glyburide appears to cross the placenta in significant amounts, and increased rates of neonatal hypoglycemia have been reported with its use. Glyburide may not work as well in women who are obese or who experienced higher levels of hyperglycemia early in pregnancy (Landon et al., 2017). Studies have shown that glyburide should be taken at least 30 minutes (preferably 1 hour) before a meal so its peak effect covers the 2-hour postmeal blood glucose level. Because episodes of hypoglycemia can occur between meals, women taking glyburide should always carry their glucose meter with them, along with glucose tablets or gel (Moore et al.).

Metformin is another oral hypoglycemic agent sometimes used in the management of GDM. Although metformin crosses the placenta, it does not appear to be teratogenic. However, glyburide may be better than metformin at controlling blood glucose levels in women with

EVIDENCE-BASED PRACTICE
Debating Gestational Diabetes Diagnosis

Ask the Question

PICOT Question: For pregnant women with hyperglycemia, at what level do diagnosis and treatment for gestational diabetes become most beneficial for the baby?

Search for the Evidence

Search Strategies: English language research-based publications since 2011 on gestational diabetes screening or diagnosis, hyperglycemia, ADA, ACOG, and NIH were included.

Databases Used: Cochrane Collaborative Database, National Guideline Clearinghouse (AHRQ), CINAHL, PubMed, UpToDate, and the professional websites for ACOG, ADA, and AWHONN

Toward a Diagnosis of Gestational Diabetes Mellitus
Background

- High serum glucose in pregnancy is associated with complications such as preeclampsia, macrosomia, operative vaginal birth, shoulder dystocia, birth injury, cesarean birth, neonatal hypoglycemia, need for neonatal intensive care, respiratory distress, and neonatal hyperbilirubinemia. A commonly accepted method of diagnosing gestational diabetes mellitus (GDM) has been a nonfasting glucose challenge test at 24–28 weeks of gestation (Moyer, 2014). For a 50-g glucose challenge test, the most common cutoff was 140 mg/dL, a level that was associated with macrosomia and gestational hypertension (Prutsky, Domecq, Sundaresh, et al., 2013). An elevated result triggered a fasting 2- or 3-hour oral glucose tolerance test (OGTT). A second abnormal result yielded a diagnosis of GDM. Using this approach, about 5% to 6% of pregnant women received treatment, including diet, exercise, glucose monitoring, and possibly oral hypoglycemic medication or insulin use..

Conflicting Guidelines

ACOG: In 2006, at least nine different criteria were used to identify gestational diabetes, using 50–100 g of glucose as the challenge. The American College of Obstetricians and Gynecologists' (ACOG) approach used two-step screening, clinical criteria, and history. Critics of this approach questioned its reliance on maternal, rather than newborn, outcomes; its acceptance of clinical criteria or history alone for diagnosis; and its ambiguous screening cutoffs (Ryan, 2013).

ADA: In 2008, the International Association of Diabetes in Pregnancy Study Group (IADPSG) set out to identify levels at which treatment would benefit the baby. They proposed a one-step approach, consisting of a 75-g OGTT. Abnormal levels were set based on their association with macrosomia and cord blood C-peptide, a marker for fetal insulin levels. One abnormal result was enough to trigger a diagnosis of GDM. This approach is estimated to

identify GDM in nearly 18% of all pregnant women. The American Diabetes Association (ADA) endorsed this approach (Ryan, 2013).

NIH Consensus Conference

- Criticism of the one-step approach includes reliance on just one abnormal result and the unintended consequences of labeling women with GDM: increase in cesarean birth and possibly labor induction, additional fetal assessments, more intensive newborn assessments, significantly increased patient costs, life disruptions, and psychologic stress. To resolve the differences between the ACOG and ADA approaches, the National Institutes of Health (NIH) convened a Consensus Conference. The NIH conference found some advantages for convenience of diagnosis within the context of one visit; however, there was insufficient evidence of clear improvement in patient outcomes to recommend the one-step approach. Therefore, the NIH group recommended continuing the current two-step approach and called for further targeted research (Vandorsten, Dodson, Espeland, et al., 2013).

Quality and Safety Competencies: Evidence-Based Practice*
Knowledge
Describe reliable sources for locating evidence reports and clinical practice guidelines.
The nurse working with pregnant women needs to understand evolving professional recommendations.

Skills
Locate evidence reports related to clinical practice topics and guidelines.
Relevant systematic reviews and professional guidelines provide recommendations for improving perinatal outcomes.

Attitudes
Value the concept of evidence-based practice as integral to determining best clinical practices.

References
Moyer, V. A. (2014). Screening for gestational diabetes mellitus: U.S. Preventive Services Task Force recommendation statement. *Annals of Internal Medicine, 160*(6), 414–420.
Ryan, E. A. (2013). Clinical diagnosis of gestational diabetes. *Clinical Obstetrics and Gynecology, 56*(4), 774–787.
Prutsky, G. J., Domecq, J. P., Sundaresh, V., et al. (2013). Screening for gestational diabetes: A systematic review and meta-analysis. *Journal of Clinical Endocrinology and Metabolism, 98*(11), 4311–4318.
Vandorsten, J. P., Dodson, W. C., Espeland, M. A., et al. (2013). NIH consensus development conference: Diagnosing gestational diabetes mellitus. *National Institutes of Health Consensus and State-of-the-Science Statements, 29*(1), 1–31.

Pat Mahaffee Gingrich

*EBP represents the best practice and its use fosters patient confidence and efficacy.

GDM because glyburide causes the maternal pancreas to produce more insulin, whereas metformin decreases hepatic glucose production and increases peripheral sensitivity to insulin (Daley, 2014; Landon et al., 2017).

Fetal Surveillance

Women with GDM whose blood glucose levels are well controlled by diet are at low risk for IUFD. Therefore, antepartum fetal testing is not performed routinely in these women unless they also have hypertension, a history of a prior stillbirth, or suspected macrosomia. Women with these complications or those who require insulin or oral hypoglycemic agents for blood glucose control may have twice-weekly fetal testing beginning at 32 weeks of gestation (Landon et al., 2017). In women

with excellent diet-controlled glucose levels and normal fetal growth, pregnancy may continue until 41 weeks of gestation. If the pregnancy extends beyond 40 weeks of gestation, twice-weekly fetal testing (NST and assessment of amniotic fluid volume) should be performed (Inturrisi, 2017). However, monitoring of fetal growth should be considered because of an apparent increasing risk for macrosomia as gestational age advances. In women whose glucose control is suboptimal, decisions regarding birth before 39 weeks of gestation should be individualized (Landon et al.).

Intrapartum

During the labor and birth process, blood glucose levels are monitored hourly to maintain levels at 80 to 110 mg/dL. Levels within this range

NURSING CARE PLAN

The Pregnant Woman With Gestational Diabetes

Case Study

Anijah is a 30-year-old African-American woman, gravida 2, para 1, in the 26th week of her second pregnancy. During her first pregnancy, 2 years ago, she had elevated blood glucose levels that she was able to control with diet. She did not lose the weight she gained during her first pregnancy and now is approximately 30 pounds over her ideal weight. She had a two-step screening for gestational diabetes last week. Her initial 1-hour glucola result was 150 mg/dL, which is a positive screen. This was followed 4 days later by a 3-hour (100 g) oral glucose tolerance test. Her obstetrician has diagnosed gestational diabetes, based on the results of her oral glucose tolerance test.

Assessment

What are the signs and symptoms of gestational diabetes mellitus (GDM)? At what stage in pregnancy should testing for GDM be done?

Defining Characteristics

Elevated blood sugar
Overweight woman

Nursing Diagnosis

Deficient Knowledge related to gestational diabetes as evidenced by the woman's questions and concerns.

Expected Outcomes

Anijah will be able to verbalize important information regarding gestational diabetes, its management, and potential effects on the pregnancy and fetus.
Anijah will follow a plan of care and maintain blood glucose levels within normal limits.

Nursing Interventions	Rationales
Address Anijah's current knowledge base regarding the disease process, management, effects on pregnancy and fetus, and potential complications.	To provide database for further teaching
Explain pathophysiologic aspects of gestational diabetes, effects on pregnancy and fetus, and potential complications.	To promote compliance with treatment plan
Explain principles of diabetic diet, and have Anijah plan her meals following these principles.	To promote self-management and compliance with treatment plan
Demonstrate procedure for blood glucose monitoring, and obtain return demonstration.	To establish Anijah's comfort and competence with procedure
Demonstrate procedure for insulin administration, should this become necessary, and obtain return demonstration.	To establish Anijah's comfort and competence with procedure
Explain importance of correctly taking oral hypoglycemic medication (right dose, right time), should this become necessary.	To promote self-management and compliance with treatment plan
Review signs and symptoms of hypoglycemia and hyperglycemia and appropriate interventions for both.	To promote prompt recognition of complications and self-management
Provide contact numbers for health care team for prompt interventions and answers to questions on ongoing basis.	To promote comfort and safety

Case Study (Continued)

Anijah is now in week 34 of her pregnancy. In speaking with her friends, she has become aware of some of the problems that can affect the fetus in a pregnancy complicated by diabetes. She has been reading about fetal anomalies and has become increasingly concerned about the status of her fetus. She said she is so worried that she is having trouble sleeping at night.

Assessment

What are the risks to the fetus in a pregnancy complicated by gestational diabetes?

Defining Characteristics

Elevated maternal glucose levels
Excessive maternal weight gain
Excessive fetal growth (macrosomia)

Nursing Diagnosis

Risk for Fetal Injury related to elevated maternal glucose levels

Expected Outcomes

The fetus will remain free from injury
The infant will be born at term in a healthy state.

Nursing Interventions	Rationales
Assess Anijah's current diabetic control.	To identify risk for fetal macrosomia
Monitor fundal height during each prenatal visit.	To identify appropriate fetal growth
Assess fetal movement and heart rate during each prenatal visit, and perform fetal assessment tests as ordered during third trimester.	To assess fetal well-being

Assessment

What are common concerns of women with GDM? What are the risks to the mother from elevated glucose levels? What are the risks to the fetus from elevated glucose levels?

Defining Characteristics

Expressed concerns due to changes in life status (diagnosis of GDM)
Irritability
Distress
Increased tension
Insomnia

Nursing Diagnosis

Anxiety related to threat to maternal and fetal well-being as evidenced by Anijah's verbal expressions of concern.

Expected Outcomes

Anijah will identify sources of anxiety and report feeling less anxious.
Anijah will be able to list risks associated with GDM and causes of problems.

Nursing Interventions	Rationales
Promote an open relationship with Anijah through therapeutic communication.	To promote trust
Listen to Anijah's feelings and concerns.	To assess for any misconceptions or misinformation that may be contributing to anxiety
Review potential dangers by providing factual information.	To correct any misconceptions or misinformation
Encourage Anijah to share her concerns with her health care team.	To promote collaboration in her care

decrease the incidence of neonatal hypoglycemia. Infusing rapid-acting insulin intravenously may be necessary during labor to maintain the desired blood glucose levels. However, it is usually possible to maintain excellent glucose control in women with GDM during labor by avoiding the use of IV fluids containing dextrose (Moore et al., 2014). If glucose-containing solutions are given, they should be administered by an infusion device so that inadvertent boluses are avoided. Although GDM is not an indication for cesarean birth, this procedure may be necessary in the presence of preeclampsia or macrosomia.

Postpartum

Although most women with GDM return to normal glucose levels after childbirth, up to one-third will be found to have diabetes or impaired glucose metabolism when they are screened postpartum. These women are also at high risk for recurrent GDM in future pregnancies (Landon et al., 2017). Additionally, women who had GDM have as high as a 60% chance of developing type 2 diabetes within 10 to 20 years. Children born to women with GDM are at risk for future health-related complications, as they may develop obesity and type 2 diabetes later in life (ADA, 2016b; Inturrisi, 2017).

ACOG recommends assessing all women who had GDM for carbohydrate intolerance with a 75-g, 2-hour OGTT or a fasting plasma glucose level at 6 to 12 weeks postpartum (Landon et al., 2017). The optimal frequency of subsequent testing has not been established. However, the ADA recommends lifelong repeat screening at least every 3 years for women with a history of GDM and normal postpartum glucose testing results. The exact frequency of screening depends on the presence of other risk factors, including family history, prepregnancy BMI, and need for insulin or oral hypoglycemic medication during pregnancy. This ongoing screening may be done using hemoglobin A1c, fasting plasma glucose, or 75-g 2-hour OGTT, using non-pregnant values (ADA, 2016b).

It is important to remember, however, that progression to type 2 diabetes is not inevitable. Women with a history of GDM who exercise, become less sedentary, and eat a healthy diet decrease their likelihood for developing type 2 diabetes in the future (Ortiz, Jimenez, Boursaw, et al., 2016).

Low-dose oral contraceptives may be safely used by women with a history of GDM. The rate of subsequent diabetes in these women is no different from that in women without a history of GDM who use low-dose oral contraceptives. Women who are also obese or have hypertension or high lipid levels in addition to a history of GDM should use a contraceptive method without the potential for causing cardiovascular side effects. For these women, the intrauterine device is a good option (Cunningham et al., 2014).

THYROID DISORDERS

HYPERTHYROIDISM

Hyperthyroidism in pregnancy is rare. The incidence varies, occurring in approximately 2 to 17 in 1000 births (Cunningham et al., 2014). In 90% to 95% of pregnant women, it is caused by Graves' disease. Clinical manifestations of hyperthyroidism include heat intolerance, diaphoresis, fatigue, anxiety, emotional lability, and tachycardia. Many of these symptoms also occur with pregnancy; thus the disorder can be difficult to diagnose. Signs that may help differentiate hyperthyroidism from normal pregnancy changes include weight loss, goiter, and a pulse rate greater than 100 beats/minute. Laboratory findings typically include elevated free thyroxine (T_4) and triiodothyronine (T_3) levels and greatly suppressed thyroid-stimulating hormone (TSH) levels (Nader, 2014). Moderate and severe hyperthyroidism must be treated during pregnancy.

Untreated or inadequately treated women have an increased risk for miscarriage, preterm birth, stillbirth, or giving birth to infants with goiter, hyperthyroidism, or hypothyroidism. However, most neonates born to women with hyperthyroidism have normal thyroid function. Women with hyperthyroidism are at increased risk for developing severe preeclampsia and heart failure (Cunningham et al.; Nader).

The primary treatment of hyperthyroidism during pregnancy is drug therapy. The medications most often prescribed in the United States are propylthiouracil (PTU) or methimazole (MMI). Both drugs are effective at controlling symptoms, but both have potentially dangerous maternal and fetal side effects. PTU can cause hepatic toxicity serious enough to require liver transplantation. When taken during the first trimester of pregnancy, MMI can cause choanal atresia or esophageal atresia, facial anomalies, hearing loss, developmental delay, and congenital cardiac malformations in exposed fetuses. Although the likelihood of maternal and fetal side effects from both drugs is low, a panel convened by the US Food and Drug Administration (FDA) and the American Thyroid Association recommended that PTU be used only in the first trimester of pregnancy. After the first trimester, women requiring drug therapy for hyperthyroidism should be switched to MMI for the remainder of pregnancy (Mestman, 2017).

The usual starting dose of PTU is 100 to 150 mg three times a day. For MMI, the initial dose is generally 20 mg/day. Women usually show clinical improvement (weight gain and less tachycardia) within 2 to 6 weeks after beginning therapy. Once clinical improvement occurs, the dose of PTU or MMI may be cut in half. If symptoms worsen, the medication dosage is doubled (Mestman, 2017). During therapy, thyroid test results are used to taper the drug to the smallest effective dose to prevent development of unnecessary fetal or neonatal hypothyroidism. In many women, the medication can be discontinued by 32 to 36 weeks of gestation. PTU readily crosses the placenta and may cause fetal hypothyroidism, which is characterized by goiter, bradycardia, and intrauterine growth restriction (IUGR) (Nader, 2014).

Both medications work well in and are well tolerated by most women. The most common maternal side effects of both PTU and MMI are pruritus and skin rash. Other possible side effects include drug-related fever, bronchospasm, migratory polyarthritis, a lupuslike syndrome, and cholestatic jaundice (Mestman, 2017; Nader, 2014). The most severe side effect is agranulocytosis, which occurs rarely and usually develops only in older women and in those taking high doses of the drug. Symptoms of agranulocytosis are fever and unexpected sore throat, which should be reported to the health care provider; and the woman should immediately stop taking the medication (Mestman; Nader). Beta-adrenergic blockers such as propranolol (Inderal) or atenolol (Tenormin) may be used in severe hyperthyroidism to control maternal symptoms, especially elevated heart rate. However, long-term use of these medications is not recommended because of the potential for IUGR, bradycardia, and hypoglycemia (Nader).

> **! NURSING ALERT**
>
> A serious but uncommon complication of undiagnosed or partially treated hyperthyroidism is thyroid storm, which can occur in response to stress such as labor and vaginal birth, infection, preeclampsia, or surgery. A woman with this emergency disorder may have fever, restlessness, tachycardia, vomiting, or stupor. Prompt treatment is essential. IV fluids and oxygen are administered, along with high doses of PTU. After administration of PTU, iodide is given. Other medications include antipyretics, dexamethasone, and beta blockers (Cunningham et al., 2014; Nader, 2014).

After birth, women taking either PTU or MMI who choose to breastfeed may do so, if their daily dose of PTU or MMI is less than 300 mg/day or 20 mg/day, respectively. Women should be informed that the medications do not appear to adversely affect the neonate's thyroid function. Antithyroid medication should be given in divided doses and taken just after breastfeeding, thus allowing a 3- to 4-hour period before nursing again (Mestman, 2017; Nader, 2014; Spencer, 2015).

Radioactive iodine must not be used in diagnosis or treatment of hyperthyroidism in pregnancy. The therapeutic doses given to treat maternal thyroid disease may also destroy the fetal thyroid gland (Cunningham et al., 2014).

In severe cases, surgical treatment of hyperthyroidism, subtotal thyroidectomy, can be performed during pregnancy. Surgery is best performed during the early second trimester of pregnancy when the risk for teratogenesis and preterm labor is lowest, although it can be done during the first or third trimester if necessary. Surgery is usually reserved for women with severe disease, those for whom drug therapy proves toxic, and those who are unable to follow the prescribed medical regimen. Risks associated with the surgery are hypoparathyroidism, recurrent laryngeal nerve paralysis, and anesthesia-related complications (Nader, 2014).

HYPOTHYROIDISM

Hypothyroidism occurs in 2 to 3 pregnancies per 1000. Because severe hypothyroidism is often associated with infertility and an increased risk for miscarriage, it is not often seen during pregnancy (Cunningham et al., 2014). Although iodine deficiency is rare in the United States, it is a common cause of maternal, fetal, and neonatal hypothyroidism in the rest of the world (Nader, 2014). Adult hypothyroidism is usually caused by glandular destruction by autoantibodies, most commonly because of Hashimoto's thyroiditis. Characteristic symptoms of hypothyroidism include weight gain, lethargy, decrease in exercise capacity, and cold intolerance. Women who are moderately symptomatic can also develop constipation, hoarseness, hair loss, brittle nails, and dry skin. Laboratory values in pregnancy include elevated levels of TSH, with or without low T_4 levels (Nader).

Pregnant women with untreated hypothyroidism are at increased risk for miscarriage, preeclampsia, gestational hypertension, placental abruption, preterm birth, and stillbirth. Infants born to mothers with hypothyroidism may also be of low birth weight (Cunningham et al., 2014; Nader, 2014). These outcomes can be improved with early treatment (Nader).

Thyroid hormone supplements are used to treat hypothyroidism. Levothyroxine (e.g., T_4 [Synthroid]) is most often prescribed during pregnancy. The usual beginning dosage is 0.1 to 0.15 mg/day, with adjustment by 25 to 50 mcg every 4 to 6 weeks as necessary based on the maternal TSH level (Cunningham et al., 2014; Nader, 2014). The aim of drug therapy is to maintain the TSH level at the lower end of the normal range for pregnant women. Women with little or no functioning thyroid tissue require higher doses of levothyroxine. In addition, as pregnancy progresses, increased doses of thyroid hormone are usually required. This increased demand during pregnancy is probably related to increased estrogen levels (Cunningham et al.; Nader).

Women with hypothyroidism will likely continue treatment with levothyroxine postpartum. This medication is considered safe for use while breastfeeding (Spencer, 2015).

🗸 MEDICATION ALERT

If taking iron supplementation, pregnant women should be told to take levothyroxine at a different time of day, at least 4 hours apart, from their iron tablets, because ferrous sulfate decreases absorption of T_4 (Nader, 2014).

The fetus depends on maternal thyroid hormones until approximately 18 weeks of gestation, when fetal production begins. Normal maternal T_4 levels early in pregnancy are important for proper fetal brain development. Results of two studies suggested that normalizing thyroid function by mid-pregnancy in women with hypothyroidism avoids neurodevelopmental deficits in their children (Mestman, 2017).

NURSING INTERVENTIONS

Education of the pregnant woman with thyroid dysfunction is essential to promote compliance with the plan of treatment. Important points to discuss with the woman and her family include the disorder and its potential effect on her, her fetus, and her family; the medication regimen and possible side effects; the need for continuing medical supervision; and the importance of compliance.

The woman often needs the nurse's help to cope with the discomforts and frustrations associated with symptoms of the disorder. For example, a woman with hyperthyroidism who has nervousness and hyperactivity along with weakness and fatigue can benefit from suggestions to channel excess energies into quiet diversional activities such as reading or crafts. Discomfort associated with hypersensitivity to heat (hyperthyroidism) or cold intolerance (hypothyroidism) can be minimized by appropriate clothing and regulation of environmental temperatures and by avoiding temperature extremes.

Nutrition counseling by a nurse or referral to a registered dietitian may provide guidance in selecting a well-balanced diet. The woman with hyperthyroidism who has increased appetite and poor weight gain and the hypothyroid woman who has anorexia and lethargy need counseling to ensure adequate intake of nutritionally sound foods to meet both maternal and fetal needs.

▋ MATERNAL PHENYLKETONURIA

Phenylketonuria (PKU), a recognized cause of cognitive impairment, is an inborn error of metabolism caused by an autosomal recessive trait that creates a deficiency in the enzyme phenylalanine hydrolase. Absence of this enzyme impairs the body's ability to metabolize the amino acid phenylalanine found in all protein foods. Consequently, toxic accumulation of phenylalanine in the blood occurs, which interferes with brain development and function. Individuals with this disorder also have hypopigmentation of hair, eyes, and skin because phenylalanine inhibits melanin production (Cunningham et al., 2014). The prevalence of PKU varies worldwide, but it is present in every racial and ethnic group. In the United States, PKU affects approximately 1 in 20,000 live births (Banta-Wright, Kodadek, Houck, et al., 2015).

PKU was the first inborn error of metabolism to be universally screened for in the United States. Since 1961, all newborns have been tested soon after birth for this disorder. Prompt diagnosis and therapy with a phenylalanine-restricted diet significantly decrease the incidence of cognitive impairment (Aminoff & Douglas, 2014). The special diet should be followed indefinitely because individuals who do not continue phenylalanine restriction have been reported to have significantly lower IQs (Cunningham et al., 2014).

The keys to the prevention of fetal anomalies caused by maternal PKU are the identification of women in their reproductive years with the disorder and dietary compliance for women who are diagnosed. Screening for undiagnosed homozygous maternal PKU at the first prenatal visit may be warranted, especially in individuals with a family history of the disorder, with low intelligence of uncertain origin, or who have given birth to microcephalic infants. Ideally women with PKU begin dietary phenylalanine restriction before conception and continue it throughout pregnancy (Aminoff & Douglas, 2014). (See

Chapter 25 for more information regarding the diet recommended for individuals with PKU.) Experts recommend that maternal phenylalanine levels be less than 6 mg/dL for at least 3 months before conception and range between 2 and 6 mg/dL throughout pregnancy. These levels are associated with a decrease in fetal sequelae (Cunningham et al., 2014). High maternal phenylalanine levels are associated with microcephaly, cognitive impairment, and congenital heart defects in their children (Aminoff & Douglas; Cunningham et al.).

Women with PKU should be advised against breastfeeding because their milk contains a high concentration of phenylalanine (Aminoff & Douglas, 2014). If these women choose to breastfeed despite the risk, their phenylalanine blood levels must be monitored closely. Breastfeeding infants diagnosed with PKU is challenging, but can usually be done safely if the mother does not also have PKU because human breast milk is a relatively low-phenylalanine food. If infants with PKU are breastfed, their blood phenylalanine levels are measured once or twice weekly and the dietary feeding plan is adjusted, based on the results. Infants are fed both breast milk and phenylalanine-free medical formula. If the infant's phenylalanine level is diminished, breastfeeding is increased. On the other hand, if the phenylalanine level is elevated, breastfeeding is decreased (Banta-Wright et al., 2015).

CARDIOVASCULAR DISORDERS

During a normal pregnancy, the maternal cardiovascular system undergoes many changes that place a physiologic strain on the heart (see Chapter 7). The major cardiovascular changes that occur during a normal pregnancy and affect the woman with cardiac disease are increased intravascular volume, decreased systemic vascular resistance, cardiac output changes occurring during labor and birth, and the intravascular volume changes that occur just after childbirth. These physiologic changes are present during pregnancy and continue for a few weeks after birth. The normal heart can compensate for the increased workload, so pregnancy, labor, and birth are generally well tolerated, but the diseased heart is hemodynamically challenged.

If the cardiovascular changes are not well tolerated, cardiac failure can develop during pregnancy, labor, or the postpartum period. In addition, if myocardial disease develops, valvular disease exists, or a congenital heart defect is present, *cardiac decompensation* (inability of the heart to maintain a sufficient cardiac output) may occur. Fever is the major cause of cardiac decompensation during pregnancy (Deen, Chandrasekaran, Stout, et al., 2017).

About 1% of pregnancies are complicated by serious heart disease. The risk for maternal morbidity and mortality ranges from low to high, depending on the cardiac defect (Roos-Hesselink, Ruys, & Johnson, 2013). The rates of congenital heart disease and mitral valve disease are increasing in women of childbearing age, whereas the incidence of rheumatic fever has diminished (Roos-Hesselink et al.). A perinatal mortality of up to 50% is anticipated with persistent cardiac decompensation. Box 11.2 lists maternal cardiac disease risk groups.

The degree of disability experienced by the woman with cardiac disease is often more important in the treatment and prognosis of cardiac disease complicating pregnancy than the diagnosis of cardiovascular disease. The New York Heart Association's (NYHA) functional classification of heart disease has been a widely accepted standard for many years:

- Class I: Asymptomatic without limitation of physical activity
- Class II: Symptomatic with slight limitation of activity
- Class III: Symptomatic with marked limitation of activity
- Class IV: Symptomatic with inability to carry on any physical activity without discomfort

No classification of heart disease can be considered rigid or absolute, but the NYHA classification offers a basic practical guide for treatment,

---

BOX 11.2   Maternal Cardiac Disease Risk Groups

Group I (Mortality Rate <1%)
- Atrial septal defect
- Ventricular septal defect (uncomplicated)
- Patent ductus arteriosus
- Pulmonic and tricuspid disease
- Biosynthetic valve prosthesis (porcine and human allograft)
- Tetralogy of Fallot (corrected)
- Mitral stenosis (New York Heart Association [NYHA] class I and II)

Group II (Mortality Rate 5%–15%)
- Mitral stenosis NYHA class III and IV or with atrial fibrillation
- Aortic stenosis
- Coarctation of aorta (uncomplicated)
- Uncorrected tetralogy of Fallot
- Previous myocardial infarction
- Marfan syndrome with normal aorta
- Artificial heart valve

Group III (Mortality Rate 25%–50%)
- Pulmonary hypertension
- Coarctation of the aorta (complicated)
- Endocarditis
- Marfan syndrome with aortic involvement
- Eisenmenger syndrome

Data from Gaddipati, S., & Troiano, N. (2013). Cardiac disorders in pregnancy. In N. Troiano, C. Harvey, & B. Chez (Eds.), *AWHONN's high risk and critical care obstetrics*, (3rd ed.). Philadelphia, PA: Wolters Kluwer/Lippincott Williams & Wilkins.

---

assuming that frequent prenatal visits, good patient cooperation, and appropriate obstetric care occur. The functional classification may change for the pregnant woman because of the hemodynamic changes that occur in the cardiovascular system during pregnancy. A 30% to 45% increase in cardiac output occurs compared with nonpregnancy resting values, with most of the increase in the first trimester and the peak at 20 to 26 weeks of gestation (Blanchard & Daniels, 2014). The functional classification of the disease is determined at 3 months and again at 7 or 8 months of gestation. Pregnant women may progress from class I or II to class III or IV during the pregnancy as cardiac output increases and more stress is placed on the heart. Women with cyanotic congenital heart disease do not fit into the NYHA classification because their exercise-induced symptoms have causes unrelated to heart failure.

A diagnosis of cardiac disease depends on the history, physical examination, radiographic and electrocardiographic findings, Holter monitoring, and, if indicated, ultrasonographic results. Most diagnostic studies are noninvasive and can be safely performed during pregnancy. The differential diagnosis of heart disease also involves ruling out respiratory problems and other potential causes of chest pain.

Pregnancy in a woman with heart disease is associated with increased risks for decompensation of maternal cardiac status and pregnancy complications, including maternal arrhythmias, heart failure, preterm birth, fetal growth restriction, and a small but significant risk for maternal and fetal death (Deen et al., 2017). The highest risk for complications or death occurs in women with pulmonary hypertension, complicated coarctation of the aorta, and Marfan syndrome with aortic involvement (Roos-Hesselink et al., 2013).

Cardiac diseases vary in their effect on pregnancy depending on whether they are acute or chronic conditions. The following discussion focuses on selected congenital and acquired cardiac conditions and other cardiac disorders. A review of the care of the pregnant woman who has had a heart transplant concludes this section.

CONGENITAL CARDIAC DISEASES

Septal Defects

Atrial Septal Defect

Atrial septal defect (ASD) is an abnormal opening between the atria. It is one of the causes of a left-to-right shunt and one of the most common congenital defects seen during pregnancy. This defect may go undetected because the woman is usually asymptomatic. The pregnant woman with an ASD usually has an uncomplicated pregnancy. However, some women may develop congestive heart failure or arrhythmias as the pregnancy progresses as a result of increased plasma volume. Another possible complication is the development of emboli (blood clots) (Gaddipati & Troiano, 2013).

Ventricular Septal Defect

Ventricular septal defect (VSD), an abnormal opening between the right and left ventricles, is another cause of a left-to-right shunt. It may occur as a single lesion or in combination with other cardiac anomalies such as tetralogy of Fallot. The defect is usually diagnosed and corrected early in life. As a result, a VSD is not very common in pregnancy. Women with small, uncomplicated VSDs usually do not have pregnancy complications. For women with a large VSD, there is a higher risk for congestive heart failure or pulmonary hypertension. Medical management includes administration of anticoagulants if indicated, along with rest and decreased physical activity (Gaddipati & Troiano, 2013).

Patent Ductus Arteriosus

Patent ductus arteriosus (PDA) is another cause of a left-to-right shunt that is usually diagnosed and corrected during infancy. Possible complications of a PDA include those of VSD as well as endocarditis and pulmonary emboli. Medical management is the same as for VSD (Blanchard & Daniels, 2014).

Acyanotic Lesions

Coarctation of the Aorta

Coarctation of the aorta is a localized narrowing of the aorta near the insertion of the ductus. Patients with this lesion have hypertension in their upper extremities but hypotension in the lower extremities. Coarctation of the aorta is an example of an acyanotic congenital heart lesion. If at all possible, the lesion should be corrected surgically before pregnancy (Blanchard & Daniels, 2014; Roos-Hesselink et al., 2013). However, pregnancy is usually relatively safe for the woman with uncomplicated, uncorrected coarctation. The maternal mortality rate is approximately 3% for uncorrected defects (Blanchard & Daniels). Complications include hypertension, heart failure, aortic dissection, rupture of associated cranial berry aneurysms and hemorrhagic stroke, ischemic heart disease associated with cephalic hypertension, and infective endocarditis (Blanchard & Daniels; Deen et al., 2017). The mainstays of treatment for uncorrected coarctation of the aorta during pregnancy are rest and antihypertensive medications, preferably beta-adrenergic–blocking agents. Vaginal birth is preferable, with epidural anesthesia and shortening of the second stage with vacuum extraction or use of forceps, if necessary. Beta blockers should be continued throughout labor. Because of the risk for endocarditis, antibiotic prophylaxis is recommended at birth (see later discussion).

Cyanotic Lesions

Tetralogy of Fallot

Tetralogy of Fallot is by far the most common cyanotic heart disease observed during pregnancy (Roos-Hesselink et al., 2013). Components of tetralogy of Fallot include a VSD, pulmonary stenosis, overriding aorta, and right ventricular hypertrophy, leading to a right-to-left shunt. Women with tetralogy of Fallot are encouraged to have surgical repair before conception because pregnancy does not cause a significant risk once the VSD and pulmonary stenosis have been repaired. On the other hand, women with uncorrected tetralogy of Fallot experience more right-to-left shunting during pregnancy, resulting in reduced blood flow through the pulmonary circulation and increasing hypoxemia, which can cause syncope or death (Gaddipati & Troiano, 2013). Maintenance of venous return in women with uncorrected tetralogy of Fallot is critical. Therefore, the most dangerous time for these women is the late third trimester of pregnancy and the early postpartum period, when venous return is reduced by the large pregnant uterus and peripheral venous pooling after birth. Use of pressure-graded support hose is recommended. Blood loss during birth may also adversely affect venous return; thus blood volume must be adequately maintained. Prophylactic antibiotics should be given during the intrapartum period (Blanchard & Daniels, 2014).

ACQUIRED CARDIAC DISEASES

Mitral Valve Prolapse

Mitral valve prolapse (MVP) is a fairly common, usually benign, condition. More specific echocardiographic diagnostic criteria have resulted in significantly reduced prevalence estimates for MVP (perhaps 1% of the female population) than previously thought (Blanchard & Daniels, 2014). In MVP, the mitral valve leaflets prolapse into the left atrium during ventricular systole, allowing some backflow of blood. Midsystolic click and late systolic murmur are hallmarks of this syndrome. Most cases are asymptomatic. A few women have atypical chest pain (sharp and located in the left side of the chest) that occurs at rest and does not respond to nitrates. They may also have anxiety, palpitations, dyspnea on exertion, and syncope. If women are symptomatic, beta-blocking drugs are given to relieve chest pain and palpitations and reduce the risk for life-threatening arrhythmias (Cunningham et al., 2014). If symptoms are unusually severe, thyroid function should also be checked (Blanchard & Daniels). Pregnancy and its associated hemodynamic changes may alter or alleviate the murmur and click of MVP, as well as symptoms. Antibiotic prophylaxis for bacterial endocarditis is no longer recommended for women with uncomplicated mitral valve prolapse. Pregnancy, labor, and birth are usually safe and well tolerated (Blanchard & Daniels; Cunningham et al.).

Mitral Stenosis

Mitral stenosis is almost always caused by rheumatic heart disease (RHD), a consequence of rheumatic fever (Deen et al., 2017). Rheumatic fever develops suddenly, often several symptom-free weeks after an inadequately treated group A beta-hemolytic streptococcal throat infection. Episodes of rheumatic fever create an autoimmune reaction in the heart tissue, leading to permanent damage of heart valves (usually the mitral valve) and the chordae tendineae cordis. This damage is classified as RHD. RHD may be evident during acute rheumatic fever or discovered years later. Recurrences of rheumatic fever are common, each with the potential to increase the severity of heart damage.

Mitral stenosis is a narrowing of the opening of the mitral valve caused by stiffening of valve leaflets, which obstructs blood flow from the atrium to the ventricle. As the mitral valve narrows, dyspnea worsens, occurring first on exertion and eventually at rest. A tight stenosis plus the increase in blood volume and cardiac output of normal pregnancy may cause pulmonary edema, atrial fibrillation, right-sided heart failure, infective endocarditis, pulmonary embolism, and massive hemoptysis (Blanchard & Daniels, 2014; Cunningham et al., 2014). Maternal mortality is related to functional capacity. Almost all maternal deaths related to mitral stenosis occur in women who are classified as NYHA class III or IV (Cunningham et al.).

Women with a history of RHD who are at risk for exposure to streptococcal infection should receive prophylaxis with daily oral penicillin G or monthly benzathine penicillin (Bicillin) injections. Pregnant women are usually considered at high risk for exposure because they generally live around groups of children (Deen et al., 2017). In addition, women with mitral stenosis may require a diuretic such as furosemide (Lasix) to prevent pulmonary edema and a beta blocker to reduce heart rate, improve diastolic blood flow across the valve, and relieve pulmonary congestion (Deen et al.). A combination of drugs will most likely be needed. Cardioversion may be needed for new-onset atrial fibrillation, a complication associated with mitral stenosis. Women who have chronic atrial fibrillation may require digoxin and beta blockers or calcium channel blockers to control the heart rate. In addition, anticoagulant therapy may be needed to prevent embolism (Blanchard & Daniels, 2014). About 25% of women with mitral valve stenosis experience cardiac failure for the first time during pregnancy (Cunningham et al., 2014).

Care of the woman with mitral stenosis typically is managed by reducing her activity, restricting dietary sodium, and monitoring weight. The pregnant woman with mitral stenosis should be assessed clinically for symptoms and with echocardiograms to monitor the atrial and ventricular size, as well as heart valve function. Prophylaxis for intrapartum endocarditis may be provided for women at high risk (Blanchard & Daniels, 2014; Deen et al., 2017).

During labor, adequate pain control is required to prevent tachycardia. Epidural analgesia for labor is preferred (Deen et al., 2017). Laboring and birthing in the side-lying position are desirable. The lithotomy position, with the woman supine and her feet in stirrups, will likely cause pulmonary edema (Blanchard & Daniels, 2014). Shortening the second stage of labor by vacuum- or forceps-assisted birth is also recommended to decrease the cardiac workload. Even with close monitoring, the woman with moderate to severe mitral stenosis is at risk for pulmonary edema and arrhythmias, the most commonly seen complications. Central hemodynamic monitoring may be necessary for some women during the intrapartum period (Deen et al.).

Medical management alone may not be adequate to control symptoms. For women with NYHA class III or IV cardiac disease, percutaneous balloon mitral valvuloplasty may be performed. Mitral balloon valvuloplasty is optimally performed after the first trimester to decrease radiation risks to the fetus. This relatively safe nonsurgical procedure is now performed more frequently during pregnancy than surgical valvotomy (Blanchard & Daniels, 2014). The balloon procedure is just as successful as surgical repair and is associated with less maternal and fetal morbidity and mortality (Cunningham et al., 2014).

Aortic Stenosis

Aortic stenosis is a narrowing of the opening of the aortic valve leading to an obstruction to left ventricular ejection. It is rarely encountered as a complication of pregnancy because most women who develop this condition do so after their childbearing years are over. In the past, the maternal mortality rate was reported to be as high as 17%, but it has decreased over the last several decades (Deen et al., 2017). Medical management is similar to that for mitral stenosis.

ISCHEMIC HEART DISEASE

Myocardial Infarction

Myocardial infarction (MI), an acute ischemic event, rarely occurs in women of childbearing age. It is estimated to occur in only 1 of 10,000

pregnancies (Blanchard & Daniels, 2014). However, experts anticipate that the incidence will rise, considering the number of women who delay childbearing until later in life (Gaddipati & Troiano, 2013). Frequently women with coronary artery disease have classic risk factors such as diabetes, hypertension, cigarette smoking, hyperlipidemia, and obesity (Cunningham et al., 2014). The cardiac changes that normally occur in a pregnant woman may provoke symptoms for the first time. It is also possible for women with a history of MI to become pregnant (Gaddipati & Troiano).

MI occurs most frequently in the last trimester of pregnancy and in women older than 33 years of age. The maternal mortality rate from an MI during pregnancy is approximately 20%. Women are most likely to die at the time of the infarction or during labor and birth (Blanchard & Daniels, 2014). The risk for maternal death increases if women give birth within 2 weeks of an MI (Deen et al., 2017).

Medical management for pregnant women with MI is the same as that for nonpregnant women and includes the administration of morphine, nitrates, lidocaine, beta blockers, aspirin, magnesium sulfate, and calcium antagonists. Coronary angioplasty and stenting procedures have been performed during pregnancy. These procedures should not be avoided if they are considered to be appropriate for treating the woman (Deen et al., 2017). Thrombolytic agents such as urokinase, streptokinase, and tissue plasminogen activator (tPA) do not appear to cross the placenta. However, their use is considered to be relatively contraindicated in pregnancy because of the risk for subsequent maternal and fetal hemorrhage (Gaddipati & Troiano, 2013). Because pain can lead to tachycardia and increased cardiac demands, pain control during labor, usually accomplished with regional anesthesia, is crucial. The side-lying position is preferred to prevent pressure on the vena cava. Vaginal birth is preferable, with avoidance of maternal pushing and a vacuum- or forceps-assisted birth (Deen et al.).

OTHER CARDIAC DISEASES AND CONDITIONS

Primary Pulmonary Hypertension

Women with primary pulmonary hypertension (PPH) have constriction of the arteriolar vessels in the lungs, leading to an increase in the pulmonary artery pressure. As a result of this pathology, there is right ventricular hypertension, right ventricular hypertrophy and dilation, and right ventricular failure with tricuspid regurgitation and systemic congestion. The major physiologic difficulty in PPH is maintaining blood flow to the lungs. Any event that significantly decreases venous return to the heart, such as hypotension, impairs the ability of the right ventricle to pump blood through the pulmonary vessels with their high, fixed vascular resistance. Because hypotension can occur quickly and is often unresponsive to medical therapy, it must be avoided at all costs (Blanchard & Daniels, 2014).

Symptoms may be nonspecific, such as fatigue and shortness of breath. Dyspnea on exertion is the most common symptom (Cunningham et al., 2014).

PPH is diagnosed by electrocardiography. Although cardiac catheterization remains the standard procedure for measuring pulmonary artery pressures, noninvasive echocardiography is often used to provide an estimate of these pressures (Cunningham et al., 2014). Mortality rates reported during pregnancy are as high as 50%, so pregnancy is not advised in women with this condition (Blanchard & Daniels, 2014). The most dangerous times for women with PPH are the intrapartum and early postpartum periods because of increases in cardiac output and fluid shifts (Roos-Hesselink et al., 2013).

Medical management of women with PPH during pregnancy includes limiting activity and avoiding supine positioning (Roos-Hesselink et al., 2013). Diuretics, supplemental oxygen, and vasodilator medications also will be ordered. During labor and birth, hypotension must be avoided by carefully establishing epidural analgesia and preventing blood loss (Cunningham et al., 2014).

Peripartum Cardiomyopathy

Peripartum cardiomyopathy (PCM) is congestive heart failure with cardiomyopathy. The classic criteria for the diagnosis of PCM include development of congestive heart failure in the last month of pregnancy or within the first 5 postpartum months, absence of heart disease before the last month of pregnancy, a left ventricular ejection fraction (EF) of less than 45%, and, most important, lack of another cause for heart failure. The cause of the disease is unknown. The incidence in the United States is 1 in 3000 to 4000 live births (Blanchard & Daniels, 2014).

Associated risk factors include maternal age older than 30 years, multiparity, African descent, obesity, tocolytic use, preeclampsia, and chronic hypertension. Clinical findings are those of congestive heart failure (left ventricular failure). Clinical manifestations include dyspnea, fatigue, edema, and radiologic findings of cardiomegaly (Gaddipati & Troiano, 2013).

Medical management of PCM includes a regimen used for congestive heart failure: diuretics, sodium and fluid restriction, afterload-reducing agents, and digoxin. Beta blockers have been shown to improve cardiac function and the chance of survival. Anticoagulation may be necessary if the cardiac chambers are significantly dilated and contract poorly because of the increased risk for clot formation. Angiotensin-converting enzyme inhibitors, often prescribed to achieve afterload reduction, can be used only in the postpartum period because they are associated with fetal renal dysfunction. During labor, epidural anesthesia is often used for pain control to reduce tachycardia and decrease the cardiac workload. Cesarean birth should be performed only for obstetric indications (Deen et al., 2017).

In one-half of all women with PCM, left ventricular dysfunction resolves within 6 months. These women generally do well. However, if left ventricular dysfunction does not resolve within 6 months, approximately 85% of women with PCM will die in the next 4 to 5 years. Death is usually the result of progressive congestive heart failure, arrhythmia, or thromboembolism (Deen et al., 2017). The recurrence rate for cardiomyopathy in a subsequent pregnancy is high—anywhere from 20% to 50%. The risk for recurrence is increased in women who did not have complete recovery of left ventricular function after the initial episode of PCM (Blanchard & Daniels, 2014).

Infective Endocarditis

Infective endocarditis is inflammation of the innermost lining—the endocardium—of the heart, caused by invasion of microorganisms. In the United States, women at greatest risk for developing infective endocarditis are those who have congenital heart lesions, degenerative valve disease, or intracardiac devices or who use drugs intravenously (Cunningham et al., 2014). Bacterial endocarditis, leading to incompetence of heart valves and thus congestive heart failure and cerebral emboli, can result in death. Treatment is with antibiotics. Prophylactic treatment with antibiotics is used only for women at highest risk for this condition.

Eisenmenger Syndrome

Eisenmenger syndrome is caused by a congenital communication between the systemic and pulmonary circulations and elevated pulmonary vascular resistance, which can result in right-to-left shunting. It is associated with an underlying structural cardiac defect, either a VSD (most common) or a patent ductus arteriosus (Blanchard & Daniels, 2014). Eisenmenger syndrome is associated with high mortality (50% in mothers and 50% in fetuses). Because of the poor pregnancy outcomes, pregnancy should be avoided by women with the syndrome. Termination (therapeutic abortion) may be recommended if pregnancy occurs (Gaddipati & Troiano, 2013). Although sudden death can occur at any time, the intrapartum period and especially the early postpartum period seem to be the most dangerous (Blanchard & Daniels). Maternal morbidity is associated with right ventricular failure and associated cardiogenic shock (Cunningham et al., 2014).

In women who continue pregnancy despite the risks, management includes measures to maintain pulmonary blood flow. Physical activity is strictly limited. Other interventions include the use of pressure-graded elastic support hose and oxygen therapy. Antepartal hospitalization may be necessary to provide optimal care (Blanchard & Daniels, 2014; Deen et al., 2017). During labor and birth, regional anesthesia using an opioid analgesic provides pain relief without causing excessive hemodynamic instability. Hypotension must be prevented at all costs because it results in more right-to-left shunting. A pulmonary artery catheter and a peripheral arterial catheter may be used to guide hemodynamic management. Cesarean birth should be performed only for obstetric indications and avoided whenever possible (Deen et al.).

Marfan Syndrome

Marfan syndrome is an autosomal dominant disorder characterized by generalized weakness of the connective tissue, resulting in the characteristic feature of the disease, aortic root dilation. Other signs and symptoms associated with Marfan syndrome include dislocation of the optic lens, deformity of the anterior thorax, scoliosis, long limbs, joint laxity, and arachnodactyly. Diagnosis is usually based on family history and physical examination, including ocular, cardiovascular, and skeletal features (Deen et al., 2017).

The majority of deaths from Marfan syndrome are caused by aortic dissection and rupture. Overall the maternal mortality rate associated with Marfan syndrome is greater than 50%. However, it is significantly increased if the aortic root diameter measures more than 4 cm (Deen et al., 2017).

Preconception counseling for women with Marfan syndrome is essential to make them aware of the risks of pregnancy with this disease. Because the condition is inherited, each child born to a woman with Marfan syndrome has a 50% chance of having the disorder (Gaddipati & Troiano, 2013). An accurate assessment of the aortic root must be obtained to assess the woman's specific risk and make management recommendations. Elective repair of the aorta prior to pregnancy is recommended when the aortic root diameter measures 4.0 cm or more. On the other hand, women with an aortic root diameter less than 4 cm can attempt pregnancy with only modest risk (Deen et al., 2017).

Management during pregnancy includes restricted activity and use of beta blockers to maintain a resting heart rate of approximately 70 beats/minute. Tachycardia should also be prevented during labor. Women with aortic root diameters less than 4 cm may give birth vaginally, reserving cesarean birth for obstetric indications. Some authorities believe that women with larger aortic root diameters should give birth by elective cesarean because of concerns about increased pressure in the aorta during labor. However, data do not exist to make this a firm recommendation (Deen et al., 2017).

Valve Replacement

Pregnant women with mechanical or bioprosthetic heart valves require specialized care for this high-risk situation. The primary medical management, anticoagulation, is both controversial and complicated. A high risk for thromboembolism exists because of the hypercoagulability of pregnancy. At the same time, the use of anticoagulants during pregnancy presents the possibility of maternal and fetal hemorrhage. Some oral anticoagulants pose a significant risk to the fetus for abnormalities and intracranial hemorrhage. However, prosthetic heart valve thrombosis is a life-threatening emergency during pregnancy and requires clot removal surgery, which carries a high mortality rate (Roos-Hesselink et al., 2013).

Women with bioprosthetic heart valves usually do not require anticoagulation during pregnancy. This type of valve may be used in women of childbearing age, because it has a relatively low rate of complications during pregnancy. However, bioprosthetic valves are not as durable as mechanical valves. In addition, pregnancy accelerates the deterioration of bioprosthetic valves (Deen et al., 2017).

Anticoagulation is required with a mechanical valve. Management of anticoagulation during pregnancy is quite controversial because commonly used medications have significant maternal and fetal adverse effects, and no single agent is safe for use throughout the entire prenatal period. Often low-molecular-weight heparin (Lovenox) is used during the first trimester. In the second and third trimesters, warfarin (Coumadin) may be used instead. If Lovenox is used during the second and third trimesters, it should be discontinued several weeks before the anticipated date of birth and the woman started on heparin. Anticoagulation therapy should be discontinued during labor and resumed in the postpartum period. Warfarin is generally used for long-term postpartum anticoagulation. Warfarin is safe for use in breastfeeding women (Deen, et al., 2017).

Heart Transplantation

Increasing numbers of heart recipients are successfully completing pregnancies. It is recommended that pregnancy be avoided for at least 1 year after the transplant because by that time the risk for acute rejection and the intensity of immunosuppression are considerably less (Blanchard & Daniels, 2014). Before conception, the woman should be assessed for quality of ventricular function and potential rejection of the transplant. Additionally, she should be stabilized on her immunosuppressant regimen. Women who have no evidence of rejection and have normal cardiac function at the beginning of the pregnancy appear to do well during pregnancy, labor, and birth. Research has shown that the transplanted heart responds normally to pregnancy-related changes. Complications that are common in women who have had a heart transplant include hypertension and at least one episode of rejection (Cunningham et al., 2014).

CARE MANAGEMENT

The presence of cardiac disease is a significant influencing factor in the decision-making process for or against becoming pregnant. Couples planning a pregnancy must understand the risks involved in their situation. If the pregnancy is unplanned, the nurse should explore the couple's desire to continue it in light of the risks involved. Pregnancy termination is one option, depending on the severity of the cardiac defect. The family may need further information to make an informed decision regarding the future of the pregnancy.

ASSESSMENT AND NURSING DIAGNOSIS

The pregnant woman with a cardiac disorder is in a high-risk situation. She requires careful assessment throughout the peripartum period to determine the potential for optimal maternal health and a viable fetus. Her care will be provided by an interprofessional health care team, including a cardiologist, obstetrician, perinatologist, and registered nurse experienced in the care of women with high-risk pregnancies. If she chooses to continue the pregnancy, the woman's condition may be assessed as often as weekly. For additional information on cardiac disease, visit the American Heart Association website at www.americanheart.org.

Potential nursing diagnoses for a woman with a cardiac disorder include the following:
- *Fear* related to
  - increased peripartum risk
- *Risk for Ineffective Coping/Compromised Family Coping* related to
  - woman's cardiac condition
  - changes in role performance
- *Ineffective Peripheral Tissue Perfusion* related to
  - hypotensive syndrome
- *Activity Intolerance* related to
  - cardiac condition
- *Deficient Knowledge* related to
  - cardiac condition
  - pregnancy and how it affects cardiac condition
  - medication dosages and possible side effects
  - requirements to alter self-care activities
- *Self-Care Deficit* (bathing, dressing, toileting) related to
  - fatigue or activity intolerance
  - need for bed rest
- *Impaired Home Maintenance* related to
  - woman's confinement to bed and/or limited activity level

INTERVENTIONS

Antepartum

Therapy for the pregnant woman with heart disease is focused on minimizing stress on the heart, which intensifies as cardiac output increases. Cardiac output begins to rise significantly early in pregnancy and probably peaks somewhere between 25 and 30 weeks of gestation (Antony, Racusin, Aagaard, et al., 2017). Factors that increase the risk for cardiac decompensation are avoided. The workload of the cardiovascular system is reduced by appropriate treatment of any coexisting emotional stress, hypertension, anemia, hyperthyroidism, or obesity.

Signs and symptoms of cardiac decompensation are taught at the first prenatal visit and reviewed at each subsequent visit (Box 11.3 and Patient Teaching Box: The Pregnant Woman at Risk for Cardiac Decompensation).

BOX 11.3   Signs of Potential Complications: Cardiac Decompensation

Pregnant Woman: Subjective Symptoms
- Increasing fatigue or difficulty breathing, or both, with her usual activities
- Feeling of smothering
- Frequent cough
- Palpitations; feeling that her heart is "racing"
- Generalized edema: Swelling of face, feet, legs, fingers (e.g., rings no longer fit)

Nurse: Objective Signs
- Irregular, weak, rapid pulse (≥100 beats/min)
- Progressive, generalized edema
- Crackles at base of lungs after two inspirations and exhalations that do not clear after coughing
- Orthopnea; increasing dyspnea
- Rapid respirations (≥25 breaths/min)
- Moist, frequent cough
- Cyanosis of lips and nail beds

PATIENT TEACHING

The Pregnant Woman at Risk for Cardiac Decompensation

Instruct the woman to do the following:
- Watch for and immediately report signs of cardiac decompensation or congestive heart failure: generalized edema; distention of neck veins; dyspnea; frequent, moist cough; or palpitations.
- Watch for and immediately report signs of thromboembolism: pain, redness, tenderness, or swelling in extremities or chest pain.
- Avoid constipation and thus straining with bowel movements (Valsalva maneuver) by taking in adequate fluids and fiber. A stool softener may also be helpful.

Teach the importance of the following:
- Daily weighing. Sudden weight gain indicates fluid retention.
- Keeping all prenatal visit appointments, although they will be scheduled more frequently than for "normal" pregnant women.
- Limiting activity (depending on classification of her heart disease). Patients with class I or II cardiac disease need 10 hours of sleep every night and 30 minutes of rest after meals. Patients with class III or IV cardiac disease usually need bed rest for most of each day.

Adapted from Gilbert, E.S. (2011). *Manual of high risk pregnancy and delivery.* (5th ed.). St. Louis, MO: Mosby.

Infections are treated promptly because they can complicate the condition by accelerating the heart rate and by direct spread of organisms (e.g., streptococci) to the heart structure. Infections are a major cause of cardiac decompensation during pregnancy. Bacteriuria screens should be performed. The woman should be instructed to notify her health care provider at the first sign of an upper respiratory infection, especially if fever is present. Vaccination against influenza and pneumococci are appropriate (Deen et al., 2017).

Many women with heart disease, especially adolescents, recent immigrants, and those living in poverty, are at risk for iron deficiency anemia. Iron and folate supplementation may help to prevent anemia, and thus decrease cardiac workload (Deen et al., 2017).

Nutrition counseling is necessary, optimally with the woman's family present. The pregnant woman needs a well-balanced diet with iron and folic acid supplementation, high protein levels, and adequate calories to gain weight. Iron supplements tend to cause constipation; thus the woman should increase her intake of fluids and fiber. A stool softener may also be prescribed. It is important that the woman with a cardiac disorder avoid straining during defecation, thus causing the Valsalva maneuver (forced expiration against a closed airway, which when released, causes blood to rush to the heart and overload the cardiac system). Sodium restriction may be necessary. The woman's intake of potassium may be monitored to prevent hypokalemia, especially if she is taking diuretics. Depending on the specific cardiac condition, some women may be limited in their total daily fluid intake. A referral to a registered dietitian may be necessary for a nutritional plan of care.

Cardiac medications are prescribed as needed, with attention to fetal well-being. The hemodynamic changes that occur during pregnancy, such as increased plasma volume and increased renal clearance of drugs, can alter the amount of medication needed to establish and maintain a therapeutic drug level. Therefore, monitoring drug levels during pregnancy is crucial to maintain effective therapy for the woman while minimizing risk to the fetus.

Anticoagulant therapy may be prescribed during pregnancy for several conditions such as recurrent venous thrombosis, pulmonary embolus, rheumatic heart disease, prosthetic valves, or cyanotic congenital heart defects. If anticoagulant therapy is required during pregnancy, several different medications may be recommended (see the section on valve disorders for more discussion of anticoagulant therapy). The woman may need to learn to self-administer injectable agents such as heparin or low-molecular-weight heparin (Lovenox). A woman taking warfarin requires specific nutritional teaching to avoid foods high in vitamin K, such as raw, dark green leafy vegetables, which counteract the effects of warfarin. In addition, she will require a folic acid supplement.

Tests for fetal maturity and well-being and placental sufficiency may be necessary. Other therapy is directly related to the functional classification of heart disease. The nurse must reinforce the need for close medical supervision.

Heart Surgery During Pregnancy

Ideally surgery to correct a cardiac lesion should be performed prior to pregnancy. In some women, however, cardiac disease is diagnosed for the first time during pregnancy. The maternal mortality risk does not increase, but there is a fetal mortality risk of 10% to 15% if heart surgery is performed, especially if cardiopulmonary bypass is used. If possible, surgery should be postponed until the third trimester of pregnancy, when the risk to the fetus is considerably decreased (Blanchard & Daniels, 2014).

Intrapartum

For all pregnant women, the intrapartum period is the one that evokes the most apprehension in patients and caregivers. The woman with impaired cardiac function has additional reasons to be anxious because labor and giving birth place an additional burden on her already compromised cardiovascular system.

Assessments include the routine assessments for all laboring women and those for cardiac decompensation. In addition, arterial blood gases (ABGs) may be needed to assess for adequate oxygenation. A pulmonary artery catheter may be inserted to monitor hemodynamic status accurately during labor and birth. Electrocardiography (ECG) monitoring and continuous monitoring of blood pressure and oxygen saturation (pulse oximetry) are usually instituted for the woman, and continuous electronic fetal heart rate monitoring is used to monitor the fetus.

! NURSING ALERT

A pulse rate of 100 beats/minute or greater or a respiratory rate of 25 breaths/minute or greater is a concern. The nurse checks the respiratory status frequently for developing dyspnea, coughing, or crackles at the base of the lungs. The color and temperature of the skin are noted, as well. Pale, cool, clammy skin may indicate cardiac shock.

Nursing care during labor and birth focuses on promoting cardiac function. A calm atmosphere in the labor and birth rooms helps to minimize anxiety. The nurse provides anticipatory guidance by keeping the woman and her family informed of labor progress and events that can occur, as well as answering any questions. It is important to support the woman's childbirth preparation method and birth plan to the degree that it is feasible for her cardiac condition. Nursing interventions that promote comfort, such as back massage, are also used.

Cardiac function is supported by keeping the woman's head and shoulders elevated and body parts resting on pillows. The side-lying position usually facilitates positive hemodynamics during labor. Discomfort is relieved with medication and supportive care. Physiologically the ideal labor for a woman with heart disease is one that is short and pain free. Therefore, use of epidural analgesia is encouraged, although care must be taken to avoid hypotension, a common side effect of regional anesthesia (Deen et al., 2017; Gaddipati & Troiano, 2013).

Beta-adrenergic agents such as terbutaline (Brethine) are associated with various side effects, including tachycardia, irregular pulse, myocardial ischemia, and pulmonary edema. Therefore these medications should not be used in women with known or suspected heart disease (Simhan, Berghella, & Iams, 2014; Simhan, Iams, & Romero, 2017).

Spontaneous or induced (with a favorable cervix) labor followed by vaginal birth is preferred for women with cardiac disease. If no obstetric problems exist, vaginal birth may be accomplished with the woman in the side-lying position to facilitate uterine perfusion. The supine position should be avoided. If it is used, a pad or small wedge is placed under one hip to displace the uterus laterally and minimize the danger of supine hypotension. The woman can flex her knees and place her feet flat on the bed. The use of stirrups is contraindicated because stirrups can compress the popliteal veins, therby increasing the blood volume in the chest and trunk as a result of the effects of gravity. Open-glottis pushing is recommended. The woman should avoid the Valsalva maneuver when pushing in the second stage of labor because it reduces diastolic ventricular filling and obstructs left ventricular outflow. Mask oxygen is important. Episiotomy and vacuum extraction or outlet forceps are often used to decrease the length of the second stage of labor and the heart's workload at that time. Cesarean birth is not routinely recommended for women who have cardiovascular disease because of the risks of dramatic fluid shifts, sustained hemodynamic changes, and increased blood loss.

Routine intrapartum antibiotic prophylaxis for the prevention of bacterial endocarditis is not recommended by the American Heart Association, but it is optional in high-risk patients who give birth vaginally. Because bacteremia is common during both vaginal and cesarean birth, many practitioners routinely give antibiotic prophylaxis to all high-risk patients. Ampicillin (vancomycin for women who are allergic to penicillin) and gentamicin are the medications recommended for prophylaxis (Deen et al., 2017; Gaddipati & Troiano, 2013). Oxytocin is usually given immediately after birth to prevent hemorrhage. Ergot products (e.g., methylergonovine [Methergine]) should not be used because they increase blood pressure. Fluid balance should be maintained, and blood loss replaced. If tubal sterilization is desired, it is best to delay surgery until the woman is hemodynamically near normal, afebrile, nonanemic, and able to ambulate normally (Cunningham et al., 2014).

Postpartum

Monitoring for cardiac decompensation in the postpartum period is essential. The first 24 to 48 hours after birth are the most hemodynamically difficult for the woman. Hemorrhage or infection or both may worsen the cardiac condition. The woman with a cardiac disorder may continue to require a pulmonary artery catheter and ABG monitoring after giving birth.

SAFETY ALERT

The immediate postbirth period is hazardous for a woman whose heart function is compromised. Cardiac output increases rapidly as extravascular fluid is remobilized into the vascular compartment. At the moment of birth, intraabdominal pressure is reduced drastically; pressure on veins is removed, the splanchnic vessels engorge, and blood flow to the heart is increased.

Care in the postpartum period is tailored to the woman's functional capacity. Postpartum assessment of the woman with cardiac disease includes vital signs, oxygen saturation levels, lung and heart auscultation, presence and degree of edema, amount and character of bleeding, uterine tone and fundal height, urinary output, pain (especially chest pain), the activity-rest pattern, dietary intake, mother-infant interactions, and emotional state. The head of the bed is elevated, and the woman is encouraged to lie on her side. Bed rest may be ordered, with or without bathroom privileges. Progressive ambulation may be permitted as tolerated. The nurse or family members may need to help the woman with her grooming and hygiene needs and other activities. Bowel movements without stress or strain are promoted with stool softeners, diet, and fluids.

The woman may need a family member to help care for the infant. Breastfeeding is not contraindicated, but some women with heart disease (particularly those with life-threatening disease) may be unable to breastfeed. The woman who chooses to breastfeed will need the support of her family and the nursing staff to be successful. For example, she may need assistance in positioning herself or the infant for feeding. Lactation consultants can assist women with breastfeeding positions and other strategies to minimize stress on the cardiovascular system. To further conserve the woman's energy, the infant can be brought to her and taken from her after the feeding. Most medications used to manage cardiac disorders are compatible with breastfeeding. However, diuretics such as furosemide and hydrocholorothiazide may decrease the milk supply (Blanchard & Daniels, 2014; Spencer, 2015). Because diuretics can cause neonatal diuresis that can lead to dehydration, lactating women must be monitored closely to determine if medication doses can be reduced and still be effective. Neonatal nurses should be alerted to watch for voiding patterns and amounts and to monitor the infant closely for signs of dehydration.

If the woman is unable to breastfeed and her energies do not allow her to bottle-feed the infant, the baby can be kept at the bedside so she can look at and touch her baby to establish an emotional bond with a low expenditure of energy. The infant should be held at the mother's eye level and near her lips and brought to her fingers. Assisting the mother to hold her baby skin-to-skin can promote maternal-infant bonding. At the same time, involving the mother passively in her infant's care helps her feel vitally important—as she is—to the infant's well-being (e.g., "You can offer something no one else can; you can provide your baby with your sounds, touch, and rhythms that are so comforting"). Perhaps the woman can be encouraged to make a recording of her talking, singing, or whispering, which can be played for the baby in the nursery to help the infant feel her presence and be in contact with her voice. This also enhances maternal-infant bonding.

Preparation for discharge is planned carefully with the woman and family. Provision of help for the woman in the home by relatives, friends, and others must be addressed. If necessary, the nurse or social worker refers the family to community resources (e.g., for assistance with household activities). Rest and sleep periods, activity, and diet must be planned. The couple may need information about reestablishing sexual relations and contraception or sterilization.

Women with congenital heart disease should be offered contraceptive counseling. In general, the complications associated with pregnancy are usually greater than the risks associated with any form of contraception (Deen et al., 2017). Women at particular risk for thromboembolism should avoid combined estrogen-progestin oral contraceptives, but progestin-only pills may be used. Parenteral progestins (e.g., medroxyprogesterone [Depo-Provera]) are safe for use by women with cardiac disease and are extremely effective. However, they cause irregular bleeding, which may be problematic for women on anticoagulant therapy. An intrauterine device (IUD) may be used by some women with congenital heart lesions (Deen et al.).

Monitoring for cardiac decompensation continues after birth. During the first 2 postpartum weeks, extravascular fluid is mobilized, diuresis begins, and vascular resistance increases, as the woman returns to a nonpregnant state (Deen et al., 2017). Women who have demonstrated little or no evidence of cardiac compromise during the antepartum or intrapartum period may do so postpartum when intravascular fluid mobilization and reduction of peripheral vascular resistance place higher demands on the heart (Cunningham et al., 2014). Maternal cardiac output usually returns to normal by 2 weeks postpartum (Deen et al.).

Men and women with congenital heart disease are at increased risk for having children who also have congenital heart disease. The risk for affected mothers is greater, approximately two to more than three times that of affected fathers. Children born with congenital heart disease to parents with congenital heart defects appear to inherit the risk for a defect in general rather than for a specific defect (Deen et al., 2017). Therefore, preconception counseling and genetic counseling before a subsequent pregnancy are essential.

OTHER MEDICAL DISORDERS IN PREGNANCY

ANEMIA

Anemia is a common medical disorder of pregnancy, affecting from 20% to 52% of pregnant women (Kilpatrick, 2014). It results in a reduction of the oxygen-carrying capacity of the blood; thus the heart tries to compensate by increasing the cardiac output. This effort increases the workload of the heart and stresses ventricular function. Therefore, anemia that occurs with any other complication (e.g., preeclampsia) may result in congestive heart failure.

An indirect index of the oxygen-carrying capacity is the packed red blood cell (RBC) volume, or hematocrit level. The normal hematocrit range in nonpregnant women is 37% to 47%. However, normal values for pregnant women with adequate iron stores may be as low as 33%. According to the Centers for Disease Control and Prevention (CDC), anemia in pregnancy is defined as hemoglobin less than 11 g/dL in the first and third trimesters and less than 10.5 g/dL in the second trimester (Kilpatrick, 2014). A hemoglobin level less than 6 to 8 mg/dL is considered severe anemia (Blackburn, 2013).

When a woman has anemia during pregnancy, the loss of blood at birth, even if minimal, is not well tolerated. She has an increased risk for requiring blood transfusions. Women with anemia have a higher incidence of postpartum complications such as infection than postpartum women with normal hematologic values.

Care of the anemic pregnant woman requires that the health care provider distinguish between the normal physiologic anemia of pregnancy and disease states. The majority of cases of anemia in pregnancy are caused by iron deficiency. The other types include a considerable variety of acquired and hereditary anemias such as folic acid deficiency, sickle cell anemia, and thalassemia.

Iron Deficiency Anemia

Iron deficiency anemia is by far the most common anemia of pregnancy, accounting for approximately 75% of cases. In developing countries, it is alarmingly common and is a major cause of maternal morbidity and mortality. It is diagnosed by checking the woman's serum ferritin level in addition to her hemoglobin and hematocrit levels. The serum ferritin level reflects iron reserves (Samuels, 2017). Serum ferritin levels below 12 mcg/L along with a low hemoglobin level indicate iron deficiency anemia (Blackburn, 2013). An association appears to exist between maternal iron deficiency anemia, especially severe anemia, and preterm birth and low-birth-weight infants, although it is uncertain whether these poor pregnancy outcomes are caused by iron deficiency anemia (Samuels). Usually even the fetus of an anemic woman receives adequate iron stores from the mother at the cost of further depleting the mother's iron level (Blackburn).

Generally iron deficiency anemia is preventable or easily treated with iron supplements. Because of the increased amounts of iron needed for fetal development and maternal stores, pregnant women are often encouraged to take prophylactic iron supplementation (Blackburn, 2013). Most women with iron deficiency anemia can absorb as much iron as they need by taking one 325-mg tablet of ferrous sulfate twice each day (Samuels, 2017). Some pregnant women cannot tolerate the prescribed oral iron because of nausea and vomiting associated with the pregnancy and as a side effect of iron therapy. Women who cannot or will not take oral iron therapy but are not anemic enough to require blood transfusion may receive parenteral iron therapy (e.g., iron dextran, iron sucrose [Venofer], or sodium ferric gluconate complex). These medications can be given either intravenously or intramuscularly, although the intramuscular injection is very painful. Women who are severely anemic may require blood transfusions (Samuels).

The nurse teaches the importance of iron supplements for preventing or treating iron deficiency anemia. In addition, the nurse teaches about increasing dietary intake of iron-rich foods and how to decrease the gastrointestinal side effects of iron therapy (see Patient Teaching box: Iron Supplementation in Chapter 9).

Folic Acid Deficiency Anemia

Folate is a water-soluble vitamin found naturally in dark green leafy vegetables, citrus fruits, eggs, legumes, and whole grains. Even in well-nourished women, folate deficiency is common. Poor diet, cooking with large volumes of water, and increased alcohol use may contribute to folate deficiency. During pregnancy, the need for folate increases, both because of fetal demands and because it is less well absorbed from the gastrointestinal tract during gestation.

Folic acid is the form of the vitamin used in vitamin supplements. The recommended daily intake of folic acid for nonpregnant women is 400 mcg. Pregnant women need 50% more, or 600 mcg/day (March of Dimes, 2017). Since 1998, the FDA has required the addition of folic acid to cereals, pasta, breads, and other foods that are labeled "enriched." However, the amount added is small, and most pregnant women need a supplement. Both prescription and nonprescription prenatal vitamins contain more than the recommended daily intake of folic acid and should be sufficient to prevent and treat folate deficiency. Women at particular risk for folate deficiency include those who have significant hemoglobinopathies, take an anticonvulsant medication, are pregnant with a multifetal gestation, or have frequent pregnancies. These women require larger than usual doses of folic acid (Samuels, 2017).

Folate deficiency is the most common cause of megaloblastic anemia during pregnancy, but a vitamin B_{12} deficiency must also be considered. Vitamin B_{12} deficiency in pregnant women is seen much more often now than in the past because of the increasing numbers of women who become pregnant after undergoing bariatric surgery. Other women at risk for developing vitamin B_{12} deficiency are those with gastrointestinal disease such as Crohn disease or who take the medication metformin (Samuels, 2017).

Megaloblastic anemia rarely occurs before the third trimester of pregnancy (Kilpatrick, 2014; Samuels, 2017). Women with megaloblastic anemia caused by folic acid deficiency have the usual presenting symptoms and signs of anemia: pallor, fatigue, and lethargy, as well as glossitis and skin roughness, which are associated specifically with megaloblastic anemia (Kilpatrick). Folate deficiency usually improves rapidly with folic acid therapy. It rarely occurs in the fetus and is not a significant cause of perinatal morbidity. Iron deficiency often occurs along with folate deficiency (Samuels).

Sickle Cell Hemoglobinopathy

Sickle cell hemoglobinopathy is a disease caused by the presence of abnormal hemoglobin in the blood. Sickle cell trait (SA hemoglobin pattern) is sickling of the RBCs but with a normal RBC life span. Most people with sickle cell trait are asymptomatic. Approximately 1 in 12 African-American adults in the United States have sickle cell trait (Samuels, 2017). Women with sickle cell trait require partner testing and genetic counseling to determine their risk for producing children with sickle cell trait or disease.

Women with sickle cell trait usually do well in pregnancy. However, they are at increased risk for preeclampsia, intrauterine fetal death, preterm birth and low-birth-weight infants, and postpartum endometritis. They are also at increased risk for UTIs and may be deficient in iron (Kilpatrick, 2014; Samuels, 2017).

Sickle cell anemia (sickle cell disease) is a recessive, hereditary, familial hemolytic anemia that affects people of African or Mediterranean ancestry. These individuals usually have abnormal hemoglobin types (SS or SC). The average life span of RBCs in a person with sickle cell anemia is only 5 to 10 days compared to the 120-day life span of a normal RBC. Sickle cell anemia occurs in 1 in 708 African-Americans in the United States (Samuels, 2017). People with sickle cell anemia have recurrent attacks (crises) of fever and pain, most often in the abdomen, joints, or extremities, although virtually all organ systems can be affected. These attacks are attributed to vascular occlusion when RBCs assume a characteristic sickled shape. Crises are usually triggered by dehydration, hypoxia, or acidosis (Samuels).

Women with sickle cell anemia require genetic counseling before pregnancy. All children born to a woman with sickle cell anemia will be affected in some way by the disease. The woman's partner must be tested to determine the couple's risk for producing children with sickle cell disease rather than sickle cell trait. Women with sickle cell anemia are at risk for poor pregnancy outcomes, including miscarriage, preterm birth, IUGR, and stillbirth. Although maternal mortality is rare, maternal morbidity is significant and includes an increased risk for preeclampsia and infection, particularly in the urinary tract and the lungs. The frequency of painful crises also appears to be increased during pregnancy (Samuels, 2017) (see Clinical Reasoning Case Study).

CLINICAL REASONING CASE STUDY

Sickle Cell Hemoglobinopathy

Latasha is a 23-year-old G1 P0 with sickle cell anemia who is hospitalized with a crisis at 16 weeks of gestation. Latasha says, "I've been in and out of the hospital all my life because of my sickle cell disease. I sure hope my baby won't have this disease!"

1. Evidence—Is there sufficient evidence to counsel Latasha regarding her baby's chance of having sickle cell disease?
2. Assumptions—Describe an underlying assumption about each of the following issues:
   a. The chance that Latasha's baby will inherit either sickle cell trait or sickle cell disease
   b. Pregnancy risks related to sickle cell disease
3. What implications and priorities for nursing care can be drawn at this time?
4. Does the evidence objectively support your argument (conclusion)?
5. Interprofessional care—Describe the roles/responsibilities of health care professionals who might be involved in Latasha's care.

Folic acid supplementation of at least 1 mg/day should begin as soon as pregnancy is diagnosed. The woman is monitored carefully during pregnancy for the development of UTI or preeclampsia. In addition, she has serial ultrasound examinations to monitor fetal growth and will likely have antepartum fetal testing performed regularly during the third trimester because of her increased risk for stillbirth. Infections are treated aggressively with antibiotics. If crises occur, they are managed with analgesia, oxygen, and hydration. Prophylactic transfusions, which replace the woman's sickle cells with normal RBCs, have not been shown to improve perinatal outcome. However, although there is no difference in perinatal morbidity or mortality, prophylactic transfusions appear to significantly decrease the incidence of painful crises (Samuels, 2017).

⚡ SAFETY ALERT

Women with sickle cell anemia are not iron deficient. Therefore routine iron supplementation, even that found in prenatal vitamins, should be avoided because these women can develop iron overload (Samuels, 2017).

If no complications occur, pregnancy can continue until term. Women with sickle cell disease should be encouraged to labor in a side-lying position. They may require supplemental oxygen. Adequate hydration should be maintained while preventing fluid overload. Regional anesthesia (e.g., epidural or combined spinal epidural anesthesia) is recommended because it provides excellent pain relief. Vaginal birth is preferred. Cesarean birth should be performed only for obstetric indications (Samuels, 2017).

Thalassemia

Thalassemia is a relatively common anemia in which an insufficient amount of hemoglobin is produced to fill the RBCs. It is a hereditary disorder that involves the abnormal synthesis of the alpha or beta chains of hemoglobin. Beta thalassemia is the more common variety in the United States and usually occurs in people of Mediterranean, North African, Middle Eastern, and Asian descent (Kilpatrick, 2014).

Beta thalassemia minor is the heterozygous form of thalassemia and has different forms of expression. Some women with this disorder are asymptomatic, while others have splenomegaly and significant anemia. They may require numerous transfusions during pregnancy (Samuels, 2017). Women with pregnancies complicated by beta thalassemia minor generally do not experience associated maternal or infant complications if their condition is stable (Blackburn, 2013). These women are managed similarly to women with sickle cell anemia during pregnancy. Iron therapy should only be prescribed for women who are iron deficient, although folic acid supplementation is recommended for all women with beta thalassemia minor (Samuels).

The homozygous form of beta thalassemia is thalassemia major, formerly called *Cooley's anemia*. People with this form of the disease usually have hepatosplenomegaly and bone deformities caused by massive marrow tissue expansion. These individuals usually die of infection or cardiovascular complications fairly early in life. If women live to reach childbearing age, infertility is common. If women with this disorder do become pregnant, they usually experience severe anemia and congestive heart failure, although successful full-term pregnancies have been reported. Women with beta thalassemia major are managed much like those with sickle cell anemia during pregnancy (Samuels, 2017).

PULMONARY DISORDERS

As pregnancy advances and the enlarged uterus presses on the thoracic cavity, any pregnant woman may experience increased respiratory difficulty. This difficulty is compounded by pulmonary disease.

Asthma

Asthma is a chronic inflammatory disorder involving the tracheobronchial airways, with increased airway responsiveness to a variety of stimuli. It is characterized by periods of exacerbations and remissions. Exacerbations are triggered by stimuli such as allergens, medications (i.e., aspirin, beta blockers), marked change in ambient temperature, or emotional tension. In many cases, the actual cause may be unknown, although a family history of allergy is common in people with asthma. In response to stimuli, there is widespread but reversible narrowing of the hyperreactive airways, making it difficult to breathe. The clinical manifestations are expiratory wheezing, productive cough, thick sputum, dyspnea, or any combination.

Asthma may be the most common potentially serious medical condition to complicate pregnancy. It affects approximately 4% to 8% of all pregnancies. The prevalence and morbidity rates are increasing, although the asthma-related mortality has dropped in recent years (Whitty & Dombrowski, 2014).

The effect of pregnancy on asthma is unpredictable. In one large study, 23% of women with asthma improved during pregnancy, whereas 30% became worse. Pregnant women with severe asthma were much more likely than those with mild or moderate asthma to have exacerbations and require hospitalization. Asthma appears to be associated with preterm birth, preeclampsia, small for gestational age fetuses, IUGR, and an increased rate of cesarean birth (Whitty & Dombrowski, 2014). While poorly controlled asthma greatly increases pregnancy risk, well-controlled asthma does not appear to adversely affect pregnancy (Mason & Dorman, 2013).

The ultimate goal of asthma therapy in pregnancy is maintaining adequate oxygenation of the fetus by preventing hypoxic episodes in the mother. Achieving this goal requires monitoring lung function objectively (e.g., peak expiratory flow rate and forced expiratory volume in one second), avoiding or controlling asthma triggers (e.g., dust mites, animal dander, pollen, wood smoke), educating women about the importance of controlling asthma during pregnancy, and drug therapy (Whitty & Dombrowski, 2017). Current drug therapy for asthma emphasizes treatment of airway inflammation to decrease airway hyperresponsiveness and prevent asthma symptoms. Decreasing airway inflammation with inhaled corticosteroids is the preferred treatment for managing persistent asthma during pregnancy (Mason & Dorman, 2013; Whitty & Dombrowski, 2014).

During pregnancy, women with poorly controlled asthma may benefit from ultrasound examinations and antenatal testing. Because asthma has been associated with IUGR and preterm birth, accurate pregnancy dating should be established by a first-trimester ultrasound if possible. Evaluation of fetal growth by serial ultrasound examinations may be considered for women who have suboptimally controlled asthma or moderate to severe asthma (beginning at 32 weeks of gestation) and after recovery from a severe asthma exacerbation. All women with asthma should be encouraged to monitor fetal activity (see Chapter 10 for information on daily fetal movement counts) (Whitty & Dombrowski, 2014). Acute exacerbations are managed with albuterol, inhaled ipratropium bromide (Atrovent), systemic corticosteroids, beta-adrenergic agents, and oxygen. Women with severe exacerbations unresponsive to treatment may require intubation and mechanical ventilation (Whitty & Dombrowski, 2017).

Although asthma attacks during labor are rare, medications for asthma are continued during labor and the postpartum period. Women who are currently taking or have received several short courses of systemic corticosteroids during pregnancy should be given stress doses of corticosteroids during labor and for the first 24 hours after birth to prevent adrenal crisis (Whitty & Dombrowski, 2017). Pulse oximetry should be instituted during labor. Epidural anesthesia reduces oxygen consumption and minute ventilation and is recommended for pain relief. Fentanyl (Sublimaze) or butorphanol (Stadol) are safer choices for systemic analgesia than morphine and meperidine (Demerol), which can cause histamine release. If tocolytic medications are necessary, indomethacin (Indocin) should be avoided because it might induce bronchospasm in aspirin-sensitive patients (Whitty & Dombrowski, 2017).

During the postpartum period women who have asthma are at increased risk for hemorrhage. If excessive bleeding occurs, prostaglandin (PGE1 or PGE2) can be given, although the patient's respiratory status should be monitored. Because carboprost (15-methyl PGF2α [Hemabate]) and ergonovine and methylergonovine (Methergine) can cause bronchospasm, their use should be avoided (Whitty & Dombrowski, 2017). In general, only small amounts of asthma medications enter breast milk; therefore their use is not considered a contraindication to breastfeeding. However, in sensitive neonates theophylline in breast milk can cause vomiting, feeding difficulties, jitteriness, and cardiac arrhythmias (Whitty & Dombrowski, 2017). The woman usually returns to her prepregnancy asthma status within 3 months after giving birth.

Cystic Fibrosis

Cystic fibrosis (CF) is a common autosomal recessive genetic disorder in which the exocrine glands produce excessive viscous secretions, which causes problems with both respiratory and digestive functions. Most people with CF have chronic obstructive pulmonary disease, pancreatic exocrine insufficiency, and elevated levels of sweat electrolytes. Morbidity and mortality are usually caused by progressive chronic bronchial pulmonary disease (Whitty & Dombrowski, 2014).

Because the gene for CF was identified in 1989, data can be collected for the purpose of genetic counseling for couples regarding carrier status. In the United States, approximately 4% of the Caucasian population are carriers of the CF gene. CF occurs in 1 in 3000 Caucasian live births. People with CF live longer than in the past because of earlier diagnosis and intervention, along with advances in antibiotic therapy and nutritional support. More than 45% of all individuals in the United States with CF are older than 18 years of age. Men tend to live a little longer (median age of survival is 29.6 years) compared with women, whose median age of survival is 27.3 years. Although most men with CF are infertile, women with the disease are often fertile. The number of women with CF who achieve pregnancy is steadily increasing (Whitty & Dombrowski, 2017).

In women with mild CF, good prepregnancy nutritional status, and less impairment of lung function, pregnancy is tolerated well (Whitty & Dombrowski, 2017). In women with severe disease, the pregnancy is often complicated by chronic hypoxemia and frequent pulmonary infections. Risk factors that may predict a poor pregnancy outcome are poor prepregnancy nutritional status, significant pulmonary disease with hypoxemia, pulmonary hypertension, liver disease, and diabetes mellitus. The incidence of preterm birth, IUGR, and uteroplacental insufficiency is increased (Whitty & Dombrowski, 2014).

Care of the pregnant woman with cystic fibrosis requires an interprofessional health team effort. Ideally the woman should lose or gain (she usually needs to gain) weight to reach 90% of her ideal body weight before becoming pregnant. A weight gain of 11 to 12 kg (24 to 26 lbs) is recommended during pregnancy. Women who are unable to achieve the recommended weight gain through oral supplements may require nasogastric tube feedings at night (Whitty & Dombrowski, 2017). Pancreatic insufficiency may put the woman at risk for malnutrition because she cannot meet the increased nutritional requirements of pregnancy. If malnutrition is severe, parenteral hyperalimentation may be necessary. Fat-soluble vitamins may not be well absorbed, resulting in deficiency in those nutrients. Throughout pregnancy, frequent monitoring of the woman's weight, blood glucose, hemoglobin, total protein, serum albumin, prothrombin time, and fat-soluble vitamins A and E is suggested. Pancreatic enzymes should be adjusted as necessary (Whitty and Dombrowski, 2014).

Women with cystic fibrosis are followed closely with serial pulmonary function testing. Test results are used both to guide management and to predict pregnancy outcome. Inhaled recombinant human deoxyribonuclease I may be given to improve lung function by decreasing sputum viscosity. Inhaled 7% saline also produces both short- and long-term benefits (Cunningham et al., 2014). Early detection and treatment of infection are critical. Management of infection includes IV antibiotics along with chest physical therapy and bronchial drainage (Whitty & Dombrowski, 2017).

Fetal assessment is essential, given that the fetus is at risk for uteroplacental insufficiency and IUGR. Maternal nutritional status and weight gain during pregnancy significantly affect fetal growth. Fundal height should be measured routinely, and ultrasound examinations performed to evaluate fetal growth and amniotic fluid volume. Fetal movement counts are often recommended, starting at 28 weeks of gestation. NSTs should be initiated at 32 weeks of gestation or sooner if evidence of fetal compromise exists (see Chapter 10 for more information on fetal assessment tests) (Whitty & Dombrowski, 2017).

During labor, increased cardiac output stresses the cardiovascular system and can lead to cardiopulmonary failure in the woman with pulmonary hypertension or cor pulmonale. These women are also more likely to develop right-sided heart failure. Epidural or local analgesia is the preferred analgesic for birth, with vaginal birth recommended. Cesarean birth should be reserved for obstetric indications. If general anesthesia is needed for cesarean birth, anticholinergic medications should not be given before surgery because they tend to promote airway drying (Whitty & Dombrowski, 2017).

Mothers with pulmonary and pancreatic disease can breastfeed, and their infants do well. It is appropriate, however to test milk samples occasionally for sodium, chloride, and total fat, and to monitor the infant's growth pattern carefully (Lawrence & Lawrence, 2016).

INTEGUMENTARY DISORDERS

Dermatologic disorders induced by pregnancy include melasma (chloasma), vascular "spiders," palmar erythema, and striae gravidarum (see Chapter 7). A number of chronic skin disorders may complicate pregnancy. These disorders may be present prior to pregnancy or appear for the first time during pregnancy. The course of these disorders varies during pregnancy. Acne, for example, may improve. Psoriasis is unpredictable during pregnancy, but postpartum flares are common. Lesions from neurofibromatosis may increase in size and number during pregnancy (Cunningham et al., 2014). Explanation, reassurance, and commonsense measures should suffice for normal skin changes. In contrast, disease processes during and soon after pregnancy may be extremely difficult to diagnose and treat.

> ⚡ **SAFETY ALERT**
>
> Isotretinoin (Accutane), commonly prescribed for cystic acne, is highly teratogenic. There is a risk for craniofacial, cardiac, and CNS malformations in exposed fetuses. This drug should not be taken during pregnancy.

Pruritus Gravidarum

Pruritus is a major symptom in several pregnancy-related skin diseases. Pruritus gravidarum, generalized itching without the presence of a rash, develops in up to 14% of pregnant women. It is often limited to the

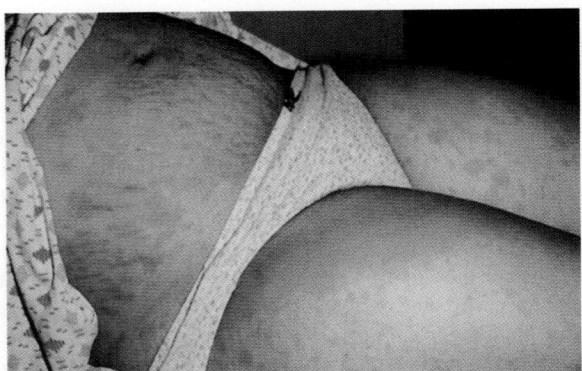

FIG 11.7 Pruritic urticarial papules and plaques of pregnancy (PUPPP). Lesions commonly begin in the abdominal striae. Confluent, erythematous urticarial papules and plaques are seen on the thighs in this woman. (From Creasy, R.K., Resnik, R., Iams, J.D., et al. [Eds.]. [2014]. *Creasy and Resnik's maternal-fetal medicine: Principles and practice*, 7th ed. Philadelphia, PA: Saunders.)

abdomen and is usually caused by skin distention and development of striae. Pruritus gravidarum is associated with twin gestation, fertility treatment, diabetes, and nulliparity. It is not associated with poor perinatal outcomes. It is treated symptomatically with skin lubrication, topical antipruritics, and oral antihistamines. Ultraviolet light and careful exposure to sunlight decrease itching. Pruritus gravidarum usually disappears shortly after birth but can recur in approximately one-half of all subsequent pregnancies (Rapini, 2014).

Pruritic Urticarial Papules and Plaques of Pregnancy

Another common pregnancy-specific cause of pruritus is pruritic urticarial papules and plaques of pregnancy (PUPPP) (Fig. 11.7), also known as *polymorphic eruption of pregnancy*. PUPPP classically appears in primigravidas during the mid to late third trimester and occurs slightly more often in women carrying male fetuses. The lesions usually appear first on the abdomen but can spread to the arms, thighs, back, and buttocks. PUPPP almost always causes pruritus, and the itching is severe in 80% of cases. It is associated with increased maternal weight gain, an increased rate of twin gestation, hypertension, and induction of labor. It is not, however, associated with poor maternal or fetal outcomes. Therefore, the goal of therapy is simply to relieve maternal discomfort. Antipruritic topical medications, topical steroids, and oral antihistamines usually provide relief. Women with severe symptoms may require oral prednisone. PUPPP usually resolves before birth or within several weeks after birth. It rarely persists or begins after birth. PUPPP does not usually recur in subsequent pregnancies (Rapini, 2014; Wang & Kroumpouzos, 2017).

Intrahepatic Cholestasis of Pregnancy

Intrahepatic cholestasis of pregnancy (ICP) is the most common liver disease of pregnancy (Gabzdyl & Schlaeger, 2015). It is characterized by generalized pruritus that usually begins in the third trimester of pregnancy. The itching commonly affects the palms and soles but can occur on any part of the body and is usually worse at night. No skin lesions are present. Women with ICP have elevated serum bile acids and elevated liver function tests. Jaundice may be present. Up to one-half of women with ICP develop dark urine and light-colored stools. The cause of ICP is unknown, but approximately one-half of women have a family history of the disorder. ICP occurs more frequently during the winter months. A geographic variance in the prevalence of the disease also exists. ICP occurs most often in Southeast Asia, Chile, Bolivia, and Scandinavia, although it is seen less frequently now in Chile and in

Scandinavia than in the past (Cappell, 2017; Williamson, Mackillop, & Heneghan, 2014).

Treatment consists of giving ursodeoxycholic acid, which effectively controls the pruritus and laboratory abnormalities associated with ICP, and continued monitoring of liver function tests and bile acid levels (Cappell, 2017; Williamson et al., 2014) Antihistamines such as diphenhydramine (Benadryl) or chlorpheniramine (Chlor-Trimeton) may be prescribed. Other comfort measures that may provide relief from itching include cool baths, oatmeal products added to a bath, oatmeal cream or lotion, baking soda baths, or an aqueous cream containing 2% menthol (Gabzdyl & Schlaeger, 2015).

The major fetal complications associated with ICP are asphyxial events, meconium staining, meconium ileus, stillbirth, and preterm birth. The cause of these complications is likely related to increased levels of fetal serum bile acids (Cappell, 2017; Williamson et al., 2014). Antepartum fetal assessment with twice-weekly NSTs will probably be performed (Cappell).

As long as fetal assessment test results remain reassuring, birth at approximately 37 weeks of gestation should be considered. Symptoms usually disappear and laboratory abnormalities resolve soon after giving birth (Cappell, 2017). ICP can recur in approximately two-thirds of subsequent pregnancies, however, or with oral contraceptive use (Cappell; Gabzdyl & Schlaeger, 2015).

NEUROLOGIC DISORDERS

The pregnant woman with a neurologic disorder must deal with potential teratogenic effects of prescribed medications, changes of mobility during pregnancy, and impaired ability to care for the baby. The nurse should be aware of all medications the woman is taking and the associated potential for producing congenital anomalies. As the pregnancy progresses, the woman's center of gravity shifts and causes balance and gait changes. The nurse should advise the woman of these expected changes and suggest safety measures as appropriate. Family and community resources may be needed to assist in providing infant care for the neurologically impaired woman.

Epilepsy

Epilepsy (often called *seizure disorder*) is a disorder of the brain that causes recurrent seizures and is the most common major neurologic disorder accompanying pregnancy. Less than 1% of all pregnant women have a seizure disorder (Aminoff & Douglas, 2014). Seizure disorders are divided into *generalized* and *focal* epilepsies. Focal epilepsy is the most common type of epilepsy in adults. The cause of most focal epilepsies remains unknown (Gerard & Samuels, 2017). Two studies found that women with epilepsy are much more likely to die during the perinatal period than are women who do not have epilepsy. However, through comprehensive care by an interprofessional health care team that includes an obstetrician, neurologist, pharmacist, nurse, and social worker, most women with a seizure disorder can have a successful pregnancy with minimal risk to mother and fetus (Gerard & Samuels).

Women with epilepsy should receive preconception counseling if at all possible. A detailed history of medication use and seizure frequency should be obtained. If the woman has frequent seizures before conception, she is likely to continue this pattern during pregnancy; therefore achieving effective seizure control is extremely important before conception. In most cases, she should be encouraged to delay pregnancy until better seizure control is established (Gerard & Samuels, 2017).

Infants born to women taking anticonvulsant medications have an increased incidence of congenital anomalies, including cleft lip and palate, congenital heart disease, neural tube defects (NTDs) and hypospadias. These anomalies are often related to the dose, type, and number of medications taken, not to epilepsy itself (Gerard & Samuels, 2017).

> ⚡ **SAFETY ALERT**
>
> Valproate (Depakote) should be avoided if possible during pregnancy because its use is associated with major congenital malformations, as well as adverse cognitive outcomes, including lower IQ and an increased risk for autism (Gerard & Samuels, 2017).

Several anticonvulsant medications have been developed for use during the past 2 decades. Lamotrigine (Lamictal) and levetiracetam (Keppra) are now the most commonly prescribed antiepileptic medications for women of childbearing age. Both appear to have relatively low major malformation rates associated with their use. More research is needed, however, regarding the fetal effects of these medications. Carbamazepine (Tegretol) is also a reasonable choice for use in women who plan to conceive, although its use is declining (Gerard & Samuels, 2017).

All women of childbearing age who take an anticonvulsant medication are advised to take a folic acid supplement of 0.4 mg to 1 mg daily, which may decrease the incidence of NTDs in their children. More research is needed to determine the optimal dose of folic acid for women with epilepsy. Many practitioners recommend a dose of 4 mg/day for women with epilepsy who are trying to conceive or are already pregnant. Vitamin D deficiency is common in women with epilepsy, because anticonvulsant medications can interfere with production of the active form of this vitamin. Therefore, pregnant women with epilepsy are encouraged to take a supplemental dose of 1000 to 2000 IU of vitamin D daily, in addition to a prenatal vitamin (Gerard & Samuels, 2017).

If possible, only one anticonvulsant medication—at the lowest dose level that is effective at keeping the woman seizure free—should be prescribed during pregnancy. The increase in plasma volume that is a normal pregnancy change can affect drug metabolism and distribution. Therefore blood levels of anticonvulsant medications should be checked throughout pregnancy, and drug dosages adjusted as necessary (Aminoff & Douglas, 2014; Gerard & Samuels, 2017). Often the dosage will need to be increased as pregnancy progresses. With patient cooperation and close monitoring, most women with epilepsy should experience no change in seizure frequency from their baseline seizure frequency (Gerard & Samuels).

In addition to congenital anomalies, the fetus of a woman with epilepsy is also at risk for IUGR. Determining an accurate gestational age as early as possible is important. This information decreases any confusion later in pregnancy regarding fetal growth issues. If the patient's weight gain and fundal height appear appropriate, serial ultrasounds for fetal weight assessment are probably unnecessary. Maternal serum alpha-fetoprotein screening around 16 weeks of gestation should be done to detect NTDs. A specialized, detailed anatomic ultrasound examination should be performed at 18 to 22 weeks of gestation to determine whether congenital malformations, including NTDs, are present. Nonstress testing later in pregnancy is not necessary for all women with epilepsy, but it should be considered for those who have seizures during the third trimester (Gerard & Samuels, 2017).

The risk for seizures during labor is small. Seizures are most likely to occur in women who have had seizures during pregnancy. They are usually treated with short-acting benzodiazepines (e.g., lorazepam [Ativan]). Most women with epilepsy successfully give birth vaginally (Gerard & Samuels, 2017).

After birth, the levels of anticonvulsant medications must be monitored frequently for the first few weeks because they can rise rapidly.

If medication dose levels were increased during pregnancy, they need to be reduced within the first 3 weeks postpartum to slightly higher than or at prepregnancy levels (Aminoff & Douglas, 2014; Gerard & Samuels, 2017). All of the major anticonvulsant medications are found in breast milk to varying degrees, but few data suggest neonatal harm from exposure through breast milk (Gerard & Samuels).

Safety measures related to the new baby should be discussed with the woman and her family members. In addition to the safety measures that apply to all newborns, specific precautions should be observed with babies whose mothers have epilepsy. The sleep deprivation that can be associated with breastfeeding a newborn may put the woman at risk for seizures. Partners or other members of the woman's support system should assist with night feedings so that the woman can have a prolonged period (typically 6 to 8 hours) of uninterrupted sleep. Bathing the baby only when another adult is present and changing diapers on a pad placed on the floor, instead of on a changing table, are other recommendations. In addition, avoiding stairs whenever possible and using a stroller to transport the baby, rather than an infant carrier strapped to the mother, are safety measures that should be considered (Gerard & Samuels, 2017).

Contraceptive counseling is an important part of postpartum and preconception planning for women with epilepsy. Drug-drug interactions are numerous between hormonal contraceptive methods and antiepileptic medications. The most reliable form of contraception is the intrauterine device (IUD). The IUD, either the copper or the levonorgestrel type, is considered the contraceptive method of choice for most women with epilepsy (Gerard & Samuels, 2017). In terms of planning for future childbearing, couples should be informed that their risk for passing epilepsy along to their children is higher than that of the general population, but still relatively low. Interestingly, mothers with epilepsy have a much greater chance of having a child with epilepsy than do fathers with epilepsy (Gerard & Samuels).

Multiple Sclerosis

Multiple sclerosis (MS), a patchy demyelinization of the spinal cord and CNS, may be a viral disorder. It affects women more often than men. Onset of symptoms, which include weakness, paresthesias, or numbness of one or both lower extremities, visual complaints, and loss of coordination, is subtle and usually occurs between 20 and 40 years of age. The disease is characterized by exacerbations and remissions. Pregnancy likely does not have any adverse long-term effect on the course of the disease (Gerard & Samuels, 2017).

Remissions during pregnancy are common. If an exacerbation occurs, it is more likely to do so during the postpartum period. The mainstay of treatment for acute MS relapses is corticosteroids and, rarely, other immunosuppressive agents. In 1993, the first disease-modifying agent (DMA), interferon-β, a new class of medications for treating MS, was introduced for use. Since then, there has been a steady increase in the number of available DMAs. Their use in pregnancy has been limited; thus few data and no controlled studies are available. Because MS exacerbations are rare during pregnancy and few data are available regarding the safety of DMA use during pregnancy, most experts recommend stopping DMA use prior to conception. A few studies have suggested that the use of DMAs prior to conception or during gestation decreases the risk for postpartum MS relapses. Postpartum relapses are also less likely to occur in women whose MS activity had been well controlled in the year prior to pregnancy (Gerard & Samuels, 2017).

No specific changes in routine obstetric care are recommended for the woman with MS, because MS in the mother does not pose significant risk to the fetus. The woman should take a prenatal vitamin. Vitamin D deficiency may affect her susceptibility to MS and MS relapses, as well as her child's subsequent risk for developing MS. Therefore, experts recommend that the woman takes 1000 to 2000 IU of vitamin D daily. Women with disturbances in bladder function are more likely to develop UTIs during pregnancy. Therefore they should be screened routinely. If an acute and severe MS relapse occurs during pregnancy, it can be treated with corticosteroids or intravenous immunoglobulin (IVIG) (Gerard & Samuels, 2017).

In the past, there were concerns that epidural use during labor and birth might somehow worsen MS or promote relapses. However, research has found that this does not seem to be the case. Cesarean birth is usually not indicated for women with MS. Only rare cases of severe or active disease that affect the spinal cord prevent a woman with MS from laboring safely (Gerard & Samuels, 2017).

Breastfeeding in women with MS is controversial. Some authorities believe that breastfeeding does not affect disease activity. Others believe that breastfeeding may reduce the likelihood of MS relapses during the postpartum period. Most experts recommend that DMAs not be used during breastfeeding because of a lack of evidence regarding their safety (Gerard & Samuels, 2017). Depression is common among women with MS; thus they should be assessed frequently for evidence of postpartum depression. All hormonal contraceptives may be used by women with MS (Stuart & Bergstrom, 2011).

Bell Palsy

Bell palsy is an acute idiopathic facial paralysis. The cause is unknown, but it may be related to the reactivation of herpes simplex virus infection or acute human immunodeficiency virus type 1 (HIV-1) retroviral infection. Bell palsy occurs fairly often, especially in women of reproductive age. An association between Bell palsy and pregnancy was first cited by Bell in 1830. Pregnant women are affected four times more often than nonpregnant women. Women who develop Bell palsy during pregnancy have an increased risk for gestational hypertension or preeclampsia (Cunningham et al., 2014).

The clinical manifestations of Bell palsy include the sudden development of a unilateral facial weakness, with maximal weakness within 48 hours after onset. Other common symptoms include pain surrounding the ear, difficulty closing the eye on the affected side, hyperacusis (abnormal acuteness of the sense of hearing), and occasionally a loss of taste (Aminoff & Douglas, 2014; Cunningham et al., 2014).

No effects of maternal Bell palsy have been observed in infants. Maternal outcome is generally good unless a complete block in nerve conduction occurs. Steroid therapy is the only medical treatment that has been shown to influence the outcome of Bell palsy. To be effective, treatment should begin within the first 3 to 5 days after the paralysis develops (Aminoff & Douglas, 2014). Supportive care includes prevention of injury to the constantly exposed cornea, facial muscle massage, careful chewing and manual removal of food from inside the affected cheek, and reassurance. Although 80% of affected men and nonpregnant women recover to a satisfactory level within 1 year, only approximately one-half of women who develop the disorder during pregnancy do so (Cunningham et al., 2014).

AUTOIMMUNE DISORDERS

Autoimmune disorders, also called *collagen vascular diseases,* make up a large group of conditions that disrupt the function of the immune system of the body. In these types of disorders, the immune system is unable to distinguish "self" from "nonself." As a result, antibodies develop that attack its normally present antigens, causing tissue damage. More women than men are affected by autoimmune disorders. Autoimmune disorders can occur during pregnancy because a large percentage of women with an autoimmune disease manifest it at some time during their reproductive years (Carpenter & Branch, 2017). Common autoimmune diseases include systemic lupus erythematosus, myasthenia gravis, antiphospholipid syndrome, rheumatoid arthritis, and systemic sclerosis.

Systemic Lupus Erythematosus

Systemic lupus erythematosus (SLE) is a multisystem chronic, inflammatory disease that affects the skin, joints, kidneys, lungs, nervous system, liver, and other body organs. The exact cause is unknown but probably involves the interaction of immunologic, environmental, hormonal, and genetic factors. SLE is the most common serious autoimmune disease affecting women of reproductive age. It occurs two to four times more often in African-American than in Caucasian women and is nine times more common in women than in men. Most cases of SLE are diagnosed in adolescence or young adulthood (Carpenter & Branch, 2017; Lockshin, Salmon, & Erkan, 2014).

Common symptoms, including myalgias, fatigue, weight change, and fevers, occur in nearly all women with SLE at some time during the course of the disease. Although a diagnosis of SLE is suspected based on clinical signs and symptoms, it is confirmed by laboratory testing that demonstrates the presence of circulating autoantibodies. As is the case with other autoimmune diseases, SLE is characterized by a series of exacerbations (flares) and remissions (Carpenter & Branch, 2017; Lockshin et al., 2014).

Pregnancy probably does not increase the likelihood of serious SLE flares (Lockshin et al., 2014). However, it appears that disease activity at the beginning of pregnancy is an important predictor of exacerbations during pregnancy. Therefore, women are advised to wait until they have been in remission for at least 6 months before attempting conception (Carpenter & Branch, 2017). In addition to exacerbations, other maternal risks include an increased rate of miscarriage, a possible need to give birth at a preterm gestation, and preeclampsia. Fetal risks include stillbirth, IUGR, and preterm birth (Carpenter & Branch).

Medical therapy during pregnancy is kept to a minimum in women who are in remission or who have a mild form of SLE. Occasional doses of nonsteroidal antiinflammatory drugs (NSAIDs) can be given to treat arthralgia. Low-dose aspirin can be used throughout pregnancy (Cunningham et al., 2014). Glucocorticoids such as prednisone are often used to treat SLE during pregnancy, either as maintenance therapy or as short-term treatment for flares. There is a small risk for fetal cleft lip and palate if glucocorticoids are used during the first trimester. Prolonged use of this group of medications also increases the risk for maternal bone loss, gestational diabetes, hypertension and preeclampsia, and adrenal suppression. Given the significant risks associated with long-term glucocorticoid use, hydroxychloroquine (Plaquenil), an antimalarial drug, may be the best medication for maintenance SLE therapy during pregnancy. It significantly reduces SLE disease activity but appears to cause no adverse effects on the fetus (Carpenter & Branch, 2017).

Prenatal care otherwise focuses on close monitoring to detect common pregnancy complications such as hypertension, proteinuria, and IUGR. Ultrasound examinations are performed monthly after 24 to 28 weeks of gestation to monitor fetal growth. Fetal assessment tests, including weekly or twice-weekly NSTs and amniotic fluid volume assessments or biophysical profiles, are performed beginning at 32 weeks of gestation unless indicated earlier in pregnancy due to IUGR (see Chapter 10) (Carpenter & Branch, 2017).

It is recommended that women with SLE give birth by 39 weeks of gestation. Birth may be necessary earlier in gestation if complications such as IUGR, preeclampsia, or worsening renal function develop. Women who have received chronic glucocorticoid therapy (more than 20 mg of prednisone daily for more than 3 weeks) should be given larger (stress) doses of steroids during labor (Carpenter & Branch, 2017).

Vaginal birth is preferred, but cesarean birth is common because of maternal and fetal complications.

Close monitoring of all women with SLE should continue after birth because some of them will experience a disease flare during the postpartum period. It is usually recommended that the woman follows up with her rheumatologist within 1 to 3 months after giving birth (Carpenter & Branch, 2017).

Women with SLE and chronic vascular or renal disease should limit their number of pregnancies because of maternal complications associated with the illness and increased adverse perinatal outcomes. If desired, the safest time for tubal sterilization is during the postpartum period or when the disease is in remission. Combined oral contraceptive pills should be avoided in women who have nephritis, antiphospholipid antibodies, or vascular disease. Progestin-only implants and injections provide effective contraception with no known effects on lupus flares. Evidence does not support concerns regarding an increased risk for infection when IUDs are prescribed for women receiving immunosuppressive therapy (Cunningham et al., 2014).

Myasthenia Gravis

Myasthenia gravis (MG), an autoimmune motor (muscle) end-plate disorder that involves acetylcholine use, affects the motor function at the myoneural junction. Muscle weakness results, particularly of the eyes, face, tongue, neck, limbs, and respiratory muscles. In addition, women may experience ptosis, diplopia, and dysphagia. Women are affected twice as often as men, and the incidence peaks between 20 and 30 years of age. Because the greatest period of risk is during the first year after diagnosis, pregnancy should probably be avoided until symptomatic improvement occurs (Cunningham et al., 2014). The response of women with MG to pregnancy is unpredictable; remission, exacerbation, or continued stability during pregnancy can occur (Aminoff & Douglas, 2014).

Pregnancy does not appear to affect the overall course of MG, but as the uterus enlarges respirations may be compromised. Also the normal fatigue experienced by many pregnant women may be tolerated poorly by those with MG (Cunningham et al., 2014). Treatment during pregnancy is the same as for nonpregnant women. Usual medications include glucocorticoids and acetylcholinesterase inhibitors. Monitoring blood glucose values is important because hyperglycemia may result from corticosteroid therapy. Thymectomy may result in remission of the disease but is best performed before or after pregnancy, if at all possible. For severe weakness, plasmapheresis or IVIG therapy may be needed (Aminoff & Douglas, 2014).

Because MG does not affect smooth muscle, most women usually tolerate labor well. Vaginal birth is desired, but vacuum or forceps assistance may be required because of muscle weakness. Oxytocin may be given, but all medications that cause muscular relaxation should be avoided if at all possible. Opioids must be used cautiously because they may cause respiratory depression, and women with MG are already at risk for respiratory muscle weakness. Regional analgesia is preferred (Aminoff & Douglas, 2014; Cunningham et al., 2014). After birth, women must be carefully supervised because relapses often occur during the puerperium.

> ⚡ **SAFETY ALERT**
>
> Magnesium sulfate must not be administered to women with MG because it inhibits the release of acetylcholine and can trigger myasthenic crisis.

Approximately 10% to 15% of neonates born to women with MG develop neonatal myasthenia. This transient disorder results from the transfer of maternal antibody against acetylcholine receptors across the placenta. Symptoms, including poor cry, respiratory difficulties, weakness in suckling, weak Moro reflex, and feeble limb movements, usually appear within the first 72 hours after birth. Neonatal myasthenia can be treated with anticholinesterase medications and usually resolves by 6 weeks after birth (Aminoff & Douglas, 2014).

SUBSTANCE ABUSE

Large numbers of women of childbearing age abuse potentially addictive and mood-altering drugs. Use of tobacco, alcohol, opioids, cocaine, methamphetamines, prescription drugs, and approximately 150 other substances can lead to chemical dependency. Chemical dependency is a chronic, relapsing, and progressive disease. Without treatment or participation in recovery activities, it can progress and result in disability or premature death.

This section discusses only substance abuse during pregnancy. Chapter 3 contains additional information related to substance abuse in the general population. See Chapter 25 for information regarding effects of maternal substance abuse on neonates.

Pregnant women who abuse drugs can display warning signs such as receiving no prenatal care, late entry into care, or sporadic care, with multiple missed appointments. They may keep prenatal appointments but leave without being seen. Another warning sign in pregnant substance abusers is noncompliance with recommended treatment (Baird, Kennedy, & Dalton, 2017). These women may also show evidence of poor nutrition, have frequent encounters with law enforcement officials, or be involved in marital and family disputes.

Drugs that affect the mother can also affect the fetus in multiple ways either directly or indirectly. Early in gestation, drugs can cause significant teratogenic effects. During the fetal period, after major structural development is complete, drugs exert more subtle effects, including abnormal growth and maturation, alterations in neurotransmitters and their receptors and brain organization. These are considered to be the direct effects of drugs (Behnke, Smith, Committee on Substance Abuse, & Committee on Fetus and Newborn, 2013). Drugs that exert a pharmacologic effect on the mother can indirectly affect the fetus. Indirect effects include altered delivery of nutrition to the fetus, either because of placental insufficiency or altered maternal health behaviors attributable to the mother's addiction.

Maternal factors can indirectly place the fetus at risk. Examples include decreased access/compliance with health care, increased exposure to violence, and increased risk for mental illness and infection (Behnke et al., 2013).

PREVALENCE

Substance use in the United States is a problem that continues to grow. Women make up about 30% of the addicted population, and many of them are in their childbearing years (Baird et al., 2017). In a national survey done in America, 5.4% of pregnant women reported illicit drug use in the previous month. Rates of use were higher in the first and second trimesters of pregnancy than in the third (Wisner, Sit, Bogen, et al., 2017). Universal screening for drug use in pregnant women is recommended. Because substance use is prevalent in all populations, providers should never make assumptions based on age, race, or socioeconomic status. Universal screening is nonbiased and nonstigmatizing (Baird et al., 2017; Wisner, et al., 2017).

Maternal and Fetal Effects of Selected Drugs of Abuse
Cigarette Smoking
Maternal effects related to cigarette smoking include thromboembolic disease and respiratory complications. Pregnancy-related complications include miscarriage, preterm birth, IUGR, placenta previa, placental abruption, and premature rupture of membranes (Wisner et al., 2017).

Alcohol
Prenatal alcohol exposure increases the chance of birth defects significantly. No amount of alcohol use during pregnancy is considered safe. Although fetal alcohol syndrome (FAS) is a known consequence of prenatal alcohol intake, other consequences include an increased risk for miscarriage, stillbirth, and preterm birth. Fetal exposure to alcohol is the most common preventable cause of cognitive impairment (Wisner et al., 2017).

Opioids
This class of drugs includes, among others, morphine, heroin, codeine, meperidine, methadone, and buprenorphine. Opioid users can develop withdrawal symptoms once the drug has been metabolized. Box 14.5 lists common signs and symptoms of opioid withdrawal in women. During pregnancy, withdrawal effects can also include preterm birth and IUFD.

Cocaine
Cocaine is a powerful central nervous system stimulant that is addictive because of the tremendous sense of euphoria that it creates. When used during pregnancy, there is an increased incidence of miscarriage, preterm labor, small-for-gestational-age babies, placental abruption, and stillbirth. Fetal anomalies have been reported with its use.

Methamphetamines
Methamphetamines are central nervous system stimulants with vasoconstrictive characteristics similar to those of cocaine, and they are used similarly. Although fewer maternal and fetal complications have been attributed to this class of substances than to cocaine, the rates of preterm birth and IUGR with smaller head circumference are higher in methamphetamine-exposed pregnant women than in pregnant women who abuse other substances.

BARRIERS TO TREATMENT

Many pregnant women who are substance abusers do not receive treatment for their addictions. Social stigma, labeling, and guilt are significant barriers to receiving necessary care. Women often do not seek help because of the fear of losing custody of their child or children or criminal prosecution. Pregnant women who abuse substances commonly have little understanding of the ways in which these substances affect them, their pregnancies, and their babies. In many instances, pregnant mothers who use psychoactive substances receive negative feedback from society and health care providers, who not only may condemn them for endangering the life of the fetus but may also even withhold support as a result. Barriers within the drug treatment system can also deter these women from receiving the help they need. Traditionally substance-abuse treatment programs have not addressed issues that affect pregnant women such as concurrent need for obstetric care and child care for other children. Long waiting lists and lack of health insurance present further barriers to treatment. Pregnant women with co-occurring substance abuse and psychiatric disorders face unique barriers because of the social stigma attached to both conditions and insufficient knowledge and training to manage coexisting disorders.

LEGAL CONSIDERATIONS

Because of the risks to the unborn children and financial concerns, pregnant women who abuse substances can now face criminal charges under expanded interpretations of child abuse and drug trafficking statutes (Guttmacher Institute, 2016). Substance abuse in pregnancy is defined as child abuse in 18 states, with 3 states defining it as reason for civil commitment. Suspected drug abuse in pregnant women is reason for reporting by health care professionals in 18 states, and prenatal drug exposure testing is required in 4 states if health care providers suspect substance abuse. Although some policymakers have proposed that pregnant women who abuse substances should be jailed or placed under house arrest, one state allows criminal charges to be filed for prenatal drug abuse. However, three states—South Carolina, Tennessee, and Alabama—do allow civil commitment (Guttmacher Institute). Health care professionals must be aware of current laws in the state(s) where they practice.

CARE MANAGEMENT

SCREENING

All pregnant women should be screened at their first prenatal visit regarding their past and present use of tobacco, alcohol, and other drugs, including the recreational use of prescription and over-the-counter medications as well as herbal remedies. Substance use information can be obtained by interview or use of a standardized screening tool. The overall approach and emotional tone of the clinician is more important than the specific wording or content used. Women are more likely to report substance use when asked in a nonjudgmental manner by an empathic interviewer and within the context of general health questions (AAP & ACOG, 2012; Wisner et al., 2017).

When questioning a woman about her drug use, it is usually best to begin by asking about her intake of over-the-counter and prescribed medications. Questions about these types of drugs are usually perceived as nonthreatening. Next, her use of legal drugs such as caffeine, nicotine, and alcohol should be determined. Finally, ask about her use of illicit drugs such as cocaine, heroin, and methamphetamines. The approximate frequency and amount should be documented for each drug used.

Use of validated screening questionnaires, along with the assurance of confidentiality, improves patient-provider communication and can increase the truthfulness of patient responses (AAP & ACOG, 2012). The *4Ps Plus* is a screening tool designed specifically to identify pregnant women who need in-depth assessment (Box 11.4). It consists of five questions and takes less than 1 minute to complete. Because women frequently deny or greatly underreport usage when asked about drug or alcohol consumption during pregnancy, asking about substance use before pregnancy is often an effective screening method (Wisner et al., 2017).

Toxicologic testing is often performed to screen for illicit drug use. Because positive test results have implications for women beyond their health, informed consent should be obtained before testing is done (AAP & ACOG, 2012). Information that should be communicated to the woman includes the test planned, purpose of the test, management

---

BOX 11.4　Screening With the *4Ps* Plus

Parents: Did either of your parents ever have a problem with alcohol or drugs?
Partner: Does your partner have a problem with alcohol or drugs?
Past: Have you ever had any beer or wine or liquor?
Pregnancy: In the month before you knew you were pregnant, how many cigarettes did you smoke? In the month before you knew you were pregnant, how much beer, wine, or liquor did you drink?

From Chasnoff, I.J., & Hung, W.C. (1999). *The 4Ps plus.* Chicago, IL: NTI Publishing.

---

based on test results, and benefits or consequences of testing (Baird et al., 2017).

> **LEGAL TIP** **Toxicologic Testing** The legal implications of testing and the need for consent from the mother can vary among states. Therefore, health care providers should be aware of local laws and legislative changes that can influence regional practice (AAP & ACOG, 2012).

Several biologic specimens can be used to screen for drug exposure. The three specimens most commonly used to establish drug exposure during the prenatal and perinatal periods are urine, meconium, and hair. There are practical limitations, however, with testing all three substances (Wisner et al., 2017).

ASSESSMENT

Because substance-abusing pregnant women are at risk for a variety of infections and medical conditions, a comprehensive medical history should be obtained, and a complete physical examination performed. Laboratory assessments will likely include screening for syphilis, hepatitis B and C, and human immunodeficiency virus (HIV). A complete blood count and a skin test to screen for tuberculosis may also be ordered. In addition, the woman may be tested for other common sexually transmitted infections such as gonorrhea and chlamydia. Initial and serial ultrasound studies are usually performed to determine gestational age because the woman may have had amenorrhea as a result of her drug use or have no idea when her last menstrual period occurred.

INTERVENTIONS

Intervention with substance-abusing pregnant women is best accomplished by an interprofessional health care team. Team members should include, at a minimum, an obstetrician, mental health provider, substance abuse counselor, nurse, and social worker.

Medical Management

Intervention with the pregnant substance abuser begins with education about specific effects on pregnancy, the fetus, and the newborn for each drug used. Consequences of perinatal drug use should be clearly communicated, and abstinence recommended as the safest course of action unless the woman is abusing opioids. Women are often more receptive to making lifestyle changes during pregnancy than at any other time in their lives. The casual, experimental, or recreational drug user is frequently able to achieve and maintain sobriety when she receives education, support, and continued monitoring throughout the remainder of the pregnancy. Periodic screening throughout pregnancy of women who have admitted to drug use may help them to continue abstinence.

Treatment for substance abuse is individualized for each woman. Specific recommendations will vary depending on the type of drug used and the frequency and amount of use.

Women are more likely to attempt to stop smoking during pregnancy than at any other time in their lives. Women who quit smoking by the first trimester have infants whose growth is comparable to those born to nonsmokers. Smoking-cessation programs during pregnancy are effective and should be offered to all pregnant smokers. These programs should continue throughout the postpartum period as well, because women who quit smoking during pregnancy tend to relapse within 1 year of giving birth. ACOG recommends the use of nicotine replacement patches in pregnant women who have been unable to stop smoking using nonpharmacologic therapy. Many smoking-cessation resources are available, both in print and online, and smoking "quitlines" (for

COMMUNITY FOCUS

Visiting a Twelve-Step Meeting

Search online to find an "open" twelve-step meeting (one that welcomes visitors) in your community. Alcoholics Anonymous, Narcotics Anonymous, and Cocaine Anonymous are all examples of twelve-step recovery groups. Attend an open meeting held by one of these groups. Discuss your experience with your clinical group. Did pregnant women or new mothers attend the meeting? What was your impression of the meeting format and the discussion that occurred? Did you notice anything at the meeting that surprised you? Do you think that attending twelve-step meetings would be helpful for pregnant women or new mothers attempting to achieve and maintain sobriety? Give reasons to support your answer to the last question.

BOX 11.5 Dealing With Pregnant Substance Abusers

Realize that the decision to become and remain sober can *only* be made by the substance abuser.

Understand that nurses do not have the power to cure anyone. They only serve as educators, supporters, and advocates.

Educate yourself about the effects of drug use in general and effects on pregnancy and the newborn specifically.

Treat substance abusers with the same respect and consideration that you show other people.

Become familiar with your local treatment centers. Learn which of them accept pregnant women. Keep an up-to-date list of groups meeting in your community.

Remember that there are no "hopeless cases." It is *never* too late to quit!

Practice patience and persistence. It may take months or years to see the effects of your work.

example, 1-800-QUIT-NOW) are effective in assisting pregnant women to quit smoking (Wisner et al., 2017). For more information on smoking cessation, visit the American Lung Association website at www.lungusa.org or the CDC website at www.cdc.gov/tobacco/quit_smoking/index.htm.

Detoxification, short-term inpatient or outpatient treatment, long-term residential treatment, aftercare services, and self-help support groups are all possible treatment options for alcohol and drug abuse. Women for Sobriety may be a more helpful organization for women than Alcoholics Anonymous or Narcotics Anonymous, which were originally developed for male substance abusers. In general, long-term treatment of any sort is becoming increasingly difficult to obtain, particularly for women who lack insurance coverage. Although some programs allow a woman to keep her children with her at the treatment facility, far too few of them are available to meet the demand (see Community Focus box: Visiting a Twelve-Step Meeting).

Pregnant women requiring withdrawal from alcohol should be admitted for inpatient management. In pregnant women, alcohol withdrawal tends to begin within 6 to 24 hours after the last drink. Alcohol withdrawal treatment during pregnancy consists of the administration of benzodiazepines. Chlordiazepoxide (Librium) and diazepam (Valium) are considered the benzodiazepine agents of choice for treatment of pregnant women (Wisner et al., 2017).

Since the 1970s, methadone maintenance therapy (MMT) has been considered the standard of care for pregnant women who are dependent on opioids. MMT is recommended because it reduces drug cravings and promotes better adherence to prenatal care and drug abuse counseling visits. Buprenorphine (Subutex or Suboxone) is another medication approved for opioid addiction treatment that is being used increasingly during pregnancy. It appears to be as effective as methadone. Neither buprenorphine nor methadone is associated with an increased risk for birth defects (Wisner et al., 2017).

Anywhere from 30% to 80% of infants exposed to opioids, including methadone or buprenorphine, in utero require treatment for neonatal abstinence syndrome (NAS). Neither the incidence nor the severity of NAS correlates directly with the maternal methadone dose at birth. Therefore, limiting the methadone dose to minimize the risk for NAS is not warranted (Wisner et al., 2017). See Chapter 25 for additional information on NAS.

Detoxification from opioids during pregnancy is currently not recommended, because of fears of maternal relapse and a potential risk for fetal distress or fetal demise. However, a study of more that 600 pregnant women who were detoxified from opioids reported no fetal harm during the process. These data highly suggest that detoxification of opioid-addicted pregnant women is not harmful. In addition, the rate of treatment for NAS is less if long-term behavioral health management is provided once women are completely off opioids (Bell, Towers, Hennessy, et al., 2016).

Pregnant women who use cocaine should be advised to stop using immediately and be referred for substance abuse treatment. Effective psychosocial and behavioral treatments have been developed for pregnant substance abusers. Communication between obstetric care providers and substance abuse treatment staff is necessary for treatment success (Wisner et al., 2017).

As is the case with cocaine users, methamphetamine users are urged to immediately stop all use during pregnancy. Unfortunately, because methamphetamine users are extremely psychologically addicted, the rate of relapse is very high.

The most effective treatments for methamphetamine addiction at this time are behavioral therapies, such as cognitive-behavioral and contingency-management interventions. There are currently no medications that counteract the specific effects of methamphetamine or that prolong abstinence from and reduce the abuse of methamphetamine (National Institute of Drug Abuse [NIDA], 2013).

Nursing Interventions

Although substance abusers can be difficult to care for at any time, they are often particularly challenging during the intrapartum and postpartum periods because of manipulative and demanding behavior. Typically these women display poor control over their behavior and a low threshold for pain. Increased dependency needs and lack of involvement with infant care may also be apparent.

Nurses must understand that substance abuse is an illness and that these women deserve to be treated with patience, kindness, consistency, and firmness when necessary (Box 11.5). Even women who are actively abusing drugs experience pain during labor and after giving birth and may need both pharmacologic and nonpharmacologic interventions. Developing a standardized plan of care so patients have limited opportunities to play staff members against one another is helpful. Mother-infant attachment should be promoted by identifying the woman's strengths and reinforcing positive maternal feelings and behaviors. Staffing should be sufficient to ensure strict surveillance of visitors and prevent unsupervised drug use.

Advice regarding breastfeeding must be individualized. Although all abused substances appear in breast milk, some in greater amounts than others, breastfeeding is definitely contraindicated in women who use methamphetamines, alcohol, cocaine, heroin, or marijuana. However, methadone use is not a contraindication to breastfeeding. The baby's nutrition and safety needs are of primary importance in this consideration. For some women, a desire to breastfeed can provide strong motivation to achieve and maintain sobriety.

Smoking can interfere with the milk ejection (let-down) reflex. Women who smoke and breastfeed should avoid smoking for 2 hours before a feeding to minimize the amount of nicotine in the milk and improve the milk-ejection reflex. All smokers should be discouraged from smoking in the same room with the infant because exposure to secondhand smoke can increase the likelihood that the infant will experience behavioral and respiratory health problems.

Follow-Up Care

Before a known substance abuser is discharged with her baby, the home situation must be assessed to determine that the environment is safe and that someone will be available to meet the infant's needs if the mother is unable to do so. The social services department of the birthing facility is usually involved in interviewing the mother before discharge to ensure that the infant's needs will be met. Family members or friends are sometimes asked to become actively involved with the mother and infant after discharge. A home care or public health nurse may be asked to make home visits to assess the mother's ability to care for the baby and provide guidance and support. If serious questions about the infant's well-being exist, the case is likely to be referred to the state child protective services agency for further action.

REFERENCES

American Academy of Pediatrics & American College of Obstetricians and Gynecologists. (2012). *Guidelines for perinatal care* (7th ed.). Washington, DC: American College of Obstetricians and Gynecologists.

American College of Obstetricians and Gynecologists. (2013, reaffirmed 2015). Practice bulletin no. 137: Gestational diabetes. *Obstetrics & Gynecology, 122*(2 pt 1), 406–416.

American College of Obstetricians and Gynecologists. (2016). Practice bulletin no. 173: Fetal macrosomia. *Obstetrics & Gynecology, 128*(5), e195–e209.

American Diabetes Association. (2016a). Classification and diagnosis of diabetes. In Standards of medical care in diabetes—2016. *Diabetes Care, 39*(1 suppl), S13–S22.

American Diabetes Association. (2016b). Management of diabetes in pregnancy. In Standards of medical care in diabetes—2016. *Diabetes Care, 39*(1 suppl), S94–S98.

Aminoff, M. J., & Douglas, V. C. (2014). Neurologic disorders. In R. K. Creasy, R. Resnik, J. D. Iams, et al. (Eds.), *Creasy and Resnik's maternal-fetal medicine: Principles and practice* (7th ed.). Philadelphia, PA: Saunders.

Antony, K. M., Racusin, D. A., Aagaard, K., et al. (2017). Maternal physiology. In S. G. Gabbe, J. R. Niebyl, J. L. Simpson, et al. (Eds.), *Obstetrics: Normal and problem pregnancies* (7th ed.). Philadelphia, PA: Elsevier.

Baird, S. M., Kennedy, B. B., & Dalton, J. (2017). Special considerations for individualized care of the laboring woman. In B. B. Kennedy & S. M. Baird (Eds.), *Intrapartum management modules: A perinatal education program* (5th ed.). Philadelphia, PA: Wolters Kluwer.

Banta-Wright, S. A., Kodadek, S. M., Houck, G. M., et al. (2015). Commitment to breastfeeding in the context of phenylketonuria. *JOGNN: Journal of Obstetric, Gynecologic, and Neonatal Nursing, 44*, 726–736.

Behnke, M., Smith, V. C., & Committee on Substance Abuse, & Committee on Fetus and Newborn. (2013). Prenatal substance abuse: Short- and long-term effects on the exposed fetus. *Pediatrics, 131*(3), e1009–e1024.

Bell, J., Towers, C. V., Hennessy, M. D., et al. (2016). Detoxification from opiate drugs during pregnancy. *American Journal of Obstetrics and Gynecology, 215*(3), 374.e1–374.e6.

Blackburn, S. (2013). *Maternal, fetal, and neonatal physiology: A clinical perspective* (4th ed.). Maryland Heights, MO: Saunders.

Blanchard, D. G., & Daniels, L. B. (2014). Cardiac diseases. In R. K. Creasy, R. Resnik, J. D. Iams, et al. (Eds.), *Creasy and Resnik's maternal-fetal medicine: Principles and practice* (7th ed.). Philadelphia, PA: Saunders.

Cappell, M. (2017). Hepatic disorders during pregnancy. In S. G. Gabbe, J. R. Niebyl, J. L. Simpson, et al. (Eds.), *Obstetrics: Normal and problem pregnancies* (7th ed.). Philadelphia, PA: Elsevier.

Carpenter, J. R., & Branch, D. W. (2017). Collagen vascular diseases in pregnancy. In S. G. Gabbe, J. R. Niebyl, J. L. Simpson, et al. (Eds.), *Obstetrics: Normal and problem pregnancies* (7th ed.). Philadelphia, PA: Elsevier.

Centers for Disease Control and Prevention. (2014). *National diabetes statistics report, 2014.* Retrieved from www.cdc.gov/diabetes/pubs;statsreport14/national-diabetes-resport-web.pdf.

Cunningham, F., Leveno, K., Bloom, S., et al. (2014). *Williams obstetrics* (24th ed.). New York, NY: McGraw-Hill Education.

Daley, J. M. (2014). Diabetes in pregnancy. In K. R. Simpson & P. Creehan (Eds.), *AWHONN's perinatal nursing* (4th ed.). Philadelphia, PA: Lippincott Willliams & Wilkins.

Deen, J., Chandrasekaran, S., Stout, K., et al. (2017). Heart disease in pregnancy. In S. G. Gabbe, J. R. Niebyl, J. L. Simpson, et al. (Eds.), *Obstetrics: Normal and problem pregnancies* (7th ed.). Philadelphia, PA: Elsevier.

Gabzdyl, E. M., & Schlaeger, J. M. (2015). Intrahepatic cholestasis of pregnancy: A critical clinical review. *Journal of Perinatal & Neonatal Nursing, 29*, 41–50.

Gaddipati, S., & Troiano, N. (2013). Cardiac disorders in pregnancy. In N. Troiano, C. Harvey, & B. Chez (Eds.), *AWHONN's high risk and critical care obstetrics* (3rd ed.). Philadelphia, PA: Wolters Kluwer/Lippincott Williams & Wilkins.

Gerard, E. E., & Samuels, P. (2017). Neurologic disorders in pregnancy. In S. G. Gabbe, J. R. Niebyl, J. L. Simpson, et al. (Eds.), *Obstetrics: Normal and problem pregnancies* (7th ed.). Philadelphia, PA: Elsevier.

Guttmacher Institute. (2016). *Substance abuse during pregnancy.* Retrieved from https://www.guttmacher.org/sites/default/files/pdfs/spibs/spib_SADP.pdf.

Inturrisi, M. (2017). Care of the laboring woman with diabetes. In B. B. Kennedy & S. M. Baird (Eds.), *Intrapartum management modules: A perinatal education program* (5th ed.). Philadelphia, PA: Wolters Kluwer.

Inturrisi, M., Lintner, N. C., & Sorem, K. (2013). Diabetic ketoacidosis and continuous insulin infusion management in pregnancy. In N. Troiano, C. Harvey, & B. Chez (Eds.), *AWHONN's high risk and critical care obstetrics* (3rd ed.). Philadelphia, PA: Wolters Kluwer/Lippincott Williams & Wilkins.

Kilpatrick, S. J. (2014). Anemia and pregnancy. In R. K. Creasy, R. Resnik, J. D. Iams, et al. (Eds.), *Creasy and Resnik's maternal-fetal medicine: Principles and practice* (7th ed.). Philadelphia, PA: Saunders.

Landon, M. B., Catalano, P. M., & Gabbe, S. G. (2017). Diabetes mellitus complicating pregnancy. In S. G. Gabbe, J. R. Niebyl, J. L. Simpson, et al. (Eds.), *Obstetrics: Normal and problem pregnancies* (7th ed.). Philadelphia, PA: Elsevier.

Lawrence, R. A., & Lawrence, R. M. (2016). *Breastfeeding: A guide for the medical profession* (8th ed.). Philadelphia, PA: Elsevier.

Lockshin, M. D., Salmon, J. E., & Erkan, D. (2014). Pregnancy and rheumatic diseases. In R. K. Creasy, R. Resnik, J. D. Iams, et al. (Eds.), *Creasy and Resnik's maternal-fetal medicine: Principles and practice* (7th ed.). Philadelphia, PA: Saunders.

March of Dimes. (2017). *Folic acid.* Retrieved from www.marchofdimes.org/pregnancy/folic-acid.aspx#.

Mason, B. A., & Dorman, K. (2013). Pulmonary disorders in pregnancy. In N. Troiano, C. Harvey, & B. Chez (Eds.), *AWHONN's high risk and critical care obstetrics* (3rd ed.). Philadelphia, PA: Wolters Kluwer/Lippincott Williams & Wilkins.

Mercer, B. M. (2014). Assessment and induction of fetal pulmonary maturity. In R. K. Creasy, R. Resnik, J. D. Iams, et al. (Eds.), *Creasy and Resnik's maternal-fetal medicine: Principles and practice* (7th ed.). Philadelphia, PA: Saunders.

Mestman, J. H. (2017). Thyroid and parathyroid diseases in pregnancy. In S. G. Gabbe, J. R. Niebyl, J. L. Simpson, et al. (Eds.), *Obstetrics: Normal and problem pregnancies* (7th ed.). Philadelphia, PA: Elsevier.

Miller, J., de Veciana, M., Turan, S., et al. (2013). First trimester detection of fetal anomalies in pregestational diabetes using nuchal translucency, ductus venosus Doppler, and maternal glycosylated hemoglobin. *American Journal of Obstetrics and Gynecology, 208*(5), 385.e1–385.e8.

Moore, T. R. H., Hauguel-deMouzon, S., & Catalano, P. (2014). Diabetes in pregnancy. In R. K. Creasy, R. Resnik, J. D. Iams, et al. (Eds.), *Creasy and Resnik's maternal-fetal medicine: Principles and practice* (7th ed.). Philadelphia, PA: Saunders.

Nader, S. (2014). Thyroid disease and pregnancy. In R. K. Creasy, R. Resnik, J. D. Iams, et al. (Eds.), *Creasy and Resnik's maternal-fetal medicine: Principles and practice* (7th ed.). Philadelphia, PA: Saunders.

National Institute of Drug Abuse. (2013). *Methamphetamine: Abuse and addiction.* www.drugabuse.gov/publications/research-reports/methamphetamine-abuse-addiction/what-methamphetamine.

Ortiz, F. M., Jimenez, E. Y., Boursaw, B., et al., (2016). Postpartum care for women with gestational diabetes. *American Journal of Maternal Child Nursing, 41*(2), 116–122.

Rapini, R. (2014). The skin and pregnancy. In R. K. Creasy, R. Resnik, J. D. Iams, et al. (Eds.), *Creasy and Resnik's maternal-fetal medicine: Principles and practice* (7th ed.). Philadelphia, PA: Saunders.

Reddy, U. M., & Spong, C. Y. (2014). Stillbirth. In R. K. Creasy, R. Resnik, J. D. Iams, et al. (Eds.), *Creasy and Resnik's maternal-fetal medicine: Principles and practice* (7th ed.). Philadelphia, PA: Saunders.

Roos-Hesselink, J. W., Ruys, P. T. E., & Johnson, M. R. (2013). Pregnancy in adult congenital heart disease. *Current Cardiology Reports, 15*(9), 401.

Sacks, D. A., & Metzger, B. E. (2013). Classification of diabetes in pregnancy: Time to reassess the alphabet. *Obstetrics and Gynecology, 121*(2 Pt. 1), 345–348.

Samuels, P. (2017). Hematologic complications of pregnancy. In S. G. Gabbe, J. R. Niebyl, J. L. Simpson, et al. (Eds.), *Obstetrics: Normal and problem pregnancies* (7th ed.). Philadelphia, PA: Elsevier.

Simhan, H. N., Berghella, V., & Iams, J. D. (2014). Preterm labor and birth. In R. K. Creasy, R. Resnik, J. D. Iams, et al. (Eds.), *Creasy and Resnik's maternal-fetal medicine: Principles and practice* (7th ed.). Philadelphia, PA: Saunders.

Simhan, H. N., Iams, J. D., & Romero, R. (2017). Preterm labor and birth. In S. G. Gabbe, J. R. Niebyl, J. L. Simpson, et al. (Eds.), *Obstetrics: Normal and problem pregnancies* (7th ed.). Philadelphia, PA: Elsevier.

Spencer, B. (2015). Medications and breastfeeding for mothers with chronic illness. *Journal of Obstetric, Gynecologic, and Neonatal Nursing, 44*(4), 543–552.

Stuart, M., & Bergstrom, L. (2011). Pregnancy and multiple sclerosis. *Journal of Midwifery & Women's Health, 56*(1), 41–47.

Wang, A. R., & Kroumpouzos, G. (2017). Skin disease and pregnancy. In S. G. Gabbe, J. R. Niebyl, J. L. Simpson, et al. (Eds.), *Obstetrics: Normal and problem pregnancies* (7th ed.). Philadelphia, PA: Elsevier.

Wapner, R. J. (2014). Prenatal diagnosis of congenital disorders. In R. K. Creasy, R. Resnik, J. D. Iams, et al. (Eds.), *Creasy and Resnik's maternal-fetal medicine: Principles and practice* (7th ed.). Philadelphia, PA: Saunders.

Whitty, J. E., & Dombrowski, M. P. (2014). Respiratory diseases in pregnancy. In R. K. Creasy, R. Resnik, J. D. Iams, et al. (Eds.), *Creasy and Resnik's maternal-fetal medicine: Principles and practice* (7th ed.). Philadelphia, PA: Saunders.

Whitty, J. E., & Dombrowski, M. P. (2017). Respiratory disease in pregnancy. In S. G. Gabbe, J. R. Niebyl, J. L. Simpson, et al. (Eds.), *Obstetrics: Normal and problem pregnancies* (7th ed.). Philadelphia, PA: Elsevier.

Williamson, C., Mackillop, L., & Heneghan, M. A. (2014). Diseases of the liver, biliary system, and pancreas. In R. K. Creasy, R. Resnik, J. D. Iams, et al. (Eds.), *Creasy and Resnik's maternal-fetal medicine: Principles and practice* (7th ed.). Philadelphia, PA: Saunders.

Wisner, K. L., Sit, D. K. Y., Bogen, D. L., et al. (2017). Mental health and behavioral disorders in pregnancy. In S. G. Gabbe, J. R. Niebyl, J. L. Simpson, et al. (Eds.), *Obstetrics: Normal and problem pregnancies* (7th ed.). Philadelphia, PA: Elsevier.

World Health Organization. (2016). *10 facts about diabetes.* Retrieved from www.who.int/features/factfiles/diabetes/en.

12

High-Risk Perinatal Care: Gestational Conditions

Kitty Cashion

e http://evolve.elsevier.com/Perry/maternal

Some women experience significant problems during the months of gestation that can greatly affect pregnancy outcome. Some of these conditions develop as a result of the pregnant state; others are problems that can happen to anyone at any time of life but occur in this case during pregnancy. This chapter discusses a variety of disorders that did not exist before pregnancy, all of which have at least one thing in common: their occurrence in pregnancy places the woman and fetus at risk. Hypertension in pregnancy, hyperemesis gravidarum, hemorrhagic complications of early and late pregnancy, urinary tract infection (UTI), surgery during pregnancy, and trauma are discussed. For each problem, management throughout the entire perinatal period (antepartum, intrapartum, and postpartum), including interprofessional care, is included in this chapter; thus all the information for each condition is located in one place in the text.

HYPERTENSION IN PREGNANCY

SIGNIFICANCE AND INCIDENCE

Hypertensive disorders are some of the most common medical complications of pregnancy, occurring in approximately 5% to 10% of all pregnancies. The incidence varies among hospitals, regions, and countries. Hypertensive disorders are a major cause of maternal and perinatal morbidity and mortality worldwide (Sibai, 2017). In the United States and Canada, they are one of the top causes of maternal morbidity and mortality (Harvey & Sibai, 2013). The three most common types of hypertensive disorders occurring in pregnancy are gestational hypertension, preeclampsia, and chronic essential hypertension (Sibai).

CLASSIFICATION

The classification of hypertensive disorders in pregnancy is confusing because standard definitions are not used consistently by all health care providers. The classification system most commonly used in the United States since 2000 was based on recommendations from the American College of Obstetricians and Gynecologists (ACOG) and the National High Blood Pressure Education Program Working Group on High Blood Pressure in Pregnancy. In 2013, ACOG convened a task force of experts in the management of hypertension in pregnancy. The Task Force on Hypertension in Pregnancy chose to continue use of this classification system, although it modified some of the system components (ACOG, 2013). The current classification system is summarized in Table 12.1.

Gestational Hypertension

Gestational hypertension is the onset of hypertension without proteinuria or other systemic findings diagnostic for preeclampsia after week 20 of pregnancy (ACOG, 2013). *Hypertension* is defined as a systolic blood pressure (BP) greater than 140 mm Hg or a diastolic BP greater than 90 mm Hg. The hypertension should be recorded on two occasions at least 4 hours apart after 20 weeks of gestation in a woman with a previously normal blood pressure (ACOG, 2013). Only one pressure (either systolic or diastolic) must be elevated to meet the definition of hypertension (Harvey & Sibai, 2013).

The definitions of gestational hypertension are the same as the definitions for blood pressure readings for preeclampsia (Table 12.2). Gestational hypertension does not persist longer than 12 weeks postpartum and usually resolves during the first postpartum week (Harvey & Sibai, 2013). Some women who are initially thought to have gestational hypertension are eventually diagnosed with chronic hypertension instead. About 25% to 50% of women with gestational hypertension go on to develop preeclampsia (Snydal, 2014).

Preeclampsia

Preeclampsia is a pregnancy-specific condition in which hypertension and proteinuria develop after 20 weeks of gestation in a woman who previously had neither condition. The signs and symptoms of preeclampsia also can develop for the first time during the postpartum period.

The 2013 ACOG Task Force on Hypertension in Pregnancy eliminated several criteria that had traditionally been used to diagnose severe features of preeclampsia. These include proteinuria, oliguria, presence of intrauterine growth restriction (IUGR), or fetal growth restriction as a requirement for the diagnosis of preeclampsia (Sibai, 2017). In the absence of proteinuria, preeclampsia may be defined as hypertension along with either thrombocytopenia, impaired liver function, new-onset renal insufficiency, pulmonary edema, or new-onset cerebral or visual disturbances (see Table 12.2) (ACOG, 2013). Table 12.3 lists common laboratory changes that occur in preeclampsia.

Eclampsia

Eclampsia is the onset of seizure activity or coma in a woman with preeclampsia who has no history of preexisting pathology that can result in seizure activity (Harvey & Sibai, 2013; Markham & Funai, 2014). In developed countries, eclampsia occurs in approximately 1 in 2000 to 1 in 3448 births. The incidence is usually higher in tertiary referral centers, with multifetal gestation, and in women who did not receive prenatal care (Sibai, 2017). Although eclamptic seizures can occur before, during, or after birth, approximately 50% of cases occur during the antepartum period (Poole, 2014).

Chronic Hypertensive Disorders
Chronic Hypertension
Chronic hypertension is defined as hypertension that is present before the pregnancy (ACOG, 2013). Hypertension initially diagnosed during pregnancy that persists longer than 12 weeks postpartum is also classified as chronic hypertension (Harvey & Sibai, 2013).

Chronic Hypertension With Superimposed Preeclampsia
Women with chronic hypertension may develop superimposed preeclampsia. This condition, which is associated with adverse maternal or fetal outcomes, can be difficult to diagnose (ACOG, 2013).

PREECLAMPSIA

ETIOLOGY

Preeclampsia is a condition unique to human pregnancy. It occurs in approximately 2% to 7% of healthy nulliparous pregnant women. The incidence and severity of preeclampsia is substantially higher in women with multifetal gestation, a history of preeclampsia, chronic hypertension, preexisting diabetes, and preexisting thrombophilias. Women with limited sperm exposure with the same partner before conception also have a greater risk for developing preeclampsia. Paternal factors also contribute to the risk for preeclampsia. Men who have fathered a preeclamptic pregnancy are nearly twice as likely to father another preeclamptic pregnancy with a different woman, regardless of whether the new partner has a history of a preeclamptic pregnancy (Sibai, 2017). Common risk factors associated with the development of preeclampsia are listed in Box 12.1.

The etiology of preeclampsia is unknown. Many theories have been suggested to explain its etiology. Current theories that are still being considered include abnormal trophoblast invasion, immunologic response to partially foreign genetic placental and fetal tissue, stimulation of the inflammatory system by cardiovascular changes of pregnancy, various dietary deficiencies, and genetic abnormalities (Harvey & Sibai, 2013).

PATHOPHYSIOLOGY

Preeclampsia is a progressive disorder, with the placenta as the root cause. Therefore, the disease begins to resolve after the placenta has been expelled. Current thought is that the pathologic changes that occur

---

TABLE 12.1   Classification of Hypertensive States of Pregnancy

Type	Description
Gestational Hypertensive Disorders	
Gestational hypertension	Development of hypertension after week 20 of pregnancy in a previously normotensive woman without proteinuria or other systemic findings (see description of Preeclampsia below)
Preeclampsia	Development of hypertension and proteinuria in a previously normotensive woman after 20 weeks of gestation or in the early postpartum period. In the absence of proteinuria, the development of new-onset hypertension with the new onset of any of the following: thrombocytopenia, renal insufficiency, impaired liver function, pulmonary edema, or cerebral or visual symptoms
Eclampsia	Development of seizures or coma not attributable to other causes in a preeclamptic woman
Chronic Hypertensive Disorders	
Chronic hypertension	Hypertension in a pregnant woman present before pregnancy
Superimposed preeclampsia	Chronic hypertension in association with preeclampsia

Data from American College of Obstetricians and Gynecologists. (2013). Executive summary: Hypertension in pregnancy. *Obstetrics & Gynecology, 122*(5), 1122-1131.

TABLE 12.2   Diagnostic Criteria for Preeclampsia and Preeclampsia With Severe Features

Component	Preeclampsia	Preeclampsia With Severe Features
Hypertension	Blood pressure (BP) reading ≥140/90 mm Hg × 2, at least 4 hours apart after 20 weeks of gestation in a previously normotensive woman	BP reading ≥160/110 mm Hg × 2, at least 4 hours apart while the woman is on bed rest (unless antihypertensive therapy has already been initiated)
Proteinuria	Proteinuria of ≥300 mg in a 24-hour specimen. Protein/creatinine ratio ≥0.3 (with each measured as mg/dL) ≥1+ on dipstick (used only if quantitative measurement is not available	Massive proteinuria (>5 g in a 24-hour specimen) is no longer used as a diagnostic criterion
Thrombocytopenia	Platelet count <100,000/μL	Platelet count <100,000/μL
Impaired liver function	Elevated blood levels of liver transaminases to twice the normal concentration	Abnormally elevated blood concentrations of liver enzymes to twice the normal concentration; severe persistent epigastric or right upper quadrant abdominal pain unresponsive to medication and not accounted for by alternative diagnoses, or both
Renal insufficiency	New development of serum creatinine >1.1 mg/dL or a doubling of the serum creatinine concentration in the absence of other renal disease	Progressive renal insufficiency (serum creatinine concentration >1.1 mg/dL or a doubling of the serum creatinine concentration) in the absence of other renal disease
Pulmonary edema		Present
Cerebral or visual disturbances		New onset

Modified from American College of Obstetricians and Gynecologists. (2013). Executive summary: Hypertension in pregnancy. *Obstetrics & Gynecology, 122*(5), 1122-1131.

TABLE 12.3 Common Laboratory Changes in Preeclampsia

	Normal Nonpregnant	Preeclampsia	HELLP
Hemoglobin, hematocrit	12–16 g/dL, 37%–47%	May ↑	↓
Platelets (cells/mm³)	150,000–400,000/mm³	<100,000/mm³	<100,000/mm³
Prothrombin time (PT), partial thromboplastin time (PTT)	12–14 sec, 60–70 sec	Unchanged	Unchanged
Fibrinogen	200–400 mg/dL	300–600 mg/dL	↓
Fibrin split products (FSPs)	Absent	Absent or present	Present
Blood urea nitrogen (BUN)	10–20 mg/dL	↑	↑
Creatinine	0.5–1.1 mg/dL	>1.1 mg/dL	↑
Lactate dehydrogenase (LDH)*	45–90 units/L	↑	↑ (>600 units/L)
Aspartate aminotransferase (AST)	4–20 units/L	↑	↑ (>70 units/L)
Alanine aminotransferase (ALT)	3–21 units/L	↑	↑
Creatinine clearance	80–125 mL/min	130–180 mL/min	↓
Burr cells or schistocytes	Absent	Absent	Present
Uric acid	2–6.6 mg/dL	>5.9 mg/dL	>10 mg/dL
Bilirubin (total)	0.1–1 mg/dL	Unchanged or ↑	↑ (>1.2 mg/dL)

*LDH values differ according to the test or assays being performed.
Data from American College of Obstetricians and Gynecologists (ACOG). (2002). *Practice bulletin no. 33: Diagnosis and management of preeclampsia and eclampsia.* Washington, DC: ACOG; American College of Obstetricians and Gynecologists. (2013). Executive summary: Hypertension in pregnancy. *Obstetrics & Gynecology, 122*(5), 1122-1131; Dildy, G. (2004). Complications of preeclampsia. In G. Dildy, M. Belfort, G. Saade, et al. (Eds.), *Critical care obstetrics* (4th ed.). Malden, MA: Blackwell Science; Harvey, C., & Sibai, B. (2013). Hypertension in pregnancy. In N.H. Troiano, C.J. Harvey, & B.F. Chez (Eds.), *AWHONN's high risk and critical care obstetrics* (3rd ed.). Philadelphia, PA: Lippincott Williams & Wilkins.

BOX 12.1 Risk Factors for Preeclampsia

- Nulliparity
- Age >40 years
- Pregnancy with assisted reproductive techniques
- Interpregnancy interval >7 years
- Family history of preeclampsia
- Woman born small for gestational age
- Obesity/gestational diabetes mellitus
- Multifetal gestation
- Preeclampsia in previous pregnancy
- Poor outcome in previous pregnancy
- Preexisting medical/genetic conditions
- Chronic hypertension
- Renal disease
- Type 1 (insulin-dependent) diabetes mellitus
- Antiphospholipid antibody syndrome
- Factor V Leiden mutation

From Sibai, B. (2017). Preeclampsia and hypertensive disorders. (2017). In S. G. Gabbe, J. R. Niebyl, J. L. Simpson, et al. (Eds.), *Obstetrics: Normal and problem pregnancies* (7th ed.). Philadelphia, PA: Elsevier.

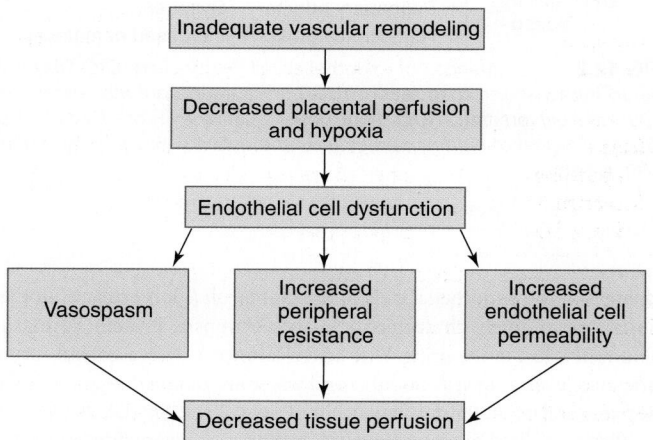

FIG 12.1 Etiology of preeclampsia: Disruptions in placental perfusion and endothelial cell dysfunction. (Data from Harvey, C., & Sibai, B. (2013). Hypertension in pregnancy. In N. Troiano, C. Harvey, & B. Chez [Eds.], *AWHONN's high risk and critical care obstetrics* (3rd ed.). Philadelphia, PA: Wolters Kluwer/Lippincott; Markham, K.B., & Funai, E.F. (2014). Pregnancy-related hypertension. In R.K. Creasy, R. Resnik, J.D. Iams, et al. [Eds.], *Creasy and Resnik's maternal-fetal medicine: Principles and practice* (7th ed.). Philadelphia, PA: Saunders; Poole, J.H. (2014). Hypertensive disorders of pregnancy. In K.R. Simpson, & P. Creehan (Eds.), *AWHONN's perinatal nursing* (4th ed.). Philadelphia, PA: Lippincott.)

in the woman with preeclampsia are caused by disruptions in placental perfusion and endothelial cell dysfunction (ACOG, 2013; Harvey & Sibai, 2013; Sibai, 2017; Snydal, 2014). These changes develop early in pregnancy, long before the signs and symptoms of preeclampsia become evident (Markham & Funai, 2014; Sibai; Snydal). Normally in pregnancy, the spiral arteries in the uterus widen from thick-walled muscular vessels to thinner, saclike vessels with much larger diameters. This change increases the capacity of the vessels, allowing them to handle the increased blood volume of pregnancy. Because this vascular remodeling does not occur or only partially develops in women with preeclampsia, decreased placental perfusion and hypoxia result (Harvey & Sibai).

Placental ischemia is thought to cause endothelial cell dysfunction by stimulating the release of a substance that is toxic to endothelial

cells. This anomaly causes generalized vasospasm, which results in poor tissue perfusion in all organ systems, increased peripheral resistance and BP, and increased endothelial cell permeability, leading to intravascular protein and fluid loss and ultimately to less plasma volume. The main pathogenic factor is not an increase in BP but poor perfusion as a result of vasospasm and reduced plasma volume (Fig. 12.1) (Markham & Funai, 2014; Poole, 2014). Fig. 12.2 demonstrates how endothelial cell dysfunction causes many of the common signs and symptoms of preeclampsia.

Reduced kidney perfusion decreases the glomerular filtration rate and can lead to degenerative glomerular changes and oliguria. Pathologic

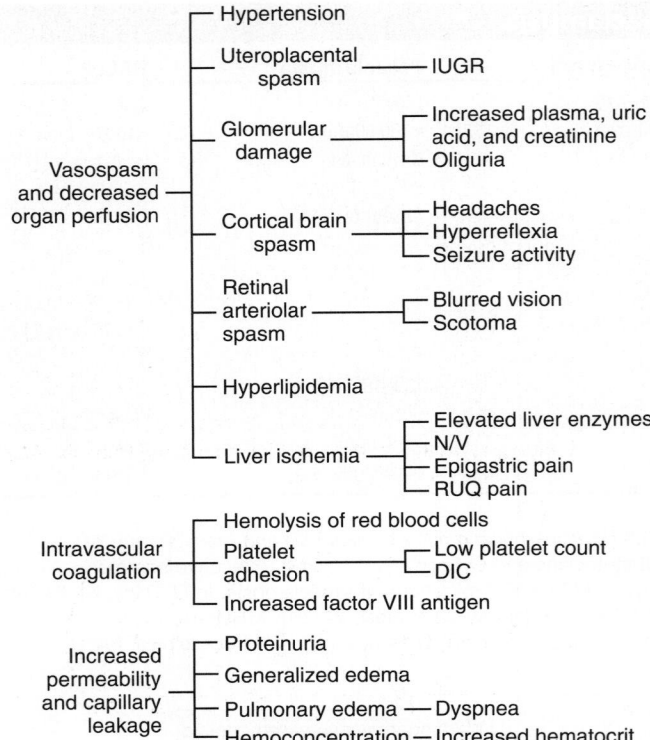

FIG 12.2 Consequences of endothelial cell dysfunction. *DIC,* Disseminated intravascular coagulation; *IUGR,* intrauterine growth restriction; *N/V,* nausea/vomiting; *RUQ,* right upper quadrant. (From Gilbert, E.S. [2011]. *Manual of high risk pregnancy and delivery* [5th ed.]. St. Louis, MO: Mosby.)

changes in the endothelial cells of the glomeruli (glomerular endotheliosis) are uniquely characteristic of preeclampsia. Protein, primarily albumin, is lost in the urine. Uric acid clearance is decreased, but serum uric acid levels increase. Sodium and water are retained. Acute tubular necrosis and renal failure may occur (Poole, 2014; Snydal, 2014).

Plasma colloid osmotic pressure decreases as serum albumin levels decrease. Intravascular volume is reduced as fluid moves out of the intravascular compartment, resulting in hemoconcentration, increased blood viscosity, and tissue edema. The hematocrit value increases as fluid leaves the intravascular space. Arteriolar vasospasm can lead to endothelial damage and increased capillary permeability, predisposing the woman to pulmonary edema (see Fig. 12.2) (Poole, 2014; Snydal, 2014).

Decreased liver perfusion can lead to impaired liver function and elevated liver enzyme levels. If hepatic edema and subcapsular hemorrhage develop, the woman may complain of epigastric or right upper quadrant abdominal pain. Hemorrhagic necrosis in the liver can result in a subcapsular hematoma, which is a rare occurrence. Rupture of a subcapsular hematoma is a life-threatening complication and a surgical emergency (Snydal, 2014) (see Fig. 12.2).

Neurologic complications associated with preeclampsia include cerebral edema and hemorrhage and increased central nervous system (CNS) irritability. CNS irritability manifests as headaches, hyperreflexia, positive ankle clonus, and seizures. Arteriolar vasospasms and decreased blood flow to the retina can lead to visual disturbances such as scotoma (dim vision or blind or dark spots in the visual field) and blurred or double vision (Poole, 2014; Snydal, 2014).

HELLP SYNDROME

HELLP syndrome is a laboratory diagnosis for a variant of preeclampsia that involves hepatic dysfunction, characterized by hemolysis *(H),* elevated liver enzymes *(EL),* and low platelet *(LP)* count. It is not a separate illness. Specific laboratory findings are needed to diagnose HELLP syndrome and distinguish it from other serious diseases that share the same signs and symptoms. HELLP syndrome occurs in 0.5% to 0.9% of all pregnancies—10% to 20% of women with preeclampsia with severe features develop it (Harvey & Sibai, 2013). Table 12.3 lists laboratory changes that occur in HELLP syndrome. Traditionally it was not diagnosed unless all three laboratory abnormalities were present. Currently, however, women who develop only one or two of the diagnostic laboratory values are being diagnosed with incomplete HELLP, partial HELLP, or the ELLP syndrome (Harvey & Sibai).

HELLP syndrome usually develops during the antepartum period. The clinical presentation is often nonspecific. Most women with the disorder report a history of malaise, influenza-like symptoms, and epigastric or right upper quadrant abdominal pain. Symptoms tend to worsen at night and improve during the daytime. HELLP syndrome can progress rapidly (Harvey & Sibai, 2013).

> **! NURSING ALERT**
>
> An extremely important point to understand is that many women with HELLP syndrome may not have signs or symptoms of preeclampsia with severe features. For example, although most women have hypertension, BP may be only mildly elevated in 15% to 50% of cases. Proteinuria may be absent. As a result, women with HELLP syndrome are often misdiagnosed with a variety of other medical or surgical disorders (Sibai, 2017).

HELLP syndrome appears to occur more frequently in Caucasian women than women of other races. A diagnosis of HELLP syndrome is associated with an increased risk for maternal death and adverse perinatal outcomes, including pulmonary edema, acute renal failure, disseminated intravascular coagulation (DIC), placental abruption, liver hemorrhage or failure, acute respiratory distress syndrome (ARDS), sepsis, and stroke (Sibai, 2017). The reported perinatal mortality rate ranges from 7.4% to 34%, with a maternal mortality rate of approximately 1% (Sibai). The rate of preterm birth in women with HELLP syndrome is approximately 70%, with 15% of these occurring before 28 weeks of gestation. Most of the perinatal deaths occur before 28 weeks of gestation in association with placental abruption or severe fetal growth restriction (Sibai).

CARE MANAGEMENT

Identifying and Preventing Preeclampsia

Numerous clinical trials have examined various interventions to prevent preeclampsia, including protein or salt restriction; zinc, magnesium, fish oil, or vitamin C and E supplementation; use of diuretics or other antihypertensive medications; and use of heparin. All of these interventions demonstrated minimal to no benefit in preventing or reducing the incidence of preeclampsia (Sibai, 2017). However, low-dose aspirin has been found to reduce preeclampsia and adverse outcomes in selected high-risk women. ACOG recommends that consideration be given to initiating daily low-dose (81 mg/day) aspirin therapy between 12 and 28 weeks of gestation for the prevention of preeclampsia. It is recommended that only women considered to be at high risk for developing preeclampsia take the low-dose aspirin. This includes women with the following risk factors: history of preeclampsia, especially if accompanied by an adverse outcome; multifetal gestation; chronic hypertension; preexisting diabetes (type 1 or type 2); renal disease; and autoimmune disease (e.g., systemic lupus erythematosus, antiphospholipid syndrome). (ACOG, 2016).

No reliable test that can be used as a routine screening tool for predicting preeclampsia has yet been developed. However, the search for biomarkers that can identify individual women who will develop hypertension during pregnancy is ongoing (Harvey & Sibai, 2013). Evaluation of maternal clinical factors and biophysical or biochemical markers measured during the first trimester is useful only for predicting women who will go on to develop preeclampsia and will need to give birth before 34 weeks of gestation. At this time, the use of first-trimester screening tests for predicting preeclampsia in clinical practice is not recommended (Sibai, 2017). Abnormal uterine artery Doppler findings in the second trimester of pregnancy have also been noted in women who go on to develop preeclampsia. At this time, however, data do not support the use of Doppler studies for routine screening of pregnant women for preeclampsia (Sibai).

Although research offers future promise, much work remains before a screening test for preeclampsia is available for widespread clinical use. Nurses should be aware of strategies that are being studied and use the most valid results so they can counsel pregnant women about interventions that are evidence-based. Meanwhile the best preeclampsia prevention methods include early prenatal care for the identification of women at risk and early detection of the disease (see Evidence-Based Practice box: Prevention of Preeclampsia).

Assessment

Accurate measurement of BP is essential in the early detection of hypertensive disorders. Many factors influence BP measurement, including accuracy of the equipment used, size of the sphygmomanometer cuff, duration of the rest period before recording the BP, posture of the patient, and the Korotkoff phase used (phase IV or phase V) for diastolic BP measurement (see Box 7.1) (Sibai, 2017).

Electronic blood pressure devices, often used in inpatient settings, produce different BP measurements from those obtained using a manual cuff and stethoscope. Electronic devices consistently underestimate diastolic BPs by approximately 10 mm Hg and overestimate systolic BP values by 4 to 6 mm Hg. Therefore, BP readings taken using different measurement devices are not interchangeable. BP assessment should focus on trends over time, rather than on a single measurement (Poole, 2014).

Assessment for edema is another component of the physical examination, although the presence of edema is no longer included in the definition of preeclampsia. Edema is assessed for distribution, degree, and pitting. Dependent edema is edema of the lowest or most dependent parts of the body, where hydrostatic pressure is greatest. If a pregnant woman is ambulatory, the edema may first be evident in the feet and ankles. If she is confined to bed, it is more likely to occur in the sacral region. Pitting edema leaves a small depression or pit after finger pressure is applied to the swollen area (Fig. 12.3). The pit, which is caused by movement of fluid to adjacent tissue away from the point of pressure, normally disappears within 10 to 30 seconds. Although the amount of edema is difficult to quantify, the method shown in Fig. 12.4 may be used to record relative degrees of edema formation.

Deep tendon reflexes (DTRs) reflect the balance between the cerebral cortex and spinal cord. They are evaluated as a baseline and to detect any changes. The biceps and patellar reflexes are assessed, and the findings recorded (Fig. 12.5 and Table 12.4). To elicit the biceps reflex, the examiner strikes a downward blow over the thumb, which is situated over the biceps tendon (see Fig. 12.5, A). Normal response is flexion of the arm at the elbow, described as a 2+ response. The patellar reflex

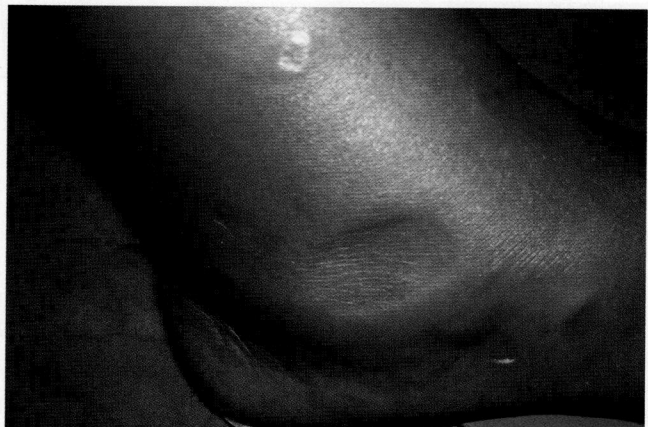

FIG 12.3 Pitting edema. (Courtesy of Shannon Perry, Phoenix, AZ.)

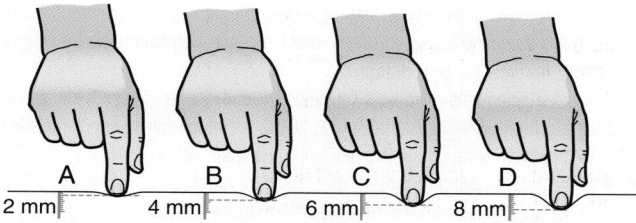

FIG 12.4 Assessment of pitting edema of lower extremities. A, +1; B, +2; C, +3; D, +4.

TABLE 12.4	**Assessing Deep Tendon Reflexes**
Grade	**Deep Tendon Reflex Response**
0	No response
1+	Sluggish or diminished
2+	Active or expected response
3+	More brisk than expected, slightly hyperactive
4+	Brisk, hyperactive, with intermittent or transient clonus

From Ball J.W., Dains J.E., Flynn J.A., et al. (2015). *Seidel's guide to physical examination*, (8th ed.) St. Louis, MO: Mosby.

is elicited with the woman's legs hanging freely over the end of the examining table or with the woman lying on her side with the knee slightly flexed (see Fig. 12.5, D). The patellar tendon (inferior to the patella) is tapped with a percussion hammer. Normal response is the extension or kicking out of the leg.

To assess for hyperactive reflexes (clonus) at the ankle joint, the examiner supports the leg with the knee flexed (see Fig. 12.5, F). With one hand, the examiner sharply dorsiflexes the foot, maintains the position for a moment, and then releases it. Normal (negative clonus) response is elicited when no rhythmic oscillations (jerks) are felt while the foot is held in dorsiflexion. When the foot is released, no oscillations are seen as the foot drops to the plantar-flexed position. Abnormal (positive clonus) response is recognized by rhythmic oscillations of one or more "beats" felt when the foot is in dorsiflexion and seen as the foot drops to the plantar-flexed position.

The presence of proteinuria is ideally determined by evaluation of a 24-hour urine collection. In a 24-hour specimen, proteinuria is defined as a concentration at or greater than 300 mg or a protein/creatinine ratio greater than 0.3. If it is not possible to obtain either of these

EVIDENCE-BASED PRACTICE
Prevention of Preeclampsia

Ask the Question

PICOT Question: For pregnant women, what are the new best practices for the prevention of preeclampsia?

Search for the Evidence

Search Strategies: English research-based publications on preeclampsia (pre-eclampsia, pre eclampsia), gestational hypertension were included.

Databases Used: Cochrane Collaborative Database, National Guideline Clearinghouse (AHRQ), CINAHL, PubMed, UpToDate, PLoS ONE, Joanna Briggs Institute, NICE, and the professional websites for ACOG and AWHONN.

Critical Appraisal of the Evidence

Risk factors for preeclampsia include smoking, young or old age, nulliparity, unmarried status, African-American race, multiple fetuses, chronic hypertension, diabetes, and history of prior preeclampsia.

In addition to management of gestational weight gain within recommendations, research has found the following to be protective against preeclampsia for pregnant women at low risk for preeclampsia:

- Calcium supplements of at least 1 g/day, especially for women with low-calcium diets (Hoffmeyr, Lawrie, Atallah, et al., 2014). An alternative to supplementation is 3–4 dairy servings daily (Magee, Pels, Helewa, et al., 2014).
- A prepregnancy Mediterranean diet, high in vegetables, fish, legumes and nuts, is associated with a protective affect against hypertensive disorders of pregnancy (Schoenaker, Soedamah-Muthu, Callaway, & Mishra, 2015).

For women at high risk for preeclampsia, the following additional measures may be beneficial (Magee, et al., 2014);

- Low-dose aspirin, started before 16 weeks of gestation.
- L-Arginine supplement.
- Increased rest at home in the third trimester

Women with prior history of preeclampsia can decrease their risk for recurrent disease by avoiding prolonged interpregnancy intervals above 4 years (Cormick, Betran, Ciapponi, et al., 2016). Longer interpregnancy intervals mean older maternal age, increased weight, and maternal disorders.

Apply the Evidence: Nursing Implications

- Preconception counseling for modifiable risk factors, such a smoking, weight gain, calcium intake, and Mediterranean diet can decrease preeclampsia risk.
- The nurse can educate women who have had preeclampsia about the benefits of interpregnancy intervals of no more than 4 years.
- Teaching stress management techniques for lifelong and pregnancy stress are important, especially in the presence of chronic hypertension.
- In addition to assessing blood pressure, alert nurses are often the first to note subtle clinical changes indicating preeclampsia, such as sudden weight gain, edema, headache, oliguria, right-sided pain, and fetal distress.

- In the event of emergent hypertensive crisis, nurses must be familiar and proficient with assessments, including reflexes and fetal monitoring, understand medications, and be proactive in environmental alteration, such as limiting visitors and lowering lights and sound in the room.
- Women with a history of recurrent preeclampsia are at twice the risk for heart disease and three times the risk for cardiovascular disease, and so should begin screening for these earlier in life (Auger, Fraser, Schnitzer, et al., 2016).

Quality and Safety Competencies: Evidence-Based Practice*
Knowledge

Describe reliable sources for locating evidence reports and clinical practice guidelines.

Use high-level evidence to guide the comprehensive preconception and prenatal care of women at risk for preeclampsia.

Skills

Locate evidence reports related to clinical practice topics and guidelines.

Relevant systematic reviews and professional guidelines provide recommendations for improving outcomes by identifying women at risk for preeclampsia and educating patients about prevention and treatment.

Attitudes

Value the concept of EBP as integral to determining best clinical practices.
EBP guides practice and fosters patient confidence and efficacy.

References

Auger, N., Fraser, W. D., Schnitzer, M., et al. (2016). Recurrent pre-eclampsia and subsequent cardiovascular risk. *Heart (British Cardiac Society)* (Online First 16 Aug 2016), 1–9. [Epub ahead of print].

Cormick, G., Betran, A. P., Ciapponi, A., et al. (2016). Inter-pregnancy interval and risk of recurrent pre-eclampsia: Systematic review and meta-analysis. *Reproductive Health*, 13(83), 1–10.

Hoffmeyr, G. J., Lawrie, T. A., et al. (2014). Calcium supplementation during pregnancy for preventing hypertensive disorders and related problems (review). *Cochrane Database of Systematic Reviews, 2014*(6), CD001059.

Magee, L. A., Pels, A., Helewa, M., et al. (2014). Diagnosis, evaluation, and management of the hypertensive disorders of pregnancy. *Pregnancy Hypertension, 4*(2), 105–145.

Schoenaker, D. A., Soedemah-Muthu, S. S., Callaway, L. K., et al. (2015). Prepregnancy dietary patterns and risk of developing hypertensive disorders of pregnancy: results from the Australian Longitudinal Study on Women's Health. *American Journal of Clinical Nutrition, 102*(1), 94–101.

Pat Mahaffee Gingrich

*Adapted from QSEN at www.qsen.org/.

measurements, proteinuria can be diagnosed by a dipstick measurement of at least 1+ on two occasions. Proteinuria is influenced by contamination with vaginal secretions, blood, bacteria, or amniotic fluid. It also varies with urine specific gravity and pH, exercise, and posture (Sibai, 2017).

Although proteinuria may still be used to define preeclampsia, studies have shown little relationship between the degree of proteinuria in women with preeclampsia and pregnancy outcome. Therefore, massive proteinuria (>5 g) is not considered to be a severe feature of preeclampsia. Because a 24-hour collection to measure the quantity of protein and creatinine clearance is more reflective of true renal status, it is preferred

over dipstick testing, which should not be used for diagnosis of preeclampsia if at all possible (ACOG, 2013).

During the examination, the woman is evaluated for signs and symptoms considered to be severe features of preeclampsia such as severe headaches (usually frontal), epigastric pain (heartburn), right upper quadrant abdominal pain, or visual disturbances such as scotoma, photophobia, or double vision.

Nursing Diagnoses

Nursing diagnoses for the woman with preeclampsia may include the following:

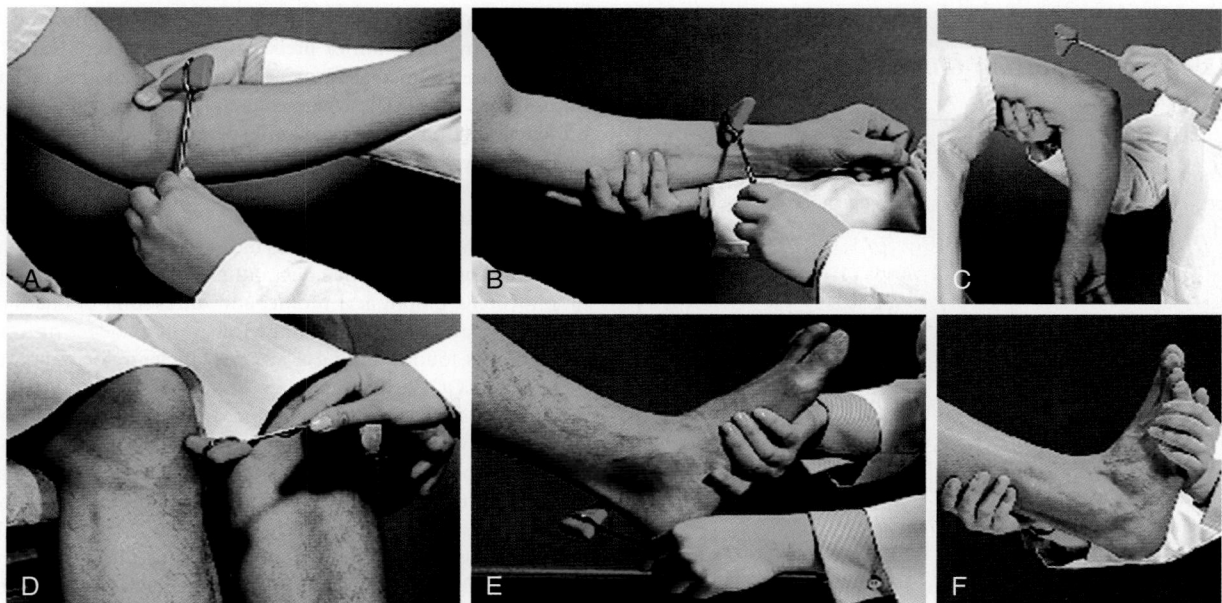

FIG 12.5 Location of tendons for evaluation of deep tendon reflexes. **A,** Biceps. **B,** Brachioradial. **C,** Triceps. **D,** Patellar. **E,** Achilles. **F,** Evaluation of ankle clonus. (From Seidel, H., Ball, J., Dains, J., et al. [2011]. *Mosby's guide to physical examination* [7th ed.]. St. Louis, MO: Mosby.)

- *Anxiety* related to
  - Preeclampsia and its effects on the woman and infant
- *Deficient Knowledge* related to
  - Management of preeclampsia (maternal and fetal assessment, medications, activity restriction, plans for labor and birth)
- *Disabled Family Coping* related to
  - Restricted activity and concern over a high-risk pregnancy
  - Financial concerns
- *Powerlessness* related to
  - Inability to prevent or control condition and outcomes
- *Risk for Injury* to woman related to
  - Hypertension
  - Central nervous system (CNS) irritability secondary to cerebral edema
  - Vasospasm
  - Decreased renal perfusion
- *Risk for Injury* to fetus related to
  - Disruption of oxygen transfer from environment to fetus
  - Intrauterine growth restriction (IUGR)
  - Placental abruption
  - Preterm birth

Interventions

Gestational Hypertension and Preeclampsia Without Severe Features

In the past, both gestational hypertension and preeclampsia were usually described as either "mild" or "severe." Because preeclampsia is a dynamic disease process, this practice is no longer recommended. A diagnosis of "mild preeclampsia" applies only at the time it is made. Women must be evaluated frequently to determine if the disease has progressed to the point that severe features are present (see Table 12.2) (ACOG, 2013).

The goals of therapy for women with gestational hypertension and preeclampsia without severe features are to ensure maternal safety and to deliver a healthy newborn as close to term as possible. Prior to 37 gestational weeks, care management is expectant with close monitoring of the maternal and fetal status. Most women with gestational hypertension or preeclampsia without severe features can be safely managed at home, provided they have frequent maternal and fetal evaluation (Sibai, 2017). Vaginal birth by induction of labor, preceded by cervical ripening (if necessary), is recommended beginning at 37 gestational weeks. At this gestational age, the risks to the fetus outweigh any potential benefits of continuing the pregnancy (ACOG, 2013; Sibai).

Outpatient management can be considered for reliable women who have a systolic BP of 155 mm Hg or less or a diastolic BP of 105 mm Hg or less and no symptoms (Sibai, 2017). A regular diet without salt restriction is recommended. Women should be taught to go to the hospital or outpatient facility immediately if they develop abdominal pain, significant headache, uterine contractions, vaginal spotting, or decreased fetal movement (Sibai). Successful home care requires the woman to be well educated about preeclampsia and highly motivated to follow the plan of care (see Patient Teaching box: Assessing and Reporting Clinical Signs of Preeclampsia). All teaching should include the woman and her family, and time must be allowed for them to absorb information, ask questions, and voice concerns. Methods for enhancing learning include visual aids, DVDs or Internet videos, handouts, and demonstrations with return demonstrations. Furthermore, the effects of illness, language, age, cultural beliefs, and support systems must be considered.

Maternal and fetal assessment. Initial laboratory evaluation for women with gestational hypertension or preeclampsia without severe features includes measurement of serum creatinine, platelet count, and liver enzymes. Thereafter, hematocrit, platelet count, serum creatinine, and liver function tests should be performed weekly. Women are also evaluated for signs or symptoms of severe features such as severe headaches, blurred or double vision, mental confusion, right upper quadrant abdominal or epigastric pain, nausea or vomiting, shortness of breath, and decreased urinary output (ACOG, 2013; Sibai, 2017). BP should be monitored twice weekly and proteinuria assessed weekly (ACOG).

Fetal evaluation generally includes daily fetal movement counts and nonstress testing or a biophysical profile once or twice weekly until birth (see Chapter 10 for more information on fetal assessment tests). Ultrasound evaluation of amniotic fluid status and determination of

PATIENT TEACHING

Assessing and Reporting Clinical Signs of Preeclampsia

- Take your blood pressure as directed. Always sit to take your blood pressure, and use your right arm each time for consistent and accurate readings. Support your arm on a table in a horizontal position at heart level.
- Report any increase in your blood pressure to your health care provider immediately.
- Dipstick test your clean-catch urine sample as directed to assess proteinuria.
- Report to your health care provider if proteinuria is 1+ or more or if you have a decrease in urine output.
- Assess your baby's activity daily. Decreased activity (four or fewer movements per hour) may indicate fetal compromise and should be reported.
- Be sure to keep your scheduled prenatal appointments so that any changes in your or your baby's condition can be detected.
- Keep a daily log or diary of your assessments for your home health care nurse, or take it with you to your next prenatal visit.
- Report any headache, dizziness, or blurred vision to your health care provider immediately.

estimated fetal weight are performed at the time preeclampsia is diagnosed and serially thereafter, depending on findings. Doppler blood flow studies are recommended if IUGR is suspected (Sibai, 2017).

Activity restriction. Complete or partial bed rest for the duration of the pregnancy is still recommended frequently by health care providers. However, no evidence has been found that this practice improves pregnancy outcomes. Moreover, prolonged bed rest is known to increase the risk for thrombophlebitis (Sibai, 2017). Other adverse physiologic outcomes related to complete bed rest include cardiovascular deconditioning; diuresis with accompanying fluid, electrolyte, and weight loss; muscle atrophy; and psychologic stress. These changes begin on the first day of bed rest and continue for the duration of therapy. Therefore, restricted activity rather than complete bed rest is recommended (ACOG, 2013; Sibai).

Women with preeclampsia generally feel reasonably well; therefore, boredom from activity restriction is common. Diversionary activities, including television and computer or smart phone use, visits from friends, and a comfortable and convenient environment are ways to cope with the boredom. Participation in online prenatal classes also may be possible. Gentle exercise (e.g., range-of-motion exercises, stretching, Kegel exercises, pelvic tilts) is important in maintaining muscle tone, blood flow, regular bowel function, and a sense of well-being (see Patient Teaching box: Coping with Activity Restriction).

A high-risk pregnancy can be very stressful for a woman and her family. Family stressors include separation from family members when hospitalized; need for activity restriction; financial concerns; and inability to manage the household, family activities, and child care. The family needs to use coping mechanisms and support systems to help them through this crisis. Relaxation techniques also may help reduce stress and prepare the woman for labor and birth. An excellent Web-based support group for pregnant women on restricted activity is Sidelines (www.sidelines.org).

Severe Gestational Hypertension and Preeclampsia With Severe Features

Women with severe gestational hypertension are at greater risk for pregnancy complications than are women who have preeclampsia without severe features. Therefore, these women should be managed as if they have preeclampsia with severe features. Women diagnosed with severe gestational hypertension or preeclampsia with severe features should be hospitalized immediately for a thorough evaluation of maternal-fetal status (Sibai, 2017). These women are placed on magnesium sulfate to prevent eclamptic seizures and antihypertensive medication if necessary to lower severe levels of hypertension. Maternal assessments include BP, urine output, cerebral status, presence of epigastric pain and/or tenderness, labor, or vaginal bleeding (Sibai). Laboratory evaluation includes a platelet count, liver enzymes, and serum creatinine (see Table 12.3). Fetal assessment includes continuous electronic fetal heart rate monitoring, a biophysical profile, and ultrasound evaluation of fetal growth and amniotic fluid volume (Sibai). If evidence of fetal growth restriction is found, umbilical artery Doppler velocimetry is recommended (ACOG, 2013; Sibai).

After this initial assessment period, an interprofessional plan of care is developed with the woman and her family. The goals of care management are to promote maternal safety, assess the degree of maternal and fetal risk, formulate a plan for giving birth, and prevent eclampsia and other serious complications such as placental abruption, HELLP syndrome, fetal growth restriction, and fetal demise. If the disease develops after 34 weeks of gestation, it is recommended that the woman give birth promptly, because severe preeclampsia has been associated with increased rates of maternal morbidity and mortality and with significant fetal risks (Sibai, 2017).

Expectant management. Women who are less than 34 0/7 weeks of gestation and have no indication for giving birth immediately may be candidates for expectant management. These women should be hospitalized at a tertiary care facility that is able to provide both maternal and neonatal intensive care. Care management decisions should be made by an interprofessional health care team that includes a **perinatologist** (a maternal fetal medicine specialist), a neonatologist, an obstetrician, a nurse, and a social worker. Patient and family counseling by a neonatologist should be provided (ACOG, 2013; Sibai, 2017).

Expectant management includes the use of oral antihypertensive medications to maintain a systolic BP between 140 and 155 mm Hg and a diastolic BP between 90 and 105 mm Hg. Management also includes ongoing maternal and fetal assessment for indicators of worsening condition (Sibai, 2017). Corticosteroids (betamethasone or dexamethasone) are ordered to enhance fetal lung maturation for gestations less than 34 weeks. The dose of betamethasone is 12 mg intramuscularly, repeated in 24 hours, while dexamethasone is given intramuscularly as four doses of 6 mg each, 12 hours apart. Neonatal benefit is maximized when the interval between the first dose and birth is longer than 48 hours. The duration of benefit after a single course of betamethasone or dexamethasone is unclear (see Medication Guide: Antenatal Glucocorticoid Therapy with Betamethasone or Dexamethasone in Chapter 17) (Sibai; Simhan, Iams, & Romero, 2017).

Most women managed expectantly develop a maternal or fetal indication for giving birth within 2 weeks, although some are able to continue their pregnancies safely for several more weeks. Immediate birth is indicated if any of the following complications are present: imminent or actual eclampsia, uncontrollable severe hypertension, pulmonary edema, placental abruption, DIC, evidence of nonreassuring fetal status, fetal gestational age less than 24 weeks, or fetal demise (ACOG, 2013; Sibai, 2017).

Intrapartum care. Intrapartum nursing care is directed toward the early identification of fetal heart rate (FHR) abnormalities and the prevention of maternal complications. Continuous FHR and uterine contraction monitoring are initiated, and the woman is assessed for signs of placental abruption such as a tense, tender uterus. Maternal evaluation also includes assessment of the central nervous, cardiovascular, pulmonary, hepatic, and renal systems (Poole, 2014). Vital signs and

PATIENT TEACHING
Coping With Activity Restriction

At Home

- Clarify with your health care provider: What is "limited" or "restricted" activity? Question your activity level, positioning, bathroom privileges, children's visits, activities, personal hygiene, mobility, diet, and visitors.
- Have your computer, tablet, or smart phone available at your bedside. These devices can be used to communicate with friends, conduct business, and shop as necessary. Also use your computer or smart phone to communicate with Internet support groups and obtain information.
- Have a television and DVD player to watch television programs or movies (can also watch on a computer or tablet) and a radio, CD player, or MP3 player to listen to music.
- Delegate responsibilities to family members or friends as much as possible (e.g., attend to the laundry, pick up groceries, drop off and pick up dry cleaning, meet repair people, attend to child care, organize meals).
- Have these available for use on your bed or couch
  - Eggcrate mattress
  - Pillows and more pillows (body pillow)
- Keep a big trash basket near your bed and daytime resting place.
- Place a box or crate near the bed/sofa to store items such as:
  - Post-it Notes
  - Cups with lids and flexible straws
  - Paper plates
  - Plastic forks, spoons, and knives
  - Baby monitor or walkie-talkie
  - Wet wipes
  - Notebook to record questions for providers, telephone numbers, and to-do lists
  - Envelopes and stationery
  - Take-out menus
  - Reading materials
  - Books
  - Audiobooks
  - Magazines
- Stock a mini-refrigerator or cooler with water or other beverages or healthy snacks.

- Plan for family time—visits and interaction, particularly with small children (see Patient Teaching box: Activities for Children of Women on Activity Restriction in Chapter 17).
- Explore your interest in a new hobby.
  - Work crossword or jigsaw puzzles.
  - Learn to embroider, smock, crochet, or knit.
  - Do mending or sewing.
- Do craft projects; make something for the baby.
- Identify relaxation exercises and activities (music) and implement.
- Arrange to have a facial, manicure/pedicure, neck massage, or other special treat when you need a lift.

In the Hospital

- Clarify with your health care provider: What is "limited" or "restricted" activity? Question your activity level, positioning, bathroom privileges, children's visits, activities, personal hygiene, mobility, diet, and visitors.
- In addition to survival tips for the home, the following may be useful in the hospital setting:
  - Bring your own pillow, shampoo, and conditioner.
  - Have a wheelchair for outside visits or visiting other antepartal women if allowed.
  - If possible, bring a laptop computer or a tablet so you can watch movies or television programs if Internet access is available.
  - Ask friends to bring healthy food and snacks rather than flowers when visiting.
  - Explore your interest in handheld games.
  - Work with staff regarding scheduling (e.g., obstetric provider examinations, vital signs, nursing assessments).
  - Bring earplugs to block the hospital noise.
  - Ask for a room with a view.
  - Have a large calendar and clock for easy viewing. Record significant events on the calendar.

---

assessments are performed as ordered and per hospital policy. Patient and family education and supportive measures are also initiated (see Nursing Care Plan: Preeclampsia with Severe Features).

The woman with preeclampsia with severe features is maintained on bed rest with the side rails up in a quiet, darkened environment. Emergency drugs, oxygen, and suction equipment should be checked and readily available (Box 12.2). To reduce the risk for pulmonary edema, total intravenous (IV) and oral fluids should not exceed 125 mL/ hr. Intensive hemodynamic monitoring with a pulmonary artery (Swan-Ganz) catheter to evaluate central venous and pulmonary artery pressures is not a routine standard of care. It is indicated only in selected women, such as those with oliguria unresponsive to a fluid challenge (Markham & Funai, 2014; Poole, 2014).

Magnesium sulfate. Magnesium sulfate is the medication of choice for preventing and treating seizure activity (eclampsia). It is almost always administered intravenously as a secondary infusion (piggyback) by a volumetric infusion pump. Per protocol or health care provider's order, an initial loading dose of 4 to 6 g of magnesium sulfate is infused over 15 to 30 minutes. This dose is followed by a maintenance dose of magnesium sulfate that is diluted in an IV solution (e.g., 40 g of magnesium sulfate in 1000 mL of lactated Ringer's solution [1 g =

BOX 12.2   Hospital Precautionary Measures for Women With Preeclampsia

- Environment
  - Quiet
  - Nonstimulating
  - Lighting subdued
- Seizure precautions
  - Suction equipment tested and ready to use
  - Oxygen administration equipment tested and ready to use
  - Call button within easy reach
- Emergency medications available on the unit
  - Hydralazine
  - Labetalol
  - Nifedipine
  - Magnesium sulfate
  - Calcium gluconate or calcium chloride
- Emergency birth pack easily accessible

◎ NURSING CARE PLAN

Preeclampsia With Severe Features

Case Study

Olga is a 38-year-old gravida 3 para 0-1-1-1 who was diagnosed with preeclampsia at 32 weeks of gestation. At that time, she was placed on restricted activity and scheduled for fetal and maternal assessments twice a week at the prenatal clinic. At a scheduled clinic visit at 35 weeks, Olga states in the interview that she has not been eating well because she feels nauseated. She complains of a headache of 2 days duration and of shortness of breath when she is out of bed for any length of time. Physical examination findings are as follows: BP 170/110, deep tendon reflexes 4+, 2 beats clonus, facial and hand edema, weight gain of 3 kg (6.6 lbs) in 1 week, bilateral breath sounds clear to auscultation, proteinuria 3+ (dipstick), fetal heart rate 140s by Doppler ultrasound. Olga was admitted to the labor and birth unit with a diagnosis of preeclampsia with severe features. IV magnesium sulfate was initiated per unit protocol, and she was placed on continuous electronic fetal heart rate monitoring.

Assessment

What are the most important signs and symptoms that the nurse should look for in a woman with preeclampsia with severe features?

Defining Characteristics

Nausea; upper right quadrant or epigastric pain
Blurred vision
Headaches unresponsive to usual treatment
Hypertension
Proteinuria
Seizure activity
Abnormal laboratory results (low platelet count, elevated liver enzymes, elevated serum creatinine level)

Nursing Diagnosis

Risk for Injury to woman related to CNS irritability (seizures) and/or magnesium sulfate treatment

Expected Outcome

Olga will show diminished signs of CNS irritability (e.g., DTRs ≤2+, absence of clonus) and have no seizure activity

Nursing Interventions	Rationales
Establish baseline data (e.g., DTRs, clonus).	To use as basis for evaluating effectiveness of treatment
Administer IV magnesium sulfate per physician's orders.	To minimize risk for seizure activity
Monitor maternal vital signs, level of consciousness, FHR, urine output, DTRs, IV flow rate, and serum levels of magnesium sulfate.	To assess for and prevent magnesium sulfate toxicity (e.g., drowsiness, lethargy, slurred speech, loss of DTRs, depressed respirations, cardiac arrest)
Have calcium gluconate or calcium chloride on the unit.	To be available if needed as an antidote for magnesium sulfate toxicity
Maintain a quiet, darkened environment.	To avoid stimuli that may precipitate seizure activity

Case Study (Continued)

Olga continues to experience headaches and blurred vision, her B/P remains elevated above 160/110 and she is voiding very small amounts infrequently.

Assessment

What evidence is there of decreased blood circulation to the periphery that occurs with vasospasm and leads to decreased tissue perfusion in all organ systems?

Defining Characteristics

Headaches
Blurred vision
Hypertension
Oliguria
Increased creatinine levels
Increased plasma uric acid levels
Decreased uteroplacental perfusion

Nursing Diagnosis

Ineffective Peripheral Tissue Perfusion related to preeclampsia secondary to arteriolar vasospasm

Expected Outcome

Olga will exhibit signs of adequate tissue perfusion (i.e., adequate urine output, normal FHR tracing).

Nursing Interventions	Rationales
Monitor Olga's urine output via indwelling urinary catheter.	To measure output accurately
Monitor creatinine and uric acid levels.	To detect potential complications
Monitor Olga's blood pressure.	To identify need for initiating antihypertensive medication, increasing the dosage, or adding an additional antihypertensive agent
Place Olga on bed rest in side-lying position.	To maximize uteroplacental blood flow, reduce blood pressure, and promote diuresis
Monitor FHR tracing for rate, baseline variability, and absence of late decelerations.	To assess for evidence of adequate uteroplacental oxygenation
Monitor Olga's urine output via indwelling urinary catheter.	To measure output accurately

Case Study (Continued)

Olga continues on bed rest with IV magnesium sulfate infusing, an indwelling urinary catheter in place, and continuous electronic fetal monitoring. Her respirations are now 22 per minute, and the nurses are auscultating her lungs every 4 hours.

Assessment

What pulmonary complications can occur in women with severe preeclampsia?

Defining Characteristics

Dyspnea
Crackles
Pulmonary edema
Hypoxemia

Nursing Diagnosis

Impaired Gas Exchange related to possible pulmonary edema secondary to endothelial damage and increased capillary permeability

Expected Outcomes

Olga will exhibit normal breath sounds, adequate oxygenation, (i.e., normal respirations; oxygen saturation values of 95% or more; full orientation to person, time, and place).
Olga will cough effectively.
Olga's intake will be sufficient to prevent dehydration but low enough to prevent fluid overload.

NURSING CARE PLAN

Preeclampsia With Severe Features—cont'd

Nursing Interventions	Rationales
Monitor Olga for signs of impaired gas exchange (i.e., increased respirations, dyspnea, altered blood gases, hypoxemia).	To detect potential complications

Olga's condition has stabilized, with decreased pain from headaches, and her affect is more positive. She expresses concern for the fetus and asks about its condition. She questions the nurse about how her illness might affect her baby.

Assessment

What fetal complications can occur when the mother has preeclampsia with severe features?

Defining Characteristics

Intrauterine growth restriction
Abnormal fetal heart rate and pattern

Iatrogenic preterm birth
Placental abruption

Nursing Diagnosis

Risk for Injury to Fetus related to uteroplacental insufficiency and the possible need for iatrogenic preterm birth

Expected Outcome

Olga's fetus will maintain well-being (i.e., adequate fetal movement, normal fetal heart rate and pattern).

Nursing Interventions	Rationales
Monitor fetus for abnormal signs (decreased fetal activity, abnormal FHR or pattern).	To detect complications and enable timely interventions.
Maintain Olga in a side-lying position.	To maintain uterine perfusion
Keep Olga informed of fetal status.	To allay anxiety

BP, blood pressure; *CNS*, central nervous system; *DTR*, deep tendon reflex; *FHR*, fetal heart rate; *IV*, intravenous.

25 mL]) and administered by an infusion pump at 2 to 3 g/hr. This dose should maintain a therapeutic serum magnesium level of 4 to 7 mEq/L. Contrary to popular belief, magnesium sulfate has little effect on maternal BP when administered in this fashion (Markham & Funai, 2014; Poole, 2014).

Magnesium sulfate is rarely given intramuscularly because the absorption rate cannot be controlled, injections are painful, and tissue necrosis may occur. However, the intramuscular (IM) route may be used in low-resource settings or with some women who are being transported to a tertiary care center. Use of the ventral gluteal site for injection is recommended. The IM dose is a 10-g loading dose (administered as two separate injections of 5 g in each buttock). The maintenance dosage is 5 g administered every 4 hours in alternating buttocks (Harvey & Sibai, 2013). Local anesthetic can be added to the solution to reduce injection pain. The Z-track technique should be used for the deep IM injection, followed by gentle massage at the site.

It is unclear how magnesium sulfate works to prevent and treat eclamptic seizures. It may cause vasodilation in the peripheral and cerebral circulation, prevent or decrease cerebral edema, or function as a central anticonvulsant (Harvey & Sibai, 2013). Because magnesium is excreted in the urine, accurate measurements of maternal urine output must be obtained. If renal function declines, excretion of magnesium sulfate is inadequate, resulting in magnesium toxicity. Common side effects of magnesium sulfate are a feeling of warmth, flushing, diaphoresis, and burning at the IV site. Symptoms of magnesium toxicity include absent deep tendon reflexes, respiratory depression, blurred vision, slurred speech, severe muscle weakness, and cardiac arrest (Harvey & Sibai). Blood can be drawn to determine the serum magnesium level if toxicity is suspected (Box 12.3) (see Medication Guide: Tocolytic Therapy for Preterm Labor in Chapter 17).

MEDICATION ALERT

High serum levels of magnesium can cause relaxation of smooth muscle, such as the uterus. However, when administered as a 4- to 6-g loading dose followed by a 1- to 2-g/hour maintenance dose, magnesium sulfate has not been shown to significantly affect the need for oxytocin (Pitocin) stimulation of labor. Other than a brief period of uterine muscle relaxation during and immediately after administration of the loading dose, no evidence of decreased uterine contractility has been observed (Cunningham, Leveno, Bloom, et al., 2014).

MEDICATION ALERT

If magnesium toxicity is suspected, prompt actions are needed to prevent respiratory or cardiac arrest. The magnesium infusion should be discontinued immediately. Calcium gluconate or calcium chloride (antidotes for magnesium sulfate) can be given intravenously (Cunningham et al., 2014).

NURSING ALERT

The effect of magnesium sulfate on FHR baseline variability is controversial. Because fetal levels of magnesium approximate those of the mother, fetal sedation is possible. However, absent or minimal baseline variability should not be assumed to be the result of magnesium sulfate therapy until other causes of fetal hypoxemia have been ruled out (Poole, 2014). Neonatal serum magnesium levels are almost identical to those of the mother (Markham & Funai, 2014).

SAFETY ALERT

Magnesium sulfate is considered a high-alert medication because it can cause patient harm when administered incorrectly. Measures to improve the safe use of this medication include developing detailed policies, procedures, protocols, and standing orders and thorough assessment and documentation. *Never* abbreviate magnesium sulfate as MgSO$_4$ anywhere in the medical record (Institute for Safe Medication Practices, 2014).

Control of blood pressure. Antihypertensive medications are indicated when the systolic BP exceeds 160 mm Hg or the diastolic BP exceeds 110 mm Hg. Maternal risks associated with severe hypertension include left ventricular failure, cerebral hemorrhage, and placental abruption. To maintain uteroplacental perfusion, antihypertensive therapy must not decrease the arterial pressure too much or too rapidly. Hydralazine (Apresoline), labetalol (Trandate), and nifedipine (Procardia) are effective drugs for treating hypertension intrapartum. They may also be used during pregnancy or in the postpartum period for BP control (ACOG, 2013; Harvey & Sibai, 2013). Table 12.5 compares antihypertensive agents commonly used to treat hypertension in pregnancy.

BOX 12.3   Care of the Woman With Preeclampsia Receiving Magnesium Sulfate

Patient and Family Teaching

- Explain technique, rationale, and reactions to expect
  - Route and rate
  - Purpose of "piggyback" infusion
- Reasons for use
  - Tailor information to woman's readiness to learn.
  - Explain that magnesium sulfate is used to prevent disease progression.
  - Explain that magnesium sulfate is used to prevent seizures, *not* to decrease blood pressure.
- Reactions to expect from medication
  - Initially the woman appears flushed and feels hot, sedated, and nauseated. She may experience burning at the IV site, especially during the bolus.
  - Sedation continues.
- Monitoring to anticipate
  - *Maternal:* Blood pressure, pulse, respiratory rate, DTRs, level of consciousness, urine output (indwelling catheter), headache, visual disturbances, epigastric pain
  - *Fetal:* FHR and activity

Administration

- Verify physician's order.
- Position woman in side-lying position.
- Prepare solution and administer with an infusion control device (pump).
- Piggyback solution of 40 g of magnesium sulfate in 1000 mL lactated Ringer's solution with infusion-control device at the ordered rate: loading dose—initial bolus of 4 g to 6 g over 15 to 30 minutes; maintenance dose—2 g/hour, according to unit protocol or specific physician's order.

Maternal and Fetal Assessments

- Vital signs and assessments are performed as ordered by the health care provider and per hospital protocol.

- Monitor blood pressure, pulse, respiratory rate every 15 to 30 minutes, depending on woman's condition.
- Monitor FHR and contractions continuously.
- Monitor level of consciousness, intake and output, proteinuria, DTRs, headache, visual disturbances, and epigastric pain at least hourly.
- Restrict hourly fluid intake to a total of no more than 125 mL/hour; urinary output should be at least 25 to 30 mL/hour.

Reportable Conditions

- Blood pressure: systolic ≥160 mm Hg or diastolic ≥110 mm Hg
- Respiratory rate: <12 breaths/minute
- Urinary output: <25 to 30 mL/hour
- Presence of headache, visual disturbances, decrease in level of consciousness, or epigastric pain
- Increasing severity or loss of DTRs, increasing edema, proteinuria
- Any abnormal laboratory values (magnesium level, platelet count, creatinine clearance, levels of uric acid, AST, ALT, prothrombin time, partial thromboplastin time, fibrinogen, fibrin split products)
- Any other significant change in maternal or fetal status

Emergency Measures

- Keep emergency drugs and intubation equipment immediately available.
- Keep side rails up.
- Keep lights dimmed, and maintain a quiet environment.

Documentation

- All of the above

ALT, Alanine aminotransferase; *AST,* aspartate aminotransferase; *DTR,* deep tendon reflex; *FHR,* fetal heart rate; *IV,* intravenous.

Postpartum care. Throughout the postpartum period, the woman needs careful assessment of her vital signs, intake and output, DTRs, and level of consciousness. The magnesium sulfate infusion is continued after birth for seizure prophylaxis as ordered, usually for 24 hours. Assessments for effects and side effects continue until the medication is discontinued. Given that magnesium sulfate potentiates the action of narcotics, CNS depressants, and calcium channel blockers, these medications must be administered with caution (Poole, 2014). The signs and symptoms of preeclampsia usually resolve within 48 hours after birth. Clinical signs that demonstrate resolution of preeclampsia include diuresis and decreased edema.

The nurse should assess the postpartum woman regularly for any symptoms of preeclampsia such as headaches, visual disturbances, or epigastric pain. Some women develop signs and symptoms of preeclampsia for the first time after giving birth. Women who develop hypertension and severe features of preeclampsia such as headaches or blurred vision or severe hypertension should be placed on IV magnesium sulfate for seizure prophylaxis. Nonsteroidal antiinflammatory pain medications should be used with caution when hypertension persists for more than 1 day after birth because these agents can contribute to an increase in BP. Women should be taught to contact their health care provider or return to the hospital immediately if they develop headaches, visual disturbances, or epigastric pain after discharge (ACOG, 2013; Sibai, 2017).

Because preeclampsia is a major cause of IUGR and preterm birth, the baby may be cared for in a neonatal intensive care unit (NICU).

Nursing care that facilitates bonding and attachment while the infant is in the NICU includes providing the family with photographs of the infant, keeping the family informed of the infant's status, encouraging the father to visit the NICU, and taking the woman to the NICU by wheelchair after her condition has stabilized (Poole, 2014). Postpartum and neonatal nurses can collaborate to provide family-centered care in this situation.

Most women with gestational hypertension become normotensive during the first week after giving birth. On the other hand, hypertension may take longer to resolve in women with preeclampsia. For women with gestational hypertension, preeclampsia, or superimposed preeclampsia, it is recommended that BP be monitored in the hospital or that equivalent outpatient surveillance be performed for at least 72 hours after birth. The BP should then be rechecked at 7 to 10 days postpartum, or earlier in women who are symptomatic. Women with a BP of 150/100 mm Hg or higher (on two occasions that are 4 to 6 hours apart) should be placed on an antihypertensive medication, often labetalol or nifedipine (ACOG, 2013). If this is the case, the BP needs to be checked frequently either at home or at the health care provider's office. Within a few weeks after birth, antihypertensive medications often can be discontinued.

Future Health Care

Women with preeclampsia with severe features have a significantly increased risk for developing preeclampsia in a future pregnancy, especially those who had early-onset (diagnosed during the second

TABLE 12.5   Pharmacologic Control of Hypertension in Pregnancy

Action	Target Tissue	Maternal Effects	Fetal Effects	Nursing Actions
Hydralazine (Apresoline, Neopresol)				
Arteriolar vasodilator	Peripheral arterioles: to decrease muscle tone, decrease peripheral resistance; hypothalamus and medullary vasomotor center for minor decrease in sympathetic tone	Headache, flushing, palpitations, tachycardia, some decrease in uteroplacental blood flow, increase in heart rate and cardiac output, increase in oxygen consumption, nausea and vomiting	Tachycardia; late decelerations and bradycardia if maternal diastolic pressure <90 mm Hg	Assess for effects of medication; alert woman (family) to expected effects of medication; assess blood pressure frequently because precipitous drop can lead to shock and perhaps placental abruption; if giving multiple doses, wait at least 20 minutes after the first dose is given to administer an additional dose to allow time to assess the effects of the initial dose; assess urinary output; maintain bed rest in lateral position with side rails up; use with caution in presence of maternal tachycardia.
Labetalol Hydrochloride (Normodyne, Trandate)				
Combined alpha- and beta-blocking agent causing vasodilation without significant change in cardiac output	Peripheral arterioles (see hydralazine)	Lethargy, fatigue, sleep disturbances; Minimal: flushing, tremulousness, orthostatic hypotension; minimal change in pulse rate	Minimal, if any. May be associated with small-for-gestational-age infant	See hydralazine; less likely to cause excessive hypotension and tachycardia; less rebound hypertension than hydralazine. Do not use in women with asthma, heart disease, or congestive heart failure. Do not exceed 80 mg in a single dose. Do not give more than 300 mg total in a 24 hour period.
Methyldopa (Aldomet)				
Maintenance therapy if needed: 250–500 mg orally every 8 hours (α_2-receptor agonist)	Postganglionic nerve endings: interferes with chemical neurotransmission to reduce peripheral vascular resistance; causes CNS sedation	Sleepiness, postural hypotension, constipation, hepatic dysfunction and necrosis, hemolytic anemia; rare: drug-induced fever in 1% of women and positive Coombs' test result in 20% of women	After 4 months of maternal therapy, positive Coombs' test result in infant	See hydralazine.
Nifedipine (Adalat, Procardia)				
Calcium channel blocker	Arterioles: to reduce systemic vascular resistance by relaxation of arterial smooth muscle	Headache, flushing, tachycardia; may interfere with labor	Minimal	See hydralazine. Avoid concurrent use with magnesium sulfate because skeletal muscle blockade can result. Avoid immediate release or sublingual form due to increased risk for profound maternal hypotension

CNS, Central nervous system.
Data from Harvey, C., & Sibai, B. (2013). Hypertension in pregnancy. In N. Troiano, C. Harvey, & B. Chez (Eds.), *AWHONN's high risk and critical care obstetrics* (3rd ed.). Philadelphia, PA: Wolters Kluwer/Lippincott Williams & Wilkins; Poole, J.H. (2014). Hypertensive disorders of pregnancy. In K. R. Simpson, & P. Creehan, (Eds.), *AWHONN's perinatal nursing* (4th ed.). Philadelphia, PA: Lippincott Williams & Wilkins; Sibai, B. (2017). Preeclampsia and hypertensive disorders. In S. G. Gabbe, J. R. Niebyl, J. L. Simpson, et al. (Eds.), *Obstetrics: Normal and problem pregnancies* (7th ed.). Philadelphia, PA: Elsevier; Witcher, P.M. (2017). Caring for the laboring woman with hypertensive disorders complicating pregnancy. In B. B. Kennedy, & S. M. Baird (Eds.), *Intrapartum management modules: A perinatal education program* (5th ed.). Philadelphia, PA: Wolters Kluwer.

trimester) preeclampsia. Even if these women remain normotensive in a subsequent pregnancy, they may have a greater likelihood of an adverse pregnancy outcome such as preterm birth, small-for-gestational-age infant, and perinatal death (Sibai, 2017).

Ideally, women who have had preeclampsia in a previous pregnancy should receive counseling during a preconception visit before the next planned pregnancy. At this visit, the previous pregnancy history should be reviewed and the prognosis for the upcoming pregnancy discussed. Potential lifestyle modifications such as weight loss and increased physical activity should be encouraged. The current status of any chronic medical conditions, such as diabetes or chronic hypertension, should be assessed, so that they are brought into the best control possible before the upcoming pregnancy. Current medications should be reviewed and their administration modified if necessary for the upcoming pregnancy (ACOG, 2013). The use of low-dose aspirin during the upcoming pregnancy will likely be recommended, especially if an adverse outcome accompanied the previous pregnancy complicated by preeclampsia (ACOG, 2016).

Women with preeclampsia (especially early-onset and preeclampsia with severe features) also have an increased risk for developing chronic hypertension and cardiovascular disease later in life. It is believed that preeclampsia does not cause cardiovascular disease but rather that preeclampsia and cardiovascular disease share common risk factors. Further research is needed to determine how to take advantage of this information relating preeclampsia to cardiovascular disease later in life. For now, women should be educated about lifestyle changes (maintaining a healthy weight, increasing physical activity, and avoiding smoking) that may decrease the risk for developing future health problems (ACOG, 2013; Sibai, 2017).

ECLAMPSIA

Eclampsia is usually preceded by premonitory signs and symptoms, including persistent headache, blurred vision, photophobia, severe epigastric or right upper quadrant abdominal pain, and altered mental status. However, seizures can appear suddenly and without warning in a seemingly stable woman with only minimal BP elevations (Sibai, 2017). Eclamptic seizures are frightening to observe. Tonic contraction of all body muscles (seen as arms flexed, hands clenched, legs inverted) precedes the tonic-clonic convulsion. During this stage muscles alternately relax and contract. Respirations are halted and then begin again with long, deep, stertorous inhalations. Hypotension follows; and muscular twitching, disorientation, and amnesia persist for a while after the seizure. The woman may also vomit or be incontinent of urine or stool.

Immediate Care

Nursing actions during a seizure are directed toward ensuring a patent airway and patient safety (see Emergency Treatment box: Preeclampsia). It is important to note the time of onset and duration of the seizure. The nurse should call for help but remain at the bedside. The side rails on the bed must be raised and should be padded with a folded blanket or pillow if possible. Women with eclampsia have been known to sustain fractures from falling out of bed during the seizure. Immediately after the seizure, the nurse should lower the head of the bed and turn the woman onto her side. This helps prevent aspiration of vomitus.

Nursing actions after a seizure are directed toward maternal stabilization. First, the status of the woman's airway, breathing, and pulse should be assessed. The nurse should suction secretions from her glottis to clear the airway, insert an oral airway, and administer oxygen at 10 L/min by face mask. If an IV infusion is not in place, one should be started with an 18-gauge needle. If an IV line was in place before the seizure, it may have infiltrated and will need to be restarted immediately. As soon as IV access is obtained, magnesium sulfate should be administered as ordered.

If eclampsia develops after initiating magnesium sulfate therapy, additional magnesium sulfate should be administered. Magnesium sulfate is the drug of choice for treating eclamptic seizures and preventing repeated seizures. One of its advantages over other antiseizure medications such as diazepam (Valium) is that it reduces the risk for aspiration because it does not depress the gag reflex (Harvey & Sibai, 2013). Occasionally a woman will experience recurrent eclamptic seizures while receiving adequate and therapeutic doses of magnesium sulfate. If this occurs, lorazepam (Ativan) 2 mg, given intravenously over 3 to 5 minutes, may be administered (Sibai, 2017).

After the woman is stabilized, uterine activity, cervical status, and fetal status must be assessed. During a seizure, the uterus becomes hypercontractile and hypertonic. As a result, the membranes may have ruptured or the cervix may have dilated rapidly, and birth may be imminent (Poole, 2014). The FHR tracing may demonstrate bradycardia, late decelerations, absent or minimal baseline variability, or compensatory

✚ EMERGENCY TREATMENT

Preeclampsia

Tonic-Clonic Convulsion Signs
- Stage of invasion: 2–3 seconds, eyes fixed, twitching of facial muscles
- Stage of contraction: 15–20 seconds, eyes protrude and are bloodshot, all body muscles in tonic contraction
- Stage of convulsion: Muscles relax and contract alternately (clonic), respirations halted and then begin again with long, deep, stertorous inhalation; coma ensues

Intervention
- Keep airway patent: turn head to one side, place pillow under one shoulder or back if possible.
- Call for assistance. Do not leave bedside.
- Raise side rails, and pad them with a folded blanket or pillow if possible.
- Observe and record convulsion activity.

After Convulsion
- Do not leave unattended until fully alert.
- Observe for postconvulsion confusion, coma, incontinence.
- Use suction as needed.
- Administer oxygen via nonrebreather face mask at 10 L/min.
- Start intravenous fluids, and monitor for potential fluid overload.
- Give magnesium sulfate or other anticonvulsant drug as ordered.
- Insert indwelling urinary catheter.
- Monitor blood pressure, pulse, and respirations frequently until stabilized.
- Monitor fetal and uterine status.
- Expedite laboratory work as ordered to monitor kidney function, liver function, coagulation system, and drug levels.
- Provide hygiene and a quiet environment.
- Support the woman and her family, and keep them informed.
- Be prepared to assist with birth when woman is in stable condition.

tachycardia. These findings usually resolve soon after the seizure ends and the woman's hypoxia is corrected (Sibai, 2017).

⚡ SAFETY ALERT

Immediately after a seizure, a woman may be very confused and combative. Restraints may be necessary temporarily. Several hours may be needed for the woman to regain her usual level of mental functioning.

After stabilizing the woman and fetus, a decision is made regarding the timing and method of birth. Eclampsia alone is not an indication for immediate cesarean birth. The route of birth (induction of labor versus cesarean birth) is determined based on the maternal and fetal condition, fetal gestational age, presence of labor, and cervical Bishop score (ACOG, 2013; Sibai, 2017).

Regional anesthesia is not recommended for eclamptic women with coagulopathy or a platelet count less than $50,000/mm^3$ (Sibai, 2017). If cesarean birth is necessary, it is performed using general anesthesia.

CHRONIC HYPERTENSION

An increasing number of women who give birth have chronic hypertension, which affects approximately 1% to 5% of all pregnancies. African-American women are much more likely to have a pregnancy complicated by chronic hypertension than are women of other races or ethnicities. In addition to race, other risk factors for chronic hypertension in pregnancy are older age and obesity. As more women delay childbearing and are obese, the number of pregnancies complicated by chronic hypertension is expected to increase (Sibai, 2017).

More than 90% of women with chronic hypertension have primary or essential hypertension. In the remaining 10%, the hypertension is secondary to a medical condition such as renal or collagen disease (Harvey & Sibai, 2013). Chronic hypertension in pregnancy is associated with maternal complications such as superimposed preeclampsia, stroke, acute kidney injury, heart failure, placental abruption, and death. Fetal risks include IUGR, death, and preterm birth (Cunningham et al., 2014; Sibai, 2017).

Ideally the management of chronic hypertension in pregnancy begins before conception. An evaluation is performed to assess the cause and severity of the hypertension and the presence of any target organ damage (e.g., heart, eye, and kidney) (Sibai, 2017). Moreover, the woman should be encouraged to make lifestyle changes before conception such as smoking and alcohol cessation, participating in aerobic exercise, and losing weight if indicated. A diet that includes a maximum of 2.4 g sodium per day is recommended (Sibai). These lifestyle modifications should continue throughout the pregnancy.

Based on the BP and presence of target organ damage, women with chronic hypertension are classified as either high or low risk for pregnancy complications. Antihypertensive medications are frequently discontinued before pregnancy in women with low-risk chronic hypertension. This decreases the risk of fetal exposure to some medications (e.g., angiotensin-converting enzyme [ACE] inhibitors) that can be teratogenic (Harvey & Sibai, 2013). Women who are high risk are managed with antihypertensive medication and frequent assessments of maternal and fetal well-being. Methyldopa (Aldomet) is most often recommended for treating chronic hypertension in pregnancy. However, because it is rarely used for treating chronic hypertension in nonpregnant women, it may not be practical to switch medications because of pregnancy. Labetalol, nifedipine, and a thiazide diuretic are other antihypertensive medications used during pregnancy (see Table 12.5). Women who are high risk are monitored closely, and the route and timing of the birth depend on the maternal and fetal status.

After giving birth, the woman should be monitored closely for complications such as pulmonary edema, hypertensive encephalopathy, and renal failure. Women with chronic hypertension can breastfeed if they desire. All antihypertensive medications are present to some degree in breast milk. Any medications given to a breastfeeding mother should be checked for safety. LactMed (https://toxnet.nlm.nih.gov/newtoxnet/lactmed.htm) is an excellent online resource.

Levels of methyldopa in breast milk appear to be low and are considered safe. Labetalol also has a low concentration in breast milk. Little is known about the transfer of calcium channel blockers such as nifedipine in breast milk, but no apparent side effects have been noted in infants. Concentrations of diuretic agents in breast milk are low, but their use may cause a decrease in milk production (Sibai, 2017).

HYPEREMESIS GRAVIDARUM

Nausea and vomiting complicate up to 70% of all pregnancies, typically beginning at 4 to 8 weeks of gestation with improvement by 16 weeks. However, 10% to 25% of women still experience symptoms at 20 to 22 weeks of gestation, and some women will have symptoms throughout pregnancy. Although nausea and vomiting are distressing, they typically do not cause significant weight loss, ketonemia, or electrolyte disturbances. The cause of nausea and vomiting in pregnancy is not well understood, although it probably involves relaxation of the smooth muscle of the stomach. Minimal data exist to show that nausea and vomiting of pregnancy is caused by elevated levels of estrogen, progesterone, and human chorionic gonadotropin (hCG) (Antony, Racusin,

Aagaard, et al., 2017). Some authorities have suggested that nausea and vomiting are evolutionary adaptations that occur during pregnancy in order to protect the woman and fetus from potentially harmful foods (Kelly & Savides, 2014). Pregnancies complicated by nausea and vomiting generally have a more favorable outcome than those without these symptoms (Antony et al.).

When vomiting during pregnancy becomes excessive enough to cause weight loss, electrolyte imbalance, nutritional deficiencies, and ketonuria, the disorder is termed hyperemesis gravidarum. This disorder occurs in approximately 0.5% of all live births. Hyperemesis gravidarum usually begins during the first trimester, but approximately 10% of women with the disorder continue to have symptoms throughout the pregnancy (Kelly & Savides, 2014). In the United States, hyperemesis gravidarum is the most common reason for hospitalization during the first half of pregnancy and the second most common reason for hospitalization during pregnancy overall (Castillo & Phillippi, 2015).

There are a number of maternal characteristics associated with an increased risk for the development of hyperemesis gravidarum, including younger maternal age, nulliparity, a body mass index (BMI) less than 18.5 or greater than 25, and low socioeconomic status. Women with asthma, migraines, preexisting diabetes, psychiatric illness, hyperthyroid disorders, gastrointestinal disorders, or a previous pregnancy complicated by hyperemesis gravidarum are also more likely to develop hyperemesis. Factors related to the current pregnancy that make a woman more likely to develop hyperemesis gravidarum are carrying a female fetus, multifetal gestation, and gestational trophoblastic disease. Also, a maternal family history of hyperemesis is associated with the disorder (Castillo & Phillippi, 2015).

Hyperemesis gravidarum can cause complications for both women and infants. Severe but rare maternal complications of hyperemesis gravidarum include esophageal rupture, pneumomediastinum, and deficiencies of vitamin K and thiamine with resulting Wernicke encephalopathy (CNS involvement) (Kelly & Savides, 2014). Infants born to women who had poor pregnancy weight gain because of hyperemesis may be small for gestational age, have a low birth weight, or be born prematurely (Castillo & Phillippi, 2015; Kelly & Savides, 2014).

ETIOLOGY

The cause of hyperemesis gravidarum remains obscure, but it probably involves many factors. Several theories have been proposed as to the cause, although none of them adequately explains the disorder. It may be related to high levels of estrogen or hCG or associated with transient hyperthyroidism during pregnancy. Gastric dysrhythmias may also contribute to the development of hyperemesis gravidarum (Castillo & Phillippi, 2015; Kelly & Savides, 2014).

CLINICAL MANIFESTATIONS

The woman with hyperemesis gravidarum usually has significant weight loss and dehydration. She may have dry mucous membranes, decreased BP, increased pulse rate, and poor skin turgor. Frequently she is unable to retain even clear liquids taken by mouth. Laboratory tests may reveal electrolyte imbalances.

CARE MANAGEMENT

Assessment and Nursing Diagnoses

Whenever a pregnant woman has nausea and vomiting, the first priority is a thorough assessment to determine the severity of the problem. In most cases, the woman should be told to come immediately to the health care provider's office, clinic, or the emergency department because the severity of the illness is often difficult to determine by telephone conversation.

The assessment should include frequency, severity, and duration of episodes of nausea and vomiting. If the woman reports vomiting, the assessment should also include the approximate amount and color of the vomitus. Other symptoms such as diarrhea, indigestion, and abdominal pain or distention also are identified. The woman is asked to report any precipitating factors relating to the onset of her symptoms. Any pharmacologic or nonpharmacologic treatment measures used should be recorded. Prepregnancy weight and documented weight gain or loss during pregnancy are important to note.

The woman's weight and vital signs are measured, and a complete physical examination is performed, with attention to signs of fluid and electrolyte imbalance and nutritional status. The most important initial laboratory test to be obtained is a determination of ketonuria. Other laboratory tests that may be ordered are a urinalysis, a complete blood cell count, electrolytes, liver enzymes, and bilirubin levels. These tests help rule out underlying diseases such as gastroenteritis, pyelonephritis, pancreatitis, cholecystitis, peptic ulcer, and hepatitis (Cunningham et al., 2014). Because of the recognized association between hyperemesis gravidarum and hyperthyroidism, thyroid levels may also be measured (Nader, 2014).

Psychosocial assessment includes asking the woman about anxiety, fears, and concerns related to her own health and the effects on pregnancy outcome. Family members should be assessed both for anxiety and their role in providing support for the woman.

Potential nursing diagnoses for women experiencing hyperemesis gravidarum include the following:
- *Deficient Fluid Volume* related to excessive vomiting as evidenced by fluid and electrolyte imbalance
- *Imbalanced Nutrition: Less Than Body Requirements* related to nausea and persistent vomiting as evidenced by weight decrease as compared with prepregnant weight
- *Anxiety* related to effects of hyperemesis on fetal well-being as evidenced by woman's statements of concern

Initial Care

Initially the woman who is unable to retain clear liquids by mouth requires IV therapy for correction of fluid and electrolyte imbalances. In the past, women requiring IV therapy were admitted to the hospital. More often they are successfully managed as outpatients or at home, even if on enteral therapy.

Medications may be used if nausea and vomiting are uncontrolled. The current ACOG guidelines for treatment of nausea and vomiting in pregnancy recommend the use of pyridoxine (vitamin B$_6$), either alone or in combination with doxylamine (Unisom) as initial medical management. Since 2013, a single drug combination of pyridoxine and doxylamine (Diclegis) has been available for use in the United States. Advantages to the use of Diclegis are that it is a single tablet and provides delayed-release effects (Castillo & Phillippi, 2015). Cost is a disadvantage to the use of Diclegis, because no generic form of the medication is currently available.

Other frequently prescribed drugs include promethazine (Phenergan), chlorpromazine (Thorazine), prochlorperazine (Compazine), and trimethobenzamide (Tigan). These medications demonstrated benefit clinically, but their safety in pregnancy has not been proven. Metoclopramide (Reglan) accelerates gastric emptying and corrects gastric dysrhythmias. It has been demonstrated in some small studies to be both safe and effective. Ondansetron (Zofran) and droperidol (Inapsine) have been used to treat postoperative nausea and vomiting, but their use in pregnancy has not been well studied (Kelly & Savides, 2014).

Corticosteroids (methylprednisolone [Medrol] or hydrocortisone) may be prescribed for women who do not respond well to the medications previously discussed. These medications have not been proven to treat hyperemesis effectively in all women, however. Because exposure to corticosteroids may increase the risk for facial clefting, they should be used with caution and avoided if possible during the first trimester, when organs and organ systems are developing (Kelly & Savides, 2014).

In addition to anti-emetic drugs, medications to control heartburn or reflux may also be prescribed. Use of antacids, histamine blockers, and proton pump inhibitors has been associated with improved symptom management and quality of life (Castillo & Phillippi, 2015).

Nursing care of the woman with hyperemesis gravidarum involves implementing the medical plan of care, whether in the hospital or home setting. Interventions may include initiating and monitoring IV therapy, administering drugs and nutritional supplements, and monitoring the woman's response to interventions. The nurse observes the woman for any signs of complications such as metabolic acidosis (secondary to starvation), jaundice, or hemorrhage and alerts the health care provider should these occur. Monitoring includes assessment of the woman's nausea, retching without vomiting (sometimes called *dry heaves*), and vomiting, given that these symptoms, although related, are separate. Intake and output, including the amount of emesis, should be measured accurately and recorded. Oral hygiene while the woman is receiving nothing by mouth and after episodes of vomiting helps allay associated discomforts. Assistance with positioning and providing a quiet, restful environment that is free from odors may increase the woman's comfort.

Once the vomiting has stopped, feedings are started in small amounts at frequent intervals. In the beginning, limited amounts of oral fluids and bland foods such as crackers, toast, or baked chicken are offered. The diet progresses slowly as tolerated by the woman until she is able to consume a nutritionally sound diet. Because sleep disturbances may accompany hyperemesis gravidarum, promoting adequate rest is important. The nurse can help coordinate treatment measures and periods of visitation to provide opportunity for rest periods.

Follow-Up Care

Most women are able to eat solid foods after several days of treatment. They should be encouraged to eat small, frequent meals and foods that sound appealing (e.g., nongreasy, dry, sweet, and salty foods). In many instances, women discover that foods they normally like have no appeal at all during this time (see Patient Teaching box: Diet for Hyperemesis for more suggestions). Many pregnant women find exposure to cooking odors nauseating. Having other family members cook may lessen the woman's nausea and vomiting, even if only temporarily. The woman is counseled to contact her health care provider immediately if the nausea and vomiting recur.

The woman with hyperemesis gravidarum needs calm, compassionate, and sympathetic care, with recognition that the manifestations of hyperemesis can be physically and emotionally debilitating to her and stressful for her family. Irritability, tearfulness, and mood changes are often consistent with this disorder. Fetal well-being is a primary concern of the woman. The nurse can provide an environment conducive to discussion of concerns and help the woman identify and mobilize sources of support. The family should be included in the plan of care whenever possible. Their participation may help alleviate some of the emotional stress associated with this disorder.

HEMORRHAGIC DISORDERS

Bleeding in pregnancy may jeopardize maternal and fetal well-being. Maternal blood loss decreases oxygen-carrying capacity, which places

PATIENT TEACHING

Diet for Hyperemesis

- Avoid an empty stomach. Eat frequently, at least every 2 to 3 hours. Separate liquids from solids, and alternate every 2 to 3 hours.
- Eat a high-protein snack at bedtime.
- Eat dry, bland, low-fat, and high-protein foods. Cold foods may be better tolerated than those served at a warm temperature.
- In general, eat what sounds good to you rather than trying to balance your meals.
- Follow the salty and sweet approach; even so-called *junk foods* are okay.
- Eat protein after sweets.
- Dairy products may stay down more easily than other foods.
- If you vomit even when your stomach is empty, try sucking on a Popsicle.
- Try ginger tea. Peel and finely dice a knuckle-sized piece of ginger and place it in a mug of boiling water. Steep for 5 to 8 minutes and add brown sugar to taste.
- Try warm ginger ale (with sugar, not artificial sweetener) or water with a slice of lemon.
- Drink liquids from a cup with a lid.

the woman at increased risk for hypovolemia, anemia, infection, and preterm labor and adversely affects oxygen delivery to the fetus. Fetal risks from maternal hemorrhage include blood loss or anemia, hypoxemia, hypoxia, anoxia, and preterm birth. Hemorrhagic disorders in pregnancy are medical emergencies. The incidence and type of bleeding vary by trimester. Ruptured ectopic pregnancy and abruptio placentae (placental abruption) have the highest incidence of maternal mortality. Prompt assessment and intervention by the health care team are essential to save the lives of both the woman and her fetus.

EARLY PREGNANCY BLEEDING

Bleeding during early pregnancy is alarming to the woman and of concern to health care providers. The common bleeding disorders of early pregnancy include miscarriage (spontaneous abortion), cervical insufficiency, ectopic pregnancy, and hydatidiform mole (molar pregnancy).

Miscarriage (Spontaneous Abortion)

A pregnancy that ends as a result of natural causes before 20 weeks of gestation is defined as a miscarriage (spontaneous abortion). This 20-week marker has traditionally been considered to be the point of viability when a fetus may survive in an extrauterine environment. A fetal weight less than 500 g also may be used to define an abortion (Cunningham et al., 2014). The term *miscarriage* rather than *abortion* is used throughout this discussion because it is more appropriate to use with patients. Abortion may be perceived as an insensitive term to use with families who are grieving a pregnancy loss. Therapeutic or elective induced abortion is discussed in Chapter 5.

Incidence and Etiology

Approximately 10% to 15% of all clinically recognized pregnancies end in miscarriage (Simpson & Jauniaux, 2017). The majority—greater than 80% of miscarriages—are early pregnancy losses, occurring before 12 weeks of gestation (Cunningham et al., 2014). Of all clinically recognized first-trimester losses, 25% result from chromosomal abnormalities (Cunningham et al.). Other possible causes of early miscarriage include endocrine imbalance (as in women who have luteal phase defects, hypothyroidism, or insulin-dependent diabetes mellitus with high blood glucose levels in the first trimester), immunologic factors (e.g.,

antiphospholipid antibodies), systemic disorders (e.g., lupus erythematosus), and genetic factors. Infections are not a common cause of early miscarriage (Cunningham et al.).

A late miscarriage, sometimes called a second-trimester loss, occurs between 12 and 20 weeks of gestation. Risk factors for a second-trimester loss include being a member of a racial or ethnic minority group, poor outcomes in previous pregnancies, and extremes of maternal age. Other factors associated with an increased risk for miscarriage are severe dietary deficiencies, morbid obesity, regular or heavy alcohol use, and excessive (about 500 mg daily) caffeine intake. Bleeding during the first trimester is also a significant risk factor (Cunningham et al., 2014). Some of these risk factors cannot be modified, but correction of maternal disorders, a healthy lifestyle, adequate early prenatal care, and treatment of pregnancy complications can do much to prevent other causes of miscarriage.

Types

The types of miscarriage include threatened, inevitable, incomplete, complete, and missed. All types of miscarriage can recur in subsequent pregnancies. All types except the threatened miscarriage can lead to infection (Fig. 12.6).

Clinical Manifestations

Signs and symptoms of miscarriage depend on the duration of pregnancy. The presence of uterine bleeding, uterine contractions, or abdominal pain is an ominous sign during early pregnancy and must be considered a threatened miscarriage until proven otherwise.

If miscarriage occurs before the sixth week of pregnancy, the woman may report what she believes is a heavy menstrual flow. Miscarriage that occurs between weeks 6 and 12 of pregnancy causes moderate discomfort and blood loss. After week 12 miscarriage is typified by severe pain similar to that of labor because the fetus must be expelled. Diagnosis of the type of miscarriage is based on the signs and symptoms present (Table 12.6).

Symptoms of a *threatened* miscarriage (see Fig. 12.6, *A)* include spotting of blood but with the cervical os closed. Mild uterine cramping may be present.

Inevitable (see Fig. 12.6, *B)* and *incomplete* (see Fig. 12.6, *C)* miscarriages involve a moderate to heavy amount of bleeding with an open cervical os. Tissue may be present with the bleeding. Mild to severe uterine cramping may be present. An inevitable miscarriage is often accompanied by rupture of membranes (ROM) and cervical dilation. Passage of the products of conception occurs. An incomplete miscarriage involves the expulsion of the fetus with retention of the placenta.

In a *complete* miscarriage (see Fig. 12.6, *D)*, the cervix has already closed after all products of conception were expelled. Slight bleeding may occur, and mild uterine cramping may also be present, as well.

The term *missed* miscarriage (see Fig. 12.6, *E)* refers to a pregnancy in which the fetus has died but the products of conception are retained in utero for days, weeks, or even months. It may be diagnosed after the uterus stops increasing in size or even decreases in size. There may be no bleeding or cramping, and the cervical os remains closed (Cunningham et al., 2014). A missed miscarriage is often simply referred to as an early pregnancy loss.

Recurrent (habitual) early miscarriage is three or more spontaneous pregnancy losses before 20 weeks of gestation. The most widely accepted causes of recurrent miscarriage are parental chromosomal abnormalities, antiphospholipid antibody syndrome, and certain uterine abnormalities (Cunningham et al., 2014).

The evaluation of couples experiencing recurrent pregnancy loss usually includes karyotyping of both partners and miscarriage specimens and assessment of the placenta; evaluating the woman's uterine cavity; and testing the woman for antiphospholipid antibody syndrome and

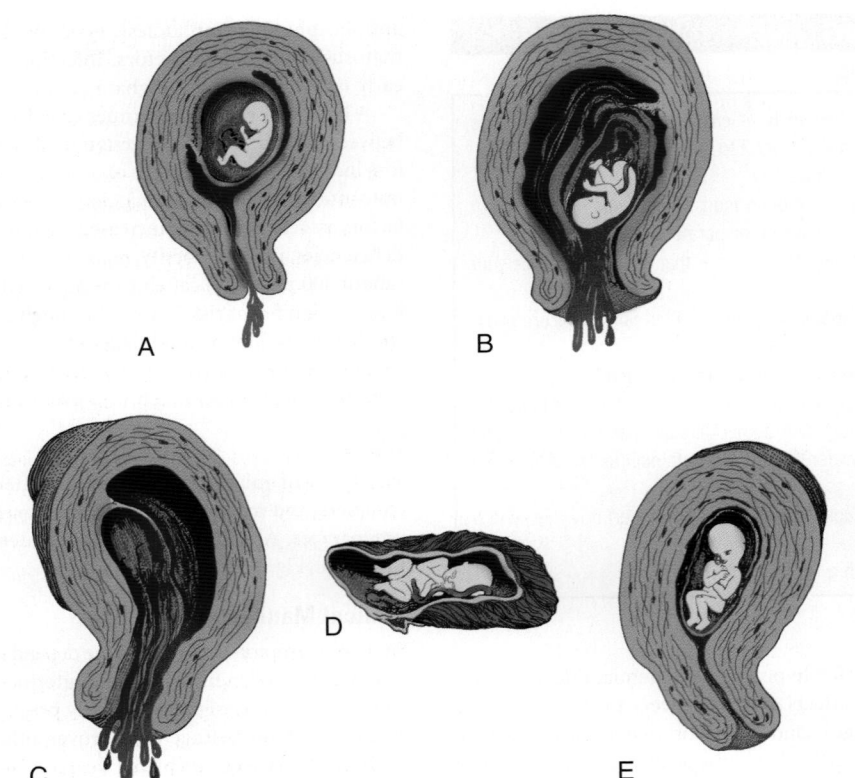

FIG 12.6 Miscarriage. **A,** Threatened. **B,** Inevitable. **C,** Incomplete. **D,** Complete. **E,** Missed.

thyroid disease. Evaluation should also address the psychologic response to this diagnosis because women and their partners often report feelings of guilt, anxiety, and depression. Thus couples experiencing recurrent pregnancy loss should be screened for depression and posttraumatic stress disorder (Rink & Lockwood, 2014).

Miscarriages can become septic, although this is uncommon. Symptoms of a septic miscarriage include fever and abdominal tenderness. Vaginal bleeding, which may be slight to heavy, is usually malodorous.

CARE MANAGEMENT

Assessment and Nursing Diagnoses

Whenever a woman has vaginal bleeding early in pregnancy, a thorough assessment should be performed. The data to be collected include pregnancy history, vital signs, type and location of pain, quantity and nature of bleeding, and emotional status. Laboratory tests may include evaluation of human chorionic gonadotropin (β-hCG) (pregnancy), hemoglobin level (anemia), and white blood cell (WBC) count (infection).

The following nursing diagnoses are appropriate for the woman experiencing a miscarriage:
- *Anxiety* related to
  - unknown outcome and unfamiliarity with medical procedures
- *Deficient Fluid Volume* related to
  - excessive bleeding secondary to miscarriage
- *Acute Pain* related to
  - uterine contractions
- *Situational Low Self-Esteem* related to
  - inability to carry a pregnancy successfully to term gestation
- *Risk for Infection* related to
  - surgical treatment
  - dilated cervix

Initial Care

Management depends on the classification of the miscarriage and on signs and symptoms (see Table 12.6). Traditionally, threatened miscarriages have been managed expectantly with supportive care. However, there are no proven effective therapies for this condition. Bed rest, although often prescribed, does not prevent progression to actual miscarriage. Repetitive transvaginal ultrasounds and measurement of human chorionic gonadotropin (hCG) and progesterone levels may be performed to determine if the fetus is alive and within the uterus (Cunningham et al., 2014).

Follow-up treatment depends on whether the threatened miscarriage progresses to actual miscarriage or symptoms subside and the pregnancy remains intact. If bleeding and infection do not occur, expectant management is a reasonable option. In approximately one-half of all threatened miscarriages managed in this way, the pregnancy continues (Cunningham et al., 2014).

Once the cervix begins to dilate, the pregnancy cannot continue, and miscarriage becomes inevitable. If all the products of conception are passed, no surgical intervention is necessary. If heavy bleeding, excessive cramping, or infection is present, however, the remaining embryonic, fetal, or placental tissue must be removed from the uterus, usually by suction curettage. In women who are clinically stable, expectant management to allow spontaneous resolution of an incomplete miscarriage is another treatment option (Cunningham et al., 2014).

In the past, because suspected fetal death could not be confirmed, expectant management was the only option for missed miscarriages, which eventually ended spontaneously. Because fetal death can now rapidly be confirmed using serial quantitative beta-human chorionic gonadotropin (β-hCG) testing and transvaginal ultrasound, many women choose to have uterine evacuation of a missed miscarriage (Cunningham et al., 2014).

TABLE 12.6   Assessing Miscarriage and the Usual Management

Type of Miscarriage	Amount of Bleeding	Uterine Cramping	Passage of Tissue	Cervical Dilation	Management
Threatened	Slight, spotting	Mild	No	No	Bed rest is often ordered but has not proven to be effective in preventing progression to actual miscarriage. Repetitive transvaginal ultrasounds and assessment of human chorionic gonadotropin and progesterone levels may be done to determine if the fetus is still alive and in the uterus. Further treatment depends on whether progression to actual miscarriage occurs.
Inevitable	Moderate	Mild to severe	No	Yes	Bed rest if no pain, bleeding, or infection If rupture of membranes, pain, bleeding, or infection is present, then prompt termination of pregnancy is accomplished, usually by dilation and curettage.
Incomplete	Heavy, profuse	Severe	Yes	Yes, with tissue in cervix	May or may not require additional cervical dilation before curettage. Suction curettage may be performed.
Complete	Slight	Mild	Yes	No (cervix has already closed after products of conception passed)	No further intervention may be needed if uterine contractions are adequate to prevent hemorrhage and no infection is present. Suction curettage may be performed to ensure no retained fetal or maternal tissue.
Missed	None, spotting	None	No	No	If spontaneous evacuation of the uterus does not occur within 1 month, pregnancy is terminated by method appropriate to duration of pregnancy. Blood clotting factors are monitored until uterus is empty. Disseminated intravascular coagulation (DIC) and incoagulability of blood with uncontrolled hemorrhage may develop in cases of fetal death after the twelfth week if products of conception are retained for longer than 5 weeks. May be treated with dilation and curettage, or misoprostol (Cytotec) given orally or vaginally.
Septic	Varies, usually malodorous	Varies	Varies	Yes, usually	Immediate termination of pregnancy by method appropriate to duration of pregnancy. Cervical culture and sensitivity studies are performed, and broad-spectrum antibiotic therapy (e.g., ampicillin) is started. Treatment for septic shock is initiated if necessary.
Recurrent (generally defined as three or more consecutive miscarriages)	Varies	Varies	Yes	Yes, usually	Varies; depends on type. Prophylactic cerclage may be performed if cervical insufficiency is the cause. Tests of value include karyotyping of both partners and miscarriage specimens and assessment of the placenta; evaluating the woman's uterine cavity; and testing the woman for antiphospholipid antibody syndrome and thyroid disease.

Data from Cunningham, F., Leveno, K., Bloom, S., et al. (2014). *William's obstetrics* (24th ed.). New York, NY: McGraw-Hill Medical; Gilbert, E. (2011). *Manual of high risk pregnancy & delivery* (5th ed.). St. Louis, MO: Mosby; Rink, B.D., & Lockwood, C.J. (2014). Recurrent pregnancy loss. In R.K. Creasy, R. Resnik, J.D. Iams, et al. (Eds.), *Creasy and Resnik's maternal-fetal medicine: Principles and practice* (7th ed.). Philadelphia, PA: Saunders.

Medical management is another treatment option if bleeding and infection are not present. Prostaglandin medications (e.g., misoprostol [Cytotec]) may be given and are usually effective in completing the miscarriage within 7 days (Cunningham et al., 2014). If medical management is chosen, nursing care is similar to the care for any woman whose labor is induced (see Chapter 17). Special care may be needed for management of side effects of prostaglandin such as nausea, vomiting, and diarrhea. If the products of conception are not passed completely, the woman may be prepared for manual or surgical evacuation of the uterus.

A third management option, and one that is often chosen, is dilation and curettage (D&C), a surgical procedure in which the cervix is dilated if necessary and a curette is inserted to scrape the uterine walls and remove uterine contents. Uterine contents may also be removed by suction curettage, using a catheter attached to an electric-powered vacuum source (Cunningham et al., 2014). Pain relief during a D&C is usually achieved by administering analgesics or sedatives intravenously or orally (conscious sedation). A paracervical block using a local anesthetic may also be administered (Cunningham et al.). Before a surgical procedure is performed, a full history should be obtained and general and pelvic examinations conducted. General preoperative and postoperative care is appropriate for the woman requiring surgical intervention for miscarriage. The nurse reinforces explanations, answers any questions or concerns, and prepares the woman for surgery.

After evacuation of the uterus, oxytocin (Pitocin) is often given to prevent hemorrhage. For excessive bleeding after the miscarriage, ergot products such as ergonovine (Methergine) or a prostaglandin derivative such as carboprost tromethamine (Hemabate) may be given to contract the uterus (see Medication Guide: Drugs Used to Manage Postpartum Hemorrhage, in Chapter 21). Antibiotics are given as necessary. Analgesics such as antiprostaglandin agents (e.g., nonsteroidal antiinflammatory drugs [NSAIDs]) may decrease discomfort from cramping. Transfusion therapy may be required for shock or anemia. The woman who is Rh negative and is not isoimmunized is given $Rh_o(D)$ immune globulin (Cunningham et al., 2014).

Psychosocial aspects of care focus on what the pregnancy loss means to the woman and her family. Grief from perinatal loss is complex and unique to each individual. Explanations are provided regarding the nature of the miscarriage, expected procedures, and possible future implications for childbearing.

As with other fetal or neonatal losses, the woman should be offered the option of seeing the products of conception. She may also want to know what the hospital does with the products of conception or whether she needs to make a decision about final disposition of fetal remains.

> ## ! NURSING ALERT
>
> Procedures for disposition of the fetal remains vary from hospital to hospital and state to state. The nurse should know what the usual procedures are in his or her setting.

Follow-Up Care

The woman will likely be discharged home within a few hours after a D&C or as soon as her vital signs are stable, vaginal bleeding remains minimal, and she has recovered from anesthesia. Discharge teaching emphasizes the need for rest. If significant blood loss has occurred, iron supplementation may be ordered. Teaching includes information about normal physical findings such as cramping, type and amount of bleeding, resumption of sexual activity, and family planning (see Patient Teaching box: Discharge Teaching for the Woman After Early Miscarriage).

Frequently the woman and her partner want to know when she should attempt to become pregnant again. Emphasis is placed on the importance of completely resolving the loss before attempting another pregnancy. Follow-up care should assess the woman's emotional as well as physical recovery. Referrals to local support groups are provided as needed. Share Pregnancy and Infant Loss Support, Inc. (www.nationalshare.org) is an excellent online resource for families who have experienced an early pregnancy loss.

Follow-up telephone calls after a loss are important. The woman may appreciate a telephone call on what would have been her due date. These calls provide opportunities for the woman to ask questions, seek advice, and receive information to help process her grief.

Cervical Insufficiency

One cause of late miscarriage is cervical insufficiency, which has traditionally been defined as passive and painless dilation of the cervix leading to recurrent preterm births during the second trimester in the absence of other causes. It was believed that these criteria defined women whose early births were caused solely by structural weakness of cervical tissue that could be corrected surgically by cerclage placement. Measurement of cervical length has been used as a way to diagnose cervical insufficiency. However, it is now known that an abnormally short cervix identified during the second trimester can also represent an early step in the process of preterm labor. Therefore, the challenge is to identify women who have cervical changes because of impaired cervical strength before conception or in early pregnancy rather than when they are beginning the process of preterm labor. However, assessment of cervical

PATIENT TEACHING

Discharge Teaching for the Woman After Early Miscarriage

- Cleanse the perineum after each voiding or bowel movement, and change perineal pads often.
- Shower (avoid tub baths) for 2 weeks.
- Avoid tampon use, douching, and vaginal intercourse for 2 weeks.
- Notify your health care provider if an elevated temperature or a foul-smelling vaginal discharge develops.
- Eat foods high in iron and protein to promote tissue repair and red blood cell replacement.
- Seek assistance from support groups, clergy, or professional counseling as needed.
- Allow yourself (and your partner) to grieve the loss before becoming pregnant again.

function to diagnose or rule out cervical insufficiency can be done only during pregnancy (Berghella & Iams, 2014).

Etiology

Cervical insufficiency may be either acquired or congenital. Congenital risk factors for cervical insufficiency include collagen disorders, uterine anomalies, and ingestion of diethylstilbestrol (DES) by the woman's mother while pregnant with the woman. Because DES has not been used since the early 1970s, however, it is now rare to encounter women who have this risk factor (Berghella & Iams, 2014). A risk factor for acquired cervical insufficiency is a history of previous cervical trauma resulting from lacerations during childbirth or mechanical dilation of the cervix during gynecologic procedures. Women who have had prior cervical surgery such as a biopsy in which a large cone specimen was removed or destroyed are also at risk for cervical insufficiency (Berghella & Iams; Ludmir, Owen, & Berghella, 2017).

Diagnosis

Cervical insufficiency is a clinical diagnosis, made by a thorough obstetric history along with speculum and digital pelvic examinations and a transvaginal ultrasound examination. Speculum and digital examinations allow identification of an opening at the internal cervical os, prolapsed fetal membranes, or both. A vaginal ultrasound examination will reveal an abnormally short (<25 mm) cervix. Often the short cervix is accompanied by *cervical funneling* (beaking), effacement of the internal cervical os, although the external cervical os remains closed (Berghella & Iams, 2014; Cunningham et al., 2014; Ludmir et al., 2017).

Management

Cervical cerclage placement has been the treatment of choice for women with cervical insufficiency due to cervical weakness. Indications for cerclage placement are a poor obstetric history (three or more previous early preterm births or second-trimester losses), a short (<25 mm) cervical length identified on transvaginal ultrasound, and an open cervix found on digital or speculum examination (Berghella & Iams, 2014). The McDonald technique is often the procedure of choice because of its proven effectiveness and ease of placement and removal. In this procedure, a suture is placed around the cervix beneath the mucosa to constrict the internal os of the cervix (Fig. 12.7) (Cunningham et al., 2014).

A cerclage may be placed either prophylactically or as a therapeutic or rescue procedure after cervical change has been identified (Berghella

& Iams, 2014; Cunningham et al., 2014). A prophylactic, or history-indicated, cerclage is usually placed at 12 to 14 weeks of gestation. An ultrasound-indicated cerclage may be placed therapeutically at 14 to 23 weeks of gestation in women with a singleton pregnancy and a history of a prior preterm birth if a short (<25 mm) cervix is identified on vaginal ultrasound. Finally, a rescue cerclage may be placed between 16 and 23 weeks of gestation in women who are found to have cervical change (>1 cm dilated or prolapsed membranes) on physical examination. The cerclage is removed if preterm premature rupture of membranes or advanced preterm labor that puts pressure on the stitch occurs. If the pregnancy progresses without further complications, the cerclage is removed when the woman reaches 36 weeks of gestation (Berghella & Iams).

The only indication for an abdominal cerclage that has been proven to be of benefit is failure of a prior history-indicated transvaginal cerclage, where spontaneous preterm birth occurred before 33 weeks of gestation. This procedure is usually done at 11 to 12 weeks of gestation or before

conception by means of a laparotomy. Suture (Mersilene tape) is placed at the junction of the lower uterine segment and the cervix (Fig. 12.8). Cesarean birth is necessary following an abdominal cerclage, and the suture is left in place if future pregnancies are desired (Ludmir et al., 2017).

The nurse assesses the woman's feelings about her pregnancy and her understanding of cervical insufficiency. Evaluating the woman's support systems is also important. Because the diagnosis of cervical insufficiency is usually not made until the woman has lost one or more pregnancies, she may feel guilty or to blame for this impending loss. Therefore assessing for previous reactions to stresses and appropriateness of coping responses is important. The woman needs the support of health care professionals and her family.

Follow-Up Care

Bed rest following cerclage was recommended in the past as a theoretical way to place less pressure on the cervix while in the recumbent position. However, the validity of bed rest has not been scientifically proven. In fact, some data suggest poorer outcomes in women on bed rest. Progesterone therapy, given either intramuscularly or vaginally, may be recommended for some women. Decisions about physical activity and intercourse are individualized, based on the status of the woman's cervix, as determined by digital and ultrasound examination (Ludmir et al., 2017).

The woman must understand the need for close observation and supervision for the remainder of the pregnancy. Additional instruction includes the need to watch for and report signs of preterm labor, rupture of membranes, and infection. Finally, the woman should know the signs that would warrant an immediate return to the hospital, including strong contractions less than 5 minutes apart, preterm premature rupture of membranes, severe perineal pressure, and an urge to push. If management is unsuccessful and the fetus is born before viability, appropriate grief support should be provided. If the fetus is born prematurely, appropriate anticipatory guidance and support including referral as needed will be necessary (see Chapter 25 for information on high-risk newborns and neonatal death and Chapter 17 for information on fetal and early neonatal loss and grief).

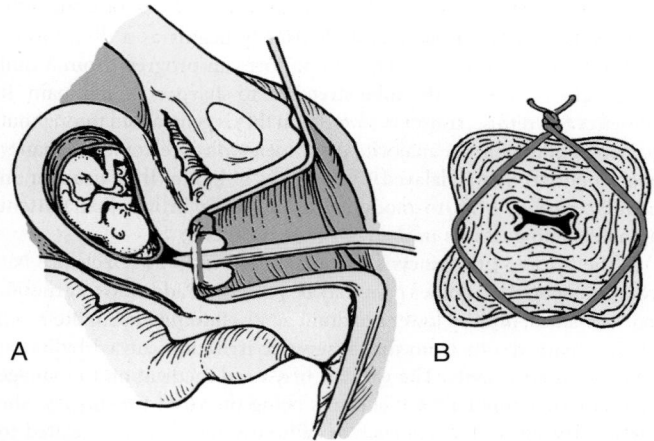

FIG 12.7 A, Cerclage correction of premature dilation of the cervical os. **B,** Cross-sectional view of closed internal os.

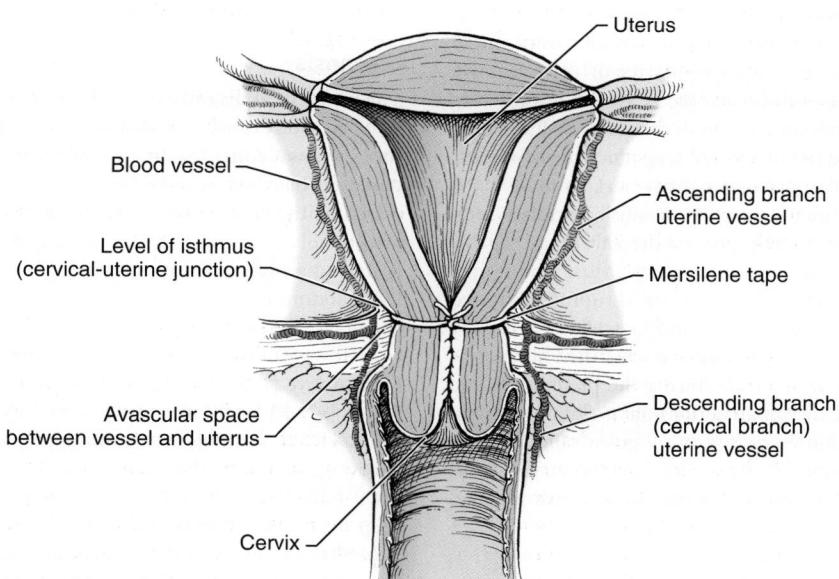

FIG 12.8 Abdominal cerclage. Surgical placement of circumferential Mersilene tape around uterine isthmus and median to uterine vessel. Knot is tied anteriorly. (In S. G. Gabbe, J. R. Niebyl, J. L. Simpson, et al. [Eds.], [2017]. *Obstetrics: Normal and problem pregnancies* [7th ed.]. Philadelphia, PA: Elsevier.)

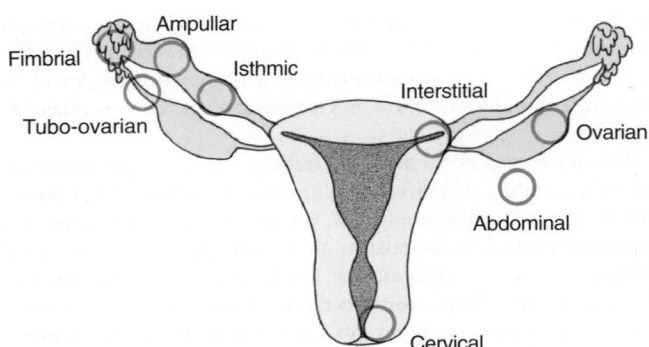

FIG 12.9 Sites of implantation of ectopic pregnancies. Order of frequency of occurrence is ampulla, isthmus, interstitium, fimbria, tubo-ovarian ligament, ovary, abdominal cavity, and cervix (external os).

Ectopic Pregnancy
Incidence and Etiology

An ectopic pregnancy is one in which the fertilized ovum is implanted outside the uterine cavity (Fig. 12.9). One to two percent of all first-trimester pregnancies in the United States are ectopic, and these account for 6% of all pregnancy-related maternal deaths. Women are less likely to have a successful subsequent pregnancy after an ectopic pregnancy (Cunningham et al., 2014). Ectopic pregnancy is also a leading cause of infertility.

Ectopic pregnancies are often called *tubal pregnancies* because at least 90% are located in the uterine (fallopian) tube (American Society for Reproductive Medicine [ASRM], 2013). Although they are much less common, ectopic pregnancies can also occur in the abdominal cavity, on an ovary, or on the cervix. Of all tubal ectopic pregnancies, approximately 80% are located in the ampulla, or largest portion of the tube (ASRM).

More than 100,000 ectopic pregnancies are reported each year in the United States. The actual number is certainly much larger, however, because only surgically managed cases are reported (ASRM, 2013). Some of the increased incidence is likely because of improved diagnostic techniques, such as more sensitive β-hCG measurement and transvaginal ultrasound, resulting in the identification of more cases. Other causes for the rise include an increased incidence of sexually transmitted infections, tubal infection and damage, popularity of contraceptive methods that predispose failures to be ectopic (e.g., the intrauterine device [IUD]), use of tubal sterilization methods that increase the chance of ectopic pregnancy, increased use of assisted reproductive techniques, and increased use of tubal surgery (Cunningham et al., 2014).

Ectopic pregnancy is classified according to site of implantation (e.g., tubal, ovarian, or abdominal). The uterus is the only organ capable of containing and sustaining a term pregnancy. Most abdominal pregnancies are thought to be the result of early tubal rupture, followed by reimplantation. Surgery to remove the embryo or fetus is usually performed as soon as an abdominal pregnancy is identified because of the high risk for hemorrhage at any time during the pregnancy (Fig. 12.10). The risk for fetal deformity in an abdominal pregnancy is high as a result of pressure deformities caused by oligohydramnios. The most common problems include facial or cranial asymmetry, various joint deformities, limb deficiency, and central nervous system anomalies (Cunningham et al., 2014).

Clinical Manifestations

Most cases of ectopic (tubal) pregnancy are diagnosed before rupture based on the three most classic symptoms: (1) abdominal pain, (2) delayed menses, and (3) abnormal vaginal bleeding (spotting). Abdominal

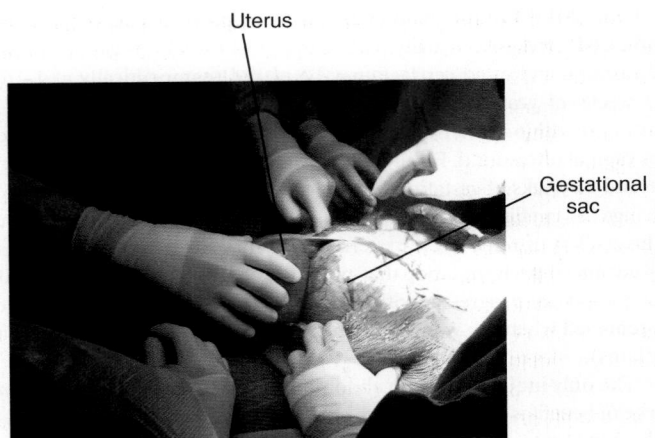

FIG 12.10 Ectopic pregnancy, abdominal, diagnosed on a routine ultrasound at 25 weeks of gestation. Note that the gestational sac is clearly outside the uterus. The placenta was attached to the right uterine tube and right ovary. (Courtesy of Danielle L. Tate, MD, Memphis, TN.)

pain occurs in almost every case. It usually begins as a dull, lower-quadrant pain on one side. The discomfort can progress from a dull to a colicky pain when the tube stretches, to sharp, stabbing, pain. It progresses to a diffuse, constant, severe pain that is generalized throughout the lower abdomen. The majority of women with an ectopic pregnancy report a period that is delayed 1 to 2 weeks or lighter than usual or an irregular period. Mild-to-moderate dark red or brown intermittent vaginal bleeding occurs in many of these women.

If the ectopic pregnancy is not diagnosed until after rupture has occurred, referred shoulder pain may be present in addition to generalized, one-sided, or deep lower quadrant acute abdominal pain. Referred shoulder pain results from diaphragmatic irritation caused by blood in the peritoneal cavity. The woman may need medication to manage severe, excruciating pain while she is being prepared for surgery. She may exhibit signs of shock such as faintness and dizziness related to the amount of bleeding in the abdominal cavity and not necessarily related to obvious vaginal bleeding. An ecchymotic blueness around the umbilicus (Cullen sign) indicating hematoperitoneum may also develop in an undiagnosed, ruptured intraabdominal ectopic pregnancy.

Diagnosis

The differential diagnosis of ectopic pregnancy involves consideration of numerous disorders that share many signs and symptoms. Many of these women come to the emergency department experiencing first-trimester bleeding or pain. Miscarriage, ruptured corpus luteum cyst, appendicitis, salpingitis, ovarian cysts, torsion of the ovary, and UTI are possible diagnoses. The key to early detection of ectopic pregnancy is having a high index of suspicion for this condition. *Every* woman with abdominal pain, vaginal spotting or bleeding, and a positive pregnancy test should undergo screening for ectopic pregnancy.

The most important screening tools for ectopic pregnancy are quantitative β-hCG levels and transvaginal ultrasound examination. When β-hCG levels are greater than 1500 to 2000 milli-International Units/mL, a normal intrauterine pregnancy should be visible on transvaginal ultrasound. Therefore, if β-hCG levels are greater than 1500 milli-International Units/mL but no intrauterine pregnancy is seen on transvaginal ultrasound, an ectopic pregnancy is very likely. β-hCG levels will probably be redrawn every 48 hours to determine if the pregnancy is viable. A transvaginal ultrasound may also be repeated to determine if the pregnancy is inside the uterus. Sometimes the location of an ectopic pregnancy will be visible on transvaginal ultrasound (Cunningham et al., 2014).

Another laboratory test that can be ordered to determine if the pregnancy is developing normally is a progesterone level. A progesterone level greater than 25 ng/mL almost always rules out the presence of an ectopic pregnancy. However, a progesterone level less than 5 ng/mL suggests either an ectopic pregnancy or an abnormal intrauterine pregnancy (Cunningham et al., 2014).

The woman should also be assessed for the presence of active bleeding, which is associated with tubal rupture. If internal bleeding is present, assessment may reveal vertigo, shoulder pain, hypotension, and tachycardia. A vaginal examination should be performed only once and then with great caution. Approximately 20% of women with a tubal pregnancy have a palpable mass on examination. Rupturing the mass is possible during a bimanual examination; thus a gentle touch is critical.

Medical management. Approximately 40% of women diagnosed with ectopic pregnancy are appropriate candidates for medical management, which involves giving methotrexate to dissolve the tubal pregnancy (ASRM, 2013). Methotrexate is an antimetabolite and folic acid antagonist that destroys rapidly dividing cells. It is classified as a hazardous drug and can cause serious toxic side effects even when given in low doses. These side effects can cause safety risks for health care providers if the drug is not handled appropriately. Additionally, the Institute for Safe Medication Practices considers methotrexate to be a high-alert drug (Box 12.4) (National Institute for Occupational Safety and Health, 2014; Shastay & Paparella, 2010).

Methotrexate therapy can prevent the need for surgery and is a safe, effective, and cost-effective way of managing many cases of tubal pregnancy. The woman must be hemodynamically stable and have normal liver and kidney function to be eligible for methotrexate therapy. The best results following methotrexate therapy are usually obtained if the mass is unruptured and measures less than 3.5 cm in diameter by ultrasound, if no fetal cardiac activity is noted on ultrasound, and if the initial serum β-hCG level is less than 1000 milli-International Units/L (Cunningham et al., 2014). The woman must also be willing to comply with posttreatment lifestyle restrictions and monitoring. She is informed of how the medication works, possible side effects, general self-care guidelines, and the importance of follow-up care (see Patient Teaching box: Teaching for Women Receiving Methotrexate Therapy).

> **! NURSING ALERT**
>
> Women receiving methotrexate to treat an ectopic pregnancy should refrain from taking any analgesic stronger than acetaminophen. Stronger analgesics can mask symptoms of tubal rupture.

Surgical management. Surgical management depends on the location and cause of the ectopic pregnancy, the extent of tissue involvement, and the woman's desires regarding future fertility. One option is removal of the entire uterine (fallopian) tube (salpingectomy). If the tube has not ruptured and the woman desires future fertility, salpingostomy may be performed instead. In this procedure, an incision is made over the pregnancy site in the tube, and the products of conception are gently and very carefully removed. The incision is not sutured but left to close by secondary intention instead, given that this method results in less scarring.

If surgery is planned, general preoperative and postoperative care is appropriate for the woman with an ectopic pregnancy. Before surgery, vital signs (pulse, respirations, and blood pressure [BP]) are assessed every 15 minutes or as needed, according to the severity of the bleeding and the woman's condition. Preoperative laboratory tests include determination of blood type and Rh status, complete blood cell count, and serum quantitative β-hCG level. Ultrasonography is used to confirm

---

BOX 12.4 Methotrexate Administration

- Obtain the woman's height and weight. These measurements are used to calculate her body surface area in order to determine the correct dose of methotrexate, so they must be accurate.
- The standard dose of methotrexate used to treat ectopic pregnancy is 50 mg/m^2 given intramuscularly, although it may also be ordered as 1 mg/kg.
- The dose of methotrexate should be prepared in the hospital pharmacy under a biologic safety cabinet. Syringe(s) containing the methotrexate should be dispensed from the pharmacy no more than three-fourths full in a sealed plastic bag without a needle attached.
- Don two pairs of gloves before removing the syringe(s) from the sealed plastic bag.
- Remove the syringe cap, and replace with an appropriate needle for intramuscular injection.
- Do not expel air from the syringe or prime the needle because these actions could aerosolize the methotrexate.
- Check the patient's identity and the medication and dosage before injecting the methotrexate. Another nurse should also perform an independent check before the injection is given.
- Dispose of any items worn or used to prepare, dispense, or administer the methotrexate injection in a waste container designated specifically for hazardous drugs.
- Wash your hands thoroughly after removing gloves.

Data from Shastay, A., & Paparella, S. (2010). Ectopic pregnancies and methotrexate: Are you prepared to manage this hazardous drug? *Journal of Emergency Nursing*, 36(1), 57-59.

PATIENT TEACHING

Teaching for Women Receiving Methotrexate Therapy

- Explain that methotrexate dissolves ectopic (tubal) pregnancies by destroying rapidly dividing cells.
- Explain that urine contains levels of drug metabolite that could be considered toxic for approximately 72 hours after receiving methotrexate. The levels are highest during the first 8 hours after treatment. Teach the woman to avoid getting urine on the toilet seat and to double flush the toilet (with the lid down) after urinating. Also explain that her stools may contain residual drug for up to 7 days.
- Inform the woman of possible side effects. Gastric distress, nausea and vomiting, stomatitis, and dizziness are common. Rare side effects include severe neutropenia, reversible hair loss, and pneumonitis.
- Advise the woman to do the following:
  - Avoid foods and vitamins containing folic acid.
  - Avoid "gas-forming" foods.
  - Avoid sun exposure.
  - Avoid sexual intercourse until the beta-human chorionic gonadotropin (β-hCG) level is undetectable.
  - Keep all scheduled follow-up appointments.
  - Contact her health care provider immediately if she has severe abdominal pain, which may be a sign of impending or actual tubal rupture.

Data from American Society for Reproductive Medicine. (2013). Medical treatment of ectopic pregnancy: A committee opinion. *Fertility and Sterility*, 100(3), 638-644; Shastay, A., & Paparella, S. (2010). Ectopic pregnancies and methotrexate: Are you prepared to manage this hazardous drug? *Journal of Emergency Nursing*, 36(1), 57-59.

an extrauterine pregnancy. Blood replacement may be necessary. The nurse verifies the woman's Rh and antibody status and administers Rh₀(D) immune globulin postoperatively if appropriate.

Follow-up care. Women who have received methotrexate therapy have their β-hCG level measured weekly to make certain that it continues to drop steadily until it becomes undetectable. Complete resolution of an ectopic pregnancy usually occurs in 2 to 3 weeks but can require as long as 6 to 8 weeks (ASRM, 2013).

Whether treated medically or surgically, the woman and her family should be encouraged to share their feelings and concerns related to the loss. Future fertility should be discussed. A contraceptive method should be used for at least three menstrual cycles to allow time for the woman's body to heal. *Every* woman who has been diagnosed with an ectopic pregnancy should be instructed to contact her health care provider as soon as she suspects that she might be pregnant because of the increased risk for recurrent ectopic pregnancy. These women may need referral to grief or infertility support groups. In addition to the loss of the current pregnancy, they are faced with the possibility of future pregnancy losses or infertility (see Chapter 17 for information on perinatal loss and grief).

Hydatidiform Mole (Molar Pregnancy)

Hydatidiform mole (molar pregnancy) is a benign proliferative growth of the placental trophoblast in which the chorionic villi develop into edematous, cystic, avascular transparent vesicles that hang in a grapelike cluster. Hydatidiform mole is a gestational trophoblastic disease (GTD). GTDs are a group of pregnancy-related trophoblastic proliferative disorders without a viable fetus that are caused by abnormal fertilization. In addition to hydatidiform mole, GTD includes invasive mole and choriocarcinoma (a rare form of cancer) (Cunningham et al., 2014).

Incidence and Etiology

Hydatidiform mole occurs in 1 in 1000 pregnancies in the United States (Cohn, Ramaswamy, & Blum, 2014). The cause is unknown, although it may be related to an ovular defect or a nutritional deficiency. Women at increased risk for hydatidiform mole formation are those who have had a prior molar pregnancy and those who are at the extremes of age for reproduction (Salani & Copeland, 2017).

Types

A hydatidiform mole may be further categorized as a complete or partial mole. The complete mole results from fertilization of an egg in which the nucleus has been lost or inactivated. The nucleus of a sperm (23,X or 23,Y) duplicates itself (resulting in the diploid number 46,XX or 46,XY) because the ovum has no genetic material or the material is inactive. It is also possible for an "empty" egg to be fertilized by two normal sperm, thereby producing either a 46,XX or 46,XY genotype (Moore, 2014). The mole resembles a bunch of white grapes. The hydropic (fluid-filled) vesicles grow rapidly, causing the uterus to be larger than expected for the duration of the pregnancy. The complete mole contains no fetus, placenta, amniotic membranes, or fluid (Fig. 12.11). Maternal blood has no placenta to receive it; therefore, hemorrhage into the uterine cavity and vaginal bleeding occur. Approximately 15% to 20% of women with a complete mole have evidence of persistent GTD (Cunningham et al., 2014).

In a partial mole, one apparently normal ovum is fertilized by two or more sperm. Triploidy (69XXY) or quadraploidy (92XXXY) genotypes then result (Moore, 2014). Partial moles often have embryonic or fetal parts and an amniotic sac (Fig. 12.12). Congenital anomalies are usually present. The risk for persistent GTD is much less than with a complete mole. If persistent GTD does occur, it is usually not a choriocarcinoma (Cunningham et al., 2014).

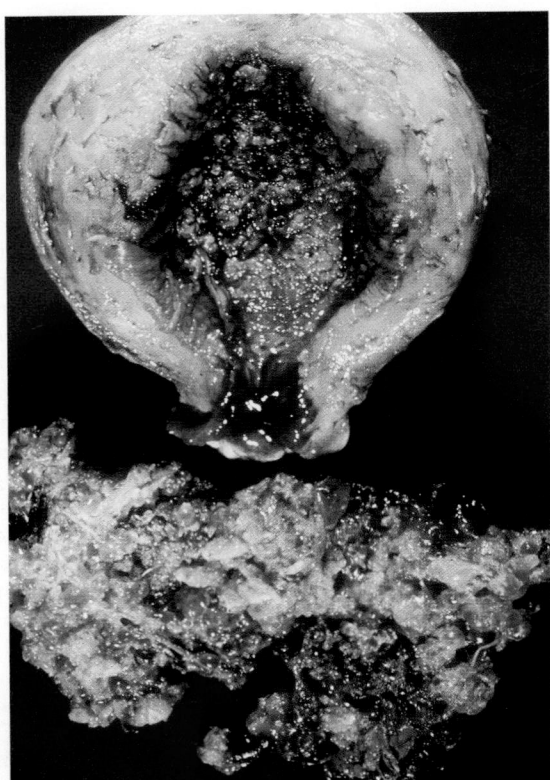

FIG 12.11 Gross specimen in a woman treated for complete hydatidiform mole with primary hysterectomy. (Courtesy of John Soper, MD. From DiSaia, P.J., & Creasman, W.T. [2012]. *Clinical gynecologic oncology* [8th ed.]. Philadelphia, PA: Mosby.)

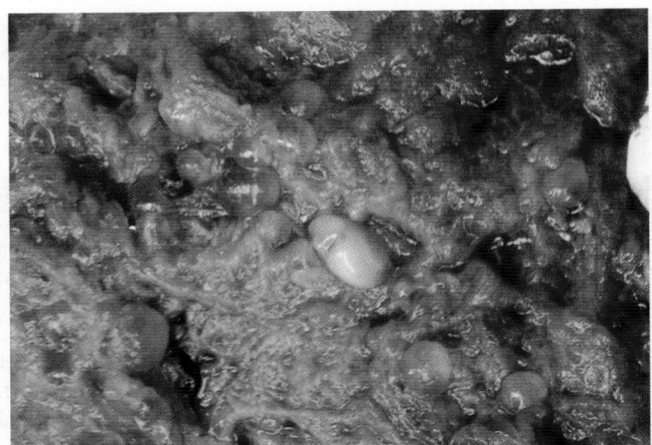

FIG 12.12 Partial hydatidiform mole. Notice the presence of grapelike vesicles. (Courtesy of Norman L. Meyer, MD, PhD, Memphis, TN.)

Clinical Manifestations

In the early stages, the clinical manifestations of a complete hydatidiform mole cannot be distinguished from those of normal pregnancy. Later, vaginal bleeding occurs in almost 95% of cases. The vaginal discharge may be dark brown (resembling prune juice) or bright red and either scant or profuse. It may continue for only a few days or intermittently for weeks. Early in pregnancy, the uterus in approximately one half of affected women is significantly larger than expected from menstrual dates. The percentage of women with an excessively enlarged uterus increases as length of time since the last menstrual period increases. Approximately 25% of affected women have a uterus smaller than would be expected from menstrual dates.

Anemia from blood loss, excessive nausea and vomiting (hyperemesis gravidarum), and abdominal cramps caused by uterine distention are relatively common findings. Women may also pass vesicles, which frequently are avascular edematous villi, from the uterus. Preeclampsia occurs in approximately 70% of women with large, rapidly growing hydatidiform moles and occurs earlier than usual in the pregnancy. If preeclampsia is diagnosed before 24 weeks of gestation, hydatidiform mole should be suspected and ruled out. Hyperthyroidism is another serious complication of hydatidiform mole. Usually treatment of the hydatidiform mole restores thyroid function to normal. Partial moles cause few of these symptoms and may be mistaken for an incomplete or missed miscarriage (Markham & Funai, 2014; Moore, 2014; Nader, 2014).

Diagnosis

Transvaginal ultrasound and serum hCG levels are used for diagnosis. Transvaginal ultrasound is the most accurate tool for diagnosing a hydatidiform mole. In the past, about half of all molar pregnancies were not diagnosed until molar tissue was passed from the vagina. Currently, however, many women are diagnosed by ultrasound while asymptomatic or by ultrasound done to evaluate vaginal bleeding or cramping symptoms. A characteristic pattern of multiple diffuse intrauterine masses, often called a *snowstorm pattern,* is seen in place of or along with an embryo or a fetus. The trophoblastic tissue secretes the hCG hormone (Cohn et al, 2014; Salani & Copeland, 2017). In a molar pregnancy, hCG levels are persistently high or rising beyond the time they would begin to decline in a normal pregnancy.

Management

Although most moles abort spontaneously, suction curettage offers a safe, rapid, and effective method of evacuating a hydatidiform mole if necessary. Older women who desire sterilization may undergo hysterectomy instead of suction curettage (Cunningham et al., 2014; Salani & Copeland, 2017). Induction of labor with oxytocic agents or prostaglandin is not recommended because of the increased risk for embolization of trophoblastic tissue (Salani & Copeland).

The nurse provides the woman and her family with information about the disease process, the necessity for a long course of follow-up, and the possible consequences of the disease. The nurse also helps the woman and her family cope with the pregnancy loss and recognize that the pregnancy was not normal. In addition, the woman and her family are encouraged to express their feelings, and information is provided about local support groups or counseling resources as needed. Internet resources such as Share: Pregnancy and Infant Loss Support, Inc. (www.nationalshare.org) and the International Society for the Study of Trophoblastic Diseases (www.isstd.org) may also be useful. Explanations about the importance of postponing a subsequent pregnancy and contraceptive counseling are provided to emphasize the need for consistent and reliable use of the method chosen.

> **! NURSING ALERT**
>
> To avoid confusion in regard to rising levels of hCG that are normal in pregnancy but could indicate GTD, pregnancy should be avoided during the follow-up assessment period. Any contraceptive method except an intrauterine device (IUD) is acceptable. Oral contraceptives are preferred because they are highly effective. Injectable medroxyprogesterone acetate (Depo Provera) is a practical option for women who have difficulty complying with the daily dosing required for oral contraceptive use.

Follow-Up Care

Follow-up care includes frequent physical and pelvic examinations along with weekly measurements of the β-hCG level until the level decreases to normal and remains normal for 3 consecutive weeks. Monthly measurements are then taken for 6 to 12 months. The follow-up assessment period usually continues for 1 year. During that time, rising β-hCG levels and an enlarging uterus may indicate GTD (Salani & Copeland, 2017).

> **🏠 COMMUNITY FOCUS**
>
> *Loss of Pregnancy*
>
> Talk with someone who has experienced an early pregnancy loss, either a miscarriage, an ectopic pregnancy, or a hydatidiform mole. What helpful things did her health care providers say or do at the time of the loss? What things did they say or do that were not helpful? Are there things that she wishes had been done or said differently? Which of her suggestions do you think would be helpful to people experiencing a different kind of loss?

LATE PREGNANCY BLEEDING

The major causes of bleeding in late pregnancy are placenta previa and premature separation of the placenta (abruptio placentae or placental abruption). Rapid assessment for and diagnosis of the cause of bleeding are essential to reduce maternal and perinatal morbidity and mortality (Table 12.7).

Placenta Previa

Because of advances in ultrasonography, especially transvaginal ultrasound, and an increased understanding of the changing relationship between the placenta and the internal cervical os as pregnancy progresses, definitions and classifications of placenta previa have changed. In **placenta previa**, the placenta is implanted in the lower uterine segment such that it completely or partially covers the cervical os or is close enough to the cervix to cause bleeding when the cervix dilates or the lower uterine segment effaces (Fig. 12.13) (Hull & Resnik, 2014). When transvaginal ultrasound is used, the placenta is classified as a *complete placenta previa* if it totally covers the internal cervical os. In a *marginal placenta previa,* the edge of the placenta is seen on transvaginal ultrasound to be 2.5 cm or closer to the internal cervical os. When the exact relationship of the placenta to the internal cervical os has not been determined or in the case of apparent placenta previa in the second trimester, the term *low-lying placenta* is used (Hull & Resnik).

Incidence and Etiology

Placenta previa affects approximately 1 in 200 pregnancies at term. Some evidence suggests that the incidence of placenta previa is increasing,

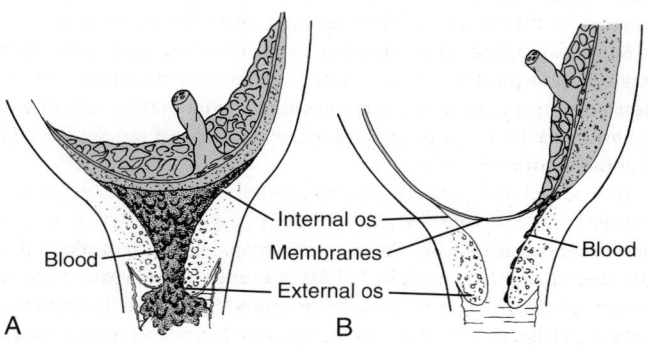

FIG 12.13 Types of placenta previa. **A,** Complete. **B,** Marginal.

TABLE 12.7   Summary of Findings: Placental Abruption and Placenta Previa

Findings	PLACENTAL ABRUPTION			Placenta Previa
	Grade 1 Mild Separation (10%–20%)	Grade 2 Moderate Separation (20%–50%)	Grade 3 Severe Separation (>50%)	
Physical and Laboratory Findings				
Bleeding, external, vaginal	Minimal	Absent to moderate	Absent to moderate	Minimal to severe and life-threatening
Total amount of blood loss	<500 mL	1000–1500 mL	>1500 mL	Varies
Color of blood	Dark red	Dark red	Dark red	Bright red
Shock	Rare; none	Mild shock	Common, often sudden, profound	Uncommon
Coagulopathy	Rare, none	Occasional DIC	Frequent DIC	None
Uterine tonicity	Normal	Increased, may be localized to one region or diffuse over uterus; uterus fails to relax between contractions	Tetanic, persistent uterine contractions, boardlike uterus	Normal
Tenderness (pain)	Usually absent	Present	Agonizing, unremitting uterine pain	Absent
Ultrasonographic Findings				
Location of placenta	Normal, upper uterine segment	Normal, upper uterine segment	Normal, upper uterine segment	Abnormal, lower uterine segment
Station of presenting part	Variable to engaged	Variable to engaged	Variable to engaged	High, not engaged
Fetal position	Usual distribution*	Usual distribution*	Usual distribution*	Commonly transverse, breech, or oblique
Gestational or chronic hypertension	Usual distribution*	Commonly present	Commonly present	Usual distribution*
Fetal effects	Normal fetal heart rate and pattern	Abnormal fetal heart rate and pattern	Abnormal fetal heart rate and pattern; fetal death can occur	Normal fetal heart rate and pattern

DIC, Disseminated intravascular coagulation.
*Usual distribution refers to the expected variations of incidence seen when there is no concurrent problem.

perhaps as a result of more cesarean births. In addition to a history of previous cesarean birth, other risk factors for placenta previa include advanced maternal age (more than 35 to 40 years of age), multiparity, history of prior suction curettage, and smoking (Hull & Resnik, 2014). Living at a higher altitude is also a risk factor for placenta previa. Like cigarette smoking, a higher altitude causes a decrease in uteroplacental oxygenation and thus a need for increased placental surface area. Maternal race is also associated with placenta previa. It appears that Asian women have the highest risk for placenta previa. Placenta previa also occurs more frequently in women carrying male fetuses. A possible explanation for this is that placentas are larger in pregnancies involving male fetuses (Francois & Foley, 2017). Multiple gestation is also a risk factor for placenta previa because of the larger placental area in these pregnancies (Cunningham et al., 2014). Women who had placenta previa in a previous pregnancy are more likely than others to develop the problem in a subsequent pregnancy, perhaps as a result of a genetic predisposition. Previous cesarean birth and curettage in the past for miscarriage or induced abortion are also risk factors for placenta previa because both result in endometrial damage and uterine scarring (Francois & Foley; Hull & Resnik).

Clinical Manifestations

Placenta previa is typically characterized by painless bright red vaginal bleeding during the second or third trimester. In the past, placenta previa was usually diagnosed after an episode of bleeding. Currently, however, most cases are diagnosed by ultrasound before significant vaginal bleeding occurs. This bleeding is associated with the disruption of placental blood vessels that occurs with stretching and thinning of the lower uterine segment. Between 70% and 80% of women with placenta previa will have at least one episode of vaginal bleeding. Of women with vaginal bleeding, one-third will present before 30 weeks of gestation, one-third between 30 and 36 weeks of gestation, and one-third after 36 weeks of gestation (Francois & Foley, 2017).

Vital signs may be normal, even with heavy blood loss, because a pregnant woman can lose up to 40% of her blood volume without showing signs of shock. Clinical presentation and decreasing urinary output may be better indicators of acute blood loss than vital signs alone. The fetal heart rate (FHR) is normal unless a major detachment of the placenta occurs.

Abdominal examination usually reveals a soft, relaxed, nontender uterus with normal tone. The presenting part of the fetus usually remains high because the placenta occupies the lower uterine segment. Thus the fundal height is often greater than expected for gestational age. Because of the abnormally located placenta, fetal malpresentation (breech and transverse or oblique lie) is common.

Maternal and Fetal Outcomes

The major maternal complication associated with placenta previa is hemorrhage. Another serious complication is development of an abnormal placental attachment (e.g., *placenta accreta, increta,* or *percreta*) (see Chapter 21). If excessive bleeding cannot be controlled, hysterectomy may be necessary (Cunningham et al., 2014; Hull & Resnik, 2014). Because most women with placenta previa give birth by cesarean, surgery-related trauma to structures adjacent to the uterus and anesthesia complications are also possible. In addition, blood transfusion reactions, anemia, thrombophlebitis, and infection may occur.

Preterm birth is a major cause of perinatal morbidity and mortality for infants born to women with placenta previa. IUGR has also been associated with placenta previa, although the risk for developing this condition is low. The incidence of fetal anomalies is increased in pregnancies complicated by placenta previa (Cunningham et al., 2014).

Diagnosis

All women with painless vaginal bleeding after 20 weeks of gestation should be assumed to have a placenta previa until proven otherwise. A transabdominal ultrasound examination should be performed initially, followed by a transvaginal scan, unless the transabdominal ultrasound clearly shows that the placenta is not located in the lower uterine segment. A transvaginal ultrasound is better than a transabdominal scan for accurately determining placental location (Hull & Resnik, 2014). If ultrasonographic scanning reveals a normally implanted placenta, a speculum examination may be performed to rule out local causes of bleeding (e.g., cervicitis, polyps, carcinoma of the cervix), and a coagulation profile is obtained to rule out other causes of bleeding.

Nursing Diagnoses and Management

Once placenta previa has been diagnosed, a management plan is developed. The woman is managed either expectantly or actively, depending on the gestational age, amount of bleeding, and fetal condition.

Potential nursing diagnoses include the following:
- *Decreased Cardiac Output* related to:
  - excessive blood loss secondary to placenta previa
- *Deficient Fluid Volume* related to:
  - excessive blood loss secondary to placenta previa
- *Ineffective Peripheral Tissue Perfusion* related to:
  - hypovolemia and shunting of blood to central circulation
- *Anxiety* related to:
  - maternal condition and pregnancy outcome
- *Grieving* related to:
  - actual or perceived threat to self, pregnancy, or infant

Expectant management. Expectant management (observation and bed rest) is implemented if the fetus is at less than 36 to 37 weeks of gestation with normal fetal growth and if no other pregnancy-associated complications exist (Francois & Foley, 2017). The woman initially is hospitalized in a labor and birth unit for continuous FHR and contraction monitoring. Large-bore IV access should be initiated immediately. Initial laboratory tests include hemoglobin, hematocrit, platelet count, and coagulation studies. A "type and screen" blood sample should be maintained at all times in the transfusion services department of the hospital to allow for immediate crossmatch of blood component therapy if necessary. If the woman is at less than 34 weeks of gestation, antenatal corticosteroids should be administered. Tocolytic medications may be given if the vaginal bleeding is preceded by or associated with uterine contractions (Francois & Foley, 2017).

If the bleeding stops, the woman will most likely be placed on bed rest with bathroom privileges and limited activity (e.g., able to use the bathroom, shower, and move around her hospital room for 15 to 30 minutes at a time, 4 times a day). No vaginal or rectal examinations are performed, and the woman is told to avoid intercourse. Ultrasound examinations are performed serially to assess placental location and fetal growth. The woman will also receive nutritional counseling and iron supplementation to avoid anemia (Francois & Foley, 2017).

Placenta previa should always be considered a potential emergency because massive blood loss with resulting hypovolemic shock can occur quickly if bleeding resumes. The possibility always exists that the woman will require an emergency cesarean birth. Placenta previa in a preterm gestation may be an indication for transfer to a tertiary-care perinatal center, given that a NICU may be necessary for care of the preterm infant. Because many community hospitals are not prepared to perform emergency surgery 24 hours per day, 7 days per week, transfer of the woman to a tertiary-care center may be necessary to ensure constant access to cesarean birth. Also, the transfusion services departments in many community hospitals do not have immediate access to large amounts of blood products, which will be necessary if massive hemorrhage occurs.

Home care. Sometimes women with placenta previa are discharged from the hospital before giving birth to be managed at home. The woman's condition should be stable, and she should have experienced no vaginal bleeding for at least 48 hours before discharge (Hull & Resnik, 2014). A candidate for home care must meet other strict criteria as well. She should be willing and able to comply with activity restrictions (bed rest with bathroom privileges and pelvic rest); live within a short distance of the hospital; have constant access to transportation; and verbalize a thorough understanding of the risks associated with placenta previa (Francois & Foley, 2017). If bleeding resumes, she needs to return to the hospital immediately. She must also be able to keep all appointments for fetal testing, laboratory assessments, and prenatal care. Visits by a perinatal home care nurse may be arranged.

If hospitalization or home care with activity restriction is prolonged, the woman can have concerns about her work- or family-related responsibilities or become bored with inactivity. She should be encouraged to participate in her own care and decisions about care as much as possible. Providing diversionary activities or encouraging her to participate in activities she enjoys and can perform while sedentary are necessary. Participating in a support group made up of other women on activity restriction while hospitalized or online if at home may be a helpful coping mechanism (see Patient Teaching box: Coping with Activity Restriction).

Active management. If the woman definitely has placenta previa and she is at or beyond 36 weeks of gestation, birth is appropriate. If bleeding is excessive or continues or there are concerns about the condition of the fetus, immediate birth is indicated, regardless of gestational age (Hull & Resnik, 2014). Almost all women with placenta previa will give birth by cesarean. If the placenta is located between 1 mm and 20 mm from the internal cervical os, however, as many as 60% of women may choose to attempt vaginal birth. If vaginal birth is attempted, health care providers must be prepared for the possibility of an emergent cesarean birth and the need for blood transfusion (Francois & Foley, 2017).

If cesarean birth is planned, the nurse continuously assesses maternal and fetal status while preparing the woman for surgery. The maternal condition is assessed frequently for decreasing BP, increasing pulse rate, changes in level of consciousness, and oliguria. Fetal assessment is maintained by continuous electronic fetal monitoring (EFM) to assess for signs of hypoxia.

Blood loss may not stop with the birth of the infant. The large vascular channels in the lower uterine segment may continue to bleed because of the diminished muscle content of that segment. The natural mechanism to control bleeding so characteristic of the upper part of the uterus (i.e., the interlacing muscle bundles, the "living ligature" contracting around open vessels) is absent in the lower part of the uterus. Therefore postpartum hemorrhage may occur even if the fundus is contracted firmly (see Chapter 21).

Emotional support for the woman and her family is extremely important. The actively bleeding woman is concerned not only for her own well-being but also for that of her fetus. All procedures should be explained, and a support person should be present. The woman should be encouraged to express her concerns and feelings. If the woman and

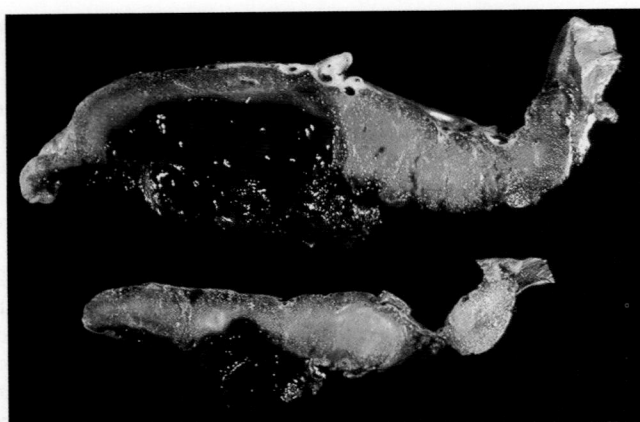

FIG 12.14 Placental abruption. Premature separation of normally implanted placenta. A large retroplacental clot is present. (From Creasy, R.K., Resnik, R., Iams, J.D., et al. [Eds.]. [2014]. *Creasy and Resnik's maternal fetal medicine: Principles and practice* [7th ed.]. Philadelphia, PA: Saunders.)

CLINICAL REASONING CASE STUDY

Third-Trimester Vaginal Bleeding

Ashley is a 29-year-old G6 P5 who presents to the emergency department with heavy vaginal bleeding and contractions. She has had no prenatal care but is at approximately 33 weeks of gestation by her LMP. During her medical screening examination, Ashley admitted to past cocaine use and reported that her boyfriend punched her in the abdomen earlier in the day.

1. Evidence—Is there sufficient evidence to determine the cause of Ashley's bleeding?
2. Assumptions—Describe an underlying assumption about each of the following issues:
   a. Possible diagnoses for Ashley
   b. Laboratory and diagnostic tests necessary to diagnose the cause of Ashley's bleeding
   c. Management options for Ashley
   d. Need for a social work consultation regarding intimate partner violence
3. What implications and priorities for nursing care can be drawn at this time?
4. Does the evidence objectively support your argument (conclusion)?
5. Interprofessional care—Describe the roles/responsibilities of health care professionals who might be involved in Ashley's care.

LMP, Last menstrual period.

her support person or family desire pastoral support, the nurse can notify the hospital chaplain service or provide information about other supportive resources.

Premature Separation of Placenta: Abruptio Placentae (Placental Abruption)

Premature separation of the placenta, or abruptio placentae, is the detachment of part or all of a normally implanted placenta from the uterus (Fig. 12.14). Separation occurs in the area of the decidua basalis after 20 weeks of gestation and before the birth of the infant.

Incidence and Etiology

Premature separation of the placenta is a serious complication that accounts for significant maternal and fetal morbidity and mortality. The overall incidence of placental abruption is 1 in 100 births, but a range of 1 in 80 to 1 in 250 pregnancies has been reported. The range in incidence likely reflects both variable criteria for diagnosis and an increased recognition of milder forms of abruption. Approximately one-third of all antepartum bleeding is caused by placental abruption (Francois & Foley, 2017) (see Clinical Reasoning Case Study: Third-Trimester Vaginal Bleeding).

Maternal hypertension, whether chronic or pregnancy related, is the most consistently identified risk factor for abruption. Cocaine use is also a risk factor because it causes vascular disruption in the placental bed. Blunt external abdominal trauma, most often the result of motor vehicle accidents (MVAs) or maternal battering, is another frequent cause of placental abruption (Cunningham et al., 2014; Francois & Foley, 2017). Other risk factors include cigarette smoking, a history of abruption in a previous pregnancy, and preterm premature rupture of membranes. There has been great interest in a possible association between thrombophilic disorders and abruption. However, both retrospective and prospective studies of women with the factor V Leiden mutation have shown no increased risk for abruption (Hull & Resnik, 2014). Abruption is more likely to occur in twin gestations than in singletons (Francois & Foley). Women who have had two previous abruptions have a recurrence risk of 25% in the next pregnancy (Hull & Resnik).

Classification

The most common classification of placental abruption is according to type and severity. This classification system is summarized in Table 12.7.

Clinical Manifestations

Clinical symptoms vary with degree of separation (see Table 12.7). Classic symptoms of placental abruption include vaginal bleeding, abdominal pain, uterine tenderness, and contractions (Cunningham et al., 2014; Hull & Resnik, 2014). Bleeding may result in maternal hypovolemia (i.e., shock, oliguria, anuria) and coagulopathy. Mild-to-severe uterine hypertonicity is present. Pain is mild to severe and localized over one region of the uterus or diffuse over the uterus with a boardlike abdomen.

Extensive myometrial bleeding damages the uterine muscle. If blood accumulates between the separated placenta and the uterine wall, it may produce a Couvelaire uterus. The uterus appears purple or blue rather than its usual "bubble-gum pink" color, and contractility is lost. Shock may occur and is out of proportion to apparent blood loss. Laboratory findings include a positive Apt test result (blood in the amniotic fluid); a decrease in hemoglobin and hematocrit levels, which may appear later; and a decrease in coagulation factor levels. Clotting defects (e.g., DIC) may be present, but most abruptions are not accompanied by maternal coagulopathy (Francois & Foley, 2017). A Kleihauer-Betke (KB) test may be ordered to determine the presence of fetal-to-maternal bleeding (transplacental hemorrhage), although it is of no diagnostic value. The KB test may be useful, however, to guide $Rh_o(D)$ immune globulin therapy in Rh-negative women who have had an abruption (Hull & Resnik, 2014).

Maternal and Fetal Outcomes

The mother's prognosis depends on the extent of placental detachment, overall blood loss, degree of coagulopathy present, and the time that passes between placental detachment and birth. Maternal complications are associated with the abruption or its treatment. Hemorrhage, hypovolemic shock, hypofibrinogenemia, and thrombocytopenia are associated with severe abruption. Renal failure and pituitary necrosis may result from ischemia. In rare cases, women who are Rh negative can become sensitized if fetal-to-maternal hemorrhage occurs and the fetal blood type is Rh positive.

Fetal complications, which include IUGR, oligohydramnios, preterm birth, hypoxemia, and stillbirth, are related to the severity and timing of the hemorrhage. Fetal survival is related to the size of the hemorrhage.

Large (>60 mL) retroplacental hemorrhages have been associated with a fetal mortality rate of 50% or greater (Francois & Foley, 2017). Risks for neurologic defects, cerebral palsy, and death from sudden infant death syndrome are greater in newborns following placental abruption (Cunningham et al., 2014; Francois and Foley).

Diagnosis

Placental abruption is primarily a clinical diagnosis. Although ultrasound can be used to rule out placenta previa, it cannot detect all cases of abruption. A retroplacental mass may be detected with ultrasonographic examination, but negative findings do not rule out a life-threatening abruption. In fact, at least 50% of abruptions cannot be identified on ultrasound (Hull & Resnik, 2014). Recent advances in imaging and interpretation have improved detection of placental abruption using ultrasound. Ultrasound can identify three main sources of abruption: *subchorionic* (between the placenta and the membranes), *retroplacental* (between the placenta and the uterine wall), and *preplacental* (between the placenta and the amniotic fluid) (Figs. 12.14 and 12.15). The location

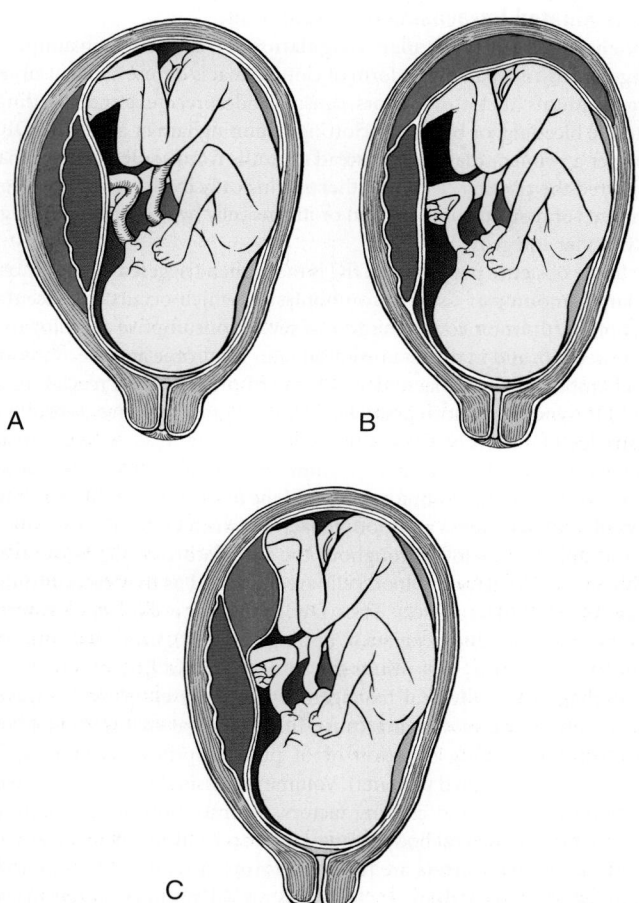

FIG 12.15 The classification system of placental abruption. **A,** Retroplacental abruption. The bright red area represents a blood collection behind the placenta *(dark red).* **B,** Subchorionic abruption. The bright red area represents subchorionic bleeding, which is observed to dissect along the chorion. **C,** Preplacental abruption. The bright red area represents a blood collection anterior to the placenta within the amnion and chorion (subamniotic). (From Gabbe, S.G., Niebyl, J.R., Simpson, J.L., et al. [Eds.]. [2017]. *Obstetrics: Normal and problem pregnancies* [7th ed.]. Philadelphia, PA: Elsevier.)

of the placental abruption is clinically significant. Retroplacental hematomas are associated with a worse fetal prognosis than is subchorionic hemorrhage (Francois & Foley, 2017). The diagnosis of abruption is confirmed after birth by visual inspection of the placenta. Adherent clot on the maternal surface of the placenta and depression of the underlying placental surface are usually present (see Fig. 12.14) (Francois & Foley, 2017).

Placental abruption should be highly suspected in the woman who experiences a sudden onset of intense, usually localized, uterine pain, with or without vaginal bleeding. Initial assessment is much the same as for placenta previa. Physical examination usually reveals abdominal pain, uterine tenderness, and contractions. The fundal height may be measured over time because an increasing fundal height indicates concealed bleeding. Approximately 60% of live fetuses exhibit abnormal FHR patterns, and elevated uterine resting tone may also be noted on the monitor tracing (Francois & Foley, 2017). Coagulopathy, as evidenced by abnormal clotting studies (fibrinogen, platelet count, partial thromboplastin time [PTT], fibrin split products), may be present if a large or complete abruption has occurred.

Management

Expectant management. Management depends on the severity of blood loss and fetal maturity and status. If the fetus is between 20 and 34 weeks of gestation and both the woman and fetus are stable, expectant management can be implemented. The woman is monitored closely because the abruption may extend at any time. The fetus is assessed regularly for evidence of appropriate growth because there is risk for IUGR. In addition, assessments of fetal well-being (e.g., nonstress testing, biophysical profile) are performed regularly. See Chapter 10 for further discussion of these tests. Corticosteroids are given to accelerate fetal lung maturity (Hull & Resnik, 2014).

Active management. Immediate birth is the management of choice if the fetus is at term gestation or the bleeding is moderate to severe and the mother or fetus is in jeopardy. At least one large-bore (16 to 18 gauge) IV line should be inserted. Maternal vital signs are monitored frequently to observe for signs of declining hemodynamic status such as increasing pulse rate and decreasing BP. Serial laboratory studies include hematocrit or hemoglobin determinations and clotting studies. Continuous EFM is mandatory. An indwelling catheter is inserted for continuous assessment of urine output, an excellent indirect measure of maternal organ perfusion. Fluid volume replacement may be necessary, along with administration of blood products to correct any coagulation defects.

Although vaginal birth is usually preferable, cesarean birth may become necessary. Cesarean birth should not be attempted when the women has severe and uncorrected coagulopathy because it can result in uncontrollable bleeding (Francois & Foley, 2017).

Nursing care of women experiencing moderate-to-severe abruption is demanding because it requires constant close monitoring of the maternal and fetal condition. Information about placental abruption, including the cause, treatment, and expected outcome, is given to the woman and her family. Emotional support is also extremely important because the woman and her family may be experiencing fetal loss and grief in addition to the woman's critical illness.

CORD INSERTION AND PLACENTAL VARIATIONS

When fetal vessels lie over the cervical os, the condition is termed **vasa previa**. In vasa previa, the vessels are implanted into the fetal membranes rather than into the placenta. Usually these vessels are protected only by the membranes (not by Wharton's jelly); thus they are at risk for rupture or compression (Hull & Resnik, 2014). In the past, vasa previa

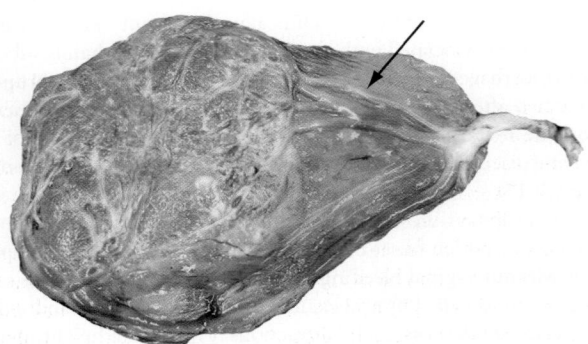

FIG 12.16 Vasa previa (velamentous insertion of cord). Arrow shows velamentous cord insertion in placenta. (From Creasy, R.K., Resnik, R., Iams, J.D. et al. [Eds.]. [2014]. *Creasy and Resnik's maternal fetal medicine: Principles and practice* [7th ed.]. Philadelphia, PA: Saunders.)

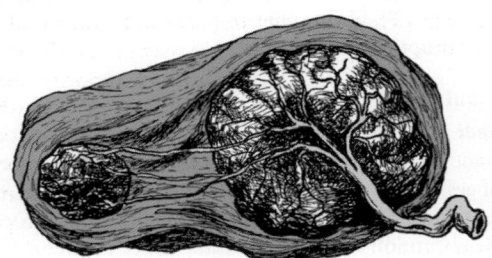

FIG 12.17 Vasa previa (succenturiate placenta).

was usually diagnosed after rupture of membranes occurred, followed by acute-onset vaginal bleeding caused by a lacerated fetal vessel. Currently, however, vasa previa is often diagnosed during pregnancy by ultrasound using color and pulsed Doppler imaging (Francois & Foley, 2017).

Vasa previa is rare, affecting between 1 in 1275 and 1 in 8333 pregnancies (Hull & Resnik, 2014). Risk factors for vasa previa include a history of second-trimester placenta previa or low-lying placenta, pregnancies resulting from assisted reproductive technology, and multiple gestations (Francois & Foley, 2017).

There are two variations of vasa previa. In both situations, artificial or spontaneous rupture of the membranes or traction on the cord may rupture one or more of the fetal vessels. As a result, the fetus may rapidly bleed to death (Francois & Foley, 2017; Sosa, 2014).

One variation of vasa previa, *velamentous insertion of the cord*, occurs when the cord vessels begin to branch at the membranes and then course onto the placenta (Fig. 12.16). The other variant of vasa previa occurs when the placenta has divided into two or more lobes rather than remaining as a single mass. This is known as a *succenturiate* placenta (Fig. 12.17). Fetal vessels then run between the lobes of the placenta. The vessels collect at the periphery, and the main trunks eventually unite to form the vessels of the cord. During the third stage of labor, one or more of the separate lobes may remain attached to the decidua basalis, preventing uterine contraction and increasing the risk for postpartum hemorrhage.

Another placental variation is *Battledore* (marginal) insertion of the cord (Fig. 12.18). This variation also increases the risk for fetal hemorrhage, especially after marginal separation of the placenta.

CLOTTING DISORDERS IN PREGNANCY

Normal Clotting

Normally a delicate balance (homeostasis) exists between the opposing hemostatic and fibrinolytic systems. The hemostatic system stops the

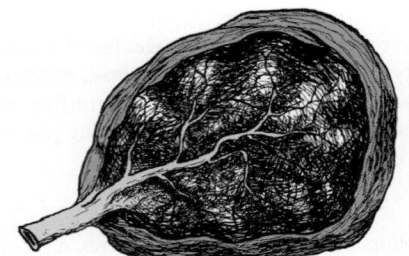

FIG 12.18 Battledore (marginal) cord insertion.

flow of blood from injured vessels, first by a platelet plug, then by the formation of a fibrin clot. The coagulation process involves an interaction of the coagulation factors that constantly circulate in the bloodstream, in which each factor sequentially activates the factor next in line (the "cascade effect" sequence). The fibrinolytic system is the process through which the fibrin clot is split into fibrinolytic degradation products and circulation is restored.

Clotting Problems
Disseminated Intravascular Coagulation

Disseminated intravascular coagulation (DIC), or consumptive coagulopathy, is a pathologic form of clotting that is diffuse and consumes large amounts of clotting factors, causing widespread external bleeding, internal bleeding, or both, and clotting (Cunningham et al., 2014). DIC is never a primary diagnosis. Instead it results from some problem that triggered the clotting cascade, either extrinsically by the release of large amounts of tissue thromboplastin or intrinsically by widespread damage to vascular integrity.

In the obstetric population, DIC is most often triggered by the release of large amounts of tissue thromboplastin, which occurs in placental abruption (the most common cause of severe consumptive coagulopathy in obstetrics), and in the retained dead fetus syndrome and the amniotic fluid embolus (anaphylactoid syndrome of pregnancy). Preeclampsia, HELLP syndrome, and gram-negative or gram-positive sepsis are examples of conditions that can trigger DIC because of widespread damage to vascular integrity (Cunningham et al., 2014). DIC is an overactivation of the clotting cascade and the fibrinolytic system, resulting in depletion of platelets and clotting factors, which causes the formation of multiple fibrin clots throughout the vasculature of the body, even in the microcirculation. Blood cells are destroyed as they pass through these fibrin-choked vessels. Thus DIC results in a clinical picture of clotting, bleeding, and ischemia (Cunningham et al). Clinical manifestations and laboratory test results are summarized in Box 12.5.

Management. Medical management in all cases of DIC involves correction of the underlying cause (e.g., removal of the dead fetus, treatment of existing infection or of preeclampsia or eclampsia, or removal of an abrupted placenta). Volume expansion, rapid replacement of blood products and clotting factors, optimization of oxygenation, achievement of normal body temperature, and continued reassessment of laboratory parameters are the usual forms of treatment. Vitamin K administration, recombinant activated factor VII, fibrinogen concentrate, prothrombin complex concentrate, tranexamic acid, and hemostatic agents should be considered as additional therapies (Francois and Foley, 2017).

Nursing interventions include assessing for signs of bleeding (see Box 12.5) and complications from the administration of blood and blood products, administering fluid or blood replacement as ordered, and protecting the woman from injury. Because renal failure is one consequence of DIC, urinary output is monitored closely by using an indwelling catheter. Vital signs are assessed frequently. If DIC develops

BOX 12.5   Clinical Manifestations and Laboratory Screening Results for Women With Disseminated Intravascular Coagulation

Possible Physical Examination Findings	Laboratory Coagulation Screening Test Results
• Spontaneous bleeding from gums, nose • Oozing, excessive bleeding from venipuncture site, intravenous access site, or site of insertion of urinary catheter • Petechiae (e.g., on arm where blood pressure cuff was placed) • Other signs of bruising • Hematuria • Gastrointestinal bleeding • Tachycardia • Diaphoresis	• Platelets: Decreased • Fibrinogen: Decreased • Factor V (proaccelerin): Decreased • Factor VIII (antihemolytic factor): Decreased • Prothrombin time: Prolonged • Partial prothrombin time: Prolonged • Fibrin degradation products: Increased • D-dimer test (specific fibrin degradation fragment): Increased • Red blood smear: Fragmented red blood cells

Data from Cunningham, F., Leveno, K., Bloom, S., et al. (2014). *William's obstetrics* (24th ed.). New York, NY: McGraw-Hill Medical; Labelle, C., & Kitchens, C. (2005). Disseminated intravascular coagulation: Treat the cause, not the lab values, *Cleveland Clinic Journal of Medicine, 72,* 377-397.

before birth, continuous EFM is necessary. The woman should be maintained in a side-lying tilt to maximize blood flow to the uterus. Oxygen may be administered through a nonrebreather face mask at 10 L/min or per hospital protocol or health care provider order. DIC usually is "cured" with the birth and as coagulation abnormalities resolve.

The woman and her family will be anxious and concerned about her condition and prognosis. The nurse offers explanations about care and provides emotional support to them through this critical time.

INFECTIONS ACQUIRED DURING PREGNANCY

SEXUALLY TRANSMITTED INFECTIONS

Sexually transmitted infections (STIs) in pregnancy are responsible for significant morbidity rates. Some consequences of maternal infection, such as infertility and sterility, last a lifetime. Psychosocial sequelae may include altered interpersonal relationships and lowered self-esteem. Congenitally acquired infections may affect the length and quality of a child's life. Chapter 4 discusses the diagnosis and management of STIs.

URINARY TRACT INFECTIONS

UTIs are a common medical complication of pregnancy, occurring in approximately 20% of all pregnancies. They are also responsible for 10% of all hospitalizations during pregnancy (Duff, 2014). UTIs include asymptomatic bacteriuria, cystitis, and pyelonephritis. They are usually caused by coliform organisms that are a normal part of the perineal flora. By far the most common cause is *Escherichia coli*, a gram-negative bacterium responsible for at least 80% of initial cases and about 70% of recurrent cases. *Klebsiella pneumoniae* and *Proteus* species are other common pathogens, particularly in women with a history of recurrent infections. Up to 10% of infections are caused by gram-positive organisms such as group B streptococci, enterococci, and staphylococci (Duff & Birsner, 2017).

Asymptomatic Bacteriuria

Asymptomatic bacteriuria refers to the persistent presence of bacteria within the urinary tract of women who have no symptoms. A clean-voided urine specimen containing more than 100,000 colonies per milliliter is diagnostic. If asymptomatic bacteriuria is not treated, about one-third of pregnant women will develop acute pyelonephritis Therefore, all women should be screened for asymptomatic bacteriuria at their first prenatal visit (Duff & Birsner, 2017). Asymptomatic bacteriuria has been associated with preterm birth and low–birth weight infants (American Academy of Pediatrics [AAP] & ACOG, 2012; Cunningham et al., 2014).

Asymptomatic bacteriuria should be treated with an antibiotic. Antibiotics that are often prescribed include amoxicillin, ampicillin, cephalexin (Keflex), ciprofloxacin (Cipro), levofloxacin (Levaquin), nitrofurantoin (Macrodantin), and trimethoprim-sulfamethoxazole (Bactrim DS). Several different regimens, including single-dose or 3-, 7-, and 10-day treatment may be used (Cunningham et al., 2014). In women who experience a prompt response to treatment of an initial infection, a urine culture for test of cure may not be clinically necessary or cost-effective. Conversely, urine cultures during or immediately after the completion of therapy are indicated for women who have a poor response to therapy or a history of recurrent infection (Duff & Birsner, 2017). Women who have persistent or frequent recurrences of bacteriuria may be placed on suppressive therapy, often nitrofurantoin, each night at bedtime, for the remainder of the pregnancy (Cunningham et al.).

Cystitis

Cystitis (bladder infection) is characterized by dysuria, urgency, and frequency, along with lower abdominal or suprapubic pain. Usually WBCs, as well as bacteria, are found in the urine. Microscopic or gross hematuria may also be present. Typically symptoms are confined to the bladder rather than becoming systemic. Cystitis is usually uncomplicated, but it may lead to ascending UTI if untreated. Approximately 40% of pregnant women with pyelonephritis experienced symptoms of bladder infection before developing pyelonephritis (Cunningham et al., 2014).

Cystitis is often treated with a 3-day course of antibiotic therapy, which is usually 90% effective in curing the infection. Antibiotics often prescribed include amoxicillin, ampicillin, cephalexin (Keflex), ciprofloxacin (Cipro), levofloxacin (Levaquin), nitrofurantoin (Macrodantin), and trimethoprim-sulfamethoxazole (Bactrim DS) (Cunningham et al., 2014). Phenazopyridine (Pyridium), a urinary analgesic, is often prescribed along with an antibiotic for relief of symptoms caused by irritation of the urinary tract. Although phenazopyridine is effective at relieving dysuria, urgency, and frequency, women should be taught that the medication colors urine and tears orange. Therefore they should be instructed to avoid wearing contact lenses while taking this medication and warned that it will stain underwear.

Pyelonephritis

Renal infection (pyelonephritis) is the most common serious medical complication of pregnancy and the leading cause of septic shock during pregnancy (Cunningham et al., 2014). The most common maternal complications associated with pyelonephritis include sepsis, ARDS, and preterm labor (Duff & Birsner, 2017).

Pyelonephritis develops most often during the second trimester of pregnancy and is usually caused by the *E. coli* organism. Infection develops only in the right kidney in more than half of all cases. The onset of pyelonephritis is often abrupt, with fever, shaking chills, and aching in the lumbar area of the back. Anorexia and nausea and vomiting also can be present. Usually one or both costovertebral angles are tender to palpation (Duff, 2014).

A woman with mild disease who is hemodynamically stable and has no evidence of preterm labor may be a candidate for outpatient management. She may be treated with oral antibiotics such as amoxicillin-clavulanic acid (Augmentin) or double-strength trimethoprim-sulfamethoxazole (Bactrim DS). Alternatively, arrangements may be made for a home care nurse to administer an antibiotic, such as ceftriaxone (Rocephin) either intravenously or intramuscularly (Duff & Birsner, 2017).

Most women diagnosed with pyelonephritis are usually admitted to the hospital immediately. Treatment with IV antibiotics is started as soon as urine and blood samples for culture and sensitivity have been collected (Cunningham et al., 2014). Ceftriaxone (Rocephin) is often prescribed because it provides excellent coverage against many of the organisms that commonly cause pyelonephritis. An additional antibiotic such as gentamicin or aztreonam (Cayston, Azactam) may be administered if the woman appears critically ill or is at high risk for a resistant organism. The woman must be monitored closely for complications such as sepsis, ARDS, and preterm labor (Duff & Birsner, 2017).

Clinical symptoms generally resolve within a couple of days after antibiotic therapy is begun. Most women are afebrile and asymptomatic after 72 hours. If no clinical improvement is seen within 48 to 72 hours, an ultrasound should be performed to assess for a urinary tract obstruction. Once the woman is afebrile, she will be changed from IV to oral antibiotics (Cunningham et al., 2014).

Usually antibiotic therapy is continued to complete a total of 7 to 10 days of treatment. Recurrent infection develops in 20% to 30% of women after completion of treatment for pyelonephritis. Many women are maintained on a prophylactic antibiotic (often nitrofurantoin [Macrodantin] daily) for the remainder of the pregnancy. Women receiving antibiotic prophylaxis should have their urine screened for bacteria at each subsequent prenatal appointment and be questioned about symptoms. If symptoms recur or the dipstick test for nitrite or leukocyte esterase is positive, a urine culture should be obtained to determine if retreatment is necessary (Duff & Birsner, 2017).

Patient Education

Nurses are often responsible for teaching pregnant women about taking medications safely and effectively. This education is especially important in regard to antibiotics because this type of medication is so often misused by the general public. The woman should be instructed to finish the entire course of prescribed antibiotic therapy rather than stopping the medication as soon as she feels better. Failure to complete treatment can lead to the creation of additional drug-resistant organisms. Antibiotics should be taken on time and around the clock so medication levels in the body remain constant. Finally, many women develop a yeast infection while taking antibiotics because the medication kills normal flora in the genitourinary tract as well as pathologic organisms. Therefore they should be encouraged to take probiotics and include yogurt, cheese, or milk containing active acidophilus cultures in their diet while on antibiotics.

The woman should also be taught simple ways to prevent future UTIs. See Box 4.5 for several suggestions.

SURGERY DURING PREGNANCY

Approximately 1 in 500 women require nonobstetric surgery during pregnancy. However, pregnancy can make the diagnosis more difficult. An enlarged uterus and displaced internal organs can make abdominal palpation more difficult, alter the position of an affected organ, and/or change the usual signs and symptoms associated with a particular disorder. Two common nonobstetric abdominal conditions requiring surgery during pregnancy are appendicitis and symptomatic cholelithiasis (Schwartz & Ludmir, 2017).

APPENDICITIS

The most common nonobstetric surgical emergency during pregnancy is appendicitis, occurring in about 1 in 1000 pregnancies (Cappell, 2017a). The diagnosis of appendicitis is often delayed because the usual signs and symptoms mimic some normal changes of pregnancy such as nausea and vomiting and increased WBC count. As pregnancy progresses, the appendix is pushed upward and to the right from its usual anatomic location (Cunningham et al., 2014). Because of these changes, rupture of the appendix and the subsequent development of peritonitis occur in up to 25% of pregnant women with appendicitis (Cappell).

The most common symptom of appendicitis in pregnant women is right lower quadrant abdominal pain, regardless of gestational age. Nausea and vomiting are often present, but loss of appetite is not a reliable indicator of appendicitis. Fever, tachycardia, a dry tongue, and localized abdominal tenderness are commonly found in nonpregnant people with appendicitis, but they are less likely indicators for the disorder in pregnant women. Because of the physiologic increase in WBCs that occurs in pregnancy, this test is not helpful in making the diagnosis. A urinalysis and a chest x-ray should be performed to rule out UTI and right lower lobe pneumonia, given that both of these conditions can cause lower abdominal pain (Kelly & Savides, 2014). Appendicitis can also be confused with other disorders such as cholecystitis, preterm labor, pyelonephritis, or placental abruption (Cunningham et al., 2014).

Radiologic imaging is necessary if appendicitis is suspected after history, physical examination, and laboratory studies have been completed. Although computed tomography (CT) is the imaging test of choice in nonpregnant patients because it is highly accurate, the use of ultrasound during pregnancy is preferred to avoid fetal exposure to radiation from CT (Cappell, 2017a). Magnetic resonance imaging (MRI) is the appropriate next step in a pregnant woman if appendicitis has not been confirmed by other imaging techniques (Cappell; Kelly & Savides, 2014).

Prompt surgical intervention to remove the appendix is still the standard treatment (Kelly & Savides, 2014). Laparoscopic surgery may be performed during the first and second trimesters of pregnancy if the appendix has not ruptured or the diagnosis is uncertain. Appendectomy is recommended even if appendicitis is not evident at surgery. Antibiotics are often administered for uncomplicated appendicitis and are definitely necessary if rupture, abscess, or peritonitis has occurred. Clindamycin and gentamicin are often prescribed because they are considered to be both effective and safe. The maternal mortality rate from ruptured appendix is about 4%. The fetal mortality rate from ruptured appendix is much higher, more than 30% (Cappell, 2017a).

CHOLELITHIASIS AND CHOLECYSTITIS

Cholelithiasis (the presence of gallstones in the gallbladder) occurs more often in women than in men. Its incidence increases during pregnancy, probably because of increased hormone levels and pressure from the enlarged uterus that interferes with the normal circulation and drainage of the gallbladder. Most gallstones are asymptomatic during pregnancy. Usually the first symptom of cholelithiasis is biliary colic presenting as, epigastric or right upper-quadrant pain that can radiate to the back or shoulders. Pain may occur spontaneously or after eating a high-fat meal. Approximately two-thirds of patients with biliary colic have recurrent attacks (Cappell, 2017b).

Cholecystitis (inflammation of the gallbladder) is usually caused when a gallstone obstructs a cystic duct. As in biliary colic that occurs with cholelithiasis, epigastric or right upper-quadrant pain is present, but the pain is usually more severe and prolonged. Nausea, vomiting,

PATIENT TEACHING

Nutrition Counseling for the Pregnant Woman With Cholecystitis or Cholelithiasis

- Assess your diet for foods that cause discomfort and gas, and omit foods that trigger episodes.
- Reduce dietary fat intake to 40 to 50 g/day.
- Limit protein to 10% to 12% of total calories.
- Choose foods so most of the calories come from carbohydrates.
- Prepare food without adding fats or oils as much as possible.
- Avoid fried foods.

BOX 12.6 Discharge Teaching for Home Care After Surgery

- Care of incision site
- Diet and elimination related to gastrointestinal (GI) function
- Signs and symptoms of developing complications (wound infection, thrombophlebitis, pneumonia)
- Equipment needed and technique for assessing temperature
- Recommended schedule for resumption of activities of daily living
- Treatments and medications ordered
- List of resource people and their telephone numbers
- Schedule of follow-up visits
- If birth has not occurred:
  Assessment of fetal activity (kick counts)
  Signs of preterm labor

---

and fever may also be present. Acute cholecystitis is the third most common indication for nonobstetric surgical intervention in pregnancy, occurring in about 4 cases per 10,000 pregnancies (Cappell, 2017b).

Often gallbladder surgery is postponed until the puerperium. The woman can usually be managed conservatively for the remainder of the pregnancy (see Patient Teaching box: Nutrition Counseling for the Pregnant Woman with Cholecystitis or Cholelithiasis:). However, women with recurrent biliary colic or acute cholecystitis generally require immediate cholecystectomy. Although the second trimester has traditionally been considered the safest time for this surgery, it is increasingly performed at any time during pregnancy because of improved surgical techniques and outcomes. Both laparoscopic and open cholecystectomy procedures are acceptable during pregnancy (Cappell, 2017b; Cunningham et al., 2014).

CARE MANAGEMENT

Assessment

Initial assessment of the pregnant woman requiring surgery focuses on her presenting signs and symptoms. A thorough history and physical examination are performed. Laboratory testing includes, at a minimum, a complete blood cell count with differential and a urinalysis. Additional laboratory and other diagnostic tests may be necessary to reach a diagnosis. In addition, FHR and activity and uterine activity should be monitored, and constant vigilance for symptoms of impending obstetric complications maintained. The extent of preoperative assessment is determined by the immediacy of surgical intervention and the specific disorder that requires surgery.

Hospital Care

When surgery becomes necessary during pregnancy, the woman and her family are concerned about the effects of the procedure and medication on fetal well-being and the course of pregnancy. An important aspect of preoperative nursing care is encouraging the woman to express her fears, concerns, and questions.

Preoperative procedures such as preparation of the operative site and time of insertion of IV lines and urinary retention catheters vary with the surgeon and the facility. However, in every instance there is a total restriction of solid foods and liquids or a clear specification of the type, amount, and time at which clear liquids may be taken before surgery. Some bowel preparation such as clear liquids and laxatives may be required before surgery. Food by mouth is restricted for several hours before a scheduled procedure. Even if she has had nothing by mouth but, more important, if surgery is unexpected, the woman is in danger of vomiting and aspirating; special precautions are taken before anesthetic is administered (e.g., administering an antacid).

Intraoperatively perinatal nurses may collaborate with the surgical staff to increase their knowledge about the special needs of pregnant women undergoing surgery. One intervention to improve fetal oxygenation is positioning the woman on the operating table with a lateral tilt to avoid compression of the maternal vena cava. Continuous FHR and uterine contraction monitoring during surgery may be performed if the fetus is considered viable. Monitoring may be accomplished by using sterile Aquasonic gel and a sterile sleeve for the transducer. During abdominal surgery, uterine contractions may be palpated manually. However, many practitioners simply monitor the fetus before and after the procedure.

In the immediate recovery period, general observations and care pertinent to postoperative recovery are initiated. Frequent assessments are carried out for several hours after surgery. Whether the woman is cared for in the surgical postanesthesia recovery area or in a labor and birth unit, continuous fetal and uterine monitoring are likely to be initiated or resumed because of the potential risk for preterm labor. Tocolysis may be necessary if preterm labor occurs (see Chapter 17).

Home Care

Plans for the woman's return home and for convalescent care should be completed as early as possible before discharge. Depending on her insurance coverage, nursing care can be provided through a home health agency. If not, the woman and other support people must be taught necessary skills and procedures such as wound care. Ideally the woman and other caregivers should have opportunities for supervised practice before discharge so they can feel comfortable with their knowledge and ability before being totally responsible for providing care. Box 12.6 lists information that should be included in discharge teaching for the postoperative patient. The woman also may need referrals to various community agencies for evaluation of the home situation, child care, home health care, and financial or other assistance.

TRAUMA DURING PREGNANCY

Trauma remains a common complication during pregnancy because most pregnant women in the United States continue their usual activities. Approximately 30,000 pregnant women in the United States experience treatable injuries each year because of trauma (Brown, 2017). Because of underreporting, the actual incidence of trauma during pregnancy is unknown. However, traumatic injury has been reported to complicate 6% to 8% of all pregnancies (Brown, 2017).

SIGNIFICANCE

As pregnancy progresses, the risk for trauma increases because more cases of trauma are reported in the third trimester than earlier in gestation. Most maternal injuries are a result of motor vehicle accidents (MVAs) and falls (Robbins, Martin, & Wilson, 2014), and most maternal deaths are caused by MVAs (Ruth & Miller, 2013). Serious injuries are more likely to occur in an MVA if the woman is not wearing a seat belt with a shoulder harness and is ejected from the vehicle. Therefore, to improve chances of survival for mother and fetus, pregnant women should wear properly positioned restraints at all times when in a motor vehicle (see Fig. 8.17). However, approximately one-third of pregnant women do not wear seat belts because of discomfort, inconvenience, or fears of hurting the baby. Other sources of trauma include intimate partner violence, assaults, and suicide attempts (Robbins et a.l).

Trauma is the leading cause of death among women of childbearing age. It is also the leading cause of nonobstetric maternal death in the United States (Mendez-Figueroa, Dahike, Vress, et al., 2013; Ruth & Miller, 2013). The effect of trauma on pregnancy is influenced by the length of gestation, type and severity of the trauma, and degree of disruption of uterine and fetal physiologic features (Robbins et al., 2014).

Fetal morbidity and mortality are also significantly affected by maternal trauma. An increased risk for fetal death is associated with maternal trauma, as well as a greater chance for other adverse maternal, fetal, and neonatal outcomes, including miscarriage, preterm birth, preterm premature rupture of membranes, uterine rupture, cesarean birth, placental abruption, and stillbirth (Brown, 2017). Fetal death rates related to maternal trauma are reported to be as high as 65% (Ruth & Miller, 2013). This information is probably underestimated because reporting of fetal death or injury resulting from maternal trauma is not standardized (Brown). Fortunately most trauma injuries during pregnancy are minor and have no effect on pregnancy outcome. However, each case must be evaluated carefully because pregnancy can mask signs of severe injury.

Special considerations for mother and fetus are necessary when trauma occurs during pregnancy because of the physiologic alterations that accompany pregnancy and because of the presence of the fetus.

MATERNAL PHYSIOLOGIC CHARACTERISTICS

Optimal care for the pregnant woman after trauma depends on understanding the physiologic state of pregnancy and its effects on trauma. The pregnant woman's body exhibits responses different from those of a nonpregnant person to the same traumatic insults. Because of the different responses to injury during pregnancy, management strategies must be adapted for appropriate resuscitation, fluid therapy, positioning, assessments, and most other interventions. Significant maternal adaptations and the relation to trauma are summarized in Table 12.8.

The uterus and bladder are confined to the bony pelvis during the first trimester of pregnancy and are at reduced risk for injury in cases of abdominal trauma. After pregnancy progresses beyond the 14th week, the uterus becomes an abdominal organ, and the risk for injury in cases of abdominal trauma increases. During the second and third trimesters, the distended bladder becomes an abdominal organ and is at increased risk for injury and rupture. Bowel injuries occur less often during pregnancy because of the protection provided by the enlarged uterus.

The elevated levels of progesterone that accompany pregnancy relax smooth muscle and profoundly affect the gastrointestinal tract. Gastrointestinal motility decreases, with a resultant increased time required for gastric emptying, whereas the production of hydrochloric acid increases in the last trimester, and the gastroesophageal sphincter relaxes (Ruth & Miller, 2013). Because of these changes, airway management of the unconscious pregnant woman is critically important.

> **! NURSING ALERT**
>
> The unconscious pregnant woman is at increased risk for regurgitation of gastric contents and aspiration whenever her head is positioned lower than her stomach or if abdominal pressure is applied.

A pregnant woman has decreased tolerance for hypoxia and apnea because of her decreased functional residual capacity and increased renal loss of bicarbonate. Acidosis develops more quickly in the pregnant than in the nonpregnant state.

Cardiac output increases 30% to 50% over prepregnancy values and is position dependent in the third trimester. Because of compression of the inferior vena cava and descending aorta by the pregnant uterus, cardiac output decreases dramatically if the woman is placed in the supine position. Therefore the supine position must be avoided, even in women with cervical spine injuries. It is a primary priority that lateral uterine displacement be accomplished without any head movement. As soon as the neck is immobilized, the stretcher should be tilted laterally (Brown, 2017; Ruth & Miller, 2013).

Circulating blood volume increases 40% to 50% during gestation. As a result, significant intraabdominal or intrauterine blood loss can occur with only minimal changes in vital signs (Robbins et al., 2014). By the time maternal tachycardia and hypotension, which are considered hallmark symptoms of blood loss, are evident, massive hemorrhage has likely already occurred (Ruth & Miller, 2013).

FETAL PHYSIOLOGIC CHARACTERISTICS

Perfusion of the uterine arteries, which provide the primary blood supply to the uteroplacental unit, depends on adequate maternal arterial pressure because these vessels lack autoregulation. Therefore maternal hypotension decreases uterine and fetal perfusion. Maternal shock results in splanchnic and uterine artery vasoconstriction, which decreases blood flow and oxygen transport to the fetus. EFM tracings can help in the evaluation of maternal status after trauma. They reflect fetal cardiac responses to hypoxia and hypoperfusion, including tachycardia or bradycardia, minimal or absent baseline variability, and/or late decelerations.

Careful monitoring of fetal status assists greatly in maternal assessment because the fetal monitor tracing works as an "oximeter" of internal maternal well-being. Hypoperfusion can be present in the pregnant woman before the onset of clinical signs of shock. The EFM tracings may show the first signs of maternal compromise (e.g., when maternal heart rate, BP, and color appear normal yet the EFM tracing shows signs of fetal hypoxia) (Brown, 2017; Miller, Miller, & Cypher, 2017).

MECHANISMS OF TRAUMA

Blunt Abdominal Trauma

Blunt abdominal trauma is most commonly the result of MVAs but also may be the result of battering or falls. Maternal and fetal mortality and morbidity rates are directly correlated with whether the mother remains inside the vehicle or is ejected. Maternal death is usually the result of a head injury or exsanguination from a major vessel rupture. Serious retroperitoneal hemorrhage after lower abdominal and pelvic trauma is reported more frequently during pregnancy. Serious maternal abdominal injuries are usually the result of splenic rupture or liver or renal injury.

Blunt trauma to the maternal abdomen is an important cause of placental abruption (Brown, 2017). Placental separation is thought to be a result of deformation of the elastic myometrium around the relatively inelastic placenta. Shearing of the placental edge from the underlying decidua basalis results and is worsened by the increased intrauterine

TABLE 12.8   **Maternal Adaptations During Pregnancy and Relation to Trauma**

System	Alteration	Clinical Responses
Respiratory	↑ Oxygen consumption	↑ Risk for acidosis
	↑ Tidal volume	↑ Risk for respiratory mismanagement
	↓ Functional residual capacity	
	Chronic compensated alkalosis	↓ Blood-buffering capacity
	↓ $PaCO_2$	
	↓ Serum bicarbonate	
Cardiovascular	↑ Circulating volume, 1600 mL	Can lose 1000 mL of blood
	↑ CO	No signs of shock until blood loss >30% of total blood volume
	↑ Heart rate	
	↓ SVR	↓ Placental perfusion in supine position
	↓ Arterial blood pressure	
	Heart displaced upward to left	Point of maximal impulse, fourth intercostal space
Renal	↑ Renal plasma flow	
	Dilation of ureters and urethra	↑ Risk for stasis, infection
	Bladder displaced forward	↑ Risk for bladder trauma
Gastrointestinal	↓ Gastric motility	↑ Risk for aspiration
	↑ Hydrochloric acid production	
	↓ Competency of gastroesophageal sphincter	Passive regurgitation of stomach acid if head lower than stomach
Reproductive	↑ Blood flow to organs	Source of ↑ blood loss
	Uterine enlargement	Vena caval compression in supine position
Musculoskeletal	Displacement of abdominal viscera	↑ Risk for injury, altered rebound response
	Pelvic venous congestion	Altered pain referral
	Cartilage softened	↑ Risk for pelvic fracture
		Center of gravity changed
	Fetal head in pelvis	↑ Risk for fetal injury
Hematologic	↑ Clotting factors	↑ Risk for thrombus formation
	↓ Fibrinolytic activity	

CO, Cardiac output; *$PaCO_2$*, arterial partial pressure of carbon dioxide; *SVR*, systemic vascular resistance.

pressure resulting from the impact. It is critical that all pregnant victims are evaluated carefully for signs and symptoms of placental abruption after even minor blunt abdominal trauma.

> **! NURSING ALERT**
>
> Signs and symptoms of placental abruption include uterine tenderness or pain, uterine irritability, uterine contractions, vaginal bleeding, leaking of amniotic fluid, or a change in FHR characteristics.

Pelvic fracture may result from severe injury and produce bladder trauma or retroperitoneal bleeding with the two-point displacement of pelvic bones that usually occurs. One point of displacement is commonly at the symphysis pubis, and the second point is posterior because of the structure of the pelvis. Careful evaluation for clinical signs of internal hemorrhage is indicated.

Direct fetal injury as a complication of trauma during pregnancy most often involves the fetal skull and brain. Most commonly this injury accompanies maternal pelvic fracture in late gestation, after the fetal head becomes engaged. When the force of the impact is great enough to fracture the maternal pelvis, the fetus often sustains a skull fracture. Evaluation for fetal skull fracture or intracranial hemorrhage is indicated.

Uterine rupture as a result of trauma is rare, occurring in less than 1% of severe cases. Rupture is more likely to occur in a previously scarred uterus. When uterine rupture occurs, it is usually associated with a direct blow delivered with substantial force (Cunningham et al.,

2014). Traumatic uterine rupture almost always results in fetal death. Maternal death occurs less frequently, in about 30% of cases (Ruth & Miller, 2013).

Penetrating Abdominal Trauma

Bullet and stab wounds are the most frequent causes of penetrating abdominal trauma in pregnant women. When the uterus sustains penetrating wounds, the fetus is more likely than the mother to be seriously injured. The enlarged uterus may protect other maternal organs, particularly the bowel, but the fetus is more vulnerable (Robbins et al., 2014).

Numerous factors determine the extent and severity of maternal and fetal injury from a bullet wound, including size and velocity of the bullet, anatomic region penetrated, angle of entry, path of the bullet, organs damaged, gestational age, and exit wound. Once the bullet enters the body, it may ricochet several times as it encounters organs or bone, or it may sever a large blood vessel. During the second half of pregnancy, the fetus usually sustains a direct injury from the bullet. Gunshot wounds require surgical exploration to determine the extent of injury and repair damage as needed.

Stab wounds are limited by the length and width of the penetrating object and are usually confined to the pathway of the weapon. Maternal and fetal injury is less if the stab wound is located in the upper abdomen and is from movement of the penetrating object from above the head downward toward the abdomen rather than from movement from the ground upward toward the lower abdomen. Stab wounds usually require surgical exploration to clean out debris, determine extent of injury, and repair damage.

Thoracic Trauma

Thoracic trauma is reported to produce 25% of all trauma deaths. Pulmonary contusion results from nearly 75% of blunt thoracic trauma and is a potentially life-threatening condition. Pulmonary contusion can be difficult to recognize, especially if flail chest also is present or if there is no evidence of thoracic injury. Pulmonary contusion should be suspected in cases of thoracic injury, especially after blunt acceleration or deceleration trauma such as that occurring when a rapidly moving vehicle crashes into an immovable object.

Penetrating wounds into the chest can result in pneumothorax or hemothorax. This type of injury is usually caused by an MVA that results in impalement by the steering column or a loose article in the vehicle that became a projectile with the force of impact. Stab wounds into the chest also may occur as a result of violence.

CARE MANAGEMENT

Immediate Stabilization

Immediate priorities for stabilization of the pregnant woman after trauma should be identical to those of the nonpregnant trauma patient. Pregnancy should not result in any restriction of the usual diagnostic, pharmacologic, or resuscitative procedures or maneuvers (AAP & ACOG, 2012). The initial response of many trauma team members when caring for the pregnant woman is to assess fetal status first because of the concern for a healthy neonate. Instead the trauma team should follow a methodic evaluation of maternal status to ensure complete assessment and stabilization of the mother. Fetal survival depends on maternal survival, and stabilization of the mother improves the chance of fetal survival.

> **! NURSING ALERT**
>
> Priorities of care for the pregnant woman after trauma must be to resuscitate the woman and stabilize her condition first and then consider fetal needs.

Primary Survey

The systematic evaluation begins with a *primary survey* and the initial *CABDs* of resuscitation: *compressions, airway, breathing,* and *defibrillation.* Increased oxygen needs during gestation necessitate a rapid response. The presence of a cervical spine injury is always assumed.

> **! NURSING ALERT**
>
> Hyperextension of the neck is avoided; instead, jaw thrust is used to establish an airway for the trauma victim.

Once an airway is established, assessment should focus on adequacy of oxygenation. The chest wall is observed for movement. If breathing is absent, ventilations and endotracheal intubation are initiated. Supplemental oxygen should be administered with a tight-fitting, nonrebreather face mask at 10 to 12 L/min to maintain adequate oxygen availability to the fetus. The chest wall is assessed for penetrating chest wound or flail chest. Breathing with a flail chest is rapid and labored; chest wall movements are uncoordinated and asymmetric; crepitus from bony fragments may be palpated.

Rapid placement of two large-bore (14 to 16 gauge) IV lines is necessary in the majority of seriously injured women. It is important to place the lines while veins are still distended. Cardiac arrest during the immediate stabilization period is usually the result of profound hypovolemia, necessitating massive fluid resuscitation. Infusion of crystalloids such as Ringer's solution or normal saline solution should be given as a 3:1 ratio; that is, 3 mL of crystalloid replacement to 1 mL of the estimated blood loss is given over the first 30 to 60 minutes of acute resuscitation. Because of the 50% increase in plasma blood volume during pregnancy, published formulas for nonpregnant adults used for estimating crystalloid and blood replacement to counter blood loss must be adjusted upward for pregnancy. When severe hemorrhage exists, transfusion with fresh frozen plasma, platelets, and packed red blood cells at a 1:1:1 ratio lowers the rate of coagulopathy and may increase the chance of survival (Mendez-Figueroa et al., 2013; Ruth & Miller, 2013).

Replacement of red blood cells and other blood components is anticipated; and blood is drawn for type, crossmatch, complete blood cell count, and platelet count. Infusion of type-specific whole blood or packed red blood cells is usually necessary to improve fetal oxygenation status and replace blood loss. During an extreme emergency, type O Rh-negative blood may be administered without matching.

Administering vasopressor drugs to treat maternal hypotension should be avoided if possible. These medications may significantly reduce uterine blood flow and thus decrease oxygen delivery to the fetus. In addition, their use does not address the cause of the hypovolemia (Ruth & Miller, 2013).

After 20 weeks of gestation, venous return to the heart is best accomplished by positioning the uterus to one side to eliminate the weight of the uterus compressing the inferior vena cava or the descending aorta. This facilitates efforts to establish the forward flow of blood through resuscitation and stabilization. If a lateral position is not possible because of resuscitative efforts or cervical spine immobilization, the uterus can be manually deflected, or a wedge should be inserted underneath one side of the backboard or stretcher.

Cardiopulmonary Resuscitation of the Pregnant Woman

Trauma, cardiac abnormalities, embolism, magnesium overdose, sepsis, intracranial hemorrhage, anesthetic complications, eclampsia, and uterine rupture are the most common causes of cardiac arrest in a pregnant woman (Robbins et al., 2014). Special modifications are necessary when cardiopulmonary resuscitation (CPR) is performed during the second half of pregnancy. In nonpregnant women, chest compressions produce a cardiac output of only about 30% of normal. Cardiac output in pregnant women may be even less as a result of aortocaval compression caused by the gravid uterus. Therefore, uterine displacement during resuscitation efforts is critical (Cunningham et al., 2014). Left lateral uterine displacement is recommended if the fundal height is at the level of the umbilicus (indicating approximately 20 weeks of gestation) or higher (Lavonas, Drennan, Gabrielli, et al., 2015). The uterus may be displaced laterally either manually or by placing a wedge, rolled blanket, or towel under one of the woman's hips. If defibrillation is needed, the paddles must be placed one rib interspace higher than usual because the heart is displaced slightly by the enlarged uterus (see Emergency Treatment box: Cardiopulmonary Resuscitation for the Pregnant Woman).

Complications, including laceration of the liver, rupture of the spleen or uterus, hemothorax, hemopericardium, or fracture of ribs or sternum may be associated with CPR on a pregnant woman. Fetal complications, including cardiac arrhythmia or asystole related to maternal defibrillation and medications and CNS depression related to antiarrhythmic drugs and inadequate uteroplacental perfusion, with possible fetal hypoxemia and acidemia, also may occur.

If the resuscitation is successful, the woman must be monitored carefully afterward. She remains at increased risk for recurrent cardiac arrest and arrhythmias (e.g., ventricular tachycardia, supraventricular tachycardia, bradycardia). Therefore her cardiovascular, pulmonary, and neurologic status should be assessed continuously. If the pregnancy

✚ EMERGENCY TREATMENT

Cardiopulmonary Resuscitation for the Pregnant Woman

Assessment
- Determine unresponsiveness and no breathing or no normal breathing.
- Activate emergency medical system and get AED if available.
- Return to victim and check for pulse.
- Begin chest compressions if no pulse is felt.

Compressions
- Position the woman on a flat, firm surface with her uterus displaced laterally with a wedge (e.g., a rolled towel placed under her hip) or manually, or place her in a lateral position.
- Begin chest compressions at a rate of 100/min to 120/min. Push hard and push fast! At the end of each compression, allow chest to recoil (reexpand) completely.
- Chest compressions should be performed to a depth of at least 5 cm (2 inches) for an average adult, but no greater than 6 cm (2.4 inches).
- Chest compressions may be performed slightly higher on the sternum if the uterus is enlarged enough to displace the diaphragm into a higher position.
- After five cycles of 30 compressions and two breaths (or approximately 2 minutes), check for a pulse. If no pulse is present, continue CPR. Rotate the compressor role every 2 minutes if possible to prevent fatigue.

Airway
- Open airway using head tilt–chin lift maneuver.

Breathing
- Deliver breaths using a face mask or bag-mask device if possible.
- Deliver each breath over 1 second, watching for chest rise.
- Deliver breaths using a ratio of 30 chest compressions to 2 breaths.

Defibrillation
- Use an AED according to standard protocol to analyze heart rhythm and deliver shock if indicated.

AED, Automated external defibrillator; *CPR,* cardiopulmonary resuscitation.
Data from Kleinman M.E., Brennan, E.E., Goldberger, Z.D., et al: (2015). Part 5: Adult basic life support and cardiopulmonary resuscitation quality: 2015 American Heart Association guidelines update for cardiopulmonary resuscitation and emergency cardiovascular care. *Circulation, 132*(2 suppl), S414–S435.

✚ EMERGENCY TREATMENT

Relief of Foreign Body Airway Obstruction

If the pregnant woman is unable to speak or cough, perform chest thrusts. Stand behind the woman, and place your arms under her armpits to encircle her chest. Press backward with quick thrusts until the foreign body is expelled (see Fig. 12.19). If the woman becomes unconscious, carefully support her to the ground, immediately activate EMS, and begin CPR.

EMS, Emergency medical services; *CPR,* cardiopulmonary resuscitation.
Data from Berg, R.A., Hemphill, R., Abella, B.S., et al. (2010). Part 5: Adult basic life support: 2010 American Heart Association guidelines for cardiopulmonary resuscitation and emergency cardiovascular care science. *Circulation, 122*(3 suppl), S685-S705.

The maternal abdomen should be evaluated carefully because a large percentage of serious injuries involve the uterus, intraperitoneal structures, and the retroperitoneum. The greatest clinical concern after severe blunt abdominal trauma is placental abruption because as many as 40% to 50% of these women have a clinically evident abruption (Brown, 2017). Assessments should focus on recognition of this complication, with careful evaluation of fetal monitor tracings, uterine tenderness, labor, or vaginal bleeding. Ultrasound examination may be performed to determine gestational age, viability of the fetus, and placental location. However, ultrasound studies cannot exclude placental abruption. Most cases of abruption that occur as a result of trauma are associated with relatively minor injuries (Robbins et al., 2014).

If trauma is the result of a penetrating wound, the woman should be completely undressed and carefully examined for all entrance and exit wounds. Focused assessment sonographic trauma (FAST) ultrasound and CT are commonly used to assess the likelihood of intraabdominal bleeding. Peritoneal lavage is less frequently used because of the availability of FAST, but it can be performed on hemodynamically unstable women to rule out bleeding or gross visceral perforation. Under direct visualization, the peritoneum is incised, and a peritoneal dialysis catheter is positioned. If aspiration yields free-flowing blood, the test is considered positive. If not, 1 L of saline is infused into the peritoneal cavity. The recovered lavage fluid is then examined for evidence of blood, bile, or bowel contents. Exploratory laparotomy is recommended if active hemorrhage or bowel perforation is suspected (Robbins et al., 2014).

Exploratory laparotomy is necessary after a gunshot wound to assess the abdominal cavity for organ damage and to repair any damage, with careful examination of all organs, the entire bowel, and posterior vessels. If uterine injury is found, a careful evaluation of the risks and benefits of cesarean birth is quickly accomplished. A cesarean birth is desirable if the fetus is alive and near term and may be necessary for the preterm fetus because of the high incidence of direct fetal injury in these cases. The fetus usually tolerates surgery and anesthesia if adequate uterine perfusion and oxygenation are maintained. Tetanus prophylaxis guidelines are not changed by pregnancy so vaccine is given if needed.

Trauma may affect numerous systems in the maternal body and may affect more than the pregnancy. External signs of maternal trauma should suggest the possibility of internal trauma. Back and neck pain suggest spine injury, abrasions on the chest suggest chest injury, and limb pain and malposition suggest limb fractures. If head injury results in nonresponsiveness, spinal, thoracic, and abdominal injuries are suspected. Hypovolemic shock can occur with internal hemorrhage, fracture of long bones, ruptured liver or spleen, hemothorax, or arterial dissection.

All female trauma victims of childbearing age should be considered pregnant until proven otherwise. Determination of the health history

remains intact, uterine activity and resting tone must be monitored. Fetal status and gestational age should also be determined and used in decision making regarding continuation of the pregnancy or the timing and route of birth.

Another common reason for performing CPR on a pregnant woman is airway obstruction caused by choking. Clearing an airway obstruction is usually accomplished by performing abdominal thrusts. However, during the second and third trimesters of pregnancy, chest thrusts rather than abdominal thrusts should be used (see Emergency Treatment box: Relief of Foreign Body Airway Obstruction and Fig. 12.19).

Secondary Survey

After immediate resuscitation and successful stabilization measures, a more detailed *secondary survey* of the mother and fetus should be completed. A complete physical assessment, including all body systems, is performed.

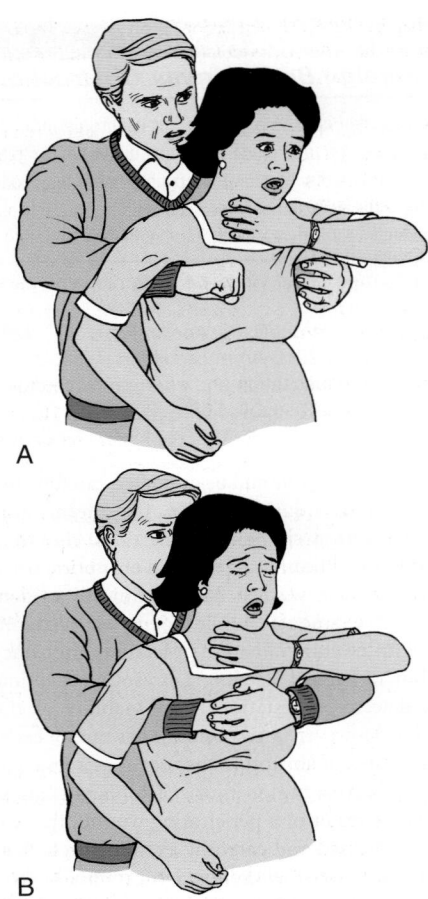

A

B

FIG 12.19 Clearing airway obstruction in woman in late stage of pregnancy. **A,** Standing behind victim, place your arms under woman's armpits and across chest. Place thumb side of your clenched fist against middle of sternum, and place other hand over fist. **B,** Perform backward chest thrusts until foreign body is expelled or woman becomes unconscious (see Emergency box: Relief of Foreign Body Airway Obstruction). (Data from Berg, R.A., Hemphill, R., Abella, B.S., et al. [2010]. Part 5: Adult basic life support: 2010 American Heart Association guidelines for cardiopulmonary resuscitation and emergency cardiovascular care science. *Circulation, 122*[3 suppl], S685-S705.)

and a history of the events preceding the trauma are important components of care. If the pregnant woman was involved in an MVA, it should be determined whether she was the driver or a passenger, if air bags were deployed, and if she was ejected from the vehicle or used a restraining device and remained within the vehicle.

Electronic Fetal Monitoring

External FHR and contraction monitoring is recommended after blunt trauma in a viable gestation for a minimum of 4 hours, regardless of injury severity. Fetal monitoring should be initiated soon after the woman is stable (Cunningham et al., 2014; Robbins et al., 2014). Continuous EFM may show early signs of placental abruption, including a change in baseline rate, loss of accelerations, or the presence of late decelerations, especially when accompanied by absent or minimal variability. The external device to monitor uterine activity, the tocodynamometer, is unable to measure pressures, so the pattern made with this device only shows the frequency and duration of contractions. Palpation is required to evaluate the intensity of contractions and the uterine resting tone.

It is important to palpate between contractions to verify that the uterus is well relaxed. If the uterus does not relax between contractions, placental abruption could be present.

The exact duration of FHR and contraction monitoring required after blunt abdominal trauma is not known. Monitoring should be continued indefinitely if uterine contractions, abnormal FHR characteristics, vaginal bleeding, uterine tenderness or irritability, serious maternal injury, or ruptured membranes are present (Cunningham et al., 2014). Most physicians recommend continuous monitoring for at least 24 hours because most serious complications appear to develop soon after the traumatic event (Robbins et al., 2014). Patients without contractions or with less than one contraction in 10 minutes may be removed from the electronic fetal monitor and discharged, as long as there is evidence of fetal movement, normal FHR characteristics, and no vaginal bleeding or indication of ruptured membranes (Miller et al., 2017).

> **LEGAL TIP** **Care of the Pregnant Woman Involved in a Minor Trauma Situation** After minor trauma, the pregnant woman may be discharged after an adequate period of EFM that demonstrates a normal (category I) tracing (see Chapter 15) and absence of uterine contractions. However, clear instructions must be given for immediate return to the health care facility if vaginal bleeding, leaking of amniotic fluid, decreased fetal movement, or severe abdominal pain occurs.

Fetal-Maternal Hemorrhage

The potential for fetomaternal hemorrhage exists after trauma. Hemorrhage can lead to fetal anemia, distress, or even death. If the pregnant trauma victim is Rh negative, fetomaternal hemorrhage can result in sensitization and hemolytic disease of the neonate. The Kleihauer-Betke assay is often performed in women following blunt abdominal trauma to estimate the amount of fetal blood within the maternal circulation. Because most cases have less than 30 mL of hemorrhage, however, Kleihauer-Betke test results seldom alter management (Cunningham et al., 2014; Robbins et al., 2014). Usually the routine administration of 300 mcg of $Rh_o(D)$ immune globulin is sufficient to protect almost all Rh-negative pregnant trauma patients from isoimmunization (Brown, 2017).

Ultrasound

Ultrasound after trauma is not as sensitive as EFM for diagnosing placental abruption. It may be useful to help establish gestational age, locate the placenta, evaluate cardiac activity (to determine whether the fetus is alive), and determine amniotic fluid volume. It may also be used to evaluate the presence of intraabdominal fluid that would suggest the presence of intraabdominal hemorrhage.

Radiation Exposure

If the pregnant woman has sustained serious injuries, any necessary radiographic examination should be performed, regardless of fetal exposure. If radiographic examination would be performed for the nonpregnant trauma victim, it also should be performed for the pregnant woman. Abdominal or pelvic CT scanning can be used to visualize extraperitoneal and retroperitoneal structures and the genitourinary tract. Radiation exposure of less than 5 rads has not been associated with fetal abnormalities or pregnancy loss, and the radiation level associated with abdominal or pelvic CT scans is far below this amount (Robbins et al., 2014). Blunt head trauma and loss of consciousness necessitate skull x-rays and CT assessment with neurosurgical consultation. MRI also can safely be used to assess injuries because it does not produce ionizing radiation (Robbins et al.).

Perimortem Cesarean Birth

In the presence of multisystem trauma, perimortem cesarean birth may be indicated. Removal of the stressor of pregnancy early in the process of resuscitation may increase the chance for an intact neonatal outcome and also improve maternal resuscitative efforts (Robbins et al., 2014). Therefore, if the pregnancy is at or beyond fetal viability (23 to 24 weeks of gestation) a cesarean birth should be performed after 4 minutes of resuscitative efforts if there is no spontaneous return of circulation (Brown, 2017; Lavonas et al., 2015; Robbins et al., 2014). It should be emphasized that perimortem cesarean birth is rarely successful, especially when the maternal arrest is related to trauma (Ruth & Miller, 2013).

REFERENCES

American Academy of Pediatrics & American College of Obstetricians and Gynecologists. (2012). *Guidelines for perinatal care* (7th ed.). Washington, DC: American College of Obstetricians and Gynecologists.

American College of Obstetricians and Gynecologists. (2013). Executive summary: Hypertension in pregnancy. *Obstetrics & Gynecology, 122*(5), 1122–1131.

American College of Obstetricians and Gynecologists. (2016). *Practice advisory on low-dose aspirin and prevention of preeclampsia: Updated recommendations.* Washington, DC: American College of Obstetricians and Gynecologists.

American Society for Reproductive Medicine. (2013). Medical treatment of ectopic pregnancy: A committee opinion. *Fertility and Sterility, 100*(3), 638–644.

Antony, K. M., Racusin, D. A., Aagaard, K., et al. (2017). Maternal physiology. In S. G. Gabbe, J. R. Niebyl, J. L. Simpson, et al. (Eds.), *Obstetrics: Normal and problem pregnancies* (7th ed.). Philadelphia, PA: Elsevier.

Berghella, V., & Iams, J. D. (2014). Cervical insufficiency. In R. K. Creasy, R. Resnik, J. D. Iams, et al. (Eds.), *Creasy and Resnik's maternal-fetal medicine: Principles and practice* (7th ed.). Philadelphia, PA: Saunders.

Brown, H. L. (2017). Trauma and related surgery in pregnancy. In S. G. Gabbe, J. R. Niebyl, J. L. Simpson, et al. (Eds.), *Obstetrics: Normal and problem pregnancies* (7th ed.). Philadelphia, PA: Elsevier.

Cappell, M. S. (2017a). Gastrointestinal disorders during pregnancy. In S. G. Gabbe, J. R. Niebyl, J. L. Simpson, et al. (Eds.), *Obstetrics: Normal and problem pregnancies* (7th ed.). Philadelphia, PA: Elsevier.

Cappell, M. S. (2017b). Hepatic disorders during pregnancy. In S. G. Gabbe, J. R. Niebyl, J. L. Simpson, et al. (Eds.), *Obstetrics: Normal and problem pregnancies* (7th ed.). Philadelphia, PA: Elsevier.

Castillo, M. J., & Phillippi, J. C. (2015). Hyperemesis gravidarum: A holistic overview and approach to clinical assessment and management. *The Journal of Perinatal & Neonatal Nursing, 29*(1), 12–22.

Cohn, D., Ramaswamy, B., & Blum, K. (2014). Malignancy and pregnancy. In R. K. Creasy, R. Resnik, J. D. Iams, et al. (Eds.), *Creasy and Resnik's maternal-fetal medicine: Principles and practice* (7th ed.). Philadelphia, PA: Saunders.

Cunningham, F., Leveno, K., Bloom, S., et al. (2014). *Williams obstetrics* (24th ed.). New York, NY: McGraw-Hill Education.

Duff, P. (2014). Maternal and fetal infections. In R. K. Creasy, R. Resnik, J. D. Iams, et al. (Eds.), *Creasy and Resnik's maternal-fetal medicine: Principles and practice* (7th ed.). Philadelphia, PA: Saunders.

Duff, P., & Birsner, M. (2017). Maternal and perinatal infection in pregnancy: Bacterial. In S. G. Gabbe, J. R. Niebyl, J. L. Simpson, et al. (Eds.), *Obstetrics: Normal and problem pregnancies* (7th ed.). Philadelphia, PA: Elsevier.

Francois, K. E., & Foley, M. R. (2017). Antepartum and postpartum hemorrhage. In S. G. Gabbe, J. R. Niebyl, J. L. Simpson, et al. (Eds.), *Obstetrics: Normal and problem pregnancies* (7th ed.). Philadelphia, PA: Elsevier.

Harvey, C., & Sibai, B. (2013). Hypertension in pregnancy. In N. Troiano, C. Harvey, & B. Chez (Eds.), *AWHONN's high risk and critical care obstetrics* (3rd ed.). Philadelphia, PA: Wolters Kluwer/Lippincott Williams & Wilkins.

Hull, A. D., & Resnik, R. (2014). Placenta previa, placenta accreta, abruptio placentae, and vasa previa. In R. K. Creasy, R. Resnik, J. D. Iams, et al. (Eds.), *Creasy and Resnik's maternal-fetal medicine: Principles and practice* (7th ed.). Philadelphia, PA: Saunders.

Institute for Safe Medication Practices. (2014). *ISMP's list of high-alert medications.* Retrieved from www.ismp.org.

Kelly, T. F., & Savides, T. J. (2014). Gastrointestinal disease in pregnancy. In R. K. Creasy, R. Resnik, J. D. Iams, et al. (Eds.), *Creasy and Resnik's maternal-fetal medicine: Principles and practice* (7th ed.). Philadelphia, PA: Saunders.

Lavonas, E. J., Drennan, I. R., Gabrielli, A., et al. (2015). Part 10: Special circumstances of resuscitation: 2015 American Heart Association guidelines update for cardiopulmonary resuscitation and emergency cardiovascular care. *Circulation, 132*(2 suppl), S501–S518.

Ludmir, J., Owen, J., & Berghella, V. (2017). Cervical insufficiency. In S. G. Gabbe, J. R. Niebyl, J. L. Simpson, et al. (Eds.), *Obstetrics: Normal and problem pregnancies* (7th ed.). Philadelphia, PA: Elsevier.

Markham, K. B., & Funai, E. F. (2014). Pregnancy-related hypertension. In R. K. Creasy, R. Resnik, J. D. Iams, et al. (Eds.), *Creasy and Resnik's maternal-fetal medicine: Principles and practice* (7th ed.). Philadelphia, PA: Saunders.

Mendez-Figueroa, H., Dahike, J. D., Vrees, R. A., et al. (2013). Trauma in pregnancy: An updated systematic review. *American Journal of Obstetrics and Gynecology, 209*(1), 1–10.

Miller, L., Miller, D., & Cypher, R. (2017). *Mosby's pocket guide to fetal monitoring: A multidisciplinary approach* (8th ed.). St. Louis, MO: Elsevier.

Moore, T. R. (2014). Placenta and umbilical cord imaging. In R. K. Creasy, R. Resnik, J. D. Iams, et al. (Eds.), *Creasy and Resnik's maternal-fetal medicine: Principles and practice* (7th ed.). Philadelphia, PA: Saunders.

Nader, S. (2014). Thyroid disease and pregnancy. In R. K. Creasy, R. Resnik, J. D. Iams, et al. (Eds.), *Creasy and Resnik's maternal-fetal medicine: Principles and practice* (7th ed.). Philadelphia, PA: Saunders.

National Institute for Occupational Safety and Health. (2014). *NIOSH list of antineoplastic and other hazardous drugs in healthcare settings (1).* Retrieved from https://www.cdc.gov/niosh/docs/2014-138/pdfs/2014-138 _v3.pdf.

Poole, J. H. (2014). Hypertensive disorders of pregnancy. In K. R. Simpson & P. Creehan (Eds.), *AWHONN's perinatal nursing* (4th ed.). Philadelphia, PA: Lippincott Willliams & Wilkins.

Rink, B. D., & Lockwood, C. J. (2014). Recurrent pregnancy loss. In R. K. Creasy, R. Resnik, J. D. Iams, et al. (Eds.), *Creasy and Resnik's maternal-fetal medicine: Principles and practice* (7th ed.). Philadelphia, PA: Saunders.

Robbins, K. S., Martin, S. R., & Wilson, W. C. (2014). Intensive care considerations for the critically ill parturient. In R. K. Creasy, R. Resnik, J. D. Iams, et al. (Eds.), *Creasy and Resnik's maternal-fetal medicine: Principles and practice* (7th ed.). Philadelphia, PA: Saunders.

Ruth, D., & Miller, R. S. (2013). Trauma in pregnancy. In N. Troiano, C. Harvey, & B. Chez (Eds.), *AWHONN's high risk and critical care obstetrics* (3rd ed.). Philadelphia, PA: Wolters Kluwer/Lippincott Williams & Wilkins.

Salani, R., & Copeland, L. J. (2017). Malignant diseases and pregnancy. In S. G. Gabbe, J. R. Niebyl, J. L. Simpson, et al. (Eds.), *Obstetrics: Normal and problem pregnancies* (7th ed.). Philadelphia, PA: Elsevier.

Schwartz, N., & Ludmir, J. (2017). Surgery during pregnancy. In S. G. Gabbe, J. R. Niebyl, J. L. Simpson, et al. (Eds.), *Obstetrics: Normal and problem pregnancies* (7th ed.). Philadelphia, PA: Elsevier.

Shastay, A., & Paparella, S. (2010). Ectopic pregnancies and methotrexate: Are you prepared to manage this hazardous drug? *Journal of Emergency Nursing, 36*(1), 57–59.

Sibai, B. (2017). Preeclampsia and hypertensive disorders. In S. G. Gabbe, J. R. Niebyl, J. L. Simpson, et al. (Eds.), *Obstetrics: Normal and problem pregnancies* (7th ed.). Philadelphia, PA: Elsevier.

Simha, H. N., Iams, J. D., & Romero, R. (2017). Preterm labor and birth. In S. G. Gabbe, J. R. Niebyl, J. L. Simpson, et al. (Eds.), *Obstetrics: Normal and problem pregnancies* (7th ed.). Philadelphia, PA: Elsevier.

Simpson, J. L. M., & Jauniaux, E. R. M. (2017). Early pregnancy loss and stillbirth. In S. G. Gabbe, J. R. Niebyl, J. L. Simpson, et al. (Eds.),

Obstetrics: Normal and problem pregnancies (7th ed.). Philadelphia, PA: Elsevier.

Snydal, S. (2014). Major changes in diagnosis and management of preeclampsia. *Journal of Midwifery & Women's Health*, *59*(6), 596–605.

Sosa, M. E. B. (2014). Bleeding in pregnancy. In K. R. Simpson & P. Creehan (Eds.), *AWHONN's perinatal nursing* (4th ed.). Philadelphia, PA: Lippincott WiIlliams & Wilkins.

13

Labor and Birth Processes

Kitty Cashion

http://evolve.elsevier.com/Perry/maternal

During late pregnancy, the woman and fetus prepare for the labor process. The fetus has grown and developed in preparation for extrauterine life. The woman has undergone various physiologic adaptations during pregnancy that prepare her for giving birth and for motherhood. Labor and birth represent the end of pregnancy, the beginning of extrauterine life for the newborn, and a change in the lives of the family. This chapter discusses the factors affecting labor, the processes involved, the normal progression of events, and the adaptations made by both the woman and the fetus.

FACTORS AFFECTING LABOR

At least five factors affect the process of labor and birth. These are easily remembered as the five *Ps*: *p*assenger (fetus and placenta), *p*assageway (birth canal), *p*owers (contractions), *p*osition of the mother, and *p*sychologic response. The first four factors are presented here as the basis of understanding the physiologic process of labor. The fifth factor is discussed in Chapter 16. Other factors can influence the woman's labor and birth experience, including place of birth, preparation, type of provider (e.g., obstetrician or family medicine physician, nurse midwife), nursing care, and procedures. These factors are discussed generally in Chapter 16 as they relate to nursing care during labor.

PASSENGER

The movement of the passenger, or fetus, through the birth canal is determined by several interacting factors: the size of the fetal head, fetal presentation, fetal lie, fetal attitude, and fetal position. Because the placenta also must pass through the birth canal, it can be considered a passenger along with the fetus; however, the placenta rarely impedes the process of labor in normal vaginal birth. An exception is the case of placenta previa (see Chapter 12).

Size of the Fetal Head

Because of its size and relative rigidity, the fetal head has a major effect on the birth process. The fetal skull is composed of two parietal bones, two temporal bones, the frontal bone, and the occipital bone (Fig. 13.1, *A*). These bones are united by connective tissue sutures: sagittal, lambdoidal, coronal, and fontanels (see Fig. 13.1, *B*). The areas where more than two bones meet are called fontanels. During labor after rupture of membranes, palpation of fontanels and sutures during vaginal examination reveals fetal presentation, position, and attitude.

The two most important fontanels are the anterior and posterior (see Fig. 13.1, *B*). The larger of these, the anterior fontanel, is diamond shaped, approximately 3 cm by 2 cm, and lies at the junction of the sagittal, coronal, and frontal sutures. It closes by 18 months after birth. The posterior fontanel lies at the junction of the sutures of the two parietal bones and the occipital bone, is triangular, and is approximately 1 cm by 2 cm. It closes 6 to 8 weeks after birth.

Sutures and fontanels make the skull flexible to accommodate the infant brain, which continues to grow for some time after birth. However, because the bones are not firmly united, slight overlapping, or molding of the shape of the head, occurs during labor. This capacity of the bones to slide over one another also permits adaptation to the various diameters of the maternal pelvis. Molding can be extensive, but the heads of most newborns assume their normal shape within 3 days after birth.

Although the size of the fetal shoulders may affect passage, their position can be altered relatively easily during labor, so one shoulder may occupy a lower level than the other. This creates a shoulder diameter that is smaller than the skull, facilitating passage through the birth canal. After the birth of the head and shoulders, the rest of the body usually emerges quickly (Cunningham, Leveno, Bloom, et al., 2014).

Fetal Presentation

Presentation refers to the part of the fetus that enters the pelvic inlet first and leads through the birth canal during labor at term. The three main presentations are *cephalic presentation* (head first), occurring in approximately 97% of births (Fig. 13.2); *breech presentation* (buttocks, feet, or both first), occurring in approximately 3% of births (Fig. 13.3, *A–C*); and *shoulder presentation*, seen in fewer than 1% of births (see Fig. 13.3, *D*) (Cunningham et al., 2014). The presenting part is that part of the fetus that lies closest to the internal os of the cervix. It is the part of the fetal body first felt by the examining finger during a vaginal examination. In a cephalic presentation the presenting part is usually the occiput; in a breech presentation it is the sacrum; in the shoulder presentation it is the scapula. When the presenting part is the occiput, the presentation is noted as *vertex* (see Fig. 13.2). Factors that determine the presenting part include fetal lie, fetal attitude, and extension or flexion of the fetal head.

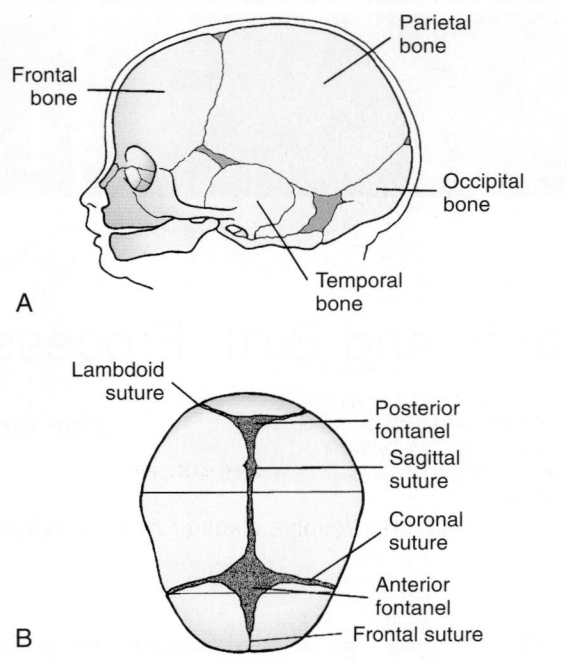

FIG 13.1 Fetal head at term. **A,** Bones. **B,** Sutures and fontanels.

Fetal Lie

Lie is the relation of the long axis (spine) of the fetus to the long axis (spine) of the mother. The two primary lies are longitudinal, or vertical, in which the long axis of the fetus is parallel with the long axis of the mother (see Fig. 13.2); and transverse, horizontal, or oblique, in which the long axis of the fetus is at a right angle diagonal to the long axis of the mother (see Fig. 13.3, *D).* Longitudinal lies are either cephalic or breech presentations, depending on the fetal structure that first enters the mother's pelvis. Vaginal birth cannot occur when the fetus stays in a transverse lie. An oblique lie, one in which the long axis of the fetus is lying at an angle to the long axis of the mother, is less common and usually converts to a longitudinal or transverse lie during labor (Cunningham et al., 2014).

Fetal Attitude

Attitude is the relation of the fetal body parts to one another. The fetus assumes a characteristic posture (attitude) in utero partly because of the mode of fetal growth and partly because of the way the fetus conforms to the shape of the uterine cavity. Normally the back of the fetus is rounded so the chin is flexed on the chest, the thighs are flexed on the abdomen, and the legs are flexed at the knees. The arms are crossed over the thorax, and the umbilical cord lies between the arms and the legs. This attitude is termed *general flexion* (see Fig. 13.2).

Deviations from the normal attitude may cause difficulties in childbirth. For example, in a cephalic presentation the fetal head may be extended or flexed in a manner that presents a head diameter that

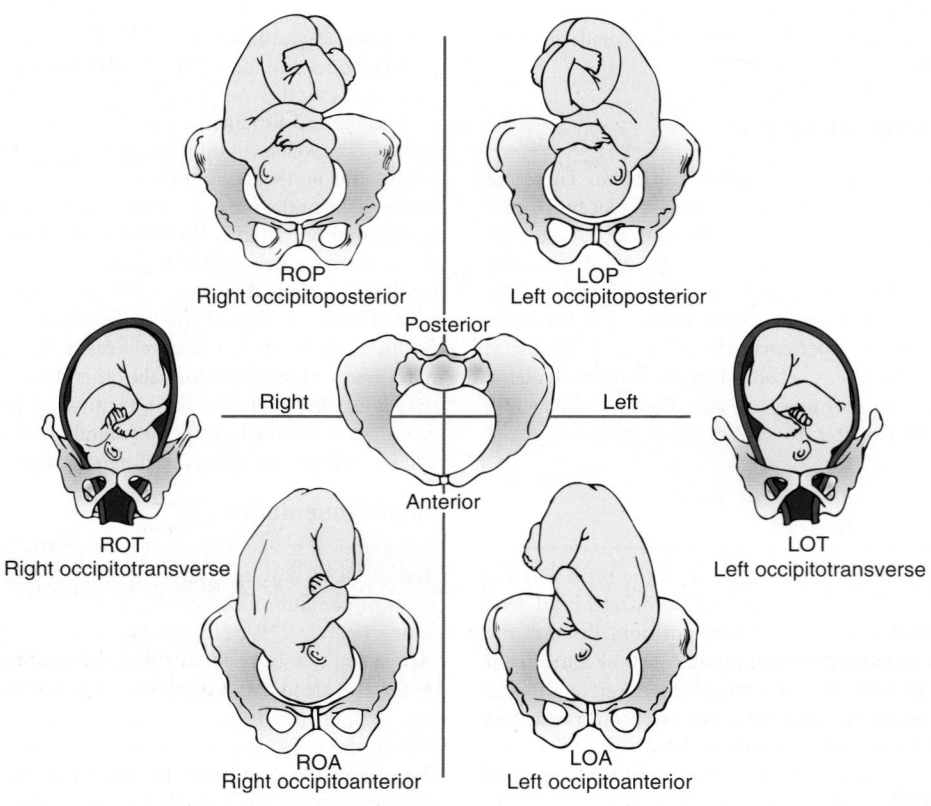

Lie: Longitudinal or vertical
Presentation: Vertex
Reference point: Occiput
Attitude: General flexion

FIG 13.2 Examples of fetal vertex (occiput) presentations in relation to front, back, or side of maternal pelvis.

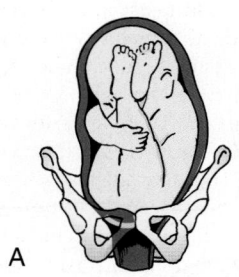

A
Frank breech

Lie: Longitudinal or vertical
Presentation: Breech (incomplete)
Presenting part: Sacrum
Attitude: Flexion, except for legs at knees

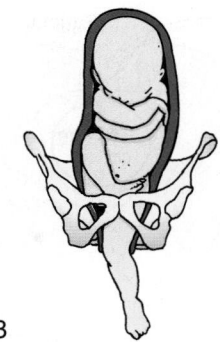

B
Single footling breech

Lie: Longitudinal or vertical
Presentation: Breech (incomplete)
Presenting part: Sacrum
Attitude: Flexion, except for one leg extended at hip and knee

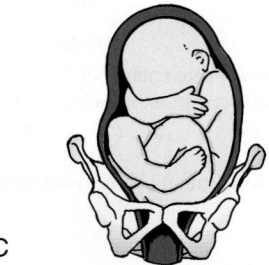

C
Complete breech

Lie: Longitudinal or vertical
Presentation: Breech (sacrum and feet presenting)
Presenting part: Sacrum (with feet)
Attitude: General flexion

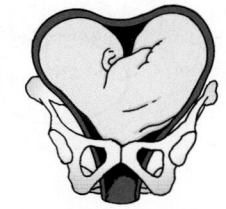

D
Shoulder presentation

Lie: Transverse or horizontal
Presentation: Shoulder
Presenting part: Scapula
Attitude: Flexion

FIG 13.3 Fetal presentations. **A–C,** Breech (sacral) presentation. **D,** Shoulder presentation.

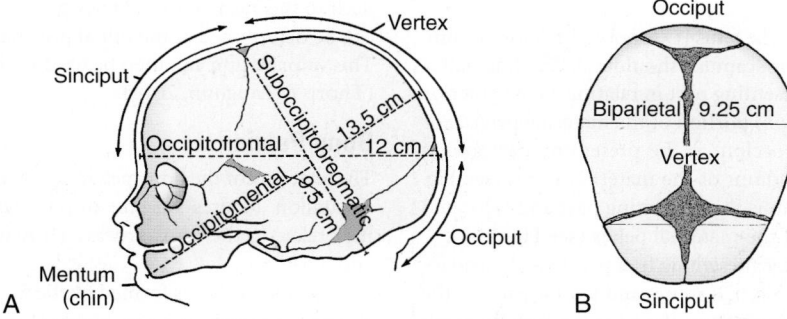

FIG 13.4 Diameters of fetal head at term. **A,** Cephalic presentations: occiput, vertex, and sinciput; and cephalic diameters: suboccipitobregmatic, occipitofrontal, and occipitomental. **B,** Biparietal diameter.

exceeds the limits of the maternal pelvis, leading to prolonged labor, forceps- or vacuum-assisted birth, or cesarean birth.

Certain critical diameters of the fetal head can be measured by ultrasound. The **biparietal diameter,** which is about 9.25 cm at term, is the largest transverse diameter and an important indicator of fetal head size (Fig. 13.4, *B*). In a well-flexed cephalic presentation, the biparietal diameter is the widest part of the head entering the pelvic inlet. Of the several anteroposterior diameters, the smallest and most critical one is the suboccipitobregmatic diameter (about 9.5 cm at term). When the head is in complete flexion, this diameter allows the fetal head to pass through the true pelvis easily (see Fig. 13.4, *A;* Fig. 13.5,

A). As the head is more extended, the anteroposterior diameter widens, and the head may not be able to enter the true pelvis (see Fig. 13.5).

Fetal Position

The presentation, or presenting part, indicates that portion of the fetus that overlies the pelvic inlet. **Position** is the relationship of a reference point on the presenting part (occiput, sacrum, mentum [chin] or sinciput [deflexed vertex]) to the four quadrants of the mother's pelvis (see Fig. 13.2). Position is denoted by a three-letter abbreviation. The first letter of the abbreviation denotes the location of the presenting part in the right (R) or left (L) side of the mother's pelvis. The middle letter stands

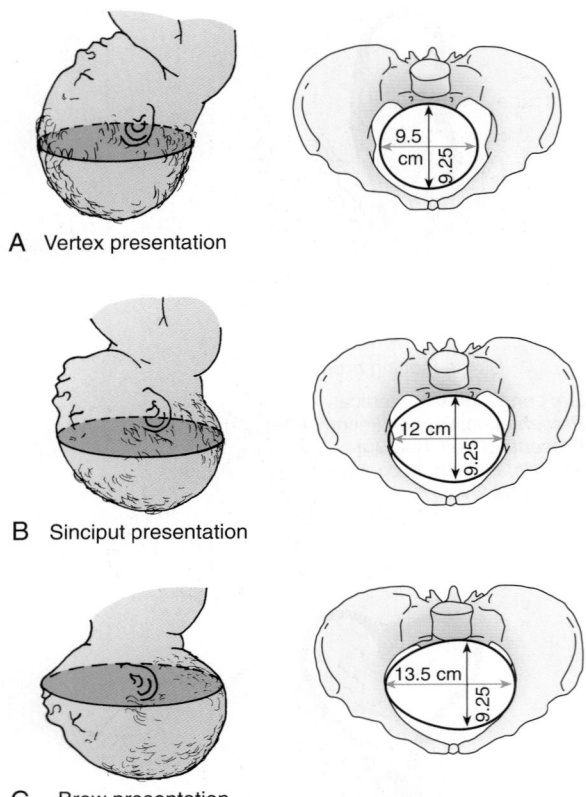

A Vertex presentation

B Sinciput presentation

C Brow presentation

FIG 13.5 Head entering pelvis. Biparietal diameter is indicated with shading (9.25 cm). **A,** Suboccipitobregmatic diameter: complete flexion of head on chest so smallest diameter enters. **B,** Occipitofrontal diameter: moderate extension (military attitude) so large diameter enters. **C,** Occipitomental diameter: marked extension (deflection) so largest diameter, which is too large to permit head to enter pelvis, is presenting.

for the specific presenting part of the fetus (*O* for occiput, *S* for sacrum, *M* for mentum [chin], and *Sc* for scapula [shoulder]). The final letter stands for the location of the presenting part in relation to the anterior *(A)*, posterior *(P)*, or transverse *(T)* portion of the maternal pelvis. For example, ROA means that the occiput is the presenting part and is located in the right anterior quadrant of the maternal pelvis (see Fig. 13.2). LSP means that the sacrum is the presenting part and is located in the left posterior quadrant of the maternal pelvis (see Fig. 13.3).

Station is the relationship of the presenting fetal part to an imaginary line drawn between the maternal ischial spines and is a measure of the degree of descent of the presenting part of the fetus through the birth canal. The placement of the presenting part is measured in centimeters above or below the ischial spines (Fig. 13.6). For example, when the lowermost portion of the presenting part is 1 cm above the spines, it is noted as being minus (−) 1. At the level of the spines, the station is referred to as 0 (zero). When the presenting part is 1 cm below the spines, the station is said to be plus (+) 1. Birth is imminent when the presenting part is at +4 to +5 cm. The station of the presenting part should be determined when labor begins so the rate of descent of the fetus during labor can be assessed accurately.

Engagement is the term used to indicate that the largest transverse diameter of the presenting part (usually the biparietal diameter) has passed through the maternal pelvic brim or inlet into the true pelvis and usually corresponds to station 0. It often occurs in the weeks just before labor begins in nulliparas and may occur before or during labor

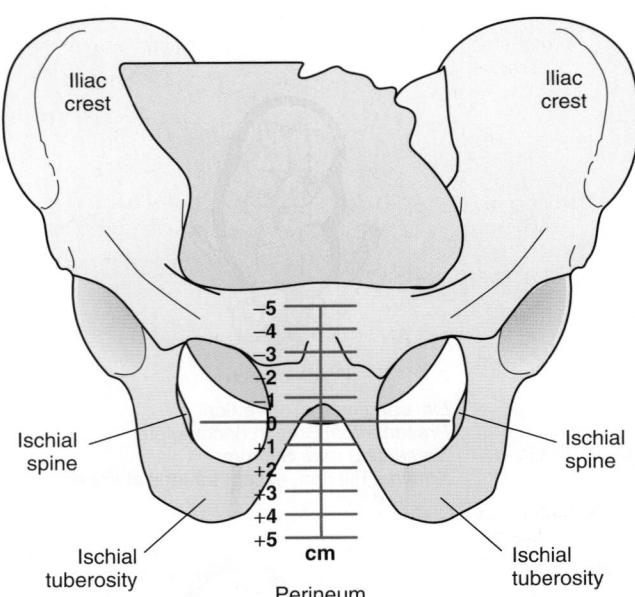

FIG 13.6 Stations of presenting part, or degree of descent. Lowermost portion of presenting part is at level of ischial spines, station 0.

in multiparas. Engagement can be determined by abdominal or vaginal examination.

PASSAGEWAY

The passageway, or birth canal, is composed of the mother's rigid bony pelvis and the soft tissues of the cervix, the pelvic floor, the vagina, and the introitus (the external opening to the vagina). Although the soft tissues, particularly the muscular layers of the pelvic floor, contribute to vaginal birth of the fetus, the maternal pelvis plays a far greater role in the labor process because the fetus must successfully accommodate itself to this relatively rigid passageway. The size and shape of the pelvis can be determined at the initial prenatal visit or on admission in labor. This information can then be used in the assessment of labor progress (Thorp & Laughon, 2014).

Bony Pelvis

The anatomy of the bony pelvis is described in Chapter 3. The following discussion focuses on the importance of pelvic configurations as they relate to the labor process. (It may be helpful to refer to Figs. 3.4 and 3.5.)

The bony pelvis is formed by the fusion of the ilium, ischium, pubis, and sacral bones. The four pelvic joints are the symphysis pubis, the right and left sacroiliac joints (Fig. 13.7, *A*), and the sacrococcygeal joint (Fig. 13.7, *B*). The bony pelvis is separated by the brim, or inlet, into two parts: the false and the true pelves. The false pelvis is the part above the brim and plays no part in childbearing. The true pelvis, the part involved in birth, is divided into three planes: the inlet, or brim; the midpelvis, or cavity; and the outlet.

The pelvic inlet, which is the upper border of the true pelvis, is formed anteriorly by the upper margins of the pubic bone, laterally by the iliopectineal lines along the innominate bones, and posteriorly by the anterior upper margin of the sacrum and the sacral promontory.

The pelvic cavity, or midpelvis, is a curved passage with a short anterior wall and a much longer concave posterior wall. It is bounded by the posterior aspect of the symphysis pubis, the ischium, a portion of the ilium, the sacrum, and the coccyx.

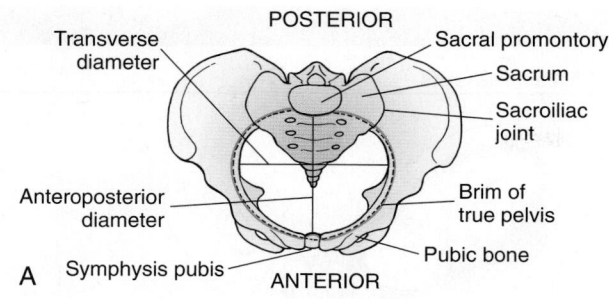

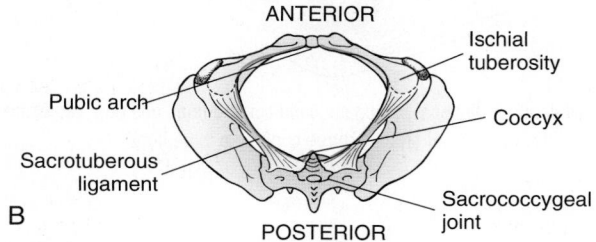

FIG 13.7 Female pelvis. **A,** Pelvic brim as viewed from above. **B,** Pelvic outlet from below, as seen by health care provider when the woman is lying supine.

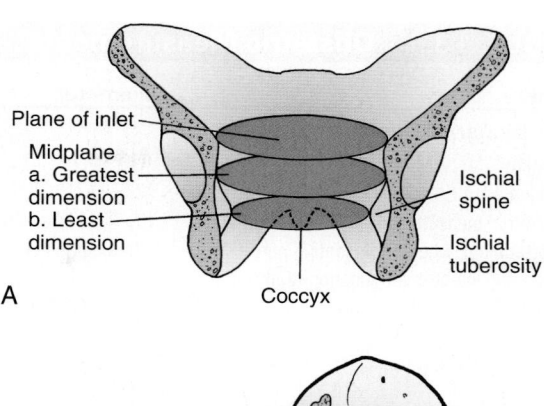

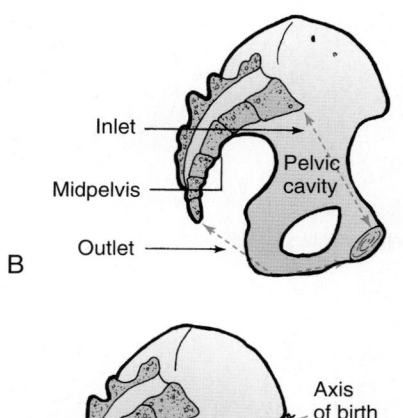

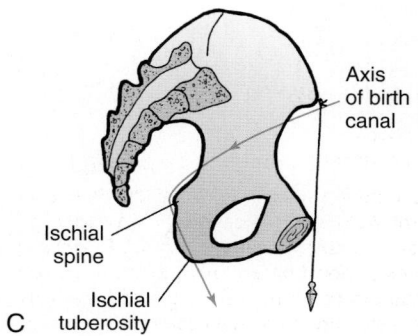

FIG 13.8 Pelvic cavity. **A,** Inlet and midplane. Outlet not shown. **B,** Cavity of true pelvis. **C,** Note curve of sacrum and axis of birth canal.

The pelvic outlet is the lower border of the true pelvis. Viewed from below it is ovoid; somewhat diamond shaped; and bounded by the pubic arch anteriorly, the ischial tuberosities laterally, and the tip of the coccyx posteriorly (see Fig. 13.7, *B*). In the latter part of pregnancy, the coccyx is movable (unless it has been previously fractured and has fused to the sacrum during healing).

The pelvic canal varies in size and shape at various levels. The diameters at the plane of the pelvic inlet, midpelvis, and outlet plus the axis of the birth canal (Fig. 13.8) determine whether vaginal birth is possible and the manner by which the fetus may pass down the birth canal.

The subpubic angle, which determines the type of pubic arch, together with the length of the pubic rami and the intertuberous diameter, is of great importance. Because the fetus must first pass beneath the pubic arch, a narrow subpubic angle is less accommodating than a rounded wide arch. The method of measurement of the subpubic arch is shown in Fig. 13.9. A summary of obstetric measurements is given in Table 13.1.

The four basic types of pelvis are classified as follows:
1. *Gynecoid* (the classic female type)
2. *Android* (resembling the male pelvis)
3. *Anthropoid* (oval shaped, with a wider anteroposterior diameter)
4. *Platypelloid* (the flat pelvis)

The gynecoid pelvis is the most common, with major gynecoid pelvic features present in 50% of all women. Anthropoid and android features are less common, and platypelloid pelvic features are the least common. Mixed types of pelves are more common than are pure types (Cunningham et al., 2014). Examples of pelvic variations and their effects on mode of birth are given in Table 13.2.

Assessment of the bony pelvis can be performed during the first prenatal evaluation and need not be repeated if the pelvis is of adequate size and suitable shape. In the third trimester of pregnancy, the examination of the bony pelvis may be more thorough, and the results more accurate because there is relaxation and increased mobility of the pelvic joints and ligaments as a result of hormonal influences. Widening of the joint of the symphysis pubis and the resulting instability may cause pain in any or all of the pelvic joints.

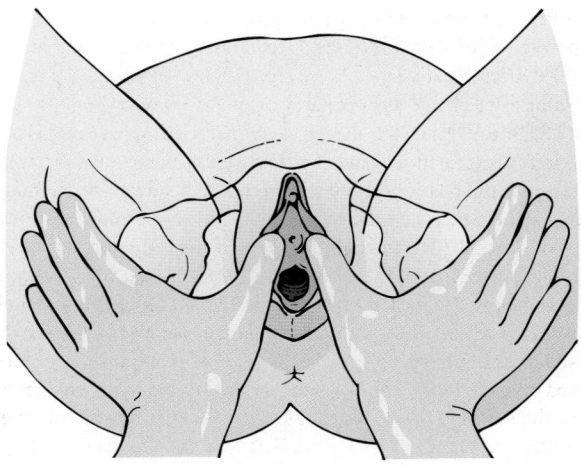

FIG 13.9 Estimation of angle of subpubic arch. With both thumbs, examiner externally traces descending rami down to tuberosities. (From Barkauskas, V.H., Baumann, L.C., & Darling-Fisher, C.S. [2002]. *Health and physical assessment*, [3rd. ed.]. St. Louis, MO: Mosby.)

TABLE 13.1   Obstetric Measurements

Plane	Diameter	Measurements
Inlet (Superior Strait)		
Conjugates		
Diagonal	12.5–13 cm	
Obstetric: measurement that determines whether presenting part can engage or enter superior strait	1.5–2 cm less than diagonal (radiographic)	
True (vera) (anteroposterior)	≥11 cm (12.5) (radiographic)	

Length of diagonal conjugate (solid colored line), obstetric conjugate (broken colored line), and true conjugate (blue line)*

Midplane		
Transverse diameter (interspinous diameter)	10.5 cm	
The midplane of the pelvis normally is its largest plane and the one of greatest diameter		

Measurement of interspinous diameter*

Outlet		
Transverse diameter (intertuberous diameter) (biischial)	≥8 cm	
The outlet presents the smallest plane of the pelvic canal		

Use of Thom's pelvimeter to measure intertuberous diameter*

*From Seidel, H.M., Ball, J.W., Dains, J.E., et al. (2011). *Mosby's guide to physical examination*, (7th ed.). St. Louis, MO: Mosby.

TABLE 13.2   Comparison of Pelvic Types

	Gynecoid (50% of Women)	Android (23% of Women)	Anthropoid (24% of Women)	Platypelloid (3% of Women)
Brim	Slightly ovoid or transversely rounded	Heart shaped, angulated	Oval, wider anteroposteriorly	Flattened anteroposteriorly, wide transversely
Shape	◯ Round	♡ Heart	〇 Oval	⬭ Flat
Depth	Moderate	Deep	Deep	Shallow
Side walls	Straight	Convergent	Straight	Straight
Ischial spines	Blunt, somewhat widely separated	Prominent, narrow interspinous diameter	Prominent, often with narrow interspinous diameter	Blunted, widely separated
Sacrum	Deep, curved	Slightly curved, terminal portion often beaked	Slightly curved	Slightly curved
Subpubic arch	Wide	Narrow	Narrow	Wide
Effects on labor/birth*	Classic female shape; associated with birth in the OA position	In theory, has an increased risk of CPD	More often associated with birth in the OP position	In theory, increases the likelihood of a transverse arrest

CPD, Cephalopelvic disproportion; OA, occipitoanterior; OP, occipitoposterior.
*Data from Kilpatrick, S., & Garrison, E. (2017). Normal labor and delivery. In Gabbe, S.G., Niebyl, J.R., Simpson, J.L., et al. (Eds.), *Obstetrics: Normal and problem pregnancies* (7th ed.). Philadelphia, PA: Elsevier.

Because the examiner does not have direct access to the bony structures and because the bones are covered with varying amounts of soft tissue, estimates of size and shape are approximate. Precise bony pelvis measurements can be determined by use of radiographic computed tomography (CT), or magnetic resonance imaging (MRI). However, these procedures are rarely performed for this purpose because evidence is lacking that they are beneficial. Indeed, some data show possible harm associated with their use because of an increase in cesarean birth rates (Kilpatrick & Garrison, 2017). Even precise measurements do not always predict a woman's ability to give birth vaginally because of the many ways the fetus can negotiate the pelvis and the accommodation of maternal soft tissues. Therefore, pelvimetry results rarely contraindicate a trial of labor.

Soft Tissues

The soft tissues of the passageway include the distensible lower uterine segment, the cervix, the pelvic floor muscles, the vagina, and the introitus. Before labor begins, the uterus is composed of the uterine body (corpus) and the cervix (neck). After labor has begun, uterine contractions cause the uterine body to have a thick and muscular upper segment and a thin-walled, passive, muscular lower segment. A *physiologic retraction ring* separates the two segments (Fig. 13.10). The lower uterine segment gradually distends to accommodate the intrauterine contents as the wall of the upper segment thickens and its accommodating capacity is reduced. The contractions of the uterine body thus exert downward pressure on the fetus, pushing it against the cervix.

The cervix effaces (thins) and dilates (opens) sufficiently to allow the first fetal portion to descend into the vagina. As the fetus descends, the cervix is actually drawn upward and over this first portion.

The pelvic floor is a muscular layer that separates the pelvic cavity above from the perineal space below. This structure helps the fetus rotate anteriorly as it passes through the birth canal. As noted earlier, the soft tissues of the vagina develop throughout pregnancy until at term the vagina can dilate to accommodate the fetus and permit its passage to the external world.

POWERS

Involuntary and voluntary powers combine to expel the fetus and placenta from the uterus. Involuntary uterine contractions, called the *primary powers*, signal the beginning of labor. Once the cervix has dilated, voluntary bearing-down efforts by the woman, called the *secondary powers*, augment the force of the involuntary contractions.

Primary Powers

The involuntary contractions originate at certain pacemaker points in the thickened muscle layers of the upper uterine segment. From the pacemaker points, contractions move downward over the uterus in waves, separated by short rest periods. Terms used to describe these involuntary contractions include *frequency* (the time from the beginning of one contraction to the beginning of the next), *duration* (length of contraction), and *intensity* (strength of contraction at its peak).

The primary powers are responsible for the effacement and dilation of the cervix and descent of the fetus. Effacement of the cervix means the shortening and thinning of the cervix during the first stage of labor. The cervix, normally 2 to 3 cm long and approximately 1 cm thick, is obliterated or "taken up" by a shortening of the uterine muscle bundles during the thinning of the lower uterine segment that occurs in advancing labor. Only a thin edge of the cervix can be palpated when effacement is complete. Effacement generally progresses significantly in first-time term pregnancy before more than slight dilation occurs. In subsequent pregnancies, effacement and dilation of the cervix tend to progress together. Degree of effacement is expressed in percentages, from 0% to 100% (e.g., a cervix is 50% effaced) (Fig. 13.11, A–C).

Dilation of the cervix is the enlargement or widening of the cervical opening and the cervical canal that occurs once labor has begun. The diameter of the cervix increases from less than 1 cm to full dilation (approximately 10 cm) to allow birth of a term fetus. When the cervix is fully dilated (and completely retracted), it can no longer be palpated (see Fig. 13.11, D). Full cervical dilation marks the end of the first stage of labor.

Dilation of the cervix occurs by the drawing upward of the musculofibrous components of the cervix caused by strong uterine contractions. Pressure exerted by the amniotic fluid while the membranes are intact or by the force applied by the presenting part can promote cervical dilation. Scarring of the cervix as a result of prior infection or surgery may slow cervical dilation.

In the first and second stages of labor, increased intrauterine pressure caused by contractions exerts pressure on the descending fetus and the cervix. When the presenting part of the fetus reaches the perineal floor,

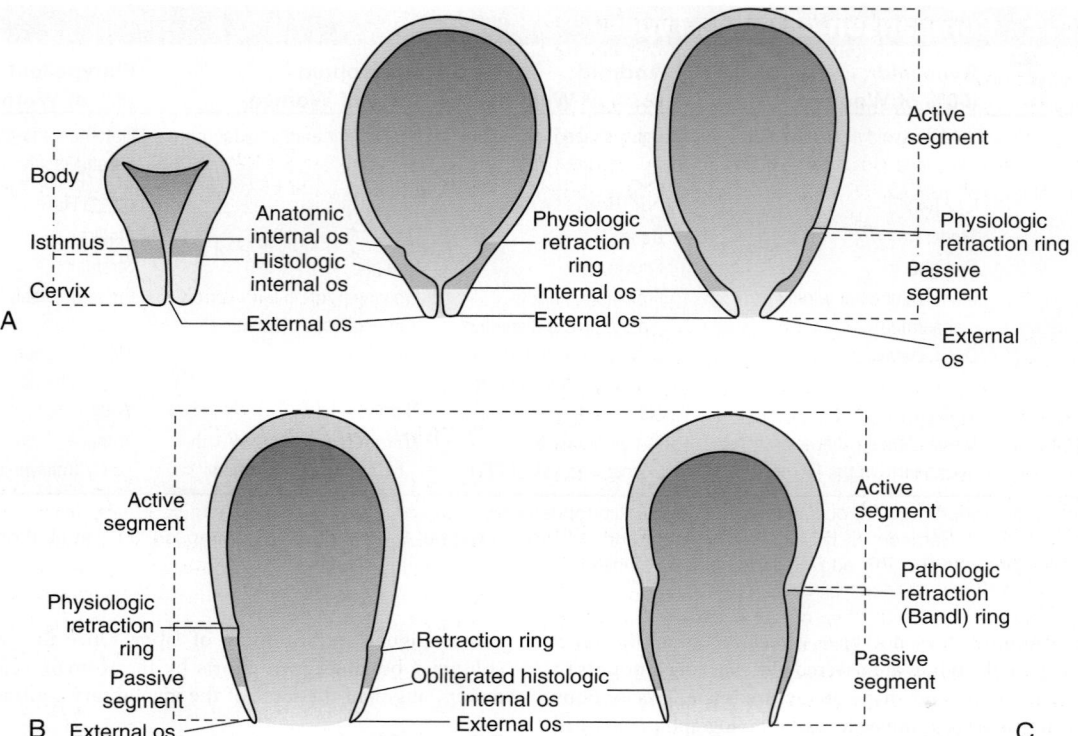

FIG 13.10 Uterus in normal labor **A,** in early first stage; and **B,** in second stage. Passive segment is derived from lower uterine segment (isthmus) and cervix, and physiologic retraction ring is derived from anatomic internal os. **C,** Uterus in abnormal labor in second-stage dystocia. Pathologic retraction (Bandl) ring that forms under abnormal conditions develops from physiologic ring.

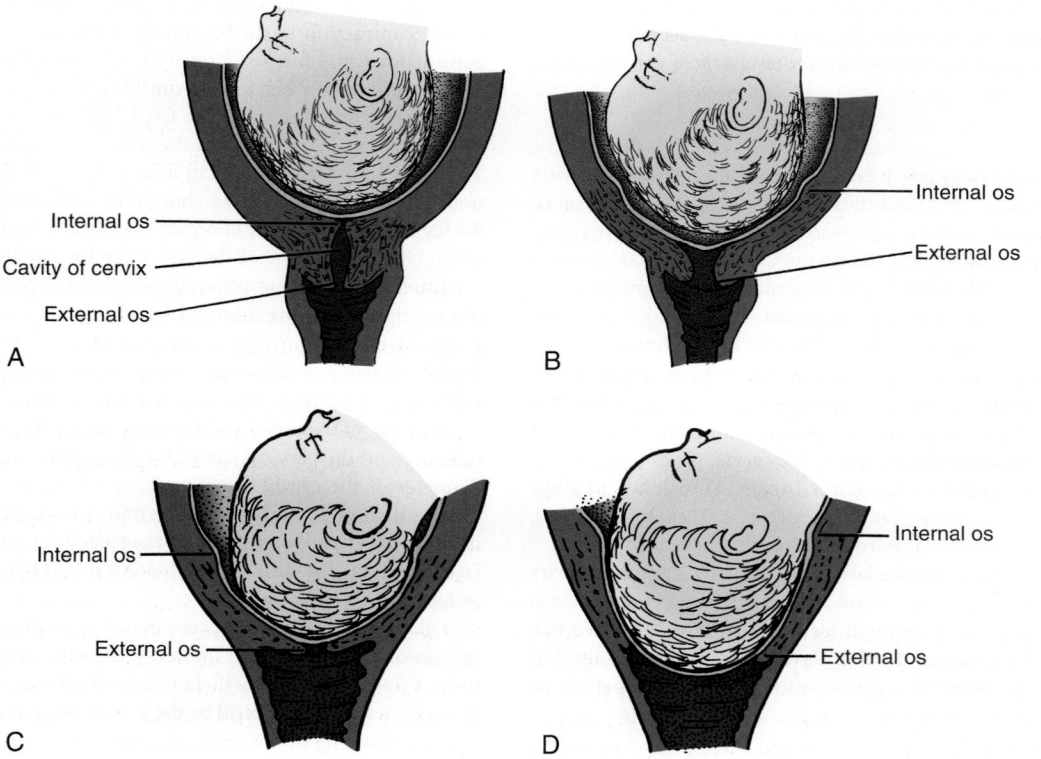

FIG 13.11 Cervical effacement and dilation. Note how cervix is drawn up around presenting part (internal os). Membranes are intact, and head is not well applied to cervix. **A,** Before labor. **B,** Early effacement. **C,** Complete effacement (100%). Head is well applied to cervix. **D,** Complete dilation (10 cm). Cranial bones overlap somewhat, and membranes are still intact.

mechanical stretching of the cervix occurs. Stretch receptors in the posterior vagina cause release of endogenous oxytocin that triggers the maternal urge to bear down, or the *Ferguson reflex.*

Uterine contractions are usually independent of external forces. For example, laboring women who are paralyzed because of spinal cord lesions above the twelfth thoracic vertebra have normal but painless uterine contractions. In addition, use of epidural analgesia during labor does not decrease the frequency or intensity of contractions (Cunningham et al. 2014).

Secondary Powers

As soon as the presenting part reaches the pelvic floor, the contractions change in character and become expulsive. The laboring woman experiences an involuntary urge to push. She uses secondary powers (bearing-down efforts) to aid in expulsion of the fetus as she contracts her diaphragm and abdominal muscles and pushes. These bearing-down efforts result in increased intraabdominal pressure that compresses the uterus on all sides and adds to the power of the expulsive forces.

The secondary powers have no effect on cervical dilation, but they are of considerable importance in the expulsion of the infant from the uterus and vagina after the cervix is fully dilated. When and how a woman pushes in the second stage of labor are much-debated topics. Continued study is needed to determine the effectiveness and appropriateness of strategies used by nurses to teach pushing techniques, the suitability and effectiveness of various pushing techniques related to abnormal fetal heart patterns, and the standards for length of pushing in terms of maternal and fetal outcomes. See Chapter 16 for further discussion regarding pushing during the second stage of labor.

POSITION OF THE LABORING WOMAN

Position affects the woman's anatomic and physiologic adaptations to labor. Frequent changes in position relieve fatigue, increase comfort, and improve circulation. Therefore a laboring woman should be encouraged to find positions that are most comfortable to her.

Positioning for second-stage labor may be determined by the woman's preference, but choices are limited by her condition or that of the fetus, the environment, and the health care provider's confidence in assisting in a birth in a specific position. See Chapter 16 for further discussion of positioning during labor and birth.

PROCESS OF LABOR

The term *labor* refers to the process of moving the fetus, placenta, and membranes out of the uterus and through the birth canal. Various changes take place in the woman's reproductive system in the days and weeks before labor begins. Labor itself can be discussed in terms of the mechanisms involved in the process and the stages through which the woman moves.

SIGNS PRECEDING LABOR

In first-time pregnancies, the uterus sinks downward and forward about 2 weeks before term, when the presenting part of the fetus (usually the fetal head) descends into the true pelvis. This settling is called *lightening,* or *dropping,* and usually happens gradually. After lightening, women feel less pressure below the ribcage and breathe more easily, but usually more bladder pressure results from this shift. Consequently, a return of urinary frequency occurs. In a multiparous woman, lightening may not take place until after uterine contractions are established and true labor is in progress.

BOX 13.1   Signs Preceding Labor

- Lightening
- Return of urinary frequency
- Backache
- Stronger Braxton Hicks contractions
- Weight loss of 0.5 to 1.5 kg (approximately 1 to 3½ pounds)
- Surge of energy
- Increased vaginal discharge; bloody show
- Cervical ripening
- Possible rupture of membranes

CLINICAL REASONING CASE STUDY
"I Think I'm in Labor"

Erica is a 15-year-old G 1 P 0 at 39 weeks of gestation. She presents by ambulance to the triage area in your labor and birth unit and announces, "I'm here to have my baby. I think I'm in labor." Erica reports that she saw a thick brownish red vaginal discharge several days ago and noticed bright red vaginal spotting when wiping after peeing earlier today. She states that she has lower abdominal cramping ("It feels like the cramps I have with my periods") but denies leakage of vaginal fluid. Erica also reports active fetal movement. She reports that her current pain level is 8 on a scale of 1 to 10, while alternating between texting on her phone and chatting with her mother, who accompanied her to the hospital.

1. Evidence—Is there sufficient evidence at this time to draw a conclusion about whether Erica is in labor?
2. Assumptions—Describe an underlying assumption about each of the following issues:
   a. Characteristics of false labor
   b. Indications of true labor
   c. Basic teaching for Erica and her mother at this time
   d. Criteria necessary for discharging Erica from the labor and birth unit
3. What implications and priorities for nursing care can be drawn at this time?
4. Does the evidence objectively support your conclusion?
5. Interprofessional care—Describe the roles/responsibilities of health care professionals who would potentially be involved in Erica's care.

The woman may complain of persistent low backache and sacroiliac distress as a result of relaxation of the pelvic joints. She may identify strong, frequent, but irregular uterine (Braxton Hicks) contractions.

The vaginal mucus becomes more profuse in response to the extreme congestion of the vaginal mucous membranes. Brownish or blood-tinged cervical mucus may be passed (*bloody show*). The cervix becomes soft (ripens) and partially effaced and may begin to dilate. The membranes may rupture spontaneously.

Other phenomena are common in the days preceding labor: (1) weight loss of 0.5 to 1.5 kg (approximately 1 to 3½ pounds) caused by water loss resulting from electrolyte shifts that in turn are produced by changes in estrogen and progesterone levels; and (2) a surge of energy. Women speak of having a burst of energy that they often use to clean the house and put everything in order. Less commonly, some women have diarrhea, nausea, vomiting, and indigestion. Box 13.1 lists signs that may precede labor (see Clinical Reasoning Case Study).

ONSET OF LABOR

The onset of true labor cannot be ascribed to a single cause. Many factors, including changes in the maternal uterus, cervix, and pituitary gland, are involved. Hormones produced by the normal fetal hypothalamus, pituitary gland, and adrenal cortex probably contribute to the onset of labor. Progressive uterine distention and increasing intrauterine pressure seem to be associated with increasing myometrial irritability. This is a result of increased concentrations of estrogen, oxytocin, and prostaglandins and decreasing progesterone levels. The mutually coordinated effects of these factors result in the occurrence of strong, regular, rhythmic uterine contractions (Blackburn, 2013; Kilpatrick & Garrison, 2017). The outcome of these factors working together is normally the birth of the fetus and the expulsion of the placenta.

STAGES OF LABOR

The course of labor at or near term gestation in a woman without complications and a fetus in vertex presentation consists of: (1) regular progression of uterine contractions, (2) effacement and progressive dilation of the cervix, and (3) progress in descent of the presenting part. Four stages of labor are recognized; an overview is discussed here. These stages are discussed in greater detail, along with nursing care for the laboring woman and family, in Chapter 16.

The *first stage of labor* is considered to last from the onset of regular uterine contractions to full dilation of the cervix. Commonly the onset of labor is difficult to establish because the woman may be admitted to the labor unit just before birth and the beginning of labor may be only an estimate. The first stage is much longer than the second and third combined. However, great variability is the rule, depending on the factors discussed previously in this chapter. The first stage of labor has traditionally been divided into three phases: a latent (early) phase, an active phase, and a transition phase. In women who labor with epidural anesthesia, however, a separate transition phase may not always be identified based on maternal physical sensations and behavior (Simpson & O'Brien-Abel, 2014). Therefore, the first stage of labor is now divided into only two phases, latent (early) and active (Kilpatrick & Garrison, 2017). During the latent phase, there is more progress in effacement of the cervix and little increase in descent. During the active phase, there is more rapid dilation of the cervix and increased rate of descent of the presenting part.

The *second stage of labor* lasts from the time the cervix is fully dilated to the birth of the fetus. It is composed of two phases: the latent (passive fetal descent) phase and the active pushing phase. During the latent phase, the fetus continues to descend passively through the birth canal and rotate to an anterior position as a result of ongoing uterine contractions. The urge to bear down during this phase is not strong, and some women do not experience it at all. During the active pushing phase, the woman has strong urges to bear down as the presenting part of the fetus descends and presses on the stretch receptors of the pelvic floor.

The *third stage of labor* lasts from the birth of the fetus until the placenta is delivered. The placenta normally separates with the third or fourth strong uterine contraction after the infant has been born. After it has separated, the placenta can be delivered with the next uterine contraction.

The *fourth stage of labor* begins with the delivery of the placenta and includes at least the first 2 hours after birth. During this stage, the woman begins to recover physically from birth, so it is an important time to observe for complications, such as abnormal bleeding (see Chapter 21).

MECHANISM OF LABOR

As already discussed, the female pelvis has varied contours and diameters at different levels, and the presenting part of the passenger is large in proportion to the passage. Therefore for vaginal birth to occur the fetus must adapt to the birth canal during the descent. The turns and other adjustments necessary in the human birth process are termed the *mechanism of labor* (Fig. 13.12). The seven cardinal movements of the mechanism of labor that occur in a vertex presentation are *engagement, descent, flexion, internal rotation, extension, external rotation (restitution),* and finally *birth by expulsion.* Although these movements are discussed separately, in actuality a combination of movements occurs simultaneously. For example, engagement involves both descent and flexion.

Engagement

When the biparietal diameter of the head passes the pelvic inlet, the head is said to be engaged in the pelvic inlet (see Fig. 13.12, *A).* In most nulliparous pregnancies, this occurs before the onset of active labor because the firmer abdominal muscles direct the presenting part into the pelvis. In multiparous pregnancies in which the abdominal musculature is more relaxed, the head often remains freely movable above the pelvic brim until labor is established.

Asynclitism

The head usually engages in the pelvis in a synclitic position (i.e., one that is parallel to the anteroposterior plane of the pelvis). Frequently *asynclitism* occurs (the head is deflected anteriorly or posteriorly in the pelvis), which can facilitate descent because the head is being positioned to accommodate to the pelvic cavity (Fig. 13.13). Extreme asynclitism can cause cephalopelvic disproportion, even in a normal-size pelvis, because the head is positioned so it cannot descend (see Chapter 17).

Descent

Descent refers to the progress of the presenting part through the pelvis. It depends on at least four forces: (1) pressure exerted by the amniotic fluid, (2) direct pressure exerted by the contracting fundus on the fetus, (3) force of the contraction of the maternal diaphragm and abdominal muscles in the second stage of labor, and (4) extension and straightening of the fetal body. The effects of these forces are modified by the size and shape of the maternal pelvic planes and the size of the fetal head and its capacity to mold.

The degree of descent is measured by the station of the presenting part (see Fig. 13.6). As mentioned, little descent occurs during the latent phase of the first stage of labor. Descent accelerates in the active phase when the cervix has dilated to 5 to 6 cm. It is especially apparent when the membranes have ruptured.

During first-time labor and birth, descent is usually slow but steady; in subsequent pregnancies, descent may be rapid. Progress in descent of the presenting part is assessed by abdominal palpation and vaginal examination until the presenting part can be seen at the introitus (see Chapter 16).

Flexion

As soon as the descending head meets resistance from the cervix, pelvic wall, or pelvic floor, it normally flexes so the chin is brought into closer contact with the fetal chest (see Fig. 13.12, *B).* Flexion permits the smaller suboccipitobregmatic diameter (9.5 cm) rather than the larger diameters to present to the outlet.

Internal Rotation

The maternal pelvic inlet is widest in the transverse diameter; therefore the fetal head passes the inlet into the true pelvis in the occipitotransverse position. The outlet is widest in the anteroposterior diameter; for the fetus to exit, the head must rotate. Internal rotation begins at the level of the ischial spines but is not completed until the presenting part reaches the lower pelvis. As the occiput rotates anteriorly, the face rotates

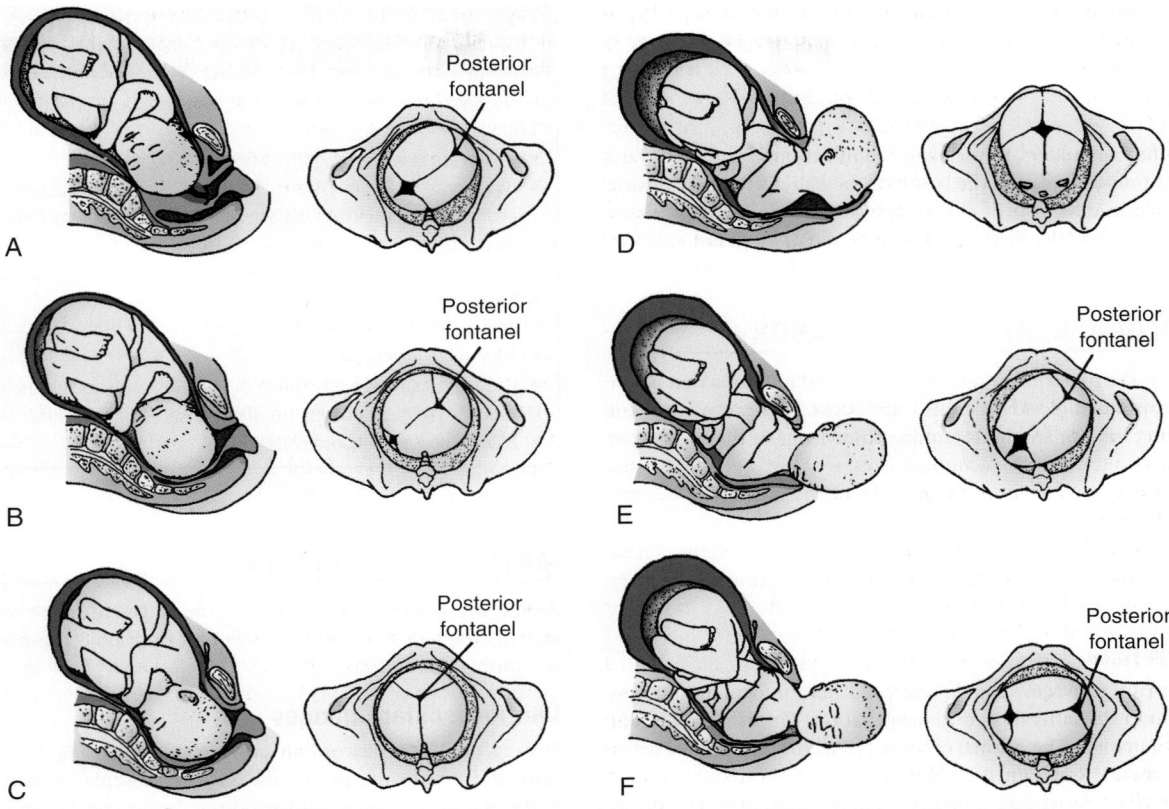

FIG 13.12 Cardinal movements of the mechanism of labor. Left occipitoanterior (LOA) position. Pelvic figures show position of fetal head as seen by birth attendant. **A,** Engagement and descent. **B,** Flexion. **C,** Internal rotation to occipitoanterior (OA) position. **D,** Extension. **E,** External rotation beginning (restitution). **F,** External rotation.

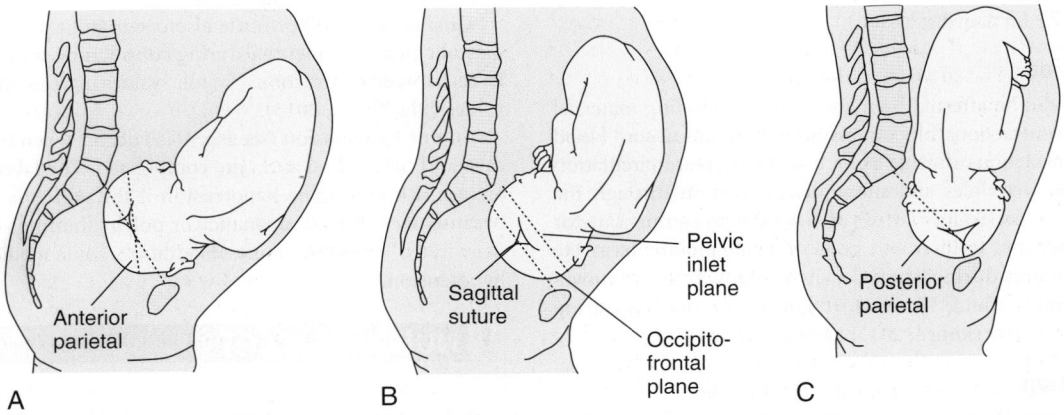

FIG 13.13 Synclitism and asynclitism. **A,** Anterior asynclitism. **B,** Normal synclitism. **C,** Posterior asynclitism.

posteriorly. With each contraction, the fetal head is guided by the bony pelvis and the muscles of the pelvic floor. Eventually the occiput will be in the midline beneath the pubic arch. The head is almost always rotated by the time it reaches the pelvic floor (see Fig. 13.12, *C*). Both the levator ani muscles and the bony pelvis are important for achieving anterior rotation. A previous childbirth injury or regional anesthesia may compromise the function of the levator sling.

Extension

When the fetal head reaches the perineum for birth, it is deflected anteriorly by the perineum. The occiput passes under the lower border of the symphysis pubis first, and the head emerges by extension: first the occiput, then the face, and finally the chin (see Fig. 13.12, *D*).

Restitution and External Rotation

After the head is born, it rotates briefly to the position it occupied when it was engaged in the inlet. This movement is referred to as *restitution* (see Fig. 13.12, *E*). The 45-degree turn realigns the infant's head with her or his back and shoulders. The head can then be seen to rotate further. This external rotation occurs as the shoulders engage and descend in maneuvers similar to those of the head (see Fig. 13.12, *F*). As noted, the anterior shoulder descends first. When it reaches the outlet, it rotates to the midline and is delivered from under the pubic arch. The posterior shoulder is guided over the perineum until it is free of the vaginal introitus.

Expulsion

After birth of the shoulders, the head and shoulders are lifted up toward the mother's pubic bone, and the trunk of the baby is born by flexing it laterally in the direction of the symphysis pubis. When the baby has emerged completely, birth is complete, and the second stage of labor ends.

PHYSIOLOGIC ADAPTATION TO LABOR

In addition to the maternal and fetal anatomic adaptations that occur during birth, physiologic adaptations must occur. Accurate assessment of the laboring woman and fetus requires knowledge of these expected adaptations.

Fetal Adaptation

Several important physiologic adaptations occur in the fetus. These changes occur in fetal heart rate (FHR), fetal circulation, respiratory movements, and other behaviors.

Fetal Heart Rate

FHR monitoring provides reliable and predictive information about the condition of the fetus related to oxygenation. The average FHR at term is 140 beats/min. The normal range is 110 to 160 beats/min. Earlier in gestation the FHR is higher, with an average of approximately 160 beats/min at 20 weeks of gestation. The rate decreases progressively as the maturing fetus reaches term. However, temporary accelerations and slight early decelerations of the FHR can be expected in response to spontaneous fetal movement, vaginal examination, fundal pressure, uterine contractions, abdominal palpation, and fetal head compression. Stresses to the uterofetoplacental unit result in characteristic FHR patterns (see Chapter 15 for further discussion).

Fetal Circulation

Fetal circulation can be affected by many factors, including maternal position, uterine contractions, blood pressure, and umbilical cord blood flow. Uterine contractions during labor tend to decrease circulation through the spiral arterioles and subsequent perfusion through the intervillous space. Most healthy fetuses are well able to compensate for this stress and exposure to increased pressure while moving passively through the birth canal during labor. Usually the umbilical cord moves freely in the amniotic fluid. However, it can be compressed during uterine contractions (Blackburn, 2013; Miller et al., 2017).

Fetal Respiration

Certain changes stimulate chemoreceptors in the aorta and carotid bodies to prepare the fetus for initiating respirations immediately after birth (Blackburn, 2013; Fraser, 2014). These changes include the following:

- Fetal lung fluid is cleared from the air passages as the infant passes through the birth canal during labor and (vaginal) birth. The process of labor itself also contributes to the absorption of some of the lung fluid before birth.
- Fetal oxygen pressure (Po_2) decreases.
- Arterial carbon dioxide pressure (Pco_2) increases.
- Arterial pH decreases.
- Bicarbonate level decreases.
- Fetal respiratory movements decrease during labor.

> ## BOX 13.2   Maternal Physiologic Changes During Labor
>
> - Cardiac output increases 10% to 15% in first stage; 30% to 50% in second stage.
> - Heart rate increases slightly in first and second stages.
> - Blood pressure (both systolic and diastolic) increases during contractions and returns to baseline levels between contractions. Systolic values increase more than diastolic values.
> - White blood cell (WBC) count increases.
> - Respiratory rate increases.
> - Temperature may be slightly elevated.
> - Proteinuria may occur.
> - Gastric motility and absorption of solid food are decreased; nausea and vomiting may occur during transition to second-stage labor.
> - Blood glucose level decreases.

MATERNAL ADAPTATION

As the woman progresses through the stages of labor, various body system adaptations cause her to exhibit both objective and subjective symptoms (Box 13.2).

Cardiovascular Changes

During each contraction, an average of 300 to 500 mL of blood is shunted from the uterus into the maternal vascular system. By the end of the first stage of labor, cardiac output during contractions is increased by 51% above baseline pregnancy values at term. Cardiac output peaks about 10 to 30 minutes after both vaginal and cesarean birth and returns to its prelabor baseline within the first postpartum hour. A drop in maternal heart rate accompanies this increase in cardiac output (Antony, Racusin, Aagaard, & Dildy, 2017).

Changes in blood pressure also occur. In general, both systolic and diastolic pressures increase during contractions and return to baseline levels between contractions. Systolic values increase more than diastolic values (Blackburn, 2013).

Supine hypotension (see Fig. 16.5) occurs when the ascending vena cava and descending aorta are compressed. The laboring woman is at greater risk for supine hypotension if the uterus is particularly large because of multifetal pregnancy or polyhydramnios or if she is obese, dehydrated, or hypovolemic. In addition, some medications can cause hypotension.

> ## ! NURSING ALERT
>
> The woman should be discouraged from using the Valsalva maneuver (holding one's breath and tightening abdominal muscles) for pushing during the second stage. This activity increases intrathoracic pressure, reduces venous return, and increases venous pressure. Cardiac output and blood pressure increase, and the pulse slows temporarily. During the Valsalva maneuver, fetal hypoxia may occur. The process is reversed when the woman takes a breath.

The white blood cell (WBC) count can increase (Blackburn, 2013). Although the mechanism leading to this increase in WBCs is unknown, it may be secondary to physical or emotional stress or tissue trauma. Labor is strenuous, and physical exercise alone can increase the WBC count.

Some peripheral vascular changes occur, perhaps in response to cervical dilation or compression of maternal vessels by the fetus passing through the birth canal. Flushed cheeks, hot or cold feet, and eversion of hemorrhoids may result.

Respiratory Changes

Increased physical activity with greater oxygen consumption is reflected in an increase in the respiratory rate. Hyperventilation may cause respiratory alkalosis (an increase in pH), hypoxia, and hypocapnia (decrease in carbon dioxide). In the unmedicated woman in the second stage, oxygen consumption almost doubles. Anxiety also increases oxygen consumption.

Renal Changes

During labor, spontaneous voiding may be difficult for various reasons such as tissue edema caused by pressure from the presenting part, discomfort, analgesia, and embarrassment. Proteinuria of 1+ is a normal finding because it can occur in response to the breakdown of muscle tissue from the physical work of labor.

Integumentary Changes

The integumentary system changes are evident, especially in the great distensibility (stretching) in the area of the vaginal introitus. The degree of distensibility varies with the individual. Despite this ability to stretch, even in the absence of episiotomy or lacerations, minute tears in the skin around the vaginal introitus do occur.

Musculoskeletal Changes

The musculoskeletal system is stressed during labor. Diaphoresis, fatigue, proteinuria (1+), and possibly an increased temperature accompany the marked increase in muscle activity. Backache and joint ache (unrelated to fetal position) occur as a result of increased joint laxity at term. The labor process itself and the woman's pointing her toes can cause leg cramps.

Neurologic Changes

Sensorial changes occur as the woman moves through the phases of the first stage of labor and from one stage to the next. Initially she may be euphoric. Euphoria gives way to increased seriousness, then to amnesia between contractions during the second stage, and finally to elation or fatigue after giving birth. Endogenous endorphins (morphine-like chemicals produced naturally by the body) raise the pain threshold and produce sedation. In addition, physiologic anesthesia of perineal tissues caused by pressure of the presenting part decreases perception of pain.

Gastrointestinal Changes

During labor, gastrointestinal motility and absorption of solid foods are decreased, and stomach-emptying time is slowed. Nausea and vomiting of undigested food eaten after the onset of labor are common. Nausea and belching also occur as a reflex response to full cervical dilation. The woman may state that diarrhea accompanied the onset of labor, or the nurse may palpate the presence of hard or impacted stool in the rectum.

Endocrine Changes

The onset of labor may be triggered by decreasing levels of progesterone and increasing levels of estrogen, prostaglandins, and oxytocin (Simpson & O'Brien-Abel, 2014). Metabolism increases, and blood glucose levels may decrease with the work of labor.

REFERENCES

Antony, K. M., Racusin, D. A., Aagaard, K., & Dildy, G. A. (2017). Maternal physiology. In S. G. Gabbe, J. R. Niebyl, J. L. Simpson, et al. (Eds.), *Obstetrics: Normal and problem pregnancies* (7th ed.). Philadelphia, PA: Elsevier.

Blackburn, S. (2013). *Maternal, fetal, and neonatal physiology: A clinical perspective* (4th ed.). Maryland Heights, MO: Saunders.

Cunningham, F., Leveno, K., Bloom, S., et al. (2014). *Williams obstetrics* (24th ed.). New York, NY: McGraw-Hill Education.

Fraser, D. (2014). Newborn adaptation to extrauterine life. In K. R. Simpson & P. Creehan (Eds.), *AWHONN's perinatal nursing* (4th ed.). Philadelphia, PA: Lippincott WiIlliams & Wilkins.

Kilpatrick, S., & Garrison, E. (2017). Normal labor and delivery. In S. G. Gabbe, J. R. Niebyl, J. L. Simpson, et al. (Eds.), *Obstetrics: Normal and problem pregnancies* (7th ed.). Philadelphia, PA: Elsevier.

Miller, L., Miller, D., & Cypher, R. (2017). *Mosby's pocket guide to fetal monitoring: A multidisciplinary approach* (8th ed.). St. Louis, MO: Elsevier.

Simpson, K., & O'Brien-Abel, N. (2014). Labor and birth. In K. R. Simpson & P. Creehan (Eds.), *AWHONN's perinatal nursing* (4th ed.). Philadelphia, PA: Lippincott.

Thorp, J. M., & Laughon, S. K. (2014). Clinical aspects of normal and abnormal labor. In R. K. Creasy, R. Resnik, J. D. Iams, et al. (Eds.), *Creasy and Resnik's maternal-fetal medicine: Principles and practice* (7th ed.). Philadelphia, PA: Saunders.

14

Maximizing Comfort for the Laboring Woman

Kitty Cashion

http://evolve.elsevier.com/Perry/maternal

Although labor and birth are considered to be natural processes, laboring women experience a significant amount of discomfort and pain, as well as a variety of other challenging sensations. Pain is a highly individualized phenomenon with sensory and emotional components. Even though most women experience discomfort or pain during labor and birth, it is the intensity of the discomfort that is unique to the individual. Pregnant women are generally concerned about the discomfort and pain they will experience during labor and birth and about how they will respond and cope. A variety of nonpharmacologic and pharmacologic methods are available to help the woman or the couple maximize her comfort during the labor process. The methods that are recommended for use by members of the interprofessional health care team depend on the situation, the availability, and the preferences of the woman and her health care providers. This chapter discusses sources of intrapartum discomfort and pain and factors that affect women's responses. It also describes nonpharmacologic and pharmacologic methods commonly used to maximize comfort during labor.

PAIN DURING LABOR AND BIRTH

NEUROLOGIC ORIGINS

The pain and discomfort of labor have two origins—visceral and somatic. During the first stage of labor, uterine contractions cause cervical dilation and effacement. Uterine ischemia (decreased blood flow and therefore local oxygen deficit) results from compression of the arteries supplying the myometrium during uterine contractions. Pain impulses during the first stage of labor are transmitted via the T10 to T12 and L1 spinal nerve segments and accessory lower thoracic and upper lumbar sympathetic nerves. These nerves originate in the uterine body and cervix (Blackburn, 2013).

The pain from distention of the lower uterine segment, stretching of cervical tissue as it effaces and dilates, pressure and traction on adjacent structures (e.g., uterine tubes, ovaries, ligaments) and nerves, and uterine ischemia during the first stage of labor is visceral pain. It is located over the lower portion of the abdomen. Referred pain occurs when pain that originates in the uterus radiates to the abdominal wall, lumbosacral area of the back, iliac areas, gluteal area, thighs, and lower back (Blackburn, 2013).

During most of the first stage of labor, the woman usually has discomfort only during contractions and is free from pain between contractions. Some women, especially those whose fetus is in a posterior position, experience continuous contraction-related lower back pain, even in the interval between contractions. As labor progresses and pain becomes more intense and persistent, women become fatigued and

discouraged, often experiencing difficulty coping with contractions (Blackburn, 2013; Burke, 2014).

During the second stage of labor, the woman has somatic pain, which is often described as intense, sharp, burning, and well localized. This pain results from the following:

- Distention and traction on the peritoneum and uterocervical supports during contractions
- Pressure against the bladder and rectum
- Stretching and distention of perineal tissues and the pelvic floor to allow passage of the fetus
- Lacerations of soft tissue (e.g., cervix, vagina, and perineum)

As women concentrate on the work of bearing down to give birth, they may report a decrease in pain intensity (Blackburn, 2013; Burke, 2014). Pain impulses during the second stage of labor are transmitted via the pudendal nerve through S2 to S4 spinal nerve segments and the parasympathetic system (Blackburn).

Pain experienced during the third stage of labor and the afterpains of the early postpartum period are uterine, similar to the pain experienced early in the first stage of labor. Areas of pain during labor are shown in Fig. 14.1.

PERCEPTION OF PAIN

The physiologic causes of pain during labor are the same for all women. However, pain is a subjective experience and is defined completely by the person who is experiencing it. Therefore, women vary in how they perceive and cope with labor pain. Factors that influence the way a woman deals with pain include her culture; age; previous personal experience with pain; parity; and the physical, psychologic, and emotional support available to her (Collins, 2017). The unique circumstances of every labor (e.g. previous surgical or diagnostic procedures that affect the responsiveness of the cervix to uterine contractions, medical and nursing procedures performed during labor, and length of labor) also influence the woman's experience of pain (Burke, 2014).

EXPRESSION OF PAIN

Pain is expressed by both physiologic and sensory or emotional (affective) reactions. During labor and birth, the pain or discomfort experienced gives rise to identifiable physiologic effects. Sympathetic nervous system activity is stimulated in response to anxiety, stress, and intensifying pain, resulting in increased catecholamine levels. Blood pressure and heart rate increase. Maternal respiratory patterns change in response to an increase in oxygen consumption. Hyperventilation, sometimes accompanied by respiratory alkalosis, can occur as pain intensifies.

fetal size, rapidity of fetal descent, maternal position, and maternal mobility during labor also affect a woman's perception of discomfort during labor and birth.

Beta (β)-endorphins are endogenous opioids secreted by the pituitary gland that act on the central and peripheral nervous systems to reduce pain. The level of β endorphins increases during pregnancy and birth in humans. β endorphins are associated with feelings of euphoria and analgesia. The pain threshold may rise as β endorphin levels increase, enabling women in labor to tolerate acute pain (Blackburn, 2013).

CULTURE

The population of pregnant women reflects the increasingly multicultural nature of society in the United States. As nurses care for women and families from a variety of cultural backgrounds, they must have knowledge and understanding of how culture mediates the response to pain. Although all women expect to experience at least some pain and discomfort during childbirth, it is their culture and religious belief system that determines how they will perceive, interpret, respond to, and manage the pain. Cultural influences may impose certain behavioral expectations regarding acceptable and unacceptable behavior when experiencing pain (Burke, 2014). For example, African-American and Puerto Rican women usually express their pain vocally, while Native Americans are often stoic (Callister, 2014).

An understanding of the beliefs, values, expectations, and practices of various cultures narrows the cultural gap and helps the nurse assess the laboring woman's pain experience more accurately. The nurse can then provide appropriate, culturally sensitive care by using pain relief measures that preserve the woman's sense of control and self-confidence (see Cultural Considerations box: Some Cultural Beliefs About Pain). Recognize that although a woman's behavior in response to pain may vary according to her cultural background, it may not accurately reflect the intensity of the pain she is experiencing. It is the nurse's role to assess the woman for the physiologic effects of pain, and listen to the words she uses to describe the sensory and affective qualities of her pain (see Community Focus box: Culture and Pain).

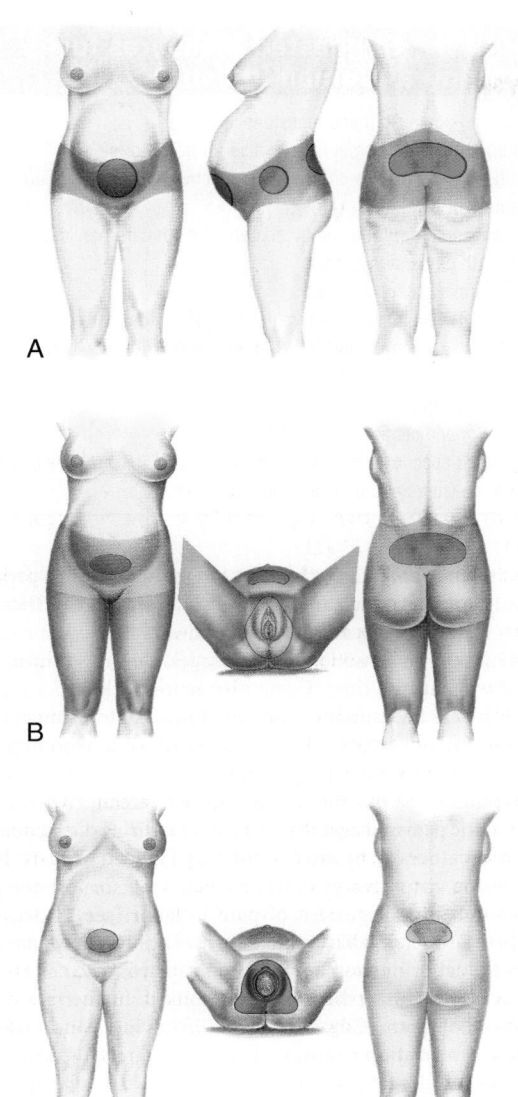

FIG 14.1 Pain during labor. **A,** Distribution of labor pain during first stage. **B,** Distribution of labor pain during active phase of first stage and early phase of second stage. **C,** Distribution of pain during late second-stage and actual birth. (*Gray areas* indicate mild discomfort; *light pink areas* indicate moderate discomfort; *dark red areas* indicate intense discomfort.)

Placental perfusion may decrease, and uterine activity may diminish, potentially prolonging labor and affecting fetal well-being (Burke, 2014).

Certain emotional (affective) expressions of pain often are seen. Such changes include increasing anxiety with lessened perceptual field, writhing, crying, groaning, gesturing (hand clenching and wringing), and excessive muscular excitability throughout the body.

FACTORS INFLUENCING PAIN RESPONSE

PHYSIOLOGIC FACTORS

A variety of physiologic factors can affect the intensity of childbirth pain. Fatigue can decrease a woman's ability to cope effectively with contraction pain (Burke, 2014). The interval and duration of contractions,

🌐 CULTURAL CONSIDERATIONS
Some Cultural Beliefs About Pain

The following examples demonstrate how women of different cultural backgrounds may react to pain. Because they are generalizations, the nurse must assess each woman experiencing pain related to childbirth.

- Chinese women may not exhibit reactions to pain, although exhibiting pain during childbirth is acceptable. They consider accepting something when it is first offered as impolite; therefore pain interventions must be offered more than once. Acupuncture may be used for pain relief.
- Arab or Middle Eastern women may be vocal in response to labor pain. They may prefer medication for pain relief.
- Japanese women may be stoic in response to labor pain, but they may request medication when pain becomes severe.
- Southeast Asian women may endure severe pain before requesting relief.
- Hispanic women may be stoic until late in labor, when they may become vocal and request pain relief.
- Native American women may use medications or remedies made from indigenous plants. They are often stoic in response to labor pain.
- African-American women may express pain openly. Use of medication for pain relief varies.

Culture and Pain

Talk to a woman and her partner from a culture different from your own who have experienced childbirth. Ask her to describe her reactions to pain, how she sought relief of pain, the atmosphere of the childbirth setting, and the attitudes of the health care providers. Ask the partner if he or she was present for the birth and to describe his/her role in the birth. How did the partner's culture influence his or her role and reaction to childbirth? How did the woman's culture influence her response to labor and the associated pain? What expressions of pain are "acceptable" in her culture? If the partner was present, how did he or she help her deal with the pain? What is the role of support persons in the labor process? Are the responses of the couple different from your responses to those same questions?

BOX 14.1   Suggested Measures for Supporting a Woman in Labor

- Provide companionship and reassurance.
- Offer positive reinforcement and praise for her efforts.
- Encourage participation in distracting activities and nonpharmacologic measures for comfort.
- Give nourishment (if allowed by obstetric health care provider).
- Assist with personal hygiene.
- Offer information and advice.
- Involve the woman in decision making regarding her care.
- Interpret the woman's wishes to other health care providers and to her support group.
- Create a relaxing environment.
- Use a calm and confident approach.
- Support and encourage the woman's support people by role-modeling labor support measures and providing time for breaks.

ANXIETY

Anxiety is commonly associated with increased pain during labor. Mild anxiety is considered normal for a woman during labor and birth. Excessive anxiety and fear, however, cause more catecholamine secretion, which increases the stimuli to the brain from the pelvis because of decreased blood flow and increased muscle tension. This action, in turn, magnifies pain perception. Thus as anxiety and fear heighten, muscle tension increases, the effectiveness of uterine contractions decreases, the experience of discomfort increases, and a cycle of increased fear and anxiety begins (Blackburn, 2013). Ultimately this cycle will slow the progress of labor. The woman's confidence in her ability to cope with pain will be diminished, potentially resulting in reduced effectiveness of the pain relief measures being used.

PREVIOUS EXPERIENCE

Previous experience with pain and childbirth may affect a woman's description of her pain and her ability to cope with the pain. Childbirth for a healthy young woman may be her first experience with significant pain, and as a result, she may not have developed effective pain coping strategies. She may describe the intensity of even early labor pain as pain "as bad as it can be." The nature of previous childbirth experiences also may affect a woman's responses to pain. For women who have had a difficult and painful previous birth experience, anxiety and fear from this past experience may lead to increased pain perception.

Sensory labor pain for nulliparous women is often greater than for multiparous women during early labor (dilation less than 5 cm) because their reproductive tract structures are less flexible. However, during the active phase of the first stage of labor and during the second stage of labor, multiparous women may experience greater sensory pain than nulliparous women because their flexible tissue increases the speed of fetal descent and thereby intensifies discomfort. The firmer tissue of nulliparous women results in a slower, more gradual fetal descent (Archie & Roman, 2013).

Parity may affect the perception of labor pain because nulliparous women often have longer labors and therefore greater fatigue. Fatigue magnifies pain, thus causing many women to have an increased perception of the intensity of pain during labor.

GATE-CONTROL THEORY OF PAIN

Intense pain stimuli can at times be ignored. This is possible because certain nerve cell groupings within the spinal cord, brainstem, and cerebral cortex have the ability to modulate the pain impulse through a blocking mechanism. This gate-control theory of pain helps explain the way hypnosis and the pain relief techniques taught in childbirth preparation classes work to relieve the pain of labor. According to this theory, pain sensations travel along sensory nerve pathways to the brain, but only a limited number of sensations, or messages, can travel through these nerve pathways at one time. Using distraction techniques reduces or completely blocks the capacity of nerve pathways to transmit pain. These distractions are thought to work by closing down a hypothetic gate in the spinal cord, thus preventing pain signals from reaching the brain. The perception of pain is thereby diminished (Dean, Gwilym, & Carr, 2013). Obstetric pain management techniques utilizing distraction include massage, aromatherapy, hypnosis, music, and guided imagery. Research into immersion virtual reality (VR) in pain management shows promise for adaptation to management of pain in labor (see Evidence-Based Practice box: Immersion Virtual Reality for Labor Pain Management).

When the laboring woman engages in neuromuscular and motor activity, activity within the spinal cord itself further modifies the transmission of pain. Cognitive work involving concentration on breathing and relaxation requires selective and directed cortical activity that activates and closes the gating mechanism as well. As labor intensifies, more complex cognitive techniques are required to maintain effectiveness. The main impetus behind the gate-control theory as it relates to pain is to introduce the brain to a positive stimulus by using all of the five senses. The brain then begins to accept the more positive stimulus, while paying less attention to negative stimuli such as discomfort or pain. Stimulating the senses will not create a pain-free environment, but it can help decrease the discomforts of labor.

COMFORT

Although the predominant medical approach to labor is that it is painful and the pain must be reduced or eliminated, an alternative view is that labor is a natural process and women can experience comfort and transcend the discomfort or pain to reach the joyful outcome of birth. Having needs and desires met promotes a feeling of comfort. The most helpful interventions in enhancing comfort are a caring nursing approach and a supportive presence.

Support

Evidence indicates that a woman's satisfaction with her labor and birth experience is determined by how well her personal expectations of childbirth are met and the quality of support and interaction she receives from her caregivers (Box 14.1). In addition, satisfaction is influenced by the degree to which she is able to stay in control of her labor and

EVIDENCE-BASED PRACTICE

Immersion Virtual Reality for Labor Pain Management?

Ask the Question

PICOT Question: For women experiencing pain in labor, could immersion virtual reality offer a nonpharmacologic distraction technique option for pain management?

Search for the Evidence

Search Strategies: English research-based publications on virtual reality, immersion, pain, labor were included

Databases Used: Cochrane Collaborative Database, National Guideline Clearinghouse (AHRQ), CINAHL, PubMed, UpToDate, PLoS ONE, and the professional websites for ACOG and AWHONN.

Critical Appraisal of the Evidence

The gate control theory utilizes stimuli to compete for attention in the brain during a painful procedure. Obstetric pain management techniques utilizing distraction have included massage, aromatherapy, hypnosis, music, and guided imagery. New research into immersion virtual reality (VR) in pain management shows promise for adaptation to management of pain in labor.

- Immersion VR is a computer-generated program that simulates a realistic three-dimensional alternate reality. Participants wear goggles and earphones, and sometimes gloves, and interact with and explore their virtual world. This lessens their attention capacity for incoming pain signals (Wiederhold, Soomro, Riva, & Wiederhold, 2014b).
- Patients with dental anxiety using VR during a dental procedure simulation were able to observe or walk around a soothing virtual restorative environment (coastal pathway). Compared to non-VR patients, the VR patients reported a less painful experience and, after 1 week, less intense memories and anxiety (Tanja-Dijkstra, Pahl, Whiote, et al., 2014). During actual (not simulated) dental procedures, the VR group showed less subjective and physiologic evidence of pain, when compared to the non-VR group (Wiederhold, Gao, & Wiederhold, 2014a).
- A systematic review of VR use, including restorative environments and games, in cancer management demonstrated improved patient well-being and support in a variety of applications, including during painful procedures and chronic and acute pain (Chirico, Lucidi, DeLautentis, et al., 2016).
- In obstetrics, VR versus non-VR use was compared during repair of episiotomy in 30 women. Pain scores were significantly improved for the VR group (JahaniShoorab, Zagmi, Nahvi, et al., 2015).

Apply the Evidence: Nursing Implications

- VR technology has become very realistic and believable. It is affordable, relative to other medical devices. It can provide control over the emotional and behavioral responses that can adversely affect treatment. It can even be configured to incorporate biofeedback to the patient (Wiederhold et al., 2014b). Such feedback could help a laboring patient with relaxation and breathing.
- VR has been shown to be safe and effective in the treatment of dental pain and anxiety, posttraumatic stress disorder (PTSD), burn wound dressing, migraine, and acute and chronic pain (Wiederhold et al., 2014b). Perhaps VR could help laboring patients suffering from PTSD, or prevent it from developing or worsening after a traumatic birth.

- Research is needed about the poossibility that women with complicated pain management issues, especially opioid addiction, could decrease their pain medication use in labor and postpartum by using VR as an adjuvant therapy.
- Research is greatly needed to evaluate the appropriateness, practicality, and efficacy of VR use in the labor setting. Side effects such as motion sickness, the isolation of the patient from the experience, and diminished communication with their partner and health care team might be unintended consequences, and even a safety concern.

Quality and Safety Competencies: Evidence-Based Practice*

Knowledge

Explain the role of evidence in determining best clinical practice.

High-quality evidence is needed to uncover the benefits and risks of adapting immersion virtual reality as an intervention for labor pain.

Skills

Locate evidence reports related to clinical practice topics and guidelines.

Seek out or suggest research of pain management techniques in obstetric settings.

Attitudes

Value the need for continuous improvement in clinical practice based on new knowledge.

As long as women still experience pain during labor, there is a need for relief options and adjuvant therapy.

References

Chirico, A., Lucidi, F., De Lautentis, M., et al. (2016). Virtual reality in health care: Beyond entertainment. A mini-review on the efficacy of VR during cancer treatment. *Journal of Cellular Physiology, 231*(2), 275–287.

JahaniShoorab, N., Zagami, S. E., Nahvi, A., et al. (2015). The effect of virtual reality on pain in primiparity women during episiotomy repair: A randomized clinical trial. *Iranian Journal of Medical Science, 40*(3), 219–224. Retrieved from http://ijms.sums.ac.ir/index.php/IJMS/article/view/1675/408.

Tanja-Dijkstra, K., Pahl, S., White, M. P., et al. (2014). Improving dental experiences by using virtual reality distraction: A simulation study. *PLoS ONE, 9*(3), e91276.

Wiederhold, M. D., Gao, K., & Wiederhold, B. K. (2014a). Clinical use of virtual reality distraction system to reduce anxiety and pain in dental procedures. *Cyberpsychology, Behavior, and Social Networking, 17*(6), 359–365.

Wiederhold, B. K., Soomro, A., Riva, G., & Wiederhold, M. D. (2014b). Future directions: Advances and implications of virtual environments designed for pain management. *Cyberpsychology, Behavior, and Social Networking, 17*(6), 414–422.

Pat Mahaffee Gingrich

*Adapted from QSEN at www.qsen.org/.

to participate in decision making regarding her labor, including the pain relief measures to be used (Collins, 2017).

The value of the continuous supportive presence of a person (e.g., partner, family member, friend, nurse, doula) during labor who provides physical comforting, facilitates communication, and offers information and guidance to the woman in labor has long been known. Emotional support is demonstrated by giving praise and reassurance and conveying a positive, calm, and confident demeanor when caring for the woman in labor (Borders, Wendland, Haozous, et al., 2013). Women who have continuous support beginning early in labor are less likely to use pain medications or epidural analgesia or anesthesia and are more likely to experience a spontaneous vaginal birth and express satisfaction with their childbirth experience. Interestingly, research findings concluded that a more positive effect was achieved when continuous support was provided by people other than hospital staff members (Hodnett, Gates, Hofmeyr, et al., 2013; Simpson & O'Brien-Abel, 2014).

ENVIRONMENT

When the childbearing woman experiences discomfort in labor, the quality of her environment can contribute to her having a more positive experience. The woman's environment includes the individuals present (e.g., how they communicate; their philosophy of care, including a belief in the value of nonpharmacologic pain relief measures; practice policies; and quality of support) and the physical space in which the labor occurs. Women who are in a supportive environment feel more in control and therefore are more likely to have a better labor and birth experience. Studies have shown a correlation between perceived control in childbirth and increased satisfaction with the entire childbirth experience (Meyer, 2013).

Women usually prefer to be cared for by familiar caregivers in a comfortable, homelike setting. The environment should be safe and private, allowing a woman to feel free to be herself as she tries out different comfort measures. Stimuli such as light, noise, and temperature should be adjusted according to her preferences. The environment should have space for movement and equipment such as birth balls. Comfortable chairs, tubs, and showers should be readily available to facilitate participation in a variety of nonpharmacologic pain relief measures. The familiarity of the environment can be enhanced by bringing items from home such as pillows, objects for a focal point, and music.

NONPHARMACOLOGIC PAIN MANAGEMENT

Relieving or reducing pain is important. Commonly it is not the amount of pain the woman experiences but whether she meets the goals she set for herself to cope with the pain that influences her perception of the birth experience as good or bad. The observant nurse looks for clues to the woman's desired level of control and her goals in the management of pain.

The labor and birth nurse can use a variety of nonpharmacologic methods for pain relief while providing support and encouragement to the laboring woman and her partner. Nonpharmacologic measures are often simple and safe; have few, if any, major adverse reactions; are relatively inexpensive; and can be used throughout labor. Additionally, they provide the woman with a sense of control over her childbirth as she makes choices about the measures that are best for her. During the prenatal period, she should explore a variety of nonpharmacologic measures. Techniques she usually finds helpful in relieving stress and enhancing relaxation (e.g., music, meditation, massage, warm baths) may be very effective as components of a plan for managing labor pain. The woman should be encouraged to communicate to her health care providers her preferences for relaxation and pain relief measures and for active participation in their implementation.

Many of the nonpharmacologic methods for relief of discomfort are taught in different types of prenatal preparation classes, or the woman or couple may have searched the internet or read various books and articles on the subject in advance. Many of these methods require practice for best results (e.g., hypnosis, patterned breathing and controlled relaxation techniques, biofeedback, focal point, distraction), although the nurse may use some of them successfully without the woman or couple having prior knowledge (e.g., slow-paced breathing, massage and touch, effleurage, counterpressure, relaxation, music, hot or cold packs, movement or positioning). Women should be encouraged to try a variety of methods and to seek alternatives, including pharmacologic methods, when the measure being used is no longer effective (Burke, 2014).

Because of the increased use of epidural analgesia or anesthesia, nurses may be less likely to encourage women to use nonpharmacologic measures, in part because these methods may be viewed as more complex and time-consuming than monitoring a woman receiving an epidural. In addition, new nurses may not have had the opportunity to develop skill in the implementation of these methods. It is imperative that perinatal nurses develop a commitment to and expertise in using a variety of nonpharmacologic pain relief strategies in order for women

---

BOX 14.2   Nonpharmacologic Strategies to Encourage Relaxation and Relieve Pain

Cutaneous Stimulation Strategies
- Counterpressure
- Effleurage (light massage)
- Therapeutic touch and massage
- Walking
- Rocking
- Changing positions
- Application of heat or cold
- Transcutaneous electrical nerve stimulation (TENS)
- Acupressure
- Water therapy (showers, baths, whirlpool baths)
- Intradermal water block

Sensory Stimulation Strategies
- Aromatherapy
- Breathing techniques
- Music
- Imagery
- Use of focal points

Cognitive Strategies
- Childbirth education
- Hypnosis
- Biofeedback

---

in labor to be comfortable using them. Although research evidence to support the effectiveness of many of these nonpharmacologic measures is limited, there are sufficient reports of their benefits from women and health care providers to recommend that nurses encourage their use. The analgesic effect of many nonpharmacologic measures is comparable to or even superior to that of opioids that are administered parenterally (Box 14.2).

CHILDBIRTH PREPARATION METHODS

The childbirth education movement began in the 1950s. Historically, popular childbirth methods taught in the United States were the Dick-Read method, the Lamaze (psychoprophylaxis) method, and the Bradley (husband-coached childbirth) method. Although these three organizations continue to exist, they are now less focused on a "method" approach. Rather, women are assisted to develop their birth philosophy and inner knowledge and then choose from a variety of skills to use to cope with the labor process.

Childbirth education has moved away from these traditional models to hospital-based classes taught by staff members. Also growing in popularity are methods developed and promoted by organizations such as Birthing From Within (www.birthingfromwithin.com), Birthworks International (www.birthworks.org), Childbirth and Postpartum Professional Association (CAPPA) (www.cappa.net), and HypnoBirthing (www.hypnobirthing.com). These methods offer classes and other services that focus on fostering a woman's confidence in her innate ability to give birth. The woman or couple are helped to recognize the uniqueness of their pregnancy and childbirth experience.

Attendance at childbirth education classes has declined in recent years. In a national survey of mothers in 2013, 59% of first-time mothers reported taking a childbirth education class (Declercq, Sakala, Corry, et al., 2013), compared with 70% of first-time mothers in 2002 (Declercq, et al.). Increasing numbers of women are utilizing online childbirth education rather than attending traditional classes because it is less expensive and more convenient for many working women and their partners.

RELAXATION AND BREATHING TECHNIQUES

Focusing and Relaxation Techniques

By reducing tension and stress, focusing and relaxation techniques allow a woman in labor to rest and conserve energy in preparation for giving birth. *Attention-focusing* and *distraction* techniques are forms of care that are effective to some degree in relieving labor pain (Jones, Othman, Dowswell, et al., 2012). Some women bring a favorite object such as a photograph or stuffed animal to the labor room and focus their attention on this object during contractions. Others choose to fix their attention on some object in the labor room. As the contraction begins, they focus on their chosen object and perform a breathing technique to reduce their perception of pain.

With *imagery* the woman focuses her attention on a pleasant scene, a place where she feels relaxed, or an activity she enjoys. She might imagine walking through a restful garden or breathing in light, energy, and a healing color, and breathing out worries and tension. Choosing the subject for the imagery and practicing the technique during pregnancy can enhance effectiveness during labor.

During childbirth preparation classes, the coach can learn how to palpate a woman's body to detect tense and contracted muscles. The woman then learns how to relax the tense muscle in response to the gentle stroking of the muscle by the coach (Fig. 14.2). In a common feedback mechanism, the woman and her coach say the word "relax" at the onset of each contraction and throughout it as needed. With practice, the coach can effectively use support, feedback, and touch to facilitate the woman's relaxation and thereby reduce tension and stress and enhance the progress of labor (Burke, 2014).

Women may find that drinking herbal tea during labor can help them to relax (e.g., chamomile), to reduce nausea (e.g., lemon balm, peppermint), and to enhance energy and reduce fatigue (e.g., ginger, ginseng). Drinking tea can have the additional benefit of maintaining fluid balance (Walls, 2009).

The nurse can assist the woman by providing a quiet and relaxed environment, offering cues as needed, and recognizing signs of tension (e.g., frowning, change in tone of voice, clenching of fists). A relaxed environment for labor is created by controlling sensory stimuli (e.g., light, noise, temperature), and reducing interruptions. Nurses should remain calm and unhurried in their approach and sit rather than stand at the bedside whenever possible (Burke, 2014).

Breathing Techniques

Different approaches to childbirth preparation stress varying breathing techniques to provide distraction, thereby reducing the perception of pain and helping the woman maintain control throughout contractions. In the first stage of labor, such breathing techniques can promote relaxation of the abdominal muscles and thereby increase the size of the abdominal cavity. This lessens discomfort generated by friction between the uterus and abdominal wall during contractions. Because the muscles of the genital area also become more relaxed, they do not interfere with fetal descent. In the second stage, breathing is used to increase abdominal pressure and thereby assist in expelling the fetus. Breathing also can be used to relax the pudendal muscles to prevent precipitate expulsion of the fetal head (Fig. 14.3).

For couples who have prepared for labor by practicing relaxing and breathing techniques, a simple review with occasional reminders may be all that is necessary to help them along. For those who have had no preparation, instruction and practice in simple breathing and relaxation techniques can be given early in labor and often are surprisingly successful. Nurses can also model breathing techniques and breathe in synchrony with the woman and her partner. Motivation is high and readiness to learn is enhanced by the reality of labor (see Clinical Reasoning Case Study: Laboring Without an Epidural).

Various breathing techniques can be used for controlling pain during contractions (Box 14.3). The nurse needs to determine what, if any, techniques the laboring couple knows before giving them instruction. Simple patterns are more easily learned. Paced breathing is most associated with prepared childbirth and includes slow-paced, modified-paced, and patterned-paced (pant-blow) breathing techniques. Each labor is different, and nursing support includes assisting couples to adapt breathing techniques to their individual labor experience.

All patterns begin with a deep, relaxing, cleansing breath to "greet the contraction" and end with another deep breath exhaled to "gently blow the contraction away." These deep breaths ensure adequate oxygen for mother and baby and signal that a contraction is beginning or has ended. As the breath is exhaled, respiratory and voluntary muscles relax (Burke, 2014). In general, *slow-paced breathing* is performed at approximately half the woman's normal breathing rate and is initiated when she can no longer walk or talk through contractions. The woman should take approximately 6 to 8 breaths per minute. Slow-paced breathing aids in relaxation and provides optimum oxygenation. The woman should continue to use this technique for as long as it is effective in reducing the perception of pain and maintaining control. As contractions increase in frequency and intensity, the woman often needs to change to a more complex breathing technique, which is shallower and faster

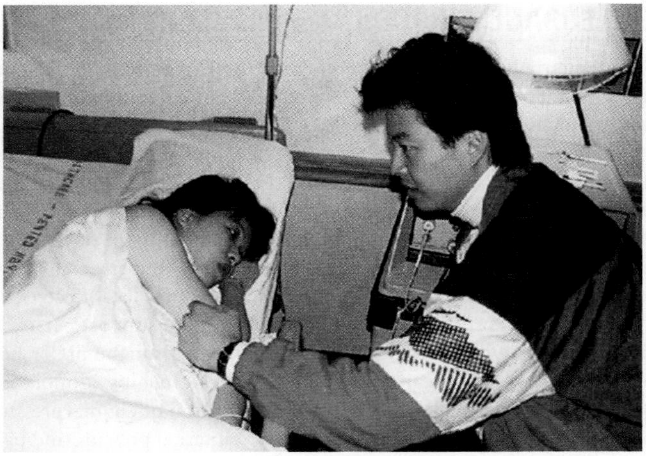

FIG 14.2 A laboring woman using focusing and breathing techniques during a uterine contraction with coaching from her partner. (Courtesy of Marjorie Pyle, RNC, Lifecircle, Costa Mesa, CA.)

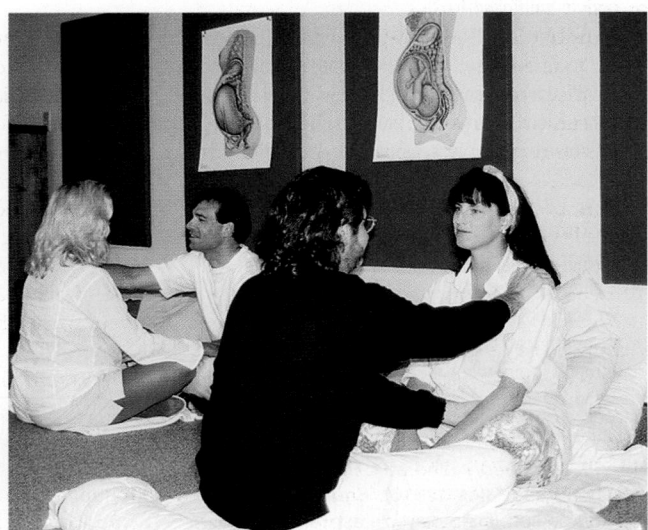

FIG 14.3 Expectant parents learning relaxation techniques. (Courtesy of Marjorie Pyle, RNC, Lifecircle, Costa Mesa, CA.)

CLINICAL REASONING CASE STUDY
Laboring Without an Epidural

Jamie is a 16-year-old G1 P0 who has been admitted with preeclampsia with severe features at 34 weeks of gestation. Jamie's physician plans to induce labor and anticipates a vaginal birth. Jamie has not attended any childbirth preparation classes and has been planning to have an epidural for labor and birth. Unfortunately, because her platelet count is very low (28,000), the anesthesia care provider refuses to place an epidural block. Jamie bursts into tears and says, "I can't make it through labor without an epidural! It's going to hurt too much! Help me!!"

1. Evidence—Is there sufficient evidence regarding avoiding neuraxial anesthesia in women who have low platelet counts?
2. Assumptions—Describe an underlying assumption about each of the following nonpharmacologic or pharmacologic methods for pain relief during labor:
   a. Breathing and relaxation techniques
   b. Application of heat and cold
   c. Systemic analgesia
   d. Presence of a support person to increase effectiveness of interventions for pain
3. What implications and priorities for nursing care can be drawn at this time?
4. Does the evidence objectively support your argument (conclusion)?
5. Interprofessional care—Describe the roles/responsibilities of health care professionals who might be involved in Jamie's care.

BOX 14.3   Paced Breathing Techniques

Cleansing Breath
- Relaxed breath in through nose and out through mouth. Used at the beginning and end of each contraction.

Slow-Paced Breathing (Approximately 6 to 8 Breaths Per Minute)
- Performed at approximately half the normal breathing rate (number of breaths per minute divided by 2)
- IN-2-3-4/OUT-2-3-4/IN-2-3-4/OUT-2-3-4…

Modified-Paced Breathing (Approximately 32 to 40 Breaths Per Minute)
- Performed at about twice the normal breathing rate (number of breaths per minute multiplied by 2)
- IN-OUT/IN-OUT/IN-OUT/IN-OUT…
- For more flexibility and variety, the woman may combine the slow and modified breathing by using the slow breathing for beginnings and ends of contractions and modified breathing for more intense peaks. This technique conserves energy, lessens fatigue, and reduces risk for hyperventilation.

Patterned-Paced or Pant-Blow Breathing (Same Rate as Modified)
- Enhances concentration
- 3:1 Patterned breathing IN-OUT/IN-OUT/IN-OUT/IN-BLOW (repeat through contraction)
- 4:1 Patterned breathing IN-OUT/IN-OUT/IN-OUT/IN-OUT/IN-BLOW (repeat through contraction)

Adapted from Nichols, F. (2000). Paced breathing techniques. In F.H. Nichols & S.S. Humenick (Eds.), *Childbirth education: Practice, research, and theory* (2nd ed.). Philadelphia, PA: Saunders; Perinatal Education Associates. (2016). *Breathing*. Retrieved from http://www.birthsource.com/scripts/article.asp?articleid=211.

than her normal rate of breathing but should not exceed twice her resting respiratory rate. This *modified-paced breathing* pattern requires that she remain alert and concentrate more fully on breathing, thus blocking more painful stimuli than the simpler slow-paced breathing pattern (Perinatal Education Associates, 2016).

The most difficult time to maintain control during contractions comes during the latter part of the active phase of the first stage of labor, when the cervix dilates from 8 cm to 10 cm. Even for the woman who has prepared for labor, concentration on breathing techniques is difficult to maintain. *Patterned-paced (pant-blow) breathing* is suggested during this time. It is performed at the same rate as modified-paced breathing and consists of panting breaths combined with soft blowing breaths at regular intervals. The patterns may vary (i.e., *pant, pant, pant, pant, blow* [4:1 pattern] or *pant, pant, pant, blow* [3:1 pattern]) (Perinatal Education Associates, 2016). An undesirable reaction to this type of breathing is hyperventilation.

> ⚡ **SAFETY ALERT**
> The woman and her support person must be aware of and watch for symptoms of the resultant respiratory alkalosis: lightheadedness, dizziness, tingling of the fingers, or circumoral numbness.

Having the woman breathe into a paper bag held tightly around her mouth and nose may eliminate respiratory alkalosis. This enables her to rebreathe carbon dioxide and replace the bicarbonate ions. The woman also can breathe into her cupped hands if no bag is available. Maintaining a breathing rate that is no more than twice her normal rate will lessen chances of hyperventilation. The partner can help the woman maintain her breathing rate with visual, tactile, or auditory cues.

As the fetal head reaches the pelvic floor, the woman may feel the urge to push and may automatically begin to exert downward pressure by contracting her abdominal muscles. During second-stage pushing, the woman should find a breathing pattern that is relaxing and feels good to her and is safe for her baby. Any regular or rhythmic breathing that avoids prolonged breath holding during pushing should maintain a good oxygen flow to the fetus (Perinatal Education Associates, 2016).

The woman can control the urge to push by taking panting breaths or by slowly exhaling through pursed lips (as though blowing out a candle or blowing up a balloon). This type of breathing can be used to overcome the urge to push when the cervix is not fully prepared (e.g., less than 8 cm dilated, not retracting) and to facilitate a slow birth of the fetal head.

EFFLEURAGE AND COUNTERPRESSURE

Effleurage (light massage) and counterpressure have brought relief to many women during the first stage of labor. The gate-control theory may supply the reason for the effectiveness of these measures. Effleurage is light stroking, usually of the abdomen, in rhythm with breathing during contractions. It is used to distract the woman from contraction pain. Often the presence of electronic fetal monitor belts makes it difficult to perform effleurage on the abdomen; therefore a thigh or the chest may be used. As labor progresses, hyperesthesia (hypersensitivity to touch) may make effleurage uncomfortable and thus less effective.

Counterpressure is steady pressure applied by a support person to the sacral area with a firm object (e.g., tennis ball) or the fist or heel of the hand. Pressure can also be applied to both hips (double hip squeeze) or to the knees (Burke, 2014). Application of counterpressure helps the woman cope with the sensations of internal pressure and pain in the lower back. It is especially helpful when back pain is caused by pressure of the occiput against spinal nerves when the fetal head is in a posterior position. Counterpressure lifts the occiput off these nerves, thereby providing pain relief. The support person will need to be relieved occasionally because application of counterpressure is hard work.

TOUCH AND MASSAGE

Touch and massage have been an integral part of the traditional care process for women in labor. A variety of massage techniques have been shown to be safe and effective during labor (Jones et al., 2012).

Touch can be as simple as holding the woman's hand, stroking her body, and embracing her. When using touch to communicate caring, reassurance, and concern, it is important that the woman's preferences for touch (e.g., who can touch her, where they can touch her, and how they can touch her) and responses to touch be determined. A woman with a history of sexual abuse or certain cultural beliefs may be uncomfortable with touch. Touch may not be desired or appreciated by some women in labor, as it may break their concentration if they are using certain prepared childbirth methods (Collins, 2017). Touch also can involve very specialized techniques that require manipulation of the human energy field.

Therapeutic touch (TT) uses the concept of energy fields within the body called *prana*. Prana are thought to be deficient in some people who are in pain. TT uses laying-on of hands by a specially trained person to redirect energy fields associated with pain. Research has demonstrated the effectiveness of TT to enhance relaxation, reduce anxiety, and relieve pain (Jones et al., 2012); however, little is known about the use or effectiveness of TT for relieving pain in labor.

Head, hand, back, and foot massage may be very effective in reducing tension and enhancing comfort. Some evidence suggests that massage may improve management of labor pain (Jones et al., 2012). Hand and foot massage may be especially relaxing in advanced labor when hyperesthesia limits a woman's tolerance for touch on other parts of her body. Combining massage with aromatherapy oil or lotion enhances relaxation both during and between contractions. The woman and her partner should be encouraged to experiment with different types of massage during pregnancy to determine which might feel best and be most relaxing during labor.

APPLICATION OF HEAT AND COLD

Warmed blankets, warm compresses, heated rice bags, a warm bath or shower, or a moist heating pad can enhance relaxation and reduce pain during labor. Heat relieves muscle ischemia and increases blood flow to the area of discomfort. Heat application is effective in reducing back pain caused by a posterior presentation or general backache from fatigue. During second-stage labor, the application of warm, moist compresses to the perineum relieves the burning sensation women often feel when the fetal head crowns (Collins, 2017).

Cold application such as cold cloths, frozen gel packs, or ice packs applied to the back, the chest, and/or the face during labor may be effective in increasing comfort when the woman feels warm. They also may be applied to areas of musculoskeletal pain. Cooling relieves pain by reducing the muscle temperature and relieving muscle spasms (Burke, 2014). However, a woman's culture may make the use of cold during labor unacceptable.

> ### ⚡ SAFETY ALERT
>
> Heat and cold may be used alternately for a greater effect. Neither heat nor cold should be applied over ischemic or anesthetized areas because tissues can be damaged (Collins, 2017). One or two layers of cloth should be placed between the skin and a hot or cold pack to prevent damage to the underlying integument.

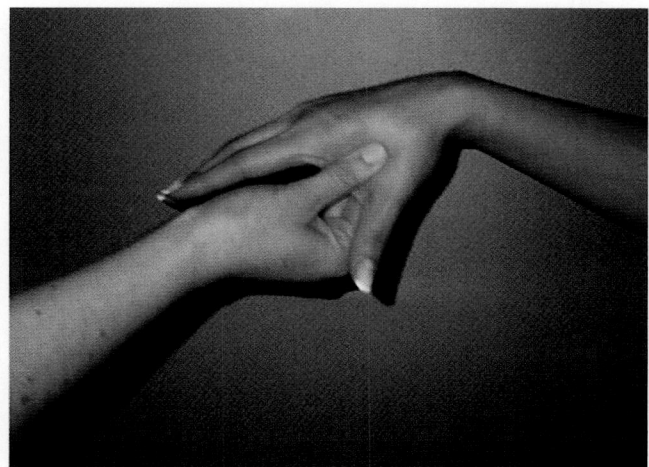

FIG 14.4 Hoku acupressure point (back of hand where thumb and index finger come together) used to enhance uterine contractions without increasing pain. (Courtesy of Julie Perry Nelson, Loveland, CO.)

ACUPRESSURE AND ACUPUNCTURE

Acupressure and acupuncture can be used in pregnancy, in labor, and postpartum to relieve pain and other discomforts. Pressure, heat, or cold is applied to acupuncture points called *tsubos*. These points have an increased density of neuroreceptors and increased electrical conductivity. Acupressure is said to promote circulation of blood, the harmony of yin and yang, and the secretion of neurotransmitters, thus maintaining normal body functions and enhancing well-being (Gisin, Poat, Fierz, et al., 2013). Acupressure is best applied over the skin without using lubricants. Pressure is usually applied with the heel of the hand, fist, or pads of the thumbs and fingers (Fig. 14.4). Tennis balls or other devices also may be used. Pressure is applied with contractions initially and then continuously as labor progresses to the end of the first stage (Gisin et al.). Synchronized breathing by the caregiver and the woman is suggested for greater effectiveness. Acupressure points are found on the neck, the shoulders, the wrists, the lower back including sacral points, the hips, the area below the kneecaps, the ankles, the nails on the small toes, and the soles of the feet. Research indicates that women may experience good pain relief with the use of acupressure (Collins, 2017).

Acupuncture is the insertion of fine needles into specific areas of the body to restore the flow of *qi* (energy) and to decrease pain, which is thought to obstruct the flow of energy. Effectiveness may be attributed to the alteration of chemical neurotransmitter levels in the body or to the release of endorphins as a result of hypothalamic activation. Acupuncture should be done by a trained, certified therapist, and arranging to have a qualified and credentialed acupuncture provider available during labor and birth may be challenging. Current evidence indicates that acupuncture relieves labor pain and reduces the use of both epidural anesthesia and systemic analgesics; however, further study is needed (Hawkins & Bucklin, 2017).

TRANSCUTANEOUS ELECTRICAL NERVE STIMULATION

Transcutaneous electrical nerve stimulation (TENS) involves the placing of two pairs of flat electrodes on either side of the woman's thoracic and sacral spine (Fig. 14.5). These electrodes provide continuous low-intensity electrical impulses or stimuli from a battery-operated device. During a contraction, the woman increases the stimulation from low

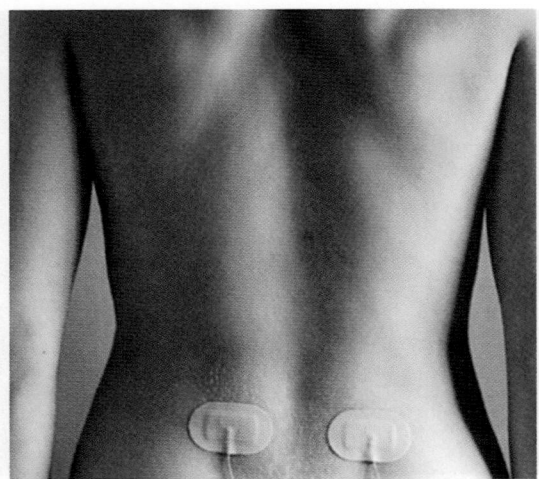

FIG 14.5 Placement of transcutaneous electrical nerve stimulation (TENS) electrodes on back for relief of labor pain.

to high intensity by turning control knobs on the device. High intensity should be maintained for at least 1 minute to facilitate release of endorphins. Women describe the resulting sensation as a tingling or buzzing. TENS is most useful for lower back pain during the early first stage of labor. Women tend to rate the device as helpful, although its use does not decrease pain. It appears that the electrical impulses or stimuli somehow make the pain less disturbing. Because women maintain control of the TENS device, this element of autonomy may increase their satisfaction with the method. No serious safety concerns are associated with the use of TENS (Collins, 2017; Hawkins & Bucklin, 2017).

WATER THERAPY (HYDROTHERAPY)

Bathing, showering, and jet hydrotherapy (whirlpool baths) with warm water (e.g., at or below body temperature) are nonpharmacologic measures that can promote comfort and relaxation during labor (Fig. 14.6). Water immersion is a specific form of hydrotherapy that involves immersion of the laboring woman in water deep enough to completely cover her abdomen. The water increases buoyancy and provides a sense of weightlessness and freedom of movement. Women who labor in water report less anxiety and pain, and increased satisfaction with their childbirth experience. Water immersion has not been associated with increases in adverse maternal, fetal, or neonatal outcomes (Brickhouse, Isaacs, Batten, et al., 2015). Additionally, hydrotherapy results in less use of pharmacologic pain relief measures, decreased use of epidural anesthesia, fewer forceps- or vacuum-assisted births, fewer episiotomies, and less perineal trauma (Arendt & Tessmer-Tuck, 2013; Burke, 2014).

Tub hydrotherapy may be contraindicated for some women. Women who require continuous electronic fetal heart rate (FHR) monitoring are not candidates for hydrotherapy unless waterproof monitors are available (see Fig. 14.6, C). Women with fever (≥38° C/100.4° F), infectious diseases (e.g. HIV+, active herpes simplex virus), and vaginal bleeding greater than a normal bloody show should not be offered water immersion. Additionally, tub hydrotherapy is contraindicated for women in preterm labor (gestational age <37 weeks) (Collins, 2017). Hydrotherapy using a shower provides comfort through the application of heat as the handheld shower head is directed to areas of discomfort (see Fig. 14.6, A and B). The coach or partner can participate in this comfort measure by holding and directing the shower head.

Women must never be left alone while using hydrotherapy. Another person should always be present to assist the woman with getting out of the tub or shower quickly if necessary. The water temperature should be maintained above 35° C (95° F) and no higher than 37.8° C (100° F). Tubs must be thoroughly cleaned after each use to prevent bacterial growth and cross-contamination between women (Brickhouse et al., 2015; Collins, 2017).

The American College of Obstetricians and Gynecologists (ACOG) has expressed concerns about actual birthing in water (waterbirth) because insufficient data are available on which to draw conclusions about its relative risks and benefits. There are concerns that waterbirth may predispose babies to potentially serious neonatal complications such as infection, water aspiration, and umbilical cord avulsion. Therefore, until sufficient data are available, ACOG recommends that birth occur out of water (ACOG, 2016).

However, a recent study using data collected from the Midwives Alliance of North America Statistics Project reported waterbirth outcomes on a large number of midwife-attended births occurring at home and in birthing centers in the United States. They found no evidence of any subsequent neonatal risk for adverse outcome (5 minute Apgar score <7, neonatal transfer to the hospital, and any hospital admission, including to the neonatal intensive care unit, during the first 6 weeks of life) in neonates born underwater. The researchers concluded that waterbirth does not confer additional risks to neonates (Bovbjerg, Cheyney, & Everson, 2016).

INTRADERMAL WATER BLOCK

An intradermal water block involves the injection of small amounts of sterile water (e.g., 0.05 to 0.1 mL) using a fine-gauge (e.g., 25-gauge) needle into four locations on the lower back to relieve lower back pain (Fig. 14.7). It is a simple procedure to perform, and there is evidence that it is effective, perhaps because of the gate-control mechanism (Collins, 2017). Other possible explanations for the effectiveness of the intradermal water block are the mechanism of counterirritation (i.e., reducing localized pain in one area by irritating the skin in an area nearby) or an increase in the level of endogenous opioids (endorphins) produced by the injections. Intense stinging will occur for about 20 to 30 seconds after injection, but relief of back pain for up to 2 hours has been reported (Burke, 2014). Although the effectiveness of this technique is largely unproven, no serious safety concerns are associated with its use (Hawkins & Bucklin, 2017).

AROMATHERAPY

Aromatherapy uses oils distilled from plants, flowers, herbs, and trees to promote health and to treat and balance the mind, body, and spirit. These essential oils are highly concentrated, complex essences and are mixed with lotions or creams before they are applied to the skin (e.g., for a back massage). Jasmine, geranium, rose, clary sage, neroli, ylang ylang, and lavender have been reported to provide good relief when used in labor. Because these oils contain medicinal properties, they should be used in the smallest amount that provides relief (Collins, 2017). Oils may also be used by adding a few drops to a warm bath, to warm water used for soaking compresses that can be applied to the body, or to an aromatherapy lamp to vaporize a room. Drops of essential oils can be put on a pillow or on a woman's brow or palms or used as

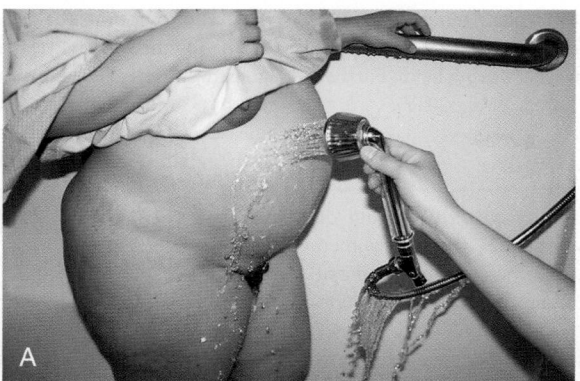

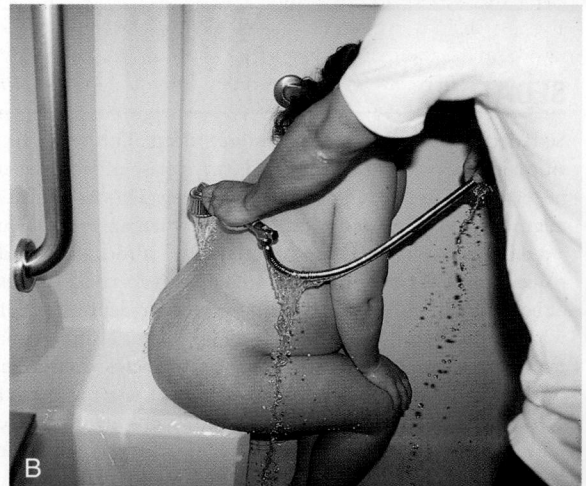

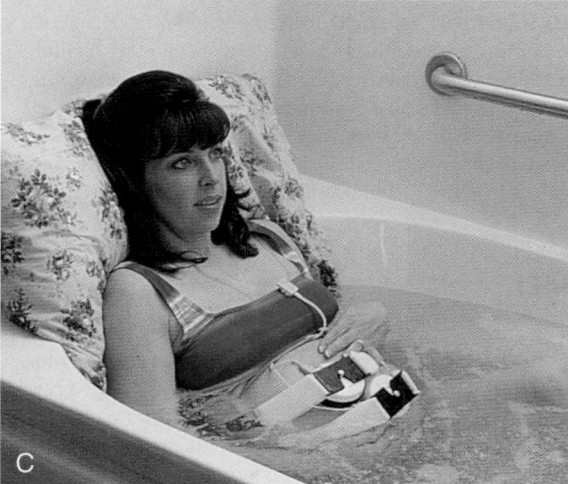

FIG 14.6 Water therapy during labor. **A,** Use of shower during labor. **B,** Woman experiencing back labor relaxes as partner sprays warm water on her back. **C,** Laboring woman relaxes in Jacuzzi. Note that fetal monitoring using waterproof monitors can continue during time in the Jacuzzi. (A and B, Courtesy of Marjorie Pyle, RNC, Lifecircle, Costa Mesa, CA; C, Courtesy of Spacelabs Medical, Redmond, WA.)

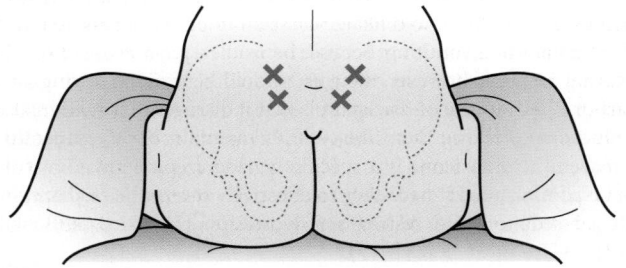

FIG 14.7 Intradermal injections of 0.1 mL of sterile water in the treatment of women with back pain during labor. Sterile water is injected into four locations on the lower back, two over each posterior superior iliac spine (PSIS) and two 3 cm below and 1 cm medial to the PSIS. The injections should raise a bleb on the skin. Simultaneous injections administered by two clinicians will decrease the pain of the injections. (From Leeman, L., Fontaine, P., King, V., et al. [2003]. The nature and management of labor pain: Part I. Nonpharmacologic pain relief. *American Family Physician, 68,* 1109–1112. Copyright 2003 by Michael Norviel.)

an ingredient in creating massage oil. They can be used with a diffuser that disperses the oils into the air. Aromatherapy has not been shown to improve labor outcomes. However, there is likely little harm associated with its use, other than the possibility of an allergic reaction (Arendt & Tessmer-Tuck, 2013).

⚡ **SAFETY ALERT**

Only a professional trained in the use of essential oils should apply them topically to laboring women, because some oils can actually be harmful when applied to the skin.

MUSIC

Music, recorded or live, can provide a distraction, enhance relaxation, and lift spirits during labor, thereby reducing the woman's level of stress, anxiety, and perception of pain. It can be used to promote relaxation in early labor and to stimulate movement as labor progresses. Music can help create a more relaxed atmosphere in the birth room, leading to a more relaxed approach by health care providers. Women should be encouraged to prepare their musical preferences in advance and to bring an electronic musical device to the hospital or birthing center. They should choose familiar music that is associated with pleasant memories, which can also facilitate the process of guided imagery and cause the release of endorphins, which can alter the perception of pain (Burke, 2014; Collins, 2017). Use of a headset or earphones may increase the effectiveness of the music because other sounds will be shut out. Live music provided at the bedside by a support person may be very helpful in transmitting energy that decreases tension and elevates mood. Changing the tempo of the music to coincide with the rate and rhythm of each breathing technique may facilitate proper pacing. Although promising, there is insufficient evidence at the present time to support the effectiveness of music as a method of pain relief during labor. Further research is recommended (Smith, Levett, Collins, et al., 2012).

HYPNOSIS

Hypnosis is a form of deep relaxation, similar to daydreaming or meditation (see www.hypnobirthing.com). While under hypnosis, women are in a state of focused concentration and the subconscious mind can be more easily accessed. Women who attend certain childbirth preparation classes may be taught to perform self-hypnosis. Hypnosis techniques used for labor and birth place an emphasis on enhancing relaxation and diminishing fear, anxiety, and perception of pain. A few negative effects of hypnosis have been reported, including mild dizziness, nausea, and headache. These negative effects seem to be associated with failure to dehypnotize the woman properly. Although some initial small studies found hypnosis to be beneficial, a Cochrane systematic review showed no difference between women who were hypnotized and those who were not in regard to their use of pain medication during labor or their satisfaction with pain relief or the overall birth experience (Arendt & Tessmer-Tuck, 2013).

BIOFEEDBACK

Biofeedback may provide another relaxation technique that can be used for labor. Biofeedback is based on the theory that if a person can recognize physical signals, certain internal physiologic events can be changed (i.e., whatever signs the woman has that are associated with her pain). For biofeedback to be effective, the woman must be educated during the prenatal period to become aware of her body and its responses and how to relax. The woman must learn how to use thinking and mental processes (e.g., focusing) to control body responses and functions. Informational biofeedback helps couples develop awareness of their bodies and use strategies to change their responses to stress. If the woman responds to pain during a contraction with tightening of muscles, frowning, moaning, and breath holding, her partner uses verbal and touch feedback to help her relax. Formal biofeedback, which uses machines to detect skin temperature, blood flow, or muscle tension, also can prepare women to intensify their relaxation responses. Biofeedback-assisted relaxation techniques are not always successful in reducing labor pain. They may initially reduce pain or discomfort in labor, but as labor progresses women often need pain medication as well. There is insufficient evidence at this time to show that biofeedback is effective for managing labor pain (Barragán Loayza, Solà, & Juandó Prats, 2011).

PHARMACOLOGIC PAIN MANAGEMENT

Pharmacologic measures for pain management should be implemented before pain becomes so severe that catecholamines increase and labor is prolonged. It is unacceptable for women in labor to endure severe pain when safe and effective relief measures are available (ACOG, 2004/2015). Pharmacologic and nonpharmacologic measures, when used together, increase the level of pain relief and create a more positive labor experience for the woman and her family. Nonpharmacologic measures can be used for relaxation and pain relief, especially in early labor. Pharmacologic measures can be implemented as labor becomes more active and discomfort and pain intensify. Less pharmacologic intervention often is required because nonpharmacologic measures enhance relaxation and potentiate the analgesic effect. However, women in the United States are increasingly using pharmacologic measures,

especially epidural analgesia, to relieve their pain during labor and birth. In one survey, nearly two-thirds of women received regional anesthesia to relieve pain during labor or during vaginal or cesarean birth (Cunningham, Leveno, Bloom, et al., 2014). Pharmacologic measures for pain management are generally used in hospital settings rather than in birthing centers or for home births.

> **⚡ SAFETY ALERT**
>
> Whenever medications are administered, nurses must remain alert for adverse reactions (e.g., difficulty breathing) and be prepared to administer antidotes or summon assistance if necessary. It is important to remember that adverse reactions can occur even if the woman has received the same medication in the past without problems.

SEDATIVES

Sedatives relieve anxiety and induce sleep. They may be given to a woman experiencing a prolonged early phase of labor when there is a need to decrease anxiety or promote sleep. They may also be given to augment analgesics and reduce nausea when an opioid is used.

Barbiturates such as secobarbital sodium (Seconal) easily cross the placenta and have a long half-life. They can cause undesirable side effects including respiratory and vasomotor depression, affecting the woman and newborn. Because of the potential for neonatal central nervous system (CNS) depression, barbiturates should be avoided if birth is anticipated within 12 to 24 hours. As a result of these disadvantages, barbiturates are seldom used in obstetrics (Burke, 2014).

Phenothiazines (e.g., promethazine [Phenergan]) do not relieve pain. In the past, promethazine was often given with opioids to enhance their analgesic effects, as well as to decrease anxiety and apprehension, increase sedation, and reduce nausea and vomiting. However, there is no research evidence to support this practice. Metoclopramide (Reglan), an antiemetic, has been found to effectively potentiate the effects of analgesics. Therefore, it may be a better choice than promethazine (Burke, 2014; Hawkins & Bucklin, 2017).

Benzodiazepines (e.g., diazepam [Valium], lorazepam [Ativan]), when given with an opioid analgesic, seem to enhance pain relief and reduce nausea and vomiting. Because benzodiazepines cause significant maternal amnesia, however, their use should be avoided during labor. A major disadvantage of diazepam is that it disrupts thermoregulation in newborns, making them less able to maintain body temperature. Flumazenil (Romazicon) is a specific benzodiazepine antagonist that can be administered if necessary to effectively reverse benzodiazepine-induced sedation and respiratory depression (Hawkins & Bucklin, 2017).

ANALGESIA AND ANESTHESIA

Nursing management of obstetric analgesia and anesthesia combines the nurse's expertise in maternity care with a knowledge and understanding of anatomy and physiology and of medications and their therapeutic effects, adverse reactions, and methods of administration.

Anesthesia encompasses analgesia, amnesia, relaxation, and reflex activity. Anesthesia abolishes pain perception by interrupting the nerve impulses to the brain. The loss of sensation may be partial or complete, sometimes with the loss of consciousness. The term analgesia refers to the alleviation of the sensation of pain or the raising of the threshold for pain perception without loss of consciousness. The type of analgesic or anesthetic chosen is determined in part by the stage of labor of the woman and by the method of birth planned (Box 14.4).

BOX 14.4   Pharmacologic Control of Discomfort by Stage of Labor and Method of Birth

First Stage
- Opioid agonist analgesics
- Opioid agonist-antagonist analgesics
- Epidural (block) analgesia
- Combined spinal-epidural (CSE) analgesia
- Nitrous oxide

- CSE analgesia
- Nitrous oxide

Vaginal Birth
- Local infiltration anesthesia
- Pudendal block
- Epidural (block) analgesia and anesthesia
- Spinal (block) anesthesia
- CSE analgesia and anesthesia
- Nitrous oxide

Second Stage
- Nerve block analgesia and anesthesia
- Local infiltration anesthesia
- Pudendal block
- Spinal (block) anesthesia
- Epidural (block) analgesia

Cesarean Birth
- Spinal (block) anesthesia
- Epidural (block) anesthesia
- General anesthesia

Systemic Analgesia

Systemic analgesics (opioids) can be administered as intermittent intravenous (IV) or intramuscular (IM) doses by health care professionals or by the woman herself using patient-controlled analgesia (PCA). With PCA, the woman self-administers small doses of an opioid analgesic by using a pump programmed for dose and frequency. Overall, a lower total amount of analgesic is used. Women appreciate the sense of autonomy provided by this method of pain relief, as well as the elimination of treatment delays while the nurse obtains and administers the medication (Hawkins & Bucklin, 2017).

Opioids provide sedation and euphoria, but their analgesic effect in labor is limited. The pain relief they provide is incomplete, temporary, and more effective in the early part of active labor. All opioids cause side effects, the most serious of which is respiratory depression. Other undesirable opioid side effects include sedation, nausea and vomiting, dizziness, altered mental status, euphoria, decreased gastric motility, delayed gastric emptying, and urinary retention (Anderson, 2011; Hawkins & Bucklin, 2017; Swart & Kelly, 2017). Prolonged gastric emptying time increases the risk for aspiration if general anesthesia becomes necessary in a woman who has received opioids (Hawkins & Bucklin). Bladder and bowel elimination can be inhibited. Because heart rate (e.g., bradycardia), blood pressure (e.g., hypotension), and respiratory effort (e.g., depression) can be adversely affected, opioid analgesics should be used cautiously in women with respiratory and cardiovascular disorders. Safety precautions should be taken after opioid administration, because several opioid side effects increase the risk for injury due to falls.

⚡ SAFETY ALERT

Opioids decrease maternal heart and respiratory rate and blood pressure, which affects fetal oxygenation. Therefore maternal vital signs and FHR and pattern must be assessed and documented before and after administration of opioids for pain relief.

Opioids readily cross the placenta. Effects on the fetus and newborn can be profound, including absent or minimal FHR variability during labor and significant neonatal respiratory depression requiring treatment after birth (Hawkins & Bucklin, 2017; Swart & Kelly, 2017).

Classifications of analgesic drugs used to relieve the pain of childbirth include opioid (narcotic) agonists and opioid (narcotic) agonist-antagonists. Choice of which medication to use often depends on the obstetric health care provider's preferences and the situation of the laboring woman, including factors such as her preferences, physical condition, and current medications. The type of systemic analgesics used therefore often varies among obstetric units. There is insufficient evidence to recommend the use of one opioid over another (Burke, 2014; Collins, 2017; Swart & Kelly, 2017). The opioids commonly used currently in obstetrics are meperidine, fentanyl, remifentanil, and nalbuphine (Hawkins & Bucklin, 2017).

Opioid Agonist Analgesics

Meperidine, fentanyl, and remifentanil are opioid (narcotic) agonist analgesics. As pure opioid agonists, they stimulate major opioid receptors, mu and kappa. They have no amnesic effect but create a feeling of well-being or euphoria and enhance a woman's ability to rest between contractions. Because opioids can inhibit uterine contractions, they should not be administered until labor is well established unless they are being used to enhance therapeutic rest during a prolonged early phase of labor (Burke, 2014).

Meperidine (Demerol) is a synthetic opioid that is the most widely used systemic medication for labor pain (Cunningham et al., 2014). Its widespread use is probably related to its low cost, the fact that care providers are quite familiar with the drug, and studies that were done many years ago that found that it caused less respiratory depression than morphine (see Medication Guide: Meperidine Hydrochloride [Demerol]). However, its use during labor is becoming more controversial because of undesirable side effects, particularly in the neonate (Anderson, 2011). Both meperidine and normeperidine, an active metabolite of meperidine, cross the placenta and cause prolonged neonatal sedation and neurobehavioral changes. These metabolite-related effects cannot be reversed with naloxone (Anderson). Because meperidine and normeperidine have long half-lives, the neonatal effects can persist for the first 2 to 3 days of life (Hawkins & Bucklin, 2017).

Fentanyl (Sublimaze) is a potent short-acting synthetic opioid agonist analgesic (see Medication Guide: Fentanyl Citrate [Sublimaze]). It rapidly crosses the placenta so is present in fetal blood within 1 minute after intravenous maternal administration. As compared with meperidine, fentanyl provides equivalent analgesia with fewer neonatal effects and less maternal sedation and nausea. Fentanyl is used as a labor analgesic because of its rapid onset of action, short half-life, and lack of a metabolite (Anderson, 2011; Hawkins, & Bucklin, 2017). A disadvantage of fentanyl is that more frequent dosing is required because of its relatively short duration of action (Hawkins & Bucklin). As a result, this medication is most commonly administered by PCA pump, although it is also administered intrathecally or epidurally alone or in combination with a local anesthetic agent.

Remifentanil (Ultiva) is an even faster-onset, shorter-acting synthetic opioid agonist with no active metabolites (see Medication Guide: Remifentanil Hydrochloride [Ultiva]). Its onset of action is approximately 1 minute. Remifentanil does cross the placenta but is metabolized rapidly in the fetus so that it does not cause neonatal depression. Because remifentanil is metabolized by plasma esterases, it is not affected by impaired renal or hepatic function. Remifentanil should be administered only by PCA pump because of its short (only 3 minute) half-life. Sedation and hypoventilation with oxygen desaturations occur more frequently with remifentanil than with other opioids, so respiratory monitoring is required with its use (Burke, 2014; Hawkins & Bucklin, 2017).

Opioid (Narcotic) Agonist-Antagonist Analgesics

An **agonist** is an agent that activates or stimulates a receptor to act; an **antagonist** is an agent that blocks a receptor or a medication designed to activate a receptor. Nalbuphine (Nubain) is a commonly used opioid (narcotic) agonist-antagonist analgesic (Hawkins & Bucklin, 2017).

MEDICATION GUIDE

Meperidine Hydrochloride (Demerol)

Classification
Opioid agonist analgesic

Action
Synthetic opioid agonist analgesic that stimulates both mu and kappa opioid receptors to decrease the transmission of pain impulses. Meperidine 100 mg is roughly equivalent in analgesic effect to morphine 10 mg, but it is reported to cause less maternal respiratory depression. Onset of action begins almost immediately after administration and lasts approximately 1.5 to 2 hours.

Indication
Moderate to severe labor pain and postoperative pain after cesarean birth

Dosage and Route
IV: 25 to 50 mg every 1 to 2 hours.
  PCA Pump: 15 mg every 10 minutes as needed until birth

Adverse Effects
Tachycardia, sedation, nausea and vomiting, dizziness, altered mental status, euphoria, decreased gastric motility, delayed gastric emptying, and urinary retention

Nursing Considerations
Implement safety measures as appropriate, including use of side rails and assistance with ambulation; continue use of nonpharmacologic pain relief measures. Do not give if birth is expected to occur within 1 to 4 hours after administration because infants born to women who received meperidine during labor may have respiratory depression, peaking at 2 to 3 hours after administration of the drug. Respiratory depression caused by normeperidine, an active metabolite of meperidine, cannot be reversed by naloxone. Both meperidine and normeperidine have long half-lives. Therefore, neonates whose mothers received meperidine during labor can exhibit sedation and neurobehavioral changes for the first 2 to 3 days of life.

Data from Anderson, D. (2011). A review of systemic opioids commonly used for labor pain relief. *Journal of Midwifery & Women's Health, 56*, 222–239; Hawkins, J.L. & Bucklin, B.A. (2017). Obstetric anesthesia. In S. G. Gabbe, J. R. Niebyl, J. L. Simpson, et al. (Eds.): *Obstetrics: Normal and problem pregnancies* (7th ed.). Philadelphia, PA: Elsevier.

Opioid agonist-antagonist analgesics are agonists at kappa opioid receptors and either antagonists or weak agonists at mu opioid receptors. In the doses used during labor, these mixed opioids provide adequate analgesia without causing significant respiratory depression in the mother or neonate. Their major advantage is their ceiling effect for respiratory depression; higher doses do not produce additional respiratory depression. They are less likely to cause nausea and vomiting, but sedation may be as great or greater when compared with pure opioid agonists (Anderson, 2011; Hawkins & Bucklin).

Nalbuphine use also has some disadvantages. Its antagonist activity may limit the amount of analgesia it can produce. Also, it is not suitable for use in women with an opioid dependence, because the antagonist activity could precipitate withdrawal symptoms (abstinence syndrome) in both the mother and her newborn (Hawkins & Bucklin, 2017) (see Medication Guide: Nalbuphine Hydrochloride [Nubain] and Box 14.5).

Opioid (Narcotic) Antagonists

Opioids such as meperidine and fentanyl can cause excessive CNS depression in the mother, the newborn, or both, although the current

MEDICATION GUIDE

Fentanyl Citrate (Sublimaze)

Classification
Opioid agonist analgesic

Action
Opioid agonist analgesic that stimulates both mu and kappa opioid receptors to decrease the transmission of pain impulses. Has a rapid onset of action with a short duration (0.5 to 1 hour IV; 1 to 2 hours IM).

Indication
Moderate to severe labor pain and postoperative pain after cesarean birth

Dosage and Route
IV: 50 to 100 mcg every hour
IM: 50 to 100 mcg every hour
PCA Pump: (sample setting) 50 mcg incremental dose with a 10 minute lockout and no basal rate.

Adverse Effects
Sedation, respiratory depression, nausea, and vomiting

Nursing Considerations
Assess for respiratory depression; naloxone should be available as an antidote. Implement safety measures as appropriate, including use of side rails and assistance with ambulation; continue use of nonpharmacologic pain relief measures. Because of its short duration of action, frequent dosing will be necessary when given intravenously. Maximum total dose for labor is usually 500 to 600 mcg.

Data from Anderson, D. (2011). A review of systemic opioids commonly used for labor pain relief. *Journal of Midwifery & Women's Health, 56*, 222–239; Hawkins, J.L. & Bucklin, B.A. (2017). Obstetric anesthesia. In S. G. Gabbe, J. R. Niebyl, J. L. Simpson, et al. (Eds.), *Obstetrics: Normal and problem pregnancies* (7th ed.). Philadelphia, PA: Elsevier.

practice of giving lower doses of opioids intravenously has reduced the incidence and severity of opioid-induced CNS depression. **Opioid (narcotic) antagonists** such as naloxone (Narcan) can promptly reverse the CNS depressant effects, especially respiratory depression, in most situations. As stated earlier, however, naloxone cannot reverse the effects of normeperidine, an active metabolite of meperidine. In addition, the antagonist counters the effect of the stress-induced levels of endorphins. An opioid antagonist is especially valuable if labor is more rapid than expected and birth occurs when the opioid is at its peak effect. The antagonist may be given intravenously, or it can be administered intramuscularly (see Medication Guide: Naloxone Hydrochloride [Narcan]). The woman should be told that the pain that was relieved with the use of the opioid analgesic will return with the administration of the opioid antagonist.

MEDICATION ALERT

An opioid antagonist (e.g., naloxone [Narcan]) is contraindicated for opioid-dependent women because it may precipitate abstinence syndrome (withdrawal symptoms). For the same reason, opioid agonist-antagonist analgesics such as nalbuphine (Nubain) should not be given to opioid-dependent women (see Box 14.5).

Nerve Block Analgesia and Anesthesia

Several different methods, referred to as *neuraxial analgesic and anesthetic techniques,* are used in obstetrics to produce sensory blockade and various

MEDICATION GUIDE
Remifentanil Hydrochloride (Ultiva)

Classification
Opioid agonist analgesic

Action
Fast-onset, short-acting synthetic opioid with no active metabolites. Has a rapid onset of action (approximately 1 minute). Because of its very short half-life (only 3 minutes), remifentanil should be administered only by PCA pump.

Indication
Moderate to severe first-stage labor pain

Dosage and Route
PCA Pump (Sample setting, as the ideal dosing regimen has not been determined): 0.5 mcg/kg every 2 to 3 minutes with no basal rate

Adverse Effects
Sedation and hypoventilation with oxygen desaturations

Nursing Considerations
Close maternal monitoring (suggested 1 : 1 nurse/patient ratio) and continuous oxygen saturation monitoring are required. Administer through a dedicated intravenous line. Implement safety measures as appropriate; continue use of nonpharmacologic pain relief measures. Can be given to patients with impaired renal or hepatic function.

Data from Burke, C. (2014). Pain in labor: Nonpharmacologic and pharmacologic management. In K.R. Simpson & P. Creehan (Eds.), *AWHONN's perinatal nursing* (4th ed.). Philadelphia, PA: Lippincott Williams & Wilkins; Hawkins, J.L. & Bucklin, B.A. (2017). Obstetric anesthesia. In S. G. Gabbe, J. R. Niebyl, J. L. Simpson, et al. (Eds.), *Obstetrics: Normal and problem pregnancies* (7th ed.). Philadelphia, PA: Elsevier.

BOX 14.5   Signs of Potential Complications: Maternal Opioid Abstinence Syndrome (Opioid/Narcotic Withdrawal)

- Yawning, rhinorrhea (runny nose), sweating, lacrimation (tearing), mydriasis (dilation of pupils)
- Anorexia
- Irritability, restlessness, generalized anxiety
- Tremors
- Chills and hot flashes
- Piloerection ("gooseflesh" or "chill bumps")
- Violent sneezing
- Weakness, fatigue, and drowsiness
- Nausea and vomiting
- Diarrhea, abdominal cramps
- Bone and muscle pain, muscle spasms, kicking movements

MEDICATION GUIDE
Nalbuphine Hydrochloride (Nubain)

Classification
Opioid agonist-antagonist analgesic

Action
Mixed agonist-antagonist analgesic that stimulates kappa opioid receptors and blocks or weakly stimulates mu opioid receptors, resulting in good analgesia but with less respiratory depression and nausea and vomiting when compared with opioid agonist analgesics. Nalbuphine's analgesic effect is similar to morphine, on a milligram-to-milligram basis. Produces a maternal ceiling effect on pain relief and respiratory depression after 30 mg of the drug has been administered. Duration of action is 2 to 4 hours when given intravenously and 4 to 6 hours when given intramuscularly.

Indication
Moderate to severe labor pain and postoperative pain after cesarean birth

Dosage and Route
IV: 5 to 10 mg every 3 hours as needed
IM: 10 mg every 3 hours as needed

Adverse Effects
Sedation, drowsiness, nausea, vomiting, dizziness, respiratory depression, temporary absent or minimal fetal heart rate (FHR) variability

Nursing Considerations
May precipitate withdrawal symptoms in opioid-dependent women and their newborns. Assess maternal vital signs, degree of pain, FHR, and uterine activity before and after administration. Observe for maternal respiratory depression, notifying obstetric health care provider if maternal respirations are ≤12 breaths per minute. Encourage voiding every 2 hours, and palpate for bladder distention. If birth occurs within 1 to 4 hours of dose administration, observe newborn for respiratory depression. Implement safety measures as appropriate, including use of side rails and assistance with ambulation. Continue use of nonpharmacologic pain relief measures.

Data from Anderson, D. (2011). A review of systemic opioids commonly used for labor pain relief. *Journal of Midwifery & Women's Health, 56,* 222–239; Hawkins, J.L. & Bucklin, B.A. (2017). Obstetric anesthesia. In S. G. Gabbe, J. R. Niebyl, J. L. Simpson, et al. (Eds.), *Obstetrics: Normal and problem pregnancies* (7th ed.). Philadelphia, PA: Elsevier.

chloroprocaine (Nesacaine), and lidocaine (Xylocaine). Rarely, people are sensitive (allergic) to one or more local anesthetics. Such a reaction may include respiratory depression, hypotension, and other serious adverse effects. Epinephrine, antihistamines, oxygen, and supportive measures should reverse these effects. Administering minute amounts of the drug to test for an allergic reaction may identify sensitivity.

Local Perineal Infiltration Anesthesia

Local perineal infiltration anesthesia may be used when an episiotomy is to be performed or when lacerations must be sutured after birth in a woman who does not have regional anesthesia. Rapid anesthesia is produced by injecting approximately 10 to 20 mL of 1% lidocaine or 2% chloroprocaine into the skin and then subcutaneously into the region to be anesthetized. Epinephrine often is added to the solution to localize and intensify the effect of the anesthesia in a region and to prevent excessive bleeding and systemic absorption by constricting local blood vessels. Injections can be repeated to keep the woman comfortable while postbirth repairs are completed.

degrees of motor blockade over a specific region of the body (Hawkins & Bucklin, 2017). A variety of local anesthetic agents are used in these techniques to produce **regional analgesia** (some pain relief and motor block) and **regional anesthesia** (complete pain relief and motor block). Most of these agents are related chemically to cocaine and end with the suffix *-caine*. This helps identify a local anesthetic.

The principal pharmacologic effect of local anesthetics is the temporary interruption of the conduction of nerve impulses, notably pain. Examples of common agents given are bupivacaine (Marcaine),

MEDICATION GUIDE

Naloxone Hydrochloride (Narcan)

Classification
Opioid antagonist

Action
Blocks both mu and kappa opioid receptors from the effects of opioid agonists

Indication
Reverses opioid-induced respiratory depression in woman or newborn; may be used to reverse pruritus from epidural opioids

Dosage and Route
Adult
Opioid overdose: 0.4 to 2 mg IV, may repeat IV at 2- to 3-minute intervals until a maximum of 10 mg has been given; if IV route unavailable, IM or subcutaneous administration may be used

Newborn
Although naloxone has been used in newborns, there is insufficient evidence to evaluate the safety and efficacy of this practice. Animal studies and case reports have raised concerns about complications from naloxone, including pulmonary edema, cardiac arrest, and seizures.

Adverse Effects
Maternal hypotension or hypertension, tachycardia, hyperventilation, nausea and vomiting, sweating, and tremulousness

Nursing Considerations
The woman should delay breastfeeding until medication is out of her system (approximately 2 hours after the last dose is given). Do not give to the woman or the newborn if the woman is opioid dependent—may cause abrupt withdrawal in the woman and newborn. If given to the woman for reversal of respiratory depression caused by opioid analgesic, pain will return suddenly. The duration of action of naloxone is shorter than that of most opioids. Therefore, the woman must be monitored closely for the return of opioid depression when the effects of naloxone are gone. Additional doses of naloxone may be necessary to maintain reversal.

Data on newborn administration from American Academy of Pediatrics & American Heart Association. (2016). *Textbook of neonatal resuscitation,* 7th ed. Elk Grove Village, IL: Author.

Pudendal Nerve Block

Pudendal nerve block, administered late in the second stage of labor, is useful if an episiotomy is to be performed or if forceps or a vacuum extractor are to be used to facilitate birth. It can also be administered during the third stage of labor if an episiotomy or lacerations must be repaired (American Academy of Pediatrics [AAP] & ACOG, 2012). A pudendal nerve block is considered to be reasonably effective for pain relief, simple to perform, and very safe (Cunningham et al., 2014; Hawkins & Bucklin, 2017). Although a pudendal nerve block does not relieve the pain from uterine contractions, it does relieve pain in the lower vagina, the vulva, and the perineum (Fig. 14.8, *A*). A pudendal nerve block should be administered 10 to 20 minutes before perineal anesthesia is needed.

The pudendal nerve traverses the sacrosciatic notch just medial to the tip of the ischial spine on each side. Injection of an anesthetic solution at or near these points anesthetizes the pudendal nerves peripherally (Fig. 14.9). The transvaginal approach is generally used because it is less painful for the woman, has a higher rate of success in

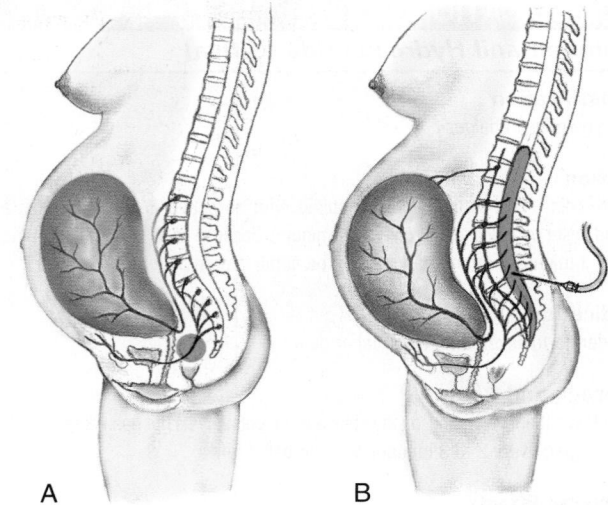

FIG 14.8 Pain pathways and sites of pharmacologic nerve blocks. **A,** Pudendal nerve block: suitable during second and third stages of labor and for repair of episiotomy or lacerations. **B,** Epidural block: suitable for all stages of labor and types of birth and for repair of episiotomy and lacerations.

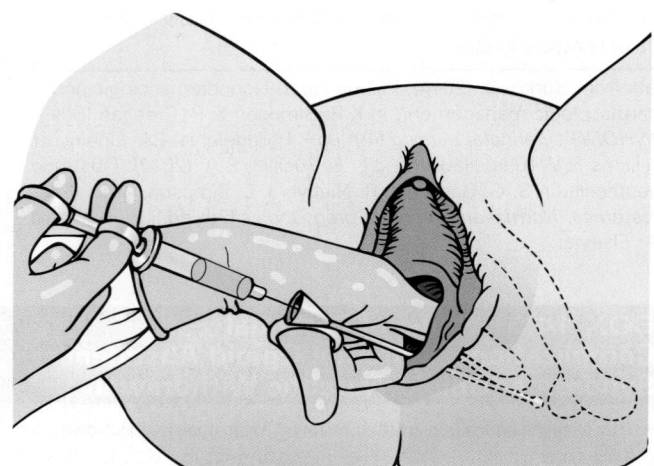

FIG 14.9 Pudendal nerve block. Use of introducer (needle guide) and Luer-Lok syringe to inject medication.

blocking pain, and tends to cause fewer fetal complications. Pudendal block does not change maternal hemodynamic or respiratory functions, vital signs, or the FHR. However, the bearing-down reflex is lessened or lost completely.

Spinal Anesthesia

In spinal anesthesia (block), an anesthetic solution containing a local anesthetic alone or in combination with an opioid agonist analgesic is injected through the third, fourth, or fifth lumbar interspace into the subarachnoid space (Fig. 14.10, *A* and *B*), where the anesthetic solution mixes with cerebrospinal fluid (CSF). Low spinal anesthesia (block) may be used for vaginal birth, but it is not suitable for labor. Spinal anesthesia (block) used for cesarean birth provides anesthesia from the nipple (T6) to the feet. If it is used for vaginal birth, the anesthesia level is from the hips (T10) to the feet (see Fig. 14.10, *C*).

For spinal anesthesia (block), the woman sits or lies on her side (e.g., modified Sims' position) with back curved to widen the intervertebral space; this position facilitates insertion of a small-gauge spinal

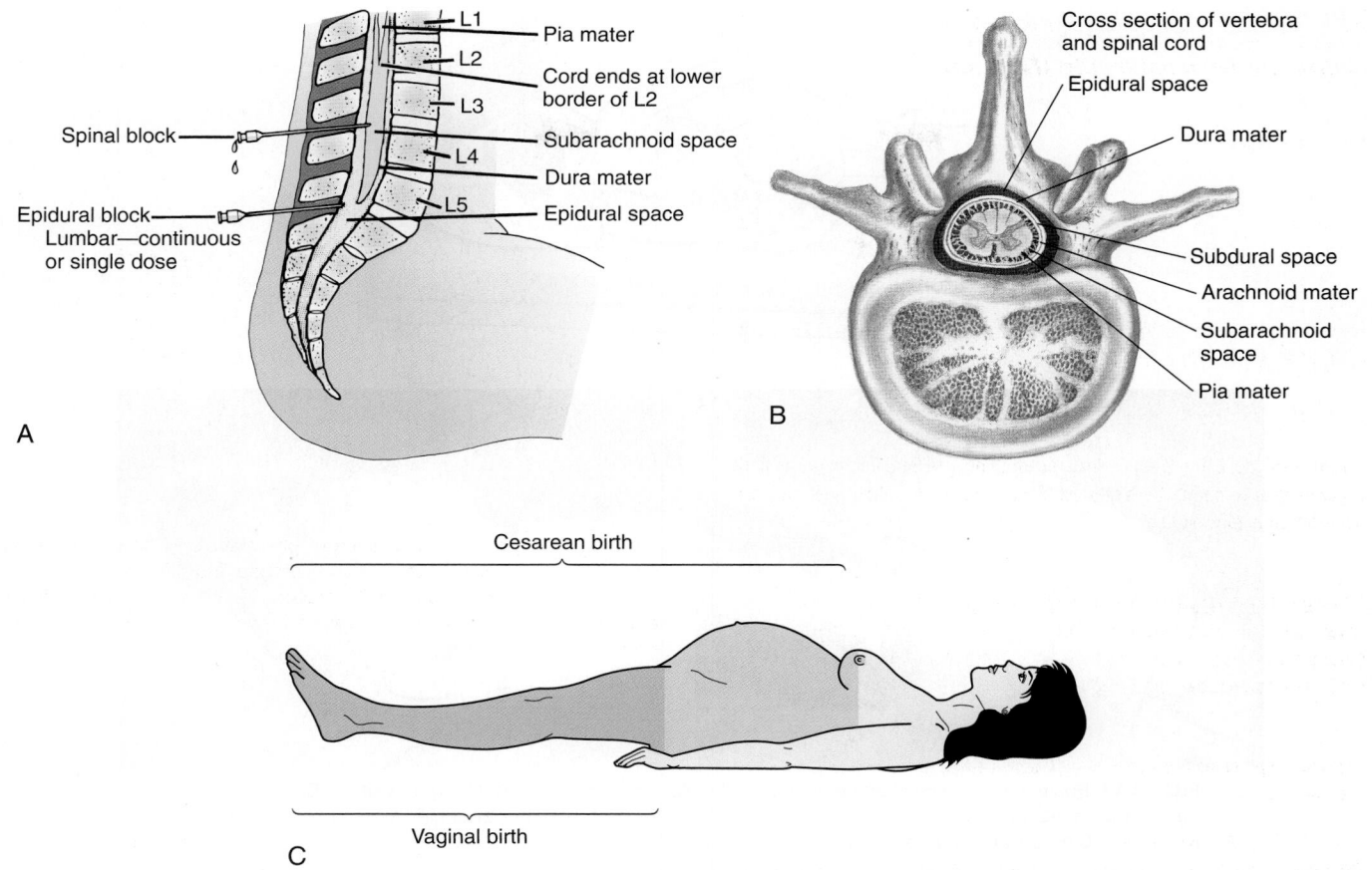

FIG 14.10 A, Membranes and spaces of spinal cord and levels of sacral, lumbar, and thoracic nerves. **B,** Cross-section of vertebra and spinal cord. **C,** Level of anesthesia necessary for cesarean birth and for vaginal birth.

needle and injection of the anesthetic solution into the spinal canal (Fig. 14.11). The nurse supports the woman and encourages her to use breathing and relaxation techniques because she must remain still during the placement of the spinal needle. The needle is inserted and the anesthetic injected between contractions. After the anesthetic solution has been injected, the woman may be positioned upright to allow the anesthetic solution to flow downward to obtain the lower level of anesthesia suitable for a vaginal birth. To obtain the higher level of anesthesia desired for cesarean birth, she will be positioned supine with head and shoulders slightly elevated. To prevent supine hypotensive syndrome, the uterus is displaced laterally by tilting the operating table or placing a wedge under one of her hips. Usually the level of the block will be complete and fixed within 5 to 10 minutes after the anesthetic solution is injected, but it can continue to creep upward for 20 minutes or longer. The anesthetic effect will last 1 to 3 hours, depending on the type and amount of agent used.

⚡ SAFETY ALERT

To reduce the risk for transmission of pathogens, the woman's back is cleansed before the procedure. Before the induction of spinal and epidural anesthesia or analgesia, the anesthesia care provider removes jewelry and washes hands; during the procedure he or she wears sterile gloves and a fresh face mask (Hawkins & Bucklin, 2017). Also, spinal or epidural anesthesia or analgesia should not be initiated if the woman has a tattoo at the site where the needle would be inserted.

Marked hypotension, impaired placental perfusion, and an ineffective breathing pattern may occur during spinal anesthesia. Before induction of the spinal anesthetic, maternal vital signs are assessed and a 20- to 30-minute electronic fetal monitoring (EFM) strip is obtained and evaluated. In addition, the woman's fluid balance is assessed. A bolus of IV fluid (usually 500 to 1000 mL of lactated Ringer's or normal saline solution) may be administered 15 to 30 minutes before induction of the anesthetic to decrease the potential for hypotension caused by sympathetic blockade (vasodilation with pooling of blood in the lower extremities decreases cardiac output). The practice guidelines published by the American Society of Anesthesiologists in 2016 state that IV fluid preloading may be used to reduce the frequency of maternal hypotension after spinal anesthesia for cesarean birth. However, the initiation of spinal anesthesia should not be delayed in order to deliver a fixed volume of fluid (American Society of Anesthesiologists Task Force on Obstetric Anesthesia & Society for Obstetric Anesthesia and Perinatology, 2016). Fluid that is used for the bolus should not contain dextrose, which could contribute to neonatal hypoglycemia (Hawkins & Bucklin, 2017).

After administration of the anesthetic, maternal blood pressure, pulse, and respirations and FHR and pattern must be assessed and documented every 5 to 10 minutes. If signs of serious maternal hypotension (e.g., a drop in systolic blood pressure to 100 mm Hg or less or below 20% of the baseline blood pressure) or fetal distress (e.g., bradycardia, minimal or absent variability, late decelerations) develop, emergency care must be given (Burke, 2014) (see the Emergency Treatment box: Maternal Hypotension with Decreased Placental Perfusion).

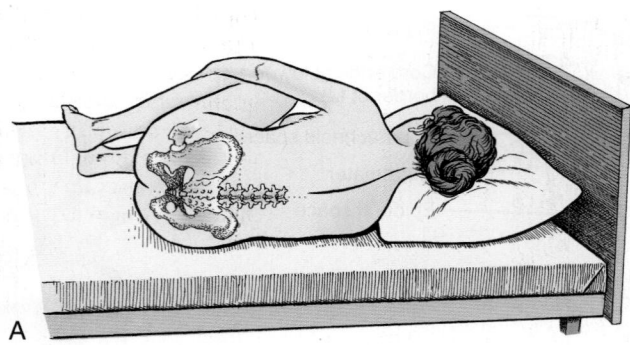

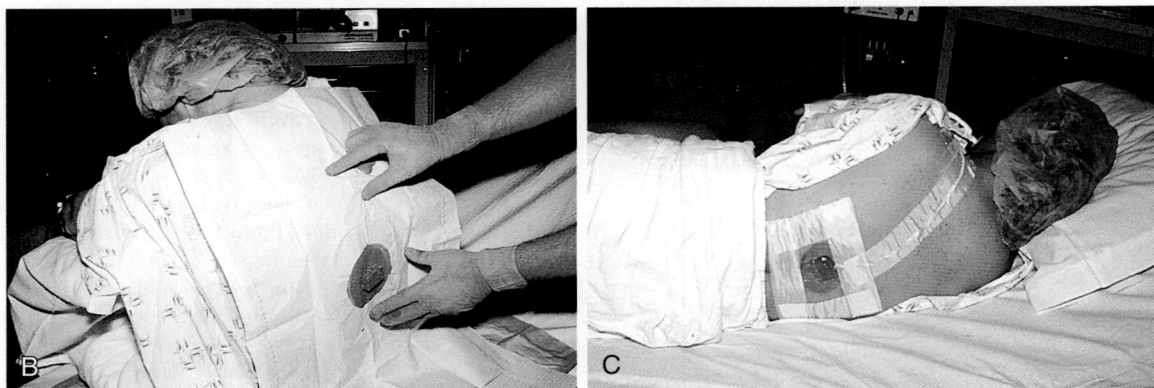

FIG 14.11 Positioning for spinal and epidural blocks. **A,** Lateral position. **B,** Upright position. **C,** Catheter for epidural is taped to woman's back with port segment located near her shoulder. (B and C, Courtesy of Michael S. Clement, MD, Mesa, AZ.)

Because the woman is unable to sense her contractions, she must be instructed when to bear down during a vaginal birth. Using a combination of a local anesthetic agent and an opioid reduces the degree of motor function loss, enhancing a woman's ability to push effectively. If the birth occurs in a delivery room (rather than a labor-delivery-recovery room), the woman will need assistance in the transfer to a recovery bed after expulsion of the placenta and perineal repair if required.

Advantages of spinal anesthesia include ease of administration and absence of fetal hypoxia with maintenance of maternal blood pressure within a normal range. Maternal consciousness is maintained, excellent muscular relaxation is achieved, and blood loss is not excessive.

Disadvantages of spinal anesthesia include possible medication reactions (e.g., allergy), hypotension, and an ineffective breathing pattern; cardiopulmonary resuscitation may be needed. When a spinal anesthetic is given, the need for operative birth (e.g., episiotomy, forceps-assisted birth, or vacuum-assisted birth) tends to increase because voluntary expulsive efforts are reduced or eliminated. After birth, the incidence of bladder and uterine atony, as well as postdural puncture headache (PDPH), is higher.

Leakage of CSF from the site of puncture of the dura mater (membranous covering of the spinal cord) is thought to be the major causative factor in PDPH, commonly referred to as a *spinal headache*. Spinal headache is much more likely to occur when the dura is accidentally punctured during the process of administering an epidural block. The needle used for an epidural block has a much larger gauge than the one used for spinal anesthesia and thus creates a bigger opening in the dura, resulting in a greater loss of CSF (i.e., "wet tap"). Presumably, postural changes cause the diminished volume of CSF to exert traction on pain-sensitive CNS structures. Characteristically, assuming an upright position triggers or intensifies the headache whereas assuming a supine

✚ EMERGENCY TREATMENT

Maternal Hypotension With Decreased Placental Perfusion

Signs and Symptoms

Maternal hypotension (20% decrease from preblock baseline level or ≤100 mm Hg systolic)

Fetal bradycardia

Absent or minimal FHR variability

Interventions

Turn woman to lateral position, or place pillow or wedge under hip to displace uterus

Maintain intravenous (IV) infusion at rate specified, or increase administration per hospital protocol

Administer oxygen by nonrebreather face mask at 10 to 12 L/minute or per protocol.

Elevate the woman's legs.

Notify the primary health care provider, anesthesiologist, or nurse anesthetist.

Administer IV vasopressor (e.g., ephedrine 5 to 10 mg or phenylephrine 50 to 100 mcg) per protocol if previous measures are ineffective.

Remain with woman; continue to monitor maternal blood pressure and fetal heart rate (FHR) every 5 minutes until her condition is stable or per primary health care provider's order.

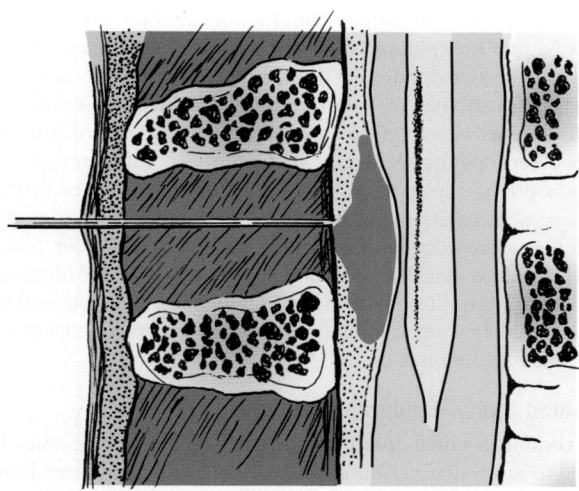

FIG 14.12 Blood-patch therapy for spinal headache.

position achieves relief (Hawkins & Bucklin, 2017). The resulting headache, auditory problems (e.g., tinnitus), and visual problems (e.g., blurred vision, photophobia) begin within 2 days of the puncture and may persist for days or weeks.

The likelihood of headache after dural puncture can be reduced if the anesthesia care provider uses a small-gauge pencil-point spinal needle. Passing an epidural catheter through the dural opening at the time of puncture to provide continuous spinal anesthesia, with removal of the catheter 24 hours later, may help prevent spinal headache. Hydration and bed rest in the prone position have been recommended as preventive measures but have proven to be of little value (Hawkins & Bucklin, 2017).

Conservative management for a PDPH includes administration of oral analgesics and methylxanthines (e.g., caffeine). Methylxanthines cause constriction of cerebral blood vessels and may provide symptomatic relief. An autologous epidural blood patch is the most rapid, reliable, and beneficial relief measure for PDPH. The woman's blood (i.e., 20 mL) is injected slowly into the lumbar epidural space, creating a clot that patches the tear or hole in the dura mater. Treatment with a blood patch is considered if the headache is severe or debilitating or does not resolve after conservative management. The blood patch is remarkably effective and is nearly complication free (Hawkins & Bucklin, 2017) (Fig. 14.12).

The woman should be observed for alteration in vital signs, pallor, clammy skin, and leakage of CSF for 1 hour after the blood patch is performed. If no complications occur, she may then resume normal activity. She should, however, be instructed to avoid coughing or straining for the first day after the blood patch (Hawkins & Bucklin, 2017).

Epidural Anesthesia or Analgesia (Block)

Relief from the pain of uterine contractions and birth (vaginal and cesarean) can be achieved by injecting a suitable local anesthetic agent (e.g., bupivacaine, ropivacaine), an opioid analgesic (e.g., fentanyl, sufentanil), or both into the epidural (peridural) space. Injection is made between the fourth and fifth lumbar vertebrae for a lumbar epidural block (see Figs. 14.8, *B*, and 14.10, *A*). Depending on the type, amount, and number of medications used, an anesthetic or analgesic effect will occur with varying degrees of motor impairment. The combination of an opioid with the local anesthetic agent reduces the dose of anesthetic required, thereby preserving a greater degree of motor function.

Epidural anesthesia and analgesia is the most effective pharmacologic pain relief method for labor that is available. As a result, it is used by the majority of women in the United States (Hawkins & Bucklin, 2017).

For relieving the discomfort of labor and vaginal birth, a block from T10 to S5 is required. For cesarean birth, a block from at least T8 to S1 is essential. The diffusion of epidural anesthesia depends on the location of the catheter tip, the dose and volume of the anesthetic agent used, and the woman's position (e.g., horizontal or head-up). The woman must cooperate and maintain her position without moving during the insertion of the epidural catheter to prevent misplacement, neurologic injury, or hematoma formation.

> ### ! NURSING ALERT
> Epidural anesthesia effectively relieves the pain caused by uterine contractions. For most women, however, it does not completely remove the pressure sensations that occur as the fetus descends in the pelvis.

For the induction of an epidural block, the woman is positioned as for a spinal block. She may sit with her back curved or assume a modified Sims' position with her shoulders parallel, legs slightly flexed, and back arched. It is important to avoid severe spinal flexion because it could compress the epidural space, increasing the risk for dural puncture (Burke, 2014) (see Fig. 14.11). A large-bore (16-, 17-, or 18-gauge) needle is inserted into the epidural space. A catheter is then threaded through the needle until its tip rests in the epidural space. The needle is then removed, and the catheter is taped in place. After the epidural catheter is inserted and secured, a small amount of medication, called a *test dose*, is injected to be sure that the catheter has not been accidentally placed in the subarachnoid (spinal) space or in a blood vessel (Hawkins & Bucklin, 2017).

Initiating neuraxial anesthesia may be difficult when the woman is obese. Early initiation may be considered, both for comfort and to decrease oxygen consumption in labor (Baird, Kennedy, & Dalton, 2017). Catheter placement can present technical challenges, however. The woman may find it harder to assume a position necessary for catheter placement. In addition, excess adipose tissue can obscure the anatomic landmarks used to identify the location of the appropriate insertion site. Up to three-fourths of women weighing more than 300 pounds may require more than one attempt at catheter placement, and there is a high risk for placement failure. Although inserted in the correct location, the catheter may later become dislodged with movement. Early initiation of neuraxial anesthesia may reduce potential problems associated with intubation during an emergent cesarean birth, since obese women are at risk for airway complications (Baird et al.). Note that epidural anesthesia presents less risk for the obese woman than does general anesthesia (AAP & ACOG, 2012).

After the epidural has been initiated, the woman is positioned preferably on her side; this is done so that the uterus does not compress the ascending vena cava and descending aorta, which can impair venous return, reduce cardiac output and blood pressure, and decrease placental perfusion. Her position should be alternated from side to side every hour. Upright positions and ambulation may be possible, depending on the degree of motor impairment. Oxygen should be available if hypotension occurs despite maintenance of hydration with IV fluid and displacement of the uterus to the side. Ephedrine or phenylephrine (vasopressors used to increase maternal blood pressure) and increased IV fluid infusion may be needed (see Emergency Treatment box: Maternal Hypotension with Decreased Placental Perfusion). The FHR and pattern, contraction pattern, and progress in labor must be monitored carefully because the woman may not be aware of changes in the strength of the uterine contractions or the descent of the presenting part.

Several methods can be used for an epidural block. An intermittent block is achieved by using repeated injections of anesthetic solution; it is the least common method. The most common method is the continuous block, achieved by using a pump to infuse the anesthetic solution

BOX 14.6 Side Effects of Neuraxial Anesthesia

- Hypotension
- Local anesthetic toxicity
  - Lightheadedness
  - Dizziness
  - Tinnitus (ringing in the ears)
  - Metallic taste
  - Numbness of the tongue and mouth
  - Bizarre behavior
  - Slurred speech
  - Convulsions
  - Loss of consciousness
- Fever
- Urinary retention
- Pruritus (itching)
- Limited movement
- Longer second-stage labor
- Increased use of oxytocin
- Increased likelihood of forceps- or vacuum-assisted birth
- High or total spinal anesthesia

through an indwelling plastic catheter. Patient-controlled epidural analgesia (PCEA) is another method; it uses an indwelling catheter and a programmed pump that allows the woman to control the dosing. PCEA has been found to provide optimal analgesia with higher maternal satisfaction and enhanced sense of control during labor while decreasing the total amount of medication, including local anesthetic, used (Capogna & Stirparo, 2013).

The advantages of an epidural block are numerous:

- The woman remains alert and is more comfortable and able to participate.
- Good relaxation is achieved.
- Airway reflexes remain intact.
- Only partial motor paralysis develops.
- Gastric emptying is not delayed.
- Blood loss is not excessive.

Fetal complications are rare but may occur in the event of rapid absorption of the medication or marked maternal hypotension. The dose, volume, type, and number of medications used can be modified (1) to allow the woman to push, to assume upright positions, and even to walk; (2) to produce perineal anesthesia; and (3) to permit forceps-assisted, vacuum-assisted, or cesarean birth if required.

The disadvantages of epidural block also are numerous. The woman's ability to move freely and to maintain control of her labor is limited, related to the use of numerous medical interventions (e.g., an intravenous infusion and electronic monitoring) and the occurrence of orthostatic hypotension and dizziness, sedation, and weakness of the legs. CNS effects (Box 14.6) can occur if a solution containing a local anesthetic agent is accidentally injected into a blood vessel or if excessive amounts of local anesthetic are given. High spinal or "total spinal" anesthesia, resulting in respiratory arrest, can occur if the relatively high dosage used with an epidural block is accidentally injected into the subarachnoid space. Women who receive an epidural have a higher rate of fever (i.e., intrapartum temperature of 38° C [100.4° F] or higher), especially when labor lasts longer than 12 hours; the temperature elevation most likely is related to thermoregulatory changes, although infection cannot be ruled out. The elevation in temperature can result in fetal tachycardia and neonatal workup for sepsis, whether or not signs of infection are present (see Box 14.6).

Hypotension as a result of sympathetic blockade can occur in about 10% to 30% of women who receive regional (spinal or epidural) analgesia during labor (Witcher & McLendon, 2013) (see Emergency Treatment box: Maternal Hypotension with Decreased Placental Perfusion). Hypotension can result in a significant decrease in uteroplacental perfusion and oxygen delivery to the fetus. Urinary retention and stress incontinence can occur in the immediate postpartum period. This

temporary difficulty in urinary elimination could be related not only to the effects of the epidural block and the need for catheterization but also to the increased duration of labor and need for forceps- or vacuum-assisted birth associated with the block. Pruritus (itching) is a side effect that often occurs with the use of an opioid, especially fentanyl. A relationship between epidural analgesia and longer second-stage labor and increased use of oxytocin and forceps- or vacuum-assisted birth has been documented (Cunningham et al., 2014; Hawkins & Bucklin, 2017). Epidural analgesia does not, however, increase the risk for cesarean birth (Hawkins & Bucklin). For some women, the epidural block is not effective and a second form of analgesia is required to establish effective pain relief. When women progress rapidly in labor, pain relief may not be obtained before birth occurs.

Combined Spinal-Epidural Analgesia

In the combined spinal-epidural (CSE) analgesia technique, sometimes referred to as a *walking epidural*, an epidural needle is inserted into the epidural space. Before the epidural catheter is placed, a smaller-gauge spinal needle is inserted through the bore of the epidural needle into the subarachnoid space. A small amount of opioid or combination of opioid and local anesthetic is then injected intrathecally to rapidly provide analgesia. Afterward the epidural catheter is inserted as usual. The CSE technique is an increasingly popular approach that can be used to block pain transmission without compromising motor ability. The concentration of opioid receptors is high along the pain pathway in the spinal cord, in the brainstem, and in the thalamus. Because these receptors are highly sensitive to opioids, a small quantity of an opioid agonist analgesic produces marked pain relief lasting for several hours. If additional pain relief is needed, medication can be injected through the epidural catheter (see Fig. 14.10, *A*). The most common side effects of opioids administered intrathecally are pruritus and nausea, which are usually mild and easily treated (Hawkins & Bucklin, 2017). CSE analgesia is also associated with a greater incidence of FHR abnormalities than is epidural analgesia alone, necessitating close assessment of FHR and pattern (Cunningham et al, 2014).

Although women can walk (hence the term *walking epidural*), they often choose not to do so because of sedation and fatigue, abnormal sensations in and weakness of the legs, and a feeling of insecurity. Often health care providers are reluctant to encourage or assist women to ambulate for fear of injury. However, women can be assisted to change positions and use upright positions during labor and birth.

Epidural and Intrathecal (Spinal) Opioids

Opioids also can be used alone, eliminating the effect of a local anesthetic altogether. The use of epidural or intrathecal opioids without the addition of a local anesthetic agent during labor has several advantages. Opioids administered in this manner do not cause maternal hypotension or affect vital signs. The woman feels contractions but not pain. Her ability to bear down during the second stage of labor is preserved because the pushing reflex is not lost and her motor power remains intact.

Fentanyl, sufentanil, or preservative-free morphine can be used. Fentanyl and sufentanil produce short-acting analgesia (i.e., 1.5 to 3.5 hours), and morphine can provide pain relief for 4 to 7 hours. Morphine can be combined with fentanyl or sufentanil. Using short-acting opioids with multiparous women and morphine with nulliparous women or women with a history of long labors is appropriate. Because opioids alone usually do not provide adequate analgesia, however, they are most often given in combination with a local anesthetic (Cunningham et al., 2014).

A more common indication for the administration of epidural or intrathecal analgesics is for the relief of postoperative pain. For example, a woman who gives birth by cesarean can receive fentanyl or morphine through a catheter. The catheter can then be removed, and the woman is usually free from pain for 24 hours. Occasionally the catheter is left in place in the epidural space in case another dose is needed.

Women receiving epidurally administered morphine after a cesarean birth can ambulate sooner than women who do not. The early ambulation and freedom from pain also facilitate bladder emptying, enhance peristalsis, and prevent clot formation (e.g., thrombophlebitis) in the lower extremities. Women may require additional medication for breakthrough pain during the first 24 hours after surgery. If so, they will usually be given an NSAID such as ketorolac (Toradol), indomethacin (Indocin), or ibuprofen (Motrin) rather than an opioid.

Side effects of opioids administered by the epidural and intrathecal routes include nausea, vomiting, diminished peristalsis, pruritus, urinary retention, and delayed respiratory depression. These effects are more common when morphine is administered. Antiemetics, antipruritics, and opioid antagonists are used to relieve these symptoms. For example, naloxone or metoclopramide may be administered. Hospital protocols or detailed physician orders should provide specific instructions for the treatment of these side effects. Use of epidural opioids is not without risk. Respiratory depression is a serious concern; for this reason the woman's respiratory status should be assessed and documented every hour for 24 hours or as designated by hospital protocol.

> **! NURSING ALERT**
>
> Naloxone should be readily available for use if the respiratory rate decreases to less than 10 breaths per minute or if the oxygen saturation rate decreases to less than 89%. Administration of oxygen by nonrebreather facemask also can be initiated, and the anesthesia care provider should be notified.

Contraindications to Subarachnoid (Spinal) and Epidural Blocks

Contraindications to spinal and epidural analgesia (Burke, 2014; Cunningham et al., 2014; Hawkins & Bucklin, 2017) include the following:

- Active or anticipated serious maternal hemorrhage. Acute hypovolemia leads to increased sympathetic tone to maintain the blood pressure. Any anesthetic technique that blocks the sympathetic fibers can produce significant hypotension that can endanger the mother and fetus.
- Maternal hypotension.
- Coagulopathy. If a woman is receiving anticoagulant therapy (e.g., last dose of low–molecular weight heparin within 12 hours) or has a bleeding disorder, injury to a blood vessel may cause the formation of a hematoma that may compress the cauda equina or the spinal cord and lead to serious CNS complications.
- Infection at the needle insertion site. Infection can be spread through the peridural or subarachnoid spaces if the needle traverses an infected area.
- Increased intracranial pressure caused by a mass lesion.
- Allergy to the anesthetic drug.
- Maternal refusal or inability to cooperate.
- Some types of maternal cardiac conditions.

Epidural Block Effects on Newborn

Analgesia or anesthesia during labor and birth has little or no lasting effect on the physiologic status of the newborn. There is no evidence that the administration of maternal analgesic or anesthetic agents during labor and birth has a significant effect on the child's later mental and neurologic development (AAP & ACOG, 2012).

Nitrous Oxide for Analgesia

Nitrous oxide, commonly called *laughing gas,* is an inhaled anesthetic gas. It was used more widely for labor analgesia in the United States in the past but never as extensively as in other countries. Recently, however, interest in using nitrous oxide during labor has increased in the United States.

Nitrous oxide is administered in a 50:50 mix with oxygen using a blender device and a mask held by the woman. Women report that nitrous oxide does not completely relieve pain but reduces their perception of pain. It causes a feeling of euphoria and decreases anxiety.

The main side effects of nitrous oxide are nausea and dizziness. Nitrous oxide is safe for both mother and fetus and does not affect uterine activity. Other advantages of nitrous oxide use include rapid onset of action, quick clearance through exhalation without accumulation in maternal or fetal tissues, and the fact that the woman can self-administer the gas while remaining awake, alert, and completely able to function. Nitrous oxide can also be used during short, painful intrapartum procedures such as perineal repair and manual removal of the placenta (Collins, 2017; Hawkins & Bucklin, 2017).

A face mask is used to self-administer the gas. The woman places the mask over her mouth and nose as soon as a contraction begins. The nurse teaches the woman how to correctly position the face mask to create a seal. When the woman inhales, a valve opens and the gas is released. When inhalation stops, the valve closes, which prevents accidental overdosing. The woman is the *only* person allowed to hold the mask. Special equipment collects the woman's exhalations to protect health care workers from repetitive occupational exposure to nitrous oxide (Collins, 2017; Hawkins & Bucklin, 2017; Rooks, 2012).

General Anesthesia

General anesthesia rarely is used for uncomplicated vaginal birth. It is used for only about 10% of cesarean births in the United States (Hawkins & Bucklin, 2017). General anesthesia may be necessary if a spinal or epidural block is contraindicated or if circumstances necessitate rapid birth (vaginal or emergent cesarean) without sufficient time or available personnel to perform a regional block (Witcher & McLendon, 2013). In addition, being awake and aware during major surgery may be unacceptable for some women having a cesarean birth. The major risks associated with general anesthesia are difficulty with or inability to intubate and aspiration of gastric contents (Cunningham et al., 2014; Hawkins & Bucklin, 2017). Anesthesia care providers are more likely to encounter difficulty with intubating morbidly obese patients, especially in an emergency situation, than women of normal weight (Witcher & McLendon).

If general anesthesia is being considered, an IV infusion is started using an 18-gauge catheter, and the woman is given nothing by mouth. If time allows, the woman is premedicated with a nonparticulate (clear) oral antacid (e.g., sodium citrate/citric acid [Bicitra]) to neutralize the acidic contents of the stomach. Aspiration of highly acidic gastric contents will damage lung tissue. Some anesthesia care providers also order the administration of a histamine (H_2)-receptor blocker such as famotidine (Pepcid) or ranitidine (Zantac) to decrease the production of gastric acid and metoclopramide (Reglan) to accelerate gastric emptying (Cunningham et al., 2014; Hawkins & Bucklin, 2017). Before the anesthesia is given, a wedge should be placed under one of the woman's hips to displace the uterus. Uterine displacement prevents compression of the aorta and vena cava, which maintains cardiac output and placental perfusion (Cunningham et al.; Hawkins & Bucklin).

Prior to anesthesia induction, the woman is preoxygenated with 100% oxygen by nonrebreather facemask for 2 to 3 minutes. This is especially important in pregnant women, who are more likely than other adults to rapidly become hypoxemic if there is a delay in successful intubation. Next, propofol (Diprivan), etomidate (Amidate), or ketamine (Ketalar) is administered intravenously to induce anesthesia by rendering the woman unconscious (Cunningham et al., 2014). After

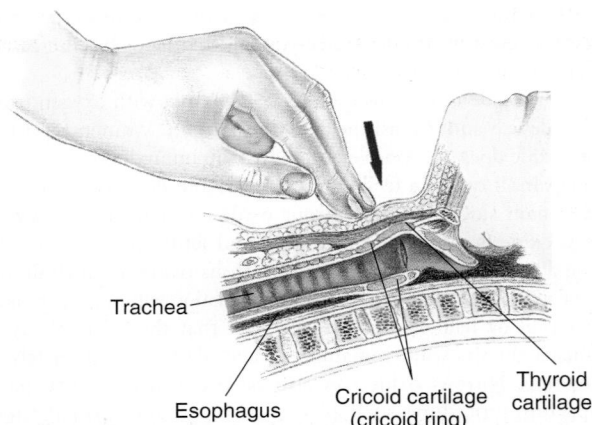

FIG 14.13 Technique of applying pressure on cricoid cartilage to occlude esophagus to prevent aspiration of gastric contents during induction of general anesthesia.

that, succinylcholine (Anectine), a muscle relaxer, is administered to facilitate passage of an endotracheal tube (Cunningham et al. 2014; Hawkins & Bucklin, 2017). Sometimes the nurse is asked to assist with applying cricoid pressure before intubation as the woman begins to lose consciousness. This maneuver blocks the esophagus and prevents aspiration should the woman vomit or regurgitate (Fig. 14.13). Pressure is released once the endotracheal tube is securely in place.

After the woman is intubated, nitrous oxide and oxygen in a 50:50 mixture are administered. A low concentration of a volatile halogenated agent (e.g., isoflurane) also may be administered to increase pain relief and to reduce maternal awareness and recall (Cunningham et al., 2014; Hawkins & Bucklin, 2017). In low concentrations, these agents do not relax the uterus, so bleeding should not increase because of their use (Hawkins & Bucklin). In higher concentrations, isoflurane or methoxyflurane relax the uterus quickly and facilitate intrauterine manipulation, version, and extraction. However, at higher concentrations, these agents cross the placenta readily and can produce narcosis in the fetus and could reduce uterine tone after birth, increasing the risk for hemorrhage. Because of the risk for neonatal narcosis, it is critical that the baby is delivered as soon as possible after inducing anesthesia to reduce the degree of fetal exposure to the anesthetic agents and the CNS depressants administered to the mother.

Priorities for post anesthesia care are to maintain an open airway and cardiopulmonary function and to prevent postpartum hemorrhage. Women who had surgery under general anesthesia will require pain medication soon after regaining consciousness. Routine postpartum care is organized to facilitate parent-infant attachment as soon as possible and to answer the mother's questions. When appropriate, the nurse assesses the mother's readiness to see her baby, as well as her response to the anesthesia and to the event that necessitated general anesthesia (e.g., emergency cesarean birth when vaginal birth was anticipated).

❙ CARE MANAGEMENT

PAIN ASSESSMENT DURING LABOR AND BIRTH

A pain scale, in which 0 represents no pain and 10 represents pain as bad as it could possibly be, is often used to evaluate a woman's pain before and after pain relief interventions are implemented. Comparing the woman's answers provides a way to objectively evaluate the effectiveness of pain relief interventions. Sometimes a coping scale, rather than a pain scale, is used to evaluate how well the woman is dealing with the discomfort of labor.

The choice of pain relief interventions depends on a combination of factors, including the woman's special needs and wishes, the availability of the desired method or methods, the knowledge and expertise in nonpharmacologic and pharmacologic methods of the health care providers involved in the woman's care, and the stage and phase of labor.

NONPHARMACOLOGIC INTERVENTIONS

The nurse supports and assists the woman as she uses nonpharmacologic interventions for pain relief and relaxation. During labor, the nurse evaluates the effectiveness of the specific pain management techniques used. Appropriate interventions can then be planned or continued for effective care, such as trying other nonpharmacologic methods or combining nonpharmacologic methods with medications (see Nursing Care Plan: Nonpharmacologic Pain Management).

PHARMACOLOGIC INTERVENTIONS

Informed Consent

Pregnant women have the right to be active participants in determining the best pain management approach to use during labor and birth. The obstetric care provider and anesthesia care provider are responsible for fully informing women of the alternative methods of pharmacologic pain relief available in the birth setting. A description of the various anesthetic techniques and what they entail is essential to informed consent, even if the woman received information about analgesia and anesthesia earlier in her pregnancy. The initial discussion of pain management options ideally should take place in the third trimester so the woman has time to consider alternatives. Nurses play a part in the informed consent by clarifying and describing procedures or by acting as the woman's advocate and asking the primary health care provider for further explanations. The three essential components of an informed consent are as follows:

- First, the procedure and its advantages and disadvantages must be thoroughly explained.
- Second, the woman must agree with the plan of labor pain management as explained to her.
- Third, her consent must be given freely without coercion or manipulation from her health care provider.

LEGAL TIP **Informed Consent for Anesthesia**   The woman receives (in an understandable manner) the following:

- Explanation of available methods of anesthesia and analgesia
- Description of the anesthetic, including its effects and the procedure for its administration
- Description of the benefits, discomforts, risks, and consequences for the mother, the fetus, and the newborn
- Explanation of how complications can be treated
- Information that the anesthetic is not always effective
- Indication that the woman may withdraw consent at any time
- Opportunity to have any questions answered
- Opportunity to have components of the consent explained in the woman's own words

The consent form will:

- Be written or explained in the woman's primary language
- Have the woman's signature
- Have the date of consent
- Carry the signature of the anesthetic care provider, certifying that the woman has received and expresses understanding of the explanation

Case Study

Brenda is a 35-year-old married woman who is pregnant for the third time (3-1-0-1-1). She has a 4-year-old daughter at home, had a miscarriage at about 3 months gestation 2 years ago, and is now at term and in the labor room in early labor. She describes her first labor as very traumatic. She had planned to labor with no analgesia but instead had an epidural, which resulted in hypotension and an abnormal fetal heart rate (FHR) tracing late in labor. Brenda says she does not want to repeat that experience during this labor and birth. She attended hypnobirthing classes and plans to have no medications during this labor. Her husband is very supportive and effectively coaches her through contractions.

Assessment

What can the nurses do to help Brenda achieve her goal of having no medications during labor? How can the nurses facilitate parental attachment to the newborn?

Defining Characteristics

Responds appropriately to the onset of labor
Is proactive in labor and birth
Uses relaxation techniques appropriate for stage of labor
Demonstrates attachment behavior to the newborn
Uses support systems appropriately

Nursing Diagnosis

Readiness for Enhanced Childbearing Process related to desire for healthy outcome of labor and birth

Expected Outcomes

Brenda and her husband will convey confidence and knowledge of pregnancy, the labor and birth process, and newborn care.
Brenda will express appropriate self-control and readily cooperate with recommendations of the health care team during labor and birth.
Brenda will express satisfaction with her performance during labor and birth.
After birth, parent-newborn attachment will be evident.
Newborn's physical, social, and nutritional needs will be met.

Nursing Interventions	Rationales
Assess Brenda's satisfaction with the amount of assistance the nurse is currently offering.	To determine whether Brenda perceives herself as performing her physical, psychosocial, and spiritual activities at a level that is comfortable for her
Discuss Brenda's birth plan and knowledge about the birth process.	To collect data for nursing plan of care
Provide information about the labor process.	To correct any misconceptions
Inform Brenda about her labor status and the well-being of the fetus.	To promote comfort and confidence
Discuss rationales for all interventions.	To incorporate Brenda into plan of care
Incorporate nonpharmacologic interventions into plan of care.	To increase Brenda's sense of control during labor
Provide emotional support and ongoing positive feedback.	To enhance positive coping mechanisms

Case Study (Continued)

Brenda is now 7 cm dilated, has received no analgesic medications, and is working very hard to deal with the contractions. She expresses concern that she will not be able to continue to labor without pharmacologic interventions and is asking what she can do to deal with the increasing intensity of the contractions. She is adamant that she does not want medication but acknowledges that she needs help. She is becoming increasingly restless and anxious.

Assessment

What nonpharmacologic measures can the nurses offer Brenda to help her cope with the contractions? What support can her husband provide?

Defining Characteristics

Expresses desire to enhance comfort
Expresses desire to enhance feeling of contentment
Expresses desire to enhance relaxation
Expresses desire to enhance resolution of complaints

Nursing Diagnosis

Anxiety related to lack of confidence in ability to cope effectively with pain during labor

Expected Outcomes

Brenda will express a decrease in anxiety and will experience satisfaction with her labor and birth performance.
With the help of the nurses, Brenda will develop plans to optimize level of comfort using nonpharmacologic measures.
Brenda will experience physical and psychologic ease as the measures are implemented.
Brenda will report an increase in relaxation as she receives support and encouragement from her husband and the nurses.

Nursing Interventions	Rationales
Since Brenda and her husband attended childbirth classes, review with them what they learned.	To plan supportive strategies that address couple's specific needs
Encourage Brenda's husband to remain with her while she is in labor.	To provide support and increase probability of positive response to comfort measures
Review or teach nonpharmacologic techniques available to decrease anxiety and pain during labor (e.g., focusing, relaxation and breathing techniques, effleurage, and sacral pressure).	To enhance chances of success in using techniques
Explore other techniques that Brenda or her husband may have learned in childbirth classes (e.g., hypnosis, hydrotherapy, acupressure, biofeedback, therapeutic touch, aromatherapy, imagery, music).	To provide more options for coping strategies
Explore use of transcutaneous electrical nerve stimulation if ordered by primary health care provider.	To provide increased perception of control over pain and increase in release of endogenous opioids (endorphins)
Assist Brenda to change positions and to use pillows.	To reduce stiffness, aid circulation, and promote comfort
Assess bladder for distention, and encourage voiding often.	To avoid bladder distention, subsequent discomfort, and potential for suppression of uterine contractions
Encourage rest between contractions.	To conserve energy and minimize fatigue
Keep Brenda and her husband informed about progress.	To allay anxiety
Guide couple through labor stages and phases, helping them use and modify comfort techniques that are appropriate to each phase.	To ensure greatest effectiveness of techniques used
Support couple if pharmacologic measures are required to increase pain relief, explaining safety and effectiveness.	To reduce anxiety and maintain self-esteem and sense of control over labor process

Timing of Administration

Nonpharmacologic measures can be used to relieve pain and stress and enhance progress at any time during labor.

It is often the nurse who notifies the primary health care provider that the woman is in need of pharmacologic measures to relieve her pain and discomfort. Orders are often written for the administration of pain medication as needed by the woman and based on the nurse's clinical judgment. In the past, pharmacologic measures for pain relief were usually not implemented until cervical dilation reached approximately 4 to 5 cm, to avoid suppressing the progress of labor. However, it is now known that epidural anesthesia in early labor does not increase the rate of cesarean birth. Whereas it may shorten the duration of first-stage labor in some women, epidural anesthesia lengthens it in others (Hawkins & Bucklin, 2017). It is no longer recommended that women in labor reach a certain level of cervical dilation or fetal station before receiving epidural anesthesia (AAP & ACOG, 2012; Cunningham et al., 2014). It is, however, still recommended that the administration of systemic opioid analgesics be delayed until labor is well established (Burke, 2014).

Preparation for Procedures

The methods of pain relief available to the woman are reviewed and information is clarified as necessary. The procedure and what will be expected of the woman (e.g., to maintain a flexed position during insertion of epidural needle) must be explained.

The woman also can benefit from knowing the way that the medication is to be given, the interval before the medication takes effect, and the expected pain relief from the medication. Skin-preparation measures are described, and an explanation is given for the need to empty the bladder before the analgesic or anesthetic is administered and the reason for keeping the bladder empty. When an indwelling catheter is to be threaded into the epidural space, the woman should be told that she may have a momentary twinge down her leg, hip, or back and that this feeling is not a sign of injury.

Administration of Medication

Accurate monitoring of the progress of labor forms the basis for the nurse's judgment that a woman needs pharmacologic control of pain. Knowledge of the medications used during childbirth is essential. The most effective route of administration is selected for each woman; then the medication is prepared and administered correctly.

Any medication can cause a minor or severe allergic reaction. As part of the assessment for such allergic reactions, the nurse should monitor the woman's vital signs, respiratory effort, cardiovascular status, integument, and platelet and white blood cell count. The woman is observed for side effects of drug therapy, especially drowsiness and dyspnea. Minor reactions can consist of rash, rhinitis, fever, shortness of breath, or pruritus. Management of the less acute allergic response is not an emergency.

Severe allergic reactions (anaphylaxis) may occur suddenly and lead to shock or death. The most dramatic form of anaphylaxis is sudden, severe bronchospasm, upper airway obstruction, and hypotension (Norred, 2012). Signs of anaphylaxis are largely caused by contraction of smooth muscles and may begin with irritability, extreme weakness, nausea, and vomiting. This may lead to dyspnea, cyanosis, convulsions, and cardiac arrest. Anaphylaxis must be diagnosed and treated immediately. Initial treatment usually consists of placing the woman in a supine position, injecting epinephrine intramuscularly, administering fluid intravenously, supporting the airway with ventilation if necessary, and giving oxygen. If the response to these measures is inadequate, intravenous epinephrine should be given (Norred). Cardiopulmonary resuscitation may be necessary (see Chapter 12).

Intravenous Route

The preferred route of administration of medications such as meperidine, fentanyl, remifentanil, or nalbuphine is through IV tubing, administered into the port nearest the point of insertion of the infusion (proximal port). The medication is given slowly, in small amounts, during a contraction. It may be given over a period of three to five consecutive contractions if needed to complete the dose. It is given during contractions to decrease fetal exposure to the medication because uterine blood vessels are constricted during contractions and the medication stays within the maternal vascular system for several seconds before the uterine blood vessels reopen. The IV infusion is then restarted slowly to prevent a bolus of medication from being administered. With this method of injection, the amount of medication crossing the placenta to the fetus is minimized. With decreased placental transfer, the mother's degree of pain relief is maximized. The IV route has the following advantages:
- Onset of pain relief is rapid and more predictable.
- Pain relief is obtained with small doses of the drug.
- Duration of effect is more predictable.

Intramuscular Route

Although analgesics are still sometimes given IM, it is not the preferred route of administration for the woman in labor. The advantages of using the IM route are quick administration and no need to start an IV line.

Disadvantages of the IM route include the following:
- Onset of pain relief is delayed.
- Higher doses of medication are required.
- Medication is released at an unpredictable rate from the muscle tissue and is available for transfer across the placenta to the fetus.

The maternal medication levels (after IM injections) are unequal because of uneven distribution (maternal uptake) and metabolism. IM injections given in the upper arm (deltoid muscle) seem to result in more rapid absorption and higher blood levels of the medication than when administered in other sites (Bricker & Lavender, 2002). If neuraxial anesthesia is planned later in labor, the deltoid muscle is the preferred site. The autonomic blockade from the neuraxial anesthesia increases blood flow to the gluteal region and accelerates absorption of medication that may be sequestered there. Administration of opioids subcutaneously in the upper arm avoids this risk and, as a result, is often used as an alternative to IM injection.

Regional (Epidural or Spinal) Anesthesia

According to professional standards (Association of Women's Health, Obstetric and Neonatal Nurses [AWHONN], 2015):

The nonanesthetist registered nurse is permitted to do the following:
- Monitor the status of the woman receiving regional anesthesia, the fetus, and the progress of labor
- Replace empty infusion syringes or bags with the same medication and concentration
- Stop the infusion if there is a safety concern or the woman has given birth
- Remove the catheter if properly educated to do so
- Initiate emergency measures if the need arises
- Communicate clinical assessments and changes in patient status to obstetric and anesthesia care providers

Only qualified, licensed anesthesia care providers should perform the following procedures:
- Insertion, initial injection, bolus injection, rebolus injection, or initiation of a continuous infusion of catheters for analgesia and anesthesia
- Preparation and programming the medication and infusion devices
- Verification of correct catheter placement
- Increasing or decreasing the rate of a continuous infusion and program doses for PCEA administration

> ⚡ **SAFETY ALERT**
>
> Safe regional or neuraxial anesthesia administration requires specialized education, experience, and competence. There is potential for significant maternal and/or fetal morbidity and mortality associated with some obstetric anesthesia complications. Therefore a licensed, credentialed anesthesia care provider should manage neuraxial anesthesia and analgesia during labor and birth and be readily available to manage obstetric anesthesia-related emergencies (AWHONN, 2015).

Because spinal nerve blocks can reduce bladder sensation, resulting in difficulty voiding, the woman should empty her bladder before the induction of the block and should be encouraged to void at least every 2 hours thereafter. The nurse should palpate for bladder distention and measure urinary output to ensure that the bladder is being completely emptied. A distended bladder can inhibit uterine contractions and fetal descent, resulting in a slowing of the progress of labor. For this reason, an indwelling urinary (Foley) catheter is often routinely inserted immediately after epidural or spinal anesthesia is initiated and left in place for the remainder of the first stage of labor.

The status of the maternal-fetal unit and the progress of labor must be established before the block is initiated. The nurse must assist the woman to assume and maintain the correct position for induction of epidural and spinal anesthesia (see Fig. 14.11, *A* and *B*).

Depending on the level of motor blockade, the woman should be assisted to remain as mobile as possible. When in bed, her position should be alternated from side to side every hour to ensure adequate distribution of the anesthetic solution and to maintain circulation to the uterus and placenta.

> ⚡ **SAFETY ALERT**
>
> After receiving a neuraxial block or opioid intravenously for pain, the woman should not be allowed to ambulate alone. She must either remain in bed or request assistance before attempting to get out of bed. The nurse assesses the woman for signs of orthostatic hypotension and return of sensation and motor function of the lower extremities prior to ambulation.

Health care providers should be aware that effective epidural anesthesia prolongs the second stage of labor by 15 to 30 minutes. A delay in the second stage of labor does not negatively affect maternal or fetal outcome, however, as long as the FHR tracing is normal, maternal hydration and analgesia are adequate, and there is ongoing progress in the descent of the fetal head. Therefore operative interventions (e.g., the use of forceps or vacuum) to hasten the birth solely because the second stage is prolonged are unnecessary. Reducing the density of the epidural block during the second stage of labor, delaying pushing until the woman feels the urge to do so, and avoiding arbitrary definitions for the "normal" duration of second-stage labor are suggested as interventions to decrease the risk for operative vaginal birth (Hawkins & Bucklin, 2017) (see Chapter 16 for a full discussion of second-stage labor management). Box 14.7 summarizes the nursing interventions for women receiving epidural or spinal anesthesia.

BOX 14.7   Nursing Interventions for the Woman Receiving Neuraxial Anesthesia

Prior to the Block
- Assist obstetric care provider and/or anesthesia care provider with explaining the procedure and obtaining the woman's informed consent.
- Assess maternal vital signs, level of hydration, labor progress, and fetal heart rate (FHR) and pattern.
- Start an intravenous (IV) line, and infuse a bolus of fluid (lactated Ringer's solution or normal saline) if ordered (e.g., 500 to 1000 mL 15 to 30 minutes before induction of the anesthesia).
- Obtain laboratory results (hematocrit or hemoglobin level, other tests as ordered).
- Assess the woman's level of pain using a pain scale (from 0 [no pain] to 10 [pain as bad as it could possibly be]).
- Assist the woman to void.

During Initiation of the Block
- Assist the woman to assume and maintain the proper position.
- Verbally guide the woman through the procedure, explaining sounds and sensations as she experiences them.
- Assist the anesthesia care provider with documentation of vital signs, time and amount of medications given, etc.
- Monitor maternal vital signs (especially blood pressure) and FHR as ordered.
- Have oxygen and suction readily available.
- Monitor for signs of local anesthetic toxicity (see Box 14.6) as the test dose of medication is administered.

While the Block Is in Effect
- Continue to monitor maternal vital signs and FHR as ordered (continuous monitoring of maternal heart rate [electrocardiogram (ECG)] and blood pressure may be ordered to monitor for accidental intravenous injection of medication).
- Continue to assess the woman's level of pain with every check of vital signs using a pain scale (from 0 [no pain] to 10 [pain as bad as it could possibly be]).
- Monitor for bladder distention:
  - Assist with spontaneous voiding on bedpan or toilet.
  - Insert a urinary catheter if necessary.
- Encourage or assist the woman to change positions from side to side every hour.
- Promote safety:
  - Keep the side rails up on the bed.
  - Place the telephone and call light within easy reach.
  - Instruct the woman not to get out of bed without help.
  - Make sure there is no prolonged pressure on anesthetized body parts.
- Keep the epidural catheter insertion site clean and dry.
- Continue to monitor for anesthetic side effects (see Box 14.6).

While the Block Is Wearing Off After Birth
- Assess regularly for the return of sensory and motor function.
- Continue to monitor maternal vital signs as ordered.
- Monitor for bladder distention:
  - Assist with spontaneous voiding on bedpan or toilet.
  - Insert a urinary catheter if necessary.
- Promote safety:
  - Keep the side rails up on the bed.
  - Place the telephone and call light within easy reach.
  - Instruct the woman not to get out of bed without help.
  - Make sure there is no prolonged pressure on anesthetized body parts.
- Keep the epidural catheter insertion site clean and dry.
- Continue to monitor for anesthetic side effects (see Box 14.6).

SAFETY AND GENERAL CARE

The nurse monitors and records the woman's response to nonpharmacologic pain relief methods and to medication(s). This includes the degree of pain relief, the level of apprehension, the return of sensations and perception of pain, and allergic or adverse reactions (e.g., hypotension, respiratory depression, fever, pruritus, and nausea and vomiting). The nurse continues to monitor maternal vital signs and FHR and pattern at frequent intervals, the strength and frequency of uterine contractions, changes in the cervix and station of the presenting part, the presence and quality of the bearing-down reflex, bladder filling, and state of hydration. Determining the fetal response after administration of analgesia or anesthesia is vital. The woman is asked if she, her partner, or other support people have any questions. The nurse also assesses the woman's and her support people's understanding of the need for ensuring her safety (e.g., keeping side rails up, calling for assistance as needed).

The time that elapses between the administration of an opioid and the baby's birth is documented. Medications given to the newborn to reverse opioid effects are recorded. After birth, the woman who has had spinal, epidural, or general anesthesia is assessed for return of sensory and motor function in addition to the usual postpartum assessments. Both the nurse and the anesthesia provider are responsible for documenting assessments and care in relation to neuraxial (epidural or spinal) anesthesia.

REFERENCES

American Academy of Pediatrics & American College of Obstetricians and Gynecologists. (2012). *Guidelines for perinatal care* (7th ed.). Washington, DC: American College of Obstetricians and Gynecologists.

American College of Obstetricians and Gynecologists. (2016). Committee opinion no. 679. Immersion in water during labor and delivery. *Obstetrics & Gynecology, 128*(5), e231–e236.

American College of Obstetricians and Gynecologists. (2004, reaffirmed 2015). Committee opinion no. 295. Pain relief during labor. *Obstetrics & Gynecology, 104*(1), 213.

American Society of Anesthesiologists Task Force on Obstetric Anesthesia & Society for Obstetric Anesthesia and Perinatology. (2016). Practice guidelines for obstetric anesthesia: An updated report. *Anesthesiology, 124*(2), 270–300.

Anderson, D. (2011). A review of systemic opioids commonly used for labor pain relief. *Journal of Midwifery & Women's Health, 56*(3), 222–239.

Archie, C. L., & Roman, A. S. (2013). Normal & abnormal labor & delivery. In A. H. DeCherney, L. Nathan, N. Laufer, & A. S. Roman (Eds.), *Current diagnosis & treatment: Obstetrics & gynecology* (11th ed.). New York, NY: The McGraw-Hill Companies, Inc.

Arendt, K. W., & Tessmer-Tuck, J. A. (2013). Nonpharmacologic labor analgesia. *Clinics in Perinatology, 40*(3), 351–371.

Association of Women's Health, Obstetric and Neonatal Nurses. (2015). Role of the registered nurse in the care of the pregnant woman receiving analgesia and anesthesia by catheter techniques. *Journal of Obstetric, Gynecologic, & Neonatal Nursing, 44*(1), 151–154.

Baird, S. M., Kennedy, B. B., & Dalton, J. (2017). Special considerations for individualized care of the laboring woman. In B. B. Kennedy & S. M. Baird (Eds.), *Intrapartum management modules: A perinatal education program* (5th ed.). Philadelphia, PA: Wolters Kluwer.

Barragán Loayza, I., Solà, I., & Juandó Prats, C. (2011). Biofeedback for pain management during labour. *Cochrane Database of Systematic Reviews, 2011*(6), CD006168.

Blackburn, S. (2013). *Maternal, fetal, and neonatal physiology: A clinical perspective* (4th ed.). Maryland Heights, MO: Saunders.

Borders, N., Wendland, C., Haozous, E., et al. (2013). Midwives' verbal support of nulliparous women in second-stage labor. *Journal of Obstetric, Gynecologic, & Neonatal Nursing, 42*(3), 311–320.

Bovbjerg, M. L., Cheyney, M., & Everson, C. (2016). Maternal and newborn outcomes following waterbirth: The Midwives Alliance of North America statistics project, 2004 to 2009 cohort. *Journal of Midwifery & Women's Health, 61*(1), 11–20.

Bricker, L., & Lavender, T. (2002). Parenteral opioids for labor pain relief: A systematic review. *American Journal of Obstetrics and Gynecology, 86* (5 suppl), S94–S109.

Brickhouse, B., Isaacs, C., Batten, M., & Price, A. (2015). Strategies for providing low-cost water immersion therapy with limited resources. *Nursing for Women's Health, 19*(6), 526–532.

Burke, C. (2014). Pain in labor: Nonpharmacologic and pharmacologic management. In K. R. Simpson & P. Creehan (Eds.), *AWHONN's perinatal nursing* (4th ed.). Philadelphia, PA: Lippincott Willliams & Wilkins.

Callister, L. C. (2014). Integrating cultural beliefs and practices when caring for childbearing women and families. In K. R. Simpson & P. Creehan (Eds.), *AWHONN's perinatal nursing* (4th ed.). Philadelphia, PA: Lippincott Willliams & Wilkins.

Capogna, G., & Stirparo, S. (2013). Techniques for the maintenance of epidural labor analgesia. *Current Opinion in Anaesthesiology, 26*(3), 261–267.

Collins, M. R. (2017). Pain in labor and nonpharmacologic modes of relief. In B. B. Kennedy & S. M. Baird (Eds.), *Intrapartum management modules: A perinatal education program* (5th ed.). Philadelphia, PA: Wolters Kluwer.

Cunningham, F., Leveno, K., Bloom, S., et al. (2014). *Williams obstetrics* (24th ed.). New York, NY: McGraw-Hill Education.

Dean, B. J. F., Gwilym, S. E., & Carr, A. J. (2013). Why does my shoulder hurt? A review of the neuroanatomical and biochemical basis of shoulder pain. *British Journal of Sports Medicine, 47*(7), 1095–1104.

Declercq, E. R., Sakala, C., Corry, M. P., et al. (2013). *Listening to mothers III: Pregnancy and birth*. New York, NY: Childbirth Connection.

Declercq, E. R., Sakala, C., Corry, M. P., et al. (2002). *Listening to mothers: Report of the first national U.S. survey of women's childbearing experiences*. New York, NY: Maternity Center Association.

Gisin, M., Poat, A., Fierz, K., & Frei, I. (2013). Women's experiences of acupuncture during labour. *British Journal of Midwifery, 21*(4), 254–262.

Hawkins, J. L. & Bucklin, B. A. (2017). Obstetric anesthesia. In S. G. Gabbe, J. R. Niebyl, J. L. Simpson, et al. (Eds.), *Obstetrics: Normal and problem pregnancies* (7th ed.). Philadelphia, PA: Elsevier.

Hodnett, E. D., Gates, S., Hofmeyr, G., & Sakala, C. (2013). Continuous support for women during childbirth. *Cochrane Database of Systematic Reviews, 2013*(7), CD003766.

Jones, L., Othman, M., Dowswell, T., et al. (2012). Pain management for women in labor: An overview of systematic reviews. *Cochrane Database of Systematic Reviews, 2012*(3), CD009234.

Meyer, S. (2013). Control in childbirth: A concept analysis and synthesis. *Journal of Advanced Nursing, 69*(1), 218–228.

Norred, C. L. (2012). Anesthetic-induced anaphylaxis. *American Association of Nurse Anesthetists Journal, 80*(2), 129–150.

Perinatal Education Associates. (2016). *Breathing*. Retrieved from http://www.birthsource.com/Scripts/article.asp?articleid=211.

Rooks, J. P. (2012). Labor pain management other than neuraxial: What do we know and where do we go next? *Birth, 39*(4), 318–322.

Simpson, K., & O'Brien-Abel, N. (2014). Labor and birth. In K. R. Simpson & P. Creehan (Eds.), *AWHONN's perinatal nursing* (4th ed.). Philadelphia, PA: Lippincott Willliams & Wilkins.

Smith, C. A., Levett, K. M., Collins, C. T., et al. (2012). Massage, reflexology and other manual methods for pain management in labour. *Cochrane Database of Systematic Reviews, 2012*(2), CD009290.

Swart, S. C., & Kelly, F. C. (2017). Pharmacologic management of labor pain. In B. B. Kennedy & S. M. Baird (Eds.), *Intrapartum management modules: A perinatal education program* (5th ed.). Philadelphia, PA: Wolters Kluwer.

Walls, D. (2009). Herbs and natural therapies for pregnancy, birth, and breastfeeding. *International Journal of Childbirth Education, 24*, 29–37.

Witcher, P., & McLendon, K. (2013). Anesthesia emergencies in the obstetric setting. In N. Troiano, C. Harvey, & B. Chez (Eds.), *AWHONN's high risk and critical care obstetrics* (3rd ed.). Philadelphia, PA: Wolters Kluwer/Lippincott Williams & Wilkins.

15

Fetal Assessment During Labor

Kitty Cashion

http://evolve.elsevier.com/Perry/maternal

The ability to assess the fetus by auscultation of the fetal heart was initially described more than 300 years ago. With the advent of the fetoscope and stethoscope after the turn of the twentieth century, the listener could hear clearly enough to count the fetal heart rate (FHR). When electronic FHR monitoring made its debut for clinical use in the early 1970s, the anticipation was that its use would result in less long-term neurologic impairment in the form of cerebral palsy (Miller, 2017). However, research has not been able to show that intrapartum FHR monitoring leads to a significant decrease in neonatal neurologic morbidity (Miller, Miller, & Cypher, 2017).

Still electronic fetal monitoring (EFM) is a useful tool for visualizing FHR and uterine contraction patterns on a monitor screen or printed tracing. A majority of the women who give birth each year in the United States will have EFM during some or all of their labor (Miller et al., 2017). Pregnant women should be informed about the equipment and procedures used and the risks, benefits, and limitations of intermittent auscultation (IA) and EFM. This chapter discusses the basis for intrapartum fetal monitoring, the types of monitoring, and nursing assessment and management of abnormal FHR and uterine contraction patterns.

BASIS FOR MONITORING

FETAL RESPONSE

Because labor is a period of physiologic stress for the fetus, frequent monitoring of fetal status is part of the nursing care during labor. The fetal oxygen supply must be maintained during labor to prevent fetal compromise and promote newborn health after birth. The fetal oxygen supply can decrease in a number of ways:

- Reduction of blood flow through the maternal vessels as a result of maternal hypertension (chronic hypertension, preeclampsia, or gestational hypertension), hypotension (caused by supine maternal position, hemorrhage, or epidural anesthesia), or hypovolemia (caused by hemorrhage)
- Reduction of the oxygen content in the maternal blood as a result of hemorrhage or severe anemia
- Alterations in fetal circulation occurring with compression of the umbilical cord (transient, during uterine contractions [UCs], or prolonged, resulting from cord prolapse), partial placental separation or complete abruption, or head compression (head compression causes increased intracranial pressure and vagal nerve stimulation with an accompanying decrease in FHR)
- Reduction in blood flow to the intervillous space in the placenta secondary to uterine hypertonus (generally caused by excessive exogenous oxytocin) or secondary to deterioration of the placental vasculature associated with maternal disorders such as hypertension or diabetes mellitus

Fetal well-being during labor can be assessed by the response of the FHR to UCs. Since 2008, a group of fetal monitoring experts, including the National Institute for Child Health and Human Development (NICHD), the American College of Obstetricians and Gynecologists (ACOG), and the Society for Maternal Fetal Medicine (SMFM) have recommended that FHR tracings demonstrating certain reassuring characteristics be described as *normal* (category I) (Macones, Hankins, Spong, et al., 2008) (Box 15.1).

UTERINE ACTIVITY

Likewise, uterine activity (UA) can also be identified as normal or abnormal. Table 15.1 describes normal UA during labor.

FETAL COMPROMISE

The goals of intrapartum FHR monitoring are to identify and differentiate the normal (reassuring) patterns from the abnormal (nonreassuring) patterns, which can indicate fetal compromise. Although the 2008 National Institute of Child Health and Human Development workshop (Macones et al., 2008) and ACOG (2009/2015) both recommend use of the terms *normal* and *abnormal* to describe FHR tracings, the terms *reassuring* and *nonreassuring* are still frequently used clinically.

Abnormal FHR patterns are those associated with fetal hypoxemia, which is a deficiency of oxygen in the blood. If uncorrected, hypoxemia can deteriorate to severe fetal hypoxia, an inadequate supply of oxygen at the cellular level that can cause metabolic acidosis. Metabolic acidosis, in turn, can lead to acidemia, or increased hydrogen ion content (decreased pH) in the blood. Metabolic acidemia may be a marker of clinically significant interruption of fetal oxygenation (Miller, 2017). See Box 15.1 for examples of abnormal (category III) FHR tracings.

MONITORING TECHNIQUES

The ideal method of fetal assessment during labor, IA or EFM, continues to be debated (see Evidence-Based Practice box: Fetal Cardiac Assessment During Labor: How Are You Doing In There?). Some clinicians prefer the use of IA in low-risk women because it promotes mobility during labor, may be used with hydrotherapy, and provides a more natural birthing experience (Miller et al., 2017). ACOG (2009/2015) suggests continuous EFM during labor for patients with high-risk conditions because the safety of IA use in high-risk pregnancies remains uncertain.

BOX 15.1 Three-Tier Fetal Heart Rate Classification System

Category I

Category I fetal heart rate (FHR) tracings include all of the following:

- Baseline rate 110 to 160 beats/min
- Baseline FHR variability: Moderate
- Late or variable decelerations: Absent
- Early decelerations: Either present or absent
- Accelerations: Either present or absent

Category II

Category II FHR tracings include all FHR tracings not categorized as category I or category III. Examples of category II tracings include any of the following:

- Baseline rate
  - Bradycardia not accompanied by absent baseline variability
  - Tachycardia
- Baseline FHR variability
  - Minimal baseline variability
  - Absent baseline variability not accompanied by recurrent decelerations
  - Marked baseline variability
- Accelerations
  - No acceleration produced in response to fetal stimulation
- Periodic or episodic decelerations
  - Recurrent variable decelerations accompanied by minimal or moderate baseline variability
  - Prolonged decelerations (≥2 minutes but <10 minutes)
  - Recurrent late decelerations with moderate baseline variability
  - Variable decelerations with other characteristics such as slow return to baseline, "overshoots," or "shoulders"

Category III

Category III FHR tracings include the following:

- Absent baseline variability and any of the following:
  - Recurrent late decelerations
  - Recurrent variable decelerations
  - Bradycardia
- Sinusoidal pattern

Data from Macones,G., Hankins, G., Spong C., et al. (2008). The 2008 National Institute of Child Health and Human Development workshop report on electronic fetal monitoring: Update on definitions, interpretation, and research guidelines. *Journal of Obstetric, Gynecologic, & Neonatal Nursing, 37*(5), 510–515.

The continued reliance on EFM in the United States is most likely because of staffing patterns, staffing mix, and the increased use of defensive practices in a litigious environment (Miller et al.).

INTERMITTENT AUSCULTATION

Intermittent auscultation involves listening to fetal heart sounds at periodic intervals to assess the FHR. IA of the fetal heart can be performed with a Pinard stethoscope (see Fig. 8.7, *C*), Doppler ultrasound (Fig. 15.1, *A*), an ultrasound stethoscope (see Fig. 15.1, *B*), or a DeLee-Hillis fetoscope (see Fig. 15.1, *C*). Doppler ultrasound and ultrasound stethoscopes transmit ultra high–frequency sound waves, reflecting movement of the fetal heart, and convert these sounds into an electronic signal that can be counted. The fetoscope is applied to the listener's forehead because bone conduction amplifies the fetal heart sounds for counting. Box 15.2 describes how to perform IA.

IA is easy to use, inexpensive, and less invasive than EFM. It is often more comfortable for the woman and gives her more freedom of

TABLE 15.1 Normal Uterine Activity During Labor

Characteristic	Description
Frequency	Contraction frequency overall generally ranges from two to five per 10 minutes during labor, with lower frequencies seen in first stage of labor and higher frequencies (up to five contractions in 10 minutes) seen in second stage.
Duration	Contraction duration remains fairly stable throughout first and second stages, ranging from 45–80 seconds, not generally exceeding 90 seconds.
Strength	Uterine contractions generally range from peaking at 40–70 mm Hg in first stage of labor to over 80 mm Hg in second stage. Contractions palpated as "mild" would likely peak at less than 50 mm Hg if measured internally, whereas contractions palpated as "moderate" or "strong" would likely peak at 50 mm Hg or greater if measured internally.
Resting tone	Average resting tone during labor is 10 mm Hg; if using palpation, should palpate as "soft" (i.e., easily indented, no palpable resistance).
Relaxation time	Relaxation time is commonly 60 seconds or more in first stage and 45 seconds or more in second stage.
Montevideo units (MVUs)	MVUs usually range from 100–250 in first stage; may rise to 300–400 in second stage. Contraction intensities of 40 mm Hg or more and MVUs of 80–120 are generally sufficient to initiate spontaneous labor. MVUs are used only with internal monitoring of contractions.

Data from Macones,G., Hankins, G., Spong C., et al. (2008). The 2008 National Institute of Child Health and Human Development workshop report on electronic fetal monitoring: Update on definitions, interpretation, and research guidelines. *Journal of Obstetric, Gynecologic & Neonatal Nurs*ing, *37*(5), 510–515; Miller, L., Miller, D., & Cypher, R. (2017). *Mosby's pocket guide to fetal monitoring: A multidisciplinary approach* (8th ed.). St. Louis, MO: Elsevier.

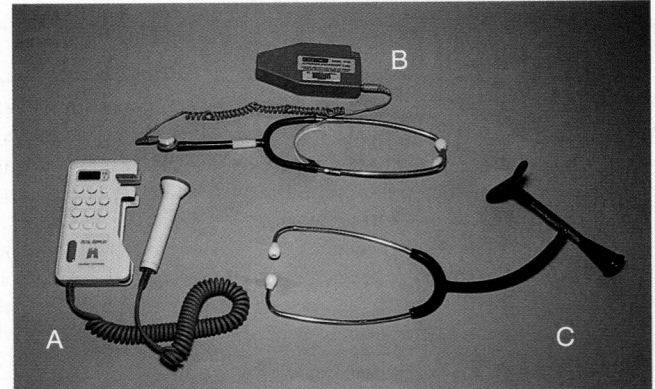

FIG 15.1 A, Ultrasound fetoscope. **B,** Ultrasound stethoscope. **C,** DeLee-Hillis fetoscope. (Courtesy of Michael S. Clement, MD, Mesa, AZ.)

movement. Other care measures such as ambulation and the use of baths or showers are easier to carry out when IA is used. However, it may be difficult to perform transabdominally in women who are obese. A transvaginal fetal Doppler probe is available that provides closer proximity to the uterus, making it easier to auscultate the FHR when the woman is obese or early in gestation (Miller et al., 2017). Because

EVIDENCE-BASED PRACTICE

Fetal Cardiac Assessment During Labor: How Are You Doing In There?

Ask the Question
PICOT Question: For low-risk women, which assessments of fetal cardiac function during labor provide better outcomes?

Search for the Evidence
Search Strategies: English research-based publications on fetal assessment, monitoring, labor, labour, cardiotocography, fetal electrocardiography, auscultation, pulse oximetry, electrocardiogram, scalp pH, scalp lactate were included. Exclusions included preterm, postterm, high risk.

Databases Used: Cochrane Collaborative Database, Joanna Briggs Institute, National Guideline Clearinghouse (AHRQ), CINAHL, PubMed, and the professional websites for AWHONN and SOGC.

Critical Appraisal of the Evidence
Intermittent auscultation utilizes regular assessment of the fetal heart rate using a handheld Doppler device or special stethoscope. It is appropriate and recommended for low-risk women (Lewis, Downe, & FIGO Intrapartum Fetal Monitoring Expert Consensus Panel, 2015).

Electronic fetal monitoring (EFM) uses ultrasound to monitor fetal heartbeats.

- As a tool, EFM has high sensitivity, meaning that the reassuring combined presence of moderate variability and accelerations nearly always mean a well-oxygenated fetus. However, it has a low specificity (many false positives), meaning that suspicious patterns may or may not indicate actual distress (Visser, Ayres-de-Campo, & FIGO Intrapartum Fetal Monitoring Expert Consensus Panel, 2015).
- Fetal electrocardiography (fECG) analyzes fetal heart tracing, on the theory that hypoxia and acidemia would show up as abnormal ECG patterns. Electrodes attach invasively to the fetal scalp, or newer noninvasive models utilize electrodes attached to the maternal abdomen, and can be used concurrently with EFM (Neilson, 2015).
- In all outcomes, fECG plus EFM is not more beneficial than EFM alone (Saccone, Schuit, Amer-Wahlin, et al., 2016). In the presence of maternal obesity, the fECG provides more accurate and reliable fetal monitoring than EFM (Cohen & Hayes-Gill, 2014).
- To address differences between practitioners in EFM interpretation, computer analysis has been developed to alert staff to patterns predictive of hypoxia and acidemia (Visser et al., 2015).

Apply the Evidence: Nursing Implications
- Even though it is not supported by strong evidence of significantly improved outcomes, EFM use is widespread in hospitals for more than a generation. As a screening tool for possible fetal distress, every member of the health care team should have appropriate training and regular updates in its interpretation.
- Overtreatment, such as unnecessary cesarean births, may be a result of fear of litigation, and create additional risks and costs. New evidence of patient

safety with intermittent auscultation should reassure caregivers and low-risk laboring women. Evaluating and communicating the evidence becomes paramount for changing long-term institutional habits.

- For obese patients, fECG offers more accurate fetal assessment than EFM. However, the cost of the single-use fECG electrodes is much greater than EFM, whose transducers are reusable.
- Both scalp fECG and scalp blood sampling require rupture of membranes. If this is not spontaneous, there is debate about the benefits versus risks of artificially rupturing membranes (increased maternal contraction pain, fetal infection, fetal distress). It falls to nurses to maintain perineal hygiene, including minimizing cervical examinations and documenting invasive procedures.

Quality and Safety Competencies: Quality Improvement*
Knowledge
Recognize that nursing and other health professions students are parts of systems of care and care processes that affect outcomes for patients and families.

Nurses can use evidence to advocate for change in institutional habits, such as interventions that lead to overtreatment.

Skills
Seek information about outcomes of care for populations served in care setting

Seek out the highest-level evidence, and demonstrate its relevance to this setting.

Attitudes
Appreciate the value of what individuals and teams can to do to improve care.

Education of the whole health care team will be necessary to improve buy-in for institutional change.

References
Cohen, W. R., & Hayes-Gill, B. (2014). Influence of maternal body mass index on accuracy and reliability of external fetal monitoring techniques. *Obstetricia et Gynecologica Scandinavica, 93*(6), 590–595.

Lewis, D., Downe, S., & F, & International Federation of Gynecology and Obstetrics (FIGO) Intrapartum Fetal Monitoring Expert Consensus Panel. (2015). FIOG consensus guidelines on intrapartum fetal monitoring: Intermittent auscultation. *International Journal of Gynecology & Obstetrics, 131*(1), 9–12.

Neilson, J. P. (2015). Fetal electrocardiogram (ECG) for fetal monitoring during labour. *Cochrane Database of Systematic Reviews, 2015*(5), CD000116.

Saccone, G., Schuit, E., Amer-Wahlin, I., et al. (2016). Electrocardiogram ST analysis during labor: A systemic review and meta-analysis of randomized controlled trials. *Obstetrics & Gynecology, 127*(1), 127–135.

Visser, G. H., Ayres-de-Campo, D., & FIGO Intrapartum Fetal Monitoring Expert Consensus Panel. (2015). FIGO consensus guidelines on intrapartum fetal monitoring: Adjunct technologies. *International Journal of Gynecology & Obstetrics, 131*(1), 25–29.

Pat Mahaffee Gingrich

*Adapted from QSEN at www.qsen.org/.

IA is intermittent, significant events may occur during a time when the FHR is not being auscultated. In addition, IA does not provide a permanent documented visual record of the FHR and cannot be used to assess visual patterns of the FHR variability or periodic changes. When using IA, the nurse can assess the baseline FHR, rhythm, and increases and decreases from baseline (Miller et al.).

There is a lack of literature to recommend the optimal intervals for FHR auscultation during latent- and active-phase labor. Therefore, several professional organizations have provided general guidelines for frequency of assessment for low- and high-risk patients during the

intrapartum period. These organizations include the Association of Women's Health, Obstetric and Neonatal Nurses (AWHONN), The American Academy of Pediatrics (AAP), ACOG, the National Institute for Health and Care Excellence (NICE), and the Society of Obstetricians and Gynaecologists of Canada (SOGC). The suggested frequencies are generally based on protocols reported in research clinical trials in which investigators compared clinical outcomes associated with IA and EFM (AWHONN, 2015a).

AWHONN recommends the following IA frequencies for low-risk women who are not receiving oxytocin: latent phase (<4 cm) at least

BOX 15.2 Procedure for Intermittent Auscultation of the Fetal Heart Rate

1. Perform Leopold's maneuvers by palpating the maternal abdomen to identify fetal presentation and position (see Box 16.5).
2. Apply ultrasonic gel to device if using Doppler ultrasound. Place listening device (see Fig. 15.1) over area of maximal intensity and clarity of fetal heart sounds to obtain clearest and loudest sound, which is easiest to count. This location is usually over the fetal back. If using fetoscope, firm pressure may be needed.
3. Count maternal radial pulse while listening to FHR to differentiate it from fetal rate.
4. Palpate abdomen for presence or absence of UA to count FHR between contractions.
5. Count FHR for 30 to 60 seconds after a uterine contraction to identify auscultated baseline rate and changes (increases or decreases) in it.
6. Auscultate FHR before, during, and after contraction to identify FHR during the contraction or as a response to the contraction and to assess for absence or presence of increases or decreases in FHR.
7. When distinct discrepancies in FHR are noted during listening periods, auscultate for a longer period during, after, and between contractions to identify significant changes that may indicate need for another mode of FHR monitoring.

FHR, Fetal heart rate; *UA,* uterine activity.
From Miller, L., Miller, D., & Cypher, R. (2017). *Mosby's pocket guide to fetal monitoring: A multidisciplinary approach* (8th ed.). St. Louis, MO: Elsevier.

hourly; latent phase (4 to 5 cm) every 15 to 30 minutes; active phase (≥6 cm) every 15 to 30 minutes; second stage, passive fetal descent every 15 minutes; and second stage, active pushing every 5 to 15 minutes (AWHONN, 2015a).

! NURSING ALERT

When the FHR is auscultated and documented, it is inappropriate to use the descriptive terms associated with EFM (e.g., moderate variability, variable deceleration) because most of the terms are visual descriptions of the patterns produced on the monitor tracing. However, terms that are numerically defined such as *bradycardia* and *tachycardia* can be used. When FHR is auscultated, it should be described as a baseline number or range and as having a regular or irregular rhythm. The presence of abrupt or gradual increases or decreases in FHR before, during, and immediately after contractions should also be noted (AWHONN, 2015b; Miller et al., 2017).

Every effort should be made to use the method of fetal assessment the woman desires if possible. However, auscultation of the FHR in accordance with the frequency guidelines suggested earlier may be difficult in today's busy labor and birth units. When used as the primary method of fetal assessment, auscultation requires a one-to-one nurse-to-patient staffing ratio. If acuity and census change so auscultation standards are no longer met, the nurse must inform the physician or nurse-midwife that continuous EFM will be used until staffing can be arranged to meet the standards.

The woman can become anxious if the examiner cannot readily count the fetal heart sounds. It often takes time for the inexperienced listener to locate the heartbeat and find the area of maximal intensity. To allay the mother's concerns, she can be told that the nurse is "finding the spot where the sounds are loudest." If it takes considerable time to locate the fetal heartbeats, the examiner can reassure the mother by offering her an opportunity to listen to them. If the examiner cannot

locate the fetal heartbeat, assistance should be requested. In some cases ultrasound can be used to help locate the fetal heartbeat. Seeing the FHR on the ultrasound screen is reassuring to the mother if there was initial difficulty in locating the best area for auscultation.

When using IA, UA is assessed by palpation. The examiner should keep his or her fingertips placed over the fundus before, during, and after contractions. The contraction intensity is usually described as mild, moderate, or strong. The contraction duration is measured in seconds, from the beginning to the end of the contraction. The frequency of contractions is measured in minutes, from the beginning of one contraction to the beginning of the next. The examiner should keep his or her hand on the fundus after the contraction is over to evaluate uterine resting tone or relaxation between contractions. Resting tone between contractions is usually described as soft or hard (Lyndon, O'Brien-Abel, & Simpson, 2014).

Accurate and complete documentation of fetal status and UA is especially important when IA and palpation are being used because no paper tracing record or computer storage of these assessments is provided as is the case with continuous EFM. Labor flow records or computer charting systems that prompt notations of all assessments are useful for ensuring such comprehensive documentation.

ELECTRONIC FETAL MONITORING

The purpose of EFM is to assess the adequacy of fetal oxygenation during labor. If the monitor demonstrates evidence of interruption, further evaluation can be initiated or interventions implemented to improve fetal oxygenation. If these actions are not successful, the monitor can provide information to assist in making decisions regarding the optimal timing and method of birth to avoid the potential consequences of fetal hypoxia (Miller, 2017). The two modes of EFM are the external mode, which uses external transducers placed on the maternal abdomen to assess FHR and UA, and the internal mode, which uses a spiral electrode applied to the fetal presenting part to assess the FHR and an intrauterine pressure catheter (IUPC) to assess UA and uterine resting tone. The differences between the external and internal modes of EFM are summarized in Table 15.2.

External Monitoring

Separate transducers are used to monitor the FHR and UCs (Fig. 15.2, *A*). The ultrasound transducer works by reflecting high-frequency sound waves off a moving interface, in this case the fetal heart and valves. It is sometimes difficult to reproduce a continuous and precise record of the FHR because of artifact introduced by fetal and maternal movement. Maternal obesity, occiput posterior position of the fetus, and anterior attachment of the placenta can cause weak or absent signals (AWHONN, 2015b). The FHR is printed on specially formatted monitor paper. The standard paper speed used in the United States is 3 cm/min. Once the area of maximal intensity of the FHR has been located, conductive gel is applied to the surface of the ultrasound transducer, and the transducer is then positioned over this area and held securely in place using an elastic belt.

The tocotransducer (tocodynamometer) measures UA transabdominally. The device is placed over the fundus above the umbilicus and held securely in place with an elastic belt (see Fig. 15.2, *B*). UCs or fetal movements depress a pressure-sensitive surface on the side next to the abdomen. The tocotransducer can measure and record the frequency and approximate duration of UCs but not their intensity. This method is especially valuable for measuring UA during the first stage of labor in women with intact membranes or for antepartum testing. If the woman is obese, the tocotransducer may be unable to detect the exact frequency and duration of UA.

Because the tocotransducer of most electronic fetal monitors is designed for assessing UA in the term pregnancy, it may not be sensitive enough to detect preterm UA. When monitoring the woman in preterm labor, the fundus may be located below the level of the umbilicus. The nurse may need to rely on the woman to indicate when UA is occurring and to use palpation as an additional way of assessing contraction frequency and validating the monitor tracing.

The external transducers are applied easily by the nurse but often must be readjusted as the woman or fetus changes position. The woman is asked to assume the semi-Fowler's or lateral position. Use of external transducers confines the woman to bed or chair.

TABLE 15.2 External and Internal Modes of Monitoring

External Mode	Internal Mode
Fetal Heart Rate	
Ultrasound transducer: High-frequency sound waves reflect mechanical action of fetal heart; noninvasive; does not require rupture of membranes or cervical dilation; used during both antepartum and intrapartum periods	*Spiral electrode:* Converts fetal ECG as obtained from presenting part to FHR via cardiotachometer; can be used only when membranes are ruptured and cervix is sufficiently dilated during intrapartum period; electrode penetrates into fetal presenting part by 1.5 mm and must be attached securely to ensure good signal
Uterine Activity	
Tocotransducer: Monitors frequency and duration of contractions by means of pressure-sensing device applied to maternal abdomen; used during both antepartum and intrapartum periods.	*Intrauterine pressure catheter (IUPC):* Monitors frequency, duration, and intensity of contractions; two types of IUPCs: fluid-filled system and solid catheter; both measure intrauterine pressure at catheter tip and convert pressure into millimeters of mercury on uterine activity panel of strip chart; both can be used only when membranes are ruptured and cervix is sufficiently dilated during intrapartum period

ECG, Electrocardiogram; *FHR,* fetal heart rate.

Portable telemetry monitors allow observation of the FHR and UC patterns by means of centrally located electronic display stations. These portable units permit the woman to walk around during electronic monitoring.

Use of another type of external monitor, which uses an integrated system of abdominally obtained electronic impulses to concurrently monitor both maternal and FHR and uterine activity, is becoming increasingly popular (Fig. 15.3, *A* and *B*). The monitor uses five electrodes placed on the woman's abdomen to directly monitor the electrocardiogram from the maternal and fetal hearts and the electromyogram from the uterine muscle. This information is transmitted wirelessly, via Bluetooth technology, to an interface device that allows the FHR and UA data to print or display on a standard fetal monitor (Miller et al., 2017).

This integrated monitoring system eliminates much of the problem caused by signal loss resulting from maternal or fetal movement or maternal obesity that often occurs with traditional external monitors. The monitor also more accurately measures the frequency, occurrence of peak, and duration of UCs than does the traditional tocotransducer, although it does not provide actual intensity measurement in millimeters of mercury (mm Hg) as an IUPC does. Other advantages of the device are that it eliminates the need for abdominal belts and frequent readjustment of the tocotransducer and ultrasound transducer and provides some patient mobility. The woman may move up to 50 feet away from the interface device without signal loss (Fig. 15.4, *A* and *B*). This type of monitor cannot be used during hydrotherapy or water birth and may not be readily available for use in all labor and birth settings (Miller et al., 2017). Also, in the United States, the device is only approved for use in monitoring singleton pregnancies at term (see Clinical Reasoning Case Study: Monitoring the Fetus of an Obese Woman) (AWHONN, 2015b).

Internal Monitoring

The technique of continuous internal FHR or UA monitoring provides a more accurate appraisal of fetal well-being during labor than external monitoring because it is not interrupted by fetal or maternal movement or affected by maternal size (Fig. 15.5). For this type of monitoring, the membranes must be ruptured, the cervix sufficiently dilated (at least 2 to 3 cm), and the presenting part low enough to allow placement of the spiral electrode or IUPC or both. Internal and external modes of monitoring may be combined (i.e., internal FHR with external UA or external FHR with internal UA) without difficulty.

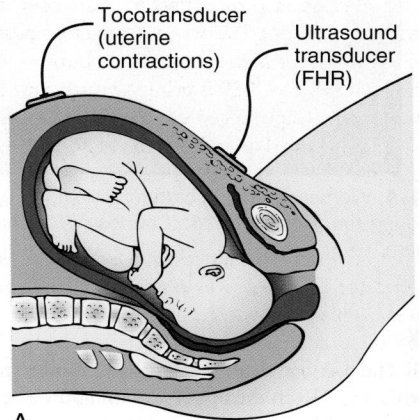
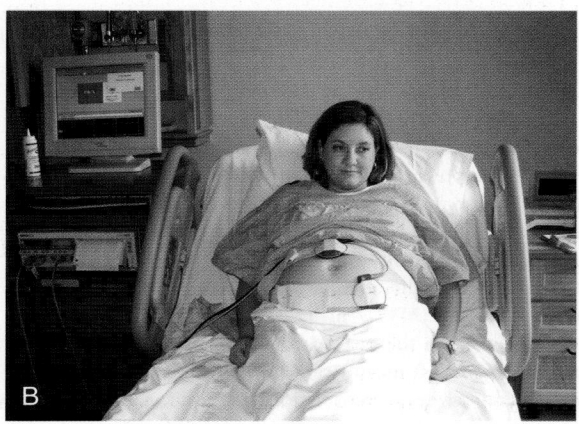

Tocotransducer (uterine contractions)

Ultrasound transducer (FHR)

A

B

FIG 15.2 A, External noninvasive fetal monitoring with tocotransducer and ultrasound transducer. **B,** Ultrasound transducer is placed below umbilicus over area where fetal heart rate is best heard, and tocotransducer is placed on uterine fundus. *FHR,* Fetal heart rate. (B, Courtesy of Julie Perry Nelson, Loveland, CO.)

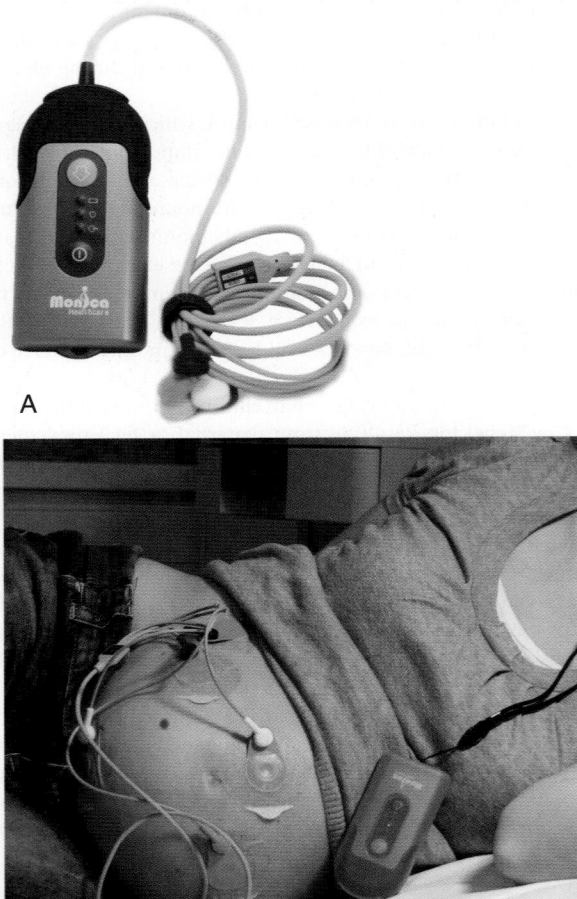

A

B

FIG 15.3 A, The Monica AN24 is a wireless and beltless device that can be used with existing monitors to obtain fetal heart rate via abdominal electrocardiogram (ECG). **B,** Electrodes placed on maternal abdomen monitor ECG from fetal and maternal heart and electromyogram (EMG) from uterine muscle. (Courtesy of Monica Healthcare Ltd, Nottingham, UK.)

Internal monitoring of the FHR is accomplished by attaching a small spiral electrode to the presenting part. For UA to be monitored internally, an IUPC is introduced into the uterine cavity. The catheter has a pressure-sensitive tip that measures changes in intrauterine pressure. As the catheter is compressed during a contraction, pressure is placed on the pressure transducer. This pressure is then converted into a pressure reading in millimeters of mercury. The IUPC can objectively measure the frequency, duration, and intensity of UCs and uterine resting tone.

Because it can measure the intensity of individual UCs precisely, the IUPC can be used to evaluate the adequacy of UA for achieving progress in labor. Montevideo units (MVUs) are calculated by subtracting the baseline uterine pressure from the peak contraction pressure for each contraction that occurs in a 10-minute window and then adding together the pressures generated by each contraction that occurs during that period of time. Spontaneous labor usually begins when MVUs are between 80 and 120. Uterine activity during the first stage of normal labor rarely exceeds 250 MVUs (see Table 15.1) (Cunningham, Leveno, Bloom, et al., 2014; Miller et al., 2017).

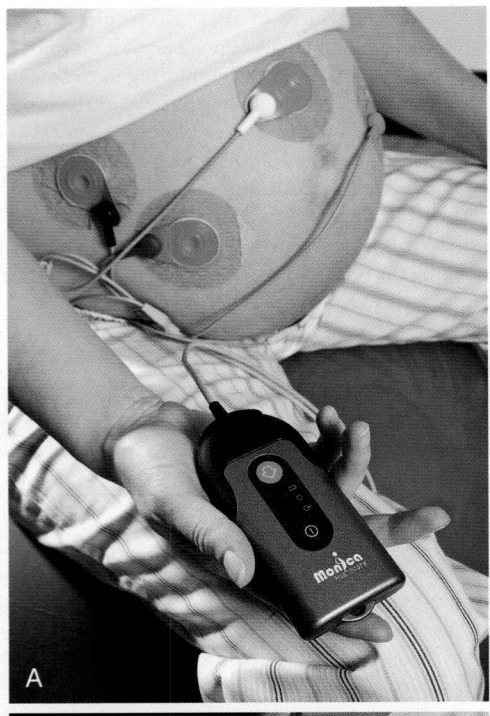

A

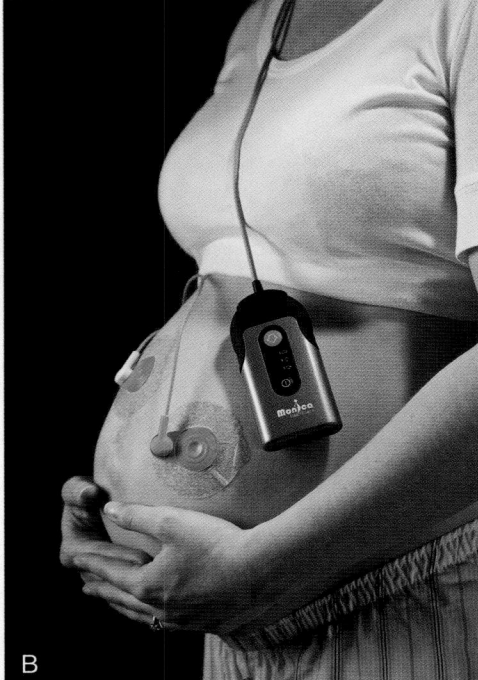

B

FIG 15.4 A, Woman sitting on birthing ball and **B,** woman ambulating, both wearing the Monica AN24. (Courtesy of Monica Healthcare Ltd, Nottingham, UK.)

Display

The FHR and UA are displayed on the monitor paper or computer screen, with the FHR in the upper section and UA in the lower section. Fig. 15.6 contrasts the internal and external modes of electronic monitoring. Note that each small square on the monitor paper or screen represents 10 seconds; each larger box of six squares equals 1 minute (when paper is moving through the monitor at the rate of 3 cm/min).

CLINICAL REASONING CASE STUDY

Monitoring the Fetus of an Obese Woman

Tameka is a 23-year-old G 4 P 2 0 1 2 at 35 weeks of gestation. She has had chronic hypertension since she was 16 years of age and is morbidly obese. Today she weighs 305 pounds. Tameka was sent from the antepartum testing area to the labor and birth unit for prolonged monitoring because she had a nonreactive nonstress test (NST) and her blood pressure was elevated at her appointment today. You are Tameka's nurse. After spending half an hour admitting her to the unit you walk out to the nurses' station and announce to your colleagues, "I am *so* frustrated! No matter what I do, I just can't keep that baby on the monitor!"

1. Evidence—Is there sufficient evidence at this time to draw a conclusion about the best way to monitor Tameka's fetus?
2. Assumptions—Describe an underlying assumption regarding use of the following modes of monitoring for Tameka's fetus:
   a. Intermittent auscultation
   b. External (ultrasound transducer)
   c. Internal (spiral electrode)
   d. Integrated abdominal fetal heart rate and uterine activity monitoring system
3. What implications and priorities for nursing care can be drawn at this time?
4. Does the evidence objectively support your conclusion?
5. Interprofessional care—Describe the roles/responsibilities of health care professionals who might be involved in Tameka's care.

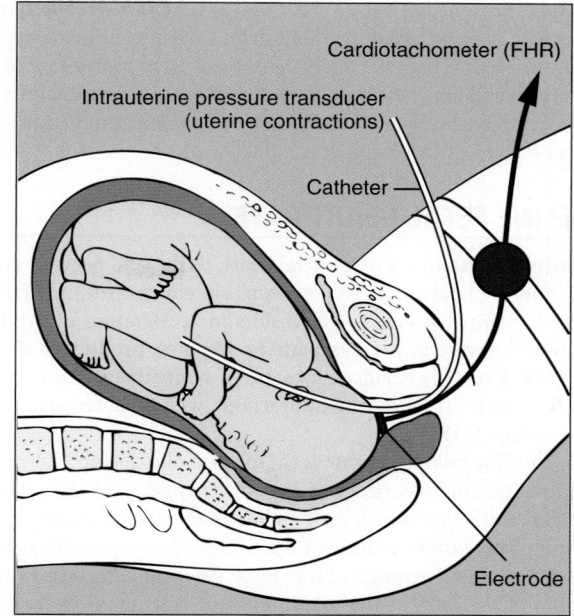

FIG 15.5 Diagrammatic representation of internal invasive fetal monitoring with intrauterine pressure catheter and spiral electrode in place (membranes ruptured and cervix dilated).

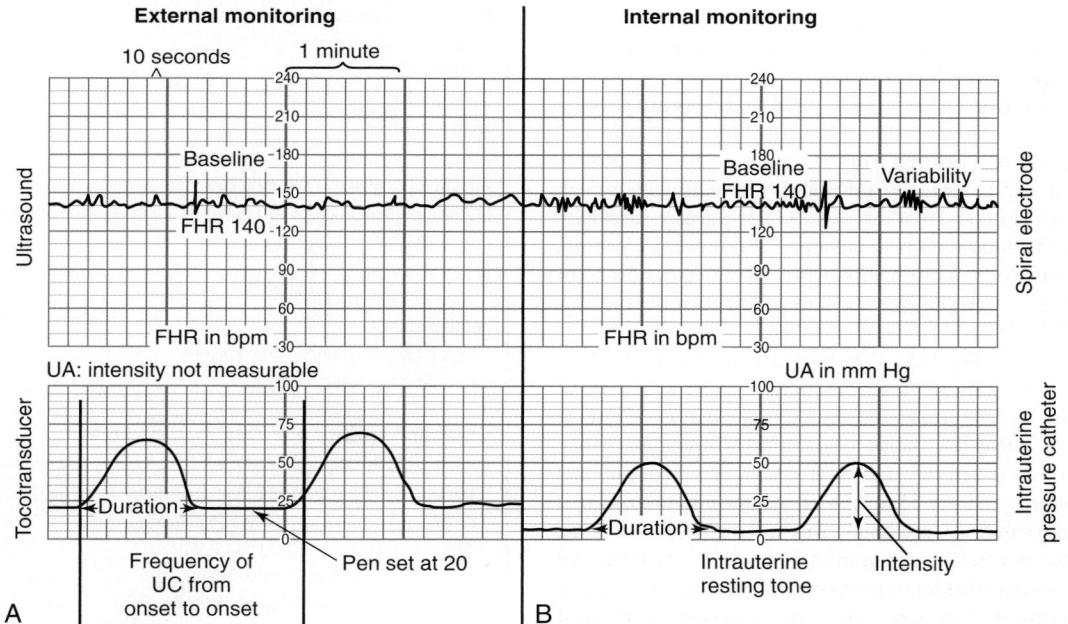

FIG 15.6 Fetal monitor display of fetal heart rate and uterine activity. **A,** Monitor strip of external mode with ultrasound and tocotransducer as the signal source. **B,** Monitor strip of internal mode with spiral electrode and intrauterine catheter as the signal source. *FHR,* Fetal heart rate; *UA,* uterine activity. (From Miller, L., Miller, D., & Cypher, R. [2017]. *Mosby's pocket guide to fetal monitoring: A multidisciplinary approach* [8th ed.]. St. Louis, MO: Elsevier.)

FETAL HEART RATE PATTERNS

Characteristic FHR patterns are associated with fetal and maternal physiologic processes and have been identified for many years. However, because EFM was introduced into clinical practice before consensus was reached regarding standardized terminology, variations in the description and interpretation of common FHR patterns were often great. In 1997, the NICHD published a proposed nomenclature system for EFM interpretation with standardized definitions for FHR monitoring (NICHD, 1997). Currently ACOG, ACNM, and AWHONN all support the use of standardized terminology (Miller et al., 2017). All three organizations cited concerns regarding patient safety and the need for improved communication among caregivers as reasons for using standard EFM definitions in clinical practice.

In April 2008 the NICHD, ACOG, and SMFM partnered to sponsor another workshop to revisit the FHR definitions recommended by the NICHD in 1997. The 1997 FHR definitions were reaffirmed at this workshop. In addition, new definitions related to UA were recommended, as well as a three-tier system of FHR pattern interpretation and categorization (see Box 15.1) (Macones et al., 2008).

BASELINE FETAL HEART RATE

The intrinsic rhythmicity of the fetal heart, the central nervous system (CNS), and the fetal autonomic nervous system control the FHR. An increase in sympathetic response results in acceleration of the FHR, whereas an increase in parasympathetic response produces a slowing of the FHR. Usually a balanced increase of sympathetic and parasympathetic response occurs during contractions, with no observable change in the baseline FHR.

The baseline fetal heart rate is the average rate during a 10-minute segment that excludes periodic or episodic changes, periods of marked variability, and segments of the baseline that differ by more than 25 beats/min. There must be at least 2 minutes of interpretable baseline data in a 10-minute segment of tracing to determine the baseline FHR (Macones et al., 2008). After 10 minutes of tracing is observed, the approximate mean rate is rounded to the closest 5 beats/min interval (AWHONN, 2015b). For example, if the FHR varies between 130 and 140 beats/min over a 10-minute period, the baseline is recorded as 135 beats/min. The normal FHR range is 110 to 160 beats/min.

Variability

Variability of the FHR can be described as irregular waves or fluctuations in the baseline FHR of two cycles per minute or greater (Macones et al., 2008). It is a characteristic of the baseline FHR and does not include accelerations or decelerations of the FHR. Variability is quantified in beats per minute and is measured from the peak to the trough of a single cycle. Four possible categories of variability have been identified: absent, minimal, moderate, and marked (Fig. 15.7). In the past, variability was described as either long-term or short-term (beat to beat). However, the NICHD definitions do not distinguish between long- and short-term variability because in actual practice they are visually determined as a unit (NICHD, 1997).

Absent variability (see Fig. 15.7, A) is defined as an amplitude range of the FHR fluctuations that is not detectable to the unaided eye. Minimal variability (see Fig. 15.7, B) has an amplitude range that is detectable to the unaided eye, but is less than 5 beats/min (Miller et al., 2017). Depending on other characteristics of the FHR tracing, absent or minimal variability is classified as either abnormal or indeterminate (Macones et al., 2008). It can result from fetal hypoxemia and metabolic acidemia. Other possible causes of absent or minimal variability include fetal sleep cycles, fetal tachycardia, extreme prematurity, medications that cause central nervous system depression, congenital anomalies, and preexisting neurologic injury (Miller et al., 2017).

Moderate variability is considered normal (see Fig. 15.7, C). Its presence reliably predicts a normal fetal acid-base balance (absence of fetal metabolic acidemia). Moderate variability indicates that FHR regulation is not affected significantly by fetal sleep cycles, tachycardia, prematurity, congenital anomalies, preexisting neurologic injury, or CNS depressant medications (Macones et al., 2008; Miller et al., 2017).

The significance of marked variability (see Fig. 15.7, D) is unclear (Macones et al., 2008). In many cases, it likely represents a normal variant (Miller et al., 2017).

A sinusoidal pattern (i.e., a regular smooth, undulating wavelike pattern) is not included in the definition of FHR variability. This uncommon pattern classically occurs with severe fetal anemia (Fig. 15.8). Variations of the sinusoidal pattern have been described in association with chorioamnionitis, fetal sepsis, and administration of opiod analgesics (Miller et al., 2017).

Tachycardia

Tachycardia is a baseline FHR greater than 160 beats/min for 10 minutes or longer (Fig. 15.9). It can be considered an early sign of fetal hypoxemia, especially when associated with late decelerations and minimal or absent variability. Fetal tachycardia can result from many other causes not directly related to fetal oxygenation. For example, tachycardia can be caused by maternal or fetal infection; by maternal hyperthyroidism or fetal anemia; or in response to medications such as atropine, hydroxyzine (Vistaril), terbutaline (Brethine), or illicit drugs such as cocaine or methamphetamines. Tachycardia can also be caused by abnormalities involving fetal cardiac pacemakers and/or the cardiac conduction system (Miller et al., 2017). Table 15.3 lists causes, clinical significance, and nursing interventions for tachycardia.

TABLE 15.3	Tachycardia and Bradycardia
Tachycardia	**Bradycardia**
Definition	
FHR >160 beats/min lasting >10 minutes	FHR <110 beats/min lasting >10 minutes
Possible Causes	
Early fetal hypoxemia	Atrioventricular dissociation (heart block)
Fetal cardiac arrhythmias	Structural defects
Maternal fever	Viral infections (e.g., cytomegalovirus)
Infection (including chorioamnionitis)	Medications
Parasympatholytic drugs (atropine, hydroxyzine)	Fetal heart failure
β-Sympathomimetic drugs (terbutaline)	Maternal hypoglycemia
Maternal hyperthyroidism	Maternal hypothermia
Fetal anemia	
Drugs (caffeine, theophylline, cocaine, methamphetamines)	
Clinical Significance	
Persistent tachycardia in absence of periodic changes does not appear serious in terms of neonatal outcome (especially true if tachycardia is associated with maternal fever); tachycardia is abnormal when associated with late decelerations, severe variable decelerations, or absent variability.	Baseline bradycardia alone is not specifically related to fetal oxygenation. Clinical significance of bradycardia depends on underlying cause and accompanying FHR patterns, including variability, accelerations, or decelerations.
Nursing Interventions	
Dependent on cause; reduce maternal fever with antipyretics as ordered and cooling measures; oxygen at 10 L/min by nonrebreather face mask may be of some value; carry out health care provider's orders based on alleviating cause.	Dependent on cause

FHR, Fetal heart rate.

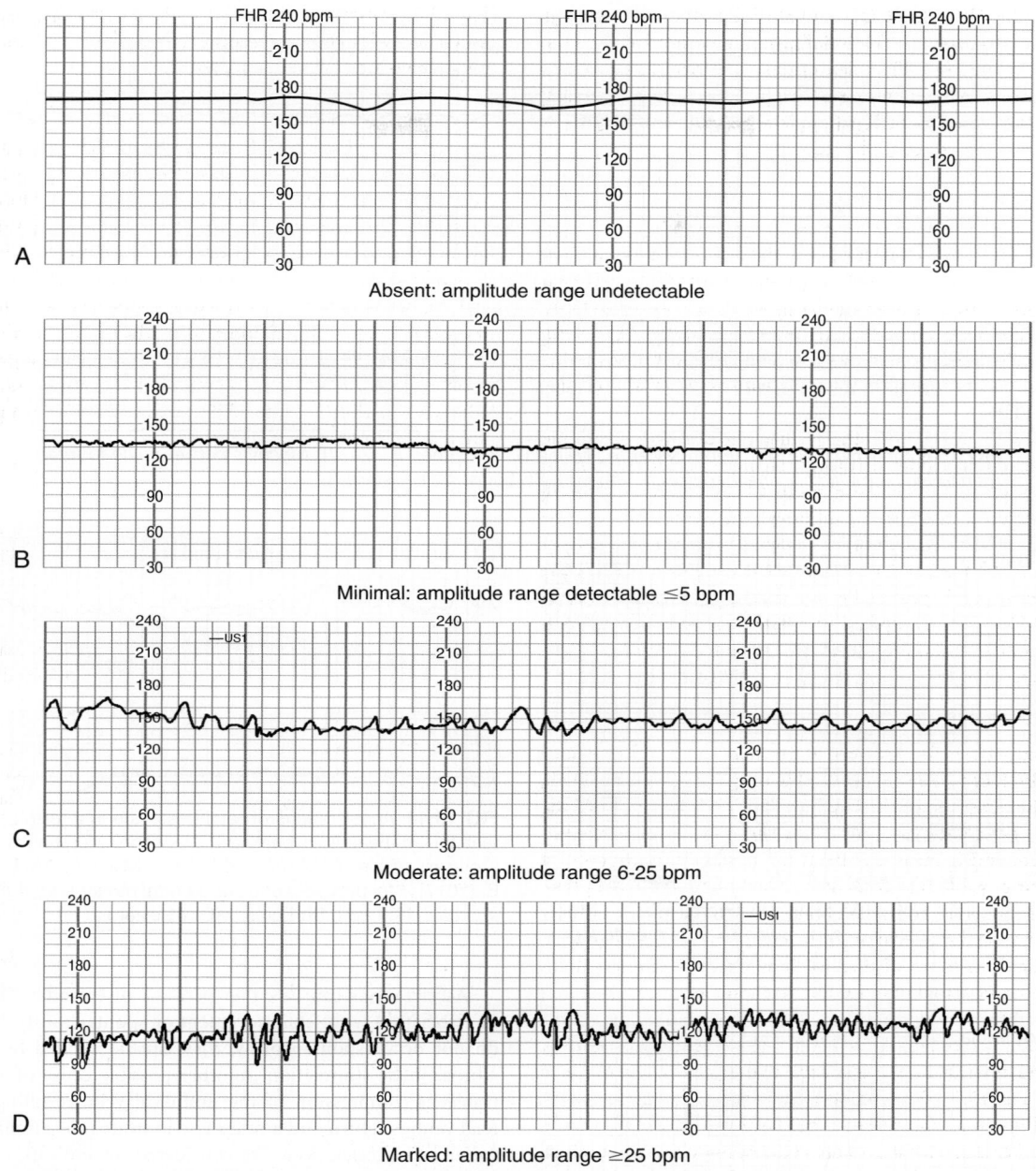

FIG 15.7 Classification of fetal heart rate variability. **A,** Absent. **B,** Minimal. **C,** Moderate. **D,** Marked. *FHR,* Fetal heart rate. (From Miller, L., Miller, D., & Cypher, R. [2017]. *Mosby's pocket guide to fetal monitoring: A multidisciplinary approach* [8th ed.]. St. Louis, MO: Elsevier.)

Bradycardia

Bradycardia is a baseline FHR less than 110 beats/min for 10 minutes or longer (Fig. 15.10). True bradycardia occurs rarely and is not specifically related to fetal oxygenation. It must be distinguished from a prolonged deceleration because the causes and management of these two conditions are very different. Bradycardia is often caused by some type of fetal cardiac problem such as structural defects involving the pacemakers or conduction system or fetal heart failure. Other causes of bradycardia include viral infections (e.g., cytomegalovirus), maternal hypoglycemia, and maternal hypothermia. Medications do not commonly cause bradycardia (Miller et al., 2017) (see Table 15.3 for a list of causes, clinical significance, and nursing interventions for bradycardia).

PERIODIC AND EPISODIC CHANGES IN FETAL HEART RATE

Changes in FHR from the baseline are categorized as periodic or episodic. Periodic changes are those that occur with UCs. Episodic changes are those that are not associated with UCs. These changes include both accelerations and decelerations (Macones et al., 2008).

Accelerations

Acceleration of the FHR is defined as a visually apparent, abrupt (onset to peak <30 seconds) increase in FHR above the baseline rate (Fig. 15.11). The peak is at least 15 beats/min above the baseline, and

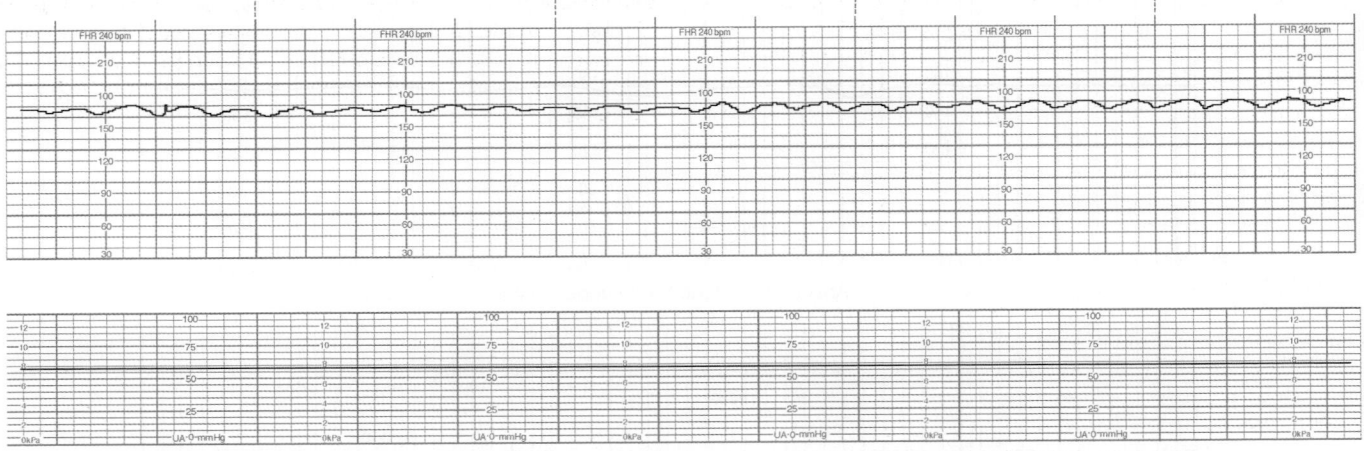

FIG 15.8 Sinusoidal pattern. (From Miller, L., Miller, D., & Cypher, R. [2017]. *Mosby's pocket guide to fetal monitoring: A multidisciplinary approach.* [8th ed.]. St. Louis, MO: Elsevier.)

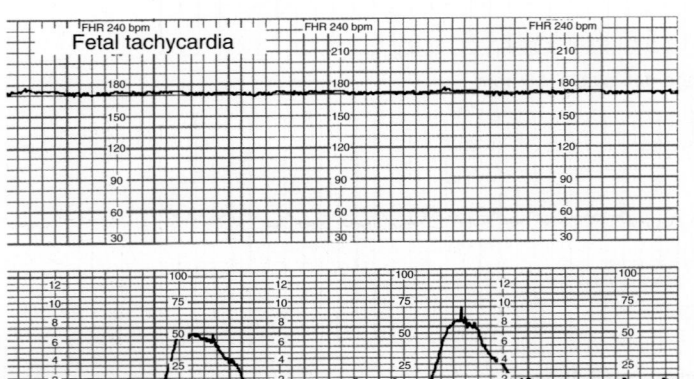

FIG 15.9 Fetal tachycardia: FHR >160 beats/min. (From Miller, L., Miller, D., & Cypher, R. [2017]. *Mosby's pocket guide to fetal monitoring: A multidisciplinary approach* [8th ed.]. St. Louis, MO: Elsevier.)

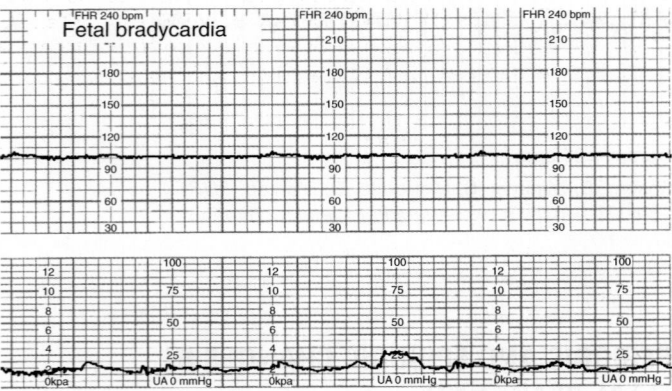

FIG 15.10 Fetal bradycardia: FHR >110 beats/min. (From Miller, L., Miller, D., & Cypher, R. [2017]. *Mosby's pocket guide to fetal monitoring: A multidisciplinary approach* [8th ed.]. St. Louis, MO: Elsevier.)

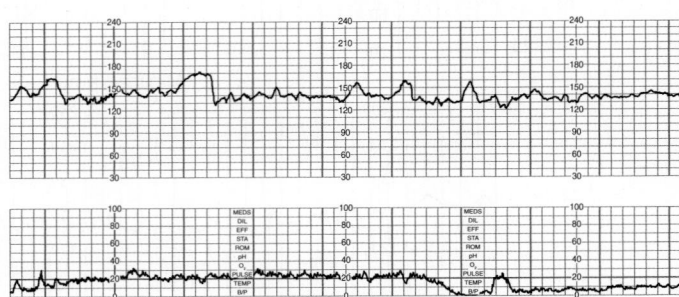

FIG 15.11 Accelerations of fetal heart rate in a term pregnancy. Note that the 15-beats/min peak and 15-second duration criteria are met. (Courtesy of Lisa A. Miller, CNM, JD. In Miller, L., Miller, D., & Cypher, R. [2017]. *Mosby's pocket guide to fetal monitoring: A multidisciplinary approach* [8th ed.]. St. Louis, MO: Elsevier.)

Accelerations can be either periodic or episodic. They may occur in association with fetal movement or spontaneously. If accelerations do not occur spontaneously, they can be elicited by fetal scalp or vibroacoustic stimulation. Another possible cause of accelerations is transient compression of the umbilical vein, resulting in decreased fetal venous return and a reflex rise in heart rate. Similar to moderate variability, accelerations are considered an indication of fetal well-being. Their presence is highly predictive of a normal fetal acid-base balance (absence of fetal metabolic acidemia) (Miller et al., 2017). Box 15.3 lists causes, clinical significance, and nursing interventions for accelerations.

Decelerations

A deceleration (caused by dominance of a parasympathetic response) may be benign or abnormal. FHR decelerations are categorized as early, late, variable, or prolonged. They are described by their visual relation to the onset and end of a contraction and by their shape.

Early Decelerations

Early deceleration of the FHR is a visually apparent, gradual (onset to lowest point ≥30 seconds) decrease in and return to baseline FHR associated with UCs. It is thought to be caused by transient fetal head compression and is considered a normal and benign finding (Macones et al., 2008; Miller et al., 2017). Generally the onset, nadir (lowest point), and recovery of the deceleration correspond to the beginning, peak,

the acceleration lasts 15 seconds or more, with the return to baseline less than 2 minutes from the beginning of the acceleration. Before 32 weeks of gestation, the definition of an acceleration is a peak of 10 beats/min or more above the baseline and a duration of at least 10 seconds. Acceleration of the FHR for more than 10 minutes is considered a change in baseline rate (Miller et al., 2017).

and end of the contraction (Figs. 15.12 and 15.13). For this reason, an early deceleration is sometimes called the *mirror image* of a contraction.

Early decelerations may occur during UCs, during vaginal examinations, as a result of fundal pressure, and during placement of the internal mode of fetal monitoring. They have no known relationship to fetal oxygenation. Instead, they are thought to represent a fetal autonomic response to changes in intracranial pressure and/or cerebral blood flow caused by fetal head compression (Miller et al., 2017). When present, they usually occur during the first stage of labor when the cervix is dilated 4 to 7 cm. However, they are sometimes seen during the second stage of labor, when the woman is pushing.

Because early decelerations are considered to be benign, interventions are not necessary. The value of identifying them is so they can be distinguished from late or variable decelerations, which can be abnormal and for which interventions are appropriate. Box 15.4 lists causes, clinical significance, and nursing interventions for early decelerations.

Late Decelerations

Late deceleration of the FHR is a visually apparent, gradual (onset to lowest point ≥30 seconds) decrease in and return to baseline FHR

associated with UCs (Macones et al., 2008). The deceleration begins after the contraction has started, and the lowest point of the deceleration occurs after the peak of the contraction. The deceleration usually does not return to baseline until after the contraction is over (Figs. 15.14 and 15.15).

BOX 15.4   Early Decelerations

Cause

Head compression resulting from the following:
- Uterine contractions
- Vaginal examination
- Fundal pressure
- Placement of internal mode of monitoring

Clinical Significance

Normal pattern; not associated with fetal hypoxemia, acidemia, or low Apgar scores

Nursing Interventions

None required

BOX 15.3   Accelerations

Causes
- Spontaneous fetal movement
- Vaginal examination
- Electrode application
- Fetal scalp stimulation
- Fetal reaction to external sounds
- Breech presentation
- Occiput posterior position
- Uterine contractions
- Fundal pressure
- Abdominal palpation

Clinical Significance
- Normal pattern: Acceleration with fetal movement signifies fetal well-being representing fetal alertness or arousal states.

Nursing Interventions
- None required

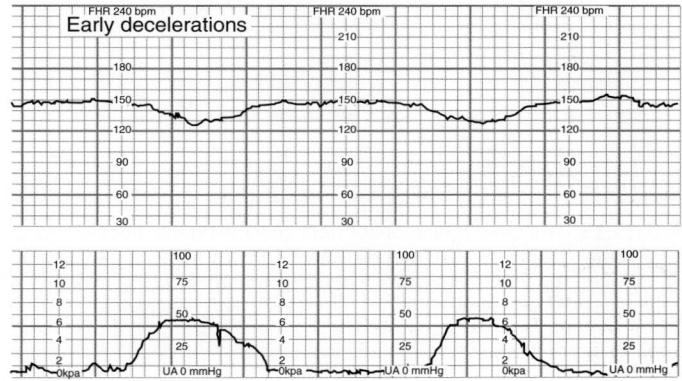

FIG 15.13 Electronic fetal monitor tracing showing early decelerations. *FHR*, Fetal heart rate; *UA*, uterine activity. (From Miller, L., Miller, D., & Cypher, R. [2017]. *Mosby's pocket guide to fetal monitoring: A multidisciplinary approach* [8th ed.]. St. Louis, MO: Elsevier.)

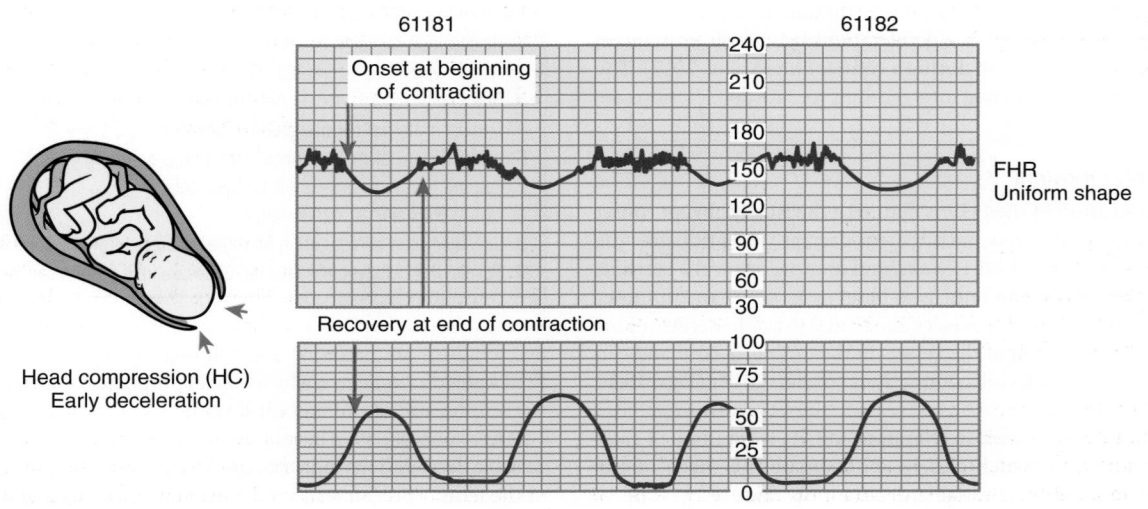

FIG 15.12 Line drawing illustrating early decelerations. *FHR*, Fetal heart rate. (From Tucker, S.M. (2004). *Pocket guide to fetal monitoring and assessment* [5th ed.]. St Louis, MO: Mosby.)

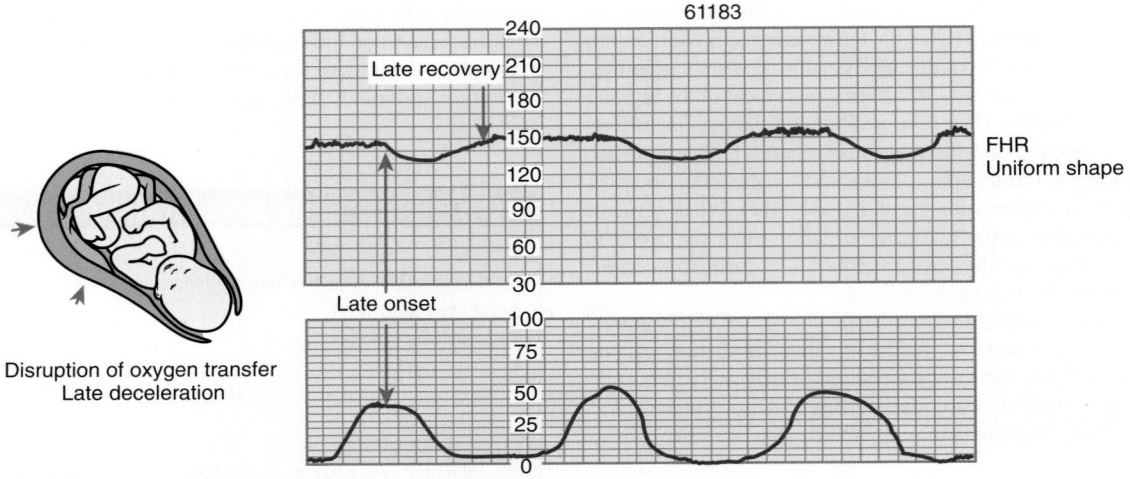

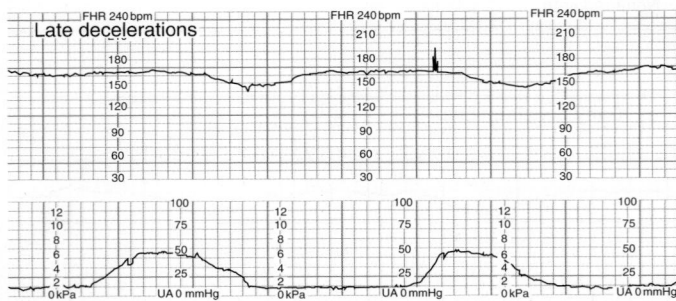

Disruption of oxygen transfer
Late deceleration

FIG 15.14 Line drawing illustrating late decelerations. *FHR,* Fetal heart rate. (From Tucker, S.M. (2004). *Pocket guide to fetal monitoring and assessment* [5th ed.]. St Louis, MO: Mosby.)

FIG 15.15 Electronic fetal monitor tracing showing late decelerations. *FHR,* Fetal heart rate; *UA,* uterine activity. (From Miller, L., Miller, D., & Cypher, R. [2017]. *Mosby's pocket guide to fetal monitoring: A multidisciplinary approach* [8th ed.]. St. Louis, MO: Elsevier.)

> ### BOX 15.5   Late Decelerations
>
> **Cause**
> Disruption of oxygen transfer from environment to fetus, resulting in transient fetal hypoxemia. Late decelerations are caused by the following:
> - Uterine tachysystole
> - Maternal supine hypotension
> - Epidural or spinal anesthesia
> - Placenta previa
> - Placental abruption
> - Hypertensive disorders
> - Postterm gestation
> - Intrauterine growth restriction
> - Diabetes mellitus
> - Intraamniotic infection
>
> **Clinical Significance**
> Abnormal pattern associated with fetal hypoxemia, acidemia, and low Apgar scores; considered ominous if persistent and uncorrected, especially when associated with absent or minimal baseline variability
>
> **Nursing Interventions**
> The usual priority is as follows:
> 1. Discontinue oxytocin if infusing.
> 2. Assist woman to lateral (side-lying) position.
> 3. Administer oxygen at 10 L/min by nonrebreather face mask.
> 4. Correct maternal hypotension by elevating legs.
> 5. Increase rate of maintenance intravenous solution.
> 6. Palpate uterus to assess for tachysystole.
> 7. Notify physician or nurse-midwife.
> 8. Consider internal monitoring for more accurate fetal and uterine assessment.
> 9. Assist with birth (vaginal assisted or cesarean) if pattern cannot be corrected.

Late decelerations are caused by a reflex fetal response to transient hypoxemia during a uterine contraction that reduces the delivery of oxygenated blood to the intervillous space of the placenta (Miller et al., 2017). A number of conditions can cause disruption of oxygen transfer from the environment to the fetus. Common causes include maternal hypotension and uterine hypertonus. If interruption of fetal oxygenation results in metabolic acidemia, late decelerations may result from direct hypoxic myocardial depression during a contraction (Miller, 2017). The clinical significance and nursing interventions for late decelerations are described in Box 15.5.

Variable Decelerations

Variable deceleration of the FHR is defined as a visually abrupt (onset to lowest point <30 seconds) and apparent decrease in FHR below the baseline. The decrease is at least 15 beats/min or more below the baseline, lasts at least 15 seconds, and returns to baseline in less than 2 minutes from the time of onset (Macones et al., 2008). Variable decelerations are caused by compression of the vessels in the umbilical cord and can occur with or without uterine contractions (Miller, 2017) (Figs. 15.16 and 15.17).

The appearance of variable decelerations differs from those of early and late decelerations, which closely approximate the shape of the corresponding UC. Instead variable decelerations have a *U, V,* or *W* shape, characterized by a rapid descent and ascent to and from the nadir of the deceleration (see Figs. 15.16 and 15.17). Some variable

decelerations are preceded and followed by brief accelerations of the FHR known as *shoulders*, which is an appropriate compensatory response to compression of the umbilical vein.

Occasional variables have little clinical significance. However, recurrent variable decelerations indicate repetitive disruption in the oxygen supply of the fetus. This can result in hypoxemia, hypoxia, metabolic acidosis, and, eventually, metabolic acidemia. Variable decelerations may also be caused by a fetal vagal response to umbilical cord stretching as the fetus

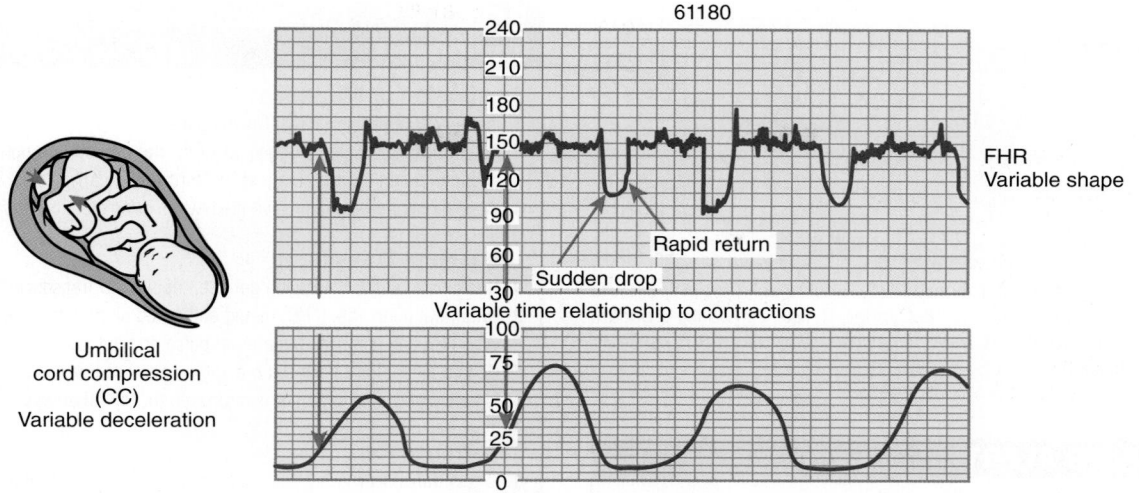

61180

FHR
Variable shape

Rapid return

Sudden drop

Variable time relationship to contractions

Umbilical
cord compression
(CC)
Variable deceleration

FIG 15.16 Line drawing illustrating variable decelerations. *FHR*, Fetal heart rate. (From Tucker, S.M. (2004). *Pocket guide to fetal monitoring and assessment.* [5th ed.] St Louis, MO: Mosby.)

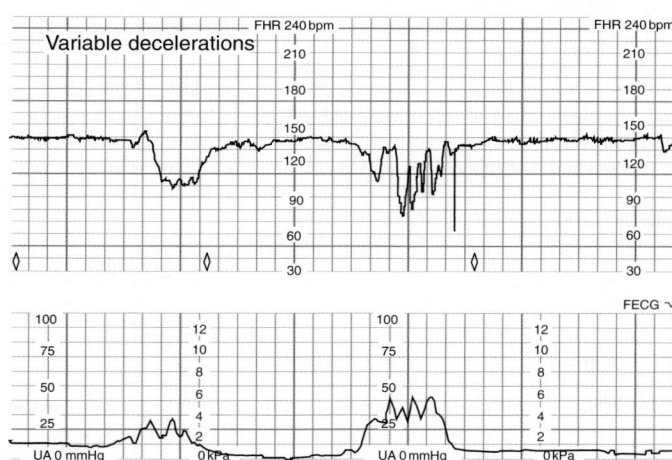

FIG 15.17 Electronic fetal monitor tracing showing variable decelerations. *FHR*, Fetal heart rate; *FECG*, fetal electrocardiogram. (From Miller, L., Miller, D., & Cypher, R. [2017]. *Mosby's pocket guide to fetal monitoring: A multidisciplinary approach* [8th ed.]. St. Louis, MO: Elsevier.)

descends in the pelvis during labor (Miller et al., 2017). Box 15.6 lists causes, clinical significance, and nursing interventions for variable decelerations.

Prolonged Decelerations

A **prolonged deceleration** is a visually apparent decrease (may be either gradual or abrupt) in FHR of at least 15 beats/min below the baseline and lasting more than 2 minutes but less than 10 minutes. A deceleration lasting more than 10 minutes is considered a baseline change (Macones, et al., 2008) (Fig. 15.19).

Prolonged decelerations are caused when the mechanisms responsible for late or variable decelerations last for an extended period (more than 2 minutes). Conditions that can cause an interruption in the fetal oxygen supply long enough to produce a prolonged deceleration can occur anywhere along the oxygen pathway. For example, at the level of the maternal lungs, a prolonged deceleration may result from maternal apnea during an eclamptic seizure. At the level of the umbilical cord, cord compression, stretch, or prolapse can result in a prolonged deceleration (Miller, 2017).

BOX 15.6 Variable Decelerations

Cause

Umbilical cord compression caused by the following:
- Maternal position with cord between fetus and maternal pelvis
- Cord around fetal neck, arm, leg, or other body part
- Short cord
- Knot in cord (Fig. 15.18)
- Prolapsed cord

Clinical Significance

Variable decelerations occur in approximately 50% of all labors and usually are transient and correctable

Nursing Interventions

The usual priority is as follows:
1. Discontinue oxytocin if infusing.
2. Change maternal position (side to side, knee chest).
3. Administer oxygen at 10 L/min by nonrebreather face mask.
4. Notify physician or nurse-midwife.
5. Assist with vaginal or speculum examination to assess for cord prolapse.
6. Assist with amnioinfusion if ordered.
7. Assist with birth (vaginal assisted or cesarean) if pattern cannot be corrected.

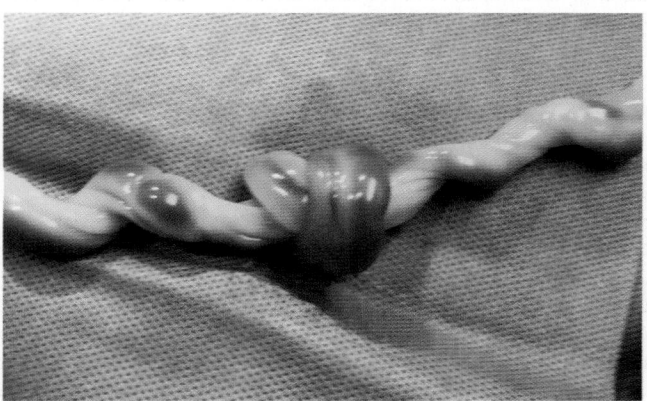

FIG 15.18 Umbilical cord containing a true knot. (Courtesy of Carshawna Knighton, Memphis, TN.)

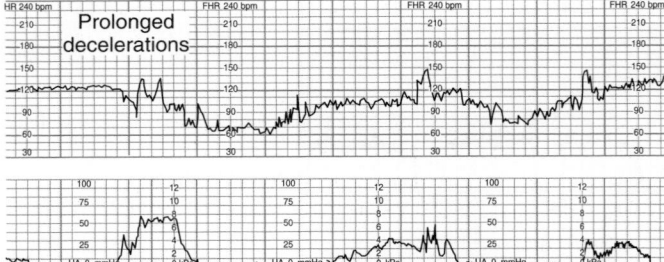

FIG 15.19 Prolonged decelerations. *FHR,* Fetal heart rate; *UA,* uterine activity. (From Miller, L., Miller, D., & Cypher, R. [2017]. *Mosby's pocket guide to fetal monitoring: A multidisciplinary approach* [8th ed.]. St. Louis, MO: Elsevier.)

! NURSING ALERT

Nurses should notify the physician or nurse-midwife immediately and initiate appropriate treatment of abnormal patterns when they see a prolonged deceleration.

CARE MANAGEMENT

Care of the woman receiving EFM in labor begins with evaluation of the EFM equipment. The nurse must ensure that the monitor is recording FHR and UA accurately and that the tracing is interpretable. If external monitoring is not adequate, changing to a fetal spiral electrode or IUPC may be necessary. A checklist for fetal monitoring equipment can be used to evaluate the equipment functions (Box 15.7).

After ensuring that the monitor is recording properly, the FHR and UA tracings are evaluated regularly throughout labor. *Guidelines for Perinatal Care,* published jointly by AAP and ACOG (2012), recommends that the FHR tracing be evaluated at least every 30 minutes during the first stage of labor and every 15 minutes during the second stage of labor in low-risk women. If risk factors are present, the FHR tracing should be evaluated more frequently: every 15 minutes in the first stage of labor and every 5 minutes in the second stage of labor.

Assessing FHR and UA patterns, implementing independent nursing interventions, documenting observations and actions according to the established standard of care, and reporting abnormal patterns to the obstetric care provider (e.g., physician, certified nurse-midwife) are the responsibilities of the nurse providing care to women in labor.

Current technology has made access to and communication regarding electronic FHR tracings much more convenient for health care providers. Many hospitals use central monitor displays, which provide the opportunity to view the tracings of several women at the same time at the nurses' station or in other locations on the nursing unit. Health care providers can also access the FHR tracings of one woman or several patients from remote locations, including office and home. It is even possible to access FHR tracings and other patient data using mobile phones (Fig. 15.20) (Miller et al., 2017).

ELECTRONIC FETAL MONITORING PATTERN RECOGNITION AND INTERPRETATION

Nurses must evaluate many factors to determine whether an FHR pattern is normal or abnormal. They evaluate these factors based on the presence of other obstetric complications, progress in labor, and use of analgesia or anesthesia. They also must consider the estimated time interval until birth. Therefore interventions are based on clinical judgment of a

BOX 15.7   Checklist for Fetal Monitoring Equipment

Preparation of Monitor
1. Is paper inserted correctly (if using paper)?
2. Are transducer cables plugged securely into appropriate port on monitor?
3. Is paper speed set to 3 cm/min (in North America)?
4. Were monitor date and time verified (when using electronic documentation)?

Ultrasound Transducer
1. Has ultrasound transmission gel been applied to transducer?
2. Was fetal heart rate (FHR) tested and noted on monitor strip?
3. Was FHR compared with maternal pulse and noted?
4. Does a signal light flash or an audible beep occur with each heartbeat?
5. Is belt secure and snug but comfortable for the laboring woman?

Tocotransducer
1. Is tocotransducer firmly positioned at site of least maternal tissue?
2. Has it been applied without gel or paste?
3. Was uterine activity (UA) baseline adjusted between contractions to print at the 20 mm Hg line?
4. Is belt secure and snug but comfortable for the laboring woman?

Spiral Electrode
1. Is connector attached firmly to electrode pad (on leg plate or abdomen)?
2. Is spiral electrode attached to presenting part of fetus?
3. Is inner surface of electrode pad pregelled or covered with electrode gel?
4. Is electrode pad properly secured to woman's thigh or abdomen?

Internal Catheter or Strain Gauge
1. Is length line on catheter visible at introitus?
2. Is it noted on monitor paper that UA test or calibration was performed?
3. Has monitor been set to zero according to manufacturer's instructions?
4. Is intrauterine pressure catheter properly secured to woman?
5. Is baseline resting tone of uterus documented?

From Miller, L., Miller, D., & Cypher, R. (2017). *Mosby's pocket guide to fetal monitoring: A multidisciplinary approach* (8th ed.). St. Louis, MO: Elsevier.

complex, integrated process. Several different organizations offer EFM courses for nurses and other health care professionals. It is also possible to earn certification in EFM.

LEGAL TIP Fetal Monitoring Standards Nurses who care for women during childbirth are legally responsible for correctly interpreting FHR patterns, initiating appropriate nursing interventions based on those patterns, and documenting the outcomes of those interventions. Perinatal nurses are responsible for the timely notification of the physician or nurse-midwife in the event of abnormal FHR patterns. They also are responsible for initiating the institutional chain of command should differences in opinion arise among health care providers concerning the interpretation of the FHR pattern and the intervention required.

Categorizing Fetal Heart Rate Tracings

As previously mentioned, a three-tier system of categorizing FHR tracings is recommended (see Box 15.1). Category I FHR tracings are normal and strongly predictive of normal fetal acid-base status at the time of observation. These tracings may be followed in a routine manner and

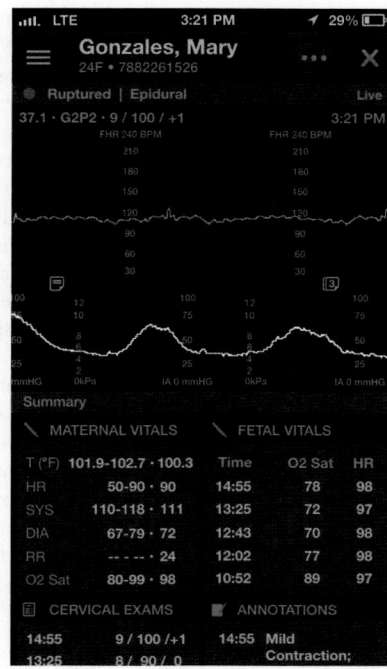

FIG 15.20 Providers can access near real-time fetal heart rate tracings and review patient data using their mobile phones. **(A)** FHR tracing, including MHR. **(B)** Patient listing. (© 2017 AirStrip Technologies. All rights reserved. iPhone is a registered trademark of Apple Inc.)

BOX 15.8   Management of Abnormal Fetal Heart Rate Patterns

Basic Interventions
- Administer oxygen by nonrebreather face mask at rate of 10 L/min for approximately 15 to 30 minutes.
- Assist woman to a side-lying (lateral) position.
- Increase maternal blood volume by increasing rate of primary IV infusion.

Interventions for Specific Problems
- Maternal hypotension
  - Increase rate of primary IV infusion.
  - Change to lateral or Trendelenburg positioning.
  - Administer ephedrine or phenylephrine if other measures are unsuccessful in increasing blood pressure.
- Uterine tachysystole
  - Reduce or discontinue dose of any uterine stimulants in use (e.g., oxytocin [Pitocin]).
  - Administer uterine relaxant (tocolytic) (e.g., terbutaline [Brethine]).
- Abnormal fetal heart rate pattern during second stage of labor
  - Use open-glottis pushing.
  - Use fewer pushing efforts during each contraction.
  - Make individual pushing efforts shorter.
  - Push only with every other or every third contraction.
  - Push only with perceived urge to push (in women with regional anesthesia).

IV, Intravenous.

---

do not require any specific action. Category II FHR tracings are indeterminate. This category includes all tracings that do not meet category I or category III criteria. Category II tracings require continued observation and evaluation. Category III FHR tracings are abnormal. Immediate evaluation and prompt intervention are required when these patterns are identified (Macones et al., 2008).

Nursing Management of Abnormal Patterns

The five essential components of the FHR tracing that must be evaluated regularly are baseline rate, baseline variability, accelerations, decelerations, and changes or trends over time. Whenever one of these five essential components is assessed as abnormal, corrective measures must be taken immediately. The purpose of these actions is to improve fetal oxygenation (Miller et al., 2017). The term *intrauterine resuscitation* is sometimes used to refer to specific interventions initiated when an abnormal FHR pattern is noted. Basic corrective measures include providing supplemental oxygen, instituting maternal position changes, and increasing intravenous fluid administration. These interventions are implemented to improve uterine and intervillous space blood flow and increase maternal oxygenation and cardiac output (Miller et al., 2017). Box 15.8 lists basic interventions to improve maternal and fetal oxygenation status.

Depending on the underlying cause of the abnormal FHR pattern, other interventions such as correcting maternal hypotension, reducing UA, and altering second-stage pushing techniques also may be instituted (Miller et al., 2017). Box 15.8 lists interventions for these specific problems. Some of the items listed are not independent nursing interventions. For example, any medications administered must be authorized either through inclusion in a unit protocol or by a verbal or written order. Some interventions are specific to the FHR pattern (see Table 15.3 and Boxes 15.5 and 15.6 for nursing interventions for tachycardia, late decelerations, and variable decelerations). Based on the FHR response to these interventions, the obstetric health care provider decides whether

additional interventions should be instituted or whether immediate vaginal or cesarean birth should be performed.

OTHER METHODS OF ASSESSMENT AND INTERVENTION

A major shortcoming of EFM is its high rate of false-positive results. Even the most abnormal patterns are poorly predictive of neonatal morbidity. Therefore other methods of assessment have been developed to evaluate fetal status. Fetal scalp stimulation, vibroacoustic stimulation, and umbilical cord acid-base determination are frequently performed assessments. Fetal scalp blood sampling is another available assessment technique. Amnioinfusion and tocolytic therapy are interventions often used in an attempt to improve abnormal FHR patterns.

Assessment Techniques

Fetal Scalp Stimulation and Vibroacoustic Stimulation

Several research studies conducted in the 1980s found that an FHR acceleration in response to digital or vibroacoustic stimulation was highly predictive of a normal scalp blood pH. The two methods of fetal stimulation used most often in clinical practice are scalp stimulation (using digital pressure during a vaginal examination) and vibroacoustic stimulation (using an artificial larynx or fetal acoustic stimulation device on the maternal abdomen over the fetal head continuously for 1 to 5 seconds). The desired result of these stimulation methods is acceleration in the FHR of at least 15 beats/min for at least 15 seconds (Miller et al., 2017). FHR acceleration indicates the absence of metabolic acidemia. If the fetus does not respond to stimulation with an acceleration, fetal compromise is not necessarily indicated; however, further evaluation of fetal well-being is needed. Fetal stimulation should be performed at times when the FHR is at baseline. Neither fetal scalp nor vibroacoustic stimulation should be instituted if FHR decelerations or bradycardia are present (Miller et al.).

TABLE 15.4   Approximate Normal Values for Cord Blood

Vessel	pH	Pco₂	Po₂	Base Deficit
Artery	7.2–7.3	45–55	15–25	<12
Vein	7.3–7.4	35–45	25–35	<12

From Miller, L., Miller, D., & Cypher, R. (2017). *Mosby's pocket guide to fetal monitoring: A multidisciplinary approach* (8th ed.). St. Louis, MO: Elsevier.

TABLE 15.5   Types of Acidemia

Value	Respiratory	Metabolic	Mixed
pH	<7.20	<7.20	<7.20
Pco₂	Elevated	Normal	Elevated
Base deficit	<12 mmol/L	≥12 mmol/L	≥12 mmol/L

From Miller, L., Miller, D., & Cypher, R. (2017). *Mosby's pocket guide to fetal monitoring: A multidisciplinary approach* (8th ed.). St. Louis, MO: Elsevier.

Umbilical Cord Acid-Base Determination

In assessing the immediate condition of the newborn after birth, a sample of cord blood is a useful adjunct to the Apgar score, especially if there has been an abnormal or confusing FHR tracing during labor or neonatal depression at birth. Generally the procedure is performed by withdrawing blood from both the umbilical artery and the umbilical vein. Both samples are then tested for pH, carbon dioxide pressure (Pco_2), oxygen pressure (Po_2), and base deficit or base excess. Umbilical arterial values reflect fetal condition, whereas umbilical vein values indicate placental function (Miller et al., 2017).

ACOG & AAP (2015) suggest obtaining umbilical artery cord blood values when a newborn has an Apgar score of ≤5 at 5 minutes of age. Normal umbilical artery and vein cord blood values are listed in Table 15.4. Normal findings preclude the presence of acidemia at or immediately before birth. If acidemia is present (e.g., pH less than 7.20), the type of acidemia is determined (respiratory, metabolic, or mixed) by analyzing the blood gas values (Table 15.5) (Miller et al., 2017).

Fetal Scalp Blood Sampling

Fetal scalp blood sampling is performed by obtaining a blood sample from the fetal scalp through the dilated cervix after the membranes have ruptured. Its use is limited by many factors, including the requirement for cervical dilation and membrane rupture, technical difficulty of the procedure, need for repetitive pH determinations, and uncertainty regarding interpretation and application of results. Fetal scalp blood sampling is now seldom used in the United States but remains a common practice in many other countries (Miller et al., 2017).

Interventions
Amnioinfusion

Amnioinfusion is infusion of room-temperature isotonic fluid (usually normal saline or lactated Ringer's solution) into the uterine cavity if the volume of amniotic fluid is low. Without the buffer of amniotic fluid, the umbilical cord can easily become compressed during contractions or fetal movement, diminishing the flow of blood between the placenta and fetus. The purpose of amnioinfusion is to relieve intermittent umbilical cord compression that results in variable decelerations and transient fetal hypoxemia by restoring the amniotic fluid volume to a normal or near-normal level. Amnioinfusion has no known effect on late decelerations and is no longer recommended as a means to dilute meconium-stained amniotic fluid (Miller et al., 2017). Women with an abnormally small amount of amniotic fluid (oligohydramnios) or no amniotic fluid (anhydramnios) are candidates for this procedure. Conditions that can result in oligohydramnios or anhydramnios include uteroplacental insufficiency and premature rupture of membranes.

Risks of amnioinfusion are overdistention of the uterine cavity and increased uterine tone. Fluid is administered through an IUPC by either gravity flow or an infusion pump. Usually a bolus of fluid is administered over 20 to 30 minutes; then the infusion is slowed to a maintenance rate. Likely no more than 1000 mL of fluid will need to be administered. The fluid can be warmed for the preterm fetus by infusing it through a blood warmer (Miller et al., 2017).

Intensity and frequency of UCs should be assessed continually during the procedure. The recorded uterine resting tone during amnioinfusion appears higher than normal because of resistance to outflow and turbulence at the end of the catheter. Uterine resting tone should not exceed 40 mm Hg during the procedure. The amount of vaginal fluid return must be estimated and documented during amnioinfusion to prevent overdistention of the uterus. The volume of fluid returned should be approximately the same as the amount infused (Miller et al., 2017).

Tocolytic Therapy

Tocolysis (relaxation of the uterus) can be achieved through the administration of drugs that inhibit UCs. This therapy can be used along with other interventions because excessive uterine activity is a common cause of interrupted fetal oxygenation. Tocolysis improves blood flow through the placenta by inhibiting UCs. It may be ordered by the obstetric health care provider when other interventions to reduce UA such as maternal position change and discontinuance of an oxytocin infusion have not diminished the UCs effectively. Tocolytics are often administered when women are having excessive UCs spontaneously. They are also frequently administered after a decision for cesarean birth has been made while preparations for surgery are under way. A commonly used tocolytic in these situations is terbutaline (Brethine) (Miller, 2017). If the FHR and UC patterns improve, the woman may be allowed to continue labor; if no improvement is seen, immediate cesarean birth may be needed.

PATIENT AND FAMILY TEACHING

Although the use of EFM can be reassuring to many parents, it can be a source of anxiety to some. Therefore the nurse must be particularly sensitive and respond appropriately to the emotional, informational, and comfort needs of the woman in labor and those of her family (Fig. 15.21; Box 15.9).

Part of the nurse's role includes partnering with other members of the interprofessional health care team, the woman, and her family to achieve a high-quality birthing experience. In addition to teaching and supporting the woman and her family with understanding of the laboring and birth process, breathing techniques, use of equipment, and pain-management techniques, the nurse can help with two factors that have an effect on fetal status: positioning and pushing. The nurse should enlist the woman's cooperation in avoiding the supine position because it can cause hypotension, which impairs placental perfusion and fetal oxygenation. Instead the woman should be encouraged to maintain the side-lying or semi-Fowler's position with a lateral tilt to the uterus. In addition, the nurse should instruct the woman to keep her mouth and glottis open and to let air escape from her lungs as she pushes. Both of these interventions help to improve fetal oxygenation. See Chapter 16 for further discussion of maternal positioning and pushing techniques.

DOCUMENTATION

Clear and complete documentation in the woman's medical record is essential. Each FHR and UA assessment must be documented completely. More and more hospitals are moving to use of the electronic medical record and computerized charting. With computerized charting, each required component usually appears on the screen so it will be addressed routinely. Computerized charting often includes forced choices that greatly increase the use of standardized FHR terminology by all members of the health care team. In the past, nurses were often encouraged to chart both on the monitor strip and in the medical record. However, charting directly on the monitor strip is unnecessary when an electronic medical record is used (Fig. 15.22). Any information that is handwritten

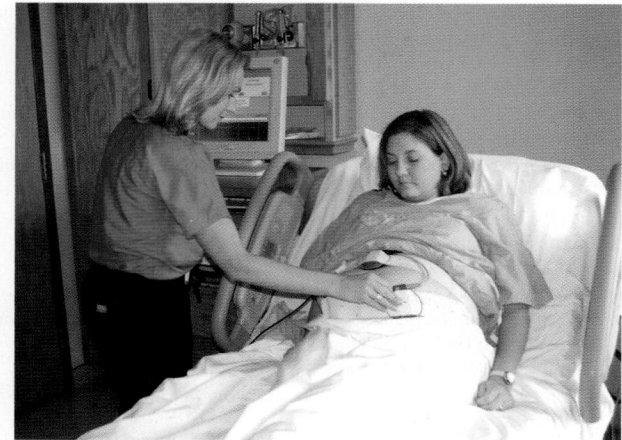

FIG 15.21 Nurse explains electronic fetal monitoring as ultrasound transducer monitors the fetal heart rate. (Courtesy of Julie Perry Nelson, Loveland, CO.)

BOX 15.9   Patient and Family Teaching When Electronic Fetal Monitor Is Used

The following guidelines relate to patient teaching and the functioning of the monitor:

- Explain purpose of monitoring.
- Explain each procedure.
- Provide rationale for maternal position other than supine.
- Explain that fetal status can be assessed continuously by electronic fetal monitoring (EFM), even during contractions.
- Explain that lower tracing on the monitor strip paper shows uterine activity (UA); upper tracing shows the fetal heart rate (FHR).
- Reassure woman and partner that prepared childbirth techniques can be implemented without difficulty.
- Explain that during external monitoring effleurage can be performed on sides of abdomen or upper portion of thighs.
- Explain that breathing patterns based on time and intensity of contractions can be enhanced by observing uterine activity on monitor strip, which shows the onset of contractions.
- Note peak of contraction; knowing that contraction will not get stronger and is halfway over is usually helpful.
- Note diminishing intensity.
- Coordinate with appropriate breathing and relaxation techniques.
- Reassure woman and partner that use of internal monitoring does not restrict movement, although she is confined to bed.*
- Explain that use of external monitoring usually requires woman's cooperation during positioning and movement.
- Reassure woman and partner that use of monitoring does not imply fetal jeopardy.

*Portable telemetry monitors permit ambulation during FHR and uterine contraction monitoring. The integrated abdominal FHR and UA monitoring system also provides some degree of patient mobility.

Fetal Monitor Integration

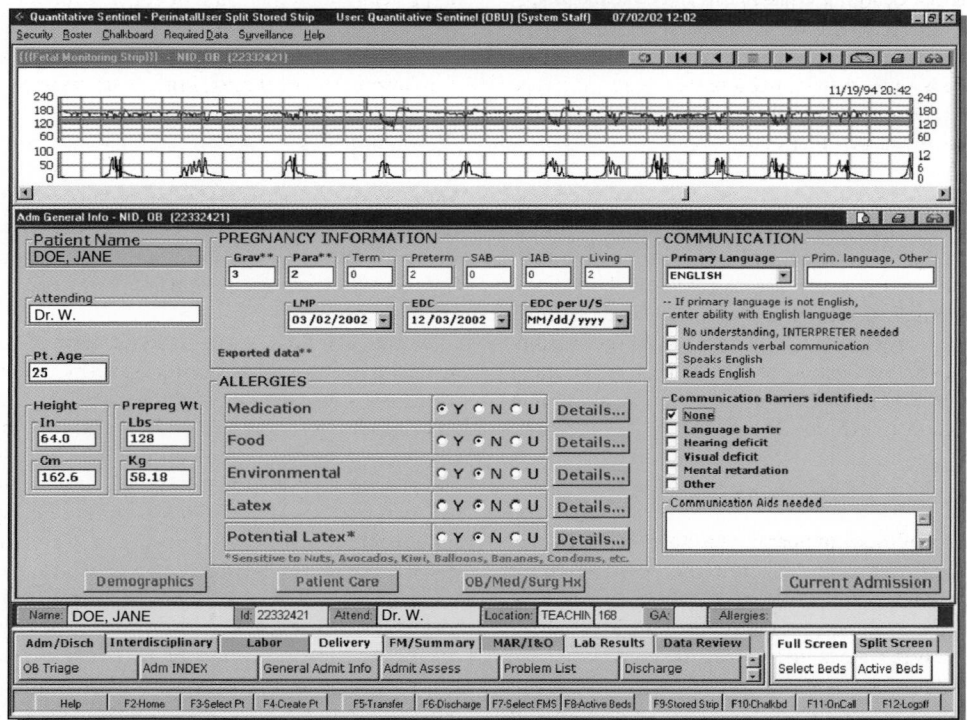

FIG 15.22 With integration of the fetal monitor tracing into the electronic medical record, the nurse can view the fetal tracing while charting. (Courtesy of General Electric Healthcare Technologies, Barrington, IL.)

on the monitor strip will not be recorded in the computer record. Furthermore, given that the EFM tracing is stored on a computer, the paper strips are destroyed after the woman is discharged. No permanent record of the handwritten charting exists.

In institutions that still use a paper chart, documentation on the woman's monitor strip is started before the initiation of monitoring and consists of identifying information plus other relevant data. This documentation is continued and updated according to institutional protocol as monitoring continues and labor progresses.

In some institutions, observations noted and interventions implemented are recorded on the monitor strip to produce a comprehensive document that chronicles the course of labor and the care rendered. In other institutions, this documentation is confined to the labor flow record. Advocates of documenting on both the medical record and the EFM strip cite as advantages of this approach the ease of writing directly on the strip while at the bedside and the improved accuracy in documenting critical events and the interventions implemented. Others believe that charting on the EFM strip constitutes duplicate documentation of the same information noted in the medical record and thus it is unnecessary additional paperwork for the nurse.

A disadvantage of documenting on both the EFM strip and in the medical record is that the times noted for events and interventions on the EFM strip frequently do not correlate with what is later documented in the medical record. These inaccuracies can lead people involved in the retrospective review process carried out during litigation to infer that documentation errors have occurred. Therefore, if institutional policy mandates documentation both on the monitor strip and in the medical record, the nurse must make sure that the times and notations of events and interventions recorded in each place agree.

REFERENCES

American Academy of Pediatrics and American College of Obstetricians and Gynecologists. (2012). *Guidelines for perinatal care* (7th ed.). Washington, DC: American College of Obstetricians and Gynecologists.

American College of Obstetricians and Gynecologists. (2009, reaffirmed 2015). Practice bulletin no. 106: Intrapartum fetal heart rate monitoring: Nomenclature, interpretation, and general management principles. *Obstetrics & Gynecology, 114*(1), 192–202.

American College of Obstetricians and Gynecologists (ACOG) and American Academy of Pediatrics. (2015). Committee opinion no. 644: The Apgar score. *Obstetrics & Gynecology, 126*(4), e52–e55.

Association of Women's Health, Obstetric and Neonatal Nurses. (2015a). AWHONN position statement: Fetal heart monitoring. *Journal of Obstetric, Gynecologic, & Neonatal Nursing, 44*(5), 683–686.

Association of Women's Health, Obstetric and Neonatal Nurses. (2015b). *Fetal heart monitoring principles and practice* (5th ed.). Dubuque, IA: Kendall/Hunt.

Cunningham, F., Leveno, K., Bloom, S., et al. (2014). *Williams obstetrics* (24th ed.). New York, NY: McGraw-Hill Education.

Lyndon, A., O'Brien-Abel, N., & Simpson, K. (2014). Fetal assessment during labor. In K. R. Simpson & P. Creehan (Eds.), *AWHONN's perinatal nursing* (4th ed.). Philadelphia, PA: Lippincott Williams & Wilkins.

Macones, G., Hankins, G., Spong, C., et al. (2008). The 2008 National Institute of Child Health and Human Development workshop report on electronic fetal monitoring: Update on definitions, interpretation, and research guidelines. *Journal of Obstetric, Gynecologic, & Neonatal Nursing, 37*(5), 510–515.

Miller, D. (2017). Intrapartum fetal evaluation. In S. G. Gabbe, J. R. Niebyl, J. L. Simpson, et al. (Eds.), *Obstetrics: Normal and problem pregnancies* (7th ed.). Philadelphia, PA: Elsevier.

Miller, L., Miller, D., & Cypher, R. (2017). *Mosby's pocket guide to fetal monitoring: A multidisciplinary approach* (8th ed.). St. Louis, MO: Elsevier.

National Institute of Child Health and Human Development Research Planning Workshop. (1997). Electronic fetal heart rate monitoring: Research guidelines for interpretation. *American Journal of Obstetrics & Gynecology, 177*(6), 1385–1390.

16

Nursing Care of the Family During Labor and Birth

Kitty Cashion

http://evolve.elsevier.com/Perry/maternal

Labor and birth are natural phenomena during which most women benefit from a philosophy of minimal intervention. The minimal intervention philosophy acknowledges that most pregnancies, labors, and births are normal and that intervention creates the potential for iatrogenic maternal-fetal injuries (Simpson & O'Brien-Abel, 2014). This is an exciting and potentially anxious time for the woman and her significant others (partner, family members, or other support people). In a relatively short period of time, they experience one of the most profound events in their lives. Birth may take place in the hospital, birth center, or home setting or unexpectedly at any number of locations. The woman and her significant others may be cared for by an interprofessional team of caregivers including nurses, doulas, nurse-midwives, and physicians (see Community Focus box: Availability of Alternative Childbirth Options in the Community).

COMMUNITY FOCUS

Availability of Alternative Childbirth Options in the Community

Search the Internet to explore options for childbearing families in your community. Is there a birthing center in your community? Are certified nurse-midwives available? Are other types of licensed midwives available? Is there an option for a home birth? For a water birth? During your clinical rotation in maternity nursing, interview a staff nurse in labor and delivery (L&D) and explore his or her views of midwives and home births. Interview a childbirth educator, and explore his or her views of midwives and home births. Compare and contrast the views of the L&D nurse and the childbirth educator. Is there a difference in their views? Discuss the findings from your interviews with your clinical group.

For most women, labor begins with the first uterine contraction, continues with hours of hard work during cervical dilation and birth, and ends as the woman and her family begin the attachment process with the newborn. Nursing care management focuses on assessment and support of the woman and her significant others throughout labor and birth, along with assessment of fetal well-being and response to labor. The goal of nursing care is to ensure the best possible outcome for all involved. The focus of this chapter is on nursing care that facilitates normal labor and birth.

FIRST STAGE OF LABOR

The **first stage of labor** begins with the onset of regular uterine contractions and ends with complete cervical effacement and dilation. Traditionally, the first stage of labor was considered to be composed of three phases: the *latent phase* (through 3 cm of dilation), the *active phase* (4 to 7 cm of dilation), and the *transition phase* (8 to 10 cm of dilation). However, these definitions have changed based on research findings. After studying the labors of thousands of contemporary women, researchers have concluded that they differ in several characteristics from the women who gave birth more than half a century ago, when Dr. E.A. Friedman published his findings regarding the length of "normal" labor. Contemporary women tend to be older and heavier than their earlier counterparts. They progress more slowly during the active phase of labor than was previously believed and experience longer labors. Active labor begins at 6 cm for both nulliparous and multiparous women. During the early phase of first-stage labor, nulliparous and multiparous women progress at similar rates. After reaching a cervical dilation of 6 cm, however, multiparous women progress more rapidly in labor (Hanson & VandeVusse, 2014; Kelly, Swart, & Baird, 2017; Kilpatrick & Garrison, 2017).

Therefore, the first stage of labor is now divided into only two phases. The **latent phase** extends from the onset of labor, characterized by regular, painful uterine contractions that cause cervical change, to the beginning of the active phase, when cervical dilation occurs more rapidly. The **active phase** is defined as the period during which the greatest rate of cervical dilation occurs, which begins at 6 cm, and ends with complete cervical dilation at 10 cm (Kelly et al., 2017; Kilpatrick & Garrison, 2017).

CARE MANAGEMENT

Most nulliparous women planning a hospital or birth center birth seek admission in the latent phase because they have not experienced labor before and are unsure of the "right" time to come in. Multiparous women usually do not come to the birth center or hospital until they are in the active phase of the first stage of labor. Even though no two labors are identical, women who have given birth before often are less anxious about the process, unless their previous experience was negative.

ASSESSMENT

Assessment begins at the first contact with the woman, whether by telephone or in person. Many women call the hospital or birthing center first for validation as to whether they should come to the hospital for evaluation or admission or whether they should remain at home. Many hospitals discourage nurses from giving advice regarding what to do because of legal liability. Nurses are often instructed to tell women who call with questions to call their nurse-midwife or physician or to come to the hospital if they feel the need to be checked. The nature of the telephone conversation, including any advice or instructions given, and the person's response to the instructions, should be documented in the patient's record (Baird, Kennedy, & Baudhuin, 2017).

A pregnant woman may first call her nurse-midwife or physician or go to the hospital or birth center while in false labor or early in the latent phase of the first stage of labor. She may feel discouraged, angry, or confused on learning that the contractions that feel so strong and regular to her do not indicate true labor because they are not causing cervical dilation or that they are still not strong or frequent enough for admission. During the third trimester of pregnancy, women should be instructed regarding the stages of labor and the signs indicating its onset. They should be informed of the possibility that they will not be admitted if they are in latent labor (see Patient Teaching box: How to Distinguish True Labor from False Labor).

If the woman lives near the hospital or birth center and has adequate support and transportation, she may be encouraged to stay home or return home to allow labor to progress (i.e., until the uterine contractions are more frequent and intense). The ideal setting for the woman at low risk for obstetric complications at this time usually is the familiar environment of her home, where she can move around freely and eat and drink at will. However, the woman who lives at a considerable distance from the hospital or birth center, who lacks adequate support and transportation, or who has a history of rapid labors in the past may be admitted in latent labor. The same measures used by the woman at home should be offered to the woman admitted in early labor.

A warm shower or bath is often calming and relaxing during early labor. Also, research has shown that water is effective at assisting irregular contractions to become more consistent (Waterbirth International, 2016). Soothing back, foot, and hand massage or a warm drink of preferred liquids such as tea or milk can help the woman rest and even sleep, especially if false or early labor is occurring at night. Diversional activities such as walking outdoors or in the house, reading, watching television, using a computer or smart phone, or talking with friends can reduce the perception of early discomfort, help time pass, and decrease anxiety.

When the woman arrives at the birth center or hospital perinatal unit, assessment is the top priority (Fig. 16.1). The nurse first performs a screening assessment by using the techniques of interview and physical assessment and reviews the laboratory and diagnostic test findings to determine the health status of the woman and her fetus and the progress of her labor. The nurse also notifies the nurse-midwife or physician. If the woman is admitted, a detailed systems assessment is done.

PATIENT TEACHING

How to Distinguish True Labor from False Labor

True Labor

Contractions

- Occur regularly, becoming stronger, lasting longer, and occurring closer together
- Become more intense with walking
- Are usually felt in the lower back, radiating to the lower portion of abdomen
- Continue despite use of comfort measures

Cervix (by Vaginal Examination)

- Shows progressive change (softening, effacement, and dilation signaled by appearance of bloody show)
- Moves to an increasingly anterior position

Fetus

- Presenting part usually becomes engaged in the pelvis, which results in increased ease of breathing; at the same time, the presenting part presses downward and compresses the bladder, resulting in urinary frequency

False Labor

Contractions

- Occur irregularly or become regular only temporarily
- Often stop with walking or position change
- Can be felt in the back or the abdomen above the umbilicus
- Can often be stopped through the use of comfort measures

Cervix (by Vaginal Examination)

- May be soft but with no significant change in effacement or dilation or evidence of bloody show
- Is often in a posterior position

Fetus

- Presenting part is usually not engaged in pelvis

LEGAL TIP Obstetric Triage and EMTALA The Emergency Medical Treatment and Active Labor Act (EMTALA) is a federal regulation enacted to protect pregnant women during an emergency regardless of their insurance status or ability to pay for care. According to the EMTALA, pregnant women who present with contractions or who may be in labor are considered unstable and must be assessed, stabilized, and treated at the hospital where they present regardless of their insurance status or ability to pay. Nurses working in labor and birth units must be familiar with their responsibilities according to the EMTALA regulations, which include providing services to pregnant women when they experience an urgent pregnancy problem (e.g., labor, decreased fetal movement, rupture of membranes, or recent trauma) and fully documenting all relevant information (e.g., assessment findings, interventions implemented, and patient responses to care measures provided). A pregnant woman presenting in an obstetric triage area is considered to be in "true" labor until a qualified health care provider certifies that she is not. Agencies need to have specific policies and procedures in place so that compliance with the EMTALA regulations is achieved while safe and efficient care is provided (Baird et al., 2017; Wilson-Griffin, 2014).

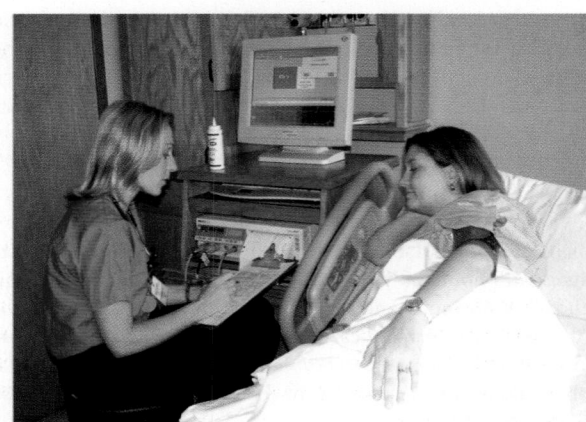

FIG 16.1 Woman being admitted. (Courtesy of Julie Perry Nelson, Loveland, CO.)

When the woman is admitted, she is usually moved from an observation area to the labor room; the labor, delivery, and recovery (LDR) room; or the labor, delivery, recovery, and postpartum (LDRP) room. If the woman wishes, the nurse includes her partner, family member, or other support person in the assessment and admission process. The nurse can direct significant other(s) not participating in this process to the appropriate waiting area. In the hospital setting, the woman undresses and puts on her own gown or a hospital gown. The nurse places an identification band on the woman's wrist. Her personal belongings are put away safely or given to family members according to agency policy. Women who participate in expectant parent classes often bring a birth bag with them. The nurse then shows the woman and her partner the layout and operation of the unit and room, how to use the call light and telephone system, how to adjust lighting in the room, and the different bed positions.

The nurse reassures the woman that she is in competent, caring hands and that she and those to whom she gives permission can ask questions related to her care and status and that of her fetus at any time during labor. The nurse can minimize the woman's anxiety by explaining terms commonly used during labor. The woman's interest, response, and prior experience guide the depth and breadth of these explanations.

Most hospitals have specific forms, whether paper or electronic, that are used to obtain important assessment information when a woman in labor is being evaluated or admitted (Fig. 16.2, A and B). More and more hospitals now use an electronic medical record; almost all charting is done on computer. Sources of data include the prenatal record, initial interview, physical examination to determine baseline physiologic parameters (e.g., vital signs), laboratory and diagnostic test results, select psychosocial and cultural factors, and clinical evaluation of labor status.

Prenatal Data

The nurse reviews the prenatal record to identify the woman's individual needs and risks. Copies of prenatal records are generally filed in the perinatal unit at some time during the woman's pregnancy (usually in the third trimester) or accessed electronically so they are readily available on admission. If the woman has had no prenatal care or her prenatal records are unavailable, the nurse must obtain certain baseline information. If the woman is having discomfort, the nurse should ask questions between contractions when she can concentrate more fully on her answers. At times the partner or support person(s) may need to be secondary sources of essential information. According to the Health Insurance Portability and Accountability Act (HIPAA), the woman must give permission for other individuals to be involved in the exchange of information regarding her care. Ideally, this permission should be obtained during pregnancy, and a signed form included in her health records.

Knowing the woman's age is important so that the nurse can individualize care to the needs of her age group. For example, a 14-year-old adolescent and a 40-year-old woman have different but specific needs, and their ages place them at risk for different problems. Accurate height and weight measurements are important. A pregnancy weight gain greater than recommended may place the woman at a higher risk for cephalopelvic disproportion and cesarean birth. This is especially true for women who are petite and have gained 16 kg (35 pounds) or more. A prepregnancy body mass index (BMI) greater than 30 is also a cause for concern. Other factors to consider are the woman's general health status, current medical conditions or allergies, respiratory status, and previous surgical procedures.

The nurse should review the woman's prenatal records carefully, taking note of her obstetric history, including gravidity; parity; and problems such as history of vaginal bleeding, gestational hypertension, anemia, pregestational or gestational diabetes, infections (e.g., bacterial, viral, sexually transmitted), and immunodeficiency status. In addition, the expected date of birth (EDB) should be confirmed. Other important data found in the prenatal record include patterns of maternal weight gain; physiologic measurements such as maternal vital signs (blood pressure, temperature, pulse, respirations); fundal height; baseline fetal heart rate (FHR); and laboratory and diagnostic test results. See Table 8.1 for a list of common prenatal laboratory tests. Common diagnostic and fetal assessment tests performed prenatally include amniocentesis, nonstress test (NST), biophysical profile (BPP), and ultrasound examination. See Chapter 10 for more information.

If this labor and birth experience is not the woman's first, the nurse needs to note the characteristics of her previous experiences. This information includes the duration of previous labors; the types of pain relief measures, including anesthesia used; the type of birth (e.g., spontaneous vaginal, forceps-assisted, vacuum-assisted, or cesarean birth); and the condition of the newborn. The nurse explores the woman's perception of her previous labor and birth experiences because this perception may influence her attitude toward her current experience.

Interview

The woman's primary reason for coming to the hospital is determined in the interview. For example, it may be that her amniotic membranes ruptured ("water broke"), with or without contractions. The woman may have come in for a period of observation reserved for women who are unsure about the onset of their labor. This allows time for the diagnosis of labor without official hospital admission and minimizes or avoids cost to the woman when used by the hospital and approved by her health insurance plan.

Even the experienced woman may have difficulty determining the onset of labor. She is asked to recall the events of the previous days and describe the following:

- Time and onset of contractions and progress in terms of frequency, duration, and intensity
- Location and character of discomfort from contractions (e.g., back pain, abdominal or suprapubic discomfort)
- Persistence of contractions despite changes in maternal position and activity (e.g., walking or lying down)
- Presence and character of vaginal discharge or "show"
- The status of amniotic membranes such as a gush or leakage of fluid (spontaneous rupture of membranes [SROM]). If there has been a discharge that may be amniotic fluid, she is asked the date and time the fluid was first noted and the fluid's characteristics (e.g., amount, color, unusual odor). In many instances, a sterile speculum examination and Nitrazine (pH) and *fern tests* can confirm that the membranes are ruptured (Box 16.1).

These descriptions help the nurse assess the degree of progress in the process of labor. Bloody show is distinguished from bleeding by the fact that it is pink and feels sticky because of its mucoid nature. There is very little bloody show in the beginning, but the amount increases with effacement and dilation of the cervix. A woman may report a small amount of brownish-to-bloody discharge that may be attributed to cervical trauma resulting from vaginal examination or coitus (intercourse) within the last 48 hours.

Assessing the woman's respiratory status is important in case general anesthesia is needed in an emergency. The nurse determines this status by asking the woman if she has a "cold" or related symptoms (e.g., stuffy nose, sore throat, or cough). The status of allergies, including allergies to latex and tape, and medications routinely used in obstetrics such as opioids (e.g., meperidine [Demerol], fentanyl [Sublimaze], remifentanil [Ultiva], and nalbuphine [Nubain]), local anesthetic agents

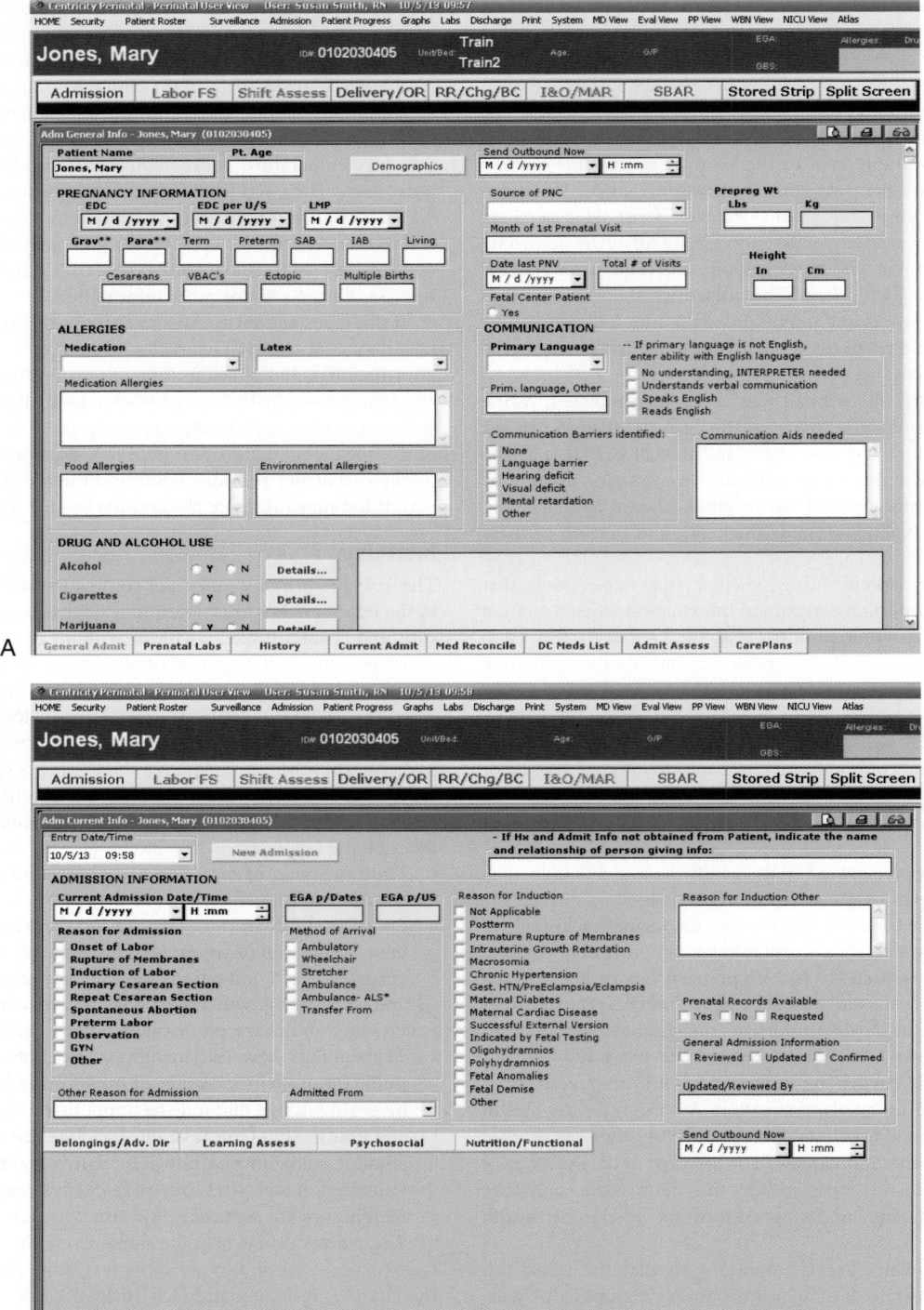

FIG 16.2 Admission screens in an electronic medical record. **A,** General admission screen. **B,** Current admission screen. (Courtesy of Kitty Cashion, RN-BC, MSN, Memphis, TN.)

(e.g., bupivacaine, lidocaine, ropivacaine), and antiseptics (Betadine) is reviewed. Some allergic responses cause swelling of the mucous membranes of the respiratory tract, which could interfere with breathing and the administration of inhalation anesthesia. Because vomiting and subsequent aspiration into the respiratory tract can complicate an otherwise normal labor, the nurse records the time and type of the woman's most recent solid and liquid intake.

The nurse obtains any information not found in the prenatal record during the admission assessment. Pertinent data include the birth plan (Box 16.2), the type of pain management (including nonpharmacologic

BOX 16.1   Procedure: Tests for Rupture of Membranes

Nitrazine Test for pH
- Explain procedure to woman or couple.

Procedure
- Wash hands and put on sterile gloves.
- Use a cotton-tipped applicator impregnated with Nitrazine dye for determining pH (differentiates amniotic fluid, which is slightly alkaline, from urine and purulent material [pus], which are acidic).
- Dip cotton-tipped applicator deep into vagina to pick up fluid. (Procedure may be performed during speculum examination.)

Read Results
- Membranes probably intact: Identifies vaginal and most body fluids that are acidic:

Yellow	pH 5.0
Olive-yellow	pH 5.5
Olive-green	pH 6.0

- Membranes probably ruptured: Identifies amniotic fluid that is alkaline:

Blue-green	pH 6.5
Blue-gray	pH 7.0
Deep blue	pH 7.5

- Realize that false test results are possible because of presence of bloody show, insufficient amniotic fluid, or semen.
- Provide pericare as needed.
- Remove gloves and wash hands.

Document Results
- Results are reported as positive or negative.

Test for Ferning or Fern Pattern
- Explain procedure to woman or couple.

Procedure
- Wash hands, put on sterile gloves, obtain specimen of fluid (usually during sterile speculum examination).
- Spread a drop of fluid from vagina on clean glass slide with sterile cotton-tipped applicator.
- Allow fluid to dry.
- Examine the slide under microscope; observe for appearance of ferning (a frond-like crystalline pattern) (do not confuse with cervical mucus test, when high levels of estrogen cause ferning).
- Observe for absence of ferning (alerts staff to possibility that amount of specimen was inadequate or that specimen was urine, vaginal discharge, or blood).
- Provide pericare as needed.
- Remove gloves and wash hands.

Document Results
- Results are reported as positive or negative.

BOX 16.2   The Birth Plan

The birth plan should include the woman's or couple's preferences related to the following:
- Presence of birth companions such as the partner, older children, parents, friends, and doula and the role each will play.
- Presence of other people such as students, male attendants, and interpreters.
- Clothing to be worn.
- Environmental modifications such as lighting, music, privacy, focal point, and items from home such as pillows.
- Labor activities such as preferred positions for labor and for birth, ambulation, birth balls, showers and whirlpool baths, oral food and fluid intake.
- List of comfort and relaxation measures.
- Labor and birth medical interventions such as pharmacologic pain relief measures, intravenous therapy, electronic monitoring, induction or augmentation measures, and episiotomy.
- Care and handling of the newborn immediately after birth such as immediate skin-to-skin contact, cutting of the cord, eye care, and breastfeeding.
- Cultural and religious requirements related to the care of the mother, newborn, and placenta.

The childbirth website (www.childbirth.org) provides couples with an interactive birth plan along with examples of birth plans and descriptions of the options that can be included.

available and determining the woman's wishes and preferences. As caregiver and advocate, the nurse integrates the woman's desires into the nursing care plan while explaining what may or may not be possible to meet all her expectations given the policies of the birthing facility. The nurse also prepares the woman for the possibility that her plan may change as labor progresses and assures her that the staff will provide information so she can make informed decisions. The woman must also understand that the more extensive her birth plan, the less is the likelihood that all her expectations will be met.

The nurse should discuss with the woman and her partner their plans for preserving childbirth memories through the use of photography and videotaping. Information should be provided about the agency's policies regarding these practices and under what circumstances they are allowed. Protection of privacy and safety and infection control are major concerns for the expectant parents and the agency. To avoid future embarrassment and distress, the nurse should clarify with the woman exactly which parts of her childbirth she wishes to have photographed and the degree of detail. The nurse reminds women and their families that photographs should not be posted on social media sites without the knowledge and consent of *every* person who appears in the picture.

> **LEGAL TIP   Recording of Childbirth** The woman's record should reflect that the childbirth was recorded. Some hospitals and health care providers do not allow videotaping of the birth because of concerns related to legal liability.

Psychosocial Factors

The woman's general appearance and behavior (and that of her partner, family member, or other support person) provide valuable clues to the type of supportive care she will need. However, keep in mind that general appearance and behavior may vary, depending on the stage and phase of labor (Table 16.1 and Box 16.3).

comfort measures) preferred, the choice of infant feeding method, and the name of the pediatric health care provider. The nurse inquires about the woman's preparation for childbirth, the support person or family members whose presence is desired during childbirth and their availability, and ethnic or cultural expectations and needs. The nurse also asks about the woman's use of alcohol, drugs, and tobacco before or during pregnancy.

The nurse reviews the birth plan. If there is no written plan, the nurse assists the woman to formulate a birth plan by describing options

TABLE 16.1   Expected Maternal Progress in First-Stage Labor

Criterion	Early Phase 0–5 cm	Active Phase 6–10 cm
*Duration[†]	Nulliparous and multiparous women progress at similar rates	Multiparous women progress more rapidly than do nulliparous women
Contractions		
**Strength	Mild to moderate by palpation	Moderate to strong by palpation
**Frequency	2–30 minutes apart; may be irregular	1.5–5 minutes apart
**Duration	30–40 seconds	40–90 seconds
Descent		
*Station of presenting part		Nulliparous women 0 by 6 cm Multiparous women −1 by 6 cm
Show		
Color	Brownish discharge, mucus plug, or pale pink mucus	Pink-to-bloody mucus
Amount	Scant	Moderate to copious
Behavior and appearance[‡]	Excited; thoughts center on self, labor, and baby; able to walk or talk through most contractions; may be talkative or silent, calm or tense; some apprehension; pain controlled fairly well; alert, follows directions readily; open to instructions	Becomes more serious, doubtful of pain control, more apprehensive; desires companionship and encouragement; attention more inwardly directed; has some difficulty following directions As active labor continues: Pain may be described as severe; backache common; frustration, fear of loss of control, and irritability may be voiced; expresses doubt about ability to continue; nausea and vomiting, especially if hyperventilating; perspiration of forehead and upper lip; shaking tremor of thighs; feeling of need to defecate, pressure on anus

[†]Duration of each phase is influenced by such factors as parity; maternal emotions; position; level of activity; and fetal size, presentation, and position.

[‡]Women who have epidural analgesia for pain relief may not demonstrate some of these behaviors.

*Data from Kennedy, B.B. & Baird, S.M. (2017). *Intrapartum management modules: A perinatal education program* (5th ed.). Philadelphia, PA: Wolters Kluwer.

**Data from Simpson, K.R. & Creehan P. (2014). *AWHONN's perinatal nursing* (4th ed.). Philadelphia, PA: Lippincott.

Women With a History of Sexual Abuse

Labor can trigger memories of sexual abuse, especially during intrusive procedures such as vaginal examinations. Monitors, intravenous (IV) lines, and epidurals can make the woman feel a loss of control or feel as if she is being confined to bed and "restrained." Being observed by students and having intense sensations in the uterus and genital area, especially at the time when she must push the baby out, can also trigger memories.

The nurse can help the abuse survivor associate the sensations she is experiencing with the process of childbirth and not with her past abuse. The nurse can help the woman maintain her sense of control by explaining all procedures and why they are needed, validating her needs, and paying close attention to her requests. It is important to wait for the woman to give permission before touching her, and to accept her often extreme reactions to labor (Simpson & O'Brien-Abel, 2014). The nurse should avoid using words and phrases that can cause the woman to recall the words of her abuser (e.g., "open your legs," "relax and it won't hurt so much"). As much as possible, health care professionals should limit the number of procedures that invade the woman's body (e.g., vaginal examinations, urinary catheter, internal monitor, forceps or vacuum extractor). Encouraging the woman to choose a person (e.g., doula, friend, family member) to be with her during labor to provide continuous support and comfort and to act as her advocate is also another suggested intervention. Nurses are advised to care for all laboring women in this manner because it is not unusual for a woman to choose not to reveal a history of sexual abuse. These care measures can help a woman perceive her childbirth experience in positive terms.

Stress in Labor

The way in which women and their support people or family members approach labor is related to the manner in which they have been prepared for and socialized to childbearing as well as how they deal with other stressors in their lives. Their reactions reflect their beliefs and life experiences regarding childbirth—physical, social, cultural, and religious. Society communicates its expectations regarding acceptable and unacceptable maternal behaviors during labor and birth. These expectations may be used by some women as the basis for evaluating their own actions during childbirth. An idealized perception of labor and birth may be a source of guilt and cause a sense of failure if the woman finds the process less than joyous, especially when the pregnancy is unplanned or is the product of a dysfunctional or terminated relationship. Often women have heard horror stories or have seen friends or relatives going through labors that appear difficult and painful. Multiparous women

BOX 16.3   Psychosocial Assessment of the Laboring Woman

Verbal Interactions

- Does the woman ask questions?
- Can she ask for what she needs?
- Does she talk to her support person(s)?
- Does she talk freely with the nurse or respond only to questions?

Body Language

- Does she change positions or lie rigidly still?
- What is her anxiety level?
- How does she react to being touched by the nurse or support person?
- Does she avoid eye contact?
- Does she look tired? If she appears tired, ask her how much rest she has had in the past 24 hours.

Perceptual Ability

- Is there a language barrier?
- Are repeated explanations necessary because her anxiety level interferes with her ability to comprehend?
- Can she repeat what she has been told or otherwise demonstrate her understanding?

Discomfort Level

- To what degree does the woman describe what she is experiencing, including her pain experience?
- How does she react to a contraction?
- How does she react to assessment and care measures?
- Are any nonverbal pain messages noted?
- Can she ask for comfort measures?

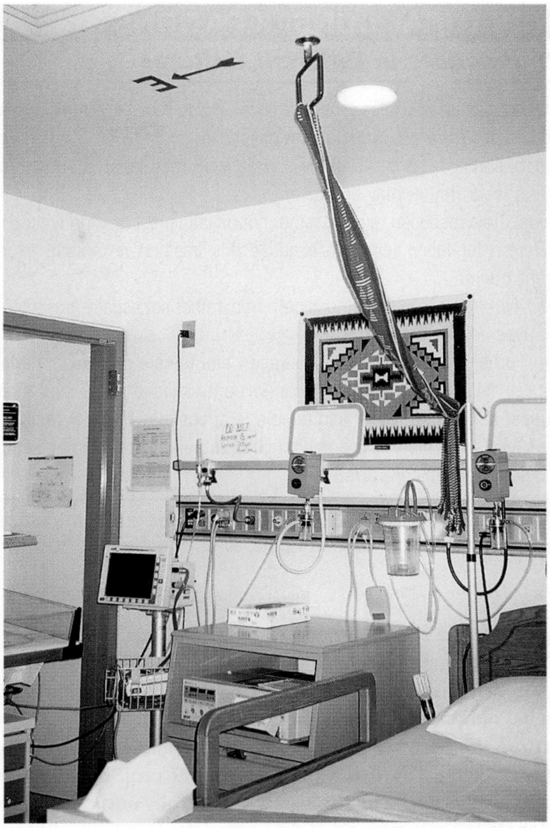

FIG 16.3 Birthing room specific to Native-American population. Note arrow pointing east, rug on wall, and rope or sash belt hanging from ceiling. (Courtesy of Patricia Hess, San Francisco, CA; Chinle Comprehensive Health Care Center, Chinle, AZ.)

often base their expectations of the current labor on their previous childbirth experiences.

The nurse encourages the woman to express her feelings about the pregnancy and her concerns and fears related to childbirth. This discussion is especially important if the woman is a primigravida who has not attended childbirth classes but has obtained information on childbirth from the Internet or reality television shows about birth or is a multiparous woman who has had a previous negative childbirth experience. Women in labor usually have a variety of concerns that they will voice if asked but may not volunteer. Major fears and concerns relate to the process and effects of childbirth, maternal and fetal well-being, and the attitude and actions of the health care staff. Every effort should be made to provide support and to encourage those with her to be supportive. Women who have continuous labor support are more likely to have a spontaneous vaginal birth and are less likely to have intrapartum analgesia or anesthesia, a cesarean or an operative vaginal birth, and a baby with a low 5-minute Apgar score; or to report dissatisfaction with their childbirth experiences (Hodnett, Gates, Hofmeyer, & Sakala, 2013).

The partner, coach, or significant other also experiences stress during labor. The nurse can assist these individuals by assessing their needs and expectations, offering support, and interpreting events that are occurring. The degree of involvement and participation in labor support varies; therefore, it is important for the nurse to determine the intended role of the support person and whether or not that person is prepared to fulfill the role. For example, has the support person attended childbirth preparation classes? Does the support person appear anxious? What is the interaction between the support person and the laboring woman?

Is the support person actively involved in labor support or sitting quietly at the bedside? If the support person is touching the woman, what is the character of the touch? Is the person watching TV or engaged in computer or smart phone activities? Is there any aggressive or hostile attitude or behavior? The nurse demonstrates sensitivity to the needs of support people, and provides teaching and support as appropriate. In many instances, the support these people provide to the laboring woman may be in direct proportion to the support they receive from the nurses and other health care professionals.

Cultural Factors

Nearly 1 million immigrants come to the United States each year, half of whom are women of childbearing age. More than 30% of the US population belongs to a cultural group other than non-Hispanic white. It is expected that by the year 2050 members of cultural groups other than non-Hispanic white will make up more than half of the US population (Callister, 2014). As the population becomes more diverse, it is increasingly important to note the woman's ethnic or cultural and religious values, beliefs, and practices in order to anticipate nursing interventions to add or eliminate from an individualized, mutually acceptable plan of care that provides a feeling of safety and control (Fig. 16.3). Nurses should be committed to providing culturally sensitive care and developing an appreciation and respect for cultural diversity (Callister). The nurse encourages the woman to request specific caregiving behaviors and practices that are important to her. If a special request contradicts usual practices in that setting, the woman or the nurse can ask the woman's nurse-midwife or physician to write an order to

🌐 CULTURAL CONSIDERATIONS

Birth Practices in Different Cultures

- *Somalia:* Because Somalis in general do not like to show any sign of weakness, women are extremely stoic during childbirth.
- *Japan:* Natural childbirth methods practiced; may labor silently; may eat during labor; father may be present
- *China:* Stoic response to pain; father not usually present; side-lying position preferred for labor and birth because this position is thought to reduce infant trauma
- *India:* Natural childbirth methods preferred; father not usually present; female relatives usually present
- *Iran:* Father not present; female support and female caregivers preferred
- *Mexico:* May be stoic about discomfort until second stage, and then may request pain relief; father and female relatives may be present
- *Laos:* May use squatting position for birth; father may or may not be present; female attendants preferred

Data from D'Avanzo, C. (2008). *Mosby's pocket guide to cultural health assessment* (4th ed.). St Louis, MO: Mosby.

accommodate the special request. For example, in many cultures it is unacceptable to have a male caregiver examine a pregnant woman. In some cultures, it is traditional to take the placenta home; in others, the woman has only certain nourishments during labor. Some women believe that cutting the body, as with an episiotomy, allows her spirit to leave her body and that rupturing the membranes prolongs, not shortens, labor. It is always important to listen respectfully and carefully explain the rationale for recommended care measures (see Cultural Considerations box: Birth Practices in Different Cultures).

Within cultures, women may have an idea of the "right" way to behave in labor and may react to the pain experienced in that way. These behaviors can range from total silence to moaning or screaming, but they do not necessarily indicate the degree of pain being experienced. A woman who moans with contractions may not be in as much physical pain as a woman who is silent but winces during contractions. Some women believe that screaming or crying out in pain is shameful if a man is present. If the woman's support person is her mother, she may perceive the need to be more stoic more strongly than if her support person is the father of the baby. She may perceive herself as failing or succeeding based on her ability to follow these "standards" of behavior. Conversely, a woman's behavior in response to pain may influence the support received from significant others. In some cultures, women who lose control and cry out in pain may be scolded, whereas in other cultures support people will become more helpful.

Culture and Father Participation

A partner or companion is an important source of support, encouragement, and comfort for women during childbirth. The woman's cultural and religious background influences her choice of birth companion as do trends in the society in which she lives. For example, in Western societies the father of the baby is often viewed as the ideal birth companion. For many years, European-American couples traditionally attended childbirth classes together as an expected activity, although this is not as common today. Laotian (Hmong) husbands also traditionally participate actively in the labor process. In some other cultures, the father may be available; but his presence in the labor room with the mother may not be considered appropriate, or he may be present but resist active involvement in her care. Such behavior could be perceived by the nursing staff to indicate a lack of concern, caring, or interest. Women from many cultures prefer female caregivers and want to have

at least one female companion present during labor and birth. They also are usually very concerned about modesty. If couples from these cultures immigrate to the United States or Canada, their roles may change. The nurse needs to talk to the woman and her support people to determine the roles they will assume.

The Non–English-Speaking Woman in Labor

A woman's level of anxiety in labor increases when she does not understand what is happening to her or what is being said. Non–English-speaking women often feel a complete loss of control over their situation if no health care professional is present who speaks their language. They can panic and withdraw or become physically abusive when someone tries to do something they perceive might harm them or their babies. A support person is sometimes able to serve as an interpreter. However, caution is warranted because the interpreter may not be able to convey exactly what the nurse or others are saying or what the woman is saying, which can increase the woman's stress level even more.

Ideally a bilingual nurse will care for the woman. Alternatively a hospital or birthing center employee or volunteer interpreter may be contacted for assistance. Ideally the interpreter is from the woman's culture. For some women, a female is more acceptable than a male interpreter. If no one in the facility is able to interpret, an interpreter may be accessed by telephone or electronic media. Even when the nurse has limited ability to communicate verbally with the woman, in most instances the woman appreciates his or her efforts to do so. Speaking slowly and avoiding complex words and medical terms can help a woman and her partner understand. Often the woman understands English much better than she speaks it.

Physical Examination

The initial physical examination includes a general systems assessment and an assessment of fetal status. During the examination, uterine contractions are assessed, and a vaginal examination is performed. The findings of the admission physical examination serve as a baseline for assessing the woman's progress in labor from that point. The information obtained from a complete and accurate assessment during the initial examination serves as the basis for determining whether the woman should be admitted and what her ongoing care should be. Expected maternal progress and minimal assessment guidelines during the first stage of labor are presented in Table 16.1 and Table 16.2.

Birth is a time when nurses, nurse midwives, physicians, and other staff members are exposed to a great deal of maternal and newborn blood and body fluids. Therefore Standard Precautions should guide all assessment and care measures (Box 16.4). Hand hygiene (e.g., washing hands with soap or application of an alcohol-based antiseptic rub) before and after assessing the woman and providing care is a critical step in the prevention of infection transmission. The nurse should explain assessment findings to the woman and her partner whenever possible. Throughout labor, accurate documentation following agency policy is done as soon as possible after a procedure has been performed (Fig. 16.4).

General Systems Assessment

On admission, the nurse should perform a general systems assessment. This includes an assessment of the heart, lungs, and skin, and an examination to determine the presence and extent of edema of the face, hands, sacrum, and legs. It also includes testing of deep tendon reflexes and assessing for clonus if indicated. The woman's weight is measured and recorded. Increasing numbers of women are overweight or obese. Excessive size can make nursing care during labor and birth more difficult and places the woman at risk for complications such as operative birth, infection, and blood clots. See Chapter 17 for further information.

TABLE 16.2   Nursing Assessments in First-Stage Labor

Labor Phase	Time Frame	Specific Assessments
Early	Every 30–60 minutes	Maternal blood pressure, pulse, and respirations *Uterine activity *Fetal heart rate (FHR) and pattern Presence of bloody show
	Every 30 minutes	Changes in maternal appearance, mood, affect, energy level, and involvement of partner or coach
	Every 2–4 hours	Temperature (every 4 hours until membranes rupture, then every 2 hours)
	As needed	Vaginal examination to identify progress in labor
Active	Every 15–30 minutes	Maternal blood pressure, pulse, and respirations
	Every 15–30 minutes	*FHR and pattern *Uterine activity Presence of bloody show
	Every 5–15 minutes	Changes in maternal appearance, mood, affect, energy level, and involvement of partner or coach
	Every 2–4 hours	Temperature (every 4 hours until membranes rupture, then every 2 hours)
	As needed	Vaginal examination to identify progress in labor

*Kennedy, B.B. & Baird, S.M. (2017). *Intrapartum management modules: A perinatal education program* (5th ed.). Philadelphia, PA: Wolters Kluwer.

BOX 16.4   Standard Precautions During Childbirth

- Perform hand hygiene by washing hands before and after putting on gloves and performing procedures; cleansing alcohol rubs can be used if hands are not visibly soiled.
- Wear gloves (clean or sterile, as appropriate) when performing procedures that require contact with the woman's genitalia and body fluids, including bloody show (e.g., during vaginal examination, amniotomy, hygienic care of the perineum, insertion of an internal scalp electrode and intrauterine pressure monitor, and urinary catheterization).
- Wear a mask that has a shield or protective eyewear and cover gown when assisting with the birth. Cap and shoe covers are worn for cesarean birth but are optional for vaginal birth in a birthing room. Gowns worn by the nurse-midwife or physician who is attending the birth should have a waterproof front and sleeves and should be sterile. Mask also should be worn during spinal puncture or insertion of an epidural catheter.
- Drape the woman with sterile towels and sheets as appropriate. Explain to the woman what can and cannot be touched.
- Help the woman's partner put on appropriate coverings for the type of birth such as cap, mask, gown, and shoe covers. Show the partner where to stand and what can and cannot be touched.
- Wear gloves and gown when handling the newborn immediately after birth.
- Use an appropriate method to suction the newborn's airway such as a bulb syringe or mechanical wall suction.

Vital Signs

The nurse assesses vital signs (temperature, pulse, respirations, and blood pressure using a correct size cuff) on admission. The initial values are used as the baseline for comparison for all future measurements. If the blood pressure is elevated, it should be reassessed 30 minutes later between contractions to obtain a reading after the woman has relaxed. The woman is encouraged to lie on her side to prevent supine hypotension and the resulting fetal hypoxemia (Fig. 16.5). Body temperature is monitored in an effort to identify signs of infection or a fluid deficit (e.g., dehydration associated with inadequate fluid intake).

Leopold Maneuvers

Leopold maneuvers are performed using abdominal palpation (Box 16.5). These maneuvers help to answer three important questions: (1)

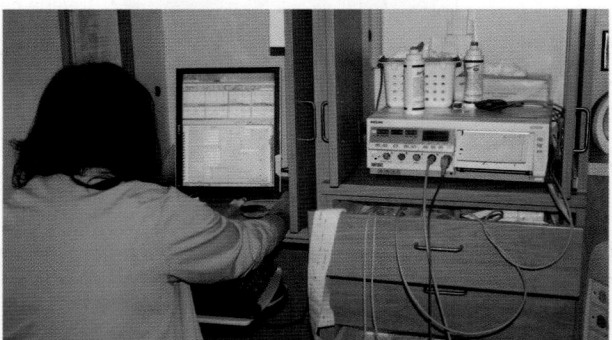

FIG 16.4 Nurse documenting assessment findings on computer in a labor, delivery, recovery, postpartum room. (Courtesy of Shannon Perry, Phoenix, AZ.)

Which fetal part is in the uterine fundus? (2) Where is the fetal back located? (3) What is the presenting fetal part?

Assessment of Fetal Heart Rate and Pattern

The point of maximal intensity (PMI) of the FHR is the location on the maternal abdomen at which the FHR is heard the loudest. It is usually directly over the fetal back. In a vertex presentation, the FHR can usually be heard below the mother's umbilicus in either the right or the left lower quadrant of the abdomen. In a breech presentation, the FHR is most easily heard above the mother's umbilicus. The PMI is where the nurse places the ultrasound transducer when the electronic fetal monitor is used to assess the FHR. Table 16.2 summarizes assessments recommended for determining fetal status during the first stage of labor. In addition, it is essential to assess the FHR after ROM because this is the most common time for the umbilical cord to prolapse, after any change in the contraction pattern or maternal status, and before and after the woman receives medication or a procedure is performed.

Assessment of Uterine Contractions

A general characteristic of effective labor is regular uterine activity (i.e., contractions becoming more frequent with increased duration), but uterine activity is not directly related to labor progress. Uterine

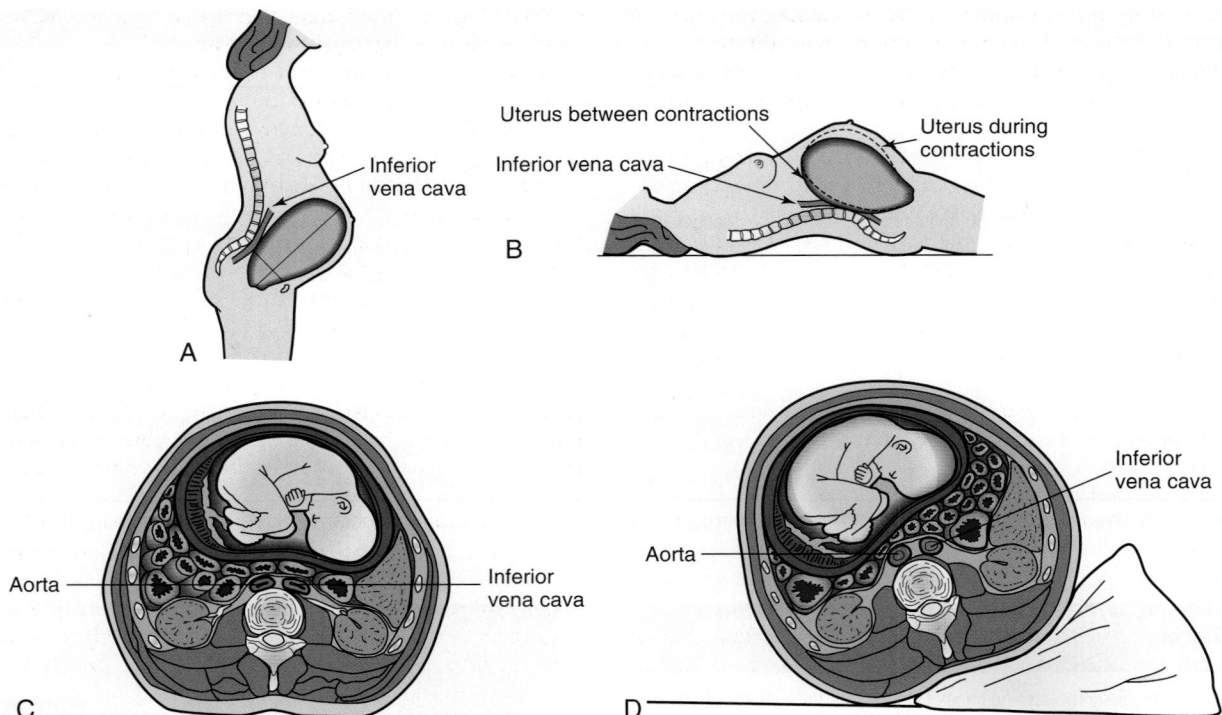

FIG 16.5 Supine hypotension. Note relationship of gravid uterus to ascending vena cava in standing posture **(A)** and supine posture **(B). C,** Compression of aorta and inferior vena cava with woman in supine position. **D,** Relieved by use of wedge pillow placed under woman's right side.

BOX 16.5   Procedure: Leopold Maneuvers

- Perform hand hygiene.
- Ask woman to empty bladder.
- Position woman supine with one pillow under her head and her knees slightly flexed.
- Place wedge pillow or small rolled towel under woman's right or left hip to displace uterus off major blood vessels (prevents supine hypotensive syndrome; see Fig. 16.5, *D*).
- If right-handed, stand on woman's right, facing her (if left-handed, stand on woman's left):
  1. Identify fetal part that occupies the fundus. The head feels round, firm, and freely movable; the breech feels less regular and softer. This maneuver identifies fetal lie (longitudinal or transverse) and presentation (cephalic or breech) (Fig. A).
  2. Using palmar surface of one hand, locate and palpate the smooth convex contour of the fetal back and the irregularities that identify the small parts (feet, hands, knees, elbows). This maneuver helps identify fetal presentation (Fig. B).
  3. With right hand, determine which fetal part is presenting over the inlet to the true pelvis. Gently grasp the lower pole of the uterus between the thumb and fingers, pressing in slightly (Fig. C). If the head is presenting and not engaged, determine the attitude of the head (flexed or extended).
  4. Turn to face the woman's feet. Using both hands, outline the fetal head (Fig. D) with the palmar surface of the fingertips. When the presenting part has descended deeply, only a small portion of it may be outlined. Palpation of the cephalic prominence helps identify the attitude of the head. If the cephalic prominence is found on the same side as the small parts, this means that the head must be flexed and the vertex is presenting (see Fig. D). If the cephalic prominence is on the same side as the back, this indicates that the presenting head is extended and the face is presenting.
- Document fetal presentation, position, and lie and whether presenting part is flexed or extended, engaged, or free floating. Use agency protocol for documentation (e.g., "Vtx, LOA, floating").

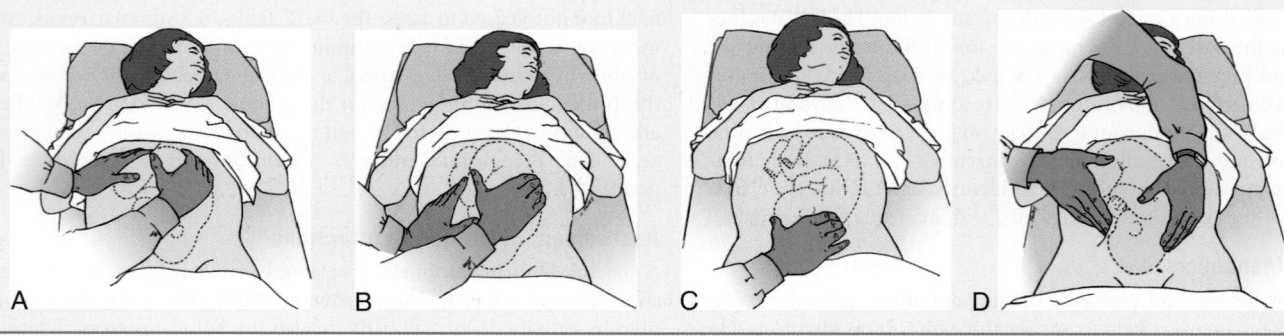

contractions are the primary powers that act involuntarily to expel the fetus and placenta from the uterus. Several methods can be used to evaluate uterine contractions, including the woman's subjective description, palpation and timing of contractions by a nurse or other health care professional, and electronic monitoring.

Each contraction exhibits a wavelike pattern. It begins with a slow increment (the increasing intensity of a contraction from its onset), gradually reaches a peak, and then diminishes rapidly (decrement, the decreasing intensity of the contraction). An interval of rest ends when the next contraction begins. The outward appearance of the woman's abdomen during and between contractions and the pattern of a typical uterine contraction are shown in Fig. 16.6.

A uterine contraction is described in terms of the following characteristics:

- *Frequency:* How often uterine contractions occur; the time that passes from the beginning of one contraction to the beginning of the next contraction
- *Intensity:* The strength of a contraction at its peak
- *Duration:* The time that passes between the onset and the end of a contraction
- *Resting tone:* The tension in the uterine muscle between contractions; relaxation of the uterus

Uterine contractions are assessed by palpation or by using external or internal electronic monitors (see Chapter 15 for further discussion). Frequency and duration can be measured by all three methods of uterine activity monitoring. The accuracy of determining intensity and resting tone varies by the method used. The woman's description and examiner's palpation are more subjective and less precise ways of determining the intensity of uterine contractions and resting tone than are the external or internal electronic monitors. The following terms describe contractions based on what is felt on palpation:

- *Mild:* Slightly tense fundus that is easy to indent with fingertips (feels like pressing finger to tip of nose)
- *Moderate:* Firm fundus that is difficult to indent with fingertips (feels like pressing finger to chin)
- *Strong:* Rigid boardlike fundus that is almost impossible to indent with fingertips (feels like pressing finger to forehead)

Women in labor tend to describe the pain of contractions in terms of the sensations they are experiencing in the lower abdomen or back, which is sometimes unrelated to the firmness of the uterine fundus. Therefore a woman's assessment of the strength of her contractions may be less accurate than that of the health care provider, although the amount of discomfort reported is valid.

External electronic monitoring provides some information about the strength of uterine contractions when the appearance of contractions on admission is compared with those that occur later in labor. However, internal electronic monitoring with an intrauterine pressure catheter is the most accurate way of assessing the intensity of uterine contractions and resting tone of the uterus.

On admission, many health care providers order that FHR and pattern be monitored electronically to obtain a baseline. However, no research suggests a difference in outcome when this is done (Kelly et al., 2017). Suggested time frames for assessing uterine activity and FHR and pattern during the phases of first-stage labor are listed in Table 16.2. The findings expected as labor progresses are summarized in Table 16.1.

⚡ **SAFETY ALERT**

If the nurse observes that the characteristics of contractions are abnormal, either exceeding or falling below what is considered acceptable in terms of the standard characteristics, this finding must be promptly reported to the nurse midwife or physician

---

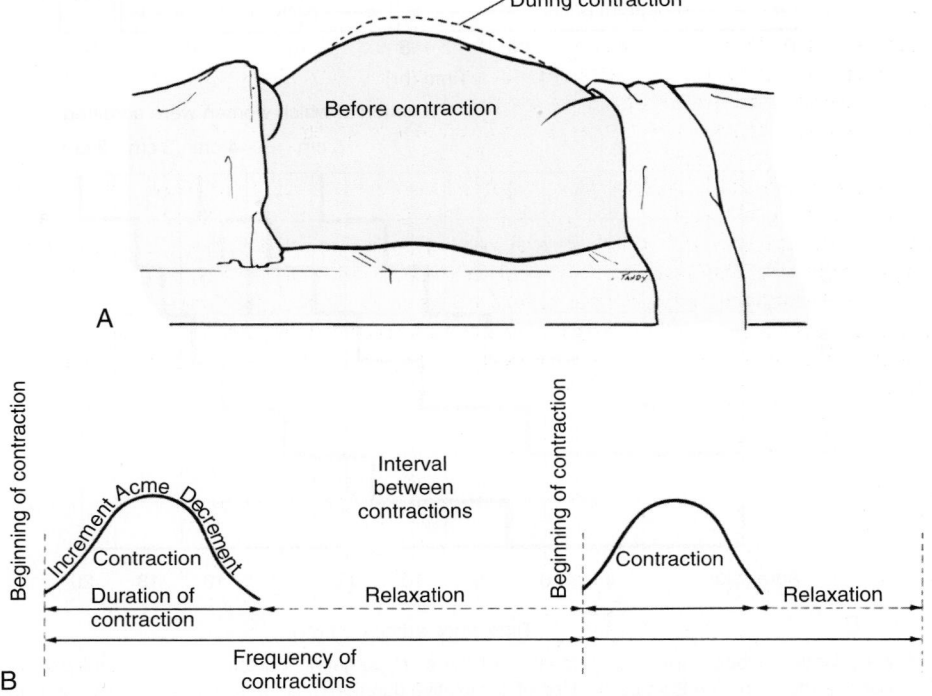

FIG 16.6 Assessment of uterine contractions. **A,** Abdominal contour before and during uterine contraction. **B,** Wavelike pattern of contractile activity.

The nurse considers uterine activity in the context of its effect on cervical effacement and dilation and the degree of descent of the presenting part (see Chapter 13). It is also important to consider the effect of uterine activity on the fetus. Progress of labor can be verified effectively through the use of graphic charts (also called *partograms* or *labor graphs*) on which cervical dilation is plotted as labor progresses. This type of graphic charting helps in early identification of deviations from expected labor patterns. Fig. 16.7 provides examples of a modern labor graph and partogram that incorporate new knowledge regarding the labor process in contemporary women. Hospitals and birthing centers may develop their own assessment graphs that may include data not only on cervical dilation but also on maternal vital signs, FHR, and uterine activity.

⚡ **SAFETY ALERT**

The nurse should recognize that active labor can actually last longer than the expected labor patterns because each woman is different. This finding is not a cause for concern unless the maternal-fetal unit exhibits signs of stress (e.g., abnormal FHR patterns, maternal fever).

Vaginal Examination

The vaginal examination reveals whether the woman is in true labor and enables the examiner to determine whether the membranes have ruptured (Fig. 16.8). Because this examination is often stressful and uncomfortable for the woman and may introduce microorganisms into

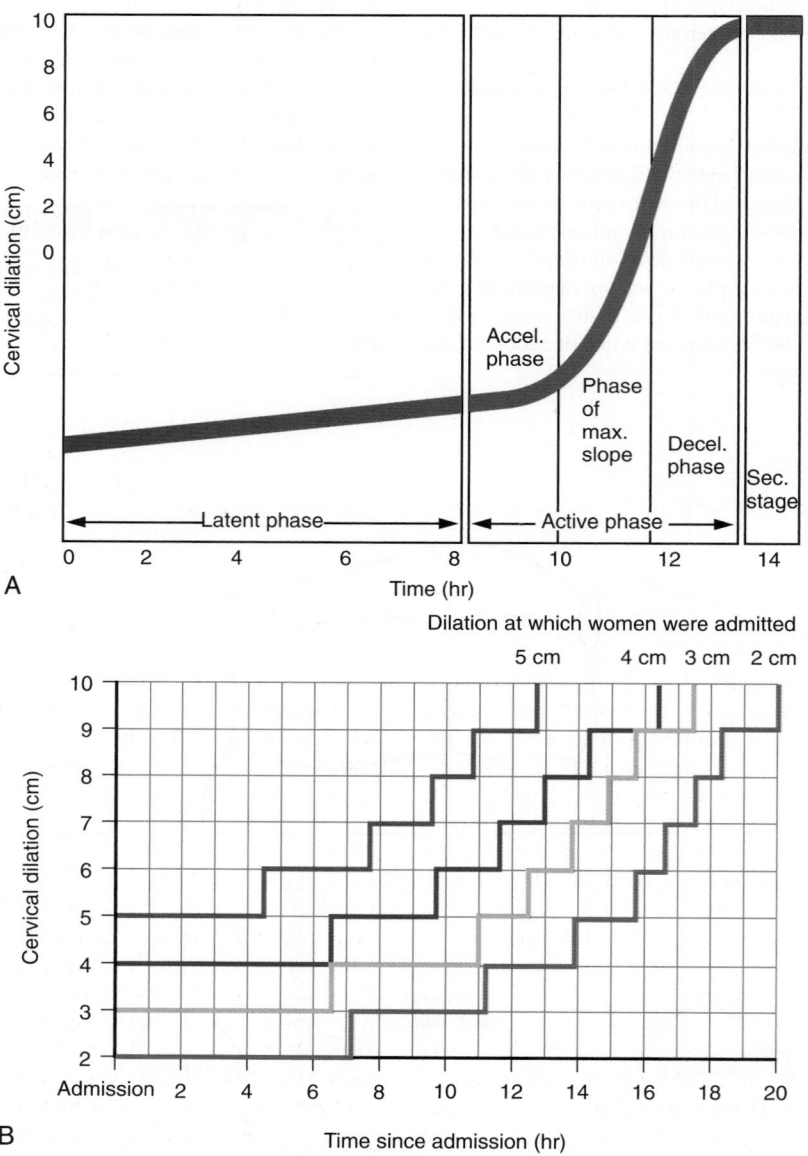

FIG 16.7 A, Modern labor graph. Characteristics of the average cervical dilation curve for nulliparous labor. **B,** Zhang labor partogram. The 95th percentiles of cumulative duration of labor from admission among singleton term nulliparous women with spontaneous onset of labor. (From Gabbe, S.G., Niebyl, J.R., Simpson, J.L., et al. [Eds.]. [2017]. *Obstetrics: Normal and problem pregnancies* [7th ed.]. Philadelphia, PA: Elsevier.)

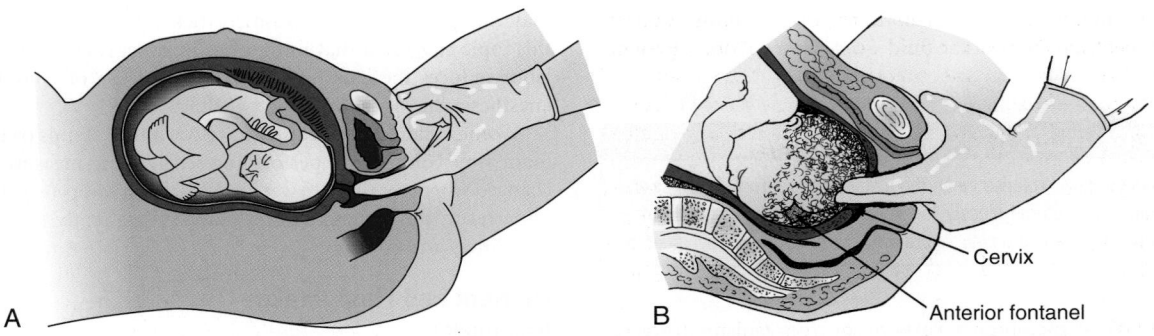

FIG 16.8 Vaginal examination. **A,** Undilated, uneffaced cervix; membranes intact. **B,** Palpation of sagittal suture line. Cervix effaced and partially dilated.

BOX 16.6   Procedure: Vaginal Examination of the Laboring Woman

- Use a sterile glove and antiseptic solution or soluble gel for lubrication.
- Position the woman to prevent supine hypotension. Drape to ensure privacy.
- Cleanse the perineum and vulva, if needed.
- After obtaining the woman's permission to touch her, gently insert the index and middle fingers into the woman's vagina.
- Determine the following:
  - Cervical dilation, effacement, and position (e.g., posterior, mid, anterior)
  - Presenting part, position, and station; molding of the head with development of caput succedaneum (may affect accuracy of determination of station)
  - Status of membranes (intact, bulging, or ruptured)
  - Characteristics of amniotic fluid (e.g., color, clarity, and odor), if membranes are ruptured
- Explain the findings of the examination to the woman.
- Document your findings, and report them to the nurse-midwife or physician.

---

the vagina if the membranes are ruptured, it is performed only when indicated by the status of the woman and her fetus. For example, a vaginal examination is performed on admission, prior to administering medications (e.g., analgesics, increasing oxytocin infusion), when significant change has occurred in uterine activity, on maternal request or perception of perineal pressure or the urge to bear down, when membranes rupture, or when variable decelerations of the FHR are noted. A full explanation of the examination and support of the woman are important in reducing the stress and discomfort associated with the examination (Simpson & O'Brien-Abel, 2014) (Box 16.6).

Laboratory and Diagnostic Tests

Urinalysis

A clean-catch urine specimen may be obtained to gather further data about the pregnant woman's health. Analysis of the specimen is a convenient and simple procedure that can provide information about her hydration status (e.g., specific gravity, color, amount); nutritional status (e.g., ketones); infection status (e.g., leukocytes); or the status of possible complications such as preeclampsia (e.g., proteinuria). In many hospitals, this test must be done in the laboratory rather than at the bedside, even if a urine dipstick is used.

Blood Tests

The blood tests performed vary with agency protocol and the woman's health status. Currently almost all blood tests must be performed in the hospital laboratory rather than on the perinatal unit. Often blood samples are obtained from the hub of the catheter when an IV line is started or a heplock or saline lock is inserted. A hematocrit will likely be ordered. More comprehensive blood assessments such as white blood cell count, red blood cell count, hemoglobin level, and platelet values are included, along with hematocrit, in a complete blood count (CBC). A CBC may be ordered for women with a history of infection, anemia, gestational hypertension, or other disorders. Any woman whose human immunodeficiency virus (HIV) status is undocumented at the time of labor should be screened with a rapid HIV test unless she declines (opts out of) testing (Centers for Disease Control and Prevention [CDC], 2016).

Most hospitals require that a "type and screen" to determine the woman's blood type and Rh status be performed on admission. Even if these tests have already been performed during pregnancy, the hospital laboratory or transfusion services department (blood bank) must verify the results in-house. If the woman had no prenatal care or if her prenatal records are not available, a prenatal screen will likely be drawn on admission. The prenatal screen includes laboratory tests that would normally have been drawn at the initial prenatal visit (see Table 8.1).

Other Tests

If the woman's group B streptococci status is not known, a rapid test may be done on admission. The rapid test results are usually available within 1 hour or so and determine if the woman must be given antibiotics during labor.

Assessment of Amniotic Membranes and Fluid

Labor is initiated at term by SROM in approximately 25% of pregnant women. A lag period, rarely exceeding 24 hours, may precede the onset of labor. Membranes also can rupture spontaneously any time during labor but most commonly in the active phase of the first stage of labor. Box 16.1 explains how to determine if membranes are ruptured. If the membranes do not rupture spontaneously, they may be ruptured artificially at some time during labor. Artificial rupture of membranes (AROM), called an *amniotomy*, is performed by the physician or nurse-midwife using a plastic AmniHook or a surgical clamp. However, this practice is discouraged if there is no medical reason because it can increase the laboring woman's sensation of pressure and pain and is not necessary for a normal birth to occur.

Whether the membranes rupture spontaneously or artificially, the time of rupture should be recorded. Other necessary documentation includes information regarding the color (clear or meconium-stained), estimated amount, and odor of the fluid. See Chapter 17 for additional information.

> ⚡ **SAFETY ALERT**
>
> The umbilical cord may prolapse when the membranes rupture. The FHR and pattern should be monitored closely for several minutes immediately after ROM to determine fetal well-being, and the findings should be documented.

Infection. When membranes rupture, microorganisms from the vagina can then ascend into the amniotic sac, causing chorioamnionitis and placentitis to develop. For this reason, vaginal examinations are limited, and maternal temperature and vaginal discharge are monitored frequently after ROM (at least every 2 hours) to quickly identify signs of infection. Even when membranes are intact, however, microorganisms can ascend and cause infection.

Assessment findings serve as a baseline for evaluating the woman's subsequent progress during labor. Although some problems can be anticipated, others may appear unexpectedly during the clinical course of labor (Box 16.7).

NURSING INTERVENTIONS

The nursing process provides the framework for the nursing care management of women in labor. The nursing care given to a woman in labor is an essential component of her care. The current emphasis on evidence-based practice supports the management of care by using this approach to enhance the safety, effectiveness, and acceptability of the physical care measures chosen to support the woman during labor and birth (Box 16.8). The various physical needs, the necessary nursing actions, and the rationale for care are presented in Table 16.3 and the Nursing Care Plan.

General Hygiene

In general, women in labor may use showers or warm-water baths, if they are available, to enhance the feeling of well-being and to minimize the discomfort of contractions. Water immersion during active labor is associated with a decrease in the use of analgesia and reports of less maternal pain (Arendt & Tessmer-Tuck, 2013). A Cochrane review of this topic suggested that immersion in water during the first stage of labor reduces the length of this stage and use of epidural or spinal anesthesia during labor (Cluett & Burns, 2009).

Women should be encouraged to wash their hands or use cleansing foam after voiding and performing self-hygiene measures. Linens are changed whenever they are wet or soiled; linen savers (e.g., Chux) placed underneath the woman can be changed frequently to help maintain cleanliness and comfort.

Nutrient and Fluid Intake
Oral Intake

Before the 1940s, women were allowed to eat and drink during labor to maintain the energy required to sustain labor and the stamina required to give birth. This practice changed, allowing the laboring woman only clear liquids or ice chips or nothing by mouth during the active phase of labor when concern arose regarding the risk for anesthesia complications and their secondary effects, if general anesthesia was required in an emergency. These secondary effects include the aspiration of gastric contents and resultant compromise in oxygen perfusion, which could endanger the lives of the mother and fetus (Collins, 2017; Simpson & O'Brien-Abel, 2014; Tillett & Hill, 2016). There have been no randomized trials evaluating the ingestion of solid foods in labor, so current management is based mostly on expert opinion. The American College of Obstetricians and Gynecologists (ACOG), the American Society of Anesthesiologists (ASA), and the Canadian Anesthesiologists' Society recommend avoiding solid food during labor (Simpson & O'Brien-Abel). This practice is being challenged by many health care providers, however, because regional anesthesia is used more often than general anesthesia, even for emergency cesarean births. Women are awake during regional anesthesia and are able to participate in their own care and protect their airways (Collins).

> ### BOX 16.7   Signs of Potential Complications
>
> - Intrauterine pressure of ≥80 mm Hg or resting tone of ≥20 mm Hg (both determined by internal monitoring with intrauterine pressure catheter [IUPC])
> - Contractions lasting ≥90 seconds
> - More than five contractions in a 10-minute period (contractions occur more frequently than every 2 minutes)
> - Relaxation between contractions lasting <30 seconds
> - Fetal bradycardia or tachycardia; absent or minimal variability not associated with fetal sleep cycle or temporary effects of central nervous system (CNS) depressant drugs given to the woman; late, variable, or prolonged fetal heart rate (FHR) decelerations
> - Irregular fetal heart rate; suspected fetal arrhythmias
> - Appearance of meconium-stained or bloody fluid from the vagina
> - Arrest in progress of cervical dilation or effacement, descent of the fetus, or both
> - Maternal temperature of ≥38° C (100.4° F)
> - Foul-smelling vaginal discharge
> - Persistent bright or dark red vaginal bleeding

> ### BOX 16.8   Evidence-Based Care Practices Designed to Promote, Protect, and Support Normal Labor and Birth
>
> - Allow labor to begin on its own: Encourage spontaneous labor rather than fostering elective labor inductions.
> - Encourage freedom of movement throughout labor to facilitate the progress of labor and enhance maternal comfort and control of the labor process.
> - Provide support beginning early in labor and continuing throughout the process of childbirth to relieve maternal anxiety and stress and decrease the use of epidural anesthesia and the likelihood of cesarean birth; support should be provided by someone not employed by the hospital (e.g., doula).
> - Avoid routine implementation of interventions (e.g., intravenous fluids, oral intake restrictions, continuous electronic fetal monitoring, labor augmentation measures [e.g., amniotomy, oxytocin administration], and epidural anesthesia).
> - Support the practice of spontaneous, nondirected pushing in nonsupine positions (e.g., lateral, squatting, standing, kneeling, and semisitting) to facilitate the progress of fetal descent and shorten the second stage of labor.
> - Avoid separation of the mother from her healthy baby after birth by encouraging skin-to-skin contact of mother and baby to keep newborn warm, prevent neonatal infection, enhance newborn's physiologic adjustment to extrauterine life, and foster early breastfeeding.
>
> Data from Hanson, L., & VandeVusse, L. (2014). Supporting labor progress toward physiologic birth, *The Journal of Perinatal & Neonatal Nursing, 28*(2), 101-107.

TABLE 16.3   Physical Nursing Care During First- and Second-Stage Labor

Need	Nursing Actions	Rationale
General Hygiene		
Showers, bed baths, tub baths, or whirlpool baths	Assess for progress in labor.	Determines appropriateness of the activity
	Supervise showers or baths closely if woman is in true labor.	Prevents injury from fall; labor may be accelerated
	Suggest allowing warm water to flow over back.	Aids relaxation; increases comfort
Perineum	Cleanse frequently, especially after rupture of membranes and when show increases.	Enhances comfort and reduces risk for infection
Oral hygiene	Offer toothbrush or mouthwash or wash teeth with ice-cold wet washcloth as needed.	Refreshes mouth; helps counteract dry, thirsty feeling
Hair	Brush, braid per woman's wishes.	Improves morale; increases comfort
Hand washing	Offer washcloths or cleansing foam before and after voiding and as needed.	Maintains cleanliness; prevents infection
Face	Offer cool washcloth.	Provides relief from diaphoresis; cools and refreshes
Gowns and linens	Change as needed.	Improves comfort; enhances relaxation
Nutrient and Fluid Intake		
Oral	Offer fluids and solid foods as ordered by nurse-midwife or physician and desired by laboring woman.	Provides hydration and calories; enhances positive emotional experience and maternal control
Intravenous (IV)	Establish and maintain IV line as ordered.	Maintains hydration; provides venous access for medications or blood products, if needed
Elimination		
Voiding	Encourage voiding at least every 2 hours.	A full bladder may impede descent of presenting part; overdistention may cause bladder atony and injury as well as postpartum voiding difficulty
Ambulatory woman	Allow ambulation to bathroom according to orders of nurse-midwife or physician, *if*:	
	The presenting part is engaged.	Reinforces normal process of urination
	The membranes are not ruptured.	Precautionary measure to protect against prolapse of umbilical cord
	The woman is not medicated.	Precautionary measure to protect against injury from a fall
Woman on bed rest	Offer bedpan	Prevents complications of bladder distention and ambulation
	Encourage upright position on bedpan, allow tap water to run; place woman's hands in warm water; pour warm water over vulva; give positive suggestion.	Encourages voiding
	Provide privacy.	Shows respect for woman
	Put up side rails on bed.	Prevents injury from a fall
	Place call bell and telephone within reach.	Reinforces safe care
	Offer washcloth or cleansing foam for hands.	Maintains cleanliness; prevents infection
	Wash vulvar area.	Maintains cleanliness; enhances comfort; prevents infection
Urinary Catheterization	Catheterize according to orders of nurse-midwife or physician or hospital protocol if measures to facilitate spontaneous voiding are ineffective.	Prevents complications of bladder distention
	Insert catheter between contractions.	Minimizes discomfort
	Avoid force if obstacle to insertion is noted.	"Obstacle" may be caused by compression of urethra by presenting part
Bowel elimination—sensation of rectal pressure	Perform vaginal examination.	Prevents misinterpretation of rectal pressure from presenting part as need to defecate
		Determines degree of descent of presenting part
	Help the woman ambulate to the bathroom or offer bedpan if rectal pressure is not from presenting part.	Reinforces normal process of bowel elimination and safe care
	Cleanse perineum immediately after passage of stool.	Reduces risk for infection and sense of embarrassment

◎ NURSING CARE PLAN

Care of the Woman in Labor

Case Study

Kamari and D'Marcus, an African-American couple, arrived at the labor and birth unit accompanied by Kamari's mother, Waneesa. They tell the nurse that this is the first pregnancy for Kamari and the baby's due date is not until 2 weeks from today. Because of this, they were surprised when Kamari started having contractions and are worried because they don't feel ready for the baby. Kamari stated that the contractions started about 6 hours ago and are getting very uncomfortable. She wants both D'Marcus and her mother to stay with her in labor.

Assessment

What are Kamari's expectations of labor? What is her ability to concentrate and listen to instructions? What are her fears and concerns? What are her usual coping methods?

Defining Characteristics

Expressed concern about labor and birth
Expressed fear of an uncertain or negative outcome
Inability to concentrate
Increased muscle tension
Fear, apprehension, wariness

Nursing Diagnosis

Anxiety related to hospitalization and birth process

Expected Outcomes

Kamari reports decreased anxiety level using an anxiety scale (from 0 [no anxiety] to 10 [anxiety as bad as it could possibly be])

Nursing Interventions	Rationales
Orient Kamari, D'Marcus, and Waneesa to the labor and birth unit and explain the admission process.	To allay initial feelings of anxiety
Assess Kamari's knowledge, experience, and expectations of labor; note any signs or expressions of anxiety, nervousness, or fear.	To establish baseline for interventions
Discuss expected progression of labor and describe what to expect during the labor process.	To decrease anxiety associated with the unknown
Identify specific source(s) of anxiety.	To better target interventions
Actively involve Kamari in care decisions during labor, interpret sights and sounds of the environment (monitor sights and sounds, unit activities), and share information on labor progression (vital signs, fetal heart rate [FHR], cervical dilation and effacement)	To increase her sense of control and lessen fears

Case Study (Continued)

On admission, Kamari's cervix was dilated to 4 cm and was 70% effaced, and her contractions were occurring every 4 to 5 minutes. She complained of increasing pain with contractions but was using controlled breathing with the help of D'Marcus. Waneesa massaged Kamari's back during contractions.

Assessment

What are characteristics of labor pain? What sociocultural and environmental variables will affect Kamari's response to pain?

Defining Characteristics

Alteration in muscle tone
Autonomic responses (diaphoresis, elevated pulse rate, elevated respiratory rate, dilated pupils)
Changes in appetite and eating
Communication (verbal or coded) of pain
Expressions of pain (such as moaning and crying)
Facial mask of pain (grimacing)

Nursing Diagnosis

Acute Pain related to physiologic response to labor

Expected Outcomes

Kamari reports decreased pain level using a pain scale (from 0 [no pain] to 10 [pain as bad as it could possibly be]), and she says she is coping effectively with the pain she is experiencing

Nursing Interventions	Rationales
Assess Kamari's level of pain and strategies that she has used to cope with it.	To establish baseline for interventions
Encourage D'Marcus and Waneesa to remain as support persons during the labor process.	To assist with support and comfort measures because measures are often more effective when delivered by a familiar person
Assist Kamari, D'Marcus, and Waneesa in the use of specific nonpharmacologic pain methods such as conscious relaxation, breathing techniques, music, distraction, imagery, massage, and touch.	To increase relaxation, decrease intensity of contractions, and promote use of controlled thought and direction of energy
Provide comfort measures such as frequent mouth care to prevent dry mouth, application of damp cloth to forehead, and changing of damp gown or bed linens.	To relieve discomfort associated with dry mouth and diaphoresis
Help Kamari to move around and change position such as squatting or using a birthing ball or birthing stool.	To reduce stiffness, promote comfort, and facilitate progress of birth
Explain which analgesics and anesthesia are available for use during labor and birth.	To provide knowledge to help Kamari make informed decisions about pain control
Administer analgesics or assist with regional anesthesia (e.g., epidural) as ordered or desired.	To provide effective pain relief during labor and birth

Case Study (Continued)

With the help of D'Marcus and Waneesa, Kamari is coping with contractions, and she is taking sips of water and ice. She has not voided since admission.

Assessment

What are signs that Kamari needs to void and cannot?

Defining Characteristics

Hesitancy
Incontinence

Continued

◎ NURSING CARE PLAN

Care of the Woman in Labor—cont'd

Retention
Urgency
Distended bladder upon palpation

Nursing Diagnosis
Impaired Urinary Elimination related to sensory impairment during labor

Expected Outcomes
Kamari's bladder is emptied at least every 2 hours, either by spontaneous voiding or urinary catheterization, and her urinary function will remain normal and free from complications.

Nursing Interventions	Rationales
Palpate Kamari's bladder above the symphysis frequently (at least every 2 hours).	To detect a full bladder that occurs from increased fluid intake and inability to feel urge to void
Encourage frequent voiding (at least every 2 hours) and catheterize if necessary.	To avoid bladder distention, which can impede fetal descent and may result in trauma to bladder
Help Kamari to bathroom or commode to void, if appropriate; provide privacy, and use techniques to stimulate voiding such as running water.	To facilitate bladder emptying with an upright position (natural) and relaxation

Case Study (Continued)
The labor has progressed and Kamari's cervix is now 9 cm dilated and 100% effaced. She is moaning with contractions and is moving back and forth in the bed. She says to Waneesa that she is scared ("What if the baby is coming too early?") but also states that she wants to get it over with ("I want him out of there!").

Assessment
What is Kamari's usual coping pattern? What is her response to analgesia? What is her current level of pain? How effective are the supportive efforts of D'Marcus and Waneesa?

Defining Characteristics
Change in communication pattern
Expressed inability to cope
Fatigue
Poor concentration
Restlessness

Nursing Diagnosis
Ineffective Individual Coping related to the uncertainty about labor and birth

Expected Outcomes
Kamari actively participates in the birth process with no evidence of injury to her or her fetus

Nursing Interventions	Rationales
Constantly monitor the events of labor and birth, including physiologic responses of Kamari and the fetus and emotional responses of Kamari, D'Marcus, and Waneesa.	To ensure well-being of mother, her support people, and the fetus
Provide ongoing feedback to Kamari, D'Marcus, and Waneesa.	To decrease anxiety and enhance participation
Continue to provide comfort measures and minimize distractions (e.g., dim the room lights, speak quietly).	To decrease discomfort and aid in focus on the birth process
Encourage Kamari to experiment with various positions.	To assist fetal descent and enhance her comfort
Ensure that Kamari takes deep cleansing breaths before and after each contraction.	To enhance gas exchange and oxygen transport to fetus
Encourage Kamari to push spontaneously when she perceives an urge to bear down during a contraction.	To aid descent and rotation of fetus
Encourage Kamari to exhale, holding her breath for only short periods of time while bearing down.	To avoid triggering the Valsalva maneuver, which would increase intrathoracic and cardiovascular pressure and decrease the amount of oxygen that reaches the uterus and placenta, thereby placing the fetus at risk
Have Kamari take deep breaths and relax between contractions.	To reduce fatigue and increase effectiveness of pushing efforts
Have Kamari pant as fetal head crowns.	To control emergence of head and reduce risk for perineal trauma or fetal head injury
Explain to Kamari, D'Marcus, and Waneesa what is expected in the third stage of labor.	To enlist cooperation
Have Kamari maintain her position.	To facilitate delivery of placenta

Case Study (Continued)
Kamari gave birth to a 6 lb. 10 oz. baby boy after almost 11 hours of labor. She had a first-degree laceration which did not need to be sutured. The nurses put the baby on Kamari's abdomen after birth, and shortly thereafter she tried to nurse the baby. Kamari, D'Marcus, and Waneesa were very excited and examined the baby thoroughly. It soon became apparent that Kamari was very tired as she had had little sleep prior to being admitted to the labor and birth unit.

Assessment
How many hours of sleep has Kamari had in the last 24 hours? What was her dietary intake during that time? How long was her labor?

Defining Characteristics
Drowsiness
Increased need for rest
Increased physical complaints
Lack of energy
Inability to maintain usual routines

Nursing Diagnosis
Fatigue related to energy expenditure required during labor and birth

Expected Outcomes
Kamari's fatigue is reduced, and her energy levels are restored.

Continued

◎ NURSING CARE PLAN

Care of the Woman in Labor—cont'd

Nursing Interventions	Rationales	Nursing Interventions	Rationales
Educate Kamari, D'Marcus, and Waneesa about the need for rest and help them plan strategies (e.g., restricting visitors, increasing role of support systems performing functions associated with daily routines) that allow specific times for rest and sleep.	To ensure that Kamari can restore her depleted energy levels in preparation for caring for the new infant	Monitor Kamari's fatigue level and amount of rest received.	To ensure restoration of energy
		Provide nourishing meal and preferred liquid nourishment.	To restore energy
		Cluster care activities as much as possible.	To allow for periods of uninterrupted rest

An adequate intake of fluids and calories is required to meet the energy demands and compensate for fluid losses associated with childbirth. The progress of labor slows, with a more rapid development of hypoglycemia and ketosis if these demands are not met and fat is metabolized. Reduced energy for bearing-down efforts (pushing) increases the risk for a forceps- or vacuum-assisted birth. This is most likely to occur in women who begin to labor early in the morning after a night without caloric intake. When women are permitted to consume fluid and food freely, they typically regulate their own oral intake, eating light foods (e.g., eggs, yogurt, ice cream, dry toast and jelly, fruit) and drinking fluids during early labor and tapering off to the intake of clear fluids and sips of water or ice chips as labor intensifies and the second stage approaches (King & Pinger, 2014; Sharts-Hopko, 2010; Tillett & Hill, 2016).

Common hospital practice is to allow clear liquids during early labor, tapering off to ice chips and sips of water as labor progresses and becomes more active. ACOG (2017) now supports the oral intake of moderate amounts of clear liquids by laboring women who do not have complications. The ASA recommends that laboring women at low risk for cesarean birth be allowed to have clear liquids during labor (Tillett & Hill, 2016). Clear fluids recommended for labor include water, fruit juices without pulp, carbonated beverages, clear teas and coffee, flavored gelatin, fruit ices, popsicles, and broth (Collins, 2017). A woman's culture may influence what she will eat and drink during labor. In addition, women who use nonpharmacologic pain relief measures and labor at home or in birthing centers are more likely to eat and drink during labor. The amount of solid and liquid carbohydrates to offer a woman in labor is still unclear. Although it is known that energy needs increase as labor becomes prolonged, there is limited evidence regarding the effect of oral carbohydrate intake on enhancing the progress of labor and reducing the risk for dystocia (Sharts-Hopko, 2010).

A Cochrane review of this topic concluded that there is no justification for restricting food or fluid intake during labor in women at low risk for complications (Singata, Tranmer, & Gyte, 2013). Nurses should follow the orders of the woman's obstetric health care provider when offering the woman food or fluid during labor. However, as advocates, nurses can facilitate change by informing others of the current research findings that support the safety and effectiveness of the oral intake of food and fluid during labor and initiating such research themselves.

Intravenous Intake

If the woman is not permitted oral intake during labor, fluids are administered intravenously to maintain hydration and meet increased energy needs. Traditionally, 125 mL/hour of intravenous fluid has been infused. However, this may not be enough volume to meet the fluid needs of the laboring woman, and the resulting dehydration may negatively affect labor progress. It may be more appropriate to infuse 250 mL/hour to ensure proper hydration (Kelly et al., 2017; King & Pinger, 2014). While somewhat controversial, some practitioners infuse intravenous fluids containing 5% dextrose in a balanced salt solution in order to meet the woman's energy needs during labor as well as ensure hydration. To help prevent maternal and fetal hyperglycemia, glucose-containing solutions should not be administered as fluid boluses in situations such as preloading before the initiation of regional anesthesia or for intrauterine resuscitation (Kelly et al.).

❗ NURSING ALERT

Nurses should carefully monitor the intake and output of laboring women receiving IV fluids because they face an increased danger of hypervolemia as a result of the fluid retention that occurs during pregnancy.

Elimination

Voiding

The woman in labor should be encouraged to void every 2 hours. A distended bladder may impede descent of the presenting part, slow or stop uterine contractions, and lead to decreased bladder tone or uterine atony after birth. Women who receive epidural analgesia or anesthesia are especially at risk for the retention of urine. Therefore the need to void should be assessed more frequently with them.

The nurse assists the woman to the bathroom to void or to use a bedside commode unless any of the following apply: the nurse-midwife or physician has ordered bed rest; the woman is receiving epidural analgesia or anesthesia; internal monitoring is being used; or ambulation will compromise the status of the laboring woman or her fetus. External monitoring can usually be interrupted long enough for the woman to go to the bathroom.

If using a bedpan is necessary, spontaneous voiding is encouraged by providing privacy and having the woman sit upright (as she would on a toilet). Other interventions to encourage urination, either in the bathroom or on the bedpan, are having the woman listen to the sound of water slowly running from a faucet, placing her hands in warm water, having her blow bubbles into a glass of water using a straw, or pouring warm water over the vulva and perineum using a plastic perineal care bottle.

Catheterization

If the woman is unable to void and her bladder is distended, she may need to be catheterized. Many hospitals have protocols or standing orders that rely on the nurse's judgment concerning the need for catheterization. Before performing the catheterization, clean the vulva and perineum because vaginal show and amniotic fluid may be present. If an obstacle prevents advancement of the catheter it is most likely the fetal presenting part. If the catheter cannot be advanced, it is withdrawn, the procedure is stopped, and the nurse midwife or physician is notified of the difficulty.

Bowel Elimination

Most women do not have bowel movements during labor because of decreased intestinal motility. Stool that has formed in the large intestine often moves downward toward the anorectal area as a result of pressure exerted by the fetal presenting part as it descends. This stool is often expelled during second-stage pushing and birth. However, the passage of stool with bearing-down efforts increases the risk for infection and may embarrass the woman, thereby reducing the effectiveness of her pushing efforts. To prevent these problems, the nurse should immediately cleanse the perineal area to remove any stool, while reassuring the woman that the passage of stool at this time is a normal and expected event because the same muscles used to expel the baby also expel stool. When the presenting part is deep in the pelvis, even in the absence of stool in the anorectal area, the woman may feel rectal pressure and think she needs to defecate.

> ## ! NURSING ALERT
>
> If the woman expresses the urge to defecate, the nurse should perform a vaginal examination to assess cervical dilation and station. When a multiparous woman experiences the urge to defecate, this often means that birth will follow quickly.

In the past, routine use of enemas on admission for women at term was suggested as a way to prevent stooling during second-stage labor and consequently, maternal embarrassment. It was also thought that enemas would reduce the length of labor and the chance of infection for both women and babies. However, a Cochrane review of this topic found that the evidence does not support the routine use of enemas during labor (Reveiz, Gaitan, & Cuervo, 2013).

Ambulation and Positioning

Upright positions and mobility during labor may be more pleasant, compared to lying in bed, for laboring women. These practices have also been associated with improved uterine contraction intensity and shorter labors, less need for pain medications, reduced rate of operative birth (e.g., cesarean birth, forceps- and vacuum-assisted birth), increased maternal autonomy and control, distraction from the discomforts of labor, and an opportunity for close interaction with the woman's partner and care provider as they help her assume upright positions and remain mobile (Kilpatrick & Garrison, 2017; King & Pinger, 2014; Lawrence, Lewis, Hofmeyr, & Styles, 2013; Simpson & O'Brien-Abel, 2014). No harmful effects have been observed from maternal activity and position changes. However, confinement to bed is the norm for laboring women in US hospitals. The increased use of epidurals during childbirth accompanied by multiple medical interventions (e.g., electronic fetal monitors, IV infusions) and reduced motor control contribute to this practice, thereby interfering with a woman's freedom of movement and often slowing labor progress. Nurses can advocate for changes in this practice in their labor and birth units.

It is important to encourage ambulation if membranes are intact, after ROM if the fetal presenting part is engaged, and if the woman has not received medication for pain (Fig. 16.9). The woman also may find it comfortable to stand and lean forward on her partner, doula, or nurse for support at times during labor (Fig. 16.10, A). In some

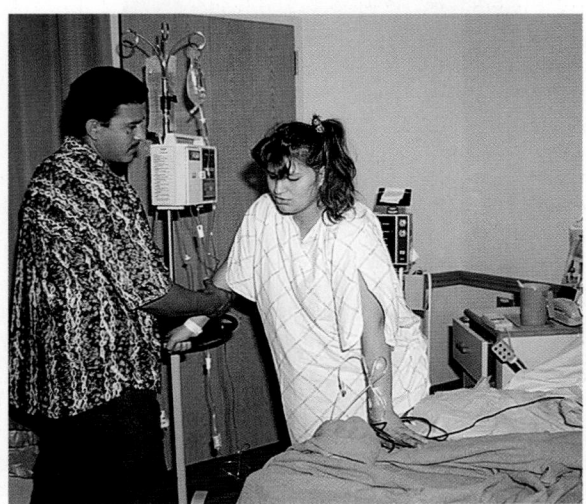

FIG 16.9 Woman preparing to walk with partner. (Courtesy of Marjorie Pyle, RNC, Lifecircle, Costa Mesa, CA.)

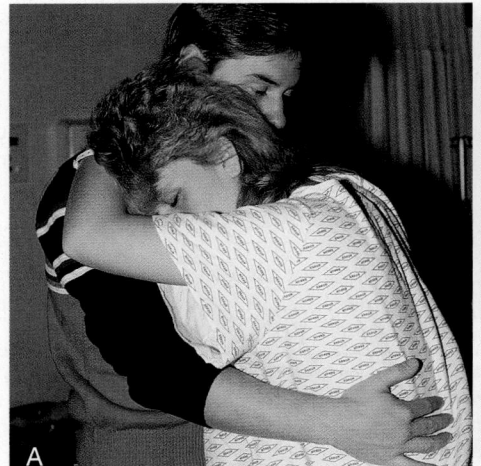
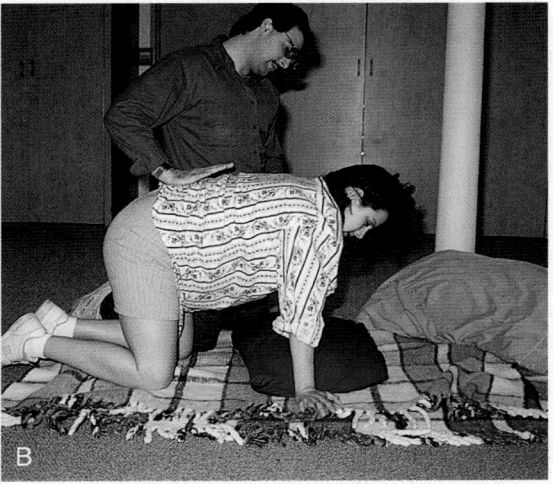

FIG 16.10 A, Woman standing and leaning forward with support. **B,** Woman in hands-and-knees position. (Courtesy of Marjorie Pyle, RNC, Lifecircle, Costa Mesa, CA.)

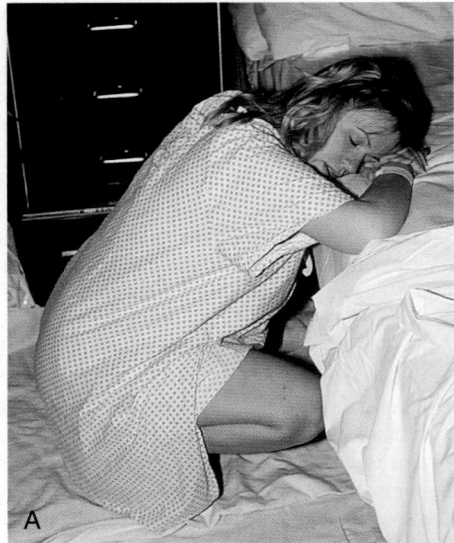

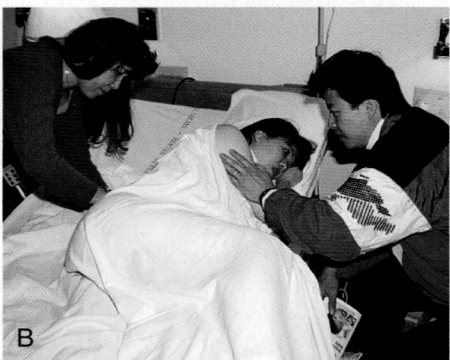

FIG 16.11 Maternal positions for labor. **A,** Squatting. **B,** Lateral position. Support person is applying sacral pressure while partner provides encouragement. (Courtesy of Marjorie Pyle, RNC, Lifecircle, Costa Mesa, CA.)

circumstances, ambulation may be contraindicated because of maternal or fetal status.

When the woman lies in bed, she usually changes her position spontaneously as labor progresses. If she does not change position every 30 to 60 minutes, the nurse assists her to do so. The side-lying (lateral) position is preferred because it promotes optimal uteroplacental and renal blood flow and increases fetal oxygen saturation (Fig. 16.11, *B*). If the woman wants to lie supine, the nurse should place a pillow under one hip as a wedge to prevent the uterus from compressing the aorta and vena cava (see Fig. 16.5). Sitting is not contraindicated unless it adversely affects fetal status, which can be determined by checking the FHR and pattern. If the fetus is in the occiput posterior position, it may be helpful to encourage the woman to squat during contractions because this position increases the pelvic diameter, allowing the head to rotate to a more anterior position (see Fig. 16.11, *A*). A hands-and-knees position during contractions (see Fig. 16.10, *B*) or a lateral position (see Fig. 16.11, *B*) on the same side as the fetal spine also are recommended to facilitate the rotation of the fetal occiput from a posterior to an anterior position, as gravity pulls the fetal back forward. These positions also provide access to the back for application of counterpressure by the partner, doula, or nurse (Collins, 2017; Kelly et al., 2017; Simpson & O'Brien-Abel, 2014) (see Fig. 16.11, *B*). Women with epidural anesthesia may not be able to squat or assume a hands-and-knees position depending on the degree of motor involvement resulting from the epidural.

BOX 16.9   Common Maternal Positions* During Labor and Birth

Semirecumbent Position (see Figs. 16.14, *B* and 16.15, *B*)
With woman sitting with her upper body elevated to at least a 30-degree angle, place wedge or small pillow under hip to prevent vena cava compression and reduce likelihood of supine hypotension (see Fig. 16.5).
- The greater the angle of elevation, the more gravity or pressure is exerted that promotes fetal descent, the progress of contractions, and the widening of pelvic dimensions.
- This position is convenient for providing care measures and for external fetal monitoring.

Lateral Position (see Figs. 16.11, *B* and 16.14, *A*)
Have the woman alternate between left and right side-lying position and provide abdominal and back support as needed for comfort.
- Removes pressure from the vena cava and back, enhances uteroplacental perfusion, and relieves backache
- Facilitates internal rotation of fetus in a posterior position to an anterior position (woman should lie on same side as fetal spine)
- Makes it easier to perform back massage or counterpressure
- Associated with less frequent, but more intense, contractions
- May be more difficult to obtain good external fetal monitor tracings
- May be used as a birthing position
- Takes pressure off perineum, allowing it to stretch gradually
- Reduces risk for perineal trauma

Upright Position
The gravity effect enhances the contraction cycle and fetal descent. The weight of the fetus places increasing pressure on the cervix; the cervix is pulled upward, facilitating effacement and dilation; impulses from the cervix to the pituitary gland increase, causing more oxytocin to be secreted; and contractions are intensified, thereby applying more forceful downward pressure on the fetus, but they are less painful.
- Fetus is aligned with pelvis, and pelvic diameters are widened slightly.
- Effective upright positions include the following:
  - Ambulation (see Fig. 16.9)
  - Standing and leaning forward with support provided by coach (see Fig. 16.10, *A*), end of bed, back of chair, or birth ball; relieves backache and facilitates application of counterpressure or back massage
  - Sitting up in bed, chair, or birthing chair or on toilet or bedside commode (see Fig. 16.14, *B*)
  - Squatting (see Fig. 16.11, *A* and Fig. 16.15, *E*)

Hands-and-Knees Position—Position for Posterior Positions of the Presenting Part (see Figs. 16.10, *B* and 16.12)
Assume an "all fours" position, or lean over an object (e.g., birth ball) while on knees in bed or on a covered floor; can also place knees on seat section of bed while leaning up over back of raised head of bed; allows for pelvic rocking.
- Relieves backache characteristic of "back labor"
- Facilitates internal rotation of the fetus by increasing mobility of the coccyx, increasing the pelvic diameters, and using gravity to turn the fetal back and rotate the head (NOTE: A side-lying position, double hip squeeze, or knee squeeze can also facilitate internal rotation.)

*Assess the effect of each position on the laboring woman's comfort and anxiety level, progress of labor, and fetal heart rate and pattern. Alternate positions every 30 to 60 minutes, allowing the woman to take control of her position changes.

Much research continues to focus on acquiring a better understanding of the physiologic and psychologic effects of maternal position in labor. Box 16.9 describes a variety of positions that are commonly used and recommended.

The woman can use a birth ball (gymnastic ball, physical therapy ball) to support her body as she assumes a variety of labor and birth positions (Fig. 16.12). She can sit on the ball while leaning over the bed or lean over the ball to support her upper body and reduce stress on her arms and hands when she assumes a hands-and-knees position. The birth ball can encourage pelvic mobility and pelvic and perineal relaxation when the woman sits on the firm yet pliable ball and rocks in rhythmic movements. Warm compresses applied to the perineum and lower back can maximize this relaxation and comfort effect. The birth ball should be large enough that, when the woman sits, her knees are bent at a 90-degree angle and her feet are flat on the floor and approximately 2 feet apart.

> ## ⚡ SAFETY ALERT
>
> A woman may experience dizziness as she changes upright positions during labor. It is essential that the nurse or support person is present to provide assistance should dizziness occur.

SUPPORTIVE CARE DURING LABOR AND BIRTH

Support during labor and birth involves emotional support, physical care and comfort measures, and advice and information. The value of the continuous supportive presence of a person (e.g., partner, family member, friend, nurse, doula) during labor has long been known. Women who have continuous support beginning in early labor are less likely to use pain medication or epidurals and are more likely to have a spontaneous vaginal birth and increased satisfaction with their birth experience. No harmful effects from continuous labor support have been identified. To the contrary, there is good evidence that labor support improves important health outcomes (Hodnett et al., 2013; Kilpatrick & Garrison, 2017; King & Pinger, 2014). Continuous labor support is associated with greater benefits when the provider of that support is not a hospital staff member (Simpson & O'Brien-Abel, 2014).

Labor rooms should be airy, clean, and homelike. The laboring woman should feel safe in this environment and free to be herself and use the comfort and relaxation measures she prefers. To enhance relaxation, the use of bright, overhead lights is avoided, and noise and intrusions are kept to a minimum. The room temperature is adjusted to ensure the laboring woman's comfort. The room should be large enough to accommodate a comfortable chair for the woman's partner,

the monitoring equipment, and hospital personnel. Some women bring their own pillows to make the hospital surroundings more homelike and facilitate position changes. Environmental modifications should reflect the preferences of the woman, including the number of visitors and availability of a telephone, television, electronic devices (e.g., computer, smartphone), and music.

Labor Support by the Nurse

Supportive nursing care for a woman in labor includes the following:
- Helping her maintain control and participate to the extent she wishes in the birth of her infant.
- Providing continuity of care by the same nurse throughout the shift.
- Providing care that is nonjudgmental and respectful of her cultural and religious values and beliefs.
- Helping the woman meet her expected outcomes for her labor.
- Listening to her concerns and encouraging her to express her feelings.
- Acting as her advocate, supporting her decisions and respecting her choices as appropriate and relating her wishes as needed to other health care providers.
- Helping her conserve her energy and cope effectively with her pain and discomfort by using a variety of comfort measures that are acceptable to her.
- Acknowledging her efforts during labor, including her strength and courage, and those of her partner, and providing positive reinforcement.
- Protecting her privacy, modesty, and dignity.

Women who have attended childbirth education classes will know something about the labor process, coaching techniques, and comfort measures. The nurse plays a supportive role and keeps the woman and her partner informed of the labor progress. If necessary, the nurse reviews the methods learned in class and practiced at home because it may be difficult for the woman to effectively use these methods and techniques now that she is in labor and in an unfamiliar setting.

Even when a laboring woman has not attended childbirth classes, the nurse can teach her simple breathing and relaxation techniques during the early phase of labor. In this case, the nurse provides more of the coaching and supportive care until the support person feels ready to take on a more active coaching role (see Chapter 14). The nurse can demonstrate comfort measures while encouraging the support person to assist. Observing the comforting approaches of the nurse can help the partner learn effective comfort measures.

Comfort measures vary with the situation (Fig. 16.13). The nurse can draw on the woman's list of comfort measures and relaxation

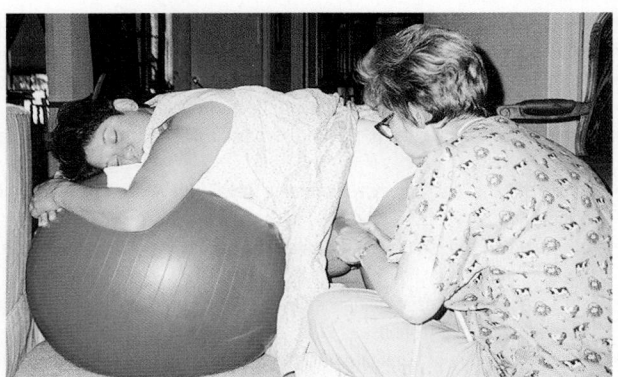

FIG 16.12 Woman laboring using birth ball. (Courtesy of Polly Perez, Cutting Edge Press, Johnson, VT.)

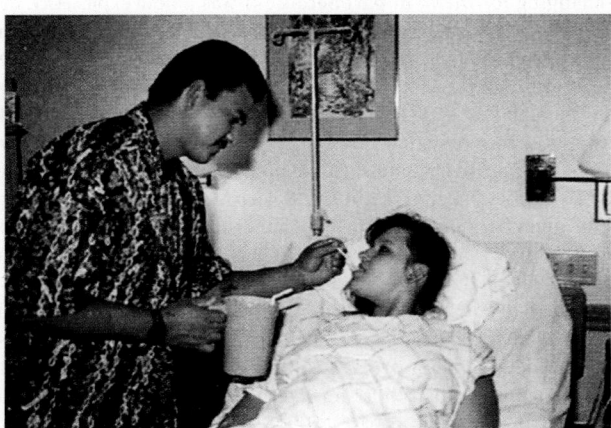

FIG 16.13 Partner providing comfort measures. (Courtesy of Marjorie Pyle, RNC, Lifecircle, Costa Mesa, CA.)

techniques learned during the pregnancy and through life experiences. Such measures include maintaining a comfortable, calm, supportive atmosphere in the labor and birth area; using touch therapeutically; providing nonpharmacologic measures to relieve discomfort (e.g., hydrotherapy, heat or cold applied to the lower back in the event of back labor, a cool cloth applied to the forehead, massage); and, most important, just being there (see Table 16.3). See Chapter 14 for a full discussion of pharmacologic and nonpharmacologic comfort measures.

Most women in labor respond positively to touch; the nurse should obtain permission before using any touching measures. Women appreciate gentle handling by staff members. Back massage and counterpressure may be offered, especially if the woman is experiencing back labor. The nurse can teach the support person to exert counterpressure against the woman's sacrum over the occiput of the head of a fetus in a posterior position (see Fig. 16.11, B). Double hip or knee squeezes can also be helpful in reducing back pain. The back pain is caused by the occiput pressing on spinal nerves; counterpressure lifts the occiput off these nerves, providing some pain relief. However, the partner needs to be relieved after a while because exerting counterpressure is hard work. Hand and foot massage also can be soothing and relaxing.

The woman's perception of the soothing qualities of touch may change as labor progresses. Many women become more sensitive to touch (hyperesthesia) as labor progresses. They may tell their coach to leave them alone or not to touch them. The partner who is unprepared for this normal response may feel rejected and react by withdrawing active support. The nurse can reassure him or her that this response is a positive indication that the first stage is ending and the second stage is approaching. Women with increased sensitivity to touch may tolerate it better on surfaces of the body where hair does not grow such as the forehead, palms of the hands, and soles of the feet.

Labor Support by the Father or Partner

The father of the baby is usually the primary support person for the laboring woman, although a same sex partner, family member, or friend may assume that role. He is often able to provide the comfort measures and touch that the laboring woman needs. When the woman becomes focused on her pain, sometimes the partner can persuade her to try nonpharmacologic variations of comfort measures. In addition, he usually is able to interpret the woman's needs and desires for staff members.

The feelings of a first-time father change as labor progresses. Although he is often calm at the onset of labor, feelings of fear and helplessness may begin to dominate as labor becomes more active and the father realizes that it is more stressful than he anticipated. First-time fathers interviewed in a recent Swedish study described childbirth as truly life-changing for them, in part because it was a new experience in an unfamiliar environment. Four factors were identified that affected their childbirth experience: preparing for childbirth, feeling vulnerable in a new situation, feeling recognized as a contributing part of a unit with the woman giving birth, and meeting their child for the first time. The study found that first-time fathers need information and support in order to participate more fully in the process and experience a positive childbirth experience (Ledenfors & Bertero, 2016).

Staff members should assure the father that his presence is helpful and encourage him to be involved in the care of the woman to the extent to which he and his partner are comfortable. He should be reassured that he is not assuming the responsibility for observation and management of his partner's labor but that his responsibility is to support her as the labor progresses. The nurse can suggest alternative comfort measures when those he is using are no longer helpful or are rejected by his partner.

The first-time father may feel excluded as birth preparations begin during the active phase. Once the second stage begins and birth nears,

the father's focus changes from the woman to the baby who is about to be born. The father will be exposed to many sights and smells he may never have experienced. Therefore the nurse needs to tell him what to expect and make him comfortable about leaving the room to regain his composure should something occur that surprises him, but make sure that someone else is available to support the woman during his absence.

Nursing actions that support the father convey several important concepts: first, he is a person of value; second, he can be a partner in the woman's care; and third, childbearing is a team effort. Box 16.10 details ways in which the nurse can support the father-partner. A well-informed father can make an important contribution to the health and well-being of the mother and child, their family interrelationship, and his self-esteem.

Labor Support by Doulas

Continuity of care has been cited by women as a critical component of a satisfying childbirth experience. A specially trained, experienced female labor attendant called a doula can meet this need. The doula is a professional or lay labor-support person who is present during labor in addition to the labor and birth nurse (Burke, 2014). The primary role of the doula is to focus on the laboring woman and to provide physical and emotional support by using soft, reassuring words of praise and encouragement; touching; stroking; and hugging. The doula also administers comfort measures to reduce pain and enhance relaxation and coping, walks with the woman, helps her to change positions, and coaches her bearing-down efforts. Doulas provide information about labor progress and explain procedures and events. They advocate for the woman's right to participate actively in managing her labor.

The doula also supports the woman's partner, who often feels unqualified to be the sole labor support and may find it difficult to watch the woman when she is experiencing pain. The doula can encourage

---

BOX 16.10   Guidelines for Supporting the Father*

- Orient him to the labor room and the unit; explain location of the cafeteria, toilet, waiting room, and nursery; give information about visiting hours; introduce personnel present by name, and describe their functions.
- Inform him of sights and smells he can expect to encounter; encourage him to leave the room if necessary.
- Respect his or the couple's decision about the degree of his involvement. Offer them freedom to make decisions.
- Tell him when his presence has been helpful, and continue to reinforce this throughout labor.
- Offer to teach him comfort measures; demonstrate or role-play these measures.
- Inform him frequently of the progress of the labor and the woman's needs. Keep him informed about procedures to be performed.
- Prepare him for changes in the woman's behavior and physical appearance.
- Remind him to eat and stay hydrated; offer him snacks and fluids if possible.
- Relieve him of the job of support person as necessary. Offer him blankets if he is to sleep in a chair by the bedside.
- Acknowledge the stress experienced by each partner during labor and birth, and identify normal responses.
- Attempt to modify or eliminate unsettling stimuli such as extra noise and extra light; create a relaxing and calm environment.

*These guidelines are appropriate for any support person or partner.

and praise the partner's efforts, create a partnership as caregivers, and provide respite care. Doulas also facilitate communication between the laboring woman and her partner as well as between the couple and the health care team (Simkin, 2012).

Doula support during labor is associated with decreased use of analgesia, decreased incidence of operative birth, increased incidence of spontaneous vaginal birth, and increased maternal satisfaction with the childbirth experience (Kilpatrick & Garrison, 2017).

The roles of the nurse and the doula are complementary. They should work together as a team, recognizing and respecting the role each plays in supporting and caring for the woman and her partner during the childbirth process. Both the nurse and the doula provide supportive care measures. The nurse also focuses on monitoring the status of the maternal-fetal unit, implementing clinical care protocols (including pharmacologic interventions), and documenting assessment findings, actions, and responses (Simkin, 2012).

Labor Support by Grandparents

When a grandparent (usually the mother of the laboring woman) is the primary support person during labor, it is especially important to support and treat her or him with respect. Grandparents may have ways to deal with pain based on their experience. Grandparents should be encouraged to help as long as their actions do not compromise the status of the mother or the fetus. The nurse treats grandparents with dignity and respect by acknowledging the value of their contributions to parental support and recognizing the difficulty parents have in witnessing the woman's discomfort or crisis. If they have never witnessed a birth, the nurse may need to provide explanations of what is happening. Many of the activities used to support fathers also are appropriate for grandparents (see Box 16.10).

Siblings During Labor and Birth

Preparing siblings for acceptance of the new child helps promote the attachment process and may help the older children accept this change. According to parents' preferences and agency policy, children may be allowed in the labor room. Older children sometimes become active participants in the birthing process. Rehearsal for the event before labor is essential.

The age and developmental level of children influence their responses; therefore preparation to be present during labor is adjusted to meet each child's needs (see Box 20.5). The child younger than 2 years shows little interest in pregnancy and labor. However, for the older child such preparation may reduce fears and misconceptions. Parents need to be prepared for labor and birth themselves and feel comfortable about the process and the presence of their children. Most parents have a "feel" for their children's maturational level and their physical and emotional ability to observe and cope with the events of the labor and birth process. Preparation can include a description of the anticipated sights, events (e.g., ROM, monitors, IV infusions), smells, and sounds; a labor and birth demonstration; a tour of the birthing unit; sibling classes (see Fig. 8.4); and an opportunity to be around a real newborn. Storybooks about the birth process can be read to or by children to prepare them for the event. Films are available for preparing preschool and school-age children to participate in the labor and birth experience. Children must learn that their mother will be working hard during labor and birth. She will not be able to talk to them during contractions. She may groan, scream, grunt, and pant at times and say things she would not say otherwise (e.g., "I can't take this anymore," "Take this baby out of me," or "This pain is killing me"). You can tell them that labor is uncomfortable, but that their mother's body is made for giving birth.

Most agencies require that a specific person is designated to watch over the children who are participating in their mother's childbirth experience to provide them with support, explanations, diversions, and comfort as needed. Health care providers involved in attending women during birth must be comfortable with the presence of children and the unpredictability of their questions, comments, and behaviors.

Emergency Interventions

Although rare, emergency conditions that require immediate nursing intervention can arise with startling speed. See Chapter 15 for information on management of abnormal FHR. Management of other emergency situations, including meconium-stained amniotic fluid, shoulder dystocia, prolapsed umbilical cord, ruptured uterus, and amniotic fluid embolus, is discussed in Chapter 17.

SECOND STAGE OF LABOR

The second stage of labor is the stage in which the infant is born. This stage begins with full cervical dilation (10 cm) and complete effacement (100%) and ends with the baby's birth (Kelly et al., 2017). The force exerted by uterine contractions, gravity, and maternal bearing-down efforts facilitates achievement of the expected outcome of a spontaneous, uncomplicated vaginal birth. The length of second-stage labor varies considerably among women and is affected by parity and the use of epidural anesthesia. As is true for first-stage labor, researchers have discovered that second-stage labor lasts longer than had been believed in the past (Kopas, 2014). Other factors that influence the length of second-stage labor include the woman's age, body mass index (BMI), emotional state and adequacy of support, and level of fatigue, along with fetal size, position, and sometimes presentation (Kelly et al., 2017; Kilpatrick & Garrison, 2017).

Historically the median duration of a stage of labor has been used to define normal (Hanson & VandeVusse, 2014). Currently it is suggested that the 95th percentile be used instead as the upper limit of normal for the length of labor stages. In other words, within a given period of time 95 of 100 women will have completed that stage of labor. The 95th percentile for second-stage labor in a nulliparous woman with epidural anesthesia is about 4 hours (Osborne & Hanson, 2014).

The following guideline lists time frames for both nulliparous and multiparous women that suggest second-stage labor may be either progressing too slowly or not at all.

- Nulliparous women   3 or more hours with no regional anesthesia
     4 or more hours with regional anesthesia
- Multiparous women   2 hours with no regional anesthesia
     3 hours with regional anesthesia

It is important to understand that as long as some progress is being made and the maternal and fetal status is reassuring, there is no need for rigid time limits or arbitrary rules related to the duration of second stage (Kelly et al., 2017).

The second stage of labor is composed of two phases: the latent phase and the active pushing phase (Osborne & Hanson, 2014). The latent phase, sometimes referred to as *delayed pushing, laboring down,* or *passive descent,* is the time from complete cervical dilation until the woman begins actively pushing (King & Pinger, 2014; Osborne & Hanson). During this phase, the fetus continues to descend passively through the birth canal and rotate to an anterior position as a result of ongoing uterine contractions. The woman is quiet and often relaxes with her eyes closed between contractions. The urge to bear down is not strong, and some women do not experience it at all or only during the acme (peak) of a contraction. Delayed pushing has been shown to result in an increase in spontaneous vaginal births, a decrease in active pushing time, a reduction in the number of operative vaginal births, and less maternal fatigue. On the other hand, delayed pushing results in a longer total second-stage labor. It has not been shown to affect the incidence of cesarean births, perineal lacerations, or episiotomies (see Clinical Reasoning Case Study: Delayed Pushing in Second-Stage Labor) (King & Pinger, 2014; Kopas, 2014).

Careful monitoring with assurance of normal fetal status should be used during delayed pushing. If descent is slow and the woman becomes anxious, she can be encouraged to try squatting or sitting, as both of these positions may be of benefit when the second stage is prolonged. Because a prolonged second stage has been associated with maternal complications such as infection, severe lacerations, and postpartum hemorrhage, the woman should be encouraged to begin pushing after 1 to 2 hours if there has been no fetal descent and she still feels no urge to push (King & Pinger, 2014; Kopas, 2014).

During the active pushing phase, the woman has strong urges to bear down as the Ferguson reflex is activated when the presenting part presses on the stretch receptors of the pelvic floor. This stimulation causes the release of oxytocin from the posterior pituitary gland, which provokes stronger expulsive uterine contractions. Physiologic management of this phase involves spontaneous, rather than directed, pushing. Instead of giving instructions, caregivers encourage the woman to push when she feels the urge to do so (Kopas, 2014). They also encourage shorter bearing down efforts using open-glottis pushes (Osborne & Hanson, 2014). Table 16.4 lists common maternal behaviors during the active pushing phase of second-stage labor.

CLINICAL REASONING CASE STUDY
Delayed Pushing in Second-Stage Labor

You are the nurse assigned to care for Emily, a 25-year-old G1 P0 at 39 weeks of gestation. You have just performed a vaginal examination and found that Emily's cervix is completely dilated. She has an epidural, which is working well. Currently Emily is feeling neither pressure nor pain. On learning that Emily's cervix is completely dilated, her health care provider exclaims, "Good! Get in there and help her push so we can have this baby! I'm ready to go home. I've had a long day!"

1. Evidence—Is there sufficient evidence to draw conclusions about effective management of second-stage labor?
2. Assumptions—Describe an underlying assumption about each of the following issues:
   a. Delayed pushing
   b. Positioning for pushing
   c. Spontaneous versus directed pushing efforts
3. What implications and priorities for nursing care can be drawn at this time?
4. Does the evidence objectively support your argument (conclusion)?
5. Interprofessional care—Describe the roles/responsibilities of health care professionals who might be involved in Emily's care.

TABLE 16.4	Expected Maternal Progress in Second-Stage Labor	
Criterion	**Latent Phase**	**Active Pushing Phase (Average Duration Varies)***
Contractions		
Intensity	Period of physiologic lull for all criteria; period of peace and rest; passive descent occurs	Significant increase becoming overwhelmingly strong and expulsive; strong by palpation
Frequency		Every 2–3 minutes progressing to every 1–2 minutes
Duration		40–60 seconds
Descent, station	0 to +2	+2 to +4; rate of descent increases, and Ferguson reflex[†] is activated; fetal head becomes visible at introitus, and birth occurs
Show: color and amount		Significant increase in dark red bloody show; bloody show accompanies emergence of head
Spontaneous bearing-down efforts	Slight to absent, except at peak of strongest contractions	Increased urge to bear down; becomes stronger as fetus descends to vaginal introitus and reaches perineum
Vocalization	Quiet	Grunting sounds or expiratory vocalizations; announces contractions; may scream or swear
Maternal behavior	Experiences sense of relief that transition to second stage is finished	Senses increased urge to push and describes increasing pain; describes *ring of fire* (burning sensation of acute pain as vagina stretches and fetal head crowns)
	Feels fatigued and sleepy	Expresses feeling of powerlessness
	Feels a sense of accomplishment and optimism because the "worst is over"	Shows decreased ability to listen to or concentrate on anything but giving birth
	Feels in control	Alters respiratory pattern: has short 4- to 5-second breath holds with regular breaths in between, 5–7 times per contraction
		Frequent repositioning
		Often shows excitement immediately after birth of head

*Duration of descent phase can vary, depending on maternal parity, effectiveness of bearing-down effort, and presence of spinal anesthesia or epidural analgesia.
[†]Pressure of presenting part on stretch receptors of pelvic floor stimulates release of oxytocin from posterior pituitary gland, resulting in more intense uterine contractions.
Data from Hanson, L. (2009). Second-stage labor care, *The Journal of Perinatal and Neonatal Nursing, 23*(1), 31-39; Roberts, J.E. (2002). The "push" for evidence: Management of the second stage, *Journal of Midwifery & Women's Health, 47*(1), 2-15; Simkin, P., & Ancheta, R. (2000). The labor progress handbook. Malden, MA: Blackwell Science; Simpson, K., Cesario, S., Morin, K., et al. (2008). *Nursing care and management of the second stage of labor: Evidence-based clinical practice guideline* (2nd ed.), Washington, DC: Association of Women's Health, Obstetric and Neonatal Nurses; K.R. Simpson & P. Creehan (Eds.). (2014). *AWHONN's perinatal nursing* (4th ed.). Philadelphia, PA; Lippincott.

CARE MANAGEMENT

Box 16.11 describes nursing care during the second stage of labor. The only certain objective sign that the second stage of labor has begun is the inability to feel the cervix during vaginal examination, indicating that it is fully dilated and effaced. The precise moment that this occurs is not easily determined because it depends on when a vaginal examination is performed to validate full dilation and effacement. This makes timing of the actual duration of the second stage difficult. Box 16.11 lists several signs that suggest the onset of second-stage labor. These signs commonly appear at the time the cervix reaches full dilation. However, they can appear earlier in labor. Women with an epidural block may not exhibit such signs.

Women who are laboring without regional anesthesia can experience an irresistible urge to bear down before full cervical dilation. For some, this occurs as early as 5 cm dilation. This is most often related to the station of the presenting part below the level of the ischial spines of the maternal pelvis. This occurrence creates a conflict between the woman, whose body is telling her to push, and her health care providers, who may believe that pushing the fetal presenting part against an incompletely dilated cervix will result in cervical edema and lacerations, as well as slow the labor progress. The premature urge to bear down may be a sign of labor progress, possibly indicating the onset of the second stage of labor. If the woman's cervix is not yet completely dilated, encouraging her to breathe through contractions using shallow, frequent panting or puffing breaths (as though she is blowing out a candle) and to assume a side-lying or hands-and-knees position may be beneficial in assisting her to avoid pushing (Kelly et al., 2017; Perinatal Education Associates, 2016).

ASSESSMENT

Assessment continues during the second stage of labor. Professional standards and agency policy determine the specific type and timing of assessments, as well as the way in which findings are documented (see Box 16.11). Signs and symptoms of impending birth (see Table 16.4) may appear unexpectedly, requiring immediate action by the nurse (Box 16.12).

The nurse continues to monitor maternal-fetal status and events of the second stage and provide comfort measures for the mother. This includes physical care measures (see Table 16.3 and Box 16.11) as well as keeping unnecessary noise, conversation, and other distractions (e.g., laughing, talking of attending personnel in or outside the labor area) to a minimum.

In the hospital, birth may occur in an LDR, LDRP, or delivery room. If the mother is to be transferred to the delivery room for birth, it is best to perform the transfer early enough to avoid rushing her. The birth area also is readied (see later discussion).

PREPARING FOR BIRTH

Maternal Position

No single ideal position for childbirth exists. Labor is a dynamic, interactive process involving the woman's uterus, pelvis, and voluntary muscles. In addition, angles between the fetus and the woman's pelvis constantly change as the fetus turns and flexes down the birth canal. The woman may want to assume various positions for childbirth. She should be encouraged to change positions frequently and to labor in any position that feels comfortable and natural (King & Pinger, 2014) (Figs. 16.14 and 16.15). The supine and lithotomy positions, however, should be avoided (Kopas, 2014; Simpson & O'Brien-Abel, 2014).

BOX 16.11   Nursing Care in Second-Stage Labor

Assessment
Signs That Suggest the Onset of the Second Stage
- Increase in frequency and intensity of uterine contractions
- Urge to push or feeling need to have a bowel movement
- An episode of vomiting
- Increased bloody show
- Uncontrolled shivering
- Verbalizations of feeling out of control or unable to cope
- Involuntary bearing-down efforts

Physical Assessment
- Perform every 5 to 30 minutes: maternal blood pressure, pulse, and respirations.
- Assess every 5 to 15 minutes, depending on risk status: fetal heart rate and pattern
- Assess every 10 to 15 minutes: vaginal show; signs of fetal descent; and changes in maternal appearance, mood, affect, energy level, and involvement of partner/coach.
- Assess every contraction and bearing-down effort.

Interventions
Latent Phase
- Help the woman to rest in a position of comfort; encourage relaxation to conserve energy.
- Promote progress of fetal descent and onset of urge to bear down by encouraging position changes, pelvic rock, ambulation, showering.

Active Pushing Phase
- Provide 1:1 nursing care (1 labor nurse to 1 laboring woman). Do not leave the woman alone.
- Help the woman to change position, and encourage spontaneous bearing-down efforts.
- Help the woman to relax and conserve energy between contractions.
- Provide comfort and pain-relief measures as needed.
- Cleanse the perineum promptly if fecal material is expelled.
- Coach the woman to pant during contractions and to gently push between contractions when head is emerging.
- Provide emotional support, encouragement, and positive reinforcement of efforts.
- Keep the woman informed regarding progress.
- Create a calm and supportive environment.
- Offer a mirror to watch birth.
- Encourage the woman to touch the fetal head when it is visible at the perineum.

Data from Kennedy, B.B. & Baird, S.M. (2017). *Intrapartum management modules: A perinatal education program* (5th ed.). Philadelphia, PA: Wolters Kluwer; American Academy of Pediatrics & American College of Obstetricians and Gynecologists. (2012). *Guidelines for perinatal care* (7th ed.). Washington, DC: American College of Obstetricians and Gynecologists.

Birth attendants play a major role in influencing a woman's choice of positions for birth, with nurse-midwives tending to suggest nonlithotomy positions (e.g., upright, lateral) for the second stage of labor. Evidence suggests that any upright or lateral position used in second-stage labor (e.g., walking, standing, sitting, kneeling, squatting, hands-and-knees, or side-lying) results in less pain, less fatigue, less perineal trauma, fewer episiotomies, fewer forceps- or vacuum-assisted births, and fewer FHR abnormalities (King & Pinger, 2014; Simpson & O'Brien-Abel, 2014). In

BOX 16.12   Guidelines for Assistance at the Emergency Birth of a Fetus in the Vertex Presentation

1. The woman usually assumes the position most comfortable for her. A lateral position is often recommended to facilitate controlled birth of the head, thereby minimizing the risk for perineal trauma and neonatal head injury.
2. Reassure the woman that birth is usually uncomplicated in these situations. Use eye-to-eye contact and a calm, relaxed manner. If there is someone else available such as the partner, that person could help support the woman in the position, assist with coaching, and provide positive reinforcement and praise of her efforts.
3. Perform hand hygiene: wash your hands or use hand sanitizer; put on gloves, if available.
4. Place under the woman's buttocks whatever clean material is available.
5. Avoid touching the vaginal area to decrease the possibility of infection.
6. As the head begins to crown, you should perform the following tasks:
   a. Tear the amniotic membranes if they are still intact.
   b. Instruct the woman to pant or pant-blow, thus minimizing the urge to push.
   c. Place the flat side of your hand on the exposed fetal head and apply *gentle* pressure toward the vagina to prevent the head from "popping out." The mother may participate by placing her hand under yours on the emerging head. CAUTION: Rapid birth of the fetal head must be prevented because a rapid change of pressure within the molded fetal skull follows, which may result in dural or subdural tears. Rapid birth also may cause vaginal or perineal lacerations.
7. After the birth of the head, check to see if the umbilical cord is around the baby's neck. If it is, *gently* try to slip it over the baby's head or pull it *gently* to get some slack so that you can slip it over the shoulders.
8. Support the baby's head as external rotation occurs. Then with one hand on each side of the baby's head, exert *gentle* pressure downward so that the anterior shoulder emerges under the symphysis pubis and acts as a fulcrum; then, as *gentle* pressure is exerted upward, the posterior shoulder, which has passed over the sacrum and coccyx, emerges.
9. Be alert! Hold the baby securely because the rest of the body may emerge quickly. The baby will be slippery!
10. Cradle the baby's head and back in one hand and the buttocks in the other. Keep the baby's head down to drain away the mucus. Use a bulb syringe, if needed, to remove mucus from the baby's mouth and then from the nose.
11. Immediately place the baby on the mother's abdomen. Dry the baby quickly to prevent rapid heat loss. Keep the baby at the same level as the mother's uterus until the cord stops pulsating. NOTE: The baby should be kept at the same level as the mother's uterus to prevent the baby's blood from flowing to or from the placenta and resulting in hypovolemia or hypervolemia. Also, do not "milk" the cord.
12. With the baby on the mother's abdomen, cover the baby (remember to keep the head warm, too) with a warmed blanket or the mother's clothing, and have her cuddle the baby. Compliment her (them) on a job well done and on the baby, if appropriate.
13. Wait for the placenta to separate. *Do not* tug on the cord. NOTE: Inappropriate traction may tear the cord, separate the placenta, or invert the uterus. Signs of placental separation include a slight gush of dark blood from the introitus, lengthening of the cord, and change in the uterine contour from a discoid to globular shape.
14. Instruct the mother to push to deliver the separated placenta. Gently ease out the placental membranes using an up-and-down motion until the membranes are removed. If birth occurs outside a hospital setting, to minimize complications do not cut the cord without proper clamps and a sterile cutting tool. Inspect the placenta for intactness. Place the baby on the placenta and wrap the two together for additional warmth.
15. Check the firmness of the uterus. Gently massage the fundus and demonstrate to the mother how she can massage her own fundus properly.
16. If supplies are available, clean the mother's perineal area and apply a peripad.
17. In addition to gentle massage of the fundus, the following measures can be taken to prevent or minimize hemorrhage:
   a. Put the baby to the mother's breast as soon as possible. Sucking or nuzzling and licking the nipple stimulates the release of oxytocin from the posterior pituitary gland. NOTE: If the baby does not or cannot nurse, manually stimulate the mother's nipples.
   b. Do not allow the mother's bladder to become distended. Assess the bladder for fullness, and encourage her to void if fullness is found.
   c. Expel any clots from the mother's uterus after ensuring that the fundus is firm.
18. Comfort or reassure the mother and her family or friends. Keep the mother and the baby warm. Give her fluids if available and tolerated.
19. If there is more than one baby, identify the infants in order of birth (using letters A, B, and so on).
20. Make notations regarding the following aspects of the birth:
   a. Fetal presentation and position
   b. Presence of cord around neck (nuchal cord) or other parts and number of times cord encircled part
   c. Color, character, and estimated amount of amniotic fluid if rupture of membranes occurred immediately before birth
   d. Time of birth
   e. Estimated time of determination of Apgar score (e.g., 1 and 5 minutes after birth), resuscitation efforts implemented, and ultimate condition of baby
   f. Gender of baby
   g. Time of placental expulsion, as well as the appearance and completeness of the placenta
   h. Maternal condition: affect, behavior, and demeanor, amount of bleeding, and status of uterine tonicity
   i. Any unusual occurrences during the birth (e.g., maternal or paternal response, verbalizations, or gestures in response to birth of baby)

an upright position, gravity can promote descent of the fetus and uterine contractions are generally stronger and more efficient in effacing and dilating the cervix, resulting in shorter labor and less need for oxytocin (Blackburn, 2013; King & Pinger; Lawrence, Lewis, Hofmeyer, & Styles, 2013; Simpson & O'Brien-Abel).

Squatting is extremely effective in facilitating the descent and birth of the fetus. Pushing efforts are maximized and gravity assists the woman's efforts (Kelly et al., 2017). The woman should assume a modified, supported squat until the fetal head is engaged, at which time a deep squat can be used. A firm surface is required for this position, and the woman will need side support (see Fig. 16.11, A). In a birthing bed, a squat bar is available that she can use to help support herself (see Fig. 16.15, E). A birth ball can also help a woman maintain the squatting position. The fetus will be aligned with the birth canal, and pelvic and perineal relaxation is facilitated as she sits on the ball or holds it in front of her for support as she squats (see Box 16.9). Women who are fatigued may find sitting on the toilet to be more comfortable than squatting (Simpson & O'Brien-Abel, 2014). In one study, however, the squatting position was associated with the largest number of perineal lacerations that required suturing, Therefore, this position may be better used for pushing, rather than for actually giving birth (Kopas, 2014).

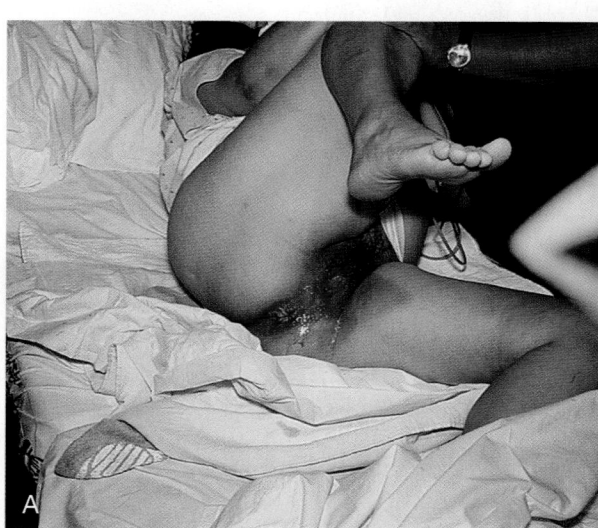
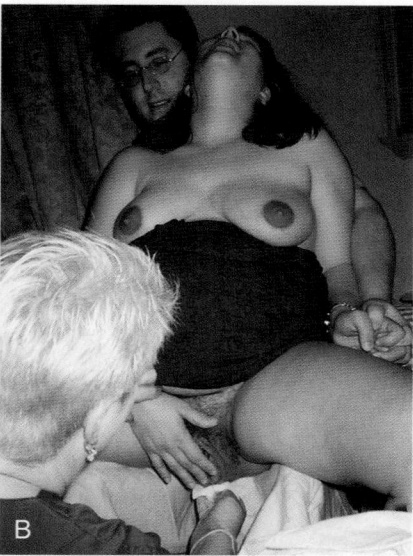

FIG 16.14 A, Pushing, side-lying position. Perineal bulging can be seen. **B,** Pushing, semisitting position. Midwife helps mother feel top of fetal head. (**A,** Courtesy of Michael S. Clement, MD, Mesa, AZ. **B,** Courtesy of Roni Wernik, Palo Alto, CA.)

When a woman uses the supported standing position for bearing down, her weight is borne on both femoral heads, allowing the pressure in the acetabulum to cause the transverse diameter of the pelvic outlet to increase by up to 1 cm. This can be helpful if descent of the head is delayed because the occiput has not rotated from the lateral (transverse diameter of pelvis) to the anterior position. Birthing chairs or rocking chairs may be used to provide women with a good physiologic position to enhance bearing-down efforts during childbirth (see Box 16.9), although some women may feel restricted by a chair. The upright position also provides a potential psychologic advantage in that it allows the mother to see the birth as it occurs and to maintain eye contact with the attendant.

Oversized beanbag chairs and large floor pillows may be used for both labor and birth. They can mold around and support the mother in whichever position she selects. These chairs are of particular value for mothers who wish to be actively involved in the birth process. Birthing stools can be used to support the woman in an upright position similar to squatting. Some women may feel more comfortable sitting on the toilet or commode during pushing because they are concerned about stool incontinence during this stage. Encourage them to empty their bladder to avoid the effects of a distended bladder. The nurse must closely monitor these women, however, and ask them to move from the toilet before birth becomes imminent. Because sitting on chairs, stools, toilets, or commodes can increase perineal edema and blood loss, it is important to help the woman change her position frequently (e.g., every 10 to 15 minutes).

The side-lying (lateral) position, with the upper part of the woman's leg held by the nurse or coach or placed on a pillow, is an effective position for the second stage of labor (see Fig. 16.14, *A,* and Box 16.9). Some women prefer a semisitting (semirecumbent) position instead (see Fig. 16.15, *B,* and Box 16.9). If the semirecumbent position is used, the woman's legs are not forced against her abdomen as she bears down. Because this position increases perineal stretching and the risk for perineal trauma and spinal and lower-extremity neurologic injuries, it is physiologically inappropriate and should be abandoned (Simpson & O'Brien-Abel, 2014). The hands-and-knees position is yet another effective position for birth, especially if the fetal position is posterior,

because it can facilitate rotation (Kelly et al., 2017) (see Fig. 16.10, *B,* and Box 16.9).

The birthing bed commonly used can be set for different positions according to the woman's needs (Figs. 16.15 and 16.16). The woman can squat, kneel, sit, recline, or lie on her side, choosing the position most comfortable for her without having to climb into bed for the birth. At the same time, the birthing bed provides excellent access and visualization for the birth attendant to perform examinations, place electrodes, and assist the woman giving birth. The bed can be positioned for the administration of anesthesia, and it is ideal to help women receiving an epidural to assume different positions to facilitate birth. The bed can also be used to transport the woman to the operating room if a cesarean birth is necessary. The woman can use squat bars, over-the-bed tables, birth balls, and pillows for support.

Bearing-Down Efforts

As the fetal head reaches the pelvic floor, most women experience the urge to bear down. Reflexively the woman begins to exert downward pressure by contracting her abdominal muscles while relaxing her pelvic floor. This bearing down is an involuntary response to the Ferguson reflex. A strong expiratory grunt or groan (vocalization) often accompanies pushing when the woman exhales as she pushes. This natural vocalization by women during open-glottis bearing-down efforts should not be discouraged.

When coaching a woman to push, she is encouraged to push as she feels the urge to do so (instinctive, spontaneous pushing) rather than to give a prolonged push on command (directed, closed-glottis pushing). Prolonged breath-holding, or sustained, directed bearing down is still a common practice, often beginning at 10 cm dilation and before the urge to bear down is perceived. The woman is coached to hold her breath, closing her glottis, and to push while the nurse or partner counts to 10. This method of bearing down is strongly discouraged because it may trigger the Valsalva maneuver, which occurs when the woman closes her glottis (closed-glottis pushing), which increases intrathoracic and cardiovascular pressure. This reduces cardiac output and decreases perfusion of the uterus and the placenta. Adverse effects associated with prolonged breath-holding and forceful pushing efforts include fetal

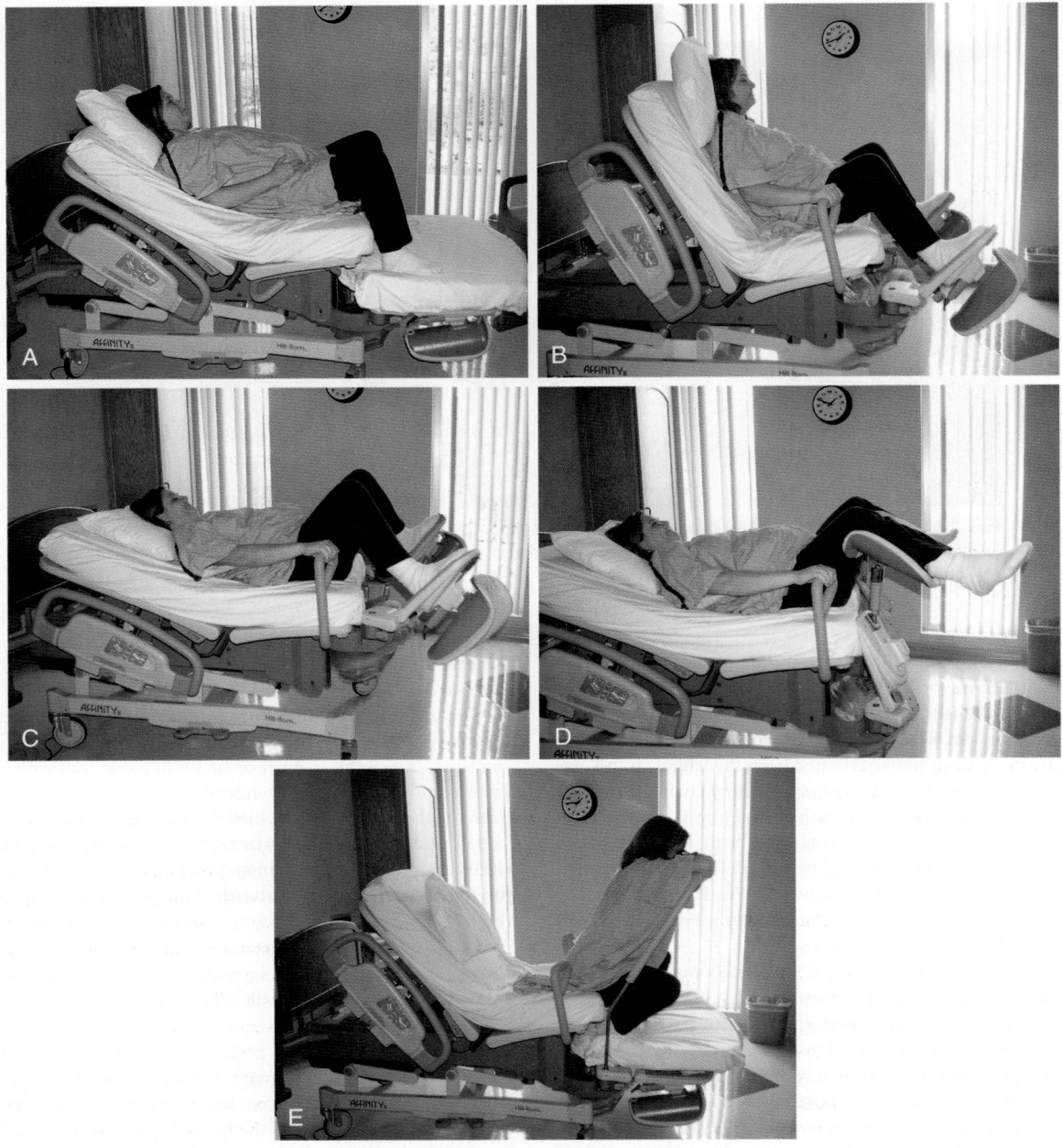

FIG 16.15 The versatility of today's birthing bed makes it practical in a variety of settings. Note: OB table used for lithotomy position. **A,** Labor bed. **B,** Birth chair. **C,** Birthing bed. **D,** OB table. **E,** Squatting or birth bar. (Courtesy of Julie Perry Nelson, Loveland, CO.)

hypoxia and subsequent acidosis, increased risk for pelvic floor damage (structural and neurogenic), and perineal trauma (Blackburn, 2013; King & Pinger, 2014; Simpson & O'Brien-Abel, 2014). Based on this evidence, it is essential that perinatal nurses advocate for the practice of delayed and spontaneous bearing-down efforts with the woman in an upright or lateral position (Kopas, 2014).

Spontaneous open glottis pushing for 6 to 8 seconds at a time is encouraged. The woman usually pushes 2 to 3 times per contraction, although she may not push at all during some contractions. The nurse or support person reminds the woman to take a cleansing breath after each contraction. Open glottis pushing helps to maintain adequate oxygen levels for the mother and fetus, thus enhancing fetal well-being. Pushing efforts become more frequent with a longer duration

as second-stage labor progresses. The woman may spontaneously bear down as the fetus crowns, even if a contraction is not occurring (Kelly et al., 2017; King & Pinger, 2014; Simpson & O'Brien-Abel, 2014).

A woman may reach the second stage of labor and then experience a lack of readiness to complete the process and give birth to her child. She may have doubts about her readiness to be a mother or desire to wait for her support person or nurse-midwife or physician to arrive. Fear, anxiety, or embarrassment regarding unfamiliar or painful sensations and behaviors during pushing (e.g., sounds made, passage of stool) may be other inhibiting factors. Fear that the baby will be in danger once it emerges from the protective intrauterine environment also may be present. By recognizing that a woman may experience a need to hold

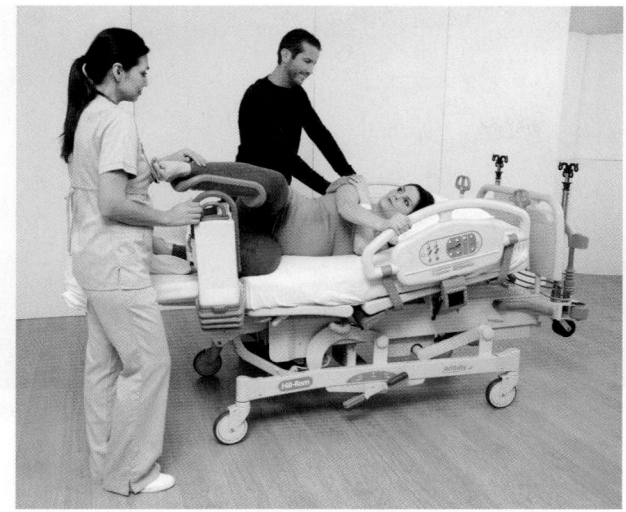

FIG 16.16 Birthing bed. (Courtesy of Hill-Rom, Batesville, IN.)

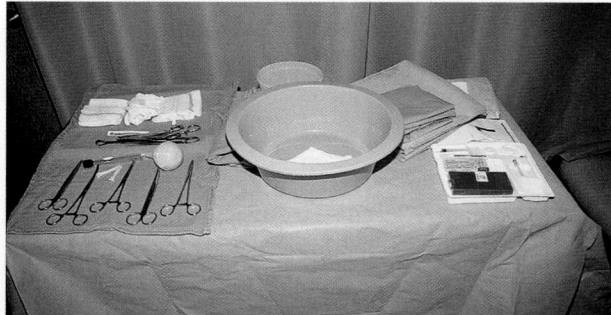

FIG 16.17 Instrument table. (Courtesy of Marjorie Pyle, RNC, Lifecircle, Costa Mesa, CA.)

back the birth of her baby, the nurse can address her concerns and effectively coach her during this stage of labor.

To ensure the slow birth of the fetal head, the woman is encouraged to control the urge to bear down by coaching her to take panting breaths or exhale slowly through pursed lips as the baby's head crowns. At this point the woman needs simple, clear directions from one person. Amnesia between contractions often occurs in the second stage; therefore the nurse may have to rouse the woman to get her to cooperate in the bearing-down process. Couples who have attended childbirth education classes may have devised a set of verbal cues for the laboring woman to follow.

Fetal Heart Rate and Pattern

The nurse must check the FHR regularly (see Chapter 15 for further discussion). If the baseline rate begins to slow, if absent or minimal variability occurs, or if abnormal (e.g., late, variable, or prolonged) deceleration patterns develop, interventions are initiated promptly. The first action is to turn the woman onto her side to reduce the pressure of the uterus against the ascending vena cava and descending aorta (see Fig. 16.5). Oxygen can be administered by nonrebreather mask at 10 L/min (Miller, Miller, & Cypher, 2017). These interventions are often all that is necessary to restore a normal pattern. If the FHR and pattern do not become normal immediately, the next step is to notify the nurse-midwife or physician because the woman may need medical intervention to give birth. See Chapter 15 for more interventions related to abnormal FHR.

> **LEGAL TIP** **Documentation** The course of labor and the maternal-fetal response may change without warning. Documentation of all observations (e.g., maternal vital signs, FHR and pattern, progress of labor) and nursing interventions, including the woman's response, must be accurate, complete, timely, and according to agency policy.

Support of the Father or Partner

During the second stage, the woman needs continuous support and coaching (see Table 16.3 and Box 16.11). Because the coaching process is often physically and emotionally tiring for support people, the nurse offers nourishment and fluids and encourages short breaks as needed (see Box 16.10). If birth occurs in an LDR or LDRP room, the support

person usually wears street clothes. The support person who attends the birth in a delivery or operating room may be asked to put on a cover gown or scrub clothes, mask, cap, and shoe covers if required by agency policy. The nurse also specifies support measures that can be used for the laboring woman and points out areas of the room in which the partner can move freely.

The nurse encourages partners to be present at the birth of their infants if doing so is in keeping with their cultural and personal expectations and beliefs. The presence of partners maintains the psychologic closeness of the family unit, and the partner can continue to provide the supportive care given during labor. The woman and her partner need to have an equal opportunity to initiate the attachment process with the baby.

Supplies, Instruments, and Equipment

Necessary supplies, instruments, and equipment should be gathered and prepared for use well before the anticipated time of birth. To prepare for birth in any setting, the birthing table is usually set up late in the active phase of first-stage labor for nulliparous women and earlier in that phase for multiparous women. Instruments are arranged according to agency protocol on the instrument table or delivery cart (Fig. 16.17). The health care team follows standard procedures for gloving, identifying and opening sterile packages, adding sterile supplies to the instrument table, unwrapping sterile instruments, and handing them to the nurse-midwife or physician. The crib or radiant warmer and equipment for the support and stabilization of the newborn are placed for ready access (Fig. 16.18). The items used for birth may vary among different facilities; therefore the nurse consults the facility's procedure manual for specific protocols

The nurse estimates the time until the birth will occur and notifies the nurse-midwife or physician if he or she is not in the woman's room. Even the most experienced nurse can inaccurately estimate the time left before birth occurs; therefore every nurse who attends a woman in labor must be prepared to assist with an emergency birth if the nurse-midwife or physician is not present (see Box 16.12).

BIRTH IN A BIRTHING ROOM OR DELIVERY ROOM

Currently, women most often give birth vaginally in a birthing room, in the same bed where they have labored, rather than in a delivery room. The maternal position for birth in a birthing room varies from a lithotomy position with the woman's feet in stirrups or resting on footrests or with her legs held and supported by the nurse or support person, to one in which her feet rest on footrests while she holds on to a squat bar, to a side-lying position with the woman's upper leg supported by the coach, nurse, or squat bar. Once the woman is

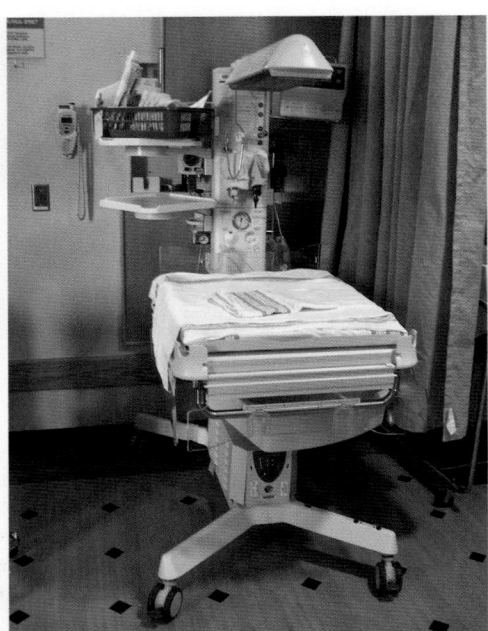

FIG 16.18 Radiant warmer for newborn. (Courtesy of Dee Lowdermilk, Chapel Hill, NC.)

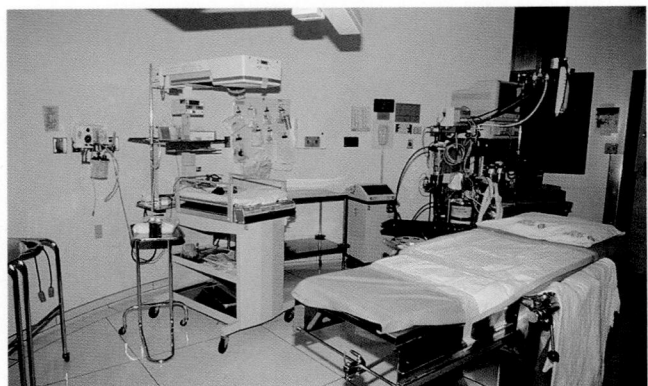

FIG 16.19 Delivery room. (Courtesy of Michael S. Clement, MD, Mesa, AZ.)

positioned, the foot of the bed is removed so that the nurse-midwife or physician attending the birth can gain better perineal access for performing an episiotomy, delivering a large baby, or using forceps or vacuum extractor. Alternately, the foot of the bed can be left in place and lowered slightly to form a ledge that allows access for birth and also serves as a place to lay the newborn (see Fig. 16.15, *A*).

The woman will need assistance if she must move from the labor bed to the delivery table (Fig. 16.19). The positions assumed for birth in a delivery room are the Sims or lateral position, in which the attendant supports the upper part of the woman's leg, the dorsal position (supine position with one hip elevated), and the lithotomy position.

The lithotomy position makes dealing with complications that arise more convenient for the nurse-midwife or physician (see Fig. 16.15, *D*). For this position, the nurse brings the woman's buttocks to the edge of the bed or table and places the legs in stirrups. Tthe nurse pads the stirrups, carefully raises and places both legs simultaneously, and then adjusts the shanks of the stirrups so the calves of the legs are supported. No pressure should be placed on the popliteal space. Stirrups that are not the same height will strain ligaments in the woman's back as she bears down, leading to considerable discomfort in the postpartum period. The lower portion of the table may be dropped down and rolled back under the table.

Once the woman is positioned for birth either in a birthing room or delivery room, the vulva and perineum are cleansed. Hospital or birthing center protocols and the preferences of nurse-midwives and physicians for cleansing may vary.

The nurse continues to coach and encourage the woman and monitor the fetal status (see Box 16.11), keeping the nurse midwife or physician informed of the FHR and pattern. The nurse obtains or prepares an oxytocic medication such as oxytocin (Pitocin) so it is ready to be administered immediately after expulsion of the baby or the placenta. Standard Precautions are always followed throughout the process of labor and birth (see Box 16.4).

In the hospital delivery room, the nurse midwife or physician may put on a cap, a mask that has a shield or protective eyewear, and shoe covers. After performing hand hygiene, the provider puts on a sterile gown (with waterproof front and sleeves) and sterile gloves. Nurses attending the birth also may need to wear caps, protective eyewear, masks, gowns, and gloves. The woman may then be draped with sterile drapes. In the birthing room the amount and types of protective coverings worn by those in attendance may vary.

During the birth process, the nurse maintains contact with the parents by touching, verbally comforting, describing progress, explaining the reasons for care, and sharing in the parents' joy at the birth of their child.

Mechanism of Birth: Vertex Presentation

The three phases of the spontaneous birth of a fetus in a vertex presentation are (1) birth of the head, (2) birth of the shoulders, and (3) birth of the body and extremities (see Chapter 13).

With voluntary bearing-down efforts, the head appears at the introitus (Fig. 16.20, *A* to *D*). **Crowning** occurs when the widest part of the head (the biparietal diameter) distends the vulva just before birth. Immediately before birth, the perineal musculature becomes greatly distended. If an episiotomy (incision into the perineum to enlarge the vaginal outlet) is necessary, it is done at this time to minimize soft-tissue damage. A local anesthetic may be administered if necessary before performing an episiotomy. Box 16.13 shows the process of normal vaginal childbirth using a series of photographs.

The physician or nurse-midwife may use a hands-on approach to control the birth of the head, believing that guarding the perineum results in a gradual birth that will prevent fetal intracranial injury, protect maternal tissues, and reduce postpartum perineal pain. This approach involves: (1) applying pressure against the rectum, drawing it downward to aid in flexing the head as the back of the neck catches under the symphysis pubis; (2) applying upward pressure from the coccygeal region (modified *Ritgen maneuver*) (Fig. 16.21) to extend the head during the actual birth, thereby protecting the musculature of the perineum; and (3) assisting the mother with voluntary control of the bearing-down efforts by coaching her to pant while letting uterine forces expel the fetus.

Some health care providers use a hands-poised (hands-off) approach when attending a birth. In this approach, hands are prepared to place light pressure on the fetal head to prevent rapid expulsion. The provider does not place hands on the perineum or use them to assist with birth of the shoulders and body.

Several studies have compared the hands-on and hands-poised approaches. Researchers found no difference between the two approaches in the rates of perineal lacerations. Women who received hands-on care, however, did report slightly less pain during the postpartum period.

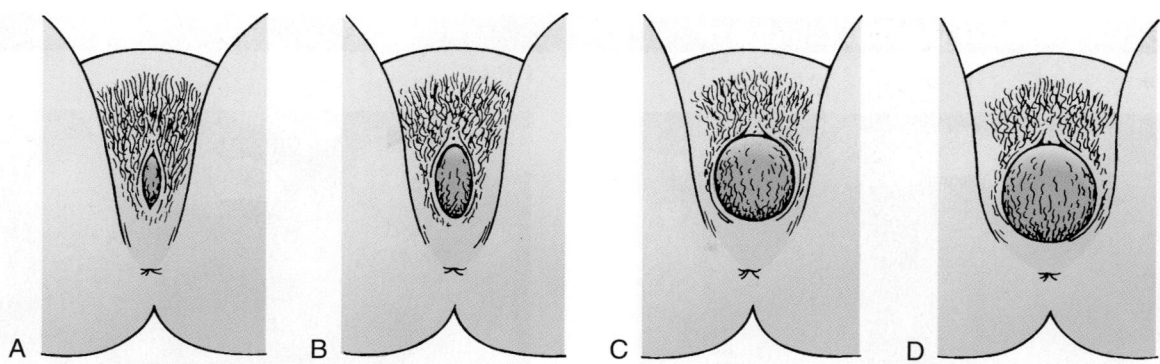

FIG 16.20 Beginning birth with vertex presenting. **A,** Anteroposterior slit. **B,** Oval opening. **C,** Circular shape. **D,** Crowning.

Until better evidence is available, the best advice for providers is to encourage slow, gentle crowning of the fetal head over the perineum by having women blow or make small pushes or by gently pushing down on the fetal head to control the rate of crowning and thus prevent a too-rapid birth (Kopas, 2014).

The umbilical cord often encircles the neck *(nuchal cord)* but rarely so tightly as to cause hypoxia. After the head is born, gentle palpation is used to feel for the cord. If present, the health care provider slips it gently over the head if possible. If the loop is tight or if there is a second loop, the provider will probably clamp the cord twice, cut between the clamps, and unwind the cord from around the neck before the birth is allowed to continue. Mucus, blood, or meconium in the nasal or oral passages may prevent the newborn from breathing. To eliminate this problem, moist gauze sponges are used to wipe the nose and mouth. A bulb syringe may be inserted first into the mouth and oropharynx and then into both nares to aspirate contents.

IMMEDIATE ASSESSMENTS AND CARE OF THE NEWBORN

The time of birth is the precise time when the entire body is out of the mother and must be recorded. In the case of multiple births, each birth is noted in the same way. If the mother's and newborn's conditions allow, immediate skin-to-skin contact and delayed cord clamping are likely to be implemented.

Skin-to-skin contact is recommended for the healthy term newborn immediately after vaginal birth and as soon as possible following cesarean birth. The baby is placed prone on the woman's bare abdomen or chest and dried. Next, a cap is placed on his or her head. The wet blankets are removed, and baby and woman are covered with fresh warm blankets. Immediate skin-to-skin contact has been shown to positively affect maternal-infant bonding, breastfeeding duration, cardiorespiratory stability, and body temperature. Blood glucose levels during the first 2 hours of life are higher in these babies compared with newborns who did not receive immediate skin-to-skin contact (Kilpatrick & Garrison, 2017; Stewart & Rodgers, 2017). It is recommended that immediate skin-to-skin contact be considered standard of care because this practice conveys many benefits and has no adverse effects. Routine assessments and procedures can be completed with the newborn on the woman's abdomen/chest (King & Pinger, 2014).

It is now recommended that the umbilical cord not be clamped until 1 to 5 minutes after birth, or until after the cord stops pulsating, to allow physiologic transfer of blood to the newborn. The optimal duration of delayed cord clamping appears to be up to 3 minutes, unless the cord stops pulsating sooner. Delayed cord clamping allows for a placental transfusion of up to 30% of the total fetal-placental blood volume. The transfusion includes many types of stem cells, red blood cells, and whole blood. It is recommended that delayed cord clamping be considered standard of care because it improves both the short- and long-term hematologic status of the newborn and has no clinically significant adverse effects (King & Pinger, 2014). At the appropriate time, the nurse-midwife or physician may ask if the woman's partner would like to cut the cord. If so, the partner is given a sterile pair of scissors and instructed to cut the cord approximately 2.5 cm above the clamp.

Immediate care given after the birth focuses on assessing and stabilizing the newborn. AWHONN (2010) recommends that at least two nurses are present for each birth. One nurse is responsible for care of the newborn, while the other nurse assists the nurse-midwife or physician with delivery of the placenta and care of the mother. The "baby nurse" must observe the infant for any signs of distress and initiate appropriate interventions. AWHONN also recommends that, in cases of multiple births, each baby has his or her own nurse (AWHONN).

The nurse performs a brief assessment of the newborn immediately, even while skin-to-skin contact is being performed. This assessment includes assigning Apgar scores at 1 and 5 minutes after birth (see Table 23.2). Major priorities for immediate newborn care include maintaining a patent airway, supporting respiratory effort, and preventing cold stress by drying and, preferably, covering the newborn with a warmed blanket while on his or her mother's abdomen/chest or, less optimally, placing him or her under a radiant warmer If the newborn appears to be stable, further examination, identification procedures, and care can be postponed until later in the third stage of labor or early in the fourth stage.

PERINEAL TRAUMA RELATED TO CHILDBIRTH

Most acute injuries and lacerations of the perineum, vagina, uterus, and their support tissues occur during childbirth. Aggressive perineal massage during labor should be avoided because it results in trauma to the perineal tissue and has not been shown to decrease the future risk for pain, pain with sexual intercourse, or urinary or fecal incontinence. Practices that help to reduce perineal trauma are perineal massage during the last trimester of pregnancy, the application of warm compresses just prior to birth, giving birth in a side-lying position, and achieving slow extension of the fetal head between contractions during birth (King & Pinger, 2014; Simpson & O'Brien-Abel, 2014).

Some degree of trauma to the soft tissues of the birth canal and adjacent structures occurs during every birth. The tendency to sustain lacerations varies with each woman; that is, the soft tissue in some women may be less distensible. Damage usually is more pronounced

BOX 16.13 Normal Vaginal Childbirth

First Stage

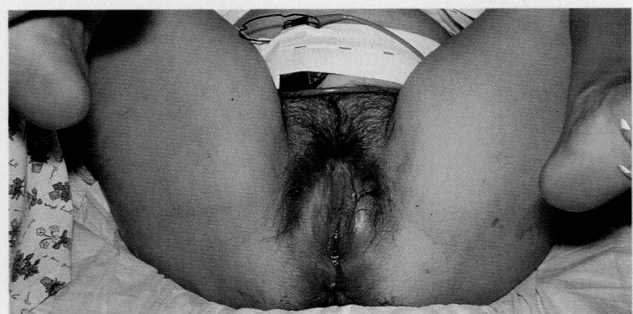

Anteroposterior slit. Vertex visible during contraction.

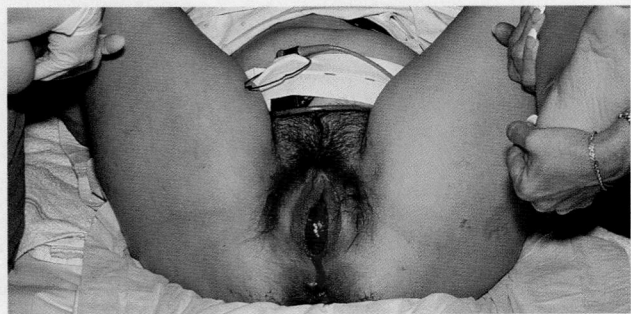

Oval opening. Vertex presenting. NOTE: Nurse *(on left)* is wearing gloves, but support person *(on right)* is not.

Second Stage

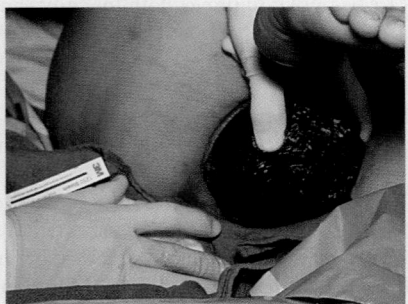

Crowning.

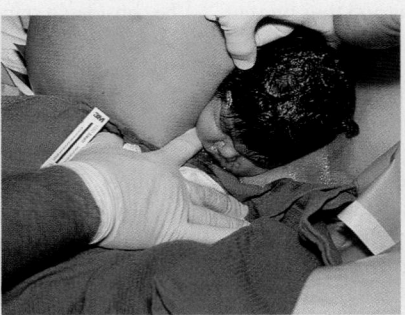

Nurse-midwife using Ritgen maneuver as head is born by extension.

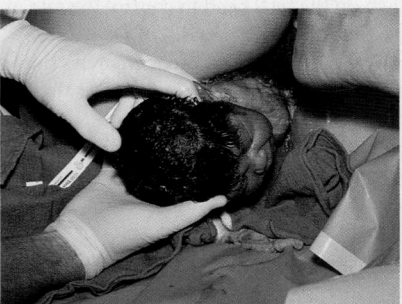

After nurse-midwife checks for nuchal cord, she supports head during external rotation and restitution.

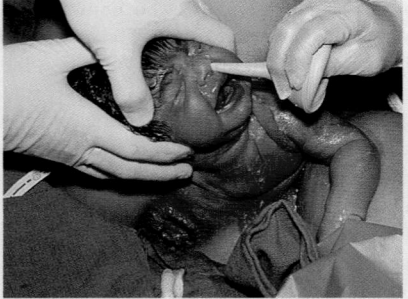

Use of bulb syringe to suction mucus.

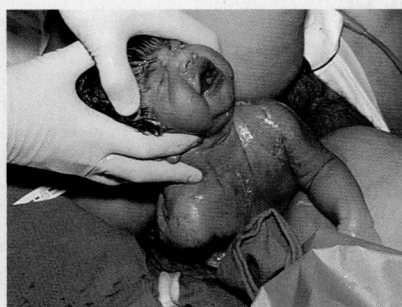

Birth of posterior shoulder.

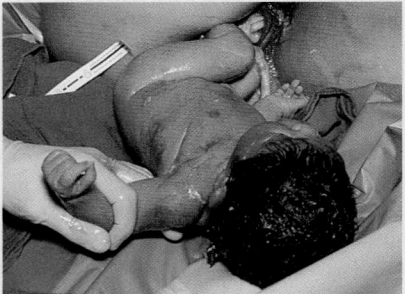

Birth of newborn by slow expulsion.

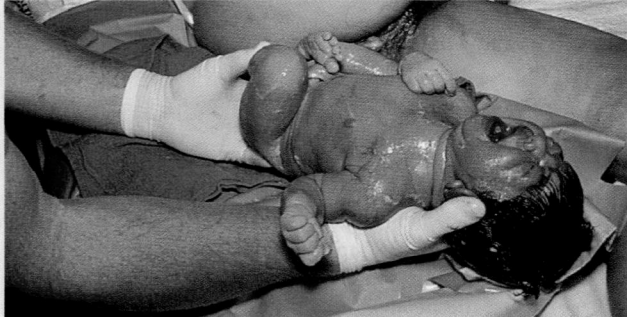

Second stage complete. Note that newborn is not completely pink yet.

Continued

BOX 16.13   Normal Vaginal Childbirth—cont'd

Third Stage

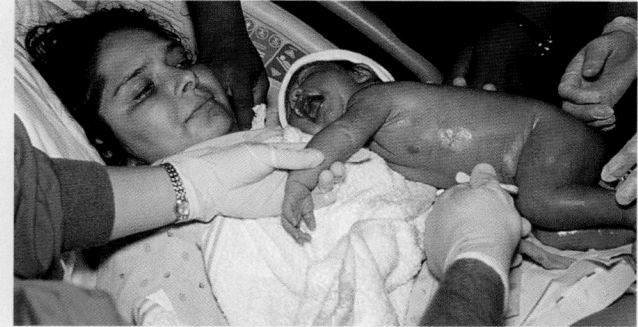

Newborn placed on mother's abdomen while cord is clamped and cut.

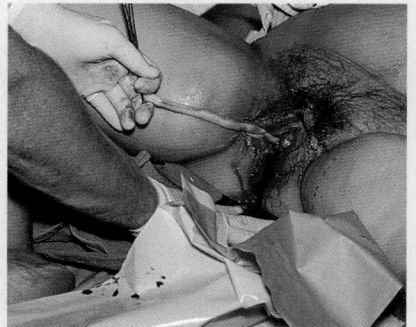

Note increased bleeding as placenta separates.

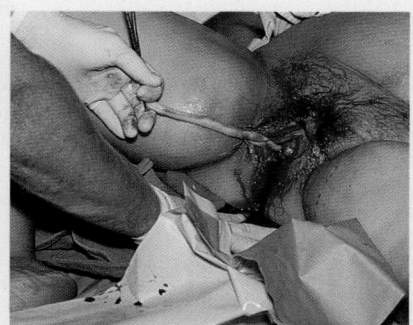

Expulsion of placenta.

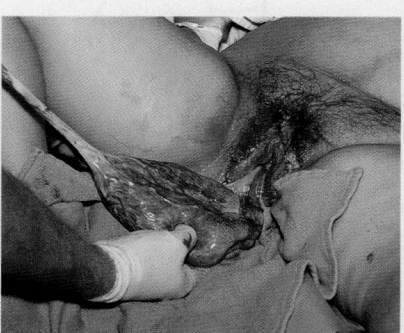

Expulsion is complete, marking end of third stage.

The Newborn

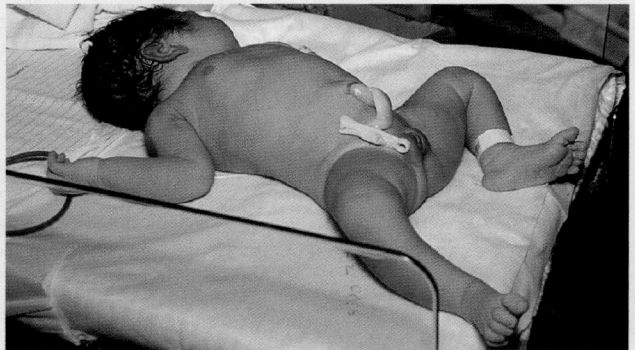

Newborn awaiting assessment. Note that color is almost completely pink.

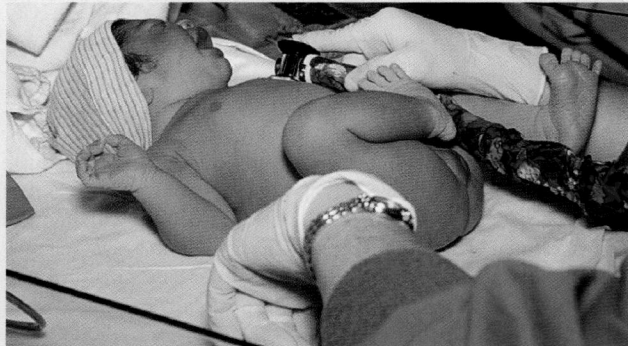

Newborn assessment under radiant warmer.

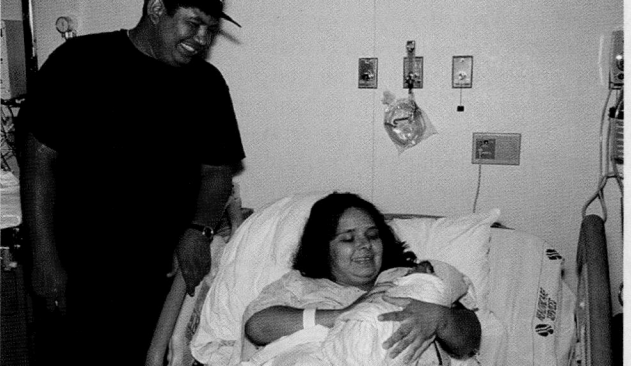

Parents admiring their newborn.

Photos courtesy of Michael S. Clement, MD, Mesa, AZ.

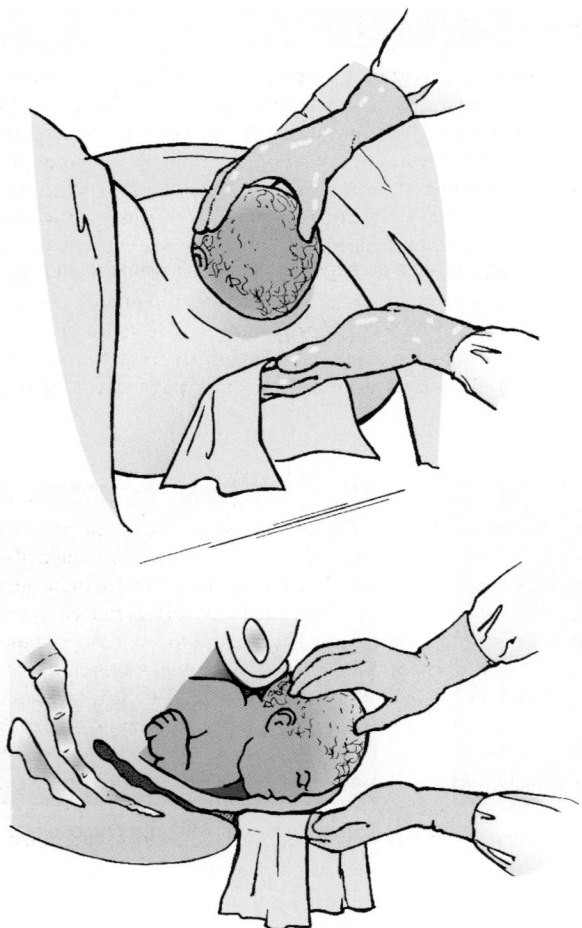

FIG 16.21 Birth of head with modified Ritgen maneuver. Note control to prevent too-rapid birth of head.

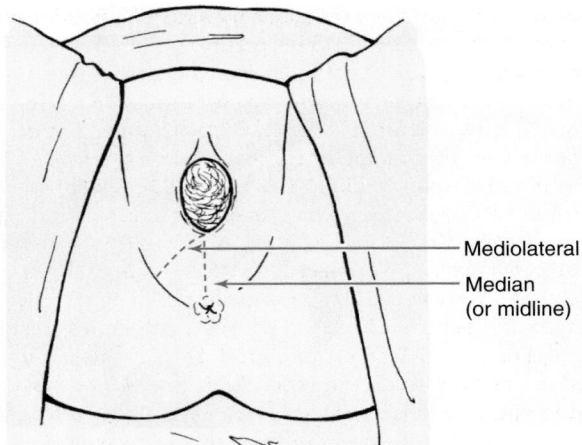

FIG 16.22 Types of episiotomies.

in nulliparous women because the tissues are firmer and more resistant than are those in multiparous women. Heredity is also a factor. For example, the tissue of light-skinned women, especially those with reddish hair, is not as readily distensible as that of darker-skinned women, and healing may be less efficient. Other risk factors associated with perineal trauma include maternal nutritional status, birth position, pelvic anatomy (e.g., narrow subpubic arch with a constricted outlet), fetal malpresentation and position (e.g., breech, occiput posterior position), large (macrosomic) infants, use of forceps or vacuum to facilitate birth, prolonged second-stage labor, and rapid labor in which there is insufficient time for the perineum to stretch.

Some injuries to the supporting tissues, whether they are acute or nonacute or are repaired or not, may lead to genitourinary and sexual problems later in life (e.g., pelvic relaxation, uterine prolapse, cystocele, rectocele, dyspareunia, urinary and bowel dysfunction). Performing Kegel exercises in the prenatal and postpartum periods improves and restores the tone and strength of the perineal muscles (see Chapter 3). Health practices, including good nutrition and appropriate hygienic measures, help maintain the integrity and suppleness of the perineal tissues, enhance healing, and prevent infection.

Perineal Lacerations

Perineal lacerations may occur as the fetal head is being born. The extent of the laceration is defined in terms of its depth (Kilpatrick & Garrison, 2017):

- *First degree:* Laceration that extends through the skin and structures superficial to muscles
- *Second degree:* Laceration that extends through muscles of the perineal body
- *Third degree:* Laceration that continues through the anal sphincter muscle
- *Fourth degree:* Laceration that extends completely through the anal sphincter and the rectal mucosa

Perineal injury often is accompanied by small lacerations on the medial surfaces of the labia minora below the pubic rami and to the sides of the urethra (periurethral) and clitoris. Lacerations in this highly vascular area often result in profuse bleeding. Third- and fourth-degree lacerations must be repaired carefully so the woman retains fecal continence. Simple perineal injuries usually heal without permanent disability, regardless of whether they were repaired. However, repairing a new perineal injury to prevent future complications is easier than correcting long-term damage.

Vaginal and Urethral Lacerations

Vaginal lacerations often occur in conjunction with perineal lacerations. Vaginal lacerations tend to extend up the lateral walls (sulci) and, if deep enough, involve the levator ani muscle. Additional injury may occur high in the vaginal vault near the level of the ischial spines. Vaginal vault lacerations are often circular and may result from use of forceps to rotate the fetal head, rapid fetal descent, or precipitous birth.

Cervical Injuries

Cervical injuries occur when the cervix retracts over the advancing fetal head. They occur at the lateral angles of the external os. Most lacerations are shallow, and bleeding is minimal. Larger lacerations may extend to the vaginal vault or beyond it into the lower uterine segment; serious bleeding may occur. Extensive lacerations may follow hasty attempts to enlarge the cervical opening artificially or to deliver the fetus before full cervical dilation is achieved. Injuries to the cervix can have adverse effects on future pregnancies and childbirths.

Episiotomy

An **episiotomy** is an incision made in the perineum to enlarge the vaginal outlet (Fig. 16.22). Its use has steadily declined in recent years due to a lack of sound, rigorous research to support its benefits. Episiotomies are performed in approximately 10% of births in the United States (Simpson & O'Brien-Abel, 2014). This practice is even less common in Europe and Canada, probably because of the more routine use in those countries of the side-lying position for birth. This position places less tension on the perineum, making possible a gradual stretching of the perineum with fewer indications for episiotomy. Whenever possible, giving birth over an intact perineum provides the best outcomes (e.g., less blood loss, less risk for infection, and less postpartum pain).

Different types of episiotomies may be performed, classified by the site and direction of the incision (see Fig. 16.22). Both types have advantages and disadvantages, and it is unclear which, if either, is a better choice (Kilpatrick & Garrison, 2017). Midline (median) episiotomy is most common in the United States. It is effective, easily repaired, and generally the least painful. However, midline episiotomies also are associated with a higher incidence of third- and fourth-degree lacerations (Cunningham, Leveno, Bloom, et al., 2014). Sphincter tone is usually restored after primary healing and a good repair. Mediolateral episiotomy is used in operative births when the need for posterior extension is likely. Although a fourth-degree laceration may be prevented, a third-degree laceration may occur. The blood loss is also greater and the repair more difficult and painful than with midline episiotomies (Cunningham et al.). It is also more painful in the postpartum period, and the pain lasts longer.

Based on the lack of consistent evidence that episiotomy is beneficial, *routine* episiotomy has no role in modern obstetric care and should be avoided whenever possible. *Indicated* episiotomy, however, may still be performed in specific situations, such as the need to hasten birth when FHR abnormalities are present (Kilpatrick & Garrison, 2017).

THIRD STAGE OF LABOR

The **third stage of labor** lasts from the birth of the baby until the placenta is expelled (Kelly et al., 2017). It is generally, by far, the shortest stage of labor.

CARE MANAGEMENT

The goal in the management of the third stage of labor is the prompt separation and expulsion of the placenta achieved in the easiest, safest manner. Under normal circumstances, the placenta is attached to the decidual layer of the basal plate's thin endometrium by numerous fibrous anchor villi—much in the same way a postage stamp is attached to a sheet of postage stamps. After the birth of the fetus, strong uterine contractions and the sudden decrease in uterine size and volume cause the placental site to shrink. This causes the anchor villi to break and the placenta to separate from its attachments. Normally the first few strong contractions that occur after the baby's birth cause the placenta to shear away from the basal plate. A placenta cannot detach itself from a flaccid (relaxed) uterus because the placental site is not reduced in size.

PLACENTAL SEPARATION AND EXPULSION

Historically, the third stage of labor was usually managed passively or expectantly in the United States, with no interventions implemented until spontaneous separation of the placenta occurred. Passive management involves patiently watching for signs that the placenta has separated from the uterine wall spontaneously and monitoring for spontaneous expulsion. Signs of placental separation include lengthening of the umbilical cord and a gush of blood from the vagina (Fig. 16.23). After separation occurs, the woman is instructed to push to aid in expelling the placenta. When passive management is practiced, the placenta is usually expelled within 15 minutes after the birth of the baby. As soon as the placenta is expelled, the uterine fundus is massaged and medication to contract the uterus (usually oxytocin [Pitocin]) is administered (Box 16.14).

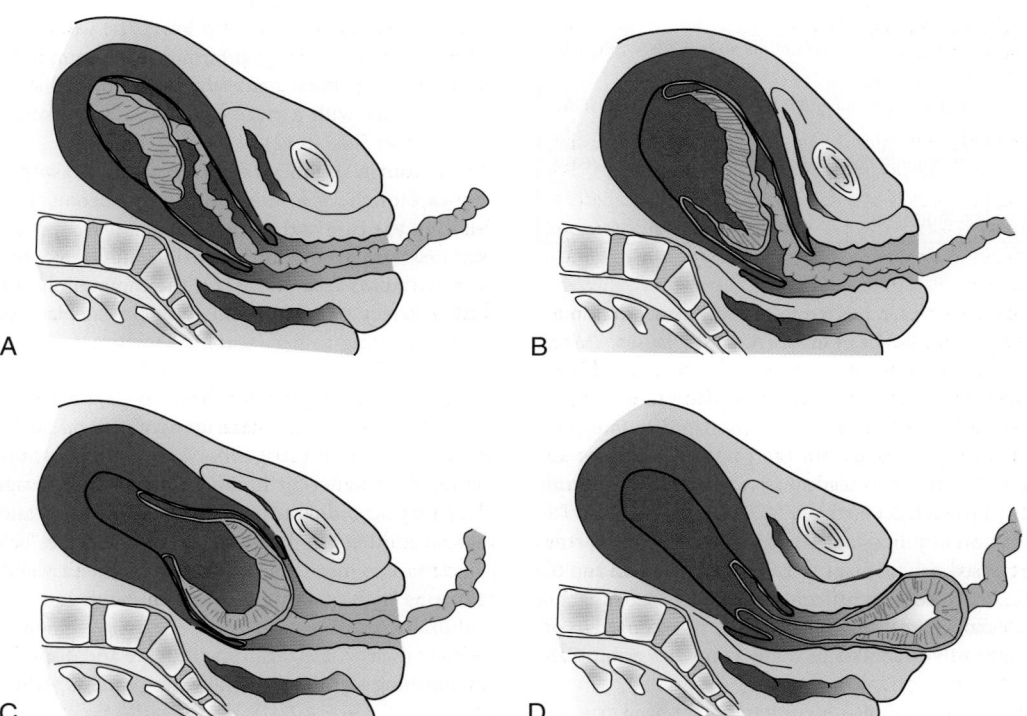

A

B

C

D

FIG 16.23 Third stage of labor. **A,** Placenta begins to separate in central portion, accompanied by retroplacental bleeding. Uterus changes from discoid to globular shape. **B,** Placenta completes separation and enters lower uterine segment. Uterus has globular shape. **C,** Placenta enters vagina, cord is seen to lengthen, and there may be an increase in bleeding. **D,** Expulsion (delivery) of placenta and completion of third stage.

BOX 16.14 Nursing Care in Third-Stage Labor

Assessment

Signs That Suggest the Onset of the Third Stage

- A firmly contracting fundus
- A change in the uterus from a discoid to a globular ovoid shape as the placenta moves into the lower uterine segment
- A sudden gush of dark blood from the introitus
- Apparent lengthening of the umbilical cord as the placenta descends to the introitus
- The finding of vaginal fullness (the placenta) on vaginal or rectal examination or of fetal membranes at the introitus

Physical Assessment

- Perform every 15 minutes: maternal blood pressure, pulse, and respirations.
- Assess for signs of placental separation and amount of bleeding.
- Assist with determination of Apgar score at 1 and 5 minutes after birth (see Table 23.2).
- Assess maternal and partner response to completion of childbirth process and their reaction to the newborn.

Interventions

- Assist mother to bear down to facilitate expulsion of the separated placenta.
- Administer an oxytocic medication as ordered to ensure adequate contraction of the uterus, thereby preventing hemorrhage.
- Provide nonpharmacologic and pharmacologic comfort and pain relief measures.
- Perform hygienic cleansing measures.
- Keep mother/partner informed of progress of placental separation and expulsion and perineal repair if appropriate.
- Explain purpose of medications administered.
- If mother's and baby's conditions permit, encourage immediate skin-to-skin contact and delayed cord clamping.
- Introduce parents to their baby, and facilitate the attachment process by delaying eye prophylaxis.
- Provide private time for parents to bond with new baby; help them create memories.
- Encourage breastfeeding if desired.

More recent research, however, has led to the recommendation for active management of the third stage of labor (AMTSL). When AMTSL is practiced, oxytocic medication (usually oxytocin) is administered immediately after the baby is born but before the placenta is expelled. Gentle continuous controlled umbilical cord traction and counterpressure are used to support the uterus until the placenta separates and is expelled. Immediately after the placenta is expelled, the uterine fundus is massaged (Kilpatrick & Garrison, 2017). Benefits of AMTSL include a shorter duration of third-stage labor, less risk for postpartum hemorrhage, and decreased risk for anemia for both the woman and the newborn (Kelly et al., 2017) (see the Evidence-Based Practice box: Active Third-Stage Labor Management for Preventing Postpartum Hemorrhage.). AMTSL is currently practiced in many countries around the world.

After the placenta and the amniotic membranes have been expelled, the nurse-midwife or physician examines them for intactness to ensure that no portion remains in the uterine cavity (i.e., no fragments of the placenta or membranes are retained) (Fig. 16.24). At this time, the nurse will obtain a sample of blood from the umbilical cord to be used for determining the baby's blood type and Rh status. Some parents will also have arranged to have blood from the cord collected for storage and possible future use.

Blood from the umbilical cord contains hematopoietic stem cells, which offer several advantages over bone marrow or stem cells obtained from other locations when transplanted. Current recommendations for cord blood transplant are limited to certain genetic, hematologic, and malignant disorders, however, and it is very unlikely that the child or another family member will develop a condition that could be treated with a transfusion of autologous umbilical cord blood. Umbilical cord blood banking is not part of routine obstetric care and is not medically indicated. If the parents still desire that it be done, blood can be collected from the umbilical cord either before or after the placenta is expelled (ACOG, 2015).

When the third stage of labor has been completed, the nurse-midwife or physician examines the woman for any perineal, vaginal, or cervical lacerations requiring repair. The nurse may need to assist by providing adequate lighting or exposure of the woman's perineum and vagina so that a thorough examination can be performed. If an episiotomy was performed, it will be sutured. Immediate repair promotes healing, limits residual damage, and decreases the possibility of infection. The woman usually feels some discomfort while the nurse-midwife or physician carries out the postbirth vaginal examination. The nurse helps the woman to use breathing and relaxation or distraction techniques to assist her in dealing with the discomfort. During this time, the "baby nurse" performs a quick assessment of the newborn's physical condition and places matching identification bands on baby and mother. Weighing the baby and administering eye prophylaxis and a vitamin K injection can be delayed until after the initial bonding time with the parents (see Chapter 24).

After any necessary repairs have been completed, the nurse cleanses the vulvar area gently with warm water or normal saline and applies a perineal pad or an ice pack to the perineum. The next step is to reposition the birthing bed or table and lower the woman's legs simultaneously from the stirrups if she gave birth in a lithotomy position. After removing any drapes, the nurse places dry linen under the woman's buttocks and provides her with a clean gown and a blanket, which is warmed if needed (see Box 16.12).

Some women and their families have culturally based beliefs regarding the care of the placenta and the manner of its disposal after birth, viewing the care and disposal of the placenta as a way of protecting the newborn from bad luck and illness. In Spanish, the placenta is referred to as *el compañero* or "the companion of the child" (Callister, 2014). A request by the woman to take the placenta home and dispose of it according to her customs sometimes conflicts with health care agency policies, especially those related to infection control and the disposal of biologic wastes. Many cultures follow specific rules regarding the disposal of the placenta in terms of method (burning, drying, burying, eating), site for disposal (in or near the home), and timing of disposal (immediately after birth, time of day, astrologic signs). Disposal rituals may vary according to the gender of the child and the length of time before another child is desired. Some cultures believe that eating the placenta is a means of restoring a woman's well-being after birth or ensuring high-quality breast milk. Health care providers can provide culturally sensitive care by encouraging women and their families to express their wishes regarding the care and disposal of the placenta and establishing a policy to fulfill these requests (D'Avanzo, 2008).

FOURTH STAGE OF LABOR

The **fourth stage of labor** begins with the expulsion of the placenta and lasts until the woman is stable in the immediate postpartum period,

EVIDENCE-BASED PRACTICE

Active Third-Stage Labor Management for Preventing Postpartum Hemorrhage

Ask the Question

PICOT Question: For third-stage labor, what management techniques are most effective for prevention of postpartum hemorrhage (PPH)?

Search for the Evidence

Search Strategies: English research-based publications on uterotonics, postpartum hemorrhage (or haemorrhage), labor (or labour) bleeding, cord clamping, active management, uterotonic were included.

Databases Used: Cochrane Collaborative Database, National Guideline Clearinghouse (AHRQ), CINAHL, PubMed, and the professional websites for ACOG, SGOC, and AWHONN.

Critical Appraisal of the Evidence

PPH is the major cause of maternal death worldwide, especially in low- and middle-income countries. In 2003, the International Confederation of Midwives, the International Federation of Gynecologists and Obstetricians, and the World Health Organization Safe Motherhood Initiative adopted a program recommending the use of active management of third-stage labor. To prevent PPH, health care providers actively manage third-stage labor by clamping the cord before pulsations have stopped, administering uterotonics (such as oxytocin or prostaglandins) to increase uterine contractions, and providing steady traction on the cord and counter-pressure on the fundus, causing earlier expulsion of the placenta.

Cochrane Database of Systematic Reviews reported the following:

- Maternal effects: (7 studies, 8000 women) When compared to expectant management, the active management protocol results in less maternal blood loss and less maternal anemia, less transfusion, and less use of additional uterotonics in the first 24 hours. Adverse effects of active management include higher maternal diastolic pressure, afterpains, use of analgesia, and postpartum vomiting. Active management is more likely to result in readmission for bleeding, for unknown reasons (Begley, Gyte, Devane, et al., 2015). The authors call for more research on the individual components of the protocol and more research in high-risk countries.
- Effects on the newborn: Birthweight is less when the cord was clamped prior to the cessation of pulsing, because there is less transfer of blood volume to the newborn. (Begley et al., 2015). The effects of this are unknown.
- Controlled cord traction (CCT) requires a skilled birth attendant to apply adequate power without causing uterine inversion. A Cochrane Review of three high-quality trials involving 28,000 women found that CCT was associated with reduced risk of having to manually extract the placenta and reduced blood loss (Hofmeyr, Mshweshwe, & Gulmezoglu, 2015). The authors recommended that CCT could be offered routinely when the birth attendant has the necessary training but cautioned that considerable investment would be necessary in training for low-resource areas. CCT can be omitted when uterotonic agents are given.

A randomized controlled trial of 934 women found that the active management group had a significantly higher postpartum hemoglobin than the expectant (non-active) management group (Yildirim, Ozyurek, Ekiz, et al., 2016).

Apply the Evidence: Nursing Implications

- In developed countries, active management of third-stage labor is beneficial and recommended. However, it may be possible to individualize the protocol for women at low risk for PPH. Patients should be educated before labor on their options for third-stage management.
- Some patients may request that the cord clamping be delayed until pulsations have ceased. This may benefit the newborn without significantly increasing the woman's risk for PPH.
- Nurses carefully assess the fundus and bleeding while recovering the immediate postpartum woman and are frequently the first to notice PPH.
- A protocol for PPH should be made clear to all staff. All staff should be able to identify excessive bleeding and implement the immediate interventions of emptying the bladder, massaging the uterus, and notifying the health care provider.
- Easily accessed kits of necessary medications should be available, along with training in their use.
- In low-resource countries, CCT should only be used by birth attendants trained in proper technique. Funding for training and further research would be a targeted investment in the prevention of the biggest risk factor for childbearing women worldwide.

Quality and Safety Competencies: Evidence-Based Practice*
Knowledge

Discriminate between valid and invalid reasons for modifying evidence-based clinical practice based on clinical expertise or patient/family preferences.

Active management of third-stage labor may be individualized to accommodate family preferences, in collaboration with the health care provider.

Skills

Consult with clinical experts before deciding to deviate from evidence-based protocols.

Delayed cord-clamping may be a safe option for the low-risk woman who desires it.

Attitudes

Acknowledge own limitations in knowledge and clinical expertise before determining when to deviate from evidence-based best practices.

Understanding the risks and benefits of active management are important for collaborative decision-making.

References

Begley, C. M., Gyte, G. M., Devane, D., et al. (2015). Active versus expectant management for women in the third stage of labour. *Cochrane Database of Systematic Reviews 2015*(3), CD007412.

Hofmeyr, G. J., Mshweshwe, N. T., & Gulmezoglu, A. M. (2015). Controlled cord traction for the third stage of labor. *Cochrane Database of Systematic Reviews 2015*(1), CD008020.

Yildirim, D., Ozyurek, S. E., Ekiz, A., et al. (2016). Comparison of active vs. expectant management of the third stage of labor in women with low risk of postpartum hemorrhage: A randomized controlled trial. *Ginekologia Polska, 87*(5), 399–404.

Pat Mahaffee Gingrich

*Adapted from QSEN at www.qsen.org/.

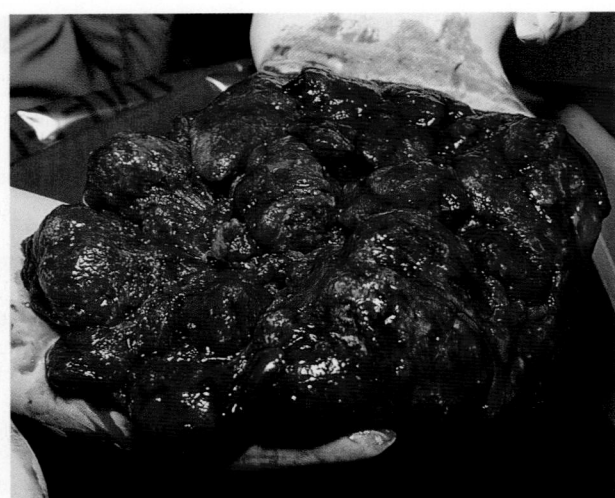

FIG 16.24 Examination of placenta. (Courtesy of Michael S. Clement, MD, Mesa, AZ.)

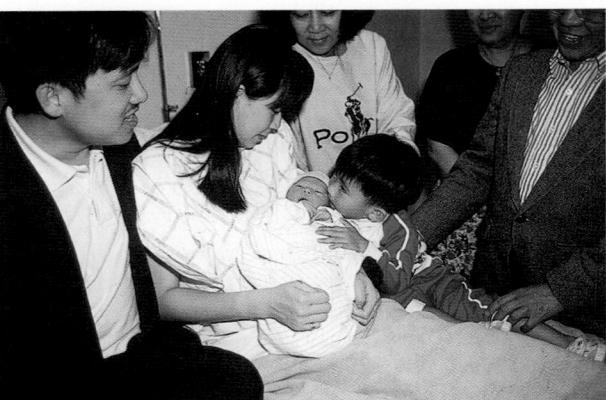

FIG 16.25 Big brother becomes acquainted with new baby sister. (Courtesy of Marjorie Pyle, RNC, Lifecircle, Costa Mesa, CA.)

usually within the first hour after birth (Simpson & O'Brien-Abel, 2014). The immediate postpartum recovery period lasts longer. It usually includes at least the first 2 hours after birth, based on maternal status (American Academy of Pediatrics [AAP] & ACOG, 2012). This is a crucial time for the mother and newborn. Both are not only recovering from the physical process of birth but are also becoming acquainted with one another and additional family members. During this time, maternal organs undergo their initial readjustment to the nonpregnant state, and the functions of body systems begin to stabilize.

CARE MANAGEMENT

In most hospitals, the mother remains in the labor and birth area during the immediate postpartum recovery period. In an institution where LDR rooms are used, the woman stays in the same room where she gave birth. In traditional settings, women are taken from the delivery room to a separate recovery area for observation. Arrangements for care of the newborn vary during the immediate postpartum recovery period. In many settings, the baby remains at the mother's bedside, and the labor or birth nurse cares for both of them. In other institutions, the baby is taken to the nursery for several hours of observation after an initial bonding period with the parents, siblings, and perhaps other family members (Fig. 16.25).

ASSESSMENT

If the recovery nurse has not previously cared for the new mother, he or she begins with an oral report from the nurse who attended the woman during labor and birth and a review of the prenatal, labor, and birth records. Of primary importance are conditions that could predispose the mother to hemorrhage such as precipitous labor, a large baby, grand multiparity (i.e., having given birth to five or more viable infants), or induced labor. For healthy women, hemorrhage is the most dangerous potential complication during the fourth stage of labor.

During the immediate postpartum recovery period, the mother is assessed frequently (Box 16.15). The AAP and ACOG recommend that blood pressure and pulse be assessed at least every 15 minutes for the first 2 hours after birth. Temperature should be assessed every 4 hours for the first 8 hours after birth and then at least every 8 hours (AAP & ACOG, 2012).

POSTANESTHESIA RECOVERY

The woman who has given birth by cesarean or received regional anesthesia for a vaginal birth requires special attention during the recovery period. Obstetric recovery areas are held to the same standard of care that would be expected of any other postanesthesia recovery (PAR) unit (AAP & ACOG, 2012). A PAR score is determined for each woman on arrival and is updated as part of every 15-minute assessment. Components of the PAR score include activity, respirations, blood pressure, level of consciousness, and color.

If the woman received general anesthesia, she should be awake and alert and oriented to time, place, and person. Her respiratory rate should be within normal limits, and her oxygen saturation level at least 95% as measured by a pulse oximeter. If the woman received epidural or spinal anesthesia, she should be able to raise her legs, extended at the knees, off the bed or flex her knees; place her feet flat on the bed; and raise her buttocks well off the bed. The numb or tingling, prickly sensation should be entirely gone from her legs. The length of time required to recover from regional anesthesia varies greatly. Often it takes several hours for these anesthetic effects to disappear completely.

> ### ! NURSING ALERT
> Regardless of her obstetric status, no woman should be discharged from the recovery area until she has recovered completely from the effects of anesthesia.

NURSING INTERVENTIONS

Care of the New Mother

If food and fluids were restricted, especially if excessive fluid loss (blood, perspiration, or emesis) occurred during labor and birth, the woman will be very hungry and thirsty soon after birth. In the absence of complications, a woman who has given birth vaginally may have fluids and a regular diet as soon as she desires (AAP & ACOG, 2012). In the immediate postpartum period, women who give birth by cesarean are usually restricted to clear liquids and ice chips.

As soon as they have had a chance to bond with the baby and eat, most new mothers are ready for a nap or at least a quiet period of rest. Following this rest period, the woman may want to shower and change clothes. Most new mothers are capable of self-management or are assisted in these activities by family members or support people.

BOX 16.15   Assessment During the Fourth Stage of Labor

Blood Pressure
- Assess every 15 minutes for the first 2 hours.*

Pulse
- Assess rate and regularity. Assess every 15 minutes for the first 2 hours.*

Temperature
- Assess at the beginning of the recovery period. Temperature should then be assessed every 4 hours for the first 8 hours after birth and then at least every 8 hours.*

Fundus
- Position woman with knees flexed and head flat.
- Just below umbilicus, cup hand and press firmly into abdomen. At the same time, stabilize uterus at symphysis with opposite hand (see Fig. 19.4).
- If fundus is firm (and bladder is empty), with uterus in midline, measure its position relative to woman's umbilicus. Lay fingers flat on abdomen under umbilicus; measure how many fingerbreadths (fb) or centimeters (cm) fit between umbilicus and top of fundus. Fundal height is documented according to agency guidelines. For example, if the fundus is 1 fb or 1 cm above the umbilicus, fundal height may be recorded as either +1, u+1, or 1/u. If the fundus is 1 fb or 1 cm below the umbilicus, fundal height may be recorded as either −1, u−1, or u/1.
- If fundus is not firm, massage it gently to contract and expel any clots before measuring distance from umbilicus.
- Place hands appropriately; massage gently only until firm.

- Expel clots while keeping hands placed as in Fig. 19.2. With upper hand, firmly apply pressure downward toward vagina; observe perineum for amount and size of expelled clots.

Bladder
- Assess distention by noting location and firmness of uterine fundus and observing and palpating bladder. A distended bladder is seen as a suprapubic rounded bulge that is dull to percussion and fluctuates like a water-filled balloon. When the bladder is distended, the uterus is usually boggy in consistency, well above umbilicus, and to the woman's right side.
- Assist woman to void spontaneously. Measure and record amount of urine voided.
- Catheterize as necessary.
- Reassess after voiding or catheterization to make sure the bladder is not palpable and the fundus is firm and in the midline.

Lochia
- Observe lochia on perineal pads and linen under the mother's buttocks. Determine amount and color; note size and number of clots; note odor.
- Observe perineum for source of bleeding (e.g., episiotomy, lacerations).

Perineum
- Ask or assist woman to turn onto her side and flex upper leg on hip.
- Lift upper buttock.
- Observe perineum in good lighting.
- Assess episiotomy or laceration repair for *r*edness (erythema), *e*dema, *ec*chymosis (bruising), *d*rainage, and *a*pproximation (REEDA).
- Assess for presence of hemorrhoids.

*Data from American Academy of Pediatrics & American College of Obstetricians and Gynecologists. (2012). *Guidelines for perinatal care* (7th ed.). Washington, DC: American College of Obstetricians and Gynecologists.

Care of the Family

Most parents enjoy being able to handle, hold, explore, and examine the baby immediately after birth. Both parents can assist with thoroughly drying the infant. Skin-to-skin contact is encouraged. The nurse places the unwrapped infant on the woman's chest or abdomen and then covers the baby and mother with a warm blanket. Holding the newborn next to her skin helps the mother maintain the baby's body heat and provides skin-to-skin contact. Stockinette caps are often used to keep the newborn's head warm and prevent heat loss (Fig. 16.26). The newborn is wrapped snugly in a receiving blanket to be held by the partner.

Many women wish to begin breastfeeding their newborns at this time to take advantage of the infant's alert state (*first period of reactivity*) and stimulate the production of oxytocin that promotes contraction of the uterus and prevents hemorrhage. In Baby-Friendly hospitals, breastfeeding is initiated within the first hour after birth, and any unnecessary separation of mother and baby is strongly discouraged. However, some women prefer to wait to breastfeed until they have had time to rest. In some cultures breastfeeding is not acceptable to some women until the milk comes in. For some women of the Hispanic culture, for example, the colostrum is thought to be bad or old milk (Callister, 2014). They typically wait until 3 or 4 days after birth to begin breastfeeding when their "milk is in" (onset of lactogenesis II) (see Chapter 24).

Family-Newborn Relationships

The woman's reaction to the sight of her newborn may range from excited outbursts of laughing, talking, and even crying to apparent apathy. A polite smile and nod may be her only acknowledgment of the comments of nurses and the nurse-midwife or physician. Occasionally the reaction is one of anger or indifference; the woman turns away from the baby, concentrates on her own pain, and sometimes makes hostile comments. These varied reactions can arise from pleasure, exhaustion, or deep disappointment. When evaluating parent-newborn interactions after birth, it is important to consider the cultural characteristics of the woman and her family and the expected behaviors of that culture. In some cultures, the birth of a male child is preferred, and women may grieve when a female child is born (Callister, 2014).

Whatever the reaction and its cause, the woman needs continuing acceptance and support from members of the health care team. Appropriate nursing actions include: making a notation regarding the parents' reaction to the newborn in the recovery record; assessing this reaction by asking questions such as, "What do the parents say?", and "What do they do?"; and conducting further assessment of the parent-newborn relationship during the recovery and postpartum period. This assessment is especially important if warning signs (e.g., passive or hostile reactions to the newborn, disappointment with the gender or appearance of the newborn, absence of eye contact, or limited interaction of parents with each other) appear immediately after birth. Nurses should discuss any warning signs with the woman's nurse-midwife or physician.

Siblings, who may have appeared only remotely interested in the final phases of the second stage, tend to experience renewed interest and excitement when the newborn appears. With supervision, they can be encouraged to hold the baby (see Fig. 16.25).

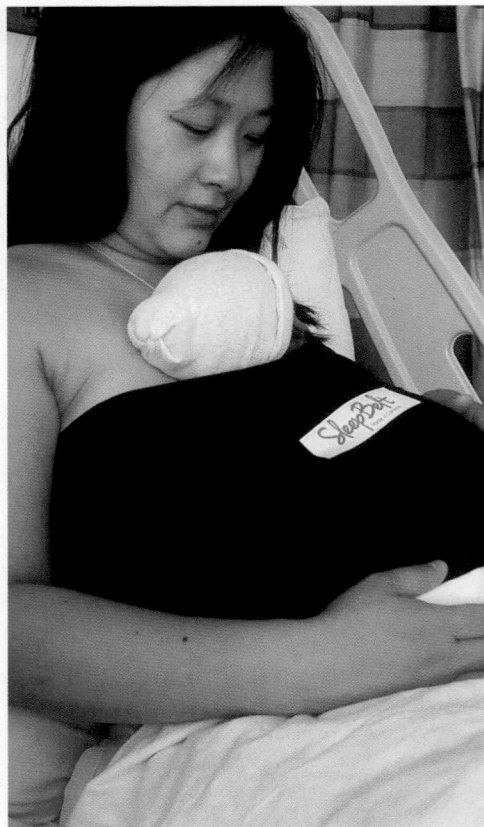

FIG 16.26 Mother and newborn enjoying skin-to-skin contact. (Courtesy of Wendy Chau, Toronto, ON.)

Parents usually respond to praise of their newborn. Many need to be reassured that the dusky appearance of their baby's hands and feet immediately after birth is normal until circulation is well established. If appropriate, the nurse explains the reason for the molding of the newborn's head. The nurse communicates information about hospital routine, recognizing, however, that the cultural background of the parents may influence their expectations regarding the care and handling of their newborn immediately after birth. For example, Korean mothers may believe that the head should not be touched because it is the most sacred part of a person's body. Hispanic mothers may believe that the "evil eye" or too much praise of the baby will cause illness, restlessness, or excessive crying (Callister, 2014). Hospital staff members, by their interest and concern, can provide the environment for making this a satisfying experience for parents, family, and significant others.

REFERENCES

American Academy of Pediatrics & American College of Obstetricians and Gynecologists. (2012). *Guidelines for perinatal care* (7th ed.). Washington, DC: American College of Obstetricians and Gynecologists.

American College of Obstetricians and Gynecologists. (2017). Committee opinion no. 687: Approaches to limit intervention during labor and birth. *Obstetrics and Gynecology, 129*(2), e20–e28.

American College of Obstetricians and Gynecologists. (2015). Committee opinion no. 648: Umbilical cord blood banking. *Obstetrics and Gynecology, 126*(6), e127–e129.

Arendt, K. W., & Tessmer-Tuck, J. A. (2013). Nonpharmacologic labor analgesia. *Clinics in Perinatology, 40*(3), 351–371.

Association of Women's Health, Obstetric and Neonatal Nurses. (2010). *Guidelines for professional registered nurse staffing for perinatal units.* Washington, DC: Association of Women's Health, Obstetric and Neonatal Nurses.

Baird, S. M., Kennedy, B. B., & Baudhuin, S. L. (2017). Liability issues in intrapartum nursing. In B. B. Kennedy & S. M. Baird (Eds.), *Intrapartum management modules: A perinatal education program* (5th ed.). Philadelphia, PA: Wolters Kluwer.

Blackburn, S. (2013). *Maternal, fetal, and neonatal physiology: A clinical perspective* (4th ed.). Maryland Heights, MO: Saunders.

Burke, C. (2014). Pain in labor: Nonpharmacologic and pharmacologic management. In K. R. Simpson & P. Creehan (Eds.), *AWHONN's perinatal nursing* (4th ed.). Philadelphia, PA: Lippincott.

Callister, L. C. (2014). Integrating cultural beliefs and practices when caring for childbearing women and families. In K. R. Simpson & P. Creehan (Eds.), *AWHONN's perinatal nursing* (4th ed.). Philadelphia, PA: Lippincott.

Centers for Disease Control and Prevention. (2016). *Rapid HIV testing of women in labor and delivery.* Retrieved from http://www.cdc.gov/hiv/testing/clinical/women.html.

Cluett, E. R., & Burns, E. (2009). Immersion in water in labour and birth. *Cochrane Database of Systematic Reviews, 2009*(2), CD000111.

Collins, M. R. (2017). Pain in labor and nonpharmacologic modes of relief. In B. B. Kennedy & S. M. Baird (Eds.), *Intrapartum management modules: A perinatal education program* (5th ed.). Philadelphia, PA: Wolters Kluwer.

Cunningham, F., Leveno, K., Bloom, S., et al. (2014). *Williams obstetrics* (24th ed.). New York, NY: McGraw-Hill Education.

D'Avanzo, C. E. (2008). *Mosby's pocket guide to cultural health assessment* (4th ed.). St. Louis, MO: Mosby.

Hanson, L., & VandeVusse, L. (2014). Supporting labor progress toward physiologic birth. *Journal of Perinatal & Neonatal Nursing, 28*(2), 101–107.

Hodnett, E. D., Gates, S., Hofmeyr, G., & Sakala, C. (2013). Continuous support for women during childbirth. *Cochrane Database of Systematic Reviews, 2013*(7), CD003766.

Kelly, F. C., Swart, S. C., & Baird, S. M. (2017). Caring for the laboring woman. In B. B. Kennedy & S. M. Baird (Eds.), *Intrapartum management modules: A perinatal education program* (5th ed.). Philadelphia, PA: Wolters Kluwer.

Kilpatrick, S., & Garrison, E. (2017). Normal labor and delivery. In S. G. Gabbe, J. R. Niebyl, J. L. Simpson, et al. (Eds.), *Obstetrics: Normal and problem pregnancies* (7th ed.). Philadelphia, PA: Elsevier.

King, T. L., & Pinger, W. (2014). Evidence-based practice for intrapartum care: The pearls of midwifery. *Journal of Midwifery & Women's Health, 59*(6), 572–585.

Kopas, M. L. (2014). A review of evidence-based practices for management of the second stage of labor. *Journal of Midwifery & Women's Health, 59*(3), 264–276.

Lawrence, A., Lewis, L., Hofmeyr, G. J., & Styles, C. (2013). Mothers' position during the first stage of labour. *Cochrane Database of Systematic Reviews, 2013*(2), CD003934.

Ledenfors, A., & Bertero, C. (2016). First-time fathers' experiences of normal childbirth. *Midwifery, 40,* 26–31.

Miller, L., Miller, D., & Cypher, R. (2017). *Mosby's pocket guide to fetal monitoring: A multidisciplinary approach* (8th ed.). St Louis, MO: Elsevier.

Osborne, K., & Hanson, L. (2014). Labor down or bear down: A strategy to translate second-stage labor evidence to perinatal practice. *Journal of Perinatal & Neonatal Nursing, 28*(2), 117–126.

Perinatal Education Associates. (2016). *Breathing.* Retrieved from http://www.birthsource.com/scripts/article.asp?articleid=211.

Reveiz, L., Gaitan, H., & Cuervo, L. (2013). Enemas during labour. *Cochrane Database of Systematic Reviews, 2013*(4), CD000330.

Sharts-Hopko, N. (2010). Oral intake during labor: A review of the evidence. *American Journal of Maternal Child Nursing 35*(4), 197–203.

Simkin, P. (2012). *Doulas of North America (DONA) international position paper: The birth doula's contribution to modern maternity care.* Retrieved from http://www.emergingbirth.com/uploads/2/4/9/7/2497446/bdpositionpaper.pdf.

Simpson, K., & O'Brien-Abel, N. (2014). Labor and birth. In K. R. Simpson & P. Creehan (Eds.), *AWHONN's perinatal nursing* (4th ed.). Philadelphia, PA: Lippincott.

Singata, M., Tranmer, J., & Gyte, G. M. L. (2013). Restricting oral fluid and food intake during labour. *Cochrane Database of Systematic Reviews, 2013*(1), CD003930.

Stewart, L. S., & Rodgers, E. (2017). Assessment and care of the term newborn transitioning to extrauterine life. In B. B. Kennedy & S. M. Baird (Eds.), *Intrapartum management modules: A perinatal education program* (5th ed.). Philadelphia, PA: Wolters Kluwer.

Tillett, J., & Hill, C. (2016). Eating and drinking in labor: Reexamining the evidence. *Journal of Perinatal & Neonatal Nursing, 30*(2), 85–87.

Waterbirth International. (2016). *Frequently asked questions.* Retrieved from http://www.waterbirth.org/faqs/.

Wilson-Griffin, J. (2014). Maternal-fetal transport. In K. R. Simpson & P. Creehan (Eds.), *AWHONN's perinatal nursing* (4th ed.). Philadelphia, PA: Lippincott.

17

Labor and Birth Complications

Kitty Cashion

http://evolve.elsevier.com/Perry/maternal

When complications arise during labor and birth, the risk for perinatal morbidity and mortality increases. Some complications are anticipated, especially if the woman is identified to be at high risk during the antepartum period; other complications are unexpected or unforeseen. It is crucial for nurses to understand the normal birth process to prevent and detect deviations from normal labor and birth and to promptly implement nursing interventions when complications arise. Optimal care of the laboring woman, fetus, and family experiencing complications is possible only when members of the interprofessional health care team use their knowledge and skills in a concerted effort to provide competent and compassionate care. This chapter focuses on the problems of preterm labor and birth, premature rupture of membranes, dystocia, obesity, postterm pregnancy, and obstetric emergencies.

PRETERM LABOR AND BIRTH

Preterm labor is generally diagnosed clinically as regular contractions along with a change in cervical effacement or dilation or both or presentation with regular uterine contractions and cervical dilation of at least 2 cm. Preterm birth is any birth that occurs between 20 0/7 and 36 6/7 weeks of gestation (American College of Obstetricians and Gynecologists [ACOG], 2016a). The preterm birth rate for all races in the United States, which had been decreasing for nearly a decade, increased just slightly to 9.63% in 2015, the most recent year for which data are available (Martin, Hamilton, Osterman, et al., 2017). Since 2014, gestational age at birth has been reported in the United States as the *obstetric estimate,* rather than according to the date of the woman's last menstrual period. The obstetric estimate represents the birth attendant's best estimate of the newborn's gestational age, as determined by using a number of sources. Thus, the gestational ages reported as national statistics now are more accurate than they have been in the past (Martin, Osterman, Kimeyer, et al., 2015). The rate of preterm birth in the United States has declined over the past decade, largely because of three major practice changes: (1) improved fertility practices that reduce the risk for higher-order multiple gestations; (2) quality improvement programs that limit scheduled late preterm and near-term births to only those with valid indications; and (3) increased use of strategies to prevent recurrent preterm birth (Simhan, Iams, & Romero, 2017).

Preterm births are categorized as *very preterm, moderately preterm* and *late preterm.* The degree of risk for an infant born prematurely is directly related to the degree of prematurity. About 75% of all preterm births in the United States are categorized as late preterm, occurring between 34 0/7 and 36 6/7 weeks of gestation. Late preterm infants are at increased risk for early death and long-term health problems when compared with infants who are born full term (see Chapter 25). Although late preterm babies do experience significant problems, the great majority of infant deaths and the most serious morbidity occur among the infants who are born before 32 weeks of gestation (very preterm birth) (Simhan, Berghella, & Iams, 2014).

Preterm birth is a worldwide problem. The rate of preterm birth is highest in Africa and North America and lowest in Europe. In the United States, African-American women have the highest rates of preterm birth, almost twice as high as those of other racial and ethnic groups (Simhan et al., 2017).

PRETERM BIRTH VERSUS LOW BIRTH WEIGHT

Although they have distinctly different meanings, the terms *preterm birth* or *prematurity* and *low birth weight* were often interchanged in the past. Preterm birth describes length of gestation (i.e., less than 37 0/7 weeks regardless of the weight of the infant), whereas low birth weight describes only weight at the time of birth (i.e., 2500 g or less). Because birth weight was far easier to determine than gestational age, in many settings and publications *low birth weight* was used as a substitute term for *preterm birth.* Preterm birth, however, is a more dangerous health condition for an infant because less time in the uterus correlates with immaturity of body systems. Low–birth-weight babies can be, but are not necessarily, preterm; low birth weight can be caused by conditions other than preterm birth, such as intrauterine growth restriction (IUGR), a condition of inadequate fetal growth not necessarily correlated with initiation of labor. Pregnant women who have various complications of pregnancy that interfere with uteroplacental perfusion, such as gestational hypertension or poor nutrition, may give birth to a baby at term who is low birth weight because of IUGR. However, infants born at a preterm gestation can weigh more than 2500 g at birth. Currently, thanks to advances in pregnancy dating, outcomes related to gestational age can increasingly be distinguished from outcomes related to birth weight. Therefore, use of birth weight as a substitute for gestational age in developed countries is no longer considered acceptable (Simhan et al. 2014).

SPONTANEOUS VERSUS INDICATED PRETERM BIRTH

Preterm births are divided into two categories: spontaneous and indicated. Spontaneous preterm births occur following an early initiation of the labor process in the apparent absence of maternal or fetal illness and make up nearly 75% of all preterm births in developed countries. Conditions such as preterm labor with intact membranes and preterm PROM often result in preterm birth (Simhan et al., 2014). Box 17.1 lists risk factors for the development of spontaneous preterm labor.

BOX 17.1 Risk Factors for Spontaneous Preterm Labor

- History of genital tract colonization, infection, or instrumentation
- African-American race
- Bleeding of uncertain origin in pregnancy
- History of a previous spontaneous preterm birth between 16 and 36 weeks of gestation*
- Uterine anomaly
- Use of assisted reproductive technology
- Multifetal gestation
- Cigarette smoking, substance abuse
- Prepregnancy underweight (BMI <19.6) and prepregnancy obesity (BMI >30)
- Periodontal disease
- Limited education and low socioeconomic status
- Late entry into prenatal care
- High levels of personal stress in one or more domains of life

Data from Simhan, H.N., Iams, J.D., & Romero, R. (2017). Preterm labor and birth. In S.G. Gabbe, J.R. Niebyl, J.L. Simpson, et al. (Eds.), *Obstetrics: Normal and problem pregnancies* (7th ed.). Philadelphia, PA: Elsevier.
BMI, body mass index.
*Strongest historic risk factor for spontaneous preterm birth

BOX 17.2 Common Causes of Indicated Preterm Birth

- Preexisting or gestational diabetes
- Chronic hypertension
- Preeclampsia
- Obstetrical disorders or risk factors in the current or a previous pregnancy
  - Previous cesarean birth via a vertical or *T*-shaped uterine incision
  - Cholestasis
  - Placental disorders (abruption or previa)
- Medical disorders
  - Seizures
  - Thromboembolism
  - Connective tissue disorders
  - Asthma and chronic bronchitis
  - Maternal HIV or active herpes infection
  - Obesity
  - Smoking
- Advanced maternal age
- Fetal disorders
  - Fetal compromise
  - Chronic (poor fetal growth)
  - Acute (abnormal results on a NST or BPP)
  - Excessive (polyhydramnios) or inadequate (oligohydramnios) amniotic fluid
  - Fetal hydrops, ascites, blood group alloimmunization
  - Birth defects
  - Fetal complications of multifetal gestation (e.g., growth deficiency, twin-to-twin transfusion syndrome)

BPP, Biophysical profile; *HIV*, human immunodeficiency virus; *NST*, nonstress test.
Data from Simhan, H.N., Iams, J.D., & Romero, R. (2017). Preterm labor and birth. In S.G. Gabbe, J.R. Niebyl, J.L. Simpson, et al. (Eds.), *Obstetrics: Normal and problem pregnancies* (7th ed.). Philadelphia, PA: Elsevier.

Indicated preterm births are *iatrogenic*, because they occur as a means to resolve maternal or fetal risk related to continuing the pregnancy. About 25% of all preterm births in the United States are indicated because of medical or obstetric conditions that affect the mother, the fetus, or both (Simhan et al., 2017). Box 17.2 lists common causes of indicated preterm birth. The remainder of this section deals with spontaneous preterm labor and birth.

CAUSES OF SPONTANEOUS PRETERM LABOR AND BIRTH

Causes of spontaneous preterm labor and birth are multifactorial. Infection is the only factor shown to be definitely associated with preterm labor. When bacterial cervical or urinary tract infections are present, the risk for preterm birth increases. Women in spontaneous preterm labor with intact membranes commonly have organisms that are normally found in the lower genital tract present in their amniotic fluid, placenta, and membranes (Simhan et al., 2014). Clinical and laboratory evidence of infection are more common when birth occurs earlier than 30 to 32 weeks of gestation rather than closer to term. Intraabdominal infections (e.g., appendicitis) also have been related to preterm birth (Simhan et al., 2017). Women with periodontal disease have been shown to have an increased risk for preterm birth. However, the risk is not reduced by periodontal care, suggesting that the link between periodontal disease and preterm birth is not a cause-and-effect relationship (Simhan et al., 2017).

Preterm labor may also be caused by congenital structural abnormalities of the uterus, which can affect the cervix, the body of the uterus, or both. Implantation of the placenta on a uterine septum may lead to preterm birth as a result of placental separation and hemorrhage. Women who experience unexplained vaginal bleeding after the first trimester of pregnancy also have an increased risk for preterm birth. The risk rises as the number of bleeding episodes increases (Simhan et al., 2017). Maternal and fetal stress, uterine overdistention, allergic reaction, and a decrease in progesterone are other factors that can play a part in initiating preterm labor. It is becoming increasingly clear that preterm labor is caused by multiple pathologic processes that eventually result in uterine contractions, cervical changes, and rupture of membranes (Buhimschi & Norman, 2014; Simhan et al., 2014).

PREDICTING SPONTANEOUS PRETERM LABOR AND BIRTH

Risk Factors

Predicting those at risk for spontaneous preterm labor and birth includes identification of risk factors. In addition to the risk factors listed in Box 17.1, living in a disadvantaged neighborhood, state, or region and lack of access to prenatal care also have been identified as risk factors. The risk for preterm birth also appears to be genetically related. For example, women who were themselves born prematurely have an increased risk for giving birth prematurely (Simhan et al., 2017). Women whose sisters gave birth prematurely are also more likely to do so, and the grandparents of women who give birth prematurely are more likely to have been born prematurely themselves than the grandparents of women who give birth at term (Simhan et al., 2014). Researchers have developed many risk scoring systems based on history, demographic characteristics, and current pregnancy risk factors in an attempt to determine which women might go into labor prematurely. No risk scoring system has been very successful in lowering the preterm birth rate, however, because at least 50% of all women who ultimately give birth prematurely have no identifiable risk factors (Simhan et al., 2017).

Cervical Length

One possible predictor of preterm labor is endocervical length. Changes in cervical length occur before uterine activity, so cervical measurement can identify women in whom the labor process has begun. However, because preterm cervical shortening occurs over a period of weeks, neither digital nor ultrasound cervical examination is very sensitive for predicting imminent preterm birth. Women whose cervical length as measured by transvaginal ultrasound is greater than 30 mm in the second and third trimester of pregnancy are unlikely to give birth prematurely even if they have symptoms of preterm labor (Simhan et al., 2014; Simhan et al., 2017).

Fetal Fibronectin Test

Fetal fibronectin (fFN) has been studied extensively and is marketed in the United States as a diagnostic test for preterm labor. fFN is a glycoprotein "glue" found in plasma and produced during fetal life. It normally appears in cervical and vaginal secretions early in pregnancy and then again in late pregnancy. The test is performed by collecting fluid from the woman's vagina using a swab during a speculum examination. The presence of fFN during the late second and early third trimesters of pregnancy may be related to placental inflammation, which is thought to be one cause of spontaneous preterm labor. The presence of fFN alone is not very sensitive as a predictor of preterm birth, however. Often the test is used to predict who will *not* go into preterm labor, because preterm labor is very unlikely to occur in women with a negative result (Simhan et al., 2014).

A combined approach to predicting preterm birth has been found to increase sensitivity and negative predictive value. Combining the evaluation of fFN levels and ultrasound measurement of cervical length was found to increase the ability to identify those at risk for preterm labor within the next 7 days as well as better identify those at low risk (DeFranco, Lewis, & Odibo, 2013).

CARE MANAGEMENT

ASSESSMENT

Because all pregnant women must be considered at risk for preterm labor, assessment for factors that contribute to this risk begins early in pregnancy and continues throughout the prenatal period. The onset of preterm labor is often insidious and can be easily mistaken for normal discomforts of pregnancy. Nursing diagnoses, expected outcomes of care, and evidence-based interventions are established for each woman based on her assessment findings (see Nursing Care Plan).

INTERVENTIONS

Prevention

Primary prevention strategies that address risk factors associated with preterm labor and birth are less costly in human and financial terms than the high-tech and often long term care required by preterm infants and their families. Programs aimed at health promotion and disease prevention that encourage healthy lifestyles for the population in general and women of childbearing age in particular should be developed. Preconception counseling and care for women, especially those with a history of preterm birth, can identify correctable risk factors and provide a means to encourage women to participate in health-promotion activities. Smoking cessation, for example, has been shown to prevent preterm labor and birth (Reedy, 2014; Simhan et al., 2017).

Preterm birth can be prevented in some women by administering prophylactic progesterone supplementation. Daily vaginal suppositories or creams or weekly intramuscular injections of 17-alpha hydroxyprogesterone caproate (17-P or 17-OHP) have been shown to decrease the rate of preterm birth by about 40% in women with a history of prior preterm birth or with a short (less than 15 mm to 20 mm length) cervix before 24 weeks of gestation. A short cervix, rather than a history of previous preterm birth, is the most appropriate reason for beginning vaginal progesterone therapy. Supplementation begins at 16 weeks and continues until 36 weeks of gestation. Progesterone supplementation does not affect the rate of preterm birth in women with multiple gestations. Exactly how progesterone works to prevent preterm birth is unclear (Simhan et al., 2017).

Early Recognition and Diagnosis

Although preterm birth often is not preventable, early recognition of preterm labor is essential to implement interventions that have been demonstrated to reduce neonatal and infant morbidity and mortality. These interventions include the following (Simhan et al., 2017):

- Transferring the mother before birth to a hospital equipped to care for her preterm infant
- Administering antibiotics during labor to prevent neonatal group B streptococci infection
- Administering antenatal glucocorticoids (e.g., betamethasone, dexamethasone) to women at risk for preterm birth to prevent or reduce neonatal and infant morbidity and mortality from health problems including respiratory distress syndrome, intraventricular hemorrhage, necrotizing enterocolitis, and other causes
- Administering magnesium sulfate to women giving birth before 32 weeks of gestation to reduce the incidence of cerebral palsy in their infants (see Evidence-Based Practice box).

In some cases, it is both wise and possible to transport pregnant women in preterm labor to a tertiary or quarternary care center (e.g., if a woman lives in a small town where there is only a community hospital with no neonatal intensive care unit). Although maternal transport helps ensure a better health outcome for the mother and the baby, it also has a downside. Women may be transported to tertiary or quarternary centers far from home, making visits by family and friends difficult and increasing the anxiety levels of the woman and her family. Attention to the needs of the woman and her family before, during, and after the transport is essential to comprehensive nursing care (see Chapter 25).

Because more than half of preterm births occur in women without obvious risk factors, it is essential that all pregnant women are taught the symptoms of preterm labor (Box 17.3). The nurse caring for women in a prenatal setting should educate them about how to recognize symptoms of preterm labor and then assess for these symptoms at each prenatal visit. Women also must be taught the significance of these symptoms of preterm labor and what to do should they occur (see Patient Teaching box: What to Do If Symptoms of Preterm Labor Occur).

In particular, patient education regarding any symptoms of uterine contractions, pain, and vaginal discharge occurring between 20 0/7 and 36 6/7 weeks of gestation must emphasize that these symptoms are not just normal discomforts of pregnancy but indications of possible preterm labor (Fig. 17.1). Waiting too long to see a health care provider could result in inevitable preterm birth without sufficient time to implement the interventions that have been shown to improve infant outcomes (see preceding discussion).

The diagnosis of preterm labor is based on three major diagnostic criteria (ACOG, 2016a):

- Gestational age between 20 0/7 and 36 6/7 weeks
- Regular uterine activity, accompanied by a change in cervical effacement, dilation, or both
- Initial presentation with regular contractions and cervical dilation of at least 2 cm.

EVIDENCE-BASED PRACTICE

Magnesium Sulfate for Neuroprotection Against Cerebral Palsy

Ask the Question
PICOT Question: For women anticipating preterm birth, can any prenatal treatment protect the premature newborn from cerebral palsy?

Search for the Evidence
Search Strategies: English research-based publications since 2011 on magnesium sulfate, neuroprotection, preterm, premature were included.
Databases Used: Cochrane Collaborative Database, National Guideline Clearinghouse (AHRQ), CINAHL, PubMed, UpToDate, and the professional websites for ACOG and AWHONN.

Critical Appraisal of the Evidence
Among the many challenges for a premature baby is the risk for cerebral palsy, the most common motor disability in children. Alert clinicians noticed that newborns whose mothers had been given magnesium sulfate for tocolysis or preeclampsia were less likely to have cerebral palsy. Further research confirmed its benefit and safety.

- Magnesium sulfate facilitates vasodilation, reduces inflammation, and reduces calcium uptake into cells. It may delay cellular injury or death and increases blood flow to the brain (Merrill, 2013).
- Although magnesium sulfate is no longer recommended for stopping preterm labor, the American College of Obstetricians and Gynecologists (ACOG) and the Society for Maternal-Fetal Medicine (SMFM) (2016) still recommend magnesium sulfate for neuroprotection against cerebral palsy in women anticipating imminent preterm birth at less than 32 weeks of gestation.
- Study protocols are in place for ongoing research into the advisability of using neuroprotective magnesium sulfate for later gestational age, up to 34 weeks (Crowther, Middleton, Wilkinson, et al., 2013).
- Administering magnesium sulfate requires intravenous infusion and close monitoring A cost-effectiveness analysis reveals that giving neuroprotective magnesium sulfate to patients with threatened preterm birth saves $1.5 million for every case of cerebral palsy that is averted (Bickford, Magee, Mitton, et al., 2013).

Apply the Evidence: Nursing Implications
- Magnesium sulfate should be given in settings where staff are familiar with its use, monitoring is available, and emergency resuscitation and ventilation equipment is available.
- Typical use in women in active preterm labor or with preterm premature rupture of membranes is a 4-g loading dose given over 30 to 60 minutes, followed by the maintenance dose of 1 g/hour, given until birth or for up to 24 hours, whichever comes first. Other tocolytics are discontinued.
- Prior to the loading dose, the nurse obtains baseline vital signs and checks patellar reflexes. These assessments are repeated at 10 minutes after initiation and at the end of the loading dose. During the maintenance dose, vitals are

repeated hourly, reflexes every 2 hours, and continuous electronic fetal monitoring is recommended.
- Signs of magnesium toxicity include a decrease in respirations of 4 breaths per minute from the baseline rate or to less than 12 per minute; a systolic blood pressure drop of 15 mm Hg from the baseline; diminished reflexes; decreased urinary output; or FHR abnormalities. If these are noted, the nurse should stop the infusion and notify the health care provider. Calcium gluconate should be available nearby as an antidote.
- To improve safety, the infusion should be given via infusion device in prepackaged concentrations clearly labeled as loading and maintenance doses, and double-checked by another nurse.
- Neonatal hypermagnesemia, although rare, can present as apnea, respiratory depression, lethargy, poor feeding, and hyporeflexia. Neonatal resuscitation should be available.

Quality and Safety Competencies: Safety*
Knowledge
Discuss effective strategies to reduce reliance on memory.
Clearly labeled standardized packaging of magnesium sulfate doses prevents medication errors.

Skills
Demonstrate effective use of technology and standardized practices that support safety and quality.
Standardized protocols and administering magnesium sulfate in facilities familiar with its use and equipped with adequate emergency equipment improve patient safety.

Attitudes
Appreciate the cognitive and physical limits of human performance.
Having another nurse double-check bags and infusion timing prevents patient injury.

References
American College of Obstetricians and Gynecologists & Society for Maternal-Fetal Medicine. (2016). Committee opinion no. 652: Magnesium sulfate use in obstetrics. *Obstetrics and Gynecology, 127*(1), e52–e53.
Bickford, C. D., Magee, L. A., Mitton, C., et al. (2013). Magnesium sulphate for fetal neuroprotection: A cost-effectiveness analysis. *BioMed Central (BMC) Health Services Research, 13*, 527.
Crowther, C. A., Middleton, P. F., Wilkinson, D., et al. (2013). Magnesium sulphate at 30 to 34 weeks' gestational age: Neuroprotection trial (MAGENTA)—Study protocol. *BioMed Central (BMC) Pregnancy and Childbirth, 13*, 91.
Merrill, L. (2013). Magnesium sulfate during anticipated preterm birth for infant neuroprotection. *Nursing for Women's Health, 17*(1), 44–50.

Pat Mahaffee Gingrich

*Adapted from QSEN at www.qsen.org/.

If the presence of fFN is used as another diagnostic criterion, a sample of cervical fluid should be obtained by sterile speculum exam. Vaginal swab collection is no longer recommended. The presence of vaginal bleeding or ruptured membranes or a history of intercourse or digital cervical examination within the past 24 hours can reduce the accuracy of the test results (Swanson & Baird, 2017).

The pregnant woman at 30 weeks of gestation with an irritable uterus but no documented cervical change is not in preterm labor, although she should be carefully evaluated during follow-up care to determine whether she has progressed to active preterm labor (e.g., effacement, dilation, or both). Women with preterm contractions without cervical change, especially those with a cervical dilation of less than 2 cm, should not be given tocolytic medications (ACOG, 2016a).

Lifestyle Modifications
Activity Restriction
Bedrest, hydration, and limited work are often recommended to reduce the risk for preterm birth in women at risk for giving birth prematurely. There is no evidence, however, to support the effectiveness of these interventions, and they should not be routinely recommended. In fact, both bed rest and excessive hydration can cause potentially harmful maternal complications. Research indicates that bed rest causes adverse

◎ NURSING CARE PLAN
Preterm Labor

Case Study
Manuela is a 42-year-old divorced woman who has had seven pregnancies. The first pregnancy ended in a term birth of a 7 lb 6 oz baby. The pregnancies were closely spaced, and the gestational periods of the next six pregnancies became progressively shorter until her last baby was born 4 years ago at 34 weeks of gestation. Manuela and her husband were divorced shortly after the last baby was born. She has since established a relationship with Juan and is currently in the 24th week of an unplanned pregnancy. Manuela smokes one-half pack of cigarettes per day. She is 4 feet, 11 inches tall and currently weighs 96 pounds. Juan is supportive of her and will continue to support her throughout the pregnancy. Currently, they have no plans to marry. Despite having several preterm infants, Manuela appears to have little understanding of preterm labor, its causes, and its treatment.

Assessment
What risk factors for preterm labor does Manuela have? What does she know about the causes, signs and symptoms, and management of preterm labor?

Defining Characteristics
History of having given birth to several preterm infants
Tobacco use
Underweight
Poor performance on test of knowledge

Nursing Diagnosis
Deficient Knowledge related to recognition of preterm labor

Expected Outcomes
Manuela and Juan will communicate desire to learn about preterm labor and will set realistic learning goals.
Manuela will express understanding of causes, signs and symptoms, and management of premature labor.
Manuela will identify and immediately report danger signals to her obstetric health care provider.
Manuela will voice emotional response to preterm labor, assuming she develops preterm labor during this pregnancy.
Manuela will use available support systems.
Pregnancy will result in positive outcome.

Nursing Interventions	Rationales
Assess what Manuela and Juan know about preterm labor and birth and how to recognize its presence.	To identify areas of deficit
Assess the couple's ability to understand, speak, and read English.	To assess need for an interpreter and/or for teaching materials written in Spanish
Discuss signs and symptoms that serve as warning signs of preterm labor so that Manuela and Juan have adequate information.	To identify problems early
Provide a list of warning signs of preterm labor and phone numbers to call if any of the listed signs occur.	For couple to reinforce and review learning and act swiftly and appropriately should a sign occur
Discuss and demonstrate how to assess and time contractions.	To provide needed skills to assess signs of labor

Case Study (Continued)
A couple of days later, Manuela tells her neighbor that she has a backache and is feeling lots of pelvic pressure. "It feels like the baby is balling up in there." Manuela noticed a larger amount than normal of clear vaginal discharge this morning. For the last several hours, Manuela has felt her "tummy tightening" regularly, although she denies pain. Manuela's neighbor says, "I think you might be going into labor."

Assessment
What are risks to mother and fetus that can be attributed to preterm labor? How can these risks be reduced?

Defining Characteristics
Change in type of vaginal discharge (watery, mucus, or bloody)
Increase in amount of vaginal discharge
Pelvic or lower abdominal pressure
Constant low, dull backache
Mild abdominal cramps, with or without diarrhea
Regular or frequent contractions or uterine tightening, often painless
Ruptured membranes

Nursing Diagnosis
Risk for Injury (Maternal/Fetal) related to recurrence of preterm labor in the current pregnancy

Expected Outcomes
Manuela demonstrates ability to assess self for signs of recurring labor
Manuela will cope successfully with preterm labor.
Maternal-fetal well-being is maintained

Nursing Interventions	Rationales
Teach Manuela and Juan to be alert for uterine contractions and how to assess their frequency, duration, and strength if they are noted.	To provide immediate evidence of worsening condition
Have Manuela and Juan report rupture of membranes, increased vaginal discharge, cramping, pelvic pressure, or low backache to obstetric health care provider.	Such symptoms can be signs of labor
Have Manuela monitor her weight, diet, fluid intake, and vital signs on a daily basis.	To evaluate for potential problems
Have Manuela limit activities to those recommended in restricted activity plan.	To decrease likelihood of onset of labor
Encourage Manuela to use side-lying position when reclining.	To enhance placental perfusion
Teach Manuela signs and symptoms of venous thromboembolism (VTE), and encourage gentle exercise of lower extremities.	Because pregnancy and limited activity increase risk for clot formation
Counsel Manuela and Juan to abstain from sexual intercourse and nipple stimulation if symptoms of preterm labor occur.	Because such activities may stimulate uterine contractions
Encourage Manuela to practice relaxation techniques.	To decrease uterine tone and decrease anxiety and stress

◎ NURSING CARE PLAN

Preterm Labor—cont'd

Nursing Interventions	Rationales
Teach Manuela to take prophylactic progesterone supplementation weekly if ordered by her physician.	To decrease the likelihood of preterm labor
Teach Manuela and Juan about and have them report any medication side effects immediately.	To prevent medication-induced complications
Have family arrange for alternate strategies in carrying out woman's usual roles and functions.	To decrease stress and limit temptations to increase activity
If small children are part of household, encourage family to make alternative arrangements for child care.	To enhance woman's adherence to her restricted activity protocol

Case Study (Continued)

Manuela has expressed a better understanding of preterm labor and the dangers to the fetus if a preterm birth occurs. Because of the increased understanding, Manuela is aware of potential risks for the fetus. Consequently, her anxiety is becoming manifest. She frequently seeks assurance that "everything will be okay" and that she is doing all she can to ensure a successful outcome of the pregnancy. Modified bed rest has been prescribed.

Assessment

What are signs and symptoms of anxiety related to preterm labor?

Defining Characteristics

Excessive attention to fetal movement or uterine activity
Expressed fear of a negative outcome
Fear, apprehension, and wariness
Inability to concentrate, understand, or remember
Restlessness, shakiness, trembling, jittery behavior, and extraneous movements

Nursing Diagnosis

Anxiety related to preterm labor and potentially premature neonate

Expected Outcomes

Manuela expresses her feelings of anxiety.
Manuela identifies causes of anxiety.
Manuela makes use of available emotional support.
Feelings and symptoms of anxiety are reduced.

Nursing Interventions	Rationales
Provide calm, soothing atmosphere, and encourage family to provide emotional support.	To facilitate coping
Encourage verbalization of fears.	To decrease intensity of emotional response
Involve Manuela and family in home management of her condition.	To promote greater sense of control
Help Manuela identify and use appropriate coping strategies and support systems.	To reduce fear/anxiety
Explore use of desensitization strategies such as progressive muscle relaxation, visual imagery, or thought stopping.	To reduce fear-related emotions and related physical symptoms

Nursing Interventions	Rationales
Provide information about online support groups.	To reduce fear and anxiety

Assessment

What are some strategies that Manuela can use to cope with activity restriction? What are some diversional activities that Manuela can use to cope with activity restriction?

Defining Characteristics

Manuela expresses frustration with her inability to prepare meals and assist with child care while on activity restriction.
She expresses boredom and loneliness while confined to her home on activity restriction.
She expresses desire for support and companionship from friends and relatives.
She expresses desire for activities to make the time pass more quickly.

Nursing Diagnosis

Deficient Diversional Activity related to activity restriction

Expected Outcomes

Manuela arranges for assistance with child care and meal preparation from her mother and neighbor. She prepares menus for daily meals.
Manuela enters a chat room of women confined to their homes on activity restriction to relieve boredom.
Manuela arranges for her children to complete their homework in the room with her.
Manuela verbalizes diminished feelings of boredom.

Nursing Interventions	Rationales
Assist Manuela to creatively explore personally meaningful activities that can be pursued while on activity restriction.	To ensure activities that have meaning, purpose, and value to individual
Maintain emphasis on Manuela's personal choices.	Because doing so promotes control and minimizes imposition of routines by others
Evaluate support and system resources that are available in environment.	To assist in providing diversional activities
Explore ways for Manuela to remain active participant in home management and decision making.	To promote control
Engage support of family and friends in carrying out chosen activities and making necessary environmental alterations.	To ensure success
Encourage Manuela to use the Internet to communicate with other women on activity restriction.	To obtain support and share feelings
Teach Manuela about stress management and relaxation techniques.	To help manage tension of confinement

BOX 17.3 Signs and Symptoms of Preterm Labor

- Change in type of vaginal discharge (watery, mucus, or bloody)
- Increase in amount of vaginal discharge
- Pelvic or lower abdominal pressure
- Constant low, dull backache
- Mild abdominal cramps, with or without diarrhea
- Regular or frequent contractions or uterine tightening, often painless
- Ruptured membranes

NOTE: A woman in preterm labor may have only one or all of these signs.

Data from Swanson, D., & Baird, S.M. (2017). Preterm labor and preterm premature rupture of membranes. In B.B. Kennedy, & S.M. Baird (Eds.), *Intrapartum management modules: A perinatal education program* (5th ed.). Philadelphia, PA: Wolters Kluwer.

PATIENT TEACHING

What to Do if Symptoms of Preterm Labor Occur

- Stop what you are doing.
- Lie down on your side.
- Drink two to three glasses of water or juice.
- Lie down on your side.
- Wait 1 hour.
- If symptoms get worse, call your health care provider.
- If symptoms go away, tell your health care provider what happened at your next prenatal visit.
- If symptoms come back, call your health care provider.

Data from Reedy, N.J. (2014). Preterm labor and birth. In K.R. Simpson, & P. Creehan (Eds.), *AWHONN's perinatal nursing* (4th ed.). Philadelphia, PA; Lippincott Williams & Wilkins.

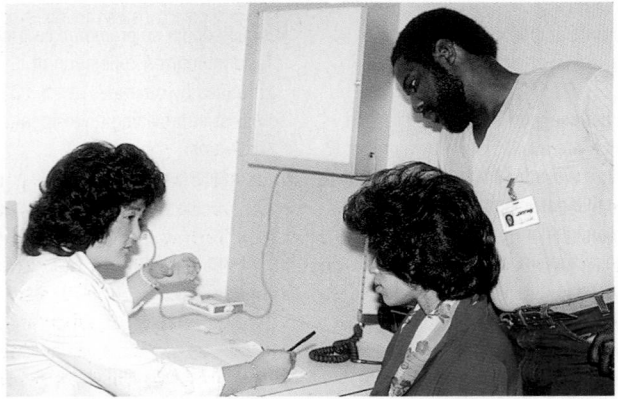

FIG 17.1 Nurse teaching a couple signs and symptoms of preterm labor. (Courtesy of Marjorie Pyle, RNC, Lifecircle, Costa Mesa, CA.)

physical effects, including risk for thrombus formation, muscle atrophy, bone loss, cardiovascular deconditioning, and endocrine system changes (Simhan et al., 2017; Swanson & Baird, 2017). In addition, bed rest affects women and their families psychologically, emotionally, socially, and financially. Many health care providers now recommend only modified bed rest.

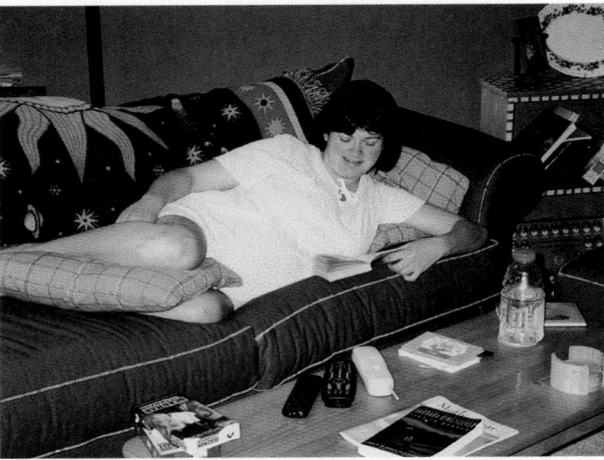

FIG 17.2 Woman at home on restricted activity for preterm labor prevention. Note how she has arranged her daytime resting area so that needed items are close at hand. (Courtesy of Amy Turner, Cary, NC.)

Restriction of Sexual Activity

Restriction of sexual activity, sometimes called *pelvic rest*, is frequently recommended for women at risk for preterm birth. Evidence is lacking that this is an effective intervention for preventing preterm birth (Simhan et al., 2017). However, sexual abstinence has not been studied in women with specific risk factors for preterm birth, such as a short cervix. Therefore, more research is indicated (Simhan et al., 2014).

Home Care

Home care of the woman at risk for preterm birth is a challenge for the nurse, who must assist the woman and her family in dealing with the many difficulties faced by families in which one member is unable to fulfill usual role responsibilities.

The woman's environment can be modified for convenience by using tables and storage units around her bed or daytime resting place to keep essential items within reach (e.g., cell or smart phone, television, radio, MP3 player, CD player, computer with Internet access, snacks, books, magazines, newspapers, and items for hobbies) (Fig. 17.2). Ensuring that the bed or couch is near a window and the bathroom is also helpful. Covering the bed with an eggcrate mattress can relieve discomfort. Women often find that a daily schedule of smaller, more frequent meals, activities (e.g., paying bills, planning and helping with meal preparation, hobbies), limited naps, and hygiene and grooming (e.g., shower, dressing in street clothes, applying makeup) reduces boredom and helps them maintain control and normalcy (see Patient Teaching box: Activities for Children of Women on Activity Restriction for additional ideas and suggestions). Also see Patient Teaching box: Coping with Activity Restriction in Chapter 12 for more information. With modified bed rest, women are usually allowed bathroom privileges for toileting and showering and can be up to the table for meals.

Suppression of Uterine Activity

Tocolytics are medications given to arrest labor after uterine contractions and cervical change have occurred. No medications that have been approved for use as tocolytics by the US Food and Drug Administration (FDA) are currently available in the United States. Ritodrine (Yutopar) was approved but has been withdrawn from the US market. However, it is still used as a tocolytic in other countries. Drugs marketed for other purposes, such as treatment of asthma or hypertension or as

PATIENT TEACHING

Activities for Children of Women on Activity Restriction

- Schedule brief play periods throughout the day.
- Keep a few favorite toys in a box or basket close to the bed or couch.
- Read to the children.
- Assemble puzzles together.
- Watch videos or play video games (remote control for television is ideal).
- Play card or board games.
- Color in coloring books.
- Cut out pictures from magazines, and paste on cardboard.
- Play bed basketball with a soft (sponge) ball or rolled up sock and a trash can or empty laundry basket.

BOX 17.4 Contraindications to Tocolytic Therapy

Maternal
- Preeclampsia or gestational hypertension with severe features
- Hemorrhage
- Significant cardiac disease

Fetal
- Gestational age of 37 weeks or more
- Fetal demise
- Lethal fetal anomaly
- Chorioamnionitis
- Evidence of acute or chronic fetal compromise

Data from Simhan, H.N., Iams, J.D., & Romero, R. (2017). Preterm labor and birth. In S.G. Gabbe, J.R. Niebyl, J.L. Simpson, et al. (Eds.), *Obstetrics: Normal and problem pregnancies* (7th ed.). Philadelphia, PA: Elsevier.

antiinflammatory or analgesic agents, are used on an "off-label" basis (i.e., drugs known to be effective for a specific purpose, although not specifically developed and tested for this purpose) to suppress preterm labor (Simhan et al., 2014). No tocolytic has been shown to reduce the rate of preterm birth. Rather, the rationale for giving these medications is to delay birth long enough to allow time for maternal transport to a Level III or Level IV neonatal care center and for corticosteroids to reach maximum benefit to reduce neonatal morbidity and mortality. Studies of individual drugs used for tocolysis rarely contain information about whether delaying birth improved infant outcomes (Simhan et al., 2017). Selecting the appropriate tocolytic medication requires consideration of each drug's effectiveness, risks, and side effects. Important contraindications exist to the use of all tocolytics. Maternal and fetal contraindications to tocolytic therapy are listed in Box 17.4. Box 17.5 describes nursing care for women receiving tocolytic therapy.

Magnesium sulfate is the most commonly used tocolytic agent because maternal, fetal, and neonatal adverse reactions are less severe and less frequent than with the beta-adrenergic agonists. Clinicians are familiar with its use as a treatment for preeclampsia and believe it is safer to use when compared with the beta-adrenergic agonists. However, although magnesium sulfate is still frequently used, its effectiveness as a tocolytic is not supported by the literature (see Medication Guide: Tocolytic Therapy for Preterm Labor) (Simhan et al., 2014; Swanson & Baird, 2017).

BOX 17.5 Nursing Care for the Woman Receiving Tocolytic Therapy

- Explain the purpose and side effects of the tocolytic medication(s) to the woman and her family.
- Position the woman on her side to enhance placental perfusion and reduce pressure on the cervix.
- Monitor maternal vital signs including lung sounds and respiratory effort, fetal heart rate and pattern, and labor status according to hospital protocol and professional standards.
- Assess mother and fetus for signs of adverse reactions related to the tocolytic medication(s) being administered (see Medication Guide: Tocolytic Therapy for Preterm Labor).
- Determine maternal fluid balance by measuring daily weight and intake and output.
- Limit fluid intake to 2500 to 3000 mL/day, especially if a beta-adrenergic agonist or magnesium sulfate is being administered.
- Provide psychosocial support and opportunities for the woman and family to express feelings and concerns.
- Offer comfort measures as needed.
- Encourage diversional activities and relaxation techniques.

⚡ SAFETY ALERT

Because magnesium sulfate depresses the function of the central nervous system (CNS), it is essential that the nurse frequently assesses the woman's respiratory status, deep tendon reflexes, and level of consciousness to identify signs that the serum level of magnesium sulfate is reaching toxic levels.

Beta$_2$-adrenergic agonists (e.g., ritodrine and terbutaline [Brethine]) have been widely used as tocolytics. They have many maternal and fetal adverse reactions, however, including beta$_1$-stimulated cardiopulmonary (e.g., tachycardia) effects and beta$_2$-stimulated metabolic (e.g., hyperglycemia) effects. Therefore, beta$_2$-adrenergic agonists are increasingly being replaced by medications that are safer and have fewer adverse reactions. They should not be used in women with known or suspected heart disease, preeclampsia with severe features or eclampsia, pregestational or gestational diabetes, or hyperthyroidism (Simhan et al., 2014; Simhan et al., 2017). These drugs are also contraindicated when preterm labor is complicated by maternal fever, fetal tachycardia, or other signs of possible chorioamnionitis (Simhan et al., 2017).

Terbutaline, the most commonly administered beta-adrenergic agonist used for tocolysis, relaxes uterine smooth muscle by stimulating beta$_2$-receptors in the uterine smooth muscle. Terbutaline is often given subcutaneously to facilitate maternal transfer to a tertiary or quartrenary center or to initiate tocolytic therapy while another agent with a slower onset of action is administered concurrently. Additionally, a subcutaneous injection of 0.25 mg may be given to suppress uterine tachysystole during labor induction or augmentation or to suppress contractions prior to cesarean birth. Long-term oral or subcutaneous administration (e.g., terbutaline pump) as maintenance therapy to suppress preterm labor has not been proven to be effective in reducing prematurity or neonatal morbidity, so terbutaline should not be used for this purpose. In addition, terbutaline has the potential to cause serious maternal cardiac problems and death (Simhan et al., 2014; Simhan et al., 2017) (see Medication Guide: Tocolytic Therapy for Preterm Labor).

Nifedipine (Adalat, Procardia), a calcium channel blocker, is a tocolytic agent that can suppress contractions. It works by preventing calcium from entering smooth muscle cells, thus reducing uterine contractions. Because of its ease of administration and low incidence of significant

r5ea

MEDICATION GUIDE
Tocolytic Therapy for Preterm Labor

Medication and Action	Dosage and Route*	Adverse Effects	Nursing Considerations
Magnesium Sulfate CNS depressant; relaxes smooth muscle, including the uterus	IV fluid should contain 40 g in 1000 mL, piggyback to primary infusion, and administer using controller pump: Loading dose: 4–6 g over 20–30 minutes Maintenance dose: 1–4 g/hour Use for stabilization only Discontinue within 24–48 hours at the maintenance dose or if intolerable adverse effects occur	**Maternal:** Hot flushes, sweating, burning at IV insertion site, nausea and vomiting, dry mouth, drowsiness, blurred vision, diplopia, headache, ileus, generalized muscle weakness, lethargy, dizziness Hypocalcemia Dyspnea Transient hypotension Some reactions may subside when loading dose is completed **Intolerable:** Respiratory rate fewer than 12 breaths/minute Pulmonary edema Absent DTRs Chest pain Severe hypotension Altered level of consciousness Extreme muscle weakness Urine output less than 25–30 mL/hour or less than 100 mL/4 hours Serum magnesium level of 10 mEq/L (9 mg/dL) or greater **Fetal (uncommon):** Decreased breathing movement Reduced FHR variability Nonreactive NST	Assess woman and fetus to obtain baseline before beginning therapy and then before and after each incremental change; follow frequency of agency protocol. Drug is almost always given IV but can also be administered IM. Monitor serum magnesium levels with higher doses; therapeutic range is 4–7.5 mEq/L or 5–8 mg/dL. Discontinue infusion and notify physician if intolerable adverse effects occur. Ensure that calcium gluconate or calcium chloride is available for emergency administration to reverse magnesium sulfate toxicity. Do not give to women with myasthenia gravis. Total IV intake should be limited to 125 mL/hour.
Beta-Adrenergic Agonist (Beta-Mimetic) Terbutaline (Brethine) Relaxes smooth muscle, inhibiting uterine activity and causing bronchodilation	Subcutaneous injection of 0.25 mg every 4 hours Treatment should last no longer than 24 hours Discontinue use if intolerable adverse effects occur	**Maternal (most are mild and of limited duration):** Tachycardia, chest discomfort, palpitations, arrhythmias Tremors, dizziness, nervousness Headache Nasal congestion Nausea and vomiting Hypokalemia Hyperglycemia Hypotension **Intolerable:** Tachycardia greater than 130 beats/minute BP less than 90/60 Chest pain Cardiac arrhythmias Myocardial infarction Pulmonary edema	Should not be used in women with known or suspected heart disease, pregestational or gestational diabetes, preeclampsia with severe features or eclampsia, hyperthyroidism, or with significant hemorrhage or possible chorioamnionitis. Myocardial infarction leading to death has been reported after use.

Continued

⬡ MEDICATION GUIDE

Tocolytic Therapy for Preterm Labor—cont'd

Medication and Action	Dosage and Route*	Adverse Effects	Nursing Considerations
		Fetal: Tachycardia Hyperinsulinemia Hyperglycemia	Assess woman and fetus according to agency protocol, being alert for adverse effects. Assess maternal glucose and potassium levels before treatment is initiated and periodically during treatment. Significant hyperglycemia (greater than 180 mg/dL) and hypokalemia (less than 2.5 mEq/L) may occur. Notify physician if the following are noted: Maternal heart rate greater than 130 beats/minute; arrhythmias, chest pain BP less than 90/60 mm Hg Signs of pulmonary edema (e.g., dyspnea, crackles, decreased SaO₂). Fetal heart rate greater than 180 beats/minute. Hyperglycemia occurs more frequently in women who are being treated simultaneously with corticosteroids. Ensure that propranolol (Inderal) is available to reverse adverse effects related to cardiovascular function.
Prostaglandin Synthetase Inhibitors (NSAIDs) Indomethacin (Indocin) Relaxes uterine smooth muscle by inhibiting prostaglandins	Loading dose: 50 mg orally, then 25–50 mg orally every 6 hours for 48 hours	**Maternal (common):** Nausea and vomiting Heartburn **Less common, but more serious:** GI bleeding Prolonged bleeding time Thrombocytopenia Asthma in aspirin-sensitive patients **Fetal:** Constriction of ductus arteriosus Oligohydramnios, caused by reduced fetal urine production Neonatal pulmonary hypertension	The long-acting formulations decrease the incidence of adverse effects. Used only if gestational age is less than 32 weeks. Administer for 2–3 days or less. Do not use in women with renal or hepatic disease, active peptic ulcer disease, poorly controlled hypertension, asthma, or coagulation disorders. Can mask maternal fever. Assess woman and fetus according to agency policy, being alert for adverse effects. Determine amniotic fluid volume and function of fetal ductus arteriosus before initiating therapy and within 48 hours of discontinuing therapy; assessment is critical if therapy continues for more than 48 hours. Administer with food to decrease GI distress. Monitor for signs of postpartum hemorrhage.

Continued

MEDICATION GUIDE

Tocolytic Therapy for Preterm Labor—cont'd

Medication and Action	Dosage and Route*	Adverse Effects	Nursing Considerations
Calcium Channel Blockers			
Nifedipine (Adalat, Procardia) Relaxes smooth muscle including the uterus by blocking calcium entry	Initial dose: 10–20 mg orally, every 3–6 hours until contractions are rare, followed by long-acting formulations of 30 or 60 mg every 8–12 hours for 48 hours while corticosteroids are being given (however, the ideal dose has not been established)	**Maternal (most effects are mild):** Hypotension Headache Flushing Dizziness Nausea **Fetal:** Hypotension (questionable)	Avoid concurrent use with magnesium sulfate because skeletal muscle blockade can result. Should not be given simultaneously with or immediately after terbutaline because of effects on heart rate and blood pressure. Assess woman and fetus according to agency protocol, being alert for adverse effects. Do not use sublingual route of administration.

NOTE: There are variations in recommended administration protocols; always consult agency protocol, which should be evidence based.
BP, Blood pressure; *CNS,* central nervous system; *DTRs,* deep tendon reflexes; *FHR,* fetal heart rate; *GI,* gastrointestinal; *IM,* intramuscular; *IV,* intravenous; *NSAIDs,* nonsteroidal antiinflammatory drugs; *NST,* nonstress test; *SaO₂,* arterial oxygen saturation; *SOB,* shortness of breath.
Data from Gilbert, E. (2011). *Manual of high risk pregnancy and delivery* (5th ed.). St. Louis, MO: Mosby; Simhan, H.N., Berghella, V., & Iams, J.D. (2014). Preterm labor and birth. In R. K. Creasy, R. Resnik, J. D. Iams, et al. (Eds.), *Creasy and Resnik's maternal-fetal medicine: Principles and practice* (7th ed.). Philadelphia, PA: Saunders; Simhan, H.N., Iams, J.D., & Romero, R. (2017). Preterm labor and birth. In S.G. Gabbe, J.R. Niebyl, J.L. Simpson, et al. (Eds.), *Obstetrics: Normal and problem pregnancies* (7th ed.). Philadelphia, PA: Elsevier.

maternal and fetal side effects, nifedipine's use is increasing (see Medication Guide: Tocolytic Therapy for Preterm Labor) (Simhan et al., 2014; Simhan et al., 2017).

⚡ SAFETY ALERT

Administering nifedipine and magnesium sulfate simultaneously can cause skeletal muscle blockade. In addition, nifedipine should not be given along with or immediately following a beta₂-adrenergic agonist (e.g., terbutaline) because of effects on maternal heart rate and blood pressure (Simhan et al., 2014; Simhan et al., 2017).

⚡ SAFETY ALERT

Because using a calcium channel blocker can result in orthostatic hypotension and dizziness, it is essential to instruct women to slowly change position from supine to upright and then sit until any dizziness disappears before standing. In addition, it is important to maintain adequate fluid balance to reduce the drop in blood pressure that can occur with the drug-related vasodilation.

Indomethacin (Indocin), a nonsteroidal antiinflammatory drug (NSAID), has been shown in some trials to suppress preterm labor by blocking the production of prostaglandins. Serious maternal side effects are uncommon, and indomethacin is usually well tolerated. However, serious fetal or neonatal side effects have caused major concerns about its use as a tocolytic. Therefore, limiting the use of indomethacin to a period of 2 to 3 days in women with preterm labor at less than 32 weeks of gestation is recommended (Simhan et al., 2014; Simhan et al., 2017) (see Medication Guide: Tocolytic Therapy for Preterm Labor).

Promotion of Fetal Lung Maturity

Antenatal glucocorticoids, given as intramuscular (IM) injections to the mother to accelerate fetal lung maturity by stimulating fetal surfactant production, are now considered one of the most effective and cost-efficient interventions for preventing morbidity and mortality associated with preterm birth. Antenatal glucocorticoids have been shown to significantly reduce the incidence of respiratory distress syndrome, intraventricular hemorrhage, necrotizing enterocolitis, and death in neonates, without increasing the risk for infection in either mothers or newborns (Mercer, 2014a; Mercer, 2017). ACOG (2016a) recommends that all women between 24 and 34 weeks of gestation be given a single course of antenatal glucocorticoids when preterm birth is threatened. Because recent data indicate that betamethasone decreases neonatal respiratory morbidity when given to women between 34 0/7 and 36 6/7 weeks of gestation who are at risk for giving birth within the next 7 days and who have not previously received glucocorticoids during the current pregnancy, ACOG (2016a) also recommends that a course of betamethasone be given to these women. A single course of steroids may also be considered for women at 23 weeks of gestation if it seems likely that they will give birth within the next 7 days (ACOG, 2016a). A single repeat (rescue) course of antenatal steroids may be given to women who received their initial course more than 2 weeks previously if their gestational age remains less than 32 6/7 weeks and they are still considered likely to give birth within the next week. More than two courses of antenatal glucocorticoids, however, are not recommended (Simhan et al., 2017). The regimen for administration of antenatal glucocorticoids is given in the Medication Guide: Antenatal Glucocorticoid Therapy with Betamethasone or Dexamethasone.

💊 MEDICATION ALERT

All women between 24 and 34 weeks of gestation who are at risk for preterm birth should receive treatment with a single course of antenatal glucocorticoids (ACOG, 2016a). Because 48 hours from the time of the first injection are required for the fetus to receive optimal benefit, timely administration of the medication is essential.

MEDICATION GUIDE

Antenatal Glucocorticoid Therapy With Betamethasone or Dexamethasone

Action
- Stimulates fetal lung maturation by promoting release of enzymes that induce production or release of lung surfactant. Glucocorticoids have similar maturational effects on other organs, including the brain, kidneys, and gut.
NOTE: The US Food and Drug Administration has not approved these medications for this use (i.e., this is an off-label use for obstetrics).

Indication
- To prevent or reduce the severity of neonatal respiratory distress syndrome by accelerating lung maturity in fetuses between 24 and 34 weeks of gestation. Infants born to women who received antenatal glucocorticoids are also less likely to experience intraventricular hemorrhage, necrotizing enterocolitis, or neonatal death.

Dosage and Route
- Betamethasone: 12 mg intramuscular (IM) for two doses 24 hours apart
- Dexamethasone: 6 mg IM for four doses 12 hours apart

Maternal Effects
- Transient (lasting 72 hours) increase in white blood cell (WBC) and platelet counts
- Hyperglycemia

Fetal Effects
- Transient (typically lasting 48 to 72 hours after the last dose) decrease in fetal breathing and body movements

Nursing Considerations
- Give deep IM in ventral gluteal or vastus lateralis muscle.
- Medication *must* be given by IM injection; oral administration is *not* an acceptable alternative.
- Injection is painful.
- Medication should *not* affect maternal blood pressure.
- Assess blood glucose levels. Women with diabetes whose blood sugars have previously been well controlled may require increased insulin doses for several days.

Data from Simhan, H.N., Iams, J.D., & Romero, R. (2017). Preterm labor and birth. In S.G. Gabbe, J.R. Niebyl, J.L. Simpson, et al. (Eds.), *Obstetrics: Normal and problem pregnancies* (7th ed.). Philadelphia, PA: Elsevier.

Management of Inevitable Preterm Birth

When preterm birth appears inevitable (i.e., is expected to occur within the next 24 hours), magnesium sulfate may be administered to reduce or prevent neonatal neurologic morbidity (e.g., cerebral palsy). The current recommendation is that magnesium sulfate for neuroprotection is given to women who are at least 24 but less than 32 weeks of gestation at the time birth is expected to occur. The magnesium sulfate infusion should not be continued longer than 24 hours if birth has not occurred. How magnesium sulfate works to provide neuroprotection is not well understood. Although it is likely that the neuroprotective effects are the result of residual concentrations of the medication in the neonate's system, data are insufficient to determine the precise maternal dose necessary to achieve the benefit (Simhan et al., 2014; Simhan et al., 2017). The recommended dose of magnesium sulfate for neuroprotection is a loading dose of 4 grams given intravenously over 30 minutes, followed by a maintenance dose of 1 g/hour (Simhan et al., 2017) (see Medication Guide: Tocolytic Therapy for Preterm Labor and Evidence Based Practice box: Magnesium Sulfate for Neuroprotection Against Cerebral Palsy).

Labor that has progressed to a cervical dilation of 4 cm or more is likely to lead to inevitable preterm birth. If birth appears imminent, members of the interprofessional health care team will make preparations to care for a small, immature neonate. Women in preterm labor can rapidly progress to birth, and a very small fetus can be born through a partially dilated cervix. Also, malpresentation (e.g., breech presentation) occurs much more frequently in preterm than in term fetuses. Therefore, nurses must be prepared to handle the emergency birth of a preterm infant, from either cephalic or breech presentation, without the woman's obstetric health care provider being present. Personnel skilled at neonatal resuscitation should be present at the time of birth. Equipment, supplies, and medications used for neonatal resuscitation should be gathered in advance and prepared for immediate use. If birth occurs in a hospital that is not prepared to provide continuing care for a preterm neonate, plans should be made for transfer of the baby as soon as possible to a facility with a higher level of care.

Fetal and Early Neonatal Loss

Preterm birth or the presence of congenital anomalies or genetic disorders incompatible with life are major reasons for intrauterine fetal demise (stillbirth) or early neonatal death. In many of these situations, the parents will already have been told that the fetus has died or that the baby has a condition that is incompatible with life and will most likely die very soon after birth. Sometimes, however, the fetal death is unexpected, diagnosed only after the woman has been admitted to the labor and birth unit. Whatever the case, labor and birth nurses must be prepared to provide sensitive care to these women and their families (see Chapter 25).

If fetal or early neonatal death is expected, the parents and members of the interprofessional health care team need to discuss the situation before the birth and decide on a management plan that is acceptable to everyone. Despite counseling about the likelihood of a poor outcome, some parents want "everything possible" to be done for the baby, including cesarean birth for an abnormal fetal heart rate (FHR) tracing. If such intervention is not desired, usually the FHR is not monitored during labor.

Another major decision is whether to attempt neonatal resuscitation. Sometimes the feasibility of neonatal resuscitation cannot be determined until the baby's size and physical appearance have been assessed. If the baby is too small, too immature, or too malformed for effective resuscitation, palliative care can be provided instead. The baby is kept warm and comfortable at the mother's bedside, in the nursery, or at home, depending on the parents' desires, until death occurs. Parents can choose to view and hold the baby as they wish.

After the birth, the woman should be given the opportunity to decide if she wants to stay on the maternity unit or be moved to another hospital unit. She may prefer to be away from the sound of crying babies and exposure to other families who have had healthy infants. However, postpartum care and grief support may not be as sensitive or effective on another hospital unit, where the staff is not experienced in postpartum and bereavement care. Whether death occurs in utero or after birth, parents are faced with the same needs. See Chapter 25 for additional information on dealing with families experiencing a perinatal loss.

PREMATURE RUPTURE OF MEMBRANES

Premature rupture of membranes (PROM) is the spontaneous rupture of the amniotic sac and leakage of amniotic fluid before the onset of labor at any gestational age. Preterm premature rupture of membranes (preterm PROM or pPROM) is membrane rupture before 37 0/7 weeks of gestation and is associated with approximately 10% of all preterm births in the United States. Preterm PROM occurs twice as often in African-Americans as in other racial groups. The frequency of preterm PROM appears to have decreased during the past decade (Mercer, 2017).

Preterm PROM most likely results from pathologic weakening of the amniotic membranes caused by inflammation, stress from uterine contractions, or other factors that cause increased intrauterine pressure. Infection of the urogenital tract is a major risk factor associated with preterm PROM (Mercer, 2014b; Mercer, 2017). Box 17.6 lists other risk factors. PROM or preterm PROM is diagnosed after the woman reports either a sudden gush of fluid or a slow leak of fluid from the vagina.

Chorioamnionitis is the most common maternal complication of preterm PROM, making it a major complication of pregnancy (see later discussion). Other less common but serious maternal complications include placental abruption, retained placenta and hemorrhage, sepsis, and death (Mercer, 2014b; Mercer, 2017). Fetal complications from preterm PROM are primarily related to intrauterine infection, cord prolapse, umbilical cord compression associated with oligohydramnios, and placental abruption. Pulmonary hypoplasia is a common complication of PROM that occurs before 20 weeks of gestation (Mercer, 2014b; Mercer, 2017).

Care Management

Management of PROM, regardless of the gestational age at which it occurs, is determined for each woman based on an assessment of the estimated risk for maternal, fetal, and neonatal complications if pregnancy is allowed to continue or immediate labor and birth are attempted. At term (at or after 37 0/7 weeks of gestation), because infection is the greatest maternal, fetal, and neonatal risk, birth is the best option. Labor will most likely be induced if it does not begin spontaneously soon after PROM occurs (Mercer, 2014b; Mercer, 2017).

Active pursuit of labor and birth, rather than expectant management, is usually recommended for women who experience preterm PROM between 34 and 36 weeks of gestation. Although infants born at this gestational age have a higher risk for complications than babies born at or after 37 0/7 weeks, serious morbidity and mortality is uncommon. Because conservative management at this gestational age prolongs pregnancy by only a few days, significantly increases the risk for chorioamnionitis, and has not been shown to improve neonatal outcomes, immediate birth is generally considered to be the best management option (Mercer, 2014b). However, a recent multicenter study found that conservative management that continued until 37 weeks of gestation was associated with less neonatal hypoglycemia and hyperbilirubinemia. Therefore, conservative management of preterm PROM that occurs at 34 to 37 weeks of gestation might be an option if the risk for intrauterine infection is considered to be low (Mercer, 2017). If pulmonary maturity can be documented, women with preterm PROM at 32 to 33 weeks of gestation may also be offered immediate birth because with conservative management they have an increased risk for complications such as umbilical cord compression (Mercer, 2014b; Mercer, 2017).

Preterm PROM before 32 weeks of gestation is usually managed expectantly or conservatively because the risks to the fetus and newborn associated with preterm birth are considered to be greater than the risk for infection. Women will likely be hospitalized in an attempt to prolong the pregnancy and allow additional time for fetal maturation unless intrauterine infection, significant vaginal bleeding, placental abruption, or advanced labor is evident, or fetal testing becomes nonreassuring. Conservative management may require transfer to a hospital that is prepared to provide 24-hour neonatal resuscitation and intensive care. Ideally transfer should occur early in the course of care, before birth

---

BOX 17.6   Risk Factors for Preterm Premature Rupture of Membranes (Preterm PROM)

- History of prior preterm birth, especially if associated with preterm PROM
- History of cervical conization or cerclage
- Urinary or genital tract infection
- Short (<25 mm) cervical length identified by transvaginal ultrasound
- Preterm labor or symptomatic contractions in the current pregnancy
- Uterine overdistention
- Second- and third-trimester bleeding
- Pulmonary disease
- Connective tissue disorders
- Low socioeconomic status
- Low body mass index
- Nutritional deficiencies (copper and ascorbic acid)
- Cigarette smoking

Data from Mercer, B. (2017). Premature rupture of the membranes. In S.G. Gabbe, J.R. Niebyl, J.L. Simpson, et al. (Eds.), *Obstetrics: Normal and problem pregnancies* (7th ed.). Philadelphia, PA: Elsevier.

---

becomes imminent or complications arise (Mercer, 2014b; Mercer, 2017). Nursing support of the woman and her family is critical at this time. They are often anxious about the health of the baby, and the woman may fear that she was responsible in some way for the membrane rupture. Other nursing interventions include encouraging expression of feelings and concerns, providing information, and making referrals as needed.

Conservative management of preterm PROM includes fetal assessment at least daily, because of the risk for FHR abnormalities as a result of umbilical cord compression. Often this assessment will be performed using the nonstress test (NST) and biophysical profile (BPP). The woman should also be taught how to assess her fetus using daily fetal movement counts (DFMCs) because a slowing of fetal movement is a warning sign of severe fetal compromise (see Chapter 10 for further discussion of these tests). In addition, the woman will be monitored for signs of labor, placental abruption, and the development of intrauterine infection.

ACOG (2016b) recommends that all women with preterm PROM between 24 0/7 and 34 0/7 weeks of gestation be given a single course of antenatal glucocorticoids. A single course of glucocorticoids may also be considered for women as early as 23 0/7 weeks of gestation if they are at risk for giving birth within the next 7 days. Current data suggest that antenatal glucocorticoid use is not associated with an increased risk for either maternal or neonatal infection. Whether to give a single rescue course of glucocorticoids to women with preterm PROM is controversial and there is insufficient evidence at this time to make a recommendation (ACOG, 2016b).

A 7-day course of broad-spectrum antibiotics (e.g., ampicillin/amoxicillin and erythromycin) is administered. Antibiotic treatment has been shown to significantly prolong the time between membrane rupture and birth, decrease the incidence of maternal chorioamnionitis, and reduce infections and gestational age-dependent complications in the neonate such as the need for oxygen or surfactant therapy and intraventricular hemorrhage (Mercer, 2017).

Administering magnesium sulfate for fetal neuroprotection to women with preterm PROM before 32 weeks of gestation who are thought to be at imminent risk for giving birth prematurely is recommended (ACOG, 2016b; Simhan et al., 2017) (see the earlier discussion for more information on magnesium sulfate administration for this reason).

Vigilance for signs of infection is a major part of the patient education and nursing care after preterm PROM. The woman must be taught how to keep her genital area clean and that nothing should be introduced into her vagina. Signs of infection (e.g., fever, foul-smelling vaginal discharge, maternal and fetal tachycardia) should be reported immediately. If chorioamnionitis develops, the woman is placed on broad-spectrum antibiotics and birth is accomplished (Mercer, 2017).

CHORIOAMNIONITIS

Chorioamnionitis, bacterial infection of the amniotic cavity, is a major cause of complications for both mothers and newborns at any gestational age. It occurs in approximately 1% to 5% of term births but in as many as 25% of preterm births (Duff & Birsner, 2017). Other terms for this condition include *amnionitis* and *intrapartum infection*. Chorioamnionitis is usually diagnosed by the clinical findings of maternal fever, maternal and fetal tachycardia, uterine tenderness, and purulent amniotic fluid in the absence of another evident source of infection (Duff & Birsner; Mercer, 2017).

Chorioamnionitis most often occurs after membranes rupture or labor begins, as organisms that are part of the normal vaginal flora ascend into the amniotic cavity. Many of the risk factors for chorioamnionitis are associated with a long labor, such as prolonged membrane rupture, multiple vaginal examinations, and use of internal FHR and contraction monitoring modes (Duff, 2014). Other risk factors include young maternal age, low socioeconomic status, nulliparity, and preexisting infections of the lower genital tract (Duff & Birsner, 2017).

Women with chorioamnionitis can develop bacteremia. They are also more likely to have dysfunctional labor, which can result in the need for cesarean birth (see later discussion). If cesarean birth is necessary, wound infection or pelvic abscess are complications that can occur (Duff & Birsner, 2017).

Neonatal risks include pneumonia, bacteremia, and meningitis. Death is more likely to occur in preterm than in term infants (Duff & Birsner, 2017). There is increasing evidence that intrauterine infection is associated with increased risks for respiratory distress syndrome, periventricular leukomalacia, and cerebral palsy. It is thought that intrauterine infection leads to fetal infection that eventually produces a fetal inflammatory response syndrome with resulting pulmonary and central nervous system damage (Duff, 2014).

In order to prevent maternal and neonatal complications, prompt treatment with intravenous broad-spectrum antibiotics and birth of the fetus are necessary. Ampicillin or penicillin and gentamicin are the antibiotics most often used to treat chorioamnionitis during labor. After cesarean birth, an antibiotic that provides coverage for anaerobic organisms, such as clindamycin (Cleocin) or metronidazole (Flagyl) should be added (Duff & Birsner, 2017; Duff, 2014). One additional dose of a combination of broad-spectrum antibiotics (e.g. ampicillin and gentamicin) given postpartum is usually sufficient treatment for women with chorioamnionitis (Duff).

The increased use of intrapartum antibiotic prophylaxis during labor in women who are group B streptococci (GBS) positive to prevent neonatal GBS infection has decreased the incidence of chorioamnionitis. Other measures that have proven to be effective in decreasing the frequency of chorioamnionitis are active management of labor (see later discussion), induction of labor, rather than expectant management, following rupture of membranes at term, and use of prophylactic antibiotics in selected women with preterm PROM (Duff, 2014).

POSTTERM PREGNANCY, LABOR, AND BIRTH

A postterm pregnancy (also sometimes referred to as a *postmature* or *prolonged pregnancy,* is one that reaches 42 0/7 weeks of gestation or more (ACOG & Society for Maternal-Fetal Medicine [SMFM], 2013/2015).

According to the Centers for Disease Control and Prevention, less than 0.5% of all births in the United States were postterm in 2015, a percentage that essentially has not changed for the past several years (Martin et al., 2017). Many pregnancies are misdiagnosed as postterm. The use of first-trimester ultrasound for pregnancy dating has confirmed that the first day of the LMP, traditionally used for pregnancy dating, is much less reliable as a predictor of true gestational age. Therefore, use of the LMP alone for pregnancy dating tends to greatly overestimate the number of postterm gestations (Rampersad & Macones, 2017).

The exact cause of true postterm pregnancy is still unknown. However, it is clear that the timing of labor is determined by complex interactions among the mother, fetus, and placenta. For example, placental sulfatase deficiency causes low estrogen production. Women with this disorder generally do not go into spontaneous labor. This is an example of a genetic cause for postterm pregnancy that supports the important role of the placenta in labor initiation. Risk factors for postterm pregnancy include a first pregnancy, prior postterm pregnancy, a male fetus, obesity, and a genetic predisposition (Rampersad & Macones, 2017).

Clinical manifestations of postterm pregnancy include maternal weight loss (more than 1.4 kg [approximately 3 lb]/week) and decreased uterine size (related to decreased amniotic fluid), meconium in the amniotic fluid, and advanced bone maturation of the fetal skeleton with an exceptionally hard fetal skull.

MATERNAL AND FETAL RISKS

A number of factors related to postterm pregnancy, including labor dystocia, severe perineal injuries, chorioamnionitis, endomyometritis, postpartum hemorrhage, and cesarean birth are associated with significant maternal risk for morbidity during the intrapartum period (Rampersad & Macones, 2017; Sheibani & Wing, 2017). Each intervention, such as induction of labor with prostaglandins or oxytocin, forceps- or vacuum-assisted birth, and cesarean birth, carries its own set of risks. The woman also may experience fatigue, physical discomfort, and psychologic reactions such as anxiety, depression, frustration, and feelings of inadequacy as she passes her estimated date of birth. Relationships with close friends and family members may become strained, and the woman's negative feelings about herself may be projected as feelings of resentment toward the fetus.

Another complication associated with postterm pregnancy is abnormal fetal growth. Although the risk for having a small for gestational age (SGA) infant is increased, only 10% to 20% of postterm fetuses are undernourished. The risk for macrosomia increases as gestational age advances. Macrosomia occurs when the placenta continues to provide adequate nutrients to support fetal growth after 40 weeks of gestation. Macrosomic infants have an increased risk for operative birth and shoulder dystocia, leading to fetal injury (Rampersad & Macones, 2017).

Other fetal risks associated with postterm gestation are related to the intrauterine environment. Decreased amniotic fluid, or *oligohydramnios*, is a common finding in postterm pregnancy. Because of the decreased amount of amniotic fluid, there is a potential for cord compression and resulting hypoxemia. Other potential complications include meconium-stained amniotic fluid and increased risk for meconium aspiration (Rampersad & Macones, 2017).

Postmaturity syndrome occurs in 10% to 20% of neonates born following postterm pregnancies. The postmature infant has decreased subcutaneous fat and lacks lanugo and vernix. Other characteristics of postmature infants include dry, cracked, peeling skin; long nails; and meconium staining of skin, nails, and umbilical cord (see Chapter 25) (Rampersad & Macones, 2017).

Care Management

Because of the increased risk for stillbirth, antepartum fetal assessment beginning at 41 0/7 weeks of gestation may be considered (ACOG, 2014/2016). There are several options for performing fetal surveillance, including the NST, contraction stress test (CST), BPP, or modified BPP. Once begun, fetal assessment is usually performed once or twice per week for the remainder of the pregnancy. Data are not sufficient to make a recommendation regarding the best assessment test or the optimal frequency of testing (ACOG, 2014/2016) (see Chapter 10 for a discussion of these tests). If the cervix is favorable, labor can be induced at 41 weeks of gestation. Studies have shown a significantly increased rate of perinatal mortality after 41 weeks of gestation (Sheibani & Wing, 2017). Currently it is recommended that birth occur after 42 0/7 weeks and by 42 6/7 weeks of gestation to decrease the risk for perinatal morbidity and mortality (ACOG, 2014/2016; Rampersad & Macones, 2017).

During the postterm period, the woman is encouraged to assess fetal activity daily, assess for signs of labor, and keep appointments with her obstetric health care provider (see Patient Teaching box: Postterm Pregnancy). The woman and her family should be encouraged to express their feelings (e.g., frustration, anger, impatience, fear) about the prolonged pregnancy and helped to realize that these feelings are normal. At times, the emotional and physical strain of a postterm pregnancy can seem overwhelming. Referral to a support group or another supportive resource may be needed.

During labor, the fetus of a woman with a postterm pregnancy should be continuously monitored electronically to accurately assess the FHR and pattern. The aging placenta in a woman with a postterm pregnancy can produce disruption in oxygen transfer to the fetus during contractions, resulting in late decelerations caused by transient fetal hypoxemia. Inadequate amniotic fluid volume, often noted in women with postterm pregnancy, can lead to compression of the umbilical cord, which results in fetal hypoxemia that is reflected in variable or prolonged deceleration patterns. If oligohydramnios is present, an amnioinfusion may be performed to restore amniotic fluid volume to maintain a cushioning of the cord. See Chapter 15 for additional information on causes and management of these FHR decelerations.

DYSFUNCTIONAL LABOR (DYSTOCIA)

Dystocia refers to a lack of progress in labor for any reason (Kilpatrick & Garrison, 2017). Dysfunctional labor is defined as a long, difficult, or abnormal labor. Dysfunctional labor is responsible for approximately 60% of all cesarean births in the United States (Cunningham, Leveno, Bloom, et al., 2014) and is the most common indication for primary cesarean birth (ACOG & SMFM, 2014). It can be caused by any of the following factors (Cunningham et al.):

- Ineffective uterine contractions or maternal bearing-down efforts (the powers)
- Fetal causes, including abnormalities of presentation, position, or development (the passenger)

- Alterations in the pelvic structure, including abnormalities of the maternal bony pelvis or soft-tissue abnormalities of the reproductive tract (the passage)

These factors are interdependent. Each may exist alone or in combination with others. In assessing the woman for an abnormal labor pattern, the nurse must consider the ways in which these factors interact and influence labor progress. Dysfunctional labor is suspected when there is an alteration in the characteristics of uterine contractions, a lack of progress in the rate of cervical dilation, or a lack of progress in fetal descent and expulsion.

ABNORMAL UTERINE ACTIVITY

Abnormal uterine activity can occur throughout first-stage labor. Ineffective contractions that are either hypertonic or hypotonic can result from abnormal uterine activity. Common labor disorders caused by abnormal uterine activity are discussed next.

Latent Phase Disorders

A common labor disorder that occurs during the latent phase of first-stage labor is *hypertonic uterine dysfunction.* The woman experiencing hypertonic uterine dysfunction, or primary dysfunctional labor, often is an anxious first-time mother who is having painful and frequent contractions that are ineffective in causing cervical dilation or effacement to progress. These contractions usually occur in the latent phase of first-stage labor (cervical dilation of <6 cm) and are usually uncoordinated. The force of the contractions may be in the midsection of the uterus rather than in the fundus; therefore the uterus cannot apply downward pressure to push the presenting part against the cervix. The uterus may not relax completely between contractions. Some women can spend days in protracted latent labor.

Women with hypertonic uterine dysfunction may be exhausted and express concern about loss of control because of the intense pain they are experiencing and the lack of progress. They can be managed expectantly, because most women will eventually enter the active phase of labor. Another management approach is to provide therapeutic rest, which is achieved with a warm bath or shower and an analgesic, such as morphine, to inhibit uterine contractions, reduce pain, and encourage sleep (Sheibani & Wing, 2017). In the absence of pain, zolpidem (Ambien) may be used to facilitate rest and sleep. After several hours of rest, these women are likely to awaken in active labor with a normal uterine contraction pattern.

Active Phase Disorders

Active-phase labor disorders can be divided into either *protraction disorders,* where progress in labor is slower than normal, or *arrest disorders,* where there is no progress in labor (ACOG & SMFM, 2014; Sheibani & Wing, 2017). The most common cause of an active-phase protraction disorder is inadequate uterine activity *(hypotonic uterine dysfunction)* (Sheibani & Wing). The woman initially makes normal progress into the active phase of first-stage labor, but then the contractions become weak and inefficient or stop altogether. The uterus is easily indented, even at the peak of contractions. Intrauterine pressure (IUP) during the contraction (usually less than 25 mm Hg) is insufficient for progress of cervical effacement and dilation. Cephalopelvic disproportion (CPD) (see later discussion) and fetal malposition are other common causes of active-phase labor protraction disorders. Examples of fetal malposition are an extended (rather than flexed) fetal head, brow or face presentation, and occiput posterior presentation (Sheibani & Wing, 2017).

Evaluation of arrest during the first stage of labor includes an assessment of uterine activity using an intrauterine pressure catheter (IUPC) (see Chapter 15 for more information on the IUPC). Fetal presentation, position, station, and estimated fetal weight must also be

TABLE 17.1 Dysfunctional Labor: Primary and Secondary Powers

PRIMARY POWERS (ABNORMAL UTERINE ACTIVITY)		SECONDARY POWERS
Hypertonic Uterine Dysfunction	Hypotonic Uterine Dysfunction	Inadequate Voluntary Expulsive Forces
Description		
Usually occurs in latent-phase labor; cause unknown, may be related to fear and tension	Cause is usually cephalopelvic disproportion or fetal malposition	Involves abdominal and levator ani muscles Occurs in second stage of labor; cause may be related to nerve block anesthetic, analgesia, exhaustion
Change in Pattern of Progress		
Pain out of proportion to intensity of contractions and to effectiveness of contractions in effacing and dilating the cervix Contractions increase in frequency and are uncoordinated Uterus is contracted between contractions, cannot be indented	Contractions decrease in frequency and intensity Uterus easily indented even at peak of contractions Uterus relaxed between contractions (normal)	No voluntary urge to push or bear down or inadequate or ineffective pushing
Potential Maternal Effects		
Loss of control related to intensity of pain and lack of progress Exhaustion Fear regarding unexpected nature of labor	Infection Exhaustion Stress regarding change in progress	Spontaneous vaginal birth prevented; assisted birth likely
Potential Fetal Effects		
Fetal asphyxia with meconium aspiration	Fetal infection Fetal and neonatal death	Fetal asphyxia
Care Management		
Initiate therapeutic rest measures Administer analgesic (e.g., morphine) if membranes are intact and pelvic adequacy is confirmed Relieve pain to permit mother to rest Assist with measures to enhance rest and relaxation (e.g., hydrotherapy, massage, music, distracting activities)	Rule out cephalopelvic disproportion Augment labor with oxytocin (Pitocin) Perform amniotomy Assist with measures to enhance the progress of labor (e.g., position changes, ambulation, hydrotherapy)	Coach mother in bearing down with contractions; assist with relaxation between contractions Position mother in favorable position for pushing Reduce epidural infusion rate Assist with forceps- or vacuum-assisted birth Prepare for cesarean birth if abnormal fetal status occurs

evaluated. If findings are normal, labor augmentation measures may be implemented (e.g., ambulation, hydrotherapy, rupture of membranes, nipple stimulation, or oxytocin infusion). Most women respond to these interventions by resuming progression of cervical dilation and are able to give birth vaginally (Sheibani & Wing, 2017).

SECONDARY POWERS

Secondary powers, or bearing-down efforts, are compromised when large amounts of analgesic medications are given. Anesthesia may also block the bearing-down reflex and, as a result, alter the effectiveness of voluntary bearing-down efforts. Exhaustion resulting from lack of sleep or long labor and fatigue resulting from inadequate hydration and food intake reduce the effectiveness of the woman's voluntary bearing-down efforts. Maternal position can work against the forces of gravity and decrease the strength and efficiency of the contractions. Table 17.1 summarizes the characteristics of dysfunctional labor.

ABNORMAL LABOR PATTERNS

Six abnormal labor patterns were identified and classified by Friedman (1989) decades ago according to the nature of the cervical dilation and fetal descent. These patterns are (1) prolonged latent phase, (2) protracted active-phase dilation, (3) secondary arrest: no change, (4) protracted descent, (5) arrest of descent, and (6) failure of descent. These patterns may result from a variety of causes, including ineffective uterine contractions, pelvic contractures, CPD, abnormal fetal presentation or position, early use of analgesics, nerve block analgesia or anesthesia, and anxiety and stress. If a woman exhibits an abnormal labor pattern, the obstetric health care provider should be notified.

Maternal morbidity and mortality from uterine rupture, infection, severe dehydration, and postpartum hemorrhage are higher for women experiencing dysfunctional labor. The fetus is at increased risk for hypoxia. A long and difficult labor also can have an adverse psychologic effect on the mother, father, and family.

Studies done within the past 2 decades indicate that the contemporary pattern of labor progression is different from what Friedman observed in the 1950s. In general, modern labor progresses at a slower rate for both nulliparous and multiparous women. The active labor phase now begins at 6 cm cervical dilation and lasts twice as long as Friedman described. It is common for more than 2 hours to pass in the active phase of labor without cervical dilation. Maternal characteristics have changed considerably since Friedman's work was published. In general, women giving birth now are older and heavier, and both of these factors are associated with longer labors. Clinical guidelines incorporating this new information are being developed by organizations such as ACOG and SMFM to assist health care providers in managing contemporary labor and birth (ACOG & SMFM, 2014).

PRECIPITOUS LABOR

Precipitous labor is defined as labor that lasts less than 3 hours from the onset of contractions to the time of birth. This abnormal labor pattern occurs in approximately 2% of all births in the United States. Precipitous birth alone is usually not associated with significant maternal or infant morbidity or mortality (Cunningham et al., 2014).

Precipitous labor may result from hypertonic uterine contractions that are tetanic in intensity. Conditions often associated with this type of uterine contractions include placental abruption, uterine tachysystole, and recent cocaine use. Maternal complications can include uterine rupture, lacerations of the birth canal, amniotic fluid embolus (anaphylactoid syndrome of pregnancy), and postpartum hemorrhage. Fetal complications include hypoxia caused by decreased periods of uterine relaxation between contractions, and, in rare instances, intracranial trauma related to rapid birth (Cunningham et al., 2014).

Women who have experienced precipitous labor often describe feelings of disbelief that their labor began so quickly, alarm that their labor progressed so rapidly, panic about the possibility they would not make it to the hospital in time to give birth, and finally, relief when they arrived at the hospital. In addition, women have expressed frustration when nurses did not believe them when they reported their readiness to push. Progress can be so rapid in some women that they may have difficulty remembering the details of their labor and birth. They should be provided with an opportunity to discuss their labor and birth experiences with caregivers who were present.

ALTERATIONS IN PELVIC STRUCTURE

Pelvic Dystocia

Pelvic dystocia can occur whenever contractures of the pelvic diameters exist that reduce the capacity of the bony pelvis, including the inlet, the midpelvis, the outlet, or any combination of these planes. Pelvic contractures may be caused by congenital abnormalities, maternal malnutrition, neoplasms, or lower spinal disorders. An immature pelvic size predisposes some adolescent mothers to pelvic dystocia. Pelvic deformities also may be the result of vehicular or other accidents or trauma.

Soft-Tissue Dystocia

Soft-tissue dystocia results from obstruction of the birth passage by an anatomic abnormality other than that involving the bony pelvis. The obstruction may result from placenta previa (low-lying placenta) that partially or completely obstructs the internal cervical os. Other causes, such as leiomyomas (uterine fibroids) in the lower uterine segment, ovarian tumors, and a full bladder or rectum, may prevent the fetus from entering the pelvis. Occasionally cervical edema occurs during labor when the cervix is caught between the presenting part and the symphysis pubis or when the woman begins bearing-down efforts prematurely, thereby inhibiting complete dilation. Sexually transmitted infections (e.g., human papillomavirus) can alter cervical tissue integrity and thus interfere with adequate effacement and dilation.

FETAL CAUSES

Dystocia of fetal origin may be caused by anomalies, excessive fetal size (macrosomia), malpresentation, malposition, or multifetal pregnancy.

Complications associated with dystocia of fetal origin include neonatal asphyxia, fetal injuries or fractures, and maternal vaginal lacerations. Although spontaneous vaginal birth is possible in these instances, a forceps-assisted, vacuum-assisted, or cesarean birth often is necessary.

Anomalies

Gross ascites, large tumors, open neural tube defects (e.g., myelomeningocele), and hydrocephalus are examples of fetal anomalies that can cause dystocia. The anomalies affect the relationship of the fetal anatomy to the maternal pelvic capacity, with the result that the fetus cannot descend through the pelvis and birth canal.

Cephalopelvic Disproportion

Cephalopelvic disproportion (CPD), also called *fetopelvic disproportion (FPD)*, is disproportion between the size of the fetus and the size of the mother's pelvis. With CPD, the fetus cannot fit through the maternal pelvis to be born vaginally. Although CPD is often related to excessive fetal size, or *macrosomia* (i.e., 4000 g or more), the problem in many cases is malposition of the fetal presenting part rather than true CPD (Sheibani & Wing, 2017). Fetal macrosomia is associated with maternal diabetes mellitus, obesity, multiparity, or the large size of one or both parents. If the maternal pelvis is too small, abnormally shaped, or deformed, CPD may be of maternal origin. In this case, the fetus may be of average size or even smaller. CPD cannot be accurately predicted (Sheibani & Wing).

Malposition

The most common fetal malposition is persistent occipitoposterior position (i.e., right occipitoposterior [ROP] or left occipitoposterior [LOP]; see Chapter 13). Labor, especially the second stage, is prolonged. The woman typically complains of severe back pain from the pressure of the fetal head (occiput) pressing against her sacrum. See Box 16.9 for suggested positions to relieve back pain and encourage rotation of the fetal occiput to an anterior position, which will facilitate birth.

Malpresentation

Malpresentation (the fetal presentation is something other than cephalic, or head first) is another commonly reported complication of labor and birth. Breech presentation is the most common form of malpresentation, occurring in 3% to 4% of all labors. The three types of breech presentation are as follows (Lanni, Gherman, & Gonik, 2017) (Fig. 17.3):
- Frank breech (hips flexed, knees extended)
- Complete breech (hips and knees flexed)
- Footling breech (one or both hips are partially or fully extended). One foot [single footling] or both feet [double footling] present before the buttocks.

Breech presentations are associated with multifetal gestation, preterm birth, fetal and maternal anomalies, polyhydramnios, and oligohydramnios. High rates of breech presentation are also noted in fetuses with certain genetic disorders (e.g., trisomies 13, 18, and 21; Potter's syndrome [renal agenesis]; and myotonic dystrophy). Fetuses with neuromuscular disorders have a high rate of breech presentation, perhaps because they are less capable of movement within the uterus. Abnormal amniotic fluid volume (both increased and decreased) also contributes to more breech presentations because it affects fetal mobility. Breech presentation is diagnosed by abdominal palpation (e.g., Leopold maneuvers) and vaginal examination and confirmed by ultrasound scan (Lanni et al., 2017; Thorp & Laughon, 2014).

During labor, the descent of the fetus in a breech presentation may be slow because the breech is not as effective a dilating wedge as is the fetal head. There is risk for prolapse of the cord if the membranes rupture in early labor. The presence of meconium in amniotic fluid is not necessarily a sign of fetal distress because it results from pressure on the fetal abdominal wall as it travels through the birth canal. Assessment of FHR and pattern should be used to determine whether the passage of meconium is an expected finding associated with breech presentation or is an abnormal sign associated with fetal hypoxia. In a breech presentation, fetal heart tones (FHTs) are best heard at or above the umbilicus.

Vaginal birth is accomplished by mechanisms of labor that manipulate the buttocks and lower extremities as they emerge from the birth canal (Fig. 17.4). Risks associated with vaginal birth from a breech presentation

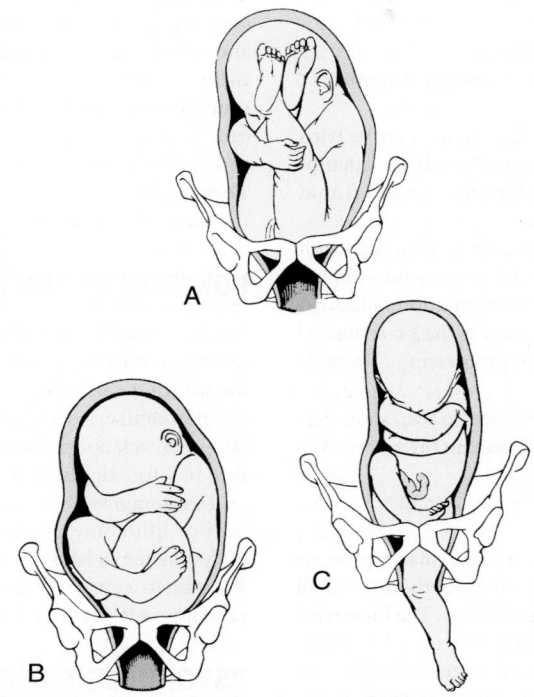

FIG 17.3 Breech presentation. **A,** Frank breech. **B,** Complete breech. **C,** Single footling breech. (From Gilbert, E. [2011]. *Manual of high risk pregnancy & delivery* [5th ed.]. St. Louis, MO: Mosby.)

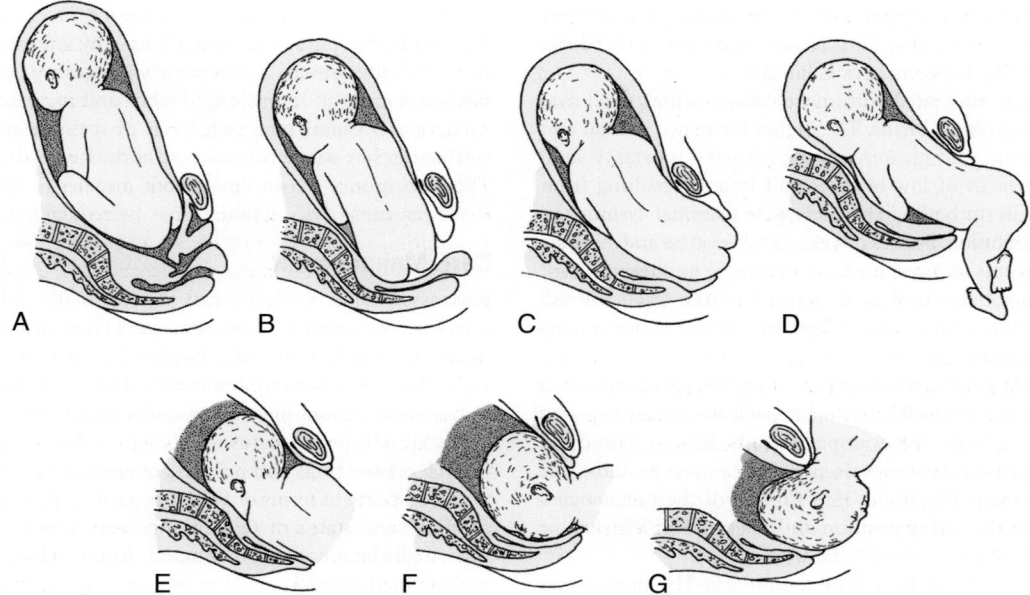

FIG 17.4 Mechanism of labor in breech presentation. **A,** Breech before onset of labor. **B,** Engagement and internal rotation. **C,** Lateral flexion. **D,** External rotation or restitution. **E,** Internal rotation of shoulders and head. **F,** Face rotates to sacrum when occiput is anterior. **G,** Head is born by gradual flexion during elevation of fetal body.

include prolapse of the umbilical cord (especially in single or double footling breech presentations), trapping of the after-coming fetal head (especially with preterm infants), and trauma resulting from extension of the fetal head or nuchal position of the arms. Safe vaginal birth from a breech presentation is largely dependent on the experience, judgment, and skill of the health care provider who assists the birth. Criteria for attempting a vaginal birth from a breech presentation are as follows (Thorp & Laughon, 2014):

- Frank or complete breech presentation
- Estimated fetal weight between 2000 and 3800 g
- Normal (gynecoid) maternal pelvis with adequate measurements
- Flexed fetal head

External cephalic version (ECV) (see later discussion) may be tried to turn the fetus from a breech to a vertex presentation. If the attempt at ECV is unsuccessful, the woman usually gives birth by cesarean (Lanni et al., 2017).

Face and brow presentations are uncommon and are associated with fetal anomalies, pelvic contractures, and CPD. Spontaneous vaginal birth is possible if the fetus flexes to a vertex presentation, although forceps often are used. Cesarean birth is indicated if the presentation persists, if fetal distress occurs, or if labor stops progressing (Thorp & Laughon, 2014).

ECV may be attempted for a fetus in a transverse lie (i.e., shoulder) presentation after 36 to 37 weeks of gestation. Cesarean birth is usually necessary, however (Thorp & Laughon, 2014).

Multifetal Pregnancy

Multifetal pregnancy is the gestation of twins, triplets, quadruplets, or more infants. Multiple gestations now account for more than 3% of all live births in the United States (Malone & D'Alton, 2014). The increasing number of twin gestations has been attributed to the use of fertility-enhancing medications and procedures and the older age of childbearing women. When compared with younger women, those 35 years of age and older are naturally more likely to have a multifetal pregnancy. The rate of triplet and higher-order multiple pregnancies peaked at an all-time high rate of 193.5 per 100,000 in 1998. Since then, the rate has generally trended downward. The decrease has been attributed to refinements in the treatments used for infertility, particularly limiting the number of embryos transferred during in vitro fertilization (IVF) procedures (Malone & D'Alton, 2014; Newman & Unal, 2017).

Multiple births are associated with more complications (e.g., dysfunctional labor) than single births. The higher incidence of fetal and newborn complications and greater risk for perinatal mortality stem primarily from the birth of low-birth-weight infants resulting from preterm birth or IUGR (or both), in part related to placental dysfunction and twin-to-twin transfusion. Fetuses can experience distress and asphyxia during the birth process as a result of cord prolapse and the onset of placental separation with the birth of the first fetus. As a result, the risk for long-term problems such as cerebral palsy is higher among infants who were part of a multiple birth.

In addition, fetal complications such as congenital anomalies and abnormal presentations can result in dysfunctional labor and an increased incidence of cesarean birth. For example, in only 40% to 45% of all twin pregnancies do both fetuses present in the vertex position, the most favorable for vaginal birth. In 35% to 40% of the pregnancies, one twin presents in the vertex position and the other in a breech or transverse lie presentation (Malone & D'Alton, 2014).

The health status of the mother can be compromised by an increased risk for hypertension, anemia, and hemorrhage associated with uterine atony, placental abruption, and multiple or adherent placentas. Duration of the phases and stages of labor can vary from the duration experienced with singleton births.

Teamwork and planning are essential components of the management of childbirth in multifetal pregnancies, especially those of higher-order multiples. The nurse plays a key role in coordinating the activities of the interprofessional health care team. Early detection and management of the maternal, fetal, and newborn complications associated with multiple births are essential to achieve a positive outcome for mother and babies. Maternal positioning and active support are used to enhance labor progress and placental perfusion. Stimulation of labor with oxytocin, epidural anesthesia, internal or external version, and forceps and vacuum assistance may be used to accomplish the vaginal birth of twins. Cesarean birth is almost always performed with higher-order multiple births. Each infant will have its own interprofessional health care team present at the birth. Nurses provide important emotional support to women and their families to help reduce anxiety and stress. They explain events as they occur and offer updates on the status of the mother and infants.

POSITION OF THE WOMAN

The functional relationship among the uterine contractions, the fetus, and the mother's pelvis are altered by the maternal position. In addition, the position can provide a mechanical advantage or disadvantage to the mechanisms of labor by altering the effects of gravity and the body-part relationships that are important to the progress of labor. See Box 16.9 for suggested positions to enhance fetal descent.

Discouraging maternal movement or restricting labor to the recumbent or lithotomy position can compromise progress. The incidence of dysfunctional labor in women confined to these positions is increased, resulting in a greater need for augmentation of labor or forceps-assisted, vacuum-assisted, or cesarean birth.

PSYCHOLOGIC RESPONSES

Hormones and neurotransmitters released in response to stress (e.g., catecholamines) can cause dysfunctional labor. Sources of stress vary for each woman, but pain and the absence of a support person are often related to dysfunctional labor. Confinement to bed and restriction of maternal movement can be a source of psychologic stress that compounds the physiologic stress caused by immobility in the unmedicated laboring woman. When anxiety is excessive, it can inhibit cervical dilation and result in prolonged labor and increased pain perception. Anxiety also causes increased levels of stress-related hormones (e.g., beta-endorphin, adrenocorticotropic hormone, cortisol, and epinephrine). These hormones act on the smooth muscles of the uterus. Increased levels can cause dysfunctional labor by reducing uterine contractility.

Care Management

Risk assessment is a continual process in the laboring woman. By reviewing the woman's history of past labor or labors and observing her physical and psychologic responses to the current labor, any factors that might contribute to dysfunctional labor should be identified. The initial and ongoing physical assessments provide information about maternal well-being; status of labor in terms of the characteristics of uterine contractions and progress of cervical effacement and dilation; fetal well-being in terms of FHR and pattern, presentation, station, and position; and status of the amniotic membranes. Nursing diagnoses that might be identified in women experiencing dysfunctional labor include the following:

- *Risk for Injury* to mother or fetus related to
  - interventions implemented for dystocia
- *Powerlessness* related to
  - loss of control

- *Ineffective Coping* related to
  - inadequate support system
  - exhaustion secondary to a prolonged labor process
  - pain
- *Risk for Impaired Parenting* related to
  - separation from infant associated with emergency cesarean birth
  - emotional responses to a traumatic childbirth experience

Nursing diagnoses, expected outcomes of care, and interventions are established for each woman based on assessment findings. Many interventions for dysfunctional labor (e.g., ECV, cervical ripening, induction or augmentation of labor, and operative procedures [forceps- or vacuum-assisted birth, cesarean birth]) are implemented collaboratively with other members of the interprofessiosnal health care team. Commonly performed interventions are discussed in detail in the Obstetric Procedures section later in the chapter. Nursing interventions are identified with each procedure.

When providing care for a woman who is experiencing labor or birth complications, all members of the health care team are responsible for complying with professional standards of care. This promotes patient safety and helps improve outcomes.

OBESITY

Excessive weight is an increasingly serious problem for children, adolescents, and adults living in affluent nations, including the United States, and pregnant women are no exception. The body mass index (BMI) is used to define obesity. Persons with a BMI of 25 or greater are categorized as overweight, whereas those with a BMI of 30 or greater are considered obese. Individuals with a BMI of 40 or greater are classified as severely or morbidly obese (Baird, Kennedy, & Dalton, 2017; Picklesimer & Dorman, 2013).

Obese women are likely to begin pregnancy with preexisting medical conditions such as chronic hypertension and type 2 diabetes. While pregnant, they can develop pregnancy-associated hypertensive disorders, or gestational diabetes may be diagnosed. Obese women also have an increased incidence of postterm pregnancy. All of these risk factors can increase the likelihood that labor will be induced (Picklesimer & Dorman, 2013). In addition to an increased risk for cesarean birth in general, obese women are also more likely to require emergency cesarean birth. During the postpartum period they are at risk for thromboembolism and wound disruption and infection after cesarean birth (Picklesimer & Dorman). Obese women also have a higher risk for postpartum hemorrhage because of an increased likelihood of induction, resulting in prolonged labor, birth of a macrosomic infant, and caregiver difficulty with locating the uterine fundus to provide effective fundal massage (Baird et al., 2017).

Care Management

Nursing care of obese women during labor and birth is challenging for a number of reasons. Sometimes standard furniture such as beds, chairs, and operating tables is simply not large enough to accommodate the woman's size. Extra-large furniture may not fit through a standard doorway, so room renovation may be necessary. Some hospitals have created rooms specifically designed to accommodate obese patients (Fig. 17.5). Continuous external FHR and contraction monitoring may be extremely difficult if not impossible to perform. Special equipment, such as extra-large blood pressure cuffs, is necessary to properly assess the woman's condition.

Even routine procedures require more time and effort to accomplish when a woman is obese. This can slow essential interventions and increase risks to the mother and fetus, such as when an emergency cesarean birth is necessary. Establishing intravenous access, for example, may require

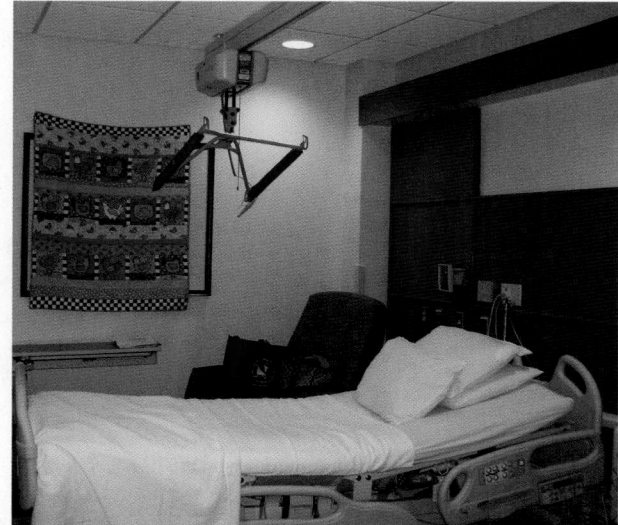

FIG 17.5 Room specifically designed to accommodate obese pregnant patients. Note lift attached to ceiling for use in transferring women from the bed to chairs or stretchers. (Courtesy of Dee Lowdermilk, Chapel Hill, NC.)

multiple attempts, sometimes by multiple people. Mobility is often a problem. Moving the woman from a labor room to the operating room and transferring her from a bed to the operating table can require the assistance of additional personnel or special equipment, especially if regional anesthesia is already in effect. If it is not, surgery may be further delayed by anesthetic complications, such as difficulty establishing an epidural or spinal block or accomplishing endotracheal intubation.

Postoperatively, obese women are at increased risk for blood clot formation. In the immediate recovery period, use of thromboembolic deterrent anti-embolism stockings (TED hose) and sequential compression devices (SCD boots) helps decrease the chance for thrombus formation. Some women may also be given heparin prophylactically to prevent thromboembolism (Simpson & O'Brien-Abel, 2014). In the postpartum period, women should also be encouraged to get out of bed and begin ambulating as soon as possible.

Keeping the incision clean and dry to prevent wound infection and promote healing is another postoperative challenge. Many obese women have a *pannus* (large roll of abdominal fat) that overlies a lower abdominal transverse skin incision made just above the pubic area. The pannus causes the area to remain moist, which encourages infection development. Women should be taught to wash the incision with soap and water several times a day, thoroughly drying the area afterward. Using a handheld hair dryer on a low setting works well for this purpose. Sutures or staples used to close the skin incision are generally left in place longer than usual to avoid possible wound disruption when they are removed. Sometimes the skin and subcutaneous layers of the incision are left open to heal by secondary intention to avoid possible dehiscence. If this course of action is chosen, the woman and other family members must be taught to do dressing changes and wound care.

OBSTETRIC PROCEDURES

VERSION

Version is the turning of the fetus from one presentation to another. It may be performed externally or internally by the health care provider.

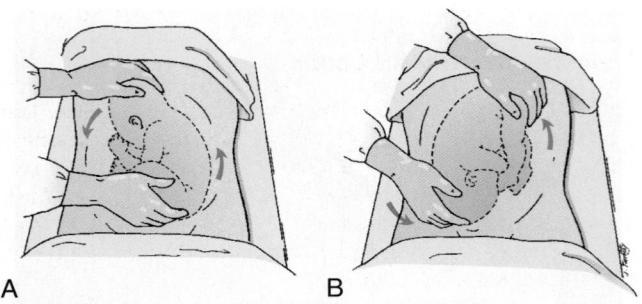

FIG 17.6 External version of fetus from breech to vertex presentation. This must be achieved without force. **A,** Breech is pushed up out of pelvic inlet while head is pulled toward inlet. **B,** Head is pushed toward inlet while breech is pulled upward.

External Cephalic Version

External cephalic version (ECV) is used in an attempt to turn the fetus from a breech or shoulder presentation to a vertex presentation for birth. It may be attempted in a labor and birth setting at 36 to 37 weeks of gestation. ECV is accomplished by the exertion of gentle, constant pressure on the abdomen (Fig. 17.6) (Lanni et al., 2017). At this gestational age, the success rate for ECV is approximately 65% and the risk for cesarean birth is reduced by 50% (Thorp & Laughon, 2014). Therefore, ECV should be offered and performed whenever possible as one strategy to safely lower the primary cesarean birth rate (ACOG & SMFM, 2014).

Before ECV is attempted, ultrasound scanning is done for the following reasons (Thorp & Laughon, 2014):
- To confirm the breech presentation
- To detect multiple gestation, oligohydramnios, or fetal abnormalities
- To measure fetal dimensions

An NST is performed to confirm fetal well-being, or the FHR and pattern are monitored for a period of time (i.e., 10 to 20 minutes). Informed consent is obtained. A tocolytic agent such as terbutaline often is given to relax the uterus and facilitate the maneuver. ECV is sometimes performed under regional anesthesia (Lanni et al., 2017; Thorp & Laughon, 2014).

Contraindications to ECV include the following (Thorp & Laughon, 2014):
- Uterine anomalies
- Third-trimester bleeding
- Multiple gestation
- Oligohydramnios
- Evidence of uteroplacental insufficiency
- A nuchal cord (identified by ultrasound)
- Previous cesarean birth or other significant uterine surgery
- Obvious CPD

ECV is most successful in a nonobese multiparous woman who has an abundant amount of amniotic fluid, and whose fetus is not yet engaged in the pelvis, and the estimated fetal weight is 2500 to 3000 g (Cunningham et al., 2014). The procedure should be performed in a hospital equipped to provide emergency surgery because 1% to 2% of women who have ECV develop placental abruption or umbilical cord compression requiring immediate cesarean birth (Thorp & Laughon, 2014).

During an attempted ECV, the nurse continuously monitors the FHR and pattern, especially for bradycardia and variable decelerations; checks the maternal vital signs; and assesses the woman's level of comfort because the procedure can be painful. After the procedure is completed, the nurse continues to monitor maternal vital signs and uterine activity and to assess for vaginal bleeding until the woman's condition is determined to be stable. FHR and pattern monitoring should continue for at least 1 hour. Women who are Rh negative should receive Rh immune globulin because the manipulation can cause fetomaternal bleeding (Thorp & Laughon, 2014).

Internal Version

With internal version, the fetus is turned by the health care provider, who inserts a hand into the uterus and changes the presentation to cephalic (head) or podalic (foot). Internal version is only rarely used, most often in twin gestations to assist with the birth of the second fetus. The safety of this procedure has not been documented; maternal and fetal injury is possible. Cesarean birth is the usual method for managing malpresentation in multifetal pregnancies. The nurse's role is to monitor the status of the fetus and to provide support to the woman.

INDUCTION OF LABOR

Induction of labor is the chemical or mechanical initiation of uterine contractions before their spontaneous onset for the purpose of bringing about birth. Labor may be induced either electively or for indicated reasons. Induction of labor is one of the most commonly performed obstetric procedures in the United States. Approximately 24% of term births (infants born between 37 and 41 weeks of gestation) result from labors that were induced (Hill & Harvey, 2013). It is likely that the rate of elective inductions is increasing more rapidly than the rate of indicated inductions (Thorp & Laughon, 2014).

Induction of labor is indicated if continuing the pregnancy could be dangerous for either the woman or the fetus, and if no contraindications exist to artificial rupture of the membranes (amniotomy) or augmenting uterine contractions with oxytocin. Prior to labor induction, gestational age should be determined and any potential risks to the maternal-fetal unit evaluated. Women must be fully counseled regarding risks, benefits, and alternatives of labor stimulation methods as part of the process for informed consent (ACOG, 2009/2016; Thorp & Laughon, 2014). Box 17.7 lists indications and contraindications for labor induction.

Elective Induction of Labor

An elective induction is one in which labor is initiated without a medical indication. Methods to ripen the cervix (e.g., application of prostaglandins or intracervical insertion of a balloon catheter) enhance the likelihood of successful induction. Many elective inductions are purely for the convenience of the woman or her obstetric health care provider. At times, however, labor may be electively induced to allay maternal fears and anxieties associated with prior perinatal losses or to ensure that an experienced interprofessional health care team is available to handle anticipated maternal or neonatal complications immediately following birth (Sheibani & Wing, 2017; Yount & Lassiter, 2013).

To prevent iatrogenic prematurity, elective induction of labor should not be initiated until the woman reaches 39 completed weeks of gestation (ACOG, 2009/2016). Information to educate pregnant women and their families about the dangers of early-term births is available from the March of Dimes (www.marchofdimes.com/pregnancy/getready_at least39weeks.html) and the Association of Women's Health, Obstetric and Neonatal Nurses (AWHONN) (www.gothefull40.com).

Birth data from the United States for 2015 indicate that the percentage of infants born early term (37 to 38 weeks) rose 2% from 2014 to 2015, from 24.76% to 24.99%, and the full-term birth rate declined slightly, from 58.72% to 58.47%. From 2007 to 2014, the early-term birth rate

BOX 17.7   Indications and Contraindications for Labor Induction

Maternal Indications

- Hypertensive complications of pregnancy: gestational hypertension, pre-eclampsia, eclampsia
- Fetal death
- Chorioamnionitis

Fetal Indications

Any condition in which a variety of fetal tests demonstrate significant fetal jeopardy in any of the following situations:

- Diabetes
- Postterm pregnancy, especially when oligohydramnios is present
- Hypertensive complications of pregnancy
- Intrauterine growth restriction
- Isoimmunization
- Chorioamnionitis
- Premature rupture of membranes with established fetal maturity

Contraindications

- Acute, severe fetal distress
- Shoulder presentation (transverse lie)
- Floating fetal presenting part
- Uncontrolled hemorrhage
- Placenta previa
- Previous uterine incision that prohibits a trial of labor

Relative Contraindications

- Grand multiparity (five or more pregnancies that ended after 20 weeks of gestation)
- Multiple gestation
- Suspected cephalopelvic disproportion (CPD)
- Breech presentation
- Inability to adequately monitor the FHR throughout labor

Data from Thorp, J.M., & Laughon, S.K. (2014). Clinical aspects of normal and abnormal labor. In R.K. Creasy, R. Resnik, J.D. Iams, et al. (Eds.), *Creasy and Resnik's maternal-fetal medicine: Principles and practice* (7th ed.). Philadelphia, PA: Saunders.

COMMUNITY FOCUS

Elective Induction of Labor

Visit the March of Dimes website (www.marchofdimes.org), and download patient teaching materials regarding the importance of avoiding an elective early-term birth by waiting until at least 39 weeks of gestation for labor induction. Then talk with a woman who is 36 to 38 weeks pregnant. Ask if she wants to have her labor induced immediately. If so, what are her reasons? Share the information you obtained from the March of Dimes website with her. Were you able to change her mind?

TABLE 17.2   Bishop Score

	SCORE			
	0	1	2	3
Dilation (cm)	0	1–2	3–4	≥5
Effacement (%)	0–30	40–50	60–70	≥80
Station (cm)	−3	−2	−1, 0	+1, +2
Cervical consistency	Firm	Medium	Soft	Soft
Cervical position	Posterior	Midposition	Anterior	Anterior

Modified from Bishop, E.H. (1964). Pelvic scoring for elective induction. *Obstetrics and Gynecology, 24*(2), 266–268.

Cervical Ripening Methods

Chemical Agents

Preparations of prostaglandins E_1 (PGE_1) and E_2 (PGE_2) have been shown to be effective when used before induction to "ripen" (soften and thin) the cervix (see Medication Guides: Prostaglandin E_1 [PGE_1]: Misoprostol [Cytotec] and Prostaglandin E_2 [PGE_2]: Dinoprostone [Cervidil Insert; Prepidil Gel]) (Hill & Harvey, 2013). In some cases, women spontaneously begin laboring after the administration of prostaglandin, thereby eliminating the need to administer oxytocin to induce labor. Additional advantages of prostaglandin use for cervical ripening include decreased oxytocin induction time and a decrease in the amount of oxytocin required for successful induction (Sheibani & Wing, 2017). PGE_1, although much less expensive and more effective than PGE_2 for inducing labor and birth, is associated with a higher risk for uterine tachysystole with abnormal FHR and pattern changes and passage of meconium into the amniotic fluid. Most of these adverse outcomes are associated with higher-dose protocols (ACOG, 2009/2016; Sheibani & Wing). Although the drug's manufacturer has acknowledged for several years that PGE_1 is effective for cervical ripening and labor induction, it has not yet been approved by the FDA for these uses (Thorp & Laughon, 2014; Yount & Lassiter, 2013). ACOG, however, considers the use of PGE_1 for preinduction cervical ripening to be a safe and effective off-label use of the medication (Sheibani & Wing). PGE_2 in the form of a vaginal insert (dinoprostone [Cervidil]), although more expensive than PGE_1, has the major advantage of easy removal should adverse reactions, including uterine tachysystole, occur (Yount & Lassiter).

Mechanical and Physical Methods

Mechanical dilators ripen the cervix by stimulating the release of endogenous prostaglandins. Balloon catheters (e.g., Foley catheter) can be inserted through the intracervical canal to ripen and dilate the cervix. The catheter balloon is inflated above the internal cervical os with 30 to 50 mL of sterile water. This process results in pressure and stretching of the lower uterine segment and the cervix, as well as the release of

had generally been on the decline, and the full-term (39 weeks of gestation or more) rate had been on the rise. Reductions in early term births from 2007 through 2014 may have been related to heightened understanding of the increased neonatal risk at this gestational age compared with full term, and with subsequent recommendations and efforts to reduce nonmedically indicated births prior to 39 weeks (Martin et al., 2017) (see Community Focus box: Elective Induction of Labor).

Chemical, mechanical, physical, and alternative methods are used to ripen the cervix and induce labor. IV oxytocin (Pitocin) and amniotomy are the most common methods used in the United States. Success rates for induction of labor are higher when the condition of the cervix is favorable, or inducible. Cervical ripeness is the most important predictor of successful induction. A rating system such as the Bishop score (Table 17.2) can be used to evaluate inducibility. For example, a score of 8 or more on this 13-point scale indicates that the cervix is soft, anterior, 50% or more effaced, and dilated 2 cm or more and that the presenting part is engaged. When the Bishop score totals 8 or more, the likelihood of vaginal birth is similar whether labor is spontaneous or induced (Sheibani & Wing, 2017). The Bishop score should be documented prior to the use of methods to ripen the cervix or induce labor.

MEDICATION GUIDE

Prostaglandin E₁ (PGE₁): Misoprostol (Cytotec)

Action

PGE₁ ripens the cervix, making it softer and causing it to begin to dilate and efface; it stimulates uterine contractions.

Indications

- PGE₁ is used for preinduction cervical ripening (ripen the cervix before oxytocin induction of labor when the Bishop score is 4 or less) and to induce labor or abortion (abortifacient agent); it has not yet been approved by the FDA for cervical ripening or labor induction (i.e., this is an off-label use for obstetrics).
- It should not be used if the woman has a history of previous cesarean birth or other major uterine surgery.

Dosage and Administration

- Misoprostol is available either as a 100- or a 200-mcg tablet. Therefore, tablets must be broken to prepare the correct dose. This preparation should take place in the pharmacy to ensure accurate doses.
- Recommended initial dose is 25 mcg. Insert intravaginally into the posterior vaginal fornix using the tips of index and middle fingers without the use of a lubricant. Repeat every 4 hours or until an effective contraction pattern is established (three or more uterine contractions in 10 minutes), the cervix ripens (Bishop score of 8 or greater), or significant adverse effects occur.

Adverse Effects

Higher doses (e.g., 50 mcg every 6 hours) are more likely to result in adverse reactions such as nausea and vomiting, diarrhea, fever, uterine tachysystole with or without an abnormal FHR and pattern, or fetal passage of meconium. The risk for adverse reactions is reduced with lower dosages and longer intervals between doses.

Nursing Considerations

- Explain the procedure to the woman and her family; ensure that an informed consent has been obtained as per agency policy.
- Assess the woman and fetus before each insertion and during treatment following agency protocol for frequency. Assess maternal vital signs and health status, FHR and pattern, and status of pregnancy, including indications for cervical ripening or induction of labor, signs of labor or impending labor, and the Bishop score. Recognize that an abnormal FHR and pattern; maternal fever, infection, vaginal bleeding, or hypersensitivity; and regular, progressive uterine contractions contraindicate the use of misoprostol.
- Avoid giving aluminum hydroxide and magnesium-containing antacids along with misoprostol.
- Use with caution in women with renal failure because the medication is eliminated through the kidneys.
- Have the woman void before insertion.
- Assist the woman to maintain a supine position with a lateral tilt or a side-lying position for 30 to 40 minutes after insertion.
- Prepare to (1) swab the vagina to remove unabsorbed medication using a saline-soaked gauze wrapped around fingers or (2) administer terbutaline 0.25 mg subcutaneously if significant adverse effects occur.
- Initiate oxytocin for induction of labor no sooner than 4 hours after the last dose of misoprostol was administered, following agency protocol, if ripening has occurred and labor has not begun.
- Document all assessment findings and administration procedures.

FDA, US Food and Drug Administration; *FHR,* fetal heart rate.
Data from Hill, W., & Harvey, C. (2013). Induction of labor. In N. Troiano, C. Harvey, & B. Chez (Eds.), *AWHONN's high risk and critical care obstetrics* (3rd ed.). Philadelphia, PA: Wolters Kluwer/Lippincott Williams & Wilkins; Moleti, C. (2009). Trends and controversies in labor induction. *American Journal of Maternal/Child Nursing, 34*(1), 40–47; Thorp, J.M., & Laughon, S.K. (2014). Clinical aspects of normal and abnormal labor. In R.K. Creasy, R. Resnik, J.D. Iams, et al. (Eds.), *Creasy and Resnik's maternal-fetal medicine: Principles and practice* (7th ed.). Philadelphia, PA: Saunders.

endogenous prostaglandins. It is especially helpful for women who cannot receive exogenous prostaglandins for cervical ripening. The balloon usually falls out within 8 to 12 hours, when cervical dilation reaches approximately 3 cm. Evidence supports the insertion of a balloon catheter as a cervical ripening method because of its low cost compared with prostaglandins, stability at room temperature, and reduced risk for uterine tachysystole with or without FHR changes (ACOG, 2009/2016; Hill & Harvey, 2013; Yount & Lassiter, 2013).

Hydroscopic dilators (substances that absorb fluid from surrounding tissues and then enlarge) also can be used for cervical ripening. Laminaria tents (natural cervical dilators made from desiccated seaweed) and synthetic dilators containing magnesium sulfate (Lamicel) are inserted into the endocervix without rupturing the membranes. As they absorb fluid, they expand and cause cervical dilation and the release of endogenous prostaglandins. These dilators are left in place for 6 to 12 hours before being removed to assess cervical dilation. Fresh dilators are inserted if further cervical dilation is necessary. Synthetic dilators swell faster than natural dilators and become larger with less discomfort. When compared with prostaglandins, these mechanical methods achieved a lower rate of birth within 24 hours, but caused no change in the cesarean birth rate. Additionally, they were less likely to cause uterine tachysystole with or without changes in the FHR (ACOG, 2009/2016; Thorp & Laughon, 2014).

Hydroscopic dilators compare favorably with prostaglandins in their effectiveness in ripening the cervix but are associated with increased discomfort at insertion and during expansion and a higher incidence of postpartum maternal and newborn infections. They are a reliable alternative when prostaglandins are contraindicated or are unavailable.

Nursing responsibilities for women who have dilators inserted include the following:

- Documenting the number of dilators and sponges inserted during the procedure, as well as the number removed
- Assessing for urinary retention, rupture of membranes, uterine tenderness or pain, contractions, vaginal bleeding, infection, and fetal distress

Amniotic membrane stripping or sweeping is a method of inducing labor through the release of prostaglandins and oxytocin. The procedure involves separation of the membrane from the wall of the cervix and lower uterine segment by inserting a finger into the internal cervical os and rotating it 360 degrees. The results of two studies suggested that membrane stripping increased the rate of spontaneous vaginal birth and shortened the induction to birth interval. Neither study reported harmful side effects that could be attributed to the procedure. Research has not demonstrated an increase in either maternal or fetal infection associated with membrane stripping. However, because there is limited data available on the risk for infection in women who

MEDICATION GUIDE

Prostaglandin E₂ (PGE₂): Dinoprostone (Cervidil Insert; Prepidil Gel)

Action

PGE_2 ripens the cervix, making it softer and causing it to dilate and efface; it stimulates uterine contractions. Dinoprostone is the only FDA-approved medication for cervical ripening or labor induction.

Indications

- PGE_2 is used for preinduction cervical ripening (ripen the cervix before oxytocin induction of labor when the Bishop score is 4 or less) and for induction of labor or abortion (abortifacient agent).
- It is not recommended for use if the woman has a history of previous cesarean birth or other major uterine surgery.

Dosage and Route

Cervidil Insert

Dosage is 10 mg of dinoprostone designed to be gradually released (approximately 0.3 mg/hour) over 12 hours. Insert is placed transvaginally into the posterior fornix of the vagina. The insert is removed after 12 hours or at the onset of active labor or earlier if tachysystole or abnormal FHR and pattern occur.

Prepidil Gel

Dosage is 0.5 mg of dinoprostone in a 2.5-mL syringe. Gel is administered through a catheter attached to the syringe into the cervical canal just below the internal cervical os. Dose may be repeated every 6 hours as needed for cervical ripening up to a maximum cumulative dose of 1.5 mg (3 doses) in a 24-hour period.

Adverse Effects

Potential adverse effects include headache, nausea and vomiting, diarrhea, fever, hypotension, uterine tachysystole with or without an abnormal FHR and pattern, or fetal passage of meconium.

Nursing Considerations

- Explain the procedure to the woman and her family. Ensure that an informed consent has been obtained per agency policy.

- Assess the woman and fetus before each insertion and during treatment following agency protocol for frequency. Assess maternal vital signs and health status, FHR and pattern, and status of pregnancy, including indications for cervical ripening or induction of labor, signs of labor or impending labor, and the Bishop score. Recognize that an abnormal FHR and pattern; maternal fever, infection, vaginal bleeding, or hypersensitivity; and regular, progressive uterine contractions contraindicate the use of dinoprostone.
- Avoid use in women with asthma, glaucoma, and hypotension or hypertension.
- Use with caution if the woman has cardiac, renal, or hepatic disease; anemia; jaundice; diabetes; epilepsy; or genitourinary (GU) infections.
- Bring the gel to room temperature just before administration. Do not force the warming process by using a warm-water bath or other source of external heat such as microwave because heat may cause inactivation.
- Keep the insert frozen until just before insertion. No warming is needed.
- Have the woman void before insertion.
- Assist the woman to maintain a supine position with a lateral tilt or a side-lying position for at least 30 minutes after insertion of the gel or for 2 hours after placement of the insert.
- Allow the woman to ambulate after the recommended period of bed rest and observation.
- Prepare to pull the string to remove the insert and to administer terbutaline 0.25 mg subcutaneously if significant adverse effects occur. There is no effective way to remove the gel from the vagina if uterine tachysystole or abnormal FHR and pattern occur.
- Delay the initiation of oxytocin for induction of labor for 6 to 12 hours after the last instillation of the gel or for 30 to 60 minutes after removal of the insert, or follow agency protocol for induction if ripening has occurred but labor has not begun.
- Document all assessment findings and administration procedures.

FDA, US Food and Drug Administration; *FHR*, fetal heart rate.
Data from Hill, W., & Harvey, C. (2013). Induction of labor. In N. Troiano, C. Harvey, & B. Chez (Eds.), *AWHONN's high risk and critical care obstetrics* (3rd ed.). Philadelphia, PA: Wolters Kluwer/Lippincott Williams & Wilkins; Moleti, C. (2009). Trends and controversies in labor induction, *American Journal of Maternal/Child Nursing, 34*(1), 40-47.

are known to be group B streptococci (GBS) positive, potential risks and benefits of the procedure should be carefully considered before performing membrane stripping on this group of women (Sheibani & Wing, 2017).

Physical methods such as sexual intercourse (prostaglandins in the semen and stimulation of contractions with orgasm), nipple stimulation (release of endogenous oxytocin from the pituitary gland), and walking (gravity applies pressure to the cervix, which stimulates the secretion of endogenous oxytocin) may be used by women to "self-induce" labor. Breast (nipple) stimulation has been shown to increase the number of women who go into labor within 72 hours, but safety issues associated with this method have not been fully evaluated. Although orgasm does stimulate uterine contractions, there is inadequate evidence to support the belief that sexual intercourse enhances cervical ripening (Thorp & Laughon, 2014). Ambulation is an effective measure to augment labor (Yount & Lassiter, 2013).

Alternative Methods

Various alternative methods have been used by women to stimulate cervical ripening and the onset of labor. For example, blue cohosh and castor oil can be used for their labor stimulation effects, and black cohosh and evening primrose oil can ripen the cervix. Nurses must be knowledgeable about these preparations and ask about their use when assessing women during prenatal visits and on admission during labor. Women may accidentally take too much of the preparation or use it incorrectly. Also these preparations may potentiate the effect of pharmacologic methods to stimulate cervical ripening and uterine contractions, thereby increasing the potential for tachysystole and precipitous labor and birth.

Acupuncture has been used effectively to induce labor and has been found, in several studies, to reduce the duration of labor, the use of oxytocin, and the rate of cesarean birth. Specific points have been identified to stimulate uterine contractions or to facilitate cervical dilation. More than one treatment may be required to establish labor.

Amniotomy

Amniotomy (i.e., artificial rupture of membranes [AROM]) can be used to induce labor when the condition of the cervix is favorable (ripe) or to augment labor if progress begins to slow. Labor usually begins within 12 hours of AROM. Amniotomy can decrease the duration of

BOX 17.8   Procedure: Assisting With Amniotomy

Procedure

- Explain to the woman what will be done.
- Assess fetal heart rate (FHR) and pattern before procedure begins to obtain a baseline reading.
- Place several underpads under the woman's buttocks to absorb the fluid.
- Position the woman on a padded bedpan, fracture pan, or rolled-up towel to elevate her hips.
- Assist the health care provider who is performing the procedure by providing sterile gloves and lubricant for the vaginal examination.
- Unwrap the sterile package containing an Amnihook or Allis clamp, and pass the instrument to the obstetric health care provider, who inserts it alongside the fingers and then hooks and tears the membranes.
- Reassess the FHR and pattern.
- Assess the color, consistency, and odor of the fluid.
- Assess the woman's temperature every 2 hours or per protocol.
- Evaluate the woman for signs and symptoms of infection.

Documentation

Record the following:

- FHR and pattern before and after the procedure
- Time of rupture
- Color, odor, and consistency of the fluid
- Maternal status (how well procedure was tolerated)

---

labor by up to 2 hours, even without oxytocin administration. However, if amniotomy does not stimulate labor, the resulting prolonged rupture may lead to chorioamnionitis. Variable FHR deceleration patterns can occur as a result of cord compression associated with umbilical cord prolapse or a decreased amount of amniotic fluid. Once an amniotomy is performed, the woman is committed to labor with an unknown outcome for how and when she will give birth. For this reason, amniotomy often is used in combination with oxytocin induction.

Before the procedure, the woman should be told what to expect. She also should be assured that the actual rupture of the membranes is painless for her and the fetus, although she may experience some discomfort when the Amnihook or other sharp instrument is inserted through the vagina and cervix (Box 17.8). The presenting part of the fetus should be engaged and well applied to the cervix prior to the procedure to prevent cord prolapse. The woman should also be free of active infection of the genital tract (e.g., herpes) and should be human immunodeficiency virus (HIV) negative. After rupture, the amniotic fluid is allowed to drain slowly. The color, odor, and consistency of the fluid are assessed (i.e., for the presence or absence of meconium or blood). The time of rupture is recorded (Simpson & O'Brien-Abel, 2014).

⚡ SAFETY ALERT

The FHR is assessed before and immediately after the amniotomy to detect any changes. Transient tachycardia is common. Bradycardia and variable decelerations can indicate cord compression or prolapse.

The woman's temperature should be checked at least every 2 hours after rupture of membranes, more frequently if signs or symptoms of infection are noted. If her temperature is 38°C (100.4°F) or higher, the nurse notifies the obstetric health care provider. The nurse assesses for other signs and symptoms of infection, such as maternal chills, uterine tenderness on palpation, foul-smelling vaginal drainage, and fetal tachycardia. Comfort measures, such as frequently changing the woman's underpads and perineal cleansing, are implemented.

LEGAL TIP   Performing Amniotomy

Performing amniotomy is outside the scope of practice of nurses. In some locations, however, nurses have been asked to perform this procedure. A policy that is consistent with professional standards of care and clearly explains the nurse's role in amniotomy should be in place in all labor and birth areas.

Oxytocin

Oxytocin is a hormone normally produced by the posterior pituitary gland. It stimulates uterine contractions and aids in milk ejection (let-down). Synthetic oxytocin (Pitocin) may be used either to induce labor or to augment a labor that is progressing slowly because of inadequate uterine contractions. Synthetic oxytocin is the most commonly used agent for labor induction in the United States (Huwe, 2017; Simpson & O'Brien-Abel, 2014). It is also the drug most commonly associated with adverse events during labor and birth. The most common errors involving oxytocin administration during labor are dose related (Simpson & O'Brien-Abel).

⚡ SAFETY ALERT

Oxytocin is included on the list of high-alert medications designated by the Institute for Safe Medication Practices because it has a heightened risk for causing significant patient harm when used in error (Institute for Safe Medication Practices [ISMP], 2014).

Oxytocin use can present hazards to the mother and fetus. Maternal hazards include placental abruption, uterine rupture, unnecessary cesarean birth because of abnormal FHR and pattern, postpartum hemorrhage, and infection. When placental perfusion is diminished by contractions that are too frequent or prolonged, the fetus can experience hypoxemia and acidemia, which eventually results in late decelerations and minimal or absent baseline variability. The goal of oxytocin use is to produce contractions of normal intensity, duration, and frequency while using the lowest dose of medication possible (Huwe, 2017).

The obstetric health care provider writes the order for the induction or augmentation of labor with oxytocin. The nurse implements the order by initiating the primary intravenous infusion and administering the oxytocin solution through a secondary line. The nurse's actions related to assessment and care of a woman whose labor is being induced are guided by hospital protocol and professional standards (see Fig. 17.7 and Medication Guide: Oxytocin [Pitocin]).

The most commonly used regimen in the United States for administering oxytocin is to begin with a starting dose of 1 milliunit/min and to increase by 1 to 2 milliunits/min no more frequently than every 30 to 40 minutes (Simpson & O'Brien-Abel, 2014). This recommendation is based on research findings related to the pharmacokinetics of oxytocin. The uterus responds to oxytocin within 3 to 5 minutes of intravenous administration. The half-life of oxytocin (the time required to metabolize and eliminate half the dose) is approximately 10 to 12 minutes. Approximately 40 minutes is required to reach a steady state of oxytocin (the point in time when the rate of oxytocin administered intravenously equals the rate of oxytocin elimination) and for the full effect of a dosage increment to be reflected in more intense, frequent, and longer contractions (Hill & Harvey, 2013; Simpson & O'Brien-Abel, 2014) (see Medication Guide: Oxytocin [Pitocin] and Fig. 17.7). Low-dose (physiologic) protocols such as the one described result in decreased risk for oxytocin-induced tachysystole. High-dose protocols, in which the initial

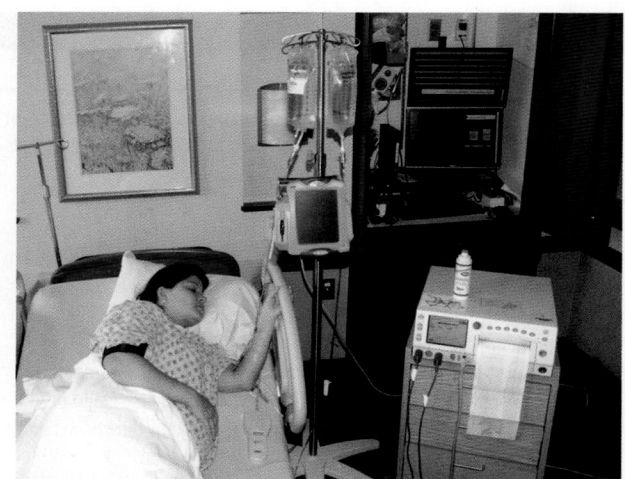

FIG 17.7 Woman in side-lying position receiving oxytocin. (Courtesy of Cheryl Briggs, RNC, Annapolis, MD.)

dose of oxytocin is larger and the dosage is increased more rapidly, have been found to result in shorter labors, fewer failed inductions, less forceps-assisted births, fewer cesarean births because of failure to progress in labor, less chorioamnionitis, and less neonatal sepsis. However, high-dose protocols have been associated with more uterine tachysystole and more cesarean births related to fetal stress (Sheibani & Wing, 2017).

Nursing Considerations

An evidence-based protocol for the preparation and administration of oxytocin should be established and utilized by the obstetric department (physicians and nurses) in each institution. Other safety measures recommended for use of this high-alert drug are using a standard concentration of oxytocin and a standard definition of uterine tachysystole that does not include an abnormal FHR or pattern or the woman's perception of pain. In addition, standardized treatment of oxytocin-induced uterine tachysystole is recommended (Huwe, 2017; Simpson & O'Brien-Abel, 2014) (see Emergency Treatment box: Uterine Tachysystole with Oxytocin [Pitocin] Infusion).

The definition of excessive uterine contractions needs to be standardized. The Eunice Kennedy Shriver National Institute of Child Health and Human Development, along with ACOG and SMFM, sponsored a workshop in April 2008 to review definitions, interpretation, and research recommendations for intrapartum fetal monitoring. Workshop participants also recommended standardizing definitions regarding uterine contractions for use in clinical practice. This group defined uterine tachysystole as more than five contractions in 10 minutes, averaged over a 30-minute window. The term tachysystole applies to both spontaneous and stimulated labor. Participants also recommended that use of the terms *hyperstimulation* and *hyperactivity* be abandoned because they are not defined (Macones, Hankins, Spong, et al., 2008).

AUGMENTATION OF LABOR

Augmentation of labor is the stimulation of uterine contractions after labor has started spontaneously and progress is unsatisfactory. Augmentation is usually implemented to manage hypotonic uterine dysfunction that resulted in a slowing of the labor process (protracted active phase). Common augmentation methods include oxytocin infusion and amniotomy. Noninvasive methods such as emptying the bladder, ambulation and position changes, relaxation measures, nourishment and hydration, and hydrotherapy should be attempted before initiating invasive interventions. The administration procedure and nursing assessment and care measures for augmenting labor with oxytocin are similar to those used for induction of labor with oxytocin (see Medication Guide: Oxytocin [Pitocin]).

Some physicians advocate active management of labor, that is, augmentation of labor to establish efficient labor with the aggressive use of oxytocin so that the woman gives birth within 12 hours of admission to the labor unit. The physicians who developed the original protocol for active management of labor found that intervening early (as soon as a nulliparous woman was not dilating her cervix at least 1 cm/hour) with use of higher (pharmacologic) oxytocin doses administered at frequent increment intervals (e.g., a starting dose of 6 milliunits/min with increases of 6 milliunits/min every 15 minutes) shortened labor for most women and significantly decreased the cesarean birth rate at their institution (Simpson & O'Brien-Abel, 2014).

Additional components of the active management of labor include (1) strict criteria to diagnose that the woman is indeed in active labor with 100% cervical effacement, (2) amniotomy within 1 hour of admission of a woman in labor if spontaneous rupture of the membranes has not occurred, and (3) continuous presence of a personal nurse who provides one-on-one care for the woman while she is in labor. Many obstetricians in the United States emphasize using high-dose oxytocin protocols but do not implement all the other components of active management (Simpson & O'Brien-Abel, 2014). At least one review of published studies on the effectiveness of active management of labor protocols concluded that the presence of a personal nurse who provides constant emotional and physical support is the only component associated with shorter labors and lower rates of cesarean birth.

OPERATIVE VAGINAL BIRTH

Operative vaginal births are performed using either forceps or a vacuum extractor. The use of both devices continues to decline. In 2012, fewer than 4% of all births in the United States were accomplished using forceps or vacuum assistance. Indications and prerequisites for the use of both instruments are identical (Nielsen, Deering, & Galan, 2017). The decision to use forceps or a vacuum extractor is based on the experience and personal preference of the physician performing the procedure. There are several types of operative vaginal births (AAP & ACOG, 2012).

Forceps-Assisted Birth

A forceps-assisted birth is one in which an instrument with two curved blades is used to assist in the birth of the fetal head. The cephalic-like curve of the forceps commonly used is similar to the shape of the fetal head, with a pelvic curve to the blades conforming to the curve of the pelvic axis. The blades are joined by a pin, screw, or groove arrangement. These locks prevent the forceps from compressing the fetal skull (Fig. 17.8). There are several types of forceps-assisted births, defined primarily by the station and position of the fetal head in relationship to the maternal pelvis (Table 17.3) (AAP & ACOG, 2012).

Maternal indications for forceps-assisted birth include a prolonged second stage of labor and the need to shorten the second stage of labor for maternal reasons (e.g., maternal exhaustion or maternal cardiopulmonary or cerebrovascular disease) (Nielsen et al., 2017). The major fetal indication is suspicion of immediate or potential fetal compromise (i.e., a nonreassuring FHR tracing). The use of forceps during birth has been decreasing, replaced by vacuum extraction or cesarean birth (Nielsen et al.; Thorp & Laughon, 2014).

Certain conditions are required for a forceps-assisted birth to be successful. The woman's cervix must be fully dilated to prevent lacerations

MEDICATION GUIDE

Oxytocin (Pitocin)

Action

Oxytocin is a hormone produced in the posterior pituitary gland that stimulates uterine contractions and aids in milk ejection (let-down). Pitocin is a synthetic form of this hormone.

Indications

Oxytocin is used primarily for labor induction and augmentation; it is also used to control postpartum bleeding.

Dosage

- The IV solution containing oxytocin should be mixed in a standard concentration. Concentrations often used are 10 units in 1000 mL of fluid, 20 units in 1000 mL of fluid, or 30 units in 500 mL of fluid.
- Oxytocin is administered intravenously through a secondary line connected to the main line at the proximal port (connection closest to the IV insertion site). Oxytocin is always administered by infusion pump.
- Begin oxytocin administration at 1 milliunit/minute. Increase the rate by 1 to 2 milliunits/minute, no more frequently than every 30 to 60 minutes based on the response of the woman and fetus and the progress of labor.
- The goal of oxytocin administration is to produce acceptable uterine contractions as evidenced by:
  - Consistent achievement of 200 to 220 MVUs *or*
  - A consistent pattern of one contraction every 2 to 3 minutes, lasting 80 to 90 seconds, and strong to palpation

Adverse Effects

- Possible maternal adverse effects include uterine tachysystole, placental abruption, uterine rupture, unplanned cesarean birth caused by abnormal FHR and pattern, postpartum hemorrhage, infection, and death from water intoxication (e.g., severe hyponatremia).
- Possible fetal adverse effects include hypoxemia and acidosis, eventually resulting in abnormal FHR and pattern.

Nursing Considerations

- Oxytocin is considered a high-alert medication because it has the potential to cause significant harm when used inappropriately.
- Patient and partner teaching and support:
  - Reasons for use of oxytocin (e.g., start or improve labor)

- Reactions to expect concerning the nature of contractions: the intensity of the contraction increases more rapidly, holds the peak longer, and ends more quickly; contractions come regularly and more often
- Monitoring to anticipate
- Continue to keep woman and her partner informed regarding progress.
- Remember that women vary greatly in their response to oxytocin; some require only very small amounts of medication to produce adequate contractions, whereas others need larger doses.
- Assessment:
  - Assess fetal status using electronic fetal monitoring; evaluate tracing every 15 minutes and with every change in dose during the first stage of labor and every 5 minutes during the active pushing phase of the second stage of labor.
  - Monitor the contraction pattern and uterine resting tone every 15 minutes and with every change in dose during the first stage of labor and every 5 minutes during the second stage of labor.
  - Monitor blood pressure, pulse, and respirations every 30 to 60 minutes and with every change in dose.
  - Assess intake and output; limit IV intake to 1000 mL in 8 hours; urine output should be 120 mL or more every 4 hours.
  - Perform a vaginal examination as indicated.
  - Monitor for side effects, including nausea, vomiting, headache, and hypotension.
  - Observe emotional responses of the woman and her partner.
- Use a standard definition for uterine tachysystole that does not include an abnormal FHR and pattern or the woman's perception of pain (see Emergency Treatment box: Uterine Tachysystole with Oxytocin [Pitocin] Infusion).
- The rate of oxytocin infusion should be continually titrated to the lowest dose that achieves acceptable labor progress. Usually the oxytocin dose can be decreased or discontinued after rupture of membranes and in the active phase of first-stage labor.
- Documentation:
  - The time the oxytocin infusion is begun, and each time the infusion is increased, decreased, or discontinued
  - Assessment data as described above
  - Interventions for uterine tachysystole and abnormal FHR and pattern and the response to the interventions
  - Notification of the obstetric health care provider and that person's response

FHR, Fetal heart rate; *IV*, intravenous; *MVUs*, Montevideo units.

Data from American College of Obstetricians and Gynecologists. (2009/2016). Practice bulletin no. 107: Induction of labor. *Obstetrics and Gynecology, 114*(2, pt 1), 386–397; Clark, S., Simpson, K., Knox, G., et al. (2009). Oxytocin: New perspectives on an old drug, *American Journal of Obstetrics and Gynecology, 200*(1), 35, e1–e6; Hill, W., & Harvey, C. (2013). Induction of labor. In N. Troiano, C. Harvey, & B. Chez (Eds.), *AWHONN's high risk and critical care obstetrics* (3rd ed.). Philadelphia, PA: Wolters Kluwer/Lippincott Williams & Wilkins; Mahlmeister, L. (2008). Best practices in perinatal care: Evidence-based management of oxytocin induction and augmentation of labor, *Journal of Perinatal and Neonatal Nursing, 22*(4), 259–263; Simpson, K.R., & O'Brien-Abel, N. (2014). Labor and birth. In K.R. Simpson, & P. Creehan (Eds.), *AWHONN's perinatal nursing* (4th ed.). Philadelphia, PA; Lippincott; Simpson, K., & Knox, G. (2009). Oxytocin as a high-alert medication: Implications for perinatal patient safety, *American Journal of Maternal/Child Nursing, 34*(1), 8–15.

and hemorrhage. The bladder should be empty. The presenting part must be engaged—vertex presentation is desired. Membranes must be ruptured so that the position of the fetal head can be precisely determined and the forceps can firmly grasp the head during birth (Fig. 17.9). In addition, the size of the maternal pelvis must be assessed as adequate for the estimated fetal head circumference and weight (Nielsen et al., 2017).

Medical Management

Both blades are positioned by the physician, and the handles are locked. Traction is usually applied during contractions. The mother may or

may not be instructed to push during contractions, depending on physician preference. If a decrease in the FHR occurs, the forceps are removed and reapplied.

⚡ SAFETY ALERT

Because compression of the cord between the fetal head and the forceps will cause a decrease in FHR, the FHR is assessed, reported, and recorded before and after application of the forceps.

✚ EMERGENCY TREATMENT

Uterine Tachysystole With Oxytocin (Pitocin) Infusion

Signs
- More than five contractions in 10 minutes *or*
- A series of single contractions lasting >2 minutes *or*
- Contractions of normal duration occurring within 1 minute of each other

Interventions (With Normal [Category I] FHR Tracing)
- Reposition or maintain woman in side-lying position (either side).
- Administer IV fluid bolus with 500 mL of lactated Ringer's solution.
- If uterine activity has not returned to normal after 10 minutes, decrease the oxytocin dose by at least half.
- If uterine activity has not returned to normal after another 10 minutes, discontinue the oxytocin infusion until fewer than five contractions occur in 10 minutes.

Interventions (With Indeterminate [Category II] or Abnormal [Category III] FHR Tracing)
- Discontinue oxytocin infusion immediately.
- Reposition or maintain woman in side-lying position (either side).
- Administer IV fluid bolus with 500 mL of lactated Ringer's solution.
- Consider giving oxygen at 10 L/min via nonrebreather face mask if the above interventions do not resolve the indeterminate or abnormal (category II or category III) FHR tracing.
- If still no response, consider giving 0.25 mg terbutaline subcutaneously according to unit protocol or standing orders.
- Notify obstetric health care provider of actions taken and maternal and fetal response.

Resumption of Oxytocin After Resolution of Tachysystole
- If the oxytocin infusion has been discontinued for less than 20 to 30 minutes, resume at no more than one-half the rate that caused the tachysystole.
- If the oxytocin infusion has been discontinued for more than 30 to 40 minutes, resume at the initial starting dose.

FHR, Fetal heart rate.
Data from Huwe, V.Y. (2017). Induction and augmentation of labor. In B.B. Kennedy, & S.M. Baird (Eds.), *Intrapartum management modules: A perinatal education program* (5th ed.). Philadelphia, PA: Wolters Kluwer; Simpson, K. (2011). Clinicians' guide to the use of oxytocin for labor induction and augmentation. *Journal of Midwifery & Women's Health, 56*(3), 214–221.

TABLE 17.3   Definitions for Forceps- and Vacuum-Assisted Births

Outlet	Fetal scalp is visible on the perineum without manually separating the labia
Low	Fetal head is at least at the +2 station
Midpelvis	Fetal head is engaged (no higher than 0 station) but above +2 station

Data from American Academy of Pediatrics, & American College of Obstetricians and Gynecologists. (2012). *Guidelines for perinatal care* (7th ed.). Washington, DC: American College of Obstetricians and Gynecologists.

Nursing Interventions

When a forceps-assisted birth is deemed necessary, the nurse obtains the type of forceps requested by the physician. The nurse can explain to the mother that the forceps blades fit the same way two tablespoons fit around an egg, with the blades placed in front of the baby's ears.

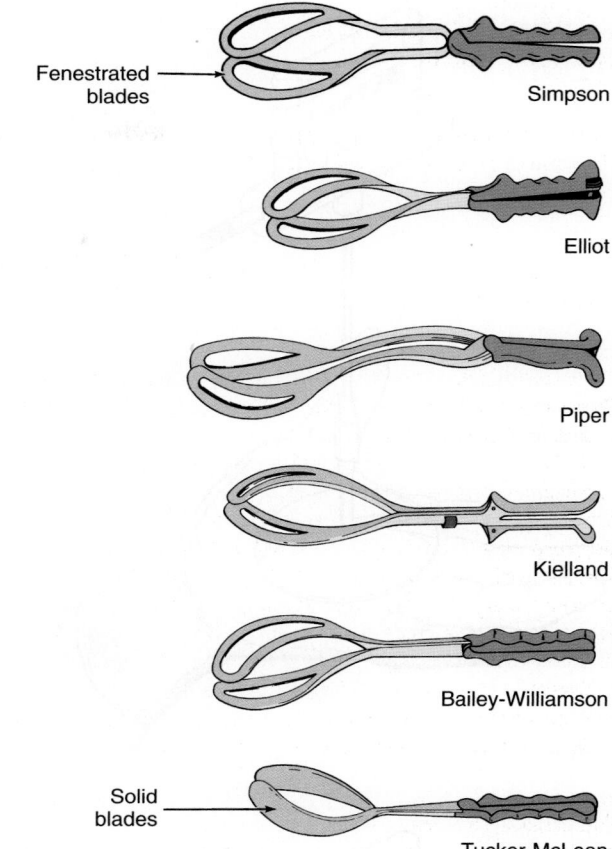

FIG 17.8 Types of forceps. Piper forceps are used to assist birth of the head in a breech birth.

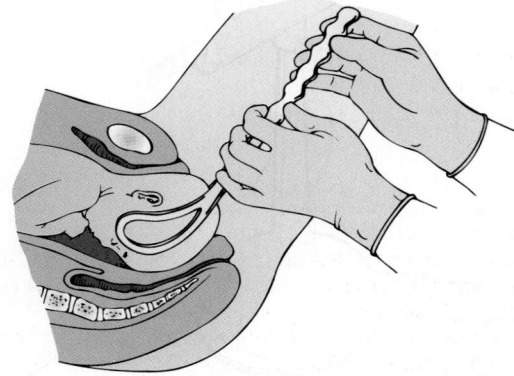

FIG 17.9 Outlet forceps-assisted extraction of the head.

After birth the mother should be assessed for vaginal or cervical lacerations, urinary retention, and hematoma formation in the pelvic soft tissues, which can result from blood vessel damage. The infant should be assessed for bruising or abrasions at the site of the blade applications, facial palsy resulting from pressure of the blades on the facial nerve, and subdural hematoma. Newborn and postpartum caregivers should be told that a forceps-assisted birth was performed.

Vacuum-Assisted Birth

Vacuum-assisted birth, or *vacuum extraction*, is a birth method involving the attachment of a vacuum cup to the fetal head, using negative pressure to assist in the birth of the head (Fig. 17.10). It is generally not used

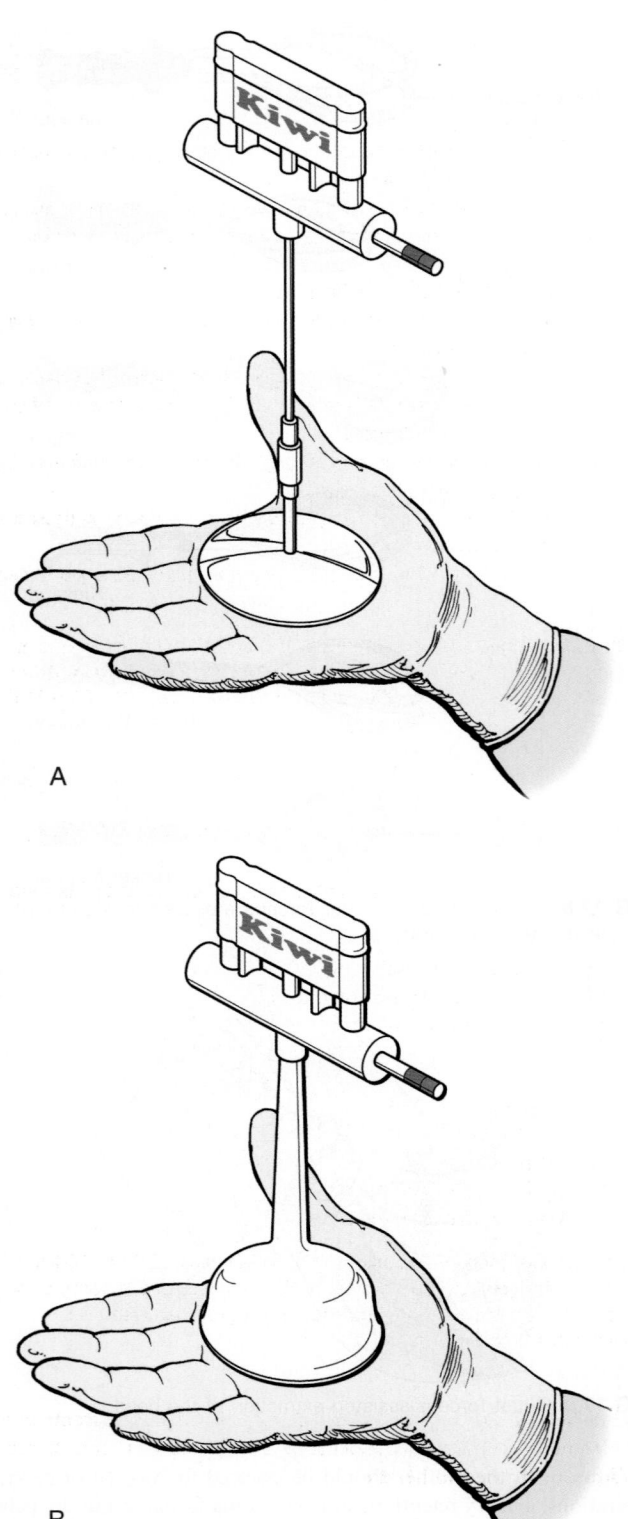

FIG 17.10 Two Kiwi vacuum devices demonstrating the handheld pump and pressure gauge device. (From Gabbe, S. G., Niebyl, J. R., Simpson, J. L., et al. (Eds.). *Obstetrics: Normal and problem pregnancies* [7th ed.]. Philadelphia, PA: Elsevier.)

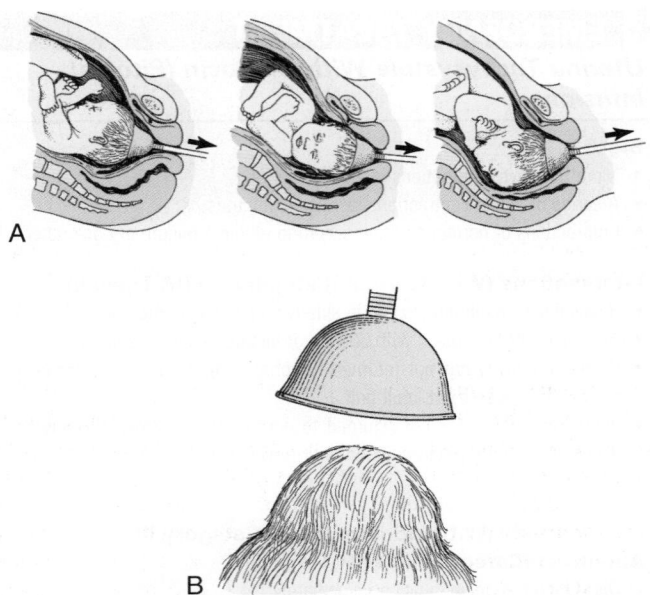

FIG 17.11 Use of vacuum extraction to rotate fetal head and assist with descent. **A,** Arrow indicates direction of traction on the vacuum cup. **B,** Caput succedaneum formed by the vacuum cup.

to assist birth before 34 weeks of gestation. Indications for its use are the same as those for outlet forceps. Prerequisites for use include a completely dilated cervix, ruptured membranes, engaged head, vertex presentation, and no suspicion of CPD (Cunningham et al., 2014). The types of vacuum-assisted births are defined the same as for forceps-assisted births—by the station and position of the fetal head in relation to the maternal pelvis (see Table 17.3) (AAP & ACOG, 2012). Advantages of vacuum-assisted birth compared with forceps-assisted birth are the ease with which the vacuum extractor can be placed and the need for less anesthesia. Also it is far easier to teach and to learn the skills necessary to safely use the vacuum extractor than to gain a similar level of skill with forceps (Thorp & Laughon, 2014).

Medical Management

The vacuum cup is applied to the fetal head by the physician. There are basically two types of vacuum devices. One is a self-contained unit, which allows the physician to both position the cup on the baby's head and generate the desired amount of negative pressure to create a vacuum. When the other type of vacuum device is used, the physician applies the cup to the baby's head, after which the nurse connects the suction tubing attached to the cup to wall suction or a separate hand pump and generates the amount of pressure requested by the physician. With both devices, a caput develops inside the cup as the pressure is initiated (Fig. 17.11). The woman is encouraged to push as traction is applied by the physician. The vacuum cup is released and removed after birth of the head. If vacuum extraction is not successful, a forceps-assisted or cesarean birth is usually performed.

Risks to the newborn include cephalhematoma, scalp lacerations, and subdural hematoma. These complications can be reduced by strict adherence to the manufacturer's recommendations for method of application, amount of pressure to be generated, and duration of application. Maternal risks include perineal, vaginal, or cervical lacerations and soft-tissue hematomas.

Nursing Interventions

The nurse provides education and support for the woman who has a vacuum-assisted birth. The nurse can prepare the woman for birth and

BOX 17.10   Recommended Measures to Safely Reduce the Primary Cesarean Birth Rate

- Encourage more expectant management of second-stage labor, considering current definitions of "normal" labor.
- Improve and standardize fetal heart rate interpretation and management.
- Increase access to nonmedical interventions during labor, such as continuous labor support.
- Offer external cephalic version for breech presentation.
- Offer a trial of labor for women with twin gestations when the first twin is in cephalic presentation.
- Avoid cesarean birth for suspected fetal macrosomia unless the estimated fetal weight is at least 5000 g in women without diabetes and at least 4500 g in women with diabetes.
- Offer operative (forceps- or vacuum-assisted) vaginal birth, performed by experienced, well-trained physicians.
- Conduct research to provide a better knowledge base to guide decisions regarding cesarean birth.
- Encourage policy changes that safely lower the rate of primary cesarean birth.

Data from American College of Obstetricians and Gynecologists & Society for Maternal-Fetal Medicine. (2014). Safe prevention of the primary cesarean delivery. *Obstetrics & Gynecology, 123,* 693–711.

encourage her to remain active in the birth process by pushing during contractions. The FHR should be assessed frequently during the procedure. Documentation of the procedure in the medical record is important and is often the nurse's responsibility (Box 17.9). Neonatal caregivers should be told that the birth was vacuum-assisted. After the birth, the newborn is observed for signs of trauma and infection at the application site and for cerebral irritation (e.g., seizures, lethargy, increased irritability, or poor feeding) (Simpson & O'Brien-Abel, 2014). The newborn can be at risk for hyperbilirubinemia and neonatal jaundice as bruising resolves. The parents need to be reassured that the caput succedaneum usually disappears in several days (see Fig. 17.11, *B*).

CESAREAN BIRTH

Cesarean birth is the birth of a fetus through a transabdominal incision of the uterus. Whether cesarean birth is planned (scheduled) or unplanned, the loss of experiencing a vaginal birth can have a negative effect on a woman's self-concept. An effort is therefore made to maintain the focus on the birth of the baby rather than on the operative procedure.

The purpose of cesarean birth is to preserve the well-being of the mother and the fetus. It may be the best choice for birth when evidence exists of maternal or fetal complications. Since the advent of modern surgical methods and care and the use of antibiotics, maternal and fetal morbidity and mortality have decreased. In addition, incisions are usually made into the lower uterine segment rather than in the muscular body of the uterus, thus promoting more effective healing. However, despite these advances, cesarean birth still poses threats to the health of the mother and infant.

Birth data for 2015, the most recent data available, indicate that the cesarean birth rate in the United States declined for the third consecutive year, to a rate of 32.0% (Martin et al., 2017). Despite this recent small decrease, the cesarean birth rate in the United States remains very high. Part of the reason is that a number of common risk factors for cesarean birth are increasing in frequency, especially in developed countries. These factors include fetal macrosomia, advanced maternal age, obesity, gestational diabetes, multifetal pregnancy, and dystocia in nulliparous women (Thorp & Laughon, 2014). Limited use of a trial of labor (TOL) after cesarean, due in part to concerns about safety and medicolegal considerations, is another reason for the high cesarean birth rate (Berghella, Mackeen, & Jauniaux, 2017).

ACOG and SMFM (2014) have recommended several measures to safely reduce the rate of primary cesarean births in the United States (Box 17.10). These measures involve the combined efforts of health care professionals and women and their families.

Indications

Few absolute indications exist for cesarean birth. Currently most are performed for conditions that might pose a threat to both the mother

BOX 17.11   Common Indications for Cesarean Birth

Maternal
- Specific cardiac disease (e.g., Marfan syndrome with dilated aortic root)

Fetal
- Nonreassuring fetal status
- Malpresentation (breech or transverse lie)
- Active maternal herpes infection

Maternal-Fetal
- Cephalopelvic disproportion
- Placental abruption
- Placenta previa
- History of previous cesarean birth
- Cesarean birth on maternal request

Data from Berghella V., Mackeen, D., & Jauniaux, E.R.M. (2017). Cesarean delivery. In S.G. Gabbe, J. R. Niebyl, J. L. Simpson, et al. (Eds.), *Obstetrics: Normal and problem pregnancies* (7th ed.). Philadelphia, PA: Elsevier.

and the fetus if vaginal birth occurred, such as complete placenta previa or placental abruption (Berghella et al., 2017). Box 17.11 lists common indications for cesarean birth.

Elective Cesarean Birth

Elective cesarean birth, sometimes referred to as *cesarean on maternal request,* refers to a primary cesarean birth without medical or obstetric indication. Reasons given for elective cesarean birth include fear of pain during labor and birth and the mistaken belief that the surgery will prevent future problems with pelvic support, bladder and bowel incontinence, or sexual dysfunction (Ecker, 2013). At this time, evidence is insufficient to recommend elective cesarean birth to prevent urinary or fecal incontinence later in life (ACOG, 2010/2015; Thorp & Laughon,

2014). Although some nulliparous women may fear the pain of labor because of no firsthand experience, multiparous women may request a cesarean birth after a previous traumatic vaginal birth. Other women desire an elective cesarean birth because of the convenience of planning a date, or having control and choice about when to give birth (Ecker). Less than 10% of women prefer a cesarean birth based solely on their own desires (Berghella et al., 2017).

Only limited data are available comparing cesarean births on request with planned vaginal births (ACOG, 2010/2015). Potential risks of cesarean birth on request include a longer hospital stay for the woman, an increased risk for mild respiratory problems for the baby, and possibly greater complications in subsequent pregnancies. Cesarean birth on request should not be performed before 39 weeks of gestation. Also, it is not recommended for women who desire several additional children, because the risks for placenta previa and placenta accreta increase with each cesarean birth and are substantial with more than three surgeries (Berghella et al., 2017).

Scheduled Cesarean Birth

Cesarean birth is scheduled or planned if any of the following occur:
- Labor and vaginal birth are contraindicated (e.g., complete placenta previa, active genital herpes, positive HIV status with a high viral load)
- Birth is necessary but labor is not inducible (e.g., hypertensive states that cause a poor intrauterine environment that threatens the fetus)
- This course of action has been chosen by the obstetric health care provider and the woman (e.g., a repeat cesarean birth)

Women who are scheduled for a cesarean birth usually have time to prepare for it psychologically. However, the psychologic responses of these women may differ. Those having a repeat cesarean birth may have disturbing memories of the conditions preceding the initial (primary) cesarean birth and of their experiences in the postoperative recovery period. They may be concerned about the added burdens of caring for the infant and perhaps other children while recovering from surgery. Others may feel glad that they have been relieved of the uncertainty about the date and time of the birth and are free of the pain of labor.

Unplanned Cesarean Birth

The psychosocial outcomes of unplanned or emergency cesarean birth are usually more pronounced and negative when compared with the outcomes associated with a scheduled or planned cesarean birth. Women and their families experience abrupt changes in their expectations for birth, postpartum care, and care of the new baby at home. This can be an extremely traumatic experience for all.

The woman may approach the procedure tired and discouraged after an ineffective and difficult labor. Fear predominates as she worries about her own safety and well-being and that of her fetus. She may be dehydrated, with low glycogen reserves. Because preoperative procedures must be done rapidly, there is often little time for explanation of the procedures and the operation itself. Because maternal and family anxiety levels are high at this time, much of what is said can be forgotten or misunderstood. The woman can experience feelings of anger or guilt in the postpartum period. Fatigue is often noticeable in these women, and they need much supportive care.

Forced Cesarean Birth

A woman's refusal to undergo cesarean birth when indicated for fetal reasons is often described as a *maternal-fetal conflict*. Health care providers are ethically obliged to protect the well-being of mother as well as fetus; a decision for one affects the other. If a woman refuses a cesarean birth that is recommended because of fetal jeopardy, health care providers

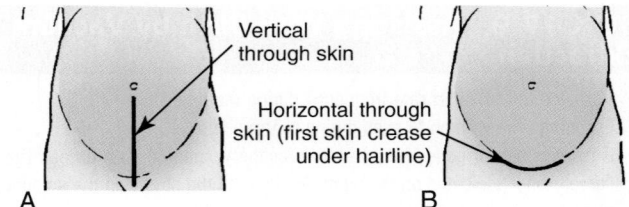

FIG 17.12 Skin incisions for cesarean birth. **A,** Vertical. **B,** Transverse (Pfannenstiel).

must make every effort to find out why she is refusing and provide information that may persuade her to change her mind. If the woman continues to refuse surgery, then health care providers must decide if it is ethical to get a court order for the surgery. Every effort, however, should be made to avoid this legal step.

Surgical Techniques

The skin incision will either be vertical, extending from near the umbilicus to the mons pubis or transverse (Pfannenstiel) in the lower abdomen (Fig. 17.12). The transverse incision, sometimes referred to as the "bikini" incision, is performed more often in the United States. The type of skin incision is generally determined by the urgency of the surgery, prior incision type, the presence of known placental disorders (i.e., anterior complete placenta previa, placenta accreta), and the possible need to explore the upper abdomen for nonobstetric pathology (Berghella et al., 2017). The type of skin incision does *not* necessarily indicate the type of uterine incision.

The two main types of uterine incisions are the low transverse (Fig. 17.13, *A*) or vertical incision, which may be either low or classical (see Fig. 17.13, *B* and *C*). Occasionally an initial low transverse incision will be extended into a *J* shape (see Fig. 17.13, *D*) or a *T* shape (see Fig. 17.13, *E*). Ideally the vertical incision is contained entirely within the lower uterine segment, but extension into the contractile portion of the uterus (e.g., a classical incision) is common. The vertical uterine incision is only rarely performed, but occasionally it is necessary. Indications for a vertical incision include an underdeveloped lower uterine segment, a transverse lie presentation, an anterior placenta previa or accreta, or if uterine leiomyomas (fibroids) obstruct the lower uterine segment (Berghella et al., 2017). Because it is associated with a higher incidence of uterine rupture in subsequent pregnancies than is lower-segment cesarean birth, vaginal birth after a classical uterine incision is contraindicated.

The low transverse uterine incision is performed in most cesarean births (see Fig. 17.13, *A*). Compared with the vertical incision, the transverse incision is preferred because it is easier to perform and repair and is associated with less blood loss. It also provides for the option of TOL and vaginal birth after cesarean (VBAC) in subsequent pregnancies (Berghella et al., 2017).

Complications and Risks

Possible maternal complications related to cesarean birth include anesthesia events (problems with intubation, drug reactions, aspiration pneumonia), hemorrhage, bowel or bladder injury, amniotic fluid embolism, and air embolism. Possible postpartum complications include atelectasis; endometritis; urinary tract infection; abdominal wound hematoma formation, dehiscence, infection, or necrotizing fasciitis; thromboembolic disease; and bowel dysfunction (Thorp & Laughon, 2014). In addition to these risks, the woman is also at economic risk because the cost of cesarean birth is higher than that of vaginal birth, and a longer recovery period may require additional expenditures.

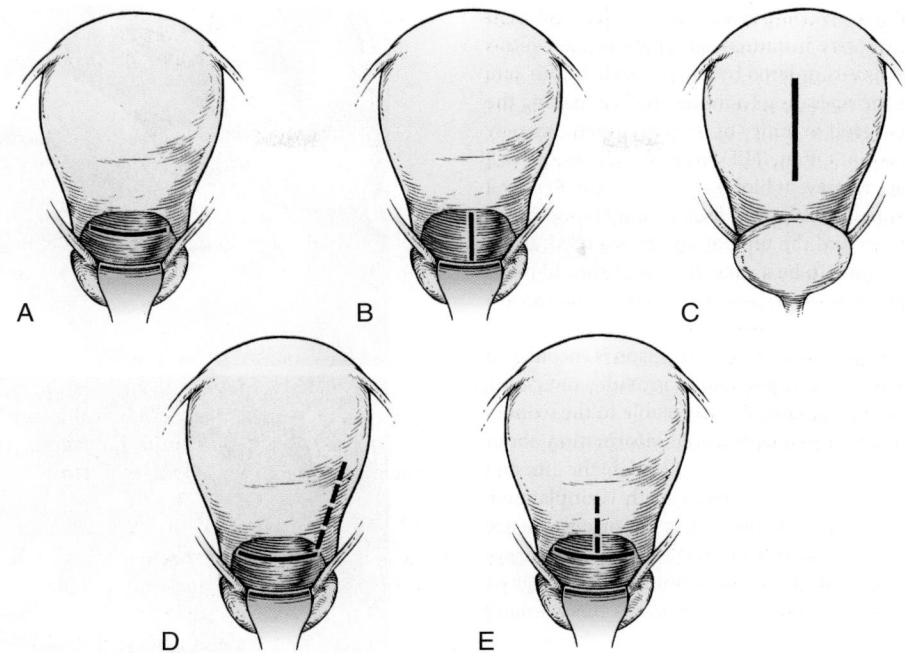

FIG 17.13 Uterine incisions for cesarean birth. **A,** Low transverse. **B** and **C,** Vertical. **D,** Low transverse *J*-shaped. **E,** Low transverse *T*-shaped. (From Gabbe, S. G., Niebyl, J. R., Simpson, J. L., et al. [2017]. *Obstetrics: Normal and problem pregnancies* [7th ed.]. Philadelphia, PA: Elsevier.)

Cesarean birth is associated with uncommon but significant dangers to the infant. The fetus may be born prematurely if the gestational age has not been accurately determined (iatrogenic prematurity). Fetal asphyxia can occur if the uterus and placenta are poorly perfused as a result of maternal hypotension caused by regional anesthesia (epidural or spinal) or maternal positioning. Fetal injuries (e.g., injuries caused by scalpel lacerations) can also occur during the surgery. The newborn is more likely to require resuscitation efforts and develop respiratory complications (Thorp & Laughon, 2014).

Anesthesia

Spinal, epidural, and general anesthetics are used for cesarean births (see Chapter 14). Epidural blocks are popular because women want to be awake for and aware of the birth experience. However, the choice of anesthetic depends on several factors. The mother's medical history or present condition, such as a spinal injury, hemorrhage, or coagulopathy, may rule out the use of regional anesthesia. Time is another factor, especially if there is an emergency and the life of the mother or infant is at stake. In an emergency, general anesthesia will most likely be used unless the woman already has an epidural block in effect. The woman herself is a factor. Either she may not know all the options or may have fears about having "a needle in her back" or about being awake and feeling pain. She needs to be fully informed about the risks and benefits of the different types of anesthesia so that she can participate in the decision whenever there is a choice.

Care Management
Prenatal Preparation

A discussion of cesarean birth should be included in all childbirth preparation classes. No woman can be guaranteed a vaginal birth, even if she is in good health and no indication of danger to the fetus exists before the onset of labor. Therefore every woman needs to be aware of and prepared for the possibility of having a cesarean birth.

Childbirth educators should emphasize the similarities and differences between a cesarean and a vaginal birth. In support of the philosophy of family-centered birth, many hospitals have instituted policies that permit fathers and other partners and family members to share in these births as they do in vaginal births. Women who have undergone cesarean birth agree that the continued presence and support of their partners helped them respond more positively to the entire experience. In addition to preparing women for the possibility of cesarean birth, childbirth educators should empower them to believe in their ability to give birth vaginally and to seek care measures during labor that will enhance the progress of their labors and reduce their risk for cesarean birth.

Preoperative Care

The preparation of the woman for cesarean birth is the same as that for other elective or emergency surgery. The obstetric health care provider discusses with the woman and her family the need for the cesarean birth and the prognosis for the mother and infant. A member of the anesthesia care team assesses the woman's cardiopulmonary status and describes the options for anesthesia. Women who are scheduled for an elective cesarean are often told to remain NPO (nothing by mouth) for at least 8 hours before the surgery. Informed consent is obtained for the procedure.

Blood tests are usually done 1 or 2 days before a planned cesarean birth or on admission to the labor and birth unit. Laboratory tests commonly ordered include a complete blood cell count and blood type and Rh status. Maternal vital signs and FHR and pattern are assessed according to hospital protocol until the operation begins. Intravenous fluids are started to maintain hydration and to provide an open line for the administration of medications and blood products, if needed. Other preoperative preparations include ensuring that an informed consent form has been signed, inserting a retention (Foley) catheter to keep the bladder empty, and administering prescribed preoperative medications. In addition to medications given to prevent aspiration pneumonia, women may also receive prophylactic antibiotics to prevent postoperative infection. In the rare instance that an abdominal-mons shave or a clipping of pubic hair is ordered by the obstetric health care provider, it is performed in the operating room just before making the incision because shaving can result in injury of the integument, thereby increasing the risk for infection. Often, TED hose or SCD boots will be placed on the woman's legs to prevent blood clot formation. Removal of contact lenses, dentures, nail polish, and jewelry may be optional, depending on hospital policies and the type of anesthesia used. If the woman wears glasses and is going to be awake, the nurse should make sure her glasses accompany her to the operating room so she can see her infant.

During the preoperative preparation, the support person is encouraged to remain with the woman as much as possible to provide continuing emotional support (if this action is culturally acceptable to the woman and support person). The nurse provides essential information about the preoperative procedures during this time. Although the nursing actions may be carried out quickly if a cesarean birth is unplanned, verbal communication, particularly explanations, is important. Silence can be frightening to the woman and her support person. The nurse's use of touch (if culturally appropriate) can communicate feelings of care and concern for the woman. The nurse can assess the woman's and her partner's perceptions about cesarean birth. As the woman expresses her feelings, the nurse may identify the potential for a disturbance in self-concept during the postpartum period that would need to be addressed. If there is time before the birth, the nurse can teach the woman about postoperative expectations and about pain relief, turning, leg exercises, coughing, and deep-breathing measures.

Intraoperative Care

Family-centered care is the goal for the woman who is undergoing cesarean birth and for her family. For the past several years, increasing efforts have been made to help women and their families optimize the cesarean birth experience while still maintaining safety. Options that can be offered to improve the cesarean birth experience include playing music chosen by the parents, softening the overhead lighting, using a surgical drape with a window if desired by the woman, and limiting extraneous conversation in the operating room. Implementing skin-to-skin care and breastfeeding in the operating room for infants who appear to be at term gestation and healthy are other interventions that are often desired by women and their families. Even seemingly "small" interventions, such as inserting the intravenous line into the woman's nondominant arm or hand, can enhance her birth experience (Schorn, Moore, Spetalnick, & Morad, 2015).

Cesarean births occur in operating rooms in the surgical suite or in the labor and birth unit. Staff members from the labor and birth unit may scrub and circulate during the surgery, or these functions may be assumed by members of the hospital's surgery staff (Fig. 17.14). If possible, the partner or another person, dressed appropriately for the operating room, accompanies the woman to the operating room and remains close to her for continued comfort and support. In unplanned cesarean birth, the nurse who cared for the woman during labor should be part of the nursing care team in the operating room if possible.

The nurse who is circulating may assist with positioning the woman on the birth (operating) table. It is important to position her so that the uterus is displaced laterally to prevent compression of the inferior vena cava, which causes decreased placental perfusion. This is usually accomplished by placing a wedge under one hip or tilting the table to one side. The woman's legs should be strapped to the table to ensure proper positioning during the surgery. A retention (Foley) catheter is inserted into the bladder at this time if one is not already in place.

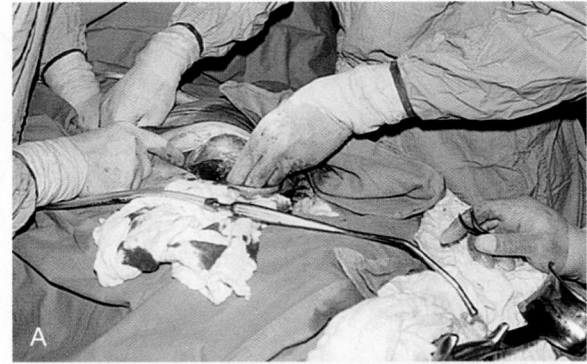
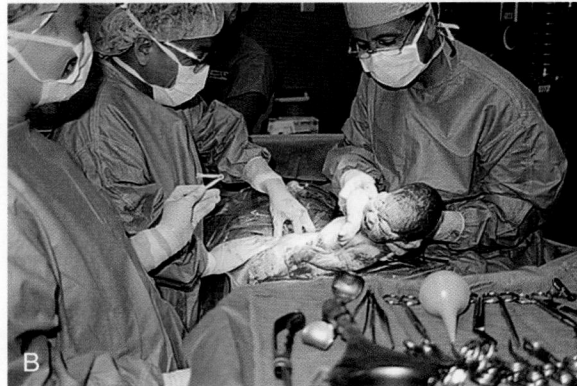
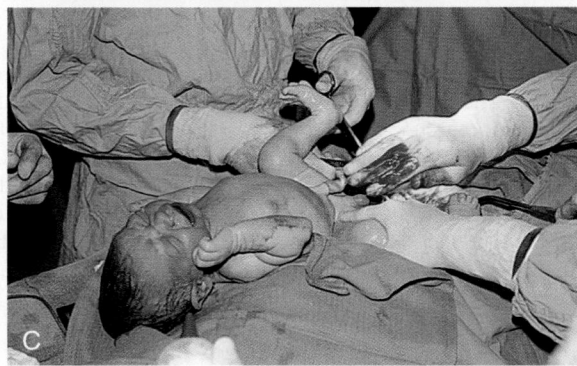

FIG 17.14 Cesarean birth. **A,** Low transverse "bikini" incision has been made, the muscle layer is separated, the abdomen is entered, and the uterus has been exposed and incised; suctioning of amniotic fluid continues as the head is brought up through the incision. Note small amount of bleeding. **B,** The neonate's birth through the uterine incision is nearly complete. **C,** A quick assessment is performed; note extreme molding of head resulting from cephalopelvic disproportion. (Courtesy of Marjorie Pyle, RNC, Lifecircle, Costa Mesa, CA.)

If the woman has general anesthesia, the partner likely will not be allowed in the operating room. If the partner or another person is not allowed or chooses not to be present, the nurse can stay in communication with him or her and give progress reports whenever possible. If the woman is awake during the birth, the nurse, anesthesia care provider, or both can tell her what is happening and provide support. She may be anxious about the sensations she is experiencing, such as the coldness of solutions used to cleanse the abdomen and pressure or pulling during the actual birth of the infant. She also may be apprehensive because of the bright lights or the presence of unfamiliar equipment and masked and gowned personnel in the room. Explanations can help decrease the woman's anxiety.

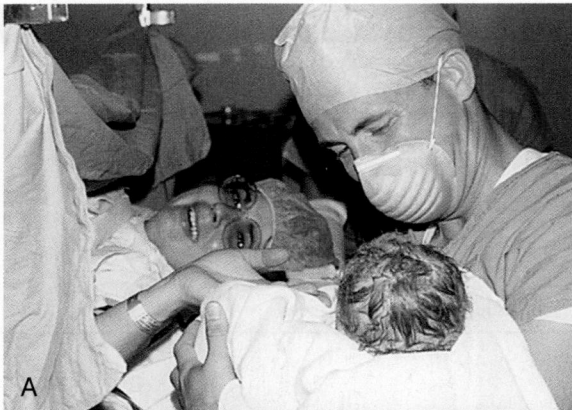

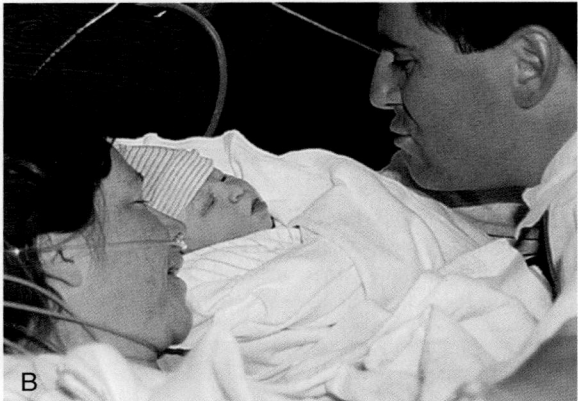

FIG 17.15 A, Parents and their newborn. The physician manually removes the placenta, suctions the remaining amniotic fluid and blood from the uterine cavity, and closes the uterine incision, peritoneum, muscle layer, fatty tissue, and finally the skin, while the new family shares some time together. **B,** Parents become better acquainted with their newborn while the mother rests after surgery. (Courtesy of Marjorie Pyle, RNC, Lifecircle, Costa Mesa, CA.)

A nurse from the labor and birth unit usually is present to provide care for the infant. A neonatal or pediatric health care provider or an interprofessional skilled in neonatal resuscitation may also be present for the surgery because these infants are considered to be at risk until evidence of physiologic stability exists after the birth. A crib with resuscitation equipment is readied before surgery. Personnel who are responsible for care are expert not only in resuscitative techniques but also in detecting normal and abnormal infant responses (AAP & American Heart Association [AHA], 2016). After the birth, if the infant's condition permits and the mother is awake, the baby can be placed skin-to-skin on the mother or can be given to the woman's partner or another person to hold (Fig. 17.15). The infant whose condition is compromised is transported after initial stabilization to the nursery for observation and the implementation of appropriate interventions. In some institutions, the partner or another person may accompany the infant; if not, personnel keep the family informed of the infant's progress, and parent-infant contacts are initiated as soon as possible.

If family members cannot accompany the woman during surgery, they are directed to the surgical or obstetric waiting room. The physician then reports on the condition of the mother and infant to the family members after the birth is completed. Family members may be allowed to accompany the infant as he or she is transferred to the nursery, giving them an opportunity to see and admire the new baby.

Immediate Postoperative Care

Once surgery is completed, the mother is transferred to a postanesthesia recovery area. After a cesarean birth, women have postoperative and postpartum needs that must be addressed. Assessments in this immediate postbirth period follow agency protocol and include recovery from the effects of anesthesia, postoperative and postbirth status, and degree of pain. A patent airway is maintained, and the woman is positioned to prevent possible aspiration. Vital signs are taken every 15 minutes for 1 to 2 hours, or until stable. The condition of the incisional dressing and the fundus and the amount of lochia are assessed, as well as the intravenous intake and the urine output through the retention (Foley) catheter. Oxytocin usually is added to at least the first liter of the intravenous infusion to ensure that the fundus remains firmly contracted, thereby reducing blood loss. The woman is helped to turn and do coughing, deep-breathing, and leg exercises. Medications for pain relief should be administered before postoperative pain becomes severe.

If the baby is present, the woman and her partner or another person are given some time alone with him or her to facilitate bonding and attachment, perhaps utilizing skin-to-skin contact. Breastfeeding can be initiated if the woman feels like trying. The woman is ready for discharge from the postanesthesia recovery area once her condition is stable and the effects of anesthesia have worn off (i.e., she is alert and oriented and able to feel and move her extremities).

Postoperative Postpartum Care

The attitude of the nurse and other interprofessional health care team members can influence the woman's perception of herself after a cesarean birth. The caregivers should stress that the woman is a new mother first and a surgical patient second. This attitude helps the woman perceive herself as having the same needs and concerns as other new mothers, while requiring supportive postoperative care.

The woman's physiologic concerns may be dominated initially by pain at the incision site and later by pain resulting from intestinal gas. For the first 24 hours after surgery, pain relief is usually provided by epidural opioids, patient-controlled analgesia (PCA), or intravenous or intramuscular injections. The most commonly used analgesics include opioids (e.g., hydromorphone, [Dilaudid], morphine sulfate, nalbuphine [Nubain]) and NSAIDs (e.g., ketorolac [Toradol]). If opioids are used, an antiemetic (e.g., metoclopramide [Reglan]) is often administered either as needed by the woman or scheduled as long as the opioid is used. Palpation of the fundus with the possibility of massage should be performed after an analgesic is given to decrease pain. By 24 hours after surgery, pain management is generally changed to oral analgesics. Other comfort measures such as position changes, splinting of the incision with pillows, and relaxation and breathing techniques (e.g., those learned in childbirth classes) may be implemented (see Patient Teaching box: Nonpharmacologic Postpartum Pain Relief After Cesarean Birth).

Women are often the best judges of what their bodies need and can tolerate, including the postoperative ingestion of foods and fluids. Some health care providers keep women NPO or allow only "sips and chips" (sips of clear fluids and teaspoons of crushed ice) until bowel sounds return. The diet is then advanced to full liquids. After women are passing

PATIENT TEACHING

Nonpharmacologic Postpartum Pain Relief After Cesarean Birth

Incisional
- Splint the incision with a pillow when moving or coughing.
- Use relaxation techniques such as music, breathing, and dim lights.

Gas
- Walk as often as you can.
- Do not eat or drink gas-forming foods, carbonated beverages, whole milk, or ice.
- Do not use straws for drinking fluids.
- Take antiflatulence medication if prescribed.
- Lie on your left side to expel gas.
- Rock in a rocking chair.

PATIENT TEACHING

Signs of Postoperative Complications After Discharge Following Cesarean Birth

Report the following signs to your health care provider:
- Temperature exceeding 38°C (100.4°F)
- Urination: painful urination, urgency, cloudy urine
- Lochia: heavier than a normal menstrual period, clots, odor
- Cesarean incision: redness, swelling, bruising, foul-smelling discharge or bleeding, wound separation
- Severe, increasing abdominal pain

flatus they can resume a regular diet. Because most women have an epidural or spinal anesthetic for surgery, most health care providers allow the early introduction of solid food if desired and tolerated. Intravenous fluids are usually continued until the woman is tolerating fluids orally. Ambulation and rocking in a rocking chair may relieve gas pains. Women should be taught to avoid gas-forming foods, ice chips, carbonated beverages, and using a straw to drink beverages to help limit gas formation, thereby minimizing the severity of gas pains (see Patient Teaching box: Nonpharmacologic Postpartum Pain Relief after Cesarean Birth).

Nursing Interventions

Nurses must be alert to a woman's physiologic needs, managing care to ensure adequate rest and pain relief. Mother-baby care (couplet care) for a cesarean birth mother may have to be modified according to her physical limitations as a surgical patient.

Daily care includes perineal care, breast care, and routine hygienic care. The woman may shower after the original incisional dressing is removed, usually on the first postoperative day (if showering is acceptable according to the woman's cultural beliefs and practices). The indwelling (Foley) catheter is also usually removed on the first postoperative day. The woman is encouraged to be out of bed and ambulating several times each day as soon as the urinary catheter is removed. Use of TED hose or SCD boots should continue as long as the woman remains in bed. They may be removed when she begins ambulating. The nurse assesses the woman's vital signs, incision, fundus, and lochia according to hospital policies, procedures, or protocols. Breath sounds, bowel sounds, circulatory status of lower extremities, and urinary and bowel elimination patterns also are assessed. It is important to observe maternal emotional status and progress of attachment to her baby.

SAFETY ALERT

The woman should be taught to seek assistance initially when getting out of bed, especially when an intravenous line and catheter are still in place. Thereafter, when rising from a supine position, she should sit on the side of the bed first to determine if dizziness will occur, then stand at the bedside, and finally ambulate.

During the postpartum period, the nurse can provide care that meets the psychologic and teaching needs of women who have had cesarean births. She or he can explain postpartum procedures to help the woman participate in her recovery from surgery. The nurse can help the woman

plan care and visits from family and friends that will allow for adequate rest periods. Providing information on and assistance with infant care can facilitate adjustment to her role as a mother. With adequate support, these women can benefit from providing baby care to facilitate attachment and enhance involvement in newborn care. The woman is supported as she breastfeeds her baby by receiving individualized assistance to comfortably hold and position the baby at her breast. Use of the side-lying or football-hold positions and supporting the newborn with pillows can enhance comfort and facilitate successful breastfeeding. The partner and other family members can be included in teaching sessions about infant care and the woman's recovery.

SAFETY ALERT

When holding her baby or breastfeeding, a woman may become drowsy and even fall asleep because of the sedation that occurs with the use of analgesics. It is important that someone be with her during these times to prevent newborn injury.

The couple also should be encouraged to express their feelings about the birth experience. Some parents are angry, frustrated, or disappointed that a vaginal birth was not possible. Some women express feelings of low self-esteem or a negative self-image. Others express relief and gratitude that the baby is healthy and safely born. It may be helpful for them to have the nurse who was present during the birth visit and help fill in "gaps" about the experience.

Discharge after cesarean birth is usually by the third postoperative day if not sooner. The nurse provides discharge teaching to prepare the woman for self-care and newborn care while trying to ensure that she is comfortable and able to rest. The nurse assesses the woman's information needs and coordinates the health care team's efforts to meet them. Discharge teaching and planning should include information about nutrition; measures to relieve pain and discomfort; exercise and specific activity restrictions; time management that includes periods of uninterrupted rest and sleep; hygiene, breast, and incision care; timing for resumption of sexual activity and contraception; signs of complications (see Patient Teaching box: Signs of Postoperative Complications After Discharge Following Cesarean Birth and Patient Teaching box: Signs of Postpartum Blues, Depression, and Psychosis in Chapter 21); and infant care. The nurse assesses the woman's need for continued support or counseling to facilitate her emotional recovery from the birth. The woman's family and friends should be educated regarding her needs during the recovery process, and their assistance should be requested before discharge. Referral to support groups (e.g., www.birthrites.org) or to community agencies may be indicated to further promote the recovery process. A postdischarge program of telephone follow-up and home visits can facilitate the woman's full recovery after cesarean birth.

BOX 17.12 Selection Criteria for Vaginal Birth After Cesarean

- One or two previous low-transverse cesarean births
- Clinically adequate pelvis
- No other uterine scars or history of previous rupture
- Physicians immediately available throughout active labor capable of monitoring labor and performing an emergency cesarean birth if necessary

Data from American College of Obstetricians and Gynecologists. (2010/2015). Practice bulletin no. 115: Vaginal birth after previous cesarean delivery. *Obstetrics and Gynecology, 116*(2, pt 1), 450–463.

TRIAL OF LABOR

A trial of labor (TOL) is the observance of a woman and her fetus for a reasonable period (e.g., 4 to 6 hours) of spontaneous active labor to assess the safety of vaginal birth for the mother and infant. It may be initiated if the mother's pelvis is of questionable size or shape or if the fetus is in an abnormal presentation or position. By far the most common reason for a TOL is if the woman wishes to have a vaginal birth after a previous cesarean birth. A woman who has had a previous cesarean birth with a low transverse uterine incision may be a candidate for a TOL. Fetal sonography, maternal pelvimetry, or both may be done before a TOL to rule out CPD. During a TOL, the woman is evaluated for active labor, including adequate contractions, engagement and descent of the presenting part, and effacement and dilation of the cervix.

The nurse assesses maternal vital signs and FHR and pattern and is alert for signs of potential complications. If complications develop, the nurse is responsible for initiating appropriate actions, including notifying the obstetric health care provider, and for evaluating and documenting the maternal and fetal responses to the interventions. Nurses must recognize that the woman and her partner are often anxious about maternal and fetal well-being. Supporting and encouraging the woman and her partner and providing information regarding progress can reduce stress and enhance the labor process and facilitate a successful outcome.

VAGINAL BIRTH AFTER CESAREAN

Indications for primary cesarean birth, such as breech presentation or abnormal FHR or pattern, often are nonrecurring. Therefore, a woman who has had a cesarean birth with a low transverse uterine incision may subsequently become pregnant, experience no contraindications to labor and vaginal birth during the pregnancy, and choose to attempt a vaginal birth after cesarean (VBAC) (see Clinical Reasoning Case Study: Trial of Labor for Vaginal Birth After Cesarean [TOL/VBAC]). Box 17.12 lists selection criteria suggested by ACOG (2010/2015) for identifying candidates for VBAC.

A VBAC is contraindicated for women at high risk for uterine rupture. It should not be attempted by women with a previous classical or *T*-shaped uterine incision or extensive transfundal uterine surgery, a previous uterine rupture, or medical or obstetric complications that prevent vaginal birth (Landon & Grobman, 2017).

The overall success rate of VBAC is approximately 60% to 80% (Landon & Grobman, 2017). The strongest predictors for a successful VBAC are a prior vaginal birth and spontaneous (rather than induced or augmented) labor (ACOG, 2010/2015). Women whose first cesarean birth was performed because of a nonrecurring indication (e.g., breech presentation) also are likely to have a successful VBAC. Women with the following characteristics are less likely to have a successful VBAC (Landon & Grobman):

CLINICAL REASONING CASE STUDY

Trial of Labor for Vaginal Birth After Cesarean (TOL/VBAC)

Heather, a 28-year-old G2 P1 gave birth by cesarean during her last pregnancy. During her routine prenatal visit at 32 weeks of gestation, Heather tells the nurse that she really wants to have a vaginal birth this time. Heather asks, "What do you think? Can I try for a VBAC?"

1. Evidence—Is there sufficient evidence to advise Heather about the safety and feasibility of a trial of labor for vaginal birth after cesarean (TOL/VBAC)?
2. Assumptions—Describe an underlying assumption about each of the following issues:
   a. Risks that Heather faces if she chooses a TOL/VBAC
   b. Criteria that must be met for Heather to attempt a TOL/VBAC
   c. Labor management practices that facilitate a successful VBAC
3. What implications and priorities for nursing care can be drawn at this time?
4. Does the evidence objectively support your argument (conclusion)?
5. Interprofessional care—Describe the roles/responsibilities of health care professionals who might be involved in Heather's care.

- Recurrent indication (e.g., labor dystocia) for initial cesarean birth
- Increased maternal age
- Non-Caucasian race or ethnicity
- Gestational age at or beyond 40 weeks
- Maternal obesity (BMI >30)
- Estimated fetal weight >4000 g
- Labor induction

Women who succeed in having a VBAC and thus avoid major abdominal surgery have less hemorrhage, fewer infections, and a shorter recovery period than women who give birth by repeat cesarean (ACOG, 2010/2015). The major risk associated with VBAC is uterine rupture (see later discussion) (Landon & Grobman, 2017). Other maternal risks include operative injury, blood transfusion, hysterectomy, endometritis, and death (ACOG).

Women are most often the primary decision makers with regard to choice of birth method. During the prenatal period, the woman should be given information about VBAC and encouraged to choose it as an alternative to repeat cesarean birth, as long as no contraindications exist. VBAC support groups (e.g., www.vbac.com) and prenatal classes can help prepare the woman psychologically for labor and vaginal birth. Women need to believe not only that their efforts during a TOL will be successful but also that they are fully capable of doing what is necessary to give birth vaginally. They must be given the opportunity to discuss their previous labor experience, including feelings of failure and loss of control, and to express concerns they may have about how they will manage during their upcoming labor and birth. Not everyone is enthusiastic about TOL and VBAC. After being fully informed about the benefits and risks, more than 25% of potential candidates choose to have a repeat cesarean birth instead (Thorp & Laughon, 2014).

If a woman chooses TOL, the nurse is attentive to her psychologic as well as physical needs during the TOL. Anxiety increases the release of catecholamines and can inhibit the release of oxytocin, thus delaying the progress of labor and possibly leading to a repeat cesarean birth. To alleviate such anxiety, the nurse can encourage the woman to use breathing and relaxation techniques and to change positions to promote labor progress. The woman's partner can be encouraged to provide comfort measures and emotional support. Collaboration among the woman in labor, her partner, the nurse, and other health care providers often results in a successful VBAC. If a TOL does not result in vaginal birth, the woman will need support and encouragement to express her feelings about having another cesarean birth. It is very important that this outcome not be labeled a "failed" VBAC.

VBAC is a reasonable option for many women who have had a previous cesarean birth. However, many women who are appropriate candidates for TOL and VBAC lack access to providers and health care facilities that are able and willing to offer this option. The ACOG continues to recommend that TOL and VBAC be offered only in facilities that have staff immediately available to provide emergency care. Because resources for immediate cesarean birth may not be available in all birthing facilities, the best alternative in some situations may be to refer interested women to other facilities that have the resources necessary to offer TOL and VBAC (Landon & Grobman, 2017).

OBSTETRIC EMERGENCIES

MECONIUM-STAINED AMNIOTIC FLUID

Meconium-stained amniotic fluid indicates that the fetus has passed meconium (first stool) before birth. Meconium-stained amniotic fluid is green. The consistency of the meconium fluid is often described as either thin (light) or thick (heavy), depending on the amount of meconium present. Three possible reasons for the passage of meconium are (1) it is a normal physiologic function that occurs with maturity (meconium passage being infrequent before weeks 23 or 24, with an increased incidence after 38 weeks) or with a breech presentation; (2) it is the result of hypoxia-induced peristalsis and sphincter relaxation; or (3) it can be a sequel to umbilical cord compression–induced vagal stimulation in mature fetuses.

The major risk associated with meconium-stained amniotic fluid is the development of meconium aspiration syndrome (MAS) in the newborn (see Table 25.9 in Chapter 25). MAS causes a severe form of aspiration pneumonia that occurs most often in term or postterm infants who have passed meconium in utero. MAS most likely results from a long-standing intrauterine process, rather than from aspiration immediately following birth as respirations are initiated (Rozance & Rosenberg, 2017).

Care Management

The presence of an interprofessional team skilled in neonatal resuscitation is required at the birth of any infant with meconium-stained amniotic fluid. When meconium-stained amniotic fluid is present, the Neonatal Resuscitation Program no longer recommends routine suctioning of the newborn's mouth and nose on the perineum (after the head is out but before the rest of the baby is born) followed by endotracheal suctioning after birth. Instead, management of a newborn with meconium-stained amniotic fluid is based only on assessment of the baby's condition at birth. No clinical studies warrant basing tracheal suctioning guidelines simply on meconium consistency (AAP & AHA, 2016). See the Emergency Treatment box: Immediate Management of the Newborn with Meconium-Stained Amniotic Fluid for specific interventions.

⚡ SAFETY ALERT

Every birth should be attended by at least one person whose only responsibility is the baby and who is capable of initiating resuscitation. Either that person or someone else who is immediately available should have the skills required to perform a complete resuscitation, including endotracheal suctioning to remove meconium, if necessary.

SHOULDER DYSTOCIA

Shoulder dystocia is an uncommon obstetric emergency that increases the risk for fetal and maternal morbidity and mortality during the

✚ EMERGENCY TREATMENT

Immediate Management of the Newborn With Meconium-Stained Amniotic Fluid

Before Birth
- Assess the amniotic fluid for the presence of meconium after rupture of membranes.
- If the amniotic fluid is meconium stained, gather equipment and supplies that might be necessary for neonatal resuscitation.
- Have at least one person capable of performing endotracheal intubation on the baby present at the birth.

Immediately After Birth
- Assess the baby's respiratory efforts, heart rate, and muscle tone.
- Suction only the baby's mouth and nose, using either a bulb syringe or a large-bore suction catheter if the baby has:
  - Strong respiratory efforts
  - Good muscle tone
  - Heart rate >100 beats/minute
- Suction the trachea using an endotracheal tube connected to a meconium aspiration device and suction source to remove any meconium present before many spontaneous respirations have occurred or assisted ventilation has been initiated if the baby has:
  - Depressed respirations
  - Decreased muscle tone
  - Heart rate <100 beats/minute

Data from American Academy of Pediatrics, & American Heart Association. (2016). *Textbook of neonatal resuscitation* (7th ed.). Elk Grove Village, IL: American Academy of Pediatrics.

attempt to accomplish birth vaginally. Shoulder dystocia is a condition in which the head is born, but the anterior shoulder cannot pass under the pubic arch. It results from a size discrepancy between the fetal shoulders and the pelvic inlet, which may be absolute or may be relative, because of malposition. It is estimated that 0.2% to 3% of all vaginal births are complicated by shoulder dystocia (Lanni et al., 2017). The incidence of shoulder dystocia has increased in recent years, perhaps because of larger birth weights or simply because more attention is now paid to documenting the condition.

Fetopelvic disproportion (FPD) related to excessive fetal size (more than 4000 g) or maternal pelvic abnormalities can cause shoulder dystocia, although up to one-half of all cases of shoulder dystocia occur with smaller fetuses (Simpson & O'Brien-Abel, 2014; Thorp & Laughon, 2014). Other risk factors for shoulder dystocia include maternal diabetes (risk for macrosomia), a history of shoulder dystocia with a previous birth, and a prolonged second stage of labor. In one-half of all cases of shoulder dystocia, however, no risk factors are identified (Thorp & Laughon). Shoulder dystocia cannot be accurately predicted or prevented (Simpson & O'Brien-Abel).

Signs that indicate the presence of shoulder dystocia include slowing of the progress of the second stage of labor and formation of a caput succedaneum that increases in size. The nurse should observe for retraction of the fetal head against the perineum immediately following its emergence (turtle sign), an early sign of shoulder dystocia. External rotation does not occur (Simpson & O'Brien-Abel, 2014; Thorp & Laughon, 2014).

Fetal injuries are usually caused either by asphyxia related to the delay in completing the birth or by trauma from the maneuvers used to accomplish the birth. The most common complications related to trauma include fracture of the clavicle or humerus and unilateral brachial

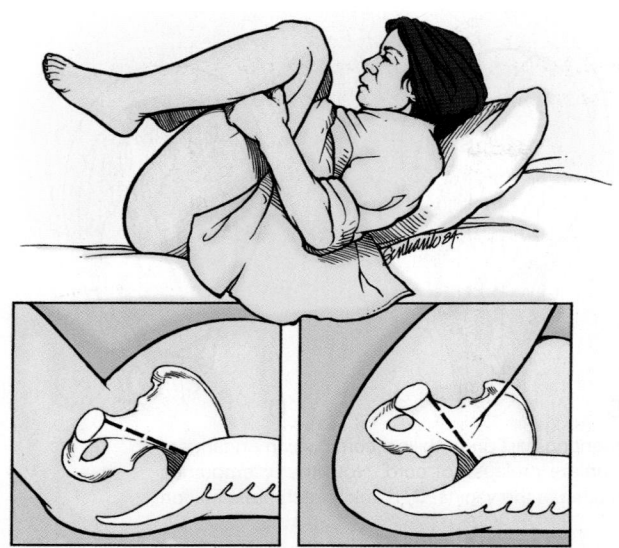

FIG 17.16 McRoberts maneuver. (From Gabbe, S. G., Niebyl, J. R., Simpson, J. L., et al. [2017]. *Obstetrics: Normal and problem pregnancies* [7th ed.]. Philadelphia, PA: Elsevier.)

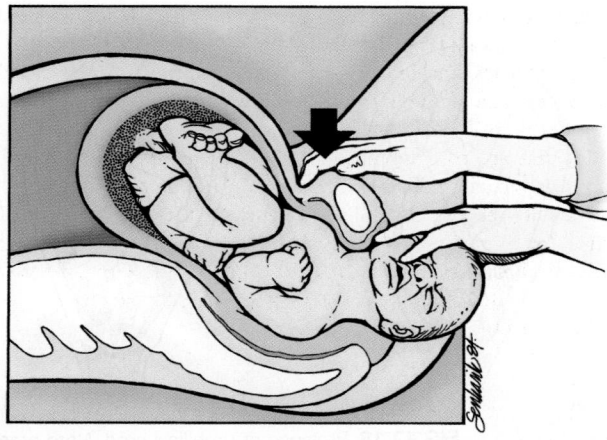

FIG 17.17 Application of suprapubic pressure. (From Gabbe, S. G., Niebyl, J. R., Simpson, J. L., et al. [2017]. *Obstetrics: Normal and problem pregnancies* [7th ed.]. Philadelphia, PA: Elsevier.)

plexus injuries. The right arm is typically the one affected. Evidence now exists that brachial plexus injuries can result from intrauterine forces during the second stage of labor rather than from the maneuvers used to accomplish birth (Lanni et al., 2017; Thorp & Laughon, 2014). If brachial plexus injuries are recognized early and treated properly, 80% to 90% heal completely. Therefore, permanent neurologic injury is rare, occurring in only 1 or 2 of every 10,000 births (Thorp & Laughon). The major maternal complications associated with shoulder dystocia are postpartum hemorrhage and rectal injuries (Lanni et al.; Thorp & Laughon).

Care Management

Many maneuvers have been suggested and tried to free the anterior shoulder. The McRoberts maneuver and suprapubic pressure are usually the first-line interventions for shoulder dystocia, because they are noninvasive, easily learned, and can be performed quickly The specific interventions used are less important than is being prepared at every vaginal birth to deal with shoulder dystocia using a planned sequence of interventions if the need arises (Lanni et al., 2017).

In the McRoberts maneuver (Fig. 17.16), the woman's legs are hyperflexed on her abdomen (Lanni et al., 2017). This maneuver causes the sacrum to straighten, and the pelvis and symphysis pubis to rotate toward the mother's head. The angle of pelvic inclination is decreased, which frees the shoulder. Suprapubic pressure can then be applied over the anterior shoulder (Fig. 17.17) in an attempt to dislodge the shoulder. Use of the McRoberts maneuver and suprapubic pressure may relieve more than one-half of all cases of shoulder dystocia. Fundal pressure as a method of relieving shoulder dystocia should be avoided because it will only further impact the anterior shoulder behind the symphysis pubis (Lanni et al., 2017). The Gaskin maneuver (having the woman move to a hands-and-knees position) has also been highly effective in resolving cases of shoulder dystocia. However, the Gaskin maneuver may be difficult to accomplish if the woman has significant loss of motor function caused by regional anesthesia (Baird & Kennedy, 2017).

When shoulder dystocia is diagnosed, the nurse should stay calm and immediately call for additional assistance (i.e., extra nurses, anesthesia care provider, and neonatal resuscitation team). The nurse then helps the woman assume the position or positions that may facilitate birth

of the shoulders, assists the obstetric health care provider with these maneuvers and techniques during birth, and documents the maneuvers, including the total amount of time required to resolve the shoulder dystocia. The nurse also provides encouragement and support to reduce the anxiety of the woman and her partner. Newborn assessment should include examination for fracture of the clavicle or humerus as well as brachial plexus injuries and asphyxia (Thorp & Laughon, 2014). Maternal assessment should focus on early detection of hemorrhage and trauma to the vagina, perineum, and rectum.

PROLAPSED UMBILICAL CORD

Prolapse of the umbilical cord occurs when the cord lies below the presenting part of the fetus. Umbilical cord prolapse may be occult (hidden, rather than visible) at any time during labor whether or not the membranes are ruptured (Fig. 17.18, *A* and *B*). It is most common to see frank (visible) prolapse directly after rupture of membranes, when gravity washes the cord in front of the presenting part (see Fig. 17.18, *C* and *D*). Contributing factors include a long cord (longer than 100 cm), malpresentation (breech or transverse lie), or an unengaged presenting part.

If the presenting part does not fit snugly into the lower uterine segment (e.g., as in polyhydramnios), when the membranes rupture, a sudden gush of amniotic fluid may cause the cord to be displaced downward. Similarly, the cord may prolapse during amniotomy if the presenting part is high. A small fetus may not fit snugly into the lower uterine segment; as a result, cord prolapse is more likely to occur.

Care Management

Prompt recognition of a prolapsed umbilical cord is important because fetal hypoxia resulting from prolonged cord compression (i.e., occlusion of blood flow to and from the fetus for more than 5 minutes) usually results in central nervous system damage or death of the fetus. Pressure on the cord may be relieved by the examiner putting a sterile gloved hand into the vagina and holding the presenting part off the umbilical cord (Fig. 17.19, *A* and *B*). The woman may also be assisted into a position such as a modified Sims' (see Fig. 17.19, *C*), Trendelenburg, or knee-chest (see Fig. 17.19, *D*) position, in which gravity keeps the pressure of the presenting part off the cord. If the cervix is fully dilated, a forceps- or vacuum-assisted birth can be performed for the fetus in a cephalic presentation; otherwise, a cesarean birth is likely to be performed. Abnormal FHR and pattern (e.g., bradycardia, absent or

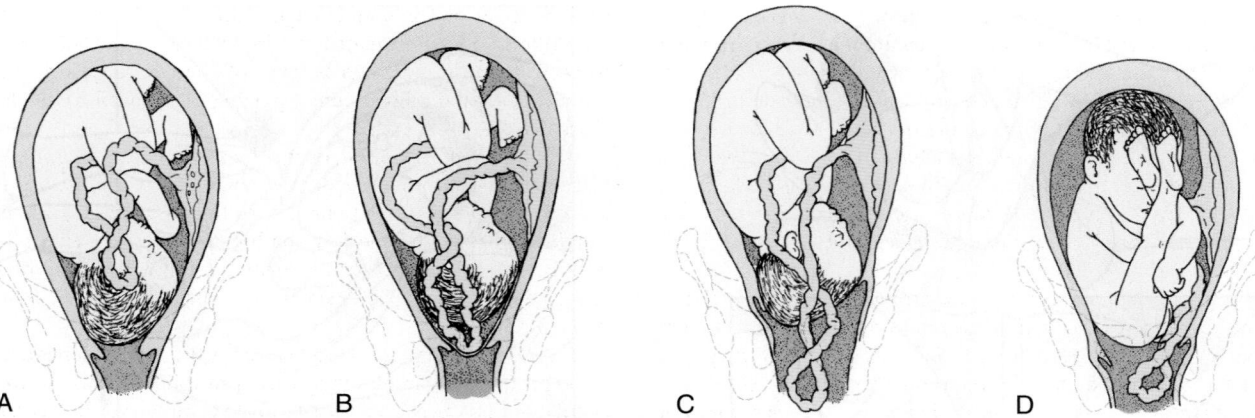

FIG 17.18 Prolapse of umbilical cord. Note pressure of presenting part on umbilical cord, which endangers fetal circulation. **A,** Occult (hidden) prolapse of cord. **B,** Complete prolapse of cord. Note that membranes are intact. **C,** Cord presenting in front of the fetal head may be seen in the vagina. **D,** Frank breech presentation with prolapsed cord.

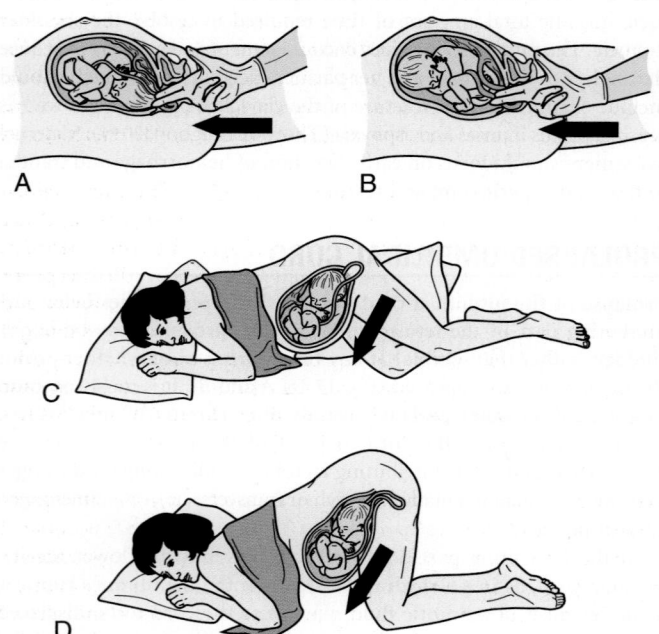

FIG 17.19 *Arrows* indicate direction of pressure against presenting part to relieve compression of prolapsed umbilical cord. Pressure exerted by the examiner's fingers in **A,** vertex presentation, and **B,** breech presentation. **C,** Gravity relieves pressure when woman is in modified Sims' position with hips elevated as high as possible with pillows. **D,** Knee-chest position.

✚ EMERGENCY TREATMENT
Prolapsed Umbilical Cord

Signs
- Variable or prolonged deceleration during uterine contractions
- Woman reports feeling the cord after membranes rupture
- Cord is seen or felt in or protruding from the vagina

Interventions
- Call for assistance. Do not leave the woman alone.
- Have someone notify the obstetric health care provider immediately.
- Glove the examining hand quickly and insert two fingers into the vagina to the cervix. With one finger on either side of the cord or both fingers to one side, exert upward pressure against the presenting part to relieve compression of the cord (see Fig. 17.19, *A* and *B*). Do *not* move your hand! Another person may place a rolled towel under the woman's right or left hip.
- Place woman into the extreme Trendelenburg or a modified Sims position (see Fig. 17.19, *C*) or a knee-chest position (see Fig. 17.19, *D*).
- If cord is protruding from vagina, wrap loosely in a sterile towel saturated with warm sterile normal saline solution. Do not attempt to replace cord into cervix.
- Administer oxygen to the woman by nonrebreather mask at 8 to 10 L/minute until birth is accomplished.
- Start intravenous (IV) fluids, or increase existing flow rate.
- Continue to monitor fetal heart rate (FHR) continuously, by internal fetal scalp electrode, if possible.
- Explain to woman and support person what is happening and the way it is being managed.
- Prepare for immediate vaginal birth if cervix is fully dilated or cesarean birth if it is not.

minimal variability, and variable or prolonged decelerations), inadequate uterine relaxation, and bleeding also can occur as a result of a prolapsed umbilical cord. Indications for immediate interventions are presented in the Emergency Treatment box: Prolapsed Umbilical Cord. Ongoing assessment of the woman and her fetus is critical to determine the effectiveness of each action taken. The woman and her family are often aware of the seriousness of the situation; therefore the nurse must provide support by giving explanations for the interventions being implemented and their effect on the status of the fetus.

RUPTURE OF THE UTERUS

Uterine rupture is defined as the symptomatic disruption and separation of the layers of the uterus or previous scar. Uterine rupture can result in the ejection of fetal parts or the entire fetus into the peritoneal cavity. The incidence of uterine rupture is approximately 1%. During labor and birth, the major risk factor for uterine rupture is a scarred uterus as a result of previous cesarean birth or other uterine surgery (Baird & Kennedy, 2017). Rupture most commonly occurs during a TOL for VBAC; symptomatic rupture is rarely observed in planned, repeat cesarean births. The likelihood of uterine rupture depends on the type and location of the previous uterine scar. Other factors that increase the risk for uterine rupture include prior uterine rupture, trauma, abortion, instrumentation injury or uterine perforation; grand multiparity; and uterine overdistension (i.e., macrosomic fetus, multiple gestation, polyhydramnios, and fetal malpresentation (Baird & Kennedy).

Uterine dehiscence, sometimes called *incomplete uterine rupture,* is separation of a prior scar. It may go unnoticed unless the woman undergoes a subsequent cesarean birth or other uterine surgery. The potential for maternal or fetal complications as a result of uterine dehiscence is negligible because separation of a prior scar does not result in hemorrhage (Landon & Grobman, 2017).

Signs and symptoms vary with the extent of the uterine rupture. The most common finding is an abnormal (category II or category III) FHR tracing, as evidenced by an abrupt decrease in FHR, late or variable decelerations, absent baseline variability, or tachycardia or bradycardia. A loss of fetal station or no fetal descent also can occur. The woman can experience sudden sharp abdominal pain or a ripping or tearing sensation that is independent of uterine contractions. She may also exhibit bright red vaginal bleeding and signs of hypovolemic shock (i.e., hypotension, tachycardia). Fetal parts may be palpable through the abdomen (Baird & Kennedy, 2017).

Care Management

Prevention is the best treatment. Women who have had a cesarean birth with a classical uterine incision are advised not to labor or attempt vaginal birth in subsequent pregnancies. Those at risk for uterine rupture are assessed closely during labor. Women whose labor is induced with oxytocin or prostaglandin (especially if their previous birth was cesarean) are monitored for signs of uterine tachysystole because this can precipitate uterine rupture. If tachysystole occurs, the oxytocin infusion is decreased or discontinued, and a tocolytic medication may be given to decrease the intensity of the uterine contractions (see Emergency Treatment box: Uterine Tachysystole with Oxytocin [Pitocin] Infusion). After giving birth, the woman is assessed for excessive bleeding, especially if the fundus is firm and signs of hemorrhagic shock are present.

If rupture occurs, management depends on the severity. A small rupture may be managed with a laparotomy and birth of the infant, repair of the laceration, and blood transfusions, if needed. Hysterectomy may be necessary if the rupture is large and difficult to repair or if the woman is hemodynamically unstable.

The nurse's role can include starting IV fluids, transfusing blood products, administering oxygen, and assisting with preparations for immediate surgery. Supporting the woman's family and providing information about the treatment are important during this emergency. The associated fetal mortality rate is high (approximately 50% to 75%), particularly if the fetus is ejected from the uterus into the abdominal cavity. Maternal morbidity and mortality also can be substantial (Cunningham et al., 2014). Providing information about spiritual support services or suggesting that the family contact their own support system may be warranted.

AMNIOTIC FLUID EMBOLUS

Amniotic fluid embolus (AFE), also known as anaphylactoid syndrome of pregnancy, is a rare but devastating complication of pregnancy characterized by the sudden, acute onset of hypoxia, hypotension,

cardiovascular collapse, and coagulopathy. The incidence of AFE in the United States is estimated at 1 in 8000 to 1 in 30,000 births. The true incidence is unknown because of the difficulty in confirming the diagnosis and inconsistent reporting of nonfatal cases (Jones & Clark, 2013).

AFE occurs during labor, during birth, or within 30 minutes after birth. This combination of sudden respiratory and cardiovascular collapse, along with coagulopathy, is similar to that observed in patients with anaphylactic or septic shock. In both conditions, a foreign substance is introduced into the circulation, resulting in disseminated intravascular coagulation (DIC), hypotension, and hypoxia (Robbins, Martin, & Wilson, 2014).

In AFE, the foreign substance that initiates the condition is presumed to be present in amniotic fluid that is introduced into the maternal circulation. However, the exact factor that initiates AFE has not been identified. In the past, particles of fetal debris (e.g., vernix, hair, skin cells, or meconium) found in amniotic fluid were thought to be responsible for initiating the syndrome; however, fetal debris can be found in the pulmonary circulation of most healthy laboring women. Also fetal debris is identified in only 78% of women diagnosed with AFE. Therefore, AFE is diagnosed clinically (Jones & Clark, 2013; Robbins et al., 2014; Simpson & O'Brien-Abel, 2014). The most recent population-based studies suggest that the mortality rate in the United States has dropped from a reported rate of 61% to a current rate of 22% (Robbins et al., 2014). Neonatal outcome in cases of AFE is poor. If the event occurs before birth, the neonatal survival rate is approximately 80%. However, only half of these fetuses survive neurologically intact (Jones & Clark).

Predisposing factors for AFE are rapid labor, meconium stained amniotic fluid, and tears into uterine and other large pelvic veins. Other maternal risk factors include older maternal age, postterm pregnancy, labor induction or augmentation, eclampsia, cesarean birth, forceps- or vacuum-assisted vaginal birth, placental abruption or previa, and polyhydramnios (Cunningham et al., 2014). Previously it was thought that the hypertonic uterine contractions that often accompany AFE actually caused the event. Instead, it appears that the physiologic response to AFE produces the hypertonic contractions (Jones & Clark, 2013).

Care Management

The immediate interventions for AFE are summarized in the Emergency Treatment box: Amniotic Fluid Embolus (Anaphylactoid Syndrome of Pregnancy). Care must be instituted immediately. Cardiopulmonary resuscitation is often necessary. If cardiopulmonary arrest occurs, a perimortem cesarean birth should be considered after 4 minutes of unsuccessful resuscitative efforts, both to improve the chances for optimal fetal survival and to facilitate maternal resuscitation (Robbins et al., 2014). The nurse's immediate responsibility is to assist with the resuscitation efforts.

If the woman survives, she is usually moved to a critical care unit. Additional interventions include replacing blood and clotting factors and maintaining adequate hydration and blood pressure. The woman is usually placed on mechanical ventilation with continuous hemodynamic monitoring (Robbins et al., 2014).

Support of the woman's partner and family is needed; they will be anxious and distressed. Brief explanations of what is happening are important during the emergency and can be reinforced after the immediate crisis is over. If the woman dies, emotional support and involvement of the perinatal loss support team or other resources for grief counseling are needed. Referral to grief and loss support groups also is appropriate (see Chapter 21). The nursing staff also may need help in coping with feelings and emotions that result from a maternal death.

✚ EMERGENCY TREATMENT

Amniotic Fluid Embolus (Anaphylactoid Syndrome of Pregnancy)

Signs
- Respiratory distress
  - Restlessness
  - Dyspnea
  - Cyanosis
  - Pulmonary edema
  - Respiratory arrest
- Circulatory collapse
  - Hypotension
  - Tachycardia
  - Shock
  - Cardiac arrest
- Hemorrhage
  - Coagulation failure: bleeding from incisions, venipuncture sites, trauma (lacerations); petechiae, ecchymoses, purpura
  - Uterine atony

Interventions
- Oxygenate
  - Administer oxygen by nonrebreather face mask (8 to 10 L/minute) or resuscitation bag delivering 100% oxygen.
  - Prepare for intubation and mechanical ventilation.
  - Initiate or assist with cardiopulmonary resuscitation. Tilt pregnant woman 30 degrees to her side to displace uterus.
- Maintain cardiac output, and replace fluid losses.
  - Position woman onto her side.
  - Administer intravenous (IV) fluids.
  - Administer blood products: packed cells, fresh-frozen plasma.
  - Insert indwelling catheter, and measure hourly urine output.
- Correct coagulation failure.
- Monitor fetal and maternal status.
- Prepare for emergency birth once woman's condition is stabilized.
- Provide emotional support to woman, her partner, and family.

REFERENCES

American Academy of Pediatrics & American College of Obstetricians and Gynecologists (2012). *Guidelines for perinatal care* (7th ed.). Washington, DC: American College of Obstetricians and Gynecologists.

American Academy of Pediatrics & American Heart Association (2016). *Textbook of neonatal resuscitation* (7th ed.). Elk Grove Village, IL: American Academy of Pediatrics.

American College of Obstetricians and Gynecologists. (2009, reaffirmed 2016). Practice bulletin no. 107: Induction of labor. *Obstetrics and Gynecology, 114*(2 pt 1), 386–397.

American College of Obstetricians and Gynecologists. (2014, reaffirmed 2016). Practice bulletin no. 146: Management of late-term and postterm pregnancies. *Obstetrics and Gynecology, 124*(2 pt 1), 390–396.

American College of Obstetricians and Gynecologists. (2016a). Practice bulletin no. 171: Management of preterm labor. *Obstetrics and Gynecology, 128*(4), e155–e164.

American College of Obstetricians and Gynecologists. (2016b). Practice bulletin no. 172: Premature rupture of membranes. *Obstetrics and Gynecology, 128*(4), e165–e177.

American College of Obstetricians and Gynecologists. (2010, reaffirmed 2015). Practice bulletin no. 115: Vaginal birth after previous cesarean delivery. *Obstetrics and Gynecology, 116*(2 pt 1), 450–463.

American College of Obstetricians and Gynecologists & Society for Maternal-Fetal Medicine. (2013, reaffirmed 2015). Committee opinion no. 579: Definition of term pregnancy. *Obstetrics and Gynecology, 122*(5), 1139–1140.

American College of Obstetricians and Gynecologists & Society for Maternal-Fetal Medicine. (2014). Safe prevention of the primary cesarean delivery. *Obstetrics and Gynecology, 123*(3), 693–711.

Baird, S. M., & Kennedy, B. B. (2017). Obstetric emergencies. In B. B. Kennedy & S. M. Baird (Eds.), *Intrapartum management modules: A perinatal education program* (5th ed.). Philadelphia, PA: Wolters Kluwer.

Baird, S. M., Kennedy, B. B., & Dalton, J. (2017). Special considerations for individualized care of the laboring woman. In B. B. Kennedy & S. M. Baird (Eds.), *Intrapartum management modules: A perinatal education program* (5th ed.). Philadelphia, PA: Wolters Kluwer.

Berghella, V., Mackeen, D., & Jauniaux, E. R. M. (2017). Cesarean delivery. In S. G. Gabbe, J. R. Niebyl, J. L. Simpson, et al. (Eds.), *Obstetrics: Normal and problem pregnancies* (7th ed.). Philadelphia, PA: Elsevier.

Buhimschi, C. S., & Norman, J. E. (2014). Pathogenesis of spontaneous preterm labor. In R. K. Creasy, R. Resnik, J. D. Iams, et al. (Eds.), *Creasy and Resnik's maternal-fetal medicine: Principles and practice* (7th ed.). Philadelphia, PA: Saunders.

Cunningham, F., Leveno, K., Bloom, S., et al. (2014). *Williams obstetrics* (24th ed.). New York, NY: McGraw-Hill Education.

DeFranco, E. A., Lewis, D. F., & Odibo, A. O. (2013). Improving the screening accuracy for preterm labor: Is the combination of fetal fibronectin and cervical length in symptomatic patients a useful predictor of preterm birth? A systematic review. *American Journal of Obstetrics and Gynecology, 208*(1), 233.e1–233.e6.

Duff, P. (2014). Maternal and fetal infections. In R. K. Creasy, R. Resnik, J. D. Iams, et al. (Eds.), *Creasy and Resnik's maternal-fetal medicine: Principles and practice* (7th ed.). Philadelphia, PA: Saunders.

Duff, P., & Birsner, M. (2017). Maternal and perinatal infection in pregnancy: Bacterial. In S. G. Gabbe, J. R. Niebyl, J. L. Simpson, et al. (Eds.), *Obstetrics: Normal and problem pregnancies* (7th ed.). Philadelphia, PA: Elsevier.

Ecker, J. (2013). Elective cesarean delivery on maternal request. *Journal of the American Medical Association, 309*(18), 1930–1936.

Friedman, E. (1989). Normal and dysfunctional labor. In W. Cohen, D. Ackers, & E. Friedman (Eds.), *Management of labor* (6th ed.). Rockville, MD: Aspen.

Hill, W., & Harvey, C. (2013). Induction of labor. In N. Troiano, C. Harvey, & B. Chez (Eds.), *AWHONN's high risk and critical care obstetrics* (3rd ed.). Philadelphia, PA: Wolters Kluwer/Lippincott Williams & Wilkins.

Huwe, V. Y. (2017). Induction and augmentation of labor. In B. B. Kennedy & S. M. Baird (Eds.), *Intrapartum management modules: A perinatal education program* (5th ed.). Philadelphia, PA: Wolters Kluwer.

Institute for Safe Medication Practices. (2014). *ISMP's list of high-alert medications.* Retrieved from http:// www.ismp.org/Tools/ highAlertMedicationLists.asp.

Jones, R., & Clark, S. (2013). Amniotic fluid embolus (anaphylactoid syndrome of pregnancy). In N. Troiano, C. Harvey, & B. Chez (Eds.), *AWHONN's high risk and critical care obstetrics* (3rd ed.). Philadelphia, PA: Wolters Kluwer/Lippincott Williams & Wilkins.

Kilpatrick, S., & Garrison, E. (2017). Normal labor and delivery. In S. G. Gabbe, J. R. Niebyl, J. L. Simpson, et al. (Eds.), *Obstetrics: Normal and problem pregnancies* (7th ed.). Philadelphia, PA: Elsevier.

Landon, M. B., & Grobman, W. A. (2017). Vaginal birth after cesarean delivery. In S. G. Gabbe, J. R. Niebyl, J. L. Simpson, et al. (Eds.), *Obstetrics: Normal and problem pregnancies* (7th ed.). Philadelphia, PA: Elsevier.

Lanni, S. M., Gherman, R., & Gonik, B. (2017). Malpresentations. In S. G. Gabbe, J. R. Niebyl, J. L. Simpson, et al. (Eds.), *Obstetrics: Normal and problem pregnancies* (7th ed.). Philadelphia, PA: Elsevier.

Macones, G., Hankins, G., Spong, C., et al. (2008). The 2008 National Institute of Child Health and Human Development workshop report on electronic fetal monitoring: Update on definitions, interpretation, and research guidelines. *Journal of Obstetric, Gynecologic, & Neonatal Nursing, 37*(5), 510–515.

Malone, F. D., & D'Alton, M. E. (2014). Multiple gestation: Clinical characteristics and management. In R. K. Creasy, R. Resnik, J. D. Iams, et al. (Eds.), *Creasy and Resnik's maternal-fetal medicine: Principles and practice* (7th ed.). Philadelphia, PA: Saunders.

Martin, J. A., Hamilton, B. E., & Osterman, M. J. K. (2017). Births: Final data for 2015. *National Vital Statistics Reports, 66*(1), 1–70.

Martin, J. A., Osterman, M. J. K., Kimeyer, S. E., & Gregory, E. C. W. (2015). Measuring gestational age in vital statistics data: Transitioning to the obstetric estimate. *National Vital Statistics Reports, 64*(5), 1–20.

Mercer, B. M. (2014a). Assessment and induction of fetal pulmonary maturity. In R. K. Creasy, R. Resnik, J. D. Iams, et al. (Eds.), *Creasy and Resnik's maternal-fetal medicine: Principles and practice* (7th ed.). Philadelphia, PA: Saunders.

Mercer, B. M. (2014b). Premature rupture of the membranes. In R. K. Creasy, R. Resnik, J. D. Iams, et al. (Eds.), *Creasy and Resnik's maternal-fetal medicine: Principles and practice* (7th ed.). Philadelphia, PA: Saunders.

Mercer, B. M. (2017). Premature rupture of the membranes. In S. G. Gabbe, J. R. Niebyl, J. L. Simpson, et al. (Eds.), *Obstetrics: Normal and problem pregnancies* (7th ed.). Philadelphia, PA: Elsevier.

Nielsen, P. E., Deering, S. P., & Galan, H. L. (2017). Operative vaginal delivery. In S. G. Gabbe, J. R. Niebyl, J. L. Simpson, et al. (Eds.), *Obstetrics: Normal and problem pregnancies* (7th ed.). Philadelphia, PA: Elsevier.

Newman, R. B. & Unal, E. R. (2017). Multiple gestations. In S. G. Gabbe, J. R. Niebyl, J. L. Simpson, et al. (Eds.), *Obstetrics: Normal and problem pregnancies* (7th ed.). Philadelphia, PA: Elsevier.

Picklesimer, A., & Dorman, K. (2013). Maternal obesity: Effects on pregnancy. In N. Troiano, C. Harvey, & B. Chez (Eds.), *AWHONN's high risk and critical care obstetrics* (3rd ed.). Philadelphia, PA: Wolters Kluwer/ Lippincott Williams & Wilkins.

Rampersad, R. & Macones, G. A. (2017). Prolonged and postterm pregnancy. In S. G. Gabbe, J. R. Niebyl, J. L. Simpson, et al. (Eds.), *Obstetrics: Normal and problem pregnancies* (7th ed.). Philadelphia, PA: Elsevier.

Reedy, N. J. (2014). Preterm labor and birth. In K. R. Simpson & P. Creehan (Eds.), *AWHONN's perinatal nursing* (4th ed.). Philadelphia, PA: Lippincott.

Robbins, K. S., Martin, S. R., & Wilson, W. C. (2014). Intensive care considerations for the critically ill parturient. In R. K. Creasy, R. Resnik, J. D. Iams, et al. (Eds.), *Creasy and Resnik's maternal-fetal medicine: Principles and practice* (7th ed.). Philadelphia, PA: Saunders.

Rozance, P. J., & Rosenberg, A. A. (2017). The neonate. In S. G. Gabbe, J. R. Niebyl, J. L. Simpson, et al. (Eds.), *Obstetrics: Normal and problem pregnancies* (7th ed.). Philadelphia, PA: Elsevier.

Schorn, M. N., Moore, E., Spetalnick, B. M., & Morad, A. (2015). Implementing family-centered cesarean birth. *Journal of Midwifery & Women's Health, 60*(6), 682–690.

Sheibani, L., & Wing, D. A. (2017). Abnormal labor and induction of labor. In S. G. Gabbe, J. R. Niebyl, J. L. Simpson, et al. (Eds.), *Obstetrics: Normal and problem pregnancies* (7th ed.). Philadelphia, PA: Elsevier.

Simhan, H. N., Berghella, V., & Iams, J. D. (2014). Preterm labor and birth. In R. K. Creasy, R. Resnik, J. D. Iams, et al. (Eds.), *Creasy and Resnik's maternal-fetal medicine: Principles and practice* (7th ed.). Philadelphia, PA: Saunders.

Simhan, H. N., Iams, J. D., & Romero, R. (2017). Preterm labor and birth. In S. G. Gabbe, J. R. Niebyl, J. L. Simpson, et al. (Eds.), *Obstetrics: Normal and problem pregnancies* (7th ed.). Philadelphia, PA: Elsevier.

Simpson, K. R., & O'Brien-Abel, N. (2014). Labor and birth. In K. R. Simpson & P. Creehan (Eds.), *AWHONN's perinatal nursing* (4th ed.). Philadelphia, PA: Lippincott.

Swanson, D., & Baird, S. M. (2017). Preterm labor and preterm premature rupture of membranes. In B. B. Kennedy & S. M. Baird (Eds.), *Intrapartum management modules: A perinatal education program* (5th ed.). Philadelphia, PA: Wolters Kluwer.

Thorp, J. M., & Laughon, S. K. (2014). Clinical aspects of normal and abnormal labor. In R. K. Creasy, R. Resnik, J. D. Iams, et al. (Eds.), *Creasy and Resnik's maternal-fetal medicine: Principles and practice* (7th ed.). Philadelphia, PA: Saunders.

Yount, S. M., & Lassiter, N. (2013). The pharmacology of prostaglandins for induction of labor. *Journal of Midwifery & Women's Health, 58*(2), 133–144.

18

Postpartum Physiologic Changes

Kathryn R. Alden

http://evolve.elsevier.com/Perry/maternal

The postpartum period is the interval between birth and the return of the reproductive organs to their normal nonpregnant state. This period is sometimes referred to as the *puerperium,* or fourth trimester of pregnancy. Although the puerperium has traditionally been considered to last 6 weeks, this time frame varies among women. The physiologic changes that occur during the reversal of the processes of pregnancy are distinctive, but they are normal. To provide care during the recovery period that is beneficial to the mother, her infant, and her family, the nurse must synthesize knowledge of maternal anatomy and physiology of the recovery period, the newborn's physical and behavioral characteristics, infant care activities, and the family's response to the birth. This chapter focuses on anatomic and physiologic changes that occur in the mother during the postpartum period.

REPRODUCTIVE SYSTEM AND ASSOCIATED STRUCTURES

UTERUS

Involution Process

The return of the uterus to a nonpregnant state after birth is called involution. This process begins immediately after expulsion of the placenta with contraction of the uterine smooth muscle.

At the end of the third stage of labor, the uterus is in the midline, approximately 2 cm below the level of the umbilicus, with the fundus resting on the sacral promontory. At this time, the uterus weighs approximately 1000 g (Isley & Katz, 2017).

Within 12 hours, the fundus can rise to approximately 1 cm above the umbilicus (Fig. 18.1). By 24 hours after birth, the uterus is about the same size as it was at 20 weeks of gestation. Involution progresses rapidly during the next few days. The fundus descends 1 to 2 cm every 24 hours. By the sixth postpartum day, the fundus is normally located halfway between the umbilicus and the symphysis pubis. The uterus should not be palpable abdominally after 2 weeks and should have returned to its nonpregnant location by 6 weeks after birth (Blackburn, 2013).

The uterus, which at full term weighs approximately 11 times its prepregnancy weight, involutes to approximately 500 g by 1 week after birth and to 300 g by 2 weeks after birth. By 4 weeks postpartum, it

weighs approximately 100g, which is the nonpregnant size (Cunningham, Leveno, Bloom, et al., 2014).

Increased estrogen and progesterone levels are responsible for stimulating the massive growth of the uterus during pregnancy. Prenatal uterine growth results from both hyperplasia (an increase in the number of muscle cells) and hypertrophy (an enlargement of the existing cells). After birth, the decrease in these hormones causes autolysis—the self-destruction of excess hypertrophied tissue. The additional cells laid down during pregnancy remain and account for the slight increase in uterine size after each pregnancy.

Subinvolution is the failure of the uterus to return to a nonpregnant state. The most common causes of subinvolution are retained placental fragments and infection (see Chapter 21).

Contractions

Postpartum hemostasis is achieved primarily by compression of intramyometrial blood vessels as the uterine muscle contracts rather than by platelet aggregation and clot formation. The hormone oxytocin, released from the pituitary gland, strengthens and coordinates these uterine contractions, which compress blood vessels and promote hemostasis. During the first 1 to 2 postpartum hours, uterine contractions can decrease in intensity and become uncoordinated. Because it is vital that the uterus remains firm and well contracted, exogenous oxytocin (Pitocin) is usually administered intravenously or intramuscularly immediately after expulsion of the placenta. The uterus is very sensitive to oxytocin during the first week or so after birth. Breastfeeding immediately after birth and in the early days postpartum increases the release of oxytocin, which promotes uterine contractions, therefore, decreasing blood loss and reducing the risk for postpartum hemorrhage (Lawrence & Lawrence, 2016).

In primiparous women, uterine tone is good, the fundus generally remains firm, and the woman usually perceives only mild uterine cramping. Periodic relaxation and vigorous contractions are more common in subsequent pregnancies and can cause uncomfortable cramping called afterpains (afterbirth pains), which typically resolve in 3 to 7 days. Afterpains are more noticeable after births in which the uterus was overdistended (e.g., macrosomic infant, multifetal gestation, polyhydramnios). Breastfeeding and exogenous oxytocic medication usually intensify afterpains because both stimulate uterine contractions.

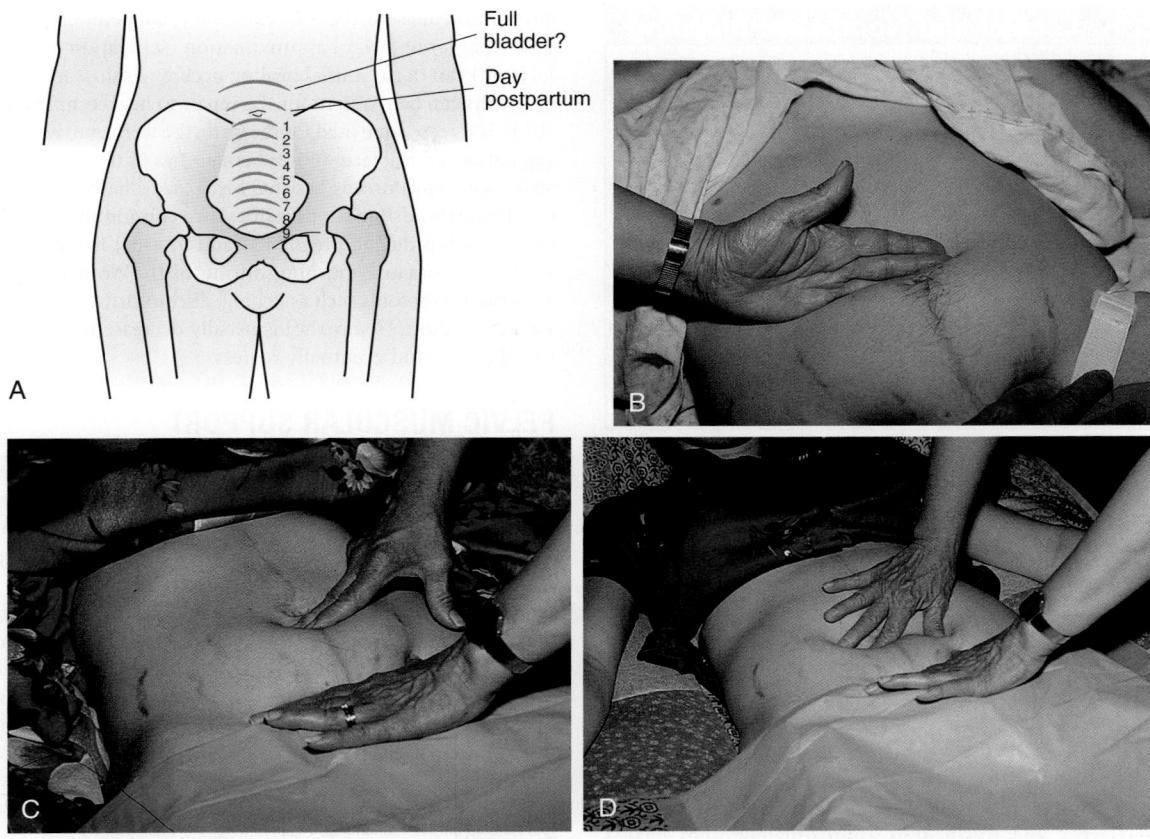

FIG 18.1 Assessment of involution of uterus after birth. **A,** Normal progress, days 1 to 9. **B,** Size and position of uterus 2 hours after birth. **C,** Two days after birth. **D,** Four days after birth. Note linea nigra and striae gravidarum ("stretch marks") in **B–D.** (B–D, Courtesy of Marjorie Pyle, RNC, Lifecircle, Costa Mesa, CA.)

Placental Site

Immediately after the placenta and membranes are expelled, vascular constriction and thromboses reduce the placental site to an irregular nodular and elevated area. Upward growth of the endometrium causes sloughing of necrotic tissue and prevents the scar formation characteristic of normal wound healing. This unique healing process enables the endometrium to resume its usual cycle of changes and permit implantation and placentation in future pregnancies. Endometrial regeneration is completed by postpartum day 16, except at the placental site. Regeneration at the placental site usually is not complete until 6 weeks after birth (Blackburn, 2013).

Lochia

Postbirth uterine discharge, commonly called lochia, initially is bright red (lochia rubra) and may contain small clots. For the first 2 hours after birth, the amount of uterine discharge should be about that of a heavy menstrual period. After that time, the lochial flow should steadily decrease.

Lochia rubra is bright red and consists mainly of blood and decidual and trophoblastic debris. The flow pales, becoming pink or brown (lochia serosa) after 3 to 4 days. Lochia serosa consists of old blood, serum, leukocytes, and tissue debris. In most women, about 10 to 14 days after birth the drainage becomes yellow to white (lochia alba). Lochia alba consists of leukocytes, decidua, epithelial cells, mucus, serum, and bacteria. Lochia can persist up to 4 to 8 weeks after birth. If the woman receives an oxytocic medication, regardless of the route of administration, the flow of lochia is often scant until the effects of the medication wear off. The amount of lochia is usually less after a cesarean birth because the surgeon suctions the blood and fluids from the uterus or wipes the uterine lining before closing the incision. Flow of lochia usually increases with ambulation and breastfeeding. Lochia tends to pool in the vagina when the woman is lying in bed; the woman then can experience a gush of blood when she stands. This gush should not be confused with hemorrhage.

Persistence of lochia rubra in the postpartum period suggests continued bleeding as a result of retained fragments of the placenta or membranes. It is not uncommon for women to experience a sudden, but brief, increase in bleeding 7 to 14 days after birth when sloughing of eschar over the placental site occurs. If this increase in bleeding does not subside within 1 to 2 hours, the woman needs to be evaluated for possible retained placental fragments (Isley & Katz, 2017).

About 10% to 15% of women still have normal lochia serosa discharge at their 6-week postpartum examination (Isley & Katz, 2017). However, the continued flow of lochia serosa or lochia alba by 3 to 4 weeks after birth can indicate endometritis, particularly if the woman has fever, pain, or abdominal tenderness. Lochia should smell like normal menstrual flow; an offensive odor usually indicates infection.

Not all postpartal vaginal bleeding is lochia; vaginal bleeding after birth can be caused by unrepaired vaginal or cervical lacerations. Box 18.1 distinguishes between lochial and nonlochial bleeding.

BOX 18.1 Lochial and Nonlochial Bleeding

Lochial Bleeding
- Lochia usually trickles from the vaginal opening. The steady flow is greater as the uterus contracts.
- A gush of lochia can appear as the uterus is massaged. If it is dark in color, it has been pooled in the relaxed vagina, and the amount soon lessens to a trickle of bright red lochia (in the early puerperium).

Nonlochial Bleeding
- If the bloody discharge spurts from the vagina, and the uterus is firmly contracted, there can be cervical or vaginal tears in addition to the normal lochia.
- If the amount of bleeding continues to be excessive and bright red, a tear can be the source.

CERVIX

The cervix is soft immediately after birth. The ectocervix (portion of the cervix that protrudes into the vagina) appears bruised and has some small lacerations, creating optimal conditions for the development of infection. Over the next 12 to 18 hours, it shortens and becomes firmer. The cervical os, which dilated to 10 cm during labor, closes gradually. Within 2 to 3 days postpartum, it has shortened, become firm, and regained its form. The cervix up to the lower uterine segment remains edematous, thin, and fragile for several days after birth. By the second or third postpartum day, the cervical dilation has decreased to 2 to 3 cm, and by 1 week after birth, it is approximately 1 cm dilated (Blackburn, 2013). The external cervical os never regains its prepregnancy appearance; it no longer has a circular shape but, instead, appears as a jagged slit often described as a "fish mouth" (see Fig. 7.2). Lactation delays the production of cervical and other estrogen-influenced mucus and affects mucosal characteristics.

VAGINA AND PERINEUM

Postpartum estrogen deprivation is responsible for the thinness of the vaginal mucosa and the absence of rugae. The smooth-walled vagina that was greatly distended during birth gradually decreases in size and regains tone, although it never completely returns to its prepregnancy state. Rugae reappear within 3 weeks, but they are never as prominent as in the nulliparous woman. Most rugae are permanently flattened. The mucosa remains atrophic in the lactating woman, at least until menstruation resumes. Thickening of the vaginal mucosa occurs with the return of ovarian function. Estrogen deficiency is responsible for a decreased amount of vaginal lubrication; vaginal dryness is more prevalent among breastfeeding mothers. Localized dryness and coital discomfort (dyspareunia) can persist until ovarian function returns and menstruation resumes. The use of a water-soluble lubricant during sexual intercourse is usually recommended.

Immediately after vaginal birth, the introitus is erythematous and edematous, especially in the area of an episiotomy or laceration repair. It is barely distinguishable from that of a nulliparous woman if lacerations or an episiotomy have been carefully repaired, hematomas are prevented or treated early, and the woman practices good hygiene during the first 2 weeks after birth.

Most episiotomies and laceration repairs are visible only if the woman is lying on her side with her upper buttock raised or if she is placed in the lithotomy position. A good light source is essential for visualization of some repairs. Healing of an episiotomy or laceration is the same as any surgical incision. Signs of infection (pain, redness, warmth, swelling, or discharge) or lack of approximation (separation of the edges of the incision) can occur. Initial healing occurs within 2 to 3 weeks, but 4 to 6 months can be required for the repair to heal completely (Blackburn, 2013). If forceps were used for the birth, the woman may have experienced vaginal or cervical lacerations; hematomas of the pelvic soft tissues can also occur with forceps-assisted birth (see Chapter 17).

Hemorrhoids (anal varicosities) are commonly seen. Hemorrhoids often develop during pregnancy, and internal hemorrhoids can evert while the woman is pushing during birth. Women often experience associated symptoms such as itching, discomfort, and bright red bleeding with defecation. Hemorrhoids usually decrease in size within 6 weeks of childbirth and eventually regress.

PELVIC MUSCULAR SUPPORT

The supporting structure (muscles and ligaments) of the uterus and vagina can be injured during birth; this can contribute to later gynecologic problems. Supportive tissues of the pelvic floor that are torn or stretched during birth can require up to 6 months to regain tone. Kegel exercises, which help strengthen perineal muscles and encourage healing, are recommended after birth (see Patient Teaching box: Kegel Exercises, Chapter 3). Later in life, women can experience pelvic relaxation—the lengthening and weakening of the fascial supports of pelvic structures. These structures include the uterus, upper posterior vaginal wall, urethra, bladder, and rectum. Although relaxation can occur in any woman, it is commonly a direct but delayed complication of birth.

ENDOCRINE SYSTEM

PLACENTAL HORMONES

Significant hormonal changes occur during the postpartum period. Expulsion of the placenta results in dramatic decreases in the hormones produced by that organ.

Estrogen and progesterone levels drop markedly after birth and reach their lowest levels 1 week after birth. Decreased estrogen levels are associated with the diuresis of excess extracellular fluid accumulated during pregnancy. In nonlactating women, estrogen levels begin to increase by 2 weeks after birth and by postpartum day 17 are higher than in women who breastfeed (Isley & Katz, 2017).

Human chorionic gonadotropin (hCG) disappears fairly quickly from maternal circulation. However, because removing hCG from the extravascular and intracellular spaces takes additional time, the hormone can be detected in the maternal system for 3 to 4 weeks after birth (Blackburn, 2013).

METABOLIC CHANGES

Decreases in human chorionic somatomammotropin (formerly called *human placental lactogen*), estrogens, cortisol, and the placental enzyme insulinase reverse the diabetogenic effects of pregnancy, resulting in significantly lower blood glucose levels in the immediate puerperium. Mothers with type 1 diabetes will likely require much less insulin for several days after birth, especially if they are breastfeeding. Because these normal hormonal changes make the puerperium a transitional period for carbohydrate metabolism, it is more difficult to interpret results of glucose tolerance tests at this time.

Thyroid volume gradually returns to normal by 3 months after birth. Levels of thyroxine and triiodothyronine decrease to prepregnant levels within 4 weeks. There is an increased risk for transient autoimmune thyroiditis in the postpartum period (Isley & Katz, 2017).

The basal metabolic rate remains elevated for the first 1 to 2 weeks after birth (James, 2014). It gradually returns to prepregnancy levels.

PITUITARY HORMONES AND OVARIAN FUNCTION

Prolactin levels in blood rise progressively throughout pregnancy. After birth, as levels of progesterone decrease, prolactin levels increase. In a woman who breastfeeds, prolactin levels are highest during the first month after birth and remain elevated above nonpregnant levels as long as she is breastfeeding. Serum prolactin levels are influenced by the frequency of breastfeeding, the duration of each feeding, and use of supplementary feedings. Individual differences in the strength of an infant's sucking stimulus also affect prolactin levels. In nonlactating women, prolactin levels decline after birth and reach the prepregnant range by the third postpartum week (Isley & Katz, 2017).

Lactating and nonlactating women differ considerably in the timing of their first ovulation and when menstruation resumes. Ovulation occurs as early as 27 days after birth in nonlactating women, with a mean time of about 7 to 9 weeks. About 70% of nonbreastfeeding women resume menstruating by 12 weeks after birth. The mean time to ovulation in women who breastfeed is about 6 months (Isley & Katz, 2017). The persistence of elevated serum prolactin levels in breastfeeding women appears to be responsible for suppressing ovulation. In lactating women, both the resumption of ovulation and the return of menses are determined in large part by breastfeeding patterns. For example, ovulation is delayed longer in women who breastfeed exclusively compared with women who breastfeed and offer supplemental infant formula to their infants. Because of the uncertainty about the return of ovulation and menstruation, discussion of contraceptive options early in the postpartum period is necessary. The first menstrual flow after birth is usually heavier than normal. Within three or four cycles, the amount of menstrual flow returns to the prepregnancy volume.

URINARY SYSTEM

The hormonal changes of pregnancy (i.e., high steroid levels) contribute to an increase in renal function; diminishing steroid levels after birth may partly explain the reduced renal function that occurs during the puerperium. Kidney function returns to normal by 8 weeks after birth. About 6 weeks are required for the pregnancy-induced hypotonia and dilation of the ureters and renal pelves to return to the nonpregnant state In a small percentage of women, dilation of the urinary tract can persist for 3 months or longer, increasing the risk for developing a urinary tract infection (Isley & Katz, 2017).

URINE COMPONENTS

The renal glycosuria induced by pregnancy disappears by 1 week postpartum, but lactosuria can occur in lactating women. The blood urea nitrogen increases during the puerperium as autolysis of the involuting uterus occurs. Plasma creatinine levels return to normal by 6 weeks postpartum. Pregnancy-associated proteinuria resolves by 6 weeks after birth (Blackburn, 2013). Ketonuria can occur in women with an uncomplicated birth or after a prolonged labor with dehydration.

FLUID LOSS

Within 12 hours of birth, women begin to lose excess tissue fluid accumulated during pregnancy. Postpartal diuresis, caused by decreased estrogen levels, removal of increased venous pressure in the lower extremities, and loss of the remaining pregnancy-induced increase in blood volume aids the body in ridding itself of excess fluid. Urine output of 3000 mL or more each day during the first 2 to 3 days is common. Profuse diaphoresis often occurs, especially at night, for the first 2 to 3 days after birth. Fluid loss through perspiration and increased urinary output accounts for a weight loss of 2 to 3 kg (5 to 6.6 lb) during the early puerperium (Cunningham et al., 2014).

URETHRA AND BLADDER

Birth-induced trauma, increased bladder capacity after birth, and the effects of conduction anesthesia can result in a decreased urge to void. In addition, pelvic soreness caused by the forces of labor, vaginal or perineal lacerations, or episiotomy can reduce or alter the voiding reflex. Decreased voiding combined with postpartal diuresis can result in bladder distention.

Immediately after birth, excessive bleeding can occur if the bladder becomes distended because it pushes the uterus up and to the side and prevents it from contracting firmly. Later in the puerperium, overdistention can make the bladder more susceptible to infection and impede the resumption of normal voiding. With adequate bladder emptying, bladder tone is usually restored by 5 to 7 days after birth.

Some women experience *stress incontinence* during the postpartum period. This is more likely to occur after vaginal than cesarean birth. Stress incontinence can be related to tissue trauma to the pelvic floor occurring with maternal expulsive efforts and increased size of the neonate. Coached pushing versus uncoached (non-Valsalva) pushing can increase the risk for damage to the pelvic floor and subsequent stress incontinence (James, 2014).

GASTROINTESTINAL SYSTEM

Most new mothers are very hungry after full recovery from analgesia, anesthesia, and fatigue. Requests for extra portions of food and frequent snacks are common.

A spontaneous bowel evacuation may not occur for 2 to 3 days after birth. This delay can be explained by slowed peristalsis related to decreased muscle tone in the intestines during labor and the immediate postpartum period, prelabor diarrhea, lack of food, or dehydration. The mother often anticipates discomfort during the bowel movement because of perineal tenderness as a result of an episiotomy, lacerations, or hemorrhoids and resists the urge to defecate. Regular bowel habits should be reestablished when bowel tone returns.

Third- and fourth-degree perineal lacerations that involve the anal sphincter are associated with an increased risk for postpartum anal incontinence. Women with this problem are more often incontinent of flatus than of stool. If anal incontinence lasts more than 6 months, studies should be conducted to determine the specific cause and appropriate treatment (Isley & Katz, 2017).

BREASTS

Promptly after birth, a decrease occurs in the concentrations of hormones (i.e., estrogen, progesterone, hCG, prolactin, cortisol, and insulin) that stimulated breast development during pregnancy. The time required for these hormones to return to prepregnancy levels is determined in part by whether or not the mother breastfeeds her infant.

BREASTFEEDING MOTHERS

During the first 24 hours after birth, there is little if any change in the breast tissue. Colostrum, or early milk, a clear yellow fluid, can be expressed from the breasts. The breasts gradually become fuller and heavier as the colostrum transitions to mature milk by about 72 to 96 hours after birth; this is often referred to as the "milk coming in," or lactogenesis II. The breasts can feel warm, firm, and somewhat tender. Bluish white milk with a skim-milk appearance (true milk) can be expressed from the nipples. As milk glands and milk ducts fill with milk, breast tissue can feel somewhat nodular or lumpy. Unlike the lumps associated with fibrocystic breast changes or cancer (which can be palpated consistently in the same location), the nodularity associated with milk production tends to shift in position. Some women experience engorgement at this time due to an increase in blood and lymphatic fluid as milk production increases. Engorged breasts are hard and uncomfortable; the fullness of the nipple tissue can make it difficult for the infant to latch on and feed. With frequent breastfeeding and proper care, engorgement is a temporary condition that typically lasts only 24 to 48 hours (see Chapter 24).

NONBREASTFEEDING MOTHERS

The breasts generally feel nodular in contrast to the granular feel of breasts in nonpregnant women. The nodularity is bilateral and diffuse. Prolactin levels drop rapidly. Colostrum is present for the first few days after birth. Palpation of the breasts on the second or third day as milk production begins can reveal tissue tenderness in some women. On the third or fourth postpartum day, engorgement can occur. The breasts are distended (swollen), firm, tender, and warm to the touch. Breast distention is caused primarily by the temporary congestion of veins and lymphatics rather than by an accumulation of milk. Milk is present but should not be expressed. Axillary breast tissue (the tail of Spence) and any accessory breast or nipple tissue along the milk line can be involved. Engorgement resolves spontaneously, and discomfort decreases usually within 24 to 36 hours. A breast binder or well-fitted supportive bra, ice packs, fresh cabbage leaves, and/or mild analgesics may be used to relieve discomfort. Nipple stimulation is avoided. If suckling or milk expression is never begun (or is discontinued), lactation ceases within a few days to 1 week.

CARDIOVASCULAR SYSTEM

BLOOD VOLUME

Changes in blood volume after birth depend on several factors, such as blood loss during birth and the amount of extravascular water (physiologic edema) mobilized and excreted. Pregnancy-induced hypervolemia (an increase in blood volume to 40% to 45% above nonpregnancy levels) allows most women to tolerate considerable blood loss during birth. The average blood loss for a vaginal birth of a single fetus ranges from 300 to 500 mL (10% of blood volume). The typical blood loss for women who give birth by cesarean is 500 to 1000 mL (15% to 30% of blood volume). During the first few days after birth, the plasma volume decreases further as a result of diuresis (Blackburn, 2013).

Maternal physiologic changes in the puerperium enable the woman to cope with the blood loss that normally occurs during birth by increasing her circulating blood volume. These changes are: (1) elimination of uteroplacental circulation that reduces the size of the maternal vascular bed by 10% to 15%; (2) loss of placental endocrine function that removes the stimulus for vasodilation; and (3) mobilization of extravascular water stored during pregnancy. By the third postpartum day, the plasma volume has been replenished as extravascular fluid returns to the intravascular space (Isley & Katz, 2017).

CARDIAC OUTPUT

Pulse rate, stroke volume, and cardiac output increase throughout pregnancy. Dramatic changes in maternal hemodynamic status occur with birth of the newborn and delivery of the placenta. The immediate blood loss reduces plasma volume without reducing cardiac output. This is due to the compensatory influx of nearly 500 mL of blood into the maternal system from the uteroplacental bed, a rapid decrease in uterine blood flow, and mobilization of extracellular fluid. Typically cardiac output is increased immediately after birth by 60% to 80% over prelabor values; it returns to prelabor values within 1 hour. By 2 weeks after birth, cardiac output decreases by 30% and gradually decreases to prepregnant levels by 6 to 8 weeks postpartum in the majority of women (Blackburn, 2013).

VITAL SIGNS

Few alterations in vital signs are seen under normal circumstances (Table 18.1). Heart rate is increased immediately after birth and can remain elevated for the first hour. Puerperal bradycardia is common, with heart rate decreasing to 40 to 50 beats/minute (James, 2014).

There is a transient increase in blood pressure of approximately 5% during the first few days after birth (Isley & Katz, 2017). It can take weeks or months for pulse and blood pressure to return to prepregnancy levels. Increase in blood pressure greater than 140/90 when measured on two or more occasions at least 6 hours apart can indicate preeclampsia.

Respiratory function rapidly returns to nonpregnant levels after birth. After the uterus is emptied, the diaphragm descends, the normal cardiac axis is restored, and the point of maximal impulse and the electrocardiogram are normalized.

Low grade fever is not uncommon during the first 24 hours after birth. However, temperature elevation of 38° C (100.4° F) or higher during the first 10 days postpartum can indicate infection and should be evaluated (Berens, 2017).

As many as 50% of women experience shivering episodes during the first few minutes up to the first hour after birth. The exact cause is unknown, and usually no treatment is needed; if the shivering is related to the effects of anesthesia, pharmacologic treatment may be needed (Berens, 2017).

BLOOD COMPONENTS

Hematocrit and Hemoglobin

In women with an average blood loss during birth, the hematocrit level drops moderately for 3 to 4 days, then begins to increase, and reaches nonpregnant levels by 8 weeks postpartum (Isley & Katz, 2017). A postpartum hematocrit can be lower than normal if the blood loss was increased or if the hypervolemia of pregnancy was less than normal.

White Blood Cell Count

Normal leukocytosis of pregnancy ranges from 5,000 to 15,000/mm³. During and after labor the white blood cell count may rise to 30,000/mm³. Leukocytosis, coupled with the increase in erythrocyte sedimentation rate that normally occurs, can obscure the diagnosis of acute infection (Antony, Racusin, Aagaard, et al., 2017).

Coagulation Factors

Clotting factors and fibrinogen are normally increased during pregnancy and remain elevated in the immediate puerperium. When combined with vessel damage and immobility, this hypercoagulable state causes an increased risk for venous thromboembolism, especially after a cesarean

TABLE 18.1   Vital Signs After Birth

Normal Findings	Deviations From Normal Findings and Probable Causes
Temperature	
During first 24 hours, temperature can increase to 38° C (100.4° F) as a result of dehydrating effects of labor. After 24 hours, the woman should be afebrile.	A diagnosis of puerperal sepsis is suggested if an increase in maternal temperature to 38° C (100.4° F) or higher is noted after the first 24 hours after birth and recurs or persists for 2 days. Other possible causes are mastitis, endometritis, urinary tract infections, and other systemic infections.
Pulse	
Pulse, along with stroke volume and cardiac output, remains elevated for the first hour or so after birth. It gradually decreases over the first 48 hours postpartum. Puerperal bradycardia (40–50 beats/min) is common.	A rapid pulse rate or one that is increasing can indicate hypovolemia as a result of hemorrhage.
Respirations	
The respiratory rate, which was unchanged or slightly increased during pregnancy, should be within the woman's normal prepregnancy range soon after birth.	Hypoventilation (respiratory depression) can occur after an unusually high subarachnoid (spinal) block or epidural opioid medication after a cesarean birth.
Blood Pressure	
Blood pressure shows a transient increase of approximately 5% over the first few days after birth, returning to prepregnancy levels over weeks or months. Orthostatic hypotension, as indicated by feelings of faintness or dizziness immediately after standing up, can develop in the first 48 hours as a result of the splanchnic engorgement that can occur after birth.	A low or decreasing blood pressure can indicate hypovolemia secondary to hemorrhage; however, it is a late sign, and other symptoms of hemorrhage usually are present. An increased reading can result from excessive use of vasopressor or oxytocic medications. Elevated BP (greater than 140/90 on two occasions 6 hours apart) can be a sign of preeclampsia and should be evaluated.

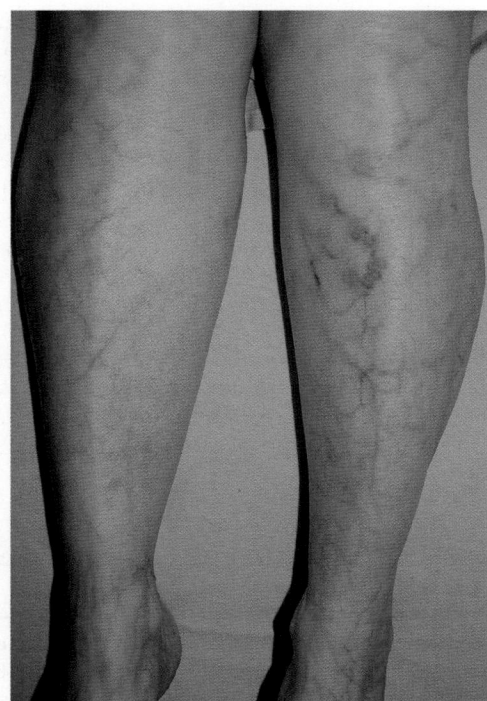

FIG 18.2 Varicosities in legs. (Courtesy of Cheryl Briggs, RNC, Annapolis, MD.)

birth. Fibrinolytic activity also increases during the first few days after birth (Isley & Katz, 2017). Factors I, II, VIII, IX, and X decrease to nonpregnant levels within a few days. Fibrin split products, probably released from the placental site, can be found in maternal blood.

VARICOSITIES

Varicosities (varices) of the legs (Fig. 18.2) and around the anus (hemorrhoids) are common during pregnancy. All varices, even the less common vulvar varices, regress (empty) rapidly immediately after birth. Total or nearly total regression of varicosities is expected in the postpartum period.

RESPIRATORY SYSTEM

When birth occurs, there is an immediate decrease in intraabdominal pressure, which allows for greater excursion of the diaphragm. With decreased pressure on the diaphragm and reduced pulmonary blood flow, chest wall compliance increases. Rib cage elasticity can take months to return to a prepregnancy state. The costal angle that was increased during pregnancy may not completely return to the prepregnancy level. The decline in progesterone that occurs with loss of the placenta causes Pa_{CO_2} levels to rise (Blackburn, 2013).

NEUROLOGIC SYSTEM

Neurologic changes during the puerperium result from a reversal of maternal adaptations to pregnancy and from trauma during labor and birth.

Pregnancy-induced neurologic discomforts disappear after birth. Elimination of physiologic edema through the diuresis that follows birth relieves carpal tunnel syndrome by easing compression of the median nerve. The periodic numbness and tingling of fingers usually disappear after the birth unless lifting and carrying the baby aggravate the condition. Nasal stuffiness, tinnitus, and laryngeal changes resolve within a few days postpartum.

Headaches are common in the first postpartum week; they are usually bilateral and frontal (Blackburn, 2013). However, headache requires careful assessment. Postpartum headaches can be caused by various conditions, including postpartum-onset preeclampsia, stress, and leakage of cerebrospinal fluid into the extradural space during placement of the needle for administration of epidural or spinal anesthesia.

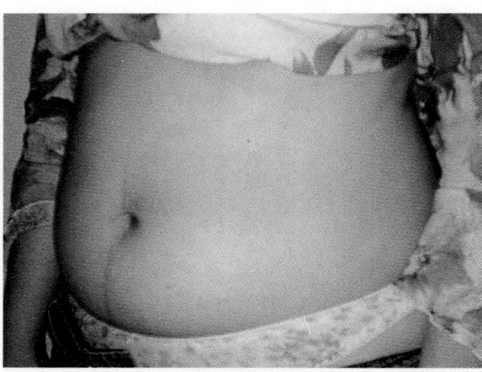

FIG 18.3 Abdominal wall 6 weeks after vaginal birth is almost back to prepregnancy appearance. Note that the linea nigra is still visible. (Courtesy of Jodi Brackett, Phoenix, AZ.)

MUSCULOSKELETAL SYSTEM

ABDOMEN

When the woman stands during the first days after birth, her abdomen protrudes and gives her a still-pregnant appearance. During the first 2 weeks after birth, the abdominal wall is relaxed. It takes about 6 weeks for the abdominal wall to return almost to its prepregnancy state (Fig. 18.3). The return of muscle tone depends on previous tone, proper exercise, and the amount of adipose tissue. Occasionally, with or without overdistention because of a large fetus or multiple fetuses, the abdominal wall muscles separate, a condition termed *diastasis recti abdominis* (see Fig. 7.13, *B*). Persistence of this separation can be disturbing to the woman, but surgical correction rarely is necessary. With time, the separation becomes less apparent.

Other adaptations of the mother's musculoskeletal system that occur during pregnancy are reversed in the puerperium. These adaptations include the relaxation and subsequent hypermobility of the joints and the change in the mother's center of gravity in response to the enlarging uterus. The joints are completely stabilized by 6 to 8 weeks after birth. Although all other joints return to their normal prepregnancy state, those in the parous woman's feet do not. The new mother may notice a permanent increase in her shoe size. Back pain usually resolves in a few weeks or months following birth.

INTEGUMENTARY SYSTEM

Melasma (chloasma or "mask of pregnancy") usually disappears in the postpartum period but persists in about 30% of women (Wang &

Kroumpouzos, 2017). Hyperpigmentation of the areolae and linea nigra may not regress completely after birth. Some women will have permanent darker pigmentation of those areas. Striae gravidarum (stretch marks) on the breasts, abdomen, hips, and thighs may fade but usually do not disappear completely.

Vascular abnormalities such as angiomatas (vascular spiders) and palmar erythema generally regress in response to the rapid decline in estrogens after birth. For some women, vascular spiders persist indefinitely.

For the first 3 months after birth, women often report hair loss when they brush or comb their hair. The abundance of fine hair seen during pregnancy usually disappears after giving birth; however, any coarse or bristly hair that appears during pregnancy usually remains. Fingernails return to their prepregnancy consistency and strength.

IMMUNE SYSTEM

In the postpartum period, the woman's immune (lymphoreticular) system, which was mildly suppressed during pregnancy, gradually returns to its prepregnant state, although the exact timeline is unclear (Blackburn, 2013). This rebound of the immune system can trigger "flare-ups" of autoimmune conditions such as multiple sclerosis or lupus erythematosus (see Chapter 11) (Isley & Katz, 2017).

REFERENCES

Antony, K. M., Racusin, D. A., Aagaard, K., & Dildy, G.A. (2017). Maternal physiology. In S. G. Gabbe, J. R. Niebyl, J. L. Simpson, et al. (Eds.), *Obstetrics: Normal and problem pregnancies* (7th ed.). Philadelphia, PA: Elsevier.

Berens, P. (2017). Overview of postpartum care. In C.J. Lockwood (Ed.), *UpToDate* (7th ed.). Waltham, MA: Wolters Kluwer.

Blackburn, S. T. (2013). *Maternal, fetal, and neonatal physiology* (4th ed.). Maryland Heights, MO: Saunders.

Cunningham, F. G., Leveno, K., Bloom, S. L., et al. (2014). *Williams obstetrics* (24th ed.). New York, NY: McGraw Hill.

James, D. C. (2014). Postpartum care. In K. R. Simpson & P. A. Creehan (Eds.), *Perinatal nursing* (4th ed.). Philadelphia, PA: Lippincott Williams & Wilkins.

Isley, M. M., & Katz, V. L. (2017). Postpartum care and long-term considerations. In S. G. Gabbe, J. R. Niebyl, J. L. Simpson, et al. (Eds.), *Obstetrics: Normal and problem pregnancies* (7th ed.). Philadelphia, PA: Elsevier.

Lawrence, R. M., & Lawrence, R. A. (2016). *Breastfeeding: A guide for the medical profession* (8th ed.). St. Louis, MO: Elsevier.

Wang, A. R., & Kroumpouzos, G. (2017). Skin disease and pregnancy. In S. G. Gabbe, J. R. Niebyl, J. L. Simpson, et al. (Eds.), *Obstetrics: Normal and problem pregnancies* (7th ed.). Philadelphia, PA: Elsevier.

19

Nursing Care of the Family During the Postpartum Period

Kathryn R. Alden

http://evolve.elsevier.com/Perry/maternal

At no other time is family-centered maternity care more important than in the postpartum period. Nursing care is provided in the context of the family unit and focuses on assessment and support of the woman's physiologic and emotional adaptation after birth. During the early postpartum period, components of nursing care include assisting the mother with rest and recovery from labor and birth, assessing physiologic and psychologic adaptation after birth, preventing complications, educating regarding self-management and infant care, and supporting the mother and her partner during the initial transition to parenthood. In addition, the nurse considers the needs of other family members and includes strategies in the nursing care plan to assist the family in adjusting to the new baby.

The approach to the care of women after birth is wellness oriented. In the United States, most women remain hospitalized no more than 1 or 2 days after vaginal birth, and some as few as 6 hours. Because so much important information needs to be shared with these women in a very short time, their care must be thoughtfully planned and provided. Ideally, discharge planning and education begins during pregnancy (American College of Obstetricians and Gynecologists [ACOG], 2016). This chapter discusses nursing care of the woman and her family in the postpartum period extending into the *fourth trimester*—the first 3 months after birth.

TRANSFER FROM THE RECOVERY AREA

After the initial recovery period has been completed (see Chapter 16), and provided that her condition is stable, the woman may be transferred to a postpartum room in the same or another nursing unit. In facilities with labor, delivery, recovery, postpartum (LDRP) rooms, the woman is not moved and the nurse who provides care during the recovery period usually continues caring for the woman. In many settings, women who have received general or regional anesthesia must be cleared for transfer from the recovery area by a member of the anesthesia care team. In other settings, a nurse makes the determination.

In preparing the transfer report or "hand-off," the labor and delivery or postanesthesia care nurse uses information from the records of admission, birth, and recovery. Information that must be communicated to the postpartum nurse includes the woman's name, age, identity of the health care provider; gravidity and parity; anesthetic used; any medications given; duration of labor and time of rupture of membranes; whether labor was induced or augmented; mode of birth (vaginal or cesarean); perineal repair or type of cesarean incision; blood type and Rh status; group B streptococcus (GBS) status; status of rubella immunity;

human immunodeficiency virus (HIV), hepatitis B, and syphilis serology test results; other infections identified during pregnancy (e.g., gonorrhea, chlamydia) and whether these were treated; type and amount of intravenous fluids; physiologic status since birth; description of fundus, lochia, bladder, and perineum; sex and weight of infant; time of birth; name of pediatric care provider; chosen method of feeding; any abnormalities noted; and assessment of initial parent-infant interaction. In addition, specific information should be provided regarding the newborn's Apgar scores (see Chapter 23), weight, voiding, stooling, feeding since birth, eye prophylaxis, and vitamin K injection.

In recent years, many inpatient nursing units, including perinatal care areas, have a bedside report. Bedside reporting is increasingly being used instead of the traditional report given at the nurses' station. Bedside reporting has been shown to improve patient safety and patient satisfaction. Patients feel more involved in their plan of care, which increases their satisfaction. Additionally, holding report at the bedside has enabled many nurses to both visualize and communicate with the patient at the time of report, which improves patient safety (Agency for Healthcare Research and Quality [AHRQ], 2013; Novak & Fairchild, 2012).

PLANNING FOR DISCHARGE

From their initial contact with the postpartum woman, nurses prepare the new mother for her return to home. Planning for discharge begins with the first interaction among the nurse, the woman, and her family and continues until they leave the hospital or birthing facility.

The length of hospital stay after giving birth depends on many factors, including the physical condition of the mother and the newborn, mental and emotional status of the mother, social support at home, patient education needs for self-care and infant care, and financial constraints.

Women who give birth in birthing centers may be discharged within a few hours, after the woman's and infant's conditions are stable. Mothers and newborns who are at low risk for complications may be discharged from the hospital within 24 to 36 hours after vaginal birth. This short time frame is often called *early postpartum discharge, shortened hospital stay,* and *1-day maternity stay.* Early discharge was popular in the late 1980s and early 1990s, but concerns related to the health and safety of mothers and newborns led to legislation promoting longer hospital stays. The passage of the Newborns' and Mothers' Health Protection Act of 1996 provided minimum federal standards for health plan coverage for mothers and their newborns. Under this act, all health plans are required to allow the new mother and newborn to remain in the hospital for a minimum of 48 hours after an uncomplicated vaginal birth and for 96 hours after a cesarean birth, unless the attending provider in consultation with the mother decides on early discharge (Center for Consumer Information and Insurance Oversight [CCIO], 2012).

CRITERIA FOR DISCHARGE

The American Academy of Pediatrics (AAP, 2015) recommends that the hospital stay for a mother with a healthy term newborn should be of sufficient length to identify early problems and determine that the mother and family are prepared and able to care for the neonate at home. The health of the mother and her newborn should be stable, the mother should be able and confident to provide care for her infant, and there should be adequate support systems in place and access to follow-up care.

It is essential that nurses consider the individual needs of the woman and her newborn and provide care that is intentionally planned to meet these needs. Hospital-based maternity nurses continue to play key roles as caregivers, teachers, and advocates for mothers, newborns, and families in developing and implementing effective home-care strategies. Postpartum order sets and maternal-newborn teaching checklists that address the mother's learning needs can be used to accomplish patient care tasks and educational outcomes.

Care Management: Physical Needs

The nursing plan of care includes the postpartum woman, her newborn, and her family. Most birth facilities use the couplet or mother/baby model of care (Association of Women's Health, Obstetric and Neonatal Nurses [AWHONN], 2010). Nurses in these settings have been educated in both mother and infant care and function as primary nurses for both mother and infant, even if the infant is kept in the nursery. This approach is a variation of rooming-in, in which the mother and infant room together and mother and nurse share in the infant's care. The organization of the mother's care must take the newborn's feeding and care needs into consideration.

ONGOING PHYSICAL ASSESSMENT

Ongoing assessments are performed throughout hospitalization. In addition to vital signs, physical assessment of the postpartum woman focuses on evaluation of the breasts, uterine fundus, lochia, perineum, bladder and bowel function, and lower extremities (Table 19.1).

ROUTINE LABORATORY TESTS

Several laboratory tests may be performed in the immediate postpartum period. Hemoglobin and hematocrit values are often evaluated on the first postpartum day to assess blood loss during birth, especially after cesarean birth. In some hospitals, a clean-catch or catheterized urine specimen is obtained and sent for routine urinalysis or culture and sensitivity, especially if an indwelling urinary catheter was inserted during the intrapartum period. In addition, if the woman's rubella immunity and Rh status are unknown, tests to determine her status and need for possible treatment should be performed at this time.

NURSING INTERVENTIONS

Based on the available data (e.g., medical record) and assessment findings, the nurse plans with the woman which nursing measures are appropriate and which are to be given priority. The nursing care plan includes periodic assessments to detect deviations from normal physical changes,

measures to relieve discomfort or pain, safety measures to prevent injury and infection, and education and counseling measures designed to promote the woman's feelings of competence in self-management and infant care. The nurse evaluates continually and is ready to change the plan if indicated. Almost all hospitals use standardized care plans as a base. Nurses individualize care of the postpartum woman and neonate according to their specific needs (see the Nursing Care Plan). Signs of potential problems that may be identified during the assessment process are listed in Table 19.1.

Nurses assume many roles while implementing the nursing care plan. They provide direct physical care, educate new mothers and their families, and provide anticipatory guidance and counseling. Perhaps most important, they nurture the woman by providing encouragement and support as she begins to assume the many tasks of motherhood. Nurses who take the time to "mother the mother" do much to increase feelings of self-confidence in new mothers. Nurses are careful to include the woman's spouse or partner and other primary support persons in education and counseling.

The first step in providing patient-centered care is to confirm the woman's identity by checking her wristband. At the same time, the infant's identification number is matched with the corresponding band on the mother's wrist and in some instances the father's or partner's wrist. The nurse determines how the mother wishes to be addressed and notes her preference in her medical record and her nursing care plan. The nurse orients the woman and her family to their surroundings. Familiarity with the unit, routines, resources, and personnel reduces one potential source of anxiety—the unknown. The mother is reassured through knowing whom and how she can call for assistance and what she can expect in the way of supplies and services. If the woman's usual daily routine before admission differs from the routine of the facility, the nurse works with the woman to develop a mutually acceptable routine. Nurses discuss infant security precautions with the mother and her family (see Chapter 23).

Preventing Excessive Bleeding

All women who have given birth are at risk for excessive bleeding that can progress to postpartum hemorrhage (see Chapter 21). The most frequent cause of excessive bleeding after birth is uterine atony (i.e., failure of the uterine muscle to contract firmly). The two most important interventions for preventing excessive bleeding are maintaining good uterine tone and preventing bladder distention. If uterine atony occurs, the relaxed uterus distends with blood and clots, blood vessels in the placental site are not clamped off, and excessive bleeding results. Although the cause of uterine atony is not always clear, it often results from retained placental fragments.

Excessive blood loss after birth can also be caused by vaginal or vulvar hematomas or unrepaired lacerations of the vagina or cervix. These potential sources might be suspected if excessive vaginal bleeding occurs in the presence of a firmly contracted uterine fundus.

A perineal pad saturated in 15 minutes or less and pooling of blood under the buttocks are indications of excessive blood loss, requiring immediate assessment, intervention, and notification of the primary health care provider.

Accurate visual estimation of blood loss is an important nursing responsibility. Blood loss is usually described subjectively as scant, light, moderate, or heavy (profuse). Fig. 19.1 shows examples of perineal pad saturation corresponding to each of these descriptions.

Although postpartum blood loss can be estimated by observing the amount of drainage on a perineal pad, judging the amount of lochia is difficult if based only on observation of perineal pads. Quantification of blood loss by weighing clots and items saturated with blood (1 mL

TABLE 19.1   Postpartum Assessment and Signs of Potential Complications

Assessment	Normal Findings	Signs of Potential Complications
Blood pressure (BP)	Consistent with BP baseline during pregnancy; transient increase of 5% first few days after birth; can have orthostatic hypotension for 48 hours	Hypertension: anxiety, preeclampsia, essential hypertension Hypotension: hemorrhage
Temperature	36.2°–38° C (97.2°–100.4° F)	>38° C (100.4° F) after 24 hours: infection
Pulse	50–90 beats/min	Tachycardia: pain, fever, dehydration, hemorrhage
Respirations	16–20 breaths/min	Bradypnea: effects of opioid medications Tachypnea: anxiety; may be sign of respiratory disease
Breath sounds	Clear to auscultation	Crackles: possible fluid overload
Breasts	Days 1–2: soft Days 2–3: filling Days 3–5: full, soften with breastfeeding (milk is "in")	Firmness, heat, pain: engorgement
Nipples	Skin intact; no soreness reported	Redness, bruising, cracks, fissures, abrasions, blisters: usually associated with latching problems
Uterus (fundus)	Firm, midline; first 24 hours at level of umbilicus; involutes ≈1 cm/day	Soft, boggy, higher than expected level: uterine atony Lateral deviation: distended bladder
Lochia	Days 1–3: rubra (dark red) Days 4–10: serosa (brownish red or pink) After 10 days: alba (yellowish white) Amount: scant to moderate Few clots Fleshy odor	Large amount of lochia, large clots: uterine atony, vaginal or cervical laceration Foul odor: infection
Perineum	Minimal edema Laceration or episiotomy: edges approximated Pain minimal to moderate: controlled by analgesics, nonpharmacologic techniques, or both	Pronounced edema, bruising, hematoma Redness, warmth, drainage: infection Excessive discomfort first 1–2 days: hematoma; after day 3: infection
Rectal area	No hemorrhoids; if hemorrhoids are present, soft and pink	Discolored hemorrhoidal tissue, severe pain: thrombosed hemorrhoid
Bladder	Able to void spontaneously; no distention; able to empty completely; no dysuria Diuresis begins ≈12 hours after birth; can void 3000 mL/day	Overdistended bladder possibly causing uterine atony, excessive lochia Dysuria, frequency, urgency burning: infection
Abdomen and bowels	Abdomen soft, active bowel sounds in all quadrants Bowel movement by day 2 or 3 after birth Cesarean: incision dressing clean and dry; suture line intact	No bowel movement by day 3 or 4: constipation; diarrhea Abdominal incision—redness, edema, warmth, drainage: infection
Legs	Deep tendon reflexes (DTRs) 1+ to 2+ Peripheral edema possibly present Homan sign* negative	DTRs ≥3+: preeclampsia Redness, tenderness, pain, thrombophlebitis
Energy level	Able to care for self and infant; able to sleep	Lethargy, extreme fatigue, difficulty sleeping: postpartum depression
Emotional status	Excited, happy, interested or involved in infant care	Sad, tearful, disinterested in infant care: postpartum blues or depression

*Homan sign was traditionally included in routine postpartum assessments; however, it is no longer common practice due to concern about its limited sensitivity and specificity in diagnosing venous thromboembolism and the potential risk for dislodging a clot when the test is performed.

◎ NURSING CARE PLAN

Postpartum Care—Vaginal Birth

Case Study

Matavia, a 22-year-old G1 P1, has been married to Elijah for 2 years and gave birth 3 hours ago to a term female infant weighing 8 lb 12 oz (3970 g) after a 13-hour labor. Matavia received no medication during labor; she managed her discomfort with relaxation and breathing and nitrous oxide. She had a second-degree tear that was repaired. She has one small hemorrhoid. The baby was placed on her chest for skin-to-skin contact immediately after birth and nursed briefly about 30 minutes later.

Assessment

What are signs of excessive bleeding after childbirth?
What assessments are critical after vaginal birth?

Defining Characteristics

Increased amounts of lochia
Passing blood clots
Decreased urine output

Continued

◎ NURSING CARE PLAN

Postpartum Care—Vaginal Birth—cont'd

Increased pulse rate
Increased urine concentration
Low blood pressure
Poor turgor of skin
Thirst

Nursing Diagnosis

Risk for Deficient Fluid Volume related to uterine atony/hemorrhage

Expected Outcomes

Fundus is firm.
Lochia is moderate.
There is no evidence of hemorrhage.
Urine output is adequate.

Nursing Interventions	Rationales
Monitor lochia (color, amount, consistency), and count or weigh sanitary pads if lochia is heavy.	To evaluate amount of bleeding
Monitor and palpate fundus for location and tone to determine status of uterus and dictate further interventions.	Because uterine atony is the most common cause of postpartum hemorrhage
Encourage oral intake of fluids.	To replace fluids lost through perspiration and blood loss
Monitor intake and output, assess for bladder fullness, and encourage voiding.	Because a full bladder interferes with involution of uterus
Monitor vital signs (increased pulse and respirations, decreased blood pressure) and skin temperature and color.	To detect signs of hemorrhage/shock
Monitor postpartum hematology studies.	To assess effects of blood loss
If fundus is boggy, apply gentle massage and assess tone response.	To promote uterine contractions and increase uterine tone. (Do not overstimulate because doing so can cause fundal relaxation.)
Express uterine clots.	To promote uterine contraction
Explain process of involution, and teach patient to assess and massage fundus and report any persistent bogginess.	To involve her in self-management and increase sense of self-control
Administer uterotonic agents (e.g., oxytocin [Pitocin]) per health care provider order, and evaluate effectiveness.	To promote continuing uterine contraction
Administer fluids, blood, blood products, or plasma expanders as ordered.	To replace lost blood volume and blood components

Case Study (Continued)

Matavia is now 8 hours postpartum. She is complaining of perineal pain at 6 on a 10-point scale. The infant has nursed twice for approximately 10 minutes each time. The nurse assisted Matavia with positioning and latch.

Assessment

What are causes of perineal pain after a vaginal birth? What nonpharmacologic and pharmacologic measures are recommended for relief of perineal pain?

Defining Characteristics

Alteration in muscle tone (listless to rigid)
Autonomic responses (diaphoresis; blood pressure, pulse rate, and respiratory rate changes; and dilated pupils)
Redness and swelling of affected part (perineum)
Reports of discomfort or pain; moaning; crying
Facial mask of pain (grimacing)
Self-focusing

Nursing Diagnosis

Acute Pain related to trauma to perineum

Expected Outcomes

Matavia will describe and implement appropriate interventions for pain relief.
Matavia will exhibit signs of decreased discomfort.
Matavia will express that the discomfort is minimal.
Vital signs remain within normal limits.

Nursing Interventions	Rationales
Assess location, type, and quality of pain.	To direct intervention
Explain to Matavia about the source and reason for pain, its expected duration, and treatments.	To decrease anxiety and increase sense of control
Administer prescribed pain medications.	To provide pain relief
Apply ice packs in first 24 hours.	To reduce edema and vulvar irritation and reduce discomfort
Encourage sitz baths using cool water the first 24 hours.	To reduce edema and discomfort
Use warm water for sitz baths after 24 hours.	To promote circulation and reduce discomfort
Apply witch hazel compresses.	To reduce edema
Teach Matavia to use prescribed perineal creams, sprays, or ointments.	To depress response of peripheral nerves
Teach Matavia to tighten buttocks before sitting and to sit on flat, hard surfaces.	To reduce pressure on perineum. (Avoid donuts and soft pillows because they separate buttocks and decrease venous blood flow, increasing pain.)

Case Study (Continued)

Matavia has not voided since the birth of the baby. She has the feeling that she needs to void but says she is afraid it will hurt and that her "bottom" will burn when the urine touches it. She is reluctant to drink any more fluids because that will make the urinary urgency increase.

Assessment

What factors interfere with voiding after birth? What nursing measures will assist Matavia to establish a normal voiding pattern?

Continued

◎ NURSING CARE PLAN

Postpartum Care—Vaginal Birth—cont'd

Defining Characteristics
Hesitancy
Urgency
Retention
Fear of causing perineal pain

Nursing Diagnosis
Risk for Impaired Urinary Elimination related to perineal trauma and fear of discomfort

Expected Outcomes
Matavia will void within 6 to 8 hours after birth and empty bladder completely.
Matavia's urinary function will remain normal and free from complications.

Nursing Interventions	Rationales
Assess position and character of uterine fundus and bladder.	To ascertain if any further interventions are indicated because of displacement of fundus or distention of bladder
Measure intake and output.	To assess adequacy of fluid intake and urine output; a full or distended bladder increases the risk for uterine atony
Administer analgesics as indicated.	To reduce perineal discomfort
Encourage voiding by assisting Matavia to bathroom, running water over perineum, running water in sink, and providing privacy.	To encourage voiding
Encourage oral fluid intake.	To replace any fluids lost during birth and prevent dehydration
Catheterize as necessary with indwelling or straight method.	To ensure bladder emptying and prevent uterine atony

Case Study (Continued)
Matavia says that she has been unable to sleep more than an hour at a time. Between waking to feed the baby, visitors, and phone calls, she cannot seem to get much sleep and is feeling very tired.

Assessment
What are signs of sleep disturbance? What can be done to assist a new mother to obtain a good night's sleep?

Defining Characteristics
Change in normal sleep pattern
Dissatisfaction with amount or quality of sleep

Decreased ability to function
Reports being awakened
Reports no difficulty falling asleep initially but has trouble getting back to sleep
Reports not feeling well rested

Nursing Diagnosis
Disturbed Sleep Pattern related to excitement, discomfort, infant feedings, and environmental interruptions

Expected Outcomes
Matavia sleeps for uninterrupted periods of time and states that she feels rested after waking.
Matavia will alter diet and habits to promote sleep by reducing caffeine intake and not eating in the late evening.
Matavia will incorporate sleep preparation measures into evening routine.
Matavia will carry out relaxation exercises that promote sleep.
Matavia will attempt to sleep when the baby is sleeping.

Nursing Interventions	Rationales
Assess Matavia's routine sleep patterns and compare with current sleep pattern, exploring things that interfere with sleep.	To determine scope of problem and direct interventions
Individualize nursing routines to fit Matavia's natural body rhythms (i.e., wake/sleep cycles); provide a sleep-promoting environment (i.e., dark, quiet, adequate ventilation, appropriate room temperature); prepare for sleep using Matavia's usual routines (i.e., back massage, soothing music, warm milk); teach use of guided imagery and relaxation techniques.	To promote optimum conditions for sleep
Teach Matavia to avoid things or routines that can interfere with sleep (i.e., caffeine, foods that induce heartburn, fluids, strenuous mental/physical activity).	To enhance quality of sleep
Administer sedative or pain medication as prescribed; assess safety of medication for breastfeeding.	To enhance quality of sleep
Advise Matavia and her partner to limit visitors and activities.	To avoid further taxation and fatigue
Suggest that Matavia uses infant nap time as a nap time for her as well.	To nap and replenish energy and decrease fatigue

equals 1 g) is recommended as the most accurate way to objectively determine blood loss.

Any estimation of lochial flow is inaccurate and incomplete without considering the time factor. The woman who saturates a perineal pad in 1 hour or less is bleeding much more heavily than the woman who saturates one perineal pad in 8 hours. When assessing blood loss, the nurse asks the woman how long it has been since her perineal pad was changed.

Nurses in general tend to overestimate rather than underestimate blood loss. Different brands of perineal pads vary in their saturation volume and soaking appearance. For example, blood placed on some brands tends to soak down into the pad, whereas on other brands it tends to spreads outward. Nurses should determine saturation volume and soaking appearance for the brands used in their institution so that they can improve accuracy of blood loss estimation.

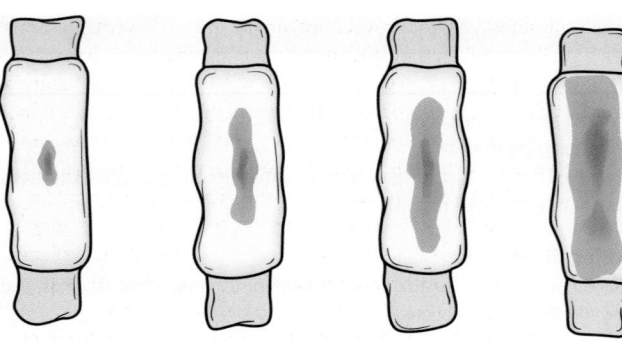

FIG 19.1 Blood loss after birth is assessed by the extent of perineal pad saturation as *(left to right)* scant (<2.5 cm), light (<10 cm), moderate (>10 cm), or heavy (one pad saturated within 2 hours).

⚡ SAFETY ALERT

The nurse always checks for blood under the mother's buttocks as well as on the perineal pad. Although the amount on the perineal pad can appear to be small, blood can flow between the buttocks onto the linens under the mother. When this happens, excessive bleeding can go undetected.

When excessive bleeding occurs, vital signs are monitored closely. Blood pressure is not a reliable indicator of impending shock from early postpartum hemorrhage because compensatory mechanisms prevent a significant drop in blood pressure until the woman has lost 30% to 40% of her blood volume (see Chapter 21). Respirations, pulse, skin condition, urinary output, and level of consciousness are more sensitive means of identifying hypovolemic shock (see the Emergency Treatment box: Hypovolemic Shock). The frequent physical assessments performed during the fourth stage of labor are designed to provide prompt identification of excessive bleeding. Nurses maintain vigilance for excessive bleeding throughout the hospital stay as they perform periodic assessment of the uterine fundus and lochia.

Maintaining Uterine Tone

A major intervention to alleviate uterine atony and restore uterine muscle tone is stimulation by gently massaging the fundus until firm (Fig. 19.2). Fundal massage can cause a temporary increase in the amount of vaginal bleeding seen as pooled blood leaves the uterus. Clots can also be expelled. The uterus can remain boggy even after massage and clot expulsion.

Fundal massage can be a very uncomfortable procedure. If the nurse explains the purpose of fundal massage as well as the causes and dangers of uterine atony, the woman will likely be more cooperative. Teaching the woman to massage her own fundus enables her to maintain some control and decreases her anxiety.

When uterine atony and excessive bleeding occur, additional interventions likely to be used are administration of intravenous fluids and oxytocic medications (drugs that stimulate contraction of the uterine smooth muscle) (see Medication Guide: Uterotonic Drugs to Manage Postpartum Hemorrhage in Chapter 21 for information about common oxytocic medications).

Preventing Bladder Distention

Uterine atony and excessive bleeding after birth can be the result of bladder distention. A full bladder causes the uterus to be displaced

---

✚ EMERGENCY TREATMENT
Hypovolemic Shock

Signs and Symptoms
- Persistent significant bleeding occurs—perineal pad is soaked within 15 minutes; may not be accompanied by a change in vital signs or maternal color or behavior.
- The woman states she feels weak, lightheaded, "funny," or nauseated or that she "sees stars."
- The woman begins to act anxious or exhibits air hunger.
- The woman's skin color turns ashen or grayish.
- Skin feels cool and clammy.
- Pulse rate increases.
- Blood pressure decreases.

Interventions
- Notify the obstetric health care provider.
- If the uterus is atonic, massage gently and expel clots to cause it to contract; compress uterus manually, as needed, using two hands. Add oxytocic agent to intravenous drip, as ordered.
- Give oxygen by nonrebreather face mask at 10 L/min.
- Tilt the woman onto her side, or elevate the right hip; elevate her legs to at least a 30-degree angle to promote venous return.
- Provide additional or maintain existing intravenous (IV) infusion of lactated Ringer's solution or normal saline solution to restore circulatory volume (woman should have two patent IV lines; insert second IV using 16- to 18-gauge IV catheter).
- Administer blood or blood products, as ordered.
- Monitor vital signs.
- Insert an indwelling urinary catheter to monitor kidney perfusion.
- Administer emergency drugs, as ordered.
- Prepare for possible surgery or other emergency treatments or procedures.
- Document the incident, medical and nursing interventions instituted, and the woman's response to interventions.

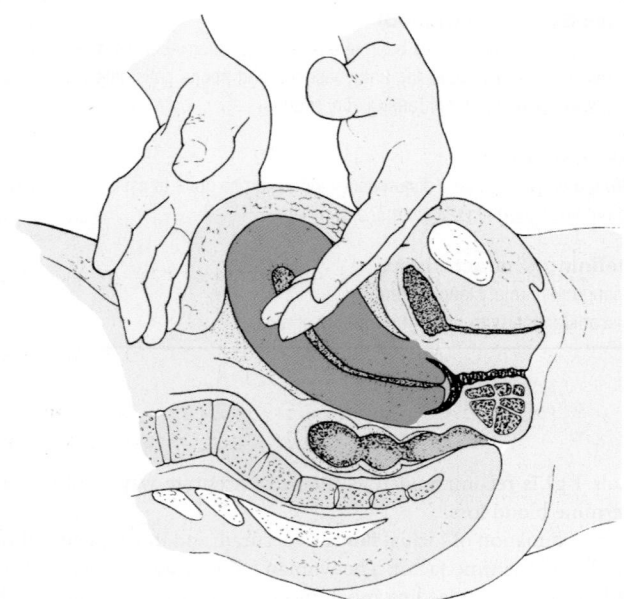

FIG 19.2 Palpating fundus of uterus during the postpartum period. Note that upper hand is cupped over fundus; lower hand dips in above symphysis pubis and supports uterus while it is massaged gently.

above the umbilicus and well to one side of midline in the abdomen. It also prevents the uterus from contracting normally.

Women can be at risk for bladder distention resulting from urinary retention based on intrapartum factors including epidural anesthesia, episiotomy, extensive vaginal or perineal lacerations, instrument-assisted birth, or prolonged labor. Women who have had indwelling catheters, such as with cesarean birth, can experience some difficulty as they initially attempt to void after the catheter is removed. Nurses who are aware of these risk factors can be proactive in preventing complications.

Nursing interventions for a postpartum woman focus on helping the woman empty her bladder spontaneously as soon as possible. The first priority is to assist the woman to the bathroom or onto a bedpan if she is unable to ambulate. Having the woman listen to running water, placing her hands in warm water, or pouring water from a squeeze bottle over her perineum may stimulate voiding. Other techniques include assisting the woman into the shower or sitz bath and encouraging her to void; relaxation techniques can also be helpful. Administering analgesics, if ordered, may be indicated because some women fear voiding because of anticipated pain. If these measures are unsuccessful, a sterile catheter may be inserted to drain the urine.

Preventing Infection

Nurses in the postpartum setting are acutely aware of the importance of preventing infection. One important means of preventing infection is by maintaining a clean environment. Bed linens should be changed as needed. Disposable pads and drawsheets are changed frequently.

Women should wear slippers when walking about to prevent contamination of the linens when they return to bed. Personnel must be conscientious about their hand hygiene to prevent cross-infection. Standard Precautions must be practiced. Staff members with colds, coughs, or skin infections (e.g., a cold sore [herpes simplex virus lesion] on the lip) must follow hospital protocol when in contact with postpartum women. In many hospitals, staff members with open herpetic lesions, strep throat, conjunctivitis, upper respiratory infections, or diarrhea are encouraged to avoid contact with mothers and infants by staying home until the condition is no longer contagious. Visitors with signs of illness are not permitted to enter the postpartum unit.

Perineal lacerations and episiotomies can increase the risk for infection as a result of interruption in skin integrity. Proper perineal care helps prevent infection in the genitourinary area and aids the healing process. Educating the woman to wipe from front to back (urethra to anus) after voiding or defecating is a simple first step. In many hospitals, a squeeze bottle filled with warm water or an antiseptic solution is used after each voiding to cleanse the perineal area. The woman should change her perineal pad from front to back each time she voids or defecates and wash her hands thoroughly before and after doing so (Box 19.1).

Promoting Comfort

Most women experience some degree of discomfort during the postpartum period. Common causes of discomfort include pain from uterine contractions (afterpains), perineal lacerations or episiotomy, hemorrhoids,

---

BOX 19.1 **Interventions for Episiotomy, Lacerations, and Hemorrhoids**

Explain procedure and rationale before implementation.

Cleansing
- Wash hands before and after cleansing perineum and changing pads.
- Wash perineum with mild soap and warm water at least once daily.
- Cleanse from symphysis pubis to anal area.
- Apply peripad from front to back, protecting inner surface of pad from contamination.
- Wrap soiled pad, and place in covered waste container.
- Change pad with each void or defecation or at least four times per day.
- Assess amount and character of lochia with each pad change.

Ice Pack
- Apply a covered ice pack to perineum from front to back:
  - During first 24 hours following birth to decrease edema formation and increase comfort
  - After first 24 hours following birth as needed to provide anesthetic effect

Squeeze Bottle
- Fill bottle with tap water warmed to approximately 38° C (100.4° F) (comfortably warm on wrist).
- Instruct woman to position nozzle between her legs so squirts of water reach perineum as she sits on toilet seat. Explain that it will take whole bottle of water to cleanse the perineum.
- Remind her to blot dry with toilet paper or clean wipes.
- Remind her to avoid contamination from anal area by wiping "front to back."
- Apply clean pad.

Sitz Bath
Built-in Type
- Prepare bath by thoroughly scrubbing with cleaning agent and rinsing.

- Pad with towel before filling.
- Fill one-third to one-half full with water of correct temperature 38°–40.6° C (100.4°–105.1° F). Some women prefer cool sitz baths. Add ice to water to lower temperature to a comfortable level.
- Encourage woman to use at least twice a day for 20 minutes.
- Place call bell within easy reach.
- Teach woman to enter bath by tightening gluteal muscles and keeping them tightened and then relaxing them after she is in bath.
- Place dry towels within reach.
- Ensure privacy.
- Check woman in 15 minutes.

Disposable Type
- Clamp tubing and fill bag with warm water.
- Raise toilet seat; place bath in bowl with overflow opening directed toward back of toilet.
- Place container above toilet bowl.
- Attach tube into groove at front of bath.
- Loosen tube clamp to regulate rate of flow; fill bath to about one-half full; continue as for built-in sitz bath.

Topical Applications
- Apply anesthetic cream or spray after cleansing perineal area: use sparingly three or four times per day.
- Apply witch hazel pads (Tucks) after cleansing perineum.
- Apply hemorrhoidal cream as ordered to anal area after cleansing.

sore nipples, and breast engorgement. The woman's description of the location, type, and severity of her pain is the best guide in choosing appropriate interventions. To confirm the location and extent of discomfort, the nurse inspects and palpates areas of pain as appropriate for redness, swelling, discharge, and heat, and observes for body tension, guarded movements, and facial tension. Blood pressure, pulse, and respirations can be elevated in response to acute pain. Diaphoresis can accompany severe pain. A lack of objective signs does not necessarily mean there is no pain because there can be a cultural component to the expression of pain. Nursing interventions are intended to eliminate the pain sensation entirely or reduce it to a tolerable level that allows the woman to care for herself and her newborn. Nurses may use nonpharmacologic and pharmacologic interventions to promote comfort. Pain relief is enhanced by using more than one method or route.

> ## ⚡ SAFETY ALERT
>
> If a postpartum woman complains of extreme perineal pain, especially after having received pain medication, the first action by the nurse should be to assess the perineum. There may be a hematoma or perineal infection that is causing the pain. Although rare, an inordinate degree of pain can be a sign of serious complications including perineal cellulitis, necrotizing fasciitis, or angioedema (Isley & Katz, 2017).

Nonpharmacologic Interventions

Various nonpharmacologic measures are used to reduce postpartum discomfort. These include distraction, imagery, therapeutic touch, relaxation, acupressure, aromatherapy, hydrotherapy, massage therapy, music therapy, and transcutaneous electrical nerve stimulation (TENS). See Chapter 14 for more information on these techniques.

For women who are experiencing discomfort associated with uterine contractions, application of warmth (e.g., heating pad) or lying prone can be helpful. Interaction with the infant can also provide distraction and decrease this discomfort. Because afterpains are more severe during and after breastfeeding, interventions are planned to provide the most timely and effective relief. A simple intervention that can decrease the discomfort associated with an episiotomy or perineal lacerations is to encourage the woman to lie on her side whenever possible. Other interventions include application of an ice pack; topical application (if ordered) of anesthetic spray or cream; cleansing with water from a squeeze bottle; and a cleansing shower, tub bath, or sitz bath. Many of these interventions are also effective for hemorrhoids, especially ice packs, sitz baths, and topical applications (such as witch hazel pads). Box 19.1 gives additional specific information about these interventions.

Sore nipples in breastfeeding mothers are most likely related to ineffective latch technique. Assessment and assistance with feeding can help alleviate the cause. To ease discomfort associated with sore nipples, the mother may apply topical preparations such as purified lanolin or hydrogel pads (see Chapter 24).

Breast engorgement can occur whether the woman is breastfeeding or formula feeding. The discomfort associated with engorged breasts may be reduced by applying ice packs or cabbage leaves (or both) to the breasts (Fig. 24.16), and wearing a well-fitted support bra. Antiinflammatory medications such as ibuprofen can also be helpful in relieving some of the discomfort. Decisions about specific interventions for engorgement are based on whether the woman chooses breastfeeding or formula feeding. Breastfeeding mothers can feed frequently and use hand expression or a breast pump to reduce engorgement and promote comfort (see Chapter 24).

Pharmacologic Interventions

Pharmacologic interventions are commonly used to relieve or reduce postpartum discomfort. Most health care providers routinely order a variety of analgesics to be administered as needed, including both opioid and nonopioid (e.g., nonsteroidal antiinflammatory drugs [NSAIDs]). NSAIDs commonly used are ibuprofen or naproxen. These medications provide better relief from uterine cramping and perineal pain than acetaminophen or propoxyphene. Ibuprofen is preferred for breastfeeding women because it has a low milk/maternal plasma drug concentration ratio and a short-half life (Isley & Katz, 2017). In some hospitals, NSAIDs are administered on a scheduled basis, especially if the woman had perineal repair. Topical application of antiseptic or anesthetic ointment or spray can be used for perineal pain. Patient-controlled analgesia (PCA) pumps and epidural analgesia are commonly used to provide pain relief after cesarean birth.

> ## ⚡ SAFETY ALERT
>
> The nurse should carefully monitor all women receiving opioids because respiratory depression and decreased intestinal motility are side effects.

Many women want to participate in decisions about analgesia. Severe pain, however, can interfere with active participation in choosing pain relief measures. If an analgesic is to be given, the nurse must make a clinical judgment of the type, appropriate dosage, and frequency from the medications ordered. The woman is informed of the prescribed analgesic and its common side effects; this teaching is documented.

Breastfeeding mothers often have concerns about the effects of an analgesic on the infant. Although nearly all drugs present in maternal circulation are also found in breast milk, many analgesics commonly used during the postpartum period are considered relatively safe for breastfeeding mothers and infants. Often the timing of medications can be adjusted to minimize infant exposure. A mother may be given pain medication immediately after breastfeeding so that the interval between medication administration and the next breastfeeding session is as long as possible. The decision to administer medications of any kind to a breastfeeding mother must always be made by carefully weighing the woman's need against actual or potential risks to the infant. Resources are readily accessible for nurses and health care providers to examine the safety of medications for breastfeeding mothers (e.g., LactMed [https://toxnet.nlm.nih.gov/newtoxnet/lactmed.htm]).

If acceptable pain relief has not been obtained in 1 hour and there is no change in the initial assessment, the nurse may need to contact the obstetric care provider for additional pain relief orders or further directions. Unrelieved pain results in fatigue, anxiety, and a worsening perception of the pain. It might also indicate the presence of a previously unidentified or untreated problem.

Promoting Rest

Lack of sleep and fatigue are common complaints of new parents. Sleep loss, feeling stressed, and physical exhaustion have been reported as the top three problems women experience within the first 2 months after birth (Declercq , Sakala, Corry, et al., 2014). The early postpartum period is the time that new parents experience the greatest disruption to their lives as they try to adjust to the nearly constant demands of a newborn (Aber, Weiss, & Fawcett, 2013). Other factors contribute to physical fatigue or exhaustion such as long labor or cesarean birth, hospital routines that interrupt periods of sleep and rest, physical discomfort, and visitors. Fatigue can also be associated with anemia, infection, or thyroid dysfunction. The excitement and exhilaration experienced after the birth of the infant makes resting difficult. Disrupted sleep and fatigue in the postpartum woman contribute to the development of postpartum depressive symptoms and increase the risk for postpartum depression (PPD) (Bhati & Richards, 2015; Okun, 2015; Park, Meltzer-Brody, & Stickgold, 2013).

Fatigue is likely to worsen over the first 6 weeks after birth, often because of situational factors. After discharge from the hospital, fatigue increases as the woman provides care and feeding for the newborn in combination with other family and household responsibilities such as caring for other children, preparing meals, and doing laundry. Many women have partners, family members, or friends to provide much-needed assistance, whereas others can be without any help at all. The nurse needs to inquire about resources available to the woman after discharge and help her plan accordingly. It is important to remember that the partner is also prone to fatigue if he or she is helping the new mother with infant care and attending to other children and household tasks.

Interventions are planned to meet the woman's individual needs for sleep and rest while she is in the hospital. Comfort measures and medications to promote sleep may be necessary. The side-lying position for breastfeeding minimizes fatigue in nursing mothers. Support and encouragement of mothering behaviors help reduce anxiety. Hospital and nursing routines can be adjusted to meet the needs of individual mothers. In addition, the nurse can help the family limit visitors and provide a comfortable chair or bed for the partner or other family member who is staying with the new mother.

Because postpartum fatigue can be very debilitating, follow-up after hospital discharge is important. Assessment for fatigue can be done with a nurse-initiated telephone call at 2 weeks, as well as at the routine 6-week postpartum visit with the health care provider. Nurses in the pediatric care provider's office or clinic should also be alert for signs of maternal fatigue. The infant will be seen within the first few days after birth—before the woman sees her obstetric care provider.

Promoting Ambulation

Early ambulation is associated with a reduced incidence of venous thromboembolism (VTE) (see Chapter 21); it also promotes the return of strength. Free movement is encouraged once anesthesia wears off unless an opioid analgesic has been administered. After the initial recovery period, the mother is encouraged to ambulate frequently.

In the early postpartum period, some women feel lightheaded or dizzy when standing. The rapid decrease in intraabdominal pressure after birth results in a dilation of blood vessels supplying the intestines (splanchnic engorgement) and causes blood to pool in the viscera. This condition contributes to the development of orthostatic hypotension when the woman who has recently given birth sits or stands up, first ambulates, or takes a warm shower or sitz bath. When assisting a woman to ambulate, the nurse needs to consider the baseline blood pressure, amount of blood loss, and type, amount, and timing of analgesic or anesthetic medications administered.

Women who have had regional (epidural or spinal) anesthesia can experience slow return of sensory and motor function in their lower extremities, increasing the risk for falls with early ambulation. Careful assessment by the postpartum nurse can prevent falls. Factors that the nurse should consider are the time lapse since epidural or spinal medication was given; the woman's ability to bend both knees, place both feet flat on the bed, and lift buttocks off the bed without assistance; medications since birth; vital signs; and estimated blood loss with birth. Before allowing the woman to ambulate, the nurse assesses the ability of the woman to stand unassisted beside her bed, simultaneously bending both knees slightly, and then standing with knees locked. If the woman

is unable to balance herself, she can be safely eased back into bed without injury (Lockwood & Anderson, 2013).

> ⚡ **SAFETY ALERT**
>
> To promote safety and prevent injury, it is important to have hospital personnel present the first time the woman gets out of bed after birth because she can feel weak, dizzy, faint, or lightheaded. The nurse instructs the woman to call for assistance before getting out of bed the first time and any time thereafter if she feels dizzy or weak. The partner or family members who are present are instructed as well.

Preventing venous thromboembolism (VTE) is important. Blood is hypercoagulable in the postpartum period, especially during the first 48 hours after birth (Isley & Katz, 2017). Women who must remain in bed after giving birth are at increased risk for this complication. Antiembolic stockings (TED hose) or a sequential compression device (SCD boots) may be ordered prophylactically. If a woman remains in bed longer than 8 hours (e.g., for postpartum magnesium sulfate therapy for preeclampsia), exercise to promote circulation in the legs is indicated, using the following routine:

- Alternate flexion and extension of the feet.
- Rotate the ankles in a circular motion.
- Alternate flexion and extension of the legs.
- Press the back of the knees to the bed surface; relax.

If the woman is susceptible to VTE, she is encouraged to walk about actively for true ambulation and is discouraged from sitting immobile in a chair. Women with varicosities are encouraged to wear support hose. If a thrombus is suspected, as evidenced by warmth, redness, or tenderness in the suspected leg, the primary health care provider should be notified. Meanwhile the woman should be confined to bed, with the affected limb elevated on pillows.

Promoting Exercise

Postpartum exercise can begin soon after birth, although the woman should be encouraged to start with simple exercises and gradually progress to more strenuous ones. Fig. 19.3 illustrates a number of exercises appropriate for the new mother. Abdominal exercises are postponed until approximately 4 to 6 weeks after cesarean birth.

Promoting Nutrition

During the hospital stay, most women have a good appetite and eat well. They may request that family members bring favorite or culturally appropriate foods. Cultural dietary preferences must be respected. This interest in food presents an ideal opportunity for nutritional counseling on dietary needs after pregnancy, with specific information related to breastfeeding, preventing constipation and anemia, promoting weight loss, and promoting healing and well-being (see Chapter 9).

A well-balanced diet helps promote healing and health in the postpartum period. The recommended caloric intake for the moderately active, nonlactating postpartum woman is 1800 to 2200 kcal/day. Lactating women need an additional 450 to 500 kcal/day, which can usually be met with simple adjustments in a normally balanced diet. Women who are underweight, exercise excessively, or are breastfeeding more than one infant need additional calories. Dietary intake for lactating women should include 200 to 300 mg of the omega-3 long-chain polyunsaturated fatty acids (docosahexaenoic acid [DHA]) so that there is adequate DHA in the breast milk. The addition of one or two portions of fish with low mercury content provides the additional DHA. Women

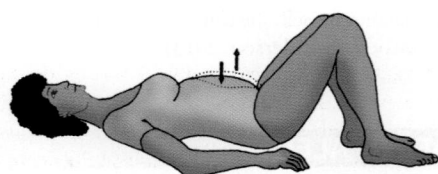

Abdominal Breathing. Lie on back with knees bent. Inhale deeply through nose. Keep ribs stationary and allow abdomen to expand upward. Exhale slowly but forcefully while contracting the abdominal muscles; hold for 3 to 5 seconds while exhaling. Relax.

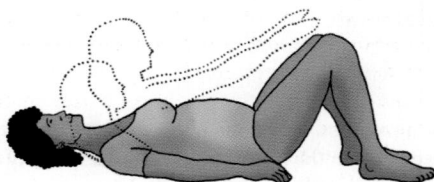

Reach for the Knees. Lie on back with knees bent. While inhaling, deeply lower chin onto chest. While exhaling, raise head and shoulders slowly and smoothly and reach for knees with arms outstretched. The body should rise only as far as the back will naturally bend while waist remains on floor or bed (about 6 to 8 inches). Slowly and smoothly lower head and shoulders back to starting position. Relax.

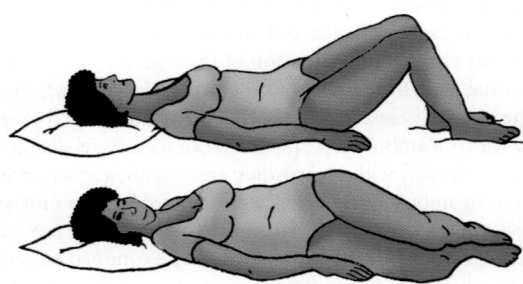

Double Knee Roll. Lie on back with knees bent. Keeping shoulders flat and feet stationary, slowly and smoothly roll knees over to the left to touch floor or bed. Maintaining a smooth motion, roll knees back over to the right until they touch floor or bed. Return to starting position and relax.

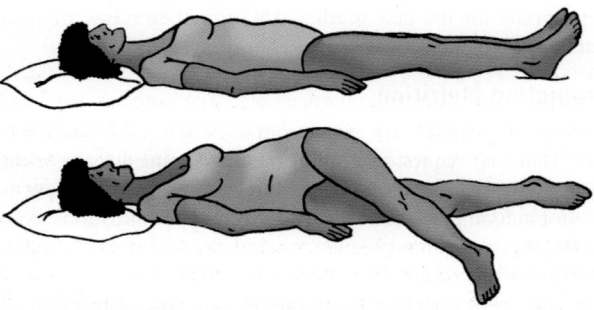

Leg Roll. Lie on back with legs straight. Keeping shoulders flat and legs straight, slowly and smoothly lift left leg and roll it over to touch the right side of floor or bed and return to starting position. Repeat, rolling right leg over to touch left side of floor or bed. Relax.

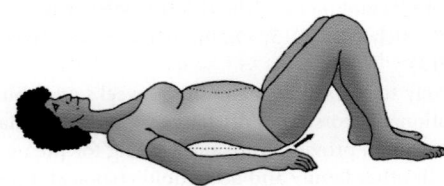

Combined Abdominal Breathing and Supine Pelvic Tilt (Pelvic Rock). Lie on back with knees bent. While inhaling deeply, roll pelvis back by flattening lower back on floor or bed. Exhale slowly but forcefully while contracting abdominal muscles and tightening buttocks. Hold for 3 to 5 seconds while exhaling. Relax.

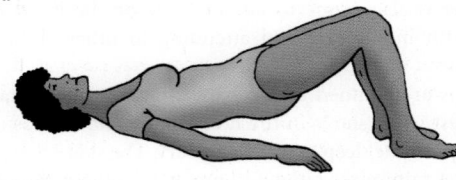

Buttocks Lift. Lie on back with arms at sides, knees bent, and feet flat. Slowly raise buttocks and arch back. Return slowly to starting position.

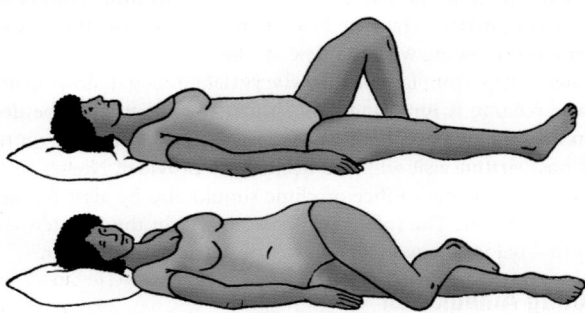

Single Knee Roll. Lie on back with right leg straight and left leg bent at the knee. Keeping shoulders flat, slowly and smoothly roll left knee over to the right to touch floor or bed and then back to starting position. Reverse position of legs. Roll right knee over to the left to touch floor or bed and return to starting position. Relax.

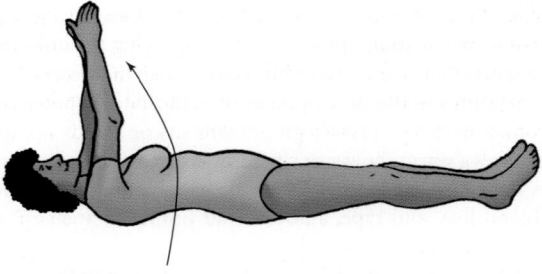

Arm Raises. Lie on back with arms extended at 90-degree angle from body. Raise arms so they are perpendicular and hands touch. Lower slowly.

FIG 19.3 Postpartum exercise should begin as soon as possible. The woman should start with simple exercises and gradually progress to more strenuous ones.

on selected vegan diets and those who are poorly nourished may need to take DHA and multivitamin supplements (AAP Section on Breastfeeding, 2012).

Prenatal vitamins may be continued until 6 weeks after birth or until the supply has been used. Iron supplements may be prescribed for women with low hemoglobin and hematocrit levels.

Promoting Normal Bladder and Bowel Patterns

Bladder Function

The mother should void spontaneously within 6 to 8 hours after giving birth. The first several voidings should be measured to document adequate emptying of the bladder. A volume of at least 150 mL is expected for each voiding. Some women experience difficulty in emptying the bladder, possibly as a result of diminished bladder tone, edema from trauma, or fear of discomfort. Nursing interventions for inability to void and bladder distention are discussed in the "Preventing Bladder Distention" section earlier in the chapter.

Urinary incontinence is not uncommon, especially if there was significant perineal trauma with birth. Pelvic floor muscle training, also known as Kegel exercises, helps to strengthen muscle tone, particularly after vaginal birth. Kegel exercises help women regain the muscle tone that is often lost as pelvic tissues are stretched and torn during pregnancy and birth. Women who maintain muscle strength benefit years later by retaining urinary continence. Women must learn to perform Kegel exercises correctly (see Guidelines box: Kegel Exercises in Chapter 3). Some women perform the exercises incorrectly and can increase the risk for incontinence, which can occur when inadvertently bearing down on the pelvic floor muscles, thrusting the perineum outward. The health care provider can assess the woman's technique during the pelvic examination at her follow-up visit by inserting two fingers intravaginally and noting whether the pelvic floor muscles correctly contract and relax.

Bowel Function

After birth, women can be at risk for constipation related to side effects of medications (opioid analgesics, iron supplements, magnesium sulfate), dehydration, immobility, or the presence of episiotomy, perineal lacerations, or hemorrhoids. The woman can be fearful of pain with the first bowel movement.

Nursing interventions to promote normal bowel elimination include educating the woman about measures to prevent constipation, such as ambulation and increasing the intake of fluids and fiber. Alerting the woman to side effects of medications such as opioid analgesics (e.g., decreased gastrointestinal tract motility) can encourage her to implement measures to reduce the risk for constipation. Stool softeners or laxatives may be necessary during the early postpartum period. These are used only at the direction of the health care provider.

⚡ SAFETY ALERT

Rectal suppositories and enemas should not be administered to women with third- or fourth-degree perineal lacerations. These measures to treat constipation can be very uncomfortable and can cause hemorrhage or damage to the suture line. They can also predispose the woman to infection.

Some mothers experience gas pains; this is more common following cesarean birth. Ambulation or rocking in a rocking chair can stimulate passage of flatus and provide relief. Antiflatulent medications may be ordered. The mother can avoid foods (e.g., legumes, beans, broccoli) that tend to produce gas.

Promoting Breastfeeding

The ideal time to initiate breastfeeding is within the first 1 to 2 hours after birth. Newborns should be placed in skin-to-skin contact with their mothers as soon as possible after birth and remain there for at least 1 hour. Nurses can encourage mothers to observe their babies for signs that they are ready to breastfeed and then assist the mothers as needed to initiate breastfeeding. During this first hour, most infants are alert and ready to nurse. Breastfeeding aids in contracting the uterus and preventing maternal hemorrhage. This initial breastfeeding session allows the nurse to assess the mother's basic knowledge of breastfeeding and the physical appearance of the breasts and nipples. Throughout the hospital stay, nurses provide education and assistance for the breastfeeding mother, making appropriate referrals to lactation consultants as needed. Nurses also provide information about community breastfeeding support groups (see Community Focus box and Chapter 24 for more information on assisting the breastfeeding woman).

🏠 COMMUNITY FOCUS

Breastfeeding Support

Women breastfeed longer if they feel supported in their breastfeeding efforts. Nurses and lactation consultants provide support during inpatient stays after birth. Women can find support in the community in various groups. Social support interventions that include peer support are successful in increasing the duration of exclusive breastfeeding and satisfaction with breastfeeding. In their discharge planning, nurses can refer breastfeeding mothers to community groups such as the La Leche League for support. Community and home health care nurses can facilitate breastfeeding efforts through organizing or facilitating support groups. Mothers experienced in breastfeeding can facilitate these efforts.

Identify sources of breastfeeding support in your community. Are these resources free and available in various parts of the community? What form does the support take? Are there group classes? Individual consultation? Who provides the consultation? Make a list of the resources you identified, and share the list with your clinical group.

Lactation Suppression

Lactation suppression is necessary when a woman has decided not to breastfeed or in the case of neonatal death. The woman wears a well-fitted support bra continuously for at least the first 72 hours after giving birth. She should avoid breast stimulation, including running warm water over the breasts, newborn suckling, or expressing milk. Some nonbreastfeeding mothers experience severe breast engorgement (swelling of breast tissue caused by increased blood and lymph supply to the breasts as the body produces milk, occurring about 72 to 96 hours after birth). Breast engorgement can usually be managed satisfactorily with nonpharmacologic interventions.

Periodic application of ice packs to the breasts can help decrease the discomfort associated with engorgement. Although there is lack of scientific evidence to support effectiveness, cabbage leaves are often recommended to help relieve engorgement; formula-feeding mothers may be told to place fresh green cabbage leaves over their breasts and to replace the leaves when they are wilted (Fig. 24.16). A mild analgesic or antiinflammatory medication can reduce discomfort associated with engorgement. Medications that were once prescribed for lactation suppression (e.g., estrogen, estrogen and testosterone, and bromocriptine) are no longer used.

Health Promotion for Future Pregnancies

Rubella Vaccination

For women who have not had rubella or who are serologically non-immune (titer of 1:8 or less or enzyme immunoassay level less than 0.8), a subcutaneous injection of rubella vaccine is recommended in the postpartum period prior to hospital discharge to prevent the possibility of contracting rubella in future pregnancies; this is given as the measles, mumps, rubella (MMR) vaccine. Women are cautioned to avoid becoming pregnant for 28 days after receiving the rubella vaccine because of the potential teratogenic risk to the fetus. The live attenuated rubella virus is not communicable in breast milk; therefore, breastfeeding mothers can be vaccinated. However, because the virus is shed in urine and other body fluids, the vaccine should not be given if the mother or other household members are immunocompromised. Fever, transient arthralgia, rash, and lymphadenopathy are common side effects of the rubella vaccine (Centers for Disease Control and Prevention [CDC], 2015a).

Varicella Vaccination

The CDC recommends that varicella vaccine be administered before discharge in postpartum women who have no immunity. A second dose is given at the postpartum follow-up visit (4 to 8 weeks after the first dose) (CDC, 2015b).

> **LEGAL TIP** **Rubella and Varicella Vaccination** Informed consent for rubella and varicella vaccination in the postpartum period includes information about possible side effects and the risk for teratogenic effects on the fetus. Women must understand that they should not become pregnant for 28 days after being vaccinated (CDC, 2015a, 2015b).

Tetanus-Diphtheria-Acellular Pertussis Vaccine

Tetanus-diphtheria-acellular pertussis (Tdap) vaccine is recommended for postpartum women who have not previously received the vaccine; it is given before discharge from the hospital or as early as possible in the postpartum period to protect women from pertussis and to decrease the risk for infant exposure to pertussis. Women should be advised that other adults and children who will be around the newborn should be vaccinated with Tdap if they have not previously received the vaccine. Women who receive the vaccine can continue to breastfeed (CDC, 2013).

Preventing Rh Isoimmunization

Injection of Rh immune globulin (a solution of gamma globulin that contains Rh antibodies) within 72 hours after birth prevents sensitization in the Rh-negative woman who has had a fetomaternal transfusion of Rh-positive fetal red blood cells (RBCs) (see the Medication Guide). Rh immune globulin promotes lysis of fetal Rh-positive blood cells before the mother forms her own antibodies against them (Aitken & Tichy, 2015). Administration of Rh immune globulin is intended to prevent problems in future pregnancies should the Rh negative woman have an Rh positive fetus.

A dose of 300 mcg (1 vial) of Rh immune globulin is usually sufficient to prevent maternal sensitization. If a large fetomaternal transfusion is suspected, however, the dosage needed should be determined by performing a Kleihauer-Betke test, which detects the amount of fetal blood in the maternal circulation. If more than 30 mL of fetal blood is present in the maternal circulation, the dosage of Rh immune globulin must be increased (AAP & ACOG, 2012).

⚡ SAFETY ALERT

Rh immune globulin suppresses the immune response. Therefore, the woman who receives both Rh immune globulin and a live virus immunization such as rubella must be tested in 3 months to see if she has developed rubella immunity. If not, she will need another dose of the vaccine.

💊 MEDICATION GUIDE

Rh Immune Globulin, RhoGAM, Gamulin Rh, HypRho-D, Rhophylac

Action
Suppression of immune response in nonsensitized women with Rh-negative blood who receive Rh-positive blood cells because of fetomaternal hemorrhage, transfusion, or accident

Indications
Routine antepartum prevention at 28 weeks of gestation in women with Rh-negative blood; suppress antibody formation after birth, miscarriage, pregnancy termination, abdominal trauma, ectopic pregnancy, amniocentesis, version, or chorionic villus sampling

Dosage and Route
Standard dose: 1 vial (300 mcg) IM in deltoid or gluteal muscle; microdose: 1 vial (50 mcg) IM in deltoid muscle; $Rh_o(D)$ immune globulin (Rhophylac) can be given IM or IV (available in prefilled syringes).

Adverse Effects
Myalgia, lethargy, localized tenderness and stiffness at injection site, mild and transient fever, malaise, headache; rarely nausea, vomiting, hypotension, tachycardia, possible allergic response

Nursing Considerations
- Give standard dose to mother at 28 weeks of gestation as prophylaxis or after an incident or exposure risk that occurs after 28 weeks of gestation (e.g., amniocentesis, second-trimester miscarriage or abortion, and after external version).
- Give standard dose within 72 hours after birth if neonate is Rh+.
- Give microdose for first-trimester miscarriage or abortion, ectopic pregnancy, chorionic villus sampling.
- Verify that the woman is Rh negative and has not been sensitized, if postpartum that Coombs' test is negative, and that baby is Rh positive. Provide explanation to the woman about the procedure, including the purpose, possible side effects, and effect on future pregnancies. Have the woman sign a consent form if required by agency. Verify correct dosage and confirm lot number and woman's identity before giving injection (verify with another registered nurse or by other procedure per agency policy); document administration per agency policy. Observe patient for at least 20 minutes after administration for allergic response.
- Document lot number and expiration date in the patient record.
- The medication is made from human plasma (a consideration if woman is a Jehovah's Witness). The risk for transmitting infectious agents, including viruses, cannot be eliminated completely.

IM, Intramuscular; *IV,* intravenous.
Data from Aitken S.L. & Tichy E.M. (2015). Rh(O)D immune globulin products for prevention of alloimmunization during pregnancy. *American Journal of Health-System Pharmacists, 72*(4), 267-276; Kedron Biopharma Inc. (2015). *Rho(D) immune globulin (human).* Biopharma Inc: Melville NY. Retrieved from http://www.kedrion.us/sites/www.kedrion.us/files/RH-0202-00-2015_RhoGAM%20Promo%20PI%2019854_Marketing-FINAL.pdf#overlay-context=user.

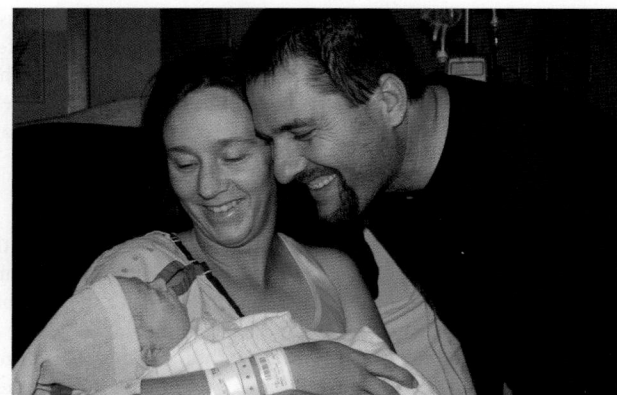

FIG 19.4 Parents getting acquainted with their new son. (Courtesy of Julie and Darren Nelson, Loveland, CO.)

There is some disagreement about whether Rh immune globulin should be considered a blood product. Health care providers need to discuss the most current information about this issue with women whose religious beliefs conflict with having blood products administered to them (e.g., Jehovah's Witnesses).

Care Management: Psychosocial Needs

Meeting the psychosocial needs of new parents involves assessing their reactions to the birth experience, feelings about themselves, and interactions with the new baby (Fig. 19.4) and other family members. Specific interventions are planned to increase the parents' knowledge and self-confidence as they assume the care and responsibility of the new baby and integrate this new member into their existing family structure in a way that meets their cultural expectations (see Chapters 20 and 23).

Taking time to assess maternal emotional needs and to address concerns before discharge can promote better psychologic health and adjustment to parenting. Ongoing support for postpartum women is also needed. Even though issues such as fatigue are often evident during the hospital stay, this type of support will likely be an ongoing concern after discharge when the woman is providing care for the newborn, herself, and other family members. Postpartum support is especially beneficial to at-risk populations such as low-income primiparas, those at risk for family dysfunction and child abuse, and those at risk for PPD. Home visitation programs for postpartum women and their families promote better outcomes.

Sometimes the psychosocial assessment indicates serious actual or potential problems that must be addressed. Box 19.2 identifies psychosocial characteristics and behaviors that warrant ongoing evaluation after hospital discharge. Women exhibiting these needs should be referred to appropriate community resources for assessment and management.

Effect of the Birth Experience

Many women need to review and reflect on labor and birth and to look retrospectively at their own intrapartal behavior. Their partners can have similar needs. If their birth experience was different from their birth plan (e.g., induction, epidural anesthesia, cesarean birth), both partners may need to mourn the loss of their expectations before they can adjust to the reality of their actual birth experience. Inviting them to review the events and describe how they feel helps the nurse assess how well they understand what happened and how well they have been able to put their birth experience into perspective.

Maternal Self-Image

An important assessment concerns the woman's self-concept, body image, and sexuality. How the new mother feels about herself and her body during the postpartum period can affect her behavior and adaptation to parenting. The woman's self-concept and body image can also affect her sexuality.

Feelings related to sexual adjustment after birth are often a cause of concern for new parents. Women who have recently given birth can be reluctant to resume sexual intercourse for fear of pain or may worry that coitus will damage healing perineal tissue. Because many new parents are anxious for information but reluctant to bring up the subject, postpartum nurses can matter-of-factly include the topic of postpartum sexuality during their routine physical assessment and teaching. Partners often have questions and concerns as well; it is helpful to include them in teaching sessions or discussions regarding sexuality in the postpartum period.

Adaptation to Parenthood and Parent-Infant Interactions

The psychosocial assessment includes assessment of adaptation to parenthood as evidenced by the parents' reactions to and interactions with the new baby. Clues indicating successful adaptation begin to appear early in the postbirth period as parents react positively to the newborn infant and continue the process of establishing a relationship with their child.

Parents are adapting well to their new roles when they exhibit a realistic perception and acceptance of their newborn's needs and limited abilities, immature social responses, and helplessness. Examples of positive parent-infant interactions include taking pleasure in the infant and in providing care, responding appropriately to infant cues, and providing comfort (see Chapter 23). If these indicators are missing, the nurse needs to investigate further in an attempt to identify what is hindering the normal adaptation process. The nurse can ask questions to determine if the woman is experiencing the normal "baby blues" or if there is a more serious underlying condition. Screening for PPD through use of a simple tool such as the Edinburgh Postnatal Depression Scale (EPDS) can be done before hospital discharge. Screening for PPD should also be done after discharge (see Chapter 21). The AAP recommends that pediatric care providers routinely perform maternal screening for PPD during infant follow-up visits at 1, 2, and 4 months (AAP, 2010) (see Clinical Reasoning Case Study).

CLINICAL REASONING CASE STUDY

Risk for Postpartum Depression

Elisabeth, a 38-year-old multipara, has just given birth to her fourth baby. The ages of her other children are 8, 4, and 2. During the morning nursing assessment, Elisabeth was noted to be tearful and stated that she was feeling "overwhelmed" and "very unsure" of herself and how to take care of the new baby, although she has three previous children. She shared that her mother was diagnosed with cancer 2 months ago and is undergoing treatment. Her husband will be starting a much-needed new job next week and will not be able to get any time off for a while. Other family members do not live close by except for her sister, who is out of town often due to her job responsibilities. Elisabeth is concerned about how she will manage taking care of a newborn and three other children with a seemingly depleted support system.

1. Evidence—Is there sufficient evidence to support counseling women with psychosocial concerns in the immediate postpartum period?
2. Assumptions—What assumptions can be made about the following issues?
   a. Elisabeth's risk for postpartum depression
   b. Elisabeth's support system
   c. Elisabeth's ability to connect with community resources after discharge
3. What implications and priorities for nursing care can be drawn at this time?
4. Interprofessional care: Describe roles/responsibilities of other health care professionals who should be involved in planning and implementing care for Elisabeth and her family.

Family Structure and Functioning

A woman's adjustment to her role as mother is affected greatly by her relationships with her partner, her mother and other relatives, and any other children (Fig. 19.5). Nurses can help ease the new mother's return home by identifying possible conflicts among family members and by helping the woman plan strategies for dealing with these problems before discharge. Such a conflict can arise when couples

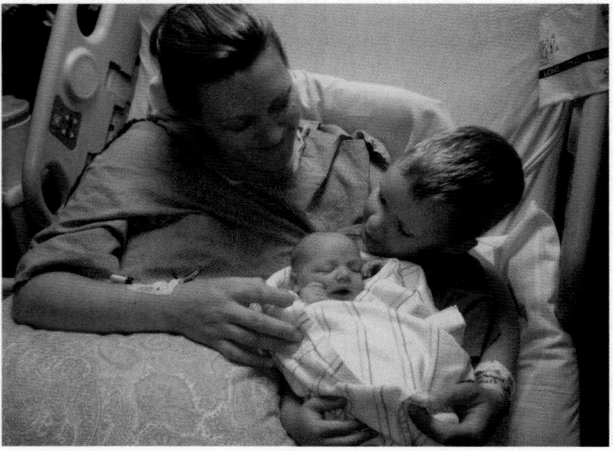

FIG 19.5 Older sibling cuddles with mother and new baby. (Courtesy of Jennifer Hobgood, Creedmoor, NC.)

have very different ideas about parenting. Dealing with the stresses of sibling rivalry and unsolicited grandparent advice also can affect the woman's transition to motherhood. Only by asking about other nuclear and extended family members can the nurse discover potential problems in such relationships and help plan workable solutions for them.

Effect of Cultural Beliefs and Practices

The final component of a complete psychosocial assessment is the woman's cultural beliefs, values, and practices. Cultural beliefs and traditions strongly influence the behaviors of the woman and her family during the postpartum period. Nurses are likely to come into contact with women from many different countries and cultures. All cultures have developed safe and satisfying methods of caring for new mothers and babies. The nurse can identify some cultural beliefs and practices through observation and interaction with the mother and her family. Only by understanding and respecting the values and beliefs of each woman can the nurse design a plan of care to meet the individual's needs.

To identify cultural beliefs and practices when planning and implementing care, the nurse conducts a cultural assessment. It can be accomplished most easily through conversation with the mother and her partner. Some hospitals have assessment tools designed to identify cultural beliefs and practices that can influence care. Components of the cultural assessment include the ability to read and write English, primary language spoken, family involvement and support, dietary preferences, infant care, attachment, religious or cultural beliefs, folk medicine practices, nonverbal communication, and personal space preferences.

Postpartum care occurs within a sociocultural context. Rest, seclusion, dietary constraints, and ceremonies honoring the mother are common traditional practices that are followed for the promotion of the health and well-being of the mother and baby. In some cultures, the postpartum period is considered a time of increased vulnerability for the mother. To protect her, there are restrictions on activity, diet, bathing, and infant caretaking.

The postpartum period is seen by some cultures as a time of impurity for the mother. For as many days or weeks as she has lochial flow, she is considered "impure" and has limited contact with others. Sexual activity is prohibited during this time.

In many Asian cultures, the balance between yin and yang (cold and hot) is necessary for balance and harmony with the environment. Postpartum practices focus on helping the mother achieve this balance. Pregnancy is considered a "hot" condition. It is believed that birth depletes the mother's body of heat through loss of blood and inner energy; this places her in a "cold" state for about 40 days until her womb is healed. The woman consumes only "hot" foods and beverages. Examples of foods that are considered "hot" include rice, eggs, beef, and chicken soup. Seaweed soup is consumed by postpartum women for the purpose of increasing milk production and helping to rid the body of lochia. Family members often bring in foods from home (Callister, 2014). To help prevent the loss of heat from the body, the mother may be discouraged from showering or bathing for several days or weeks; however, there is attention to perineal care and hygiene. The temperature of the hospital room is warmer than usual. The mother likely spends most of the time in bed to prevent cold air from entering the body, and she has minimal contact with the infant. Family members provide care for the mother and the newborn. For example, in the Korean culture, the mother-in-law is charged with caring for her daughter-in-law and newly born grandchild during the postpartum period (Callister, 2014).

Hispanic and Latino women who have immigrated to the United States or other Western nations often observe the period of 40 days (6 weeks) after birth as *la cuarentena*. During this time, the woman's body is perceived to be "open" and vulnerable to drafts; la cuarentena is about "closing the body." Traditional practices associated with la cuarentena include a liquid diet of nutritious drinks, soups, and broths in the early postpartum period; binding the abdomen; avoiding cool air; and maintaining sexual abstinence. Activity is restricted, and the mother stays at home (Waugh, 2011). A common concern of Hispanic and Latino women is the "evil eye" or *mal de ojo*. They believe that if someone admires or covets the infant but does not touch him or her, it can cause bad luck, illness, or even death. In an attempt to ward off the evil eye, some mothers place a bracelet with a black onyx hand, la manita de azabache, on or near the newborn (Callister, 2014) (see Cultural Considerations box in Chapter 23).

The nurse should not assume that a mother desires to use traditional health practices that represent a particular cultural group merely because she is a member of that culture. Many young women who are first- or second-generation Americans follow their cultural traditions only when older family members are present or not at all.

It is important that nurses consider all cultural aspects when planning care and not use their own cultural beliefs as the framework for that care. Although the beliefs and behaviors of other cultures can seem different or strange, they should be encouraged as long as the mother wants to conform to them and she and the baby have no ill effects.

The Cultural Considerations box: Examples of Cultural Beliefs and Practices in the Postpartum Period lists some common cultural beliefs about the postpartum period and family planning.

DISCHARGE TEACHING

Self-Care and Signs of Complications

Discharge planning begins at the time of admission to the unit and should be reflected in the nursing care plan developed for each woman. For example, a great deal of time during the hospital stay is usually spent in teaching about maternal self-management and care of the newborn because the goal is for all women to be capable of providing basic care for themselves and their infants at the time of discharge. In addition, every woman must be taught to recognize physical and psychologic signs and symptoms that might indicate problems and how to obtain advice and assistance quickly if these signs appear. Table 19.1

and Box 19.2 list several common indications of maternal physical and psychosocial problems in the postpartum period (see Chapter 21 for more information on postpartum complications). Before discharge, women need basic instruction regarding a variety of self-management topics such as nutrition, exercise, family planning, the resumption of sexual intercourse, prescribed medications, and routine mother-baby follow-up care.

Because of the limited time available for teaching, nurses must target their teaching on expressed needs of the woman. Giving the woman a list of topics and asking her to indicate her learning needs help the nurse maximize teaching efforts and can increase retention of information. Providing written materials on postpartum self-management, breastfeeding, and infant care that the woman can consult after discharge is helpful. Nurses can direct women to on-line resources; some hospitals and birth centers provide information for new parents on their websites.

Just before the time of discharge, the nurse reviews the woman's records to see that laboratory reports, medications, signatures, and other items are in order. Some facilities have a checklist to use before the woman's discharge. The nurse verifies that medications, if ordered, have arrived on the unit; that any valuables kept secured during the woman's stay have been returned to her and that she has signed a receipt for them; and that the infant is ready to be discharged. The woman's and the baby's identification bands are checked carefully.

⚡ SAFETY ALERT

No medication that can cause drowsiness should be administered to the mother before discharge if she is the one who will be holding the baby when they leave the hospital. In most instances, the woman is seated in a wheelchair and given the baby to hold. Some families leave unescorted and ambulatory, depending on hospital protocol. The newborn must be secured in a car seat for the drive home.

In many birthing facilities, new mothers (breastfeeding and formula feeding) are routinely presented with gift bags that contain samples of infant formula. This practice is not consistent with the Baby-Friendly Hospital USA Initiative (2016) and is contrary to the International Code of Marketing of Breast-Milk Substitutes (World Health Organization, 1981). Prepackaged formula should not be given to mothers who are breastfeeding. Such "gifts" are associated with earlier cessation of breastfeeding.

Sexual Activity and Contraception

Discussing sexual activity with women and their partners before they leave the hospital is important because many couples resume sexual activity before the traditional postpartum follow-up visit with the health care provider 6 weeks after birth. For most women, the risk for hemorrhage or infection is minimal by approximately 2 weeks postpartum. Couples may be anxious about the topic but uncomfortable and unwilling to bring it up. The nurse needs to discuss the physical and psychologic effects that giving birth can have on sexual activity (see Patient Teaching box: Resuming Sexual Activity After Birth).

Many factors can influence the timing and quality of sexual activity after birth. Postpartum perineal pain and dyspareunia (painful intercourse) are common among women with perineal lacerations or episiotomy. Some women who had an episiotomy report discomfort with intercourse for months after birth.

Discomfort is more severe and lasts longer with third- and fourth-degree lacerations (see Evidence-Based Practice box: When an OASIS is Not a Scenic Travel Destination: Minimizing Anal Sphincter Injury in Childbirth). Breastfeeding mothers often experience vaginal dryness related to high prolactin levels and low estrogen levels. Changes in family structure and altered sleep patterns can make it difficult for a couple to find time for privacy and intimacy. PPD is associated with decreased sexual desire; medication used to treat PPD can reduce sexual desire and inhibit orgasm.

PATIENT TEACHING
Resuming Sexual Activity After Birth

- Unless your health care provider indicates otherwise, you can safely resume sexual activity (intercourse) by the second to fourth week after birth, when bleeding has stopped and the perineum is healed. Most women resume sexual activity by 5 to 6 weeks after birth, although this varies and is often related to perineal discomfort. Perineal lacerations or episiotomy increase the chances of discomfort with intercourse. For the first 6 weeks to 6 months, vaginal lubrication might be decreased, especially among breastfeeding women. Your physiologic reactions to sexual stimulation for the first 3 months after birth may be slower and less intense. The strength of the orgasm may be reduced.
- A water-soluble gel or contraceptive cream or jelly might be recommended for lubrication. If some vaginal tenderness is present, your partner can be instructed to insert one or more clean, lubricated fingers into the vagina and rotate them to help the vagina relax and identify possible areas of discomfort. A position in which you have control of the depth of the insertion of the penis also is useful. The side-by-side or female-on-top position may be most comfortable.
- The presence of the baby influences sexual activity and enjoyment. Parents hear every sound made by the baby; conversely you may be concerned that the baby hears every sound you make. In either case, any phase of the sexual response cycle can be interrupted by hearing the baby cry or move, leaving both of you frustrated and unsatisfied. In addition, the amount of psychologic energy expended by you in child-care activities can lead to fatigue. Newborns require a great deal of attention and time.
- Some women have reported feeling sexual stimulation and orgasms when breastfeeding their babies. This is not abnormal. Breastfeeding mothers often are interested in returning to sexual activity before nonbreastfeeding mothers.
- You should be instructed to perform the Kegel exercises correctly to strengthen your pubococcygeal muscle. This muscle is associated with bowel and bladder function and vaginal feeling during intercourse.

Contraceptive options should also be discussed with women (and their partners, if present) before discharge so that they can make informed decisions about fertility management before resuming sexual activity. Waiting to discuss contraception at the 6-week checkup can be too late. Ovulation can occur as soon as 1 month after birth, particularly in women who formula-feed their infants. Breastfeeding mothers should be informed that breastfeeding is not a reliable means of contraception and that other methods should be used; nonhormonal methods are best because oral contraceptives can interfere with milk production. Women who are undecided about contraception at the time of discharge need information about using condoms with spermicidal foam or creams until the first postpartum checkup. Contraceptive options are discussed in detail in Chapter 5.

Medications

Women routinely continue to take their prenatal vitamins during the postpartum period. Breastfeeding mothers may continue prenatal vitamins for the duration of breastfeeding. Supplemental iron may be prescribed for mothers with lower than normal hemoglobin levels. Women with extensive episiotomies or perineal lacerations (third or fourth degree) are usually prescribed stool softeners to take at home. Pain medications (opioid and nonopioid) may be prescribed, especially for women who had cesarean births. The nurse should make certain

EVIDENCE-BASED PRACTICE

When an OASIS Is Not a Scenic Travel Destination: Minimizing Anal Sphincter Injury in Childbirth

Ask the Question
PICOT Question: For women in labor, what perinatal interventions to minimize perineal trauma are safe and effective?

Search for the Evidence
Search Strategies: English research-based publications on perineal trauma, birth, postpartum, anal sphincter, lacerations.

Databases Used: Cochrane Collaborative Database, National Guideline Clearinghouse (AHRQ), CINAHL, PubMed, and the professional website for ACOG.

Critical Appraisal of the Evidence
Perineal lacerations that reach the anal sphincter (third degree) and the rectal wall (fourth degree) are called *obstetrical anal sphincter injuries (OASIS)*. Risk factors include large baby (>4 kg), nulliparity, induction or augmentation of labor, operative/instrumental delivery, prolonged second-stage labor, epidural anesthesia, shoulder dystocia, and maternal position (upright/squatting).

- OASIS is associated with long-term postpartum anal incontinence and urgency, pelvic pain, and dyspareunia (LaCross, Grodd, & Smaldone, 2015).
- OASIS may be a complication of an episiotomy, which compromises the integrity of the perineum and may allow further tearing. Of all the risk factors for anal injury and incontinence, episiotomy is the most modifiable (LaCross et al., 2015).
- Although obesity is on many lists as a risk factor, it may be significantly protective against third- and fourth-degree lacerations (Garretto, Lin, Syn, et al., 2016). This may be due to stretchier tissue, dispersement of contraction force, and/or less frequent use of squatting in second-stage labor. Decreased ability by the provider to visualize the perineum due to maternal obesity may also mask the true extent of perineal damage (Garretto et al.).
- Perineal support during crowning involves the provider using one hand to press the tissue under the crown, between the vagina and rectum, in order to support some weight of the fetal head as it lays the heaviest upon the opening. Some practices include using the other hand to apply gentle counterpressure against the fetal skull, to slow down birth of the head. Evidence regarding the practice of provider support of the perineum during crowning is mixed. A systematic review and meta-analysis found no difference between perineal support and hands-off during delivery in three randomized controlled trials (RCTs), but a protective effect of perineal support against OASIS in three nonrandomized studies (NRSs). The RCTs were the higher-quality evidence, but the NRSs were much larger (6647 vs 74,000 women). The authors did not find the evidence sufficient to make a recommendation (Bulchandani, Watts, Sucharitha et al., 2015).

Apply the Evidence: Nursing Implications
The American College of Obstetricians and Gynecologists (2016) recommends the following to prevent lacerations:
- Use of warm compresses and perineal massage during first- and second-stage birth significantly decreases third- and fourth-degree tears. In addition, perineal massage during the final 6 weeks of pregnancy may decrease perineal trauma.
- Use of episiotomy should be restricted, not routine. When necessary, the mediolateral cut is less associated with OASIS; however, the mediolateral episiotomy is more likely to result in dyspareunia and pelvic pain.

- Women with OASIS should be given antibiotics, stool softeners, and laxatives, as well as counseling on avoiding constipation.
- Women who have had prior OASIS have a low risk for recurrence, but may reasonably be offered a cesarean birth, if they request it.

Women may be deeply embarrassed discussing dyspareunia and incontinence with their partners and/or with their health care team. Nurses are ideally placed to initiate and keep the dialogue going throughout childbearing.

- Discussion of anatomy, physiology, and sexual function should begin in early pregnancy and continue throughout the postpartum period, including a brief valid and reliable sexual function survey.
- Prior to hospital discharge, the nurse can initiate discussions with the patient and her partner regarding pain, dyspareunia, resumption of intercourse, and contraception. Patients should know the hypoestrogenic and sensitivity changes they may experience due to breastfeeding, and the need for additional vaginal lubrication.
- At postpartum visits, the nurse assesses bladder, bowel, and sexual function; inspects the perineum; and assesses and discusses mood and intimacy challenges such as fatigue and timing issues. Suggesting alternate positions may help increase comfort during intercourse. The nurse evaluates patient satisfaction with the selected contraceptive method.

Quality and Safety Competencies: Evidence-Based Practice*
Knowledge
Describe EBP to include the components of research evidence, clinical expertise, and patient/family values.
Perineal trauma may be minimized by using best practices.

Skills
Base individualized care plan on patient values, clinical expertise, and evidence.
The nurse models a view of human sexuality as a healthy and normal part of one's quality of life.

Attitudes
Value the concept of EBP as integral to determining best clinical practice.
The nurse can educate the patient and partner about the challenges of OASIS repair and recovery, and sexual concerns.

References
American College of Obstetricians and Gynecologists. (2016). Practice bulletin #165: Prevention and management of obstetric lacerations at vaginal delivery. *Obstetrics and Gynecology*, *128*(1), e1–e15.

Bulchandani, S., Watts, E., Sucharitha, A., et al. (2015). Manual perineal support at the time of childbirth: A systematic review and meta-analysis. *British Journal of Obstetrics and Gynaecology*, *122*(9), 1157–1165.

Garretto, D., Lin, B.B., Syn, H.L., et al. (2016). Obesity may be protective against severe perineal lacerations. *Journal of Obesity*, *2016*, Article ID 9376592, 5 pages.

LaCross, A., Grodd, M., & Smaldone, A. (2015). Obstetric anal sphincter injury and anal incontinence following vaginal birth: A systematic review and meta-analysis. *Journal of Midwifery & Women's Health*, *60*(1), 37–47.

Pat Mahaffee Gingrich

*Adapted from QSEN at www.qsen.org/.

that the woman knows the route, dosage, frequency, and common side effects of all medications that she will be taking at home. Written information about the medications is usually included in the discharge instructions.

Follow-Up After Discharge
Routine Schedule of Care
Follow-up with the obstetric health care provider is important to the health of the woman. It is a time for comprehensive evaluation of the new mother's physical, emotional, mental, and social well-being. Important components of the postpartum visit are review of the woman's postpartum concerns; routine screening for PPD; review of the labor and birth experience and any complications that occurred; counseling for women with ongoing health concerns such as diabetes; contraceptive planning; anticipatory guidance related to return to employment, weight loss, and so on; and planning for ongoing care under the supervision of a primary health care provider (ACOG, 2016).

Women who have experienced uncomplicated vaginal births are commonly scheduled for the traditional 6-week postpartum examination. Women who have had a cesarean birth are usually seen in the health care provider's office or clinic within 2 weeks after hospital discharge. Early follow-up is warranted for women who experienced complications such as hypertensive disorders of pregnancy, those with chronic health conditions, women at high risk for depression, and breastfeeding mothers who are experiencing lactation problems (ACOG, 2016). The date and time for the follow-up appointment should be included in the discharge instructions. If an appointment has not been made before the woman leaves the hospital, she should be encouraged to call the health care provider's office or clinic to schedule one. The nurse should explain the importance of postpartum follow-up care and encourage the new mother to be compliant.

As many as 40% of new mothers forego the postpartum visit (ACOG, 2016). There are a variety of reasons for this, including thinking that they are feeling fine and do not need to follow-up, believing that their maternity care was already completed, difficulty getting to an appointment, and lack of insurance (Declercq et al., 2014). In an effort to increase compliance with postpartum visits, discussions related to discharge planning should begin during pregnancy with providers and nurses talking with expectant parents about the importance of follow-up care. A postpartum plan of care can be developed during pregnancy in collaboration with the woman and her partner, considering the mother's physical and mental health, individual and family needs and desires, support system, and available resources. The plan of care should be reviewed after birth, prior to hospital discharge, and revised as needed at the postpartum follow-up visit. An interprofessional team for postpartum care may include the obstetric and pediatric health care providers, lactation consultants, home visitation nurses or peer counselors, public health nurses, nutritionists, mental health care providers, and other specialists based on the specific needs of the mother and infant.

Prior to discharge from the birthing facility, the nurse emphasizes the need for follow-up care for the newborn. Breastfeeding infants are routinely seen by the pediatric health care provider or clinic within 3 to 5 days after birth or 48 to 72 hours after hospital discharge and again at approximately 2 weeks of age (AAP Section on Breastfeeding, 2012). Formula-feeding infants may be seen for the first time at 2 weeks of age. If an appointment was not scheduled for the infant's follow-up visit before leaving the hospital, the parents should be encouraged to call the office or clinic soon after their arrival home. This visit is essential for evaluating the status of the infant, and provides an opportunity for assessing the mother for PPD, even before she returns to her obstetric health care provider.

Home Visits
Home visits to mothers and babies within a few days of discharge can help bridge the gap between hospital care and routine visits to health care providers. In the United States, home visitation programs often target special populations such as low-income, first-time mothers; patients who were discharged early from the birthing facility; patients with special needs related to complications during pregnancy or birth; victims of intimate partner violence; or families with preterm infants. Nurses can assess the mother, infant, family, and home environment; answer questions and provide education and emotional support; and make referrals to community resources if necessary. The support provided by nurses and other trained community health care workers such as peer counselors can enhance parent-infant interaction and parenting skills; home visits also help to promote mutual support between the mother and her partner. Breastfeeding outcomes can be enhanced through home visitation programs.

Home nursing care may not be available, even if needed, because no agencies are available to provide the service or no coverage is in place for payment by third-party payers. If care is available, a referral form containing information about the mother and baby should be completed at discharge from the birthing facility and sent immediately to the home care agency.

The home visit is most commonly scheduled on the woman's second day home from the hospital, but it can be scheduled on any of the first 4 days at home, depending on the individual family's situation and needs. Additional visits are planned throughout the first week, as needed. The home visits may be extended beyond that time if the family's needs warrant it and if a home visit is the most appropriate option for carrying out the follow-up care required to meet the specific needs identified.

During the home visit, the nurse conducts a systematic assessment of mother and newborn to determine physiologic adjustment and identify any existing complications. The assessment also focuses on the mother's emotional adjustment and her knowledge of self-management and infant care. Conducting the assessment in a private area of the home provides an opportunity for the mother to ask questions on potentially sensitive topics such as breast care, constipation, sexual activity, or family planning. The nurse assesses family adjustment to the newborn and addresses any concerns during the home visit. See Chapter 2 for more information on home visits.

During the newborn assessment, the nurse can demonstrate and explain normal newborn behavior and capabilities and encourage the mother and family to ask questions or express concerns they have. The home care nurse verifies if the blood sample for newborn screening has been drawn (see Chapter 23). If the baby was discharged from the hospital before 24 hours of age, a blood sample for the newborn screen may be drawn by the home care nurse, or the family will need to take the infant to the health care provider's office or clinic to have the blood sample drawn.

Telephone Follow-Up
In addition to or instead of a home visit, postpartum telephone follow-up calls are sometimes used for assessment, health teaching, and identification of complications to facilitate timely intervention and referrals. Telephone follow-up may be offered by hospitals, private physicians, clinics, or private agencies. It may be either a separate service or combined with other strategies for extending postpartum care. Telephone nursing assessments are frequently used as follow-up to postpartum home visits to reassess a woman's knowledge about the signs and symptoms of adequate intake by the breastfeeding infant or, after initiating home phototherapy, to assess the caregiver's knowledge regarding equipment complications. There is evidence that phone support for new mothers

during the postpartum period is beneficial; it can contribute to improved breastfeeding outcomes, reduced depression scores, and increased patient satisfaction (Lavender, Richens, Milan, et al., 2013; Miller, Dane, Thompson, et al., 2014).

Warm Lines

The warm line is another type of telephone link between the new family and concerned caregivers or experienced parent volunteers. A warm line is a help line or consultation service, not a crisis intervention line. The warm line is appropriately used for dealing with less extreme concerns that seem urgent at the time the call is placed but are not actual emergencies. Calls to warm lines commonly relate to infant feeding, prolonged crying, or sibling rivalry. Families are encouraged to call when concerns arise. Telephone numbers for warm lines should be given to parents before hospital discharge.

Support Groups

The woman adjusting to motherhood may desire interaction and conversation with other women who are having similar experiences. Postpartum women who have met earlier in prenatal clinics or on the hospital unit can begin to associate for mutual support. Members of childbirth classes who attend a postpartum reunion may decide to extend their relationship during the fourth trimester. Fathers or partners also benefit from participation in support groups.

A postpartum support group enables mothers and partners/fathers to share experiences and concerns and support one another as they adjust to parenting. Many new parents find it reassuring to discover that they are not alone in their feelings of confusion and uncertainty. An experienced parent can often impart concrete information that is valuable to other group members. Inexperienced parents can imitate the behavior of others in the group whom they perceive as particularly capable. There are local support groups for a variety of postpartum topics and concerns. For example, women can find breastfeeding support through local meetings of La Leche League (http://www.llli.org/webus.html).

Internet technology can help women connect with support groups. Women can find support through groups on social media. They can participate in virtual meetings while in the comfort of their own homes, and they can participate in forums on specific topics. One example of an on-line support group is through Postpartum Support International. This organization provides weekly on-line support group meetings for women with PPD and other mental health issues (http://www.postpartum.net/psi-online-support-meetings/).

Referral to Community Resources

To develop an effective referral system, the nurse should have an understanding of the needs of the woman and family and of the organization and community resources available for meeting those needs. Locating and compiling information about available community services contributes to the development of a referral system. The nurse also needs to develop his or her own resource file of local and national services that are frequently useful to postpartum families. This list should be updated regularly as services and/or providers change frequently.

REFERENCES

Aber, C., Weiss, M., & Fawcett, J. (2013). Contemporary women's adaptation to motherhood: The first 3 to 6 weeks postpartum. *Nursing Science Quarterly, 26*(4), 344–351.

Agency for Healthcare Research and Quality. (2013). *Strategy 3: Nurse bedside shift report.* Agency for Healthcare Research and Quality: Rockville, MD. Retrieved from http://www.ahrq.gov/professionals/systems/hospital/engagingfamilies/strategy3/index.html.

Aitken, S. L., & Tichy, E. M. (2015). RhO (D) immune globulin products for prevention of alloimmunization during pregnancy. *American Journal of Health-System Pharmacy, 72*(4), 267–276.

American Academy of Pediatrics. (2010). Incorporating recognition and management of perinatal and postpartum depression into pediatric practice. *Pediatrics, 126*(5), 1032–1039.

American Academy of Pediatrics. (2015). Hospital stay for healthy term newborn infants. *Pediatrics, 135*(5), 948–953.

American Academy of Pediatrics & American College of Obstetricians and Gynecologists. (2012). *Guidelines for perinatal care* (7th ed.). Washington, DC: Author.

American Academy of Pediatrics. (2012). Breastfeeding and the use of human milk. *Pediatrics, 129*(3), e827–e841.

American College of Obstetricians and Gynecologists. (2016). Committee Opinion no. 666: Optimizing postpartum care. *Obstetrics and Gynecology, 127*(6), e187–e192.

Association of Women's Health, Obstetric and Neonatal Nurses. (2010). *Guidelines for professional registered nurse staffing for perinatal units.* Washington, DC: Author.

Baby-Friendly USA. (2016). *Guidelines and evaluation criteria for facilities seeking Baby-Friendly designation.* Baby-Friendly USA: Sandwich, MA. Retrieved from www.babyfriendlyusa.org/get-started/the-guidelines-evaluation-criteria.

Bhati, S., & Richards, K. (2015). A systematic review of the relationship between postpartum sleep disturbance and postpartum depression. *Journal of Obstetric, Gynecologic, and Neonatal Nursing, 44*(3), 350–357.

Callister, L. C. (2014). Integrating cultural beliefs and practices when caring for childbearing women and families. In K. R. Simpson & P. A. Creehan (Eds.), *Perinatal nursing* (4th ed.). Philadelphia, PA: Wolters Kluwer/Lippincott.

Center for Consumer Information and Insurance Oversight. (2012). *Newborns' and mothers' health protection act.* Retrieved from https://www.cms.gov/CCIIO/Programs-and-Initiatives/Other-Insurance-Protections/nmhpa_factsheet.html.

Centers for Disease Control and Prevention. (2013). Updated recommendations for use of tetanus toxoid, reduced diphtheria toxoid, and acellular pertussis vaccine (Tdap) in pregnant women—Advisory Committee on Immunization Practices, 2012. *Morbidity and Mortality Weekly Report, 62*(7), 131–135.

Centers for Disease Control and Prevention. (2015a). Rubella. In J. Hamborsky, A. Kroger, & S. Wolfe (Eds.), *Epidemiology and prevention of vaccine-preventable diseases* (13th ed.). Washington, DC: Public Health Foundation.

Centers for Disease Control and Prevention. (2015b). Varicella. In J. Hamborsky, A. Kroger, & S. Wolfe (Eds.), *Epidemiology and prevention of vaccine-preventable diseases* (13th ed.). Washington, DC: Public Health Foundation.

Declercq, R., Sakala, C., Corry, M. P., et al. (2014). Major survey findings of Listening to Mothers III: New mothers speak out. *Journal of Perinatal Education, 23*(1), 17–24.

Isley, M. M., & Katz, V. L. (2017). Postpartum care and long-term health considerations. In S. G. Gabbe, J. R. Niebyl, J. L. Simpson, et al. (Eds.), *Obstetrics: Normal and problem pregnancies* (7th ed.). Philadelphia, PA: Elsevier.

Lavender, T., Richens, Y., Milan, S. J., et al. (2013). Telephone support for women during pregnancy and the first six weeks postpartum. *The Cochrane Database of Systematic Reviews, 2013*(7), CD009338.

Lockwood, S., & Anderson, K. (2013). Postpartum safety: A patient-centered approach to fall prevention. *American Journal of Maternal Child Nursing, 38*(1), 15–18.

McLean, H. Q., Fiebelkorn, A. P., Temte, J. L., & Wallace, G. S. (2013). Prevention of measles, rubella, congenital rubella syndrome, and mumps, 2013: Summary recommendations of the Advisory Committee on Immunization Practices. *Morbidity and Mortality Weekly Report, 62*(RR04), 1–34.

Miller, Y. D., Dane, A. C., & Thompson, R. (2014). A call for better care: The impact of postnatal contact services on women's parenting confidence and experiences of postpartum care in Queensland, Australia. *BMC Health Services Research, 14*(1), 1–13.

Novak, K., & Fairchild, R. (2012). Bedside reporting and SBAR: Improving patient communication and satisfaction. *Journal of Pediatric Nursing, 27*(6), 760–762.

Okun, M. L. (2015). Sleep and postpartum depression. *Current Opinion in Psychiatry, 28*(6), 490–496.

Park, E. M., Meltzer-Brody, S., & Stickgold, R. (2013). Poor sleep maintenance and subjective sleep quality are associated with postpartum maternal depression symptom severity. *Archives of Women's Mental Health, 16*(6), 539–547.

Waugh, L. J. (2011). Beliefs associated with Mexican immigrant families' practice of la cuarentena during postpartum recovery. *Journal of Obstetric, Gynecologic, and Neonatal Nursing, 40*(6), 732–741.

World Health Organization. (1981). *International code of marketing breast-milk substitutes.* WHO: Geneva, Switzerland. Retrieved from http://www.who.int/nutrition/publications/code_english.pdf.

20

Transition to Parenthood

Ellen F. Olshansky

 http://evolve.elsevier.com/Perry/maternal

Becoming a parent creates a period of change and instability for men and women who decide to rear children. This period occurs whether parenthood is biologic or adoptive and whether the parents are married husband-wife couples, cohabiting couples, single mothers, single fathers, lesbian couples with one woman as biologic mother, or gay male couples who adopt a child. Parenting is a process of role attainment and role transition. The transition is an ongoing process as the parents and infant develop and change.

PARENTAL ATTACHMENT, BONDING, AND ACQUAINTANCE

The process by which a parent comes to love and accept a child and a child comes to love and accept a parent is known as attachment. Using the terms *attachment* and *bonding,* Klaus and Kennell (1976) originally proposed that there is a sensitive period during the first few minutes or hours after birth when mothers and fathers must have close contact with their infant to optimize the child's later development. Klaus and Kennell (1982) later revised their theory of parent-infant bonding, modifying their claim of the critical nature of immediate contact with the infant after birth. They acknowledged the adaptability of human parents, stating that more than minutes or hours were needed for parents to form an emotional relationship with their infants. The terms *attachment* and *bonding* continue to be used interchangeably.

Attachment is developed and maintained by proximity and interaction with the infant through which the parent becomes acquainted with the infant, identifies the infant as an individual, and claims the infant as a member of the family. Attachment is facilitated by positive feedback (i.e., social, verbal, and nonverbal responses, whether real or perceived, that indicate acceptance of one partner by the other). Attachment occurs through a mutually satisfying experience. A mother commented on her son's grasp reflex, "I put my finger in his hand, and he grabbed right on. It is just a reflex, I know, but it felt good anyway" (Fig. 20.1).

The concept of attachment includes *mutuality*; that is, the infant's behaviors and characteristics elicit a corresponding set of parental behaviors and characteristics. The infant displays signaling behaviors such as crying, smiling, and cooing that initiate the contact and bring the caregiver to the child. These behaviors are followed by executive behaviors such as rooting, grasping, and postural adjustments that maintain the contact. Most caregivers are attracted to an alert, responsive, cuddly infant but find it less desirable to interact with an irritable, apparently disinterested infant. Attachment occurs more readily with the infant whose temperament, social capabilities, appearance, and sex fit the parent's expectations. If the child does not meet these expectations, the parent's disappointment can delay the attachment process. Table 20.1 presents a comprehensive list of classic infant behaviors affecting parental attachment. Table 20.2 presents a corresponding list of parental behaviors that affect infant attachment.

An important part of attachment is *acquaintance*. Parents use eye contact (Fig. 20.2), touching, talking, and exploring to become acquainted with their infant during the immediate postpartum period. Adoptive parents undergo the same process when they first meet their new child.

During this period, families engage in the *claiming process*, which is the identification of the new baby (Fig. 20.3). The child is first identified in terms of "likeness" to other family members, then in terms of "differences," and finally in terms of "uniqueness." The unique newcomer is thus incorporated into the family. Mother and father examine their infant carefully and point out characteristics that the child shares with other family members and that are indicative of a relationship between them. The claiming process is revealed by maternal comments such as "Daniel held him close and said, 'He's the image of his father,' but I found one part like me—his toes are shaped like mine."

Conversely, some mothers react negatively. They "claim" the infant in terms of the discomfort or pain the baby causes. The mother interprets the infant's normal responses as being negative toward her and reacts to her child with dislike or indifference. She does not hold the child close or touch the child to be comforting. For example, "The nurse put the baby into Marie's arms. She promptly laid him across her knees and glanced up at the television. 'Stay still until I finish watching—you've been enough trouble already.'"

Nursing interventions to facilitate parental attachment are numerous and varied (Table 20.3). They can enhance positive parent-infant contacts by heightening parental awareness of an infant's responses and ability to communicate. As the parent attempts to become competent and loving in that role, nurses can bolster the parent's self-confidence and ego.

Nurses can identify actual and potential problems and collaborate with other health care professionals who will provide care for the parents after discharge. Nursing considerations for fostering maternal-infant bonding among special populations may vary (see Cultural Considerations box: Fostering Bonding in Women of Varying Ethnic and Cultural Groups).

Nurses should become knowledgeable of the childbearing beliefs and practices of diverse cultural and ethnic groups. Because individual cultural variations exist within groups, nurses need to clarify with the patient and family members or friends what cultural norms the patient follows. Incorrect judgments may be made about mother-infant bonding if nurses do not practice culturally sensitive care.

ASSESSMENT OF ATTACHMENT BEHAVIORS

One of the most important areas of assessment is careful observation of specific behaviors thought to indicate the formation of emotional bonds between the newborn and family, especially the mother. Unlike physical assessment of the neonate, which has concrete guidelines to

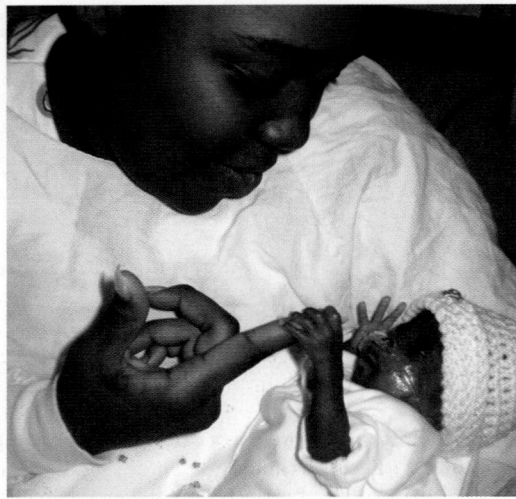

FIG 20.1 Hands. (Courtesy of Cheryl Briggs, RNC, Annapolis, MD.)

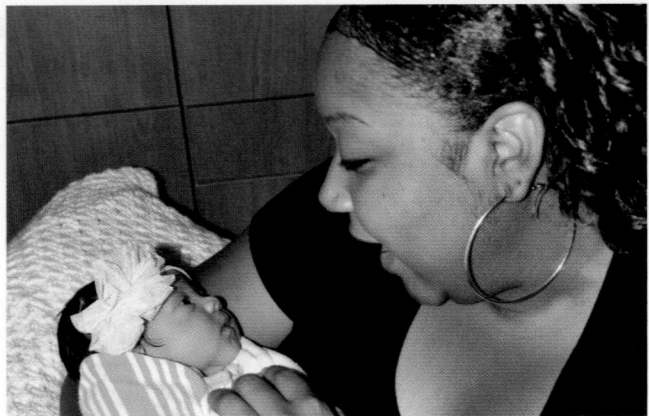

FIG 20.2 Eye-to-eye contact. (Courtesy of Cheryl Briggs, RNC, Annapolis, MD.)

TABLE 20.1   Infant Behaviors Affecting Parental Attachment

Facilitating Behaviors	Inhibiting Behaviors
Visually alert; eye-to-eye contact; tracking or following of parent's face	Sleepy; eyes closed most of the time; gaze aversion
Appealing facial appearance; randomness of body movements reflecting helplessness	Resemblance to person parent dislikes; hyperirritability or jerky body movements when touched
Smiles	Bland facial expression; infrequent smiles
Vocalization; crying only when hungry or wet	Crying for hours on end; colicky
Grasp reflex	Exaggerated motor reflex
Anticipatory approach behaviors for feedings; sucks well; feeds easily	Feeds poorly; regurgitates; vomits often
Enjoys being cuddled and held	Resists holding and cuddling by crying, stiffening body
Easily consolable	Inconsolable; unresponsive to parenting, caregiving tasks
Activity and regularity somewhat predictable	Unpredictable feeding and sleeping schedule
Attention span sufficient to focus on parents	Inability to attend to parent's face or offered stimulation
Differential crying, smiling, and vocalizing; recognizes and prefers parents	Shows no preference for parents over others
Approaches through locomotion	Unresponsive to parent's approaches
Clings to parent; puts arms around parent's neck	Seeks attention from any adult in room
Lifts arms to parents in greeting	Ignores parents

Data from Gerson, E. (1973). *Infant behavior in the first year of life.* New York, NY: Raven Press.

TABLE 20.2   Parental Behaviors Affecting Infant Attachment

Facilitating Behaviors	Inhibiting Behaviors
Looks; gazes; takes in physical characteristics of infant; assumes en face position; eye contact	Turns away from infant; ignores infant's presence
Hovers; maintains proximity; directs attention to, points to infant	Avoids infant; does not seek proximity; refuses to hold infant when given opportunity
Identifies infant as unique individual	Identifies infant with someone parent dislikes; fails to recognize any of infant's unique features
Claims infant as family member; names infant	Fails to place infant in family context or identify infant with family member; has difficulty naming
Touches; progresses from fingertip to fingers to palms to encompassing contact	Fails to move from fingertip touch to palmar contact and holding
Smiles at infant	Maintains bland countenance or frowns at infant
Talks to, coos, or sings to infant	Wakes infant when infant is sleeping; handles roughly; hurries feeding by moving nipple continuously
Expresses pride in infant	Expresses disappointment, displeasure in infant
Relates infant's behavior to familiar events	Does not incorporate infant into life
Assigns meaning to infant's actions and sensitively interprets infant's needs	Makes no effort to interpret infant's actions or needs
Views infant's behaviors and appearance in positive light	Views infant's behavior as exploiting, deliberately uncooperative; views appearance as distasteful, ugly

Data from Mercer, R. (1983). Parent-infant attachment. In L. Sonstegard, K. Kowalski, & B. Jennings. (Eds.), *Women's health* (vol. 2). New York, NY: Grune & Stratton.

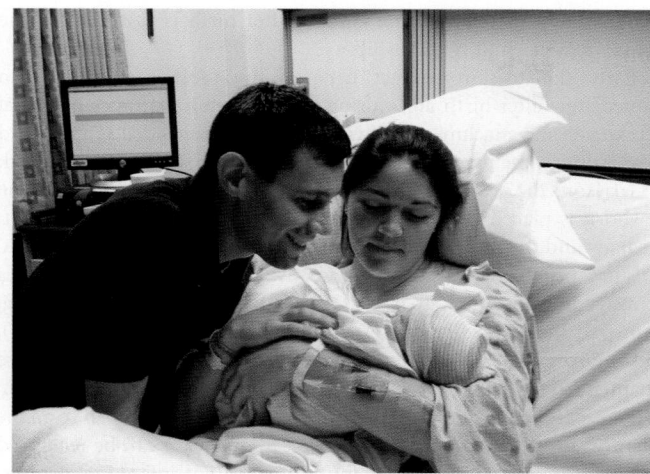

FIG 20.3 Early acquaintance between parents and infant. (Courtesy of Kathryn Alden, Chapel Hill, NC.)

follow, assessment of parent-infant attachment relies more on skillful observation and interviewing. Rooming-in of mother and infant and liberal visiting privileges for father or partner, siblings, and grandparents provide nurses with excellent opportunities to observe interactions and identify behaviors that demonstrate positive or negative attachment. Attachment behaviors can be easily observed during infant feeding sessions. Box 20.1 presents guidelines for assessment of attachment behaviors.

During pregnancy and often even before conception, parents develop an image of the "ideal" or "fantasy" infant. At birth, the fantasy infant becomes the real infant. How closely the dream child resembles the real child influences the bonding process. Assessing such expectations during pregnancy and at the time of the infant's birth allows identification of discrepancies in the parents' view of the fantasy child and the real child.

The labor process significantly affects the immediate attachment of mothers to their newborn infants. Factors such as a long labor, feeling tired or "drugged" after birth, problems with breastfeeding (Tharner, Luijk, Raat, et al., 2012), premature birth, and being separated from the infant at birth (Flacking, Lehtonen, Thomson, et al., 2012; Hoffenkamp, Tooten, Hall, et al., 2012) can delay the development of initial positive feelings toward the newborn. Referral to groups such as La Leche League International (www.llli.org) or Postpartum Support International (www.postpartum.net) can be useful in helping parents develop positive feelings toward their newborn.

TABLE 20.3	**Examples of Parent-Infant Attachment Interventions**
Intervention Label and Definition	**Activities**
Attachment Promotion Facilitation of the development of an affective, enduring relationship between infant and parent	Discuss with parent(s) culture-based expressions of attachment prior to and after birth. Place newborn skin-to-skin with parent immediately after birth. Provide opportunity for parents to see, hold, and examine newborn immediately after birth (i.e., delay unnecessary procedures and provide privacy). Discuss infant behavioral characteristics with parents. Assist parents of multiples in recognizing individuality of each infant. Instruct parents on attachment development, emphasizing its complexity, ongoing nature, and opportunities.
Family Integrity Promotion: Childbearing Family Facilitation of the growth of individuals or families who are adding an infant to family unit	Respect and support family's cultural value system. Assist family in developing adaptive coping mechanisms to deal with the transition to parenthood. Prepare parent(s) for expected role changes involved in becoming a parent. Prepare parent(s) for responsibilities of parenthood. Reinforce positive parenting behaviors. Identify effect of newborn on family dynamics and equilibrium.
Parent Education: Infant Instruction on nurturing and physical care needed during the first year of life	Determine parent(s)' knowledge and readiness and ability to learn about infant care. Provide anticipatory guidance about developmental changes during first year of life. Teach parent(s) skills to care for newborn. Demonstrate ways in which parent(s) can stimulate infant's development. Discuss infant's capabilities for interaction. Demonstrate quieting techniques.
Risk Identification: Childbearing Family Identification of individual or family likely to experience difficulties in parenting, and prioritization of strategies to prevent parenting problems	Ascertain understanding of English or other language used in communication. Determine developmental stage of parents. Review prenatal history for factors that predispose patient to complications. Monitor parent-infant interactions, noting behaviors thought to indicate attachment. Plan for risk-reduction activities, in collaboration with the individual or family. Refer to the appropriate community agency for follow-up if risk for parent problems or a lag in attachment has been identified.

Data from Bulechek, G., Butcher, H., Dochterman, J., et al. (2013). *Nursing interventions classification* (NIC) (6th ed.). St. Louis, MO: Mosby.

BOX 20.1   Assessing Attachment Behaviors

- When the infant is brought to the parents, do they reach out for the infant and call the infant by name? (Recognize that in some cultures parents may not name the infant in the early newborn period.)
- Do the parents speak about the infant in terms of identification—whom the infant resembles, and what appears special about their infant over other infants?
- When parents are holding the infant, what kind of body contact is seen? Do parents feel at ease in changing the infant's position, are fingertips or whole hands used, and does the infant have parts of the body they avoid touching or parts of the body they investigate and scrutinize?
- When the infant is awake, what kinds of stimulation do the parents provide? Do they talk to the infant, to each other, or to no one, and how do they look at the infant—direct visual contact, avoidance of eye contact, or looking at other people or objects?
- How comfortable do the parents appear in terms of caring for the infant? Do they express any concern regarding their ability or disgust for certain activities, such as changing diapers?
- What type of affection do they demonstrate to the newborn, such as smiling, stroking, kissing, or rocking?
- If the infant is fussy, what kinds of comforting techniques do the parents use, such as rocking, swaddling, talking, or stroking?

PARENT-INFANT CONTACT

EARLY CONTACT

Early close contact may facilitate the attachment process between parent and child. Although a delay in contact does not necessarily mean that attachment will be inhibited, additional psychologic energy may be necessary to achieve the same effect. To date, no scientific evidence has demonstrated that immediate contact after birth is essential for the human parent-child relationship.

Early skin-to-skin contact between the mother and newborn immediately after birth and during the first hour facilitates maternal affectionate and attachment behaviors and is recommended as a standard of care due to the many benefits and lack of adverse effects (Kilpatrick & Garrison, 2017; King & Pinger, 2014; Stewart & Rodgers, 2017). The newborn is placed in the prone position on the mother's bare chest; the baby and the mother's chest are covered with a warm, dry blanket. This practice promotes early and effective breastfeeding and increases breastfeeding duration. It is also associated with less infant crying, improved thermoregulation (especially in low–birth weight infants), and improved cardiorespiratory stability in late preterm infants (see Chapter 16) (Kilpatrick & Garrison, 2017; Stewart & Rodgers, 2017).

Parents who cannot have early contact with their newborn (e.g., the infant was transferred to the intensive care nursery) can be reassured that such contact is not essential for optimal parent-infant interactions. Otherwise, adopted infants would not form affectionate ties with their parents. Nurses need to stress that the parent-infant relationship is a process that develops over time.

EXTENDED CONTACT

Rooming-in is common in family-centered care. With this practice, the infant stays in the room with the mother. In some facilities, the newborn never leaves the mother's presence; nurses perform the initial and ongoing assessments and care in the room with the parents. In other hospitals, the infant is transferred to the postpartum or mother-baby unit from the transitional nursery (if the facility uses one) after showing satisfactory extrauterine adjustment. Nurses encourage the father or partner to participate in caring for the infant in as active a role as desired. They can also encourage siblings and grandparents to visit and become acquainted with the infant. Whether the method of family-centered care is rooming-in, mother-baby or couplet care, or a family birth unit, mothers, their partners, and family members are equal and integral parts of the developing family.

Extended contact with the infant should be available for all parents but especially for those at risk for parenting inadequacies, such as adolescents and low-income women. Postpartum nurses need to consider and encourage activities that optimize family-centered care (Welch, Hofer, Brunelli, et al., 2012). Baby-friendly status for a hospital is one means to promote family-centered care (Perrine, Scanlon, Li, et al., 2012). Baby-friendly hospitals originated through the Baby-Friendly Hospital Initiative (BFHI), which encouraged hospitals to create space that is conducive to new mothers to bond with their babies and to be supportive of breastfeeding.

COMMUNICATION BETWEEN PARENT AND INFANT

The parent-infant relationship is strengthened through the use of sensual responses and abilities by both partners in the interaction. The nurse should keep in mind that cultural variations are often seen in these interactive behaviors.

THE SENSES

Touch

Touch, or the tactile sense, is used extensively by parents as a means of becoming acquainted with the newborn. Many mothers reach out for their infants as soon as they are born and the cord is cut. Mothers lift their infants to their breasts, enfold them in their arms, and cradle

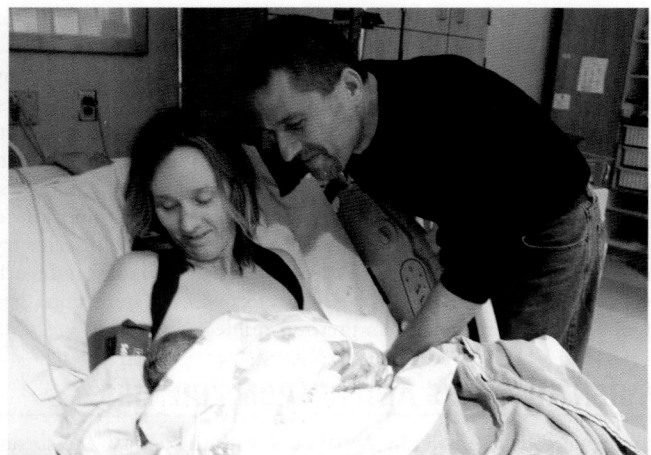

FIG 20.4 Breastfeeding in first hour after birth. (Courtesy of Julie and Darren Nelson, Loveland, CO.)

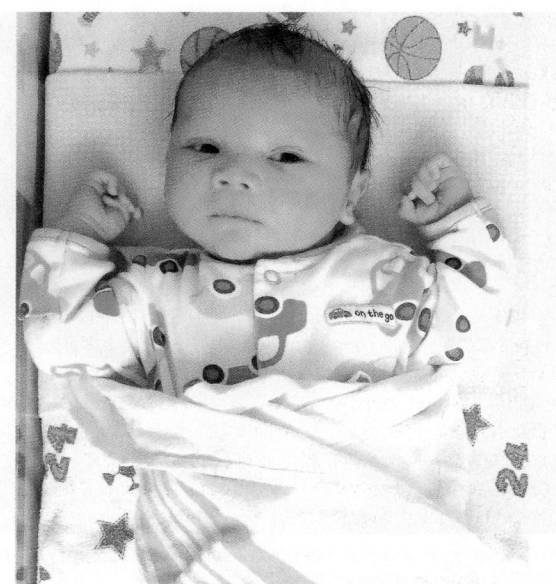

FIG 20.5 Infant in alert state. (Courtesy of Cheryl Briggs, RNC, Annapolis, MD.)

them. Once the infant is close, the mother begins the exploration process with her fingertips, one of the most touch-sensitive areas of the body. Within a short time, she uses her palm to caress the baby's trunk and eventually enfolds the infant. Gentle stroking motions are used to soothe and quiet the infant; patting or gently rubbing the infant's back is a comfort after feedings. Infants also pat the mother's breast as they nurse. Both seem to enjoy sharing each other's body warmth. Parents seem to have an innate desire to touch, pick up, and hold the infant (Fig. 20.4). They comment on the softness of the baby's skin and note details of the baby's appearance. As parents become increasingly sensitive to the infant's like or dislike of different types of touch, they draw closer to the baby.

Touching behaviors of mothers vary in different cultural groups. For example, minimal touching and cuddling is a traditional Southeast Asian practice thought to protect the infant from evil spirits. Because of tradition and spiritual beliefs, women in India and Bali have practiced infant massage since ancient times. Field (2017) described the benefits of the worldwide practice of infant massage, such as mitigating painful procedures like heel sticks.

Eye Contact

Parents repeatedly demonstrate interest in having eye contact with the baby. Some mothers remark that once their babies have looked at them, they feel much closer to them. Parents spend much time getting their babies to open their eyes and look at them. In North American culture, eye contact appears to reinforce the development of a trusting relationship and is an important factor in human relationships at all ages. In other cultures, eye contact is perceived differently. For example, in Mexican culture, sustained direct eye contact is considered to be rude, immodest, and dangerous for some. This danger may arise from the *mal de ojo* (evil eye), resulting from excessive admiration. Women and children are thought to be more susceptible to the *mal de ojo* than men (D'Avanzo, 2008).

As newborns become functionally able to sustain eye contact with their parents, they spend time in mutual gazing, often in the **en face** position. In this position, the parent's face and the infant's face are approximately 8 inches apart and on the same plane (see Fig. 20.2). Nurses and nurse-midwives/physicians can facilitate eye contact immediately after birth by positioning the infant on the mother's abdomen or breasts with the mother's and the infant's faces on the same plane. Dimming the lights encourages the infant's eyes to open.

To promote eye contact, instillation of prophylactic antibiotic ointment into the infant's eyes can be delayed until the infant and parents have had some time together in the first hour after birth.

Voice

The shared response of parents and infants to each other's voices is remarkable. Parents wait tensely for the first cry. Once that cry has reassured them of the baby's health, they begin comforting behaviors. As the parents speak, the infant is alerted and turns toward them. Infants respond to higher-pitched voices and can distinguish the mother's voice from others soon after birth.

Odor

Another behavior shared by parents and infants is a response to each other's odor. Mothers comment on the smell of their babies when first born and have noted that each infant has a unique odor. Infants learn rapidly to distinguish the odor of their mother's breast milk.

ENTRAINMENT

Newborns move in time with the structure of adult speech, which is termed **entrainment**. They wave their arms, lift their heads, and kick their legs, seemingly "dancing in tune" to a parent's voice. Culturally determined rhythms of speech are ingrained in the infant long before he or she uses spoken language to communicate. This shared rhythm also gives the parent positive feedback and establishes a positive setting for effective communication.

BIORHYTHMICITY

The fetus is in tune with the mother's natural rhythms, referred to as *biorhythmicity,* such as her heartbeat. After birth, the mother's heartbeat or a recording of a heartbeat can sooth a crying infant. One task of a newborn is to establish a personal biorhythm. Parents can help in this process by giving consistent loving care and by using their infant's alert state to develop responsive behavior and increase social interactions and opportunities for learning (Fig. 20.5). The more quickly parents become competent in child care activities, the more quickly they can

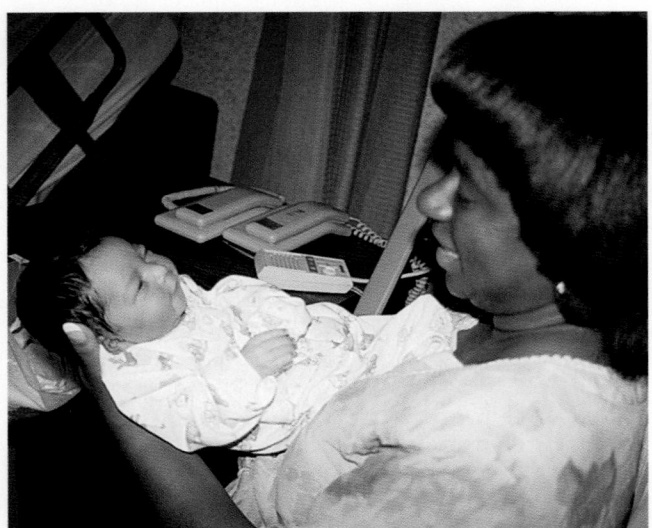

FIG 20.6 Sharing a smile; an example of synchrony. (Courtesy of Marjorie Pyle, RNC, Lifecircle, Costa Mesa, CA.)

direct their psychologic energy toward observing the communication cues the infant gives them.

RECIPROCITY AND SYNCHRONY

Reciprocity is a type of body movement or behavior that provides the observer with cues. The observer or receiver interprets those cues and responds to them. Reciprocity often takes several weeks to develop with a new baby. For example, when the newborn fusses and cries, the mother responds by picking up and cradling the infant; the baby becomes quiet and alert and establishes eye contact; the mother verbalizes, sings, and coos while the baby maintains eye contact. The baby then averts the eyes and yawns; the mother decreases her active response. If the parent continues to stimulate the infant, the baby may again become fussy.

Synchrony refers to the "fit" between the infant's cues and the parent's response. When parent and infant have a synchronous interaction, it is mutually rewarding (Fig. 20.6). Parents need time to learn to interpret the infant's cues correctly. For example, the infant develops a specific cry in response to different situations such as boredom, loneliness, hunger, and discomfort. The parent may need assistance in interpreting these cries, along with trial-and-error interventions, before synchrony develops.

PARENTAL ROLE AFTER BIRTH

Adaptation involves a stabilizing of tasks and a coming to terms with commitments. Parents demonstrate growing competence in child care activities and become increasingly attuned to their infant's behavior. Typically, the period from the decision to conceive through the first months of having a child is termed the transition to parenthood.

TRANSITION TO PARENTHOOD

Historically, the transition to parenthood was viewed as a crisis. The current perspective is that parenthood is a developmental transition rather than a major life crisis. The transition to parenthood is described as a time of disorder and disequilibrium, as well as satisfaction, for mothers and their partners. Usual methods of coping often seem ineffective during this time. Some parents are so distressed that they cannot support each other. Because men typically identify their spouses as their primary or only source of support, the transition can be harder for the fathers. They often feel deprived when the mothers, who are also experiencing stress, cannot provide their usual level of support. Many parents are unprepared for the strong emotions such as the helplessness, inadequacy, and anger that arise when dealing with a crying infant. However, parenthood allows adults to develop and display a selfless, warm, and caring side that may not be expressed in other adult roles.

For the majority of mothers and their partners, the transition to parenthood is an opportunity rather than a time of danger. Parents try new coping strategies as they work to master their new roles and reach new developmental levels. As they work through the transition, they often find personal strength and resourcefulness.

PARENTAL TASKS AND RESPONSIBILITIES

Parents need to reconcile the actual child with the fantasy and dream child. This process means coming to terms with the infant's physical appearance, sex, innate temperament, and physical status. If the real child differs greatly from the fantasy child, parents may delay acceptance of the child. In some instances, they never accept the child.

Many parents know the sex of the infant before birth because of the results of prenatal testing (e.g. ultrasonography, amniocentesis). For those who do not have this information, disappointment over the sex of the infant can take time to resolve. The parents can provide adequate physical care but find it difficult to be sincerely involved with the infant until this internal conflict has been resolved. As one mother remarked, "I really wanted a boy. I know it is silly and irrational, but when they said, 'She's a lovely little girl,' I was so disappointed and angry—yes, angry—I could hardly look at her. Oh, I looked after her okay, her feedings and baths and things, but I couldn't feel excited. To tell the truth, I felt like a monster not liking my child. Then one day she was lying there and she turned her head and looked right at me. I felt a flooding of love for her come over me, and we looked at each other a long time. It's okay now. I wouldn't trade her for all the boys in the world."

The normal appearance of the neonate—size, color, molding of the head, or bowed appearance of the legs—is startling for some parents. Nurses can encourage parents to examine their babies and to ask questions about newborn characteristics.

Parents need to become adept in the care of the infant, including caregiving activities, noting the communication cues the infant gives to indicate needs and responding appropriately to those needs. Self-esteem grows with competence. Breastfeeding helps mothers feel they are contributing in a unique way to the welfare of the infant. The parent may interpret the infant's response to his or her parental care and attention as a comment on the quality of that care. Infant behaviors that parents interpret as positive responses to their care include being consoled easily, enjoying being cuddled, and making eye contact. Spitting up frequently after feedings, crying, and being unpredictable may be perceived as negative responses to parental care. Continuation of these infant responses that parents view as negative can result in alienation of parent and infant.

Some people view assistance, including advice by husbands, partners, wives, mothers, mothers-in-law, and health care professionals, as supportive. Others view advice as criticism or an indication of how inept these others judge the new parents to be. Criticism, real or imagined, of the new parents' ability to provide adequate physical care, nutrition, or social stimulation for the infant can be devastating. By providing encouragement and praise for parenting efforts, nurses can bolster the new parents' confidence.

Parents must establish a place for the newborn within the family group. Whether the infant is the firstborn or the last born, all family members must adjust their roles to accommodate the newcomer.

BECOMING A MOTHER

Rubin (1961) identified three phases of maternal role attainment in which the mother adjusts to her parental role. Mercer (2004) suggested that the concept of maternal role attainment be replaced with becoming a mother to signify the transformation and growth of the mother's identity. Becoming a mother implies more than attaining a role. It includes learning new skills and increasing her confidence in herself as she meets new challenges in caring for her child or children.

The transition to motherhood requires adjustment for the mother and her family. Not all mothers experience the transition to motherhood in the same way. For some women, becoming a mother entails multiple losses. For example, for some single women, there may be a loss of the family of origin when the family does not accept her decision to have the child. There may be loss of a relationship with the father of the baby, with friends, and with their own sense of self. Some women describe a loss of dreams including loss of job, financial security, and a future profession.

Reality-based perinatal education programs help to prepare mothers and decrease their anxiety. Live classes allow time for questions to be answered and for mothers to lend support to one another. Mothers need to know during the first months of parenthood it is common to feel overwhelmed and insecure and to experience physical and mental fatigue. They need to be assured that this situation is temporary and that 3 to 6 months may be needed to become comfortable in caregiving and in being a mother. Maternal support by health care professionals should not end with hospital discharge but, instead, extend over the next 4 to 6 months; long-term interventions tend to be more successful than one-time encounters. Nurses can advocate for the extension of such support services well into the postpartum period. Nurses can also advocate the use of doulas, who are laypersons who provide ongoing support to pregnant and postpartum women.

During pregnancy and after birth, nurses can discuss the usual postpartum concerns that mothers experience. They can provide anticipatory guidance on coping strategies, such as resting when the infant sleeps and planning with an extended family member or friend to do the housework for the first week or two after the baby is born. Once a mother is home, periodic telephone calls from a nurse who cared for her in the birth setting can provide the mother with an opportunity to vent her concerns and get support and advice from "her" nurse. Nurses should plan additional supportive counseling for first-time mothers inexperienced in child care; women whose careers had provided outside stimulation; women who lack friends or family members with whom to share delights and concerns; and adolescent mothers. When possible, postpartum home visits are included in the plan of care.

In summary, nurses have the unique opportunity to experience the miracle of a birth and provide valuable patient and family education and emotional support that will help during and after this exciting and overwhelming time of transition to parenthood (Husmillo, 2013).

Postpartum Blues

The "pink" period surrounding the first day or two after birth, characterized by heightened joy and feelings of well-being, is often followed by a "blue" period. Many women of all ethnic and racial groups experience the postpartum blues or "baby blues." During the blues, women are emotionally labile and often cry easily for no apparent reason. This lability seems to peak around the fifth day and subside by the tenth day. Other symptoms of postpartum blues include a let-down feeling, restlessness, fatigue, insomnia, headache, anxiety, sadness, and anger. Biochemical, psychologic, social, and cultural factors have been explored as possible causes of the postpartum depressive state; however, the etiology remains unknown.

BOX 20.2 Coping With Postpartum Blues

- Remember that the "blues" are normal and that both the mother and the father or partner may experience them.
- Get plenty of rest; nap when the baby does if possible. Go to bed early, and let friends and family know when to visit and how they can help. (Remember, you are not "Supermom.")
- Use relaxation techniques learned in childbirth classes (or ask the nurse to teach you and your partner some techniques).
- Do something for yourself. Take advantage of the time your partner or family members care for the baby. Soak in the tub (a 20-minute soak can be the equivalent of a 2-hour nap), or go for a walk.
- Plan a day out of the house. Go to the mall with the baby, being sure to take a stroller or carriage, or go out to eat with friends without the baby. Many communities have churches or other agencies that provide child care programs such as Mothers' Morning Out.
- Talk to your partner about the way you feel—for example, about feeling tied down, how the birth met your expectations, and things that will help you (do not be afraid to ask for specifics).
- If you are breastfeeding, give yourself and your baby time to learn.
- Seek out and use community resources such as La Leche League or community mental health centers. One nationally recognized resource is:
Postpartum Support International
927 North Kellogg Avenue
Santa Barbara, CA 93111
(805) 967-7636
www.postpartum.net

Whatever the cause, the early postpartum period appears to be one of emotional and physical vulnerability for new mothers, who are often psychologically overwhelmed by the reality of parental responsibilities. Mothers feel deprived of the supportive care they received from family members and friends during pregnancy. Some mothers regret the loss of the mother–unborn child relationship and mourn its passing. Still others experience a let-down feeling when labor and birth are complete. The majority of women experience fatigue after childbirth, which is compounded by the around-the-clock demands of the new baby. Postpartum fatigue increases the risk for postpartum depressive symptoms and can have a negative effect on maternal role attainment. During the postpartum period, it is common for women to experience disrupted sleep. While breastfeeding mothers may be awake more frequently during the night to breastfeed compared with mothers who formula-feed, there is evidence to suggest that breastfeeding, which enhances maternal role attainment, can also help improve maternal sleep (Shaver, 2015). To help mothers cope with postpartum blues, nurses can suggest various strategies (Box 20.2).

Although the postpartum blues are usually mild and short-lived, approximately 8% to 20% of women experience a more severe syndrome called *postpartum depression (PPD)* (Isley & Katz, 2017) (see Chapter 21). It is likely, however, that the actual occurrence of PPD is greater than the reported numbers because it is often unrecognized and undiagnosed (American College of Obstetricians and Gynecologists [ACOG], 2015). Symptoms of PPD can range from mild to severe, with women having good days and bad days. Fathers can also experience PPD. Screening for PPD should be performed with both mothers and fathers. PPD can go undetected because new parents generally do not voluntarily admit to this kind of emotional distress out of embarrassment, guilt, or fear. Nurses need to include teaching about how to differentiate symptoms of the "blues" and PPD and urge parents to report depressive symptoms promptly if they occur.

BECOMING A FATHER

The realities of the first few weeks at home with a newborn cause fathers to change their expectations, set new priorities, and redefine their role. First-time fathers perceive the first 4 to 10 weeks of parenthood in much the same way that mothers do. It is a period characterized by uncertainty, increased responsibility, disruption of sleep, and inability to control time needed to care for the infant and reestablish the relationship with their partner (Yu, Hung, Chan, et al., 2012). Fathers express concerns about decreased attention from their partners relative to their personal relationship, the mother's lack of recognition of the father's desire to participate in decision making for the infant, and limited time available to establish a relationship with the infant (de Montigny, Lacharité, & Devault, 2012). These concerns can precipitate feelings of jealousy of the infant. The father should discuss his individual concerns and needs with the mother and become more involved with the infant. This can help alleviate feelings of jealousy.

Father-Infant Relationship

In North American culture, neonates have a powerful effect on their fathers who become intensely involved with them. The term used for the father's absorption, preoccupation, and interest in the infant is engrossment. Characteristics of engrossment include some of the sensual responses relating to touch and eye-to-eye contact that were discussed earlier and the father's keen awareness of features both unique and similar to himself that validate his claim to the infant. An outstanding response is one of strong attraction to the newborn. This relationship between a father and his newborn is beneficial to both (Ramchandani, Domoney, Sethna, et al., 2013). Fathers spend considerable time "communicating" with the infant and taking delight in the infant's response to them (Fig. 20.7). Fathers experience increased self-esteem and a sense of being proud, bigger, more mature, and older after seeing their baby for the first time.

Fathers spend less time than mothers with infants, and their interactions with infants tend to be characterized by stimulating social play rather than caregiving. The variations in infant stimulation from both parents provide a wider social experience for the infant.

Fathers receive less interpersonal and professional support compared with mothers and can feel excluded from antenatal appointments and antenatal classes (Steen, Downe, Bamford, et al., 2012). They need information and encouragement during pregnancy and in the postnatal

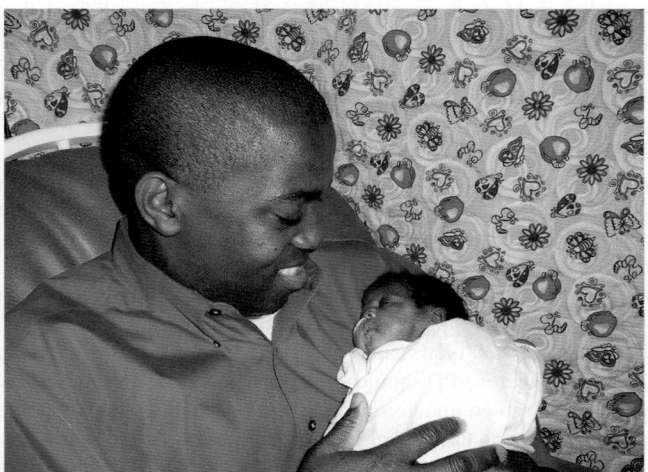

FIG 20.7 Father interacts with his newborn son. (Courtesy of Cheryl Briggs, RNC, Annapolis, MD.)

period related to infant care, parenting, and relationship changes. During the postpartum hospital stay, nurses can arrange to teach infant care when the father is present and provide anticipatory guidance for fathers about the transition to parenthood. Separate prenatal and parenting classes and parenting support groups for fathers can provide them with an opportunity to discuss their concerns and have some of their needs met. To prepare fathers for the transition to parenthood, perinatal education should include information on role changes associated with parenting, the importance of parenting "teamwork," the increased risk for mental distress and depression, the mother's experience and how to provide support, how to interpret and respond to infant behaviors, and how to deal with infant crying (May & Fletcher, 2013). Postpartum telephone calls and home visits by the nurse should include time for assessment of the father's adjustment and needs.

ADJUSTMENT FOR THE COUPLE

The transition to parenthood brings about changes in the relationship between the mother and her partner. A strong, healthy marriage or couple relationship is the best foundation for parenthood, although even the best relationships are often shaken with the addition of a baby. During the first few weeks after birth, parents experience a plethora of emotions. Even though they may feel an overwhelming love and a sense of amazement toward their newborn, they also feel a great responsibility. Even if the mother and her partner have been to prenatal classes, read books, or sought advice from family or friends, they are usually surprised by the realities of life with a new baby and the changes in their relationship. Because men and women experience pregnancy and birth differently, the expectation is that they will also vary in their adjustment to parenthood.

Common issues that couples face as they become parents include changes in their relationship with one another, division of household and infant care responsibilities, financial concerns, balancing work and parental responsibilities, and social activities. To assist new parents in their transition, nurses can encourage them during pregnancy and in the postpartum period to share personal expectations with each other and to assess their relationship periodically. Couples need to schedule time into their busy lives for one-on-one conversation and try to have regular "dates" or time apart from the infant. The mother and her partner need to express appreciation for one another as well as for their baby. Support from family, friends, and community health professionals should be identified early and used as needed during pregnancy and in the postpartum period and beyond. The couple who is willing to experiment with new approaches to their lifestyle and habits can find the transition to parenthood less difficult.

RESUMING SEXUAL INTIMACY

Nurses can provide opportunities for parents to discuss concerns and ask questions about resuming sexual intimacy. The couple may begin to engage in sexual intercourse during the second to fourth week after the baby is born. Some couples begin earlier, as soon as it can be accomplished without discomfort, depending on factors such as timing and vaginal dryness. Sexual intimacy enhances the adult aspect of the family, and the adult pair shares a closeness denied to other family members. Changes in a woman's sexual desire after birth are related to hormonal shifts, increased breast size, uneasiness with a body that has yet to return to a prepregnant size, chronic fatigue related to sleep deprivation, and physical exhaustion. Partners can feel alienated when they observe the intimate mother-infant relationship, and some are frank in expressing feelings of jealousy toward the infant. The resumption of sexual intimacy seems to bring the parents' relationship back into focus. Before and after birth, nurses should review with new parents their plans for other pregnancies and their preferences for contraception (see Chapter 21).

INFANT-PARENT ADJUSTMENT

Newborns participate actively in shaping their parents' reaction to them. Behavioral characteristics of the infant influence parenting behaviors. The infant and the parent each have unique rhythms, behaviors, and response styles that are brought to every interaction. Infant-parent interactions can be facilitated in at least three ways: (1) modulation of rhythm, (2) modification of behavioral repertoires, and (3) mutual responsivity. Nurses can teach parents about these three aspects of infant-parent interaction through discussions, written materials, and video recordings demonstrating infant capabilities. A creative approach is to record the parent-infant pair during an interaction and then use the individualized recording to discuss the pair's rhythm, behavioral repertoire, and responsivity.

Rhythm

To modulate rhythm, both parent and infant must be able to interact. Therefore the infant must be in the quiet alert state, one of the most difficult of the sleep-wake states to maintain. The alert state (Fig. 20.8) occurs most often during a feeding or in face-to-face play. The parent must work hard to help the infant maintain the alert state long enough and often enough for interactions to take place. The en face position is usually assumed (see Fig. 20.8, *D*). Multiparous mothers in particular are very sensitive and responsive to the infant's feeding rhythms. Mothers learn to reserve stimulation for pauses in sucking activity and not to talk or smile excessively while the infant is sucking because the infant will stop feeding to interact with her. With maturity, the infant can sustain longer interactions by modulating activity rhythms (i.e., limb movement, sucking, gaze alternation, and habituation). Meanwhile, the parent becomes more attuned to the infant's rhythms and learns to modulate the rhythms, facilitating a rhythmic turn-taking interaction.

Behavioral Repertoires

Both the infant and the parent have a repertoire of behaviors they can use to facilitate interactions. Fathers and mothers engage in these behaviors depending on the extent of contact and caregiving of the infant. Nurses can teach parents to recognize, interpret, and respond to infant behaviors. An innovative program called HUG Your Baby (Help, Understanding and Guidance for Young Families: www.hugyourbaby.org) is designed to prepare health care professionals to teach parents how to understand their newborns and prevent problems related to crying, sleeping, eating, attachment, and bonding (See Chapter 23: Patient Teaching Box: Helping Parents Recognize, Interpret, and Respond to Newborn Behaviors).

The infant's behavioral repertoire includes gazing, vocalizing, and facial expressions. The infant is able to focus and follow the human face from birth and is able to alternate the gaze voluntarily, looking away from the parent's face when understimulated or overstimulated (see Fig. 20.8, *F*). Parents need to learn to be sensitive to the infant's capacity for attention and inattention and to recognize states and signs of overstimulation. Developing this sensitivity is especially important when interacting with preterm infants.

Body gestures form a part of the infant's early "language." Babies greet parents with waving hands (see Fig. 20.8, *E*) or a reaching out of hands. They can raise an eyebrow or soften their expression to elicit loving attention. Game playing can stimulate them to smile or laugh. Pouting or crying, arching of the back, and general squirming usually signal the end of an interaction.

The parents' repertoire includes various types of interactive behaviors such as constantly looking at the infant and noting the infant's response. New parents often remark that they are exhausted from looking at the baby and smiling. Adults also "infantilize" their speech to help the infant "listen." They do this by slowing the tempo, speaking loudly and rhythmically, and emphasizing key words. Phrases are repeated frequently. Infantilizing does not mean using "baby talk," which involves distortion of sounds.

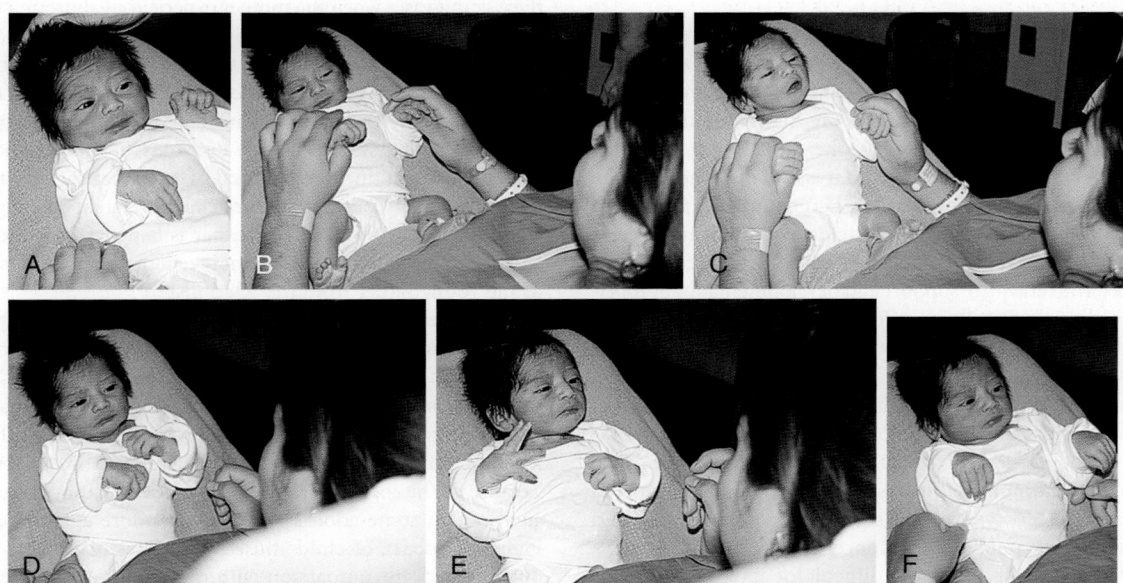

FIG 20.8 Holding newborn in the en face position, mother works to alert her daughter, 6 hours old. **A,** Infant is quiet and alert. **B,** Mother begins talking to daughter. **C,** Infant responds, opens mouth like her mother. **D,** Infant gazes at her mother. **E,** Infant waves hand. **F,** Infant glances away, resting. Hand relaxes. (Courtesy of Marjorie Pyle, RNC, Lifecircle, Costa Mesa, CA.)

To communicate emotions to the infant, parents often use facial expressions such as slow and exaggerated looks of surprise, happiness, and confusion. Games such as "peek-a-boo" and imitation of the infant's behaviors are other means of interaction. For example, if the baby smiles, so does the parent; if the baby frowns, the parent responds in kind.

Responsivity

Contingent responses (responsivity) are those that occur within a specific time and are similar in form to a stimulus behavior. The adult has the feeling of having an influence on the interaction. Infant behaviors such as smiling, cooing, and sustained eye contact, usually in the en face position, are viewed as contingent responses. The infant's responses act as rewards to the initiator and encourage the adult to continue with the game when the infant responds positively. When the adult imitates the infant, the infant appears to enjoy it. A progression occurs in the types of behaviors that parents present for the baby to imitate; for example, in early interactions, the parent will grimace rather than laugh, which is in keeping with the infant's developmental level. Such "turn-about" behaviors sustain interactions and promote harmony in the relationship.

DIVERSITY IN TRANSITIONS TO PARENTHOOD

Various factors, including age, social networks, socioeconomic conditions, and personal aspirations for the future, influence how parents respond to the birth of a child. Cultural beliefs and practices also affect parenting behaviors. Factors that influence the risk for parenting problems include age (adolescent or older than 35 years of age), same-sex parenting, social support, culture, socioeconomic conditions, and personal aspirations.

AGE

Maternal age has a definite effect on the outcome of pregnancy. The mother, fetus, and newborn are at highest risk when the mother is an adolescent or older than 35 years of age (see Clinical Reasoning Case Study: Postpartum Adjustment for the Adolescent and the Older Mother).

The Adolescent Mother

Although becoming a parent is biologically possible for the adolescent female, her egocentricity and concrete thinking can interfere with her ability to parent effectively. Mortality rates are higher among infants of adolescent mothers. This can be related to inherent problems associated with preterm birth or other conditions, but it is also influenced by the mother's inexperience, lack of knowledge, and immaturity. In the United States, adolescent mothers are often poorer, less educated, and receive less prenatal care than older mothers (Geoghegan, 2013). Nevertheless, in most instances, with adequate support and developmentally appropriate teaching, adolescents can learn effective parenting skills. Strong social and functional support promote positive outcomes for adolescent mothers.

Contrary to popular beliefs related to the detrimental effects of adolescent pregnancy, research evidence suggests that the life course for adolescent mothers is similar to that of their socioeconomic peers. In some families or communities, adolescent parenthood is considered a normal or positive life event. Even so, adolescent pregnancy and parenting are important public health concerns.

The transition to parenthood can be difficult for adolescent parents. Because many adolescents have their own unmet developmental needs, coping with the developmental tasks of parenthood is often difficult. Some young parents experience difficulty accepting a changing self-image and adjusting to new roles related to the responsibilities of infant care.

CLINICAL REASONING CASE STUDY
Postpartum Adjustment for the Adolescent and the Older Mother

You are a home care nurse and have had two patients referred to you. Carol is a 15-year-old first-time mother of a 5-day-old girl; she lives with her mother. The father of the baby, Robert, is 17 years old and attended childbirth classes with Carol. She is breastfeeding the baby but says that the baby sucks too slowly and takes too much time to eat. She said she thinks the baby should know enough to sleep longer at night. Robert would like to feed the baby some cereal, since he heard that will make a baby sleep longer at night.

Audrey is a 36-year-old attorney who has been practicing law for 7 years. She just gave birth to her first baby; she and her husband delayed parenting by choice until their careers were well established. She had an uneventful pregnancy, labor, and birth. During a telephone call 48 hours after discharge, when she was asked how things were going, Audrey burst into tears and said, "I didn't expect it to be like this! Nothing is going right."

1. Evidence—Is there sufficient evidence to draw conclusions about both Carol's condition and Audrey's condition?
2. Assumptions—What assumptions can be made about the following?
   a. The relationship of maternal age and postpartum adjustment
   b. The need for social support in the postnatal period
   c. The need for perinatal education
   d. Long-term prognosis for positive outcomes
3. What is the nursing priority in these two situations?
4. Does the evidence objectively support your argument (conclusion)?
5. Interprofessional care—Describe roles and responsibilities of other health care professionals who would potentially be involved in the care of both of these patients.

Adolescent mothers are at increased risk for postpartum depression (Jeha, Usta, Ghulmiyya, et al., 2015). This is often associated with a lack of social support and poor relations with their partner. There is an increased risk for child abuse and neglect by adolescent mothers; the risk increases when the mother experienced abuse as a child (Bartlett & Easterbrooks, 2015).

As adolescent parents move through the transition to parenthood, they may feel "different" from their peers, excluded from "fun" activities, and prematurely forced to enter an adult social role. The conflict between their own desires and the infant's demands, in addition to the low tolerance for frustration that is typical of adolescence, further contributes to the normal psychosocial stress of childbirth and parenting. Maintaining a relationship with the baby's father is beneficial for the teen mother and her infant, although adolescent pregnancy often heralds the departure of the young father from the relationship.

Adolescent mothers provide warm and attentive physical care; however, they use less verbal interaction than do older parents, and adolescents tend to be less responsive and to interact less positively with their infants than do older mothers. Interventions emphasizing verbal and nonverbal communication skills between mother and infant are important. Such intervention strategies must be concrete and specific because of the cognitive level of adolescents. Although some observers suggest that some adolescents may use more aggressive behaviors, a higher incidence of child abuse by adolescent mothers has not been documented. In comparison with older mothers, adolescent mothers have a limited knowledge of child development. They tend to expect too much of their infants too soon and often characterize their infants as being fussy. This limited knowledge may cause adolescents to respond to their infants inappropriately.

Many young mothers pattern their maternal role on what they themselves experienced. Therefore, nurses need to determine the type of support that people close to the young mother are able and prepared to give, as well as the kinds of community assistance available to supplement this support. Many adolescent mothers can identify a source of social support, with the predominant source being their own mothers.

Continued assessment of the new mother's parenting abilities during this postbirth period is essential. Continued support should be provided by involving the grandparents and other family members, as well as through home visits and group sessions for discussion of infant care and parenting concerns. Community-based programs for pregnant adolescents and adolescent parents improve access to health care, education, and other support services. Serious problems can be prevented through outreach programs concerned with self-management, parent-child interactions, infant development, child injuries, and failure to thrive. As the adolescent performs her mothering role within the framework of her family, she may need to address dependency versus independency issues. The adolescent's family members also need help adapting to their new roles. Some mothers and fathers of adolescents feel they are too young and unprepared to be grandparents.

The Adolescent Father

The adolescent father and mother face immediate developmental crises, which include completing the developmental tasks of adolescence, making a transition to parenthood, and sometimes adapting to marriage. These transitions are stressful.

The nurse can initiate interaction with the adolescent father if he is present during prenatal visits or if he is with his partner during labor and birth. The nurse can assess the relationship between the two adolescents and encourage them to discuss their plans for the father's involvement with the mother and infant after birth (Fagan, 2013). During the hospital stay, the nurse can include the adolescent father in teaching sessions about infant care and parenting. The nurse can ask him to be present during postpartum home visits and to accompany the mother and the baby to well-baby checkups at the clinic or pediatrician's office. With the adolescent mother's agreement, the nurse may contact the father directly.

Adolescent fathers need support to discuss their emotional responses to the pregnancy, birth, and fatherhood. The nurse needs to be aware of the father's feelings of guilt, powerlessness, or bravado because these feelings may have negative consequences for both the parents and the child. Counseling of adolescent fathers needs to be reality oriented and should include topics such as finances, child care, parenting skills, and the father's role in the parenting experience. Adolescent fathers also need to know about reproductive physiology and contraceptive options, as well as sex practices that lower the risk for pregnancy and sexually transmitted infections.

The adolescent father may or may not continue to be involved in an ongoing relationship with the young mother and his baby. If he does, he can play an important role in the decisions about child care and raising the child. He may need help to develop realistic perceptions of his role as "father to a child" and is encouraged to use coping mechanisms that are not harmful to his own, his partner's, or his child's well-being. The nurse enlists support systems, parents, and professional agencies on his behalf.

Maternal Age Older Than 35 Years

Women older than 35 years of age have always continued their childbearing either by choice or because of a lack of or a failure of contraception during the perimenopausal years. Added to this group are women who have postponed pregnancy because of careers or other reasons, as well as women of infertile couples who finally become pregnant with the aid of technologic advances.

Support from partners aids in the adjustment of older mothers to changes involved in becoming a parent and seeing themselves as competent. Support from other family members and friends is also important for positive self-evaluation of parenting, a sense of well-being and satisfaction, and help in dealing with stress. Women who are older can experience social isolation. Older mothers may have less family and social support than younger mothers. They are less likely to live near family, and their own parents, if still living, may be unable to provide assistance or support because of age or health issues. These mothers are often caught in the "sandwich generation," taking on responsibility for care of aging parents while parenting young children. Social support may be lacking because their peers are busy with their careers and have limited time to help. Their friends are likely to have older children and have less in common with the new mother.

Changes in the sexual aspect of a relationship can create stress for new midlife parents. Mothers report that it is difficult to find time and energy for a romantic rendezvous. They attribute much of this difficulty to the reality of caring for an infant, but the decreasing libido that normally accompanies getting older also contributes.

Work and career issues are sources of conflict for older mothers. Conflicts emerge over being disinterested in work, worrying about giving enough attention to work with the distractions of a new baby, and anticipating what returning to work will entail. Child care is a major factor in causing stress about work.

Another major issue for older mothers with careers is the perception of loss of control. Mothers older than 35 years, when compared with younger mothers, are at a different stage in their careers, having attained high levels of education, career, and income. The loss of control experienced when going from the consistency of a work role to the inconsistency of the parent role comes as a surprise to many older women. Helping the older mother have realistic expectations of herself and of parenthood is essential.

New mothers who are also perimenopausal may have difficulty understanding that fatigue, loss of sleep, decreased libido, or other physiologic symptoms are the causes of the change in their sex drives. Although many women view menopause as a natural stage of life, for midlife mothers, this cessation of menstruation coincides with the state of parenthood. The changes of midlife and menopause can add more emotional and physical stress to older mothers' lives because of the time- and energy-consuming aspects of rearing a young child.

Paternal Age Older Than 35 Years

Although many older fathers describe their experience of midlife parenting as wonderful, they also recognize drawbacks. Positive aspects of parenthood in older years include increased love and commitment between the two parents, a reinforcement of why one married in the first place, a feeling of being complete, experiencing of "the child" in oneself again, more financial stability than in younger years, and more freedom to focus on parenting rather than on career. Drawbacks of midlife parenting include having a young child and not being physically fit to participate in activities, being much older than other fathers, and the change that it makes in the relationship with their partner.

PARENTING IN SAME-SEX COUPLES

The transition to parenting for same-sex couples can present unique challenges. Whether the couple consists of two women or two men, issues such as a lack of family acceptance and support, public ignorance, and social and legal invisibility influence their ability to adapt as new parents. The health care environment is heteronormative; for example, educational materials for new parents include information for mothers and fathers, and photos depict the traditional heterosexual couple.

Attitudes of health care professionals can either positively or negatively affect the care provided to same-sex couples.

Lesbian Couples

The decision for lesbian couples to conceive is intentional. Factors that influence the decision include the age, health, fertility, and career considerations of each partner. In addition, one partner may have a greater desire to experience the pregnancy and birth and to be genetically related to the infant.

Several pathways are available for two women in a same-sex or lesbian relationship who wish to become parents. The couple may decide for one of the women to conceive a child who is genetically related to her; this is usually done through donor insemination. Alternatively, the fertilized egg of one partner can be implanted into the uterus of the other partner, who carries the pregnancy. In some cases, a woman is implanted with the fertilized egg from a donor so the child is not biologically related to either partner. Another option is for a lesbian couple to adopt an infant born to a surrogate mother. They can also choose to adopt an infant through an adoption agency or by private arrangement.

Health care professionals demonstrate a variety of reactions to lesbian couples, ranging from rejection and exclusion to complete acceptance and inclusion. Some couples attempt to hide their relationship because they fear a homophobic response. Judgmental attitudes, confusion, or lack of understanding can affect the quality of care provided to these families (Dahl, Fylkesnes, Sorlie, et al., 2013). Although the traditional roles of the mother and father in heterosexual relationships are well recognized, the role of the lesbian coparent can be questioned, misunderstood, and ignored by society and by health care providers. Intentionally or accidentally, health care providers can exclude partners or fail to acknowledge their roles in pregnancy, birth, and parenting. Integration of the nonchildbearing partner into care includes offering opportunities afforded male partners of heterosexual women, such as cutting the cord and rooming in with the mother and baby during hospitalization.

An option not available to male partners is to actually breastfeed the infant. The nonchildbearing female partner can stimulate milk production through induced lactation using medications and regular pumping. A supplemental feeding device containing expressed breast milk or formula can be used to provide additional milk to the breastfeeding infant. Women who choose not to induce lactation yet desire to have the breastfeeding experience can put the baby to breast using a supplemental feeding device containing formula or expressed breast milk.

Similar to heterosexual parents, lesbian couples face challenges in adjusting to life with a new baby. After birth, the birth mother tends to be the one most responsible for child care because she is likely to be working fewer hours than her partner. Tensions can arise between the partners in relation to their roles. This can be compounded by the lack of a formal, recognized relationship between the coparent and the infant and the issues surrounding her legal rights in relation to her partner and the infant.

Lesbian couples face strong social sanctions regarding pregnancy and parenting. Their families may not have resolved the initial dismay and guilt over learning of their daughters' homosexuality, or they may disagree with the lesbian couple's decision to conceive and be parents. Alternatively, a pregnancy or adoption can transform family relationships and open the door to acceptance by grandparents. In situations in which family support is limited or absent, the nurse can help lesbian couples locate supportive social groups, lesbian or heterosexual.

Gay Couples

Men in same-sex relationships, or gay couples, can become parents by adoption or by impregnating a surrogate by artificial insemination or sexual intercourse. Female-to-male transgender individuals in gay relationships have been known to become pregnant. Same-sex male couples face the same social sanctions regarding pregnancy and parenting that lesbian couples encounter. Both lesbian and gay couples can have children from previous heterosexual relationships.

Nurses are likely to encounter gay couples in the hospital setting if they are present for birth by a surrogate or if they are adopting a newborn and visit the hospital to spend time with the infant and learn about infant care. Nurses can help these men locate support groups that will address their needs. They need to ensure that these families receive effective health care. Data on gay parenting are limited and focus more on developmental outcomes of the children than on parenting styles or parental caregiving. Research is needed to identify the needs of gay parents and ways to support them in their parenting. Research is also needed on transgender parents.

SOCIAL SUPPORT

Social support is strongly related to positive adaptation by new parents, including adolescent parents, during the transition to parenthood. Social support is multidimensional and includes the number of members in a person's social network, types of support, perceived general support, actual support received, and satisfaction with support available and received. Partner support in pregnancy has a positive influence on emotional distress in the postpartum period (Stapleton, Schetter, Westling, et al., 2012). The type and satisfaction of support seem to be more important than the total number of support network members.

Across cultural groups, families and friends of new parents form an important dimension of the parents' social network. Through seeking help within the social network, new mothers learn culturally valued practices and develop role competency.

Social networks provide a support system on which parents can rely for assistance, but they also can be a source of conflict. Sometimes a large network can cause problems because it results in conflicting advice that comes from numerous people. Grandparents or in-laws are most appreciated when they assist with household responsibilities and do not intrude into the parents' privacy or judge them critically.

Because of the extent of restructuring and reorganization that occur in a family with the birth of another child, the mother's moods and fatigue in the postpartum period can be helped more by situation-specific support from family and friends than by general support. General support addresses feeling loved, respected, and valued. Situation-specific support relates to practical concerns such as physical needs and child care. For example, the practical support of a grandparent bathing the infant can help lessen a second-time mother's feelings of loss by providing her time to be with her firstborn child.

CULTURE

Cultural beliefs and practices are important determinants of parenting behaviors. Culture influences the interactions with the baby as well as the parent's or family's caregiving style. For example, the provision for a period of rest and recuperation for the mother after birth is prominent in several cultures. Asian mothers remain at home with the baby up to 30 days after birth and are not supposed to engage in household chores, including care of the baby. Often the grandmother takes over the baby's care immediately, even before discharge from the hospital (D'Avanzo, 2008). Jordanian mothers have a 40-day lying-in after birth, during which their mothers or sisters care for the baby (D'Avanzo). Japanese mothers rest for the first 2 months after childbirth. Hispanics practice an intergenerational family ritual, *la cuarentena*. For 40 days after birth, the mother is expected to recuperate and get acquainted with her infant.

All cultures place importance on desiring and valuing children. In Asian families, children are a source of family strength and stability, are perceived as wealth, and are objects of parental love and affection. Infants are almost always given an affectionate "cradle" name that is used during the first years of life; for example, a Filipino girl might be called "Ling-Ling" and a boy "Bong-Bong."

Knowledge of cultural beliefs can help the nurse make more accurate assessments and diagnoses of observed parenting behaviors. For example, nurses may become concerned when they observe cultural practices that appear to reflect poor maternal-infant bonding. Algerian mothers may not unwrap and explore their infants as part of the acquaintance process because in Algeria, babies are wrapped tightly in swaddling clothes to protect them physically and psychologically (D'Avanzo, 2008). The nurse may observe a Vietnamese woman who gives minimal care to her infant but refuses to cuddle or further interact with her baby. This apparent lack of interest in the newborn is this cultural group's attempt to ward off "evil spirits" and actually reflects an intense love and concern for the infant (Galanti, 2015). An Asian mother might be criticized for almost immediately relinquishing the care of the infant to the grandmother and not even attempting to hold her baby when it is brought to her room. However, in Asian extended families, members show their support for a new mother's rest and recuperation by assisting with the care of the baby. Contrary to the guidance given to mothers in the United States about "nipple confusion," a mix of breastfeeding and bottle-feeding is standard practice for Japanese mothers. This tradition is related to concern for the mother's rest during the first 2 to 3 months and does not usually lead to any problems with lactation; breastfeeding is widespread and successful among Japanese women.

Cultural beliefs and values give perspective to the meaning of childbirth for a new mother and a new father. Nurses can provide an opportunity for new mothers and fathers to talk about their perceptions of the meaning of childbearing. In helping new families adjust to parenthood, nurses must provide culturally competent care by following principles that facilitate nursing practice within transcultural situations.

SOCIOECONOMIC CONDITIONS

Socioeconomic conditions often determine access to available resources. Parents whose economic condition is made worse with the birth of each child and who cannot use an effective method of fertility management may find childbirth complicated by concern for their own health and a sense of helplessness. Mothers who are single, separated or divorced from their husbands, or without a partner, family, and friends can view the birth of a child with dread. Serious financial problems may override any desire for mothering the infant. Similarly, fathers who are overwhelmed with financial stresses may lack effective parenting skills and behaviors.

PERSONAL ASPIRATIONS

For some women, parenthood interferes with or blocks their plans for personal freedom or advancement in their careers. Unresolved resentment can affect caregiving activities and adjustment to parenting. This situation may result in indifference and neglect of the infant or in excessive concerns; the mother may set impossibly high standards for her own behavior or the child's performance.

Nursing intervention includes providing opportunities for mothers to express their feelings freely to an objective listener, to discuss measures to permit personal growth, and to learn about the care of their infant.

Referring the woman to a support group of other mothers who are in similar circumstances may also be helpful.

Nurses can be proactive in influencing changes in work policies related to maternity and paternity leaves, varying models of work sharing, and family-friendly work environments. Some corporations already structure their work sites to support new mothers (e.g., by providing on-site day care facilities and lactation rooms).

PARENTAL SENSORY IMPAIRMENT

In the early interactions between the parent and child, each uses all senses—sight, hearing, touch, taste, and smell—to initiate and sustain the attachment process. A parent who has an impairment of one or more of the senses needs to maximize use of the remaining senses. Mothers with disabilities tend to value the importance of performing parenting tasks in the perceived culturally usual way.

VISUALLY IMPAIRED PARENT

Visual impairment alone does not seem to have a negative effect on parents' early parenting experiences. These parents, just as sighted parents, express the wonders of parenthood and encourage other visually impaired persons to become parents.

Although visually impaired parents initially feel a pressure to conform to traditional, sighted ways of parenting, they soon adapt these ways and develop methods better suited to themselves. Examples of activities that visually impaired parents do differently include preparation of the infant's nursery, clothes, and supplies. Some parents put an entire clothing outfit together and hang it in the closet rather than keeping the items separate in drawers. Some develop a labeling system for the infant's clothing and put diapering, bathing, and other care supplies where these will be easy to locate. A strength that visually impaired parents have is a heightened sensitivity to other sensory outputs. Visually impaired parents can tell when their infant is facing them because they can feel the baby's breath on their face.

One of the major difficulties that visually impaired parents experience is the skepticism, open or hidden, of health care professionals. Visually impaired people sense reluctance on the part of others to acknowledge that they have a right to be parents. Too often, nurses and other health care providers lack the experience to deal with the childbearing and childrearing needs of visually impaired parents, as well as parents with other disabilities (e.g., the hearing impaired, physically impaired, and mentally challenged). The nurse's best approach is to assess the parent's capabilities. From that basis, the nurse can make plans to assist the parent, often in much the same way as for a parent without impairment. Visually impaired mothers have made suggestions for providing care for women such as themselves during childbearing (Box 20.3). Such approaches can help avoid a sense of increased vulnerability on the parent's part. Childbirth education and other materials are available in Braille (www.loc.gov/nls).

Eye contact is important in North American culture. With a parent who is visually impaired, this critical factor in the parent-child attachment process is obviously missing. However, the visually impaired parent, who may never have experienced this method of strengthening relationships, does not miss it. The infant will need other sensory input from that parent. An infant looking into the eyes of a parent who is visually impaired may be unaware that the eyes are unseeing. Other people in the newborn's environment can participate in active eye-to-eye contact to supply this need. A problem may arise, however, if the visually impaired parent has an impassive facial expression. The infant, making repeated unsuccessful attempts to engage in face play with the mother, will abandon the behavior with her and intensify it with the father or other people

BOX 20.3 Nursing Approaches for Working With Visually Impaired Parents

- Parents who are visually impaired need oral teaching by health care providers because pregnancy and childbirth information is usually not accessible to visually impaired people.
- A visually impaired parent needs an orientation to the hospital room that allows the parent to move about the room independently. For example, "Go to the left of the bed and trail the wall until you feel the first door. That is the bathroom."
- Parents who are visually impaired need explanations of routines.
- Parents who are visually impaired need to feel devices (e.g., portable sitz bath equipment, breast pump) and to hear descriptions of the devices.
- Visually impaired parents need a chance to ask questions.
- Visually impaired parents need the opportunity to hold and touch the baby after birth.
- Nurses need to demonstrate baby care by touch and to follow with, "Now show me how you would do it."
- Nurses need to give instructions such as "I'm going to give you the baby. The head is to your left side."

BOX 20.4 Nursing Approaches for Working With Hearing-Impaired Parents

- Before initiating communication, be aware of the parents' preferences and capabilities. Do they wear a hearing aid? Do they read lips? Do they wish to have an interpreter?
- Make certain that the parent(s) sees you approaching to avoid startling the parent.
- Before speaking, be directly in front of the parent and have that person's full attention.
- When speaking, face the parent directly and be at the same level.
- Avoid standing in front of a light or a window while speaking to the parent.
- Keep your hands away from your face while speaking to minimize distractions.
- If the parent relies on lip reading, sit close enough so that the parent can easily see your lip movements.
- Speak clearly with a regular voice volume and lip movements, while maintaining eye contact.
- Speak in short, simple sentences to facilitate understanding.
- If the parent does not understand something, it is better to find a different way to say what needs to be communicated rather than repeating the same words over and over.
- Written messages aid in communication. A small white or black erasable board can be useful.
- Give educational materials to hearing-impaired parents, and ask them to read the materials before doing parent teaching. They can refer to the materials after discharge.
- Use visual aids such as pictures, diagrams, or other devices when doing parent teaching.
- When doing parent teaching, it is helpful for a hearing person (partner or family member) to be present.
- Allow ample time to communicate with the hearing-impaired parent; being in a rush can evoke stress and create barriers to effective communication.

in the household. Nurses can provide anticipatory guidance regarding this situation and help the mother learn to nod and smile while talking and cooing to the infant.

HEARING-IMPAIRED PARENT

A parent who has a hearing impairment faces challenges in caregiving and parenting, particularly if the deafness dates from birth or early childhood. Whether one or both parents are hearing impaired, they are likely to have established an independent household. Devices that transform sound into light flashes can be fitted into the infant's room to permit immediate detection of crying. Even if the parent is not speech trained, vocalizing can serve as both a stimulus and a response to the infant's early vocalizing. Deaf parents can provide additional vocal training by use of recordings and television, so that from birth, the child is aware of the full range of the human voice. Young children acquire sign language readily, and the first sign used is as varied as the first word.

Section 504 of the Rehabilitation Act of 1973 requires that hospitals and other institutions receiving funds from the US Department of Health and Human Services use various communication techniques and resources with the deaf, including having staff members or certified interpreters who are proficient in sign language. Providing written materials with demonstrations and having nurses stand where the parent can read their lips (if the parent practices lipreading) are two techniques that can be used. A creative approach is for the nursing unit to develop videos in which information on postpartum care, infant care, and parenting issues is signed by an interpreter and spoken by a nurse. A video in which a nurse signs while speaking would be ideal. With the advent of the Internet, many resources are available to the deaf parent. Box 20.4 lists suggestions for working with hearing-impaired parents.

SIBLING ADAPTATION

Because the family is an interactive, open unit, the addition of a new family member affects everyone in the family. Siblings have to assume new positions within the family hierarchy. Parents often face the task of caring for a new child while not neglecting the others and need to

distribute their attention equitably. When the newborn was born prematurely or has special needs, this task can be difficult.

Reactions of siblings result from temporary separation from the mother, changes in the mother's or father's behavior, or the infant coming home. Positive behavioral changes of siblings include interest in and concern for the baby (Fig. 20.9) and increased independence. Regression in toileting and sleep habits, aggression toward the baby, and increased seeking of attention and whining are examples of negative behaviors.

The parents' attitudes toward the arrival of the baby can set the stage for the other children's reactions (see Fig. 20.9). Because the baby absorbs the time and attention of the important people in the other children's lives, jealousy (sibling rivalry) is common once the initial excitement of having a new baby in the home is over.

Parents, especially mothers, spend much time and energy promoting sibling acceptance of a new baby. Participating in sibling preparation classes makes a difference in the ability of parents to cope with sibling behavior (see Fig. 8.4). Older children are actively involved in preparing for the infant, and this involvement intensifies after the birth of the child. Parents have to manage their feelings of guilt that the older children are being deprived of parental time and attention and monitor the behavior of older children toward the more vulnerable infant and divert aggressive behavior. Strategies that parents have used to facilitate siblings' acceptance of a new baby are presented in Box 20.5).

Siblings demonstrate acquaintance behaviors with the newborn. The acquaintance process depends on the information given to the child before the baby is born and on the child's cognitive development level.

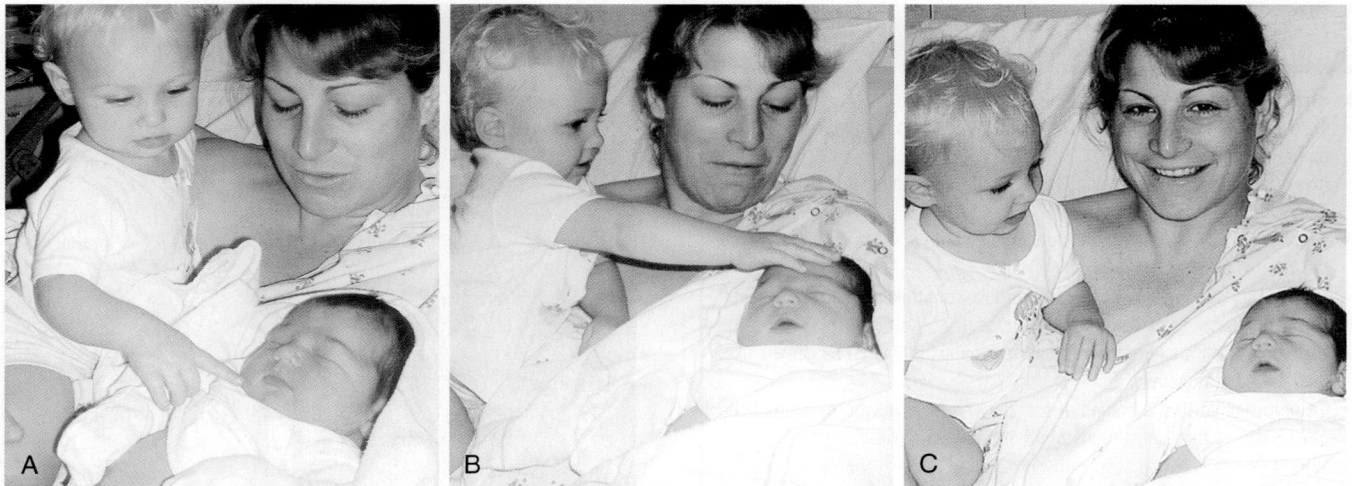

FIG 20.9 First meeting. **A,** Sister touching new sibling with fingertip. **B,** Touching with whole hand. **C,** Smiles indicate acceptance. (Courtesy of Sara Kossuth, Los Angeles, CA.)

The initial behaviors of siblings with the newborn include looking at the infant and touching the head (see Fig. 20.9). The adjustment of older children to a newborn takes time, and parents should allow children to interact at their own pace rather than forcing them to interact. To expect a young child to accept and love a rival for the parents' affection assumes an unrealistic level of maturity. Sibling love grows as does other love, that is, by being with another person and sharing experiences. This bond between siblings involves a secure base in which one child provides support for the other, is missed when absent, and is looked to for comfort and security.

GRANDPARENT ADAPTATION

Becoming a grandparent is usually associated with great joy and happiness. Yet it is a time of transition as roles and relationships are changing and new opportunities arise. Emotions are varied and can change from day to day; feelings of joy, anticipation, and excitement are often intermingled with some degree of anxiety and uncertainty. Circumstances surrounding the pregnancy and birth influence the feelings, reactions, and responses of grandparents.

Pregnancy and birth necessitate redefining intergenerational roles and relationships within the family. A primary role of the grandparents is to support, nurture, and empower their child in his or her parenting role. Grandparents must acknowledge that things have changed since they first became parents as they deal with changes in practices and attitudes toward childbirth, childrearing, and men's and women's roles at home and in the workplace. The degree to which grandparents understand and accept current practices can influence how supportive they are to their adult children.

At the same time that they are adjusting to grandparenthood, the majority of grandparents are experiencing normative middle- and old-age life transition issues, such as retirement and a move to smaller housing, and they need support from their adult children. Some may feel regret about their limited involvement because of poor health or geographic distance.

The extent of involvement of grandparents in the care of the newborn depends on many factors, for example, the willingness of the grandparents to become involved, the proximity of the grandparents, and ethnic and cultural expectations of the grandparent's role (Fig. 20.10). If the new

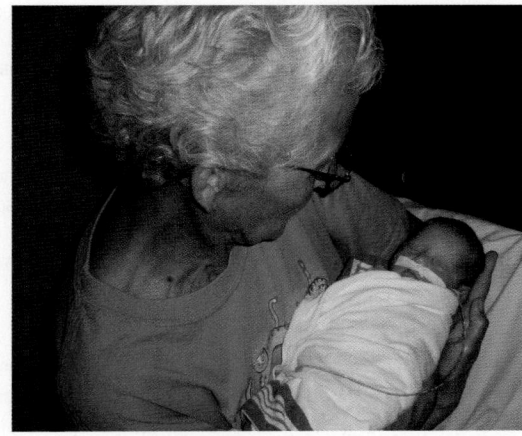

FIG 20.10 Great-grandmother and great-granddaughter get acquainted. (Courtesy of Sharon Tallon, Bloomington, IL.)

parents live in the United States, Asian grandparents typically are asked to come to the United States to care for the baby and the mother after birth and to care for the children once the parents return to work. In the United States, paternal grandparents, in contrast to those in other cultures, frequently consider themselves secondary to the maternal grandparents. Less seems expected of them, and they are initially less involved. Nevertheless, these grandparents are eager to help and express great pleasure in their son's fatherhood and his involvement with the baby (Fig. 20.11).

Relationships between grandparents and parents may change with the birth of a new baby. For first-time parents, pregnancy and parenthood can reawaken old issues related to dependence versus independence. Couples often do not plan on their parents' help immediately after the baby arrives. They want time "to be a family," implying a couple-baby unit, not the intergenerational family network. Contrary to their expectations, however, new parents do call on their parents for help, especially the maternal grandmother. Many grandparents are aware of their adult children's wishes for autonomy, respect these wishes, and remain available to help when asked.

BOX 20.5   Sibling Adaptation: Tips for Sibling Preparation

Prenatal

- Take your child on a prenatal visit. Let the child listen to the fetal heartbeat and feel the baby move.
- Involve the child in preparations for the baby, such as helping decorate the baby's room.
- Move the child to a bed (if still sleeping in a crib) at least 2 months before the baby is due.
- Read books, show videos or DVDs, and/or take your child to sibling preparation classes, including a hospital tour.
- Answer your child's questions about the coming birth, what babies are like, and any other questions.
- Take your child to the homes of friends who have newborns so that the child has realistic expectations of what babies are like.

During the Hospital Stay

- Have someone bring the child to the hospital to visit you and the baby (unless you plan to have the child attend the birth).
- When the child arrives, make sure your arms are open to embrace the child.
- Do not force interactions between the child and the baby. Often the child will be more interested in seeing you and being reassured of your love.
- Help the child explore the infant by showing how and where to touch the baby.
- Give the child a gift (from you or from you, the father or your partner, and baby).

Going Home

- Leave the child at home with a relative or babysitter or have someone such as the grandmother available to focus on the child during hospital discharge and on the trip home.
- Have someone else carry the baby from the car so that you can hug the child first.

Adjustment After the Baby Is Home

- Arrange for a special time for the child to be alone with each parent.
- Do not exclude the child during infant feeding times. The child can sit with you and the baby and feed a doll or drink juice or milk or sit quietly with a game. You can read aloud to the child while you are feeding the infant.
- Prepare small gifts for the child so that when the baby gets gifts, the sibling will not feel left out. The child can also help open the baby gifts.
- Praise the child for acting age appropriately (so that being a baby does not seem better than being older).

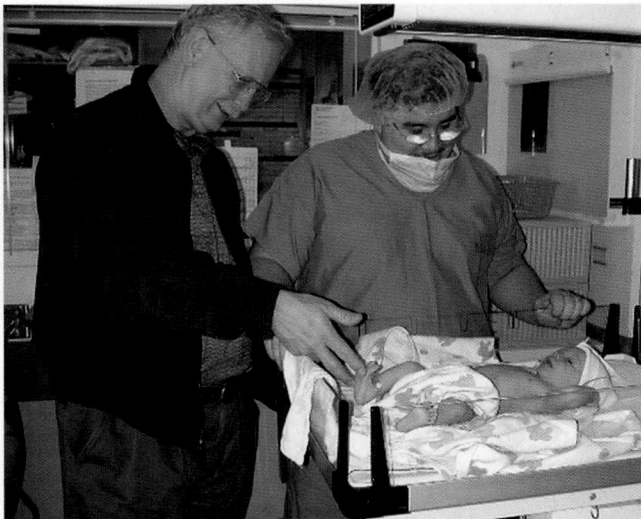

FIG 20.11 Father and grandfather becoming acquainted with new family member. (Courtesy of Sharon Johnson, Petaluma, CA.)

🏠 COMMUNITY FOCUS

Helping Grandparents Bridge the Generation Gap

Interview a grandfather and a grandmother about their experiences with childbirth and infant care. The purpose is to understand grandparents' experiences and perspectives. Ask them how they feel about their new roles; their description of their involvement in helping their son or daughter with a new baby; their description of how they view rewards and challenges of being a grandparent; and what they would like their grandchild to call them. Students can discuss findings in clinical conference and learn from one another about the various perspectives of being a grandparent

CARE MANAGEMENT

Numerous changes occur during the first weeks of parenthood. Care management should be directed toward helping parents cope with infant care, role changes, altered lifestyle, and change in family structure resulting from the addition of a new baby. During the first weeks of parenthood, care management involves the interprofessional health care team. For example, neonatal or pediatric care providers and nurses in the hospital setting teach new parents about infant behaviors and expectations for incorporating the baby in the existing family. Social workers may be involved if the family has limited resources. Developing skill and confidence in caring for an infant can be anxiety provoking. Anticipatory guidance can help prevent a shock of reality in the transition from hospital or birthing center to home that might negate the parents' joy or cause them undue stress.

Through education, support, and encouragement, nurses are instrumental in assisting mothers and their partners in the transition to parenthood, whether they are first-time parents or parents of several other children. Early and ongoing assessment and intervention promote positive outcomes for parents, infants, and family members (see Community Focus box: Identifying Parenting Resources on the Web and Nursing Care Plan box: Home Care Follow-Up: Transition to Parenthood).

Grandparents' classes can be used to bridge the generation gap and to help the grandparents understand their adult children's parenting concepts. The classes include information on up-to-date childbearing practices; family-centered care; infant care, feeding, and safety (e.g. car seats, safe sleep); and exploration of roles that grandparents play in the family unit (see Community Focus box: Helping Grandparents Bridge the Generation Gap).

Increasing numbers of grandparents are providing permanent care for their grandchildren as a result of divorce, substance abuse, child abuse or neglect, abandonment, adolescent pregnancy, death, human immunodeficiency virus (HIV) and acquired immunodeficiency syndrome (AIDS), unemployment, incarceration, and mental health problems. This emerging trend requires the nurse to evaluate the role of the grandparent in parenting the infant. Educational and financial considerations must be addressed and available support systems identified for these families.

COMMUNITY FOCUS

Identifying Parenting Resources on the Web

- Visit the website of a hospital that provides maternity services in your community. Does the hospital offer prepared childbirth, parenting, sibling, or infant/child cardiopulmonary resuscitation (CPR) classes? Are group tours of the birthing center provided for expectant parents?
- Visit the website *babycenter.com*, which provides information for parents about pregnancy, parenting, and children's health. Review the information about postpartum emotional health, causes and treatments of baby blues, and baby blues versus postpartum depression.
- Visit the website *familyandhome.org*, and research the availability of support groups for parents in your community.

NURSING CARE PLAN

Home Care Follow-Up: Transition to Parenthood

Case Study

Nicole and Robert were discharged with their newborn infant, Timothy, from the birthing site 26 hours after Timothy was born. They are first-time parents, attended childbirth classes, and received infant care instructions before discharge. Nicole is breastfeeding and Robert has a week of parental leave to assist Nicole in adjusting to new parenthood and care of Timothy. Their insurance supports a home visit by a nurse within the first 2 weeks after birth.

Assessment

What are signs that Nicole and Robert are adjusting to new parenthood and providing adequate and safe care for Timothy? What are signs that Timothy is being adequately cared for?

Defining Characteristics

Willingness to enhance parenting
Satisfaction with home environment
Fulfillment of physical and emotional needs
Realistic expectations of Timothy and themselves

Nursing Diagnosis

Readiness for Enhanced Parenting related to lack of experience or lack of support.

Expected Outcomes

Nicole and Robert will express satisfaction in role of parent.
Nicole and Robert will express confidence in ability to parent.
Home will exhibit signs of safe and functional environment.
Child care routines will be adequate.

Nursing Interventions	Rationales
Discuss with Nicole and Robert their perceptions and philosophy related to the role of parents in a family.	Verbalizing perceptions and beliefs provides an opportunity to clarify Nicole and Robert's thinking
Support efforts of Nicole and Robert as they adapt to the ever-changing issue of family needs.	Recognition of and appreciation for one's efforts enhances motivation to continue to improve skills
Observe the home environment and discuss the issues of safety and cleanliness, if needed.	Nicole, Robert and Timothy need to have an environment that is free from environmental hazards, both chemical and physical
Ask Nicole and Robert to describe a typical day with normal routines related to family dynamics and functioning.	This provides a concrete example for reflection of family functioning

Nursing Interventions	Rationales
Observe Timothy's appearance (height-weight ratio, head circumference, fontanels, skin tone and turgor), and assess vital signs, overall tone, reflexes, and age-appropriate developmental skills.	To evaluate for signs indicative of inadequate care
Explore available support systems for infant care.	To determine adequacy of existing system
Provide ongoing follow-up and referrals as needed.	To ensure that identified potential and actual care deficits are addressed and resolved

Case Study (Continued)

On the 2-week postpartum visit, the nurse notes that Timothy is lying in his crib looking around, and is dressed in clean clothes and a dry diaper. There are dirty dishes piled in the sink, waste baskets are overflowing, dirty linen is piled in a basket, and Nicole appears tired and frustrated. She apologized for the messy appearance of the home and states that Robert has gone back to work and she is having a hard time feeding Timothy as often as he demands and keeping up with the housework.

Assessment

What are signs that Nicole is maintaining a safe and growth-promoting environment?

Defining Characteristics

Difficulty in maintaining home in a comfortable environment
Disorderly surroundings
Unwashed or unavailable cooking equipment, clothes or linens

Nursing Diagnosis

Impaired Home Maintenance related to addition of new family member; inadequate support

Expected Outcomes

Nicole will express concern about poor home maintenance.
Home exhibits signs of safe and functional environment.
Nicole will identify resources to maintain home.

Continued

NURSING CARE PLAN

Home Care Follow-up: Transition to Parenthood—cont'd

Nursing Interventions	Rationales
Observe home environment (e.g., available living space and sleeping arrangements; adequacy of facilities for food preparation and storage, hygiene, and toileting; overall state of repair; cleanliness; presence of safety hazards).	To determine adequacy and effective use of resources
Observe arrangements for infant, such as sleeping space, care equipment, and supplies (bathing, changing, feeding, transportation).	To determine adequacy of resources
Explore how Robert might participate more in home maintenance.	To provide respite and assistance for Nicole
Explore who is responsible for cooking, cleaning, child care, and infant care, and determine whether Nicole seems adequately rested.	To determine adequacy of support systems
Identify and arrange referrals to needed social agencies (e.g., Temporary Assistance for Needy Families [TANF]; Special Supplemental Nutrition Program for Women, Infants and Children [WIC] program; food pantries).	To address resource deficits (e.g., in finances, supplies, equipment)

Case Study (Continued)

Nicole comments to the nurse that she is so busy taking care of Timothy who requires a lot of care that she and Robert rarely have any time for themselves. "Timothy just takes so long to nurse that I don't have time to do anything else."

Assessment

What are signs that Nicole and Robert are adjusting to new parenthood, supporting each other, and sharing household tasks?

Defining Characteristics

Adequate communication
Family adaptation to change
Flexible family roles
Energy level that supports activities of daily living

Nursing Diagnosis

Readiness for Enhanced Family Processes related to inclusion of new family member

Expected Outcomes

Robert and Nicole will maintain open communication.
Robert and Nicole will maintain a safe home environment.
Robert and Nicole will contact community resources for help, if needed.
Timothy is successfully incorporated into family structure.

Nursing Interventions	Rationales
Explore with Nicole and Robert ways that birth and infant have changed family structure and function.	To evaluate functional and role adjustment
Observe Nicole and Robert's interaction with Timothy, and note degree of bonding and involvement in infant care.	To evaluate acceptance of newest family member
Clarify identified misinformation and misperceptions.	To promote clear communication
Assist Nicole and Robert in exploring options for solutions to identified problems.	To promote effective problem resolution
Support Nicole and Robert's efforts as they move to incorporate Timothy into the family.	To reinforce new functions and roles
If needed, make referrals to appropriate social services or community agencies.	To ensure ongoing support and care

REFERENCES

American College of Obstetricians and Gynecologists. (2015). Screening for perinatal depression. *Obstetrics and Gynecology*, *125*(5), 1268–1271.

Bartlett, J. D., & Easterbrooks, M. A. (2015). The moderating effect of relationships on intergenerational risk for infant neglect by young mothers. *Child Abuse and Neglect*, *45*, 21–34.

D'Avanzo, C. (2008). *Mosby's pocket guide to cultural assessment* (4th ed.). St Louis: Mosby.

de Montigny, F., Lacharité, C., & Devault, A. (2012). Transition to fatherhood: modeling the experience of fathers of breastfed infants. *Advances in Nursing Science*, *35*(3), E11–E22.

Dahl, B., Fylkesnes, A. M., Sorlie, V., et al. (2013). Lesbian women's experiences with healthcare providers in the birthing context: A meta-ethnography. *Midwifery*, *29*(6), 674–681.

Fagan, J. (2013). Adolescent parents' partner conflict and parenting alliance, fathers' prenatal involvement, and fathers' engagement with infants. *Journal of Family Issues*, *35*(11), 1415–1439.

Field, T. (2017). Newborn massage therapy. *International Journal of Pediatrics and Neonatal Health*, *1*(2), 54–64.

Galanti, C. A. (2015). *Caring for patients from different cultures* (5th ed.). Philadelphia, PA: University of Pennsylvania Press.

Geoghegan, T. (2013). Surviving the first day: State of the world's mothers 2013. Retrieved from www.savethechildrenweb.org/SOWM-2013/files/assets/common/downloads/State%20of%20the%20WorldOWM-2013.pdf.

Hoffenkamp, H. N., Tooten, A., Hall, R. A., et al. (2012). The impact of premature childbirth on parental bonding. *Evolutionary Psychology*, *10*(3), 542–561.

Husmillo, M. (2013). Maternal role attainment theory. *International Journal of Childbirth Education*, *28*(2), 46–48.

Isley, M. M., & Katz, V. L. (2017). Postpartum care and long-term health considerations. In S. G. Gabbe, J. R. Neibyl, J. L. Simpson, et al. (Eds.), *Obstetrics: Normal and problem pregnancies* (7th ed.). Philadelphia, PA: Elsevier.

Jeha, D., Usta, I., Ghulmiyyah, L., et al. (2015). A review of the risks and consequences of adolescent pregnancy. *Journal of Neonatal & Perinatal Medicine*, *8*(1), 1–8.

Kilpatrick, S., & Garrison, E. (2017). Normal labor and delivery. In S. G. Gabbe, J. R. Neibyl, J. L. Simpson, et al. (Eds.), *Obstetrics: Normal and problem pregnancies* (7th ed.). Philadelphia, PA: Elsevier.

King, T. L., & Pinger, W. (2014). Evidence-based practice for intrapartum care: The pearls of midwifery. *Journal of Midwifery and Women's Health*, *59*, 572–585.

Klaus, M., & Kennell, J. (1976). *Maternal-infant bonding*. St Louis, MO: Mosby.

Klaus, M., & Kennell, J. (1982). *Parent-infant bonding* (2nd ed.). St Louis, MO: Mosby.

May, C., & Fletcher, R. (2013). Preparing fathers for the transition to parenthood: Recommendations for the content of antenatal education. *Midwifery*, *29*(5), 474–478.

Mercer, R. (2004). Becoming a mother versus maternal role attainment. *Journal of Nursing Scholarship*, *36*(3), 226–232.

Perrine, C. G., Scanlon, K. S., Li, R., et al. (2012). Baby-friendly hospital practices and meeting exclusive breastfeeding intention. *Pediatrics*, *130*(1), 54–60.

Ramchandani, P. G., Domoney, J., Sethna, V., et al. (2013). Do early father-infant interactions predict the onset of externalizing behaviours in young children? Findings from a longitudinal cohort study. *Journal of Child Psychology and Psychiatry*, *54*(1), 56–64.

Rubin, R. (1961). Basic maternal behavior. *Nursing Outlook*, *9*, 683–686.

Shaver, J. L. F. (2015). Promoting healthy sleep. In E. F. Olshansky (Ed.), *Women's health and wellness across the lifespan*. Philadelphia, PA: Wolters Kluwer.

Stapleton, L. R., Schetter, C. D., Westling, E., et al. (2012). Perceived partner support in pregnancy predicts lower maternal and infant distress. *Journal of Family Psychology*, *26*(3), 453–463.

Steen, M., Downe, S., Bamford, N., et al. (2012). Not-patient and not-visitor: A metasynthesis of fathers' encounters with pregnancy, birth and maternity care. *Midwifery*, *28*(4), 362–371.

Stewart, L. S., & Rodgers, E. (2017). Assessment and care of the term newborn transitioning to extrauterine life. In B. B. Kennedy & S. M. Baird (Eds.), *Intrapartum management modules: A perinatal education program* (5th ed.). Philadelphia, PA: Wolters Kluwer.

Tharner, A., Luijk, M. P., Raat, H., et al. (2012). Breastfeeding and its relation to maternal sensitivity and infant attachment. *Journal of Developmental and Behavioral Pediatrics*, *33*(5), 396–404.

Welch, M. G., Hofer, M. A., Brunelli, S. A., et al. (2012). Family Nurture Intervention (FNI) Trial Group: Family nurture intervention (FNI): methods and treatment protocol of a randomized controlled trial in the NICU. *BMC Pediatrics*, *12*, 14.

Yu, C. Y., Hung, C. H., Chan, T. F., et al. (2012). Prenatal predictors of father-infant attachment after childbirth. *Journal of Clinical Nursing*, *21*(11-12), 1577–1583.

21

Postpartum Complications

Kathryn R. Alden

http://evolve.elsevier.com/Perry/maternal

The postpartum period is a time of change and transition for mothers and newborns. Mothers experience incredible physiologic shifts and emotional adjustments in the hours and days following birth. Perinatal nurses provide education, care, and support for mothers and newborns during this important time. In addition, nurses have the responsibility to pay careful attention to signs and symptoms of complications. The nurse works collaboratively with the interprofessional health care team to provide safe and effective care to women experiencing postpartum physiologic complications. In most instances, women respond to treatment, and outcomes are positive. However, in some cases this does not occur; a woman may die as a result of the postpartum complication she is experiencing. This is devastating for the family as well as for the health care professionals involved in her care. This chapter focuses on the postpartum complications of hemorrhage, infection, thromboembolic disorders, and psychologic complications.

POSTPARTUM HEMORRHAGE

DEFINITION AND INCIDENCE

Postpartum hemorrhage (PPH) continues to be a leading cause of maternal morbidity and mortality in the United States and throughout the world (World Health Organization [WHO], 2015). Postpartum hemorrhage is a life-threatening event that can occur with little warning and is often not recognized until the mother has profound symptoms.

Definitions of PPH in the literature are varied. PPH is often defined as the loss of 500 mL or more of blood after vaginal birth and 1000 mL or more after cesarean birth, although normal blood loss for some women approaches these amounts. PPH may be defined as a 10% change in hematocrit from the time of admission to the birthing facility for labor until postpartum; or it may be defined by the need for erythrocyte transfusion. Diagnosis is often based on subjective observations, with blood loss often being underestimated by as much as 50% (Cunningham, Leveno, Bloom, et al., 2014). PPH may be more practically defined as excessive blood loss that causes the woman to become hemodynamically symptomatic and possibly develop hypovolemic shock (Francois & Foley, 2017). (See Clinical Reasoning Case Study: Postpartum Hemorrhage.)

Postpartum hemorrhage is classified as early or late with respect to the birth. Early, acute, or primary PPH occurs within 24 hours of the birth. Late or secondary PPH occurs more than 24 hours but less than 6 weeks after the birth (Francois & Foley, 2017). Today's health care environment encourages shortened hospital stays after birth, which increases the potential for acute episodes of PPH to occur outside the traditional hospital or birth center setting.

ETIOLOGY AND RISK FACTORS

When excessive bleeding is observed, it is important to note the color and consistency of the blood as well as the stage of labor. From birth of the infant until separation of the placenta, the character and quantity of blood expelled from the vagina can suggest excessive bleeding. For example, dark red blood is likely of venous origin, perhaps from varices or superficial lacerations of the birth canal. Bright blood is arterial and can indicate deep lacerations of the cervix. Spurts of blood with clots can indicate partial placental separation. Failure of blood to clot or remain clotted indicates a pathologic condition or coagulopathy such as disseminated intravascular coagulation (DIC) (see Chapter 12).

Excessive bleeding can occur during the period from the separation of the placenta to its expulsion or removal. This can result from incomplete placental separation, undue manipulation of the fundus, or excessive traction on the cord. After the placenta has been expelled or removed, persistent or excessive blood loss usually is the result of uterine atony or prolapse of the uterus into the vagina. Late PPH can be the result of subinvolution of the uterus, endometritis, or retained placental fragments (Francois & Foley, 2017). Predisposing factors for PPH are listed in Box 21.1.

Uterine Atony

The greatest risk for early postpartum hemorrhage is during the first hour after birth. During this time, large venous areas are exposed after the placenta separates from the uterine wall. The corpus or body of the uterus is essentially a basket-weave of strong, interlacing smooth muscle bundles through which many large maternal blood vessels pass (see Fig. 3.3). Bleeding is controlled by the contraction of smooth muscle in the uterus. If the uterus is flaccid after detachment of all or part of the placenta, brisk venous bleeding occurs, and normal coagulation of the open vasculature is impaired and continues until the uterine muscle is contracted. This marked hypotonia of the uterus is called **uterine atony**.

Uterine atony is the leading cause of early PPH. It is associated with high parity, polyhydramnios, fetal macrosomia, obesity, and multiple gestation. In such conditions, the uterus is "overstretched" and contracts poorly after birth. Other causes of atony include traumatic birth, use of halogenated anesthetic (e.g., halothane), magnesium sulfate, rapid or prolonged labor, chorioamnionitis, use of oxytocin for labor induction or augmentation, and uterine atony in a previous pregnancy (Francois & Foley, 2017).

Retained Placenta

When the placenta has not been delivered within 30 minutes after birth despite gentle traction on the umbilical cord and uterine massage, it is

CLINICAL REASONING CASE STUDY
Postpartum Hemorrhage

You are the mother-baby nurse assigned to Ms. Avery. She is a G4 P3 who gave birth to a 9-lb (4082-g) baby boy this morning. Ms. Avery had an uncomplicated but precipitous vaginal birth. Her perineum is intact. She is breastfeeding. All labs are normal. She is now 3 hours postpartum. A family member calls out from the patient's room for assistance. When you walk into the room Ms. Avery is standing up on her way to the bathroom with a large pool of blood on the floor. She states, "I don't know what happened; it all just came when I stood up. I am so dizzy and lightheaded." What do you, as the nurse, do next?

1. Evidence—Is there sufficient evidence to draw conclusions about what the nurse should do?
2. Assumptions—Describe underlying assumptions about each of the following:
   a. Risk factors for early postpartum hemorrhage (PPH) and specifically those described for Ms. Avery.
   b. Need for frequent assessments in the early postpartum period
   c. Use of oxytocics for prevention and management of PPH
3. What implications and priorities for nursing care can be made at this time?
4. Interprofessional care: Describe roles/responsibilities of health care professionals who would potentially be involved in care management for Ms. Avery.

BOX 21.1 Risk Factors and Causes of Postpartum Hemorrhage

- Uterine atony
  - Overdistended uterus
  - Large fetus
  - Multiple fetuses
  - Hydramnios
  - Distention with clots
- Anesthesia and analgesia
  - General or halogenated anesthesia
- Previous history of uterine atony
- High parity
- Obesity
- Prolonged labor, oxytocin-induced labor
- Trauma during labor and birth
  - Forceps-assisted birth
  - Vacuum-assisted birth
  - Cesarean birth
- Unrepaired lacerations of the birth canal
- Retained placental fragments
- Ruptured uterus
- Inversion of the uterus
- Placenta accreta, increta, percreta
- Coagulation disorders
- Placental abruption
- Placenta previa
- Manual removal of a retained placenta
- Magnesium sulfate administration during labor or the postpartum period
- Chorioamnionitis
- Uterine subinvolution

described as "retained." Initial management of a retained placenta consists of manual separation and removal by the physician or nurse-midwife. This involves the provider reaching into the uterus and gently separating the placenta from the uterine wall and removing it manually. When the mother has regional anesthesia for labor, supplementary anesthesia is usually not needed. For other women, administration of light nitrous oxide and oxygen inhalation anesthesia or intravenous (IV) pain medications should be considered (Francois & Foley, 2017). After removal of a retained placenta, the woman is at continued risk for PPH and infection.

Fragments of the placenta can remain in the uterus after spontaneous separation of the placenta during the third stage of labor. In this case, the woman will have excessive bleeding and the uterus feels boggy (soft) due to uterine atony. Ultrasonography can be used to detect placental fragments. The physician or nurse-midwife may attempt manual exploration to remove the fragments; uterine curettage (removal of uterine contents using a curette or vacuum suction) may be necessary.

Postpartum hemorrhage can be due to abnormally implanted, invasive, or adhered placenta; this is known as *placenta accrete syndrome*. It is unknown why this occurs, but it is thought to result from zygote implantation in an area of defective endometrium so that no zone of separation exists between the placenta and the decidua. Unusual placental adherence can be total, partial, or focal, depending on how much placental tissue is involved. The following degrees of abnormal placental attachment are recognized:

Placenta accreta—Slight penetration of myometrium
Placenta increta—Deep penetration of myometrium
Placenta percreta—Perforation of myometrium and uterine serosa, possibly involving adjacent organs

Placenta accrete syndrome has demonstrated an increased incidence in association with the rise in cesarean birth rates (Cunningham, Leveno, Bloom, et al., 2014). Other risk factors include placenta previa, prior uterine surgery, endometrial defects, submucosal fibroids, multiparity, and older maternal age (Francois & Foley, 2017). Placenta accrete syndrome can be diagnosed before birth using ultrasound and magnetic resonance imaging (MRI), but often it is not recognized until there is excessive bleeding after birth. Cesarean birth is recommended when the diagnosis is made prenatally. Bleeding may not occur unless manual removal of the placenta is attempted. With more extensive involvement, bleeding becomes profuse when removal of the placenta is attempted. Less blood is lost if the diagnosis is made antenatally and no attempt is made to manually remove the placenta. Treatment includes blood component replacement therapy. Hysterectomy can be indicated for all three types of placental adherence if bleeding is uncontrolled (Cunningham et al). Attempts to remove the placenta in the usual manner are unsuccessful, and laceration or perforation of the uterine wall can result, putting the woman at great risk for severe PPH and infection (Francois & Foley, 2017).

Lacerations of the Genital Tract

Lacerations of the cervix, vagina, and perineum also are causes of PPH. Hemorrhage related to lacerations should be suspected if bleeding continues despite a firm, contracted uterine fundus. This bleeding can be a slow trickle, an oozing, or frank hemorrhage. Factors that influence the causes and incidence of obstetric lacerations of the lower genital tract include operative birth, precipitous birth, congenital abnormalities of the maternal soft tissue, and contracted pelvis. Other possible causes of lacerations are increased size, abnormal presentation, and position of the fetus; relative size of the presenting part and the birth canal; previous scarring from infection, injury, or operation; and vulvar, perineal, and vaginal varicosities.

Lacerations of the perineum are the most common of all injuries in the lower portion of the genital tract. These are classified as first, second, third, and fourth degree (see Chapter 16). An episiotomy can extend to become either a third- or fourth-degree laceration.

Prolonged pressure of the fetal head on the vaginal mucosa ultimately interferes with the circulation and may produce ischemic or pressure necrosis. The state of the tissues in combination with the type of birth can result in deep vaginal lacerations, with consequent predisposition to vaginal hematomas.

Cervical lacerations usually occur at the lateral angles of the external os. Most are shallow, and bleeding is minimal. More extensive lacerations may extend into the vaginal vault or into the lower uterine segment.

Lacerations are usually identified and sutured immediately after birth. After the bleeding has been controlled, the care of the woman with lacerations of the perineum is similar to that for women with episiotomies (i.e., analgesia as needed for pain and application of hot or cold applications as necessary). The need for increased fiber in the diet and increased intake of fluids is emphasized to reduce the risk for constipation. Stool softeners may be used to assist the woman in reestablishing bowel habits without straining and putting stress on the suture lines.

> **NURSING ALERT**
>
> To avoid injury to the suture line, a woman with third- or fourth-degree lacerations is not given rectal suppositories or enemas.

Hematomas

Pelvic hematomas (i.e., a collection of blood in the connective tissue) can be vulvar, vaginal, or retroperitoneal in origin. Vulvar hematomas are the most common. Pain is the most common symptom, and most vulvar hematomas are visible. Vaginal hematomas occur more commonly in association with a forceps-assisted birth, an episiotomy, or primigravidity (Francois & Foley, 2017).

Retroperitoneal hematomas are the least common but life-threatening. They are caused by laceration of one of the vessels attached to the hypogastric artery, usually associated with rupture of a cesarean scar during labor. During the postpartum period, if the woman reports persistent perineal or rectal pain or a feeling of pressure in the vagina, a careful examination is made. However, a retroperitoneal hematoma can cause minimal pain and the initial symptoms can be signs of shock (Francois & Foley, 2017).

Hematomas are usually surgically evacuated. Once the bleeding has been controlled, usual postpartum care is provided with careful attention to pain relief, monitoring the amount of bleeding, replacing fluids, and reviewing laboratory results (hemoglobin and hematocrit).

Inversion of the Uterus

Inversion of the uterus (turning inside out) after birth is a rare but potentially life-threatening complication. The incidence of uterine inversion varies from 1 in 2000 to 1 in 20,000 births and differs depending on whether the birth was vaginal or cesarean (Cunningham et al., 2014). Uterine inversion can recur with a subsequent birth. Uterine inversion can be incomplete, complete, or prolapsed. Incomplete inversion cannot be seen; a smooth mass can be palpated through the dilated cervix. In complete inversion, the lining of the fundus crosses through the cervical os and forms a mass in the vagina. Prolapsed inversion of the uterus is obvious—a large, red, rounded mass (perhaps with the placenta attached) protrudes 20 to 30 cm outside the introitus.

Contributing factors to uterine inversion include fundal implantation of the placenta, vigorous fundal pressure, excessive traction applied to the cord, fetal macrosomia, short umbilical cord, tocolysis, prolonged labor, uterine atony, nulliparity, and abnormally adherent placental tissue (Francois & Foley, 2017). The primary presenting signs of uterine inversion are sudden and include hemorrhage, shock, and pain. The uterus is not palpable abdominally. The uterus must be replaced into its proper position by the obstetric health care provider.

Prevention—always the easiest, least expensive, and most effective therapy—is especially appropriate for uterine inversion. The umbilical cord should not be pulled unless there are clear signs of placental separation.

Uterine inversion is an emergency situation requiring immediate interventions that include maternal fluid resuscitation, replacement of the uterus within the pelvic cavity, and correction of associated clinical conditions. Tocolytics or halogenated anesthetics may be given to relax the uterus before attempting replacement (Francois & Foley, 2017). Oxytocic agents are administered after the uterus is repositioned; broad-spectrum antibiotics are initiated. The woman's response to treatment is monitored closely to prevent shock or fluid overload. If the uterus has been repositioned manually, care must be taken to avoid aggressive fundal massage.

Subinvolution of the Uterus

Late postpartum bleeding can result from subinvolution of the uterus (delayed return of the enlarged uterus to normal size and function). Recognized causes of subinvolution include retained placental fragments and pelvic infection. Signs and symptoms include prolonged lochial discharge, irregular or excessive bleeding, and sometimes hemorrhage. A pelvic examination usually reveals a larger-than-normal uterus that can be boggy.

Treatment of subinvolution depends on the cause. Ergonovine (Ergotrate) or methylergonovine (Methergine), 0.2 mg every 3 to 4 hours for 24 to 48 hours, is often used. Dilation and curettage (D&C) may be performed to remove retained placental fragments or to debride the placental site. If the cause of subinvolution is infection, antibiotic therapy is needed (Cunningham et al., 2014).

CARE MANAGEMENT

Care of women experiencing postpartum hemorrhage requires the collaboration of an interprofessional health care team. Nurses and obstetric care providers work closely with personnel from the transfusion services department (blood bank), pharmacy, and laboratory to manage the emergent situation that occurs when a woman begins to bleed excessively after birth. Each birthing facility should have an obstetric hemorrhage team that is called into action when hemorrhage occurs. This team is separate from the woman's obstetric health care provider, although her provider may be involved. The hemorrhage team should include health care providers who can perform surgical procedures (e.g., general obstetrics, maternal-fetal medicine, anesthesia), critical care nursing, blood bank, and laboratory (Fleischer & Meirowitz, 2016; Lyndon, Lagrew, Shields, et al., 2015).

In order for the health care team to be optimally prepared for obstetric hemorrhage, institutions must develop standardized management protocols and regularly conduct emergency drills. The California Maternal Quality Care Collaborative (www.cmqcc.org) has developed best practice approaches that can be adopted by other institutions (Lyndon et al., 2015). The use of obstetric rapid response teams and massive transfusion protocols is vital to promoting safe, effective care and improving outcomes.

The National Partnership for Maternal Safety, representing all major professional organizations dealing with women's health, developed a safety bundle for obstetric hemorrhage. This bundle consists of evidence-based recommendations for care management and is organized in four action domains: (1) Readiness—hemorrhage cart, immediate access to hemorrhage medications, a response team, massive and emergency-release transfusion protocols, and unit-based education with drills; (2) Recognition and Prevention—assessment of risk for hemorrhage, measurement of blood loss, and active management of third stage of labor; (3) Response—emergency management plan with checklists and support program for patients, families, and staff when significant hemorrhage occurs; and (4) Reporting and Systems Learning—huddling and postevent debriefs, multidisciplinary review of serious hemorrhages, and monitoring outcomes and processes (http://www.safehealthcareforeverywoman.org/) (Main, Goffman, Scavone, et al., 2015).

ASSESSMENT

Early recognition and treatment of PPH are critical to care management (Fig. 21.1). Risk assessment beginning during pregnancy and continuing during the intrapartum and postpartum periods is important in identifying women who are at risk for postpartum hemorrhage. This increases the awareness of the health care team in planning and implementing care and in preventing hemorrhage and its sequelae. Team members should be made aware whenever a woman with identified risk factors is admitted to the birthing facility (Fleischer & Meirowitz, 2016).

Excessive blood loss is the clinical finding that warrants prompt action. In general, health care professionals are highly inaccurate in estimating blood loss in terms of volume (Hancock, Weeks, & Lavender,

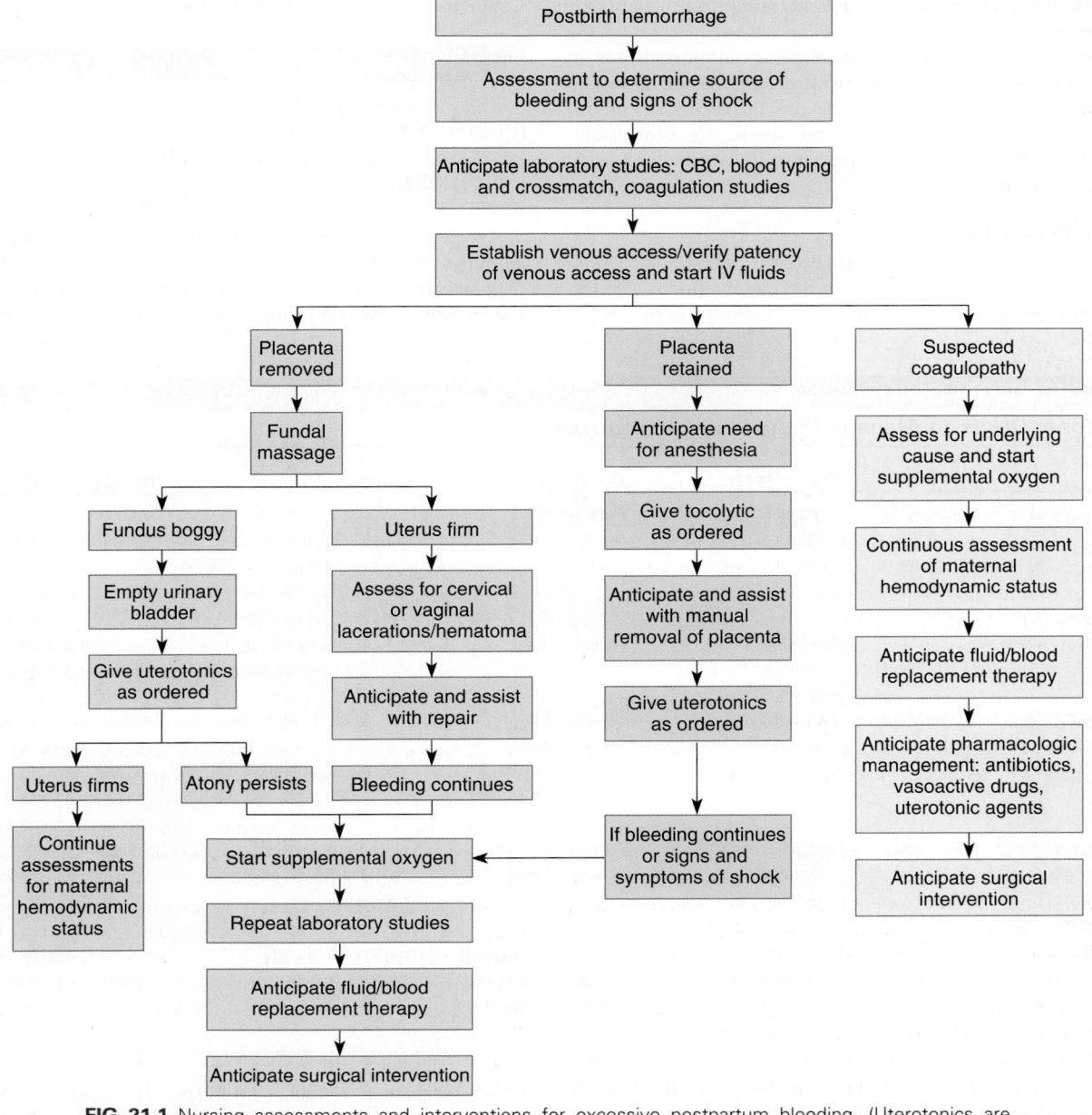

FIG 21.1 Nursing assessments and interventions for excessive postpartum bleeding. (Uterotonics are medications to contract the uterus; tocolytics are medications to relax the uterus.) *CBC,* Complete blood count; *IV,* intravenous.

2015). Most often blood loss is estimated by visual assessment and results in low estimates compared to actual blood loss. Accuracy of estimating blood loss can be improved by interventions that can quantify the amount of blood the woman loses during and after birth. The Association of Women's Health, Obstetric and Neonatal Nurses (AWHONN, 2015b) published a Practice Brief on quantification of blood loss (QBL), recommending that cumulative blood loss is measured with every birth, whether vaginal or cesarean. For vaginal birth, QBL should begin immediately after birth, prior to delivery of the placenta, using a calibrated under-buttocks drape and weighing all blood-soaked items. With cesarean birth, QBL begins when the membranes are ruptured or after birth of the neonate, measuring fluids in suction canisters (subtracting irrigation fluid) and weighing all blood-soaked materials and clots.

Whenever blood loss appears to be excessive, the first step is to evaluate the contractility of the uterus. If the uterus is hypotonic or boggy, management is directed toward increasing contractility and minimizing blood loss.

If the uterus is firmly contracted and bleeding continues, the source of bleeding still must be identified and treated. Assessment may include visual or manual inspection of the perineum, the vagina, the uterus, the cervix, or the rectum, as well as laboratory studies (e.g., hemoglobin, hematocrit, coagulation studies, platelet count). Treatment depends on the source of the bleeding.

Medical Management

The initial intervention in management of excessive postpartum bleeding due to uterine atony is firm massage of the uterine fundus (see Fig. 19.2). Expression of any clots in the uterus, elimination of bladder distention, and continuous IV infusion of 10 to 40 units of oxytocin added to 1000 mL of lactated Ringer's or normal saline solution also are primary interventions. If the uterus fails to respond to oxytocin, other uterotonic medications are administered. Misoprostol (Cytotec), a synthetic prostaglandin E_1 analog, is often used. An advantage is that it can be given rectally, sublingually, or orally. Methylergonovine may be given intramuscularly to produce sustained uterine contractions. A derivative of prostaglandin $F_{2\alpha}$ (carboprost tromethamine [Carboprost; Hemabate]) may be given intramuscularly. It can also be given intramyometrially at cesarean birth or intraabdominally after vaginal birth. Prostaglandin E_2 (Dinoprostone) vaginal or rectal suppository can be used for postpartum hemorrhage. (See Medication Guide: Uterotonic Drugs to Manage Postpartum Hemorrhage for a comparison of uterotonic drugs and common dosages used to manage PPH). In addition to the medications used to contract the uterus, rapid administration of crystalloid solutions or blood or blood products or both will be needed to restore the woman's intravascular volume (Francois & Foley, 2017).

MEDICATION ALERT

Use of ergonovine or methylergonovine is contraindicated in the presence of hypertension or cardiovascular disease. Prostaglandin $F_{2\alpha}$ should not be given to women with a history of asthma as it can cause bronchoconstriction (Francois & Foley, 2017).

Oxygen can be given by nonrebreather face mask to enhance oxygen delivery to the cells. An indwelling urinary catheter is usually inserted to monitor urine output as a measure of intravascular volume. Laboratory studies usually include a complete blood count with platelet count,

MEDICATION GUIDE

Uterotonic Drugs to Manage Postpartum Hemorrhage

Drug	Action	Side Effects	Contraindications	Dosage and Route	Nursing Considerations
Oxytocin (Pitocin)	Contraction of uterus; decreases bleeding	Infrequent: water intoxication, nausea and vomiting	None for PPH	10 to 20 units/L up to 80 units/L diluted in lactated Ringer's solution or normal saline at 125–200 milliunits/min IV; or 10–20 units IM	Continue to monitor vaginal bleeding and uterine tone.
Misoprostol (Cytotec)	Contraction of uterus	Headache, nausea, vomiting, diarrhea, fever, chills	None	600–1000 mcg rectally once or 400 mcg sublingually or PO once	Continue to monitor vaginal bleeding and uterine tone.
Methylergonovine (Methergine)	Contraction of uterus	Hypertension, hypotension, nausea, vomiting, headache	Hypertension, preeclampsia, cardiac disease	0.2 mg IM q2–4h up to five doses; may also be given intrauterine or orally	Check blood pressure before giving, and do not give if >140/90 mm Hg; continue monitoring vaginal bleeding and uterine tone.
15-Methylprostaglandin $F_{2\alpha}$ (Prostin/15 m; Carboprost, Hemabate)	Contraction of uterus	Headache, nausea and vomiting, fever, chills, tachycardia, hypertension, diarrhea	Avoid with asthma or hypertension	250 mcg IM or intrauterine injection q15–90 min up to eight doses	Continue to monitor vaginal bleeding and uterine tone.
Dinoprostone (Prostin E_2)	Contraction of uterus	Headache, nausea and vomiting, fever, chills, diarrhea	Use with caution with history of asthma, hypertension, or hypotension	20 mg vaginal or rectal suppository q2h	Continue to monitor vaginal bleeding and uterine tone.

IM, Intramuscular; *IV,* intravenous; *PO,* by mouth; *PPH,* postpartum hemorrhage.
Data from Francois, K.E., & Foley, M.R. (2017). Antepartum and postpartum hemorrhage. In S.G. Gabbe, J.R. Niebyl, J.L. Simpson, et al. (Eds.), *Obstetrics: Normal and problem pregnancies* (7th ed.). Philadelphia, PA: Elsevier; Lyndon, A., Lagrew, D., Shields, L., et al. (Eds.). (2015). *California maternal quality care collaborative toolkit to transform maternity care: Improving health care response to obstetric hemorrhage version 2.0.* Stanford, CA: California Maternal Quality Care Collaborative (CMQCC). Retrieved from https://www.cmqcc.org/ob_hemorrhage.

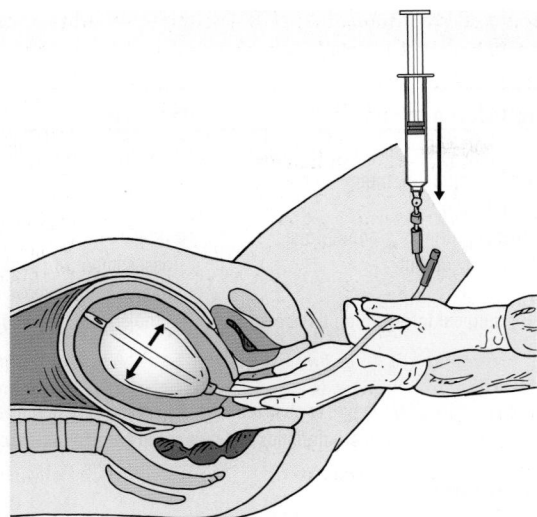

FIG 21.2 Bakri tamponade balloon. (From Bakri, Y.N., & Arulkumaran, S. [2015]. *Intrauterine balloon tamponade for control of postpartum hemorrhage.* Retrieved from http://www.uptodate.com/contents/intrauterine-balloon-tamponade-for-control-of-postpartum-hemorrhage.)

BOX 21.2 Noninvasive Assessments of Cardiac Output in Postpartum Women With Excessive Bleeding

Palpation of Pulses (Rate, Quality, Equality)
- Arterial

Auscultation
- Heart sounds/murmurs
- Breath sounds

Inspection
- Skin color, temperature, turgor
- Level of consciousness
- Capillary refill
- Neck veins
- Mucous membranes

Observation
- Presence or absence of anxiety, apprehension, restlessness, disorientation

Measurement
- Blood pressure
- Pulse oximetry
- Urinary output

fibrinogen, fibrin split products, prothrombin time, and partial thromboplastin time. Blood type and antibody screen are done if not previously performed (Cunningham et al., 2014).

If bleeding persists, bimanual compression may be performed by the obstetrician or nurse-midwife. This procedure involves inserting a fist into the vagina and pressing the knuckles against the anterior side of the uterus, and then placing the other hand on the abdomen and massaging the posterior uterus with it. If the uterus still does not become firm, the health care provider performs manual exploration of the uterine cavity for retained placental fragments.

Surgical Management

If the preceding procedures are ineffective, surgical management is needed. Surgical management options include uterine tamponade (uterine packing or an intrauterine tamponade balloon), bilateral uterine artery ligation, ligation of utero-ovarian arteries and infundibulopelvic vessels, and selective arterial embolization. Uterine compression suturing (e.g., B-Lynch or Hayman vertical sutures) may be performed and is sometimes combined with a tamponade balloon (Fig. 21.2). If these treatment measures are ineffective, hysterectomy likely is needed (Cunningham et al., 2014; Francois & Foley, 2017).

Nursing Interventions

The nurse must be alert to the symptoms of hemorrhage and be prepared to act quickly to minimize blood loss (see Fig. 21.1). Astute assessment of circulatory status can be done with noninvasive monitoring (Box 21.2). This means the nurse must monitor the woman's vital signs frequently. Nursing diagnoses, expected outcomes of care, and interventions are based on the cause of PPH as previously discussed (see Nursing Care Plan: Postpartum Hemorrhage).

The woman and her family will be anxious about her condition. In an emergent care situation, the nurse can provide brief explanations about interventions being performed and the need to act quickly. Family members will likely be asked to leave the room while the hemorrhage team is intervening. After the event, the nurse can help the woman and her family to understand what occurred and the interventions that were needed.

Once the woman's condition is stabilized and she has begun the recovery process, preparations for discharge are made. Discharge instructions for the woman who experienced PPH are similar to those for any postpartum woman. In addition, the woman should be told that she will probably feel fatigue, even exhaustion, and will need to limit her physical activities to conserve her strength. She may need instructions about increasing her dietary iron and protein intake and iron supplementation to rebuild lost red blood cell (RBC) volume. She may need assistance with infant care and household activities until she has regained strength. The nurse should assess the mother's anticipated level of support from family and friends and help the mother plan how to ask for help when returning home. Some mothers experiencing a PPH have problems with delayed lactogenesis, insufficient milk production, or postpartum depression (PPD). Interprofessional care for the woman may include lactation consultants, obstetric and pediatric health care providers, mental health providers, social workers, and home care nurses. Referrals for home care follow-up or to community resources may be needed, including lactation support or a postpartum doula service.

HEMORRHAGIC (HYPOVOLEMIC) SHOCK

Hemorrhage can result in **hemorrhagic (hypovolemic) shock**. Shock is an emergency situation in which the perfusion of body organs can become severely compromised and death can occur. Physiologic compensatory mechanisms are activated in response to hemorrhage. The adrenal glands release catecholamines, causing arterioles and venules in the skin, lungs, gastrointestinal tract, liver, and kidneys to constrict. The available blood flow is diverted to the brain and heart and away from other organs, including the uterus. If shock is prolonged, the continued reduction in cellular oxygenation results in an accumulation of lactic acid and acidosis (from anaerobic glucose metabolism). Acidosis (lowered serum pH) causes arteriolar vasodilation; venule vasoconstriction persists. A circular pattern is established (i.e., decreased perfusion, increased tissue anoxia and acidosis, edema formation, and pooling of blood further decrease the perfusion). Cellular death occurs. See

◎ NURSING CARE PLAN
Postpartum Hemorrhage

Case Study

Marti, a 25-year-old, gave birth to twins at 38 weeks of gestation after being induced with IV oxytocin for preeclampsia. This is Marti's fourth pregnancy; she has three children, ages 2, 4, and 6 years old. The first twin was delivered spontaneously, but forceps were used to deliver the second one. Marti is 8 hours postpartum on magnesium sulfate 1 g/hour IV. Postpartum oxytocin was discontinued at the 7-hour postpartum check as the fundus was firm and lochia was moderate.

At this postpartum check, the fundus is boggy and located 3 cm above the umbilicus. It did not respond to fundal massage. The peripad was soaked completely, and more lochia was noted on the underpad. Marti says she feels weak and dizzy and worried that something is wrong. Vital signs are BP 90/60, pulse 90 and thready, respirations 22, temperature 37.8° C (100.1° F), O$_2$ saturation 95%, and urine output 50 mL since giving birth 8 hours ago. Marti appears pale, and her skin is cool.

The nurse notified the physician using the SBAR technique and is initiating the unit's protocol for postpartum hemorrhage.

Assessment

What are the important risk factors and signs of postpartum hemorrhage present in this situation?

Risk Factors

Overdistended uterus with twin pregnancy
Postpartum magnesium sulfate IV for 8 hours
Forcep delivery with second twin
Oxytocin-induced labor

Defining Characteristics

Uterine atony unresponsive to massage
Increased bleeding
Increased pulse rate
Increased respirations
Pale, cool skin
Change in sensorium: dizzy, anxious

Nursing Diagnosis

Deficient Fluid Volume related to postpartum hemorrhage

Expected Outcomes

Marti will demonstrate fluid balance as evidenced by stable vital signs, prompt capillary refill time, and balanced intake and output.

Nursing Interventions	Rationales
Monitor vital signs, oxygen saturation, urine specific gravity, and capillary refill.	To provide baseline data and detect changes
Activate postpartum hemorrhage team or rapid response team.	To provide emergent interprofessional care
Measure and record amount and type of bleeding by weighing and counting saturated pads; save any clots and tissue for further examination.	To estimate type and amount of blood loss for fluid replacement
Provide quiet environment.	To promote rest and decrease metabolic demands
Give explanation of all procedures.	To reduce anxiety
Begin intravenous (IV) access with 18-gauge or larger catheter for infusion of isotonic solution as ordered.	To provide fluid or blood replacement

Nursing Interventions	Rationales
Administer medications as ordered, such as oxytocin, misoprostol, methylergonovine, or prostaglandin F$_{2\alpha}$.	To increase contractility of uterus
Insert indwelling urinary catheter, and monitor hourly output.	To provide most accurate assessment of renal function and hypovolemia
Prepare for surgical intervention as needed.	To stop source of bleeding

Assessment

Anxiety is characterized by vague, uneasy feelings of discomfort or apprehension. What kind of feeling or characteristics are present in Marti's situation?

Defining Characteristics

Worry
Apprehension
Fear
Altered respiratory pattern
Increased pulse rate
Faintness
Threat to current status
Awareness of physiologic symptoms

Nursing Diagnosis

Anxiety related to sudden change in health status

Expected Outcomes

Marti will verbalize that anxious feelings are diminished.

Nursing Interventions	Rationales
Using therapeutic communication, evaluate Marti's understanding of events.	To provide clarification of any misconceptions
Provide calm, competent attitude and quiet environment.	To aid in decreasing anxiety
Explain all procedures.	To decrease anxiety about the unknown
Encourage Marti to verbalize feelings.	To permit clarification of information and promote trust
Continue to assess vital signs or other clinical indicators of hypovolemic shock.	To evaluate if psychologic response of anxiety intensifies physiologic indicators

Assessment

What cardiovascular or pulmonary responses can occur due to postpartum hemorrhage?

Defining Characteristics

Hypovolemia
Hypoxia
Vasoconstriction
Acidosis

Nursing Diagnosis

Risk for Altered Tissue Perfusion related to hypovolemia

◉ NURSING CARE PLAN

Postpartum Hemorrhage—cont'd

Expected Outcomes

Marti will have stable vital signs, and oxygen saturation, arterial blood gases, and hematocrit and hemoglobin will be within normal limits.

Nursing Interventions	Rationales
Monitor vital signs, oxygen saturation, arterial blood gases, and hematocrit and hemoglobin.	To assess for hypovolemic shock, decreased tissue perfusion, acidosis, or hypoxia
Assess capillary refill, mucous membranes, and skin temperature.	To note indicators of vasoconstriction
Give supplementary oxygen by nonrebreather face mask as ordered.	To provide additional oxygenation to tissues
Administer sodium bicarbonate if ordered.	To reverse metabolic acidosis

Assessment

What are the signs of infection that the nurse should look for after stabilization of Marti's condition?

Defining Characteristics

Increased temperature
Increased pulse rate
Foul-smelling lochia
Perineal redness, warmth
Chills

Nursing Diagnosis

Risk for Infection related to blood loss and invasive procedures as result of postpartum hemorrhage

Expected Outcomes

Marti will demonstrate no signs of infection.
Marti will verbalize understanding of risk factors.

Nursing Interventions	Rationales
Maintain Standard Precautions, and use proper hand hygiene technique when providing care.	To prevent introduction of or spread of infection
Teach Marti to maintain proper hand hygiene (particularly before handling her newborn) and to maintain scrupulous perineal care with frequent change and careful disposal of perineal pads.	To avoid spread of microorganisms
Monitor vital signs.	To detect signs of systemic infection
Monitor level of fatigue and lethargy, evidence of chills, loss of appetite, nausea and vomiting, and abdominal pain.	To indicate extent of infection and serve as indicators of status of infection
Monitor lochia for foul smell.	To detect signs of infection
Assist with collection of intrauterine cultures or other specimens for laboratory analysis.	To identify specific causative organism
Monitor laboratory values (i.e., white blood cell [WBC] count, cultures).	To indicate type and status of infection
Ensure adequate fluid and nutritional intake.	To promote healthy recovery
Administer and monitor broad-spectrum antibiotics as ordered.	To prevent or treat infection
Administer antipyretics as ordered and necessary.	To reduce elevated temperature

BP, Blood pressure.

Emergency Treatment: Hemorrhagic Shock for assessments and interventions for hemorrhagic shock.

CARE MANAGEMENT

Interprofessional teamwork and collaboration are key to managing care of postpartum women who experience hemorrhagic shock. The woman is likely to be transferred to a critical care unit for stabilization and ongoing care and monitoring.

MEDICAL MANAGEMENT

Vigorous treatment is necessary to prevent adverse outcomes. Management of hypovolemic shock involves restoring circulating blood volume and eliminating the cause of the hemorrhage (e.g., lacerations, uterine atony, or inversion). Venous access with a large-bore IV catheter is critical to successful care management of the woman with a hemorrhagic complication. Establishing two IV lines facilitates fluid resuscitation. Fluid resuscitation includes administering crystalloids (lactated Ringer's, normal saline solution), colloids (albumin), blood, and blood components. To restore circulating blood volume, a rapid IV infusion of crystalloid solution is given at a rate of 3 mL infused for every 1 mL of estimated blood loss (e.g., 3000 mL infused for 1000 mL of blood loss). Packed red blood cells (RBCs) are usually infused if the woman

is still actively bleeding and no improvement in her condition is noted after the initial crystalloid infusion. Infusion of fresh frozen plasma may be needed if clotting factors and platelet counts are below normal values (Cunningham et al., 2014; Francois & Foley, 2017).

NURSING INTERVENTIONS

Hemorrhagic shock can occur rapidly, but the classic signs of shock may not appear until the postpartum woman has lost 30% to 40% of blood volume. By the time vital signs are abnormal, the woman may be in an advanced stage of shock. The shock index has been proposed as a parameter to identify early stages of hypovolemic shock. Shock index is the ratio of heart rate to systolic blood pressure; with shock, as the heart rate increases, the blood pressure decreases. For example, with a heart rate of 120 and a systolic BP of 90, the shock index is 1.3. A shock index >1.1 suggests significant blood loss, even before there are notable changes in the vital signs (Fleischer & Meirowitz, 2016).

Major goals of care are to restore oxygen delivery to the tissues and to maintain cardiac output. Fluid resuscitation must be monitored carefully because fluid overload can occur. Intravascular fluid overload occurs most often with colloid therapy.

If the woman is actively bleeding and unstable despite fluid boluses, transfusion of blood products is needed. There should be protocols in

✚ EMERGENCY TREATMENT

Hemorrhagic Shock

Assessments	Characteristics
• Respirations	• Rapid and shallow
• Pulse	• Rapid, weak, irregular
• Blood pressure	• Decreasing (late sign)
• Skin	• Cool, pale, clammy
• Urinary output	• Decreasing
• Level of consciousness	• Lethargy → coma
• Mental status	• Anxiety → coma
• Central venous pressure	• Decreased

Interventions

• Summon assistance and equipment.
• Start intravenous infusion per standing orders.
• Ensure patent airway; administer oxygen.
• Continue to monitor status.

place for emergency release of blood products; these products may be universally compatible (e.g., O-negative red blood cells or AB plasma) or type-specific if the woman's blood type is known and the supply is available. A massive transfusion protocol facilitates timely access to and administration of blood products (Fleischer & Meirowitz, 2016).

Transfusion reactions can follow administration of blood or blood components, including cryoprecipitate. Even in an emergency, each unit of blood or blood products should be carefully checked per hospital protocol. Complications of fluid or blood replacement therapy include hemolytic reactions, febrile reactions, allergic reactions, circulatory overload, and air embolism.

The nurse continues to monitor the woman's pulse and blood pressure. If invasive hemodynamic monitoring is ordered, the nurse may assist with placement of a central venous pressure (CVP) or pulmonary artery (Swan-Ganz) catheter. Subsequently, the nurse monitors CVP, pulmonary artery pressure, or pulmonary artery wedge pressure as ordered.

Additional assessments include evaluating skin temperature, color, and turgor and mucous membranes. Breath sounds should be auscultated before fluid volume replacement to provide a baseline for future assessment. Inspection for signs of DIC such as oozing at the sites of incisions or injections, and assessment for the presence of petechiae or ecchymosis in areas not associated with surgery or trauma are critical in evaluating for DIC (see Chapter 12).

Oxygen is administered, preferably by a nonrebreather face mask, at 10 to 12 L/min to maintain oxygen saturation. Oxygen saturation should be monitored with a pulse oximeter, although measurements are not always accurate in a patient with hypovolemia or decreased perfusion. Level of consciousness is assessed frequently and provides additional indications of blood volume and oxygen saturation. In early stages of decreased blood flow, the woman may report "seeing stars" or feeling dizzy or nauseated. She can become restless and orthopneic. As cerebral hypoxia increases, she can become confused and react slowly to stimuli or not at all. Some women complain of headaches.

Continuous electrocardiographic monitoring may be indicated for the woman who is hypotensive or tachycardic or continues to bleed profusely. A Foley catheter is inserted and a urometer is attached to allow hourly assessment of urine output. The most objective and least invasive assessment of adequate organ perfusion and oxygenation is a

urine output of at least 30 mL/hour (Cunningham et al., 2014). Hemoglobin and hematocrit levels, platelet count, and coagulation studies are closely monitored.

COAGULOPATHIES

When bleeding is continuous and there is no identifiable source, a coagulopathy can be the cause. The woman's coagulation status must be assessed quickly and continuously. Abnormal results depend on the cause and can include increased prothrombin time, increased partial thromboplastin time, decreased platelets, decreased fibrinogen level, increased fibrin degradation products, and prolonged bleeding time. Causes of coagulopathies can include pregnancy complications such as idiopathic or immune thrombocytopenic purpura, von Willebrand disease, or DIC.

IDIOPATHIC THROMBOCYTOPENIC PURPURA

Idiopathic or immune thrombocytopenic purpura (ITP) is an autoimmune disorder in which antiplatelet antibodies decrease the life span of the platelets. Thrombocytopenia, capillary fragility, and increased bleeding time are diagnostic findings. ITP can cause severe hemorrhage after cesarean birth or cervical or vaginal lacerations. The incidence of postpartum uterine bleeding and vaginal hematomas is also increased. Neonatal thrombocytopenia can result, but serious bleeding is unusual (Samuels, 2017).

Medical management focuses on control of platelet stability. If ITP was diagnosed during pregnancy, the woman likely was treated with corticosteroids or IV immunoglobulin. Platelet transfusions are usually given when there is significant bleeding. A splenectomy may be needed if the ITP does not respond to medical management (Cunningham et al., 2014).

VON WILLEBRAND DISEASE

von Willebrand disease (vWD), a type of hemophilia, is the most common congenital bleeding disorder. It results from a deficiency or defect in a blood clotting protein called *von Willebrand factor (vWF)*. There are as many as 20 variations of vWD, most of which are inherited as autosomal dominant traits; types I and II are the most common. Symptoms include recurrent bleeding episodes such as nosebleeds or after tooth extraction, bruising easily, prolonged bleeding time (the most important test), factor VIII deficiency (mild to moderate), and bleeding from mucous membranes. Although factor VIII increases during pregnancy, a risk for PPH still exists as levels of vWF begin to decrease (Cunningham et al., 2014). The woman can be at risk for bleeding for up to 4 weeks after birth.

The treatment of choice is administration of desmopressin, which promotes the release of vWF and factor VIII. It can be given nasally, intravenously, or orally. Transfusion therapy with plasma products that have been treated for viruses and contain factor VIII and vWF also may be used. Concentrates of antihemophiliac factor (Humate-P or Alphanate) can be administered (Cunningham et al., 2014).

VENOUS THROMBOEMBOLIC DISORDERS

Venous thromboembolism (VTE) results from the formation of a blood clot or clots inside a blood vessel and is caused by inflammation (**thrombophlebitis**) or partial obstruction of the vessel (Fig. 21.3). Three thromboembolic conditions are of concern in the postpartum period: *Superficial venous thrombosis*—Involvement of the superficial saphenous venous system

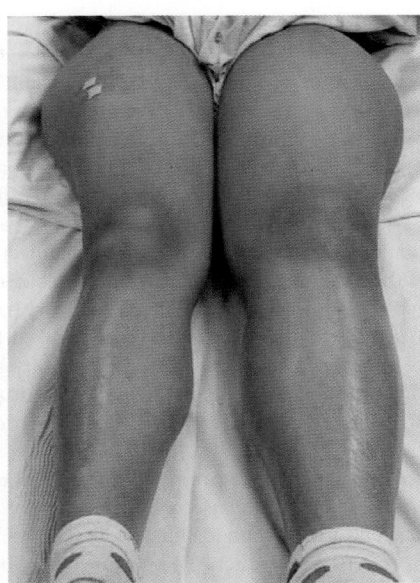

FIG 21.3 Deep vein thrombophlebitis. (From Murphy, E.H., Davis, C.M., Journeycake, J.M., et al. [2009]. Symptomatic ileofemoral DVT after onset of oral contraceptive use in women with previously undiagnosed May-Thurner Syndrome. *Journal of Vascular Surgery, 49*(3), 697–703.)

Deep vein thrombosis (DVT)—Occurs most often in the lower extremities; involvement varies but can extend from the foot to the iliofemoral region

Pulmonary embolism (PE)—Complication of DVT occurring when part of a blood clot dislodges and is carried to the pulmonary artery, where it occludes the vessel and obstructs blood flow to the lungs

INCIDENCE AND ETIOLOGY

The incidence of venous thromboembolism (VTE) is approximately 1 in 1500 pregnancies (Pettker & Lockwood, 2017). VTE can occur in any trimester of pregnancy and in the postpartum period. The highest incidence of postpartum VTE is during the first 3 weeks after birth (Tepper, Boulet, Whiteman, et al., 2014). DVT occurs most often during pregnancy, and PE is more common in the postpartum period. The incidence of VTE in the postpartum period has declined since early ambulation after childbirth has become standard practice. However, PE is a major cause of maternal death.

The primary causes of thromboembolic disease are venous stasis and hypercoagulation, both of which are present in pregnancy and continue into the postpartum period. Cesarean birth nearly doubles the risk for VTE; therefore, routine preoperative placement of pneumatic compression devices is recommended. For women with risk factors such as obesity, immobility, malignancy, or other chronic medical conditions, prophylactic low-dose heparin may be administered prior to cesarean birth. Other risk factors include operative vaginal birth; history of venous thrombosis, pulmonary embolism, or varicosities; maternal age older than 35 years; multiparity; and smoking (Pettker & Lockwood, 2017). Women who experience complications such as preeclampsia, hemorrhage, or postpartum infection have an increased risk for VTE (Tepper et al., 2014).

CLINICAL MANIFESTATIONS

Superficial venous thrombosis is the most common form of postpartum thrombophlebitis. It is characterized by pain and tenderness in the lower extremity. Physical examination may reveal warmth; redness; and an enlarged, hardened vein over the site of the thrombosis.

Deep vein thrombosis is more common during pregnancy than in the postpartum period and is characterized by unilateral leg pain, calf tenderness, and swelling. Physical examination may reveal redness, warmth, and a positive Homan sign, although women can have a large clot with few symptoms (Leung & Lockwood, 2014).

Acute pulmonary embolism (PE) usually results from dislodged deep vein thrombi. The most common presenting symptoms are dyspnea and chest pain. Other signs of PE include tachypnea (more than 20 breaths/minute), tachycardia (more than 100 beats/minute), apprehension, cough, hemoptysis, elevated temperature, and syncope (Cunningham et al., 2014; Leung & Lockwood, 2014).

Physical examination is not a sensitive diagnostic indicator for thrombosis. Compression ultrasonography with or without color Doppler is the most commonly used diagnostic test. MRI and D-dimer assays also may be used (Leung & Lockwood, 2014). With PE, echocardiographic abnormalities may be seen in right ventricular size or function. Pregnancy limits the usefulness of arterial blood gases and oxygen saturation in diagnosis. A ventilation-perfusion scan, spiral computed tomography scan, magnetic resonance angiography, and pulmonary arteriogram may be used for diagnosis (Leung & Lockwood, 2014).

MEDICAL MANAGEMENT

Superficial venous thrombosis is treated with analgesia (nonsteroidal antiinflammatory agents), rest with elevation of the affected leg, and elastic compression stockings (Cunningham et al., 2014). Heat may also be applied locally.

DVT is initially treated with anticoagulant therapy (usually continuous IV heparin), bed rest with the affected leg elevated, and analgesia. After the symptoms have decreased, the woman may be fitted with elastic compression stockings to wear when she is allowed to ambulate. She is taught how to put on the stockings before getting out of bed. IV heparin therapy continues for 3 to 5 days or until symptoms resolve. Oral anticoagulant therapy (warfarin [Coumadin]) is started during this time and will be continued for about 3 months. If a breastfeeding mother is on long-term anticoagulant therapy, the infant's prothrombin time should be monitored at least monthly and vitamin K given to the infant if necessary (Lawrence & Lawrence, 2016).

Acute PE is an emergent situation that requires prompt treatment. Massive pulmonary emboli can lead to pulmonary hypertension and right ventricular dysfunction; if right ventricular dysfunction is present, mortality can be as high as 25% (Cunningham et al., 2014). Immediate treatment of PE is anticoagulant therapy. Continuous IV heparin therapy is used for PE until symptoms have resolved. Intermittent subcutaneous heparin or oral anticoagulant therapy is often continued for up to 6 months (Pettker & Lockwood, 2017).

NURSING INTERVENTIONS

In the birthing facility, nursing care of the woman with a thrombosis consists of ongoing assessments: inspecting and palpating the affected area; palpating the peripheral pulses; and measuring and comparing leg circumferences. Signs of PE, including chest pain, coughing, dyspnea, and tachypnea, and respiratory status for presence of crackles are also assessed. Laboratory reports are monitored for prothrombin or partial thromboplastin times. The nurse assesses for unusual bleeding. Increased lochia, generalized petechiae, hematuria, or oozing from venipuncture sites should be immediately reported to the health care provider (James, 2014). In addition, the woman and her family are assessed for their level of understanding about the diagnosis and their ability to cope during the unexpected extended period of recovery.

Interventions include explanations and education about diagnosis and treatment. The woman will need assistance with personal care as long as she is on bed rest; the family should be encouraged to participate in the care if that is what she and they wish. While the woman is on bed rest, she should be encouraged to change positions frequently but to avoid placing her knees in a sharply flexed position that could cause pooling of blood in the lower extremities. She also should be cautioned to avoid rubbing the affected area because this action could cause the clot to dislodge. Heparin and warfarin are administered as ordered, and the health care provider is notified if clotting times are outside the therapeutic level. If the woman is breastfeeding, she is informed that neither heparin nor warfarin is excreted in significant quantities in breast milk (Lawrence & Lawrence, 2016). If the infant has been discharged, the family is encouraged to bring the infant for feedings as permitted by hospital policy; the woman also can express milk to be sent home.

Pain can be managed with a variety of measures. Changing positions, elevating the leg, and applying moist heat may decrease discomfort. It may be necessary to administer analgesics and antiinflammatory medications.

The woman is usually discharged home on oral anticoagulants and will need an explanation of the treatment schedule and possible side effects. If subcutaneous injections are to be given, the woman and family are taught how to administer the medication and about site rotation. They should also be given information about dietary restrictions (e.g., limited intake of green, leafy vegetables) and safe care practices to prevent bleeding and injury while she is on anticoagulant therapy (e.g., using a soft toothbrush and an electric razor). She will need information about follow-up with her health care provider to monitor clotting times and regulate the correct dosage of anticoagulant therapy. The woman should also use a reliable form of contraception if taking warfarin because this medication is considered teratogenic. Oral contraceptives are contraindicated because of the increased risk for thrombosis (Cunningham et al., 2014).

MEDICATION ALERT

Medications containing aspirin are not given to women on anticoagulant therapy because aspirin inhibits synthesis of clotting factors and can lead to prolonged clotting time and increased risk for bleeding.

POSTPARTUM INFECTION

Postpartum infection, or *puerperal infection,* is any clinical infection of the genital tract that occurs within 28 days after miscarriage, induced abortion, or birth. The definition used in the United States continues to be the presence of a fever of 38° C (100.4° F) or more on 2 successive days of the first 10 postpartum days (not counting the first 24 hours after birth).

Endometritis is the most common puerperal infection (Isley & Katz, 2017). Other common postpartum infections include wound infections, urinary tract infections (UTIs), and respiratory tract infections. Mastitis, or breast infection, should also be considered as a possible diagnosis among breastfeeding mothers, with symptoms such as fever, malaise, flu-like symptoms, and a sore area in a breast (Lawrence & Lawrence, 2016) (Fig. 21.4). (See Chapter 24 for further discussion of mastitis.)

The most common infecting organisms are the numerous streptococcal and anaerobic organisms. *Staphylococcus aureus, gonococci,* coliform bacteria, and *clostridia* are less common but serious pathogenic organisms that can cause puerperal infection. Postpartum infections are more common in women who have concurrent medical or immunosuppressive conditions or who had a cesarean or other operative birth. Intrapartal factors such as prolonged rupture of membranes, prolonged labor, and intrauterine monitoring of uterine contractions or fetal heart rate and pattern increase the risk for infection (Cunningham et al., 2014). Factors that predispose the woman to postpartum infection are listed in Box 21.3.

ENDOMETRITIS

Endometritis (infection of the lining of the uterus) usually begins as a localized infection at the placental site but can spread to the entire endometrium. The highest incidence occurs in women who gave birth by cesarean after prolonged labor and rupture of membranes. Prophylactic antibiotics administered during labor and during cesarean surgery can help reduce the incidence and severity of endometritis.

Signs of endometritis include fever (usually greater than 38° C [100.4° F]), increased pulse, chills, anorexia, nausea, fatigue and lethargy, pelvic pain, uterine tenderness, and foul-smelling, profuse lochia. Leukocytosis and a markedly increased RBC sedimentation rate are typical laboratory findings. Anemia can also be present. Blood cultures or intracervical or intrauterine bacterial cultures (aerobic and anaerobic) should

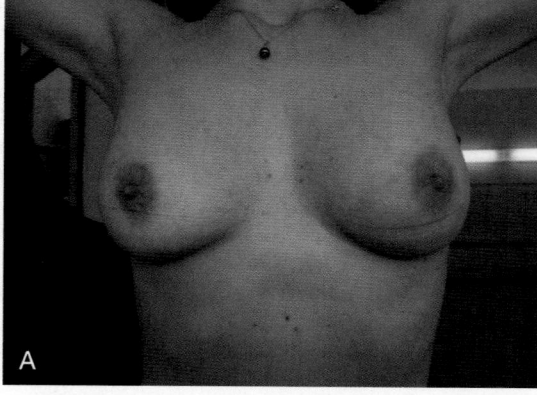
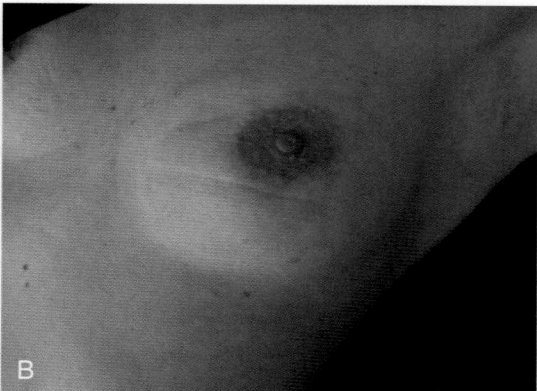

FIG 21.4 Mastitis. **A,** Comparison of left breast with mastitis to normal right breast. **B,** Closer view of inflamed right lower quadrant of left breast. (From Boutet, G. [2012]. Breast inflammation: Clinical examination, aetiological pointers. *Diagnostic and Interventional Imaging, 93*[2], 78–84.)

BOX 21.3 Predisposing Factors for Postpartum Infection

Preconception or Antepartal Factors

- History of previous venous thrombosis, urinary tract infection, mastitis, pneumonia
- Diabetes mellitus
- Alcoholism
- Drug abuse
- Immunosuppression
- Anemia
- Malnutrition
- Obesity
- Preeclampsia

Intrapartal Factors

- Cesarean birth
- Operative vaginal birth
- Prolonged rupture of membranes
- Chorioamnionitis
- Prolonged labor
- Bladder catheterization
- Internal fetal heart rate/uterine contraction monitoring
- Multiple vaginal examinations after rupture of membranes
- Epidural analgesia/anesthesia
- Retained placental fragments
- Postpartum hemorrhage
- Episiotomy or lacerations
- Hematomas

reveal the offending pathogens within 36 to 48 hours (Cunningham et al., 2014).

Management

Management of endometritis consists of IV broad-spectrum antibiotic therapy (cephalosporins, penicillins, or clindamycin and gentamicin) and supportive care, including hydration, rest, and pain relief. Antibiotic therapy is usually discontinued 24 hours after the woman is asymptomatic. Assessments of lochia, vital signs, and changes in the woman's condition continue during treatment. Comfort measures depend on the symptoms and may include cool compresses, warm blankets, perineal care, and sitz baths. Patient education should include side effects of therapy, prevention of spread of infection, signs and symptoms of worsening condition, adherence to the treatment plan, and the need for follow-up care. Women may need to be encouraged or assisted to maintain mother-infant interactions and breastfeeding.

WOUND INFECTIONS

Wound infections are common postpartum infections that often develop after mothers are discharged home. Rates of wound infection after cesarean birth are 3% to 5%. Women can also develop infection in the perineum in a repaired laceration or episiotomy site. Predisposing factors are similar to those for endometritis (see Box 21.3). Signs of wound infection include fever, erythema, edema, warmth, tenderness, pain, seropurulent drainage, and wound separation.

Management

Culture of wound exudate is performed to identify the causative organism. Wound infections are treated with intravenous antibiotic therapy. When pus is present in the incision, the wound is opened and drained. Wounds are irrigated with normal saline and re-dressed several times daily; healing occurs by secondary intention. In some cases, a wound vacuum device is used. Antibiotic treatment is continued until the base of the wound appears clear and there are no apparent signs of cellulitis (Duff & Birsner, 2017).

Nursing care includes frequent assessments of temperature and vital signs; wound assessment and care; and comfort measures such as analgesics, sitz baths, warm compresses, and perineal care. Teaching includes hygienic care techniques (e.g., changing perineal pads front to back, hand hygiene before and after perineal care), self-care measures, and signs of worsening conditions to report to the obstetric health care provider. Wound care and assessment will continue after discharge from the birthing facility. The woman and her family are instructed in how to perform wound care and dressing changes. Home visits by nurses may be provided to assess the wound, reinforce teaching, and offer support. If intravenous antibiotic therapy is continued in the home, it is likely to be administered by the family with regular monitoring by the visiting nurse.

URINARY TRACT INFECTIONS

Urinary tract infections (UTIs) occur in 2% to 4% of postpartum women. Risk factors include urinary catheterization, frequent pelvic examinations, regional (epidural or spinal) anesthesia, genital tract injury, history of UTI, and cesarean birth. Signs and symptoms include dysuria, frequency and urgency, low-grade fever, urinary retention, hematuria, and pyuria. Costovertebral angle tenderness or flank pain can indicate upper UTI. The most common infecting organism is *Escherichia coli*, although other gram-negative aerobic bacilli can cause UTIs.

Management

Medical management for UTIs consists of antibiotic therapy, analgesia, and hydration. Postpartum women are usually treated on an outpatient basis; therefore, teaching should include instructions on how to monitor temperature, bladder function, and appearance of urine. The woman should also be taught about signs of potential complications and the importance of taking all antibiotics as prescribed. Other suggestions for prevention of UTIs include proper perineal care, wiping from front to back after urinating or having a bowel movement, and increasing fluid intake. Unsweetened cranberry juice or cranberry supplements may be beneficial in preventing UTI.

CARE MANAGEMENT

ASSESSMENT AND NURSING DIAGNOSES

Women who are predisposed to postpartum infection (see Box 21.3) should be assessed carefully. Signs and symptoms associated with postpartum infection were discussed with each infection. Elevation of temperature, redness, and swelling are common signs. The mother may also complain of chills, fever, localized tenderness, or pain. Depending on the type of infection, laboratory tests usually include a complete blood count, venous blood cultures, urine cultures, and uterine tissue cultures. Assessment includes a review of the woman's history, and the laboratory results should be included in the assessment. Nursing diagnoses for women experiencing postpartum infection are listed in Box 21.4.

Interventions

The most effective and least expensive treatment of postpartum infection is prevention. Preventive measures include good prenatal nutrition to reduce the risk for anemia. Proper maternal perineal hygiene with thorough hand hygiene is emphasized. Strict adherence to aseptic techniques by all health care personnel caring for women during labor, birth, and the postpartum period is very important. Specific medical, surgical, and nursing interventions were discussed with each infection.

Postpartum women are usually discharged to home by 48 hours after birth. This is often before signs of infection are evident. Nurses in birth centers and hospital settings must be able to identify women at risk for postpartum infection and provide anticipatory teaching and counseling before discharge. This teaching should include the signs of infection and when to notify the health care provider. After discharge, telephone follow-up, hotlines, support groups, lactation counselors, home visits by nurses, and teaching materials (videos, written materials) can be used to quickly identify postpartum infection. Home care nurses must be able to recognize the signs and symptoms of postpartum infection and then contact the mother's primary health care provider or have her make the contact. Home care nurses must also be able to provide the appropriate nursing care for women who need follow-up care at home. See Chapter 2 for more information about home visits.

POSTPARTUM MOOD DISORDERS

The weeks after birth are a time of vulnerability to psychologic complications for many women, causing significant distress for the mother, disrupting family life, and, if prolonged, negatively affecting the child's emotional and social development. Preexisting mood and anxiety disorders are particularly likely to recur or worsen during these weeks. Such conditions can interfere with attachment to the newborn and family integration, and some may threaten the safety and well-being of the mother, the newborn, and other children. Because birth is usually thought to be a happy event, a new mother's emotional distress can puzzle and immobilize family and friends. When she most needs the caring attention of loved ones, they may either criticize or withdraw because of their anxiety. Nurses can offer anticipatory guidance, assess the mental health of new mothers, offer therapeutic interventions, and make referrals when necessary. Failure to do so can result in tragic consequences. In rare cases, a disturbed mother may kill her infant, other family members, or herself.

Mood disorders are the predominant mental health disorder in the postpartum period (American Psychiatric Association [APA], 2013).

Up to 85% of women experience a mild depression or "baby blues" after the birth of a child; however, the woman's functioning is usually not impaired. Baby blues are characterized by mood swings, feelings of sadness and anxiety, crying, difficulty sleeping, and loss of appetite. The symptoms resolve within a few days, and treatment is not needed (Paschetta, Berrisford, Coccia, et al., 2014).

POSTPARTUM DEPRESSION

Prevalence estimates of postpartum depression vary based on the definition and the period of time included. PPD is experienced by approximately 8% to 20% of women during the postpartum period (Isley & Katz, 2017). It is likely that the actual occurrence of PPD exceeds the reported estimates because it is often unrecognized and undiagnosed (American College of Obstetricians and Gynecologists [ACOG], 2015).

The cause of PPD can be biologic, psychologic, situational, or multifactorial. The change from the high levels of estrogen and progesterone at the end of pregnancy to the much lower levels of both hormones that are present after birth are important etiologic factors in the development of PPD. While all women experience these hormonal changes, there are some who are more sensitive to the mood-destabilizing effects of withdrawal from the pregnancy hormones and are therefore at risk for PPD (O'Hara & Wisner, 2014). Poor nutrition may also be a contributing factor. Folate and vitamin B_{12} are needed for the synthesis of serotonin and other neurotransmitters. Marginal or low folate also increases the likelihood of a poor response to antidepressant medication as well as the potential for relapse in people who initially responded well to pharmacologic therapy (Wisner, Sit, Bogen, et al., 2017).

Women at greatest risk for PPD are those with a history of anxiety or depression and especially those who had a previous episode of major depressive disorder in the past, including during or after pregnancy (Cunningham et al., 2014). Other risk factors include younger age, unintended pregnancy, personal history of severe premenstrual dysphoria, family history of mood disorder, unmarried status, marital discord, lack of social support, socioeconomic deprivation, lower education, substance abuse, low self-esteem, and stressful life events (O'Hara & McCabe, 2013; Wisner et al., 2017). Women facing multiple or severe psychosocial problems or chronic interpersonal difficulties are at increased risk for PPD. Complications of pregnancy and birth increase the risk for PPD. Having a preterm, low–birth weight, and ill neonate is associated with higher rates of PPD (Alkozei, McMahon, & Lahav, 2014). Women who are victims of intimate partner violence are at increased risk for PPD (Beydoun, Beydoun, Kaufman, et al., 2012; Kothari, Liepman, Tareen, et al., 2016; Woolhouse, Gartland, Hegarty, et al., 2012). Cultural practices can positively or negatively affect the development of PPD.

Paternal Postpartum Depression

It is estimated that paternal perinatal depression (PPND) occurs in approximately 8% to 10% of men during the period of time from the first trimester of pregnancy through the first year after birth. During the first 6 months after birth, the incidence increases to approximately 25% (Cameron, Sedov, & Tomfohr-Madsen, 2016; Paulson & Bazemore, 2010).

The best predictor of PPND is having a partner with postpartum depression. Other risk factors are a history of depression, age younger than 25 years, low socioeconomic status, being unmarried, an inadequate support system, and family and social stressors. Men may not exhibit classic symptoms of PPD but are likely to display fatigue, frustration, anger, irritability, indecisiveness, withdrawal from social situations, alcohol/drug use, marital conflict, partner violence, and somatic symptoms (Musser, Ahmed, Foli, & Coddington, 2013). (See Evidence-Based Practice: Paternal Peripartum Depression.)

Men are not routinely screened for perinatal depressive symptoms. There is no depression scale designed for this specific use. Some experts recommend using the Edinburgh Postnatal Depression Scale in combination with the Gotland Male Depression Scale to identify men with signs of PPND (Habib, 2012).

When both the father and the mother are depressed, life can be very difficult. Routine tasks of caring for the newborn and maintaining a household can present significant challenges. Interaction with the infant can be affected, and there can be negative effects on parenting.

Nurses should include partners in discussions about postpartum depression, raising awareness that fathers can also suffer from depression, describing symptoms, and providing information about resources for

EVIDENCE-BASED PRACTICE

Paternal Perinatal Depression

Ask the Question

PICOT Question: For new fathers, what are the risk and protective factors for depression? What are the best ways to screen for depression?

Search for the Evidence

Search Strategies: English research-based publications on depression, father, anxiety, paternal, perinatal, peripartum, and postpartum depression

Databases Used: Cochrane Collaborative Database, National Guideline Clearinghouse (AHRQ), CINAHL, PubMed, and the professional website for ACOG.

Critical Appraisal of the Evidence

When a mother suffers perinatal (first trimester until the infant is 1 year of age) depression, the evidence for poorer growth, cognitive, and behavioral outcomes for her baby is indisputable. Much research continues to understand the decreased maternal responsiveness to her infant's cues. Because family dynamics extend beyond the mother-baby dyad, new research is investigating the implications of paternal depression to the family system (Freitas, Williams-Reade, Distelberg, et al., 2016):

- Incidence of paternal depression (10%) is about half that of maternal depression (up to 20%), but about twice the male baseline rate of 5%.
- Experts from many fields reached structured consensus about defining paternal depression markers as low mood, negative thoughts, feeling inadequate, weight loss, sleep deprivation, and "masked" male depressive symptoms of irritability, isolation or withdrawal, substance abuse, cheating, or gambling.
- Risk factors for paternal depression include prior depression, poor social and relationship support, partner experiencing depression, and financial and work stress. Young paternal age, first child, and unrealistic expectations may also be risk factors.

Massoud, Hwang, and Wickberg (2016) surveyed 885 Swedish couples at 3 months postpartum with the Edinburgh Postnatal Depression Scale (EPDS), which is also validated for fathers:

- Risk for depression doubled when the partner had depression, regardless which partner was the first.
- Other risk factors included prior depression, lower education, lack of support from partner, sleep deprivation, work stress, or conflicts. High EPDS scores for fathers were more likely to represent general distress, worry, anxiety, or unhappiness than actual depression.
- Paternal depressive symptoms are associated with behavioral and relational problems in their offspring, and increased conflict and violence in the home.

Apply the Evidence: Nursing Implications

Nurses who encounter new fathers, especially young and first-time fathers, in any setting should be alert to symptoms of distress, and understand that depression may manifest differently in fathers than in mothers.

- Reaching out to fathers should be a routine part of family-based care, beginning at pregnancy or before. Assessment begins with questions about physical issues such as sleep quality and diet changes, and proceeds sensitively into questions about relational and life distress. Universal screening with validated

screening tools and psychosocial interviews are recommended (Siu & US Preventive Services Task Force, 2016).

- Starting with prenatal visits and continuing with well-child visits, nurses who reach out and include fathers may be in the best position to screen for depression in both parents, and refer for early intervention (Vismara, Rolle, Agostini, et al., 2016).
- Discussing the transition to parenthood, life balance, and distress, and teaching open communication, partner support, and self-care, especially adequate sleep, may be preventive.
- Fathers do not like to be labeled. To avoid stigma, the health care team can call it whatever he wants (Freitas et al., 2016).
- Spreading awareness in society at large, and education for perinatal families in particular, can foster increased open communication, and increase identification of problems early. Advocating for strong health care team relationships with parents and supportive employer, community, and government policies can help, especially with unexpected stressors such as the special needs baby.

Quality and Safety Competencies: Evidence-Based Practice*
Knowledge

Describe EBP to include the components of research evidence, clinical expertise, and patient/family values.

Spread awareness and decrease stigma about the importance of the mental health of both mother and father for the child.

Skills

Participate in structuring the work environment to facilitate integration of new evidence into standards of practice

Include new fathers in family care. Screen for symptoms of depression in both parents.

Attitudes

Value the need for continuous improvement in clinical practice based on new knowledge.

Use validated screening tools, such as the EPDS, and psychosocial interviews.

References

Freitas, C. J., Williams-Reade, J., Distelberg, B., et al. (2016). Paternal depression during pregnancy and postpartum: An international Delphi study. *Journal of Affective Disorders*, 202(15), 128–136.

Massoud, P., Hwang, C. P., & Wickberg, B. (2016). Father's depressive symptoms in the postnatal period: Prevalence and correlates in a population-based Swedish study. *Scandinavian Journal of Public Health*, August 24, 2016. doi:10.1177/1403494816661652. [Epub ahead of print].

Siu, A. L., & US Preventive Services Task Force. (2016). Screening for depression in adults: US Preventive Services Task Force recommendation statement. *Journal of the American Medical Association*, 315(4), 380–387.

Vismara, L., Rolle, L., Agostini, F., et al. (2016). Perinatal parenting stress, anxiety, and depression outcomes in first-time mothers and fathers: A 3- to 6-months postpartum follow-up study. *Frontiers in Psychology, 7,* 938.

Pat Mahaffee Gingrich

*Adapted from QSEN at www.qsen.org/

help if the symptoms occur. During interactions with fathers, nurses can assess for signs of PPND, provide support and encouragement, and offer information about resources for further assessment and treatment (Letourneau, Tryphonopoulos, Duffett-Leger, et al., 2012). The nurse can direct fathers to online resources such as www.postpartummen.com or http://postpartumhealthalliance.org (Stadtlander, 2015).

Signs of Postpartum Depression

Postpartum depression, also known as PPD without psychotic features, is an intense and pervasive sadness with severe and labile mood swings. It is more serious and persistent than postpartum blues, lasting more than 2 weeks. Intense fears, anger, anxiety, and despondency that persist past the baby's first few weeks are not a normal part of postpartum blues. These symptoms rarely disappear without outside help. Most of these mothers seek help only after reaching a "crisis point."

The symptoms of postpartum major depression are very similar to those of adult depression except that the mother's ruminations of guilt and inadequacy feed her worries about being an incompetent and inadequate parent. In PPD, there can be loss of appetite or odd food cravings (often sweet desserts) and binges with abnormal appetite and weight gain. Sleep disturbance is common. Sleep deprivation is a factor in the development of PPD, and it can worsen the symptoms (Park, Meltzer-Brody, & Stickgold, 2013). (See Clinical Reasoning Case Study: Postpartum Depression.)

A distinguishing feature of PPD is irritability. These episodes of irritability can flare up with little provocation, and they sometimes escalate to violent outbursts or dissolve into uncontrollable sobbing. Many of these outbursts are directed against significant others. Women with postpartum major depressive episodes often have severe anxiety, panic attacks, and spontaneous crying long after the usual duration of baby blues.

Feelings of detachment toward the newborn or not feeling love for the newborn are common symptoms of PPD. Women feel guilt and shame for having these feelings and are not likely to verbalize or discuss this with anyone. Many women feel especially guilty about having depressive feelings at a time when they believe they should be happy. They can be reluctant to discuss their symptoms or their negative feelings toward the infant. A woman with PPD may have obsessive thoughts about harming the infant, and this can be very frightening to her. Often she does not share these thoughts because of embarrassment; when she does, other family members become very frightened. On the other hand, some women feel very emotionally attached and connected to their infants; this can prevent them from experiencing total despair (Puryear, 2014).

Medical Management

The natural course is one of gradual improvement over the 6 months after birth. Treatment options for PPD include psychotherapy and antidepressant medication. Antidepressants are the most commonly used treatment; one explanation for this is that primary care providers can prescribe these medications and monitor the woman's progress. In some communities, access to mental health care providers is limited and primary care providers treat women with PPD.

Psychotherapy without the use of medication can be effective for mild cases of PPD. It is often used in combination with antidepressants for moderate to severe cases. Psychotherapy methods include general counseling (listening visits), interpersonal psychotherapy (IPT), cognitive-behavioral therapy (CBT), and psychodynamic therapy (O'Hara & McCabe, 2013). Peer support may be helpful; some women find that postpartum support groups are very beneficial (www.postpartum.net). Internet-based and telephone-based psychotherapy are increasing in use; there is a need for more evidence to support their effectiveness (Stuart & Koleva, 2014). For some women with severe PPD, hospitalization is necessary.

For more severe PPD, antidepressant medication is combined with some form of psychotherapy. Often, an SSRI is prescribed initially and if symptoms improve during a 6-week trial period, the medication is continued for at least 6 months to prevent relapse. If response to the medication is less than optimal, another SSRI may be prescribed instead (Cunningham et al., 2014).

Sleep deprivation must be resolved; 4 to 5 hours of uninterrupted sleep for several days may help the woman to begin the road to recovery from PPD. Planning with the woman and her family to protect her sleep as much as possible is essential to the plan of care (Puryear, 2014).

Other treatments for PPD include hormone therapy, complementary or alternative therapies (herbs, dietary supplements, massage, aromatherapy, acupuncture, exercise, bright light therapy), and electroconvulsive therapy (ECT). The safety and efficacy of these treatment modalities relative to standard treatments must still be systematically determined (Deligiannidis & Freeman, 2014).

POSTPARTUM PSYCHOSIS

The most severe of the perinatal mood disorders, postpartum psychosis, also known as *postpartum depression with psychotic features*, occurs in 1 to 2 per 1000 births during the first month, although it usually manifests within the first 2 weeks postpartum (Wisner et al., 2017).

Because the recurrence rate of postpartum psychosis is 50%, women with a history of postpartum psychosis are at significant risk. Other risk factors include bipolar disorder, family history of bipolar disorder or postpartum psychosis, and recent discontinuation of lithium or other mood stabilizers. Primiparous women are more likely to suffer from postpartum psychosis, especially if they experienced obstetric complications (Cunningham et al., 2014).

Postpartum psychosis can be due to major depression. However, it is most commonly associated with bipolar disorder (or manic-depressive

---

CLINICAL REASONING CASE STUDY
Postpartum Depression

Jennifer is a 35-year-old G1, P1 who gave birth by emergency cesarean 2 weeks ago, to a 7-lb 6-oz baby boy. She has come to the OB clinic for her 2-week follow-up visit and is accompanied by her husband and her mother. Jennifer appears tired, her color is pale, and she has dark circles under both eyes. Her affect is flat. Jennifer's husband reports that she is not sleeping, she cries often, her appetite is poor, and she seems to be constantly worried about breastfeeding. Jennifer's mother states that the baby cries much of the time and never seems satisfied after breastfeeding. She says that there have been times in the past when Jennifer was depressed and she took antidepressant medication, although she did not want to take any medication during pregnancy.

1. Evidence—Is there sufficient evidence to draw conclusions about Jennifer's current condition?
2. Assumptions—What assumptions can be made about the following?
   a. Jennifer's risk factors for PPD
   b. Jennifer's support system
   c. Jennifer's concern with breastfeeding
   d. Jennifer's reluctance to take antidepressant medication
3. Priority: What is the nursing priority in this situation?
4. Interprofessional care—Describe roles/responsibilities of health care professionals who would potentially be involved in care management for Jennifer.

disorder) and presents with symptoms of mania, depression, or both (Wisner et al., 2017). Postpartum psychosis is defined by the presence of abnormally elevated energy levels, cognition, and mood; and one or more depressive episodes. The elevated moods are generally referred to as *mania*. Clinical manifestations of a manic episode include at least three of the following: grandiosity, decreased need for sleep, pressure speech, flight of ideas, distractibility, psychomotor agitation, and excessive involvement in pleasurable activities without regard for negative consequences (APA, 2013). Individuals who experience manic episodes also commonly experience depressive episodes or symptoms of mixed episodes in which features of both mania and depression are present at the same time. These episodes are usually separated by periods of normal mood, but in some individuals, depression and mania rapidly alternate. These rapid changes in mood are known as *rapid cycling*.

In general, postpartum psychosis is characterized by rapid onset of bizarre behavior, auditory or visual hallucinations, paranoid or grandiose delusions, elements of delirium or disorientation, and extreme deficits in judgment accompanied by high levels of impulsivity that can contribute to increased risk for suicide or infanticide (O'Hara & Wisner, 2014). Initially the woman may complain of fatigue, insomnia, and restlessness and can have episodes of tearfulness and emotional lability. Later, suspiciousness, confusion, incoherence, irrational statements, and obsessive concerns about the baby's health and welfare can be present. Hallucinations and delusions are common. Auditory hallucinations that command the mother to kill the infant can occur in severe cases. When delusions are present, they are often related to the infant. The mother may think the infant is possessed by the devil, has special powers, or is destined for a terrible fate. Grossly disorganized behavior can be manifested as a disinterest in the infant or an inability to provide care. Some women will insist that something is wrong with the baby or accuse nurses or family members of hurting or poisoning their child.

> **! NURSING ALERT**
>
> Nurses are advised to be alert for mothers who are agitated, overactive, confused, complaining, or suspicious.

Medical Management

Women with postpartum psychosis usually need inpatient psychiatric care. Antipsychotics, mood stabilizers, and benzodiazepines are the treatments of choice. Other psychotropic medications such as antidepressants may be used based on the underlying diagnosis (e.g., bipolar mania, bipolar depression). ECT, especially when bilaterally administered, has also been shown to be highly effective in the treatment of postpartum psychosis. It is usually advantageous for the mother to have contact with her baby if she so desires, but visits must be closely supervised. Psychotherapy is indicated after the period of acute psychosis has passed.

CARE MANAGEMENT

An interprofessional team approach to care is needed for the woman who presents with signs and symptoms of postpartum depression. A nurse in the role of case manager can coordinate care management. The obstetric health care provider assesses her physical condition in relation to postbirth recovery as well as her current symptoms. The provider may order pharmacologic treatment (e.g., antidepressant medications) or may refer the woman to a psychiatric care provider for treatment of the depression. A pharmacist may consult with the provider regarding the optimal medications and their safety during breastfeeding and may provide education to the woman about the medications (dose, schedule, side effects, when to expect improvement

in symptoms). If the woman is experiencing a loss of appetite, a nutritionist may be a part of care management. A lactation consultant and pediatric health care provider may need to be consulted if the woman is experiencing breastfeeding difficulties. The pediatric health care provider will monitor the infant's weight and health status. Close follow-up and ongoing monitoring of the woman's mental and physical status and the infant's health, growth, and development are vital to optimizing outcomes.

SCREENING FOR POSTPARTUM DEPRESSION

When PPD is identified early, it is highly treatable. Screening for depression during pregnancy and the postpartum period may reduce the prevalence and symptoms of depression (O'Connor, Rossom, Henninger, et al., 2016). Screening for anxiety and depression during pregnancy and in the postpartum period is recommended by the American College of Obstetricians and Gynecologists (ACOG, 2015), the US Preventive Services Task Force (Siu & USPSTF, 2016), and the Association of Women's Health, Obstetric, and Neonatal Nursing (AWHONN, 2015a).

Postpartum nurses can screen for PPD before women are discharged from the birth setting. Although this identifies some who are at risk, it is important that follow-up screening is also done. PPD is most likely to occur around 4 weeks after birth. Follow-up assessments for risks and signs of PPD can be done by primary care providers during pediatric care visits for the infant and during postpartum follow-up visits for the mother. The American Academy of Pediatrics (AAP) recommends maternal depression screening at the infant's 1-, 2-, and 4-month visits (Earls & AAP Committee on Psychosocial Aspects of Child and Family Health, 2010). Women with a positive screen should be referred appropriately for evaluation and treatment.

In perinatal populations the most widely used and validated tools are the Edinburgh Postnatal Depression Scale (EPDS) and the Postpartum Depression Screening Scale (PDSS). Both are brief, self-report questionnaires specifically developed for use with perinatal women, which take between 5 and 10 minutes to complete (Milgrom & Gemmill, 2014).

The EPDS tool asks the woman to respond to 10 statements about the common symptoms of depression. The woman is asked to choose the response that is closest to describing how she has felt for the past week. A maximum score on the EPDS is 30; women with scores of 12 or higher may possibly have depression and need further assessment. One item on the tool addresses suicidal thoughts; responses to this item should be carefully examined (Cox, Holden, & Henshaw, 2014).

The PDSS is a 35-item Likert response scale that assesses for seven dimensions of depression: sleeping or eating disturbances, anxiety or insecurity, emotional lability, mental confusion, loss of self, guilt or shame, and suicidal thoughts (Myers, Aubuchon-Endsley, & Bastian, 2013). Both published tools are designed to be used by nurses and other health care professionals to elicit information from the woman during an interview to assess risk.

In addition, a simple two-item tool has been shown to be effective in identifying women at risk for PPD. If the woman answers yes to either of the two questions, the screen is considered to be positive. The questions are as follows: "Over the past 2 weeks have you ever felt down, depressed, or hopeless?" and "Over the past 2 weeks have you felt little interest or pleasure in doing things?" (Earls & AAP Committee on Psychosocial Aspects of Child and Family Health, 2010).

The effectiveness of screening for postpartum depression is related to the follow-up for positive screening results (Agency for Healthcare Research and Quality [AHRQ], 2013). If PPD screening results are positive or if the woman's self-report shows signs that she might be depressed, a formal screening is needed to determine the urgency of the referral and the type of provider. Also important is the need to assess the woman's family because they may be able to offer valuable information, as well as need to express how they have been affected by the woman's emotional disorder.

NURSING CONSIDERATIONS

Postpartum nurses carefully observe all new mothers for signs of depression and conduct further assessments as necessary. Prior to discharge from the birthing facility, nurses educate the mother and her partner about signs of postpartum blues, PPD, and postpartum psychosis; as well as when and where to seek help (see Patient Teaching box: Signs of Postpartum Blues, Depression, and Psychosis). Nurses also provide information about how to prevent PPD (Logsdon, Tomasulo, Eckert, et al., 2012) (see Patient Teaching box: Preventing Postpartum Depression). Nurses should provide women and their families with a current list of available community resources for treating postpartum depression (AWHONN, 2015a).

Before the mother is discharged from the birthing facility and in follow-up visits to clinics or health care provider offices, nurses are key to identifying symptoms of PPD. The nurse should be an active listener and demonstrate a caring attitude. Nurses cannot depend on women to volunteer unsolicited information about their depression or ask for help. Examples of ways to initiate conversation include the following: "Now that you've had your baby, how are things going for you? Have you had to change many things in your life since having the baby?" If the nurse believes that the new mother is showing signs of depression, the next step is to ask if the mother has thought about hurting herself or the baby. The woman may be more willing to answer honestly if the nurse says, "Many women feel depressed after having a baby, and some feel so badly that they think about hurting themselves or the baby. Have you had these thoughts?" (see Nursing Care Plan: Postpartum Depression).

Whenever a woman exhibits signs of postpartum depression, the nurse notifies the obstetric or primary health care provider. Women with moderate to severe cases of PPD should be referred to a mental health professional such as a psychiatric nurse practitioner or psychiatrist for evaluation and therapy. Inpatient psychiatric hospitalization may be necessary. This decision is made when the safety of the mother, her infant, or other children is threatened.

Women who are at risk for postpartum depression and those showing early signs of depression may be followed after discharge from the birthing facility through home visits or telephone calls. Postpartum home visits can reduce the incidence of or complications from depression (Dennis & Dowswell, 2013).

Supervision of the mother with emotional complications can become a prime concern. Depression can greatly interfere with a woman's ability to care for herself, her infant, and other children. This is a time for family and friends to provide assistance; the nurse can work with them to ensure adequate supervision and their understanding of the woman's mental illness.

When the woman has PPD, her partner often reacts with confusion, shock, denial, and anger and feels neglected and blamed. The nurse can provide nonjudgmental opportunities for the partner to verbalize feelings and concerns, help the partner identify positive coping strategies, and be a source of encouragement for the partner to continue supporting the woman. Suggestions for partners of women with PPD include helping around the house, setting limits with family and friends, going with her to appointments with the health care provider, educating himself or herself, writing down concerns and questions to take to the primary care provider or therapist, and just being with her—sitting quietly, hugging her, and demonstrating concern and compassion. Both the woman and her partner need an opportunity to express their needs, fears, thoughts, and feelings in a nonjudgmental environment.

Even if the woman is severely depressed, hospitalization may be avoided if adequate resources can be mobilized to ensure safety for mother and infant. The nurse in home health care needs to make frequent telephone calls or home visits for assessment and counseling.

PATIENT TEACHING

Signs of Postpartum Blues, Depression, and Psychosis

Signs of baby blues (these should go away in a few days or 1 week):
- Sad, anxious, or overwhelmed feelings
- Crying spells
- Loss of appetite
- Difficulty sleeping

Signs of postpartum depression (can begin any time in the first year):
- Same signs as baby blues, but they last longer and are more severe
- Thoughts of harming yourself or your baby
- Not having any interest in the baby

Signs of postpartum psychosis:
- Seeing or hearing things that are not there
- Feelings of confusion
- Rapid mood swings
- Trying to hurt yourself or your baby

When to call your health care provider:
- The baby blues continue for more than 2 weeks
- Symptoms of depression get worse
- Difficulty performing tasks at home or at work
- Inability to care for yourself or your baby
- Thoughts of harming yourself or your baby

PATIENT TEACHING

Preventing Postpartum Depression

- Share knowledge about postpartum emotional problems with close family and friends.
- At least once each day or every other day, purposely relax for 15 minutes by deep breathing, meditating, or taking a hot bath.
- Take Eat a balanced diet.
- Exercise on a regular basis, at least 30 minutes a day.
- Sleep as much as possible; make a promise to yourself to try to sleep when the baby sleeps.
- Get out of the house: try to leave home for 30 minutes a day; take a walk outdoors, or walk at the mall.
- Share your feelings with someone close to you; don't isolate yourself at home with the TV.
- Don't overcommit yourself or feel like you need to be a superwoman. Ask for help from family and friends.
- Don't place unrealistic expectations on yourself; no mother is perfect!
- Be flexible with your daily activities.
- Go to a new mothers' support group: for example, take a postpartum exercise class, or attend a breastfeeding support group.

Data from US Department of Health and Human Services Office of Women's Health. (2009). *Depression during and after pregnancy fact sheet*. Retrieved from http://www.womenshealth.gov/publications/our-publications/fact-sheet/depression-pregnancy.html.

⊚ NURSING CARE PLAN

Postpartum Depression

Case Study

Cara, age 25, G2 P2, gave birth 3 days ago to a full-term baby boy by cesarean section. She has a history of prenatal depression and substance abuse. She is in an "on and off" relationship with the father of the baby who has not yet visited her in the hospital. Cara says her parents don't want anything to do with her since she got pregnant, and she lives with an aunt. The pregnancy was unintended, and Cara states she is worried about being a mother and she does not know how she is going to support herself and the baby. Cara's mood alternates between being very irritable about everything and everybody to bouts of crying and saying she is sorry for being bad and really feeling down about being a mother. Once when her baby cried, Cara said she felt like hitting him to give him a reason to cry. She hardly ever holds him, even though the nurses are encouraging her to breastfeed. Cara was evaluated by a mental health care provider who diagnosed her with postpartum depression and prescribed citalopram, a selective serotonin reuptake inhibitor.

Assessment

What are the risk factors and signs of postpartum depression in this situation?

Risk Factors

History of substance abuse
History of prenatal depression
Lack of social support
Unintended pregnancy
Single status

Defining Characteristics

Irritability
Bouts of crying
Disinterest/annoyance with the infant—leaves baby in bassinet, and complains about his crying
Inability to meet role expectations—worried about how to be a mother
Inadequate confidence to deal with situation—how will she care for self and baby

Nursing Diagnosis

Risk for Injury to Cara and/or infant related to Cara's emotional state

Expected Outcomes

Cara and her infant will remain free from injury.
Cara's aunt will verbalize understanding of the need to supervise Cara and the infant and have a plan to provide that supervision.

Nursing Interventions	Rationales
Assess for risk factors for depression (before discharge).	To determine if Cara is at risk and in need of prompt interventions or referral
Provide information about signs of postpartum depression (PPD), when to call health care provider, and available resources to Cara and her aunt.	To promote prompt recognition of problems
Observe maternal-infant interactions before discharge.	To determine appropriateness
Maintain frequent contact with Cara by telephone calls and home visits after discharge.	To monitor maternal physical and mental health, and to determine if further interventions are necessary
Counsel Cara and her aunt to contact health care provider if behaviors indicating depression, such as crying, increase.	To provide prompt care and referral if necessary and avoid injury to infant and Cara

Nursing Interventions	Rationales
Provide opportunities for Cara and her aunt to verbalize feelings and concerns in a nonjudgmental setting.	To promote a trusting relationship
Assist Cara's aunt to develop a plan for maternal and infant supervision.	To provide for safety of Cara and infant
Provide information about community resources for assistance.	To obtain assistance if Cara is unable to care for herself or infant
Reinforce teaching about antidepressant medication (effects, side effects, dosage).	To help Cara understand her treatment regimen
Reinforce teaching, or refer Cara to lactation consultant.	To obtain information regarding effects of antidepressant medication on breastfeeding
Provide opportunity for Cara to verbalize feelings and concerns.	To establish a trusting relationship
Give information regarding postpartum depression to Cara.	To correct any misconceptions or misinformation
Assist Cara to identify positive coping mechanisms that have been effective during past crises.	To promote active participation in care
Assist Cara to identify community sources of support.	To provide additional resources as needed
Refer Cara to mental health care provider as needed.	To provide further expertise from a mental health professional
Observe maternal-infant interactions.	To assess quality of interactions and to determine need for interventions
Encourage Cara to express her anxiety, fears, or other feelings.	To allow Cara to verbalize her concerns and have them accepted
Encourage Cara to have as much contact with the infant as possible.	To minimize separation, and to promote attachment
Demonstrate infant care, and explain infant behaviors.	To enhance Cara's care abilities and understanding of infant's abilities
Make referrals to community resources as needed.	To assist Cara in developing parenting skills or promoting confidence in infant care

Nursing Diagnosis

Risk for Impaired Parenting related to inability of Cara to attach to her infant because of insufficient resources (i.e., knowledge, social), maternal depression

Expected Outcomes

Cara demonstrates appropriate attachment behaviors in infant interactions.
Cara expresses satisfaction with infant.

Nursing Interventions	Rationales
Observe maternal-infant interactions.	To assess quality of interactions and to determine need for interventions
Encourage Cara to express her anxiety, fears, or other feelings.	To allow Cara to ventilate her concerns and have them accepted
Encourage Cara to have as much contact with the infant as possible.	To minimize separation, and to promote attachment
Demonstrate infant care and explain infant behaviors.	To enhance Cara's care abilities and understanding of infant's abilities
Make referrals to community resources as needed.	To assist Cara in developing parenting skills or promoting confidence in infant care

Community resources that may be helpful are temporary child care or foster care, homemaker services, parenting guidance centers, mother's-day-out programs, and support groups such as Postpartum Support International (http://postpartum.net) and Depression After Delivery (www.depressionafterdelivery.com).

SAFETY CONCERNS

When a woman is suffering from depression, there can be safety concerns related to risk for self-harm or harm to the infant. If delusional thinking about the baby is suspected, the nurse asks, "Have you thought about hurting your baby?" When depression is suspected, the nurse asks, "Have you thought about hurting yourself?" Four criteria can be used to measure the seriousness of a suicidal plan: method, availability, specificity, and lethality. Has the woman specified a method? Is the method of choice available? How specific is the plan? If the method is concrete and detailed, with access to carry it out at hand, the suicide risk increases. How lethal is the method? The most lethal method is shooting, with hanging a close second. The least lethal is slashing one's wrists.

> **! NURSING ALERT**
>
> Suicidal or homicidal ideations and/or attempt to cause harm to self or others (including the infant) are among the most serious symptoms of PPD. This is considered a psychiatric emergency and warrants immediate assessment, evaluation, and intervention by a mental health care professional.

> **LEGAL TIP** **Commitment for Psychiatric Care** If a woman with PPD or postpartum psychosis is experiencing active suicidal ideation or harmful delusions about the baby and is unwilling to seek treatment, legal intervention may be necessary to commit the woman to an inpatient setting for treatment.

When a mother is hospitalized, she is separated from her infant. After her condition is stabilized, and if allowed within the inpatient psychiatric setting, the reintroduction of the baby to the mother can occur at the mother's own pace. A schedule is set for increasing the number of hours the mother cares for the baby over several days, culminating in the infant's staying overnight in the mother's room. This method allows the mother to experience meeting the infant's needs and giving up sleep for the baby, a situation difficult for new mothers even under ideal conditions. The mother's readiness for discharge and caring for the baby is assessed. Her interactions with her baby are carefully supervised and guided. A postpartum nurse is often asked to assist the psychiatric nursing staff in assessment of the mother-infant interactions.

Nurses should observe the mother for signs of bonding with the baby. Attachment behaviors are defined as eye-to-eye contact; physical contact that involves holding, touching, cuddling, and talking to the baby and calling the baby by name; and the initiation of appropriate care. A staff member is assigned to observe the baby at all times. Praise and encouragement are used to bolster the mother's self-esteem and self-confidence.

PSYCHOTROPIC MEDICATIONS

Antidepressant medications are the most widely used treatment for PPD. Paroxetine, sertraline, fluoxetine, venlafaxine, nortriptyline, and nefazodone have been evaluated and are associated with improvement in PPD symptoms over 2 to 3 months of treatment (O'Hara & Wisner, 2014). If the woman with PPD is not breastfeeding, in most cases antidepressants can be prescribed without special precautions. A variety of medications can be prescribed for these women, including TCAs, SSRIs, SNRIs, MAOIs, mood stabilizers, and antipsychotic medications.

Mood stabilizers are used in the treatment of severe psychiatric syndromes such as schizophrenia, bipolar disorder, or psychotic depression. Women taking mood stabilizers must be taught about the many side effects, and especially for those taking lithium, the need to have serum lithium levels determined every 6 months. Most of the mood-stabilizing medications can cause sedation and orthostatic hypotension—both of which can interfere with the mother being able to care safely for her baby. They also can cause peripheral nervous system (PNS) effects such as constipation, dry mouth, blurred vision, tachycardia, urinary retention, weight gain, and agranulocytosis. CNS effects may include akathisia, dystonias, parkinsonian-like symptoms, tardive dyskinesia (irreversible), and neuroleptic malignant syndrome (potentially fatal). Medication education is especially important when caring for women who are taking antipsychotic medications. The nurse should use discretion in selecting the content to be shared because of the women's altered thought processes and the large number of side/toxic effects. The nurse may choose to do more extensive education with a close family member. The newer, atypical antipsychotic medications such as aripiprazole, olanzapine, quetiapine, risperidone, and ziprasidone are usually safer and have fewer side effects than the older, more traditional antipsychotics. Their safety in breastfeeding women, however, has not been established.

PSYCHOTROPIC MEDICATIONS AND LACTATION

Use of any psychotropic medication in a breastfeeding mother is done with consideration of risks and benefits. The risk of not treating the mother versus not breastfeeding the infant prompts providers to prescribe medications that reduce maternal symptoms without harming the infant. Concerns about many psychotropic drugs are related to the long-term use and potential effects on the infant (Lawrence & Lawrence, 2016; Sriraman, Melvin, Meltzer-Brody, et al., 2015) (Table 21.1).

Factors that affect the passage of a medication through breast milk include the size of the molecule, the solubility in lipids and water, the protein-binding capacity, the drug's pH, and the rate of diffusion. Infant factors to consider relate to the gestational and chronologic age of the infant, weight, health, and frequency and amount of feeding (Lawrence & Lawrence, 2016). To minimize the infant's exposure to maternal medication, the mother should avoid breastfeeding when the blood levels of the medication are peaking.

SSRIs are the most common pharmacologic treatment for PPD; they are also prescribed for anxiety disorders. Research has shown that the majority of the SSRIs taken by breastfeeding mothers pass through the milk to the infant in small amounts and have no untoward effects on the infant. Paroxetine (Paxil), sertraline (Zoloft), and nortriptyline (Pamelor) provide less infant exposure than fluoxetine (Prozac) and citalopram (Celexa). All breastfeeding mothers who take SSRIs should be taught to monitor their infants for signs of irritability, poor feeding, and alterations in sleep pattern (Hudak, Tan, & AAP Committee on Fetus and Newborn, 2012; Sriraman et al., 2015).

Benzodiazepines, mood stabilizers, and antipsychotic medications are used frequently in the treatment of postpartum psychiatric disorders despite the lack of research in this population. No long-term effects have been reported in exclusively breastfed infants whose mothers were taking benzodiazepines on a regular basis. The shorter-acting agents (alprazolam [Xanax], lorazepam [Ativan]) are favored over those with

TABLE 21.1   Medications for Perinatal Mood Disorders

Class	Drug	Indications	Maternal Side Effects	Infant Exposure Effects	Comments
SSRIs	Citalopram, escitalopram, fluoxetine, fluvoxamine, paroxetine, sertraline	Anxiety disorders, depression	Gastrointestinal distress, nervousness, headache, sexual dysfunction, sedation	All SSRIs are detectable in human milk. Paroxetine and sertraline usually undetectable in infant serum; fluoxetine and citalopram >10% maternal level. Infant effects: irritability, uneasy sleep, drowsiness, colic, feeding problems. Fluoxetine contraindicated during lactation.	Sertraline most common; undetectable to low levels in human milk. Long-term effects of SSRI exposure on infants: more evidence needed; recent evidence is reassuring
SNRIs	Venlafaxine, duloxetine, desvenlafaxine	Depression	Galactorrhea	Detectable in human milk and infant serum. No proven side effects; assess weight gain and sedation	Lack of evidence on outcomes for breastfed infants
Other antidepressants (norepinephrine/dopamine/serotonin reuptake blockers)	Bupropion, mirtazapine	Depression	Drowsiness, increased appetite, weight gain, dizziness, dry mouth; dose-dependent	Limited data; concerns range from possible irritability to seizures	Not a reason to stop breastfeeding; another drug may be preferable.
TCAs/heterocyclics	Amitryptyline, amoxapine, clomipramine, desipramine, doxepin, maprotiline, nortriptyline, protriptyline, trimipramine	Anxiety disorders, depression	Hypotension, sedation, urinary retention, dry mouth, weight gain, sexual dysfunction, constipation; overdose can cause cardiac arrhythmias and death	Lack of evidence on most drugs; nortriptyline undetectable in infant serum, no adverse effects reported	Older class of drugs
Antipsychotic	Quetiapine	Bipolar disorder, schizophrenia	Sedation	Sedation	
Mood stabilizer	Lithium	Postpartum psychosis	Diarrhea, vomiting	Elevated TSH	Dosage based on maternal blood levels, which should be checked frequently
Herbal/natural remedy	St. John's wort	Depression		Poorly excreted into human milk; possible drowsiness, lethargy	Used in Europe for many years to treat depression; use in United States is controversial

Adapted from Sriraman N.K., Melvin K., Meltzer-Brody S., & Academy of Breastfeeding Medicine. (2015). ABM clinical protocol no. 18: Use of antidepressants in breastfeeding mothers. *Breastfeeding Medicine, 10*(6), 290–299.

longer half-lives (clonazepam [Klonopin], diazepam [Valium]) (Lawrence & Lawrence, 2016).

Mood-stabilizing medications are present in the breast milk of women who take these drugs. Lithium has been the most extensively studied. Lithium can be used safely in breastfeeding mothers with dosing based on maternal serum drug levels (Sriraman et al., 2015). Infants should be monitored for signs of toxicity (hypotonia, lethargy, feeding problems) (Wisner et al., 2017). Valproic acid (Depakote) and carbamazepine (Tegretol) are considered reasonably safe while breastfeeding, although careful monitoring for infant hepatotoxicity is recommended. The benefits of breastfeeding and the potential risks must be carefully considered before using mood stabilizers.

In summary, all psychotropic medications studied to date are excreted in breast milk. The best psychotropic medications for breastfeeding women are those with the greatest documentation of prior use, few or no metabolites, and fewer side effects.

When breastfeeding women have emotional complications and need psychotropic medications, referral to a mental health care provider who specializes in postpartum disorders is preferred. The woman should be informed of the risks and benefits to her and her infant of the medications to be taken. Depressed women will need the nurse to reinforce the importance of taking antidepressants as ordered. Because antidepressants usually do not exert any significant effect for approximately 2 weeks and usually do not reach full effect for 4 to 6 weeks, many women discontinue taking the medication on their own. Patient and family teaching should reinforce the need for taking medications until therapeutic effects are present and for as long as prescribed by the health care provider.

Current information about breastfeeding and drug compatibility can be found at the Drugs and Lactation Database (LactMed; http://toxnet.nlm.nih.gov/cgi-bin/sis/htmlgen?LACT). This is a peer-reviewed and fully referenced database of drugs to which breastfeeding mothers may be exposed. Among the data included are maternal and infant levels of drugs, possible effects on breastfed infants and on lactation, and alternate drugs to consider (Anderson, 2016).

BIPOLAR DISORDER

Women with bipolar disorder are at high risk for relapse during the postpartum period. (Wesseloo, Kamperman, Munk-Olsen, et al., 2016). Bipolar disorder involves unusual changes in mood, energy, activity, and cognition. It can present as mania, hypomania, depression, or as a mixed state. Depression is the most common mood state, and it is easily confused with severe postpartum depression. Severe anxiety and/or panic attacks are common with postpartum depressive episodes. Postpartum psychosis occurs most frequently in women with bipolar disorder and can be the initial presentation of the disorder. Co-morbidities are common in women with bipolar disorder, including anxiety disorders; substance abuse; and medical problems such as migraines, pain disorders, hypothyroidism, and metabolic syndrome (Wisner et al., 2017).

Women with bipolar disorder should be monitored closely for symptoms of relapse in the postpartum period. Attempts to reduce stress and avoid disrupted sleep cycle may help prevent recurrence. Some experts recommend prophylactic treatment with mood stabilizers during pregnancy and in the early postpartum period (Wesseloo et al., 2016). Lithium, valproic acid, and lamotrigine are mood stabilizers commonly used to treat bipolar disorder. Olanzapine and quetiapine are newer antipsychotics that are sometimes used as mood stabilizers (Khan, Fersh, Ernst, et al., 2016).

POSTPARTUM ANXIETY DISORDERS

Anxiety disorders are common during the postpartum period; these include generalized anxiety, panic, obsessive-compulsive, and social anxiety disorders. Women with a history of anxiety disorder are at greatest risk. Anxiety disorders and PPD are likely to occur at the same time (O'Hara & Wisner, 2014).

With generalized anxiety disorder, women have a pervasive feeling of anxiety most of the time and worry excessively about multiple concerns. Anxiety symptoms can interfere with the mother's ability to care for herself, the infant, and her family. Women with generalized anxiety disorder may experience chest tightness, shortness of breath, tachycardia, dizziness or lightheadedness, sweating, trembling, nausea, abdominal pain, fatigue, constant worry, sense of doom, and difficulty concentrating (Puryear, 2014; Wisner et al., 2017).

Panic disorder consists of unpredictable, intermittent episodes (attacks) of symptoms similar to those of generalized anxiety disorder. Women with panic disorder may develop agoraphobia or fear of leaving home because they fear having another panic attack (Wisner et al., 2017).

Women with a history of obsessive-compulsive disorder (OCD) often find that their symptoms increase during the postpartum period. For some women with no history of OCD, the first episode occurs postpartum. Women with postpartum OCD tend to have obsessive, intrusive thoughts, and they perform compulsive actions that temporarily reduce or alleviate the distress caused by the intrusive thoughts. In the postpartum period, obsessive thoughts are likely to involve contamination and fear of germs; women often fear harm will come to the infant, either inflicted by themselves or others. The obsessive thoughts can be incapacitating. Women fear they will lose control and act on their thoughts. Women with OCD are afraid they will harm their infants, but are unlikely to do so. Women with postpartum psychosis who have the same thoughts are more apt to actually cause harm (Puryear, 2014; Wisner et al., 2017).

Postpartum posttraumatic stress disorder (PTSD) is the result of exposure to trauma, either during the prenatal or intrapartum period, or it may be related to previous life experiences and events such as childhood sexual abuse or intimate partner violence. Risk factors for postpartum PTSD include history of pregnancy loss, high-risk pregnancy, preterm birth, infant in the NICU, painful and/or difficult vaginal birth, instrument-assisted vaginal birth, and emergency cesarean (Vesel & Nickasch, 2015–2016).

Anxiety disorders may be treated with psychotherapy; CBT and exposure response prevention (ERP) are often used effectively. Medications include SSRIs and antianxiety drugs, although it can take 2 weeks for these medications to be effective. Benzodiazepines provide short-term relief from anxiety symptoms, but should be used judiciously as they can be addictive. There is a lack of evidence related to use in breastfeeding mothers (Wisner et al., 2017).

MATERNAL DEATH

Maternal death can be caused by a variety of complications, including embolism, hypertension, hemorrhage, infection, and cardiomyopathy (see Chapter 1). In many cases, the death of a mother is sudden and unexpected. Any instance of maternal death is tragic for the family as well as for the nurses and other health care professionals who were involved in her care.

When a woman dies of a complication related to childbearing, the husband or partner and extended family are faced with mourning the death of a wife or partner and mother. The loss and grief are greatly compounded when there is also the death of a fetus or neonate. When the infant survives, the husband or partner is faced with parenting a baby without a surviving mother. The responsibilities of infant care can be overwhelming during this time of intense loss and grief.

Because most maternal deaths are unexpected, the grief that follows a maternal death is usually unplanned. This differs from anticipatory grief in which the loss is expected, such as with cancer. The shock and disbelief associated with unplanned grief can be engulfing and debilitating, overwhelming the normal coping abilities and creating difficulties with everyday functioning and decision making.

Nurses and other health care professionals working with families who experience maternal loss need to consider the context and implications of the maternal death on the remaining family members. Young parents may never have experienced a significant personal loss or tragedy; in many cases, their parents and grandparents are still living. Cultural beliefs and customs surrounding death can influence a family's response to maternal death (Hill, 2012). The grief response of each family member will vary; grief is an individual response, and the grieving process does not always proceed in a predictable manner.

Hospital protocols regarding maternal death are varied. When a maternal death occurs, the hospital chaplain and social worker may provide the initial contact with the family, taking them into a private room. As soon as possible, they are joined by the obstetrician, perinatologist, and nurse. This first meeting with the family is often short, providing brief explanations about the events leading up to the maternal death and attempting to answer the family's questions. The primary goal of this meeting is to show empathy and compassion for the family and to assure them of updates as soon as information becomes available (Hill, 2012). If there is a surviving infant, the family will likely want to see and hold the infant. If the neonate is in the intensive care nursery, the family can be escorted to the baby's bedside. The family will need assistance with the "next steps" in terms of making arrangements for funeral services; the nurse, chaplain, or social worker can provide the family with information and offer support during this difficult time.

Families who experience maternal loss are at risk for developing complicated bereavement and altered parenting of the surviving infant and other children in the family. A referral to social services to help the family mobilize support systems and for counseling can help combat potential problems before they develop and can be beneficial not only at the time of the loss but also in the future. Follow-up care for grieving families is essential as they progress through the stages of grief and adjust to life without the mother.

The emotional toll that a maternal death can take on the nursing and medical staff must also be addressed. Guilt, anger, fear, sadness, and depression are all common responses to a maternal death. The staff may want to participate in a debriefing session in which they can review the situation surrounding the events, their participation in caring for the mother, and their response to the death. Attending memorial or funeral services can benefit staff and family. Follow-up conferences with a social worker or grief counselor can help staff members work through their grief.

REFERENCES

Agency for Healthcare Research and Quality. (2013). *Efficacy and safety of screening for postpartum depression.* Retrieved from https://effectivehealthcare.ahrq.gov/ehc/products/379/1437/postpartum-screening-report-130409.pdf.

Alkozei, A., McMahon, E., & Lahav, A. (2014). Stress levels and depressive symptoms in NICU mothers in the early postpartum period. *Journal of Maternal, Fetal, and Neonatal Medicine, 27*(17), 1738–1743.

American College of Obstetricians and Gynecologists. (2015). Screening for perinatal depression. *Obstetrics and Gynecology, 125*(5), 1268–1271.

American Psychiatric Association. (2013). *Diagnostic and statistical manual of mental disorders* (5th ed.). Washington, DC: American Psychiatric Association.

Anderson, P. O. (2016). LactMed update: An introduction. *Breastfeeding Medicine, 11*(2), 54–55.

Association of Women's Health, Obstetric and Neonatal Nurses. (2015a). AWHONN position statement: Mood and anxiety disorders in pregnant and postpartum women. *Journal of Obstetric, Gynecologic, and Neonatal Nursing, 44*(5), 561–563.

Association of Women's Health, Obstetric and Neonatal Nurses. (2015b). AWHONN practice brief no. 1: Quantification of blood loss. *Journal of Obstetric, Gynecologic, and Neonatal Nursing, 44*(1), 158–160.

Beydoun, H. A., Beydoun, M. A., Kaufman, J. S., et al. (2012). Intimate partner violence against adult women and its association with major depressive disorder, depressive symptoms and postpartum depression: A systematic review and meta-analysis. *Social Science & Medicine, 75*(6), 959–975.

Cameron, E. E., Sedov, I. D., & Tomfohr-Madsen, L. M. (2016). Prevalence of paternal depression in pregnancy and the postpartum: An updated meta-analysis. *Journal of Affective Disorders, 206,* 189–203.

Cox, J., Holden, J., & Henshaw, C. (2014). *Perinatal mental health: The Edinburgh postnatal depression scale (EPDS) manual.* London, UK: RCPsych Publications.

Cunningham, F., Leveno, K., Bloom, S., et al. (2014). *Williams obstetrics* (24th ed.). New York, NY: McGraw-Hill.

Deligiannidis, K. M., & Freeman, M. P. (2014). Complementary and alternative medicine therapies for perinatal depression. *Best Practice & Research. Clinical Obstetrics & Gynaecology, 28*(1), 85–95.

Dennis, C. L., & Dowswell, T. (2013). Psychosocial and psychological interventions for preventing postpartum depression (review). *Cochrane Database of Systematic Reviews, 2013*(2), CD001134.

Duff, P., & Birsner, M. (2017). Maternal and perinatal infection in pregnancy: Bacterial. In S. G. Gabbe, J. R. Niebyl, J. L. Simpson, et al. (Eds.), *Obstetrics: Normal and problem pregnancies* (7th ed.). Philadelphia, PA: Elsevier.

Earls, M. F., & American Academy of Pediatrics Committee on Psychosocial Aspects of Child and Family Health. (2010). Incorporating recognition and management of perinatal and postpartum depression into pediatric practice. *Pediatrics, 126*(5), 1032–1039.

Fleischer, A., & Meirowitz, N. (2016). Care bundles for management of postpartum hemorrhage. *Seminars in Perinatology, 40*(2), 99–108.

Francois, K. E., & Foley, M. R. (2017). Antepartum and postpartum hemorrhage. In S. G. Gabbe, J. R. Niebyl, J. L. Simpson, et al. (Eds.), *Obstetrics: Normal and problem pregnancies* (7th ed.). Philadelphia, PA: Elsevier.

Habib, C. (2012). Paternal perinatal depression: An overview and suggestions towards an intervention model. *Journal of Family Studies, 18*(1), 4–16.

Hancock, A., Weeks, A. D., & Lavender, D. T. (2015). Is accurate and reliable blood loss estimation the "crucial step" in early detection of postpartum haemorrhage: An integrative review of the literature. *BMC Pregnancy and Childbirth, 15,* 1–9.

Hill, P. E. (2012). Support and counseling after maternal death. *Seminars in Perinatology, 36*(1), 84–88.

Hudak, M. L., Tan, R. C., & American Academy of Pediatrics Committee on Fetus and Newborn. (2012). Neonatal drug withdrawal. *Pediatrics, 129*(2), e540–e560.

Isley, M. M., & Katz, V. L. (2017). Postpartum care and long-term health considerations. In S. G. Gabbe, J. R. Niebyl, J. L. Simpson, et al. (Eds.), *Obstetrics: Normal and problem pregnancies* (7th ed.). Philadelphia, PA: Elsevier.

James, D. C. (2014). Postpartum care. In K. R. Simpson & P. A. Creehan (Eds.), *AWHONN's perinatal nursing* (4th ed.). Philadelphia, PA: Lippincott Williams & Wilkins.

Khan, S. J., Fersh, M. E., Ernst, C., et al. (2016). Bipolar disorder in pregnancy and postpartum: Principles of management. *Current Psychiatry Reports, 18*(2), 1–11.

Kothari, C. L., Liepman, M. R., Tareen, R. S., et al. (2016). Intimate partner violence associated with postpartum depression, regardless of socioeconomic status. *Maternal and Child Health Journal, 20*(6), 1237–1246.

Lawrence, R. A., & Lawrence, R. M. (2016). *Breastfeeding: A guide for the medical profession* (8th ed.). St. Louis, MO: Elsevier.

Letourneau, N., Tryphonopoulos, P. D., Duffett-Leger, L., et al. (2012). Support intervention needs and preferences of fathers affected by postpartum depression. *Journal of Perinatal & Neonatal Nursing, 26*(1), 69–80.

Leung, A. N., & Lockwood, C. J. (2014). Thromboembolic disorders in pregnancy. In R. K. Creasy, R. Resnik, J. D. Iams, et al. (Eds.), *Creasy and Resnik's maternal fetal-medicine: Principles and practice* (7th ed.). Philadelphia, PA: Elsevier.

Logsdon, M. C., Tomasulo, R., Eckert, D., et al. (2012). Identification of mothers at risk for postpartum depression by hospital-based perinatal nurses. *American Journal of Maternal Child Nursing, 37*(4), 218–225.

Lyndon, A., Lagrew, D., Shields, L., et al. (2015). *A California toolkit to transform maternity care: Improving health care response to obstetric hemorrhage version 2.0.* Stanford, CA: California Maternal Quality Care Collaborative (CMQCC). Retrieved from http://www.cmqcc.org/ob_hemorrhage.

Main, E. K., Goffman, D., & Scavone, B. M. (2015). National Partnership for Maternal Safety: Consensus bundle on obstetric hemorrhage. *Obstetrics and Gynecology, 126*(5), 155–162.

Milgrom, J., & Gemmill, A. W. (2014). Screening for perinatal depression. *Best Practice & Research: Clinical Obstetrics & Gynaecology, 28*(1), 13–23.

Musser, A. K., Ahmed, A. H., Foli, K. J., & Coddington, J. A. (2013). Paternal postpartum depression: What health care providers should know. *Journal of Pediatric Health Care, 27*(6), 479–485.

Myers, E. R., Aubuchon-Endsley, N., & Bastian, L. A. (2013). *Efficacy and safety of screening for postpartum depression. Comparative effectiveness review 106.* Rockville, MD: Agency for Healthcare Research and Quality.

O'Connor, E., Rossom, R. C., Henninger, M., et al. (2016). Primary care screening for and treatment of depression in pregnant and postpartum women: Evidence report and systematic review for the U.S. Preventive Services Task Force. *Journal of the American Medical Association, 315*(4), 388–406.

O'Hara, M. W., & McCabe, J. E. (2013). Postpartum depression: Current status and future directions. *Annual Review of Clinical Psychology, 9,* 379–407.

O'Hara, M. W., & Wisner, K. L. (2014). Perinatal mental illness: Definition, description, aetiology. *Best Practice & Research: Clinical Obstetrics & Gynaecology, 28*(1), 3–12.

Park, E. M., Meltzer-Brody, S., & Stickgold, R. (2013). Poor sleep maintenance and subjective sleep quality are associated with postpartum maternal depression symptom severity. *Archives of Women's Mental Health, 16*(6), 539–547.

Paulson, J. F., & Bazemore, S. D. (2010). Prenatal and postnatal depression in fathers and its association with maternal depression: A meta-analysis. *Journal of the American Medical Association, 303*(19), 1961–1969.

Paschetta, E., Berrisford, G., Coccia, F., et al. (2014). Perinatal psychiatric disorders: An overview. *American Journal of Obstetrics and Gynecology, 210*(6), 501–509, e6.

Pettker, C. M., & Lockwood, C. J. (2017). Thromboembolic disorders. In S. G. Gabbe, J. R. Niebyl, J. L. Simpson, et al. (Eds.), *Obstetrics: Normal and problem pregnancies* (7th ed.). Philadelphia, PA: Elsevier.

Puryear, L. J. (2014). Postpartum adjustment: What is normal and what is not? In D. L. Barnes (Ed.), *Women's reproductive mental health across the lifespan.* Cham, Switzerland: Springer International.

Samuels, P. (2017). Hematologic complications of pregnancy. In S. G. Gabbe, J. R. Niebyl, J. L. Simpson, et al. (Eds.), *Obstetrics: Normal and problem pregnancies* (7th ed.). Philadelphia, PA: Elsevier.

Siu, A. L., & US Preventive Services Task Force. (2016). Screening for depression in adults: US Preventive Services Task Force recommendation statement. *Journal of the American Medical Association, 315*(4), 380–387.

Sriraman, N. K., Melvin, K., Meltzer-Brody, S., & Academy of Breastfeeding Medicine. (2015). ABM clinical protocol no. 18: Use of antidepressants in breastfeeding mothers. *Breastfeeding Medicine, 10*(6), 290–299.

Stadtlander, L. (2015). Paternal postpartum depression. *International Journal of Childbirth Education, 30*(2), 11–13.

Stuart, S., & Koleva, H. (2014). Psychological treatments for perinatal depression. *Best Practice and Research: Clinical Obstetrics and Gynaecology, 28*(1), 61–70.

Tepper, N. K., Boulet, S. L., Whiteman, M. K., et al. (2014). Postpartum venous thrombosis: Incidence and risk factors. *Obstetrics and Gynecology, 123*(5), 987–996.

Vesel, J., & Nickasch, B. (2015-2016). An evidence review and model for prevention and treatment of postpartum posttraumatic stress disorder. *Nursing for Women's Health, 19*(6), 504–525.

Wesseloo, R., Kamperman, A. M., Munk-Olsen, T., et al. (2016). Risk of postpartum relapse in bipolar disorder and postpartum psychosis: A systematic review and meta-analysis. *American Journal of Psychiatry, 173*(2), 117–127.

Wisner, K. L., Sit, D. K. T., Bogen, D. L., et al. (2017). Mental health and behavioral disorders in pregnancy. In S. G. Gabbe, J. R. Niebyl, J. L. Simpson, et al. (Eds.), *Obstetrics: Normal and problem pregnancies* (7th ed.). Philadelphia, PA: Elsevier.

Woolhouse, H., Gartland, D., Hegarty, K., et al. (2012). Depressive symptoms and intimate partner violence in the 12 months after childbirth: A prospective pregnancy cohort study. *British Journal of Obstetrics and Gynaecology, 119*(3), 315–323.

World Health Organization. (2015). *Maternal mortality fact sheet no. 348.* Retrieved from http://www.who.int/mediacentre/factsheets/fs348/en.

22

Physiologic and Behavioral Adaptations of the Newborn

Kathryn R. Alden

ⓔ http://evolve.elsevier.com/Perry/maternal

The neonatal period includes the time from birth through day 28 of life. During this time, the neonate must make many physiologic and behavioral adaptations to extrauterine life. Physiologic adjustment tasks are those that involve: (1) establishing and maintaining respirations; (2) adjusting to circulatory changes; (3) regulating temperature; (4) ingesting, retaining, and digesting nutrients; (5) eliminating waste; and (6) regulating weight. Behavioral tasks include: (1) establishing a regulated behavioral tempo independent of the mother, which involves self-regulating arousal, self-monitoring changes in state, and patterning sleep; (2) processing, storing, and organizing multiple stimuli; and (3) establishing a relationship with caregivers and the environment. The term infant usually makes these adjustments with little or no difficulty. This chapter describes the physiologic and behavioral adaptations required by the neonate for transition to extrauterine life.

TRANSITION TO EXTRAUTERINE LIFE

The major adaptations associated with transition from intrauterine to extrauterine life occur during the first 6 to 8 hours after birth. The predictable series of events during transition are mediated by the sympathetic nervous system and result in changes that involve heart rate, respirations, temperature, and gastrointestinal function. This transition period represents a time of vulnerability for the neonate and warrants careful observation. To detect disorders in adaptation soon after birth, nurses must be aware of normal features of the transition period. In their classic work on newborn adaptation to extrauterine life.

Desmond, Rudolph, and Phitaksphraiwan (1966) proposed three stages of newborn transition. The stages are still considered valid today. The first stage of the transition period lasts up to 30 minutes after birth and is called the *first period of reactivity*. The newborn's heart rate increases rapidly to 160 to 180 beats/minute but gradually falls after 30 minutes or so to a baseline rate of 100 to 120 beats/minute. Respirations are irregular, with a rate between 60 and 80 breaths/minute. Fine crackles can be present on auscultation. Audible grunting, nasal flaring, and retractions of the chest also can be present, but these should cease within the first hour of birth. The infant is alert and may have spontaneous startles, tremors, crying, and head movement from side to side. Bowel sounds are audible, and meconium may be passed.

After the first period of reactivity, the newborn either sleeps or has a marked decrease in motor activity. This *period of decreased responsiveness* lasts from 60 to 100 minutes. During this time the infant is pink, and respirations are rapid (up to 60 breaths/minute) and shallow but unlabored. Bowel sounds are audible, and peristaltic waves may be noted over the rounded abdomen.

The *second period of reactivity* occurs roughly between 2 and 8 hours after birth and lasts from 10 minutes to several hours. Brief periods of tachycardia and tachypnea occur, associated with increased muscle tone, changes in skin color, and mucus production. Meconium is commonly passed at this time. Most healthy newborns experience this transition, regardless of gestational age or type of birth; very preterm infants do not because of physiologic immaturity.

PHYSIOLOGIC ADJUSTMENTS

RESPIRATORY SYSTEM

As the infant emerges from the intrauterine environment and the umbilical cord is clamped and severed, profound adaptations are necessary for survival. The most critical of these is the establishment of effective respirations. Most newborns breathe spontaneously after birth and are able to maintain adequate oxygenation. Preterm infants often encounter respiratory difficulties related to their immature lungs.

Initiation of Breathing

During intrauterine life, oxygenation of the fetus occurs through transplacental gas exchange. At birth, the lungs must be established as the site of gas exchange. In utero fetal blood was shunted away from the lungs, but when birth occurs the pulmonary vasculature must be fully perfused for this purpose. Clamping the umbilical cord causes a rise in blood pressure (BP), which increases circulation and lung perfusion.

There is no single trigger for newborn respiratory function. The initiation of respirations in the neonate is the result of a combination of chemical, mechanical, thermal, and sensory factors (Blackburn, 2013).

Chemical Factors

The activation of chemoreceptors in the carotid arteries and aorta results from the relative state of hypoxia associated with labor. With each labor contraction there is a temporary decrease in uterine blood flow and transplacental gas exchange, resulting in transient fetal hypoxia and hypercarbia. Although the fetus is able to recover between contractions, there appears to be a cumulative effect that results in progressive decline in P_{O_2}, increased P_{CO_2}, and lowered blood pH. Decreased levels of oxygen and increased levels of carbon dioxide seem to have a cumulative effect that is involved in initiating neonatal breathing by stimulating the respiratory center in the medulla. Another chemical factor may also play a role; it is thought that as a result of clamping the cord, there is a drop in levels of a prostaglandin that can inhibit respirations.

Mechanical Factors

Respirations in the newborn can be stimulated by changes in intrathoracic pressure resulting from compression of the chest during vaginal birth. As the infant passes through the birth canal, the chest is compressed. With birth this pressure on the chest is released, and the negative intrathoracic pressure helps draw air into the lungs. Crying increases the distribution of air in the lungs and promotes expansion of the alveoli. The positive pressure created by crying helps keep the alveoli open.

Thermal Factors

With birth the newborn enters the extrauterine environment, in which the temperature is significantly lower. The profound change in environmental temperature stimulates receptors in the skin, resulting in stimulation of the respiratory center in the medulla.

Sensory Factors

Sensory stimulation occurs in a variety of ways with birth. Some of these include handling by the obstetric health care provider, suctioning the mouth and nose, and drying by the nurses. Environmental factors (lights, sounds, smells) stimulate the respiratory center.

At term the lungs hold approximately 20 mL of fluid per kilogram. Air must be substituted for the fluid that filled the fetal respiratory tract. Traditionally it had been thought that the thoracic squeeze occurring during normal vaginal birth resulted in significant clearance of lung fluid. However, it appears that this event plays a minor role. In the days preceding labor, there is reduced production of fetal lung fluid and concomitant decreased alveolar fluid volume. Shortly before the onset of labor, there is a catecholamine surge that seems to promote fluid clearance from the lungs, which continues during labor. The movement of lung fluid from the air spaces occurs through active transport into the interstitium, with drainage occurring through the pulmonary circulation and lymphatic system. Retention of lung fluid can interfere with the infant's ability to maintain adequate oxygenation, especially if other factors that compromise respirations (e.g., meconium aspiration, congenital diaphragmatic hernia, esophageal atresia with fistula, choanal atresia, congenital cardiac defect, immature alveoli) are present. Infants born by cesarean in which labor did not occur before birth can experience some lung fluid retention, although it typically clears without harmful effects on the infant (Hillman, Kallapur, & Jobe, 2012). These infants are also more likely to develop transient tachypnea of the newborn (TTN) (Fraser, 2015).

The alveoli of the term infant's lungs are lined with surfactant, a protein manufactured in type II lung cells. Lung expansion depends largely on chest wall contraction and adequate surfactant secretion. Surfactant lowers surface tension, therefore reducing the pressure required to keep the alveoli open with inspiration, and prevents total alveolar collapse on exhalation, thereby maintaining alveolar stability. The decreased surface tension results in increased lung compliance, helping to establish the functional residual capacity of the lungs (Blackburn, 2013). With absent or decreased surfactant, more pressure must be generated for inspiration, which can soon tire or exhaust preterm or sick term infants.

Breathing movements that began in utero as intermittent become continuous after birth, although the mechanism for this is not well understood. Once respirations are established, breaths are shallow and irregular, ranging from 30 to 60 breaths/minute, with periods of breathing that include pauses in respirations lasting less than 20 seconds. These episodes of periodic breathing occur most often during the active (rapid eye movement [REM]) sleep cycle and decrease in frequency and duration with age. Apneic periods longer than 20 seconds are abnormal and should be evaluated.

Newborn infants are by preference nose breathers. The reflex response to nasal obstruction is to open the mouth to maintain an airway. This response is not present in most infants until 3 weeks after birth; therefore cyanosis or asphyxia can occur with nasal blockage.

In most newborns, auscultation of the chest reveals loud, clear breath sounds that seem very near because little chest tissue intervenes. Breath sounds should be clear and equal bilaterally, although fine rales for the first few hours are not unusual. The ribs of the infant articulate with the spine at a horizontal rather than a downward slope; consequently the rib cage cannot expand with inspiration as readily as that of an adult. Because neonatal respiratory function is largely a matter of diaphragmatic contraction, abdominal breathing is characteristic of newborns. The newborn infant's chest and abdomen rise simultaneously with inspiration. Characteristics of the respiratory system of the neonate and the effects of these characteristics on respiratory function are listed in Table 22.1.

Signs of Respiratory Distress

Signs of respiratory distress can include nasal flaring, intercostal or subcostal retractions (in-drawing of tissue between the ribs or below the rib cage), or grunting with respirations. Suprasternal or subclavicular retractions with stridor or gasping most often represent an upper airway obstruction. Seesaw or paradoxical respirations (exaggerated rise in abdomen with respiration as the chest falls) instead of abdominal respirations are abnormal and should be reported. A respiratory rate of less than 30 or greater than 60 breaths/minute with the infant at rest must be evaluated. The respiratory rate of the infant can be slowed, depressed, or absent as a result of the effects of analgesics or anesthetics administered to the mother during labor and birth. Apneic episodes can be related to events such as rapid increase in body temperature, hypothermia, hypoglycemia, or sepsis that require thorough evaluation. Tachypnea can result from inadequate clearance of lung fluid, or it can be an indication of newborn respiratory distress syndrome (RDS). Tachypnea can be the first sign of respiratory, cardiac, metabolic, or infectious illnesses (Gardner, Enzman-Hines, & Nyp, 2016).

Changes in the infant's color can indicate respiratory distress. Acrocyanosis, the bluish discoloration of hands and feet, is a normal finding in the first 24 hours after birth. Transient periods of duskiness while crying are common immediately after birth; however, central cyanosis is abnormal and signifies hypoxemia. With central cyanosis, the lips and mucous membranes are bluish (circumoral cyanosis). It can be the result of inadequate delivery of oxygen to the alveoli, poor perfusion of the lungs that inhibits gas exchange, or cardiac dysfunction. Because central cyanosis is a late sign of distress, newborns usually have significant hypoxemia when cyanosis appears.

Infants who experience mild TTN often have signs of respiratory distress during the first 1 to 2 hours after birth as they transition to extrauterine life. Tachypnea with rates up to 100 breaths/minute can be present along with intermittent grunting, nasal flaring, and mild retractions. Supplemental oxygen may be needed. TTN usually resolves in 24 to 48 hours (Soltau & Carlo, 2014).

TABLE 22.1   Characteristics of the Respiratory System of the Neonate

Characteristic	Effect on Function
Immature alveoli; decreased size and number of alveoli	Risk for respiratory insufficiency and pulmonary problems
Thicker alveolar wall; decreased alveolar surface area	Less efficient gas transport and exchange
Continued development of alveoli until childhood	Possible opportunity to reduce effects of discrete lung injury
Decreased lung elastic tissue and recoil	Decreased lung compliance requiring higher pressures and more work to expand; increased risk for atelectasis
Reduced diaphragm movement and maximal force potential	Less effective respiratory movement; difficulty generating negative intrathoracic pressures; risk for atelectasis
Tendency to nose breathe; altered position of larynx and epiglottis	Enhanced ability to synchronize swallowing and breathing; risk for airway obstruction; possibly more difficult to intubate
Small compliant airway passages with higher airway resistance; immature reflexes	Risk for airway obstruction and apnea
Increased pulmonary vascular resistance with sensitive pulmonary arterioles	Risk for ductal shunting and hypoxemia with events such as hypoxia, acidosis, hypothermia, hypoglycemia, and hypercarbia
Increased oxygen consumption	Increased respiratory rate and work of breathing; risk for hypoxia
Increased intrapulmonary right-left shunting	Increased risk for atelectasis with wasted ventilation; lower Pco_2
Immaturity of pulmonary surfactant system in immature infants	Increased risk for atelectasis and respiratory distress syndrome; increased work of breathing
Immature respiratory control	Irregular respirations with periodic breathing; risk for apnea; inability to rapidly alter depth of respirations

Pco_2, Partial pressure of carbon dioxide.
From Blackburn, S. (2013). *Maternal, fetal, and neonatal physiology: A clinical perspective* (4th ed.). Maryland Heights, MO: Saunders.

In neonates with more serious respiratory problems, symptoms of distress are more pronounced and tend to last beyond the first 2 hours after birth. Respiratory rates can exceed 120 breaths/minute. Moderate to severe retractions, grunting, pallor, and central cyanosis can occur. The respiratory symptoms can be accompanied by hypotension, temperature instability, hypoglycemia, acidosis, and signs of cardiac problems. Common respiratory complications affecting neonates include RDS, meconium aspiration, pneumonia, and persistent pulmonary hypertension of the newborn (PPHN). Congenital defects such as anomalies of the great vessels, diaphragmatic hernia, or chest wall defects can cause severe respiratory problems. Blood incompatibilities such as hydrops fetalis can result in respiratory compromise (Gardner, Enzman-Hines, and Nyp, 2016) (see Chapter 25).

CARDIOVASCULAR SYSTEM

The cardiovascular system changes significantly after birth. The infant's first breaths, combined with increased alveolar capillary distention, inflate the lungs and reduce pulmonary vascular resistance to pulmonary blood flow from the pulmonary arteries. Pulmonary artery pressure drops, and pressure in the right atrium declines. Increased pulmonary blood flow from the left side of the heart increases pressure in the left atrium, which causes a functional closure of the foramen ovale. During the first few days of life, crying can temporarily reverse the flow through the foramen ovale and lead to mild cyanosis. Soon after birth, cardiac output nearly doubles and blood flow increases to the lungs, heart, kidneys, and gastrointestinal (GI) tract (Hillman et al., 2012).

In utero fetal Po_2 is 20 to 30 mm Hg. After birth, when the Po_2 level in the arterial blood approximates 50 mm Hg, the ductus arteriosus constricts in response to increased oxygenation. Circulating prostaglandin E (PGE_2) levels also have an important role in closing the ductus arteriosus. In term infants, it functionally closes within the first 24 hours after birth; permanent (anatomic) closure usually occurs within 3 to 4 weeks, and the ductus arteriosus becomes a ligament. The ductus arteriosus can open in response to low oxygen levels in association with hypoxia, asphyxia, or prematurity. With auscultation of the chest, a patent ductus arteriosus can be detected as a heart murmur (Lott, 2014).

When the cord is clamped and severed, the umbilical arteries, the umbilical vein, and the ductus venosus are functionally closed; they are converted into ligaments within 2 to 3 months. The hypogastric arteries also occlude and become ligaments. Table 22.2 summarizes the cardiovascular changes at birth.

Heart Rate and Sounds

The heart rate for a term newborn ranges from 120 to 160 beats/minute, with brief fluctuations greater and less than these values usually noted during sleeping and waking states. The range of the heart rate in the term infant is about 80 to 100 beats/minute during deep sleep and can increase to 180 beats/min or higher when the infant cries. A heart rate that is either high (more than 160 beats/minute) or low (fewer than 100 beats/minute) should be reevaluated within 30 minutes to 1 hour or when the activity of the infant changes.

The apical impulse (point of maximal impulse [PMI]) in the newborn is at the fourth intercostal space and to the left of the midclavicular line. The PMI is often visible and easily palpable because of the thin chest wall; this is also called *precordial activity*.

Irregular heart rate or sinus dysrhythmia is common in the first few hours of life but thereafter may need to be evaluated. Heart sounds during the neonatal period are of higher pitch, shorter duration, and greater intensity than during adult life. The first sound (S_1) is typically louder and duller than the second sound (S_2), which is sharp. The third and fourth heart sounds are not audible in newborns. Most heart murmurs heard during the neonatal period have no pathologic significance, and more than one-half of the murmurs disappear by 6 months of age. However, the presence of a murmur and accompanying signs such as poor feeding, apnea, cyanosis, or pallor is considered abnormal and should be investigated. There can be significant cardiac defects without a murmur or other symptoms (Smith, 2012). This reinforces the importance of ongoing assessment.

Blood Pressure

Values for newborn blood pressure vary with gestational age, weight, state of alertness, and cuff size. The term newborn infant's average systolic BP is 60 to 80 mm Hg, and average diastolic BP is 40 to 50 mm Hg. The mean arterial pressure (MAP) should be equivalent to the weeks of gestation. For example, an infant born at 40 weeks of gestation should have a MAP of at least 40. The BP increases by the second day of life, with minor variations noted during the first month of life. A drop in systolic BP (about 15 mm Hg) in the first hour of life is common. Crying and movement usually cause increases in the systolic BP.

TABLE 22.2   Cardiovascular Changes at Birth

Prenatal Status	Postbirth Status	Associated Factors
Primary Changes		
Pulmonary circulation: High pulmonary vascular resistance, increased pressure in right ventricle and pulmonary arteries	Low pulmonary vascular resistance; decreased pressure in right atrium, ventricle, and pulmonary arteries	Expansion of collapsed fetal lung with air
Systemic circulation: Low pressures in left atrium, ventricle, and aorta	High systemic vascular resistance; increased pressure in left atrium, ventricle, and aorta	Loss of placental blood flow
Secondary Changes		
Umbilical arteries: Patent, carrying of blood from hypogastric arteries to placenta	Functionally closed at birth; obliteration by fibrous proliferation possibly taking 2 to 3 months, distal portions becoming lateral vesicoumbilical ligaments, proximal portions remaining open as superior vesicle arteries	Closure preceding that of umbilical vein, probably accomplished by smooth muscle contraction in response to thermal and mechanical stimuli and alteration in oxygen tension Mechanically severed with cord at birth
Umbilical vein: Patent, carrying of blood from placenta to ductus venosus and liver	Closed; becoming ligamentum teres hepatis after obliteration	Closure shortly after umbilical arteries; hence blood from placenta possibly entering neonate for short period after birth Mechanically severed with cord at birth
Ductus venosus: Patent, connection of umbilical vein to inferior vena cava	Closed; becoming ligamentum venosum after obliteration	Loss of blood flow from umbilical vein
Ductus arteriosus: Patent, shunting of blood from pulmonary artery to descending aorta	Functionally closed almost immediately after birth; anatomic obliteration of lumen by fibrous proliferation requiring 1 to 3 months, becoming ligamentum arteriosum	Increased oxygen content of blood in ductus arteriosus creating vasospasm of its muscular wall High systemic resistance increasing aortic pressure; low pulmonary resistance reducing pulmonary arterial pressure
Foramen ovale: Formation of a valve opening that allows blood to flow directly to left atrium (shunting of blood from right to left atrium)	Functionally closed at birth; constant apposition gradually leading to fusion and permanent closure within a few months or years in majority of persons	Increased pressure in left atrium and decreased pressure in right atrium, causing closure of valve over foramen

Data from Blackburn, S. (2013). *Maternal, fetal, and neonatal physiology: A clinical perspective* (4th ed.). Maryland Heights, MO: Saunders.

Blood Volume

Blood volume in the term newborn ranges from 80 to 100 mL/kg of body weight. In the preterm infant, the range is 90 to 105 mL/kg (Diehl-Jones & Fraser, 2015). The preterm infant has a relatively greater blood volume than the term newborn. This occurs because the preterm infant has a proportionately greater plasma volume, not a greater red blood cell (RBC) mass.

Delayed clamping of the umbilical cord changes the circulatory dynamics of the newborn. Delayed cord clamping (DCC) expands the blood volume from the so-called *placental transfusion* of blood to the newborn by as much as 100 mL, depending on the length of time to cord clamping and cutting. Delayed cord clamping has been associated with increased blood volume and blood pressure, and reduced risk for intraventricular hemorrhage and necrotizing enterocolitis (Perlman, Wyllie, Kattwinkel, et al., 2015). These benefits are most important for preterm infants. Polycythemia that occurs with delayed clamping is usually not harmful, although there can be an increased risk for hyperbilirubinemia that requires phototherapy. The American College of Obstetricians and Gynecologists (ACOG, 2012) and the American Academy of Pediatrics (AAP, 2013) recommend that DCC is practiced whenever possible. DCC is reasonable for term and preterm newborns who do not need resuscitation; there is a lack of evidence regarding DCC for neonates who require immediate resuscitation (Perlman et al.).

Signs of Cardiovascular Problems

Variations in vital signs can be indicative of cardiovascular problems. Persistent tachycardia (more than 160 beats/minute) can be associated with anemia, hypovolemia, hyperthermia, or sepsis. Persistent bradycardia (less than 80 beats/minute) can be a sign of a congenital heart block or hypoxemia. Unequal or absent pulses, bounding pulses, and decreased or elevated blood pressure can indicate cardiovascular problems (Verklan, 2015).

The newborn's skin color can reflect cardiovascular problems. Pallor in the immediate postbirth period is often a sign of underlying problems such as anemia or marked peripheral vasoconstriction as a result of intrapartum asphyxia or sepsis. Cyanosis other than in the hands or feet, with or without increased work of breathing, can indicate respiratory and/or cardiac problems. The presence of jaundice can indicate ABO or Rh factor incompatibility problems (see Chapter 25).

Congenital heart defects are the most common types of congenital malformations (Centers for Disease Control and Prevention [CDC], 2015) (see Chapter 25). Although the more serious defects such as tetralogy of Fallot are likely to have clinical manifestations such as cyanosis, dyspnea, and hypoxia, others such as small ventricular septal defects can be asymptomatic. The prenatal history can provide information regarding risk factors for congenital heart defects so the nurse knows to be more alert for symptoms. Maternal illness such as rubella, metabolic disease such as diabetes, and drug ingestion are associated with an increased risk for cardiac defects.

HEMATOPOIETIC SYSTEM

Red Blood Cells

Because fetal circulation is less efficient at oxygen exchange than the lungs, the fetus needs additional RBCs for transport of oxygen in utero.

Therefore, at birth the average levels of RBCs, hemoglobin, and hematocrit are higher than those in the adult; these levels fall slowly over the first month. At birth, the RBC count ranges from 4.6 to 5.2 million/mm³ (Blackburn, 2013). The term newborn can have a hemoglobin concentration of 14 to 24 g/dL at birth, decreasing gradually to 12 to 20 g/dL during the first 2 weeks (Pagana, Pagana, & Pagana, 2017). Hematocrit at birth ranges from 51% to 56%, increases slightly in the first few hours or days as fluid shifts from intravascular to interstitial spaces (Blackburn, 2013), and by 8 weeks is between 39% and 59% (Pagana et al.). Polycythemia (central venous hematocrit greater than 65%) can occur in term and preterm infants as a result of delayed cord clamping, maternal hypertension or diabetes, or intrauterine growth restriction.

The source of the sample is a significant factor in levels of RBCs, hemoglobin, and hematocrit. Capillary blood yields higher values than venous blood.

The timing of blood sampling is also significant; the slight rise in RBCs after birth is followed by a substantial drop. At birth the infant's blood contains an average of 70% fetal hemoglobin; however, because of the shorter life span of the cells containing fetal hemoglobin, the percentage falls rapidly, so that by the age of 6 to 12 months there is only a trace of fetal hemoglobin remaining (Christensen & Ohls, 2016). Iron stores generally are sufficient to sustain normal RBC production for approximately 4 months in the term infant, at which time a transient physiologic anemia can occur.

Leukocytes

Leukocytosis, with a white blood cell (WBC) count ranging from 9000 to 30,000/mm³, is normal at birth (Pagana et al., 2017). The number of WBCs increases up to 24,000/mm³ during the first day after birth. The initial high WBC count of the newborn decreases rapidly, and a stable level of 12,000/mm³ is normally maintained during the neonatal period (Blackburn, 2013). Newborns are susceptible to infection. Leukocytes, especially the polymorphonuclear neutrophils, are limited in their ability to recognize foreign protein and localize and fight infection early in life (Benjamin, Mezu-Ndubuisi, & Maheshwari, 2015). Sepsis can be accompanied by a concomitant rise in neutrophils; however, some infants initially have clinical signs of sepsis without a significant elevation in WBCs. In addition, events other than infection (i.e., prolonged crying, maternal hypertension, asymptomatic hypoglycemia, hemolytic disease, meconium aspiration syndrome, labor induction with oxytocin, surgery, difficult labor, high altitude, and maternal fever) can cause neutrophilia in the newborn.

Platelets

Platelets appear to be activated during the birth process and demonstrate improved aggregation in the first hours after birth. The platelet count ranges between 150,000 and 300,000/mm³ and is essentially the same in newborns as in adults. Levels of vitamin K–dependent clotting factors II, VII, IX, and X increase slowly after birth and reach adult levels by 6 months of age (Monagle, 2017).

Blood Groups

The infant's blood group is determined genetically and established early in fetal life. However, during the neonatal period the strength of the agglutinogens present in the RBC membrane gradually increases. Cord blood samples can be used to identify the infant's blood type and Rh status.

THERMOGENIC SYSTEM

Next to establishing respirations and effective extrauterine circulation, heat regulation is most critical to the newborn's survival. During the first 12 hours after birth, the neonate attempts to achieve thermal balance in adjusting to the extrauterine environmental temperature. Thermoregulation is the maintenance of balance between heat loss and heat production. Newborns attempt to stabilize their core body temperatures within a narrow range. Hypothermia from excessive heat loss is a common and potentially serious problem.

Anatomic and physiologic characteristics of neonates place them at risk for heat loss. Newborns have a thin layer of subcutaneous fat. The blood vessels are close to the surface of the skin. Newborns have larger body surface–to–body weight (mass) ratios than children and adults. Changes in environmental temperature alter the temperature of the blood, thereby influencing temperature regulation centers in the hypothalamus (Blackburn, 2013).

Heat Loss

The body temperature of newborn infants depends on the heat transfer between the infant and the external environment. Factors that influence heat loss to the environment include the temperature and humidity of the air, the flow and velocity of the air, and the temperature of surfaces in contact with and around the infant. The goal of care is to provide a neutral thermal environment for the neonate in which heat balance is maintained. The neutral thermal environment is the ideal environmental temperature that allows the neonate to maintain a normal body temperature to minimize oxygen and glucose consumption (Ringer, 2013a). Heat loss in the newborn occurs by four modes:

1. *Convection* is the flow of heat from the body surface to cooler ambient air. Because of heat loss by convection, the ambient temperature in newborn care areas should range between 22° and 26°C (72° to 78°F) and the humidity between 30% and 60% (AAP & ACOG, 2012). Newborns in open bassinets are wrapped to protect them from the cold. A cap may be worn to decrease heat loss from the infant's head.
2. *Radiation* is the loss of heat from the body surface to a cooler solid surface not in direct contact but in relative proximity. To prevent this type of loss, bassinets and examining tables are placed away from outside windows, and care is taken to avoid direct air drafts.
3. *Evaporation* is the loss of heat that occurs when a liquid is converted to a vapor. In the newborn, heat loss by evaporation occurs as a result of moisture vaporization from the skin. This heat loss is intensified by failing to completely dry the newborn after birth or with bathing. Evaporative heat loss, as a component of insensible water loss, is the most significant cause of heat loss in the first few days of life.
4. *Conduction* is the loss of heat from the body surface to cooler surfaces in direct contact. During the initial assessment, the newborn is placed on a prewarmed bed under a radiant warmer to minimize heat loss. The scales used for weighing the newborn should have a protective cover to minimize conductive heat loss.

Heat loss must be controlled to protect the infant. Control of such modes of heat loss is the basis of caregiving policies and techniques. Drying the infant quickly after birth is essential to prevent hypothermia. Skin-to-skin contact with the mother is an effective means of reducing conductive and radiant heat loss and enhancing newborn temperature control and maternal-infant interaction. The naked newborn is placed on the mother's bare chest and covered with a warm blanket; a cap may be placed on the infant's head to help conserve heat (Fig. 22.1). Alternatively, the neonate is placed under a radiant warmer to reduce heat loss and promote thermoregulation.

Thermogenesis

In response to cold, the neonate attempts to generate heat (thermogenesis) by increasing muscle activity. Cold infants may cry and appear

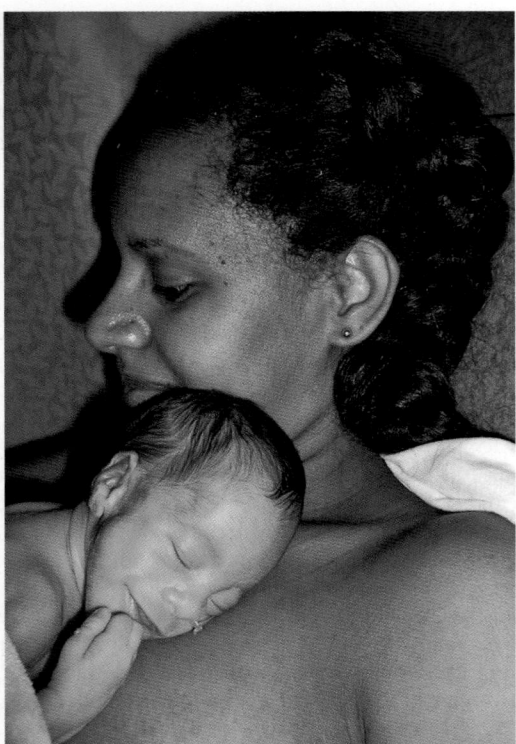

FIG 22.1 Infant in skin-to-skin contact with mother. Note infant smile. (Courtesy of Cheryl Briggs, RNC, Annapolis, MD.)

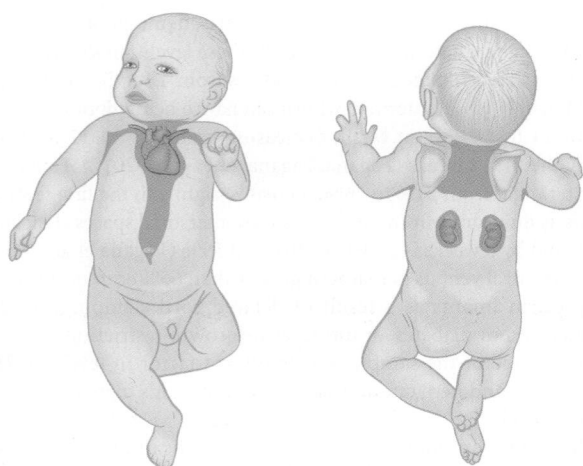

FIG 22.2 Distribution of brown fat in the newborn. (Modified from Murray S.S., & McKinney E.S. [2010]. *Foundations of maternal-newborn and women's health nursing* (6th ed.). St. Louis, MO: Elsevier.)

restless. Because of vasoconstriction the skin can feel cool to touch, and acrocyanosis can be present. There is an increase in cellular metabolic activity, primarily in the brain, heart, and liver; this also increases oxygen and glucose consumption.

In an effort to conserve heat, term newborns assume a position of flexion that helps guard against heat loss because it diminishes the amount of body surface exposed to the environment. Infants also can reduce the loss of internal heat through the body surface by constricting peripheral blood vessels.

Adults are able to produce heat through shivering; however, the shivering mechanism of heat production is rarely operable in the newborn unless there is prolonged cold exposure (Blackburn, 2013). Newborns produce heat through nonshivering thermogenesis. This is accomplished primarily by metabolism of brown fat, which is unique to the newborn; and secondarily by increased metabolic activity in the brain, heart, and liver. Brown fat is located in superficial deposits in the interscapular region and axillae and in deep deposits at the thoracic inlet, along the vertebral column, and around the kidneys (Fig. 22.2). Brown fat has a richer vascular and nerve supply than ordinary fat. Heat produced by intense lipid metabolic activity in brown fat can warm the newborn by increasing heat production as much as 100%. Reserves of brown fat, usually present for several weeks after birth, are rapidly depleted with cold stress. The amount of brown fat reserve increases with the weeks of gestation. A full-term newborn has greater stores than a preterm infant (Ringer, 2013a).

Hypothermia and Cold Stress

When the neonate's temperature drops, vasoconstriction occurs as a mechanism to conserve heat. The infant can appear pale and mottled; the skin feels cool, especially on the extremities. If the hypothermia is not corrected, it will progress to cold stress, which imposes metabolic and physiologic demands on all infants, regardless of gestational age and condition. The respiratory rate increases in response to the increased need for oxygen. In the cold-stressed infant, oxygen consumption and energy are diverted from maintaining normal brain and cardiac function and growth to thermogenesis for survival. If the infant cannot maintain an adequate oxygen tension, vasoconstriction follows and jeopardizes pulmonary perfusion. As a consequence, the Po_2 is decreased, and the blood pH drops (Ringer, 2013b). Surfactant synthesis can be altered. These changes can prompt a transient respiratory distress or aggravate existing RDS. Moreover, decreased pulmonary perfusion and oxygen tension can maintain or reopen the right-to-left shunt across the ductus arteriosus.

The basal metabolic rate increases with cold stress. If cold stress is protracted, anaerobic glycolysis occurs, resulting in increased production of acids. Metabolic acidosis develops, and, if a defect in respiratory function is present, respiratory acidosis also develops (Fig. 22.3). Excessive fatty acids can displace the bilirubin from the albumin-binding sites and exacerbate hyperbilirubinemia. Hypoglycemia is another metabolic consequence of cold stress. The process of anaerobic glycolysis can deplete existing stores. If the infant is sufficiently stressed and low glucose stores are not replaced, hypoglycemia, which can be asymptomatic in the newborn, can develop (Gardner & Hernández, 2016).

Hyperthermia

Although occurring less frequently than hypothermia, hyperthermia can occur and must be corrected. A body temperature greater than 37.5°C (99.5°F) is considered to be abnormally high and is typically caused by excess heat production related to sepsis or a decrease in heat loss. Hyperthermia can result from the inappropriate use of external heat sources such as radiant warmers, phototherapy, sunlight, increased environmental temperature, and the use of excessive clothing or blankets (Gardner & Hernández, 2016). The clinical appearance of the infant who is hyperthermic often indicates the causative mechanism. Infants who are overheated because of environmental factors such as being swaddled in too many blankets exhibit signs of heat-losing mechanisms: skin vessels dilate, skin appears flushed, hands and feet are warm to touch, and the infant assumes a posture of extension. The newborn who is hyperthermic because of sepsis appears stressed: vessels in the skin are constricted, color is pale, and hands and feet are cool. Hyperthermia develops more rapidly in a newborn than in an adult because of the relatively larger surface area of an infant. Sweat glands do not function well. Hyperthermia can cause neurologic injury and increased

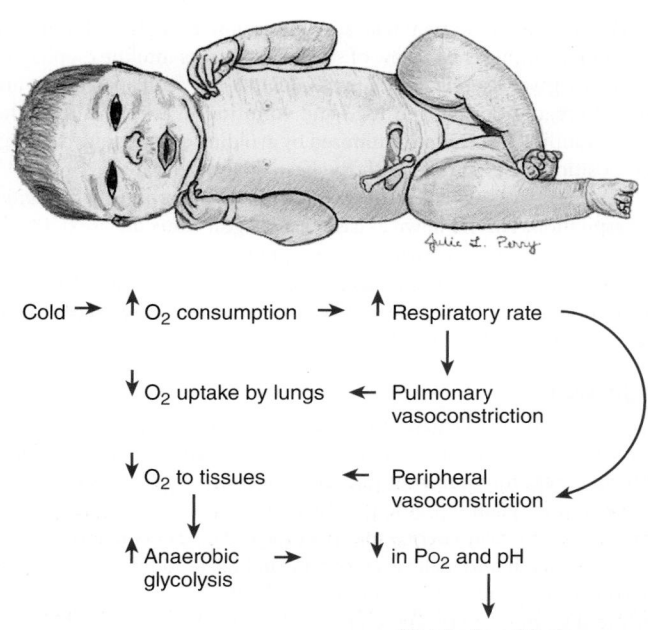

FIG 22.3 Effects of cold stress. When an infant is stressed by cold, oxygen consumption increases, and pulmonary and peripheral vasoconstriction occur, thereby decreasing oxygen uptake by the lungs and oxygen to the tissues; anaerobic glycolysis increases, and there is a decrease in P_{O_2} and pH, leading to metabolic acidosis.

risk for seizures; severe cases can result in heat stroke and death (Gardner & Hernández, 2016; Ringer, 2013b).

RENAL SYSTEM

At term, the kidneys occupy a large portion of the posterior abdominal wall. The bladder lies close to the anterior abdominal wall and is both an abdominal and a pelvic organ. In the newborn, almost all palpable masses in the abdomen are renal in origin.

At birth, a small quantity (approximately 40 mL) of urine is usually present in the bladder of a full-term infant. Many newborns void at the time of birth, although this is easily missed and may not be recorded. During the first few days, term infants generally excrete 15 to 60 mL/kg/day of urine; output gradually increases over the first month (Blackburn, 2013). The frequency of voiding varies from 2 to 6 times per day during the first and second days of life and increases during the subsequent 24 hours. After day 4, approximately 6 to 8 voidings per day of pale straw-colored urine indicate adequate fluid intake.

> **! NURSING ALERT**
>
> Noting and recording the first voiding are important. An infant who has not voided by 24 hours should be assessed for adequacy of fluid intake, bladder distention, restlessness, and signs of discomfort. The neonatal health care provider should be notified.

Full-term newborns have limited capacity to concentrate urine; therefore, the specific gravity is usually low (less than 1.004) (Cadnapaphornchai, Schoenbein, Woloschuk, et al., 2016). The ability to concentrate urine fully is attained by about 3 months of age. After the first voiding, the infant's urine can appear cloudy (because of mucus content) and have a much higher specific gravity. This decreases as fluid intake increases. Normal urine during early infancy is usually straw colored and almost odorless. Sometimes pink-tinged uric acid crystals or "brick dust" appear on the diaper. Uric acid crystals are normal during the first week, but thereafter can be a sign of inadequate intake (Janke, 2014). Loss of fluid through urine, feces, lungs, increased metabolic rate, and limited fluid intake can result in a 5% to 10% loss of the birth weight over the first 3 to 5 days. Excessive weight loss can be related to feeding difficulties or other issues. The neonate should regain the birth weight within 10 to 14 days, depending on the feeding method (breastfeeding, breast milk feeding, or infant formula).

Fluid and Electrolyte Balance

In the term neonate, approximately 75% of body weight consists of total body water (extracellular and intracellular). A reduction in extracellular fluid occurs with diuresis during the first few days after birth. The weight loss experienced by most newborns during the first few days after birth is caused primarily by extracellular water loss (Cadnapaphornchai et al., 2016).

The daily fluid requirement for neonates weighing more than 1500 g is 60 to 80 mL/kg during the first 2 days of life. From 3 to 7 days the requirement is 100 to 150 mL/kg/day, and from 8 to 30 days it is 120 to 180 mL/kg/day (Dell, 2015).

At birth, the glomerular filtration rate (GFR) of a newborn is significantly lower than in the adult. This results in a decreased ability to remove nitrogenous and other waste products from the blood. The GFR rapidly increases during the 2 to 4 weeks after birth as a result of postnatal physiologic changes, including decreased renal vascular resistance, increased renal blood flow, and increased filtration pressure. The GFR gradually rises to adult levels by 2 years of age (Blackburn, 2013; Vogt & Dell, 2015).

Sodium reabsorption is decreased as a result of a lowered sodium- or potassium-activated adenosine triphosphatase activity. The decreased ability to excrete excess sodium results in hypotonic urine compared with plasma, leading to a higher concentration of sodium, phosphates, chloride, and organic acids and a lower concentration of bicarbonate ions. The infant has a higher renal threshold for glucose than adults.

Tubular reabsorption of glucose in the term neonate is similar to that of an adult. While the renal threshold for glucose is lower, newborns do not typically exhibit glycosuria.

Because of a lower renal threshold for bicarbonate and a limited capacity for reabsorption, the neonate's serum bicarbonate and plasma pH levels are lower. Buffering capacity is decreased. This reduces the newborn's ability to cope with events (e.g., cold stress) that produce acidosis (Blackburn, 2013).

Signs of Renal System Problems

The renal system has a wide range of functions. Dysfunction resulting from physiologic abnormalities can range from the lack of a steady stream of urine to gross anomalies such as hypospadias and exstrophy of the bladder, which can be identified easily at birth. Enlarged or cystic kidneys can be identified as masses during abdominal palpation. Some kidney anomalies also can be detected by ultrasound examination during pregnancy (see Chapter 25).

GASTROINTESTINAL SYSTEM

The full-term newborn is capable of swallowing, digesting, metabolizing, and absorbing proteins and simple carbohydrates and emulsifying fats. With the exception of pancreatic amylase, the characteristic digestive enzymes are present even in low-birth-weight neonates.

In the adequately hydrated infant, the mucous membrane of the mouth is moist and pink; the hard and soft palates are intact. The presence of moderate to large amounts of mucus is common in the first few hours after birth. Small whitish areas (Epstein pearls) may be found on the gum margins and at the juncture of the hard and soft palates. The cheeks are full because of well-developed sucking pads. These, like the labial tubercles (sucking calluses) on the upper lip, disappear at around 12 months of age when the sucking period is over.

Feeding behavior is related to gestational age and is influenced by neuromuscular maturity, maternal medications during labor and birth, and the type of initial feeding. Feeding requires that the neonate is able to coordinate sucking, swallowing, and breathing. Sucking is a reflex behavior that begins in utero as early as 15 to 16 weeks. By 28 weeks, some infants can coordinate sucking and swallowing. By 32 to 34 weeks most are able to coordinate sucking, swallowing, and breathing; this is well developed by 36 to 38 weeks (Blackburn, 2013). Sucking takes place in small bursts of 3 or 4 and up to 8 to 10 sucks at a time, with a brief pause between bursts. The neonate is unable to move food from the lips to the pharynx; therefore placing the nipple (breast or bottle) well inside the baby's mouth is necessary. Peristaltic activity in the esophagus is uncoordinated in the first few days of life. It quickly becomes a coordinated pattern in healthy full-term infants, and they swallow easily.

Teeth begin developing in utero, with enamel formation continuing until about 10 years of age. Tooth development is influenced by neonatal or infant illnesses and medications and by maternal illnesses or medications taken by the mother during pregnancy. The fluoride level in the water supply also influences tooth development. Occasionally an infant may be born with one or more teeth. These natal teeth have poorly formed roots and as they loosen place the infant at risk for aspiration. Therefore, they are usually extracted.

The mucosal barrier in the intestines is not fully mature until 4 to 6 months of age, which allows antigens and other macromolecules such as bacteria to be transported across the intestinal wall into the systemic circulation. This increases the risk for allergies and infection (Blackburn, 2013).

Intestinal flora, or gut microbiota, are established within the first week after birth; and normal intestinal flora help synthesize vitamin K, folate, and biotin. Traditionally it was thought that the fetus grows and develops in a sterile environment. Research on the human microbiome suggests that the pregnant woman and the developing fetus coexist with a variety of commensal and symbiotic microbes that have important influences on the health of both the mother and her infant. Research evidence of microbial presence in amniotic fluid, placenta, and meconium indicates that the fetus is exposed to microbes during pregnancy. The mode of birth (vaginal or cesarean) seems to play a major role in the microbial colonization of the neonate. Infants born vaginally appear to be initially colonized by the maternal vaginal microbes, whereas infants born by cesarean section are first colonized by maternal skin microbes. This initial colonization plays a major role in establishing intestinal flora; research is ongoing to identify the implications for the child's future health. The microbiome of the infant is also influenced by diet, antibiotics, and environmental factors (Bäckhed, Roswall, Peng, et al., 2015; Mueller, Bakacs, Combellick, et al., 2015; Neu, 2017).

Breastfeeding is important in establishing the intestinal microbiome of the newborn. Human milk contains a variety of microbes that appear to originate in the mother's gastrointestinal tract, Oligosaccharides in human milk may have a prebiotic function that facilitates the growth of beneficial bacteria in the neonatal gastrointestinal tract (Neu, 2017).

The capacity of the newborn stomach varies widely, depending on the size of the infant, from less than 10 mL on day 1 to nearly 30 mL on day 3 and expanding to 60 mL on day 7. After birth, the newborn stomach becomes increasingly more compliant and relaxed to accommodate larger volumes. Several factors such as time and volume of feedings or type and temperature of food can affect the emptying time.

The normal intermittent relaxation of the lower esophageal sphincter results in involuntary backflow of stomach contents into the esophagus, known as gastroesophageal reflux (GER). As a result, newborns are prone to regurgitation, "spitting," and vomiting, especially during the first 3 months. GER can be minimized by avoiding overfeeding, burping, and positioning the infant with the head slightly elevated.

In some infants, GER is severe enough to cause dysphagia, esophagitis, and aspiration. This is known as gastroesophageal reflux disease (GERD). Treatment may include medications to reduce gastric acidity such as antacids, histamine-blocking agents, or proton-pump inhibitors; and medication to increase gastric motility. In severe cases, surgical treatment may be considered (Hibbs, 2015).

Digestion

The infant's ability to digest carbohydrates, fats, and proteins is regulated by the presence of certain enzymes. Most of these enzymes are functional at birth except for pancreatic amylase and lipase. Amylase is produced by the salivary glands after approximately 3 months of age and by the pancreas at approximately 6 months of age. This enzyme is necessary to convert starch into maltose and occurs in high amounts in colostrum. The other exception is lipase, also secreted by the pancreas; it is necessary for the digestion of fat. Therefore, the normal newborn is capable of digesting simple carbohydrates and proteins but has a limited ability to digest fats. Mammary lipase in human milk aids in digestion of fats by the neonate.

Lactase levels in newborns are higher than in older infants. This enzyme is necessary for digestion of lactose, the major carbohydrate in human milk and commercial infant formula.

Stools

Meconium fills the lower intestine at birth. It is formed during fetal life from the amniotic fluid and its constituents, intestinal secretions (including bilirubin), and cells (shed from the mucosa). Meconium is greenish black and viscous and contains occult blood. Most healthy term infants pass meconium within the first 12 to 24 hours of life, and almost all do so by 48 hours. The number of stools passed varies during the first week, being most numerous between the third and sixth days. Newborns fed early pass stools sooner. The colostrum consumed by breastfed neonates during the first 2 to 3 days after birth promotes stooling. Progressive changes in the stooling pattern indicate a properly functioning GI tract (Box 22.1).

Feeding Behaviors

Variations occur among infants regarding interest in food, signs of hunger, and amount ingested at one time. The amount the infant consumes at any feeding depends on gestational and chronologic age, weight, hunger level, and alertness. When put to breast some infants feed immediately, whereas others require a longer learning period. Random hand-to-mouth movement and sucking of fingers are well developed at birth and intensify when the infant is hungry. Caregivers should be alert and responsive to these hunger cues (Lawrence & Lawrence, 2016).

Signs of Gastrointestinal Problems

The time, color, and character of the infant's first stool should be noted. Failure to pass meconium can indicate bowel obstruction related to conditions such as an inborn error of metabolism (e.g., cystic fibrosis) or a congenital disorder (e.g., Hirschsprung's disease or an imperforate anus). An active rectal "wink" reflex (contraction of the anal sphincter muscle in response to touch) is a sign of good sphincter tone. Passage of meconium from the vagina or urinary meatus is a sign of a possible fistulous tract from the rectum.

Fullness of the abdomen above the umbilicus can be caused by hepatomegaly, duodenal atresia, or distention. Abdominal distention at birth usually indicates a serious disorder such as a ruptured viscus (from abdominal wall defects) or tumors. Distention that occurs later can be the result of overfeeding or can be a sign of a GI disorder. A scaphoid (sunken) abdomen, with bowel sounds heard in the chest and signs of respiratory distress, indicates a diaphragmatic hernia. Fullness below the umbilicus can indicate a distended bladder.

Some infants are intolerant of certain commercial infant formulas. If an infant is allergic or unable to digest a formula, the stools can become very soft with a high water content that is signaled by a distinct water ring around the stool on the diaper. Forceful ejection of stool and a water ring around the stool are signs of diarrhea. Care must be taken to avoid misinterpreting transitional stools for diarrhea. The loss of fluid in diarrhea can rapidly lead to fluid and electrolyte imbalance.

The amount and frequency of regurgitation, "spitting," or vomiting after feedings should be documented. Color change, gagging, and projectile (very forceful) vomiting occur in association with esophageal and tracheoesophageal anomalies. Vomiting in large amounts, especially if it is projectile, can be a sign of pyloric stenosis. Bilious (green) emesis is suggestive of intestinal obstruction or malrotation of the bowel.

HEPATIC SYSTEM

In the newborn, the liver can be palpated about 1 to 2 cm below the right costal margin because it is enlarged and occupies about 40% of the abdominal cavity. The infant's liver plays an important role in iron storage, glucose and fatty acid metabolism, bilirubin synthesis, and coagulation. Although the liver is relatively immature at birth, healthy term infants do not typically experience problems.

Iron Storage

The fetal liver, which serves as the site for production of hemoglobin after birth, begins storing iron in utero. The infant's iron store is proportional to total body hemoglobin content and length of gestation. At birth, the term infant has an iron store sufficient to last approximately 4 months. Iron stores of preterm and small-for-gestational-age infants are often lower and are depleted sooner than in healthy term infants.

Although both breast milk and cow's milk contain iron, the bioavailability of iron in breast milk (lactoferrin) is far superior.

Glucose Homeostasis

The liver is responsible for regulation of blood glucose levels. In utero, the glucose concentration in the umbilical vein is approximately 70% of the maternal level. At birth, the newborn is removed from the maternal glucose supply resulting in an initial drop in blood glucose from fetal levels of 70 to 90 mg/dL to levels of 55 to 60 mg/dL between 30 and 90 minutes after birth. During this time, glucagon levels increase while insulin levels decrease and the limited hepatic glycogen stores are mobilized. The initiation of feedings helps to stabilize blood glucose levels as milk lactose is metabolized. Glucose production also occurs through glycogenolysis and gluconeogenesis (Grijalva & Vakili, 2013). Glucose levels rise gradually and stabilize by the second or third day at levels greater than 70 mg/dL (Hawkes & Stanley, 2017).

Glucose levels are not routinely assessed in newborns unless there are risk factors or symptoms of hypoglycemia. Risk factors include small or large for gestational age, preterm, and infant of a diabetic mother. The hypoglycemic infant can be asymptomatic or can display the classic symptoms of jitteriness, lethargy, apnea, feeding problems, or seizures. Hypoglycemia in the initial newborn period is most often transient and easily corrected through feeding. Persistent or recurrent hypoglycemia necessitates intravenous glucose therapy and possible pharmacologic intervention.

Fatty Acid Metabolism

Fatty acid metabolism is an additional source of energy for the neonate in the initial hours after birth. Catecholamine release increases the rate of lipolysis, which produces fatty acids for oxidation and ketone body synthesis. Hepatic ketogenesis is increased in term newborns for the first 3 days (Grijalva & Vakili, 2013).

Bilirubin Synthesis

The liver is responsible for the conjugation of bilirubin, which results from the breakdown of RBCs. When RBCs reach the end of their life span, their membranes rupture, and hemoglobin is released. The hemoglobin is phagocytosed by macrophages; it then splits into heme and globin. The heme is broken down by the reticuloendothelial cells, converted to bilirubin, and released in an unconjugated form. The unconjugated (indirect) bilirubin is relatively insoluble and almost entirely bound to circulating albumin, a plasma protein. Bilirubin that is not bound to albumin, or free bilirubin, can easily cross the blood-brain barrier and cause neurotoxicity (acute bilirubin encephalopathy or kernicterus).

The unconjugated bilirubin must be conjugated so it becomes soluble and excretable. In the liver, the unbound bilirubin is conjugated with glucuronic acid in the presence of the enzyme glucuronyl transferase. The conjugated form of bilirubin (direct bilirubin) is soluble and excreted from liver cells as a constituent of bile. Along with other components of bile, direct bilirubin is excreted into the biliary tract system that carries the bile into the duodenum. Bilirubin is converted to urobilinogen and stercobilinogen within the duodenum through the action of the bacterial flora. Urobilinogen is excreted in urine and feces; stercobilinogen is excreted in the feces. The effectiveness of bilirubin excretion through the feces depends on the stooling pattern of the newborn and the substances in the intestine that break down conjugated bilirubin. In the newborn intestine, the enzyme β-glucuronidase is able to convert conjugated bilirubin into the unconjugated form, which is subsequently reabsorbed by the intestinal mucosa and transported to the liver; this is called *enterohepatic circulation*. Feeding is important in reducing serum bilirubin levels because it stimulates peristalsis and produces

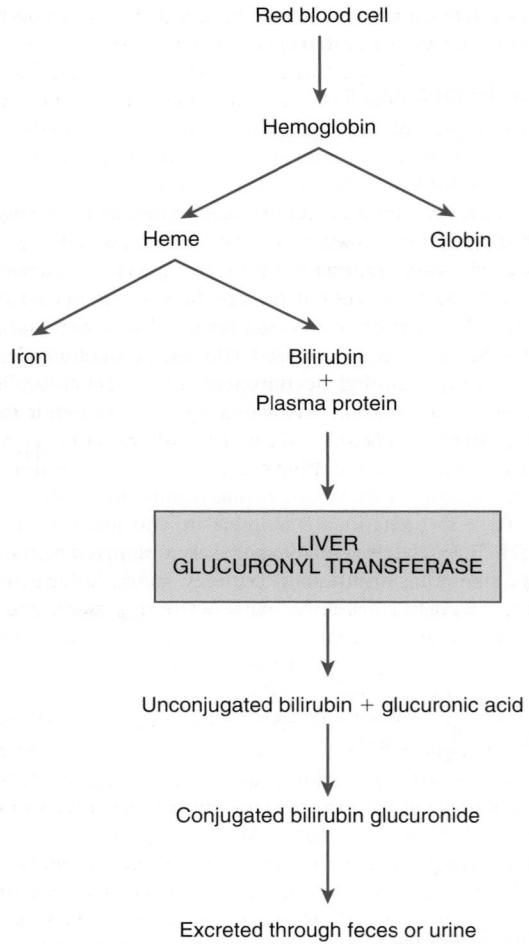

Red blood cell

↓

Hemoglobin

Heme   Globin

Iron   Bilirubin
            +
        Plasma protein

↓

**LIVER
GLUCURONYL TRANSFERASE**

↓

Unconjugated bilirubin + glucuronic acid

↓

Conjugated bilirubin glucuronide

↓

Excreted through feces or urine

FIG 22.4 Formation and excretion of bilirubin.

Basis	Causes
Increased Production of Bilirubin	
Increased hemoglobin destruction	Fetomaternal blood group incompatibility (Rh, ABO)
	Congenital red blood cell abnormalities
	Congenital enzyme deficiencies (G6PD, galactosemia)
	Enclosed hemorrhage (cephalhematoma, bruising)
	Sepsis
Increased amount of hemoglobin	Polycythemia (maternal-fetal or twin-twin transfusion, SGA)
	Delayed cord clamping
Increased enterohepatic circulation	Delayed passage of meconium, meconium ileus, or plug
	Fasting or delayed initiation of feeding
	Intestinal atresia or stenosis
Altered Hepatic Clearance of Bilirubin	
Alteration in uridine diphosphate glucuronyl transferase production or activity	Immaturity
	Metabolic/endocrine disorders (e.g., Crigler-Najjar disease, hypothyroidism, disorders of amino acid metabolism)
Alteration in hepatic function and perfusion (and thus conjugating ability)	Asphyxia, hypoxia, hypothermia, hypoglycemia
	Sepsis (also causes inflammation)
	Drugs and hormones (e.g., novobiocin, pregnanediol)
Hepatic obstruction (associated with direct hyperbilirubinemia)	Congenital anomalies (biliary atresia, cystic fibrosis)
	Biliary stasis (hepatitis, sepsis)
	Excessive bilirubin load (often seen with severe hemolysis)

TABLE 22.3 Causes of Neonatal Unconjugated (Indirect) Hyperbilirubinemia

G6PD, Glucose-6-phosphate dehydrogenase; *SGA,* small for gestational age.
From Blackburn, S. (2013). *Maternal, fetal, and neonatal physiology: A clinical perspective* (4th ed.). Maryland Heights, MO: Saunders.

more rapid passage of meconium, thus diminishing the amount of reabsorption of unconjugated bilirubin. Feeding also introduces bacteria to aid in the reduction of bilirubin to urobilinogen. Colostrum, a natural laxative, facilitates the passage of meconium in breastfed infants (Fig. 22.4).

When levels of unconjugated bilirubin exceed the ability of the liver to conjugate it, plasma levels of bilirubin increase, and jaundice appears. Jaundice, the visible yellowish color of the skin and sclera, is likely to appear when the total serum bilirubin (TSB) level exceeds 6 to 7 mg/dL. Jaundice is generally noticeable first in the head, especially in the sclera and mucous membranes, and progresses gradually to the thorax, abdomen, and extremities. The degree of jaundice is determined by serum total bilirubin measurements (Kamath-Rayne, Thilo, Deacon, et al., 2016).

The newborn is at risk for hyperbilirubinemia because of distinctive aspects of normal neonatal physiology. The higher RBC mass at birth and shorter life span of neonatal RBCs create the need for greater bilirubin synthesis. The ability of the liver to conjugate bilirubin is reduced during the first few days after birth; it can metabolize and excrete only about two-thirds of the circulating bilirubin. In addition, there are fewer bilirubin binding sites because newborns have lower serum albumin levels. In the intestines, conjugated bilirubin becomes unconjugated and recirculated through the enterohepatic circulation, which increases serum bilirubin levels.

Traditionally newborn jaundice has been categorized as either *physiologic* or *pathologic* (nonphysiologic), depending primarily on the

time it appears and on serum bilirubin levels. Controversy surrounds the definitions of normal or physiologic ranges of TSB. TSB levels in newborns are affected by variables such as gestational age, chronologic age, weight, race, nutritional status, mode of feeding, and presence of extravasated blood (e.g., cephalhematoma or severe bruising) (Blackburn, 2013). The time of onset of jaundice is a key factor in evaluating its cause and determining if treatment is needed. Table 22.3 lists the varying causes of neonatal hyperbilirubinemia.

Among the factors that increase the risk for hyperbilirubinemia, preterm birth is the most significant. Prematurity affects liver and brain metabolism and albumin binding sites, placing preterm and late preterm infants at greater risk for hyperbilirubinemia. Infants of Asian, Native-American, and Eskimo ethnicity have higher bilirubin levels. Breastfeeding infants are at greater risk for hyperbilirubinemia (see later discussion).

Physiologic Jaundice

Physiologic or nonpathologic jaundice (unconjugated hyperbilirubinemia) occurs in approximately 60% of term newborns. It appears after 24 hours of age and usually resolves without treatment.

In normal full-term newborns, TSB levels progressively increase from 2 mg/dL in cord blood to an average peak of 5 to 6 mg/dL by 72 to 96 hours of life. From that point, TSB levels gradually decrease to a plateau of approximately 3 mg/dL by 1 week of age, reaching normal adult levels of 2 mg/dL or less by 2 weeks of age. This pattern varies according to racial group, method of feeding (breast vs. formula), and gestational age (Kamath-Rayne et al., 2016).

> ⚡ **SAFETY ALERT**
>
> The appearance of jaundice during the first 24 hours of life or persistence beyond the ages previously delineated usually indicates a potential pathologic process that requires investigation.

Pathologic Jaundice

Although physiologic jaundice is usually considered benign, unconjugated (indirect) bilirubin can accumulate to hazardous levels and lead to a pathologic condition. Pathologic or nonphysiologic jaundice is unconjugated hyperbilirubinemia that is either pathologic in origin or severe enough to warrant further evaluation and treatment. Jaundice is usually considered pathologic or nonphysiologic if it appears within 24 hours after birth, TSB levels increase by more than 0.2 mg/dL per hour, TSB is greater than the 95th percentile for age in hours, direct serum bilirubin levels exceed 1.5 to 2 mg/dL, or clinical jaundice lasts for more than 2 weeks (Kamath-Rayne et al., 2016). High levels of unconjugated bilirubin are usually caused by excessive production of bilirubin through hemolysis. Hemolytic disease of the newborn caused by maternal/newborn blood group incompatibility (Rh, ABO, or minor blood groups) is the most common cause. It can also be caused by glucose-6-phosphate dehydrogenase (G6PD) deficiency, a genetic disorder that is more common among Asian and Native-American populations. Other causes are listed in Table 22.3.

If increased levels of unconjugated bilirubin are left untreated, neurotoxicity can result as bilirubin is transferred into the brain cells. Acute bilirubin encephalopathy refers to the acute manifestations of bilirubin toxicity that occur during the first weeks after birth. This can include a range of symptoms such as lethargy, hypotonia, irritability, seizures, coma, and death. Kernicterus refers to the irreversible, long-term consequences of bilirubin toxicity such as hypotonia, delayed motor skills, hearing loss, cerebral palsy, and gaze abnormalities (AAP Subcommittee on Hyperbilirubinemia, 2004) (see Chapter 25).

Jaundice Related to Breastfeeding

Two forms of breastfeeding-related jaundice are recognized: breastfeeding-associated jaundice and breast milk jaundice. These typically occur in otherwise healthy infants. Both types can occur in the same infant and are not easily differentiated (Kamath-Rayne et al., 2016).

Breastfeeding-associated jaundice (early-onset jaundice) begins at 2 to 5 days of age. Breastfeeding does not cause the jaundice; rather it is a lack of effective breastfeeding that contributes to the hyperbilirubinemia. If the infant is not feeding effectively, there is less caloric and fluid intake and possible dehydration. Hepatic clearance of bilirubin is reduced. With less intake, there are fewer stools. As a result, bilirubin is reabsorbed from the intestine back into the bloodstream and must be conjugated again so it can be excreted (Blackburn, 2013; Lawrence & Lawrence, 2016).

Breast milk jaundice (late-onset jaundice) usually occurs at 5 to 10 days of age. Infants are typically feeding well and gaining weight appropriately. Rising levels of unconjugated bilirubin peak during the second week and gradually diminish. Despite high levels of bilirubin that can persist for 3 to 12 weeks, these infants have no signs of hemolysis or liver dysfunction. The etiology of breast milk jaundice is uncertain.

However, it seems to be related to factors in the breast milk (e.g., pregnanediol, fatty acids, and β-glucuronidase) that either inhibit the conjugation of bilirubin or decrease the excretion of bilirubin (Blackburn, 2013). (See Chapter 24 for a discussion of these conditions in relation to newborn nutrition.)

Coagulation

The liver plays an important role in blood coagulation. Coagulation factors, which are synthesized in the liver, are activated by vitamin K. The lack of intestinal bacteria needed to synthesize vitamin K results in transient blood coagulation deficiency between the second and fifth days of life. The levels of coagulation factors slowly increase to reach adult levels by 9 months of age. The administration of intramuscular vitamin K shortly after birth helps prevent vitamin deficiency bleeding (VKDB) which can occur suddenly and can be catastrophic (Shearer, 2017). Any bleeding problems noted in the newborn should be reported immediately, and tests for clotting ordered.

Drug Metabolism

The immaturity of the liver and depressed liver enzyme systems at birth result in slower biotransformation and elimination of drugs. This can result in slower drug clearance, increased serum levels, and longer half-lives (Blackburn, 2013).

Signs of Hepatic System Problems

Hypoglycemia and hyperbilirubinemia are the most common liver-related problems experienced by newborns. In most cases, the problems are transient and require little, if any treatment. Preterm infants are at increased risk for hepatic system problems because of the immaturity of the liver.

The hematologic status of all newborns should be assessed for anemia. For the first week of life, neonates are at risk for bleeding until the coagulation factors are well-established. Male newborns who are circumcised prior to discharge from the birthing facility must be monitored carefully for bleeding.

IMMUNE SYSTEM

Beginning early in gestation, the immune system of the fetus is developing the capacity to respond to foreign antigens. The development of the immune system is necessary to equip the neonate to meet the numerous environmental challenges (e.g., microorganisms) associated with life in the extrauterine world. Compared to adults, the immune response at birth is reduced, leading to increased susceptibility to pathogens.

Neonatal levels of circulating immunoglobins are low in comparison to adult levels. Most of the circulating antibodies in the newborn are immunoglobulin G (IgG) antibodies that were transported across the placenta from the maternal circulation. This transfer of antibodies from the mother begins as early as 14 weeks of gestation and is greatest during the third trimester. By term, the IgG levels in the cord blood of the infant are higher than those in maternal blood. The passive immunity afforded the infant through the placental transfer of IgG usually provides sufficient antimicrobial protection during the first 3 months of life. Production of adult concentrations of IgG is reached by 4 to 6 years of age (Benjamin et al., 2015).

The fetus is capable of producing IgM by the eighth week of gestation, and low levels (less than 10% of adult levels) are present at term. IgM is important for immunity to blood-borne infections and is the major immunoglobulin synthesized during the first month. By 2 years of age, IgM reaches adult levels. The production of IgA, IgD, and IgE is much more gradual, and maximal levels are not attained until early childhood (Benjamin et al., 2015).

The membrane-protective IgA is missing from the respiratory and urinary tracts, and, unless the newborn is breastfed, it also is absent from the GI tract. The secretory IgA in human milk acts locally in the intestines to neutralize bacterial and viral pathogens. It can also lessen the risk for allergy and food intolerance through modulation of exposure to foreign milk protein antigens (Turfkruyer & Verhasselt, 2015).

Other components of breast milk strengthen the neonate's immune system. Antimicrobial factors such as oligosaccharides, lysozyme, and lactoferrin aid in microbial clearance. Infants who are breastfed have enhanced antibody responses to vaccines. Long-term effects of breastmilk on the immune system are demonstrated by lower risk for immune-mediated conditions such as allergies, inflammatory bowel disease, and type I diabetes mellitus (Turfkruyer & Verhasselt, 2015).

The WBCs of the newborn display a delayed response to invading bacteria. Neutrophil levels are low, and therefore their key functions of phagocytosis, chemotaxis, and intracellular killing are limited (Greenberg, Narendran, Schibler, et al., 2014). The influx of phagocytic cells to areas of inflammation is somewhat slowed, although the ability of these cells to attack and destroy bacteria is equivalent to that of adults. B cells and T cells are present in the newborn, although their function is immature (Benjamin et al., 2015).

Risk for Infection

All newborns, and preterm newborns especially, are at high risk for infection during the first several months of life. During this period, infection is one of the leading causes of morbidity and mortality. The newborn cannot limit the invading pathogen to the portal of entry because of the generalized hypofunctioning of the inflammatory and immune mechanisms.

Early signs of infection must be recognized so prompt diagnosis and treatment can occur. Temperature instability or hypothermia can be symptomatic of serious infection; newborns do not typically exhibit fever, although hyperthermia can occur (temperature greater than 38°C [100.4°F]). Lethargy, irritability, poor feeding, vomiting or diarrhea, decreased reflexes, and pale or mottled skin color are some of the clinical signs that suggest infection. Respiratory symptoms such as apnea, tachypnea, grunting, or retracting can be associated with infection such as pneumonia (Bodin, 2014). Any unusual discharge from the infant's eyes, nose, mouth, or other orifice must be investigated. If a rash appears, it must be evaluated closely; many normal rashes in the newborn are not associated with any infection. Infants must be protected from infections by the use of proper hand hygiene.

The greatest risk factor for neonatal infection is prematurity because of immaturity of the immune system. Other risk factors include premature rupture of membranes, chorioamnionitis, maternal fever, antenatal or intrapartal asphyxia, invasive procedures, stress, and congenital anomalies.

INTEGUMENTARY SYSTEM

All skin structures are present at birth. The epidermis and dermis are loosely bound and extremely thin. After 35 weeks of gestation, the skin is covered by **vernix caseosa** (a cheeselike, whitish substance) that is fused with the epidermis and serves as a protective covering. Vernix caseosa is a complex substance that contains sebaceous gland secretions. It has emollient and antimicrobial properties and prevents fluid loss through the skin; it also has antioxidant properties. Removal of the vernix is followed by desquamation of the epidermis in most infants. There is evidence that leaving residual vernix intact after birth has positive benefits for neonatal skin such as decreasing the skin pH, decreasing skin erythema, and improving skin hydration (Association

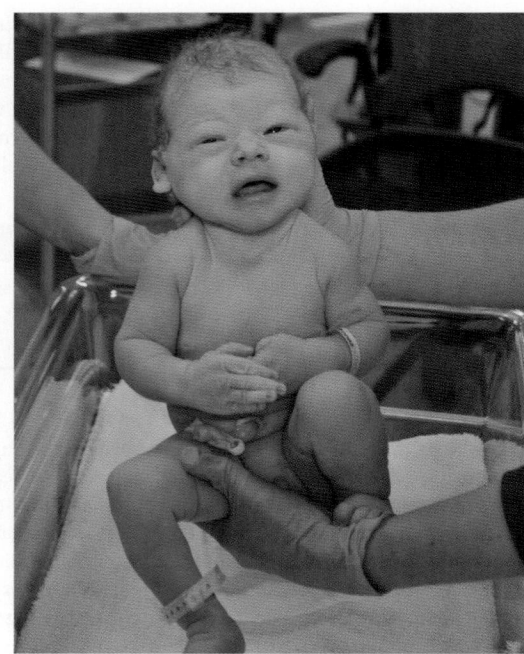

FIG 22.5 Newborn infant with acrocyanosis of upper and lower extremities. (Courtesy of Barbara Wilson, West Jordan, UT.)

of Women's Health, Obstetric, and Neonatal Nurses [AWHONN], 2013; Visscher, Adam, Brink, et al., 2015).

The skin of a term infant is erythematous (red) for a few hours after birth, and then it fades to its normal color. The skin often appears blotchy or mottled, especially over the extremities. The hands and feet appear slightly cyanotic (acrocyanosis); this is caused by vasomotor instability and capillary stasis. Acrocyanosis is normal and appears intermittently over the first 7 to 10 days, especially with exposure to cold (Fig. 22.5).

The healthy term infant usually has a plump appearance because of large amounts of subcutaneous tissue and extracellular water content. Subcutaneous fat accumulated during the last trimester acts as insulation. Fine lanugo hair may be noted over the face, shoulders, and back. Edema of the face and ecchymosis (bruising) or petechiae may be noted as a result of face presentation, forceps-assisted birth, or vacuum extraction.

Creases are located on the palms of the hands and the soles of the feet. The simian line, a single palmar crease, is often seen in Asian infants and infants with Down syndrome. The soles of the feet should be inspected for the number of creases during the first few hours after birth; as the skin dries, more creases appear. More creases correlate with a greater maturity rating. Preterm newborns have few, if any, creases.

Sweat Glands

Distended, small, white sebaceous glands noticeable on the newborn face are known as milia. Although sweat glands are present at birth, term infants usually do not sweat for the first 24 hours. By day 3 sweating begins on the face, then progresses to the palms. Infants can sweat as a function of body or environmental temperature; there can also be emotional sweating from crying or pain (Hoath & Narendran, 2015).

Desquamation

Desquamation (peeling) of the skin of the term infant does not occur until a few days after birth. Large generalized areas of skin desquamation present at birth can be an indication of postmaturity.

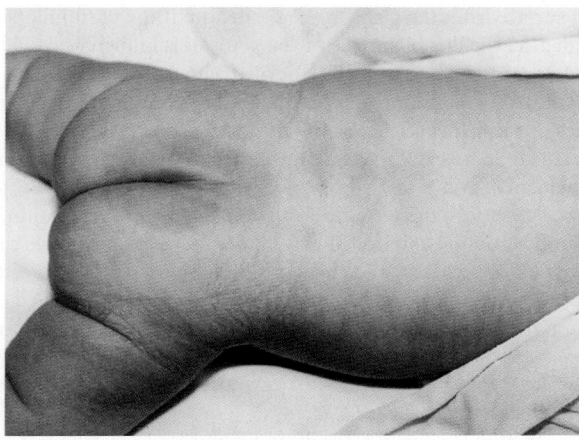

FIG 22.6 Mongolian spot.

Mongolian Spots

Mongolian spots, bluish black areas of pigmentation, can appear over any part of the exterior surface of the body, including the extremities. They are most common on the back and buttocks (Fig. 22.6). These pigmented areas occur most frequently in newborns whose ethnic origins are Latin America, Asia, Africa, or the Mediterranean area. They are more common in dark-skinned individuals but can occur in 5% to 13% of Caucasians (Blackburn, 2013). Mongolian spots fade gradually over months or years.

The presence of Mongolian spots on the newborn should be documented carefully in the medical record. These normal skin pigmentations can be mistaken for bruises once the infant is discharged, and this can raise suspicion of physical abuse.

Nevi

Nevus simplex, also known as salmon patches, telangiectatic nevi, "stork bites," or "angel kisses," are the result of a superficial capillary defect and occur in up to 80% of newborns. They are usually small, flat, and pink and are easily blanched (Fig. 22.7, *A*). The most common sites are the upper eyelids, nose, upper lip, and nape of the neck. Salmon patches tend to be symmetric, with lesions occurring on both eyelids or both sides of midline. They have no clinical significance and require no treatment. Facial lesions usually fade between the first and second years of life, whereas neck lesions can be visible into adulthood (Hoath & Narendran, 2015).

A port-wine stain, or nevus flammeus, is usually visible at birth and is due to an asymmetric postcapillary venule malformation. It is usually pink and flat at birth, but darkens with time, becoming red or purple and pebbly in consistency. True port-wine stains do not blanch on pressure or disappear. They are found most commonly on the face and neck (Hoath & Narendran, 2015).

Infantile Hemangioma

Infantile hemangiomas consist of dilated newly formed capillaries occupying the entire dermal and subdermal layers with associated connective tissue hypertrophy. The typical lesion is a raised, sharply demarcated, bright or dark red rough-surfaced swelling that may be present at birth or may appear during the early weeks after birth. Common sites are the scalp, face, back, and anterior chest. These lesions are sometimes called *strawberry hemangiomas,* although experts deem that term inappropriate. Most lesions reach maximum growth in about 6 months and then begin a slow process of involution that can take 5 to 10 years (Martin, 2016).

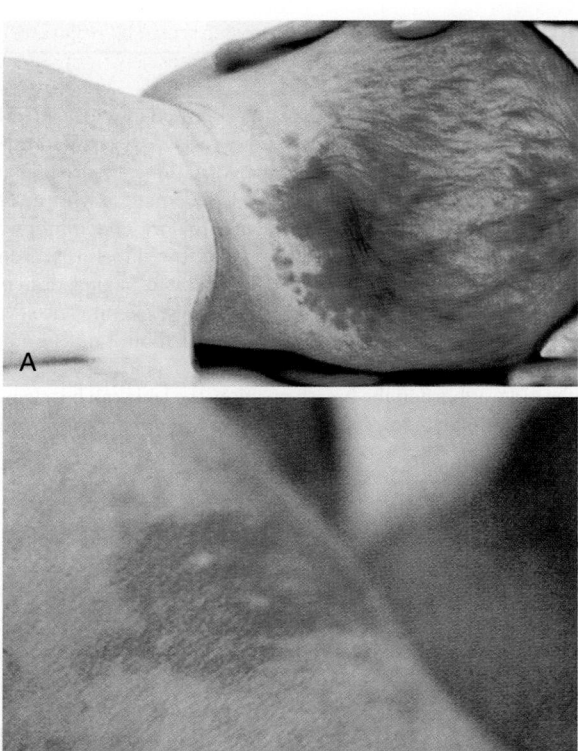

FIG 22.7 A, Nevus simplex or telangiectatic nevi (stork bite). **B,** Erythema toxicum. (Courtesy of Mead Johnson & Company, Evansville, IN.)

Erythema Toxicum

Erythema toxicum, a transient rash, is also called *erythema neonatorum, newborn rash,* or *flea bite dermatitis.* It first appears in term neonates during the first 24 to 72 hours after birth and can last up to 3 weeks of age (Blackburn, 2013). It has lesions in different stages: erythematous macules, papules, and small vesicles (see Fig. 22.7, *B*). The lesions can appear suddenly anywhere on the body. The rash is thought to be an inflammatory response. Eosinophils, which help decrease inflammation, are found in the vesicles. Although the appearance is alarming, the rash has no clinical significance and requires no treatment.

Signs of Integumentary Problems

Close observation of the newborn's skin color can lead to early detection of potential problems. Any pallor, plethora (deep purplish color from increased circulating RBCs), petechiae, central cyanosis, or jaundice should be noted and documented. The skin should be examined for signs of birth injuries such as forceps marks and lesions related to fetal monitoring. Bruises or petechiae can be present on the head, neck, and face of an infant born with a nuchal cord (cord around the neck) or who had a face presentation at birth. Bruising can increase the risk for hyperbilirubinemia. Petechiae can be present if increased pressure was applied to an area. Petechiae scattered over the infant's body should be reported to the health care provider because petechiae can indicate underlying problems such as low platelet count or infection.

Unilateral or bilateral periauricular papillomas (skin tags) occur fairly frequently. Their occurrence is usually a family trait and of no consequence.

REPRODUCTIVE SYSTEM

Female

An increase in estrogen during pregnancy followed by a drop after birth causes female newborns to have mucoid vaginal discharge and even some slight bloody spotting (pseudomenstruation). External genitalia (i.e., labia majora and minora) are usually edematous with increased pigmentation. In term neonates, the labia majora and minora cover the vestibule (Fig. 22.8, *A*). In preterm infants, the clitoris is prominent, and the labia majora are small and widely separated. Vaginal or hymenal tags are common findings and have no clinical significance. Vernix caseosa can be present between the labia and should not be forcibly removed during bathing.

If the girl was born in the breech position, the labia can be edematous and bruised. The edema and bruising resolve in a few days; no treatment is necessary.

Male

In the uncircumcised newborn, the foreskin or prepuce completely covers the glans. The foreskin adheres to the glans and is not fully retractable for 3 to 4 years. The position of the urethra should be at the tip of the penis. With *hypospadias,* the urethral opening is located in an abnormal position, at any point on the ventral surface of the penile surface from the glans to the perineum. If the urethral opening is located on the dorsal surface of the penis, it is known as *epispadias;* this is less common and is often associated with extrophy of the bladder (Elder, 2016). A common finding in newborn males is small, white, firm lesions called *epithelial pearls* at the tip of the prepuce.

By 28 to 36 weeks of gestation, the testes can be palpated in the inguinal canal, and a few rugae appear on the scrotum. At 36 to 40 weeks of gestation, the testes are palpable in the upper scrotum, and rugae appear on the anterior portion. After 40 weeks, the testes can be palpated in the scrotum, and rugae cover the scrotal sac. The postterm neonate has deep rugae and a pendulous scrotum. Undescended testes (cryptorchidism) occur in approximately 4% of term newborn males; in most cases, the testes gradually descend without intervention (Lissauer, 2015). The primary risk factors for cryptorchidism are preterm birth and low birth weight (Lee, 2017).

The scrotum is usually more deeply pigmented than the rest of the skin (see Fig. 22.8, *B*), particularly in darker-skinned infants. A bluish discoloration of the scrotum suggests testicular torsion, which needs immediate attention. If the male infant is born in a breech presentation, the scrotum can be very edematous and bruised (Fig. 22.9). The swelling and discoloration subside within a few days.

Hydrocele, caused by an accumulation of fluid around the testes, can be present. Hydroceles can be easily transilluminated with a light and usually resolve without treatment (Fig. 22.10).

Swelling of Breast Tissue

Swelling of the breast tissue in term infants of both sexes is caused by the hyperestrogenism of pregnancy. In a few infants, a thin discharge ("witch's milk") can be seen. This finding has no clinical significance, requires no treatment, and subsides within a few days as the maternal hormones are eliminated from the infant's body.

The nipples should be symmetric on the chest. Breast tissue and areola size increase with gestation. The areola appears slightly elevated at 34 weeks of gestation. By 36 weeks, a breast bud of 1 to 2 mm is palpable; this increases to 12 mm by 42 weeks.

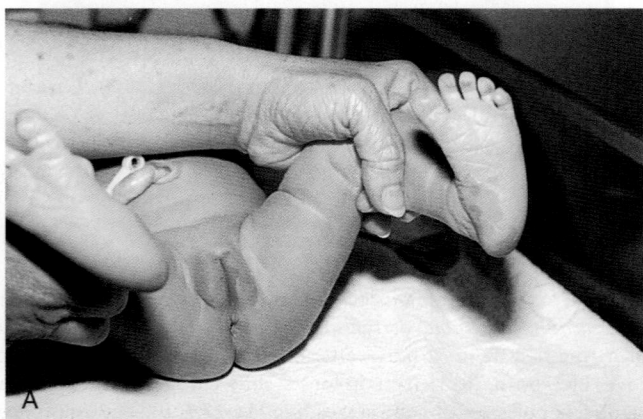

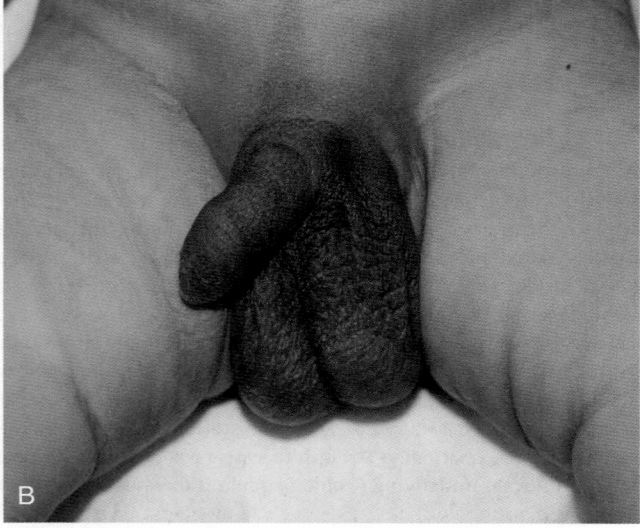

FIG 22.8 External genitalia. **A,** Genitalia in female term infant. **B,** Genitalia in uncircumcised male infant. Rugae cover scrotum, indicating term gestation. (Courtesy of Marjorie Pyle, RNC, Lifecircle, Costa Mesa, CA.)

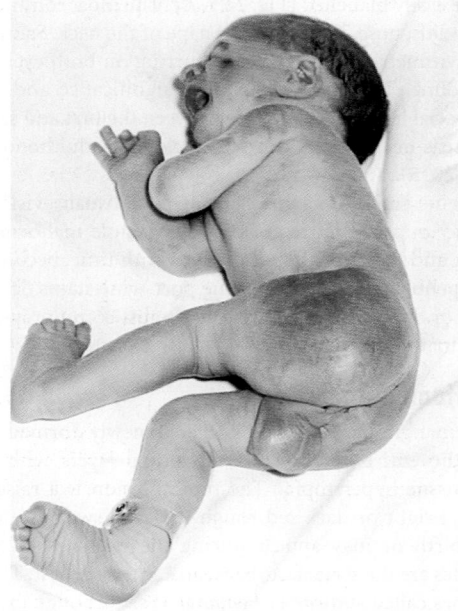

FIG 22.9 Swelling of the genitals and bruising of the buttocks after a breech birth. (From O'Doherty, N. [1986]. *Neonatology: Micro atlas of the newborn*. Nutley, NJ: Hoffman-LaRoche.)

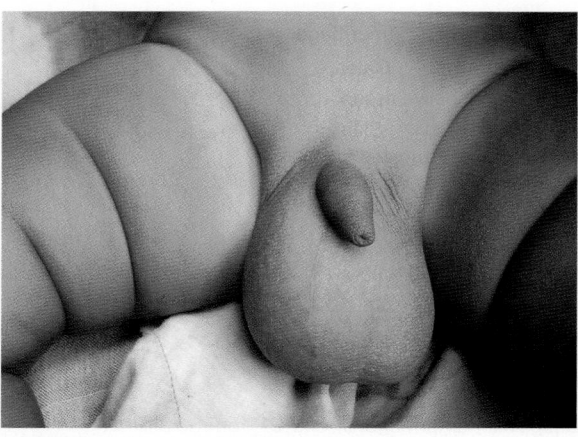

FIG 22.10 Bilateral hydrocele in the newborn. The scrotum is distended by fluid. (From Poenaru D. [2012]. Abdominal wall problems. In Gleason, C.A., Devaskar, S.U. [Eds.], *Avery's diseases of the newborn* [9th ed.]. Philadelphia, PA: Saunders.)

Signs of Reproductive System Problems

The infant must be inspected closely for ambiguous genitalia and other abnormalities. Normally in a female infant the urethral opening is located behind the clitoris. Any deviation from this can incorrectly suggest that the clitoris is a small penis, which can occur in conditions such as adrenal hyperplasia. Nearly all female infants are born with hymenal tags; absence of such tags can indicate vaginal agenesis. Fecal discharge from the vagina indicates a rectovaginal fistula. Any of these findings must be reported to the neonatal or pediatric health care provider for further evaluation.

Hypospadias, undescended testes, or other abnormalities of the male genitalia must be reported. Circumcision is contraindicated in the presence of hypospadias because the foreskin is used in repair of this anomaly.

Inguinal hernias can be present and become more obvious when the infant cries. They are common, especially in African-American neonates, and usually require no treatment because they resolve with time.

SKELETAL SYSTEM

The infant's skeletal system undergoes rapid development during the first year of life. At birth, more cartilage is present than ossified bone.

Because of cephalocaudal (head-to-rump) development, the newborn looks somewhat out of proportion. The head at term is approximately one-fourth of the total body length. The arms are slightly longer than the legs. In the newborn, the legs are about one-third of the total body length. As growth proceeds, the midpoint in head-to-toe measurements gradually descends from the level of the umbilicus at birth to the level of the symphysis pubis at maturity.

The face appears small in relation to the skull. The skull appears large and heavy. Cranial size and shape can be distorted by molding (the shaping of the fetal head by overlapping of the cranial bones to facilitate movement through the birth canal during labor) (Fig. 22.11).

Caput Succedaneum

Caput succedaneum is a generalized, easily identifiable edematous area of the scalp, most often on the occiput (Fig. 22.12, *A*). With vertex presentation, the sustained pressure of the presenting part against the cervix results in compression of local vessels, slowing venous return. The slower venous return causes an increase in tissue fluids within the

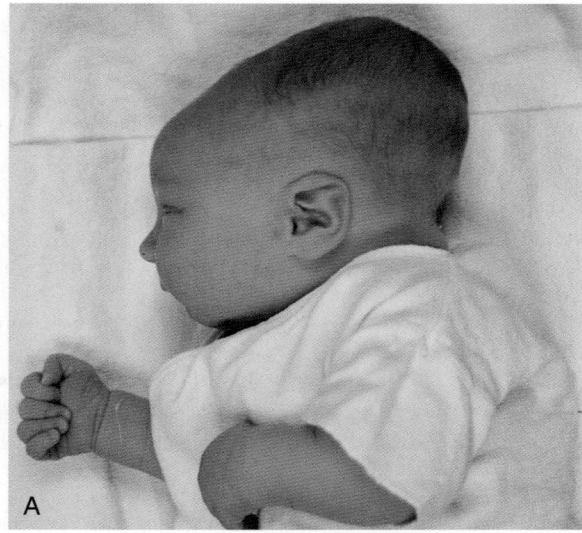

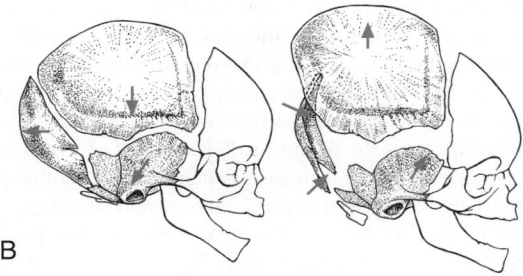

FIG 22.11 Molding. **A,** Significant molding after vaginal birth. **B,** Schematic of bones of skull when molding is present. (A, Courtesy of Kim Molloy, Knoxville, IA.)

skin of the scalp, and edema develops. This edematous area, present at birth, extends across suture lines of the skull and usually disappears spontaneously within 3 to 4 days. Infants who are born with the assistance of vacuum extraction usually have a caput in the area where the cup was applied. Bruising of the scalp is often seen in the presence of caput succedaneum.

Cephalhematoma

Cephalhematoma is a collection of blood between a skull bone and its periosteum. Therefore, a cephalhematoma does not cross a cranial suture line (see Fig. 22.12, *B*). A cephalhematoma is firmer and better defined than a caput. Often caput succedaneum and cephalhematoma occur simultaneously. A cephalhematoma usually resolves in 2 to 8 weeks. As the hematoma resolves, hemolysis of RBCs occurs, and hyperbilirubinemia can result (Bonifacio, Gonzalez, & Ferriero, 2012).

Subgaleal Hemorrhage

Subgaleal hemorrhage is bleeding into the subgaleal compartment (see Fig. 22.12, *C*). The subgaleal compartment is a potential space that contains loosely arranged connective tissue; it is located beneath the galea aponeurotica, the tendinous sheath that connects the frontal and occipital muscles and forms the inner surface of the scalp. Subgaleal hemorrhage is the result of traction or application of shearing forces to the scalp, commonly associated with difficult operative vaginal birth, especially vacuum extraction. The scalp is pulled away from the bony calvarium; the vessels are torn, and blood collects in the subgaleal space. Blood loss can be severe, resulting in hypovolemic shock, disseminated

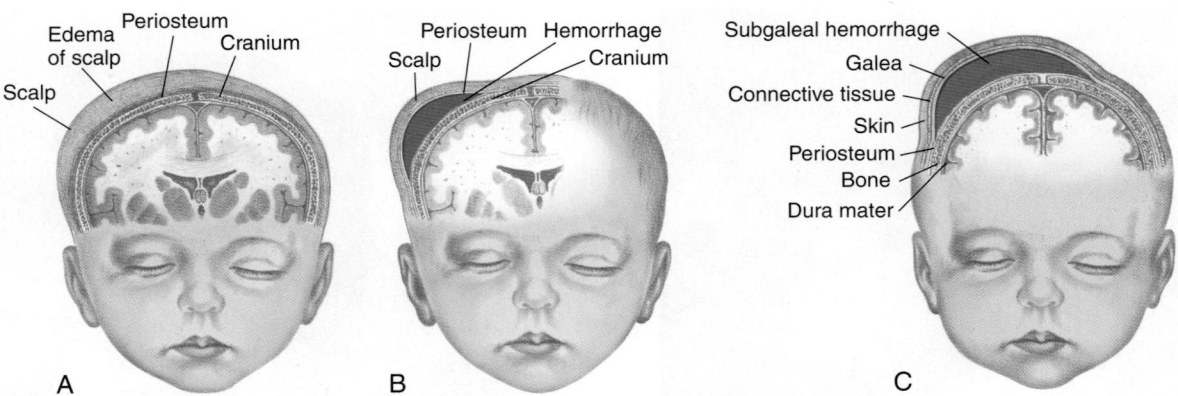

FIG 22.12 A, Caput succedaneum. **B,** Cephalhematoma. **C,** Subgaleal hemorrhage. (A and C, From Seidel, H., Ball, J., Dains, J., & Benedict, G. [2006]. *Mosby's guide to physical examination* [6th ed.]. St. Louis. MO: Mosby.)

intravascular coagulation (DIC), and death (Mangurten, Puppala, & Prazad, 2015).

Early detection of the hemorrhage is vital; serial head circumference measurements and inspection of the back of the neck for increasing edema and a firm mass are essential. A boggy scalp, pallor, tachycardia, and increasing head circumference can be early signs of a subgaleal hemorrhage. Computed tomography or magnetic resonance imaging is useful in confirming the diagnosis. Replacement of lost blood and clotting factors is required in acute cases of hemorrhage. Another possible early sign of subgaleal hemorrhage is a forward and lateral positioning of the newborn's ears because the hematoma extends posteriorly. Monitoring the infant for changes in level of consciousness and decreases in hematocrit is also key to early recognition and management. An increase in serum bilirubin level may be seen as a result of the degradation of blood cells within the hematoma (Mangurten et al., 2015).

Spine

The bones in the vertebral column of the newborn form two primary curvatures—one in the thoracic region and one in the sacral region. Both are forward, concave curvatures. As the infant gains head control at approximately 3 months of age, a secondary curvature appears in the cervical region. The newborn's spine appears straight and can be flexed easily. The newborn can lift the head and turn it from side to side when prone. The vertebrae should appear straight and flat. If a pilonidal dimple is noted, further inspection is required to determine whether a sinus is present. A pilonidal dimple, especially with a sinus and nevus pilosis (hairy nevus), can be associated with spina bifida.

Extremities

The infant's extremities should be symmetric and of equal length. Fingers and toes should be equal in number (five fingers on each hand and five toes on each foot) and should have nails present. Digits may be missing *(oligodactyly)*. Extra digits *(polydactyly)* are sometimes found on the hands or feet. Fingers or toes may be fused *(syndactyly)*.

The infant is examined for developmental dysplasia of the hips (DDH). In newborns with DDH, the affected hip is unlikely to be dislocated at birth; instead it is easily dislocatable. Postnatal factors determine whether the hip dislocates, subluxates, or remains stable. DDH occurs more often in first-born infants, female infants, in breech presentations (Fig. 22.13), and in infants with a family history of DDH (Son-Hing & Thompson, 2015).

Signs of DDH are asymmetric gluteal and thigh skinfolds, uneven knee levels, a positive Ortolani test, and a positive Barlow test. The hips are inspected for symmetry. Gluteal and thigh skinfolds should be equal

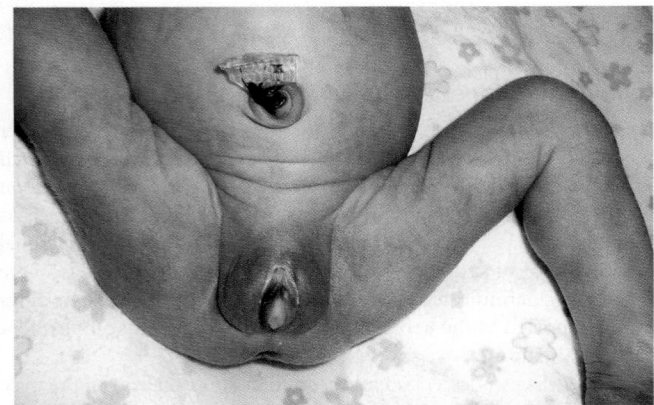

FIG 22.13 Position of infant's legs after breech birth. Note preterm genitalia. (Courtesy of Cheryl Briggs, RNC, Annapolis, MD.)

and symmetric, and legs should be of equal length (Fig. 22.14, *A*). The level of the knees in flexion should be equal (see Fig. 22.14, *C*). Hip integrity is assessed by using the Barlow test and the Ortolani maneuver. For the Barlow test, the examiner places the middle finger over the greater trochanter and the thumb along the midthigh. The hip is flexed to 90 degrees and adducted, followed by gentle downward pushing of the femoral head. If the hip can be dislocated with this maneuver, the femoral head moves out of the acetabulum, and the examiner feels a "clunk." The hip is then checked to determine if the femoral head can be returned into the acetabulum using the Ortolani maneuver. As the hip is abducted and upward leverage is applied, a dislocated hip returns to the acetabulum with a clunk that is felt by the examiner (White & Goldberg, 2012) (see Fig. 22.14, *B* and *D*).

> ⚡ **SAFETY ALERT**
>
> Only expert examiners (physicians, nurse practitioners) should perform the Barlow test and Ortolani maneuver to assess for DDH. An unskilled examiner can cause injury to the newborn.

Signs of Skeletal Problems

Abnormalities of the skeletal system can be congenital, developmental, drug induced, or the result of intrapartum or postnatal factors. Signs of DDH, additional digits or webbing of digits, and any other abnormality should be documented and reported to the primary health care provider.

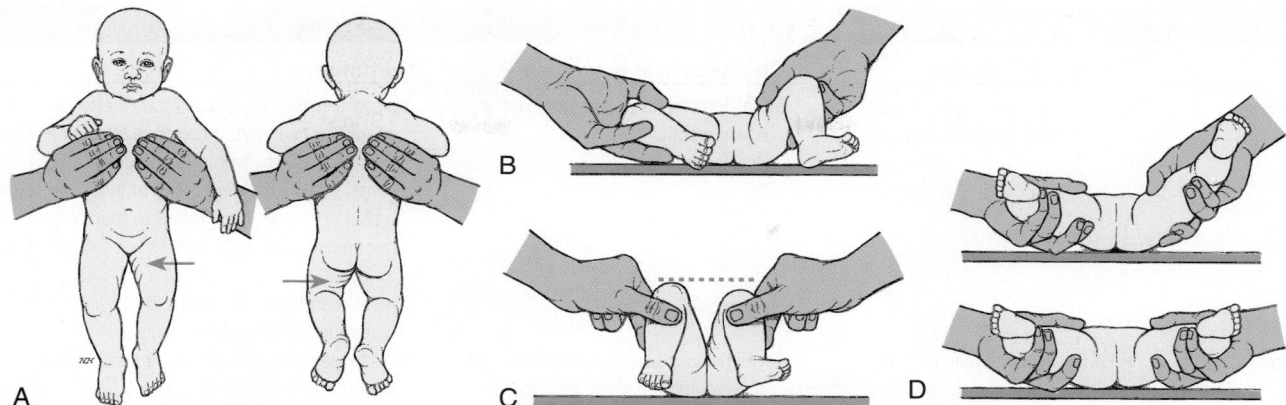

FIG 22.14 Signs of developmental dysplasia of the hip. **A,** Asymmetry of gluteal and thigh folds with shortening of the thigh (Galeazzi sign). **B,** Limited hip abduction, as seen in flexion (Ortolani test). **C,** Apparent shortening of the femur, as indicated by the level of the knees in flexion (Allis sign). **D,** Ortolani maneuver with femoral head moving in and out of acetabulum (in infants 1 to 2 months of age). (From Hockenberry, M. J., & Wilson, D. [2013]. *Wong's essentials of pediatric nursing* [9th ed.]. St. Louis, MO: Mosby.)

A fractured clavicle often occurs in macrosomic infants and in those who had a difficult birth (e.g., shoulder dystocia). Unequal movement of the upper extremities or crepitus over the clavicular area can indicate fracture.

The newborn's feet can appear to be abnormally positioned. This can indicate congenital deformity or can be related to fetal positioning in utero. For example, clubfoot (talipes equinovarus), a deformity in which the foot turns inward and is fixed in a plantar-flexion position, is a congenital condition that warrants attention. If the foot is turned inward in the plantar-flexion position but can be moved into the normal position, it is likely caused by fetal positioning and should gradually resolve.

NEUROMUSCULAR SYSTEM

The neuromuscular system is almost completely developed at birth. The term newborn is a responsive and reactive being with remarkable capacity for social interaction and self-organization.

Growth of the brain after birth follows a predictable pattern of rapid growth during infancy and early childhood; it becomes more gradual during the remainder of the first decade and minimal during adolescence. By the end of the first year, the cerebellum ends its growth spurt, which began at approximately 30 weeks of gestation.

The brain requires glucose as a source of energy and a relatively large supply of oxygen for adequate metabolism. The necessity for glucose requires careful assessment of neonates who are at risk for hypoglycemia (e.g., infants of mothers who have diabetes; infants who are macrosomic or small for gestational age; and newborns who experienced prolonged birth, hypoxia, or preterm birth).

Spontaneous motor activity can be seen as transient tremors of the mouth and chin, especially during crying episodes, and of the extremities, notably the arms and hands. Transient tremors are normal and can be observed in nearly every newborn. They most often involve the mouth and chin or the arms and hands. These tremors should not be present when the infant is quiet and should not persist beyond 1 month of age. Persistent tremors or tremors involving the total body can indicate pathologic conditions. Normal tremors, tremors (jitteriness) of hypoglycemia, and seizure activity must be differentiated so corrective care can be instituted as necessary (Ditzenberger & Blackburn, 2014).

To differentiate between tremors or jitteriness and seizure activity, the nurse can consider the following signs (Ditzenberger & Blackburn, 2014; Scher, 2012):

- Tremors or jitteriness are easily elicited by motions or voice and cease with gentle restraint of the body part, whereas seizure activity continues.
- Passive flexion and repositioning of the tremulous extremity reduces or stops the movement.
- Seizure activity is associated with ocular changes (eyes deviating or staring) and autonomic changes (apnea, tachycardia, pupil changes, increased salivation); these signs are not associated with jitteriness or tremors.

The posture of the term newborn demonstrates flexion of the arms at the elbows and the legs at the knees. Hips are abducted and partially flexed. Intermittent fisting of the hands is common.

Muscle tone and strength are directly related. The infant with normal tone and strength exhibits some resistance to passive movement such as when being pulled to sit or when the arm or leg is extended by the examiner. The hypotonic neonate shows little resistance and can feel like a "rag doll." Hypertonia is evidenced by increased resistance to passive movement.

Although neuromuscular control is very limited, it can be noted. If newborns are placed face down on a firm surface, they will turn their heads to the side. They attempt to hold their heads in line with their bodies if they are raised by their arms. Various reflexes serve to promote safety and adequate food intake.

Newborn Reflexes

The newborn has many primitive reflexes. The times at which these reflexes appear and disappear reflect the maturity and intactness of the developing nervous system. The most common reflexes found in the normal term newborn are described in Table 22.4.

BEHAVIORAL ADAPTATIONS

The healthy infant must accomplish behavioral and biologic tasks to develop normally. Behavioral characteristics form the basis of the social capabilities of the infant. Newborns progress through a hierarchy of developmental challenges as they adapt to their environment and caregivers. They must first be able to regulate their physiologic or

TABLE 22.4   Assessment of Newborn Reflexes

Reflex	Eliciting the Reflex	Characteristic Response	Comments
Sucking and rooting	Touch infant's lip, cheek, or corner of mouth with nipple or finger.	Infant turns head toward stimulus and opens mouth.	Response is difficult if not impossible to elicit after infant has been fed; if response is weak or absent, consider preterm birth or neurologic defect. Parental guidance: Avoid trying to turn head toward breast or nipple; allow infant to root; response disappears after 3–4* months but can persist up to 1 year. If response is weak or absent, it can indicate prematurity or neurologic defect.
Swallowing	Feed infant; swallowing usually follows sucking and obtaining fluids.	Swallowing is usually coordinated with sucking and breathing and usually occurs without gagging, coughing, apnea, or vomiting.	If response is weak or absent, it can indicate preterm birth, effects of maternal analgesics, or illness that needs investigation. Sucking, swallowing, and breathing are often uncoordinated in preterm infant.
Grasp			
Palmar	Place finger in palm of hand.	Infant's fingers curl around examiner's fingers.	Palmar response lessens by 3–4 months; parents enjoy this contact with infant.
Plantar	Place finger at base of toes.	Toes curl downward.	Plantar response lessens by 8 months.

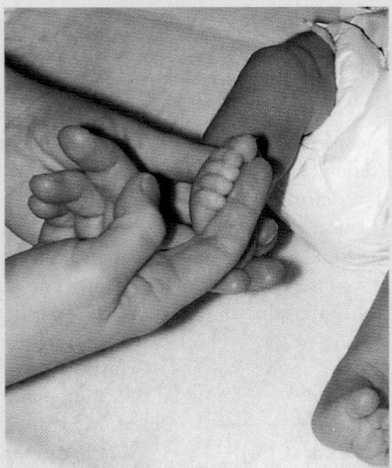

Plantar grasp reflex. (From Zitelli, B. J., & Davis, H. W. [2007]. *Atlas of pediatric physical diagnosis* [5th ed.]. St. Louis, MO: Mosby.)

Reflex	Eliciting the Reflex	Characteristic Response	Comments
Extrusion	Touch or depress tip of tongue.	Newborn forces tongue outward.	Response disappears by about 4–5 months.
Glabellar (Myerson)	Tap over forehead, bridge of nose, or maxilla of newborn whose eyes are open.	Newborn blinks for first four or five taps.	Continued blinking with repeated taps is consistent with extrapyramidal signs.
Tonic neck or "fencing"	With infant in supine neutral position, turn head quickly to one side.	With infant facing left side, arm and leg on that side extend; opposite arm and leg flex (turn head to right, and extremities assume opposite postures).	Responses in leg are more consistent. Complete response disappears by 3–4 months; incomplete response may be seen until 3–4 years. After 6 weeks, persistent response is sign of possible cerebral palsy.

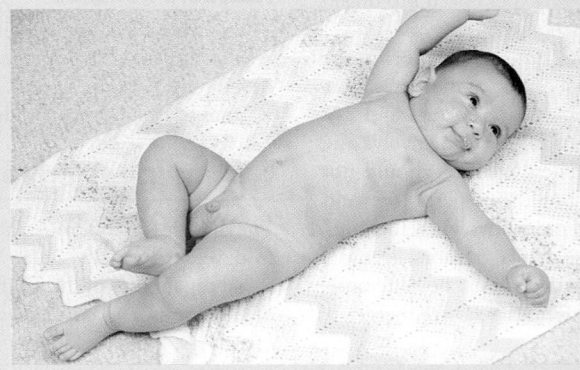

Classic pose in tonic neck reflex. (Courtesy of Marjorie Pyle, RNC, Lifecircle, Costa Mesa, CA.)

TABLE 22.4   Assessment of Newborn Reflexes—cont'd

Reflex	Eliciting the Reflex	Characteristic Response	Comments
Moro	Hold infant in semisitting position, allow head and trunk to fall backward to angle of at least 30 degrees (with support). Place infant supine on flat surface; perform sharp hand clap.	Symmetric abduction and extension of arms are seen; fingers fan out and form a *C* with thumb and forefinger; slight tremor may be noted; arms are adducted in embracing motion and return to relaxed flexion and movement. A cry may accompany or follow motor movement. Legs may follow similar pattern of response. Preterm infant does not complete "embrace"; instead arms fall backward because of weakness.	Response is present at birth; complete response may be seen until 8 weeks; body jerk only is seen between 8 and 18 weeks; response is absent by 6 months if neurologic maturation is not delayed; response may be incomplete if infant is in deep sleep state; give parental guidance about normal response. Asymmetric response can connote injury to brachial plexus, clavicle, or humerus. Persistent response after 6 months indicates possible neurologic abnormality.

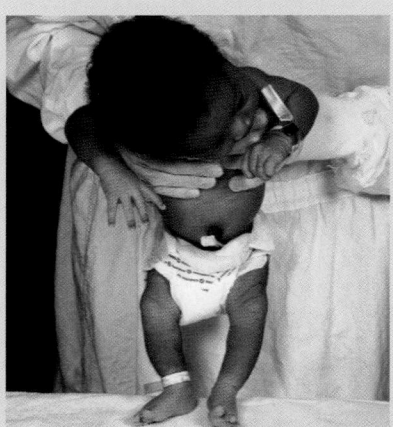

Moro reflex. (Courtesy of Paul Vincent Kuntz, Texas Children's Hospital, Houston.)

Reflex	Eliciting the Reflex	Characteristic Response	Comments
Stepping or "walking"	Hold infant vertically under arms or on trunk, allowing one foot to touch table surface.	Infant will simulate walking, alternating flexion and extension of feet; term infants walk on soles of their feet, and preterm infants walk on their toes.	Response is normally present for 3–4 weeks.

Stepping reflex. (From Dickason, E. J., Silverman, B. L., & Kaplan, J. A. [1998]. *Maternal-infant nursing care* [3rd ed.]. St. Louis, MO: Mosby.)

Continued

TABLE 22.4   Assessment of Newborn Reflexes—cont'd

Reflex	Eliciting the Reflex	Characteristic Response	Comments
Crawling	Place newborn on abdomen.	Newborn makes crawling movements with arms and legs.	Response should disappear by about 6 weeks of age.

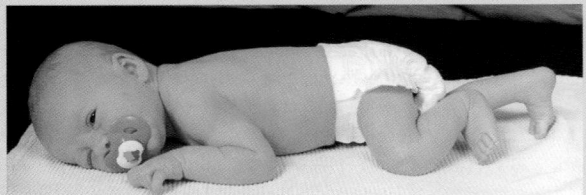

Crawling reflex. (Courtesy of Paul Vincent Kuntz, Texas Children's Hospital, Houston, TX.)

Reflex	Eliciting the Reflex	Characteristic Response	Comments
Deep tendon	Use finger instead of percussion hammer to elicit patellar, or knee-jerk, reflex; newborn must be relaxed.	Reflex jerk is present; even with newborn relaxed, nonselective overall reaction may occur.	It is usually more difficult to elicit upper extremity reflexes than lower extremity reflexes.
Crossed extension	With infant in supine position, examiner extends one leg of infant and presses down knee. Stimulation of sole of foot of fixated limb should cause free leg to flex, adduct, and extend as if attempting to push away stimulating agent.	Opposite leg flexes, adducts, and then extends.	This reflex should be present during newborn period.

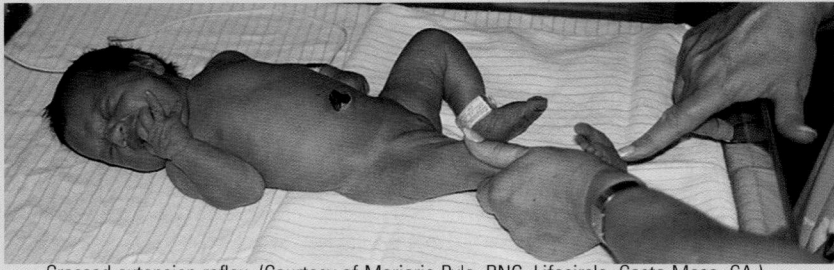

Crossed extension reflex. (Courtesy of Marjorie Pyle, RNC, Lifecircle, Costa Mesa, CA.)

Reflex	Eliciting the Reflex	Characteristic Response	Comments
Babinski (plantar)	On sole of foot, beginning at heel, stroke upward along lateral aspect of sole; then move finger across ball of foot.	All toes hyperextend, with dorsiflexion of big toe—recorded as a positive sign.	Absence requires neurologic evaluation; should disappear after 1 year of age. Response depends on infant's general muscle tone, maturity, and condition.

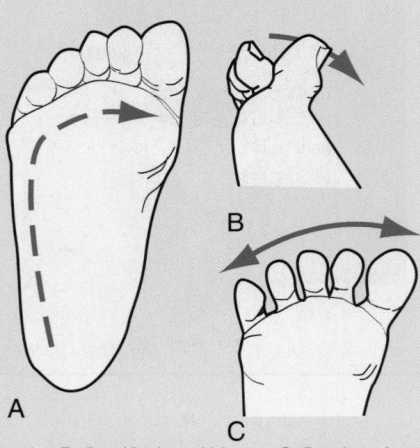

Babinski reflex. **A,** Direction of stroke. **B,** Dorsiflexion of big toe. **C,** Fanning of toes.
(From Hockenberry, M. J., & Wilson, D. [2013]. *Wong's nursing care of infants and children* [9th ed.]. St. Louis, MO: Mosby.)

TABLE 22.4	**Assessment of Newborn Reflexes—cont'd**		
Reflex	**Eliciting the Reflex**	**Characteristic Response**	**Comments**
Pull-to-sit (traction response); postural tone	Pull infant up by wrists from supine position with head in midline.	Head lags until infant is in upright position; then head is held in same plane with chest and shoulder momentarily before falling forward; infant attempts to right head.	Response depends on general muscle tone and maturity and condition of infant.
Truncal incurvation (Galant)	Place infant prone on flat surface; run finger down back about 4–5 cm lateral to spine, first on one side and then down the other.	Trunk is flexed, and pelvis is swung toward stimulated side.	Response disappears by 4 weeks. Response varies but should be obtainable in all infants, including preterm. Absence suggests general depression of nervous system. With transverse lesions of cord, no response below level of lesion is present.

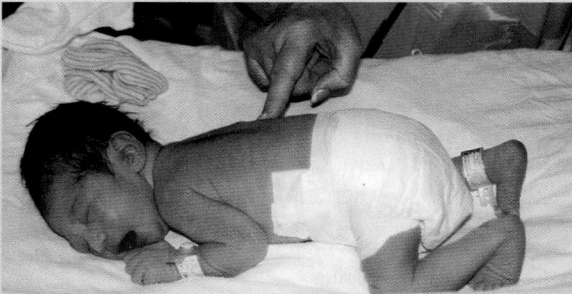

Trunk incurvation reflex. (Courtesy of Marjorie Pyle, RNC, Lifecircle, Costa Mesa, CA.)

Magnet	Place infant in supine position, partially flex both lower extremities, and apply light pressure with fingers to soles of feet (Fig. A). Normally, while examiner's fingers maintain contact with soles of feet, lower limbs extend.	Both lower limbs should extend against examiner's pressure (Fig. B).	Absence suggests damage to central nervous system. Weak reflex may be seen after breech presentation *without* extended legs or may indicate sciatic nerve stretch syndrome. Breech presentation *with* extended legs may evoke exaggerated response.

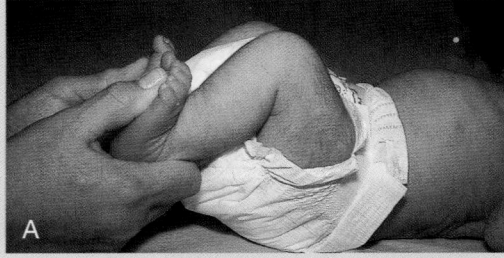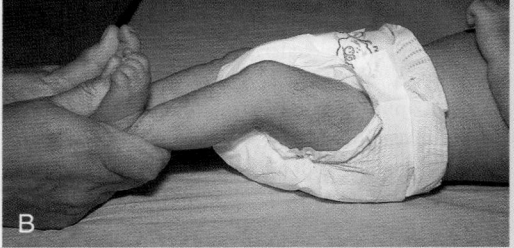

Magnet reflex. (Courtesy of Michael S. Clement, MD, Mesa, AZ.)

Additional newborn responses: yawn, stretch, burp, hiccup, sneeze	These are spontaneous behaviors.	Responses can be slightly depressed temporarily because of maternal analgesia or anesthesia, fetal hypoxia, or infection.	Parental guidance: Most of these behaviors are pleasurable to parents. Parents need to be assured that behaviors are normal. Sneeze is usually a response to mucus in the nose and not an indicator of a cold (upper respiratory tract infection). No treatment is needed for hiccups; sucking may help. In a preterm infant, these are signs of neurodevelopmental immaturity and physiologic stress.

*All durations for persistence of reflexes are based on time elapsed after 40 weeks of gestation (i.e., if newborn was born at 36 weeks of gestation, add 1 month to all time limits given).

autonomic system, including involuntary physiologic functions such as heart rate, respiration, and temperature. The next level is motor organization, in which infants regulate or control their motor behavior. This includes controlling random movements, improving muscle tone, and reducing excessive activity. The third level of behavior is *state regulation*, which refers to the ability to modulate the state of consciousness. The infant develops predictable sleep and wake states and is able to react to stress through self-regulation or communicating with the caregiver by crying and then being consoled. Finally the infant reaches the fourth level of attention and social interaction. He or she is able to attend to visual and auditory stimulation, stay alert for long periods, and engage in social interaction (Brazelton & Nugent, 2011).

This progression in behavior is the basis for the Brazelton Neonatal Behavioral Assessment Scale (NBAS) (Brazelton & Nugent, 2011). The NBAS is an interactive examination that assesses the infant's response to 28 areas organized according to the clusters in Box 22.2. It is generally used as a research or diagnostic tool and requires special training. The NBAS helps the practitioner identify where the infant falls along the continuum of behaviors and determine the type of support needed.

SLEEP-WAKE STATES

Healthy newborns differ in their activity levels, feeding patterns, sleeping patterns, and responsiveness. Parents' reactions to their newborns are often determined by these differences. Showing parents the unique characteristics of their infant helps them develop a more positive perception of the infant and promotes increased interaction between infant and parent. Infant responses to environmental stimuli and to their caregivers depend on the infant's state or state of consciousness.

In the early newborn period, infants tend to alternate periods of sleep and wakefulness that resemble their fetal inactivity and activity patterns. Variations in the state of consciousness of infants are called sleep-wake states. The six states form a continuum from deep sleep to extreme irritability (Fig. 22.15): two sleep states (deep sleep and light sleep) and four wake states (drowsy, quiet alert, active alert, and crying) (Brazelton & Nugent, 2011). Each state has specific characteristics and state-related behaviors. The optimal state of arousal is the quiet alert state. During this state, infants smile, vocalize, move in synchrony with speech, watch their parents' faces, and respond to people talking to them. They respond to internal and external environmental factors by controlling sensory input and regulating the sleep-wake states; the ability to make smooth transitions between states is called *state modulation*. The ability to regulate sleep-wake states is essential in the infant's neurobehavioral development. Term infants are better able than preterm infants to cope with external or internal factors that affect the sleep-wake patterns.

Infants use purposeful behavior to maintain the optimal arousal state as follows: (1) actively withdrawing by increasing physical distance, (2) rejecting by pushing away with hands and feet, (3) decreasing sensitivity by falling asleep or breaking eye contact by turning the head, or (4) using signaling behaviors such as fussing and crying. These behaviors permit infants to quiet themselves and reinstate readiness to interact.

The first 6 weeks of life involve a steady decrease in the proportion of active REM sleep to total sleep. A steady increase in the proportion of quiet sleep to total sleep also occurs. Periods of wakefulness increase. For the first few weeks, the wakeful periods seem dictated by hunger, but soon a need for socializing appears. The newborn sleeps approximately 16 to 19 hours per day, with periods of wakefulness gradually increasing. By the fourth week of life, some infants stay awake from one feeding to the next (Gardner, Goldson, & Hernández, 2016).

BOX 22.2   Clusters of Neonatal Behaviors in Brazelton Neonatal Behavioral Assessment Scale

- Habituation—Ability to respond to and then inhibit responding to discrete stimulus (e.g., light, rattle, bell, pinprick) while asleep
- Orientation—Quality of alert states and ability to attend to visual and auditory stimuli while alert
- Motor performance—Quality of movement and tone
- Range of state—Measure of general arousal level or arousability of infant
- Regulation of state—How infant responds when aroused
- Autonomic stability—Signs of stress (e.g., tremors, startles, skin color) related to homeostatic (self-regulator) adjustment of the nervous system
- Reflexes—Assessment of several neonatal reflexes

From Brazelton, T., & Nugent, J. (2011). *Neonatal behavioral assessment scale* (4th ed.). London. UK: MacKeith.

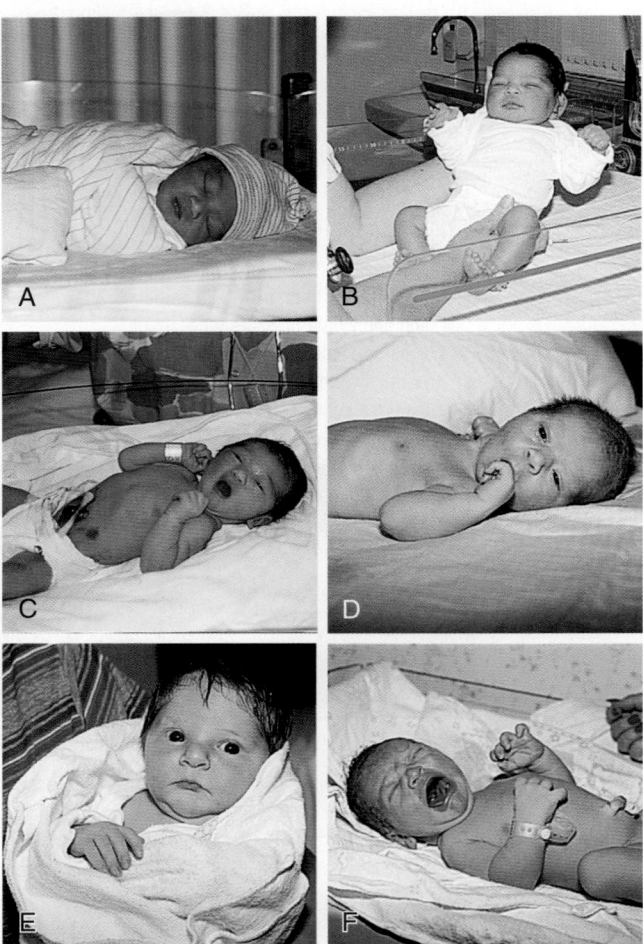

FIG 22.15 Newborn sleep-wake states. **A,** Deep sleep. **B,** Light sleep. **C,** Drowsy. **D,** Quiet alert. **E,** Active alert. **F,** Crying. (Courtesy of Marjorie Pyle, RNC, Lifecircle, Costa Mesa, CA.)

OTHER FACTORS INFLUENCING NEWBORN BEHAVIOR

Gestational Age

Gestational age and level of central nervous system (CNS) maturity affect infant behavior. In the preterm neonate with an immature CNS, the entire body responds to a pinprick of the foot, although the response may not be observed by an untrained observer. The more mature infant withdraws only the foot. CNS immaturity is reflected in reflex development, sleep-wake states, and ability (or lack thereof) to regulate or modulate a smooth transition between different states. Preterm infants have brief periods of alertness but have difficulty maintaining alertness without becoming overstimulated, which leads to autonomic instability unless intervention is implemented. Premature or sick infants show signs of fatigue or physiologic stress sooner than full-term healthy infants.

Time

The time elapsed since birth affects the behavior of infants as they attempt to become organized initially. Time elapsed since the previous feeding and time of day also can influence infants' responses.

Stimuli

Environmental events and stimuli affect the infant's behavioral responses. The newborn responds to animate and inanimate stimuli. Nurses in intensive care nurseries observe that infants respond to loud noises, bright lights, monitor alarms, and tension in the unit. If a mother is tense, nervous, or uncomfortable while feeding her infant, the infant may sense her tension and demonstrate difficulty feeding.

Medication

No conclusive evidence exists regarding the effects of maternal analgesia or anesthesia during labor on neonatal behavior. Researchers who have studied the effects of epidural medications on breastfeeding behaviors have been unable to show a cause-and-effect relationship (Hoyt & Pages-Arroyo, 2015).

SENSORY BEHAVIORS

From birth, infants possess sensory capabilities that indicate a state of readiness for social interaction. They effectively use behavioral responses in establishing their first dialogues. These responses, coupled with the newborns' "baby appearance" (e.g., facial proportions of forehead, eyes larger than the lower portion of the face) and their small size and helplessness, rouse feelings of wanting to hold, protect, and interact with them.

Vision

At birth the eye is structurally incomplete, and the muscles are immature. The process of accommodation is not present but improves over the first 3 months of life. The pupils react to light, the blink reflex is stimulated easily, and the corneal reflex is activated by light touch. Term newborns can see objects as far away as 50 cm (2.5 feet). The clearest visual distance is 17 to 20 cm (8 to 12 inches), which is approximately the distance between the mother's and infant's faces during breastfeeding or cuddling. Newborns seem to have a preference for faces and can recognize the mother's face. This facilitates interaction and promotes bonding. They will engage the mother or caregiver with eye contact. Newborns can imitate facial expressions and motions such as protruding the tongue (Gardner, Goldson, & Hernández, 2016). Newborns prefer complex patterns over nonpatterned stimuli. They prefer black and white, possibly because of the greater contrast. Within 2 to 3 months, they can discriminate colors (Nugent & Morell, 2011).

Hearing

Term newborns can hear and differentiate among various sounds. They will turn toward a sound and attempt to locate the source. The neonate recognizes and responds readily to the mother's voice and shows a preference for high-pitched intonation. Newborns respond to rhythmic sounds. They are accustomed to hearing the regular rhythm of the mother's heartbeat, which was a constant sound during intrauterine

life. As a result, they respond by relaxing and ceasing to fuss and cry if a regular heartbeat simulator is placed in their cribs; a lullaby can have the same effect (Nugent & Morell, 2011). Hearing is integral to bonding and attachment and may be more important than vision (Gardner, Goldson, & Hernández, 2016).

Routine hearing screening is recommended for all newborns before hospital discharge. See Chapter 23 and Fig. 23.11 for a discussion about newborn hearing screening.

Smell

Newborns have a highly developed sense of smell and can detect and discriminate distinct odors. It has been shown that preterm infants as early as 28 weeks are capable of reacting to odors. They react to strong odors such as alcohol or vinegar by turning their heads away but are attracted to sweet smells. By the fifth day of life, newborn infants can recognize their mother's smell. Breastfed infants are able to smell breast milk and can differentiate their mothers from other lactating women (Lawrence & Lawrence, 2016).

Taste

Young infants are particularly oriented toward the use of their mouths, both for meeting their nutritional needs for rapid growth and for releasing tension through sucking. The early development of circumoral sensation, muscle activity, and taste would seem to be preparation for survival in the extrauterine environment. The newborn can distinguish among tastes and has a preference for sweet solutions (Gardner, Goldson, & Hernández, 2016).

Touch

The infant is responsive to touch on all parts of the body. The face (especially the mouth), the hands, and the soles of the feet seem to be the most sensitive. Reflexes can be elicited by stroking the infant. The newborn's responses to touch suggest that this sensory system is well prepared to receive and process tactile messages (Gardner, Goldson, & Hernández, 2016). Touch and motion are essential to normal growth and development. However, each infant is unique, and variations can be seen in newborns' responses to touch. Birth trauma or stress and depressant drugs taken by the mother decrease the infant's sensitivity to touch or painful stimuli.

RESPONSE TO ENVIRONMENTAL STIMULI

Temperament

Each neonate has a unique repertoire of behaviors that are influenced by various factors including temperament, sensory threshold, ability to habituate, and consolability. Temperament refers to individual variations in the reaction pattern of newborns. Newborns possess individual characteristics that affect selective responses to various stimuli present in the internal and external environments. Some infants appear to be quiet by nature and can remain still for extended periods. Their movements may be smooth and relaxed most of the time, and they have little difficulty settling down for feeding, Other infants are more active and seem to be in constant motion; they seem to be excited and interested in exploring the faces and sounds around them. These infants often need help to settle; containment (swaddling), physical contact, and boundaries surrounding the neonate in the crib can facilitate a quiet alert state (Nugent & Morell, 2011).

Habituation

Habituation is a protective mechanism that allows the infant to become accustomed to environmental stimuli. It is a psychologic and physiologic phenomenon in which the response to a constant or repetitive stimulus is decreased. In the term newborn, this can be demonstrated in several ways. Shining a bright light into a newborn's eyes causes a startle or squinting the first two or three times. The third or fourth flash elicits a diminished response, and by the fifth or sixth flash the infant ceases to respond (Brazelton & Nugent, 2011). The same response pattern holds true for the sounds of a rattle or stroking the bottom of the foot.

The ability to habituate allows the healthy term newborn to select stimuli that promote continued learning about the social world, thus avoiding overload. The intrauterine environment seems to have programmed the newborn to be especially responsive to human voices, soft lights, soft sounds, and sweet tastes.

The newborn quickly learns the sounds in the home environment and is able to sleep in their midst. The selective responses of the newborn indicate cerebral organization capable of memory and making choices. The ability to habituate depends on the state of consciousness, hunger, fatigue, and temperament. These factors also affect consolability, cuddliness, irritability, and crying.

Consolability

Newborns vary in the ability to console themselves or be consoled. In the crying state, most newborns initiate one of several ways to reduce their distress. Hand-to-mouth movements with or without sucking and being alert to voices, noises, or visual stimuli are common. Some infants are consoled only if they are held and rocked (Brazelton & Nugent, 2011).

Cuddliness

Cuddliness is especially important to parents because they often gauge their ability to care for the child by the child's responses to their actions. The degree to which newborns relax and mold into the contours of the person holding them varies. One extreme is the infant who always resists being held with thrashing and stiffening of the body. This is in contrast to the infant who immediately relaxes when held and molds to the body of the person. Less extreme behavior is demonstrated by infants who are passive when held and those who gradually mold after being held for a while (Brazelton & Nugent, 2011).

Irritability

Some newborns cry longer and harder than others. For some, the sensory threshold seems low. They are easily upset by unusual noises, hunger, wetness, or new experiences and thus respond intensely. Others with a high sensory threshold require a great deal more stimulation and variation to reach the active, alert state.

Crying

Crying is the language an infant uses most often to communicate needs. It can signal hunger, discomfort, pain, desire for attention, or fussiness. Infants may cry in response to environmental stimuli such as cold, being overstimulated, or being held by multiple persons. Responsiveness of the caregiver to the crying creates trust as the infant learns to associate the caregiver with comfort.

The amount and tone of crying vary based on gestational age, weight, and the reason for the cry (e.g., hunger, pain). A high-pitched cry can be a sign of a neurologic disorder. Some mothers state that they learn to distinguish among the cries. The breastfeeding mother's body responds physiologically to infant crying by stimulating the milk-ejection reflex ("let-down").

The duration of crying also varies greatly in each infant; newborns may cry for as little as 5 minutes or as much as 2 hours or more per day. The amount of crying peaks in the second month and then decreases. There is a diurnal rhythm of crying, with more crying occurring in the evening hours.

REFERENCES

American Academy of Pediatrics. (2013). Statement of endorsement: Timing of umbilical cord clamping after birth. *Pediatrics, 131*(4), e1323.

American Academy of Pediatrics and American College of Obstetricians and Gynecologists (2012). *Guidelines for perinatal care* (7th ed.). Washington, DC: Author.

American Academy of Pediatrics Subcommittee on Hyperbilirubinemia. (2004). Clinical practice guideline: Management of hyperbilirubinemia in the newborn infant 35 or more weeks of gestation. *Pediatrics, 114*(1), 297–316.

American College of Obstetricians and Gynecologists. (2012). Timing of umbilical cord clamping after birth. *Obstetrics and Gynecology, 120*(6), 1522–1526.

Association of Women's Health, Obstetric, and Neonatal Nurses (2013). *Neonatal skin care* (3rd ed.). Washington, DC: Author.

Bäckhed, F., Roswall, J., Peng, Y., et al. (2015). Dynamics and stabilization of the human gut microbiome during the first year of life. *Cell Host and Microbe, 17*(5), 690–703.

Benjamin, J. T., Mezu-Ndibuisi, O. J., & Maheshwari, A. (2015). Developmental immunology. In R. J. Martin, A. A. Fanaroff, & M. C. Walsh (Eds.), *Fanaroff & Martin's neonatal-perinatal medicine* (10th ed.). Philadelphia, PA: Saunders.

Blackburn, S. T. (2013). *Maternal, fetal, and neonatal physiology* (4th ed.). Maryland Heights, MO: Saunders.

Bodin, M. B. (2014). Immune system. In C. Kenner & J. W. Lott (Eds.), *Comprehensive neonatal nursing care* (5th ed.). New York, NY: Springer.

Bonifacio, S. L., Gonzalez, F., & Ferriero, D. M. (2012). Central nervous system injury and neuroprotection. In C. A. Gleason & S. U. Devaskar (Eds.), *Avery's diseases of the newborn* (9th ed.). Philadelphia, PA: Saunders.

Brazelton, T., & Nugent, J. (2011). *Neonatal behavioral assessment scale* (4th ed.). London, UK: MacKeith.

Cadnapaphornchai, M. A., Schoenbein, M. B., Woloschuk, R., et al. (2016). Neonatal nephrology. In S. L. Gardner, B. S. Carter, M. Enzman-Hines, et al. (Eds.), *Merenstein & Gardner's handbook of neonatal intensive care* (8th ed.). St. Louis, MO: Elsevier.

Centers for Disease Control and Prevention. (2015). *Congenital heart defects: Data and statistics.* Retrieved from http://www.cdc.gov/ncbddd/heartdefects/data.html.

Christensen, R. D., & Ohls, R. K. (2016). Development of the hematopoietic system. In R. M. Kliegman, B. F. Stanton, J. W. St Geme III, et al. (Eds.), *Nelson textbook of pediatrics* (20th ed.). Philadelphia, PA: Elsevier.

Dell, K. M. (2015). Fluids, electrolytes, and acid-base homeostasis. In R. J. Martin, A. A. Fanaroff, & M. C. Walsh (Eds.), *Fanaroff & Martin's neonatal-perinatal medicine* (10th ed.). St. Louis, MO: Saunders.

Diehl-Jones, W., & Fraser, D. (2015). Hematologic disorders. In M. T. Verklan & M. Walden (Eds.), *Core curriculum for neonatal intensive care nursing* (5th ed.). St. Louis, MO: Elsevier.

Desmond, M., Rudolph, A., & Phitaksphraiwan, P. (1966). The transitional care nursery: A mechanism for preventive medicine in the newborn. *Pediatric Clinics of North America, 13*(3), 651–668.

Ditzenberger, G. R., & Blackburn, S. T. (2014). Neurologic system. In C. Kenner & J. W. Lott (Eds.), *Comprehensive neonatal nursing care* (5th ed.). New York, NY: Springer.

Elder, J. S. (2016). Anomalies of the penis and urethra. In R. M. Kliegman, B. F. Stanton, J. W. St. Geme III, et al. (Eds.), *Nelson textbook of pediatrics* (20th ed.). Philadelphia, PA: Elsevier.

Fraser, D. (2015). Respiratory distress. In M. T. Verklan & M. Walden (Eds.), *Core curriculum for neonatal intensive care nursing* (5th ed.). St. Louis, MO: Elsevier.

Gardner, S. L., Enzman Hines, M., & Nyp, M. (2016). Respiratory diseases. In S. L. Gardner, B. S. Carter, M. Enzman-Hines, et al. (Eds.), *Merenstein & Gardner's handbook of neonatal intensive care* (8th ed.). St. Louis, MO: Elsevier.

Gardner, S. L., Goldson, E., & Hernández, J. A. (2016). The neonate and the environment: Impact on development. In S. L. Gardner, B. S. Carter, M. Enzman-Hines, et al. (Eds.), *Merenstein & Gardner's handbook of neonatal intensive care* (8th ed.). St. Louis, MO: Elsevier.

Gardner, S. L., & Hernández, J. A. (2016). Heat balance. In S. L. Gardner, B. S. Carter, M. Enzman-Hines, et al. (Eds.), *Merenstein & Gardner's handbook of neonatal intensive care* (8th ed.). St. Louis, MO: Elsevier.

Greenberg, J. M., Narendran, V., Schibler, K. R., et al. (2014). Neonatal morbidities of prenatal and perinatal origin. In R. K. Creasy, R. Resnik, J. D. Iams, et al. (Eds.), *Creasy & Resnik's maternal-fetal medicine: Principles and practice* (7th ed.). Philadelphia, PA: Saunders.

Grijalva, J., & Vakili, K. (2013). Neonatal liver physiology. *Seminars in Pediatric Surgery, 22*(4), 185–189.

Hawkes, C. P., & Stanley, C. A. (2017). Pathophysiology of neonatal hypoglycemia. In R. A. Polin, S. H. Abman, D. H. Rowitch, et al. (Eds.), *Fetal and neonatal physiology* (5th ed.). Philadelphia, PA: Elsevier.

Hibbs, A. M. (2015). Gastroesophageal reflux and gastroesophageal reflux disease in the neonate. In R. J. Martin, A. A. Fanaroff, & M. C. Walsh (Eds.), *Fanaroff & Martin's neonatal-perinatal medicine* (10th ed.). Philadelphia, PA: Saunders.

Hillman, N. H., Kallapur, S. G., & Jobe, A. H. (2012). Physiology of transition from intrauterine to extrauterine life. *Clinics in Perinatology, 39*(4), 769–783.

Hoath, S. B., & Narendran, V. (2015). The skin of the neonate. In R. J. Martin, A. A. Fanaroff, & M. C. Walsh (Eds.), *Fanaroff & Martin's neonatal-perinatal medicine* (10th ed.). Philadelphia, PA: Saunders.

Hoyt, M. R., & Pages-Arroyo, E. M. (2015). Anesthesia for labor and delivery. In R. J. Martin, A. A. Fanaroff, & M. C. Walsh (Eds.), *Fanaroff & Martin's neonatal-perinatal medicine* (10th ed.). Philadelphia, PA: Saunders.

Janke, J. (2014). Newborn nutrition. In K. R. Simpson & P. A. Creehan (Eds.), *Perinatal nursing* (4th ed.). Philadelphia, PA: Wolters Kluwer/Lippincott.

Kamath-Rayne, B. D., Thilo, E. H., Deacon, J., et al. (2016). Neonatal hyperbilirubinemia. In S. L. Gardner, B. S. Carter, M. Enzman-Hines, et al. (Eds.), *Merenstein & Gardner's handbook of neonatal intensive care* (8th ed.). St. Louis, MO: Elsevier.

Lawrence, R. A., & Lawrence, R. M. (2016). *Breastfeeding: A guide for the medical profession* (8th ed.). St. Louis, MO: Mosby.

Lee, M. M. (2017). Testicular development and descent. In R. A. Polin, S. H. Abman, D. H. Rowitch, et al. (Eds.), *Fetal and neonatal physiology* (5th ed.). Philadelphia, PA: Elsevier.

Lissauer, T. (2015). Physical examination of the newborn. In R. J. Martin, A. A. Fanaroff, & M. C. Walsh (Eds.), *Fanaroff & Martin's neonatal-perinatal medicine* (10th ed.). Philadelphia, PA: Saunders.

Lott, J. W. (2014). Cardiovascular system. In C. Kenner & J. W. Lott (Eds.), *Comprehensive neonatal care* (5th ed.). New York, NY: Springer.

Mangurten, H. H., Puppala, B. L., & Prazad, R. A. (2015). Birth injuries. In R. J. Martin, A. A. Fanaroff, & M. C. Walsh (Eds.), *Fanaroff & Martin's neonatal-perinatal medicine* (10th ed.). Philadelphia, PA: Saunders.

Martin, K. L. (2016). Vascular disorders. In R. M. Kliegman, B. F. Stanton, J. W. St. Geme III, et al. (Eds.), *Nelson textbook of pediatrics* (20th ed.). Philadelphia, PA: Elsevier.

Monagle, P. (2017). Developmental hemostasis. In R. A. Polin, S. H. Abman, D. H. Rowitch, et al. (Eds.), *Fetal and neonatal physiology* (5th ed.). Philadelphia, PA: Elsevier.

Mueller, N. T., Bakacs, E., Combellick, J., et al. (2015). The infant microbiome development: Mom matters. *Trends in Molecular Medicine, 21*(2), 109–117.

Neu, J. (2017). The developing microbiome of the fetus and newborn. In R. A. Polin, S. H. Abman, D. H. Rowitch, et al. (Eds.), *Fetal and neonatal physiology* (5th ed.). Philadelphia, PA: Elsevier.

Nugent, K., & Morell, A. (2011). *Your baby is speaking to you.* Boston, MA: Houghton Mifflin Harcourt.

Pagana, K. D., Pagana, T. J., & Pagana, T. N. (2017). *Mosby's diagnostic and laboratory test reference* (13th ed.). St. Louis, MO: Elsevier.

Perlman, J. M., Wyllie, J., Kattwinkel, J., et al. (2015). Part 7: Neonatal resuscitation: 2015 international consensus on cardiopulmonary resuscitation and emergency cardiovascular care science with treatment recommendations. *Circulation, 132*(16 Suppl. 1), S204–S241.

Ringer, S. A. (2013a). Core concepts: Thermoregulation in the newborn part I: Basic mechanisms. *Neoreviews, 14*(4), c161–c167.

Ringer, S. A. (2013b). Core concepts: Thermoregulation in the newborn part II: Prevention of aberrant body temperature. *Neoreviews, 14*(5), c221–c226.

Scher, M. S. (2012). Neonatal seizures. In C. A. Gleason & S. U. Devaskar (Eds.), *Avery's diseases of the newborn* (9th ed.). Philadelphia, PA: Saunders.

Shearer, M. J. (2017). Vitamin K metabolism in the fetus and neonate. In R. A. Polin, S. H. Abman, D. H. Rowitch, et al. (Eds.), *Fetal and neonatal physiology* (5th ed.). Philadelphia, PA: Elsevier.

Smith, J. B. (2012). Initial evaluation: History and physical examination of the newborn. In C. A. Gleason & S. U. Devaskar (Eds.), *Avery's diseases of the newborn* (9th ed.). Philadelphia, PA: Saunders.

Soltau, T. D., & Carlo, W. A. (2014). Respiratory system. In C. Kenner & J. W. Lott (Eds.), *Comprehensive neonatal care* (5th ed.). New York, NY: Springer.

Son-Hing, J. P., & Thompson, G. H. (2015). Congenital abnormalities of the upper and lower extremities and spine. In R. J. Martin, A. A. Fanaroff, & M. C. Walsh (Eds.), *Fanaroff & Martin's neonatal-perinatal medicine* (10th ed.). Philadelphia, PA: Saunders.

Turfkruyer, M., & Verhasselt, V. (2015). Breast milk and its impact on the maturation of the neonatal immune system. *Current Opinions in Infectious Diseases, 28*(3), 199–206.

Verklan, M. T. (2015). Adaptation to extrauterine life. In M. T. Verklan & M. Walden (Eds.), *Core curriculum for neonatal intensive care nursing* (5th ed.). St. Louis, MO: Elsevier.

Visscher, M. O., Adam, R., Brink, S., et al. (2015). Newborn infant skin: Physiology, development. *Clinics in Dermatology, 33*(3), 271–280.

Vogt, B. A., & Dell, K. M. (2015). The kidney and urinary tract of the neonate. In R. J. Martin, A. A. Fanaroff, & M. C. Walsh (Eds.), *Fanaroff & Martin's neonatal-perinatal medicine* (10th ed.). Philadelphia, PA: Saunders.

White, K. K., & Goldberg, M. J. (2012). Common neonatal orthopedic ailments. In C. A. Gleason & S. U. Devaskar (Eds.), *Avery's diseases of the newborn* (9th ed.). Philadelphia, PA: Saunders.

23

Nursing Care of the Newborn and Family

Kathryn R. Alden

http://evolve.elsevier.com/Perry/maternal

Although most newborns make the necessary biopsychosocial adjustments to extrauterine existence without undue difficulty, their well-being depends on the care they receive. This chapter describes the assessment and care of the neonate immediately after birth until discharge from the birth setting, as well as important anticipatory guidance for parents related to ongoing infant care.

CARE MANAGEMENT: BIRTH THROUGH THE FIRST 2 HOURS

Care begins immediately after birth and focuses on assessing and stabilizing the newborn's condition. Interprofessional care is key to optimizing outcomes for newborns. While the obstetric health care provider is focused on the mother, the labor and delivery nurse is responsible for care of the neonate immediately after birth. There may be a second labor and delivery nurse who is available for newborn care. In some hospitals, a "stork nurse" from the newborn nursery is assigned to do newborn care and administer medications. The nurse must be alert for any signs of distress and initiate appropriate interventions.

When risk factors or birth events are likely to affect the well-being of the neonate, the labor and delivery nurse notifies the neonatal or pediatric care team to request their attendance at the birth, or may call for them once the infant is born. Depending on the status of the neonate, additional health team members from other professions such as respiratory therapy and pharmacy may be needed.

The foundation for providing comprehensive, family-centered newborn care is awareness of the mother's preconception and prenatal history as well as intrapartal events. Recognition of risk factors (Box 23.1) enables the nurse to be more astute in observations and assessments and more likely to identify early signs of complications. This allows for earlier intervention and promotes positive outcomes.

⚡ SAFETY ALERT

With the possibility of transmission of viruses such as hepatitis B virus (HBV) and human immunodeficiency virus (HIV) through maternal blood and blood-stained amniotic fluid, the newborn must be considered a potential contamination source until proved otherwise. As part of Standard Precautions, nurses wear gloves when handling the newborn until blood and amniotic fluid are removed by bathing.

IMMEDIATE CARE AFTER BIRTH

The primary goal of care in the first moments after birth is to assist the neonate to successfully transition to extrauterine life. The first priority for the newborn is to establish effective respirations. If the infant is at term, has good muscle tone, and is crying or breathing, routine care may begin. The infant is placed prone skin-to-skin on the mother's abdomen or chest and is positioned with the head slightly extended. Nasal and oral secretions are wiped away, and the bulb syringe may be used if secretions appear to be blocking the airway. The nurse begins ongoing assessment of the neonate's breathing, color, and activity. Vigorously drying the infant provides tactile stimulation to stimulate respiratory effort and removes moisture to prevent evaporative heat loss. Wet linens are removed. A cap is placed on the neonate's head; the mother and her newborn are covered with a warm blanket (Wyckoff, Aziz, Escobedo, et al., 2015).

A neonate who is not term, has poor muscle tone, or is not crying or breathing is placed immediately under a radiant warmer. Assessments and interventions are accomplished under the warmer until the infant is stable and can be safely placed skin-to-skin with the mother or transported to a nursery or neonatal intensive care (NICU) setting (Wyckoff et al., 2015).

The newborn should be breathing spontaneously. The trunk and lips should be pink; acrocyanosis is a normal finding (see Fig. 22.5). If the neonate is apneic or has gasping respirations, positive-pressure ventilation is needed.

The heart rate is quickly assessed by grasping the base of the cord or by auscultating the chest with a stethoscope. The nurse counts for 6 seconds and multiplies by 10 to calculate the heart rate. It should be greater than 100 beats/minute. If the newborn requires respiratory or circulatory support, the nurse and other members of the health care team (e.g., neonatologist, respiratory therapist) follow the American Heart Association guidelines for neonatal resuscitation (Wyckoff et al., 2015). The neonatal resuscitation algorithm directs the care (Fig. 23.1).

As soon as possible after birth, the nurse places identically numbered bands on the infant's wrist and ankle, on the mother, and in some birth settings, on the father or significant other. An electronic infant security tag or abduction system alarm should be placed on all newborns to aid in protecting against infant abduction. The infant is footprinted with ink or a scanning device within 2 hours of birth (see the "Preventing Infant Abduction" section later in the chapter).

INITIAL ASSESSMENT AND APGAR SCORING

The initial assessment of the neonate is performed immediately after birth (Table 23.1). This is followed by Apgar scoring at 1 and 5 minutes (Table 23.2). A gestational age assessment is completed within the first hours of birth (Fig. 23.2).

BOX 23.1   Assessment of Preconception, Prenatal, and Intrapartum Risk Factors

Preconception

- Age
- Preexisting medical conditions: diabetes, hypertension, cardiac disease, anemia, thyroid disorder, renal disease, obesity
- Genetic factors: family history
- Obstetric history: gravidity, parity, number of living children and their ages, history of stillbirth, previous infant with congenital anomalies, habitual abortion, use of assisted reproductive technology, interpregnancy spacing
- Blood type and Rh status

Prenatal

- Prenatal care: when started
- Nutrition: weight gain, diet, obesity, eating disorders
- Health-compromising behaviors: smoking, alcohol use, substance abuse
- Blood group or Rh sensitization
- Medications: prescription, over-the-counter, and complementary and alternative medications
- History of infection: sexually transmitted infections, TORCH* infections, group B streptococcus status

Intrapartum

- Length of gestation: preterm, late preterm, early term, term, or postterm
- First stage of labor: length, electronic fetal monitoring—internal or external, rupture of membranes (time, presence of meconium), signs of fetal distress (decelerations)
- Group B streptococcus status: treatment during labor
- Second stage of labor: length, vaginal or cesarean, instrument assisted—forceps or vacuum extractor, complications (shoulder dystocia, bleeding [abruptio placentae or placenta previa]), cord prolapse, maternal analgesia and/or anesthesia

*TORCH is the collective name for toxoplasmosis, other infections (e.g., hepatitis), rubella virus, cytomegalovirus (CMV), and herpes simplex virus.
Adapted from Hurst, H.M. (2015). Antepartum-intrapartum complications. In T.M. Verklan, & M. Walden (Eds.), *Core curriculum for neonatal intensive care nursing* (5th ed.). St. Louis, MO: Saunders.

TABLE 23.1   Initial Physical Assessment of the Newborn

General appearance	☐ Color pink
	☐ Acrocyanosis present
	☐ Flexed posture
	☐ Alert
	☐ Active
Respiratory system	☐ Airway patent
	☐ No upper airway congestion
	☐ No retractions or nasal flaring
	☐ Respiratory rate, 30–60 breaths/min
	☐ Lungs clear to auscultation bilaterally
	☐ Chest expansion symmetric
Cardiovascular system	☐ Heart rate >100 beats/min; strong and regular
	☐ No murmurs heard
	☐ Pulses strong and equal bilaterally
Neurologic system	☐ Moves extremities
	☐ Normotonic
	☐ Symmetric features, movement
	Reflexes present:
	☐ Sucking ☐ Rooting
	☐ Moro ☐ Grasp
	☐ Anterior fontanel soft and flat
Gastrointestinal system	☐ Abdomen soft, no distention
	☐ Cord attached and clamped
	☐ Anus appears patent
Eyes, nose, mouth	☐ Eyes clear
	☐ Palate intact
	☐ Nares patent
Skin	☐ No signs of birth trauma
	☐ No lesions or abrasions
Genitourinary system	☐ Normal genitalia
Comments:	

Initial Physical Assessment

The initial examination of the newborn (see Table 23.1) may be accomplished while the infant is lying on the mother's abdomen or chest or in her arms immediately after birth, or alternatively while the neonate is lying on the radiant warmer bed. Efforts should be directed toward minimizing interference in the initial parent-infant acquaintance process. If the infant is breathing effectively, is pink, and has no apparent life-threatening anomalies or risk factors requiring immediate attention, further examination may be delayed until after the parents have had an opportunity to interact with the infant. Ideally, the newborn remains skin-to-skin with the mother for at least the first 1 to 2 hours after birth, and breastfeeding is initiated during that time. Routine procedures and the admission process can be carried out in the mother's room or in a separate nursery.

Apgar Score

The Apgar score done at 1 and 5 minutes after birth permits a rapid assessment of the newborn's transition to extrauterine life based on five signs that indicate the physiologic state of the neonate: (1) heart rate, based on auscultation with a stethoscope or palpation of the umbilical cord; (2) respiratory effort, based on observed movement of

TABLE 23.2   Apgar Score

Sign	SCORE		
	0	1	2
Heart rate	Absent	Slow (<100/min)	≥100/min
Respiratory effort	Absent	Slow, weak cry	Good cry
Muscle tone	Flaccid	Some flexion of extremities	Well flexed
Reflex irritability	No response	Grimace	Cry
Color	Blue, pale	Body pink, extremities blue	Completely pink

the chest wall; (3) muscle tone, based on degree of flexion and movement of the extremities; (4) reflex irritability, based on response to suctioning of the nares or nasopharynx; and (5) generalized skin color, described as pallid, cyanotic, or pink (see Table 23.2). Evaluations can be completed by the nurse or birth attendant. Scores of 0 to 3 indicate severe distress, scores of 4 to 6 indicate moderate difficulty, and scores of 7 to 10 indicate that the infant is having minimal or no difficulty adjusting to extrauterine life. For scores less than 7 at 5 minutes, the assessment

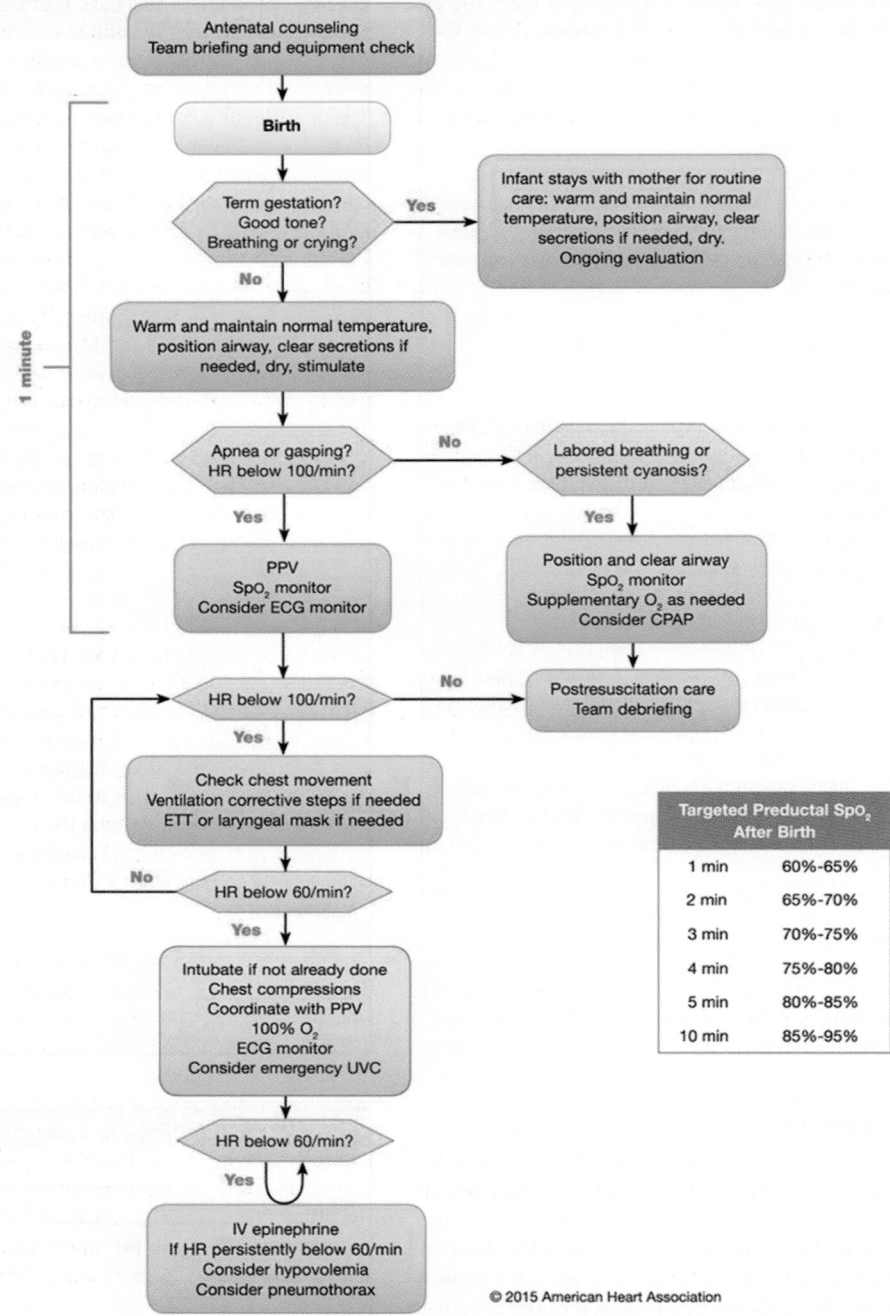

Neonatal Resuscitation Algorithm—2015 Update

Antenatal counseling
Team briefing and equipment check

Birth

Term gestation?
Good tone?
Breathing or crying?

Yes → Infant stays with mother for routine care: warm and maintain normal temperature, position airway, clear secretions if needed, dry. Ongoing evaluation

No

Warm and maintain normal temperature, position airway, clear secretions if needed, dry, stimulate

Apnea or gasping?
HR below 100/min?

No → Labored breathing or persistent cyanosis?

Yes → Position and clear airway
SpO₂ monitor
Supplementary O₂ as needed
Consider CPAP

Yes

PPV
SpO₂ monitor
Consider ECG monitor

HR below 100/min?

No → Postresuscitation care
Team debriefing

Yes

Check chest movement
Ventilation corrective steps if needed
ETT or laryngeal mask if needed

HR below 60/min?

No

Yes

Intubate if not already done
Chest compressions
Coordinate with PPV
100% O₂
ECG monitor
Consider emergency UVC

HR below 60/min?

Yes

IV epinephrine
If HR persistently below 60/min
Consider hypovolemia
Consider pneumothorax

1 minute

Targeted Preductal SpO₂ After Birth	
1 min	60%-65%
2 min	65%-70%
3 min	70%-75%
4 min	75%-80%
5 min	80%-85%
10 min	85%-95%

© 2015 American Heart Association

FIG 23.1 Neonatal resuscitation algorithm. *CPAP*, Continuous positive airway pressure; *HR*, heart rate; *IV*, intravenous; *PPV*, positive-pressure ventilation; *SpO₂*, blood oxygen saturation. (From Wyckoff, M.H., Aziz, K., Escobedo, M.B., et al. [2015]. Part 13: Neonatal resuscitation: 2015 American Heart Association guidelines update for cardiopulmonary resuscitation and emergency cardiovascular care. *Circulation, 132*[18; suppl 2], S543–S560. Reprinted with permission from the American Heart Association.)

should be repeated every 5 minutes for up to 20 minutes. Apgar scores do not predict future neurologic outcome but are useful for describing the newborn's transition to the extrauterine environment and the need for and response to resuscitative efforts. If resuscitation is required, it should be initiated before the 1-minute Apgar score is determined (American Academy of Pediatrics [AAP] & American College of Obstetricians and Gynecologists [ACOG], 2015).

PHYSICAL ASSESSMENT

Although the initial assessment after birth can reveal significant anomalies, birth injuries, and cardiopulmonary problems that have immediate implications, a more detailed, thorough physical examination should follow within 12 to 18 hours after birth (AAP & ACOG, 2012) (Table 23.3). The parents' presence during this and other examinations encourages discussion of their concerns and actively involves them in the health care of their infant from birth. It also affords the nurse an opportunity to observe parental interactions with the infant. The findings provide data for planning nursing care of the newborn and education for the parents. Ongoing assessments are made throughout the stay in the birthing facility; another detailed physical examination is performed before discharge.

General Appearance

Features to assess in the general survey include color, posture, activity, any overt signs of anomalies that can cause initial distress, presence of bruising or other birth trauma, and state of alertness. The neonate's maturity level can be gauged by assessing general appearance. The normal resting position of the neonate is one of general flexion.

Vital Signs

The temperature, heart rate, and respiratory rate are assessed. Blood pressure (BP) is not routinely measured unless cardiac problems are suspected. An irregular, very slow, or very fast heart rate, or a heart murmur can indicate a need for further evaluation of circulatory status including BP measurement.

The axillary temperature is a safe, accurate measurement of temperature. Electronic thermometers have expedited this task and provide a reading within 1 minute. Taking an infant's temperature can cause the infant to cry and struggle against the placement of the thermometer in the axilla. Before assessing the temperature, the examiner can determine the apical heart rate and respiratory rate while the infant is quiet and at rest. The desired range for axillary temperature is 36.5° to 37.5°C (97.7° to 99.5°F).

> ## ⚡ SAFETY ALERT
>
> Rectal temperatures should not routinely be performed on a newborn because of the risk for perforation and vagal stimulation.

The respiratory rate varies with the state of alertness and activity after birth. Respirations are abdominal in nature and can be counted by observing or lightly feeling the rise and fall of the abdomen. Neonatal respirations are shallow and irregular. The nurse counts respirations for a full minute to obtain an accurate assessment because there are periods of apnea when respirations can cease for seconds (≤20) and resume again. The nurse also observes for symmetry of chest movement. The normal range for newborn respirations is 30 to 60 breaths/minute; respiratory rate can exceed 60 breaths/minute if the newborn is very active or crying.

An apical pulse rate should be obtained on all newborns. Auscultation is done for a full minute, preferably when the infant is asleep or in a quiet alert state. The infant may need to be held and comforted during assessment. The normal heart rate ranges from 110 to 160 beats/minute when the infant is awake. It is common to detect brief irregularities in the heart rate. Heart rate varies with the newborn's behavioral state. Bradycardia is a heart rate less than 80 beats/minute. However, a term infant in deep sleep can have a heart rate in the 80s or 90s; the rate should increase when the infant awakens. Tachycardia is a heart rate exceeding 160 beats/minute (Gardner & Hernández, 2016). It is not unusual for a crying infant to have a heart rate greater than 160; the heart rate should decrease when the crying ceases.

Assessment of neonatal blood pressure is based on agency policy. If BP is measured, an oscillometric monitor calibrated for neonatal pressures is preferred. An appropriate-size cuff (width-to-arm or width-to-calf ratio of 0.45 to 0.70, or approximately ½ to ¾) is essential for accuracy. Neonatal BP usually is highest immediately after birth,

decreasing over the next 3 hours, and then rising steadily until it reaches a plateau between 4 and 6 days after birth. This measurement is usually equal to that of the immediate postbirth BP. The BP varies with the neonate's activity; accurate measurement is best obtained while the newborn is at rest. Blood pressure varies with gestational age, chronologic age, and weight. Systolic pressure in a term neonate ranges from 60 to 80 mm Hg; diastolic pressure averages 40 to 50 mm Hg. The mean arterial pressure should approximate the neonate's week of gestation. According to agency protocol, four extremity blood pressures may be assessed routinely or only when a murmur is auscultated. If the upper extremity systolic pressures are more than 20 mm Hg greater than those in the lower extremities, the infant may have a cardiac defect such as coarctation of the aorta (Gardner & Hernández, 2016). Peripheral pulses are also palpated as part of the assessment in any infant with a heart murmur. Additionally, if a murmur is present, oxygen saturation is usually measured using pulse oximetry.

Baseline Measurements of Physical Growth

Baseline measurements are done and recorded to help assess the progress and determine the growth patterns of the neonate. These measurements may be recorded on growth charts.

Weight

The newborn is weighed soon after birth. This assessment is performed in the labor and birthing area, the mother's room, or in the nursery. The nurse ensures that the scales are balanced. The totally unclothed neonate is placed in the center of the scale, which is usually covered with a disposable pad or cloth to prevent heat loss via conduction and to prevent cross-infection. The nurse should place one hand over (but not touching) the neonate to be prepared to prevent the infant from falling off the scales. Weighing the infant at the same time every day is common during the hospital stay. Birth weight of a term infant typically ranges from 2500 to 4000 g (5.5 to 8.8 lb).

Head Circumference and Body Length

The head is measured at the widest part, which is the occipitofrontal diameter. The tape measure is placed around the head just above the infant's eyebrows. The term neonate's head circumference ranges from 32 to 38 cm (12.6 to 14.7 in.). Accuracy of the head circumference can be altered by temporary swelling due to pressure on the head during labor and birth (Gardner & Hernández, 2016).

Length can be difficult to measure accurately because of the flexed posture of the newborn. The nurse places the newborn on a flat surface and extends the leg until the knee is flat against the surface. Placing the head against a perpendicular surface and extending the leg can assist with obtaining this measurement. In the term neonate, head-to-heel length ranges from 45 to 55 cm (17.7 to 21.7 in.).

Neurologic Assessment

The physical examination includes a neurologic assessment of newborn reflexes (see Table 22.4). This assessment provides useful information about the infant's nervous system and state of neurologic maturation. Many reflex behaviors (e.g., sucking, rooting) are important for proper development. Other reflexes such as gagging and sneezing act as primitive safety mechanisms. The assessment needs to be carried out as early as possible because abnormal signs in the early neonatal period can require further investigation before the newborn is discharged home.

GESTATIONAL AGE ASSESSMENT

Assessment of gestational age is important because perinatal morbidity and mortality rates are related to gestational age and birth weight. A

ESTIMATION OF GESTATIONAL AGE BY MATURITY RATING

NEUROMUSCULAR MATURITY

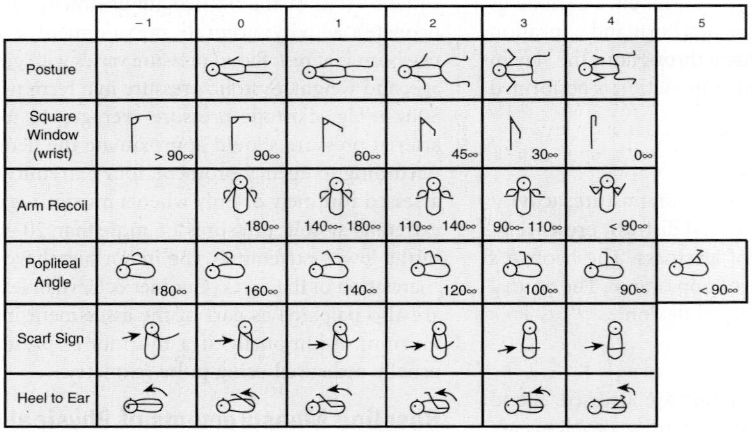

	−1	0	1	2	3	4	5
Posture							
Square Window (wrist)	> 90∞	90∞	60∞	45∞	30∞	0∞	
Arm Recoil		180∞	140∞–180∞	110∞–140∞	90∞–110∞	< 90∞	
Popliteal Angle	180∞	160∞	140∞	120∞	100∞	90∞	< 90∞
Scarf Sign							
Heel to Ear							

PHYSICAL MATURITY

Skin	sticky friable transparent	gelatinous red, translucent	smooth pink, visible veins	superficial peeling &/or rash, few veins	cracking pale areas rare veins	parchment deep cracking no vessels	leathery cracked wrinkled
Lanugo	none	sparse	abundant	thinning	bald areas	mostly bald	
Plantar Surface	heel-toe 40-50 mm: -1 <40 mm: -2	>50 mm no crease	faint red marks	anterior transverse crease only	creases ant. 2/3	creases over entire sole	
Breast	imperceptible	barely perceptible	flat areola no bud	stippled areola 1-2 mm bud	raised areola 3-4 mm bud	full areola 5-10 mm bud	
Eye/Ear	lids fused loosely: -1 tightly: -2	lids open pinna flat stays folded	slightly curved pinna; soft; slow recoil	well-curved pinna; soft but ready recoil	formed & firm instant recoil	thick cartilage ear stiff	
Genitals (male)	scrotum flat, smooth	scrotum empty faint rugae	testes in upper canal rare rugae	testes descending few rugae	testes down good rugae	testes pendulous deep rugae	
Genitals (female)	clitoris prominent labia flat	prominent clitoris small labia minora	prominent clitoris enlarging minora	majora & minora equally prominent	majora large minora small	majora cover clitoris & minora	

MATURITY RATING

score	weeks
-10	20
-5	22
0	24
5	26
10	28
15	30
20	32
25	34
30	36
35	38
40	40
45	42
50	44

A

FIG 23.2 Estimation of gestational age. **A,** New Ballard score for newborn maturity rating. Expanded scale includes extremely premature infants and has been refined to improve accuracy in more mature infants.

frequently used method of determining gestational age is the New Ballard Score, which can be used to measure gestational ages of infants as young as 20 weeks of gestation (see Fig. 23.2). It assesses six external physical and six neuromuscular signs. Each sign has a numeric score, and the cumulative score correlates with a maturity rating (gestational age). The examination of infants with a gestational age of 26 weeks or less should be performed at a postnatal age of less than 12 hours. For infants with a gestational age of at least 26 weeks, the examination can be performed up to 96 hours after birth. To ensure accuracy, experts recommend that the initial examination is performed within the first 48 hours of life. Neuromuscular adjustments after birth in extremely immature neonates require a follow-up examination to further validate neuromuscular criteria (Ballard, Khoury, Wedig, et al., 1991). Box 23.2 highlights specific maneuvers used in gestational age assessment.

CLASSIFICATION OF NEWBORNS BY GESTATIONAL AGE AND BIRTH WEIGHT

Classification of infants at birth by both birth weight and gestational age provides a more satisfactory method for predicting mortality risks

and providing guidelines for management of the neonate than estimating gestational age or birth weight alone. The infant's birth weight, length, and head circumference are plotted on standardized graphs that identify normal values for gestational age. A normal range of birth weights exists for each gestational week (see Fig. 23.2, *B*).

The infant whose weight is **appropriate for gestational age (AGA)** (between the 10th and 90th percentiles) can be presumed to have grown at a normal rate regardless of the length of gestation—preterm, term, or postterm. The infant who is **large for gestational age (LGA)** (more than the 90th percentile) can be presumed to have grown at an accelerated rate during fetal life; the **small for gestational age (SGA)** infant (less than the 10th percentile) can be presumed to have grown at a restricted rate during intrauterine life. When gestational age is determined according to the New Ballard Score, the newborn will fall into one of the following nine possible categories for birth weight and gestational age: AGA—term, preterm, postterm; SGA—term, preterm, postterm; or LGA—term, preterm, postterm. Birth weight influences mortality: the lower the birth weight, the higher the mortality. The same is true for gestational age: the lower the gestational age, the higher the mortality (Gardner & Hernández, 2016).

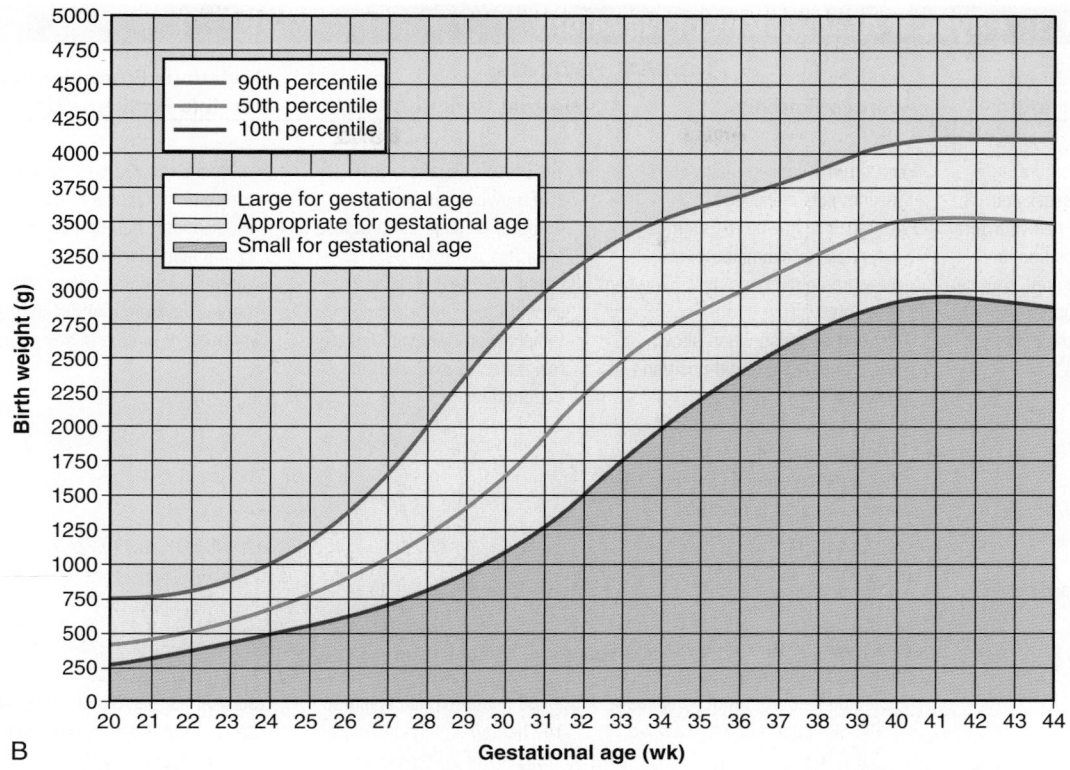

B

FIG 23.2, cont'd B, Intrauterine growth: birth weight percentiles based on live single births at gestational ages 20 to 44 weeks. (A, From Ballard, J., Khoury, J., Wedig, K., et al. [1991]. New Ballard score, expanded to include extremely premature infants. *Journal of Pediatrics, 119*[3], 417–423.)

BOX 23.2 Maneuvers Used in Assessing Gestational Age

Posture

With infant quiet and in supine position, observe degree of flexion in arms and legs. Muscle tone and degree of flexion increase with maturity. Full flexion of the arms and legs = score 4.*

Square Window

With thumb supporting back of arm below wrist, apply gentle pressure with index and third fingers on dorsum of hand without rotating infant's wrist. Measure angle between base of thumb and forearm. Full flexion (hand lies flat on ventral surface of forearm) = score 4.*

Arm Recoil

With infant supine, fully flex both forearms on upper arms and hold for 5 seconds; pull down on hands to extend fully, and rapidly release arms. Observe rapidity and intensity of recoil to a state of flexion. A brisk return to full flexion = score 4.*

Popliteal Angle

With infant supine and pelvis flat on a firm surface, flex lower leg on thigh and then flex thigh on abdomen. While holding knee with thumb and index finger, extend lower leg with index finger of other hand. Measure degree of angle behind knee (popliteal angle). An angle of less than 90 degrees = score 5.*

Scarf Sign

With infant supine, support head in midline with one hand; use other hand to pull infant's arm across the shoulder so that infant's hand touches shoulder. Determine location of elbow in relation to midline. Elbow does not reach midline = score 4.*

Heel to Ear

With infant supine and pelvis flat on a firm surface, pull foot as far as possible (without using force) up toward ear on same side. Measure distance of foot from ear and degree of knee flexion (same as popliteal angle). Knees flexed with a popliteal angle of less than 10 degrees = score 4.*

*See Fig. 23.2 for scale and interpretation of scores.
From Hockenberry, M.J., & Wilson, D. (2015). *Wong's nursing care of infants and children* (10th ed.). St. Louis, MO: Mosby.

Infants may also be classified in the following ways according to gestation (ACOG & Society for Maternal-Fetal Medicine, 2013):
- **Preterm,** *or premature*—born before 37 0/7 weeks of gestation, regardless of birth weight
- **Late preterm**—34 0/7 through 36 6/7 weeks
- **Early term**—37 0/7 through 38 6/7 weeks

- **Full term**—39 0/7 through 40 6/7 weeks
- **Late term**—41 0/7 through 41 6/7 weeks
- **Postterm**—42 0/7 weeks and beyond
- **Postmature**—born after completion of week 42 of gestation and showing the effects of progressive placental insufficiency

Text continued on p. 571

TABLE 23.3   Physical Assessment of Newborn

Area Assessed and Appraisal Procedure	NORMAL FINDINGS		Deviations From Normal Range: Possible Problems (Etiology)
	Average Findings	Normal Variations	
Posture Inspect newborn before disturbing for assessment. Refer to maternal chart for fetal presentation, position, and type of birth (vaginal, surgical), given that newborn readily assumes in utero position.	Vertex: arms, legs in moderate flexion; fists clenched Resistance to having extremities extended for examination or measurement, crying possible when attempted Cessation of crying when allowed to resume curled-up fetal position (lateral) Normal spontaneous movement bilaterally asynchronous (legs moving in bicycle fashion) but equal extension in all extremities	Frank breech: legs straighter and stiff, newborn assuming intrauterine position in repose for a few days Prenatal pressure on limb or shoulder possibly causing temporary facial asymmetry or resistance to extension of extremities	Hypotonia, relaxed posture while awake (preterm or hypoxia in utero, maternal medications, neuromuscular disorder such as spinal muscular atrophy) Hypertonia (chemical dependence, central nervous system [CNS] disorder) Limitation of motion in any extremity
Vital Signs Check heart rate and pulses: Thorax (chest) Inspection	Visible pulsations in left midclavicular line, fifth intercostal space		
Palpation	Apical pulse, fourth intercostal space 110–160 beats/min when awake	80–100 beats/min (sleeping) to 160 beats/min (crying); possibly irregular for brief periods, especially after crying	Tachycardia: persistent, ≥160 beats/min (respiratory distress syndrome [RDS]; pneumonia) Bradycardia: persistent, ≤80 beats/min (congenital heart block, maternal lupus)
Auscultation Apex: mitral valve Second interspace, left of sternum: pulmonic valve Second interspace, right of sternum: aortic valve Junction of xiphoid process and sternum: tricuspid valve	Quality: first sound (closure of mitral and tricuspid valves) and second sound (closure of aortic and pulmonic valves) sharp and clear	Murmur, especially over base or at left sternal border in interspace 3 or 4 (foramen ovale anatomically closing at approximately 1 year of age)	Murmur (possibly functional) Dysrhythmias: irregular rate Sounds: Distant (pneumopericardium) Poor quality Extra Heart on right side of chest (dextrocardia, often accompanied by reversal of intestines)
Peripheral pulses: femoral, brachial, popliteal, posterior tibial	Peripheral pulses equal and strong		Weak or absent peripheral pulses (decreased cardiac output, thrombus, possible coarctation of aorta if weak on left and strong on right) Bounding
Assess temperature: Axillary: method of choice Temporal and intraauricular thermometers not effective in measuring newborn temperature	Axillary: 37° C (98.6° F) Temperature stabilized by 8–10 hours of age	36.5°–37.5° C (97.7°–99.5° F) Heat loss: from evaporation, conduction, convection, radiation	Subnormal (preterm birth, infection, low environmental temperature, inadequate clothing, dehydration) Increased (infection, high environmental temperature, excessive clothing, proximity to heating unit or in direct sunshine, chemical dependence, diarrhea and dehydration) Temperature not stabilized by 6–8 hours after birth (if mother received magnesium sulfate, newborn less able to conserve heat by vasoconstriction; maternal analgesics possibly reducing thermal stability in newborn)

TABLE 23.3 Physical Assessment of Newborn—cont'd

Area Assessed and Appraisal Procedure	NORMAL FINDINGS		Deviations From Normal Range: Possible Problems (Etiology)
	Average Findings	Normal Variations	
Observe and monitor respiratory rate and effort:			
Observe respirations when infant is at rest. Observe respiratory effort. Count respirations for full minute. Auscultate breath sounds. Listen for sounds audible without stethoscope.	40/min Tendency to be shallow and irregular in rate, rhythm, and depth when infant is awake Crackles may be heard after birth No adventitious sounds audible on inspiration and expiration Breath sounds: bronchial; loud, clear	30–60/min Short periodic breathing episodes and no evidence of respiratory distress or apnea (>20 sec); periodic breathing First period (reactivity): 50–60/min Second period: 50–70/min Stabilization (1–2 days): 30–40/min Crackles (fine)	Apneic episodes: >20 sec (preterm infant: rapid warming or cooling of infant; CNS or blood glucose instability) Bradypnea: <30/min (maternal narcosis from analgesics or anesthetics, birth trauma) Tachypnea: >60/min (RDS, transient tachypnea of the newborn, congenital diaphragmatic hernia) Breath sounds: Crackles (coarse), rhonchi, wheezing Expiratory grunt (narrowing of bronchi) Distress evidenced by nasal flaring, grunting, retractions, labored breathing Stridor (upper airway occlusion)
Obtain blood pressure (BP) (usually not assessed in normal term infant).			
Check oscillometric monitor BP cuff: BP cuff width affects readings, use appropriate-size cuff and palpate brachial, popliteal, or posterior tibial pulse (depending on measurement site).	60–80/40–50 mm Hg (approximate ranges) At birth Systolic: 60–80 mm Hg Diastolic: 40–50 mm Hg At 2 weeks Systolic: 68–88 mm Hg Diastolic: 40–60 mm Hg	Variation with change in activity level: awake, crying, sleeping	Difference between upper and lower extremity pressures (coarctation of aorta) Hypotension (sepsis, hypovolemia) Hypertension (coarctation of aorta, renal involvement, thrombus)
Weight			
Put cloth or paper protective liner in place, and adjust scale to 0 g or pounds and ounces. Weigh at same time each day. Protect newborn from heat loss.	Female: 3400 g (7.5 lb) Male: 3500 g (7.7 lb) Regaining of birth weight within first 2 weeks	2500–4000 g (5.5-8.8 lb) Acceptable weight loss: 5% to 10% or less in first 3–5 days Second baby weighing more than first (on average)	Weight ≤2500 g (preterm, small for gestational age, rubella syndrome) Weight ≥4000 g (large for gestational age, maternal diabetes, heredity—normal for these parents) Weight loss more than 10% (growth failure, dehydration); assess breastfeeding success

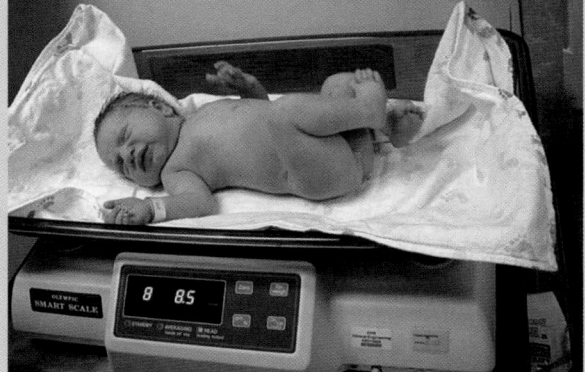

Weighing the infant. The nurse never leaves the infant alone on a scale. The scale is covered to protect against cross-infection. (Courtesy of Wendy and Marwood Larson-Harris, Roanoke, VA.)

Continued

TABLE 23.3   Physical Assessment of Newborn—cont'd

Area Assessed and Appraisal Procedure	NORMAL FINDINGS		Deviations From Normal Range: Possible Problems (Etiology)
	Average Findings	**Normal Variations**	
Length Measure length from top of head to heel; measuring is difficult in term infant because of presence of molding, incomplete extension of knees.	50 cm (19.7 in.)	45–55 cm (17.7–21.7 in.)	<45 cm (17.7 in.) or >55 cm (21.7 in.) (chromosomal abnormality, heredity—normal for these parents); some syndromes present shorter than average limb length (skeletal dysplasias, achondroplasia)

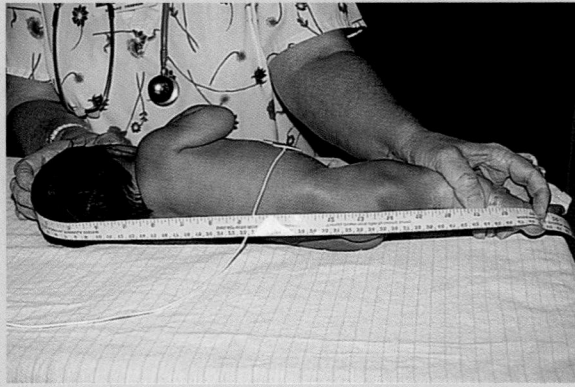

Measuring length crown to heel. To determine total length, include length of legs. If measurements are taken before the infant's initial bath, wear gloves. (Courtesy of Marjorie Pyle, RNC, Lifecircle, Costa Mesa, CA.)

Head Circumference Measure head at greatest diameter: occipitofrontal circumference May need to remeasure on second or third day after resolution of molding and caput succedaneum	33–35 cm (13–13.8 in.) Circumference of head and chest approximately the same for first 1 or 2 days after birth Chest rarely measured on routine basis	32–36.8 cm (12.6–14.5 in.)	Microcephaly, head ≤32 cm: (maternal rubella, toxoplasmosis, cytomegalovirus, fused cranial sutures [craniosynostosis]) Hydrocephaly: sutures widely separated, circumference ≥4 cm more than chest circumference (infection) Increased intracranial pressure (hemorrhage, space-occupying lesion)

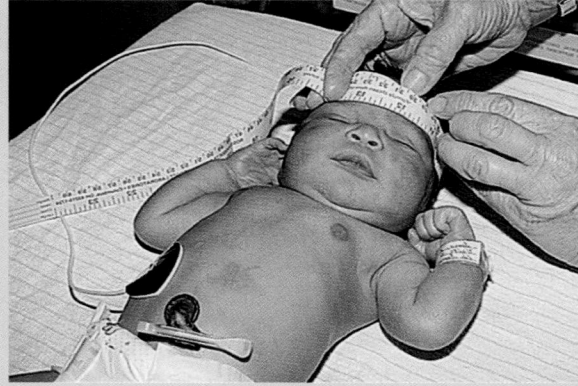

Measuring head circumference. (Courtesy of Marjorie Pyle, RNC, Lifecircle, Costa Mesa, CA.)

TABLE 23.3 Physical Assessment of Newborn—cont'd

Area Assessed and Appraisal Procedure	NORMAL FINDINGS		Deviations From Normal Range: Possible Problems (Etiology)
	Average Findings	Normal Variations	
Chest Circumference			
Measure at nipple line	2–3 cm (0.8–1.2 in.) less than head circumference; average 30–33 cm (11.8-13 in.)	≤30 cm	Prematurity

Measuring chest circumference. (Courtesy of Marjorie Pyle, RNC, Lifecircle, Costa Mesa, CA.)

Skin			
Check color: Inspect and palpate. Inspect semi-naked newborn in well-lighted, warm area without drafts; natural daylight best. Inspect newborn when quiet and alert.	Generally pink Varies with ethnic origin, skin pigmentation beginning to deepen right after birth in basal layer of epidermis Acrocyanosis common after birth	Mottling Harlequin sign Plethora Telangiectases ("stork bites" or infantile hemangiomas) (see Fig. 22.7, *A*) Erythema toxicum/neonatorum ("newborn rash") (see Fig. 22.7, *B*) Milia Petechiae over presenting part Ecchymoses from forceps in vertex births or over buttocks, genitalia, and legs in breech births	Dark red (preterm, polycythemia) Gray (hypotension, poor perfusion) Pallor (cardiovascular problem, CNS damage, blood dyscrasia, blood loss, twin-to-twin transfusion syndrome, infection) Cyanosis (hypothermia, infection, hypoglycemia, cardiopulmonary diseases, neurologic or respiratory malformations) Generalized petechiae (clotting factor deficiency, infection) Generalized ecchymoses (hemorrhagic disease)
Observe for jaundice.	None at birth	Physiologic jaundice in up to 60% of term infants in first week of life	Jaundice within first 24 hours (increased hemolysis, Rh isoimmunization, ABO incompatibility)
Observe for birthmarks or bruises: Inspect and palpate for location, size, distribution, characteristics, color, if obstructing airway or oral cavity.		Mongolian spot (see Fig. 22.6) in infants of African-American, Asian, Native American, and (rarely) Caucasian origin	Nevus flammeus: port-wine stain Infantile hemangioma

Continued

TABLE 23.3 Physical Assessment of Newborn—cont'd

Area Assessed and Appraisal Procedure	NORMAL FINDINGS		Deviations From Normal Range: Possible Problems (Etiology)
	Average Findings	Normal Variations	
Check skin condition: Inspect and palpate for intactness, smoothness, texture, edema, pressure points if ill or immobilized.	Edema confined to eyelid (result of eye prophylaxis) Opacity: few large blood vessels visible indistinctly over abdomen	Slightly thick; superficial cracking, peeling, especially of hands, feet No visible blood vessels, a few large vessels clearly visible over abdomen Some fingernail scratches	Edema on hands, feet; pitting over tibia; periorbital (overhydration; hydrops) Texture thin, smooth, or of medium thickness; rash or superficial peeling visible (preterm, postterm) Numerous vessels visible over abdomen (preterm) Texture thick, parchment-like; cracking, peeling (postterm) Skin tags, webbing Papules, pustules, vesicles, ulcers, maceration (impetigo, candidiasis, herpes, diaper rash)
Weigh infant routinely. Gently pinch skin between thumb and forefinger over abdomen and inner thigh to check for turgor.	Dehydration: loss of weight best indicator After pinch released, skin returns to original state immediately	Normal weight loss after birth: less than 10% by 3–5 days	Loose, wrinkled skin (prematurity, postmaturity, dehydration: fold of skin persisting after release of pinch) Tense, tight, shiny skin (edema, extreme cold, shock, infection)
Note presence of subcutaneous fat deposits (adipose pads) over cheeks, buttocks.		Variation in amount of subcutaneous fat	Lack of subcutaneous fat, prominence of clavicle or ribs (preterm, malnutrition)
Check for vernix caseosa: Observe color, amount, and odor before bath.	Whitish, cheesy, odorless	Usually more found in creases, folds	Absent or minimal (postmature) Abundant (preterm) Green color (possible in utero release of meconium or presence of bilirubin) Odor (possible intrauterine infection)
Assess lanugo: Inspect for this fine, downy hair, amount and distribution.	Over shoulders, pinnae of ears, forehead	Variation in amount	Absent (postmature) Abundant (preterm, especially if lanugo abundant, long, and thick over back)
Head			
Palpate skin.	(See "Skin")	Caput succedaneum, possibly showing some ecchymosis (see Fig. 22.12, *A*)	Cephalhematoma (see Fig. 22.12, *B*) Subgaleal hemorrhage (see Fig. 22.12 *C*)
Inspect shape, size.	Making up one-fourth of body length Molding (see Fig. 22.11)	Slight asymmetry from intrauterine position Lack of molding (preterm, breech presentation, cesarean birth)	Severe molding (birth trauma) Indentation (fracture from trauma)
Palpate, inspect, and note size and status of fontanels (open vs. closed).	Anterior fontanel 5-cm diamond, increasing as molding resolves Posterior fontanel triangle, smaller than anterior	Variation in fontanel size with degree of molding Difficulty in feeling fontanels possible because of molding	Fontanels: Full, bulging (tumor, hemorrhage, infection) Large, flat, soft (malnutrition, hydrocephaly, delayed bone age, hypothyroidism) Depressed (dehydration)
Palpate sutures.	Palpable and separated sutures	Possible overlap of sutures with molding	Sutures: Widely spaced (hydrocephaly) Premature closure (fused) (craniosynostosis)
Inspect pattern, distribution, amount of hair; feel texture.	Silky, single strands lying flat; growth pattern toward face and neck	Variation in amount	Fine, wooly (preterm) Unusual swirls, patterns, or hairline; or coarse, brittle (endocrine or genetic disorders)

TABLE 23.3 Physical Assessment of Newborn—cont'd

Area Assessed and Appraisal Procedure	NORMAL FINDINGS		Deviations From Normal Range: Possible Problems (Etiology)
	Average Findings	Normal Variations	
Eyes			
Check placement on face.	Eyes and space between eyes each one-third the distance from inner to outer canthus	Epicanthal folds: characteristic in some ethnicities	Epicanthal folds when present with other signs (chromosomal disorders such as Down, cri du chat syndromes)

Eyes. In pseudostrabismus, inner epicanthal folds cause the eyes to appear misaligned; however, corneal light reflexes are perfectly symmetric. Eyes are symmetric in size and shape and are well placed.

Area Assessed and Appraisal Procedure	Average Findings	Normal Variations	Deviations From Normal Range: Possible Problems (Etiology)
Check for symmetry in size, shape.	Symmetric in size, shape		
Check eyelids for size, movement, blink.	Blink reflex	Edema if eye prophylaxis drops or ointment instilled	
Assess for discharge.	None No tears	Some discharge if silver nitrate used Occasional presence of tears	Discharge: purulent (infection) Chemical conjunctivitis from eye medication is common—requires no treatment
Evaluate eyeballs for presence, size, shape.	Both present and of equal size, both round, firm	Subconjunctival hemorrhage	Agenesis or absence of one or both eyeballs Lens opacity or absence of red reflex (congenital cataracts, possibly from rubella, retinoblastoma [cat's-eye reflex]) Lesions: coloboma, absence of part of iris (congenital) Pink color of iris (albinism) Jaundiced sclera (hyperbilirubinemia)
Check pupils.	Present, equal in size, reactive to light		Pupils: unequal, constricted, dilated, fixed (intracranial pressure, medications, tumor)
Evaluate eyeball movement.	Random, jerky, uneven, focus possible briefly, following to midline	Transient strabismus or nystagmus until third or fourth month	Persistent strabismus Doll's eyes (increased intracranial pressure) Sunset (increased intracranial pressure)
Assess eyebrows: amount of hair, pattern.	Distinct (not connected in midline)		Connection in midline (Cornelia de Lange syndrome)
Nose			
Observe shape, placement, patency, configuration.	Midline Some mucus but no drainage Preferential nose breather Sneezing to clear nose	Slight deformity (flat or deviated to one side) from passage through birth canal	Copious drainage (rarely congenital syphilis); membranous or bony blockage with cyanosis at rest and return of pink color with crying (choanal atresia) Malformed (congenital syphilis, chromosomal disorder) Flaring of nares (respiratory distress)

Continued

TABLE 23.3   Physical Assessment of Newborn—cont'd

Area Assessed and Appraisal Procedure	NORMAL FINDINGS		Deviations From Normal Range: Possible Problems (Etiology)
	Average Findings	Normal Variations	
Ears			
Observe size, placement on head, amount of cartilage, open auditory canal.	Correct placement line drawn through inner and outer canthi of eyes reaching to top notch of ears (at junction with scalp) Well-formed, firm cartilage	Size: small, large, floppy Darwin tubercle (nodule on posterior helix)	Agenesis Lack of cartilage (preterm) Low placement (chromosomal disorder, intellectual disability, kidney disorder) Preauricular tag or sinus Size: possibly overly prominent or protruding ears

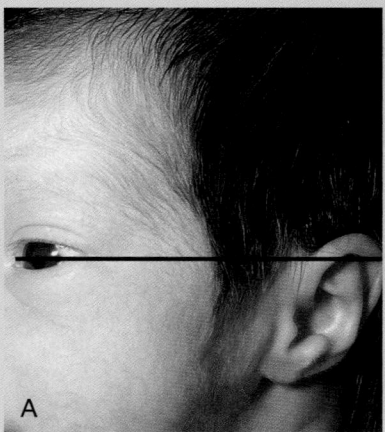 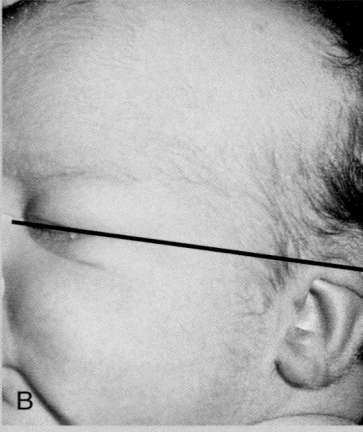 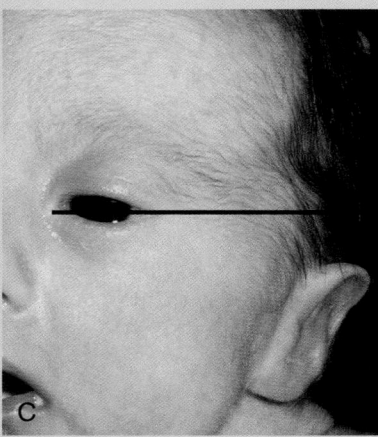

Placement of ears on the head in relation to a line drawn from the inner to the outer canthus of the eye. **A,** Normal position. **B,** Abnormally angled ear. **C,** True low-set ear. (Courtesy of Mead Johnson Nutritionals, Evansville, IN.)

Assess hearing.	Responds to voice and other sounds	State (e.g., alert, asleep) influencing response	Lack of response to loud noise should not imply deafness
Perform universal newborn hearing screening to identify deficits (see Fig. 23.11).	Both ears pass		One or both ears fail
Facies			
Observe overall appearance and symmetry of face.	Rounded and symmetric; influenced by birth type, molding, or both	Positional deformities	Usually accompanied by other features such as low-set ears, other structural disorders (hereditary, chromosomal aberration)
Mouth			
Inspect and palpate. Assess buccal mucosa: Dry or moist Pink Status intact Assess lips for color, configuration, movement.	Symmetry of lip movement	Transient circumoral cyanosis	Gross anomalies in placement, size, shape (cleft lip or palate [or both], gums) Cyanosis, circumoral pallor (respiratory distress, hypothermia) Asymmetry in movement of lips (seventh cranial nerve paralysis)
Check gums.	Pink gums	Inclusion cysts (Epstein pearls— Bohn nodules, whitish, hard nodules on gums or roof of mouth)	Teeth: predeciduous or deciduous (hereditary)
Assess tongue for color, mobility, movement, size.	Tongue not protruding, freely movable, symmetric in shape, movement Sucking pads inside cheeks	Short lingual frenulum (ankyloglossia)	Macroglossia (preterm, chromosomal disorder) Thrush: white plaques on cheeks or tongue that bleed if touched *(Candida albicans)*
Assess palate (soft, hard): Arch Uvula	Soft and hard palates intact Uvula in midline	Anatomic groove in palate to accommodate nipple, disappearance by 3–4 years of age Epstein pearls	Cleft hard or soft palate

TABLE 23.3 Physical Assessment of Newborn—cont'd

Area Assessed and Appraisal Procedure	NORMAL FINDINGS		Deviations From Normal Range: Possible Problems (Etiology)
	Average Findings	Normal Variations	
Assess chin.	Distinct chin		Micrognathia—recessed chin with prominent overbite (Pierre Robin or other syndrome)
Evaluate saliva for amount, character.	Mouth moist, pink		Excessive salivation and choking or turning blue (esophageal atresia, tracheoesophageal fistula)
Check reflexes: Rooting Sucking Extrusion	Reflexes present	Reflex response dependent on state of wakefulness and hunger	Absent (preterm)
Neck			
Inspect and palpate for movement, flexibility, masses, bruising.	Short, thick, surrounded by skin folds; no webbing		Webbing (Turner syndrome)
Check sternocleidomastoid muscles, movement and position of head.	Head held in midline (sternocleidomastoid muscles equal), no masses Freedom of movement from side to side and flexion and extension, no movement of chin past shoulder	Transient positional deformity apparent when newborn is at rest: passive movement of head possible	Restricted movement, holding of head at angle (torticollis [wryneck], opisthotonos) Absence of head control (preterm birth, Down syndrome, hypotonia [spinal muscular atrophy])
Assess trachea for position and thyroid gland.	Thyroid not palpable		Masses (enlarged thyroid) Distended veins (cardiopulmonary disorder) Skin tags
Chest			
Inspect and palpate shape.	Almost circular, barrel shaped	Tip of sternum possibly prominent	Bulging of chest, unequal movement (pneumothorax, pneumomediastinum) Malformation (funnel chest—pectus excavatum)
Observe respiratory movements.	Symmetric chest movements, chest and abdominal movements synchronized during respirations	Occasional retractions, especially when crying	Retractions with or without respiratory distress (preterm, RDS) Paradoxic breathing
Evaluate clavicles.	Clavicles intact		Fracture of clavicle (trauma); crepitus
Assess ribs.	Rib cage symmetric, intact; moves with respirations		Poor development of rib cage and musculature (preterm)
Assess nipples for size, placement, number.	Nipples prominent, well formed; symmetrically placed		Nipples Supernumerary, along nipple line Malpositioned or widely spaced
Check breast tissue.	Breast nodule: approximately 6 mm in term infant	Breast nodule: 3–10 mm Secretion of witch's milk	Lack of breast tissue (preterm)
Auscultate: Heart sounds and rate and breath sounds (see "Vital Signs")			Sounds: bowel sounds may be heard in diaphragmatic hernia (see "Abdomen")
Abdomen			
Inspect and palpate umbilical cord.	Two arteries, one vein Whitish gray Definite demarcation between cord and skin, no intestinal structures within cord Dry around base, drying Odorless Cord clamp in place for 24–48 hours	Reducible umbilical hernia	One artery (renal anomaly) Meconium stained (intrauterine distress) Bleeding or oozing around cord (hemorrhagic disease) Redness or drainage around cord (infection, possible persistence of urachus) Hernia: herniation of abdominal contents through cord opening (e.g., omphalocele); defect covered with thin, friable membrane, possibly extensive

Continued

TABLE 23.3   Physical Assessment of Newborn—cont'd

Area Assessed and Appraisal Procedure	NORMAL FINDINGS		Deviations From Normal Range: Possible Problems (Etiology)
	Average Findings	Normal Variations	
Inspect size of abdomen and palpate contour.	Rounded, prominent, dome shaped because abdominal musculature not fully developed Liver possibly palpable 1–2 cm (0.4–0.8 in.) below right costal margin No other masses palpable No distention Few visible veins on abdominal surface	Some diastasis recti (separation) of abdominal musculature	Gastroschisis: herniation of abdominal contents to the side or above the cord, contents not covered by membranous tissue and may include liver Distention at birth: ruptured viscus, genitourinary masses or malformations: hydronephrosis, teratomas, abdominal tumors Mild (overfeeding, high gastrointestinal tract obstruction) Marked (lower gastrointestinal tract obstruction, anorectal malformation, anal stenosis), often with bilious emesis Intermittent or transient (overfeeding) Partial intestinal obstruction (stenosis of bowel) Visible peristalsis (obstruction) Malrotation of bowel or adhesions Sepsis (infection)
Auscultate bowel sounds, and note number, amount, and character of stools.	Sounds present within minutes after birth in healthy term infant Meconium stool passing within 24–48 hours after birth		Scaphoid, with bowel sounds in chest and severe respiratory distress (congenital diaphragmatic hernia)
Assess color.		Linea nigra possibly apparent and caused by hormone influence during pregnancy	
Observe movement with respiration.	Respirations primarily diaphragmatic, abdominal and chest movement synchronous		Decreased or absent abdominal movement with breathing (phrenic nerve palsy, congenital diaphragmatic hernia)
Genitalia **Female (see Fig. 22.8, _A_)** Inspect and palpate:			
General appearance		Increased pigmentation caused by pregnancy hormones	Ambiguous genitalia—wide variation (small phallus not well distinguished from enlarged clitoris)
Clitoris	Usually edematous		Virilized female—extremely large clitoris (congenital adrenal hyperplasia)
Labia majora	Usually edematous, covering labia minora in term newborns	Edema and ecchymosis after breech birth Some vernix caseosa between labia possible	
Labia minora	Possible protrusion over labia majora		Enlarged clitoris with urinary meatus on tip, absent scrotum, micropenis, fused labia Stenosed meatus Labia majora widely separated and labia minora prominent (preterm)
Discharge	Smegma	Blood-tinged discharge from pseudomenstruation caused by pregnancy hormones	Fecal discharge (fistula)
Vagina	Open orifice Mucoid discharge Hymenal/vaginal tag		Absence of vaginal orifice
Urinary meatus	Beneath clitoris, difficult to see		Bladder exstrophy (bladder outside abdominal cavity and turned inside out)
Urination	Void within 24 hours; voiding 2–6 times per 24 hours for first 1–2 days; voiding 6–8 times per 24 hours by day 4 or 5	Rust-stained urine (uric acid crystals)	No void within first 24 hours (renal agenesis; Potter syndrome)

TABLE 23.3 Physical Assessment of Newborn—cont'd

Area Assessed and Appraisal Procedure	NORMAL FINDINGS		Deviations From Normal Range: Possible Problems (Etiology)
	Average Findings	Normal Variations	
Male (see Fig. 22.8, *B*)			
Inspect and palpate:			
General appearance		Increased size and pigmentation caused by pregnancy hormones (wide variation in size of genitalia)	Ambiguous genitalia Micropenis
Penis			
Urinary meatus appearance Prepuce (foreskin)—do not forcibly retract foreskin if uncircumcised	Foreskin covers glans (if uncircumcised), meatus at tip of penis Prepuce covering glans penis and not retractable	Prepuce removed if circumcised	Urinary meatus not on tip of glans penis (hypospadias, epispadias, foreskin may be retracted or absent) Round meatal opening
Scrotum: Rugae (wrinkles)	Large, edematous, pendulous in term infant; covered with rugae	Scrotal edema and ecchymosis if breech birth Hydrocele, small, noncommunicating	Scrotum smooth and testes undescended (preterm, cryptorchidism) Bifid scrotum Hydrocele Inguinal hernia
Testes	Palpable on each side	Bulge palpable in inguinal canal	Undescended (preterm)
Urination	Voiding within 24 hours, stream adequate; voiding 2–6 times per 24 hours for first 1–2 days; voiding 6–8 times per 24 hours by day 4 or 5	Rust-stained urine (uric acid crystals)	No void in first 24 hours (renal agenesis; Potter syndrome)
Check reflexes:			
Cremasteric	Testes retracted, especially when newborn is chilled		
Extremities			
Make a general check: Inspect and palpate Degree of flexion Range of motion Symmetry of motion Muscle tone	Assuming of position maintained in utero Attitude of general flexion Full range of motion, spontaneous movements	Transient positional deformities	Limited motion (malformations) Poor muscle tone (preterm, maternal medications, CNS anomalies)
Check arms and hands: Inspect and palpate: Color Intactness Appropriate placement	Longer than legs in newborn period Contours and movements symmetric	Slight tremors sometimes apparent Some acrocyanosis	Asymmetry of movement (fracture/crepitus, brachial nerve trauma, malformations) Asymmetry of contour (malformations, fracture) Amelia or phocomelia (teratogens) Palmar creases Simian line with short, incurved little fingers (Down syndrome)
Count number of fingers.	Five on each hand Fist often clenched with thumb under fingers		Webbing of fingers: syndactyly Absence or excess of fingers Strong, rigid flexion; persistent fists; positioning of fists in front of mouth constantly (CNS disorder) Yellowed nailbeds (meconium staining)
Evaluate joints: Shoulder Elbow Wrist Fingers	Full range of motion, symmetric contour		Increased tonicity, clonus, prolonged tremors (CNS disorder)
Check reflexes (see Table 22.4) Palmar grasp	Infant's fingers tightly flex around examiner's finger when palm is stimulated	May occur spontaneously when sucking	Weak or absent reflexes can indicate CNS depression
Plantar grasp	Infant's toes flex and curl around examiner's finger when sole of foot at base of toes is stimulated		

Continued

TABLE 23.3 Physical Assessment of Newborn—cont'd

Area Assessed and Appraisal Procedure	NORMAL FINDINGS		Deviations From Normal Range: Possible Problems (Etiology)
	Average Findings	Normal Variations	
Check legs and feet:			
Inspect and palpate	Appearance of bowing because lateral muscles more developed than medial muscles	Feet appearing to turn in but can be easily rotated externally, positional defects tending to correct while infant is crying	Amelia, phocomelia (chromosomal defect, teratogenic effect)
Color			Temperature of one leg differing from that of the other (circulatory deficiency, CNS disorder)
Intactness			
Length in relation to arms and body and to each other		Acrocyanosis	
Number of toes	Five on each foot		Webbing, syndactyly (chromosomal defect)
			Absence or excess of digits (chromosomal defect, familial trait)
Femur	Intact femur		Femoral fracture (difficult breech birth)
Head of femur as legs are flexed and abducted, placement in acetabulum (see Fig. 22.14)			Developmental dysplasia of the hip (DDH)
Major gluteal folds	Major gluteal folds even		Gluteal folds uneven: DDH
Soles of feet	Soles well lined (or wrinkled) over two-thirds of foot in term infants		Soles of feet:
			Few creases (preterm)
	Plantar fat pad giving flat-footed effect		Covered with creases (postmature)
			Congenital clubfoot
Evaluate joints:	Full range of motion, symmetric contour		Hypermobility of joints (Down syndrome)
Hip			
Knee			
Ankle			
Toes			
Check reflexes (see Table 22.4)			Asymmetric movement (trauma, CNS disorder)
Back			
Assess anatomy:		Temporary minor positional deformities, correction with passive manipulation	Limitation of movement (fusion or deformity of vertebra)
Inspect and palpate			
Spine	Spine straight and easily flexed		Spina bifida cystica (meningocele, myelomeningocele)
	Infant able to raise and support head momentarily when prone		Pigmented nevus with tuft of hair, location anywhere along the spine often associated with spina bifida occulta
Shoulders	Shoulders, scapulae, and iliac crests line up in same plane		
Scapulae			
Iliac crests			
Base of spine—pilonidal dimple or sinus			Sinus (opening to spinal cord)
Check reflexes (spinal related).			
Test trunk incurvation reflex.	Trunk flexed and pelvis swings to stimulated side	May not be apparent in first few days but is usually present in 5–6 days	If transverse lesion is present, no response below lesion; absence of response: CNS abnormality or CNS depression
Test magnet reflex.	Lower limbs extend as pressure applied to feet with legs in semiflexed position	Weak or exaggerated response with breech presentation	Absence: suggestive of CNS damage or malformation
Anus			
Inspect and palpate:	One anus with good sphincter tone	Passage of meconium within 48 hours of birth	Imperforate anus without fistula
Placement	Passage of meconium within 24 hours after birth		Rectal atresia and stenosis
Patency			Absence of anal opening; drainage of fecal material from vagina in female or urinary meatus in male (rectal fistula) or along perineal raphe (midline area between base of penis and anus)—anorectal malformation
Test for sphincter response (active "wink" reflex)	Anal "wink" present, anal opening patent		
Observe for the following:			
Abdominal distention			
Passage of meconium from anal opening			
Fecal drainage from perineum, penis, vagina			
Stools			
Observe frequency, color, consistency.	Meconium followed by transitional and soft yellow stool		No stool (obstruction)
			Frequent watery stools (infection, phototherapy)

Early Term Infant

"Early term" (37 0/7 through 38 6/7 weeks) is a recent addition to the categories describing newborns according to gestational age. In 2015, 24.99% of births were considered early term; this is a decline from 29.46% in 2007 and is likely related to increased awareness of the risks associated with birth prior to 39 weeks of gestation (Martin, Hamilton, Osterman et al., 2017). Compared with full-term infants, early-term infants are at increased risk for morbidity and mortality. Early-term birth is associated with higher risk for hypoglycemia, respiratory problems such as respiratory distress syndrome and transient tachypnea of the newborn (TTN), and a greater likelihood of NICU admission (Parikh, Reddy, Männistö, et al., 2014; Sengupta, Carrion, Shelton, et al., 2013). Currently there is a lack of evidence about the long-term effects of early term birth (Vohr, 2013). Nurses and other health care providers need to be aware of the vulnerability of this population of neonates and monitor them closely (Craighead, 2012).

Late-Preterm Infant

The rate of preterm birth in the United States was 9.63% in 2015. The majority of preterm births are considered late preterm, occurring from 34 0/7 through 36 6/7 weeks of gestation. These late-preterm infants account for 6.87% of all births (Martin et al., 2017). Elective vaginal and cesarean births before 39 weeks have contributed significantly to late-preterm birth rates in the United States.

Late preterm infants have been called "the great impostors" because they are often the size and weight of term infants. Despite their appearance as term infants, late preterm infants are at increased risk for respiratory distress, temperature instability, hypoglycemia, apnea, feeding difficulties, and hyperbilirubinemia. Nurses and health care providers must be cognizant of the risk factors for late preterm infants and be continually vigilant for the development of problems related to the infant's immaturity (Phillips, Goldstein, Hougland, et al., 2013). In an effort to identify these infants, a gestational age assessment should be performed on all newborns soon after birth. The late preterm infant's care is further addressed in Chapter 25.

Postterm or Postmature Infant

Infants born at 42 0/7 weeks of gestation or beyond are considered postterm, regardless of birth weight. Some infants are appropriate for gestational age, but show characteristics of progressive placental insufficiency. These infants are labeled as postmature and are likely to have little if any vernix caseosa, absence of lanugo, abundant scalp hair, and long fingernails. The skin is often cracked, parchment-like, and peeling. A common finding in postmature infants is a wasted physical appearance that reflects placental insufficiency. Depletion of subcutaneous fat gives them a thin, elongated appearance. The little vernix caseosa that remains in the skinfolds may be stained deep yellow or green, which is usually an indication of meconium in the amniotic fluid.

There is a significant increase in fetal and neonatal mortality in postmature infants compared with those born at term. They are especially prone to fetal distress associated with placental insufficiency, macrosomia, and meconium aspiration syndrome.

IMMEDIATE INTERVENTIONS

Changes can occur quickly in newborns immediately after birth. Assessment must be followed by prompt implementation of appropriate care.

Airway Maintenance

Generally the healthy term infant born vaginally has little difficulty clearing the airway. Most secretions are moved by gravity and brought

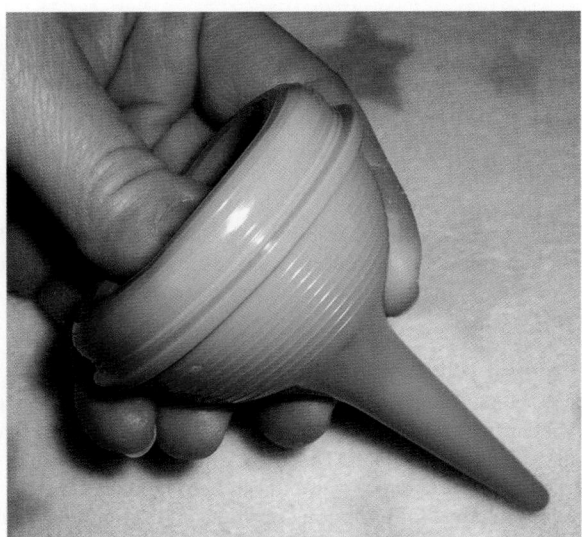

FIG 23.3 Bulb syringe. Bulb is compressed before inserting tip into mouth. (Courtesy of Cheryl Briggs, RNC, Annapolis, MD.)

by the cough reflex to the oropharynx to be drained or swallowed or wiped away. If the infant has excess mucus in the respiratory tract, the mouth and nasal passages can be gently suctioned with a bulb syringe (see Patient Teaching box: Suctioning with a Bulb Syringe and Fig. 23.3). Routine chest percussion and suctioning of healthy term or late-preterm infants are avoided; evidence is insufficient to support anything other than gentle nasopharyngeal and oropharyngeal suctioning to clear secretions. The nurse should auscultate the infant's chest with a stethoscope to assess for adventitious breath sounds or inspiratory stridor. Fine crackles may be auscultated for several hours after birth, especially in neonates born by cesarean. If the bulb syringe does not clear mucus interfering with respiratory effort, mechanical suction may be used.

If the newborn has an obstruction that is not cleared with suctioning, the neonatal or pediatric care provider should be notified. Further investigation may be needed to determine if a mechanical defect (e.g., tracheoesophageal fistula or choanal atresia [see Chapter 25]) is causing the obstruction.

Deeper suctioning may be needed to remove mucus from the newborn's nasopharynx or posterior oropharynx. However, this type

BOX 23.3 Signs of Potential Complications
Abnormal Newborn Breathing

- Bradypnea (<30 respirations/min)
- Tachypnea (>60 respirations/min)
- Abnormal breath sounds: coarse or fine crackles, wheezes
- Audible expiratory grunt
- Respiratory distress: nasal flaring, retractions, stridor, gasping, chin tug
- Seesaw or paradoxical respirations
- Skin color: central cyanosis, mottling
- Pulse oximetry value: <95%

of suctioning should be performed only after an assessment of the risks involved.

Maintaining an Adequate Oxygen Supply

Four conditions are essential for maintaining an adequate oxygen supply:
- A clear airway
- Effective establishment of respirations
- Adequate circulation, adequate perfusion, and effective cardiac function
- Adequate thermoregulation

Newborns who encounter respiratory problems are likely to exhibit signs and symptoms that indicate some degree of distress. Preterm infants are at greatest risk for respiratory distress (Box 23.3; see also Chapter 25).

Maintaining Body Temperature

Effective neonatal care includes maintenance of a neutral thermal environment (see Chapter 22). Cold stress increases the need for oxygen and can deplete glucose stores. The infant can react to exposure to cold by increasing the respiratory rate and can become cyanotic.

The ideal method for promoting warmth and maintaining neonatal body temperature is early skin-to-skin contact (SSC) with the mother (see Fig. 16.26). The unclothed infant is placed prone directly on the mother's chest; both mother and infant are then covered with a warm blanket, and a cap is placed on the infant's head. Early SSC has distinct short- and long-term benefits including temperature stabilization, reduced crying, improved breastfeeding initiation and duration, and enhanced maternal attachment (Moore, Anderson, Bergman, et al., 2012). Additionally, SSC and breastfeeding at birth can reduce the risk for postpartum hemorrhage (Saxton, Fahy, Rolfe, et al., 2015). Other interventions to promote warmth include drying and wrapping the newborn in warm blankets immediately after birth, keeping the head well covered, and keeping the ambient temperature of the nursery or mother's room at 22° to 26°C (72° to 78°F) (AAP & ACOG, 2012).

If the infant does not remain skin-to-skin with the mother during the first 1 to 2 hours after birth, the nurse places the thoroughly dried infant under a radiant warmer or in a warm incubator until the body temperature stabilizes. The infant's skin temperature is used as the point of control in a warmer with a servo-controlled mechanism. The control panel is usually maintained between 36° and 37°C (96.8° and 98.6°F). This setting should maintain the healthy term newborn's skin temperature at approximately 36.5° to 37°C (97.7° to 98.6°F). A thermistor probe (automatic sensor) is usually placed on the upper quadrant of the abdomen immediately below the right or left costal margin (never

over a bone). A reflector adhesive patch can be used over the probe to provide adequate warming. This probe is designed to detect minor temperature changes resulting from external environmental factors or neonatal factors (peripheral vasoconstriction, vasodilation, or increased metabolism) before a dramatic change in core body temperature develops. The servo-controller adjusts the temperature of the warmer to maintain the infant's skin temperature within the preset range. The sensor needs to be checked periodically to make sure it is securely attached to the infant's skin. The nurse assesses the axillary temperature of the newborn every hour (or more often as needed) until the newborn's temperature stabilizes. The length of time to stabilize and maintain body temperature varies; therefore, care should be individualized so that each newborn is allowed to achieve thermoregulation.

During all procedures, heat loss must be avoided or minimized for the newborn; therefore, examinations and activities are performed with the newborn under a radiant warmer. The initial bath is postponed until the newborn's skin temperature is stable and can adjust to heat loss from a bath. Even a healthy term infant can become hypothermic. Inadequate drying and wrapping immediately after birth, a cold birthing room, or birth in a car on the way to the birthing facility can cause the newborn's temperature to fall below the normal range (hypothermia). The hypothermic infant should be warmed gradually because rapid warming can cause apneic spells and acidosis.

Eye Prophylaxis

The American Academy of Pediatrics (AAP Committee on Infectious Diseases, 2015) and the US Preventive Services Task Force (USPSTF, 2011) recommend instilling a prophylactic agent in the eyes of all newborns to prevent ophthalmia neonatorum or neonatal conjunctivitis, which is an inflammation caused by sexually transmitted bacteria acquired during passage through the mother's birth canal. Because ascending infection can occur, eye prophylaxis is recommended for all neonates, including those born by cesarean. The Canadian Paediatric Society (CPS) no longer recommends routine eye prophylaxis for newborns, although some jurisdictions still require it (Moore, MacDonald, & CPS Infectious Diseases and Immunization Committee, 2015).

In the United States, erythromycin 0.5% ophthalmic ointment is the recommended prophylactic medication to prevent infection from *Neisseria gonorrhoeae* (see Medication Guide: Eye Prophylaxis: Erythromycin Ophthalmic Ointment, 0.5%). Without prompt treatment, this infection can lead to blindness (Fig. 23.4). Eye prophylaxis is usually administered within the first hour after birth. It may be delayed up to 2 hours until after the first breastfeeding so that eye contact and parent-infant attachment and bonding are facilitated. Eye prophylaxis for every newborn is mandated by law in the majority of US states without regard to the mode of birth. In some states, parents may refuse eye prophylaxis by signing a form that becomes part of the newborn record (AAP Committee on Infectious Diseases, 2015).

Topical antibiotics such as erythromycin are not effective in preventing chlamydial conjunctivitis. Oral erythromycin or azithromycin is used to treat chlamydial conjunctivitis (AAP Committee on Infectious Diseases, 2015).

Vitamin K Prophylaxis

At birth, neonates have low vitamin K levels related to limited transplacental transfer of vitamin K and the lack of normal intestinal flora necessary for vitamin K synthesis. The establishment of normal intestinal flora begins with early feedings, and by 7 days of age, healthy newborns are able to produce their own vitamin K.

💊 MEDICATION GUIDE

Eye Prophylaxis: Erythromycin Ophthalmic Ointment, 0.5%

Action
Bacteriostatic and bactericidal for *Neisseria gonorrhoeae*.

Indication
To prevent ophthalmia neonatorum in newborns of mothers who are infected with *Neisseria gonorrhoeae*. Eye prophylaxis for ophthalmia neonatorum is required by law in all US states and in some Canadian provinces.

Neonatal Dosage
Apply a 1- to 2-cm ribbon of ointment to the lower conjunctival sac of each eye.

Adverse Reactions
Can cause chemical conjunctivitis that lasts 24 to 48 hours; vision can be blurred temporarily

Nursing Considerations
Administer within 1 to 2 hours of birth. Wear gloves. Use a sterile cotton ball to wipe each eyelid prior to administering the ointment. Open the eyes by putting a thumb and finger at the corner of each lid and gently pressing on the periorbital ridges. Squeeze the tube, and spread the ointment from the inner canthus of the eye to the outer canthus. Do not touch the tube to the eye. Gently massage the closed eyelids to disperse the ointment. After 1 minute, excess ointment may be wiped away. Observe eyes for irritation. Explain the treatment to the parents.

Data from American Academy of Pediatrics Committee on Infectious Diseases. (2015). Section 5: Antimicrobial prophylaxis. In D.W. Kimberlin, M.T. Brady, M.A. Jackson, et al. (Eds.). *Red book: 2015 report of the Committee on Infectious Diseases* (30th ed.). Elk Grove Village, IL: Author.

💊 MEDICATION GUIDE

Vitamin K: Phytonadione (AquaMEPHYTON, Konakion)

Action
Provides vitamin K because the newborn does not have the intestinal flora to produce this vitamin for approximately 1 week after birth. It also promotes formation of clotting factors (II, VII, IX, X) in the liver.

Indication
To prevent vitamin K deficiency bleeding (hemorrhagic disease) of the newborn.

Neonatal Dosage
Administer a 0.5-mg (0.25-mL) dose to newborns weighing less than 1500 g and a 1-mg (0.5-mL) dose to newborns weighing more than 1500 g) intramuscularly soon after birth; the injection can be delayed until after initial breastfeeding.* Vitamin K is never administered by the intravenous (IV) route for the prevention of hemorrhagic disease of the newborn except in some cases of a preterm infant who has no muscle mass. In such instances, the medication is diluted and given over 10 to 15 minutes while closely monitoring the infant with a cardiorespiratory monitor. Rapid IV administration of vitamin K can cause cardiac arrest.

Adverse Reactions
Edema, erythema, and pain at the injection site occur rarely; hemolysis, jaundice, and hyperbilirubinemia have been reported, particularly in preterm infants.

Nursing Considerations
Follow the procedure for intramuscular injection (see Fig. 23.15). Encourage parents to use comfort measures for neonate such as skin-to-skin contact before, during, and after injection.

*Administration may be delayed for up to 6 hours in Canada.
Data from American Academy of Pediatrics Committee on Fetus and Newborn. (2003, reaffirmed 2014). Controversies concerning vitamin K and the newborn. *Pediatrics, 112*(1 pt 1), 191–192; McMillan, D., & Canadian Paediatric Society Fetus and Newborn Committee. (1997, reaffirmed 2016). *Position statement: Routine administration of vitamin K to newborns*. Retrieved from www.cps.ca/documents/position/administration-vitamin-K-newborns.

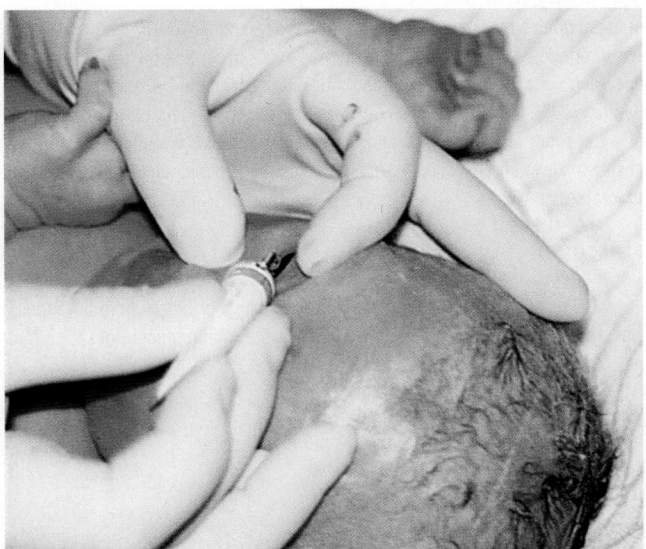

FIG 23.4 Instillation of medication into eye of newborn. Thumb and forefinger are used to open the eye; medication is placed in the lower conjunctiva from the inner to the outer canthus. (Courtesy of Marjorie Pyle, Lifecircle, Costa Mesa, CA.)

Administering vitamin K intramuscularly is routine in the newborn period in the United States and Canada. A single intramuscular (IM) injection of 0.5 to 1 mg of vitamin K is given soon after birth to prevent vitamin K deficiency bleeding (VKDB) or hemorrhagic disease of the newborn (see Medication Guide: Vitamin K: Phytonadione [AquaME-PHYTON, Konakion]). In the United States, administration may be delayed until after the first breastfeeding in the birthing room (AAP & ACOG, 2012). In Canada, newborns should receive the injection within 6 hours after birth when the infant is stable and there has been opportunity for interaction with the parents (McMillan & CPS Fetus and Newborn Committee, 2016).

Increasingly, parents are refusing vitamin K injections, related to concerns about synthetic or toxic ingredients, excessive dose, side effects, and neonatal pain with administration (Hamrick, Gable, Freeman et al., 2016). Neonatal or pediatric care providers should explain benefits versus risks related to vitamin K administration. Providers and nurses can encourage parents to use comfort measures such as SSC before, during, and after the injection.

Promoting Parent-Infant Interaction

Contemporary birthing practices are family-centered. Parents generally desire to share in the birth process and have early and continuous contact with their newborn. SSC with the mother beginning immediately after birth and breastfeeding within the first 1 to 2 hours after birth are important in promoting maternal-infant attachment. Early mother-infant contact produces physiologic benefits for the neonate and the mother. SSC promotes physiologic stability of the newborn. Maternal levels of oxytocin and prolactin rise with SSC and early breastfeeding. Rooming-in after birth until discharge from the birthing facility promotes parent-infant interaction.

CARE MANAGEMENT: FROM 2 HOURS AFTER BIRTH UNTIL DISCHARGE

Depending on the model of care delivery, the mother-baby nurse or newborn nursery nurse is responsible for ongoing assessment and care of the newborn. Astute assessment skills and appropriate interventions promote positive outcomes, especially for newborns who experience any problems before going home. Newborn care is family centered—the nurse provides education and support for the new parents throughout the stay in the birthing facility and assists them in preparing for discharge (see the Nursing Care Plan).

COMMON NEWBORN PROBLEMS

Birth Injuries

Birth trauma includes any physical injury sustained by a newborn during labor and birth. Although most injuries are minor and resolve during the neonatal period without treatment, some types of trauma require intervention; a few are serious enough to be fatal (see Chapter 25 for more information on birth injuries).

Retinal and subconjunctival hemorrhages result from rupture of capillaries caused by increased pressure during birth. These hemorrhages usually clear within 5 days and present no further problems. Parents need explanation and reassurance that these injuries are harmless.

◉ NURSING CARE PLAN

The Normal Newborn

Case Study

Timothy is 24 hours old. He was born at 38 weeks gestation to Nicole and Robert after an 18-hour labor. He weighs 6 lb 8 oz (2948 g) and is 18 inches (46 cm) long. Since birth, his temperature has been in the low normal range (97.7° F; 36.5° C);his respiratory rate ranges from 30 to 60 with lower rates when he is asleep and higher rates when he is awake and active. He has had several episodes of choking and spitting up mucus. He is restless, and circumoral cyanosis has been noted on several occasions. He breastfeeds well and sleeps after feedings.

Assessment

What are signs of ineffective airway clearance? What is the significance of spitting up mucus? How can the airway be cleared?

Defining Characteristics

Changes in respiratory rate and rhythm
Adventitious breath sounds, such as crackles, rhonchi, and wheezes or stridor
Cyanosis
Dyspnea
Excess mucus
Restlessness
Wide-eyed appearance

Nursing Diagnosis

Ineffective Airway Clearance related to excess mucus production or improper positioning

Expected Outcomes

Timothy's airway will be patent.
Adventitious breath sounds, such as crackles, rhonchi, and wheezes or stridor will be absent.
Breath sounds will be clear, and no respiratory distress will be evident.
Oxygen saturation level will be in normal range.

Nursing Interventions	Rationales
Teach parents that gagging, coughing, and sneezing are normal neonatal responses.	These responses are to assist neonate in clearing airways.

Nursing Interventions	Rationales
Teach parents feeding techniques that prevent overfeeding and distention of abdomen.	Proper feeding techniques will help prevent regurgitation and aspiration.
Position neonate on back when sleeping.	To prevent suffocation
Teach parents how to use bulb syringe and how to relieve airway obstruction.	To enable parents to clear airway safely
Suction mouth and nasopharynx with bulb syringe as needed; clean nares of crusted secretions.	To clear airway and prevent aspiration and airway obstruction

Case Study (Continued)

The nurse does a routine axillary check of Timothy's temperature and notes that he is wrapped in two blankets with a stocking cap in place. He is wearing a diaper, tee-shirt, and fleece pajamas that his grandmother gave him. His temperature is 38° C (100.4° F). His mother says that she is afraid that the air conditioning in the room is too cold for him, so she dressed him warmly and wrapped him in two blankets. His temperature has been within normal ranges at all previous temperature checks.

Assessment

What are signs that Timothy's temperature is not within normal limits? What factors can cause a temperature that is either above or below normal ranges? What teaching do parents need in relation to maintenance of a normal temperature?

Defining Characteristics

Clothing not appropriate for environmental temperature
Inactivity or vigorous activity
Dehydration
Exposure to cold or hot environment
Body temperature outside of desired range

Nursing Diagnosis

Risk for Imbalanced Body Temperature related to larger body surface relative to body mass

NURSING CARE PLAN

The Normal Newborn—cont'd

Expected Outcomes

Timothy's temperature remains in range of 36.5° to 37.5°C (97.7° to 99.5°F). Timothy will maintain a balanced intake and output within normal limits. Parents will verbalize understanding of infant thermoregulation.

Nursing Interventions	Rationales
Maintain neutral thermal environment.	To identify any changes in Timothy's temperature that may be related to other causes
Monitor Timothy's axillary temperature frequently.	To identify any changes promptly and to prevent hyperthermia or hypothermia and cold stress
Bathe Timothy efficiently when his temperature is stable, using warm water, drying carefully, and avoiding exposing him to drafts.	To avoid heat loss from evaporation and convection
Report any alterations in temperature findings promptly.	To assess for signs of infection or hypoglycemia and facilitate prompt treatment
Dress Timothy appropriately for the ambient temperature.	To maintain Timothy's temperature within normal limits
Teach Timothy's parents to dress him appropriately for the ambient temperature.	To enable parents to care for Timothy safely

Assessment

What are signs of infection? How can the parents and other caregivers reduce the risk for infection?

Defining Characteristics

Elevated or subnormal temperature
Listlessness; flaccid muscles
Poor feeding
Regurgitation
Increased heart rate
Increased respiratory rate

Nursing Diagnosis

Risk for Infection related to immature immunologic defenses and environmental exposure

Expected Outcomes

Tiimothy's vital signs will remain within normal range.
Timothy will be alert and active.
Timothy will remain free from signs of infection.
Timothy's umbilical cord will heal properly and remain free from infection.
Family members will demonstrate hand hygiene technique before handling Timothy.

Nursing Interventions	Rationales
Review maternal record for evidence of any risk factors.	To ascertain whether neonate is predisposed to infection
Monitor temperature and other vital signs.	To identify early evidence of possible infection, especially temperature instability
Have all care providers, including parents, perform proper hand hygiene before handling newborn.	To protect Timothy from infection
Provide prescribed eye prophylaxis.	To prevent infection

Nursing Interventions	Rationales
Keep genital area clean and dry using proper cleansing techniques.	To promote drying and to minimize chance of infection
Keep umbilical stump clean and dry.	To promote drying and to minimize chance of infection
If infant is circumcised, keep site clean and apply diaper loosely.	To prevent infection and to prevent trauma
Teach parents to keep Timothy away from crowds and environmental irritants.	To reduce potential sources of infection

Assessment

What are common conditions or hazards in which a neonate can suffer injury? What teaching do the parents require to provide a safe environment for Timothy?

Defining Characteristics

Unsafe sleep positioning
Extremes in environmental temperatures
Litter or liquid spills on floor
Parents' or caregivers' lack of information and experience in infant care
Unsafe handling of Timothy
Water at improper temperature for bathing Timothy
Improper or no use of car seat
Jaundice

Nursing Diagnosis

Risk for Injury related to environmental conditions interacting with Timothy's adaptive and defensive reserves

Expected Outcomes

Timothy will have his physical and safety needs met.
Family members will provide safe environment for Timothy after discharge.
Family members will recognize and report dangerous or potentially dangerous situations.
Timothy will remain free from injury.

Nursing Interventions	Rationales
Teach parents about safe sleep practices such as supine position, no cosleeping, crib safety.	To prevent suffocation (sudden infant death syndrome)
Monitor environment for hazards such as sharp objects (e.g., long fingernails, jewelry of caregiver)	To prevent injury
Handle neonate gently and support head, ensure use of car seat by parents, teach parents to avoid placing neonate on high surface unsupervised, and to supervise pet and sibling interactions.	To prevent injury
Assess neonate frequently for any evidence of jaundice, and teach parents to monitor for jaundice.	To identify rising bilirubin levels, treat promptly, and prevent complications such as acute bilirubin encephalopathy and kernicterus

Case Study (Continued)

Nicole and Robert have been home with Timothy for 2 weeks. At their 2-week well-baby check in the pediatrician's office, they meet with the pediatric nurse practitioner. While Nicole and Robert report that Timothy is healthy, gaining weight, and sleeping for longer periods at night, they are frustrated with the

Continued

NURSING CARE PLAN

The Normal Newborn—cont'd

frequency of Timothy's crying and have difficulty quieting him. They are having difficulty understanding why he is crying and what he wants or needs.

Assessment
What is the meaning of an infant cry? What are some reasons that infants cry? What are effective soothing techniques?

Defining Characteristics
Parents ask questions and seek understanding of reasons Timothy cries.
Parents report relief in learning that for an infant, crying is a means of communication.
Parents learn five new soothing techniques.
Frequency of episodes of infant crying are lessened.

Nursing Diagnosis
Readiness for Enhanced Family Coping related to anticipatory guidance regarding responses to Timothy's crying

Expected Outcomes
Parents will verbalize their understanding of methods of coping with Timothy's crying and describe increased success in interpreting his cries.

Parents will acknowledge their feelings of frustration.
Parents will seek additional support resources as necessary.

Nursing Interventions	Rationales
Alert parents to crying as Timothy's form of communication and that cries can be differentiated to indicate hunger, wetness, pain, and loneliness.	To provide reassurance that crying is not indicative of Timothy's rejection of parents and that parents will learn to interpret his different cries
Teach parents normal patterns of infant crying (e.g., Period of PURPLE Crying), and alert them to the danger of shaking a baby	To provide anticipatory guidance and to prevent injury to Timothy
Differentiate self-consoling behaviors from fussing or crying.	To give parents concrete examples of interventions
Discuss methods of consoling Timothy when he is crying, such as changing diapers, talking softly to him, holding his arms close to his body, swaddling, picking him up, rocking, using a pacifier, or feeding.	To provide anticipatory guidance and promote parental confidence

Erythema, ecchymoses, petechiae, abrasions, lacerations, or edema of the buttocks and extremities can be present. Localized discoloration can appear over the presenting part as a result of forceps- or vacuum-assisted birth. Ecchymoses and edema can appear anywhere on the body. Petechiae (pinpoint hemorrhagic areas) acquired during birth can extend over the upper trunk and face. These lesions are benign if they disappear within 2 or 3 days of birth and no new lesions appear. Ecchymoses and petechiae can be signs of a more serious disorder, such as thrombocytopenic purpura. To differentiate hemorrhagic areas from a skin rash or discolorations, the nurse attempts to blanch the skin by pressing with two fingers, lifting the fingers off the skin, and waiting for the return of blood. Petechiae and ecchymoses will not blanch because extravasated blood remains within the tissues, whereas skin rashes and discolorations will blanch.

Trauma to the presenting fetal part can occur during labor and birth. Caput succedaneum and cephalhematoma are discussed in Chapter 22 (see Fig. 22.12). Forceps injury and bruising from the vacuum cup occur at the site of application of the instruments. A forceps injury commonly produces a linear mark across both sides of the face in the shape of forceps blades. The affected areas are kept clean to minimize the risk for infection. These injuries usually resolve spontaneously within several days with no specific therapy.

Bruises over the face can be the result of face presentation (Fig. 23.5). In a breech presentation, bruising and swelling may be seen over the buttocks or genitalia (see Fig. 22.9). The skin over the entire head can be ecchymotic and covered with petechiae caused by a tight nuchal cord. If the hemorrhagic areas do not disappear spontaneously in 2 days or if the infant's condition changes, the primary health care provider is notified.

Accidental lacerations can be inflicted with a scalpel during a cesarean birth. These cuts can occur on any part of the body but are most often found on the scalp, buttocks, and thighs. They are usually superficial and need only to be kept clean. If skin closure is needed, an adhesive substance or strips may be applied. Sutures are rarely needed.

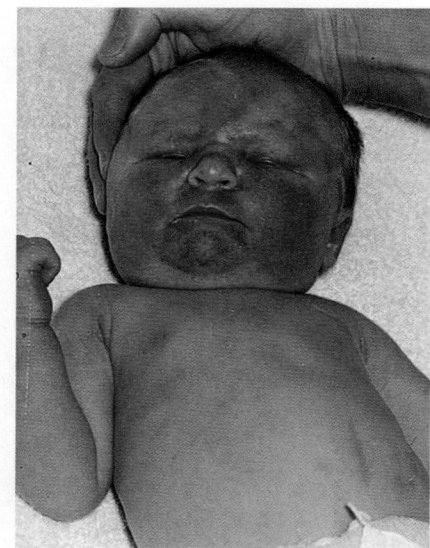

FIG 23.5 Marked bruising on the entire face of an infant born vaginally after face presentation. Less severe ecchymoses were present on the extremities. Phototherapy was required for treatment of jaundice resulting from the breakdown of accumulated blood. (From O'Doherty, N. [1986]. *Neonatology: Micro atlas of the newborn.* Nutley, NJ: Hoffman-La Roche.)

Physiologic Problems

Hyperbilirubinemia

Assessment and screening. A majority of newborn infants experience some level of jaundice due to hyperbilirubinemia during the first few days of life, usually occurring after 24 hours. In most cases, it is physiologic jaundice caused by increased levels of unconjugated bilirubin; physiologic jaundice is usually self-limiting and requires no treatment. It peaks at about 3 to 5 days in term infants and resolves after 1 to 2

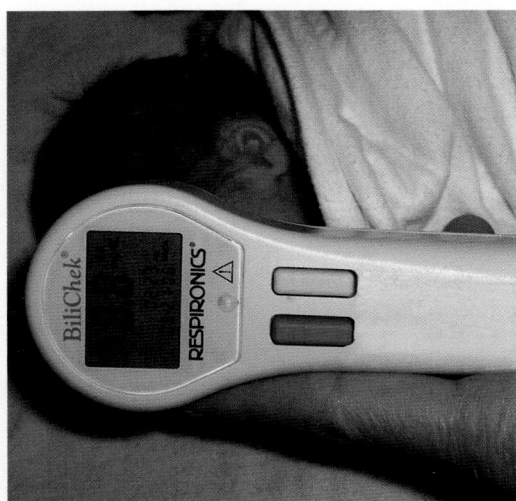

FIG 23.6 Transcutaneous monitoring of bilirubin with a transcutaneous bilirubinometry (TcB) monitor. (Courtesy of Cheryl Briggs, RNC, Annapolis, MD.)

weeks. In some cases, phototherapy is needed to lower bilirubin levels to within an acceptable range. Physiologic jaundice must be differentiated from pathologic jaundice, which is associated with higher levels of unconjugated bilirubin (see Chapter 22). Jaundice can also be associated with breastfeeding (see Chapters 22 and 24).

Every newborn should be assessed for jaundice at least every 8 to 12 hours; this can be easily done when vital signs are assessed. To differentiate cutaneous jaundice from normal skin color, the nurse applies pressure with a finger over a bony area (e.g., the nose, forehead, sternum) for several seconds to empty all the capillaries in that spot, then releases the pressure by lifting the finger. If jaundice is present, the blanched area will appear yellowish before the capillaries refill. The conjunctival sacs and buccal mucosa also are assessed, especially in darker-skinned infants. Assessing for jaundice in natural light is recommended because artificial lighting and reflection from walls can distort the actual skin color.

Visual assessment of jaundice alone does not provide an accurate assessment of hyperbilirubinemia, especially in dark-skinned newborns (Burgos, Flaherman, & Newman, 2012). A more accurate noninvasive assessment of hyperbilirubinemia is accomplished using transcutaneous bilirubinometry [TcB] (Fig. 23.6). TcB levels correlate well with serum bilirubin levels in full-term infants (Dijk & Hulzebos, 2012). Recent developments in this technology have increased the accuracy of TcB measurement in dark-skinned neonates (Kamath-Rayne, Thilo, Deacon, et al., 2016). TcB monitors can be used to screen for clinically significant jaundice and decrease the need for serum bilirubin measurements. However, TcB measurement is not considered reliable at levels greater than 15 mg/dL, and total serum bilirubin (TSB) measurement is needed. TcB measurement is not reliable during phototherapy (Kamath-Rayne et al., 2016).

If an infant appears jaundiced in the first 24 hours of life, a TcB or TSB level should be measured and results interpreted based on the newborn's age in hours according to the hour-specific nomogram for infants born at 35 weeks of gestation or later (AAP Subcommittee on Hyperbilirubinemia, 2004) (Fig. 23.7). Repeat testing is based on the risk level (low, intermediate, or high), the age of the neonate, and the progression of jaundice.

In an effort to prevent severe hyperbilirubinemia and the neurologic complications of acute bilirubin encephalopathy and kernicterus, the AAP and the CPS recommend routine screening of all newborns before hospital discharge using TcB or TSB measurement (AAP Subcommittee on Hyperbilirubinemia, 2004; Barrington, Sankaran, & CPS Fetus and Newborn Committee, 2011). In general, if the TcB level is greater than 12 mg/dL, a serum bilirubin check is done and levels are interpreted according to the hour-specific nomogram (AAP Subcommittee on Hyperbilirubinemia, 2004). A tool available at www.bilitool.org facilitates calculating the risk for neonatal hyperbilirubinemia.

Infants in the low-risk category are less likely to develop hyperbilirubinemia. However, the AAP warns that all infants should be considered as being at potential risk for hyperbilirubinemia, even if they were identified as being in the low-risk category. This means that all newborns should be followed after discharge from the birthing facility for the development of unexpected jaundice and that parents should be given printed and oral information about newborn jaundice (Bromiker, Bin-Nun, Schimmel, et al., 2012).

Adequate feeding is essential in preventing hyperbilirubinemia. Newborns should breastfeed early (within 1 to 2 hours after birth) and often (at least 8 to 12 times/24 hours) (AAP Section on Breastfeeding, 2012; AAP Subcommittee on Hyperbilirubinemia, 2004). Colostrum acts as a laxative to promote stooling, which helps rid the body of bilirubin. Formula-fed infants should be fed after birth when their physiologic status has stabilized and thereafter at least every 3 to 4 hours.

Newborns should be assessed for risk factors for severe hyperbilirubinemia. The most common risk factors include gestational age less than 38 weeks, exclusive breastfeeding (especially in association with breastfeeding difficulties and excessive weight loss), significant jaundice in a sibling, isoimmune or other hemolytic disease (e.g., glucose-6-phosphate dehydrogenase [G6PD] deficiency), cephalhematoma, significant bruising, and East Indian race (AAP Subcommittee on Hyperbilirubinemia, 2004).

Close follow-up of infants at risk for hyperbilirubinemia is essential; parents should be educated and encouraged to follow postdischarge recommendations (AAP Subcommittee on Hyperbilirubinemia, 2004). Follow-up should occur 48 to 72 hours after discharge from the birthing facility or sooner based on the length of stay and presence of risk factors for hyperbilirubinemia (Burgos et al., 2012).

Therapy for hyperbilirubinemia. The decision to treat an infant for hyperbilirubinemia is based on total serum bilirubin levels, the infant's gestational age, and the presence of risk factors. Using a nomogram that plots bilirubin levels according to gestational age, the provider determines the appropriate management plan (Maisels, 2010). The AAP provides guidelines that provide direction for health care providers in determining the need for phototherapy or exchange transfusion (AAP Committee on Hyperbilirubinemia, 2004).

The goal of treatment of hyperbilirubinemia is to reduce the newborn's serum levels of unconjugated bilirubin. There are two ways to reduce unconjugated bilirubin levels: phototherapy and exchange blood transfusion.

Phototherapy. The most common treatment for hyperbilirubinemia is phototherapy. Its purpose is to reduce the level of circulating unconjugated bilirubin or keep it from increasing. Phototherapy uses light energy to change the shape and structure of unconjugated bilirubin, converting it into a conjugated form that can be excreted through urine and stool. Phototherapy is delivered through lamp, blanket, pad, or cover-body devices. The severity of the newborn's hyperbilirubinemia determines the type of phototherapy device and strength of light, duration of treatment, and venue (hospital or home). The neonate's response to phototherapy depends on the bilirubin level, the effectiveness of the phototherapy device, and the infant's ability to excrete the bilirubin (Bhutani & Committee on Fetus and Newborn, 2011).

The dose and effectiveness of phototherapy are affected by the source of light. Phototherapy units vary in the spectrum of light they deliver

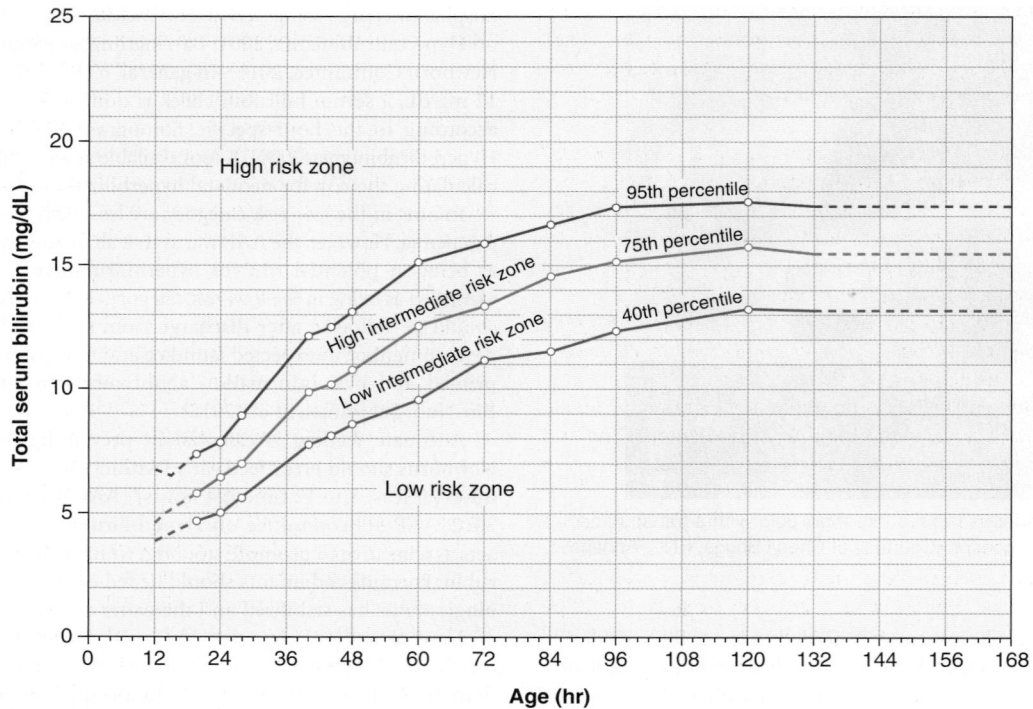

FIG 23.7 Nomogram for designation of risk in 2840 well newborns at 36 or more weeks of gestational age with birth weight of 2000 g or more or 35 or more weeks of gestational age with birth weight of 2500 g or more based on the hour-specific serum bilirubin values. (This nomogram should not be used to represent the natural history of neonatal hyperbilirubinemia.) (From Bhutani, V., Johnson, L., & Sivieri, E.M. [1999]. Predictive ability of a predischarge hour-specific serum bilirubin for subsequent significant hyperbilirubinemia in healthy term and near-term newborns. *Pediatrics, 103*[1], 6–14.)

and in the filters used. The most effective therapy is achieved with special blue fluorescent tubes or a specially designed light-emitting diode (LED). Phototherapy lights do not emit significant ultraviolet radiation; the small amount that is emitted does not cause erythema. Most of the ultraviolet light is absorbed by the glass wall of the fluorescent tube and by the plastic cover of the light (Bhutani & Committee on Fetus and Newborn, 2011; Kamath-Rayne et al., 2016). Phototherapy is usually effective in treating hyperbilirubinemia that has not reached levels associated with acute bilirubin encephalopathy or kernicterus.

The effectiveness of phototherapy is related to the distance between the light and the neonate and to the surface area of skin that is exposed. To maximize skin exposure, multiple devices may be used simultaneously. For example, a neonate may be placed under a phototherapy lamp while also lying on a fiberoptic pad or LED mattress (Bhutani & Committee on Fetus and Newborn, 2011).

During phototherapy using a lamp, the neonate, wearing only a diaper, is placed under a bank of lights approximately 45 to 50 cm from the light source. Phototherapy can be used for the infant in an incubator (Fig. 23.8) or in an open crib. The distance varies according to unit protocol and type of light used. The irradiance of the light is monitored routinely with a radiometer, with measurements at several sites over the neonate's body surface during treatment to ensure efficacy of therapy (Bhutani & Committee on Fetus and Newborn, 2011).

If phototherapy is effective, the bilirubin level should begin to decrease within 4 to 6 hours after phototherapy is initiated and within 24 hours should decrease by 30% to 40% (Kamath-Rayne et al., 2016). Phototherapy is used until the infant's serum bilirubin level decreases to within an acceptable range. The decision to discontinue therapy is based on the observation of a definite downward trend in the bilirubin values.

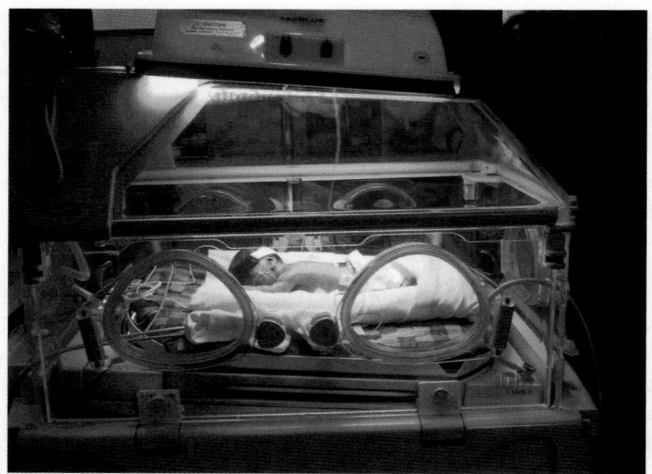

FIG 23.8 Infant under phototherapy lights while in an incubator. (Courtesy of Cheryl Briggs, RNC, Annapolis, MD.)

⚡ SAFETY ALERT

When a phototherapy lamp is used, the infant's eyes must be protected by an opaque mask to prevent retinal damage. The eye shield should cover the eyes completely but not occlude the nares. Before the mask is applied, the infant's eyes should be closed gently to prevent excoriation of the corneas. The mask should be removed periodically and during infant feedings so that the eyes can be assessed and cleansed with water and the parents can have visual contact with the infant (Kamath-Rayne et al., 2016).

Phototherapy can cause changes in the infant's temperature, depending partially on the bed used—bassinet, incubator, or radiant warmer. When under a phototherapy light, infants are usually clothed only with a diaper. The infant's temperature should be closely monitored for hypothermia and hyperthermia.

Phototherapy lights, especially if the newborn is low birth weight or under a radiant warmer, can increase the rate of insensible water loss, which contributes to fluid loss and dehydration. Therefore, the infant must be adequately hydrated. Hydration maintenance in the healthy newborn is accomplished through breastfeeding, pasteurized donor milk, or infant formula. Feedings of glucose water or plain water have no advantage or benefit because these liquids do not promote excretion of bilirubin in the stools and can actually perpetuate enterohepatic circulation, thus delaying bilirubin excretion.

The nurse closely monitors urinary output as an indicator of hydration status while the infant is receiving phototherapy. Urine output can be decreased or unaltered; the urine can have a dark gold or brown appearance.

The number and consistency of stools are monitored. Bilirubin is excreted primarily through the stool, so it is important that the infant is having bowel movements. Bilirubin breakdown increases gastric motility, which can result in loose stools that can cause skin excoriation and breakdown. The infant's buttocks must be cleaned after each stool to help maintain skin integrity.

> ⚡ **SAFETY ALERT**
>
> No ointments, creams, or lotions should be applied to the newborn's skin during phototherapy because they can absorb heat and cause burns.

Infants under phototherapy lights need to be repositioned at least every 2 to 3 hours to maximize skin exposure. Transient skin rashes or tanning of the skin can occur during phototherapy. In rare instances, there can be bullous eruptions or the development of bronze baby syndrome in which the skin appears grayish brown (Kamath-Rayne et al., 2016). There is a lack of evidence regarding long-term effects of phototherapy (Bhutani & Committee on Fetus and Newborn, 2011).

In addition to phototherapy lights, other systems are used for phototherapy. A bassinet system provides special blue light above and beneath the infant. Another phototherapy device is a fiberoptic blanket that is connected to a light source. The blanket is flexible and can be placed around the infant's torso or underneath the infant in the bassinet. There are also bilirubin beds with LED lights in a pad that covers the surface of the bassinet (Fig. 23.9). The LEDs do not produce heat and

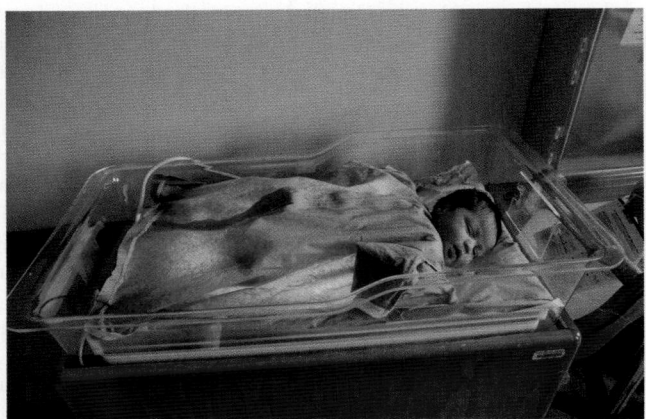

FIG 23.9 Infant receiving phototherapy using a bilirubin bed. (Courtesy of Cheryl Briggs, RNC, Annapolis, MD.)

can be used with radiant warmers. These devices are usually less effective when used alone as compared with conventional phototherapy lights. They can be very useful in combination with overhead phototherapy lights. In certain instances, the infant's bilirubin levels increase rapidly and intensive phototherapy is required; this situation involves the use of a combination of conventional lights and fiberoptic blankets to maximize bilirubin reduction. Although fiberoptic lights do not produce heat as do conventional lights, staff should ensure that a covering pad is placed between the infant's skin and the fiberoptic device to prevent skin burns, especially in preterm infants. The newborn can remain in the mother's room in an open crib or in her arms during treatment. The use of eye patches depends on whether the devices are used alone or in combination with phototherapy lights.

The use of home phototherapy should be reserved for healthy term infants with bilirubin levels in the "optional phototherapy" range according to the nomogram. The concern is that home phototherapy units do not provide the same level of irradiance or body surface coverage as phototherapy devices used in the hospital (AAP Committee on Hyperbilirubinemia, 2004).

Phototherapy treatment is associated with concerns related to psychobehavioral issues, including parent-infant separation, potential social isolation, decreased sensorineural stimulation, altered biologic rhythms, altered feeding patterns, and activity changes. Parental anxiety can be greatly increased, particularly at the sight of the newborn with eyes covered and under special lights. The interruption of breastfeeding for phototherapy is a potential deterrent to successful maternal-infant attachment and interaction. Although there are conflicting opinions about continuous versus intermittent phototherapy, for most infants phototherapy can safely be interrupted for feedings, parental interaction, assessments, and laboratory draws (Kamath-Rayne et al., 2016).

Close follow-up is needed for infants who have been treated for hyperbilirubinemia. Repeat testing of serum bilirubin levels and follow-up visits with the pediatric health care provider are expected. In some cases, a nurse may conduct a home visit to evaluate the infant's condition, draw blood for bilirubin testing, and monitor the mother's health.

Exchange transfusion. When phototherapy is not effective in reducing serum bilirubin levels or with severe hyperbilirubinemia such as in hemolytic disease, or for treatment of acute bilirubin encephalopathy, exchange transfusion may be needed. This procedure is done in an intensive care setting and can reduce bilirubin levels by 45% to 85%. A portion of the infant's blood is replaced with donor blood (Kamath-Rayne et al., 2016) (see Chapter 25).

Hypoglycemia

Hypoglycemia in a term infant during the early newborn period is defined as a blood glucose concentration inadequate to support neurologic, organ, and tissue function; however, there is a lack of consensus among experts regarding the precise level at which this concentration occurs. Similarly, there is no consensus about when to screen for hypoglycemia or the level at which treatment should be instituted (Adamkin & Committee on Fetus and Newborn, 2011). The lower limit for normal plasma glucose levels during the first 72 hours after birth is often cited as 40 to 45 mg/dL. There is concern about neurologic injury as a result of severe or prolonged hypoglycemia, especially in combination with ischemia (Rozance, McGowan, Price-Douglas, et al., 2016).

At birth, the maternal source of glucose is eliminated when the umbilical cord is clamped. Most healthy term newborns experience a transient decrease in glucose levels to as low as 30 mg/dL during the first 1 to 2 hours after birth, with a subsequent mobilization of free fatty acids and ketones to help maintain adequate glucose levels (Blackburn, 2013). Early and regular feeding promotes normoglycemia. There is no need to routinely assess glucose levels of healthy term infants.

Infants considered to be at risk for hypoglycemia include those who are preterm or late preterm; SGA or LGA; low birth weight; infants of mothers with diabetes; and infants who experienced perinatal stress such as asphyxia, cold stress, or respiratory distress (Wight, Marinelli, & Academy of Breastfeeding Medicine, 2014).

Screening and treatment protocols vary across institutions. Glucose levels should be measured in all newborns with risk factors for hypoglycemia and in any newborn with clinical manifestations of hypoglycemia. The frequency of glucose testing is determined by the risk factors for each individual newborn. All neonates at-risk for hypoglycemia should be fed within the first hour, with glucose testing done 30 minutes after feeding. For at least the first 24 hours after birth, late-preterm and SGA neonates should be fed every 2 to 3 hours, with glucose levels measured before each feeding. LGA infants and infants of mothers with diabetes should have glucose screening before feedings for at least the first 12 hours after birth; further testing is done if glucose levels are less than 45 mg/dL (Adamkin & Committee on Fetus and Newborn, 2011). Early and frequent breastfeeding and SSC with the mother for as long as possible after birth promote thermoregulation and stabilization of glucose levels (Wight et al., 2014).

Nurses should observe all newborns for signs of hypoglycemia. Glucose testing should be done on any infant with clinical signs of hypoglycemia. These signs can be transient or recurrent and include jitteriness, lethargy, poor feeding, abnormal cry, hypotonia, temperature instability (hypothermia), respiratory distress, apnea, and seizures (Rozance et al., 2016). It is important to remember that hypoglycemia can be present in the absence of clinical manifestations.

Bedside glucose monitoring is performed using reagent test strips with or without a reflectance colorimeter. Because of variations in devices and operator techniques, it is recommended that any level less than 45 mg/dL should be followed up with a stat serum glucose level prior to initiating treatment, especially in asymptomatic newborns. However, treatment of hypoglycemia should not be delayed while awaiting serum glucose results (Rozance et al., 2016; Wight et al., 2014).

! NURSING ALERT

A heel warmer should be applied prior to every glucose assessment via heelstick. If the extremity is cool, the test result can be falsely low.

Protocols for treatment of hypoglycemia vary. The at-risk asymptomatic neonate with hypoglycemia should be fed, either by breastfeeding or feeding 1 to 5 mL/kg of expressed colostrum, pasteurized donor human milk, or infant formula (Wight et al., 2014). For exclusively breastfed infants, when expressed colostrum or donor milk is not available, some hospitals use dextrose gel (40%) administered buccally or sublingually (Bennett, Fagan, Chaharbakhshi, et al., 2016; Harris, Weston, Signal, et al., 2013–2014). Glucose testing should be repeated before subsequent feedings until the glucose level is stable at greater than 40 mg/dL. If levels remain low despite feeding, IV dextrose is warranted. In such infants, treatment should be aimed at maintaining the blood glucose levels greater than 45 mg/dL. For the neonate with symptomatic hypoglycemia, regardless of cause or age, the health care provider is notified; IV dextrose infusion is recommended. For any infant with hypoglycemia, follow-up glucose testing at specified intervals is needed until glucose levels are stable (Adamkin & Committee on Fetus and Newborn, 2011; Wight et al., 2014).

Hypocalcemia

Hypocalcemia is defined as serum calcium levels of less than 7 mg/dL (Nyp, Brunkhorst, Reavey, et al., 2016). Hypocalcemia is common in critically ill neonates but also can occur in infants of mothers with diabetes or in those who had perinatal asphyxia or trauma and in low–birth-weight and preterm infants. Infants born to mothers treated with anticonvulsants during pregnancy also are at risk (Halbardier, 2015). Early-onset hypocalcemia occurs within the first 24 to 72 hours after birth and is usually asymptomatic; jitteriness or twitching can occur. Late-onset hypocalcemia is more severe and usually presents between 5 and 10 days after birth with jitteriness, seizures, or apnea. Jitteriness can be a sign of hypoglycemia and hypocalcemia; therefore, if treatment for hypoglycemia is ineffective, hypocalcemia should be considered.

In most instances, early-onset hypocalcemia is self-limiting and resolves within 1 to 3 days. Treatment usually includes early feeding of an appropriate source of calcium such as fortified human milk or preterm infant formula. Treatment of late-onset hypocalcemia varies according to the underlying cause; immediate treatment with intravenous calcium is needed (Nyp et al., 2016).

LABORATORY AND DIAGNOSTIC TESTS

Because newborns experience many transitional events in the first 28 days of life, blood samples are often collected to determine adequate physiologic adaptation and to identify disorders that can adversely affect the child's life beyond the neonatal period. Blood samples for most laboratory tests can be obtained from the neonate with a heel puncture, also known as a *heelstick*. Tests commonly performed other than blood glucose and bilirubin levels include newborn screening tests and serum drug levels. Standard laboratory values for a term newborn are listed in Table 23.4.

Universal Newborn Screening

Mandated by US law, newborn screening is an important public health program aimed at early detection of genetic diseases that result in severe health problems if not treated early. The universal screening program is state-based and involves a variety of components including education, screening, follow-up, treatment, and a system for monitoring and evaluation. The US Department of Health and Human Services (USDHHS) Committee on Heritable Disorders in Newborns and Children (2015) recommends screening for 34 core disorders and 26 secondary disorders. The core disorders include hemoglobinopathies (e.g., sickle cell disease), inborn errors of metabolism (e.g., phenylketonuria [PKU], galactosemia), severe combined immunodeficiency, hearing loss, and critical congenital heart disease. The majority of disorders included in the screening are not symptomatic at birth. Individual states select additional disorders to include in the screening.

In Canada, universal newborn screening policies and practices are varied. Individual provinces in Canada determine the disorders included in newborn screening; however, all provinces screen for PKU and congenital hypothyroidism (Canadian Organization for Rare Disorders, 2015).

Capillary blood samples are obtained using a heelstick; blood is collected on a special filter paper and sent to a designated state laboratory for analysis (Fig. 23.10). Samples are usually collected in the hospital after 24 hours of age and before discharge; testing may be delayed for sick or preterm infants or those born outside the hospital. The screening test should be repeated at 1 to 2 weeks of age if the initial specimen was obtained when the infant was younger than 24 hours of age.

The American College of Medical Genetics (2009) recommends that states retain the residual dried blood filter spots. These blood samples are useful for future testing and research purposes. However, ethical concerns are related to the need for parental consent to retain blood samples and use them for biomedical research. Nurses need to be aware of policies and procedures regarding retention and use of newborn screening samples in the state where they practice so they are able to provide information to parents (Tluczek & De Luca, 2013).

Families should be educated about universal newborn screening during the prenatal period (ACOG Committee on Genetics, 2015). However, this is not common practice; newborn screening is not usually discussed with parents prior to birth. This may be related to the fact that in the majority of states informed consent is not required for newborn screening (Tarini & Goldenberg, 2012). In many cases, discussion about newborn screening occurs in the hospital setting at the time of blood sample collection. Nurses can provide education for parents regarding the purpose of the screening, the procedure for blood sampling, when to expect results, and the importance of follow-up (Araia, Wilson, Chakraborty, et al., 2012; Tluczek & De Luca, 2013) (see the Community Focus box).

Newborn Hearing Screening

Hearing loss is the most commonly diagnosed genetic disorder of all the core conditions in the universal screening program (Howell, Terry, Tait, et al., 2012). The Joint Committee on Infant Hearing (2007) recommends routine hearing screening for all newborns before hospital discharge or no later than 1 month of age. The Canadian Paediatric Society recommends hearing screening for all newborns (Patel, Feldman, & CPS Community Paediatrics Committee, 2014). Through early hearing detection and intervention programs, the outcome for infants who are deaf or hard of hearing can be maximized.

Using noninvasive technology, newborn hearing screening provides information about the pathways from the external ear to the cerebral cortex. Two tests commonly are used to assess hearing function in the newborn. Initial screening is done with the evoked otoacoustic emissions (EOAE) test. The auditory brainstem response (ABR) test is used as follow-up if the initial screening is abnormal. Neither test is definitive in diagnosing hearing loss; they are used to determine whether further, more accurate hearing testing is needed through audiologic evaluation. For the EOAE test, a soft rubber earpiece that makes a soft clicking noise is placed in the baby's outer ear (Fig. 23.11, A). A healthy ear will "echo" the click sound back to a microphone inside the earpiece. The ABR test is performed by attaching sensors to the baby's forehead and behind each ear. An earphone is placed in the baby's outer ear and sends a series of quiet sounds into the sleeping baby's ear (see

TABLE 23.4 Standard Laboratory Values in a Term Neonate

Hematology	Values
Hemoglobin (g/dL)	14 to 24
Hematocrit (%)	44 to 64
Red blood cells (RBCs)/µL	4.8×10^6 to 7.1×10^6
Reticulocytes (%)	1.8 to 4.6
Fetal hemoglobin (% of total)	50 to 70
Platelet count/mm³	150,000 to 300,000
White blood cells (WBCs)/µL	9000 to 30,000
Bilirubin, total (mg/dL)*	
24 hours	2 to 6
48 hours	6 to 7
3 to 5 days	4 to 6
Serum glucose (mg/dL)	
<1 day	40 to 60
>1 day	50 to 90
Arterial blood gases	
pH	7.35 to 7.45
Pco_2	35 to 45 mm Hg
Po_2	60 to 80 mm Hg
HCO_3	18 to 26 mEq/L
Base excess	(−5) to (+5)
O_2 saturation	92% to 94%

dL, Deciliter; *µL,* microliter; *Pco₂,* partial pressure of carbon dioxide; *Po₂,* partial pressure of oxygen.

*Bilirubin levels should be interpreted according to the hour-specific nomogram (AAP Subcommittee on Hyperbilirubinemia, 2004).
Data from American Academy of Pediatrics (AAP) Subcommittee on Hyperbilirubinemia. (2004). Clinical practice guideline: Management of hyperbilirubinemia in the newborn infant 35 or more weeks of gestation. *Pediatrics, 114*(1):297–316; Blackburn, S.T. (2013). *Maternal, fetal, and neonatal physiology* (4th ed.). Maryland Heights, MO: Elsevier Saunders; Pagana, K.D., & Pagana, T.J. (2014). *Mosby's manual of diagnostic and laboratory tests* (5th ed.). St. Louis, MO: Elsevier; Barry, J.S., Deacon, J., Hernández, C., et al. (2016). Acid-base homeostasis and oxygenation. In S. L. Gardner, B. S. Carter, M. Enzman-Hines, et al. (Eds.), *Merenstein & Gardner's handbook of neonatal intensive care* (8th ed.). St. Louis, MO: Elsevier.

🏠 COMMUNITY FOCUS
Newborn Screening

Visit the National Newborn Screening and Genetics Resource Center (NNSGRC) website (http://genes-r-us.uthscsa.edu). Review the information for parents and family about resources, disorders tested, and screening programs.

At the NNSGRC website, visit the newborn screening program site for your state. What types of disorders are including in newborn screening? Does your state require newborn hearing screening? Review the information for parents about diagnostic testing and community support services.

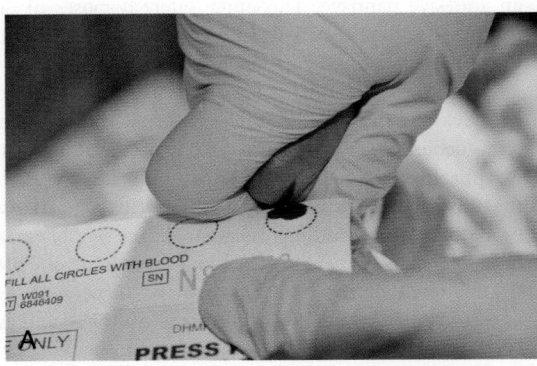
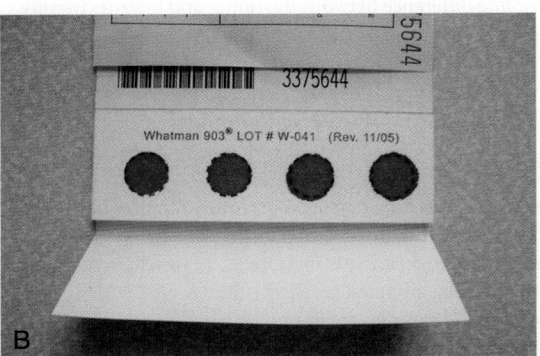

FIG 23.10 **A,** Nurse obtaining blood sample from newborn's heel for universal screening. Sample is applied to filter paper. **B,** All circles on the filter paper must be filled in completely. (Courtesy of Cheryl Briggs, RNC, Annapolis, MD.)

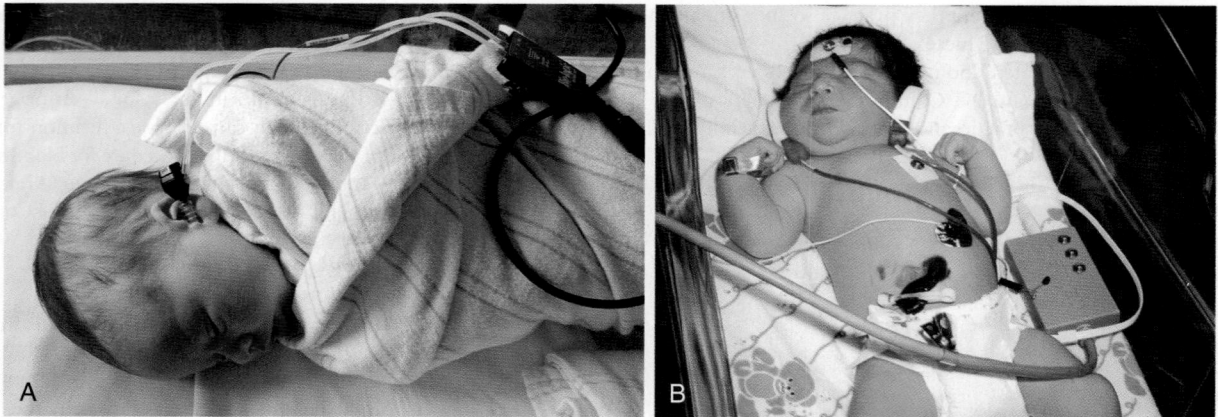

FIG 23.11 Newborn hearing screening. **A,** Evoked otoacoustic emissions (EOAE) test. **B,** Auditory brain response (ABR) test. (A, Courtesy of Julie and Darren Nelson, Loveland, CO. B, Courtesy of Dee Lowdermilk, Chapel Hill, NC.)

Fig. 23.11, *B*). The sensors measure the responses of the baby's acoustic nerve. The responses are recorded and stored in a computer.

Newborns who do not pass the initial screening test should have the hearing screening test repeated as part of follow-up care. If the infant still does not pass, a comprehensive audiologic evaluation should be done by 3 months of age. Regardless of the outcome of hearing testing, all infants should have regular and ongoing surveillance of developmental, hearing, and speech-language skills through regular well-child visits beginning at 2 months of age so that any hearing loss can be promptly identified and treated (Joint Committee on Infant Hearing, 2007).

Screening for Critical Congenital Heart Disease

Critical congenital heart disease (CCHD) was added to the uniform screening panel in the United States in 2011 and is endorsed by the AAP (AAP Section on Cardiology and Cardiac Surgery Executive Committee, 2012). The noninvasive screening test is performed using pulse oximetry to measure oxygen saturation for the purpose of detecting hypoxemia. Pulse oximetry testing can detect some critical congenital heart defects that present with hypoxemia in the absence of other physical symptoms. Hypoxemia can be the first sign that a congenital heart defect is present and other symptoms can develop once the newborn has been discharged. Screening is performed at 24 to 48 hours of age. Oxygen saturation is measured in the right hand and one foot. A "passing" result is oxygen saturation of greater than 95% in either extremity, with a less than 3% absolute difference between the upper and lower extremity readings. Immediate evaluation is needed if the oxygen saturation is less than 90%. The baby is evaluated for hemodynamic stability and hypoxemia; an echocardiogram is usually performed (AAP Section on Cardiology and Cardiac Surgery Executive Committee).

Collection of Specimens

Ongoing evaluation and screening of a newborn often requires obtaining blood by heelstick or venipuncture or the collection of a urine specimen. Laboratory tests may be ordered routinely (e.g., newborn screening) or for a specific purpose as directed by the health care provider.

Heelstick. Most blood samples are drawn by laboratory technicians. Nurses, however, may be required to perform heelsticks to obtain blood for glucose monitoring, newborn screening, or other tests.

Blood samples should be collected in a manner that minimizes pain and trauma to the infant and maximizes the accuracy of test results. If a laboratory technician is collecting the specimen, the nurse assists as needed to maximize safety and infant comfort.

It is helpful to warm the heel before the sample is taken; application of heat for 5 to 10 minutes helps dilate the vessels in the area. A cloth soaked with warm water and wrapped loosely around the foot provides effective warming (Fig. 23.12, *A*). Disposable heel warmers are available from a variety of companies but should be used with care to prevent burns. Nurses should wear gloves when collecting any specimen. The nurse cleanses the area with an appropriate skin antiseptic, restrains the infant's foot with a free hand, and then punctures the site. A spring-loaded automatic puncture device causes less pain and requires fewer punctures than a manual lance blade.

The most serious complication of an infant heelstick is necrotizing osteochondritis resulting from lancet penetration of the bone. To prevent this problem, the puncture is made at the outer aspect of the heel and penetrates no deeper than 2.4 mm. To identify the appropriate puncture site, the nurse draws an imaginary line from between the fourth and fifth toes and parallel to the lateral aspect of the foot to the heel, where the puncture is made; a second line can be drawn from the great toe to the medial aspect of the heel (see Fig. 23.12, *B*). Repeated trauma to the walking surface of the heel can cause fibrosis and scarring that can lead to problems with walking later in life.

After the specimen has been collected, gentle pressure is applied with a dry gauze pad. No further skin cleanser should be applied because it will cause the site to continue to bleed. The site is then covered with an adhesive bandage. The nurse safely disposes of equipment used, reviews the laboratory requisition for correct identification, and checks the specimen for accurate labeling and routing.

A heelstick is traumatic for the infant and causes pain. After several heelsticks, infants have been observed to withdraw their feet when they are touched. The nurse can reduce procedural pain using a variety of nonpharmacologic techniques including allowing the mother to hold the neonate skin to skin, using nonnutritive sucking with or without oral sucrose, or swaddling the neonate (see the "Neonatal Pain" section later in the chapter) (McNair, Yeo, Johnston, et al., 2013). To reassure the infant and promote feelings of safety, the neonate should be cuddled and comforted when the procedure is complete and appropriate pain management measures taken to minimize the pain.

Venipuncture. Occasionally laboratory tests are ordered that require larger samples of blood than can be collected with a heelstick. Venous blood samples can be drawn from antecubital, saphenous, superficial

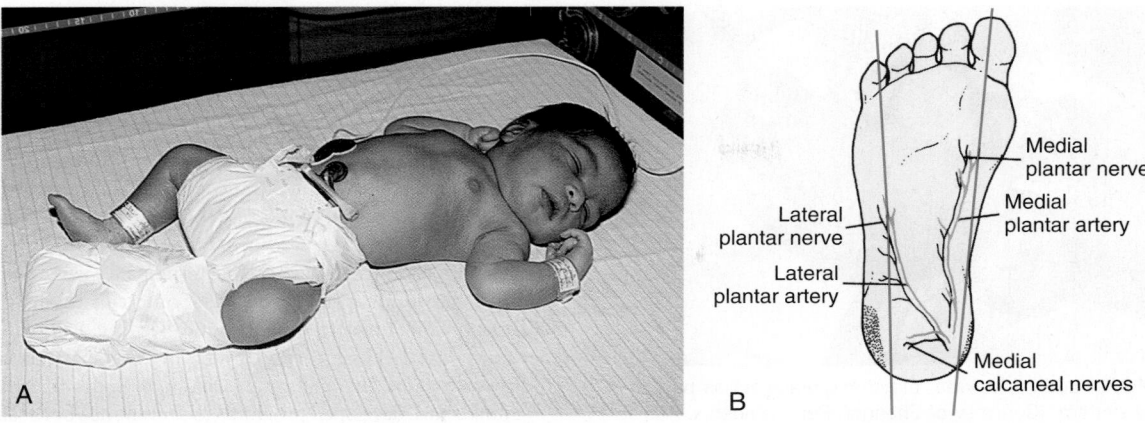

FIG 23.12 Heelstick. **A,** Newborn with foot wrapped for warmth to increase blood flow to extremity before heelstick. **B,** Heelstick sites *(shaded areas)* on infant's foot for obtaining samples of capillary blood. (A, Courtesy of Marjorie Pyle, RNC, Lifecircle, Costa Mesa, CA.)

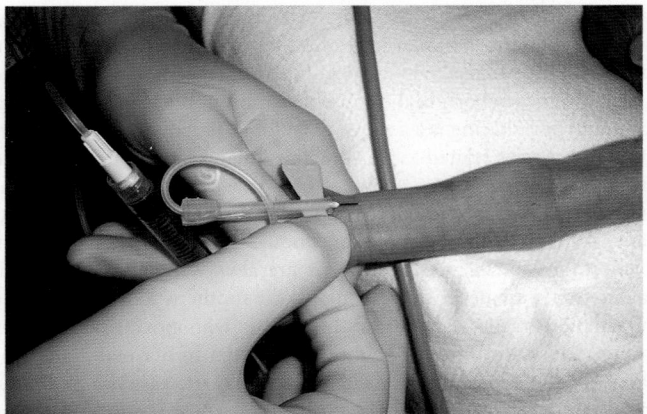

FIG 23.13 Venipuncture using a butterfly needle. (Courtesy of Cheryl Briggs, RNC, Annapolis, MD.)

wrist, and rarely, scalp veins. When venipuncture is required, positioning of the needle is extremely important. A 23- or 25-gauge butterfly needle or hypodermic needle with a syringe is used (Fig. 23.13). Patience is required during the procedure because the blood return in small veins is slow and consequently the small needle must remain in place longer than a larger needle. A tourniquet is optional but can help increase blood flow with venipuncture. The infant is carefully restrained during the procedure to prevent injury. If venipuncture or arterial puncture is performed for blood gas studies, crying, fear, and agitation will affect the values; therefore, every effort must be made to keep the infant quiet during the procedure. Pressure must be maintained over an arterial or femoral vein puncture with a dry gauze square for 3 to 5 minutes to prevent bleeding from the site.

For 1 hour after any venipuncture, the nurse observes the infant frequently for evidence of bleeding or hematoma formation at the puncture site. The infant is cuddled and comforted when the procedure is completed, and appropriate pain management measures are taken. The nurse assesses and documents the infant's tolerance of the procedure.

Urine specimen. Analysis of urine is a valuable laboratory tool for infant assessment; the way in which the specimen is collected can influence the results. The urine sample should be fresh and analyzed within 1 hour of collection. A urine collection bag is often used to obtain a specimen.

INTERVENTIONS

Protective Environment

The provision of a protective environment is basic to the care of the newborn. The construction, maintenance, and operation of nurseries in accredited hospitals are monitored by national professional organizations such as the AAP, The Joint Commission (TJC), the Occupational Safety and Health Administration (OSHA), and local or state governing bodies. In addition, hospital personnel develop their own policies and procedures for protecting the newborns under their care. Prescribed standards cover areas such as environmental factors, measures to control infection, and safety factors.

Current health care trends and the focus on nonseparation of mothers and babies (rooming-in) have prompted some hospitals to abandon having a separate newborn nursery. In the mother-baby model of care, the infant stays in the mother's room, which reduces the need for a separate nursery.

Environmental Factors

Environmental factors include provision of adequate lighting, elimination of potential fire hazards, safety of electrical appliances, adequate ventilation, and controlled temperature and humidity (AAP & ACOG, 2012).

Infection-Control Factors

Measures to control infection in newborn nurseries include adequate floor space to permit the positioning of bassinets at least 3 feet apart in all directions, hand hygiene facilities, and areas for cleaning and storing equipment and supplies. Only specified personnel directly involved in the care of mothers and infants are allowed in these areas, thereby reducing the opportunities for the transmission of pathogenic organisms.

> ⚡ **SAFETY ALERT**
>
> Proper hand hygiene is essential to prevent the spread of health care–associated infection. Personnel should wash hands with soap and water or use an alcohol-based handrub in accordance with hospital infection-control policies. Hand hygiene should be performed before and after touching the infant, before an invasive procedure or medication administration, after contact with potentially contaminated objects (e.g., computer keyboards, telephone, countertop surfaces), and after removing sterile or nonsterile gloves (World Health Organization [WHO], 2009).

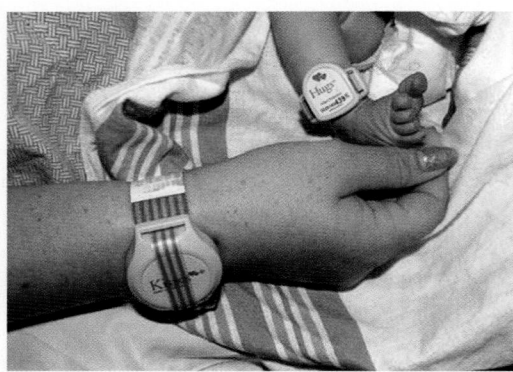

FIG 23.14 Mother and infant wear electronic bracelets as part of an infant security system. (Courtesy of Shannon Perry, Phoenix, AZ.)

Health care workers must wear gloves when handling infants until blood and amniotic fluid have been removed from the skin, when drawing blood (e.g., heelstick), when caring for a fresh wound (e.g., circumcision), and during diaper changes.

Visitors such as siblings and grandparents are expected to perform hand hygiene before having contact with infants or equipment. Individuals with infectious conditions are excluded from contact with newborns or must take special precautions when working with infants. This group includes people with upper respiratory tract infections, gastrointestinal tract infections, and infectious skin conditions.

Preventing infant abduction. Nurses discuss infant security precautions with the mother and her family because infant abductions are an ongoing concern. Many birthing facilities have special limited-entry systems. Nurses teach mothers and their families to check the identity of any person who comes to remove the baby from their room. Personnel are required to wear picture identification badges. On some units, all staff members wear matching scrubs or special badges. Other units use closed-circuit television, computer monitoring systems, fingerprint identification pads, or infant bracelet security systems (Fig. 23.14) that alarm if the newborn is separated from the mother or is taken outside the boundaries of the unit. Nurses and new parents must work together to ensure the safety of newborns in the hospital environment (Hiner, Pyka, Burks, et al., 2012).

⚡ SAFETY ALERT

Nurses play a critical role in educating parents about measures to prevent infant abduction. Parents should be instructed how to identify legitimate hospital personnel and to request a second staff member to verify the identity of any questionable person who wants to take the baby from the mother's room. Parents should never leave the newborn in the birthing facility room without direct supervision. Parents should be instructed to use caution when posting photos of the new baby on the Internet and publishing public notices about the birth (AAP & ACOG, 2012).

Preventing Newborn Injury

Newborn infants are at risk for injury as a result of falling. Infants who fall, even from low level surfaces such as beds or chairs, are at risk for sustaining head injury that can include skull fracture. Parents may hesitate to report falls due to feelings of guilt and fear of reproach from staff members.

Although newborn falls are likely underreported, it has been estimated that approximately 600 to 1600 falls occur each year in US hospitals (Helsey, McDonald, & Stewart, 2010). Currently there is no standardized system for reporting newborn falls, and, furthermore, there is no standardized tool for assessing newborn fall risk (Ainsworth, Summerlin-Long, & Mog, 2016).

Based on the available information, it appears that most falls or "near misses" occur when the mother falls asleep while holding the newborn in her bed or in a reclining chair, although some falls occur at birth or when the infant is transported. Exhaustion from labor and birth and sleep deprivation increase the chances of a new mother falling asleep while holding her newborn. Other factors that increase the risk for newborn falls include cesarean birth and pain medications or sedatives within 2 to 3 hours prior to the fall. Some falls occur when mothers fall asleep while breastfeeding or bottle-feeding. Falls can occur when newborns are held or carried by family members or hospital staff (Ainsworth et al., 2016; Slogar, Gargiulo, & Bodrock, 2013).

Nurses have developed programs to prevent newborn falls by increasing awareness of the problem through staff and parent education, assessing for fall risk, and implementing policies targeting fall prevention (Ainsworth et al., 2016; Slogar et al., 2013).

Nurses can help prevent newborn falls by identifying risk factors such as maternal medications (e.g., opioids) that cause drowsiness and can increase the risk for the mother falling asleep while holding the infant. A specially designed wrap may be used to secure the newborn in place on the parent's chest (see Fig. 16.26). Parents should be instructed to place their newborn in the supine position in the bassinet for sleep. Although bed-sharing is a controversial topic, parents need to be aware of potential risks related to this practice. Infants should not be placed on couches or armchairs, whether or not a parent is present. Some hospitals ask parents and staff to sign an infant safety pledge to promote patient safety. Staff members conduct hourly rounds, especially at night, to monitor for fall risks. Newborns are always transported in their bassinets and are never carried outside the mother's room. Nurses can inform mothers that staff are available to assist with moving the newborn to the bassinet from being held by the mother in her bed. Educating parents using a nonjudgmental approach may increase the likelihood that a parent will report a newborn fall (Ainsworth et al., 2016; Matteson, Henderson-Williams, & Nelson, 2013; Slogar et al., 2013).

Another concern is related to sudden unexpected postnatal collapse (SUPC). This term describes any condition that results in temporary or permanent cessation of respirations or cardiorespiratory failure. By definition, SUPC occurs during the first week of life in any term or near-term infant who is well at birth, collapses suddenly to the point of needing intermittent positive-pressure ventilation, and either dies, requires intensive care, or develops encephalopathy (Feldman, Goldsmith, Committee of Fetus and Newborn, et al., 2016; Nassi, Piumelli, Nardini, et al., 2013). The vast majority of SUPC cases occur during the first 2 hours after birth and appear to often be related to suffocation or entrapment. It has occurred when newborns are held prone on the mother's chest or abdomen during SSC and when mothers are not paying close attention to the infant as they are breastfeeding or holding the infant (Feldman et al).

⚡ SAFETY ALERT

Nurses need to closely observe mothers and newborns in SSC, especially during the first few hours after birth (Box 23.4).

Therapeutic and Surgical Procedures
Intramuscular Injection

Newborns routinely receive IM injections before discharge. A single dose of vitamin K is administered shortly after birth, and hepatitis B (Hep B) vaccine is administered before discharge. Under specific

BOX 23.4 Safe Skin-to-Skin Positioning

- The newborn's face is visible.
- The newborn's nose and mouth are uncovered.
- The newborn's neck is straight and the head is turned to one side, in "sniffing position."
- The newborn's chest and shoulders face the mother.
- The newborn's legs are flexed.
- The newborn's back is covered with blankets.
- Labor and delivery nursing staff continuously monitor the mother and newborn in skin-to-skin contact after birth.
- Postpartum or mother-baby nurses provide regular monitoring of mothers and newborns in skin-to-skin contact.
- When the mother is finished with skin-to-skin contact, a staff member or support person who is awake and alert places the newborn in the bassinet.

Data from Feldman-Winter, L., Goldsmith, J.P., & Committee on Fetus and Newborn, Task Force on Sudden Infant Death Syndrome. (2016). Safe sleep and skin-to-skin care in the neonatal period for healthy term newborns. *Pediatrics, 138*(3), e1–e10; Ludington-Hoe, S., & Morgan, K. (2014). Infant assessment and reduction of sudden unexpected postnatal collapse risk during skin-to-skin contact. *Newborn and Infant Nursing Reviews, 14*(1), 28–33.

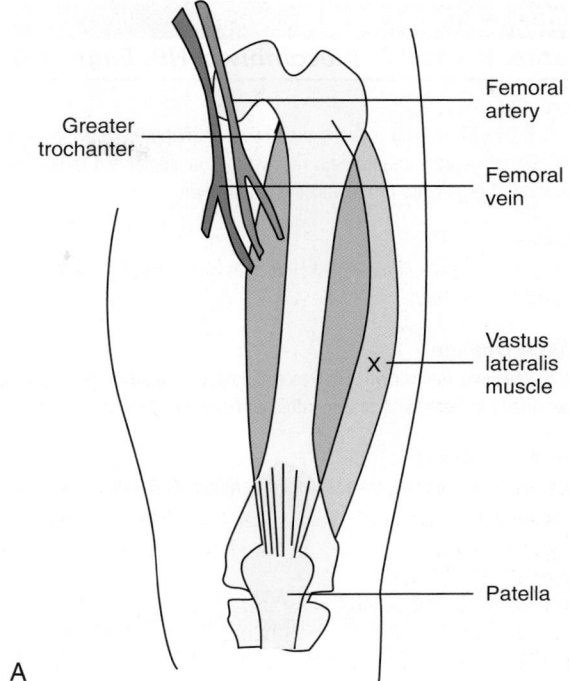

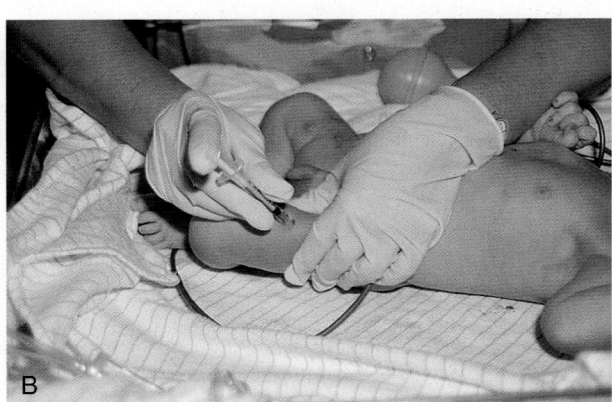

FIG 23.15 Intramuscular injection. **A,** Acceptable intramuscular injection site for newborn infant. *X,* injection site. **B,** Infant's leg stabilized for intramuscular injection. Nurse is wearing gloves to give injection. (B, Courtesy of Marjorie Pyle, Lifecircle, Costa Mesa, CA.)

circumstances, other IM injections may be ordered, such as a dose of HepB immune globulin for infants born to mothers who are positive for HepB.

Selection of the appropriate equipment and site for IM injection is important. In most cases, a 25-gauge, ⅝-inch needle is used. Injections must be given in muscles large enough to accommodate the medication, and major nerves and blood vessels must be avoided. The muscles of newborns may not tolerate more than 0.5 mL per IM injection. The preferred injection site for newborns is the vastus lateralis (Fig. 23.15). The dorsogluteal muscle is very small, poorly developed, and dangerously close to the sciatic nerve, which occupies a proportionately larger area in infants than in older children. Therefore, it is not recommended as an injection site in small children. The deltoid muscle has inadequate muscle mass for IM administration. A key factor in preventing and minimizing local reaction to IM injections is adequate deposition of the medication deep within the muscle; therefore, muscle size, needle length, and amount of medication injected should be carefully considered.

The nurse wears nonsterile gloves when administering an injection. The neonate's leg should be stabilized. The nurse cleanses the injection site with an appropriate skin antiseptic and then stabilizes the infant's muscle between the thumb and forefinger. The needle is inserted into the vastus lateralis at a 90-degree angle. The medication is injected slowly. After the medication is injected, the nurse withdraws the needle quickly and places a dry gauze pad over the site, applying gentle pressure to minimize pain and bleeding.

The nurse discards equipment properly. Needles are never recapped but are properly discarded in an appropriate safety container. The name of the medication, date and time, amount, route, and site of injection are documented in the newborn's record.

The nurse uses nonpharmacologic techniques to decrease the newborn's pain response during the injection. This may include administering the injection while the mother is holding the infant skin-to-skin. Oral sucrose administered prior to the injection and/or nonnutritive sucking during the procedure can reduce discomfort. After the injection, the mother or nurse uses comfort measures to calm the infant.

Immunizations. IM injections are used to administer immunizations such as the hepatitis B (HepB) vaccine. HepB vaccination is recommended for all infants before discharge (see Medication Guide: Hepatitis B Vaccine [Recombivax HB, Engerix-B]). Prior to administering the vaccine, the nurse obtains parental consent and notes the mother's HepB status. Infants at highest risk for contracting HepB are those born to women who have HepB or whose HepB status is unknown. If the mother is positive for HepB, the infant should receive the HepB vaccine and HepB immune globulin (HBIG) within 12 hours after birth (see Medication Guide: Hepatitis B Immune Globulin) (Centers for Disease Control and Prevention [CDC], 2016).

Circumcision

Policies and recommendations. Circumcision is the removal of all or part of the foreskin (prepuce) of the penis. Usually it is performed during the first few days of life but is sometimes done at a later time for preterm or ill neonates or for religious or cultural reasons.

The CDC reports that rates of newborn circumcision performed in US hospitals peaked at 64.5% in 1981, dropping to a low of 55.4 in 2007. Rates increased slightly to 58.3% in 2010 (Owings, Uddin, & Williams, 2013).

MEDICATION GUIDE
Hepatitis B Vaccine (Recombivax HB, Engerix-B)

Action

Hepatitis B (HepB) vaccine induces protective antihepatitis B antibodies in 95% to 99% of healthy infants who receive the recommended three doses. The duration of protection of the vaccine is unknown.

Indication

HepB vaccine is for immunizing against infection caused by all known subtypes of hepatitis B virus (HBV).

Neonatal Dosage

The usual dosage is Recombivax HB 5 mcg/0.5 mL or Engerix-B 10 mcg/0.5 mL intramuscularly at birth, at 1 to 2 months, and at 6 to 18 months.

Adverse Reactions

Common adverse reactions are rash, fever, erythema, swelling, and pain at the injection site.

Nursing Considerations

- Parental consent must be obtained before administration. Follow proper procedure for administration of intramuscular (IM) injection (see Fig. 23.15). If infant also needs hepatitis B immune globulin (HBIG), use separate sites for the two injections.
- For infants of mothers with negative HepB status, administer HepB vaccine before discharge from birthing facility.
- For infants born to hepatitis B surface antigen (HBsAg)–positive mothers, administer HepB vaccine and HBIG within 12 hours after birth.
- For infants born to mothers whose HepB status is unknown:
  - ≤2000 g: administer HepB vaccine and HBIG within 12 hours after birth
  - ≥2000 g: administer HepB vaccine within 12 hours; if mother's HepB results are positive, give HBIG by 1 week of age
- Document the date, time, and site of injection, the lot number, and expiration date according to agency protocol.

Data from Centers for Disease Control and Prevention (2016). Advisory Committee on Immunization Practices recommended immunization schedule for persons aged 0 through 18 years—United States, 2016. *Morbidity and Mortality Weekly Report, 65*(4), 86–87.

MEDICATION GUIDE
Hepatitis B Immune Globulin

Action

Hepatitis B immune globulin (HBIG) provides a high titer of antibody to hepatitis B surface antigen (HBsAg).

Indication

The HBIG vaccine provides prophylaxis against infection in infants born to HBsAg-positive mothers.

Neonatal Dosage

Administer one 0.5-mL dose intramuscularly within 12 hours of birth.

Adverse Reactions

Hypersensitivity may occur.

Nursing Considerations

- Administer within 12 hours of birth.
- Follow proper procedure for administration of intramuscular injection (see Fig. 23.15). (See guidelines for administration in Medication Guide: Hepatitis B Vaccine.)
- The HBIG vaccine can be given at the same time as the HepB vaccine but at a different site.
- Document the date, time, and site of injection, as well as the lot number and expiration date of the vaccine, according to agency policy.

Data from Centers for Disease Control and Prevention. (2016). Advisory Committee on Immunization Practices recommended immunization schedule for persons aged 0 through 18 years—United States, 2016. *Morbidity and Mortality Weekly Report 65*(4), 86–87.

Changes in recommendations from the AAP regarding newborn male circumcision (NMC) have likely influenced US circumcision rates. The AAP policy on circumcision that was issued in 1999 and reaffirmed in 2005 recognized potential benefits of NMC, although the AAP did not deem them sufficient to recommend routine newborn circumcision (AAP Task Force on Circumcision, 2005). In 2012, the AAP issued a new policy statement regarding newborn male circumcision. The policy states: "Evaluation of current evidence indicates that the health benefits of newborn male circumcision outweigh the risks and that the procedure's benefits justify access to this procedure for families who choose it" (AAP Task Force on Circumcision, 2012, p. 585). The health benefits of NMC cited by the AAP include prevention of urinary tract infection in male infants younger than 1 year of age, reduced risk for penile cancer, and reduced risk for heterosexual acquisition of sexually transmitted infections, particularly HIV (AAP Task Force on Circumcision, 2012). In spite of the new evidence, the AAP does not recommend the practice of routine newborn circumcision. Similarly, the Canadian Paediatric Society (CPS) revised the policy on newborn circumcision in 2015; while recognizing the potential benefits to certain at-risk populations, the CPS does not recommend routine newborn circumcision (Sorokan, Finlay, Jefferies, et al., 2015).

The World Health Organization (WHO) (2012) recognizes male circumcision as an important intervention in reducing the risk for heterosexually acquired HIV in men. The organization recommends early infant circumcision for newborn males weighing more than 2500 grams and without medical contraindication (World Health Organization and Jhpiego, 2010).

Ethical and legal issues surrounding newborn male circumcision create ongoing controversy about this procedure. Opponents of circumcision feel that newborn circumcision is unnatural and unnecessary and that it violates basic human rights. They cite concerns about acute pain; risks related to acute complications such as hemorrhage, infection, and penile injury (removal of excessive skin, damage to the meatus or glans); and long-term implications such as adverse effects on sexual function and pleasure. Websites such as www.intactamerica.org discourage parents from circumcising their newborn sons.

Parental decision. Circumcision is a matter of personal parental choice. Parents usually decide to have their newborn circumcised for one or more of the following reasons: hygiene, religious conviction, tradition, culture, or social norms. Cost and insurance coverage are considerations in the parents' decision-making process. Parents need to make an informed choice regarding newborn circumcision based on the most current evidence and recommendations. Health care providers and nurses who care for childbearing families can help parents make an informed choice about newborn circumcision by providing factual, unbiased, evidence-based information. They can provide opportunities for discussion about the benefits and risks of the procedure.

Expectant parents need to begin learning about circumcision during the prenatal period, but circumcision often is not discussed with the parents. In many instances, it is only when the mother is being admitted to the hospital or birthing unit that she is first confronted with the

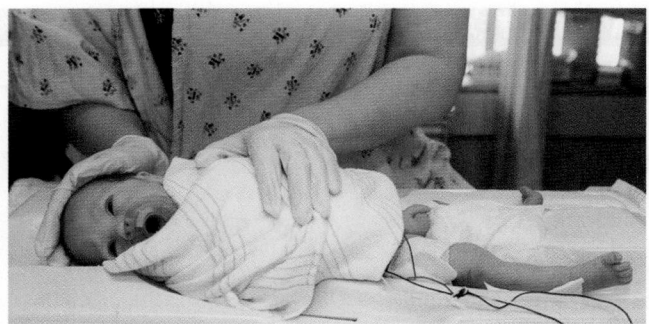

FIG 23.16 Positioning of infant in Circumstraint immobilizer. (Courtesy of Paul Vincent Kuntz, Texas Children's Hospital, Houston, TX.)

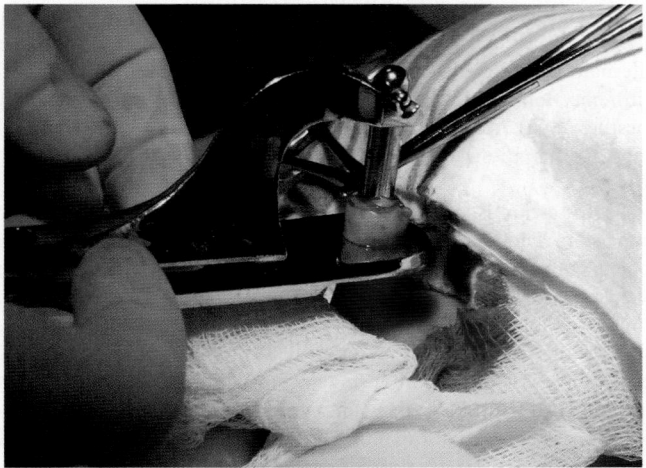

FIG 23.17 Circumcision with the Gomco (Yellen) clamp. After hemostasis occurs, the foreskin (over the metal dome) is cut away. (Courtesy of Cheryl Briggs, RNC, Annapolis, MD.)

decision regarding circumcision. Because the stress of the intrapartum period makes this a difficult time for parental decision-making, this is not an ideal time to broach the topic of circumcision and expect a well-informed decision.

Circumcision requires informed consent. Although the health care provider who will perform the procedure is legally responsible for educating parents about newborn circumcision so they can make an informed decision, nurses are often involved in discussions on this topic and should provide parents with current evidence-based information.

Procedure. Circumcision is not performed immediately after birth because of the danger of cold stress and decreased clotting factors but is usually done in the hospital before discharge. The circumcision of a Jewish male infant is commonly performed on the eighth day after birth at home in a ceremony called a *bris*. This timing is logical from a physiologic standpoint because clotting factors decrease somewhat immediately after birth and do not return to prebirth levels until the end of the first week.

Feedings may be withheld up to 2 to 3 hours before the circumcision to prevent vomiting and aspiration, although in some hospitals, infants are allowed to breastfeed until they are taken to the nursery for the procedure. To prepare the infant for the circumcision, he is positioned on a plastic restraint form (Fig. 23.16) and the penis is cleansed with soap and water or an antiseptic solution such as povidone-iodine. The infant is draped to provide warmth and a sterile field, and the sterile equipment is readied for use.

In the hospital setting, newborn circumcision is usually performed using the Gomco (Yellen) or Mogen clamp or the PlastiBell device. The technique is usually based on health care provider training and preference. The procedure takes only a few minutes to perform. Use of the Gomco or Mogen clamp involves surgical removal of the foreskin. The clamp technique minimizes blood loss (Fig. 23.17). After the circumcision is completed, a small petrolatum gauze dressing is applied to the penis for the first 24 hours; thereafter, parents are instructed to apply petrolatum with each diaper change for 7 to 10 days to keep the penis from adhering to the diaper (Association of Women's Health, Obstetric, and Neonatal Nurses [AWHONN], 2013).

With the PlastiBell technique, the plastic bell is first fitted over the glans, a suture is tied around the rim of the bell, and excess foreskin is cut away. The plastic rim remains in place for about 1 week; it falls off after healing has taken place, usually within 5 to 7 days (Fig. 23.18). Petrolatum or dressings are not applied to the penis following circumcision with the PlastiBell (AWHONN, 2013).

Procedural pain management. Circumcision is painful. The pain is characterized by both physiologic and behavioral changes in the infant (see discussion that follows). Commonly used anesthetics for circumcision include dorsal penile nerve block (DPNB), ring block, and topical anesthetic cream such as eutectic mixture of local anesthetic (EMLA)

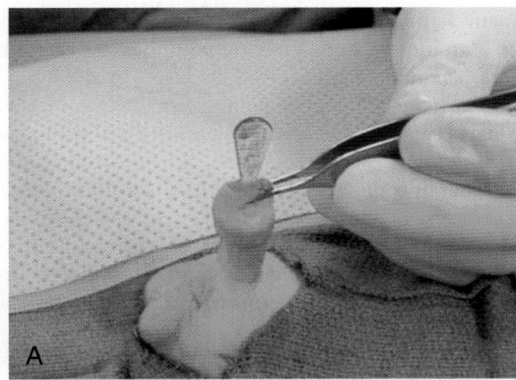

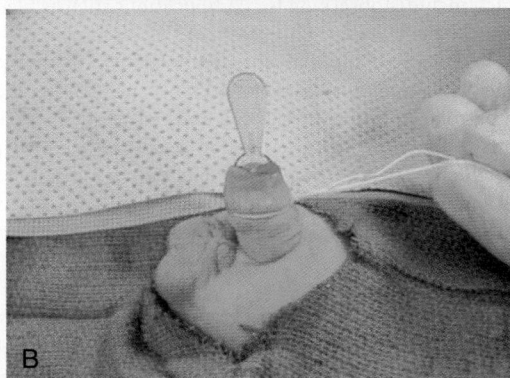

FIG 23.18 The PlastiBell technique. **A,** The PlastiBell is placed over the glans inside the prepuce. **B,** A string is then tied around the prepuce and positioned in the groove of the bell. The excess foreskin is trimmed, and the handle is broken off the bell. The foreskin remnant and bell are expected to slough in 1 to 2 weeks. (From Holcomb, G.W., Murphy, J.P., & Ostlie D.J. [2014]. *Ashcraft's pediatric surgery* [6th ed.]. Philadelphia, PA: Elsevier.)

(prilocaine-lidocaine) or LMX4 (4% lidocaine). Nonpharmacologic methods such as concentrated oral sucrose, nonnutritive sucking, and swaddling can be used to enhance pain management. Pain during circumcision is most effectively managed using a combination of pharmacologic and nonpharmacologic measures (Bellieni, Alagna, & Buonocore, 2013).

A DPNB consists of subcutaneous injections of buffered lidocaine at the 2 o'clock and 10 o'clock positions on the dorsum of the penis. Alternatively, buffered lidocaine may be administered using a ring block with injections around the base of the penis. To ensure adequate anesthesia, circumcision should not be performed for at least 5 to 8 minutes after these injections (Gardner, Enzman-Hines, & Agarwal, 2016).

EMLA cream is applied to the penis at least 1 hour before the circumcision. The area where the prepuce attaches to the glans is well coated with 1 g of the cream and then covered with a transparent occlusive dressing or finger cot. Just before the procedure, the cream is removed. Blanching or redness of the skin can occur.

After the circumcision the infant is comforted until he is quiet. If the parents were not present during the procedure, the infant is returned to them. The infant can be fussy for several hours and can have disturbed sleep-wake states and disorganized feeding behaviors. Some infants will go into a deep sleep after circumcision until they are awakened for feeding. Liquid acetaminophen may be administered orally after the procedure and repeated every 4 to 6 hours for the first 24 hours as ordered by the health care provider (Gardner et al., 2016).

Care of the newly circumcised infant. Postcircumcision protocols vary. In many settings, the circumcision site is assessed for bleeding every 15 to 30 minutes for the first hour and then hourly for the next 4 to 6 hours. The nurse monitors the infant's urinary output, noting the time and amount of the first voiding after the circumcision.

If bleeding occurs from the circumcision site, the nurse applies gentle pressure with a folded sterile gauze pad. A hemostatic agent such as Gelfoam powder or sponge can be applied to help control bleeding. If bleeding is not easily controlled, a blood vessel may need to be ligated. In this event, one nurse notifies the health care provider and prepares the necessary equipment (i.e., circumcision tray and suture material) while another nurse maintains intermittent pressure until the provider arrives.

Nurses provide education for parents related to care of the circumcised infant, which includes observing for complications such as bleeding or infection (see Patient Teaching box: Care of the Circumcised Newborn at Home). Parents need support and encouragement as they perform postcircumcision care. Newborns typically cry when the diaper is changed and when petrolatum gauze is removed and reapplied. This can make new parents feel anxious because they do not want to inflict pain on the infant. Nurses can inform parents that the discomfort is usually temporary and will soon subside. Additionally, nurses can teach parents a variety of nonpharmacologic comfort measures.

NEONATAL PAIN

Neonatal Responses to Pain

There is clear evidence that neonates can feel pain, despite previous thinking that the immaturity of the nervous system prevented or blunted pain sensation and that neonates were incapable of remembering painful experiences. Pain in the neonate and pain in later life can be qualitatively different, but research has substantiated that newborns do experience pain (Blackburn, 2013).

Pain has physiologic and psychologic components. Its psychologic component and the diffuse total body response to pain exhibited by the neonate led many health care providers in the past to believe that infants, especially preterm infants, do not experience pain. The central nervous system is well developed, however, as early as 24 weeks of gestation. The peripheral and spinal structures that transmit pain information are present and functional between the first and second trimesters. The pituitary-adrenal axis is also well developed at this time,

---

PATIENT TEACHING

Care of the Circumcised Newborn at Home

Wash hands before touching the newly circumcised penis.

Check for Bleeding
- Check circumcision site for bleeding with each diaper change.
- If bleeding occurs, apply gentle pressure with a folded sterile gauze square. If bleeding does not stop with pressure, notify primary health care provider.

Observe for Urination
- Check to see that the infant urinates after being circumcised.
- Infant should have a wet diaper 2 to 6 times per 24 hours the first 1 to 2 days after birth and then at least 6 to 8 times per 24 hours after 3 to 4 days.

Keep Area Clean
- Change the diaper and inspect the circumcision at least every 4 hours.
- Wash the penis gently with warm water to remove urine and feces. Apply petrolatum to the glans with each diaper change (omit petrolatum if a PlastiBell was used). Do not use baby wipes because they can contain alcohol.
- Do not wash the penis with soap until the circumcision is healed (5 to 6 days).
- Apply the diaper loosely over the penis to prevent pressure on the circumcised area.

Check for Infection
- The glans penis is dark red after circumcision and then becomes covered with yellow exudate in 24 hours, which is normal and will persist for 2 to 3 days. Do not attempt to remove it.
- Redness, swelling, discharge, or odor indicates infection. Notify the pediatric health care provider if you think the circumcision area is infected.

Provide Comfort
- Circumcision is painful. Handle the area gently.
- Provide comfort measures such as holding the baby skin-to-skin, breastfeeding, cuddling, swaddling, or rocking.

---

and a fight-or-flight reaction is observed in response to the catecholamines released in response to stress.

The physiologic response to pain in neonates can be life-threatening. Pain response can decrease tidal volume, increase demands on the cardiovascular system, increase metabolism, and cause neuroendocrine imbalance. The hormonal-metabolic response to pain in a term infant has greater magnitude and shorter duration than in adults. The newborn's sympathetic response to pain is less mature and therefore less predictable than an adult's.

Pain response is influenced by a variety of factors including characteristics of the painful stimulus, gestational age, biologic factors, and behavioral state. The source, location, and timing of the pain affect the response; newborns respond differently to acute pain than to prolonged or recurrent pain. Pain perception and stress can be greater in preterm infants, although they often display less vigorous pain responses than term infants (Maxwell, Malavolta, & Fraga, 2013). There can be genetic differences in pain responses related to the amounts and types of neurotransmitters and receptors available to mediate pain. The behavioral state of the neonate also affects the pain response. Those who are more awake tend to have more robust pain responses than those in sleep states (Gardner et al., 2016).

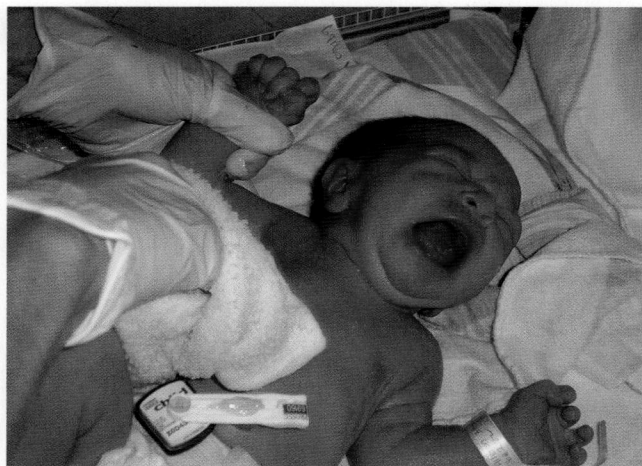

FIG 23.19 Signs of discomfort: note eye squeeze, brow bulge, nasolabial furrow, and wide-spread mouth. (Courtesy of Kathryn Alden, Chapel Hill, NC.)

The most common behavioral sign of pain is a vocalization or crying, ranging from a whimper to a distinctive high-pitched, shrill cry. Facial expressions include grimacing, eye squeeze, brow contraction, deepened nasolabial furrows, a taut and quivering tongue, and an open mouth (Fig. 23.19) (Box 23.5). The infant will flex and adduct the upper body and lower limbs in an attempt to withdraw from the painful stimulus. The preterm infant has a lower than normal threshold for initiation of this response (Gardner et al., 2016).

Pain can result in significant changes in heart rate, blood pressure (increased or decreased), intracranial pressure, vagal tone, respiratory rate, and oxygen saturation. Neonates respond to painful stimuli with release of epinephrine, norepinephrine, glucagon, corticosterone, cortisol, 11-deoxycorticosterone, lactate, pyruvate, and glucose (Blackburn, 2013).

Assessment of Neonatal Pain

In assessing pain, the nurse needs to consider the health of the neonate, the type and duration of the painful stimulus, environmental factors, and the infant's state of alertness. For example, severely compromised neonates may be unable to generate a pain response although they are, in fact, experiencing pain.

Every neonate should have an initial pain assessment as well as a pain management plan. The National Association of Neonatal Nurses (NANN) developed practice guidelines stating that all nurses who care for newborns should have education and competency validation in pain assessment. Pain should be assessed and documented on a regular basis (Walden & Gibbins, 2012).

Pain assessment tools include the following:
- Neonatal Infant Pain Scale (NIPS) (Lawrence, Alcock, McGrath, et al., 1993)
- Premature Infant Pain Profile (PIPP) (Stevens, Johnston, Petryshen, et al., 1996)
- Neonatal Pain Agitation and Sedation Scale (NPASS) (Hummel, Puchalski, Creech, et al., 2008)
- CRIES (Krechel & Bildner, 1995) (Table 23.5)

Healthy term newborns are exposed to fewer sources of pain than preterm infants in an NICU where painful procedures are inherent to care management. Even in low-risk newborns, nurses need to assess for signs of discomfort as part of routine assessments and especially during and after routine procedures such as heelsticks, injections, and circumcisions (Maxwell et al., 2013).

BOX 23.5   Manifestations of Acute Pain in the Neonate

Physiologic Responses
- Vital signs
  - Increased heart rate
  - Increased blood pressure
  - Rapid, shallow respirations
- Oxygenation
  - Decreased transcutaneous oxygen saturation ($tcPO_2$)
  - Decreased arterial oxygen saturation (SaO_2)
- Skin
  - Pallor or flushing
  - Diaphoresis
  - Palmar sweating
- Laboratory evidence of metabolic or endocrine changes
  - Hyperglycemia
  - Lowered pH
  - Elevated corticosteroids
- Other observations
  - Increased muscle tone
  - Dilated pupils
  - Decreased vagal nerve tone
  - Increased intracranial pressure

Behavioral Responses
- Vocalizations
  - Crying
  - Whimpering
  - Groaning
- Facial expression
  - Grimaces
  - Brow furrowed
  - Chin quivering
  - Eyes tightly closed
  - Mouth open and squarish
- Body movements and posture
  - Limb withdrawal
  - Thrashing
  - Rigidity
  - Flaccidity
  - Fist clenching
- Changes in state
  - Changes in sleep-wake cycles
  - Changes in feeding behavior
  - Changes in activity level
  - Fussiness, irritability
  - Listlessness

Data from Blackburn, S. (2013). *Maternal, fetal, and neonatal physiology: A clinical perspective* (4th ed.). Maryland Heights, MO: Saunders; Gardner, S.L., Enzman-Hines, M., & Agarwal, R. (2016). Pain and pain relief. In S.L. Gardner, B.S. Carter, M. Enzman-Hines, et al. (Eds.), *Merenstein & Gardner's handbook of neonatal intensive care* (8th ed.). St. Louis, MO: Elsevier.

Management of Neonatal Pain

The goals of pain management are to (1) minimize the intensity, duration, and physiologic cost of the pain and (2) maximize the neonate's ability to cope with and recover from the pain. Nonpharmacologic and pharmacologic strategies are used. It is important to note that despite

TABLE 23.5   CRIES Neonatal Postoperative Pain Scale*

	0	1	2
Crying	No	High pitched	Inconsolable
Requires oxygen for saturation >95%	No	<30%	>30%
Increased vital signs	Heart rate and blood pressure equal to or less than preoperative state	Heart rate and blood pressure <20% of preoperative state	Heart rate and blood pressure >20% of preoperative state
Expression	None	Grimace	Grimace and grunt
Sleepless	No	Wakes at frequent intervals	Constantly awake

Coding Tips for Using CRIES

Crying	The characteristic cry of pain is high pitched.
	If no cry or cry that is not high pitched, score 0.
	If cry is high pitched but infant is easily consoled, score 1.
	If cry is high pitched and infant is inconsolable, score 2.
Requires oxygen for saturation >95%	Look for changes in oxygenation. Infants experiencing pain manifest decreases in oxygenation as measured by total carbon dioxide or oxygen saturation. (Consider other causes of changes in oxygenation, such as atelectasis, pneumothorax, oversedation.)
	If no oxygen is required, score 0.
	If <30% oxygen is required, score 1.
	If >30% oxygen is required, score 2.
Increased vital signs	Note: Measure blood pressure last because this may wake the infant, causing difficulty with other assessments. Use baseline preoperative parameters from a nonstressed period.
	Multiply baseline heart rate (HR) × 0.2; then add this to baseline HR to determine the HR that is 20% over baseline. Do likewise for blood pressure (BP). Use mean BP.
	If HR and BP are both unchanged or less than baseline, score 0.
	If HR or BP is increased but increase is <20% of baseline, score 1.
	If either one is increased >20% over baseline, score 2.
Expression	The facial expression most often associated with pain is a grimace. This may be characterized by brow lowering, eyes squeezed shut, deepening of the nasolabial furrow, open lips and mouth.
	If no grimace is present, score 0.
	If grimace alone is present, score 1.
	If grimace and noncry vocalization grunt are present, score 2.
Sleepless	This is scored based on the infant's state during the hour preceding this recorded score.
	If the child has been continuously asleep, score 0.
	If he or she has awakened at frequent intervals, score 1.
	If he or she has been awake constantly, score 2.

*Neonatal pain assessment tool developed at the University of Missouri—Columbia.
From Krechel, S.W., & Bildner, J. (1995). CRIES: A new neonatal postoperative pain measurement score. Initial testing of validity and reliability. *Paediatric Anaesthesia, 5*(1), 53–61.

research evidence, policies, and standards of practice focused on assessing and managing pain in newborns, acute infant pain remains undermanaged and, in some cases, unmanaged (Gardner et al., 2016).

Nonpharmacologic Management

A variety of nonpharmacologic pain management techniques are used with neonates. Combining two or more nonpharmacologic methods can result in more effective pain reduction (Gabriel, de Mendoza, Figueroa, et al., 2013).

One of the most common measures is swaddling or snugly wrapping the infant with a blanket. Swaddling limits the neonate's boundaries, aids in self-regulation, and reduces physiologic and behavioral stress resulting from acute pain (Riddell, Racine, Turcotte, et al., 2012). Swaddling is popular among nurses and parents as a comfort measure for calming a fussy baby and for promoting sleep. However, it is important that it is done properly. Safe swaddling involves wrapping the infant snugly in a lightweight blanket with the arms extended, legs flexed, and hips in neutral position without rotation (Fig. 23.20, *A*) (AAP, 2014). In the early newborn period, nurses often swaddle infants with the arms flexed (see Fig. 23.20, *B*).

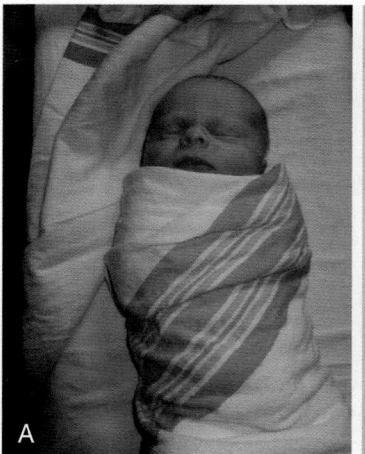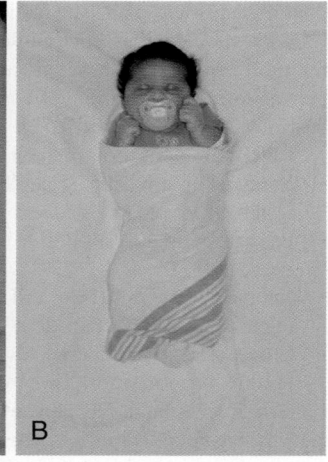

FIG 23.20 A, Newborn is swaddled with arms extended. **B,** Newborn is swaddled with arms flexed. (A, Courtesy of Jennifer and Travis Alderman, Durham, NC. B, Courtesy of Cheryl Briggs, RNC, Annapolis, MD.)

Swaddling an infant tightly with legs extended is associated with increased risk for hip dislocation (developmental dysplasia of the hip [DDH]). The correct way to swaddle an infant is with the hips in slight flexion and abducted and allowing freedom of movement of the knees. It is important that the blanket is not wrapped too tightly as it can cause overheating or respiratory compromise. There should be space for two to three adult fingers between the infant's chest and the swaddle. A swaddled infant should be lying on his or her back. Swaddling is not recommended after approximately 2 months of age when the infant is capable of rolling over (AAP, 2014).

Other nonpharmacologic pain relief measures are used by nurses and parents. Facilitated tucking, a hand-swaddling technique in which the care provider holds the neonate in a flexed, side-lying position, is effective for reducing pain and distress in preterm infants (Riddell et al., 2012).

Nonnutritive sucking (NNS) on a pacifier is a common comfort measure used with newborns. Oral sucrose in small amounts given with a syringe with or without a pacifier for sucking is safe and effective in reducing neonatal pain during painful procedures such as venipunctures or heelsticks (Cignacco, Sellam, Stoffel, et al., 2012; Kassab, Roydhouse, Fowler, et al., 2012; Riddell et al., 2012; Stevens, Yamada, Lee, et al., 2013). Oral sucrose and NNS used in combination before or during a painful procedure can help reduce discomfort (Naughton, 2013).

SSC with the mother who holds the infant prone on her chest, also known as *kangaroo care,* during a painful procedure can help reduce pain (Johnston, Campbell-Yeo, Fernandes, et al., 2014; Kostandy, Anderson, & Good, 2013; Riddell et al., 2012). Breastfeeding or breast milk helps reduce pain during heel lancing and blood collection (Academy of Breastfeeding Medicine Protocol Committee, 2010; Shah, Herbozo, Aliwalas, et al., 2012).

Distraction with visual, oral, auditory, or tactile stimulation can be helpful in term neonates or older infants (see Evidence-Based Practice box: Nonpharmacologic Pain Relief for Newborns). Sensorial saturation uses multiple senses to diminish minor pain. This technique involves speaking softly to the infant, massaging the face, and providing oral sucrose solution on the tongue (Bellieni, Tei, Coccina, et al., 2012).

Other nonpharmacologic measures for reducing pain in newborns include touch, massage, rocking, holding, and environmental modification (e.g., low noise and lighting).

Pharmacologic Management

Pharmacologic agents are used to alleviate pain associated with procedures. Local anesthesia is routinely used during procedures such as circumcision. Topical anesthesia is used for circumcision, lumbar puncture, venipuncture, and heelsticks. Nonopioid analgesia (oral liquid acetaminophen) is effective for mild to moderate pain from inflammatory conditions. Morphine and fentanyl are the most widely used opioid analgesics for pharmacologic management of neonatal pain. Continuous or bolus IV infusion of opioids provides effective and safe pain control. Other methods for managing neonatal pain are epidural infusion, local and regional nerve blocks, and intradermal or topical anesthetics (Gardner et al., 2016).

PROMOTING PARENT-INFANT INTERACTION

Nurses play an important role in promoting early social interaction between parents and their newborn infant. From birth throughout the hospital stay, nurses assess attachment behaviors (see Chapter 20) and provide support and education to parents as they become acquainted with the neonate. Nurses working in outpatient settings or home care provide follow-up assessments and care related to parent-child

🌐 **CULTURAL CONSIDERATIONS**

Cultural Beliefs and Practices Related to Infant Care

Nurses working with childbearing families from other cultures and ethnic groups must be aware of cultural beliefs and practices that are important to individual families. People with a strong sense of heritage may hold on to traditional health beliefs long after adopting other U.S. lifestyle practices. These health beliefs can involve practices regarding the newborn. For example, some Asians, Hispanics, Eastern Europeans, and Native Americans delay breastfeeding until the mother's milk is "in" (day 3 or 4) because they believe that colostrum is "bad." Some Hispanics and African-Americans place a belly band over the infant's umbilicus. In some Hispanic cultures, infants wear a special bracelet to help protect them from the evil eye (mal de ojo) (see photo). The birth of a male child is generally preferred by Asians and Eastern Indians, and some Asians and Haitians delay naming their infants. Families of Hindu heritage name the baby on the 11th day during a "cradle ceremony." Some women from India keep the cord of a male infant as a good omen that will ward off evil and will bring them more male infants in the future. The practice of skin-to-skin contact after birth may conflict with cultural beliefs about thermoregulation; some women from Africa prefer that the newborn is wrapped prior to being placed on the mother's chest. On the other hand, women from Mexico are wrapped in warm blankets after birth and wrap the newborn inside their blankets. Cultural beliefs influence when the newborn is taken out of the house, such as after the cord falls off, or after the mother's confinement period is over (approximately 30 days after birth). Weighing the infant can raise concerns for some women such as those from rural India, who may believe that frequent weighing will slow the infant's growth.

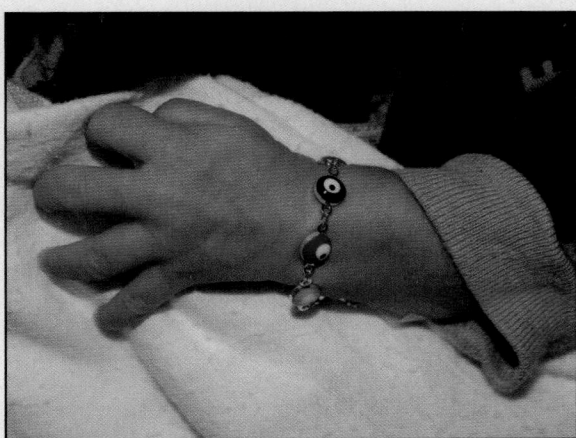

Newborn wearing "evil eye" bracelet. (Courtesy of Cheryl Briggs, RNC, Annapolis, MD.)

Data from Giger, J.N. (2013). *Transcultural nursing* (6th ed.). St. Louis, MO: Mosby; Purnell, L.D. (2014). *Culturally competent health care* (3rd ed.). Philadelphia, PA: FA Davis.

interactions. By teaching parents to recognize infant cues and respond appropriately, the nurse facilitates development of the parents' confidence in meeting the needs of their newborn (see Patient Teaching box: Helping Parents Recognize, Interpret, and Respond to Newborn Behaviors).

The sensitivity of the parent to the social responses of the infant is basic to the development of a mutually satisfying parent-child relationship. Sensitivity increases over time as parents become more aware of their infant's social capabilities. In supporting parents, nurses need to consider cultural beliefs and traditions that influence parenting behaviors and infant care practices (see Cultural Considerations box: Cultural Beliefs and Practices Related to Infant Care).

EVIDENCE-BASED PRACTICE
Nonpharmacologic Pain Relief for Newborns

Ask the Question

PICOT Question: For term newborns, what complementary or alternative pain relief is effective for minor painful procedures, such as heelstick?

Search for the Evidence

Search Strategies: English language research-based publications on newborn, pain, kangaroo care, skin-to-skin contact (SSC), breastfeeding, heelstick, sucrose were included.

Databases Used: Cochrane Collaborative Database, National Guidelines Clearinghouse (AHRQ), CINAHL, and PubMed.

Critical Appraisal of the Evidence

Pain scales in newborns are used to assess physical and behavioral changes to determine pain levels. Physical measures typically include heart rate, respiratory rate, and peripheral oxygen saturation. Other physiologic measures include gas exchange across skin, skin sensitivity measures, and electroencephalogram (EEG). Ways to measure behavioral changes include various scales utilizing breathing patterns, states of arousal, facial tension, leg movement, activity, cry and consolability.

Cochrane Database systematic analyses revealed the following:

- Sucrose is effective at decreasing pain response for single painful procedures, especially when paired with sucking (Stevens, Yamada, & Ohlsson, 2016).
- Skin-to-skin contact during painful procedures, such as heelstick, decreases behavioral pain scores, but not physiologic measures, and is safe. SSC with breastfeeding is the first choice for single painful procedures, for the multisensorial and synergistic comfort it brings. It also provides the parents a caretaking role (Johnston, Campbell-Yeo, Fernandes, et al., 2014).
- For preterm infants until 3 years of age, pain reactivity and immediate pain regulation were significantly improved with nonnutritive sucking, swaddling, and holding/rocking (Pillai Riddell, Racine, Gennis, et al., 2015).

A randomized control study of 102 newborns found that the smells of lavender and breast milk decreased both physiologic and behavioral responses to pain during heelstick more than control (Akcan & Polat, 2016).

Apply the Evidence: Nursing Implications

- For newborns who experienced a painful stimuli, subsequent painful procedures caused increased response (Gokulu, Bigen, Ozdemir, et al., 2016). This has implications for decreasing the initial pain response as much as possible, especially in the neonatal critical care setting where multiple painful stimuli may be necessary.
- Nonpharmacologic pain relief methods for newborns utilize the gate-control theory to distract the newborn's attention by using strong single or multisensorial

stimulation. Warmth, touch, sensory attention, swaddling, rocking, sucking a sweet solution, and smells decrease pain scores.

- Parents who are taught these techniques become active participants in their newborn's procedural care. However, they need clear education that using sucrose is not an appropriate long-term strategy for use at home.
- Comfort measures may work best when initiated a few minutes prior to the procedure, to allow the newborn time to relax and reorganize.
- Procedures other than single heelstick or needlestick should be evaluated for pharmacologic analgesia.

Quality and Safety Competencies: Evidence-Based Practice*
Knowledge

Describe how the strength and relevance of available evidence influences the choice of interventions in provision of patient-centered care.

Multisensorial stimulation which includes SSC, sucrose, and sucking have the best evidence for pain relief for newborns receiving a painful stimulus.

Skills

Participate in structuring the work environment to facilitate integration of new evidence into standards of practice.

Nurses can use various methods to provide comfort and reduce pain during painful procedures.

Parents can learn skills to manage their newborn's pain.

Attitudes

Value the need for continuous improvement in clinical practice based on new knowledge.

Nurses can explain to parents the evidence for pain relief in newborns, and advocate for effective pain relief measures.

References

Akcan, E., & Polat, S. (2016). Comparative effect of the smells of amniotic fluid, breast milk, and lavender on newborns' pain during heel lance. *Breastfeeding Medicine, 11*(6), 309–314.

Gokulu, G., Bigen, H., Ozdemir, H., et al. (2016). Comparative heel stick study showed that newborn infants who had undergone repeated painful procedures showed increased short-term pain responses. *Acta Paediatrica, 105*(11), e520–e525.

Johnston, C., Campbell-Yeo, M., Fernandes, A., et al. (2014). Skin-to-skin care for procedural pain in neonates. *Cochrane Database of Systematic Reviews, 2014*(1), CD008435.

Pillai Riddell, R. R., Racine, N. M., Gennis, H. G., et al. (2015). Non-pharmacological management of infant and young child procedural pain. *Cochrane Database of Systematic Reviews, 2015*(12), CD006275.

Stevens, B., Yamada, J., & Ohlsson, A. (2016). Sucrose for analgesia in newborn infants undergoing painful procedures. *Cochrane Database of Systematic Reviews, 2016*(7), CD001069.

Pat Mahaffee Gingrich

*Adapted from QSEN at www.qsen.org/

The activities of daily care during the neonatal period are ideal for infant and family interactions. While caring for their newborn, the mother and father (or other family member) can talk to the infant, play baby games, caress and cuddle the baby, and perhaps use infant massage. Feeding is an optimal time for interaction because the infant is usually awake and alert, at least at the beginning of the feeding. Too much stimulation should be avoided after feeding and before a sleep period. In Fig. 23.21, a great-grandmother and infant are shown engaging in arousal, imitation of facial expression, and smiling. Older children's contact with a newborn is encouraged and supervised based on the developmental level of the child (Fig. 23.22). Parents often keep memento books that record the birth, the hospital stay, and their infant's progress. Other parents create blogs to share their development as a family.

DISCHARGE PLANNING AND PARENT EDUCATION

Infant care activities can cause anxiety for new parents. Support from nurses influences whether new parents seek and accept help in the future. It is best for the nurse to avoid trying to cover all the content about newborn care at one time because the parents can be overwhelmed by too much information and become more anxious. Instead, parent education should occur throughout the hospital stay. Printed materials about newborn care are usually given to parents to augment the teaching done by the mother-baby or postpartum nurses. Some birthing facilities provide information about newborn care on their websites (e.g., www.mombaby.org). Nurses can direct parents to reliable websites for information on infant care (e.g., www.healthychildren.org). Some facilities

PATIENT TEACHING

Helping Parents Recognize, Interpret, and Respond to Newborn Behaviors

Learning to read a baby's body language can enable parents to be more effective in preventing and solving problems around the infant's sleeping, eating, and crying and enhances parent-infant interaction. Nurses can teach new parents the following:

1. Identify three newborn "zones" (traditionally referred to as *newborn states*).
   - "Resting zone": also known as *sleep states*
     - *Still/deep sleep:* Baby is completely still. Breathing is regular. No spontaneous activity. No movement of eyes, and eyelids stay shut. No vocalizing. Muscles are totally relaxed.
     - *Active/light sleep:* Baby may wiggle or vocalize. Eyes may flash open. Baby may make sucking movements—but still be asleep.
   - "Ready zone": *alert state*
     - Baby's eyes are bright. Baby can focus on an object or person. Baby reacts to stimulation. Motor activity is minimal.
   - "Rebooting zone": *fussy/crying state*
     - Baby's motor activity increases and is jerky. Baby is less responsive and moves from fussing to crying.
2. Identify signs of stress.
   - When babies are stressed or overstimulated, they show changes in their body and behavior. These changes are called *SOSs* (Signs of Over-Stimulation), traditionally referred to as a baby's *stress response*.
     - *Body SOSs:* changes in color (becoming more red or pale); changes in breathing (becoming more irregular or choppy); changes in movement (becoming jerky or having more tremors)
     - *Behavioral SOSs:* "spacing out" (going from an alert state to a drowsy state); "switching off" (gaze aversion, or looking away from parent); "shutting down" (going from drowsy to a sleep state)
   - When baby shows an SOS, parents should *decrease* stimulation and *increase* support by doing one or several of the following:
     - Quiet one's voice.
     - Glance away from baby.
     - Encourage baby to suck a finger or mother's breast.
     - Swaddle baby.
     - Place baby skin-to-skin.

3. Help baby sleep well.
   - Distinguish active/light sleep from still/deep sleep.
   - Parent's care:
     - *Prepare baby to sleep:* swaddling may help; feed in quiet, dark room at night and active, light environment during day.
     - *Get baby to sleep:* put baby down for sleep while he or she is still awake.
     - *Help baby stay asleep:* don't pick up during active/light sleep.
     - After breastfeeding is well established, notice when sleeping baby moves into active/light sleep. Wait and see if baby will transition from active/light sleep back to deep/still sleep—and sleep a bit longer.
4. Help baby eat well.
   - Recognize early signs of hunger during the first few weeks: wiggling, making sucking movements, bringing hand to mouth.
   - Notice if a fragile baby "spaces out" or "shuts down" when trying to eat. Bring this baby skin-to-skin and decrease stimulation before resuming feeding.
   - If a parent needs to wake a fragile or small baby to eat, do so from active/light sleep, not from still/deep sleep.
5. Help crying baby: consider what "TO DO."
   - **T:** *Talk* quietly to baby in sing-song voice.
   - **O:** *Observe* to see if baby takes self-calming actions: brings his or her hand to his or her mouth, making sucking movements, or moves into the fencing reflex position.
   - **DO:** *Bring* baby's hands to his or her chest; encourage sucking; make gentle "shooshing" sounds; swaddle baby; and/or bring baby skin-to-skin.
6. Play with baby so he or she can learn and grow.
   - Demonstrate baby's ability to look at a parent's face, watch a toy move, or turn to parent's voice.
   - Watch for an SOS during play. If an SOS occurs, decrease stimulation and increase support as described previously.
   - Observe baby's developing process of interaction: first, getting quiet and still; second, turning toward parent; third, turning toward and looking at parent.
   - Reinforce benefits of sensitive, face-to-face parent interaction with baby.

Data from Tedder, J.L. (2008). Give them the HUG: An innovative approach to helping parents understand the language of their newborn. *Journal of Perinatal Education, 17*(2), 14–20; Tedder, J.L. (2017). *H.U.G.: Help-understanding-guidance for young families.* Retrieved from hugyourbaby.org.

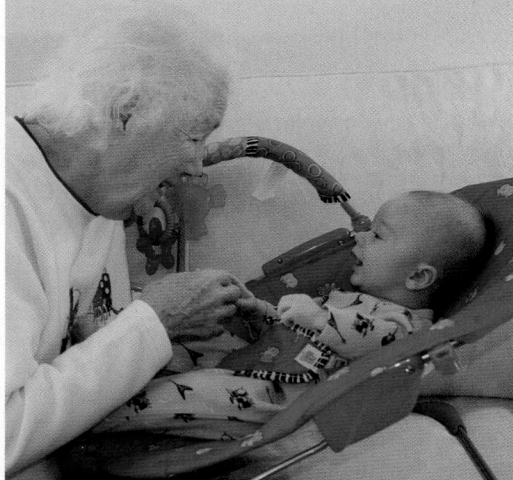

FIG 23.21 Great-grandmother and infant enjoying social interaction. (Courtesy of Freida Belding, Bird City, KS.)

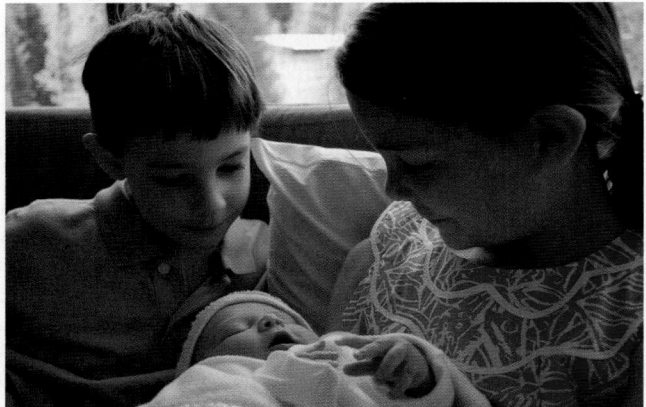

FIG 23.22 Older siblings meet their newborn sister. (Courtesy of Allison and Matthew Wyatt, Eagle, CO.)

have around-the-clock television programming on topics related to newborn and postpartum care. Postpartum and newborn home visitation programs may be available; the home visit nurse assesses the parents' learning needs and provides appropriate information.

To set priorities for teaching, the nurse follows parental cues. Knowledge deficits or gaps should be identified before beginning to teach. Normal growth and development and the changing needs of the infant (e.g., for personal interaction and stimulation, growth milestones, exercise, injury prevention, and social contacts), as well as the topics that follow, should be included during discharge planning with parents. Safety issues should be addressed (see Patient Teaching box: Infant Safety).

Temperature

Parents need to understand practical information related to thermoregulation. The nurse discusses the following topics in parent teaching:

- The causes of changes in body temperature (e.g., overwrapping, cold stress with resultant vasoconstriction, or minimal response to infection) and the body's response to extremes in environmental temperature
- Ways to promote normal body temperature, such as dressing the infant appropriately for the environmental air temperature and protecting the infant from exposure to direct sunlight
- Technique for taking the newborn's axillary temperature, and normal values for axillary temperature
- Signs to be reported to the primary health care provider such as high or low temperatures with accompanying fussiness, lethargy, irritability, poor feeding, and excessive crying

Respirations

The nurse provides information to parents regarding the normal characteristics of newborn respirations, emergency procedures, and measures to protect the infant. It is helpful to discuss signs of respiratory infection and to offer suggestions related to care of the infant who experiences symptoms. The following points are included in teaching about respirations:

- Normal variations in the rate and rhythm of respirations
- Reflexes such as sneezing to clear the airway
- Use of the bulb syringe
- Steps to take if the infant appears to be choking
- The need to protect the infant from the following:
  - Exposure to people with upper respiratory tract infections and respiratory syncytial virus
  - Exposure to secondhand tobacco smoke
  - Suffocation from loose bedding, water beds, and beanbag chairs; drowning (in bath water); entrapment under excessive bedding or in soft bedding; anything tied around the infant's neck; poorly constructed playpens, bassinets, or cribs
- Avoid the use of baby powder or corn starch; these substances can cause lung irritation
- Notify the health care provider if the infant develops symptoms such as difficulty breathing or swallowing, nasal congestion, excess drainage of mucus, coughing, sneezing, decreased interest in feeding, or fever.
- If the infant has a respiratory illness such as the "common cold," the following suggestions can be helpful:
  - Feed smaller amounts more often to prevent overtiring the infant.
  - Hold the infant in an upright position to feed.
  - For sleeping, raise the infant's head and chest by raising the mattress 30 degrees (do *not* use a pillow).
  - Avoid drafts; do not overdress the baby.
  - Use only medications prescribed by a pediatric health care provider. Do not use over-the-counter medications without provider approval.

PATIENT TEACHING
Infant Safety

- Always lay the baby flat in bed (in the bassinet or crib) on his or her back for sleep, for naps, and at night. Do not place your infant on the abdomen for sleep.
- Room-sharing, but not bed-sharing, is recommended during the early weeks.
- Never put your baby on a cushion, pillow, beanbag, or waterbed to sleep. Your baby may suffocate.
- There should be no bumper pads, blankets, stuffed toys, or other soft objects in the baby's crib because of the risk for suffocation.
- Do not cover the baby with blankets or quilts; dress the baby in light sleep clothing such as a sleep sack or one-piece sleeper.
- Check your baby's crib for safety. Slats should be no more than $2\frac{1}{4}$ inches apart. The space between the mattress and sides should be less than 2 fingerwidths. The bedposts should have no decorative knobs.
- The crib mattress should be firm and should fit snugly against the crib rails.
- Do not use a crib with drop rails.
- Never leave your baby alone on a bed, couch, or table. Even newborns can move enough to eventually reach the edge and fall off.
- When using an infant carrier, place the carrier on the floor in a place where you can see the baby. It should never be on a high place, such as a table, sofa, or store counter.
- Infant carriers do not keep your baby safe in a car. Always place your baby in an approved car safety seat when traveling in a motor vehicle (car, truck, bus, or van). Car safety seats are recommended for travel on trains and airplanes as well. Use the car safety seat for every ride. Your baby should be in a rear-facing infant car safety seat from birth until 2 years of age or until exceeding the car seat's limits for height and weight. The car safety seat should be in the back seat of the car (see Fig. 23.26). This precaution is especially important in vehicles with front passenger air bags because when air bags inflate, they can be fatal for infants and toddlers. If an infant must ride in the front seat, disable the air bag.
- When bathing your baby, never leave him or her alone. Newborns and infants can drown in 1 to 2 inches of water.
- Be sure that your hot water heater is set at 49° C (120° F) or less. Always check bath water temperature with your elbow before putting your baby in the bath.
- Do not tie anything around your baby's neck. Pacifiers, for example, tied around the neck with a ribbon or string can strangle your baby.
- Keep the crib or playpen away from window blinds and drapery cords; your baby could strangle on them.
- Keep the crib and playpen well away from radiators, heat vents, and portable heaters. Linens in the crib or playpen can catch fire if they come into contact with these heat sources.
- Install smoke detectors on every floor of your home. Check them once a month to be sure they are working properly. Change batteries twice a year.
- Avoid exposing your baby to cigarette or cigar smoke in your home or other places. Passive exposure to tobacco smoke greatly increases the likelihood that your infant will have respiratory symptoms and illnesses. It also increases the risk for sudden infant death syndrome (SIDS).
- Be gentle with your baby. Do not pick up your baby or swing your baby by the arms or throw him or her up in the air. Never shake the baby.

Data from American Academy of Pediatrics Task Force on Sudden Infant Death Syndrome. (2011). SIDS and other sleep-related infant deaths: Expansion of recommendations for a safe infant sleeping environment. *Pediatrics, 128*(5), e1341-e1367; National Institute of Child Health and Human Development. (2014). *Sudden infant death (SIDS) and other sleep-related causes of infant death: Questions and answers for health care providers.* Rockville, MD: Author; National Highway Traffic Safety Administration (NHTSA) Parents Central. (2012). *From car seats to car keys: Keeping kids safe.* Washington, DC: Author.

- Use nasal saline drops in each nostril and suction well with bulb syringe to decrease and relieve secretions.

Feeding Patterns

Nurses instruct parents about infant feeding and provide assistance based on whether they have chosen breastfeeding, expressed milk feeding, formula feeding, or a combination. Feeding patterns and practices for newborns are discussed in Chapter 24.

Elimination

Awareness of the normal elimination patterns of newborns helps parents recognize problems related to voiding or stooling. The following points are included in teaching about elimination:

- Color of normal urine and number of voidings to expect each day: at least two to six for the first 1 to 3 days; then a minimum of six to eight voidings per day thereafter. Urine should be pale yellow (like lemonade).
- Changes to be expected in the color and consistency of the stool (i.e., meconium to transitional to soft yellow or golden yellow) and the number of bowel movements, plus the odor of stools for breastfed or bottle-fed infants (see Box 22.1).
  - Formula-fed infants may have as few as one stool every other day after the first few weeks of life; stools are pasty to semi-formed.
  - Breastfed infants should have at least three stools every 24 hours for the first few weeks. The stools are looser and resemble mustard mixed with cottage cheese; the odor is less offensive than stools of infants who are formula fed.

Sleeping, Positioning, and Holding

Infants should be placed in the supine position for sleep during the first year of life to prevent sudden infant death syndrome (SIDS). Infants should lie on a firm surface, specifically on a firm crib mattress covered by a fitted sheet. Soft materials such as bumper pads, comforters, quilts, pillows, sheepskins, or stuffed toys should not be placed in the crib. Room sharing, but not bed sharing, is recommended during infant sleep for at least the first 6 months and ideally for the first year. Bed sharing can increase the risk for suffocation and falls. Infants may be brought into the parent's bed for comforting or for breastfeeding but should be returned to the crib or bassinet before the parent goes to sleep (AAP Task Force on Sudden Infant Death Syndrome [SIDS], 2016; National Institute of Child Health and Human Development [NICHD], 2014) (see Patient Teaching box: Infant Safety).

Parent education prior to hospital discharge should include specific information about safe sleep practices. The Safe to Sleep campaign from the National Institute of Child Health and Human Development provides materials for health care professionals and parents (http://safetosleep.nichd.nih.gov). The educational resources are designed to reach culturally diverse audiences with messages about promoting a safe sleep environment and preventing SIDS. (See Clinical Reasoning Case Study: Safe Infant Sleep Practices.)

Anatomically, the infant's shape—a barrel chest and flat, curveless spine—facilitates the infant to roll from the side to the prone position; therefore, the side-lying position for sleep is not recommended. When the infant is awake, "tummy time" can be provided under parental supervision so the infant can begin to develop appropriate muscle tone for eventual crawling; placing the infant prone at intervals when awake aids in preventing a misshapen head (positional plagiocephaly) (AAP Task Force on SIDS, 2016).

Care must be taken to prevent the infant from rolling off flat, unguarded surfaces. When an infant is on such a surface, the parent or nurse who must turn away from the infant even for a moment should always keep one hand placed securely on the infant.

Safe Infant Sleep Practices

The mother-baby nurse is teaching the new parents, Allison and Matt, about safe sleep practices for their healthy term newborn son. The grandmother is listening and insists that all her babies slept most soundly when they were on their "tummies." Allison proudly shows the nurse a photo of the baby's nursery at home, including an antique crib with colorful fabric-covered bumper pads and a matching fluffy quilt. There are several stuffed animals in the crib. What information should the nurse provide related to safety concerns for the newborn?

1. Evidence—Is there sufficient evidence to draw conclusions about the safety of the sleep environment in terms of preventing sudden infant death syndrome or infant injury?
2. Assumptions—What assumptions can be made about the following factors related to safe infant sleep?
   a. Infant positioning for sleep
   b. Risk for suffocation
   c. Risk for injury
3. What implications and priorities for nursing care can be drawn at this time?
4. Does the evidence objectively support your conclusion?
5. Interprofessional care—Describe the roles/responsibilities of members of the interprofessional health care team who may be involved in care management of this mother and her infant.

The infant is always held securely with the head supported because newborns are unable to maintain an erect head posture for more than a few moments. Fig. 23.23 illustrates various positions for holding an infant with adequate support.

Rashes
Diaper Rash

Many infants develop a diaper rash at some time. This is usually irritant contact dermatitis or skin inflammation appearing as redness, scaling, blisters, or papules. Various factors contribute to diaper rash including infrequent diaper changes, diarrhea, use of plastic pants to cover the diaper, a change in the infant's diet such as when solid foods are added, or when breastfeeding mothers eat certain foods.

Parents are instructed in measures to help prevent diaper rash. Diapers should be checked often and changed as soon as the infant voids or stools. Plain water with mild soap, if needed, is used to cleanse the diaper area; if baby wipes are used, they should be unscented and contain no alcohol. The infant's skin should be allowed to dry completely before applying another diaper.

When diaper rash occurs, it is helpful to use emollients, creams, or other protectants such as zinc oxide ointment to restore skin integrity while providing some protection from the irritants of urine and stool (Visscher, Adam, Brink, et al., 2015). Although diaper rash can be alarming to parents and annoying to babies, most cases resolve within a few days with simple home treatments. There are instances when diaper rash is more serious and requires medical treatment.

The warm, moist atmosphere in the diaper area provides an optimal environment for Candida albicans growth; dermatitis appears in the perianal area, inguinal folds, and lower abdomen. The affected area is intensely erythematous with a sharply demarcated, scalloped edge, often with numerous satellite lesions that extend beyond the larger lesion (AWHONN, 2013). Therapy consists of applications of an anticandidal ointment, such as clotrimazole or miconazole, with each diaper change. Sometimes the infant is given an oral antifungal preparation such as nystatin or fluconazole to eliminate any gastrointestinal source of infection.

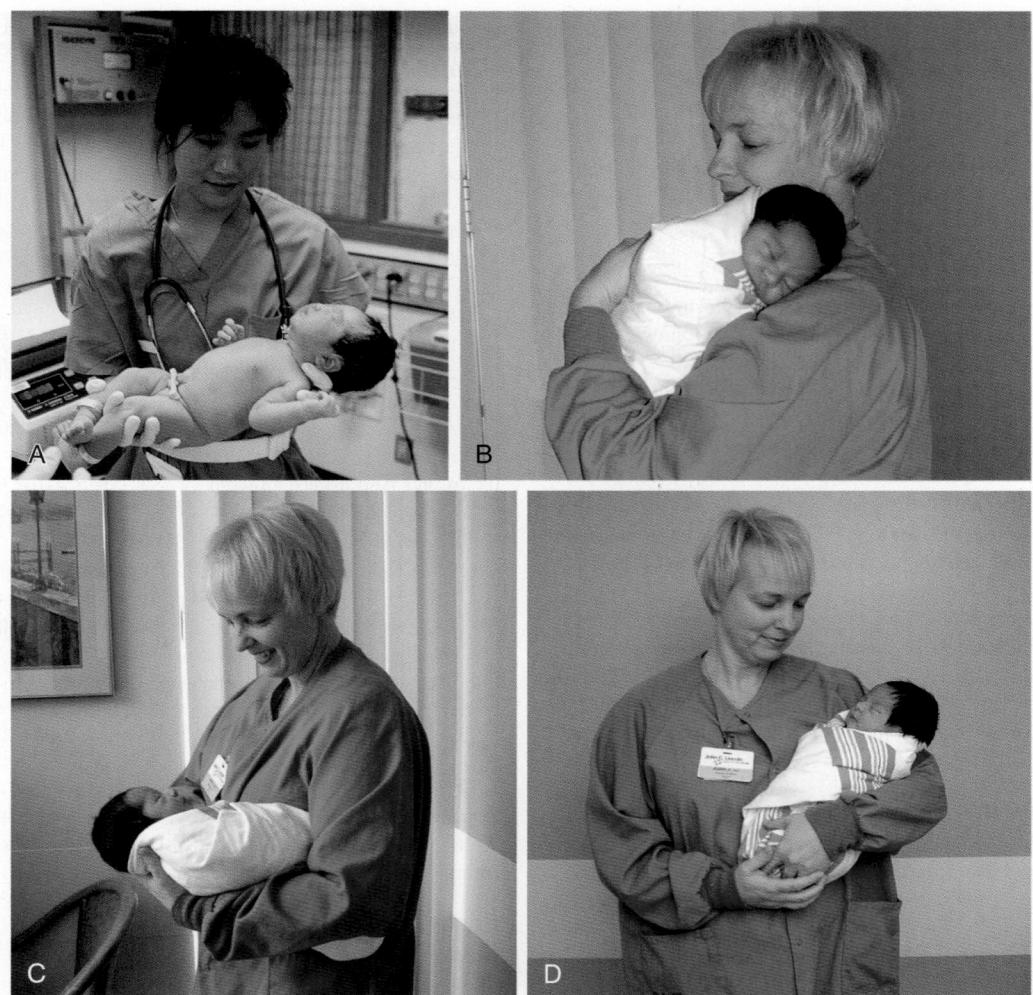

FIG 23.23 Holding the baby securely with support for head. **A,** Holding infant while moving infant from scale to bassinet. Baby is undressed to show posture. **B,** Holding baby upright in "burping" position. C, "Football" (under the arm) hold. D, Cradling hold. (A, Courtesy of Kim Molloy, Knoxville, IA. B, C, and D, Courtesy of Julie Perry Nelson, Loveland, CO.)

Other Rashes

A rash on the cheeks can result from the infant's scratching with long unclipped fingernails or from rubbing the face against the crib sheets, particularly if regurgitated stomach contents are not washed off promptly. The newborn's skin begins a natural process of peeling and sloughing after birth. Dry skin may be treated with an emollient applied once or twice daily (AWHONN, 2013). Newborn rash, erythema toxicum, is a common finding (see Fig. 22.7, *B*) and needs no treatment.

Clothing

Parents commonly ask how warmly they should dress their infant. A simple suggestion is to dress the child for the environment as they dress themselves, adding no more than one layer more than they would be wearing as adults. Overheating should be avoided (AAP Task Force on SIDS, 2016). A cap or bonnet is needed to protect the scalp and minimize heat loss if the weather is cool or to protect against sunburn. Overdressing in warm temperatures can cause discomfort, as can underdressing in cold weather. Parents are encouraged to dress the infant at all times in flame-retardant clothing. The eyes should be shaded if it is sunny and

hot. Infant sunglasses are available to protect the infant's eyes when outdoors (Fig. 23.24).

For sleep, infants can be placed in a safe sleeping bag or sleep sack with fitted neck and arm openings and no hood. Some hospitals use sleep sacks for all newborns (Fig. 23.25). A safe sleep sack prevents the infant from rolling over on the abdomen and keeps the legs contained so they do not go through the crib rails. For additional warmth, the infant can be dressed in fitted clothing in layers as needed prior to being placed in the sleep sack.

For the first 2 to 3 months until the infant is able to roll over, safe swaddling for sleep can be done using a lightweight blanket or wrap (not in combination with a sleep sack). The head, neck, and chin are not covered, and the wrap should not be tight around the chest or legs.

Car Seat Safety

Infants should travel only in federally approved rear-facing safety seats secured in the rear seat using the vehicle safety belt or an anchor and tether system (Fig. 23.26). The infant is secured in the car seat with a 5-point safety harness that goes over both shoulders, both hips, and buckles at the crotch. Shoulder harnesses are placed in the slots at or below the level of the infant's shoulders. The harness is snug, and the retainer clip is placed at the level of the infant's armpits as opposed to on the abdomen or neck area.

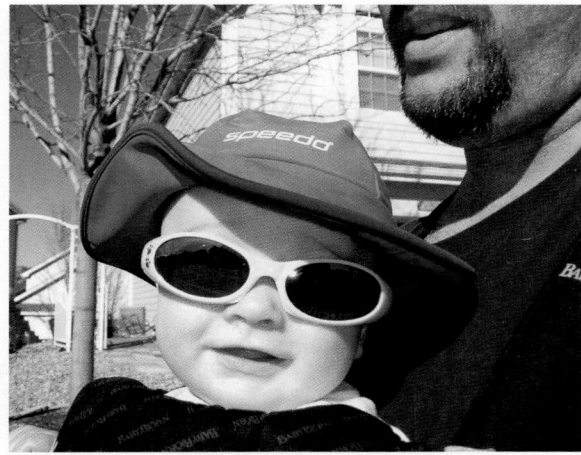

FIG 23.24 Sunglasses protect the infant's eyes. (Courtesy of Julie Perry Nelson, Loveland, CO.)

> ### ⚡ SAFETY ALERT
>
> Infants and toddlers should use a rear-facing car seat at least until the age of 2 years. The safest area of the car is the back seat. A car safety seat that faces the rear gives the best protection for an infant's disproportionately weak neck and heavy head. In this position, the force of a frontal crash is spread over the head, neck, and back; the back of the car safety seat supports the spine (AAP, 2017).

In cars equipped with front air bags, rear-facing infant seats should never be placed in the front seat. Serious injury can occur if the air bag inflates because these types of infant seats fit close to the dashboard. If the infant must ride in the front seat, the air bag must be turned off. For cars with side air bags, parents should read the vehicle owner's manual for information about placement of car seats next to a side air bag (AAP, 2017).

Infants are positioned at a 45-degree angle in a car seat to prevent slumping and subsequent airway obstruction. Many seats allow for adjustment of the seat angle. If the infant slouches down or to the side of the seat, a tightly rolled receiving blanket may be placed on each side of the infant (AAP, 2017).

Bulky clothing such as a coat or snow suit can compress if there is a car accident, causing the straps of the harness to loosen and placing the infant at risk for injury. Parents should dress their infant in thinner layers; for warmth, they can place a blanket or coat over the buckled harness straps (AAP, 2017).

Parents need to know that the most appropriate and safest car seat for their infant is based on the infant's age as well as on the type of vehicle in which the car seat will be installed. If parents need help or have questions, there are National Child Passenger Safety Certified Technicians located in most communities (http://cert.safekids.org/). Some hospitals have staff members with the certification.

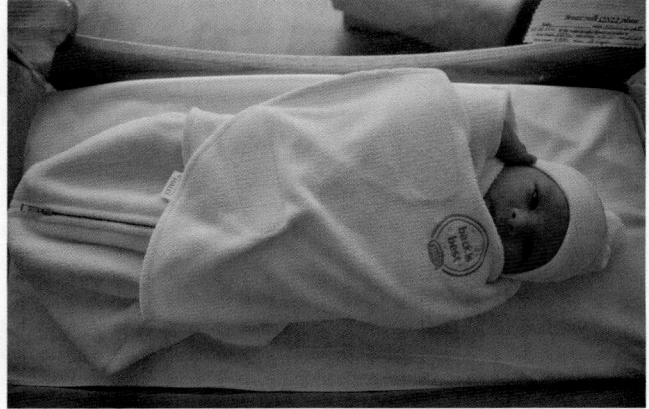

FIG 23.25 Newborn in sleep sack. (Courtesy of Allison and Matthew Wyatt, Eagle, CO.)

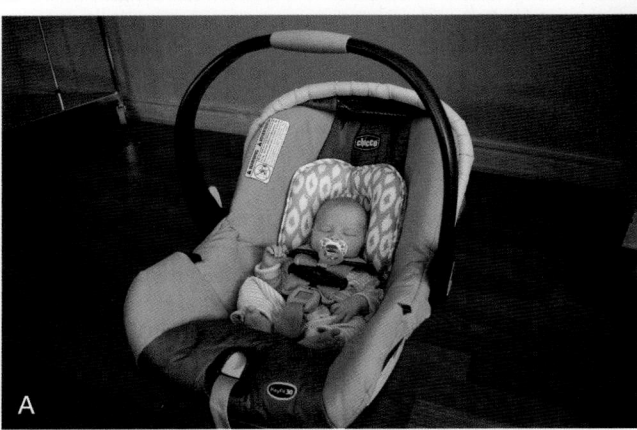
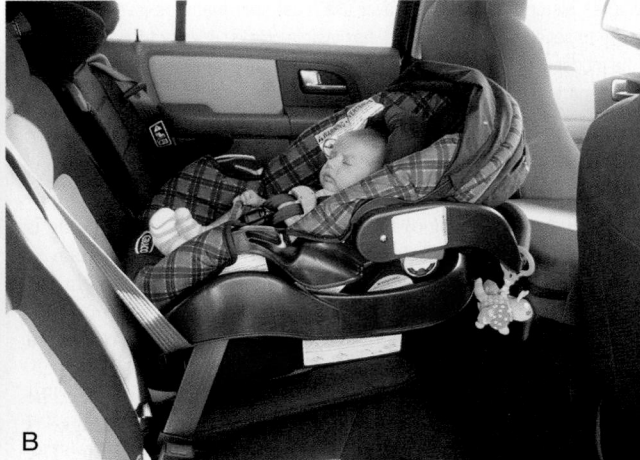

FIG 23.26 A, Newborn secured in car seat ready for hospital discharge. B, Rear-facing car seat in rear seat of car. Infant is placed in seat when going home from the hospital. (A, Courtesy of Allison and Matthew Wyatt, Eagle, CO. B, Courtesy of Brian and Mayannyn Sallee, Minot, ND.)

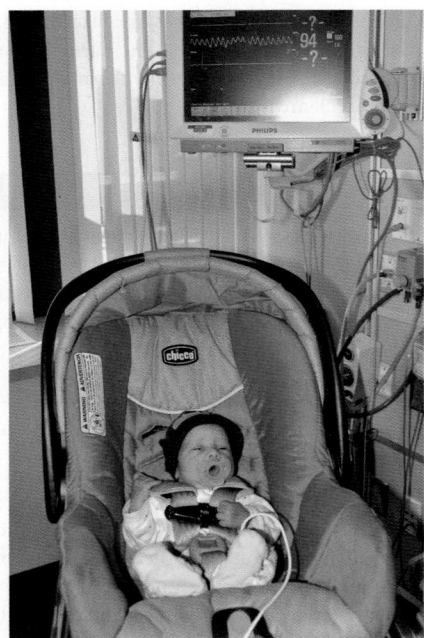

FIG 23.27 Infant Car Seat Challenge: testing is done before discharge from the birthing facility. Preterm infant is in car seat with pulse oximetry monitoring. (Courtesy of Cheryl Briggs, RNC, Annapolis, MD.)

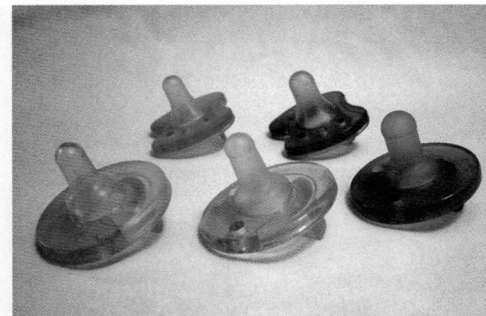

FIG 23.28 Safe pacifiers for term and preterm infants. Note one-piece construction, easily grasped handle, and large shield with ventilation holes. (Courtesy of Julie Perry Nelson, Loveland, CO.)

Before discharge from the birth institution, infants born at less than 37 weeks of gestation should be observed in a car seat (preferably their own) for at least 90 to 120 minutes or a period of time equal to the length of the car ride home. This is known as the Infant Car Seat Challenge. The infant is monitored for apnea, bradycardia, and a decrease in oxygen saturation (Fig. 23.27). If the infant exhibits any of these clinical signs, travel home should be in a Federal Motor Vehicle Safety Standard No. 213 (FMVSS 213)–approved car bed (Bull, Engle, & AAP, 2009).

> **⚡ SAFETY ALERT**
>
> If the parents do not have a car safety seat, arrangements should be made to make an appropriate seat available for purchase, loan, or donation. Parents need to be cautioned about purchasing a secondhand car safety seat without knowing its history. They should never use a car seat that was involved in a moderate to severe crash, is too old, has visible cracks, does not have a label with the model number and manufacture date, does not come with instructions, is missing parts, or was recalled (AAP, 2017).

Nonnutritive Sucking

Sucking provides pleasure for infants. However, sucking needs may not be satisfied by breastfeeding or bottle-feeding alone. In fact, sucking is such a strong need that infants who are deprived of sucking, such as those with a cleft lip, will suck on their tongues. Several benefits of nonnutritive sucking have been demonstrated, such as an increased weight gain in preterm infants, increased ability to maintain an organized state, and decreased crying.

There is compelling evidence that pacifiers help prevent SIDS. The AAP Task Force on Sudden Infant Death Syndrome (2016) suggests that parents consider offering a pacifier for naps and bedtime. The pacifier should be used when the infant is placed supine for sleep, and it should not be reinserted once the infant falls asleep. No infant should be forced to take a pacifier. Pacifiers must be cleaned often and replaced regularly and should not be coated with any type of sweet solution. Pacifier use for breastfeeding infants should be delayed for 3 to 4 weeks to ensure that breastfeeding is well established.

Problems arise when parents are concerned about the sucking of fingers, thumb, or pacifier and try to restrain this natural tendency. Before giving advice, nurses should investigate the parents' feelings and base the guidance they give on the information solicited. For example, some parents see no problem with the infant sucking on a thumb or finger but find the use of a pacifier objectionable. In general, either practice need not be restrained unless thumb sucking or pacifier use persists past 4 years of age or past the time when the permanent teeth erupt. Parents are advised to consult with their pediatric health care provider or pediatric dentist about this topic.

A parent's excessive use of the pacifier to calm the infant should also be explored, however. Placing a pacifier in the infant's mouth as soon as the infant begins to cry can reinforce a pattern of distress and relief.

> **⚡ SAFETY ALERT**
>
> If parents choose to let their infant use a pacifier, they need to be aware of certain safety considerations before purchasing one. A homemade or poorly designed pacifier can be dangerous because the entire object can be aspirated if it is small or a portion can become lodged in the pharynx. Improvised pacifiers, such as those made from a padded nipple, also pose dangers because the nipple can separate from the plastic collar and be aspirated. Safe pacifiers are made of one piece that includes a shield or flange large enough to prevent entry into the mouth and a handle that can be grasped (Fig. 23.28).

Bathing and Umbilical Cord Care
Bathing

Bathing serves several purposes. It provides opportunities for (1) cleansing the skin, (2) observing the infant's condition, (3) promoting comfort, and (4) parent-child-family interaction.

An important consideration in skin cleansing is the preservation of the skin's acid mantle, which is formed from the uppermost horny layer of the epidermis, sweat, superficial fat, metabolic products, and external substances such as amniotic fluid and microorganisms. To protect the newborn's skin, it is best to use a cleanser with a neutral pH and preferably without preservatives or with preservatives recognized as safe and well tolerated in neonates. Antimicrobial cleansers should not be used (AWHONN, 2013).

Neonatal skin care guidelines from AWHONN (2013) indicate that bathing should be performed according to agency protocols using sponge bathing, immersion, or swaddled bathing. Traditionally, sponge baths

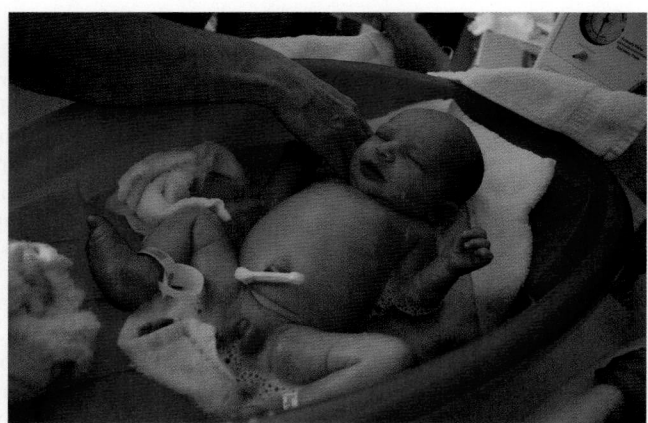

FIG 23.29 Initial newborn bath by immersion. (Courtesy of Allison and Matthew Wyatt, Eagle, CO.)

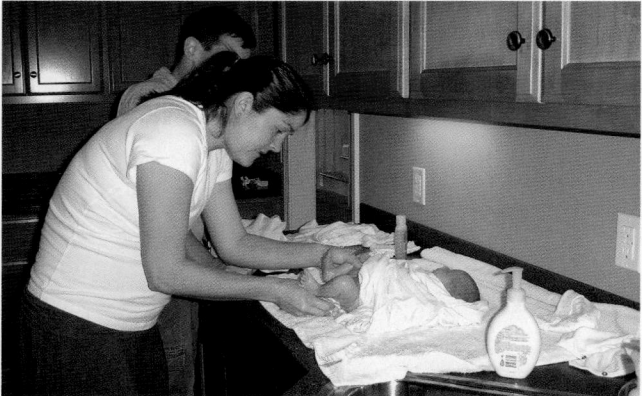

FIG 23.30 Mother and father giving newborn a sponge bath at home. (Courtesy of Allison and Matthew Wyatt, Eagle, CO.)

are given until the infant's umbilical cord falls off and the umbilicus is healed. For immersion bathing, the neonate is placed in warm water (38°C [100.4°F]) deep enough to cover the shoulders, but not the head and neck (Lund & Durand, 2016) (Fig. 23.29). Bathing by immersion has been found to allow less heat loss and provoke less crying. It has not been shown to increase the risk for bacterial colonization of the cord. Swaddled bathing is a type of immersion bathing in which the newborn is swaddled in a blanket or towel and immersed in a tub of warm water. One body part at a time is unwrapped and washed (AWHONN, 2013).

Ideally the initial bath is delayed for at least 2 hours after birth until the neonate has reached thermal and cardiorespiratory stability. In some birthing facilities, the bath is delayed for as long as 24 hours. This bath should be quick (5 to 10 minutes) and can be performed at the mother's bedside or in the nursery. Tap water and a minimal amount of pH neutral or slightly acidic cleanser are recommended. Following the bath, the infant should be immediately dried, diapered, and wrapped in warm blankets; a cap is placed on the head. Ten minutes later, the newborn is dressed, wrapped in warm blankets, and the cap is changed (AWHONN, 2013).

A daily bath is not necessary for achieving cleanliness and can do harm by disrupting the integrity of the newborn's skin. Cleansing the perineum after a soiled diaper and daily cleansing of the face are usually sufficient. In general, infants should not be bathed more frequently than every other day; the hair should be shampooed once or twice a week (AWHONN, 2013).

Bath time is an ideal time for parent-infant social interaction (Fig. 23.30). While bathing the baby, parents can talk to the infant, caress and cuddle the infant, and engage in arousal and imitation of facial expressions and smiling. Parents can pick a time for the bath that is easy for them and when the baby is awake, usually before a feeding.

Umbilical Cord Care

The goal of cord care is to prevent or decrease the risk for hemorrhage and infection. The umbilical cord stump is an excellent medium for bacterial growth and can easily become infected. Hospital protocol determines the technique for routine cord care. AWHONN (2013) recommendations for cord care include cleaning the cord with water (using cleanser sparingly if needed to remove debris) during the initial bath. Evidence does not support the routine use of antiseptic or antimicrobial preparations for cord care (AWHONN; Lund & Durand, 2016). However, the American Academy of Pediatrics recognizes the benefit of applying selected antimicrobial agents to the umbilical cords

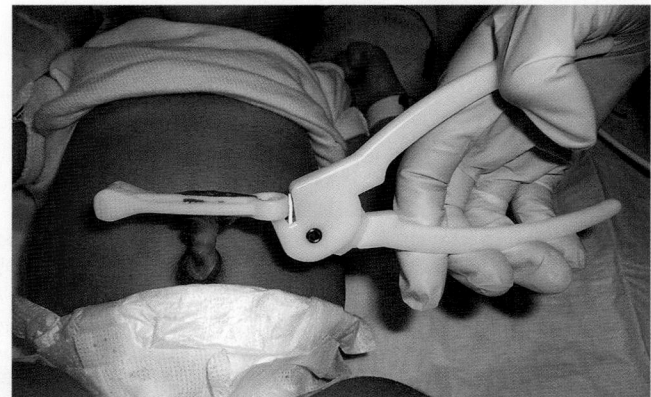

FIG 23.31 With special tool, nurse removes clamp after cord dries (approximately 24 to 48 hours after birth). (Courtesy of Cheryl Briggs, RNC, Annapolis, MD.)

of infants born at home in resource-limited countries, for births occurring outside of hospitals or birth centers, and in resource-limited populations such as Native American communities (Stewart, Benitz, Committee on Fetus and Newborn, 2016).

The plastic cord clamp that was applied at birth is removed once the stump has dried (Fig. 23.31), typically in 24 to 48 hours. The stump and base of the cord should be assessed for edema, redness, and purulent drainage with each diaper change. The area should be kept clean and dry and open to air or loosely covered with clothing. If soiled, the area is cleansed with plain water and dried thoroughly. The diaper is folded down and away from the stump (AWHONN, 2013). The umbilical cord begins to dry, shrivel, and blacken by the second or third day of life. The stump deteriorates through the process of dry gangrene; therefore, odor alone is not a positive indicator of omphalitis (infection of the umbilical stump). Cord separation time is influenced by several factors, including type of cord care, type of birth, and other perinatal events. The average cord separation time is 10 to 14 days, although it can take up to 3 weeks. Some dried blood may be seen in the umbilicus at separation (Fig. 23.32). Parents are instructed in appropriate home cord care (per pediatric health care practitioner or institution protocol) and the expected time of cord separation (see Patient Teaching box: Home Care: Bathing, Cord Care, Skin Care, and Nail Care for information regarding bathing, skin care, cord care, nail care, and dressing the infant).

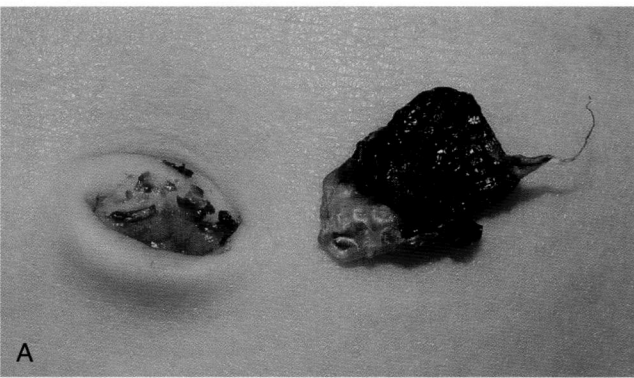

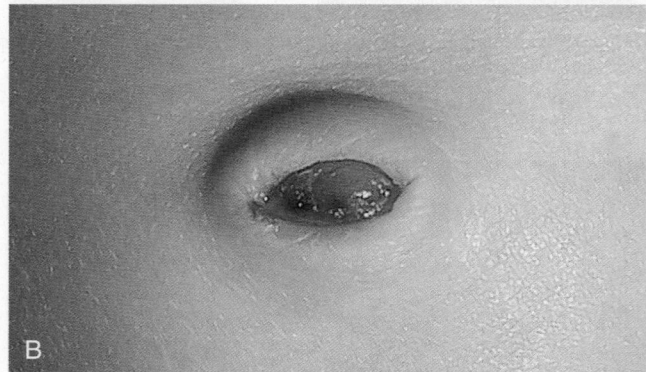

FIG 23.32 Cord separation. **A,** Cord separated with some dried blood still in the umbilicus. **B,** Umbilicus cleansed and beginning to heal. (Courtesy of Cheryl Briggs, RNC, Annapolis, MD.)

Infant Follow-Up Care

Follow-up care after discharge from the birthing facility usually occurs within 72 hours at the clinic or health care provider's office. This is especially important for breastfed newborns for monitoring their weight and hydration status. When infants are discharged at less than 48 hours of age, home care follow-up is an essential component of care. Home care may be provided either by a nurse as part of the routine follow-up care of infants or through a visiting nurse or community health nurse referral service.

Cardiopulmonary Resuscitation

All personnel working with infants must have current infant cardio-pulmonary resuscitation (CPR) certification. Additionally, health care personnel working in birth settings should be certified in neonatal resuscitation.

Parents should receive instruction in relieving airway obstruction and CPR. Classes are often offered in hospitals and clinics during the prenatal period or to parents of newborns. Such instruction is especially important for parents whose infants were preterm or have a history of cardiac or respiratory problems. Some grandparents take CPR classes. Babysitters should also learn CPR.

Practical Suggestions for the First Weeks at Home

Numerous changes occur during the first weeks of parenthood. Care management should be directed toward helping parents cope with infant care, role changes, altered lifestyle, and changes in family structure resulting from the addition of a new baby.

Parents must be helped to anticipate events during the transition from birthing facility to home. This is especially important for first-time

---

PATIENT TEACHING

Home Care: Bathing, Cord Care, Skin Care, and Nail Care

Timing
- Newborns do not need a bath every day. Every 2 or 3 days is often enough.
- Fit bath time into the family's schedule.
- Give a bath at any time convenient to you but not immediately after a feeding period because the increased handling can cause regurgitation.

Prevent Heat Loss
- The temperature of the room should be 26° to 27°C (79° to 81°F), and the bathing area should be free of drafts (close the door in the room where the bath is performed).
- The water temperature should be between 38° and 40°C (100° to <104°F). A water thermometer is useful for determining appropriate water temperature.
- Control heat loss during the bath to conserve the infant's energy. Bathe the infant quickly; with a sponge bath, expose only a portion of the body at a time; and dry thoroughly.

Gather Supplies and Clothing Before Starting
- Tub for water placed in a safe place on a sturdy surface
- Towels for drying the infant and a clean washcloth
- Mild cleanser with a neutral pH and preferably with no preservatives
- Diaper
- Clothing suitable for wearing indoors: shirt; stretch suit or nightgown optional
- Cotton balls
- Lightweight blanket

Bathe the Baby
- Take the infant to the bathing area when all supplies are ready.

- Never leave the infant alone on bath table or in the bathwater, not even for a second! If you have to leave, take the infant with you or place the infant back into the crib.
- Test the temperature of the water. Do not hold the infant under running water—the water temperature can change, and the infant can be scalded or chilled rapidly. For immersion bathing (tub bath), carefully lower the infant into the tub; the head and neck should be above the water. The tub should be filled with enough water to keep the baby's shoulders covered; this helps reduce heat loss. First wash the baby's face with a soft washcloth and plain water. Then proceed to wash the rest of the body, going from top to bottom.
- If sponge bathing is to be performed, undress the baby and wrap in a towel with the head exposed. Uncover and gently wash one part of the body at a time, taking care to keep the rest of the baby covered as much as possible to prevent heat loss.
- Begin by washing the baby's face with water; do not use soap on the face. Cleanse the eyes from the inner canthus outward using separate parts of a clean washcloth for each eye. For the first 2 to 3 days, a discharge can result from the reaction of the conjunctiva to the substance (erythromycin) used as a prophylactic measure against infection. After 2 to 3 days of age, any discharge should be considered abnormal and reported to the pediatric health care provider.
- Cleanse the ears and nose with twists of moistened cotton or a corner of the washcloth. Do not use cotton-tipped swabs because they can cause injury. The areas behind the ears need daily cleansing.
- Wash between the skinfolds. Place your hand under the baby's shoulders and lift gently to expose the neck, lift the chin, and wash the neck, taking care to cleanse between the skinfolds.

PATIENT TEACHING

Home Care: Bathing, Cord Care, Skin Care, and Nail Care—cont'd

- Wash the genital area last.
- If the hair is to be washed, begin by wrapping the infant in a towel with the head exposed. Hold the infant in a football position (under the arm) with one hand, using the other hand to wash the hair. Wash the scalp with water and shampoo that is mild for the eyes and safe for babies. Massage the scalp gently, rinse well, and dry thoroughly. A blow dryer is never used on an infant because the temperature is too hot for a baby's skin.
- Wash hair with baby wrapped to limit heat loss.

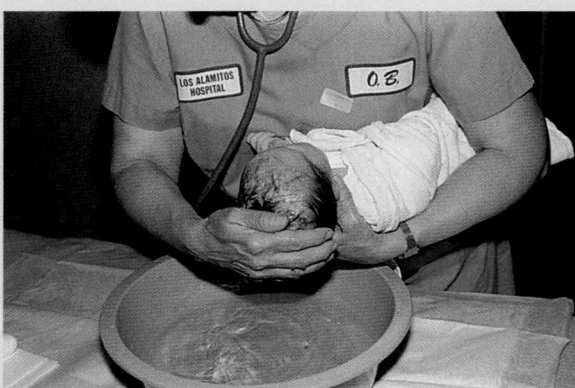

(Courtesy Marjorie Pyle, RNC, Lifecircle, Costa Mesa, CA.)

Skin Care

- If the skin appears dry or cracking, apply an emollient (lotion) once or twice daily. Check with your pediatric health care provider about the type of emollient to use.
- The fragile skin can be injured by too vigorous cleansing. If stool or other debris has dried and caked on the skin, soak the area to remove it. Do not attempt to rub it off because abrasion can result. Cleanse gently using a mild cleanser, and pat dry.
- Babies are very prone to sunburn and should be kept out of direct sunlight. Use of sunscreens should be discussed with the health care provider. For infants younger than 6 months of age, sunscreen is applied to areas not covered by protective clothing or shade such as the face and backs of the hands.
- Babies often develop rashes that are normal. Neonatal acne resembles pimples and can appear at 2 to 4 weeks of age, resolving without treatment by 6 to 8 months. Heat rash is common in warm weather, which appears as a fine red rash around creases or folds where the baby sweats.

Cord Care

- Cleanse with plain water around base of the cord where it joins the skin. Notify the pediatric health care provider of any odor, discharge, or skin inflammation (redness) around the cord. The clamp is removed by the nurse when the cord is dry (approximately 24 to 48 hours after birth). Keep the diaper folded down so that it does not cover the cord. A wet or soiled diaper will slow or prevent drying of the cord and foster infection. When the cord drops off after 10 to 14 days, a few small drops of blood may be seen. If there is active bleeding, notify the pediatric health care provider.

Nail Care

- Do not cut fingernails and toenails immediately after birth. The nails have to grow out far enough from the skin so that the skin is not cut by mistake. If the baby scratches himself or herself, apply loosely fitted mitts over each of the baby's hands. Do so as a last resort, however, because it interferes with the baby's ability for self-consolation sucking on thumb or finger. When the nails have grown, the fingernails and toenails can be trimmed with manicure scissors or clippers; nails should be cut straight across. The ideal time to trim the nails is when the infant is sleeping. Soft emery boards may be used to file the nails. Nails should be kept short.

Genital Care

- Cleanse the genitalia of infants daily and after voiding or stooling using disposable diaper wipes or soft cloths and water (with gentle cleanser if needed). For girls, the genitalia are cleansed by gently separating the labia and gently washing from the pubic area to the anus. For uncircumcised boys, wash and rinse the penis with soap and warm water. Do not attempt to retract the foreskin. The health care provider will inform you when the foreskin can safely be retracted. By 3 years of age in the majority of boys, the foreskin can be retracted easily without causing pain or trauma. For others, the foreskin is not retractable until adolescence. As soon as the foreskin is partly retractable and the child is old enough, he can be taught self-care. Once healed, the circumcised penis does not require any special care other than cleansing with diaper changes.
- The infant's skin should be allowed to dry completely before applying another diaper.
- Exposing the buttocks to air can help dry up diaper rash. Because bacteria thrive in moist dark areas, exposing the skin to dry air decreases bacterial proliferation. Zinc oxide ointments can be used to protect the infant's skin from moisture and further excoriation.

Data from American Academy of Pediatrics. (2013). *Baby 0–12 mos.* Retrieved from https://www.healthychildren.org/english/ages-stages/baby/bathing-skin-care/Pages/default.aspx; Association of Women's Health, Obstetric, and Neonatal Nurses. (2013). *Neonatal skin care* (3rd ed.). Washington, DC: Author.

parents. Even the simplest strategies can provide enormous support. Printed materials reinforcing education topics are helpful, as is a list of available community resources and websites that provide reliable information about child care. Classes in the prenatal period or during the postpartum stay are helpful. Instructions for the first days at home include relevant topics such as activities of daily living, dealing with visitors, and activity and rest.

Interpretation of Crying and Use of Quieting Techniques

Crying is an infant's first social communication. Some babies cry more than others, but all babies cry. They cry to communicate that they are hungry, uncomfortable, wet, ill, or bored and sometimes for no apparent reason at all. The longer parents are around their infants, the easier it becomes to interpret the meaning of infant cries and to respond appropriately. Many infants have a fussy period during the day, often in the late afternoon or early evening when everyone is naturally tired. Environmental tension adds to the length and intensity of crying spells. Babies also have periods of vigorous crying when no comforting can help. These periods of crying can last for long stretches until the infants seem to cry themselves to sleep. The nurse informs new parents that time and infant maturation will take care of these types of cries. Many hospitals distribute a DVD on infant crying to new parents. It is intended to help parents understand that crying is normal and help them cope with infant crying. If parents have greater understanding of infant crying,

PATIENT TEACHING

Signs of Illness

Notify the pediatric health care provider if any of the following signs occur:

- Fever: temperature greater than 38° C (100.4° F) axillary; also a continual rise in temperature (Note: Tympanic [ear] thermometers are not recommended for infants younger than 3 months of age.)
- Hypothermia: temperature less than 36.5° C (97.7° F) axillary
- Poor feeding or little interest in food: refusing two feedings in a row
- Vomiting: more than one episode of forceful vomiting or frequent vomiting (over a 6-hour period)
- Diarrhea: two consecutive green, watery stools (Note: Stools of breastfed infants are normally looser than stools of formula-fed infants. Diarrhea leaves a water ring around the stool, whereas breastfed stools do not.)
- Decreased bowel movement: in a breastfed infant, fewer than three stools per day; in a formula-fed infant, less than one stool every other day
- Decreased urination: fewer than six to eight wet diapers per day after 3 to 4 days of age
- Breathing difficulties: labored breathing with flared nostrils or absence of breathing for more than 15 seconds (Note: A newborn's breathing is normally irregular and between 30 to 40 breaths/minute. Count the breaths for a full minute.)
- Cyanosis (bluish skin color) whether accompanying a feeding or not
- Lethargy: sleepiness, difficulty waking, or periods of sleep longer than 6 hours (most newborns sleep for short periods, usually from 1 to 4 hours, and wake to be fed)
- Inconsolable crying (attempts to quiet not effective) or continuous high-pitched cry
- Bleeding or purulent (yellowish) drainage from umbilical cord or circumcision; foul odor or redness at the site
- Drainage from the eyes

they may be less likely to inflict harm such as occurs with shaken-baby syndrome.

Nurses should instruct new parents about strategies to calm a crying or fussy baby. Certain types of sensory stimulation can calm and quiet infants and help them get to sleep. Important characteristics of this sensory stimulation—whether tactile, vestibular, auditory, or visual—appear to be that the stimulation is mild, slow, rhythmic, and consistently and regularly presented. Tactile stimulation can include SSC, warmth, patting, and back massage. Swaddling provides widespread and constant tactile stimulation and a sense of security. Vestibular stimulation is especially effective and can be accomplished by mild rhythmic movement such as rocking or by holding the infant upright, as on the parent's shoulder. Some infants respond to being held in a body carrier. Rhythmic sounds can provide auditory stimulation; parents can use devices that provide white noise or sounds resembling the mother's heartbeat.

Recognizing Signs of Illness

In addition to explaining the need for well-baby follow-up visits, the nurse should discuss with parents the signs of illness in newborns (see Patient Teaching box: Signs of Illness). Of particular importance is the parents' assessment of jaundice in newborns discharged early. Parents should be advised to call their pediatric care provider immediately if they notice increasing jaundice or signs of illness.

REFERENCES

Academy of Breastfeeding Medicine Protocol Committee. (2010). ABM clinical protocol no. 23: Non-pharmacologic management of procedure-related pain in the breastfeeding infant. *Breastfeeding Medicine,* 5(6), 315–319.

Adamkin, D. H., & Committee on Fetus and Newborn. (2011). Clinical report—Postnatal glucose homeostasis in late-preterm and term infants. *Pediatrics,* 127(3), 575–579.

Ainsworth, R. M., Summerlin-Long, S., & Mog, C. (2016). A comprehensive initiative to prevent falls among newborns. *Nursing for Women's Health,* 20(3), 248–257.

American Academy of Pediatrics. (2014). *Swaddling: Is it safe?* Elk Grove Village, IL: Author.

American Academy of Pediatrics. (2017). *Car seats: Information for families.* Elk Grove Village, IL: Author. Retrieved from https://www.healthychildren.org/English/safety-prevention/on-the-go/Pages/Car-Safety-Seats-Information-for-Families.

American Academy of Pediatrics & American College of Obstetricians and Gynecologists. (2012). *Guidelines for perinatal care* (7th ed.). Elk Grove Village, IL: Author.

American Academy of Pediatrics & American College of Obstetricians and Gynecologists. (2015). The Apgar score. *Pediatrics,* 136(4), 819–822.

American Academy of Pediatrics Committee on Infectious Diseases. (2015). Section 5: Antimicrobial prophylaxis. In D. W. Kimberlin, M. T. Brady, M. A. Jackson, et al. (Eds.), *Red book: 2015 report of the Committee on Infectious Diseases* (30th ed.). Elk Grove Village, IL: Author.

American Academy of Pediatrics Section on Breastfeeding. (2012). Breastfeeding and the use of human milk—Policy statement. *Pediatrics,* 129(3), e827–e841.

American Academy of Pediatrics Section on Cardiology and Cardiac Surgery Executive Committee. (2012). Endorsement of Health and Human Services recommendation for pulse oximetry screening for critical congenital heart disease. *Pediatrics,* 129(1), 190–192.

American Academy of Pediatrics Subcommittee on Hyperbilirubinemia. (2004). Clinical practice guideline: Management of hyperbilirubinemia in the newborn infant 35 or more weeks of gestation. *Pediatrics,* 114(1), 297–316.

American Academy of Pediatrics Task Force on Circumcision. (1999, reaffirmed 2005). Circumcision policy statement. *Pediatrics,* 103(3), 686–693.

American Academy of Pediatrics Task Force on Circumcision. (2012). Circumcision policy statement. *Pediatrics,* 130(3), 585–586.

American Academy of Pediatrics Task Force on Sudden Infant Death Syndrome. (2016). SIDS and other sleep-related infant deaths: Updated 2016 recommendations for a safe infant sleeping environment. *Pediatrics,* 138(5), e1–e12.

American College of Medical Genetics. (2009). *Position statement on importance of residual newborn screening dried blood spots.* Retrieved from https://www.acmg.net/staticcontent/newsreleases/blood_spot_position_statement2009.pdf.

American College of Obstetricians and Gynecologists. (2015). Newborn screening. *Obstetrics and Gynecology,* 125(1), 256–260.

American College of Obstetricians and Gynecologists & Society for Maternal-Fetal Medicine. (2013). Definition of term pregnancy. *Obstetrics and Gynecology,* 122(5), 1139–1140.

Araia, M. H., Wilson, B. J., Chakraborty, P., et al. (2012). Factors associated with knowledge of and satisfaction with newborn screening education: A survey of mothers. *Genetics in Medicine,* 14(12), 963–970.

Association of Women's Health, Obstetric, and Neonatal Nurses. (2013). *Neonatal skin care: Evidence-based clinical practice guideline* (3rd ed.). Washington, DC: Author.

Ballard, J., Khoury, J., Wedig, K., et al. (1991). New Ballard score, expanded to include extremely premature infants. *Journal of Pediatrics,* 119(3), 417–423.

Barrington, K. J., Sankaran, K., & Canadian Paediatric Society Fetus and Newborn Committee. (2007, reaffirmed 2011). Guidelines for detection, management, and prevention of hyperbilirubinemia in term and late preterm newborn infants. *Paediatrics & Child Health,* 12(B suppl), 1B–12B.

Bellieni, C. V., Alagna, M. G., & Buonocore, G. (2013). Analgesia for infants' circumcision. *Italian Journal of Pediatrics,* 39(38), 1–7.

Bellieni, C. V., Tei, M., Coccina, F., & Buonocore, G. (2012). Sensorial saturation for infants' pain. *Journal of Maternal-Fetal & Neonatal Medicine*, 25(S1), 79–81.

Bennett, C., Fagan, E., Chaharbakhshi, E., et al. (2016). Using glucose gel to treat neonatal hypoglycemia. *Nursing for Women's Health*, 20(1), 64–74.

Bhutani, V. K., & Committee on Fetus and Newborn. (2011). Phototherapy to prevent severe neonatal hyperbilirubinemia in the newborn infant 35 or more weeks of gestation. *Pediatrics*, 128(4), e1046–e1052.

Blackburn, S. T. (2013). *Maternal, fetal, and neonatal physiology: A clinical perspective* (4th ed.). Maryland Heights, MO: Saunders.

Bromiker, R., Bin-Nun, A., Schimmel, M. S., et al. (2012). Neonatal hyperbilirubinemia in the low-intermediate-risk category on the bilirubin nomogram. *Pediatrics*, 130(3), e470–e475.

Bull, M., Engle, W. A., & American Academy of Pediatrics (AAP) Committee on Injury, Violence, and Poison Prevention, and Committee on Fetus and Newborn. (2009). Safe transportation of preterm and low birth weight infants at hospital discharge. *Pediatrics*, 123(5), 1424–1429.

Burgos, A. E., Flaherman, V. J., & Newman, T. B. (2012). Screening and follow-up for neonatal hyperbilirubinemia: A review. *Clinical Pediatrics*, 51(1), 7–16.

Canadian Organization for Rare Disorders. (2015). *Newborn screening in Canada status report*. Retrieved from https://www.raredisorders.ca/content/uploads/Canada-NBS-status-updated-Sept.-3-2015.pdf.

Centers for Disease Control and Prevention. (2016). Advisory Committee on Immunization Practices recommended immunization schedule for persons aged 0 through 18 years—United States, 2016. *Morbidity and Mortality Weekly Report*, 65(4), 86–87.

Cignacco, E. L., Sellam, G., Stoffel, L., et al. (2012). Oral sucrose and "facilitated tucking" for repeated pain relief in preterms: A randomized control trial. *Pediatrics*, 129(2), 299–308.

Craighead, D. V. (2012). Early term birth: Understanding the health risks to infants. *Nursing for Women's Health*, 16(2), 136–145.

Dijk, P., & Hulzebos, C. (2012). An evidence-based review on hyperbilirubinemia. *Acta Paediatrica*, 101(464 suppl), 3–10.

Feldman-Winter, L., Goldsmith, J. P., & Committee on Fetus and Newborn, Task Force on Sudden Infant Death Syndrome. (2016). Safe sleep and skin-to-skin care in the neonatal period for healthy term newborns. *Pediatrics*, 138(3), e1–e10.

Gabriel, M. A. M., de Mendoza, B. R. H., Figueroa, L. J., et al. (2013). Analgesia with breastfeeding in addition to skin-to-skin contact during heel prick. *Archives of Diseases in Childhood. Fetal and Neonatal Edition*, 98(6), F499–F503.

Gardner, S. L., Enzman-Hines, M., & Dickey, L. A. (2016). Pain and pain relief. In S. L. Gardner, B. S. Carter, M. Enzman-Hines, et al. (Eds.), *Merenstein & Gardner's handbook of neonatal intensive care* (8th ed.). St. Louis, MO: Elsevier.

Gardner, S. L., & Hernández, J. A. (2016). Initial nursery care. In S. L. Gardner, B. S. Carter, M. Enzman-Hines, et al. (Eds.), *Merenstein & Gardner's handbook of neonatal intensive care* (8th ed.). St. Louis, MO: Elsevier.

Halbardier, B. H. (2015). Fluid and electrolyte management. In M. T. Verklan & M. Walden (Eds.), *Core curriculum for neonatal intensive care nursing* (5th ed.). St. Louis, MO: Elsevier.

Hamrick, H. J., Gable, E. K., Freeman, E. H., et al. (2016). Reasons for refusal of newborn vitamin K prophylaxis: Implications for management and education. *Hospital Pediatrics*, 6(1), 15–21.

Harris, D. L., Weston, P. J., Signal, M., et al. (2013-2014). Dextrose gel for neonatal hypoglycaemia (the Sugar Babies study): A randomized, double-blind, placebo-controlled study. *Lancet*, 382(9910), 2077–2083.

Helsey, L., McDonald, J. V., & Stewart, V. T. (2010). Addressing in-hospital falls of newborn infants. *Joint Commission Journal on Quality and Patient Safety*, 36(7), 327–333.

Hiner, J., Pyka, J., Burks, C., et al. (2012). Preventing infant abductions: An infant security program transitioned into an interdisciplinary model. *Journal of Perinatal & Neonatal Nursing*, 26(1), 47–56.

Howell, R. R., Terry, S., Tait, V. F., et al. (2012). CDC grand rounds: Newborn screening and improved outcomes. *Morbidity and Mortality Weekly Report*, 61(21), 390–393.

Hummel, P., Puchalski, M., Creech, S. D., et al. (2008). Clinical reliability and validity of the N-PASS: Neonatal pain, agitation, and sedation scale with prolonged pain. *Journal of Perinatology*, 28(1), 55–60.

Johnston, C., Campbell-Yeo, M., Fernandes, A., et al. (2014). Skin-to-skin care for procedural pain in neonates. *Cochrane Database of Systematic Reviews*, 2014(1), CD008435.

Joint Committee on Infant Hearing. (2007). Year 2007 position statement: Principles and guidelines for early hearing detection and intervention programs. *Pediatrics*, 120(4), 898–921.

Kamath-Rayne, B. D., Thilo, E. H., Deacon, J., et al. (2016). Neonatal hyperbilirubinemia. In S. L. Gardner, B. S. Carter, M. Enzman-Hines, et al. (Eds.), *Merenstein & Gardner's handbook of neonatal intensive care* (8th ed.). St. Louis, MO: Elsevier.

Kassab, M. I., Roydhouse, J. K., Fowler, C., & Foureur, M. (2012). The effectiveness of glucose in reducing needle-related procedural pain in infants. *Journal of Pediatric Nursing*, 27(1), 3–17.

Kostandy, R., Anderson, G. C., & Good, M. (2013). Skin-to-skin contact diminishes pain from hepatitis B vaccine injection in healthy full-term infants. *Neonatal Network*, 32(4), 274–280.

Krechel, S., & Bildner, J. (1995). CRIES: A new neonatal postoperative pain measurement score—Initial testing of validity and reliability. *Paediatric Anaesthesia*, 5(1), 53–61.

Lawrence, J., Alcock, D., McGrath, P., et al. (1993). The development of a tool to assess neonatal pain. *Neonatal Network*, 12(6), 59–66.

Lund, C. H., & Durand, D. J. (2016). Skin and skin care. In S. L. Gardner, B. S. Carter, M. Enzman-Hines, et al. (Eds.), *Merenstein & Gardner's handbook of neonatal intensive care* (8th ed.). St. Louis, MO: Elsevier.

Maisels, M. J. (2010). Screening and early postnatal management strategies to prevent hazardous hyperbilirubinemia in newborns of 35 or more weeks of gestation. *Seminars in Fetal and Neonatal Medicine*, 15(3), 129–135.

Martin, J. A., Hamilton, B. E., Osterman, M. J. K., et al. (2017). Births: Final data for 2015. *National Vital Statistics Report*, 66(1), 1–69.

Matteson, T., Henderson-Williams, A., & Nelson, J. (2013). Preventing in-hospital newborn falls. *American Journal of Maternal Child Nursing*, 38(6), 359–366.

Maxwell, L. G., Malavolta, C. P., & Fraga, M. V. (2013). Assessment of pain in the neonate. *Clinics in Perinatology*, 40(3), 457–469.

McMillan, D., & Canadian Paediatric Society (CPS) Fetus and Newborn Committee (1997, reaffirmed 2016). *Position statement: Routine administration of vitamin K to newborns*. Retrieved from https://www.cps.ca/documents/position/administration-vitamin-K-newborns.

McNair, C., Yeo, M. C., Johnston, C., & Taddio, A. (2013). Nonpharmacologic management of pain during common needle puncture procedures in infants: Current evidence and practical considerations. *Clinics in Perinatology*, 40(3), 493–508.

Moore, E. R., Anderson, G. C., Bergman, N., & Dowswell, T. (2012). Early skin-to-skin contact for mothers and their healthy newborn infants. *Cochrane Database of Systematic Reviews*, 2012(5), CD003519.

Moore, D. L., MacDonald, N. E., & Canadian Paediatric Society Infectious Diseases and Immunization Committee. (2015). Position statement: Preventing ophthalmia neonatorum. *Paediatrics & Child Health*, 20(2), 93–96.

Nassi, N., Piumetti, R., Nardini, V., et al. (2013). Sudden unexpected perinatal collapse and sudden unexpected early neonatal death. *Early Human Development*, 89(4 suppl), S25–S26.

National Institute of Child Health and Human Development. (2014). *Sudden unexplained infant death (SIDS) and other sleep-related causes of infant death: Questions and answers for health care providers*. Rockville, MD: Author.

Naughton, K. A. (2013). The combined use of sucrose and nonnutritive sucking for procedural pain in both term and preterm neonates. *Advances in Neonatal Care*, 13(1), 9–19.

Nyp, M., Brunkhorst, J. L., Reavey, D., et al. (2016). Fluid and electrolyte management. In S. L. Gardner, B. S. Carter, M. Enzman-Hines, et al. (Eds.), *Merenstein & Gardner's handbook of neonatal intensive care* (8th ed.). St. Louis, MO: Elsevier.

Owings, M., Uddin, S., & Williams, S. (2013). *Trends in circumcision for male newborns in US hospitals: 1979-2010.* Health E-Stats. Retrieved from www.cdc.gov/nchs/data/hestat/circumcision_2013/circumcision_2013.htm.

Parikh, L. I., Reddy, U. M., Männistö, T., et al. (2014). Neonatal outcomes of early term birth. *American Journal of Obstetrics and Gynecology, 211*(3), e1–e265.

Patel, H., Feldman, M., & Canadian Paediatric Society (CPS) Community Paediatrics Committee. (2011, reaffirmed 2014). Universal newborn hearing screening. *Paediatrics & Child Health, 16*(5), 301–305.

Phillips, R. M., Goldstein, M., Hougland, K., et al. (2013). Multidisciplinary guidelines for the care of late preterm infants. *Journal of Perinatology, 33*(S2), S5–S22.

Pillai Riddell, R. P., Racine, N. M., Turcotte, K., et al. (2012). Non-pharmacological management of infant and young child procedural pain. *Evidence-Based Child Health, 7*(6), 1905–2121.

Rozance, P. J., McGowan, J. E., Price-Douglas, W., et al. (2016). Glucose homeostasis. In S. L. Gardner, B. S. Carter, M. Enzman-Hines, et al. (Eds.), *Merenstein & Gardner's handbook of neonatal intensive care* (8th ed.). St. Louis, MO: Elsevier.

Saxton, A., Fahy, K., Rolfe, M., et al. (2015). Does skin-to-skin and breastfeeding at birth affect the rate of primary postpartum haemorrhage: Results of a cohort study. *Midwifery, 31*(11), 1110–1117.

Sengupta, S., Carrion, V., Shelton, J., et al. (2013). Adverse neonatal outcomes associated with early-term birth. *JAMA Pediatrics, 167*(11), 1053–1059.

Shah, P. S., Herbozo, C., Aliwalas, L. L., et al. (2012). Breastfeeding or breast milk for procedural pain in neonates. *Cochrane Database of Systematic Reviews, 2012*(12), CD004950.

Slogar, A., Gargiulo, D., & Bodrock, J. (2013). Tracking "near misses" to keep newborns safe from falls. *Nursing for Women's Health, 17*(3), 219–223.

Sorokan, S. T., Finlay, J. C., Jefferies, A. L., et al. (2015). Newborn male circumcision. *Paediatrics & Child Health, 20*(6), 311–315.

Stevens, B., Johnston, C., Petryshen, P., & Taddio, A. (1996). Premature infant pain profile: Development and initial validation. *Clinical Journal of Pain, 12*(1), 13–22.

Stevens, B., Yamada, J., Lee, G. Y., & Ohlsson, A. (2013). Sucrose for analgesia in newborn infants undergoing painful procedures. *Cochrane Database of Systematic Reviews, 2013*(1), CD001069.

Stewart, D., Benitz, W., & Committee on Fetus and Newborn. (2016). Umbilical cord care in the newborn infant. *Pediatrics, 138*(3), e1–e5.

Tarini, B. A., & Goldenberg, A. J. (2012). Ethical issues and newborn screening in the genomics era. *Annual Review of Genomics and Human Genetics, 13*, 381–393.

Tluczek, A., & De Luca, J. M. (2013). Newborn screening policy and practice issues for nurses. *Journal of Obstetric, Gynecologic, and Neonatal Nursing, 42*(6), 718–727.

United States Department of Health and Human Services (USDHHS) Committee on Heritable Disorders in Newborns and Children. (2015). *Recommended uniform screening panel.* Retrieved from http://www.hrsa.gov/advisorycommittees/mchbadvisory/heritabledisorders/recommendedpanel/index.html.

United States Preventive Services Task Force (USPSTF). (2011). *Ocular prophylaxis for gonococcal ophthalmia neonatorum.* Preventive medication. Retrieved from www.uspreventiveservicestaskforce.org/uspstf10/gonoculproph/gonocupsum.htm.

Visscher, M. O., Adam, R., Brink, S., & Odio, M. (2015). Newborn infant skin care: Physiology, development, and care. *Clinics in Dermatology, 33*(3), 271–280.

Vohr, B. (2013). Long-term outcomes of moderately preterm, late preterm, and early term infants. *Clinics in Perinatology, 40*(4), 739–751.

Walden, M., & Gibbins, S. (2012). *Newborn pain assessment & management: Guideline for practice* (3rd ed.). Glenview, IL: National Association of Neonatal Nurses.

Wight, N., & Marinelli, K. A., & Academy of Breastfeeding Medicine. (2014). ABM protocol no. 1: Guidelines for blood glucose monitoring and treatment of hypoglycemia in term and late preterm neonates, revised 2014. *Breastfeeding Medicine, 9*(4), 173–179.

World Health Organization & Jhpiego. (2010). *Manual for early infant male circumcision under local anesthesia.* Geneva, Switzerland: WHO Press. Retrieved from http://whqlibdoc.who.int/publications/2010/9789241500753_eng.pdf?ua=1.

World Health Organization (WHO). (2012). *Voluntary medical male circumcision for HIV prevention.* Retrieved from www.who.int/hiv/topics/malecircumcision/fact_sheet/en/.

World Health Organization (WHO). (2009). *WHO guidelines on hand hygiene in health care: A summary.* Geneva, Switzerland: WHO Press.

Wyckoff, M. H., Aziz, K., Escobedo, M. B., et al. (2015). Part 13: Neonatal resuscitation: 2015 American Heart Association guidelines update for cardiopulmonary resuscitation and emergency cardiovascular care. *Circulation, 132*(18; suppl 2), S543–S560.

24

Newborn Nutrition and Feeding

Kathryn R. Alden

ⓔ http://evolve.elsevier.com/Perry/maternal

Good nutrition in infancy fosters optimal growth and development. Infant feeding is more than providing nutrition; it is an opportunity for social, psychologic, and even educational interaction between parent and infant. It can establish a basis for developing good eating habits that last a lifetime.

Through preconception and prenatal education and counseling, nurses play an instrumental role in helping parents make an informed decision about infant feeding. Scientific evidence is clear that human milk provides the best nutrition for infants, and parents should be strongly encouraged to choose breastfeeding (American Academy of Pediatrics [AAP] Section on Breastfeeding, 2012). Although many consider commercial infant formula to be equivalent to breast milk, this belief is erroneous. Human milk is the gold standard for infant nutrition. It is species specific, uniquely designed to meet the needs of human infants. The composition of human milk changes to meet the nutritional needs of growing infants. It is highly complex, with antiinfective and nutritional components combined with growth factors, enzymes that aid in digestion and absorption of nutrients, and fatty acids that promote brain growth and development. Infant formulas are usually adequate in providing nutrition to maintain infant growth and development within normal limits, but they are not equivalent to human milk.

Breastfeeding is defined as the transfer of human milk from the mother to the infant; the infant receives milk directly from the mother's breast. *Exclusive breastfeeding* means that the infant receives no other liquid or solid food (AAP Section on Breastfeeding, 2012). If the infant is fed expressed breast milk from the mother or a donor milk bank, it is called *human milk feeding*.

Whether the parents choose breastfeeding, human milk feeding, or formula-feeding, nurses provide support and ongoing education. Parent education and care management are necessarily based on current research findings and standards of practice. Nurses and lactation consultants (who are most often nurses) provide education, assistance, and support for mothers, infants, and families prior to discharge from the birthing facility. After discharge, nurses and lactation consultants in primary care and community health settings provide ongoing support and assistance to promote optimal feeding practices and positive health outcomes.

This chapter focuses on meeting nutritional needs for normal growth and development from birth to 6 months of age, with emphasis on the neonatal period when feeding practices and patterns are established. Breastfeeding and formula-feeding are addressed. Information on breastfeeding is focused on the direct transfer of milk from mother to infant.

RECOMMENDED INFANT NUTRITION

The American Academy of Pediatrics (AAP) recommends exclusive breastfeeding for the first 6 months of life and that breastfeeding continues as complementary foods are introduced. Breastfeeding should continue for 1 year and thereafter as desired by the mother and her infant (AAP Section on Breastfeeding, 2012). According to the World Health Organization (WHO, 2016), infants should be exclusively breastfed for 6 months, receive safe and nutritionally adequate complementary foods beginning at 6 months, and continue breastfeeding until 2 years of age or beyond.

Exclusive breastfeeding for the first 6 months of life is also recommended by other professional health care organizations such as the American College of Nurse-Midwives (ACNM, 2016), American Academy of Family Physicians (AAFP, 2012), Academy of Breastfeeding Medicine (Chantry, Eglash, & Labbok, 2015), the American College of Obstetricians and Gynecologists (ACOG, 2016), and the American Dietetic Association (ADA, 2009). The Association of Women's Health, Obstetric, and Neonatal Nurses (AWHONN, 2014; 2015) actively supports breastfeeding as the ideal form of infant nutrition and provides guidelines for nurses in promoting breastfeeding and supporting breastfeeding families.

BREASTFEEDING RATES

Breastfeeding rates in the United States have risen steadily over the past decade. The Centers for Disease Control and Prevention (CDC, 2016b) reported that the US breastfeeding initiation rate for infants born in 2013 was 81.1%, which is the highest ever reported. The 6-month breastfeeding rate was 51.8%, and the 12-month rate was 30.7%. The rate of exclusive breastfeeding at 3 months was 44.4% and at 6 months, 22.3%. One factor that may be related to the increase in breastfeeding rates is a rise in the percentage of births at Baby-Friendly hospitals, which rose from 7.8% in 2014 to 18.3% in 2016 (CDC).

With the increase in breastfeeding rates, the United States is close to meeting the Healthy People 2020 goal of 81.9% of infants ever breastfed. More than 50% of states have already met or exceeded this goal. The United States continues to fall short of meeting Healthy People goals of 60.6% breastfeeding at 6 months, and 34.1% at 12 months as well as goals for exclusive breastfeeding of 46.2% through 3 months and 25.5% through 6 months (CDC, 2016b; US Department of Health and Human Services [USDHHS], 2016). The CDC (2016b) suggests that the low breastfeeding continuation rates may be related to lack of

TABLE 24.1   Benefits of Breastfeeding

Benefits for the Infant/Child	Benefits for the Mother	Benefits for Families and Society

• Reduced infant and child mortality
• Reduced risk for:
  • Nonspecific gastrointestinal infections
  • Celiac disease
  • Childhood inflammatory bowel disease
  • Necrotizing enterocolitis in preterm infants
  • Asthma
  • Atopic dermatitis
  • Lower respiratory tract infection
  • Otitis media
  • SIDS
  • Obesity in childhood, adolescence, and adulthood
  • Type 2 diabetes
  • Acute lymphocytic and myeloid leukemia
  • Dental malocclusions
• Enhanced neurodevelopmental outcomes, including higher intelligence
	• Decreased postpartum bleeding and more rapid uterine involution
	• Reduced risk for:
	  • Ovarian cancer and breast cancer
	  • Type 2 diabetes
	  • Hypertension, hypercholesterolemia, and cardiovascular disease
	  • Rheumatoid arthritis
	• More rapid postpartum weight loss
	• Delayed return of menses
	• Unique bonding experience
	• Increased maternal role attainment
		• Convenient; ready to feed
		• No bottles or other necessary equipment
		• Less expensive than infant formula
		• Reduced annual health care costs
		• Less parental absence from work because of ill infant
		• Reduced environmental burden related to disposal of formula packaging and equipment

SIDS, Sudden infant death syndrome.
Data from American Academy of Pediatrics Section on Breastfeeding. (2012). Breastfeeding and the use of human milk—Policy statement. *Pediatrics, 129*(3), e827–e841; Chowdhury R, Sinha B, Sankar M.J., et al. (2015). Breastfeeding and maternal health outcomes: A systematic review and meta-analysis. *Acta Paediatrica, 104*(S467), 96–113; Grummer-Strawn, L.M., & Rollins, N. (2015). Summarising the health benefits of breastfeeding. *Acta Paediatrica, 104*(S467), 1–2; Horta, B.L., de Mola, C.L., & Victora, C.G. (2015). Breastfeeding and intelligence: A systematic review and meta-analysis. *Acta Paediatrica, 104*(S467), 14–19; Sankar, M.J., Sinha, B., Chowdhury, R., et al. (2015). Optimal breastfeeding practices and infant and child mortality: A systematic review and meta-analysis. *Acta Paediatrica, 104*(S467), 3–13; Victora, C.G., Bahl, R., Barros, A.J., et al. (2016). Breastfeeding in the 21st century: Epidemiology, mechanisms, and lifelong effect. *Lancet, 387*(10017), 473–490.

support offered to breastfeeding mothers by family members, health care providers, and employers.

In 2013, the highest breastfeeding initiation rates in the United States were among non-Hispanic white women (84.3%) and lowest rates were among non-Hispanic black women (66.3%). Rates were similar among Hispanic and non-Hispanic Asian women, although the non-Hispanic Asian women had higher rates at 6 and 12 months (CDC, 2016a).

Breastfeeding rates are lower among low-income families and those who live in rural communities. Historically, breastfeeding rates have been lower among women participating in the Special Supplemental Nutrition Program for Women, Infants, and Children (WIC). However, breastfeeding rates in this population are gradually rising. Data for 2014 indicate that 69.8% of 6- to 13-month-old infants participating in the WIC program were currently breastfeeding or had been breastfed; this was an increase from 67.1% in 2012 (Thorn, Tadler, Huret, et al., 2015).

BENEFITS OF BREASTFEEDING

Extensive evidence exists concerning the health benefits of breastfeeding and human milk for infants, with some of the benefits extending into adulthood (Table 24.1). For example, breastfed infants have a decreased incidence of respiratory tract infections, otitis media, gastrointestinal infections, and sudden infant death syndrome (SIDS). Benefits are optimized when infants are breastfed exclusively and when the duration of breastfeeding is increased (AAP Section on Breastfeeding, 2012; Grummer-Strawn & Rollins, 2015; Sankar, Sinha, Chowdhury et al., 2015; Victora, Bahl, Barros, et al., 2016).

Breastfeeding is associated with health benefits for mothers such as reduced risk of breast cancer and ovarian cancer (AAP Section on Breastfeeding, 2012; Chowdhury, Sinha, Sankar, et al., 2015). The benefits are increased with the number of children who were breastfed and the total length of time of lactation.

The psychologic benefits for mothers include enhanced bonding and attachment. For many women, breastfeeding is associated with a sense of empowerment in the ability to provide nutrition for the infant.

Breastfeeding is convenient. The milk is ready to feed and at the proper temperature. In most cases, there is no need for bottles or other equipment.

The economic benefits of breastfeeding affect families, employers, insurers, and the entire nation. Because infant formula is expensive, breastfeeding represents a significant savings for families. It reduces health care costs and decreases employee absenteeism because breastfed infants are ill less often and need fewer visits to health care providers and because parents miss work less often to stay home to care for ill infants.

Breastfeeding has environmental benefits. It reduces the waste that is deposited in landfills, including formula packaging, bottles, nipples, and other equipment. There is no need for fuel to prepare or transport human milk, which saves energy resources.

INFANT FEEDING DECISION-MAKING

The choice of infant feeding method is influenced by a variety of personal and sociocultural factors. The decision may not be as simple as choosing whether to breastfeed or formula-feed; it often is about weighing the positive and negative aspects of breastfeeding (Roll & Cheater, 2016). The evidence supporting breastfeeding as the ideal form of infant nutrition is so strong that health care professionals may need to present information about it from two perspectives: benefits of breastfeeding and risks of not breastfeeding.

For some women, there is a clear choice to either breastfeed or formula-feed. In some cases women decide to combine breastfeeding and formula-feeding. However, this practice can be associated with a shorter duration of breastfeeding. Some women want their infants to receive breast milk but prefer not to feed directly from their breasts. These women express their milk and bottle-feed it to their infants.

The majority of women make the infant feeding decision either before or during pregnancy. Women tend to select the same method of infant feeding for each of their children. If the first child was breastfed, subsequent children will likely also be breastfed. Older mothers and women with intended versus unintended pregnancies are more likely to breastfeed (Hedburg, 2013). Women with higher levels of education and socioeconomic status are more likely to breastfeed than women with less education and less income. Women living in rural areas are less likely to breastfeed. Adolescent mothers are less likely to breastfeed, and those who initiate breastfeeding are likely to stop within 1 month after birth (Kanhadilok & McGrath, 2015).

Women most often choose to breastfeed because they are aware of the benefits to the infant (Nelson, 2012). This is evidence of the effectiveness of health promotion efforts and activities that have raised public awareness of the benefits of breastfeeding for infants, mothers, and families (Roll & Cheater, 2016).

The concept of the maternal role is important in the decision to breastfeed. Women who decide to breastfeed are likely to view breastfeeding as a natural extension of pregnancy and childbirth; it is much more than simply a means of supplying nutrition. Many women seek the unique bonding experience between mother and infant that is characteristic of breastfeeding (Kanhadilok & McGrath, 2015; Roll & Cheater, 2016).

Partner and family support is a major factor in the mother's decision to breastfeed. Women who perceive their partners and family members (especially the maternal grandmother) to prefer breastfeeding are more likely to breastfeed. Women are more likely to breastfeed successfully when partners and family members provide encouragement and support (Kanhadilok & McGrath, 2015; Mueffelmann, Racine, Warren-Findlow et al., 2015; Odom, Li, Scanlon et al., 2014; Roll & Cheater, 2016).

Female role models and their transfer of information and sharing of experiences about breastfeeding, either positive or negative, influence the mother's infant feeding decision. Mothers who have observed others breastfeeding may be more likely to breastfeed (Nelson, 2012; Roll & Cheater, 2016).

Cultural factors influence infant feeding decisions. For example, in the Hispanic culture breastfeeding is the norm, whereas formula-feeding is more common among African-American families (see the "Cultural Influences on Infant Feeding" section later in the chapter).

For some women and their partners, perceptions of breast function influence the decision to formula-feed. The breast may be seen as a sexual object. There can be modesty issues; women fear the embarrassment of having to breastfeed in public. Some women fear pain related to breastfeeding or worry that they will not produce sufficient milk for their infants (Hedburg, 2013; Roll & Cheater, 2016).

The mother's perception of the practical aspects of feeding influence her decision. Some view breastfeeding as more convenient, while others choose to formula-feed because people other than the mother can bottle-feed the infant. They may think that breastfeeding is time-consuming. They consider formula-feeding as imposing fewer restrictions on family and social life (Hedburg, 2013; Roll & Cheater, 2016).

Some women initiate breastfeeding in response to pressure from family members, health care professionals, or their own perception of being a "good mother." These women may say they plan to "try breastfeeding," while lacking commitment and determination (Roll & Cheater, 2016). These women benefit from care by nurses who will help them explore their feelings and concerns and will provide information, support, and assistance.

There appears to be a relationship between maternal weight and infant feeding decisions. Women who are overweight or obese are less likely to breastfeed than women who are underweight or of average weight (Turcksin, Bel, Galjaard, et al., 2014).

Other factors influence decisions about infant nutrition. The widespread marketing by infant formula companies including free samples through the mail can encourage women to formula-feed. In addition, there is a lack of prenatal breastfeeding education for expectant parents and insufficient training and education of health care professionals about breastfeeding. In some institutions, the policies and practices do not support exclusive breastfeeding.

A major obstacle to breastfeeding for some women is employment and the need to return to work after birth. Access to breast pumps, pumping facilities, and time for pumping impact a mother's ability to continue breastfeeding when she returns to work or to school. This is especially problematic for women employed in lower-income jobs such as waitressing (Hedburg, 2013). Employers are acknowledging the value of providing space and time for pumping and storage of breastmilk, recognizing that employee absenteeism is reduced among breastfeeding mothers.

Awareness of the availability of breastfeeding resources can influence a mother's decision to breastfeed. For example, women who participate in the WIC program may benefit from information about in-hospital breastfeeding support, peer counseling programs, and breast pump programs (Hedburg, 2013).

Health care professionals are influential in the infant feeding decision. Strategies that promote breastfeeding decisions in the prenatal setting include a breastfeeding-friendly office or clinic environment; intentional promotion, education, and support for breastfeeding throughout prenatal care; and discussion of breastfeeding at each prenatal visit (Rosen-Carole, Hartman, & Academy of Breastfeeding Medicine, 2015). Because of their significant influence on the mother's decision to breastfeed, partners and family members should be included in discussions about breastfeeding. Through the education, support, and encouragement of health care professionals during the prenatal period, women and their families can make informed decisions about infant feeding (ACOG, 2016; AWHONN, 2015).

CONTRAINDICATIONS TO BREASTFEEDING

Breastfeeding is contraindicated in a few circumstances. Newborns who have galactosemia should not receive human milk. Breastfeeding is contraindicated for mothers who are positive for human T-cell lymphotropic virus types I or II and those with untreated brucellosis. Women should not breastfeed if they have active tuberculosis (TB) or if they have active herpes simplex lesions on the breasts. However, neither of these conditions precludes a mother from expressing milk for her infant. Women with active TB can breastfeed when they have been treated for at least 2 weeks and are deemed noninfectious. Varicella that occurs 5 days before or 2 days after birth and acute H1N1 infection require temporary separation of mother and infant. In both instances, it is safe for infants to receive expressed milk (AAP Section on Breastfeeding, 2012).

In the United States, maternal human immunodeficiency virus (HIV) infection is considered a contraindication for breastfeeding (AAP Section on Breastfeeding, 2012). However, this is not true in other countries. In developing countries where HIV is prevalent, the benefits of breastfeeding for infants outweigh the risk for contracting HIV from infected mothers (WHO, 2013).

CULTURAL INFLUENCES ON INFANT FEEDING

Cultural beliefs and practices are significant influences on infant feeding methods. Although recognized cultural norms exist, one cannot assume that generalized observations about any cultural group hold true for all members of that group. Many regional and ethnic cultures are found within the United States. Dealing effectively with these groups requires that nurses are knowledgeable and sensitive to the cultural factors influencing infant feeding practices.

In general, people who have immigrated to the United States from poorer countries often choose to formula-feed their infants because they believe it is a better, more "modern" method or because they want to adapt to US culture and perceive that formula-feeding is the custom. Hispanic women who are more acculturated may be less likely to breastfeed and, if they do, tend to breastfeed for a shorter duration (Ahluwalia, D'Angelo, Morrow, et al., 2012).

Breastfeeding beliefs and practices vary across cultures. For example, among the Muslim culture, breastfeeding for 24 months is customary. Before the first feeding, rubbing a small piece of softened date on the newborn's palate is a ritual. Because of the cultural emphasis on privacy and modesty, Muslim women may choose to bottle-feed formula or expressed breast milk while in the hospital.

Because of beliefs about the harmful nature or inadequacy of colostrum, some cultures apply restrictions on breastfeeding for a period of days after birth. Such is the case for many cultures in southern Asia, the Pacific Islands, and parts of sub-Saharan Africa. Before the mother's milk is deemed to be "in," babies are fed prelacteal food such as honey or clarified butter in the belief that these substances will help clear out meconium. Other cultures begin breastfeeding immediately and offer the breast each time the infant cries.

A common practice among Mexican women is *las dos cosas* ("both things"). This refers to combining breastfeeding and commercial infant formula. It is based on the belief that by combining the two methods, the mother and infant receive the benefits of breastfeeding, and the infant receives the additional vitamins from infant formula (Bartick & Reyes, 2012). This practice can result in problems with milk supply and babies refusing to latch on to the breast, which can lead to early termination of breastfeeding.

Cultural expectations influence breastfeeding patterns and behaviors. In many Western cultures, women are more likely to try to "schedule" feeding sessions. This is in contrast to more frequent breastfeeding in some developing countries where mothers "wear" their babies close against their bodies as they go about daily activities. Those babies have constant or frequent access to the breast to feed on demand (Mohrbacher, 2013).

Some cultures have specific beliefs and practices related to the mother's intake of foods that foster milk production. Korean mothers often eat seaweed soup and rice to enhance milk production. Hmong women believe that boiled chicken, rice, and hot water are the only appropriate nourishments during the first postpartum month. The balance between energy forces, hot and cold, or yin and yang is integral to the diet of the lactating mother. Hispanics, Vietnamese, Chinese, East Indians, and Arabs often use this belief in choosing foods. "Hot" foods are considered best for new mothers. This belief does not necessarily relate to the temperature or spiciness of foods. For example, chicken and broccoli are considered "hot," whereas many fresh fruits and vegetables are considered "cold." Families often bring desired foods into the health care setting.

LACTATION AND LGBTQ FAMILIES

Increasingly, members of the lesbian, gay, bisexual, transgender, queer/questioning, intersex (LGBTQI) community are becoming parents and providing human milk to their infants through a variety of methods. There is a lack of research, clinical papers, and commentaries in the literature on the topic of lactation and the LGBT community. These families face lactation and family adjustment issues similar to those of heterosexual mothers while also dealing with unique challenges (Farrow, 2015). For example, in lesbian couples who become parents, one woman may give birth and breastfeed, and the co-parent may choose

to induce lactation so that she can also nurse the baby. Induction of lactation involves medications and pumping. The co-parent may decide to breastfeed using a supplemental feeding device with expressed milk from the mother who gave birth. Transgender men may give birth and provide human milk through breastfeeding (also known as *chest feeding*) (Wolfe-Roubatis & Spatz, 2015); the female partner may also breastfeed by induced lactation or the use of a supplementary feeding device. Same-sex mothers may adopt a newborn who was born to a surrogate; the surrogate may provide expressed milk, and the two adoptive mothers may also breastfeed or feed expressed milk from induced lactation (Wilson, Perrin, Fogleman, et al., 2015). Nurses, lactation consultants, and other health care professionals who care for LGBT families can provide more effective care if they are familiar with needs of these parents. Information on resources about lactation and LGBT families can be found at http://dianawest.com/lgbtqia-resources/.

■ NUTRIENT NEEDS

FLUIDS

During the first 2 days of life, the fluid requirement for healthy infants (more than 1500 g) is 60 to 80 mL/kg of body weight per day. From day 3 to day 7, the requirement is 100 to 150 mL/kg/day; from day 8 to day 30, it is 120 to 180 mL/kg/day (Dell, 2015). In general, neither breastfed nor formula-fed infants need to be given water, not even those living in very hot climates. Breast milk contains 87% water, which easily meets fluid requirements. Feeding water to infants can decrease caloric consumption at a time when they are growing rapidly.

Infants have room for little fluctuation in fluid balance and should be monitored closely for fluid intake and water loss. They lose water through excretion of urine and insensibly through respiration. Under normal circumstances, they are born with some fluid reserve, and some of the weight loss during the first few days is related to fluid loss. However, in some cases they do not have this fluid reserve, possibly because of inadequate maternal hydration during labor or birth.

ENERGY

Infants require adequate caloric intake to provide energy for growth, digestion, physical activity, and maintenance of organ metabolic function. Energy needs vary according to age, maturity level, thermal environment, growth rate, health status, and activity level. For the first 3 months, the infant needs 110 kcal/kg/day. From 3 months to 6 months, the requirement is 100 kcal/kg/day. This level decreases slightly to 95 kcal/kg/day from 6 months to 9 months and increases to 100 kcal/kg/day from 9 months to 1 year (AAP Committee on Nutrition, 2014).

Human milk provides an average of 67 kcal/100 mL or 20 kcal/oz. The fat portion of the milk provides the greatest amount of energy. Infant formulas simulate the caloric content of human milk. Usually standard commercial infant formula contains 20 kcal/oz, although the composition differs among brands.

CARBOHYDRATE

According to the Institute of Medicine (IOM, 2005), the recommended adequate intake (AI) for carbohydrate in the first 6 months of life is 60 g/day and 95 g/day for the second 6 months. Because newborns have only small hepatic glycogen stores, carbohydrates should provide at least 40% to 50% of the total calories in the diet. Moreover, newborns may have a limited ability to carry out gluconeogenesis (the formation of glucose from amino acids and other substrates) and ketogenesis (the formation of ketone bodies from fat), the mechanisms that provide alternative sources of energy.

As the primary carbohydrate in human milk and commercial infant formula, lactose is the most abundant carbohydrate in the diet of infants up to 6 months of age. Lactose provides calories in an easily available form. Its slow breakdown and absorption also increase calcium absorption. Corn syrup solids or glucose polymers are added to infant formulas to supplement the lactose in the cow's milk and thereby provide sufficient carbohydrates.

Oligosaccharides, another form of carbohydrate found in breast milk, are critical in the development of microflora in the intestinal tract of the newborn. These prebiotics promote an acidic environment in the intestines, preventing the growth of gram-negative and other pathogenic bacteria, thus increasing the infant's resistance to gastrointestinal (GI) illness.

FAT

Fats provide a major energy source for infants, supplying as much as 50% of the calories in breast milk and formula. The recommended AI of fat for infants younger than 6 months of age is 31 g/day (IOM, 2005). The fat content of human milk is composed of lipids, triglycerides, and cholesterol; cholesterol is an essential element for brain growth. Human milk contains the essential fatty acids (EFAs) linoleic acid and linolenic acid and the long-chain polyunsaturated fatty acids arachidonic acid (ARA) and docosahexaenoic acid (DHA). Fatty acids are important for growth, neurologic development, and visual function. Cow's milk contains fewer of the EFAs and no polyunsaturated fatty acids. Most formula companies add DHA to their products, although there is a lack of evidence supporting the benefit (Lawrence & Lawrence, 2016). Modified cow's milk is used in most infant formulas, but the milk fat is removed, and another fat source such as corn oil, which the infant can digest and absorb, is added in its place. If whole milk or evaporated milk without added carbohydrate is fed to infants, the resulting fecal loss of fat (and therefore loss of energy) can be excessive because the milk moves through the infant's intestines too quickly for adequate absorption to take place. This can lead to poor weight gain.

PROTEIN

High-quality protein from breast milk, infant formula, or other complementary foods is necessary for infant growth. The protein requirement per unit of body weight is greater in the newborn period than at any other time of life. For infants younger than 6 months of age, the recommended AI for protein is 9.1 g/day (IOM, 2005).

Human milk contains the two proteins whey and casein in a ratio of approximately 70:30 compared with the ratio of 20:80 in most cow's milk–based formulas (Blackburn, 2013). This whey-to-casein ratio in human milk makes it more easily digestible and produces the soft stools seen in breastfed infants. The primary whey protein in human milk is α-lactalbumin; this protein is high in essential amino acids needed for growth. The whey protein lactoferrin in human milk has iron-binding capabilities and bacteriostatic properties, particularly against gram-positive and gram-negative aerobes, anaerobes, and yeasts. The casein in human milk enhances the absorption of iron, thus preventing iron-dependent bacteria from proliferating in the GI tract (Lawrence & Lawrence, 2016). The amino acid components of human milk are uniquely suited to the newborn's metabolic capabilities. For example, cystine and taurine levels are high, whereas phenylalanine and methionine levels are low.

VITAMINS

With the exception of vitamin D, human milk contains all of the vitamins required for infant nutrition, with individual variations based on maternal diet and genetic differences. Vitamins are added to cow's-milk formulas

to resemble levels found in breast milk. Although cow's milk contains adequate amounts of vitamins A and B complex, vitamin C (ascorbic acid), vitamin E, and vitamin D must be added.

Vitamin D facilitates intestinal absorption of calcium and phosphorus, bone mineralization, and calcium resorption from bone. According to the AAP, all infants who are breastfed or partially breastfed should receive 400 International Units of vitamin D daily, beginning the first few days of life. Nonbreastfeeding infants and older children who consume less than 1 quart per day of vitamin D–fortified milk should also receive 400 International Units of vitamin D each day (Wagner, Grier, & AAP Section on Breastfeeding and Committee on Nutrition, 2008).

Vitamin K, required for blood coagulation, is produced by intestinal bacteria. However, the gut is sterile at birth, and a few days are required for intestinal flora to become established and produce vitamin K. To prevent hemorrhagic problems in the newborn, an injection of vitamin K is given at birth to all newborns in the United States and Canada, regardless of feeding method (AAP Section on Breastfeeding, 2012; McMillan & Canadian Paediatric Society Fetus and Newborn Committee, 1997/2016). (See the Medication Guide: Vitamin K: Phytonandione [AquaMEPHYTON, Konakion]) in Chapter 23.)

The breastfed infant's vitamin B_{12} intake depends on the mother's dietary intake and stores. Mothers who are on strict vegetarian (vegan) diets and those who consume few dairy products, eggs, or meat are at risk for vitamin B_{12} deficiency. Mothers who have had bariatric surgery are also at risk for vitamin B_{12} deficiency. Breastfeeding infants may need vitamin B_{12} supplements in these instances.

Minerals

The mineral content of commercial infant formula is designed to reflect that of breast milk. Unmodified cow's milk is much higher in mineral content than human milk, which also makes it unsuitable for infants during the first year of life. Minerals are typically highest in human milk during the first few days after birth and decrease slightly throughout lactation.

The ratio of calcium to phosphorus in human milk is 2:1, an optimal proportion for bone mineralization. Although cow's milk is high in calcium, the calcium-to-phosphorus ratio is low, resulting in decreased calcium absorption. Consequently, young infants fed unmodified cow's milk are at risk for hypocalcemia, seizures, and tetany. The calcium-to-phosphorus ratio in commercial infant formula is between that of human milk and cow's milk.

Iron levels are low in all types of milk; however, iron from human milk is better absorbed than iron from cow's milk, iron-fortified formula, or infant cereals. Breastfed infants draw on iron reserves deposited in utero and benefit from the high lactose and vitamin C levels in human milk that facilitate iron absorption. Full-term infants have enough iron stores from the mother to last for the first 4 to 5 months. After 4 months of age, infants who are exclusively breastfed are at risk for iron deficiency. The AAP recommends giving exclusively breastfed infants an iron supplement (1 mg/kg/day) beginning at 4 months and continuing until the infant is consuming iron-containing complementary foods such as iron-fortified cereals. Infants who are partially breastfed should receive the same iron supplement if more than half of their daily feedings consist of human milk and they are not consuming iron-rich foods. Formula-feeding infants should receive an iron-fortified commercial infant formula until 12 months of age. Infants younger than 1 year of age should never be fed whole milk (Baker, Greer, & AAP Committee on Nutrition, 2010).

Fluoride levels in human milk and commercial formulas are low. This mineral, which is important in preventing dental caries, can cause spotting of the permanent teeth (fluorosis) in excess amounts. Experts recommend that no fluoride supplements are given to infants younger than 6 months of age. From 6 months to 3 years of age, fluoride supplements are based on the concentration of fluoride in the water supply (AAP Section on Breastfeeding, 2012).

ANATOMY AND PHYSIOLOGY OF LACTATION

ANATOMY OF THE LACTATING BREAST

Each female breast is composed of approximately 15 to 20 segments (lobes) embedded in fat and connective tissues and well supplied with blood vessels, lymphatic vessels, and nerves (Fig. 24.1). Within each lobe is glandular tissue consisting of alveoli, the milk-producing cells, surrounded by myoepithelial cells that contract to send the milk forward to the nipple during milk ejection. Each nipple has multiple pores that transfer milk to the suckling infant. The ratio of glandular to adipose tissue in the lactating breast is approximately 2 : 1 compared with a 1 : 1 ratio in the nonlactating breast. Within each breast is a complex, intertwining network of milk ducts that transport milk from the alveoli to the nipple. The milk ducts dilate and expand at milk ejection (Fig. 24.2).

The size and shape of the breast are not accurate indicators of its ability to produce milk. Although nearly every woman can lactate, a small number have insufficient mammary gland development to breastfeed their infants exclusively. Typically, these women experience few breast changes during puberty or early pregnancy. In some cases,

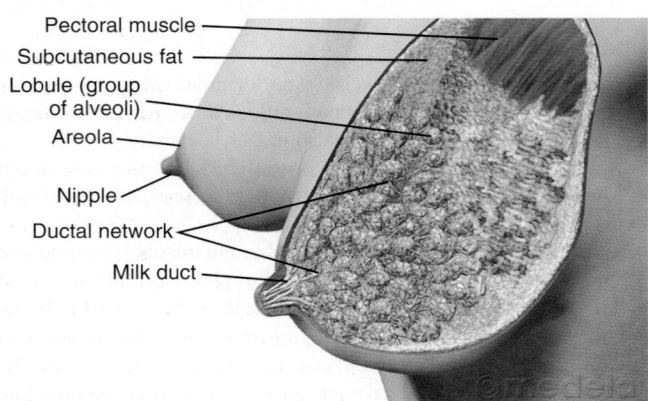

FIG 24.1 Anatomy of the lactating breast. (Copyright 2017 by Medela LLC.)

- Pectoral muscle
- Subcutaneous fat
- Lobule (group of alveoli)
- Areola
- Nipple
- Ductal network
- Milk duct

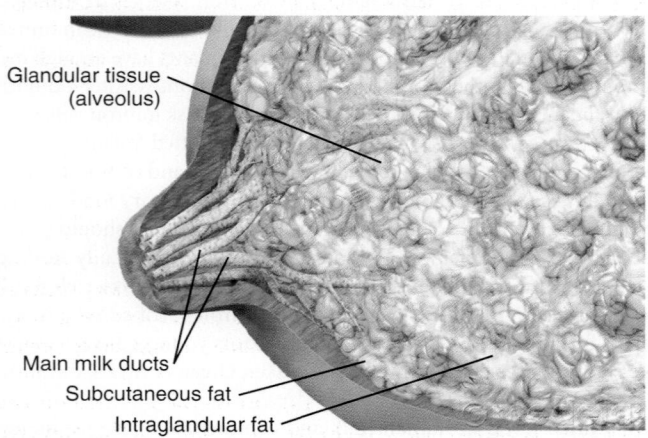

FIG 24.2 Enhanced view of milk glands and ducts. (Copyright 2017 by Medela LLC.)

- Glandular tissue (alveolus)
- Main milk ducts
- Subcutaneous fat
- Intraglandular fat

they are still able to produce some breast milk, although the quantity is not likely to be sufficient to meet the nutritional needs of the infant. These mothers can offer supplemental nutrition to support optimal infant growth.

Because of the effects of estrogen, progesterone, human placental lactogen, and other hormones of pregnancy, changes occur in the breasts in preparation for lactation. Breasts increase in size due to growth of glandular and adipose tissue. Blood flow to the breasts nearly doubles during pregnancy. Sensitivity of the breasts increases, and veins become more prominent. The nipples become more erect, and the areolae darken. Nipples and areola enlarge. At around week 16 of gestation, the alveoli begin producing prepartum milk, or colostrum. Montgomery glands on the areola enlarge. The oily substance secreted by these sebaceous glands helps provide protection against the mechanical stress of sucking and invasion by pathogens. The odor of the secretions can be a means of communication with the infant.

LACTOGENESIS

After the mother gives birth, a precipitous fall in progesterone triggers the release of prolactin from the anterior pituitary gland. During pregnancy, prolactin prepares the breasts to secrete milk and during lactation to synthesize and secrete milk. Prolactin levels are highest during the first 10 days after birth, gradually declining over time but remaining above baseline levels for the duration of lactation. Prolactin is produced in response to infant suckling and emptying of the breasts (Fig. 24.3, *A*). Milk production is a **supply-meets-demand system** (i.e., as milk is removed from the breast, more is produced). Incomplete removal of milk from the breasts can lead to decreased milk supply.

Oxytocin is essential to lactation. As the nipple is stimulated by the suckling infant, the posterior pituitary gland is prompted by the hypothalamus to produce oxytocin. This hormone is responsible for the **milk ejection reflex (MER)**, or **let-down reflex** (see Fig. 24.3, *B*). The myoepithelial cells surrounding the alveoli respond to oxytocin by contracting and sending the milk forward through the ducts to the nipple. The MER is triggered multiple times during a feeding session. Thoughts, sights, sounds, or odors that the mother associates with her baby (or other babies), such as hearing the baby cry, can trigger the MER. Many women report a tingling "pins and needles" sensation in the breasts as milk ejection occurs, although some mothers can detect milk ejection only by observing the sucking and swallowing of the infant. The MER also can occur during sexual activity because oxytocin is released during orgasm. The reflex can be inhibited by fear, stress, and alcohol consumption.

Oxytocin is the same hormone that stimulates uterine contractions during labor. Consequently, the MER can be triggered during labor, as evidenced by leakage of colostrum. This reflex readies the breasts for immediate feeding by the infant after birth. Oxytocin has the important function of contracting the mother's uterus after birth to control postpartum bleeding and promote uterine involution. Thus mothers who breastfeed are at decreased risk for postpartum hemorrhage. Uterine contractions that occur with breastfeeding are often painful during and after feeding for the first 3 to 5 days. These afterpains are more common in multiparas and tend to resolve completely within 1 week after birth.

Prolactin and oxytocin have been called the "mothering hormones" because they affect the postpartum woman's emotions and her physical state. Many women report feeling thirsty or very relaxed during breastfeeding, probably as a result of these hormones.

The nipple-erection reflex is an important part of lactation. When the infant cries, suckles, or rubs against the breast, the nipple becomes erect, which aids in the propulsion of milk through the ducts to the nipple pores. Nipple sizes, shapes, and ability to become erect vary with

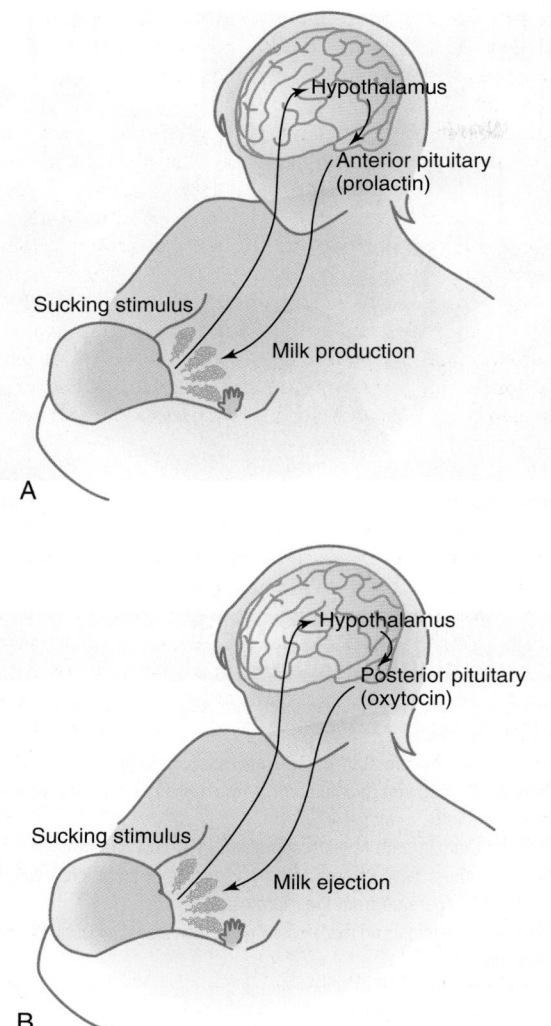

FIG 24.3 Maternal breastfeeding reflexes. **A,** Milk production. **B,** Milk ejection (let-down).

Breast milk promotes colonization and maturation of the infant's intestinal microbiome, which is essential to development of the immune system. The bacteria in human milk vary according to the stage of lactogenesis and gestational age of the infant. Maternal health status and mode of birth affect breast milk microbiota. The predominant flora of breastfed infants are *L. bifidus* and *Bifidobacterium* spp., which metabolize milk saccharides and lower the pH of infant stool; this limits the growth of pathogenic bacteria such as *E. coli, Bacteroides,* and *Staphylococcus* In contrast, the gut microbiota of the formula-fed infant are predominantly gram-negative bacteria, especially *Bacteroides Clostridium, Enterobacter,* and *Enterococcus* (Lawrence & Lawrence, 2016; Mueller, Bakacs, Combellick, et al., 2015). Antibiotics, cesarean birth, and formula-feeding can alter the gut microbiome and may be causally associated with development of autoimmune and metabolic diseases (Mueller et al.).

Human milk composition and volumes vary according to the stage of lactation. In lactogenesis stage I, beginning at approximately 16 to 18 weeks of pregnancy, the breasts prepare for milk production by producing prepartum milk, or colostrum. Stage II of lactogenesis begins with birth as progesterone levels drop sharply when the placenta is removed. For the first 2 to 3 days after birth, the baby receives colostrum, a clear, yellowish fluid that is rich in antibodies and higher in protein but lower in fat than mature milk. The high protein level of colostrum facilitates binding of bilirubin, and the laxative action of colostrum promotes early passage of meconium. Colostrum is important in establishing normal *Lactobacillus bifidus* flora in the infant's digestive tract. It gradually changes to transitional milk. By 3 to 5 days after birth, the woman experiences a noticeable increase in milk production. This is often referred to as *the milk coming in.* Breast milk continues to change in composition for approximately 10 days, when the mature milk is established. This is stage III of lactogenesis (Lawrence & Lawrence, 2016).

The composition of human milk changes over time as the infant grows and develops. Fat is the most variable component of human milk with changes in concentration over a feeding, over a 24-hour period, and across time. Variations in fat content exist between breasts and among individuals. During each feeding, the concentration of fat gradually increases from the lower fat foremilk to the richer hindmilk. The hindmilk contains the denser calories from fat necessary for ensuring optimal growth and contentment between feedings. Because of this changing composition of human milk during each feeding, breastfeeding the infant long enough to supply a balanced feeding is important.

Milk production gradually increases as the baby grows. Infants have fairly predictable growth spurts (at approximately 10 days, 3 weeks, 6 weeks, 3 months, and 6 months), when more frequent feedings stimulate increased milk production. These growth spurts usually last 24 to 48 hours, after which the infants resume their usual feeding pattern as the mother's milk supply increases.

individuals. Some women have flat or inverted nipples that do not become erect with stimulation; these women likely need assistance with effective latch. Their infants should not be offered bottles or pacifiers until breastfeeding is well established.

UNIQUENESS OF HUMAN MILK

Human milk is the ideal food for human infants. It is a dynamic substance with a composition that changes to meet the changing nutritional and immunologic needs of the growing infant. Breast milk is specific to the needs of each infant; for example, the milk produced by mothers of preterm infants differs in composition from that of mothers who give birth at term.

Human milk contains immunologically active components that provide some protection against a broad spectrum of bacterial, viral, and protozoal infections. The major immunoglobulin (Ig) in human milk is secretory IgA; IgG, IgM, IgD, and IgE are also present. Human milk also contains T lymphocytes and B lymphocytes, epidermal growth factor, cytokines, interleukins, bifidus factor, complement (C3 and C4), and lactoferrin, all of which have a specific role in preventing localized and systemic bacterial and viral infections (Lawrence & Lawrence, 2016).

CARE MANAGEMENT

SUPPORTING BREASTFEEDING MOTHERS AND INFANTS

Nurses interact with women in a variety of preconception, prenatal, intrapartum, and postpartum settings. These interactions are strategic opportunities to provide breastfeeding education and support to women and their families (AWHONN, 2015).

The key to encouraging mothers to breastfeed is education and anticipatory guidance, beginning as early as possible during and even before pregnancy. Each encounter with an expectant mother is an opportunity to educate, dispel myths, clarify misinformation, and address concerns. Prenatal education and preparation for breastfeeding influence feeding decisions, breastfeeding success, and the amount of time that women breastfeed. Prenatal preparation ideally includes the father of the baby, partner, or another significant support person and provides information about benefits of breastfeeding and how he or she can participate in infant care and nurturing. Nurses begin by assessing knowledge of the woman and her family about breastfeeding, providing information, and helping them to develop breastfeeding goals and a breastfeeding plan (AWHONN, 2015). Education about breastfeeding is provided through a variety of methods including one-on-one or group sessions, printed materials, videos, and electronic media including websites and phone apps.

As part of the admission assessment to the birthing unit, the nurse asks the woman if she is planning to breastfeed and if she and her partner or family members are knowledgeable about the benefits. The nurse assesses the breasts and nipples and examines the obstetric and medical history for factors that may influence lactation. The events during labor and birth, including medications and any complications that occur such as emergent cesarean or neonatal resuscitation, can influence breastfeeding and should be communicated to the postpartum nurse who can share this information with the lactation consultant (AWHONN, 2015). The labor and delivery nurse assists the mother with initial breastfeeding after birth while the infant is skin-to-skin, providing encouragement and support.

For women with limited access to health care, the postpartum period may provide the first opportunity for education about breastfeeding. Even women who have indicated the desire to formula-feed can benefit from information about the benefits of breastfeeding. Offering these women the chance to try breastfeeding with the assistance of a nurse or lactation consultant can influence a change in infant feeding practices.

Promoting feelings of competence and confidence in the breastfeeding mother and reinforcing the unequaled contribution she is making toward the health and well-being of her infant are the responsibility of the nurse and other health care professionals. The first 2 weeks of breastfeeding can be the most challenging as mothers are adjusting to life with a newborn, the baby is learning to latch on and feed effectively, and the mother may be experiencing nipple or breast discomfort. This is a time when support is critical. Anticipatory guidance during the prenatal period and especially during the hospital stay after birth can provide the mother with information and increase her confidence in her ability to successfully breastfeed her infant. New mothers need access to lactation support following discharge through primary care offices or outpatient lactation services.

Connecting expectant mothers with women from similar backgrounds who are breastfeeding or have successfully breastfed is often helpful. Nursing mothers' support groups such as La Leche League provide information about breastfeeding along with opportunities for breastfeeding mothers to interact with one another and share concerns (Fig. 24.4). Community-based peer counseling programs such as those instituted by the WIC program are beneficial (Chapman & Perez-Escamilla, 2012).

The most common reasons for breastfeeding cessation are insufficient milk supply, painful nipples, and problems getting the infant to feed (Lawrence & Lawrence, 2016; Wagner, Chantry, Dewey, et al., 2013). Early and ongoing assistance and support from health care professionals to prevent and address problems with breastfeeding can help promote a successful and satisfying breastfeeding experience for mothers and infants. Many health care agencies have certified lactation consultants on staff. These health care professionals, who are usually nurses, have specialized training and experience in helping breastfeeding mothers and infants.

The US Breastfeeding Committee (USBC, 2010a) has identified key competencies for health care professionals related to breastfeeding care

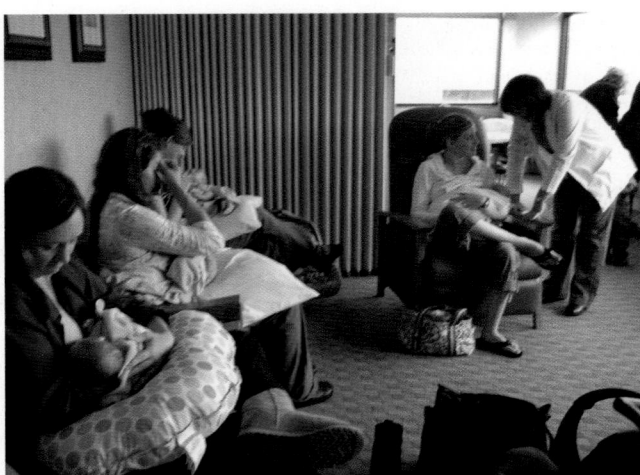

FIG 24.4 Breastfeeding mothers support group with lactation consultant. (Courtesy of Shannon Perry, Phoenix, AZ.)

BOX 24.1 Ten Steps to Successful Breastfeeding for Hospitals

1. Have a written breastfeeding policy that is routinely communicated to all health care staff.
2. Train all health care staff in skills necessary to implement this policy.
3. Inform all pregnant women about the benefits and management of breastfeeding.
4. Help mothers initiate breastfeeding within $\frac{1}{2}$ hour of birth.
5. Show mothers how to breastfeed and maintain lactation, even if they should be separated from their infants.
6. Give newborn infants no food or drink other than breast milk unless medically indicated.
7. Practice rooming-in (i.e., allow mothers and infants to remain together 24 hours a day).
8. Encourage breastfeeding on demand.
9. Give no pacifiers or artificial nipples to breastfeeding infants.
10. Foster the establishment of breastfeeding support groups, and refer mothers to them on discharge from the hospital or clinic.

From Baby-Friendly USA. (2012). *The ten steps to successful breastfeeding*. Retrieved from www.babyfriendlyusa.org/about-us/baby-friendly-hospital-initiative/the-ten-steps.

---

and services. The competencies include knowledge, skills, and attitudes to promote and support breastfeeding. The USBC identifies specific competencies for those who provide more "hands-on" care (e.g., nurses and lactation consultants). The competencies are to "assist in early initiation of breastfeeding, assess the lactating breast, perform an infant feeding observation, recognize normal and abnormal infant feeding patterns, and develop and appropriately communicate a breastfeeding care plan" (USBC, 2010a, p. 5).

All parents are entitled to a birthing environment that promotes and supports breastfeeding. The Baby-Friendly Hospital Initiative (BFHI), sponsored by the WHO and UNICEF, was founded in 1991 to encourage institutions to offer optimal levels of care for lactating mothers. When a hospital achieves the "Ten Steps to Successful Breastfeeding for Hospitals," it is recognized as a Baby-Friendly hospital (Box 24.1). As of August 2016, 369 hospitals and birthing centers in the United States were designated as Baby-Friendly (Baby-Friendly USA, 2016); many hospitals and birthing facilities are working toward the designation. Approximately 18% of live births in the United States occur at Baby-Friendly facilities (CDC, 2016a). More than 20,000 facilities in more than 150 countries have achieved Baby-Friendly status (BFUSA). Women are more likely to achieve their goals for exclusive breastfeeding if they give birth in facilities where all or most of the 10 steps are in place (Perrine, Scanlon, Li, et al., 2012).

The Joint Commission (TJC) issued a set of Perinatal Core Measures that includes exclusive breast milk feeding. In implementing the core measures, hospitals strive to improve their adherence to evidence-based best practices that can result in increased rates of exclusive breastfeeding (TJC, 2012; USBC, 2010b). Care management of the breastfeeding mother and infant requires that nurses and other health care professionals are knowledgeable about the benefits and basic anatomic and physiologic aspects of breastfeeding. They also need to know how to help the mother with feedings and discuss interventions for common problems. Ongoing support of the mother enhances her self-confidence and promotes a satisfying and successful breastfeeding experience. Mothers should be encouraged to ask for help with breastfeeding, especially while they are in the hospital. Women most likely to need assistance are primiparas as well as multiparas who formula-fed their other children. In many facilities these women are routinely seen by lactation consultants.

BREASTFEEDING INITIATION

The mother needs to understand infant behaviors in relation to breastfeeding and recognize signs that the baby is ready to feed. Infants exhibit feeding-readiness cues or early signs of hunger. Instead of waiting to feed until the infant is crying in a distraught manner or withdrawing into sleep, the mother should attempt to breastfeed when the baby exhibits feeding cues (see Evidence-Based Practice box: Interventions for Early Postpartum Breast Pain):

- Hand-to-mouth or hand-to-hand movements
- Sucking motions
- Rooting reflex—infant moves toward whatever touches the area around the mouth and attempts to suck
- Mouthing

Babies normally consume small amounts of milk with feedings during the first 3 days of life. As the baby adjusts to extrauterine life and the digestive tract is cleared of meconium, milk intake increases from 15 to 30 mL per feeding in the first 24 hours to 60 to 90 mL by the end of the first week.

In the postpartum period, interventions focus on helping the mother and the newborn initiate successful breastfeeding. An important goal is to build maternal confidence in breastfeeding. Interventions to promote successful breastfeeding include educating and assisting mothers and their partners with basics such as latch and positioning, signs of adequate feeding, and self-care measures such as prevention of engorgement. It is important to provide the parents with a list of resources that they can contact after discharge from the birthing facility.

The ideal time to begin breastfeeding is within the first hour after birth. Newborns without complications should be allowed to remain in direct skin-to-skin contact with the mother until the baby is able to breastfeed for the first time (AAP Section on Breastfeeding, 2012). This is true both for mothers who gave birth by cesarean section and for those who gave birth vaginally. Early skin-to-skin contact is associated with higher rates of exclusive breastfeeding and increased duration of breastfeeding (Augustin, Donovan, Lozano, et al., 2013; Moore, Anderson, Bergman, et al., 2012; Suzuki, 2013). Routine procedures such as vitamin K injection, eye prophylaxis, weighing, and bathing should be delayed until the neonate has completed the first feeding (AAP Section on Breastfeeding, 2012).

POSITIONING

For the initial feedings, it can be advantageous to encourage and assist the mother to breastfeed in a semi-reclining position with the newborn lying prone, skin-to-skin on the mother's bare chest. Her body supports the baby. The mother is more relaxed, nipple pain is reduced or eliminated, and she has more freedom of movement to use her hands. The baby is able to use inborn reflexes to latch onto the breast and feed effectively. This approach to breastfeeding is based on the concept of "biological nurturing" (Colson, 2012).

The four traditional positions for breastfeeding are the football or clutch hold (under the arm), modified cradle, cross-cradle or across the lap, cradle, and side-lying (Fig. 24.5). The mother should be encouraged to use the position that most easily facilitates latch while allowing maximal comfort. The football or clutch hold is often recommended for early feedings because the mother can see the baby's mouth easily as she guides the infant onto the nipple. Mothers who gave birth by cesarean often prefer the football or clutch hold. The modified cradle or across-the-lap hold works well for early feedings, especially with smaller babies. The side-lying position allows the mother to rest while breastfeeding. Women with perineal pain and swelling often prefer this position. Cradling is the most common breastfeeding position for infants who have learned to latch easily and feed effectively. Before discharge from the birth institution, the nurse can help the mother try all of the positions so she will be confident in trying these positions at home.

During breastfeeding, the mother should be as comfortable as possible. After arranging for privacy, the nurse might suggest that she empty her bladder and attend to other needs before starting a feeding session. The nurse or lactation consultant who is assisting with breastfeeding should be at the mother's eye level. The mother holds the infant securely at the level of the breast, supported by firm pillows or folded blankets, facing toward her. The baby's mouth is directly in front of the nipple. The mother should support the baby's neck and shoulders with her hand and not push on the occiput. The baby's body is held in alignment (ears, shoulders, and hips are in a straight line) during latch and feeding.

LATCH

Latch, or latch-on, is defined as placement of the infant's mouth over the nipple, areola, and breast, making a seal between the mouth and breast to create adequate suction for milk removal. In preparation for latch during early feedings, the mother should manually express a few drops of colostrum or milk and spread it over the nipple. This action lubricates the nipple and entices the baby to open the mouth as the milk is tasted.

To facilitate latch, the mother supports her breast in one hand with the thumb on top and four fingers underneath at the back edge of the areola. The breast is compressed slightly with the fingers parallel to the infant's lips, as one might compress a large sandwich in preparing to take a bite, so an adequate amount of breast tissue is taken into the mouth with latch. Most mothers need to support the breast during feeding for at least the first days until the infant is adept at feeding.

The mother holds the baby close to the breast with the infant's mouth directly in front of the nipple. The infant who is displaying the rooting reflex with the mouth opening widely may easily latch on. If the infant is not readily opening the mouth, the mother tickles the baby's lips with her nipple, stimulating the mouth to open. When the mouth is open wide and the tongue is down, the mother quickly "hugs" the baby to the breast, bringing him or her onto the nipple (Fig. 24.6). The amount of areola in the baby's mouth with correct latch depends

EVIDENCE-BASED PRACTICE
Interventions for Early Postpartum Breast Pain

Ask the Question

PICOT Question: For postpartum women, could education on techniques to decrease breast engorgement help improve breastfeeding duration?

Search for the Evidence

Search Strategies: English language research-based publications on engorgement, breast pain, nipple pain, breastfeeding, hand expression, breast massage were included

Databases Used: Cochrane Collaborative Database, JoAnna Briggs Institute, National Guideline Clearinghouse (AHRQ), CINAHL, PubMed, and the professional websites for ACOG, AWHONN, and the Academy of Breastfeeding Medicine.

Critical Appraisal of the Evidence

Women are encouraged to exclusively breastfeed for the first 6 months of life, but without support and education, they may face challenges that cause them to stop early. Nipple pain is one of the early challenges (Newby & Davies, 2016).

- A Cochrane Database review examined four trials involving 656 women with nipple pain, and found insufficient evidence to recommend lanolin, lanolin shells, glycerin gel dressings, or all-purpose nipple cream. They suggested using breast milk or nothing on sore nipples, and found that, regardless of treatment, symptoms got better by 7 to 10 days postpartum (Dennis, Jackson, & Watson, 2014).

Another early challenge is breast engorgement, peaking around day 5 postpartum. As colostrum production transitions to milk, postpartum women may find that painful and swollen breasts make it more difficult for the newborn to latch on.

- New mothers who were given education about breast engorgement management techniques at their child's postdischarge visit on day 5 reported increased use of hand expression, massage towards the axilla, reverse pressure softening (description below), ice packs, and more frequent feeding. Painful engorgement was significantly decreased, and patients appreciated being empowered to self-manage (Witt, Bolman, & Kredit, 2016). The authors suggest that education provided solely during the hospitalization may have been forgotten after discharge, and skills taught at the time when needed have the best uptake.
- Women who experience luteal (premenstrual) breast engorgement are at greater risk to experience postpartum engorgement. Those women can decrease their symptoms by hand expressing their colostrum thoroughly at least once before the transitional milk appears (Alekseev, Vladimir, & Nadezhda, 2015).

Apply the Evidence: Nursing Implications

Teaching women to manage breastfeeding is one of the 10 steps for Baby-Friendly hospitals.

- Massaging the breast tissue allows the let-down reflex to engage. This is accomplished using a circular or rhythmic massage or tapping of the breast tissue. Hand expression is the technique of removing milk from the breasts, and involves compressing behind the areola toward the nipple (Witt et al., 2016).
- When the breasts are engorged, ice packs between feedings and reverse pressure softening decreases excess swelling. Reverse pressure softening consists of applying oil to the skin and lightly massaging the tissue towards the axilla. The engorged nipple can be compressed gently for up to 1 minute, in order to make it less swollen and easier for the newborn to latch (for technique, see http://bfmedneo.com/resources/video) (Witt et al., 2016).

Quality and Safety Competencies: Evidence-Based Practice*
Knowledge

Describe how the strength and relevance of available evidence influences the choice of interventions in provision of patient-centered care.

Breast massage and hand expression education provide improved outcomes and a better chance for prolonged breastfeeding.

Skills

Locate evidence reports related to clinical practice topics and guidelines.

Skills learned about breast massage and reverse pressure softening of the areola improve newborn latch.

Attitudes

Value the need for continuous improvement in clinical practice based on new knowledge.

New knowledge about ice packs and massage techniques may improve comfort and breastfeeding efficacy during engorgement.

References

Alekseev, N. P., Vladimir, I. I., & Nadezhda, T. E. (2015). Pathological postpartum breast engorgement: Prediction, prevention, and resolution. *Breastfeeding Medicine, 10*(4), 203–208.

Dennis, C., Jackson, K., & Watson, J. (2014). Interventions for treating painful nipples among breastfeeding women. *Cochrane Database of Systematic Reviews, 2014*(12), CD007366.

Newby, R. M., & Davies, P. S. (2016). Why do women stop breastfeeding? Results from a contemporary prospective study in a cohort of Australian women. *European Journal of Clinical Nutrition, 70*(12), 1428–1432.

Witt, A. M., Bolman, M., & Kredit, S. (2016). Mothers value and utilize outpatient education on breast massage and hand expression in their self-management of engorgement. *Breastfeeding Medicine, 11*(9), 1–7.

Pat Mahaffee Gingrich

*Adapted from QSEN at www.qsen.org/

---

on the size of the baby's mouth and the size of the areola and nipple. If breastfeeding is painful, the baby likely has not taken enough of the breast into the mouth, and the tongue is pinching the nipple.

Mothers may use the *asymmetric latch technique*. When the baby's mouth opens widely, the mother moves the baby in toward her body so the chin and lower mandible make contact with the breast first, followed by the top lip. When the baby is latched on, the nose is tilted slightly away from the mother's breast, and the chin is pressed into the underside of the breast. The infant's mouth placement is asymmetric on the areola; the lower part is covered by the baby's mouth, but the top is clearly visible above the top lip.

Once the infant is latched on and sucking, there are signs that the feeding is going well. These include (1) the mother reports a firm tugging sensation on her nipple but feels no pinching or pain; (2) the baby sucks with cheeks rounded, not dimpled; (3) the baby's jaw glides smoothly with sucking; and (4) swallowing is usually audible. Sucking creates a vacuum in the intraoral cavity as the breast is compressed between the tongue and the palate. When the infant is latched on and sucking correctly, breastfeeding is not painful. If the mother feels pinching or pain after the initial sucks or does not feel a strong tugging sensation on the nipple, the latch and positioning are evaluated. Any time the signs of adequate latch and sucking are not present, the baby should

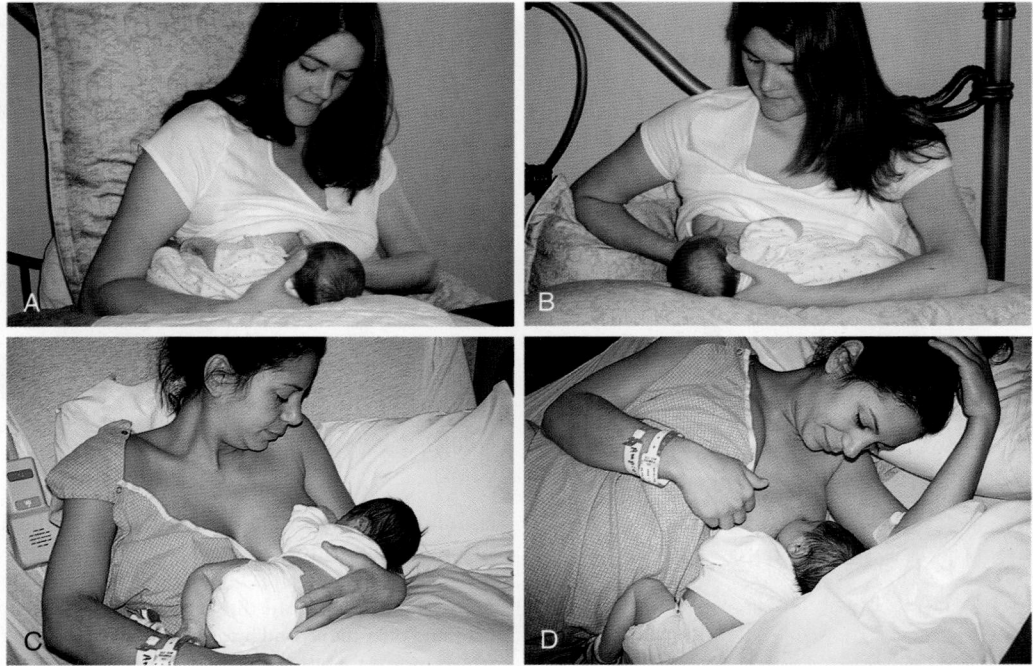

FIG 24.5 Breastfeeding positions. **A,** Football or clutch (under the arm) hold. **B,** Across the lap (modified cradle). **C,** Cradling. **D,** Side-lying. (A and B, Courtesy of Kathryn Alden, Chapel Hill, NC; C and D, Courtesy of Marjorie Pyle, RNC, Lifecircle, Costa Mesa, CA.)

be taken off the breast, and latch attempted again. To prevent nipple trauma as the baby is taken off the breast, the mother is instructed to break the suction by inserting a finger in the side of the baby's mouth between the gums and leaving it there until the nipple is completely out of the mouth (Fig. 24.7) (see Nursing Care Plan: Breastfeeding and Infant Nutrition).

The nurse should observe at least one feeding every 8 to 12 hours while the mother and newborn are in the hospital (Holmes, McLeod, & Bunik, 2013). Using a standard breastfeeding scoring tool such as the LATCH tool (Jenson, Wallace, & Kelsay, 1994) to document observations provides consistency in assessment criteria. With the LATCH assessment tool, each letter represents a scored item: *L*atch, *A*udible swallowing, *T*ype of nipple, *C*omfort level of the mother, and *H*old (positioning). During the feeding assessment, the nurse can provide education about breastfeeding, help with feeding techniques, and offer support. If the mother's partner or other family members are present, the nurse can include them in the teaching and demonstrate how they can help the mother and provide support.

MILK EJECTION OR LET-DOWN

As the baby begins sucking on the nipple, the milk ejection, or let-down, reflex is stimulated (see Fig. 24.3, *B*). The following signs indicate that milk ejection has occurred:

- The mother may feel a tingling sensation in the nipples and breasts, although many women never feel when milk ejection occurs.
- The baby's suck changes from quick, shallow sucks to a slower, more drawing sucking pattern.
- Audible swallowing is heard as the baby sucks.
- In the early days, the mother feels uterine cramping and can have increased lochia during and after feedings.
- The mother feels relaxed or drowsy during feedings.
- The opposite breast may leak.

FREQUENCY OF FEEDINGS

Feeding patterns vary because every mother-infant dyad is unique. Breastfeeding frequency is influenced by a variety of factors, including the infant's age, weight, maturity level, stomach capacity and gastric emptying time, and the storage capacity of the breast (i.e., the milk available when the breast is full).

Newborns need to breastfeed at least 8 to 12 times in a 24-hour period (AAP Section on Breastfeeding, 2012). Some infants breastfeed every 2 to 3 hours throughout a 24-hour period. Others cluster-feed, breastfeeding every hour or so for three to five feedings and then sleeping for 3 to 4 hours between clusters. During the first 24 to 48 hours after birth, most babies do not awaken often enough to feed. Parents need to understand that they should awaken the baby to feed at least every 3 hours during the day and at least every 4 hours at night. (Feeding frequency is determined by counting from the beginning of one feeding to the beginning of the next.) Once the infant is feeding well and gaining weight adequately, going to **demand feeding** is appropriate, in which case the infant determines the frequency of feedings. (With demand feeding, the infant should still receive at least eight feedings in 24 hours.)

> **⚡ SAFETY ALERT**
>
> Nurses should caution parents against attempting to place newborn infants on strict feeding schedules. Strict scheduling of feedings (forcing the baby to wait for a set amount of time before feeding) can result in failure to meet the nutritional needs of infants.

Infants should be fed whenever they exhibit feeding cues. Keeping the baby close is the best way to observe and respond to these cues. Newborns should remain with mothers during the recovery period after birth and room-in during the hospital stay. At home, babies should be kept nearby so parents can observe signs that the baby is ready to

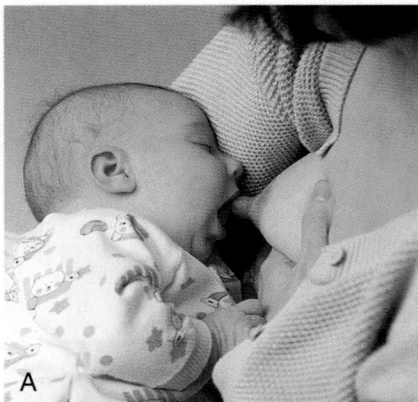

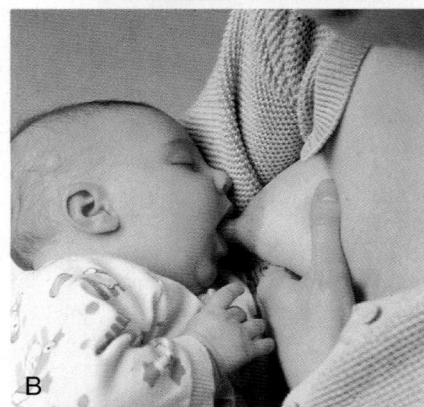

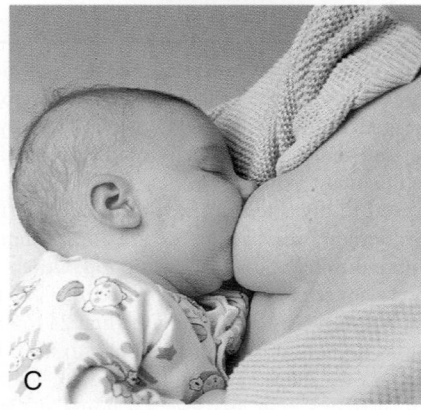

FIG 24.6 Latch. **A,** Mother tickles baby's lips with nipple until he or she opens wide. **B,** Once baby's mouth is opened wide, she quickly "hugs" baby to breast. **C,** Baby should have as much areola (dark area around nipple) in his or her mouth as possible, not just the nipple. (Courtesy of Medela, Inc., McHenry, IL.)

feed. The mother and breastfeeding infant should sleep in proximity (in the same room but not in the same bed) to promote breastfeeding (AAP Section on Breastfeeding, 2012).

DURATION OF FEEDINGS

The duration of breastfeeding sessions varies greatly because the timing of milk transfer differs for each mother-baby pair. The average time for early feedings is 30 to 40 minutes or approximately 15 to 20 minutes per breast. As infants grow, they become more efficient at breastfeeding, and consequently the length of feedings decreases. The amount of time an infant spends breastfeeding is not a reliable indicator of the amount

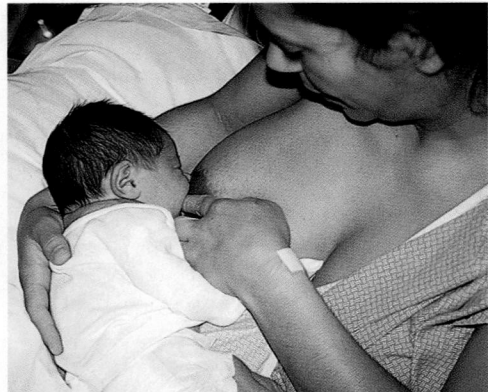

FIG 24.7 Removing infant from breast by inserting a finger to break suction. (Courtesy of Marjorie Pyle, RNC, Lifecircle, Costa Mesa, CA.)

of milk the infant consumes because some of the time at the breast is spent in nonnutritive sucking.

In the early days after birth, the mother may be instructed to feed on the first breast until the neonate falls asleep and try to wake the baby and offer the second breast. Some mothers prefer one-sided nursing, which means that the baby nurses only one breast at each feeding. The first breast offered should be alternated at each feeding to ensure that each breast receives equal stimulation and emptying.

Instead of instructing mothers to feed for a set number of minutes, nurses should teach them to look for signs that the baby has finished feeding (e.g., the baby's sucking and swallowing pattern has slowed, the breast is softened, the baby appears content and may fall asleep or release the nipple).

If a baby seems to be feeding effectively and urine output and bowel movements are adequate but the weight gain is not satisfactory, the mother may be switching to the second breast too soon. Feeding on the first breast until it softens ensures that the baby receives the higher-fat hindmilk, which usually results in increased weight gain.

INDICATORS OF EFFECTIVE BREASTFEEDING

One of the most common concerns of breastfeeding mothers is how to determine if the baby is getting enough milk. In the newborn period, when breastfeeding is becoming established, parents should be taught about the signs that breastfeeding is going well. Awareness of these signs helps them recognize when problems arise so they can seek appropriate assistance (Box 24.2).

During the early days of breastfeeding, keeping a feeding diary can be helpful. This involves recording the time and length of feedings and infant urine output and bowel movements. The data from the diary provide evidence of the effectiveness of breastfeeding and are useful to health care providers in assessing adequacy of feeding. Parents are instructed to take this feeding diary to the follow-up visit with the infant's health care provider. There are smartphone apps that parents can use to track infant feedings and urine/stool output.

The infant's output is highly indicative of feeding adequacy. It is important that parents are aware of the expected changes in the characteristics of urine output and bowel movements during the early newborn period. As the volume of breast milk increases, urine becomes more dilute and should be light yellow; dark, concentrated urine can be associated with inadequate intake and possible dehydration. (Note: Infants with jaundice often have darker urine as bilirubin is excreted.) Infants should have at least six to eight sufficiently wet diapers (light yellow urine) every 24 hours after day 4. The first 1 to 2 days after birth,

◎ NURSING CARE PLAN

Breastfeeding and Infant Nutrition

Case Study

Nikki is G2 P2 with a 3-year-old son, Alex, at home. She gave birth to a healthy baby girl yesterday at 40 weeks gestation after an uneventful vaginal birth. Nikki did not breastfeed Alex, but decided to breastfeed her daughter, Molly, after learning the benefits of breastfeeding. Nikki has seen several of her friends successfully breastfeed babies; they made it look easy. Nikki is optimistic about breastfeeding, although she does express some apprehension about getting her baby to latch correctly so breastfeeding is not painful.

Assessment

What are signs of ineffective breastfeeding? What are signs of correct positioning and latching? What information and support is needed for a mother who is breastfeeding for the first time?

Defining Characteristics

Actual or perceived inadequate milk supply (mother)
Arching and crying when at breast (infant)
Inability to latch on to nipple correctly (infant)
Inadequate opportunity for suckling (infant)
Evidence of inadequate intake (infant)
Insufficient emptying of each breast (mother)
Unsatisfactory breastfeeding process (mother and infant)

Nursing Diagnosis

Risk for Ineffective Breastfeeding related to knowledge deficit of the mother as evidenced by her stated concerns about latch technique

Expected Outcomes

Nikki will demonstrate correct latch techniques; Molly will latch correctly and suck with gliding jaw movements and audible swallowing.
Nikki will report "tugging" but no nipple pain with infant suckling.
Nikki will express increased satisfaction with breastfeeding, and Molly will exhibit satisfaction of hunger and sucking needs.

Nursing Interventions	Rationales
Assess Nikki's knowledge and motivation for breastfeeding.	To provide starting point for teaching
Observe breastfeeding session at least once each shift and document findings.	To provide baseline assessment for positive reinforcement and problem identification
Describe and demonstrate ways to stimulate sucking reflex, various positions for breastfeeding, and use of pillows during session.	To promote maternal and neonatal comfort and effective latch
Monitor position of Molly's mouth on areola and position of head and body; observe for gliding movements of jaw and audible swallowing.	To give positive reinforcement for correct latch position or to correct poor latch position and to monitor for milk transfer
Teach Nikki ways to stimulate Molly to maintain an awake state by diapering, unwrapping, or massaging.	To complete breastfeeding session thoroughly and satisfactorily
Give Nikki information regarding her diet while breastfeeding, expression of milk by hand or pump, and storage of expressed breast milk.	To provide basic information
Provide Nikki with printed information on all aspects of breastfeeding and refer her to reliable Web-based resources.	To reinforce verbal instructions and demonstrations

Nursing Interventions	Rationales
Provide Nikki with information about follow-up care and support after discharge, including support groups, lactation consultants, and other community resources.	To provide further information and group support

Case Study (Continued)

It is now 24 hours after birth, and Nikki has breastfed her newborn daughter, Molly, every 3 hours since birth as instructed by the nurses, although sometimes Molly falls asleep after a few sucks. She has experienced difficulty in getting Molly to latch. Her nipples appear reddened. The nurse adjusts Molly's position, shows Nikki how to safely remove the baby from the breast, and assists Nikki with latching the baby to the breast. Nikki says that she is more comfortable but that her nipples are already sore and that breastfeeding is much harder than she thought it would be. Molly has not yet voided or stooled since birth. Nikki begins to cry and says she is very worried about whether she can breastfeed her baby.

Assessment

What are signs that Nikki is having difficulty with breastfeeding? How can you determine whether Molly is receiving adequate nutrition? What assistance and education does Nikki need to successfully breastfeed her baby?

Defining Characteristics

Nipple discomfort
Reddened nipples
Difficulty with positioning and latch
Inability to initiate or sustain effective suck
Infant falls asleep while feeding
Lack of output

Nursing Diagnosis

Ineffective Breastfeeding related to incorrect latch and sleepy baby as evidenced by lack of urinary output and bowel movement since birth

Expected Outcomes

Molly will void at least 2 to 3 times in the next 24 hours and will have at least one bowel movement.
Molly will lose no more than 10% of her birth weight within the first week of life.
Molly will gain 4 to 7 oz (114 to 199 g) per week after the first week of life.
Molly will not become dehydrated.
Nikki will identify signs that milk transfer is occurring.
Nikki will express increased confidence in her ability to breastfeed and to identify signs that the baby is receiving adequate intake.
Molly will establish an effective feeding pattern.

Nursing Interventions	Rationales
Observe feeding session, assessing positioning, latch, infant sucking, and signs of milk transfer.	To identify cause of sore nipples and to assess for signs that milk transfer is occurring
Assess for factors that can contribute to ineffective sucking and swallowing.	To provide basis for plan of care
Teach Nikki to observe feeding-readiness cues.	To enhance effective feeding

Continued

NURSING CARE PLAN
Breastfeeding and Infant Nutrition—cont'd

Nursing Interventions	Rationales
Assess Molly's oral anatomy and ability to suck.	To identify signs of ankyloglossia or other factors that can inhibit effective sucking and milk transfer
Monitor infant output and weight; assess for signs of dehydration.	To determine adequacy of feeding and prevent dehydration.
Teach Nikki about signs of effective feeding (i.e., signs that breastfeeding is going well).	To prevent dehydration and excessive weight loss
Assist Nikki to modify positioning and latch techniques as needed.	To maintain hydration status and nutritional requirements
Teach Nikki how to treat sore nipples.	To promote comfort
Promote calm, relaxed atmosphere.	To provide pleasant breastfeeding experience for Nikki and Molly
Refer to lactation consultant.	To provide specialized support

Assessment

What are signs of maternal anxiety? What measures can the nurse use to assist Nikki to relieve her anxiety?

Defining Characteristics

Irritability
Fearfulness
Uncertainty
Shakiness
Increased tension
Impaired attention

Nursing Diagnosis

Anxiety related to ineffective infant feeding pattern

Expected Outcomes

Nikki will identify factors that elicit anxious behaviors.
Nikki will discuss activities that tend to decrease anxious behaviors.
Nikki and Molly will establish a satisfactory feeding pattern.
Nikki will report a decrease in anxiety level and express satisfaction with breastfeeding.

Nursing Interventions	Rationales
Assess Nikki's feelings and anxieties about breastfeeding.	To identify specific concerns
Monitor Nikki's anxiety level during feeding sessions.	To provide basis for care planning
Provide education about breastfeeding	To help mother increase her knowledge about breastfeeding and improve her confidence
Provide positive reinforcement to Nikki for feeding pattern improvement.	To decrease anxiety
Monitor Molly's weight, intake, and output.	To assess milk transfer
Enlist assistance of support persons.	To provide positive feedback for increasing skill
Provide information for lactation support.	To decrease anxiety after discharge
Initiate follow-up (telephone calls, follow-up with health care provider, outpatient lactation consultant) as needed.	To assess progress, detect problems, and provide support

BOX 24.2   Signs of Effective Breastfeeding

Mother
- Onset of copious milk production (milk is "in") by day 3 or 4
- Firm tugging sensation on nipple as infant sucks but no pain
- Uterine contractions and increased vaginal bleeding while feeding (first week or less)
- Feels relaxed and drowsy while feeding
- Increased thirst
- Breasts soften or feel lighter while feeding
- With milk ejection (let-down), can feel warm rush or tingling in breasts, leaking of milk from opposite breast

Infant
- Latches without difficulty
- Has bursts of 15 to 20 sucks/swallows at a time
- Audible swallowing is present
- Easily releases breast at end of feeding
- Infant appears content after feeding
- Has at least three substantive bowel movements and six to eight wet diapers every 24 hours after day 4

newborns pass meconium stools, which are greenish black, thick, and sticky. By day 2 or 3, the stools become greener, thinner, and less sticky. If the mother's milk has come in by day 3 or 4, the stools start to appear greenish yellow and are looser. By the end of the first week, breast milk stools are yellow, soft, and seedy (they resemble a mixture of mustard and cottage cheese). If an infant is still passing meconium stool by day 3 or 4, breastfeeding effectiveness and milk transfer should be assessed.

Infants should have at least three stools (quarter-size or larger) per day for the first month. Some babies stool with every feeding. The stooling pattern gradually changes; breastfed infants can continue to stool more than once per day, or they may stool only every 2 or 3 days. As long as the baby continues to gain weight and appears healthy, this decrease in the number of bowel movements is normal.

SUPPLEMENTS, BOTTLES, AND PACIFIERS

Unless a medical indication exists, no supplements should be given to breastfeeding infants (AAP Section on Breastfeeding, 2012). With sound breastfeeding knowledge and practice, supplements are rarely needed. Early supplementation by hospital staff undermines a new mother's confidence and models behavior that is counterproductive to establishing breastfeeding.

When supplementation is deemed necessary, giving the baby expressed breast milk is best. If the mother is not able to provide the milk, the recommended alternative is pasteurized donor milk from a milk bank. However, in many cases donor milk is not readily accessible and a commercial infant formula is used. Before supplementation, it is important to perform a careful evaluation of the mother-infant dyad.

Possible indications for supplementary feeding include infant factors such as hypoglycemia, dehydration, weight loss of more than 7% associated with delayed lactogenesis, delayed passage of bowel movements or meconium stool continued to day 5, poor milk transfer, or hyperbilirubinemia (ABM Protocol Committee, 2009).

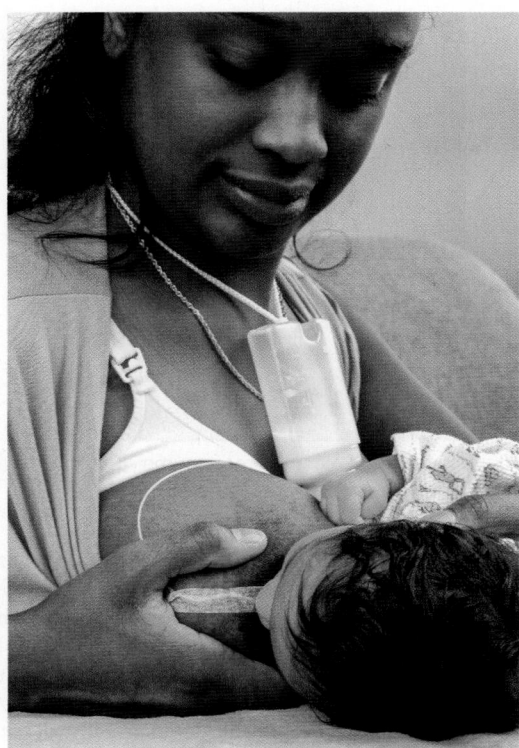

FIG 24.8 Supplemental nursing device. (Copyright 2017 by Medela LLC.)

Maternal indications for possible supplementation include delayed lactogenesis and intolerable pain during feedings. Women who have had previous breast surgery such as augmentation or reduction may need to provide supplementary feedings for their infants (ABM Protocol Committee, 2009).

Newborns can become confused going from breast to bottle or bottle to breast when breastfeeding is first being established. Breastfeeding and bottle-feeding require different oral motor skills. It is best to avoid bottles until breastfeeding is well established, usually after 3 or 4 weeks.

If supplemental feeding is needed, nurses or lactation consultants can help parents use supplemental nursing devices. This allows the baby to be supplemented with expressed breast milk or infant formula while still breastfeeding (Fig. 24.8). Infants can also be fed with a spoon, dropper, cup, or syringe. If parents choose to use bottles, a slow-flow nipple is recommended. Although some parents combine breastfeeding and bottle-feeding, some infants never take a bottle and go directly from the breast to a cup.

Because of the correlation between pacifier use and a decreased risk for sudden infant death syndrome (SIDS), experts recommend pacifier use for healthy term infants at nap or sleep time, but only after breastfeeding is well established at about 3 or 4 weeks of age (AAP Section on Breastfeeding, 2012).

SPECIAL CONSIDERATIONS

Sleepy Baby

Some babies need to be awakened for feedings for the first few days after birth. If the infant is awakened from a sound sleep, attempts at feeding may be unsuccessful. Babies are more likely to feed if they are awakened from a light or active sleep state. Signs that the infant is in this sleep state are movements of the eyelids, body movements, and making sounds while sleeping. Unwrapping the baby, changing the diaper, sitting the baby upright, talking to him or her with variable

pitch, gently massaging his or her chest or back, and stroking the palms or soles may bring the baby to an alert state. It is helpful to place the sleepy baby skin-to-skin with the mother; she can move the infant to the breast when feeding-readiness cues are apparent.

Fussy Baby

Babies sometimes awaken from sleep crying frantically. Although they are hungry, they cannot focus on feeding until they are calmed. Parents can swaddle the baby, hold him or her close, talk soothingly, and allow him or her to suck on a clean finger until calm enough to latch on to the breast. Placing the baby skin-to-skin with the mother can be very effective in calming a fussy infant. Fussiness during feeding can be the result of birth injury such as bruising of the head or fractured clavicle. Changing the feeding position can help alleviate this problem.

Infants who were suctioned extensively or intubated at birth can demonstrate an aversion to oral stimulation. The baby may scream and stiffen if anything approaches the mouth. Parents need to spend time holding and cuddling the baby before attempting to breastfeed.

An infant can become fussy and appear discontented when sucking if the nipple does not extend far enough into the mouth. The feeding can begin with well-organized sucks and swallows, but the infant soon begins to pull off the breast and cry. The mother should support her breast throughout the feeding so the nipple stays in the same position as the feeding proceeds and the breast softens.

Fussiness can be related to GI distress (e.g., cramping, gas pains, gastroesophageal reflux). It can occur in response to an occasional feeding of infant formula, or it can be related to something the mother has ingested, although most women are able to eat a normal diet without causing GI distress to the breastfeeding infant. Persistent crying or refusing to breastfeed can indicate illness. Parents are instructed to notify the health care provider if either circumstance occurs.

Some mothers find that their babies are less fussy when placed in a sling or carrier. Some slings make it easy to breastfeed without removing the baby from the sling (Fig. 24.9).

Slow Weight Gain

Newborn infants typically lose 5% to 10% of body weight after birth before they begin to gain weight. Weight loss of more than 7% in a breastfeeding infant during the first 3 days of life needs to be investigated (Lawrence & Lawrence, 2016). After the early milk has transitioned to mature milk, infants should gain approximately 110 to 200 g (3.9 to 7 oz) per week or 20 to 28 g (0.7 to 1 oz) per day for the first 3 months. Breastfed infants usually do not gain weight as quickly as formula-fed infants.

Parents are taught the warning signs of ineffective breastfeeding, including inadequate weight gain, minimal output, and feeding constantly. If any of these warning signs is present, the parent should notify the health care provider.

At times, slow weight gain is related to inadequate breastfeeding. Feedings can be short or infrequent, or the infant can be latching incorrectly or sucking ineffectively or inefficiently. Other possibilities are illness or infection; malabsorption; or circumstances that increase the baby's energy needs such as congenital heart disease, cystic fibrosis, or being small for gestational age. Slow weight gain must be differentiated from failure to thrive; this can be a serious problem that warrants medical intervention.

Maternal factors can be the cause of slow weight gain. The mother can have a problem with inadequate emptying of the breasts, pain with feeding, or inappropriate timing of feedings. Inadequate glandular breast tissue or previous breast surgery can affect milk supply. Severe intrapartum or postpartum hemorrhage (Sheehan syndrome), illness, or medications can decrease milk supply. Stress and fatigue also negatively affect milk production (Lawrence & Lawrence, 2016).

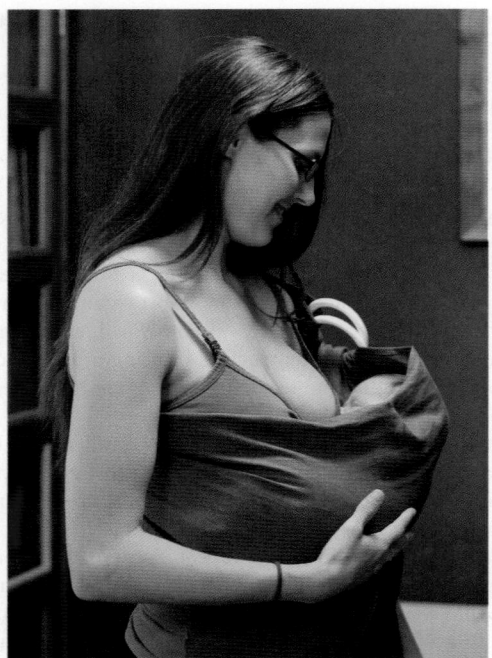

FIG 24.9 Baby breastfeeding while in sling. (Courtesy of Julie Perry Nelson, Loveland, CO.)

In most instances, the solution to slow weight gain is to increase feeding frequency and to improve the feeding technique. Positioning and latch are evaluated, and adjustments are made. Adding a feeding or two in a 24-hour period can help. If the problem is a sleepy baby, parents are instructed in waking techniques.

Using alternate breast massage during feedings can help increase the amount of milk going to the infant. With this technique, the mother massages her breast from the chest wall to the nipple whenever the baby has sucking pauses. This technique also can increase the fat content of the milk, which aids in weight gain.

When babies are calorie deprived and need supplementation, they can receive expressed breast milk or formula with a supplemental nursing device (see Fig. 24.8), spoon, cup, syringe, or bottle. In most cases, supplementation is necessary only for a short time until the baby gains weight and is feeding adequately.

Jaundice

Chapter 22 and Chapter 23 discuss jaundice (hyperbilirubinemia) in the newborn in detail. Breastfeeding infants can develop early-onset jaundice or breastfeeding-associated jaundice, which is associated with insufficient feeding and infrequent stooling. Colostrum has a natural laxative effect and promotes early passage of meconium. Bilirubin is excreted from the body primarily through the intestines. Infrequent stooling allows bilirubin in the stool to be resorbed into the infant's system, thus increasing bilirubin levels (Blackburn, 2013).

To prevent early-onset, breastfeeding-associated jaundice, newborns should breastfeed frequently (at least 8 to 12 times in 24 hours) during the first several days of life. Increased frequency of feedings is associated with decreased bilirubin levels (Kamath-Rayne, Thilo, Deacon, et al., 2016).

To treat early-onset jaundice, breastfeeding is evaluated in terms of frequency and length of feedings, positioning, latch, and milk transfer. Factors such as a sleepy or lethargic infant or maternal breast engorgement can interfere with effective breastfeeding and should be corrected. If the infant is not breastfeeding effectively, the mother can use a mechanical

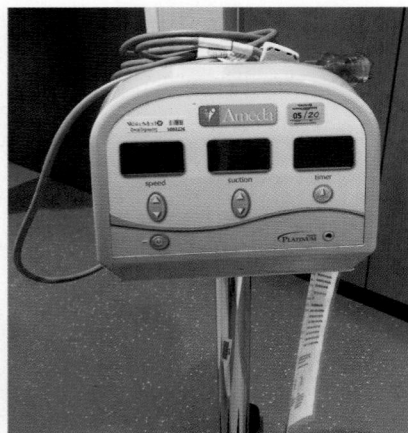

FIG 24.10 Hospital-grade electric breast pump. (Courtesy of Kathryn Alden, Chapel Hill, NC.)

breast pump to stimulate her milk supply and the expressed milk can be fed to the infant. In some cases, donor milk or formula supplementation is needed. Bilirubin levels are closely monitored (Kamath-Rayne et al., 2016).

Late-onset jaundice or breast milk jaundice affects a small number of breastfed infants and develops between 5 and 10 days of age. Affected infants typically thrive, gain weight, and stool normally; all pathologic causes of jaundice have been ruled out. In the presence of other risk factors, hyperbilirubinemia can be severe enough to require phototherapy. In most cases of breast milk jaundice, no intervention is necessary. Some health care providers recommend temporary interruption of breastfeeding for 12 to 24 hours to allow bilirubin levels to decrease (Newton, 2017).

Any breastfeeding infant who develops jaundice should be evaluated carefully for weight loss greater than 7%, decreased milk intake, infrequent stooling (fewer than three stools per day), and decreased urine output (fewer than four to six wet diapers per day). Bilirubin levels should be assessed by serum testing or transcutaneous monitoring (see Chapter 23).

Preterm Infants

Human milk is the ideal food for preterm infants, with benefits that are unique and in addition to those received by term healthy infants. Breast milk enhances retinal maturation in the preterm infant and improves neurocognitive outcomes; it also decreases the risk for sepsis and necrotizing enterocolitis. Greater physiologic stability occurs with breastfeeding compared to bottle-feeding (AAP Section on Breastfeeding, 2012; Lawrence & Lawrence, 2016).

Initially preterm milk contains higher concentrations of protein, sodium, chloride, potassium, iron, and magnesium than term milk. It is more similar to term milk by approximately 4 to 6 weeks. Depending on gestational age and physical condition, many preterm infants are capable of breastfeeding for at least some feedings each day. Mothers of preterm infants who are not able to breastfeed their infants should begin pumping their breasts as soon as possible after birth with a hospital-grade electric pump (Fig. 24.10). Pumping frequency depends on the mother's breastfeeding goals but may be recommended 8 to 10 times every 24 hours to establish the milk supply. These women are taught proper handling and storage of breast milk to minimize bacterial contamination and growth. Kangaroo care (skin-to-skin contact) is encouraged until the baby is able to breastfeed and while breastfeeding is established because it enhances milk production (Meier, Patel, Bigger, et al., 2013).

Mothers of preterm infants often receive specific emotional benefits in breastfeeding or providing breast milk for their babies. They find rewards in knowing that they can provide the healthiest nutrition for the infant and believe that breastfeeding enhances feelings of closeness to the infant.

Late Preterm Infants

Neonates born at 34 0/7 to 36 6/7 weeks of gestation are categorized as late preterm infants. These newborns are at risk for feeding difficulties because of their low energy stores and high energy demands. Additionally, they are more prone to hypothermia, hypoglycemia, and hyperbilirubinemia (ABM Protocol Committee, 2011a; Cooper, Holditch-Davis, Verklan, et al., 2012). They tend to be sleepy, with minimal and short wakeful periods. Late preterm infants often tire easily while feeding and have a weak suck and low tone; these factors can contribute to inadequate milk intake resulting in dehydration and poor weight gain (Meier, Patel, Wright, et al., 2013). This predisposes mothers to delayed onset of lactogenesis II and inadequate milk supply.

Goals of care are to nourish the infant and protect the mother's milk supply. A lactation consultant should be involved in planning and providing appropriate care that usually includes milk expression with a hospital-grade pump and supplementation of the infant with expressed breast milk or infant formula (Meier, Patel, Wright, et al., 2013).

Early and extended skin-to-skin contact promotes breastfeeding and helps prevent hypothermia. Because these infants are more prone to positional apnea than term infants, mothers are advised to use the clutch (under the arm or football) or cross-cradle hold for feeding, and avoid flexing the head, which can impede breathing. When supplementation is needed, expressed breast milk is the optimal supplement. Due to their weak suck, many infants are fed with a bottle, although in some cases a supplemental feeding device can be used (see Fig. 24.8) (Lanese & Cross, 2013; Meier, Patel, Wright, et al., 2013).

Breastfeeding Multiple Infants

Breastfeeding is especially beneficial to twins, triplets, and other higher-order multiples because of the immunologic and nutritional advantages and the opportunity for the mother to interact with each baby frequently. Most mothers are capable of producing an adequate milk supply for multiple infants. Parenting multiples can be overwhelming; mothers and their husbands or partners need extra support and help to learn how to manage feedings (Fig. 24.11). Parents of multiples can find breastfeeding information and support through groups such as La Leche League International (www.lalecheleague.org/nb/nbmultiples.html).

EXPRESSING AND STORING BREAST MILK

Breast milk expression is a common practice, typically performed to obtain breast milk for someone other than the mother to feed to the baby. It is most often associated with maternal employment. In some situations, expression of breast milk is necessary or desirable such as when engorgement occurs, when the mother's nipples are sore or damaged, when the mother and baby are separated as in the case of a preterm infant who remains in the hospital after the mother is discharged, or when the mother leaves the infant with a caregiver and will not be present for feeding. Some women express milk to have an emergency supply. Some women choose to pump exclusively, providing breast milk for their infants but never allowing the baby to suckle at the breast. Because pumping and hand expression are rarely as efficient as a baby in removing milk from the breast, the milk supply is never judged based solely on the volume expressed. Milk volume can be more accurately assessed using prefeeding and postfeeding infant weights, also known as test weights.

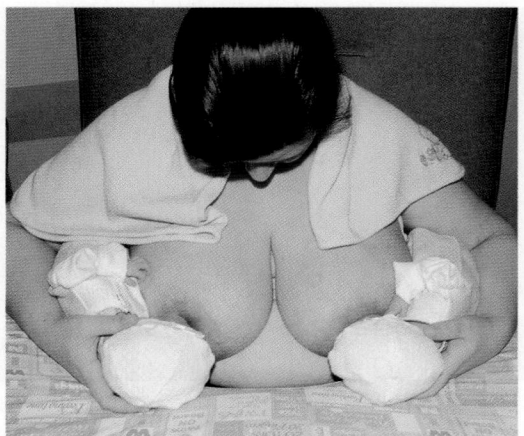

FIG 24.11 Breastfeeding twins. (Courtesy of Cheryl Briggs, RNC, Annapolis, MD.)

Hand Expression

All mothers should be instructed in hand expression. This simple technique can actually be more effective than an electric breast pump for expressing colostrum, which tends to be thicker than mature milk (Flaherman, Gay, Scott, et al., 2012; Morton, Hall, & Pessl, 2013–2014). Hand expression during the first 3 days after birth can have a positive effect on milk production during the early weeks. Morton and colleagues report that combining hand expression and hands-on pumping (breast massage before and during pumping) with the use of an electric breast pump can increase milk production and enhance fat content and caloric value of milk (Morton, Wong, Hall, et al., 2012). A video of hand expression of breast milk is available at http://newborns.stanford.edu/Breastfeeding/HandExpression.html.

Mechanical Milk Expression (Pumping)

For most women, recommendations are to initiate pumping only after the milk supply is well established and the infant is latching and breastfeeding well. However, when breastfeeding is delayed after birth such as when babies are ill or preterm, mothers should begin pumping with an electric breast pump as soon as possible and continue to pump regularly until the infant is able to breastfeed effectively. Early pumping may be initiated if the baby is too sleepy to feed effectively or if there are issues with latching or milk transfer. Milk expression is essential to maintaining milk supply if breastfeeding is interrupted. Double pumping (pumping both breasts at the same time) saves time and can stimulate the milk supply more effectively than single pumping (Fig. 24.12).

The amount of milk obtained when pumping depends on the type of pump being used, the time of day, the time since the baby breastfed, the mother's milk supply, how practiced she is at pumping, and her comfort level (pumping is uncomfortable for some women). Breast milk can vary in color and consistency, depending on the time of day, the age of the baby, and foods the mother has eaten.

Types of Pumps

Many types of breast pumps are available, varying in price and effectiveness. Before purchasing or renting a breast pump, the mother will benefit from professional advice from a nurse, lactation consultant, or health care provider to determine which pump best suits her needs (Meier, Patel, Hoban, et al., 2016).

The flange (funnel-shaped device that fits over the nipple or areola) should fit the nipple to prevent nipple pain, trauma, and possible reduction in milk supply. Mothers are advised to use the lowest suction

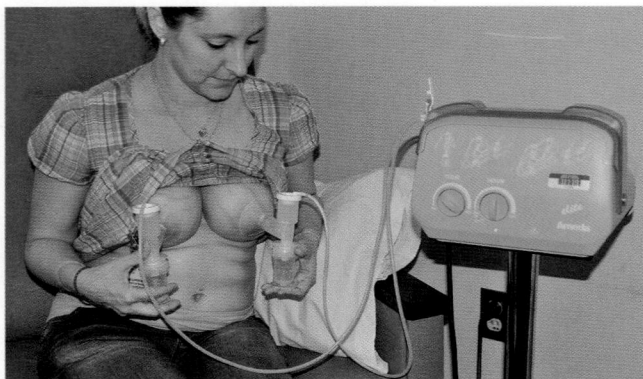

FIG 24.12 Bilateral breast pumping. (Courtesy of Cheryl Briggs, RNC, Annapolis, MD.)

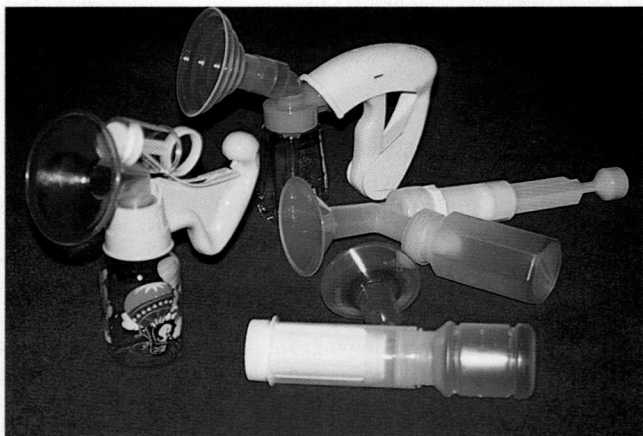

FIG 24.13 Manual breast pumps. (Courtesy of Marjorie Pyle, RNC, Lifecircle, Costa Mesa, CA.)

setting on electric pumps, increasing gradually if needed. Breast massage before and during pumping can increase the amount of milk obtained.

Manual, battery-operated, or mini-electric pumps are the least expensive and can be the most appropriate when portability and quietness of operation are important. These pumps are most often used by mothers who are pumping for an occasional bottle (Fig. 24.13).

Full-service electric pumps, or hospital-grade pumps (see Figs. 24.10 and 24.12), most closely duplicate the sucking action and pressure of the breastfeeding infant. When breastfeeding is delayed after birth (e.g., preterm or ill newborn) or when the mother and baby are separated for lengthy periods, these pumps are most appropriate (Meier et al., 2016). Portable versions of these pumps are available to rent for home use.

Electric self-cycling double pumps are efficient and easy to use. They are designed for working mothers or for use during brief periods (1 to 2 days) of separation by women with established lactation (Meier et al., 2016). Some of these pumps come with carry bags containing coolers to store pumped milk.

Storage of Breast Milk

Mothers who express and feed breast milk to their infants need to be educated about safe practices for handling, storing, and feeding. Attention to hand hygiene and proper cleaning of equipment reduces the risk for bacterial contamination. This is especially important when mothers are providing milk for preterm or ill neonates (Labiner-Wolfe & Fein, 2013; Meier, Patel, Bigger et al., 2013). Guidelines for storing expressed breast milk for a healthy term infant are listed in the Patient Teaching box: Breast Milk Storage Guidelines for Home Use for Term Infants.

PATIENT TEACHING

Breast Milk Storage Guidelines for Home Use for Term Infants

- Before expressing or pumping breast milk, wash your hands.
- Containers for storing milk should be washed in hot, soapy water and rinsed thoroughly; they can also be washed in a dishwasher. If the water supply may not be clean, boil containers after washing. Plastic bags designed specifically for breast milk storage can be used for short-term storage (<72 hours).
- Write the date of expression on the container before storing milk. A waterproof label is best.
- Store milk in serving sizes of 2 to 4 ounces to prevent waste.
- Storing breast milk in the refrigerator or freezer with other food items is acceptable.
- You can combine milk from pumping sessions in the same day; cool freshly expressed milk before adding it to the refrigerated container. Do not add warm milk to a container of refrigerated milk.
- When storing milk in a refrigerator or freezer, place containers in the middle or back of the freezer, not on the door.
- When filling a storage container that will be frozen, fill only three quarters full, allowing space at the top of the container for expansion.
- To thaw frozen breast milk, place container in the refrigerator for gradual thawing or under warm, running water for quicker thawing. Never boil or microwave.
- Milk thawed in the refrigerator can be stored for 24 hours.
- Thawed breast milk should never be refrozen.
- Shake milk container before feeding baby, and test the temperature of the milk on the inner aspect of your wrist.
- Any unused milk left in the bottle after feeding is discarded.

Location of Storage	Temperature	Recommended Safe Duration for Storage
Room temperature	16°–29°C (60°–85°F)	3–4 hours optimal 6–8 hours acceptable*
Refrigerator	4°C (39°F) or lower	72 hours optimal 5–8 days acceptable*
Freezer	Less than –4°C (24°F)	6 months optimal 12 months acceptable

*Under very clean conditions.
Modified from Academy of Breastfeeding Medicine. (2010). ABM clinical protocol no. 8: Human milk storage information for home use for full-term infants. *Breastfeeding Medicine, 5*(3), 127–130.

The preferred containers for long-term storage of breast milk have hard sides such as hard plastic or glass with an airtight seal. Flexible polyethylene bags are not recommended for long-term milk storage (>72 hours) because there is a greater chance of leakage, puncture, and loss of immune cells.

⚡ SAFETY ALERT

Breast milk is never thawed or heated in a microwave oven. Microwaving does not heat evenly and can cause encapsulated boiling bubbles to form in the center of the liquid, which may not be detected when drops of milk are checked for temperature. Babies have sustained severe burns to the mouth, throat, and upper GI tract as a result of microwaved milk. In addition, microwaving significantly decreases the antiinfective properties and vitamin C content. The safety of low-temperature microwaving is questionable (ABM Protocol Committee, 2010; Lawrence & Lawrence, 2016).

MATERNAL EMPLOYMENT

Returning to work after birth is associated with a decrease in the duration of breastfeeding. Women who return to work often face workplace challenges in breastfeeding such as lack of flexibility in work schedules, inadequate breaks to allow time for pumping, lack of privacy, lack of space for pumping, and lack of support from supervisors or coworkers. Mothers who are students in educational settings face similar challenges. Issues that can affect continued breastfeeding include fatigue, child care concerns, competing demands, and household responsibilities.

Employed mothers can continue breastfeeding with appropriate guidance and support (Robertson, 2014). They are encouraged to set realistic goals for employment and breastfeeding, with accurate information regarding the costs, risks, and benefits of available feeding options. Women need information about planning for their return to work; nurses and lactation consultants can provide guidance. Websites such as www.workandpump.com include information about choosing pumps and other supplies, making a plan for breastfeeding and expressing milk, and preparing for their return to work.

Women who are able to breastfeed their infants during the workday tend to breastfeed longer. With increasing numbers of women having the option of working from home, this situation is becoming more common. In some settings, mothers are able to breastfeed during the workday, either by going to an on-site daycare center or by having a friend or relative bring the baby to her for some feedings. Many working mothers pump their milk while they are at work and save the milk for later feedings. Working mothers who are unable to pump or breastfeed their infants during the workday have the shortest duration of breastfeeding.

Because women are a significant proportion of the workforce, many companies make provisions for breastfeeding women returning to work. Ideally, employers should provide accommodations for breastfeeding mothers, specifically reasonable breaks during the workday and a non-bathroom space for milk expression until the child's first birthday. Breastfeeding programs typically include on-site lactation rooms (Fig. 24.14) and education and consulting services. Some employers provide on-site child care and high-quality breast pumps for their employees (Marinelli, Moren, Taylor, et al., 2013). Workplace support for breastfeeding mothers has improved significantly in recent years. However, further efforts are needed to educate employers about the importance of supporting their breastfeeding employees. Employers need to realize that breastfeeding programs can provide short- and long-term cost savings with significant health benefits for mothers, infants, and families. The Health Resources and Services Administration offers a free toolkit for employers: the "Business Case for Breastfeeding" outlines steps that employers can take to support breastfeeding employees (https://www.womenshealth.gov/breastfeeding/business-case-for-breastfeeding.html).

WEANING

Weaning may be defined as the process of transferring the infant's dependence on the mother's milk for nutrition to other sources of nutrition (Lawrence & Lawrence, 2016). For infants who are exclusively breastfed, the process of weaning is initiated when babies are introduced to foods other than breast milk and concludes with the last breastfeeding, which ideally continues until the infant is 1 year of age and beyond as desired. Gradual weaning over weeks or months is easier for mothers and infants than abrupt weaning. Abrupt weaning is likely to be distressing for mother and baby and physically uncomfortable for the mother because it can cause engorgement and mastitis (Mohrbacher, 2013).

Weaning is initiated by either the infant or the mother. With infant-led weaning, the infant moves at his or her own pace in omitting feedings, which usually facilitates a gradual decrease in the mother's milk supply. In most cases, the mother determines when weaning will occur. Mother-led weaning means that the mother decides which feedings to drop. This approach is most easily undertaken by omitting the feeding of least interest to the baby or the one through which the infant is most likely to sleep. Every few days thereafter, the mother drops another feeding until the infant is gradually weaned from the breast.

Infants can be weaned directly from the breast to a cup. Bottles are usually offered to infants younger than 6 months of age. If the infant is weaned before 1 year of age, he or she should receive iron-fortified formula instead of cow's milk (AAP Section on Breastfeeding, 2012).

If abrupt weaning is necessary, breast engorgement can occur. To relieve the discomfort, the mother can take mild analgesics such as ibuprofen, wear a supportive bra, apply ice packs or cabbage leaves to the breasts, and pump small amounts if needed. When possible, it is best to avoid pumping because the breasts should remain full enough to promote a decrease in the milk supply.

Weaning is often a very emotional time for mothers; many believe that it is the end to a special, satisfying relationship with the infant and experience feelings of sadness or depression. Some women go through a grieving period after weaning. Sudden weaning can evoke feelings of guilt and disappointment. Nurses and others can help the mother by discussing other ways to continue this nurturing relationship with the infant such as skin-to-skin contact while bottle-feeding or holding and cuddling the baby. Support from the father or partner and other family members is essential at this time.

MILK BANKING

The AAP recommends pasteurized donor milk for preterm infants if the mother's own milk is not available despite substantial lactation support (AAP Section on Breastfeeding, 2012). For infants who cannot be breastfed but who also cannot survive except on human milk, banked donor milk is critically important. Because of the antiinfective and growth-promoting properties of human milk and its superior nutrition, processed donor milk is used in some neonatal intensive care units, primarily for very low–birth weight infants as well as for other preterm or sick infants when the mother's own milk is not available. Donor milk may be used therapeutically in other situations such as for infants with short gut syndrome, formula intolerance, metabolic disorders, or congenital anomalies. It is also used for infants with IgA deficiency who

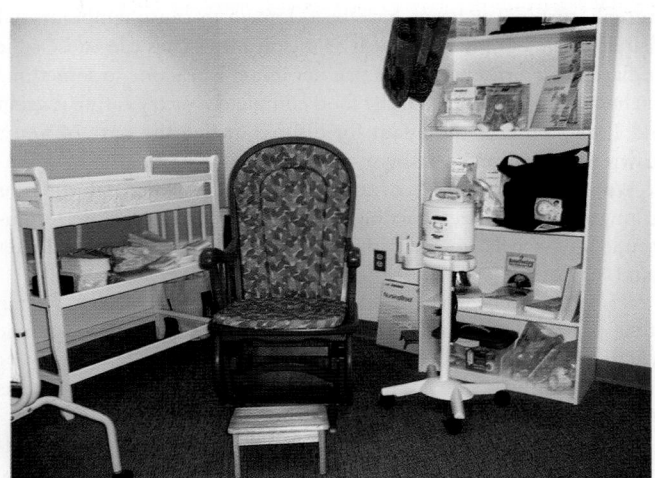

FIG 24.14 Lactation room. Note breast pump, rocking chair, nursing foot stool, changing table, books, and supplies. (Courtesy of Cheryl Briggs, RNC, Annapolis, MD.)

Milk Donation

The Human Milk Banking Association of North America is a nonprofit organization that provides donor milk that has been safely pasteurized and tested. It is dispensed only by hospital purchase order or health care provider prescription. Visit the website www.hmbana.org, and read about how milk is processed. Also explore how a woman can become a milk donor. Examine websites that offer milk sharing via the Internet: Eats on Feets (www.eatsonfeets.org) and Human Milk 4 Human Babies (http://hm4hb.net). What is the process for procuring human milk? What is the cost? What information is available about potential risks?

are not breastfed, and older children or adults with IgA deficiency (ABM Protocol Committee, 2009; Lawrence & Lawrence, 2016).

The Human Milk Banking Association of North America (HMBANA) (www.hmbana.org) has established annually reviewed guidelines for the operation of not-for-profit donor human milk banks (HMBANA, 2015). There is no federal oversight or regulation of milk banking in the United States. However, some states have laws and regulations that specify how donor milk is to be procured, processed, and distributed (Landers & Hartmann, 2012). Currently there are 26 HMBANA milk banks in the United States and Canada, with more in various stages of planning and development (www.hmbana.org/locations). The milk banks collect, screen, process, and distribute the milk donated by lactating mothers. All donors are screened both by interview and serologically for communicable diseases. Donor milk is stored frozen until it is pasteurized (heat processed) to kill potential pathogens; it is then refrozen for storage until it is dispensed for use. The heat processing adds a level of protection for the recipient that is not possible with any other donor tissue or organ. Banked milk is dispensed only by prescription. A per-ounce fee is charged by the bank to pay for the processing costs, but the HMBANA guidelines prohibit payment to donors (Updegrove, 2013).

The demand for human milk far exceeds the supply that is available through the non-profit HMBANA facilities. There are for-profit companies who offer payment to women who donate their breast milk. There is controversy surrounding the sale of human milk, the compensation to donors, and diverting the supply of donor milk from nonprofit milk banks. There is also concern about the safety of the milk. Another concern about for-profit milk banking is the potential for predatory recruitment of low-income women as donors (http://www.cbsnews.com/news/the-battle-for-control-of-the-human-breast-milk-industry/). (See Community Focus box.)

MILK SHARING

In some situations when a mother is unable to provide breast milk in sufficient quantity for her infant, or is unable to breastfeed because of a contraindication such as HIV, or in the case of maternal death when the family wants human milk for the surviving infant, women and families may turn to alternative sources for human milk. In such cases, the family is unlikely to be considered a priority for milk from a human milk bank, or they may not have the financial resources to purchase the milk. They may resort to cross-nursing or wet-nursing, where the infant is breastfed by a woman other than the birth mother. Some families acquire donor milk for their babies through Internet-based milk sharing or community sharing of donor human milk (see Community Focus box). In these cases, there is a lack of screening of milk donors in terms of diseases, medications, or illicit substances (Martino & Spatz, 2014). The US Food and Drug Administration (FDA, 2015) warns against milk sharing, recommending that potential users should

consult a health care provider before obtaining milk from a source other than the baby's own mother. They warn individuals against feeding donor milk procured directly from individuals or through the Internet, citing safety risks including exposing the infant to infectious diseases or chemical contaminants in donor milk. Samples of milk purchased through the Internet have been shown to have high overall bacterial growth and contamination with pathogenic bacteria; this is likely related to improper techniques for collecting, storing, and shipping the milk (Keim, Hogan, McNamara, et al., 2013).

⚡ **SAFETY ALERT**

Nurses and lactation consultants should be aware of the safety concerns associated with milk sharing. Parents who indicate an interest in obtaining donor human milk for their infant should be directed to one of the HMBANA milk banks and should be cautioned about the safety risks associated with feeding donor milk from an alternative source.

CARE OF THE MOTHER

Nutrition

In general the breastfeeding mother should eat a healthy, well-balanced diet. Caloric intake during lactation should be sufficient to achieve the goal of balancing energy intake and expenditure. Most women are able to achieve that balance by adding 450 to 500 calories per day (AAP Section on Breastfeeding, 2012). Even with the increased caloric intake, women who are breastfeeding tend to lose weight more quickly than those who are formula-feeding (Lawrence & Lawrence, 2016).

Medications or diets that promote weight loss are not recommended for breastfeeding mothers. Rapid loss of large amounts of weight can be detrimental, given that fat-soluble contaminants to which the mother has been exposed are stored in body fat reserves, and these can be released into the breast milk. Another potential consequence of weight loss is reduced milk production (Newton, 2017). For most women, a weight loss of 1 to 2 kg (2.2 to 4.4 lb) per month is safe; however, if weight loss exceeds this amount, careful evaluation of infant weight and feeding pattern is recommended. The mother's diet is also evaluated.

No specific foods that the breastfeeding mother should avoid have been identified. In most cases, the woman can consume a normal diet, according to her personal preferences and cultural practices. However, there is clinical evidence that some breastfeeding infants are sensitive to specific foods in the mother's diet; for example, garlic, onions, cabbage, broccoli, turnips, or beans have been known to cause temporary GI distress (colic). Some fruits such as melon or peaches can cause colic or diarrhea. If a mother thinks that her infant is reacting to something she has eaten, she can avoid the food completely, or try eating it again and closely observe the infant for distress during the next 24 hours (Lawrence & Lawrence, 2016).

Women may be told to continue taking their prenatal vitamins as long as they are breastfeeding. Vitamin D supplements are recommended, especially for women with limited sun exposure or darker skin (Newton, 2017).

It is recommended that breastfeeding mothers consume 200 to 300 mg of the omega-3 long-chain polyunsaturated fatty acids (docosahexaenoic acid [DHA]) daily. A DHA supplement and a multivitamin may be needed for women who are undernourished and those on vegan diets (AAP Section on Breastfeeding, 2012).

Women on vegetarian diets are at risk for dietary deficiencies including B vitamins (especially B_{12}), total protein, and some amino acids. Recommendations for lactating women on vegetarian diets include: (1) supplementing protein intake with soy flour, nuts, and molasses; and using complementary protein combinations; (2) avoiding excessive intake of phylates and bran; and (3) taking vitamin supplements of B_{12}, B_2, and D (Lawrence & Lawrence, 2016; Newton, 2017).

Mothers are encouraged to drink fluids in response to thirst (women often report feeling thirsty when they are breastfeeding). It can be helpful for the mother to know that if her urine appears light yellow (like lemonade), she is probably consuming adequate fluids. Excessive consumption of water or other fluids by the mother does not increase milk supply, and overhydration can actually decrease milk production.

Rest

The breastfeeding mother should rest as much as possible, especially in the first 1 or 2 weeks after birth. Fatigue, stress, and worry can negatively affect milk production and ejection (let-down). The nurse can encourage the mother to sleep when the baby sleeps. Breastfeeding in a side-lying position promotes rest for the mother. The father or partner, grandparents, other relatives, and friends can help with household chores and caring for other children.

Breast Care

The breastfeeding mother's normal routine bathing is all that is necessary to keep her breasts clean. Soap can have a drying effect on nipples; therefore, the mother should avoid washing the nipples with soap. Breast creams should not be used routinely because they can block the natural oil secreted by the Montgomery glands on the areola.

The mother with flat or inverted nipples may benefit from wearing breast shells in her bra. It is thought that these hard plastic devices exert mild pressure around the base of the nipple to encourage nipple eversion. Breast shells are also useful for sore nipples to keep the mother's bra or clothing from touching the nipples (Fig. 24.15).

If a mother needs breast support, she will likely be uncomfortable unless she wears a bra because otherwise the ligament that supports the breast (Cooper ligament) will stretch and be painful. Bras should fit well and provide nonbinding support. Underwire or improperly fitting bras can cause clogged milk ducts.

If milk leakage between feedings is a problem, mothers can wear breast pads (disposable or washable) inside the bra. Plastic-lined breast pads are not recommended because they trap moisture and can contribute to sore nipples. Pads should be changed when they are damp.

Breastfeeding and Contraception

Although breastfeeding confers a period of infertility, it is not considered an effective method of contraception unless the mother is strictly following guidelines for the lactational amenorrhea method of contraception (see Chapter 5). Breastfeeding delays the return of ovulation and menstruation; however, ovulation can occur before the first menstrual period after birth.

The contraceptives least likely to affect breastfeeding and milk production are the nonhormonal methods such as the lactational amenorrhea

method, natural family planning, barrier methods (diaphragm/cap, spermicides, condoms), and intrauterine devices (Berens, Labbok, & Academy of Breastfeeding Medicine, 2015).

Hormonal contraceptives containing estrogen, including combined estrogen-progesterone pills or injectables, are not recommended for breastfeeding mothers because of the potential for reducing milk supply. Progestin-only contraceptives (pill, injection, or implant) are better options for breastfeeding mothers, although their use is not recommended during the first 6 weeks after birth (Berens et al., 2015) (see Chapter 5).

Breastfeeding During Pregnancy

Breastfeeding women who become pregnant can continue to breastfeed if there are no medical contraindications (e.g., risk for preterm labor). For pregnant women who are breastfeeding, adequate nutrition is especially important to promote normal fetal growth.

Nipple tenderness associated with early pregnancy can cause discomfort when breastfeeding the older child. The taste and composition of breast milk are altered during pregnancy, which can prompt some children to self-wean (Lawrence & Lawrence, 2016).

When the baby is born, colostrum is produced. The practice of breastfeeding a newborn and an older child is called **tandem nursing**. The nurse should remind the mother always to feed the infant first to ensure that he or she is receiving adequate nutrition. The supply-meets-demand principle works in this situation, just as with breastfeeding multiples.

Breastfeeding After Breast Surgery

Any type of previous breast or chest surgery (biopsy, augmentation, reduction, reconstructive surgery) can affect the ability to produce breast milk and transfer it to the infant. Surgical procedures can damage nerves and interrupt milk ducts (Newton, 2017). Before undergoing breast surgery, all women should discuss their lactation potential with their surgeon. During preconception or prenatal care, obstetric health care providers should identify women who have had breast surgery, discuss potential concerns related to breastfeeding, and refer women to lactation professionals for further counseling and assistance.

Women who have had augmentation mammoplasty (breast implants) may be able to breastfeed successfully. Many women have breast augmentation surgery purely for cosmetic reasons. However, if the procedure was done because of hypoplastic or asymmetric breasts or for breast reconstruction following cancer surgery, there can be concerns about adequate milk production. Submuscular implants are less likely to cause these problems; implants placed through periareolar incisions are more likely to result in breastfeeding problems. Large implants can impede milk flow by compressing milk ducts. Women with silicone implants can safely breastfeed without adverse effects on the infant (Newton, 2017). Women who have had hyaluronic acid injections for breast enhancement can safely breastfeed (Smith & Heads, 2013).

Reduction mammoplasty causes problems with milk production and transfer because of interference with milk ducts, removal of glandular tissue, and nerve damage (Newton, 2017). Even so, many women are still able to breastfeed while also supplementing with infant formula or banked donor milk.

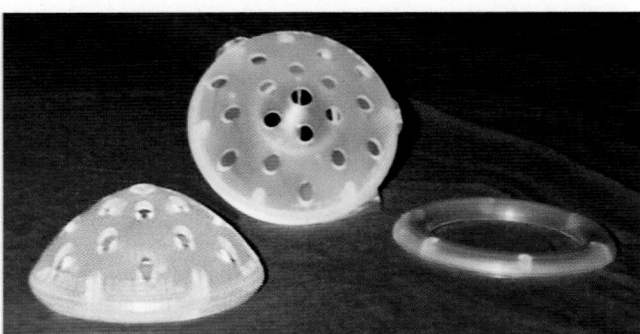
FIG 24.15 Breast shells.

> ## ! NURSING ALERT
>
> Women may not self-report previous breast or chest surgery such as breast biopsy, augmentation, or reduction mammoplasty. If surgical scars are present on the breast, the nurse should inquire about the type of surgery and the reason it was performed. Mothers with a history of breast surgery should be informed about the risk for interference with milk production and transfer. They are instructed to monitor their infants carefully for signs of adequate feeding.

It is possible for some women with a history of breast cancer to breastfeed. However, treatment for breast cancer (surgery, radiation, chemotherapy) can result in reduced milk supply or absence of lactation in the affected breast.

Breastfeeding and Nipple Piercing

Women who have nipple piercings can safely breastfeed. It can take as long as a year after piercing for the nipples to completely heal, placing the woman at risk for infection such as mastitis. Therefore, it is best if the piercing is done 18 to 24 months prior to pregnancy or at least 3 months after weaning. Piercings can damage milk ducts, obstructing the flow of milk. There can be leakage of milk from the piercing sites or fast flow of milk through the holes. Pierced nipples may have increased sensitivity. To prevent infant choking, breastfeeding mothers who have nipple piercings must remove the jewelry from the nipples before breastfeeding (Roche-Paull, 2016).

Breastfeeding and Obesity

Women who are overweight or obese are less likely to breastfeed, and the duration of breastfeeding tends to be shortened. These women are more likely to experience delayed onset of lactogenesis stage II and to experience problems with insufficient milk production compared with women of average weight (Turcksin et al., 2014).

For women who have had bariatric surgery and plan to breastfeed, nutritional deficiencies are a primary concern. Monitoring of the breastfeeding mother's micronutrient levels is recommended as frequently as every 3 months (Kominiarek & Rajan, 2016). Breastfeeding mothers who have had a malabsorptive procedure such as a Roux-en-Y gastric bypass should take daily dietary supplements, including a prenatal vitamin, vitamin B_{12}, iron with vitamin C (to maximize absorption), and calcium (La Leche League International, 2012; Lamb, 2011). It is important to monitor infant weight gain. Vitamin B_{12} deficiency or decreased milk production can cause failure to thrive. In addition, vitamin B_{12} deficiency can result in infant anemia, developmental delays, and neurologic problems (Lamb). Women with a history of bariatric surgery can benefit from referrals to registered dieticians and lactation consultants during pregnancy and in the postpartum period to discuss optimizing their nutritional status in preparation for and while breast-feeding (Caplinger, Cooney, Bledsoe et al., 2015).

Medications, Alcohol, Smoking, and Caffeine

Although much concern exists about the compatibility of drugs and breastfeeding, few drugs are absolutely contraindicated during lactation (Sachs & Committee on Drugs, 2013). Considerations in evaluating the safety of a specific medication during breastfeeding include the pharmacokinetics of the drug in the maternal system and the absorption, metabolism, distribution, storage, and excretion in the infant. The gestational and chronologic age of the infant, body weight, and breastfeeding pattern are also considered. In general, any medication that is given to an infant routinely is safe for a mother who is breastfeeding. The benefits of breastfeeding should be weighed against any risks of the medication to the infant (Sachs & Committee on Drugs).

MEDICATION ALERT

Breastfeeding mothers should be cautioned about taking any medications except those that are deemed essential. They are advised to check with their health care provider before taking any medication, even over-the-counter drugs.

Information about the safety of medications and breastfeeding can be accessed through the Drugs and Lactation Database (LactMed), a website provided by National Library of Medicine: http://toxnet.nlm.nih.gov/cgi-bin/sis/htmlgen?LACT (Anderson, 2016). The AAP recommends that providers consult this resource for the most current evidence-based information about specific medications for breastfeeding mothers (Sachs & Committee on Drugs, 2013).

Breastfeeding should be discontinued temporarily when the mother undergoes imaging procedures that use radiopharmaceuticals. Mothers are advised to pump and discard milk for a period of time based on the properties of the specific radioactive agent (Sachs & Committee on Drugs, 2013).

Drugs that are associated with adverse effects on the breastfeeding infant include antimetabolite and cytotoxic medications and drugs of abuse such as cocaine, heroin, amphetamines, and phencyclidine. These substances are not compatible with breastfeeding.

Women with a history of opioid use (prescription medications or heroin) who are on a medication-assisted treatment program may be encouraged to breastfeed as long as they are not using other illicit substances. Methadone and buprenorphine are considered safe during breastfeeding. Infants may have decreased severity of neonatal abstinence symptoms when they are receiving breast milk from mothers taking these medications (Reece-Stremtan & Marinelli, 2015; Sachs & Committee on Drugs, 2013).

Pain in postpartum breastfeeding mothers is most safely managed with nonopioid analgesics such as ibuprofen. When opioid analgesia is used, breastfeeding infants are at risk for sedation and sucking difficulties. Parenteral doses of morphine or butorphanol are preferred over meperidine. Oral hydrocodone is often used; however, frequent administration and doses greater than 10 mg can result in neonatal sedation (Montgomery, Hale, & Academy of Breastfeeding Medicine, 2012). Oxycodone is considered less desirable because relatively high amounts are transferred to the nursing infant and can lead to central nervous system depression (Sachs & Committee on Drugs, 2013).

As the use of antidepressant, antianxiety, and mood stabilizing medications rises among childbearing women, there are increasing concerns about the effects of these medications on breastfeeding infants (see Chapter 21). There is a lack of evidence about the long-term effects on infants and children. Psychotropic medications are prescribed for breastfeeding mothers based on risk/benefit considerations. Commonly used antidepressant medications that are considered safe during lactation include nortriptyline, sertraline, and paroxetine (Sriraman, Melvin, Meltzer-Brody, et al., 2015).

Although there is no standard recommendation about avoiding alcohol use when breastfeeding, it is important for mothers to be aware of potential risks. The AAP Section on Breastfeeding (2012) recommends that alcohol intake by breastfeeding women should be minimal. Intake of alcohol should be limited to occasional consumption of less than 0.5 g/kg of body weight. Alcohol passes freely from the blood into breast milk, with peak levels occurring in 30 to 60 minutes on an empty stomach and 60 to 90 minutes when consumed with food. The MER and milk production can be adversely affected by maternal alcohol intake. If a breastfeeding mother chooses to have one or two drinks, she should not breastfeed for at least 2 hours. Contrary to popular belief, pumping and discarding milk do not accelerate removal of alcohol from the milk (Lawrence & Lawrence, 2016). Some mothers use test strips for alcohol content of breast milk; however, there is a lack of evidence to support the accuracy or reliability of these strips.

Smoking by breastfeeding mothers should be strongly discouraged (AAP Section on Breastfeeding, 2012). It can impair milk production; it also exposes the infant to the risks of secondhand smoke. Nicotine is transferred to the infant in breast milk, whether the mother smokes or uses a nicotine patch, although the effect on the infant is uncertain. Lactating mothers who continue to smoke should be advised not to smoke within 2 hours before breastfeeding and never to smoke in the same room with the infant.

Moderate intake of caffeine by breastfeeding mothers appears to pose no risk to normal full-term infants. Minimal amounts of caffeine pass through to the infant in the breast milk. However, caffeine accumulates in infants, especially if they are preterm (Lawrence & Lawrence, 2016).

Herbal Preparations

Herbs and herbal preparations such as teas are often recommended for breastfeeding women, especially when there is a need to increase milk supply. Although these herbal preparations may seem to be effective for some women, the recommendations are based on anecdotal information. There is a lack of evidence related to the prevalence, effectiveness, and safety of herbs during breastfeeding (Budzynska, Gardner, Dugoua, et al., 2012). Herbals are not regulated by the FDA because they are considered dietary supplements. Consequently, there is a lack of quality control; unknown additives in and unknown side effects from herbal preparations can be harmful to the infant. Although some herbs may be considered safe, others contain pharmacologically active compounds that can have unfavorable effects. A thorough maternal history should include the use of any herbal remedies. Each remedy should then be evaluated for its compatibility with breastfeeding. LactMed provides information about the safety of herbal preparations and breastfeeding. Additionally, regional poison control centers can provide information on the active properties of herbs (Lawrence & Lawrence, 2016; Sachs & Committee on Drugs, 2013).

Common Concerns of the Breastfeeding Mother

The breastfeeding mother can experience some common problems. In most cases, these complications are preventable if the mother receives appropriate education about breastfeeding and assistance as needed. Early recognition and prompt resolution of these problems are important to prevent interruption of breastfeeding and to promote the mother's comfort and sense of well-being. Emotional support provided by nurses or lactation consultants is essential to help allay maternal frustration and anxiety and prevent early cessation of breastfeeding.

Engorgement

Engorgement is a common response of the breasts to the sudden change in hormones and the onset of significantly increased milk volume in lactogenesis stage II. It usually occurs 3 to 5 days after birth when the milk "comes in." At this time, there is increased blood flow to the breasts, and increased uptake of glucose and oxygen by the breasts. Milk production is copious (Newton, 2017). As milk production rapidly increases, the volume can exceed the storage capacity of the alveoli in the breasts. If milk is not removed, the alveoli become distended, causing impairment of capillary blood flow surrounding the alveolar cells. As the blood vessels become more congested, fluid leaks into the surrounding tissue, resulting in edema. The milk ducts can be compressed by the tissue edema so milk cannot flow easily from the breasts. The breasts can become firm, tender, and hot and can appear shiny and taut. The areolae are firm, and the nipples can flatten, making it difficult for the infant to latch on to the breast (see Clinical Reasoning Case Study: Breastfeeding: Engorgement). Because back pressure on full milk glands inhibits milk production, if milk is not removed from the breasts, the milk supply can diminish.

Engorgement does not occur in all breastfeeding mothers. The frequency and effectiveness of feedings during the first 2 to 3 days after birth seem to affect the development of engorgement. Early and frequent feedings may help to prevent engorgement. Emptying one breast at each feeding and alternating which breast is offered first at each feeding

---

CLINICAL REASONING CASE STUDY
Breastfeeding: Engorgement

The nurse on the mother-baby unit is caring for Johanna, a 37-year-old primipara who gave birth to a baby girl by emergency cesarean 3 days ago. During the morning assessment, the nurse observes that Johanna's breasts are engorged. Johanna sent the baby to the nursery during the night for feeding because she was exhausted. The engorgement seems to have happened overnight while Johanna was sleeping. Johanna is scheduled for discharge today.

1. Evidence—Does the nurse have enough evidence at this time to draw conclusions about the engorgement and feeding issues facing this mother and infant?
2. Assumptions—What assumptions can be made about the following issues?
   a. The need to relieve the engorgement
   b. Johanna's understanding of milk production
   c. The infant's ability to feed effectively
   d. Johanna's commitment to breastfeeding
3. What implications and priorities for nursing care can be identified at this time?
4. Interprofessional care—Describe interprofessional health care roles/responsibilities in optimizing care for Johanna and her infant after discharge.

---

may also help to prevent engorgement. The risk for engorgement appears to be increased among primiparas, women who received large amounts of IV fluids during labor and birth, and women who had previous breast surgery (Berens, Brodribb, & Academy of Breastfeeding Medicine, 2016).

When engorgement occurs it is a temporary condition that is usually resolved within 24 hours. The mother is instructed to feed every 2 hours, softening at least one breast and pumping the other breast as needed to soften it. Pumping during engorgement does not cause a problematic increase in milk supply.

A variety of interventions are used to treat engorgement, although there is a lack of research evidence confirming the effectiveness of any specific treatment regimen (Berens, Brodribb, & Academy of Breastfeeding Medicine, 2016; Mangesi & Zakarija-Grkovic, 2016). Frequently used interventions for engorgement include the use of cold (ice packs, gel packs, cold compresses), warmth (warm compresses, warm showers), cabbage leaves, antiinflammatory medications, breast massage, and hand expression or pumping. Other treatment techniques for engorgement include the use of ultrasound, acupressure, acupuncture, and Gua sha (usually part of acupuncture therapy). Gua sha is an East Asian healing technique believed to increase microperfusion of surface tissue and is performed by applying unidirectional press-stroking to a lubricated area with the intention of creating temporary petechiae (Nielsen, 2013).

To reduce swelling of breast tissue surrounding the milk ducts, ice packs are often recommended in a 15- to 20-minutes-on, 45-minutes-off rotation between feedings. The ice packs should cover both breasts. Large bags of frozen peas make easy packs and can be refrozen between uses.

Fresh, raw cabbage leaves placed over the breasts between feedings can help relieve engorgement. It is thought that the effect of the cabbage leaves is related to the coolness of the leaves and phytoestrogens within them. They are washed, dried, chilled in the refrigerator or freezer, and then placed over the breasts for 15 to 20 minutes (Fig. 24.16). Some clinicians recommend crushing the leaves slightly to break up the veins in the leaves prior to placing them over the breasts. This treatment can be repeated for two or three sessions. Frequent application of cabbage leaves can decrease milk supply. Cabbage leaves should not be used if the mother is allergic to cabbage or develops a skin rash.

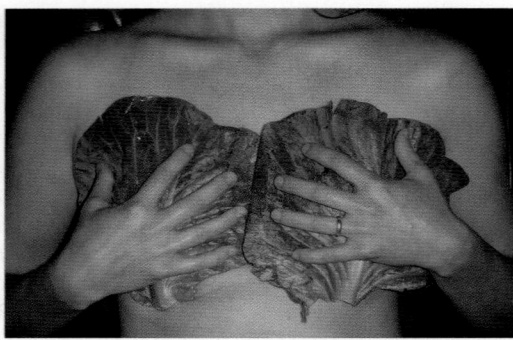

FIG 24.16 Cabbage leaves to treat engorgement. (Courtesy of Kathryn Alden, Chapel Hill, NC.)

Antiinflammatory medications such as ibuprofen can help reduce the pain and swelling associated with engorgement. Ibuprofen also helps reduce fever and aching in the breasts that are often associated with engorgement.

Because heat increases blood flow, its application to an already congested breast is usually counterproductive. However, occasionally standing in a warm shower starts the milk leaking, or the mother may be able to manually express enough milk to soften the areola sufficiently to allow the baby to latch and breastfeed.

As a result of engorgement, excessive intravenous fluids during labor, or oxytocin for labor induction or augmentation, the nipple and areola can become distended, making it difficult for the newborn to latch successfully. A technique called *reverse pressure softening* manually displaces the areolar interstitial fluid inward, softening the areola and making it easier for the infant's mouth to grasp the nipple and areola with latch (Berens, Brodribb, & Academy of Breastfeeding Medicine, 2016).

Sore Nipples

Mild nipple tenderness during the first few days of breastfeeding is common. Severe soreness or painful, abraded, cracked, or bleeding nipples are not normal and most often result from poor positioning, incorrect latch, improper suck, or infection. Suboptimal positioning can result in a shallow latch and abnormal nipple compression with sucking. Latch and sucking difficulties can be related to infant issues such as prematurity, oral and mandibular anatomy, muscle tone, congenital anomalies, ankyloglossia (tongue-tie), biting, or jaw-clenching. Latch problems can also be due to maternal issues such as nipple size or anatomy (e.g., flat or inverted nipples), breast size, engorgement, or milk flow. Painful nipples can be due to eczematous conditions such as atopic dermatitis, contact dermatitis, psoriasis, or in rare cases, Paget's disease. Severe nipple pain can be related to vasospasm or Raynaud's phenomenon. Bacterial, viral, or candida infections of the nipple and/or breast can cause pain (Berens, Eglash, Malloy, et al., 2016).

The key to preventing sore nipples is correct breastfeeding technique. Limiting the time at the breast does not prevent sore nipples. They are often the result of the mother allowing the baby to latch on to the breast before the mouth is open wide.

For the first few days after birth, the mother can experience some mild discomfort with the infant's initial sucks. This should quickly dissipate as the milk begins to flow and acts as a lubricant. To make the initial sucks less painful, the mother can express a few drops of colostrum or milk to moisten the nipple and areola before latch. If the mother continues to experience nipple pain or discomfort after the first few sucks, the nurse or lactation consultant helps her evaluate the latch and baby's position at the breast. If the nipple pain continues, the mother needs to remove the baby from the breast, breaking suction

with her finger in the baby's mouth (see Fig. 24.7). Repositioning the mother or infant can be helpful in resolving the nipple discomfort. The mother then proceeds to attempt latch again, making sure that the baby's mouth is open wide before latching him or her on to the breast (see Fig. 24.6).

The nurse or lactation consultant can assess the infant's suck by inserting a clean, gloved finger into the mouth and stimulating the infant to suck. If the tongue is not extruding over the lower gum and the mother reports pain or pinching with sucking, the baby may have ankyloglossia, which is a short or tight frenulum (commonly known as *tongue-tie*). In some instances, this condition is corrected surgically to free the tongue for less painful, more effective breastfeeding (Lawrence & Lawrence, 2016).

The treatment for sore nipples is first to identify the cause and then attempt to correct the problem. Early assessment and intervention are essential to increase the likelihood that the mother will continue to breastfeed. Once the problem is identified and corrected, sore nipples should heal within a few days, even though the baby continues to breastfeed regularly. When sore nipples occur, the woman is advised to start the feeding on the least sore nipple. It is important to assess the nipples for cracking or other damage to the skin integrity, which increases the risk for infection. If there is any break in the skin, the mother is advised to wipe the nipples with water after feeding to remove the baby's saliva. Expressing a few drops of colostrum or breast milk and rubbing it into the nipples may be recommended. A thin coating of a topical antibiotic on damaged nipples may help reduce the risk for infection and promote healing (the antibiotic cream or ointment should be removed before breastfeeding). Sore nipples should be open to air as much as possible. To promote comfort, breast shells can be worn inside the bra; these devices allow air to circulate while keeping clothing off sore nipples (see Fig. 24.15).

Rapid healing of sore nipples is critical to relieve the mother's discomfort, maintain breastfeeding, and prevent mastitis. Although numerous creams, ointments, gels, and gel pads have been used to treat sore nipples, there is a lack of conclusive evidence related to the effectiveness of any particular method (Dennis, Jackson, & Watson, 2014). However, because they have not been shown to cause harm, many health care professionals recommend their use. Some women report increased comfort for sore nipples with the application of purified lanolin, petroleum jelly, or hydrogel pads. If nipples are extremely sore or damaged and if the mother cannot tolerate breastfeeding, she may need to use an electric breast pump for 24 to 48 hours to allow the nipples to begin healing before resuming breastfeeding. She should use a pump that effectively empties the breasts (see Figs. 24.10 and 24.12).

Insufficient Milk Supply

A common reason that women stop breastfeeding is perceived or actual insufficient milk supply (Odom, Li, Scanlon, et al., 2013; Stuebe, 2014). This often leads to formula supplementation and early weaning. Careful evaluation of the mother-infant dyad is needed, including assessment of infant weight gain or loss, feeding technique, milk transfer, and consideration of possible medical causes for low supply (e.g., medications, glandular insufficiency, previous breast surgery). Stress and fatigue can cause decreased milk production.

The key to establishing and maintaining milk supply is frequent emptying of the breasts. Interventions for increasing milk supply are based on causative factors. In many cases, the mother is told to spend time with the baby skin-to-skin, increase feeding frequency, express milk using an electric pump, rest as much as possible, consume a healthy diet, and reduce stress. If nonpharmacologic measures to increase milk supply are not effective, **galactagogues** (medications or other substances that are believed to increase milk supply) may be recommended. Mothers often use herbal galactagogues such as fenugreek, blessed thistle, goat's rue, and shatavari to increase milk production. However, there is a lack of evidence to support the use of these substances (Sachs & Committee on Drugs, 2013).

Pharmaceutical galactagogues must be prescribed by the health care provider. Metoclopramide and domperidone are the most commonly prescribed medications; both are dopamine antagonists typically used to treat gastroesophageal reflux. It is thought that they increase prolactin levels, which enhances milk production. There is a lack of evidence to support the use of these medications in breastfeeding women (Sachs & Committee on Drugs, 2013).

> ### ✏ MEDICATION ALERT
>
> Metoclopramide clearance in neonates is prolonged, which increases the risk for conditions resulting from overdose such as methemoglobinemia. Mothers are at risk for adverse reactions to metoclopramide including depression, suicidal ideation, and GI disturbances (Sachs & Committee on Drugs, 2013).

Domperidone is often prescribed for lactating women in Canada and other countries (Flanders, Lowe, Kramer, et al., 2012), although it is not available in the United States except through some compounding pharmacies (ABM Protocol Committee, 2011b). Domperidone has been associated with increased risk for sudden cardiac death. The FDA issued a warning against the use of domperidone, stating that "the importation of this drug presents a public health risk and violates the Federal Food, Drug, and Cosmetic Act (the Act)" (FDA, 2012).

Plugged Milk Ducts

A milk duct can become plugged or clogged, causing an area of the breast to become swollen and tender. This area typically does not empty or soften with feeding or pumping. A small white pearl may be visible on the tip of the nipple; this pearl is the curd of milk blocking the flow. The mother is afebrile and has no generalized symptoms.

Plugged milk ducts are most often the result of inadequate removal of milk from the breast, which can be caused by clothing that is too tight, a poorly fitting or underwire bra, or always using the same position for feeding. Application of warm compresses to the affected area and to the nipple before feeding helps promote emptying of the breast and release of the plug.

Frequent feeding is recommended, with the baby beginning the feeding on the affected side to foster more complete emptying. The mother is advised to massage the affected area while the infant nurses or while she is pumping. Varying feeding positions and feeding without wearing a bra may be useful in resolving a plugged duct. Plugged milk ducts can increase susceptibility to breast infection. For recurrent plugged ducts, taking lecithin, a fat emulsifier, may be useful (Lawrence & Lawrence, 2016).

Mastitis

Although the term mastitis means inflammation of the breast, it is most often used to refer to infection of the breast. It is characterized by the sudden onset of influenza-like symptoms, including fever, chills, malaise, body aches, headache, nausea, and vomiting. The woman usually has localized breast pain and tenderness and a hot, reddened area on the breast. Mastitis most commonly occurs in the upper outer quadrant of the breast; one or both breasts can be affected. Most cases occur during the first 2 to 4 weeks postpartum, although mastitis can occur at any time (Newton, 2017).

Certain factors can predispose a woman to mastitis. Inadequate emptying of the breasts is common; this can be related to engorgement,

plugged ducts, a sudden decrease in the number of feedings, abrupt weaning, or wearing underwire bras. Sore, cracked nipples can lead to mastitis by providing a portal of entry for causative organisms (*Staphylococcus, Streptococcus,* and *Escherichia coli* are most common). Stress, fatigue, maternal illness, ill family members, breast trauma, and poor maternal nutrition also are predisposing factors for mastitis (Amir & Academy of Breastfeeding Medicine, 2014). Breastfeeding mothers should be taught the signs of mastitis before they are discharged from the hospital after birth, and they need to know to call the health care provider promptly if the symptoms occur.

Treatment includes antibiotics such as cephalexin or dicloxacillin for 10 to 14 days and analgesic and antipyretic medications such as ibuprofen. The mother is advised to rest as much as possible and breastfeed or pump frequently, striving to empty the affected side adequately. Warm compresses to the breast before feeding or pumping can be useful. Adequate fluid intake and a balanced diet are important for the mother with mastitis (Newton, 2017).

Complications of mastitis include breast abscess, chronic mastitis, and fungal infections of the breast. Most complications can be prevented by early recognition and treatment.

FOLLOW-UP AFTER DISCHARGE

Problems with sore nipples, engorgement, and jaundice are likely to occur after discharge from the birthing facility. Nurses and lactation consultants educate the mother about potential problems she may encounter once she is home. She should be given a list of resources for help with breastfeeding concerns. Community resources for breastfeeding mothers include lactation consultants in hospitals, primary care offices, or private practice; nurses in pediatric or obstetric offices; support groups such as La Leche League; and peer counseling programs (e.g., those offered through WIC). The Internet has many websites containing current and correct information about breastfeeding (e.g., www.breastfeeding.com). The National Breastfeeding Helpline (1-800-994-9662) through the Office of Women's Health provides breastfeeding information and counseling by English- and Spanish-speaking counselors.

Telephone follow-up by nurses or lactation consultants in hospitals, birth centers, clinics, or offices within the first day or two after discharge can help identify problems and offer needed advice and support. It often takes at least 2 weeks for breastfeeding to become established, so on-going contact with the mother is important in providing her with needed support.

Follow-up care of the breastfeeding mother and infant is interprofessional. Breastfeeding infants should be seen by a pediatric health care provider at 3 to 5 days of age and again at 2 to 3 weeks of age to assess weight gain and offer encouragement and support to the mother (AAP Section on Breastfeeding, 2012). A lactation consultant or a nurse in the pediatric office or clinic will assess breastfeeding and provide education and counseling. Referral may be made to a home health agency or peer counselor for further lactation assistance and support. If the mother encounters problems such as mastitis, she will need to be evaluated by her obstetric or primary health care provider. If the mother is taking any medications, a pharmacist can help in evaluating safety of use in lactation.

▌FORMULA-FEEDING

PARENT EDUCATION

Most infants receive at least some amount of commercial infant formula during their first year of life. Some parents choose formula-feeding instead of breastfeeding; others combine the two methods. If the infant is weaned from breastfeeding before the first birthday, iron-fortified infant formula should be given (AAP Section on Breastfeeding, 2012).

It is important for nurses and other health care professionals to be intentional about providing education for parents related to formula preparation, feeding, and common problems they can encounter. Because of the lack of clear information about the practical aspects of formula-feeding, parents often rely on advice from friends and family. If that advice is incorrect and the parents use unsafe practices for formula preparation and feeding, the infant is at risk for foodborne illness and burns (see Patient Teaching box: Formula Preparation and Feeding).

READINESS FOR FEEDING

Ideally the first feeding of formula is given after the neonate's initial transition to extrauterine life. Feeding-readiness cues include stability of vital signs, effective breathing pattern, presence of bowel sounds, an active sucking reflex, and signs described earlier for breastfed infants.

FEEDING PATTERNS

In the first 24 to 48 hours of life, a newborn typically consumes 15 to 30 mL of formula at a feeding. Intake gradually increases during the first week of life. Most newborns are drinking 90 to 150 mL at a feeding by the end of the second week or sooner. Many parents do not understand about the capacity of the newborn stomach and will tend to overfeed the newborn infant. In explaining to parents about how the stomach capacity gradually increases, it can be helpful to use analogies. This is also helpful in teaching parents of breastfeeding infants. On day 1 the newborn stomach is about the size of a cherry or a shooter marble and can hold about 5 to 7 mL (approximately 1 to 1½ teaspoons). By the third day, the stomach is about the size of a walnut or ping-pong ball, and the capacity increases to 22 to 27 mL (approximately 1 oz). By one week, the stomach is about the size of an apricot with a capacity of 45 to 60 mL (1.5 to 2 oz). By 2 weeks, the stomach is about the size of a large egg with a capacity of 80 to 150 mL (2.5 to 5 oz) (http://blog.medelabreastfeedingus.com/2015/04/the-size-of-your-babys-stomach-breastfeeding-in-the-early-days/).

The newborn infant should be fed at least every 3 to 4 hours, even if it is necessary to wake him or her for the feedings; however, rigid feeding schedules are not recommended. The infant showing an adequate weight gain may be allowed to sleep at night and be fed only on awakening. Most newborns need six to eight feedings in 24 hours; the number of feedings decreases as the infant matures and consumes more at each feeding. By 3 to 4 weeks after birth, a fairly predictable feeding pattern has usually developed. Scheduling feedings arbitrarily at predetermined intervals may not meet a newborn's needs, but initiating feedings at convenient times often moves the feedings to times that work for the family.

Mothers usually notice increases in the infant's appetite at the age of approximately 10 days, 3 weeks, 6 weeks, 3 months, and 6 months. These appetite spurts correspond to growth spurts. Mothers should increase the amount of formula per feeding by approximately 30 mL to meet the baby's needs at these times.

FEEDING TECHNIQUE

Infants should be held for all feedings. During feedings parents are encouraged to sit comfortably, holding the infant close in a semi-upright position with good head support. Feedings provide opportunities to bond with the baby through touching, talking, singing, or reading to the infant. Parents should consider feedings a time of peaceful relaxation

with the infant. Mothers who bottle-feed should be encouraged to spend some time with their newborns in skin-to-skin contact.

> ## ⚡ SAFETY ALERT
>
> A bottle should never be propped with a pillow or other inanimate object and left with the infant. This practice can result in choking, and it deprives the infant of important interaction during feeding. Moreover, propping the bottle has been implicated in causing nursing-bottle caries or decay of the first teeth resulting from continuous bathing of the teeth with carbohydrate-containing fluid as the infant sporadically sucks the nipple.

Newborns must learn to coordinate sucking, swallowing, and breathing as they feed. The typical fast flow of milk from bottles can create difficulty for an infant trying to learn to feed. A slow-flow nipple is often used for the first few weeks.

Traditionally parents are told to position the infant in a semi-reclining position and to hold the bottle so that fluid fills the nipple and none of the air in the bottle is allowed to enter it (Fig. 24.17, *A*). A more physiologic approach to bottle-feeding is called paced bottle-feeding. With this method of feeding, the bottle is held at more of a horizontal angle (approximately 45 degrees); when the baby pauses between bursts of sucking, the parent withdraws the nipple, allowing it to rest on the baby's lip until he or she is ready to resume sucking (Lauwers & Swisher, 2016). This position slows the flow of milk from the bottle so the infant is more in control. Paced bottle-feeding works well for infants who are primarily breastfeeding but are occasionally fed from a bottle.

If the infant falls asleep, spits out the nipple, seals the lips, turns the head away, or ceases to suck, it usually indicates that he or she has consumed enough formula to feel satiated. Teach parents to look for these cues and avoid overfeeding, which can contribute to obesity.

Instruct parents to observe the infant for signs of stress during feeding, including turning the head, arching the back, choking, sputtering, changing color, moving the arms, and tensing fists. When these signs occur, the parent should stop feeding and attempt to calm the infant before resuming. The signs can indicate that the infant is finished with the feeding and does not want to drink any more.

Most infants swallow air when fed from a bottle and need a chance to burp several times during a feeding. Parents are taught various positions that can be used for burping (Fig. 24.18).

COMMON CONCERNS

Parents need to know what to do if the infant spits up. They may need to decrease the amount of feeding or feed smaller amounts more frequently. Burping the infant several times during a feeding such as when the infant's sucking slows down or stops can decrease spitting. Holding the baby upright for 30 minutes after feeding and avoiding bouncing or placing him or her on the abdomen soon after the feeding is finished also can help. Spitting can be a result of overfeeding, or it can be symptomatic of gastroesophageal reflux. Parents should report vomiting one third or more of the feeding at most feeding sessions or projectile vomiting to the health care provider and should be cautioned to refrain from changing the infant's formula without consulting the health care provider.

BOTTLES AND NIPPLES

Various brands and styles of bottles and nipples are available. Most babies feed well with any bottle and nipple. The bottles, nipples, rings, and caps should be washed in warm soapy water, using a bottle and

PATIENT TEACHING
Formula Preparation and Feeding

Formula Preparation

- Using warm soapy water, wash your hands, arms, and under your nails; rinse well. Clean and sanitize the surface where you will be preparing the bottles.
- Thoroughly wash bottles, nipples, rings, caps, can opener, and other preparation utensils in hot soapy water and rinse thoroughly. Squeeze water through nipples to make sure that the holes are open. If using canned formula, wash the top of the can with soap and water, rinse, and dry.
- Place bottles, nipples, rings, and caps in a pot, and cover with water; boil for 5 minutes; remove items from pot with sanitized tongs, and allow them to air dry. (Do this before using items the first time; thereafter you can continue to do this or place items in the dishwasher.)
- Note the expiration date on the formula container. It should be used before the expiration date. Any unopened expired formula should be returned to the place of purchase.
- Read the label on the container of formula, and mix it exactly according to the directions.
- Mix formula with tap water deemed safe by the local health department. Allow cold water to run for 2 minutes before collecting it. Then bring it to a rolling boil and continue boiling for 1 to 2 minutes. If using bottled water, make sure that it is labeled as "sterile"; unsterile bottled water must be boiled. After boiling, allow water to cool before mixing the formula but not for longer than 30 minutes.
- If using a can of ready-to-feed or concentrated formula, wash the top of the can with hot soapy water and rinse well. Shake the can before opening.
- Mixing formula
  - Ready-to-feed: No mixing is needed; do not add water. Pour desired amount of formula into clean bottle; add nipple and ring.
  - Concentrate: Pour desired amount of formula into clean bottle and add equal amount of cooled boiled water. Add nipple and ring and shake well.
  - Powder: When first opening the container of powder, write the date on the lid. Using the scoop from the container, add 1 scoop of powdered formula for each 2 oz of boiled, cooled water in a clean bottle. For example, if 6 oz of water is in the bottle, add three scoops of powder. Add nipple and ring, and shake well.
- If preparing multiple bottles at the same time, place nipple right side up on each bottle and cover with a clean nipple cap. Use bottles within 48 hours.
- Opened cans of ready-to-feed or concentrated formula should be covered and refrigerated. Any unused portions must be discarded after 48 hours.
- Bottles or cans of unopened formula can be stored at room temperature.
- If the formula is refrigerated, warm it by placing the bottle in a pan of hot water. Never use a microwave to warm any food to be given to a baby. Test the temperature of the formula by letting a few drops fall on the inside of your wrist. If the formula feels comfortably warm to you, the temperature is correct.
- A bottle of formula should be discarded within 1 hour after being fed to an infant; do not save the "leftovers" for another feeding.

Feeding Techniques and Tips

- Wash your hands with soap and water before feeding.
- Newborns should be fed at least every 3 to 4 hours and should never go longer than 4 hours without feeding until a satisfactory pattern of weight gain is established. This period can be as long as 2 weeks. If a baby cries or fusses between feedings, check to see if the diaper should be changed and if the baby needs to be picked up and cuddled. If the baby continues to cry and acts hungry, feed him or her. Babies do not get hungry on a regular schedule.
- Infants gradually increase the amount of milk they drink with each feeding. The first day or so, most newborns consume 15 to 30 mL (0.5 to 1 oz) with each feeding. This amount increases as the infant grows. If any formula remains in the bottle as the feeding ends, it must be thrown away because saliva from the baby's mouth can cause the formula to spoil. To avoid wasting formula, fill the bottle with no more than 30 mL (1 oz) more than you expect the baby to drink at that feeding. For the first 1 to 2 weeks of life, 120 mL (4 oz) should provide plenty of formula for each feeding.
- Keep a feeding diary, writing down the amount of formula the infant drinks with each feeding for the first week or so. Also record the number of the baby's wet diapers and bowel movements. Take this diary with you to the baby's first follow-up visit with the primary health care provider.
- For feeding, hold the infant close in a semi-reclining position. Talk to him or her during the feeding. This time is ideal for social interaction and cuddling.
- Place the nipple in the infant's mouth on the tongue. It should touch the roof of the mouth to stimulate the baby's sucking reflex. Hold the bottle like a pencil. Keep it tipped so the nipple stays filled with milk and the baby does not suck in air.
- Taking a few sucks and then pausing briefly before continuing to suck again is normal for infants. Some infants take longer to feed than others. Be patient. Keep the baby awake; encouraging sucking may be necessary. Moving the nipple gently in the infant's mouth may stimulate sucking.
- Another technique that can be used for bottle-feeding is *paced bottle-feeding*. The infant is placed in a more upright position, and the bottle is held at a more horizontal angle. When the baby pauses between bursts of sucking, withdraw the nipple and allow it to rest on the baby's lip until he or she is ready to resume sucking. This slows the flow of milk from the bottle so the infant is more in control. Paced bottle-feeding works well for infants who are primarily breastfeeding but are occasionally fed from a bottle.
- Newborns are apt to swallow air when sucking. Give the infant opportunities to burp several times during a feeding. As he or she gets older, you will know better when to stop for burping.
- Watch for signs that the infant is getting full: spitting out the nipple, sealing the lips together, slower sucking, or turning away from the nipple.
- After the first 2 or 3 days, the stools of a formula-fed infant are yellow and soft but formed. The infant may have a stool with each feeding in the first 2 weeks, although this amount can decrease to one or two stools each day. It is not abnormal for formula-fed infants to have a stool every other day.

Safety Tips

- Infants should be held and never left alone while feeding. Never prop the bottle. The infant might inhale formula or choke on any that was spit up. Infants who fall asleep with a propped bottle of milk or juice can be prone to cavities when the first teeth come in.
- Know how to use the bulb syringe and help an infant who is choking.

Data from American Academy of Pediatrics Committee on Nutrition. (2014). Feeding the infant. In R.E. Kleinman, & F.R. Greer (Eds.), *Pediatric nutrition* (7th ed.). Elk Grove, IL: American Academy of Pediatrics; World Health Organization & Food and Agriculture Organization of the United Nations. (2007). *Safe preparation, storage, and handling of powdered infant formula: Guidelines.* Geneva, Switzerland: World Health Organization; US Department of Agriculture. (2008). *Infant nutrition and feeding.* Washington, DC: USDA.

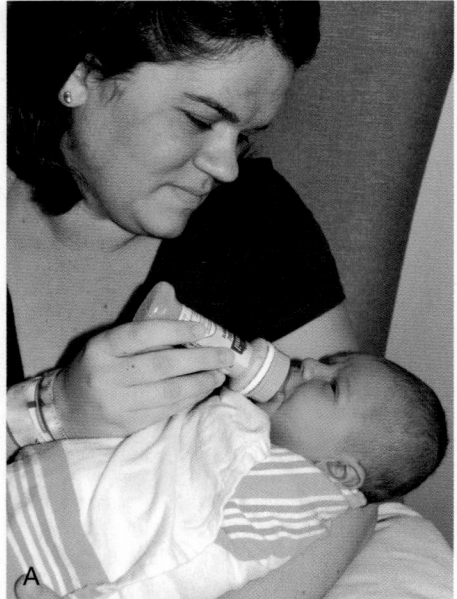

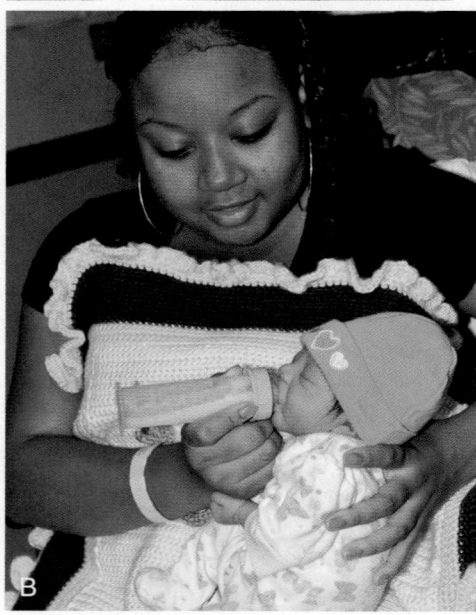

FIG 24.17 A, Bottle-feeding: traditional technique with infant semi-reclining **B,** Paced bottle-feeding: infant is more upright. (Courtesy of Cheryl Briggs, RNC, Annapolis, MD.)

nipple brush to facilitate thorough cleansing. They should be placed in boiling water for 5 minutes and allowed to air dry; this should be done at least before the first use and thereafter unless they are cleaned in a dishwasher (see Patient Teaching box: Formula Preparation and Feeding). Boiling of feeding equipment is recommended if the infant has oral thrush.

INFANT FORMULAS

Commercial Formulas

Commercial infant formulas are designed to resemble human milk as closely as possible, although none has ever duplicated it. The exact composition of infant formula varies with the manufacturer, but all must meet specific standards.

Infants who are not breastfed should be given commercial iron-fortified formulas. Families with limited income may be eligible for services through the WIC program, which provides iron-fortified infant formula.

The most widely used commercially prepared formulas are cow's milk–based formulas that have been modified to closely resemble the nutritional content of human milk. The caloric content of standard infant formula is 20 kcal/oz. These formulas are altered from cow's milk by removing butterfat, decreasing the protein content, and adding vegetable oil and carbohydrate. Regardless of the commercial brand, the standard cow's milk–based formulas have essentially the same compositions of vitamins, minerals, protein, carbohydrates, and essential amino acids, with minor variations such as the source of carbohydrate; nucleotides to enhance immune function; and long-chain polyunsaturated fatty acids (DHA and ARA), which are thought to improve visual and cognitive function. Furthermore, the FDA regulates the manufacture of infant formula in the United States to ensure product safety. Standard cow's milk–based formulas are sold as low-iron and iron-fortified formulas; however, only the iron-fortified formulas meet infants' requirements.

Four main categories of commercially prepared infant formulas are available: (1) cow's milk–based formulas; (2) soy-based formulas, commonly used for children who are lactose or cow's milk–protein intolerant; (3) casein- or whey-hydrolysate formulas, used primarily for children who cannot tolerate or digest cow's milk– or soy-based formulas; and (4) amino acid formulas, used for infants with multiple food protein intolerances.

The AAP Committee on Nutrition indicates that few solid indications exist for the use of soy protein–based formulas instead of cow's milk–based formulas (Bhatia, Greer, & AAP Committee on Nutrition, 2008). Soy protein–based formulas are recommended for infants with galactosemia and congenital lactase deficiency; infants with secondary lactase deficiency may benefit as well. Infants with documented IgE allergies caused by cow's milk should be fed an extensively hydrolyzed protein formula. Soy protein–based formulas have not been proven to be effective against colic or in the prevention of allergy in healthy or high-risk infants.

Alternate milk sources such as goat's milk; skim or low-fat milk; condensed milk; or raw, unpasteurized milk from any animal source should not be fed to infants because they are inadequate to support growth and can contain excess protein or an inadequate calcium-to-phosphorus ratio, which can cause seizures.

⚡ **SAFETY ALERT**

Because of concerns about potential harmful effects of bisphenol A (BPA), parents should be cautioned about using hard plastic polycarbonate baby bottles or containers. BPA is a chemical that is used to harden plastics, prevent bacterial contamination of foods, and prevent can rusting. It is in many food and liquid containers, including baby bottles. The AAP (2012) recommends avoiding clear plastic bottles or containers imprinted with the recycling number 7 and the letters PC and purchasing bottles that are certified or identified as BPA-free. Glass bottles are an alternative, but parents must be aware of the risk for injury if the bottle is dropped or broken. Because heat can cause the release of BPA from plastic, polycarbonate bottles should never be boiled, heated in the microwave, or washed in a dishwasher (AAP, 2012).

Formula Preparation

Commercial formulas are available in three forms: powder, concentrate, and ready to feed. All forms are equivalent in terms of nutritional content, but they vary considerably in cost.

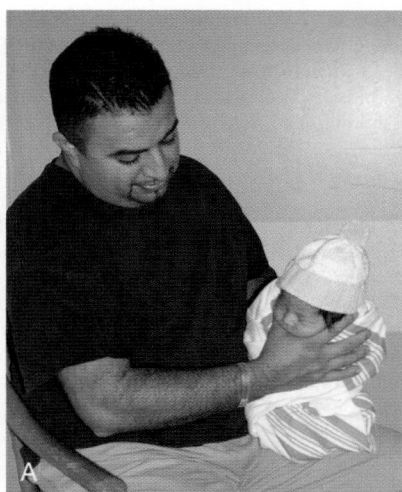 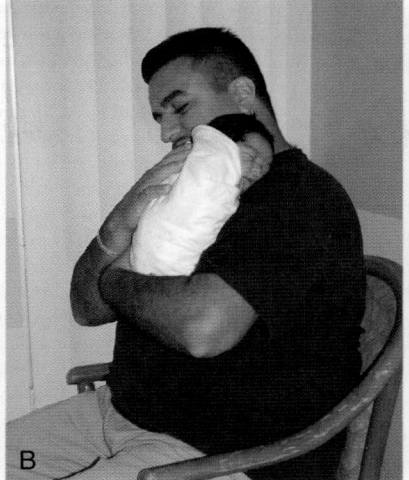 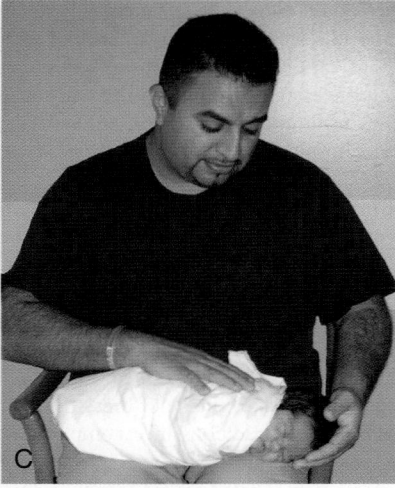

FIG 24.18 Positions for burping an infant. **A,** Sitting. **B,** On shoulder. **C,** Across lap. (Courtesy of Julie Perry Nelson, Loveland, CO.)

Ready-to-feed formula is the most expensive but the easiest to use. The desired amount is poured into the bottle. The opened can is refrigerated safely for 48 hours. This type of formula can be purchased in individual disposable bottles for the most convenient feeding.

Concentrated formula is less expensive than ready to feed. It is diluted with equal parts of water and can be stored in the refrigerator for 48 hours after opening.

Powdered formula is the least expensive. It is easily mixed by using 1 scoop for every 60 mL of water.

The commercial infant formula must include label directions for preparation and use of the formula with pictures and symbols for the benefit of individuals who cannot read. Some manufacturers translate the directions into languages such as Spanish, French, Vietnamese, Chinese, and Arabic to prevent misunderstanding and errors in formula preparation.

⚡ SAFETY ALERT

An important aspect to impress on families is that the proportions must not be altered (i.e., neither diluted to extend the amount of formula nor concentrated to provide more calories). The newborn's kidneys are immature; giving the infant overly concentrated formula can provide protein and minerals in amounts that exceed the excretory ability of the kidneys. In contrast, if the formula is diluted too much (sometimes done to save money), the infant does not consume sufficient calories to grow appropriately.

The water used to mix either powdered or concentrated liquid formula need not contain any fluoride, especially in the first 6 months of life. Excess fluoride can permanently stain the teeth once they appear.

Sterilization of formula rarely is recommended when families have access to a safe public water supply. Instead formula is prepared with attention to cleanliness. When water from a private well is used, parents should be advised to contact the health department to have a chemical and bacteriologic analysis of the water performed before using the water in formula preparation. The presence of nitrates, excess fluoride, or bacteria can be harmful to the infant.

It is usually safe to mix infant formula with cold tap water that has been boiled for 1 to 2 minutes and allowed to cool. Bottled water that is labeled as "sterile" is safe for mixing formula. However, nonsterile bottled water should be boiled for 1 to 2 minutes and cooled.

If the conditions in the home appear unsanitary, the nurse should recommend the use of ready-to-feed formula or teach the mother to sterilize the formula. The two traditional methods for sterilization are terminal heating and the aseptic method. In the terminal heating method, the prepared formula is placed in the bottles, which are topped with the nipples placed upside down and covered with the caps and sealed loosely with the rings. The bottles are then boiled together in a water bath for 25 minutes. In the aseptic method the bottles, rings, caps, nipples, and any other necessary equipment such as a funnel are boiled separately, after which the formula is poured into the bottles. Instructions for formula preparation and feeding are provided in the Patient Teaching box: Formula Preparation and Feeding.

VITAMIN AND MINERAL SUPPLEMENTATION

Commercial iron-fortified formula has all of the nutrients that infants need for the first 6 months of life. After 6 months of age, fluoride supplementation is recommended based on levels in the water supply.

WEANING

The bottle-fed infant gradually learns to use a cup, and the parents find that they are preparing fewer bottles. The bottle-feeding before bedtime is often the last one to remain. Babies have a strong need to suck, and the baby who has the bottle taken away too early or abruptly compensates with nonnutritive sucking on his or her fingers, thumb, a pacifier, or even the tongue. Therefore, weaning from a bottle should be attempted gradually because the baby has learned to rely on the comfort that sucking provides.

COMPLEMENTARY FEEDING: INTRODUCING SOLID FOODS

Complementary feedings are defined as foods or liquids given to the infant in addition to breast milk or formula. The American Academy of Pediatrics recommends introducing solid foods after 6 months of age (AAP Committee on Nutrition, 2014; AAP Section on Breastfeeding, 2012). First foods should include iron- and zinc-fortified cereals and meats. New foods should be introduced slowly to assess for any allergic reaction or intolerance. It is best to wait 3 to 5 days before introducing a new food. Infants should be consuming foods from all food groups by 7 to 8 months of age. Fruit juices are not recommended before 6 months of age, and juice consumption should be limited because it is possible that the infant who drinks juice will consume less breast milk or formula. Consumption of low-nutrient foods such as fatty or sugary foods or restaurant foods should be limited (AAP Committee on Nutrition).

In spite of the recommendations from the AAP, many parents begin complementary feedings earlier than 4 months of age. They need to be informed that the infant receives the right balance of nutrients from breast milk or formula during the first 4 to 6 months. The notion that the feeding of solids helps the infant sleep through the night is not true. Parents should not put cereal into the infant's bottle. Introduction of solid foods before the infant is 4 to 6 months of age can result in overfeeding and decreased intake of breast milk or formula.

Cultural beliefs and traditions affect complementary feeding practices. First foods given to infants vary widely. For example, first foods for Egyptian infants include bread soaked in milk and tea or yogurt sweetened with honey. Chinese and Vietnamese infants are sometimes fed prechewed rice paste, rice, or sweetened porridge.

Nurses and other health care professionals educate parents regarding complementary feedings. This most often occurs during well-baby supervision visits with the pediatric health care provider. Early feeding practices have implications for long-term dietary patterns; therefore, it is essential to teach parents about proper nutrition.

REFERENCES

Academy of Breastfeeding Medicine. (2009). ABM clinical protocol #3: Hospital guidelines for the use of supplementary feedings in the healthy term breastfed infant. *Breastfeeding Medicine, 4*(3), 175–182.

Academy of Breastfeeding Medicine. (2010). ABM clinical protocol #8: Human milk storage information for home use for full-term infants. *Breastfeeding Medicine, 5*(3), 127–130.

Academy of Breastfeeding Medicine. (2011a). ABM Clinical Protocol #10: Breastfeeding the late preterm infant. *Breastfeeding Medicine, 6*(3), 151–156.

Academy of Breastfeeding Medicine. (2011b). ABM clinical protocol #9: Use of galactogogues in initiating or augmenting the rate of maternal milk secretion. *Breastfeeding Medicine, 6*(1), 41–49.

Ahluwalia, I. B., D'Angelo, D., Morrow, B., et al. (2012). Association between acculturation and breastfeeding among Hispanic women: Data from the Pregnancy Risk Assessment and Monitoring System. *Journal of Human Lactation, 28*(2), 167–173.

American Academy of Family Physicians. (2012). *Breastfeeding policy statement.* Retrieved from www.aafp.org/online/en/home/policy/policies/b/breastfeedingpolicy.html.

American Academy of Pediatrics. (2012). *Ages and stages: Baby bottles and bisphenol A (BPA).* Retrieved from www.healthychildren.org/English/ages-stages/baby/feeding-nutrition/Pages/Baby-Bottles-And-Bisphenol-A-BPA.aspx.

American Academy of Pediatrics Committee on Nutrition (2014). Feeding the infant. In R. E. Kleinman & F. R. Greer (Eds.), *Pediatric nutrition* (7th ed.). Elk Grove Village, IL: American Academy of Pediatrics.

American Academy of Pediatrics Section on Breastfeeding. (2012). Breastfeeding and the use of human milk—Policy statement. *Pediatrics, 129*(3), e827–e841.

American College of Nurse-Midwives. (2016). *Position statement: Breastfeeding.* Retrieved from http://www.midwife.org/ACNM/files/ACNMLibraryData/UPLOADFILENAME/000000000248/Breastfeeding-statement-Feb-2016.pdf.

American College of Obstetricians and Gynecologists. (2016). Optimizing support for breastfeeding as part of obstetric practice. *Obstetrics and Gynecology, 127*(2), e86–e92.

American Dietetic Association. (2009). Position of the American Dietetic Association: Promoting and supporting breastfeeding. *Journal of the American Dietetic Association, 109*(11), 1926–1942.

Amir, L. H., & Academy of Breastfeeding Medicine Protocol Committee. (2014). ABM clinical protocol no. 4: Mastitis, revised March 2014. *Breastfeeding Medicine, 9*(5), 239–243.

Anderson, P. O. (2016). LactMed update: An introduction. *Breastfeeding Medicine, 11*(2), 54–55.

Association of Women's Health, Obstetric and Neonatal Nurses. (2014). AWHONN position statement: Breastfeeding. *Journal of Obstetric, Gynecologic, and Neonatal Nursing, 44*(1), 145–150.

Association of Women's Health, Obstetric, and Neonatal Nurses (2015). *Breastfeeding support: Preconception care through the first year* (3rd ed.). Washington, DC: Author.

Augustin, A. L., Donovan, K., Lozano, E. A., et al. (2013). Still nursing at 6 months: A survey of breastfeeding mothers. *American Journal of Maternal Child Nursing, 39*(1), 50–55.

Baby-Friendly USA. (2016). *Baby-Friendly USA: Find facilities.* Retrieved from http://www.babyfriendlyusa.org/find-facilities.

Baker, R. D., Greer, F. R., & American Academy of Pediatrics Committee on Nutrition. (2010). Clinical report: Diagnosis and prevention of iron-deficiency and iron-deficiency anemia in infants and young children (0–3 years of age). *Pediatrics, 126*(5), 1–11.

Bartick, M., & Reyes, C. (2012). Las dos cosas: An analysis of attitudes of Latina women on non-exclusive breastfeeding. *Breastfeeding Medicine, 7*(1), 19–24.

Berens, P., Brodribb, W., & Academy of Breastfeeding Medicine. (2016). ABM clinical protocol no. 20: Engorgement, revised 2016. *Breastfeeding Medicine, 11*(4), 159–163.

Berens, P., Eglash, A., & Malloy, M. (2016). ABM clinical protocol no. 26: Persistent pain with breastfeeding. *Breastfeeding Medicine, 11*(2), 46–53.

Berens, P., Labbok, M., & Academy of Breastfeeding Medicine. (2015). ABM protocol no. 13: Contraception during breastfeeding, revised 2015. *Breastfeeding Medicine, 10*(1), 3–12.

Bhatia, J., Greer, F., & American Academy of Pediatrics Committee on Nutrition. (2008). Use of soy protein-based formulas in infant feeding. *Pediatrics, 121*(5), 1062–1068.

Blackburn, S. T. (2013). *Maternal, fetal, and neonatal physiology* (4th ed.). Maryland Heights, MO: Saunders.

Budzynska, K., Gardner, Z. E., Dugoua, J., et al. (2012). Systematic review of breastfeeding and herbs. *Breastfeeding Medicine, 7*(6), 489–503.

Caplinger, P., Cooney, A. T., Bledsoe, C., Hagan, P., Smith, A., et al. (2015). Breastfeeding outcomes following bariatric surgery. *Clinical Lactation, 6*(4), 144–152.

Centers for Disease Control and Prevention. (2016a). *Breastfeeding among U.S. children born 2002–2013, CDC National Immunization Survey.* Retrieved from http://www.cdc.gov/breastfeeding/data/NIS%5Fdata/.

Centers for Disease Control and Prevention. (2016b). *Breastfeeding report card: Progressing toward national breastfeeding goals.* Retrieved from http://www.cdc.gov/breastfeeding/pdf/2016breastfeedingreportcard.pdf.

Chantry, C. J., Eglash, A., & Labbok, M. (2015). Position on breastfeeding—Revised 2015. *Breastfeeding Medicine, 10*(9), 407–411.

Chapman, D. J., & Perez-Escamilla, R. (2012). Breastfeeding among minority women: Moving from risk factors to interventions. *Advances in Nutrition, 3*(1), 95–104.

Chowdhury, R., Sinha, B., Sankar, M. J., et al. (2015). Breastfeeding and maternal health outcomes: A systematic review and meta-analysis. *Acta Paediatrica, 104*(467), 96–113.

Colson, S. (2012). The laid-back breastfeeding revolution. *Midwifery Today With International Midwife, 101*, 9–11. and 66.

Cooper, B. M., Holditch-Davis, D., Verklan, M. T., et al. (2012). Newborn clinical outcomes of the AWHONN late preterm infant research-based practice project. *Journal of Obstetric, Gynecologic, and Neonatal Nursing, 41*(6), 774–785.

Dell, K. M. (2015). Fluid, electrolytes, and acid-base homeostasis. In R. J. Martin, A. A. Fanaroff, & M. C. Walsh (Eds.), *Fanaroff and Martin's neonatal-perinatal medicine: Diseases of the fetus and infant* (10th ed.). St. Louis, MO: Mosby.

Dennis, C., Jackson, K., & Watson, J. (2014). Interventions for treating painful nipples among breastfeeding women. *Cochrane Database of Systematic Reviews, 2014*(12), CD007366.

Farrow, A. (2015). Lactation support and the LGBTQI community. *Journal of Human Lactation, 31*(1), 26–28.

Flaherman, V. J., Gay, B., Scott, C., et al. (2012). Randomised control trial comparing hand expression with breast pumping for mothers of term newborns feeding poorly. *Archives of Diseases in Childhood. Fetal and Neonatal Edition, 97*(1), F18–F23.

Flanders, D., Lowe, A., Kramer, M., et al. (2012). *A consensus statement on the use of domperidone to support lactation. Canadian Lactation Consultant Association.* Retrieved from http://rcp.nshealth.ca/sites/default/files/Domperidone_Consensus_Statement_May_11_2012.pdf.

Grummer-Strawn, L. A., & Rollins, N. (2015). Summarising the health benefits of breastfeeding. *Acta Paediatrica, 104*(467), 1–2.

Hedburg, I. C. (2013). Barriers to breastfeeding in the WIC population. *Maternal-Child Nursing Journal, 38*(4), 244–249.

Holmes, A. V., McLeod, A. Y., & Bunik, M. (2013). ABM clinical protocol no. 5: Peripartum breastfeeding management for the healthy mother and infant at term, revision 2013. *Breastfeeding Medicine, 8*(6), 469–473.

Human Milk Banking Association of North America. (2015). *Guidelines for the establishment and operation of a donor human milk bank.* Ft. Worth, TX: Author. Retrieved from https://www.hmbana.org/publications.

Institute of Medicine (2005). *Dietary reference intakes for energy, carbohydrate, fiber, fatty acids, cholesterol, protein, and amino acids.* Washington, DC: National Academies Press.

Jenson, D., Wallace, S., & Kelsay, P. (1994). LATCH: A breastfeeding charting system and documentation tool. *Journal of Obstetric, Gynecologic, and Neonatal Nursing, 23*(1), 27–32.

The Joint Commission. (2012). *Specifications manual for Joint Commission national quality core measures* (version 2013A1). Washington, DC: Author. Retrieved from https://manual.jointcommission.org/releases/TJC2013A/MIF0170.html.

Kamath-Rayne, B. D., Thilo, E. H., Deacon, J., et al. (2016). Neonatal hyperbilirubinemia. In S. L. Gardner, B. S. Carter, M. Enzman Hines, et al. (Eds.), *Merenstein & Gardner's handbook of neonatal intensive care* (8th ed.). St. Louis, MO: Elsevier.

Kanhadilok, S., & McGrath, J. M. (2015). An integrative review of factors influencing breastfeeding in adolescent mothers. *Journal of Perinatal Education, 24*(2), 119–127.

Keim, S. A., Hogan, J. S., McNamara, K. A., et al. (2013). Microbial contamination of human milk purchased via the internet. *Pediatrics, 132*(5), e1227–e1235.

Kominiarek, M. A., & Rajan, P. (2016). Nutrition recommendations in pregnancy and lactation. *Medical Clinics of North America, 100*(6), 1199–1215.

Labiner-Wolfe, J., & Fein, S. B. (2013). How US mothers store and handle their expressed breast milk. *Journal of Human Lactation, 29*(1), 54–58.

La Leche League International. (2012). *Bariatric surgery and lactation. Update to the breastfeeding answer book.* Schaumburg, IL: Author.

Lamb, M. (2011). Weight-loss surgery and breastfeeding. *Clinical Lactation, 2*(2-3), 17–21.

Landers, S. L., & Hartmann, B. T. (2012). Donor human milk banking and the emergence of milk sharing. *Pediatric Clinics of North America, 60*(1), 247–260.

Lanese, M. G., & Cross, M. (2013). Breastfeeding a preterm infant. In R. Mannel, P. J. Martens, & M. Walker (Eds.), *Core curriculum for lactation consultant practice* (3rd ed.). Burlington, MA: Jones and Bartlett.

Lauwers, J., & Swisher, A. (2016). *Breastfeeding techniques and devices. Counseling the nursing mother* (6th ed.). Burlington MA: Jones & Bartlett.

Lawrence, R. M., & Lawrence, R. A. (2016). *Breastfeeding: A guide for the medical profession* (8th ed.). St. Louis, MO: Elsevier.

Mangesi, L., & Zakarija-Grkovic, I. (2016). Treatments for breast engorgement during lactation. *Cochrane Database of Systematic Reviews, 2016*(6), CD006946.

Marinelli, K. A., Moren, K., Taylor, J. S., et al. (2013). Breastfeeding support for mothers in workplace employment or educational settings: Summary statement. *Breastfeeding Medicine, 8*(1), 137–142.

Martino, K., & Spatz, D. (2014). Informal milk sharing: What nurses need to know. *Maternal-Child Nursing Journal, 39*(6), 369–374.

McMillan, D., & Canadian Paediatric Society Fetus and Newborn Committee. (1997, reaffirmed 2016). *Position statement: Routine administration of vitamin K to newborns.* Retrieved from www.cps.ca/documents/position/administration-vitamin-K-newborns.

Meier, P. P., Patel, A. L., Bigger, H. R., et al. (2013). Supporting breastfeeding in the neonatal intensive care unit: Rush Mother's Milk Club as a case study of evidence-based care. *Pediatric Clinics of North America, 60*(1), 209–226.

Meier, P. P., Patel, A. L., Hoban, R., et al. (2016). Which breast pump for which mother: An evidence-based approach to individualizing breast pump technology. *Journal of Perinatology, 36*(7), 493–499.

Meier, P. P., Patel, A. L., Wright, K., et al. (2013). Management of breastfeeding during and after the maternity hospitalization for late preterm infants. *Clinics in Perinatology, 40*(4), 689–705.

Mohrbacher, N. (2013). Breastfeeding and growth: Birth through weaning. In R. Mannel, P. J. Martens, & M. Walker (Eds.), *Core curriculum for lactation consultant practice* (3rd ed.). Burlington, MA: Jones and Bartlett.

Montgomery, A., Hale, T. W., & Academy of Breastfeeding Medicine. (2012). ABM protocol no. 15: Analgesia and anesthesia for the breastfeeding mother, revised 2012. *Breastfeeding Medicine, 7*(6), 547–553.

Moore, E. R., Anderson, G. C., Bergman, N., et al. (2012). Early skin-to-skin contact for mothers and their healthy newborn infants. *Cochrane Database of Systematic Reviews, 2012*(5), CD003519.

Morton, J., Hall, J. Y., & Pessl, M. (2013–2014). Five steps to improve bedside breastfeeding care. *Nursing for Women's Health, 17*(6), 478–488.

Morton, J., Wong, R. J., Hall, J. Y., et al. (2012). Combining hand techniques with electric pumping increases the caloric content of milk in mothers of preterm infants. *Journal of Perinatology, 32*(10), 791–796.

Mueffelmann, R. E., Racine, E. F., Warren-Findlow, J., et al. (2015). Perceived infant feeding preferences of significant family members and mothers' intentions to exclusively breastfeed. *Journal of Human Lactation, 31*(3), 479–489.

Mueller, N. T., Bakacs, E., Combellick, J., et al. (2015). The infant microbiome development: Mom matters. *Trends in Molecular Medicine, 21*(2), 109–117.

Nelson, A. M. (2012). A meta-synthesis related to infant feeding decision making. *American Journal of Maternal Child Nursing, 37*(4), 247–252.

Newton, E. R. (2017). Lactation and breastfeeding. In S. G. Gabbe, J. R. Niebyl, J. L. Simpson, et al. (Eds.), *Obstetrics: Normal and problem pregnancies* (7th ed.). Philadelphia, PA: Elsevier.

Nielsen, A. (2013). *Gua sha: A traditional technique for modern practice* (2nd ed.). London, UK: Elsevier Churchill Livingstone.

Odom, E. C., Li, R., Scanlon, K. S., et al. (2013). Reasons for earlier than desired cessation of breastfeeding. *Pediatrics, 131*(3), e726–e732.

Odom, E. C., Li, R., Scanlon, K. S., et al. (2014). Association of family and health care provider opinion on infant feeding with mother's breastfeeding decision. *Journal of the Academy of Nutrition and Dietetics, 114*(8), 1203–1207.

Perrine, C. G., Scanlon, K. S., Li, R., et al. (2012). Baby-friendly hospital practices and meeting exclusive breastfeeding intention. *Pediatrics, 130*(1), 54–60.

Reece-Stremtan, S., & Marinelli, K. A. (2015). ABM clinical protocol no. 21: Guidelines for breastfeeding and substance use or substance use disorder. *Breastfeeding Medicine, 10*(3), 135–141.

Robertson, B. D. (2014). Working and breastfeeding: Practical ways you can support employed and breastfeeding mothers. *Clinical Lactation, 5*(4), 137–140.

Roche-Paull, R. (2016). *Can you breastfeed with nipple piercings?* Retrieved from breastfeeding.support/breastfeeding-with-nipple-piercings/.

Roll, C. L., & Cheater, F. (2016). Expectant parents' views of factors influencing infant feeding decisions in the antenatal period: A systematic review. *International Journal of Nursing Studies, 60*(2016), 145–155.

Rosen-Carole, C., Hartman, S., & Academy of Breastfeeding Medicine. (2015). ABM clinical protocol no. 19: Breastfeeding promotion in the prenatal setting. *Breastfeeding Medicine, 10*(10), 451–457.

Sachs, H. C., & Committee on Drugs. (2013). The transfer of drugs and therapeutics into human breast milk: An update on selected topics. *Pediatrics, 132*(3), e796–e809.

Sankar, M. J., Sinha, B., Chowdhury, R., et al. (2015). Optimal breastfeeding practices and infant and child mortality: A systematic review and meta-analysis. *Acta Paediatrica, 104*(467), 3–13.

Smith, A., & Heads, J. (2013). Breast pathology. In R. Mannel, P. J. Martens, & M. Walker (Eds.), *Core curriculum for lactation consultant practice* (3rd ed.). Burlington, MA: Jones and Bartlett.

Sriraman, N. K., Melvin, K., Meltzer-Brody, S., & Academy of Breastfeeding Medicine. (2015). ABM clinical protocol no. 18: Use of antidepressants in breastfeeding mothers. *Breastfeeding Medicine, 10*(6), 290–299.

Stuebe, A. M. (2014). Enabling women to achieve their breastfeeding goals. *Obstetrics and Gynecology, 123*(3), 643–652.

Suzuki, S. (2013). Effect of early skin-to-skin contact on breastfeeding. *Journal of Obstetrics and Gynaecology, 33*(7), 695–696.

Thorn, B., Tadler, C., Huret, N., et al. (2015). *WIC participant and program characteristics 2014*. Alexandria, VA: USDA. Retrieved from http://www.fns.usda.gov/sites/default/files/ops/WICPC2014-Summary.pdf.

Turcksin, R., Bel, S., Galjaard, S., et al. (2014). Maternal obesity and breastfeeding intention, initiation, intensity and duration: A systematic review. *Maternal and Child Nutrition, 10*(2), 166–183.

Updegrove, K. (2013). Nonprofit human milk banking in the United States. *Journal of Midwifery and Women's Health, 58*(5), 502–508.

US Breastfeeding Committee. (2010a). *Core competencies in breastfeeding care and services for all health care professionals* (rev. ed.). Washington, DC: Author.

US Breastfeeding Committee. (2010b). *Implementing the Joint Commission perinatal care core measure on exclusive breast milk feeding* (rev. ed.). Washington, DC: Author.

US Department of Health and Human Services. (2016). *Healthy People 2020: Maternal, infant, and child health*. Washington, DC: Author. Retrieved from www.healthypeople.gov/2020/topics-objectives/topic/maternal-infant-and-child-health/objectives.

US Food and Drug Administration. (2012). *Import alert 61-07*. Retrieved from www.accessdata.fda.gov/cms_ia/importalert_166.html.

US Food and Drug Administration. (2015). *Use of donor milk*. Retrieved from http://www.fda.gov/ScienceResearch/SpecialTopics/PediatricTherapeuticsResearch/ucm235203.htm.

Victora, C. G., Bahl, R., Barros, A. J., et al. (2016). Breastfeeding in the 21st century: Epidemiology, mechanisms, and lifelong effect. *Lancet, 387*(10017), 475–490.

Wagner, E. A., Chantry, C. J., Dewey, K. G., et al. (2013). Breastfeeding concerns at 3 and 7 days postpartum and feeding status at 2 months. *Pediatrics, 132*(4), e865–e875.

Wagner, C., Grier, F., & American Academy of Pediatrics Section on Breastfeeding, and Committee on Nutrition. (2008). Prevention of rickets and vitamin D deficiency in infants, children and adolescents. *Pediatrics, 122*(5), 1142–1152.

Wilson, E., Perrin, M. T., Fogleman, A., et al. (2015). The intricacies of induced lactation for same-sex mothers of an adopted child. *Journal of Human Lactation, 31*(1), 64–67.

Wolfe-Roubatis, E., & Spatz, D. L. (2015). Transgender men and lactation. *Maternal-Child Nursing Journal, 40*(1), 32–38.

World Health Organization. (2013). *Essential nutrition actions: Improving maternal, newborn, infant, and young child health and nutrition*. Geneva, Switzerland: Author. Retrieved from http://www.who.int/nutrition/publications/infantfeeding/essential_nutrition_actions/en/.

World Health Organization. (2016). *Exclusive breastfeeding. E-library of evidence for nutrition actions*. Geneva, Switzerland: Author. Retrieved from http://www.who.int/elena/titles/exclusive_breastfeeding/en/.

25

The High-Risk Newborn

Debbie Fraser

http://evolve.elsevier.com/Perry/maternal

A high-risk neonate can be defined as a newborn, regardless of gestational age or birth weight, who has a greater-than-average chance of morbidity or mortality because of conditions or circumstances associated with birth and the adjustment to extrauterine existence.

High-risk infants are most often classified according to birth weight, gestational age, and predominant pathophysiologic problems. The more common problems related to physiologic status are closely associated with the state of maturity of the infant and usually involve chemical disturbances (e.g., hypoglycemia, hypocalcemia) or consequences of immature organs and systems (e.g., hyperbilirubinemia, respiratory distress, hypothermia). Because high-risk factors are common to several specialty areas—particularly obstetrics, pediatrics, and neonatology—specific terminology is needed to describe the developmental status of the newborn (Box 25.1).

An infant may be considered high risk because of birth trauma, maternal substance abuse, infection, or congenital anomalies. Infants born preterm and postterm and those born to mothers with conditions such as diabetes are also considered high risk and warrant careful monitoring. Birth trauma includes physical injuries that a neonate sustains during labor and birth. Congenital anomalies include conditions such as gastrointestinal (GI) malformations, cleft lip and cleft palate, genitourinary defects, neural tube defects, abdominal wall defects, and cardiac defects.

At times, the nurse is able to anticipate problems such as when a woman is admitted in preterm labor or a congenital anomaly is diagnosed by ultrasound before birth. At other times, the birth of a high-risk infant is unanticipated. In either case, the interprofessional health care team and equipment necessary for immediate care of the infant must be available.

BIRTH INJURIES

Birth trauma (injury) is physical injury sustained by a neonate during labor and birth. It remains an important source of neonatal morbidity. Many birth injuries are avoidable, especially with careful assessment of risk factors and appropriate planning of the birth. The use of fetal ultrasonography allows antepartum diagnosis of certain fetal conditions that may be treated in utero or shortly after birth. Elective cesarean birth can be chosen for some pregnancies to prevent significant birth injury. Some injuries cannot be anticipated until the specific circumstances are encountered during birth. The same injury might be caused in several ways (e.g., a cephalhematoma could result from an obstetric technique such as forceps- or vacuum-assisted birth or from pressure of the fetal skull against the maternal pelvis).

Many injuries are minor and resolve in the neonatal period without treatment. Other trauma requires some degree of intervention; few injuries cause long-term morbidity or mortality.

CARE MANAGEMENT

At birth, the nurse makes a rapid inspection and physical assessment of the neonate to identify any life-threatening conditions that require immediate medical or surgical attention. A comprehensive physical assessment of the newborn is performed after the parents have had the opportunity to interact with their new baby (see Table 23.3). Because evidence of some birth injuries may not be apparent at the initial examination, assessment continues during each contact with the neonate. Promptly reporting deviations from normal permits early initiation of appropriate therapy. Table 25.1 provides an overview of neurologic birth injuries and the sites in which they occur. Soft tissue injuries that commonly occur at birth (i.e., caput succedaneum and cephalhematoma) are discussed in Chapter 22. Nursing and medical interventions are discussed in the following sections.

SKELETAL INJURIES

The newborn's immature, flexible skull can withstand a great degree of deformation (molding) before fracture results. Skull fractures in the newborn are usually linear or depressed fractures. The location of the fracture and involvement of underlying structures determine its significance.

If an artery lying in a groove on the undersurface of the skull is torn as a result of the fracture, increased intracranial pressure (ICP) follows. Unless a blood vessel is involved, linear fractures heal without special treatment. The soft skull can become indented without laceration of either the skin or the dural membrane. These depressed fractures, or "ping pong ball" indentations, can occur during difficult births from pressure of the head on the bony pelvis. They can also occur as a result of application of forceps (Parsons, Seay, & Jacobson, 2016).

The clavicle is the bone most often fractured during birth. Generally the break is in the middle third of the bone (Fig. 25.1). Dystocia, particularly shoulder impaction, may be the predisposing problem. Limited arm motion, crepitus over the bone, and absence of the Moro reflex on the affected side are often present. Except for use of gentle handling and containment of the limb against the chest, no treatment for fractured clavicle of the newborn is required, and the prognosis is good. The humerus and femur are other bones that may be fractured during a difficult birth. Fractures in newborns generally heal rapidly.

BOX 25.1   Classification of High-Risk Infants

Classification According to Size

- **Low–birth weight (LBW) infant**—Infant whose birth weight is less than 2500 g (5 lbs 8 oz), regardless of gestational age
- **Very low–birth weight (VLBW) infant**—Infant whose birth weight is less than 1500 g (3 lbs 5 oz)
- **Extremely low–birth weight (ELBW) infant**—Infant whose birth weight is less than 1000 g (2 lb 3 oz)
- **Appropriate-for-gestational-age (AGA) infant**—Infant whose weight falls between the 10th and 90th percentiles on intrauterine growth curves
- **Small-for-date (SFD) or small-for-gestational age (SGA) infant**—An infant whose rate of intrauterine growth was slowed and whose birth weight falls below the 10th percentile on intrauterine growth curves
- **Intrauterine growth restriction (IUGR)**—Found in infants whose intrauterine growth is restricted (sometimes used as a more descriptive term for SGA infants)
- **Symmetric IUGR**—Growth restriction in which the weight, length, and head circumference are all affected
- **Asymmetric IUGR**—Growth restriction in which the head circumference remains within normal parameters while the birth weight falls below the 10th percentile
- **Large-for-gestational-age (LGA) infant**—Infant whose birth weight falls above the 90th percentile on intrauterine growth charts

Classification According to Gestational Age

- **Preterm (premature) infant**—Infant born before 37 0/7 weeks of gestation
- **Late-preterm infant**—Infant born between 34 0/7 and 36 6/7 weeks of gestation
- **Early-term infant** – Infant born between 37 0/7 weeks and 38 6/7 weeks of gestation
- **Full-term infant**—Infant born between 39 0/7 weeks and 40 6/7 weeks of gestation
- **Late-term infant:** Infant born between 41 0/7 weeks and 41 6/7 weeks of gestation
- **Postterm (postmature) infant**—Infant born after 42 0/7 weeks of gestation

Classification According to Mortality

- **Live birth**—Birth in which neonate manifests any heartbeat, breathes, or displays voluntary movement, regardless of gestational age
- **Fetal death**—Death of fetus after 20 weeks of gestation and before birth with absence of any signs of life at birth
- **Neonatal death**—Death that occurs in the first 28 days of life; early neonatal death occurs in the first week of life; late neonatal death occurs at 8 to 28 days
- **Perinatal mortality**—Total number of fetal and early neonatal deaths per 1000 live births
- **Infant death** – Death that occurs before the first birthday
- **Infant mortality** – Total number of infant deaths per 1000 live births

Data from American College of Obstetricians and Gynecologists Committee on Obstetric Practice & Society for Maternal-Fetal Medicine. (2013). Definition of term pregnancy. *Obstetrics and Gynecology, 122*(5), 1139–1140; Centers for Disease Control and Prevention. (2016). *Infant mortality.* Retrieved from http://www.cdc.gov/reproductivehealth/maternalinfanthealth/infantmortality.htm.

TABLE 25.1   Types of Birth Injuries

Site of Injury	Type of Injury
Scalp	Caput succedaneum
	Subgaleal hemorrhage
	Cephalhematoma
Skull	Linear fracture
	Depressed fracture
	Occipital osteodiastasis
Intracranial	Epidural hematoma
	Subdural hematoma (laceration of falx, tentorium, or superficial veins)
	Subarachnoid hemorrhage
	Cerebral contusion
	Cerebellar contusion
	Intracerebellar hematoma
Spinal cord (cervical)	Vertebral artery injury
	Intraspinal hemorrhage
	Spinal cord transection or injury
Plexus	Erb's palsy
	Klumpke paralysis
	Total (mixed) brachial plexus injury
	Horner syndrome
	Diaphragmatic (phrenic nerve) paralysis
	Lumbosacral plexus injury
Cranial and peripheral nerve	Radial nerve palsy
	Medial nerve palsy
	Sciatic nerve palsy
	Laryngeal nerve palsy
	Diaphragmatic paralysis
	Facial nerve palsy

Data from Parsons, J.A., Seay, A.R., & Jacobson, M. (2016). Neurologic disorders. In S.L. Gardner, B.S. Carter, M. Enzman-Hines, et al. (Eds.), *Merenstein and Gardner's handbook of neonatal intensive care* (8th ed.). St. Louis, MO: Elsevier.

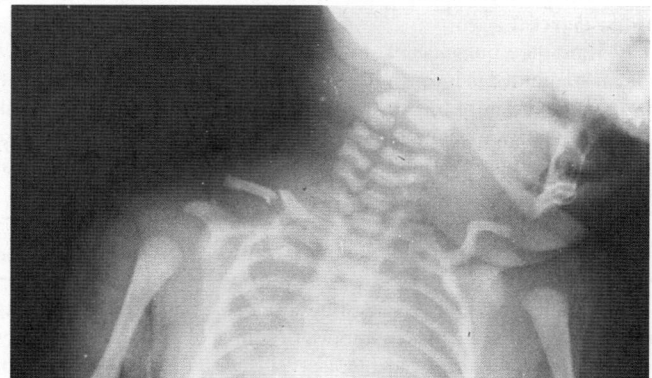

FIG 25.1 Fractured clavicle after shoulder dystocia. (From O'Doherty, N. [1986]. *Neonatology: Micro atlas of the newborn.* Nutley, NJ: Hoffmann-La Roche.)

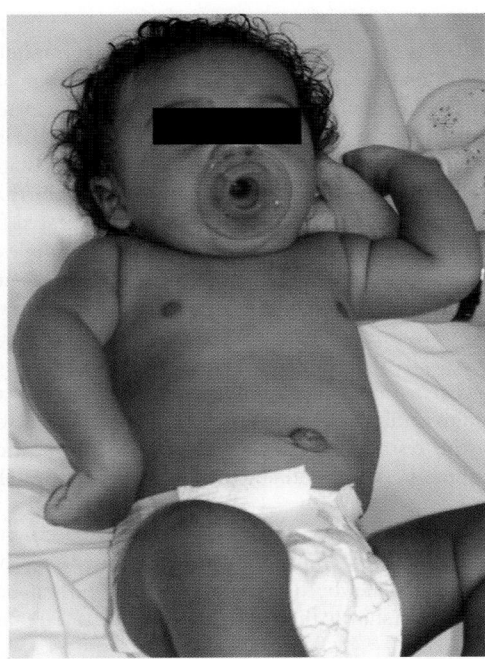

FIG 25.2 Erb-Duchenne paralysis in a newborn infant. Moro reflex is absent in right upper extremity. Recovery was complete. (From Chung, K.C., Yang, L.J.S., & McGillicuddy, J.E. [2012]. *Practical management of pediatric and adult brachial plexus palsies*. Philadelphia, PA: Saunders.)

Immobilization is accomplished with slings, splints, swaddling, and other devices.

The parents need support in handling these infants because they are often afraid of hurting them. They are encouraged to practice handling, changing, and feeding the affected neonate under the guidance of nursery personnel. This increases their confidence and knowledge and facilitates attachment. A plan for follow-up therapy is developed with the parents so the times and arrangements for therapy are acceptable to them.

PERIPHERAL NERVOUS SYSTEM INJURIES

Plexus injury results from forces that alter the normal position and relationship of the arm, shoulder, and neck. Erb's palsy (Erb-Duchenne paralysis) is caused by damage to the upper plexus nerve and usually results from a stretching or pulling of the shoulder away from the head, such as might occur with shoulder dystocia or a difficult vertex or breech birth. The less common lower plexus palsy, or Klumpke palsy, results from stretching of the upper extremity while the trunk is relatively less mobile (Parsons et al., 2016).

The clinical manifestations of Erb's palsy are related to the paralysis of the affected extremity and muscles. The arm hangs limp alongside the body. The shoulder and arm are adducted and rotated internally. The elbow is extended, and the forearm is pronated with the wrist and fingers flexed; a grasp reflex may be present because finger and wrist movement remains normal (Carlo & Ambalavanan, 2016b) (Fig. 25.2). In lower plexus palsy, the muscles of the hand are paralyzed, with consequent wrist drop and relaxed fingers. In a third and more severe form of brachial palsy, the entire arm is paralyzed and hangs limp and motionless at the side. The Moro reflex is absent on the affected side for all of the forms of brachial palsy. Total plexus is the second most common type of plexus injury (Verklan, 2015).

Treatment of the affected arm is aimed at preventing contractures of the paralyzed muscles and maintaining correct placement of the humeral head within the glenoid fossa of the scapula. Complete recovery

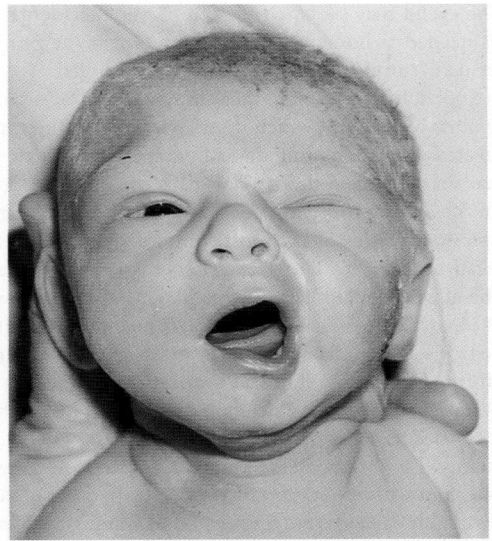

FIG 25.3 Facial paralysis 15 minutes after forceps birth. Absence of movement on affected side is especially noticeable when infant cries. (From O'Doherty, N. [1986]. *Neonatology: Micro atlas of the newborn*. Nutley, NJ: Hoffmann-La Roche.)

from stretched nerves usually takes 3 to 6 months. However, avulsion of the nerves (complete disconnection of the ganglia from the spinal cord that involves both anterior and posterior roots) results in permanent damage. For injuries that do not improve by 3 months, surgical intervention may be needed to relieve pressure on the nerves or repair the nerves with grafting (Carlo & Ambalavanan, 2016b).

Nursing care of the newborn with brachial palsy is concerned primarily with proper positioning of the affected arm. The affected arm should be abducted 90 degrees with external shoulder rotation, forearm supination, and extension at the wrist with the palm facing the infant's face. Passive range-of-motion exercises of the shoulder, wrist, elbow, and fingers are initiated in the latter part of the first week. Wrist flexion contractures may be prevented with the use of a wrist splint with padding in the fist. In dressing the infant, preference is given to the affected arm. Undressing begins with the unaffected arm, and redressing begins with the affected arm to prevent unnecessary manipulation and stress on the paralyzed muscles. Parents are instructed to use the football position when holding the infant and to avoid picking the child up from under the axillae or pulling on the arms.

Pressure on the facial nerve (cranial nerve VII) during birth can result in injury. The primary clinical manifestations are loss of movement on the affected side such as an inability to completely close the eye, drooping of the corner of the mouth, and absence of wrinkling of the forehead and nasolabial fold (Fig. 25.3). Facial palsy or paralysis is most noticeable when the infant cries. The mouth is drawn to the unaffected side, the wrinkles are deeper on the normal side, and the eye on the involved side remains open. Often the condition is temporary, resolving within hours or days of birth. Permanent paralysis is rare unless the nerve fibers were torn, in which case surgical intervention may be necessary.

Nursing care of the infant with facial nerve paralysis involves assisting the mother with feeding techniques. The infant's ability to suck effectively can be impaired, and drooling is common. The infant may require gavage feeding to prevent aspiration (Parsons et al., 2016). Breastfeeding is not contraindicated, but the mother needs additional assistance from a lactation consultant or infant feeding specialist to help the infant grasp and compress the areolar area.

If the eyelid on the affected side does not close completely, artificial tears may be instilled to prevent drying of the conjunctiva, sclera, and cornea. The eyelid may be taped shut to prevent accidental injury. If eye care is needed at home, the parents are taught the procedure for administering eyedrops before the infant is discharged.

Phrenic nerve injury results in diaphragmatic paralysis as demonstrated by ultrasonography, which shows paradoxical chest movement and an elevated diaphragm. Initially radiography may not demonstrate an elevated diaphragm if the neonate is receiving positive-pressure ventilation. The injury sometimes occurs in conjunction with brachial palsy. Respiratory distress is the most common and important sign of injury. Because injury to the phrenic nerve is usually unilateral, the lung on the affected side does not expand, and respiratory efforts are ineffective (Carlo & Ambalavanan, 2016b). The infant is positioned on the affected side to facilitate maximum expansion of the uninvolved lung. Breathing is primarily thoracic; cyanosis, tachypnea, or complete respiratory failure may be seen. Pneumonia and atelectasis on the affected side may also occur.

The infant with phrenic nerve paralysis requires the same nursing care as any infant with respiratory distress. As with other birth injuries, the family's emotional needs are similar to those discussed for soft-tissue injury (see Chapter 22). Follow-up is also essential because of the extended length of recovery.

NEUROLOGIC INJURIES

Neurologic injury in newborn infants is common with the increased survival of low–birth weight (LBW) and very low–birth weight infants (VLBW); in addition, the lower the gestational age, the higher the risk for certain neurologic injuries. Such infants are particularly vulnerable to ischemic injury caused by variable (both increased and decreased) cerebral blood flow subsequent to asphyxia; and preterm infants, with a fragile cerebrovascular network, are highly prone to periventricular or intraventricular hemorrhage. Fragility and increased permeability of capillaries and prolonged prothrombin time predispose preterm infants to trauma when delicate structures are subjected to the forces of labor (Parsons et al., 2016). The more common cerebral complications and nursing care are outlined in Table 25.2.

The highest incidence of abnormal neurologic findings occurs in VLBW infants and those with intracranial hemorrhage. Major neurologic problems such as cerebral palsy, seizures, and hydrocephalus are usually diagnosed in the first 2 years of life. Less severe deficits such as learning disorders, attention deficit hyperactivity disorder (ADHD), and fine- and gross-motor incoordination may not be diagnosed until preschool or school age. Cerebral palsy is one of the most common neurologic deficits in survivors of preterm birth (Parsons et al., 2016) (see Chapter 49).

Therapeutic hypothermia provided by cooling either the infant's head or the whole body reduces the severity of the neurologic damage in hypoxic ischemic encephalopathy when it is applied in the early stages of injury (first 6 hours after birth) in term or late preterm infants (Azzopardi, Strohm, Marlow, et al., 2014; McAdams & Juul, 2016; Shankaran, 2012; Zubcevic, Heljic, Catibusic, et al., 2015).

NEONATAL INFECTIONS

SEPSIS

Sepsis (the presence of microorganisms or their toxins in the blood or other tissues) continues to be one of the most significant causes of neonatal morbidity and mortality. Septicemia refers to a generalized infection in the bloodstream. Pneumonia, the most common form of neonatal infection, is one of the leading causes of perinatal death. Bacterial meningitis occurs in approximately 0.2 to 0.4 cases per 1000 live births, with a higher rate in preterm infants (Stoll & Shane, 2016).

Gastroenteritis is sporadic, depending on epidemic outbreaks. Local infections such as conjunctivitis and thrush occur commonly.

Newborn infants are at risk for sepsis for a number of reasons. Maternal immunoglobulin M (IgM) does not cross the placenta. IgG levels in term infants are equal to maternal levels; however, in preterm infants the amount of IgG is directly proportional to gestational age. IgA and IgM require time to reach optimum levels after birth. Neonatal neutrophils are present in term infants but have decreased functional capabilities; response to infections is sluggish. Phagocytosis is less efficient. Serum complement levels are low in term infants and even lower in the preterm infant; serum complement is involved in immunologic reactions, some of which kill or lyse bacteria and enhance phagocytosis. The gut mucosal barrier is initially immature in both term and preterm infants; this barrier is enhanced by the ingestion of human colostrum, which contains antiinfective properties. Dysmaturity seen with intrauterine growth restriction (IUGR) and preterm and postterm birth further compromises the immune system of the neonate (Stoll & Shane, 2016).

Table 25.3 outlines risk factors for neonatal sepsis. Special precautions for preventing infection and prompt recognition when it occurs are necessary for optimal newborn care. Neonatal infections can be acquired in utero, at birth or shortly thereafter, and as a health care–associated infection (HAI).

Neonatal bacterial infection is classified into two patterns according to the time of presentation. Early onset or congenital sepsis usually manifests within 72 hours of birth, progresses more rapidly than later-onset infection, and carries a mortality rate as high as 20% to 30% in preterm infants. Early-onset sepsis is acquired in the perinatal period; infection can occur from direct contact with organisms from the maternal GI and genitourinary tracts. The most common infecting organisms are gram-negative organisms, specifically *Escherichia coli* and group B streptococcus (GBS) (Pammi, Brand, & Weisman, 2016; Stoll, Hansen, Sanchez, et al., 2011). GBS is an extremely virulent organism in neonates, with a high death rate in affected infants. Other bacteria noted to cause early onset infection include *Haemophilus influenzae*, *Citrobacter* and *Enterobacter* organisms, coagulase-negative staphylococci, and *Streptococcus viridans*. Other pathogens that are harbored in the vagina and may infect the infant include gonococci, *Candida albicans*, herpes simplex virus (HSV) type 2, and chlamydia. Early onset sepsis is associated with a history of obstetric events such as preterm birth, prolonged rupture of membranes (more than 18 hours), maternal fever during labor, and chorioamnionitis. Early onset infection is also inversely related to infant birth weight (Polin & AAP Committee on Fetus and Newborn, 2012).

Late onset sepsis, occurring at approximately 7 to 30 days of age, is considered primarily to be an infection acquired in the hospital or community; the offending organisms are usually staphylococci, *Klebsiella* organisms, GBS, enterococci, *E. coli*, and *Pseudomonas* or *Candida* species (Pammi et al., 2016). Coagulase-negative staphylococci, considered to be primarily a contaminant in older children and adults, are commonly found to be the cause of septicemia in extremely low birth weight (ELBW) and VLBW infants. Additional infections of concern include methicillin-resistant *Staphylococcus aureus* (MRSA), vancomycin-resistant enterococci (VRE), and multidrug-resistant gram-negative pathogens. Bacterial invasion can occur through sites such as the umbilical stump; the skin; mucous membranes of the eye, nose, pharynx, and ear; and internal systems such as the respiratory, nervous, urinary, and GI systems.

Perinatally acquired infections can cause spontaneous abortion (miscarriage), stillbirth, intrauterine infection, congenital malformations, and acute neonatal disease. Other viral infections such as respiratory syncytial virus (RSV), rotavirus, herpes simplex, influenza, and varicella may occur in the neonatal intensive care unit (NICU). These pathogens also may cause chronic infection, with subtle manifestations that may

TABLE 25.2   Neurologic Complications

Description	Clinical Manifestations	Therapeutic Management	Care Management
Hypoxic-Ischemic Brain Injury			
Nonprogressive neurologic (brain) impairment caused by intrauterine or postnatal asphyxia resulting in hypoxemia or cerebral ischemia Hypoxic-ischemic encephalopathy—the resultant cellular damage that causes the clinical manifestations Stage I to stage III (mild to severe encephalopathy)	Appears within first 6–12 hours after hypoxic episode Seizures Abnormal muscle tone (usually hypotonia) Disturbance of sucking and swallowing Apneic episodes Stupor or coma Muscular weakness in hips and shoulders (full- term), lower-limb weakness (preterm)	Prevent hypoxia. Provide supportive care. Provide adequate ventilation. Maintain cerebral perfusion. Prevent cerebral edema. Treat underlying cause. Administer antiseizure drugs. Initiate therapeutic hypothermia if criteria met (see Neurologic Injuries).	See Care of the High-Risk Newborn and Family. Observe for signs that indicate cerebral hypoxia. Monitor ventilatory and intravenous therapy. Observe for and manage seizures. Support family. Provide guidelines for family management of potential mild-to-severe neurologic damage.
Germinal Matrix or Intraventricular Hemorrhage			
Hemorrhage into and around ventricles caused by ruptured vessels as a result of an event that increases cerebral blood flow to area	Most bleeds initially asymptomatic Sudden deterioration in condition if bleed is large: • Oxygen desaturation • Bradycardia • Hypotonia • Metabolic acidosis • Shock • Significant drop in hematocrit • Tense anterior fontanel Signs of worsening hemorrhage: • Twitching • Decreased level of consciousness, stupor • Apnea • Seizures • Full, tense fontanels Evident on cranial ultrasonography or magnetic resonance imaging	Provide supportive care. Provide ventilatory support. Maintain oxygenation. Regulate fluid, electrolytes, acid-base balance. Provide ventricular shunting or drainage.	See Care of the High-Risk Newborn and Family. Prevent increased cerebral blood pressure. Avoid events that may increase or decrease cerebral blood flow (e.g., pain, unnecessary stimulation, endotracheal suctioning, hypoxia, hyperosmolar drugs, rapid volume expansion). Elevate head of bed 20–30 degrees; keep head in midline. Support family. Monitor for posthemorrhagic hydrocephalus after diagnosis. Provide developmental care and enhancement.
Intracranial Hemorrhage			
Subdural Subarachnoid Intracerebellar	Sudden decrease in hematocrit Change in sensorium Seizures Poor feeding See Chapter 45	See Chapter 46.	Same as for germinal matrix or intraventricular hemorrhage

Data from Parsons, J.A., Seay, A.R., & Jacobson, M. (2016). Neurologic disorders. In S.L. Gardner, B.S. Carter, M. Enzman-Hines, et al. (Eds.), *Merenstein and Gardner's handbook of neonatal intensive care* (8th ed.). St. Louis, MO: Elsevier; Verklan, M.T. (2015). Neurologic disorders. In M.T. Verklan, & M. Walden (Eds.), *Core curriculum for neonatal intensive care nursing* (5th ed.). St. Louis, MO: Elsevier.

be recognized only after a prolonged period. It is important to recognize the manifestations of infections in the neonatal period to be able to treat the acute infection, prevent HAIs in other infants, and anticipate effects on the infant's subsequent growth and development.

Fungal infection is a major concern in the immunocompromised or preterm infant. Occasionally fungal infections such as thrush are found in otherwise healthy term infants.

Care Management

The nurse reviews the prenatal record for risk factors associated with infection and the signs and symptoms suggestive of infection. Maternal vaginal or perineal infection may be transmitted directly to the infant during passage through the birth canal. Psychosocial history and history

of sexually transmitted infections (STIs) may indicate possible human immunodeficiency virus (HIV), hepatitis B virus (HBV), herpes (type 2), or cytomegalovirus (CMV) infection.

Perinatal events should also be reviewed. Premature rupture of membranes (PROM) can be caused by maternal or intrauterine infection. Ascending infection can occur after prolonged PROM, prolonged labor, or intrauterine fetal monitoring. In some cases, infection occurs with intact membranes or contributes to early rupture. A maternal history of fever during labor or the presence of foul-smelling amniotic fluid can also indicate infection. Antibiotic therapy initiated during labor should be noted. The neonate's gestational age, maturity, birth weight, and sex affect the incidence of infection. Sepsis occurs about twice as often and results in a higher mortality in male than in female infants.

TABLE 25.3 Risk Factors for Neonatal Sepsis

Source	Risk Factors
Maternal	Low socioeconomic status
	Poor prenatal care
	Poor nutrition
	Substance abuse
Intrapartum	Premature rupture of membranes
	Maternal group B streptococcus colonization
	Maternal fever
	Chorioamnionitis
	Prolonged labor
	Rupture of membranes >18 hours
	Premature labor
	Maternal urinary tract infection
Neonatal	Twin or multiple gestation
	Male
	Birth asphyxia
	Meconium aspiration
	Congenital anomalies of skin or mucous membranes
	Galactosemia
	Absence of spleen
	Low birth weight or preterm birth
	Malnourishment
	Prolonged hospitalization
	Invasive procedures

Data from Bodin, M.B. (2014). Immune system. In C. Kenner, & J.W. Lott (Eds.), *Comprehensive neonatal nursing care* (5th ed.). New York, NY: Springer; Leonard, E.G., & Dobbs, K. (2015). Postnatal bacterial infections. In R.J. Martin, A.A. Fanaroff, & M.C. Walsh (Eds.), *Fanaroff and Martin's neonatal-perinatal medicine: Diseases of the fetus and infant* (10th ed.). St. Louis, MO: Elsevier.

TABLE 25.4 Clinical Manifestations of Neonatal Sepsis*

System	Signs
Respiratory	Apnea
	Tachypnea
	Grunting
	Nasal flaring
	Retractions
	Cyanosis
	Decreased oxygen saturation
	Metabolic acidosis
Cardiovascular	Decreased cardiac output
	Tachycardia or bradycardia
	Arrhythmias
	Hypotension
	Decreased perfusion: poor peripheral pulses, delayed capillary refill; cold, clammy, or mottled skin
Neurologic	Temperature instability, hypothermia, fever
	Lethargy
	Hypotonia
	Jitteriness
	Irritability, seizures
	Bulging fontanels
	High-pitched or abnormal cry
Gastrointestinal	Feeding intolerance (decreased suck strength and intake; increasing residuals)
	Vomiting, diarrhea
	Abdominal distention
	Hypoactive bowel sounds

*Laboratory findings include neutropenia, increased bands, hypoglycemia or hyperglycemia, metabolic acidosis, and thrombocytopenia.
Data from Wilson, D.J., & Tyner, C.I. (2015). Infectious diseases in the neonate. In M.T. Verklan, & M. Walden (Eds.), *Core curriculum for neonatal intensive care nursing* (5th ed.). St. Louis, MO: Elsevier; Wynn, J.L., Wong, H.R., Shanley, T.P., et al. (2014). Time for a neonatal-specific consensus definition for sepsis. *Pediatric Critical Care Medicine, 15*(6), 523–528.

The nurse assesses the neonate for respiratory distress, skin abscesses, petechial rashes, and other indications of infection.

During the postnatal period, the nurse notes the time of onset of suspicious clinical signs. Onset within the first 48 hours of life is more often associated with prenatal or perinatal predisposing factors; onset after 2 or 3 days more often reflects an HAI.

The earliest clinical signs of neonatal sepsis are often nonspecific and can include lethargy, poor feeding, poor weight gain, and irritability. The nurse or parent may simply note that the infant is not doing as well as before. Differential diagnosis can be difficult because signs of sepsis are similar to signs of noninfectious neonatal problems such as hypoglycemia and respiratory distress. Additional clinical and laboratory information, including cultures, supplement the findings described. Table 25.4 outlines the clinical manifestations associated with neonatal sepsis.

Laboratory studies are important. Specimens for cultures include blood, cerebrospinal fluid (CSF), stool, and urine. A complete blood cell count with differential is performed to determine the presence of bacterial infection or increased or decreased white blood cell count (the latter is an ominous sign). The total neutrophil count, immature-to-total (I/T) neutrophil ratio, absolute neutrophil count, platelet count, procalcitonin, and C-reactive protein may be used to determine the presence of sepsis. It is important to note that these tests are likely adjuncts for the confirmation of neonatal sepsis; a combination of these tests and clinical signs often alerts the practitioner to the need for treatment. Additional diagnostic tests that may be used to identify or exclude neonatal sepsis include sedimentation rate, interleukins (IL-8, IL-2, IL-6, and IL-1β), and nucleic acid amplification testing (NAAT).

Antepartum infection can be treated successfully with a number of antiviral medications to decrease viral replication and fetal transmission of disease; neonates may also be treated with antiviral medications such as acyclovir and ganciclovir. In high risk infants with significant illness, antiviral or antibiotic treatment may begin once cultures are obtained. Once the pathogen is identified, antibiotic, antiviral, or antifungal therapy may be modified.

Vigilant assessment continues during and after treatment. Prolonged administration of antibiotics to ELBW neonates without positive cultures in the first week of life is associated with an increased incidence of necrotizing enterocolitis (NEC), mortality, and late-onset infection; therefore, careful use of antibiotics and close observation of such infants are recommended (Kuppala, Meinzen-Derr, Morrow, et al., 2011). The newborn continues to be assessed for sequelae to septicemia, which include meningitis, disseminated intravascular coagulation (DIC), NEC, pneumonia, and septic shock. Septic shock results from the toxins released into the bloodstream. The most common signs include decreasing oxygen saturation, poor perfusion (prolonged capillary refill, cool extremities, mottling), tachycardia, respiratory distress, and hypotension.

Breastfeeding or feeding the newborn expressed breast milk from the mother or alternatively, donor milk from a milk bank, is encouraged. Breast milk provides protective mechanisms. Colostrum contains IgA, which offers protection against infection in the GI tract. Human milk contains iron-binding protein that exerts a bacteriostatic effect on *E. coli*. Human milk also contains macrophages and lymphocytes. The vulnerability of infants to common mucosal pathogens such as RSV may be reduced by passive transfer of maternal immunity in the colostrum and breast milk. There is evidence that early enteral feedings with human milk are beneficial in establishing a natural barrier to infection in ELBW and VLBW infants (Hamilton, Massey, Ross, et al., 2014).

Administering medications, taking precautions when performing treatments, and following isolation procedures are also interventions to consider in the prevention and treatment of neonatal sepsis. Monitoring an intravenous (IV) infusion and administering antibiotics are important nursing responsibilities. It is important to administer the prescribed dose of antibiotic immediately after it is prepared to avoid loss of drug stability. If the IV fluid that the infant is receiving contains electrolytes, vitamins, or other medications, the nurse should check with the hospital pharmacy before adding antibiotics. The antibiotic (or other medication) may be deactivated or may form a precipitate when combined with other medications.

Efforts should also be taken to prevent ventilator-associated pneumonia in infants on mechanical ventilation (see Chapter 40). Isolation procedures are implemented as indicated according to hospital policy. Isolation protocols change rapidly, and the nurse is urged to participate in continuing education and in-service programs to remain up to date.

Prevention

Nursing staff are directly or indirectly responsible for minimizing or eliminating environmental sources of microbes in the nursery. Measures to be taken include Standard Precautions, careful and thorough cleaning of contaminated equipment, frequent replacement of used equipment (e.g., changing IV and nasogastric [NG] tubing per hospital protocol and cleaning resuscitation and ventilation equipment, IV pumps, and incubators), and appropriate disposal of contaminated linens and diapers. Overcrowding must be avoided in nurseries. Guidelines for space, visitation, and general infection control in areas where newborns receive care have been established and published (American Academy of Pediatrics [AAP] & American College of Obstetricians and Gynecologists [ACOG], 2012).

Hand hygiene is the single most effective measure to reduce HAI. However, the rate of compliance with standards for hand hygiene is reported to be generally poor (Shlomai, Rao, & Patole, 2015). The combined use of hand hygiene and gloves is effective in reducing the incidence of systemic infection. It is incumbent on caregivers to strictly adhere to recommended guidelines for hand hygiene.

Antibiotic ointment is instilled into a newborn's eyes within 1 to 2 hours after birth to prevent infection (see Fig. 23.4). The skin, its secretions, and normal flora are natural defenses that protect against invading pathogens. Warm water may be used to remove blood and meconium from the neonate's face, head, and body. A mild nonmedicated soap (in a single-use container) can be used with careful water rinsing. Vernix caseosa is not scrubbed vigorously for removal, since this further disrupts the skin barrier properties (see Guidelines box: Neonatal Skin Care). No single method of cord care has been shown to be more effective in the promotion of drying, separating, and preventing colonization. Current recommendations for cord care by the Association of Women's Health, Obstetric, and Neonatal Nurses (AWHONN, 2013) include cleaning the cord with sterile water or a neutral pH cleanser; subsequent care entails cleaning the cord with water. Nurses must follow agency protocols for cord care, but they can recommend revision of protocols based on research evidence (see the "Umbilical Cord Care" section in Chapter 23). Polin, Denson, Brady, and associates (2012) provide additional strategies for the prevention of HAI in the NICU.

📋 GUIDELINES

Neonatal Skin Care

General Skin Care
Assessment
- Assess skin every day or more often as needed.
- Identify risk factors for skin injury: gestational age ≤30 weeks, adhesive use, nutritional compromise, high-frequency ventilation, extracorporeal membrane oxygenation, hypotension requiring vasopressors.
- Use a valid assessment tool to provide reliable and objective measurement of skin condition.
- Evaluate/report abnormal skin findings, and analyze for possible causes.

Bathing
Initial Bath
- Assess to ensure that the infant has a stable temperature for a minimum of 2 to 4 hours before first bath.
- Use cleansing agents with neutral pH or minimal dyes or perfume.
- Use Standard Precautions; wear gloves.
- Do not completely remove vernix; allow it to wear off with normal care and handling.
- Bathe preterm infant less than 32 weeks of gestational age in warm water only for the first week.

Routine
- Use pH-neutral cleanser or soaps no more than 2 or 3 times per week.
- Avoid rubbing skin during bathing or drying.

- Immerse stable infants fully (except head) in an appropriate-size tub.
- Use swaddled immersion bathing technique: slowly unwrap after gently lowering into water for sensitive but stable infants needing assistance with motor system reactivity.

Emollients
- Apply sparingly to dry, flaking, fissured areas as needed.
- Choose petrolatum-based products that are free of preservatives, dyes, and perfumes.
- Observe neonates ≤750 g (1 lb 10 oz) receiving emollient therapy for increased risk for coagulase-negative *Staphylococcus* infections.
- Consider dispensing emollients from hospital pharmacy, unit dose, or patient-specific container to reduce contamination.

Adhesives
- Decrease use as much as possible.
- Use semipermeable dressings to secure intravenous (IV) lines, nasogastric or orogastric tubes, silicone catheters, and central lines.
- Use hydrogel or limb electrodes.
- Consider hydrocolloid barriers beneath adhesives to protect skin.
- Secure pulse oximeter probe or electrodes with elasticized dressing material.
- Do not use adhesive remover, solvents, or bonding agents.
- Avoid removing adhesives for at least 24 hours after application.

Continued

GUIDELINES

Neonatal Skin Care—cont'd

- Adhesive removal can be facilitated using water, mineral oil, or petrolatum.
- Remove adhesives or skin barriers slowly, supporting the skin underneath with one hand and gently peeling away the product from the skin with the other hand.

Antiseptic Agents
- Apply before invasive procedures.
- Consider the potential for skin breakdown or irritation with disinfectant.
- No specific disinfectant is recommended over another for all neonates.
- Avoid use of isopropyl alcohol for skin preparation or removal of other disinfectants.

Transepidermal Water Loss
- Minimize transepidermal water loss (TEWL) and heat loss in small preterm infants at less than 30 weeks of gestational age:
  - Monitor ambient humidity during first weeks of life.
  - Apply occlusive polyethylene body bag immediately at birth and removing after infant is stabilized in the neonatal intensive care unit.
  - Consider increasing humidity to 70% to 90% by using a humidified incubator for first 7 days; gradually decrease to 50% thereafter.
  - Use supplemental conductive heat and reducing radiant heat source.
  - Apply semipermeable transparent dressings to skin surfaces.
  - Consider use of emollients (see Emollients above).

Skin Breakdown
Prevention
- Decrease pressure from externally applied forces using water, air, or gel mattresses; sheepskin; or cotton bedding.
- Provide adequate nutrition, including protein, fat, and zinc.
- Apply transparent adhesive dressings to protect arms, elbows, and knees from friction injury.
- Use emollient in diaper area (groin and thighs) to reduce urine irritation.

Treating Skin Breakdown
- Irrigate wound with warm half-strength normal saline.
- Culture wound, and treat if signs of infection are present.
- Use transparent adhesive dressing for uninfected wounds.
- Apply hydrogel with or without antibacterial or antifungal ointments (as ordered) for infected wounds (may need to moisten before removal).
- Use hydrocolloid for deep, uninfected wounds or as an ostomy barrier and to improve appliance adhesion.
- Avoid use of antiseptic solutions for wound cleansing (use for intact skin only).

Treating Diaper Dermatitis
- Maintain clean, dry skin; use absorbent diapers and change often.
- If mild irritation occurs, use petrolatum barrier or zinc oxide ointment.
- For developing dermatitis, apply a generous quantity of zinc-oxide barrier (remove only soiled matter, leaving original barrier in place).
- For severe dermatitis, identify cause and treat.
- Treat *Candida albicans* with antifungal ointment or cream.
- Avoid powders and antibiotic ointments (See the "Umbilical Cord Care" and "Care of the Newly Circumcised Infant" sections in Chapter 23).

Other Skin Care Concerns
Use of Substances on Skin
- Evaluate all substances that come in contact with infant's skin.
- Before using any topical agent, analyze components of preparation and:
  - Use sparingly and only when necessary.
  - Whenever possible and appropriate, wash off with water.
  - Monitor infant carefully for signs of toxicity and systemic effects.

Use of Thermal Devices
- Avoid heat lamps because of increased potential for burns. If needed, measure actual temperature of exposed skin every 15 minutes.
- When using preheated transcutaneous electrodes:
  - Avoid use on extremely low–birth-weight infants.
  - Set at lowest possible temperature.
- Use pulse oximetry rather than transcutaneous monitoring whenever possible.
- When prewarming heels before phlebotomy, avoid temperatures over 40° C (104° F).
- Provide warm ambient humidity directed away from infant; use aerosolized sterile water, and maintain ambient temperature not to exceed 40° C (104° F).
- Document use of all heating devices.

Use of Fluid Therapy and Hemodynamic Monitoring
- Be certain that fingers or toes are visible whenever extremity is used for peripheral IV or arterial line.
- Secure catheter or needle with transparent dressing and tape to promote easy visualization of site.
- Assess site hourly for signs of ischemia, infiltration, and inadequate perfusion (check capillary refill, pulses, color).
- Avoid use of restraints (e.g., arm boards); if used, check that they are secured safely and not restricting circulation or movement (check for pressure areas).
- Use commercial IV protector (e.g., I.V. House) with minimal tape.

Data from Ness, M.J., Davis, D.M.R., & Carey, W.A. (2013). Neonatal skin care: A concise review. *International Journal of Dermatology, 52*(1), 14–22; Lund, C. (2014). Medical adhesives in the NICU. *Newborn and Infant Nursing Reviews, 14*(4), 160–165; Danby, S.G., Bedwell, C., & Cork, M.J. (2014). Neonatal skin care and toxicology. In L.F. Eichenfield, I.J. Frieden, A. Zaenglein, et al. (Eds.), *Neonatal and infant dermatology* (3rd ed.). London, UK: Elsevier; Association of Women's Health, Obstetric and Neonatal Nurses. (2013). *Evidence-based clinical practice guideline: Neonatal skin care* (3rd ed.). Washington, DC: Author.

CONGENITAL INFECTIONS

The range of pathologic conditions produced by infectious agents is large, and the difference between the maternal and fetal effects caused by any one agent is also great. Some maternal infections, especially during early gestation, can result in fetal loss or malformations because the fetus's ability to handle infectious organisms is limited and the fetal immunologic system is unable to prevent the dissemination of infectious organisms to the various tissues.

Not all prenatal infections produce teratogenic effects. Furthermore, the clinical picture of disorders caused by transplacental transfer of infectious agents is not always well defined. Some viral agents can cause remarkably similar manifestations, and it is common to test for all of them when a prenatal infection is suspected. This is the so-called *TORCH* complex, an acronym for the following:
- *T*—Toxoplasmosis
- *O*—Other (e.g., HBV, parvovirus, HIV, West Nile virus)
- *R*—Rubella

- *C*—CMV infection
- *H*—Herpes simplex

To determine the causative agent in a symptomatic infant, tests are performed to rule out each of these infections. The *O* category may involve testing for several viral infections (e.g., HBV, varicella zoster, measles, mumps, HIV, syphilis, human parvovirus, and Zika virus). Bacterial infections are not included in the TORCH workup because they are usually identified by clinical manifestations and readily available laboratory tests. The incidence of gonococcal conjunctivitis (ophthalmia neonatorum) has been reduced significantly by prophylactic measures at birth (see Clinical Reasoning Case Study: Neonate with Chlamydia Infection and Chapter 23). The major maternal infections, their possible effects, and specific nursing considerations are outlined in Table 25.5.

CARE MANAGEMENT

One of the major goals in the care of infants suspected of having an infectious disease is identification of the causative organism. Pregnant health care personnel are cautioned to avoid contact with infants with suspected CMV and rubella infections. HSV is easily transmitted from one infant to another; therefore the risk for cross-contamination is reduced or eliminated by wearing gloves for patient contact. The *Red Book: 2015 Report of the Committee on Infectious Diseases* (Kimberlin & AAP Committee on Infectious Diseases, 2015) provides guidelines for the type and duration of precautions for most bacterial and viral exposures. Careful hand hygiene is the most important nursing intervention in reducing the spread of any infection.

TABLE 25.5 Infections Acquired From the Mother Before, During, or After Birth*

Fetal or Newborn Effect	Transmission	Nursing Considerations†
Human Immunodeficiency Virus		
No significant difference between infected and uninfected infants at birth in some instances Embryopathy reported by some observers: • Depressed nasal bridge • Mild upward or downward obliquity of eyes • Long palpebral fissures with blue sclerae • Patulous lips • Ocular hypertelorism • Prominent upper vermilion border See also Chapter 43	Transplacental; during vaginal birth; potentially in breast milk	Administer combination antiretroviral prophylaxis to human immunodeficiency (HIV)–positive mother; prophylaxis to prevent perinatal transmission may begin in first trimester. Choice of regimens is determined by examining a number of factors, including mother's current treatment. Detailed recommendations can be obtained from HHS Panel on Treatment of HIV-Infected Pregnant Women and Prevention of Perinatal Transmission (2016) (https://aidsinfo.nih.gov/contentfiles/lvguidelines/PerinatalGL.pdf.). Four weeks of ZDV prophylaxis are recommended for full-term neonates whose mothers received ART regimen during pregnancy with sustained viral suppression. HIV-exposed neonates born to mothers who had no antepartum or intrapartum ARV drugs, intrapartum ARV only, or combination ARV drugs without sustained viral suppression should receive a 6-week course of ZDV starting as soon after birth as possible but preferably within 6–12 hours; nevirapine may also be given in 3 doses during the first week of life. ZDV dosing varies according to infant gestational age and route of administration (HHS Panel on Treatment of HIV-Infected Pregnant Women and Prevention of Perinatal Transmission, 2016). In developed countries, avoid breastfeeding in HIV-positive mother. For chemoprophylaxis against *Pneumocystis carinii* pneumonia in HIV-exposed infants, drug of choice is trimethoprim-sulfamethoxazole (Bactrim, Septra). Documented routine HIV education and routine testing with consent for all pregnant women in United States are recommended.
Chickenpox (Varicella-Zoster Virus [VZV])		
Intrauterine exposure—congenital varicella syndrome: limb dysplasia, microcephaly, cortical atrophy, chorioretinitis, cataracts, cutaneous scars, other anomalies, auditory nerve palsy, motor and cognitive delays Severe symptoms (rash, fever) and higher mortality in infant whose mother develops varicella 5 days before to 2 days after birth	First trimester (fetal varicella syndrome); perinatal period (infection)	Use varicella zoster immune globulin or IVIg to treat infants born to mothers with onset of disease within 5 days before or 2 days after birth. Healthy term infants exposed postnatally to varicella (especially if mother's rash does not appear until after 48 hours after birth) should not receive varicella zoster immune globulin (AAP Committee on Infectious Diseases, 2015). Institute isolation precautions in newborn born to mother with varicella up to 21–28 days (latter time if newborn received varicella zoster immune globulin or IVIg after birth (if hospitalized).† Prevention—Immunize all children with varicella vaccine.

Continued

TABLE 25.5 Infections Acquired From the Mother Before, During, or After Birth*—cont'd

Fetal or Newborn Effect	Transmission	Nursing Considerations[†]
Chlamydia Infection (Chlamydia trachomatis)		
Conjunctivitis, pneumonia	Last trimester or perinatal period	Standard ophthalmic prophylaxis for gonococcal ophthalmia neonatorum (topical antibiotics, silver nitrate, or povidone-iodine) is *not effective* in treatment or prevention of chlamydial ophthalmia. Treat with oral erythromycin or azithromycin; a second course of erythromycin may be required, and follow-up of exposed infant is recommended (see Clinical Reasoning Case Study: Neonate with Chlamydia Infection).
Coxsackievirus (Group B Enterovirus [Nonpolio], Parechovirus)		
Poor feeding, vomiting, diarrhea, fever; cardiac enlargement, arrhythmias, congestive heart failure; lethargy, seizures, meningoencephalitis, pneumonitis Mimics bacterial sepsis	Peripartum	Treatment is supportive. Provide IVIg in neonatal infections.
Cytomegalovirus (CMV)		
Variable manifestation from asymptomatic to severe Microcephaly, cerebral calcifications, chorioretinitis Jaundice, hepatosplenomegaly Petechial or purpuric rash (Fig. 25.4) Neurologic sequelae—seizure disorders, sensorineural hearing loss, cognitive impairment	Throughout pregnancy	Infection acquired at birth, shortly thereafter, or via human milk is not associated with clinical illness in term infants. Exposed preterm infants may have systemic infection, including interstitial pneumonia. Affected individuals excrete virus. Virus is detected in urine or tissue by electron microscopy. Pregnant women should avoid close contact with known cases. To treat infection, administer antivirals such as IV ganciclovir or oral valganciclovir for 6 weeks to newborn (Kimberlin & AAP Committee on Infectious Diseases, 2015).
Parvovirus B19 (Erythema Infectiosum)		
Fetal hydrops and death from anemia and heart failure with early exposure Anemia with later exposure No teratogenic effects established Ordinarily low risk for adverse effects for fetus	Transplacental	First-trimester infection has most serious effects. Aggressive cardiovascular and respiratory support is required in newborns with hydrops. Pregnant health care workers should not care for patients who might be highly contagious (e.g., child with sickle cell anemia, aplastic crisis). Routine exclusion of pregnant women from workplace where disease is occurring is not recommended.
Gonococcal Disease (Neisseria gonorrhoeae)		
Ophthalmitis Neonatal gonococcal arthritis, septicemia, meningitis	Last trimester or perinatal period	Preventive—Apply prophylactic medication to eyes at time of birth. Infant with confirmed ophthalmia, scalp abscess, or disseminated infection should be hospitalized, and cultures obtained to determine antimicrobial treatment. Consider testing infant for *Chlamydia*, HIV, and syphilis. Irrigate infant's eyes with saline until discharge is eliminated. Obtain smears for culture. To treat ophthalmia and nondisseminated infection, administer IV or IM ceftriaxone once. Disseminated disease requires cefotaxime treatment for 1 week.
Hepatitis B Virus (HBV)		
May be asymptomatic at birth; more than 90% of infants infected perinatally develop chronic Hepatitis B infection Clinical hepatitis, jaundice, changes in liver function; possible fulminant hepatitis	Transplacental; contaminated maternal fluids or secretions during birth	Administer HBIG to all infants of HBsAG-positive mothers within 12 hours of birth; in addition, administer HepB vaccine at separate site. Prevention—Immunize all infants with HepB vaccine. Infants born to HBsAG-positive mothers and weighing <2000 g (4 lbs 7 oz) should receive three-dose vaccine series *in addition* to birth dose (see "Immunizations" section in Chapter 31).

TABLE 25.5   Infections Acquired From the Mother Before, During, or After Birth*—cont'd

Fetal or Newborn Effect	Transmission	Nursing Considerations†
Listeriosis (Listeria monocytogenes)		
Maternal infection associated with spontaneous abortion, preterm birth, and fetal death Preterm birth, sepsis, and pneumonia seen in early onset disease; late onset disease usually manifests as meningitis	Transplacental by ascending infection or exposure at birth	Hand washing is essential to prevent nosocomial spread. Treat infected newborn with antibiotics—ampicillin and an aminoglycoside such as gentamicin (14- to 21-day treatment is recommended for meningitis).
Rubella, Congenital (Rubella Virus)		
Congenital rubella syndrome Eyes—retinopathy, cataracts (unilateral or bilateral), microphthalmia, retinitis, glaucoma CNS signs—microcephaly, seizures, severe cognitive impairment Congenital heart defects—patent ductus arteriosus Auditory defects—sensorineural hearing loss Dermal erythropoiesis—blueberry muffin lesions IUGR—hyperbilirubinemia, meningitis, thrombocytopenia, hepatomegaly	First trimester; early second trimester	Pregnant women should avoid contact with all affected persons, including infants with rubella syndrome. Emphasize vaccination of all unimmunized prepubertal children, susceptible adolescents, and women of childbearing age (nonpregnant). Caution women against becoming pregnant for at least 28 days after vaccination.
Syphilis, Congenital (Treponema pallidum)		
Stillbirth, prematurity, hydrops fetalis May be asymptomatic at birth and in first few weeks of life or may have multisystem manifestations: hepatosplenomegaly, lymphadenopathy, hemolytic anemia, pneumonia, and thrombocytopenia Copper-colored maculopapular cutaneous lesions (Fig. 25.5) (usually after first few weeks of life), mucous membrane patches, hair loss, nail exfoliation, snuffles (syphilitic rhinitis), profound anemia, poor feeding, pseudoparalysis of one or more limbs, dysmorphic teeth (older child)	Transplacental; can be anytime during pregnancy or at birth	This is most severe form of syphilis. Treatment consists of IV aqueous penicillin or IM procaine penicillin. Diagnostic evaluation depends on maternal serology testing, maternal therapy and response, maternal and infant serologic titers, results of nontreponemal infant tests, and infant physical examination (including ophthalmologic examinations and long-bone radiographs) and laboratory examination results (e.g., LFTs, CBC, platelets, CSF protein and cell count). Monitor closely for development of complications of disease during first year of life.
Toxoplasmosis, Congenital (Toxoplasma gondii)		
May be asymptomatic at birth (70%–90% of cases) or have maculopapular rash, lymphadenopathy, hepatosplenomegaly, jaundice, thrombocytopenia In some cases, severely infected fetus may die in utero or shortly after birth Later developments— hydrocephaly, cerebral calcifications, chorioretinitis (classic triad), microcephaly, seizures, cognitive impairment, deafness, encephalitis, myocarditis, hepatosplenomegaly, anemia, jaundice, diarrhea, vomiting, purpura	Throughout pregnancy Predominant host for organism is cats May be transmitted through cat feces or poorly cooked or raw infected meats	Caution pregnant women to avoid contact with cat feces (e.g., emptying cat litter boxes) and to avoid eating raw or undercooked meat (e.g., rare beef). Administer sulfadiazine (with folinic acid) and pyrimethamine (Daraprim). Spiramycin may be administered to infected pregnant female to reduce transmission to fetus but has no effect if fetal infection has occurred.
Herpes Simplex Virus (HSV)		
Neonatal herpes manifests in one of three ways: (1) with SEM involvement; (2) as localized CNS disease; or (3) as disseminated disease involving multiple organs. In skin and eye disease, rash appears as vesicles or pustules on erythematous base. Clusters of lesions are common. Lesions ulcerate and crust over rapidly (Fig. 25.6) Ophthalmologic clinical findings include chorioretinitis and microphthalmia; neurologic involvement such as microcephaly and encephalomalacia may also develop. Disseminated infections may involve virtually every organ system; but liver, adrenal glands, and lungs are most commonly affected. In HSV meningitis, infants develop multiple lesions of cortical hemorrhagic necrosis. It can occur alone or with SEM lesions. Presenting symptoms, which may occur in second to fourth weeks of life, include lethargy, poor feeding, irritability, and local or generalized seizures. Neonatal HSV has high mortality rate.	Most often transmitted at time of birth; can also be from ascending infection through ruptured membranes	Absence of skin lesions in neonate exposed to maternal herpes virus does not indicate absence of disease. Contact Precautions (in addition to Standard Precautions) should be instituted. It is recommended that swabs of mouth, nasopharynx, conjunctivae, rectum, and any skin vesicles be obtained from exposed neonate; in addition, urine, stool, blood, and CSF specimens should be obtained for culture. Therapy with IV acyclovir is initiated if culture results are positive or if there is strong suspicion of herpesvirus infection; ophthalmic treatment (e.g., 1% trifluridine or 3% vidarabine) is required for ocular involvement in addition to acyclovir. Therapy with oral acyclovir for 6 months is recommended for neonates with HSV CNS disease (Kimberlin & AAP Committee on Infectious Diseases, 2015).

Continued

TABLE 25.5 Infections Acquired From the Mother Before, During, or After Birth*—cont'd

Fetal or Newborn Effect	Transmission	Nursing Considerations[†]
Group B *Streptococcus*		
Early-onset infection (birth to 6 days of age)—pneumonia, respiratory distress, shock, apnea, and meningitis Late-onset infection—(7 days to 3 months of age)—bacteremia or meningitis; may occur later in LBW infants	Acquired perinatally; intrapartum antibiotics decrease early onset but not late onset disease Risk factors include preterm birth, maternal GBS (untreated), previous birth of GBS-infected newborn, maternal chorioamnionitis	Administer ampicillin plus an aminoglycoside such as gentamicin in infant with presumptive GBS infection; in infant with positive GBS, administer penicillin G. Observe Standard Precautions, including strict hand hygiene for handling all infants.

CNS, Central nervous system; *CBC,* complete blood count; *CSF,* cerebrospinal fluid; *GBS,* group B streptococcus; *HBIg,* hepatitis B immunoglobulin; *HBsAG,* hepatitis B surface antigen; *IUGR,* intrauterine growth restriction; *IM,* intramuscular; *IV,* intravenous; *IVIg,* intravenous immunoglobulin; *LBW,* low–birth weight; *LFT,* liver function test; *SEM,* skin, eye, and mouth; *ZDV,* zidovudine.

*This table is not an exhaustive representation of all perinatally transmitted infections. For further information regarding specific diseases or treatment, refer to Kimberlin, D. W., & American Academy of Pediatrics Committee on Infectious Diseases (2015). *Red book: 2015 report of the Committee on Infectious Diseases* (30th ed.). Elk Grove Village, IL: Author; HHS Panel on Treatment of HIV-Infected Women and Prevention of Perinatal Transmission. (2016). *Recommendations for the use of antiretroviral drugs in pregnant HIV-1-infected women and interventions to reduce perinatal HIV transmission in the United States.* Retrieved from http://aidsinfo.nih.gov/contentfiles/lvguidelines/PerinatalGL.pdf.

[†]Isolation precautions depend on institutional policy.

CLINICAL REASONING CASE STUDY
Neonate With Chlamydia Infection

An 8-day-old male infant is brought to the pediatric urgent care center on a Sunday morning by Maggie, an 18 year old single mother, who reports the baby has had eye drainage for 2 days. Maggie is breastfeeding and states that she was diagnosed and partially treated for a couple of sexually transmitted infections late in pregnancy; she does not remember the name but says one started with a *C*. The medications made her nauseous, so she quit taking them after 2 days. The practitioner examines the infant, who has a purulent yellowish discharge from both eyes but otherwise appears healthy; she suspects chlamydial conjunctivitis and orders cultures of the eye drainage. The retrieved medical record from the infant's birth indicates that eye prophylaxis with erythromycin ophthalmic ointment was administered.

1. Evidence—Is there sufficient evidence to draw conclusions about the cause of the infant's eye drainage?
2. Assumptions—What assumptions can be made about the following factors:
   a. Treatment for neonatal chlamydia infection.
   b. Neonatal sequelae of inadequate chlamydia treatment in the newborn.
   c. The mother's health status and possible treatment (she is not allergic to penicillin).
3. What implications and priorities for nursing care can be drawn at this time?
4. Does the evidence objectively support your conclusion?
5. Interprofessional care—Describe the roles/responsibilities of the members of the interprofessional health care team who would be involved in care management of Maggie and her baby.

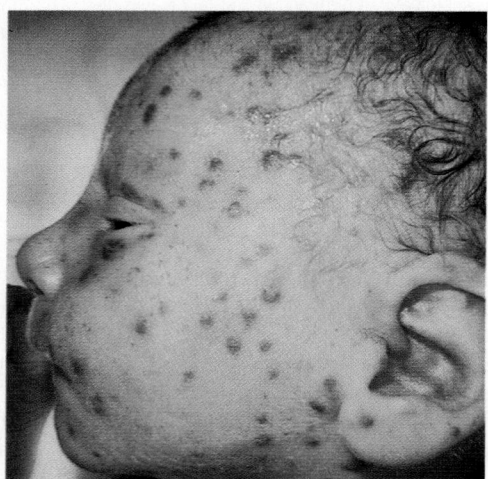

FIG 25.4 Neonatal cytomegalovirus infection. Typical rash seen in a severely affected infant. (Courtesy of David A. Clarke, Philadelphia, PA.*)*

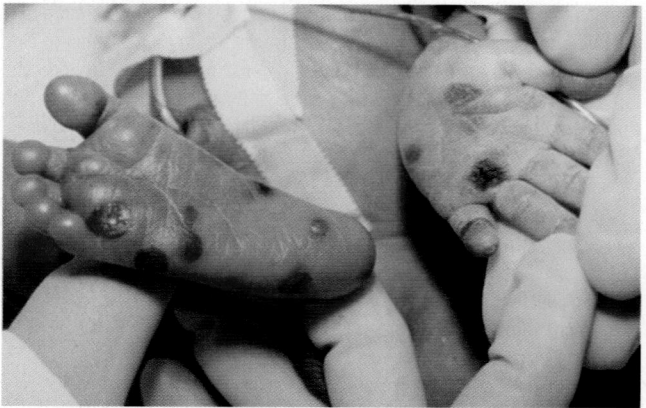

FIG 25.5 Neonatal syphilis lesions on hands and feet. (Courtesy of Mahesh Kotwal, MD, Phoenix, AZ.)

Specimens need to be obtained for laboratory examinations, and the infant and parents need to be prepared for diagnostic procedures. When possible, long-term disabilities are prevented by early evaluation and implementation of therapy. Nurses teach families about any special handling techniques needed for the care of their infant and signs of complications or possible sequelae. If sequelae are inevitable, the family needs assistance in determining how they can best cope with the problems such as assistance with home care, referral to appropriate agencies, or placement in an institution for care. The major goal of nursing care is to prevent these disorders through provision of adequate prenatal care

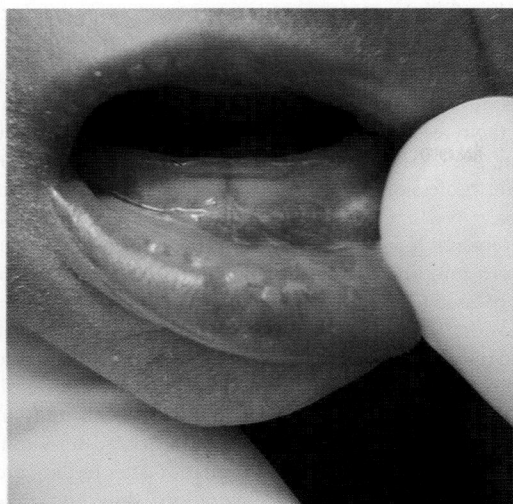

FIG 25.6 Herpes simplex virus oral lesions. (Courtesy of David A. Clarke, Philadelphia, PA.)

BOX 25.2   **Signs of Neonatal Abstinence Syndrome**

Neurologic
- Irritability
- Seizures
- Hyperactivity
- High-pitched cry
- Tremors
- Exaggerated Moro reflex
- Hypertonicity of muscles

Gastrointestinal
- Poor feeding
- Diarrhea
- Dehydration
- Vomiting
- Frantic, uncoordinated sucking
- Gastric residuals

Autonomic
- Diaphoresis
- Fever
- Mottled skin

Respiratory
- Tachypnea (>60 breaths/min)
- Nasal flaring
- Nasal stuffiness

Miscellaneous
- Disrupted sleep patterns
- Diaphoresis
- Excoriations (knees, face)
- Temperature instability

Data from Kocherlakota, P. (2014). Neonatal abstinence syndrome. *Pediatrics, 134*(2), e547–e561.

for the expectant mother and precautions regarding exposure to teratogenic infections.

DRUG-EXPOSED INFANTS*

Maternal habits hazardous to the fetus and neonate include substance use and addiction, smoking or use of electronic cigarettes (vaping), and alcohol abuse. Occasional withdrawal reactions have been reported in neonates of mothers who use to excess such drugs as barbiturates, alcohol, amphetamines, or antidepressants. Serious reactions are seen in neonates whose mothers abuse psychoactive drugs or are treated with methadone or buprenorphine.

Opioids, which have a low molecular weight, readily cross the placental membrane and enter the fetal system. Illicit substances can also be transmitted to the newborn through breast milk. When the mother is a habitual user of opioid drugs, especially OxyContin, heroin, or methadone, the fetus can also become chemically dependent on the drug, which places such infants at risk during the perinatal and early neonatal periods. Neonatal abstinence syndrome (NAS) is the term used to describe the set of behaviors exhibited by infants exposed to opioids in utero (Weiner & Finnegan, 2016).

The adverse effects of exposure of a fetus to drugs are varied. They include transient changes such as alterations in fetal breathing movements and irreversible effects such as fetal death, intrauterine growth restriction (IUGR), structural malformations, behavioral problems, or cognitive impairment. Determining the specific effects of individual drugs on an individual fetus is complicated by polydrug use, which is common; errors or omissions in reporting drug use; and variations in the strength, purity, and types of additives found in street drugs. Maternal conditions such as poverty, malnutrition, and comorbid conditions such as STIs further compound the difficulty in identifying intrauterine drug exposure and the sequelae. Most infants who are exposed to drugs in utero demonstrate no immediate untoward effects and appear normal at birth. Infants exposed only to heroin may begin to exhibit signs of drug withdrawal within 12 to 24 hours. If mothers have been taking

methadone, the signs appear somewhat later (i.e., anywhere from 1 or 2 days to 2 to 3 weeks or more after birth). The clinical manifestations can fall into any one or all of the following categories: CNS, GI, respiratory, and autonomic nervous system signs (Jones & Fielder, 2015; Weiner & Finnegan, 2016). The manifestations become most pronounced between 48 and 72 hours of age and can last from 6 days to 8 weeks, depending on the severity of the withdrawal (Box 25.2). Although these infants suck avidly on fists and display an exaggerated rooting reflex, they are poor feeders with uncoordinated and ineffective sucking and swallowing reflexes.

Approximately 55% to 94% of infants born to mothers using opioids show signs of withdrawal (AAP Committee on Drugs, 2016). Because of irregular and varying degrees of drug use, quality of drug, and mixed-drug usage by the mother, some infants display mild or variable manifestations. Most manifestations are the vague, nonspecific signs characteristic of all infants in general; therefore it is important to differentiate between drug withdrawal and other disorders before specific therapy is instituted. Other conditions (e.g., hypocalcemia, hypoglycemia, sepsis) often coexist with the drug withdrawal. Additional signs seen in drug-exposed newborns include loose stools; tachycardia; fever; projectile vomiting; crying; nasal stuffiness; and generalized perspiration, which is unusual in newborns.

Newborn urine, hair, or meconium sampling may be required to identify drug exposure and implement appropriate early interventional therapies aimed at minimizing the consequences of intrauterine drug exposure. Meconium sampling for fetal drug exposure is reported to provide more screening accuracy than urine screening because drug metabolites accumulate in meconium. Urine toxicology screening reflects only recent substance intake by the mother (Kocherlakota, 2014). Meconium and hair testing for drug metabolites has the advantages of being noninvasive, more accurate, and easy to collect.

The treatment of drug-exposed infants initially consists of early identification through maternal history, presenting symptoms of NAS, or toxicology screening when substance abuse is strongly suspected. Early identification and intervention are essential to prevent further adverse effects. Early discharge from the birth institution should be postponed until the maternal situation is assessed further and a treatment plan for the mother and infant is established. Drug therapies to decrease withdrawal effects include parenteral or oral administration of

---

*Unless otherwise noted, the information presented throughout this section refers to drug-exposed neonates in general, regardless of the drug to which they have been exposed.

phenobarbital, buprenorphine, clonidine, methadone, and morphine. A combination of these drugs may be necessary to treat infants exposed to multiple drugs in utero, and careful attention should be given to possible adverse effects of the treatment drugs (Kraft & van den Anker, 2012).

The prognosis for drug-exposed infants depends on the type and amount of drug(s) taken by the mother and the stage(s) of fetal development in which the drug was taken. The overall mortality rate of infants born to narcotic-addicted mothers is increased; but with early recognition, proper treatment, and long-term follow-up the morbidity and mortality associated with drug exposure are decreased.

Often drug-exposed infants exhibit poor brain and body growth at birth. However, sometimes infants do not exhibit any signs that indicate exposure to harmful agents; therefore their condition can be overlooked until symptoms appear later in life. Drug-exposed infants may have chronic feeding problems; irritability; abnormal neurologic responses; abnormal parent-infant interactions; developmental and cognitive delays; learning disabilities in childhood; and behavioral problems, including ADHD.

CARE MANAGEMENT

One of the key factors in the treatment of drug-exposed neonates is early identification of substance use in the pregnant woman so that treatment can be initiated and side effects minimized (see Evidence-Based Practice box: Nonpharmacologic Interventions for Neonatal Abstinence Syndrome [NAS]). This is especially problematic from a social and legal standpoint because the pregnant woman is often aware of the consequences of admitting to substance abuse and therefore may be less likely to readily admit to the problem for fear of social and legal repercussions. If the mother has had good prenatal care, the practitioner is likely aware of the problem and may have instituted therapy before birth. However, a number of mothers deliver their infants without the benefit of adequate prenatal care, and the condition is unknown to health care personnel at the time of birth.

The degree of withdrawal is closely related to the type and amount of drug the mother has habitually taken, the length of time she has been taking the drug, and her drug level at the time of birth. The most severe symptoms are observed in the infants of mothers who have taken large amounts of drugs over a long period of time. In addition, the nearer to the time of birth that the mother takes the drug, the longer it takes the child to develop withdrawal, and the more severe the manifestations. The infant may not exhibit withdrawal symptoms until 7 to 10 days after birth, by which time most newborns have been discharged from the birthing facility, and caregivers are less likely to recognize signs of irritability and poor feeding as withdrawal, thus predisposing the newborn to abuse or neglect and growth failure (failure to thrive). The infant may be at further risk for subsequent abuse or neglect because of home conditions that preclude adequate newborn care and follow-up.

When NAS is identified, nursing care is directed toward treating the presenting signs, decreasing stimuli that can precipitate hyperactivity and irritability (e.g., dimming the lights, decreasing noise levels), providing adequate nutrition and hydration, and promoting mother-infant attachment. Appropriate individualized developmental care is implemented to facilitate self-consoling and self-regulating behaviors. Irritable and hyperactive infants are likely to respond to physical comforting, movement, and close contact. Wrapping infants snugly and rocking and holding them tightly limit their ability to self-stimulate. Arranging nursing activities to reduce the amount of disturbance helps decrease exogenous stimulation.

Breastfeeding is encouraged in mothers who are not using illicit substances, do not have HIV infection, and are compliant with a treatment program; breastfeeding promotes mother-infant bonding, and small quantities of methadone or buprenorphine passed through breast milk is not harmful (Sriraman, Melvin, & Meltzer-Brody, 2015).

The Neonatal Abstinence Scoring System or Finnegan tool (Fig. 25.7) was developed to monitor infants in an objective manner and evaluate their response to clinical and pharmacologic interventions (Finnegan, 1985). This system is also designed to help nurses and other health care professionals evaluate the severity of infants' withdrawal symptoms.

The Neonatal Intensive Care Unit Network Neurobehavioral Scale (NNNS) is a comprehensive neurologic and behavioral assessment tool that may be used to identify newborns at risk as a result of intrauterine drug exposure. The tool measures stress or abstinence, state, neurologic status, and muscle tone in the context of the newborn's medical condition at the time of examination. The NNNS may be used for medically stable newborns who are at least 30 weeks of gestation and up to 48 weeks of corrected or conceptional age (Lester, Tronick, & Brazelton, 2004).

Loose stools, poor intake, and regurgitation after feeding predispose these infants to malnutrition, dehydration, skin breakdown, and electrolyte imbalance. In addition, they burn up energy with continual activity and increased oxygen consumption at the cellular level. Frequent weighing, careful monitoring of intake and output and electrolytes, and additional caloric supplementation may be necessary. Hyperactive infants must be protected from skin abrasions on the knees, toes, and cheeks that are caused by rubbing on bed linens while in a prone position during waking periods.. Monitoring and recording the activity level and its relationship to other activities such as feeding and preventing complications are important nursing responsibilities (Weiner & Finnegan, 2016).

A valuable aid to anticipating problems in the newborn is recognizing substance abuse in the mother. In the absence of prenatal care, infants and mothers are exposed to the additional hazards of obstetric and medical complications. Moreover, the nature of substance use and addiction makes the user susceptible to disorders such as infection (HBV, HIV), and the hazards of inadequate nutrition and preterm birth. Methadone treatment does not prevent withdrawal reaction in neonates, but the clinical course may be modified. In addition, the intensive psychologic support of mothers is a factor in the treatment and reduction of perinatal mortality. Experience has indicated that these mothers may be anxious and depressed, lack confidence, have a poor self-image, and have difficulty with interpersonal relationships. They may have a psychologic need for the pregnancy and an infant.

Initial symptoms or the recurrence of withdrawal symptoms can develop after discharge from the hospital and last up to 6 months; therefore it is important to establish rapport and maintain contact with the family so they will return for treatment if this occurs. The demands of the drug-exposed infant on the caregiver are enormous and unrewarding in terms of positive feedback. The infants are difficult to comfort, and they cry for long periods, which can be especially trying for the caregiver after the infant's discharge from the hospital. Long-term follow-up to evaluate the status of the infant and family is very important (Weiner & Finnegan, 2016). Sudden infant death syndrome (SIDS) (see Chapter 31) and HIV infection (see Chapter 43) are observed more commonly in infants born to users of methadone and heroin.

ALCOHOL EXPOSURE

Alcohol ingestion during pregnancy is associated with both short- and long-term effects on the fetus and newborn. The quantity of alcohol required to produce fetal effects is unclear, but it is known that infants born to heavy drinkers have twice the risk for congenital abnormalities than those born to moderate drinkers (Carlo & Ambalavanan, 2016a). Alcohol withdrawal can occur in neonates, particularly when maternal

EVIDENCE-BASED PRACTICE

Nonpharmacologic Interventions for Neonatal Abstinence Syndrome (NAS)

Ask the Question

PICOT Question: For newborns withdrawing from maternal substances, what nonpharmacologic and relational interventions can improve outcomes?

Search for the Evidence

Search Strategies: English-language research-based publications since 2013 on neonatal abstinence, NAS, Finnegan, substance abuse in pregnancy were included

Databases Used: Cochrane Collaborative Database, National Guideline Clearinghouse (AHRQ), CINAHL, PubMed, and the professional websites for ACOG and AWHONN.

Critical Appraisal of the Evidence

Newborns exposed to maternal substances in utero may develop neonatal abstinence syndrome (NAS) as they go through withdrawal, sometimes requiring medication, prolonged length of stay, and NICU admission. Long accepted interventions have included swaddling, low light, quiet environment, minimal handling, and pacifier use, but not all are evidence-based.

- An integrative review of fourteen articles on nonpharmacologic interventions reveals that breastfeeding, rooming-in, prone position, acupressure, and use of a nonoscillating newborn bed resulted in improved outcomes that included shorter length of stay, decrease in NAS scores, better sleep, and less pharmacologic treatment (Edwards & Brown, 2016).
- A systematic review of six studies found that providing multidisciplinary, integrated, and comprehensive perinatal services for substance-addicted women and caring relationships with their providers resulted in better neonatal outcomes of greater gestational age at birth, higher birth weight, shorter length of stay, lower NAS score, and discharge to home with mother (Kramlich & Kronk, 2015).
- A multidisciplinary quality improvement team implemented a protocol for standardized care that included training the nurses for interrater reliability when using the NAS scoring tool, scoring only after on-demand breastfeeding and skin-to-skin contact, rooming-in, standardizing the physician interpretation of NAS scores and medical decision-making, increasing prenatal teaching and family involvement in monitoring symptoms, and providing comfort care. Improved outcomes included shorter stays, less NICU admissions, less medication, and lower costs (Holmes, Atwood, Whalen, et al., 2016).

Apply the Evidence: Nursing Implications

- The nurse can utilize standardized NAS scoring by watching training videos and practicing scoring with coworkers and managers. Assessing the baby after breastfeeding and skin-to-skin contact ensures accurate equivalency.
- Family-centered care begins prenatally, and includes education about the newborn's symptoms, coping strategies, and nonpharmacologic interventions. Institutional interdisciplinary commitment to rooming-in and breastfeeding is even more important for NAS babies.

- Prone position, if used, is contrary to what is taught for SIDS prevention, and should be explained to the family as a temporary measure, to be used only until symptoms improve. Pulse and oxygen levels should be monitored.
- Relationships matter, both between the family and caregivers and within the health team. A qualitative study of 16 NICU RNs identified six themes about caring for NAS newborns: "Learning the baby" via trial-and-error; core team support; role satisfaction; grief for the baby's present and future; making a difference; and caring for the mother (Nelson, 2016). Judgment and stigma were identified as toxic, and barriers to family-centered care.
- The nurse needs to know the state laws regarding maternal substance abuse. The Association of Women's Health, Obstetric, and Neonatal Nurses has taken a position opposed to criminalization of substance abuse during pregnancy, because the threat of incarceration is ineffective and counterproductive to getting women the interventions they need (AWHONN, 2015).

Quality and Safety Competencies: Evidence-Based Practice*
Knowledge

Describe how the strength and relevance of available evidence influences the choice of interventions in provision of patient-centered care.

Standardizing the use of NAS scoring improves team coordination and patient care.

Skills

Participate in structuring the work environment to facilitate integration of new evidence into standards of practice.

A report of a protocol in another institution improving outcomes invites the adaptation of it to your health care team.

Attitudes

Value the need for continuous improvement in clinical practice based on new knowledge.

Identify the importance of nonjudgmental and open communication between patient and family and within the health team to directly improve patient outcomes.

References

Association of Women's Health, Obstetric, and Neonatal Nurses. (2015). Criminalization of pregnant women with substance use disorders. *Journal of Obstetric, Gynecologic, and Neonatal Nursing, 44*(1), 155–157.

Edwards, L. & Brown, L. F. (2016). Nonpharmacologic management of neonatal abstinence syndrome: An integrative review. *Neonatal Network, 35*(5), 305–313.

Holmes, A. V., Atwood, E. C., Whalen, B., et al. (2016). Rooming-in to treat neonatal abstinence syndrome: Improved family-centered care at lower cost. *Pediatrics, 137*(6).

Kramlich, D. & Kronk, R. (2015). Relational care for perinatal substance use: A systematic review. *American Journal of Maternal Child Nursing, 40*(5), 320–326.

Nelson, M. M. (2016). NICU culture of care for infants with neonatal abstinence syndrome: A focused ethnography. *Neonatal Network, 35*(5), 287–296.

Pat Mahaffee Gingrich

*Adapted from QSEN at www.qsen.org/.

ingestion occurs near the time of birth. Signs and symptoms include jitteriness, increased tone and reflex responses, and irritability. Seizures are common. Fetal effects of alcohol exposure vary from subtle learning disabilities to obvious facial features and growth abnormalities. The term *fetal alcohol spectrum disorder* (FASD) is an umbrella term that describes the range of clinical effects; there are three types of FASDs, based on the symptoms. *Fetal alcohol syndrome* (FAS) is the most severe type; affected individuals have abnormal facial features (e.g., small eyes or short palpebral fissures, a thin upper lip, a flat midface, and an

indistinct philtrum) (Fig. 25.8), growth restriction, and neurodevelopmental deficits, with or without a confirmed history of maternal alcohol consumption (Senturias & Asamoah, 2014). Neurologic problems in persons with FAS can include some degree of cognitive deficit, ADHD, diminished fine-motor skills, and poor speech. They have been shown to lack inhibition, have no stranger anxiety, and lack appropriate judgment skills. Persons with *alcohol-related neurodevelopmental disorder* (ARND) are likely to have cognitive and learning disabilities and behavioral problems such as poor impulse control. Alcohol-related birth

NEONATAL ABSTINENCE SCORING SYSTEM

System	Signs and Symptoms	Score	AM					PM					Comments
Central Nervous System Disturbances	Excessive high-pitched (or other) cry	2											Daily weight:
	Continuous high-pitched (or other) cry	3											
	Sleeps <1 hour after feeding	3											
	Sleeps <2 hours after feeding	2											
	Sleeps <3 hours after feeding	1											
	Hyperactive Moro reflex	2											
	Markedly hyperactive Moro reflex	3											
	Mild tremors disturbed	1											
	Moderate-severe tremors disturbed	2											
	Mild tremors undisturbed	3											
	Moderate-severe tremors undisturbed	4											
	Increased muscle tone	2											
	Excoriation (specific area)	1											
	Myoclonic jerks	3											
	Generalized convulsions	5											
Metabolic/Vasomotor/Respiratory Disturbances	Sweating	1											
	Fever <101° (99–100.8° F/37.2–38.2° C)	1											
	Fever >101° (38.4° C and higher)	2											
	Frequent yawning (>3 or 4 times/interval)	1											
	Mottling	1											
	Nasal stuffiness	1											
	Sneezing (>3 or 4 times/interval)	1											
	Nasal flaring	2											
	Respiratory rate >60/min	1											
	Respiratory rate >60/min with retractions	2											
Gastrointestinal Disturbances	Excessive sucking	1											
	Poor feeding	2											
	Regurgitation	2											
	Projectile vomiting	3											
	Loose stools	2											
	Watery stools	3											
	Total Score												
	Initials of Scorer												

FIG 25.7 Neonatal Abstinence Scoring (NAS) system developed by L. Finnegan. (From Nelson, N. [1990]. *Current therapy in neonatal-perinatal medicine* (2nd ed.). St. Louis, MO: Mosby.)

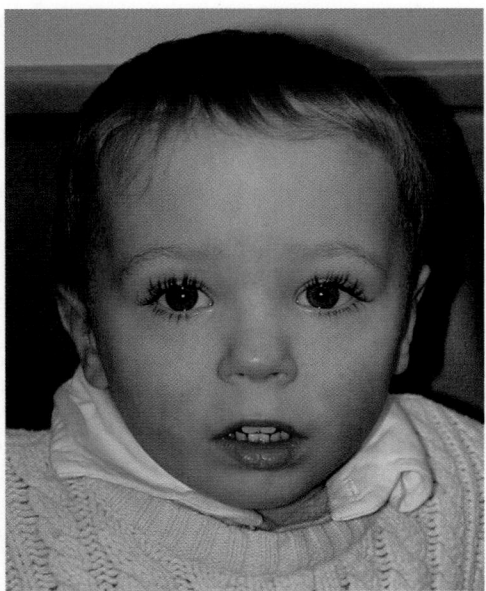

FIG 25.8 Child with fetal alcohol syndrome. (From Jorde, L.B., Carey, J.C., & Bamshad, M.J. [2016]. *Medical genetics* [5th ed.]. St. Louis, MO: Elsevier.)

defects (ARBD) refers to persons with cardiac, renal, musculoskeletal, or hearing problems, or any combination of these (CDC, 2016).

Infants who do not display the signs of FAS but are born to mothers who are also heavy alcohol drinkers have significantly more tremors, hypertonia, restlessness, excessive mouthing movements, crying, and inconsolability than infants of substance-abusive mothers who do not consume alcohol during pregnancy. An added concern regarding substance abuse is that many of the mothers often use several drugs such as tranquilizers, sedatives, amphetamines, phencyclidine, marijuana, and other psychotropic agents. These drugs can alter the mother's perception of the newborn's cues and physical and emotional needs.

For additional details regarding diagnosis and treatment of FASD see the Centers for Disease Control and Prevention FAS website: www.cdc.gov/ncbddd/fasd/index.html.

COCAINE EXPOSURE

Cocaine is a CNS stimulant and peripheral sympathomimetic. Legally it is classified as a narcotic, but it is not an opioid. The effects on fetuses are secondary to maternal effects, which include increased blood pressure (BP), decreased uterine blood flow, and increased vascular resistance. Consequently, the fetus experiences decreased blood flow and oxygenation because of placental and fetal vasoconstriction. Researchers have concluded that variables such as the mother's lack of prenatal care; poor nutrition; and use of tobacco, alcohol, and other drugs during pregnancy compound the effects of cocaine exposure in the infant (Cain, Bornick, & Whiteman, 2013).

Infants can appear normal or show neurologic problems at birth that continue during the neonatal period. In much of the research literature these findings were transient, and evidence demonstrating permanent sequelae has varied. Either of two types of behavior may emerge as a result of the effects of cocaine on fetal development: neurobehavioral depression or excitability. The behaviors of a depressed infant include lethargy, hypotonia, and difficulty in arousing. The behaviors of an excitable neonate can include hypertonicity, irritability, an inability to be consoled, and an intolerance to changes in routine (Fallone, LaGasse, Lester, et al., 2014; Martin, Graham, McCarthy, et al., 2016).

Sequelae of prenatal cocaine exposure include preterm birth, a smaller head circumference, decreased birth length, and decreased weight. Head growth may be one of the best predictors of long-term deficits (Martin et al., 2016). Early studies of cocaine exposure identified an increased incidence of gastroschisis, genitourinary anomalies, and stroke; however, meta-analyses have not confirmed these complications (Holbrook & Rayburn, 2014; Mactier, 2013). Heavy cocaine exposure has reported to result in elevated or irregular heart rate after birth (Ramirez, Femenia, Simpson, et al., 2012).

Some studies found that long-term sequelae for newborns exposed to cocaine include lower language, motor, and cognitive scores and an increased risk for learning disabilities, although these effects are moderated by the child's environment (Fraser, Walker, & Green, 2016). In a study that controlled for other prenatal drug exposures, a dose-related effect of cocaine was found on expressive, receptive, and total language scores at 3, 5, and 12 years of age (Bandstra, Morrow, Accornero, et al., 2011). Studies using the Brazelton Neonatal Assessment Scale have shown inconsistent results with subtle abnormalities in neurobehavioral clusters varying in timing of severity and according to levels of exposure (Minnes, Lang, & Singer, 2011).

Nursing and Medical Interventions

Nursing care of cocaine-exposed infants is the same as that for other drug-exposed infants. Because they have increased flexor tone, these infants respond to swaddling (Sublett, 2013). Positioning, infant massage, and limited tactile stimulation have been shown to be effective interventions. Significant amounts of cocaine have been found in breast milk (D'Apolito, 2013), therefore mothers should be cautioned regarding this hazard to their infants.

Referral to early intervention programs, including child health care, parental drug treatment, individualized developmental care, and parenting education, is essential in promoting optimum outcomes for these children. Because they often live in impoverished environments, they are at high risk for cognitive delays, lack of child health care, and inadequate nutrition and benefit from early intervention programs.

METHAMPHETAMINE EXPOSURE

Methamphetamine use has increased significantly in certain regions of the United States. National estimates on the prevalence of methamphetamine use during pregnancy suggest that between 0.7% and 5.2% of mothers use the substance (Forray & Foster, 2015).

The fetal and neonatal effects of maternal use of methamphetamines in pregnancy are not well known, and findings are often confounded by polydrug use and the effects of the newborn or child's environment. A higher incidence of placental abruption, preterm birth, and IUGR is associated with methamphetamine use during pregnancy (Geary & Wells, 2013; Narkowicz, Plotka, Polkowska, et al., 2013). Infants exposed to methamphetamine can experience signs of withdrawal such as agitation, tremors, hypertonia, poor feeding, and state disorganization (Shah, Diaz, Arria, et al., 2012).

The long-term effects of methamphetamine exposure on children remain unclear; however, some studies have shown problems with mathematics and language skills. It is postulated that, similar to cocaine, methamphetamine exposure may affect areas of the brain responsible for higher-order functioning, with effects more likely to be manifest when the child reaches school age (Roos, Kwiatkowski, Fouche, et al., 2015).

MARIJUANA EXPOSURE

Marijuana is the most common illicit drug used by pregnant women in the United States (Conner, Carter, Tuuli, et al., 2015). Marijuana crosses the placenta; however, specific effects on the fetus have been difficult to determine. Data on effects of marijuana on the fetus are confounded by maternal use of tobacco and other substances and issues with maternal self-reporting of use and biologic sampling. Marijuana use is associated with increased risk for preterm birth, stillbirth, and IUGR. There is increasing evidence that marijuana can cause problems with neurologic development including hyperactivity, lower cognitive function, and attention problems (Conner et al., 2015; Metz & Stickrath, 2015). More subtle effects of major exposure such as an increase in attention problems have also been identified. Long-term follow-up studies on exposed infants are needed.

SELECTIVE SEROTONIN REUPTAKE INHIBITORS

Studies estimate that between 1% and 20% of pregnant women experience major depression (Sie, Wennink, van Driel, et al., 2012). For many of these women, selective serotonin reuptake inhibitors (SSRIs) provide an important therapeutic benefit; however, these drugs may result in side effects in their newborns. Signs of withdrawal are present in up to one-third of infants exposed to SSRIs in utero (Sie et al.). Findings include hypertonia, tremulousness, wakefulness, high-pitched crying, and feeding problems. An increased risk for persistent pulmonary hypertension has been reported in neonates exposed to SSRIs late in pregnancy (Kieler, Artama, Engeland, et al., 2012). Some SSRIs are transferred into breast milk. Breastfeeding infants whose mothers are taking SSRIs should be monitored for sleep disturbances, irritability, and poor feeding (Sriraman et al., 2015).

Nursing Interventions

The general nursing care of the newborn exposed to these drugs is directed toward identification of substance use in the mother and vigilance for signs of withdrawal in the neonate. Nurses may use the NAS tool to identify the severity of narcotic withdrawal for the implementation of specific drug treatment. Identifying specific signs and symptoms associated with drug withdrawal also assists in developing a plan of care to benefit the mother-infant pair. The nurse has an important role in helping the mother with caretaking abilities to promote self-esteem and meet the newborn's individual needs. Referral to special developmental care programs may be required to prevent serious cognitive and behavioral problems at the time of school entry.

▌HEMOLYTIC DISORDERS

Hyperbilirubinemia in the first 24 hours of life is most often the result of hemolytic disease of the newborn (HDN) (erythroblastosis fetalis), an abnormally rapid rate of red blood cell (RBC) destruction. Anemia caused by this destruction stimulates the production of RBCs, which in turn provides increasing numbers of cells for hemolysis. Major causes of increased erythrocyte destruction are isoimmunization (primarily Rh) and ABO incompatibility.

BLOOD INCOMPATIBILITY

The membranes of human blood cells contain a variety of antigens, also known as agglutinogens, substances capable of producing an immune response if recognized by the body as foreign. The reciprocal relationship between antigens on RBCs and antibodies in the plasma causes agglutination (clumping). In other words, antibodies in the plasma of one blood group (except the AB group, which contains no antibodies) produce agglutination when mixed with antigens of a different blood group. In the ABO blood group system, the antibodies occur naturally. In the Rh system, the person must be exposed to the Rh antigen before significant

antibody formation takes place and causes a sensitivity response known as isoimmunization.

Rh Incompatibility (Isoimmunization)

The Rh blood group consists of several antigens (with D being the most prevalent). For simplicity only, the terms *Rh positive* (presence of antigen) and *Rh negative* (absence of antigen) are used in this discussion. The presence or absence of the naturally occurring Rh factor determines the blood type.

Ordinarily no problems are anticipated when the Rh blood types are the same in both the mother and the fetus or when the mother is Rh positive and the infant is Rh negative. Difficulty can arise when the mother is Rh negative and the infant is Rh positive. Although the maternal and fetal circulations are separate, there is evidence of a bidirectional trafficking of fetal RBCs and cell-free DNA to the maternal circulation (Solomonia, Playforth, & Reynolds, 2012). However, more commonly fetal RBCs enter into the maternal circulation at the time of birth. The mother's natural defense mechanism responds to these alien cells by producing anti-Rh antibodies. Other factors that increase the risk for isoimmunization include spontaneous or therapeutic abortion, chorionic villus sampling, amniocentesis, cordocentesis, external cephalic version, manual removal of the placenta, abruptio placentae, and maternal abdominal trauma (Moise, 2017).

Under normal circumstances, this process of isoimmunization has no effect during the first pregnancy with an Rh-positive fetus because the initial sensitization to Rh antigens rarely occurs before the onset of labor. However, with the increased risk for fetal blood being transferred to the maternal circulation during placental separation, maternal antibody production is stimulated. During a subsequent pregnancy with an Rh-positive fetus, these previously formed maternal antibodies to Rh-positive blood cells can enter the fetal circulation, where they attack and destroy fetal erythrocytes (Fig. 25.9).

Because the condition begins in utero, the fetus attempts to compensate for the progressive hemolysis and anemia by accelerating the rate of erythropoiesis. As a result, immature RBCs (erythroblasts) appear in the fetal circulation; thus the term erythroblastosis fetalis.

There is wide variability in the development of maternal sensitization to Rh-positive antigens. Inhibitory antibodies in the maternal circulation influence the degree and severity of maternal-fetal response, and in some cases there is no hemolytic reaction in the newborn (Moise, 2017).

In the most severe form of erythroblastosis fetalis, hydrops fetalis, the progressive hemolysis causes fetal hypoxia; cardiac failure; generalized edema (anasarca); and fluid effusions into the pericardial, pleural, and peritoneal spaces (hydrops). The fetus may be delivered stillborn or in severe respiratory distress. Maternal RhIg administration, early intrauterine detection of fetal anemia by ultrasonography (serial Doppler assessment of the peak velocity in the fetal middle cerebral artery), and subsequent treatment by fetal blood transfusions or high-dose intravenous immunoglobulin (IVIg) have dramatically improved the outcome of affected fetuses (Houston, Govia, Abou-Setta, et al., 2015).

ABO Incompatibility

Hemolytic disease can also occur when the major blood group antigens of the fetus are different than those of the mother. The most common blood group incompatibility in the neonate is between a mother with O blood group and an infant with A or B blood group (see Table 25.6 for possible ABO incompatibilities). Naturally occurring anti-A or anti-B antibodies already present in the maternal circulation cross the placenta and attack the fetal RBCs, causing hemolysis. Usually the hemolytic reaction is less severe than in Rh incompatibility; however, rare cases of hydrops have been reported (Mundy & Bhatia, 2015). Unlike the Rh reaction, ABO incompatibility can occur in the first pregnancy. The

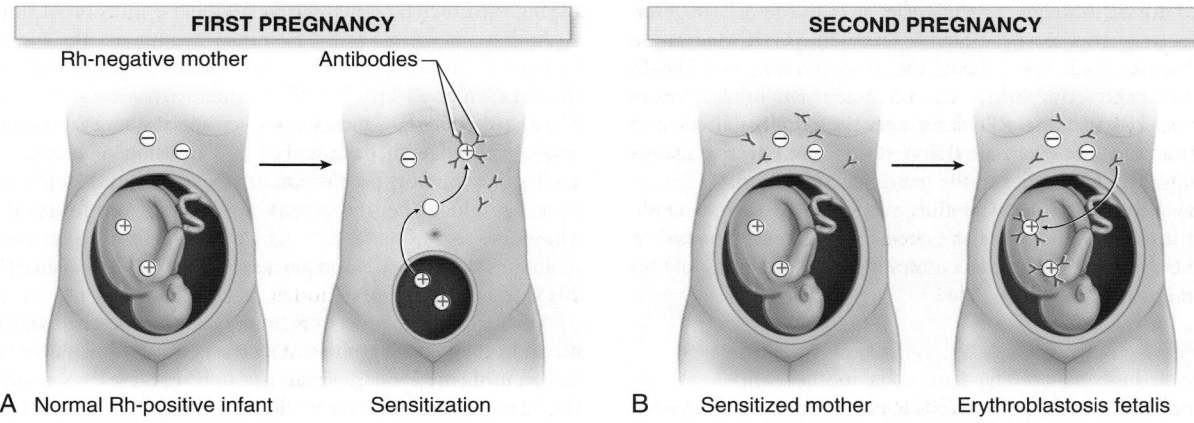

FIG 25.9 Development of maternal sensitization to Rh antigens. **A,** Fetal Rh-positive erythrocytes enter the maternal system. Maternal anti-Rh antibodies are formed. **B,** Anti-Rh antibodies cross the placenta and attack fetal erythrocytes. (From Silvestri, L.A. [2017]. *Saunders comprehensive review for the NCLEX-RN examination* (7th ed.). St. Louis, MO: Elsevier.)

TABLE 25.6 Potential Maternal-Fetal ABO Incompatibilities

Maternal Blood Group	Incompatible Fetal Blood Group
0	A or B
B	A or AB
A	B or AB

risk for significant hemolysis in subsequent pregnancies is higher when the first pregnancy is complicated by ABO incompatibility (Egbor, Knott, & Bhide, 2012).

Jaundice can appear shortly after birth (during the first 24 hours) in newborns affected by HDN, and serum levels of unconjugated bilirubin rise rapidly. Anemia results from the hemolysis of large numbers of erythrocytes, and hyperbilirubinemia and jaundice result from the inability of the liver to conjugate and excrete the excess bilirubin. Most newborns with HDN are not jaundiced at birth. However, hepatosplenomegaly and varying degrees of hydrops may be evident. If the infant is severely affected, signs of anemia (notably marked pallor) and hypovolemic shock are apparent. Hypoglycemia can occur as a result of pancreatic cell hyperplasia.

Early identification and diagnosis of Rh(D) sensitization are important in the management and prevention of fetal complications. A maternal antibody titer (indirect Coombs' test) should be drawn at the first prenatal visit. Genetic testing allows early identification of paternal zygosity at the Rh(D) gene locus, thus allowing earlier detection of the potential for isoimmunization (Egbor et al., 2012). Amniocentesis may be used to test the fetal blood type of a woman whose antibody screen result is positive; the use of polymerase chain reaction (PCR) may determine the fetal blood type and presence of maternal antibodies. The fetal hemoglobin and hematocrit may also be measured. Chorionic villus sampling has drawbacks that preclude its use, including possible spontaneous abortion of the fetus and fetomaternal hemorrhage, which would essentially make the situation worse. With either method, if the fetus is found to be Rh negative, no further treatment is required. The detection of cell-free fetal DNA in the maternal plasma of Rh(D)-negative women to detect an Rh(D)-positive fetus has been used successfully in Europe. Such testing usually negates the necessity of amniocentesis for fetal blood type (Moise & Argoti, 2012).

Ultrasonography is considered an important adjunct in the detection of isoimmunization; alterations in the placenta, umbilical cord, and amniotic fluid volume and the presence of fetal hydrops can be detected with high-resolution ultrasonography and allow early treatment before the development of erythroblastosis. Doppler ultrasonography of fetal middle cerebral artery peak velocity has been used to detect and measure fetal hemoglobin and subsequently fetal anemia (Moise & Argoti, 2012). Erythroblastosis fetalis caused by Rh incompatibility can also be monitored by evaluating rising anti-Rh antibody titers in the maternal circulation or testing the optical density of amniotic fluid (delta OD450 test) because bilirubin discolors the fluid.

The disease in the newborn is suspected on the basis of the timing and appearance of jaundice and can be confirmed postnatally by detecting antibodies attached to the circulating erythrocytes of affected infants (direct antiglobulin test [DAT]). The DAT can be performed on umbilical cord blood samples from infants born to Rh-negative mothers if there is a history of incompatibility or further investigation is warranted.

Postnatal therapy is usually phototherapy for mild cases of hemolysis and exchange transfusion for more severe forms. Although phototherapy may control bilirubin levels in mild cases, the hemolytic process may continue, causing severe anemia between 7 and 21 days of life. In some institutions, a metalloporphyrin is administered intramuscularly to decrease the formation of bilirubin in neonates with ABO incompatibility.

Prevention

The primary aim of therapeutic management of isoimmunization is prevention. The administration of Rh immune globulin (RhIg), a human gamma globulin concentrate of anti-D, to all unsensitized Rh-negative mothers after birth or abortion of an Rh-positive infant or fetus prevents the development of maternal sensitization to the Rh factor. The injected anti-Rh antibodies are thought to destroy (by subsequent phagocytosis and agglutination) fetal RBCs passing into the maternal circulation before they can be recognized by the mother's immune system. Because the immune response is blocked, anti-D antibodies and memory cells (which produce the primary and secondary immune responses, respectively) are not formed (Bagwell, 2014; Blackburn, 2013). The inhibition of memory cell formation is especially important because memory cells provide long-term immunity by initiating a rapid immune response after the antigen is reintroduced (McCance & Huether, 2014).

To be effective, RhIg (e.g., RhoGAM) must be administered to unsensitized mothers during first pregnancies and within 72 hours after the first birth or spontaneous or therapeutic abortion; it is also administered during subsequent pregnancies at 26 to 28 weeks of gestation and after pregnancy losses (Aitken & Tichy, 2015) (see Medication Guide: Rh Immune Globulin, RhoGAM, Gamulin Rh, HypRho-D, Rhophylac in Chapter 19). RhIg is also given after any other event in which there is a risk that fetal RBCs can enter the maternal circulation such as amniocentesis or external version. RhIg is not effective against existing Rh-positive antibodies in the maternal circulation.

IVIg may be used to decrease the severity of RBC destruction (hemolysis) in HDN and reduce the need for exchange transfusion. However, there is a lack of evidence to support the efficacy of this intervention (Louis et al., 2014).

Management

Intrauterine transfusion. The fetus of a mother who is already sensitized may be treated by intrauterine transfusion, which consists of infusing blood into the umbilical vein. The need for therapy is based on the antenatal diagnosis of fetal anemia by serial Doppler assessments of peak systolic velocity of the middle cerebral artery (Moise & Argoti, 2012). With advances in ultrasound technology, fetal transfusion may be accomplished directly via the umbilical vein, infusing type O Rh-negative packed RBCs to raise the fetal hematocrit to 40% to 50%; fetal movement and transfusion risks are minimized by administering vecuronium bromide for temporary fetal paralysis. The frequency of intrauterine transfusions varies according to institution and fetal hydropic status, but one recommendation is for intervals of 10 days, 2 weeks, and then 3 weeks for subsequent procedures until the fetus reaches pulmonary maturity at approximately 37 to 38 weeks of gestation (Moise & Argoti). Intraperitoneal blood transfusions are used less commonly for isoimmunization because of higher associated fetal risks; however, they may be used when intravascular access is impossible.

Exchange transfusion. Exchange transfusion, in which the infant's blood is removed in small amounts (usually 5 to 10 mL at a time) and replaced with compatible blood (e.g., Rh-negative blood), is a standard mode of therapy for treatment of severe hyperbilirubinemia and is the treatment of choice for hyperbilirubinemia and hydrops caused by Rh incompatibility. Exchange transfusion removes the sensitized erythrocytes, lowers the serum bilirubin level to prevent bilirubin encephalopathy, corrects the anemia, and prevents cardiac failure. Indications for exchange transfusion in full-term infants may include a rapidly increasing serum bilirubin level and hemolysis despite intensive phototherapy. The criteria for exchange transfusions in preterm infants vary according to associated illness factors. The AAP Subcommittee on Hyperbilirubinemia (2004) practice parameter guidelines provide recommendations for initiating phototherapy and exchange transfusion in infants at 35 weeks of gestation or more. An infant born with hydrops fetalis or signs of cardiac failure is a candidate for immediate exchange transfusion with fresh whole blood.

For exchange transfusion, fresh whole blood is typed and cross-matched to the mother's serum. The amount of donor blood used is usually double the blood volume of the infant, which is approximately 85 mL/kg body weight but is limited to no more than 500 mL. A single-volume exchange transfusion replaces approximately 63% of the neonate's blood, and a two-volume exchange transfusion replaces approximately 86% (Kamath-Rayne, Thilo, Deacon, et al., 2016).

An exchange transfusion is a sterile surgical procedure. A catheter is inserted into the umbilical vein and threaded into the inferior vena cava. Depending on the infant's weight, 5 to 10 mL of blood is withdrawn within 15 to 20 seconds, and the same volume of donor blood is infused over 60 to 90 seconds.

The nurse prepares the infant and the family and assists the practitioner with the procedure. The infant receives nothing by mouth (NPO)

during the procedure; therefore a peripheral infusion of dextrose and electrolytes is established. The nurse documents the blood volume exchanged, including the amount of blood withdrawn and infused, the time of each procedure, and the cumulative record of the total volume exchanged. Vital signs monitored electronically are evaluated frequently and correlated with the removal and infusion of blood. If signs of cardiac or respiratory problems occur, the procedure is stopped temporarily and resumed after the infant's cardiorespiratory function stabilizes. The nurse also observes for signs of blood transfusion reaction and maintains the infant's blood glucose levels and fluid balance (Bradshaw, 2015).

Throughout the procedure, attention must be given to the infant's thermoregulation. Hypothermia increases oxygen and glucose consumption, causing metabolic acidosis. Not only do these consequences hinder the infant's overall physical ability to withstand the long procedure, but they also inhibit the binding capacity of albumin and bilirubin and the hepatic enzymatic reactions, thus increasing the risk for kernicterus. Conversely, hyperthermia damages the donor erythrocytes, elevating the free potassium content and predisposing the infant to cardiac arrest. The exchange transfusion is performed with the infant in a radiant warmer. However, he or she is usually covered with sterile drapes that may prevent the radiant heat from sufficiently warming the skin. The blood may also be warmed (using specially designed blood-warming devices only) before infusion (Bradshaw, 2015).

After the procedure is completed, the nurse inspects the umbilical site for evidence of bleeding. The catheter may remain in place in case repeated exchanges are required. The nurse monitors the infant for signs of complications such as thrombocytopenia, infection, feeding intolerance, and abdominal distension. High intensity phototherapy is continued, and bilirubin levels are closely monitored.

INFANTS OF DIABETIC MOTHERS

Maternal diabetes increases the risk for fetal and neonatal complications and contributes to perinatal mortality due to congenital anomalies, respiratory distress syndrome (RDS), and extreme prematurity (see Chapter 11) (Inturrisi, 2017; Reddy & Spong, 2014). There is a two- to six-fold increase in the incidence of major anomalies associated with type I and type II diabetes mellitus; cardiac and CNS anomalies are the most common (Landon, Catalano, & Gabbe, 2017).

The severity of maternal diabetes affects infant survival. It is determined by the duration of the disease before pregnancy; age of onset; extent of vascular complications; and abnormalities of the current pregnancy such as pyelonephritis, diabetic ketoacidosis, pregnancy-associated hypertension, and noncompliance. The single most important factor influencing fetal well-being is the euglycemic status of the mother. It has been found that reasonable metabolic control that begins before conception and continues during the first weeks of pregnancy can prevent malformation in an IDM. Elevated levels of hemoglobin A1c during the periconception period appear to be associated with a higher incidence of congenital malformations. In the case of gestational diabetes, macrosomia is the most common finding (Hay, 2012).

Hypoglycemia may appear a short time after birth and in IDMs is associated with increased insulin activity in the blood. The serum glucose level that corresponds to clinical hypoglycemia has not been well defined. Because some infants experience metabolic complications at higher levels than previously thought, some researchers recommend that serum glucose levels be maintained above 40 mg/dL (2.5 mmol/L) in infants with abnormal clinical symptoms and as high as 55 to 65 mg/dL in other infants (Adamkin & Polin, 2016). The AAP recommends that symptomatic infants receive treatment if their blood glucose is less than 40 mg/dL (Adamkin & AAP Committee on Fetus and Newborn, 2011).

Hypoglycemia in IDMs is related to hypertrophy and hyperplasia of the pancreatic islet cells and the transient state of hyperinsulinism. High maternal blood glucose levels during fetal life provide a continual stimulus to the fetal islet cells for insulin production (glucose easily passes the placental barrier from maternal to fetal side; however, insulin does not cross the placental barrier). Historically, maternal hyperglycemia was believed to contribute to fetal macrosomia. However, maternal hyperlipidemia and increased lipid transfer to the fetus are more likely responsible for the excessive weight gain and fat deposition seen in such infants. IDMs also have an increased risk for shoulder dystocia and birth injury (Hay, 2012). When the neonate's glucose supply is removed abruptly at the time of birth, the continued production of insulin soon depletes the blood of circulating glucose, creating a state of hyperinsulinism and hypoglycemia within 0.5 to 4 hours, especially in infants of mothers with poorly controlled diabetes. Precipitous drops in blood glucose levels can cause serious neurologic damage or death.

IDMs have a characteristic appearance (Box 25.3 and Fig. 25.10). Infants of mothers with advanced diabetes may be small for gestational age, have IUGR, or be the appropriate size for gestational age because of the maternal vascular (placental) involvement.

IDMs are highly susceptible to hypoglycemia, hypocalcemia, hypomagnesemia, polycythemia, hyperbilirubinemia, cardiomyopathy, and respiratory disorders. Hyperinsulinemia and hyperglycemia in the diabetic mother may be factors in reducing fetal surfactant synthesis, thus contributing to the development of respiratory distress syndrome (RDS). Although large, these infants may be delivered before term as a result of maternal complications or increased fetal size (Landon et al., 2017).

Some IDMs are also at increased risk for deep vein thrombosis, with renal vein thrombosis and hematuria being the most common presentation. Additional problems in IDMs include perinatal iron deficiency and neurologic impairments (seizures, lethargy, jitteriness, and changes in tone) (Hay, 2012).

BOX 25.3 Clinical Manifestations of Infants of Diabetic Mothers

- Large for gestational age
- Very plump and full faced
- Abundant vernix caseosa
- Plethora
- Listless and lethargic
- Possibly meconium stained at birth
- Hypotonia

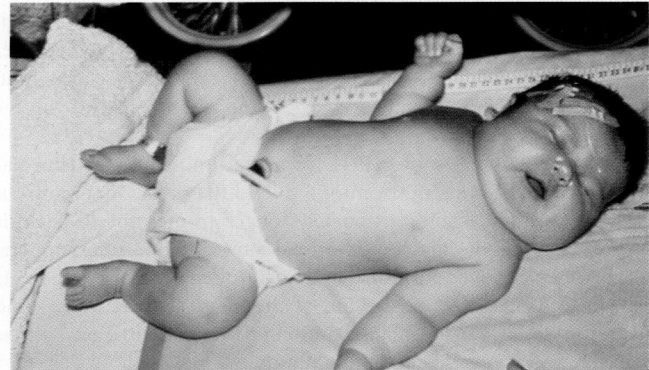

FIG 25.10 Large-for-gestational-age infant. This infant of a diabetic mother weighed 5 kg (11 lbs) at birth and exhibits the typical round facies. (From Zitelli, B.J., McIntire, S.C., Nowalk, A.J. [2012]. *Zitelli and Davis' atlas of pediatric physical diagnosis* (6th ed.). Philadelphia, PA: Elsevier.)

The most important management of IDMs is careful monitoring of serum glucose levels and observation for accompanying complications such as RDS and cardiac anomalies. The infants are examined for the presence of any anomalies or birth injuries; and blood studies for determination of glucose, calcium, hematocrit, and bilirubin are done on a regular basis.

Because the hypertrophied pancreas is so sensitive to blood glucose concentrations, the administration of oral glucose may trigger a massive insulin release, resulting in rebound hypoglycemia. Therefore feedings of breast milk or formula begin within the first hour after birth if the infant's cardiorespiratory condition is stable. Approximately one-half of these infants do well and adjust without complications. Infants born to mothers with poorly controlled diabetes may require IV dextrose infusions. Treatment with 10% dextrose and water intravenously is initiated with the goal of maintaining serum blood glucose levels between 40 and 50 mg/dL (Adamkin & AAP Committee on Fetus and Newborn, 2011). Oral and IV intake may be titrated to maintain adequate blood glucose levels. Frequent blood glucose determinations are needed for the first 2 to 4 days of life to assess the degree of hypoglycemia present at any given time. Testing blood taken from the heel with calibrated portable reflectance meters (e.g., glucometers) is a simple and effective screening evaluation; however, it is essential that any abnormal values are followed with immediate blood glucose determination by laboratory examination (Rozance, McGowan, Price-Douglas, et al., 2016).

CARE MANAGEMENT

The nursing care of IDMs involves early examination for congenital anomalies and signs of possible respiratory or cardiac problems, maintenance of adequate thermoregulation, early introduction of carbohydrate feedings as appropriate, and monitoring of serum blood glucose levels. The latter is of particular importance because many infants with hypoglycemia may remain asymptomatic. Symptomatic IDMs who are unable to feed should be started on a continuous intravenous infusion of 10% dextrose at 4 to 6 mg/min/kg unless blood glucose is below 20 mg/dL. In such cases, a one-time bolus infusion of 10% dextrose (2 mL/kg) should be given over 2 to 4 minutes, followed by a constant intravenous infusion of 10% dextrose and water as noted previously (Hay, 2012). IV glucose infusion requires careful monitoring of the site and the neonate's reaction to therapy; high glucose concentrations (≥12.5%) should be infused via a central line instead of a peripheral site.

Because macrosomic infants are at risk for problems associated with a difficult birth, they are monitored for birth injuries such as brachial plexus injury and palsy, fractured clavicle, and phrenic nerve palsy. Additional monitoring of the infant for problems associated with this condition (polycythemia, hypocalcemia, poor feeding, and hyperbilirubinemia) is also a vital nursing function.

Some evidence indicates that IDMs have an increased risk for acquiring type 2 diabetes and metabolic syndrome in childhood or early adulthood (Hay, 2012). Nursing care should also focus on healthy lifestyle and prevention later in life with IDMs.

CONGENITAL ANOMALIES

Congenital defects are reported to occur in 3% of all births in the United States, and 6% worldwide (Mburia-Mwalili & Yang, 2014), but this number increases to about 6% by the time children reach 5 years of age, as more anomalies are diagnosed. In addition, the incidence of congenital malformations in aborted fetuses is higher than that in infants who are born alive, thus adding to the overall incidence

(Parikh & Mitchell, 2015). Congenital malformations, deformations, and chromosomal abnormalities are the leading cause of death in infants younger than 1 year of age in the United States and account for 20% of infant deaths within the first year of life (Xu, Murphy, Kochanek, et al., 2016). Between 1999 and 2013, rates of cleft lip and cleft palate had the highest prevalence followed by Down syndrome, omphalocele or gastroschisis, spina bifida or myelomeningocele, and anencephaly. Prevalence of Down syndrome was highest among mothers 40 to 54 years of age, and rates of omphalocele or gastroschisis were highest among mothers younger than 20 years of age (Environmental Protection Agency Report on the Environment, 2015). Although the incidences of other causes of neonatal mortality have decreased, the death rate associated with most congenital anomalies has essentially remained stable since 1932.

The most common major congenital anomalies that cause serious problems in the neonate are congenital heart disease, abdominal wall defects, imperforate anus, neural tube defects (NTDs), cleft lip or palate, clubfoot, and developmental dysplasia of the hip. These are thought to result from the interaction of multiple genetic and environmental factors.

Most congenital anomalies are detected at birth or shortly thereafter. Although surgical techniques and treatments have made a significant difference in the morbidity of some anomalies, these continue to be a major source of chronic illness and morbidity in the first year of life.

An interprofessional team approach is vital for providing holistic care: the surgical treatment, rehabilitation, and education of the child and psychosocial and financial assistance for the parents. Parental disappointment and disillusion add to the complexity of the nursing care needed for these infants.

A number of congenital anomalies are discussed in the following pediatric systems and conditions chapters:
- Cleft lip and cleft palate, Chapter 41
- Esophageal atresia and tracheoesophageal fistula, Chapter 41
- Omphalocele and gastroschisis, Chapter 41
- Congenital cardiac defects, Chapter 42
- Congenital diaphragmatic hernia and choanal atresia, Chapter 40
- Neural tube defects and myelomeningocele, Chapter 49
- Developmental dysplasia of the hip and clubfoot, Chapter 48
- Hypospadias, disorders of sex development, and bladder exstrophy, Chapter 45

PRETERM AND POSTTERM INFANTS

PRETERM INFANTS

Prematurity accounts for the largest number of admissions to NICUs. Immaturity of most organ systems places infants at risk for a variety of neonatal complications (e.g., hyperbilirubinemia, RDS, cognitive and motor delays). Disorders related to LBW and prematurity were the second leading cause of infant mortality in the United States in 2013 (Xu et al., 2016). The actual cause of prematurity is not known in most instances. Factors such as previous preterm birth, maternal infections, multiple gestation, pregnancy-associated hypertension, and placental problems are responsible for a large number of preterm births.

The outlook for preterm infants is primarily related to the state of physiologic and anatomic immaturity of the various organs and systems at the time of birth. There is a significant difference between a 24 week preterm infant and one born at 36 weeks, yet both are considered preterm. Therefore in the context of this discussion of prematurity, the term is relative to the gestational age of the infant. Infants at term have advanced to a state of maturity sufficient to allow a successful transition to the extrauterine environment. Preterm infants must make the same

adjustments but with functional immaturity proportional to the stage of development reached at the time of birth. However, these adjustments may be limited or even hindered by the external environment to which the preterm infant is exposed. Exposure to excessive stimuli, bacteria, and viruses make the environment less conducive for preterm infants to grow and develop. The degree to which infants are prepared for extrauterine life can be predicted to some extent by birth weight and estimated gestational age.

Preterm infants have a number of distinct characteristics at various stages of development. Identification of these characteristics provides valuable clues to the gestational age and thus to the infant's physiologic capabilities. The general outward physical appearance changes as the fetus progresses to maturity. Characteristics of skin, general attitude (or posture) when supine, appearance of hair, and amount of subcutaneous fat provide cues to a newborn's physical development. Observation of spontaneous, active movements and response to stimulation and passive movement contributes to the assessment of neurologic status. The appraisal is made as soon as possible after admission to the nursery because much of the observation and management of infants depend on this information (see Chapter 23).

On inspection, preterm infants are very small and appear scrawny because they have minimal subcutaneous fat deposits (or none in some cases) and a proportionately large head in relation to the body, which reflects the cephalocaudal direction of growth. The skin is bright pink (often translucent, depending on the degree of immaturity), smooth, and shiny, with small blood vessels clearly visible underneath the thin epidermis. The fine lanugo hair is abundant over the body (depending on gestational age) but is sparse, fine, and fuzzy on the head. The ear cartilage is soft and pliable, and the soles and palms have minimal creases, resulting in a smooth appearance. The bones of the skull and the ribs feel soft, and the eyes may be closed. Male infants have few scrotal rugae, and the testes are undescended; in girls the labia and clitoris are prominent.

In contrast to full term infants' overall attitude of flexion and continuous activity, preterm infants may be inactive and listless. The extremities maintain an attitude of extension and remain in any position in which they are placed. Reflex activity is only partially developed; sucking is absent, weak, or ineffectual; swallow, gag, and cough reflexes are absent or weak; and other neurologic signs are absent or diminished. Physiologically immature preterm infants are unable to maintain body temperature, have limited ability to excrete solutes in the urine, and have increased susceptibility to infection. A pliable thorax, immature lung tissue, and an immature regulatory center lead to periodic breathing, hypoventilation, and frequent periods of apnea. They are more susceptible to biochemical alterations such as hyperbilirubinemia and hypoglycemia, and they have a higher extracellular water content that renders them more vulnerable to fluid and electrolyte derangements. Preterm infants exchange fully half of their extracellular fluid volume every 24 hours compared with one seventh of the volume in adults.

The soft cranium is subject to characteristic unintentional deformation caused by positioning from one side to the other on a mattress. The head appears disproportionately longer from front to back, is flattened on both sides, and lacks the usual convexity seen at the temporal and parietal areas. This positional molding is often a concern to parents and can influence their perception of the infant's attractiveness and their responsiveness to the infant. Positioning the infant on a gel mattress can reduce or minimize cranial molding.

Neurologic impairment (e.g., from intraventricular hemorrhage) and serious sequelae correlate with the size and gestational age of infants at birth and the severity of neonatal complications. The greater the degree of immaturity, the greater is the degree of potential disability.

An increased incidence of cerebral palsy, ADHD, visual-motor deficits, and altered intellectual functioning is observed in preterm infants compared with full-term infants. However, behavioral development can be enhanced when families are provided with support and infants are referred to appropriate services for neurologic and developmental interventions. Parental interest and involvement are important variables in the developmental progress of infants.

When the birth of a preterm infant is anticipated, the NICU is alerted, and an interprofessional care team including a neonatologist, an advanced practice nurse, a staff nurse, and a respiratory therapist are usually present for the birth. Infants who do not require resuscitation are immediately transferred in a heated incubator to the NICU, where they are weighed and IV lines, oxygen therapy, and other therapeutic interventions are initiated as needed. Resuscitation is conducted in the birthing area until infants can be safely transported to the NICU.

Subsequent care is determined by the infant's status. The general care of preterm infants differs from that of full term infants primarily in the areas of respiratory support, thermoregulation, nutrition, susceptibility to infection, activity intolerance, neurodevelopmental care, and other consequences of physical immaturity.

Care Management

The nursing care, similar to the therapeutic management, is individualized for each infant. For additional details of care, see appropriate discussions in the "Care of the High Risk Newborn and Family" section later in the chapter.

LATE-PRETERM INFANTS

Late-preterm infants are born between 34 0/7 and 36 6/7 weeks of gestation. Although they are preterm, they often have the appearance of term infants and may receive the same care. Late-preterm infants experience morbidities similar to those of preterm infants, including respiratory distress, hypoglycemia requiring treatment, temperature instability, poor feeding, jaundice, and discharge delays as a result of illness. Therefore assessment and prompt intervention in life-threatening perinatal emergencies often make the difference between a favorable outcome and a lifetime of disability. It is estimated that late preterm infants represent 70% of the total preterm infant population and that the mortality rate for this group is significantly higher than that of term infants (7.1 per 1000 live births at 34 weeks vs. 0.8 per 1000 live births at 39 weeks) (Horgan, 2015). Because late-preterm infants' birth weights often range from 2000 to 2500 g (4.4 to 5.5 lbs) and they appear relatively mature compared with smaller preterm infants, they may be cared for in the same manner as healthy term infants while risk factors for late preterm infants are overlooked. Late preterm infants are often discharged early from the birth institution and have a significantly higher rate than term infants of rehospitalization within 2 weeks of being discharged (National Perinatal Association, 2012; Young, Korgensky, & Buichi, et al., 2013). Discussions regarding high-risk infants in this chapter also refer to late-preterm infants who are experiencing a delayed transition to extrauterine life. Nurses in newborn nurseries should be familiar with the characteristics of late-preterm infants and recognize the significance of serious deviations from expected observations (see Clinical Reasoning Case Study: Late-Preterm Infant). When providers can anticipate the need for specialized care and plan for it, the probability of successful outcome is increased.

The Association of Women's Health, Obstetric, and Neonatal Nurses (AWHONN, 2014) published *Assessment and Care of the Late Preterm Infant* for the education of perinatal nurses regarding assessment and care of the late-preterm infant (Table 25.7). The National Perinatal

CLINICAL REASONING CASE STUDY

Late-Preterm Infant

A 2013-g (4 lb 7 oz) male infant is born at an estimated gestational age of 35 weeks. The parents are excited about this birth because they have been trying to become pregnant for 6 years. The baby is placed on the mother's abdomen after birth for skin-to-skin contact but does not breastfeed. The nurse assessing the baby notes that he has some mild grunting, nasal flaring, and intercostal retractions; he is taken to the transitional nursery for further evaluation and treatment. The father speaks little English but asks when they will be able to hold their son again; the mother is crying and asks to have her baby brought back to her as soon as his condition is stable because she really wants to breastfeed him.

1. Evidence—Is there sufficient evidence to draw conclusions about what to tell the new parents about their newborn son?
2. Assumptions—What assumptions can be made about the following?
   a. The mother's and father's reaction to their son's birth
   b. The infant's expected progress
   c. The possibility of the mother breastfeeding the baby
3. What implications and priorities for nursing care can be drawn at this time?
4. Interprofessional care—Describe the roles and responsibilities of the interprofessional health care members who can contribute to optimizing outcomes for this mother, newborn, and family.

Association (2012) published an extensive multidisciplinary guideline for the care of late-preterm infants.

COMPLICATIONS OF PRETERM BIRTH

Respiratory Distress Syndrome

Respiratory distress is a name applied to respiratory dysfunction in neonates and is primarily a disease related to developmental delay in lung maturation. The terms respiratory distress syndrome (RDS) and *hyaline membrane disease* are most often applied to this severe lung disorder, which not only is responsible for more infant deaths than any other disease but also carries the highest risk in terms of long-term respiratory and neurologic complications. It is seen almost exclusively in preterm infants and occurs twice as often in male as in female infants. The disorder is rare in drug-exposed infants and infants who have been subjected to chronic intrauterine stress (e.g., maternal preeclampsia or hypertension) (Gardner, Enzman-Hines, & Nyp, 2016). Respiratory distress of a nonpulmonary origin in neonates may also be caused by sepsis, cardiac defects (structural or functional), hemolytic disease, CNS defects, exposure to cold, airway obstruction (atresia), intraventricular hemorrhage, hypoglycemia, metabolic acidosis, acute blood loss, and drugs. Pneumonia in the neonatal period can result in respiratory distress caused by bacterial or viral agents and may occur alone or as a complication of RDS (Gardner et al., 2016).

Preterm infants are born before the lungs are fully prepared to serve as efficient organs for gas exchange. The effects of lung immaturity are compounded by the presence of more cartilage in the chest wall, leading to increased compliance of the chest wall, which collapses inward in response to less compliant (stiffer) lung tissue.

There is evidence of fetal respiratory activity before birth. The lungs make feeble respiratory movements, and fluid is excreted through the alveoli. Because the final unfolding of the alveolar septa, which increases the surface area of the lungs, occurs during the last trimester of pregnancy, preterm infants are born with numerous underdeveloped and many uninflatable alveoli. Pulmonary blood flow is limited as a result of the collapsed state of the fetal lungs, particularly poor vascular development in general, and an immature capillary network. Because

TABLE 25.7   Late-Preterm Infant Assessment and Interventions

Risk Factors	Assessment	Interventions*
Respiratory distress	Assess for cardinal signs of respiratory distress (nasal flaring, grunting, tachypnea, central cyanosis, retractions) and presence of apnea, especially during feedings. Assess for hypothermia, hypoglycemia.	Perform gestational age assessment. Observe for signs of respiratory distress; monitor oxygenation by pulse oximetry; provide supplemental oxygen judiciously.
Thermal instability	Monitor axillary temperature every 30 minutes immediately after birth until stable; thereafter every 1–4 hours, depending on gestational age and ability to maintain thermal stability.	Provide skin-to-skin care in immediate postpartum period for stable infant. Implement measures to avoid excess heat loss (adjust environmental temperature, avoid drafts). Bathe only after thermal stability has been maintained for 1 hour.
Hypoglycemia	Monitor for signs and symptoms of hypoglycemia. Assess feeding ability (latch-on, nipple feeding). Assess thermal stability and signs and symptoms of respiratory distress. Monitor bedside glucose in infants with additional risk factors (IDM, prolonged labor, respiratory distress, poor feeding).	Initiate early feedings of human milk or formula. Avoid dextrose water or water feedings. Provide IV dextrose as necessary for hypoglycemia.
Jaundice	Observe for jaundice in first 24 hours. Evaluate maternal-fetal history for additional risk factors that may cause increased hemolysis and circulating levels of unconjugated bilirubin (Rh, ABO, spherocytosis, bruising). Assess feeding method, voiding and stooling patterns.	Monitor transcutaneous bilirubin, and note risk zone on hour-specific nomogram (see Figs. 23.6 and 23.7).
Feeding problems	Assess suck-swallow and breathing. Assess for respiratory distress, hypoglycemia, thermal stability. Assess latch-on, maternal comfort with feeding method. Determine weight loss (should be ≤10% of birth weight).	Initiate early feedings (human milk or formula). Ensure maternal knowledge of feeding method and signs of inadequate feeding (sleepiness, lethargy, color changes during feeding, apnea during feeding, decreased or absent urine output).
Neurodevelopmental problems	Assess for respiratory distress, neonatal jaundice, hypoglycemia, and thermal instability. Assess neurodevelopmental status. Assess for seizure activity.	Perform newborn screening, including hearing test. Implement individualized developmental care. Encourage parents to keep follow-up appointments with health care provider for evaluation of growth and development (including cognitive function and achievement of appropriate milestones).
Infection	Evaluate maternal-fetal history for risk factors that may contribute to neonatal septicemia. Assess for signs and symptoms of neonatal infection (see Tables 25.4 and 25.5).	Use Standard Precautions, especially hand washing between infants and after contact with surfaces that may harbor bacteria (e.g., keyboards, telephones). Maintain thermal stability. Administer hepatitis B vaccine. Encourage breastfeeding and assist mother-baby pair with breastfeeding. Encourage parents to decrease infant exposure to respiratory viruses after discharge and obtain vaccines as appropriate to prevent development of respiratory infections (e.g., influenza).

IDM, Infant of diabetic mother; *IV,* intravenous.

*This is not an exhaustive list of nursing interventions; additional interventions include those discussed under the care of the high risk infant in this chapter.

Portions adapted from Association of Women's Health, Obstetric, and Neonatal Nurses (2014). *Assessment and care of the late preterm infant: Evidence-based clinical practice guideline,* Washington, DC: Author.

of increased pulmonary vascular resistance (PVR), the major portion of fetal blood is shunted from the lungs by way of the ductus arteriosus and foramen ovale.

At birth, infants must initiate breathing and keep the previously fluid-filled lungs inflated with air. At the same time, the pulmonary capillary blood flow must be increased approximately 10-fold to provide for adequate lung perfusion and alter the intracardiac pressure that closes the fetal cardiac structures. Most full term infants successfully accomplish these adjustments, but preterm infants with respiratory distress are unable to do so.

Surfactant deficiency appears to be the principal factor in the development of RDS. Surfactant is a surface-active phospholipid secreted by the alveolar epithelium. Acting much like a detergent, this substance reduces the surface tension of fluids that line the alveoli and respiratory passages, resulting in uniform expansion and maintenance of lung expansion at low intraalveolar pressure. Immature development of these functions produces consequences that seriously compromise respiratory efficiency. Deficient surfactant production causes unequal inflation of alveoli on inspiration and the collapse of alveoli on end expiration. Without surfactant, infants are unable to keep their lungs inflated and therefore exert a great deal of effort to re-expand the alveoli with each breath. With increasing exhaustion, infants are able to open fewer and fewer alveoli. This inability to maintain lung expansion produces widespread atelectasis.

In the absence of alveolar stability (normal functional residual capacity) and with progressive atelectasis, PVR increases; with normal lung expansion it would decrease. Consequently hypoperfusion to the lung tissue occurs, with a decrease in effective pulmonary blood flow. The increase in PVR causes partial reversion to the fetal circulation, with a right-to-left shunting of blood through the persisting fetal communications (i.e., the ductus arteriosus and foramen ovale).

Inadequate pulmonary perfusion and ventilation produce hypoxemia and hypercapnia. Pulmonary arterioles, with their thick muscular layer, are markedly reactive to diminished oxygen concentration. Thus a decrease in oxygen tension causes vasoconstriction in the pulmonary arterioles that is exacerbated by a decrease in blood pH. Vasoconstriction creates a marked increase in PVR. In normal ventilation with increased oxygen concentration, the ductus arteriosus constricts, and the pulmonary vessels dilate to decrease PVR.

Prolonged hypoxemia activates anaerobic glycolysis, which produces increased amounts of lactic acid. An increase in lactic acid causes metabolic acidosis; an inability of the atelectatic lungs to blow off excess carbon dioxide produces respiratory acidosis. Acidosis causes further vasoconstriction. With deficient pulmonary circulation and alveolar perfusion, partial pressure of oxygen in arterial blood continues to fall, pH falls, and the materials needed for surfactant production are not circulated to the alveoli.

The diagnosis of RDS is made on the basis of clinical manifestations (Box 25.4) and radiographic studies. Radiographic findings characteristic of RDS include (1) a diffuse granular pattern over both lung fields that closely resembles ground glass and represents alveolar atelectasis; and (2) dark streaks, or bronchograms, within the ground glass areas that represent dilated, air-filled bronchioles. It is often difficult to distinguish between RDS and pneumonia in infants with respiratory distress. The extent of respiratory function and acid-base balance is determined by blood gas analysis. Pulse oximetry, carbon dioxide monitoring, and pulmonary function studies help to differentiate pulmonary and extrapulmonary illness and are used in the management of RDS (Fraser, 2015).

The treatment of RDS involves immediate establishment of adequate oxygenation and ventilation, supportive care and measures required for any preterm infant, and those instituted to prevent further complications associated with preterm birth. The goals of supportive measures most crucial to a favorable outcome are as follows:
- Maintain adequate ventilation and oxygenation.
- Maintain acid-base balance.
- Maintain a neutral thermal environment.
- Maintain adequate tissue perfusion and oxygenation.
- Prevent hypotension.
- Maintain adequate hydration and electrolyte status.

Nipple and gavage feedings are contraindicated in any situation that creates a marked increase in respiratory rate because of the greater hazards of aspiration. Nutrition is provided by parenteral therapy during the acute stage of the disease, and minimal enteral feeding is provided to enhance maturation of the neonate's GI system.

The administration of exogenous surfactant to preterm neonates with RDS has become an accepted and common therapy in most neonatal centers worldwide. Clinical trials involving the administration of exogenous surfactant to infants with or at high risk for RDS demonstrate reduction in severity of RDS, decreased incidence of pulmonary air leaks and pneumothorax, and an overall decreased infant mortality rate (Sweet, Halliday, & Speer, 2013). The overall rates of some associated comorbidities (bronchopulmonary dysplasia, NEC, patent ductus arteriosus) have not decreased with surfactant replacement. Currently exogenous surfactant is derived from a natural source (e.g., porcine, bovine). In 2012 a synthetic surfactant, Lucinactant, was approved for use in infants with RDS. However, clinical trials have yet to establish its effectiveness over an animal-derived surfactant (Piehl & Fernandez-Bustamante, 2012; Walsh, Daigle, Diblasi, et al., 2013).

Complications of surfactant administration can include pulmonary hemorrhage and mucus plugging. Surfactant therapy is also being used in infants with meconium aspiration, infectious pneumonia, sepsis, persistent pulmonary hypertension, and pulmonary hemorrhage. Surfactant may be administered at birth as a preventive or prophylactic treatment of RDS or later in the course of RDS as a rescue treatment; however, research has demonstrated improved clinical outcomes and fewer adverse effects when surfactant is administered prophylactically to infants at risk for developing RDS (Bahadue & Soll, 2012; Sweet et al., 2013). Surfactant is administered via an endotracheal (ET) tube directly into the infant's trachea (Fig. 25.11). Nursing responsibilities with surfactant administration include assisting with the administration

---

> ### BOX 25.4 Clinical Manifestations of Respiratory Distress Syndrome
>
> - Tachypnea (≥60 breaths/min) initially*
> - Dyspnea
> - Pronounced intercostal or substernal retractions
> - Fine inspiratory crackles
> - Audible expiratory grunt
> - Flaring of the external nares
> - Cyanosis or pallor
> - Apnea
> - With progression of condition, deteriorating vital signs including blood pressure, apnea, body temperature instability

*Not all infants born with respiratory distress syndrome manifest these characteristics; very low–birth weight and extremely low–birth weight infants may have respiratory failure and shock at birth because of physiologic immaturity.

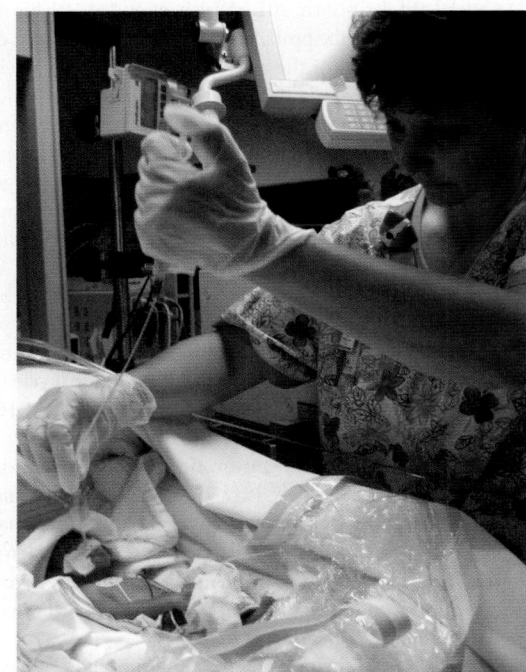

FIG 25.11 Exogenous surfactant administration via endotracheal tube. (Courtesy of E. Jacobs, Texas Children's Hospital, Houston, TX.)

TABLE 25.8	**Common Methods for Assisted Ventilation in Neonatal Respiratory Distress**	
Method	**Description**	**How Provided**
Conventional Methods		
Continuous positive airway pressure (CPAP)	Provides constant distending pressure to airway in spontaneously breathing infant	Nasal prongs Face mask Nasal cannula
Intermittent mandatory ventilation (IMV)*	Allows infant to breathe spontaneously at own rate but provides mechanical cycled respirations and pressure at regular preset intervals	Endotracheal intubation and ventilator
Synchronized intermittent mandatory ventilation (SIMV)	Mechanically delivered breaths are synchronized to onset of spontaneous patient breaths; assist/control mode facilitates full inspiratory synchrony; involves signal detection of onset of spontaneous respiration from abdominal movement, thoracic impedance, and airway pressure or flow changes	Patient-triggered infant ventilator with signal detector and assist/control mode; endotracheal tube
Volume-guarantee ventilation	Delivers predetermined volume of gas using inspiratory pressure that varies according to infant's lung compliance (often used in conjunction with SIMV)	Volume-guarantee ventilator with flow sensor; endotracheal tube
Alternative Methods		
High-frequency oscillation (HFO)	Application of high-frequency, low-volume, sine-wave flow oscillations to airway at rates between 480 and 1200 breaths/min	Variable-speed piston pump (or loudspeaker, fluidic oscillator); endotracheal tube
High-frequency jet ventilation (HFJV)	Uses separate, parallel, low-compliant circuit and injector port to deliver small pulses or jets of fresh gas deep into airway at rates between 250 and 900 breaths/min	May be used alone or with low-rate IMV; endotracheal tube

*Also referred to as *conventional ventilation* (vs. high-frequency ventilation [HFV]).

of the product, collection and monitoring of arterial blood gases, careful monitoring of oxygenation with pulse oximetry, and assessment of the infant's tolerance of the procedure. After surfactant is absorbed, respiratory compliance usually increases, which requires adjustment of ventilator settings to decrease mean airway pressure and prevent overinflation or hyperoxemia. Suctioning is usually delayed for approximately 1 hour (depending on the type of surfactant and unit protocol) to allow maximum effects to occur. Although an aerosolized surfactant is now available and is being used in adults, further research is needed to establish protocols for the dose, preparation, and route of administration in infants (Abdel-Latif & Osborn, 2012; Walsh, et al, 2013). This method would theoretically decrease the problems associated with current delivery systems (i.e., contamination of the airway, interruption of mechanical ventilation, and loss of the drug in the ET tubing from reflux).

The goals of oxygen therapy are to provide adequate oxygen to the tissues, prevent lactic acid accumulation resulting from hypoxia, and at the same time avoid the potentially negative effects of oxygen and barotrauma. Numerous methods have been devised to improve oxygenation (Table 25.8). All require that the gas is warmed and humidified before entering the respiratory tract. If the infant does not require intubation and mechanical ventilation, oxygen can be supplied by nasal cannula or via nasal prongs in conjunction with continuous positive airway pressure (CPAP). If oxygen saturation of the blood cannot be maintained at a satisfactory level and the carbon dioxide level ($PaCO_2$) rises, infants require ventilatory assistance (Gardner et al., 2016).

RDS is a self-limiting disease. Before the use of surfactant, infants typically experienced a period of deterioration ($\approx$48 hours) and, in the absence of complications, improved by 72 hours. Often heralded by the onset of diuresis, this improvement was attributed primarily to increased production and greater availability of surfactant. With the administration of surfactant, lung compliance begins to improve almost immediately, resulting in lower oxygen requirements and a decreased need for ventilatory support (Polin et al., 2014).

Infants with RDS who survive the first 96 hours have a reasonable chance of recovery. However, complications of RDS include associated respiratory conditions and problems associated with prematurity,

including patent ductus arteriosus and congestive heart failure, intraventricular hemorrhage, bronchopulmonary dysplasia, retinopathy of prematurity (ROP), pneumonia, air leak syndrome, sepsis, NEC, and neurologic sequelae (Fraser, 2015).

Care Management

Care of infants with RDS involves all of the observations and interventions previously described for high-risk infants and involves an interprofessional health care team. Care management is focused on the complex problems related to respiratory therapy and the constant threat of hypoxemia and acidosis that complicates the care of patients in respiratory difficulty.

The respiratory therapist, an important member of the NICU team, is often responsible for maintaining respiratory equipment. Although it may be the respiratory therapist's responsibility to regulate the apparatus, nurses should understand the equipment and be able to recognize when it is not functioning correctly. The most essential nursing function is to observe and assess the infant's response to therapy. Continuous monitoring and close observation are mandatory because an infant's status can change rapidly and oxygen concentration and ventilation parameters are prescribed according to the infant's blood gas measurements and pulse oximetry readings.

Changes in oxygen concentration are based on these observations. The amount of oxygen administered, expressed as the fraction of inspired air (FIO_2), is determined on an individual basis according to pulse oximetry or direct or indirect measurement of arterial oxygen concentration. Capillary samples collected from the heel are useful for pH and $PaCO_2$ determinations but not for oxygenation status. Continuous transcutaneous or pulse oximetry readings are recorded at least hourly.

Mucus can collect in the respiratory tract as a result of the infant's pulmonary condition. Secretions interfere with gas flow and predispose the infant to obstruction of the passages, including the endotracheal tube. Suctioning should be performed only when necessary and should be based on individual infant assessment, which includes auscultation of the chest, evidence of decreased oxygenation, excess moisture in the

ET tube, or increased infant irritability. During suctioning, a variety of techniques can be used to minimize complications such as increased intracranial pressure (ICP) and health care–associated pneumonia, including using a closed suctioning system, placing the infant in a lateral instead of a supine position, and maintaining the ventilator circuit in a horizontal position to reduce the draining of oropharyngeal secretions into the lower respiratory tract (Polin et al., 2012).

When nasopharyngeal passages, the trachea, or the ET tube is being suctioned, the catheter should be inserted gently but quickly; intermittent suction is applied as the catheter is withdrawn. Negative airway pressure should be applied for no more than 10 to 15 seconds because continuous suction removes air from the lungs along with the mucus. It is recommended that the "two-person" suctioning procedure be used on infants who are acutely ill and who do not tolerate any procedure without profound decreases in oxygen saturation, BP, and heart rate. The object of suctioning an artificial airway is to maintain patency of that airway, not the bronchi. Suction applied beyond the ET tube can cause traumatic lesions of the trachea. The use of in-line suction catheters may decrease airway contamination and hypoxia (Gardner et al., 2016).

The most advantageous positions for facilitating an infant's open airway are side-lying with the head supported in alignment by a small folded blanket or, when supine, positioned to keep the neck slightly extended. With the head in the "sniffing" position, the trachea is opened at its maximum; hyperextension reduces the tracheal diameter in neonates.

Inspection of the skin is part of routine infant assessment. Position changes and the use of water pillows are helpful in guarding against skin breakdown.

Mouth care is especially important when infants are NPO: the problem is often aggravated by the drying effect of oxygen therapy. Drying and cracking can be prevented by careful oral hygiene using sterile water. Irritation to the nares or mouth that occurs from appliances used to administer oxygen (e.g., nasal CPAP) may be reduced by the use of a water-soluble ointment. Routine oral hygiene care in intubated adults and older children has been shown to decrease the incidence of ventilator-associated pneumonia (see Chapter 40).

The nursing care of an infant with RDS is demanding; meticulous attention must be given to subtle changes in the infant's oxygenation status. The importance of attention to detail cannot be overemphasized, particularly in regard to medication administration.

◎ NURSING CARE PLAN

The High-Risk Preterm Infant

Case Study

Anthony was born at 33 weeks of gestation, weighing 2575 g (5 lbs 10 oz) to 24 year old Leslie, whose first pregnancy ended in a miscarriage at 18 weeks. Leslie is single but in a committed relationship with her boyfriend, Sean. Soon after birth, Anthony exhibited signs of respiratory distress. When he displayed increasing distress, he was transported by air ambulance to a neonatal intensive care unit (NICU) in a hospital located approximately 50 miles from where he was born. Leslie was discharged from the hospital after 24 hours; she is very upset and anxious about Anthony's condition. She had planned to breastfeed, so the nurses gave her an electric breast pump with instructions about expressing and storing the milk.

Assessment

What are signs of respiratory distress? What factors contribute to respiratory distress?

Defining Characteristics

Decreased inspiratory and expiratory pressure
Decreased minute ventilation
Use of accessory muscles to breathe
Retractions
Nasal flaring
Grunting
Apnea
Tachypnea
Altered chest excursion
Respiratory rate <30/min or >60/min

Nursing Diagnosis

Ineffective Breathing Pattern related to pulmonary, neurologic, vascular, alveolar, and muscular immaturity.

Expected Outcomes

Anthony will maintain a patent airway and ventilatory status adequate for oxygenation.

Nursing Interventions	Rationales
Position to facilitate airway expansion and prevent collection of secretions.	To allow oxygen entry into bronchial tree and alveoli
Closely monitor for deviations from desired breathing pattern—pulse oximetry, arterial blood gases, clinical signs of poor oxygenation, grunting, nasal flaring, apnea, tachypnea, retractions, and cyanosis.	To facilitate proper oxygenation by implementing appropriate therapy as needed, such as supplemental oxygen, mechanical ventilation, or change of position
Monitor vital signs for change in condition or status such as decreased cardiac output (poor perfusion, mottling, deteriorating respiratory status).	To implement appropriate therapy such as suctioning, supplemental oxygen, or vasopressor drugs
Assist with exogenous surfactant administration, and monitor patient tolerance or change in status.	To increase alveolar expansion and enhance oxygen–carbon dioxide exchange
Suction oropharynx, nasopharynx, trachea, or endotracheal tube only as necessary and based on respiratory assessment.	To remove secretions that may interfere with adequate ventilation and oxygenation

Case Study (Continued)

Soon after birth, the nurse noted that Anthony's axillary temperature was 35.8° C (96.4° F).

Assessment

What are signs of ineffective thermoregulation? What is the normal temperature range for a newborn infant? What factors contribute to unstable temperatures?

Defining Characteristics

Fluctuations in body temperature above or below normal range
Cyanotic nail beds
Flushed or mottled skin
Increased respirations or heart rate
Moderate pallor

Continued

NURSING CARE PLAN

The High-Risk Preterm Infant—cont'd

Warm or cool skin
Slow capillary refill time

Nursing Diagnosis
Ineffective Thermoregulation related to immature neurologic and metabolic temperature control

Expected Outcomes
Infant will maintain stable body temperature of 36.5° C to 37.2° C (97.6° F to 99° F).

Nursing Interventions	Rationales
Place Anthony in thermally controlled incubator or radiant warmer.	To control environmental temperature and keep Anthony's temperature stable
Use environmental controls for decreasing body heat loss (plastic heat shield, increased ambient temperature, servo control on warmer or incubator).	To regulate body temperature within acceptable range and minimize heat loss
Place knitted or cloth cap on head.	To prevent heat loss from exposed scalp
Monitor axillary or skin temperature as often as necessary or per unit protocol.	To detect necessity for environmental temperature regulation and to determine Anthony's response to environmental thermoregulation
Check temperature of newborn in relation to environmental temperature and temperature of heating element.	To detect change in thermoregulatory status, which may indicate significant disease process such as sepsis
Monitor vital signs and skin color, perfusion, pulses, and respiratory status.	To detect changes in status that require additional intervention for stabilization
Monitor for signs of hyperthermia (flushing, tachycardia, altered level of consciousness) and hypothermia (decreased activity; respiratory distress [deterioration]; cool, mottled extremities).	To prevent untoward effects of hyperthermia (fluctuating cerebral perfusion, apnea, increased metabolism with decreased available glucose for vital functions) or hypothermia (increased glucose use, lactic acidosis, respiratory compromise)
Monitor serum glucose levels as necessary or per unit protocol.	To ensure that euglycemia is maintained

Case Study (Continued)
Leslie is increasingly concerned about Anthony's condition. Anthony's respiratory distress is increasing; if his condition does not improve within the next couple of hours, they will intubate him and begin ventilation. Sean is working and is unable to take time off to drive her the 50 miles to the NICU to see Anthony.

Leslie is expressing minimal amounts of colostrum or milk when using the electric breast pump; she is very discouraged and is ready to give up the effort to pump. Leslie says she is afraid to love Anthony because of what happened with her first pregnancy and that Anthony doesn't seem real since she only saw him briefly before he was transferred to the NICU.

Assessment
What are characteristics of attachment? What are characteristics of impaired attachment? What factors interfere with attachment? What can facilitate attachment?

Defining Characteristics
Anxiety over parental role
Anxiety over infant's condition
Illness in infant that doesn't allow contact with parents
Physical barriers
Parent-child separation
Premature infant

Nursing Diagnosis
Risk for Impaired Parent-Infant Attachment related to condition of infant and separation from him

Expected Outcomes
Leslie and Sean will initiate positive interactions with Anthony.
Leslie and Sean will form an emotional bond or attachment with Anthony.
Parents will recognize when they need assistance.

Nursing Interventions	Rationales
Refer Leslie to a social worker for assistance in finding transportation to the NICU.	To provide opportunity for Leslie (and Sean) to see and touch Anthony.
Encourage parent(s) to hold and make eye contact with Anthony as physical status allows.	To minimize effects of physical separation from Anthony
Encourage parent-newborn skin-to-skin contact as condition of newborn allows.	To facilitate parent-infant interaction that is meaningful and comforting
Explain to parents the newborn's illness and expectations for recovery in terms they can understand.	To enhance parental knowledge and decrease potential fear of unknown regarding Anthony's survival and recovery
Encourage parent participation in newborn care activities such as touching Anthony, expressing and storing breast milk, and talking to Anthony.	To facilitate parental involvement in attaining the role of parents and decrease feelings of helplessness

ELBW, Extremely low–birth weight; *VLBW,* very low–birth weight.

Other Respiratory Disorders

Newborn infants are vulnerable to a variety of pulmonary complications, some requiring oxygen therapy (Table 25.9). For example, the preterm infant is subject to periods of apnea; and in term and postterm infants, intrauterine stress often causes fetuses to pass meconium, which can be aspirated before or during birth. Oxygen therapy, although lifesaving, is not without its hazards. Positive pressure introduced by mechanical apparatus has created an increase in the incidence of ruptured alveoli and subsequent pneumothorax and bronchopulmonary dysplasia (BPD) (chronic lung disease). The use of nasal CPAP (Fig. 25.13) decreases the incidence of adverse effects associated with intubation and positive-pressure ventilation in preterm infants with RDS (Gardner et al., 2016). Retinopathy of prematurity is observed almost exclusively in preterm infants and is related primarily to prematurity and oxygen therapy (see Table 25.9). Some evidence supports the resuscitation of asphyxiated newborns with 21% oxygen rather than 100% oxygen. Proponents for room air resuscitation suggest that fewer complications are associated with oxidative stress and hyperoxemia when room air is administered (Vento, 2015). The 2016 Neonatal Resuscitation Guidelines recommend the initiation of neonatal resuscitation using room air (no supplemental oxygen); if the neonate does not improve within 90 seconds, the use of supplemental oxygen is recommended (see Evidence-Based Practice box: Use of Room Air or Low Oxygen for Newborn Stabilization and Resuscitation in the Delivery Room). Pulse oximetry is recommended to monitor the infant's oxygenation status during resuscitation and prevent excessive use of oxygen in both term and preterm infants (AAP & American Heart Association [AHA], 2016).

Inhaled nitric oxide (INO) and extracorporeal membrane oxygenation (ECMO) are additional therapies used in the treatment of respiratory distress and respiratory failure in neonates. INO is used in term and late-preterm infants with conditions such as persistent pulmonary hypertension, meconium aspiration syndrome (see Table 25.9), pneumonia, sepsis, and congenital diaphragmatic hernia to decrease or reverse pulmonary hypertension, pulmonary vasoconstriction, acidosis, and hypoxemia. Nitric oxide is a colorless, highly diffusible gas that can be administered through the ventilator circuit blended with oxygen. INO may be used in conjunction with surfactant replacement therapy, high-frequency ventilation, or ECMO. Although INO is used in preterm infants with respiratory distress and respiratory failure, its use has not proved to be significantly effective in decreasing rates of bronchopulmonary dysplasia or improving survival rates in preterm infants (Dani & Pratesi, 2013; Donohue, Gilmore, Cristofalo, et al., 2011).

TABLE 25.9   Respiratory Complications

Description	Clinical Manifestations	Therapeutic Management	Care Management
Meconium Aspiration Syndrome			
Aspiration of amniotic fluid containing meconium into fetal or newborn trachea in utero or at first breath	Meconium stained at birth Tachypnea Hypoxia Acidemia Hyperventilation (early) Hypoventilation (later)	Routine intubation for the removal of meconium is no longer recommended (Fig. 25.12). Infants should be evaluated according to the Neonatal Resuscitation Program (American Academy of Pediatrics [AAP] & American Heart Association [AHA], 2016). Monitor for respiratory distress; manage with supplemental oxygen. Prevent acidosis and hypoxemia. Exogenous surfactant, high-frequency ventilation, inhaled nitric oxide, or extracorporeal membrane oxygenation (ECMO) may be used	See Respiratory Distress Syndrome.
Apnea of Prematurity			
Lapse of spontaneous breathing for ≥20 seconds, which may or may not be followed by bradycardia, oxygen desaturation, and color change	Persistent apneic spells, bradycardia, oxygen desaturation, and cyanosis	Observe for apnea. Check for thermal stability and metabolic problem such as hypoglycemia. Administer caffeine as prescribed. Administer nasal continuous positive airway pressure (CPAP).	Provide continuous electronic monitoring (respiratory and heart rates). Observe for presence of respirations. Observe color. Provide gentle tactile stimulation. Suction nose and oropharynx if still apneic. Apply artificial ventilation with bag-valve-mask using minimum of pressure needed to gently lift rib cage. Assess for and manage any precipitating factors (e.g., temperature instability, abdominal distention, ambient oxygen). Observe for signs of caffeine toxicity: tachycardia (rate ≥180 beats/min) and (later) vomiting, restlessness, irritability. Assess skin (with use of nasal CPAP) for breakdown, irritation at nasal septum.

Continued

TABLE 25.9 Respiratory Complications—cont'd

Description	Clinical Manifestations	Therapeutic Management	Care Management
Pneumothorax			
Presence of extraneous air in pleural space as a result of alveolar rupture	Tachypnea or apnea Systemic hypotension Sudden or persistent oxygen desaturation Grunting, nasal flaring Retractions Absent or diminished breath sounds Shift in point of maximum impulse of heart sounds Bradycardia, cyanosis	Evacuate trapped air in pleural space through needle aspiration or insertion of chest tube. In otherwise healthy term infants who do not require high oxygen concentration or mechanical ventilation, a nitrogen "washout" may be performed with 100% oxygen; this accelerates resorption of free air in pleura into blood; consider benefits and risks of hyperoxygenation.	Maintain close vigilance of infants with respiratory distress and those on assisted ventilation. Provide appropriate care of closed chest drainage apparatus. Ensure that emergency needle aspiration set-up is available.
Bronchopulmonary Dysplasia			

Pathologic process related to alveolar damage from lung disease, prolonged exposure to mechanical ventilation, high peak inspiratory pressures and oxygen, and immature alveoli and respiratory tract	Dyspnea
	Barrel chest
	Inability to wean from oxygen or mechanical ventilation after course of respiratory distress syndrome (surfactant deficiency)
	Wheezing
		Prevention—Administer maternal steroids; administer exogenous surfactant postnatally.
		Provide early detection with pulmonary function tests.
		Use synchronized or volume guarantee ventilation, decreased inspiratory pressures, or nasal CPAP.
		Prevent air leaks.
		Use high-frequency ventilation.
		Prevent or control respiratory or systemic infections.
		Minimize use of high oxygen concentrations in neonatal resuscitation and with mechanical ventilation; monitor oxygen saturation and implement resuscitation according to neonate response to low oxygen administration.
		Diagnosis established:
		  Support respiratory efforts.
		  Maintain adequate oxygenation, and avoid hypoxemia.
		  Administer diuretics, bronchodilators.
		  Provide supplemental oxygen in hospital or home.
		  Prevent upper respiratory infections (e.g., RSV).
		  Administer age-appropriate immunizations (e.g., pneumococcal).
			Provide individualized developmental care and enhancement.
			Monitor oxygen saturations closely in preterm infants, and avoid hyperoxemia.
			Provide opportunities for additional rest during feedings.
			Observe for signs of fluid overload or pulmonary edema.
			Assist with home oxygen therapy as needed.
			Assess susceptibility to upper respiratory tract infections and need for frequent hospitalization for respiratory dysfunction.
			Provide increased caloric density (feedings) with human milk fortifier or protein supplements.

Persistent Pulmonary Hypertension of the Newborn			
Severe pulmonary hypertension and large right-to-left shunt through foramen ovale and ductus arteriosus; often associated with conditions such as meconium aspiration, congenital diaphragmatic hernia, congenital cardiac anomalies	Hypoxia Marked cyanosis Tachypnea with grunting and retractions Decreased peripheral pulses and prolonged capillary refill (poor perfusion) Shock	Provide supplemental oxygen and assisted ventilation. Administer systemic vasodilators such as sildenafil to increase pulmonary perfusion and systemic oxygenation. Maintain acid-base balance. Prevent hypoxemia and hypercarbia. Regulate intravenous fluids. Administer inhaled nitric oxide or ECMO.	See Care of the High-Risk Newborn and Family and Respiratory Distress Syndrome. Provide nursing care to reduce stress to infant, especially noxious stimuli that cause increased oxygen demands. Decrease physical manipulation and disturbance. Monitor oxygenation status.

TABLE 25.9 Respiratory Complications—cont'd

Description	Clinical Manifestations	Therapeutic Management	Care Management
Retinopathy of Prematurity			
Severe vascular constriction in immature retinal vasculature followed by hypoxemia in retina, which in turn stimulates abnormal vascular proliferation of retinal capillaries into hypoxic area; as retinal veins dilate and multiply in direction of lens, retinal detachment may occur if untreated Multifactorial etiology—preterm birth major risk factor	Progressive vascular growth of retina Eventual blindness if not treated Diagnosed by ophthalmologic examination	Prevent preterm birth. Provide early screening and detection in infants who are born at <30 weeks of gestation and weigh <1500 g (3 lbs 5 oz) and those with a birth weight between 1500 (3 lbs 5 oz) and 2000 g (4 lbs 6.5 oz) with an unstable clinical course (AAP Section on Ophthalmology, American Academy of Ophthalmology, American Association for Pediatric Ophthalmology and Strabismus, & American Association of Certified Orthoptists, 2013). Decrease exposure to bright, direct lighting; although exposure to bright light has not been proven to contribute to retinopathy of prematurity, such exposure is undesirable from a neurobehavioral developmental perspective. Use supplemental oxygen judiciously, and monitor oxygen blood levels carefully; prevent wide fluctuations in oxygen blood levels (hyperoxia and hypoxia). Arrest vascular proliferation process—cryotherapy or laser photocoagulation; surgical repair of detached retina. Recently there has been increased interest in administration of an antivascular endothelial growth factor drug bevacizumab, which arrests proliferation of vessels and prevents retinal detachment commonly seen in retinopathy of prematurity. This therapy is an alternative treatment to the use of laser therapy (Hwang, Hubbard, Hutchinson, et al., 2015).	See Care of the High-Risk Newborn and Family. Provide preventive care by monitoring blood oxygen levels closely, responding promptly to saturation alarms, and preventing fluctuations in blood oxygen levels. Provide postoperative pain management if surgery is performed. Provide parental education and support. Provide nursing care using principles of individualized developmental care.

Data from American Academy of Pediatrics, & American Heart Association. (2016). *Textbook of neonatal resuscitation* (7th ed.). Elk Grove Village IL: Author; American Academy of Pediatrics Section on Ophthalmology, American Academy of Ophthalmology, American Association for Pediatric Ophthalmology and Strabismus, et al. (2013). Screening examination of premature infants for retinopathy of prematurity. *Pediatrics, 131*(1), 189–195; Hwang, C. K., Hubbard, G. B., Hutchinson, A. K., et al. (2015). Outcomes after intravitreal bevacizumab versus laser photocoagulation for retinopathy of prematurity. *Ophthalmology, 122*(5), 1008–1015.

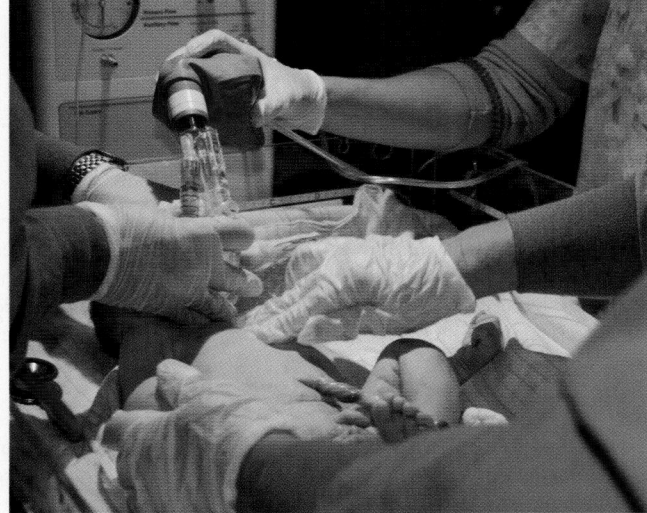

FIG 25.12 Infant being resuscitated at birth. Note presence of meconium on abdomen and umbilical cord. (Courtesy of Shannon Perry, Phoenix, AZ.)

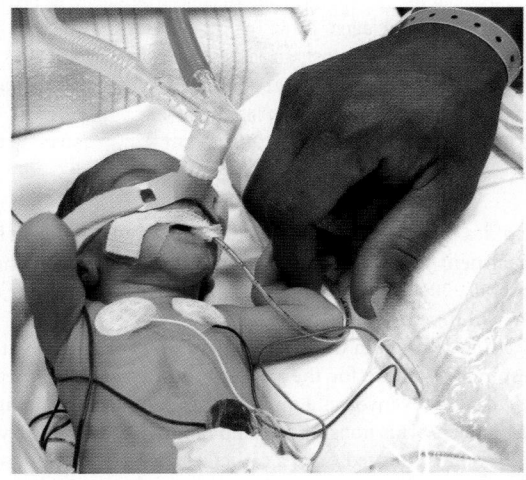

FIG 25.13 Infant on nasal continuous positive airway pressure with father's finger in hand. (Courtesy of E. Jacobs, Texas Children's Hospital, Houston, TX.)

EVIDENCE-BASED PRACTICE

Use of Room Air or Low Oxygen for Newborn Stabilization and Resuscitation in the Delivery Room

Ask the Question

PICOT Question: Is room air or low oxygen (O_2) better for newborn stabilization and resuscitation in the delivery room?

Search for Evidence

Search Strategies: Search selection included English-language publications on room air or low O_2 use for newborn stabilization and resuscitation in delivery room in past 5 years.
Databases Used: PubMed

Critical Appraisal of the Evidence

- Stabilization or resuscitation in the delivery room with fraction of inspired oxygen (FiO_2) below 100% or room air can be initiated without contributing to morbidity (Davis & Dawson, 2012).
- Systematic review of optimal initial FiO_2 use for stabilization or resuscitation of preterm newborns found a significant reduction in mortality when a low initial FiO_2 was used (Saugstad, Aune, Aguar, et al., 2014).
- In neonates born at less than 32 weeks of gestational age, resuscitation with 100% O_2 was associated with significantly more oxidative stress (Tataranno, Oei, Perrone, et al., 2015).
- In neonates 24 to 34 weeks of gestational age, use of a low FiO_2 (≤30%) for resuscitation was found to be safe. The supply of O_2 should be adjusted, depending on the response of the newborn (Kapadia, Chalak, Sparks, et al., 2013).
- In neonates less than or equal to 27 weeks of gestational age, those that received 21% to 40% oxygen had a higher risk for neurologic injury than those receiving 100% oxygen (Rabi, Lodha, Soraisham, et al., 2015).
- Use of heated and humidified air in neonates less than or equal to 32 weeks of gestational age during resuscitation or stabilization in the delivery room minimized postnatal heat loss (Meyer, Hou, Ishrar, et al., 2015).
- Initial use of 30% oxygen for preterm infants showed no difference in incidence of bronchopulmonary dysplasia or oxidative stress versus 65% oxygen (Rook, Schierbeek, Vento, et al., 2014)
- Blended oxygen with a low starting FiO_2 achieves oxygen saturation targets faster than either room air or 100% oxygen (Goldsmith & Kattwinkel, 2012).
- A meta-analysis showed no difference in risk for preterm morbidities after resuscitation with lower or higher FiO_2 (Oei, Vento, Rabi, et al., 2017).

Apply the Evidence: Nursing Implications

- There is good evidence with strong recommendations for initiating resuscitation with room air in term neonates (American Academy of Pediatrics, & American Heart Association, 2016). The optimal level of oxygen for initiating resuscitation in preterm infants remains to be determined. Factors such as newborn gestational age and heart rate should be taken into consideration when determining O_2 concentration for neonatal resuscitation.

Quality and Safety Competencies: Evidence-Based Practice*
Knowledge
Differentiate clinical opinion from research and evidence-based summaries.
Describe the various interventions for newborn stabilization and delivery room resuscitations with room air or low O_2.

Skills
Base individualized care plan on patient values, clinical expertise, and evidence.
Integrate evidence into practice by using interventions for newborn stabilization and delivery room resuscitations with room air or low O_2.

Attitudes
Value the concept of evidence-based practice as integral in determining best clinical practice.
Appreciate strengths and weakness of evidence for newborn stabilization and delivery room resuscitations with room air or low oxygen.

References
American Academy of Pediatrics & American Heart Association. (2016). *Textbook of neonatal resuscitation* (7th ed.). Elk Grove Village IL: Author.
Davis, P. G., & Dawson, J. A. (2012). New concepts in neonatal resuscitation. *Current Opinion in Pediatrics, 24*(2), 147–153.
Goldsmith, J. P., & Kattwinkel, J. (2012). The role of oxygen in the delivery room. *Clinics in Perinatology, 39*(4), 803–815.
Kapadia, V. S., Chalak, L. F., Sparks, J. E., et al. (2013). Resuscitation of preterm neonates with limited versus high oxygen strategy. *Pediatrics, 132*(6), e1488–e1496.
Meyer, M. P., Hou, D., Ishrar, N. N., et al. (2015). Initial respiratory support with cold, dry gas versus heated humidified gas and admission temperature of preterm infants. *Journal of Pediatrics, 166*(2), 245–250.
Oei, J. L., Vento, M., Rabi, Y., et al. (2017). Higher or lower oxygen for delivery room resuscitation of preterm infants below 28 completed weeks: A meta-analysis. *Archives of Disease in Childhood. Fetal and Neonatal Edition, 102*(1), F24–F30.
Rabi, Y., Lodha, A., Soraisham, A., et al. (2015). Outcomes of preterm infants following the introduction of room air resuscitation. *Resuscitation, 96*, 252–259.
Rook, D., Schierbeek, H., Vento, M., et al. (2014). Resuscitation of preterm infants with different inspired oxygen fractions. *Journal of Pediatrics, 164*(6), 1322–1326.
Saugstad, O. D., Aune, D., Aguar, M., et al. (2014). Systematic review and meta-analysis of optimal initial fraction of oxygen levels in the delivery room at ≤32 weeks. *Acta Paediatrica, 103*(7), 744–751.
Tataranno, M. L., Oei, J. L., Perrone, S., et al. (2015). Resuscitating preterm infants with 100% oxygen is associated with higher oxidative stress than room air. *Acta Paediatrica, 104*(8), 759–765.

Olga A. Taylor

*Adapted from QSEN at www.qsen.org.

Sildenafil, a potent vasodilator, has demonstrated significant benefits in the treatment of persistent pulmonary hypertension in neonates (Gardner et al., 2016; Shah & Ohlsson, 2011). The drug may be administered by NG tube or via IV route.

ECMO may be used in the management of term infants with acute severe respiratory failure for the same conditions as those mentioned for INO. This therapy involves a modified heart-lung machine, although with ECMO the heart is not stopped, and blood does not entirely bypass the lungs. Blood is shunted from a catheter in the right atrium or right internal jugular vein by gravity to a servo-regulated roller pump, pumped through a membrane lung where it is oxygenated and through a small heat exchanger, and then returned to the systemic circulation via a major artery such as the carotid artery to the aortic arch. ECMO provides oxygen to the circulation; allows the lungs to "rest"; and decreases pulmonary hypertension and hypoxemia in such conditions as persistent pulmonary hypertension of the newborn, congenital diaphragmatic hernia, sepsis, meconium aspiration, and severe pneumonia (Gardner et al., 2016).

Necrotizing Enterocolitis

Necrotizing enterocolitis (NEC) is an acute inflammatory disease of the bowel with increased incidence in preterm infants. The precise cause of NEC remains uncertain, but it appears to occur in infants whose GI tracts have experienced vascular compromise. Intestinal ischemia of unknown etiology, immature GI host defenses, bacterial proliferation, and feeding substrate are now believed to have a multifactorial role in the etiology of NEC. Preterm birth remains the most prominent risk factor in the development of NEC (Bucher, Pacetti, Lovvorn, et al., 2016).

The damage to mucosal cells lining the bowel wall can be significant. Diminished blood supply to these cells causes their death in large numbers; they stop secreting protective, lubricating mucus; and the thin, unprotected bowel wall is attacked by proteolytic enzymes. Thus the bowel wall continues to swell and break down; it is unable to synthesize protective IgM; and the mucosa is permeable to macromolecules (e.g., exotoxins), which further hampers intestinal defenses. Gas-forming bacteria invade the damaged areas to produce pneumatosis intestinalis, the presence of gas in the submucosal or subserosal surfaces of the bowel.

A consistent relationship has been observed between the development of NEC and enteric feeding of hypertonic substances (e.g., formula, hyperosmolar medications). It is unclear whether this connection is a result of the formula imposing a stress on an ischemic bowel or serving as a substrate for bacterial growth or possibly a combination of these factors. It has also been suggested that the absence of protective factors found in breast milk may account for the higher incidence of NEC in infants who receive formula feedings (Lawrence & Lawrence, 2016).

Radiographic studies show a sausage-shaped dilation of the intestine that progresses to marked distention and the characteristic pneumatosis intestinalis (i.e., "soapsuds," or the bubbly appearance of thickened bowel wall and ultralumina). There may be air in the portal circulation or free air observed in the abdomen, indicating perforation. Laboratory findings may include anemia, leukopenia, leukocytosis, metabolic acidosis, and electrolyte imbalance. In severe cases, coagulopathy (DIC) or thrombocytopenia may be evident. Organisms are often cultured from blood, although bacteremia or septicemia may not be prominent early in the course of the disease (Bucher et al., 2016).

Treatment of NEC begins with prevention. Minimal enteral feedings may be used for infants who are believed to have experienced birth asphyxia. Breast milk is the preferred enteral nutrient because it confers some passive immunity (IgA), macrophages, and lysozymes. The early clinical signs of NEC are subtle and nonspecific and may often be overlooked for other conditions; the earliest clinical signs include lethargy, abdominal distention, and high gastric residuals (Kastenberg & Sylvester, 2013).

Minimal enteral feedings (trophic feeding, GI priming) have gained acceptance with no evidence of increased incidence of NEC. In particular, the use of fresh human milk has been shown to decrease the risk for NEC (Senterre, 2014). Systematic reviews of the role of probiotics such as *Lactobacillus acidophilus* and *Bifidobacterium infantis* administered with enteral feedings for the prevention of NEC have demonstrated a reduced incidence of severe NEC and mortality in preterm infants (Alfaleh, Anabrees, Bassler, et al., 2011; Patel & Denning, 2013). The preferred type and optimal dosing of probiotics remain to be determined. There is evidence that the use of standardized feeding protocols that guide decisions about the initiation of feedings in preterm infants, advancement of feedings, and management of feeding intolerance may help prevent NEC (Gephart & Hanson, 2013). The role of lactoferrin (the major whey protein in human milk) in combination with lysozyme (also found in human milk) may have a significant role in the prevention of NEC and neonatal sepsis in high-risk preterm infants; both act in the intestine to kill harmful bacteria and enhance intestinal immune properties (Sherman, 2013).

Medical treatment of infants with confirmed NEC consists of discontinuation of all oral feedings; institution of abdominal decompression via NG suction; administration of IV antibiotics; and correction of extravascular volume depletion, electrolyte abnormalities, acid–base imbalances, and hypoxia. Replacing oral feedings with parenteral fluids decreases the need for oxygen and circulation to the bowel. Serial abdominal radiographs (supine and left lateral decubitus) are taken in the acute phase to monitor for possible progression of the disease to intestinal perforation.

With early recognition and treatment, medical management is increasingly successful. If there is progressive deterioration under medical management or evidence of perforation, surgical intervention is considered. Extensive involvement may necessitate surgical intervention and establishment of an ileostomy, jejunostomy, or colostomy. Sequelae in surviving infants include short-bowel syndrome (see Chapter 41), colonic stricture with obstruction, fat malabsorption, and growth failure secondary to intestinal dysfunction. A variety of surgical interventions for NEC are available and depend on the extent of bowel necrosis, associated illness factors, and infant stability (Bucher et al., 2016). Intestinal transplantation has been successful in some former preterm infants with NEC-associated short-bowel syndrome who had already developed life-threatening total parenteral nutrition–related complications. Transplantation may be a lifesaving option for infants who previously faced high morbidity and mortality (Amin, Pappas, Iyengar, 2013).

Care Management

Nursing responsibilities begin with the prompt recognition of the early warning signs of NEC. Because the signs are similar to those observed in many other disorders of newborns, nurses must constantly be aware of the possibility of this disease in infants who are at high risk for NEC (Box 25.5).

When the disease is suspected, the nurse assists with diagnostic procedures and implements the therapeutic regimen. Vital signs, including BP, are monitored for changes that might indicate bowel perforation, septicemia, or cardiovascular shock; and measures are instituted to prevent possible transmission to other infants. It is especially important to avoid rectal temperatures because of the increased risk for perforation. To avoid pressure on the distended abdomen and facilitate continuous observation, infants are often left undiapered and positioned supine or side-lying.

Nurses observe for indications of early development of NEC. Assessment of high-risk infants includes checking the appearance of the abdomen for distention, measuring abdominal girth, measuring residual gastric contents before feedings, and listening for bowel sounds.

Conscientious attention to nutrition and hydration needs is essential; antibiotics are administered as prescribed. The time at which oral feedings are reinstituted varies considerably but is usually at least 7 to 10 days after diagnosis and treatment. Feeding is usually reestablished using human milk if available.

Because NEC is an infectious disease, one of the most important nursing functions is control of infection. Strict hand hygiene is the

---

BOX 25.5   Clinical Manifestations of Necrotizing Enterocolitis

Nonspecific Clinical Signs
- Lethargy
- Poor feeding
- Hypotension
- Vomiting
- Apnea
- Decreased urinary output
- Unstable body temperature
- Jaundice

Specific Signs
- Distended (often shiny) abdomen
- Blood in stools or gastric contents
- Gastric retention (undigested formula)
- Localized abdominal wall erythema or induration
- Bilious vomitus

primary barrier to its spread, and confirmed multiple cases of NEC are isolated. Persons with symptoms of a GI disorder should not care for these or any other infants.

Infants who require surgery require the same careful postoperative attention and observation as any infant who had abdominal surgery, including ostomy care (as applicable). This condition is one of the most common reasons for performing ostomies on newborns. Throughout the medical and surgical management of infants with NEC, the nurse should be continually alert to signs of complications such as septicemia, DIC, hypoglycemia, and other metabolic derangements.

POSTTERM INFANTS

Infants born after 42 0/7 weeks of gestation are considered to be postterm, or postmature, regardless of birth weight. The cause of delayed birth is unknown. In some cases, the placenta continues to function and fetal growth continues, resulting in macrosomia. Other postterm infants appear appropriate for gestational age but show the characteristics of progressive placental dysfunction; this is also known as *dysmaturity syndrome*. These infants display characteristics such as absence of lanugo, little if any vernix caseosa, abundant scalp hair, and long fingernails. The skin is often cracked, parchment-like, and peeling. A common finding in postterm infants is a wasted physical appearance that reflects intrauterine deprivation. Depletion of subcutaneous fat gives them a thin, elongated appearance. The minimal vernix caseosa that remains in the skinfolds may be stained a deep yellow or green, which is usually an indication of meconium in the amniotic fluid (Blickstein & Flidel-Rimon, 2015).

There is a significant increase in fetal and neonatal mortality in postterm infants compared with those born at term. Macrosomic infants are at increased risk for birth injury, neurologic damage, and death. Infants with dysmaturity syndrome are especially prone to fetal distress associated with the decreasing efficiency of the placenta, macrosomia, and meconium aspiration syndrome. The greatest risk occurs during the stresses of labor and birth, particularly in infants of primigravidas. Close surveillance with fetal assessment and induction of labor is usually recommended when pregnancy extends beyond 40 weeks (Blickstein & Flidel-Rimon, 2015).

CARE OF THE HIGH RISK NEWBORN AND FAMILY

ASSESSMENT

A thorough systematic physical assessment is an essential component in the care of high risk infants. Subtle changes in feeding behavior, activity, color, oxygen saturation (Sao_2), or vital signs often indicate an underlying problem. LBW preterm infants, especially VLBW or ELBW infants, are ill equipped to withstand prolonged physiologic stress and may die within minutes of exhibiting abnormal symptoms if the underlying pathologic process is not corrected. Alert nurses are aware of subtle changes and react promptly to implement interventions that promote optimal functioning in high-risk neonates. Changes in the infant's status are noted through ongoing observations of adaptation to the extrauterine environment.

Observational assessments of high risk infants are made according to each infant's acuity; critically ill infants require close observation and assessment of respiratory function, including continuous pulse oximetry, electrolytes, and evaluation of blood gases. Accurate documentation of the infant's status is an integral component of nursing care. With the aid of continuous, sophisticated cardiopulmonary monitoring, nursing assessments and daily care can be coordinated to allow for minimal handling of the infant (especially VLBW or ELBW infants) to decrease the effects of environmental stress.

Most neonates under intensive observation are placed in a controlled thermal environment and monitored for heart rate, respiratory activity, and temperature. The monitoring devices are equipped with an alarm system that indicates when the vital signs are above or below preset limits.

Blood pressure (BP) is monitored routinely in sick neonates by either internal or external means. Direct recording with arterial catheters is often used but carries the risks inherent in any procedure in which a catheter is introduced into an artery. BP values gradually increase over the first month of life in preterm and term infants. BP norms vary by gestational age and weight, medications such as corticosteroids, and disease process. One of the primary considerations in the preterm infant is the relationship between systemic BP and the determination of adequate cerebral blood flow. In the NICU, frequent laboratory examinations and their interpretation are integral parts of the ongoing assessment of infants' progress. Accurate intake and output records are kept on all acutely ill infants. An accurate output can be obtained by collecting urine in a plastic urine collection bag specifically made for preterm infants or by weighing the diapers, which is the simplest and least traumatic means of measuring urinary output. The preweighed wet diaper is weighed on a gram scale, and the gram weight of the urine is converted directly to milliliters (e.g., 1 g = 1 mL).

Blood testing is a necessary part of the ongoing assessment and monitoring of the high-risk newborn's progress. The tests most often performed are CBC, blood glucose, bilirubin, calcium, serum electrolytes, and blood gases. Samples may be obtained from the heel; by venipuncture; by arterial puncture; or by an indwelling catheter in an umbilical vein, an umbilical artery, or a peripheral artery. When numerous blood samples must be drawn, it is important to maintain an accurate record of the amount of blood being removed, especially in ELBW and VLBW infants, who can ill afford to have their blood supply depleted during the acute phase of their illness. There is an increased emphasis on drawing as little blood as possible from high-risk neonates to minimize the depletion of blood volume and avoid blood transfusions and associated complications. To avoid the need for repeated arterial punctures, pulse oximetry, which measures the saturation or percentage of oxygen in the hemoglobin, is typically used. Although used less frequently than pulse oximetry, transcutaneous carbon dioxide ($tcPco_2$) is monitored in some situations. The nurse notes changes in oxygenation (or other aspects being monitored) associated with handling and adjusts the infant's care accordingly. The frequency of vital signs is determined by the infant's acuity level and response to handling.

RESPIRATORY SUPPORT

The primary objective in the care of high-risk infants is to establish and maintain respiration. Many infants require supplemental oxygen and assisted ventilation. All infants require appropriate positioning to maximize oxygenation and ventilation. Oxygen therapy is provided on the basis of the infant's requirements and illness (see the "Respiratory Distress Syndrome" section earlier in the chapter).

THERMOREGULATION

After or concurrent with the establishment of respiration, the most crucial need of LBW infants is application of external warmth. Preventing heat loss in distressed infants is absolutely essential for survival, and maintaining a neutral thermal environment is a challenging aspect of neonatal intensive care nursing. Heat production is a complicated process that involves the cardiovascular, neurologic, and metabolic systems;

and immature neonates have all of the problems related to heat production that are faced by full term infants (see the "Thermogenic System" section in Chapter 22). However, LBW infants are placed at further disadvantage by a number of additional problems. They have an even smaller muscle mass and fewer deposits of brown fat for producing heat, lack insulating subcutaneous fat, and have poor reflex control of skin capillaries.

To delay or prevent the effects of cold stress, at-risk newborns are placed in a heated environment immediately after birth, where they remain until they are able to maintain thermal stability (i.e., the capacity to balance heat production and conservation with heat dissipation). Because overheating produces an increase in oxygen and calorie consumption, infants are also jeopardized in a hyperthermic environment. A neutral thermal environment is one at which oxygen consumption is minimal but adequate to maintain body temperature (Blackburn, 2013). Studies indicate that optimum thermoneutrality cannot be predicted for every high-risk infant's needs. In healthy term infants, it is recommended that axillary temperatures be maintained at 36.5° to 37.5° C (97.7° to 99.5° F); in preterm infants, axillary temperatures of 36.3° to 36.9° C (97.3° to 98.4° F) are considered appropriate (Gardner & Hernández, 2016).

VLBW and ELBW infants, with thin skin and almost no subcutaneous fat, can control body heat loss or gain only within a limited range of environmental temperatures. In these infants, heat loss from radiation, evaporation, and transepidermal water loss is 3 to 5 times greater than in larger infants, and a decrease in body temperature is associated with an increase in mortality. Further research is needed to define a neutral thermal environment for ELBW infants.

The consequences of cold stress that produce additional hazards to neonates are (1) hypoxia, (2) metabolic acidosis, and (3) hypoglycemia. Increased metabolism in response to chilling creates a compensatory increase in oxygen and calorie consumption. If available oxygen is not increased to accommodate this need, arterial oxygen tension is decreased. This is further complicated by a smaller lung volume in relation to the metabolic rate, which creates diminished oxygen in the blood and concurrent pulmonary disorders. A small advantage is gained by the presence of fetal hemoglobin because its increased capacity to carry oxygen allows the infant to exist for longer periods in conditions of lowered oxygen tension.

The three primary methods for maintaining a neutral thermal environment are the use of an incubator (Fig. 25.14), a radiant warming panel, and an open bassinet with cotton blankets. A dressed infant under blankets can maintain a certain temperature within a wider range of environmental temperatures; however, the close observations required with a high-risk infant are best accomplished if the infant remains partially unclothed. The incubator should always be prewarmed before placing an infant in it. Inside or outside the incubator, head coverings are effective in preventing heat loss. A fabric-insulated or wool cap is more effective than one fashioned from stockinette. The use of a heated gel mattress with radiant heat has been shown to decrease the incidence of radiation heat loss significantly and preserve an adequate neutral thermal environment for the VLBW neonate (Fastman, Howell, Holzman, et al., 2014; Lewis, Sanders, & Brockopp, 2011). An effective means for maintaining the desired range of temperature in the infant is the use of a manually adjusted or automatically controlled (servo-controlled) incubator. The latter mechanism, when set at the upper and lower limits of the desired circulating air temperature range, adjusts automatically in response to signals from a thermal sensor attached to the abdominal skin. If the infant's temperature drops, the warming device is triggered to increase heat output. The servo control is usually set to a desired skin temperature between 36° and 36.5° C (96.8° and 97.7° F) (Gardner & Hernández, 2016).

A high-humidity atmosphere contributes to maintaining body temperature by reducing evaporative heat loss. A number of "microenvironments" may be used with VLBW and ELBW infants to minimize evaporative and insensible water losses. These include items such as food-grade plastic bags or plastic wrap, humidified reservoirs for incubators, and humidified plastic heat shields covered with plastic wrap. When such environments are used, special care must be taken to avoid bacterial contamination of the warm and humid environment by organisms such as *Pseudomonas* and *Serratia,* which have an affinity for moist environments. Postnatally acquired pneumonia from such organisms may be fatal, particularly in VLBW infants. A systematic review found that plastic wraps (polyethylene) or bags lead to higher temperatures on admission to neonatal units and less hypothermia (Lewis et al., 2011; Li, Guo, Zou, et al., 2016). This practice is now recommended in the Neonatal Resuscitation Program guidelines published by the American Academy of Pediatrics and American Heart Association (AAP & AHA, 2016).

Skin-to-skin (kangaroo) contact (Fig. 25.15) between a stable preterm infant and parent is also a viable option for interaction because of the maintenance of appropriate body temperature by the infant. Other benefits of skin-to-skin contact are discussed later in this chapter.

PROTECTION FROM INFECTION

Protection from infection is an integral part of all newborn care, but it is critical for preterm and sick neonates because they are at increased risk for infection. Thorough, meticulous, and frequent hand hygiene is the foundation of a preventive program. This includes *all* people who come in contact with infants and their equipment. After handling another infant or equipment, no one should ever touch an infant without first performing hand hygiene (AAP & ACOG, 2012).

Personnel with infectious disorders are either excluded from the unit until they are no longer infectious or are required to wear suitable shields such as masks or gloves to reduce the likelihood of contamination. An annual influenza vaccination is recommended for NICU personnel. Standard Precautions as a method of infection control are instituted in all nursery areas to protect the infants and staff. The benefit of "gowning" by visitors and hospital staff to control infection is not supported by research. Sibling visitation in the NICU has not been shown to increase HAIs; however, appropriate screening for upper respiratory illness in siblings is recommended (AAP & ACOG, 2012).

The sources of infection rise in direct relationship to the number of persons and pieces of equipment coming in contact with the infants.

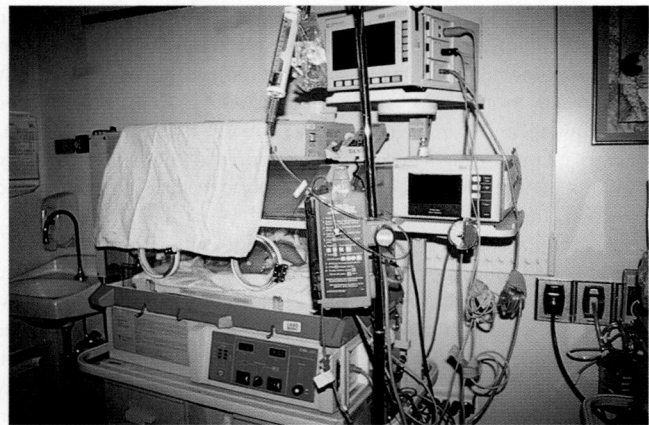

FIG 25.14 Infant in double-walled incubator with a blanket for a light shield. (Courtesy of Marjorie Pyle, RNC, Lifecircle, Costa Mesa, CA.)

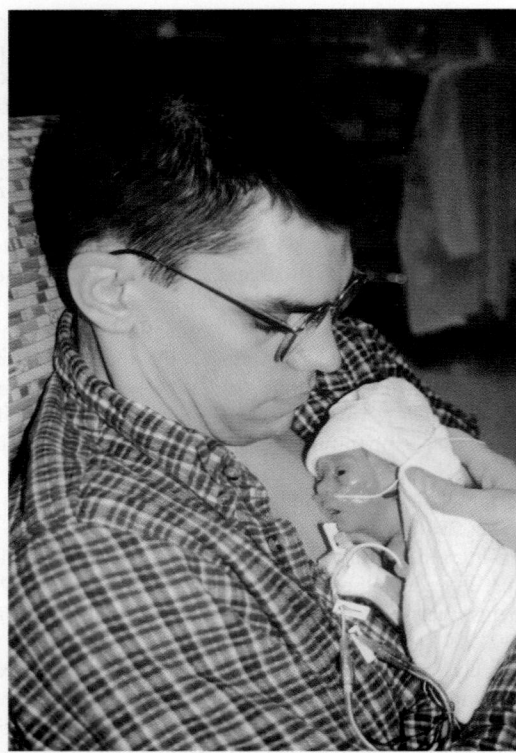

FIG 25.15 Father providing skin-to-skin care (kangaroo care). (Courtesy of Judy Meyr, St Louis, MO).

Equipment used in the care of infants is cleaned on a regular basis in accordance with manufacturer recommendations or institutional protocol; this includes cleaning cribs, mattresses, incubators, radiant warmers, cardiorespiratory monitors, pulse oximeters, and vital sign–monitoring equipment after usage with one infant and before usage with another. Because organisms thrive best in water, plumbing fixtures and humidifying equipment are particularly hazardous. Disposable equipment used for water-related therapies such as nebulizers and plastic tubing is changed regularly.

HYDRATION

High-risk infants often receive supplemental parenteral fluids to supply additional calories, electrolytes, and water. Adequate hydration is particularly important in preterm infants because their extracellular water content is higher than in term infants, their body surface is larger, and the capacity for handling fluid shifts is limited in preterm infants' underdeveloped kidneys. Therefore these infants are highly vulnerable to fluid depletion (Nyp, Brunkhorst, Reavey, et al., 2016).

Parenteral fluids may be given to the high-risk neonate via several routes, depending on the nature of the illness, the duration and type of fluid therapy, and unit preference. Common routes of fluid infusion include peripheral, peripherally inserted central venous (or percutaneous central venous) catheters; and surgically inserted central venous and umbilical venous catheters. The preferred sites for peripheral IV infusions in neonates are the peripheral veins on the dorsal surfaces of the hands or feet. Alternative sites are scalp veins and antecubital veins. Special precautions and frequent observations must accompany the use of peripheral lines (Restieaux, Maw, Broadbent, et al., 2013). In many neonatal centers, the percutaneous central venous catheter is used for parenteral therapy and medication administration because it reduces the need for frequent IV starts.

In most facilities, NICU nurses insert peripheral IV catheters and maintain the infusions. Intravenous fluids must always be delivered by continuous infusion pumps that deliver minute volumes at a preset flow rate. The catheter is secured to the skin with a transparent dressing or minimum amount of tape (see the "Skin Care" section later in the chapter), with care taken not to cause undue pressure from the catheter hub and tubing. Because all infants, especially those who are ELBW and VLBW, are highly vulnerable to any fluid shifts, infusion rates are regulated carefully and checked hourly to prevent tissue damage from extravasation, fluid overload, or dehydration. Pulmonary edema, congestive heart failure, patent ductus arteriosus, and intraventricular hemorrhage can occur with fluid overload. Dehydration can cause electrolyte disturbances with potentially serious CNS effects.

Infants who are ELBW, tachypneic, receiving phototherapy, or in a radiant warmer have increased insensible water losses that require appropriate fluid adjustments (Halbardier, 2015). Nurses must monitor fluid status by daily (or more frequent) weights and accurate measurement of intake and output of all fluids, including medications and blood products. Serum electrolytes are monitored per unit protocol, and urine electrolytes are obtained as warranted by the infant's condition. ELBW infants often require more frequent monitoring of these parameters because of their inordinate transepidermal fluid loss, immature renal function, and propensity to dehydration or overhydration. Intolerance of even dextrose 5% is not uncommon in ELBW infants, with subsequent glycosuria and osmotic diuresis. Alterations in behavior, alertness, or activity level in these infants receiving IV fluids may signal an electrolyte imbalance, hypoglycemia, or hyperglycemia. Nurses should also be observant for tremors or seizures in VLBW or ELBW infants because these may be a sign of hyponatremia or hypernatremia (Nyp et al., 2016).

NUTRITION

Optimum nutrition is critical in the management of LBW and preterm infants, but there are difficulties in providing for their nutritional needs. The various mechanisms for ingestion and digestion of foods are not fully developed; the more immature the infant, the greater the problem. In addition, the nutritional requirements for this group of infants are not known with certainty. It is known that all preterm infants are at risk because of poor nutritional stores and several physical and developmental characteristics.

An infant's nutritional needs for rapid growth and daily maintenance must be met in the presence of physiologic challenges. Although some sucking and swallowing activities are demonstrated before birth and in preterm infants, coordination of these mechanisms does not occur until approximately 32 to 34 weeks of gestation, and they are not fully synchronized until 36 to 37 weeks. Initial sucking is not accompanied by swallowing, and esophageal contractions are uncoordinated. Consequently, infants are highly prone to aspiration and its attendant dangers. As infants mature, the suck-swallow pattern develops but is slow and ineffectual, and these reflexes may also become easily exhausted.

The amount and method of feeding are determined by the infant's size and condition. Nutrition can be provided by either the parenteral or enteral route or by a combination of the two. Infants who are ELBW, VLBW, or critically ill often obtain most of their nutrients by the parenteral route because of their inability to digest and absorb enteral nutrition. Illness factors resulting in hypoxia and major organ immaturity further preclude the use of enteral feeding until the infant's condition has stabilized. NEC has previously been associated with enteral feedings in acutely ill or distressed infants (see the "Necrotizing Enterocolitis" section earlier in the chapter). Total parenteral nutritional support of acutely ill infants may be accomplished successfully with commercially available IV solutions specifically designed to meet the infant's nutritional needs, including protein, amino acids, trace minerals, vitamins, carbohydrates (dextrose), and fat (lipid emulsion).

Studies have shown that there are benefits to the early introduction of small amounts of enteral feedings in metabolically stable preterm infants. These minimal enteral (trophic gastrointestinal priming) feedings have been shown to stimulate the infant's GI tract, preventing mucosal atrophy and subsequent enteral feeding difficulties. Enteral feedings with as little as 0.1 to 4 mL/kg of breast milk or preterm formula may be given by gavage as soon as the infant is medically stable. Parenteral hydration and nutrition are continued until the infant is able to tolerate an amount of enteral feeding sufficient to sustain growth. An increased incidence of NEC in VLBW infants receiving minimal enteral nutrition has not been substantiated (Ramani & Ambalavanan, 2013). Minimal enteral feedings increase mineral absorption, increase serum calcium and alkaline phosphatase activity, and substantially decrease the incidence of bilious gastric residuals and feeding intolerance in preterm infants. Minimal enteral feedings are recommended as the standard of care for feeding VLBW infants.

Although the timing of the first feeding has been a matter of controversy, most authorities now believe that early feeding (provided that the infant is medically stable) reduces the incidence of complicating factors such as hypoglycemia, dehydration, and the degree of hyperbilirubinemia. The feeding regimen used varies across neonatal intensive care units.

Breastfeeding

Ample evidence indicates that human milk is the best source of nutrition for term and preterm infants. Studies indicate that small preterm infants are able to breastfeed if they have adequate sucking and swallowing reflexes and there are no other contraindications such as respiratory complications or concurrent illness (Smith & Lucas, 2016). Mothers who wish to breastfeed their preterm infants are encouraged to express breast milk until their infants are sufficiently stable to tolerate breastfeeding. Appropriate guidelines for the storage of expressed mother's milk should be followed to decrease the risk for milk contamination and destruction of its beneficial properties (Lawrence & Lawrence, 2016).

Milk produced by mothers whose infants are born before term contains higher concentrations of protein, sodium, chloride, and IgA. Growth factors, hormones, prolactin, calcitonin, thyroxine (T_4), steroids, and taurine (an essential amino acid) are also present in human milk. Secretory IgA concentration is higher in the milk from mothers of preterm infants than in the milk from mothers of full term infants. IgA is important in the control of bacteria in the intestinal tract, where it inhibits adherence and proliferation of bacteria on epithelial surfaces. Additional protection from infection is provided by leukocytes, lactoferrin, and lysozyme, all of which are present in human milk. The milk produced by mothers for their infants changes in content over the first 30 days postnatally, at which time it is similar to full term human milk. Despite its benefits, LBW infants (<1500 g [3 lbs 5 oz]) who are fed unfortified human milk exclusively demonstrate decreased growth rates and nutritional deficiencies even beyond the hospitalization period. These infants often have inadequacies of calcium, phosphorus, protein, sodium, vitamins, and energy. Specially designed supplements for human milk have been developed to address these deficits. Fortifiers are commercially available, usually as a liquid or powder containing protein; carbohydrate; calcium; phosphorus; magnesium; sodium; and varied amounts of zinc, copper, and vitamins. Because fortifiers do not contain

sufficient iron, an exogenous source must be administered after enteral feedings (Lawrence & Lawrence, 2016).

Preterm infants may be able to breastfeed successfully earlier than previously believed (28 to 36 weeks); in addition, preterm infants who are breastfed rather than bottle-fed demonstrate fewer incidences of oxygen desaturation; absence of bradycardia; warmer skin temperature; and better coordination of breathing, sucking, and swallowing (Gardner & Lawrence, 2016). Preterm infants should be evaluated carefully for readiness to breastfeed, including assessment of behavioral state, ability to maintain body temperature outside an artificial heat source, respiratory status, and readiness to suckle at the mother's breast. Readiness to suckle may be accomplished with nonnutritive suckling at the breast during skin-to-skin (kangaroo) contact so the mother and newborn may become accustomed to one another (Gardner & Lawrence, 2016). Nasal cannula oxygen may also be provided during preterm breastfeeding on the basis of the infant's assessed requirements.

Transition to Oral Feedings

Vigorous infants feed by breast or bottle with little difficulty, but compromised preterm infants require alternative methods. The amount to be fed orally is determined largely by the infant's weight gain and tolerance of previous feedings and is increased by small increments until a satisfactory caloric intake is ensured.

The rate of progression to oral feedings that is well tolerated varies from one infant to another. Preterm infants require more time and patience to feed compared with full-term infants, and the oropharyngeal mechanism can be stressed by an attempt to feed too rapidly. It is important to not tire the infants or overtax their capacity to retain the feedings. When infants require a prolonged time to complete a feeding, gavage feeding may be considered for the next feeding.

A developmental approach to feeding considers the individual infant's readiness rather than initiating feedings based on weight and age or a predetermined time schedule. Feeding readiness is determined by each infant's medical status, energy level, ability to sustain a brief quiet alert state, spontaneous rooting and sucking behaviors, and hand-to-mouth behaviors (Kish, 2013). A preterm infant may experience difficulty coordinating sucking, swallowing, and breathing, with resultant apnea, bradycardia, and decreased oxygen saturation. The infant's ability to suck on a pacifier does not indicate complete readiness for nipple feeding or ability to coordinate the previously mentioned activities without some degree of stress; a gradual introduction of nippling in preterm infants is based on careful evaluation of their ability to maintain adequate cardiopulmonary functions while feeding.

Bottle Feeding

When selecting a feeding system, the nipple used should be relatively firm and stable. Although a high-flow, pliable nipple requires less energy to use, it may provide a flow rate that is too rapid for some preterm infants to manage without a risk for aspiration. A firmer nipple facilitates a more "cupped" tongue configuration and allows for a more controlled, manageable flow rate.

The infant is positioned in the feeder's arms or placed semi-upright in the lap and held with the back curved slightly to simulate the position assumed naturally by most full term newborns. The use of gentle cheek and jaw support for preterm infants has been shown to facilitate feedings. Stroking the infant's lips, cheeks, and tongue before feeding helps promote oral sensitivity. Inward and upward support to the infant's cheeks and a slightly upward lift to the chin are provided by the fingers to assist nipple compression during feeding.

Bottle feedings are continued if infants are able to tolerate the feedings and take the required amount. Some preterm infants respond more slowly than full term infants; therefore the feeding interval and the amount of the feeding are individualized. Preterm infants are often slow feeders and require patience, frequent rest periods, and frequent burping (or bubbling).

Gavage Feeding

Gavage feeding is a safe means of meeting the nutritional requirements of infants who are unable to feed orally. These infants are usually too weak to suck effectively, are unable to coordinate swallowing, and lack a gag reflex. Gavage feedings may be provided by continuous drip regulated via infusion pump or by intermittent bolus feedings. Studies have demonstrated an overall decrease in total milk fat concentration delivery when continuous gavage infusions are administered, which suggests that intermittent or bolus gavage of expressed mother's milk should be administered when possible (Rayyan, Rommel & Allegaert, 2015). Intermittent gavage feeding is used as an energy-conserving technique for infants learning to nipple feed who become excessively tired, listless, or cyanotic.

A size 3.5-, 5-, 6-, or 8-Fr feeding tube is used to instill the feeding; and the methods for determining correct placement are described later in the chapter (Fig. 25.16). Although the more relaxed lower esophageal sphincter makes passage of the tube easier, there may be changes in heart rate and BP in response to vagal stimulation. When an indwelling tube is required, consideration should be given to using a product made of Silastic rather than polyvinyl chloride (PVC) because PVC becomes stiff when exposed to body fluids.

The stomach is aspirated, the contents measured, and the aspirate returned as part of the feeding. However, this practice may vary, depending on circumstances and individual unit protocols. The amount of aspirate depends on the time since the previous feeding or concurrent illness.

With intermittent feedings, the milk or formula is allowed to flow by gravity, and the length of time varies. This procedure is not used as a timesaving method for the nurse. Complications of indwelling tubes include aspiration, obstructed nares, mucus plugs, purulent rhinitis, epistaxis, infection, and possible stomach perforation. Current best practice dictates a radiograph as the only certain way to determine NG tube placement in the stomach. Methods such as auscultation of an air bubble, neck-ear-xiphoid (NEX) measurements for insertion depth, or pH measurements are considered imprecise when used as the only method for determination of placement of feeding tubes in infants (Freeman, Saxton, & Holberton, 2012). Ellett, Cohen, Perkins, and associates (2011) developed an age-related, height-based regression equation for determining adequate gastric tube insertion length for use in neonates less than 1 month of age (corrected age). Others have developed guidelines for correct NG tube insertion and placement in LBW and term infants based on the infant's weight (Freeman et al.). Further research is needed to determine optimal positioning of feeding tubes in high-risk infants on intermittent bolus or continuous gavage feedings.

The infant may be held during gavage feedings by the caregiver or parent. If necessary, oxygen may be supplied via nasal cannula to facilitate handling. It is not recommended that the infant be removed from a primary source of oxygen for feedings because doing so decreases oxygen availability. Nonnutritive sucking (NNS) on a pacifier may help bring the infant to a quiet alert state in preparation for feeding. Proposed benefits of NNS include improved weight gain, improved milk intake, more stable heart rate and oxygen saturation, earlier age at full oral feedings, and improved behavioral state.

ENERGY CONSERVATION

One of the major goals of care for the high-risk infant is conservation of energy. Much of the care described in this section is directed toward

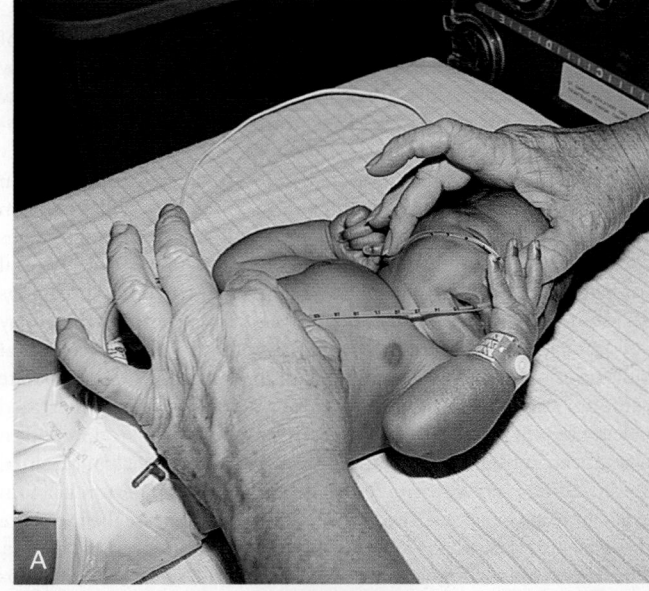

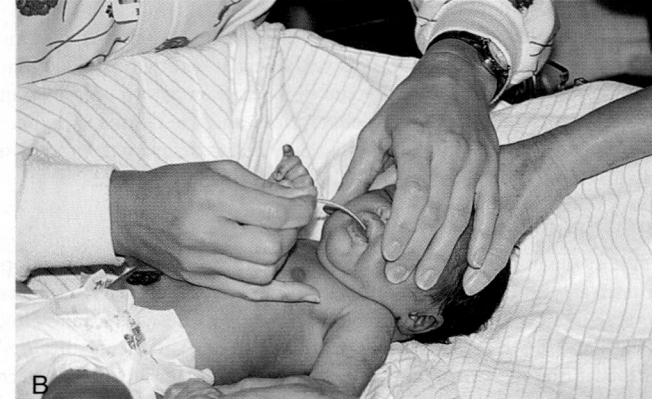

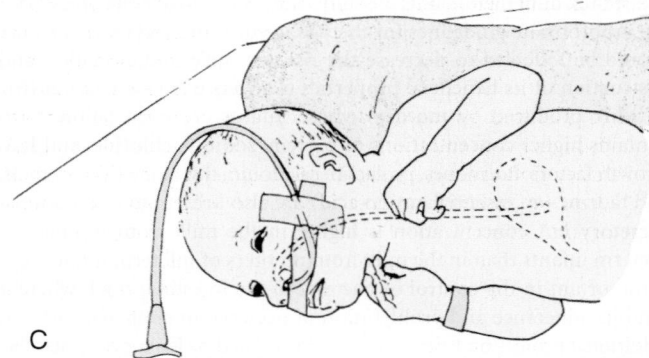

FIG 25.16 Gavage feeding. **A,** Measurement of gavage feeding tube from tip of nose to earlobe and to midpoint between end of xiphoid process and umbilicus. Tape may be used to mark correct length on tube. **B,** Insertion of gavage tube using orogastric route. **C,** Indwelling gavage tube, nasogastric route. After feeding by orogastric or nasogastric tube, infant is propped on right side or placed prone (preterm infant) for 1 hour to facilitate emptying of stomach into small intestine. Note rolled towel for support (see the column at left for methods to determine adequate feeding tube placement). (A and B, Courtesy of Marjorie Pyle, RNC, Lifecircle, Costa Mesa, CA.)

this goal (e.g., disturbing the infant as little as possible, maintaining a neutral thermal environment, gavage feeding as appropriate, promoting oxygenation, and judiciously implementing any caregiving activities that increase oxygen intake and caloric consumption). An infant who is not required to expend excess energy to breathe, eat, or maintain body temperature can use this energy for growth and development. Diminishing environmental noise levels and shading the infant from bright lights also promote rest (see the "Developmental Considerations" section later in the chapter).

SKIN CARE

The skin of preterm infants is characteristically immature relative to that of full term infants. In most preterm infants, the skin barrier properties resemble those of the term infant by 2 to 4 weeks' postnatal age, regardless of gestational age at birth. Because of its increased sensitivity and fragility, no alkaline-based soap that might destroy the acid mantle of the skin is used. The increased permeability of the skin facilitates absorption of ingredients. All skin products (e.g., alcohol, chlorhexidine, povidone-iodine) should be used with caution; the skin is rinsed with water afterward because these substances can cause severe irritation and chemical burns in VLBW and ELBW infants.

The skin is easily excoriated and denuded; therefore care must be taken to avoid damage to the delicate structure. The total skin is thinner than that of full term infants and lacks rete pegs, appendages that anchor the epidermis to the dermis. Therefore there is less cohesion between the thinner skin layers. The use of adhesive tape or bandages can excoriate the skin or adhere to the skin surface so well that the epidermis can be separated from the dermis and pulled away with the tape, thus altering skin barrier function. Pectin barriers and hydrocolloid adhesives may be useful because these products mold well to skin contours and adhere in moist conditions. Recommendations for protecting the integrity of the skin of preterm infants include using minimal adhesive tape, backing the tape with a skin barrier or hydrocolloid dressing, and delaying adhesive removal until adherence is reduced. Emollients such as Eucerin or Aquaphor have been used to promote skin integrity and prevent dry, cracking, and peeling skin in infants at risk for skin breakdown. Emollients may also reduce transepidermal water loss and protect infants from HAIs. However, in some studies these agents have been shown to increase the risk for coagulase-negative infections in preterm infants and therefore should be used with caution. The use and effectiveness of emollients in high-risk neonates is controversial, and further studies are needed (Telofski, Morello, Mack Correa, et al., 2012). Guidelines for skin care are listed in the Guidelines box: Neonatal Skin Care.

> ### ⚡ SAFETY ALERT
>
> It is unsafe to use scissors to remove dressings or tape from the extremities of very small and immature infants because it is easy to snip off tiny extremities or nick loosely attached skin. Solvents used to remove tape are avoided because they tend to dry and burn the skin.

During skin assessment of preterm infants, nurses are alert to the subtle signs that indicate zinc deficiency, a problem sometimes seen in infants who have inadequate intake or abnormal losses of zinc. Breakdown usually occurs in the areas around the mouth, buttocks, fingers, and toes. In preterm and VLBW infants, it can also occur in the creases of the neck, wrists, and ankles and around wounds. Zinc deficiency is most likely to appear in preterm infants with inadequate zinc intake, an ileostomy, short-bowel syndrome, or chronic diarrhea. Suspicious lesions are reported to the practitioner so that zinc supplements can

be prescribed. Skin injuries have been reported during the use of phototherapy blankets. Caution is warranted in using these products in ELBW infants and infants who are at risk for skin breakdown.

DEVELOPMENTAL CONSIDERATIONS

Much attention has been focused on the effects of early developmental intervention on both normal and preterm infants. Infants respond to a great variety of stimuli, and the atmosphere and activities of the NICU are overstimulating. Consequently, infants in NICUs are subjected to inappropriate stimulation that can be harmful. For example, the noise level that results from monitoring equipment, alarms, and general unit activity has been correlated with the incidence of intracranial hemorrhage, especially in ELBW and VLBW infants. Personnel should reduce noise-generating activities such as closing doors (including incubator portholes), listening to loud radios, talking loudly, and handling equipment (e.g., trash containers). Sound levels in the NICU can be monitored to identify problem areas, and appropriate measures can be instituted to reduce noise (Laubach, Wilhelm, & Carter, 2014). Nursing care activities such as taking vital signs, changing the infant's position, weighing, and changing diapers are associated with frequent periods of hypoxia, oxygen desaturation, and elevated ICP. The more immature the infant, the less able he or she is to habituate to a single procedure such as taking an oscillometric BP without becoming overstimulated.

Twenty-four hour surveillance of sick infants implies maximum visibility and the use of bright lights. Units should establish a night-day sleep pattern by darkening the room, covering cribs with blankets, or placing eye patches over the infant's eyes at night. Infants need scheduled rest periods during which the lights are dimmed, the incubators are covered with blankets, and the infants are not disturbed for handling of any kind. Sleep periods should be undisturbed for at least 50 minutes to allow complete sleep cycles. Clustering of care can promote longer uninterrupted periods of sleep (Legendre, Burtner, Martinez, et al., 2011).

Infants' eyes should be shielded from bright procedure lights to prevent potential harm. Many experts suggest that the human face, especially the parent's, is the best visual stimulus and that visual stimuli be kept to a minimum early in development. Developmental care, accentuating the infant's unique ability to achieve behavioral state organization, is tailored to the developmental level and tolerance of each infant based on a comprehensive behavioral assessment. During the early stages of development (especially before 33 weeks of gestation), external stimulation produces uncoordinated, random activity such as jerky limb extension, hyperflexion, and irregular vital signs. At this stage, infants need to have minimal environmental stimulation. Using the developmental model of supportive care, the nurse closely monitors physiologic and behavioral signs to promote organization and well-being of the high-risk infant during handling. Softly calling the infant by name and then gently placing a hand on the body signal that care is beginning and alleviate the abrupt interruption that precedes caregiving. Infants are handled with slow, controlled movements (some infants are unstable if moved abruptly), and their random movements are controlled with limbs held flexed close to their bodies during turning or other position changes. This containment or facilitated tucking may also be used before invasive procedures such as heelstick to alleviate distress. Blanket swaddling and nesting or containment have been shown to decrease physiologic and behavioral stress during routine care procedures such as bathing, weighing, and heelstick. A nest constructed by placing blanket rolls underneath the bed sheet helps infants maintain an attitude of flexion when prone or side lying.

Although it must be individually adjusted, skin-to-skin contact (kangaroo care) and short periods of gentle massage can help reduce stress in preterm infants. Regular skin-to-skin contact between parents (mother or father) and LBW infants has been shown to alleviate stress. The parent wears a loose-fitting, open-front top; the undressed (except for diaper) infant is placed in a vertical position on the parent's bare chest, which permits direct eye contact, skin-to-skin sensations, and close proximity (see Fig. 25.15). In addition to being a safe and effective method for VLBW infant-parent acquaintance, skin-to-skin contact between the parent and infant can have a positive effect for the mother who had a high-risk pregnancy. Mothers may experience psychologic healing related to preterm birth and regain the mothering role through early skin-to-skin contact with their VLBW infants. Major neonatal benefits of skin-to-skin care include a reduced risk for mortality, fewer HAIs, decreased length of hospital stay, maintenance of neonatal thermal stability and oxygen saturation, increased feeding vigor, and improved growth (Boundy, Dastjerdi, Spiegelman, et al., 2016; Conde-Agudelo, Belizán, & Diaz-Rossello, 2011). In full-term newborns, skin-to-skin contact has a strong analgesic effect during procedures such as heel lance (Cong, Cusson, Walsh, et al., 2012). LBW infants receiving skin-to-skin contact with breastfeeding mothers maintained higher oxygen saturation and were less likely to have desaturations below 90%, and their mothers were more likely to continue breastfeeding both in the hospital and for 1 month after discharge. Kangaroo care of preterm infants fosters appropriate neurobehavioral development by reducing stress, improving quality of movement, improving the infant's attention and behavioral state, and permitting maternal-infant bonding (Silva, Barros, Pessoa, et al., 2016).

The arena of developmental care for preterm infants has expanded to include a wide variety of interventions such as infant massage, soothing soft music, recordings of parents reading stories, positioning to enhance self-regulatory abilities, enhancement of hand-to-mouth activities, uninterrupted sleep periods, decreased environmental light and noise, and even the use of stuffed animals to facilitate infant positioning. As a result of such interventions, parents may perceive the NICU environment as less threatening. Active participation in providing such an environment for their special infant also involves the parents in the provision of daily care when the newborn is critically ill and cannot be fed or held.

When infants have reached sufficient developmental organization and stability, interventions are designed and implemented to support their growing abilities. Nurses and parents become adept at learning to read infants' behavioral cues and supplying appropriate interventions (Table 25.10). Cues include both approach and avoidance behaviors. Approach behaviors that are supported and enhanced include tongue extension, hand clasp, hand-to-mouth movements, sucking, looking, and cooing. Signs of stress or fatigue that signal the infant's need for "time-out" are described in Table 25.10.

When infants are recovering and are free from support systems, medically stable, and on room air or smaller amounts of oxygen, they are assessed to document behavioral state organization and ability to self-regulate. When the infant is stable and mature enough to begin developmental intervention, activities are individualized according to each infant's cues, temperament, state, behavioral organization, and

TABLE 25.10   Signs of Stress or Fatigue in Neonates

Subsystem	Signs of Stress
Respiratory	Tachypnea, pauses, gasping, sighing
Color	Mottled, dusky, pale or gray
Visceral	Hiccups, gagging, choking, spitting up, grunting and straining as if having a bowel movement, coughing, sneezing, yawning
Autonomic	Tremors, startles, twitches
Motor	Fluctuating tone; lack of control over movement, activity, and posture; increased motor activity; progressively frantic diffuse activity if stimulation continues
Flaccidity	Low tone in trunk; limp, floppy upper and lower extremities; limp, drooping jaw (gape face)
Hypertonicity	Arm or leg extensions, arm(s) outstretched with fingers splayed in salute gesture, fingers stiffly outstretched, trunk arching, neck hyperextended
Hyperflexion	Trunk, extremities, fisting
Activity	Frantic, diffuse activity or little or no activity or responsiveness
State	Disorganized quality to state behaviors, including available states, maintenance of state control, and transition from one state to another; roving eyes; gaze averting; glazed, unfocused look or worried, panicked expression; weak cry; irritability; closed eyes and sleeplike withdrawal; abrupt state changes; signs of stress when presented with more than one type of stimulus at a time
Sleep	Whimpering sounds, facial twitching, irregular respirations, fussing, grimacing, restless appearance
Awake	Glazed, unfocused look; staring; worried or pained expression; hyperalert or panicked appearance; eye roving; crying; actively averting gaze or closing eyes; irritability; prolonged awake periods; inconsolability
	Abrupt or rapid state changes
Other state-related behaviors and attention interaction	Efforts to attend to and interact with environmental stimulation eliciting signs of stress and disorganized subsystem functioning
Autonomic	Physiologic instability of varying degrees with autonomic, respiratory, color, and visceral responses

Data from Alvarez-Garcia, A., Fornieles-Deu, A., Costas-Moragas, C., & Botet-Mussons, F. (2014). Maturational changes associated with neonatal stress in preterm infants hospitalized in the NICU. *Journal of Reproductive and Infant Psychology, 32*(4), 412–422; Lin, H.C., Huang, L.C., Li, T.C., et al. (2014). Relationship between energy expenditure and stress behaviors of preterm infants in the neonatal intensive care unit. *Journal for Specialists in Pediatric Nursing, 19*(4), 331–338; Sweeney, J., & Blackburn, S. (2013). Neonatal physiological and behavioral stress during neurological assessment. *Journal of Perinatal and Neonatal Nursing, 27*(3), 242–252.

particular needs. Intervention periods are short (e.g., 2 to 3 minutes of voices, 5 minutes of quiet music). Hearing and vestibular interventions are initiated earlier than visual stimulation. One type of intervention at a time is applied to document the infant's tolerance and response. An intervention program for convalescing infants includes parents and siblings early in the infant's hospitalization; teaching parents to be responsive to the infant's individual cues is an important function of the NICU nurse. Parents, siblings, and health care providers are encouraged to adhere to the established developmental care plan to avoid disruption in sleep-wake cycles and minimize inappropriate stimuli.

Developmental care of preterm neonates is an ongoing process in the NICU and is incorporated into the daily care given to each infant. The nurse is cognizant of the preterm infant's developmental needs, temperament, and newborn state and environmental conditions that adversely affect the infant; nursing care is planned accordingly to enhance optimal physical, psychosocial, and neurologic development. This task is often difficult to accomplish when invasive treatments or interventions are required to stabilize the critically ill neonate.

FAMILY SUPPORT AND INVOLVEMENT

The significance of early parent-child interaction and infant stimulation has been documented by reliable research. Nurses must be aware of these infant and family needs and incorporate activities that facilitate family interaction into the nursing care plan.

The birth of a preterm infant is an unexpected and stressful event for which families are emotionally unprepared. They find themselves simultaneously coping with their own needs, the needs of their infant, and the needs of their family (especially when they have other children). To compound the situation, their infant's precarious condition engenders an atmosphere of apprehension and uncertainty. They are faced with multiple crises and overwhelming feelings of responsibility, helplessness, and frustration.

All parents have some anxieties about the outcome of a pregnancy, but after a preterm birth the concern is heightened regarding both the viability and normalcy of their infant. Mothers may see their infant only briefly before the newborn is removed to the NICU or even to another hospital, leaving them with just the recollection of the infant's very small size and unusual appearance. They often feel alone or lost on the mother-baby unit, belonging neither with mothers who have lost their infants nor with those who have delivered healthy, full-term infants. The staff and physicians are often guarded in discussing the infant's condition; mothers are continually expecting to hear that their infant has died, and they are sensitive to the anxieties of other mothers and staff members. Going home without their infant only compounds their feelings of disappointment, failure, and deprivation.

When an infant is to be transported to another hospital, the parents need a description of the facility where the infant is going. They need to know the location, reputation, and nature of the facility and the care that the infant is expected to receive. The name of the infant's physician and the telephone number of the nursery should be given to them, and unfamiliar terms such as *neonatologist, ventilator, infusion,* and *incubator* should be explained. Explanations should be kept simple, and parents should be given the opportunity to ask questions. If booklets are available that describe the facility, they are given to the family.

Perhaps most important, the parents should have some contact with the infant before the transport. Being able to see, touch, and (if possible) hold their infant may help decrease parents' anxiety. Often a photograph or even a video of their infant can serve as tangible evidence of the newborn's existence until the parents are able to travel to the regional facility. When possible, the mother should be transferred to the same institution as her infant.

Parents need to be informed of their infant's progress and reassured that he or she is receiving proper care. They need to understand the smallest aspects of the infant's condition and treatment. Parents need a realistic, honest, and direct assessment of the situation. Using nonmedical terminology, moving at a pace that is comfortable for parents to assimilate the information, and avoiding lengthy technical explanations facilitate communication with family members. Psychologic tasks that must be accomplished by parents during their infant's care are presented in Box 25.6.

FACILITATING PARENT-INFANT RELATIONSHIPS

Because of their physiologic instability, infants are separated from their mothers immediately and surrounded by a complex, impenetrable barrier of glass windows, mechanical equipment, and special caregivers. There is some evidence indicating that the emotional separation that accompanies the physical separation of mothers and infants may interfere with the normal mother-infant attachment process discussed in Chapter 20. Maternal attachment is a cumulative process that begins before conception, grows stronger during pregnancy, and matures through mother-infant contact during the neonatal period and infancy.

When an infant is sick, the necessary physical separation appears to be accompanied by an emotional estrangement by the parents, which can seriously damage the capacity for parenting their infant (see Nursing Care Plan). This detachment is further hampered by the tenuous nature of the infant's condition. When survival is in doubt, parents may be reluctant to establish a relationship with their infant. They prepare themselves for the infant's death while continuing to hope for recovery. This anticipatory grief and hesitancy to embark on a relationship are evidenced by behaviors such as delay in giving the infant a name, reluctance in visiting the nursery (or when they do visit, focusing on equipment and treatments rather than on their infant), and hesitancy to touch or handle the infant when given the opportunity.

Family-centered care of high-risk newborns includes encouraging and facilitating parental involvement rather than isolating parents from their infant and associated care. This is particularly important for mothers; to reduce the effects of physical separation, mothers are united with their newborn at the earliest opportunity.

Preparing the parents to see their infant for the first time is an important nursing responsibility. The nurse prepares them for their infant's appearance, the equipment attached to the child, and the general atmosphere of the unit. The initial encounter with the NICU is a stressful experience; and the frightening array of people, equipment, and activity

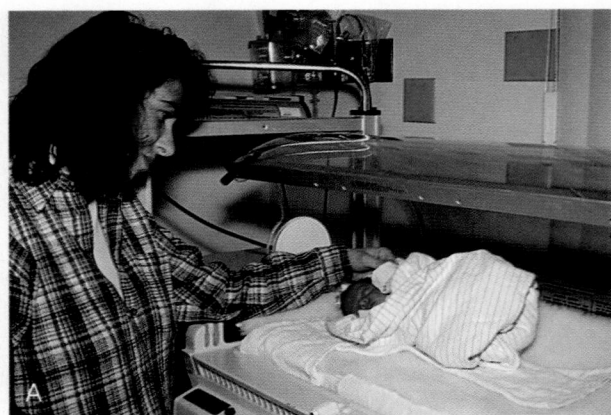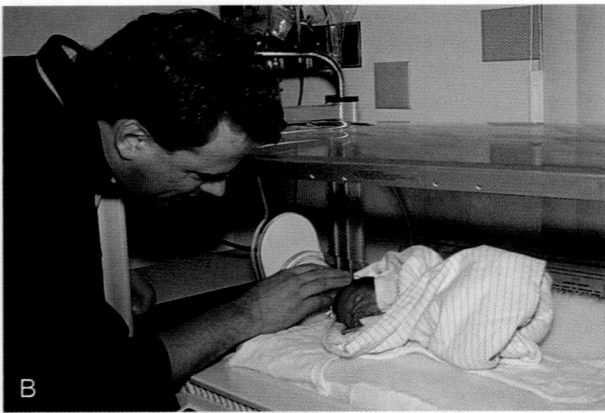

FIG 25.17 A, Mother interacts with her preterm infant by touch. **B,** Father interacts with his newborn by stroking and touching infant with fingertips. (Courtesy of Michael S. Clement, MD, Mesa, AZ.)

is likely to be overwhelming. A book of photographs or pamphlets describing the NICU environment (infants in incubators or under radiant warmers, monitors, mechanical ventilators, and IV equipment), or a video can provide a useful and nonthreatening introduction to the NICU.

Parents are encouraged to visit their infant as soon as possible. Even if they saw the infant at the time of transport or shortly after birth, he or she may have changed considerably, especially if a number of medical and equipment requirements are associated with the hospitalization. At the bedside, the nurse should explain the function of each piece of equipment and the role it plays in facilitating recovery. Explanations may often need to be patiently repeated because parents' anxiety over the infant's condition and the surroundings may prevent them from really "hearing" what is being said. When possible, some items related to therapy can be removed (e.g., phototherapy can be discontinued temporarily, and eye patches removed to permit eye-to-eye contact).

Parents appreciate the support of a nurse during the initial visit with their infant, but they may also appreciate some time alone with the infant. It is important during the early visits to emphasize the positive aspects of their infant's behavior and development so the parents can focus on their child as an individual rather than on the equipment that surrounds him or her. For example, the nurse may describe the infant's spontaneous behaviors during care such as the grasp reflex or make comments about the infant's biologic functions. Most institutions have open visiting policies so parents and siblings may visit their infant as often as they wish.

Parents vary greatly in the degree to which they are able to interact with their infant. Some may wish to touch or hold him or her during the first visit, but others may not feel comfortable enough to even enter the nursery. These reactions depend on a variety of prenatal and postnatal factors such as the parity of the mother and her preparation before birth; the infant's size, condition, and physical appearance; and the type of treatment the infant is receiving. It is essential to recognize that the individualized pacing and quality of the interactions are more important than an early onset of these interactions. Parents may not be receptive to early and extended infant contact because they need time to adjust to the impact of an infant with problems and must be helped to grieve before they can accept the child.

The parents' inability to focus on their infant is a clue for the nurse to help them express and deal with feelings of guilt, anxiety, helplessness, inadequacy, anger, and ambivalence. Nurses can help them recognize that they are experiencing normal responses shared by other parents. It is important to point out and reinforce the positive aspects of parents' behavior and interactions with their infant.

Most parents feel anxious and insecure about initiating interaction with their infant. Nurses can sense parents' level of readiness and offer encouragement in these initial efforts. Parents of preterm infants follow the same acquaintance process as do parents of term infants. They may quickly proceed through the process or may require several days or even weeks to complete it. They begin by touching their infant's extremities with their fingertips and poking the infant tenderly and then proceed to caresses (Fig. 25.17). Touching is the first act of communication between parents and child. Parents need to be prepared for their infant's exaggerated and generalized startle responses to touch so they do not interpret these as negative reactions to their overtures. It may be necessary to limit tactile stimuli when the infant is critically ill and labile, but the nurse can offer other options such as containing the infant or sitting at the bedside.

Parents of acutely ill preterm infants may express feelings of helplessness and lack of control. Involving the parent in some type of caregiving activity, no matter how minor it may seem to the nurse, enables the parent to "take on" a more active role. Examples of such caregiving for an acutely ill infant who cannot be held and is seemingly not responding positively include moistening the infant's lips with a small amount of sterile water on a cotton-tipped swab or expressing and storing breast milk.

Eventually parents begin to endow their infant with an identity—as part of the family. When an infant no longer appears as a foreign object and begins to take on aspects of family members such as the father's chin or the sister's nose, nurses can facilitate this incorporation. Parents are encouraged to bring in clothes or a family snapshot for their infant; and the nurse can help them set goals for themselves and the child. Parents may become involved by reading a children's storybook or nursery rhymes in a soft, soothing voice. Some families record the parents' voices telling or reading stories and play the recording when the infant is able to cope with such stimuli. The nurse must discuss feeding schedules, and parents are encouraged to visit at times when they can become involved in the care of their infant. Throughout the parent-infant acquaintance process, the nurse listens carefully to what the parents say to assess their concerns and their progress toward incorporating their infant into their lives. The manner in which parents refer to their infant and the questions they ask reveal their worries and feelings and can serve as valuable clues to future relationships with the child. The alert nurse is attuned to these subtle indications of parents' needs, which provide guidelines for nursing intervention. Often all that they need is reassurance that they will have the support of the nurse during caregiving activities and that the behaviors about which they are concerned are normal reactions and will disappear as the infant matures.

Parents need guidance in their relationships with their infant and help in their efforts to meet the child's physical and developmental needs. The nursing staff can help parents understand that their preterm infant offers few behavioral rewards and show them how to accept small rewards. The infant's reactions and behaviors are explained to parents, who take their infant's jerky, rejective behavior personally. They need reassurance that these behaviors are not a reflection on their parenting skills. Parents are taught to recognize their infant's cues regarding stimulation, handling, and other interaction, especially aversive behaviors that indicate a need for rest. Nurses need to include parents in planning their infant's care.

Above all, nurses encourage and support parents during their caregiving activities and interactions with their infant to promote healthy parent-child relationships. It is also helpful for the parents to have contact and communication with a consistent group of nurses. This promotes consistency of information given to them and often instills confidence that, although they cannot be at their infant's bedside 24 hours a day, there are competent and caring nurses whom they may call to inquire about the infant's status. Periodic parent conferences involving the staff caring for the infant serve to clarify misunderstandings or problems related to the infant's condition.

DISCHARGE PLANNING AND HOME CARE

Parents become apprehensive and excited as the time for discharge approaches. They have many concerns and insecurities regarding the care of their infant. They fear that the child may still be in danger, that they will be unable to recognize signs of distress or illness in their infant, and that the infant may not yet be ready for discharge. Nurses need to begin early to help parents acquire or increase their skills in the care of their infant. Appropriate instruction must be provided, and sufficient time allowed for the family to assimilate the information and learn the continuing special care requirements. Where rooming-in or other live-in arrangements are available, parents can stay for a few days and nights and assume the care of their infant with the supervision and support of the nursing staff.

There should be appropriate medical and nursing follow-up and referrals to services that can benefit the family, including developmental follow-up. Parents of preterm infants should also be given adequate information about immunizations with other discharge planning information. With the trend toward earlier discharge, many hospital-based home health care agencies become involved in the follow-up and care of NICU "graduates" in the home. For the parents of an infant being discharged with equipment such as an oxygen tank, apnea monitor, or even a ventilator, discharge planning requires interprofessional collaborative practice to ensure that the family has not only the appropriate resources but also the available assistance for dealing with the infant's needs. Many communities have organized support groups, including those discussed previously; other support groups target specific needs such as parents of infants who require special care because of specific defects or disabilities, and parents of multiple births.

Since preterm infants remain at high risk for SIDS following discharge to the home environment, nurses should discuss safe infant sleep practices with the parents and other potential caregivers, including guidelines for safe sleep for infants with special needs (gastroesophageal reflux, mechanical ventilation, oroesophageal malformations) (see "SIDS" section in Chapter 31). Parents and other caregivers should be trained in infant CPR prior to taking a preterm infant home from the hospital.

Car seat safety is an essential aspect of discharge planning. The AAP recommends that infants born before 37 weeks of gestation should have a period of observation in an appropriate car seat to monitor for

---

BOX 25.7   Preterm and Late-Preterm Infant Car Seat Evaluation

Suggestions for providing a car seat evaluation of infants born before 37 weeks of gestation include the following:

- Use the parents' car seat for the evaluation.
- Perform the evaluation 1 to 7 days before the infant's anticipated discharge.
- Secure the infant in the car seat per guidelines using blanket rolls on the side.
- Set the pulse oximeter low alarm at 88% (or per unit protocol).
- Set the heart rate low alarm limit at 80 beats/min and apnea alarm at 20 seconds (cardiorespiratory monitor).
- Leave the infant undisturbed semi-upright in the car seat for a minimum of 90 to 120 minutes or for the time period parents state it takes (whichever is longer) to arrive at their home.
- Document the infant's tolerance to the car seat evaluation.
- Repeat the test after 24 hours after modifications have been made to the car seat, car bed, or infant's position in either restraint system.
- If the infant is being discharged on an apnea or cardiorespiratory monitor, this equipment should be used during the trip home.
- A certified car-seat technician technician demonstrates appropriate positioning of the infant in the restraint device to the parents and has the parents do a return demonstration.
- Document the interventions, the infant's tolerance, and the parents' return demonstration.

Modified from American Academy of Pediatrics. (1996). Safe transportation of premature and low birth weight infants. *Pediatrics, 97*(5), 758–760; American Academy of Pediatrics. (1999). Transporting children with special health care needs. *Pediatrics, 104*(4), 988–992; Bull, M.J., Engle, W.A., Committee on Injury, Violence, and Poison Prevention and the Committee on Fetus and Newborn. (2009). Safe transportation of preterm and low birth weight infants at hospital discharge, *Pediatrics, 123*(54), 1424–1429.

---

possible apnea, bradycardia, and decreased SaO_2 (Bull, Engle, & AAP Committee on Injury, Violence, and Poison Prevention & Committee on Fetus and Newborn, 2009; Davis, Zenchenko, Lever, et al., 2013) (see Box 25.7). Several models of car seats can be adapted for small infants with the placement of blanket rolls on each side of the infant to support the head and trunk. For adequate support without slumping, the seat back–to-crotch strap distance must be 14 cm (5.5 inches) or less; a small rolled blanket may be placed between the crotch strap and the infant to reduce slouching. The distance from the lower harness strap to the seat bottom should be 25.5 cm (10 inches) or less to decrease the potential for the harness straps to cross the infant's ears. The rear-facing semi-upright position provides support for the head, neck, and back, thereby reducing the stress to the neck and spinal cord in a vehicle crash. Car seat manufacturers must specify recommended minimum and maximum weights for the occupant; therefore it is important to check the manufacturer recommendations before purchasing a car seat for a smaller infant. Additional guidelines are available from the AAP (Durbin & AAP Committee on Injury, Violence, and Poison Prevention, 2011).

An important part of discharge planning and care of preterm infants is nutrition for continued growth; thus the choice of feeding must be addressed carefully. Human milk should be fortified according to the infant's corrected age and physiologic needs. Human milk with fortifier (protein, phosphorus, and calcium) is recommended for LBW infants because it increases weight gain and improves bone mineralization (Gardner & Lawrence, 2016). Full term infant formulas are not considered adequate for proper growth in preterm infants.

Knowing that staff members are available for telephone or personal contact when the parents take the infant home provides a measure of security to anxious parents. Many NICU facilities maintain a policy of open communication between staff and parents both during the infant's hospitalization and after discharge. It is the responsibility of the NICU staff to make certain that parents are prepared to care for their infant both emotionally and physically. At the same time, it is important that parents establish a trusting relationship with the infant's primary care provider in the community before discharge from the acute care facility.

NEWBORN SCREENING FOR DISEASE

A number of genetic disorders can be detected in the newborn period. There is no national policy for such detection in the United States; therefore the extent of neonatal screening is determined by state laws and voluntary guidelines. The US Department of Health and Human Services (USDHHS Advisory Committee on Heritable Disorders in Newborns and Children, 2016) recommends screening for at least 34 core conditions including for phenylketonuria (PKU), congenital hypothyroidism (CH), galactosemia, hemoglobin defects such as sickle cell disease, and hearing loss (see Chapters 23 and 43). In Canada, universal newborn screening policies and practices are varied. Individual provinces in Canada determine the disorders included in newborn screening; however, all provinces screen for PKU and congenital hypothyroidism (Canadian Organization for Rare Disorders, 2015).

The purpose of screening is to identify infants who may have a condition that benefits from early identification and treatment to prevent cognitive impairment. The screening test is most reliable if the blood sample is taken after the infant has ingested a source of protein for 24 hours. Because of early discharge of newborns, recommendations for screening include (1) collecting the initial specimen as close as possible to discharge or no later than 7 days after birth, (2) obtaining a subsequent sample by 2 weeks of age if the initial specimen is collected before the newborn is 24 hours of age, and (3) designating a primary care provider to all newborns before discharge for adequate newborn screening follow-up. A major concern is that many infants are *not* rescreened for metabolic disorders after early discharge and are at risk for a missed or delayed diagnosis of a treatable disorder. Special consideration must be given to screening infants born at home who have no hospital contact. It is always necessary to confirm the screening results with diagnostic testing.

The nurse's responsibilities are to educate parents regarding the importance of screening and collect appropriate specimens at the recommended time (after 24 hours of age). If the blood sample was collected before 24 hours, the nurse stresses to the parents the importance of follow-up with the pediatric care provider for repeat testing (Tluczek & De Luca, 2013). Accurate screening depends on high-quality blood spots on approved filter paper forms. The blood should completely saturate the filter paper spot on one side only. The paper should not be handled, placed on wet surfaces, or contaminated with any substance (See Fig. 23.10).

The use of pulse oximetry to screen for critical congenital heart disease in healthy term infants has been endorsed by the US Department of Health and Human Services and is being implemented in numerous states; this screening should be incorporated into the recommended uniform newborn screening panel (Bradshaw & Martin, 2012; Mahle, Martin, Beekman, et al., 2012). Recommendations for screening healthy term newborns include the following (Kemper, Mahle, Martin, et al., 2011):

- Screen healthy term newborns after 24 hours of life or as close to discharge from the birth hospital as possible.
- Use a motion-tolerant pulse oximeter.

- Avoid false-positive results by screening while the infant is alert.
- Obtain pulse oximeter readings from the right hand and one foot.
- Pulse oximetry ≤90% in the right hand or foot is considered a positive screening, and additional evaluation is warranted (e.g., echocardiogram).
- 90% to 95% in the right hand or foot or >3% difference between the two extremities warrants a repeat test in 1 hour. If screening values remain the same as the first time, consider repeating the screen in 1 hour. If parameters remain unchanged after the second screen, repeat a third time. If unchanged, consider it a positive screen.
- ≥95% in the right hand or foot and ≤3% difference between the two extremities is a negative screen (no further testing is required).

The AAP and ACOG (2012) also recommend routine prenatal and perinatal HIV counseling and testing for all pregnant women and their newborns. Benefits of early identification of HIV-infected infants are early antiretroviral therapy and aggressive nutritional supplementation; appropriate changes in their immunization schedule; monitoring and evaluation of immunologic, neurologic, and neuropsychologic functions for possible changes caused by antiretroviral therapy; initiation of interventions for special educational needs; evaluation for the need of other therapies such as IVIg for the prevention of bacterial infections; tuberculosis screening and treatment; and management of communicable disease exposures. See Chapter 3 for more information on HIV. For information on additional diseases that may be screened in the newborn period, see Newborn Screening Fact Sheets (https://www.aap.org/en-us/advocacy-and-policy/aap-health-initiatives/PEHDIC/Documents/Newbornscreeningdisorders.pdf).

INBORN ERRORS OF METABOLISM

Inborn errors of metabolism (IEMs) constitute a large number of inherited diseases caused by the absence or deficiency of a substance essential to cellular metabolism, usually an enzyme. When the normal metabolic process is interrupted as a result of a missing enzyme, an accumulation of substances precedes the interruption, the end product of the process is absent, or the process takes an alternate metabolic pathway. The consequence is manifested as an illness. Most IEMs are characterized by abnormal protein, carbohydrate, or fat metabolism.

Newborn screening for IEMs varies from state to state; but all states test for at least seven core disorders, (i.e., PKU, CH, galactosemia, sickle cell disease, thalassemia, congenital adrenal hyperplasia [CAH], and cystic fibrosis [CF]. See Chapter 23 for information on universal newborn screening.

Congenital Hypothyroidism

Congenital hypothyroidism may have a number of causes and can be either permanent or transient. Transient CH is frequently associated with maternal Graves' disease that was treated with anti-thyroid drugs. Congenital hypothyroidism is most often due to thyroid dysgenesis: absent, hypolastic, and/or ectopic thyroid gland (LaFranchi & Huang, 2016); in most cases the cause is unknown. Approximately 10% to 20% of cases of CH are due to inherited defects of thyroid hormone metabolism (Stokowski, 2015). Worldwide the most common cause of CH resulting in hypothyroidism is iodine deficiency. However, no matter what the cause, the manifestations (Box 25.8) and management are similar. In some conditions the thyroid deficiency is severe, and manifestations develop early; in others the symptoms may be delayed for months or years. Early detection and prompt initiation of treatment are essential because their delay results in varying degrees of cognitive impairment (LaFranchi & Huang).

Results of screening tests in the United States indicate that CH occurs in approximately 1 in 1400 to 1 in 2800 newborns (Wassner & Brown,

BOX 25.8 Clinical Manifestations of Congenital Hypothyroidism

Birth*
- Poor feeding
- Lethargy
- Prolonged jaundice (>2 weeks)
- Respiratory difficulties
- Cyanosis
- Constipation
- Bradycardia
- Hoarse cry
- Large anterior and posterior fontanels
- Postterm
- Birth weight over 4000 g (8 lbs 13 oz)

Ages 6 to 9 Weeks†
- Depressed nasal bridge
- Short forehead
- Puffy eyelids
- Large tongue
- Thick, dry, mottled skin
- Coarse, dry, lusterless hair
- Abdominal distention
- Umbilical hernia
- Hyporeflexia
- Bradycardia
- Hypothermia
- Hypotension
- Anemia
- Widely patent cranial sutures

*Clinical manifestations may not be obvious at birth, possibly because of maternal transfer of thyroid hormone to the fetus. Manifestations may be delayed in infants with certain types of familial hypothyroidism and in breastfed infants (may show after weaning).
†If untreated, classical features.
Data from Chuang, J., Gutmark-Little, I., Rose, S.R. (2015): Thyroid disorders in the neonate. In R.J. Martin, A.A. Fanaroff, & M.C. Walsh (Eds.), *Fanaroff and Martin's neonatal-perinatal medicine: Diseases of the fetus and infant* [10th ed.]. St. Louis, MO: Mosby.

2015). It affects all races and ethnicities, but it is more prevalent among Hispanic and American Indian or Alaskan Native people (1 in 700 to 1 in 2000 newborns) and less prevalent among African-Americans (1 in 3200 to 1 in 17,000 newborns). Infants with Down syndrome have a much higher rate of either permanent or transient forms of the disorder, with a reported prevalence of 1.5% to 6.1% (King, O'Gorman, & Gallagher, 2014). In addition, a higher incidence of other congenital abnormalities has been observed in infants with CH. Many preterm infants have transient hypothyroidism (hypothyroxinemia) at birth as a result of hypothalamic and pituitary immaturity. Infants born before 28 weeks of gestation may require temporary thyroid hormone replacement. Some screening programs target both primary (thyroid-based) and secondary (pituitary-based) hypothyroidism.

Because CH is one of the most common preventable causes of cognitive impairment, early diagnosis and treatment of this disease are essential interventions. Screening for CH is mandatory in all U.S. states and territories. Neonatal screening consists of an initial filter paper blood spot measurement of thyroid-stimulating hormone (TSH) followed by measurement of T_4 in specimens with low values; alternatively, screening may first assess T_4, followed by TSH if the T_4 is abnormal. Although a blood sample obtained by heelstick for the spot test is best obtained between 2 and 4 days of age, specimens are usually taken within the first 24 to 48 hours or before discharge as part of a concurrent screen for other metabolic defects (American Academy of Pediatrics, American Thyroid Association, & Lawson Wilkins Pediatric Endocrine Society, 2006/2011; Stokowski, 2015).

CH is likely if the T_4 is less than 6 mcg/dL and the TSH is greater than 50 mU/L. Additional tests include serum measurement of T_4, triiodothyronine (T_3), resin uptake, free T_4, and thyroid-bound globulin. Tests of thyroid gland function (thyroid scan and uptake) usually involve oral administration of a radioactive isotope of iodine (^{131}I) and measurement of iodine uptake by the thyroid gland, usually within 24 hours. In CH protein-bound iodine, T_4, T_3, and free T_4 levels are low; and

thyroid uptake of ^{131}I is decreased. Skeletal radiography is used to assess age (Stokowski, 2015).

In newborns, thyroid function studies are elevated in comparison with values in older children; therefore it is important to document the timing of the tests. In preterm and sick full term infants, thyroid hormone levels are usually lower than in healthy full term infants; a repeat T_4 and TSH may be evaluated after 30 weeks (corrected age) in newborns born before that time and after resolution of the acute illness in sick full term infants.

Treatment involves lifelong thyroid hormone replacement therapy beginning as soon as possible after diagnosis to abolish all signs of hypothyroidism and reestablish normal physical and mental development. The drug of choice is synthetic levothyroxine sodium (Synthroid, Levothroid). Optimum dosage of levothyroxine should be able to maintain blood TSH concentration between 0.5 and 2 mU/L during the first 3 years of life (Agrawal et al., 2015). Regular measurement of T_4 levels is important to ensure optimum treatment. Bone age surveys are also performed to ensure optimum growth.

The most important nursing objective is early identification of the disorder. Nurses caring for neonates must be certain that screening is performed, especially in infants who are preterm, discharged early, or born at home. Some cases are detected only by a second screening at 2 to 6 weeks of age. Nurses in community health need to be aware of the earliest signs of the disorder. Parental remarks about an unusually "quiet and good" baby and demonstrated symptoms such as prolonged jaundice, constipation, and umbilical hernia should lead to a suspicion of hypothyroidism.

After the diagnosis is confirmed, parents need an explanation of the disorder and the necessity of lifelong treatment. The child should be referred to a pediatric endocrinologist for care. The importance of compliance with the drug regimen for the child to achieve normal development must be stressed (Shanholtz, 2013). Because the thyroid medication is tasteless, it can be crushed and added to formula, water, or food. If a dose is missed, twice the dose should be given the next day. Unless there are maternal contraindicative factors, breastfeeding is acceptable and encouraged in infants with hypothyroidism (Lawrence & Lawrence, 2016). Parents also need to be aware of signs indicating overdose such as a rapid pulse, dyspnea, irritability, insomnia, fever, sweating, and weight loss. Ideally they should know how to count the pulse and be instructed to withhold a dose and consult their practitioner if the pulse rate is above a certain value. Signs of inadequate treatment are fatigue, sleepiness, decreased appetite, and constipation.

If the diagnosis was delayed past early infancy, the chance of permanent cognitive impairment is great. Parents need the same guidance in caring for their child as do others who have an offspring with cognitive impairment. They need an opportunity to discuss their feelings regarding late recognition of the disorder. Although treatment will not reverse the intellectual deficit, it may prevent further damage. Genetic counseling is important for the rare families in whom the etiology of CH is thyroid dyshormonogenesis, which is inherited in an autosomal recessive manner.

Phenylketonuria

PKU, an inborn error of metabolism inherited as an autosomal recessive trait (the *PAH* gene is located on chromosome 12q22-q24.1), is caused by a deficiency or absence of the enzyme needed to metabolize the essential amino acid phenylalanine. Classic PKU is at one end of a spectrum of conditions known as *hyperphenylalaninemia*. Within the spectrum of hyperphenylalaninemia are conditions with varying degrees of severity, depending on the degree of enzyme deficiency. Because rarer forms are a result of a deficiency in other enzymes and are diagnosed and treated differently, the following discussion of PKU is limited to the severe, classic form.

In PKU the hepatic enzyme phenylalanine hydroxylase, which normally controls the conversion of phenylalanine to tyrosine, is deficient. This results in the accumulation of phenylalanine in body fluids and in the brain. Excess phenylalanine is excreted in the urine as phenylketones (phenylacetic and phenylpyruvic acid); thus, the term *phenylketonuria* (PKU) (Rezvani & Ficicioglu, 2016).

Tyrosine, the amino acid produced by the metabolism of phenylalanine, is absent in PKU. Tyrosine is needed to form the pigment melanin and the hormones epinephrine and T_4. Decreased melanin production results in similar phenotypes of most individuals with PKU; an affected individual has a lighter complexion that is particularly susceptible to eczema and other dermatologic problems (Rezvani & Ficicioglu, 2016).

The prevalence of PKU varies widely in the United States because different states have different definition criteria for what constitutes hyperphenylalaninemia and PKU. The reported figures for PKU in the United States are 1 case per 15,000 live births. The incidence of the disease varies widely by ethnic group. In Europe, the incidence is 1 per 10,000 births; in South Asia and Africa, the prevalence is quite low (Blau, Shen, & Carducci, 2014).

Clinical manifestations in untreated PKU include failure to thrive (growth failure); frequent vomiting; irritability; hyperactivity; and unpredictable, erratic behavior. Cognitive impairment is thought to be caused by the accumulation of phenylalanine and presumably by decreased levels of the neurotransmitters dopamine and tryptophan, which affect the normal development of the brain and CNS, resulting in defective myelinization, cystic degeneration of the gray and white matter, and disturbances in cortical lamination. Older children commonly display behavior patterns such as fright reactions, screaming episodes, head banging, arm biting, disorientation, failure to respond to strong stimuli, and catatonia-like positions (Rezvani & Ficicioglu, 2016).

The objective in diagnosing and treating the disorder is to prevent cognitive impairment. Every newborn should be screened for PKU. The screening method with the best accuracy and precision is tandem mass spectrometry, which detects all forms of hyperphenylalaninemia and has limited false-positive results. Only fresh heel blood, not cord blood, can be used for the test.

> **! NURSING ALERT**
>
> When collecting the blood specimen for screening, "layering" the blood specimen on the special paper is avoided. Layering is placing one drop of blood on top of the other or overlapping the specimen. This practice results in a falsely high reading, or false positive, which will lead the newborn screening department to call the family and health care provider to arrange for a diagnostic blood phenylalanine test to determine whether the newborn truly has PKU. Best results are obtained by collecting the specimen with a pipette from the heelstick and spreading the blood uniformly over the blot paper.

If the screening test is positive, measurement of plasma phenylalanine is done (Rezvani & Ficicioglu, 2016). Because of the possibility of variant forms of hyperphenylalaninemia, PKU cofactor variant screen should be performed in all children diagnosed with PKU. A major concern is that a significant number of infants are not rescreened for PKU after early discharge and are at risk for a missed or delayed diagnosis. Give special consideration to screening infants born at home who have no hospital contact and infants adopted internationally.

Treatment of PKU involves restricting phenylalanine in the diet. Because the genetic enzyme is intracellular, systemic administration of phenylalanine hydroxylase is of no value. Phenylalanine cannot be eliminated from the diet because it is an essential amino acid in tissue growth. Therefore dietary management must meet two criteria: (1) meet the child's nutritional need for optimum growth and (2) maintain phenylalanine levels within a safe range (2 to 6 mg/dL) (Boyer, Barclay, & Burrage, 2015).

Infants with blood phenylalanine levels higher than 10 mg/dL should be started on treatment to establish metabolic control as soon as possible (Rezvani & Ficicioglu, 2016). The daily amounts of phenylalanine are individualized for each child and require frequent changes on the basis of appetite, growth and development, and blood phenylalanine and tyrosine levels.

Because all natural food proteins contain phenylalanine and are limited, the diet must be supplemented with a specially prepared phenylalanine-free formula (e.g., Phenex-1 for infants or Phenex-2 for children and adults). The phenylalanine-free formula is an amino acid–modified formula essential in the low phenylalanine diet to provide the appropriate protein, vitamins, minerals, and calories for optimal growth and development. Because tyrosine becomes an essential amino acid, the phenylalanine-free formula supplies an adequate amount; but in some cases additional supplementation may be needed (Rezvani & Ficicioglu, 2016). The phenylalanine-free amino acid–modified formula for infants has all the nutrients necessary for adequate infant growth. Because of the low phenylalanine content of breast milk, total or partial breastfeeding may be possible with close monitoring of phenylalanine levels (Lawrence & Lawrence, 2016).

Most clinicians now agree that, to achieve optimal metabolic control and outcome, a restricted phenylalanine diet, including medical foods and low-protein products, most likely is medically required for virtually all individuals with classic PKU for their entire lives (Berry, Brown, Grant, et al., 2013). Such lifetime reduction of phenylalanine intake is necessary to prevent neuropsychologic and cognitive deficits because even mild hyperphenylalaninemia (20 mg/dL) would produce such effects. To evaluate the effectiveness of dietary treatment, frequent monitoring of blood phenylalanine and tyrosine levels is necessary.

The principal nursing considerations involve teaching the family regarding the dietary restrictions. Although the treatment may sound simple, the task of maintaining such a strict dietary regimen is demanding, especially for older children and adolescents. In addition, mothers of children with PKU may have to spend many hours preparing special foods such as low-phenylalanine snacks. Foods with low phenylalanine levels (e.g., vegetables; fruits; juices; some cereals, breads, and starches) must be measured to provide the prescribed amount of phenylalanine. High-protein foods such as meat and dairy products are eliminated from the diet. The sweetener aspartame should be avoided because it is composed of two amino acids, aspartic acid and phenylalanine, and if used decreases the amount of natural phenylalanine that is prescribed for the day. However, medications that use aspartame as the sweetener may be used if no other nonaspartame medications are available because the content of the artificial sweetener is minimal or can be counted in the total daily phenylalanine allowance.

Maintaining the diet during infancy presents few problems. Solid foods such as cereal, fruits, and vegetables are introduced as usual to the infant. Difficulties arise as the child gets older. Studies show a decline in diet compliance with consequent increases in blood phenylalanine levels during early adolescence and young adulthood (Demirkol, Gizewska, Giovannini, et al., 2011).

A decreased appetite and refusal to eat may reduce intake of the calculated phenylalanine requirement. The child's increasing independence may also inhibit absolute control of what he or she eats. Either factor can result in decreased or increased phenylalanine levels. During the school years, peer pressure becomes a major force in deterring the child from eating the prescribed foods or abstaining from high-protein foods such as milkshakes and ice cream. Limitations of this diet are best illustrated by an example: a quarter-pound hamburger may provide a 2-day phenylalanine allowance for a school-age child.

The assistance of a registered dietitian is essential. Parents need a basic understanding of the disorder and practical suggestions regarding food selection and preparation. Meal planning is based on weighing the food on a gram scale; a less accurate method is the exchange list. As soon as children are old enough, usually by early preschool, they should be involved in the daily calculation, menu planning, and formula preparation. Using a computer, voice-activated calculator, cards, or colored beads can help them keep track of the daily allowance of phenylalanine foods. A system of goal setting, self-monitoring, contracts, and rewards can promote compliance in adolescents.

Preparation of the phenylalanine-free formula can present some challenges. The formula tends to be lumpy; mixing the powder with a small amount of water to make a paste and then adding the rest of the required liquid helps to alleviate this problem. A blender or mixer dissolves the powder more easily; a rechargeable hand mixer can be used when traveling. Although the taste is virtually impossible to camouflage, many new products are on the market today. Some of the complete formulas are chocolate, vanilla, strawberry, and orange flavored. Incomplete formulas that do not contain the vitamins and minerals and are plain tasting are also available; these can be added to cold foods instead of mixing them as a formula. Formula bars are convenient for active adolescents. Formula capsules are also available, but the patient would need to take 20 or more capsules per day.

Galactosemia

Galactosemia is a rare autosomal recessive disorder that results from various gene mutations leading to three distinct enzymatic deficiencies. The most common type of galactosemia (classic galactosemia) results from a deficiency of a hepatic enzyme, galactose 1-phosphate uridyl-transferase (GALT), and affects approximately 1 in 60,000 births. The other two varieties of galactosemia involve deficiencies in the enzymes galactokinase (GALK) and galactose 4-epimerase (GALE); these are extremely rare disorders. All three enzymes (GALT, GALK, and GALE) are involved in the conversion of galactose into glucose (Kishnani & Chen, 2016).

As galactose accumulates in the blood, several organs are affected. Hepatic dysfunction leads to cirrhosis, resulting in jaundice in the infant by the second week of life. The spleen subsequently becomes enlarged as a result of portal hypertension. Cataracts are usually recognizable by 1 or 2 months of age; cerebral damage, manifested by the symptoms of lethargy and hypotonia, is evident soon afterward. Infants with galactosemia appear normal at birth, but within a few days of ingesting milk (which has a high lactose content) they begin to experience vomiting and diarrhea, leading to weight loss. *E. coli* sepsis is also a common presenting clinical sign. Death during the first month of life is frequent in untreated infants. Occasionally a clinical variant galactosemia is seen with milder, chronic manifestations such as growth failure, feeding difficulty, and developmental delay. This presentation is more frequent among African-American children with galactosemia (Berry, 2017).

Diagnosis is made on the basis of the infant's history, physical examination, galactosuria, increased levels of galactose in the blood, and decreased levels of GALT activity in erythrocytes. The infant may display characteristics of malnutrition (i.e., hypoglycemia, jaundice, sepsis, and cataracts) (Berry, 2017). Newborn screening for this disease is required in most states. Heterozygotes can also be identified because heterozygotic individuals have significantly lower levels of the essential enzyme.

During infancy, treatment consists of eliminating all milk and lactose-containing formula, including breast milk. Traditionally lactose-free formulas are used, with soy-protein formula being the feeding of choice; however, some research suggests that elemental formula (galactose-free) may be more beneficial than soy formulas (Van Calcar, Bernstein, Rohr, et al., 2014). The AAP recommends the use of soy protein–based formula for infants with galactosemia, and it is considerably less expensive than elemental formula (Bhatia, Greer, & AAP Committee on Nutrition, 2008). As the infant progresses to solids, only foods low in galactose should be consumed. Certain fruits are high in galactose, and some dietitians recommend that they be avoided. Food lists should be given to the family to ensure that appropriate foods are chosen.

If galactosemia is suspected, supportive treatment and care are implemented, including monitoring for hypoglycemia, liver failure, bleeding disorders, and *E. coli* sepsis.

Nursing interventions are similar to those for PKU except that dietary restrictions are easier to maintain because many more foods are allowed. However, reading food labels carefully for the presence of any form of lactose, especially dairy products, is mandatory. Many drugs such as some of the penicillin preparations contain lactose as filler and also must be avoided. Unfortunately lactose is an unlabeled ingredient in many pharmaceuticals. Therefore parents should be instructed to ask their local pharmacist about galactose content of any over-the-counter or prescription medications.

GENETIC EVALUATION AND COUNSELING

Nurses are often the first health care professionals to whom parents turn for information and guidance about genetic counseling. Genetic counseling is usually provided by an interprofessional health care team with expertise in clinical and medical genetics; this may include clinical and medical geneticists, genetics counselors, and advanced practice genetics nurse specialists. They provide education and support to families with actual or potential genetic health concerns, relaying information about the diagnosis, treatment options, recurrence risk, and availability of prenatal diagnosis for potential or actual genetic disease (Van Riper, 2016). Nurses working in maternity, women's health, and neonatal settings need to understand the basic principles of heredity and how heredity contributes to disorders and to be aware of the types of genetic testing available so that they are able to answer questions and make appropriate referrals.

Nurses frequently encounter children with genetic diseases and families in which there is a risk that a disorder may be transmitted to or occur in an offspring. It is their responsibility to be alert to situations in which people could benefit from a genetic evaluation and counseling, be aware of the local genetic resources, aid families in finding services, and offer support and care for children and families affected by genetic conditions. Local genetic clinics can be located through several sites. The Genetic Alliance (www.geneticalliance.org) is a nonprofit organization that has a database of support groups for genetic conditions. Another resource is GeneTests (www.ncbi.nlm.nih.gov/sites/GeneTests), a publicly funded medical genetics information resource developed for physicians and other health care providers that is available at no cost to all interested people. A third resource is the National Society of Genetic Counselors (www.nsgc.org), which lists genetic counselors by state in the United States.

Maintaining contact with the family or referring them to an agency that can provide a sustained relationship, usually the public health agency in their locality, is one of the most important aspects in the care of the patient and family. In a disorder that requires conscientious diet management such as PKU or galactosemia, it is important to make certain that the family understands and follows the advice. A vital role for nurses is to advocate for the child and family as they make their way through the various specialty clinics. This is especially important for families who are more vulnerable because of cognitive, hearing, language, or financial issues and those who otherwise may have difficulty accessing health services. Nurses can reinforce the genetic information or arrange for additional genetic counseling if a family has additional questions or misunderstandings (see the "Genetic Counseling" section in Chapter 6).

NEONATAL LOSS

The precarious nature of many high-risk infants makes death a real and ever-present possibility. Although infant mortality has been reduced sharply with improved technology, the mortality rate is still greatest during the neonatal period. Nurses in the NICU are usually the people who must prepare the parents for an inevitable death, provide end-of-life care for the infant and family, and facilitate a family's grieving process after an expected or unexpected death. In the event of a stillbirth or infant death shortly after birth, nurses in the labor and birth unit and the postpartum unit provide care for the infant and family.

The loss of an infant has special meaning for the grieving parents. It represents a loss of a part of themselves (especially for mothers), a loss of the potential for immortality that offspring represent, and the loss of the dream child that has been fantasized about throughout the pregnancy. There is often a sense of emptiness and failure. In addition, when an infant has lived for such a short time, there may be few, if any, pleasant memories to serve as a basis for the identification and idealization that are part of the resolution of a loss.

To help parents understand that the death is a reality and to facilitate their grieving, it is important that they be offered the opportunity to hold their infant before death and, if possible, be present at the time of death so their infant can die in their arms if they choose. Many who decide not to hold their infant may later regret the decision.

Parents are given the opportunity to actually "parent" the infant in any manner they wish or are able to do before and after the death. This may include seeing, touching, holding, caressing, and talking to their infant privately; the parents may also wish to bathe and dress the infant. If parents are hesitant about seeing their dead infant, it is advisable to keep the body in the unit for a few hours because many parents change their minds after the initial shock of the death.

Parents may need to see and hold the infant more than once—the first time to say "hello" and the last time to say "good-bye." If parents wish to see the infant after the body has been taken to the morgue, the infant should be retrieved, wrapped in a blanket, rewarmed, and taken to the mother's room or other private place. The family needs private time alone with their dead infant; the nurse should be available if needed. Some families need a few minutes, while others wish to have the infant with them for hours. The nurse can be alert for verbal and nonverbal cues that the family is ready to say "good-bye" and allow the nurse to take the baby out of the room. Individual grief responses of the mother and father should be recognized and handled appropriately; gender differences and cultural and religious beliefs will affect the parents' grief responses (Black, 2016).

A hospice approach may be implemented for families with infants for whom the decision has been made to not prolong life and who are receiving only palliative care. Another approach is to send the family home with the infant and allow them to spend time together until the eventual death; hospice services may be available, and supportive care is provided in the home setting. Some families find this option less restrictive and more family oriented than being in the hospital setting (see Chapter 36 for further discussion of hospice care).

Tangible momentos of the infant are important for families. Photographs can provide special memories. With the family's permission, nurses may take photos of the infant before and after death; photos of the family spending time with the infant prior to death can be very comforting. Parents may wish to have a special family portrait taken with the infant and other family members; this often helps personalize and make the experience more tangible. In some communities, there are professional photographers who volunteer their services without charge to take photos of families and their deceased infant. The organization, Now I Lay Me Down to Sleep is an example of this (www.nowilaymedowntosleep.org). Some hospitals take digital photos of the baby and give the memory card to parents for viewing when they feel ready. The parents may not wish to see photographs at the time of death, but the chance to view them later may help make their infant seem more real, which is a part of the normal grieving process. A photograph of their infant being held by the hand or touched by an adult offers a more positive image than a morgue type of photograph. A bereavement or memory packet can be given to the grieving parents and family and may include the infant's handprints and footprints, a lock of hair, the bedside name card, the ID bracelet or armbands and, as appropriate to the family's religious beliefs, a certificate of baptism (Black, 2016).

Naming the deceased infant is an important step in the grieving process. Some parents may hesitate to give the newborn a name that had been chosen during the pregnancy for their "special baby." However, having a tangible person for whom to grieve is an important component of the grieving process.

A nurse who is familiar to the family should be present during discussions regarding autopsies, organ donation, and disposition of the infant's body. The nurse should talk with parents openly and honestly about funeral arrangements because few parents have had experience with this aspect of death. Many funeral homes offer inexpensive arrangements in these special situations. Someone from the NICU should take the responsibility for acquiring this type of information. It is often helpful to parents for the NICU to have a list of local funeral homes, services offered, and prices. Families need to be informed of the options available, but a funeral service is preferable because the ritual provides an opportunity for parents to feel the support of friends and relatives. The hospital chaplain, the family's minister, or a member of the clergy of the appropriate faith may be notified if the parents wish; their presence with the family can be very helpful during this difficult time, and there can be discussion about spiritual rituals that are very important to some families. Issues regarding an autopsy or organ donation (when appropriate) are approached with respect, sensitivity to cultural and religious beliefs, tact, and consideration of the family's wishes (Black, 2016). Gardner and Carter (2016) provide additional suggestions for helping families who experience neonatal loss.

Before the parents leave the hospital, they are given the telephone number of the unit and are invited to call any time they have questions. Many intensive care units contact the parents several weeks after a neonatal death to assess the parents' coping mechanisms, evaluate the grieving process, and provide support as needed. Several organizations are available to offer support and understanding to families who have lost a newborn; these organizations include the Compassionate Friends (http://www.compassionatefriends.org/home.aspx); Aiding Mothers and Fathers Experiencing Neonatal Death (AMEND) (http://www.amendgroup.com); and Share Pregnancy and Infant Loss Support, Inc. (http://nationalshare.org/) (see Chapter 36 for further discussion of end-of-life care).

Nurses who care for critically ill infants also experience grief; NICU nurses may feel helpless and sorrowful. It is important that such grief be allowed and that nurses attend the funeral or memorial service as a part of working through their own grief. Nurses may fear that showing emotion is unprofessional and that the expression of grief indicates "loss of control." These fears are unfounded. Studies have demonstrated that to continue to be effective managers and providers of care, nurses must be allowed to grieve and support each other through the process (Gardner & Carter, 2016).

BAPTISM

Because many Christian parents wish to have their child baptized if death is anticipated or is a decided possibility, this may become a nursing responsibility. Whenever possible, it is most desirable that a representative of the parents' faith (e.g., a Roman Catholic priest or a Protestant minister) perform such a ritual. When death is imminent, a nurse or health care provider can perform the baptism by simply pouring water on the infant's forehead (a medicine dropper is a convenient means) while repeating the words, "I baptize you in the name of the Father and of the Son and of the Holy Spirit." This includes a birth of any gestational age, particularly when the parents are Roman Catholic.

When the parents' faith is uncertain, a conditional baptism can be carried out by saying, "If you are capable of receiving baptism, I baptize you in the name of the Father and of the Son and of the Holy Spirit." The baptism is recorded in the infant's chart, and a notice is placed on the crib or incubator. Parents are informed at the first opportunity.

REFERENCES

Abdel-Latif, M. E., & Osborn, D. A. (2012). Nebulised surfactant in preterm infants with or at risk of respiratory distress syndrome. *Cochrane Database of Systematic Reviews, 2012*(10), CD008310.

Adamkin, D. H., & American Academy of Pediatrics Committee on Fetus and Newborn. (2011). Postnatal glucose homeostasis in late-preterm and term infants. *Pediatrics, 127*(3), 575–579.

Adamkin, D. H., & Polin, R. (2016). Neonatal hypoglycemia: Is 60 the new 40? The questions remain the same. *Journal of Perinatology, 36*(1), 10–12.

Agrawal, P., Philip, R., Saran, S., et al. (2015). Congenital hypothyroidism. *Indian Journal of Endocrinology and Metabolism, 19*(2), 221–227.

Alfaleh, K., Anabrees, J., Bassler, D., et al. (2011). Probiotics for prevention of necrotizing enterocolitis in preterm infants. *Cochrane Database of Systematic Reviews, 2011*(3), CD005496.

Aitken, S. L., & Tichy, E. M. (2015). RhO D Immune globulin products for prevention of alloimmunization during pregnancy. *American Journal of Health-System Pharmacists, 72*(4), 267–276.

American Academy of Pediatrics, & American College of Obstetricians and Gynecologists. (2012). *Guidelines for perinatal care* (7th ed.). Elk Grove Village, IL: Author.

American Academy of Pediatrics, & American Heart Association. (2016). *Textbook of neonatal resuscitation* (7th ed.). Elk Grove Village, IL: Author.

American Academy of Pediatrics, American Thyroid Association, & Lawson Wilkins Pediatric Endocrine Society. (2006, reaffirmed 2011). Update of newborn screening and therapy for congenital hypothyroidism. *Pediatrics, 117*(6), 2290–2303.

American Academy of Pediatrics Committee on Drugs. (2016). Neonatal drug withdrawal. *Pediatrics, 101*(6), 1079–1088.

American Academy of Pediatrics Section on Ophthalmology, American Association for Pediatric Ophthalmology and Strabismus, & American Association of Certified Orthoptists. (2013). Screening examination of premature infants for retinopathy of prematurity. *Pediatrics, 131*(1), 189–195.

American Academy of Pediatrics Subcommittee on Hyperbilirubinemia. (2004). Management of hyperbilirubinemia in the newborn infant 35 or more weeks of gestation (clinical practice guideline). *Pediatrics, 114*(1), 297–316.

Amin, S. C., Pappas, C., Iyengar, H., et al. (2013). Short bowel syndrome in the NICU. *Clinics in Perinatology, 40*(1), 58–63.

Association of Women's Health, Obstetric, and Neonatal Nurses (2013). *Evidence-based clinical practice guideline: Neonatal skin care* (3rd ed.). Washington, DC: Author.

Association of Women's Health, Obstetric, and Neonatal Nurses (2014). *Assessment and care of the late preterm infant: Evidence-based clinical practice guideline* (updated ed.). Washington, DC: Author.

Azzopardi, D., Strohm, B., Marlow, N., et al. (2014). Effects of hypothermia for perinatal asphyxia on childhood outcomes. *New England Journal of Medicine, 371*(2), 140–149.

Bagwell, G. A. (2014). Hematologic system. In C. Kenner & J. Lott (Eds.), *Comprehensive neonatal care: An interdisciplinary approach* (5th ed.). St. Louis, MO: Saunders.

Bahadue, F. L., & Soll, R. (2012). Early versus delayed selective surfactant treatment for neonatal respiratory distress syndrome. *Cochrane Database of Systematic Reviews, 2012*(11), CD001456.

Bandstra, E. S., Morrow, C. E., Accornero, V. H., et al. (2011). Estimated effects of in utero cocaine exposure on language development through early adolescence. *Neurotoxicology and Teratology, 33*(1), 25–35.

Berry, G. T. (2017). Classic galactosemia and clinical variant galactosemia. In R. A. Pagon, M. P. Adam, H. H. Ardinger, et al. (Eds.), *GeneReviews*. Seattle, WA: University of Washington.

Berry, S. A., Brown, C., Grant, M., et al. (2013). Newborn screening 50 years later: Access issues faced by adults with PKU. *Genetics in Medicine, 15*(8), 591–599.

Bhatia, J., Greer, F., & AAP Committee on Nutrition. (2008). Use of soy protein-based formulas in infant feeding. *Pediatrics, 121*(5), 1062–1068.

Black, B. P. (2016). Perinatal loss, bereavement, and grief. In D. L. Lowdermilk, S. E. Perry, K. Cashion, et al. (Eds.), *Maternity and Women's Health Care* (11th ed.). St. Louis, MO: Elsevier.

Blackburn, S. T. (2013). *Maternal, fetal, and neonatal physiology: A clinical perspective* (4th ed.). Maryland Heights, MO: Saunders.

Blau, N., Shen, N., & Carducci, C. (2014). Molecular genetics and diagnosis of phenylketonuria: State of the art. *Expert Review of Molecular Diagnostics, 14*(6), 655–671.

Blickstein, I., & Flidel Rimon, O. (2015). Post-term pregnancy. In R. J. Martin, A. A. Fanaroff, & M. C. Walsh (Eds.), *Fanaroff and Martin's neonatal-perinatal medicine* (10th ed.). St. Louis, MO: Elsevier.

Boundy, E. O., Dastjerdi, R., Spiegelman, D., et al. (2016). Kangaroo mother care and neonatal outcomes: A meta-analysis. *Pediatrics, 137*(1), e20152238.

Boyer, S. W., Barclay, L. J., & Burrage, L. C. (2015). Inherited metabolic disorders—Aspects of chronic nutrition management. *Nutrition in Clinical Practice, 30*(4), 502–510.

Bradshaw, W. T. (2015). Gastrointestinal disorders. In M. T. Verklan & M. Walden (Eds.), *Core curriculum for neonatal intensive care nursing* (5th ed.). St. Louis, MO: Elsevier.

Bradshaw, E. A., & Martin, G. R. (2012). Screening for critical congenital heart disease: Advancing detection in the newborn. *Current Opinion in Pediatrics, 24*(5), 603–608.

Bucher, B. T., Pacetti, A. S., Lovvorn III, H. N., et al. (2016). Neonatal surgery. In S. L. Gardner, B. S. Carter, M. Enzman-Hines, et al. (Eds.), *Merenstein and Gardner's handbook of neonatal intensive care* (8th ed.). St. Louis, MO: Elsevier.

Bull, M. J., Engle, W. A., & AAP Committee on Injury, Violence, and Poison Prevention & Committee on Fetus and Newborn. (2009). Safe transportation of preterm and low-birth-weight infants at hospital discharge. *Pediatrics, 123*(5), 1424–1429.

Cain, M. A., Bornick, P., & Whiteman, V. (2013). The maternal, fetal, and neonatal effects of cocaine exposure in pregnancy. *Clinical Obstetrics and Gynecology, 56*(1), 124–132.

Canadian Organization for Rare Disorders. (2015). *Newborn screening in Canada status report*. Retrieved from https://www.rarediseases.ca/content/uploads/Canada-NBS-status-updated-Sept.-3-2015.pdf.

Carlo, W. A., & Ambalavanan, N. (2016a). Metabolic disorders. In R. M. Kliegman, B. F. Stanton, J. W. St Geme, et al. (Eds.), *Nelson textbook of pediatrics* (20th ed.). Philadelphia, PA: Elsevier.

Carlo, W. A., & Ambalavanan, N. (2016b). Nervous system disorders. In R. M. Kliegman, B. F. Stanton, J. W. St Geme, et al. (Eds.), *Nelson textbook of pediatrics* (20th ed.). Philadelphia, PA: Elsevier.

Centers for Disease Control and Prevention. (2016). *Alcohol and pregnancy*. Retrieved from http://www.cdc.gov/vitalsigns/fasd/index.html.

Conde-Agudelo, A., Belizán, J. M., & Diaz-Rossello, J. (2011). Kangaroo mother care to reduce morbidity and mortality in low birthweight infants. *Cochrane Database of Systematic Reviews, 2011*(3), CD002771.

Cong, X., Cusson, R. M., Walsh, S., et al. (2012). Effects of skin-to-skin on autonomic pain responses in preterm infants. *Journal of Pain, 13*(7), 636–645.

Conner, S. N., Carter, E. B., Tuuli, M. G., et al. (2015). Maternal marijuana use and neonatal morbidity. *American Journal of Obstetrics & Gynecology, 213*(3), 422e1–422e4.

Dani, C., & Pratesi, S. (2013). Nitric oxide for the treatment of preterm infants with respiratory distress syndrome. *Expert Opinion on Pharmacotherapy, 14*(1), 97–103.

D'Apolito, K. (2013). Breastfeeding and substance abuse. *Clinical Obstetrics and Gynecology, 56*(1), 202–211.

Davis, N. L., Zenchenko, Y., Lever, A., et al. (2013). Car seat safety for preterm neonates: Implementation and testing parameters of the Infant Car Seat Challenge. *Academic Pediatrics, 13*(3), 272–277.

Demirkol, M., Gizewska, M., Giovannini, M., & Walter, J. (2011). Follow up of phenylketonuria patients. *Molecular Genetics and Metabolism, 104*(S1), S31–S39.

Donohue, P. K., Gilmore, M. M., Cristofalo, E., et al. (2011). Inhaled nitric oxide in preterm infants: A systematic review. *Pediatrics, 127*(2), e414–e422.

Durbin, D. R., & AAP Committee on Injury, Violence, and Poison Prevention. (2011). Child passenger safety. *Pediatrics, 127*(4), e1050–e1066.

Egbor, M., Knott, P., & Bhide, A. (2012). Red-cell and platelet alloimmunisation in pregnancy. *Best Practice & Research: Clinical Obstetrics & Gynaecology, 26*(1), 119–132.

Ellett, M. L., Cohen, M. D., Perkins, S. M., et al. (2011). Predicting the insertion length for gastric tube placement for neonates. *Journal of Obstetric, Gynecologic, and Neonatal Nursing, 40*(4), 412–421.

Environmental Protection Agency Report on the Environment (2015). *Birth defects prevalence and mortality.* Washington, DC: US EPA. Retrieved from https://cfpub.epa.gov/roe/indicator.cfm?i=72.

Fallone, M. D., LaGasse, L. L., Lester, B. M., et al. (2014). Reactivity and regulation of motor responses in cocaine-exposed infants. *Neurotoxicology and Teratology, 43*, 25–32.

Fastman, B. R., Howell, E. A., Holzman, I., et al. (2014). Current perspectives on temperature management and hypothermia in low birth weight infants. *Newborn and Infants Nursing Reviews, 14*(2), 50–55.

Finnegan, L. P. (1985). Neonatal abstinence. In N. Nelson (Ed.), *Current therapy in neonatal perinatal medicine 1985–1986.* Toronto, Canada: Decker.

Forray, A., & Foster, D. (2015). Substance use in the perinatal period. *Current Psychiatry Reports, 17*(11), 91.

Fraser, A., Walker, K., & Green, J. (2016). Maternal cocaine abuse—An evidence review. *Journal of Neonatal Nursing, 22*(2), 56–60.

Fraser, D. (2015). Respiratory distress. In M. T. Verklan & M. Walden (Eds.), *Core curriculum for neonatal intensive care nursing* (5th ed.). St. Louis, MO: Elsevier.

Freeman, D., Saxton, V., & Holberton, J. (2012). A weight-based formula for the estimation of gastric tube insertion length in newborns. *Advances in Neonatal Care, 12*(3), 179–182.

Gardner, S. L., & Carter, B. S. (2016). Grief and perinatal loss. In S. L. Gardner, B. S. Carter, M. Enzman-Hines, et al. (Eds.), *Merenstein and Gardner's handbook of neonatal intensive care* (8th ed.). St. Louis, MO: Elsevier.

Gardner, S. L., Enzman-Hines, M., & Nyp, M. (2016). Respiratory diseases. In S. L. Gardner, B. S. Carter, M. Enzman-Hines, et al. (Eds.), *Merenstein and Gardner's handbook of neonatal intensive care* (8th ed.). St. Louis, MO: Elsevier.

Gardner, S. L., & Hernández, J. A. (2016). Heat balance. In S. L. Gardner, B. S. Carter, M. Enzman-Hines, et al. (Eds.), *Merenstein and Gardner's handbook of neonatal intensive care* (8th ed.). St. Louis, MO: Elsevier.

Gardner, S. L., & Lawrence, R. A. (2016). Breast feeding the neonate with special needs. In S. L. Gardner, B. S. Carter, M. Enzman-Hines, et al. (Eds.), *Merenstein and Gardner's handbook of neonatal intensive care* (8th ed.). St. Louis, MO: Elsevier.

Geary, F., & Wells, M. (2013). Management of the patient in labor who has abused substances. *Clinical Obstetrics, 56*(1), 166–172.

Gephart, S. M., & Hanson, C. K. (2013). Preventing necrotizing enterocolitis with standardized feeding protocols: Not only possible, but imperative. *Advances in Neonatal Care, 13*(1), 48–54.

Halbardier, B. H. (2015). Fluid and electrolyte management. In M. T. Verklan & M. Walden (Eds.), *Core curriculum for neonatal intensive care nursing* (5th ed.). St. Louis, MO: Elsevier.

Hamilton, E., Massey, C., Ross, J., & Taylor, S. (2014). Early enteral feeding in very low birth weight infants. *Early Human Development, 90*(5), 227–230.

Hay, W. W. (2012). Care of the infant of the diabetic mother. *Current Diabetes Reports, 12*(1), 4–15.

Holbrook, B. D., & Rayburn, W. F. (2014). Teratogenic risks from exposure to illicit drugs. *Obstetrics & Gynecology Clinics of North America, 41*(2), 229–239.

Horgan, M. J. (2015). Management of the late preterm infant: Not quite ready for prime time. *Pediatric Clinics of North America, 62*(2), 439–451.

Houston, B. L., Govia, R., Abou-Setta, A. M., et al. (2015). Severe Rh alloimmunization and hemolytic disease of the fetus managed with plasmapheresis, intravenous immunoglobulin and intrauterine transfusion: A case report. *Transfusion and Apheresis Science, 53*(3), 399–402.

Hwang, C. K., Hubbard, G. B., Hutchinson, A. K., et al. (2015). Outcomes after intravitreal bevacizumab versus laser photocoagulation for retinopathy of prematurity. *Ophthalmology, 122*(5), 1008–1015.

Inturrisi, M. (2017). Care of the laboring woman with diabetes. In B. B. Kennedy & S. M. Baird (Eds.), *Intrapartum management modules: A perinatal education program* (5th ed.). Philadelphia, PA: Wolters Kluwer.

Jones, H. E., & Fielder, A. (2015). Neonatal abstinence syndrome: Historical perspective, current focus, future directions. *Preventative Medicine, 80*, 12–17.

Kamath-Rayne, B. D., Thilo, E. H., Deacon, J., et al. (2016). Neonatal hyperbilirubinemia. In S. L. Gardner, B. S. Carter, M. Enzman-Hines, et al. (Eds.), *Merenstein and Gardner's handbook of neonatal intensive care* (8th ed.). St. Louis, MO: Elsevier.

Kastenberg, Z. J., & Sylvester, K. G. (2013). The surgical management of necrotizing enterocolitis. *Clinics in Perinatology, 40*(1), 135–148.

Kemper, A. R., Mahle, W. T. Martin, G. R. et al. (2011). Strategies for implementing screening for critical congenital heart disease. *Pediatrics, 128*(5), e1259–e1267.

Kieler, H., Artama, M., Engeland, A., et al. (2012). Selective serotonin reuptake inhibitors during pregnancy and risk of persistent pulmonary hypertension in the newborn: Population based cohort study from the five Nordic countries. *British Medical Journal, 344*, d8012.

Kimberlin, D. W., & AAP Committee on Infectious Diseases (2015). *Red book: 2015 report of the Committee on Infectious Diseases* (30th ed.). Elk Grove Village, IL: Author.

King, K., O'Gorman, C., & Gallagher, S. (2014). Thyroid dysfunction in children with Down syndrome: A literature review. *Irish Journal of Medical Science, 183*(1), 1–6.

Kish, M. Z. (2013). Oral feeding readiness in preterm infants: A concept analysis. *Advances in Neonatal Care, 13*(4), 230–237.

Kishnani, P. S., & Chen, Y. (2016). Defects on galactose metabolism. In R. M. Kliegman, B. F. Stanton, J. W. St. Geme, et al. (Eds.), *Nelson textbook of pediatrics* (20th ed.). Philadelphia, PA: Elsevier.

Kraft, W. K., & van den Anker, J. N. (2012). Pharmacologic management of the opioid neonatal abstinence syndrome. *Pediatric Clinics of North America, 59*(5), 1147–1165.

Kocherlakota, P. (2014). Neonatal abstinence syndrome. *Pediatrics, 134*(2), e547–e561.

Kuppala, V. S., Meinzen-Derr, J., Morrow, A. L., et al. (2011). Prolonged initial empirical antibiotic treatment is associated with adverse outcomes in premature infants. *Journal of Pediatrics, 159*(5), 720–725.

LaFranchi, S. H., & Huang, S. A. (2016). Hypothyroidism. In R. M. Kliegman, B. F. Stanton, J. W. St Geme, et al. (Eds.), *Nelson textbook of pediatrics* (20th ed.). Philadelphia, PA: Elsevier.

Landon, M. B., Catalano, P. M., & Gabbe, S. G. (2017). Diabetes mellitus complicating pregnancy. In S. G. Gabbe, J. R. Niebyl, J. L. Simpson, et al.

(Eds.), *Obstetrics: Normal and problem pregnancies* (7th ed.). Philadelphia, PA: Elsevier.

Laubach, V., Wilhelm, P., & Carter, K. (2014). Shhh…I'm growing: Noise in the NICU. *Nursing Clinics of North America, 49*(3), 329–344.

Lawrence, R. A., & Lawrence, R. M. (2016). *Breastfeeding: A guide for the medical profession* (8th ed.). St. Louis, MO: Elsevier.

Legendre, V., Burtner, P., Martinez, K., & Crowe, T. (2011). The evolving practice of developmental care in the neonatal unit: A systematic review. *Occupational Therapy in Pediatrics, 31*(3), 315–338.

Lester, B. M., Tronick, E. Z., & Brazelton, T. B. (2004). The Neonatal Intensive Care Unit Network Neurobehavioral Scale procedures. *Pediatrics, 113* (3 suppl), 641–667.

Lewis, D. A., Sanders, L. P., & Brockopp, D. Y. (2011). The effect of three nursing interventions on thermoregulation in low-birth-weight infants. *Neonatal Network, 30*(3), 160–164.

Li, S., Guo, P., Zou, Q., et al. (2016). Efficacy and safety of plastic wrap for prevention of hypothermia after birth and during NICU in preterm infants: A systematic review and meta-analysis. *PLoS ONE, 11*(6), e0156960.

Louis, D., More, K., Oberoi, S., & Shah, P. S. (2014). Intravenous immunoglobulin in isoimmune haemolytic disease of newborn: An updated systematic review and meta-analysis. *Archives of Disease in Childhood. Fetal and Neonatal Edition, 99*(4), F325–F331.

Mactier, H. (2013). Neonatal and longer term management following substance misuse in pregnancy. *Early Human Development, 89*(11), 887–892.

Mahle, W. T., Martin, G. R., Beekman 3rd, W. R., et al. (2012). Endorsement of Health and Human Services recommendation for pulse oximetry screening for critical congenital heart disease. *Pediatrics, 129*(1), 190–192.

Mantagou, L., Fouzas, S., Skylogianni, E., et al. (2012). Trends of transcutaneous bilirubin in neonates who develop significant hyperbilirubinemia. *Pediatrics, 130*(4), e898–e904.

Martin, M. M., Graham, D. L., McCarthy, D. M., et al. (2016). Cocaine-induced neurodevelopmental deficits and underlying mechanisms. *Embryo Today Reviews, 108*(2), 147–173.

Mburia-Mwalili, A., & Yang, W. (2014). Birth defects surveillance in the United States. *International Scholarly Research Notices, 2014*, 212874.

McAdams, R. M., & Juul, S. E. (2016). Neonatal encephalopathy: Update on therapeutic hypothermia and other novel therapeutics. *Clinics in Perinatology, 43*(3), 485–500.

McCance, K., & Huether, S. (2014). *Pathophysiology: The biological basis for disease in infants and children* (7th ed.). St. Louis, MO: Elsevier.

Metz, T. D., & Stickrath, E. H. (2015). Marijuana use in pregnancy and lactation: A review of the evidence. *American Journal of Obstetrics and Gynecology, 213*(6), 761–778.

Minnes, S., Lang, A., & Singer, L. (2011). Prenatal tobacco, marijuana, stimulant and opiate exposure: Outcomes and practice implications. *Addict Science & Clinical Practice, 6*(1), 57–70.

Moise, K. J. (2017). Red cell alloimmunization. In S. G. Gabbe, J. R. Niebyl, J. L. Simpson, et al. (Eds.), *Obstetrics: Normal and problem pregnancies* (7th ed.). Philadelphia, PA: Elsevier.

Moise, K. J., & Argoti, P. S. (2012). Management and prevention of red cell alloimmunization in pregnancy: A systematic review. *Obstetrics & Gynecology, 120*(5), 1132–1139.

Mundy, C. A., & Bhatia, J. (2015). Variable clinical presentations of ABO incompatibility in dizygotic twins. *Neonatal Network, 34*(6), 317–319.

Narkowicz, S., Plotka, J., Polkowska, Z., et al. (2013). Prenatal exposure to substance of abuse: A worldwide problem. *Environment International, 54*, 141–163.

National Perinatal Association (2012). *Multidisciplinary guidelines for the care of late preterm infants.* Binghamton, NY: Author. Retrieved from www.nationalperinatal.org/Resources/LatePretermGuidelinesNPA.pdf.

Ness, M. J., Davis, D. M. R., & Carey, W. A. (2013). Neonatal skin care: A concise review. *International Journal of Dermatology, 52*(1), 14–22.

Nyp, M., Brunkhorst, J. L., Reavey, D., & Pallotto, E. K. (2016). Fluid and electrolyte management. In S. L. Gardner, B. S. Carter, M. Enzman-Hines, et al. (Eds.), *Merenstein and Gardner's handbook of neonatal intensive care* (8th ed.). St. Louis, MO: Elsevier.

Pammi, M., Brand, M. C., & Weisman, L. E. (2016). Infection in the neonate. In S. L. Gardner, B. S. Carter, M. Enzman-Hines, et al. (Eds.), *Merenstein and Gardner's handbook of neonatal intensive care* (8th ed.). St. Louis, MO: Elsevier.

Panel on Treatment of HIV-Infected Pregnant Women and Prevention of Perinatal Transmission (2011). *Recommendations for use of antiretroviral drugs in pregnant HIV-infected women for maternal health and interventions to reduce perinatal HIV transmission in the United States.* Washington, DC: National Institutes of Health.

Parikh, A. S., & Mitchell, A. L. (2015). Congenital anomalies. In R. J. Martin, A. A. Fanaroff, & M. C. Walsh (Eds.), *Fanaroff and Martin's neonatal-perinatal medicine: Diseases of the fetus and infant* (10th ed.). St. Louis, MO: Elsevier.

Parsons, J. A., Seay, A. R., & Jacobson, M. (2016). Neurologic disorders. In S. L. Gardner, B. S. Carter, M. Enzman-Hines, et al. (Eds.), *Merenstein and Gardner's handbook of neonatal intensive care* (8th ed.). St. Louis, MO: Elsevier.

Patel, R. M., & Denning, P. W. (2013). Therapeutic use of prebiotics, probiotics, and postbiotics to prevent necrotizing enterocolitis: What is the current evidence? *Clinics in Perinatology, 40*(1), 11–25.

Piehl, E., & Fernandez-Bustamante, A. (2012). Lucinactant for the treatment of respiratory distress syndrome in neonates. *Drugs Today (Barcelona), 48*(9), 587–593.

Polin, R. A., & AAP Committee on Fetus and Newborn. (2012). Management of neonates with suspected or proven early-onset bacterial sepsis. *Pediatrics, 129*(5), 1006–1015.

Polin, R. A., Carlo, W. A., & AAP Committee on Fetus and Newborn. (2014). Surfactant replacement therapy for preterm and term neonates with respiratory distress. *Pediatrics, 133*(1), 156–163.

Polin, R. A., Denson, S., Brady, M. T., et al. (2012). Strategies for prevention of health care–associated infections in the NICU. *Pediatrics, 129*(4), e1085–e1093.

Ramani, M., & Ambalavanan, N. (2013). Feeding practices and NEC. *Clinics in Perinatology, 40*(1), 1–10.

Ramirez, F. D., Femenia, F., Simpsons, C. S., et al. (2012). Electrocardiographic findings associated with cocaine use in humans: A systematic review. *Expert Review of Cardiovascular Therapy, 10*(1), 105–127.

Rayyan, M., Rommel, N., & Allegaert, K. (2015). The fate of fat: Pre-exposure fat losses during nasogastric tube feeding in preterm newborns. *Nutrients, 7*(8), 6213–6223.

Reddy, U. M., & Spong, C. Y. (2014). Stillbirth. In R. K. Creasy, R. Resnik, J. D. Iams, et al. (Eds.), *Creasy and Resnik's maternal-fetal medicine: Principles and practice* (7th ed.). Philadelphia, PA: Saunders.

Restieaux, M., Maw, A., Broadbent, R., et al. (2013). Neonatal extravasation injury: Prevention and management in Australia and New Zealand— A survey of current practice. *BMC Pediatrics, 13*, 34.

Rezvani, I., & Ficicioglu, C. H. (2016). Defects in metabolism of amino acids. In R. M. Kliegman, B. F. Stanton, J. W. St Geme, et al. (Eds.), *Nelson textbook of pediatrics* (20th ed.). Philadelphia, PA: Elsevier.

Roos, A., Kwiatkowski, M. A., Fouche, J.-P., et al. (2015). White matter integrity and cognitive performance in children with prenatal methamphetamine exposure. *Behavioural Brain Research, 279*, 62–67.

Rozance, P. J., McGowan, J. E., Price-Douglas, W., et al. (2016). Glucose homeostasis. In S. L. Gardner, B. S. Carter, M. Enzman-Hines, et al. (Eds.), *Merenstein and Gardner's handbook of neonatal intensive care* (8th ed.). St. Louis, MO: Elsevier.

Senterre, T. (2014). Practice of enteral nutrition in very low birth weight and extremely low birth weight infants. *World Review of Nutrition and Dietetics, 110*, 201–214.

Senturias, Y., & Asamoah, A. (2014). Fetal alcohol spectrum disorders: Guidance for recognition, diagnosis, differential diagnosis and referral. *Current Problems in Pediatric and Adolescent Health Care, 44*(4), 88–95.

Shah, R., Diaz, S. D., Arria, A., et al. (2012). Prenatal methamphetamine exposure and short-term maternal and infant medical outcomes. *American Journal of Perinatology, 29*(5), 391–400.

Shah, P. S., & Ohlsson, A. (2011). Sildenafil for pulmonary hypertension in neonates. *Cochrane Database of Systematic Reviews, 2011*(8), CD005494.

Shanholtz, H. J. (2013). Congenital hypothyroidism. *Journal of Pediatric Nursing, 28*(2), 200–202.

Shankaran, S. (2012). Therapeutic hypothermia for neonatal encephalopathy. *Current Treatment Options in Neurology, 14*(6), 608–619.

Sherman, M. P. (2013). Lactoferrin and necrotizing enterocolitis. *Clinics in Perinatology, 40*(1), 79–91.

Shlomai, N. O., Rao, S., & Patole, S. (2015). Efficacy of interventions to improve hand hygiene compliance in neonatal units: A systematic review and meta-analysis. *European Journal of Clinical Microbiology & Infectious Diseases, 34*(5), 887–897.

Sie, S. D., Wennink, J. M. B., van Driel, J. J., et al. (2012). Maternal use of SSRIs, SNRIs and NaSSAs: Practical recommendations during pregnancy and lactation. *Archives of Disease in Childhood. Fetal and Neonatal Edition, 97*(6), F472–F476.

Silva, M. G., Barros, M. C., Pessoa, U. M. L., & Guinsburg, R. (2016). Kangaroo-mother care method and neurobehavior of preterm infants. *Early Human Development, 95*, 55–59.

Smith, R. L., & Lucas, R. (2016). Evaluation of nursing knowledge of early initiation of breastfeeding in preterm infants in a hospital setting. *Journal of Neonatal Nursing, 22*(3), 138–143.

Solomonia, N., Playforth, K., & Reynolds, E. (2012). Fetal-maternal hemorrhage: A case and literature review. *American Journal of Perinatology Reports, 2*(1), 7–14.

Sriraman, N. K., Melvin, K., Meltzer-Brody, S., et al. (2015). ABM clinical protocol no. 18: Use of antidepressants in breastfeeding mothers. *Breastfeeding Medicine, 10*(6), 290–299.

Stokowski, L. (2015). Endocrine disorders. In M. T. Verklan & M. Walden (Eds.), *Core curriculum for neonatal intensive care nursing* (5th ed.). St. Louis, MO: Elsevier.

Stoll, B. J., & Shane, A. L. (2016). Infections of the neonatal infant. In R. M. Kliegman, B. F. Stanton, J. W. St. Geme, et al. (Eds.), *Nelson textbook of pediatrics* (20th ed.). Philadelphia, PA: Elsevier.

Stoll, B. J., Hansen, N. I., Sanchez, P. J., et al. (2011). Early-onset neonatal sepsis: The burden of group B streptococcal and *E. coli* disease continues. *Pediatrics, 127*(5), 817–826.

Sublett, J. (2013). Neonatal abstinence syndrome: Therapeutic interventions. *American Journal of Maternal/Child Nursing, 38*(2), 102–107.

Sweet, D. G., Halliday, H. L., & Speer, C. P. (2013). Surfactant therapy for neonatal respiratory distress syndrome in 2013. *Journal of Maternal-Fetal & Neonatal Medicine, 26*(s2), 27–29.

Telofski, L. S., Morello, A. P., Mack Correa, M. C., et al. (2012). The infant skin barrier: Can we preserve, protect, and enhance the barrier? *Dermatology Research and Practice, 2012*, 198789.

Tluczek, A., & De Luca, J. M. (2013). Newborn screening policy and practice issues for nurses. *Journal of Obstetric, Gynecologic, and Neonatal Nursing, 42*(6), 718–729.

US Department of Health and Human Services Advisory Committee on Heritable Disorders in Newborns and Children. (2016). *Recommended uniform screening panel core conditions.* Retrieved from https://www.hrsa.gov/advisorycommittees/mchbadvisory/heritabledisorders/recommendedpanel/uniformscreeningpanel.pdf.

Van Calcar, S. C., Bernstein, L. E., Rohr, F. J., et al. (2014). A re-evaluation of life-long severe galactose restriction for the nutrition management of classic galactosemia. *Molecular Genetics and Metabolism, 112*(3), 191–197.

Van Riper, M. (2016). Nursing and genomics. In D. L. Lowdermilk, S. E. Perry, K. Cashion, et al. (Eds.), *Maternity and women's health care* (11th ed.). St. Louis, MO: Elsevier.

Vento, M. (2015). Oxygen therapy in neonatal resuscitation. In R. J. Martin, A. A. Fanaroff, & M. C. Walsh (Eds.), *Fanaroff and Martin's neonatal-perinatal medicine: Diseases of the fetus and infant* (10th ed.). St. Louis, MO: Elsevier.

Verklan, M. T. (2015). Neurologic disorders. In M. T. Verklan & M. Walden (Eds.), *Core curriculum for neonatal intensive care nursing* (5th ed.). St. Louis, MO: Elsevier.

Walsh, B. K., Daigle, B., Diblasi, R. M., et al. (2013). AARC clinical practice guideline: Surfactant replacement therapy. *Respiratory Care, 58*(2), 367–375.

Wassner, A. J., & Brown, R. S. (2015). Congenital hypothyroidism: Recent advances. *Current Opinion in Endocrinology, Diabetes & Obesity, 22*(5), 407–412.

Weiner, S. M., & Finnegan, L. P. (2016). Drug withdrawal in the neonate. In S. L. Gardner, B. S. Carter, M. Enzman-Hines, et al. (Eds.), *Merenstein & Gardner's handbook of neonatal intensive care* (8th ed.). St. Louis, MO: Elsevier.

Xu, J., Murphy, S. L., Kochanek, M. A., et al. (2016). Deaths: Final data for 2013. *National Vital Statistics Reports, 64*(2), 1–118. Retrieved from http://www.cdc.gov/nchs/data/nvsr/nvsr64/nvsr64_02.pdf.

Young, P. C., Korgenski, K., & Buchi, K. F. (2013). Early readmission of newborns in a large health care system. *Pediatrics, 131*(5), e1538–e1544.

Zubcevic, S., Heljic, S., Catibusic, F., et al. (2015). Neurodevelopmental follow up after therapeutic hypothermia for perinatal asphyxia. *Medical Archives, 69*(6), 362–366.

26

21st Century Pediatric Nursing

Marilyn J. Hockenberry

http://evolve.elsevier.com/Perry/maternal

HEALTH CARE FOR CHILDREN

The major goal for pediatric nursing is to improve the quality of health care for children and their families. In 2014, almost 75 million children 0 to 17 years of age lived in the United States, composing 23% of the population (Federal Interagency Forum on Child and Family Statistics, 2016). The health status of children in the United States has improved in a number of areas, including increased immunization rates for all children, decreased adolescent birth rate, and improved child health outcomes. The 2016 America's Children in Brief—Indicators of Well-Being reveals that preterm births declined for the seventh straight year and that the adolescent birth rate reached a record low. Average mathematics scores for 4th- and 8th-grade students increased, and the violent crime victimization rate among youth decreased. Although the number of children living in poverty decreased slightly in 2015, overall the rate remain high at 23%.

Millions of children and their families have no health insurance, which results in a lack of access to care and health-promotion services. In addition, disparities in pediatric health care are related to race, ethnicity, socioeconomic status, and geographic factors (Flores & Lesley, 2014). Patterns of child health are shaped by medical progress and societal trends. Urgent priorities for health and health care of children in the United States are the focus for action toward new policy priorities (Box 26.1).

HEALTH PROMOTION

Child health promotion provides opportunities to reduce differences in current health status among members of different groups and to ensure equal opportunities and resources to enable all children to achieve their fullest health potential. The Healthy People 2020 Leading Health Indicators (Box 26.2) provide a framework for identifying essential components for child health-promotion programs designed to prevent future health problems in our nation's children. Bright Futures is a national health-promotion initiative with a goal to improve the health of our nation's children (Bright Futures, 2014). Major themes of the Bright Futures guideline are promoting family support, child development, mental health, healthy nutrition that leads to healthy weight, physical activity, oral health, healthy sexual development and sexuality, safety and injury prevention, and the importance of community relationships and resources.* Throughout this text, developmentally appropriate health-promotion strategies are discussed. Key examples of child health-promotion themes essential for all age-groups include promoting development, nutrition, and oral health. Bright Futures recommendations for preventive health care during infancy, early childhood, and adolescents are found in Chapters 31 to 34.

Development

Health promotion integrates surveillance of the physical, psychologic, and emotional changes that occur in human beings between birth and the end of adolescence. Developmental processes are unique to each stage of development, and continuous screening and assessment are essential for early intervention when problems are found. The most dramatic time of physical, motor, cognitive, emotional, and social development occurs during infancy. Interactions between the parent and infant are central to promoting optimal developmental outcomes and are a key component of infant assessment. During early childhood, early identification of developmental delays is critical for establishing early interventions. Anticipatory guidance strategies ensure that parents are aware of the specific developmental needs of each developmental stage. Ongoing surveillance during middle childhood provides opportunities to strengthen cognitive and emotional attributes, communication skills, self-esteem, and independence. Recognition that adolescents differ greatly in their physical, social, and emotional maturity is important for surveillance throughout this developmental period.

An important consideration for health promotion during early years of a child's development is to be aware of changing recommendations that address the fast-changing world of technology in our society. An important example is the changes in the latest American Academy of Pediatrics (2016) policy statement on screen viewing by infants and children. New guidelines for screen viewing (laptop or phone) shift the importance from what is on the screen to who is viewing the information with the young child (AAP, 2016). For infants younger than 18 months of age, no screen time is recommended except for FaceTime-visiting a grandparent or loved one. Parents should be advised to use technology sparingly before 5 years of age and to always participate during screen-time viewing.

---

*Bright Futures is supported by the American Academy of Pediatrics and can be found at http://brightfutures.aap.org/about.html.

689

BOX 26.1   **Health and Health Care Priorities for Children in the United States**

Poverty	Firearm deaths and injuries
Hunger	Mental health
Lack of health insurance	Racial and ethnic disparities
Child abuse and neglect	Immigration
Overweight and obesity	

Adapted from Flores, G., & Lesley, B. (2014). Children and US federal policy on health and health care: seen but not heard, *JAMA Pediatrics, 168*(12), 1155–1163.

BOX 26.2   **Healthy People 2020**

Goals
Increase quality and length of healthy life
Eliminate health disparities

Leading Health Indicators
Physical activity
Overweight and obesity
Tobacco use
Substance abuse
Responsible sexual behavior
Mental health
Injury and violence
Environmental quality
Immunization
Access to health care

From US Department of Health and Human Services, Office of Disease Prevention and Health Promotion. (2013). *Healthy People 2020*. Retrieved from http://www.healthypeople.gov/.

Nutrition

Nutrition is an essential component for healthy growth and development. Human milk is the preferred form of nutrition for all infants. Breastfeeding provides the infant with micronutrients, immunologic properties, and several enzymes that enhance digestion and absorption of these nutrients. A recent resurgence in breastfeeding has occurred due to the education of mothers and fathers regarding its benefits and increased social support.

Children establish lifelong eating habits during the first 3 years of life, and the nurse is instrumental in educating parents on the importance of nutrition. Most eating preferences and attitudes related to food are established by family influences and culture. During adolescence, parental influence diminishes and the adolescent makes food choices related to peer acceptability and sociability. Occasionally these choices are detrimental to adolescents with chronic illnesses like diabetes, obesity, chronic lung disease, hypertension, cardiovascular risk factors, and renal disease.

Families that struggle with lower incomes, homelessness, and migrant status generally lack the resources to provide their children with adequate food intake, nutritious foods such as fresh fruits and vegetables, and appropriate protein intake (Flores & Lesley, 2014). The result is nutritional deficiencies with subsequent growth and developmental delays, depression, and behavior problems.

Oral Health

Oral health is an essential component of health promotion throughout infancy, childhood, and adolescence. Preventing dental caries and developing healthy oral hygiene habits must occur early in childhood.

Dental caries is the single most common chronic disease of childhood. In the most recent National Surveys of Children's Health, minority children experience disparities in oral health care and were much more likely to have dental disease (Flores & Lin, 2013). The most common form of early dental disease is early childhood caries, which may begin before the first birthday and progress to pain and infection within the first 2 years of life (Kagihara, Niederhauser, & Stark, 2009). Preschoolers of low-income families are twice as likely to develop tooth decay and only half as likely to visit the dentist as other children. Early childhood caries is a preventable disease, and nurses play an essential role in educating children and parents about practicing dental hygiene, beginning with the first tooth eruption; drinking fluoridated water, including bottled water; and instituting early dental preventive care. Oral health care practices established during the early years of development prevent destructive periodontal disease and dental decay.

CHILDHOOD HEALTH PROBLEMS

Changes in modern society, including advancing medical knowledge and technology, the proliferation of information systems, struggles with insurance disparities, economically troubled times, and various changes and disruptive influences on the family, are leading to significant medical problems that affect the health of children (Berdahl, Friedman, McCormick, et al., 2013; Leslie, Slaw, Edwards, et al., 2010). The new morbidity, also known as *pediatric social illness*, refers to the behavior, social, and educational problems that children face. Problems that can negatively impact a child's development include poverty, violence, aggression, noncompliance, school failure, and adjustment to parental separation and divorce. In addition, mental health issues cause challenges in childhood and adolescence. Recent concern has focused on groups of children who are at highest risk, such as children born prematurely or with very low birth weight (VLBW) or low birth weight (LBW), children attending child care centers, children who live in poverty or are homeless, children of immigrant families, and children with chronic medical and psychiatric illnesses and disabilities. In addition, these children and their families face multiple barriers to adequate health, dental, and psychiatric care. A perspective of several health problems facing children and the major challenges for pediatric nurses is discussed in the following sections.

Obesity and Type 2 Diabetes

Childhood obesity, the most common nutritional problem among children in the United States, is increasing in epidemic proportions (Martin, Saunders, Shenkin et al., 2014; Giannini & Caprio, 2012). Obesity in children and adolescents is defined as a body mass index (BMI) at or greater than the 95th percentile for youth of the same age and gender. Overweight is defined as a BMI at or above the 85th percentile and below the 95th percentile for children and teens of the same age and sex. Over 30% of children in the United States are overweight, and 17% are obese (Flores & Lesley, 2014).

Advancements in entertainment and technology, such as television, computers, and video games, have contributed to the growing childhood obesity problem in the United States. In the National Longitudinal Study of Adolescent Health, screen times (TV, video, computer use) interact with genetic factors to influence BMI changes (Graff, North, Monda et al., 2011). Lack of physical activity related to limited resources, unsafe environments, and inconvenient play and exercise facilities, combined with easy access to television and video games, increases the incidence of obesity among low-income minority children. Overweight youth have an increased risk for cardiometabolic changes (a cluster of cardiovascular factors that include hypertension, altered glucose metabolism, dyslipidemia, and abdominal obesity) in the future (Weiss, Bremer, & Lustig, 2013) (Fig. 26.1). The US Department of Health and

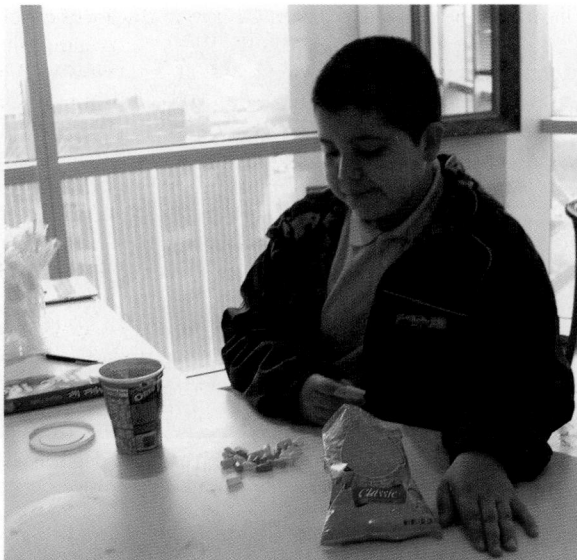

FIG 26.1 The American culture's intake of high-caloric, fatty food contributes to obesity in children.

Human Services (2013a) suggests that nurses focus on prevention strategies to reduce the incidence of overweight children from the current 20% in all ethnic groups to less than 6%. Emphasis is on preventive strategies that start in infancy or even begin in the prenatal period. Lifestyle interventions show promise in preventing obesity and decreasing occurrence if targeted at children 6 to 12 years of age (Martin, Saunders, Shenkin et al., 2014; Waters, de Silva-Sanigorski, Hall et al., 2011).

Childhood Injuries

Injuries are the most common cause of death and disability to children in the United States (Centers for Disease Control and Prevention [CDC], 2013) (Table 26.1). Mortality rates for suicide, poisoning, and falls rose substantially over the past decade. Suicide has surpassed motor vehicle injuries (MVAs) as the leading cause of injury mortality (Rockett, Regier, Kapusta, et al., 2012). Other unintentional injuries (head injuries, drowning, burns, and firearm injuries) take the lives of children every day. Implementing programs of injury prevention and health promotion could prevent many childhood injuries and fatalities.

The type of injury and the circumstances surrounding it are closely related to normal growth and development (Box 26.3). As children develop, their innate curiosity compels them to investigate the environment and to mimic the behavior of others. This is essential to acquire competency as an adult, but it can also predispose children to numerous hazards.

The child's developmental stage partially determines the types of injuries that are most likely to occur at a specific age and helps provide clues to preventive measures. For example, small infants are helpless in any environment. When they begin to roll over or propel themselves, they can fall from unprotected surfaces. The crawling infant, who has a natural tendency to place objects in the mouth, is at risk for aspiration or poisoning. The mobile toddler, with the instinct to explore and investigate and the ability to run and climb, may experience falls, burns, and collisions with objects. As children grow older, their absorption with play makes them oblivious to environmental hazards such as street traffic or water. The need to conform and gain acceptance compels older children and adolescents to accept challenges and dares. Although the rate of injuries is high in children younger than 9 years of age, most fatal injuries occur in later childhood and adolescence.

TABLE 26.1 Mortality from Leading Types of Unintentional Injuries, United States*

Type of Injury	<1	1–4	5–14	15–24
	AGE (YEARS)			
Males				
All causes	716.4	31.2	15.9	108.8
Unintentional injuries (all types)	33.3	10.5	5.8	48.1
Motor vehicle	2.8 (2)	3.0 (2)	3.0 (1)	29.5 (1)
Drowning	1.1 (4)	3.4 (1)	0.9 (2)	2.3 (3)
Fires and burns	0.5 (5)	1.1 (3)	0.5 (3)	0.4 (5)
Firearms	—	—	—	—
Choking	1.7 (3)	0.5 (5)	—	—
Falls	—	—	—	0.9 (4)
Mechanical suffocation	25.0 (1)	0.6 (4)	0.2 (4)	—
Poisoning	—	—	0.1 (5)	11.2 (2)
All other unintentional injuries	4.6	1.9	1.0	3.8
Injuries as a percent of all deaths	4.6%	33.7%	36.5%	44.2%
Females				
All causes	591.7	24.7	12.0	39.2
Unintentional injuries (all types)	28.0	6.9	3.4	16.6
Motor vehicle	2.0 (2)	2.4 (1)	2.0 (1)	11.7 (1)
Drowning	0.9 (4)	1.8 (2)	0.4 (2)	0.3 (3)
Fires and burns	0.4 (5)	0.9 (3)	0.4 (2)	0.3 (3)
Firearms	—	—	—	—
Choking	1.1 (3)	0.3 (4)	—	—
Falls	—	—	—	0.2 (5)
Mechanical suffocation	21.4 (1)	0.3 (4)	0.1 (4)	—
Poisoning	—	—	0.1 (4)	3.4 (2)
All other unintentional injuries	2.1	1.1	0.4	0.8
Injuries as a percent of all deaths	4.7%	27.9%	28.3%	42.3%

*Rate per 100,000 population in each age-group. Adapted from National Safety Council. (2012). *Injury facts, 2012* edition. Istaska, IL: Author.
Data from National Center for Health Statistics and US Census Bureau.

The pattern of deaths caused by unintentional injuries, especially from MVAs, drowning, and burns, is remarkably consistent in most Western societies. The leading causes of death from injuries for each age group according to sex are presented in Table 26.1. The majority of deaths from injuries occur in boys. It is important to note that injuries continue to account for more than three times as many teen deaths as any other cause (Annie E. Casey Foundation, 2014). Fortunately, prevention strategies such as the use of car restraints, bicycle helmets, and smoke detectors have significantly decreased fatalities for children. Nevertheless, the overwhelming causes of death in children are MVAs, including occupant, pedestrian, bicycle, and motorcycle deaths; these account for more than one-half of all injury deaths (CDC, 2014) (Fig. 26.2).

Pedestrian injuries involving children account for significant numbers of motor vehicle–related deaths. Most of these injuries occur at midblock, at intersections, in driveways, and in parking lots. Driveway injuries typically involve small children and large vehicles backing up.

Bicycle-associated injuries also cause a number childhood deaths. Children 5 to 9 years of age are at greatest risk for bicycling fatalities. The majority of bicycling deaths are from traumatic head injuries (CDC, 2014). Helmets greatly reduce the risk for head injury, but few children wear helmets. Community-wide bicycle helmet campaigns and mandatory-use laws have resulted in significant increases in helmet

BOX 26.3   Childhood Injuries: Risk Factors

- Sex—Preponderance of males; difference mainly the result of behavioral characteristics, especially aggression
- Temperament—Children with difficult temperament profile, especially persistence, high activity level, and negative reactions to new situations
- Stress—Predisposes children to increased risk-taking and self-destructive behavior; general lack of self-protection
- Alcohol and drug use—Associated with higher incidence of motor vehicle injuries, drownings, homicides, and suicides
- History of previous injury—Associated with increased likelihood of another injury, especially if initial injury required hospitalization
- Developmental characteristics
  - Mismatch between child's developmental level and skill required for activity (e.g., all-terrain vehicles)
  - Natural curiosity to explore environment
  - Desire to assert self and challenge rules
  - In older child, desire for peer approval and acceptance
- Cognitive characteristics (age-specific)
  - Infant—Sensorimotor: explores environment through taste and touch
  - Young child—Object permanence: actively searches for attractive object; cause and effect: lacks awareness of consequential dangers; transductive reasoning: may fail to learn from experiences (e.g., perceives falling from a step as a different type of danger from climbing a tree); magical and egocentric thinking: is unable to comprehend danger to self or others
  - School-age child—Transitional cognitive processes: is unable to fully comprehend causal relationships; attempts dangerous acts without detailed planning regarding consequences
  - Adolescent—Formal operations: is preoccupied with abstract thinking and loses sight of reality; may lead to feeling of invulnerability
- Anatomic characteristics (especially in young children)
  - Large head—Predisposes to cranial injury
  - Large spleen and liver with wide costal arch—Predisposes to direct trauma to these organs
  - Small and light body—May be thrown easily, especially inside a moving vehicle
- Other factors—Poverty, family stress (e.g., maternal illness, recent environmental change), substandard alternative child care, young maternal age, low maternal education, multiple siblings

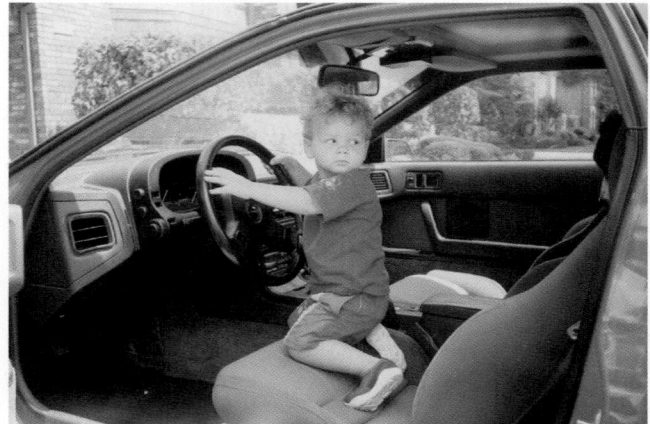

FIG 26.2 Motor vehicle injuries are the leading cause of death in children older than 1 year of age. The majority of fatalities involve occupants who are unrestrained.

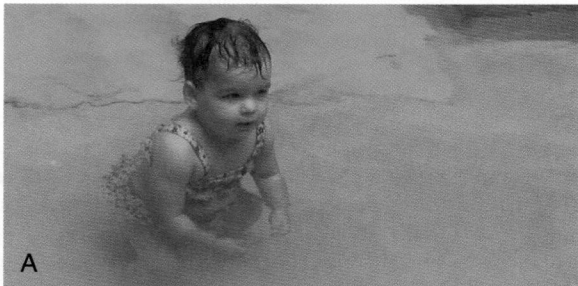

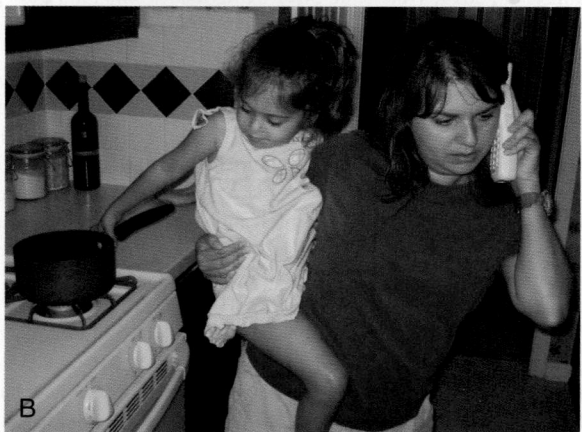

FIG 26.3 **A,** Drowning is one of the leading causes of death. Children left unattended are unsafe even in shallow water. **B,** Burns are among the top three leading causes of death from injury in children 1 to 14 years of age.

use. Still, issues such as stylishness, comfort, and social acceptability remain important factors in noncompliance. Nurses can educate children and families about pedestrian and bicycle safety. In particular, school nurses can promote helmet wearing and encourage peer leaders to act as role models.

Drowning and burns are among the top three leading causes of deaths for males and females throughout childhood (Fig. 26.3). In addition, improper use of firearms is a major cause of death among males (Fig. 26.4). During infancy, more boys die from aspiration or suffocation than do girls (Fig. 26.5). Each year, more than 500,000 children 5 years of age and younger experience a potential poisoning related to medications (Bond, Woodward, & Ho, 2011). Currently, more children are brought to emergency departments for unintentional medication overdoses. Approximately 95% of medication-related emergency department visits in children younger than 5 years of age are due to ingesting medication while unsupervised (Budnitz & Salis, 2011) (Fig. 26.6). Intentional poisoning, associated with drug and alcohol abuse and suicide attempt, is the second leading cause of death in adolescent females and the third leading cause in adolescent males.

Violence

Youth violence is a high-visibility, high-priority concern in every sector of US society (US Department of Health and Human Services, 2013b). Strikingly higher homicide rates are found among minority populations, especially African-American children. The causes of violence against children and self-inflicted violence are not fully understood. Violence seems to permeate US households through television programs, commercials, video games, and movies, all of which tend to desensitize the child toward violence. Violence also permeates the schools with the availability of guns, illicit drugs, and gangs. The problem of child

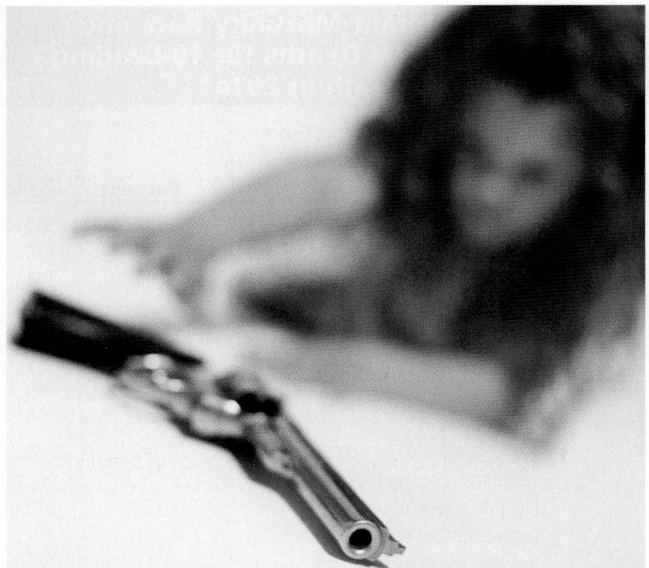

FIG 26.4 Improper use of firearms is the fourth leading cause of death from injury in children 5 to 14 years of age. (Copyright 2012 by Photos. com, a division of Getty Images. All rights reserved.)

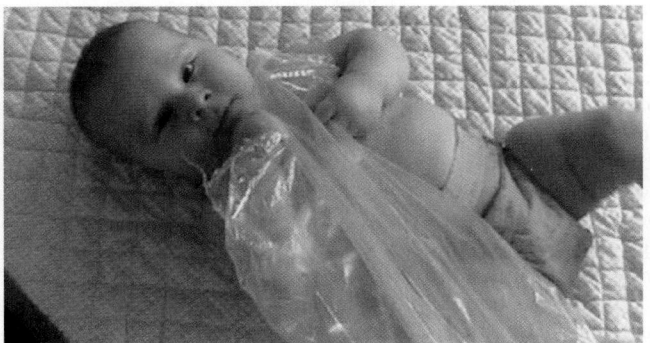

FIG 26.5 Mechanical suffocation is the leading cause of death from injury in infants.

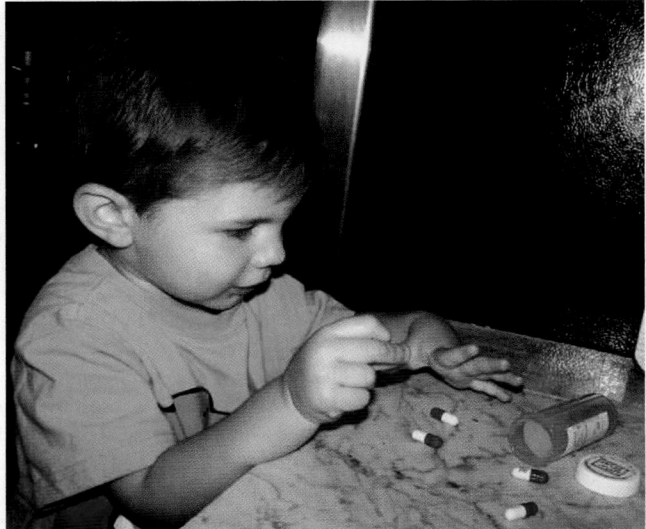

FIG 26.6 Poisoning causes a considerable number of injuries in children younger than 4 years of age. Medications should never be left where young children can reach them.

COMMUNITY FOCUS

Violence in Children

Community violence has reached epidemic proportions in the United States. The serious problem of community violence affects the lives of many children and expands throughout the family, schools, and the workplace. Nurses working with children, adolescents, and families have a critical role in reducing violence through early identification and symptom recognition of the mental-emotional stress that can result from these experiences.

Violent crimes continue to be a significant health issue for children, with homicide being the third leading cause of death in 15- to 19-year-olds (Annie E. Casey Foundation, 2014). The multifaceted origins of violence include developmental factors, gang involvement, access to firearms, drugs, the media, poverty, and family conflict. Often the silent and underrecognized victims are the children who witness acts of community violence. Studies suggest that chronic exposure to violence has a negative effect on a child's cognitive, social, psychologic, and moral development. Also, multiple exposures to episodes of violence do not inoculate children against the negative effects; continued exposure can result in lasting symptoms of stress.

National concern about the increasing prevalence of violent crimes has prompted nurses to actively participate in ensuring that children grow up in safe environments. Pediatric nurses are positioned to assess children and adolescents for signs of exposure to violence and well-known risk factors; nurses also can provide nonviolent problem-solving strategies, counseling, and referrals. These activities affect community practice and expand the nurse's role in the future health environment. Professional resources include the following:

National Domestic Violence Hotline
PO Box 161810
Austin, TX 78716
800-799-SAFE
www.ndvh.org

Child Trends
www.childtrends.org

Data from Child Trends Databank: *Teen homicide, suicide, and firearm deaths,* 2015. Retrieved from http://www.childtrends.org/?indicators=teen -homicide-suicide-and-firearm-deaths.

homicide is extremely complex and involves numerous social, economic, and other influences. Prevention lies in a better understanding of the social and psychologic factors that lead to the high rates of homicide and suicide. Nurses need to be especially aware of young people who harm animals or start fires, are depressed, are repeatedly in trouble with the criminal justice system, or are associated with groups known to be violent. Prevention requires early identification and rapid therapeutic intervention by qualified professionals.

Pediatric nurses can assess children and adolescents for risk factors related to violence. Families that own firearms must be educated about their safe use and storage. The presence of a gun in a household increases the risk for suicide by about fivefold and the risk for homicide by about threefold. Technologic changes such as childproof safety devices and loading indicators could improve the safety of firearms (see Community Focus box: Violence in Children).

Bullying

Bullying can be a serious problem and can involve emotional, physical, verbal, and cyber-related abuse. Bullying behaviors are used to assert domination and can occur in the school, home, or neighborhood settings (Juvonen & Graham, 2014). When youth are not well accepted by their peers, they are vulnerable to bullying; physical disabilities, obesity, and sexual orientation can be risk factors creating vulnerability. Peer victimization can result in adjustment and health problems in the future for these individuals.

Mental Health Problems

One out of five children experience mental health problems, and one out of 10 has a serious emotional problem that affects daily functioning (Flores & Lesley, 2014). Currently the top five chronic conditions are related to mental health issues (Slomski, 2012). Psychosocial problems in children seen in primary care settings in rural areas are common (Polaha, Dalton, & Allen, 2011). Many adolescents with anxiety disorders and impulse-control disorders (such as conduct disorder or attention-deficit/hyperactivity disorder [ADHD]) develop these during adolescence. Nurses should be alert to the symptoms of mental illness and potential suicidal ideation and be aware of potential resources for high-quality integrated mental health services.

INFANT MORTALITY

The infant mortality rate is the number of deaths during the first year of life per 1000 live births. It may be further divided into neonatal mortality (<28 days of life) and postneonatal mortality (28 days to 11 months). In the United States, infant mortality has decreased dramatically; the rate is approximately 200 infant deaths per 1000 live births (CDC, 2014).

From a worldwide perspective, however, the United States lags behind other nations in reducing infant mortality. In 2013, the United States ranked last among 30 nations that have a population of at least 2.5 million and at least 40 thousand births. Finland, Japan, and Norway have the three lowest rates, with the United States ranked last behind Hungary and the Slovak Republic (Murphy, S.L., Mathews, T.J., Martin, J.A., et. al., 2017).

Birth weight is considered the major determinant of neonatal death in technologically developed countries. The relatively high incidence of LBW (<2500 g [5.5 pounds]) in the United States is considered a key factor in its higher neonatal mortality rate when compared with other countries. Access to and the use of high-quality prenatal care are promising preventive strategies to decrease early delivery and infant mortality.

As Table 26.2 demonstrates, many of the leading causes of death during infancy continue to occur during the perinatal period. The first four causes—congenital anomalies, disorders relating to short gestation and unspecified LBW, newborn affected by maternal complications of pregnancy, and sudden infant death syndrome—accounted for about one-half (52%) of all deaths of infants younger than 1 year of age. Many birth defects are associated with LBW, and reducing the incidence of LBW will help prevent congenital anomalies. Infant mortality resulting from human immunodeficiency virus (HIV) infection decreased significantly during the 1990s.

When infant death rates are categorized according to race, a disturbing difference is seen. Infant mortality for Caucasians is considerably lower than for all other races in the United States, with African-Americans having twice the rate of Caucasians. The LBW rate is also much higher for African-American infants than for any other group. One encouraging note is that the gap in mortality rates between Caucasian and non-Caucasian races (other than African-Americans) has narrowed in recent years. Infant mortality rates for Hispanics and Asian–Pacific Islanders have decreased dramatically during the past 2 decades.

CHILDHOOD MORTALITY

Death rates for children older than 1 year of age have always been lower than those for infants. Children 5 to 14 years of age have the lowest

TABLE 26.2   Infant Mortality Rate and Percentage of Total Deaths for 10 Leading Causes of Infant Death in 2014*

Rank	Cause of Death (Based on International Classification of Diseases, 10th Revision)	Percent	Rate
	All races, all causes	100.00%	582.1
1	Congenital anomalies	20.4	119.0
2	Disorders relating to short gestation and unspecified low birth weight	18.0	104.6
3	Newborn affected by maternal complications of pregnancy	6.8	39.5
4	Sudden infant death syndrome	6.7	38.7
5	Accidents (unintentional injuries)	5.0	29.1
6	Newborn affected by complications of placenta, cord and membranes	4.2	24.2
7	Bacterial sepsis of newborn	2.3	13.6
8	Respiratory distress of newborn	2.0	11.5
9	Diseases of circulatory system	1.9	11.1
10	Neonatal hemorrhage	1.9	11.1

*Rate per 1000 live births.
Modified from Kochanek, K.D., Murphy, S.L., Xu, J., et al. (2016). Deaths: Final data for 2014. *National Vital Statistics Report, 65*(4), 1–122.

rate of death. However, a sharp rise occurs during later adolescence, primarily from injuries, homicide, and suicide (Table 26.3). In 2014, accidental injuries accounted for 38.8% of all deathss in teens ages 15–19. The second leading cause of death amongst teens was suicide, accounting for 19.2% of all death. The trend in racial differences that occurs in infant mortality is also apparent in childhood deaths for all ages and for both sexes. Caucasians have fewer deaths for all ages, and male deaths outnumber female deaths.

After 1 year of age, the cause of death changes dramatically, with unintentional injuries (accidents) being the leading cause from the youngest ages to the adolescent years. Violent deaths have been steadily increasing among young people 10 to 25 years of age, especially African-Americans and males. Homicide is the third leading cause of death in the 15- to 19-year age group (see Table 26.3). Children 12 years of age and older tend to be killed by nonfamily members (acquaintances and gangs, typically of the same race) and most frequently by firearms. Suicide, a form of self-violence, is the second leading cause of death among children and adolescents 10 to 19 years of age.

CHILDHOOD MORBIDITY

Acute illness is defined as an illness with symptoms severe enough to limit activity or require medical attention. Respiratory illness accounts for approximately 50% of all acute conditions, 11% are caused by infections and parasitic disease, and 15% are caused by injuries. The chief illness of childhood is the common cold.

The types of diseases that children contract during childhood vary according to age. For example, upper respiratory tract infections and diarrhea decrease in frequency with age, whereas other disorders, such as acne and headaches, increase. Children who have had a particular type of problem are more likely to have that problem again. Morbidity is not distributed randomly in children. Recent concern has focused on groups of children who have increased morbidity: homeless children, children living in poverty, LBW children, children with chronic illnesses, foreign-born adopted children, and children in day care centers. A

TABLE 26.3   Five Leading Causes of Death in Children in the United States: Selected Age Intervals, 2002*

Rank	1–4 YEARS OF AGE		5–9 YEARS OF AGE		10–14 YEARS OF AGE		15–19 YEARS OF AGE	
	Cause	Rate	Cause	Rate	Cause	Rate	Cause	Rate
	All causes	24.0	All causes	11.5	All causes	14.0	All causes	45.5
1	Injuries	7.6	Injuries	3.6	Injuries	3.6	Injuries	17.7
2	Congenital anomalies	2.5	Cancer	2.1	Suicide	2.1	Suicide	8.7
3	Homicide	2.3	Congenital anomalies	0.9	Cancer	2.0	Homicide	6.7
4	Cancer	2.0	Homicide	0.6	Congenital anomalies	0.8	Cancer	2.9
5	Heart disease	0.9	Heart disease	0.3	Homicide	0.8	Heart disease	1.4

*Rate per 100,000 population.
Modified from Murphy, S.L., Mathews, T.J., Martin, J.A., et.al. (2017). Annual summary of vital statistics: 2013-2014, *Pediatrics 139*(6), e20163239.

number of factors place these groups at risk for poor health. A major cause is barriers to health care, especially for the homeless, the poverty stricken, and those with chronic health problems. Other factors include improved survival of children with chronic health problems, particularly VLBW infants.

THE ART OF PEDIATRIC NURSING

PHILOSOPHY OF CARE

Nursing of infants, children, and adolescents is consistent with the American Nurses Association (2015) definition of nursing as the protection, promotion, and optimization of health and abilities, prevention of illness and injury, alleviation of suffering through the diagnosis and treatment of human response, and advocacy in the care of individuals, families, and populations.

Family-Centered Care

The philosophy of family-centered care recognizes the family as the constant in a child's life. Family-centered care is an approach to the planning, delivery, and evaluation of health care that is grounded in mutually beneficial partnerships among health care providers, patients, and families (Institute for Patient- and Family-Centered Care, 2017). Nurses support families in their natural caregiving and decision-making roles by building on their unique strengths and acknowledging their expertise in caring for their child both within and outside the hospital setting. The nurse considers the needs of all family members in relation to the care of the child (Box 26.4). The philosophy acknowledges diversity among family structures and backgrounds; family goals, dreams, strategies, and actions; and family support, service, and information needs.

Two basic concepts in family-centered care are enabling and empowerment. Professionals enable families by creating opportunities and means for all family members to display their current abilities and competencies and to acquire new ones to meet the needs of the child and family. *Empowerment* describes the interaction of professionals with families in such a way that families maintain or acquire a sense of control over their family lives and acknowledge positive changes that result from helping behaviors that foster their own strengths, abilities, and actions.

Although caring for the family is strongly emphasized throughout this text, it is highlighted in features such as Cultural Considerations and Family-Centered Care boxes.

Atraumatic Care

Atraumatic care is the provision of therapeutic care in settings, by personnel, and through the use of interventions that eliminate or minimize the psychologic and physical distress experienced by children and their

BOX 26.4   Key Elements of Family-Centered Care

- Incorporating into policy and practice the recognition that the family is the constant in a child's life, whereas the service systems and support personnel within those systems fluctuate
- Facilitating family-professional collaboration at all levels of hospital, home, and community care:
  - Care of an individual child
  - Program development, implementation, and evaluation
  - Policy formation
- Exchanging complete and unbiased information between family members and professionals in a supportive manner at all times
- Incorporating into policy and practice the recognition and honoring of cultural diversity, strengths, and individuality within and across all families, including ethnic, racial, spiritual, social, economic, educational, and geographic diversity
- Recognizing and respecting different methods of coping and implementing comprehensive policies and programs that provide developmental, educational, emotional, environmental, and financial support to meet the diverse needs of families
- Encouraging and facilitating family-to-family support and networking
- Ensuring that home, hospital, and community service and support systems for children needing specialized health and developmental care and their families are flexible, accessible, and comprehensive in responding to diverse family-identified needs
- Appreciating families as families and children as children, recognizing that they possess a wide range of strengths, concerns, emotions, and aspirations beyond their need for specialized health and developmental services and support

From Shelton, T.L., & Stepanek, J.S. (1994). *Family-centered care for children needing specialized health and developmental services.* Bethesda, MD: Association for the Care of Children's Health.

families in the health care system. Therapeutic care encompasses the prevention, diagnosis, treatment, or palliation of acute or chronic conditions. *Setting* refers to the place in which that care is given—the home, the hospital, or any other health care setting. Personnel include anyone directly involved in providing therapeutic care. Interventions range from psychologic approaches, such as preparing children for procedures, to physical interventions, such as providing space for a parent to room in with a child. Psychologic distress may include anxiety, fear, anger, disappointment, sadness, shame, or guilt. Physical distress may range from sleeplessness and immobilization to disturbances from sensory stimuli, such as pain, temperature extremes, loud noises, bright lights, or darkness. Thus atraumatic care is concerned with the where, who, why, and how of any procedure performed on a child for the purpose of preventing or minimizing psychologic and physical stress (Wong, 1989).

The overriding goal in providing atraumatic care is: First, do no harm. Three principles provide the framework for achieving this goal: (1) prevent or minimize the child's separation from the family, (2) promote a sense of control, and (3) prevent or minimize bodily injury and pain. Examples of providing atraumatic care include fostering the parent-child relationship during hospitalization, preparing the child before any unfamiliar treatment or procedure, controlling pain, allowing the child privacy, providing play activities for expression of fear and aggression, providing choices to children, and respecting cultural differences.

ROLE OF THE PEDIATRIC NURSE

The pediatric nurse is responsible for promoting the health and well-being of the child and family. Nursing functions vary according to regional job structures, individual education and experience, and personal career goals. Just as patients (children and their families) have unique backgrounds, each nurse brings an individual set of variables that affect the nurse-patient relationship. No matter where pediatric nurses practice, their primary concern is the welfare of the child and family. The pediatric nurse plays a role as a member of the interprofessional care team. Throughout the pediatric section of this text, the importance of interprofessional care is emphasized.

Therapeutic Relationship

The establishment of a therapeutic relationship is the essential foundation for providing high-quality nursing care. Pediatric nurses need to have meaningful relationships with children and their families and yet remain separate enough to distinguish their own feelings and needs. In a therapeutic relationship, caring, well-defined boundaries separate the nurse from the child and family. These boundaries are positive and professional and promote the family's control over the child's health care. Both the nurse and the family are empowered and maintain open communication. In a nontherapeutic relationship, these boundaries are blurred, and many of the nurse's actions may serve personal needs, such as a need to feel wanted and involved, rather than the family's needs.

Exploring whether relationships with patients are therapeutic or nontherapeutic helps nurses identify problem areas early in their interactions with children and families (see Guidelines box: Exploring Your Relationships With Children and Families). Although questions regarding the nurse's involvement may label certain actions negative or positive, no one action makes a relationship therapeutic or nontherapeutic. For example, a nurse may spend additional time with the family but still recognize his or her own needs and maintain professional separateness. An important clue to nontherapeutic relationships is the staff's concerns about their peer's actions with the family.

Family Advocacy and Caring

Although nurses are responsible to themselves, the profession, and the institution of employment, their primary responsibility is to the consumer of nursing services: the child and family. The nurse must work with family members, identify their goals and needs, and plan interventions that best address the defined problems. As an advocate, the nurse assists the child and family in making informed choices and acting in the child's best interest. Advocacy involves ensuring that families are aware of all available health services, adequately informed of treatments and procedures, involved in the child's care, and encouraged to change or support existing health care practices.

As nurses care for children and families, they must demonstrate caring, compassion, and empathy for others. Aspects of caring embody

the concept of atraumatic care and the development of a therapeutic relationship with patients. Parents perceive caring as a sign of quality in nursing care, which is often focused on the nontechnical needs of the child and family. Parents describe "personable" care as actions by the nurse that include acknowledging the parent's presence, listening, making the parent feel comfortable in the hospital environment, involving the parent and child in the nursing care, showing interest in and concern for their welfare, showing affection and sensitivity to the parent and child, communicating with them, and individualizing the nursing care. Parents perceive personable nursing care as being integral to establishing a positive relationship.

Disease Prevention and Health Promotion

Every nurse involved in caring for children must understand the importance of disease prevention and health promotion. A nursing care plan must include a thorough assessment of all aspects of child growth and development, including nutrition, immunizations, safety, dental care, socialization, discipline, and education. If problems are identified, the nurse intervenes directly or refers the family to other health care providers or agencies.

The best approach to prevention is education and anticipatory guidance. In this text, each chapter on health promotion includes sections on anticipatory guidance. An appreciation of the hazards or conflicts of each developmental period enables the nurse to guide parents regarding childrearing practices aimed at preventing potential problems. One significant example is safety. Because each age-group is at risk for special types of injuries, preventive teaching can significantly reduce injuries, lowering permanent disability and mortality rates.

Prevention also involves less obvious aspects of caring for children. The nurse is responsible for providing care that promotes mental well-being (e.g., enlisting the help of a child life specialist during a painful procedure, such as an immunization).

Health Teaching

Health teaching is inseparable from family advocacy and prevention. Health teaching may be the nurse's direct goal, such as during parenting classes, or may be indirect, such as helping parents and children understand a diagnosis or medical treatment, encouraging children to ask questions about their bodies, referring families to health-related professional or lay groups, supplying patients with appropriate literature, and providing anticipatory guidance.

Health teaching is one area in which nurses often need preparation and practice with competent role models, because it involves transmitting information at the child's and family's level of understanding and desire for information. As an effective educator, the nurse focuses on providing the appropriate health teaching with generous feedback and evaluation to promote learning.

Injury Prevention

Each year, injuries kill or disable more children older than 1 year of age than all childhood diseases combined. The nurse plays an important role in preventing injuries by using a developmental approach to safety counseling for parents of children of all ages. Realizing that safety concerns for a young infant are completely different than injury risks of adolescents, the nurse discusses appropriate injury preventions tips to parents and children as part of routine patient care.

Support and Counseling

Attention to emotional needs requires support and, sometimes, counseling. The role of child advocate or health teacher is supportive by virtue of the individualized approach. The nurse can offer support by listening, touching, and being physically present. Touching and physical presence

GUIDELINES

Exploring Your Relationships With Children and Families

To foster therapeutic relationships with children and families, you must first become aware of your caregiving style, including how effectively you take care of yourself. The following questions should help you understand the therapeutic quality of your professional relationships.

Negative Actions
- Are you overinvolved with children and their families?
  - Do you work overtime to care for the family?
  - Do you spend off-duty time with children's families, either in or out of the hospital?
  - Do you call frequently (either the hospital or home) to see how the family is doing?
  - Do you show favoritism toward certain patients?
  - Do you buy clothes, toys, food, or other items for the child and family?
  - Do you compete with other staff members for the affection of certain patients and families?
  - Do other staff members comment to you about your closeness to the family?
  - Do you attempt to influence families' decisions rather than facilitate their informed decision making?
- Are you underinvolved with children and families?
  - Do you restrict parent or visitor access to children, using excuses such as the unit is too busy?
  - Do you focus on the technical aspects of care and lose sight of the person who is the patient?
- Are you overinvolved with children and underinvolved with their parents?
  - Do you become critical when parents do not visit their children?
  - Do you compete with parents for their children's affection?

Positive Actions
- Do you strive to empower families?
  - Do you explore families' strengths and needs in an effort to increase family involvement?
  - Have you developed teaching skills to instruct families rather than doing everything for them?
  - Do you work with families to find ways to decrease their dependence on health care providers?
  - Can you separate families' needs from your own needs?

- Do you strive to empower yourself?
  - Are you aware of your emotional responses to different people and situations?
  - Do you seek to understand how your own family experiences influence reactions to patients and families, especially as they affect tendencies toward overinvolvement or underinvolvement?
  - Do you have a calming influence, not one that will amplify emotionality?
  - Have you developed interpersonal skills in addition to technical skills?
  - Have you learned about ethnic and religious family patterns?
  - Do you communicate directly with people with whom you are upset or take issue?
  - Are you able to "step back" and withdraw emotionally, if not physically, when emotional overload occurs, yet remain committed?
  - Do you take care of yourself and your needs?
  - Do you periodically interview family members to determine their current issues (e.g., feelings, attitudes, responses, wishes), communicate these findings to peers, and update records?
  - Do you avoid relying on initial interview data, assumptions, or gossip regarding families?
  - Do you ask questions if families are not participating in care?
  - Do you assess families for feelings of anxiety, fear, intimidation, worry about making a mistake, a perceived lack of competence to care for their child, or fear of health care professionals overstepping their boundaries into family territory, or vice versa?
  - Do you explore these issues with family members and provide encouragement and support to enable families to help themselves?
  - Do you keep communication channels open among self, family, physicians, and other care providers?
  - Do you resolve conflicts and misunderstandings directly with those who are involved?
  - Do you clarify information for families or seek the appropriate person to do so?
- Do you recognize that from time to time a therapeutic relationship can change to a social relationship or an intimate friendship?
  - Are you able to acknowledge the fact when it occurs and understand why it happened?
  - Can you ensure that there is someone else who is more objective who can take your place in the therapeutic relationship?

---

are most helpful with children, because they facilitate nonverbal communication. Counseling involves a mutual exchange of ideas and opinions that provides the basis for mutual problem solving. It involves support, teaching, techniques to foster the expression of feelings or thoughts, and approaches to help the family cope with stress. Optimally, counseling not only helps resolve a crisis or problem but also enables the family to attain a higher level of functioning, greater self-esteem, and closer relationships. Although counseling is often the role of nurses in specialized areas, counseling techniques are discussed in various sections of this text to help students and nurses cope with immediate crises and refer families for additional professional assistance.

Coordination and Collaboration

The nurse, as a member of the health care team, collaborates and coordinates nursing care with the care activities of other professionals. A nurse working in isolation rarely serves the child's best interests. The concept of holistic care can be realized through a unified, interdisciplinary approach by being aware of individual contributions and limitations and collaborating with other specialists to provide high-quality health

services. Failure to recognize limitations can be nontherapeutic at best and destructive at worst. For example, the nurse who feels competent in counseling but who is really inadequate in this area may not only prevent the child from dealing with a crisis but also impede future success with a qualified professional. Nursing should be seen as a major contributor to assuring a health care team focuses on high-quality, safe care.

Ethical Decision Making

Ethical dilemmas arise when competing moral considerations underlie various alternatives. Parents, nurses, physicians, and other health care team members may reach different but morally defensible decisions by assigning different weights to competing moral values. These competing moral values may include autonomy, the patient's right to be self-governing; nonmaleficence, the obligation to minimize or prevent harm; beneficence, the obligation to promote the patient's well-being; and justice, the concept of fairness. Nurses must determine the most beneficial or least harmful action within the framework of societal mores, professional practice standards, the law, institutional rules, the family's value system and religious traditions, and the nurse's personal values.

Nurses must prepare themselves systematically for collaborative ethical decision making. They can accomplish this through formal course work, continuing education, contemporary literature, and work to establish an environment conducive to ethical discourse.

The nurse also uses the professional code of ethics for guidance and as a means for professional self-regulation. Nurses may face ethical issues regarding patient care, such as the use of lifesaving measures for VLBW newborns or the terminally ill child's right to refuse treatment. They may struggle with questions regarding truthfulness, balancing their rights and responsibilities in caring for children with acquired immune deficiency syndrome (AIDS), whistle-blowing, or allocating resources. Throughout this text, such dilemmas are addressed in boxes titled Ethics in Practice. Conflicting ethical arguments are presented to help nurses clarify their value judgments when confronted with sensitive issues.

RESEARCH AND EVIDENCE-BASED PRACTICE

Nurses should contribute to research because they are the individuals observing human responses to health and illness. The current emphasis on measurable outcomes to determine the efficacy of interventions (often in relation to the cost) demands that nurses know whether clinical interventions result in positive outcomes for their patients. This demand has influenced the current trend toward evidence-based practice (EBP), which implies questioning why something is effective and whether a better approach exists. The concept of EBP also involves analyzing and translating published clinical research into the everyday practice of nursing. When nurses base their clinical practice on science and research and document their clinical outcomes, they will be able to validate their contributions to health, wellness, and cure, not only to their patients, third-party payers, and institutions but also to the nursing profession. Evaluation is essential to the nursing process, and research is one of the best ways to accomplish this.

EBP is the collection, interpretation, and integration of valid, important, and applicable patient-reported, nurse-observed, and research-derived information. Using the PICOT (population/patient problem, intervention, comparison, outcome and time) question to clearly define the problem of interest, nurses are able to obtain the best evidence to impact care. Evidence-based nursing practice combines knowledge with clinical experience and intuition. It provides a rational approach to decision-making that facilitates best practice (Melnyk & Fineout-Overholt, 2014). EBP is an important tool that complements the nursing process by using critical-thinking skills to make decisions based on existing knowledge. The traditional nursing process approach to patient care can be used to conceptualize the essential components of EBP nursing. During the assessment and diagnostic phases of the nursing process, the nurse establishes important clinical questions and completes a critical review of existing knowledge. EBP also begins with identification of the problem. The nurse asks clinical questions in a concise, organized way that allows for clear answers. Once the specific questions are identified, extensive searching for the best information to answer the question begins. The nurse evaluates clinically relevant research, analyzes findings from the history and physical examinations, and reviews the specific pathophysiology of the defined problem. The third step in the nursing process is to develop a care plan. In evidence-based nursing practice, the care plan is established on completion of a critical appraisal of what is known and not known about the defined problem. Next, in the traditional nursing process, the nurse implements the care plan. By integrating evidence with clinical expertise, the nurse focuses care on the patient's unique needs. The final step in EBP is consistent with the final phase of the nursing process—to evaluate the effectiveness of the care plan.

TABLE 26.4 The GRADE Criteria to Evaluate the Quality of the Evidence

Quality	Type of Evidence
High	Consistent evidence from well-performed RCTs or exceptionally strong evidence from unbiased observational studies
Moderate	Evidence from RCTs with important limitations (inconsistent results, flaws in methodology, indirect evidence, or imprecise results) or unusually strong evidence from unbiased observational studies
Low	Evidence for at least one critical outcome from observational studies, from RCTs with serious flaws, or from indirect evidence
Very Low	Evidence for at least one of the critical outcomes from unsystematic clinical observations or very indirect evidence

Quality	Recommendation
Strong	Desirable effects clearly outweigh undesirable effects, or vice versa
Weak	Desirable effects closely balanced with undesirable effects

RCT, Randomized controlled clinical trial.
Adapted from Guyatt, G.H., Oxman, A.D., Vist, G.E., et al. (2008). GRADE: An emerging consensus on rating quality of evidence and strength of recommendations, *British Medical Journal, 336,* 924–926.

For nurses to implement EBP, they must have access to appropriate, recent resources such as online search engines and journals. In many institutions, computer terminals are available on patient care units, with the Internet and online journals easily accessible. Another important resource for the implementation of EBP is time. The nursing shortage and ongoing changes in many institutions have compounded the issue of nursing time allocation for patient care, education, and training. In some institutions, nurses are given paid time away from performing patient care to participate in activities that promote EBP. This requires an organizational environment that values EBP and its potential impact on patient care. As knowledge is generated regarding the significant impact of EBP on patient care outcomes, it is hoped that the organizational culture will change to support the staff nurse's participation in EBP. As the amount of available evidence increases, so does our need to critically evaluate the evidence.

Throughout this text, Evidence-Based Practice boxes summarize the existing evidence that promotes excellence in clinical care. The GRADE criteria are used to evaluate the quality of research articles used to develop practice guidelines (Guyatt, Oxman, Vist, et al., 2008). Table 26.4 defines how the nurse rates the quality of the evidence using the GRADE criteria and establishes a strong versus weak recommendation. Each Evidence-Based Practice box rates the quality of existing evidence and the strength of the recommendation for practice change.

THE PROCESS OF PROVIDING NURSING CARE TO CHILDREN AND FAMILIES

NURSING PROCESS

The nursing process is a method of problem identification and problem solving that describes what the nurse actually does. The nursing process model includes assessment, diagnosis outcomes/planning, implementation, and evaluation (American Nurses Association, 2015).

Assessment

Assessment is a continuous process that operates at all phases of problem solving and is the foundation for decision-making. Assessment involves multiple nursing skills and consists of the purposeful collection, classification, and analysis of data from a variety of sources. To provide an accurate and comprehensive assessment, the nurse must consider information about the patient's biophysical, psychologic, sociocultural, and spiritual background.

Diagnosis

The next stage of the nursing process is problem identification and nursing diagnosis. At this point, the nurse must interpret and make decisions about the data gathered. Not all children have actual health problems; some have a potential health problem, which is a risk state that requires nursing intervention to prevent the development of an actual problem. Potential health problems may be indicated by risk factors or signs, predispose a child and family to a dysfunctional health pattern, and are limited to individuals at greater risk than the population as a whole. Nursing interventions are directed toward reducing risk factors. To differentiate actual from potential health problems, the word *risk* is included in the nursing diagnosis statement (e.g., *Risk for Infection*).

Signs and symptoms refer to a cluster of cues and defining characteristics that are derived from patient assessment and indicate actual health problems. When a defining characteristic is essential for the diagnosis to be made, it is considered critical. These critical defining characteristics help differentiate between diagnostic categories. For example, in deciding between the diagnostic categories related to family function and coping, the nurse uses defining characteristics to choose the most appropriate nursing diagnosis (see Family-Centered Care box: Using Defining Characteristics to Select an Appropriate Nursing Diagnosis).

Outcomes/Planning

The goal for outcomes identification is to establish priorities and select expected patient outcomes or goals. The nurse organizes information during assessment and diagnosis and clusters these data into categories to identify significant areas and makes one of the following decisions:

- No dysfunctional health problems are evident; health promotion is emphasized.
- Risk for dysfunctional health problems exists; interventions are needed for health promotion and illness prevention.
- Actual dysfunctional health problems are evident; interventions are needed for illness management, illness prevention, and health promotion.
- Specific outcomes are formulated to address the realistic patient- and family-focused goals.

After identifying specific patient- and family-focused goals, the nurse develops a care plan specific to the identified outcomes. The outcome is the projected or expected change in a patient's health status, clinical condition, or behavior that occurs after nursing interventions have been instituted. The care plan must be established before specific nursing interventions are developed and implemented.

Implementation

The implementation phase begins when the nurse puts the selected intervention into action and accumulates feedback data regarding its effects (or the patient's response to the intervention). The feedback returns in the form of observation and communication and provides a database on which to evaluate the outcome of the nursing intervention. It is imperative that continual assessment of the patient's status occurs throughout all phases of the nursing process, thus making the process a dynamic rather than static problem-solving method. Throughout the implementation stage, the main concerns are the patient's physical safety and psychologic comfort in terms of atraumatic care.

FAMILY-CENTERED CARE

Using Defining Characteristics to Select an Appropriate Nursing Diagnosis

An 18-month-old only child is admitted with respiratory distress and a presumptive diagnosis of epiglottitis. Initial nursing actions focus on the child's physiologic status. As the condition stabilizes, the nurse gathers family assessment data. The child's immunizations are current, he is clean and well nourished, and his developmental age is appropriate. The parents are both present at admission. The mother is distraught about the sudden onset of respiratory distress. She states that earlier her child had only a "runny nose," and she thought it was just a cold. When the child suddenly began to have difficulty breathing, she felt helpless and unable to relieve her child's discomfort. She states, "Nothing I did made him any better. If I had known this could happen, I would have brought him to the hospital sooner. I feel like a bad mother." In the hospital, after explanations by the nurses, the mother understands that epiglottitis is a sudden illness that typically follows symptoms of a cold. She is cooperative and asks what she can do to make her child more comfortable. She implements all the suggestions of the health care team. The father supports both the child and mother, although he assumes a more passive "listening" role.

Three nursing diagnoses that relate to family and parent situations may be relevant. The first step is to review the diagnoses and the defining characteristics and decide which one is most appropriate:

1. *Parenting, Impaired*—Inability of the primary caretaker to create, maintain, or regain an environment that nurtures the child's growth and development
   Selected defining characteristics:
   - Insecure (or lack of) attachment to infant
   - Poor or inappropriate caretaking skills

2. *Conflict, Parental Role*—Parent experience of role confusion and conflict in response to crisis
   Selected defining characteristics:
   - Parent expressing concerns about changes in parental role
   - A demonstrated disruption in care or caretaking routines
   - Parent expressing concerns or feelings of inadequacy to provide for the child's physical and emotional needs during hospitalization or in the home
   - Parent verbalizing or demonstrating feelings of guilt, anger, fear, anxiety, or frustration about effect of child's illness on family process

3. *Family Processes, Interrupted*—A change in family relationships or functioning
   Selected defining characteristics:
   - Expressions of conflict within the family
   - Changes in communication patterns among family members

Of these three diagnoses, the most relevant one is *Conflict, Parental Role*. The parents demonstrate attachment behavior to their child and are attentive to his needs. They appear to have appropriate parenting skills and are able to communicate effectively with each other. Neither parent expressed any conflict within the family. The sudden onset of this child's illness has interrupted the mother's usual role and caused her to feel inadequate, anxious, and guilty. However, the mother is able to adapt to this crisis. She demonstrates an ability to cope by learning and implementing new comforting skills for her child. The defining characteristics of the other two diagnoses require maladaptive characteristics that are clearly not demonstrated by these parents.

GUIDELINES

Documentation of Nursing Care

- Initial assessments and reassessments
- Nursing diagnoses and/or patient care needs
- Interventions identified to meet the patient's nursing care needs
- Nursing care provided
- Patient's response to, and the outcomes of, the care provided
- Abilities of patient and/or, as appropriate, significant other(s) to manage continuing care needs after discharge

Evaluation

Evaluation is the last step in the nursing care process. The nurse gathers, sorts, and analyzes data to determine whether (1) the established outcome has been met, (2) the nursing interventions were appropriate, (3) the plan requires modification, or (4) other alternatives should be considered. The evaluation phase either completes the nursing process (outcome is met) or serves as the basis for selecting alternative interventions to solve the specific problem.

With the current focus on patient outcomes in health care, the patient's care is evaluated not only at discharge but thereafter as well to ensure that the outcomes are met and there is adequate care for resolving existing or potential health problems. One federal agency that has developed clinical guidelines is the Agency for Healthcare Research and Quality.*

Documentation

Although documentation is not one of the steps of the nursing process, it is essential for evaluation. The nurse can assess, diagnose, and identify problems; plan; and implement without documentation; however, evaluation is best performed with written evidence of progress toward outcomes. The patient's medical record should include evidence of those elements listed in the Guidelines box: Documentation of Nursing Care.

QUALITY OUTCOME MEASURES

Quality of care refers to the degree to which health services for individuals and populations increase the likelihood of desired health outcomes and are consistent with current professional knowledge (Pelletier & Beaudin, 2008).

To provide a perspective on the importance of quality in health care, in March 2011, the US Department of Health and Human Services released the inaugural report to Congress on the National Strategy for Quality Improvement in Health Care (National Strategy for Quality Improvement in Health Care, 2012). The National Quality Strategy** focuses on six domains that establish the priorities for health care quality improvement. These domains areas follows:

- Patient and family engagement
- Patient safety
- Care coordination
- Population/public health
- Efficient use of health care resources

- Clinical process/effectiveness

A 2013 Hastings Center Report stresses the importance of viewing health care institutions as learning health care systems committed to carrying out quality patient care activities. As health care systems continue to evolve, it is evident that clinical practice cannot be of the highest quality if it is independent of its connection with ongoing, systematic learning (Kass, Faden, & Goodman, 2013). Learning health care systems, described in the Hastings Center Report, view clinical practice as an ongoing source of data to be used for continuously changing and improving patient care. Because nurses are the principal caregivers within health care institutions, high-quality outcomes that are specific to direct nursing care are used as a nursing-sensitive indicator of the ability to provide excellence in patient care.

The Quality and Safety Education for Nurses Institute has defined quality and safety competencies for nursing. The Quality and Safety Education for Nurses Institute is now being hosted by faculty at the Case Western Reserve University and provides a comprehensive overview for the development of knowledge, skills, and attitudes related to quality and safety in health care.* In this text, each Evidence-Based Practice box includes the Quality and Safety Education for Nurses Institute competencies related to knowledge, skills, and attitudes for evidence-based nursing practice.

Throughout the chapters that focus on serious health problems, we have developed examples of quality outcome measures for specific diseases that reflect patient-centered outcomes. Quality outcome measures promote interdisciplinary teamwork, and the boxes throughout this text exemplify measures of effective collaboration to improve care. Quality Patient Outcomes boxes throughout this text are developed to assist nurses in identifying appropriate measures that evaluate the quality of patient care.

REFERENCES

American Academy of Pediatrics. (2016). *American Academy of Pediatrics announces new recommendations for Children's media use.* Retrieved from https://www.aap.org.

American Nurses Association. (2015). *The nursing process.* Retrieved from http://www.nursingworld.org/EspeciallyForYou/What-is-Nursing/Tools-You-Need/Thenursingprocess.html.

Annie E. Casey Foundation. (2014). *2014 Kids count data book: State profiles of child well-being.* Baltimore, MD: Author.

Berdahl, T. A., Friedman, B. S., McCormick, M. C., et al. (2013). Annual report on health care for children and youth in the United States: Trends in racial/ethnic, income, and insurance disparities over time, 2002-2009. *Academic Pediatrics, 13*(3), 191–293.

Bond, G. R., Woodward, R. W., & Ho, M. (2011). The growing impact of pediatric pharmaceutical poisoning. *Journal of Pediatrics, 160*(2), 265–270.

Bright Futures. (2014). *Prevention and health promotion for infants, children, adolescents, and their families.* Retrieved from http://brightfutures.aap.org/index.html.

Budnitz, D. S., & Salis, S. (2011). Preventing medication overdoses in young children: An opportunity for harm elimination. *Pediatrics, 127*(6), e1597–e1599.

Centers for Disease Control and Prevention. (2014). *Injury and violence prevention and control.* Retrieved from http://www.cdc.gov/injury.

Centers for Disease Control and Prevention. (2013). *Put your medicines up and away and out of sight.* Retrieved from http://www.cdc.gov/features/medicationstorage/.

---

*540 Gaither Road, Suite 2000, Rockville, MD 20850; 301-427-1364; email: info@ahrq.gov; www.ahrq.gov.
**National Quality Strategy information can be found at: http://www.ahrq.gov/workingforquality/about.htm#priorities

---

*Quality and Safety Education for Nurses Institute, Frances Payne Bolton School of Nursing, Case Western Reserve University, email: qsen.institute@gmail.com

Federal Interagency Forum on Child and Family Statistics. (2016). *America's children: Key national indicators of well-being.* Washington, DC: US Government Printing Office. Retrieved from http://www.childstats.gov/americaschildren/index.asp.

Flores, G., & Lesley, B. (2014). Children and US federal policy on health and health care. *Journal of the American Medical Association Pediatrics, 168*(12), 1155–1163.

Flores, G., & Lin, H. (2013). Trends in racial/ethnic disparities in medical and oral health, access to care and use of services in US children: Has anything changed over the years? *International Journal for Equity in Health, 12,* 10. Retrieved from http://www.equityhealthj.com/content/12/1/10.

Giannini, C., & Caprio, S. (2012). Islet function in obese adolescents. *Diabetes, Obesity and Metabolism, 14*(3 suppl), 40–45.

Graff, M., North, K. E., Monda, K. L., et al. (2011). The combined influence of genetic factors and sedentary activity on body mass changes from adolescence to young adulthood: The National Longitudinal Adolescent Health Study. *Diabetes/Metabolism Research and Reviews, 27*(1), 63–69.

Guyatt, G. H., Oxman, A. D., Vist, G. E., et al. (2008). GRADE: An emerging consensus on rating quality of evidence and strength of recommendations. *British Medical Journal, 336*(7650), 924–926.

Institute for Patient- and Family-Centered Care. (2017). *Advancing the practice of patient-and-family-centered care in hospitals: How to get started.* Bethesda, MD: Institute for Patient- and Family-Centered Care. Retrieved from www.ipfcc.org/resources/getting_started.pd.

Juvonen, J., & Graham, S. (2014). Bullying in schools: The power of bullies and the plight of victims. *Annual Review of Psychology, 65,* 159–185.

Kagihara, L. E., Niederhauser, V. P., & Stark, M. (2009). Assessment, management, and prevention of early childhood caries. *Journal of the American Academy of Nurse Practitioners, 21*(1), 1–10.

Kass, N. E., Faden, R. R., Goodman, S. N., et al. (2013). The research-treatment distinction: A problematic approach for determining which activities should have ethical oversight. *Hastings Center Report,* S4–S15.

Leslie, L. K., Slaw, K. M., Edwards, A., et al. (2010). Peering into the future: Pediatrics in a changing world. *Pediatrics, 126*(5), 982–988.

Martin, A., Saunders, D. H., Shenkin, S. D., et al. (2014). Lifestyle intervention for improving school achievement in overweight or obese children and adolescents. *Cochrane Database of Systematic Review, 2014*(3), CD009728.

Melnyk, B. M., & Fineout-Overholt, E. (2014). *Evidence-based practice in nursing and healthcare: A guide to best practice.* Philadelphia, PA: Lippincott.

Murphy, S. L., Mathews, T. J., Martin, J. A., et al. (2017). Annual summary of vital statistics: 2013-2014. *Pediatrics, 139*(6), e20163239.

National Strategy for Quality Improvement in Health Care. (2012). *Annual progress report to congress.* Washington, DC: US Department of Health and Human Services.

Pelletier, L. R., & Beaudin, C. L. (2008). *Q solutions: Essential resources for the healthcare quality professional* (2nd ed.). Glenview, IL: National Association for Healthcare Quality.

Polaha, J., Dalton, W. T., 3rd, & Allen, S. (2011). The prevalence of emotional and behavior problems in pediatric primary care serving rural children. *Journal of Pediatric Psychology, 36*(6), 652–660.

Rockett, I. R., Regier, M. D., Kapusta, N. D., et al. (2012). Leading causes of unintentional and intentional injury mortality: United States, 2000-2009. *American Journal of Public Health, 102*(11), e84–e92.

Slomski, A. (2012). Chronic mental health issues in children now loom larger than physical problems. *Journal of the American Medical Association, 308*(3), 223–225.

US Department of Health and Human Services. (2013a). *Healthy People 2020.* Retrieved from http://www.healthypeople.gov/.

US Department of Health and Human Services. (2013b). *Youth violence: A report of the surgeon general.* Retrieved from http://www.ncbi.nlm.nih.gov/books/NBK44294/.

Waters, E., de Silva-Sanigorski, A., Hall, B. J., et al. (2011). Intervention for preventing obesity in children. *Cochrane Database of Systematic Reviews, 2011*(12), CD001871.

Weiss, R., Bremer, A. A., & Lustig, R. H. (2013). What is metabolic syndrome, and why are children getting it? *Annals of the New York Academy of Sciences, 1281,* 123–140.

Wong, D. (1989). Principles of atraumatic care. In V. Feeg (Ed.), *Pediatric nursing: Forum on the future: Looking toward the 21st century.* Pitman, NJ: Anthony J Jannetti.

27

Family, Social, Cultural, and Religious Influences on Child Health Promotion

Marilyn J. Hockenberry

http://evolve.elsevier.com/Perry/maternal

GENERAL CONCEPTS

DEFINITION OF FAMILY

The term family has been defined in many different ways according to the individual's own frame of reference, values, or discipline. There is no universal definition of family; a family is what an individual considers it to be. Biology describes the family as fulfilling the biologic function of perpetuation of the species. Psychology emphasizes the interpersonal aspects of the family and its responsibility for personality development. Economics views the family as a productive unit providing for material needs. Sociology depicts the family as a social unit interacting with the larger society, creating the context within which cultural values and identity are formed. Others define family in terms of the relationships of the people who make up the family unit. The most common type of relationships are consanguineous (blood relationships), affinal (marital relationships), and family of origin (family unit a person is born into).

Earlier definitions of family emphasized that family members were related by legal ties or genetic relationships and lived in the same household with specific roles. Later definitions have been broadened to reflect both structural and functional changes. A family can be defined as an institution where individuals, related through biology or enduring commitments, and representing similar or different generations and genders, participate in roles involving mutual socialization, nurturance, and emotional commitment (Kaakinen, Gedaly-Duff, & Hanson, 2009).

Considerable controversy has surrounded the newer concepts of family, such as communal families, single-parent families, and homosexual families. To accommodate these and other varieties of family styles, the descriptive term household is frequently used.

> ### ! NURSING ALERT
>
> The nurse's knowledge and the sensitivity with which he or she assesses a household will determine the types of interventions that are appropriate to support family members.

Nursing care of infants and children is intimately involved with care of the child and the family. Family structure and dynamics can have an enduring influence on a child, affecting the child's health and well-being (American Academy of Pediatrics, 2003). Consequently, nurses must be aware of the functions of the family, various types of family structures, and theories that provide a foundation for understanding the changes within a family and for directing family-oriented interventions.

FAMILY THEORIES

A family theory can be used to describe families and how the family unit responds to events both within and outside the family. Each family theory makes assumptions about the family and has inherent strengths and limitations (Kaakinen, Gedaly-Duff, & Hanson, 2009). Most nurses use a combination of theories in their work with children and families. Commonly used theories are family systems theory, family stress theory, and developmental theory (Table 27.1).

Family Systems Theory

Family systems theory is derived from general systems theory, a science of "wholeness" that is characterized by interaction among the components of the system and between the system and the environment (Bomar, 2004; Papero, 1990). The family is viewed as a whole that is different from the sum of the individual members. For example, a household of parents and one child consists of not only three individuals, but also four interactive units. These units include three dyads (the marital relationship, the mother-child relationship, and the father-child relationship) and a triangle (the mother-father-child relationship). In this ecologic model, the family system functions within a larger system, with the family dyads in the center of a circle surrounded by the extended family, the subculture, and the culture, with the larger society at the periphery.

Bowen's family systems theory emphasizes that the key to healthy family function is the members' ability to distinguish themselves from one another both emotionally and intellectually (Kaakinen, Gedaly-Duff, & Hanson, 2009; Papero, 1990). The family unit has a high level of adaptability. When problems arise within the family, change occurs by altering the interaction or feedback messages that perpetuate disruptive behavior. *Feedback* refers to processes in the family that help identify strengths and needs and determine how well goals are accomplished. Positive feedback initiates change; negative feedback resists change (Goldenberg & Goldenberg, 2008). When the family system is disrupted, change can occur at any point in the system.

A major factor that influences a family's adaptability is its boundary, an imaginary line that exists between the family and its environment (Kaakinen, Gedaly-Duff, & Hanson, 2009). Families have varying degrees of openness and closure in these boundaries. For example, one family has the capacity to reach out for help, whereas another considers help threatening. Knowledge of boundaries is critical when teaching or counseling families. Families with open boundaries may demonstrate a greater receptivity to interventions, whereas families demonstrating

TABLE 27.1   Summary of Family Theories and Application

Assumptions	Strengths	Limitations	Applications
Family Systems Theory			
A change in any one part of a family system affects all other parts of the family system (circular causality). Family systems are characterized by periods of rapid growth and change and periods of relative stability. Both too little change and too much change are dysfunctional for the family system; therefore, a balance between morphogenesis (change) and morphostasis (no change) is necessary. Family systems can initiate change, as well as react to it.	Applicable for family in normal everyday life, as well as for family dysfunction and pathology. Useful for families of varying structure and various stages of life cycle.	More difficult to determine cause-and-effect relationships because of circular causality.	Mate selection, courtship processes, family communication, boundary maintenance, power and control within family, parent-child relationships, adolescent pregnancy and parenthood.
Family Stress Theory			
Stress is an inevitable part of family life, and any event, even if positive, can be stressful for the family. Family encounters both normative expected stressors and unexpected situational stressors over life cycle. Stress has a cumulative effect on family. Families cope with and respond to stressors with a wide range of responses and effectiveness.	Potential to explain and predict family behavior in response to stressors and to develop effective interventions to promote family adaptation. Focuses on positive contribution of resources, coping, and social support to adaptive outcomes. Can be used by many disciplines in health field.	Relationships between all variables in framework not yet adequately described. Not yet known if certain combinations of resources and coping strategies are applicable to all stressful events.	Transition to parenthood and other normative transitions, single-parent families, families experiencing work-related stressors (dual-earner family, unemployment), acute or chronic childhood illness or disability, infertility, death of a child, divorce, and adolescent pregnancy and parenthood.
Developmental Theory			
Families develop and change over time in similar and consistent ways. Family and its members must perform certain time-specific tasks set by themselves and by people in the broader society. Family role performance at one stage of family life cycle influences family's behavioral options at next stage. Family tends to be in stage of disequilibrium when entering a new life cycle stage and strives toward homeostasis within stages.	Provides a dynamic, rather than static, view of family. Addresses both changes within family and changes in family as a social system over its life history. Anticipates potential stressors that normally accompany transitions to various stages and when problems may peak because of lack of resources.	Traditional model more easily applied to two-parent families with children. Use of age of oldest child and marital duration as marker of stage transition sometimes problematic (e.g., in stepfamilies, single-parent families).	Anticipatory guidance, educational strategies, and developing or strengthening family resources for management of transition to parenthood; family adjustment to children entering school, becoming adolescents, leaving home; management of "empty nest" years and retirement.

closed boundaries often require increased sensitivity and skill on the part of the nurse to gain their trust and acceptance. The nurse who uses family systems theory should assess the family's ability to accept new ideas, information, resources, and opportunities and to plan strategies.

Family Stress Theory

Family stress theory explains how families react to stressful events and suggests factors that promote adaptation to stress (Kaakinen, Gedaly-Duff, & Hanson, 2009). Families encounter stressors (events that cause stress and have the potential to effect a change in the family social system), including those that are predictable (e.g., parenthood) and those that are unpredictable (e.g., illness, unemployment). These stressors are cumulative, involving simultaneous demands from work, family, and community life. Too many stressful events occurring within a relatively short period (usually 1 year) can overwhelm the family's ability to cope and place it at risk for breakdown or physical and emotional health problems among its members. When the family experiences too many stressors for it to cope adequately, a state of crisis ensues. For adaptation to occur, a change in family structure or interaction is necessary.

The resiliency model of family stress, adjustment, and adaptation emphasizes that the stressful situation is not necessarily pathologic or detrimental to the family but demonstrates that the family needs to make fundamental structural or systemic changes to adapt to the situation (McCubbin & McCubbin, 1994).

Developmental Theory

Developmental theory is an outgrowth of several theories of development. Duvall (1977) described eight developmental tasks of the family throughout its life span (Box 27.1). The family is described as a small group, a semiclosed system of personalities that interacts with the larger cultural social system. As an interrelated system, the family does not have changes in one part without a series of changes in other parts.

Developmental theory addresses family change over time using Duvall's family life cycle stages, based on the predictable changes in the family's structure, function, and roles, with the age of the oldest child as the marker for stage transition. The arrival of the first child marks the transition from stage I to stage II. As the first child grows and develops, the family enters subsequent stages. In every stage, the family faces certain developmental tasks. At the same time, each family member

---

BOX 27.1 Duvall's Developmental Stages of the Family

Stage I: Marriage and an Independent Home: The Joining of Families
Re-establish couple identity.
Realign relationships with extended family.
Make decisions regarding parenthood.

Stage II: Families With Infants
Integrate infants into the family unit.
Accommodate to new parenting and grandparenting roles.
Maintain marital bond.

Stage III: Families With Preschoolers
Socialize children.
Parents and children adjust to separation.

Stage IV: Families With Schoolchildren
Children develop peer relations.
Parents adjust to their children's peer and school influences.

Stage V: Families With Teenagers
Adolescents develop increasing autonomy.
Parents refocus on midlife marital and career issues.
Parents begin a shift toward concern for the older generation.

Stage VI: Families as Launching Centers
Parents and young adults establish independent identities.
Parents renegotiate marital relationship.

Stage VII: Middle-Aged Families
Reinvest in couple identity with concurrent development of independent interests.
Realign relationships to include in-laws and grandchildren.
Deal with disabilities and death of older generation.

Stage VIII: Aging Families
Shift from work role to leisure and semiretirement or full retirement.
Maintain couple and individual functioning while adapting to the aging process.
Prepare for own death and dealing with the loss of spouse and/or siblings and other peers.

Modified from Wright, L.M., & Leahey, M. (1984). *Nurses and families: A guide to family assessment and intervention.* Philadelphia, PA: Davis.

BOX 27.2 Family Nursing Intervention

- Behavior modification
- Case management and coordination
- Collaborative strategies
- Contracting
- Counseling, including support, cognitive reappraisal, and reframing
- Empowering families through active participation
- Environmental modification
- Family advocacy
- Family crisis intervention
- Networking, including use of self-help groups and social support
- Providing information and technical expertise
- Role modeling
- Role supplementation
- Teaching strategies, including stress management, lifestyle modifications, and anticipatory guidance

From Friedman, M.M., Bowden, V.R., & Jones, E.G. (2003). *Family nursing: research theory and practice* (5th ed.). Upper Saddle River, NJ: Prentice Hall.

---

must achieve individual developmental tasks as part of each family life cycle stage.

Developmental theory can be applied to nursing practice. For example, the nurse can assess how well new parents are accomplishing the individual and family developmental tasks associated with transition to parenthood. New applications should emerge as more is learned about developmental stages for nonnuclear and nontraditional families.

FAMILY NURSING INTERVENTIONS

In working with children, the nurse must include family members in their care plan. Research confirms parents' desire and expectation to participate in their child's care (Power & Franck, 2008). To discover family dynamics, strengths, and weaknesses, a thorough family assessment is necessary (see Chapter 29). The nurse's choice of interventions depends on the theoretic family model that is used (Box 27.2). For example, in family systems theory, the focus is on the interaction of family members within the larger environment (Goldenberg & Goldenberg, 2008). In this case, using group dynamics to involve all members in the intervention process and being a skillful communicator are essential. Systems theory also presents excellent opportunities for anticipatory guidance. Because each family member reacts to every stress experienced by that system, nurses can intervene to help the family prepare for and cope with changes. In family stress theory, the nurse employs crisis intervention strategies to help family members cope with the challenging event. In developmental theory, the nurse provides anticipatory guidance to prepare members for transition to the next family stage. Nurses who think family involvement plays a key role in the care of a child are more likely to include families in the child's daily care (Fisher, Lindhorst, Matthews, et al., 2008).

FAMILY STRUCTURE AND FUNCTION

FAMILY STRUCTURE

The family structure, or family composition, consists of individuals, each with a socially recognized status and position, who interact with one another on a regular, recurring basis in socially sanctioned ways (Kaakinen, Gedaly-Duff, & Hanson, 2009). When members are gained or lost through events such as marriage, divorce, birth, death, abandonment, or incarceration, the family composition is altered and roles must be redefined or redistributed.

Traditionally, the family structure was either a nuclear or extended family. In recent years, family composition has assumed new configurations, with the single-parent family and blended family becoming prominent forms. The predominant structural pattern in any society depends on the mobility of families as they pursue economic goals and as relationships change. It is not uncommon for children to belong to several different family groups during their lifetime.

Nurses must be able to meet the needs of children from many diverse family structures and home situations. A family's structure affects the direction of nursing care. The US Census Bureau uses four definitions for families: (1) the traditional nuclear family, (2) the nuclear family, (3) the blended family or household, and (4) the extended family or household. In addition, numerous other types of families have been defined, such as single-parent, binuclear, polygamous, communal, and

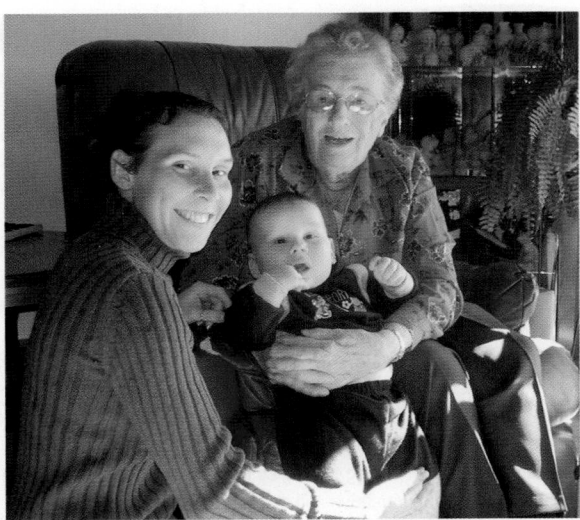

FIG 27.1 Children benefit from interaction with grandparents, who sometimes assume the parenting role.

lesbian, gay, transgender, queer, questioning, and intersex (LGBTQI) families.

Traditional Nuclear Family

A traditional nuclear family consists of a married couple and their biologic children. Children in this type of family live with both biologic parents and, if siblings are present, only full brothers and sisters (i.e., siblings who share the same two biologic parents). No other people are present in the household (i.e., no step relatives, foster or adopted children, half-siblings, other relatives, or nonrelatives).

Nuclear Family

The nuclear family is composed of two parents and their children. The parent-child relationship may be biologic, step, adoptive, or foster. Sibling ties may be biologic, step, half, or adoptive. The parents are not necessarily married. No other relatives or nonrelatives are present in the household.

Blended Family

A blended family or household, also called a reconstituted family, includes at least one stepparent, stepsibling, or half-sibling. A stepparent is the spouse of a child's biologic parent but is not the child's biologic parent. Stepsiblings do not share a common biologic parent; the biologic parent of one child is the stepparent of the other. Half-siblings share only one biologic parent.

Extended Family

An extended family or household includes at least one parent, one or more children, and one or more members (related or unrelated) other than a parent or sibling. Parent-child and sibling relationships may be biologic, step, adoptive, or foster.

In many nations and among many ethnic and cultural groups, households with extended families are common. Within the extended family, grandparents often find themselves rearing their grandchildren (Fig. 27.1). Young parents are often considered too young or too inexperienced to make decisions independently. Often, the older relative

holds the authority and makes decisions in consultation with the young parents. Sharing residence with relatives also assists with the management of scarce resources and provides child care for working families. A resource for extended families is the Grandparent Information Center.*

Single-Parent Family

In the United States, an estimated 24.6 million children live in single-parent families (Annie E. Casey Foundation, 2015a). The contemporary single-parent family has emerged partially as a consequence of the women's rights movement and also as a result of more women (and men) establishing separate households because of divorce, death, desertion, or single parenthood. In addition, a more liberal attitude in the courts has made it possible for single people, both male and female, to adopt children. Although mothers usually head single-parent families, it is becoming more common for fathers to be awarded custody of dependent children in divorce settlements. With women's increased psychologic and financial independence and the increased acceptability of single parents in society, more unmarried women are deliberately choosing mother-child families. Frequently, these mothers and children are absorbed into the extended family.

Binuclear Family

The term binuclear family refers to parents continuing the parenting role while terminating the spousal unit. The degree of cooperation between households and the time the child spends with each can vary. In joint custody, the court assigns divorcing parents equal rights and responsibilities concerning the minor child or children. These alternate family forms are efforts to view divorce as a process of reorganization and redefinition of a family rather than as a family dissolution. Joint custody and co-parenting are discussed later in this chapter.

Polygamous Family

Although it is not legally sanctioned in the United States, the conjugal unit is sometimes extended by the addition of spouses in polygamous matings. Polygamy refers to either multiple wives (polygyny) or, rarely, husbands (polyandry). Many societies practice polygyny that is further designated as sororal, in which the wives are sisters, or nonsororal, in which the wives are unrelated. Sororal polygyny is widespread throughout the world. Most often, mothers and their children share a husband and father, with each mother and her children living in the same or a separate household.

Communal Family

The communal family emerged from disenchantment with most contemporary life choices. Although communal families may have divergent beliefs, practices, and organization, the basic impetus for formation is often dissatisfaction with the nuclear family structure, social systems, and goals of the larger community. Relatively uncommon today, communal groups share common ownership of property. In cooperatives, property ownership is private, but certain goods and services are shared and exchanged without monetary consideration. There is strong reliance on group members and material interdependence. Both provide collective security for nonproductive members, share homemaking and childrearing functions, and help overcome the problem of interpersonal isolation or loneliness.

Lesbian, Gay, Transgender, Queer, Questioning, and Intersex (LGBTQI) Families

A same-sex, homosexual, or LGBTQI family is one in which there is a legal or common-law tie between two people of the same sex who have children (Blackwell, 2007). There are a growing number of families with same-sex parents in the United States, with an estimated one-fifth

---

*For information, contact the local AARP representative or office; http://www.aarp.org/relationships/friends-family/.

of all same-sex couples raising children (O'Connell & Feliz, 2011; US Census Bureau, 2011). Although some children in LGBTQI households are biologic from a former marriage relationship, children may be present in other circumstances. They may be foster or adoptive parents, lesbian mothers may conceive through artificial fertilization, or a gay male couple may become parents through use of a surrogate mother.

When children are brought up in LGBTQI families, the relationships seem as natural to them as heterosexual parents do to their offspring. In other cases, however, disclosure of parental homosexuality ("coming out") to children can be a concern for families. There are a number of factors to consider before disclosing this information to children. Parents should be comfortable with their own sexual preference and should discuss this with the children as they become old enough to understand relationships. Discussions should be planned and take place in a quiet setting where interruptions are unlikely.

Nurses need to be nonjudgmental and to learn to accept differences rather than demonstrate prejudice that can have a detrimental effect on the nurse-child-family relationship (Blackwell, 2007). Moreover, the more nurses know about the child's family and lifestyle, the more they can help the parents and the child.

FAMILY STRENGTHS AND FUNCTIONING STYLE

Family function refers to the interactions of family members, especially the quality of those relationships and interactions (Bomar, 2004). Researchers are interested in family characteristics that help families to function effectively. Knowledge of these factors guides the nurse throughout the nursing process and helps the nurse to predict ways that families may cope and respond to a stressful event, to provide individualized support that builds on family strengths and unique functioning style, and to assist family members in obtaining resources.

Family strengths and unique functioning styles are significant resources that nurses can use to meet family needs (Box 27.3). Building on qualities that make a family work well and strengthening family resources make the family unit even stronger. All families have strengths as well as vulnerabilities.

FAMILY ROLES AND RELATIONSHIPS

Each individual has a position, or status, in the family structure and plays culturally and socially defined roles in interactions within the family. Each family also has its own traditions and values and sets its own standards for interaction within and outside the group. Each determines the experiences the children should have, those they are to be shielded from, and how each of these experiences meets the needs of family members. When family ties are strong, social control is highly effective, and most members conform to their roles willingly and with commitment. Conflicts arise when people do not fulfill their roles in ways that meet other family members' expectations, either because they are unaware of the expectations or because they choose not to meet them.

PARENTAL ROLES

In all family groups, the socially recognized status of father and mother exists with socially sanctioned roles that prescribe appropriate sexual behavior and childrearing responsibilities. The guides for behavior in these roles serve to control sexual conflict in society and provide for prolonged care of children. The degree to which parents are committed and the way they play their roles are influenced by a number of variables and by the parents' unique socialization experience.

Parental role definitions have changed as a result of the changing economy and increased opportunities for women (Bomar, 2004). As the woman's role has changed, the complementary role of the man has

---

> **BOX 27.3   Qualities of Strong Families**
>
> - A belief and sense of commitment toward promoting the well-being and growth of individual family members, as well as the family unit
> - Appreciation for the small and large things that individual family members do well and encouragement to do better
> - Concentrated effort to spend time and do things together, no matter how formal or informal the activity or event
> - A sense of purpose that permeates the reasons and basis for "going on" in both bad and good times
> - A sense of congruence among family members regarding the value and importance of assigning time and energy to meet needs
> - The ability to communicate with one another in a way that emphasizes positive interactions
> - A clear set of family rules, values, and beliefs that establishes expectations about acceptable and desired behavior
> - A varied repertoire of coping strategies that promote positive functioning in dealing with both normative and nonnormative life events
> - The ability to engage in problem-solving activities designed to evaluate options for meeting needs and procuring resources
> - The ability to be positive and see the positive in almost all aspects of their lives, including the ability to see crisis and problems as an opportunity to learn and grow
> - Flexibility and adaptability in the roles necessary to procure resources to meet needs
> - A balance between the use of internal and external family resources for coping and adapting to life events and planning for the future

From Dunst, C., Trivette, C., & Deal, A. (1988). *Enabling and empowering families: principles and guidelines for practice*, Cambridge, MA: Brookline Books.

also changed. Many fathers are more active in childrearing and household tasks. As the redefinition of sex roles continues in families in the United States, role conflicts may arise in many families because of a cultural lag of the persisting traditional role definitions.

ROLE LEARNING

Roles are learned through the socialization process. During all stages of development, children learn and practice, through interaction with others and in their play, a set of social roles and the characteristics of other roles. They behave in patterned and more or less predictable ways, because they learn roles that define mutual expectations in typical social relationships. Although role definitions are changing, the basic determinants of parenting remain the same. Several determinants of parenting infants and young children are parental personality and mental well-being, systems of support, and child characteristics. These determinants have been used as consistent measurements to determine a person's success in fulfilling the parental role.

Parents, peers, authority figures, and other socializing agents who use positive and negative sanctions to ensure conformity to their norms transmit role conceptions. Role behaviors positively reinforced by rewards such as love, affection, friendship, and honors are strengthened. Negative reinforcement takes the form of ridicule, withdrawal of love, expressions of disapproval, or banishment.

In some cultures, the role behavior expected of children conflicts with desirable adult behavior. One of the family's responsibilities is to develop culturally appropriate role behavior in children. Children learn to perform in expected ways consistent with their position in the family and culture. The observed behavior of each child is a single manifestation—a combination of social influences and individual psychologic processes. In this way, the uniting of the child's intrapersonal system (the self) with the interpersonal system (the family) is simultaneously understood as the child's conduct.

Role structuring initially takes place within the family unit, in which the children fulfill a set of roles and respond to the roles of their parents and other family members (Kaakinen, Gedaly-Duff, & Hanson, 2009). Children's roles are shaped primarily by the parents, who apply direct or indirect pressures to induce or force children into the desired patterns of behavior or direct their efforts toward modification of the role responses of the child on a mutually acceptable basis. Parents have their own techniques and determine the course that the socialization process follows.

Children respond to life situations according to behaviors learned in reciprocal transactions. As they acquire important role-taking skills, their relationships with others change. For instance, when a teenager is also the mother but lives in a household with the grandmother, the teenager may be viewed more as an adolescent than as a mother. Children become proficient at understanding others as they acquire the ability to discriminate their own perspectives from those of others. Children who get along well with others and attain status in the peer group have well-developed role-taking skills.

PARENTING

PARENTING STYLES

Children respond to their environment in a variety of ways. A child's temperament heavily influences his or her responses, but styles of parenting have also been shown to affect a child and lead to particular behavioral responses. Parenting styles are often classified as authoritarian, permissive, or authoritative (Baumrind, 1971; 1996). Authoritarian parents try to control their children's behavior and attitudes through unquestioned mandates. They establish rules and regulations or standards of conduct that they expect to be followed rigidly and unquestioningly. The message is: "Do it because I say so." Punishment need not be corporal but may be stern withdrawal of love and approval. Careful training often results in rigidly conforming behavior in the children who tend to be sensitive, shy, self-conscious, retiring, and submissive. They are more likely to be courteous, loyal, honest, and dependable but docile. These behaviors are more typically observed when close supervision and affection accompany parental authority. If not, this style of parenting may be associated with both defiant and antisocial behaviors.

Permissive parents exert little or no control over their children's actions. They avoid imposing their own standards of conduct and allow their children to regulate their own activity as much as possible. These parents consider themselves to be resources for the children, not role models. If rules do exist, the parents explain the underlying reason, elicit the children's opinions, and consult them in decision-making processes. They employ lax, inconsistent discipline; do not set sensible limits; and do not prevent the children from upsetting the home routine. These parents rarely punish the children.

Authoritative parents combine practices from both of the previously described parenting styles. They direct their children's behavior and attitudes by emphasizing the reason for rules and negatively reinforcing deviations. They respect the individuality of each child and allow the child to voice objections to family standards or regulations. Parental control is firm and consistent but tempered with encouragement, understanding, and security. Control is focused on the issue, not on withdrawal of love or the fear of punishment. These parents foster "inner-directedness," a conscience that regulates behavior based on feelings of guilt or shame for wrongdoing, not on fear of being caught or punished. Parents' realistic standards and reasonable expectations produce children with high self-esteem who are self-reliant, assertive, inquisitive, content, and highly interactive with other children.

There are differing philosophies in regard to parenting. Childrearing is a culturally bound phenomenon, and children are socialized to behave in ways that are important to their family. In the authoritative style, authority is shared and children are included in discussions, fostering an independent and assertive style of participation in family life. When working with individual families, nurses should give these differing styles equal respect.

LIMIT SETTING AND DISCIPLINE

In its broadest sense, discipline means "to teach" or refers to a set of rules governing conduct. In a narrower sense, it refers to the action taken to enforce the rules after noncompliance. Limit setting refers to establishing the rules or guidelines for behavior. For example, parents can place limits on the amount of time children spend watching television or chatting online. The clearer the limits that are set and the more consistently they are enforced, the less need there is for disciplinary action.

Nurses can help parents establish realistic and concrete "rules." Limit setting and discipline are positive, necessary components of childrearing and serve several useful functions as they help children do the following:

- Test their limits of control
- Achieve in areas appropriate for mastery at their level
- Channel undesirable feelings into constructive activity
- Protect themselves from danger
- Learn socially acceptable behavior

Children want and need limits. Unrestricted freedom is a threat to their security and safety. By testing the limits imposed on them, children learn the extent to which they can manipulate their environment and gain reassurance from knowing that others are there to protect them from potential harm.

MINIMIZING MISBEHAVIOR

The reasons for misbehavior may include attention, power, defiance, and a display of inadequacy (e.g., the child misses classes because of a fear that he or she is unable to do the work). Children may also misbehave because the rules are not clear or consistently applied. Acting-out behavior, such as a temper tantrum, may represent uncontrolled frustration, anger, depression, or pain. The best approach is to structure interactions with children to prevent or minimize unacceptable behavior (see Family-Centered Care box: Minimizing Misbehavior).

GENERAL GUIDELINES FOR IMPLEMENTING DISCIPLINE

Regardless of the type of discipline used, certain principles are essential to ensure the efficacy of the approach (see Family-Centered Care box: Implementing Discipline). Many strategies, such as behavior modification, can only be implemented effectively when principles of consistency and timing are followed. A pattern of intermittent or occasional enforcement of limits actually prolongs the undesired behavior, because children learn that if they are persistent, the behavior is permitted eventually. Delaying punishment weakens its intent, and practices such as telling the child, "Wait until your father comes home," are not only ineffectual but also convey negative messages about the other parent.

TYPES OF DISCIPLINE

To deal with misbehavior, parents need to implement appropriate disciplinary action. Many approaches are available. Reasoning involves explaining why an act is wrong and is usually appropriate for older children, especially when moral issues are involved. However, young

FAMILY-CENTERED CARE
Minimizing Misbehavior

- Set realistic goals for acceptable behavior and expected achievements.
- Structure opportunities for small successes to lessen feelings of inadequacy.
- Praise children for desirable behavior with attention and verbal approval.
- Structure the environment to prevent unnecessary difficulties (e.g., place fragile objects in an inaccessible area).
- Set clear and reasonable rules; expect the same behavior regardless of the circumstances; if exceptions are made, clarify that the change is for one time only.
- Teach desirable behavior through own example, such as using a quiet, calm voice rather than screaming.
- Review expected behavior before special or unusual events, such as visiting a relative or having dinner in a restaurant.
- Phrase requests for appropriate behavior positively, such as "Put the book down," rather than "Don't touch the book."
- Call attention to unacceptable behavior as soon as it begins; use distraction to change the behavior or offer alternatives to annoying actions, such as exchanging a quiet toy for one that is too noisy.
- Give advance notice or "friendly reminders," such as "When the TV program is over, it is time for dinner," or "I'll give you to the count of three, and then we have to go."
- Be attentive to situations that increase the likelihood of misbehaving, such as overexcitement or fatigue, or decreased personal tolerance to minor infractions.
- Offer sympathetic explanations for not granting a request, such as "I am sorry I can't read you a story now, but I have to finish dinner. Then we can spend time together."
- Keep any promises made to children.
- Avoid outright conflicts; temper discussions with statements, such as "Let's talk about it and see what we can decide together," or "I have to think about it first."
- Provide children with opportunities for power and control.

FAMILY-CENTERED CARE
Implementing Discipline

- Consistency: Implement disciplinary action exactly as agreed on and for each infraction.
- Timing: Initiate discipline as soon as child misbehaves; if delays are necessary, such as to avoid embarrassment, verbally disapprove of the behavior and state that disciplinary action will be implemented.
- Commitment: Follow through with the details of the discipline, such as timing of minutes; avoid distractions that may interfere with the plan, such as telephone calls.
- Unity: Make certain that all caregivers agree on the plan and are familiar with the details to prevent confusion and alliances between child and one parent.
- Flexibility: Choose disciplinary strategies that are appropriate to child's age and temperament and the severity of the misbehavior.
- Planning: Plan disciplinary strategies in advance, and prepare child if feasible (e.g., explain use of time-out); for unexpected misbehavior, try to discipline when you are calm.
- Behavior orientation: Always disapprove of the behavior, not the child, with statements, such as "That was a wrong thing to do. I am unhappy when I see behavior like that."
- Privacy: Administer discipline in private, especially with older children, who may feel ashamed in front of others.
- Termination: After the discipline is administered, consider child as having a "clean slate," and avoid bringing up the incident or lecturing.

children cannot be expected to "see the other side" because of their egocentrism. Children in the preoperative stage of cognitive development (toddlers and preschoolers) have a limited ability to distinguish between their point of view and that of others. Sometimes children use "reasoning" as a way of gaining attention. For example, they may misbehave, thinking the parents will give them a lengthy explanation of the wrongdoing and knowing that negative attention is better than no attention. When children use this technique, parents should end the explanation by stating, "This is the rule, and this is how I expect you to behave. I won't explain it any further."

Unfortunately, reasoning is often combined with scolding, which sometimes takes the form of shame or criticism. For example, the parent may state, "You are a bad boy for hitting your brother." Children take such remarks seriously and personally, believing that they are bad.

! NURSING ALERT

When reprimanding children, focus only on the misbehavior, not on the child. Use of "I" messages rather than "you" messages expresses personal feelings without accusation or ridicule. For example, an "I" message attacks the behavior ("I am upset when Johnny is punched; I don't like to see him hurt") not the child.

Positive and negative reinforcement is the basis of behavior modification theory—behavior that is rewarded will be repeated; behavior that

is not rewarded will be extinguished. Using rewards is a positive approach. By encouraging children to behave in specified ways, the parents can decrease the tendency to misbehave. With young children, using paper stars is an effective method. For older children, the "token system" is appropriate, especially if a certain number of stars or tokens yields a special reward, such as a trip to the movies or a new book. In planning a reward system, the parents must explain expected behaviors to the child and establish rewards that are reinforcing. They should use a chart to record the stars or tokens and always give an earned reward promptly. Verbal approval should always accompany extrinsic rewards.

Consistently ignoring behavior will eventually extinguish or minimize the act. Although this approach sounds simple, it is difficult to implement consistently. Parents frequently "give in" and resort to previous patterns of discipline. Consequently, the behavior is actually reinforced because the child learns that persistence gains parental attention. For ignoring to be effective, parents should (1) understand the process, (2) record the undesired behavior before using ignoring to determine whether a problem exists and to compare results after ignoring is begun, (3) determine whether parental attention acts as a reinforcer, and (4) be aware of "response burst." *Response burst* is a phenomenon that occurs when the undesired behavior increases after ignoring is initiated because the child is "testing" the parents to see if they are serious about the plan.

The strategy of consequences involves allowing children to experience the results of their misbehavior. It includes the following three types:
1. Natural: Those that occur without any intervention, such as being late and having to clean up the dinner table
2. Logical: Those that are directly related to the rule, such as not being allowed to play with another toy until the used ones are put away
3. Unrelated: Those that are imposed deliberately, such as no playing until homework is completed or the use of time-out

Natural or logical consequences are preferred and effective if they are meaningful to children. For example, the natural consequence of living in a messy room may do little to encourage cleaning up, but

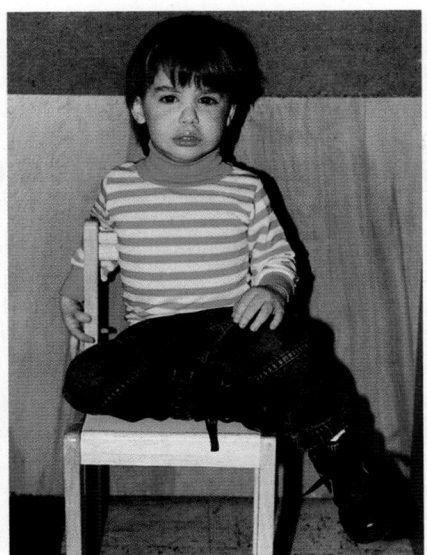

FIG 27.2 Time-out is an excellent disciplinary strategy for young children.

allowing no friends over until the room is neat can be motivating! Withdrawing privileges is often an unrelated consequence. After the child experiences the consequence, the parent should refrain from any comment, because the usual tendency is for the child to try to place blame for imposing the rule.

Time-out is a refinement of the common practice of sending the child to his or her room and is a type of unrelated consequence. It is based on the premise of removing the reinforcer (i.e., the satisfaction or attention the child is receiving from the activity). When placed in an unstimulating and isolated place, children become bored and consequently agree to behave in order to re-enter the family group (Fig. 27.2). Time-out avoids many of the problems of other disciplinary approaches. No physical punishment is involved; no reasoning or scolding is given; and the parent does not need to be present for all of the time-out, thus facilitating consistent application of this type of discipline. Time-out offers both the child and the parent a "cooling-off" time. To be effective, however, time-out must be planned in advance (see Family-Centered Care box: Using Time-Out). Implement time-out in a public place by selecting a suitable area, or explain to children that time-out will be spent immediately on returning home.

Corporal or physical punishment most often takes the form of spanking (Larzelere, 2008). Based on the principles of aversive therapy, inflicting pain through spanking causes a dramatic short-term decrease in the behavior. However, this approach has serious flaws: (1) it teaches children that violence is acceptable; (2) it may physically harm the child if it is the result of parental rage; and (3) children become "accustomed" to spanking, requiring more severe corporal punishment over time. Spanking can result in severe physical and psychologic injury, and it interferes with effective parent-child interaction (Cain, 2008). In addition, when the parents are not around, children are likely to misbehave, because they have not learned to behave well for their own sake. Parental use of corporal punishment may also interfere with the child's development of moral reasoning.

SPECIAL PARENTING SITUATIONS

Parenting is a demanding task under ideal circumstances, but when parents and children face situations that deviate from "the norm," the potential for family disruption is increased. Situations that are encountered frequently are divorce, single parenthood, blended families, adoption, and dual-career families. In addition, as cultural diversity increases in our communities, many immigrants are making the transition to parenthood and a new country, culture, and language simultaneously. Other situations that create unique parenting challenges are parental alcoholism, homelessness, and incarceration. Although these topics are not addressed here, the reader may wish to investigate them further.

PARENTING THE ADOPTED CHILD

Adoption establishes a legal relationship between a child and parents who are not related by birth but who have the same rights and obligations that exist between children and their biologic parents. In the past, the biologic mother alone made the decision to relinquish the rights to her child. In recent years, the courts have acknowledged the legal rights of the biologic father regarding this decision. Concerned child advocates have questioned whether decisions that honor the father's rights are in the best interest of the child. As the child's rights have become recognized, older children have successfully dissolved their legal bond with their biologic parents to pursue adoption by adults of their choice. Furthermore, there is a growing interest and demand within the LGBTQI community to adopt.

Unlike biologic parents, who prepare for their child's birth with prenatal classes and the support of friends and relatives, adoptive parents have fewer sources of support and preparation for the new addition to their family. Nurses can provide the information, support, and reassurance needed to reduce parental anxiety regarding the adoptive process and refer adoptive parents to state parental support groups. Such sources can be contacted through a state or county welfare office.

Siblings, adopted or biologic, who are old enough to understand, should be included in decisions regarding the commitment to adopt with reassurance that they are not being replaced. Ways that the siblings can interact with the adopted child should be stressed (Fig. 27.3).

ISSUES OF ORIGIN

The task of telling children that they are adopted can be a cause of deep concern and anxiety. There are no clear-cut guidelines for parents to follow in determining when and at what age children are ready for

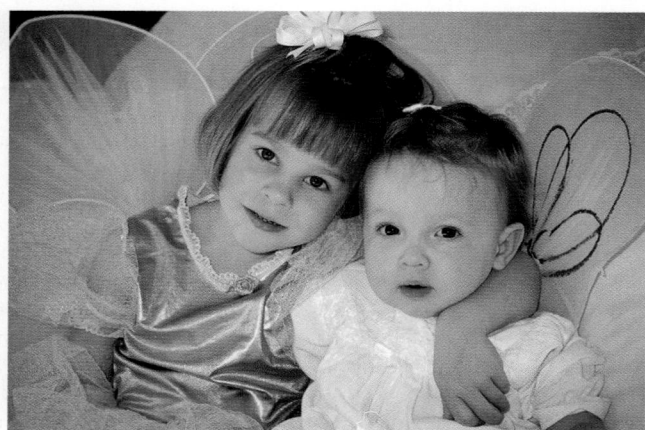

FIG 27.3 An older sister lovingly embraces her adopted sister.

the information. Parents are naturally reluctant to present such potentially unsettling news. However, it is important that parents not withhold the adoption from the child, because it is an essential component of the child's identity.

The timing arises naturally as parents become aware of the child's readiness. Most authorities believe that children should be informed at an age young enough so that, as they grow older, they do not remember a time when they did not know they were adopted. The time is highly individual, but it must be right for both the parents and the child. It may be when children ask where babies come from, at which time children can also be told the facts of their adoption. If they are told in a way that conveys the idea that they were active participants in the selection process, they will be less likely to feel that they were abandoned victims in a helpless situation. For example, parents can tell children that their personal qualities drew the parents to them. It is wise for parents who have not previously discussed adoption to tell children that they are adopted before the children enter school to avoid having them learn it from third parties. Complete honesty between parents and children strengthens the relationship.

Parents should anticipate behavior changes after the disclosure, especially in older children. Children who are struggling with the revelation that they are adopted may benefit from individual and family counseling. Children may use the fact of their adoption as a weapon to manipulate and threaten parents. Statements such as, "My real mother would not treat me like this," or "You don't love me as much because I'm adopted," hurt parents and increase their feelings of insecurity. Such statements may also cause parents to become overpermissive. Adopted children need the same undemanding love, combined with firm discipline and limit setting, as any other child.

ADOLESCENCE

Adolescence may be an especially trying time for parents of adopted children. The normal confrontations of adolescents and parents assume more painful aspects in adoptive families. Adolescents may use their adoption to defy parental authority or as a justification for aberrant behavior. As they attempt to master the task of identity formation, they may begin to have feelings of abandonment by their biologic parents. Gender differences in reacting to adoption may surface.

Adopted children fantasize about their biologic parents and may feel the need to discover their parents' identity to define themselves and their own identity. It is important for parents to keep the lines of communication open and to reassure their child that they understand the need to search for their identity. In some states, birth certificates

are made legally available to adopted children when they come of age. Parents should be honest with questioning adolescents and tell them of this possibility. (The parents themselves are unable to obtain the birth certificate; it is the children's responsibility if they desire it.)

CROSS-RACIAL AND INTERNATIONAL ADOPTION

Adoption of children from racial backgrounds different from that of the family is commonplace. In addition to the problems faced by adopted children in general, children of a cross-racial adoption must deal with physical and sometimes cultural differences. It is advised that parents who adopt children with different ethnic background do everything to preserve the adopted children's racial heritage.

> ### ! NURSING ALERT
>
> As a health care provider, it is important not to ask the wrong questions, such as:
> - "Is she yours, or is she adopted?"
> - "What do you know about the 'real' mother?"
> - "Do they have the same father?"
> - "How much did it cost to adopt him?"

Although the children are full-fledged members of an adopting family and citizens of the adopted country, if they have a strikingly different appearance from other family members or exhibit distinct racial or ethnic characteristics, challenges may be encountered outside the family. Bigotry may appear among relatives and friends. Strangers may make thoughtless comments and talk about the children as though they were not members of the family. It is vital that family members declare to others that this is their child and a cherished member of the family.

In international adoptions, the medical information the parents receive may be incomplete or sketchy; weight, height, and head circumference are often the only objective information present in the child's medical record. Many internationally adopted children were born prematurely, and common health problems, such as infant diarrhea and malnutrition, delay growth and development. Some children have serious or multiple health problems that can be stressful for the parents.

PARENTING AND DIVORCE

Since the mid-1960s, a marked change in the stability of families has been reflected in increased rates of divorce, single parenthood, and remarriage. In 2011, the divorce rate for the United States was 3.2 per 1000 total population (Centers for Disease Control and Prevention [CDC], 2017). The divorce rate has changed little since 1987. In the decade before that, the rate increased yearly, with a peak in 1979. Although almost half of all divorcing couples are childless, it is estimated that more than 1 million children experience divorce each year.

The process of divorce begins with a period of marital conflict of varying length and intensity, followed by a separation, the actual legal divorce, and the re-establishment of different living arrangements (Box 27.4). Because a function of parenthood is to provide for the security and emotional welfare of children, disruption of the family structure often engenders strong feelings of guilt in the divorcing parents (Fig. 27.4).

During a divorce, parents' coping abilities may be compromised. The parents may be preoccupied with their own feelings, needs, and life changes and be unavailable to support their children. Newly employed parents, usually mothers, are likely to leave children with new caregivers, in strange settings, or alone after school. The parent may also spend more time away from home, searching for or establishing new relationships. Sometimes, however, the adult feels frightened and alone and

BOX 27.4 The Divorce Process

Acute Phase
- The married couple makes the decision to separate.
- This phase includes the legal steps of filing for dissolution of the marriage and, usually, the departure of the father from the home.
- This phase lasts from several months to more than 1 year and is accompanied by familial stress and a chaotic atmosphere.

Transitional Phase
- The adults and children assume unfamiliar roles and relationships within a new family structure.
- This phase is often accompanied by a change of residence, a reduced standard of living and altered lifestyle, a larger share of the economic responsibility being shouldered by the mother, and radically altered parent-child relationships.

Stabilizing Phase
- The post-divorce family re-establishes a stable, functioning family unit.
- Remarriage frequently occurs with concomitant changes in all areas of family life.

Modified from Wallerstein, J.S. (1988). Children of divorce: Stress and developmental tasks. In N. Garmezy, & N. Rutter (Eds.), *Stress, coping, and development in children.* New York: McGraw-Hill.

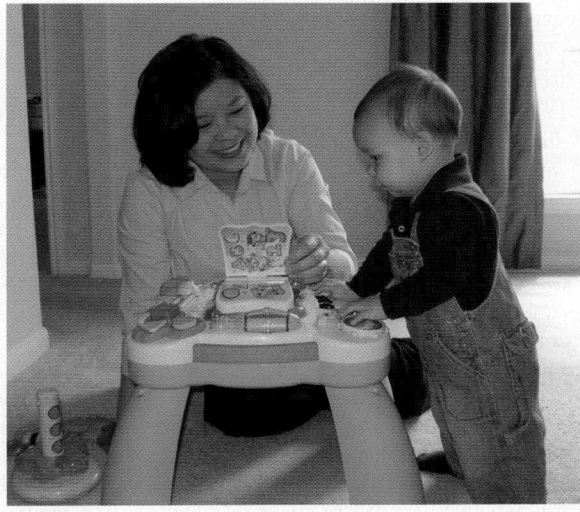

FIG 27.4 Quality time spent with a child during a divorce is essential to a family's health and well-being.

begins to depend on the child as a substitute for the absent parent. This dependence places an enormous burden on the child.

Common characteristics in the custodial household after separation and divorce include disorder, coercive types of control, inflammable tempers in both parents and children, reduced parental competence, a greater sense of parental helplessness, poorly enforced discipline, and diminished regularity in household routines. Noncustodial parents are seldom prepared for the role of visitor, may assume the role of recreational and "fun" parent, and may not have a residence suitable for children's visits. They may also be concerned about maintaining the arrangement over the years to follow.

Impact of Divorce on Children

Parental divorce is an additional childhood adversity that contributes to poor mental health outcomes, especially when combined with child abuse. Parental psychopathology may be one possible mechanism to explain the relationships between child abuse, parental divorce, and psychiatric disorders and suicide attempts (Afifi, Boman, Fleisher, et al., 2009). Even when a divorce is amicable and open, children recall parental separation with the same emotions felt by victims of a natural disaster: loss, grief, and vulnerability to forces beyond their control.

The impact of divorce on children depends on several factors, including the age and sex of the children, the outcome of the divorce, and the quality of the parent-child relationship and parental care during the years following the divorce. Family characteristics are more crucial to the child's well-being than specific child characteristics, such as age or sex. High levels of ongoing family conflict are related to problems of social development, emotional stability, and cognitive skills for the child.

A major problem occurs when children are "caught in the middle" between the divorced parents. They become the message bearer between the parents, are often quizzed about the other parent's activities, and have to listen to one parent criticize the other. A nurse may be able to help the child get out of the middle by stating "I messages" based on the formula of "I feel (state the feeling) when you (state the source). I would like it if you…" An example of an "I message" is: "I do not feel comfortable when you ask me questions about mom; maybe you could ask her yourself." This approach enables the child to feel in control.

Feelings of children toward divorce vary with age (Box 27.5). Previously, researchers believed that divorce had a greater impact on younger children, but recent observations indicate that divorce constitutes a major disruption for children of all ages. The feelings and behaviors of children may be different for various ages and gender, but all children suffer stress second only to the stress produced by the death of a parent. Although considerable research has looked at sex differences in children's adjustments to divorce, the findings are not conclusive.

Some children feel a sense of shame and embarrassment concerning the family situation. Sometimes children see themselves as different, inferior, or unworthy of love, especially if they feel responsible for the family dissolution. Although the social stigma attached to divorce no longer produces the emotions it did in the past, such feelings may still exist in small towns or in some cultural groups and can reinforce children's negative self-image. The lasting effects of divorce depend on the children's and the parents' adjustment to the transition from an intact family to a single-parent family and, often, to a reconstituted family.

Although most studies have concentrated on the negative effects of divorce on youngsters, some positive outcomes of divorce have been reported. A successful postdivorce family, either a single-parent or a reconstituted family, can improve the quality of life for both adults and children. If conflict is resolved, a better relationship with one or both parents may result, and some children may have less contact with a disturbed parent. Greater stability in the home setting and the removal of arguing parents can be a positive outcome for the child's long-term well-being.

Telling the Children

Parents are understandably hesitant to tell children about their decision to divorce. Most parents neglect to discuss either the divorce or its inevitable changes with their preschool child. Without preparation, even children who remain in the family home are confused by the parental separation. Frequently, children are already experiencing vague, uneasy feelings that are more difficult to cope with than being told the truth about the situation.

If possible, the initial disclosure should include both parents and siblings, followed by individual discussions with each child. Sufficient time should be set aside for these discussions, and they should take place during a period of calm, not after an argument. Parents who

BOX 27.5   Feelings and Behaviors of Children Related to Divorce

Infancy
- Effects of reduced mothering or lack of mothering
- Increased irritability
- Disturbance in eating, sleeping, and elimination
- Interference with attachment process

Early Preschool Children (2 to 3 Years of Age)
- Frightened and confused
- Blame themselves for the divorce
- Fear of abandonment
- Increased irritability, whining, tantrums
- Regressive behaviors (e.g., thumb sucking, loss of elimination control)
- Separation anxiety

Later Preschool Children (3 to 5 Years of Age)
- Fear of abandonment
- Blame themselves for the divorce; decreased self-esteem
- Bewilderment regarding all human relationships
- Become more aggressive in relationships with others (e.g., siblings, peers)
- Engage in fantasy to seek understanding of the divorce

Early School-Age Children (5 to 6 Years of Age)
- Depression and immature behavior
- Loss of appetite and sleep disorders
- May be able to verbalize some feelings and understand some divorce-related changes
- Increased anxiety and aggression
- Feelings of abandonment by departing parent

Middle School-Age Children (6 to 8 Years of Age)
- Panic reactions
- Feelings of deprivation: loss of parent, attention, money, and secure future
- Profound sadness, depression, fear, and insecurity
- Feelings of abandonment and rejection

- Fear regarding the future
- Difficulty expressing anger at parents
- Intense desire for reconciliation of parents
- Impaired capacity to play and enjoy outside activities
- Decline in school performance
- Altered peer relationships: become bossy, irritable, demanding, and manipulative
- Frequent crying, loss of appetite, sleep disorders
- Disturbed routine, forgetfulness

Later School-Age Children (9 to 12 Years of Age)
- More realistic understanding of divorce
- Intense anger directed at one or both parents
- Divided loyalties
- Ability to express feelings of anger
- Ashamed of parental behavior
- Desire for revenge; may wish to punish the parent they hold responsible
- Feelings of loneliness, rejection, and abandonment
- Altered peer relationships
- Decline in school performance
- May develop somatic complaints
- May engage in aberrant behavior, such as lying, stealing
- Temper tantrums
- Dictatorial attitude

Adolescents (12 to 18 Years of Age)
- Able to disengage themselves from parental conflict
- Feelings of a profound sense of loss: of family, childhood
- Feelings of anxiety
- Worry about themselves, parents, siblings
- Expression of anger, sadness, shame, embarrassment
- May withdraw from family and friends
- Disturbed concept of sexuality
- May engage in acting-out behaviors

physically hold or touch their children provide them with a feeling of warmth and reassurance. The discussions should include the reason for the divorce, if age appropriate, and reassurance that the divorce is not the fault of the children.

Parents should not fear crying in front of the children, because their crying gives the children permission to cry also. Children need to ventilate their feelings. Children may feel guilt, a sense of failure, or that they are being punished for misbehavior. They normally feel anger and resentment and should be allowed to communicate these feelings without punishment. They also have feelings of terror and abandonment. They need consistency and order in their lives. They want to know where they will live, who will take care of them, if they will be with their siblings, and if there will be enough money to live on. Children may also wonder what will happen on special days such as birthdays and holidays, whether both parents will come to school events, and whether they will still have the same friends. Children fear that if their parents stopped loving each other, they could stop loving them. Their need for love and reassurance is tremendous at this time.

Custody and Parenting Partnerships

In the past, when parents separated, the mother was given custody of the children with visitation agreements for the father. Now both parents and the courts are seeking alternatives. Current belief is that neither fathers nor mothers should be awarded custody automatically. Custody should be awarded to the parent who is best able to provide for the children's welfare. In some cases, children experience severe stress when living or spending time with a parent. Many fathers have demonstrated both their competence and their commitment to care for their children.

Often overlooked are the changes that may occur in the children's relationships with other relatives, especially grandparents. Grandparents are increasingly involved in the care of young children (Fergusson, Maughan, & Golding, 2008). Grandparents on the noncustodial side are often kept from their grandchildren, whereas those on the custodial side may be overwhelmed by their adult child's return to the household with grandchildren.

Two other types of custody arrangements are divided custody and joint custody. Divided custody, or split custody, means that each parent is awarded custody of one or more of the children, thereby separating siblings. For example, sons might live with the father and daughters with the mother.

Joint custody takes one of two forms. In joint physical custody, the parents alternate the physical care and control of the children on an agreed-on basis while maintaining shared parenting responsibilities legally. This custody arrangement works well for families who live close to each other and whose occupations permit an active role in the care and rearing of the children. In joint legal custody, the children reside with one parent, but both parents are the children's legal guardians, and both participate in childrearing.

Co-parenting offers substantial benefits for the family. Children can be close to both parents, and life with each parent can be more normal (as opposed to having a disciplinarian mother and a recreational father). To be successful, parents in these arrangements must be highly committed to provide normal parenting and to separate their marital conflicts from their parenting roles. No matter what type of custody arrangement is awarded, the primary consideration is the welfare of the children.

SINGLE PARENTING

An individual may acquire single-parent status as a result of divorce, separation, death of a spouse, or birth or adoption of a child. In 2013, 35% of children younger than 18 years of age lived in single-parent families, and the majority of single parents were women (Annie E. Casey Foundation, 2015a; Kreider & Elliott, 2009). Although some women are single parents by choice, most never planned on being single parents, and many feel pressure to marry or remarry.

Managing shortages of money, time, and energy is often a concern for single parents. Studies repeatedly confirm the financial difficulties of single-parent families, particularly single mothers. In 13, 34 percent of single-parent families had household incomes below the poverty line (Annie E. Casey Foundation, 2015a). In fact, the stigma of poverty may be more keenly felt than the discrimination associated with being a single parent. These families are often forced by their financial status to live in communities with inadequate housing and personal safety concerns. Single parents often feel guilty about the time spent away from their children. Divorced mothers, from marriages in which the father assumed the role of breadwinner and the mother the household maintenance and parenting roles, have considerable difficulty adjusting to their new role of breadwinner. Many single parents have trouble arranging for adequate child care, particularly for a sick child.

Social supports and community resources needed by single-parent families include health care services that are open on evenings and weekends; high-quality child care; respite child care to relieve parental exhaustion and prevent burnout; and parent enhancement centers for advancing education and job skills, providing recreational activities, and offering parenting education. Single parents need social contacts separate from their children for their own emotional growth and that of their children.

Single Fathers

Fathers who have custody of their children have many of the same problems as divorced mothers. They feel overburdened by the responsibility; depressed; and concerned about their ability to cope with the emotional needs of the children, especially girls. Some fathers lack homemaking skills. They may find it difficult at first to coordinate household tasks, school visits, and other activities associated with managing a household alone (Fig. 27.5).

PARENTING IN RECONSTITUTED FAMILIES

In the United States, many of the children living in homes where parents have divorced will experience another major change in their lives, such as the addition of a stepparent or new siblings (Kaakinen, Gedaly-Duff, and Hanson, 2009). The entry of a stepparent into a ready-made family requires adjustments for all family members. Some obstacles to the role adjustments and family problem solving include disruption of previous lifestyles and interaction patterns, complexity in the formation of new ones, and lack of social supports. Despite these problems, most children from divorced families want to live in a two-parent home.

Cooperative parenting relationships can allow more time for each set of parents to be alone to establish their own relationship with the

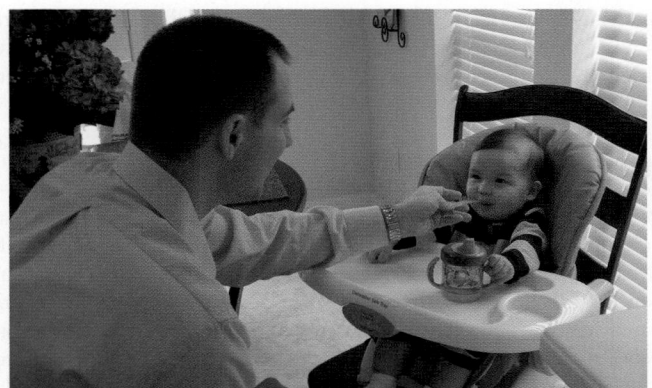

FIG 27.5 Fathers who assume care of their children may feel more comfortable and successful in their parenting role.

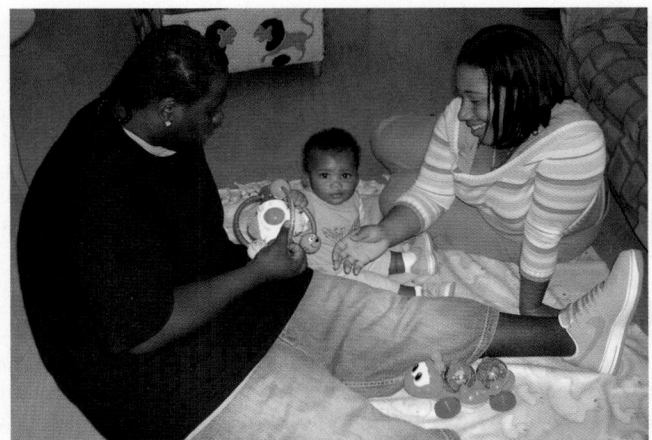

FIG 27.6 Learning new roles in reconstituted families as a mother and father can enhance parenting relationships.

children. Under ideal circumstances, power conflicts between the two households can be reduced, and tension and anxiety can be lessened for all family members. In addition, the children's self-esteem can be increased, and there is a greater likelihood of continued contact with grandparents. Flexibility, mutual support, and open communication are critical in successful relationships in stepfamilies and stepparenting situations (Fig. 27.6).

PARENTING IN DUAL-EARNER FAMILIES

No change in family lifestyle has had more impact than the large numbers of women moving away from the traditional homemaker role and entering the workplace (Kaakinen, Gedaly-Duff, & Hanson, 2009). The trend toward increased numbers of dual-earner families is unlikely to diminish significantly. As a result, the family is subject to considerable stress as members attempt to meet often competing demands of occupational needs and those regarded as necessary for a rich family life.

Role definitions are frequently altered to arrange a more equitable division of time and labor, as well as to resolve conflict, especially conflict related to traditional cultural norms. Overload is a common source of stress in a dual-earner family, and social activities are significantly curtailed. Time demands and scheduling are major problems for all individuals who work. When the individuals are parents, the demands can be even more intense. Dual-earner couples may increase the strain on themselves to avoid creating stress for their children. Although there is no evidence to indicate that the dual-earner lifestyle is stressful to children, the stress experienced by the parents may affect the children indirectly.

WORKING MOTHERS

Working mothers have become the norm in the United States. Maternal employment may have variable effects on preschool children's health (Mindlin, Jenkins, & Law, 2009). The quality of child care is a persistent concern for all working parents. Determinants of child care quality are based on health and safety requirements, responsive and warm interaction between staff and children, developmentally appropriate activities, trained staff, limited group size, age-appropriate caregivers, adequate staff-to-child ratios, and adequate indoor and outdoor space. Nurses play an important role in helping families find suitable sources of child care and prepare children for this experience.

KINSHIP CARE

Since the 1980s, the proportion of children in out-of-home care placed with relatives has increased rapidly. More than 2.7 million American children are cared for by extended family or close family friends at some time in their lives (Annie E. Casey Foundation, 2012). According to US Census Bureau data, kinship caregivers are more likely to be poor, single, older, less educated, and unemployed than families in which at least one parent is present.

FOSTER PARENTING

Foster care can be defined as the placement of a child in a stable and approved environment with a nonrelated family. The living situation may be an approved foster home, possibly with other children, or a pre-adoptive home. Each state provides a standard for the role of foster parent and a process by which to become one. These "parents" contract with the state to provide a home for children for a limited duration. Most states require about 27 hours of training before being on contract and at least 12 hours of continuing education per year. Foster parents may be required to attend a foster parent support group that is often separate from a state agency. Each state has guidelines regarding the relative health of the prospective foster parents and their families, background checks regarding legal issues for the adults, personal interviews, and a safety inspection of the residence and surroundings (Chamberlain, Price, Leve, et al., 2008).

Foster homes include both kinship and nonrelative placements. Since the 1980s, the proportion of children in out-of-home care placed with relatives has increased rapidly and been accompanied by a decrease in the number of foster families. As with their nonfoster counterparts, much of the child's adjustment depends on the family's stability and available resources. Even though foster homes are designed to provide short-term care, it is not unusual for children to stay for many years.

Nurses should be aware that on any given day over 55,000 children are in the child welfare system (Annie E. Casey Foundation, 2015b). Children from lower-income, single-mother, and mother-partner families are considerably more likely to be living in foster care (Berger & Waldfogel, 2004). Children in foster care tend to have a higher than normal incidence of acute and chronic health problems and may experience feelings of isolation or confusion. Foster children are often at risk because of their previous caretaking environment. Nurses should strive to implement strategies to improve the health care for this group of children. In particular, assessment and case management skills are required to involve other disciplines in meeting their needs.

SOCIOCULTURAL INFLUENCES UPON THE CHILD AND FAMILY

A child and his or her immediate family are nested within a local community of school, peers, and extended family and within a larger community that may be bound by common geography, background, traditions, and an even broader community that incorporates the social, political, and economic elements that influence many aspects of family life. This section of this chapter delves into a deeper discussion of such factors.

Bronfenbrenner (1979) offers a perspective of viewing children and their families within the context of various circles of influence, called an ecologic framework. This framework posits that individuals adapt in response to changes in their surrounding environments, whether that be the environment of the immediate family, the school, the neighborhood in which the family lives, or the socioeconomic forces that may shape job availability in their geographic area. In addition, he argues that a person's behavior results from the interaction of his or her traits and abilities with the environment. No single factor can explain the totality of a child and his or her family's health behaviors. Children possess their own factors that influence their behavior (i.e., personal history or biologic factors). In turn, they are surrounded by relationships with family, friends, and peers who influence their behavior. Children and their families are then situated within a community that establishes the context in which social relationships develop. Finally, wider sociocultural factors exist that influence whether a behavior is encouraged or prohibited (i.e., social policy on smoking, cultural norms of mothers as primary caregivers of young children, media that can influence how an adolescent thinks he or she should look) (CDC, 2009; Perry-Jenkins, Newkirk, & Ghunney, 2013) (Fig. 27.7).

Promoting the health of children requires a nurse to understand social, cultural, and religious influences on children and their families. The population in the United States is constantly evolving. Patients experience negative health outcomes when social, cultural, and religious factors are not considered as influencing their health care (Chavez, 2012; Williams, 2012). Educating health care providers is one way to reduce disparities in health care.

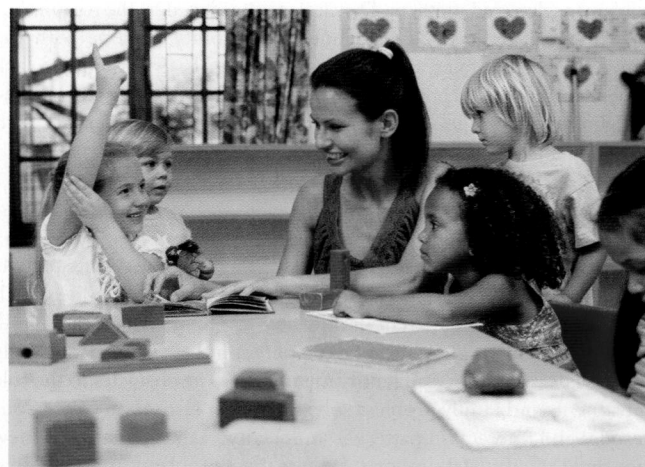

FIG 27.7 Children from a variety of cultural and ethnic backgrounds begin to socialize in the child care setting. (Copyright 2012 by Photos. com, a division of Getty Images. All rights reserved.)

INFLUENCES IN THE SURROUNDING ENVIRONMENT

SCHOOLS

When children enter school, their radius of relationships extends to include a wider variety of peers and a new source of authority. Although parents continue to exert the major influence on children, in the school environment, teachers have the most significant psychologic impact on children's development and socialization. In addition to academic and cognitive progress, teachers are concerned with the emotional and social development of the children in their care. Both parents and teachers act to model, shape, and promote positive behavior, constrain negative behavior, and enforce standards of conduct. Ideally, parents and teachers work together for the benefit of the children in their care.

Schools serve as a major source of socialization for children. Next to the family, schools exert a major force in providing continuity and passing down culture from one generation to the next. This, in turn, prepares children to carry out the social roles they are expected to assume as they develop into adults. School is the center of cultural diffusion wherein the cultural standards of the larger group are disseminated into the community. It governs what is taught and, to a great extent, how it is taught. School rules and regulations regarding attendance, authority relationships, and the system of rewards and penalties based on achievement transmit to children the expectations of the adult world of employment and relationships. School is an important institution in which children systematically learn about the negative consequences of behavior that departs from social expectations. School also serves as an avenue for children to participate in the larger society in rewarding ways, to promote social mobility, and to connect the family with new knowledge and services. Like parents, teachers are responsible for transmitting knowledge and culture (i.e., values on which there is a broad consensus) to the children in their care. Teachers are also expected to stimulate and guide children's intellectual development and creative problem solving. Traditionally, the socialization process of school began when children entered kindergarten. However, this process is starting at younger ages as children enter various child care settings with more than 60% of mothers working outside the home.

PEER CULTURES

Peer groups also have an impact on the socialization of children. Peer relationships become increasingly important and influential as children proceed through school. In school, children have what can be regarded as a culture of their own. This is even more apparent in unsupervised playgroups because the culture in school is partly produced by adults.

During their lives, children are subjected to many influential factors, such as family, religious community, and social class. In peer-group interactions, they confront a variety of these sets of values. The values imposed by the peer group are especially compelling because children must accept and conform to them to be accepted as members of the group. When the peer values are not too different from those of family and teachers, the mild conflict created by these small differences serves to separate children from the adults in their lives and to strengthen the feeling of belonging to the peer group.

Although the peer group has neither the traditional authority of the parents nor the legal authority of the schools for teaching information, it manages to convey a substantial amount of information to its members, especially on taboo subjects such as sex and drugs. Children's need for the friendship of their peers brings them into an increasingly complex social system. Through peer relationships, children learn to deal with dominance and hostility and to relate with people in positions of leadership and authority. Other functions of the peer subculture are to relieve boredom and to provide recognition that individual members do not receive from teachers and other authority figures.

The peer-group culture has secrets, mores, and codes of ethics that promote group solidarity and detachment from adults. They have traditions, including age-related games and other activities that are transferred from "generation to generation" of schoolchildren and that have a great influence over the behavior of all group members. As children move from one level to the next, they discard the folkways of the younger group as they adopt those of the new group. For example, a school-age child rides a bicycle to school, whereas the high school student prefers a car. As they advance, children are forward oriented only—they look forward with anticipation but may look backward with contempt.

SOCIAL ROLES

Much of children's self-concept comes from their ideas about their social roles. Roles are cultural creations; therefore, the culture prescribes patterns of behavior for people in a variety of social positions. All people who hold similar social positions have an obligation to behave in a particular manner. A role prohibits some behaviors and allows others. Because culture outlines and clarifies roles, it is a significant influence on the development of children's self-concept (i.e., attitudes and beliefs they have about themselves). To establish their place in the group, children learn to follow a mode of behavior that is in agreement with the standards specific to the group and learn how they can expect others to behave toward them. They take their cues by observing and imitating those to whom they are exposed consistently.

CO-CULTURAL OR SUBCULTURAL INFLUENCES

Except in rare circumstances, children grow and develop in a blend of cultures. Subcultures or co-cultures are groups within a cultural group that possess their own standards and mores (Dysart-Gale, 2006). For example, nursing or medicine constitutes a subculture or co-culture. In a large, complex society like the United States, different groups have their own sets of standards, values, and expectations within the collective ways of the larger culture. Most of these co-cultures were formed when groups of people clustered together by preferences, external pressure from the majority culture, or geographic isolation. Although cultural differences may be related to geographic boundaries, co-cultures are not always restricted by location, especially in the context of Internet support groups and social media. Considering children, in particular, some subcultures are even related to the stages of development. For example, the behavior of school-age children and adolescents demonstrate age-related subcultures. Although there are countless subcultures or co-cultures within the United States, those that seem to exert great influence upon children and their families are ethnicity, social class, minority group membership, religion/spirituality, schools, communities, and peer groups.

COMMUNITIES

Communities can be sites of opportunity and growth for children and families. Communities can also be a site where poverty and disenfranchisement are minimized through connections with high-quality early childhood education, job training for adolescents and parents, and safe, effective schools. Communities can also contribute to toxic stress if violence and poverty are pervasive and resources absent (Annie E. Casey Foundation, 2013). Recent research with over 1 million youth in the United States has shown that assets within a community can bolster healthy decision-making, minimize high-risk behaviors, and support positive child and adolescent development (Search Institute, 2009). The child's or adolescent's community is made up of family, school, neighborhood, youth organizations, and other members.

Four categories of external assets that youth receive from the community are as follows (Search Institute, 2009):

1. Support: Young people need to feel support, care, and love from their families, neighbors, and others. They also need organizations and institutions that offer positive, supportive environments.
2. Empowerment: Young people need to feel valued by their community and be able to contribute to others. They need to feel safe and secure.
3. Boundaries and expectations: Young people need to know what is expected of them and what activities and behaviors are within the community boundaries and what are outside of them.
4. Constructive use of time: Young people need opportunities for growth through constructive, enriching opportunities and through quality time at home.

Internal assets must also be nurtured in the community's young members. These internal qualities guide choices and create a sense of centeredness, purpose, and focus. The four categories of internal assets are as follows (Search Institute, 2009):

1. Commitment to learning: Young people need to develop a commitment to education and lifelong learning.
2. Positive values: Youth need to have a strong sense of values that direct their choices.
3. Social competencies: Young people need competencies that help them make positive choices and build relationships.
4. Positive identity: Young people need a sense of their own power, purpose, worth, and promise.

BROADER SOCIOCULTURAL INFLUENCES UPON THE CHILD AND FAMILY

RACE AND ETHNICITY

Race and ethnicity are socially constructed terms used to group people who share similar characteristics, traditions, or historical experience together. Race is a term that groups together people by their outward, physical appearance. Ethnicity is a classification aimed at grouping "individuals who consider themselves, or are considered by others, to share common characteristics that differentiate them from the other collectivities in a society, and from which they develop their distinctive cultural behavior" (Scott & Marshall, 2009). Ethnicities may be differentiated from one another by customs and language and may influence family structure, food preferences, and expressions of emotion. The composition and definition of ethnic and racial groups can be fluid in response to changes in geography (i.e., moving from one country to another) and changing social definitions over time (Roberts, 2011). Race and ethnicity influence a family's health when they are used as criteria by which a child or family is discriminated against. There is a significant body of work that describes this. In fact, 100 years of research describe racial gaps in health (Williams, 2012).

Racism remains an important social determinant of health (Smedley, 2012). According to Williams (2012), for minority or other groups who experience stigmatization, "inequalities in health are created by larger inequalities in society," meaning that prevailing social conditions and obstacles to equal opportunities for all influences the health of all individuals. For example, from birth forward, African-American and Native American children have a higher mortality rate than Caucasian children in general. There is also a higher death rate for babies of African-American and Hispanic women versus Caucasian women. Even when controlling for maternal levels of education, the infant mortality rate for college-educated African-American women is 2.5 times higher

than for Hispanic and Caucasian women of similar education level (Williams, 2012). These numbers demonstrate that children and families ultimately feel the effects of such health disparities.

Children and families may also experience perceived racism, which also has negative consequences. For example, in a study of more than 5000 fifth-graders, 15% of Hispanic youth and 20% of African-American youth reported that they had experienced racial discrimination. Such experiences were then associated with a higher risk for mental health symptoms (Coker, Elliot, Kanouse, et al., 2009). Teens also report racial discrimination through online communities, social networking sites, and texting, which is related to increased anxiety and depression (Tynes, Giang, Williams, et al., 2008).

Ethnocentrism is the emotional attitude that one's own ethnic group is superior to others; that one's values, beliefs, and perceptions are the correct ones; and that the group's ways of living and behaving are the best (Spector, 2009). Ethnocentrism implies that all other groups are inferior. Stereotyping or labeling stems from ethnocentric beliefs. It is a common attitude among the dominant ethnic group and strongly influences a person's ability to evaluate objectively the beliefs and behaviors of others. Nurses must overcome the natural tendency to have ethnocentric attitudes when caring for people from backgrounds different from their own (Scott & Marshall, 2009).

SOCIAL CLASS

The influence of social class cannot be overlooked. This relates to the family's economic and educational levels and their ability to access resources needed to thrive in daily life. Strength of family relationships is not tied to social class. A family of lower socioeconomic status may have fewer resources, but they may be well connected to the broader family network and rely on them for support to meet physical and emotional needs. Families in higher socioeconomic groups may have access to resources that reach beyond their extended family but may be disconnected because of pressures of work and outside obligations (i.e., children's activities).

POVERTY

Consider the following statistics. More than 25% of all children in the United States are receiving Supplemental Nutrition Assistance program (i.e., food stamps). In the United States, in 2011, more than 16 million children were poor (Isaacs & Healy, 2012). The United States has the second largest share of children living under the relative poverty line among wealthy nations (UNICEF, 2013), and less than 8% of the federal US budget is invested in children. An absolute standard of poverty attempts to delimit a basic set of resources needed for adequate existence. A relative standard reflects the median standard of living in a society and is the term used in referring to childhood poverty in the United States—in other words, what appears to be deprivation in one area may be the standard or norm in another. Growth in the number of poor children over the past decade has not been attributable to an increase in the number of families receiving government assistance but to the growing ranks of the working poor. Approximately 20% of children in the United States live below the national poverty threshold, which is currently estimated at $23,550 for two adults and two children (US Department of Health and Human Services, 2013). In addition, 20% of children live in neighborhoods where more than 20% of the population lives below the federal poverty threshold. Taken together, such information tells us that not only might resources be limited in a family home but also the community surrounding that home, which can affect opportunities for child growth and development (i.e., safe, thriving schools and places to play).

A high correlation between poverty and illness has long been observed. Impoverished families suffer from poor nutrition, and without medical insurance, families have little access to preventive health care and services. More than 14 million children are underinsured, meaning that their parents report spending a significant amount of money on out-of-pocket expenses related to their children's health. Day-to-day needs for clothing, food, and lodging take precedence over health care as long as the ill person is able to perform his or her daily tasks. The passage of major health care legislation, both the Children's Health Insurance Plan Reauthorization Act and the Affordable Care Act, has expanded health insurance to 3.7 million children (Harrington, Smith, Trenholm, et al., 2014). Hopefully, this will lead to improved health of children and families.

EVOLVING DEMOGRAPHICS IN THE UNITED STATES

The United States has more racial and ethnic diversity than any other nation. By 2018, no one racial/ethnic group will be a majority group (Annie E. Casey Foundation, 2014). For example, the 2010 US Census revealed that more than 300 million people live in the United States. In 2010, individuals who identified as Hispanic made up over 16% of the population (Humes, Jones, & Ramirez, 2011); this will be one of the fastest-growing groups in the United States. Individuals who identify as Asian are expanding at an even faster rate in the United States (Hoeffel, Rastogi, Kim, et al., 2012). In addition, the 2010 Census data demonstrated that almost one-half of all children 1 year of age in the United States were from a racial ethnic minority (Frey, 2011). In light of these findings, it becomes even more important for pediatric nurses to care for children and families in an open, culturally humble manner.

RELIGIOUS INFLUENCES

The family's religious orientation dictates a code of behavior and influences the family's attitudes toward education, male and female role identity, and their ultimate destiny. It may also influence the school that the children attend or the community in which the family embeds itself. Religious beliefs are such an integral part of many cultures that it is difficult to distinguish the culture from the religion. In a few instances, such as in the Mennonite and Amish communities, religion is the basis for a common way of life that determines where the children are raised and their lifestyle. It is also important to remember that families that do not subscribe to a particular religion or that are atheist also have beliefs and convictions about family, the surrounding world, and life in general that influence the children in these families.

Religious Beliefs

Religious and spiritual dimensions are among the most important influences in many people's lives (Fig. 27.8). The terms religion and spirituality are often used interchangeably, but this is incorrect. According to Mercer (2006), spirituality is "concerned with the deepest levels of human experiencing, the places of deepest … meaning in and for our lives." According to Yates (2011), spirituality is "a dynamic and personal experiential process." For children in particular, spirituality possesses a relational consciousness; it concerns the child in relation to the source of power (God, Allah) that gives meaning to the relationship, other people, the surrounding world, and within oneself (Mercer, 2006). Religion, on the other hand, is a particular and culturally influenced representation of human spirituality. Children and teens who are supported in their spiritual expression can develop a foundation for understanding social relationships, making lifestyle decisions, and demonstrating resilience. Spirituality and religion can also have

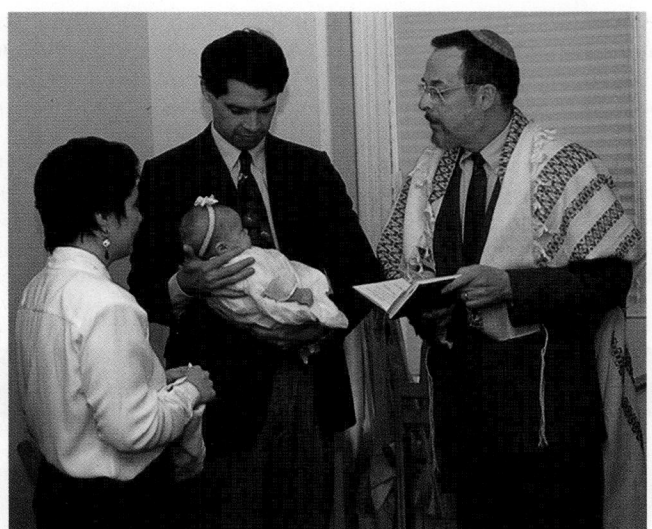

FIG 27.8 Soon after an infant is born, many families have special religious ceremonies.

deleterious effects on children's health if preventive health care or treatment of health conditions is discouraged or if it promotes or allows abusive behavior (Mueller, 2010). Nurses promote holistic nursing care through an integration of spiritual and psychosocial care. The care focuses on activities that support a person's system of beliefs and worship, such as praying, reading religious materials, and performing religious rituals. In addition, it means being attentive and open to children's unique spiritual experiences and insights. Mueller (2010) states, "Children are spiritual beings, but may be limited by adults' ability to understand them." Unfortunately, as Mercer (2006) reports, "such insights may be dismissed as cute or the product of an overactive imagination." Meeting the spiritual needs of both the child and the family can provide strength and promote connection between the family and the nurse, whereas unmet spiritual needs can result in spiritual distress and debilitation and challenge the nurse-family relationship (Yates, 2011). It is also important to remember children may have different spiritual needs across the illness experience. For example, Petersen (2014) notes that nurses can help seriously ill children meet their spiritual needs through assessment, helping the child express feelings and strengthen relationships, helping the child with legacy work to be remembered by family and friends, and helping the child find meaning in the illness experience. In practice, application of the nursing process for spiritual care (Box 27.6) can enhance the spiritual well-being of both the child and the family.

MASS MEDIA

Fifty years of research has demonstrated that the media is an influential teacher and can exert a significant impact upon the health of children and adolescents. The message conveyed in and through the media can be both positive and negative. The adults in society and in the life of children are charged with increasing the positive, pro-social effect of media and diminishing its ill effects, which can influence important health problems that afflict children across the spectrum (Strasburger, Jordan, & Donnerstein, 2012).

Children in the United States spend approximately 7 hours per day interfacing with media of some sort (i.e., television, computer, video games, smart phones). From a public health perspective, media contributes to 10% to 20% of health problems in the United States

(Strasburger, Jordan, & Donnerstein, 2012). Thus, although certain media may not be a direct cause of health care problems in children, a relationship exists that nurses and other health care providers should be aware of in order to provide the best evidence-based care to children and families.

What is the effect of this media on children and adolescents? Research has demonstrated that media can be quite influential, impacting attitudes, beliefs, and behaviors. There may be a "displacement effect" whereby the time that is spent interacting with media competes with time the child could be running, playing, or participating in a sport or creative

activity. Three additional theories that conceptualize how children and teens experience media are: (1) social learning theory, which emphasizes learning through observation and imitation; (2) script theory, which posits that media provide youth with a "script" or directions for how to behave in new situations; and (3) "super-peer" theory, which describes media as an extreme source of peer pressure on youth to participate in what is shown to be normal behavior (i.e., adolescents not practicing safe sex).

Both old and new media are thought to play a role in various health issues that are particularly relevant to youth. Table 27.2 describes these in greater detail. Media also has great potential to exert a positive effect upon children and their families. Properly used, media can introduce young children to learning and promote school-readiness (i.e., *Sesame Street*), can serve as an outlet for adolescent expression of individuality, can connect youth who may otherwise feel isolated (i.e., those with specialized health care needs), or can be a source of exercise and activity (i.e., video games, exercise videos).

Box 27.7 discusses some recommendations that nurses can make to families and other adults charged with promoting the well-being of youth and families. Families may find it difficult to limit the use of technology in their homes for a number of reasons, including the potential for greater conflict in the family (especially between siblings and between parent and child) and may lack the resources to provide other safe entertainment (Evans, Jordan, & Horner, 2011).

UNDERSTANDING CULTURES IN THE HEALTH CARE ENCOUNTER

BRIDGING THE GAP

Some health care institutions may depend on teachings about cultural competence to ensure that holistic care is provided to their patients. Teachings based on cultural competence, while informative, do not

---

BOX 27.6   Guidelines for Integrating Spiritual Care Into Pediatric Nursing Practice

- Respect the child and family's religious beliefs and practices.
- Consider the child's development when talking about spiritual concerns.
- Contact the institution's chaplaincy department for patients and families who have symptoms of spiritual distress, or ask for specific religious rituals.
- Become knowledgeable about the religious worldviews of cultural groups found in the patients you care for.
- Encourage visitation with family members, members of the patient's spiritual community, and spiritual leaders.
- Allow children and families to teach you about the specifics of their religious beliefs.
- Develop awareness of your own spiritual perspective.
- Listen for understanding rather than agreement or disagreement.

Adapted from Brooks, B. (2004). Spirituality. In Kline, N. (Ed.), *Essentials of pediatric oncology nursing: a core curriculum*, 2nd ed. Glenview, IL: Association of Pediatric Oncology Nurses; Barnes, L.L., Plotnikoff, G.A., Fox, K., et al. (2000). Spirituality, religion, and pediatrics: Intersecting worlds of healing. *Pediatrics* 106(4 Suppl):899-908.

TABLE 27.2   Media Effects on Children and Adolescents

Media Effect	Potential Consequences
Violence	Government, medical, and public health data show exposure to media violence as one factor in violent and aggressive behavior. Both adults and children become desensitized by violence witnessed through various media, including television (including children's programming), movies (including G-rated movies), music, and video games. In addition, cyber-bullying and harassment via text messages are a growing concern among middle school and high school students.
Sex	A significant body of research shows that sexual content in the media can contribute to beliefs and attitudes about sex, sexual behavior, and initiation of intercourse. Teens access sexual content through a variety of media: television, movies, music, magazines, Internet, social media, and mobile devices. Current issues receiving attention for the role they play in adolescent sexual behavior include sending of sexual images via mobile devices (i.e., sexting), impact of violent media on youth views of women and forced sex/rape, and cyber-bullying LGBTQI youth. Media can also serve as a positive source of sexual information (i.e., information, apps, social media about sexually transmitted infections, adolescent pregnancy, and promoting acceptance and support of LGBTQI youth).
Substance use and abuse	Although the causes of adolescent substance use and abuse are numerous, media plays a significant role. Alcohol and tobacco are still heavily marketed to adolescents/young adults. Television and movies featuring the use of these substances can influence initiation of use. Media also shows substance use to be pervasive and without consequences. Finally, content shared over social networking sites can serve as a form of peer pressure and can influence likelihood of use.
Obesity	Obesity is a highly prevalent public health issue among children of all ages, and rates are increasing around the world. A number of studies have demonstrated a link between the amount of screen time and obesity. Advertising of unhealthy food to children is a long-standing marketing practice, which may increase snacking in the face of decreased activity. In addition, both increased screen time and unhealthy eating may also be related to unhealthy sleep.
Body image	Media may play a significant role in the development of body image awareness, expectations, and body dissatisfaction among young and older adolescent girls. Their beliefs may be influenced by images on television, movies, and magazines. New media also contributes to this through Internet images, social network sites, and websites that encourage disordered eating (e.g., pro-Ana sites) (Strasburger, Jordan, & Donnerstein, 2012).

LGBTQI, Lesbian, gay, bisexual, transgender, queer, questioning, and intersex.

provide nurses with the skills to effectively engage with families and are a short-sighted way to approach this contextualized part of children's lives. Cultural competence does spur reflection upon elements of society that perpetuate social inequity or injustices, such as racism, ageism, or homophobia. Cultural humility, on the other hand, recognizes that children and families are affected by the intersection of social elements of society, and this can contribute to health inequity or poor health outcomes. For example, migrant children may face special challenges because of poverty or low-wage work, the family's undocumented status, and community attitudes toward immigration. Cultural humility is a "commitment and active engagement in a lifelong process that individuals enter into for an ongoing basis with patients, communities, colleagues, and themselves" (Tervalon & Murray-Garcia, 1998). It requires that health care providers participate in a continual process of self-reflection and self-critique that recognizes the power of the health care provider role, views the patient and family as full members of the health care team, and does not end after reading one chapter or attending one course; it is an evolving aspect of being a health care provider. Similarly, Furlong and Wright (2011) encourage health care providers to be "critically aware." This means that nurses should engage with children and families from a stance of curiosity and "informed not-knowing" by changing the dynamic of the encounter to learn from the family, rather than only being the expert clinician (Furlong & Wright, 2011). This liberates the nurse from a reliance on static knowledge that may not be relevant for the patient, and it allows the nurse to be a "knowledge-seeker" who tries to understand what life is like for the child and family. This critical awareness also calls nurses to assess their own history and the contextual factors that have shaped their own life. Critical awareness draws us to reflect on aspects of North American culture that may be invisible or taken-for-granted, such as emphasis on independence and individualism, and the ways in which this doesn't match the needs of children and families.

A family's religious and sociocultural backgrounds can influence their decisions about health care and the religious traditions and clergy they want to include during their loved one's illness. It also influences how they discuss serious topics with their children, for example, their own health conditions; the significance of illness, suffering, pain, death, and dying; and the rituals and traditions associated with important life events, such as birth and death (Weiner, McConnell, Latella, et al., 2013).

CULTURAL DEFINITIONS

Culture characterizes a particular group with its values, beliefs, norms, patterns, and practices that are learned, shared, and transmitted from one generation to another (Leininger, 2002). Culture is not the same as race or ethnicity. **Race** is a socially constructed term with roots in anthropology, distinguishing variety in humans by physical traits. **Ethnicity** is the affiliation of a set of people who share a unique cultural, social, and linguistic heritage. **Gender** is an individual's self-identification as man or woman, and *sex* is the biologic designation of male or female. **Social class** is a complex social construction that usually incorporates levels of education in the family, occupation, income, and access to resources. Culture is a complex whole in which each part is interrelated. It is an umbrella term that holds together many interrelated yet unique aspects of humanity, including beliefs, tradition, lifeways, and heritage. It is much more than a country of origin or a demographic designation, such as African-American or Caucasian. Meeting the needs of children and families from a variety of backgrounds requires fluidity in understanding the many layers of influence within a family and understanding that a child and family must be understood contextually.

Cultures and co-cultures contribute to the uniqueness of child members in such a subtle way and at such an early age that children grow up believing their beliefs, attitudes, values, and practices are the "correct" or "normal" ones. A set of values learned in childhood may characterize children's attitudes and behaviors for life, influencing long-range goals and short-range impulses. Thus every ongoing society socializes each succeeding generation to its cultural heritage.

COMPONENTS OF CULTURAL HUMILITY

Cultural humility includes the following tenets (Chavez, 2012; Tervalon & Murray-Garcia, 1998):

- Lifelong commitment to self-reflection and critique
- Addressing the power imbalances in the nurse-patient relationship
- Developing mutually beneficial and nonpaternalistic partnerships with the community in which one is working

The manner and sequence of the growth and development phenomenon are universal and fundamental features of all children; however, children's varied behavioral responses to similar events are often determined by their culture. Culture plays a critical role in the parenting behaviors that facilitate children's development (Melendez, 2005). Children acquire the skills, knowledge, beliefs, and values that are important to their own family and culture.

Cultures may also differ in whether status in a group is based on age or skill. Even children's play and their types of games are culturally determined. In some cultures, children play in groups composed of members of the same gender; and in others, they play in mixed-gender groups. In some cultures, team games predominate; and in others, most play is limited to individual games.

Standards and norms vary from culture to culture and from location to location; a practice that is accepted in one area may meet with disapproval or create tension in another. The extent to which cultures tolerate divergence from the established norm also varies among cultures and subcultural groups. Although conforming to cultural norms provides a degree of security, it is a decided deterrent to change.

BOX 27.8   **Exploring a Family's Culture, Illness, and Care**

- What do you think caused your child's health problem?
- Why do you think it started when it did?
- How severe is your child's sickness? Will it have a short or long course?
- How do you think your child's sickness affects your family?
- What are the chief problems your child's sickness has caused?
- What kind of treatment do you think your child should receive?
- What are the most important results you hope to receive from your child's treatment?
- What do you fear most about your child's sickness?

! NURSING ALERT

American cultures and co-cultures can be so diverse that it is essential that nurses be aware of and knowledgeable about the predominant groups in their work community and apply this knowledge in their practice. It is also essential that nurses practice with an openness to learning about cultures and co-cultures different from their own and have a few open-ended questions that they can use to ask families about what shapes their lives, what they find meaningful, and how they carry that out in their lives. These questions should be simple and open-ended, such as "What is important to you in caring for your child?" "Please tell me a little bit about your family," and "What is important to you as a family?"

Observing the various influences on the child's and the family's lives can help us understand how these factors affect their health and how they make decisions about their own health.

HEALTH BELIEFS AND PRACTICES

For many families, traditional practices and beliefs are an integral part of their daily lives. Health care workers should be aware that other people might live by different rules and priorities that decisively influence their health-related behaviors. Guidelines for exploring a family's culture are provided in Box 27.8.

A model for learning about health traditions that differ from the Western, or modern, health care system is based on the following three dimensions:

1. What are the physical aspects of caring for the body (e.g., are there special clothes, foods, medicines)?
2. What are the mental parts of caring for health (e.g., feelings, attitudes, rituals, actions)?
3. What are the spiritual aspects of health (e.g., who I am, spiritual customs, prayers, healers)?

For each of these dimensions, one must consider the cultural traditions used to maintain health, protect health, and restore health (Spector, 2009).

HEALTH BELIEFS

The beliefs related to the causes of illness and the maintenance of health are integral parts of a family's cultural heritage. Often related to religious beliefs, they influence the way families cope with health problems and respond to health care providers. Predominant among most cultures are beliefs related to natural forces, supernatural forces, and an imbalance between forces.

Natural and Supernatural Forces

The most common natural forces blamed for ill health if the body is not adequately protected are cold air entering the body and impurities in the air. For example, a Chinese parent may overdress an infant in an effort to keep cold wind from entering the child's body. The innate energy, chi, is an example of this. A lack of chi is believed to cause fatigue and a variety of ailments. Alternatively, some cultures view supernatural forces as a cause of illness, especially illnesses that cannot be explained by other means. Examples of such forces include voodoo, witchcraft, or evil spirits. Belief in the "evil eye" is another example of this. It stems from a belief in health as a state of balance and illness as a state of imbalance. As long as an individual's strength and weakness remain in balance, he or she is unlikely to become a victim of the evil eye. Weaknesses are not necessarily physical. For example, an excess of some emotion, such as envy, can create weakness. Infants and small children, because of immature development of their internal strength-weakness states, are especially vulnerable to the gaze of the evil eye.

Imbalance of Forces

The concept of balance or equilibrium is widespread throughout the world. One of the most common imbalances is the one between "hot" and "cold." This belief derived from the ancient Greek concept of body humors, which states that illness is caused by imbalance of the four humors. Such imbalance is thought to cause internal damage or altered function. Treatment of the illness is directed at restoring balance. The hot and cold understanding of disease is based in this concept. Diseases, areas of the body, foods, and illnesses are classified as either "hot" or "cold." Foods and beverages are designated hot or cold based on the effect they exert, not their actual temperature. In Chinese health belief, the forces are termed yin (cold) and yang (hot) (Spector, 2009).

Health care workers who are aware of this belief are better able to understand why some people refuse to eat certain foods. It is often useful to discuss the diet with the family to determine their beliefs regarding food choices. It is possible to help families devise a diet that contains the necessary balance of basic food groups prescribed by the medical subculture while conforming to the beliefs of the ethnic subculture. By determining a family's preferences during well-child visits or prior to discharge, the nurse can help prevent any adverse effects.

HEALTH PRACTICES

Cultures have numerous similarities regarding prevention and treatment of illness. Folk healers are powerful members of the community and can acquire information about an illness without resorting to probing questions. They "speak the language" of the family who seeks help and often combine their rituals with the family or community spirituality. They also are able to create an atmosphere conducive to successful management. Furthermore, they exhibit a sincere interest in the family and their problems.

Some folk remedies are compatible with the medical regimen and are useful to reinforce the treatment plan. For example, aspirin (a "hot" medication) is an appropriate therapy for "cold" diseases, such as arthritis. It is common to discover that a folk prescription has a scientific basis. In any case, nurses must respect practices that do not harm patients. A folk healer may also be requested to perform certain rituals. For example, the Chicano curandero ascertains that the condition is truly the result of the evil eye by performing an assessment ritual and then performs a curative ritual. Sometimes faith in the folk practitioner delays obtaining needed medical treatment, although the practitioner usually suggests medical care if his or her efforts are unsuccessful.

Health practices of different cultures may also present problems of assessment and interpretation. For example, certain cultural practices or remedies can be mistakenly judged as evidence of child abuse by uninformed professionals (Box 27.9). It is important to keep the lines of communication open with families and approach the situation with a sense of cultural humility.

Faith healing and religious rituals are closely allied with many folk-healing practices. Wearing of amulets, medals, and other religious relics believed by the culture to protect the individual and facilitate healing is a common practice. It is important for health workers to recognize the value of this practice and keep the items where the family has placed them or nearby. It offers comfort and support and rarely impedes medical and nursing care. If an item must be removed during a procedure, it should be replaced, if possible, when the procedure is completed. The nurse should explain the reason for its temporary removal to the family to reassure them that their wishes will be respected (see Family-Centered Care box: Cultural Awareness).

Concepts that come from medical anthropology can provide a framework for addressing health care issues. These concepts can have a direct impact on patient care. They lead the nurse away from an ethnocentric or medicine-based view of the health care encounter into the health care reality as constructed by the patient and family. This is relevant for addressing many of the problems that plague the health care system in the United States, including patient dissatisfaction with the health care they receive, unequal distribution of high-quality health care, and excessive costs (Kleinman & Benson, 2006).

It is also important for nurses to recognize that disease and illness are distinct entities. Clinicians diagnose and treat diseases, abnormalities in the structure and function of body organs and systems. Illness and disease are not interchangeable; illness may occur even when disease is not present, and the course of a disease may vary substantially from the experience of illness.

Illness is culturally constructed; an individual's culture influences how a sickness is perceived, labeled, and explained. Culture also influences

FAMILY-CENTERED CARE

Cultural Awareness

A 15-month-old Bosnian girl in status epilepticus was carried in by her parents. They were frightened and spoke little English. I learned that the child had received a measles, mumps, and rubella (MMR) immunization the day before. As I proceeded to unwrap her from the blanket she was in, I quickly assessed the ABCs (airway, breathing, and circulation). I noticed that she was warm (probably a febrile seizure) and that a rag soaked in alcohol was tied around each thigh. Focusing on her potential airway compromise and trying to calm the parents, I put an oxygen mask on her, undressed her for a full assessment, and removed the alcohol rags. I spoke to the parents all the while in a calm, soothing voice. Once I had established an intravenous line and given her lorazepam (Ativan), the seizures stopped. So did the communication between her parents and me. I noticed that they would no longer give me eye contact, and the mother would not even speak to me after the seizures stopped. It wasn't until I was returning to the department from admitting her that I realized why they might have stopped communicating with me: I had removed the rags! Had I only thought to replace the rags or asked their permission to remove the rags, things might have been different.

Laura L. Kuensting, MSN(R), RN
Cardinal Glennon Children's Hospital
St. Louis, Missouri

the meaning assigned to the illness, the role the individual with the sickness adopts, and the response of the family and community to the sickness.

REFERENCES

Afifi, T. O., Boman, J., Fleisher, W., et al. (2009). The relationship between child abuse, parental divorce, and lifetime mental disorders and suicidality in a nationally representative adult sample. *Child Abuse & Neglect*, 33(3), 139–147.

American Academy of Pediatrics. (2003). Family pediatrics: Report of the Task Force on the Family. *Pediatrics*, 111(6), 1541–1571.

Annie E. Casey Foundation. (2012). *Stepping up for kids*. Retrieved from http://www.aecf.org/m/resourcedoc/AECF-SteppingUpForKids-2012.pdf.

Annie E. Casey Foundation. (2013). *Lessons learned: community change lessons from making connections*. Retrieved from http://www.aecf.org/m/blogdoc/aecf-CommunityChangeLessonsLearnedFromMakingConnections-2013.pdf.

Annie E. Casey Foundation. (2014). *Race for results: Building a path to opportunity for all children*. Retrieved from http://www.aecf.org/m/resourcedoc/AECF-RaceforResults-2014.pdf.

Annie E. Casey Foundation. (2015a). *2015 kids count data book: State profiles of child well-being*. Retrieved from http://datacenter.kidscount.org/data#USA/1/23/2488,24,2592,26,2721.

Annie E. Casey Foundation. (2015b). *Every kid needs a family*. Retrieved from http://www.aecf.org/resources/every-kid-needs-a-family/.

Baumrind, D. (1971). Harmonious parents and their preschool children. *Developmental Psychology*, 41, 92–102.

Baumrind, D. (1996). The discipline controversy revisited. *Family Relations*, 45, 405–414.

Berger, L., & Waldfogel, J. (2004). Out-of-home placement of children and economic factors: An empirical analysis. *Review of Economics of the Household*, 2(4), 387–411.

Blackwell, C. W. (2007). Belief in the "free choice" model of homosexuality: a correlate of homophobia in registered nurses. *Journal of LGBT Health Research*, 3(3), 31–40.

Bomar, P. J. (2004). *Promoting health in families* (3rd ed.). Philadelphia, PA: Saunders.

Bronfenbrenner, U. (1979). *The ecology of human development: Experiments by nature and design.* Cambridge, MA: Harvard University Press.

Cain, D. S. (2008). Parenting online and lay literature on infant spanking: information readily available to parents. *Social Work in Health Care, 47*(2), 174–184.

Centers for Disease Control and Prevention. (2009). *The social-ecological model: A framework for prevention.* Retrieved from http://www.cdc.gov/violenceprevention/overview/social-ecologicalmodel.html.

Centers for Disease Control and Prevention. (2017). *National marriage and divorce rate trends.* Retrieved from http://www.cdc.gov/nchs/nvss/marriage_divorce_tables.htm.

Chamberlain, P., Price, J., Leve, L. D., et al. (2008). Prevention of behavior problems for children in foster care: Outcomes and mediation effects. *Prevention Science, 9*(1), 17–27.

Chavez, V. (2012). *Cultural humility: People, principles, and practices (documentary film).* Retrieved from https://www.youtube.com/watch?v=SaSHLbS1V4w.

Coker, T. R., Elliot, M. N., Kanouse, D. K., et al. (2009). Perceived racial/ethnic discrimination among fifth-grade students and its association with mental health. *American Journal of Public Health, 99*(5), 878–884.

Duvall, E. R. (1977). *Family development* (5th ed.). Philadelphia, PA: Lippincott.

Dysart-Gale, D. (2006). Cultural sensitivity beyond ethnicity: A universal precautions model. *Internet Journal of Allied Health Sciences and Practice, 4*(1), 1–5.

Evans, C. A., Jordan, A., & Horner, J. (2011). Only two hours? A qualitative study of the challenges parents perceive in restricting child television time. *Journal of Family Issues, 32*(9), 1223–1244.

Fergusson, E., Maughan, B., & Golding, J. (2008). Which children receive grandparental care and what effect does it have? *Journal of Child Psychology and Psychiatry, 49*(2), 161–169.

Fisher, C., Lindhorst, H., Matthews, T., et al. (2008). Nursing staff attitudes and behaviors regarding family presence in the hospital setting. *Journal of Advanced Nursing, 64*(6), 615–624.

Frey, W. H. (2011). *America reaches its demographic tipping point.* Retrieved from http://www.brookings.edu/blogs/up-front/posts/2011/08/26-census-race-frey.

Friedman, M. M., Bowden, V. R., & Jones, E. G. (2003). *Family nursing: research Theory and practice* (5th ed.). Upper Saddle River, NJ: Prentice Hall.

Furlong, M., & Wright, J. (2011). Promoting critical awareness and critiquing cultural competence: towards disrupting received professional knowledge. *Australian Social Work, 64*(1), 38–54.

Goldenberg, I., & Goldenberg, H. (2008). *Family theory: An overview* (7th ed.). Pacific Grove, CA: Brooks-Cole Cengage Learning.

Harrington, A., Smith, K., Trenholm, C., et al. (2014). *CHIPRA Mandated Evaluation of the Children's Health Insurance Program: Final Findings.* Report submitted to the Office of the Assistant Secretary for Planning and Evaluation. Ann Arbor, MI: Mathematica Policy Research.

Hoeffel, E. M., Rastogi, S., Kim, M. O., et al. (2012). *The Asian population: 2010: 2010 census briefs.* Retrieved from www.census.gov/prod/cen2010/briefs/c2010br-11.pdf.

Humes, K. R., Jones, N. A., & Ramirez, R. R. (2011). *Overview of race and Hispanic origin: 2010: 2010 census briefs.* Retrieved from http://www.census.gov/prod/cen2010/briefs/c2010br-02.pdf.

Isaacs, J., & Healy, O. (2012). *The recession's ongoing impact on children.* Retrieved from https://firstfocus.org/resources/report/recessions-ongoing-impact-children-2012/.

Kaakinen, J. R., Gedaly-Duff, V., & Hanson, S. M. H. (2009). *Family health care nursing* (4th ed.). Philadelphia, PA: Davis.

Kleinman, A., & Benson, P. (2006). Anthropology in the clinic: The problem of cultural competency and how to fix it. *PLoS Medicine, 3*(10), 1673–1676.

Kreider, R. M., & Elliott, D. B. (2009). America's families and living arrangements: 2007. *In U.S. Census Bureau: Current population reports.* Washington, DC: The Bureau.

Larzelere, R. E. (2008). Disciplinary spanking: The scientific evidence. *Journal of Developmental & Behavioral Pediatrics, 29*(4), 334–335.

Leininger, M. J. (2002). Culture care theory: A major contribution to advance transcultural nursing knowledge and practices. *Journal of Transcultural Nursing, 13*(3), 189–192.

McCubbin, M. A., & McCubbin, H. I. (1994). Families coping with illness: The resiliency model of family stress, adjustment, and adaptation. In C. B. Danielson, B. H. Bissel, & P. Winstead-Fry (Eds.), *Families, health, and illness.* St. Louis, MO: Mosby.

Melendez, L. (2005). Parental beliefs and practices around early self-regulation: The impact of culture and immigration. *Infants & Young Children, 18*(2), 136–146.

Mercer, J. A. (2006). Children as mystics, sages, and holy fools: Understanding the spirituality of children and its significance for clinical work. *Pastoral Psychology, 54*(5), 497–515.

Mindlin, M., Jenkins, R., & Law, C. (2009). Maternal employment and indicators of child health: A systemic review in pre-school children in OECD countries. *Journal of Epidemiology and Community Health, 63*(5), 340–350.

Mueller, C. R. (2010). Spirituality in children: Understanding and developing interventions. *Pediatric Nursing, 36*(4), 197–208.

O'Connell, M., & Feliz, S. (2011). *Same-sex couple household statistics from the 2010 Census: SEHSD working paper number 2011-26.* Washington, DC: Fertility and Family Statistics Branch Social, Economic and Housing Statistics Division, US Census Bureau.

Papero, D. V. (1990). *Bowen family systems theory.* Boston, MA: Pearson.

Perry-Jenkins, M., Newkirk, K., & Ghunney, A. K. (2013). Family work through time: An ecological perspective. *Journal of Family Theory and Review, 5*(2), 105–123.

Petersen, C. L. (2014). Spiritual care of the child with cancer at end of life: A concept analysis. *Journal of Advanced Nursing, 70*(6), 1243–1253.

Power, N., & Franck, L. (2008). Parent participation in the care of hospitalized children: A systematic review. *Journal of Advanced Nursing, 62*(6), 622–641.

Roberts, D. (2011). *Fatal invention: How science, politics, and big-business recreate race in the twenty-first century.* The New Press.

Scott, J., & Marshall, G. (2009). Ethnicity. In *Oxford dictionary of sociology.* Oxford, UK: Oxford University Press.

Search Institute. (2009). *Developmental assets.* Retrieved from http://www.search-institute.org.

Smedley, B. D. (2012). The lived experience of race and its health consequences. *American Journal of Public Health, 102*(5), 933–935.

Spector, R. E. (2009). *Cultural diversity in health and illness* (7th ed.). Upper Saddle River, NJ: Prentice-Hall.

Strasburger, V., Jordan, A., & Donnerstein, E. (2012). Children, adolescents, and the media: Health effects. *Pediatric Clinics of North America, 59*(3), 533–587.

Tervalon, M., & Murray-Garcia, J. (1998). Cultural humility versus cultural competence: A critical distinction in defining physician training outcomes in multicultural education. *Journal of Health Care for the Poor and Underserved, 9*(2), 117–125.

Tynes, B. M., Giang, M. T., Williams, D. R., et al. (2008). Online racial discrimination and psychological adjustment among adolescents. *Journal of Adolescent Health, 43*(6), 565–569.

UNICEF. (2013). *Child well-being in rich countries: A comparative overview.* Retrieved from http://www.unicef-irc.org/publications/pdf/rc11_eng.pdf.

US Census Bureau. (2011). *Same sex couple households: American community survey briefs.* Retrieved from https://www.census.gov/prod/2011pubs/acsbr10-03.pdf.

US Department of Health and Human Services. (2013). *ASPE: 2013 poverty guidelines.* Retrieved from http://aspe.hhs.gov/poverty/13poverty.cfm.

Weiner, L., McConnell, D. G., Latella, L., et al. (2013). Cultural and religious considerations in pediatric palliative care. *Palliative & Supportive Care, 11*(1), 47–67.

Williams, D. R. (2012). Miles to go before we sleep: Racial inequities in health. *Journal of Health and Social Behavior, 53*(3), 279–295.

Yates, F. D., Jr. (2011). Ethics for the pediatrician: Religion and spirituality in pediatrics. *Pediatrics in Review, 32*(9), e91–e94.

28

Developmental and Genetic Influences on Child Health Promotion

Marilyn J. Hockenberry

ⓔ http://evolve.elsevier.com/Perry/maternal

GROWTH AND DEVELOPMENT

FOUNDATIONS OF GROWTH AND DEVELOPMENT

Growth and development, usually referred to as a unit, express the sum of the numerous changes that take place during the lifetime of an individual. The entire course is a dynamic process that encompasses several interrelated dimensions:

Growth: an increase in number and size of cells as they divide and synthesize new proteins; results in increased size and weight of the whole or any of its parts

Development: a gradual change and expansion; advancement from lower to more advanced stages of complexity; the emerging and expanding of the individual's capacities through growth, maturation, and learning

Maturation: an increase in competence and adaptability; aging; usually used to describe a qualitative change; a change in the complexity of a structure that makes it possible for that structure to begin functioning; to function at a higher level

Differentiation: processes by which early cells and structures are systematically modified and altered to achieve specific and characteristic physical and chemical properties; sometimes used to describe the trend of mass to specific; development from simple to more complex activities and functions

All of these processes are interrelated, simultaneous, and ongoing; none occurs apart from the others. The processes depend on a sequence of endocrine, genetic, constitutional, environmental, and nutritional influences (Ball, Dains, Flynn, et al., 2015). The child's body becomes larger and more complex; the personality simultaneously expands in scope and complexity. Very simply, growth can be viewed as a *quantitative* change and development as a *qualitative* change.

Stages of Development

Most authorities in the field of child development categorize child growth and behavior into approximate age stages or in terms that describe the features of a developmental age period. The age ranges of these stages are arbitrary, because they do not take into account individual differences and cannot be applied to all children with any degree of precision. Categorization does provide a convenient means to describe the characteristics associated with the majority of children at periods when distinctive developmental changes appear and specific developmental tasks must be accomplished. (A developmental task is a set of skills and competencies specific to each developmental stage that children must accomplish or master to function effectively within their environment.) It is also significant for nurses to know that there are characteristic health problems related to each major phase of development. The

sequence of descriptive age periods and subperiods that are used here and elaborated in subsequent chapters is listed in Box 28.1.

Patterns of Growth and Development

There are definite and predictable patterns in growth and development that are continuous, orderly, and progressive. These patterns, or trends, are universal and basic to all human beings, but each human being accomplishes these in a manner and time unique to that individual.

Directional Trends

Growth and development proceed in regular, related directions or gradients and reflect the physical development and maturation of neuromuscular functions (Fig. 28.1). The first pattern is the cephalocaudal, or head-to-tail, direction. The head end of the organism develops first and is large and complex, whereas the lower end is small and simple and takes shape at a later period. The physical evidence of this trend is most apparent during the period before birth, but it also applies to postnatal behavior development. Infants achieve control of the heads before they have control of their trunks and extremities, hold their backs erect before they stand, use their eyes before their hands, and gain control of their hands before they have control of their feet.

Second, the proximodistal, or near-to-far, trend applies to the midline-to-peripheral concept. A conspicuous illustration is the early embryonic development of limb buds, which is followed by rudimentary fingers and toes. In infants, shoulder control precedes mastery of the hands, the whole hand is used as a unit before the fingers can be manipulated, and the central nervous system develops more rapidly than the peripheral nervous system.

These trends or patterns are bilateral and appear symmetric; each side develops in the same direction and at the same rate as the other. For some of the neurologic functions, this symmetry is only external because of unilateral differentiation of function at an early stage of postnatal development. For example, by approximately 5 years of age, children have demonstrated a decided preference for the use of one hand over the other, although previously either one had been used.

The third trend, *differentiation,* describes development from simple operations to more complex activities and functions, from broad, global patterns of behavior to more specific, refined patterns. All areas of development (physical, cognitive, social, and emotional) proceed in this direction. Through the process of development and differentiation, early embryonal cells with vague, undifferentiated functions progress to an immensely complex organism composed of highly specialized and diversified cells, tissues, and organs. Generalized development precedes specific or specialized development; gross, random muscle movements take place before fine muscle control.

BOX 28.1   Developmental Age Periods

Prenatal Period: Conception to Birth

Germinal: Conception to approximately 2 weeks of age

Embryonic: 2 to 8 weeks of age

Fetal: 8 to 40 weeks of age (birth)

A rapid growth rate and total dependency make this one of the most crucial periods in the developmental process. The relationship between maternal health and certain manifestations in the newborn emphasizes the importance of adequate prenatal care to the health and well-being of the infant.

Infancy Period: Birth to 12 Months of Age

Neonatal: Birth to 27 or 28 days of age

Infancy: 1 to approximately 12 months of age

The infancy period is one of rapid motor, cognitive, and social development. Through mutuality with the caregiver (parent), the infant establishes a basic trust in the world and the foundation for future interpersonal relationships. The critical first month of life, although part of the infancy period, is often differentiated from the remainder because of the major physical adjustments to extrauterine existence and the psychologic adjustment of the parent.

Early Childhood: 1 to 6 Years of Age

Toddler: 1 to 3 years of age

Preschool: 3 to 6 years of age

This period, which extends from the time children attain upright locomotion until they enter school, is characterized by intense activity and discovery. It is a time of marked physical and personality development. Motor development advances steadily. Children at this age acquire language and wider social relationships, learn role standards, gain self-control and mastery, develop increasing awareness of dependence and independence, and begin to develop a self-concept.

Middle Childhood: 6 to 11 or 12 Years of Age

Frequently referred to as the *school age*, this period of development is one in which the child is directed away from the family group and centered around the wider world of peer relationships. There is steady advancement in physical, mental, and social development with emphasis on developing skill competencies. Social cooperation and early moral development take on more importance with relevance for later life stages. This is a critical period in the development of a self-concept.

Later Childhood: 11 to 19 Years of Age

Prepubertal: 10 to 13 years of age

Adolescence: 13 to approximately 18 years of age

The tumultuous period of rapid maturation and change known as *adolescence* is considered to be a transitional period that begins at the onset of puberty and extends to the point of entry into the adult world—usually high school graduation. Biologic and personality maturation are accompanied by physical and emotional turmoil, and there is redefining of the self-concept. In the late adolescent period, the young person begins to internalize all previously learned values and to focus on an individual, rather than a group, identity.

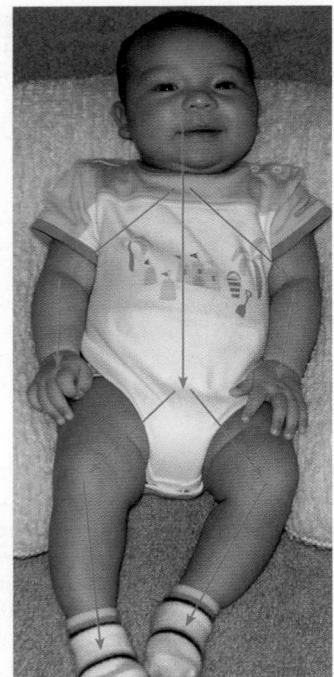

FIG 28.1 Directional trends in growth.

Developmental Pace

Although development has a fixed, precise order, it does not progress at the same rate or pace. There are periods of accelerated growth and periods of decelerated growth in both total body growth and the growth of subsystems. Not all areas of development progress at the same pace. When a spurt occurs in one area (e.g., gross motor), minimal advances may take place in language, fine motor, or social skills. After the gross motor skill has been achieved, the focus will shift to another area of development. The rapid growth before and after birth gradually levels off throughout early childhood. Growth is relatively slow during middle childhood, markedly increases at the beginning of adolescence, and levels off in early adulthood. Each child grows at his or her own pace. Distinct differences are observed among children as they reach developmental milestones.

! NURSING ALERT

Research suggests that normal growth, particularly height in infants, may occur in brief (possibly even 24-hour) bursts that punctuate long periods in which no measurable growth takes place. The researchers noted sex differences, with girls growing in length during the week they gained weight and boys growing in the week after a significant weight gain. Sex-specific growth hormone pulse patterns may coordinate body composition, weight gain, and linear growth (Lampl, Johnson, & Frongillo, 2001; 2005). Furthermore, findings indicate a stuttering or saltatory pattern of growth that follows no regular cycle and can occur after "quiet" periods that last as long as 4 weeks.

Sequential Trends

In all dimensions of growth and development, there is a definite, predictable sequence, with each child passing through every stage. For example, children crawl before they creep, creep before they stand, and stand before they walk. Later facets of the personality are built on the early foundation of trust. The child babbles, then forms words, and finally sentences; writing emerges from scribbling.

Sensitive Periods

There are limited times during the process of growth when the organism interacts with a particular environment in a specific manner. Periods termed *critical, sensitive, vulnerable,* and *optimal* are the times in the lifetime of an organism when it is more susceptible to positive or negative influences.

The quality of interactions during these sensitive periods determines whether the effects on the organism will be beneficial or harmful. For example, physiologic maturation of the central nervous system is influenced by the adequacy and timing of contributions from the environment, such as stimulation and nutrition. The first 3 months of prenatal life is a sensitive period in the physical growth of fetuses.

Psychosocial development also appears to have sensitive periods when an environmental event has maximal influence on the developing personality. For example, primary socialization occurs during the first year when the infant makes the initial social attachments and establishes a basic trust in the world. A warm and consistently responsive relationship with a parent figure is fundamental to a healthy personality. The same concept might be applied to readiness for learning skills, such as toilet training or reading. In these instances, there appears to be an opportune time when the skill is best learned.

Individual Differences

Each child grows in his or her own unique and personal way. The sequence of events is predictable; the exact timing is not. Rates of growth vary, and measurements are defined in terms of ranges to allow for individual differences. Periods of fast growth, such as the pubescent growth spurt, may begin earlier or later in some children than in others. Children may grow fast or slowly during the spurt and may finish sooner or later than other children. Gender is an influential factor because girls seem to be more advanced in physiologic growth at all ages.

BIOLOGIC GROWTH AND PHYSICAL DEVELOPMENT

As children grow, their external dimensions change. These changes are accompanied by corresponding alterations in structure and function of internal organs and tissues that reflect the gradual acquisition of physiologic competence. Each part has its own rate of growth, which may be directly related to alterations in the size of the child (e.g., the heart rate). Skeletal muscle growth approximates whole body growth; brain, lymphoid, adrenal, and reproductive tissues follow distinct and individual patterns (Fig. 28.2). When growth deficiency has a secondary cause, such as severe illness or acute malnutrition, recovery from the illness or the establishment of an adequate diet will produce a dramatic acceleration of the growth rate that usually continues until the child's individual growth pattern is resumed.

External Proportions

Variations in the growth rate of different tissues and organ systems produce significant changes in body proportions during childhood. The cephalocaudal trend of development is most evident in total body growth as indicated by these changes. During fetal development, the head is the fastest growing body part, and at 2 months of gestation, the head constitutes 50% of total body length. During infancy, growth of the trunk predominates; the legs are the most rapidly growing part during childhood; in adolescence, the trunk again elongates. In newborn infants, the lower limbs are one-third the total body length but only 15% of the total body weight; in adults, the lower limbs constitute one-half of the total body height and 30% or more of the total body weight. As growth proceeds, the midpoint in head-to-toe measurements gradually descends from a level even with the umbilicus at birth to the level of the symphysis pubis at maturity.

Biologic Determinants of Growth and Development

The most prominent feature of childhood and adolescence is physical growth (Fig. 28.3). Throughout development, various tissues in the body undergo changes in growth, composition, and structure. In some

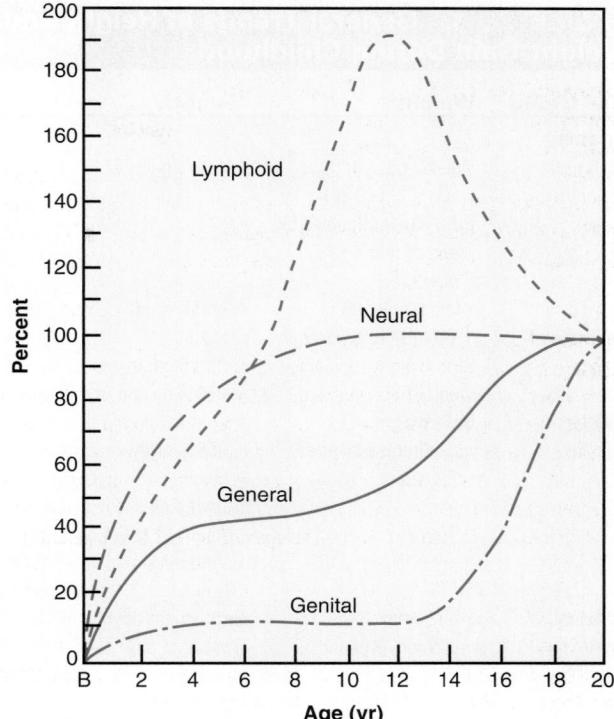

FIG 28.2 Growth rates for the body as a whole and three types of tissues. General—body as a whole; external dimension; and respiratory, digestive, renal, circulatory, and musculoskeletal systems. Lymphoid—thymus, lymph nodes, and intestinal lymph masses. Neural—brain, dura, spinal cord, optic apparatus, and head dimensions. (Data from Jackson, J.A., Patterson, D.G., & Harris, R.E. [1930]. *The measurement of man.* Minneapolis, MN: University of Minnesota Press.)

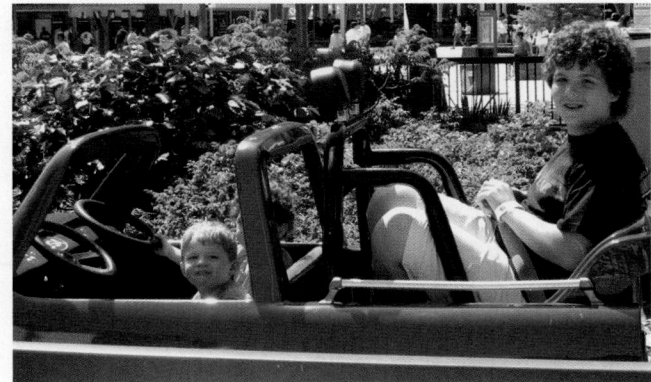

FIG 28.3 Changes in body proportions occur dramatically during childhood.

tissues, the changes are continuous (e.g., bone growth and dentition); in others, significant alterations occur at specific stages (e.g., appearance of secondary sex characteristics). When these measurements are compared with standardized norms, a child's developmental progress can be determined with a high degree of confidence (Table 28.1). Growth in children with Down syndrome differs from that in other children. They have slower growth velocity between 6 months and 3 years of age and then again in adolescence. Puberty occurs earlier, and they achieve shorter stature. In this population, patients are frequent users of the health care system, often with multiple providers, and benefit from the use of the Down syndrome growth chart to monitor their growth (Cronk, Crocker, Pueschel, et al., 1988; Myrelid, Gustafsson, Ollars, et al., 2002).

TABLE 28.1   General Trends in Height and Weight Gain During Childhood

Age Group	Weight*	Height*
Infants		
Birth to 6 months of age	Weekly gain: 140 to 200 g (5 to 7 oz) Birth weight doubles by end of first 4 to 7 months[†]	Monthly gain: 2.5 cm (1 inch)
6 to 12 months of age	Weight gain: 85 to 140 g (3 to 5 ounces) Birth weight triples by end of first year	Monthly gain: 1.25 cm (0.5 inch) Birth length increases by ≈50% by end of first year
Toddlers	Birth weight quadruples by age 2½ years	Height at 2 years of age is ≈50% of eventual adult height Gain during second year: About 12 cm (4.7 inches) Gain during third year: About 6 to 8 cm (2.4 to 3.1 inches)
Preschoolers	Yearly gain: 2 to 3 kg (4.5 to 6.5 pounds)	Birth length doubles by 4 years of age Yearly gain: 5 to 7.5 cm (2 to 3 inches)
School-age children	Yearly gain: 2 to 3 kg (4.5 to 6.5 pounds)	Yearly gain after 7 years: 5 cm (2 inches) Birth length triples by about 13 years of age
Pubertal Growth Spurt		
Females: 10 to 14 years of age	Weight gain: 7 to 25 kg (15.5 to 55 pounds) Mean: 17.5 kg (38.5 pounds)	Height gain: 5 to 25 cm (2 to 10 inches); ≈95% of mature height achieved by onset of menarche or skeletal age of 13 years of age Mean: 20.5 cm (8 inches)
Males: 11 to 16 years of age	Weight gain: 7 to 30 kg (15.5 to 66 pounds) Mean: 23.7 kg (52.2 pounds)	Height gain: 10 to 30 cm (4 to 12 inches); ≈95% of mature height achieved by skeletal age of 15 years of age Mean: 27.5 cm (11 inches)

*Yearly height and weight gains for each age group represent averaged estimates from a variety of sources.
[†]Jung, F.E., & Czajka-Narins, D.M. (1985). Birth weight doubling and tripling times: An updated look at the effects of birth weight, sex, race, and type of feeding. *American Journal of Clinical Nutrition*, 42(2), 182–189.

Linear growth, or *height,* occurs almost entirely as a result of skeletal growth and is considered a stable measurement of general growth. Growth in height is not uniform throughout life but ceases when maturation of the skeleton is complete. The maximum rate of growth in length occurs before birth, but newborns continue to grow at a rapid, although slower, rate.

! NURSING ALERT

Double the child's height at 2 years of age to estimate how tall he or she may be as an adult.

At birth, *weight* is more variable than height and is, to a greater extent, a reflection of the intrauterine environment. The average newborn weighs from 3175 to 3400 g (7 to 7.5 pounds). In general, the birth weight doubles by 4 to 7 months of age and triples by the end of the first year. By 2 to 2½ years of age, the birth weight usually quadruples. After this point, the "normal" rate of weight gain, just as the growth in height, assumes a steady annual increase of approximately 2 to 2.75 kg (4.4 to 6 pounds) per year until the adolescent growth spurt.

Both bone age determinants and state of dentition are used as indicators of development. Because both are discussed elsewhere, neither is elaborated here (see the next section for bone age).

Skeletal Growth and Maturation

The most accurate measure of general development is *skeletal* or *bone age*, the radiologic determination of osseous maturation. Skeletal age appears to correlate more closely with other measures of physiologic maturity (e.g., onset of menarche) than with chronologic age or height. Bone age is determined by comparing the mineralization of ossification centers and advancing bony form to age-related standards.

Bone formation begins during the second month of fetal life when calcium salts are deposited in the intercellular substance (matrix) to form calcified cartilage first and then true bone. Bone formation exhibits some differences. In small bones, the bone continues to form in the center, and cartilage continues to be laid down on the surfaces. In long bones, the ossification begins in the *diaphysis* (the long central portion of the bone) and continues in the *epiphysis* (the end portions of the bone). Between the diaphysis and the epiphysis, an *epiphyseal cartilage plate* (or *growth plate*) unites with the diaphysis by columns of spongy tissue, the *metaphysis*. Active growth in length takes place in the epiphyseal growth plate. Interference with this growth site by trauma or infection can result in deformity.

The first centers of ossification appear in 2-month-old embryos; and at birth, the number is approximately 400, about one-half the number at maturity. New centers appear at regular intervals during the growth period and provide the basis for assessment of bone age. Postnatally, the earliest centers to appear (at 5 to 6 months of age) are those of the capitate and hamate bones in the wrist. Therefore, radiographs of the hand and wrist provide the most useful areas for screening to determine skeletal age, especially before 6 years of age. These centers appear earlier in girls than in boys.

Nurses must understand that the growing bones of children possess many unique characteristics. Bone fractures occurring at the growth plate may be difficult to discover and may significantly affect subsequent growth and development (Urbanski & Hanlon, 1996). Factors that may influence skeletal muscle injury rates and types in children and adolescents include the following (Caine, DiFiori, & Maffulli, 2006; Kaczander, 1997):

- Less protective sports equipment for children
- Less emphasis on conditioning, especially flexibility
- In adolescents, fractures that are more common than ligamentous ruptures because of the rapid growth rate of the physeal (segment of tubular bone that is concerned mainly with growth) zone of hypertrophy

Neurologic Maturation

In contrast to other body tissues, which grow rapidly after birth, the nervous system grows proportionately more rapidly before birth. Two periods of rapid brain cell growth occur during fetal life, a dramatic increase in the number of neurons between 15 and 20 weeks of gestation and another increase at 30 weeks, which extends to 1 year of age. The rapid growth of infancy continues during early childhood and then slows to a more gradual rate during later childhood and adolescence.

Postnatal growth consists of increasing the amount of cytoplasm around the nuclei of existing cells, increasing the number and intricacy of communications with other cells, and advancing their peripheral axons to keep pace with expanding body dimensions. This allows for increasingly complex movement and behavior. Neurophysiologic changes also provide the foundation for language, learning, and behavior development. Neurologic or electroencephalographic development is sometimes used as an indicator of maturational age in the early weeks of life.

Lymphoid Tissues

Lymphoid tissues contained in the lymph nodes, thymus, spleen, tonsils, adenoids, and blood lymphocytes follow a growth pattern unlike that of other body tissues. These tissues are small in relation to total body size, but they are well developed at birth. They increase rapidly to reach adult dimensions by 6 years of age and continue to grow. At about 10 to 12 years of age, they reach a maximum development that is approximately twice their adult size. This is followed by a rapid decline to stable adult dimensions by the end of adolescence.

Development of Organ Systems

All tissues and organ systems undergo changes during development. Some are striking; others are subtle. Many have implications for assessment and care. Because the major importance of these changes relates to their dysfunction, the developmental characteristics of various systems and organs are discussed throughout the book as they relate to these areas. Physical characteristics and physiologic changes that vary with age are included in age-group descriptions.

PHYSIOLOGIC CHANGES

Physiologic changes that take place in all organs and systems are discussed as they relate to dysfunction. Other changes, such as pulse and respiratory rates and blood pressure, are an integral part of physical assessment. In addition, there are changes in basic functions, including metabolism, temperature, and patterns of sleep and rest.

Metabolism

The rate of metabolism when the body is at rest (**basal metabolic rate**, or BMR) demonstrates a distinctive change throughout childhood. Highest in newborn infants, the BMR closely relates to the proportion of surface area to body mass, which changes as the body increases in size. In both sexes, the proportion decreases progressively to maturity. The BMR is slightly higher in boys at all ages and further increases during pubescence over that in girls.

The rate of metabolism determines the caloric requirements of the child. The basal energy requirement of infants is about 108 kcal/kg of body weight and decreases to 40 to 45 kcal/kg at maturity. Water requirements throughout life remain at approximately 1.5 mL/calorie of energy expended. Children's energy needs vary considerably at different ages and with changing circumstances. The energy requirement to build tissue steadily decreases with age following the general growth curve; however, energy needs vary with the individual child and may be considerably higher. For short periods (e.g., during strenuous exercise) and more prolonged periods (e.g., illness), the needs can be very high.

> **! NURSING ALERT**
>
> Each degree of fever increases the basal metabolism 10%, with a correspondingly increased fluid requirement.

Temperature

Body temperature, reflecting metabolism, decreases over the course of development. Thermoregulation is one of the most important adaptation responses of infants during the transition from intrauterine to extrauterine life. In healthy neonates, hypothermia can result in several negative metabolic consequences, such as hypoglycemia, elevated bilirubin levels, and metabolic acidosis. Skin-to-skin care, also referred to as *kangaroo care,* is an effective way to prevent neonatal hypothermia in infants. Unclothed, diapered infants are placed on the parent's bare chest after birth, promoting thermoregulation and attachment (Galligan, 2006). After the unstable regulatory ability in the neonatal period, heat production steadily declines as the infant grows into childhood. Individual differences of 0.5° F to 1° F are normal, and occasionally a child normally displays an unusually high or low temperature. Beginning at approximately 12 years of age, girls display a temperature that remains relatively stable, but the temperature in boys continues to fall for a few more years. Females maintain a temperature slightly above that of males throughout life.

Even with improved temperature regulation, infants and young children are highly susceptible to temperature fluctuations. Body temperature responds to changes in environmental temperature and is increased with active exercise, crying, and emotional stress. Infections can cause a higher and more rapid temperature increase in infants and young children than in older children. In relation to body weight, an infant produces more heat per unit than adolescents. Consequently, during active play or when heavily clothed, an infant or small child is likely to become overheated.

Sleep and Rest

Sleep, a protective function in all organisms, allows for repair and recovery of tissues after activity. As in most aspects of development, there is wide variation among individual children in the amount and distribution of sleep at various ages. As children mature, there is a change in the total time they spend in sleep and the amount of time they spend in deep sleep.

Newborn infants sleep much of the time that is not occupied with feeding and other aspects of their care. As infants grow older, the total time spent sleeping gradually decreases, they remain awake for longer periods, and they sleep longer at night. For example, the length of a sleep cycle increases from approximately 50 to 60 minutes in newborn infants to approximately 90 minutes in adolescents (Anders, Sadeh, & Appareddy, 2005). During the latter part of the first year, most children sleep through the night and take one or two naps during the day. By the time they are 12 to 18 months of age, most children have eliminated the second nap. After 3 years of age, children have usually given up daytime naps except in cultures in which an afternoon nap or siesta is customary. Sleep time declines slightly from 4 to 10 years of age and then increases somewhat during the pubertal growth spurt.

The quality of sleep changes as children mature. As children develop through adolescence, their need for sleep does not decline, but their opportunity for sleep may be affected by social, activity, and academic schedules.

NUTRITION

Nutrition is probably the single most important influence on growth. Dietary factors regulate growth at all stages of development, and their effects are exerted in numerous and complex ways. During the rapid prenatal growth period, poor nutrition may influence development from the time of implantation of the ovum until birth. During infancy and childhood, the demand for calories is relatively great, as evidenced

---

BOX 28.2   Attributes of Temperament

Activity: Level of physical motion during activity, such as sleep, eating, play, dressing, and bathing

Rhythmicity: Regularity in the timing of physiologic functions, such as hunger, sleep, and elimination

Approach-withdrawal: Nature of initial responses to a new stimulus, such as people, situations, places, foods, toys, and procedures (**Approach** responses are positive and are displayed by activity or expression; **withdrawal** responses are negative expressions or behaviors.)

Adaptability: Ease or difficulty with which the child adapts or adjusts to new or altered situations

Threshold of responsiveness (sensory threshold): Amount of stimulation, such as sounds or light, required to evoke a response in the child

Intensity of reaction: Energy level of the child's reactions regardless of quality or direction

Mood: Amount of pleasant, happy, friendly behavior compared with unpleasant, unhappy, crying, unfriendly behavior exhibited by the child in various situations

Distractibility: Ease with which a child's attention or direction of behavior can be diverted by external stimuli

Attention span and persistence: Length of time a child pursues a given activity (**attention**) and the continuation of an activity despite obstacles (**persistence**)

---

by the rapid increase in both height and weight. At this time, protein and caloric requirements are higher than at almost any period of postnatal development. As the growth rate slows, with its concomitant decrease in metabolism, there is a corresponding reduction in caloric and protein requirements.

Growth is uneven during the periods of childhood between infancy and adolescence, when there are plateaus and small growth spurts. Children's appetites fluctuate in response to these variations until the turbulent growth spurt of adolescence, when adequate nutrition is extremely important but may be subjected to numerous emotional influences. Adequate nutrition is closely related to good health throughout life, and an overall improvement in nourishment is evidenced by the gradual increase in size and early maturation of children in this century (see Community Focus box: Healthy Food Choices).

TEMPERAMENT

Temperament is defined as "the manner of thinking, behaving, or reacting characteristic of an individual" (Chess and Thomas, 1999) and refers to the way in which a person deals with life. From the time of birth, children exhibit marked individual differences in the way they respond to their environment and the way others, particularly the parents, respond to them and their needs. A genetic basis has been suggested for some differences in temperament. Nine characteristics of temperament have been identified through interviews with parents (Box 28.2). Temperament refers to behavioral tendencies, not to discrete behavioral acts. There

are no implications of good or bad. Most children can be placed into one of three common categories based on their overall pattern of temperamental attributes:

The easy child: Easygoing children are even tempered, are regular and predictable in their habits, and have a positive approach to new stimuli. They are open and adaptable to change and display a mild to moderately intense mood that is typically positive. Approximately 40% of children fall into this category.

The difficult child: Difficult children are highly active, irritable, and irregular in their habits. Negative withdrawal responses are typical, and they require a more structured environment. These children adapt slowly to new routines, people, and situations. Mood expressions are usually intense and primarily negative. They exhibit frequent periods of crying, and frustration often produces violent tantrums. This group represents about 10% of children.

The slow-to-warm-up child: Slow-to-warm-up children typically react negatively and with mild intensity to new stimuli and, unless pressured, adapt slowly with repeated contact. They respond with only mild but passive resistance to novelty or changes in routine. They are inactive and moody but show only moderate irregularity in functions. Fifteen percent of children demonstrate this temperament pattern.

Thirty-five percent of children either have some, but not all, of the characteristics of one of the categories or are inconsistent in their behavioral responses. Many normal children demonstrate this wide range of behavioral patterns.

Significance of Temperament

Observations indicate that children who display the difficult or slow-to-warm-up patterns of behavior are more vulnerable to the development of behavior problems in early and middle childhood. Any child can develop behavior problems if there is dissonance between the child's temperament and the environment. Demands for change and adaptation that are in conflict with the child's capacities can become excessively stressful. However, authorities emphasize that it is not the temperament patterns of children that place them at risk; rather, it is the *degree of fit* between children and their environment, specifically their parents, that determines the degree of vulnerability. The potential for optimum development exists when environmental expectations and demands fit with the individual's style of behavior and the parents' ability to navigate this period (Chess and Thomas, 1999).

DEVELOPMENT OF PERSONALITY AND COGNITIVE FUNCTION

Personality and cognitive skills develop in much the same manner as biologic growth; new accomplishments build on previously mastered skills. Many aspects depend on physical growth and maturation. This is not a comprehensive account of the multiple facets of personality and behavior development. Many aspects are integrated with the child's social and emotional development in later discussion of various age groups. Table 28.2 summarizes some of the developmental theories.

Theoretical Foundations of Personality Development
Psychosexual Development (Freud)

According to Freud, all human behavior is energized by psychodynamic forces, and this psychic energy is divided among three components of personality: the *id, ego,* and *superego* (Freud, 1933). The id, the unconscious mind, is the inborn component that is driven by instincts. The id obeys the pleasure principle of immediate gratification of needs, regardless of whether the object or action can actually do so. The ego, the conscious mind, serves the reality principle. It functions as the

TABLE 28.2 Summary of Personality, Cognitive, and Moral Development Theories

Psychosexual (Freud)	Psychosocial (Erikson)	Cognitive (Piaget)	Moral Judgment (Kohlberg)
Oral	Trust vs. mistrust	Sensorimotor (birth to 2 years of age)	
Anal	Autonomy vs. shame and doubt	Preoperational thought, preconceptual phase (transductive reasoning [e.g., specific to specific]) (2 to 4 years of age)	Preconventional (premoral) level Punishment and obedience orientation
Phallic	Initiative vs. guilt	Preoperational thought, intuitive phase (transductive reasoning) (4 to 7 years of age)	Preconventional (premoral) level Naive instrumental orientation
Latency	Industry vs. inferiority	Concrete operations (inductive reasoning and beginning logic) (7 to 11 years of age)	Conventional level Good-boy, nice-girl orientation Law-and-order orientation
Genital	Identity vs. role confusion	Formal operations (deductive and abstract reasoning) (11 to 15 years of age)	Postconventional or principled level Social-contract orientation

conscious or controlling self that is able to find realistic means for gratifying the instincts while blocking the irrational thinking of the id. The superego, the conscience, functions as the moral arbitrator and represents the ideal. It is the mechanism that prevents individuals from expressing undesirable instincts that might threaten the social order.

Freud considered the sexual instincts to be significant in the development of the personality (Freud, 1964). However, he used the term *psychosexual* to describe any sensual pleasure. During childhood, certain regions of the body assume a prominent psychologic significance as the source of new pleasures and new conflicts gradually shifts from one part of the body to another at particular stages of development:

Oral stage (birth to 1 year of age): During infancy, the major source of pleasure seeking is centered on oral activities, such as sucking, biting, chewing, and vocalizing. Children may prefer one of these over the others, and the preferred method of oral gratification can provide some indication of the personality they develop.

Anal stage (1 to 3 years of age): Interest during the second year of life centers in the anal region as sphincter muscles develop and children are able to withhold or expel fecal material at will. At this stage, the climate surrounding toilet training can have lasting effects on children's personalities.

Phallic stage (3 to 6 years of age): During the phallic stage, the genitalia become an interesting and sensitive area of the body. Children recognize differences between the sexes and become curious about the dissimilarities. This is the period around which the controversial issues of the Oedipus and Electra complexes, penis envy, and castration anxiety are centered.

Latency period (6 to 12 years of age): During the latency period, children elaborate on previously acquired traits and skills. Physical and psychic energy are channeled into acquisition of knowledge and vigorous play.

Genital stage (12 years of age and older): The last significant stage begins at puberty with maturation of the reproductive system and production of sex hormones. The genital organs become the major source of sexual tensions and pleasures, but energies are also invested in forming friendships and preparing for marriage.

Psychosocial Development (Erikson)

The most widely accepted theory of personality development is that advanced by Erikson (1963). Although built on Freudian theory, it is known as *psychosocial* development and emphasizes a healthy personality as opposed to a pathologic approach. Erikson also uses the biologic concepts of critical periods and epigenesis, describing key conflicts or core problems that the individual strives to master during critical periods in personality development. Successful completion or mastery of each

of these core conflicts is built on the satisfactory completion or mastery of the previous stage.

Each psychosocial stage has two components—the favorable and the unfavorable aspects of the core conflict—and progress to the next stage depends on resolution of this conflict. No core conflict is ever mastered completely but remains a recurrent problem throughout life. No life situation is ever secure. Each new situation presents the conflict in a new form. For example, when children who have satisfactorily achieved a sense of trust encounter a new experience (e.g., hospitalization), they must again develop a sense of trust in those responsible for their care in order to master the situation. Erikson's life-span approach to personality development consists of eight stages; however, only the first five relating to childhood are included here:

Trust versus mistrust (birth to 1 year of age): The first and most important attribute to develop for a healthy personality is basic trust. Establishment of basic trust dominates the first year of life and describes all of the child's satisfying experiences at this age. Corresponding to Freud's oral stage, it is a time of "getting" and "taking in" through all the senses. It exists only in relation to something or someone; therefore, consistent, loving care by a mothering person is essential for development of trust. Mistrust develops when trust-promoting experiences are deficient or lacking or when basic needs are inconsistently or inadequately met. Although shreds of mistrust are sprinkled throughout the personality, from a basic trust in parents stems trust in the world, other people, and oneself. The result is faith and optimism.

Autonomy versus shame and doubt (1 to 3 years of age): Corresponding to Freud's anal stage, the problem of autonomy can be symbolized by the holding on and letting go of the sphincter muscles. The development of autonomy during the toddler period is centered on children's increasing ability to control their bodies, themselves, and their environment. They want to do things for themselves using their newly acquired motor skills of walking, climbing, and manipulating and their mental powers of selecting and decision making. Much of their learning is acquired by imitating the activities and behavior of others. Negative feelings of doubt and shame arise when children are made to feel small and self-conscious, when their choices are disastrous, when others shame them, or when they are forced to be dependent in areas in which they are capable of assuming control. The favorable outcomes are self-control and willpower.

Initiative versus guilt (3 to 6 years of age): The stage of initiative corresponds to Freud's phallic stage and is characterized by vigorous, intrusive behavior; enterprise; and a strong imagination. Children explore the physical world with all their senses and powers (Fig. 28.4). They develop a conscience. No longer guided only by outsiders,

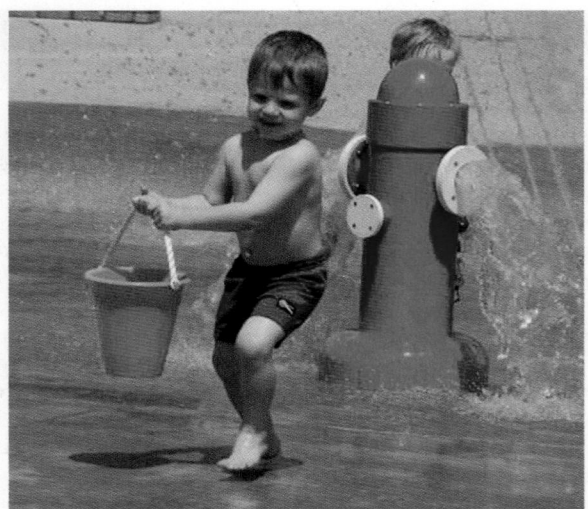

FIG 28.4 The stage of initiative is characterized by physical activity and imagination while children explore the physical world around them.

they have an inner voice that warns and threatens. Children sometimes undertake goals or activities that are in conflict with those of parents or others, and being made to feel that their activities or imaginings are bad produces a sense of guilt. Children must learn to retain a sense of initiative without impinging on the rights and privileges of others. The lasting outcomes are direction and purpose.

Industry versus inferiority (6 to 12 years of age): The stage of industry is the latency period of Freud. Having achieved the more crucial stages in personality development, children are ready to be workers and producers. They want to engage in tasks and activities that they can carry through to completion; they need and want real achievement. Children learn to compete and cooperate with others, and they learn the rules. It is a decisive period in their social relationships with others. Feelings of inadequacy and inferiority may develop if too much is expected of them or if they believe that they cannot measure up to the standards set for them by others. The ego quality developed from a sense of industry is competence.

Identity versus role confusion (12 to 18 years of age): Corresponding to Freud's genital period, the development of identity is characterized by rapid and marked physical changes. Previous trust in their bodies is shaken, and children become overly preoccupied with the way they appear in the eyes of others compared with their own self-concept. Adolescents struggle to fit the roles they have played and those they hope to play with the current roles and fashions adopted by their peers, to integrate their concepts and values with those of society, and to come to a decision regarding an occupation. An inability to solve the core conflict results in role confusion. The outcome of successful mastery is devotion and fidelity to others and to values and ideologies.

THEORETICAL FOUNDATIONS OF COGNITIVE DEVELOPMENT

The term *cognition* refers to the process by which developing individuals become acquainted with the world and the objects it contains. Children are born with inherited potentials for intellectual growth, but they must develop that potential through interaction with the environment. By assimilating information through the senses, processing it, and acting on it, they come to understand relationships between objects and between themselves and their world. With cognitive development, children acquire

the ability to reason abstractly, to think in a logical manner, and to organize intellectual functions or performances into higher-order structures. Language, morals, and spiritual development emerge as cognitive abilities advance.

Cognitive Development (Piaget)

Jean Piaget (1969), a Swiss psychologist, developed a stage theory to better understand the way a child thinks. According to Piaget, intelligence enables individuals to make adaptations to the environment that increase the probability of survival, and through their behavior, individuals establish and maintain equilibrium with the environment. Each stage of cognitive development is derived from and builds on the accomplishments of the previous stage in a continuous, orderly process. This course of development is both maturational and invariant and is divided into the following four stages (ages are approximate):

Sensorimotor (birth to 2 years of age): The sensorimotor stage of intellectual development consists of six substages that are governed by sensations in which simple learning takes place. Children progress from reflex activity through simple repetitive behaviors to imitative behavior. They develop a sense of cause and effect as they direct behavior toward objects. Problem solving is primarily by trial and error. They display a high level of curiosity, experimentation, and enjoyment of novelty and begin to develop a sense of self as they are able to differentiate themselves from their environment. They become aware that objects have *permanence*—that an object exists even though it is no longer visible. Toward the end of the sensorimotor period, children begin to use language and representational thought.

Preoperational (2 to 7 years of age): The predominant characteristic of the preoperational stage of intellectual development is *egocentrism,* which in this sense does not mean selfishness or self-centeredness but the inability to put oneself in the place of another. Children interpret objects and events not in terms of general properties but in terms of their relationships or their use to them. They are unable to see things from any perspective other than their own; they cannot see another's point of view, nor can they see any reason to do so. Preoperational thinking is concrete and tangible. Children cannot reason beyond the observable, and they lack the ability to make deductions or generalizations. Thought is dominated by what they see, hear, or otherwise experience. However, they are increasingly able to use language and symbols to represent objects in their environment. Through imaginative play, questioning, and other interactions, they begin to elaborate concepts and to make simple associations between ideas. In the latter stage of this period, their reasoning is *intuitive* (e.g., the stars have to go to bed just as they do), and they are only beginning to deal with problems of weight, length, size, and time. Reasoning is also *transductive;* because two events occur together, they cause each other, or knowledge of one characteristic is transferred to another (e.g., all women with big bellies have babies).

Concrete operations (7 to 11 years of age): At this age, thought becomes increasingly logical and coherent. Children are able to classify, sort, order, and otherwise organize facts about the world to use in problem solving. They develop a new concept of permanence: conservation; that is, they realize that physical factors (such as, volume, weight, and number) remain the same even though outward appearances are changed. They are able to deal with a number of different aspects of a situation simultaneously. They do not have the capacity to deal in abstraction; they solve problems in a concrete, systematic fashion based on what they can perceive. Reasoning is *inductive.* Through progressive changes in thought processes and relationships with others, thought becomes less self-centered. They can consider points of view other than their own. Thinking has become socialized.

Formal operations (11 to 15 years of age): Formal operational thought is characterized by adaptability and flexibility. Adolescents can think in abstract terms, use abstract symbols, and draw logical conclusions from a set of observations. For example, they can solve the following question: If *A* is larger than *B* and *B* is larger than *C*, which symbol is the largest? (The answer is *A*.) They can make hypotheses and test them; they can consider abstract, theoretic, and philosophic matters. Although they may confuse the ideal with the practical, most contradictions in the world can be dealt with and resolved.

Language Development

Children are born with the mechanism and capacity to develop speech and language skills. However, they do not speak spontaneously. The environment must provide a means for them to acquire these skills. Speech requires intact physiologic structure and function (including respiratory, auditory, and cerebral) plus intelligence, a need to communicate, and stimulation.

The rate of speech development varies from child to child and is directly related to neurologic competence and cognitive development. Gesture precedes speech. As speech develops, gesture recedes but never disappears entirely. Research suggests that infants can learn sign language before vocal language and that it may enhance the development of vocal language (Thompson, Cotner-Bichelman, McKerchar, et al., 2007). At all stages of language development, children's comprehension vocabulary (what they understand) is greater than their expressed vocabulary (what they can say), and this development reflects a continuing process of modification that involves both the acquisition of new words and the expanding and refining of word meanings previously learned. By the time they begin to walk, children are able to attach names to objects and people.

The first parts of speech used are nouns, sometimes verbs (e.g., "go"), and combination words (e.g., "bye-bye"). Responses are usually structurally incomplete during the toddler period, although the meaning is clear. Next, they begin to use adjectives and adverbs to qualify nouns followed by adverbs to qualify nouns and verbs. Later, pronouns and gender words are added (e.g., "he" and "she"). By the time children enter school, they are able to use simple, structurally complete sentences that average five to seven words.

Moral Development (Kohlberg)

Children also acquire moral reasoning in a developmental sequence. Moral development, as described by Kohlberg (1968), is based on cognitive developmental theory and consists of three major levels, each of which has two stages:

Preconventional level: The preconventional level of moral development parallels the preoperational level of cognitive development and intuitive thought. Culturally oriented to the labels of good/bad and right/wrong, children integrate these in terms of the physical or pleasurable consequences of their actions. At first, children determine the goodness or badness of an action in terms of its consequences. They avoid punishment and obey without question those who have the power to determine and enforce the rules and labels. They have no concept of the basic moral order that supports these consequences. Later, children determine that the right behavior consists of that which satisfies their own needs (and sometimes the needs of others). Although elements of fairness, give and take, and equal sharing are evident, they are interpreted in a practical, concrete manner without loyalty, gratitude, or justice.

Conventional level: At the conventional stage, children are concerned with conformity and loyalty. They value the maintenance of family, group, or national expectations regardless of consequences. Behavior that meets with approval and pleases or helps others is considered

good. One earns approval by being "nice." Obeying the rules, doing one's duty, showing respect for authority, and maintaining the social order are the correct behaviors. This level is correlated with the stage of concrete operations in cognitive development.

Postconventional, autonomous, or principled level: At the postconventional level, the individual has reached the cognitive stage of formal operations. Correct behavior tends to be defined in terms of general individual rights and standards that have been examined and agreed on by the entire society. Although procedural rules for reaching consensus become important, with emphasis on the legal point of view, there is also emphasis on the possibility for changing law in terms of societal needs and rational considerations.

The most advanced level of moral development is one in which self-chosen ethical principles guide decisions of conscience. These are abstract and ethical but universal principles of justice and human rights with respect for the dignity of people as individuals. It is believed that few people reach this stage of moral reasoning.

DEVELOPMENT OF SELF-CONCEPT

Self-concept is how an individual describes himself or herself. The term *self-concept* includes all of the notions, beliefs, and convictions that constitute an individual's self-knowledge and that influence that individual's relationships with others. It is not present at birth but develops gradually as a result of unique experiences within the self, significant others, and the realities of the world. However, an individual's self-concept may or may not reflect reality.

In infancy, the self-concept is primarily an awareness of one's independent existence learned in part as a result of social contacts and experiences with others. The process becomes more active during toddlerhood as children explore the limits of their capacities and the nature of their impact on others. School-age children are more aware of differences among people, are more sensitive to social pressures, and become more preoccupied with issues of self-criticism and self-evaluation. During early adolescence, children focus more on physical and emotional changes taking place and on peer acceptance. Self-concept is crystallized during later adolescence as young people organize their self-concept around a set of values, goals, and competencies acquired throughout childhood.

Body Image

A vital component of self-concept, *body image* refers to the subjective concepts and attitudes that individuals have toward their own bodies. It consists of the physiologic (the perception of one's physical characteristics), psychologic (values and attitudes toward the body, abilities, and ideals), and social nature of one's image of self (the self in relation to others). All three of the components interrelate with one another. Body image is a complex phenomenon that evolves and changes during the process of growth and development. Any actual or perceived deviation from the "norm" (no matter how this is interpreted) is cause for concern. The extent to which a characteristic, defect, or disease affects children's body image is influenced by the attitudes and behavior of those around them.

The significant others in their lives exert the most important and meaningful impact on children's body image. Labels that are attached to them (e.g., "skinny," "pretty," or "fat") or body parts (e.g., "ugly mole," "bug eyes," or "yucky skin") are incorporated into the body image. Because they lack the understanding of deviations from the physical standard or norm, children notice prominent differences in others and unwittingly make rude or cruel remarks about such minor deviations as large or widely spaced front teeth, large or small eyes, moles, or extreme variations in height.

Infants receive input about their bodies through self-exploration and sensory stimulation from others. As they begin to manipulate their environment, they become aware of their bodies as separate from others. Toddlers learn to identify the various parts of their bodies and are able to use symbols to represent objects. Preschoolers become aware of the wholeness of their bodies and discover the genitalia. Exploration of the genitalia and the discovery of differences between the sexes become important. At this age, children have only a vague concept of internal organs and function (Stuart & Laraia, 2000).

School-age children begin to learn about internal body structure and function and become aware of differences in body size and configuration. They are highly influenced by the cultural norms of society and current fads. Children whose bodies deviate from the norm are often criticized or ridiculed. Adolescence is the age when children become most concerned about the physical self. The unfamiliar body changes, and the new physical self must be integrated into the self-concept. Adolescents face conflicts over what they see and what they visualize as the ideal body structure. Body image formation during adolescence is a crucial element in the shaping of identity, the psychosocial crisis of adolescence.

Self-Esteem

Self-esteem is the value that an individual places on oneself and refers to an overall evaluation of oneself (Willoughby, King, & Polatajko, 1996). Whereas self-esteem is described as the affective component of the self, self-concept is the cognitive component; however, the two terms are almost indistinguishable and are often used interchangeably.

The term *self-esteem* refers to a personal, subjective judgment of one's worthiness derived from and influenced by the social groups in the immediate environment and individuals' perceptions of how they are valued by others. Self-esteem changes with development. Highly egocentric toddlers are unaware of any difference between competence and social approval. On the other hand, preschool and early school-age children are increasingly aware of the discrepancy between their competencies and the abilities of more advanced children. Being accepted by adults and peers outside the family group becomes more important to them. Positive feedback enhances their self-esteem; they are vulnerable to feelings of worthlessness and are anxious about failure.

As children's competencies increase and they develop meaningful relationships, their self-esteem rises. Their self-esteem is again at risk during early adolescence when they are defining an identity and sense of self in the context of their peer group. Unless children are continually made to feel incompetent and of little worth, a decrease in self-esteem during vulnerable times is only temporary.

ROLE OF PLAY IN DEVELOPMENT

Through the universal medium of play, children learn what no one can teach them. They learn about their world and how to deal with this environment of objects, time, space, structure, and people. They learn about themselves operating within that environment—what they can do, how to relate to things and situations, and how to adapt themselves to the demands society makes on them. Play is the work of children. In play, children continually practice the complicated, stressful processes of living, communicating, and achieving satisfactory relationships with other people.

CLASSIFICATION OF PLAY

From a developmental point of view, patterns of children's play can be categorized according to content and social character. In both, there is an additive effect; each builds on past accomplishments, and some

element of each is maintained throughout life. At each stage in development, the new predominates.

CONTENT OF PLAY

The content of play involves primarily the physical aspects of play, although social relationships cannot be ignored. The content of play follows the directional trend of the simple to the complex:

Social-affective play: Play begins with social-affective play, wherein infants take pleasure in relationships with people. As adults talk, touch, nuzzle, and in various ways elicit responses from an infant, the infant soon learns to provoke parental emotions and responses with such behaviors as smiling, cooing, or initiating games and activities. The type and intensity of the adult behavior with children vary among cultures.

Sense-pleasure play: Sense-pleasure play is a nonsocial stimulating experience that originates from without. Objects in the environment (light and color, tastes and odors, textures and consistencies) attract children's attention, stimulate their senses, and give pleasure. Pleasurable experiences are derived from handling raw materials (water, sand, food), body motion (swinging, bouncing, rocking), and other uses of senses and abilities (smelling, humming) (Fig. 28.5).

Skill play: After infants have developed the ability to grasp and manipulate, they persistently demonstrate and exercise their newly acquired abilities through skill play, repeating an action over and over again. The element of sense-pleasure play is often evident in the practicing of a new ability, but all too frequently, the determination to conquer the elusive skill produces pain and frustration (e.g., putting paper in and taking it out of a toy car) (Fig. 28.6).

Unoccupied behavior: In unoccupied behavior, children are not playful but focus their attention momentarily on anything that strikes their interest. Children daydream, fiddle with clothes or other objects, or walk aimlessly. This role differs from that of onlookers, who actively observe the activity of others.

Dramatic, or pretend, play: One of the vital elements in children's process of identification is dramatic play, also known as *symbolic* or *pretend play*. It begins in late infancy (11 to 13 months of age) and is the predominant form of play in preschool children. After children begin to invest situations and people with meanings and to attribute affective significance to the world, they can pretend and fantasize almost anything. By acting out events of daily life, children

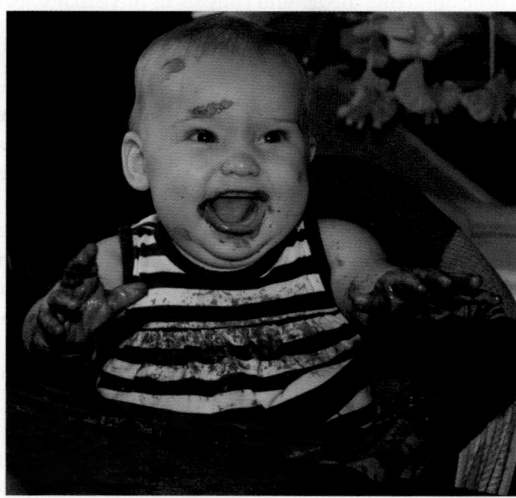

FIG 28.5 Children derive pleasure from handling raw materials. (Paints in this picture are nontoxic.)

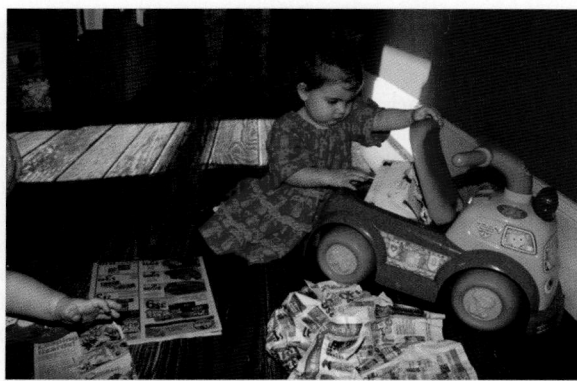

FIG 28.6 After infants develop new skills to grasp and manipulate, they begin to conquer new abilities, such as putting paper in a toy car and taking it out.

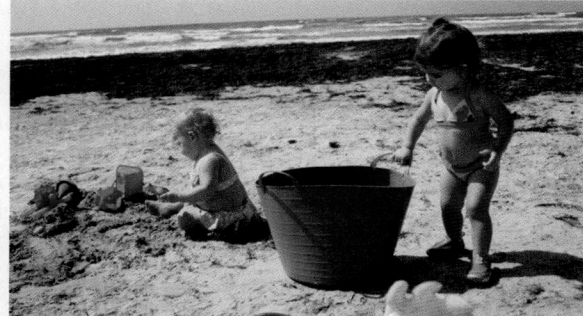

FIG 28.7 Parallel play at the beach.

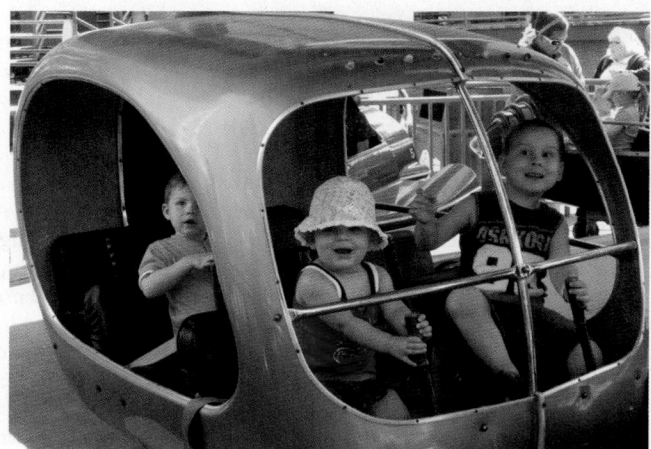

FIG 28.8 Associative play.

learn and practice the roles and identities modeled by the members of their family and society. Children's toys, replicas of the tools of society, provide a medium for learning about adult roles and activities that may be puzzling and frustrating to them. Interacting with the world is one way children get to know it. The simple, imitative, dramatic play of toddlers, such as using the telephone, driving a car, or rocking a doll, evolves into more complex, sustained dramas of preschoolers, which extend beyond common domestic matters to the wider aspects of the world and the society, such as playing police officer, storekeeper, teacher, or nurse. Older children work out elaborate themes, act out stories, and compose plays.

Games: Children in all cultures engage in games alone and with others. Solitary activity involving games begins as very small children participate in repetitive activities and progress to more complicated games that challenge their independent skills, such as puzzles, solitaire, and computer or video games. Very young children participate in simple, *imitative games* such as pat-a-cake and peek-a-boo. Preschool children learn and enjoy *formal games,* beginning with ritualistic, self-sustaining games, such as ring around the rosy and London Bridge. With the exception of some simple board games, preschool children do not engage in *competitive games.* Preschoolers hate to lose and try to cheat, want to change rules, or demand exceptions and opportunities to change their moves. School-age children and adolescents enjoy competitive games, including cards, checkers, and chess, and physically active games, such as baseball.

SOCIAL CHARACTER OF PLAY

The play interactions of infancy are between the child and an adult. Children continue to enjoy the company of adults but are increasingly able to play alone. As age advances, interaction with age-mates increases in importance and becomes an essential part of the socialization process. Through interaction, highly egocentric infants, unable to tolerate delay or interference, ultimately acquire concern for others and the ability to delay gratification or even to reject gratification at the expense of another. A pair of toddlers will engage in considerable combat because their personal needs cannot tolerate delay or compromise. By the time they reach 5 or 6 years of age, children are able to arrive at compromises or make use of arbitration, usually after they have attempted but failed to gain their own way. Through continued interaction with peers and the growth of conceptual abilities and social skills, children are able to increase participation with others in the following types of play:

Onlooker play: During onlooker play, children watch what other children are doing but make no attempt to enter into the play activity. There

is an active interest in observing the interaction of others but no movement toward participating. Watching an older sibling bounce a ball is a common example of the onlooker role.

Solitary play: During solitary play, children play alone with toys different from those used by other children in the same area. They enjoy the presence of other children but make no effort to get close to or speak to them. Their interest is centered on their own activity, which they pursue with no reference to the activities of the others.

Parallel play: During parallel activities, children play independently but among other children. They play with toys similar to those the children around them are using but as each child sees fit, neither influencing nor being influenced by the other children. Each plays beside, but not with, other children (Fig. 28.7). There is no group association. Parallel play is the characteristic play of toddlers, but it may also occur in other groups of any age. Individuals who are involved in a creative craft with each person separately working on an individual project are engaged in parallel play.

Associative play: In associative play, children play together and are engaged in a similar or even identical activity, but there is no organization, division of labor, leadership assignment, or mutual goal. Children borrow and lend play materials, follow each other with wagons and tricycles, and sometimes attempt to control who may or may not play in the group. Each child acts according to his or her own wishes; there is no group goal (Fig. 28.8). For example, two children play with dolls, borrowing articles of clothing from each other and engaging in similar conversation, but neither directs the other's actions or establishes rules regarding the limits of the play session. There is a great deal of behavioral contagion: When one child initiates an activity, the entire group follows the example.

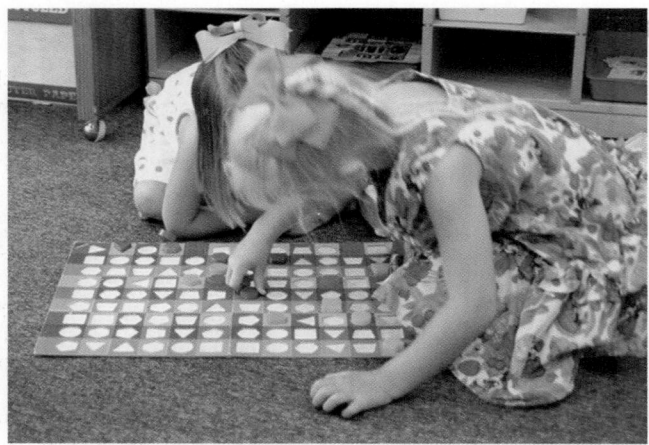

FIG 28.9 Cooperative play.

Cooperative play: Cooperative play is organized, and children play in a group with other children (Fig. 28.9). They discuss and plan activities for the purposes of accomplishing an end: to make something, attain a competitive goal, dramatize situations of adult or group life, or play formal games. The group is loosely formed, but there is a marked sense of belonging or not belonging. The goal and its attainment require organization of activities, division of labor, and role playing. The leader-follower relationship is definitely established, and the activity is controlled by one or two members who assign roles and direct the activity of the others. The activity is organized to allow one child to supplement another's function to complete the goal.

FUNCTIONS OF PLAY

Sensorimotor Development

Sensorimotor activity is a major component of play at all ages and is the predominant form of play in infancy. Active play is essential for muscle development and serves a useful purpose as a release for surplus energy. Through sensorimotor play, children explore the nature of the physical world. Infants gain impressions of themselves and their world through tactile, auditory, visual, and kinesthetic stimulation. Toddlers and preschoolers revel in body movement and exploration of objects in space. With increasing maturity, sensorimotor play becomes more differentiated and involved. Whereas very young children run for the sheer joy of body movement, older children incorporate or modify the motions into increasingly complex and coordinated activities, such as races, games, roller skating, and bicycle riding.

Intellectual Development

Through exploration and manipulation, children learn colors, shapes, sizes, textures, and the significance of objects. They learn the significance of numbers and how to use them; they learn to associate words with objects; and they develop an understanding of abstract concepts and spatial relationships, such as *up, down, under,* and *over.* Activities such as puzzles and games help them develop problem-solving skills. Books, stories, films, and collections expand knowledge and provide enjoyment as well. Play provides a means to practice and expand language skills. Through play, children continually rehearse past experiences to assimilate them into new perceptions and relationships. Play helps children comprehend the world in which they live and distinguish between fantasy and reality.

Socialization

From very early infancy, children show interest and pleasure in the company of others. Their initial social contact is with the mothering person, but through play with other children, they learn to establish social relationships and solve the problems associated with these relationships. They learn to give and take, which is more readily learned from critical peers than from more tolerant adults. They learn the sex role that society expects them to fulfill, as well as approved patterns of behavior and deportment. Closely associated with socialization is development of moral values and ethics. Children learn right from wrong, the standards of the society, and to assume responsibility for their actions.

Creativity

In no other situation is there more opportunity to be creative than in play. Children can experiment and try out their ideas in play through every medium at their disposal, including raw materials, fantasy, and exploration. Creativity is stifled by pressure toward conformity; therefore, striving for peer approval may inhibit creative endeavors in school-age or adolescent children. Creativity is primarily a product of solitary activity; yet creative thinking is often enhanced in group settings where listening to others' ideas stimulates further exploration of one's own ideas. After children feel the satisfaction of creating something new and different, they transfer this creative interest to situations outside the world of play.

Self-Awareness

Beginning with active explorations of their bodies and awareness of themselves as separate from their mothers, the process of developing a self-identity is facilitated through play activities. Children learn who they are and their place in the world. They become increasingly able to regulate their own behavior, to learn what their abilities are, and to compare their abilities with those of others. Through play, children are able to test their abilities, assume and try out various roles, and learn the effects their behavior has on others. They learn the sex role that society expects them to fulfill, as well as approved patterns of behavior and deportment.

Therapeutic Value

Play is therapeutic at any age (Fig. 28.10). In play, children can express emotions and release unacceptable impulses in a socially acceptable fashion. Children are able to experiment and test fearful situations and can assume and vicariously master the roles and positions that they are unable to perform in the world of reality. Children reveal much about themselves in play. Through play, children are able to communicate to the alert observer the needs, fears, and desires that they are unable to express with their limited language skills. Throughout their play, children need the acceptance of adults and their presence to help them control aggression and to channel their destructive tendencies.

Morality

Although children learn at home and at school those behaviors considered right and wrong in the culture, the interaction with peers during play contributes significantly to their moral training. Nowhere is the enforcement of moral standards as rigid as in the play situation. If they are to be acceptable members of the group, children must adhere to the accepted codes of behavior of the culture (e.g., fairness, honesty, self-control, consideration for others). Children soon learn that their peers are less tolerant of violations than are adults and that to maintain a place in the play group, they must conform to the standards of the group (Fig. 28.11).

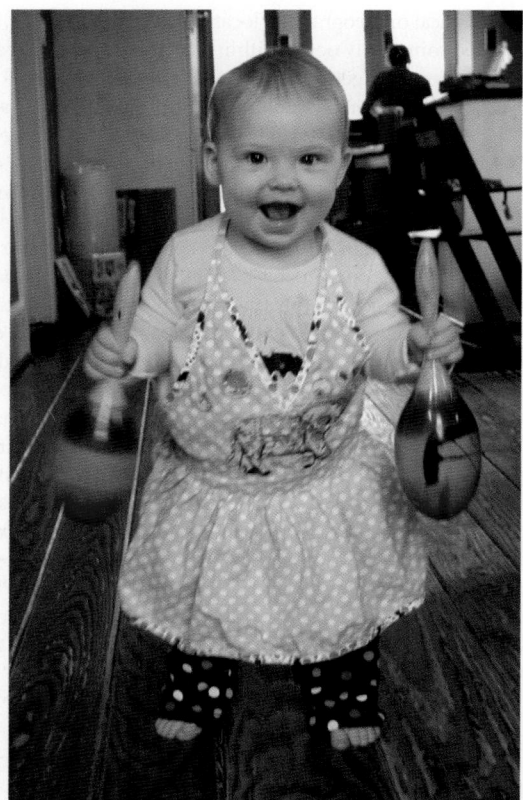

FIG 28.10 Play is therapeutic at any age and provides a means for release of tension and stress.

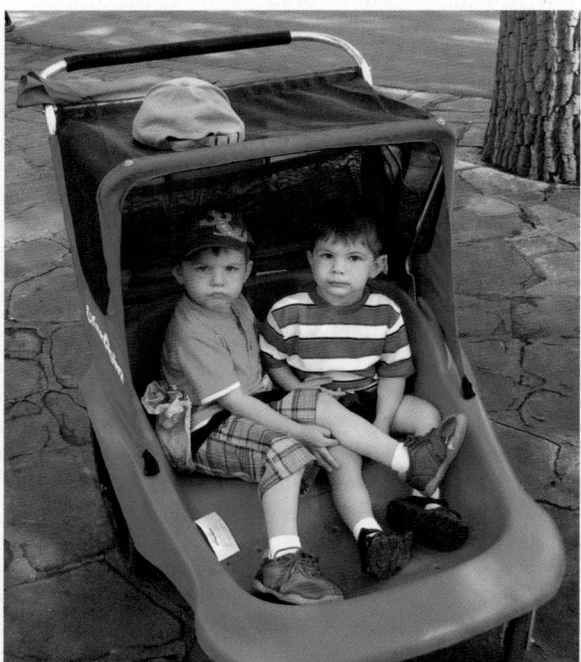

FIG 28.11 Peers become increasingly important as children develop friendships outside the family group.

TOYS

The type of toys chosen by or provided for children can support and enhance children's development in the areas just described. Although no scientific evidence shows that any toy is necessary for optimal learning, toys offer an opportunity to bring children and parents together. Research has indicated that a positive parent-child interaction can enhance early childhood brain development (Glassy, Romano, & Committee on Early Childhood, Adoption, and Dependent Care, et al., 2003). Toys that are small replicas of the culture and its tools help children assimilate into their culture. Toys that require pushing, pulling, rolling, and manipulating teach them about physical properties of the items and help develop muscles and coordination. Rules and the basic elements of cooperation and organization are learned through board games.

Because they can be used in a variety of ways, raw materials with which children can exercise their own creativity and imaginations are sometimes superior to ready-made items. For example, building blocks can be used to construct a variety of structures, count, and learn shapes and sizes.

DEVELOPMENTAL ASSESSMENT

One of the most essential components of a complete health appraisal is assessment of developmental function. Screening procedures are designed to identify quickly and reliably children whose developmental level is below normal for their age and who therefore require further investigation. They also provide a means of recording objective measurements of present developmental function for future reference. Since the passage of Public Law 99-457, the Education of the Handicapped Act Amendments of 1986, much greater emphasis is placed on developmental assessment of children with disabilities, and nurses can play a vital role in providing this service. It is estimated that 16% of children are affected by developmental disabilities, but fewer than 30% of these children are identified before kindergarten (Wagner, Jenkins, & Smith, 2006). There are numerous developmental screening tools, and each uses a different approach.

In the past, the most widely used developmental screening tests for young children are the series of tests known as the Denver Developmental Screening Test (DDST) and its revision, the DDST-R, that have been revised, re-standardized, and renamed the Denver II. The American Academy of Neurology and the Child Neurology Society state that research has found that the Denver-II is insensitive and lacks specificity, and neither the American Academy of Neurology nor the Child Neurology Society recommends use of the Denver-II for primary care developmental screening (Filipek, Accardo, Ashwal, et al., 2000). A comprehensive list of child development assessment tools has been developed by the National Early Childhood Technical Assistance Center as part of its cooperative agreement with the US Office of Special Education Programs. The pediatric health-promotion chapters include detailed information on developmental assessment that is unique to the age and each developmental stage of the child.

AGES AND STAGES

Ages and stages is a term used to broadly outline key periods in the human development timeline. During each stage, growth and development occur in the primary developmental domains, including physical, intellectual, language, and social-emotional. The Ages & Stages Questionnaires (ASQ)* are high-quality screening tools that include 19 age-specific

---

*The ASQ can be found at www.agesandstages.com.

surveys that ask parents about developmental skills common in daily life for children 1 month to 5½ years of age (Box 28.3). Parents or other caregivers answer questions regarding their child's abilities (e.g., "Does your child climb on an object such as a chair to reach something he wants?" "When your child wants something, does she tell you by pointing at it?"). Children whose development appears to fall significantly below results of other children their age are flagged for further evaluation. The ASQ can be used as a universal screening tool in pediatric clinics to identify children at risk for social-emotional developmental delays (Briggs, Stettler, Silver, et al., 2012).

There are several additional parent report developmental screening tools that are reliable and valid. Some of the most common in addition to the ASQ, Parents' Evaluation of Developmental Status (PEDS), Child Development Inventory, and the Pediatric Symptom Checklist. Although it is beyond the scope of this chapter to describe each screening tool, using a tool can aid the nurse in providing anticipatory guidance and appropriate referral (Wagner, Jenkins, & Smith, 2006). Throughout this text, each of the health-promotion chapters include detailed information on development unique to the age and stage of the child.

GENETIC FACTORS THAT INFLUENCE DEVELOPMENT

OVERVIEW OF GENETICS AND GENOMICS

Nurses and other health care providers are increasingly faced with incorporating genetic and genomic information into their practice. In response to this need, the Consensus Panel on Genetic/Genomic Nursing Competencies was established in 2006. This independent panel of nurse leaders from clinical, research, and academic settings established essential minimal competencies necessary for nurses to deliver competent genetic- and genomic-focused nursing care (Consensus Panel on Genetic/Genomic Nursing Competencies, 2009). In a similar manner, genetic and genomic competencies were created and published for nurses with graduate degrees (Greco, Tinley, & Seibert, 2012). This brief overview identifies key terms and concepts and highlights essential genetics and genomics competencies for all nurses.

GENES, GENETICS, AND GENOMICS

Genes are segments of deoxyribonucleic acid (DNA) that contain genetic information necessary to control a certain physiologic function or characteristic. These segments are often referred to as *sites* or *loci*,

indicating a physical or "geographic" location on a chromosome. Variant forms of a gene commonly occur within a population. When referring to a particular form of a gene, the term *allele* is used. Variant forms of a gene (variant alleles) may lead to no measureable or observable differences, may cause the person to be susceptible to clinically recognizable pathology within specific environmental contexts, may cause a clinically recognized disease or disorder, or may prove advantageous within a particular environmental context.

In earlier times, human diseases were thought to be either clearly genetic or typically environmental. However, the observation that some genetic disorders are congenital (present at birth) but others are expressed later in life has led scientists to conclude that many, if not most, diseases are caused by a genetic predisposition that can be activated by an environmental trigger. Examples of such interactions are found in single-gene disorders, such as phenylketonuria (PKU) and sickle cell disease, and *multifactorial conditions,* such as cancer and neural tube defects (NTDs). PKU is a disorder resulting from the (genetically determined) absence of an enzyme that metabolizes the amino acid phenylalanine. However, the deleterious effects in the infant are expressed only after sufficient ingestion of phenylalanine-containing substances, such as milk (environmental trigger). Even in the case of a "classic" genetic condition, such as sickle cell disease, its acute symptoms are precipitated by certain conditions, such as lowered oxygen tension, infection, or dehydration.

CONGENITAL ANOMALIES

Embryogenesis and fetal development are an intricate and precisely timed series of events in which all parts must be properly integrated to ensure a coordinated whole. Insults during development or abnormalities in differentiation or in the proper timing of organogenesis may result in a variety of congenital anomalies. *Congenital anomalies,* or birth defects, occur in 2% to 4% of all live-born children and are often classified as deformations, disruptions, dysplasias, or malformations. *Deformations* are often caused by extrinsic mechanical forces on normally developing tissue. Club foot is an example of a deformation often caused by uterine constraint. *Disruptions* result from the breakdown of previously normal tissue. Congenital amputations caused by amniotic bands (fibrous strands of amnion that wrap around different body parts during development) are examples of disruption anomalies. *Dysplasias* result from abnormal organization of cells into a particular tissue type. Congenital abnormalities of the teeth, hair, nails, or sweat glands may be manifestations of one of the more than 100 different ectodermal dysplasia syndromes (National Foundation for Ectodermal Dysplasias, 2017). *Malformations* are abnormal formations of organs or body parts resulting from an abnormal developmental process. Most malformations occur before 12 weeks of gestation. Cleft lip, an example of a malformation, occurs at approximately 5 weeks of gestation when the developing embryo naturally has two clefts in the area. Normally, between 5 and 7 weeks, cells rapidly divide and migrate to fill in those clefts. If there is an abnormality in this developmental process, the embryo is left with either a unilateral or bilateral cleft lip that may also involve the palate.

The types of anomalies that can result from genetic or prenatal environmental causes can be major structural abnormalities with serious medical, surgical, or quality-of-life consequences, or they can be minor anomalies or normal variants with no serious consequences, such as a sacral dimple, an extra nipple, or a café-au-lait spot. Congenital anomalies can occur in isolation, such as congenital heart defect, or multiple anomalies may be present. A recognized pattern of anomalies resulting from a single specific cause is called a *syndrome* (e.g., Down syndrome, fetal alcohol syndrome). A nonrandom pattern of malformations for which a cause has not been determined is called an *association* (e.g.,

VACTERL [vertebral defects, anal atresia, cardiac defect, tracheoesophageal fistula, and renal and limb defects] association). When a single anomaly leads to a cascade of additional anomalies, the pattern of defects is referred to as a *sequence*. Pierre Robin sequence begins with the abnormal development of the mandible, resulting in abnormal placement of the tongue during development. The normal developmental process for the palate is prevented because the tongue obstructs the migration of the palatal shelves toward the midline, and a cleft palate remains. Consequently, infants born with Pierre Robin sequence have a recessed mandible and an abnormally placed tongue and are at risk for obstructive apnea. NTDs, cleft lip and palate, deafness, congenital heart defects, and cognitive impairment are examples of congenital malformations that can occur in isolation or as part of a syndrome, association, or sequence and can have different causes, such as single-gene or chromosome abnormalities, prenatal exposures, or multifactorial causes.

DISORDERS OF THE INTRAUTERINE ENVIRONMENT

The intrauterine environment can have a profound and permanent effect on developing fetuses with or without chromosome or single-gene abnormalities. Intrauterine growth restriction, for example, can occur with many genetic syndromes, such as Down, Russell-Silver, Prader-Willi, and Turner syndromes (Rimoin, Pyeritz, & Korf, 2013), or it can be caused by nongenetic factors, such as maternal alcohol ingestion. Placental abnormalities are increasingly being found to be the etiologic factor in neurodevelopmental disorders (e.g., cerebral palsy and cognitive impairment) that were previously attributed to asphyxia during delivery (McIntyre, Taitz, Keogh, et al., 2013).

Teratogens, agents that cause birth defects when present in the prenatal environment, account for the majority of adverse intrauterine effects not attributable to genetic factors. Types of teratogens include drugs (phenytoin [Dilantin], warfarin [Coumadin], isotretinoin [Accutane]), chemicals (ethyl alcohol, cocaine, lead), infectious agents (rubella, cytomegalovirus), physical agents (maternal ionizing radiation, hyperthermia), and metabolic agents (maternal PKU). Many of these teratogenic exposures and the resulting effects are completely preventable. For example, pregnant women can avoid having a child with one of the fetal alcohol spectrum disorders by not ingesting alcohol during pregnancy.

GENETIC DISORDERS

Genetic disorders can be caused by chromosome abnormalities as seen in Turner syndrome, Down syndrome, or velocardiofacial syndrome (VCFS); single-gene mutations as seen in sickle cell anemia, neurofibromatosis, or Duchenne muscular dystrophy; a combination of genetic and environmental factors as seen in NTDs or maturity-onset diabetes in the young; and mitochondrial deoxyribonucleic acid (mtDNA) mutations as seen in nonsyndromic deafness susceptibility caused by aminoglycoside sensitivity.

Both numeric and large structural abnormalities of autosomes (all chromosomes except the X and Y chromosomes) account for a variety of syndromes usually characterized by cognitive deficiencies. Nurses often note dysmorphic facial features, behavioral characteristics such as an unusual cry and poor feeding behavior, and other neurologic manifestations such as hypotonia or abnormal reflex responses, which may alert them to these and other chromosome abnormalities.

Somatic cells contain 44 autosomes (the 22 pairs of chromosomes that do not greatly influence sex determination at conception) and two sex chromosomes, XX in females and XY in males. For the purpose of cytogenetic studies, chromosomes are usually displayed in a karyotype, the laboratory-made arrangement of specially prepared chromosomes according to their size, centromere position, and band pattern. Numeric chromosome abnormalities occur whenever entire chromosomes are added or deleted. Down syndrome is an example of a condition caused by having an extra autosome, chromosome 21. Turner syndrome is the only example of a condition compatible with life that is caused by the absence of a chromosome. Children with Turner syndrome have one X chromosome. Chromosomes are subject to structural alterations resulting from breakage and rearrangement. A chromosome deletion occurs when chromosome breakage results in loss of the broken fragment at a chromosome's terminal end or within the chromosome. Some structural chromosome abnormalities are too small to reliably visualize under a light microscope but are still clinically relevant. Fragile, or weak, sites associated with expanded triplet repeats have been identified on both the autosomes and the X chromosome. A classic example is fragile X syndrome. Contiguous gene syndromes are disorders characterized by a microdeletion or microduplication of smaller chromosome segments, which may require special analysis techniques or molecular testing to detect (Bar-Shira, Rosner, Rosner, et al., 2006).

Chromosome anomalies typically affect large numbers of genes; however, a single-gene disorder is caused by an abnormality within a gene or in a gene's regulatory region. Single-gene disorders can affect all body systems and may have mild to severe expressions. Single-gene disorders display a Mendelian pattern of dominant or recessive inheritance that was first delineated in the mid-nineteenth century by Gregor Mendel's experiments with plants.

Mendelian inheritance laws allow for risk prediction in single-gene disorders; however, phenotypic expression may be altered by incomplete penetrance or variable expressivity of the responsible allele. An allele is said to have reduced or incomplete penetrance in a population when a proportion of people who possess that allele do not express the phenotype. An allele is said to have variable expressivity when individuals possessing that allele display the features of the syndrome in various degrees, from mild to severe. If a person expresses even the mildest possible phenotype, the allele is penetrant in that individual.

ROLE OF NURSES IN GENETICS

All nurses need to be prepared to use genetic and genomic information and technology when providing care. The professional practice domains of the essential genetic and genomic competencies include applying and integrating genetic knowledge into nursing assessment; identifying and referring patients who may benefit from genetic information or services; identifying genetics resources and services to meet patients' needs; and providing care and support before, during, and after providing genetic information and services (Consensus Panel on Genetic/Genomic Nursing Competencies, 2009). Often a nurse is the first one to recognize the need for genetic evaluation by identifying an inherited disorder in a family history or by noting physical, cognitive, or behavioral abnormalities when performing a nursing assessment (Box 28.4).

Nursing Assessment: Applying and Integrating Genetic and Genomic Knowledge

Family health history is an important tool to identify individuals and families at increased risk for disease, risk factors for disease (e.g., obesity), and inheritance patterns of diseases. Because of its importance, all nurses need to be able to elicit family history information and, when feasible, document the collected information in pedigree format.

When eliciting a family health history, nurses should collect information about all family members within a minimum of three generations. This process usually takes 20 to 30 minutes. When possible, it is best

BOX 28.4   Pediatric Indications for Genetic Consultation

Family History
- Family history of hereditary diseases, birth defects, or developmental problems
- Family history of sudden cardiac death or early-onset cancer
- Family history of mental illness

Medical History
- Abnormal newborn screen
- Abnormal genetic test result ordered by a nongenetics professional who lacks the knowledge and experience to discuss the implications of results
- Excessive bleeding or excessive clotting
- Progressive neurologic condition
- Recurrent infection or immunodeficiency

Developmental History
- Behavioral disorders
- Cognitive impairment or autism
- Developmental and speech delays or loss of developmental milestones

Physical Assessment
- Major congenital anomaly
- Minor anomalies and dysmorphic features
- Growth abnormalities
- Skeletal abnormalities
- Visual or hearing problems
- Metabolic disorder (unusual odor of breath, urine, or stool)
- Sexual development abnormalities or delayed puberty
- Skin disorders or abnormalities

Parental Requests
- Parent requests that child be evaluated by a genetics professional

Adapted from Pletcher, B.A., Toriello, H.V., Noblin, S.J., et al. (2007). Indications for genetic referral: A guide for healthcare providers. *Genetics in Medicine, 9*(6), 385–389.

to include both parents in the interview to elicit information about relatives on both sides of the family. Medical records, birth and death records, family Bibles, and photograph albums are helpful resources, and people being interviewed should be instructed to bring such items if they are available. It may be necessary to consult other members of the family. The level of education and the degree of understanding vary widely among informants and influence their reliability. The informants may be reticent, particularly if they view the disorder as something to be ashamed of or in some way threatening. Sometimes true relationships may be concealed, such as adoption or misattributed paternity.

In addition to family history, nurses caring for children and families need to collect pregnancy, labor and delivery, perinatal, medical, and developmental histories. Although it is common for genetics nurses to obtain all of these histories before or during an initial genetics consultation, not all nurses are expected to obtain all of these assessment data from each patient during a pediatric encounter. Electronic health records are making it more practical to construct a comprehensive set of histories even when many health care professionals contribute only a portion of the total history.

All nurses are taught to perform physical assessments, but they are seldom taught to recognize minor anomalies and dysmorphology that may suggest a genetic disorder. Yet nurses are keen in recognizing delays in development, behavior differences, and global appearances that raise concern that a newborn, infant, child, or adolescent needs further evaluation (Prows, Hopkin, Barnoy, et al., 2013). Although dysmorphology is beyond the scope of this chapter, readers are encouraged to review

the January 2009 issue of *American Journal of Medical Genetics* (Carey, Cohen, Curry, et al., 2009). Drawings and photographs of normal and abnormal morphologic characteristics are provided for the head, face, and extremities together with accepted dysmorphology terminology. Nurses knowledgeable in dysmorphology are able to articulate specific concerns about a child's appearance rather than relying on the outdated and offensive phrase "funny-looking kid." When a major anomaly is identified, nurses should raise suspicion that the child could have additional congenital anomalies. When three or more minor anomalies are identified, nurses should suspect the possibility of an underlying syndrome. However, it is important to consider the biologic parents' physical appearance, development, and behavior when considering the relevance of the child's combination of minor anomalies.

Identification and Referral

It is nurses' responsibility to learn basic genetic principles, to be alert to situations in which families could benefit from genetic evaluation and counseling, to know about special services that can help manage and support affected children, and to be familiar with facilities in their areas where these services are available. In this way, nurses are able to direct individuals and families to needed services and be active participants in the genetic evaluation and counseling process. A regularly updated resource for locating genetics clinics can be found at http://ghr.nlm.nih.gov/handbook/ (click on link for Genetic Consultation). In addition, state health departments either offer services or can help identify health professionals with specialty training in genetics.

Early identification of a genetic disorder allows anticipation of associated conditions and implementation of available preventive measures and therapy to avoid potential complications and to enhance the child's health. It may also prevent the unexpected birth of another affected child in the immediate or extended family. Nurses have an important role in identifying patients and families who have or are at risk for developing or transmitting a genetic condition (see Box 28.4). When facilitating genetics consultations, nurses should share with the genetics professional the findings in the histories they collected that triggered the consultation. Nurses can also help the referral process by determining and communicating the family's initial concerns, their state of knowledge about the reason for referral, and their attitudes and beliefs concerning genetics.

Genetic evaluation for diagnostic purposes may occur at any point in the life span. In the newborn period, birth defects and abnormal newborn screen results are obvious reasons for referral. Beyond the newborn period, indicators for referral include metabolic disorders, developmental delays, growth delays, behavioral problems, cognitive delays, abnormal or delayed sexual development, and medical problems known to be associated with genetic diseases. For example, a preschooler with hyperactivity and autistic-like behaviors may need evaluation for fragile X syndrome, and a 17-year-old girl with primary amenorrhea and short stature should be evaluated for Turner syndrome.

With so many recent advances in genetic testing, it is not unusual for a child or adult with longstanding medical problems, including cognitive impairment, to be referred for re-evaluation of his or her condition as a possible genetic disorder that might not have been diagnosable a few years earlier, such as microdeletion disorders or single-gene mutations. If a genetic diagnosis is made, the patient is usually referred back to the primary care physician with recommendations for routine management.

Providing Education, Care, and Support

Maintaining contact with the family or making a referral to a health care practice or an agency that can provide a sustained relationship is critical. It is becoming more common for genetics health care professionals to provide regular follow up and management, particularly for children with rare genetic disorders. However, some families choose not to have follow-up visits with genetic experts.

Regardless of whether families choose to receive continued care with a genetics center, clinic, or professional, nurses can help patients and families process and clarify the information they receive during a genetics visit. Misunderstanding of this information can have many causes, including cultural differences, the disparity of knowledge between the counselor and the family, and the heightened emotion surrounding genetic counseling. Family members have difficulty absorbing all of the information presented during a genetics evaluation and counseling session. Knowing this, genetics professionals write and send clinic summary letters to families. The nurse may need to help the family understand terminology in the letter, help them identify and articulate remaining questions or areas of clarification, and coach them through the process of accessing genetics health professionals to get remaining questions and concerns answered. Information often needs to be repeated several times before the family understands the content and its implications.

Nurses must assess for and address parents' feelings of guilt about carrying "bad genes" or having "made my child sick." Depending on the type of cytogenetic disorder, the nurse may be able to absolve the parents of guilt by explaining the random nature of segregation during both gamete formation and fertilization. If the condition is a Mendelian-inherited or mitochondrial disorder, it is important to assess parents' understanding of recurrence risk, help them understand the chances that a subsequent pregnancy will be affected and will not be affected, and ensure they have been given information about their options for future children (preimplantation diagnosis, use of donor egg or sperm, prenatal diagnosis, or adoption). Families often try to reason that some unrelated event caused the abnormality (e.g., a fall, a urinary tract infection, or "one glass of wine") before the mother was aware that she was pregnant. These misconceptions need to be assessed and dispelled.

After a genetics visit, and sometimes before the visit, parents often use the Internet to find answers to their questions. During the initial genetics evaluation, a diagnosis may not be possible. Instead, findings in medical, developmental, and family histories lead the professional to order genetic tests and other diagnostic procedures. Diagnoses under consideration are discussed briefly with the parents. Some parents are satisfied with the brief information and do not care to find out more until the actual diagnosis is established. Other parents go home and seek as much information as they can about the diagnoses under consideration. The information they find can be terrifying and overwhelming and inaccurate or misleading. Nurses can play an important role in helping parents identify reliable, accurate resources for information at whatever time they desire it. It is also important to stress that everything that is described for a genetic condition may not be relevant to their child. Before the follow-up genetics visit when test and procedure results are discussed, nurses can help parents identify and write down the questions and concerns they need addressed before leaving the clinic.

After a genetic diagnosis is made or a genetic predisposition to a delayed-onset disorder is identified, nurses need to have frequent contact with patients and families as they attempt to incorporate recommended therapies or disease-prevention strategies into their daily lives. For example, a disorder such as PKU requires conscientious diet management; therefore, it is important to make certain that the family understands and follows instructions and is able to navigate the health care system to access the essential formula and low-phenylalanine food products. An infant evaluated for cleft palate and cardiac defect and subsequently found to have VCFS requires surgical intervention for the congenital malformations. Such an infant also benefits from early intervention services and eventually an individualized education plan in school because developmental delays and eventual learning problems are common.

Initial and ongoing assessment of the family's coping abilities, resources, and support systems is vital to determine their need for additional assistance and support. As with any family who has a child with chronic health care needs, nurses must teach the family to become the child's advocate. Nurses can help families locate agencies and clinics specializing in a specific disorder or its consequences that can provide services (e.g., equipment, medication, and rehabilitation), educational programs, and parent support groups. Referral to local and national support groups or contact with a local family that has a child with the same condition can be helpful for new parents. Privacy and confidentiality are imperative, and both families must give permission before their contact information is given. Nurses can also be instrumental in helping parents start a support group when none is available.

Parental attachment and adjustment to the baby can be supported and facilitated by nursing interventions. Assessing the parents' understanding of the child's disorder and providing simple and truthful explanations can help them begin to understand their child's health issues. Guiding the parents in recognizing their child's cues, responses, and strengths can be helpful even for experienced parents. A caring attitude conveys the value of their child and, by extension, their value as parents. The nurse can help the parents identify their strengths as a family and identify support that is available to them.

Giving birth to and raising a child with a genetic disorder is not necessarily a lifetime burden. It is important for nurses to ask parents to describe their experience raising their child with a particular genetic condition. What has been the impact on their family? Although parents may initially experience negative outcomes, such as shock, emotional distress, and grief, families can adapt and thrive. Resources for managing stress and restoring balance in the lives of families affected by a genetic condition can help. Van Riper's (2007) research has identified nursing interventions that can promote resilience and adaptation in families of children with Down syndrome. Van Riper's recommendations are useful for families of children with any type of genetic disorder:

- Recognize multiple stressors, strains, and transitions in their lives (e.g., unmet family needs).
- Discuss and implement strategies for reducing family demands (e.g., setting priorities and reducing the number of outside activities family members are involved in).
- Identify and use individual, family, and community resources (e.g., humor, family flexibility, supportive extended family, respite care, local support groups, and Internet resources).
- Expand the range and efficacy of their coping strategies (e.g., increase the use of active strategies such as reframing, mobilize their ability to acquire and accept help, and decrease the use of passive appraisal).
- Encourage the use of an affirming style of family problem-solving communication (e.g., one that conveys support and caring and exerts a calming influence).

Some families do struggle after learning their child has a genetic disorder. Families may feel ashamed of a hereditary disorder and seek to blame their partner for transmitting a faulty gene or chromosome. Intra-familial strife, hostility, and marital or couple disharmony, sometimes to the point of family disintegration, can occur. Nurses should be alert for evidence of risk factors that indicate poor adjustment (e.g., child abuse, divorce, or other maladaptive behaviors). Referral to psychosocial professionals for crisis intervention may be necessary.

REFERENCES

Anders, T. F., Sadeh, A., & Appareddy, V. (2005). Normal sleep in neonates and children. In S. Sheldon, R. Ferber, & M. Kryger (Eds.), *Principles and practice of sleep medicine in the child*. Philadelphia, PA: Saunders.

Ball, J. W., Dains, J. E., Flynn, J. A., et al. (2015). *Mosby's guide to physical examination* (8th ed.). St. Louis, MO: Mosby/Elsevier.

Bar-Shira, A., Rosner, G., Rosner, S., et al. (2006). Array-based comparative genome hybridization in clinical genetics. *Pediatric Research, 60*(3), 353–358.

Briggs, R. D., Stettler, E. M., Silver, E. J., et al. (2012). Social-emotional screening for infants and toddlers in primary care. *Pediatrics, 129*(2), e377–e384.

Caine, D., DiFiori, J., & Maffulli, N. (2006). Physeal injuries in children's and youth sports: Reasons for concern? *British Journal of Sports Medicine, 40*(9), 749–760.

Carey, J. C., Cohen, M. M., Curry, C. J., et al. (2009). Elements of morphology: Standard terminology for the lips, mouth, and oral region. *American Journal of Medical Genetics. Part A, 149A*(1), 77–92.

Chess, S., & Thomas, A. (1999). *Goodness of fit: Clinical applications from infancy through adult life.* London: Routledge.

Consensus Panel on Genetic/Genomic Nursing Competencies (2009). *Essentials of genetic and genomic nursing: Competencies, curricula guidelines, and outcome indicators* (2nd ed.). Silver Spring, MD: American Nurses Association.

Cronk, C., Crocker, A. C., Pueschel, S. M., et al. (1988). Growth charts for children with Down syndrome: 1 month to 18 years of age. *Pediatrics, 81*(1), 102–110.

Delva, J., O'Malley, P. M., & Johnston, L. D. (2007). Availability of more-healthy and less-healthy food choices in American schools: A national study of grade, racial/ethnic, and socioeconomic differences. *American Journal of Preventive Medicine, 33*(4 suppl), S226–S239.

Erikson, E. H. (1963). *Childhood and society* (2nd ed.). New York, NY: Norton.

Filipek, P. A., Accardo, P. J., Ashwal, S., et al. (2000). Practice parameter: Screening and diagnosis of autism: Report of the Quality Standards Subcommittee of the American Academy of Neurology and the Child Neurology Society. *Neurology, 55*(4), 468–479.

Freud, S. (1933). *New introductory lectures in psychoanalysis.* New York, NY: Norton.

Freud, S. (1964). An outline of psychoanalysis. In J. Strachey (Ed. and translator), *The standard edition of the complete psychological works of Sigmund Freud* (vol. 23). London: Hogarth Press.

Galligan, M. (2006). Proposed guidelines for skin-to-skin treatment of neonatal hypothermia. *American Journal of Maternal Child Nursing, 31*(5), 298–304.

Glassy, D., Romano, J., Committee on Early Childhood, Adoption, and Dependent Care, et al. (2003). Selecting appropriate toys for young children: The pediatrician's role. *Pediatrics, 111*(4 pt 1), 911–913.

Greco, K. E., Tinley, S., & Seibert, D. (2012). *Essential genetic and genomic competencies for nurses with graduate degrees,* Silver Spring, MD, American Nurses Association and International Society of Nurses in Genetics.

Kaczander, B. I. (1997). Pediatric sports medicine: A unique perspective. *Podiatry Management, 16*(2), 53–60.

Kohlberg, L. (1968). Moral development. In D. L. Sills (Ed.), *International encyclopedia of the social sciences.* New York, NY: Macmillan.

Lampl, M., Johnson, M. L., & Frongillo, E. A. (2001). Mixed distribution analysis identifies saltation and stasis growth. *Annals of Human Biology, 28*(4), 403–411.

Lampl, M., Thompson, A., & Frongillo, E. A. (2005). Sex differences in the relationships among weight gain, subcutaneous skinfold tissue and salutatory length growth spurts in infancy. *Pediatric Research, 58*(6), 1238–1242.

Matvienko, O. (2007). Impact of a nutrition education curriculum on snack choices of children ages six and seven years. *Journal of Nutrition Education and Behavior, 39*(5), 281–285.

Mcintyre, S., Taitz, D., Keogh, J., et al. (2013). A systematic review of risk factors for cerebral palsy in children born at term in developed countries. *Developmental Medicine and Child Neurology, 55*(6), 499–508.

Myrelid, A., Gustafsson, J., Ollars, B., et al. (2002). Growth charts for Down's syndrome from birth to 18 years of age. *Archives of Disease in Childhood, 87*(2), 97–103.

National Foundation for Ectodermal Dysplasias. (2017). *About ectodermal dysplasias,* Retrieved from http://nfed.org/index.php/about_ed/abou t-ectodermal-dysplasias.

Piaget, J. (1969). *The theory of stages in cognitive development.* New York, NY: McGraw-Hill.

Prows, C. A., Hopkin, R. J., Barnoy, S., et al. (2013). An update of childhood genetic disorders. *Journal of Nursing Scholarship, 45*(1), 34–42.

Rimoin, D. L., Pyeritz, R. E., & Korf, B. (Eds.), (2013). *Principles and practice of medical genetics* (6th ed.). New York, NY: Elsevier Science.

Stuart, G. W., & Laraia, M. T. (2000). *Principles and practice of psychiatric nursing* (7th ed.). St Louis, MO: Mosby.

Thompson, R., Cotner-Bichelman, N., McKerchar, P., et al. (2007). Enhancing early communication through infant sign training. *Journal of Applied Behavior Analysis, 40*(1), 15–23.

Urbanski, L. F., & Hanlon, D. P. (1996). Pediatric orthopedics. *Topics in Emergency Medicine, 18*(2), 73–90.

Van Riper, M. (2007). Families of children with Down syndrome: Responding to "a change in plans" with resilience. *Journal of Pediatric Nursing, 22*(2), 116–128.

Wagner, J., Jenkins, B., & Smith, J. (2006). Nurses' utilization of parent questionnaires for developmental screening. *Pediatric Nursing, 32*(5), 409–412.

Willoughby, C., King, G., & Polatajko, H. (1996). A therapist's guide to children's self-esteem. *American Journal of Occupational Therapy, 50*(2), 124–132.

29

Communication and Physical Assessment of the Child and Family

Marilyn J. Hockenberry

http://evolve.elsevier.com/Perry/maternal

GUIDELINES FOR COMMUNICATION AND INTERVIEWING

The most widely used method of communicating with parents on a professional basis is the interview process. Unlike social conversation, interviewing is a specific form of goal-directed communication. As nurses converse with children and adults, they focus on the individuals to determine the kind of people they are, their usual mode of handling problems, whether they need help, and the way they react to counseling. Developing interviewing skills requires time and practice, but following some guiding principles can facilitate this process. An organized approach is most effective when using interviewing skills in patient teaching.

ESTABLISHING A SETTING FOR COMMUNICATION

Appropriate Introduction

Introduce yourself, and ask the name of each family member who is present. Address parents or other adults by their appropriate titles, such as "Mr." and "Mrs.," unless they specify a preferred name. Record the preferred name on the medical record. Using formal address or their preferred names, rather than using first names or "mother" or "father," conveys respect and regard for the parents or other caregivers (Ball, Dains, Flynn, et al., 2014).

At the beginning of the visit, include children in the interaction by asking them their name, age, and other information. Nurses often direct all questions to adults even when children are old enough to speak for themselves. This only terminates one extremely valuable source of information—the patient. When including the child, follow the general rules for communicating with children given in the Guidelines box: Communicating with Children.

Assurance of Privacy and Confidentiality

The place where the nurse conducts the interview is almost as important as the interview itself. The physical environment should allow for as much privacy as possible with distractions (such as, interruptions, noise, or other visible activity) kept to a minimum. At times, it is necessary to turn off a television, radio, or mobile phone. The environment should also have some play provision for young children to keep them occupied during the parent-nurse interview (Fig. 29.1). Parents who are constantly interrupted by their children are unable to concentrate fully and tend to give brief answers to finish the interview as quickly as possible.

Confidentiality is another essential component of the initial phase of the interview. Because the interview is usually shared with other members of the health care team or the teacher (in the case of students), be certain to inform the family of the limits regarding confidentiality. If confidentiality is a concern in a particular situation, such as when talking to a parent suspected of child abuse or a teenager contemplating suicide, deal with this directly and inform the person that in such instances, confidentiality cannot be ensured. However, the nurse judiciously protects information of a confidential nature.

COMPUTER PRIVACY AND APPLICATIONS IN NURSING

The use of computer technology to store and retrieve health information has become widespread; most clinics and hospitals now maintain electronic health records for patients. The health care community is increasingly concerned about the privacy and security of this health information, and all nurses are engaged in protecting confidentiality of health care records. Any person accessing confidential health information is charged with managing safeguards for disclosure including password protection to prevent violation of patient privacy and confidentiality.

TELEPHONE TRIAGE AND COUNSELING

Telephone triage care management has increased access to high-quality health care services and empowered parents to participate in their child's health care. Consequently, patient satisfaction has significantly improved. Unnecessary emergency department and clinic visits have decreased, saving health care costs and time (with less absence from work) for families in need of health care.

Telephone triage is more than "just a phone call" because a child's life is a high price to pay for poorly managed or incompetent telephone assessment skills. Typically, guidelines for telephone triage include asking screening questions; determining when to immediately refer to emergency medical services (dial 911) or the emergency department; and determining when to refer to same-day appointments, appointments in 24 to 72 hours, appointments in 4 days or more, or home care (Box 29.1).

741

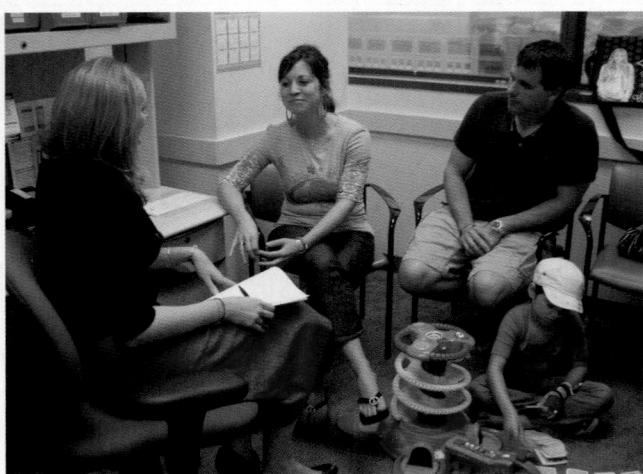

FIG 29.1 Child plays while nurse interviews parents.

BOX 29.1   Telephone Triage Guidelines

Date and time
Background
- Name, age, sex, contact information
- Chronic illness
- Allergies, current medications, treatments, or recent immunizations

Chief complaint
General symptoms
- Severity
- Duration
- Other symptoms
- Pain

Systems review
Steps taken
- Advised to call emergency medical services (911)
- Advised to go to emergency department
- Advised to see practitioner (today, tomorrow, or later appointment)
- Advised regarding home care
- Advised to call back if symptoms worsen or fail to improve

Resources for Telephone Triage Protocols

Beaulieu, R., & Humphreys, J. (2008). Evaluation of a telephone advice nurse in a nursing faculty managed pediatric community clinic. *Journal of Pediatric Health Care, 22*(3), 175–181.

Marklund, B., Ström, M., Månsson, J., et al. (2007). Computer-supported telephone nurse triage: An evaluation of medical quality and costs. *Journal of Nursing Management, 15*(2), 180–187.

Schmitt, B. D. (2012). *Pediatric telephone protocols: Office version* (14th ed.). Elk Grove Village, IL: American Academy of Pediatrics.

Simonsen, S. M. (2001). *Telephone assessment: Guidelines for practice* (2nd ed.). St Louis: Mosby.

Successful outcomes are based on the consistency and accuracy of the information provided. A systematic review of 49 studies where nurses triaged calls found that the appropriateness of a decision and subsequent compliance often varied (Blank, Coster, O'Cathain, et al., 2012). A meta-analysis of 13 studies provided further insight and found patient compliance with triage recommendations were influenced by the quality of provider communication (Purc-Stephenson & Thrasher, 2012). The importance of nurse-patient communication is reinforced as an essential aspect of telephone triage training. Training of communication skills that are patient- and family-centered and specifically address active listening and advising skills offers the greatest opportunity for success. Assessment skills used in direct nurse-to-patient interactions are not directly transferable to the telephone and provide further support for training in decision-making skills for phone triage (Purc-Stephenson & Thrasher, 2010). Evidence-based clinical protocols for telephone triage can provide a structured method for assessment (Stacey, Macartney, Carley, et al., 2013).

COMMUNICATING WITH FAMILIES

COMMUNICATING WITH PARENTS

Although the parent and the child are separate and distinct individuals, the nurse's relationship with the child is frequently mediated by the parent, particularly with younger children. For the most part, nurses acquire information about the child by direct observation and through communication with the parents. Usually it can be assumed that because of the close contact with the child, the parent gives reliable information. Assessing the child requires input from the child (verbal and nonverbal), information from the parent, and the nurse's own observations of the child and interpretation of the relationship between the child and the parent. When children are old enough to be active participants in their own health care, the parent becomes a collaborator.

Encouraging the Parents to Talk

Interviewing parents not only offers the opportunity to determine the child's health and developmental status but also offers information about factors that influence the child's life. Whatever the parent sees as a problem should be a concern of the nurse. These problems are not always easy to identify. Nurses need to be alert for clues and signals by which a parent communicates worries and anxieties. Careful phrasing with broad, open-ended questions (such as, "What is Jimmy eating now?") provides more information than several single-answer questions (such as, "Is Jimmy eating what the rest of the family eats?").

Sometimes the parent will take the lead without prompting. At other times, it may be necessary to direct another question on the basis of an observation, such as "Connie seems unhappy today," or "How do you feel when David cries?" If the parent appears to be tired or distraught, consider asking, "What do you do to relax?" or "What help do you have with the children?" A comment such as "You handle the baby very well. What kind of experience have you had with babies?" to new parents who appear comfortable with their first child gives positive reinforcement and provides an opening for questions they might have on the infant's care. Often all that is required to keep parents talking is a nod or saying "yes" or "uh-huh."

Directing the Focus

Directing the focus of the interview while allowing maximum freedom of expression is one of the most difficult goals in effective communication. One approach is the use of open-ended or broad questions followed by guiding statements. For example, if the parent proceeds to list the other children by name, say, "Tell me their ages, too." If the parent continues to describe each child in depth, which is not the purpose of the interview, redirect the focus by stating, "Let's talk about the other children later. You were beginning to tell me about Paul's activities at school." This approach conveys interest in the other children but focuses the assessment on the patient.

Listening and Cultural Awareness

Listening is the most important component of effective communication. When the purpose of listening is to understand the person being interviewed, it is an active process that requires concentration and

CULTURAL CONSIDERATIONS
Interviewing Without Judgment

It is easy to inject one's own attitudes and feelings into an interview. Often nurses' own prejudices and assumptions, which may include racial, religious, and cultural stereotypes, influence their perceptions of a parent's behavior. What the nurse may interpret as a parent's passive hostility or lack of interest may be shyness or an expression of anxiety. For example, in Western cultures, eye contact and directness are signs of paying attention. However, in many non-Western cultures, including that of Native Americans, directness (e.g., looking someone in the eye) is considered rude. Children are taught to avert their gaze and to look down when being addressed by an adult, especially one with authority (Ball, Dains, Flynn, et al., 2014). Therefore, nurses must make judgments about "listening," as well as verbal interactions, with an appreciation of cultural differences.

BOX 29.2   Blocks to Communication

Communication Barriers (Nurse)
Socializing
Giving unrestricted and sometimes unsought advice
Offering premature or inappropriate reassurance
Giving over-ready encouragement
Defending a situation or opinion
Using stereotyped comments or clichés
Limiting expression of emotion by asking directed, closed-ended questions
Interrupting and finishing the person's sentence
Talking more than the interviewee
Forming prejudged conclusions
Deliberately changing the focus

Signs of Information Overload (Patient)
Long periods of silence
Wide eyes and fixed facial expression
Constant fidgeting or attempting to move away
Nervous habits (e.g., tapping, playing with hair)
Sudden interruptions (e.g., asking to go to the bathroom)
Looking around
Yawning, eyes drooping
Frequently looking at a watch or clock
Attempting to change the topic of discussion

attention to all aspects of the conversation—verbal, nonverbal, and abstract. Major blocks to listening are environmental distraction and premature judgment.

Although it is necessary to make some preliminary judgments, listen with as much objectivity as possible by clarifying meanings and attempting to see the situation from the parent's point of view. Effective interviewers consciously control their reactions and responses and the techniques they use (see Cultural Considerations box: Interviewing Without Judgment).

Careful listening relies on the use of clues, verbal leads, or signals from the interviewee to move the interview along. Frequent references to an area of concern, repetition of certain key words, or a special emphasis on something or someone serve as cues to the interviewer for the direction of inquiry. Concerns and anxieties are often mentioned in a casual, offhand manner. Even though they are casual, they are important and deserve careful scrutiny to identify problem areas. For example, a parent who is concerned about a child's habit of bedwetting may casually mention that the child's bed was "wet this morning."

Using Silence

Silence as a response is often one of the most difficult interviewing techniques to learn. The interviewer requires a sense of confidence and comfort to allow the interviewee space in which to think without interruptions. Silence permits the interviewee to sort out thoughts and feelings and search for responses to questions. Silence can also be a cue for the interviewer to go more slowly, re-examine the approach, and not push too hard (Ball, Dains, Flynn, et al., 2014).

Sometimes it is necessary to break the silence and reopen communication. Do this in a way that encourages the person to continue talking about what is considered important. Breaking a silence by introducing a new topic or by prolonged talking essentially terminates the interviewee's opportunity to use the silence. Suggestions for breaking the silence include statements such as the following:
- "Is there anything else you wish to say?"
- "I see you find it difficult to continue. How may I help?"
- "I don't know what this silence means. Perhaps there is something you would like to put into words but find difficult to say."

Being Empathic

Empathy is the capacity to understand what another person is experiencing from within that person's frame of reference; it is often described as the ability to put oneself in another's shoes. The essence of empathic interaction is accurate understanding of another's feelings. Empathy differs from sympathy, which is having feelings or emotions similar to those of another person, rather than understanding those feelings.

Providing Anticipatory Guidance

The ideal way to handle a situation is to deal with it before it becomes a problem. The best preventive measure is anticipatory guidance. Traditionally, anticipatory guidance focused on providing families information on normal growth and development and nurturing childrearing practices. For example, one of the most significant areas in pediatrics is injury prevention. Beginning prenatally, parents need specific instructions on home safety. Because of the child's maturing developmental skills, parents must implement home safety changes early to minimize risks to the child.

Unprepared parents can be disturbed by many normal developmental changes, such as a toddler's diminished appetite, negativism, altered sleeping patterns, and anxiety toward strangers. Anticipatory guidance should extend beyond giving general information to empowering families to use the information as a means of building competence in their parenting abilities (Dosman & Andrews, 2012). To achieve this level of anticipatory guidance, the nurse should do the following:
- Base interventions on needs identified by the family, not by the professional
- View the family as competent or as having the ability to be competent
- Provide opportunities for the family to achieve competence

Avoiding Blocks to Communication

A number of blocks to communication can adversely affect the quality of the helping relationship. The interviewer introduces many of these blocks, such as giving unrestricted advice or forming prejudged conclusions. Another type of block occurs primarily with the interviewees and concerns information overload. When individuals receive too much information or information that is overwhelming, they often demonstrate signs of increasing anxiety or decreasing attention. Such signals should alert the interviewer to give less information or to clarify what has been said. Box 29.2 lists some of the more common blocks to communication, including signs of information overload.

The nurse can correct communication blocks by careful analysis of the interview process. One of the best methods for improving interviewing skills is audiotape or videotape feedback. With supervision and guidance, the interviewer can recognize the blocks and consciously avoid them.

Communicating With Families Through an Interpreter

Sometimes communication is impossible because two people speak different languages. In this case, it is necessary to obtain information through a third party: the interpreter. When using an interpreter, the nurse follows the same interviewing guidelines. Specific guidelines for using an interpreter are given in the Guidelines box: Using an Interpreter.

Communicating with families through an interpreter requires sensitivity to cultural, legal, and ethical considerations (see Cultural Considerations box: Using Children as Interpreters). In some cultures, class differences between the interpreter and the family may cause the family to feel intimidated and less inclined to offer information. Therefore, it is important to choose the interpreter carefully and provide time for the interpreter and family to establish rapport.

In obtaining informed consent through an interpreter, the nurse should fully inform the family of all aspects of the particular procedure to which they are consenting. Issues of confidentiality may arise when family members related to another patient are asked to interpret for the family, thus revealing sensitive information that may be shared with other families on the unit. With increased sensitivity toward patient rights and confidentiality, many institutions now require consent forms translated in the patient's primary language.

! NURSING ALERT

When using translated materials, such as a health history form, be certain the informant is literate in the foreign language.

📋 GUIDELINES

Using an Interpreter

- Explain to interpreter the reason for the interview and the type of questions that will be asked.
- Clarify whether a detailed or brief answer is required and whether the translated response can be general or literal.
- Introduce the interpreter to the family, and allow some time before the interview for them to become acquainted.
- Communicate directly with family members when asking questions to reinforce interest in them and to observe nonverbal expressions, but do not ignore the interpreter.
- Pose questions to elicit only one answer at a time, such as "Do you have pain?" rather than "Do you have any pain, tiredness, or loss of appetite?"
- Refrain from interrupting family members and the interpreter while they are conversing.
- Avoid commenting to the interpreter about family members, because they may understand some English.
- Be aware that some medical words, such as *allergy*, may have no similar word in another language; avoid medical jargon whenever possible.
- Be aware that cultural differences may exist regarding views on puberty, sex, marriage, or pregnancy.
- Allow time after the interview for the interpreter to share something that he or she thought could not be said earlier; ask about the interpreter's impression of nonverbal clues to communication and family members' reliability or ease in revealing information.

Arrange for the family to speak with the same interpreter on subsequent visits whenever possible.

COMMUNICATING WITH CHILDREN

Although the greatest amount of verbal communication is usually carried out with the parent, do not exclude the child during the interview. Pay attention to infants and younger children through play or by occasionally directing questions or remarks to them. Include older children as active participants so that they can share their own experiences and perspectives.

In communication with children of all ages, the nonverbal components of the communication process convey the most significant messages. It is difficult to disguise feelings, attitudes, and anxiety when relating to children. They are alert to surroundings and attach meaning to every gesture and move that is made; this is particularly true of very young children.

Active attempts to make friends with children before they have had an opportunity to evaluate an unfamiliar person tend to increase their anxiety. Continue to talk to the child and parent, but go about activities that do not involve the child directly, thus allowing the child to observe from a safe position. If the child has a special toy or doll, "talk" to the doll first. Ask simple questions, such as "Does your teddy bear have a name?" to ease the child into conversation. Other guidelines for communicating with children are in the Guidelines box: Communicating with Children.

🌐 CULTURAL CONSIDERATIONS

Using Children as Interpreters

When no one else is readily available to interpret, there may be temptation to use a bilingual child within the family as an interpreter. However, the use of children in health care interpreting is strongly discouraged, because they are often not mature enough to understand health care questions, answers, or messages (American Academy of Pediatrics, 2011). Children may inadvertently commit interpretive errors, such as inaccuracies, omissions, or substitutions. In addition, children can be adversely affected by serious or sensitive information that may be discussed. In some cultures, using a child as an interpreter is considered an insult to an adult because children are expected to show respect by not questioning their elders. Note that some institutions prohibit the use of children as interpreters; check institutional policy for compliance. If a trained on-site or community-based interpreter is not available, a *language line* using a telephonic interpreter may be an option.

📋 GUIDELINES

Communicating With Children

- Allow children time to feel comfortable.
- Avoid sudden or rapid advances, broad smiles, extended eye contact, and other gestures that may be seen as threatening.
- Talk to the parent if the child is initially shy.
- Communicate through transition objects (such as dolls, puppets, and stuffed animals) before questioning a young child directly.
- Give older children the opportunity to talk without the parents present.
- Assume a position that is at eye level with the child (Fig. 29.2).
- Speak in a quiet, unhurried, and confident voice.
- Speak clearly, be specific, and use simple words and short sentences.
- State directions and suggestions positively.
- Offer a choice only when one exists.
- Be honest with children.
- Allow children to express their concerns and fears.
- Use a variety of communication techniques.

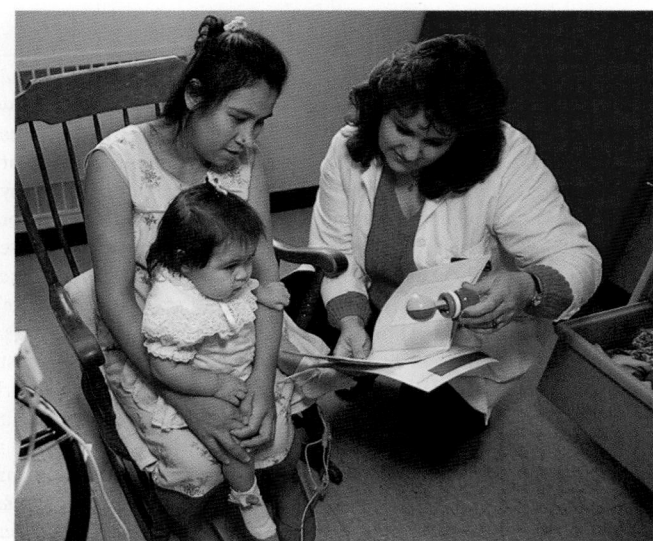

FIG 29.2 Nurse assumes position at child's level.

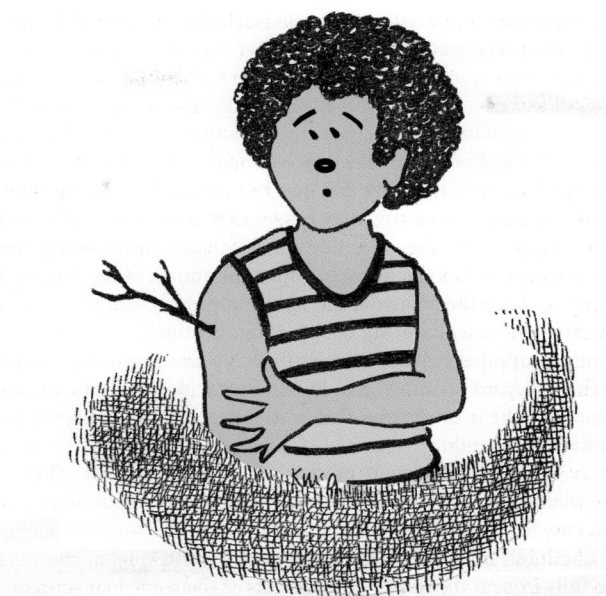

FIG 29.3 A young child may take the expression "a little stick in the arm" literally.

Communication Related to Development of Thought Processes

The normal development of language and thought offers a frame of reference for communicating with children. Thought processes progress from sensorimotor to perceptual to concrete and finally to abstract, formal operations. An understanding of the typical characteristics of these stages provides the nurse with a framework to facilitate social communication.

Infancy

Because they are unable to use words, infants primarily use and understand nonverbal communication. Infants communicate their needs and feelings through nonverbal behaviors and vocalizations that can be interpreted by someone who is around them for a sufficient time. Infants smile and coo when content and cry when distressed. Crying is provoked by unpleasant stimuli from inside or outside, such as hunger, pain, body restraint, or loneliness. Adults interpret this to mean that an infant needs something and consequently try to alleviate the discomfort by meeting their physical needs, speaking softly, and communicating through touch.

Infants respond to adults' nonverbal behaviors. They become quiet when they are cuddled, rocked, or receive other forms of gentle physical contact. They receive comfort from the sound of a soft voice even though they do not understand the words that are spoken. Until infants reach the age at which they experience stranger anxiety, they readily respond to any firm, gentle handling and quiet, calm speech. Loud, harsh sounds and sudden movements are frightening.

Early Childhood

Children younger than 5 years of age are *egocentric*. They see things only in relation to themselves and from their point of view. Therefore, focus communication on them. Tell them what they can do or how they will feel. Experiences of others are of no interest to them. It is futile to use another child's experience in an attempt to gain the cooperation of small children. Allow them to touch and examine articles they will come in contact with. A stethoscope bell will feel cold; palpating a neck might tickle. Although they have not yet acquired sufficient language skills to express their feelings and wants, toddlers can effectively use their hands to communicate ideas without words. They push an

unwanted object away, pull another person to show them something, point, and cover the mouth that is saying something they do not wish to hear.

Everything is direct and concrete to small children. They are unable to work with abstractions and interpret words literally. Analogies escape them because they are unable to separate reality from fantasy. For example, they attach literal meaning to such common phrases as "two-faced," "sticky fingers," and "coughing your head off." Children who are told they will get "a little stick in the arm" may not be able to envision an injection (Fig. 29.3). Therefore, use simple, direct language rather than phrases that might be misinterpreted by a small child.

School-Age Years

Younger school-age children rely less on what they see and more on what they know when faced with new problems. They want explanations and reasons for everything but require no verification beyond that. They are interested in the functional aspect of all procedures, objects, and activities. They want to know why an object exists, why it is used, how it works, and the intent and purpose of its user. They need to know what is going to take place and why it is being done to them specifically. For example, to explain a procedure such as taking blood pressure, show the child how squeezing the bulb pushes air into the cuff and makes the "arrow" move. Let the child operate the bulb. An explanation for the procedure might be as simple as, "I want to see how far the arrow moves when the cuff squeezes your arm." Consequently, the child becomes an enthusiastic participant.

School-age children have a heightened concern about body integrity. Because of the special importance they place on their body, they are sensitive to anything that constitutes a threat or suggestion of injury to it. This concern extends to their possessions, so they may appear to overreact to loss or threatened loss of treasured objects. Encouraging children to communicate their needs and voice their concerns enables the nurse to provide reassurance, to dispel myths and fears, and to implement activities that reduce their anxiety. For example, if a shy child dislikes being the center of attention, ignore that particular child by talking and relating to other children in the family or group. When children feel more comfortable, they will usually interject personal ideas, feelings, and interpretations of events.

Adolescence

As children move into adolescence, they fluctuate between child and adult thinking and behavior. They are riding a current that is moving them rapidly toward a maturity that may be beyond their coping ability. Therefore, when tensions rise, they may seek the security of the more familiar and comfortable expectations of childhood. Anticipating these shifts in identity allows the nurse to adjust the course of interaction to meet the needs of the moment. No single approach can be relied on consistently, and encountering cooperation, hostility, anger, bravado, and a variety of other behaviors and attitudes is common. It is as much a mistake to regard an adolescent as an adult with an adult's wisdom and control as it is to assume that a teenager has the concerns and expectations of a child.

Interviewing an adolescent presents some special issues. The first may be whether to talk with the adolescent alone or with the adolescent and parents together. If the parents and teenager are together, talking with the adolescent first has the advantage of immediately identifying with the young person, thus fostering the interpersonal relationship. However, talking with the parents initially may provide insight into the family relationship. In either case, give both parties an opportunity to be included in the interview. If time is limited, such as during history taking, clarify this at the onset to avoid appearing to "take sides" by talking more with one person than with the other.

Privacy and confidentiality are of great importance when communicating with adolescents because it is consistent with developmental maturity and autonomy. Explain to parents and teenagers the legal and ethical protections and limits of confidentiality. Nurses need to know and understand the state and federal consent and confidentiality laws pertaining to adolescent circumstances, such as suspected abuse, alcohol or other drug use, suicidal or homicidal ideation, contraceptive care, pregnancy, sexually transmitted infections, and sexual assault (Broner, Embry, Gremminger, et al., 2013).

Another dilemma in interviewing adolescents is that two views of a problem frequently exist: the teenager's and the parents'. Clarification of the problem is a major task. However, providing both parties an opportunity to discuss their perceptions in an open and unbiased atmosphere can, by itself, be therapeutic. Demonstrating positive communication skills can help families with adolescents to communicate more effectively (see Guidelines box: Communicating With Adolescents).

📋 GUIDELINES

Communicating With Adolescents

Build a Foundation	Communicate Effectively
Spend time together.	Give undivided attention.
Encourage expression of ideas and feelings.	Listen, listen, listen.
	Be courteous, calm, honest, and open-minded.
Respect their views.	Try not to overreact. If you do, take a break.
Tolerate differences.	Avoid judging or criticizing.
Praise good points.	Avoid the "third degree" of continuous questioning.
Respect their privacy.	
Set a good example.	Choose important issues when taking a stand.
	After taking a stand:
	• Think through all options.
	• Make expectations clear.

HISTORY TAKING

PERFORMING A HEALTH HISTORY

The format used for history taking may be (1) direct, in which the nurse asks for information via direct interview with the informant, or (2) indirect, in which the informant supplies the information by completing some type of questionnaire. The direct method is superior to the indirect approach or a combination of both. However, because time is limited, the direct approach is not always practical. If the nurse cannot use the direct approach, he or she should review the parents' written responses and question them regarding any unusual answers. The categories listed in Box 29.3 encompass children's current and past health status and information about their psychosocial environment.

Identifying Information

Much of the identifying information may already be available from other recorded sources. However, if the parent and child seem anxious, use this opportunity to ask about such information to help them feel more comfortable.

Informant

One of the important elements of identifying information is the *informant,* the person(s) who furnishes the information. Record (1) who the person is (child, parent, or other), (2) an impression of reliability and willingness to communicate, and (3) any special circumstances such as the use of an interpreter or conflicting answers by more than one person.

Chief Complaint

The *chief complaint* is the specific reason for the child's visit to the clinic, office, or hospital. It may be the theme, with the present illness viewed as the description of the problem. Elicit the chief complaint by asking open-ended, neutral questions (such as, "What seems to be the matter?" "How may I help you?" or "Why did you come here today?"). Avoid labeling-type questions (such as, "How are you sick?" or "What is the problem?"). It is possible that the reason for the visit is not an illness or problem.

Occasionally, it is difficult to isolate one symptom or problem as the chief complaint because the parent may identify many. In this situation, be as specific as possible when asking questions. For example, asking informants to state which *one* problem or symptom prompted them to seek help now may help them focus on the most immediate concern.

Present Illness

The history of the present illness* is a narrative of the chief complaint from its earliest onset through its progression to the present. Its four major components are the details of onset, a complete interval history, the present status, and the reason for seeking help now. The focus of the present illness is on all factors relevant to the main problem even if they have disappeared or changed during the onset, interval, and present.

Analyzing a Symptom

Because pain is often the most characteristic symptom denoting the onset of a physical problem, it is used as an example for analysis of a symptom. Assessment includes type, location, severity, duration, and

---

*The term *illness* is used in its broadest sense to denote any problem of a physical, emotional, or psychosocial nature. It is actually a history of the chief complaint.

BOX 29.3   Outline of a Pediatric Health History

Identifying information
1. Name
2. Address
3. Telephone
4. Birth date and place
5. Race or ethnic group
6. Sex
7. Religion
8. Date of interview
9. Informant

Chief complaint (CC): To establish the major specific reason for the child's and parents' seeking of health care

Present illness (PI): To obtain all details related to the chief complaint

Past history (PH): To elicit a profile of the child's previous illnesses, injuries, or surgeries
1. Birth history (pregnancy, labor and delivery, perinatal history)
2. Previous illnesses, injuries, or surgeries
3. Allergies
4. Current medications
5. Immunizations
6. Growth and development
7. Habits

Review of systems (ROS): To elicit information concerning any potential health problem
1. Constitutional
2. Integument
3. Eyes
4. Ears/nose/mouth/throat
5. Neck
6. Chest
7. Respiratory
8. Cardiovascular
9. Gastrointestinal
10. Genitourinary
11. Gynecologic
12. Musculoskeletal
13. Neurologic
14. Genitourinary
15. Gynecologic
16. Musculoskeletal
17. Neurologic
18. Endocrine

Family medical history: To identify genetic traits or diseases that have familial tendencies and to assess exposure to a communicable disease in a family member and family habits that may affect the child's health, such as smoking and chemical use

Psychosocial history: To elicit information about the child's self-concept

Sexual history: To elicit information concerning the child's sexual concerns or activities and any pertinent data regarding adults' sexual activity that influences the child

Family history: To develop an understanding of the child as an individual and as a member of a family and a community
1. Family composition
2. Home and community environment
3. Occupation and education of family members
4. Cultural and religious traditions
5. Family function and relationships

Nutritional assessment: To elicit information on the adequacy of the child's nutritional intake and needs
1. Dietary intake
2. Clinical examination

---

influencing factors (see Guidelines box: Analyzing the Symptom: Pain; see also the "Pain Assessment" section in Chapter 30).

History

The history contains information relating to all previous aspects of the child's health status and concentrates on several areas that are ordinarily passed over in the history of an adult, such as birth history, detailed feeding history, immunizations, and growth and development. Because this section includes a great deal of information, use a combination of open-ended and fact-finding questions. For example, begin interviewing for each section with an open-ended statement (e.g., "Tell me about your child's birth") to provide the informants the opportunity to relate what they think is most important. Ask fact-finding questions related to specific details whenever necessary to focus the interview on certain topics.

Birth History

The *birth history* includes all data concerning (1) the mother's health during pregnancy, (2) the labor and delivery, and (3) the infant's condition immediately after birth. Because prenatal influences have significant effects on a child's physical and emotional development, a thorough investigation of the birth history is essential. Because parents may question what relevance pregnancy and birth have on the child's present condition, particularly if the child is past infancy, explain why such questions are included. An appropriate statement may be, "I will be asking you some questions about your pregnancy and ____'s [refer to

child by name] birth. Your answers will give me a more complete picture of his [or her] overall health."

Because emotional factors also affect the outcome of pregnancy and the subsequent parent-child relationship, investigate concurrent crises during pregnancy and prenatal attitudes toward the fetus. It is best to approach the topic of parental acceptance of pregnancy through indirect questioning. Asking the parents if the pregnancy was planned is a leading statement, because they may respond affirmatively for fear of criticism if the pregnancy was unexpected. Rather, encourage parents to state their true reactions by referring to specific facts relating to the pregnancy, such as the spacing between offspring, an extended or short interval between marriage and conception, or a pregnancy during adolescence. The parent can choose to explore such statements with further explanations or, for the moment, may not be able to reveal such feelings. If the parent remains silent, return to this topic later in the interview.

Dietary History

Because parental concerns are common and nursing interventions are important in ensuring optimum nutrition, the dietary history is discussed in detail later in the "Nutritional Assessment" section later in this chapter.

Previous Illnesses, Injuries, and Surgeries

When inquiring about past illnesses, begin with a general question (such as, "What other illnesses has your child had?"). Because parents are most likely to recall serious health problems, ask specifically about colds, earaches, and childhood diseases, such as measles, rubella (German

GUIDELINES

Analyzing the Symptom: Pain

Type
Be as specific as possible. With young children, asking the parents how they know the child is in pain may help describe its type, location, and severity. For example, a parent may state, "My child must have a severe earache because she pulls at her ears, rolls her head on the floor, and screams. Nothing seems to help." Help older children describe the "hurt" by asking them if it is sharp, throbbing, dull, or stabbing. Record whatever words they use in quotes.

Location
Be specific. "Stomach pain" is too general a description. Children can better localize the pain if they are asked to "point with one finger to where it hurts" or to "point to where mommy or daddy would put a Band-Aid." Determine if the pain radiates by asking, "Does the pain stay there or move? Show me with your finger where the pain goes."

Severity
Severity is best determined by finding out how it affects the child's usual behavior. Pain that prevents a child from playing, interacting with others, sleeping, and eating is most often severe. Assess pain intensity using a rating scale, such as a numeric or Wong-Baker FACES Pain Rating Scale (see Chapter 30).

Duration
Include the duration, onset, and frequency. Describe these in terms of activity and behavior, such as "pain reported to last all night; child refused to sleep and cried intermittently."

Influencing Factors
Include anything that causes a change in the type, location, severity, or duration of the pain: (1) precipitating events (those that cause or increase the pain), (2) relieving events (those that lessen the pain, such as medications), (3) temporal events (times when the pain is relieved or increased), (4) positional events (standing, sitting, lying down), and (5) associated events (meals, stress, coughing).

GUIDELINES

Taking an Allergy History

- Has your child ever taken any prescription or over-the-counter medications that have disagreed with him or her or caused an allergic reaction? If yes, can you remember the name(s) of this medication(s)?
- Can you describe the reaction?
- Was the medication taken by mouth (as a tablet or syrup), or was it an injection?
- How soon after starting the medication did the reaction happen?
- How long ago did this happen?
- Did anyone tell you it was an allergic reaction, or did you decide for yourself?
- Has your child ever taken this medication, or a similar one, again? If yes, did your child experience the same problems?
- Have you told the physicians or nurses about your child's reaction or allergy?

Current Medications

Inquire about current medications, including vitamins, antipyretics (especially aspirin), antibiotics, antihistamines, decongestants, nutritional supplements, or herbs and homeopathic medications. List all medications, including name, dose, schedule, duration, and reasons for use. Often parents are unaware of a medication's actual name. Whenever possible, ask the parents to bring the containers with them to the next visit, or ask for the name of the pharmacy and call for a list of all the child's recent prescription medications. However, this list will not include over-the-counter medications, which are important to know.

Immunizations

A record of all immunizations is essential. As many parents are unaware of the exact name and date of each immunization, sources of information include the child's health care provider, school record, and the state's centralized immunization registry. All immunizations and "boosters" are listed, stating (1) the name of the specific disease, (2) the number of injections, (3) the dosage (sometimes lesser amounts are given if a reaction is anticipated), (4) the date when administered, and (5) the occurrence of any reaction following immunization. Children should be screened for contraindications and precautions before every vaccine is administered.

Growth and Development

Review the child's growth including the following:
- Measurements of weight, length, and head circumference at birth
- Patterns of growth on the growth chart and any significant deviations from previous percentiles
- Concerns about growth from the family or child
- Developmental milestones include:
  - Age of holding up head steadily
  - Age of sitting alone without support
  - Age of walking without assistance
  - Age of saying first words with meaning
  - Age of achieving bladder and bowel control
- Present grade in school
- Scholastic performance
- If the child has a best friend
- Interactions with other children, peers, and adults

Use specific and detailed questions when inquiring about each developmental milestone. For example, "sitting up" can mean many different activities, such as sitting propped up, sitting in someone's lap, sitting with support, sitting up alone but in a hyperflexed position for

measles), chickenpox, mumps, pertussis (whooping cough), diphtheria, tuberculosis, scarlet fever, strep throat, recurrent ear infections, gastroesophageal reflux, tonsillitis, or allergic manifestations.

In addition to illnesses, ask about injuries that required medical intervention, surgeries, procedures, and hospitalizations, including the dates of each incident. Focus on injuries (such as, accidental falls, poisoning, choking, concussion, fractures, or burns) because these may be potential areas for parental guidance.

Allergies

Ask about commonly known allergic disorders, such as hay fever and asthma; unusual reactions to drugs, food, or latex products; and reactions to other contact agents, such as poisonous plants, animals, household products, or fabrics. If asked appropriate questions, most people can give reliable information about drug reactions (see Guidelines box: Taking an Allergy History).

! NURSING ALERT

Information about allergic reactions to drugs or other products is essential. Failure to document a serious reaction places the child at risk if the agent is given.

BOX 29.4   Habits to Explore During a Health Interview

- Behavior patterns, such as nail biting, thumb sucking, pica (habitual ingestion of nonfood substances), rituals ("security" blanket or toy), and unusual movements (head banging, rocking, overt masturbation, walking on toes)
- Activities of daily living, such as hours of sleep and arising, duration of nighttime sleep and naps, type and duration of exercise, regularity of stools and urination, age of toilet training, and daytime or nighttime bedwetting
- Unusual disposition; response to frustration
- Use or abuse of alcohol, drugs, coffee, or tobacco

BOX 29.5   Anticipatory Guidance—Sexuality

12 to 14 Years of Age
Have adolescent identify a supportive adult with whom to discuss sexuality issues and concerns.
Discuss the advantages of delaying sexual activity.
Discuss making responsible decisions regarding normal sexual feelings.
Discuss the roles of gender, peer pressure, and the media in sexual decision making.
Discuss contraceptive options (advantages and disadvantages).
Provide education regarding sexually transmitted infections (STIs), including human immunodeficiency virus (HIV) infection; clarify risks, and discuss condoms.
Discuss abuse prevention, including avoiding dangerous situations, the role of drugs and alcohol, and the use of self-defense.
Have the adolescent clarify his or her values, needs, and ability to be assertive.
If the adolescent is sexually active, discuss limiting partners, use of condoms, and contraceptive options.
Have a confidential interview with the adolescent (including a sexual history).
Discuss the evolution of sexual identity and expression.
Discuss breast examination or testicular examination.

15 to 18 Years of Age
Support delaying sexual activity.
Discuss alternatives to intercourse.
Discuss "When are you ready for sex?"
Clarify values; encourage responsible decision making.
Discuss consequences of unprotected sex: Early pregnancy; STIs, including HIV infection.
Discuss negotiating with partners and barriers to safer sex.
If the adolescent is sexually active, discuss limiting partners, use of condoms, and contraceptive options.
Emphasize that sex should be safe and pleasurable for both partners.
Have a confidential interview with the adolescent.
Discuss concerns about sexual expression and identity.

Data from Wright, K. (1997). Anticipatory guidance: Developing a healthy sexuality. *Pediatric Annals, 26*(2 suppl), S142–S144, C3; Fonseca, H., & Greydanus, D. (2007). Sexuality in the child, teen and young adult: Concepts for the clinician. *Primary Care: Clinics in Office Practice, 34*, 275–292.

assisted balance, or sitting up unsupported with the back slightly rounded. A clue to misunderstanding of the requested activity may be an unusually early age of achievement.

Habits

Habits are an important area to explore (Box 29.4). Parents frequently express concerns during this part of the history. Encourage their input by saying, "Please tell me any concerns you have about your child's habits, activities, or development." Investigate further any concerns that parents express.

One of the most common concerns relates to sleep. Many children develop a normal sleep pattern, and all that is required during the assessment is a general overview of nighttime sleep and nap schedules. However, a number of children develop sleep problems. When sleep problems occur, the nurse needs a more detailed sleep history to guide appropriate interventions.

Habits related to use of chemicals apply primarily to older children and adolescents. If a child admits to smoking, drinking, or using drugs, ask about the quantity and frequency. Questions such as "Many kids your age are experimenting with drugs and alcohol; have you ever had any drugs or alcohol?" may give more reliable data than questions such as "How much do you drink?" or "How often do you drink or take drugs?" Clarify that "drinking" includes all types of alcohol, including beer and wine. When quantities such as a "glass" of wine or a "can" of beer are given, ask about the size of the container.

If older children deny use of chemical substances, inquire about past experimentation. Asking, "You mean you never tried to smoke or drink?" implies that the nurse expects some such activity, and the child may be more inclined to answer truthfully. Be aware of the confidential nature of such questioning, the adverse effect that the parents' presence may have on the adolescent's willingness to answer, and the fact that self-reporting may not be an accurate account of chemical abuse.

Reproductive Health History

The reproductive health history is an essential component of adolescents' health assessment. The history uncovers areas of concern related to sexual activity, alerts the nurse to circumstances that may indicate screening for sexually transmitted infections or testing for pregnancy, and provides information related to the need for reproductive health counseling, such as safer sex practices. Box 29.5 gives guidelines for anticipatory guidance topics for parents and adolescents.

One approach to initiating a conversation about reproductive health concerns is to begin with a history of peer interactions. Open-ended statements and questions (such as, "Tell me about your social life" or "Who are your closest friends?") generally lead into a discussion of dating and sexual issues. To probe further, include questions about the adolescent's attitudes on such topics as sex education, "going steady," "living together," and premarital sex. Phrase questions to reflect concern rather than judgment or criticism of sexual practices.

In any conversation regarding reproductive health history, be aware of the language that is used in either eliciting or conveying sexual information. For example, avoid asking whether the adolescent is "sexually active," because this term is broadly defined. "Are you having sex with anyone?" is probably the most direct and best understood question. Because same-sex experimentation may occur, refer to all sexual contacts in non-gender terms, such as "anyone" or "partners," rather than "girlfriends" or "boyfriends."

Family Health History

The family health history is used primarily to discover any genetic or chronic diseases affecting the child's family members. Assess for the presence or absence of consanguinity (if anyone in the family is related to their spouse's/partner's family). Family health history is generally confined to first-degree relatives (parents, siblings, grandparents, and immediate aunts and uncles). Information includes age, marital status, health status, cause of death if deceased, and any evidence of conditions, such as early heart disease, stroke, sudden death from unknown cause, hypercholesterolemia, hypertension, cancer, diabetes mellitus, obesity, congenital anomalies, allergies, asthma, seizures, tuberculosis, abnormal bleeding, sickle cell disease, cognitive impairment, hearing or visual deficits, and psychiatric disorders (e.g., depression, psychosis, or emotional problems). Confirm the accuracy of the reported disorders by inquiring about the symptoms, course, treatment, and sequelae of each diagnosis.

Geographic Location

One of the important areas to explore when assessing the family health history is geographic location, including the birthplace and travel to different areas in or outside of the country, for identification of possible exposure to endemic diseases. Include current and past housing, whether they rent or own, whether they reside in an urban or rural location, the age of the home, and whether there are significant threats such as molds or pests within the housing structure. Although the primary interest is the child's temporary residence in various localities, also inquire about close family members' travel, especially during tours of military service or business trips. Children are especially susceptible to parasitic infestation in areas of poor sanitary conditions and to vector-borne diseases, such as those from mosquitoes or ticks in warm and humid or heavily wooded regions.

Family Structure

Assessment of the family, both its structure and function, is an important component of the history-taking process. Because the quality of the functional relationship between the child and family members is a major factor in emotional and physical health, family assessment is discussed separately and in greater detail apart from the more traditional health history.

Family assessment is the collection of data about the composition of the family and the relationships among its members. In its broadest sense, *family* refers to all those individuals who are considered by the family member to be significant to the nuclear unit, including relatives, friends, and social groups (e.g., school and church). Although family assessment is not family therapy, it can and frequently is therapeutic. Involving family members in discussing family characteristics and activities can provide insight into family dynamics and relationships.

Because of the time involved in performing an in-depth family assessment as presented here, be selective in deciding when knowledge of family function may facilitate nursing care (see Guidelines box: Initiating a Comprehensive Family Assessment). During brief contacts with families, a full assessment is not appropriate, and screening with one or two questions from each category may reflect the health of the family system or the need for additional assessment.

GUIDELINES
Initiating a Comprehensive Family Assessment

Perform a comprehensive assessment on the following:
- Children receiving comprehensive well-child care
- Children experiencing major stressful life events (e.g., chronic illness, disability, parental divorce, death of a family member)
- Children requiring extensive home care
- Children with developmental delays
- Children with repeated accidental injuries and those with suspected child abuse
- Children with behavioral or physical problems that could be caused by family dysfunction

---

The most common method of eliciting information on the family structure is to interview family members. The principal areas of concern are family composition, home and community environment, occupation and education of family members, and cultural and religious traditions.

Psychosocial History

The traditional medical history includes a personal and social section that concentrates on children's personal status, such as school adjustment and any unusual habits, and the family and home environment. Because several personal aspects are covered under development and habits, only those issues related to children's ability to cope and their self-concept are presented here.

Through observation, obtain a general idea of how children handle themselves in terms of confidence in dealing with others, answering questions, and coping with new situations. Observe the parent-child relationship for the types of messages sent to children about their coping skills and self-worth. Do the parents treat the child with respect, focusing on strengths, or is the interaction one of constant reprimands with emphasis on weaknesses and faults? Do the parents help the child learn new coping strategies or support the ones the child uses?

Parent-child interactions also convey messages about body image. Do the parents label the child and body parts (such as, "bad boy," "skinny legs," or "ugly scar")? Do the parents handle the child gently, using soothing touch to calm an anxious child, or do they treat the child roughly, using force or restraint to make the child obey? If the child touches certain parts of the body, such as the genitalia, do the parents make comments that suggest a negative connotation?

With older children, many of the communication strategies discussed earlier in this chapter are useful in eliciting more definitive information about their coping and self-concept. Children can name or write down five things they like and dislike about themselves. The nurse can use sentence completion statements, such as "The thing I like best (or worst) about myself is _____;" "If I could change one thing about myself, it would be _____;" or "When I am scared, I _____."

Review of Systems

The review of systems is a specific review of each body system, following an order similar to that of the physical examination (see Guidelines box: Review of Systems). Often the history of the present illness provides a complete review of the system involved in the chief complaint. Because asking questions about other body systems may appear irrelevant to the parents or child, precede the questioning with an explanation of why the data are necessary (similar to the explanation concerning the relevance of the birth history) and reassure the parents that the child's main problem has not been forgotten.

Begin the review of a specific system with a broad statement (such as, "How has your child's general health been?" or "Has your child had any problems with his eyes?"). If the parent states that the child has had problems with some body function, pursue this with an encouraging statement, such as "Tell me more about that." If the parent denies any problems, query for specific symptoms (e.g., "Any headaches, bumping into objects, or squinting?"). If the parent confirms the absence of such symptoms, record positive statements in the history, such as "Mother denies headaches, bumping into objects, and squinting." In this way, anyone who reviews the health history is aware of exactly what symptoms were investigated.

NUTRITIONAL ASSESSMENT
Dietary Intake

Knowledge of the child's dietary intake is an essential component of a nutritional assessment. However, it is also one of the most difficult

GUIDELINES
Review of Systems

Constitutional: Overall state of health, fatigue, recent or unexplained weight gain or loss (period of time for either), contributing factors (change of diet, illness, altered appetite), exercise tolerance, fevers (time of day), chills, night sweats (unrelated to climatic conditions), general ability to carry out activities of daily living

Integument: Pruritus, pigment or other color changes (including birthmarks), acne, eruptions, rashes (location), bruises, petechiae, excessive dryness, general texture, tattoos or piercings, disorders or deformities of nails, hair growth or loss, hair color change (for adolescents, use of hair dyes or other potentially toxic substances, such as hair straighteners)

Eyes: Visual problems (behaviors indicative of blurred vision, such as bumping into objects, clumsiness, sitting close to television, holding a book close to face, writing with head near desk, squinting, rubbing the eyes, bending head in an awkward position), cross-eyes (strabismus), eye infections, edema of lids, excessive tearing, use of glasses or contact lenses, date of last vision examination

Ears/nose/mouth/throat: Earaches, ear discharge, evidence of hearing loss (ask about behaviors such as the need to repeat requests, loud speech, inattentive behavior), results of any previous auditory testing, nosebleeds (epistaxis), constant or frequent runny or stuffy nose, nasal obstruction (difficulty breathing), alteration or loss of sense of smell, mouth breathing, gum bleeding, number of teeth and pattern of eruption/loss, toothaches, tooth brushing, use of fluoride, difficulty with teething (symptoms), last visit to the dentist (especially if temporary dentition is complete), sore throats, difficulty swallowing, choking, hoarseness or other voice irregularities

Neck: Pain, limitation of movement, stiffness, difficulty holding head straight (torticollis), thyroid enlargement, enlarged nodes or other masses

Chest: Breast enlargement, discharge, masses; for adolescent girls, ask about breast self-examination

Respiratory: Chronic cough, wheezing, shortness of breath at rest or on exertion, difficulty breathing, snoring, sputum production, infections (pneumonia, tuberculosis), skin reaction from tuberculin testing

Cardiovascular: Cyanosis or fatigue on exertion, history of heart murmur or rheumatic fever, tachycardia, syncope, edema

Gastrointestinal: Appetite, nausea, vomiting (not associated with eating; may be indicative of brain tumor or increased intracranial pressure), abdominal pain, jaundice or yellowing skin or sclera, belching, flatulence, distention, diarrhea, constipation, recent change in bowel habits, blood in stools

Genitourinary: Pain on urination, frequency, hesitancy, urgency, hematuria, nocturia, polyuria, enuresis, unpleasant odor to urine, force of stream, discharge, change in size of scrotum, date and result of last urinalysis; for adolescents, sexually transmitted infection and type of treatment; for adolescent boys, ask about testicular self-examination

Gynecologic: Menarche, date of last menstrual period, regularity or problems with menstruation, vaginal discharge, pruritus; if sexually active, type of contraception, sexually transmitted infection and type of treatment; if sexually active with weakened immune system or if 21 years of age and older, date and result of last Papanicolaou (Pap) smear; obstetric history (as discussed under birth history, when applicable)

Musculoskeletal: Weakness, clumsiness, lack of coordination, unusual movements, scoliosis, back pain, joint pain or swelling, muscle pains or cramps, abnormal gait, deformity, fractures, serious sprains, activity level

Neurologic: Headaches, seizures, tremors, tics, dizziness, loss of consciousness episodes, loss of memory, developmental delays or concerns

Endocrine: Intolerance to heat or cold, excessive thirst or urination, excessive sweating, salt craving, rapid or slow growth, signs of early or late puberty

Hematologic/lymphatic: Easy bruising or bleeding, anemia, date and result of last blood count, blood transfusions, swollen or painful lymph nodes (cervical, axillary, inguinal)

Allergic/immunologic: Allergic responses, anaphylaxis, eczema, rhinitis, unusual sneezing, autoimmunity, recurrent infections, infections associated with unusual complications

Psychiatric: General affect, anxiety, depression, mood changes, hallucinations, attention span, tantrums, behavior problems, suicidal ideation, substance abuse

---

factors to assess. Individuals' recall of food consumption, especially amounts eaten, is frequently unreliable. The food intake history of children and adolescents is prone to reporting error, mostly in the form of underreporting. People from different cultures may have difficulty adequately describing the types of food they eat. Despite these obstacles, a dietary evaluation is a vital element of the child's health assessment.

The *Dietary Reference Intakes (DRIs)* are a set of four evidence-based nutrient reference values that provide quantitative estimates of nutrient intake for use in assessing and planning dietary intake (US Department of Agriculture, National Agricultural Library, 2014). The specific DRIs are as follows:

Estimated Average Requirement (EAR): Estimated to meet the nutrient requirement of one-half of healthy individuals for a specific age and gender group

Recommended Dietary Allowance (RDA): Sufficient to meet the nutrient requirement of nearly all healthy individuals for a specific age and gender group

Adequate Intake (AI): Based on estimates of nutrient intake by healthy individuals

Tolerable Upper Intake Level (UL): Highest nutrient intake level likely to pose no risk for adverse health effects

The US Department of Agriculture has an online interactive DRI tool for health care professionals to calculate nutrient requirements based on age, gender, height, weight, and activity (http://fnic.nal.usda.gov/ fnic/interactiveDRI/), although it is important to note that individual requirements may vary.

Fig. 29.4 illustrates ChooseMyPlate.gov, which describes the five food groups forming the foundation for a healthy diet. MyPlate Kids' Place provides resources to help families build healthy meals and be active. Specific questions used to conduct a nutritional assessment are given in Box 29.6. Every nutritional assessment should begin with a dietary history. The exact questions used to elicit a dietary history vary with the child's age. In general, the younger the child, the more specific and detailed the history should be. The overview elicited from the dietary history can be helpful in evaluating food frequency records. The history is also concerned with financial and cultural factors that influence food selection and preparation (see Cultural Considerations box: Food Practices).

Clinical Examination of Nutrition

A significant amount of information regarding nutritional deficiencies comes from a clinical examination, especially from assessing the skin, hair, teeth, gums, lips, tongue, and eyes. Hair, skin, and mouth are vulnerable because of the rapid turnover of epithelial and mucosal tissue. Table 29.1 summarizes some clinical signs of possible nutritional deficiency or excess. Few are diagnostic for a specific nutrient, and if suspicious signs are found, they must be confirmed with dietary and biochemical data.

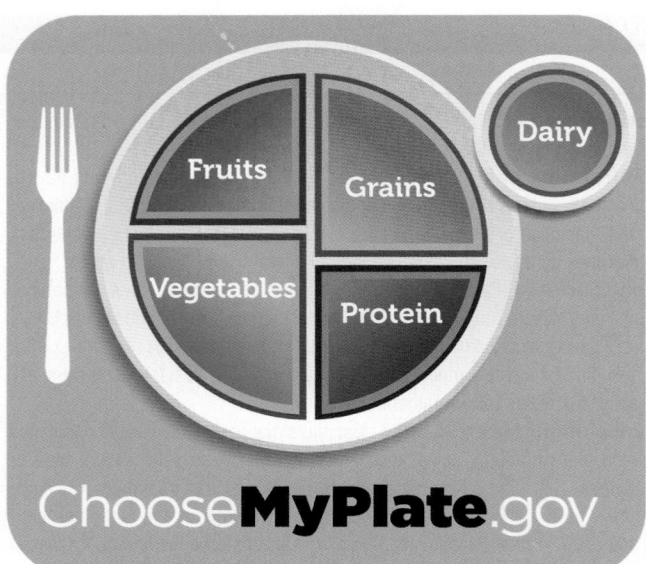

FIG 29.4 MyPlate. MyPlate advocates building a healthy plate by making half of your plate fruits and vegetables and the other half grains and lean protein. Avoiding oversized portions, making half your grains whole grains, and drinking fat-free or low-fat (1%) milk are among the recommendations for a healthy diet. (From US Department of Agriculture, Center for Nutrition Policy and Promotion. (2015). *MyPlate.* Retrieved from www.ChooseMyPlate.gov.)

🌐 CULTURAL CONSIDERATIONS
Food Practices

Because cultural practices are prevalent in food preparation, consider carefully the kinds of questions that are asked and the judgments made during counseling. For example, some cultures, such as Hispanic, African-American, and Native American, include many vegetables, legumes, and starches in their diet that together provide sufficient essential amino acids even though the actual amount of meat or dairy protein is low.

The most common and probably easiest method of assessing daily intake is the 24-hour recall. The child or parent recalls every item eaten in the past 24 hours and the approximate amounts. The 24-hour recall is most beneficial when it represents a typical day's intake. Some of the difficulties with a daily recall are the family's inability to remember exactly what was eaten and inaccurate estimation of portion size. To increase accuracy of reporting portion sizes, the use of food models and additional questions are recommended. In general, this method is most useful in providing qualitative information about the child's diet.

To improve the reliability of the daily recall, the family can complete a **food diary** by recording every food and liquid consumed for a certain number of days. A 3-day record consisting of 2 weekdays and 1 weekend day is representative for most people. Providing specific charts to record intake can improve compliance. The family should record items immediately after eating.

Anthropometry, an essential parameter of nutritional status, is the measurement of height, weight, head circumference, proportions, skinfold thickness, and arm circumference in children. Height and head circumference reflect past nutrition, whereas weight, skinfold thickness, and arm circumference reflect present nutritional status, especially of protein and fat reserves. Skinfold thickness is a measurement of the body's fat content because approximately one-half the body's total fat stores are

directly beneath the skin. The upper arm muscle circumference is correlated with measurements of total muscle mass. Because muscle serves as the body's major protein reserve, this measurement is considered an index of the body's protein stores. Ideally, growth measurements are recorded over time, and comparisons are made regarding the velocity of growth and weight gain based on previous and present values.

Numerous biochemical tests are available for assessing nutritional status. The most common laboratory studies to assess children for undernutrition are hemoglobin, red blood cell indices, and serum albumin or prealbumin. For obese children, fasting serum glucose, lipids, and liver function studies may be performed to assess for complications.

Evaluation of Nutritional Assessment

After collecting the data needed for a thorough nutritional assessment, evaluate the findings to plan appropriate counseling. From the data, assess whether the child is malnourished, at risk for becoming malnourished, well-nourished with adequate reserves, or overweight or obese.

Analyze the daily food diary for the variety and amounts of foods suggested in MyPlate (see Fig. 29.4). For example, if the list includes no vegetables, inquire about this rather than assuming that the child dislikes vegetables, because it is possible that none were served that day. Also, evaluate the information in terms of the family's ethnic practices and financial resources. Encouraging increased protein intake with additional meat is not always feasible for families on a limited budget and may conflict with food practices that use meat sparingly, such as in Asian meal preparation.

GENERAL APPROACHES TOWARD EXAMINING THE CHILD

SEQUENCE OF THE EXAMINATION

Ordinarily, the sequence for examining patients follows a head-to-toe direction. The main function of such a systematic approach is to provide a general guideline for assessment of each body area to avoid omitting segments of the examination. The standard recording of data also facilitates exchange of information among different professionals. In examining children, this orderly sequence is frequently altered to accommodate the child's developmental needs, although the examination is recorded following the head-to-toe model. Using developmental and chronologic age as the main criteria for assessing each body system accomplishes several goals:

- Minimizes stress and anxiety associated with assessment of various body parts
- Fosters a trusting nurse-child-parent relationship
- Allows for maximum preparation of the child
- Preserves the essential security of the parent-child relationship, especially with young children
- Maximizes the accuracy and reliability of assessment findings

PREPARATION OF THE CHILD

Although the physical examination consists of painless procedures, for some children the use of a tight arm cuff, probes in the ears and mouth, pressure on the abdomen, and a cold piece of metal to listen to the chest are stressful. In addition to that discussion, general guidelines related to the examining process are given in the Guidelines box: Performing Pediatric Physical Examination.

The physical examination should be as pleasant as possible, as well as educational. The paper-doll technique is a useful approach to teaching children about the body part that is being examined (Fig. 29.5). At the

BOX 29.6   Dietary Reference Intakes for an Individual

Estimated Average Requirement (EAR): Used to examine the possibility of inadequacy.

Recommended Dietary Allowance (RDA): Dietary intake at or above this level usually has a low probability of inadequacy.

Adequate Intake (AI): Dietary intake at or above this level usually has a low probability of inadequacy.

Tolerable Upper Intake Level (UL): Dietary intake above this level usually places an individual at risk for adverse effects from excessive nutrient intake.

Dietary History

What are the family's usual mealtimes?

Do family members eat together or at separate times?

Who does the family grocery shopping and meal preparation?

How much money is spent to buy food each week?

How are most foods prepared (baked, broiled, fried, other)?

How often does the family or your child eat out?
- What kinds of restaurants do you go to?
- What kinds of food does your child typically eat at restaurants?

Does your child eat breakfast regularly?

Where does your child eat lunch?

What are your child's favorite foods, beverages, and snacks?
- What are the average amounts eaten per day?
- What foods are artificially sweetened?
- What are your child's snacking habits?
- When are sweet foods usually eaten?
- What are your child's tooth brushing habits?

What special cultural practices are followed? What ethnic foods are eaten?

What foods and beverages does your child dislike?

How would you describe your child's usual appetite (hearty eater, picky eater)?

What are your child's feeding habits (breast, bottle, cup, spoon, eats by self, needs assistance, any special devices)?

Does your child take vitamins or other supplements? Do they contain iron or fluoride?

Does your child have any known or suspected food allergies? Is your child on a special diet?

Has your child lost or gained weight recently?

Are there any feeding problems (excessive fussiness, spitting up, colic, difficulty sucking or swallowing)? Are there any dental problems or appliances, such as braces, that affect eating?

What types of exercise does your child do regularly?

Is there a family history of cancer, diabetes, heart disease, high blood pressure, or obesity?

Additional Questions for Infants

What was the infant's birth weight? When did it double? Triple?

Was the infant premature?

Are you breastfeeding, or have you breastfed your infant? For how long?

If you use a formula, what is the brand?
- How long has the infant been taking it?
- How many ounces does the infant drink per day?

Are you giving the infant cow's milk (whole, low-fat, skim)?
- When did you start?
- How many ounces does the infant drink per day?

Do you give your infant extra fluids (water, juice)?

If the infant takes a bottle to bed at nap or nighttime, what is in the bottle?

At what age did the child start on cereal, vegetables, meat or other protein sources, fruit or juice, finger food, and table food?

Do you make your own baby food or use commercial foods, such as infant cereal?

Does the infant take a vitamin or mineral supplement? If so, what type?

Has the infant had an allergic reaction to any food(s)? If so, list the foods and describe the reaction.

Does the infant spit up frequently; have unusually loose stools; or have hard, dry stools? If so, how often?

How often do you feed your infant?

How would you describe your infant's appetite?

Adapted from Murphy, S.P., Poos, M.I. (2002). Dietary reference intakes: summary of applications in dietary assessment. *Public Health Nutrition, 5*(6A suppl), 843–849.

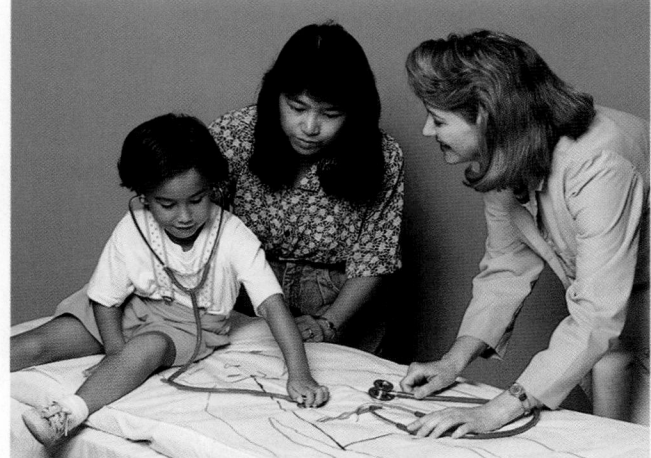

FIG 29.5 Using the paper-doll technique to prepare a child for physical examination.

conclusion of the visit, the child can bring home the paper doll as a memento.

Table 29.2 summarizes guidelines for positioning, preparing, and examining children at various ages. Because no child fits precisely into one age category, it may be necessary to vary the approach after a preliminary assessment of the child's developmental achievements and needs. Even with the best approach, many toddlers are uncooperative and inconsolable for much of the physical examination. However, some seem intrigued by the new surroundings and unusual equipment and respond more like preschoolers than toddlers. Likewise, some early preschoolers may require more of the "security measures" used with younger children, such as continued parent-child contact, and less of the preparatory measures used with preschoolers, such as playing with the equipment before and during the actual examination (Fig. 29.6).

PHYSICAL EXAMINATION

Although the approach to and sequence of the physical examination differ according to the child's age, the following discussion outlines the traditional model for physical assessment. The focus includes all pediatric age groups. Because the physical examination is a vital part of preventive pediatric care, Fig. 29.7 gives a schedule for periodic health visits.

TABLE 29.1   Clinical Assessment of Nutritional Status

Evidence of Adequate Nutrition	Evidence of Deficient or Excess Nutrition	Deficiency or Excess*
General Growth		
Normal weight gain, growth velocity, and head growth for age and gender	Weight loss or poor weight gain, growth failure	Protein, calories, fats, and other essential nutrients, especially vitamin A, pyridoxine, niacin, calcium, iodine, manganese, zinc
	Excess weight gain	Excess calories
Sexual development appropriate for age	Delayed sexual development	Excess vitamins A, D
Skin		
Smooth, slightly dry to touch	Hardening and scaling	Vitamin A
Elastic and firm	Seborrheic dermatitis	Excess niacin
Absence of lesions	Dry, rough, petechiae	Riboflavin
Color appropriate to genetic background	Delayed wound healing	Vitamin C
	Scaly dermatitis on exposed surfaces	Riboflavin, vitamin C, zinc
	Wrinkled, flabby	Niacin
	Crusted lesions around orifices, especially nares	Protein, calories, zinc
	Pruritus	Excess vitamin A, riboflavin, niacin
	Poor turgor	Water, sodium
	Edema	Protein, thiamine
		Excess sodium
	Yellow tinge (jaundice)	Vitamin B_{12}
		Excess vitamin A, niacin
	Depigmentation	Protein, calories
	Pallor (anemia)	Pyridoxine, folic acid, vitamins B_{12}, C, E (in premature infants), iron
		Excess vitamin C, zinc
	Paresthesia	Excess riboflavin
Hair		
Lustrous, silky, strong, elastic	Stringy, friable, dull, dry, thin	Protein, calories
	Alopecia	Protein, calories, zinc
	Depigmentation	Protein, calories, copper
	Raised areas around hair follicles	Vitamin C
Head		
Even molding, occipital prominence, symmetric facial features	Softening of cranial bones, prominence of frontal bones, skull flat and depressed toward middle	Vitamin D
Fused sutures after 18 months	Delayed fusion of sutures	Vitamin D
	Hard, tender lumps in occiput	Excess vitamin A
	Headache	Excess thiamine
Neck		
Thyroid not visible, palpable in midline	Thyroid enlarged, may be grossly visible	Iodine
Eyes		
Clear, bright	Hardening and scaling of cornea and conjunctiva	Vitamin A
Good night vision	Night blindness	Vitamin A
Conjunctiva: pink, glossy	Burning, itching, photophobia, cataracts, corneal vascularization	Riboflavin
Ears		
Tympanic membrane: pliable	Calcified (hearing loss)	Excess vitamin D
Nose		
Smooth, intact nasal angle	Irritation and cracks at nasal angle	Riboflavin
		Excess vitamin A
Mouth		
Lips: smooth, moist, darker color than skin	Fissures and inflammation at corners	Riboflavin
		Excess vitamin A
Gums: firm, coral pink, stippled	Spongy, friable, swollen, bluish red or black, bleed easily	Vitamin C
Mucous membranes: bright pink, smooth, moist	Stomatitis	Niacin

TABLE 29.1   Clinical Assessment of Nutritional Status—cont'd

Evidence of Adequate Nutrition	Evidence of Deficient or Excess Nutrition	Deficiency or Excess*
Tongue: rough texture, no lesions, taste sensation	Glossitis	Niacin, riboflavin, folic acid
	Diminished taste sensation	Zinc
Teeth: uniform white color, smooth, intact	Brown mottling, pits, fissures	Excess fluoride
	Defective enamel	Vitamins A, C, D, calcium, phosphorus
	Caries	Excess carbohydrates
Chest		
In infants, shape almost circular	Depressed lower portion of rib cage	Vitamin D
In children, lateral diameter increased in proportion to anteroposterior diameter	Sharp protrusion of sternum	Vitamin D
Smooth costochondral junctions	Enlarged costochondral junctions	Vitamins C, D
Breast development: normal for age	Delayed development	See under General Growth; especially zinc
Cardiovascular System		
Pulse and BP within normal limits	Palpitations	Thiamine
	Rapid pulse	Potassium
		Excess thiamine
	Arrhythmias	Magnesium, potassium
		Excess niacin, potassium
	Increased BP	Excess sodium
	Decreased BP	Thiamine
		Excess niacin
Abdomen		
In young children, cylindric and prominent	Distended, flabby, poor musculature	Protein, calories
	Prominent, large	Excess calories
In older children, flat	Potbelly, constipation	Vitamin D
Normal bowel habits	Diarrhea	Niacin
		Excess vitamin C
	Constipation	Excess calcium, potassium
Musculoskeletal System		
Muscles: firm, well-developed, equal strength bilaterally	Flabby, weak, generalized wasting	Protein, calories
	Weakness, pain, cramps	Thiamine, sodium, chloride, potassium, phosphorus, magnesium
		Excess thiamine
	Muscle twitching, tremors	Magnesium
	Muscular paralysis	Excess potassium
Spine: cervical and lumbar curves (double *S* curve)	Kyphosis, lordosis, scoliosis	Vitamin D
Extremities: symmetric; legs straight with minimum bowing	Bowing of extremities, knock knees	Vitamin D, calcium, phosphorus
	Epiphyseal enlargement	Vitamins A, D
	Bleeding into joints and muscles, joint swelling, pain	Vitamin C
Joints: flexible, full range of motion, no pain or stiffness	Thickening of cortex of long bones with pain and fragility, hard tender lumps in extremities	Excess vitamin A
	Osteoporosis of long bones	Calcium
		Excess vitamin D
Neurologic System		
Behavior: alert, responsive, emotionally stable	Listless, irritable, lethargic, apathetic (sometimes apprehensive, anxious, drowsy, mentally slow, confused)	Thiamine, niacin, pyridoxine, vitamin C, potassium, magnesium, iron, protein, calories
		Excess vitamins A, D, thiamine, folic acid, calcium
Absence of tetany, convulsions	Masklike facial expression, blurred speech, involuntary laughing	Excess manganese
	Convulsions	Thiamine, pyridoxine, vitamin D, calcium, magnesium
		Excess phosphorus (in relation to calcium)
Intact peripheral nervous system	Peripheral nervous system toxicity (unsteady gait, numb feet and hands, fine motor clumsiness)	Excess pyridoxine
Intact reflexes	Diminished or absent tendon reflexes	Thiamine, vitamin E

BP, Blood pressure.

*Nutrients listed are deficient unless specified as excess.

GUIDELINES
Performing Pediatric Physical Examination

Perform the examination in an appropriate, nonthreatening area:
- Have room well-lit and decorated with neutral colors.
- Have room temperature comfortably warm.
- Place all strange and potentially frightening equipment out of sight.
- Have some toys, dolls, stuffed animals, and games available for the child.
- If possible, have rooms decorated and equipped for different-age children.
- Provide privacy, especially for school-age children and adolescents.
- Provide time for play and becoming acquainted.

Observe behaviors that signal the child's readiness to cooperate:
- Talking to the nurse
- Making eye contact
- Accepting the offered equipment
- Allowing physical touching
- Choosing to sit on the examining table rather than the parent's lap

If signs of readiness are not observed, use the following techniques:
- Talk to the parent while essentially "ignoring" the child; gradually focus on the child or a favorite object, such as a doll.
- Make complimentary remarks about the child, such as about his or her appearance, dress, or a favorite object.
- Tell a funny story, or play a simple magic trick.
- Have a nonthreatening "friend" available, such as a hand puppet, to "talk" to the child for the nurse (see Fig. 4.26, A).

If the child refuses to cooperate, use the following techniques:
- Assess reason for uncooperative behavior; consider that a child who is unduly afraid may have had a traumatic experience.
- Try to involve the child and parent in the process.
- Avoid prolonged explanations about the examining procedure.
- Use a firm, direct approach regarding expected behavior.
- Perform the examination as quickly as possible.
- Have an attendant gently restrain the child.
- Minimize any disruptions or stimulation.
- Limit the number of people in the room.
- Use an isolated room.
- Use a quiet, calm, confident voice.

Begin the examination in a nonthreatening manner for young children or children who are fearful:
- Use activities that can be presented as games, such as test for cranial nerves (see Table 29.11 or parts of developmental screening tests (see Chapter 28).
- Use approaches such as Simon Says to encourage the child to make a face, squeeze a hand, stand on one foot, and so on.
- Use the paper-doll technique:
  1. Lay the child supine on an examining table or floor that is covered with a large sheet of paper.
  2. Trace around the child's body outline.
  3. Use the body outline to demonstrate what will be examined, such as drawing a heart and listening with a stethoscope before performing activity on the child.

If several children in the family will be examined, begin with the most cooperative child to model desired behavior.

Involve the child in the examination process:
- Provide choices, such as sitting on table or in parent's lap.
- Allow the child to handle or hold equipment.
- Encourage the child to use equipment on a doll, family member, or examiner.
- Explain each step of the procedure in simple language.
- Examine the child in a comfortable and secure position:
  - Sitting in parent's lap
  - Sitting upright if in respiratory distress

Proceed to examine the body in an organized sequence (usually head to toe) with the following exceptions:
- Alter sequence to accommodate needs of different-age children (see Table 29.2).
- Examine painful areas last.
- In an emergency situation, examine vital functions (airway, breathing, and circulation) and injured area first.

Reassure the child throughout the examination, especially about bodily concerns that arise during puberty.

Discuss findings with the family at the end of the examination.

Praise the child for cooperation during the examination; give a reward such as a small toy or sticker.

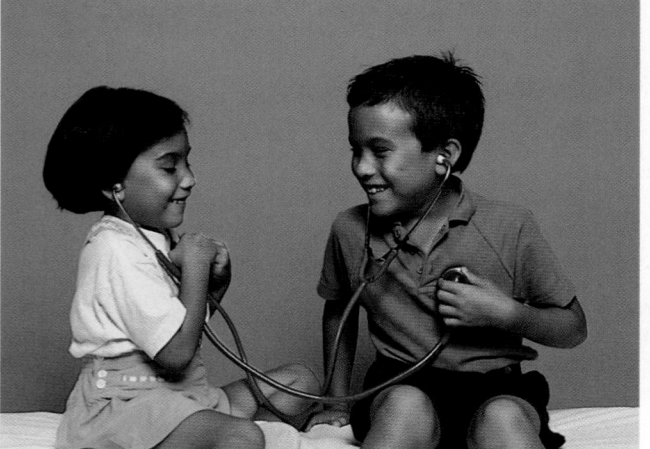

FIG 29.6 Preparing children for physical examination.

GROWTH MEASUREMENTS

Measurement of physical growth in children is a key element in evaluating their health status. Physical growth parameters include weight, height (length), skinfold thickness, arm circumference, and head circumference. Values for these growth parameters are plotted on percentile charts, and the child's measurements in percentiles are compared with those of the general population.

Growth Charts

Growth charts use a series of percentile curves to demonstrate the distribution of body measurements in children. The Centers for Disease Control and Prevention recommend that the World Health Organization growth standards be used to monitor growth for infants and children between 0 and 2 years of age. Because breastfeeding is the recommended standard for infant feeding, the World Health Organization growth charts are used; they reflect growth patterns among children who were predominately breastfed for at least 4 months and are still breastfeeding at 12 months of age. The Centers for Disease Control and Prevention growth charts (www.cdc.gov/growthcharts) are used for children 2 years of age and older.

TABLE 29.2   Age-Specific Approaches to Physical Examination During Childhood

Position	Sequence	Preparation
Infant		
Before able to sit alone—supine or prone, preferably in parent's lap; before 4 to 6 months, can place on examining table After able to sit alone—sitting in parent's lap whenever possible; if on table, place with parent in full view	If quiet, auscultate heart, lungs, and abdomen. Record heart and respiratory rates. Palpate and percuss same areas. Proceed in usual head-to-toe direction. Perform traumatic procedures last (eyes, ears, mouth [while crying]). Elicit reflexes as body part is examined. Elicit Moro reflex last.	Completely undress if room temperature permits. Leave diaper on male infant. Gain cooperation with distraction, bright objects, rattles, talking. Smile at infant; use soft, gentle voice. Pacify with bottle of sugar water or feeding. Enlist parent's aid for restraining to examine ears, mouth. Avoid abrupt, jerky movements.
Toddler		
Sitting or standing on or near parent Prone or supine in parent's lap	Inspect body area through play: "Count fingers," "tickle toes." Use minimum physical contact initially. Introduce equipment slowly. Auscultate, percuss, palpate whenever quiet. Perform traumatic procedures last (same as for infant).	Have parent remove outer clothing. Remove underwear as body part is examined. Allow toddler to inspect equipment; demonstrating use of equipment is usually ineffective. If uncooperative, perform procedures quickly. Use restraint when appropriate; request parent's assistance. Talk about examination if cooperative; use short phrases. Praise for cooperative behavior.
Preschool Child		
Prefer standing or sitting Usually cooperative prone or supine Prefer parent's closeness	If cooperative, proceed in head-to-toe direction. If uncooperative, proceed as with toddler.	Request self-undressing. Allow to wear underpants if shy. Offer equipment for inspection; briefly demonstrate use. Make up story about procedure (e.g., "I'm seeing how strong your muscles are" [blood pressure]). Use paper-doll technique. Give choices when possible. Expect cooperation; use positive statements (e.g., "Open your mouth").
School-Age Child		
Prefer sitting Cooperative in most positions Younger child prefers parent's presence Older child may prefer privacy	Proceed in head-to-toe direction. May examine genitalia last in older child.	Respect need for privacy. Request self-undressing. Allow to wear underpants. Give gown to wear. Explain purpose of equipment and significance of procedure, such as otoscope to see eardrum, which is necessary for hearing. Teach about body function and care.
Adolescent		
Same as for school-age child Offer option of parent's presence	Same as older school-age child. May examine genitalia last.	Allow to undress in private. Give gown. Expose only area to be examined. Respect need for privacy. Explain findings during examination (e.g., "Your muscles are firm and strong"). Matter-of-factly comment about sexual development (e.g., "Your breasts are developing as they should be"). Emphasize normalcy of development. Examine genitalia as any other body part; may leave to end.

Children whose growth may be questionable include the following:

- Children whose height and weight percentiles are widely disparate (e.g., height in the 10th percentile and weight in the 90th percentile, especially with above-average skinfold thickness)
- Children who fail to follow the expected growth velocity in height and weight, especially during the rapid growth periods of infancy and adolescence
- Children who show a sudden increase (except during normal puberty) or decrease in a previously steady growth pattern (i.e., crossing two major percentile lines after 3 years of age)
- Children who are short in the absence of short parents

Because growth is a continuous but uneven process, the most reliable evaluation lies in comparing growth measurements over time because they reflect change. It is important to remember that normal growth patterns vary among children the same age (Fig. 29.8).

Clinical Preventive Services for Normal-Risk Children*

	Infancy							Early Childhood							Middle Childhood						Adolescence							
Age	Newborn	3-5 d	By1mo	2 mo	4 mo	6 mo	9 mo	12mo	15mo	18mo	24mo	30mo	3 y	4 y	5 y	6 y	7 y	8 y	9 y	10 y	11 y	12 y	13 y	14 y	15 y	16 y	17 y	18 y
History Initial/Interval	•	•	•	•	•	•	•	•	•	•	•	•	•	•	•	•	•	•	•	•	•	•	•	•	•	•	•	•
Measurements																												
Length/Height and Weight	•	•	•	•	•	•	•	•	•	•	•	•	•	•	•	•	•	•	•	•	•	•	•	•	•	•	•	•
Head Circumference	•	•	•	•	•	•	•	•	•	•	•																	
Weight for Length	•	•	•	•	•	•	•	•	•	•																		
Body Mass Index											•	•	•	•	•	•	•	•	•	•	•	•	•	•	•	•	•	•
Blood Pressure	★	★	★	★	★	★	★	★	★	★	★	★	•	•	•	•	•	•	•	•	•	•	•	•	•	•	•	•
Sensory Screening																												
Vision	★	★	★	★	★	★	★	★	★	★	★	★	•	•	•	•	★	•	★	•	★	•	★	★	•	★	★	•
Hearing	•	★	★	★	★	★	★	★	★	★	★	★	★	•	•	•	★	•	★	•	★	★	★	★	★	★	★	★
Developmental/ Behavioral Assessment																												
Developmental Screening							•			•		•																
Autism Screening										•	•																	
Developmental Surveillance	•	•	•	•	•	•		•	•		•		•	•	•	•	•	•	•	•	•	•	•	•	•	•	•	•
Psychosocial/ Behavioral Assessment	•	•	•	•	•	•	•	•	•	•	•	•	•	•	•	•	•	•	•	•	•	•	•	•	•	•	•	•
Alcohol and Drug Use Assessment																					★	★	★	★	★	★	★	★
Physical Examination	•	•	•	•	•	•	•	•	•	•	•	•	•	•	•	•	•	•	•	•	•	•	•	•	•	•	•	•
Procedures																												
Newborn Metabolic/ Hemoglobin Screening	◄——	•	——►																									
Immunization	•	•	•	•	•	•	•	•	•	•	•	•	•	•	•	•	•	•	•	•	•	•	•	•	•	•	•	•
Hematocrit or Hemoglobin					★			•			★		★	★	★	★	★	★	★	★	★	★	★	★	★	★	★	★
Lead Screening						★	★	● or ★		★	● or ★		★	★	★	★												
Tuberculin Test			★			★		★		★	★		★	★	★	★	★	★	★	★	★	★	★	★	★	★	★	★
Dyslipidemia Screening											★			★		★		★	•	•		★	★	★	★	★	•	★
STI Screening																							★	★	★	★	★	★
Cervical Dysplasia Screening																							★	★	★	★	★	★
Oral Health						★	★	● or ★		● or ★	● or ★	● or ★	•			•												
Anticipatory Guidance	•	•	•	•	•	•	•	•	•	•	•	•	•	•	•	•	•	•	•	•	•	•	•	•	•	•	•	•

Key: • = To be performed; ★ = risk assessment to be performed, with appropriate action to follow, if positive; ◄—•—► = range during which a service may be provided, with the symbol indicating the preferred age.

*For current immunization schedules, see Chapter 31.

FIG 29.7 Preventive pediatric health care chart. (Adapted from American Academy of Pediatrics Committee on Practice and Ambulatory Medicine, Bright Futures Periodicity Schedule Workgroup. [2016]. 2016 Recommendations for preventive pediatric health care. *Pediatrics, 137*[1], 25–27.).

Length

The term length refers to measurements taken when children are supine (also referred to as *recumbent length*). Until children are 2 years of age and able to stand alone (or 36 months of age if using a chart for birth to 36 months), measure recumbent length using a length board and two measurers (Fig. 29.9, *A;* see the Evidence-Based Practice box: Linear Growth Measurement in Pediatrics). Because of the normally flexed position during infancy, fully extend the body by (1) holding the head in midline, (2) grasping the knees together gently, and (3) pushing down on the knees until the legs are fully extended and flat against the table. Place the head touching the headboard and the footboard firmly against the heels of the feet. A tape measure should not be used to measure the length of infants and children due to inaccuracy and unreliability (Foote, Brady, Burke, et al., 2014).

Height

The term height (or stature) refers to the measurement taken when a child is standing upright. Wall charts and flip-up horizontal bars (floppy-arm devices) mounted to weighing scales should not be used to measure the height of children (Foote, Brady, Burke, et al., 2014). These devices are not steady and do not maintain a right angle to the vertical ruler, preventing an accurate and reliable height. Measure height by having the child, with the shoes removed, stand as tall and straight as possible with the head in midline and the line of vision parallel to the ceiling and floor. Be certain the child's back is to the wall or other vertical flat surface, with the head, shoulder blades, buttocks, and heels touching the vertical surface (see Fig. 29.9, *B*). Check for and correct slumping of the shoulders, positional lordosis, bending of the knees, or raising of the heels.

> **! NURSING ALERT**
>
> Normally height is less if measured in the afternoon than in the morning. The time of day should be recorded when measurements are taken (Foote, Brady, Burke, et al., 2014). For children in whom there are concerns about growth, serial measurements should be taken at the same time of day, when possible, to establish an accurate growth velocity (see Evidence-Based Practice box: Linear Growth Measurement in Pediatrics).

For the most accurate measurement, use a wall-mounted unit (stadiometer; see Fig. 29.9). To improvise a flat, vertical surface for measuring height, attach a paper or metal tape or yardstick to the wall, position the child adjacent to the tape, and place a three-dimensional object, such as a thick book or box, on top of the head. Rest the side

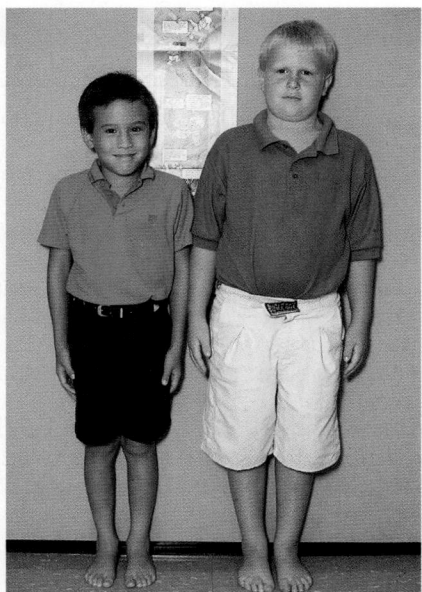

FIG 29.8 These children of identical age (8 years) are markedly different in size. The child on the left, of Asian descent, is at the 5th percentile for height and weight. The child on the right is above the 95th percentile for height and weight. However, both children demonstrate normal growth patterns.

of the object firmly against the wall to form a right angle. Measure length or stature to the nearest 1 mm or $\frac{1}{16}$ inch.

Weight

Weight is measured with an electronic or appropriately sized balance beam scale, which measures weight to the nearest 10 g (0.35 oz) for infants and 100 g (0.22 lb) for children. Before weighing the child, balance the scale by setting it at 0 and noting if the scale registers at exactly 0 or in the middle of the mark. If the end of the balance beam rises to the top or bottom of the mark, more or less weight, respectively, is needed. Some scales are designed to self-correct, but others need to be recalibrated by the manufacturer. Scales vary in their accuracy; infant scales tend to be more accurate than adult platform scales, and newer scales tend to be more accurate than older ones, especially at the upper levels of weight measurement. When precise measurements are necessary, two nurses should take the weight independently; if there is a discrepancy, take a third reading and use the mean of the measurements in closest agreement.

Take measurements in a comfortably warm room. When the birth–to–2-year or birth–to–36-month growth charts are used, children should be weighed nude. Older children are usually weighed while wearing their underpants, a gown, or light clothing, depending on the setting. However, always respect the privacy of all children. If the child must be weighed wearing some type of special device, such as a prosthesis or an armboard for an intravenous device, note this when recording the weight. Children who are measured for recumbent length are usually

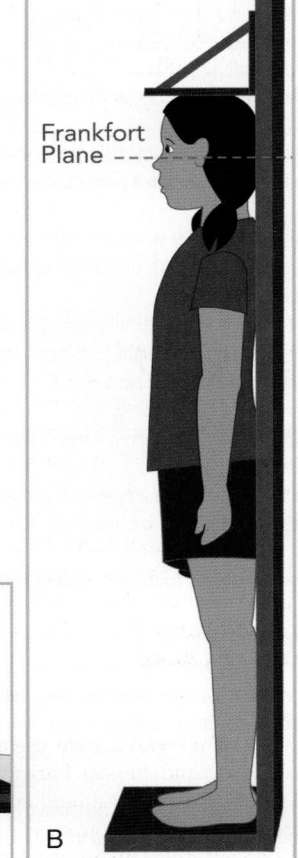

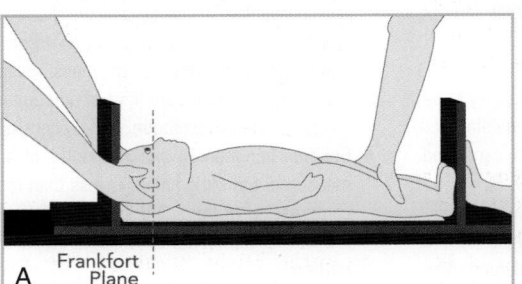

FIG 29.9 Measurement of linear growth. **A,** Infant. **B,** Child. (Courtesy of Jan M. Foote.)

EVIDENCE-BASED PRACTICE
Linear Growth Measurement in Pediatrics

Ask the Question
PICOT Question: In children, what are the best instruments and techniques to measure linear growth (length and height)?

Search for the Evidence
Search Strategies
Search Selection Criteria: English language, research-based and review articles and expert opinion from databases, anthropometric and endocrinology textbooks, contact with experts in the field, and informal discovery
Key Terms: Length, height, stature, infant, child, adolescent, measurement, instrument, length board, stadiometer, calibration, technique, accuracy, reliability, diurnal variation
Exclusion Criteria: Other types of anthropometric measurements, adults

Databases Used
MEDLINE, CINAHL, COCHRANE, EMBASE, OCLC, ERIC, National Guideline Clearinghouse (AHRQ)

Critical Appraisal of the Evidence
An interdisciplinary team systematically and critically appraised the evidence to develop these clinical practice recommendations using an evidence-based practice rating scheme (US Preventive Services Task Force, 1996).

Measure recumbent length in children younger than 24 to 36 months of age and children who cannot stand alone (Foote, Brady, Burke, et al., 2011, 2014) (see Fig. 29.9, *A*).

- Use a length board with these components: Flat, horizontal surface with stationary headboard and smoothly movable footboard, both at 90-degree angles to the horizontal surface, and attached ruler marked in millimeter and/or $\frac{1}{16}$-inch increments. Tape measures should never be used.
- Cover length board with soft, thin cloth or paper.
- Remove all clothing and shoes. Remove or loosen diaper. Remove hair ornaments on crown of head.
- Two measurers are required to accomplish correct positioning; one measurer (assistant) can be a parent or other caregiver when procedures are explained and understood.
- Place the child supine on length board. Never leave the child unattended.
- Assistant holds the child's head in midline with the crown of head against headboard, compressing the hair.
- Position the child's head in the Frankfort vertical plane (imaginary line from the lower border of the orbit through the highest point of the auditory meatus; the line is parallel to the headboard and perpendicular to the length board).
- Lead measurer positions the child's body on length board with one hand placed on both legs to fully extend the body.
- Ensure that the child's head remains against headboard, shoulders and hips are not rotated, back is not arched, and legs are not bent. Reposition as necessary.
- Using the other hand, lead measurer moves footboard against heels of both feet with toes pointing upward.
- Read measurement to the nearest millimeter or $\frac{1}{16}$ inch.
- Reposition the child and repeat procedure. Measure at least twice (ideally three times). Average the measurements for the final value. Record immediately.
- Measure height in children 24 to 36 months of age and older who can stand alone well (Foote, Brady, Burke, et al., 2011; 2014) (see Fig. 29.9, *B*).
- Use a stadiometer with these components: Vertical surface to stand against, footboard or firm surface to stand on, movable horizontal headboard at 90-degree angle to the vertical surface, and attached ruler marked in millimeter and/or

$\frac{1}{16}$-inch increments. Wall charts and flip-up horizontal bars (floppy-arm devices) mounted to weighing scales should never be used.
- Remove shoes and heavy outer clothing. Remove hair ornaments on crown of head.
- Stand the child on flat surface with back against vertical surface of stadiometer.
- Weight is evenly distributed on both feet with heels together.
- Occiput, scapulae, buttocks, and heels are in contact with vertical surface.
- Encourage the child to maintain fully erect position with positional lordosis minimized, knees fully extended, and heels flat. Reposition as necessary.
- Child continues normal breathing with shoulders relaxed and arms hanging down freely.
- Position the child's head in the horizontal Frankfort plane (imaginary line from the lower border of the orbit through the highest point of the auditory meatus; the line is parallel to the headboard and perpendicular to the vertical surface).
- Move headboard down to crown of head, compressing the hair.
- Read measurement at eye level to the nearest millimeter or $\frac{1}{16}$ inch to avoid a parallax error.
- Reposition the child, and repeat procedure. Measure at least twice (ideally three times). Average the measurements for the final value. Record immediately.

Special Considerations (Foote, Brady, Burke, et al., 2014; Lohman, Roche, & Martorell, 1988)
- Some children, such as those who are obese, may not be able to place their occiput, scapulae, buttocks, and heels all in one vertical plane while maintaining their balance, so use at least two of the four contact points.
- If the child has a leg length discrepancy, place a block or wedge of suitable height under the shortest leg until the pelvis is level and both knees are fully extended before measuring height. To measure length, keep the legs together and measure to the heel of the longest leg.
- Children with special health care needs may require alternative measurements, such as arm span, crown-rump length, sitting height, knee height, or other segmental lengths. In general, when recumbent length is measured in a child with spasticity or contractures, measure the side of the body that is unaffected or less affected.
- Always document the presence of any condition that may interfere with accurate and reliable linear growth measurement.

Quality Control Measures (Foote, Brady, Burke, et al., 2014)
- Personnel who measure the growth of infants, children, and adolescents need proper education. Competency should be demonstrated. Refresher sessions should occur when a lack of standardization occurs.
- Length boards and stadiometers must be assembled and installed properly and calibrated at regular intervals (ideally daily, at least monthly, and every time they are moved) due to frequent inaccuracy and the variability between different instruments. Calibration can be performed by measuring a rod of known length and adjusting the instrument accordingly.
- All children should be measured at least twice (ideally three times) during each encounter. The measurements should agree within 0.5 cm (ideally 0.3 cm). Use the mean value. If the variation exceeds the limit of agreement, measure again and use the mean of the measures in closest agreement. If none of the measures are within the limit of agreement, then (1) have another measurer assist, (2) check technique, and (3) consider another education session.
- Children between 24 and 36 months of age may have length and/or height measured. Standing height is less than recumbent length due to gravity and compression of the spine. Plot length measurements on a length curve and height measurements on a height curve to avoid misinterpreting the growth pattern.

EVIDENCE-BASED PRACTICE
Linear Growth Measurement in Pediatrics—cont'd

Apply the Evidence: Nursing Implications

Growth is well established as an important and sensitive indicator of health in children. Abnormal growth is a common consequence of many conditions; therefore, its measurement can be a useful warning of possible pathology. In a study of 55 primary care practices within eight geographic areas in the United States, only 30% of children were measured accurately due to faulty instruments and casual techniques; an educational intervention increased measurement accuracy to 70% (Lipman, Hench, Benyi, et al., 2004). Measurement error influences growth assessment and can result in delayed evaluation and treatment of some children, as well as apparent growth deviation in others who are actually growing normally (Foote, Brady, Burke, et al., 2011). There is good evidence with strong recommendations for using length boards and stadiometers, the described measurement techniques, and the quality control measures. There is fair evidence to recommend procedures for children with special needs (Foote, Brady, Burke, et al., 2014; Lohman, Roche, & Martorell, 1988).

Quality and Safety Competencies: Evidence-Based Practice*
Knowledge

Differentiate clinical opinion from research and evidence-based summaries.

Describe the appropriate instruments and techniques to obtain accurate and reliable linear growth measurement of children.

Skills

Base individualized care plan on patient values, clinical expertise, and evidence.

Integrate evidence into practice by using the instruments and techniques for linear growth measurement in clinical care.

Attitudes

Value the concept of evidence-based practice as integral to determining best clinical practice.

Appreciate strengths and weaknesses of evidence for measuring the linear growth of children.

References

Foote, J. M. (2014). Optimizing linear growth measurement in children. *Journal of Pediatric Health Care, 28*(5), 413–419.

Foote, J. M., Brady, L. H., Burke, A. L., et al. (2011). Development of an evidence-based clinical practice guideline on linear growth measurement of children. *Journal of Pediatric Nursing, 26*(4), 312–324.

Foote, J. M., Brady, L. H., Burke, A. L., et al. (2014). *Evidence-based clinical practice guideline on linear growth measurement of children.* Retrieved from https://www.pedsendo.org/assets/education_training/PENSpositionstatement_linear_growth_measurement2014.pdf (to access full-text guideline and implementation tools).

Lipman, T. H., Hench, K. D., Benyi, T., et al. (2004). A multicentre randomised controlled trial of an intervention to improve the accuracy of linear growth measurement. *Archives of Disease in Childhood, 89,* 342–346.

Lohman, T. J., Roche, A. F., & Martorell, R. (Eds.), (1988). *Anthropometric standardization reference manual.* Champaign, IL: Human Kinetics Books.

US Preventive Services Task Force. (1996). *Guide to clinical preventive services: report of the U.S. Preventive Services Task Force* (2nd ed.). Philadelphia, PA: Lippincott.

*Adapted from the Quality and Safety Education for Nurses (QSEN) Institute.

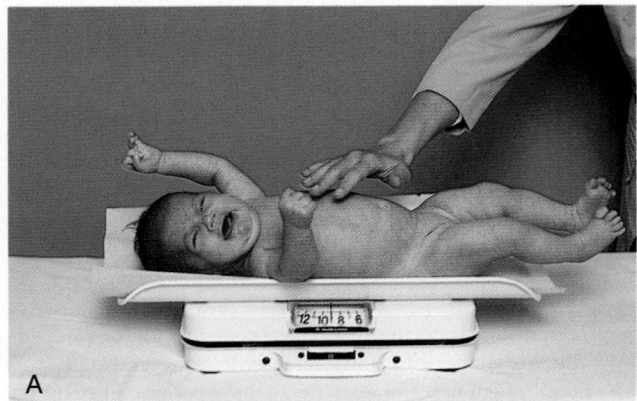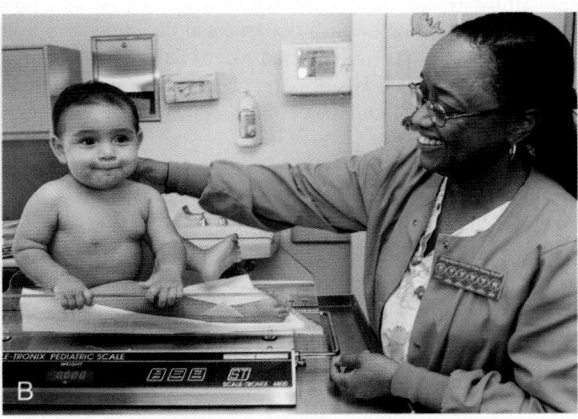

FIG 29.10 A, Infant on scale. **B,** Toddler on scale. Note the presence of the nurse to prevent falls. (B, Courtesy of Paul Vincent Kuntz, Texas Children's Hospital, Houston, TX.)

weighed on an infant platform scale and placed in a lying or sitting position. When weighing a child, place your hand slightly above the infant to prevent him or her from accidentally falling off the scale (Fig. 29.10, *A*), or stand close to the toddler, ready to prevent a fall (see Fig. 29.10, *B*). For maximum asepsis, cover the scale with a clean sheet of paper between each child's weight measurement.

Nurses need to become familiar with determining body mass index (BMI), which requires accurate information about the child's weight and height.

$$BMI = (Weight\ in\ pounds \div [Height\ in\ inches]^2) \times 703$$

or

$$BMI = Weight\ in\ kilograms \div (Height\ in\ meters)^2$$

With the increasing number of overweight children in the United States, the BMI charts are a critical component of children's physical assessment.

! NURSING ALERT

BMI for sex and age may be used to identify children and adolescents who are either underweight (<5th percentile), healthy weight (5th percentile to <85th percentile), overweight (≥85th percentile and <95th percentile), or obese (≥95th percentile).

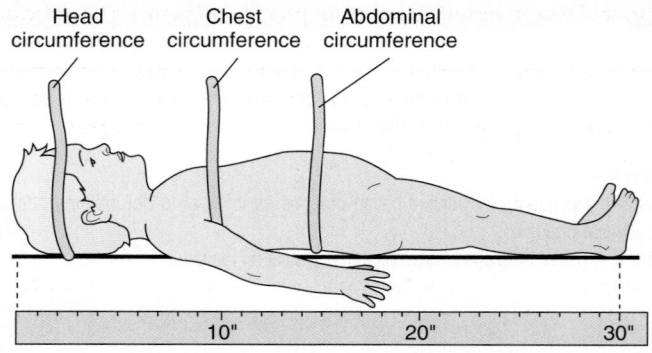
Head circumference   Chest circumference   Abdominal circumference

10"   20"   30"
Crown-to-heel recumbent length

FIG 29.11 Measurement of head circumference. (From Seidel, H.M., Ball, J.W., Dains, J.E., et al. [1999]. *Mosby's guide to physical examination* [4th ed.]. St. Louis, MO: Mosby.)

Skinfold Thickness and Arm Circumference

Measures of relative weight and stature cannot distinguish between adipose (fat) tissue and muscle. One convenient measure of body fat is *skinfold thickness,* which is increasingly recommended as a routine measurement. Measure skinfold thickness with special calipers, such as the Lange calipers. The most common sites for measuring skinfold thickness are the triceps (most practical for routine clinical use), subscapular, suprailiac, abdomen, and upper thigh. For greatest reliability, follow the exact procedure for measurement and record the average of at least two measurements of one site.

Arm circumference is an indirect measure of muscle mass. Measurement of arm circumference follows the same procedure as for skinfold thickness except the midpoint is measured with a paper or steel tape. Place the tape vertically along the posterior aspect of the upper arm from the acromial process and to the olecranon process; half of the measured length is the midpoint. World Health Organization growth curves are available for triceps skinfold and arm circumference measurements.

Head Circumference

Head circumference is a reflection of brain growth. Measure head circumference in children up to 36 months of age and in any child whose head size is questionable. Measure the head at its greatest frontooccipital circumference, usually slightly above the eyebrows and pinna of the ears and around the occipital prominence at the back of the skull (Fig. 29.11). Use a paper or non-stretchable tape because a cloth tape can stretch and give a falsely small measurement. Because head shape can affect the location of the maximum circumference, more than one measurement is necessary to obtain the most accurate measure. Measure head circumference to the nearest 1 mm or $\frac{1}{16}$ inch.

Plot the head size on the appropriate growth chart under head circumference. Generally, head and chest circumferences are equal at about 1 to 2 years of age. During childhood, chest circumference exceeds head size by about 5 to 7 cm (2 to 2.75 inches).

PHYSIOLOGIC MEASUREMENTS

Physiologic measurements, key elements in evaluating physical status of vital functions, include temperature, pulse, respiration, and blood pressure. Compare each physiologic recording with normal values for that age group. In addition, compare the values taken on preceding health visits with present recordings. For example, a falsely elevated blood pressure (BP) reading may not indicate hypertension if previous recent readings have been within normal limits. The isolated recording may indicate some stressful event in the child's life.

BOX 29.7   Recommended Temperature Screening Routes in Infants and Children

Birth to 2 Years of Age
Axillary
Rectal: if definitive temperature reading is needed for infants older than 1 month of age

2 to 5 Years of Age
Axillary
Tympanic
Oral: when child can hold thermometer under tongue
Rectal: if definitive temperature reading is needed

Older Than 5 Years of Age
Oral
Axillary
Tympanic

As in most procedures carried out with children, treat older children and adolescents much the same as adults. However, give special consideration to preschool children (see Atraumatic Care box: Reducing Young Children's Fears). For best results in taking vital signs of infants, count respirations first (before the infant is disturbed), take the pulse next, and measure temperature last. If vital signs cannot be taken without disturbing the child, record the child's behavior (e.g., crying) along with the measurement.

Temperature

Temperature is the measure of heat content within an individual's body. The core temperature most closely reflects the temperature of the blood flow through the carotid arteries to the hypothalamus. Core temperature is relatively constant despite wide fluctuations in the external environment. When a child's temperature is altered, receptors in the skin, spinal cord, and brain respond in an attempt to achieve normothermia, a normal temperature state. In pediatrics, there is a lack of consensus regarding what temperature constitutes normothermia for every child. For rectal temperatures in children, a value of 37° to 37.5°C (98.6° to 99.5°F) is an acceptable range, where heat loss and heat production are balanced. For neonates, a core body temperature between 36.5° and 37.6°C (97.7° to 99.7°F) is a desirable range. In the neonate, obtain temperature measurements for monitoring adequacy of thermoregulation, not just for fever; therefore, temperature measurements in each infant should be carefully considered in the context of the purpose and the environment.

The nurse can measure temperature in healthy children at several body sites via oral, rectal, axillary, ear canal, tympanic membrane, temporal artery, or skin route (Box 29.7). For the ill child, other sites for temperature measurement have been investigated. The pulmonary

BOX 29.8   Alternative Temperature Measurement Sites for Ill Children

Skin

A probe is placed on the skin to determine heat output in response to changes in the patient's skin temperature.

Skin temperature sensors are most often used for neonates and infants placed in radiant heat warmers or isolettes (using servo control feature of the apparatus). In turn, the heater unit warms to a set point to maintain the infant's temperature within a specified range.

ThermoSpot is an example of a device allowing continuous thermal monitoring in neonates.

Urinary Bladder

A thermistor or thermocouple is placed within the indwelling bladder catheter. The catheter tip immersed in the bladder provides a continuous temperature read-out on the bedside monitor.

This is not a true measure of core temperature but responds better than rectal and skin temperatures to core body changes.

Because of thermistor sizes, this method is unusable with neonates and small infants.

Pulmonary Artery

A catheter is placed into the heart to obtain a reading in the pulmonary artery.

It is used in critical care settings or operating rooms only in patients requiring aggressive monitoring.

Catheters are not available in sizes for neonates or small infants.

Esophageal Site

A probe is inserted into the lower third of the esophagus at the level of the heart.

This is used in critical care settings or operating rooms.

Several companies have esophageal stethoscopes with temperature probe monitors for patients in the operating room that show a continuous temperature reading.

Nasopharyngeal Site

A probe is inserted into the nasopharynx, posterior to the soft palate, and provides an estimate of hypothalamic temperature.

This is used in critical care settings or operating rooms.

Data from Kumar, P.R., Nisarga, R., & Gowda, B. (2004). Temperature monitoring in newborns using ThermoSpot. *Indian Journal of Pediatrics, 71*(9), 795–796; Martin, S.A., & Kline, A.M. (2004). Can there be a standard for temperature measurement in the pediatric intensive care unit? *AACN Clinical Issues, 15*(2), 254–266; Maxton, F.J.C., Justin, L., & Gilles, D. (2004). Estimating core temperature in infants and children after cardiac surgery: A comparison of six methods. *Journal of Advanced Nursing, 45*(2), 214–222.

artery is the closest to the hypothalamus and best reflects the core temperature (Batra, Saha, & Faridi, 2012). Other sites used are the distal esophagus, urinary bladder, and nasopharynx (Box 29.8). All of these methods are invasive and difficult to use in clinical practice. One of the most important influences on the accuracy of temperature is improper temperature-taking technique. Detailed discussion of temperature-taking methods and visual examples of proper techniques are given in Table 29.3. For a critical review of the evidence on temperature-taking methods, see the Evidence-Based Practice box.

The most frequently used temperature measurement devices in infants and children include the following:

Electronic intermittent thermometers: measure the patient's temperature at oral, rectal, and axillary sites and are used as primary diagnostic indicators

Infrared thermometers: measure the patient's temperature by collecting emitted thermal radiation from a particular site (e.g., ear canal)

Electronic continuous thermometers: measure the patient's temperature during the administration of general anesthesia, treatment of hypothermia or hyperthermia, and other situations that require continuous monitoring

---

! NURSING ALERT

The belief that core temperature can be estimated by adding 1°C to the temperature taken in the axilla is incorrect. Do not add a degree to the finding obtained by taking a temperature by the axillary route.

Pulse

A satisfactory pulse can be taken radially in children older than 2 years of age. However, in infants and young children, the apical impulse (AI) (heard through a stethoscope held to the chest at the apex of the heart) is more reliable (see Fig. 29.33 for location of pulses). Count the pulse for 1 full minute in infants and young children because of possible irregularities in rhythm. However, when frequent apical rates are necessary, use shorter counting times (e.g., 15- or 30-second intervals). For greater accuracy, measure the apical rate while the child is asleep; record the child's behavior along with the rate. Grade pulses according to the criteria in Table 29.4. Compare radial and femoral pulses at least once during infancy to detect the presence of circulatory impairment, such as coarctation of the aorta.

Respiration

Count the respiratory rate in children in the same manner as for adult patients. However, in infants, observe abdominal movements, because respirations are primarily diaphragmatic. Because the movements are irregular, count them for 1 full minute for accuracy (see also the "Chest" section later in this chapter).

Blood Pressure

BP should be measured annually in children 3 years of age through adolescence and in children with symptoms of hypertension, children in emergency departments and intensive care units, and high-risk infants (National High Blood Pressure Education Program Working Group on High Blood Pressure in Children and Adolescents, 2004). Auscultation remains the gold standard method of BP measurement in children, under most circumstances. Use of the automated devices is acceptable for BP measurement in newborns and young infants, in whom auscultation is difficult, and in the intensive care setting where frequent BP measurement is needed.

Oscillometric devices measure mean arterial BP and then calculate systolic and diastolic values. The algorithms used by companies are proprietary and differ from company to company and device to device. These devices can yield results that vary widely when one is compared with another, and they do not always closely match BP values obtained by auscultation. An elevated BP reading obtained with an automated or oscillometric device should be repeated using auscultation.

BP readings using oscillometry, such as Dinamap, are generally higher (10 mm Hg higher) than measurements using auscultation (Park, Menard, and Schoolfield, 2005). Differences between Dinamap and auscultatory readings prevent the interchange of the readings by the two methods.

Selection of Cuff

No matter what type of noninvasive technique is used, the most important factor in accurately measuring BP is the use of an appropriately sized

TABLE 29.3 Temperature Measurement Locations for Infants and Children

Temperature Site

Oral

Place tip under tongue in right or left posterior sublingual pocket, not in front of tongue. Have child keep mouth closed without biting on thermometer.

Pacifier thermometers measure intraoral or supralingual temperature and are available but lack support in the literature.

Several factors affect mouth temperature: Eating and mastication, hot or cold beverages, open-mouth breathing, and ambient temperature.

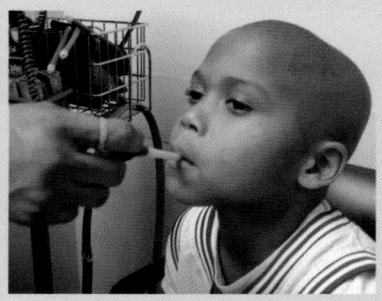

Axillary

Place tip under arm in center of axilla and keep close to skin, not clothing. Hold child's arm firmly against side. Temperature may be affected by poor peripheral perfusion (results in lower value), clothing or swaddling, use of radiant warmer, or amount of brown fat in cold-stressed neonate (results in higher value).

Advantage: Avoids intrusive procedure and eliminates risk for rectal perforation.

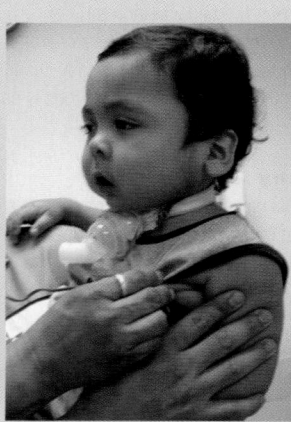

Ear Based (Aural)

Insert small infrared probe deeply into canal to allow sensor to obtain measurement.

Size of probe (most are 8 mm) may influence accuracy of result. In young children, this may be a problem because of small diameter of canal.

Proper placement of ear is controversial related to whether the pinna should be pulled in manner similar to that used during otoscopy.

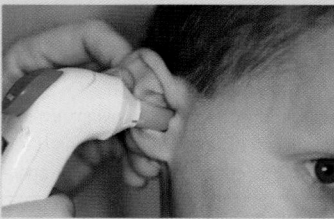

Rectal

Place well-lubricated tip at maximum 2.5 cm (1 inch) into rectum for children and 1.5 cm (0.6 inch) for infants; securely hold thermometer close to anus.

Child may be placed in side-lying, supine, or prone position (i.e., supine with knees flexed toward abdomen); cover penis because procedure may stimulate urination. A small child may be placed prone across parent's lap.

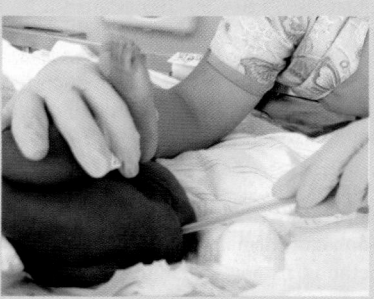

TABLE 29.3   Temperature Measurement Locations for Infants and Children—cont'd

Temperature Site

Temporal Artery

An infrared sensor probe scans across forehead, capturing heat from arterial blood flow.

Temporal artery is the only artery close enough to skin's surface to provide access for accurate
temperature measurement.

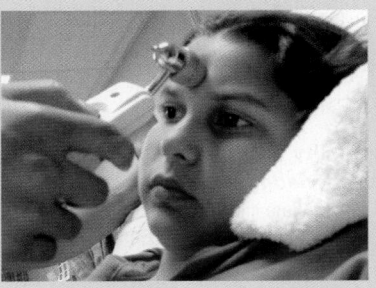

Data from Martin, S.A., & Kline, A.M. (2004). Can there be a standard for temperature measurement in the pediatric intensive care unit? *AACN Clinical Issues, 15*(2), 254–266; Falzon, A., Grech, V., Caruana, B., et al. (2003). How reliable is axillary temperature measurement? *Acta Paediatrica, 92*(3), 309–313. Oral, axillary, rectal, and temporal artery images courtesy of Paul Vincent Kuntz, Texas Children's Hospital, Houston, TX.

EVIDENCE-BASED PRACTICE

Temperature Measurement in Pediatrics

Ask the Question

PICOT Question: In infants and children, what is the most accurate method for measuring temperature in febrile children?

Search for the Evidence

Search Strategies

Clinical research studies related to this issue were identified by searching for English publications within the past 15 years for infant and child populations; comparisons with gold standard: rectal thermometry.

Databases Used

PubMed, Cochrane Collaboration, MD Consult, Joanna Briggs Institute, National Guideline Clearinghouse (AHRQ), TRIP Database Plus, PedsCCM, BestBETs

Critical Appraisal of the Evidence

- **Rectal temperature:** Rectal measurement remains the clinical gold standard for the precise diagnosis of fever in infants and children compared with other methods (Fortuna, Carney, Macy, et al., 2010; Holzhauer, Reith, Sawin, et al., 2009). However, this procedure is more invasive and is contraindicated for infants younger than 1 month of age due to risk for rectal perforation (Batra, Saha, & Faridi, 2012). Children with recent rectal surgery, diarrhea, or anorectal lesions, or who are receiving chemotherapy (cancer treatment usually affects the mucosa and causes neutropenia) should not undergo rectal thermometry.

- **Oral temperature (OT):** OT indicates rapid changes in core body temperature, but accuracy may be an issue compared with the rectal site (Batra, Saha, & Faridi, 2012). OTs are considered the standard for temperature measurement (Gilbert, Barton, & Counsell, 2002), but they are contraindicated in children who have an altered level of consciousness, are receiving oxygen, are mouth breathing, are experiencing mucositis, had recent oral surgery or trauma, or are younger than 5 years of age (El-Radhi & Barry, 2006). Limitations of OTs include the effects of ambient room temperature and recent oral intake (Martin & Kline, 2004).

- **Axillary temperature:** This is inconsistent and insensitive in infants and children older than 1 month of age (Falzon, Grech, Caruana, et al., 2003; Jean-Mary, Dicanzio, Shaw, et al., 2002; Stine, Flook, & Vincze, 2012). A systematic review of 20 studies concluded that axillary thermometers showed variation in findings and are not a good method for accurate temperature assessment (Craig, Lancaster, Williamson, et al., 2005). In neonates with fever, the axillary temperature should not be used interchangeably with rectal measurement (Hissink Muller, van Berkel, de Beaufort, 2008). It can be used as a screening tool for fever in young infants (Batra, Saha, & Faridi, 2012).

- **Ear (aural) temperature:** This is not a precise measurement of body temperature. A meta-analysis of 101 studies comparing tympanic membrane temperatures with rectal temperatures in children concluded that the tympanic method demonstrated a wide range of variability, limiting its application in a pediatric setting (Craig, Lancaster, Taylor, et al., 2002). Other published reviews continue to find poor sensitivity using infrared ear thermometry (Devrim, Kara, Ceyhan, et al., 2007; Dodd, Lancaster, Craig, et al., 2006). Diagnosis of fever without a focus should not be made based on tympanic thermometry, because it is not an accurate measure of core temperature (Batra, Saha, & Faridi, 2012; Devrim, Kara, Ceyhan, et al., 2007; Dodd, Lancaster, Craig, et al., 2006).

- **Temporal artery temperature (TAT):** TAT is not predictable for fever in young children but can be used as a screening tool for detecting fever less than 38° C (100.4° F) in children 3 months to 4 years of age (Al-Mukhaizeem, Allen, Komar, et al., 2004; Callanan, 2003; Fortuna, Carney, Macy, et al., 2010; Hebbar, Fortenberry, Rogers, et al., 2005; Holzhauer, Reith, Sawin, et al., 2009; Schuh, Komar, Stephens, et al., 2004; Siberry, Diener-West, Schappell, et al., 2002; Titus, Hulsey, Heckman, et al., 2009). However, a study by Batra and Goyal (2013) found that temporal artery temperature correlated better with rectal temperature than axillary and tympanic measures in a group of 50 afebrile children between 2 and 12 years of age.

Apply the Evidence: Nursing Implications

- No single site used for temperature assessment provides unequivocal estimates of core body temperature.
- Studies show that the axillary and tympanic measures demonstrate poor agreement when these modes are compared with more accurate core temperature methods. The differences are more evident as temperature increases, regardless of age.
- TAT is not predictable for fever and should be only used as a screening tool in young children.

Continued

EVIDENCE-BASED PRACTICE

Temperature Measurement in Pediatrics—cont'd

- When an accurate method for obtaining a correct reflection of core temperature is needed, the rectal temperature is recommended in younger children and the oral route in older children.

  For infants younger than 1 month of age, axillary temperatures are recommended for screening.

Quality and Safety Competencies: Evidence-Based Practice*

Knowledge

Differentiate clinical opinion from research and evidence-based summaries.
Demonstrate understanding of thermometry selection based on the developmental age of the child.

Skills

Base individualized care plan on patient values, clinical expertise, and evidence.
Integrate evidence into practice by using the correct type of thermometry to screen for fever compared with measures used for accurate determination of the degree of fever.

Attitudes

Value the concept of evidence-based practice as integral to determining best clinical practice.
Recognize strengths and weaknesses of evidence for the most accurate method for measuring temperature and fever in infants and children.

References

Al-Mukhaizeem, F., Allen, U., Komar, L., et al. (2004). Comparison of temporal artery, rectal and esophageal core temperatures in children: Results of a pilot study. *Paediatrics & Child Health, 9*(7), 461–465.

Batra, P., & Goyal, S. (2013). Comparison of rectal, axillary, tympanic, and temporal artery thermometry in the pediatric emergency room. *Pediatric Emergency Care, 29*(7), 877.

Batra, P., Saha, A., & Faridi, M. M. (2012). Thermometry in children. *Journal of Emergencies, Trauma, and Shock, 5*(3), 246–249.

Callanan, D. (2003). Detecting fever in young infants: Reliability of perceived, pacifier, and temporal artery temperatures in infants younger than 3 months of age. *Pediatric Emergency Care, 19*(4), 240–243.

Craig, J. V., Lancaster, G. A., Taylor, S., et al. (2002). Infrared ear thermometry compared with rectal thermometry in children: A systemic review. *Lancet, 360*, 603–609.

Craig, J. V., Lancaster, G. A., Williamson, P. R., et al. (2005). Temperature measured at the axilla compared with rectum in children and young people: Systematic review. *British Medical Journal, 320*(7243), 1174–1178.

Devrim, I., Kara, A., Ceyhan, M., et al. (2007). Measurement accuracy of fever by tympanic and axillary thermometry. *Pediatric Emergency Care, 23*(1), 16–19.

Dodd, S. R., Lancaster, G. A., Craig, J. V., et al. (2006). In a systematic review, infrared ear thermometry for fever diagnosis in children finds poor sensitivity. *Journal of Clinical Epidemiology, 59*, 354–357.

El-Radhi, A. S., & Barry, W. (2006). Thermometry in paediatric practice. *Archives of Disease in Childhood, 91*(4), 351–356.

Falzon, A., Grech, V., Caruana, B., et al. (2003). How reliable is axillary temperature measurement? *Acta Paediatrica, 92*(3), 309–313.

Fortuna, E. L., Carney, M. M., Macy, M., et al. (2010). Accuracy of non-contact infrared thermometry versus rectal thermometry in young children evaluated in the emergency department for fever. *Journal of Emergency Nursing, 36*(2), 101–104.

Gilbert, M., Barton, A. J., & Counsell, C. M. (2002). Comparison of oral and tympanic temperatures in adult surgical patients. *Applied Nursing Research, 15*(1), 42–47.

Hebbar, K., Fortenberry, J. D., Rogers, K., et al. (2005). Comparison of temporal artery thermometer to standard temperature measurement in pediatric intensive care unit patients. *Pediatric Critical Care Medicine, 6*(5), 557–561.

Hissink Muller, P. C. E., van Berkel, L. H., & de Beaufort, A. J. (2008). Axillary and rectal temperature measurements poorly agree in newborn infants. *Neonatology, 94*(1), 31–34.

Holzhauer, J. K., Reith, V., Sawin, K., et al. (2009). Evaluation of temporal artery thermometry in children 3–36 months old. *Journal for Specialists in Pediatric Nursing, 14*(4), 239–244.

Jean-Mary, M. B., Dicanzio, J., Shaw, J., et al. (2002). Limited accuracy and reliability of infrared axillary and aural thermometers in a pediatric outpatient population. *The Journal of Pediatrics, 141*(5), 671–676.

Martin, S. A., & Kline, A. M. (2004). Can there be a standard for temperature measurement in the pediatric intensive care unit? *AACN Clinical Issues, 15*(2), 254–266.

Schuh, S., Komar, L., Stephens, D., et al. (2004). Comparison of the temporal artery and rectal thermometry in children in the emergency department. *Pediatric Emergency Care, 20*(11), 736–741.

Siberry, G. K., Diener-West, M., Schappell, E., et al. (2002). Comparison of temple temperatures with rectal temperatures in children under 2 years of age. *Clinical Pediatrics, 41*(6), 405–414.

Stine, C. A., Flook, D. M., & Vincze, D. L. (2012). Rectal versus axillary temperatures: Is there a significant difference in infants less than 1 years of age? *Journal of Pediatric Nursing, 3*, 265–270.

Titus, M. O., Hulsey, T., Heckman, J., et al. (2009). Temporal artery thermometry utilization in pediatric emergency care. *Clinical Pediatrics, 48*(2), 190–193.

*Adapted from the Quality and Safety Education for Nurses (QSEN) Institute.

TABLE 29.4   Grading of Pulses

Grade	Description
0	Not palpable
+1	Difficult to palpate, thready, weak, easily obliterated with pressure
+2	Difficult to palpate, may be obliterated with pressure
+3	Easy to palpate, not easily obliterated with pressure (normal)
+4	Strong, bounding, not obliterated with pressure

TABLE 29.5   Recommended Dimensions for Blood Pressure Cuff Bladders

Age	Width (cm)	Length (cm)	Maximum Arm Circumference (cm)*
Newborn	4	8	10
Infant	6	12	15
Child	9	18	22
Small adult	10	24	26
Adult	13	30	34
Large adult	16	38	44
Thigh	20	42	52

*Calculated so that largest arm would still allow bladder to encircle arm by at least 80%.
From National High Blood Pressure Education Program Working Group on High Blood Pressure in Children and Adolescents. (2004). The fourth report on the diagnosis, evaluation, and treatment of high blood pressure in children and adolescents. *Pediatrics, 114*(2 suppl, 4th report), 555–576.

cuff (cuff size refers only to the inner inflatable bladder, not the cloth covering) (Table 29.5). A technique to establish an appropriate cuff size is to choose a cuff with a bladder width that is at least 40% of the arm circumference midway between the olecranon and the acromion (Clark, Kieh-Lai, Sarnaik et al., 2002). This will usually be a cuff bladder that covers 80% to 100% of the circumference of the arm (Fig. 29.12). Cuffs that are either too narrow or too wide affect the accuracy of BP measurements. If the cuff size is too small, the reading on the device is falsely high. If the cuff size is too large, the reading is falsely low.

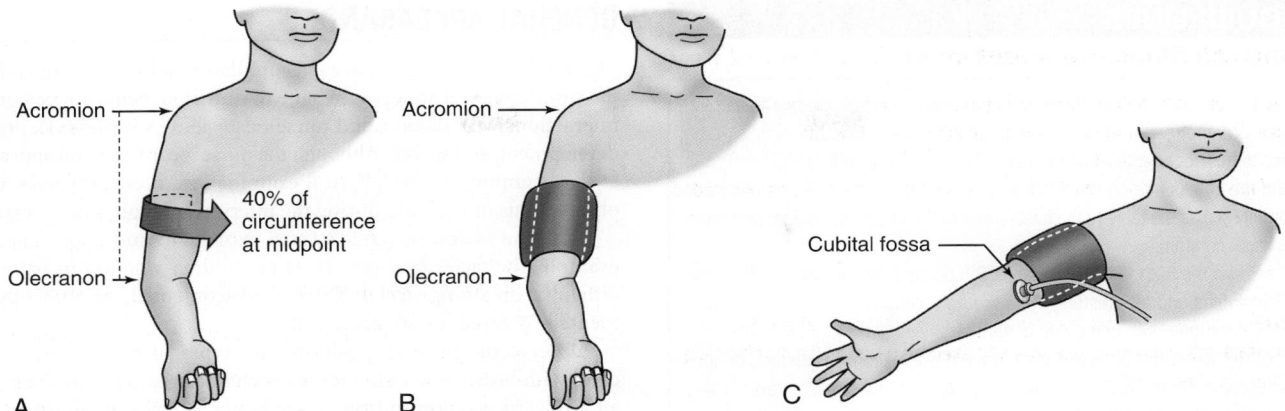

FIG 29.12 Determination of proper cuff size. **A,** Cuff bladder width should be approximately 40% of circumference of arm measured at a point midway between olecranon and acromion. **B,** Cuff bladder length should cover 80% to 100% of arm circumference. **C,** Blood pressure (BP) should be measured with the cubital fossa at the heart level. The arm should be supported. The stethoscope bell is placed over the brachial artery pulse proximal and medial to the cubital fossa and below the bottom edge of the cuff. (From National Institutes of Health, National Heart, Lung, and Blood Institute. [1996]. *Update on the Task Force Report [1987] on high blood pressure in children and adolescents: A working group report from the National High Blood Pressure Education Program.* NIH Pub No 96-3790, Bethesda, MD: Author.)

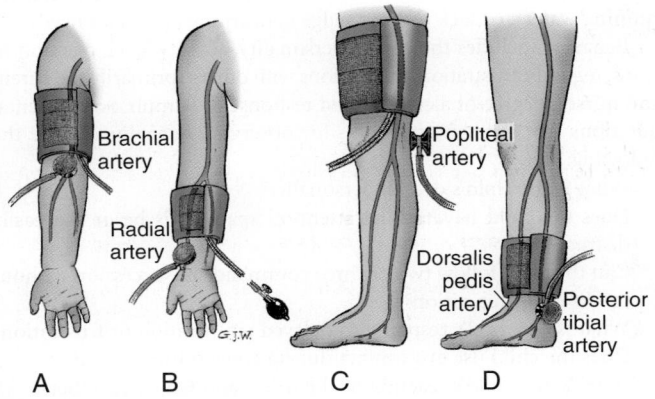

FIG 29.13 Sites for measuring blood pressure. **A,** Upper arm. **B,** Lower arm or forearm. **C,** Thigh. **D,** Calf or ankle.

When using a site other than the arm, BP measurements using noninvasive techniques may differ. Generally, systolic BP in the lower extremities (thigh or calf) is greater than pressure in the upper extremities, and systolic BP in the calf is higher than that in the thigh (Schell, Briening, Lebet, et al., 2011) (Fig. 29.13).

> **! NURSING ALERT**
>
> When taking blood pressure (BP), use an appropriately sized cuff. When the correct size is not available, use an oversized cuff rather than an undersized one, or use another site that more appropriately fits the cuff size. Do not choose a cuff based on the name of the cuff (e.g., an "infant" cuff may be too small for some infants).

> **! NURSING ALERT**
>
> Compare blood pressure (BP) in the upper and lower extremities to detect abnormalities, such as coarctation of the aorta, in which the lower extremity pressure is less than the upper extremity pressure.

Measurement and Interpretation

Measuring and interpreting BP in infants and children requires attention to correct procedure because (1) limb sizes vary and cuff selection must accommodate the circumference; (2) excessive pressure on the antecubital fossa affects the Korotkoff sounds; (3) children easily become anxious, which can elevate BP; and (4) BP values change with age and growth. In children and adolescents, determine the normal range of BP by body size and age. BP standards that are based on gender, age, and height provide a more precise classification of BP according to body size. This approach avoids misclassifying children who are very tall or very short. The revised BP tables include the 50th, 90th, 95th, and 99th percentiles (with standard deviations) by gender, age, and height.

To use the tables in a clinical setting, determine the height percentile by using the Centers for Disease Control and Prevention growth charts (www.cdc.gov/growthcharts). The child's measured systolic BP and diastolic BP are compared with the numbers provided in the table (boys or girls) according to the child's age and height percentile. The child is normotensive if the BP is below the 90th percentile. If the BP is at or above the 90th percentile, repeat the BP measurement at that visit to verify an elevated BP. BP measurements between the 90th and 95th percentiles indicate prehypertension and necessitate reassessment ar consideration of other risk factors. In addition, if an adolescent's B′ more than 120/80 mm Hg, consider the patient prehypertensive if this value is below the 90th percentile. This BP level typically for systolic BP at 12 years of age and for diastolic BP at 16 yea If the child's BP (systolic or diastolic) is at or above the 95th the child may be hypertensive, and the measurement mus on at least two occasions to confirm diagnosis (Natior Pressure Education Program Working Group on Hig′ in Children and Adolescents, 2004) (see Guidelines b′ Pressure Tables).

Orthostatic Hypotension

Orthostatic hypotension (OH), also calle′ *orthostatic intolerance,* often manifests as (dizziness), or lightheadedness and is c′ to the brain (cerebral hypoperfusion). ′ is maintained at a constant level

GUIDELINES

Using the Blood Pressure Tables

1. Use the standard height charts to determine the height percentile.
2. Measure and record the child's systolic BP and diastolic BP.
3. Use the correct gender table for systolic BP and diastolic BP.
4. Find the child's age on the left side of the table. Follow the age row horizontally across the table to the intersection of the line for the height percentile (vertical column).
5. Then, find the 50th, 90th, 95th, and 99th percentiles for systolic BP in the left columns and for diastolic BP in the right columns.
   - BP less than 90th percentile is normal.
   - BP between the 90th and 95th percentiles is prehypertension. In adolescents, BP of 120/80 mm Hg or greater is prehypertension even if this figure is less than the 90th percentile.
   - BP over the 95th percentile may be hypertension.
6. If the BP is over the 90th percentile, the BP should be repeated twice at the same office visit, and an average systolic BP and diastolic BP should be used.
7. If the BP is over the 95th percentile, the BP should be staged. If BP is stage 1 (95th to 99th percentile plus 5 mm Hg), BP measurements should be repeated on two more occasions. If hypertension is confirmed, evaluation should proceed. If BP is stage 2 (>99th percentile plus 5 mm Hg), prompt referral should be made for evaluation and therapy. If the patient is symptomatic, immediate referral and treatment are indicated.

BP, Blood pressure.
From National High Blood Pressure Education Program Working Group on High Blood Pressure in Children and Adolescents. (2004). The fourth report on the diagnosis, evaluation, and treatment of high blood pressure in children and adolescents. *Pediatrics, 114*(2 suppl, 4th report), 555–576.

mechanisms that regulate systemic BP. When one assumes a sitting or standing position from a supine or recumbent position, peripheral capillary vasoconstriction occurs, and blood that was pooling in the lower vasculature is returned to the heart for redistribution to the head and remainder of the body. When this mechanism fails or is slow to respond, the person may experience vertigo or syncope. One of the most common causes of OH is hypovolemia, which may be induced by medications, such as diuretics, vasodilator medications, and prolonged immobility or bed rest. Other causes of OH include dehydration, diarrhea, emesis, fluid loss from sweating and exertion, alcohol intake, dysrhythmias, diabetes mellitus, sepsis, and hemorrhage.

BP measurements taken with the child first supine and then standing (at least 2 minutes in each position) may demonstrate variability and assist in the diagnosis of OH. The child with a sustained drop in systolic BP of more than 20 mm Hg or in diastolic pressure of more than 10 mm Hg after standing for 2 minutes without an increase in heart rate of more than 15 beats/min most likely has an autonomic deficit. Nonneurogenic causes of OH have a compensatory increase in pulse of more than 15 beats/min, as well as a drop in BP, as noted previously. For children and adolescents with vertigo, lightheadedness, nausea, syncope, diaphoresis, and pallor, it is important to monitor BP and heart rate to determine the original cause. BP is an important diagnostic measurement in children and adolescents and must be a part of the routine monitoring of vital signs.

NURSING ALERT

...hed norms for blood pressure (BP) are valid only if you use the same ...d of measurement (auscultation and cuff size determination) in clinical

GENERAL APPEARANCE

The child's general appearance is a cumulative, subjective impression of the child's physical appearance, state of nutrition, behavior, personality, interactions with parents and nurse (also siblings if present), posture, development, and speech. Although the nurse records general appearance at the beginning of the physical examination, it encompasses all the observations of the child during the interview and physical assessment.

Note the facies, the child's facial expression and appearance. For example, the facies may give clues to children who are in pain; have difficulty breathing; feel frightened, discontented, or unhappy; are mentally delayed; or are acutely ill.

Observe the posture, position, and types of body movement. A child with hearing or vision loss may characteristically tilt the head in an awkward position to hear or see better. A child in pain may favor a body part. The child with low self-esteem or a feeling of rejection may assume a slumped, careless, and apathetic pose. Likewise, a child with confidence, a feeling of self-worth, and a sense of security usually demonstrates a tall, straight, well-balanced posture. While observing such body language, do not interpret too freely but rather record objectively.

Note the child's hygiene in terms of cleanliness; unusual body odor; the condition of the hair, neck, nails, teeth, and feet; and the condition of the clothing. Such observations are excellent clues to possible instances of neglect, inadequate financial resources, housing difficulties (e.g., no running water), or lack of knowledge concerning children's needs.

Behavior includes the child's personality, activity level, reaction to stress, requests, frustration, interactions with others (primarily the parent and nurse), degree of alertness, and response to stimuli. Some mental questions that serve as reminders for observing behavior include the following:

- What is the child's overall personality?
- Does the child have a long attention span, or is he or she easily distracted?
- Can the child follow two or three commands in succession without the need for repetition?
- What is the child's response to delayed gratification or frustration?
- Does the child use eye contact during conversation?
- What is the child's reaction to the nurse and family members?
- Is the child quick or slow to grasp explanations?

SKIN

Assess skin for color, texture, temperature, moisture, turgor, lesions, acne, and rashes. Examination of the skin and its accessory organs primarily involves inspection and palpation. Touch allows the nurse to assess the texture, turgor, and temperature of the skin. The normal color in light-skinned children varies from a milky white and rose to a deeply hued pink. Dark-skinned children, such as those of Native American, Hispanic, or African descent, have inherited various brown, red, yellow, olive green, and bluish tones in their skin. Asian persons have skin that is normally of a yellow tone. Several variations in skin color can occur, some of which warrant further investigation. The types of color change and their appearance in children with light or dark skin are summarized in Table 29.6.

Normally, the skin texture of young children is smooth, slightly dry, and not oily or clammy. Evaluate skin temperature by symmetrically feeling each part of the body and comparing upper areas with lower ones. Note any difference in temperature.

Determine tissue turgor, or elasticity in the skin, by grasping the skin on the abdomen between the thumb and index finger, pulling it taut, and quickly releasing it. Elastic tissue immediately resumes its normal position without residual marks or creases. In children with

TABLE 29.6   Differences in Color Changes of Racial Groups

Description	Appearance in Light Skin	Appearance in Dark Skin
Cyanosis: bluish tone through skin; reflects reduced (deoxygenated) hemoglobin	Bluish tinge, especially in palpebral conjunctiva (lower eyelid), nail beds, earlobes, lips, oral membranes, soles, and palms	Ashen gray lips and tongue
Pallor: paleness; may be sign of anemia, chronic disease, edema, or shock	Loss of rosy glow in skin, especially face	Ashen gray appearance in black skin More yellowish brown color in brown skin
Erythema: redness; may be result of increased blood flow from climatic conditions, local inflammation, infection, skin irritation, allergy, or other dermatoses or may be caused by increased numbers of red blood cells as compensatory response to chronic hypoxia	Redness easily seen anywhere on body	Much more difficult to assess; rely on palpation for warmth or edema
Ecchymosis: large, diffuse areas, usually black and blue, caused by hemorrhage of blood into skin; typically result of injuries	Purplish to yellow-green areas; may be seen anywhere on skin	Very difficult to see unless in mouth or conjunctiva
Petechiae: same as ecchymosis except for size: small, distinct, pinpoint hemorrhages ≤2 mm in size; can denote some type of blood disorder, such as leukemia	Purplish pinpoints most easily seen on buttocks, abdomen, and inner surfaces of arms or legs	Usually invisible except in oral mucosa, conjunctiva of eyelids, and conjunctiva covering eyeball
Jaundice: yellow staining of skin usually caused by bile pigments	Yellow staining seen in sclerae of eyes, skin, fingernails, soles, palms, and oral mucosa	Most reliably assessed in sclerae, hard palate, palms, and soles

poor skin turgor, the skin remains suspended or tented for a few seconds before slowly falling back on the abdomen. Skin turgor is one of the best estimates of adequate hydration and nutrition.

ACCESSORY STRUCTURES

Inspection of the accessory structures of the skin may be performed while examining the skin, scalp, or extremities. Inspect the hair for color, texture, quality, distribution, and elasticity. Children's scalp hair is usually lustrous, silky, strong, and elastic. Genetic factors affect the appearance of hair. For example, the hair of African-American children is usually curlier and coarser than that of Caucasian children. Hair that is stringy, dull, brittle, dry, friable, and depigmented may suggest poor nutrition. Record any bald or thinning spots. Loss of hair in infants may indicate lying in the same position and may be a cue to counsel parents concerning the child's stimulation needs.

Inspect the hair and scalp for general cleanliness. Persons in some ethnic groups condition their hair with oils or lubricants that, if not thoroughly washed from the scalp, clog the sebaceous glands, causing scalp infections. Also examine the area for lesions, scaliness, evidence of infestation (e.g., lice or ticks), and signs of trauma (e.g., ecchymosis, masses, or scars).

In children who are approaching puberty, look for growth of secondary hair as a sign of normally progressing pubertal changes. Note precocious or delayed appearance of hair growth because, although not always suggestive of hormonal dysfunction, it may be of great concern to the early- or late-maturing adolescent.

Inspect the nails for color, shape, texture, and quality. Normally, the nails are pink, convex, smooth, and hard but flexible (not brittle). The edges, which are usually white, should extend over the fingers. Dark-skinned individuals may have more deeply pigmented nail beds. Short, ragged nails are typical of habitual biting. Uncut, dirty nails are a sign of poor hygiene.

The palm normally shows three flexion creases (Fig. 29.14, *A*). In some conditions such as Down syndrome, the two distal horizontal creases may be fused to form a single horizontal crease (the single palmar crease, or transpalmar crease) (see Fig. 29.14, *B*). If grossly abnormal lines or folds are observed, sketch a picture to describe them, and refer the finding to a specialist for further investigation.

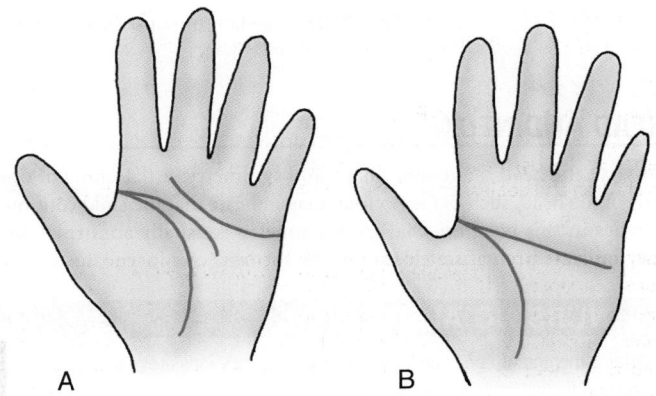

FIG 29.14 Examples of flexion creases on palm. **A,** Normal. **B,** Transpalmar crease.

LYMPH NODES

Lymph nodes are usually assessed during examination of the part of the body in which they are located. The body's lymphatic drainage system is extensive. Fig. 29.15 shows the usual sites for palpating accessible lymph nodes.

Palpate nodes using the distal portion of the fingers and gently but firmly pressing in a circular motion along the regions where nodes are normally present. During assessment of the nodes in the head and neck, tilt the child's head upward slightly but without tensing the sternocleidomastoid or trapezius muscles. This position facilitates palpation of the submental, submandibular, tonsillar, and cervical nodes. Palpate the axillary nodes with the child's arms relaxed at the sides but slightly abducted. Assess the inguinal nodes with the child in the supine position. Note size, mobility, temperature, and tenderness, as well as reports by the parents regarding any visible change of enlarged nodes. In children, small, nontender, movable nodes are usually normal. Tender, enlarged, warm, erythematous lymph nodes generally indicate infection or inflammation close to their location. Report such findings for further investigation.

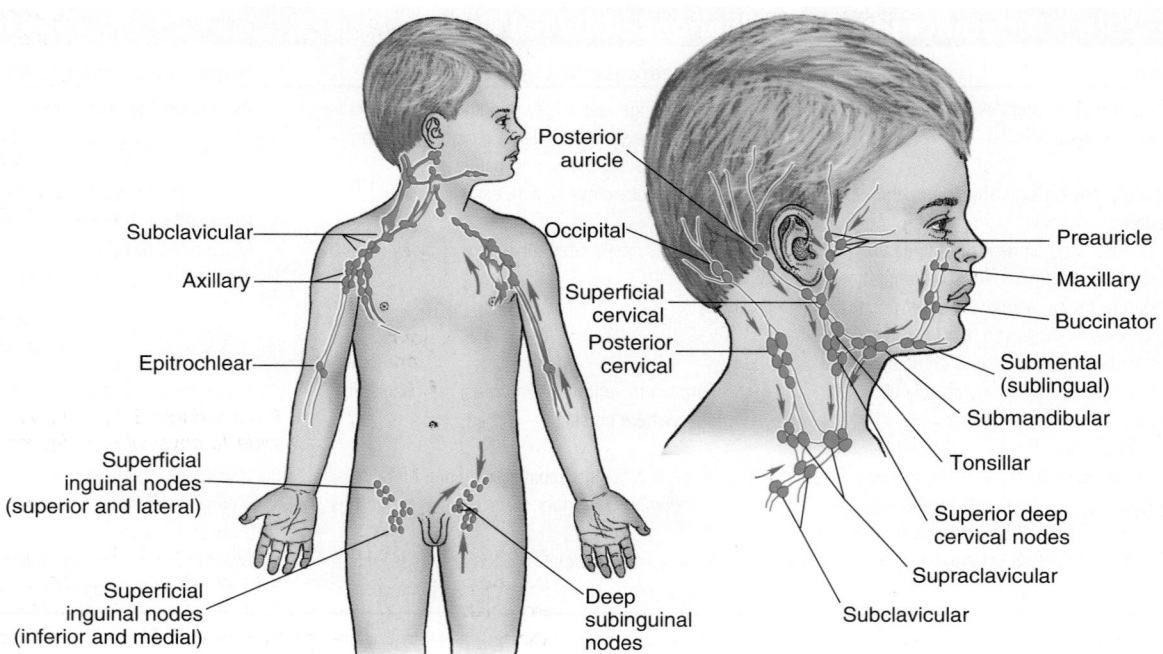

FIG 29.15 Location of superficial lymph nodes. *Arrows* indicate directional flow of lymph.

HEAD AND NECK

Observe the head for general shape and symmetry. A flattening of one part of the head, such as the occiput, may indicate that the child continually lies in this position. Marked asymmetry is usually abnormal and may indicate premature closure of the sutures (craniosynostosis).

> **! NURSING ALERT**
>
> After 6 months of age, significant head lag strongly indicates cerebral injury and is referred for further evaluation.

Note head control in infants and head posture in older children. By 4 months of age, most infants should be able to hold the head erect and in midline when in a vertical position.

Evaluate range of motion by asking the older child to look in each direction (to either side, up and down) or by manually putting the younger child through each position. Limited range of motion may indicate wry neck, or torticollis, in which the child holds the head to one side with the chin pointing toward the opposite side as a result of injury to the sternocleidomastoid muscle.

> **! NURSING ALERT**
>
> Hyperextension of the head (opisthotonos) with pain on flexion is a serious indication of meningeal irritation and is referred for immediate medical evaluation.

Palpate the skull for patent sutures, fontanels, fractures, and swellings. Normally, the posterior fontanel closes by 2 months of age, and the anterior fontanel fuses between 12 and 18 months of age. Early or late closure is noted, because either may be a sign of a pathologic condition.

While examining the head, observe the face for symmetry, movement, and general appearance. Ask the child to "make a face" to assess symmetric movement and disclose any degree of paralysis. Note any unusual facial proportion, such as an unusually high or low forehead; wide- or close-set eyes; or a small, receding chin.

In addition to assessment of the head and neck for movement, inspect the neck for size, and palpate its associated structures. The neck is normally short, with skinfolds between the head and shoulders during infancy; however, it lengthens during the next 3 to 4 years.

> **! NURSING ALERT**
>
> If any masses are detected in the neck, report them for further investigation. Large masses can block the airway.

EYES

Inspection of External Structures

Inspect the lids for proper placement on the eye. When the eye is open, the upper lid should fall near the upper iris. When the eyes are closed, the lids should completely cover the cornea and sclera (Fig. 29.16).

Determine the general slant of the palpebral fissures or lids by drawing an imaginary line through the two points of the medial canthus and across the outer orbit of the eyes and aligning each eye on the line. Usually the palpebral fissures lie horizontally. However, in Asians, the slant is normally upward.

Also inspect the inside lining of the lids, the palpebral conjunctivae. To examine the lower conjunctival sac, pull the lid down while the child looks up. To evert the upper lid, hold the upper lashes and gently pull down and forward as the child looks down. Normally the conjunctiva appears pink and glossy. Vertical yellow striations along the edge are the meibomian glands, or sebaceous glands, near the hair follicle. Located in the inner or medial canthus and situated on the inner edge of the upper and lower lids is a tiny opening, the *lacrimal punctum*. Note any excessive tearing, discharge, or inflammation of the lacrimal apparatus.

The bulbar conjunctiva, which covers the eye up to the limbus, or junction of the cornea and sclera, should be transparent. The sclera,

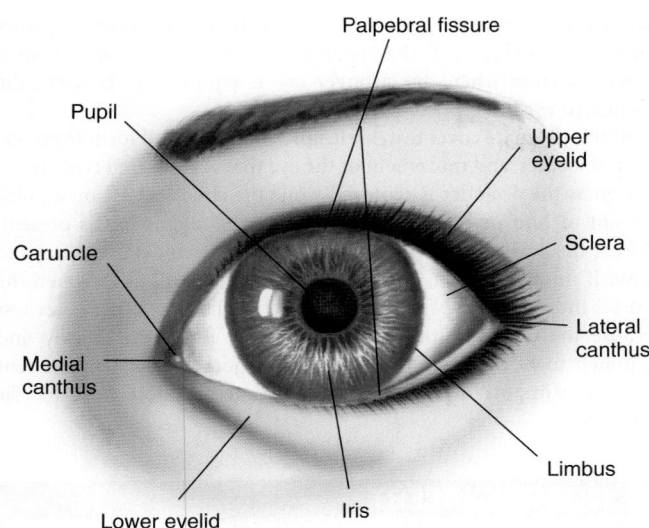

FIG 29.16 External structures of the eye.

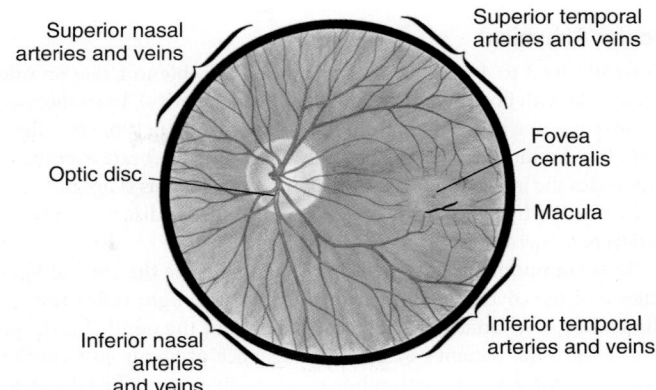

FIG 29.17 Structures of the fundus. (From Ball, J.W., Dains, J.E., Flynn, J.A., et al. [2015]. *Seidel's guide to physical examination* (8th ed.). St. Louis, MO: Elsevier.)

or white covering of the eyeball, should be clear. Tiny black marks in the sclera of heavily pigmented individuals are normal.

The cornea, or covering of the iris and pupil, should be clear and transparent. Record opacities, because they can be signs of scarring or ulceration, which can interfere with vision. The best way to test for opacities is to illuminate the eyeball by shining a light at an angle (obliquely) toward the cornea.

Compare the pupils for size, shape, and movement. They should be round, clear, and equal. Test their reaction to light by quickly shining a light toward the eye and removing it. As the light approaches, the pupils should constrict; as the light fades, the pupils should dilate. Test the pupil for any response of accommodation by having the child look at a bright, shiny object at a distance and quickly moving the object toward the face. The pupils should constrict as the object is brought near the eye. Record normal findings on examination of the pupils as PERRLA, which stands for "Pupils Equal, Round, React to Light, and Accommodation."

Inspect the iris and pupil for color, size, shape, and clarity. Permanent eye color is usually established by 6 to 12 months of age. While inspecting the iris and pupil, look for the lens. Normally, the lens is not visible through the pupil.

Inspection of Internal Structures

The ophthalmoscope permits visualization of the interior of the eyeball with a system of lenses and a high-intensity light. The lenses permit clear visualization of eye structures at different distances from the nurse's eye and correct visual acuity differences in the examiner and child. Use of the ophthalmoscope requires practice to know which lens setting produces the clearest image.

The ophthalmic and otic heads are usually interchangeable on one "body" or handle, which encloses the power source—either disposable or rechargeable batteries. The nurse should practice changing the heads, which snap on and are secured with a quarter turn, and replacing the batteries and light bulbs. Nurses who are not directly involved in physical assessment are often responsible for ensuring that the equipment functions properly.

Preparing the Child

The nurse can prepare the child for the ophthalmoscopic examination by showing the child the instrument, demonstrating the light source

and how it shines in the eye, and explaining the reason for darkening the room. For infants and young children who do not respond to such explanations, it is best to use distraction to encourage them to keep their eyes open. Forcibly parting the eyelids results in an uncooperative, watery-eyed child and a frustrated nurse. Usually, with some practice, the nurse can elicit a red reflex almost instantly while approaching the child and may also gain a momentary inspection of the blood vessels, macula, or optic disc.

Funduscopic Examination

Figure 29.17 shows the structures of the back of the eyeball, or the fundus. The fundus is immediately apparent as the red reflex. The intensity of the color increases in darkly pigmented individuals.

> **! NURSING ALERT**
>
> A brilliant, uniform red reflex is an important sign because it rules out many serious defects of the cornea, aqueous chamber, lens, and vitreous chamber. Any dark shadows or opacities are recorded because they indicate some abnormality in any of these structures.

As the ophthalmoscope is brought closer to the eye, the most conspicuous feature of the fundus is the optic disc, the area where the blood vessels and optic nerve fibers enter and exit the eye. The disc is orange to creamy pink with a pale center and lighter in color than the surrounding fundus. Normally, it is round or vertically oval.

After locating the optic disc, inspect the area for blood vessels. The central retinal artery and vein appear in the depths of the disc and emanate outward with visible branching. The veins are darker and about one-fourth larger than the arteries. Normally, the branches of the arteries and veins cross each other.

Other structures that are common are the macula, the area of the fundus with the greatest concentration of visual receptors, and in the center of the macula, a minute glistening spot of reflected light called the *fovea centralis;* this is the area of most perfect vision.

Vision Testing

The US Preventive Services Task Force (2011) recommends vision screening for the presence of amblyopia and its risk factors for all children 3 to 5 years of age. Several tests are available for assessing vision. This discussion focuses on ocular alignment, visual acuity, peripheral vision, and color vision. Nurses can provide accurate vision screening with appropriate training (Mathers, Keyes, & Wright, 2010).

Ocular Alignment

Normally, by 3 to 4 months of age, children are able to fixate on one visual field with both eyes simultaneously (binocularity). In *strabismus,* or cross-eye, one eye deviates from the point of fixation. If the misalignment is constant, the weak eye becomes "lazy," and the brain eventually suppresses the image produced by that eye. If strabismus is not detected and corrected by 4 to 6 years of age, blindness from disuse, known as *amblyopia,* may result.

Tests commonly used to detect misalignment are the corneal light reflex and the cover tests. To perform the corneal light reflex test, or Hirschberg test, shine a flashlight or the light of the ophthalmoscope directly into the patient's eyes from a distance of about 40.5 cm (16 inches). If the eyes are orthophoric, or normal, the light falls symmetrically within each pupil (Fig. 29.18, *A*). If the light falls off-center in one eye, the eyes are misaligned. Epicanthal folds, excess folds of skin that extend from the roof of the nose to the inner termination of the eyebrow and that partially or completely overlap the inner canthus of the eye, may give a false impression of misalignment (pseudostrabismus) (see Fig. 29.18, *B*). Epicanthal folds are often found in Asian children.

In the cover test, one eye is covered, and the movement of the uncovered eye is observed while the child looks at a near (33 cm [13 inches]) or distant (6 m [20 feet]) object. If the uncovered eye does not move, it is aligned. If the uncovered eye moves, a misalignment is present because when the stronger eye is temporarily covered, the misaligned eye attempts to fixate on the object.

In the alternate cover test, occlusion shifts back and forth from one eye to the other, and movement of the eye that was covered is observed as soon as the occluder is removed while the child focuses on a point in front of him or her (Fig. 29.19). If normal alignment is present, shifting the cover from one eye to the other will not cause the eye to move. If misalignment is present, eye movement will occur when the cover is moved. This test takes more practice than the other cover test because the occluder must be moved back and forth quickly and accurately to see the eye move. Because deviations can occur at different ranges, it is important to perform the cover tests at both close and far distances.

> ### ! NURSING ALERT
>
> The cover test is usually easier to perform if the examiner uses his or her hand rather than a card-type occluder (see Fig. 29.19). Attractive occluders fashioned like an ice cream cone or happy-face lollipop cut from cardboard are also well received by young children.

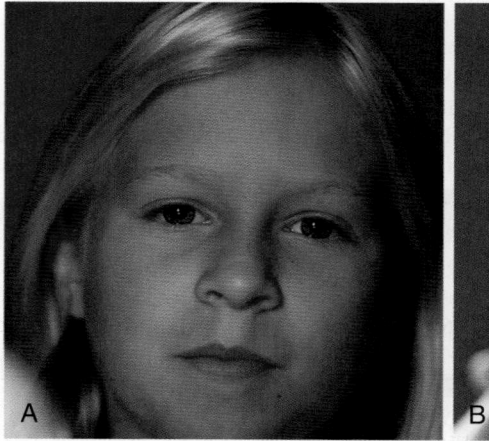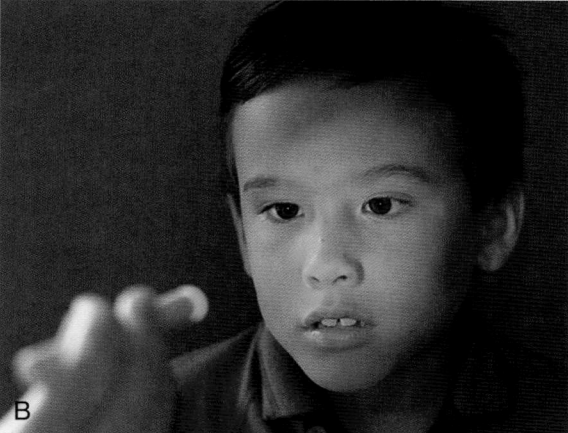

FIG 29.18 A, Corneal light reflex test demonstrating orthophoric eyes. **B,** Pseudostrabismus. Inner epicanthal folds cause the eyes to appear misaligned; however, the corneal light reflexes fall perfectly symmetrically.

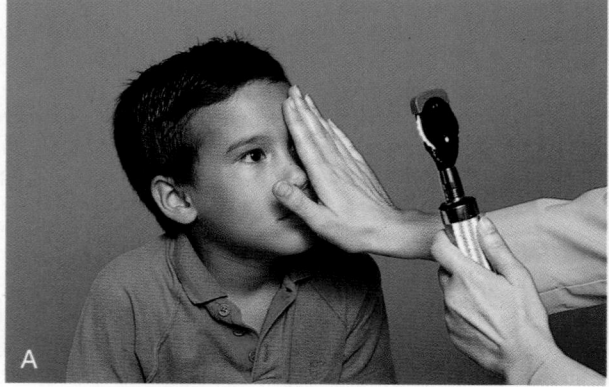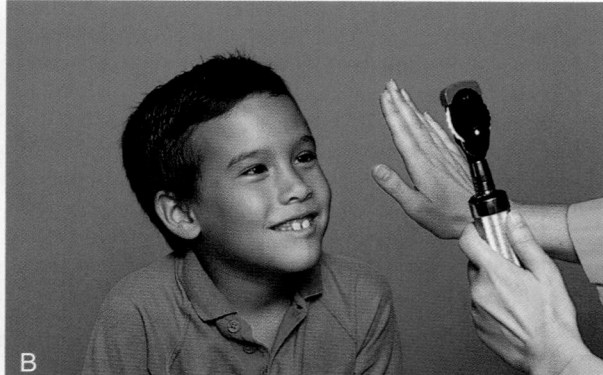

FIG 29.19 Alternate cover test to detect amblyopia in a patient with strabismus. **A,** The eye is occluded, and the child is fixating on light source. **B,** If the eye does not move when uncovered, the eyes are aligned.

Visual Acuity Testing in Children

The most common test for measuring visual acuity is the Snellen letter chart, which consists of lines of letters of decreasing size. The child stands with his or her heels at a line 10 feet away from the chart. When screening for visual acuity in children, the nurse tests the child's right eye first by covering the left. Children who wear glasses should be screened with them on. Tell the child to keep both eyes open during the examination. If the child fails to read the current line, move up the chart to the next larger line. Continue up the chart until the child is able to read the line. Then begin moving down the chart again until the child fails to read the line. To pass each line, the child must correctly identify four of six symbols on the line. Repeat the procedure, covering the right eye. Table 29.7 provides a list of visual screening tests for children and guidelines for referral.

For children unable to read letters and numbers, the tumbling E or HOTV test is useful. The tumbling E test uses the capital letter *E* pointing in four different directions. The child is asked to point in the direction

TABLE 29.7 Eye Examination Guidelines*

Function	Recommended Tests	Referral Criteria	Comments
3 to 5 Years of Age			
Distance visual acuity	Snellen letters Snellen numbers Tumbling E HOTV Picture test: • Allen figures • LEA symbols	1. Less than four of six correct on 20-foot (6-m) line with either eye tested at 10 feet (3 m) monocularly (i.e., <10/20 or 20/40) *or* 2. Two-line difference between eyes, even within passing range (i.e., 10/12.5 and 10/20 or 20/25 and 20/40)	1. Tests are listed in decreasing order of cognitive difficulty; highest test that child is capable of performing should be used; in general, tumbling E or HOTV test should be used for children 3 to 5 years of age and Snellen letters or numbers for children 6 years of age and older. 2. Testing distance of 10 feet (3 m) is recommended for all visual acuity tests. 3. Line of figures is preferred over single figures. 4. Non-tested eye should be covered by occluder held by examiner or by adhesive occluder patch applied to eye; examiner must ensure that it is not possible to peek with non-tested eye.
Ocular alignment	Cross cover test at 10 feet (3 m) Random dot E stereo test at 18 inches (40 cm) Simultaneous red reflex test (Bruckner test)	Any eye movement Less than four of six correct Any asymmetry of pupil color, size, brightness	Child must be fixing on a target while cross cover test is performed. Use direct ophthalmoscope to view both red reflexes simultaneously in a darkened room from 2 to 3 feet (0.6 to 0.9 m) away; detects asymmetric refractive errors as well.
Ocular media clarity (e.g., cataracts, tumors)	Red reflex	White pupil, dark spots, absent reflex	Use direct ophthalmoscope in a darkened room. View eyes separately at 12 to 18 inches (30 to 45 cm); white reflex indicates possible retinoblastoma.
6 Years of Age and Older			
Distance visual acuity	Snellen letters Snellen numbers Tumbling E HOTV Picture test: • Allen figures • LEA symbols	1. Less than four of six correct on 15-foot (4.5-m) line with either eye tested at 10 feet (3 m) monocularly (i.e., <10/15 or 20/30) *or* 2. Two-line difference between eyes, even within the passing range (i.e., 10/10 and 10/15 or 20/20 and 20/30)	1. Tests are listed in decreasing order of cognitive difficulty; highest test that child is capable of performing should be used; in general, tumbling E or HOTV test should be used for children 3 to 5 years of age and Snellen letters or numbers for children 6 years of age and older. 2. Testing distance of 10 feet (3 m) is recommended for all visual acuity tests. 3. Line of figures is preferred over single figures. 4. Non-tested eye should be covered by occluder held by examiner or by adhesive occluder patch applied to eye; examiner must ensure that it is not possible to peek with non-tested eye.
Ocular alignment	Cross cover test at 10 feet (3 m) Random dot E stereo test at 18 inches (40 cm) Simultaneous red reflex test (Bruckner test)	Any eye movement Less than four of six correct Any asymmetry of pupil color, size, brightness	Child must be fixing on target while cross cover test is performed. Use direct ophthalmoscope to view both red reflexes simultaneously in a darkened room from 2 to 3 feet (0.6 to 0.9 m) away; detects asymmetric refractive errors as well.
Ocular media clarity (e.g., cataracts, tumors)	Red reflex	White pupil, dark spots, absent reflex	Use direct ophthalmoscope in a darkened room. View eyes separately at 12 to 18 inches (30 to 45 cm); white reflex indicates possible retinoblastoma.

*Assessing visual acuity (vision screening) is one of the most sensitive techniques for detection of eye abnormalities in children. The American Academy of Pediatrics Section on Ophthalmology, in cooperation with the American Association for Pediatric Ophthalmology and Strabismus and the American Academy of Ophthalmology, has developed these guidelines to be used by physicians, nurses, educational institutions, public health departments, and other professionals who perform vision evaluation services.

From American Academy of Pediatrics, Committee on Practice and Ambulatory Medicine, Section on Ophthalmology. (2003). Eye examination in infants, children, and young adults by pediatricians, *Pediatrics, 111*(4), 902–907.

the *E* is facing. The HOTV test consists of a wall chart composed of the letters H, O, T, and V. The child is given a board containing a large H, O, T, and V. The examiner points to a letter on the wall chart, and the child matches the correct letter on the board held in his or her hand. The tumbling E and HOTV are excellent tests for preschool-age children.

Visual Acuity Testing in Infants and Difficult-to-Test Children

In newborns, vision is tested mainly by checking for light perception by shining a light into the eyes and noting responses, such as pupillary constriction, blinking, following the light to midline, increased alertness, or refusal to open the eyes after exposure to the light. Although the simple maneuver of checking light perception and eliciting the pupillary light reflex indicates that the anterior half of the visual apparatus is intact, it does not confirm that the infant can see. In other words, this test does not assess whether the brain receives the visual message and interprets the signals.

Another test of visual acuity is the infant's ability to fix on and follow a target. Although any brightly colored or patterned object can be used, the human face is excellent. Hold the infant upright while moving your face slowly from side to side. Other signs that may indicate visual loss or other serious eye problems include fixed pupils, strabismus, constant nystagmus, the setting-sun sign, and slow lateral movements. Unfortunately, it is difficult to test each eye separately; the presence of such signs in one eye could indicate unilateral blindness.

Special tests are available for testing infants and other difficult-to-test children to assess acuity or confirm blindness. For example, in visually evoked potentials, the eyes are stimulated with a bright light or pattern, and electrical activity to the visual cortex is recorded through scalp electrodes.

> **! NURSING ALERT**
>
> If visual fixation and following are not present by 3 to 4 months of age, further ophthalmologic evaluation is necessary.

Peripheral Vision

In children who are old enough to cooperate, estimate peripheral vision, or the visual field of each eye, by having the children fixate on a specific point directly in front of them while an object, such as a finger or a pencil, is moved from beyond the field of vision into the range of peripheral vision. As soon as children see the object, have them say "Stop." At that point, measure the angle from the anteroposterior axis of the eye (straight line of vision) to the peripheral axis (point at which the object is first seen). Check each eye separately and for each quadrant of vision. Normally children see about 50 degrees upward, 70 degrees downward, 60 degrees nasalward, and 90 degrees temporally. Limitations in peripheral vision may indicate blindness from damage to structures within the eye or to any of the visual pathways.

Color Vision

The tests available for color vision include the Ishihara test and the Hardy-Rand-Rittler test. Each consists of a series of cards (pseudoisochromatic) containing a color field composed of spots of a certain "confusion" color. Against the field is a number or symbol similarly printed in dots but of a color likely to be confused with the field color by a person with a color vision deficit. As a result, the figure or letter is invisible to an affected individual but is clearly seen by a person with normal vision.

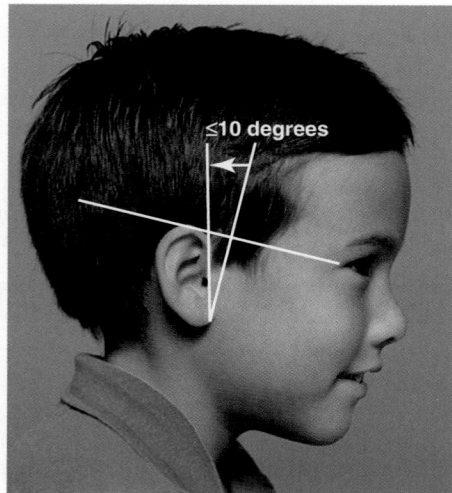

FIG 29.20 Ear alignment.

EARS

Inspection of External Structures

The entire external ear is called the *pinna*, or *auricle*; one is located on each side of the head. Measure the height alignment of the pinna by drawing an imaginary line from the outer orbit of the eye to the occiput, or most prominent protuberance of the skull. The top of the pinna should meet or cross this line. Low-set ears are commonly associated with renal anomalies or cognitive impairment. Measure the angle of the pinna by drawing a perpendicular line from the imaginary horizontal line and aligning the pinna next to this mark. Normally the pinna lies within a 10-degree angle of the vertical line (Fig. 29.20). If it falls outside this area, record the deviation and look for other anomalies.

Normally the pinna extends slightly outward from the skull. Except in newborn infants, ears that are flat against the head or protruding away from the scalp may indicate problems. Flattened ears in an infant may suggest a frequent side-lying position and, just as with isolated areas of hair loss, may be a clue to investigate parents' understanding of the child's stimulation needs.

Inspect the skin surface around the ear for small openings, extra tags of skin, sinuses, or earlobe creases. If a sinus is found, note this because it may represent a fistula that drains into some area of the neck or ear. Note if an earlobe crease is found, because it may be associated with a rare, inherited syndrome. However, having one small abnormality is not uncommon and is often not associated with a serious condition. Cutaneous tags represent no pathologic process but may cause parents concern in terms of the child's appearance.

Also assess the ears for hygiene. An otoscope is not necessary for looking into the external canal to note the presence of cerumen, a waxy substance produced by the ceruminous glands in the outer portion of the canal. Cerumen is usually yellow-brown and soft. If an otoscope is used and any discharge is visible, note its color and odor. Avoid transmitting potentially infectious material to the other ear or to another child through hand washing and using disposable specula or sterilizing reusable specula between each examination.

Inspection of Internal Structures

The head of the otoscope permits visualization of the tympanic membrane by use of a bright light, a magnifying glass, and a speculum. Some otoscopes have an attachment for a pneumonic device to insert

ATRAUMATIC CARE

Reducing Distress From Otoscopy in Young Children

Make examining the ear a game by explaining that you are looking for a "big elephant" in the ear. This kind of make-believe is an absorbing distraction and usually elicits cooperation. After examining the ear, clarify that "looking for elephants" was only pretend and thank the child for letting you look in his or her ear. Another great distraction technique is asking the child to put a finger on the opposite ear to keep the light from getting out.

air into the canal to determine membrane compliance (movement). The speculum, which is inserted into the external canal, comes in a variety of sizes to accommodate different canal widths. The largest speculum that fits comfortably into the ear is used to achieve the greatest area of visualization. The lens, or magnifying glass, is movable, allowing the examiner to insert an object, such as a curette, into the ear canal through the speculum while still viewing the structures through the lens.

Positioning the Child

Before beginning the otoscopic examination, position the child properly and gently restrain (sit on parent's lap and hold parent's hands) if necessary. Older children usually cooperate and do not need restraint. However, prepare them for the procedure by allowing them to play with the instrument, demonstrating how it works, and stressing the importance of remaining still. A helpful suggestion is to let them observe you examining the parent's ear. Restraint is needed for younger children, because the ear examination upsets them (see Atraumatic Care box: Reducing Distress from Otoscopy in Young Children).

As you insert the speculum into the meatus, move it around the outer rim to accustom the child to the feel of something entering the ear. If examining a painful ear, examine the unaffected ear first, then return to the painful ear, and touch a nonpainful part of the affected ear first. By this time, the child is usually less fearful of anything causing discomfort to the ear and will cooperate more.

For their protection and safety, restrain infants and toddlers for the otoscopic examination. There are two general positions of restraint. In one, the child is seated sideways in the parent's lap with one arm hugging the parent and the other arm at the side. The ear to be examined is toward the nurse. With one hand the parent holds the child's head firmly against his or her chest and hugs the child with the other arm, thereby securing the child's free arm (Fig. 29.21, A). Examine the ear using the same procedure for holding the otoscope as described later.

The other position involves placing the child on the side, back, or abdomen with the arms at the side and the head turned so that the ear to be examined points toward the ceiling. Lean over the child, use the upper part of the body to restrain the arms and upper trunk movements, and use the examining hand to stabilize the head. This position is practical for young infants and for older children who need minimum restraint, but it may not be feasible for other children who protest vigorously. For safety, enlist the parent's or an assistant's help in immobilizing the head by firmly placing one hand above the ear and the other on the child's side, abdomen, or back (see Fig. 29.21, B).

With cooperative children, examine the ear with the child in a side-lying, sitting, or standing position. One disadvantage to standing is that the child may "walk away" as the otoscope enters the canal. If the child is standing or sitting, tilt the head slightly toward the child's opposite shoulder to achieve a better view of the eardrum (Fig. 29.22).

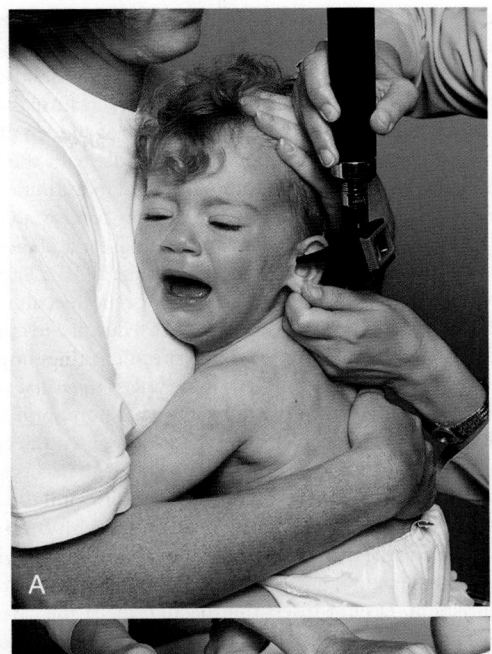
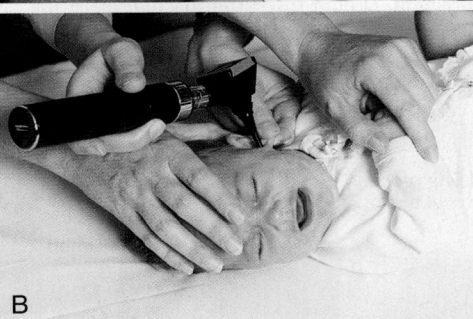

FIG 29.21 Position for restraining a child **(A)** and an infant **(B)** during otoscopic examination.

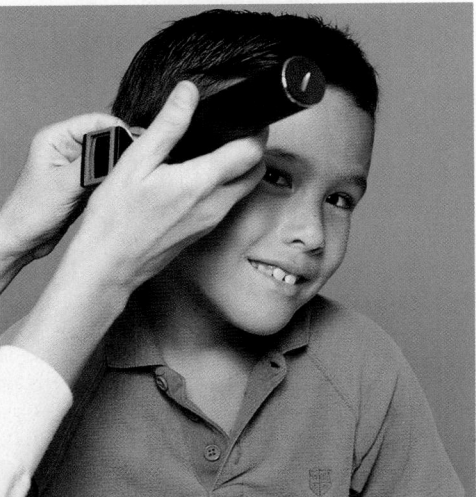

FIG 29.22 Positioning the head by tilting it toward the opposite shoulder for full view of the tympanic membrane.

With the thumb and forefinger of the free (usually nondominant) hand, grasp the auricle. For the two positions of restraint, hold the otoscope upside down at the junction of its head and handle with the thumb and index finger. Place the other fingers against the skull to allow the otoscope to move with the child in case of sudden movement. In examining a cooperative child, hold the handle with the otic head upright or upside down. Use the dominant hand to examine both ears or reverse hands for each ear, whichever is more comfortable.

Before using the otoscope, visualize the external ear and the tympanic membrane as being superimposed on a clock (Fig. 29.23). The numbers are important geographic landmarks. Introduce the speculum into the meatus between the 3 and 9 o'clock positions in a downward and forward position. Because the canal is curved, the speculum does not permit a panoramic view of the tympanic membrane unless the canal is straightened. In infants, the canal curves upward. Therefore, pull the pinna down and back to the 6 to 9 o'clock range to straighten the canal (Fig. 29.24, A). With older children, usually those older than 3 years of age, the canal curves downward and forward. Therefore, pull the pinna up and back toward the 10 o'clock position (see Fig. 29.24, B). If you have difficulty visualizing the membrane, try repositioning the head, introducing the speculum at a different angle, and pulling the pinna in a slightly different direction. Do not insert the speculum past the cartilaginous (outermost) portion of the canal, usually a distance of 0.60 to 1.25 cm (0.23 to 0.5 inch) in older children. Insertion of the speculum into the posterior or bony portion of the canal causes pain.

In neonates and young infants, the walls of the canal are pliable and floppy because of the underdeveloped cartilaginous and bony structures. Therefore, the very small 2-mm speculum usually needs to be inserted deeper into the canal than in older children. Exercise great care not to damage the walls or eardrum. For this reason, only an experienced examiner should insert an otoscope into the ears of very young infants.

Otoscopic Examination

As you introduce the speculum into the external canal, inspect the walls of the canal, the color of the tympanic membrane, the light reflex, and the usual landmarks of the bony prominences of the middle ear. The walls of the external auditory canal are pink, although they are more pigmented in dark-skinned children. Minute hairs are evident in the outermost portion, where cerumen is produced. Note signs of irritation, foreign bodies, or infection.

Foreign bodies in the ear are common in children and range from erasers to beans. Symptoms may include pain, discharge, and affected hearing. Remove soft objects, such as paper or insects, with forceps. Remove small, hard objects, such as pebbles, with a suction tip, a hook, or irrigation. However, irrigation is contraindicated if the object is vegetative matter, such as beans or pasta, which swells when in contact with fluid.

> **! NURSING ALERT**
>
> If there is any doubt about the type of object in the ear and the appropriate method to remove it, refer the child to the appropriate practitioner.

The tympanic membrane is a translucent, light pearly pink or gray. Note marked erythema (which may indicate suppurative otitis media); a dull, nontransparent grayish color (sometimes suggestive of serous otitis media); or ashen gray areas (signs of scarring from a previous perforation). A black area usually suggests a perforation of the membrane that has not healed.

The characteristic tenseness and slope of the tympanic membrane cause the light of the otoscope to reflect at about the 5 or 7 o'clock position. The light reflex is a fairly well-defined, cone-shaped reflection, which normally points away from the face.

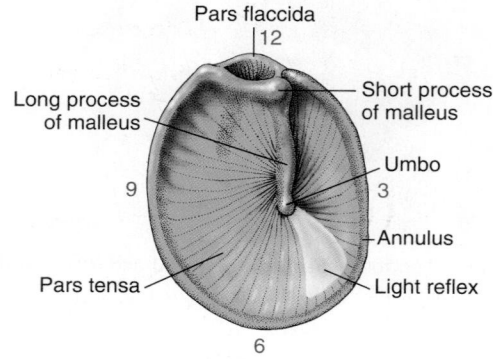

FIG 29.23 Landmarks of the tympanic membrane. (From Ignatavicius, D.D., & Workman, M.L. [2013]. *Medical-surgical nursing: Patient-centered collaborative care* [7th ed.]. St. Louis, MO: Saunders.)

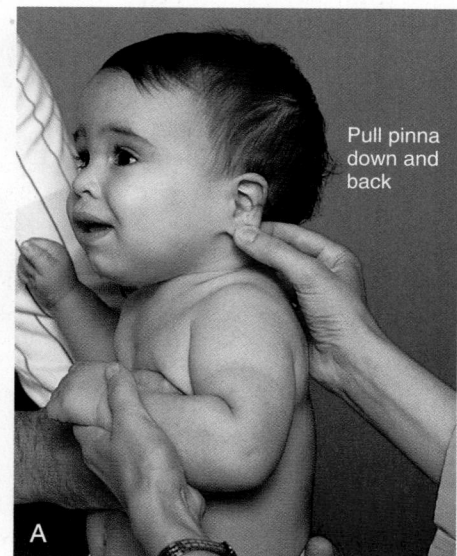
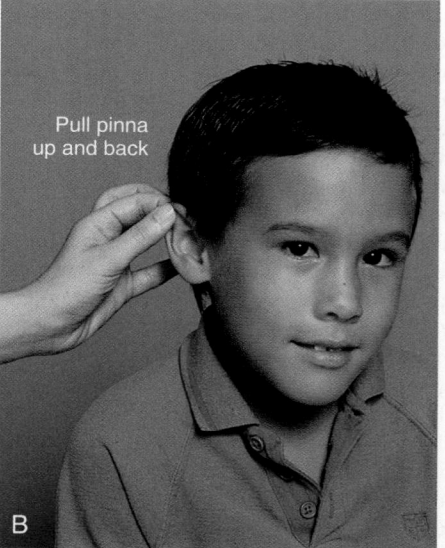

FIG 29.24 Positioning for visualizing the eardrum in an infant **(A)** and in a child older than 3 years of age **(B)**.

TABLE 29.8   Auditory Tests for Infants and Children

Age	Auditory Test and Average Time	Type of Measurement	Procedure
Newborns	Auditory brainstem response (ABR)	Electrophysiologic measurement of activity in auditory nerve and brainstem pathways	Placement of electrodes on child's head detects auditory stimuli presented though earphones one ear at a time.
Infants	Behavioral audiometry	Used to observe their behavior in response to certain sounds heard through speakers or earphones	The child's responses are observed to the sounds heard.
Toddlers	Play audiometry	Uses an audiometer to transmit sounds at different volumes and pitches	The toddler is asked to do something with a toy (i.e., touch a toy, move a toy) every time the sound is heard.
Children and adolescents	Pure tone audiometry	Uses an audiometer that produces sounds at different volumes and pitches in the child's ears	The child is asked to respond in some way when the tone is heard in the earphone.
	Tympanometry (also called *impedance* or *admittance*)	Determines how the middle ear is functioning and detects any changes in pressure in the middle ear	A soft plastic tip is placed over the ear canal and the tympanometer measures eardrum movement when the pressure changes.
All ages	Evoked optoacoustic emissions (EOAE)	Physiologic test specifically measuring cochlear (outer hair cell) response to presentation of stimulus	Small probe containing sensitive microphone is placed in ear canal for stimulus delivery and response detection.

The bony landmarks of the eardrum are formed by the umbo, or tip of the malleus. It appears as a small, round, opaque, concave spot near the center of the eardrum. The manubrium (long process or handle) of the malleus appears to be a whitish line extending from the umbo upward to the margin of the membrane. At the upper end of the long process near the 1 o'clock position (in the right ear) is a sharp, knoblike protuberance, representing the short process of the malleus. Note the absence or distortion of the light reflex or loss or abnormal prominence of any of these landmarks.

Auditory Testing

Several types of hearing tests are available and recommended for screening in infants and children (Table 29.8). The American Academy of Pediatrics recommends pure tone audiometry testing at 500, 1000, 2000, and 4000 Hz, with children failing if they cannot hear the tones at 20 dB (Harlor, Bower, & Committee on Practice and Ambulatory Medicine, Section on Otolaryngology–Head and Neck Surgery, 2009). Universal newborn hearing screening is available in most US states. The nurse must operate under a high index of suspicion for those children who may have conditions associated with hearing loss, whose parents are concerned about hearing loss, and who may have developed behaviors that indicate auditory impairment.

NOSE

Inspection of External Structures

The nose is located in the middle of the face just below the eyes and above the lips. Compare its placement and alignment by drawing an imaginary vertical line from the center point between the eyes down to the notch of the upper lip. The nose should lie exactly vertical to this line, with each side exactly symmetric. Note its location, any deviation to one side, and asymmetry in overall size and in diameter of the nares (nostrils). The bridge of the nose is sometimes flat in Asian and African-American children. Observe the alae nasi for any sign of flaring, which indicates respiratory difficulty. Always report any flaring of the alae nasi. Fig. 29.25 illustrates the landmarks used in describing the external structures of the nose.

Inspection of Internal Structures

Inspect the anterior vestibule of the nose by pushing the tip upward, tilting the head backward, and illuminating the cavity with a flashlight or otoscope without the attached ear speculum. Note the color of the mucosal lining, which is normally redder than the oral membranes, as

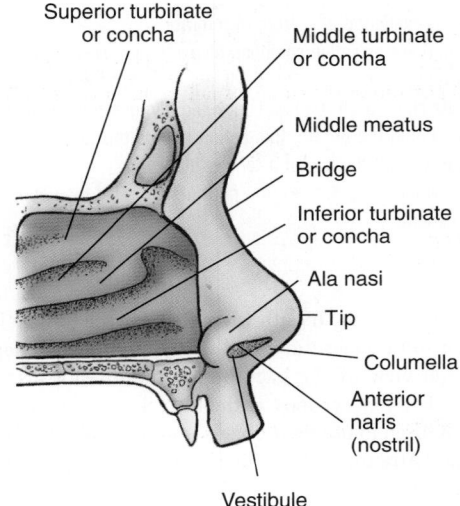

FIG 29.25 External landmarks and internal structures of the nose.

Labels: Superior turbinate or concha; Middle turbinate or concha; Middle meatus; Bridge; Inferior turbinate or concha; Ala nasi; Tip; Columella; Anterior naris (nostril); Vestibule

well as any swelling, discharge, dryness, or bleeding. There should be no discharge from the nose.

On looking deeper into the nose, inspect the turbinates, or concha, plates of bone that jut into the nasal cavity and are enveloped by the mucous membranes. The turbinates greatly increase the surface area of the nasal cavity as air is inhaled. The spaces or channels between the turbinates are called the *meatus* and correspond to each of the three turbinates. Normally, the front end of the inferior and middle turbinate and the middle meatus are seen. They should be the same color as the lining of the vestibule.

Inspect the septum, which should divide the vestibules equally. Note any deviation, especially if it causes an occlusion of one side of the nose. A perforation may be evident within the septum. If this is suspected, shine the light of the otoscope into one naris and look for admittance of light to the other. Because olfaction is an important function of the nose, testing for smell may be done at this point or as part of cranial nerve assessment (see Table 29.11).

MOUTH AND THROAT

With a cooperative child, the nurse can accomplish almost the entire examination of the mouth and throat without the use of a tongue blade.

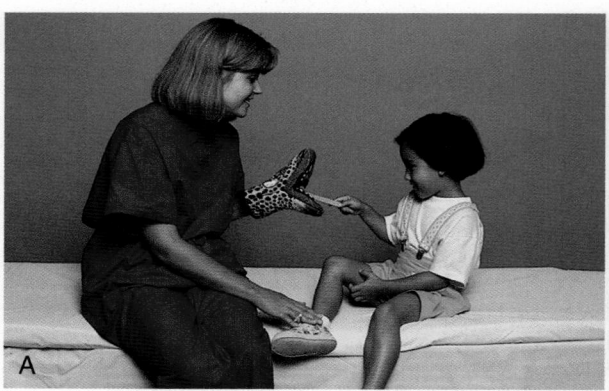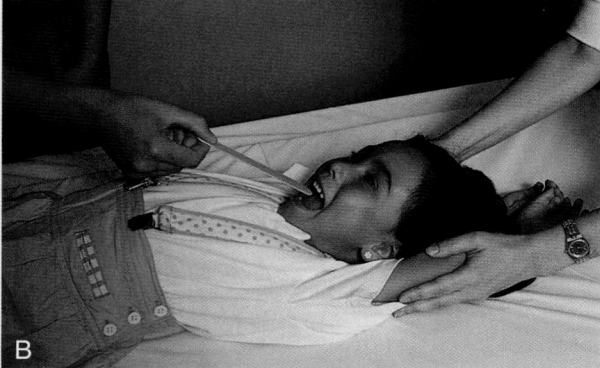

FIG 29.26 A, Encouraging a child to cooperate. **B,** Positioning a child for examination of the mouth.

ATRAUMATIC CARE

Encouraging Opening the Mouth for Examination

- Perform the examination in front of a mirror.
- Let the child first examine someone else's mouth, such as the parent, the nurse, or a puppet (see Fig. 29.26, *A*), and then examine the child's mouth.
- Instruct the child to tilt the head back slightly, breathe deeply through the mouth, and hold the breath; this action lowers the tongue to the floor of the mouth without the use of a tongue blade.
- Lightly brushing the palate with a cotton swab also may open the mouth for assessment.

Ask the child to open the mouth wide; to move the tongue in different directions for full visualization; and to say "ahh," which depresses the tongue for full view of the back of the mouth (tonsils, uvula, and oropharynx). For a closer look at the buccal mucosa, or lining of the cheeks, ask children to use their fingers to move the outer lip and cheek to one side (see Atraumatic Care box: Encouraging Opening the Mouth for Examination).

Infants and toddlers usually resist attempts to keep the mouth open. Because inspecting the mouth is upsetting, leave it for the end of the physical examination (along with examination of the ears) or do it during episodes of crying. However, the use of a tongue blade (preferably flavored) to depress the tongue may be needed. Place the tongue blade along the side of the tongue, not in the center back area where the gag reflex is elicited. Fig. 29.26, *B*, illustrates proper positioning of the child for the oral examination.

The major structure of the exterior of the mouth is the lips. The lips should be moist, soft, smooth, and pink, or a deeper hue than the surrounding skin. The lips should be symmetric when relaxed or tensed. Assess symmetry when the child talks or cries.

Inspection of Internal Structures

The major structures that are visible within the oral cavity and oropharynx are the mucosal lining of the lips and cheeks, gums (or gingiva), teeth, tongue, palate, uvula, tonsils, and posterior oropharynx (Fig. 29.27). Inspect all areas lined with mucous membranes (inside the lips and cheeks, gingiva, underside of the tongue, palate, and back of the pharynx) for color, any areas of white patches or ulceration, bleeding, sensitivity, and moisture. The membranes should be bright pink, smooth, glistening, uniform, and moist.

Inspect the teeth for number (deciduous, permanent, or mixed dentition) in each dental arch, for hygiene, and for occlusion or bite. Discoloration of tooth enamel with obvious plaque (whitish coating

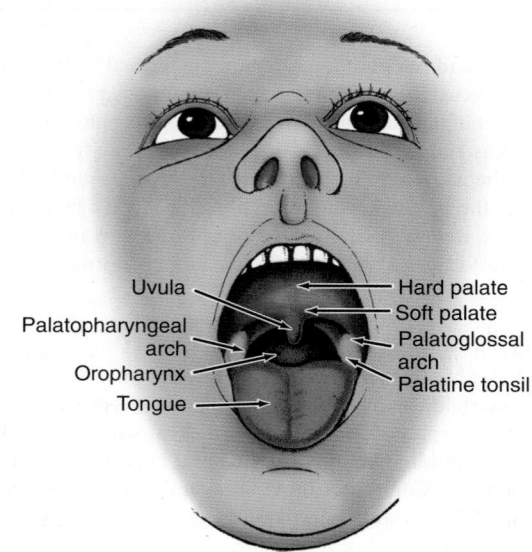

FIG 29.27 Interior structures of the mouth.

on the surface of the teeth) is a sign of poor dental hygiene and indicates a need for counseling. Brown spots in the crevices of the crown of the tooth or between the teeth may be caries (cavities). Chalky white to yellow or brown areas on the enamel may indicate fluorosis (excessive fluoride ingestion). Teeth that appear greenish black may be stained temporarily from ingestion of supplemental iron.

Examine the gums (gingiva) surrounding the teeth. The color is normally coral pink, and the surface texture is stippled, similar to the appearance of an orange peel. In dark-skinned children, the gums are more deeply colored, and a brownish area is often observed along the gum line.

Inspect the tongue for papillae, small projections that contain several taste buds and give the tongue its characteristic rough appearance. Note the size and mobility of the tongue. Normally the tip of the tongue should extend to the lips or beyond.

The roof of the mouth consists of the hard palate, which is located near the front of the oral cavity, and the soft palate, which is located toward the back of the pharynx and has a small midline protrusion called the *uvula*. Carefully inspect the palates to ensure they are intact. The arch of the palate should be dome shaped. A narrow, flat roof or a high, arched palate affects the placement of the tongue and can cause feeding and speech problems. Test movement of the uvula by eliciting

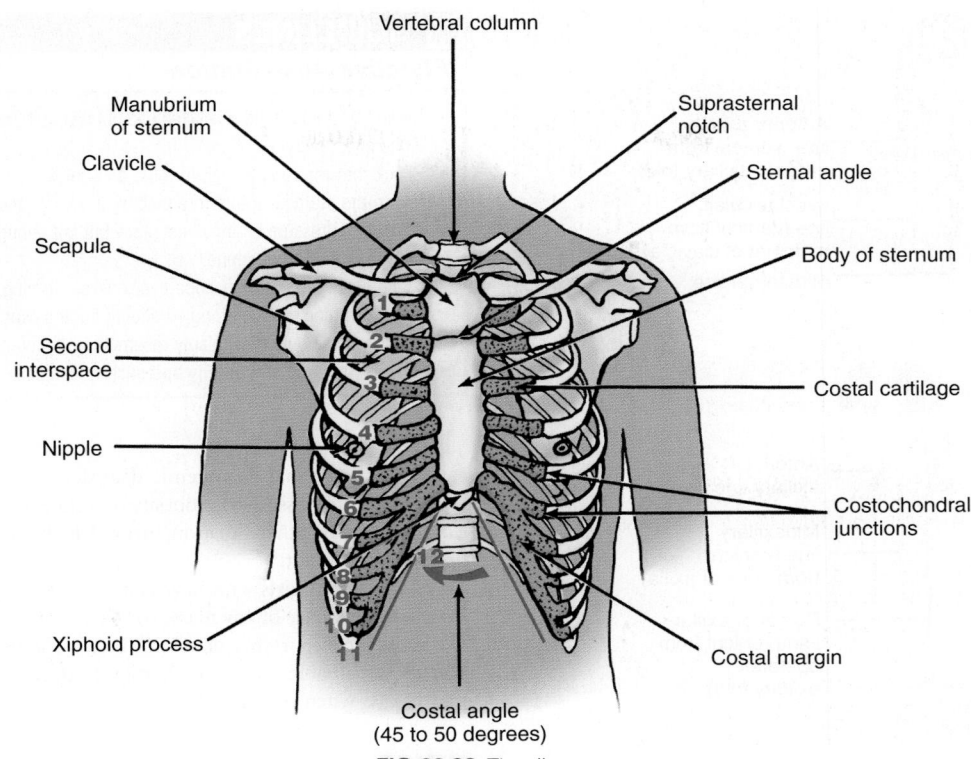

FIG 29.28 The rib cage.

a gag reflex. It should move upward to close off the nasopharynx from the oropharynx.

Examine the oropharynx, and note the size and color of the palatine tonsils. They are normally the same color as the surrounding mucosa; glandular, rather than smooth in appearance; and barely visible over the edge of the palatoglossal arches. The size of the tonsils varies considerably during childhood. However, report any swelling, redness, or white areas on the tonsils.

CHEST

Inspect the chest for size, shape, symmetry, movement, breast development, and the bony landmarks formed by the ribs and sternum. The rib cage consists of 12 ribs on each side and the sternum, or breast bone, located in the midline of the trunk (Fig. 29.28). The sternum is composed of three main parts. The manubrium, the uppermost portion, can be felt at the base of the neck at the suprasternal notch. The largest segment of the sternum is the body, which forms the sternal angle (angle of Louis) as it articulates with the manubrium. At the end of the body is a small, movable process called the *xiphoid*. The angle of the costal margin as it attaches to the sternum is called the *costal angle* and is normally about 45 to 50 degrees. These bony structures are important landmarks in the location of ribs and intercostal spaces (ICSs), which are the spaces between the ribs. They are numbered according to the rib directly above the space. For example, the space immediately below the second rib is the second ICS.

The thoracic cavity is also divided into segments by drawing imaginary lines on the chest and back. Fig. 29.29 illustrates the anterior, lateral, and posterior divisions.

Measure the size of the chest by placing the measuring tape around the rib cage at the nipple line. For greatest accuracy, take two measurements (one during inspiration and the other during expiration), and record the average. Chest size is important mainly in relation to head

circumference (see the "Head Circumference" section earlier in this chapter). Always report marked disproportions because most are caused by abnormal head growth, although some may be a result of altered chest shape, such as barrel chest (chest is round), pectus excavatum (sternum is depressed), or pectus carinatum (sternum protrudes outward).

During infancy, the chest's shape is almost circular, with the anteroposterior (front-to-back) diameter equaling the transverse, or lateral (side-to-side), diameter. As the child grows, the chest normally increases in the transverse direction, causing the anteroposterior diameter to be less than the lateral diameter. Note the angle made by the lower costal margin and the sternum, and palpate the junction of the ribs with the costal cartilage (costochondral junction) and sternum, which should be fairly smooth.

Movement of the chest wall should be symmetric bilaterally and coordinated with breathing. During inspiration, the chest rises and expands, the diaphragm descends, and the costal angle increases. During expiration, the chest falls and decreases in size, the diaphragm rises, and the costal angle narrows (Fig. 29.30). In children younger than 6 or 7 years of age, respiratory movement is principally abdominal or diaphragmatic. In older children, particularly girls, respirations are chiefly thoracic. In either case, the chest and abdomen should rise and fall together. Always report any asymmetry of movement.

While inspecting the skin surface of the chest, observe the position of the nipples and any evidence of breast development. Normally the nipples are located slightly lateral to the midclavicular line between the fourth and fifth ribs. Note symmetry of nipple placement and normal configuration of a darker pigmented areola surrounding a flat nipple in prepubertal children.

Pubertal breast development usually begins in girls between 8 and 12 years of age (see Chapter 35). Record early (precocious) or delayed breast development, as well as evidence of any other secondary sexual characteristics. In males, breast enlargement (gynecomastia) may be

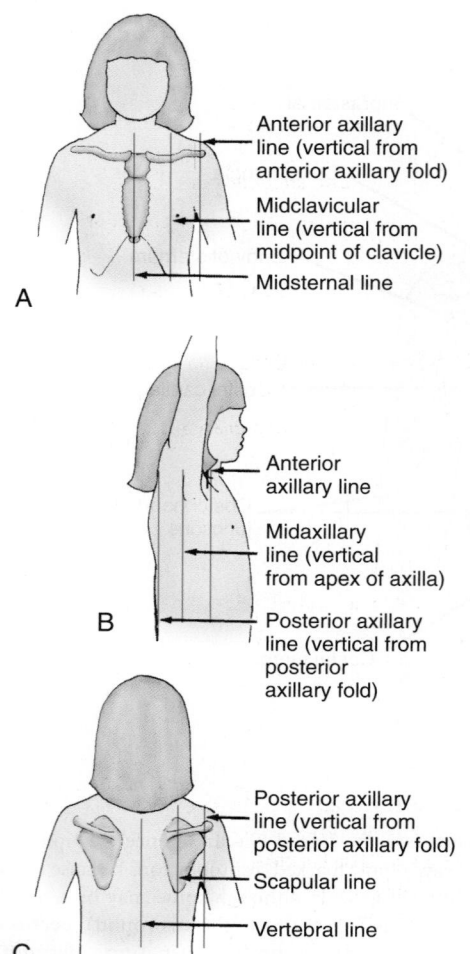

FIG 29.29 Imaginary landmarks of the chest. **A,** Anterior. **B,** Right lateral. **C,** Posterior.

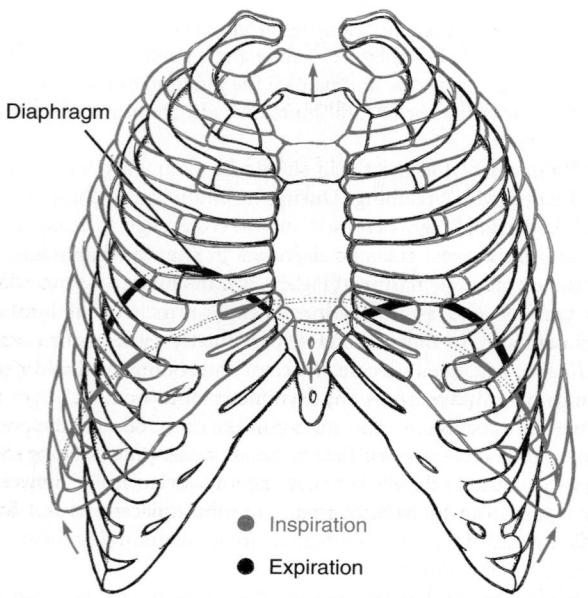

FIG 29.30 Movement of the chest during respiration.

GUIDELINES
Effective Auscultation

- Make certain the child is relaxed and not crying, talking, or laughing. Record if the child is crying.
- Check that the room is comfortable and quiet.
- Warm the stethoscope before placing it against the child's skin.
- Apply firm pressure on the chest piece but not enough to prevent vibrations and transmission of sound.
- Avoid placing the stethoscope over hair or clothing, moving it against the skin, breathing on the tubing, or sliding fingers over the chest piece, which may cause sounds that falsely resemble pathologic findings.
- Use a symmetric and orderly approach to compare sounds.

---

caused by hormonal or systemic disorders, but more commonly is a result of adipose tissue from obesity or a transitory body change during early puberty. In either situation, investigate the child's feelings regarding breast enlargement.

In adolescent girls who have achieved sexual maturity, palpate the breasts for evidence of any masses or hard nodules. Use this opportunity to discuss the importance of routine breast self-examination. Emphasize that most palpable masses are benign to decrease any fear or concern that results when a mass is felt.

LUNGS

The lungs are situated inside the thoracic cavity, with one lung on each side of the sternum. Each lung is divided into an apex, which is slightly pointed and rises above the first rib; a base, which is wide and concave and rides on the dome-shaped diaphragm; and a body, which is divided into lobes. The right lung has three lobes: the upper, middle, and lower. The left lung has only two lobes, the upper and lower, because of the space occupied by the heart (Fig. 29.31).

Inspection of the lungs primarily involves observation of respiratory movements. Evaluate respirations for (1) rate (number per minute), (2) rhythm (regular, irregular, or periodic), (3) depth (deep or shallow), and (4) quality (effortless, automatic, difficult, or labored). Note the character of breath sounds, such as noisy, grunting, snoring, or heavy.

Evaluate respiratory movements by placing each hand flat against the back or chest with the thumbs in midline along the lower costal margin of the lungs. The child should be sitting during this procedure and, if cooperative, should take several deep breaths. During respiration your hands will move with the chest wall. Assess the amount and speed of respiratory excursion, and note any asymmetry of movement.

Experienced examiners may percuss the lungs. Percuss the anterior lung from apex to base, usually with the child in the supine or sitting position. Percuss each side of the chest in sequence to compare the sounds. When percussing the posterior lung, the procedure and sequence are the same, although the child should be sitting. Resonance is heard over all the lobes of the lungs that are not adjacent to other organs. Record and report any deviation from the expected sound.

Auscultation

Auscultation involves using the stethoscope to evaluate breath sounds (see Guidelines box: Effective Auscultation). Breath sounds are best heard if the child inspires deeply (see Atraumatic Care box: Encouraging Deep Breaths). In the lungs, breath sounds are classified as vesicular, bronchovesicular, or bronchial (Box 29.9).

Absent or diminished breath sounds are always an abnormal finding warranting investigation. Fluid, air, or solid masses in the pleural space

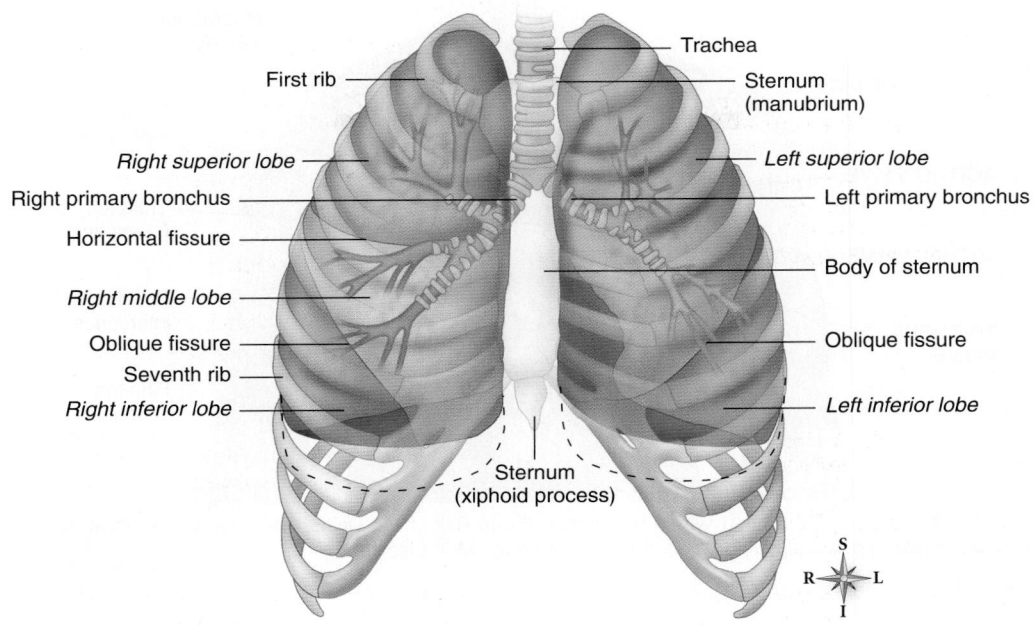

FIG 29.31 Location of the lobes of the lungs within the thoracic cavity. (From Patton, K.T., Thibodeau, G.A. [2016] Anatomy and physiology, 9th ed. St Louis: Elsevier.)

BOX 29.9   Classification of Normal Breath Sounds

Vesicular Breath Sounds
Heard over the entire surface of the lungs with the exception of the upper intrascapular area and area beneath the manubrium.
Inspiration is louder, longer, and higher pitched than expiration.
The sound is a soft, swishing noise.

Bronchovesicular Breath Sounds
Heard over the manubrium and in the upper intrascapular regions where the trachea and bronchi bifurcate.
Inspiration is louder and higher pitched than in vesicular breathing.

Bronchial Breath Sounds
Heard only over trachea near suprasternal notch.
The inspiratory phase is short, and the expiratory phase is long.

BOX 29.10   Various Patterns of Respiration

Tachypnea: Increased rate
Bradypnea: Decreased rate
Dyspnea: Distress during breathing
Apnea: Cessation of breathing
Hyperpnea: Increased depth
Hypoventilation: Decreased depth (shallow) and irregular rhythm
Hyperventilation: Increased rate and depth
Kussmaul respiration: Hyperventilation, gasping and labored respiration; usually seen in diabetic coma or other states of respiratory acidosis
Cheyne-Stokes respiration: Gradually increasing rate and depth with periods of apnea
Biot respiration: Periods of hyperpnea alternating with apnea (similar to Cheyne-Stokes except that depth remains constant)
Seesaw (paradoxic) respirations: Chest falls on inspiration and rises on expiration
Agonal: Last gasping breaths before death

ATRAUMATIC CARE

Encouraging Deep Breaths

- Ask the child to "blow out" the light on an otoscope or pocket flashlight; discreetly turn off the light on the last try so the child feels successful.
- Place a cotton ball in the child's palm; ask the child to blow the ball into the air and have parent catch it.
- Place a small tissue on the top of a pencil, and ask the child to blow the tissue off.
- Have child blow a pinwheel, a party horn, or bubbles.

interfere with the conduction of breath sounds. Diminished breath sounds in certain segments of the lung can alert the nurse to pulmonary areas that may benefit from chest physiotherapy. Increased breath sounds after pulmonary therapy indicate improved passage of air through the respiratory tract. Box 29.10 lists terms used to describe various respiration patterns.

Various pulmonary abnormalities produce adventitious sounds that are not normally heard over the chest. These sounds occur in addition to normal or abnormal breath sounds. They are classified into two main groups: (1) crackles, which result from the passage of air through fluid or moisture, and (2) wheezes, which are produced as air passes through narrowed passageways, regardless of the cause, such as exudate, inflammation, spasm, or tumor. Considerable practice with an experienced tutor is necessary to differentiate the various types of lung sounds. Often it is best to describe the type of sound heard in the lungs rather than trying to label it. Always report any abnormal sounds for further medical evaluation.

HEART

The heart is situated in the thoracic cavity between the lungs in the mediastinum and above the diaphragm (Fig. 29.32). About two-thirds

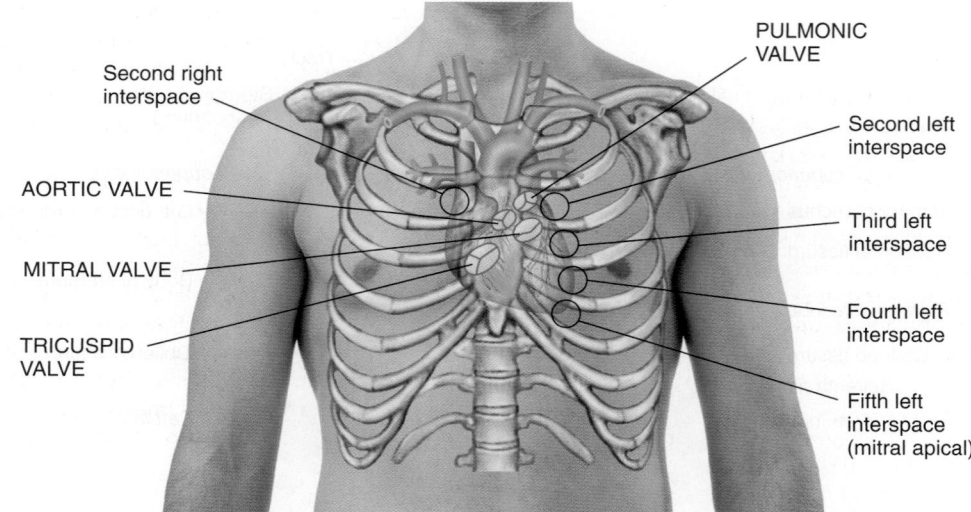

FIG 29.32 Position of the heart within the thorax. (From Ball, J.W., Dains, J.E., Flynn, J.A., et al. [2015]. *Seidel's guide to physical examination* (8th ed.). St Louis, MO: Elsevier.)

of the heart lies within the left side of the rib cage, with the other one-third on the right side as it crosses the sternum. The heart is positioned in the thorax like a trapezoid:

Vertically along the right sternal border (RSB) from the second to the fifth rib

Horizontally (long side) from the lower right sternum to the fifth rib at the left midclavicular line (LMCL)

Diagonally from the left sternal border (LSB) at the second rib to the LMCL at the fifth rib

Horizontally (short side) from the RSB and LSB at the second ICS—base of the heart

Inspection is easiest when the child is sitting in the semi-Fowler position. Look at the anterior chest wall from an angle, comparing both sides of the rib cage with each other. Normally they should be symmetric. In children with thin chest walls, a pulsation may be visible. Because comprehensive evaluation of cardiac function is not limited to the heart, also consider other findings, such as the presence of all pulses (especially the femoral pulses) (Fig. 29.33), distended neck veins, clubbing of the fingers, peripheral cyanosis, edema, blood pressure, and respiratory status.

Use palpation to determine the location of the AI, the most lateral cardiac impulse that may correspond to the apex. The AI is found:

• At the fifth ICS and LMCL in children older than 7 years of age
• At the fourth ICS and just lateral to the LMCL in children younger than 7 years of age

Although the AI gives a general idea of the size of the heart (with enlargement, the apex is lower and more lateral), its normal location is variable, making it an unreliable indicator of heart size.

The **point of maximum intensity (PMI)**, as the name implies, is the area of most intense pulsation. Usually the PMI is located at the same site as the AI, but it can occur elsewhere. For this reason, the two terms should not be used synonymously.

Assess the **capillary refill time**, an important test for circulation and hydration, by pressing the skin lightly on a central site, such as the forehead, or a peripheral site, such as the top of the hand, to produce a slight blanching. The time it takes for the blanched area to return to its original color is the capillary refill time.

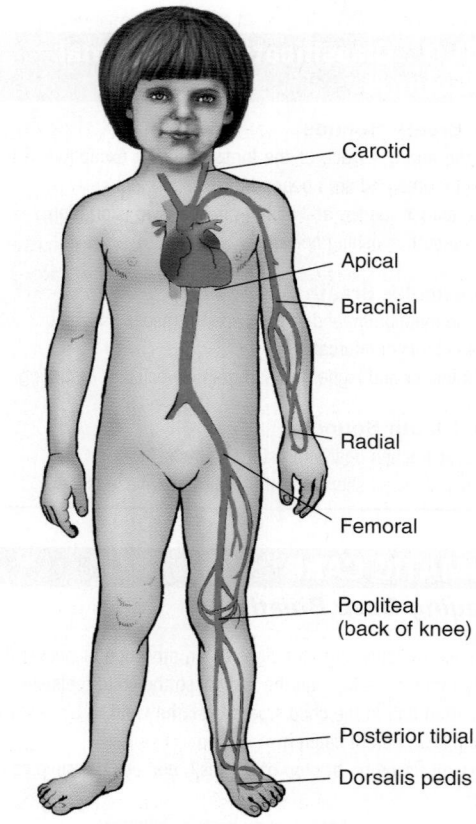

FIG 29.33 Location of pulses.

> **! NURSING ALERT**
>
> Capillary refill should be brisk—less than 2 seconds. Prolonged refill may be associated with poor systemic perfusion or a cool ambient temperature.

Auscultation

Origin of Heart Sounds

The heart sounds are produced by the opening and closing of the valves and the vibration of blood against the walls of the heart and vessels. Normally, two sounds—S_1 and S_2—are heard, which correspond, respectively, to the familiar "lub dub" often used to describe the sounds. S_1 is caused by closure of the tricuspid and mitral valves (sometimes called the atrioventricular valves). S_2 is the result of closure of the pulmonic and aortic valves (sometimes called semilunar valves). Normally the split of the two sounds in S_2 is distinguishable and widens during inspiration. Physiologic splitting is a significant normal finding.

> **! NURSING ALERT**
>
> Fixed splitting, in which the split in S_2 does not change during inspiration, is an important diagnostic sign of atrial septal defect.

Two other heart sounds, S_3 and S_4, may be produced. S_3 is normally heard in some children; S_4 is rarely heard as a normal heart sound; it usually indicates the need for further cardiac evaluation.

Differentiating Normal Heart Sounds

Fig. 29.34 illustrates the approximate anatomic position of the valves within the heart chambers. Note that the anatomic location of valves does not correspond to the area where the sounds are heard best. The auscultatory sites are located in the direction of the blood flow through the valves.

Normally S_1 is louder at the apex of the heart in the mitral and tricuspid area, and S_2 is louder near the base of the heart in the pulmonic and aortic area (Table 29.9). Listen to each sound by inching down the chest. Auscultate the following areas for sounds, such as murmurs, which may radiate to these sites: sternoclavicular area above the clavicles and manubrium, area along the sternal border, area along the left midaxillary line, and area below the scapulae.

> **! NURSING ALERT**
>
> To distinguish between S_1 and S_2 heart sounds, simultaneously palpate the carotid pulse with the index and middle fingers and listen to the heart sounds; S_1 is synchronous with the carotid pulse.

Auscultate the heart with the child in at least two positions: sitting and reclining. If adventitious sounds are detected, further evaluate them with the child standing, sitting and leaning forward, and lying on the left side. For example, atrial sounds (such as, S_4) are heard best with the person in a recumbent position and usually fade if the person sits or stands.

Evaluate heart sounds for (1) quality (they should be clear and distinct, not muffled, diffuse, or distant); (2) intensity, especially in relation to the location or auscultatory site (they should not be weak or pounding); (3) rate (they should have the same rate as the radial pulse); and (4) rhythm (they should be regular and even). A particular arrhythmia that occurs normally in many children is sinus arrhythmia, in which the heart rate increases with inspiration and decreases with expiration. Differentiate this rhythm from a truly abnormal arrhythmia by having children hold their breath. In sinus arrhythmia, cessation of breathing causes the heart rate to remain steady.

Heart Murmurs

Another important category of the heart sounds is murmurs, which are produced by vibrations within the heart chambers or in the major

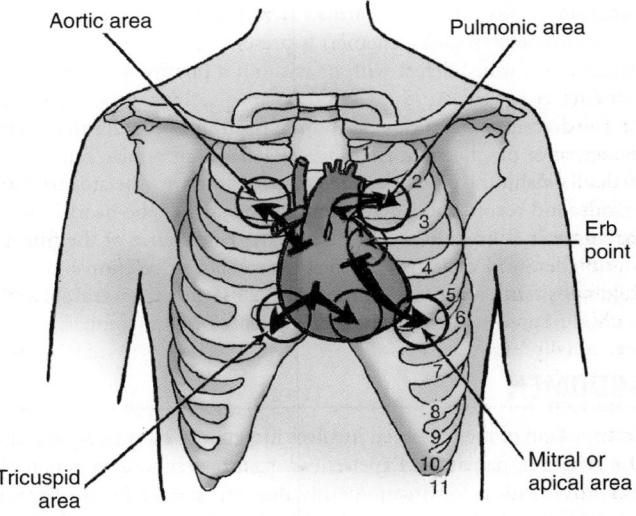

FIG 29.34 Direction of heart sounds for anatomic valve sites and areas *(circled)* for auscultation.

TABLE 29.9	Sequence of Auscultating Heart Sounds*	
Auscultatory Site	**Chest Location**	**Characteristics of Heart Sounds**
Aortic area	Second right ICS close to sternum	S_2 heard louder than S_1; aortic closure heard loudest
Pulmonic area	Second left ICS close to sternum	Splitting of S_2 heard best, normally widens on inspiration; pulmonic closure heard best
Erb point	Second and third left ICSs close to sternum	Frequent site of innocent murmurs and those of aortic or pulmonic origin
Tricuspid area	Fifth right and left ICSs close to sternum	S_1 heard as louder sound preceding S_2 (S_1 synchronous with carotid pulse)
Mitral or apical area	Fifth ICS, LMCL (third to fourth ICS and lateral to LMCL in infants)	S_1 heard loudest; splitting of S_1 may be audible because mitral closure is louder than tricuspid closure
		S_3 heard best at beginning of expiration with child in recumbent or left side-lying position; occurs immediately after S_2; sounds like word S_1 S_2 S_3: "Ken-tuck-y"
		S_4 heard best during expiration with child in recumbent position (left side-lying position decreases sound); occurs immediately before S_1; sounds like word S_4 S_1 S_2: "Ten-nes-see"

ICS, Intercostal space; LMCL, left midclavicular line.
*Use both diaphragm and bell chest pieces when auscultating heart sounds. Bell chest piece is necessary for low-pitched sounds of murmurs, S_3, and S_4.

TABLE 29.10 Grading the Intensity of Heart Murmurs

Grade	Description
I	Very faint; often not heard if child sits up
II	Usually readily heard; slightly louder than grade I; audible in all positions
III	Loud, but not accompanied by a thrill
IV	Loud, accompanied by a thrill
V	Loud enough to be heard with a stethoscope barely touching the chest; accompanied by a thrill
VI	Loud enough to be heard with the stethoscope not touching the chest; often heard with the human ear close to the chest; accompanied by a thrill

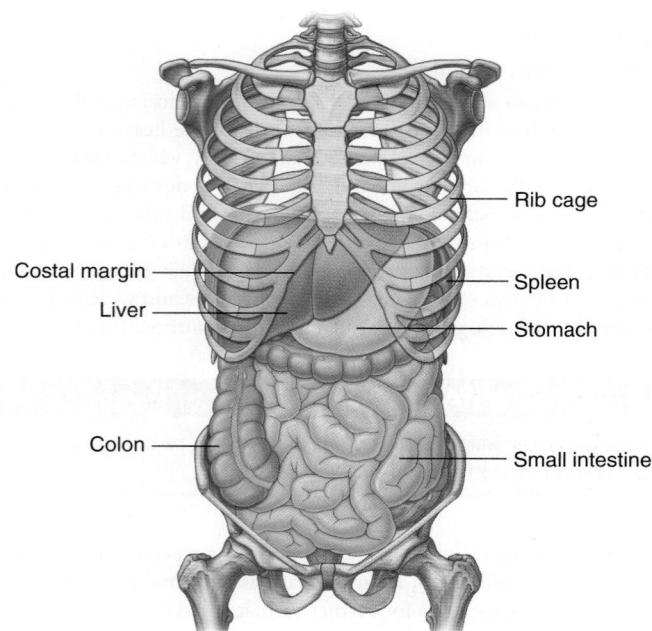

FIG 29.35 Location of structures in the abdomen. (From Drake, R.L., Vogl, W., Mitchell, A.W.M. [2015]. *Gray's anatomy for students* [3rd ed.]. New York, NY: Churchill Livingstone.)

arteries from the back-and-forth flow of blood. (For a more detailed discussion, see the "Cardiovascular Dysfunction" section in Chapter 42.) Murmurs are classified as:

Innocent: No anatomic or physiologic abnormality exists.

Functional: No anatomic cardiac defect exists, but a physiologic abnormality (such as, anemia) is present.

Organic: A cardiac defect with or without a physiologic abnormality exists.

The description and classification of murmurs are skills that require considerable practice and training. In general, recognize murmurs as distinct swishing sounds that occur in addition to the normal heart sounds, and record the (1) location, or the area of the heart in which the murmur is heard best; (2) time of the occurrence of the murmur within the S_1–S_2 cycle; (3) intensity (evaluate in relationship to the child's position); and (4) loudness. Table 29.10 lists the usual subjective method of grading the loudness or intensity of a murmur.

ABDOMEN

Examination of the abdomen involves inspection followed by auscultation and then palpation. Experienced examiners may also percuss the abdomen to assess for organomegaly, masses, fluid, and flatus. Perform palpation last because it may distort the normal abdominal sounds. Knowledge of the anatomic placement of the abdominal organs is essential to differentiate normal, expected findings from abnormal ones (Fig. 29.35).

For descriptive purposes, the abdominal cavity is divided into four quadrants by drawing a vertical line midway from the sternum to the symphysis pubis and a horizontal line across the abdomen through the umbilicus. The sections are named:

- Left upper quadrant
- Left lower quadrant
- Right upper quadrant
- Right lower quadrant

Inspection

Inspect the contour of the abdomen with the child erect and supine. Normally the abdomen of infants and young children is cylindric and, in the erect position, fairly prominent because of the physiologic lordosis of the spine. In the supine position, the abdomen appears flat. A midline protrusion from the xiphoid to the umbilicus or symphysis pubis is usually diastasis recti, or failure of the rectus abdominis muscles to join in utero. In a healthy child, a midline protrusion is usually a variation of normal muscular development.

! NURSING ALERT

A tense, boardlike abdomen is a serious sign of paralytic ileus and intestinal obstruction.

The skin covering the abdomen should be uniformly taut, without wrinkles or creases. Sometimes silvery, whitish striae ("stretch marks") are seen, especially if the skin has been stretched as in obesity. Superficial veins are usually visible in light-skinned, thin infants, but distended veins are an abnormal finding.

Observe movement of the abdomen. Normally chest and abdominal movements are synchronous. In infants and thin children, **peristaltic waves** may be visible through the abdominal wall; they are best observed by standing at eye level to and across from the abdomen. Always report this finding.

Examine the umbilicus for size, hygiene, and evidence of any abnormalities, such as hernias. The umbilicus should be flat or only slightly protruding. If a herniation is present, palpate the sac for abdominal contents and estimate the approximate size of the opening. **Umbilical hernias** are common in infants, especially in African-American children.

Hernias may exist elsewhere on the abdominal wall (Fig. 29.36). An inguinal hernia is a protrusion of peritoneum through the abdominal wall in the inguinal canal. It occurs mostly in boys, is frequently bilateral, and may be visible as a mass in the scrotum. To locate a hernia, slide the little finger into the external inguinal ring at the base of the scrotum, and ask the child to cough. If a hernia is present, it will hit the tip of the finger.

! NURSING ALERT

If the child is too young to cough, have the child blow a pinwheel or bubbles or laugh to raise the intraabdominal pressure sufficiently to demonstrate the presence of an inguinal hernia.

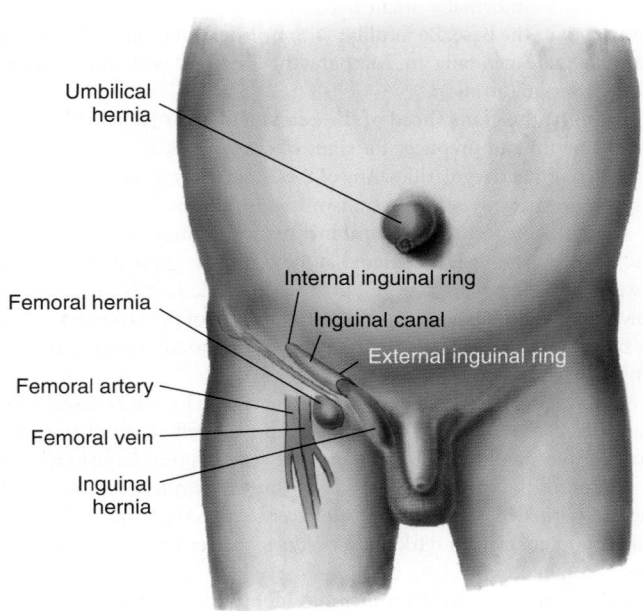

FIG 29.36 Location of hernias.

Umbilical hernia

Internal inguinal ring

Inguinal canal

External inguinal ring

Femoral hernia

Femoral artery

Femoral vein

Inguinal hernia

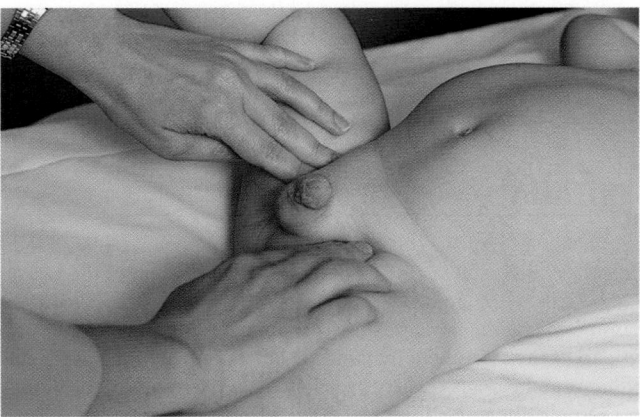

FIG 29.37 Palpating for femoral pulses.

A femoral hernia, which occurs more frequently in girls, is felt or seen as a small mass on the anterior surface of the thigh just below the inguinal ligament in the femoral canal (a potential space medial to the femoral artery). Feel for a hernia by placing the index finger of your right hand on the child's right femoral pulse (left hand for left pulse) and the middle finger flat against the skin toward the midline. The ring finger lies over the femoral canal, where the herniation occurs. Palpation of hernias in the pelvic region is often part of the genital examination.

Auscultation

The most important finding to listen for is peristalsis, or bowel sounds, which sound like short metallic clicks and gurgles. Record their frequency per minute (e.g., 5 sounds/min). Listen for up to 5 minutes before determining that bowel sounds are absent. Stimulate bowel sounds by stroking the abdominal surface with a fingernail. Report absence of bowel sounds or hyperperistalsis, because either usually denotes an abdominal disorder.

Palpation

There are two types of palpation: superficial and deep. For superficial palpation, lightly place your hand against the skin and feel each quadrant, noting any areas of tenderness, muscle tone, and superficial lesions, such as cysts. Because superficial palpation is often perceived as tickling, use several techniques to minimize this sensation and relax the child (see Atraumatic Care box: Promoting Relaxation during Abdominal Palpation). Admonishing the child to stop laughing only draws attention to the sensation and decreases cooperation.

Deep palpation is for palpating organs and large blood vessels and for detecting masses and tenderness that were not discovered during superficial palpation. Palpation usually begins in the lower quadrants and proceeds upward to avoid missing the edge of an enlarged liver or spleen. Except for palpating the liver, successful identification of other organs such as the spleen, kidney, and part of the colon requires considerable practice with tutored supervision. Report any questionable mass. The lower edge of the liver is sometimes felt in infants and young children as a superficial mass 1 to 2 cm (0.4 to 0.8 inch) below the right

costal margin (the distance is sometimes measured in fingerbreadths). Normally the liver descends during inspiration as the diaphragm moves downward. Do not mistake this downward displacement as a sign of liver enlargement.

! NURSING ALERT

If the liver is palpable 3 cm (1.2 inch) below the right costal margin or the spleen is palpable more than 2 cm (0.8 inch) below the left costal margin, these organs are enlarged—a finding that is always reported for further medical investigation.

Palpate the femoral pulses by placing the tips of two or three fingers (index, middle, or ring) along the inguinal ligament about midway between the iliac crest and symphysis pubis. Feel both pulses simultaneously to make certain that they are equal and strong (Fig. 29.37).

GENITALIA

Examination of genitalia conveniently follows assessment of the abdomen while the child is still supine. In adolescents, inspection of the genitalia may be left to the end of the examination. The best approach is to examine the genitalia matter-of-factly, placing no more emphasis on this part of the assessment than on any other segment. It helps to relieve children's and parents' anxiety by telling them the results of the findings; for example, the nurse might say, "Everything looks fine here."

If it is necessary to ask questions, such as about discharge or difficulty urinating, respect the child's privacy by covering the lower abdomen with the gown or underpants. To prevent embarrassing interruptions, keep the door or curtain closed and post a "do not disturb" sign. Have a drape ready to cover the genitalia if someone enters the room.

In examining the genitalia, wear gloves when touching the child. It might be helpful for the adolescent to know that wearing gloves also prevents skin-to-skin contact.

The genital examination is an excellent time for eliciting questions or concern about body function or sexual activity. Also use this opportunity to increase or reinforce the child's knowledge of reproductive anatomy by naming each body part and explaining its function. This part of the health assessment is an opportune time to teach testicular self-examination to boys.

Male Genitalia

Note the external appearance of the glans and shaft of the penis, the prepuce, the urethral meatus, and the scrotum (Fig. 29.38). The penis is generally small in infants and young boys until puberty, when it begins to increase in both length and width. In an obese child, the penis

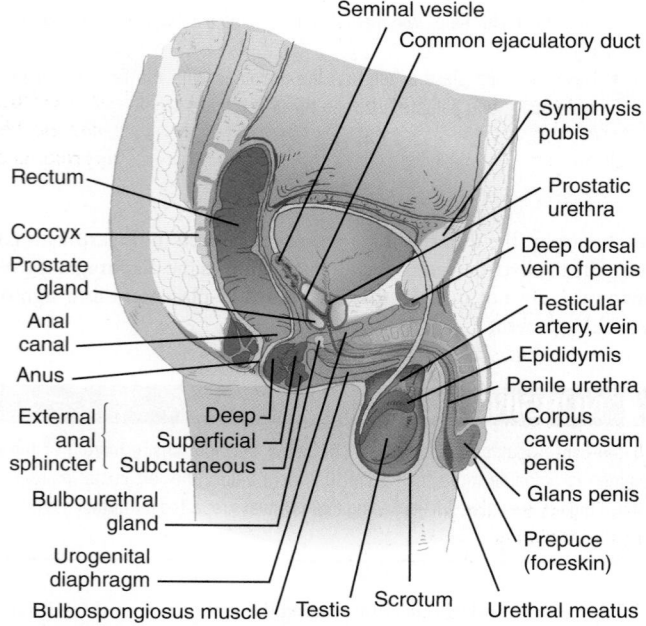

FIG 29.38 Major structures of genitalia in an uncircumcised postpubertal male. (From Douglas, G., Nicol, F., & Robertson, C. [2013]. *Macleod's clinical examination* [13th ed.]. Philadelphia, PA: Elsevier.)

often looks abnormally small because of the folds of skin partially covering it at the base. Be familiar with normal pubertal growth of the external male genitalia to compare the findings with the expected sequence of maturation.

Examine the glans (head of the penis) and shaft (portion between the perineum and prepuce) for signs of swelling, skin lesions, inflammation, or other irregularities. Any of these signs may indicate underlying disorders, especially sexually transmitted infections.

Carefully inspect the urethral meatus for location and evidence of discharge. Normally it is centered at the tip of the glans. Also note hair distribution. Normally, before puberty, no pubic hair is present. Soft, downy hair at the base of the penis is an early sign of pubertal maturation. In older adolescents, hair distribution is diamond-shaped from the umbilicus to the anus.

Note the location and size of the scrotum. The scrota hang freely from the perineum behind the penis, and the left scrotum normally hangs lower than the right. In infants, the scrota appear large in relation to the rest of the genitalia. The skin of the scrotum is loose and highly rugated (wrinkled). During early adolescence, the skin normally becomes redder and coarser. In dark-skinned boys, the scrota are usually more deeply pigmented.

Palpation of the scrotum includes identification of the testes, epididymis, and, if present, inguinal hernias. The two testes are felt as small, ovoid bodies about 1.5 to 2 cm (0.6 to 0.8 inch) long (one in each scrotal sac). They do not enlarge until puberty. Pubertal testicular development usually begins in boys between 9 and 13 years of age. Record early (precocious) or delayed pubertal development, as well as evidence of any other secondary sexual characteristics.

When palpating for the presence of the testes, avoid stimulating the cremasteric reflex, which is stimulated by cold, touch, emotional excitement, or exercise. This reflex pulls the testes higher into the pelvic cavity. Several measures are useful in preventing the cremasteric reflex during palpation of the scrotum. First, warm the hands. Second, if the child is old enough, examine him in a tailor or "Indian" position, which stretches the muscle, preventing its contraction (Fig. 29.39, *A*). Third, block the normal pathway of ascent of the testes by placing the thumb and index finger over the upper part of the scrotal sac along the inguinal canal (see Fig. 29.39, *B*). If there is any question concerning the existence of two testes, place the index and middle fingers in a scissors fashion to separate the right and left scrota. If, after using these techniques, you have not palpated the testes, feel along the inguinal canal and perineum to locate masses that may be undescended testes. Although undescended testes may descend at any time during childhood and are checked at each visit, report any failure to palpate the testes.

Female Genitalia

The examination of female genitalia is limited to inspection and palpation of external structures. If a vaginal examination is required, the nurse should make an appropriate referral unless he or she is qualified to perform the procedure.

A convenient position for examination of the genitalia involves placing the young girl supine on the examining table or in a semireclining position on the parent's lap with the feet supported on your knees as you sit facing the child. Divert the child's attention from the examination by instructing her to try to keep the soles of her feet pressed against each other. Separate the labia majora with the thumb and index finger, and retract outward to expose the labia minora, urethral meatus, and vaginal orifice.

Examine the female genitalia for size and location of the structures of the vulva, or pudendum (Fig. 29.40). The mons pubis is a pad of adipose tissue over the symphysis pubis. At puberty, the mons is covered with hair, which extends along the labia. The usual pattern of female hair distribution is an inverted triangle. The appearance of soft, downy hair along the labia majora is an early sign of sexual maturation. Note the size and location of the clitoris, a small, erectile organ located at the anterior end of the labia minora. It is covered by a small flap of skin, the prepuce.

The labia majora are two thick folds of skin running posteriorly from the mons to the posterior commissure of the vagina. Internal to the labia majora are two folds of skin called the *labia minora*. Although the labia minora are usually prominent in newborns, they gradually atrophy, which makes them almost invisible until their enlargement during puberty. The inner surface of the labia should be pink and moist. Note the size of the labia and any evidence of fusion, which may suggest male scrota. Normally, no masses are palpable within the labia.

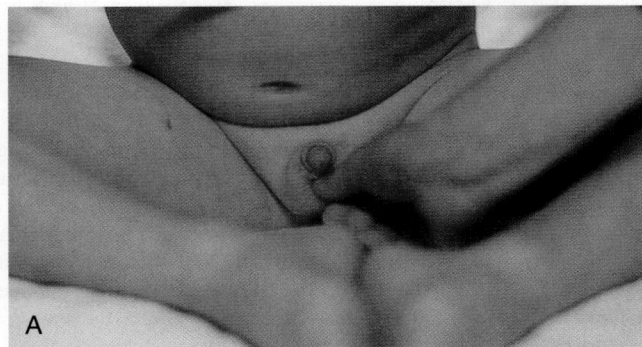
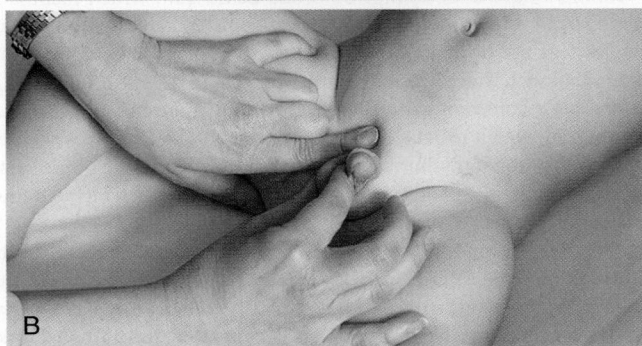

FIG 29.39 A, Preventing the cremasteric reflex by having the child sit in the tailor position. **B,** Blocking the inguinal canal during palpation of the scrotum for descended testes.

The **urethral meatus** is located posterior to the clitoris and is surrounded by the Skene glands and ducts. Although not a prominent structure, the meatus appears as a small V-shaped slit. Note its location, especially if it opens from the clitoris or inside the vagina. Gently palpate the glands, which are common sites of cysts and sexually transmitted lesions.

The **vaginal orifice** is located posterior to the urethral meatus. Its appearance varies depending on individual anatomy and sexual activity. Ordinarily, examination of the vagina is limited to inspection. In virgins, a thin crescent-shaped or circular membrane, called the *hymen,* may cover part of the vaginal opening. In some instances, it completely occludes the orifice. After rupture, small rounded pieces of tissue called caruncles remain. Although an imperforate hymen denotes lack of penile intercourse, a perforate one does not necessarily indicate sexual activity.

> **! NURSING ALERT**
>
> In girls who have been circumcised, the genitalia will appear different. Do not show surprise or disgust, but note the appearance and discuss the procedure with the young woman.

Surrounding the vaginal opening are Bartholin glands, which secrete a clear, mucoid fluid into the vagina for lubrication during intercourse. Palpate the ducts for cysts. Also note the discharge from the vagina, which is usually clear or white.

ANUS

After examination of the genitalia, it is easy to identify the anal area, although the child should be placed on the abdomen. Note the general firmness of the buttocks and symmetry of the gluteal folds. Assess the tone of the anal sphincter by eliciting the anal reflex (anal wink). Gently scratching the anal area results in an obvious quick contraction of the external anal sphincter.

BACK AND EXTREMITIES

Spine

Note the general curvature of the spine. Normally, the back of a newborn is rounded or *C* shaped from the thoracic and pelvic curves. The development of the cervical and lumbar curves approximates

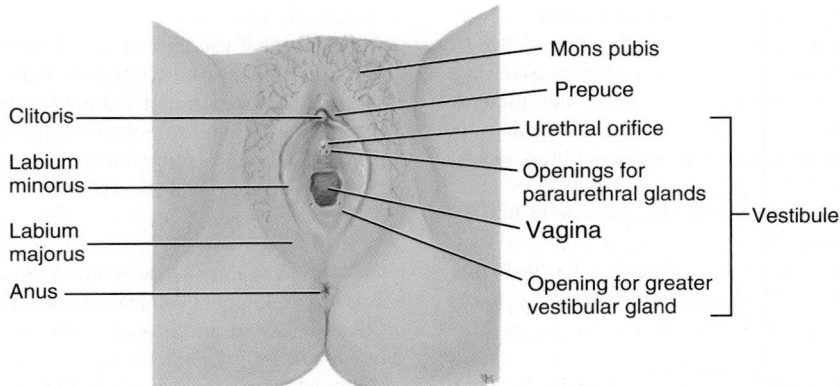

FIG 29.40 External structures of the genitalia in a postpubertal female. The labia are spread to reveal deeper structures. (From Paulsen, F., & Waschke, J. [2013]. *Sobotta atlas of human anatomy* [vol 2; 15th ed.]. Munich, Germany: Elsevier.)

development of various motor skills, such as cervical curvature with head control, and gives older children the typical double *S* curve.

Marked curvatures in posture are abnormal. Scoliosis, lateral curvature of the spine, is an important childhood problem, especially in girls. Although scoliosis may be identified by observing and palpating the spine and noting a sideways displacement, more objective tests include the following:

- With the child standing erect, clothed only in underpants (and bra if an older girl), observe from behind, noting asymmetry of the shoulders and hips.
- With the child bending forward so the back is parallel to the floor, observe from the front and side, noting asymmetry or prominence of the rib cage.

A slight limp, a crooked hemline, or complaints of a sore back are other signs and symptoms of scoliosis.

Inspect the back, especially along the spine, for any tufts of hair, dimples, or discoloration. Mobility of the vertebral column is easy to assess in most children because of their tendency to be in constant motion during the examination. However, you can test mobility by asking the child to sit up from a prone position or to do a modified sit-up exercise.

Movement of the cervical spine is an important diagnostic sign of neurologic problems, such as meningitis. Normally movement of the head in all directions is effortless.

> ### ❗ NURSING ALERT
> Hyperextension of the neck and spine, or opisthotonos, which is accompanied by pain when the head is flexed, is always referred for immediate medical evaluation.

Extremities

Inspect each extremity for symmetry of length and size; refer any deviation for orthopedic evaluation. Count the fingers and toes to be certain of the normal number. This is so often taken for granted that an extra digit (polydactyly) or fusion of digits (syndactyly) may go unnoticed.

Inspect the arms and legs for temperature and color, which should be equal in each extremity, although the feet may normally be colder than the hands.

Assess the shape of bones. There are several variations of bone shape in children. Although many of them cause parents concern, most are benign and require no treatment. Bowleg, or *genu varum,* is lateral bowing of the tibia. It is clinically present when the child stands with an outward bowing of the legs, giving the appearance of a bow. Usually, there is an outward curvature of both femur and tibia (Fig. 29.41, *A*). Toddlers are usually bowlegged after beginning to walk until all of their lower back and leg muscles are well developed. Unilateral or asymmetric bowlegs that are present beyond 2 to 3 years of age, particularly in African-American children, may represent pathologic conditions requiring further investigation.

Knock knee, or genu valgum, appears as the opposite of bowleg, in that the knees are close together but the feet are spread apart. It is determined clinically by using the same method as for genu varum but by measuring the distance between the malleoli, which normally should be less than 7.5 cm (3 inches) (see Fig. 29.41, *B*). Knock knee is normally present in children from about 2 to 7 years of age. Knock knee that is excessive, asymmetric, accompanied by short stature, or evident in a child nearing puberty requires further evaluation.

Next inspect the feet. Infants' and toddlers' feet appear flat because the foot is normally wide and the arch is covered by a fat pad.

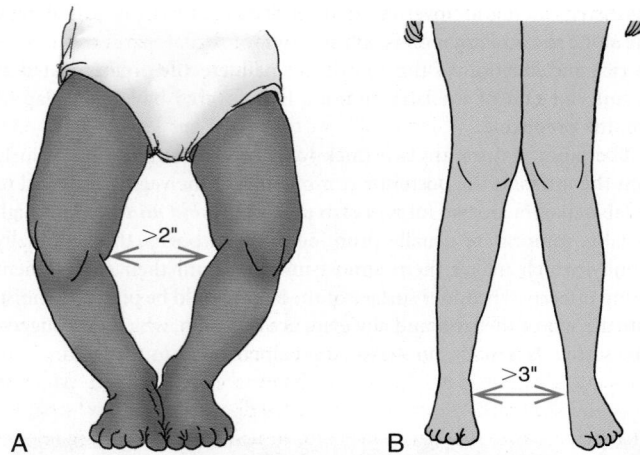

FIG 29.41 A, Genu varum. **B,** Genu valgum.

Development of the arch occurs naturally from the action of walking. Normally at birth the feet are held in a valgus (outward) or varus (inward) position. To determine whether a foot deformity at birth is a result of intrauterine position or development, scratch the outer, then inner, side of the sole. If the foot position is self-correctable, it will assume a right angle to the leg. As the child begins to walk, the feet turn outward less than 30 degrees and inward less than 10 degrees.

Toddlers have a "toddling" or broad-based gait, which facilitates walking by lowering the center of gravity. As the child reaches preschool age, the legs are brought closer together. By school age, the walking posture is much more graceful and balanced.

The most common gait problem in young children is pigeon toe, or toeing in, which usually results from torsional deformities, such as internal tibial torsion (abnormal rotation or bowing of the tibia). Tests for tibial torsion include measuring the thigh-foot angle, which requires considerable practice for accuracy.

Elicit the plantar or grasp reflex by exerting firm but gentle pressure with the tip of the thumb against the lateral sole of the foot from the heel upward to the little toe and then across to the big toe. The normal response in children who are walking is flexion of the toes. The Babinski sign, dorsiflexion of the big toe and fanning of the other toes, is normal during infancy but abnormal after about 1 year of age or when locomotion begins.

Joints

Evaluate the joints for range of motion. Normally this requires no specific testing if you have observed the child's movements during the examination. However, routinely investigate the hips in infants for congenital dislocation by checking for subluxation of the hip. Report any evidence of joint immobility or hyperflexibility. Palpate the joints for heat, tenderness, and swelling. These signs, as well as redness over the joint, warrant further investigation.

Muscles

Note symmetry and quality of muscle development, tone, and strength. Observe development by looking at the shape and contour of the body in both a relaxed and a tensed state. Estimate tone by grasping the muscle and feeling its firmness when it is relaxed and contracted. A common site for testing tone is the biceps muscle of the arm. Children are usually willing to "make a muscle" by clenching their fists.

Estimate strength by having the child use an extremity to push or pull against resistance, as in the following examples:

Arm strength: Child holds the arms outstretched in front of the body and tries to raise the arms while downward pressure is applied.

Hand strength: Child shakes hands with nurse and squeezes one or two fingers of the nurse's hand.

Leg strength: Child sits on a table or chair with the legs dangling and tries to raise the legs while downward pressure is applied.

Note symmetry of strength in the extremities, hands, and fingers, and report evidence of paresis, or weakness.

NEUROLOGIC ASSESSMENT

The assessment of the nervous system is the broadest and most diverse part of the examination process, because every human function, both physical and emotional, is controlled by neurologic impulses. Much of the neurologic examination has already been discussed, such as assessment of behavior, sensory testing, and motor function. The following focuses on a general appraisal of cerebellar function, deep tendon reflexes, and the cranial nerves.

Cerebellar Function

The cerebellum controls balance and coordination. Much of the assessment of cerebellar function is included in observing the child's posture, body movements, gait, and development of fine and gross motor skills. Tests to assess balance include balancing on one foot and the heel-to-toe walk. Test coordination by asking the child to reach for a toy, button clothes, tie shoes, or draw a straight line on a piece of paper (provided the child is old enough to do these activities). Coordination can also be tested by any sequence of rapid, successive movements, such as quickly touching each finger with the thumb of the same hand.

Several tests for cerebellar function can be performed as games (Box 29.11). When a Romberg test is done, stay beside the child if there is a possibility that he or she might fall. School-age children should be able to perform these tests, although in the finger-to-nose test, preschoolers normally can only bring the finger within 5 to 7.5 cm (2 to 3 inches) of the nose. Difficulty in performing these exercises indicates a poor sense of position (especially with the eyes closed) and incoordination (especially with the eyes open).

Reflexes

Testing reflexes is an important part of the neurologic examination. Persistence of primitive reflexes, loss of reflexes, or hyperactivity of deep tendon reflexes is usually a result of a cerebral insult.

Elicit reflexes by using the rubber head of the reflex hammer, flat of the finger, or side of the hand. If the child is easily frightened by equipment, use your hand or finger. Although testing reflexes is a simple procedure, the child may inhibit the reflex by unconsciously tensing the muscle. To avoid tensing, distract younger children with toys or talk to them. Older children can concentrate on the exercise of grasping their two hands in front of them and trying to pull them apart. This

diverts their attention from the testing and causes involuntary relaxation of the muscles.

Deep tendon reflexes are stretch reflexes of a muscle. The most common deep tendon reflex is the knee-jerk reflex, or patellar reflex (sometimes called the quadriceps reflex). Figs. 29.42 to 29.45 illustrate the reflexes normally elicited. Report any diminished or hyperreflexive response for further evaluation.

Cranial Nerves

Assessment of the cranial nerves is an important area of neurologic assessment (Fig. 29.46; Table 29.11). With young children, present the tests as games to foster trust and security at the beginning of the examination. Also include the cranial nerve test when examining each system, such as tongue movement and strength, gag reflex, swallowing, cardinal positions of gaze (Fig. 29.47), and position of the uvula during examination of the mouth.

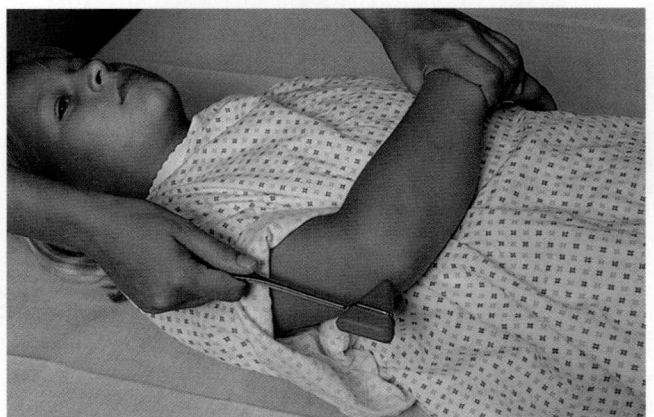

FIG 29.42 Testing for the triceps reflex. The child is placed supine, with the forearm resting over the chest, and the triceps tendon is struck. Alternate procedure: The child's arm is abducted with the upper arm supported and the forearm allowed to hang freely. The triceps tendon is struck. Normal response is partial extension of the forearm.

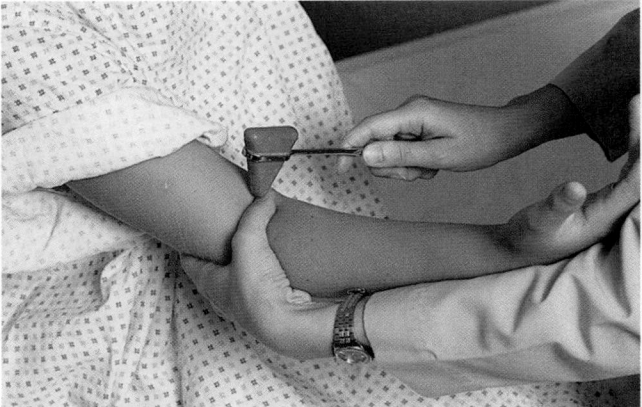

FIG 29.43 Testing for the biceps reflex. The child's arm is held by placing the partially flexed elbow in the examiner's hand with the thumb over the antecubital space. The examiner's thumbnail is struck with a hammer. Normal response is partial flexion of the forearm.

BOX 29.11   Tests for Cerebellar Function

Finger-to-nose test: With the child's arm extended, ask the child to touch the nose with the index finger with the eyes open and then closed.

Heel-to-shin test: Have the child stand and run the heel of one foot down the shin or anterior aspect of the tibia of the other leg, both with the eyes opened and then closed.

Romberg test: Have the child stand with the eyes closed and heels together; falling or leaning to one side is abnormal and is called the *Romberg sign.*

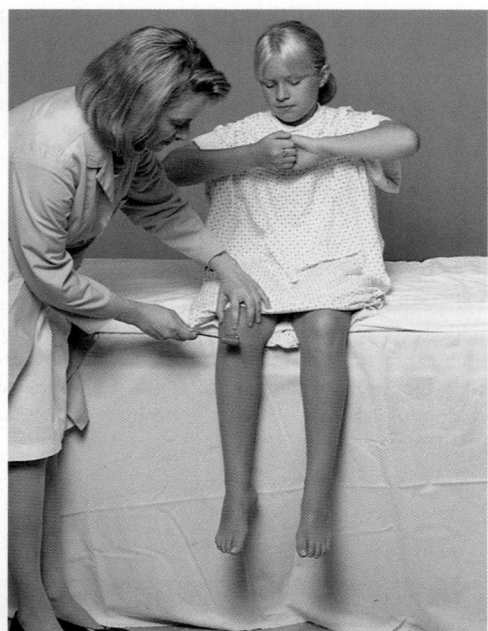

FIG 29.44 Testing for the patellar, or knee-jerk, reflex, using distraction. The child sits on the edge of the examining table (or on the parent's lap) with the lower legs flexed at the knee and dangling freely. The patellar tendon is tapped just below the kneecap. Normal response is partial extension of the lower leg.

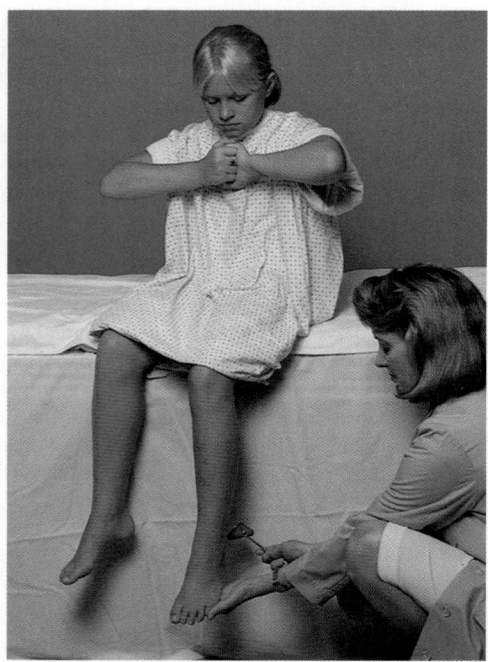

FIG 29.45 Testing for the Achilles reflex. The child should be in the same position as for the knee-jerk reflex. The foot is supported lightly in the examiner's hand, and the Achilles tendon is struck. Normal response is plantar flexion of the foot (the foot pointing downward).

PATHOPHYSIOLOGY REVIEW

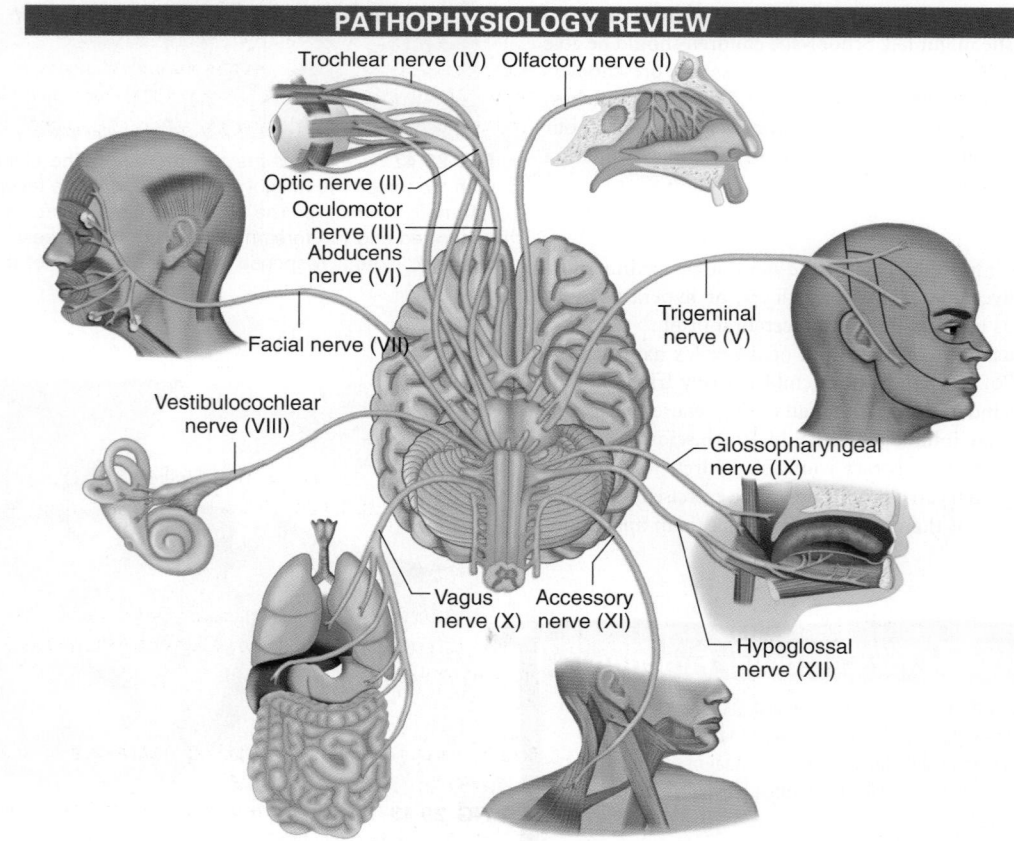

FIG 29.46 Cranial nerves. (From Patton, K.T., & Thibodeau, G.A. [2016]. *Anatomy and physiology* [9th ed.]. St. Louis, MO: Elsevier.)

TABLE 29.11   Assessment of Cranial Nerves

Description and Function	Tests
I—Olfactory Nerve Olfactory mucosa of nasal cavity Smell	With eyes closed, have child identify odors, such as coffee, alcohol from a swab, or other smells; test each nostril separately.
II—Optic Nerve Rods and cones of retina, optic nerve Vision	Check for perception of light, visual acuity, peripheral vision, color vision, and normal optic disc.
III—Oculomotor Nerve Extraocular muscles of eye: • Superior rectus: moves eyeball up and in • Inferior rectus: moves eyeball down and in • Medial rectus: moves eyeball nasally • Inferior oblique: moves eyeball up and out Pupil constriction and accommodation Eyelid closing	Have child follow an object (toy) or light in six cardinal positions of gaze (see Fig. 29.47). Perform PERRLA (Pupils Equal, Round, React to Light, and Accommodation). Check for proper placement of eyelid.
IV—Trochlear Nerve Superior oblique (SO) muscle: moves eye down and out	Have child look down and in (see Fig. 29.47).
V—Trigeminal Nerve Muscles of mastication Sensory: face, scalp, nasal and buccal mucosa	Have child bite down hard and open jaw; test symmetry and strength. With child's eyes closed, see if child can detect light touch in mandibular and maxillary regions. Test corneal and blink reflex by touching cornea lightly with a whisk of cotton ball twisted into a point (approach from side so the child does not blink before cornea is touched).
VI—Abducens Nerve Lateral rectus (LR) muscle: moves eye temporally	Have child look toward temporal side (see Fig. 29.47).
VII—Facial Nerve Muscles for facial expression Anterior two-thirds of tongue (sensory)	Have child smile, make funny face, or show teeth to see symmetry of expression. Have child identify sweet or salty solution; place each taste on anterior section and sides of protruding tongue; if child retracts tongue, solution will dissolve toward posterior part of tongue.
VIII—Auditory, Acoustic, or Vestibulocochlear Nerve Internal ear Hearing and balance	Test hearing; note any loss of equilibrium or presence of vertigo.
IX—Glossopharyngeal Nerve Pharynx, tongue Posterior third of tongue Sensory	Stimulate posterior pharynx with a tongue blade; child should gag. Test sense of sour or bitter taste on posterior segment of tongue.
X—Vagus Nerve Muscles of larynx, pharynx, some organs of gastrointestinal system, sensory fibers of root of tongue, heart, and lung	Note hoarseness of voice, gag reflex, and ability to swallow. Check that uvula is in midline; when stimulated with tongue blade, it should deviate upward and to stimulated side.
XI—Accessory Nerve Sternocleidomastoid and trapezius muscles of shoulder	Have child shrug shoulders while applying mild pressure; with examiner's palms placed laterally on child's cheeks, have child turn head against opposing pressure on either side; note symmetry and strength.
XII—Hypoglossal Nerve Muscles of tongue	Have child move tongue in all directions; have child protrude tongue as far as possible; note any midline deviation. Test strength by placing tongue blade on one side of tongue and having child move it away.

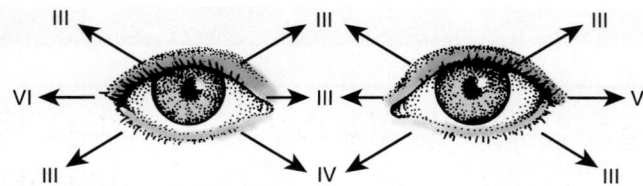

FIG 29.47 Checking extraocular movements in the six cardinal positions indicates the functioning of cranial nerves III, IV, and VI. (From Ignatavicius, D.D., Workman, M.L. [2016]. Medical-surgical nursing: patient-centered collaborative care, 8th ed. St Louis: Saunders.)

REFERENCES

American Academy of Pediatrics. (2011). *Culturally effective care toolkit.* Retrieved from http://www.aap.org/en-us/professional-resources/practice-support/Patient-Management/Pages/Culturally-Effective-Care-Toolkit.aspx.

Ball, J. W., Dains, J. E., Flynn, J. A., et al. (2014). *Seidel's guide to physical examination* (8th ed.). St Louis, MO: Elsevier.

Batra, P., Saha, A., & Faridi, M. M. (2012). Thermometry in children. *Journal of Emergencies, Trauma, and Shock, 5*(3), 246–249.

Blank, L., Coster, J., O'Cathain, A., et al. (2012). The appropriateness of, and compliance with, telephone triage decisions: A systematic review and narrative synthesis. *Journal of Advanced Nursing, 68*(12), 2610–2621.

Broner, N., Embry, V. V., Gremminger, M. G., et al. (2013). *Mandatory reporting and keeping youth safe.* Washington, DC: Administration on Children, Youth and Families, Family and Youth Services Bureau.

Clark, J. A., Kieh-Lai, M. W., Sarnaik, A., et al. (2002). Discrepancies between direct and indirect blood pressure measurements using various recommendations for arm cuff selection. *Pediatrics, 110*(5), 920–923.

Dosman, C., & Andrews, D. (2012). Anticipatory guidance for cognitive and social-emotional development: Birth to five years. *Paediatrics & Child Health, 17*(2), 75–80.

Harlor, A. D., Jr., Bower, C., & Committee on Practice and Ambulatory Medicine, Section on Otolaryngology–Head and Neck Surgery. (2009). Hearing assessment in infants and children: Recommendations beyond neonatal screening. *Pediatrics, 124*(4), 1252–1263.

Mathers, M., Keyes, M., & Wright, M. (2010). A review of the evidence on the effectiveness of children's vision screening. *Child: Care, Health and Development, 36*(6), 754–780.

National High Blood Pressure Education Program Working Group on High Blood Pressure in Children and Adolescents. (2004). The fourth report on the diagnosis, evaluation, and treatment of high blood pressure in children and adolescents. *Pediatrics, 114*(2 suppl, 4th report), 555–576.

Park, M. K., Menard, S. W., & Schoolfield, J. (2005). Oscillometric blood pressure standards for children. *Pediatric Cardiology, 26*(5), 601–607.

Purc-Stephenson, R. J., & Thrasher, C. (2010). Nurses' experiences with telephone triage and advice: A meta-ethnography. *Journal of Advanced Nursing, 66*(3), 482–494.

Purc-Stephenson, R. J., & Thrasher, C. (2012). Patient compliance with telephone triage recommendations: A meta-analytic review. *Patient Education and Counseling, 87*(2), 135–142.

Schell, K., Briening, E., Lebet, R., et al. (2011). Comparison of arm and calf automatic noninvasive blood pressures in pediatric intensive care patients. *Journal of Pediatric Nursing, 26*(1), 3–12.

Stacey, D., Macartney, G., Carley, M., et al. (2013). Development and evaluation of evidence-informed clinical nursing protocols for remote assessment, triage and support of cancer treatment-induced symptoms. *Nursing Research and Practice, 2013,* 171872. [Epub].

US Department of Agriculture, National Agricultural Library. (2014). *Food and nutrition information center: Interactive DRI for healthcare professionals.* Retrieved from http://fnic.nal.usda.gov/fnic/interactiveDRI/.

US Preventive Services Task Force. (2011). Vision screening for children 1 to 5 years of age: U.S. Preventive Task Force recommendation statement. *Pediatrics, 127*(2), 340–346.

30

Pain Assessment and Management in Children

Marilyn J. Hockenberry

http://evolve.elsevier.com/Perry/maternal

The evidence-based literature on pediatric pain assessment and management grows considerably each year. Treatment options for pediatric acute and chronic pain are continually being evaluated, and new technologies and administration options become available every day (Tobias, 2014a). Unfortunately, despite advances in acute and chronic pediatric pain management, many children and adolescents continue to suffer from inadequately treated pain of all types. Pain is a frequent occurrence in children with more than 25% of children experiencing pain during hospitalization (Kozlowski, Kost-Byerly, Colantuoni, et al., 2014). Effective management of pain in children requires a comprehensive approach of assessment, pain intervention, and reassessment (Habich, Wilson, Thielk, et al., 2012). Nurses play a major role as the member of an interprofessional team involved in managing pain in children.

PAIN ASSESSMENT

The purpose of a pediatric pain assessment is to determine how much pain the child is feeling. The Pediatric Initiative on Methods, Measurement, and Pain Assessment in Clinical Trials (PedIMMPACT) recommends specific core domains to assess pain in children that include pain intensity, global judgment of satisfaction with treatment, symptoms and adverse events, physical recovery, and emotional response (McGrath, Walco, Turk, et al., 2008). Although pain assessment includes more than a number rating, understanding the intensity of the pain experienced by the child is essential for effective pain management. Numerous pediatric pain scales exist and are most commonly identified as behavioral pain measures, self-report pain rating scales, and multidimensional pain assessment tools.

BEHAVIORAL PAIN MEASURES

Behavioral or observational measures of pain are generally used for children from infancy to 4 years of age (Table 30.1). Behavioral pain assessment may provide a more complete picture of the total pain experience when administered in conjunction with a subjective self-report measure. Behavioral pain measurement tools may be more time-consuming than self-reports because they depend on a trained observer to watch and record children's behaviors, such as vocalization, facial expression, and body movements that suggest discomfort. Distress behaviors, such as vocalization of sounds associated with pain, changes in facial expression, and unexpected or unusual body movements, have been associated with pain (Figs. 30.1 and 30.2). Understanding that these behaviors are associated with pain makes assessing pain in infants and small children with no or limited communication skills a little easier. However, discriminating between pain behaviors and reactions

to other sources of distress, such as hunger, anxiety, or other types of discomfort, is not always easy. Behavioral pain measures are most reliable when used to measure short, sharp procedural pain, such as during injections or lumbar punctures, or when assessing pain in infants and young children. They are less reliable when measuring recurrent or chronic pain and when assessing pain in older children, where pain scores on behavioral measures do not always correlate with the children's own reports of pain intensity. Box 30.1 describes pain responses by infants and children of various ages.

The FLACC Pain Assessment Tool is an interval scale that includes the five categories of behavior: Facial expression, Leg movement, Activity, Cry, and Consolability (Babl, Crellin, Cheng, et al., 2012; Merkel, Voepel-Lewis, Shayevitz, et al., 1997). It measures each behavior on a 0 to 10 scale, with total scores ranging from 0 (no pain behaviors) to 10 (most possible pain behaviors).

The only behavior pain measurement tool recommended for use with children in critical care settings is the COMFORT scale (Ambuel, Hamlett, Marx, et al., 1992). The COMFORT scale is a behavioral, unobtrusive method of measuring distress in unconscious and ventilated infants, children, and adolescents. This scale has eight indicators: alertness, calmness/agitation, respiratory response, physical movement, blood pressure, heart rate, muscle tone, and facial tension. Each indicator is scored between 1 and 5 based on the behaviors exhibited by the patient. The provider observes the patient unobtrusively for 2 minutes and derives the total score by adding the scores of each indicator. The total scores can range between 8 and 40. A score of 17 to 26 generally indicates adequate sedation and pain control. The COMFORT behavior (COMFORT-B) scale is able to detect specific changes in pain or distress intensity in critically ill children and in young children with burns (Boerlage, Ista, Duivenvoorden, et al., 2015; de Jong, Tuinebreijer, Bremer, et al., 2012). The COMFORT scale performed best when compared to the CHIPPS, CRIESS, and PIPP in assessing behavioral and physiologic components of pain in newborns following cardiac surgery (Franck, Ridout, Howard, et al., 2011).

SELF-REPORT PAIN RATING SCALES

Self-report measures are most often used for children older than 4 years of age (Table 30.2). There are many different "faces" scales for the measurement of pain intensity. Although children at 4 or 5 years of age are able to use self-report measures, cognitive characteristics of the preoperational stage influence their ability to separate feelings of pain and mood. Smiling faces on pain assessment scales can result in inadequacies of the pain rating (Quinn, Sheldon, & Cooley, 2014). Simple, concrete anchor words, such as "no hurt" to "biggest hurt," are more appropriate

TABLE 30.1	**Summary of Selected Behavioral Pain Assessment Scales for Young Children**		
Ages of Use	**Reliability and Validity**	**Variables**	**Scoring Range**
FLACC Postoperative Pain Tool			
2 months of age to 7 years of age	Validity using analysis of variance for repeated measures to compare FLACC scores before and after analgesia; preanalgesia FLACC scores significantly higher than postanalgesia scores at 10, 30, and 60 minutes ($p <0.001$ for each time) Correlation coefficients used to compare FLACC pain scores and OPS pain scores; significant positive correlation between FLACC and OPS scores ($r = 0.80$; $p <0.001$); positive correlation also found between FLACC scores and nurses' global ratings of pain ($r[47] = 0.41$; $p <0.005$)	Face (0–2) Legs (0–2) Activity (0–2) Cry (0–2) Consolability (0–2)	0 = no pain; 10 = worst pain

FLACC Scale			
FLACC	**0**	**1**	**2**
Face	No particular expression or smile	Occasional grimace or frown, withdrawn, disinterested	Frequent to constant frown, clenched jaw, quivering chin
Legs	Normal position or relaxed	Uneasy, restless, tense	Kicking, or legs drawn up
Activity	Lying quietly, normal position, moves easily	Squirming, shifting back and forth, tense	Arched, rigid, or jerking
Cry	No cry (awake or asleep)	Moans or whimpers, occasional complaint	Crying steadily, screams or sobs, frequent complaints
Consolability	Content, relaxed	Reassured by occasional touching, hugging, or talking to; distractible	Difficult to console or comfort

From Merkel, S.I., Voepel-Lewis, T., Shayevitz, J.R., et al. (1997). The FLACC: A behavioral scale for scoring postoperative pain in young children. *Pediatric Nursing, 23*(3), 293–297. Used with permission of Jannetti Publications, Inc., and the University of Michigan Health System. Can be reproduced for clinical and research use.

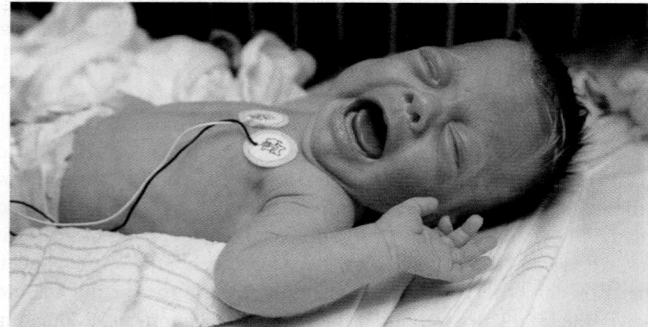

FIG 30.1 Full, robust crying of preterm infant after heel stick. (Courtesy of Halbouty Premature Nursery, Texas Children's Hospital, Houston, TX; photo by Paul Vincent Kuntz.)

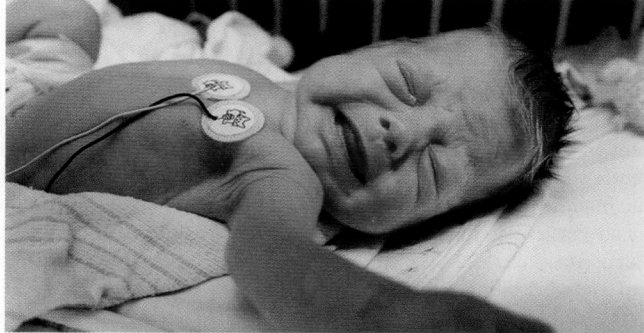

FIG 30.2 The face of pain after heel stick. Note eye squeeze, brow bulge, nasolabial furrow, and wide-spread mouth. (Courtesy of Halbouty Premature Nursery, Texas Children's Hospital, Houston, TX; photo by Paul Vincent Kuntz.)

than "least pain sensation to worst intense pain imaginable." The ability to discriminate degrees of pain in facial expressions appears to be reasonably established by 3 years of age (see Table 30.2). Faces scales provide a series of facial expressions depicting gradations of pain. The faces are appealing because children can simply point to the face that represents how they feel.

The Faces Pain Scale–Revised (FPS-R; Hicks, von Baeyer, Spafford, et al., 2001) and the Wong-Baker FACES Pain Rating Scale (Wong & Baker, 1988) are the most widely used faces pain measurement tools. The FPS-R scale consists of six faces depicting increasing gradation of pain severity from 0 = "no pain" on the left face to 5 = "most pain possible" on the right face. In developing this scale, the authors did not include a smiling face at the "no pain" end or tears at the "most pain" end and validated it so that it is equivalent to a 0 to 10 metric system. The Wong-Baker FACES Pain Rating Scale consists of six cartoon faces

ranging from a smiling face for "no pain" to a tearful face for "worst pain." The child is asked to choose a face that describes his or her pain. The Wong-Baker FACES Pain Rating Scale is able to differentiate pain from fear in school-age children (Garra, Singer, Domingo, et al., 2013). The Wong-Baker FACES Pain Rating Scale is the most preferred and widely used in children's hospitals across the United States and has been translated into many languages (Oakes, 2011).

For children 8 years of age and older, the Numeric Rating Scale (NRS), specifically the 0 to 10 scale, is most widely used in clinical practice because it is easy to use. The Visual Analogue Scale (VAS) uses descriptors along a line that provides a highly subjective evaluation of a pain or other symptom. VASs are often used with older children and adults. Although the VAS requires a higher degree of abstraction than the NRS, the PedIMMPACT group recommends the VAS because of

BOX 30.1   Children's Responses to Pain at Various Ages

Newborn and Young Infant

- Uses crying
- Reveals facial appearance of pain (brows lowered and drawn together, eyes tightly closed, and mouth open and squarish)
- Exhibits generalized body response of rigidity or thrashing, possibly with local reflex withdrawal from what is causing the pain
- Shows no relationship between what is causing the pain and subsequent response

Older Infant

- Uses crying
- Shows a localized body response with deliberate withdrawal from what is causing the pain
- Reveals expression of pain or anger
- Demonstrates a physical struggle, especially pushing away from what is causing the pain

Young Child

- Uses crying and screaming
- Uses verbal expressions, such as "Ow," "Ouch," or "It hurts"
- Uses thrashing of arms and legs to combat pain
- Attempts to push what is causing the pain away before it is applied
- Displays lack of cooperation; need for physical restraint
- Begs for the procedure to end
- Clings to parent, nurse, or other significant person
- Requests physical comfort, such as hugs or other forms emotional support
- Becomes restless and irritable with ongoing pain
- Worries about the anticipation of the actual painful procedure

School-Age Child

- Demonstrates behaviors of the young child, especially during actual painful procedure, but less before the procedure
- Exhibits time-wasting behavior, such as "Wait a minute" or "I'm not ready"
- Displays muscular rigidity, such as clenched fists, white knuckles, gritted teeth, contracted limbs, body stiffness, closed eyes, wrinkled forehead

Adolescent

- Less vocal with less physical resistance
- More verbal in expressions, such as "It hurts" or "You're hurting me"
- Displays increased muscle tension and body control

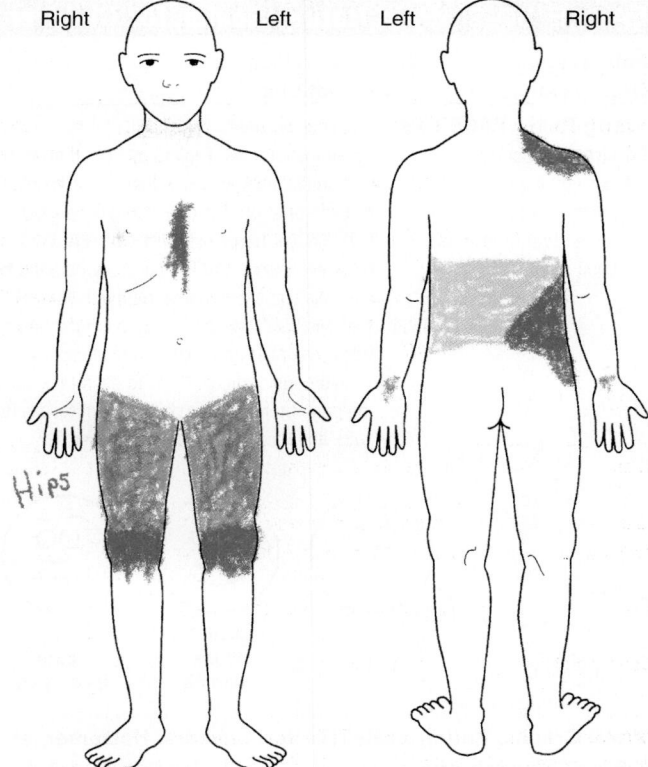

FIG 30.3 Adolescent Pediatric Pain Tool (APPT): Body outlines for pain assessment. Instructions: "Color in the areas on these drawings to show where you have pain. Make the marks as big or as small as the place where the pain is." Tool has been completed by a child with sickle cell disease. (From Savedra, M.C., Tesler, M.D., Holzemer, W.L., & Ward, J.A., University of California School of Nursing, San Francisco; copyright 1989, 1992.)

the lack of supportive evidence through psychometric studies with the NRS in children and adolescents.

The number of pain measures available for use in infants, young children, and adolescents has increased dramatically and adds a layer of complexity to the assessment of pain in children. The current trend supports a common metric for measurement of pain in children. Most instruments consist of 0 for no pain to a range of 4 to 160 for the top anchors in pain measures. A pain score of 5 may mean a lot of pain (if a 0 to 5 scale is used) or very little (if a 0 to 100 scale is used), and it may not be clearly specified which score corresponds to which scale. Other health care providers who do not specialize in pediatric pain may be confused by the available instruments and scoring methods and may not be able to determine the effectiveness of interventions by the pain score documented. An advantage to using a common metric is that a certain score may be considered as the point at which an intervention is required, or a point at which relief may be considered effective. The 0 to 10 system as the common metric was reported to be preferred by health care providers and would make pain scores easier to read, interpret, and integrate into research and practice.

MULTIDIMENSIONAL MEASURES

Several cognitive skills, such as measurement, classification, and seriation (the ability to accurately place in ascending or descending order), become apparent between 7 and 10 years of age. Older children are able to use a 0 to 10 NRS used by adolescents and adults. Other dimensions (such as pain quality, pain location, and spatial distribution of pain) may change without a change in pain intensity.

Pain charts or pain drawings are used to obtain information regarding the location of pain and have been well validated for children 8 years of age and older (von Baeyer, Lin, Seidman, et al., 2011). The Adolescent Pediatric Pain Tool (APPT), modeled after the McGill Pain Questionnaire (Melzack, 1975), is a multidimensional pain measurement instrument used with children and adolescents to assess pain location, intensity, and quality (Fernandes, De Campos, Batalha, et al., 2014) (Fig. 30.3). The APPT is an instrument with an anterior and posterior body outline on one side and a 100-mm word-graphing rating scale with a pain descriptor on the other side (Savedra, Holzemer, Tesler, et al., 1993; Savedra, Tesler, Holzemer, et al., 1989; Tesler, Savedra, Holzemer, et al., 1991). Each of the three components of the APPT is scored separately. The body outline is scored by placing a clear plastic template overlay with 43 body areas on the body outline diagram. An estimate of the pervasiveness of the pain is made by counting the number of body

TABLE 30.2 Pain Rating Scales for Children

Pain Scale, Description	Instructions	Recommended Age, Comments
Wong-Baker FACES Pain Rating Scale*		
Consists of six cartoon faces ranging from smiling face for "no pain" to tearful face for "worst pain"	Original instructions: Explain to child that each face is for a person who feels happy because there is no pain (hurt) or sad because there is some or a lot of pain. FACE 0 is very happy because there is no hurt. FACE 1 hurts just a little bit. FACE 2 hurts a little more. FACE 3 hurts even more. FACE 4 hurts a whole lot, but FACE 5 hurts as much as you can imagine, although you don't have to be crying to feel this bad. Ask child to choose face that best describes own pain. Record number under chosen face on pain assessment record. Brief word instructions: Point to each face using the words to describe the pain intensity. Ask child to choose face that best describes own pain, and record appropriate number.	For children as young as 3 years of age. Using original instructions without affect words, such as *happy* or *sad,* or brief words resulted in same range of pain rating, probably reflecting child's rating of pain intensity. For coding purposes, numbers 0, 2, 4, 6, 8, and 10 can be substituted for 0 to 5 system to accommodate 0 to 10 system. The Wong-Baker FACES Pain Rating Scale provides three scales in one: facial expressions, numbers, and words. Research supports cultural sensitivity of FACES for Caucasian, African-American, Hispanic, Thai, Chinese, and Japanese children.

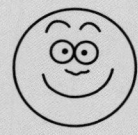 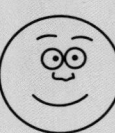 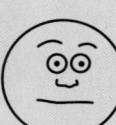 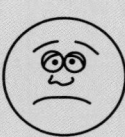 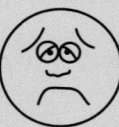 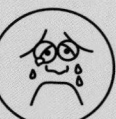

0	1 or 2	2 or 4	3 or 6	4 or 8	5 or 10
No hurt	Hurts little bit	Hurts little more	Hurts even more	Hurts whole lot	Hurts worst

Word-Graphic Rating Scale† (Tesler, Savedra, Holzemer, et al., 1991)

Uses descriptive words (may vary in other scales) to denote varying intensities of pain	Explain to child, "This is a line with words to describe how much pain you may have. This side of the line means no pain, and over here the line means worst possible pain." (Point with your finger where "no pain" is, and run your finger along the line to "worst possible pain," as you say it.) "If you have no pain, you would mark like this." (Show example.) "If you have some pain, you would mark somewhere along the line, depending on how much pain you have." (Show example.) "The more pain you have, the closer to worst pain you would mark. The worst pain possible is marked like this." (Show example.) "Show me how much pain you have right now by marking with a straight, up-and-down line anywhere along the line to show how much pain you have right now." With millimeter rule, measure from the "no pain" end to mark, and record this measurement as pain score.	For children from 4 to 17 years of age.

No pain	Little pain	Medium pain	Large pain	Worst possible pain

Numeric Scale

Uses straight line with end points identified as "no pain" and "worst pain" and sometimes "medium pain" in the middle; divisions along line marked in units from 0 to 10 (high number may vary)	Explain to child that at one end of line is 0, which means that person feels no pain (hurt). At the other end is usually a 5 or 10, which means the person feels worst pain imaginable. The numbers 1 to 5 or 1 to 10 are for very little pain to a whole lot of pain. Ask child to choose number that best describes own pain.	For children as young as 5 years of age, as long as they can count and have some concept of numbers and their values in relation to other numbers. Scale may be used horizontally or vertically. Number coding should be same as other scales used in facility.

No pain   Worst pain

0 1 2 3 4 5 6 7 8 9 10

TABLE 30.2   Pain Rating Scales for Children—cont'd

Pain Scale, Description	Instructions	Recommended Age, Comments
Visual Analog Scale (VAS) (Cline, Herman, Shaw, et al., 1992)		
Defined as vertical or horizontal line that is drawn to certain length, such as 10 cm (4 inches), and anchored by items that represent extremes of the subjective phenomenon being measured, such as pain	Ask child to place mark on line that best describes amount of own pain. With centimeter ruler, measure from "no pain" end to mark, and record this measurement as pain score.	For children as young as 4½ years of age, preferably 7 years of age. Vertical or horizontal scale may be used. Research shows that children from 3 to 18 years of age least prefer VAS compared with other scales (Luffy & Grove, 2003; Wong & Baker, 1988).

No pain   Worst pain

Oucher (Villarruel and Denyes, 1991)		
Consists of six photographs of a white child's face representing "no hurt" to "biggest hurt you could ever have;" also includes vertical scale with numbers from 0 to 100; scales for African-American and Hispanic children have been developed	*Numeric scale:* Point to each section of scale to explain variations in pain intensity: "0 means no hurt." "This means little hurts" (pointing to lower part of scale, 1 to 29). "This means middle hurts" (pointing to middle part of scale, 30 to 69). "This means big hurts" (pointing to upper part of scale, 70 to 99). "100 means the biggest hurt you could ever have." Score is actual number stated by child. *Photographic scale:* Point to each photograph, and explain variations in pain intensity using the following language: First picture from the bottom is "no hurt," second is "a little hurt," third is "a little more hurt," fourth is "even more hurt than that," fifth is "pretty much or a lot of hurt," and sixth is "biggest hurt you could ever have." Score pictures from 0 to 5, with bottom picture scored as 0. *General:* Practice using Oucher by recalling and rating previous pain experiences (e.g., falling off bike). Child points to number or photograph that describes pain intensity associated with experience. Obtain current pain score from child by asking, "How much hurt do you have right now?"	For children from 3 to 13 years of age. Use numeric scale if child can count off any two numbers or by tens (Jordan-Marsh, Yoder, Hall, et al., 1994). Determine whether child has cognitive ability to use photographic scale; child should be able to rate six geometric shapes from largest to smallest. Determine which ethnic version of Oucher to use; allow child to select version of Oucher, or use version that most closely matches physical characteristics of child. *Note:* Ethnically similar scale may not be preferred by child when given choice of ethnically neutral cartoon scale (Luffy & Grove, 2003).

*Copyright 1983 by Wong-Baker FACES Foundation, www.WongBakerFACES.org. Used with permission. Originally published in *Whaley & Wong's nursing care of infants and children.* Copyright Elsevier Inc.
†Instructions for Word-Graphic Rating Scale from Acute Pain Management Guideline Panel. (1992). Acute pain management in infants, children, and adolescents: Operative and medical procedures; quick reference guide for clinicians, ACHPR Pub. No. 92-0020, Rockville, MD: Agency for Health Care Research and Quality, US Department of Health and Human Services. Word-Graphic Rating Scale is part of the Adolescent Pediatric Pain Tool and is available from Pediatric Pain Study, University of California, School of Nursing, Department of Family Health Care Nursing, San Francisco, CA 94143-0606; 415-476-4040.

areas marked. A ruler or micrometer preprinted on the APPT is used to score the word-graphic rating scale. The number of millimeters from the left side of the scale to the point marked by the child is measured; and the numeric value provides an overall evaluation of the amount of pain the child is experiencing. The total number of words on the descriptor list is counted, and scores range from 0 to 56. The clinician then counts the number of words selected in each of three categories— evaluative (0–8), sensory (0–37), and affective (0–11)—and calculates a percentage score for each one (Savedra, Holzemer, Tesler, et al., 1993). A systematic review of the APPT found that it can be helpful in customizing pain management interventions for adolescents (Fernandes, De Campos, Batalha, et al., 2014).

The Pediatric Pain Questionnaire (PPQ) is a multidimensional pain instrument to assess patient and parental perceptions of the pain experience in a manner appropriate for the cognitive-developmental level of children and adolescents (Lootens & Rapoff, 2011). The PPQ consists of eight areas of inquiry: pain history, pain language, the colors children associate with pain, emotions children experience, the worst pain experiences, the ways children cope with pain, the positive aspects of pain, and the location of their current pain. The three components of the PPQ include (1) VASs; (2) color-coded rating scales; and (3) verbal descriptors to provide information about the sensory, affective, and evaluative dimensions of chronic pain. There is also information about the child and family's pain history, symptoms, pain relief interventions, and socio-environmental situations that may influence pain. The child, parent, and physician each complete the form separately.

CHRONIC AND RECURRENT PAIN ASSESSMENT

Pain that persists for 3 months or more or beyond the expected period of healing is defined as chronic pain. Complex regional pain syndrome and chronic daily headache are the most common types of chronic pain conditions in children. Pain that is episodic and recurs is defined as recurrent pain—the time frame within which episodes of pain recurs every 3 months or more frequently. Recurrent pain syndromes in children include migraine headache, episodic sickle cell pain, recurrent abdominal pain (RAP), and recurrent limb pain.

For children and adolescents with chronic pain, a measure such as the Functional Disability Inventory (FDI) (Walker & Greene, 1991) provides a more comprehensive evaluation of the influence of pain on physical functioning. The FDI assesses the child's ability to perform everyday physical activities and has established psychometric properties with different populations (Claar & Walker, 2006; Kashikar-Zuck, Flowers, Claar, et al., 2011). For children younger than 7 years of age, the Pediatric Quality of Life Scale (PedsQL), developed by Varni, Seid, and Rode (1999), is a multidimensional scale with both parent and child versions that is recommended for assessing physical, emotional, social, and academic functioning as they relate to the child's pain. The PedsQL and the PedMIDAS (Gold, Mahrer, Yee, et al., 2009; Hershey, Powers, Vockell, et al., 2001; 2004) have been validated for measurement of role functioning in children with chronic or recurrent pain. The PedMIDAS is specifically designed to evaluate pain caused by migraines in children.

Pain diaries are commonly used to assess pain symptoms and response to treatment in children and adolescents with recurrent or chronic pain (Fortier, Wahi, Bruce, et al., 2014; Stinson, Stevens, Feldman, et al., 2008). Diary studies have included children as young as 6 years of age. Conventional paper-and-pencil measures have been associated with several limitations, such as poor compliance, missing data, hoarding of responses, and back and forward filling. An electronic diary to assess pediatric chronic pain is a developing area that holds promise for the future.

Sleep disruption is also common in those with chronic or recurrent pain (Valrie, Bromberg, Palermo, et al., 2013). A sleep diary can be useful in keeping a record of activities surrounding sleep, including bedtime, time to fall asleep, number of night awakenings, waking in the morning, and especially any pain or other circumstance that interfered with sleeping. The sleep diary was validated using sleep actigraphy in healthy 13- to 14-year-old children (Gaina, Sekine, Chen, et al., 2004). The Sleep Habits Questionnaire, which is useful for assessing sleep behaviors in school-age children with chronic or recurrent pain, has also been evaluated for use in preschool and toddlers using parent proxy (Sneddon, Peacock, & Crowly, 2013).

ASSESSMENT OF PAIN IN SPECIFIC POPULATIONS

PAIN IN NEONATES

The impact of early pain exposure greatly affects the developing nervous system, with persistent long-term effects. This makes neonatal assessment extremely important, although difficult, because the most reliable indicator of pain, self-report, is not possible. Evaluation must be based on physiologic changes and behavioral observations with validated instruments (Hatfield & Ely, 2015) (Box 30.2). Although behaviors (such as vocalizations, facial expressions, body movements, and general relaxation state) are common to all infants, they vary with different situations. Crying associated with pain is more intense and sustained

---

BOX 30.2 Manifestations of Acute Pain in the Neonate

Physiologic Responses

Vital signs: Observe for variations
- Increased heart rate
- Increased blood pressure
- Rapid, shallow respirations

Oxygenation
- Decreased transcutaneous oxygen saturation (TcPO$_2$)
- Decreased arterial oxygen saturation (SaO$_2$)

Skin: Observe color and character
- Pallor or flushing
- Diaphoresis
- Palmar sweating

Other observations
- Increased muscle tone
- Dilated pupils
- Decreased vagal nerve tone
- Increased intracranial pressure
- Laboratory evidence of metabolic or endocrine changes: Hyperglycemia, lowered pH, elevated corticosteroids

Behavioral Responses

Vocalizations: Observe quality, timing, and duration
- Crying
- Whimpering
- Groaning

Facial expression: Observe characteristics, timing, orientation of eyes and mouth
- Grimaces
- Brow furrowed
- Chin quivering
- Eyes tightly closed
- Mouth open and squarish

Body movements and posture: Observe type, quality, and amount of movement or lack of movement; relationship to other factors
- Limb withdrawal
- Thrashing
- Rigidity
- Flaccidity
- Fist clenching

Changes in state: Observe sleep, appetite, activity level
- Changes in sleep-wake cycles
- Changes in feeding behavior
- Changes in activity level
- Fussiness, irritability
- Listlessness

SaO$_2$, Arterial oxygen saturation; *TcPO$_2$*, transcutaneous oxygen pressure.

(see Fig. 30.1). Facial expression is the most consistent and specific characteristic; scales are available to systematically evaluate facial features, such as eye squeeze, brow bulge, open mouth, and taut tongue. Most infants respond with increased body movements, but the infant may be experiencing pain even when lying quietly with eyes closed. The preterm infant's response to pain may be behaviorally blunted or absent; however, there is ample evidence that such infants are neurologically capable of feeling pain. In addition, infants in awake or alert states demonstrate a more robust reaction to painful stimuli than infants in sleep states. Also, an infant receiving a muscle-paralyzing agent (vecuronium) is incapable of a behavioral or visible pain response.

Although regular use of pain assessment tools can assist caregivers in determining whether the infant is in pain, caregivers must consider the infant's maturity, behavioral state, energy resources available to respond, and risk factors for pain. In infants with diminished ability to respond robustly to pain, it is imperative to presume that pain exists in all situations that are usually considered painful for adults and children, even in the absence of behavioral or physiologic signs.

Several pain assessment tools for neonates have been developed (Table 30.3). One tool used by nurses who work with premature and full-term infants in the neonatal intensive care setting is called *CRIES*,

TABLE 30.3   Summary of Pain Assessment Scales for Infants

Ages of Use	Reliability and Validity	Variables	Scoring Range
Neonatal Infant Pain Scale (NIPS) (Lawrence, Alcock, McGrath, et al., 1993)			
Average gestational age: 33.5 weeks	Interrater reliability: 0.92 and 0.97 Construct validity using analysis of variance between scores before, during, and after procedure: F = 18.97, df = 2.42, p <0.001 Concurrent validity between NIPS and visual analog scale (VAS) using Pearson correlations: 0.53–0.84 Internal consistency using Cronbach alpha: 0.95, 0.87, and 0.88 for before, during, and after procedure scores	Facial expression (0–1) Arms (0–1) Cry (0–2) Legs (0–1) Breathing patterns (0–1) State of arousal (0–1)	0 = no pain; 7 = worst pain
CRIES (Krechel & Bildner, 1995)			
32–60 weeks of gestational age	Concurrent validity between CRIES and POPS: 0.73 (p <0.0001, n = 1382); Spearman correlation between subjective report and POPS and CRIES: 0.49 (p <0.0001, n >1300) Discriminant validity using before and after analgesia scores: Wilcoxon sign rank test; mean decline of 3.0 units (p <0.0001, n = 74) Interrater reliability using Spearman correlation coefficient: r = 0.72 (p <0.0001, n = 680)	Crying (0–2) Requires increased oxygen (0–2) Increased vital signs (0–2) Expression (0–2) Sleepless (0–2)	0 = no pain; 10 = worst pain
Premature Infant Pain Profile (PIPP) (Stevens, Johnston, Petryshen, et al., 1996)			
28–40 weeks of gestational age	Internal consistency using Cronbach alpha: 0.75–0.59; standardized item alpha for six items: 0.71 Construct validity using handling versus painful situations: Statistically significant differences (paired t = 12.24, two-tailed p <0.0001, and Mann-Whitney U = 765.5, p <0.00001) and using real versus sham heel stick procedures with infants ages 28–30 weeks of gestational age (t = 2.4, two-tailed p <0.02, and Mann-Whitney U = 132, p <0.016) and with full-term boys undergoing circumcision with topical anesthetic versus placebo (t = 2.6, two-tailed p <0.02, or nonparametric equivalent Mann-Whitney U test, U = 145.7, two-tailed p <0.02)	Gestational age (0–3) Eye squeeze (0–3) Behavioral state (0–3) Nasolabial furrow (0–3) Heart rate (0–3) Oxygen saturation (0–3) Brow bulge (0–3)	0 = no pain; 21 = worst pain
Neonatal Pain, Agitation, and Sedation Scale (NPASS) (Puchalski & Hummel, 2002)			

Birth (23 weeks of gestational age) and full-term newborns up to 100 days	Interrater reliability using ICC: 0.95 CI for preintervention and postintervention pain scale; 0.95 CI for preintervention and postintervention sedation scale
	Internal consistency (Cronbach alpha):
	    Preintervention pain scale, 0.75 and 0.71 raters 1 and 2
	    Postintervention pain scale, 0.25 and 0.27 raters 1 and 2
	    Preintervention sedation scale, 0.88 and 0.81 raters 1 and 2
	    Postintervention sedation scale, 0.86 and 0.89 raters 1 and 2
		Cry/irritability (0–2)
		Behavior/state (0–2)
		Facial expression (0–2)
		Extremities/tone (0–2)
		Vital signs: heart rate, respiratory rate, blood pressure, SaO_2 (0–2)
			Pain score: 0 = no pain; 10 = intense pain
			Sedation score: 0 = no sedation; 10 = deep sedation

CRIES NEONATAL POSTOPERATIVE PAIN SCALE

CRIES	0	1	2
Crying	No	High pitched	Inconsolable
Requires oxygen for saturation >95%	No	<30%	>30%
Increased vital signs	Heart rate and blood pressure ≤ preoperative state	Heart rate and blood pressure increase <20% of preoperative state	Heart rate and blood pressure increase >20% of preoperative state
Expression	None	Grimace	Grimace, grunt
Sleepless	No	Wakes at frequent intervals	Constantly awake

SaO₂, Arterial oxygen saturation.

which is an acronym for the tool's physiologic and behavioral indicators of pain: **C**rying, **R**equiring increased oxygen, **I**ncreased vital signs, **E**xpression, and **S**leeplessness. Each indicator is scored from 0 to 2, with a total possible pain score, representing the worst pain, of 10. A pain score greater than 4 is considered significant. This tool has been tested for reliability and validity for postoperative pain in infants between the ages of 32 weeks of gestation up to 20 weeks postterm (60 weeks) (Sweet & McGrath, 1998).

The Premature Infant Pain Profile (PIPP and PIPP-R) were developed specifically for preterm infants (Sweet & McGrath, 1998; Stevens, Gibbins, Yamada, et al., 2014). The category "gestational age at time of observation" gives a higher pain score to infants with lower gestational age. Infants who are asleep 15 seconds before the painful procedure also receive additional points for their blunted behavioral responses to painful stimuli.

The Neonatal Pain, Agitation, and Sedation Scale (NPASS) was originally developed to measure pain or sedation in preterm infants after surgery (Hillman, Tabrizi, Gauda, et al., 2015). It measures five criteria (see Table 30.3) in two dimensions (pain and sedation) and is used in neonates as young as 23 weeks of gestation up to infants 100 days of age. Extra points are added in the pain scale dimension for preterm infants based on gestational age.

CHILDREN WITH COMMUNICATION AND COGNITIVE IMPAIRMENT

The assessment of pain in children with communication and cognitive impairment can be challenging (Crosta, Ward, Walker, et al., 2014). Children who have significant difficulties in communicating with others about their pain include those who have significant neurologic impairments (e.g., cerebral palsy), cognitive impairment, metabolic disorders, autism, severe brain injury, and communication barriers (e.g., critically ill children who are on ventilators or heavily sedated or have neuromuscular disorders, loss of hearing, or loss of vision) and consequently are at greater risk for undertreatment of pain. Children with communication and cognitive deficits often experience spasticity, contractures, injury, infection, and orthopedic surgical treatment that may be painful. Behaviors include moaning, inconsistent patterns of play and sleep, changes in facial expression, and other physical problems that may mask expression of pain and be difficult to interpret.

The revised FLACC observational pain scale uses a behavioral approach that observes the child's face, legs, activity, cry, and consolability and is supported for use in clinical practice for children with cognitive impairment (Voepel-Lewis, Malviya, Tait, et al., 2008).

The Non-Communicating Children's Pain Checklist- Revised (NCCPC) is a pain measurement tool specifically designed for children with cognitive impairments (Breau, McGrath, Camfield, et al., 2002). The scale discriminates between periods of pain and calm and can predict behavior during subsequent episodes of pain (Fig. 30.4). The scale consists of six subscales (vocal, social, facial, activity, body and limbs, physiologic signs), which are scored based on the number of times the items are observed over a 10-minute period (0 = not at all; 1 = just a little; 2 = fairly often; 3 = very often). The NCCPC has been used during the postoperative period and was effective in measuring pain in the clinical setting (Massaro, Ronfani, Ferrara, et al., 2014).

CULTURAL DIFFERENCES

Expression of pain can be greatly affected by communication barriers (Azize, Humphreys, Cattani, 2011). A major challenge in the assessment and management of pain in children is the cultural appropriateness of pain assessment tools that have been validated only in Caucasian and

⊕ CULTURAL CONSIDERATIONS
Pain Scales

Observational scales and interview questionnaires for pain may not be as reliable for pain assessment as self-report scales in children of Hispanic origin. Children of Asian descent, who may learn to read Chinese characters vertically downward and from right to left, may have difficulty using horizontally-oriented scales.

English-speaking children (see Cultural Considerations box: Pain Scales). Cultural background may influence the validity and reliability of pain assessment tools developed in a single cultural context.

CHILDREN WITH CHRONIC ILLNESS AND COMPLEX PAIN

Questionnaires and pain assessment scales do not always provide the most meaningful means of assessing pain in children, particularly for those with complex pain. Some children cannot relate to a face or a number that describes their pain. Other children, such as those with cancer, are experiencing multiple symptoms and may find it difficult to isolate the pain from other symptoms. Rating the pain is only one aspect of assessment and does not always accurately convey to others how they really feel (Oakes, 2011).

The most important aspect of pain assessment for children with chronic illness, particularly those with complex pain, is the relationship that develops between the child and the family. This relationship offers health care providers a sense of what the pain experience means to the child and family. The pain experience can interfere with the child's ability to eat, sleep, and perform daily activities and routines and may be complicated by side effects of medical treatments, and complications associated with disease management.

Other important components of assessment include the onset of pain; pain duration or pattern; the effectiveness of the current treatment; factors that aggravate or relieve the pain; other symptoms and complications concurrently felt; and interference with the child's mood, function, and interactions with family (Pasero & McCaffrey, 2011). In addition to asking the child or parent when the pain started and how long the pain lasts, the nurse can assess variations and rhythms by asking whether the pain is better or worse at certain times of the day or night. If the child has had pain for a while, the child or parent may know which medications and doses are helpful. They may also have found some nonpharmacologic methods that have helped. The nurse may ask the child or parent to keep a diary of activities, positions, and other events that may increase or decrease the pain. Pain may be accompanied by other symptoms (e.g., nausea and poor appetite), and it may interfere with sleep and other activities. A diary can help families identify triggers that may cause pain and interventions that work.

Other aspects warranting careful assessment that may pose barriers to effective management include family issues and relationships, fears and concerns about addictions, the clinician's and family's lack of knowledge about pain, inappropriate use of pain medications, ineffective management of adverse effects from medications, and the use of different pain management modalities.

PAIN MANAGEMENT

Children may experience pain as a result of surgery, injuries, acute and chronic illnesses, and medical or surgical procedures. Unrelieved pain may lead to potential long-term physiologic, psychosocial, and behavioral

Non-communicating Children's Pain Checklist — Postoperative Version (NCCPC-PV)

NAME:_____   UNIT/FILE #: _____   DATE:_____ (dd/mm/yy)

OBSERVER:_____   START TIME:_____ AM/PM   STOP TIME:_____AM/PM

How often has this child shown these behaviors in the last 10 minutes? Please circle a number for each behavior. If an item does not apply to this child (for example, this child cannot reach with his/her hands), then indicate "not applicable" for that item.

| 0 = NOT AT ALL | 1 = JUST A LITTLE | 2 = FAIRLY OFTEN | 3 = VERY OFTEN | NA = NOT APPLICABLE |

I. Vocal

1. Moaning, whining, whimpering (fairly soft)... 0	1	2	3	NA
2. Crying (moderately loud).. 0	1	2	3	NA
3. Screaming/yelling (very loud)... 0	1	2	3	NA
4. A specific sound or word for pain (e.g., a word, cry, or type of laugh).......... 0	1	2	3	NA

II. Social

5. Not cooperating, cranky, irritable, unhappy... 0	1	2	3	NA
6. Less interaction with others, withdrawn.. 0	1	2	3	NA
7. Seeking comfort or physical closeness.. 0	1	2	3	NA
8. Being difficult to distract, not able to satisfy or pacify............................. 0	1	2	3	NA

III. Facial

9. A furrowed brow.. 0	1	2	3	NA
10. A change in eyes, including squinching of eyes, eyes opened wide, eyes frowning 0	1	2	3	NA
11. Turning down of mouth, not smiling.. 0	1	2	3	NA
12. Lips puckering up, tight, pouting, or quivering... 0	1	2	3	NA
13. Clenching or grinding teeth, chewing, or thrusting tongue out 0	1	2	3	NA

IV. Activity

14. Not moving, less active, quiet.. 0	1	2	3	NA
15. Jumping around, agitated, fidgety... 0	1	2	3	NA

V. Body and Limbs

16. Floppy.. 0	1	2	3	NA
17. Stiff, spastic, tense, rigid 0	1	2	3	NA
18. Gesturing to or touching part of the body that hurts 0	1	2	3	NA
19. Protecting, favoring, or guarding part of the body that hurts 0	1	2	3	NA
20. Flinching or moving the body part away, being sensitive to touch................. 0	1	2	3	NA
21. Moving the body in a specific way to show pain (e.g., head back, arms down, curls up, etc.) 0	1	2	3	NA

VI. Physiologic

22. Shivering... 0	1	2	3	NA
23. Change in color, pallor.. 0	1	2	3	NA
24. Sweating, perspiring.. 0	1	2	3	NA
25. Tears... 0	1	2	3	NA
26. Sharp intake of breath, gasping.. 0	1	2	3	NA
27. Breath holding... 0	1	2	3	NA

SCORE SUMMARY

Category	I	II	III	IV	V	VI	TOTAL
Score							

FIG 30.4 Non-communicating Children's Pain Checklist—Postoperative Version (NCCPC-PV). (Copyright 2004 by Lynn Breau, Patrick McGrath, Allen Finley, and Carol Camfield. Reprinted with permission.)   *Continued*

USING THE NCCPC-PV

The NCCPC-PV was designed to be used for children age 3 to 18 years who are unable to speak because of cognitive (mental/intellectual) impairments or disabilities. It can be used *whether or not* a child has physical impairments or disabilities. Descriptions of the types of children used to validate the NCCPC-PV can be found in: Breau, L.M., Finley, G.A., McGrath, P.J., & Camfield, C.S. (2002). Validation of the Non-communicating Children's Pain Checklist — Postoperative Version. *Anesthesiology, 96* (3), 528-535. The NCCPC-PV was designed to be used without training by parents and caregivers (carers), or by other adults who are not familiar with a specific child (do not know them well).

The NCCPC-PV may be freely copied for clinical use or use in research funded by not-for-profit agencies. For-profit agencies should contact Lynn Breau: Pediatric Pain Research, IWK Health Centre, 5850 University Avenue, Halifax, Nova Scotia, Canada, B3J 3G9 (lbreau@ns.sympatico.ca).

The NCCPC-PV was intended for use for pain after surgery or due to other procedures conducted in hospital. If short- or long-term pain is suspected for a child at home or in a long-term residential setting, the **Non-communicating Children's Pain Checklist — Revised** may be used. It can be obtained by contacting Lynn Breau. Information regarding the NCCPC-R can be found in: Breau, L.M., McGrath, P.J., Camfield, C.S. & Finley, G.A. (2002). Psychometric Properties of the Non-communicating Children's Pain Checklist—Revised. *Pain, 99,* 349-357.

ADMINISTRATION

To complete the NCCPC-R, base your observations on the child's behavior over <u>10 minutes</u>. *It is not necessary to watch the child continuously for this period*. However, it is recommended that the observer be in the child's presence for the majority of this time (e.g., be in the same room with the child). Although shorter observation periods may be used, the cut-off scores described below may not apply.

At the end of the observation time, indicate how frequently (how often) each item was seen or heard. This should not be based on the child's typical behavior or in relation to what he or she usually does. A guide for deciding the frequency of items is below:

> 0 = Not present at all during the observation period. (Note: If the item is not present because the child is not capable of performing that act, it should be scored as "NA").
> 1 = Seen or heard rarely (hardly at all), but is present.
> 2 = Seen or heard a number of times, but not continuous (not all the time).
> 3 = Seen or heard often, almost continuous (almost all the time); anyone would easily notice this if they saw the child for a few moments during the observation time.
> NA = Not applicable. This child is not capable of performing this action.

SCORING

1. Add up the scores for each subscale and enter below that subscale number in the Score Summary at the bottom of the sheet. Items marked "NA" are scored as "0" (zero).
2. Add up all subscale scores for Total Score.
3. Check whether the child's score is greater than the cut-off score.

CUT-OFF SCORE

Based on the scores of 24 children age 3 to 18 (Breau, Finley, McGrath, & Camfield, 2002), a **Total Score of <u>11 or more</u>** indicates a child has <u>moderate to severe pain</u>. Based on unpublished data from this same sample, a *Total score of 6-10* indicates a child has <u>mild pain</u>. When parents and caregivers completed the NCCPC-PV in hospital for the study group, this was accurate 88% of the time. When other observers completed the NCCPC-PV, this was accurate 75% of the time. A Total Score of 10 or less indicates less than moderate/severe pain. This was correct in the study group for parents and caregivers 81% of the time and for other observers 63% of the time.

USE OF CUT-OFF SCORES

As with all observational tools, caution should be taken in using cut-off scores, because they may not be 100% accurate. They should not be used as the only basis for deciding whether a child should be treated for pain. In some cases children may have lower scores when pain is present. For more detailed instructions for use of the NCCPC-PV in such situations, please refer to the full manual, available from Lynn Breau: Pediatric Pain Research, IWK Health Centre, 5850 University Avenue, Halifax, Nova Scotia, Canada, B3J 3G9 (lbreau@ns.sympatico.ca).

FIG 30.4, cont'd

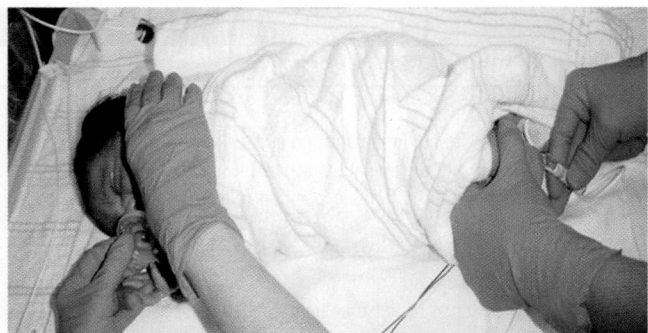

FIG 30.5 Sucking following oral sucrose can enhance analgesia before a heel stick in a preterm infant.

consequences. Improving pain management requires a multifactorial approach encompassing education, institutional support, attitude shifts, and change leaders (Twycross, 2010). Nonpharmacologic interventions and adequate pain medications are both essential to providing optimal pain management.

NONPHARMACOLOGIC MANAGEMENT

Pain is often associated with fear, anxiety, and stress. A number of nonpharmacologic techniques, such as distraction, relaxation, guided imagery, and cutaneous stimulation, can help with pain control (see Guidelines box: Nonpharmacologic Strategies for Pain Management). It is also important to provide coping strategies that help reduce pain perception, make pain more tolerable, decrease anxiety, and enhance the effectiveness of analgesics or reduce the dosage required.

There is strong evidence that distraction and hypnosis are effective interventions for needle-related pain and distress in children and adolescents (Uman, Birnie, Noel, et al., 2013). There is less evidence that cognitive-behavioral therapy (CBT), parent coaching plus distraction, suggestion, or virtual reality are effective for needle-related pain. Environmental and psychologic factors may exert a powerful influence on children's pain perceptions and may be modified by using psychosocial strategies, education, parental support, and cognitive-behavioral interventions. CBT is an evidence-based psychologic approach for managing pediatric pain (Logan, Coakley, & Garcia, 2014). CBT uses strategies that focus on thoughts and behaviors that modify negative beliefs and enhance the child's ability to solve pain-related problems that result in better pain management.

Nonnutritive sucking (pacifier) (Fig. 30.5), kangaroo care (Fig. 30.6), swaddling/facilitated tucking interventions reduce behavioral, physiologic, and hormonal responses to pain from procedures, such as heel punctures, in preterm and newborn infants (Meek & Huertas, 2012; Pillai Riddell, Racine, Turcotte, et al., 2011).

If the child cannot identify a familiar coping technique, the nurse can describe several strategies (e.g., distraction, breathing, guided imagery) and let the child select the most appealing one. Experimentation with several strategies that are suitable to the child's age, pain intensity, and abilities is often necessary to determine the most effective approach. Parents should be involved in the selection process; they may be familiar with the child's usual coping skills and can help identify potentially successful strategies. Involving parents also encourages their participation in learning the skill with the child and acting as coach. If the parent cannot assist the child, other appropriate people may include a grandparent, older sibling, nurse, or child-life specialist.

Children should learn to use a specific strategy before pain occurs or before it becomes severe. To reduce the child's effort, instructions

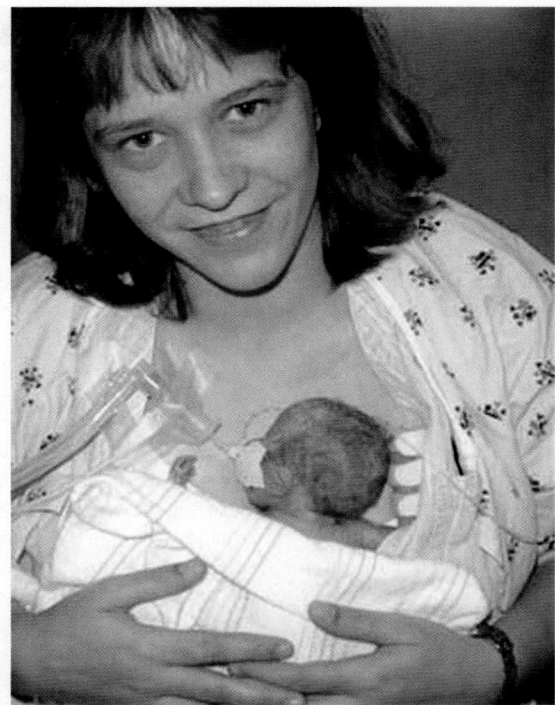

FIG 30.6 Mother using kangaroo hold with her newborn infant. Note placement of the infant directly on the mother's skin.

for a strategy, such as distraction or relaxation, can be audiotaped and played during a period of comfort. However, even after they have learned an intervention, children often need help using it during a painful procedure. The intervention can also be used after the procedure. This gives the child a chance to recover, feel mastery, and cope more effectively.

COMPLEMENTARY PAIN MEDICINE

Many terms are used to describe approaches to health care that are outside the realm of conventional medicine as practiced in the United States. Complementary and alternative medicine (CAM), as defined by the National Center for Complementary and Alternative Medicine, is a group of diverse medical and health care systems, practices, and products that are not currently considered part of conventional medicine. Although some scientific evidence exists regarding some CAM therapies, for most, key questions are yet to be answered through well-designed scientific studies—questions such as whether these therapies are safe and whether they work for the diseases or medical conditions for which they are used.

Classification of Complementary and Alternative Medicine

CAM therapies are grouped into five classes:
- Biologically based: foods, special diets, herbal or plant preparations, vitamins, other supplements
- Manipulative treatments: chiropractic, osteopathy, massage
- Energy based: Reiki, bioelectric or magnetic treatments, pulsed fields, alternating and direct currents
- Mind-body techniques: mental healing, expressive treatments, spiritual healing, hypnosis, relaxation
- Alternative medical systems: homeopathy; naturopathy; ayurveda; traditional Chinese medicine, including acupuncture and moxibustion

GUIDELINES

Nonpharmacologic Strategies for Pain Management

General Strategies

Consult child-life specialist.

Use nonpharmacologic interventions to supplement, not replace, pharmacologic interventions, and use for mild pain and pain that is reasonably well controlled with analgesics.

Form a trusting relationship with child and family.

Express concern regarding their reports of pain, and intervene appropriately.

Take an active role in seeking effective pain management strategies.

Use general guidelines to prepare child for procedure.

Prepare child before potentially painful procedures, but avoid "planting" the idea of pain.

- For example, instead of saying, "This is going to (or may) hurt," say, "Sometimes this feels like pushing, sticking, or pinching, and sometimes it doesn't bother people. Tell me what it feels like to you."
- Use "nonpain" descriptors when possible (e.g., "It feels like heat" rather than "It's a burning pain"). This allows for variation in sensory perception, avoids suggesting pain, and gives the child control in describing reactions.
- Avoid evaluative statements or descriptions (e.g., "This is a terrible procedure" or "It really will hurt a lot").

Stay with child during a painful procedure.

Allow parents to stay with child if child and parent desire; encourage parent to talk softly to child and to remain near child's head.

Involve parents in learning specific nonpharmacologic strategies and in assisting child with their use.

Educate child about the pain, especially when explanation may lessen anxiety (e.g., that pain may occur after surgery and does not indicate something is wrong); reassure the child that he or she is not responsible for the pain.

For long-term pain control, offer the child a doll, which represents "the patient," and allow child to do everything to the doll that is done to him or her; emphasize pain control through the doll by stating, "Dolly feels better after the medicine."

Teach procedures to child and family for later use.

Specific Strategies

Distraction

Involve parent and child in identifying strong distractors.

Involve child in play; use radio, smartphone, tablet, or computer game; have child sing or use rhythmic breathing.

Have child take a deep breath and blow it out until told to stop.

Have child blow bubbles to "blow the hurt away."

Have child concentrate on yelling or saying "ouch," with instructions to "yell as loud or soft as you feel it hurt; that way I know what's happening."

Have child look through kaleidoscope (type with glitter suspended in fluid-filled tube) and encourage him or her to concentrate by asking, "Do you see the different designs?"

Use humor, such as watching cartoons, telling jokes or funny stories, or acting silly with child.

Have child read, play games, or visit with friends.

Relaxation

With an infant or young child:

- Hold in a comfortable, well-supported position, such as vertically against the chest and shoulder.
- Rock in a wide, rhythmic arc in a rocking chair, or sway back and forth, rather than bouncing child.
- Repeat one or two words softly, such as "Mommy's here."

With a slightly older child:

- Ask child to take a deep breath and "go limp as a rag doll" while exhaling slowly; then ask child to yawn (demonstrate if needed).
- Help child assume a comfortable position (e.g., pillow under neck and knees).
- Begin progressive relaxation: starting with the toes, systematically instruct child to let each body part "go limp" or "feel heavy." If child has difficulty relaxing, instruct child to tense or tighten each body part and then relax it.
- Allow child to keep eyes open, since children may respond better if eyes are open rather than closed during relaxation.

Guided Imagery

Have child identify some highly pleasurable real or imaginary experience.

Have child describe details of the event, including as many senses as possible (e.g., "feel the cool breezes," "see the beautiful colors," "hear the pleasant music").

Have child write down or record script.

Encourage child to concentrate only on the pleasurable event during the painful time; enhance the image by recalling specific details by reading the script or playing the tape.

Combine with relaxation and rhythmic breathing.

Positive Self-Talk

Teach child positive statements to say when in pain (e.g., "I will be feeling better soon," or "When I go home, I will feel better, and we will eat ice cream").

Thought Stopping

Identify positive facts about the painful event (e.g., "It does not last long").

Identify reassuring information (e.g., "If I think about something else, it does not hurt as much").

Condense positive and reassuring facts into a set of brief statements, and have child memorize them (e.g., "Short procedure, good veins, little hurt, nice nurse, go home").

Have child repeat the memorized statements whenever thinking about or experiencing the painful event.

Behavioral Contracting

Informal: May be used with children as young as 4 or 5 years of age:

- Use stars, tokens, or cartoon character stickers as rewards.
- Give a child who is uncooperative or procrastinating during a procedure a limited time (measured by a visible timer) to complete the procedure.
- Proceed as needed if child is unable to comply.
- Reinforce cooperation with a reward if the procedure is accomplished within specified time.

Formal: Use written contract, which includes the following:

- Realistic (seems possible) goal or desired behavior
- Measurable behavior (e.g., agrees not to hit anyone during procedures)
- Contract written, dated, and signed by all people involved in any of the agreements
- Identified rewards or consequences that are reinforcing
- Goals that can be evaluated
- Commitment and compromise requirements for both parties (e.g., while timer is used, nurse will not nag or prod child to complete procedure)

The therapies that are increasingly used include herbal medicine, massage, megavitamins, self-help groups, folk remedies, energy healing, and homeopathy (Myers, Stuber, Bonamer-Rheingans, et al., 2005). CAM options are used frequently with children at the end of life and are found by their caregivers to be beneficial (Heath, Oh, Clarke, et al., 2012).

PHARMACOLOGIC MANAGEMENT

The World Health Organization (2012) states that the principles for pharmacologic pain management should include the following:
- Using a two-step strategy
- Dosing at regular intervals
- Using the appropriate route of administration
- Adapting treatment to the individual child

The traditional World Health Organization stepladder has been replaced with a two-step approach for use with children. The interprofessional care team uses this strategy to develop appropriate pain management interventions. This two-step strategy consists of a choice of category of analgesic medications, according to the child's level of pain severity. For children older than 3 months of age with mild pain, the first step is to administer a nonopioid; nonsteroidal antiinflammatory drugs (NSAIDs) are frequently used for mild pain. A strong opioid is usually administered to children with moderate or severe pain. Morphine is the medicine of choice for the second step, although other opioids may be considered (World Health Organization, 2012). The following sections discuss the most common pain medications used in children in the nonopioid and opioid categories.

Nonopioids

Nonopioids, including acetaminophen (Tylenol, paracetamol) and NSAIDs are suitable for mild to moderate pain (Table 30.4). These agents are known for the antipyretic, antiinflammatory, and/or analgesic actions (Tobias, 2014a). Nonopioids are usually the first analgesics for pain related to tissue injury, also known as *nociceptive pain*. NSAIDs can provide safe and effective pain relief when dosed at appropriate levels with adequate frequency. Most NSAIDs take about 1 hour for effect, so timing is crucial.

Opioids

Opioids are needed for moderate to severe pain (Tables 30.5 to 30.7). Morphine remains the standard agent used for comparison to other opioid agents. When morphine is not a suitable opioid, drugs such as hydromorphone hydrochloride (Dilaudid) and fentanyl citrate (Sublimaze) are used. Codeine, a once commonly used oral opiate analgesic, is a weak opioid and has well-known safety and efficacy problems related to genetic variability in biotransformation (Yellon, Kenna, Cladis, et al., 2014; Racoosin, Roberson, Pacanowski, et al., 2013; World Health Organization, 2012). For this reason, codeine is excluded as a recommendation for treatment of moderate pain in the *WHO Guidelines on the Pharmacological Treatment of Persisting Pain in Children with Medical Illnesses*. Dilaudid has a longer duration of action than morphine (4 to 6 hours) and is less associated with nausea and pruritus than morphine. Sublimaze is a synthetic product that is 100 times more potent than morphine (Tobias, 2014b).

> ⚡ **SAFETY ALERT**
>
> The optimum dosage of an analgesic is one that controls pain without causing undesirable side effects. This usually requires titration, the gradual adjustment of drug dosage (usually by increasing the dose) until optimum pain relief without excessive sedation is achieved. Dosage recommendations are only safe initial dosages (see Tables 30.5 to 30.7), not optimum dosages.

Coanalgesic Drugs

Several drugs, known as *coanalgesic drugs* or *adjuvant analgesics*, may be used alone or with opioids to control pain symptoms and opioid side effects (Table 30.8). Drugs frequently used to relieve anxiety, cause sedation, and provide amnesia are diazepam (Valium) and midazolam (Versed); however, these drugs are not analgesics and should be used to enhance the effects of analgesics, not as a substitute for analgesics. Other adjuvants include tricyclic antidepressants (e.g., amitriptyline, imipramine) and antiepileptics (e.g., gabapentin, carbamazepine, clonazepam) for neuropathic pain (Rastogi & Campbell, 2014). Other medications commonly prescribed include stool softeners and laxatives for constipation, antiemetics for nausea and vomiting, diphenhydramine for

TABLE 30.4   Nonsteroidal Antiinflammatory Drugs for Children

Drug	Dosage	Comments
Acetaminophen (Tylenol)	10–15 mg/kg/dose q 4-6 h PO not to exceed five doses in 24 h or 75 mg/kg/day, or 4000 mg/day	Available in numerous preparations Nonprescription Higher dosage range may provide increased analgesia
Choline magnesium trisalicylate (Trilisate)	10–15 mg/kg q 8–12 h PO Maximum dose 3000 mg/day	Available in suspension, 500 mg/5 mL Prescription
Ibuprofen (children's Motrin, children's Advil)	Children >6 months of age: 5–10 mg/kg/dose q 6–8 h Maximum dose 30 mg/kg/day or 3200 mg/day	Available in numerous preparations Available in suspension, 100 mg/5 mL, and drops, 100 mg/2.5 mL Nonprescription
Naproxen (Naprosyn)	Children >2 years of age: 5–7 mg/kg/dose every 12 h Maximum 20 mg/kg/day or 1250 mg/day	Available in suspension, 125 mg/5 mL, and several different dosages for tablets Prescription
Indomethacin	1–2 mg/kg q 6–12 h Maximum 4g/kg/day or 200 mg/day	Available in 25-mg and 50-mg capsules and suspension 25 mg/5 mL Prescription
Diclofenac	0.5–0.75 mg/kg q 6–12 h PO Maximum 3 mg/kg day or 200 mg/day	Available in 50-mg tablet and extended-release 100-mg tablets Prescription

PO, By mouth.
Data from McAuley, D.F. (2013). *GlobalRPh: NSAIDs*. Retrieved from http://www.globalrph.com/nsaids.htm.

TABLE 30.5   Starting Dosages for Opioid Analgesics in Opioid-Naïve Children (1 to 12 Years of Age)

Medicine	Route of Administration	Starting Dosage
Morphine	Oral (immediate release)	1–2 years of age: 200–400 mcg/kg every 4 h 2–12 years of age: 200–500 mcg/kg every 4 h (maximum: 5 mg)
	Oral (prolonged release)	200–800 mcg/kg every 12 h
	IV injection* SC injection	1–2 years of age:100 mcg/kg every 4 h 2–12 years of age: 100–200 mcg/kg every 4 h (maximum: 2.5 mg)
	IV infusion	Initial IV dose: 100–200 mcg/kg*, then 20–30 mcg/kg/h
	SC infusion	20 mcg/kg/h
Fentanyl	IV injection	1–2 mcg/kg,[†] repeated every 30–60 min
	IV infusion	Initial IV dose 1–2 mcg/kg,[†] then 1 mcg/kg/h
Hydromorphone[‡]	Oral (immediate release)	30–80 mcg/kg every 3–4 h (maximum: 2 mg/dose)
	IV injection[§] or SC injection	15 mcg/kg every 3–6 h
Methadone[‖]	Oral (immediate release)	100–200 mcg/kg
	IV injection[a] and SC injection	Every 4 h for the first 2–3 doses, then every 6–12 h (maximum: 5 mg/dose initially)[¶]
Oxycodone	Oral (immediate release)	125–200 mcg/kg every 4 h (maximum: 5 mg/dose)
	Oral (prolonged release)	5 mg every 12 h

IV, Intravenous; *SC*, subcutaneous.
*Administer IV morphine slowly over at least 5 minutes.
[†]Administer IV fentanyl slowly over 3 to 5 minutes.
[‡]Hydromorphone is a potent opioid, and significant differences exist between oral and IV dosing. Use extreme caution when converting from one route to another. In converting from parenteral hydromorphone to oral hydromorphone, doses may need to be titrated up to five times the IV dose.
[§]Administer IV hydromorphone slowly over 2 to 3 minutes.
[‖]Due to the complex nature and wide interindividual variation in the pharmacokinetics of methadone, methadone should only be commenced by practitioners experienced with its use.
[¶]Methadone should initially be titrated like other strong opioids. The dosage may need to be reduced by 50% 2 to 3 days after the effective dose has been found to prevent adverse effects due to methadone accumulation. From then on, dosage increases should be performed at intervals of 1 week or over and with a maximum increase of 50%.
[a]Administer IV methadone slowly over 3 to 5 minutes.
From World Health Organization. (2012). *WHO guidelines on the pharmacological treatment of persisting pain in children with medical illnesses.* Geneva, Switzerland: World Health Organization.

TABLE 30.6   Starting Dosages for Opioid Analgesics for Opioid-Naïve Neonates

Medicine	Route of Administration	Starting Dosage
Morphine	IV injection* SC injection	25–50 mcg/kg every 6 h
	IV infusion	Initial IV dose* 25–50 mcg/kg, then 5–10 mcg/kg/h
		100 mcg/kg every 4–6 h
Fentanyl	IV injection[†] IV infusion[†]	1–2 mcg/kg every 2–4 h[‡] Initial IV dose[‡] 1–2 mcg/kg, then 0.5–1 mcg/kg/h

IV, Intravenous; *SC*, subcutaneous.
*Administer intravenous (IV) morphine slowly over at least 5 minutes.
[†]The IV doses for neonates are based on acute pain management and sedation dosing information. Lower doses are required for nonventilated neonates.
[‡]Administer IV fentanyl slowly over 3 to 5 minutes.
From World Health Organization. (2012). *WHO guidelines on the pharmacological treatment of persisting pain in children with medical illnesses.* Geneva, Switzerland: World Health Organization.

TABLE 30.7   Starting Dosages for Opioid Analgesics in Opioid-Naïve Infants (1 Month to 1 Year of Age)

Medicine	Route of Administration	Starting Dosage
Morphine	Oral (immediate release)	80–200 mcg/kg every 4 h
	IV injection* SC injection	1–6 months of age: 100 mcg/kg every 6 h 6–12 months of age: 100 mcg/kg every 4 h (maximum: 2.5 mg/dose)
	IV infusion*	1–6 months of age: Initial IV dose: 50 mcg/kg, then 10–30 mcg/kg/h 6–12 months of age: Initial IV dose: 100–200 mcg/kg, then 20–30 mcg/kg/h
	SC infusion	1–3 months of age: 10 mcg/kg/h 3–12 months of age: 20 mcg/kg/h
Fentanyl[†]	IV injection	1–2 mcg/kg every 2–4 h[‡]
	IV infusion	Initial IV dose 1–2 mcg/kg[‡], then 0.5–1 mcg/kg/h
Oxycodone	Oral (immediate release)	50–125 mcg/kg every 4 h

IV, Intravenous; *SC*, subcutaneous.
*Administer intravenous (IV) morphine slowly over at least 5 minutes.
[†]The IV doses of fentanyl for infants are based on acute pain management and sedation dosing information.
[‡]Administer IV fentanyl slowly over 3 to 5 minutes.
From World Health Organization. (2012). *WHO guidelines on the pharmacological treatment of persisting pain in children with medical illnesses.* Geneva, Switzerland: World Health Organization.

TABLE 30.8   Coanalgesic Adjuvant Drugs

Drug	Dosage	Indications	Comments
Antidepressants			
Amitriptyline	0.2–0.5 mg/kg PO hs Titrate upward by 0.25 mg/kg q 5–7 days prn Available in 10- and 25-mg tablets Usual starting dose: 10–25 mg	Continuous neuropathic pain with burning, aching, dysesthesia with insomnia	Provides analgesia by blocking reuptake of serotonin and norepinephrine, possibly slowing transmission of pain signals Helps with pain related to insomnia and depression (use nortriptyline if patient is oversedated) Analgesic effects seen earlier than antidepressant effects
Nortriptyline	0.2–1 mg/kg PO AM or bid Titrate up by 0.5 mg q 5–7 days Maximum: 25 mg/dose	Neuropathic pain as above without insomnia	Side effects include dry mouth, constipation, urinary retention
Anticonvulsants			
Gabapentin	5 mg/kg PO hs Increase to bid on day 2, tid on day 3 Maximum: 300 mg/day	Neuropathic pain	Mechanism of action unknown Side effects include sedation, ataxia, nystagmus, dizziness
Carbamazepine	<6 years of age: 2.5–5 mg/kg PO bid initially Increase 20 mg/kg/24 h, divide bid every week prn Maximum: 100 mg bid 6–12 years of age: 5 mg/kg PO bid initially Increase 10 mg/kg/24 h; divide bid every week prn to usual Maximum: 100 mg/dose bid >12 years of age: 200 mg PO bid initially Increase 200 mg/24 h, divide bid every week prn to maximum: 1.6–2.4 g/24 h	Sharp, lancinating neuropathic pain Peripheral neuropathies Phantom limb pain	Similar analgesic effect to amitriptyline Monitor blood levels for toxicity only Side effects include decreased blood counts, ataxia, gastrointestinal irritation
Anxiolytics			
Lorazepam	0.03–0.1 mg/kg q 4–6 h PO or IV Maximum: 2 mg/dose	Muscle spasm Anxiety	May increase sedation in combination with opioids Can cause depression with prolonged use
Diazepam	0.1–0.3 mg/kg q 4–6 h PO or IV Maximum: 10 mg/dose		
Corticosteroids			
Dexamethasone	Dose dependent on clinical situation; higher bolus doses in cord compression, then lower daily dose Try to wean to NSAIDs if pain allows Cerebral edema: 1–2 mg/kg load, then 1–1.5 mg/kg/day divided q 6 h Maximum: 4 mg/dose Antiinflammatory: 0.08–0.3 mg/kg/day divided q 6–12 h	Pain from increased intracranial pressure Bony metastasis Spinal or nerve compression	Side effects include edema, gastrointestinal irritation, increased weight, acne Use gastro protectants such as H₂ blockers (ranitidine) or proton pump inhibitors, such as omeprazole for long-term administration of steroids or NSAIDs in end-stage cancer with bony pain
Others			
Clonidine	2–4 mcg/kg PO q 4–6 h May also use a 100-mcg transdermal patch q 7 days for patients >40 kg (88 lbs)	Neuropathic pain Lancinating, sharp, electrical, shooting pain Phantom limb pain	α_2-adrenoreceptor agonist modulates ascending pain sensations Routes of administration: oral, transdermal, and spinal Management of withdrawal symptoms Monitor for orthostatic hypertension, decreased heart rate Sedation common
Mexiletine	2–3 mg/kg/dose PO tid, may titrate 0.5 mg/kg q 2–3 wk prn Maximum: 300 mg/dose		Similar to lidocaine, longer acting Stabilizes sodium conduction in nerve cells, reduces neuronal firing Can enhance action of opioids, antidepressants, anticonvulsants Side effects include dizziness, ataxia, nausea, vomiting May measure blood levels for toxicity

bid, Twice a day; *hs,* at bedtime; *IV,* intravenous; *NSAID,* nonsteroidal antiinflammatory drug; *PO,* by mouth; *prn,* as needed; *q,* every; *tid,* three times a day.

itching, steroids for inflammation and bone pain, and dextroamphetamine and caffeine for possible increased pain and sedation (Table 30.9).

⚡ SAFETY ALERT

The use of placebos to determine whether the patient is having pain is unjustified and unethical; a positive response to a placebo, such as a saline injection, is common in patients who have a documented organic basis for pain. Therefore, the deceptive use of placebos does not provide useful information about the presence or severity of pain. The use of placebos can cause side effects similar to those of opioids, can destroy the patient's trust in the health care staff, and raises serious ethical and legal questions. The American Society of Pain Management Nursing has issued a position statement against the use of placebos to treat pain (Arnstein, Broglio, Wuhrman, et al., 2011).

Choosing the Pain Medication Dose

Children (except infants younger than 3 to 6 months of age) metabolize drugs more rapidly than adults and show great variability in drug elimination and side effects (Oakes, 2011). Younger children may require higher doses of opioids to achieve the same analgesic effect. Therefore, the therapeutic effect and duration of analgesia vary. Children's dosages are usually calculated according to body weight, except in children with a weight greater than 50 kg (110 lbs), where the weight formula may exceed the average adult dose. In this case, the adult dose is used.

A reasonable starting dose of an opioid for infants younger than 6 months of age who are not mechanically ventilated is one-fourth to one-third of the recommended starting dose for older children. The infant is monitored closely for signs of pain relief and respiratory depression. The dose is titrated to effect. Because tolerance can develop rapidly, large doses may be needed for continued severe pain. If pain relief is inadequate, the initial dose is increased (usually by 25% to 50% if pain is moderate, or by 50% to 100% if pain is severe) to provide greater analgesic effectiveness. Decreasing the interval between doses may also provide more continuous pain relief.

A major difference between opioids and nonopioids is that nonopioids have a *ceiling effect*, which means that doses higher than the recommended dose will not produce greater pain relief. Opioids do not have a ceiling

TABLE 30.9   Management of Opioid Side Effects

Side Effect	Adjuvant Drugs	Nonpharmacologic Techniques

Constipation	Senna and docusate sodium
	Tablet:
	  2–6 years of age: Start with ½ tablet once a day; maximum: 1 tablet twice a day
	  6–12 years of age: Start with 1 tablet once a day; maximum: 2 tablets twice a day
	  >12 years of age: Start with 2 tablets once a day; maximum: 4 tablets twice a day
	Liquid:
	  1 month of age to 1 year of age: 1.25–5 mL q hs
	  1–5 years of age: 2.5–5 mL q hs
	  5–15 years of age: 5–10 mL q hs
	  >15 years of age: 10–25 mL q hs
	Casanthranol and docusate sodium
	Liquid: 5–15 mL q hs
	Capsules: 1 cap PO q hs
	Bisacodyl: PO or PR
	  3–12 years of age: 5 mg/dose/day
	  >12 years of age: 10–15 mg/dose/day
	Lactulose
	  7.5 mL/day after breakfast
	  Adult: 15–30 mL/day PO
	Mineral oil: 1–2 tsp/day PO
	Magnesium citrate
	  <6 years of age: 2–4 mL/kg PO once
	  6–12 years of age: 100–150 mL PO once
	  >12 years of age: 150–300 mL PO once
	Milk of magnesia
	  <2 years of age: 0.5 mL/kg/dose PO once
	  2–5 years of age: 5–15 mL/day PO
	  6–12 years of age: 15–30 mL PO once
	  >12 years of age: 30–60 mL PO once
		Increase water intake
		Prune juice, bran cereal, vegetables
		Exercise

Sedation	Caffeine: Single dose of 1–1.5 mg PO Dextroamphetamine: 2.5–5 mg PO in AM and early afternoon Methylphenidate: 2.5–5 mg PO in AM and early afternoon Consider opioid switch if sedation persists	Caffeinated drinks (e.g., Mountain Dew, cola drinks)
Nausea, vomiting	Promethazine: 0.5 mg/kg q 4–6 h; maximum: 25 mg/dose Ondansetron: 0.1–0.15 mg/kg IV or PO q 4 h; maximum: 8 mg/dose Granisetron: 10–40 mcg/kg q 2–4 h; maximum: 1 mg/dose Droperidol: 0.05–0.06 mg/kg IV q 4–6 h; can be very sedating	Imagery, relaxation Deep, slow breathing

TABLE 30.9 Management of Opioid Side Effects—cont'd

Side Effect	Adjuvant Drugs	Nonpharmacologic Techniques
Pruritus	Diphenhydramine: 1 mg/kg IV or PO q 4–6 h prn; maximum: 25 mg/dose Hydroxyzine: 0.6 mg/kg/dose PO q 6 h; maximum: 50 mg/dose Naloxone: 0.5 mcg/kg q 2 min until pruritus improves (diluted in solution of 0.1 mg of naloxone per 10 mL of saline) Butorphanol: 0.3–0.5 mg/kg IV (use cautiously in opioid-tolerant children; may cause withdrawal symptoms); maximum: 2 mg/dose because mixed agonist-antagonist	Oatmeal baths, good hygiene Exclude other causes of itching Change opioids
Respiratory depression—mild to moderate	Hold dose of opioid Reduce subsequent doses by 25%	Arouse gently, give oxygen, encourage to deep breathe
Respiratory depression—severe	Naloxone During disease pain management: 0.5 mcg/kg in 2-minute increments until breathing improves (Pasero & McCaffrey, 2011) Reduce opioid dose if possible Consider opioid switch During sedation for procedures: 5–10 mcg/kg until breathing improves Reduce opioid dose if possible Consider opioid switch	Oxygen, bag and mask if indicated
Dysphoria, confusion, hallucinations	Evaluate medications, eliminate adjuvant medications with central nervous system effects as symptoms allow Consider opioid switch if possible Haloperidol (Haldol): 0.05–0.15 mg/kg/day divided in two to three doses; maximum: 2–4 mg/day	Rule out other physiologic causes

Urinary retention	Evaluate medications, eliminate adjuvant medications with anticholinergic effects (e.g., antihistamines, tricyclic antidepressants)
	Occurs more frequently with spinal analgesia than with systemic opioid use
	Oxybutynin
	   1 year of age: 1 mg tid
	   1–2 years of age: 2 mg tid
	   2–3 years of age: 3 mg tid
	   4–5 years of age: 4 mg tid
	   >5 years of age: 5 mg tid
		Rule out other physiologic causes
		In/out or indwelling urinary catheter

hs, At bedtime; *IV*, intravenous; *PO*, by mouth; *PR*, by rectum; *prn*, as needed; *q*, every; *tid*, three times a day.

TABLE 30.10 Approximate Dose Ratios for Switching Between Parenteral and Oral Dosage Forms

Medicine	Dosage Ratio (Parenteral:Oral)
Morphine	1:2 to 1:3
Hydromorphone	1:2 to 1:5*
Methadone	1:1 to 1:2

*Hydromorphone is a potent opioid, and significant differences exist between oral and intravenous (IV) dosing. Use extreme caution when converting from one route to another. In converting from parenteral hydromorphone to oral hydromorphone, doses may need to be titrated up to 5 times the IV dose.
From World Health Organization. (2012). *WHO guidelines on the pharmacological treatment of persisting pain in children with medical illnesses*. Geneva, Switzerland: World Health Organization.

effect other than that imposed by side effects; therefore, larger dosages can be safely given for increasing severity of pain.

Parenteral and oral dosages of opioids are not the same. Because of the first-pass effect, an oral opioid is rapidly absorbed from the gastrointestinal tract and is partially metabolized in the liver before reaching the central circulation. Therefore, oral dosages must be larger to compensate for the partial loss of analgesic potency to achieve an equal analgesic effect. Conversion factors (Table 30.10) for selected opioids must be used when a change is made from intravenous (IV) (preferred) or intramuscular (IM) to oral. Immediate conversion from IM or IV to the suggested equianalgesic oral dose may result in a substantial error. For example, the dose may be significantly more or less than what the child requires. Small changes ensure small errors.

Choosing the Timing of Analgesia

The right timing for administering analgesics depends on the type of pain. For continuous pain control, such as for postoperative or cancer pain, a preventive schedule of medication around the clock (ATC) is effective. The ATC schedule avoids the low plasma concentrations that permit breakthrough pain. If analgesics are administered only when pain returns (a typical use of the prn, or "as needed," order), pain relief may take several hours. This may require higher doses, leading to a cycle of undermedication of pain alternating with periods of overmedication and drug toxicity. This cycle of erratic pain control also promotes "clock watching," which may be erroneously equated with addiction. Nurses can effectively use prn orders by giving the drug at regular intervals, because "as needed" should be interpreted as "as needed to prevent pain," not "as little as possible."

Choosing the Method of Administration

Several routes of analgesic administration can be used (Box 30.3), and the most effective and least traumatic route of administration should be selected. Continuous analgesia is not always appropriate, because not all pain is continuous. Frequently, temporary pain control or

BOX 30.3 Routes and Methods of Analgesic Drug Administration

Oral

Oral route preferred because of convenience, cost, and relatively steady blood levels

Higher dosages of oral form of opioids required for equivalent parenteral analgesia

Peak drug effect occurring after 1 to 2 hours for most analgesics

Delay in onset a disadvantage when rapid control of severe or fluctuating pain is desired

Sublingual, Buccal, or Transmucosal

Tablet or liquid placed between cheek and gum (buccal) or under tongue (sublingual)

Highly desirable because more rapid onset than oral route

- Produces less first-pass effect through liver than oral route, which normally reduces analgesia from oral opioids (unless sublingual or buccal form is swallowed, which occurs often in children)

Few drugs commercially available in this form

Many drugs can be compounded into sublingual troche or lozenge.*

- Actiq: Oral transmucosal fentanyl citrate in hard confection base on a plastic holder; indicated only for management of breakthrough cancer pain in patients with malignancies who are already receiving and are tolerant to opioid therapy, but can be used for preoperative or preprocedural sedation and analgesia

Intravenous (Bolus)

Preferred for rapid control of severe pain

Provides most rapid onset of effect, usually in about 5 minutes

Advantage for acute pain, procedural pain, and breakthrough pain

Needs to be repeated hourly for continuous pain control

Drugs with short half-life (morphine, fentanyl, hydromorphone) preferable to avoid toxic accumulation of drug

Intravenous (Continuous)

Preferred over bolus and intramuscular (IM) injection for maintaining control of pain

Provides steady blood levels

Easy to titrate dosage

Subcutaneous (Continuous)

Used when oral and intravenous (IV) routes not available

Provides equivalent blood levels to continuous IV infusion

Suggested initial bolus dose to equal 2-hour IV dose; total 24-hour dose usually requires concentrated opioid solution to minimize infused volume; use smallest-gauge needle that accommodates infusion rate

Patient-Controlled Analgesia

Generally refers to self-administration of drugs, regardless of route

Typically uses programmable infusion pump (IV, epidural, subcutaneous [SC]) that permits self-administration of boluses of medication at preset dose and time interval (lockout interval is time between doses)

Patient-controlled analgesia (PCA) bolus administration often combined with initial bolus and continuous (basal or background) infusion of opioid

Optimum lockout interval not known but must be at least as long as time needed for onset of drug

- Should effectively control pain during movement or procedures
- Longer lockout provides larger dose

Family-Controlled Analgesia

One family member (usually a parent) or other caregiver designated as child's primary pain manager with responsibility for pressing PCA button

Guidelines for selecting a primary pain manager for family-controlled analgesia:

- Spends a significant amount of time with the patient
- Is willing to assume responsibility of being primary pain manager
- Is willing to accept and respect patient's reports of pain (if able to provide) as best indicator of how much pain the patient is experiencing; knows how to use and interpret a pain rating scale
- Understands the purpose and goals of patient's pain management plan
- Understands concept of maintaining a steady analgesic blood level
- Recognizes signs of pain and side effects and adverse reactions to opioid

Nurse-Activated Analgesia

Child's primary nurse designated as primary pain manager and is only person who presses PCA button during that nurse's shift

Guidelines for selecting primary pain manager for family-controlled analgesia also applicable to nurse-activated analgesia

May be used in addition to basal rate to treat breakthrough pain with bolus doses; patient assessed every 30 minutes for need for bolus dose

May be used without a basal rate as a means of maintaining analgesia with around-the-clock bolus doses

Intramuscular

Note: Not recommended for pain control; not current standard of care

Painful administration (hated by children)

Tissue and nerve damage caused by some drugs

Wide fluctuation in absorption of drug from muscle

Faster absorption from deltoid than from gluteal sites

Shorter duration and more expensive than oral drugs

Time-consuming for staff and unnecessary delay for child

Intranasal

Available commercially as butorphanol (Stadol NS); approved for those older than 18 years of age

Should not be used in patient receiving morphine-like drugs because butorphanol is partial antagonist that will reduce analgesia and may cause withdrawal

Intradermal

Used primarily for skin anesthesia (e.g., before lumbar puncture, bone marrow aspiration, arterial puncture, skin biopsy)

Local anesthetics (e.g., lidocaine) cause stinging, burning sensation

Duration of stinging dependent on type of "caine" used

To avoid stinging sensation associated with lidocaine:

- Buffer the solution by adding 1 part sodium bicarbonate (1 mEq/mL) to 9 to 10 parts 1% or 2% lidocaine with or without epinephrine

Normal saline with preservative, benzyl alcohol, anesthetizes venipuncture site

Same dose used as for buffered lidocaine

Topical or Transdermal

EMLA (eutectic mixture of local anesthetics [lidocaine and prilocaine]) cream and anesthetic disk or LMX4 (4% liposomal lidocaine cream)

- Eliminates or reduces pain from most procedures involving skin puncture
- Must be placed on intact skin over puncture site and covered by occlusive dressing or applied as anesthetic disc for 1 hour or more before procedure

Lidocaine-tetracaine (Synera, S-Caine)

- Apply for 20 to 30 minutes
- Do not apply to broken skin

LAT (lidocaine-adrenaline-tetracaine), tetracaine-phenylephrine (tetraphen)

- Provides skin anesthesia about 15 minutes after application on nonintact skin
- Gel (preferable) or liquid placed on wounds for suturing
- Adrenaline not for use on end arterioles (fingers, toes, tip of nose, penis, earlobes) because of vasoconstriction

BOX 30.3   Routes and Methods of Analgesic Drug Administration—cont'd

Transdermal fentanyl (Duragesic)
- Available as patch for continuous pain control
- Safety and efficacy not established in children younger than 12 years of age
- Not appropriate for initial relief of acute pain because of long interval to peak effect (12 to 24 hours); for rapid onset of pain relief, give an immediate-release opioid
- Orders for "rescue doses" of an immediate-release opioid recommended for breakthrough pain, a flare of severe pain that breaks through the medication being administered at regular intervals for persistent pain
- Has duration of up to 72 hours for prolonged pain relief
- If respiratory depression occurs, possible need for several doses of naloxone

Vapo-coolant
- Use of prescription spray coolant, such as Fluori-Methane or ethyl chloride (Pain-Ease); applied to the skin for 10 to 15 seconds immediately before the needle puncture; anesthesia lasts about 15 seconds
- Some children dislike cold; may be more comfortable to spray coolant on a cotton ball and then apply this to the skin
- Application of ice to the skin for 30 seconds found to be ineffective

Rectal
Alternative to oral or parenteral routes
Variable absorption rate
Generally disliked by children
Many drugs able to be compounded into rectal suppositories*

Regional Nerve Block
Use of long-acting local anesthetic (bupivacaine or ropivacaine) injected into nerves to block pain at site

Provides prolonged analgesia postoperatively, such as after inguinal herniorrhaphy
May be used to provide local anesthesia for surgery, such as dorsal penile nerve block for circumcision or for reduction of fractures

Inhalation
Use of anesthetics, such as nitrous oxide, to produce partial or complete analgesia for painful procedures
Side effects (e.g., headache) possible from occupational exposure to high levels of nitrous oxide

Epidural or Intrathecal
Involves catheter placed into epidural, caudal, or intrathecal space for continuous infusion or single or intermittent administration of opioid with or without a long-acting local anesthetic (e.g., bupivacaine, ropivacaine)
Analgesia primarily from drug's direct effect on opioid receptors in spinal cord
Respiratory depression rare but may have slow and delayed onset; can be prevented by checking level of sedation and respiratory rate and depth hourly for initial 24 hours and decreasing dose when excessive sedation is detected
Nausea, itching, and urinary retention common dose-related side effects from the epidural opioid
Mild hypotension, urinary retention, and temporary motor or sensory deficits common unwanted effects of epidural local anesthetic
Catheter for urinary retention inserted during surgery to decrease trauma to child; if inserted when child is awake, anesthetize urethra with lidocaine

*For further information about compounding drugs in troche or suppository form, contact Professional Compounding Centers of America (PCCA), 9901 S. Wilcrest Drive, Houston, TX 77009; 800-331-2498; www.pccarx.com.
Data from Pasero, C., & McCaffrey, M. (2011). *Pain assessment and pharmacologic management.* St. Louis, MO: Elsevier.

conscious sedation is needed to provide analgesia before a scheduled procedure. When pain can be predicted, the drug's peak effect should be timed to coincide with the painful event. For example, with opioids the peak effect is approximately a half hour for the IV route; with nonopioids the peak effect occurs about 2 hours after oral administration. For rapid onset and peak of action, opioids that quickly penetrate the blood-brain barrier (e.g., IV fentanyl) provide excellent pain control.

Severe pain that is uncontrolled by large variations in plasma concentrations of opioids is best controlled through continuous IV infusion rather than intermittent boluses. If intermittent boluses are given, make certain the intervals between doses do not exceed the drug's expected duration of effectiveness. For extended pain control with fewer administration times, drugs that provide longer duration of action (e.g., some NSAIDs, time-released morphine or oxycodone, methadone) can be used.

Patient-Controlled Analgesia

A significant advance in the administration of IV, epidural, or subcutaneous analgesics is the use of patient-controlled analgesia (PCA). As the name implies, the patient controls the amount and frequency of the analgesic, which is typically delivered through a special infusion device. Children who are physically able to "push a button" (i.e., 5 to 6 years of age) and who can understand the concept of pushing a button to obtain pain relief can use PCA. Although it is controversial, parents and nurses have used the IV PCA system for the child. Nurses can

efficiently use the infusion device on a child of any age to administer analgesics to avoid signing for and preparing opioid injections every time one is needed (Fig. 30.7). When PCA is used as "nurse- or parent-controlled" analgesia, the concept of patient control is negated, and the inherent safety of PCA needs to be monitored. Research has reported safe and effective analgesia in children when the patient, parent, or nurse controlled the PCA (Oakes, 2011). The interprofessional care team works closely together to establish the most appropriate method for drug administration.

PCA infusion devices typically allow for three methods or modes of drug administration to be used alone or in combination:
1. Patient-administered boluses that can be infused only according to the preset amount and lockout interval (time between doses). More frequent attempts at self-administration may mean the patient needs the dose and time adjusted for better pain control.
2. Nurse-administered boluses that are typically used to give an initial loading dose to increase blood levels rapidly and to relieve breakthrough pain (pain not relieved with the usual programmed dose).
3. Continuous basal rate infusion that delivers a constant amount of analgesic and prevents pain from returning during those times, such as sleep, when the patient cannot control the infusion.

As with any type of analgesic management plan, continued assessment of the child's pain relief is essential for the greatest benefit from PCA. Typical uses of PCA are for controlling pain from surgery, sickle cell crisis, trauma, and cancer. Morphine is the drug of choice for PCA and

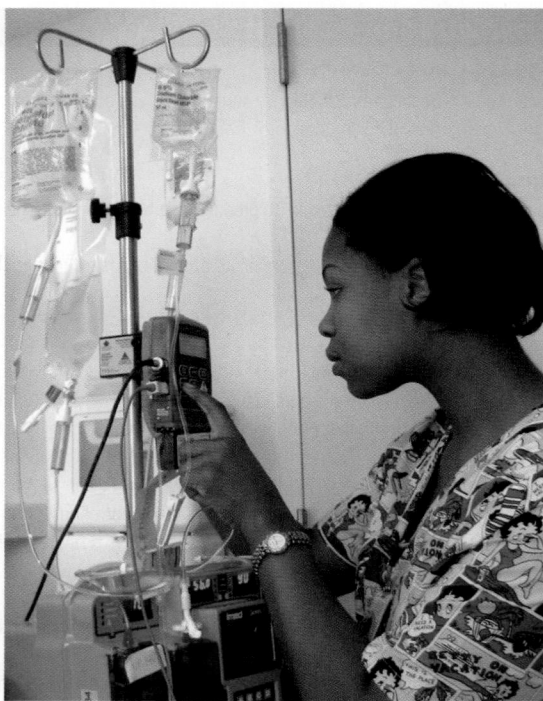

FIG 30.7 Nurse programming a patient-controlled analgesia (PCA) pump to administer analgesia.

TABLE 30.11	Initial Patient-Controlled Analgesia Settings for Opioid-Naïve Children	
Drug	**Continuous Infusion Dosage**	**Bolus Dosage/ Frequency**
Morphine	0–0.02 mg/kg/h	0.02 mg/kg q 15–30 min
Hydromorphone	0–0.004 mg/kg/h	0.004 mg/kg q 15–30 min
Fentanyl	0–0.5 to 1 mcg/kg/h	0.5–1 mcg/kg q 10–15 min

usually comes in a concentration of 1 mg/mL. Other options are hydromorphone (0.2 mg/mL) and fentanyl (0.01 mg/mL). Hydromorphone is often used when patients are not able to tolerate side effects, such as pruritus and nausea from the morphine PCA. Table 30.11 provides initial PCA settings for opioid-naïve children.

Epidural Analgesia

Epidural analgesia is used to manage pain in selected cases by the interprofessional care team. Although an epidural catheter can be inserted at any vertebral level, it is usually placed into the epidural space of the spinal column at the lumbar or caudal level (Suresh, Birmingham, & Kozlowski, 2012). The thoracic level is usually reserved for older children or adolescents who have had an upper-abdominal or thoracic procedure, such as a lung transplant. An opioid (usually fentanyl, hydromorphone, or preservative-free morphine, which is often combined with a long-acting local anesthetic, such as bupivacaine or ropivacaine) is instilled via single or intermittent bolus, continuous infusion, or patient-controlled epidural analgesia. Analgesia results from the drug's effect on opiate receptors in the dorsal horn of the spinal cord, rather than the brain. As a result, respiratory depression is rare, but if it occurs, it develops slowly, typically 6 to 8 hours after administration. Careful monitoring of sedation level and respiratory status is critical to prevent opioid-induced

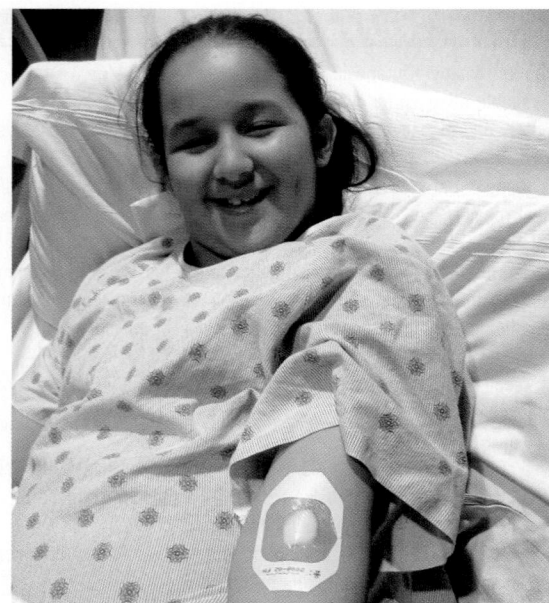

FIG 30.8 LMX (liposomal lidocaine cream) is an effective analgesic before intravenous (IV) insertion or blood draw.

respiratory depression. Assessment of pain and the skin condition around the catheter site are important aspects of nursing care.

Transmucosal and Transdermal Analgesia

Oral transmucosal fentanyl (Oralet) and intranasal fentanyl (Mudd, 2011) provides nontraumatic preoperative and preprocedural analgesia and sedation. Fentanyl is also available as a transdermal patch (Duragesic). Duragesic is contraindicated for acute pain management, but it may be used for older children and adolescents who have cancer pain or sickle cell pain or for patients who are opioid tolerant.

One of the most significant improvements in the ability to provide atraumatic care to children undergoing procedures is the anesthetic cream (Zempsky, 2014; Oakes, 2011). LMX4 (a 4% liposomal lidocaine cream) or EMLA (a eutectic mixture of local anesthetics) are the most well-studied topical anesthetics found to be effective in children. The EMLA (lidocaine 2.5% and prilocaine 2.5%), whose melting point is lower than that of the two anesthetics alone, permits effective concentrations of the drug to penetrate intact skin (Fig. 30.8). Transdermal patches, such as Synera (lidocaine and tetracaine), are effective methods to administer topical analgesia before painful procedures.

In emergency situations, there is not enough time for topical preparations like LMX or EMLA to take effect, and refrigerant sprays, such as ethyl chloride and fluoromethane can be used. When sprayed on the skin, these sprays vaporize, rapidly cool the area, and provide superficial anesthesia. Hospital formularies may have other products with lidocaine, prilocaine, or amethocaine topical preparations that require less time for application.

The intradermal route is sometimes used to inject a local anesthetic, typically lidocaine, into the skin to reduce the pain from a lumbar puncture, bone marrow aspiration, or venous or arterial access. One problem with the use of lidocaine is the stinging and burning that initially occur. However, the use of buffered lidocaine with sodium bicarbonate reduces the stinging sensation.

Monitoring Side Effects

Both NSAIDs and opioids have side effects, although the major concern is with those from opioids (Box 30.4). Respiratory depression is the

BOX 30.4 Side Effects of Opioids

General
Constipation (possibly severe)
Respiratory depression
Sedation
Nausea and vomiting
Agitation, euphoria
Mental clouding
Hallucinations
Orthostatic hypotension
Pruritus
Urticaria
Sweating
Miosis (may be sign of toxicity)
Anaphylaxis (rare)

Signs of Tolerance
Decreasing pain relief
Decreasing duration of pain relief

Signs of Withdrawal Syndrome in Patients With Physical Dependence
Initial Signs of Withdrawal
Lacrimation
Rhinorrhea
Yawning
Sweating

Later Signs of Withdrawal
Restlessness
Irritability
Tremors
Anorexia
Dilated pupils
Gooseflesh
Nausea, vomiting

GUIDELINES

Managing Opioid-Induced Respiratory Depression

If Respirations Are Depressed
Assess sedation level.
Reduce Infusion by 25% When Possible.
Stimulate patient (shake shoulder gently, call by name, ask to breathe).
Administer oxygen.

If Patient Cannot Be Aroused or Is Apneic
Initiate resuscitation efforts as appropriate.
Administer naloxone (Narcan):
- For children weighing less than 40 kg (88 lbs), dilute 0.1 mg naloxone in 10 mL sterile saline to make 10 mcg/mL solution, and give 0.5 mcg/kg.
- For children weighing more than 40 kg (88 lbs), dilute 0.4-mg ampule in 10 mL sterile saline and give 0.5 mL.

Administer bolus by slow intravenous (IV) push every 2 minutes until effect is obtained.
Closely monitor patient. Naloxone's duration of antagonist action may be shorter than that of the opioid, requiring repeated doses of naloxone.

Note: Respiratory depression caused by benzodiazepines (e.g., diazepam [Valium] or midazolam [Versed]) can be reversed with flumazenil (Romazicon). Pediatric dosing experience suggests 0.01 mg/kg (0.1 mL/kg); if no (or inadequate) response after 1 to 2 minutes, administer same dose and repeat as needed at 60-second intervals for maximum dose of 1 mg (10 mL).

COMMUNITY FOCUS
Fear of Opioid Addiction

One of the reasons for the unfounded but prevalent fear of addiction from opioids used to relieve pain is a misunderstanding of the differences between physical dependence, tolerance, and addiction. Health care professionals and the community often confuse addiction with the physiologic effects of opioids, when in reality these three events are unrelated.

The American Society of Addiction Medicine defines these three terms as follows:
- **Physical dependence** on an opioid is a physiologic state in which abrupt cessation of the opioid, or administration of an opioid antagonist, results in a withdrawal syndrome. Physical dependence on opioids is an expected occurrence in all individuals who continuously use opioids for therapeutic or nontherapeutic purposes. It does not, in and of itself, imply addiction.
- **Tolerance** is a form of neuroadaptation to the effects of chronically administered opioids (or other medications) that is indicated by the need for increasing or more frequent doses of the medication to achieve the initial effects of the drug. A person may develop tolerance both to the analgesic effects of opioids and to some of the unwanted side effects, such as respiratory depression, sedation, or nausea. Tolerance is variable in occurrence, but it does not, in and of itself, imply addiction.
- **Addiction** in the context of pain treatment with opioids is characterized by a persistent pattern of dysfunctional opioid use that may involve any or all of the following:
  - Adverse consequences associated with the use of opioids
  - Loss of control over the use of opioids
  - Preoccupation with obtaining opioids, despite the presence of adequate analgesia

Unfortunately, individuals who have severe, unrelieved pain may become intensely focused on finding relief. Sometimes behaviors such as "clock watching" make patients appear to others to be preoccupied with obtaining opioids. However, this preoccupation focuses on finding relief of pain, not on using opioids for reasons other than pain control. This phenomenon has been termed *pseudoaddiction* and must not be confused with real addiction.

Nurses must educate older children, parents, and health care professionals about the extremely low risk for real addiction (>1%) from the use of opioids to treat pain. Infants, young children, and comatose or terminally ill children simply cannot become addicted because they are incapable of a consistent pattern of drug-seeking behavior, such as stealing, drug dealing, prostitution, and use of family income, to obtain opioids for nonanalgesic reasons.

Data from American Society of Addiction Medicine. (2001). *Public policy statement: Definitions related to the use of opioids for pain treatment.* Retrieved from http://www.asam.org and http://www.asam.org/public-resources/pain-and-addiction).

most serious complication and is most likely to occur in sedated patients. The respiratory rate may decrease gradually, or respirations may cease abruptly; lower limits of normal are not established for children, but any significant change from a previous rate calls for increased vigilance. A slower respiratory rate does not necessarily reflect decreased arterial oxygenation; an increased depth of ventilation may compensate for the altered rate. If respiratory depression or arrest occurs, be prepared to intervene quickly (see Guidelines box: Managing Opioid-Induced Respiratory Depression).

Although respiratory depression is the most dangerous side effect, constipation is a common, and sometimes serious, side effect of opioids,

which decrease peristalsis and increase anal sphincter tone. Prevention with stool softeners and laxatives is more effective than treatment once constipation occurs. Dietary treatment, such as increased fiber, is usually not sufficient to promote regular bowel evacuation. However, dietary measures, such as increased fluid and fruit intake, and physical activity are encouraged. Pruritus from epidural or IV infusion is treated with low doses of IV naloxone, nalbuphine, or diphenhydramine. Nausea, vomiting, and sedation usually subside after 2 days of opioid administration, although oral or rectal antiemetics are sometimes necessary.

Both tolerance and physical dependence can occur with prolonged use of opioids (see Community Focus box: Fear of Opioid Addiction). Physical dependence is a normal, natural, physiologic state of "neuroadaptation." When opioids are abruptly discontinued without weaning, withdrawal symptoms occur 24 hours later and reach a peak within 72 hours. Symptoms of withdrawal include signs of neurologic excitability (irritability, tremors, seizures, increased motor tone, insomnia), gastrointestinal dysfunction (nausea, vomiting, diarrhea, abdominal cramps), and autonomic dysfunction (sweating, fever, chills, tachypnea, nasal congestion, rhinitis). Withdrawal symptoms can be anticipated and prevented by weaning patients from opioids that were administered for more than 5 to 10 days. Adherence to a weaning protocol to prevent or minimize withdrawal symptoms from opioids is required.

Tolerance occurs when the dose of an opioid needs to be increased to achieve the same analgesic effect that was previously achieved at a lower dose (see Community Focus box: Fear of Opioid Addiction). Tolerance may develop after 10 to 21 days of morphine administration. Treatment of tolerance involves increasing the dose or decreasing the duration between doses.

Parents and older children may fear addiction when opioids are prescribed. The nurse should address these concerns with assurance that any such risk is extremely low. It may be helpful to ask the question, "If you did not have this pain, would you want to take this medicine?" The answer is invariably no, which reinforces the solely therapeutic nature of the drug. It is also important to avoid making statements to the family, such as "We don't want you to get used to this medicine," or "By now you shouldn't need this medicine," which may reinforce the fear of becoming addicted. Whereas both physical dependence and tolerance are physiologic states, addiction or psychologic dependence is a psychologic state and implies a "cause-effect" mode of thinking, such as "I need the drug because it makes me feel better." Infants and children do not have the cognitive ability to make the cause-effect association and therefore cannot become addicted. The use of opioid analgesics early in life has not been demonstrated to increase the risk for addiction later in life. Nurses need to explain to parents the differences among physical dependence, tolerance, and addiction and allow them to express concerns about the use and duration of use of opioids. Infants and children, when treated appropriately with opioids, may be at risk for physical tolerance and physical dependence but not psychologic dependence or addiction.

Decreasing opioids in children requires a systematic approach. For children on opioids for less than 5 days, decrease the opioid dose by 20% to 30% every 1 to 2 days (Oakes, 2011). For children who have been on opioids for longer than 5 to 7 days, a slower weaning is recommended: Wean by a 20% reduction on the first day, follow with opioid reductions of 5% to 10% each day as tolerated until a total daily dose of morphine (or its equivalent) of 30 mg for an adolescent or a dose of 0.6 mg/kg/day is reached (Oakes, 2011).

CONSEQUENCES OF UNTREATED PAIN IN INFANTS

Despite current research on the neonate's experience of pain, infant pain often remains inadequately managed. The mismanagement of infant pain is partially the result of misconceptions regarding the effects of pain on the neonate and the lack of knowledge of immediate and long-term consequences of untreated pain. Infants respond to noxious stimuli through physiologic indicators (increased heart rate and blood pressure, variability in heart rate and intracranial pressure, and decreases in arterial oxygen saturation [SaO_2] and skin blood flow) and behavioral indicators (muscle rigidity, facial expression, crying, withdrawal, and sleeplessness) (Clark, 2011; Oakes, 2011). The physiologic and behavioral changes, as well as a variety of neurophysiologic responses to noxious stimulation, are responsible for acute and long-term consequences of pain.

BOX 30.5 Consequences of Untreated Pain in Infants

Acute Consequences
Periventricular-intraventricular hemorrhage
Increased chemical and hormone release
Breakdown of fat and carbohydrate stores
Prolonged hyperglycemia
Higher morbidity for neonatal intensive care unit patients
Memory of painful events
Hypersensitivity to pain
Prolonged response to pain
Inappropriate innervation of the spinal cord
Inappropriate response to nonnoxious stimuli
Lower pain threshold

Potential Long-Term Consequences
Higher somatic complaints of unknown origin
Greater physiologic and behavioral responses to pain
Increased prevalence of neurologic deficits
Psychosocial problems
Neurobehavioral disorders
Cognitive deficits
Learning disorders
Poor motor performance
Behavioral problems
Attention deficits
Poor adaptive behavior
Inability to cope with novel situations
Problems with impulsivity and social control
Learning deficits
Emotional temperament changes in infancy or childhood
Accentuated hormonal stress responses in adult life

Several harmful effects occur with unrelieved pain, particularly when pain is prolonged. Pain triggers a number of physiologic stress responses in the body, and they lead to negative consequences that involve multiple systems. Unrelieved pain may prolong the stress response and adversely affect an infant or child's recovery, whether it is from trauma, surgery, or disease.

Poorly controlled acute pain can predispose patients to chronic pain syndromes. Box 30.5 provides a list of numerous complications of untreated pain in infants. A guiding principle in pain management is that prevention of pain is always better than treatment. Pain that is established and severe is often more difficult to control. When pain is unrelieved, sensory input from injured tissues reaches spinal cord neurons and may enhance subsequent responses. Long-lasting changes in cells within spinal cord pain pathways may occur after a brief painful stimulus and may lead to the development of chronic pain conditions.

An experience known as the *windup phenomenon* has been attributed to a decreased pain threshold and chronic pain. Central and peripheral mechanisms that occur in response to noxious tissue injury have been studied in an attempt to explain a prolonged neonatal response to pain characteristic of the windup phenomenon. After exposure to noxious stimuli, multiple levels of the spinal cord experience an altered excitability. This altered excitability may cause nonnoxious stimuli, such as routine nursing care and handling, to be perceived as noxious stimuli. Nurses who care for infants and children should consider the potential acute and long-term effects of pain on their young patients and be advocates in treating and preventing pain.

TABLE 30.12 Local Anesthetics Given by Systems Without Needles

Agents	Time for Effective Analgesia	Concerns
EMLA (eutectic mixture of local anesthetics) (2.5% lidocaine and 2.5% prilocaine)	60–90 min	Use with caution for young infants (<3 months of age) because of possible methemoglobinemia related to metabolism of prilocaine Not effective for heel lancing or finger sticks Vasoconstriction decreases vein visibility May be applied by parent
LMX4 (4% liposomal lidocaine cream)	30 min	Available over the counter May be applied by parent
Synera (lidocaine [70 mg] and tetracaine [70 mg])	20–30 min	Not approved for parent application
Needle-free lidocaine injection device (J-tip) (1% buffered lidocaine)	1 min	Creates a disconcerting "pop" when activated Local hyperemia and minor bleeding Not approved for parent application

Adapted from Oakes, L.L. (2011). *Infant and child pain management*, New York, NY: Springer Publishing; Pasero, C., & McCaffrey, M. (2011). *Pain assessment and pharmacologic management*. St. Louis, MO: Elsevier.

COMMON PAIN STATES IN CHILDREN

PAINFUL AND INVASIVE PROCEDURES

Procedures that infants and children must experience as part of routine medical care often cause pain and distress. For example, infants and children experience a substantial amount of pain due to routine immunizations.

Combining pharmacologic and nonpharmacologic interventions provides the best approach for reducing pain. Local anesthetic administration is crucial to minimize pain from the procedure and is discussed in the "Transmucosal and Transdermal Analgesia" section earlier in this chapter. Common systems that do not require needles for providing local analgesics are found in Table 30.12.

Procedural Sedation and Analgesia

Severe pain associated with invasive procedures and anxiety associated with diagnostic imaging can be managed with sedation and analgesia. Sedation involves a wide range of levels of consciousness (Box 30.6). A thorough patient assessment including the child's history is essential before procedural sedation.

Key components to include in the patient history include the following:

- Past medical history: Major illnesses, such as asthma, psychiatric disorders, cardiac disease, hepatic or renal impairment; previous hospitalizations or surgeries; history of previous anesthesia or sedation
- Allergies: Opiates, benzodiazepines, barbiturates, local anesthetics, or others
- Current medications: Cardiovascular medications, central nervous system depressants; use caution with chronic benzodiazepine and

BOX 30.6 Levels of Sedation

Minimal Sedation (Anxiolysis)
Patient responds to verbal commands.
Cognitive function may be impaired.
Respiratory and cardiovascular systems are unaffected.

Moderate Sedation (Previously Conscious Sedation)
Patient responds to verbal commands but may not respond to light tactile stimulation.
Cognitive function is impaired.
Respiratory function is adequate; cardiovascular system is unaffected.

Deep Sedation
Patient cannot be easily aroused except with repeated or painful stimuli.
Ability to maintain airway may be impaired.
Spontaneous ventilation may be impaired; cardiovascular function is maintained.

General Anesthesia
Loss of consciousness, patient cannot be aroused with painful stimuli.
Airway cannot be maintained adequately, and ventilation is impaired.
Cardiovascular function may be impaired.

From Meredith, J.R., O'Keefe, K.P., & Galwankar, S. (2008). Pediatric procedural sedation and analgesia. *Journal of Emergencies, Trauma and Shock, 1*(2), 88–96.

opiate users; administration of reversal agents may induce withdrawal or seizures
- Drug use: Narcotics, benzodiazepines, barbiturates, cocaine, and alcohol
- Last oral intake: For nonemergent cases, some guidelines recommend more than 6 hours for solid food and more than 2 hours for clear liquid
- Volume status: Vomiting, diarrhea, fluid restriction, urinary output, making tears

A physical status evaluation using the American Society of Anesthesiologists Physical Status Classification (Meredith, O'Keefe, & Galwankar, 2008) is documented before administering analgesia and sedation:

- Class I: A normally healthy patient
- Class II: A patient with mild systemic disease
- Class III: A patient with severe systemic disease
- Class IV: A patient with severe systemic disease that is a constant threat to life
- Class V: A moribund patient who is not expected to survive without the operation

To provide a safe environment for procedural sedation and analgesia (PSA), equipment should be readily available to prevent or manage adverse events and complications (Box 30.7). The patient should have an IV access for titration of sedation and analgesic medications and for administration of possible antagonists and fluids. Trained personnel who are members of the interprofessional care team, (physician, registered nurse, respiratory therapist) whose sole responsibility is to monitor the patient (rather than performing or assisting with the procedure) should be present to monitor for adverse events and complications.

POSTOPERATIVE PAIN

Surgery and traumatic injuries (fractures, dislocations, strains, sprains, lacerations, burns) generate a catabolic state as a result of increased secretion of catabolic hormones and lead to alterations in blood flow,

- High-flow oxygen and delivery method
- Airway management materials: endotracheal tubes, bag valve masks, and laryngoscopes
- Pulse oximetry, blood pressure monitor, electrocardiography,* capnography*
- Suction and large-bore catheters
- Vascular access supplies
- Resuscitation drugs, intravenous (IV) fluids
- Reversal agents, including flumazenil and naloxone

*May be optional devices.

coagulation, fibrinolysis, substrate metabolism, and water and electrolyte balance and increase the demands on the cardiovascular and respiratory systems. The major endocrine and metabolic changes occur during the first 48 hours after surgery or trauma. Local anesthetics and opioid neural blockade may effectively mitigate the physiologic responses to surgical injury.

Pain associated with surgery to the chest (e.g., repair of congenital heart defects, chest trauma) or abdominal regions (e.g., appendectomy, cholecystectomy, splenectomy) may result in pulmonary complications. Pain leads to decreased muscle movement in the thorax and abdominal area and leads to decreased tidal volume, vital capacity, functional residual capacity, and alveolar ventilation. The patient is unable to cough and clear secretions, and the risk for complications (such as, pneumonia and atelectasis) is high. Severe postoperative pain also results in sympathetic overactivity that leads to increases in heart rate, peripheral resistance, blood pressure, and cardiac output. The patient eventually experiences an increase in cardiac demand and myocardial oxygen consumption and a decrease in oxygen delivery to the tissues.

The basis for good postoperative pain control in children is preemptive analgesia (Michelet, Andreu-Gallien, Bensalah, et al., 2012). Preemptive analgesia involves administration of medications (e.g., local and regional anesthetics, analgesics) before the child experiences the pain or before surgery is performed so that the sensory activation and changes in the pain pathways of the peripheral and central nervous system can be controlled. Preemptive analgesia lowers postoperative pain, lowers analgesic requirement, lowers hospital stay, lowers complications after surgery, and minimizes the risks for peripheral and central nervous system sensitization that can lead to persistent pain.

A combination of medications (multimodal or balanced analgesia) is used for postoperative pain and may include NSAIDs, local anesthetics, nonopioids, and opioid analgesics to achieve optimum relief and minimize side effects. Opioids (see Tables 5.5 to 5.7) administered ATC during the first 48 hours or administered via PCA are commonly prescribed (see Table 30.8). Perioperative NSAID administration is shown to reduce opioid consumption and postoperative nausea and vomiting in children (Michelet, Andreu-Gallien, Bensalah, et al., 2012). Scheduled acetaminophen is supported as the preferred medication in children after tonsillectomy; codeine is not recommended because of the risk for children who may be ultra-rapid metabolizers due to abnormal function of the CYP2D6 enzyme (Yellon, Kenna, Cladis, et al., 2014).

The combination of the IV NSAID ketorolac and morphine using a PCA device is frequently prescribed after thoracic surgery. Morphine delivered by PCA leads to a lower total dosage of opioid analgesia when compared with the administration of intermittent doses of analgesic as required. After bowel surgery, a mixture of a local anesthetic (bupivacaine) and a low-dose opioid (fentanyl) delivered by epidural route

improves the rate of recovery and minimizes the gastrointestinal effects (e.g., bowel stasis, nausea, vomiting). Once bowel function has been restored, oral opioids (e.g., immediate-release and controlled-release preparations) are preferred in older children. Controlled-release opioids facilitate ATC dosing and improve sleep. They are also associated with a lower incidence of nausea, sedation, and breakthrough pain.

BURN PAIN

Because burn pain has multiple components, involves repeated manipulations over the injured painful sites, and has changing patterns over time, it is difficult and challenging to control. Burn pain includes a constant background pain that is felt at the wound sites and surrounding areas. Burn pain is exacerbated (breakthrough pain) by movements, such as changing position, turning in bed, walking, or even breathing. Areas of normal skin that have been harvested for skin grafts (donor sites) also are painful. Pain is commonly experienced with intense tingling or itching sensations when skin grafting is required. During the healing process, when the tissue and nerve regenerate, the necrotic tissue (eschar) is excised until viable tissue is reached. The healing process may last for months to years. Pain or paresthetic sensations (itching, tingling, cold sensations, and so on) may persist. In addition, discomfort may be associated with immobilization of limbs in splints or garments, as well as multiple surgical interventions such as skin grafting and reconstructive surgery.

Multiple therapeutic procedures are carried out during the course of treatment. These procedures (dressing changes, wound débridement and cleansing, physical therapy sessions) occur daily or even several times per day (see Chapter 47). Providing proper analgesia without interfering with the patient's awareness during and after the procedure is the biggest challenge in the management of burn pain. Fentanyl or alfentanil has a major advantage over morphine because of the short duration. Fentanyl can prevent oversedation after the procedure. For less painful procedures, premedication with oral morphine, oral ketamine, or milder opioids 15 minutes before the procedure may be sufficient. Depending on the patient's anxiety level, a benzodiazepine (e.g., lorazepam) before the procedure may be beneficial. For longer procedures, morphine is the mainstay of treatment. Some patients may require moderate to deep sedation and analgesia. Oral oxycodone with midazolam and acetaminophen, in addition to nitrous oxide, may be needed. IV ketamine administered at subtherapeutic doses has been one of the most extensively used anesthetics for burn patients. The dysphoria and unpleasant reactions associated with ketamine administration may be minimized with premedication with a benzodiazepine. If ketamine is used with either morphine or fentanyl, the regimen could have opioid-sparing actions and reduce the opioid-related side effects.

Psychologic interventions are helpful in the treatment of burn pain. These interventions include hypnosis, relaxation training (breathing exercises, progressive muscle relaxation), biofeedback, stress inoculation training, cognitive-behavioral strategies (guided imagery, distraction, coping skills), and group and individual psychotherapy. They can be used alone or in combination. All these techniques can help the patient relax and maintain a sense of control. A major disadvantage of these interventions is they require time and discipline and often patients are too stressed, fatigued, disoriented, or sick to engage in them.

RECURRENT HEADACHES IN CHILDREN

Recurrent headaches in children can be caused by several factors, including tension, dental braces, imbalance or weakness of eye muscles causing deviation in alignment and refractive errors, sequelae to accidents, sinusitis and other cranial infection or inflammation, increased intracranial pressure, epileptic attacks, drugs, obstructive sleep apnea, and, rarely, hypertension (see Chapter 35). Other causes may include arteriovenous malformations, disturbances in cerebrospinal fluid flow or absorption, intracranial hemorrhages, ocular and dental diseases, bacterial infections, and brain tumors.

Severe pain is the most disturbing symptom in migraine. Tension-type headache is usually mild or moderate, often producing a pressing feeling in the temples, like a "tight band around the head." Continuous, daily, or near-daily headache with no specific cause occurs in a small subgroup of children. In epilepsy, headaches commonly occur immediately before, during, or after a seizure attack.

Treatment of recurrent headaches requires an understanding of the antecedents and consequences of headache pain. A headache diary can allow the child to record the time of onset, activities before the onset, any worries or concerns as far back as 24 hours before the onset, severity and duration of pain, pain medications taken, and activity pattern during headache episodes. The headache diary allows ongoing monitoring of headache activity, indicates the effects of interventions, and guides treatment planning.

Headache management involves two main behavioral approaches: (1) teaching patients self-control skills to prevent headache (biofeedback techniques and relaxation training), and (2) modifying behavior patterns that increase the risk for headache occurrence or reinforce headache activity (cognitive-behavioral stress management techniques). Families may be able to identify factors that trigger the headache and avoid the triggers in the future. Biofeedback is a technology-based form of relaxation therapy and can be useful in assessing and reinforcing learning of relaxation skills, such as progressive muscle relaxation, deep breathing, and imagery. Children as young as 7 years of age are able to learn these skills and with 2 to 3 weeks of practice are able to decrease the time needed to achieve relaxation.

To modify behavior patterns that increase the risk for headache or reinforce headache activity, the nurse instructs parents to avoid giving excessive attention to their child's headache and to respond matter-of-factly to pain behavior and requests for special attention. Parents learn to assess whether the child is avoiding school or social performance demands because of headache. Parents are taught to focus attention on adaptive coping, such as the use of relaxation techniques and maintenance of normal activity patterns. When using cognitive-behavioral stress management techniques, the parents identify negative thoughts and situations that may be associated with increased risk for headache. The parent teaches the child to activate positive thoughts and engage in adaptive behavior appropriate to the situation.

RECURRENT ABDOMINAL PAIN IN CHILDREN

RAP or functional abdominal pain is defined as pain that occurs at least once per month for 3 consecutive months, accompanied by pain-free periods, and is severe enough that it interferes with a child's normal activities (see Chapter 34). Management of RAP is highly individualized to reflect the causes of the pain and the psychosocial needs of the child and family. A clear understanding of the child's characteristics (anxiety, physical health, temperament, coping skills, experience, learned response, depression), child's disability (school attendance, activities with family, social interactions, pain behaviors), environmental factors (family attitudes and behavioral patterns, school environment, community, friendships), and the pain stimulus (disease, injury, stress) is important in planning management strategies (Oakes, 2011).

Before any workup of the pain, the nurse informs the family that RAP is common in children and only 10% of children with RAP have an identifiable organic cause for their pain symptom. Medical workup is dictated by the child's symptoms and signs in combination with knowledge about common organic causes of RAP. If an organic cause is found, it will be treated appropriately. Even if no organic cause is found, the nurse needs to communicate to the child and family a belief that the pain is real. Usually the abdominal pain goes away, but even if problems are identified, they may not be the actual cause, and pain may persist, may be replaced by another symptom, or may go away on its own. The management plan includes regular follow-up at 3- to 4-month intervals, a list of symptoms that call for earlier contact, and biobehavioral pain management techniques. The goal is to minimize the impact of the pain on the child's activities and the family's life.

The use of CBT has been documented to reduce or eliminate pain in children with RAP and highlights the involvement of parents in supporting their child's self-management behavior. Case reports have demonstrated the effectiveness of implementing a time-out procedure, token systems, and positive reinforcement based on operant theory treatment modalities. Stress management and cognitive-behavioral strategies have also been successful. Parent training in how to avoid positive reinforcement of sick behaviors and focus on rewarding healthy behaviors is important. Over the course of several sessions, parents are educated about RAP, how to distinguish between sick and well behaviors, a reward system for well behaviors, and the importance of reinforcing relaxation and coping skills taught to children for pain management. Treatment may consist of a varying number of sessions over 1 to 6 months and may include various components, such as monitoring symptoms, limiting parent attention, relaxation training, increasing dietary fiber, and requiring school attendance. No negative side effects of symptom substitution occurred with the interventions.

PAIN IN CHILDREN WITH SICKLE CELL DISEASE

A painful episode is the most frequent cause for emergency department visits and hospital admissions among children with sickle cell disease (see Chapter 43). The acute painful episode in sickle cell disease is the only pain syndrome in which opioids are considered the major therapy and are started in early childhood and continued throughout adult life. A source of frustration for patients and clinicians is that most current analgesic regimens are inadequate in controlling some of the most severe painful episodes. A multidisciplinary approach that involves both pharmacologic and nonpharmacologic modalities (cognitive-behavioral intervention, heat, massage, physical therapy) is needed but not often implemented. The goals of treatment of the acute episode may not be to take all the pain away, which is usually impossible, but to make the pain tolerable to the patient until the episode resolves and to increase function and patient participation in activities of daily living (Oakes, 2011).

Patients coming to an emergency department for acute painful episodes usually have exhausted all home care options or outpatient therapy. The nurse should ask patients what the usual medication, dosage, and side effects were in the past; the usual medication taken at home; and medication taken since the onset of present pain. The patient may be on long-term opioid therapy at home and therefore may have developed some degree of tolerance. A different potent opioid or a larger dose of the same medication may be indicated. Because mixed opioid-agonist-antagonists may precipitate withdrawal syndromes, avoid these if patients were taking long-term opioids at home. A "passport" card with patient information about the diagnosis, previous complications, suggested pain management regimen, and name and contact information of the primary hematologist is helpful for parents and facilitates management of pain in the emergency department.

The patient is admitted for inpatient management of severe pain if adequate relief is not achieved in the emergency department. For severe pain, IV administration with bolus dosing and continuous infusion using a PCA device may be necessary. Patients requiring more than 5 to 7 days of opioids should have tapering doses to avoid the physiologic symptoms of withdrawal (dysphoria, nasal congestion, diarrhea, nausea and vomiting, sweating, and seizures). Appropriate weaning of the PCA schedules start with reduction of the continuous infusion rate before discontinuation while the patient continues to use demand doses for analgesia. Morphine-equivalent equianalgesic conversions may be used to convert continuous infusion rates to equivalent oral analgesics (see Table 30.10). Doses of long-acting oral analgesics, such as sustained-release oral morphine, may also be used to replace continuous infusion dosing. The demand doses can be subsequently reduced if analgesia remains adequate.

Patients who are administered doses of opioids that are inadequate to relieve their pain or whose doses are not tapered after a course of treatment may develop iatrogenic pseudoaddiction, which resembles addiction. Pseudoaddiction or clock-watching behavior may be resolved by communicating with patients to ensure accurate assessment, involving them in decisions about their pain management, and administering adequate opioid doses.

CANCER PAIN IN CHILDREN

Pain in children with cancer is present before diagnosis and treatment and may resolve after initiation of anticancer therapy. However, treatment-related pain is common (Table 30.13). Pain may be related to an operation, mucositis, a phantom limb, or infection. Pain can also be related to chemotherapy and procedures, such as bone marrow aspiration, needle puncture, and lumbar puncture. Tumor-related pain frequently occurs when the child relapses or when tumors become resistant to treatment. Intractable pain may occur in patients with solid tumors that metastasize to the central or peripheral nervous system. In young adult survivors of childhood cancer, chronic pain conditions may develop, including complex regional pain syndrome of the lower extremity, phantom limb pain, avascular necrosis, mechanical pain related to bone that failed to unite after tumor resection, and postherpetic neuralgia.

Oral mucositis (ulceration of the oral cavity and throat) may occur in patients undergoing chemotherapy or radiotherapy and in patients undergoing bone marrow transplant. No present therapy adequately relieves the pain of these lesions. Antihistamines, local anesthetics, and opioids provide only temporary relief, may block taste perception, or may produce additional side effects, such as lethargy and constipation. Initial treatment includes single agents (saline, opioids, sodium bicarbonate, hydrogen peroxide, sucralfate suspension, clotrimazole, nystatin, viscous lidocaine, amphotericin B, dyclonine) or mouthwash mixtures using a combination of agents (lidocaine, diphenhydramine, Maalox or Mylanta, nystatin). The mucositis after bone marrow transplantation may be prolonged, continuously intense, exacerbated by mouth care and swallowing, or worse during waking hours. The patient may be unable to eat or swallow. Morphine administered as a continuous infusion

TABLE 30.13   Cancer Pain in Children

Type	Clinical Presentation	Causes
Bone Skull Vertebrae Pelvis and femur	Aching to sharp, severe pain generally more pronounced with movement; point tenderness common Skull: headaches, blurred vision Spine: tenderness over spinous process Extremities: pain associated with movement or lifting Pelvis and femur: pain associated with movement; pain with weight bearing and walking	Infiltration of bone Skeletal metastases: irritation and stretching of pain receptors in periosteum and endosteum Prostaglandins released from bone destruction
Neuropathic Peripheral Plexus Epidural Cord compression	Complaints of pain without any detectable tissue damage Abnormal or unpleasant sensations, generally described as tingling, burning, or stabbing Often a delay in onset Brief, shooting pain Increased intensity of pain with receptive stimuli	Nerve injury caused by tumor infiltration; can also be caused by injury from treatment (e.g., vincristine toxicity) Infiltration or compression of peripheral nerves Surgical interruption of nerves (phantom pain after amputation)
Visceral Soft tissue Tumors of bowel Retroperitoneum	Poorly localized Varies in intensity Pressure, deep or aching	Obstruction: bowel, urinary tract, biliary tract Mucosal ulceration Metabolic alteration Nociceptor activation, generally from distention or inflammation of visceral organs
Treatment Related Mucositis Infection Post–lumbar puncture headaches Radiation dermatitis Postsurgical	Difficulty swallowing, pain from lesions in oropharynx; may extend throughout entire gastrointestinal tract Infection may be localized pain from focused infection or generalized (i.e., tissue infection versus septicemia) Severe headache after lumbar puncture Skin inflammation causing redness and breakdown Pain related to tissue trauma secondary to surgery	Direct side effects of treatment for cancer: Chemotherapy Radiation Surgery

or delivered by PCA device may be required until mucositis is resolved (Hickman, Varadarajan, & Weisman, 2014).

Other treatment-related pain includes (1) abdominal pain after allogeneic bone marrow transplantation, which may be associated with acute graft-versus-host disease; (2) abdominal pain associated with typhlitis (infection of the cecum), which occurs when the patient is immunocompromised; (3) phantom sensations and phantom limb pain after an amputation; (4) peripheral neuropathy after administration of vincristine; and (5) medullary bone pain, which may be associated with administration of granulocyte colony-stimulating factor.

Survivors of childhood cancer describe vivid memories of their experience with repeated painful procedures during treatment. These procedures include needle puncture for IM chemotherapy (L-asparaginase), IV lines, port access, and blood draws, lumbar puncture, bone marrow aspiration and biopsy, removal of central venous catheters, and other invasive diagnostic procedures. Fear and anxiety related to these procedures may be minimized with parent and child preparation. The preparation starts with obtaining information from the parent about the child's coping styles, explaining the procedure, and enlisting their support, followed by an age-appropriate explanation to the child. CBT (guided imagery, relaxation, music therapy, hypnosis), conscious sedation, and general anesthesia have been effective in decreasing pain and distress during the procedure. Topical analgesics (cold sprays, EMLA, amethocaine gels), as discussed previously, are effective in providing analgesia before needle procedures.

Lumbar puncture for administration of chemotherapy (e.g., cytarabine, methotrexate) and collection of cerebrospinal fluid may lead to a leak at the puncture site and low intracranial pressure. Some children may experience postdural puncture headache, which may be treated by administering nonopioid analgesics and placing the patient in the supine position for 1 hour after the procedure. The pain related to bone marrow aspiration is due to the insertion of a large needle into the posterior iliac space and the unpleasant sensation experienced at the time of marrow aspiration.

If the patient is neutropenic (absolute neutrophil count <500/mm³), the antipyretic action of acetaminophen may mask a fever. In patients with thrombocytopenia (platelet count <50,000/mm³), who may be at risk for bleeding, NSAIDs are contraindicated. Morphine is the most widely used opioid for moderate to severe pain and may be administered via the oral (including sustained-release formulations, such as MS Contin), IV, subcutaneous, epidural, and intrathecal routes.

The most common clinical syndrome of neuropathic pain is painful peripheral neuropathy caused by chemotherapeutic agents, particularly vincristine and cisplatin, and rarely cytarabine (Hickman, Varadarajan, & Weisman, 2014). After withdrawal of the chemotherapy, the neuropathy may resolve over weeks to months, or it may persist even after withdrawal. Neuropathic pain is associated with at least one of the following: (1) pain that is described as electric or shocklike, stabbing, or burning; (2) signs of neurologic involvement (paralysis, neuralgia, pain hypersensitivity) other than those associated with the progression of the tumor; and (3) the location of the solid organ cancer consistent with neurologic damage that could give rise to neuropathic pain. An epidural or subarachnoid infusion may be initiated if the patient experiences dose-limiting side effects of opioids or if pain is resistant to opioids. Tricyclic antidepressants (amitriptyline, desipramine) and anticonvulsants (gabapentin, carbamazepine) have demonstrated effectiveness in neuropathic cancer pain.

PAIN AND SEDATION IN END-OF-LIFE CARE

Many patients at the end of life require doses of opioids that make them sedated but arousable as their disease progresses (cancer, human immunodeficiency virus, cystic fibrosis, neurodegenerative disease). Patients achieve comfort with a combination of opioids and adjuvant analgesics in most situations. Parents need reassurance that the opioids are treating pain but not causing the child's death and that the child's advancing disease is the cause of death.

A small group of patients have intolerable side effects or inadequate analgesia despite extremely aggressive use of medications to relieve pain and side effects. Continuous sedation may be a means of relieving suffering when there is no feasible or acceptable means of providing analgesia that preserves alertness. A continuing high-dose infusion of opioids along with sedation is prescribed to reduce the possibility that a child might experience unrelieved pain but be too sedated to report it. Sedation in these situations is widely regarded as providing comfort, not euthanasia. Clinicians and ethicists have a range of views regarding assisted suicide and euthanasia, but they all agree that no child or parent should choose death because of inadequate efforts to relieve pain and suffering.

REFERENCES

Ambuel, B., Hamlett, K. W., Marx, C. M., et al. (1992). Assessing distress in pediatric intensive care environments: The COMFORT scale. *Journal of Pediatric Psychology, 17*(1), 95–109.

Arnstein, P., Broglio, K., Wuhrman, E., et al. (2011). Use of placebos in pain management. *Pain Management Nursing, 12*(4), 225–229.

Azize, P. M., Humphreys, A., & Cattani, A. (2011). The impact of language on the expression and assessment of pain in children. *Intensive Critical Care Nursing, 27*(5), 235–243.

Babl, F. E., Crellin, D., Cheng, J., et al. (2012). The use of faces, legs, activity, cry and consolability scale to assess procedural pain and distress in young children. *Pediatric Emergency Care, 28*(12), 1281–1296.

Boerlage, A. A., Ista, E., Duivenvoorden, H. J., et al. (2015). The COMFORT behavior scale detects clinically meaningful effects of analgesic and sedative treatment. *European Journal of Pain, 19*(4), 473–479.

Breau, L. M., McGrath, P. J., Camfield, C. S., et al. (2002). Psychometric properties of the non-communicating children's pain checklist—Revised. *Pain, 99*(1-2), 349–357.

Claar, R. L., & Walker, L. S. (2006). Functional assessment of pediatric pain patients: Psychometric properties of the functional disability inventory. *Pain, 121*(1-2), 77–84.

Clark, L. (2011). Pain management in the pediatric population. *Critical Care Nursing Clinics of North America, 23*(2), 291–301.

Cline, M. E., Herman, J., Shaw, E. R., et al. (1992). Standardization of the visual analogue scale. *Nursing Research, 41*(6), 378–380.

Crosta, Q. R., Ward, T. M., Walker, A. J., et al. (2014). A review of pain measures for hospitalized children with cognitive impairment. *Journal for Specialists in Pediatric Nursing, 19*(2), 109–118.

de Jong, A. E., Tuinebreijer, W. E., Bremer, M., et al. (2012). Construct validity of two pain behavior observation measurement instruments for young children with burns by Rasch analysis. *Pain, 153*(11), 2260–2266.

Fernandes, A. M., De Campos, C., Batalha, L., et al. (2014). Pain assessment using the adolescent pediatric pain tool: A systematic review. *Pain Research and Management, 19*(4), 212–218.

Fortier, M. A., Wahi, A., Bruce, C., et al. (2014). Pain management at home in children with cancer: A daily diary study. *Pediatric Blood & Cancer, 61*(6), 1029–1033.

Franck, L. S., Ridout, D., Howard, R., et al. (2011). A comparison of pain measures in newborn infants after cardiac surgery. *Pain, 152*(8), 1758–1765.

Gaina, A., Sekine, M., Chen, X., et al. (2004). Validity of child sleep diary questionnaire among junior high school children. *Journal of Epidemiology, 14*(1), 1–4.

Garra, F., Singer, A. J., Domingo, A., et al. (2013). The Wong-Baker pain FACES scale measures pain, not fear. *Pediatric Emergency Care, 29*(1), 17–20.

Gold, J. I., Mahrer, N. E., Yee, J., et al. (2009). Pain, fatigue and health-related quality of life in children and adolescents with chronic pain. *Clinical Journal of Pain, 25*(5), 407–412.

Habich, M., Wilson, D., Thielk, D., et al. (2012). Evaluating the effectiveness of pediatric pain management guidelines. *Journal of Pediatric Nursing, 27*(4), 336–345.

Hatfield, L. A., & Ely, E. A. (2015). Measurement of acute pain in infants: A review of behavioural and physiological variables. *Biological Research for Nursing, 17*(1), 100–111.

Heath, J. A., Oh, L. J., Clarke, N. E., et al. (2012). Complementary and alternative medicine use in children with cancer at the end of life. *Journal of Palliative Medicine, 15*(11), 1218–1221.

Hershey, A. D., Powers, S. W., Vockell, A. L., et al. (2001). PedMIDAS: Development of a questionnaire to assess disability of migraines in children. *Neurology, 57*(11), 2034–2039.

Hershey, A. D., Powers, S. W., Vockell, A. L., et al. (2004). Development of a patient-based grading scale for PedMIDAS. *Cephalalgia: An International Journal of Headache, 24*(10), 844–849.

Hickman, J., Varadarajan, J., & Weisman, S. J. (2014). Paediatric cancer pain. In P. C. McGrath, B. J. Stevens, S. M. Walker, et al. (Eds.), *Oxford textbook of paediatric pain*. Oxford UK: Oxford University Press.

Hicks, C. L., von Baeyer, C. L., Spafford, P. A., et al. (2001). The Faces Pain Scale–Revised: Toward a common metric in pediatric pain measurement. *Pain, 93*(2), 173–183.

Hillman, B. A., Tabrizi, M. N., Gauda, E. B., et al. (2015). The neonatal pain, agitation and sedation scale and the bedside nurse's assessment of neonates. *Journal of Perinatology, 35*(2), 128–131.

Jordan-Marsh, M., Yoder, L., Hall, D., et al. (1994). Alternate Oucher form testing gender ethnicity and age variations. *Research in Nursing & Health, 17*(2), 111–118.

Kashikar-Zuck, S., Flowers, S. R., Claar, R. L., et al. (2011). Clinical utility and validity of the Functional Disability Inventory among a multicenter sample of youth with chronic pain. *Pain, 152*(7), 1600–1607.

Kozlowski, L. J., Kost-Byerly, S., Colantuoni, E., et al. (2014). Pain prevalence, intensity, assessment and management in a hospitalized pediatric population. *Pain Management Nursing, 15*(1), 22–35.

Krechel, S. W., & Bildner, J. (1995). CRIES: A new neonatal postoperative pain measurement score: Initial testing of validity and reliability. *Paediatric Anaesthesia, 5*(1), 53–61.

Lawrence, J., Alcock, D., McGrath, P., et al. (1993). The development of a tool to assess neonatal pain. *Neonatal Network, 12*(6), 59–66.

Logan, D. E., Coakley, R. M., & Garcia, B. N. B. (2014). Cognitive-behavioural interventions. In P. C. McGrath, B. J. Stevens, S. M. Walker, et al. (Eds.), *Oxford textbook of paediatric pain*. Oxford UK: Oxford University Press.

Lootens, C. C., & Rapoff, M. A. (2011). Measures of pediatric pain: 21-numbered circle visual analog scale (VAS), E-Ouch electronic pain diary, oucher, pain behavior observation method, pediatric pain assessment tool (PPAT), and pediatric pain questionnaire (PPQ). *Arthritis Care & Research, 63*(11 suppl), S253–S262.

Luffy, R., & Grove, S. K. (2003). Examining the validity, reliability, and preference of three pediatric pain measurement tools in African-American children. *Pediatric Nursing, 29*(1), 54–60.

Massaro, M., Ronfani, L., Ferrara, G., et al. (2014). A comparison of three scales for measuring pain in children with cognitive impairment. *Acta Paediatrica, 103*(11), e495–e500.

McGrath, P. J., Walco, G. A., Turk, D. C., et al. (2008). Core outcome domains and measures for pediatric acute and chronic/recurrent pain clinical trials: PedIMMPACT recommendations. *Journal of Pain, 9*(9), 771–783.

Meek, J., & Huertas, A. (2012). Cochrane review: Non-nutritive sucking, kangaroo care and swaddling/facilitated tucking are observed to reduce procedural pain in infants and young children. *Evidence-Based Nursing, 15*(3), 84–85.

Melzack, R. (1975). The McGill pain questionnaire: Major properties and scoring methods. *Pain, 1*(3), 277–299.

Meredith, J. R., O'Keefe, K. P., & Galwankar, S. (2008). Pediatric procedural sedation and analgesia. *Journal of Emergencies, Trauma, and Shock, 1*(2), 88–96.

Merkel, S. I., Voepel-Lewis, T., Shayevitz, J. R., et al. (1997). The FLACC: A behavioral scale for scoring postoperative pain in young children. *Pediatric Nursing, 23*(3), 293–297.

Michelet, D., Andreu-Gallien, J., Bensalah, T., et al. (2012). A meta-analysis of the use of nonsteroidal antiinflammatory drugs for pediatric postoperative pain. *Anesthesia & Analgesia, 114*(2), 393–406.

Mudd, S. (2011). Intranasal fentanyl for pain management in children: A systematic review of the literature. *Journal of Pediatric Health Care, 25*(5), 316–322.

Myers, C., Stuber, M. L., Bonamer-Rheingans, J. I., et al. (2005). Complementary therapies and childhood cancer. *Cancer Control: Journal of the Moffitt Cancer Center, 12*(3), 172–180.

Oakes, L. L. (2011). *Infant and child pain management*. New York: Springer.

Pasero, C., & McCaffrey, M. (2011). *Pain assessment and pharmacologic management*. St Louis: Elsevier.

Pillai Riddell, R., Racine, N., Turcotte, K., et al. (2011). Nonpharmacological management of procedural pain in infants and young children: An abridged Cochrane review. *Pain Research and Management, 16*(5), 321–330.

Puchalski, M., & Hummel, P. (2002). The reality of neonatal pain. *Advances in Neonatal Care, 2*(5), 233–244.

Quinn, B. L., Sheldon, L. K., & Cooley, M. E. (2014). Pediatric pain assessment by drawn faces scales: A review. *Pain Management Nursing, 15*(4), 909–918.

Racoosin, J. A., Roberson, D. W., Pacanowski, M. A., et al. (2013). New evidence about an old drug—Risk with codeine after adenotonsillectomy. *New England Journal of Medicine, 368*(23), 2155–2157.

Rastogi, S., & Campbell, F. (2014). Drugs for neuropathic pain. In P. C. McGrath, B. J. Stevens, S. M. Walker, et al. (Eds.), *Oxford textbook of paediatric pain*. Oxford UK: Oxford University Press.

Savedra, M. C., Holzemer, W. L., Tesler, M. D., et al. (1993). Assessment of postoperation pain in children and adolescents using the adolescent pediatric pain tool. *Nursing Research, 42*(1), 5–9.

Savedra, M. C., Tesler, M. D., Holzemer, W. L., et al. (1989). Pain location: Validity and reliability of body outline markings by hospitalized children and adolescents. *Research in Nursing & Health, 12*(5), 307–314.

Sneddon, P., Peacock, G. G., & Crowley, S. L. (2013). Assessment of sleep problems in preschool aged children: An adaptation of the children's sleep habits questionnaire. *Behavioral Sleep Medicine, 11*(4), 283–296.

Stevens, B. J., Gibbins, S., Yamada, J., et al. (2014). The premature infant pain profile-revised (PIPP-R): Initial validation and feasibility. *Clinical Journal of Pain, 30*(3), 238–243.

Stevens, B., Johnston, C., Petryshen, P., et al. (1996). Premature Infant Pain Profile: Development and initial validation. *Clinical Journal of Pain, 12*(1), 13–22.

Stinson, J. N., Stevens, B. J., Feldman, B. M., et al. (2008). Construct validity of a multidimensional electronic pain diary for adolescents with arthritis. *Pain, 136*(3), 281–292.

Suresh, S., Birmingham, P. K., & Kozlowski, R. J. (2012). Pediatric pain management. *Anesthesiology Clinics, 30*(1), 101–117.

Sweet, S., & McGrath, P. (1998). Physiological measures of pain. In G. A. Finley & P. J. McGrath (Eds.), *Measurement of pain in infants and children*. Seattle: IASP Press.

Tesler, M. D., Savedra, M. C., Holzemer, W. L., et al. (1991). The word-graphic rating scale as a measure of children's and adolescents' pain intensity. *Research in Nursing & Health, 14*(5), 361–371.

Tobias, J. D. (2014a). Acute pain management in infants and children-Part 1: Pain pathways, pain assessment, and outpatient pain management. *Pediatric Annals, 43*(7), e163–e168.

Tobias, J. D. (2014b). Acute pain management in infants and children—Part 2: Intravenous opioids, intravenous nonsteroidal anti-inflammatory drugs, and managing adverse effects. *Pediatric Annals, 43*(7), e169–e175.

Twycross, A. (2010). Managing pain in children: Where to from here? *Journal of Clinical Nursing, 19*(15-16), 2090–2099.

Uman, L. S., Birnie, K. A., Noel, M., et al. (2013). Psychological interventions for needle-related procedural pain and distress in children and adolescents. *Cochrane Database of Systematic Reviews, (10)*, CD005179.

Valrie, C. R., Bromberg, M. H., Palermo, T., et al. (2013). A systematic review of sleep in pediatric pain populations. *Journal of Developmental and Behavioral Pediatrics, 34*(2), 120–128.

Varni, J. W., Seid, M., & Rode, C. A. (1999). The PedsQL: Measurement model for the pediatric quality of life inventory. *Medical Care, 37*(2), 126–139.

Villarruel, A. M., & Denyes, M. J. (1991). Pain assessment in children: Theoretical and empirical validity. *Advances in Nursing Science, 14*(2), 32–41.

Voepel-Lewis, T., Malviya, S., Tait, A. R., et al. (2008). A comparison of the clinical utility of pain assessment tools for children with cognitive impairment. *Anesthesia & Analgesia, 106*(1), 72–78.

von Baeyer, C. L., Lin, V., Seidman, L. C., et al. (2011). Pain charts (body maps or manikins) in assessment of the location of pediatric pain. *Pain Management, 1*(1), 61–68.

Walker, L. S., & Greene, J. W. (1991). The functional disability inventory: Measuring a neglected dimension of child health status. *Journal of Pediatric Psychology, 16*(1), 39–58.

Wong, D. L., & Baker, C. M. (1988). Pain in children: Comparison of assessment scales. *Pediatric Nursing, 14*(1), 9–17.

World Health Organization. (2012). *WHO guidelines on the pharmacological treatment of persisting pain in children with medical illnesses.* Geneva: World Health Organization.

Yellon, R. F., Kenna, M. A., Cladis, F. P., et al. (2014). What is the best non-codeine post adenotonsilectomy pain management for children? *The Laryngoscope, 124*(8), 1737–1738.

Zempsky, W. T. (2014). Topical anesthetics and analgesics. In P. C. McGrath, B. J. Stevens, S. M. Walker, et al. (Eds.), *Oxford textbook of paediatric pain.* Oxford UK: Oxford University Press.

31

The Infant and Family

Cheryl C. Rodgers

e http://evolve.elsevier.com/Perry/maternal

PROMOTING OPTIMAL GROWTH AND DEVELOPMENT

BIOLOGIC DEVELOPMENT

At no other time in life are physical changes and developmental achievements as dramatic as during infancy. All major body systems undergo progressive maturation, and there is concurrent development of skills that increasingly allow infants to respond to and cope with the environment. Acquisition of these fine and gross motor skills occurs in an orderly head-to-toe and center-to-periphery (cephalocaudal and proximodistal) sequence.

Proportional Changes

Growth is very rapid during the first year, especially the initial 6 months. Infants gain 150 to 210 g (5 to 7 oz) weekly until approximately 5 to 6 months of age, when the birth weight has at least doubled. An average weight for a 6-month-old child is 7.3 kg (16 pounds). Weight gain slows during the second 6 months. By 1 year of age, the infant's birth weight has tripled, for an average weight of 9.75 kg (21.5 pounds). Height increases by 2.5 cm (1 inch) per month during the first 6 months of life and also slows during the second 6 months. Increases in length occur in sudden spurts, rather than in a slow, gradual pattern. The average height is 65 cm (25.5 inches) at 6 months of age and 74 cm (29 inches) at 12 months of age. By 1 year of age, the birth length has increased by almost 50%. This increase occurs mainly in the trunk, rather than in the legs, and contributes to the infant's characteristic physique.

Head growth is also rapid. During the first 3 months, head circumference increases approximately 2 cm (0.75 inch) per month, 1 cm (0.4 inch) per month from 4 to 6 months, then the rate of growth declines to only 0.5 cm (0.2 inch) monthly during the second 6 months. The average size is 43 cm (17 inches) at 6 months of age and 46 cm (18 inches) at 12 months of age. By 1 year of age, head size has increased by almost 33%. Closure of the cranial sutures occurs, with the posterior fontanel closing by 6 to 8 weeks of age and the anterior fontanel closing by 12 to 18 months of age (the average being 14 months).

Expanding head size reflects the growth and differentiation of the nervous system. By the end of the first year, the brain has increased in weight about 2.5 times. Maturation of the brain is exhibited in the

dramatic developmental achievements of infancy (Table 31.1). Primitive reflexes are replaced by voluntary, purposeful movement, and new reflexes that influence motor development appear. Although all milestones are important, some represent essential integrative aspects of development that lay the foundation for achievement of more advanced skills. These essential milestones are designated by an asterisk in Table 31.1. It must be remembered that although the sequence is the same, the rate will vary among children.

The chest assumes a more adult contour, with the lateral diameter becoming larger than the anteroposterior diameter. The chest circumference approximately equals the head circumference by the end of the first year. The heart grows less rapidly than the rest of the body. Its weight is usually doubled by 1 year of age; in comparison, body weight triples during the same period. The size of the heart is still large in relation to the chest cavity; its width is approximately 55% of the chest width.

Maturation of Systems

Other organ systems also change and grow during infancy. The respiratory rate slows somewhat and is relatively stable. Respiratory movements continue to be abdominal. Several factors predispose infants to more severe and acute respiratory problems than older children. The close proximity of the trachea to the bronchi and its branching structures rapidly transmits infectious agents from one anatomic location to another. The short, straight eustachian tube closely communicates with the ear, allowing infection to ascend from the pharynx to the middle ear. In addition, the inability of the immune system to produce immunoglobulin A (IgA) in the mucosal lining provides less protection against infection in infancy than during later childhood.

The heart rate slows, and the rhythm is often sinus arrhythmia (rate increases with inspiration and decreases with expiration). Blood pressure also changes during infancy. Systolic pressure rises during the first 2 months as a result of the increasing ability of the left ventricle to pump blood into the systemic circulation. Diastolic pressure decreases during the first 3 months and then gradually rises to values close to those at birth. Fluctuations in blood pressure occur during varying states of activity and emotion.

Significant hematopoietic changes occur during the first year. Fetal hemoglobin (HgbF) is present for the first 5 months, with adult

Text continued on p. 827

TABLE 31.1 Growth and Development During Infancy

Age (Mo)	Physical	Gross Motor	Fine Motor	Sensory	Vocalization	Socialization/ Cognition
1	Weight gain of 150–210 g (5–7 oz) weekly for first 6 months Height gain of 2.5 cm (1 inch) monthly for first 6 months Head circumference increases by 1.5 cm (0.5 inch) monthly for first 6 months Primitive reflexes present and strong Doll's eye reflexes and dance reflex fading Obligatory nose breathing (most infants)	Assumes flexed position with pelvis high but knees not under abdomen when prone (at birth, knees flexed under abdomen)* Can turn head from side to side when prone; lifts head momentarily from bed (see Fig. 31.3, A)* Has marked head lag, especially when pulled from lying to sitting position (see Fig. 31.2, A) Holds head momentarily parallel and in midline when suspended in prone position Assumes asymmetric tonic neck reflex position when supine When held in standing position, body is limp at knees and hips In sitting position, back is uniformly rounded, absence of head control	Hands predominantly closed Grasp reflex strong Hand clenches on contact with rattle	Able to fixate on moving object in range of 45 degrees when held at a distance of 20–25 cm (8–10 inches) Visual acuity approaches 20/100† Follows light to midline Quiets when hears a voice	Cries to express displeasure Makes small, throaty sounds Makes comfort sounds during feeding	Is in sensorimotor phase—stage I, use of reflexes (birth–1 month), and stage II, primary circular reactions (1–4 months) Watches parent's face intently as parent talks to infant
2	Posterior fontanel closed Crawling reflex disappears	Assumes less flexed position when prone—hips flat, legs extended, arms flexed, head to side* Less head lag when pulled to sitting position (see Fig. 31.2, B) Can maintain head in same plane as rest of body when held in ventral suspension When prone, can lift head almost 45 degrees off table When moved to sitting position, head is held up but bends forward (see Fig. 31.5, B) Assumes asymmetric tonic neck reflex position intermittently	Hands often open Grasp reflex fading	Binocular fixation and convergence to near objects beginning When supine, follows dangling toy from side to point beyond midline Visually searches to locate sounds Turns head to side when sound is made at level of ear	Vocalizes, distinct from crying* Crying becomes differentiated Coos Vocalizes to familiar voice	Demonstrates social smile in response to various stimuli*
3	Primitive reflexes fading	Able to hold head more erect when sitting, but still bobs forward Has only slight head lag when pulled to sitting position Assumes symmetric body positioning Able to raise head and shoulders from prone position to a 45- to 90-degree angle from table; bears weight on forearms When held in standing position, able to bear slight fraction of weight on legs Regards own hand	Actively holds rattle but will not reach for it* Grasp reflex absent Hands kept loosely open Clutches own hand; pulls at blankets and clothes	Follows object to periphery (180 degrees)* Locates sound by turning head to side and looking in same direction* Begins to have ability to coordinate stimuli from various sense organs	Squeals aloud to show pleasure* Coos, babbles, chuckles Vocalizes when smiling "Talks" a great deal when spoken to Less crying during periods of wakefulness	Displays considerable interest in surroundings Ceases crying when parent enters room Can recognize familiar faces and objects, such as feeding bottle Shows awareness of strange situations

Continued

TABLE 31.1   Growth and Development During Infancy—cont'd

Age (Mo)	Physical	Gross Motor	Fine Motor	Sensory	Vocalization	Socialization/Cognition
4	Drooling begins Moro, tonic neck, and rooting reflexes have disappeared*	Has almost no head lag when pulled to sitting position (see Fig. 31.2, C)* Balances head well in sitting position (see Fig. 31.5, C)* Back less rounded, curved only in lumbar area Able to sit erect if propped up Able to raise head and chest off surface to angle of 90 degrees (see Fig. 31.3, B) Assumes predominant symmetric position Rolls from back to side*	Inspects and plays with hands; pulls clothing or blanket over face in play* Tries to reach objects with hand but overshoots Grasps object with both hands Plays with rattle placed in hand, shakes it, but cannot pick it up if dropped Can carry objects to mouth	Able to accommodate to near objects Binocular vision fairly well established Can focus on a 1.25-cm (½-inch) block Beginning eye-hand coordination	Makes consonant sounds n, k, g, p, b Laughs aloud* Vocalization changes according to mood	Is in stage III, secondary circular reactions Demands attention by fussing; becomes bored if left alone Enjoys social interaction with people Anticipates feeding when sees bottle or mother if breastfeeding Shows excitement with whole body, squeals, breathes heavily Shows interest in strange stimuli Begins to show memory
5	Beginning signs of tooth eruption Birth weight doubles	No head lag when pulled to sitting position When sitting, able to hold head erect and steady Able to sit for longer periods when back is well supported Back straight When prone, assumes symmetric positioning with arms extended Can turn over from abdomen to back* When supine, puts feet to mouth	Able to grasp objects voluntarily* Uses palmar grasp, bidextrous approach Plays with toes Takes objects directly to mouth Holds one cube while regarding a second one	Visually pursues a dropped object Is able to sustain visual inspection of an object Can localize sounds made below ear	Squeals Makes cooing vowel sounds interspersed with consonant sounds (e.g., ah-goo)	Smiles at mirror image Pats bottle or breast with both hands More enthusiastically playful, but may have rapid mood swings Is able to discriminate strangers from family Vocalizes displeasure when object is taken away Discovers parts of body
6	Growth rate may begin to decline Weight gain of 90–150 g (3–5 oz) weekly for next 6 months Height gain of 1.25 cm (0.5 inch) monthly for next 6 months Teething may begin with eruption of two lower central incisors* Chewing and biting occur*	When prone, can lift chest and upper abdomen off surface, bearing weight on hands (see Fig. 31.3, C) When about to be pulled to a sitting position, lifts head Sits in high chair with back straight Rolls from back to abdomen When held in standing position, bears almost all of weight Hand regard absent	Resecures a dropped object Drops one cube when another is given Grasps and manipulates small objects Holds bottle Grasps feet and pulls to mouth	Adjusts posture to see an object Prefers more complex visual stimuli Can localize sounds made above ear Will turn head to the side, then look up or down	Begins to imitate sounds* Babbling resembles one-syllable utterances—ma, mu, da, di, hi* Vocalizes to toys, mirror image Takes pleasure in hearing own sounds (self-reinforcement)	Recognizes parents; begins to fear strangers Holds arms out to be picked up Has definite likes and dislikes Begins to imitate (cough, protrusion of tongue) Excites on hearing footsteps Briefly searches for a dropped object (object permanence beginning)* Frequent mood swings—from crying to laughing with little or no provocation

TABLE 31.1 Growth and Development During Infancy—cont'd

Age (Mo)	Physical	Gross Motor	Fine Motor	Sensory	Vocalization	Socialization/Cognition
7	Eruption of upper central incisors	When supine, spontaneously lifts head off surface Sits, leaning forward on hands (see Fig. 31.5, *D*)* When prone, bears weight on one hand Sits erect momentarily Bears full weight on feet (see Fig. 31.6, *A*) When held in standing position, bounces actively	Transfers objects from one hand to the other (see Fig. 31.5, *E*)* Has unidextrous approach and grasp Holds two cubes more than momentarily Bangs cube on table Rakes at a small object	Can fixate on very small objects* Responds to own name Localizes sound by turning head in a curving arch Beginning awareness of depth and space Has taste preferences	Produces vowel sounds and chained syllables—*baba, dada, kaka** Vocalizes four distinct vowel sounds "Talks" when others are talking	Increasing fear of strangers; shows signs of fretfulness when parent disappears* Imitates simple acts and noises Tries to attract attention by coughing or snorting Plays peekaboo Demonstrates dislike of food by keeping lips closed Exhibits oral aggressiveness in biting and mouthing Demonstrates expectation in response to repetition of stimuli
8	Begins to show regular patterns in bladder and bowel elimination Parachute reflex appears (see Fig. 31.4) Eruption of upper central incisors	Sits steadily unsupported (see Fig. 31.5, *E*)* Readily bears weight on legs when supported; may stand holding onto furniture Adjusts posture to reach an object	Has beginning pincer grasp using index, fourth, and fifth fingers against lower part of thumb Releases objects at will Rings bell purposely Retains two cubes while regarding third cube Secures an object by pulling on a string Reaches persistently for toys out of reach		Makes consonant sounds *t, d, w* Listens selectively to familiar words Utterances signal emphasis and emotion Combines syllables, such as *dada,* but does not ascribe meaning to them	Increasing anxiety over loss of parent, particularly mother, and fear of strangers Responds to word "no" Dislikes dressing, undressing, and diaper change
9	Eruption of upper lateral incisor may begin	Creeps on hands and knees Sits steadily on floor for prolonged time (10 min) Recovers balance when leaning forward but cannot do so when leaning sideways Pulls self to standing position and stands holding onto furniture (see Fig. 31.6, *B* and *C*)*	Uses thumb and index fingers in crude pincer grasp (see Fig. 31.1)* Preference for use of dominant hand now evident Grasps third cube Compares two cubes by bringing them together	Localizes sounds by turning head diagonally and directly toward sound Depth perception increasing	Responds to simple verbal commands Comprehends "no-no"	Parent (mother) is increasingly important for own sake Shows increasing interest in pleasing parent Begins to show fears of going to bed and being left alone Puts arms in front of face to avoid having it washed

Continued

TABLE 31.1   Growth and Development During Infancy—cont'd

Age (Mo)	Physical	Gross Motor	Fine Motor	Sensory	Vocalization	Socialization/ Cognition
10	Labyrinth-righting reflex is strongest—when infant is in prone or supine position, is able to raise head	Can change from prone to sitting position Stands while holding onto furniture, sits by falling down Recovers balance easily while sitting While standing, lifts one foot to take a step (see Fig. 31.6, *D*)	Crude release of an object beginning Grasps bell by handle		Says "dada," "mama" with meaning* Comprehends "bye-bye" May say one word (e.g., "hi," "bye," "no")	Inhibits behavior to verbal command of "no-no" or own name Imitates facial expressions; waves bye-bye Extends toy to another person but will not release it Develops object permanence* Repeats actions that attract attention and cause laughter Pulls clothes of another to attract attention Plays interactive game such as pat-a-cake Reacts to adult anger; cries when scolded Demonstrates independence in dressing, feeding, locomotive skills, and testing of parents Looks at and follows pictures in a book
11	Eruption of lower lateral incisor may begin	When sitting, pivots to reach toward back to pick up an object Cruises or walks holding onto furniture or with both hands held*	Explores objects more thoroughly (e.g., clapper inside bell) Has neat pincer grasp Drops object deliberately for it to be picked up Puts one object after another into a container (sequential play) Able to manipulate an object to remove it from tight-fitting enclosure		Imitates definite speech sounds	Experiences joy and satisfaction when a task is mastered Reacts to restrictions with frustration Rolls ball to another on request Anticipates body gestures when a familiar nursery rhyme or story is being told (e.g., holds toes and feet in response to "This little piggy went to market") Plays game up-down, "so big," or peekaboo Shakes head for "no"

TABLE 31.1   Growth and Development During Infancy—cont'd

Age (Mo)	Physical	Gross Motor	Fine Motor	Sensory	Vocalization	Socialization/Cognition
12	Birth weight tripled* Birth length increased by 50%* Head and chest circumference equal (head circumference 46 cm [18 inches]) Has six to eight deciduous teeth Anterior fontanel almost closed Landau reflex fading Babinski reflex disappears Lumbar curve develops; lordosis evident during walking	Walks with one hand held* Cruises well May attempt to stand alone momentarily; may attempt first step alone* Can sit down from standing position without help	Releases cube in cup Attempts to build two-block tower but fails Tries to insert a pellet into a narrow-necked bottle but fails Can turn pages in a book, many at a time	Discriminates simple geometric forms (e.g., circle) Amblyopia may develop with lack of binocularity Can follow rapidly moving object Controls and adjusts response to sound; listens for sound to recur	Says three to five words besides "dada," "mama"* Comprehends meaning of several words (comprehension always precedes verbalization) Recognizes objects by name Imitates animal sounds Understands simple verbal commands (e.g., "Give it to me," "Show me your eyes")	Shows emotions such as jealousy, affection (may give hug or kiss on request), anger, fear Enjoys familiar surroundings and explores away from parent Is fearful in strange situation; clings to parent May develop habit of "security blanket" or favorite toy Has increasing determination to practice locomotor skills Searches for an object even if it has not been hidden, but searches only where object was last seen*

*Milestones that represent essential integrative aspects of development that lay the foundation for the achievement of more advanced skills.
†Degree of visual acuity varies according to vision measurement procedure used.

hemoglobin steadily increasing through the first half of infancy. Fetal hemoglobin has a shorter life span than adult hemoglobin; therefore there is an increased turnover of these cells resulting in a decrease in hemoglobin. This process results in a physiologic anemia around 3 to 6 months of age. High levels of HgbF depress the production of erythropoietin, a hormone released by the kidney that stimulates red blood cell production. Maternally derived iron stores are present for the first 5 to 6 months and gradually diminish, which also accounts for lowered hemoglobin levels toward the end of the first 6 months. The occurrence of physiologic anemia is not affected by an adequate supply of iron. However, when erythropoiesis is stimulated, iron supplies are necessary for the formation of hemoglobin.

The digestive processes are immature at birth. Although term newborn infants have some limitations in digestive function, human milk has properties that partially compensate for decreased digestive enzymatic activity, thus enabling breastfed infants to receive optimal nutrition during the first several months of life. The enzyme amylase (also called *ptyalin*) is present in small amounts but usually has little effect on the foodstuffs because of the small amount of time the food stays in the mouth. Gastric digestion in the stomach consists primarily of the action of hydrochloric acid and rennin, an enzyme that acts specifically on the casein in milk to cause the formation of curds (coagulated semisolid particles of milk). The curds cause the milk to be retained in the stomach long enough for digestion to occur.

Digestion also takes place in the duodenum, where pancreatic enzymes and bile begin to break down protein and fat. Secretion of the pancreatic enzyme amylase, which is needed for digestion of complex carbohydrates, is deficient until about the fourth to sixth month of life. Lipase is also limited, and infants do not achieve adult levels of fat absorption until 4 to 5 months of age. Trypsin is secreted in sufficient quantities to catabolize protein into polypeptides and some amino acids.

The immaturity of the digestive processes is evident in the appearance of stools. During infancy, solid foods (e.g., peas, carrots, corn, raisins) are passed incompletely broken down in the feces. An excess quantity of fiber easily disposes infants to loose, bulky stools. During infancy, the stomach enlarges to accommodate a greater volume of food. By the end of the first year, infants are able to tolerate three meals per day and an evening bottle and may have one or two bowel movements daily. With any type of gastric irritation, however, the infant is vulnerable to diarrhea, vomiting, and dehydration (see Chapter 41).

The liver is the most immature of all the gastrointestinal (GI) organs throughout infancy. The ability to conjugate bilirubin and secrete bile is achieved after the first couple of weeks of life. However, the capacities for gluconeogenesis, formation of plasma protein and ketones, storage of vitamins, and deaminization of amino acids remain relatively immature for the first year of life.

Maturation of the suckling, sucking, and swallowing reflexes and the eruption of teeth (see the "Teething" section later in this chapter) parallel the changes in the GI tract and prepare infants for the introduction of solid foods.

The immunologic system undergoes numerous changes during the first year. Full-term newborns receive significant amounts of maternal immunoglobulin G (IgG), which, for approximately 3 months, confers immunity against antigens to which their mothers were exposed. During this time, infants begin to synthesize IgG; approximately 40% of adult levels are reached by 1 year of age. Significant amounts of immunoglobulin M (IgM) are produced at birth, and adult levels are reached by 9 months of age. Prebiotic oligosaccharides found in breast milk produce probiotic bacteria such bifidobacteria and lactobacilli, which in turn stimulate synthesis and secretion of secretory IgA (sIgA). Secretory IgA is present in large amounts in colostrum; IgA confers protection to the mucous membranes of the GI tract (Durand, Ochoa, Bellomo, et al., 2013) against many bacteria, such as *Escherichia coli*, and viruses such as rubella, poliovirus, and the enteroviruses. The development of the mucosa-associated lymphoid tissue occurs during infancy; in part, this system is believed to prevent colonization and passage of bacteria across the infant's mucosal barrier. The function and quantity of T-lymphocytes, lymphokines, interferon-γ, interleukins, tumor necrosis factor-α, and complement are reduced in early infancy, thus preventing optimal response to certain bacteria and viruses. The production of IgA and immunoglobulins D and E (IgD and IgE) is much more gradual, and maximum levels are not attained until early childhood. Probiotics may have a significant role in helping the GI tract establish a "good" bacterial colonization in the gut to prevent many illnesses, including antibiotic-induced diarrhea and possibly *Helicobacter pylori* gastritis (Vitetta, Briskey, Alford, et al., 2014).

Evidence indicates that vernix caseosa, a white oily substance that coats the term infant's body and is often found in abundance in creases of the axilla and groin, has innate immunologic properties that serve to protect the newborn from infection (Visscher & Narendran, 2014). Vernix also appears to have a role in maintaining the integrity of the stratum corneum and facilitating acid mantle development (Visscher & Narendran). The epidermis of the full-term infant undergoes maturation during the first month of life; the newborn's skin acts as a barrier to infection, assists in thermal regulation, and prevents transepidermal water loss in term infants.

During infancy, thermoregulation becomes more efficient; the ability of the skin to contract and of muscles to shiver in response to cold increases. The peripheral capillaries respond to changes in ambient temperature to regulate heat loss. The capillaries constrict in response to cold, conserving core body temperature and decreasing potential evaporative heat loss from the skin surface. The capillaries dilate in response to heat, decreasing internal body temperature through evaporation, conduction, and convection. Shivering (thermogenesis) causes the muscles and muscle fibers to contract, generating metabolic heat that is distributed throughout the body. Increased adipose tissue during the first 6 months insulates the body against heat loss.

A shift in the total body fluid occurs. At birth, 78% of the term infant's body weight is water, with a large percentage being extracellular fluid (ECF). As the percentage of body water decreases, so does the amount of ECF—from 44% at term to 20% in adulthood. The high proportion of ECF, which is composed of blood plasma, interstitial fluid, and lymph, predisposes infants to a more rapid loss of total body fluid and, consequently, dehydration. The loss of 5% to 10% of the term newborn's initial birth weight in the first 5 days of life is attributed to ECF compartment contraction, enhanced renal tubular function, and rapidly increasing glomerular filtration rate (Blackburn, 2013).

The immaturity of the renal structures also predisposes infants to dehydration and electrolyte imbalance. Complete maturity of the kidney occurs during the latter half of the second year, when the cuboidal epithelium of the glomeruli becomes flattened. Before this time, the glomeruli's filtration capacity is reduced. Urine is voided frequently and has a low specific gravity (i.e., 1.008 to 1.012). At term, most infants produce and excrete approximately 15 to 60 mL/kg/24 hours, and an output of less than 0.5 mL/kg/hour after 48 hours of age is considered to be oliguria (Blackburn, 2013).

Auditory acuity is at adult levels during infancy. Visual acuity begins to improve, and binocular fixation is established. Binocularity, or the fixation of two ocular images into one cerebral picture (fusion), begins to develop by 6 weeks of age and should be well established by 4 months

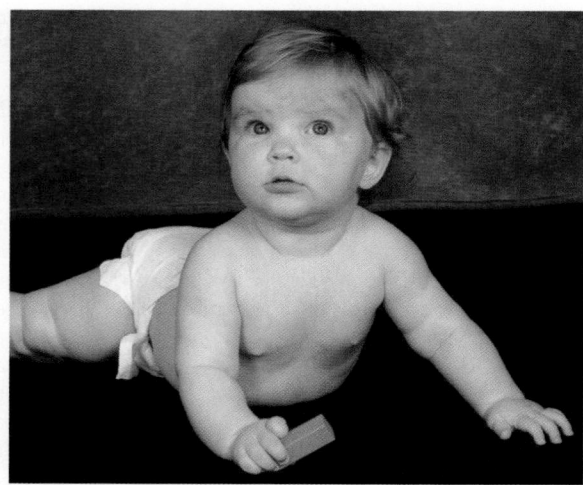

FIG 31.1 Crude pincer grasp at 8 to 10 months. (Photo by Paul Vincent Kuntz, Texas Children's Hospital, Houston, TX.)

of age. Depth perception (stereopsis) begins to develop by 7 to 9 months of age but may not be fully mature until 2 to 3 years of age, thus increasing the infant's and younger toddler's risk for falling.

Fine Motor Development

Fine motor behavior includes the use of the hands and fingers in the prehension (grasp) of an object. Grasping occurs during the first 2 to 3 months as a reflex and gradually becomes voluntary. At 1 month of age, the hands are predominantly closed, and by 3 months of age, they are mostly open. By this time, infants demonstrate a desire to grasp an object, but they "grasp" it more with the eyes than with the hands. If a rattle is placed in the hand, infants will actively hold onto it. By 4 months of age, infants regard both a small ball and the hands and then look from the object to the hands and back again. By 5 months, infants are able to voluntarily grasp an object.

By 6 months of age, infants have increased manipulative skill: they hold their bottle, grasp their feet and pull them to their mouth, and feed themselves a cracker. By 7 months of age, they transfer objects from one hand to the other, use one hand for grasping, and hold a cube in each hand simultaneously. Gradually the palmar grasp (using the whole hand) is replaced with a pincer grasp (using the thumb and index finger). Infants use a crude pincer grasp by 8 to 9 months of age and progress to a neat pincer grasp by 10 months of age (Fig. 31.1). The neat pincer grasp is sufficiently established to enable infants to pick up a raisin and other finger foods, and deliberately let go of an object. By 11 months of age, they put objects into a container and like to remove them. By 1 year of age, infants try to build a tower of two blocks but fail.

Gross Motor Development
Head Control

The full-term newborn can momentarily hold the head in midline and parallel when the body is suspended ventrally and can lift and turn the head from side to side when prone. This is not the case when infants are lying prone on a pillow or soft surface; infants do not have the head control to lift their head out of the depression of the object and therefore risk possible suffocation in the prone position early in infancy (see the "Sudden Infant Death Syndrome" section later in this chapter). Marked head lag is evident when infants are pulled from a lying to a sitting position. By 3 months of age, infants can hold their head well beyond the plane of the body. By 4 months of age, infants can lift the head and

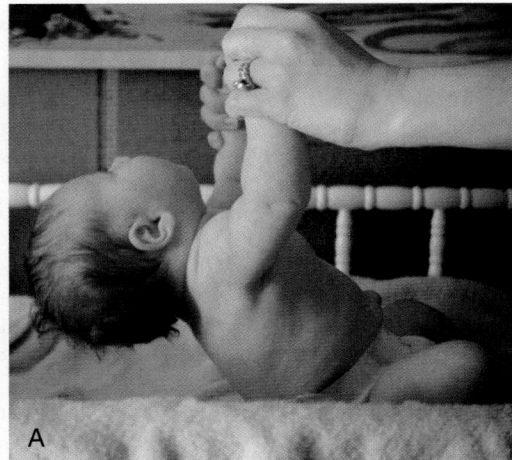
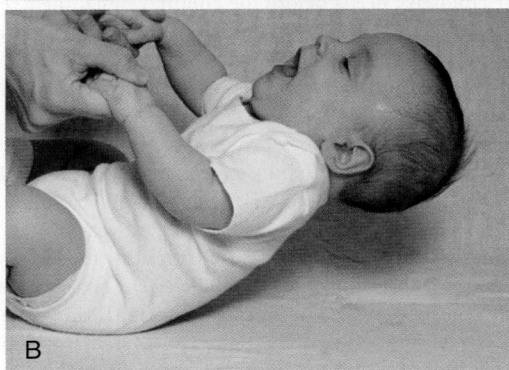
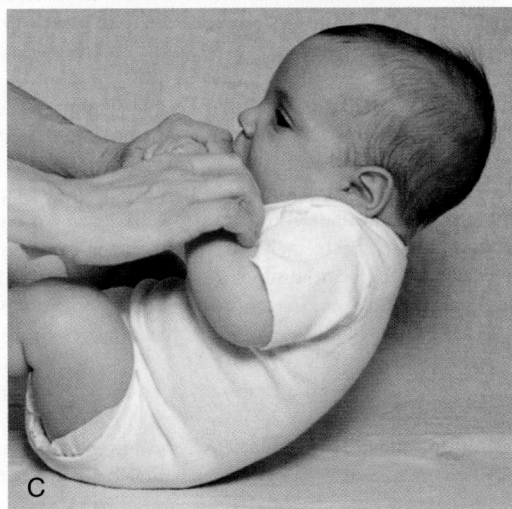

FIG 31.2 Head control while pulled to sitting position. **A,** Complete head lag at 1 month. **B,** Partial head lag at 2 months. **C,** Almost no head lag at 4 months.

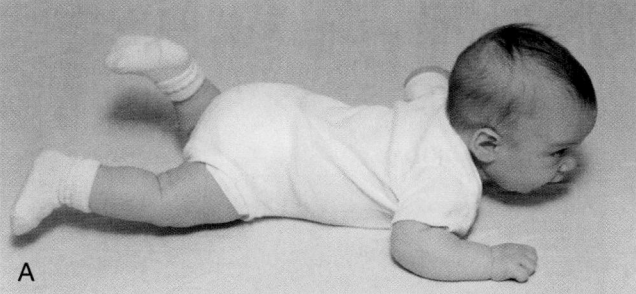
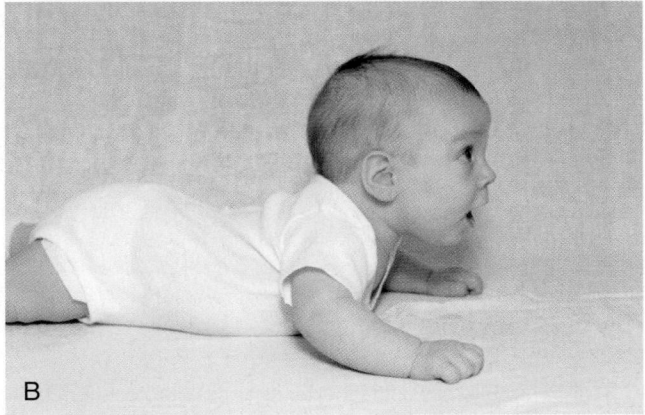
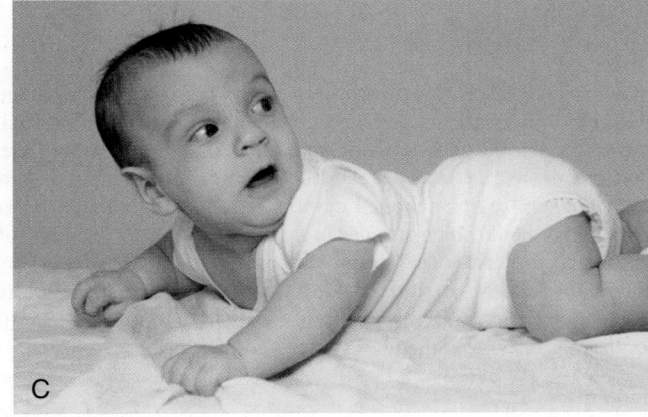

FIG 31.3 Head control while prone. **A,** Infant momentarily lifts head at 1 month. **B,** Infant lifts head and chest 90 degrees and bears weight on forearms at 4 months. **C,** Infant lifts head, chest, and upper abdomen and can bear weight on hands at 6 months. Note how this position facilitates turning from abdomen to back.

front portion of the chest approximately 90 degrees above the table, bearing their weight on the forearms. Only slight head lag is evident when infants are pulled from a lying to a sitting position, and by 4 to 6 months of age, head control is well established (Figs. 31.2 and 31.3).

> **! NURSING ALERT**
>
> An infant who displays head lag at 6 months of age should have a developmental and neurologic evaluation.

Rolling Over

Newborns may roll over accidentally because of their rounded back. The ability to willfully turn from the abdomen to the back occurs at 5 months of age, and the ability to turn from the back to the abdomen occurs at approximately 6 months of age. Infants put to sleep on their sides may easily roll over to a prone (face-down) position, thus placing them at higher risk for sudden infant death syndrome (SIDS). It is therefore important to place infants in a supine position for sleep. While infants are awake, a prone position (tummy time) is acceptable to enhance achievement of milestones such as head control, crawling, creeping, and turning over. It is noteworthy that the parachute reflex (Fig. 31.4), a protective response to falling, appears at approximately 7 months of age.

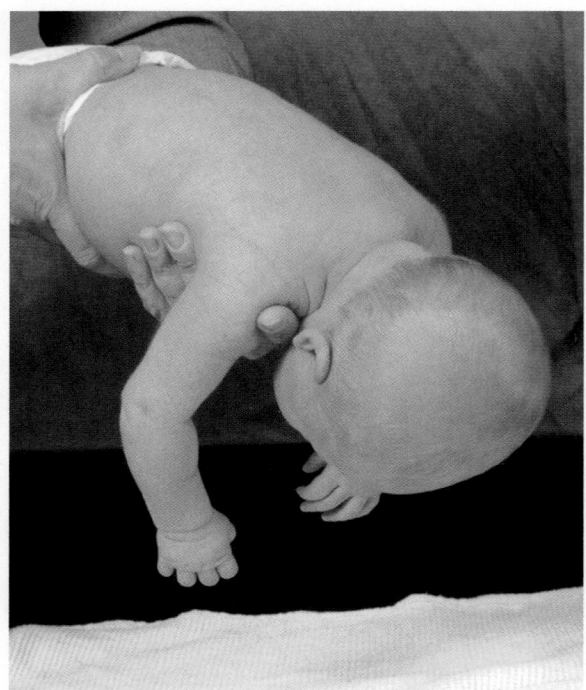

FIG 31.4 Parachute reflex. Infant extends arms to protect from falling. (Photo by Paul Vincent Kuntz, Texas Children's Hospital, Houston, TX.)

Sitting

The ability to sit follows progressive head control and straightening of the back (Fig. 31.5). For the first 2 to 3 months, the back is uniformly rounded. The convex cervical curve forms at approximately 3 to 4 months of age, when head control is established. The convex lumbar curve appears when the child begins to sit, at about 4 months of age. As the spinal column straightens, infants can be propped in a sitting position. By 7 months of age, infants can sit alone, leaning forward on their hands for support. By 8 months of age, they can sit well while unsupported and begin to explore their surroundings in this position rather than in a lying position. By 10 months of age, they can maneuver from a prone to a sitting position.

Locomotion

Locomotion involves acquiring the ability to bear weight, propel forward on all four extremities, stand upright with support, cruise by holding onto furniture, and, finally, walk alone (Fig. 31.6). Following a cephalocaudal pattern, infants 4 to 6 months of age have increasing coordination in their arms. Initial locomotion results in infants propelling themselves backward by pushing with the arms. By 6 to 7 months of age, they are able to bear all their weight on their legs with assistance. *Crawling* (propelling forward with the belly on the floor) progresses to *creeping* (on hands and knees with belly off the floor) by 9 months. At this time, they stand while holding on to furniture and can pull themselves to the standing position, but they are unable to maneuver back down except by falling. By 11 months of age, they walk while holding onto furniture or with both hands held, and by 1 year of age, they may be able to walk with one hand held. A number of infants attempt their first independent steps by their first birthday.

> **! NURSING ALERT**
>
> An infant who does not pull to a standing position by 11 to 12 months of age should be further evaluated for possible developmental dysplasia of the hip (see Chapter 48).

PSYCHOSOCIAL DEVELOPMENT: DEVELOPING A SENSE OF TRUST (ERIKSON)

Erikson's (1963) phase I (birth to 1 year) is concerned with *acquiring a sense of trust* while *overcoming a sense of mistrust*. The trust that develops is a trust of self, of others, and of the world. Infants "trust" that their feeding, comfort, stimulation, and caring needs will be met. The crucial element for the achievement of this task is the quality of both the parent-child (or caregiver-child) relationship and the care the infant receives. The provision of food, warmth, and shelter by itself is inadequate for the development of a strong sense of self. The infant and parent must jointly learn to satisfactorily meet their needs in order for mutual regulation of frustration to occur. When this synchrony fails to develop, mistrust is the eventual outcome.

Failure to learn *delayed gratification* leads to mistrust. Mistrust can result from either too much or too little frustration. If parents always meet their children's needs before the children signal their readiness, infants will never learn to test their ability to control the environment. If the delay is prolonged, infants experience constant frustration and eventually mistrust others in their efforts to satisfy them. Therefore consistency of care is essential.

The trust acquired in infancy provides the foundation for all succeeding phases. Trust allows infants a feeling of physical comfort and security, which assists them in experiencing unfamiliar situations with a minimum of fear. Erikson has divided the first year of life into two oral-social stages. During the first 3 to 4 months, food intake is the most important social activity in which the infant engages. Newborns can tolerate little frustration or delay of gratification. Primary narcissism (total concern for oneself) is at its height. However, as bodily processes such as vision, motor movements, and vocalization become better controlled, infants use more advanced behaviors to interact with others. For example, rather than cry, infants may put their arms up to signify a desire to be held.

The next social modality involves a mode of reaching out to others through grasping. Grasping is initially reflexive, but even as a reflex, it has a powerful social meaning for the parents. The reciprocal response to the infant's grasping is the parents' holding on and touching. There is pleasurable tactile stimulation for both the child and the parents.

Tactile stimulation is extremely important in the total process of acquiring trust. The degree of mothering skill, the quantity of food, or the length of sucking does not determine the quality of the experience. Rather, it is the overall quality of the interpersonal relationship that influences the infant's formulation of trust.

During the second stage, the more active and aggressive modality of biting occurs. Infants learn that they can hold onto what is their own and can more fully control their environment. During this stage, infants may be confronted with one of their first conflicts. If they are breastfeeding, they quickly learn that biting causes the mother to become upset and withdraw the breast. Yet biting also brings internal relief from teething discomfort and a sense of power or control.

This conflict may be solved in a variety of ways. The mother may wean the infant from the breast and begin bottle-feeding, or the infant may learn to bite substitute "nipples," such as a pacifier, and retain pleasurable breastfeeding. The successful resolution of this conflict strengthens the mother-child relationship because it occurs at a time when infants are recognizing the mother as the most significant person in their life.

COGNITIVE DEVELOPMENT: SENSORIMOTOR PHASE (PIAGET)

The theory most commonly used to explain *cognition,* or the ability to know, is that of Piaget (1952). The period from birth to 24 months is

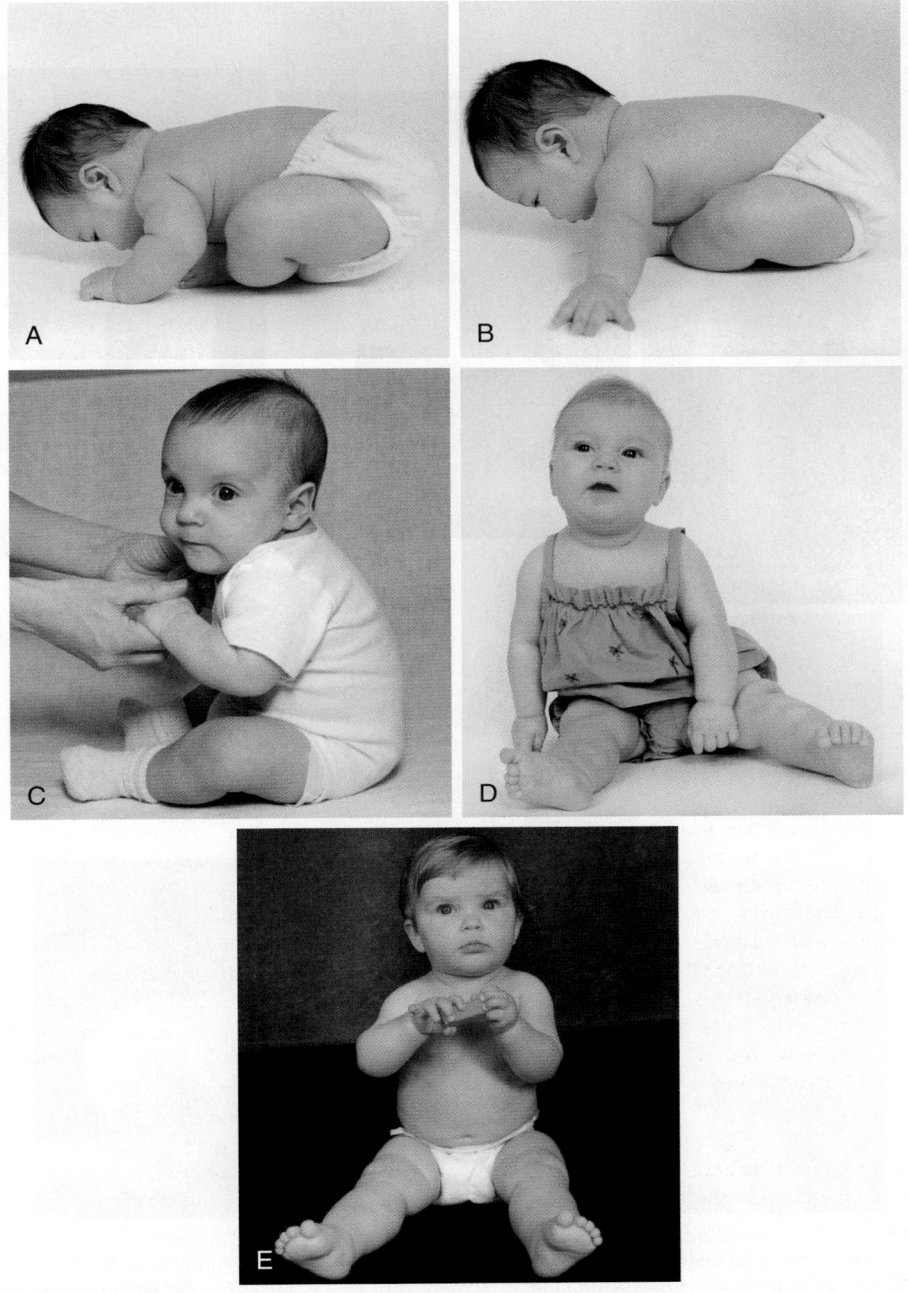

FIG 31.5 Development of sitting. **A,** Back is completely rounded, and infant has no ability to sit upright at 1 month of age. **B,** At 2 months of age, infant exhibits more control; back is still rounded, but infant can sit up momentarily with some head control. **C,** Back is rounded only in lumbar area, and infant is able to sit erect with good head control at 4 months of age. **D,** Infant can sit alone, leaning on hands for support, at 7 months of age. **E,** Infant sits without support at 8 months of age. Note the transferring of objects that occurs beginning at 7 months of age. (Photos by Paul Vincent Kuntz, Texas Children's Hospital, Houston, TX.)

termed the *sensorimotor phase* and is composed of six stages; however, because this discussion is concerned with birth to 12 months of age, only the first four stages are discussed. The last two stages occur during the toddler period of 12 to 24 months of age and are discussed in Chapter 32.

During the sensorimotor phase, infants progress from reflex behaviors to simple repetitive acts to imitative activity. Three crucial events take place during this phase. The first event involves separation, in which infants learn to separate themselves from other objects in the environment. They realize that others besides themselves control the environment and that certain readjustments must take place for mutual satisfaction to occur. This coincides with Erikson's concept of the formation of trust.

The second major accomplishment is achieving the concept of object permanence, or the realization that objects that leave the visual field still exist. A typical example of the development of object permanence is when infants are able to pursue objects they observe being hidden under a pillow or behind a chair (Fig. 31.7). This skill develops at

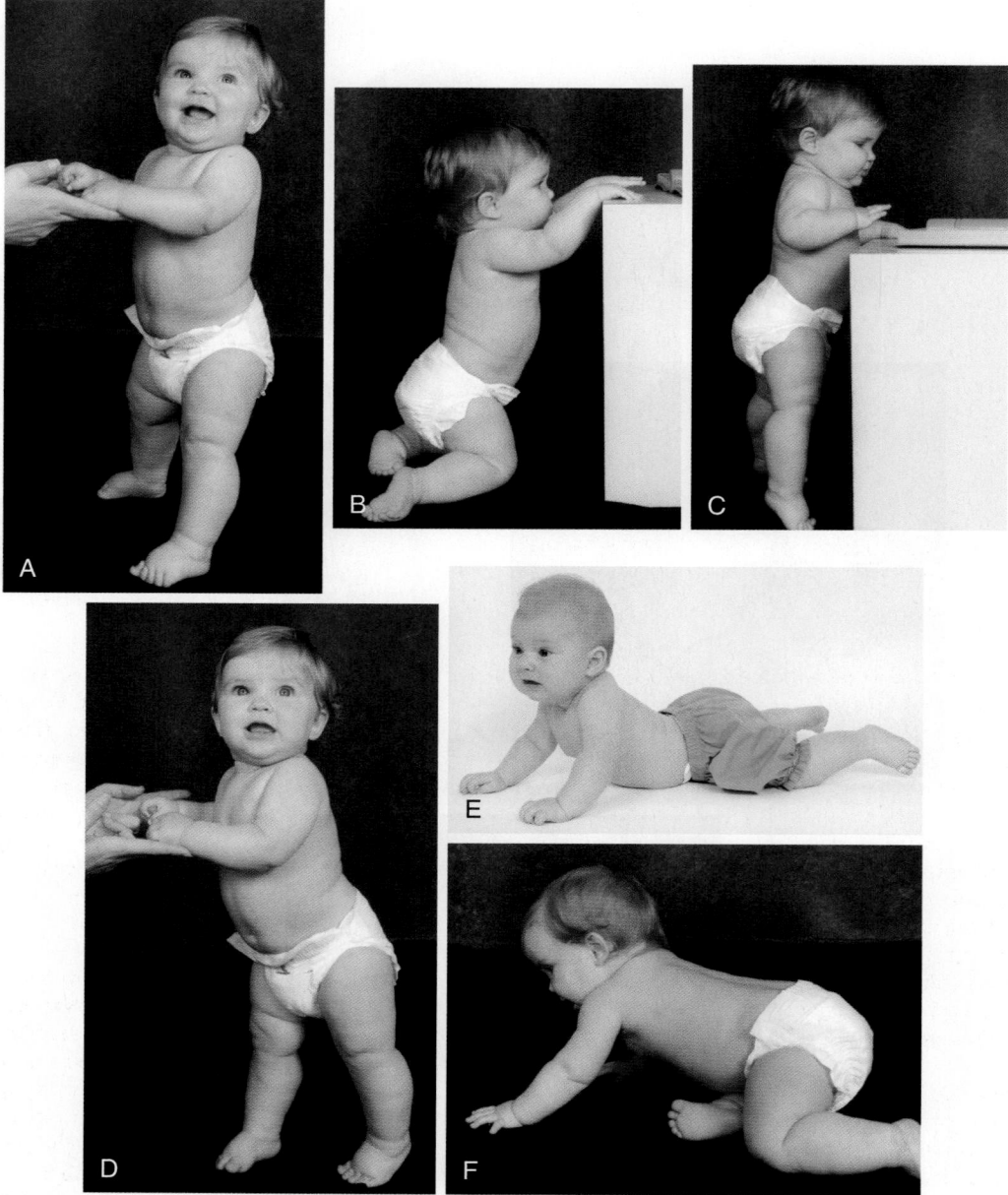

FIG 31.6 Development of locomotion. **A,** Infant bears full weight on feet by 7 months of age. **B,** Infant can maneuver from sitting to kneeling position. **C,** Infant can stand holding onto furniture at 9 months of age. **D,** While standing, infant takes deliberate step at 10 months of age. **E,** Infant crawls with abdomen on floor and pulls self forward, and then, **F,** creeps on hands and knees at 9 months of age. (Photos by Paul Vincent Kuntz, Texas Children's Hospital, Houston, TX.)

approximately 9 to 10 months of age, which corresponds to the time of increased locomotion skills.

The last major intellectual achievement of this period is the ability to use symbols, or mental representation. The use of symbols allows the infant to think of an object or situation without actually experiencing it. The recognition of symbols is the beginning of the understanding of time and space.

The first stage, from birth to 1 month, is identified by the infant's use of reflexes. At birth, infants' individuality and temperament are expressed through the physiologic reflexes of sucking, rooting, grasping, and crying. The repetitious nature of the reflexes is the beginning of associations between an act and a sequential response. When infants

cry because they are hungry, a nipple is put in the mouth and they suck, feel satisfaction, and sleep. They are assimilating this experience while perceiving auditory, tactile, and visual cues. This experience of perceiving certain patterns, or "ordering," provides a foundation for the subsequent stages.

The second stage, primary circular reactions, marks the beginning of the replacement of reflexive behavior with voluntary acts. During the period from 1 to 4 months of age, activities such as sucking or grasping become deliberate acts that elicit certain responses. The beginning of accommodation is evident. Infants incorporate and adapt their reactions to the environment and recognize the stimulus that produced a response. Previously they cried until the nipple was brought to the

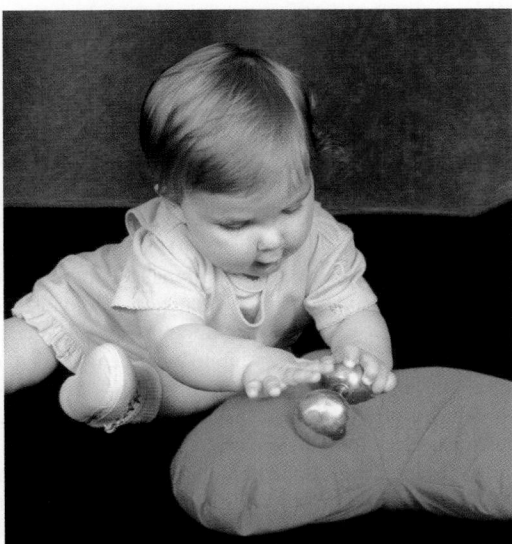

FIG 31.7 Nine-month-old infant actively searches for object hidden behind pillow. (Photo by Paul Vincent Kuntz, Texas Children's Hospital, Houston, TX.)

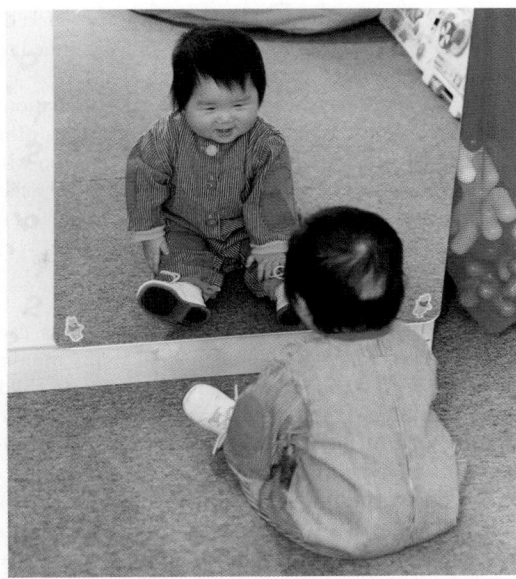

FIG 31.8 Nine-month-old infant enjoying own image in mirror.

mouth. Now they associate the nipple with the sound of the parent's voice. They accommodate this new piece of information and adapt by ceasing to cry when they hear the voice—before receiving the nipple. What is taking place is a realization of causality and a recognition of an orderly sequence of events. The environment is taken in with all of the senses and with whatever motor ability is present.

The secondary circular reactions stage is a continuation of primary circular reactions and lasts until 8 months of age. In this stage, the primary circular reactions are repeated and prolonged for the response that results. Grasping and holding now become shaking, banging, and pulling. Shaking is performed to hear a noise, not solely for the pleasure of shaking. The quality and quantity of an act become evident. More or less shaking produces different responses. Understanding of causality, time, deliberate intention, and separateness from the environment begins to develop.

Three new processes of human behavior occur. Imitation requires the differentiation of selected acts from several events. By the second half of the first year, infants can imitate sounds and simple gestures. Play becomes evident as they take pleasure in performing an act after they have mastered it. Many of the infant's waking hours are absorbed in sensorimotor play. Affect (the outward manifestation of emotion and feeling) is seen as infants begin to develop a sense of permanency. During the first 6 months, infants believe that an object exists only for as long as they can visually perceive it. In other words, out of sight, out of mind. Affect to external objects is evident when the object continues to be present or remembered even though it is beyond the range of perception. Object permanence is a critical component of parent-child attachment and is seen in the development of separation anxiety at 6 to 8 months of age.

During the fourth sensorimotor stage, coordination of secondary schemas and their application to new situations, infants use previous behavioral achievements primarily as the foundation for adding new intellectual skills to their expanding repertoire. This stage is largely transitional. Increasing motor skills allow for greater exploration of the environment. They begin to discover that hiding an object does not mean that it is gone but that removing an obstacle will reveal the object. This marks the beginning of intellectual reasoning. Furthermore, they can experience an event by observing it, and they begin to associate

symbols with events (e.g., "bye-bye" with "Mommy or Daddy goes to work"), but the classification is purely their own. In this stage, they learn from the object itself; this is in contrast to the second stage, in which infants learn from the type of interaction between objects or individuals. Intentionality is further developed in that infants now actively attempt to remove a barrier to the desired (or undesired) action (see Fig. 31.7). If something is in their way, they attempt to climb over it or push it away. Previously, an obstacle would cause them to give up any further attempt to achieve the desired goal.

DEVELOPMENT OF BODY IMAGE

The development of body image parallels sensorimotor development. Infants' kinesthetic and tactile experiences are the first perceptions of their bodies, and the mouth is the principal area of pleasurable sensations. Other parts of the body are primarily objects of pleasure—the hands and fingers to suck and the feet to play with. As physical needs are met, they feel comfort and satisfaction with their body. Messages conveyed by the caregivers reinforce these feelings. For example, when infants smile, they receive emotional satisfaction from others who smile back.

Achieving the concept of object permanence is basic to the development of self-image. By the end of the first year, infants recognize that they are distinct from their parents. At the same time, they have increasing interest in their image, especially in the mirror (Fig. 31.8). As motor skills develop, they learn that parts of the body are useful; for example, the hands bring objects to the mouth and the legs help them move to different locations. All of these achievements transmit messages to them about themselves. Therefore it is important to transmit positive messages to infants about their bodies.

SOCIAL DEVELOPMENT

Infants' social development is initially influenced by their reflexive behavior, such as the grasp, and eventually depends primarily on the interaction between them and the principal caregivers. *Attachment* to their parents is increasingly evident during the second half of the first year. In addition, tremendous strides are made in communication and personal-social behavior. Whereas crying and reflexive behavior are methods to meet one's needs in early infancy, the social smile is an early step in social communication. This has a profound effect on family members and is a tremendous stimulus for evoking continued responses from others. By 4 months of age, infants laugh aloud.

Play is a major socializing agent and provides stimulation needed to learn from and interact with the environment. By 6 months of age, infants are personable. They play games such as peekaboo when their heads are hidden in a towel, they signal their desire to be picked up by extending their arms, and they show displeasure when a toy is removed or their faces are washed.

Attachment

The importance of human physical contact to infants cannot be overemphasized. Parenting is not an instinctual ability but, instead, a learned, acquired process. The attachment of parent and child, which begins before birth, assumes even more importance at birth and continues during the first year. In the following discussion of attachment, the term *mother* is used in the broad context of the consistent caregiver with whom the child relates more than anyone else. However, in society's changing social climate and gender-role stereotypes, this person may very well be the father or a grandparent. Studies on paternal-infant attachment demonstrate that stages similar to those in maternal attachment occur and that fathers are often more involved in child care when mothers are employed (although many mothers continue to do the majority of infant care). Additional research has shown that inexperienced, first-time fathers are as capable as experienced fathers of developing a close attachment with their infants. Fathers verbalized more positive feelings of love and affection toward their newborns when they were able to have close physical contact, such as holding their infant (Feeley, Sherrard, Waitzer, et al., 2013). Research demonstrates that fathers develop feelings of attachment with their offspring and that their relationship with the infant is an important factor in the mother's emotional well-being. It is important for nurses to recognize that infant-parent attachments may be present or absent in situations wherein caregiver roles are less well defined by those involved.

When the infant is not provided a safe haven and consistent and loving care, an insecure attachment develops; such infants do not feel they can trust the world in which they live. This insecure attachment may result in psychosocial difficulties as the child grows and may persist even into adulthood. Insecure attachment may also exist in homes where there is domestic violence and maternal postnatal depression.

Attachment progresses during infancy, with the child assuming an increasingly significant role. Two components of cognitive development are required for attachment: (1) the ability to discriminate the mother from other individuals, and (2) the achievement of object permanence. Both of these processes prepare infants for an equally important aspect of attachment: separation from the parent. Separation-individuation should occur as a harmonious, parallel process with emotional attachment.

During the formation of attachment to the parent, the infant progresses through four distinct but overlapping stages. For the first few weeks, infants respond indiscriminately to anyone. Beginning at approximately 8 to 12 weeks of age, they cry, smile, and vocalize more to the mother than to anyone else but continue to respond to others, whether familiar or not. At approximately 6 months of age, infants show a distinct preference for the mother. They follow her more, cry when she leaves, enjoy playing with her more, and feel most secure in her arms. About 1 month after showing attachment to the mother, many infants begin attaching to other members of the family, most often the father.

Infants acquire other developmental behaviors that influence the attachment process. These include the following:
- Differential crying, smiling, and vocalization (more to the mother than to anyone else)
- Visual-motor orientation (looking more at the mother, even if she is not close)
- Crying when the mother leaves the room
- Approaching through locomotion (crawling, creeping, or walking)
- Clinging (especially in the presence of a stranger)
- Exploring away from the mother while using her as a secure base

Severe attachment disorders are psychologic and developmental problems that stem from maladaptive or absent attachment between the infant and parent (Zeanah & Gleason, 2015). There are two different patterns of attachment disorders: the emotionally withdrawn–inhibited pattern and an indiscriminate-disinhibited pattern (Zeanah & Gleason). These two subtypes have been classified into separate disorders: reactive attachment disorder (RAD) and disinhibited social engagement disorder (DSED) of infancy or early childhood. Infants at risk for severe attachment disorders include those who have been victims of physical or sexual abuse or neglect; infants exposed to parental alcoholism, mental illness, and substance abuse; and infants who have experienced the absence of a consistent primary caregiver as a result of foster care, institutionalization, parental abandonment, or parental incarceration (Zeanah & Gleason). Children with RAD may manifest behaviors such as not being cuddly with parents, failing to seek and respond to comfort when distressed, showing minimal social and emotional reciprocity, and emotional deregulation such unexplained fearfulness or irritability (Zeanah & Gleason). Children with DSED may exhibit behaviors such as inappropriate approach to unfamiliar adults, lack of suspicion of strangers, and poor impulse control (Zeanah & Gleason). Without early intervention, some of these children fail to develop a conscience and develop an antisocial personality disorder that may lead to criminal acts. Children with autism or other pervasive developmental disorders have behaviors that are categorically different from those with RAD (Zeanah & Gleason).

Separation Anxiety

Between 4 and 8 months of age, infants progress through the first stage of separation-individuation and begin to have some awareness of self and mother as separate beings. At the same time, object permanence is developing and the infant is aware that the parent can be absent. Therefore *separation anxiety* develops and is manifested through a predictable sequence of behaviors.

During the early second half of the first year, infants protest when placed in their crib, and a short time later they object when the mother leaves the room. Infants may not notice the mother's absence if they are absorbed in an activity. However, when they realize her absence, they protest. From this point on, they become alert to her activities and whereabouts. By 11 to 12 months of age, they are able to anticipate her imminent departure by watching her behaviors, and they begin to protest before she leaves. At this point, many parents learn to postpone alerting the child to their departure until just before leaving.

Stranger Fear

As infants demonstrate attachment to one person, they correspondingly exhibit less friendliness to others. Between 6 and 8 months of age, fear of strangers and stranger anxiety become prominent and are related to infants' ability to discriminate between familiar and unfamiliar people. Behaviors such as clinging to the parent, crying, and turning away from the stranger are common (Fig. 31.9).

Language Development

Infants' first means of verbal communication is crying. Crying as a biologic sign conveys a message of urgency and signals displeasure, such as hunger. However, crying is also a social event that affects the development of the parent-infant relationship—either by its absence,

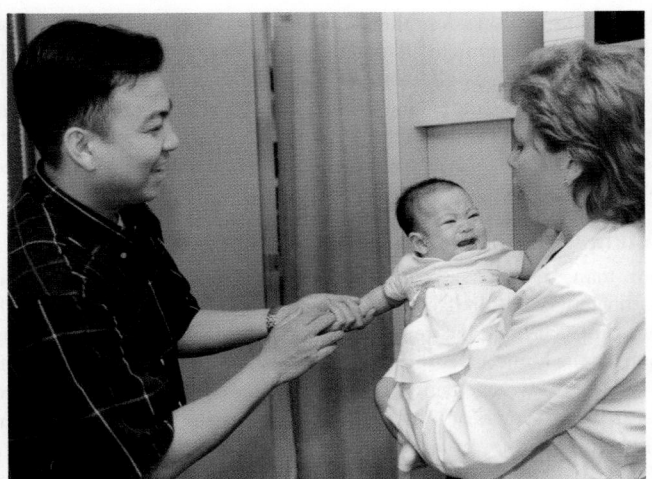

FIG 31.9 Behaviors related to fear of strangers include clinging to the parent and turning away from the stranger. (Photo by Paul Vincent Kuntz, Texas Children's Hospital, Houston, TX.)

which usually has a positive effect on parents, or its presence, which may involve a negative response or persuade parents to minister to the child's physical or emotional needs.

In the first few weeks of life, crying has a reflexive quality and is mostly related to physiologic needs. Infants cry for 1 to 1.5 hours a day up to 3 weeks of age and then build up to 2 and even 4 hours by 6 weeks of age. Crying tends to decrease by 12 weeks of age. It is thought that the increase in crying for no apparent reason during the first few months may be related to the discharge of energy and the maturational changes in the central nervous system. During the end of the first year, infants cry for attention; from fear (especially stranger fear); and from frustration, usually in response to their developing but inadequate motor skills.

> **! NURSING ALERT**
>
> Be alert to parents' reports about maternal postpartum depression and infant crying, since these concerns may indicate a stressed mother-infant relationship.

Vocalizations heard during crying eventually become syllables and words (e.g., the "mama" heard during vigorous crying). Infants vocalize as early as 5 to 6 weeks of age by making small throaty sounds. By 2 months of age, they make single vowel sounds such as *ah, eh,* and *uh.* By 3 to 4 months of age, the consonants *n, k, g, p,* and *b* are added and the infants coo, gurgle, and laugh aloud. By 8 months of age, they imitate sounds; add the consonants *t, d,* and *w;* and combine syllables (e.g., "dada"), but they do not ascribe meaning to the word until 10 to 11 months of age. By 9 to 10 months of age, they comprehend the meaning of the word "no" and obey simple commands. By 1 year of age, they can say three to five words with meaning. Because language development is based on expressive skills (ability to make thoughts, ideas, and desires known to others) and receptive skills (ability to understand the words being spoken), it is important that infants are exposed to expressive speech and infants with delays in achieving milestones are evaluated for potential hearing loss.

Play

Play during infancy represents the various social modalities observed during cognitive development. Infants' activity is primarily narcissistic and revolves around their own body. As discussed in the "Development

of Body Image" section earlier in this chapter, body parts are primarily objects of play and pleasure.

During the first year, play becomes more sophisticated and interdependent. From birth to 3 months of age, infants' responses to the environment are global and largely undifferentiated. Play is dependent; pleasure is demonstrated by a quieting attitude (1 month), a smile (2 months), or a squeal (3 months). From 3 to 6 months of age, infants show more discriminate interest in stimuli and begin to play alone with a rattle or a soft stuffed toy or with someone else. There is much more interaction during play. By 4 months of age, they laugh aloud, show a preference for certain toys, and become excited when food or a favorite object is brought to them. They recognize an image in a mirror, smile at it, and vocalize to them.

By 6 months to 1 year of age, play involves sensorimotor skills. Actual games such as peekaboo and pat-a-cake are played. Verbal repetition and imitation of simple gestures occur in response to demonstration. Play is much more selective, not only in terms of specific toys but also in terms of "playmates." Although play is solitary or one-sided, infants choose with whom they will interact. At 6 to 8 months of age, they usually refuse to play with strangers. Parents are definite favorites, and infants know how to attract their attention. At 6 months of age, they extend the arms to be picked up; at 7 months of age, they cough or squeal to make their presence known; at 10 months of age, they pull their parent's clothing; and at 12 months of age, they call them by name. This represents a tremendous advance from the newborn, who signaled biologic needs by crying to express displeasure.

Stimulation is as important for psychosocial growth as food is for physical growth. Knowledge of developmental milestones allows nurses to guide parents regarding proper play for infants. It is not sufficient to place a mobile over a crib and toys in a play yard for a child's optimal social, emotional, and intellectual development. Likewise, the television or recorded videos, for the most part, do not provide infants with appropriate sensory stimulation, do not increase language skills, and should therefore be restricted in children younger than 2 years of age (AAP Council on Communications and Media, 2011). Play must provide interpersonal contact and recreational and educational stimulation. Infants need to be *played with,* not merely allowed to play. Although the type of play infants engage in is called *solitary,* this is a figurative, not literal, term to denote one-sided play. The type of toys given to the child is much less important than the quality of personal interaction that occurs.

TEMPERAMENT

The infant's temperament or behavioral style influences the type of interaction that occurs between the child and parents, especially the mother, and other family members (see general discussion of temperament in Chapter 28). In assessment of a child's temperament, it is the parents' perception of the child and the degree of fit between their expectations and the child's actual temperament that are important. The more dissonance, or lack of harmony, between the child's temperament and the parent's ability to accept and deal with the behavior, the more risk for subsequent parent-child conflicts.

Although most behavioral researchers agree that there is a strong biologic component to temperament, researchers also suggest that temperament may be modified by the environment, particularly the family (Gallitto, 2015). Family interaction with the infant is perceived as a circular process wherein each family member affects others and the family as a unit. With these concepts in mind, the nurse has an important role in helping the family understand the infant's temperament as it relates to family dynamics and the eventual well-being of the child and family unit.

Some researchers speculate that infant temperament may contribute to parents' depression. Depressed mothers and fathers (vs. nondepressed mothers and fathers) rate their infant's temperament as more difficult at 3 and 18 months of age (Kerstis, Engström, Edlund, et al., 2013). When reciprocity is lacking between the infant and the parent or when the infant's behavior does not meet expectations, there is increased risk for discord. Researchers have correlated fussy infant temperament with the introduction of early complementary feedings (at 3 months of age) (Wasser, Bentley, Borja, et al, 2011) and feeding infants foods that may contribute to obesity (Vollrath, Tonstad, Rothbart, et al., 2011).

Several instruments can measure infant temperament. These instruments include the Revised Infant Temperament Questionnaire (Carey & McDevitt, 1978), the Infant Behavior Questionnaire (Gartstein & Rothbart, 2003), and the Early Infancy Temperament Questionnaire (Medoff-Cooper, Carey, & McDevitt, 1993). In discussing test results to parents, it is best to avoid descriptors (such as, "difficult"); instead, infants can be described in terms of characteristics (such as, "intense" or "less predictable").

With knowledge of the infant's temperament, nurses are better able to (1) provide parents with background information that will help them see their child in a better perspective, (2) offer a more organized picture of their child's behavior and possibly reveal distortions in their perceptions of the behavior, and (3) guide parents regarding appropriate childrearing techniques. Appropriate counseling based on awareness of the child's temperament can greatly enhance the quality of interaction between parents and infant.

Knowledge of the developmental sequence allows the nurse to assess normal growth and minor or abnormal deviations. It also helps parents gain realistic expectations of their child's ability and provides guidelines for suitable play and stimulation. Parents who lack knowledge of child growth and development may set inappropriate behavioral expectations for their child. Emphasizing the child's developmental rather than chronologic age strengthens the parent-child relationship by fostering trust and lessening frustration.

COPING WITH CONCERNS RELATED TO NORMAL GROWTH AND DEVELOPMENT

Separation and Stranger Fear

A number of fears can appear during infancy. However, the fear that causes parents the most concern is fear related to strangers and separation. Although erroneously interpreted by some as a sign of undesirable, antisocial behavior, stranger fear and separation anxiety are important components of a strong, healthy, parent-child attachment. Nevertheless, this period can present difficulties for the parent and child. Parents may experience guilt at having to leave the infant because he or she violently protests being separated from the parents. To accustom the infant to new people, parents are encouraged to have close friends or relatives visit often. This provides other people with whom the child is comfortable and who can give parents time for themselves. Usually toward the end of the first year, infants begin to venture away from the parent and demonstrate curiosity about strangers. If allowed to explore at their own rate, many infants eventually "warm up."

The best approach for the stranger (including nurses) is to talk softly; meet the child at eye level (to appear smaller); maintain a safe distance from the infant; and avoid sudden, intrusive gestures, such as holding the arms out and smiling broadly. If parents hold the child away from their face, the infant can observe while maintaining close physical contact.

Parents also may wonder whether they should encourage the child's clinging, dependent behavior, especially if there is pressure from others who view this as "spoiling." Parents need to be reassured that such

behavior is healthy, desirable, and necessary for the child's optimal emotional development. If parents can reassure the infant of their presence, the infant will learn to realize that they are still there even if not physically present. Talking to infants when leaving the room, allowing them to hear one's voice on the telephone, and using transitional objects (e.g., a favorite blanket or toy) reassures them of the parent's continued presence.

Alternative Child Care Arrangements

For many parents, especially working mothers, locating safe and competent child care facilities for the infant is an increasingly difficult problem—one that is compounded by the number of mothers working outside the home. Over the past 40 years, there has been a marked shift in child care arrangements; whereas the majority of children are cared for in group centers or other settings, an increasing number of children are being cared for in home settings.

The basic types of care are (1) in-home care, either in the parents' or caregivers' home (family day care) and (2) center-based care, usually in a day care center. In-home care may consist of a full-time baby-sitter who lives in the home, a full-time baby-sitter who comes to the home, cooperative arrangements such as exchange baby-sitting, or family day care. A licensed small family child day care home typically provides care and protection for up to six children for part of a day and does not include informal arrangements such as exchange baby-sitting or caregivers in the child's own home. Large family child day care homes may provide care for eight to twelve children. Unfortunately, many family child day care homes operate without a license and may care for large numbers of infants without adequate staff and facilities.

Child center-based care usually refers to a licensed day care facility that provides care for six or more children for 6 or more hours per day. Work-based group care is another option that is becoming increasingly popular as employers recognize the benefit of providing high-quality and convenient child care to their employees. Sick-child care may also be available for times when the child is ill. Such programs are often located in community hospitals or in work settings.

Nurses may fulfill a unique role in guiding parents in locating suitable facilities that have well-qualified staff. State licensing agencies can help parents identify day care centers that accept children of specific age-groups and that are convenient to home and work. Their records are available to the public and provide reports from the health, safety, and fire departments; periodic evaluations from the licensing agency; complaints filed against the center; and qualifications of the center's employees. Early childhood programs may also belong to a voluntary accreditation system, the National Association for the Education of Young Children, which serves as a model for optimal care.*

The same attention should be applied to locating competent baby-sitters. References from other parents are essential, and there is no substitute for observing the interaction between the individual and the child. Although very young infants need little if any preparation for the introduction of a new caregiver, older infants may benefit from a gradual placement to reduce stranger anxiety. At all times, the parent should have the right to visit the child, and regular conferences should be established to review the child's progress. Some child care centers provide a service whereby the parent may log on to the Internet from work and view the child's activity at the center for reassurance that the child is well.

---

*Information about accreditation criteria and procedures of the National Academy for Early Childhood Program Accreditation/NAEYC is available from the National Association for the Education of Young Children, 1313 L Street NW, Suite 500, Washington, DC 20005; 800-424-2460 or 202-232-8777; www.naeyc.org.

Important areas for parents to evaluate are the center's daily program, teacher qualifications, nurturing qualities of caregivers, child-to-staff ratio, discipline policy, environmental safety precautions, provision of meals, sanitary conditions, adequate indoor and outdoor space per child, and fee schedule. Although fees vary considerably, a program that charges a minimum fee may also be providing minimum services. Parents should arrange to meet the director and some of the employees, especially those who would be caring for the child. Resources to familiarize parents with characteristics of quality child care and checklists to systematically evaluate the center and compare it with other facilities can help parents make successful choices.

One of the areas that is increasingly important in selecting child care is the center's health practices. Evidence shows that children, especially those younger than 6 years of age in day care centers, have more illnesses—especially diarrhea, otitis media, respiratory tract infections (especially if the caregiver smokes), hepatitis A, meningitis, and cytomegalovirus—than children cared for in their home. The strongest predictor of risk for illness is the number of unrelated children in the room. Proactive infection control measures and education of staff have been effective in reducing the incidence of upper respiratory tract infections, diarrhea, and rotavirus. It has been reported that families who have children in out-of-home child care lose an estimated 6 to 29 days of work per year as a result of children's illnesses (Shope & Hashikawa, 2012).

Limit Setting and Discipline

As infants' motor skills advance and mobility increases, parents face the need to set safe limits to protect the child and establish a positive and supportive parent-child relationship (see the "Nurse's Role in Injury Prevention" section later in this chapter). Although there are numerous disciplinary techniques, some are more appropriate for this age than others. An effective approach used in disciplining a child is the use of "time-out." The important principle to consider is that the place for time-out needs to be commensurate with the child's abilities. For example, the play yard is better for most infants than a chair. Although parents may be concerned with instituting discipline during infancy, it is important to stress that the earlier effective disciplinary methods are employed, the easier it is to continue these approaches.

Parents must recognize the child's cognitive and behavioral limitations; adequate protection from hazards must be implemented because infants and toddlers do not understand a cause-effect relationship between dangerous objects and physical harm. Children will innately test limits and explore during the exploratory phase of growth; instead of discouraging exploration, parents should provide safe alternatives, put away dangerous household items, and provide consistent discipline and nurturing.

Effective teaching for injury prevention optimally begins in infancy by helping parents understand the nature of their child's normal development. It must be reiterated continually that infants cry because a need is not being met, not to intentionally irritate an adult. A fussy or irritable infant is a potential victim of shaken baby syndrome (or other bodily harm) because adults and caregivers may not understand the nature of the infant's crying.

Thumb-Sucking and Use of a Pacifier

Sucking is the infant's chief pleasure and may not be satisfied by breastfeeding or bottle-feeding. It is such a strong need that infants who are deprived of sucking, such as those with a cleft lip repair, suck on their tongues. Some newborns are born with sucking blisters on their hands from in utero sucking activity.

Problems arise when parents are overly concerned about the sucking of the fingers, thumb, or pacifier and attempt to restrain this natural tendency. Before giving advice, nurses should investigate the parents' feelings and base guidance on this information. Nelson (2012) suggests that it cannot be stated with absolute certainty that pacifier use is bad in every situation.

The American Academy of Pediatrics Task Force on Sudden Infant Death Syndrome (2016) cites strong evidence for a protective effect in SIDS reduction when pacifiers are used at bedtime and nap time. The exact mechanism involved in the protection for SIDS is not known. Still, pacifiers should be cleaned and replaced regularly, and there should be an emphasis on allowing the infant to control the pace, frequency, and termination of feeding rather than allowing the pacifier (or anything else) to become the focus of the interaction. Pacifier use during painful procedures in neonates has been shown to produce an analgesic effect (see Chapter 30). However, pacifier use has been associated with an increased risk for otitis media (Salah, Abdel-Aziz, Al-Farok, et al., 2013). Because of this, the American Academy of Pediatrics Subcommittee on the Management of Acute Otitis Media recommended that parents reduce pacifier usage in the second 6 months of life (Nelson, 2012).

A systematic review found an association between pacifier use in infancy and a reduction in breastfeeding and exclusive breastfeeding (Nelson, 2012). However, the authors concluded that pacifier use and poor breastfeeding outcomes may not have a causal effect; rather, it may be related to a marker for socioeconomic, demographic, psychosocial, and cultural factors that determine pacifier use and breastfeeding. A Cochrane review found that pacifier use in full-term healthy infants started from birth or after lactation did not significantly affect the prevalence of duration of exclusive and partial breastfeeding up to 4 months of age (Jaafar, Jahanfar, Angolkar, et al., 2011). Nonnutritive sucking should not be withheld from preterm infants, especially when used in conjunction with concentrated sucrose for pain management.

To decrease dependence on nonnutritive sucking in young infants, sucking pleasure can be increased by prolonging feeding time. Also, the parent's excessive use of the pacifier to calm the child should be explored. It is not unusual for parents to place a pacifier in the infant's mouth as soon as crying begins, thus reinforcing a pattern of distress-relief.

During infancy and early childhood, there is no need to restrain nonnutritive sucking of the fingers. Malocclusion may occur if thumb sucking persists past approximately 4 years of age, or when the permanent teeth erupt. Some parents may perceive pacifiers as less damaging because they are discarded by 2 to 3 years of age, whereas thumb sucking may persist well into school-age years. Because of the limited number of studies correlating pacifier use and increased risk for infections or dental malocclusion, there are no recommendations for or against pacifier use related to oral health (Nelson, 2012). Both pacifier use and thumb sucking may also have significant cultural variations. Thumb sucking reaches its peak at 18 to 20 months of age and is most prevalent when the child is hungry, tired, or feeling insecure. Persistent thumb sucking in a listless, apathetic child always warrants investigation. It may be a sign of an emotional problem between parent and child or of boredom, isolation, and lack of stimulation.

Teething

One of the more difficult periods in the infant's (and parents') life is the eruption of the deciduous (primary) teeth, often referred to as *teething*. The age of tooth eruption shows considerable variation among children, but the order of their appearance is fairly regular and predictable (Fig. 31.10). The first primary teeth to erupt are the lower central incisors, which appear at approximately 6 to 10 months of age (average 8 months). These are followed closely by the upper central incisors. The following is a quick guide to assessment of deciduous teeth during the first 2 years: Age of the child in months − 6 = Number of teeth. For example: 8 months of age − 6 = 2 teeth at this time.

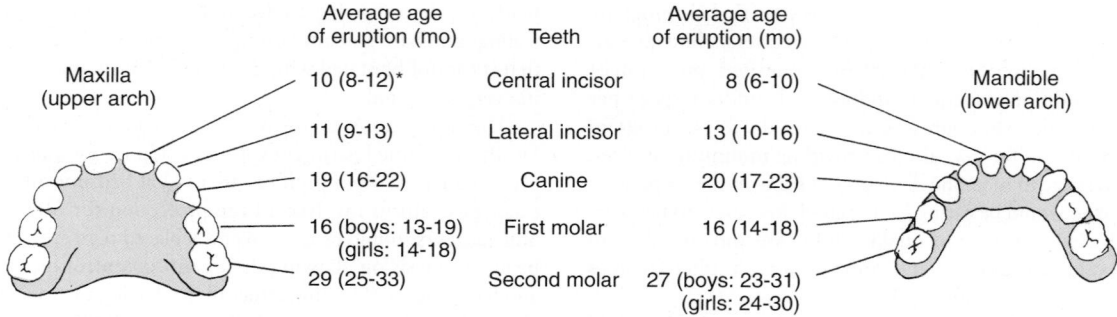

Maxilla (upper arch)	Average age of eruption (mo)	Teeth	Average age of eruption (mo)	Mandible (lower arch)
	10 (8-12)*	Central incisor	8 (6-10)	
	11 (9-13)	Lateral incisor	13 (10-16)	
	19 (16-22)	Canine	20 (17-23)	
	16 (boys: 13-19) (girls: 14-18)	First molar	16 (14-18)	
	29 (25-33)	Second molar	27 (boys: 23-31) (girls: 24-30)	

FIG 31.10 Sequence of eruption of primary teeth. *Range represents ±1 standard deviation, or 67% of subjects studied. (Data from American Dental Association. Retrieved from http://www.mouthhealthy.org/en/az-topics/e/eruption-charts.aspx.)

Teething is a physiologic process; some discomfort is common as the crown of the tooth breaks through the periodontal membrane. Some children show minimal evidence of teething, such as drooling, increased finger sucking, or biting on hard objects. Others are very irritable, have difficulty sleeping, ear rubbing, and decreased interest in solid foods. Generally, signs of illness such as fever, vomiting, or diarrhea are not symptoms of teething but of illness and may warrant further investigation. Because teething pain is a result of inflammation, cold is soothing. Giving the child a cold teething ring helps relieve the inflammation, but do not freeze teething rings filled with gels or nonsterile water because they may crack and leak into the infant's mouth. Several nonprescription topical anesthetic ointments are available, although parents and health care workers should be aware that the active ingredient in most of them is benzocaine, which may rarely cause methemoglobinemia. Therefore, the US Food and Drug Administration recommends use of such products only under the advice and supervision of a health care provider (US Food and Drug Administration, 2014). In the event of persistent irritability that affects sleeping and feeding, systemic analgesics such as acetaminophen or ibuprofen can be given (if age appropriate) for no more than 3 days; however, parents should know that this is a temporary measure and should contact the practitioner if symptoms persist or if the child's condition changes.

The use of teething powders or procedures such as cutting or rubbing the gums with salicylates (aspirin) is discouraged because ingestion of the powder, infection or irritation of the tissue, and ingestion or aspiration of the aspirin can occur. Hard candy may cause accidental choking or aspiration and should be avoided at this age.

PROMOTING OPTIMAL HEALTH DURING INFANCY

NUTRITION

Ideally, discussion of optimal nutrition should begin prenatally with a discussion regarding maternal intake of adequate nutrition in the form of a balanced diet and adequate amounts of protein, vitamins, and minerals, all of which have an impact on the growing fetus. Nurses should encourage and provide information for parents to discuss the options of breastfeeding or bottle-feeding the infant well in advance of the birth date. The choice for either is highly individual and is discussed in Chapter 24. This section is concerned primarily with infant nutrition during the months when growth needs and developmental milestones ready the child for the introduction of solid foods.

Despite adequate availability of optimal nutrient sources, health care experts are concerned that infants are not fed appropriately. Infants may be given solid foods when their digestive system is not ready to completely absorb such foods. In addition, drinks that are inappropriate for growing infants may be given in place of enriched infant milk and may only provide "empty" calories; these drinks contribute to childhood and adult cardiovascular disease and obesity, and place the infant at risk for iron deficiency anemia, vitamin D deficiency, and rickets. A survey of infant feeding practices found that about 20% of infants had consumed solid foods before 4 months of age, despite recommendations that such foods not be introduced until 4 to 6 months of age (Aronsson, Uusitalo, Vehik, et al., 2015). Infant health practices, including nutrition, may have a far-reaching, long-term impact on the child's life. Growth and development could be negatively affected, as could the risk for acquiring certain chronic health conditions. There is some evidence that childhood obesity is significantly decreased when breastfeeding is continued and solid food introduction is delayed until at least 4 months of age (Moss & Yeaton, 2014). Nurses must be proactive in teaching parents what constitutes appropriate infant nutrition and nutritional habits, which provide the child with an optimal opportunity to grow and develop into a healthy child and adult.

The First 6 Months

Human milk is the most desirable complete diet for the infant during the first 6 months. A healthy term infant receiving breast milk from a well-nourished mother usually requires no specific vitamin and mineral supplements, with a few exceptions. Daily supplements of vitamin D and vitamin B_{12} may be indicated if the mother's intake of these vitamins is inadequate. The American Academy of Pediatrics (Wagner, Greer, American Academy of Pediatrics Section on Breastfeeding, et al., 2008) recommends that all infants (including those exclusively breastfed) receive a daily supplement of 400 IU of vitamin D beginning in the first few days of life to prevent rickets and vitamin D deficiency. Vitamin D supplementation should occur until the infant is consuming at least 1 L/day (or 1 qt/day) of vitamin D–fortified formula (Wagner et al., 2008). Non-breastfed infants who are taking less than 1 L/day of vitamin D–fortified formula should also receive a daily vitamin D supplement of 400 IU (see Safety Alert). If the infant is being exclusively breastfed after 4 months (when fetal iron stores are depleted), iron supplementation (1 mg/kg/day) is recommended until appropriate iron-containing complementary foods such as iron-fortified cereal are introduced (Baker, Greer, & AAP Committee on Nutrition, 2010) (see Community Focus box: Administration of Oral Iron Supplements). Infants, whether breastfed or bottle-fed, do not require additional fluids, especially water or juice, during the first 4 months of life. Excessive intake of water in infants may result in water intoxication and hyponatremia.

🏠 COMMUNITY FOCUS

Administration of Oral Iron Supplements

- Ideally, iron supplements should be administered between meals for greater absorption.
- Liquid iron supplements may stain the teeth; therefore administer with a dropper toward the back of the mouth (side). In older children, administer liquid iron supplements through a straw, or rinse mouth thoroughly after ingestion.
- Avoid administration of liquid iron supplements with whole cow's milk or milk products because these bind free iron and prevent absorption.
- Educate parents that iron supplements will turn stools black or tarry green.
- Iron supplements may cause transient constipation. Caution parents not to switch to a low-iron–containing formula or whole milk, which are poor sources of iron and may lead to iron deficiency anemia (see the "Iron Deficiency Anemia" section in Chapter 43).
- In older children, follow liquid iron supplement with a citrus fruit or juice drink (no more than 3–4 oz).
- Avoid administration of iron supplements with foods or drinks that bind iron and prevent absorption (see information earlier in this chapter).

⚡ SAFETY ALERT

There are reports of accidental overdoses of liquid vitamin D in infants caused by packaging errors; the syringe for liquid administration may not be labeled clearly for 400 IU. Nurses should educate parents to read the syringe and to avoid administering more than 400 IU of vitamin D (US Food and Drug Administration Consumer Health Information, 2010).

❗ NURSING ALERT

Warming expressed milk in a microwave decreases the availability of anti-infective properties and nutrients (Labiner-Wolfe & Fein, 2013). To prevent oral burns from uneven warming of the milk, breast milk should never be thawed or rewarmed in a microwave oven. To thaw the frozen milk, either place the container under a lukewarm water bath (<40.5° C [105° F]), or place in a refrigerator overnight.

An alternative to breastfeeding is commercial iron-fortified formula. Similar to human milk, it supplies all nutrients needed by infants for the first 6 months. Unmodified whole cow's milk, low-fat cow's milk, skim milk, other animal milks, and imitation milk drinks are not acceptable as a major source of nutrition for infants because of their limited digestibility, increased risk for contamination, and lack of components needed for appropriate growth. Whole milk can cause iron deficiency anemia in infants, possibly as a result of occult GI blood loss. Pasteurized whole cow's milk is deficient in iron, zinc, and vitamin C and has a high renal solute load, which makes it undesirable for infants younger than 12 months of age (American Academy of Pediatrics, Committee on Nutrition, 2014).

❗ NURSING ALERT

Dietary fat in infants younger than 6 months of age should not be restricted unless on specific medical advice. Substituting skim or low-fat milk is unacceptable, since the essential fatty acids are inadequate and the solute concentration of protein and electrolytes, such as sodium, is too high.

🌐 CULTURAL CONSIDERATIONS

Multicultural Feeding Practices

Cultural beliefs and values often influence infant feeding practices. Health care professionals may benefit from understanding the multicultural feeding practices that parents choose for their infant. Traditional feeding practices include offering a variety of liquids or foods, such as sugared wine, water, or honey during the first few days of life and thereafter.

The amount of formula per feeding and the number of feedings per day vary among infants. Infants being fed on demand usually determine their own feeding schedule, but some infants may need a more planned schedule based on average feeding patterns to ensure sufficient nutrients. In general, the number of feedings decreases from six at 1 month of age to four or five at 6 months of age. Regardless of the number of feedings, the total amount of formula ingested will usually level off at about 32 ounces (946 mL) per day.

Honey should be avoided in the first 12 months because of the risk for botulism (see Chapter 49); a pacifier should not be coated with honey to encourage the infant to take it. Socializing the infant to food flavors of the family's culture is common in addition to continuing breastfeeding for 2 to 4 years (see Cultural Considerations box: Multicultural Feeding Practices).

Bottled water for mixing powdered or concentrated formula is a relatively safe alternative to tap water if available tap water has a high content of contaminants such as lead. Do not assume, however, that bottled water is sterile unless specifically stated on the container. Fluoridated bottled water is not necessary for mixing powdered formula unless the local water source is low in fluoride, in which case fluoride supplementation is recommended after 6 months of age (see the "Dental Health" section later in this chapter).

The addition of solid foods before 4 to 6 months of age is not recommended. During the early months, solid foods are not compatible with the ability of the GI tract and infant's nutritional needs. Feeding solids to young infants exposes them to food antigens that may produce food protein allergy. There is ample evidence that early introduction of foods other than maternal milk in the first 6 months of life predisposes children to an increased risk for food allergy development; foods known to be allergenic (e.g., peanuts, eggs, fish, seafood) should be introduced later than 12 months according to the child's risk for atopy (Heinrich, Koletzko, & Koletzko, 2014).

Developmentally, infants are not ready for solid food. The extrusion (protrusion) reflex is strong and often causes them to push food out of the mouth. Infants instinctively suck when given food. Parents should be cautioned concerning the use of juices and nonnutritive drinks such as fruit-flavored drinks or carbonated beverages (soda or pop) during this period. Many juices and nonnutritive drinks, although readily available to consumers, do not provide sufficient and appropriate caloric intake for infants younger than 12 months of age; such drinks may replace the nutrients in breast milk or formula and lead to growth or health problems.

The Second 6 Months

During the second half of the first year, human milk or formula should continue to be the primary source of nutrition. The use of fluoride supplementation depends on the infant's intake of fluoride tap water (see the "Dental Health" section later in this chapter). If breastfeeding is discontinued, a commercial iron-fortified formula should be substituted. Follow-up or transition formulas marketed for older infants offer no special advantages over other infant formulas and provide excessive protein (American Academy of Pediatrics, Committee on Nutrition, 2014).

The major change in feeding habits is the addition of solid foods to the infant's diet. Physiologically and developmentally, infants 6 months of age are in a transition period. By this time, the GI tract has matured sufficiently to handle more complex nutrients and is less sensitive to potentially allergenic foods. Tooth eruption is beginning and facilitates biting and chewing. The extrusion reflex has disappeared, and swallowing is more coordinated to allow the infant to accept solids easily. Head control is well developed, which permits infants to sit with support and purposely turn the head away to communicate lack of interest in food. Voluntary grasping and improved eye-hand coordination gradually allow infants to pick up finger foods and feed themselves. Their increasing sense of independence is evident in their desire to hold the bottle and try to "help" during feeding.

Selection and Preparation of Solid Foods

The choice of solid foods to introduce first is variable but should meet the reasons for feeding solids, such as supplying nutrients not found in formula or breast milk. Iron-fortified infant cereal is generally introduced first because of its high iron content (7 mg/3 Tbsp of prepared dry cereal). Commercially prepared ready-to-serve dry cereals for infants include rice, barley, oatmeal, and high-protein cereals; rice is usually suggested as an initial food because of its easy digestibility and low allergenic potential. Cereals such as cream of farina should not be used, because infant commercial cereals are a better source of iron. Some of the commercial baby cereals are combined with fruit. There is little nutritional benefit from these preparations, and they are more expensive. New foods should be added one at a time; therefore parents should avoid cereal combinations when beginning a new grain.

Infant cereal (iron fortified) may be mixed with expressed breast milk or water until whole milk is given. After 6 months of age, small amounts of 100% fruit juices can be mixed with the dry cereal; the vitamin C content of the juice enhances the absorption of iron in the cereal. Because of their benefit as a source of iron, infant cereals should be continued until the child is 18 months of age.

Fruit juice can be offered from a cup for its rich source of vitamin C. Avoid fruit-flavored drinks, which may be marketed as juices but contain high concentrations of complex sugars. White grape juice (no more than 5 oz/day) may be better absorbed and safe for infants this age without causing GI distress. The American Academy of Pediatrics, Committee on Nutrition (2014) recommends that fruit juice intake not exceed 4 to 6 ounces per day and that juices not be given to infants younger than 6 months of age. Juice containers are always kept covered and refrigerated to prevent vitamin loss.

The addition of other foods is arbitrary. A common sequence is to introduce strained fruits followed by vegetables and, finally, meats; however, some practitioners prefer to add vegetables before fruit. Commercially prepared baby foods are the most common type of food served to infants in the United States. An alternative is to prepare baby foods at home, which is a simple and inexpensive process. By 1 year of age, well-cooked table foods are served.

The introduction of solid foods into the infant's diet at this age is primarily for taste and chewing experience, not for growth. The majority of the infant's caloric needs are derived from the primary milk source (human or formula); therefore solids should not be perceived as a substitute for milk until the child is older than 12 months of age. Portion sizes may vary according to the infant's taste. In general, 1 tablespoon per year of age (i.e., $\frac{1}{2}$ to $\frac{3}{4}$ tablespoon for most infants younger than 12 months of age) is adequate for most infants. The addition of solid foods to the exclusively breastfed infants' diet does not significantly increase overall caloric intake or weight gain.

Parents are cautioned to avoid reliance on food supplements marketed as iron- or vitamin-fortified as primary sources of minerals. Instead, encourage parents to offer the child a variety of fruits, vegetables, and whole grains, including those known to naturally be rich in iron.

Introduction of Solid Foods

When the spoon is first introduced, infants often push it away and appear dissatisfied. Patience and skill are required to overcome this initial response. Food that is placed on the front of the tongue and pushed out is simply scooped up and refed. As infants become accustomed to the spoon, they more eagerly accept the food and eventually will open the mouth in anticipation (or keep it closed in dislike).

One food item is introduced at intervals of 4 to 7 days to allow for identification of food allergies. New foods are fed in small amounts. As the amount of solid food increases, the quantity of milk is decreased to less than 1 liter daily to prevent overfeeding.

Because feeding is a learning process as well as a means of nutrition, new foods are given alone to allow the child to learn new tastes and textures. Food should not be mixed in the bottle and fed through a nipple with a large hole. This deprives the child of the pleasure of learning new tastes and of developing a discriminating palate. It can also cause problems with poor chewing of food later in life because of lack of experience.

Parents are encouraged to interpret the infant's signals of discomfort and intervene in ways other than through feeding. Crying, fussiness, and sucking do not necessarily indicate hunger. Rocking, stroking, holding, and offering a toy or a pacifier may be more appropriate than automatically responding with food.

Weaning

Defined as the process of giving up one method of feeding for another, *weaning* usually refers to relinquishing the breast or bottle for a cup. In Western societies, this is generally regarded as a major task for infants and is often seen as a potentially traumatic experience. It is psychologically significant because the infant is required to give up a major source of oral pleasure and gratification. Other cultural groups define weaning in relation to significant life events (e.g., teething) or reaching a specific age. No one time for weaning is best for every child, but generally, most infants show signs of readiness during the second half of the first year. It is recommended that weaning be accomplished with the infant's needs as a guide (Lawrence & Lawrence, 2011). Their increasing desire for freedom of movement may lessen their desire to be held close for feedings. They are acquiring more control over their actions and can easily manipulate a cup to their lips. Imitation becomes a powerful motivator by 8 or 9 months of age, and they enjoy using a cup or glass like others do.

Weaning should be gradual, replacing one bottle-feeding or breastfeeding session at a time. The nighttime feeding is usually the last feeding to be discontinued. It is advisable never to begin allowing a child to take a bottle of milk to bed; this is a major cause of early childhood caries in deciduous teeth. If breastfeeding is terminated before 5 or 6 months of age, weaning should be to a bottle to provide for the infant's continued sucking needs. If breastfeeding is discontinued later, weaning can be directly to a cup, especially by 12 to 14 months of age. Any sweet liquid, such as fruit juice, should be given in a cup and should not be given at bedtime.

SLEEP AND ACTIVITY

Sleep patterns vary among infants, with active infants typically sleeping less than placid children. The total daily sleep for 2-month-old infants is approximately 15 hours (range 10 to 20 hours), whereas the total daily sleep for 6- to 12-month-old infants is approximately 13 hours (range 9 to 17 hours) (Galland, Taylor, Elder, et al., 2012). Consolidation of nocturnal sleep hours occurs during the first 12 months with decreasing daytime sleep and increasing nighttime sleep. The number of naps per day varies, but infants typically take two naps by the end of the first year. Breastfed infants usually sleep for shorter periods, with more frequent waking, especially during the night, compared with bottle-fed infants (Middlemiss, Yaure, & Huey, 2015).

Most infants are naturally active and need no encouragement to be mobile. Problems can arise when devices such as play yards, strollers, commercial swings, and mobile walkers are used excessively. These items restrict movement and prevent infants from exploring and developing gross motor skills. Contrary to popular belief, mobile walkers do not enhance coordination and are dangerous if tipped over or placed near stairs, porches, in-ground pools, furnaces, and other hazardous surfaces.

DENTAL HEALTH

Good dental hygiene begins with appropriate maternal dental health before and during the pregnancy and counseling during early infancy regarding dietary intake for the promotion of optimal oral hygiene. Counsel parents early regarding feeding practices that increase the risk for poor dental health. Some of these, as previously mentioned, include propping the milk bottle, giving the milk bottle in the bed, or giving fruit juices in a bottle. These contribute to enamel erosion and *early childhood caries* (previously called *baby bottle tooth decay*). Parents should also be made aware that dental caries is contagious and can be prevented with optimal oral hygiene starting in infancy (Okunseri, Gonzalez, & Hodgson, 2015).

Once the primary teeth erupt, cleaning should begin. The teeth and gums are initially cleaned by wiping with a damp cloth; toothbrushing is too harsh for the tender gingiva. The caregiver can stabilize the infant by cradling the child with one arm and using the free hand to cleanse the teeth. Oral hygiene can be made pleasant by singing or talking to the infant. It is recommended that the infant have a brief oral health examination by 6 months of age from a qualified pediatric health care practitioner; infants at high risk for caries are identified, and oral health counseling is implemented. It is also recommended that the infant have an established dental home by 1 year of age (American Academy of Pediatric Dentistry, 2014). It is generally recommended that a small, soft-bristled toothbrush be used as more teeth erupt and the infant adjusts to the routine of cleaning. Water is preferred to toothpaste, which the infant will swallow (and if the toothpaste is fluoridated, the infant may ingest excessive amounts of fluoride).

Fluoride, an essential mineral for building caries-resistant teeth, is needed beginning at 6 months of age if the infant does not receive water with adequate fluoride content. The American Academy of Pediatric Dentistry (2014) recommends that the determination of fluoride administration be based on the individual needs of each child. Systemic fluoride administration should be considered for all children at risk for dental caries who drink fluoride-deficient water (<0.6 ppm) but only after determining all dietary sources of fluoride.

IMMUNIZATIONS

One of the most dramatic advances in pediatrics has been the decline of infectious diseases during the twentieth century because of the widespread use of immunization for preventable diseases. This trend has continued into the twenty-first century with the development of newer vaccines. Although many of the immunizations can be given to individuals of any age, the recommended primary schedule begins during infancy and, with the exception of boosters, is completed during early childhood.

Therefore, health promotion during infancy includes a discussion of childhood immunizations for diphtheria, tetanus, and acellular pertussis (DTaP); poliovirus; measles, mumps, and rubella (MMR); *Haemophilus influenzae* type b (Hib); hepatitis A virus (HAV); hepatitis B virus (HBV); pneumococcal conjugate vaccine (PCV); influenza; meningococcal; and varicella-zoster virus (VZV; chickenpox).

Schedule for Immunizations

In the United States, two organizations—the Advisory Committee on Immunization Practices of the Centers for Disease Control and Prevention and the Committee on Infectious Diseases of the American Academy of Pediatrics—govern the recommendations for immunization policies and procedures. In Canada, recommendations are from the National Advisory Committee on Immunization under the authority of the Minister of Health and Public Health Agency of Canada. The policies of each committee are recommendations, not rules, and they change as a result of advances in the field of immunology. Nurses need to be knowledgeable about the purpose of each organization, view immunization practices in light of the needs of each individual child and the community, and keep informed of the latest advances and changes in policy.

In the United States, the recommended age for beginning primary immunizations of infants is at birth. Infants born preterm should receive the full dose of each vaccine at the appropriate chronologic age. Recommended schedules for children not immunized during infancy are available at the Centers for Disease Control and Prevention website (http://www.cdc.gov/vaccines/schedules/index.html). Immunization recommendation schedules for Canadian children are available at http://www.phac-aspc.gc.ca/im/is-cv/index-eng.php.

Children who began primary immunizations at the recommended age but fail to receive all of the doses do not need to begin the series again but, instead, receive only the missed doses. For situations in which there is doubt that the child will return for immunization according to the optimal schedule, HBV vaccine (HepB), DTaP, IPV (poliovirus vaccine), MMR, varicella, and Hib vaccines can be administered simultaneously at separate injection sites. Parenteral vaccines are given in separate syringes in different injection sites (American Academy of Pediatrics, Committee on Infectious Diseases, 2015).

Recommendations for Routine Immunizations*
Hepatitis a Virus

Hepatitis A has been recognized as a significant child health problem, particularly in communities with unusually high infection rates. HAV is spread by the fecal-oral route and from person-to-person contact, by ingestion of contaminated food or water, and rarely by blood transfusion. The illness has an abrupt onset, with fever, malaise, anorexia, nausea, abdominal discomfort, dark urine, and jaundice being the most common clinical signs of infection. In children younger than 6 years of age, who represent approximately one-third of all cases of hepatitis A, the disease may be asymptomatic, and jaundice is rarely evident.

HepA vaccine is now recommended for all children beginning at 1 year of age (i.e., 12 months to 23 months). The second dose in the two-dose series may be administered no sooner than 6 months after the first dose.

---

*Because of constant changes in the pharmaceutical industry, trade names of single and combination vaccines in this section may differ from those currently available. The reader is encouraged to access the vaccine page of the Center for Biologics Evaluation and Research (CBER) of the Food and Drug Administration for the latest licensed vaccine trade names: http://www.fda.gov/BiologicsBloodVaccines/default.htm.

Hepatitis B Virus

Hepatitis B (HBV) is a significant pediatric disease because HBV infections that occur during childhood and adolescence can lead to fatal consequences from cirrhosis or liver cancer during adulthood. Up to 90% of infants infected perinatally and 25% to 50% of children infected before 5 years of age become HBV carriers. In addition, the incidence of HBV infection increases rapidly during adolescence (American Academy of Pediatrics, Committee on Infectious Diseases, 2015). It is recommended that newborns receive the HepB vaccine before hospital discharge if the mother is hepatitis B surface antigen (HBsAg) negative. Monovalent HepB vaccine should be given as the birth dose, whereas a combination vaccine containing HepB may be given for subsequent doses in the series. Both full-term and preterm infants born to mothers whose HBsAg status is positive or unknown should receive HepB vaccine and hepatitis B immune globulin (HBIG) within 12 hours of birth at two different injection sites. Because the immune response to the HepB vaccine is not optimal in newborns weighing less than 2000 g (4.4 pounds), the first HepB vaccine dose should be given to such infants at a chronologic age of 1 month, as long as the mother's HBsAg status is negative (American Academy of Pediatrics, Committee on Infectious Diseases, 2015). In the event that the preterm infant is given a dose at birth, the current recommendation is that the infant be given the full series (three additional doses) at 1, 2, and 6 months of age. The American Academy of Pediatrics Committee on Infectious Diseases (2015) also encourages immunization of all children by 11 years of age.

The vaccine is given intramuscularly in the vastus lateralis in newborns or in the deltoid for older infants and children. Regardless of age, avoid the dorsogluteal site because it has been associated with low antibody seroconversion rates, indicating a reduced immune response. No data exist regarding the seroconversion when the ventrogluteal site is used. The vaccine can be safely administered simultaneously at a separate site with DTaP, MMR, and Hib vaccines.

Diphtheria

Although cases of diphtheria are rare in the United States, the disease can result in significant morbidity. Respiratory manifestations include respiratory nasopharyngitis or obstructive laryngotracheitis with upper airway obstruction. The cutaneous manifestations of the disease include vaginal, otic, conjunctival, or cutaneous lesions, which are seen primarily in urban homeless people and in the tropics (American Academy of Pediatrics, Committee on Infectious Diseases, 2015). Administer a single dose of equine antitoxin intravenously to the child with clinical symptoms because of the often fulminant progression of the disease (American Academy of Pediatrics, Committee on Infectious Diseases, 2015). Diphtheria vaccine is commonly administered as follows:

1. In combination with tetanus and pertussis vaccines (DTaP) or DTaP and Hib vaccines for children younger than 7 years of age
2. In combination with a conjugate Hib vaccine
3. In a combined vaccine with tetanus (DT) for children younger than 7 years of age who have some contraindication to receiving pertussis vaccine
4. In combination with tetanus and acellular pertussis (Tdap) for children 11 years of age and older

OR

5. As a single antigen when combined antigen preparations are not indicated

Although the diphtheria vaccine does not produce absolute immunity, protective antitoxin persists for 10 years or more when given according to the recommended schedule, and boosters are given every 10 years for life (see later discussion for adolescent diphtheria and acellular pertussis and tetanus toxoid recommendation). Several vaccines contain diphtheria toxoid (Hib, meningococcal, pneumococcal), but this does not confer immunity to the disease.

Tetanus

Three forms of tetanus vaccine—tetanus toxoid, tetanus immunoglobulin (TIG) (human), and tetanus antitoxin (equine antitoxin)—are available; however, tetanus antitoxin is no longer available in the United States. Tetanus toxoid is used for routine primary immunization, usually in one of the combinations listed for diphtheria, and provides protective antitoxin levels for approximately 10 years.

Tetanus and diphtheria toxoids along with acellular pertussis vaccine (Tdap, adolescent formulation) are now recommended for children 11 to 12 years of age who have completed the recommended DTaP/DTP vaccine series but have not received the tetanus (Td) booster dose. Adolescents 13 to 18 years of age who have not received the Td/Tdap booster should receive a single Tdap booster, provided the routine DTaP/DTP childhood immunization series has been previously received. In response to the increase in cases of pertussis in children, adolescents, and adults, the Centers for Disease Control and Prevention (Advisory Committee on Immunization Practices) now recommend administration of a Tdap booster regardless of the time interval from the last tetanus- or diphtheria-toxoid containing vaccine (DTaP, DTP, Td, or Tdap). In addition, children 7 to 10 years of age who are not fully vaccinated for pertussis (did not receive five doses of DTaP or four doses of DTaP with the fourth dose being administered on or after the fourth birthday) should receive a dose of Tdap (Centers for Disease Control and Prevention, 2011). It is recommended that children receive subsequent Td boosters every 10 years (American Academy of Pediatrics, Committee on Infectious Diseases, 2015).

For wound management, passive immunity is available with TIG. People with a history of two previous doses of tetanus toxoid can receive a booster dose of the toxoid. Separate syringes and different sites are used when tetanus toxoid and TIG are given concurrently.

For children older than 7 years of age who require wound prophylaxis, tetanus immunization may be accomplished by administering Td (adult-type diphtheria and tetanus toxoids). If TIG is not available, the equine antitoxin (not available in the United States) may be administered after appropriate testing for sensitivity. The antitoxin is administered in a separate syringe and at a separate intramuscular site if given concurrently with tetanus toxoid.

Pertussis

Pertussis vaccine is recommended for all children 6 weeks to 6 years of age (up to the seventh birthday) who have no neurologic contraindications to its use. Concerns over outbreaks of the disease in the past decade have prompted discussion about vaccinating infants and adults. Many cases of pertussis have occurred in those younger than 6 months of age or older than 7 years of age, both groups falling in the category for which pertussis immunization previously was not recommended. The tetanus and diphtheria toxoids and acellular pertussis vaccine (Tdap) is now recommended at 11 to 12 years of age for children who have completed the DTaP/DTP childhood series. The Tdap is also recommended for adolescents 13 to 18 years of age who have not received a tetanus booster (Td) or Tdap dose and have completed the childhood DTaP/DTP series. When the Tdap is used as a booster dose, it may be administered regardless of the interval from the previous tetanus, diphtheria, and pertussis-containing vaccine. In addition, children 7 to 10 years of age who are not fully vaccinated for pertussis (i.e., did not receive five doses of DTaP or four doses of DTaP, with the fourth dose being administered on or after the fourth birthday) should receive a dose of Tdap (Centers for Disease Control and Prevention, 2011) (see discussion in the "Tetanus" section earlier in the chapter).

Currently, two forms of pertussis vaccine are available in the United States. The whole-cell pertussis vaccine is prepared from inactivated cells of *Bordetella pertussis* and contains multiple antigens. In contrast, the acellular pertussis vaccine contains one or more immunogens derived from the *B. pertussis* organism. The highly purified acellular vaccine is associated with fewer local and systemic reactions than those occurring with the whole-cell vaccine in children of similar age. The acellular pertussis vaccine is recommended by the American Academy of Pediatrics (2015) for the first three immunizations and is usually given at 2, 4, and 6 months of age with diphtheria and tetanus (DTaP). Several forms of acellular pertussis vaccine are currently licensed for use in infants: Daptacel, Pediarix, Kinrix (DTaP and IPV), and Infanrix (diphtheria, tetanus toxoid, and acellular pertussis conjugate). Pentacel is licensed for use in infants 4 weeks of age and older; in addition to acellular pertussis, diphtheria, and tetanus, this vaccine also contains inactivated poliovirus (IPV) and Hib conjugate. Either the acellular or whole-cell vaccine may be given for the fourth and fifth doses, but the acellular vaccine is preferred. It is also recommended that the first three DTaP vaccinations be from the same manufacturer. The fourth dose may be from a different manufacturer. The child who has received one or more whole-cell vaccines may complete the series of five with the acellular vaccine.

Health care workers who may be susceptible to pertussis as a result of waning immunity and who have potential exposure to children or adults with pertussis should receive a single dose of Tdap (if not previously vaccinated with same) and take the necessary protective precautions against droplet contamination (wear procedural or surgical masks and practice hand washing). The diagnosis of pertussis may be missed or delayed in unvaccinated infants, who often are seen with respiratory distress and apnea without the typical cough. Additional guidelines for prevention and treatment of pertussis among health care workers and close contacts are available from the Centers for Disease Control and Prevention website (www.cdc.gov/vaccines/).

Polio

An all-IPV (inactivated poliovirus) vaccine schedule for routine childhood polio vaccination is now recommended for children in the United States. All children should receive four doses of IPV at 2 months, 4 months, 6 to 18 months, and 4 to 6 years of age (American Academy of Pediatrics, Committee on Infectious Diseases, 2015).

The change from the exclusive use of oral polio vaccine (OPV) to the exclusive use of the IPV vaccine is related to the rare risk for vaccine-associated polio paralysis (VAPP) from OPV. The exclusive use of the IPV vaccine eliminates the risk for VAPP but is associated with an increased number of injections and increased cost. Since IPV vaccine usage was instituted in the United States in 2000, no new indigenously acquired cases of VAPP have occurred. PEDIARIX is a combination vaccine containing DTaP, hepatitis B, and IPV; this may be used as the primary immunization beginning at 2 months of age (American Academy of Pediatrics, Committee on Infectious Diseases, 2015). KINRIX contains DTaP and IPV, and it may be used as the fifth dose in the DTaP series and the fourth dose in the IPV series in children 4 to 6 years of age whose previous vaccine doses have been with INFANRIX and/or PEDIARIX for the first three doses and INFANRIX for the fourth dose. As noted earlier, Pentacel is also licensed for use in infants 4 weeks of age and older and contains DTaP, Hib, and IPV. PEDIARIX has been licensed for use in children as young as 6 weeks of age and contains DTaP, Hep B, and IPV.

Measles

The measles (rubeola) vaccine is given at 12 to 15 months of age. During the course of measles outbreaks, the vaccine can be given at 6 to 11 months of age, followed by a second inoculation after 12 months of age. The second measles immunization is recommended at 4 to 6 years of age (at school entry) but may be given earlier provided that 4 weeks have elapsed since the previous dose. Revaccination should occur by 11 to 12 years of age if the measles vaccine was not administered at school entry (4 to 6 years of age). Any child who is vaccinated before 12 months of age should receive two additional doses beginning at 12 to 15 months and separated by at least 4 weeks (American Academy of Pediatrics, Committee on Infectious Diseases, 2015). Revaccination should include all individuals born after 1956 who have not received two doses of measles vaccine after 12 months of age. Individuals born before this date are thought to be immune from exposure to natural measles virus. Because of the continuing occurrence of measles in older children and young adults, identify potentially susceptible individuals and immunize them if two doses of measles vaccine have not been administered previously or the person had a confirmed case of the illness.

The measles, mumps, rubella, and varicella (MMRV) vaccine is an attenuated live virus vaccine and may be given to children 12 to 15 months of age and before or at 4 to 6 years of age concurrent with other vaccines. Children with immune deficiencies should not receive the MMRV vaccine because of a lack of evidence of its safety in this population.

Mumps

Mumps virus vaccine is recommended for children 12 to 15 months of age and is typically given in combination with measles and rubella. It should not be administered to infants younger than 12 months of age because persisting maternal antibodies can interfere with the immune response.

Because of recent outbreaks of the disease, especially in children 10 to 19 years of age, mumps immunization is recommended for all individuals born after 1957 who may be susceptible to mumps (i.e., those who have no history of having had the disease or vaccine and who have no laboratory evidence of immunity).

Rubella

Rubella is a relatively mild infection in children, but in a pregnant woman the actual infection presents serious risks to the developing fetus. Therefore the aim of rubella immunization is actually protection of the unborn child rather than the recipient of the immunization.

Rubella immunization is recommended for all children at 12 to 15 months of age and at the age of school entry or 4 to 6 years of age, according to the routine recommendations for MMRV vaccine (American Academy of Pediatrics, Committee on Infectious Diseases, 2015). Increased emphasis should also be placed on vaccinating all unimmunized prepubertal children and susceptible adolescents and adult women in the childbearing age-group. Because the live attenuated virus may cross the placenta and theoretically present a risk to the developing fetus, rubella vaccine is currently not given to any pregnant woman. Postpubertal females without evidence of rubella immunity should be immunized unless they are pregnant; they should be counseled not to become pregnant for 28 days after receiving the rubella-containing vaccine (American Academy of Pediatrics, Committee on Infectious Diseases, 2015).

Pneumococcal Infections

Streptococcal pneumococci are responsible for a number of bacterial infections in children younger than 2 years of age, which may cause serious morbidity and mortality. Among these are generalized infections such as septicemia and meningitis or localized infections such as otitis media, sinusitis, and pneumonia. These illnesses are particularly problematic in children who attend day care facilities (the incidence in day care children is two or three times higher than in children not attending out-of-home day care) and in those who are immuno-compromised. A 13-valent pneumococcal conjugate vaccine (PCV 13 [Prevnar 13]) has been licensed for use and is currently recommended as the standard pneumococcal vaccine for children 6 weeks to 24 months of age. Children who have started the PCV series with PCV 7 may complete the vaccine series with PCV 13 (American Academy of Pediatrics, Committee on Infectious Diseases, 2015; Centers for Disease Control and Prevention, 2013).

The PCV 13 vaccine is administered at 2, 4, and 6 months of age, with a fourth dose at 12 to 15 months of age. A single supplemental dose of PCV 13 is recommended for children 14 to 59 months of age who have received an age-appropriate series of PCV 7. PCV 13 is also recommended for all children younger than 24 months of age and for older children (24 to 71 months of age) with sickle cell disease; functional or anatomic asplenia; nephrotic syndrome or chronic renal failure; conditions associated with immunosuppression (e.g., solid organ transplantation); diabetes mellitus; cochlear implants; congenital immunodeficiency; human immunodeficiency virus (HIV) infection; cerebrospinal fluid leaks; chronic cardiovascular disease (e.g., congestive heart failure or cardiomyopathy); chronic pulmonary disease (e.g., emphysema or cystic fibrosis, but not asthma); chronic liver disease (e.g., cirrhosis); or exposure to living environments or social settings in which the risk for invasive pneumococcal disease or its complications is very high (e.g., Alaskan Native, African-American, and certain Native American populations). The PCV 13 vaccine may be administered in conjunction with all other immunizations in a separate syringe and at a separate intramuscular site. The PPSV23 (pneumococcal polysaccharide [23-valent] vaccine) is not recommended for children younger than 24 months of age who do not have one of the high-risk conditions described previously. One dose of PPSV23 is recommended in children older than 23 months of age who have one of the high-risk conditions after primary immunization with PCV 13.

Haemophilus influenzae Type B

Hib conjugate vaccines protect against a number of serious infections caused by *H. influenza* type b, especially bacterial meningitis, epiglottitis, bacterial pneumonia, septic arthritis, and sepsis (Hib is not associated with the viruses that cause influenza, or "flu"). Hib vaccines that are currently available include PedvaxHIB, Pentacel, and Comvax, which are combination vaccines; Hiberix; and ActHIB. Pentacel is described in the "Pertussis" section earlier in this chapter. MenHibrix has been licensed for administration to children 6 weeks to 18 months of age and provides protection against meningococcal (groups A, C, Y, and W-135) as well as *Haemophilus influenzae* type b (Hib) infections. MenHibrix is administered in a four-dose series at 2, 4, 6, and 12 to 15 months of age. These conjugate vaccines connect Hib to a nontoxic form of another organism, such as meningococcal protein, tetanus toxoid, or diphtheria protein. There is no antibody response to these nontoxic proteins, but they significantly improve the antibody response to Hib, especially in infants. The use of combination vaccines provides equivalent immunogenicity and decreases the number of injections an infant receives. However, it is important that they be given to the appropriate-age child. Hiberix is a conjugate vaccine licensed for use as the booster (final) dose of the Hib vaccine series for children 15 months to 4 years of age (Briere, Rubin, Moro, et al., 2014). In 2013, the American Academy of Pediatrics Committee on Infectious Diseases clarified that only one dose of Hib vaccine should be given to children 15 months of age or older who have not been previously vaccinated (American Academy of Pediatrics, Committee on Infectious Diseases, 2013).

When possible, the Hib conjugate vaccine used at the first vaccination should be used for all subsequent vaccinations in the primary series.

All Hib vaccines are administered by intramuscular injection using a separate syringe and at a site separate from any concurrent vaccinations.

> **! NURSING ALERT**
>
> The use of meningococcal and diphtheria proteins in combination vaccines does not mean the child has received adequate immunization for meningococcal or diphtheria illnesses; the child must be given the appropriate vaccine for that specific disease.

Varicella

Administration of the cell-free live-attenuated varicella vaccine is recommended for any susceptible child (one who lacks proof of varicella vaccination or has a reliable history of varicella infection). A single dose of 0.5 mL should be given by subcutaneous injection. The first dose of varicella vaccine is recommended for children 12 to 15 months of age, and to ensure adequate protection, a second varicella vaccine is recommended for children 4 to 6 years of age. The second varicella vaccine may be administered before 4 years of age as long as a period of 3 months occurs between the first and second dose. Children 13 years of age or older who are susceptible should receive two doses administered at least 4 weeks apart. Children in the same age-group (13 to 18 years of age) who have received only one previous varicella vaccine should receive a second varicella vaccine. The combination vaccine MMRV (ProQuad) is licensed for use in children 12 months to 12 years of age.

According to the American Academy of Pediatrics Committee on Infectious Diseases (2015), children who have received two doses of the varicella vaccine are one-third less likely to have breakthrough illness in the first 10 years of immunization in comparison with those who have received one dose. Children who do contract varicella after immunization reportedly have milder cases with fewer vesicles, lower degree of fever, and faster recovery. Antibodies persist for at least 8 years.

Varicella vaccine may be administered simultaneously with MMR. However, separate syringes and injection sites should be used. If they are not administered simultaneously, the interval between administration of varicella vaccine and MMR should be at least 1 month. Varicella vaccine may also be given simultaneously with DTaP, IPV, HepB, or Hib vaccine (American Academy of Pediatrics, Committee on Infectious Diseases, 2015).

Influenza

The influenza vaccine is recommended annually for children starting at 6 months of age. Influenza vaccine (inactivated influenza vaccine [IIV*]) may be given to healthy children 6 months of age and older. The vaccine is administered in early fall before the flu season begins and is repeated yearly for ongoing protection. The intramuscular vaccine is administered as two separate doses 4 weeks apart in first-time recipients younger than 9 years of age. The dose is 0.25 mL for children 6 to 35 months of age and 0.5 mL for children 3 years of age and older. The vaccine may be given simultaneously with other vaccines but in a separate syringe and at a separate site. The vaccine is administered yearly because different strains of influenza are used each year in the manufacture of the vaccine. The Advisory Committee on Immunization Practices

---

*The trivalent inactivated influenza vaccine (TIV) was changed to inactivated influenza vaccine (IIV) because of the anticipated quadrivalent influenza vaccine in the 2013–2014 season (AAP Committee on Infectious Diseases, 2013).

(Grohskopf, Sokolow, Olsen, et al., 2015) recommends an assessment of the egg allergenic reaction prior to making a decision about the vaccine administration to children who have a history of egg allergy. Several options for administering the influenza vaccine are described in the literature, and individuals should discuss the risks and benefits with a knowledgeable health care practitioner.

The live attenuated influenza vaccine (LAIV) is an acceptable alternative to the intramuscular vaccine in specific age-groups. The vaccine is given nasally as two doses at least 28 days apart in healthy people 2 to 49 years of age. The LAIV form is not recommended for children 2 to 4 years of age with wheezing in the previous 12 months or those diagnosed with asthma (Grohskopf et al., 2015; American Academy of Pediatrics, Committee on Infectious Diseases, 2013). Although the LAIV is an alternative to the injection, it costs more and may not be covered by insurance companies. Either IIV or LAIV may be given to healthy, nonpregnant individuals 2 to 49 years of age (American Academy of Pediatrics, Committee on Infectious Diseases, 2015). Yearly influenza vaccine should be administered to health care workers and to children 6 to 59 months of age with medical conditions (including asthma, cardiac disease, HIV, diabetes, and sickle cell disease) that place them at risk for influenza-related complications.

Meningococcal Infections

Invasive meningococcal disease continues to be the cause of high morbidity in children in the United States. Infants younger than 1 year of age are particularly susceptible, yet the highest fatalities occur in adolescents (approximately 20%). There is also evidence that the risk for meningococcal infections is high in college freshmen living in dormitories. Meningococcal infections are also responsible for significant morbidities, including limb or digit amputation, skin scarring, hearing loss, and neurologic disabilities.

Neisseria meningitidis is the leading cause of bacterial meningitis in the United States. It is not recommended that children 9 months to 10 years of age routinely receive the meningococcal conjugate vaccines because the infection rate is low in this age-group. Children at increased risk for meningococcal infection should receive a two-dose series of either MenACY-D (Menactra) or MenACY-CRM (Menveo), both of which are MCV-4 vaccines, or the infant series of MenHibrix (Hib-MenCY) given at least 2 months apart. These include children with terminal complement component deficiency, anatomic or functional asplenia, or HIV. Children 2 to 18 years of age who travel to or reside in countries where *N. meningitidis* is hyperendemic or epidemic or who are at risk during a community outbreak should receive one dose of MCV-4 (either Menveo or Menactra). Menactra is licensed for administration in children as young as 9 months of age, whereas Menveo is licensed only for children 2 years of age and older.

Children and adolescents 11 to 12 years of age should receive a single immunization of MCV-4 (either Menactra or Menveo) and a booster of the same at 16 to 18 years of age. Others at high risk who should receive MCV-4 include college freshmen living in dormitories and military recruits. MenHibrix has been licensed for administration to children 6 weeks to 18 months of age and provides protection against meningococcal (groups A, C, Y, and W-135) as well as Hib infections. MenHibrix is administered in a four-dose series at 2, 4, 6, and 12 to 15 months of age.

People who are at high risk for the disease and previously received MPSV4 (meningococcal polysaccharide vaccine) 3 or more years previously should be reimmunized with MCV-4. MCV-4 (Menveo or Menactra) is administered as an intramuscular injection (0.5 mL) and may be administered in conjunction with other vaccines in a separate syringe and at a separate site. Immunization with MCV-4 is contraindicated in people with hypersensitivity to any components of the vaccine, including diphtheria toxoid, and to rubber latex (part of vial stopper).

Recommendations for Selected Immunizations

Two additional vaccines are recommended for children and adolescents at high risk for particular diseases. Two rotavirus vaccines, RotaTeq (RV5) and Rotarix (RV1), have received a license from the US Food and Drug Administration for distribution in the United States. Rotavirus is one of the leading causes of severe diarrhea in infants and young children. RotaTeq is licensed for administration to infants 6 to 12 weeks of age, with two additional doses administered at 4- to 10-week intervals but not after 32 weeks of age; the dose is 2 mL, and the product must be protected from light until administration (American Academy of Pediatrics, Committee on Infectious Diseases, 2015). Rotarix may be administered beginning at 6 weeks of age with a second dose at least 4 weeks after the first dose but before 24 weeks of age. Both vaccines are administered orally.

Three human papillomavirus (HPV) vaccines have been licensed for use in adolescents; a bivalent HPV vaccine (HPV2), a quadrivalent HPV vaccine (HPV4), and a nine-valent HPV vaccine (HPV9) have been approved and recommended for female children and adolescents to prevent HPV-related cervical cancer. The vaccine is administered intramuscularly in three separate doses; the first dose in the series may be given at 11 to 12 years of age (minimum age, 9 years), and the second dose is administered 2 months after the first, with the third dose being given 6 months after the first dose. The HPV4 or HPV9 vaccine may also be administered to boys and men 9 to 26 years of age in a three-dose series to reduce the likelihood of genital warts (Petrosky, Bocchini, Hariri, et al., 2015; American Academy of Pediatrics, Committee on Infectious Diseases, 2015). The bivalent vaccine (HPV2), Cervarix, is licensed for use in girls and women 10 to 25 years of age for the prevention of HPV-related cervical cancer; this vaccine is given in a three-dose series.

Reactions

Vaccines for routine immunizations are among the safest and most reliable drugs available. However, minor side effects do occur after many of the immunizations, and, rarely, a serious reaction may result from the vaccine. A number of inactive components are incorporated in vaccines to enhance their effectiveness and safety. Some of these components include preservatives, stabilizers, adjuvants, antibiotics (e.g., neomycin), and purified culture medium proteins (e.g., egg) to enhance effectiveness. A child may react to the preservative in the vaccine rather than the vaccine component; an example of this is the hepatitis B vaccine, which is prepared from yeast cultures.

Some vaccines contain a preservative, thimerosal, that contains ethyl mercury. Concerns regarding possible mercury poisoning in the 1990s prompted many to put off vaccination of infants and small children for fear of childhood developmental problems, such as autism. A number of manufacturers have since stopped producing vaccines containing thimerosal. Studies on thimerosal and the potential link to autism or any other pervasive developmental disorder failed to establish a causal relationship between the two (Price, Thompson, Goodson, et al., 2010; Schultz, 2010). A recent systematic review concluded that there was no link between autism and the MMR vaccine (Maglione, Das, Raaen, Smith, et al., 2014).

With inactivated antigens, such as DTaP, side effects are most likely to occur within a few hours or days of administration and are usually limited to local tenderness, erythema, and swelling at the injection site; low-grade fever; and behavioral changes (drowsiness, fretfulness, eating less, prolonged or unusual cry). Rarely, more severe reactions may occur, especially with pertussis and varicella. Reactions to DTaP tend to be more severe if they occurred with a previous immunization.

Hib vaccine is one of the safest vaccines available but may be associated with low-grade fever and mild local reactions at the site of injection, which resolve rapidly. Unlike the inactivated antigens, live attenuated virus vaccines such as MMR and MMRV multiply for days or weeks, and unfavorable reactions such as fever and rash and vaccine-associated disorders can occur up to 30 to 60 days later.

Contraindications and Precautions

Nurses need to be aware of the reasons for withholding immunizations—both for the child's safety in terms of avoiding reactions and for the child's maximum benefit from receiving the vaccine. Unfounded fears and lack of knowledge regarding contraindications can needlessly prevent a child from having protection from life-threatening diseases. Issues that have surfaced regarding vaccines include the misconception that administering combination vaccines may overload the child's immune system; the combined vaccines have undergone rigorous study in relation to side effects and immunogenicity rates following administration. Others may express concern that vaccines are not a part of the individual's natural immunity and that administering too many vaccines may decrease the child's immunity to such diseases. Parents may also voice concerns that vaccines may cause diseases such as asthma, arthritis, or diabetes mellitus (Luthy, Burningham, Eden, et al., 2015). Another concern of parents is the number of vaccines or "shots" given to infants at any given time and the pain and discomfort this may cause.

A contraindication is considered as a condition in an individual that increases the risk for a serious adverse reaction (e.g., not administering a live virus vaccine to a severely compromised child). Thus one would not administer a vaccine when a contraindication is present. A precaution is a condition in a recipient that might increase the risk for a serious adverse reaction or that might compromise the ability of the vaccine to produce immunity. If conditions are such that the benefit of receiving the vaccine would outweigh the risk for an adverse event or incomplete response, a precaution would not prevent vaccine administration (American Academy of Pediatrics, Committee on Infectious Diseases, 2015).

The general contraindication for all immunizations is a severe febrile illness. This precaution avoids adding the risk for adverse side effects from the vaccine to an already ill child or mistakenly identifying a symptom of the disease as having been caused by the vaccine. The presence of minor illnesses, such as the common cold, is not a contraindication.

Live virus vaccines such as varicella and MMR should not be administered to people who are severely immunocompromised (National Center for Immunization and Respiratory Diseases, 2011). Another contraindication to live virus vaccines (e.g., MMR and varicella) is the presence of recently acquired passive immunity through blood transfusions, immunoglobulin, or maternal antibodies. Administration of MMR and varicella vaccines should be postponed for a minimum of 3 months after passive immunization with immunoglobulins and blood transfusions

(except washed red blood cells, which do not interfere with the immune response). Suggested intervals between administration of immunoglobulin preparations and MMR and varicella vaccines depend on the type of immune product and dosage. If the vaccine and immunoglobulin are given simultaneously because of imminent exposure to disease, the two preparations are injected at sites far from each other. Vaccination should be repeated after the suggested intervals unless there is serologic evidence of antibody production.

A final contraindication is a known allergic response to a previously administered vaccine or a substance in the vaccine. An anaphylactic reaction to a vaccine or its component is a true contraindication. MMR vaccines contain minute amounts of neomycin; measles and mumps vaccines, which are grown on chick embryo tissue cultures, are not believed to contain significant amounts of egg cross-reacting proteins. Therefore only a history of anaphylactic reaction to neomycin, gelatin, or the vaccine itself is considered a contraindication to their use.

Pregnancy is a contraindication to MMR vaccines, although the risk for fetal damage is primarily theoretical. Breastfeeding is not a contraindication for any vaccine. The only vaccine virus that has been isolated in human milk is rubella, and there is no indication this is harmful to infants. Rubella infection in an infant as a result of exposure to the rubella virus in human milk would likely be well tolerated because the vaccine is attenuated (American Academy of Pediatrics, Committee on Infectious Diseases, 2015). See also Family-Centered Care box: Communicating with Parents About Immunizations.

Administration

The principal precautions in administering immunizations include proper storage of the vaccine to protect its potency and institution of recommended procedures for injection. The nurse must be familiar with the manufacturer's directions for storage and reconstitution of the vaccine. Because subcutaneous or intracutaneous injection can cause local irritation, inflammation, or abscess formation, excellent intramuscular injection technique must be used (see Atraumatic Care box: Immunizations).

One of the most important features of injecting vaccines is adequate penetration of the muscle for deposition of the drug intramuscularly and not subcutaneously (depending on the manufacturer's recommendation for administration). The use of appropriate needle length is an essential component of administering vaccines. A recent systematic review found the use of longer needles significantly decreased the incidence of localized edema and tenderness when vaccines were administered to a group of infants (Beirne, Hennessy, Cadogan, et al., 2015) (see Evidence-Based Practice box: Appropriate Site, Technique,

Needle Size, and Dose for Intramuscular Injections in Infants, Toddlers, and Small Children). Similar findings have been recorded for children 4 to 6 years of age receiving the fifth DTaP vaccine (Jackson, Yu, Nelson, et al., 2011). In some studies, the site of administration influenced pain perception and localized reactions. Cook and Murtagh (2006) found that administration of the pertussis vaccine in the ventrogluteal muscle

ATRAUMATIC CARE
Immunizations

Needle length is an important factor and must be considered for each individual child; fewer reactions to immunizations are observed when the vaccine is given deep into the muscle rather than into subcutaneous tissue. Deep intramuscular tissue has a better blood supply and fewer pain receptors than adipose tissue, thus providing an optimum site for immunizations with fewer side effects (Taddio, Ilersich, Ipp, et al., 2009).

EVIDENCE-BASED PRACTICE

Appropriate Site, Technique, Needle Size, and Dose for Intramuscular Injections in Infants, Toddlers, and Small Children

Ask the Question
PICOT Question: In infants, toddlers, and small children, what is the best site, technique, needle size and gauge, and dosage for intramuscular (IM) injections?

Search for the Evidence
Search Strategies
Literature from 2000 to 2009 was reviewed to obtain clinical research studies related to this issue.

Databases Used
CINAHL, PubMed

Critical Appraisal of the Evidence
Searches reviewed were small studies. There were no randomized trials, double-blind trials, or large clinical studies addressing the subject of IM injections in children.

Infants and Toddlers
- A 16-mm needle was sufficient to penetrate the anterolateral thigh muscle if the needle is inserted at a 90-degree angle without pinching the muscle in children 2, 4, 6, and 18 months of age (Cook & Murtagh, 2002).
- A 25-mm needle was necessary to penetrate the thigh muscle when a 45-degree injection technique was employed. Longer needle length is needed to fully deposit the medication into the muscle in children 2, 4, 6, and 18 months of age (Cook & Murtagh, 2002).
- Vaccines containing adjuvant such as alum (e.g., DTaP, hepatitis A and hepatitis B, diphtheria-tetanus [DT or Td]) should be given deep into the muscle to prevent local reactions (American Academy of Pediatrics [AAP], 2012; Centers for Disease Control and Prevention [CDC], 2002; Petousis-Harris, 2008; Taddio, Ilersich, Ipp, et al., 2009).
- Injecting adjuvant-containing vaccines into subcutaneous tissue increases the incidence of local reactions (Taddio et al., 2009).
- 4-month-old infants experienced fewer local side effects (redness, tenderness, and swelling) when immunizations were administered into the anterior aspect of the thigh with a 25-mm (1-inch) needle versus shorter 16-mm (⅝-inch) needle (Diggle & Deeks, 2000).
- Localized vaccine reactions were significantly reduced when long needles (25 mm) were used for infant immunizations (Diggle, Deeks, & Pollard, 2006; Petousis-Harris, 2008).

- A 16-mm needle may be adequate for injections in small infants, and a 22- to 25-mm (⅞- to 1-inch) needle can be used in infants 2 months of age and older (AAP, 2012).
- A 22- to 32-mm (⅞- to 1¼-inch) needle is recommended for injections in toddlers if deltoid muscle size is adequate (CDC, 2002).
- A minimum of 25-mm needle is recommended for anterolateral thigh injection in toddlers (CDC, 2002).
- The dorsogluteal muscle should be avoided in infants and toddlers, and in smaller preschoolers with smaller muscle mass, because of the possibility of damaging the sciatic nerve (AAP, 2012).
- In children older than 1 year of age, the deltoid muscle is recommended for IM injections. When multiple vaccines are given, two may be given in the thigh (anterior and lateral) because of its larger size (Diggle, 2003).
- Injections in the anterolateral thigh should be given at least 2.5 cm (1 inch) apart so local reactions are less likely to overlap (AAP, 2012).
- No research or supportive data were found regarding the amount of medication to be given at the different sites in infants and toddlers.

Children and Adolescents
- A 22- to 25-gauge needle for all IM childhood immunizations is recommended (AAP, 2012; CDC, 2002).
- The deltoid muscle may be used for immunizations in toddlers, older children, and adolescents (AAP, 2012; CDC, 2002).
- 16-mm needle for children who weigh less than 60 kg and a 25-mm needle for children 60–70 kg are appropriate for IM injections in the deltoid injection site (Koster, Stellato, Kohn, et al., 2009).
- Needle length was found to be the most significant variable for local reactions in children after injection: A 25-mm needle was associated with fewer localized reactions versus a 16-mm needle (Davenport, 2004).
- In children older than 1 year of age, the deltoid muscle is recommended for IM injections. When multiple vaccines are given, two may be given in the thigh (anterior and lateral) because of its larger size (Diggle, 2003).
- Injections in the anterolateral thigh should be given at least 2.5 cm (1 inch) apart so local reactions are less likely to overlap (AAP, 2012).
- IM injections in the buttocks with longer needles and a 90-degree angle are associated with less reactogenicity (Petousis-Harris, 2008).

Continued

EVIDENCE-BASED PRACTICE

Appropriate Site, Technique, Needle Size, and Dose for Intramuscular Injections in Infants, Toddlers, and Small Children—cont'd

Apply the Evidence: Nursing Implications

There is low quality evidence with strong recommendation to continue administering IM injections to children in the anterolateral thigh (up to 12 months of age), deltoid (12 months and older), and ventrogluteal site (Guyatt, Oxman, Vist, et al., 2008). Needle length is an important factor in decreasing local reactions; the length should be adequate to deposit the medication into the muscle for IM injections. Recommendations are for a 25-mm (1-inch) needle in infants, a 25- to 32-mm (1- to 1¼-inch) needle for toddlers, and a 38- to 51-mm (1½- to 2-inch) needle for older children; preterm and small emaciated infants may require a shorter needle (16 to 25 mm [⅝ to 1 inch]) based on weight and muscle mass size.

Quality and Safety Competencies: Evidence-Based Practice*
Knowledge
Differentiate clinical opinion from research and evidence-based summaries.

Describe various methods for identifying appropriate site, technique, needle size, and dose for intramuscular injections in infants, toddlers, and small children.

Skills
Base individualized care plan on patient values, clinical expertise, and evidence.

Integrate evidence into practice by using the techniques for intramuscular injections in clinical care.

Attitudes
Value the concept of evidence-based practice (EBP) as integral to determining best clinical practice.

Appreciate strengths and weakness of evidence for identifying appropriate site, technique, needle size, and dose for intramuscular injections in infants, toddlers, and small children.

References

American Academy of Pediatrics Committee on Infectious Diseases (2012). L. Pickering (Ed.), *Red book: report of the Committee on Infectious Diseases* (29th ed.). Elk Grove Village, IL: Author.

Centers for Disease Control and Prevention. (2002). General recommendations on immunization. *Morbidity and Mortality Weekly Report Recommdations and Reports, 51*(RR-2), 12–14.

Cook, I. F., & Murtagh, J. (2002). Needle length required for intramuscular vaccination of infants and toddlers: an ultrasonographic study. *Australian Family Physician, 31*(3), 295–297.

Davenport, J. M. (2004). A systematic review to ascertain whether the standard needle is more effective than a longer or wider needle in reducing the incidence of local reaction in children receiving primary immunization. *Journal of Advanced Nursing, 46*(1), 66–77.

Diggle, L. (2003). The administration of child vaccines, part 11, Childhood vaccinations. *Practice Nurse, 25*(12), 63–69.

Diggle, L., & Deeks, J. (2000). Effect of needle length on incidence of local reactions to routine immunisation in infants aged 4 months: randomised controlled trial. *British Medical Journal, 321*(7266), 931–933.

Diggle, L., Deeks, J. J., & Pollard, A. J. (2006). Effect of needle size on immunogenicity and reactogenicity of vaccines in infants: randomized controlled trial. *British Medical Journal, 333*(7568), 571.

Guyatt, G. H., Oxman, A. D., Vist, G. E., et al. (2008). GRADE: an emerging consensus on rating quality of evidence and strength of recommendations. *British Medical Journal, 336*(7650), 924–926.

Koster, M., Stellato, N., Kohn, N., et al. (2009). Needle length for immunizations of early adolescents as determined by ultrasound. *Pediatrics, 124,* 667–672.

Petousis-Harris, H. (2008). Vaccine injection technique and reactogenicity: evidence for practice. *Vaccine, 26,* 6299–6304.

Taddio, A., Ilersich, A. L., Ipp, M., et al. (2009). Physical interventions and injection techniques for reducing injection pain during routine childhood immunizations: systematic review of randomized controlled trials and quasi-randomized controlled trials. *Clinical Therapeutics, 31,* S48–S76.

*Adapted from the Quality and Safety Education for Nurses (QSEN) Institute.

in children 2 to 18 months of age was safe and had few localized reactions compared with anterolateral thigh administration. Junqueira, Tavares, Martins, and colleagues (2010) found that administration of the hepatitis B vaccine in the ventrogluteal muscle (vs. anterolateral thigh) of 580 infants resulted in a lower incidence of fever and localized reactions (see the "Intramuscular Administration" section in Chapter 39).

The total series requires several injections, and every attempt is made to rotate the sites and administer the injections as painlessly as possible. When two or more injections are given at separate sites, the order of injections is arbitrary. Because allergic reactions can occur after injection of vaccines, appropriate precautions are taken (see the "Anaphylaxis" section in Chapter 42).

Nurses administer vaccines and thus have the responsibility for adequately informing parents of the nature, prevalence, and risks of the disease; the type of immunization product to be used; the expected benefits and the risk for side effects of the vaccine; and the need for accurate immunization records. Referring to immunizations as "baby shots" and limiting the discussion to vague statements about the vaccines are unacceptable practices.

Another important nursing responsibility is accurate documentation. Each child should have an immunization record for parents to keep, especially for families who move frequently. Although immunization rates have increased significantly, health care professionals should use every opportunity to encourage complete immunization of all children (see Family-Centered Care box: Communicating with Parents About Immunizations). Blank immunization records may be downloaded from a number of websites, including the Immunization Action Coalition (www.immunize.org), which has vaccine information and records in a number of languages.

The following information is documented on the medical record: day, month, and year of administration; manufacturer and lot number of vaccine; and the name, address, and title of the person administering the vaccine. Additional data to record are the site and route of administration and evidence that the parent or legal guardian gave informed consent before the immunization was administered. Any adverse reactions after the administration of any vaccine are reported to the Vaccine Adverse Event Reporting System (www.vaers.hhs.gov; 1-800-822-7967).

An additional source of vaccine information that must be given to parents by law (National Childhood Vaccine Injury Act of 1986) before the administration of vaccines is the vaccine information statement (VIS) for the particular vaccine being administered. Practitioners are required by law to fully inform families of the risks and benefits of the vaccines. VISs are designed to provide updated information regarding the risks and benefits of each vaccine to the adult being vaccinated or the parents or legal guardians of the children being vaccinated. Questions regarding the information in the VISs should be answered by the practitioner. VISs are available for the following vaccines: adenovirus, anthrax, tetanus, diphtheria, pertussis, MMR, MMRV, IPV, HPV, varicella, Hib, influenza, meningococcal, pneumococcal (13 and 23), rabies, rotavirus, shingles, smallpox, yellow fever, Japanese encephalitis, typhoid, HepA, and HepB.

An updated VIS should be provided, and documentation in the patient's chart should state that the VIS was given and include the publication date of the VIS; this represents informed consent once the parent or caregiver gives permission to administer the vaccines. VISs are available from state or local health departments or from the Immunization Action Coalition* and Centers for Disease Control and Prevention.†

SAFETY PROMOTION AND INJURY PREVENTION

Injuries are a major cause of death during infancy, especially for children 6 to 12 months of age. The three leading causes of accidental death in infants were suffocation, motor vehicle–related injuries, and drowning (Centers for Disease Control and Prevention, 2012a). During 2000 to 2009, unintentional infant suffocation death rates increased by 54% (Centers for Disease Control and Prevention, 2012a). During 2010 to

---

*www.immunize.org/vis.
†www.cdc.gov/vaccines.

2011, unintentional injuries (accidents) were the leading cause of death in children 1 to 4 years of age, while accidents were the fifth leading cause of death in infants birth to 12 months of age (Hamilton, Hoyert, Martin, Strobino, & Guyer, 2013). Fall-related injuries were the most common cause of unintentional injuries resulting in emergency department (ED) visits among infants 0 to 12 months of age, with 59% of the ED visits attributed to this cause (Centers for Disease Control and Prevention, 2012b). In a study of infants treated for accidents, causes of injuries included beds, car seats, and stairs (Mack, Gilchrist, & Ballesteros, 2008). One-third of all injuries occur in the home, yet there is insufficient evidence to demonstrate that modification of the home environment has an impact on the rate of injuries (Turner, Arthur, Lyons, et al., 2011). Constant vigilance, awareness, and supervision are essential as the child gains increased locomotor and manipulative skills that are coupled with an insatiable curiosity about the environment. Box 31.1 lists the major developmental achievements of each period during infancy and the appropriate injury prevention plan. Table 31.2 lists common types of injuries and associated objects that predispose to such injuries. Suggestions

---

BOX 31.1   Safety Promotion and Injury Prevention During Infancy

Birth to 4 Months of Age
Major Developmental Accomplishments
- Exhibits involuntary reflexes (e.g., crawling reflex may propel infant forward or backward; startle reflex may cause the body to jerk)
- May roll over
- Has increasing eye-hand coordination and voluntary grasp reflex

Injury Prevention
Aspiration
- Aspiration is not as great a danger to this age-group, but parents should begin practicing safeguarding early (see under 4 to 7 Months of Age).
- Never shake baby powder directly on infant; place powder in hand and then on infant's skin; store container closed and out of infant's reach.
- Hold infant for feeding; do not prop bottle.
- Know emergency procedures for choking.
- Use pacifier with one-piece construction and loop handle.

Burns
- Install smoke detectors in home.
- Do not microwave infant formula or breast milk because this can cause burns because of uneven warming.
- Check bathwater temperature.
- Do not pour hot liquids when infant is close by, such as sitting on lap.
- Beware of cigarette ashes that may fall on infant.
- Do not leave infant in sun for more than a few minutes; keep skin covered.
- Wash flame-retardant clothes according to label directions.
- Use cool-mist vaporizers.
- Do not leave child in parked car.
- Check surface heat of car restraint before placing child in seat.

Suffocation and Drowning
- Keep all plastic bags stored out of infant's reach; discard large plastic garment bags after tying in a knot.
- Do not cover mattress with plastic.
- Use firm mattress and loose blankets, with no pillows.
- Make certain crib design follows federal regulations and mattress fits snugly—crib slats 2.375 inches (6 cm) apart.*
- Position crib away from other furniture and away from heat radiators.
- Do not tie pacifier on a string around infant's neck.
- Remove bibs at bedtime.

- Never leave infant alone in bath.
- Do not leave infant younger than 12 months of age alone on adult or youth mattress or "beanbag" type seats.
- Install carbon monoxide monitor.

Motor Vehicles
- Transport infant in federally approved, rear-facing car seat, preferably in back seat.
- Do not place infant on seat (of car) or in lap.
- Do not place child in a carriage or stroller behind a parked car.
- Do not place infant or child in front passenger seat with an air bag.
- Do not leave infant unattended in car, especially in environmental temperatures above 70° F.

Falls
- Crib rails are fixed and firmly latched. As of 2011, only beds with fixed rails are recommended, but some older models may be in use (suggest purchasing a rail-latching mechanism for older models).
- Never leave infant alone on a raised, unguarded surface.
- When in doubt as to where to place child, use floor.
- Restrain child in infant seat, and never leave child unattended while the seat is resting on a raised surface.
- Avoid using a high chair until child can sit well with support.

Poisoning
- Poisoning is not as great a danger to this age-group, but parents should begin practicing safeguards early (see under 4 to 7 Months of Age).

Bodily Damage
- Keep sharp or jagged objects such as knives and broken glass out of child's reach.
- Keep diaper pins closed and away from infant.

4 to 7 Months of Age
Major Developmental Accomplishments
- Rolls over
- Sits momentarily
- Grasps and manipulates small objects
- Resecures a dropped object
- Has well-developed eye-hand coordination
- Can focus on and locate very small objects

Continued

BOX 31.1 Safety Promotion and Injury Prevention During Infancy—cont'd

- Has prominent mouthing (oral fixation)
- Can push up on hands and knees
- Crawls backward

Injury Prevention
Aspiration
- Keep buttons, beads, syringe caps, and other small objects out of infant's reach.
- Keep floor free of any small objects.
- Do not feed infant hard candy, nuts, food with pits or seeds, or whole or circular pieces of hot dog.
- Exercise caution when giving teething biscuits, since large chunks may be broken off and aspirated.
- Do not feed infant while he or she is lying down.
- Inspect toys for removable parts.
- Keep baby powder, if used, out of reach.
- Avoid storing large quantities of cleaning fluid, paints, pesticides, and other toxic substances.
- Discard used containers of poisonous substances.
- Do not store toxic substances in food or drink containers.
- Discard used button-size batteries; store new batteries in a safe area.
- Know telephone number of local poison control center (800-222-1222).

Suffocation
- Keep all latex balloons out of reach.
- Remove all crib toys that are strung across crib or play yard when child begins to push up on hands or knees or is 5 months of age.

Burns
- Keep water faucets out of reach.
- Place hot objects (cigarettes, candles, incense) on high surface out of child's reach.
- Limit exposure to sun; apply sunscreen.

Falls
- Restrain in a high chair.
- Crib rails are fixed and firmly latched. As of 2011, only beds with fixed rails are recommended.

Motor Vehicles
- See under Birth to 4 Months of Age.

Poisoning
- Make certain that paint for furniture or toys does not contain lead.
- Place toxic substances on a high shelf or in locked cabinet.
- Hang plants, or place on high surface rather than on floor.
- Know telephone number of local poison control center (800-222-1222).

Bodily Damage
- Give toys that are smooth and rounded, preferably made of wood or plastic.
- Avoid long, pointed objects as toys.
- Avoid toys that are excessively loud.
- Keep sharp objects out of infant's reach.

8 to 12 Months of Age
Major Developmental Accomplishments
- Crawls or creeps
- Stands, holding onto furniture
- Stands alone

- Cruises around furniture
- Walks
- Climbs
- Pulls on objects
- Throws objects
- Is able to pick up small objects; has pincer grasp
- Explores by putting objects in mouth
- Dislikes being restrained
- Explores away from parent
- Increasingly understands simple commands and phrases

Injury Prevention
Aspiration
- Keep small objects off floor, off furniture, and out of reach of children.
- Take care in feeding solid table food to give very small pieces.
- Do not use beanbag toys or allow child to play with dried beans.
- See also under 4 to 7 Months of Age.

Bodily Damage
- See under 4 to 7 Months of Age.
- Avoid placing televisions or other large objects on top of furniture, which may be overturned when infant pulls self to standing position.

Falls
- Avoid walkers, especially near stairs.*
- Ensure that furniture is sturdy enough for child to pull self to standing position and cruise.
- Fence stairways at top and bottom if child has access to either end.*
- Dress infant in safe shoes and clothing (soles that do not "catch" on floor, tied shoelaces, pant legs that do not touch floor).

Suffocation and Drowning
- Keep doors of ovens, dishwashers, refrigerators, coolers, and front-loading clothes washers and dryers closed at all times.
- If storing an unused large appliance, such as a refrigerator, remove the door.
- Supervise contact with inflated balloons; immediately discard popped balloons, and keep uninflated balloons out of reach.
- Fence swimming pools and other bodies of standing water such as decorative fountains; lock gate to swimming pools so only adult can access.
- Always supervise when near any source of water, such as cleaning buckets, drainage areas, ponds, toilets.
- Keep bathroom doors closed.
- Eliminate unnecessary pools of water.
- Keep one hand on child at all times when in bathtub.

Poisoning
- Administer medications as a drug, not as a candy.
- Do not administer medications unless prescribed by a practitioner.
- Return medications and poisons to safe storage area immediately after use; replace caps properly if a child-protector cap is used.
- Have poison control center number (800-222-1222) on telephone and refrigerator.

Burns
- Place guards in front of or around any heating appliance, fireplace, or furnace.
- Keep electrical wires hidden or out of reach.
- Place plastic guards over electrical outlets; place furniture in front of outlets.
- Keep hanging tablecloths out of reach (child may pull down hot liquids or heavy or sharp objects).

*Information on many items such as cribs or walkers is available from US Consumer Product Safety Commission, 800-638-2772; www.cpsc.gov/.

TABLE 31.2	**Common Infant Injuries, Associated Risk Factors, and Safety Promotion**	
Safe Pad	**Risk Factors**	**Suggested Safety Interventions**
S—Suffocation, Sleep position	Latex balloons	Avoid latex balloons except with close adult supervision.
	Plastic bags	Tie unused plastic bags in a knot and dispose of in a safe container.
	Bed surface (noninfant) such as sofa or adult bed	Avoid placing infants to sleep on sofas, soft bedding, or adult bed.
	Pillows	Avoid use of pillows for sleep.
	Soft cushions and blankets	Clear bedding of soft cushions and blankets.
	Prone sleeping	Place infant to sleep on back at all times.
A—Asphyxia, animal bites	Food items: cylindric items such as hot dogs, hard candy, nuts	Cut hot dogs lengthwise; avoid hard candy in infants and toddlers. Infants should completely chew up each food item in mouth; do not feed more until item is swallowed.
	Toys: small toys such as Legos	As a general rule of thumb, if the toy fits into a toilet paper cardboard roll, it can be swallowed by a small child.
	Small objects: batteries, buttons, beads, dried beans, syringe caps, safety pins	Keep out of reach of infants, who are naturally inquisitive.
	Pacifiers	Pacifiers should be one piece.
	Baby (talc) powder	Avoid shaking powder over infant; if used, place on adult's hand and then place on infant's skin.
	Domestic dogs, cats	Supervise child around domestic animals; teach not to approach dog that is eating, has puppies, or is not feeling well. Animals that are "tame" can be unpredictable. Small children are the right size for most domesticated animals to come face to face. Closely supervise child around visiting pets.
F—Falls	Stairs	Infants like to climb; place childproof gate at top and bottom of stairs.
	Diaper changing table	Infants do not have depth perception and cannot perceive a dangerous height from one that is safe. Never leave infants unattended on a flat surface, even if not rolling over.
	Crib, bed-crib sides can fall when infant leans on them	In 2011, a mandate was made to stop selling drop-side infant cribs.*
	Infant carriers	Never leave infant unattended in a carrier on top of a surface such as a shopping cart, clothes dryer, washer, kitchen cabinet; place carrier on floor.
	Car seat restraints	Secure infant in car seat restraint and never leave unattended if unrestrained.
	High chair	Restrain infant in high chair; avoid using high chair except for feeding and only if adult supervision is adequate; even restrained infants can squirm out of some restraints and fall.
	Infant walkers	Use only stationary walkers. There is no evidence that walkers help infants "walk" any sooner. Wheeled walkers can easily be propelled off stairs and other platforms such as porches or decks, causing significant injury.
	Windows, screens	Avoid placing furniture next to a window. Infants learn to climb and can fall out of open windows, even with screens.
	Television, stereos, sound systems	These must be secured to the stand; infants can pull the stand over, causing the TV or sound system to land on their heads, causing significant injury.
E—Electrical burns or burns	Electrical outlets	Place safety cap over electrical outlets; infants may be burned by placing conductive object into outlet.
	Hot hair styling appliances (curlers, flat irons)	Keep out of reach of infant and keep turned off when not in use.
	Water	Infants may turn on tap or faucet in bathtub and burn self. Lower the water heater to a safe temperature of 49° C (120° F). Before placing infant in tub, check temperature of water and completely turn off faucet so child cannot alter temperature of water. NEVER leave infant unattended in tub or sink of water.
	Fireplace	Place a childproof screen in front of fireplace.
	Stove, hot liquids	Keep top front burners off and keep pot handles turned toward back to avoid infant pulling hot pot onto self and causing burn injuries.
	Cigarettes	Avoid smoking and holding infant on lap while smoking cigar or cigarette.

Continued

TABLE 31.2	Common Infant Injuries, Associated Risk Factors, and Safety Promotion—cont'd	
Safe Pad	**Risk Factors**	**Suggested Safety Interventions**
P—Poisoning, ingestions	Medication, ointments, cream, lotions	Medications left in purses or handbags or on a table top can often be ingested by the curious infant. Keep Poison Control Center number readily available ([800]-222-1222).
	Plants: household plants may be a source of accidental poisoning	Keep plants out of child's reach.
	Cleaning solutions	Store in locked cabinet or in top cabinet where there are no drawers or shelves for infant to climb on. Avoid storing cleaning and caustic solutions in containers such as a soda bottle or jar—infants and toddlers cannot differentiate a soda from a caustic drain cleaner.
	Inhalation or oral or nasal ingestion of poisonous or harmful chemicals such as methamphetamine, gasoline, turpentine	Keep gasoline and turpentine stored in a locked cabinet or closet out of child's reach. Avoid storing in containers that are also used to keep drinks or food.
A—Automobile safety	Car or truck and hot weather	An automobile-related hazard for infants is overheating (hyperthermia) and subsequent death when left in a vehicle in hot weather (>26.4° C [80° F]). Infants dissipate heat poorly, and an increase in body temperature may cause death in a few hours. Caution parents against leaving infants in a vehicle alone for *any reason*.
	Air bags	Avoid placing infant in a car restraint behind an air bag. Deactivate the air bag (available in certain models) or place the infant in the back seat in a proper car seat restraint.
	Car seat restraint	See discussion later in this chapter.
D—Drowning	Bath tub	NEVER leave infant unattended in tub or sink of water.
	Swimming pools, bird baths, decorative ponds of water, splash pads	Place fence around pools with gate lock that is out of child's reach. Supervise infants in water at ALL times; an infant may drown in as little as 2 inches of water. Swimming lessons are encouraged but are not foolproof for drowning if infant or child hits head on hard object and becomes unconscious as falling into the water.
	5-gal buckets	Keep 5-gal buckets empty of water and elevated out of child's reach.

*A number of parent education pamphlets—such as *Crib Safety Tips* and *Is Your Used Crib Safe?*—are available in English and Spanish from the US Consumer Product Safety Commission, 4330 East West Highway, Bethesda, MD 20814; 800-638-2772; www.cpsc.gov/.

for promoting safety in the home environment are given for specific types of injuries. The acronym *SAFE PAD* shown in Table 31.2 may be used to identify common types of injuries to infants and older children.

Motor Vehicle Safety

A significant number of infants are injured or die from improper restraint within vehicles. Desapriya, Joshi, Subwarzi, and Nolan (2008) found that falls accounted for a significant proportion of injuries (98%) in infants from birth to 4 months of age as a result of inappropriate use of a car restraint system. Reports indicate that child restraint use decreases with increasing age of children and increasing number of occupants. Lack of proper child restraint continues to be a major factor in fatal accidents involving children. One observational report of newborns being placed in a car seat restraint by their family found a 52% incidence of newborn infants placed incorrectly in car seat restraints and a 48% incidence of errors in the placement of infant car seat restraints with 29% of the car seat restraints not attached to the vehicle (Rogers, Gallo, Saleheen,et al., 2012). All infants must be secured in a federally approved restraint rather than held or placed on the seat of the car. There is no safe alternative.

Infant restraints are designed either as an infant-only model or as a convertible infant-toddler model. Either restraint is a semireclined seat that faces the rear of the car. A rear-facing car seat provides the best protection for the disproportionately heavy head and weak neck of an infant (Fig. 31.11). This position minimizes the stress on the neck by spreading the forces of a frontal crash over the entire back, neck, and head; the spine is supported by the back of the car seat. If the seat were faced forward, the head would whip forward because of the force of the crash, creating enormous stress on the neck. It is now recommended that all infants and toddlers ride in rear-facing

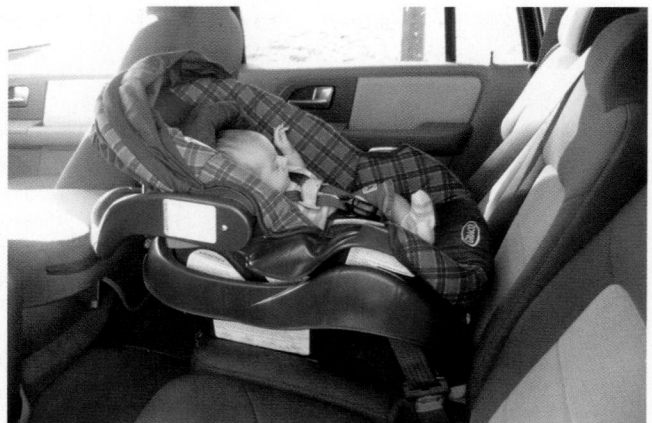

FIG 31.11 Rear-facing infant seat in rear seat of car. The infant is placed in the seat when going home from the hospital. (Courtesy of Brian and Mayannyn Sallee, Anchorage, AK.)

car safety seats until they reach 2 years of age or until they surpass the maximum height and weight recommended for the car seat (AAP, 2011).* Studies indicate that toddlers up to 24 months of age are safer

*Car seat information is available from the AAP (www.healthychildren. org/carseatguide) and the Insurance Institute for Highway Safety (http:// www.iihs.org/iihs/brochures/keeping-children-safe), 1005 N. Glebe Road, Suite 800, Arlington, VA 22201, 703-247-1500, fax: 703-247-1588. The National Highway Traffic Safety Administration (www.nhtsa.gov/ document/car-seat-recommendations-children) also provides child passenger safety and air bag safety information for parents.

riding in convertible seats in the rear-facing position (Bull & Durbin, 2008; Truong, Hill, & Cole, 2013).

The restraint is anchored to the vehicle with the vehicle's seat belt, and the restraint has a harness system for securing the infant. Some harness systems require a clip to keep the shoulder straps correctly positioned. Vehicles manufactured after 1999 have tether straps that attach to anchors in the car seat to better secure the seat and minimize forward movement of the forward-facing convertible seats in the event of an accident. The LATCH (lower anchors and tethers for children) system provides car seat anchors between the front cushion and backrest so that the seat belt does not have to be used. Although many infant restraints can be recliners, they are used in the car only in the position specified by the manufacturer. In 2014, the National Highway Traffic Safety Administration changed the LATCH system rule, which now states if the combined weight of the child and the car seat is more than 65 pounds, parents will be instructed to use the shoulder-lap belt restraint to restrain the child in the car seat instead of relying on the LATCH system for maximum protection.

Severe injuries and deaths in children have occurred from air bags deploying on impact in the front passenger seat. The back seat is the safest area of the car for children. For restraints to be effective, they must be used properly. Dressing the infant in an outfit with sleeves and legs allows the harness to hold the child securely in the seat. A small blanket or towel rolled tightly can be placed on either side of the head to minimize movement and keep the infant's hips against the back of the seat. Padding between the infant's legs and crotch is added to prevent slouching. Thick, soft padding is not placed under the infant or behind the back because during the impact, the padding will compress, leaving the harness straps loose. Preterm infants being discharged home from the hospital should be placed in an appropriate car seat restraint as it would be placed in the car, and their heart rate and oxygen saturation are monitored for 90 to 120 minutes to detect any potential problems with airway occlusion. (For further discussion of car seat restraints, see Chapter 23.)

! NURSING ALERT

Rear-facing infant safety seats must not be placed in the front seats of cars equipped with an air bag on the passenger side. If an infant safety seat is placed in the passenger seat with an air bag, the child could be seriously injured if the air bag is released, since rear-facing infant seats extend closer to the dashboard.

Another automobile-related hazard for infants is *overheating* (hyperthermia) and subsequent death when left in a vehicle in hot weather (over 26.4° C [80° F]). Infants dissipate heat poorly, and an increase in body temperature may cause death in a few hours. Parents are cautioned against leaving infants in a vehicle alone for *any reason*. Busy parents may forget the child in the back when preoccupied with errands, children's school and extracurricular activities, and busy work schedules. A small sign or placard has been designed to hang in the rear-view mirror to remind the parent that there is a child in the back seat.

Nurse's Role in Injury Prevention

The task of injury prevention begins to be appreciated only when the potential environmental dangers to which infants are vulnerable are considered. Injury prevention and parent education should be handled on a growth and developmental basis. It is simply impossible to completely protect infants and small children from all potential dangers without placing them in a sterile, impractical environment. However,

a large percentage of childhood deaths continue to occur as a result of *preventable* injuries. Nurses must be aware of the possible causes of injury in each age-group to provide anticipatory, preventive teaching. For example, the nurse should discuss guidelines for injury prevention during infancy (see Box 31.1) before the child reaches the susceptible age-group. Preventive teaching ideally begins during pregnancy.

One-third of all injuries to children occur in the home, and therefore the importance of safety cannot be overemphasized. The Family-Centered Care box: Child Home Safety Checklist summarizes a home safety checklist that can be presented to parents to increase their awareness of danger areas in the home and assist them in implementing safety devices and practices before their absence can inflict injury on infants. Hands-on displays such as cabinet latches or toilet seat locks can familiarize parents with inexpensive, commercial devices that can be used in the home to prevent injuries.

Injury prevention requires protection of the child and education of the caregiver. Nurses in ambulatory care settings, health maintenance centers, and visiting nurse agencies are in the most favorable position for injury education. This does not exclude nurses in inpatient facilities, who could use visiting times as an excellent opportunity for discussing this topic. Although early discharge after birth may be restrictive for parent teaching, this is an excellent opportunity to introduce the family to infant safety and safety for other children as well. Injury prevention must be practical. For instance, parents are taught bathroom cleaning agents, cosmetics, and personal care items can be placed on a top shelf in the linen closet, and towels or sheets can be stored on the lower shelves and floor. Parents should be encouraged to take an infant cardiopulmonary resuscitation (CPR) class to deal effectively with potential problems. If an injury has occurred, the nurse should not be too quick to admonish the parent. Injuries do not always indicate neglect. It is a difficult task to watch children carefully without overprotecting or unnecessarily confining them. Allowing children to explore while maintaining consistent, age-appropriate limits is sound advice.

Parents need to remember that infants and young children cannot anticipate danger or understand when it is or is not present. Also, infants have no cognitive concept of cause and effect and therefore cannot relate meaning to experiences or potential dangers. A dead electrical wire may present no actual harm, but if the child is allowed to play with it, a poor behavior is enforced and will be practiced when the child encounters a live wire. Although it is always wise to explain why something is dangerous, it must be remembered that small children need to be physically removed from the situation.

It is not easy to teach safety, supervise closely, and refrain from saying "no" a hundred times a day. Parents become acutely aware of this dilemma as soon as the infant learns to crawl. Preventing injuries to children is usually the first reason for limit setting and discipline, but limits are also set to prevent damage to valuable household objects. When small children are in the home, dangerous objects must be removed or guarded and valuable articles placed out of reach.

When children are taught the meaning of "no," they should also be taught what "yes" means. Children should be praised for playing with suitable toys, their efforts at behaving or listening should be reinforced, and innovative and creative recreational toys should be provided for them. Infants love to tear paper and avidly pursue books, magazines, or newspapers left on the floor. Instead of scolding them for destroying a valued book, parents should provide child-safe books (e.g., those constructed of fabric) for them to play with. If they enjoy pots and pans, a cabinet can be arranged with safe utensils for them to explore.

One additional factor must be stressed concerning injury prevention and education. Children are imitators; they copy what they see and hear. Practicing safety teaches safety, which applies to parents and their children

FAMILY-CENTERED CARE
Child Home Safety Checklist

Safety: Fire, Electrical, Burns
- Guards in front of or around any heating appliance, fireplace, or furnace (including floor furnace)*
- Electrical wires hidden or out of reach*
- No frayed or broken wires; no overloaded sockets
- Plastic guards or caps over electrical outlets; furniture in front of outlets*
- Hanging tablecloths out of reach, away from open fires*
- Smoke detectors tested and operating properly
- Kitchen matches stored out of child's reach*
- Large, deep ashtrays throughout house (if used)
- Small stoves, heaters, and other hot objects (cigarettes, candles, coffee pots, slow cookers) placed where they cannot be tipped over or reached by children
- Hot water heater set at 49° C (120° F) or lower
- Pot handles turned toward back of stove, center of table
- No loose clothing worn near stove
- No cooking or eating hot foods or liquids with child standing nearby or sitting in lap
- All small appliances, such as iron, turned off, disconnected, and placed out of reach when not in use
- Cool, not hot, mist vaporizer if used
- Fire extinguisher available on each floor and checked periodically
- Electrical fuse box and gas shutoff accessible
- Family escape plan in case of a fire practiced periodically; fire escape ladder available on upper-level floors
- Telephone number of fire or rescue squad and address of home with nearest cross street posted near phone

Safety: Suffocation and Aspiration
- Small objects stored out of reach*
- Toys inspected for small removable parts or long strings*
- Hanging crib toys and mobiles placed out of reach
- Plastic bags stored away from young child's reach; large plastic garment bags discarded after tying in knots*
- Mattress or pillow not covered with plastic or in manner accessible to child*
- Crib design according to federal regulations (crib slats less than 2.375 inches [6 cm] apart) with snug-fitting mattress*†
- Crib positioned away from other furniture or windows*
- Portable play yard gates up at all times while in use*
- Accordion-style gates not used*
- Bathroom doors kept closed and toilet lids down*
- Faucets turned off firmly*
- Pool fenced with locked gate
- Proper safety equipment at poolside
- Electronic garage door openers stored safely, and garage door adjusted to rise when door strikes object
- Doors of ovens, trunks, dishwashers, refrigerators, and front-loading clothes washers and dryers kept closed*
- Unused appliance, such as a refrigerator, securely closed with lock or doors removed*
- Food served in small, non-cylindric pieces*

- Toy chests without lids or with lids that securely lock in open position*
- Buckets and wading pools kept empty when not in use*
- Clothesline above head level
- At least one member of household trained in basic life support (cardiopulmonary resuscitation), including first aid for choking

Safety: Poisoning
- Toxic substances, including batteries, placed on a high shelf, preferably in locked cabinet
- Toxic plants hung or placed out of reach*
- Excess quantities of cleaning fluid, paints, pesticides, drugs, and other toxic substances not stored in home
- Used containers of poisonous substances discarded where child cannot obtain access
- Telephone number of local poison control center (800-222-1222) and home address with nearest cross street posted near phone
- Medicines clearly labeled in childproof containers and stored out of reach
- Household cleaners, disinfectants, and insecticides kept in their original containers, separate from food and out of reach
- Smoking in areas away from children

Safety: Falls
- Nonskid mats, strips, or surfaces in tubs and showers
- Exits, halls, and passageways in rooms kept clear of toys, furniture, boxes, or other items that could be obstructive
- Stairs and halls well lighted, with switches at both top and bottom
- Sturdy handrails for all steps and stairways
- Nothing stored on stairways
- Treads, risers, and carpeting in good repair
- Glass doors and walls marked with decals
- Safety glass used in doors, windows, and on walls
- Gates on top and bottom of staircases and elevated areas, such as porch, fire escape*
- Guardrails on upstairs windows with locks that limit height of window opening and access to areas such as fire escape*
- Crib side rails raised to full height; mattress lowered as child grows*
- Restraints used in high chairs, walkers, or other baby furniture; preferably walkers not used*
- Scatter rugs secured in place or used with nonskid backing
- Walks, patios, and driveways in good repair

Safety: Bodily Injury
- Knives, power tools, and unloaded firearms stored safely or placed in locked cabinet
- Garden tools returned to storage racks after use
- Pets properly restrained and immunized for rabies
- Swings, slides, and other outdoor play equipment kept in safe condition
- Yard free of broken glass, nail-studded boards, other litter
- Cement birdbaths placed where young child cannot tip them over*
- Furniture anchored so child cannot pull down on top of self when climbing or pulling to stand

*Safety measures are specific for homes with young children. All safety measures should be implemented in homes where children reside and visit frequently, such as those of grandparents or baby-sitters.
†Federal regulations are available from the US Consumer Product Safety Commission, 800-638–2772; www.cpsc.gov.

FAMILY-CENTERED CARE

Guidance During the Infant's First Year

First 6 Months

- Teach parents car safety with use of federally approved restraint, facing rearward, in the middle of the back seat—not in a front seat with an air bag.
- Understand each parent's adjustment to the newborn, especially mother's emotional needs after birth.
- Teach care of infant, and help parents understand his or her individual needs and temperament and that the infant expresses wants through crying.
- Reassure parents that infant cannot be spoiled by too much attention during the first 4 to 6 months.
- Encourage parents to establish a schedule that meets needs of child and themselves.
- Help parents understand infant's need for stimulation in environment.
- Support parents' pleasure in seeing child's growing friendliness and social response, especially smiling.
- Plan anticipatory guidance for safety.
- Stress need for childhood immunizations.
- Prepare for introduction of solid foods.

Second 6 Months

- Prepare parents for child's "stranger anxiety."
- Encourage parents to allow child to cling to them and avoid long separation from either.
- Guide parents concerning discipline because of infant's increasing mobility.
- Encourage use of negative voice and eye contact rather than physical punishment as a means of discipline.
- Encourage showing most attention when infant is behaving well, rather than when infant is crying.
- Teach injury prevention because of child's advancing motor skills and curiosity.
- Encourage parents to leave child with suitable caregiver to allow some free time.
- Discuss readiness for weaning.
- Explore parents' feelings regarding infant's sleep patterns.

and to nurses and their patients. Saying one thing but doing another confuses children and can lead to difficulties as the child grows older.

ANTICIPATORY GUIDANCE—CARE OF FAMILIES

Childrearing is no easy task; it presents challenges to both new and seasoned parents. Society's changing roles, combined with a highly mobile population, leave little stability for traditional role models and time-honored methods of raising children. As a result, parents look to health care professionals for guidance. Nurses are in an advantageous position to render assistance and offer suggestions. Every phase of a child's life has its particular traumas—toilet training for toddlers, unexplained fears for preschoolers, and identity crises for adolescents. For parents of an infant, some challenges center around dependency, discipline, increased mobility, and safety. Major areas for parental guidance during the first year are listed in the Family-Centered Care box: Guidance during the Infant's First Year.

SPECIAL HEALTH PROBLEMS

COLIC (PAROXYSMAL ABDOMINAL PAIN)

Colic is reported to occur in 5% to 20% of all infants (Savino, Ceratto, Poggi, et al., 2015; Milidou, Sondergaard, Jensen, et al., 2014). An organic

cause may be identified in fewer than 5% of infants seen by physicians because of excessive crying (Akhnikh, Engelberts, van Sleuwen, et al., 2014). The condition is defined by the rule of threes: crying and fussing for more than 3 hours per day occurring more than 3 days per week and for more than 3 weeks in a healthy infant (Johnson, Cocker, & Chang, 2015). Infants commonly develop an increase in symptoms (fussiness and crying) in the evening that is unprovoked (Johnson et al., 2015); however, in some infants, the onset of symptoms occurs at another time. Colic is more common in infants younger than 3 months of age than in older infants, and infants with difficult temperaments are more likely to be colicky.

Despite the obvious behavioral indications of pain, the infant with colic gains weight and usually thrives. There is no evidence of a residual effect of colic on older children except perhaps a strained parent-child relationship in some cases. In other words, infants who are colicky grow up to be normal children and adults. Colic is self-limiting and in most cases resolves as infants mature, generally around 12 to 16 weeks of age (Akhnikh, Engelberts, van Sleuwen, L'Hoir, & Benninga, 2014).

Among the theories investigated as potential causes are too rapid feeding, overeating, swallowing excessive air, poor feeding technique (especially in positioning and burping), and emotional stress or tension between the parent and child. Although all of these may occur, there is no evidence that one factor is consistently present. Infants with cow's milk allergy (CMA) symptoms have a high rate of colic (44%), and eliminating cow's milk products from the infant's diet can reduce the symptoms. The exact cause of colic is not fully understood, but some experts believe maternal smoking, inadequate parent-infant interaction, lactase deficiency, difficult infant temperament, fecal microflora, and abnormal GI motility are potential causes of colic (Drug and Therapeutics Bulletin, 2013; Johnson, Cocker, & Chang, 2015). Some experts have suggested that inadequate amounts of lactobacilli in the GI tract influences gut motor function and gas production (Drugs and Therapeutics Bulletin, 2013). The consensus of many experts who study colic is that it is multifactorial and that no single treatment for every colicky infant will be effective in alleviating the symptoms.

Therapeutic Management

Management of colic should begin with an investigation of possible organic causes, such as CMA, intussusception, or another GI problem. If a sensitivity to cow's milk is strongly suspected, a trial substitution of another formula such as an extensively hydrolyzed (Nutramigen, Alimentum, Pregestimil), whey hydrolysate, or amino acid (Neocate, EleCare) formula is warranted. Soy formulas are usually avoided because of the possibility of sensitivity to soy protein as well (Drugs and Therapeutics Bulletin, 2013). A position statement by the Canadian Paediatric Society, Nutrition and Gastroenterology Committee concluded that dietary modifications are beneficial in some cases but not all (Critch, 2011). A systematic review and randomized placebo-controlled trial noted that the probiotic *Lactobacillus reuteri* significantly decreased colic in infants who were breastfed (Urbanska & Szajewska, 2014; Szajewska, Gyrczuk, & Horvath, 2013).

When no specific inciting agent can be found, the supportive measures discussed in the Care Management section are used. The use of drugs, including sedatives, antispasmodics, antihistamines, and antiflatulents, is sometimes recommended. However, in most controlled studies, none of these drugs completely reduced the symptoms of colic. Behavioral interventions have not proved effective at reducing the symptoms of colic but have helped parents deal with their crying infants in a more positive manner. The use of complementary medicines for infantile colic, namely fennel extract, herbal tea, and sugar solutions, reportedly lack sufficient evidence to recommend their use (Perry, Hunt, & Ernst, 2011).

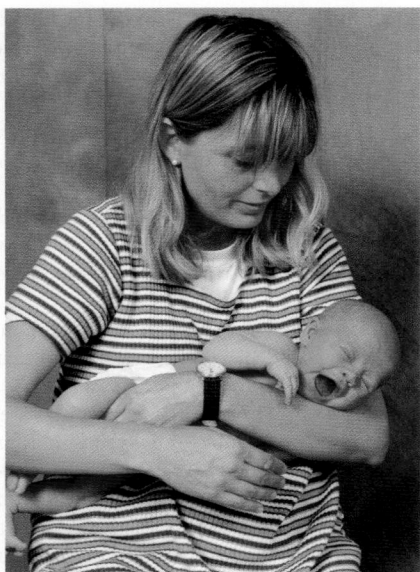

FIG 31.12 The "colic carry" may be comforting to an infant with colic. (Photo by Paul Vincent Kuntz, Texas Children's Hospital, Houston, TX.)

Care Management

The initial step in managing colic is to take a thorough, detailed history of the usual daily events. Areas that should be stressed include (1) the infant's diet; (2) the diet of the breastfeeding mother; (3) the time of day when crying occurs; (4) the relationship of crying to feeding time; (5) the presence of specific family members during crying and habits of family members, such as smoking; (6) the activity of the mother or usual caregiver before, during, and after crying; (7) the characteristics of the cry (duration, intensity); (8) the measures used to relieve crying and their effectiveness; and (9) the infant's stooling, voiding, and sleeping patterns. Of special emphasis is a careful assessment of the feeding process via demonstration by the parent.

If CMA is suspected, breastfeeding mothers should follow a milk-free diet for a minimum of 3 to 5 days in an attempt to reduce the infant's symptoms. Caution mothers that some nondairy creamers may contain calcium caseinate, a cow's milk protein. If a milk-free diet is helpful, lactating mothers may need calcium supplements to meet the body's requirement. Bottle-fed infants may improve with the same dietary modifications as for infants with CMA. Additional approaches for managing colic are listed in the Family-Centered Care box: Managing the Colicky Infant (see also Fig. 31.12).

One important nursing intervention (before or after an organic cause has been eliminated) is reassuring both parents that they are not doing anything wrong and that the infant is not experiencing any physical or emotional harm. Parents become easily frustrated with their infant's crying and perceive this as a sign that something is horribly wrong. In addition, colicky infants may be at increased risk for being shaken or otherwise abused by their caregivers and experiencing traumatic brain injury. A survey of fathers of colicky infants described the experience of having a colicky infant as similar to falling into an abyss from which they had to climb with the assistance of family and friends (Ellett, Appleton, & Sloan, 2009). An empathetic, gentle, and reassuring attitude, in addition to suggestions for treatment, will help allay parents' anxieties, which are usually exacerbated by loss of sleep and preoccupation over the infant's welfare. Colic disappears spontaneously, usually by 3 to 4 months of age, although guarantees should never be given since it may continue for much longer. Other support people and extended family members may be enlisted to support the parents during this difficult time.

FAMILY-CENTERED CARE
Managing the Colicky Infant

- Place infant prone over a covered hot-water bottle or heated towel.
- Massage infant's abdomen.
- Respond immediately to the crying.
- Change infant's position frequently; walk with child's face down and with body across parent's arm, with parent's hand under infant's abdomen, applying gentle pressure.
- Use a front carrier for transporting infant.
- Swaddle infant tightly with a soft, stretchy blanket.
- Take infant for car rides or outside for a change in environment.
- Use bottles that minimize air swallowing (curved bottle or inner collapsible bag).
- Use a commercial device in the crib that stimulates the vibration and sound of a car ride or plays soothing "noise," in utero sounds, or music.
- Provide smaller, frequent feedings; burp infant during and after feedings using the shoulder position or sitting upright, and place infant in an upright seat after feedings.
- Introduce a pacifier for added sucking.
- If household members smoke, avoid smoking near infant; preferably confine smoking activity to outside of home.
- If nothing reduces the crying, place infant in crib and allow to cry; periodically hold and comfort child, and put down again.
- Maintain a brief diary of the time of day the crying starts; events going on in household; time, amount, and type of last feeding; length of crying; and characteristics of cry. Although this will not stop the crying, it may help the practitioner identify a possible cause.

FAILURE TO THRIVE (GROWTH FAILURE)

Failure to thrive (FTT), or growth failure, is a sign of inadequate growth resulting from an inability to obtain or use calories required for growth. FTT has no universal definition, although one of the more common criteria is a weight (and sometimes height) that falls below the 5th percentile for the child's age. Another definition of FTT includes a weight for age (height) z value of less than −2.0 (a z value is a standard deviation value that represents anthropometric data normalizing for sex and age with greater precision than growth percentile curves [Atalay & McCord, 2012]). A third way to define FTT is a weight curve that crosses more than 2 percentile lines on a standardized growth chart after previous achievement of a stable growth pattern. Weight for length is reported to be a better indicator of acute undernutrition (Becker, Carney, Corkins, Monczka, Smith et al., 2015). Growth measurements alone are not used to diagnose children with FTT. Rather, the finding of a pattern of persistent deviation from established growth parameters is cause for concern. In addition to lack of consensus on the precise definition of FTT, some advocate for a change in terminology; thus terms such as *growth failure* and *pediatric undernutrition* are used in the literature for FTT. The term *FTT* will be used in the following discussion. According to Cole and Lanham (2011), approximately 5% to 10% of children in primary care in the United States have FTT, with the majority presenting before 18 months of age.

Some experts suggest that the previously used classifications of organic FTT and nonorganic FTT are too simplistic because most cases of growth failure have mixed causes; they suggest that FTT be classified according to pathophysiology in the categories in Box 31.2.

The cause of FTT is often multifactorial and may involve a combination of infant organic disease, subtle neurologic or behavioral problems, and complex parent-child interactions (McLean & Price, 2016). However, the primary etiology is inadequate caloric intake, regardless of the cause.

BOX 31.2 Pathophysiologic Causes of Failure to Thrive

Inadequate caloric intake: Incorrect formula preparation, neglect, food fads, excessive juice consumption, lack of food availability, breastfeeding problems, behavioral problems affecting eating, or central nervous system problems affecting intake

Inadequate absorption: Food allergy, malabsorption, pyloric stenosis, GI atresia, inborn errors of metabolism

Excessive caloric expenditure: Hyperthyroidism, malignancy, congenital heart disease, chronic pulmonary disease, or chronic immunodeficiency

Adapted from Cole, S.Z., Lanham, J.S. (2011). Failure to thrive: An update. *American Family Physician, 83*(7), 829–834.

Infants who are born preterm and with very low birth weight (VLBW) or extremely low birth weight (ELBW), as well as those with intrauterine growth restriction (IUGR), are often referred for FTT within the first 2 years of life because they typically do not grow physically at the same rate as term cohorts, even after discharge from the acute care facility. Catch-up growth has been shown to be much more difficult to achieve in ELBW and VLBW infants. As young adults, former VLBW infants are more likely to have small stature (both height and weight) and lower rates of tertiary education than term cohorts (Darlow, Horwood, Pere-Bracken, et al., 2013).

Other factors that can lead to inadequate caloric intake in infancy include poverty, health or childrearing beliefs such as fad diets, child neglect, inadequate nutritional knowledge, family stress, feeding resistance, and insufficient breast milk intake. In infants younger than 8 weeks of age, breastfeeding problems as a result of inadequate latch or uncoordinated sucking and swallowing may occur (Cole & Lanham, 2011). One account reports a 6-month-old term infant with FTT as a result of severe ankyloglossia (tongue tie) (Forlenza, Paradise Black, McNamara, et al., 2010).

Diagnostic Evaluation

Diagnosis is initially made from evidence of growth failure. If FTT is recent, the weight but not the height is below accepted standards (usually the 5th percentile); if FTT is longstanding, both weight and height are low, indicating chronic malnutrition. Perhaps as important as anthropometric measurements are a complete health and dietary history (including perinatal history), physical examination for evidence of organic causes, developmental assessment, and family assessment. A dietary intake history, either a 24-hour food intake or a history of food consumed over a 3- to 5-day period, is also essential. In addition, explore the child's activity level, perceived food allergies, and dietary restrictions. An assessment of household organization and mealtime behaviors and rituals is important in the collection of pertinent data. It is often helpful to obtain the growth patterns of the affected child's parents and siblings; these can be compared with norm-referenced standards to evaluate the child's growth. Other tests (lead toxicity, anemia, stool-reducing substances, occult blood, ova and parasites, alkaline phosphatase, and zinc levels) are selected only as indicated to rule out organic problems. In most cases, laboratory studies are of little diagnostic value (Cole & Lanham, 2011).

Therapeutic Management

The primary management of FTT is aimed at reversing the cause of the growth failure. If malnutrition is severe, the initial treatment is directed at reversing the malnutrition. The goal is to provide sufficient calories to support "catch-up" growth—a rate of growth greater than the expected rate for age. In addition to adding caloric density to feedings, the child may require multivitamin supplements and dietary supplementation with high-calorie foods and drinks. Any coexisting medical problems are treated.

Prognosis

The prognosis for children with FTT is related to the cause. Few long-term studies provide data on the prognosis for children with FTT; however, experts indicate that children who had FTT as infants are at risk for shorter heights, and delayed development than peers (Nangia & Tiwari, 2013). Factors related to poor prognosis are severe feeding resistance, lack of awareness in and cooperation from the parent(s), low family income, low maternal educational level, adolescent mother, preterm birth, IUGR, and early age of onset of FTT. Because later cognitive and motor function are affected by malnourishment in infancy, many of these children are below normal in intellectual development, with childhood IQ scores significantly lower than peers without a history of malnourishment (Romano, Hartman, Privitera, et al., 2015). In addition, there is a higher likelihood of eating and behavioral issues among children with a history of malnutrition when compared to peers (Romano, et al., 2015). Such findings indicate that a long-term plan and follow-up care are needed for the optimal development of these children.

Interprofessional Care of Failure to Thrive

In most cases of FTT, an interdisciplinary team of physician, nurse, dietitian, child life specialist, occupational therapist, pediatric feeding specialist, and social worker or mental health professional is needed to deal with the multiple problems. Make efforts to relieve any additional stresses on the family by offering referrals to welfare agencies or supplemental food programs. In some cases, family therapy may be required. Temporary placement in a foster home may relieve the family's stress, protect the child, and allow the child some stability if insurmountable obstacles are preventing appropriate family function. Behavior modification aimed at mealtime rituals (or lack thereof) and family social time may be required. Hospitalization admission is indicated for (1) evidence (anthropometric) of severe acute malnutrition, (2) child abuse or neglect, (3) significant dehydration, (4) caregiver substance abuse or psychosis, (5) outpatient management that does not result in weight gain, and (6) serious intercurrent infection (American Academy of Pediatrics, Committee on Nutrition, 2014).

In addition to attending to the child's physical needs, the interdisciplinary team must plan care for appropriate developmental stimulation. After an approximate developmental age is established, a planned program of play is begun. Ideally, a child life specialist is involved to implement and supervise the stimulation program. Every effort is made to teach the parent how to play and interact with the child.

Care Management

Nurses play a critical role in the diagnosis of FTT through their assessment of the child, parents, and family interactions. Having a primary core of nurses is beneficial in understanding the family dynamics (Fig. 31.13). Knowledge of the characteristics of children with FTT and their families is essential in helping identify these children and hastening the confirmation of a diagnosis (Box 31.3). Accurate assessment of initial weight and height and daily weight, as well as recording of all food intake, is imperative. The nurse documents the child's feeding behavior and the parent-child interaction during feeding, other caregiving activities, and play.

Some parents are at increased risk for attachment problems because of (1) isolation and social crisis; (2) inadequate support systems, such as teenage and single mothers; and (3) poor parenting role models as

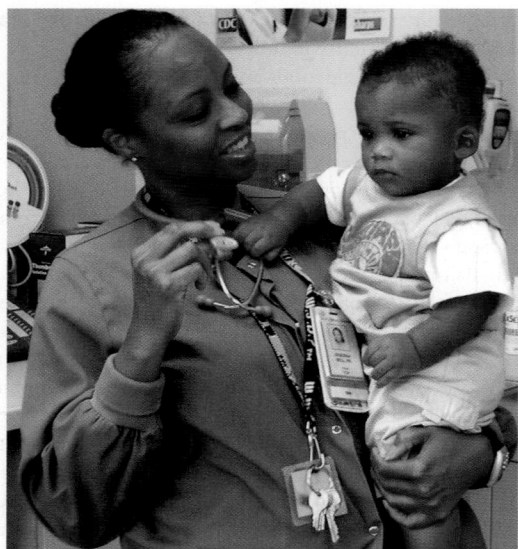

FIG 31.13 Consistent nursing contact is important in developing trust in infants with failure to thrive.

BOX 31.3   Clinical Manifestations of Failure to Thrive

- Growth failure (see earlier in this chapter for definitions)
- Developmental delays—social, motor, adaptive, language
- Undernutrition
- Apathy
- Withdrawn behavior
- Feeding or eating disorders, such as vomiting, feeding resistance, anorexia, pica, rumination
- No fear of strangers (at age when stranger anxiety is normal)
- Avoidance of eye contact
- Wide-eyed gaze and continual scan of the environment ("radar gaze")
- Stiff and unyielding or flaccid and unresponsive
- Minimal smiling

---

a child. Other factors that should be considered are lack of education; physical and mental health problems such as physical and sexual abuse, depression, or drug dependence; immaturity, especially in adolescent parents; and lack of commitment to parenting, such as giving priority to entertainment or employment. Often these parents and their families are under stress and in multiple chronic emotional, social, and financial crises.

Children with FTT may use feeding as a control mechanism or attention-seeking mechanism in a poorly organized or chaotic family situation; parents may allow the child to dictate the norms for behavior and feeding because of inexperience with parenting or poor parenting role models. Thus refusing to eat or eating only sweets and snacks with nonnutritive value may be the child's norm based on food availability and family tradition. General guidelines for the feeding process are outlined in the Guidelines box: Failure to Thrive.

Four primary goals in the nutritional management of children with FTT are to (1) correct nutritional deficiencies and achieve the ideal weight for height, (2) provide adequate calories for catch-up growth, (3) restore optimal body composition, and (4) educate the parents or primary caregivers regarding the child's nutritional requirements and appropriate feeding methods. For infants, 24 kcal/oz formulas may be

---

 GUIDELINES

Feeding the Child With Failure to Thrive

Provide a primary core of staff to feed the child. The same nurses are able to learn the child's cues and respond consistently.

Provide a quiet, unstimulating atmosphere. A number of children with failure to thrive (FTT) are very distractible, and their attention is diverted with minimal stimuli. Older children do well at a feeding table; bottle-fed infants and children should always be held.

Maintain a calm, even temperament throughout the meal. Negative outbursts may be commonplace in this child's habit formation. Limits on eating behavior definitely need to be provided, but they should be stated in a firm, calm tone. If the nurse is hurried or anxious, the feeding process will not be optimized.

Talk to the child by giving directions about eating. "Take a bite, Lisa" is appropriate and directive. The more distractible the child, the more directive the nurse should be to refocus attention on feeding. Positive comments about feeding are actively given.

Be persistent. This is perhaps one of the most important guidelines. Parents often give up when the child begins negative feeding behavior. Calm perseverance through 10 to 15 minutes of food refusal will eventually diminish negative behavior. Although forced feeding is avoided, "strictly encouraged" feeding is essential.

Maintain a face-to-face posture with the child when possible. Encourage eye contact, and remain with the child throughout the meal.

Introduce new foods slowly. Often these children have been exclusively bottle-fed. If acceptance of solid foods is a problem, begin with pureed food and, after it is accepted, advance to junior and regular solid foods.

Follow the child's rhythm of feeding. The child will set a rhythm when the previous conditions are met.

Develop a structured routine. Disruption in other activities of daily living has great impact on feeding responses, so bathing, sleeping, dressing, playing, and feeding are structured. The nurse should feed the child in the same way and place as often as possible. The length of the feeding should also be established (usually 30 minutes).

---

provided to increase caloric intake; older children (1 to 6 years) may benefit from a 30-kcal/oz formula (American Academy of Pediatrics, Committee on Nutrition, 2014). Other carbohydrate additives include fortified rice cereal and vegetable oil. Because vitamin and mineral deficiencies may occur, multivitamin supplementation, including zinc and iron, is recommended. Usually only in extreme cases of malnourishment are tube feedings or intravenous therapy required. Restrict juice intake in children with FTT until adequate weight gain has been achieved with appropriate milk sources; thereafter give no more than 4 oz/day of juice.

POSITIONAL PLAGIOCEPHALY

Since the Back to Sleep campaign began in 1994 advocating nonprone sleeping for infants to prevent sudden infant death syndrome (SIDS), an increase in the incidence of positional plagiocephaly has been observed (Laughlin, Luerssen, Dias, et al., 2011). Approximately 20% of infants have a skull that is most prevalent between 2 and 4 months of age (van Wijk, van Vlimmeren, Groothuis-Oudshoorn, et al., 2014). The term *plagiocephaly* connotes an oblique or asymmetric head; *positional plagiocephaly*, *deformational plagiocephaly*, or *nonsynostotic plagiocephaly* implies an acquired condition that occurs as a result of cranial molding during infancy, usually as a result of lying in the supine position (van Wijk et al., 2014). Because infants' sutures are not closed, the skull is

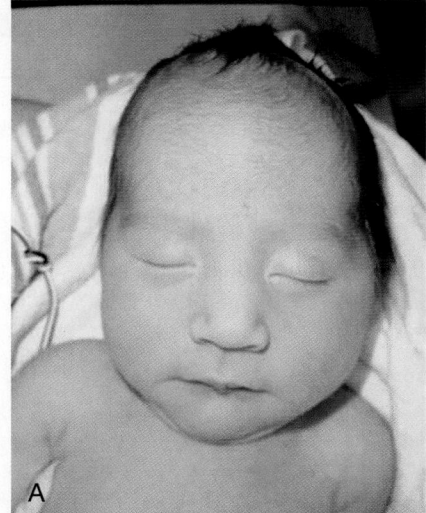
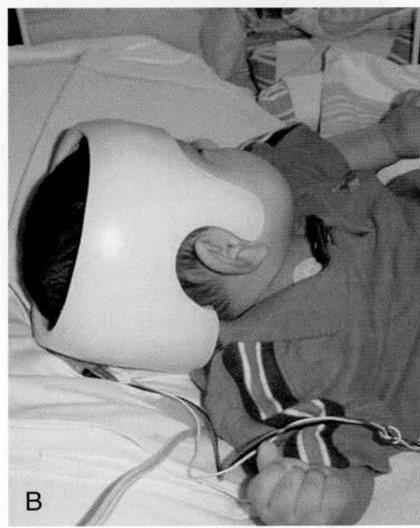

FIG 31.14 A, Plagiocephaly. B, Helmet used to correct plagiocephaly. (Courtesy of Dr. Gerardo Cabrera-Meza, Department of Neonatology, Baylor College of Medicine, Houston, TX.)

pliable and, when infants are placed on their backs to sleep, the posterior occiput flattens over time (Fig. 31.14, A). A typical bald spot develops, which is usually transient. As a result of prolonged pressure on one side of the skull, that side becomes misshapen; mild facial asymmetry may develop. The sternocleidomastoid muscle may tighten on the preferential side, and torticollis may also develop. Congenital or acquired torticollis may cause plagiocephaly; other causes of deformational plagiocephaly include certain craniofacial syndromes. This discussion centers only on positional plagiocephaly caused by the supine sleeping position.

Diagnostic Evaluation

The diagnosis of positional plagiocephaly may be made on physical examination of the infant's head; the infant's head is viewed frontally and from above. The typical infant's head shape will resemble a parallelogram, with unilateral flattening of the occiput, frontal and parietal bossing, a prominent cheekbone, and an anterior ear displacement. An evaluation of neck movement and range of motion is also made to determine the presence of torticollis. In most cases, skull films and further radiologic studies (computed tomographic scan) are used only

to rule out craniosynostosis or other cranial deformity that may affect brain growth.

Therapeutic Management

Prevention of positional plagiocephaly may begin shortly after birth by placing the infant to sleep supine and alternating the infant's head position nightly, avoiding prolonged placement in car safety seats and swings, and using prone positioning or "tummy time" for approximately 30 to 60 minutes per day when the infant is awake (Laughlin, Luerssen, Dias, et al., 2011).

Treatment of torticollis and plagiocephaly initially involves exercises to loosen the tight muscle and switching head position sides during feeding, carrying, and sleep. If the plagiocephaly is not resolved within 4 to 8 weeks of physical therapy, a customized helmet may be worn to decrease the pressure on the affected side of the skull (see Fig. 31.14, B). If no improvement occurs with physical therapy or a molded helmet over a period of 2 to 3 months, the infant may be referred to a pediatric neurosurgeon or craniofacial surgeon; the referral should optimally occur by 4 to 6 months of age (Laughlin, Luerssen, Dias, et al., 2011).

The helmet is worn 23 hours per day for a prescribed period (usually 3 months). Repositioning and physical therapy are said to be more effective when used before the infant can roll over or move his or her head alone (i.e., before approximately 3 to 4 months of age) (Robinson & Proctor, 2009).

Care Management

Minor skull flattening is not considered significant, but parents should learn to prevent plagiocephaly by altering the infant's head position during sleep. Infants should be placed prone on a firm surface during awake time (tummy time), which prevents plagiocephaly and facilitates development of upper shoulder girdle strength; the latter helps in the progressive development of movements such as rolling over and starting to rise up on all fours, which are precursors to crawling and eventually walking. A total of 30 to 60 minutes of supervised tummy time per day in infants younger than 6 months of age is recommended (Laughlin, Luerssen, Dias et al., 2011).

Despite the perceived increase in the incidence of positional plagiocephaly, the supine sleeping position is still recommended because it has led to a significant decrease in loss of infant lives from SIDS (American Academy of Pediatrics, Task Force on Sudden Infant Death Syndrome, 2016). Additional measures to prevent positional plagiocephaly include avoiding excessive time spent in car restraint seats, infant seats, and bouncers. Alternating the infant's head position for sleep times can also prevent unilateral molding. When a nurse or parent notices plagiocephaly, a consultation with the primary health care practitioner is recommended to evaluate the head shape and ascertain the need for early intervention.

SUDDEN INFANT DEATH SYNDROME

Sudden infant death syndrome (SIDS) is defined as the sudden death of an infant younger than 1 year of age that remains unexplained after a complete postmortem examination, including an investigation of the death scene and a review of the case history. Since 1994, the incidence of SIDS in the United States has decreased due to the Safe to Sleep campaign (formerly known as the Back to Sleep campaign).* SIDS is

---

*Safe to Sleep materials may be ordered by contacting the National Institute of Child Health and Human Development Information Resource Center, Safe to Sleep, PO Box 3006, Rockville, MD 20847; 800-505-CRIB (2742); fax: 866-760-5947; www.nichd.nih.gov/sids.

TABLE 31.3   Epidemiology of Sudden Infant Death Syndrome

Factor	Occurrence
Incidence	1545 per 100,000 live births (2014)*
Peak age	2–3 months; 95% occur by 6 months; preterm infants die from sudden infant death syndrome (SIDS) at mean age of 6 weeks later than mean age of death from SIDS for term infants
Sex	Higher percentage of boys affected
Time of death	During sleep
Time of year	Increased incidence in winter
Racial	Greater incidence in African-Americans and Native Americans (see the "Sudden Infant Death Syndrome" section earlier in this chapter)
Birth	Higher incidence in the following: • Preterm infants, especially infants of extremely and very low birth weight • Multiple births† • Neonates with low Apgar scores • Infants with central nervous system disturbances and respiratory disorders such as bronchopulmonary dysplasia • Increasing birth order (subsequent siblings as opposed to firstborn child)
Health status	Infants with a recent history of illness; lower incidence in immunized infants
Sleep habits	Highest risk associated with prone position; use of soft bedding; overheating (thermal stress); cosleeping with adult, especially on sofa or noninfant bed; higher incidence in cosleeping with adult smoker Infants cosleeping with adult at higher risk if younger than 11 weeks of age
Feeding habits	Lower incidence in breastfed infants
Pacifier	Lower incidence in infants put to sleep with pacifier
Siblings	May have greater incidence in siblings of SIDS victims
Maternal	Young age; cigarette smoking, especially during pregnancy; poor prenatal care; substance abuse (heroin, methadone, cocaine). A few studies have shown an increased risk in infants exposed to second-hand environmental tobacco smoke.

*Heron, M. (2016). Deaths: Leading causes for 2014. *National Vital Statistics Reports, 65*(5), 1–96.
†Although a rare event, simultaneous death of twins from SIDS can occur.
Adapted from American Academy of Pediatrics Task Force on Sudden Infant Death Syndrome. (2005). The changing concept of sudden infant death syndrome: diagnostic coding shifts, controversies regarding the sleeping environment, and new variables to consider in reducing risk. *Pediatrics, 116*(5), 1245–1255; American Academy of Pediatrics. (2016). Task Force on Sudden Infant Death Syndrome: SIDS and other sleep-related infant deaths: Updated 2016 recommendations for a safe infant sleeping environment. *Pediatrics, 138*(5), 1–14.

the third leading cause of infant deaths (birth to 12 months of age) and the leading cause of postneonatal deaths (between 1 and 12 months of age). SIDS claimed the lives of 2063 infants in the United States in 2010, a 4% decrease from 2009 (Murphy, Xu, & Kochanek, 2013). Despite dramatic decreases in SIDS rates, rates for African-American, Native American, and American-Alaskan infants remain disproportionately higher (two to three times higher) than for the rest of the population (Hunt & Hauck, 2016). It is also important to note that the percentage of infants born preterm (<37 weeks) was significantly higher (18.5%) in African-American women than in Caucasian women (11.7%) (MacDorman & Mathews, 2011). Preterm births rank second as a cause of infant death; this trend has been constant since the mid-1990s, when the rates of SIDS deaths significantly decreased in the United States.

The SIDS rate has remained fairly static since 2009. This has been attributed to determination of non-SIDS causes of postneonatal mortality, such as suffocation and asphyxia (Moon & Fu, 2012). Table 31.3 summarizes the major epidemiologic characteristics of SIDS.

There has been considerable debate over the term *SIDS*, yet the definition noted above remains for the time being. Other terms have been developed to explain sudden death in infants. *Sudden unexpected early neonatal death* (SUEND) and *sudden unexpected infant death* (SUID) share similar features but differ in regard to the timing of death: whereas SUID is considered a death in the postneonatal period, SUEND occurs in the first week of life.

Etiology

There are numerous theories regarding the etiology of SIDS; however, the cause remains unknown. One hypothesis is that SIDS is related to a brainstem abnormality in the neurologic regulation of cardiorespiratory

control. This maldevelopment affects arousal and physiologic responses to a life-threatening challenge during sleep (Bejjani, Machaalani, & Waters, 2013). Abnormalities include prolonged sleep apnea, increased frequency of brief inspiratory pauses, excessive periodic breathing, and impaired arousal responsiveness to increased carbon dioxide or decreased oxygen. However, *sleep apnea is not the cause of SIDS.* The vast majority of infants with apnea do not die, and only a minority of SIDS victims have documented apparent life-threatening events (ALTEs) (see the "Apparent Life-Threatening Event" section later in this chapter). Numerous studies indicate that no association exists between SIDS and any childhood vaccine (Moon & Fu, 2012).

A genetic predisposition to SIDS has been postulated as a cause. A deficiency of the complement component C4 is associated with SIDS cases (Opdal & Rognum, 2011). In addition, polymorphisms among interleukin genes, transforming growth factor, tumor necrosis factor, and interferon gamma are closely associated with cases of SIDS (Opdal & Rognum, 2011).

A number of triple-risk model hypotheses have been proposed to explain the etiology of SIDS. Some of the proposed factors include an underlying infant vulnerability factor such as a brain abnormality, a critical incident in the fetal developmental period or in early neonatal life, and an environmental stressor such as prone sleep positioning (Matthews & Moore, 2013).

Risk Factors for SIDS

Maternal smoking during pregnancy has emerged in numerous epidemiologic studies as a major factor in SIDS, and tobacco smoke in the infant's environment after birth has also been shown to have a possible relationship to the incidence of SIDS (American Academy of Pediatrics,

Task Force on Sudden Infant Death Syndrome, 2016). A meta-analysis shows that exposure to tobacco smoke significantly increases an infant's risk for SIDS with an odds ratio of 2.25 for prenatal maternal smoking and 1.97 for postnatal maternal smoking (Zhang & Wang, 2013).

Cosleeping, or an infant sharing a bed with an adult or older child on a non-infant bed, has been reported to have a positive association with SIDS. Two meta-analyses found a significant increase in the risk for SIDS among infants that bed shared compared to infants who slept alone (Das, Sankar, Agarwal, et al., 2014; Carpenter, McGarvey, Mitchell, et al., 2013). However, room-sharing is now recommended with an infant on a sleeping surface separate from the adult (American Academy of Pediatrics, Task Force on Sudden Infant Death Syndrome, 2016). Studies correlated higher incidences of SIDS and infant co-sleeping with maternal smoking, co-sleeping with multiple family members, sleeping on a couch, use of a pillow in the infant's bed, soft bedding, loose bedding, and unintentional asphyxiation resulting from adult intoxication (overlaying) (American Academy of Pediatrics, Task Force on Sudden Infant Death Syndrome, 2016; Blair, Sidebotham, Pease, et al., 2014; Rechtman, Colvin, Blair, & Moon, 2014; Li, Zhang, Zielke, et al., 2009). Bedding items such as stuffed animals and toys should be removed from the crib while the infant is asleep.

Prone sleeping may cause oropharyngeal obstruction or affect thermal balance or arousal state. Rebreathing of carbon dioxide by infants in the prone position is also a possible cause of SIDS. Infants sleeping prone and on soft bedding may not be able to move their heads to the side, thus increasing the risk for suffocation and lethal rebreathing. Thus *the side-lying position is no longer recommended* for infants (unless medically indicated).

Another postulated cause of SIDS has been a prolonged Q-T interval or other arrhythmias (Hunt & Hauck, 2016).

Infant Risk Factors

Certain groups of infants are at increased risk for SIDS:
- Low birth weight or preterm birth
- Low Apgar scores
- Recent viral illness
- Siblings of two or more SIDS victims
- Male gender
- Infants of Native American or African-American ethnicity

No diagnostic tests exist to predict which infants, including those in the above groups, will survive, and home apnea monitoring is no guarantee of survival (American Academy of Pediatrics, Task Force on Sudden Infant Death Syndrome, 2016). Whether subsequent siblings of one SIDS infant are at increased risk for SIDS is unclear. Even if the risk is increased, families have a 99% chance that their subsequent child will *not* die of SIDS.

Protective Factors for SIDS

A meta-analysis confirmed that exclusive breastfeeding for any period of time decreased the overall risk for SIDS (Hauck, Thompson, Tanabe, et al., 2011). Several studies have found pacifier use in infants to be a protective factor against the occurrence of SIDS; the pacifier should be used when the infant is falling asleep and does not need to be reinserted if it falls out (American Academy of Pediatrics, Task Force on Sudden Infant Death Syndrome, 2016). Therefore the American Academy of Pediatrics recommends using a pacifier at naptime and bedtime, using a pacifier only if the infant is breastfeeding successfully, not using a sweetened coating on the pacifier, and avoiding forcing the infant to use the pacifier.

Although the cause of SIDS is unknown, autopsies reveal consistent pathologic findings, such as pulmonary edema and intrathoracic hemorrhages that confirm the diagnosis. Consequently, autopsies should be performed on all infants suspected of dying of SIDS, and findings should be shared with the parents as soon as possible after the death.

Care Management

Nurses have a vital role in preventing SIDS by educating families about the risk for prone sleeping position in infants from birth to 6 months of age, the use of appropriate bedding surfaces, the association with maternal smoking, and the dangers of cosleeping on noninfant surfaces with adults or other children. Also, nurses have an important role in modeling behaviors for parents to foster practices that decrease the risk for SIDS, including placing infants in a supine sleeping position in the hospital. Many health care workers are concerned that infants placed on the back to sleep will aspirate emesis or mucus, yet studies fail to show an increase in infant deaths, spitting up during sleep, aspiration, asphyxia, or respiratory failure as a result of supine sleep positioning (American Academy of Pediatrics, Task Force on Sudden Infant Death Syndrome, 2016).

Education can change practice. After an educational session and laminated reminder card on safe sleep recommendations, neonatal intensive care unit (NICU) nurses had a significant increase in rate of supine positioning (39% before and 83% after), providing a firm sleeping surface (5% before and 96% after), and removal of soft objects in bed (45% before and 75% after) for their NICU patients (Gelfer, Cameron, Masters, et al., 2013). Role modeling safe sleep practices and providing education to parents is imperative before hospital discharge because limited opportunities exist for parents to receive information about caring for their infant (Ateah, 2013). Nurses must be proactive in further decreasing the incidence of SIDS; postpartum discharge planning, newborn discharges, follow-up home visits, well-baby clinic visits, and immunization visits provide excellent opportunities to educate parents on these matters. Nurses must continue to take every opportunity to advocate for infants by providing information for parents and caregivers about the modifiable risk factors for SIDS that can be implemented to prevent its occurrence across all sectors of the population.

Interprofessional Care of the Family of a SIDS Infant

Loss of a child from SIDS presents several crises with which the parents must cope. In addition to grief and mourning the death of their child, the parents must face a tragedy that was sudden, unexpected, and unexplained. The psychologic intervention for the family must deal with these additional variables. This discussion focuses primarily on the objectives of care for families experiencing SIDS rather than on the process of grief and mourning, which is explored in Chapter 36.

The first people to arrive at the scene may be the police and emergency medical service personnel. They should handle the situation by asking few questions; giving no indication of wrongdoing, abuse, or neglect; making sensitive judgments concerning any resuscitation efforts for the child; and comforting the family members as much as possible. A compassionate, sensitive approach to the family during the first few minutes can help spare them some of the overwhelming guilt and anguish that commonly follow this type of death.

The medical examiner or coroner may go to the home or place of death and make the death pronouncement; until then, the sleep environment should remain as it was when the infant was initially found. If the infant is not pronounced dead at the scene, he or she may be transported to the ED to be pronounced by a physician. Usually there is no attempt at resuscitation in the ED. While they are in the ED, the parents should be asked only factual questions, such as when they found the infant, how he or she looked, and whom they called for help. The nurse should avoid any remarks that may suggest responsibility, such as "Didn't you hear the infant cry out?" or "Was the head buried in a blanket?" It is the investigators' responsibility to document these findings at the scene rather than have parents recount the experience in the ED.

At this time, the physician should initiate the discussion of an autopsy, often with the nurse being present to support the family. The physician or medical examiner, depending on the circumstances, should emphasize that a diagnosis cannot be confirmed until the postmortem examination is completed. Requesting an autopsy may be difficult because of the parents' emotional state; however, an autopsy may clear up possible misconceptions regarding the death. Instructions about the autopsy and funeral arrangements may need to be repeated or put in writing. If the mother was breastfeeding, she needs information about abrupt discontinuation of lactation. The nurse or physician should contact the primary care practitioner for the infant and the mother to avoid any miscommunications or telephone calls at a later date.

Parents experiencing perinatal death perceive health care workers' responses as having a significant impact on the parents' grieving process. A family-centered approach that involves the sociocultural context and unique needs of the family is essential for perinatal bereavement care (Flenady, Boyle, Koopmans, Wilson, Stones et al., 2014). An important aspect of compassionate care for these parents is allowing them to say good-bye to their child. These are the parents' last moments with their child, and they should be as quiet, meaningful, peaceful, and undisturbed as possible. Encourage parents to hold their infant before leaving the ED. Because the parents leave the hospital without their infant, it is helpful to accompany them to the car or arrange for someone else to take them home.

When the parents return home, a competent, qualified professional should visit them as soon after the death as possible. They should receive printed material that contains excellent information about SIDS (available from national organizations*). When the unexpected death of a child occurs, it is common for one parent to blame the other for the child's death. Parents may also experience guilt over the child's death; if they had checked earlier, the child might still be alive. It is important that the health care team assist parents in working through these feelings to prevent marital disruption in addition to the loss of the loved child.

A debriefing session may help health care workers who dealt with the family and deceased infant to cope with emotions that are often engendered when a SIDS victim is brought into the acute care facility. Comprehensive guidelines have been published for health care professionals involved in SIDS investigations to assist the family and at the same time to determine that the infant's death was not the result of other factors, such as child maltreatment (American Academy of Pediatrics, Task Force on Sudden Infant Death Syndrome, 2016).

APPARENT LIFE-THREATENING EVENT

An apparent life-threatening event (ALTE), formerly referred to as *aborted SIDS death* or *near-miss SIDS*, generally refers to an event that is sudden and frightening to the observer in which the infant exhibits a combination of apnea, change in color (pallor, cyanosis, redness), change in muscle tone (usually hypotonia), and choking, gagging, or coughing and that usually involves a significant intervention and even CPR by the caregiver who witnesses the event. The definition of *ALTE* may include apnea, but ALTE may occur without apnea (Silvestri, 2012). It is erroneous to

characterize ALTE as a near-miss SIDS incident; however, infants with ALTE are at increased risk for SIDS. The risk for SIDS may be three to five times greater in infants who experienced an ALTE (Hunt & Hauck, 2016).

Diagnostic Evaluation

An essential component of the diagnostic process includes a detailed description of the event, including who witnessed the event; where the infant was during the event; and what, if any, activities were involved (e.g., during or after a feeding, riding in a car seat restraint, presence of siblings or any minor children, what clothing the infant was wearing). In addition, a prenatal and postnatal history must be obtained. A short period of observation in the ED may be appropriate to observe the infant's respiratory pattern and response to feeding. A careful evaluation of late preterm and preterm infants in the car restraints currently in use is essential; upper airway occlusion and subsequent apnea and cyanosis may occur if the infant is not positioned properly. Reported diagnoses in infants with ALTE include a neurologic event such as a seizure (10% to 20% of cases seen); GI problem, including gastroesophageal reflux (48%); respiratory conditions (20% to 30%); cardiac conditions (10% to 20%); and other concerns such as ear, nose, and throat (ENT) abnormalities, ingestions, Munchausen syndrome by proxy, or child abuse (each <5%) (Chu & Hagemen, 2013). In some cases, multiple diagnoses may be made.

In the event that an underlying diagnosis such as those mentioned previously is not established, home monitoring may be recommended. The most commonly used monitoring is continuous recording of cardiorespiratory patterns (cardiopneumogram or pneumocardiogram). A more sophisticated test, polysomnography (sleep study), also records brain waves, eye and body movements, esophageal manometry, and end-tidal carbon dioxide measurements. However, none of these tests can predict risk. Some children with normal results may still have subsequent apneic episodes.

Therapeutic Management

The treatment of an infant with an ALTE depends on the underlying condition. Treatment of recurrent apnea (without an underlying organic problem) usually involves continuous home monitoring of cardiorespiratory rhythms and, in some cases, the use of methylxanthines (respiratory stimulant drugs, such as caffeine). The decision to discontinue the monitoring is based on the infant's clinical condition. A general guideline for discontinuation is when infants with ALTEs have gone 2 or 3 months without significant numbers of episodes requiring intervention. Newer home apnea monitors allow download of information that assists the practitioner in deciding when to discontinue home monitoring.

Care Management

The diagnosis of an ALTE causes great anxiety and concern in parents, and the institution of home monitoring presents additional physical and emotional burdens. Parents of infants on home apnea monitors report experiencing emotional distress, especially depression and hostility, during the first few weeks after hospital discharge. Home apnea monitoring may offer some predictability and control over the current child's survival through the period of uncertainty.

If home monitoring is required, the nurse can be a major source of support to the family in terms of education about the equipment; education regarding observation of the infant's status; and instructions regarding immediate intervention during apneic episodes, including CPR. To help the family cope with the numerous procedures they must learn, adequate preparation before discharge and written instructions are essential. In the first few weeks after discharge, parents may benefit

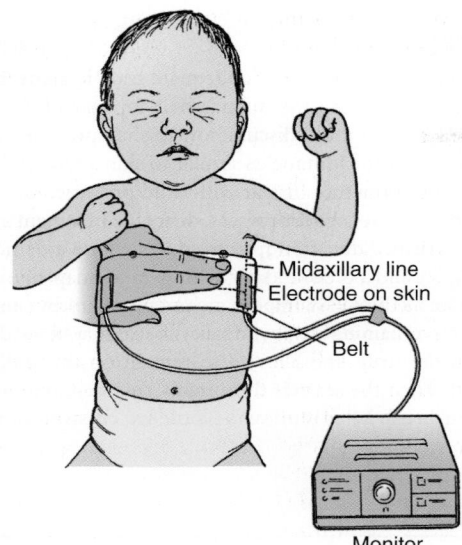

FIG 31.15 Placement of electrodes or belt for apnea monitoring. In small infants, one fingerbreadth below the nipple line may be used to determine correct placement of the monitor belt.

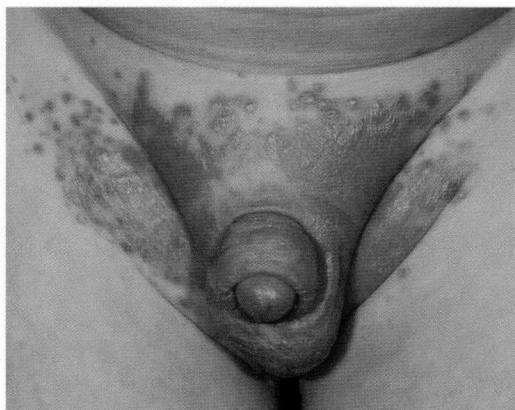

FIG 31.16 Irritant diaper dermatitis. Note the sharply demarcated edges. (From Habif, T.P. [2016]. *Clinical dermatology: a color guide to diagnosis and therapy* [6th ed.]. St. Louis, MO: Elsevier.)

by having a practitioner readily available to answer questions regarding false alarms and for other technical assistance. Safety is a major concern with monitor use. The following precautions are recommended:
- Remove leads from infant when not attached to the monitor.
- Unplug the power cord from the electrical outlet when the cord is not plugged into the monitor.
- Use safety covers on electrical outlets to discourage children from inserting objects into sockets.

Siblings should also be supervised when near the infant and taught that the monitor is not a toy. Other safety practices include informing local utility and rescue squads (fire and/or emergency services) of the home monitoring in case of an emergency, especially if the family lives in a remote rural area. Telephone numbers for these services should be posted in the home or set up as speed dial. If a cellular phone is the main house phone, make sure it stays in a central location for all family members to access in an emergency.

Caregivers need detailed information regarding proper attachment of the electrodes to the infant's chest with impedance monitors that detect chest movement. The electrodes are placed in the midaxillary line at a space one or two fingerbreadths below the nipple. For home use, electrodes attached to a belt that is placed around the child's trunk are preferred (Fig. 31.15). The belt is positioned so that the electrodes contact the skin in the same area. Monitors may have memory chips that allow for event recording, which can be an effective tool in evaluating the use of the monitor, events immediately before and after the ALTE, and reported frequency of alarms.

Monitors are effective only if they are used. They do not prevent death but alert the caregiver to the ALTE in time to intervene. The need to use the monitor and to respond appropriately to alarms must be stressed. Noncompliance can result in the infant's death.

DIAPER DERMATITIS

Diaper dermatitis is common in infants and one of several acute inflammatory skin disorders caused either directly or indirectly by wearing diapers. The peak age of occurrence is 9 to 12 months of age, and the incidence is greater in bottle-fed infants than in breastfed infants.

Pathophysiology and Clinical Manifestations

Diaper dermatitis is caused by prolonged and repetitive contact with an irritant (e.g., urine, feces, soaps, detergents, ointments, friction). Although the irritant in the majority of cases is urine and feces, a combination of factors contributes to irritation. Prolonged contact of the skin with diaper wetness produces higher friction, greater abrasion damage, increased transepidermal permeability, and increased microbial counts. The irritant quality of urine is related to an increase in pH from the breakdown of urea in the presence of fecal urease. The increased pH promotes the activity of fecal enzymes, principally the proteases and lipases, which act as irritants. Fecal enzymes also increase the permeability of skin to bile salts, another potential irritant in feces.

The eruption of diaper dermatitis is manifested primarily on convex surfaces or in folds. Eruptions involving the skin in most intimate contact with the diaper (e.g., the convex surfaces of buttocks, inner thighs, mons pubis, scrotum) but sparing the folds are likely to be caused by chemical irritants, especially from urine and feces (Fig. 31.16). Other causes are detergents or soaps from inadequately rinsed cloth diapers or the chemicals in disposable wipes. Perianal involvement is usually the result of chemical irritation from feces, especially diarrheal stools. *Candida albicans* infection produces perianal inflammation and a maculopapular rash with satellite lesions that may cross the inguinal fold (Fig. 31.17).

Care Management

Nursing interventions are aimed at altering the three factors that produce dermatitis: wetness, pH, and fecal irritants. The most significant factor amenable to intervention is the moist environment created in the diaper area. Changing the diaper as soon as it becomes wet eliminates a large part of the problem, and removing the diaper to expose healthy skin to air facilitates drying. The use of a hair dryer or heat lamp is not recommended because these devices can cause burns.

Guidelines for controlling diaper rash are presented in the Family-Centered Care box: Controlling Diaper Rash. A common misconception about using cornstarch on skin is that it promotes the growth of *C. albicans*. Neither cornstarch nor talc promotes the growth of fungi under conditions normally found in the diaper area. Cornstarch is more effective in reducing friction and tends to cake less than talc when the skin is wet. On the basis of these properties and its safety in terms of inhalation injury, cornstarch is the preferred product. Talc should not be used.

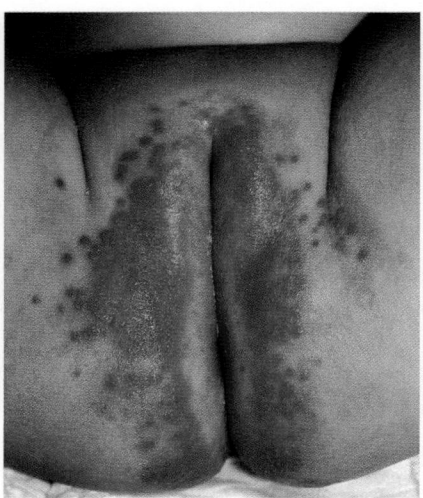

FIG 31.17 Candidiasis of diaper area. Note the beefy red central erythema with satellite pustules. (From Paller, A.S., Mancini, A.J. [2016]. *Hurwitz clinical pediatric dermatology* [5th ed.]. St. Louis, MO: Elsevier.)

👪 FAMILY-CENTERED CARE

Controlling Diaper Rash

Keep skin dry.*
Use superabsorbent disposable diapers to reduce skin wetness.
Change diapers as soon as soiled—especially with stool—whenever possible, preferably once during the night.
Expose healthy or only slightly irritated skin to air, not heat, to dry completely.
Apply ointment, such as zinc oxide or petrolatum, to protect skin, especially if skin is very red or has moist, open areas.
Avoid removing skin barrier cream with each diaper change; remove waste material and reapply skin barrier cream.
To completely remove ointment, especially zinc oxide, use mineral oil; do not wash vigorously.
Avoid overwashing the skin, especially with perfumed soaps or commercial wipes, which may be irritating.
May use a moisturizer or non-soap cleanser, such as cold cream or Cetaphil, to wipe urine from skin.
Gently wipe stool from skin using a soft cloth and warm water.
Use disposable diaper wipes that are detergent- and alcohol-free.

*Powder helps keep the skin dry, but talc is dangerous if breathed into the lungs. Plain cornstarch or cornstarch-based powder is safer. When using any powder product, first shake it into your hand and then apply it to the diaper area. Store the container away from the infant's reach, and keep the container closed when not in use.

SEBORRHEIC DERMATITIS

Seborrheic dermatitis is a chronic, recurrent, inflammatory reaction of the skin that occurs most commonly on the scalp (cradle cap) but may involve the eyelids (blepharitis), external ear canal (otitis externa), nasolabial folds, and inguinal region. The cause is unknown, although it is more common in early infancy, when sebum production is increased. The lesions are characteristically thick, adherent, yellowish, scaly, oily patches that may or may not be mildly pruritic. Unlike atropic dermatitis, seborrheic dermatitis is not associated with a positive family history for allergy. Diagnosis is made primarily by the appearance and the location of the crusts or scales.

Care Management

Cradle cap may be prevented with adequate scalp hygiene. Frequently, parents omit shampooing the infant's hair for fear of damaging the fontanels. The nurse should discuss how to shampoo the infant's hair and emphasize that the fontanel is similar to skin anywhere else on the body; it does not puncture or tear with mild pressure.

When seborrheic lesions are present, direct the treatment at removing the scales or crusts. Education may need to include a demonstration. Shampooing should be done daily with a mild soap or commercial baby shampoo; medicated shampoos are not necessary, but an antiseborrheic shampoo containing sulfur and salicylic acid may be used. Shampoo is applied to the scalp and allowed to remain on the scalp until the crusts soften. Then the scalp is thoroughly rinsed. A fine-tooth comb or a soft facial brush helps remove the loosened crusts from the strands of hair after shampooing.

REFERENCES

Akhnikh, S., Engelberts, A. C., van Sleuwen, B. E., et al. (2014). The excessively crying infant: Etiology and treatment. *Pediatric Annals, 43*(4), e69–e75.

American Academy of Pediatrics, Committee on Infectious Diseases. (2013). Recommended childhood and adolescent immunization schedule—United States, 2013. *Pediatrics, 131*(2), 397–398.

American Academy of Pediatrics, Committee on Infectious Diseases (2015). L. Pickering (Ed.), *2015 Red Book: Report of the Committee on Infectious Diseases* (30th ed.). Elk Grove Village, IL: The Academy.

American Academy of Pediatrics, Committee on Nutrition (2014). *Pediatric nutrition handbook* (7th ed.). Elk Grove Village, IL: American Academy of Pediatrics.

American Academy of Pediatrics (AAP). (2011). Council on Communications and Media: Media use by children younger than 2 years. *Pediatrics, 128*(5), 1040–1045.

American Academy of Pediatric Dentistry (2014). *Guideline on infant oral health care.* Retrieved from http://www.aapd.org/media/Policies_Guidelines/G_InfantOralHealthCare.pdf.

American Academy of Pediatrics, Task Force on Sudden Infant Death Syndrome. (2016). SIDS and other sleep-related infant deaths: Updated 2016 recommendations for a safe infant sleeping environment. *Pediatrics, 138*(5), 1–14.

Aronsson, C. A., Uusitalo, U., Vehik, K., et al. (2015). Age at first introduction to complementary foods is associated with sociodemographic factors in children with increased genetic risk of developing type 1 diabetes. *Maternal & Child Nutrition, 11*(4), 803–814.

Atalay, A., & McCord, M. (2012). Characteristics of failure to thrive in a referral population: Implications for treatment. *Clinical Pediatrics, 51*(3), 219–225.

Ateah, C. A. (2013). Prenatal parent education for first-time expectant parents: "Making it through labor is just the beginning…". *Journal of Pediatric Health Care, 27*(2), 91–97.

Baker, R. D., & Greer, F. R. (2010). American Academy of Pediatrics (AAP) Committee on Nutrition: Clinical report—Diagnosis and prevention of iron deficiency and iron-deficiency anemia in infants and young children (0-3 years of age). *Pediatrics, 126*(5), 1040–1050.

Becker, P., Carney, L. N., Corkins, M. R., et al. (2015). Consensus statement of the Academy of Nutrition and Dietetics/American Society for Parenteral and Enteral Nutrition: Indicators recommended for the identification and documentation of pediatric malnutrition (undernutrition). *Nutrition in Clinical Practice, 30*(1), 147–161.

Bejjani, C., Machaalani, R., & Waters, K. A. (2013). The dorsal motor nucleus of the vagus (DMNV) in sudden infant death syndrome (SIDS): Pathways leading to apoptosis. *Respiratory Physiology & Neurobiology, 185*(2), 203–210.

Beirne, P. V., Hennessy, S., Cadogan, S. L., et al. (2015). Needle size for vaccination procedures in children and adolescents. *Cochrane Database of Systematic Reviews, 2015*(6), CD010720.

Blackburn, S. T. (2013). *Maternal, fetal, and neonatal physiology: A clinical perspective* (4th ed.). Maryland Heights, MO: Saunders.

Blair, P. S., Sidebotham, P., Pease, A., et al. (2014). Bed-sharing in the absence of hazardous circumstances: Is there a risk of sudden infant death syndrome? An analysis from two case-control studies conducted in the UK. *PLoS ONE, 9*(9), e107799.

Briere, E. C., Rubin, L., Moro, P. L., et al. (2014). Prevention and control of *Haemophilus influenzae* type B disease: Recommendations of the advisory committee on immunization practices (ACIP). *Morbidity and Mortality Weekly Report Recommendations and Reports, 63*(RR-01), 1–14.

Bull, M. J., & Durbin, D. R. (2008). Rear-facing car safety seats: Getting the message right. *Pediatrics, 121*(3), 619–620.

Carey, W. B., & McDevitt, S. C. (1978). Revision of the infant temperament questionnaire. *Pediatrics, 61*(5), 735–739.

Carpenter, R., McGarvey, C., Mitchell, E. A., et al. (2013). Bed-sharing when parents do not smoke: Is there a risk of SIDS? An individual level analysis of five major case-control studies. *British Medical Journal Open, 2013*(3), 1–12.

Centers for Disease Control and Prevention. (2013). Use of 13-valent pneumococcal conjugate vaccine and 23-valent pneumococcal polysaccharide vaccine among children aged 6-18 years with immunocompromising conditions: Recommendation of the advisory committee on immunization practices (ACIP). *Morbidity and Mortality Weekly Report, 62*(25), 521–524.

Centers for Disease Control and Prevention. (2012a). Unintentional injury deaths among persons aged 0-19 years—United States, 2000-2009. *Morbidity and Mortality Weekly Report, 61*(15), 270–276.

Centers for Disease Control and Prevention (2012b). *Protect the ones you love: child injuries are preventable.* Retrieved from http://www.cdc.gov/safechild/.

Centers for Disease Control and Prevention. (2011). Updated recommendations for use of tetanus toxoid, reduced diphtheria toxoid and acellular pertussis (Tdap) vaccine from the Advisory Committee on Immunization Practices, 2010. *Morbidity and Mortality Weekly Report, 60*(1), 13–15.

Chu, A., & Hagemen, J. R. (2013). Apparent life-threatening events in infancy. *Pediatric Annals, 42*(2), 78–83.

Cole, S. Z., & Lanham, J. S. (2011). Failure to thrive: An update. *American Family Physician, 83*(7), 829–834.

Cook, I. F., & Murtagh, J. (2006). Ventrogluteal area: A suitable site for intramuscular vaccination in infants and toddlers. *Vaccine, 24*(13), 2403–2408.

Critch, J. N. (2011). Infantile colic: Is there a role for dietary interventions? *Paediatrics and Child Health, 16*(1), 47–49.

Darlow, B. A., Horwood, J., Pere-Bracken, H. M., et al. (2013). Psychosocial outcomes of young adults born very low birth weight. *Pediatrics, 132*(6), e1521–e1528.

Das, R. R., Sankar, M. J., Agarwal, R., et al. (2014). Is "bed sharing" beneficial and safe during infancy? A systematic review. *International Journal of Pediatrics,* 468538. Epub ahead of print].

Desapriya, E. B., Joshi, P., Subwarzi, S., et al. (2008). Infant injuries from child restraint safety seat misuse at British Columbia Children's Hospital. *Pediatrics International, 50*(5), 674–678.

Drug and Therapeutics Bulletin. (2013). Management of infantile colic. *British Medical Journal, 347,* 4102.

Durand, D., Ochoa, T. J., Bellomo, S. M., et al. (2013). Detection of secretory immunoglobulin A in human colostrum as mucosal immune response against proteins of the type III secretion system of *Salmonella, Shigella* and enteropathogenic *Escherichia coli. Pediatric Infectious Disease Journal, 32*(10), 1122–1126.

Ellett, M. L., Appleton, M. M., & Sloan, R. S. (2009). Out of the abyss of colic: A view through the father's eyes. *American Journal of Maternal/Child Nursing, 34*(3), 164–171.

Erikson, E. H. (1963). *Childhood and society* (2nd ed.). New York, NY: Norton.

Feeley, N., Sherrard, K., Waitzer, E., et al. (2013). The father at the bedside: Patterns of involvement in the NICU. *Journal of Perinatal & Neonatal Nursing, 27*(1), 72–80.

Flenady, V., Boyle, F., Koopmans, L., et al. (2014). Meeting the needs of parents after a stillbirth or neonatal death. *International Journal of Obstetrics and Gynaecology, 121*(Suppl. 4), 137–140.

Forlenza, G. P., Paradise Black, N. M., McNamara, E. G., et al. (2010). Ankyloglossia, exclusive breastfeeding, and failure to thrive. *Pediatrics, 125*(6), e1500–e1504.

Galland, B. C., Taylor, B. J., Elder, D. E., et al. (2012). Normal sleep patterns in infants and children: A systematic review of observational studies. *Sleep Medicine Reviews, 16*(3), 213–222.

Gallitto, E. (2015). Temperament as a moderator of the effects of parenting on children's behavior. *Development and Psychopathology, 27*(3), 757–773.

Gartstein, M. A., & Rothbart, M. K. (2003). Studying infant temperament via the Revised Infant Behavior Questionnaire. *Infant Behavior and Development, 26*(1), 64–86.

Gelfer, P., Cameron, R., Masters, K., et al. (2013). Integrating "back to sleep" recommendations into neonatal ICU practice. *Pediatrics, 131*(4), e1264–e1270.

Grohskopf, L. A., Sokolow, L. Z., Olsen, S. J., Bresee, J. S., Broder, K. R., & Karron, R. A. (2015). Prevention and control of influenza with vaccines: Recommendations of the Advisory Committee on Immunization Practices, United States, 2015-16 influenza season. *Morbidity and Mortality Weekly Report, 64*(30), 818–825.

Hamilton, B. E., Hoyert, D. L., Martin, J. A., et al. (2013). Annual summary of vital statistics: 2010-2011. *Pediatrics, 131*(3), 548–558.

Hauck, F. R., Thompson, J. M., Tanabe, K. O., et al. (2011). Breastfeeding and reduced risk of sudden infant death syndrome: A meta-analysis. *Pediatrics, 128*(1), 103–110.

Heinrich, J., Koletzko, B., & Koletzko, S. (2014). Timing and diversity of complementary food introduction for prevention of allergic diseases. How early and how much? *Expert Review of Clinical Immunology, 10*(6), 701–704.

Hunt, C. E., & Hauck, F. R. (2016). Sudden infant death syndrome. In R. M. Kliegman, B. F. Stanton, J. W. St. Geme, et al. (Eds.), *Nelson textbook of pediatrics* (20th ed.). Philadelphia, PA: Elsevier/Saunders.

Jaafar, S. H., Jahanfar, S., Angolkar, M., et al. (2011). Pacifier use versus no pacifier use in breastfeeding term infants for increasing duration of breastfeeding. *Cochrane Database of Systematic Reviews, 2011*(3), CD007202.

Jackson, L. A., Yu, O., Nelson, J. C., et al. (2011). Injection site and risk of medically attended local reactions to acellular pertussis vaccine. *Pediatrics, 127*(3), e681–e687.

Johnson, J. D., Cocker, K., & Chang, E. (2015). Infantile colic: Recognition and treatment. *American Family Physician, 92*(7), 577–582.

Junqueira, A. L. N., Tavares, V. R., Martins, R. M. B., et al. (2010). Safety and immunogenicity of hepatitis B vaccine administered into ventrogluteal vs. anterolateral thigh sites in infants: A randomized controlled trial. *International Journal of Nursing Studies, 47*(9), 1074–1079.

Kerstis, B., Engström, G., Edlund, B., et al. (2013). Association between mothers' and fathers' depressive symptoms, sense of coherence and perception of their child's temperament in early parenthood in Sweden. *Scandanavian Journal of Public Health, 41*(3), 233–239.

Labiner-Wolfe, J., & Fein, S. B. (2013). How US mothers store and handle their expressed breast milk. *Journal of Human Lactation, 29*(1), 54–58.

Laughlin, J., Luerssen, T. G., Dias, M. S., et al. (2011). Prevention and management of positional skull deformities in infants. *Pediatrics, 128*(6), 1236–1241.

Lawrence, R. A., & Lawrence, R. M. (2011). *Breastfeeding: A guide for the medical profession* (7th ed.). St. Louis, MO: Mosby.

Li, L., Zhang, Y., Zielke, R. H., et al. (2009). Observations on increased accidental asphyxia deaths in infancy while cosleeping in the state of Maryland. *American Journal of Forensic Medicine and Pathology, 30*(4), 318–321.

Luthy, K. E., Burningham, J., Eden, L. M., et al. (2015). Addressing parental vaccination questions in the school setting: An integrative literature review. *Journal of School Nursing, 32*(1), 47–57. 2016.

MacDorman, M. F., & Mathews, T. J. (2011). Centers for Disease Control and Prevention: Infant deaths—United States, 2000-2007. *Morbidity and Mortality Weekly Report. Surveillance Summaries, 60*(suppl), 49–51.

Mack, K. A., Gilchrist, J., & Ballesteros, M. F. (2008). Injuries among infants treated in the emergency departments in the United States, 2001-2004. *Pediatrics*, 121(5), 930–937.

Maglione, M. A., Das, L., Raaen, L., et al. (2014). Safety of vaccines used for routine immunization of US children; A systematic review. *Pediatrics*, 134(2), 325–337.

Matthews, R., & Moore, A. (2013). Babies are still dying of SIDS. *American Journal of Nursing*, 113(2), 59–64.

McLean, H. S., & Price, D. T. (2016). Failure to thrive. In R. M. Kliegman, B. F. Stanton, J. W. St. Geme, et al. (Eds.), *Nelson textbook of pediatrics* (20th ed.). Philadelphia, PA: Elsevier/Saunders.

Medoff-Cooper, B., Carey, W. B., & McDevitt, S. C. (1993). The early infancy temperament questionnaire. *Journal of Development and Behavioral Pediatrics*, 14(4), 230–235.

Middlemiss, S., Yaure, R., & Huey, E. (2015). Translating research-based knowledge about infant sleep into practice. *Journal of the American Association of Nurse Practitioners*, 27(6), 328–337.

Milidou, I., Sondergaard, C., Jensen, M. S., 2014). Gestational age, small for gestational age, and infantile colic. *Paediatric and Perinatal Epidemiology*, 28(2), 138–145.

Moon, R. Y., & Fu, L. (2012). Sudden infant death syndrome: An update. *Pediatrics in Review*, 33(7), 314–320.

Moss, B. G., & Yeaton, W. H. (2014). Early childhood healthy and obese weight status: Potentially protective benefits of breastfeeding and delaying solid foods. *Maternal and Child Health Journal*, 18(5), 1224–1232.

Murphy, S. L., Xu, J., & Kochanek, K. D. (2013). Deaths: Final data for 2010. *National Vital Statistics Report*, 61(4), 1–118.

Nangia, S., & Tiwari, S. (2013). Failure to thrive. *Indian Journal of Pediatrics*, 80(7), 585–589.

National Center for Immunization and Respiratory Diseases. (2011). General recommendations on immunization: Recommendations of the Advisory Committee on Immunization Practices (ACIP). *Morbidity and Mortality Weekly Report Recommendations and Reports*, 60(2), 1–64.

Nelson, A. M. (2012). A comprehensive review of evidence and current recommendations related to pacifier usage. *Journal of Pediatric Nursing*, 27(6), 690–699.

Okunseri, C., Gonzalez, C., & Hodgson, B. (2015). Children's oral health assessment, prevention, and treatment. *Pediatric Clinics of North America*, 62, 1215–1226.

Opdal, S. H., & Rognum, T. O. (2011). Gene variants predisposing to SIDS: Current knowledge. *Forensic Science, Medicine, and Pathology*, 7(1), 26–36.

Petrosky, E., Bocchini, J. A., Hariri, S., et al. (2015). Use of 9-valent human papillomavirus (HPV) vaccine: Updated HPV vaccination recommendations of the Advisory Committee on Immunization Practices. *Morbidity and Mortality Weekly Report*, 64(11), 300–304.

Perry, R., Hunt, K., & Ernst, E. (2011). Nutritional supplements and other complementary medicines for infantile colic: A systematic review. *Pediatrics*, 127(4), 720–733.

Piaget, J. (1952). *The origins of intelligence in children*. New York, NY: International Universities Press.

Price, C. S., Thompson, W. W., Goodson, B., et al. (2010). Prenatal and infant exposure to thimerosal from vaccines and immunoglobulins and risk of autism. *Pediatrics*, 126(4), 656–664.

Rechtman, L. R., Colvin, J. D., Blair, P. S., et al. (2014). Sofas and infant mortality. *Pediatrics*, 134(5), e1293–e1300.

Robinson, S., & Proctor, M. (2009). Diagnosis and management of deformational plagiocephaly: A review. *Journal of Neurosurgery. Pediatrics*, 3(4), 284–295.

Rogers, S. C., Gallo, K., Saleheen, H., et al. (2012). Wishful thinking: safe transportation of newborns at hospital discharge. *Journal of Trauma and Acute Care Surgery*, 73(4 Suppl. 3), S262–S264.

Romano, C., Hartman, C., Privitera, C., et al. (2015). Current topics in the diagnosis and management of the pediatric non organic feeding disorders (NOFEDs). *Clinical Nutrition*, 34(2), 195–200.

Salah, M., Abdel-Aziz, M., Al-Farok, A., et al. (2013). Recurrent acute otitis media in infants: Analysis of risk factors. *International Journal of Pediatric Otorhinolaryngology*, 77(10), 1665–1669.

Savino, F., Ceratto, S., Poggi, E., et al. (2015). Preventive effects of oral probiotic on infantile colic: a prospective, randomized blinded, controlled trial using *Lactobacillus reuteri* DSM 17938. *Beneficial Microbes*, 6(3), 245–251.

Schultz, S. T. (2010). Does thimerosal or other mercury exposure increase the risk for autism? *Acta Neurobiologiae Experimentalis (Wars)*, 70(2), 187–195.

Shope, T. R., & Hashikawa, A. N. (2012). Exclusion of mildly ill children from childcare. *Pediatric Annals*, 41(5), 204–208.

Silvestri, J. (2012). Indications for home monitoring (or not). *Clinics in Perinatology*, 36(1), 87–99.

Szajewska, H., Gyrczuk, E., & Horvath, A. (2013). *Lactobacillus reuteri* DSM 17938 for the management of infantile colic in breastfed infants: A randomized, double-blind, placebo-controlled trial. *Journal of Pediatrics*, 162(2), 257–262.

Truong, W. H., Hill, B. W., & Cole, P. A. (2013). Automobile safety in children: A review of North American evidence and recommendations. *Journal of the American Academy of Orthopaedic Surgeons*, 21(6), 323–331.

Turner, S., Arthur, G., Lyons, R. A., et al. (2011). Modification of the home environment for the reduction of injuries. *Cochrane Database of Systematic Reviews*, 2013(2), CD003600.

Urbanska, M., & Szajewska, H. (2014). The efficacy of *Lactobacillus reuteri* DSM 17938 in infants and children: a review of the current evidence. *European Journal of Pediatrics*, 173(10), 1327–1337.

US Food and Drug Administration. (2014). *Do teething babies need medicine on their gums?* Retrieved from http://www.fda.gov/ForConsumers/ConsumerUpdates/ucm385817.htm.

US Food and Drug Administration Consumer Health Information. (2010). *Infant overdose risk with liquid vitamin D*. Retrieved from http://www.fda.gov/downloads/ForConsumers/ConsumerUpdates/UCM215586.pdf.

van Wijk, R. M., van Vlimmeren, L. A., Groothuis-Oudshoorn, C. G., et al. (2014). Helmet therapy in infants with positional skull deformation: Randomized controlled trial. *British Medical Journal*, 348, g2741.

Vitetta, L., Briskey, D., Alford, H., et al. (2014). Probiotics, prebiotics and the gastrointestinal tract in health and disease. *Inflammopharmacology*, 22(3), 135–154.

Visscher, M., & Narendran, V. (2014). The ontogeny of skin. *Advanced Wound Care*, 3(4), 291–303.

Vollrath, M. E., Tonstad, S., Rothbart, M. K., et al. (2011). Infant temperament is associated with potentially obesogenic diet at 18 months. *International Journal of Pediatric Obesity*, 6(2-2), e408–e414.

Wagner, C. L., Greer, F. R., American Academy of Pediatrics Section on Breastfeeding, et al. (2008). Prevention of rickets and vitamin D deficiency in infants, children, and adolescents. *Pediatrics*, 122(5), 1142–1152.

Wasser, H., Bentley, M., Borja, J., et al. (2011). Infants perceived as "fussy" are more likely to receive complementary foods before 4 months. *Pediatrics*, 127(2), 229–237.

Zeanah, C. H., & Gleason, M. M. (2015). Attachment disorders in early childhood—Clinical presentation, causes, correlates, and treatment. *Journal of Child Psychology and Psychiatry*, 56(3), 207–222.

Zhang, K., & Wang, X. (2013). Maternal smoking and increased risk of sudden infant death syndrome: A meta-analysis. *Legal Medicine*, 15(3), 115–121.

The Toddler and Family

Cheryl C. Rodgers

http://evolve.elsevier.com/Perry/maternal

PROMOTING OPTIMAL GROWTH AND DEVELOPMENT

The term *terrible twos* has often been used to describe the toddler years, the period from 12 to 36 months of age. Although the term may be used often to describe the toddler's behavior, it is not meant to typify or label the child. It is a time of intense exploration of the environment as children attempt to find out how things work and the power of temper tantrums, negativism, and obstinacy. Although this can be a challenging time for parents and child as each learns to know the other better, it is an extremely important period for developmental achievement and intellectual growth. Toddlers are very lovable at times; however, because of their search for autonomy, they may test parents' and caregivers' patience.

BIOLOGIC DEVELOPMENT

Proportional Changes

Physical growth slows considerably during toddlerhood. The average weight gain is 1.8 to 2.7 kg (4 to 6 pounds) per year. The birth weight is quadrupled by 2½ years of age. The rate of increase in height also slows. The usual increment is an addition of 7.5 cm (3 inches) per year and occurs mainly in elongation of the legs rather than the trunk. The average height of a 2-year-old is 86.6 cm (34 inches). In general adult height is about twice the 2-year-old child's height. Accurate measurement of height and weight during the toddler years should reveal a steady growth curve that is steplike in nature rather than linear (straight), which is characteristic of the growth spurts during the early childhood years.

The rate of increase in head circumference slows somewhat by the end of infancy, and head circumference is usually equal to chest circumference by 1 to 2 years of age. The usual total increase in head circumference during the second year is 2.5 cm (1 inch). Then the rate of increase slows until 5 years of age, when the increase is less than 1.25 cm (0.5 inch) per year. The anterior fontanel closes between 12 and 18 months of age.

Chest circumference continues to increase in size and exceeds head circumference during the toddler years. The chest's shape also changes as the transverse, or lateral, diameter exceeds the anteroposterior diameter. After the second year the chest circumference exceeds the abdominal measurement; this, in addition to the growth of the lower extremities, gives the child a taller, leaner appearance. However, toddlers retain a squat and "pot-bellied" appearance because of their less well-developed abdominal musculature and short legs. The legs remain slightly bowed or curved during the second year from the weight of the relatively large trunk.

Sensory Changes

Visual acuity of 20/40 is considered acceptable during the toddler years. Full binocular vision is well developed, and any evidence of persistent strabismus requires professional attention as early as possible to prevent amblyopia. Depth perception continues to develop but, because of the child's lack of motor coordination, falls from heights are a persistent danger.

The senses of hearing, smell, taste, and touch become increasingly well developed, coordinated with one another, and associated with other experiences. All of the senses are used to explore the environment. Toddlers visually inspect an object by turning it over; they may taste it, smell it, and touch it several times before they are satisfied with their investigation. They shake it to see if it makes noise and vigorously test its durability.

Another example of the integrated function of the senses is the toddler's development of specific taste preferences. Toddlers are much less likely than infants to try new foods because of their appearance, texture, or smell, not just their taste.

Maturation of Systems

Most of the physiologic systems are relatively mature by the end of toddlerhood. Volume of the respiratory tract and growth of associated structures continue to increase during early childhood, lessening some of the factors that predisposed the child to frequent and serious infections during infancy. The internal structures of the ear and throat continue to be short and straight, and the lymphoid tissue of the tonsils and adenoids continues to be large. As a result, otitis media, tonsillitis, and upper respiratory tract infections are common. The respiratory and heart rates slow, and the blood pressure increases. Respirations continue to be abdominal.

Under conditions of moderate variation in temperature, the toddler rarely has the difficulties of the young infant in maintaining body temperature. The mature functioning of the renal system serves to conserve fluid under times of stress, decreasing the risk of dehydration.

The digestive processes are fairly complete by the beginning of toddlerhood. The acidity of the gastric contents continues to increase and has a protective function because it is capable of destroying many types of bacteria. Stomach capacity increases to allow for the usual schedule of three meals per day.

One of the more prominent changes of the gastrointestinal system is the voluntary control of elimination. With complete myelination of the spinal cord, control of the anal and urethral sphincters is gradually achieved. The physiologic ability to control the sphincters probably occurs somewhere between 18 and 24 months of age. Bladder capacity also increases considerably, and by 14 to 18 months of age the child is able to retain urine for up to 2 hours or longer.

The defense mechanisms of the skin and blood, particularly phagocytosis, are much more efficient in toddlers than in infants. The production of antibodies is well established. However, many young children have a sudden increase in colds and minor infections when they enter preschool or other group situations such as day care because of their exposure to new pathogens.

Rapid growth in neurobehavioral organization contributes to greater regularity of sleep-wake cycles, the diminishing of crying and unexplained fussiness, and the enhanced predictability in mood. Valuable stimulants of early brain development include the various interactions (talking, singing, and playing) between the toddler and caregivers.

Gross and Fine Motor Development

The major gross motor skill during the toddler years is the development of locomotion. By 12 to 13 months of age, toddlers walk alone using a wide stance for extra balance, and by 18 months of age they try to run but fall easily (Fig. 32.1). At 2 years of age, toddlers can walk up and down stairs; by 2½ years of age they can jump using both feet, stand on one foot for 1 or 2 seconds, and manage a few steps on tiptoe. By the end of the second year, they can stand on one foot, walk on tiptoe, and climb stairs with alternate footing.

Fine motor development is demonstrated in increasingly skillful manual dexterity. For example, by 12 months of age, toddlers are able to grasp a very small object but are unable to release it at will. At 15 months of age, they can drop a pellet into a narrow-necked bottle. Casting or throwing objects and retrieving them become almost obsessive activities at about 15 months of age. By 18 months of age, toddlers can throw a ball overhand without losing their balance.

Mastery of gross and fine motor skills is evident in all phases of the child's activity such as play, dressing, language comprehension, response to discipline, social interaction, and propensity for injuries. Activities occur less in isolation and more in conjunction with other physical and mental abilities to produce a purposeful result. For example, the toddler walks to reach a new location, releases a toy to pick it up or to choose a new one, and scribbles to look at the image produced. The possibilities of the exploration, investigation, and manipulation of the environment—and its hazards—are endless.

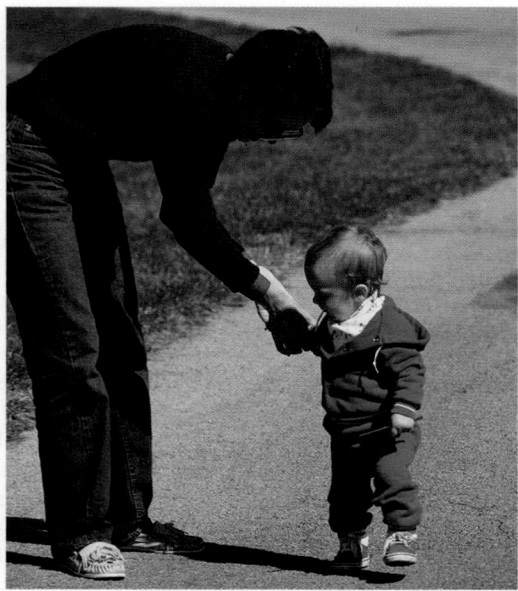

FIG 32.1 Typical toddling gait.

PSYCHOSOCIAL DEVELOPMENT

Toddlers are faced with the mastery of several important tasks. If the need for basic trust has been satisfied, they are ready to give up dependence for control, independence, and autonomy. Some of the specific tasks to be dealt with include the following:

- Differentiation of self from others, particularly the mother
- Toleration of separation from parent
- Ability to withstand delayed gratification
- Control over bodily functions
- Acquisition of socially acceptable behavior
- Verbal means of communication
- Ability to interact with others in a less egocentric manner

Mastery of these goals is only begun during late infancy and the toddler years, and tasks such as developing interpersonal relationships with others may not be completed until adolescence. However, crucial foundations for successful completion of such developmental tasks are established during these early formative years.

Developing a Sense of Autonomy (Erikson)

According to Erikson (1963), the developmental task of toddlerhood is acquiring a sense of *autonomy* while overcoming a sense of *doubt and shame*. As infants gain trust in the predictability and reliability of their parents, environment, and interaction with others, they begin to discover that their behavior is their own and that it has a predictable, reliable effect on others. Although they realize their will and control over others, they are confronted with the conflict of exerting autonomy and relinquishing the much-enjoyed dependence on others. Exerting their will has definite negative consequences, whereas retaining dependent, submissive behavior is generally rewarded with affection and approval. At the same time, continued dependency creates a sense of doubt regarding their potential capacity to control their actions. This doubt is compounded by a sense of shame for feeling this urge to revolt against others' will and a fear that they will exceed their own capacity for manipulating the environment. Skillful monitoring and balance of controls by parents allows a growing rate of realistic successes and the emergence of autonomy.

Just as infants have the social modalities of grasping and biting, toddlers have the newly gained modality of holding on and letting go. To hold on and let go is evident with the use of the hands, mouth, eyes, and eventually the sphincters when toilet training is begun. These social modalities are expressed constantly in the child's play activities such as throwing objects; taking objects out of boxes, drawers, or cabinets; holding on tighter when someone says, "No, don't touch"; and refusing to eat certain foods as taste preferences become strong.

Several characteristics, especially negativism and ritualism, are typical of toddlers in their quest for autonomy. As they attempt to express their will, they often act with *negativism*, the persistent negative response to requests. The words "no" or "me do" can be the sole vocabulary. Emotions become strongly expressed, usually in rapid mood swings. One minute toddlers can be engrossed in an activity, and the next minute they might be extremely frustrated because they are unable to manipulate a toy or open a door. If scolded for doing something wrong, they can have a temper tantrum and almost instantaneously pull at the parent's legs to be picked up and comforted. Understanding and coping with these swift changes in behavior is often difficult for parents. Many parents find the negativism exasperating and, instead of dealing constructively with it, give in to it, which further threatens children in their search for learning acceptable methods of interacting with others (see the "Temper Tantrums" section later in this chapter).

In contrast to negativism, which frequently disrupts the environment, ritualism, the need to maintain sameness and reliability, provides a sense of comfort. Toddlers can venture out with security when they know that familiar people, places, and routines still exist. One can easily understand why any change in the daily routine represents such a threat to these children. Without comfortable rituals, they have little opportunity to exert autonomy. Consequently dependency and regression occur (see the "Regression" section later in this chapter).

Erikson focuses on the development of the *ego*, which may be thought of as reason or common sense, during this phase of psychosocial development. The child struggles to deal with the impulses of the id, tolerate frustration, and learn socially acceptable ways of interacting with the environment. The ego is evident as the child is able to tolerate delayed gratification.

Toddlers also have a rudimentary beginning of the *superego*, or conscience, which is the incorporation of the morals of society and the process of acculturation. With the development of the ego, children further differentiate themselves from others and expand their sense of trust within themselves. However, as they begin to develop awareness of their own will and capacity to achieve, they also become aware of their ability to fail. This ever-present awareness of potential failure creates doubt and shame. Successful mastery of the task of autonomy necessitates opportunities for self-mastery while withstanding the frustration of necessary limit setting and delayed gratification. Opportunities for self-mastery are present in appropriate play activities, toilet training, the crisis of sibling rivalry, and successful interactions with significant others.

COGNITIVE DEVELOPMENT

Sensorimotor and Preoperational Phase (Piaget)

The period from 12 to 24 months of age is a continuation of the final two stages of the sensorimotor phase. During this time, the cognitive processes develop rapidly and at times seem similar to those of mature thinking. However, reasoning skills are still primitive and need to be understood to effectively deal with the typical behaviors of a child of this age.

In the fifth stage of the sensorimotor phase (13 to 18 months of age), tertiary circular reactions, the child uses active experimentation to achieve previously unattainable goals. Newly acquired physical skills are increasingly important for the function they serve rather than for the acts themselves. The child incorporates the old learning of secondary circular reactions with new skills and applies the combined knowledge to new situations, with emphasis on the results of the experimentation. In this way, there is the beginning of rational judgment and intellectual reasoning. During this stage, the child further differentiates self from objects. This is evident in the child's increasing ability to venture away from their parents and tolerate longer periods of separation.

Awareness of a *causal relationship* between two events is apparent. After flipping a light switch, toddlers are aware that a reciprocal response occurs. However, they are not able to transfer that knowledge to new situations. Therefore, every time they see what appears to be a light switch, they must reinvestigate its function. Such behavior demonstrates the beginning of categorizing data into distinct classes and subclasses. Examples of this type of behavior are innumerable as toddlers continuously explore the same object each time it appears in a new place.

Because classification of objects is basic, the appearance of an object denotes its function. For example, if the child's toys are stored in a paper bag or large container, that toy receptacle is no different from the garbage pail or laundry basket. If allowed to turn over the toy receptacle, the child will just as quickly do the same to other similar containers because in the child's mind, there is no difference. Expecting the child to judge which receptacles are permissible to explore and which are not is inappropriate for this age-group. Instead the forbidden

object, such as the garbage pail, should be placed out of reach. This has significant implications for prevention of accidents and accidental ingestion of injurious agents.

The discovery of objects as objects leads to the awareness of their spatial relationships. Children are able to recognize different shapes and their relationship to one another. For example, they can fit slightly smaller boxes into one another (nesting) and can place a round object into a hole, even if the board is turned around, upside down, or reversed. Children are also aware of space and the relationship of their body to dimensions, such as height. They stretch, stand on a low stair or stool, and pull a string to reach an object.

Object permanence has also advanced. Although they still cannot find an object that has been invisibly displaced or moved from under one pillow to another without actually seeing the change, toddlers are increasingly aware of the existence of objects behind closed doors, in drawers, on countertops, and under tables. Parents are usually acutely aware of this developmental achievement and find high places and locked cabinets to be the only places inaccessible to toddlers.

From 19 to 24 months of age, the child is in the final sensorimotor stage. This stage completes the more primitive, autistic-like thought processes of infancy and prepares the way for more complex mental operations that occur during the phase of preoperational thought. One of the most dramatic achievements of this stage is in the area of object permanence. Toddlers will now actively search for an object in several potential hiding places. In addition, they can infer a cause when only experiencing the effect. They can infer that an object was hidden in any number of places even if they only saw the original hiding place.

Imitation displays deeper meaning and understanding. There is greater symbolization to imitation. Children are acutely aware of others' actions and attempt to copy them in gestures and words. *Domestic mimicry* (imitating household activities) and gender-role behavior become increasingly common during this stage, especially during the second year. Identification with the parent of the same gender becomes apparent by the second year and represents the child's intellectual ability to identify different models of behavior and imitate them appropriately (Fig. 32.2).

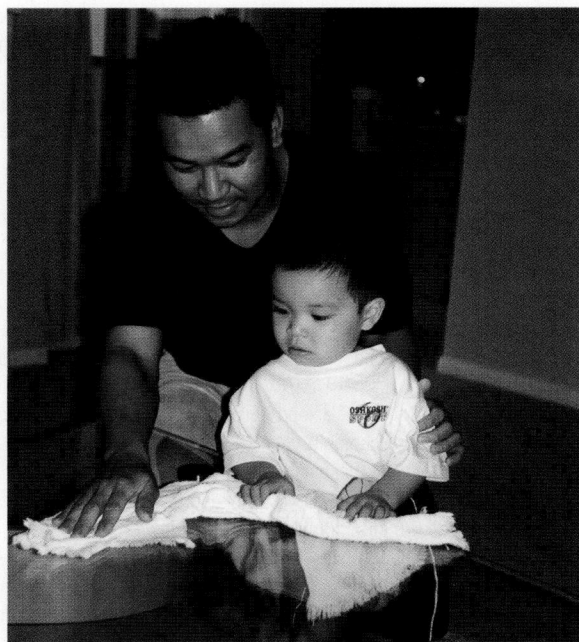

FIG 32.2 Domestic mimicry and sex-role behavior are common during toddlerhood.

The concept of time is still embryonic; but children have some sense of timing in terms of anticipation, memory, and a limited ability to wait. They may listen to the command, "Just a minute," and behave appropriately. However, their sense of time is exaggerated; 1 minute can seem like 1 hour. Toddlers' limited attention spans also indicate their sense of immediacy and concern for the present.

Preoperational Phase (Piaget)

At approximately 2 years of age, the child enters the preconceptual phase of cognitive development, which lasts until about 4 years of age. The preconceptual phase is a subdivision of the preoperational phase, which spans 2 to 7 years of age. It is primarily one of transition that bridges the purely self-satisfying behavior of infancy and the rudimentary socialized behavior of latency. *Preoperational thinking* implies that children cannot think in terms of operations (i.e., the ability to manipulate objects in relation to one another in a logical fashion). Rather toddlers think primarily on the basis of their perception of an event. Problem solving is based on what they see or hear directly rather than on what they recall about objects and events. Several characteristics are unique to preoperational thought (Box 32.1).

Within the second year, the child increasingly uses language symbolically and is concerned with the "why" and "how" of things. For example, a pencil is "something to write with," and food is "something to eat." However, such mental symbolization is closely associated with prelogical reasoning. For instance, a needle is "something that hurts." Such painful experiences take on new significance because memory is associated with the specific event, and fears are likely to develop such as resistance to people who wear a uniform or rooms that look like the practitioner's office. Because of the vulnerability of these early years, it is essential to prepare children for any new experience, whether it is a new baby-sitter or a visit to the dentist.

SPIRITUAL DEVELOPMENT

Spiritual development in children is often discussed in terms of the child's developmental level because the evolution of spirituality often parallels cognitive development (Mueller, 2010). The child's family and environment strongly influence the child's perception of the world around him or her, and this often includes spirituality. Furthermore, family values, beliefs, customs, and expressions of these influence the child's perception of his or her spiritual self (Mueller, 2010). Neuman (2011) proposes that Fowler's (1981) stages of faith be used to better understand children and spirituality; she provides an excellent overview of the stages of faith in childhood. The relationship between spirituality, illness in childhood, and nursing has been studied in the context of suffering, terminal illness such as cancer, and end-of-life care. In the past decade, there has been an increased interest in and focus on spiritual care in adults and children as further understanding of the influence of one's spirituality on health, illness, and well-being has progressed.

Toddlers learn about God through the words and actions of those closest to them. They have only a vague idea of God and religious teachings because of their immature cognitive processes; however, if

---

BOX 32.1 Characteristics of Preoperational Thought

Egocentrism: Inability to envision situations from perspectives other than one's own
Example: If a person is positioned between the toddler and another child, the toddler, who is facing the person, will explain that both children can see the middle person's face. The young child is unable to realize that the other person views the middle person from a different perspective, the back.
Implication: Avoid moralizing about "why" something is wrong if it requires an understanding of someone else's feelings or opinion. Telling a child to stop hitting because hitting hurts the other person is often ineffective because to the aggressor it feels good to hit someone else. Instead emphasize that hitting is not allowed.

Transductive reasoning: Reasoning from the particular to the particular
Example: Child refuses to eat a food because something previously eaten did not taste good.
Implication: Accept child's reasoning; offer refused food at a different time.

Global organization: Reasoning that changing any one part of the whole changes the entire whole
Example: Child refuses to sleep in room because location of bed is changed.
Implication: Accept child's reasoning; use same bed position or introduce change slowly.

Centration: Focusing on one aspect rather than considering all possible alternatives
Example: Child refuses to eat a food because of its color, even though its taste and smell are acceptable.
Implication: Accept child's reasoning.

Animism: Attributing lifelike qualities to inanimate objects
Example: Child scolds stairs for making child fall down.
Implication: Join child in the "scolding." Keep frightening objects out of view.

Irreversibility: Inability to undo or reverse actions initiated physically
Example: When told to stop doing something such as talking, child is unable to think of positive activity.
Implication: State requests or instructions positively (e.g., "Be quiet.")

Magical thinking: Believing that thoughts are all-powerful and can cause events
Examples: Child wishes someone died; then if the person dies, child feels at fault because of the "bad" thought that made the death happen.
- Calling children "bad" because they did something wrong makes them feel as if they are bad.
Implications: Clarify that thoughts do not make things happen and that the child is not responsible.
- Use "I" rather than "you" messages to communicate thoughts, feelings, expectations, or beliefs without imposing blame or criticism. Emphasize that the act is bad, not the child.

Inability to conserve: Inability to understand the idea that a mass can be changed in size, shape, volume, or length without losing or adding to the original mass (instead children judge what they see by the immediate perceptual clues given to them)
Example: If two lines of equal length are presented in such a way that one appears longer than the other, child will state that one line is longer even if child measures both lines with a ruler or yardstick and finds that each has the same length.
Implications: Change the most obvious perceptual clue to reorient child's view of what is seen. For example, give medicine in a small medicine cup rather than a large cup because child will imagine that the large vessel contains more liquid. If child refuses the medicine in the small cup, pour it into a large cup, because the liquid will appear to be less in a tall, wide container.
- Give a large, flat cookie rather than a thick, small one, or do the reverse with meat or cheese; child will usually eat larger size of favorite food and smaller size of less favorite food.

God is spoken about with reverence, young children associate God with something special. During this period, the assignment of powerful religious symbols and images is strongly influenced by the manner in which it is presented usually in the form of rituals, games, and songs (Mueller, 2010). God may be described as being around like air by the toddler because of the fluidity in dividing fantasy and reality (Neuman, 2011).

Toddlers begin to assimilate behaviors associated with the divine (folding hands in prayer). Routines such as saying prayers before meals or at bedtime can be important and comforting. Because toddlers tend to find solace in ritualistic behavior and routines, they incorporate routines associated with religious practices into their behavioral patterns without understanding all of the implications of the rituals until later. Near the end of toddlerhood, when children use preoperational thought, there is some advancement of their understanding of God. Religious teachings such as reward or fear of punishment (heaven or hell) and moral development (see Chapter 28), may influence their behavior.

DEVELOPMENT OF BODY IMAGE

As in infancy, the development of body image closely parallels cognitive development. During the second year, children recognize themselves in a mirror and make verbal references to themselves ("Me big"). With increasing motor ability, toddlers recognize the usefulness of body parts and gradually learn their names. They also learn that certain parts of the body have various meanings (e.g., during toilet training, the genitalia become significant, and cleanliness is emphasized). By 2 years of age, they recognize gender differences and refer to self by name and then by pronoun. Gender identity is developed by 3 years of age. By this time, the child also begins to remember events with reference to their personal significance, forming an autobiographic memory that helps establish a continuous identity throughout the events of life.

Once they begin preoperational thought, toddlers can use symbols to represent objects, but their thinking may lead to inaccuracies. For example, if someone who is pregnant is called "fat," they describe all "fat" women as having babies. They begin to recognize words used to describe physical appearance such as "pretty," "handsome," or "big boy." Such expressions eventually influence how children view their own bodies.

It is evident that body integrity is poorly understood and intrusive experiences are threatening. For example, toddlers forcefully resist procedures such as examining the ear or mouth and taking an axillary temperature. The procedure itself (e.g., taking vital signs) does not hurt the child, but it represents an intrusion into the child's personal space, which elicits a strong protest. Toddlers also have unclear body boundaries and may associate nonviable parts such as feces with essential body parts. This can be seen in a toddler who is upset by flushing the toilet and watching the stool disappear.

Nurses can assist parents in fostering a positive body image in their child by encouraging them to avoid negative labels such as "skinny arms" or "chubby legs"; such self-perceptions are internalized and can last a lifetime. Body parts, especially those related to elimination and reproduction, should be called by their correct names. Respect for the body should be practiced.

DEVELOPMENT OF GENDER IDENTITY

Just as toddlers explore their environment, they also explore their bodies and find that touching certain body parts is pleasurable. Genital fondling (masturbation) can occur and involves manual stimulation and posturing movements (especially in young girls) such as tightening the thighs or applying mechanical pressure to the pubic or suprapubic area. Other demonstrations of pleasurable activities include rocking, swinging, and hugging people and toys. Parental reactions to toddlers' behavior influence the children's own attitudes and should be accepting rather than critical. If such acts are performed in public, parents should not condone or bring attention to the behavior but should teach the child that it is more acceptable to perform the behavior in private.

Children in this age-group are learning vocabulary associated with anatomy, elimination, and reproduction. Certain associations between words and functions become significant and can influence future sexual attitudes. For example, if parents refer to the genitalia as dirty, especially in the context of elimination, this association between "genitalia" and "dirty" may be transferred to sexual functions later in life. Sex-role differences become obvious to children and are evident in much of toddlers' imitative play. Although research indicates that prenatal exposure to testosterone strongly influences the individual's gender identity, researchers also indicate that there are sensitive periods (e.g., puberty) that may influence the development of gender identity (Berenbaum & Beltz, 2011; Hines, 2011; Savic, Garcia-Falqueras, & Swaab, 2010). A sense of maleness or femaleness, or *gender identity,* begins by 24 months of age when children are able to label their own and other's gender (Steensma, Kreukels, de Vries, et al., 2013). Early attitudes are formed about affectionate behaviors between adults from observing parental and other adult intimate or sensual activities. (See also the "Sex Education" section in Chapter 33.) The quality of relationships with parents is important to the child's capacity for sexual and emotional relationships later in life.

SOCIAL DEVELOPMENT

A major task of the toddler period is differentiation of self from significant others, usually the mother. The differentiation process consists of two phases: *separation* (i.e., the child's emergence from a symbiotic fusion with the mother) and *individuation* (i.e., achievements that mark the child's expressions of his or her individual characteristics in the environment). Although the process begins during the latter half of infancy, the major achievements occur during the toddler years.

Toddlers have an increased understanding and awareness of object permanence and some ability to withstand delayed gratification and tolerate moderate frustration. As a result, toddlers react differently to strangers than do infants. The appearance of unfamiliar people does not represent such a significant threat to their attachment to mother. They have learned from experience that parents still exist when physically absent. Repetition of events such as going to bed without the parents but waking to find them there again (in the household) reinforces the reliability of such brief separations. Consequently, toddlers are able to venture away from their parents for brief periods because of the security of knowing that the parents will be there when they return.

The separation-individuation phase of the toddler encompasses the phenomenon of rapprochement; as the toddler separates from the mother and begins to make sense of experiences in the environment, the child is drawn back to the mother for assistance in verbally articulating the meaning of the experiences (Meissner, 2009). Developmentally the term *rapprochement* means the child moves away and returns for reassurance. If the mother's response to the toddler is inappropriate, the toddler may experience insecurity and confusion.

Transitional objects such as a favorite blanket or toy provide security for children, especially when they are separated from parents, dealing with a new stress, or just fatigued (Fig. 32.3). Security objects often become so important to toddlers that they refuse to have them taken away. Such behavior is normal; there is no need to discourage this tendency. During separations such as day care, hospitalization, or even overnight stays with relatives, transitional objects should be provided to minimize any feelings of fear or loneliness.

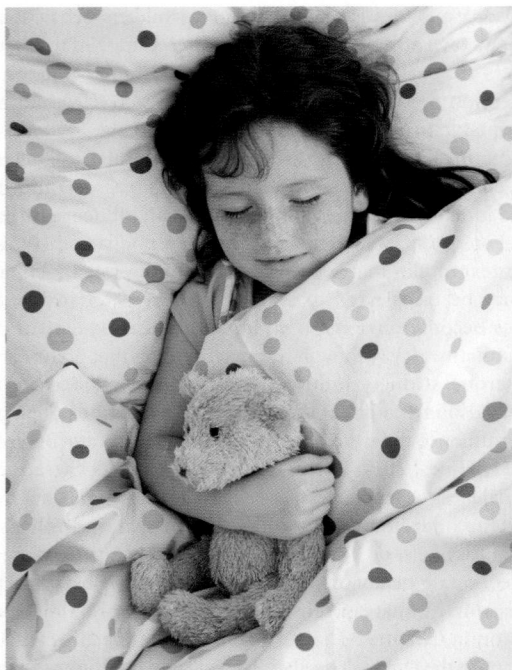

FIG 32.3 Transitional objects such as a fuzzy stuffed animal are sources of security to a toddler. (Copyright 2011 by Photos.com, a division of Getty Images. All rights reserved.)

Learning to tolerate and master brief periods of separation are important developmental tasks for children in this age-group. In addition, it is a necessary component of parenting because brief periods of separation allow parents to regain their energy and patience and minimize any tendency to direct their irritations and frustrations at the children.

Language

The most striking characteristic of language development during early childhood is the increasing level of comprehension. Although the number of words acquired (i.e., from about four at 1 year of age to approximately 300 at 2 years of age is notable, the ability to comprehend and understand speech is much greater than the number of words the child can say. Bilingual children can also achieve their early linguistic milestones in each of the languages at the same time and produce a substantial number of semantically corresponding words in each of their two languages from the very first words or signs.

At 1 year of age, children use one-word sentences or holophrases. The word "up" can mean "pick me up" or "look up there." For children, the one word conveys the meaning of a sentence, but to others it may mean many things or nothing. At this age, about 25% of the vocalizations are intelligible. By 2 years of age, children use multiword sentences by stringing together two or three words, such as the phrases "mama go bye-bye" or "all gone," and approximately 65% of their speech is understandable. By 3 years of age, children put words together into simple sentences, begin to master grammatical rules, know their age and gender, and can count three objects correctly (Feigelman, 2016). Reading books together during this period provides an ideal setting for further language development. Researchers have evaluated the impact of television viewing on toddler language development and found that those who started watching television at younger than 12 months of age and who watched longer than 2 hours per day had a six-fold increase in the likelihood of significant language delays (Christakis, 2010).

Adult-child conversations with infants and toddlers have been shown to positively affect language development; the researchers recommend reading, storytelling, and interactive adult-child communication (Zimmerman, Gilkerson, Richards, et al., 2009). The American Academy of Pediatrics Council on Communications and Media (2016) reaffirms that televised or recorded media usage in children younger than 2 years of age decreases language skills and the time parents interact with the child. Furthermore, excessive television viewing in early childhood decreases cognitive, language, and social skills in young children (American Academy of Pediatrics, Council on Communications and Media, 2016).

Gestures precede or accompany each of the language milestones up to 30 months of age (putting phone to ear, pointing). After sufficient language development, gestures phase out, and the pace of word learning increases.

Personal-Social Behavior

Perhaps one of the most dramatic aspects of development in the toddler is personal-social interaction. Personal-social behaviors are evident in such areas as dressing, feeding, playing, and establishing self-control. Parents wonder why their manageable, docile, lovable infant has turned into a determined, strong-willed, volatile little tyrant. In addition, the tyrant of the terrible twos can swiftly and unpredictably revert back to the adorable, cuddly child. All of this is part of growing up as toddlers acquire a more sophisticated awareness that others' feelings and desires can be different from their own. Through interactions with caregivers, children are able to explore these differences and their consequences.

Toddlers are developing skills of independence, and these are evident in all areas of behavior. By 15 months of age, children feed themselves, drink well from a covered cup, and manage a spoon with considerable spilling. By 24 months of age they use a spoon well, and by 36 months of age may be using a fork. Between 2 and 3 years of age, they eat with the family and like to help with chores such as setting the table or removing dishes from the dishwasher. However, they lack table manners and may find it difficult to sit through the family's entire meal.

In dressing, toddlers also demonstrate strides in independence. The 15-month-old child helps by putting the arm or foot out for dressing and pulls shoes and socks off. The 18-month-old child removes gloves, helps with pullover shirts, and may be able to unzip. By 2 years of age, the toddler removes most articles of clothing and puts on socks, shoes, and pants without regard to right or left and back or front. Help is still needed to fasten clothes.

Toddlers also begin to develop concern for the feelings of others and an understanding of how adult expectations for behavior apply to specific situations (e.g., causing a sibling to cry while playing rough). As their understanding increases, they develop control. Age-appropriate discipline contributes to healthy social and emotional development. Positive reinforcement, redirecting, and time-out are appropriate for most toddlers. Social and emotional problems can develop in the youngest children. Early screening and intervention promote more positive developmental outcomes as the young child grows and develops.

Play

Play magnifies toddlers' physical and psychosocial development. Interaction with people becomes increasingly important. The solitary play of infancy progresses to *parallel play* (i.e., toddlers play alongside, not with, other children). Although sensorimotor play is still prominent, there is much less emphasis on the exclusive use of one sensory modality. Toddlers inspect toys, talk to toys, test toys' strength and durability, and invent several uses for toys. Imitation is one of the most distinguishing characteristics of play and enriches children's opportunity to engage in fantasy. With less emphasis on gender-stereotyped toys, play objects

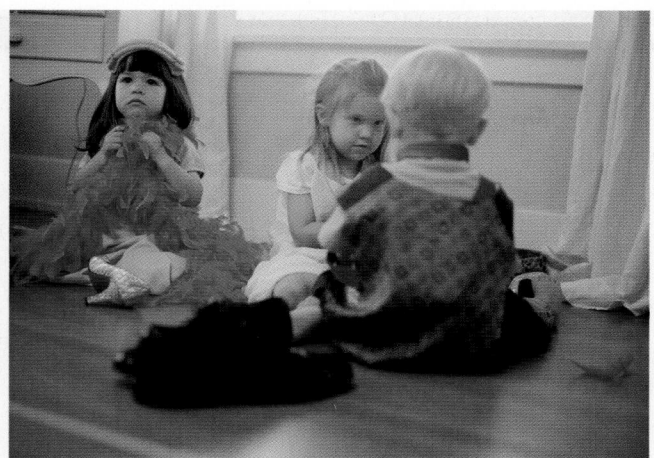

FIG 32.4 Young children enjoy dressing up. (Copyright 2011 by Photos. com, a division of Getty Images. All rights reserved.)

such as dolls, carriages, dollhouses, balls, dishes, cooking utensils, child-size furniture, trucks, and dress-up clothes are suitable for both genders (Fig. 32.4); however, boys may be more interested than girls in activities related to trucks, trailers, action figures, and building blocks, and girls may prefer doll-related activities.

Increased locomotive skills make push-pull toys, straddle trucks or cycles, a small gym and slide, balls of various sizes, and riding toys appropriate for energetic toddlers. Finger paints; thick crayons; chalk; blackboard; paper; and puzzles with large, simple pieces use toddlers' developing fine motor skills. Interlocking blocks in various sizes and shapes provide hours of fun and during later years are useful objects for creative and imaginative play. The most educational toy is the one that fosters the interaction of an adult with a child in supportive, unconditional play. Parents and other providers are encouraged to allow children to play with a variety of simple toys that foster creative thinking (e.g., blocks, dolls, and clay) rather than passive toys that the child observes (battery-operated or mechanical). Active play time should also be encouraged over the use of computer or video games. Toys should not be substitutes for the attention of devoted caregivers, but toys can enhance these interactions.

Certain aspects of play are related to emerging linguistic abilities. Talking is a form of play for toddlers, who enjoy musical toys such as "talking" dolls and animals, and toy telephones. Toddlers also enjoy "reading" stories from a picture book and imitating the sounds of animals. Children's television programs are appropriate for some children older than 18 months of age who learn to associate words with visual images. However, parents should choose high-quality programming, watch the program together, and reteach the content (American Academy of Pediatrics, Council on Communications and Media, 2016). In addition, for children 2 to 5 years of age, total media time should be limited to 1 hour per day of quality programming, and parents should view the programs with the child (American Academy of Pediatrics, Council on Communications and Media). Parents are encouraged to allow the child to engage in unstructured playtime and parent-child interactions, which is considered much more beneficial than any electronic media exposure (American Academy of Pediatrics, Council on Communications and Media).

Tactile play is also important for exploring toddlers. Water toys, a sandbox with a pail and shovel, finger paints, soap bubbles, and clay provide excellent opportunities for creative and manipulative recreation. Adults sometimes forget the fascination of feeling textures such as slippery cream, mud, or pudding; catching air bubbles; squeezing and reshaping clay; or smearing paints. These types of unstructured activities are as important as educational play to allow children the freedom of expression.

Selection of appropriate toys must involve safety factors, especially in relation to size and sturdiness. The oral activity of toddlers puts them at risk for aspirating small objects and ingesting toxic substances. Parents need to be especially vigilant of toys played with in other children's homes and those of older siblings. Toys are a potential source of serious bodily damage to toddlers, who may have the physical strength to manipulate them but not the knowledge to appreciate their danger. Ride-on toys (i.e., tricycles, wagons, scooters) and early exploratory toys (i.e., blocks, stacking toys, building sets) were the most common type of toy causing injury to children younger than 5 years of age (Abraham, Gaw, Chounthirath, et al., 2015). Government agencies do not inspect and police all toys on the market. Therefore adults who purchase play equipment, supervise purchases, or allow children to use play equipment need to evaluate its safety, including toys that are gifts or those that are purchased by the children themselves. Adults should also be alert to notices of toys determined to be defective and recalled by the manufacturers. Parents and health care workers can obtain information on a variety of recalled products and report potentially dangerous toys and child products to the US Consumer Product Safety Commission* or, in Canada, the Canadian Toy Testing Council.† Printable tips on toy safety are also available from Safe Kids Worldwide (www.safekids.org).

Table 32.1 summarizes the major features of growth and development for the age-groups of 15, 18, 24, and 30 months.

COPING WITH CONCERNS RELATED TO NORMAL GROWTH AND DEVELOPMENT

Toilet Training

One of the major tasks of toddlerhood is toilet training. Anticipatory guidance and clinical intervention for families surrounding toilet training should begin during routine well-child visits before the child's developmental readiness to toilet train. Preparation and education reveal and allay misconceptions; lead to the development of appropriate expectations; and provide information, guidance, and support to parents for managing this potentially frustrating process.

Voluntary control of the anal and urethral sphincters is achieved sometime after the child is walking, probably between 18 and 24 months of age. However, complex psychophysiologic factors are required for readiness. The child must be able to recognize the urge to let go and hold on and communicate this sensation to the parent. In addition, some motivation is probably involved in the desire to please the parent by holding on rather than pleasing oneself by letting go. Cultural beliefs may also affect the age at which children demonstrate readiness (Feigelman, 2016).

Trends in toilet training have changed, likely due to the availability of disposable diapers. In the 1920s, toilet training began around 12 months of age, which changed to at least 18 months of age in the 1960s, and is now initiated around 21 months of age with approximately one-half of children toilet trained by 36 months of age (Rogers, 2013). Four markers signal a child's readiness to toilet train: (1) waking up dry from a nap or overnight sleep, (2) being aware of the urge to void or stool, (3) communicating the need to go, and (4) being dry for at

---

*800-638-2772; http://www.cpsc.gov (assistance is also available in Spanish).
†1973 Baseline Road, Ottawa, Ontario K2C 0C7 Canada; 613-228-3155; www.toy-testing.org.

TABLE 32.1   Growth and Development During Toddler Years

Age (Months)	Physical	Gross Motor	Fine Motor	Sensory	Language	Socialization
15	Steady growth in height and weight Head circumference 48 cm (19 inches) Weight 11 kg (24 pounds) Height 78.7 cm (31 inches)	Walks without help (usually since age 13 months) Creeps up stairs Kneels without support Cannot walk around corners or stop suddenly without losing balance Cannot throw ball without falling	Constantly casting objects to floor Builds tower of two cubes Holds two cubes in one hand Releases pellet into narrow-necked bottle Scribbles spontaneously Uses cup well, but rotates spoon before it reaches mouth	Able to identify geometric forms; places round object into appropriate hole Binocular vision well developed Displays intense and prolonged interest in pictures	Uses expressive jargon Says four to six words, including names "Asks" for objects by pointing Understands simple commands May use head-shaking gesture to denote "no" Uses "no" even while agreeing to the request Uses common gestures such as putting cup to mouth when empty	Tolerates some separation from parent Less likely to fear strangers Beginning to imitate parents such as cleaning house (sweeping, dusting), folding clothes May discard bottle Kisses and hugs parents; may kiss pictures in a book Expresses emotions; has temper tantrums
18	Physiologic anorexia from decreased growth needs Anterior fontanel closed Physiologically able to control sphincters	Runs clumsily; falls often Walks up stairs with one hand held Pulls and pushes toys Jumps in place with both feet Seats self on chair Throws ball overhand without falling	Builds tower of three or four cubes Release, prehension, and reach well developed Turns two or three pages in a book at a time In drawing makes stroke imitatively Manages spoon without rotation		Says 10 or more words Points to common object such as shoe or ball and to two or three body parts Forms word combinations Forms gesture-word combinations Forms gesture-gesture combinations	Great imitator (domestic mimicry) Takes off gloves, socks, and shoes and unzips zippers Temper tantrums may be more evident Beginning awareness of ownership ("my toy") May develop dependence on transitional objects such as security blanket
24	Head circumference 49 to 50 cm (19.5 to 20 inches) Chest circumference exceeds head circumference Lateral diameter of chest exceeds anteroposterior diameter Usual weight gain of 1.8 to 2.7 kg (4 to 6 pounds) per year Usual gain in height of 10 to 12.5 cm (4 to 5 inches) per year Adult height approximately double height at 2 years of age Primary dentition of 16 teeth May demonstrate readiness for beginning daytime control of bowel and bladder	Goes up and down stairs alone with two feet on each step Runs fairly well, with wide stance Picks up object without falling Kicks ball forward without overbalancing	Builds tower of six or seven cubes Aligns two or more cubes like a train Turns pages of book one at a time In drawing imitates vertical and circular strokes Turns doorknob; unscrews lids	Accommodation well developed in geometric discrimination; able to insert square block into oblong space	Has vocabulary of approximately 300 words Uses two- or three-word phrases Uses pronouns "I," "me," "you" Understands directional commands Gives first name; refers to self by name Verbalizes need for toileting, food, or drink Talks incessantly Able to remember and imitate arbitrary sequences of manual actions and gestures	Stage of parallel play Has sustained attention span Temper tantrums decreasing Pulls people to show them something Increased independence from parent Dresses self in simple clothing Develops visual recognition and verbal self-reference ("Me big") Develops awareness that feelings and desires of others may be different and begins to explore implications and consequences

TABLE 32.1	Growth and Development During Toddler Years—cont'd					
Age (Months)	Physical	Gross Motor	Fine Motor	Sensory	Language	Socialization
30	Birth weight quadrupled Primary dentition (20 teeth) completed May have daytime bowel and bladder control	Jumps with both feet Jumps from chair or step Stands on one foot momentarily Takes a few steps on tiptoe	Builds tower of eight cubes Adds chimney to train of cubes Good hand-finger coordination; holds crayon with fingers rather than fist In drawing imitates vertical and horizontal strokes; makes two or more strokes for cross; draws circles		Gives first and last name Refers to self by appropriate pronoun Uses plurals Names one color	Separates more easily from parent In play helps put things away; can carry breakable objects; pushes with good steering Begins to notice gender differences; knows own gender May attend to toilet needs without help except for wiping Emotions expand to include pride, shame, guilt, embarrassment

least 2 hours during the day (Wu, 2010). According to some experts, physiologic and psychologic readiness is not complete until 24 to 30 months of age (Rogers, 2013); however, parents should begin preparing their children for toilet training earlier than 30 months. By this time, children have mastered most essential gross motor skills, can communicate intelligibly, are in less conflict with their parents in terms of self-assertion and negativism, and are aware of the ability to control the body and please their parents. There is no universal right age to begin toilet training or an absolute deadline to complete it. An important role for the nurse is to help parents identify the readiness signs in their children (see Guidelines box: Assessing Toilet Training Readiness).* On average, girls are developmentally ready to begin toilet training before boys (Elder, 2016).

Nighttime bladder control normally takes several months to years after daytime training begins. This is because the sleep cycle needs to mature so that the child can awake in time to urinate. Feigelman (2016) indicates that bedwetting is normal in girls up to 4 years of age and boys up to 5 years of age. Few children have night wetting episodes after daytime dryness is totally achieved; however, children who do not have nighttime dryness by 6 years of age are likely to require intervention.

Bowel training is usually accomplished before bladder training because of its greater regularity and predictability. The sensation for defecation is stronger than that for urination and easier for children to recognize. A well-balanced diet that includes dietary fiber helps keep stool soft and supports the development and maintenance of regular bowel movements.

A number of techniques are helpful when initiating training, and cultural differences should be considered. In the United States, some of the options recommended by practitioners include the Brazelton child-oriented approach, the AAP guidelines (which are similar to the Brazelton method), Dr. Spock's training method, and the intensive "toilet-training-in-a-day" (operant conditioning) approach by Azrin

---

*A helpful book is *Guide to Toilet Training*, available from the AAP; 847-434-4000; https://shop.aap.org/guide-to-toilet-training-2nd-edition -paperback.

GUIDELINES
Assessing Toilet Training Readiness

Physical Readiness
- Voluntary control of anal and urethral sphincters, usually by 24 to 30 months of age
- Ability to stay dry for 2 hours; decreased number of wet diapers; waking dry from nap
- Regular bowel movements
- Gross motor skills of sitting, walking, and squatting
- Fine motor skills to remove clothing

Mental Readiness
- Recognizing urge to defecate or urinate
- Verbal or nonverbal communicative skills to indicate when wet or has urge to defecate or urinate
- Cognitive skills to imitate appropriate behavior and follow directions

Psychologic Readiness
- Expressing willingness to please parent
- Ability to sit on toilet for 5 to 8 minutes without fussing or getting off
- Curiosity about adults' or older sibling's toilet habits
- Impatience with soiled or wet diapers; desire to be changed immediately

Parental Readiness
- Recognizing child's level of readiness
- Willingness to invest time required for toilet training
- Absence of family stress or change such as a divorce, moving, new sibling, or imminent vacation

and Foxx (Wu, 2010). A systematic review concluded that the child-oriented method and the Azrin and Foxx methods are effective at toilet training healthy children (Kiddoo, 2012). The following discussion of toilet training methods includes suggestions from the child-oriented approach.

Parents should begin the readiness phase of toilet training by teaching the child about how the body functions in relation to voiding and having a stool. Keep toilet training as easy and simple as possible. Important considerations are the selection of the child's clothing and the potty chair or use of the toilet. A freestanding potty chair allows children a feeling of security (Fig. 32.5, *A*). Planting the feet firmly on the floor also facilitates defecation. Another option is a portable seat attached to the regular toilet, which may ease the transition from potty chair to regular toilet. Placing a small bench under the feet helps stabilize the child's position. It is probably best to keep the potty in the bathroom and let the child observe the excreta being flushed down the toilet to associate these activities with usual practices. If a potty chair is not available, having the child sit facing the toilet tank provides added support (see Fig. 32.5, *B*). Practice sessions should be limited to 5 to 8 minutes, and a parent should stay with the child, practicing

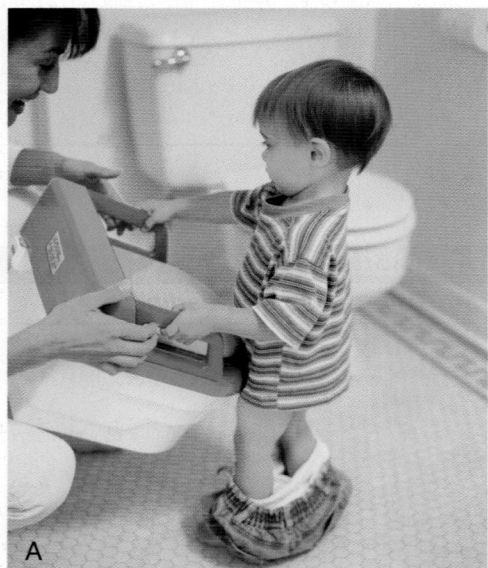

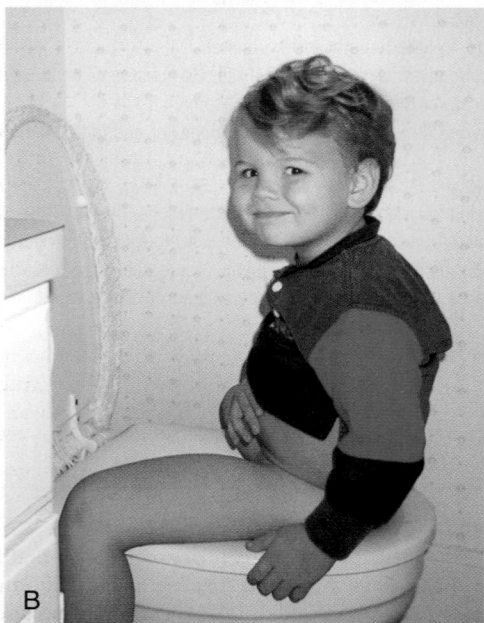

FIG 32.5 A, Children may begin toilet training sitting on a small potty chair. **B,** Sitting in reverse fashion on a regular toilet provides additional support to a young child. (A, Copyright 2011 by Photos.com, a division of Getty Images. All rights reserved.)

sanitary habits after every session. Children should be praised for cooperative behavior and successful evacuation. Dressing children in easily removed clothing; using training pants, "pull-on" diapers, or underwear; and encouraging imitation by watching others are other helpful suggestions.

When the child begins to experience regular daytime dryness, parents may experiment with underwear during the day. Daytime accidents are common, particularly during periods of intense activity. Young children become so engrossed in play activity that, if they are not reminded, they will wait until it is too late to reach the bathroom. Therefore frequent reminders and trips to the toilet are necessary. Parents often forget to plan ahead when their toddlers are being toilet trained; before trips outside the house, it is important to remind children to at least try to urinate to decrease the chance of needing to use the toilet while the car is stuck in traffic.

As the child masters each step of toileting (discussion, undressing, going, wiping, dressing, flushing, and hand washing), he or she gains a sense of accomplishment that parents should reinforce. If the parent-child relationship becomes strained, both may need a break to focus on enjoyable activities together. Regression may coincide with a stressful family situation or the child being pushed too hard and too fast. Regression is a normal part of toilet training and does not mean failure but should be viewed as a temporary setback to a more comfortable place for the child.

Daycare providers also play a role in the support and education of parents regarding toilet training practices. It is important for parents to inform all caregivers of their individual family values and the child's specific needs when planning for training away from home. Ensuring consistency in care of toddlers and healthy practices in a sanitary environment allow for safe and effective toilet practices in all settings.

Sibling Rivalry

The natural jealousy and resentment of children to a new child in the family is referred to as *sibling rivalry.* The arrival of a new infant represents a crisis for even the best-prepared toddlers. It is not the infant that toddlers resent but the changes that this additional sibling produces, especially the separation from mother during the birth. The parents now share their love and attention with someone else, the usual routine is disrupted, and toddlers may lose their crib or room, all at a time when they thought they were in control of their world. Sibling rivalry tends to be most pronounced in the firstborn, who experiences *dethronement* (i.e., loss of sole parental attention). It also seems to be most difficult for young children, particularly in terms of mother-child interaction.

Preparation of children for the birth of a sibling is individual, but age dictates some important considerations. Time for toddlers is a vague concept. Tomorrow could be yesterday or next week, and a month from now could be never. Preparing children too soon for the birth may lessen their interest by the time the event occurs. A good time to start talking about the new baby is when the toddler becomes aware of the pregnancy and the changes taking place in the home in anticipation of the new member. To avoid additional stresses when the newborn arrives, parents should perform anticipated changes, such as moving the toddler to a different room or bed, well in advance of the birth.

Toddlers need to have a realistic idea of what the newborn will be like. Telling them that a new playmate will come home soon sets up unrealistic expectations. Rather parents should stress the activities that will take place when the baby arrives home such as diapering, bottle-feeding or breastfeeding, bathing, and dressing. At the same time, parents should emphasize which routines will stay the same such as reading stories or going to the park. If toddlers have had no contact with an infant, it is a good idea to introduce them to one if feasible.

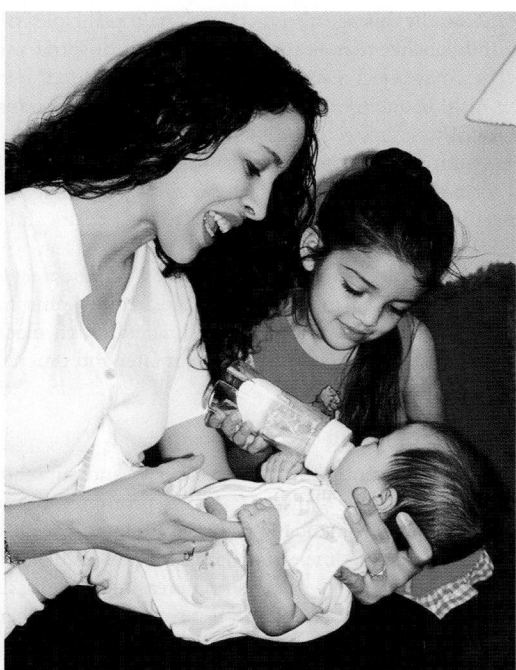

FIG 32.6 To minimize sibling rivalry, parents should include the toddler during caregiving activities.

When the newborn arrives, toddlers keenly feel the changed focus of attention. Visitors may initiate problems when they inadvertently shower the infant with attention and presents while neglecting the older child. Parents can minimize this by alerting visitors to the toddler's needs and including the child in the visits as much as possible. The toddler can also help with the care of the newborn by getting diapers and doing other small tasks (Fig. 32.6).

How children exhibit jealousy is complex. Some overtly hit the infant, push the child off the mother's lap, or pull the bottle or breast from the infant's mouth. For this reason, infants must be protected by parental supervision of the interaction between the siblings. More often the expressions of hostility and resentment are more subtle and covert. Toddlers may verbally express a wish that the infant "go back inside mommy"; or they revert to more infantile forms of behavior such as demanding a bottle, soiling their underpants, clinging for attention, using baby talk, or aggressively acting out toward others.

Temper Tantrums

Toddlers may assert their independence by violently objecting to discipline. They may lie down on the floor, kick their feet, and scream as loud as possible. Some have learned the effectiveness of holding their breath until the parent relents. Although holding one's breath may cause fainting from lack of oxygen, the accumulation of carbon dioxide stimulates the respiratory control center, resulting in no physical harm. Tantrums are an indication of the child's inability to control emotions; toddlers are particularly prone to tantrums because their strong drive for mastery and autonomy is frustrated by adult figures or lack of motor and cognitive skills.

The best approach toward tapering temper tantrums requires consistency and developmentally appropriate expectations and rewards. Ensuring consistency among all caregivers in expectations, prioritizing which rules are important, and developing consequences that are reasonable for the child's level of development help manage the behavior. For example, a popular time for a tantrum is before bed. Active toddlers

often have trouble slowing down and, when placed in bed, resist staying there. Parents can reinforce consistency and expectations by stating, "After this story, it is bedtime." Starting at 18 months, time-outs work well for managing temper tantrums. One key to handling the child's behavior is to demonstrate consistency in dealing with both the behavior and the situation that seemingly precipitated the tantrum; inconsistency reinforces the negative behavior because the child cannot cognitively comprehend the ambiguous messages being received from the parents. During tantrums, stay calm and ignore the behavior, provided it is not injurious to the child such as violently banging the head on the floor. Continue to be present to provide a feeling of control and security to the child once the tantrum has subsided. When the child starts demonstrating appropriate behavior, provide positive feedback about that behavior. During periods of no tantrums, practice developmentally appropriate positive reinforcement.

Other suggestions for handling tantrums include (Luangrath, 2011):
- Offer the child options instead of an "all or none" position.
- Set clear boundaries and expectations with all caregivers.
- Ensure a consistent response to the child's behavior by all caregivers.
- Praise the child for positive behavior when he or she is not having a tantrum, or provide a reward system (i.e., sticker chart).

Temper tantrums are common during the toddler years and essentially represent normal developmental behaviors. However, temper tantrums can be signs of serious problems. Temper tantrums that occur past 5 years of age, last longer than 15 minutes, or occur more than five times per day are considered abnormal and may indicate a serious problem (Daniels, Mandleco, & Luthy, 2012). Nurses should be alert to situations that require further evaluation.

Negativism

One of the more difficult aspects of rearing children in this age-group is their persistent negative response to every request. The negativism is not an expression of being stubborn or insolent but a necessary assertion of self-control. Children test limits to gain understanding of the world and to learn to modify their behavior to fit the expectations of society. Negativism begins to subside as most children prepare to enter kindergarten.

One method of dealing with the negativism is to reduce the opportunities for a "no" answer. Asking the child, "Do you want to go to sleep now?" is an example of a question that will almost certainly be answered with an emphatic "no." Instead, tell the child that it is time to go to sleep and proceed accordingly. In their attempt to exert control, children like to make choices. When confronted with appropriate choices such as, "You may have a peanut butter and jelly sandwich or chicken noodle soup for lunch," they are more likely to choose one rather than automatically say no. However, if their response is negative, parents should make the choice for the child.

Nurses working with children and parents can help parents understand this concept by role modeling. For example, when the nurse approaches the toddler to take vital signs, instead of asking, "Can I listen to your heart?" the nurse can say, "I'm going to listen to your heart." Because of normal developmental behavior, toddlers vigorously resist first attempts at taking vital signs because it is an intrusion on their bodies. Second, they are most likely going to answer "no," not because they necessarily fear the procedure itself but because of the tendency to answer all questions with a negative response. If the nurse asks the question, and the toddler says, "No," but the nurse proceeds anyway, the toddler starts to mistrust the nurse's actions because they contradict his or her words.

Regression

The retreat from one's present pattern of functioning to past levels of behavior is referred to as *regression*. It usually occurs in instances of discomfort or stress when one attempts to conserve psychic energy by reverting to patterns of behavior that were successful in earlier stages of development. Regression is common in toddlers because almost any additional stress hinders their ability to master present developmental tasks. Any threat to their autonomy, such as illness, hospitalization, separation, or adjustment to a new sibling represents a need to revert to earlier forms of behavior such as increased dependency. This can include refusal to use the potty chair; temper tantrums; demand for the bottle or pacifier; and loss of newly learned motor, language, social, and cognitive skills.

At first, such regression appears acceptable and comfortable for children, but the loss of newly acquired achievements is actually frightening and threatening because they are aware of their helplessness. Parents become concerned about regressive behavior and often, in their efforts to deal with it, force the child to cope with an additional source of stress (i.e., the pressure to live up to expected standards). Brazelton (1999) suggests that these predictable times of regression, or touchpoints, are an opportunity to prepare parents for the next step in their child's development.

When regression does occur, the best approach is to ignore it while praising existing patterns of appropriate behavior. Regression is a child's way of saying, "I can't cope with this present stress and perfect this skill as well, but I will if given patience and understanding." For this reason, it is advisable not to attempt new areas of learning when an additional crisis is present or expected, such as beginning toilet training shortly before a sibling is born or during a brief period of hospitalization.

PROMOTING OPTIMAL HEALTH DURING TODDLERHOOD

NUTRITION

During the period from 12 to 18 months of age, the growth rate slows, decreasing the child's need for calories, protein, and fluid. However, the protein (16 g/day) and energy requirements are still relatively high to meet the demands for muscle tissue growth and high activity level. The need for minerals, such as iron, calcium, and phosphorus may be difficult to meet, considering the characteristic food habits of children in this age-group. Parents may be tempted to rely on vitamin supplementation rather than a well-balanced diet to meet these requirements. Toddlers usually require three meals and two snacks per day; however, the portions consumed are generally much smaller compared with those of older children.

The Feeding Infants and Toddlers Study (FITS) (Butte, Fox, Briefel et al., 2010) found that in general toddlers met or exceeded the requirements for daily energy and protein requirements. However, intake of a variety of foods was seen with advancing age in toddlers as their food preferences changed. The FITS recommended that toddlers be fed a more balanced diet of vegetables, fruits, and whole grains.

At approximately 18 months of age, most toddlers manifest this decreased nutritional need with a decreased appetite, a phenomenon known as *physiologic anorexia*. They become picky, fussy eaters with strong taste preferences. They may eat large amounts one day and almost nothing the next. They are increasingly aware of the nonnutritive function of food (i.e., the pleasure of eating, the social aspect of mealtime, and the control of refusing food). They are influenced by factors other than taste when choosing food. If a family member refuses to eat something, toddlers are likely to imitate that response. If the plate is overfilled, they are likely to push it away, overwhelmed by its size. If food does not appear or smell appetizing, they will probably not agree to try it. In essence, mealtime is more closely associated with psychologic rather than nutritional components.

The *ritualism* of this age also dictates certain principles in feeding practices. Toddlers like to have the same dish, cup, or spoon every time they eat. They may reject a favorite food simply because it is served in a different dish. If one food touches another, they often refuse to eat it. Mixed foods such as stews or casseroles are rarely favorites. Because toddlers have unpredictable table manners, it is best to use plastic dishes and cups for both economic and safety reasons. For some children, a regular mealtime schedule also contributes to their desire and need for predictability and ritualism.

Developmentally by 12 months of age most children eat many of the same foods prepared for the rest of the family. Some may have mastered using a cup with occasional spilling, although most cannot use a spoon adeptly until 18 months of age or later and generally prefer using their fingers.

Nutritional Counseling

The emphasis on preventing childhood obesity and subsequent cardiovascular disease in the United States has prompted a number of changes in dietary recommendations for children and adults alike. It is now recognized that lifetime eating habits may be established in early childhood, and health care workers are increasingly emphasizing the role of food selection choices, exercise, stress reduction, and other lifestyle choices (tobacco and alcohol use) on the quality of adult life and survival. Conditions such as obesity and cardiovascular disease can be prevented by encouraging healthy eating habits in toddlers and their families.

If food is used as a reward or sign of approval, a child may overeat for nonnutritive reasons. If food is forced and mealtime is consistently unpleasant, the usual pleasure associated with eating may not develop. Mealtimes should be enjoyable rather than times for discipline or family arguments. The social aspect of mealtime may be distracting for young children; therefore an earlier feeding hour may be appropriate. Young children are unable to sit through a long meal and become restless and disruptive. This is particularly common when children are brought to the table just after active play. Calling them in from play 15 minutes before mealtime allows them ample opportunity to get ready for eating while settling down their active minds and bodies.

The method of serving food also takes on more importance during this period. Toddlers need to have a sense of control and achievement in their abilities. Giving them large, adult-size portions can overwhelm them. In general, what is eaten is much more significant than how much is consumed. Toddlers usually restrict their food preference to four or five main foods and rarely try new foods; in some cases, a toddler may insist on one food such as mashed potatoes for lunch and dinner. Small amounts of meat and vegetables supply greater food value than a large consumption of bread or potato. Serving sizes need to be appropriate for age. Young children tend to like less spicy, bland food, although this is a culturally determined preference. Substitutions can be provided for foods that they do not enjoy, although parents need not cater to all of their desires. Frequent nutritious snacks can replace a meal. Grazing (i.e., nibbling and snacking) is a good way to ensure proper nutrition, provided that appropriate foods are offered.

To determine serving size for young children, use the following guidelines:
- A general guide to the serving size of food is 1 tablespoon of solid food per year of age, or one-fourth to one-third of the adult portion size.
- Use the tablespoon guide for easily measured foods such as vegetables or rice.
- Use the fraction guide for bread or milk.

Mastication skills continue to mature, putting children at risk for choking; therefore large round foods (e.g., hot dogs, grapes, peas, carrots, popcorn, and fruit gel snacks) should be avoided until the child is able to chew them effectively. Active play while eating should be discouraged to prevent choking. Appetite and food preferences are sporadic. Often the interest in food parallels a growth spurt; thus periods of good eating are interspersed with phases of poor eating. If exposed to the same food every day, a young toddler does not learn how to manage the complex sensory information needed to eat new, more difficult foods (e.g., vegetables with a different texture versus pureed, slippery fruits). To help prevent "food jags," it is recommended that parents present food in various physical forms. The child may need to progress to eating new foods in a stepwise fashion such as visually tolerating the food, interacting with it, smelling it, touching it, tasting it, and then eating it.

Many authorities consider it to be a developmental phase, and growth charts can be used to demonstrate growth to parents who are often concerned (Parks, Shaikhkhalil, Groleau, et al., 2016). Parents should be encouraged to plan a nutritionally balanced week instead of day because of the way toddlers restrict food intake in their effort to exert control over their environment (Schwartz & Benuck, 2013).

Dietary Guidelines

Dietary guidelines are necessary to promote adequate energy and nutrient intake to support physical, emotional, psychologic, and cognitive development. A number of new dietary guidelines have been developed to address the issues of childhood obesity, sedentary lifestyles, and increase in cardiovascular disease mortality in the United States.

The Institute of Medicine (2005) has developed guidelines for nutritional intake that encompass the Recommended Daily Allowances (RDAs) yet extend their scope to include additional parameters related to nutritional intake. The Dietary Reference Intakes (DRIs)* are composed of four categories: estimated average requirements (EARs) for age and gender categories, tolerable upper-limit (UL) nutrient intakes that are associated with a low risk for adverse effects, adequate intakes (AIs) of nutrients, and new standard RDAs. The guidelines present information about lifestyle factors that may affect nutrient function such as caffeine intake and exercise and about how the nutrient may be related to chronic disease. An important factor in the development of the DRIs that affects children, particularly infants from birth to 6 months of age, is that the AIs are based on the nutrient intake of full-term, healthy, breastfed infants (by well-nourished mothers), which now represents the gold standard for infant nutrition in this age-group. In 2010, new DRIs for vitamin D and calcium were released by the Institute of Medicine.

The 2010 Dietary Guidelines for Americans may also be used to encourage healthy dietary intakes and regular exercise designed to decrease obesity, cardiovascular risk factors, and subsequent cardiovascular disease, which is now known to occur in both young children and adults. The 2010 Dietary Guidelines recommend a caloric intake for a moderately active boy, 2 to 3 years of age, of 1000 to 1400 calories per day. The emphasis in the Dietary Guidelines is in decreasing overall fat and sodium intakes and increasing the amount of daily exercise to reduce the incidence of obesity and cardiovascular disease. The 2010 Dietary Guidelines† are for children 2 years of age and older. They encourage a variety of fruits, vegetables, whole grains, and low-fat and nonfat dairy products in addition to fish, beans, and lean meat.

Additional resources for dietary counseling include MyPlate,‡ recently developed by the US Department of Agriculture to replace MyPyramid. This colorful plate shows the five main food groups (i.e., fruits, grains, vegetable, protein, and dairy) with the intended purpose to involve children and their families in making appropriate food choices for meals and decrease the incidence of overweight and obesity in the United States. MyPlate provides an online interactive feature that allows the individual to select (click on) an individual food group and see choices for foods in that group. Approximate serving sizes are suggested, and vegetarian substitutions are also provided.

Nutrition during toddlerhood involves a transition as a young toddler is weaned off milk- or formula-based diets. Milk intake, the chief source of calcium and phosphorus, should average two or three servings (24 to 30 oz) per day. Consuming more than 1 quart of milk daily considerably limits the intake of solid foods, resulting in a deficiency of dietary iron and other nutrients. After 2 years of age, children can be given low-fat milk to reduce daily total fat to less than 30% of calories, saturated fatty acids to less than 10% of calories, and cholesterol to less than 300 mg. Other measures to reduce dietary fat include using lean meats, fat-modified products (e.g., low-fat cheese), and low-fat cooking. Because less fat in children's diets can also mean fewer calories and nutrients, caregivers must know what kinds of food to choose. However, *trans* fatty acids and saturated fats should be avoided.

Iron-fortified cereals and iron-rich foods are recommended for all children older than 6 months of age. Parents should be encouraged to provide an iron-rich diet that includes heme and nonheme iron sources (red meats, poultry, fish, green leafy vegetables, dried fruit, and beans) and limits whole-milk consumption. Iron supplementation may be necessary in some cases.

Calcium and vitamin D are essential for healthy bone development. Adequate intake of calcium for children 1 to 3 years of age is 500 mg per day. Whole milk, cheese, yogurt, legumes (beans), and vegetables (broccoli, collard greens, and kale) are good sources of calcium. Popular calcium-fortified foods include waffles, cereals and cereal bars, orange juice, and some white breads. Adequate vitamin D intake is essential to prevent rickets; it is now recommended that children and adolescents have an intake of at least 400 IU of vitamin D daily (Institute of Medicine, 2010). Multivitamin preparations containing 400 IU of vitamin D (by tablet or liquid) are adequate if food intake is poor or exposure to sunlight is minimal; vitamin D–only preparations containing 400 IU are also available commercially. Sources of vitamin D include fish, fish oils, and egg yolks. Fortified cereals, dairy products, and meat are also good sources of zinc and vitamin E.

It is also recommended that toddlers have 1 cup of fruit each day. Vitamin C enhances iron absorption. Toddlers should consume approximately 4 to 6 ounces of juice per day. It tastes good to toddlers and is readily available. A 6-ounce glass of fruit juice equals one fruit serving; however, juices lack the fiber of whole fruit and should not be a substitution for whole fruit. High intake of juice can contribute to diarrhea, overnutrition or undernutrition, and the development of caries; thus only 4 to 6 ounces of 100% fruit juice per day is recommended for toddlers (American Academy of Pediatrics, Committee on Nutrition, 2014). Fruit-flavored drinks advertised as juices may not actually contain 100% juice and should be avoided.

Vegetarian Diets

Vegetarian diets have become increasingly popular in the United States because people are concerned about hypertension; cholesterol; obesity; cardiovascular disease; cancer of the stomach, intestine, and colon; and the influence of the animal rights movement. The American Dietetic Association issued a statement endorsing vegetarian diets for adults and children (Craig, Mangels, & American Dietetic Association, 2009); the statement further notes that well-planned vegetarian diets are adequate for all stages of the life cycle and promote normal growth. Children and adolescents on vegetarian diets have the potential for lifelong healthy diets and have been shown to have lower intakes of cholesterol, saturated fat, and total fat and higher intakes of fruits, fiber,

*https://www.nal.usda.gov/fnic/dietary-reference-intakes.
†www.cnpp.usda.gov/DietaryGuidelines.htm.
‡www.choosemyplate.gov/.

and vegetables than non-vegetarians (Craig, Mangels, & American Dietetic Association, 2009).

The major types of vegetarianism are as follows:
- Lacto-ovo vegetarians, who exclude meat from their diet but consume dairy products and rarely fish
- Lactovegetarians, who exclude meat and eggs but drink milk
- Pure vegetarians (vegans), who eliminate all foods of animal origin, including milk and eggs
- Macrobiotics, who are even more restrictive than pure vegetarians, allowing only a few types of fruits, vegetables, and legumes
- Semi-vegetarians, who consume a lacto-ovo vegetarian diet with some fish and poultry. This is an increasingly popular form of vegetarianism and poses little or no nutritional risk to infants unless dietary fat and cholesterol intake is severely restricted.

Many individuals who are concerned about healthy diets subscribe to vegetarian diets that may not be typified by the previous categories. Therefore during nutritional assessment, it is necessary to clearly list exactly what the diet includes and excludes.*

The major deficiencies that may occur in the stricter vegan diets are inadequate protein for growth; inadequate calories for energy and growth; poor digestibility of many of the bulky natural, unprocessed foods, especially for infants; and deficiencies of vitamin B_6, niacin, riboflavin, vitamin D, iron, calcium, and zinc. Vitamin D is essential if exposure to sunlight is inadequate ($\approx$5 to 15 min/day on the hands, arms, and face of light-skinned persons; slightly more in darker-pigmented individuals) or in people who are dark skinned or who live in northern latitudes or cloudy or smoky areas. Many of these deficiencies can be avoided with a multivitamin and mineral supplement in children who are not consuming 100% of the RDA of vitamins and minerals.

Evaluate for *iron-deficiency anemia* and *rickets* in children on strict vegetarian and macrobiotic diets; this may occur as a result of consuming plant foods such as unrefined cereals, which impair the absorption of iron, calcium, and zinc. The American Academy of Pediatrics, Committee on Nutrition (2014) recommend iron supplementation of 1 mg/kg/day in infants exclusively breastfed after 4 to 6 months of age by vegetarian mothers and no dietary fat restrictions in vegetarian children younger than 2 years of age. Other factors that affect iron absorption are listed in Box 32.2.

Achieving a nutritionally adequate vegetarian diet is not difficult (except with the strictest diets), but it requires careful planning and knowledge of nutrient sources (American Academy of Pediatrics, Committee on Nutrition, 2014). For children, the lacto-ovo vegetarian diet is nutritionally adequate; however, the vegan diet requires supplementation with vitamins D and B_{12} for children 2 to 12 years of age.

To ensure sufficient protein in the diet, foods with incomplete proteins (i.e., those that do not have all the essential amino acids) must be eaten at the same meal with other foods that supply the missing amino acids. The three basic combinations of foods consumed by vegetarians that generally provide the appropriate amounts of essential amino acids are as follows:
1. Grains (cereal, rice, pasta) and legumes (beans, peas, lentils, peanuts)
2. Grains and milk products (milk, cheese, yogurt)
3. Seeds (sesame, sunflower) and legumes

COMPLEMENTARY AND ALTERNATIVE MEDICINE

There are four complementary and alternative medicine (CAM) domains according to the National Center for Complementary and Integrative

---

*Additional information regarding vegetarian diets may be found at the Vegetarian Resource Group; 410-366-8343; www.vrg.org. Another helpful resource is the KidsHealth website: http://kidshealth.org.

BOX 32.2   Factors That Affect Iron Absorption

Increase
- Acidity (low pH)—Administer iron between meals (gastric hydrochloric acid).
- Ascorbic acid (vitamin C)—Administer iron with juice, fruit, or multivitamin preparation.
- Vitamin A
- Tissue (cellular) need
- Meat, fish, poultry
- Cooking in cast iron pots

Decrease
- Alkalinity (high pH)—Avoid any antacid preparation.
- Phosphates—Milk is unfavorable vehicle for iron administration.
- Phytates—Found in cereals
- Oxalates—Found in many fruits and vegetables (plums, currants, green beans, spinach, sweet potatoes, tomatoes)
- Tannins—Found in tea, coffee
- Tissue (cellular) saturation
- Malabsorptive disorders
- Disturbances that cause diarrhea or steatorrhea
- Infection

Health; this discussion centers only on one of those biologically based practices that include herbs, vitamins, and foods. The National Center for Complementary and Integrative Health (2014) classifies probiotics as a type of natural product and CAM. Many CAM products are sold over the counter as dietary supplements, but the use of some dietary supplements such as calcium for bone health or a multivitamin supplement are not considered to be CAM (National Center for Complementary and Integrative Health, 2014). The National Center for Complementary and Integrative Health (2014) reports that natural products are the most commonly used CAM products in children, and most often these products are used for chronic conditions, such as neck and back pain, and for head and chest colds. Other surveys confirm that CAM is often used for children's chronic remedies for which traditional therapy is not effective (Huillet, Erdie-Lalena, Norvell, et al., 2011).

The misuse of vitamins as a part of CAM has the potential for placing some children at risk for health problems. Zuzak and colleagues (2010) noted that of persons reportedly using CAM, the most common CAM remedies used in children seen in an emergency department were homeopathy (77%), herbs (64%), and traditional Chinese medicine (13%). A survey in a Women, Infants, and Children clinic found that child herbal use was common, especially among Hispanic children attending the clinic. Some of the herbs used by the children in the survey (ma huang, foxglove, anise tea, and mistletoe) have questionable safety (Kemper & Gardiner, 2016). A study of CAM use in children on a military base found that 23% of parents reported using CAM in their children, with herbal therapy being the most common type of CAM reported; 50% of the parents who used CAM for their children reported the use of vitamins and minerals in amounts that exceeded the RDA (Huillet et al., 2011).

There is concern that terms often used to market supplements such as megavitamins may mislead parents regarding the actual benefits (or harm) of such therapies. The intention herein is not to discredit the use of CAM such as vitamin supplements; rather it is to ensure safety and efficacy in children who may experience inadvertent harm. The use of various herbal therapies, or intake of herbs, is also becoming more popular; many of these have been a part of medicine since early days and are beneficial in some cases. Many mind-body CAM therapies (e.g., guided imagery, distraction) have proved beneficial for children undergoing cancer treatment, but the small sample sizes of the groups being studied may preclude generalization to a larger population group until further studies are undertaken (Landier & Tse, 2010).

Herbs known to have adverse effects in children include ephedra, comfrey, and pennyroyal; some herbs may not be harmful taken alone but may counteract or potentiate prescription medications when taken together. Parents should be fully informed of the use of herbs to ensure that there is more benefit than potential harm in the ingredients being used. Health care workers also need to be knowledgeable of the benefits or potential harm in herbs to counsel parents and address their concerns appropriately. Little research has been performed in children on many over-the-counter herbal medicines, yet some herbs are known to cause harm (Kemper & Gardiner, 2016). Parents should be cautioned not to exceed the upper limits of vitamin intake according to the new DRIs.*

SLEEP AND ACTIVITY

Total sleep decreases only slightly during the second year and averages about 11 to 12 hours per day. Most children take one nap per day but may relinquish this habit by the end of the second or third year.

Toddlers are more prone to having bedtime resistance (refusal to go to bed) and frequent night waking. Sleep problems, especially going to bed and falling asleep, are common and probably related to fears. Fears can be provoked by a child's daily stressors such as pressure to toilet train, moves, sibling birth, experiences of loss, or separation from parents. A recent study found that a consistent nightly bedtime routine is associated with better sleep patterns, such as shorter sleep onset latency, decreased waking, longer total sleep, and decreased daytime behavior problems (Mindell, Li, Sadeh, et al., 2015). In addition, providing transitional objects, such as a favorite stuffed animal or blanket, can ease the child's insecurity at bedtime (see Fig. 32.3). Children may need a light snack before bedtime; a heavy meal immediately before bedtime may interfere with sleep. Other suggestions to help small children sleep better include keeping the television out of the child's room, making the hour before bedtime a quiet time of reading stories, and avoiding stimulating activities such as computer games and roughhousing (Owens, 2016). Toddlers no longer sleeping in a crib may come out of their rooms after being put to bed. Limit prolonged bedtime rituals by defining a length of time and set of activities (one more story, one more drink of water). Toddlers who are too immature to respond to the measures identified may need their doorways gated.

A toddler's activity level is high, and there is rarely a problem with too little physical exercise, provided inappropriate restrictions are not instituted. However, recently there has been concern that decreased time spent in actual physical play and more time involved with computers and television watching have increased the tendency toward being overweight. This is especially true in large urban centers during the winter months where there may not be adequate "safe" play and physical exercise space. With increasing numbers of young children being cared for outside the home, attention to the kinds of activity provided is important. For example, children with high activity levels may benefit from an environment that encourages vigorous play, whether outside or in a large indoor play area.

Sleep Problems

A number of sleep problems are identified in small children. Children may have trouble going to sleep, wake during the night, have difficulty

resuming sleep after waking during the night, have nightmares or sleep terrors, or prolong the inevitable bedtime through elaborate rituals. Such sleep disturbances are typically related to increasing autonomy, negative sleep associations, nighttime fears, inconsistent bedtime routines, and lack of limit setting (Babcock, 2011).

Minor sleep issues in toddlers such as refusal to go to sleep and frequent waking during the night are reviewed in Table 32.2.

Concerns regarding sleep are common during childhood. Sometimes these concerns are as basic as parents' questioning whether the infant needs additional sleep. In this case, it is best to investigate the reason for their concern, stressing the individual needs of each child. When a sleeping problem is presented, a careful assessment is essential. Charting sleep habits both before and after interventions is also an important strategy. Questions regarding the frequency and duration of waking, the usual bedtime routine, the number of nighttime feedings, the perceived problem (e.g., how much disruption the behavior generates), and the attempted interventions are important in planning effective approaches designed for the specific sleep problem.

The best way to prevent sleep problems is to encourage parents to establish bedtime rituals that do not foster problematic patterns. One of the most constructive is placing infants awake in their own crib. When infants are accustomed to falling asleep somewhere else such as in their parent's arms and then being transferred to their crib, they awaken in unfamiliar surroundings and are unable to fall asleep until the routine is repeated. In addition, the bed should be used for sleeping only—not as a play yard. It is advisable not to hang playthings over or on the bed so the child associates the bed with sleep and not with activity. Although the interventions described previously and in Table 32.2 are usually successful, it is much easier to prevent the problem with appropriate counseling during the early months of the infant's life.

Consequences of inadequate sleep include daytime tiredness, behavior changes, hyperactivity, difficulty concentrating, impaired learning ability, poor control of emotions and impulses, and strain on family relationships (Bhargava, 2011). Nurses should incorporate assessment of sleep patterns and education about the development of healthy sleep behaviors into every well-child visit. Recommendations for handling a sleep disturbance are offered only after a thorough assessment. Cultural traditions may dictate sleep practices contrary to certain well-accepted professional recommendations. Thus, parents may not perceive particular sleep habits as problematic (see Cultural Considerations box: Co-Sleeping).

CULTURAL CONSIDERATIONS
Co-Sleeping

Many experts recommend that infants and children be trained to always sleep in their own crib or bed. However, co-sleeping, or the "family bed" (in which parents allow the children to sleep with them) is an accepted cultural practice among many African-American and Asian families (Ward & Doering, 2014; Mindell, Sadeh, Kohyama, et al., 2010). Others who have adopted co-sleeping include parents who believe that co-sleeping promotes parent-child bonding, parents who think that co-sleeping diminishes their child's nighttime fears or other sleep disturbances, and mothers who are breastfeeding. Co-sleeping may be a practical solution to limited numbers of bedrooms or beds in lower-socioeconomic families. Controversy exists regarding the medical, developmental, and social advantages and disadvantages of co-sleeping. Studies have indicated that co-sleeping is associated with sleep problems, such as frequent night wakings, poor sleep quality, and decreased length of sleep (Mindell et al.). Parents who are considering co-sleeping should fully investigate the potential risks and benefits. Health care providers should be proactive in discussing sleeping arrangements with families at each visit to ensure children's safety and healthy sleep habits.

---

*Helpful websites for health care and consumer information concerning herbs are National Center for Complementary and Integrative Health, https://nccih.nih.gov; American Botanical Council, http://abc.herbalgram.org; and Herb Research Foundation, http://www.herbs.org.

TABLE 32.2 Selected Sleep Disturbances During Infancy and Early Childhood

Condition and Description	Management
Nighttime Feeding Child has prolonged need for middle-of-night bottle or breastfeeding. Child goes to sleep at breast or with bottle. Awakenings are frequent (may be hourly). Child returns to sleep after feeding; other comfort measures (e.g., rocking or holding) are usually ineffective.	Increase daytime feeding intervals to 4 hours or more (may need to be done gradually). Offer last feeding as late as possible at night; may need to gradually reduce amount of formula or length of breastfeeding. Offer no bottles in bed. Put to bed awake. When child is crying, check at progressively longer intervals each night; reassure child but do not hold, rock, take to parent's bed, or give bottle or pacifier.
Developmental Nighttime Crying Child 6–12 months of age with undisturbed nighttime sleep now awakens abruptly; may be accompanied by nightmares.	Reassure parents that this phase is temporary. Enter room immediately to check on child, but keep reassurances brief. Avoid feeding, rocking, taking to parent's bed, or any other routine that may initiate trained nighttime crying.
Refusal to Go to Sleep Child resists bedtime and comes out of room repeatedly. Nighttime sleep may be continuous, but frequent awakenings and refusal to return to sleep may occur and become a problem if parent allows child to deviate from usual sleep pattern.	Evaluate if hour of sleep is too early (child may resist sleep if not tired). Help parents establish consistent before-bedtime routine and enforce consistent limits regarding child's bedtime behavior. If child persists in leaving bedroom, close door for progressively longer periods. Use reward system with child to provide motivation.
Trained Nighttime Crying (Inappropriate Sleep Associations) Child typically falls asleep in place other than own bed (e.g., rocking chair or parent's bed) and is brought to own bed while asleep; on awakening, cries until usual routine is instituted (e.g., rocking).	Put child in own bed when awake. If possible, arrange sleeping area separate from other family members. When child is crying, check at progressively longer intervals each night; reassure child, but do not resume usual routine.
Nighttime Fears Child resists going to bed or wakes during night because of fears. Child seeks parent's physical presence and falls asleep easily with parent nearby unless fear is overwhelming.	Evaluate if hour of sleep is too early (child may fantasize when nothing to do but think in dark room). Calmly reassure frightened child; keeping night light on may be helpful. Use reward system with child to provide motivation to deal with fears. Avoid patterns that can lead to additional problems (e.g., sleeping with child or taking child to parent's room). If child's fear is overwhelming, consider desensitization (e.g., progressively spending longer periods of time alone; consult professional help for protracted fears). Distinguish between nightmares and sleep terrors (confused partial arousals).

Adapted from Ferber, R. (1987). Behavioral "insomnia" in the child. *Psychiatric Clinics of North America, 10*(4), 641–653.

Interventions differ greatly; for example, *nightmares* and *sleep terrors* require different approaches (Table 32.3). For children who delay going to bed, a recommended approach involves counseling consistent bedtime ritual and emphasizing the normalcy of this type of behavior in young children. Parents should ignore attention-seeking behavior, and the child should not be taken into the parents' bed or allowed to stay up past a reasonable hour. Other measures that may be helpful include keeping a light on in the room, providing transitional objects such as a favorite toy, or leaving a drink of water by the bed.

Helping children slow down before bedtime also reduces resistance to going to bed. One approach is to establish soothing, limited rituals that signal readiness for bed, such as a bath or story. Parents can reinforce the pattern by stating, "After this story, it is bedtime," and consistently carrying through the routine. If anticipated extra stimulation (e.g., having visitors arrive at the children's bedtime) disrupts this routine, it is advisable to settle children in bed beforehand.

DENTAL HEALTH

Regular Dental Examinations

The American Academy of Pediatric Dentistry (2014a) recommends that every child have an oral health examination by a practitioner by 6 months of age; if the child is in a high-risk category for caries, it is recommended that an initial visit to a dentist or pedodontist (pediatric dentist) occur by 6 months of age or within 6 months of the eruption of the first tooth. Every child should have an established dental home by 12 months of age (American Academy of Pediatric Dentistry, 2014a). Initial visits to the dentist should be nontraumatizing. Because toddlers react negatively to new and potentially frightening experiences, the initial visit can center around meeting the dentist, seeing the equipment, and sitting in the chair. If the child is cooperative, the dentist may just look at the teeth but reserve a more thorough examination for another visit. Modeling, in which the child observes procedures performed on

TABLE 32.3 Comparison of Nightmares to Sleep Terrors

Characteristics	Nightmares	Sleep Terrors
Description	A scary dream; takes place during REM sleep and is followed by full waking	A partial arousal from very deep sleep (state IV, non-REM) sleep
Time of distress	After dream is over, child wakes and cries or calls; not during nightmare itself	During terror itself, as child screams and thrashes; afterward is calm
Time of occurrence	In second half of night, when dreams are most intense	Usually 1 to 4 hours after falling asleep, when non-REM sleep is deepest
Child's behavior	Crying in younger children, fright in all; behaviors persistent even though child is awake	Initially may sit up, thrash, or run in bizarre manner, with eyes bulging, heart racing, and profuse perspiring; may cry, scream, talk, or moan; shows apparent fright, anger, or obvious confusion, which disappears when child is fully awake
Responsiveness to others	Is aware of and reassured by another's presence	Is not very aware of another's presence, is not comforted, and may push person away and scream and thrash more if held or restrained
Return to sleep	May be considerably delayed because of persistent fear	Usually rapid; often difficult to keep child awake
Description of dream	Yes (if old enough)	No memory of dream or of yelling or thrashing
interventions	Accept dream as real fear	Observe child for a few minutes, without interfering, until child becomes calm or wakes fully
	Sit with child; offer comfort, assurance, and sense of protection	Intervene only if necessary to protect child from injury
	Avoid forcing child back to his or her own bed	Guide child back to bed if needed
	Consider professional counseling for recurrent nightmares unresponsive to above approaches	Stress to parents that sleep terrors are a normal, common phenomenon in preschoolers that requires relatively little intervention

Adapted from Haupt, M., Sheldon, S.H., & Loghmanee, D. (2013). Just a scary dream? A brief review of sleep terrors, nightmares, and rapid eye movement sleep behavior disorder. *Pediatric Annals, 42*(10), 211–216.
REM, Rapid eye movement.

the parent or a cooperative sibling, can also be effective but may not work on all toddlers.

Plaque Removal

Oral hygiene measures should be implemented in toddlers to remove plaque (i.e., soft bacterial deposits that adhere to the teeth and cause dental caries [decay or cavities] and periodontal [gum] disease). Poor oral hygiene and dietary habits are associated with the development of caries in children.

The most effective methods for plaque removal are brushing and flossing. Several brushing techniques exist, although there is no universal agreement regarding the best method. One that is suitable for cleaning the primary teeth is the scrub method. The tips of the bristles are placed firmly at a 45-degree angle against the teeth and gums and moved back and forth in a vibratory motion. The ends of the bristles should be wiggling but not moving forcefully back and forth, which can damage the gums and enamel. All the surfaces of the teeth are cleaned in this manner except the lingual (inner) surfaces of the anterior teeth. To clean these surfaces the toothbrush is placed vertical to the teeth and moved up and down. Only a few teeth are brushed at one time, using six to eight strokes for each section. A systematic approach is used so all surfaces are thoroughly cleaned (Fig. 32.7).

For young children, the most effective cleaning is done by parents (Fig. 32.8). Several positions can be used that facilitate access to the mouth and help stabilize the head for comfort:

- Stand with the child's back toward the adult. (When done in front of a bathroom mirror, both the child and adult can see what is being done in the mirror.)
- Sit on a couch or bed with the child's head resting in the adult's lap.
- Sit on the floor or a stool with the child's head resting between the adult's thighs.

Use one hand to cup the chin and one to brush the teeth. For easier access to back teeth, hold the mouth partially open. After brushing with an appropriate amount of fluoridated paste or gel, avoid rinsing the mouth to maximize the beneficial effects of the fluoride.

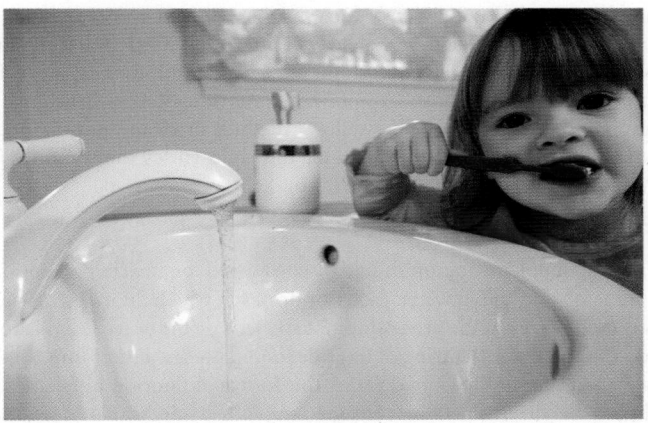

FIG 32.7 Young children can participate in toothbrushing, but parents need to brush all the child's teeth thoroughly. (Copyright 2011 by Photos.com, a division of Getty Images. All rights reserved.)

For effective cleaning, a small toothbrush with soft, rounded, multi-tufted nylon bristles that are short and uniform in length is recommended. Nylon bristles dry more rapidly after use and retain their shape better than natural bristles. Toothbrushes are replaced as soon as the bristles are frayed or bent. With young children, brushing may be accomplished more easily using only water because many children dislike the foam from toothpaste, and the foam interferes with visibility. Introduce toothpaste around 2 years of age, and allow children to select the flavor they like to encourage the brushing habit. Use a "smear" or "rice-size" amount of toothpaste for children younger than 3 years of age (apply across the narrow width of the toothbrush, rather than along its length, to decrease the chance of applying an excessive amount); use a "pea-size" amount of toothpaste for children 3 to 6 years of age (American Academy of Pediatric Dentistry, 2014b).

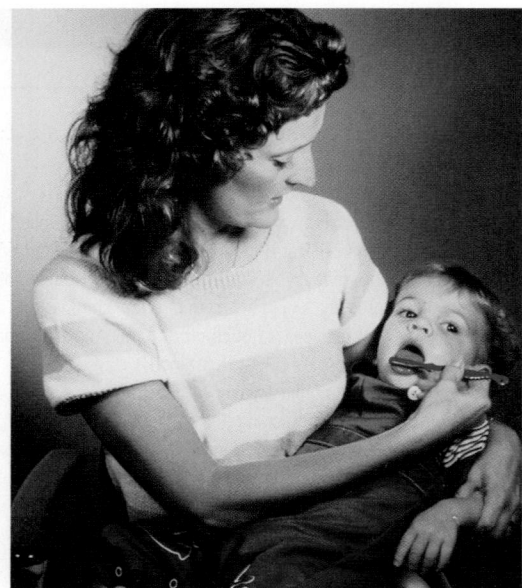

FIG 32.8 The most effective teeth cleaning is done by parents.

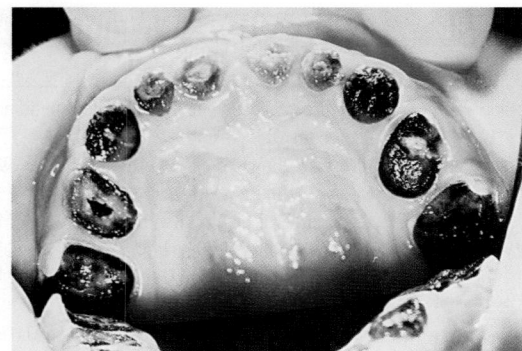

FIG 32.9 Nursing caries. Note extensive carious involvement of maxillary primary incisors. (Courtesy of Bruce Carter, DDS, Texas Children's Hospital, Houston, TX.)

After the teeth have been cleaned, they are flossed to remove plaque and debris from between the teeth and below the gum margin, where brushing is ineffective. Because young children do not have the dexterity to manipulate dental floss, parents must perform the procedure.

Ideally the teeth should be cleaned after each meal and especially before bedtime, and the child should be given nothing to eat or drink after the night brushing except water. At times when brushing is impractical, the "swish-and-swallow" method of cleaning the mouth is taught; with a mouthful of water the child rinses the mouth and swallows, repeating the procedure 3 or 4 times.*

Fluoride

Fluoride supplementation should be considered for any child. Fluoride, a mineral, is found in water, foods, or drinks in which fluoridated water was used as part of the processing system. Because the water fluoridation process and manufacturing of fluoride toothpaste are almost impossible to standardize in the United States, the dosage of fluoride supplements should be determined in consultation with a medical professional (American Academy of Pediatric Dentistry, 2014b). Increased fluoride ingestion leads to enamel protein retention, hypomineralization of the enamel and dentin, and disturbance of crystal formation. The effects caused by this change range from barely discernible white fiberlike lines or spots to gray-brown stains or pitted areas. Parents should be cautioned against regular use of fluoridated water or beverages such as bottled water containing fluoride if the community water supply already has an adequate amount of fluoride. Topical fluoride treatments (e.g., fluoride varnish) performed in the dental home is also effective in decreasing caries (American Academy of Pediatric Dentistry, 2014c).

Dietary Factors

Diet is critical to developing good teeth because the carious process depends primarily on fermentable sugars, especially sucrose, and other carbohydrates. Refined table sugar, honey, molasses, corn syrup, and dried fruits such as raisins are highly cariogenic. Complex carbohydrates such as breads, potatoes, and pasta also contribute to caries because

they lower the plaque pH. Beverages and snacks that are commonly consumed by children and adolescents are also highly cariogenic and may contribute to the incidence of overweight and obesity (American Academy of Pediatric Dentistry, 2014d).

Ideally highly cariogenic foods, especially those containing complex sugars, should be eliminated. However, because this is impractical some suggestions can be helpful. First, the frequency with which sugar is consumed is more important than the total amount eaten. Therefore, when sweets are eaten, they are less damaging if consumed immediately after a meal rather than as a snack between meals. When they are served as the dessert, the teeth can be cleaned afterward, decreasing the amount of time the sugar is in the mouth.

Second, the form of sugar (sucrose) is important. The more cariogenic foods are those that are sticky or hard because they remain in the mouth longer. Consequently, sucking on lollipops is more cariogenic than eating a chocolate bar. Sometimes the source of the sugar is "hidden," as in numerous prescription and nonprescription drugs and many popular cereals, including the "all-natural" variety. Reading food labels is essential in eliminating sources of sucrose.

Some snacks do not contribute to tooth decay. Aged cheeses such as cheddar may alter the pH and delay bacterial growth. Sugarless gum chewed after eating may actually protect against cavities by stimulating saliva that neutralizes acid.

A special form of tooth decay in children between 18 months and 3 years of age is early childhood caries (ECC) (historically called *nursing caries* or *baby bottle tooth decay*) (Fig. 32.9). This often occurs when a child is routinely given a bottle of milk or juice at naptime or bedtime or uses the bottle as a pacifier while awake. Frequent nocturnal breastfeeding for prolonged periods also leads to extensive destruction of the teeth. The practice of coating pacifiers in honey can also contribute to caries and may be a potential source of botulism. As the sweet liquid pools in the mouth, the teeth are bathed for several hours in this cariogenic environment. Prolonged bottle-feeding well into toddler years in some cultures may contribute to significant ECC (Brotanek, Schroer, Valentyn, et al., 2009). The maxillary (upper) incisors and molars are affected most because the mandibular (lower) incisors are protected by the lower lip, tongue, and saliva. Severely decayed teeth may require the application of stainless steel bands to preserve the spacing until the permanent teeth erupt.

Early childhood caries is now considered to be an infectious disease of childhood. There is evidence that *Streptococcus mutans* is a highly cariogenic bacteria (American Academy of Pediatric Dentistry, 2014b). One of the early origins of *S. mutans* is the mother's saliva; infants of mothers with high counts of the bacteria have a greater incidence of

*More detailed information can be obtained from the American Academy of Pediatric Dentistry, www.aapd.org.

ECC. Therefore it is important to discuss oral hygiene with pregnant women because of its impact on their children's tooth development.

Prevention involves eliminating the bedtime bottle completely, feeding the last bottle before bedtime, substituting a bottle of water for milk or juice, not using the bottle as a pacifier, and never coating pacifiers in sweet substances. Juice in bottles, especially commercially available ready-to-use bottles, is discouraged; these beverages are especially damaging because the sugar is more readily converted to acid. Juice should always be offered in a cup to avoid prolonging the bottle-feeding habit. Toddlers should be encouraged to drink from a cup at the first birthday and weaned from a bottle by 14 months of age. Nurses are in an excellent position to counsel parents regarding the dangers of this habit and other aspects of dental care.*

ATOPIC DERMATITIS (ECZEMA)

Eczema or eczematous inflammation of the skin refers to a descriptive category of dermatologic diseases and not to a specific etiology. Atopic dermatitis (AD) is a type of pruritic eczema that usually begins during infancy and is associated with an allergic contact dermatitis with a hereditary tendency (atopy) (Jacob, Yang, Herro, & Zhang, 2010). AD manifests in three forms based on the child's age and the distribution of lesions:

Infantile (infantile eczema): Usually begins at 2 to 6 months of age; generally undergoes spontaneous remission by 3 years of age

Childhood: May follow the infantile form; occurs at 2 to 3 years of age; 90% of children have manifestations by 5 years of age

Preadolescent and adolescent: Begins at about 12 years of age; may continue into the early adult years or indefinitely

The diagnosis of AD is based on a combination of history, clinical manifestations, and in some cases, morphologic findings (Box 32.3). The majority of children with infantile AD have a family history of eczema, asthma, food allergies, or allergic rhinitis, which strongly supports a genetic predisposition. The cause is unknown but appears to be related to abnormal function of the skin, including alterations in perspiration, peripheral vascular function, and heat tolerance. Manifestations of the chronic disease improve in humid climates and get worse in the fall and winter, when homes are heated and environmental humidity is lower. The disorder can be controlled but not cured.

Therapeutic Management

The major goals of management are to hydrate the skin, relieve pruritus, prevent and minimize flare-ups or inflammation, and prevent and control secondary infection. The general measures for managing AD focus on reducing pruritus and other aspects of the disease. Management strategies include avoiding exposure to skin irritants or allergens; avoiding overheating; and administrating medications such as antihistamines, topical immunomodulators, topical steroids, and (sometimes) mild sedatives, as indicated.

Enhancing skin hydration and preventing dry, flaky skin are accomplished in a number of ways, depending on the child's skin characteristics

---

*Sources of information about nursing caries and other aspects of child dental health include the National Institute of Dental and Craniofacial Research, National Institutes of Health, Bethesda, MD 20892-2190, 301-496-4261, www.nidcr.nih.gov; American Academy of Pediatric Dentistry, 211 E. Chicago Avenue, Suite 1700, Chicago, IL 60611, 312-337-2169, www.aapd.org; American Dental Association, 211 E. Chicago Avenue, Chicago, IL 60611, 312-440-2500, www.ada.org/; and Canadian Dental Association, 1815 Alta Vista Drive, Ottawa, Ontario K1G 3Y6, 613-523-1770, www.cda-adc.ca.

> ## BOX 32.3   Clinical Manifestations of Atopic Dermatitis
>
> **Distribution of Lesions**
>
> **Infantile form:** Generalized, especially cheeks, scalp, trunk, and extensor surfaces of extremities
>
> **Childhood form:** Flexural areas (antecubital and popliteal fossae, neck), wrists, ankles, and feet
>
> **Preadolescent and adolescent form:** Face, sides of neck, hands, feet, face, and antecubital and popliteal fossae (to a lesser extent)
>
> **Appearance of Lesions**
> **Infantile Form**
> Erythema
> Vesicles
> Papules
> Weeping
> Oozing
> Crusting
> Scaling
> Often symmetric
>
> **Childhood Form**
> Symmetric involvement
> Clusters of small erythematous or flesh-colored papules or minimally scaling patches
> Dry and may be hyperpigmented
> Lichenification (thickened skin with accentuation of creases)
> Keratosis pilaris (follicular hyperkeratosis) common
>
> **Adolescent or Adult Form**
> Same as childhood manifestations
> Dry, thick lesions (lichenified plaques) common
> Confluent papules
>
> **Other Physical Manifestations**
> Intense itching
> Unaffected skin dry and rough
> African-American children likely to exhibit more papular or follicular lesions than are white children
> May exhibit one or more of the following:
>   Lymphadenopathy, especially near affected sites
>   Increased palmar creases (many cases)
>   Atopic pleats (extra line or groove of lower eyelid)
>   Prone to cold hands
>   Pityriasis alba (small, poorly defined areas of hypopigmentation)
>   Facial pallor (especially around nose, mouth, and ears)
>   Bluish discoloration beneath eyes ("allergic shiners")
>   Increased susceptibility to unusual cutaneous infections (especially viral)

and individual needs. A tepid bath with a mild soap (Dove or Neutrogena), no soap, or an emulsifying oil followed immediately by application of an emollient (within 3 minutes) assists in trapping moisture and preventing its loss. Bubble baths and harsh soaps should be avoided. Some lotions are not effective, and emollients should be chosen carefully to prevent excessive skin drying. Aquaphor, Cetaphil, and Eucerin are acceptable lotions for skin hydration. A nighttime bath followed by emollient application and dressing in soft cotton pajamas may help alleviate most nighttime pruritus.

Sometimes colloid baths, such as the addition of 2 cups of cornstarch to a tub of warm water, provide temporary relief of itching and may help the child sleep if given before bedtime.

Oral antihistamine drugs (e.g., hydroxyzine or diphenhydramine) usually relieve moderate or severe pruritus. Nonsedating antihistamines, such as loratadine (Claritin) or fexofenadine (Allegra), may be preferred for daytime pruritus relief. Fingernails and toenails are cut short, kept clean, and filed frequently to prevent sharp edges. Gloves or cotton stockings can be placed over the hands. One-piece outfits with long sleeves and long pants also decrease direct contact with the skin. If gloves or socks are used, the child needs time to be free from such restrictions.

Occasional flare-ups require the use of topical steroids to diminish inflammation. Low-, moderate-, or high-potency topical corticosteroids are prescribed, depending on the degree of involvement, the area of the body to be treated, the child's age, the potential for local side effects (striae, skin atrophy, and pigment changes), and the type of vehicle to be used (e.g., cream, lotion, ointment). Topical immunomodulators, a new nonsteroidal treatment for AD, are best used at the beginning of a "flare-up" just as the skin becomes red and itches. Two immunomodulator medications used in children with AD are tacrolimus and pimecrolimus (Schneider, Tilles, Lio, et al., 2013). Both drugs can be used freely on the face without worrying about steroid side effects.

If secondary skin infections occur in children with AD, these infections are managed with appropriate antibiotics. Topical and oral antibiotics are used; however, areas of active infection are first cultured to ensure appropriate therapy (Wolter & Price, 2014).

Interprofessional Care of AD

Assessment of the child with AD includes a family history for evidence of atopy, a history of previous involvement, and any environmental or dietary factors associated with the present and previous exacerbations. The skin lesions are examined for type, distribution, and evidence of secondary infection. Parents are interviewed regarding the child's behavior, especially in relation to scratching, irritability, and sleeping patterns. Exploration of the family's feelings and methods of coping is also important.

Wet soaks and compresses are applied and medications for pruritus or infection are administered as directed. The family is given explicit instructions on the preparation and use of soaks, special baths, and topical medications, including the order of application if more than one is prescribed. It is important to emphasize that one thick application of topical medication is not equivalent to several thin applications and that excessive use of an agent (particularly steroids) can be hazardous.

When a hypoallergenic diet is prescribed, parents need help to understand the reason for the diet and the guidelines for avoiding hyperallergenic foods. Consultation with a dietician is recommended. Because hypoallergenic diets take time before visible effects are apparent, parents need reassurance that results may not be seen immediately.

During acute phases, emotional stress can become intense for the family. They need time to discuss negative feelings and to be reassured that these feelings are normal. Refer to psychosocial services if further support is needed. Stress tends to aggravate the severity of the condition. Therefore, efforts to relieve as much anxiety as possible in both the parents and the child have a beneficial emotional and physical effect. Parents are assured that the disease is not contagious; however, the child may have repeated exacerbations and remissions. Spontaneous and permanent remission takes place at approximately 2 to 3 years of age in most children with the infantile disorder.

SAFETY PROMOTION AND INJURY PREVENTION

Unintentional childhood injury was the leading cause of death among children 1 to 19 years of age in 2009, accounting for 37% of all deaths in this age-group (Gilchrist, Ballesteros, & Parker, 2012). Unintentional death rates among newborns and infants from suffocation nearly doubled from 2000 to 2009. Likewise, unintentional poisoning death rates doubled for adolescents 15 to 19 years of age during the same time period (Gilchrist et al.). These deaths and injuries are preventable, and they highlight the need for public health action and education. There is evidence that one-on-one and face-to-face education as well as safety interventions and safety equipment are effective in reducing the number of unintentional childhood injuries that can have catastrophic results (Kendrick, Young, Mason-Jones, et al., 2012).

A major factor in the critical increase of injuries during early childhood is the unrestricted freedom achieved through locomotion combined with an unawareness of danger within the environment. Toddlers delight in the repetitive use of gross motor skills, and with increasing age these skills are refined. This age-group is also very curious about how things work, and exploration of previously unknown or unseen objects and places is common. Toddlers also have not fully developed or do not understand the cause-and-effect principles that older children have and often are unable to gauge danger; poorly developed depth perception may also contribute to falls and tumbles as does the general bodily structure of toddlers.

Specific categories of injuries and appropriate prevention are best understood by associating them with the major growth and developmental achievements of this age (Table 32.4). The discussions of injuries in Chapters 31 and 33 are also relevant to safety concerns at this age.

Motor Vehicle Safety

Motor vehicle injuries cause more accidental deaths in all pediatric age-groups after 1 year of age than any other type of injury or disease and are responsible for almost one-half of all accidental deaths among children 1 to 4 years of age. Many of the deaths are caused by injuries within the car when restraints have not been used or have been used improperly. Unrestrained children riding in the front seat of the vehicle are at highest risk for injury. Approved restraints properly installed and applied can prevent many fatalities and injuries (Weaver, Brixey, Williams, et al., 2013).

Car Restraints

Nurses are responsible for educating parents regarding the importance of car restraints and their proper use. Five types of restraints are available: (1) infant-only devices, (2) convertible models for both infants and toddlers, (3) boosters, (4) safety belts, and (5) devices for children with disabilities. Chapter 31 discusses the infant-type restraints; convertible restraints and boosters are included here. Convertible restraints are suitable for infants and toddlers in the rearward-facing position (Fig. 32.10). The American Academy of Pediatrics and National Highway Traffic Safety Administration recommended that children up to 2 years of age ride in a rear-facing car safety seat until the child has outgrown the manufacturer's weight and height recommendation (Durbin & Committee on Injury, Violence, and Poison Prevention, 2011). Many rear-facing car safety seats can accommodate children weighing up to a maximum of 35 pounds (according to manufacturer specifications).*

---

*www.carseat.org.

Studies indicate that toddlers up to 24 months of age are safer riding in convertible seats in the rear-facing position (American Academy of Pediatrics, 2015).

Children 2 years of age and older (or those younger than 2 years of age) who have outgrown the rear-facing height or weight limit for their car safety seat should use a forward-facing car safety seat with a harness up to the maximum height or weigh recommended by the manufacturer (Durbin & Committee on Injury, Violence, and Poison Prevention, 2011). Convertible restraints use different types of harness systems: a five-point harness that consists of a strap over each shoulder, one on each side of the pelvis, and one between the legs (all five come together at a common buckle) and a padded overhead shield that uses shoulder

---

TABLE 32.4 Injury Prevention During Early Childhood

Developmental Abilities Related to Risk for Injury	Injury Prevention
Motor Vehicles	
Walks, runs, and climbs	Use federally approved car restraint per manufacturer's recommendations for weight and height.
Able to open doors and gates	Supervise child while playing outside.
Can ride tricycle and other toy vehicles	Do not allow child to play on curb or behind parked car.
	Do not permit child to play in pile of leaves, snow, or large cardboard container in trafficked area.
	Supervise tricycle riding; have child wear helmet.
	Lock fences and doors if not directly supervising children.
	Teach child to obey pedestrian safety rules:
	• Obey traffic regulations; cross only at crosswalks and only when traffic signal indicates that it is safe.
	• Stand back a step from curb until it is time to cross.
	• Look left, right, and left again and check for turning cars before crossing street.
	• Use sidewalks; when there is no sidewalk, walk on left, facing traffic.
	• Wear light colors at night and attach fluorescent material to clothing.
Drowning	
Able to explore if left unsupervised	Supervise closely when near any source of water regardless of depth, including buckets.
Has great curiosity	Keep bathroom doors closed and lid down on toilet (or install latch).
Helpless in water; unaware of its danger—may consider "play" in any body of water same as in bath; depth of water has no significance	Have fence around swimming pool and lock gate.
	Teach swimming and water safety (however, this is not a substitute for safety).
	Supervise small children when swimming by "touch" (adult can reach out and touch child at all times).
Burns	
Able to reach heights by climbing, stretching, and standing on toes	Turn pot handles toward back of stove.
Pulls objects	Place electrical appliances such as coffee maker and toaster toward back of counter.
Explores any holes or opening	Place guardrails in front of radiators, fireplaces, or other heating elements.
Can open drawers and closets	Store matches and cigarette lighters in locked or inaccessible area; discard carefully.
Unaware of potential sources of heat or fire	Place burning candles, incense, hot foods, and cigarettes out of reach.
Plays with mechanical objects	Do not let tablecloth hang within child's reach.
	Do not let electric cord from iron, curling iron, or other appliance hang within child's reach.
	Cover electrical outlets with protective plastic caps.
	Keep electrical wires hidden or out of reach.
	Do not allow child to play with electrical appliance, wires, or lighters.
	Stress danger of open flames; teach what "hot" means.
	Always check bath-water temperature; adjust water heater temperature to 49° C (120° F) or lower; do not allow children to play with faucets.
	Apply sunscreen when child is exposed to sunlight (all year round).
Accidental Poisoning	
Explores by putting objects in mouth	Place all potentially toxic agents, including cosmetics, cleaning products, pesticides, and medications, out of reach or in locked cabinet.
Can open drawers, closets, boxes, and most containers	Caution against eating nonedible items such as plants.
Climbs	Replace medications or poisons immediately in locked cabinet; replace child-guard caps properly.
Cannot read labels	Administer medications as drug, not as candy.
Does not know safe dose or amount	Do not store surplus toxic agents.
	Promptly discard empty poison containers; never reuse to store food item or other poison.
	Teach child not to play in trash containers.
	Never remove labels from containers of toxic substances.
	Know number of nearest poison control center (800-222-1222).

Continued

TABLE 32.4   Injury Prevention During Early Childhood—cont'd

Developmental Abilities Related to Risk for Injury	Injury Prevention
Falls	
Able to open doors and some windows	Use window guards; do not rely on screens to stop falls.
Goes up and down stairs	Place gates at top and bottom of stairs.
Depth perception unrefined	Keep doors locked or use child-proof doorknob covers at entry to stairs, high porch, or other elevated area, including laundry chute.
	Remove unsecured or scatter rugs.
	Apply nonskid decals in bathtub or shower.
	Keep crib rails fully raised and mattress at lowest level.
	Place carpeting under crib and in bathroom.
	Keep large toys and bumper pads out of crib or play yard (child can use these as "stairs" to climb out); move child to youth bed when he or she is able to climb out of crib.
	Avoid using wheeled walkers, especially near stairs.
	Dress in safe clothing (soles that do not "catch" on floor, tied shoelaces, pant legs that do not touch floor).
	Keep child restrained in vehicles; never leave unattended in shopping cart.
	Supervise at playgrounds; select play areas with soft ground cover and safe equipment.
Choking and Suffocation	
Puts things in mouth	Avoid large, round chunks of meat such as whole hot dogs (slice lengthwise into short pieces).
May swallow hard or nonedible pieces of food	Avoid fruit with pits, fish with bones, hard candy, chewing gum, nuts, popcorn, grapes, and marshmallows.
	Choose large, sturdy toys without sharp edges or small removable parts.
	Discard old refrigerators, ovens, and other appliances after removing door.
	Install smoke and carbon monoxide alarms; change batteries every 6 months.
	Develop a fire escape plan for the entire family, and have drills.
	Select safe toy boxes or chests without heavy, hinged lids.
	Keep Venetian blind (or shade) cords out of child's reach.
	Remove drawstrings from clothing; shorten essential drawstrings to 15.24 cm (6 inches) or less.
Bodily Injury	
Still clumsy in many skills	Avoid giving sharp or pointed objects such as knives, scissors, or toothpicks, especially when walking or running.
Easily distracted from tasks	Do not allow lollipops or similar objects in mouth when walking or running.
Unaware of potential danger from strangers or other people	Teach safety precautions (e.g., to carry knife or scissors with pointed end away from face).
	Store all dangerous tools, garden equipment, and firearms in locked cabinet.
	Be alert to danger of supervised animals and household pets.
	Use safety glass and decals on large glassed areas such as sliding glass doors.
	Teach child name, address, and phone number and to ask for help from appropriate people (cashier, security guard, policeman) if lost; have identification on child (sewn in clothes, inside shoe).
	Teach stranger safety:
	• Avoid personalized clothing in public places.
	• Never go with a stranger.
	• Tell parents if anyone makes child feel uncomfortable in any way.
	Always listen to child's concerns regarding others' behavior.
	Teach child to say "no" when confronted with uncomfortable situations.

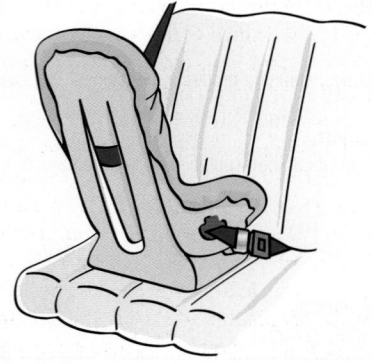

FIG 32.10 Rear-facing convertible car seat.

straps attached to a shield that is held in place by a crotch strap. With both the infant and toddler restraints, it is important not to add extra blankets, head cushions, or padding between the child and the restraint straps that did not come as original equipment because these "add-ons" create spaces of air between the child and the restraint and decrease support for the back, head, and neck. Cars with free-sliding latch plates on the lap or shoulder belt require the use of a metal locking clip to keep the belt in a tight-holding position. The locking clip is threaded onto the belt above the latch plate (Fig. 32.11, *A*). If parents have newer cars with automatic lap and shoulder belts, they need to have additional lap belts installed to properly secure the restraint. Booster seats are not restraint systems like the convertible devices because they depend on the vehicle belts to hold the child and booster seat in place. Three

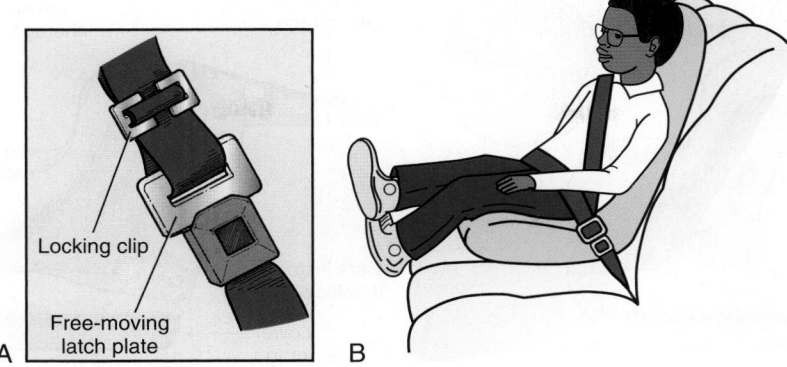

FIG 32.11 A, Locking clip used with free-sliding lap or shoulder belt to keep the belt in a tight-holding position. **B,** Automobile booster seat. Note placement of the shoulder strap (away from the neck and face).

booster models have been approved by the National Highway Traffic Safety Administration (2010): the high-back belt-positioning seat (see Fig. 32.11, *B*), which provides head and neck support for the child riding in a vehicle seat without a headrest; the no-back belt-positioning seat, which should be used only if the vehicle seat has a headrest; and a combination seat, which converts from a forward-facing toddler seat to a booster seat. This last model is equipped with a harness for use by toddlers; the harness may be removed, and a shoulder-lap belt used when the child outgrows the harness. The belt-positioning booster seats are used for children who are less than 145 cm (4 feet, 9 inches) tall and weigh 15.9 kg to 36.3 kg (35 to 80 pounds, depending on the type of booster seat). In general, school-age children should ride in a belt-positioning booster seat until approximately 7 to 8 years of age. However, note that, because children's sizes vary considerably, manufacturer recommendations should be followed regarding height and weight limitations. A booster seat should be used until the child is able to sit against the back of the seat with feet hanging down and legs bent at the knees. Children who outgrow the convertible restraint may still be able to ride safely in a booster seat until the midpoint of the head is higher than the vehicle seat back.

Children should use specially designed car restraints until they are 145 cm (4 feet, 9 inches) in height and 8 to 12 years of age (American Academy of Pediatrics, 2015). Shoulder-lap safety belts should be worn low on the hips, snug, and not on the abdominal area. Children should be taught to sit up straight to allow for proper fit. The shoulder belt is used only if it does not cross the child's neck or face.

Shoulder-only automatic belts are designed to protect adults. Children should use the manual shoulder belts in the rear seat. Air bags do not take the place of child safety seats or seat belts and can be lethal to young children. The safest area of the car for children is the back seat. Children who must ride in the passenger side of the front seat with an air bag should be positioned as far back as possible or have the air bag disabled.

For any restraint to be effective, it must be used consistently and properly. Examples of misuse include misrouting the vehicle seat belt through the restraint; failing to use the vehicle seat belt to secure the restraint; failing to use a tether strap; failing to use the restraint harness system; and incorrectly positioning the child, especially by facing infants forward instead of rearward. To address these issues, nurses must stress correct use of car restraints and rules that ensure compliance (see Family-Centered Care box: Using Car Safety Restraints). Children riding in car safety seats are generally much better behaved than children left unrestrained, which can be a major benefit to parents and should be emphasized as an additional advantage of restraints.

FAMILY-CENTERED CARE

Using Car Safety Restraints

- Read manufacturer directions, and follow them exactly.
- Anchor safety seat securely to automobile seat, and apply harness snugly to child.
- Do not start the car until everyone is properly restrained.
- *Always* use the restraint, even for short trips.
- If child begins to climb out or undo the harness, firmly say, "No." It may be necessary to stop the car to reinforce the expected behavior. Use rewards to encourage cooperative behavior.
- Encourage child to help attach buckles, straps, and shields, but always double-check fastenings.
- Decrease boredom on long trips. Keep soft toys in the car for quiet play; talk to child; point out objects, and teach child about them. Stop periodically. If child wishes to sleep, make certain that he or she stays in the restraint.
- Insist that others who transport children also follow these safety rules.

The LATCH (lower anchors and tethers for children) universal child safety seat system was implemented as a requirement starting in 2002 for all new automobiles and child safety seats. This system provides uniform anchorage consisting of two lower anchorages and one upper anchorage in the rear seat of the vehicle (Fig. 32.12). When used appropriately, the top anchor (tether) strap prevents the child from pitching forward in a crash. If the tether strap is not used, up to 90% of the protection of the restraint is lost. Instructions for proper installation of the tether strap and permanent bracket are included with the car restraint. New child safety seats have a hook, buckle, strap, or other connector that attaches to the anchorage. Concerns about the increased weight of children in the United States has led some to question the safety of the LATCH system with child restraints (car seats) and the child whose combined weight is more than 29.5 kg (65 lbs). The National Highway Traffic Safety Administration recently changed the rule about the use of the LATCH system; if the child's weight and that of the car seat weighs more than 65 lbs, then parents will be instructed to use the shoulder-lap belt restraint to restrain the child in the car.

Children with disabilities may require a restraint system that secures them appropriately in the event of a crash. Examples of such devices include car bed restraints for infants who cannot tolerate a semi-reclining position and specially adapted molded-plastic chairs for children who have spica casts. The E-Z-On vest is a special safety harness for larger children with poor trunk control. A HIPPO (Spica Cast) car seat is

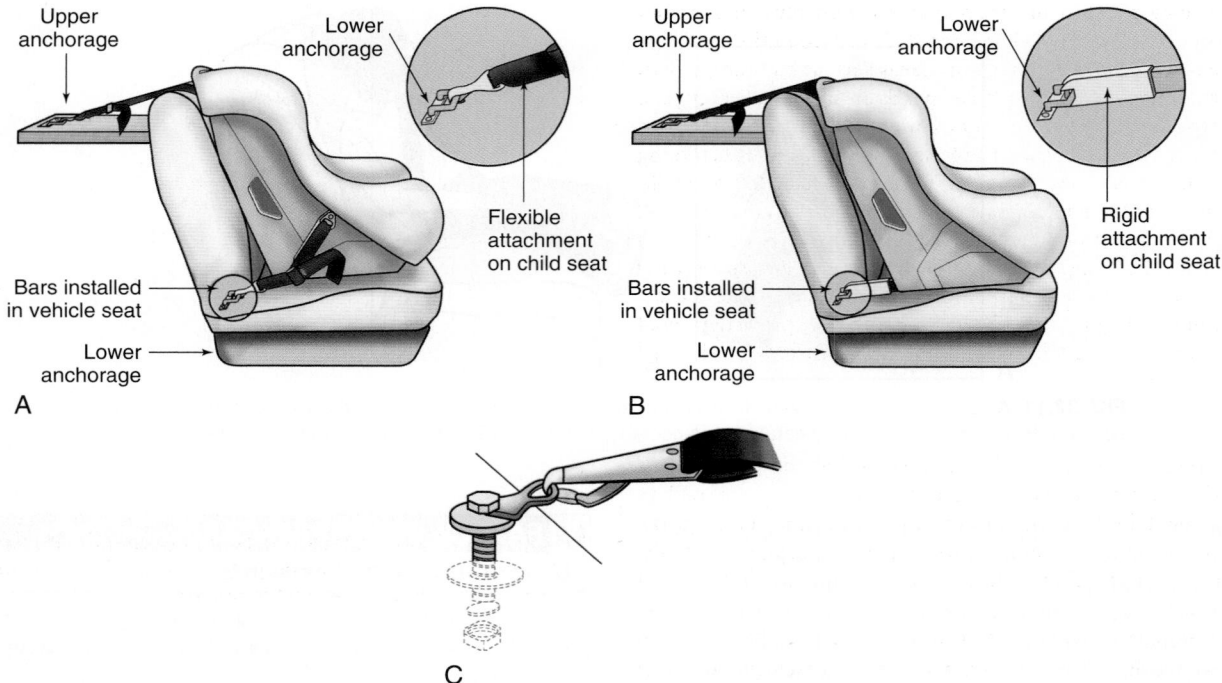

FIG 32.12 Lower anchors and tethers for children (LATCH). **A,** Flexible two-point attachment with top tether. **B,** Rigid two-point attachment with top tether. **C,** Top tether. (Courtesy of US Department of Transportation, National Highway Traffic Safety Administration.)

available for transporting children with spica casts; these are sold only in the United States. Additional safety restraints and a list of distributors are available at the SafetyBeltSafe U.S.A. website.* See also Chapter 25 for a discussion of preterm infants being discharged home and car-seat evaluation.

Children should not ride in the open back of a truck. The danger of falls can be compounded by another vehicle striking the child or by the truck rolling over. In addition, leaving children unsupervised in a parked vehicle provides an opportunity for a child to release the brake or put the car in gear.

Motor Vehicle–Related Injuries

Toddlers are often involved in pedestrian traffic injuries. Because of their gross motor skills of walking, running, and climbing and their fine motor skills of opening doors and fence gates, they are likely to be in hazardous areas when unsupervised. Unaware of danger and unable to approximate the speed of cars, they are hit by moving vehicles. Running after a ball, riding a tricycle, and playing behind a parked car are common activities that may result in a vehicular tragedy.

Toddlers playing in driveways or farmyards are at risk for back-over injury from vehicles in reverse gear. A precaution when children are playing in driveways is attaching a pole to the tricycle with a bright flag that is high enough to be visible through the back window of an automobile. Another safeguard is the use of a device that beeps when the vehicle is driven in reverse to alert children to the oncoming car, van, tractor, or truck. Many vehicles now come equipped with rearview motion cameras so the driver can see the driveway clearly while backing out. Physical barriers (fences or barricades) limiting children from playing near vehicles help prevent these injuries.

One type of injury that has become more commonplace occurs when children crawl into an open trunk and pull it closed. Asphyxia

may occur in such cases; therefore car trunks should not be left open when children are not being supervised. Some cars are equipped with a safety switch that can be activated from inside the trunk to open a closed trunk door.

Another automobile-related hazard for toddlers is overheating (hyperthermia) and subsequent death when left in a vehicle in hot weather (>27°C [80°F]). Small children dissipate heat poorly, and an increase in body temperature can cause death in a few hours. Since 1998, a total of 661 children died from hyperthermia when left alone in parked cars; in 2014, the total number of child deaths was 41, and it is estimated that an average of 37 children die each year from overheating in cars (Null, 2015). It is estimated that, with the ambient temperature at 22° to 35.5°C (72° to 96°F), the vehicle interior temperature rises by 10.5° to 11°C (19° to 20°F) for each 10 minutes, even with a window cracked (Duzinski, Barczyk, Wheeler, et al., 2014). Approximately 50% of adults who left a child in a car either forgot or were unaware that the child was still in the car (Duzinski et al., 2014). Parents are cautioned against leaving infants alone in a vehicle for any reason.

Preventing vehicular injuries involves protecting and educating children about the danger of moving and parked vehicles. Although preschool children are too young to be trusted to always obey, parents should emphasize looking for moving vehicles before crossing the street, recognizing the stop and go colors of traffic lights, and following traffic officers' signals. Physical barriers limiting children from playing near vehicles help prevent these injuries. Most important, what is preached must be practiced. Children learn through imitation, and consistency reinforces learning.

Drowning

The highest rate of drowning from 2000 to 2006 was in children 0 to 4 years of age; children 12 to 36 months of age were at highest risk for drowning during the same time period (Weiss & American Academy of Pediatrics, Committee on Injury, Violence, and Poison Prevention,

*www.carseat.org.

2010). Drowning deaths in infants occur most commonly in the bathtub and large buckets. With well-developed skills of locomotion, toddlers are able to reach potentially dangerous areas such as bathtubs, toilets, buckets, swimming pools, hot tubs, and ponds or lakes. Toddlers' intense drive for exploration and investigation combined with an unawareness of the danger of water and their helplessness in water makes drowning always a viable threat. It is also one category of injury that results in death within minutes, diminishing the chance for rescue and survival. Close adult supervision of children when near any source of water is essential; many drownings in this age-group occur when a supervising adult becomes distracted. Teaching swimming and water safety can be helpful but cannot be regarded as sufficient protection. Pool fencing, although critical, does not always deter fast-moving children (see Table 32.4).

Burns

Toddlers' ability to climb, stretch, and reach objects above their heads makes any hot surface a potential source of danger. Scalds from children pulling pots with hot liquids on top of themselves are a major source of burns. As a precaution, pot handles should be turned toward the back of the stove, and electric pots including cords should be placed out of reach.

Other sources of heat, such as radiators, fireplaces, accessible furnaces, kerosene heaters, and wood-burning stoves, should have guards placed in front of them. Portable electric heaters must be placed in a high area, well out of reach of climbing young children. Hair curling irons and hot curlers may also be reached easily and can burn the hands of curious toddlers.

Hot objects such as candles, incense, cigarettes, and irons must be placed away from children. The flame of a candle and the smoke of a cigarette invite investigation. Flame burns represent one of the most fatal types of burns and commonly occur when children play with matches and accidentally set themselves (and the home) on fire. To prevent flame burns, matches and lighters must be stored safely away from children, and parents need to teach children the dangers of playing with such objects. In addition, all homes, apartments, and any other type of dwelling where people sleep should have smoke detectors installed to alert the occupants of a fire. A safety plan for immediate escape is also essential.

Electrical burns represent an immediate danger to children. Young toddlers may explore outlets with conductive articles and wires by mouthing them. Because water is an excellent conductor, the chance for a severe circumoral electrical burn is great. Electrical outlets should have protective guards (or sliding guards) plugged into them when not in use (Fig. 32.13) or be made inaccessible by having furniture placed in front of them when feasible. Children should not be allowed to play with electrical cords, appliances, or batteries.

Scald burns are the most common type of thermal injury in children. A scalding burn is often caused by high-temperature tap water, with which children come in contact as a result of turning on the hot-water faucet, falling into a bathtub of hot water, pulling hot pots onto themselves, or suffering deliberate abuse. Limiting household water temperatures to less than 49°C (120°F) is highly recommended. At this temperature, it takes 10 minutes of exposure to the water to cause a full-thickness burn. Conversely, water temperatures of 54°C (130°F), the usual setting of most water heaters, expose household members to the risk for full-thickness burns within 30 seconds. Nurses can help prevent such burns by advising parents of this common household danger and recommending that they readjust their water heaters to a safe temperature.

Sunburns are a year-round concern in certain regions. Children spend a large amount of time outdoors, and their increased mobility

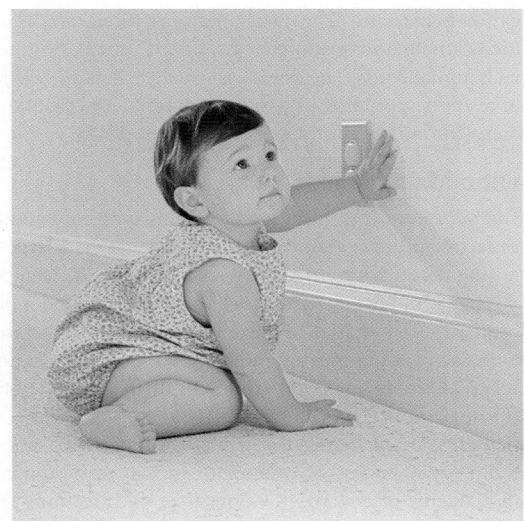

FIG 32.13 Special plastic caps in electrical sockets prevent young fingers from exploring dangerous areas. (Copyright 2011 by Photos.com, a division of Getty Images. All rights reserved.)

makes it difficult to prevent sun exposure. Sunburn can be prevented by applying a sunscreen with a sun protection factor (SPF) of 15 or greater, dressing in protective clothing (wide-brimmed hat, protective cotton clothing with a tight weave), and avoiding sun exposure between 10 AM and 2 PM.

SKIN DISORDERS RELATED TO ANIMAL CONTACTS

ARTHROPOD BITES AND STINGS

Arthropods include insects and arachnids, such as mites, ticks, spiders, and scorpions. Most arthropods in the United States, including tarantulas, are relatively harmless. Only scorpions and two spiders—the brown recluse and the black widow—inject venom deadly enough to require immediate attention. Children bitten by these arachnids must receive medical attention as soon as possible.

When a hymenopteran (bees in particular) stings, its barbed stinger penetrates the skin. As long as the stinger remains in the skin, the muscles push the stinger deeper, and the venom is pumped into the wound. The best approach is to remove the stinger as quickly as possible. Children who have become sensitized to hymenopteran bites may demonstrate a severe systemic response including urticaria, respiratory difficulty (from laryngeal edema), hypotension, and death. Intramuscular administration of epinephrine (i.e., Epi Pen) provides immediate relief.

ANIMAL BITES

Animal bites are common in childhood. The discussion is directed primarily toward dog bites, because most animal bites to children are caused by dogs. Small children are likely to be bitten or scratched on the head, face, and neck because they tend to put their heads near the animal's head and flail their arms rather than protecting their heads. Injuries vary in intensity from small puncture wounds to complete evulsion of tissue that is associated with significant crush injury.

Cat bites are less frequent, although cat scratches are common. Cat scratch disease usually follows the scratch or bite of an animal (a cat or kitten in 90% of cases) and is caused by *Bartonella henselae*, a gram-negative bacterium. The usual manifestations are a painless, nonpruritic erythematous papule at the site of inoculation, followed by regional lymphadenitis. The disease is usually a benign, self-limiting illness that resolves spontaneously in 4 to 6 weeks (American Academy of Pediatrics, Committee on Infectious Diseases, 2015).

Therapeutic Management

General wound care consists of rinsing the wound with copious amounts of saline or lactated Ringer's solution under pressure via a large syringe and of washing the surrounding skin with mild soap. A clean pressure dressing is applied, and the extremity is elevated if the wound is bleeding. Medical evaluation is advised because of the danger of tetanus and rabies. Prophylactic antibiotics are indicated for puncture wounds and wounds in areas where infection could result in cosmetic (face) or functional impairment (hand).

Treatment of cat scratch disease is primarily supportive. Some experts recommend a 5-day course of oral azithromycin to hasten recovery (American Academy of Pediatrics, Committee on Infectious Diseases, 2015). Antibiotics do not shorten the duration or prevent progression to suppuration but may be helpful in severe forms of the disease. Analgesics may be given for discomfort.

Care Management

The most important aspect related to animal bites is prevention. Children should understand animal behavior and develop respect for animals. Parents should monitor their children's behavior with pets and instruct them not to tease or surprise animals, invade their territory, interfere with their feeding or sleeping, or interact with sick or injured animals.

HUMAN BITES

Children often acquire lacerations from the teeth of other humans in rough play, during fights, or as victims of child abuse. Because human dental plaque and gingiva harbor pathogenic organisms, all human bites should receive immediate medical attention. Delayed treatment increases the risk for infection.

The wound is washed vigorously with soap and water, and a pressure dressing is applied to stop bleeding. Ice applications minimize discomfort and swelling. Tetanus toxoid is needed if the child is insufficiently immunized. Wounds larger than 6 mm should receive medical attention.

INGESTION OF INJURIOUS AGENTS

Since the passage of the Poison Prevention Packaging Act of 1970, which requires that certain potentially hazardous drugs and household products be sold in child-resistant containers, the incidence of poisonings in children has decreased dramatically. However, despite these advances poisoning remains a significant health concern, with most cases (49% in 2011) occurring in children younger than 6 years of age (Bronstein, Spyker, Cantilena, et al., 2012). Although pharmaceuticals such as analgesics, cough and cold preparations, topical preparations, antibiotics, vitamins, gastrointestinal preparations, hormones, and antihistamines are frequently the agents of poisonings, a variety of other substances can also poison children. The most frequently ingested poisons include the following (Bond, Woodward, & Ho, 2012; Bronstein et al., 2012):*

- Cosmetics and personal care products (deodorants, makeup, perfume, cologne, mouthwash)

*The most common substances in each category are in parentheses. Substances ingested are not necessarily the most toxic but often are readily available.

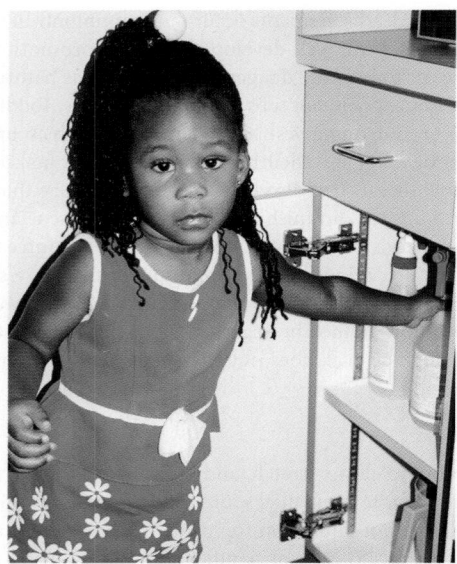

FIG 32.14 Children are most likely to ingest substances that are on their level such as cleaning agents stored under sinks, rat poison, plants, or diaper pail deodorants.

- Medications (acetaminophen, acetylsalicylic acid, ibuprofen, opioids)
- Household cleaning products (bleaches, laundry pods, disinfectants)
- Plants (nontoxic GI irritants, oxalates)
- Foreign bodies, toys, and miscellaneous substances (desiccants, thermometers, bubble-blowing solutions)

Disk or button battery ingestion has recently emerged as the primary cause of fatal ingestions in children younger than 5 years of age; lithium batteries are reported to cause the most harm (Centers for Disease Control and Prevention [CDC], 2012; Panella, Kirse, Pranikoff, et al., 2013; Sharpe, Rochette, & Smith, 2012). Acute tissue injury can occur within 2 hours of any battery ingestion resulting in serious harm, and emergent removal is recommended (Glenn, 2015).

Many poisonings reflect the ready accessibility of the products in the home, where more than 90% of poisonings occur (Bronstein et al., 2012). Improper storage is a common reason for poisoning (Fig. 32.14). The developmental characteristics of young children predispose them to poisoning by ingestion. Infants and toddlers explore their environment through oral experimentation. Because their sense of taste is not discriminating at this age, they ingest many unpalatable substances. In addition, toddlers and preschoolers are developing autonomy and initiative, which increase their curiosity and noncompliant behavior. Imitation is also a powerful motivator, especially when combined with a lack of awareness of danger.

This section is concerned primarily with the immediate emergency treatment of ingestion of injurious agents. Box 32.4 summarizes specific management of corrosive, hydrocarbon, acetaminophen, salicylate, iron, and plant poisoning. Because of the importance of lead poisoning among young children, ingestion of lead is discussed separately.

PRINCIPLES OF EMERGENCY TREATMENT

A poisoning may or may not require emergency intervention, but in every instance medical evaluation is necessary to initiate appropriate action. Advise parents to call the poison control center (PCC) *before* initiating any intervention. Parents should post the local PCC telephone number near each phone in the house (see Emergency Treatment box: Poisoning).

BOX 32.4 Selected Accidental Poisonings in Children

Corrosives (Strong Acids or Alkalis)
- Drain, toilet, or oven cleaners
- Electric dishwasher detergent (liquid, because of higher pH, is more hazardous than granular)
- Mildew remover
- Batteries
- Clinitest tablets
- Denture cleaners
- Bleach

Clinical Manifestations
- Severe burning pain in mouth, throat, and stomach
- White, swollen mucous membranes; edema of lips, tongue, and pharynx (respiratory obstruction)
- Coughing, hemoptysis
- Drooling and inability to clear secretions
- Signs of shock
- Anxiety and agitation

Comments
- Household bleach is a frequently ingested corrosive but rarely causes serious damage.
- Liquid corrosives cause more damage than granular/solid preparations. Liquids may also be aspirated, causing upper airway injury. Solid products tend to stick to and burn tissues, causing localized damage.

Treatment
- Inducing emesis is contraindicated (vomiting redamages the mucosa).
- Assess child's breathing and level of consciousness.
- Contact poison control center (800-222-1222) immediately. If the PCC or medical advice and treatment is not immediately available, it may be appropriate to dilute corrosive with water or milk (usually ≤120 mL [4 oz]).
- *Do not neutralize.* Neutralization can cause an exothermic reaction (which produces heat and causes increased symptoms or produces both a thermal and a chemical burn).
- Maintain patent airway as needed.
- Administer analgesics (under medical supervision).
- Esophageal stricture may require repeated dilations or surgery.

Hydrocarbons
- Gasoline
- Kerosene
- Lamp oil
- Mineral seal oil (found in furniture polish)
- Lighter fluid
- Turpentine
- Paint thinner and remover (some types)

Clinical Manifestations
- Gagging, choking, and coughing
- Burning throat and stomach
- Nausea
- Vomiting
- Alterations in sensorium, such as lethargy
- Weakness
- Respiratory symptoms of pulmonary involvement, such as tachypnea, cyanosis, retractions, and grunting

Comments
- Immediate danger is aspiration (even small amounts can cause bronchitis and chemical pneumonia).
- Gasoline, kerosene, lighter fluid, mineral seal oil, and turpentine cause severe pneumonia.

Treatment
- Contact poison control center (800-222-1222).
- Inducing emesis is generally contraindicated.
- Gastric decontamination and emptying are questionable, even when the hydrocarbon contains a heavy metal or pesticide; if gastric lavage must be performed, a cuffed endotracheal tube should be in place before lavage because of a high risk for aspiration.
- Symptomatic treatment of chemical pneumonia includes high humidity, oxygen, hydration, and antibiotics for secondary infection.

Acetaminophen
Clinical Manifestations
Occurs in four stages:
1. Initial period (0 to 24 hours after ingestion)
   - Nausea
   - Vomiting
   - Sweating
   - Pallor
2. Latent period (24 to 72 hours)
   - Patient improves
   - May have right upper quadrant abdominal pain
3. Hepatic involvement (72 to 96 hours)
   - Pain in right upper quadrant
   - Jaundice
   - Vomiting
   - Confusion
   - Stupor
   - Coagulation abnormalities
   - Sometimes renal failure, pancreatitis
4. Patients who do not die in hepatic stage gradually recover.

Comments
- It is the most common accidental drug poisoning in children.
- Toxicity occurs from acute ingestion. Toxic dose is 150 mg/kg or greater in children.

Treatment
- Antidote *N*-acetylcysteine (Mucomyst) is equally effective given intravenously or orally. When given orally, may first be diluted in fruit juice or soda because of the antidote's offensive odor. An antiemetic may be given if vomiting occurs.
- It is given as 1 loading dose followed by 17 additional doses in different dosages. Intravenous administration is given as a continuous infusion.

Aspirin (Acetylsalicylic Acid [ASA])
Clinical Manifestations
Acute poisoning (early symptoms)
- Nausea
- Hyperventilation
- Vomiting
- Tinnitus
- Diaphoresis

Continued

BOX 32.4 Selected Accidental Poisonings in Children—cont'd

Acute poisoning (later symptoms):
- Hyperactivity
- Fever
- Confusion
- Seizures
- Renal failure
- Respiratory failure

Chronic poisoning
- Same as above but subtle onset and nonspecific symptoms (often mistaken for viral illness)
- Bleeding tendencies

Comments
- It may be caused by acute ingestion (severe toxicity occurs with 300 to 500 mg/kg).
- It may be caused by chronic ingestion (i.e., more than 100 mg/kg/day for 2 or more days) and can be more serious than acute ingestion.
- Time to peak serum salicylate level can vary with enteric aspirin or the presence of concretions (bezoars).

Treatment
- Hospitalization is required for severe toxicity.
- Activated charcoal is given as soon as possible (unless contraindicated by altered mental status). If bowel sounds are present, may be repeated every 4 hours until charcoal appears in the stool.
- Lavage will not remove concretions of ASA.
- Sodium bicarbonate (intravenous) is used to correct metabolic acidosis, and urinary alkalinization may be effective in enhancing elimination; hypokalemia may interfere with achieving urinary alkalinization.
- Be aware of the risk for fluid overload and pulmonary edema.
- Use external cooling for hyperpyrexia.
- Administer anticonvulsants if seizures are present.
- Provide oxygen and ventilation for respiratory depression.
- Administer vitamin K for bleeding.
- In severe cases, hemodialysis (not peritoneal dialysis) is used.

Iron
- Mineral supplement or vitamin containing iron

Clinical Manifestations
Occurs in five stages (may have significant variation in symptoms and their progression):
1. Within 6 hours after ingestion (if child does not develop gastrointestinal symptoms in 6 hours, toxicity is unlikely)
   - Vomiting
   - Hematemesis
   - Diarrhea
   - Hematochezia (bloody stools)
   - Abdominal pain
   - Severe toxicity may have tachypnea, tachycardia, hypotension, coma
2. Latency (up to 24 hours)
   - Patient improves

3. Systemic toxicity (12 to 24 hours after ingestion)
   - Metabolic acidosis
   - Fever
   - Hyperglycemia
   - Bleeding
   - Seizures
   - Shock
   - Death (may occur)
4. Hepatic injury (2 to 5 days)
   - Jaundice
   - Liver failure
   - Coma
5. Rarely pyloric stenosis develops at 2 to 5 weeks

Comments
Factors related to frequency of iron poisoning:
- Widespread availability
- Packaging of large quantities in individual containers
- Lack of parental awareness of iron toxicity
- Resemblance of iron tablets to candy (e.g., M&M's)
- Toxic dose is based on the amount of elemental iron ingested. Common preparations include ferrous sulfate (20% elemental iron), ferrous gluconate (12%), and ferrous fumarate (33%). Ingestions of 20 to 60 mg/kg are considered mildly to moderately toxic, and >60 mg/kg is severely toxic and may be fatal.

Treatment
- Hospitalization is required when more than mild gastroenteritis is present.
- Use whole bowel irrigation if radiopaque tablets are visible on abdominal x-ray; may need to be given via nasogastric tube.
- Emesis empties the stomach more effectively than lavage.
- Chelation therapy with deferoxamine is used in severe intoxication (may turn urine a red to orange color).
- If intravenous deferoxamine is given too rapidly, hypotension, facial flushing, rash, urticaria, tachycardia, and shock may occur; stop the infusion, maintain the intravenous line with normal saline, and notify the practitioner immediately.

Plants
Clinical Manifestations
- Depends on type of plant ingested
- May cause local irritation of oropharynx and entire gastrointestinal tract
- May cause respiratory, renal, and central nervous system symptoms
- Topical contact with plants can cause dermatitis

Comments
- Plants are some of the most frequently ingested substances.
- Plant ingestions rarely cause serious problems, although some can be fatal.
- Plants can also cause choking and allergic reactions.

Treatment
- Wash from skin or eyes.
- Provide supportive care as needed.

Based on the initial telephone assessment, the PCC counsels the parents to begin treatment at home or to take the child to an emergency facility. When a call is taken, the name and telephone number of the caller are recorded to reestablish contact if the connection is interrupted. Because most poisonings are managed in the home, expert advice is essential to minimize adverse effects. When the exact quantity or type of ingested toxin is not known, admission to a health care facility with

pediatric emergency treatment services for laboratory evaluation and surveillance during the time after ingestion is critical.

Assessment

The first and most important principle in dealing with a poisoning is to treat the child first, not the poison. This requires an immediate concern for life support. Vital signs are taken, and respiratory or circulatory

✚ EMERGENCY TREATMENT

Poisoning

1. Assess the victim:
   - Initiate cardiorespiratory support if needed (circulation, airway, breathing).
   - Take vital signs; reevaluate routinely.
   - Evaluate for possibility of concomitant trauma or illness; treat prior to initiation of gastric decontamination.
2. Terminate exposure:
   - Empty mouth of pills, plant parts, or other material.
   - Flush any body surface (including the eyes) exposed to a toxin with large amounts of moderately warm water or saline.
   - Remove contaminated clothes, including socks, shoes, and jewelry. Ensure protection of rescuers and health care workers from exposure.
   - Bring victim of an inhalation poisoning into fresh air.
3. Identify the poison:
   - Question the victim and witnesses.
   - Look for environmental clues (empty container, nearby spill, odor on breath), and save all evidence of poison (container, vomitus, urine).
   - In absence of other evidence, be alert to signs and symptoms of potential poisoning in the absence of other evidence, including symptoms of ocular or dermal exposure.
   - Call the *poison control center* or other competent emergency facility for immediate advice regarding treatment.
4. Prevent poison absorption:
   - Place the child in a side-lying, sitting, or kneeling position with the head below the chest to prevent aspiration.

❗ NURSING ALERT

The national number for the poison control center is 800-222-1222; online at American Association of Poison Control Centers, www.aapcc.org.

support is instituted as needed. The child's condition is reevaluated routinely. Because shock is a complication of several types of household poisons, particularly corrosives, measures to reduce the effects of shock are important, beginning with the CABs (circulation, airway, and breathing). Establishing and maintaining vascular access for rapid intravascular volume expansion is vital in the treatment of pediatric shock.

The emergency department nurse's responsibility is to be prepared for immediate intervention with all of the necessary equipment. Because time and speed are critical factors in recovery from serious poisonings, anticipation of potential problems and complications may mean the difference between life and death.

Gastric Decontamination

Although pediatric poison ingestions are common, they rarely result in significant morbidity or mortality (Bronstein et al, 2012). Consider using *GI decontamination (GID)* only after careful evaluation of the potential toxicity of the poison and the risks versus benefits. GID, such as ipecac, activated charcoal, and gastric lavage, are not routinely recommended for most childhood poisonings. Because of continuing controversy regarding the use of these methods, treat each toxic ingestion individually (Albertson, Owen, Sutter, et al., 2011). Specific antidotes may be administered for certain poisonings.

Syrup of ipecac, an emetic that exerts its action through irritation of the gastric mucosa and by stimulation of the vomiting center, is no longer recommended for routine treatment of poison ingestion (Theurer & Bhavsar, 2013; Glenn, 2015).

❗ NURSING ALERT

Ipecac is not recommended for routine poison treatment intervention in the home (Theurer & Bhavsar, 2013; Glenn, 2015).

A commonly used method of GID is the use of *activated charcoal* (AC), an odorless, tasteless, fine black powder that adsorbs many compounds, creating a stable complex. AC is mixed with water or a saline cathartic to form slurry. Slurries are neither gritty nor distasteful but resemble black mud. To increase the child's acceptance of AC, the nurse should mix it with small amounts of chocolate milk, fruit syrup, or cola drinks and serve it through a straw in an opaque container with a cover (e.g., a disposable coffee cup and lid) or an ordinary cup covered with aluminum foil. For small children, an NG tube may be required to administer AC. However, recent data indicate that, except in cases of severe poisoning, the use of AC has not significantly improved clinical outcomes (Buckley, Dawson, Juurlink, et al., 2016). Best results are achieved when AC is administered within 30 to 60 minutes of a poison ingestion. Potential complications from the use of AC include aspiration (usually in patients with impaired gag reflexes), constipation, and intestinal obstruction (in multiple doses) (Albertson et al., 2011).

If the child is admitted to an emergency facility, gastric lavage may be performed to empty the stomach of the toxic agent; however, this procedure can be associated with serious complications (gastrointestinal perforation, hypoxia, aspiration). There is no conclusive evidence that gastric lavage decreases morbidity (Benson, Hoppu, Troutman, et al., 2013). In addition, gastric lavage may be of little benefit if used later than 1 hour after ingestion (Albertson et al., 2011). Conditions that may be appropriate for the use of gastric lavage include presentation within 1 hour of ingestion of a toxin, ingestion in a patient who has decreased gastrointestinal motility, ingestion of a toxic amount of sustained-release medication, and a large or life-threatening amount of poison (Albertson et al., 2011). When gastric lavage is used, the patient requires a protected airway, possible sedation, and the largest-diameter tube that can be inserted to facilitate passage of gastric contents.

In a minority of poisonings, specific antidotes are available to counteract the poison. They are highly effective and should be available in all emergency facilities. The supply of antidotes should be checked routinely and replaced as used or according to expiration dates. Antidotes available to treat toxin ingestion include *N*-acetylcysteine for acetaminophen poisoning, oxygen for carbon monoxide inhalation, naloxone for opioid overdose, flumazenil (Romazicon) for benzodiazepine (diazepam [Valium], midazolam [Versed]) overdose, digoxin immune Fab (Digibind) for digoxin toxicity, amyl nitrate for cyanide poisoning, and antivenin for certain poisonous bites.

Prevention of Recurrence

The ultimate objective is to prevent poisonings from occurring or recurring. Home safety education improves poison prevention practices (Glenn, 2015). Research supports the effectiveness of parent education on preventing unintentional injuries (Kendrick, Mulvaney, Ye, et al., 2013). One effective counseling method is first to discuss the difficulties of constantly watching and safeguarding young children (see Family-Centered Care box: Accidental Poisoning). In this way, the challenging task of raising children can lead to a discussion of injury prevention as part of the parental role. This approach also incorporates contributory causes for the incident such as inadequate support systems; marital discord; discipline techniques (especially use of physical punishment); and any disruption in the family or family activities such as vacations, moves, visitors, illnesses, or births. A visit to the home, especially after repeat poisonings, is recommended as part of the follow-up care to assess hazards, including family factors, and to evaluate appropriate

FAMILY-CENTERED CARE
Accidental Poisoning

An accidental poisoning is more than a physical emergency for the child; it usually represents an emotional crisis for the parents, particularly in terms of guilt, self-reproach, and insecurity in the parenting role. The emergency department is no place to admonish the family for negligence, lack of appropriate supervision, or failure to injury-proof the home. Rather it is a time to calm and support the child and parents while unaccusingly exploring the circumstances of the injury. If the nurse prematurely attempts to discuss ways of preventing such an incident from recurring, the parents' anxiety will block out any suggestions or offered guidance. Therefore it is preferable for the nurse to delay the discussion until the child's condition is stabilized or, if the child is discharged immediately after emergency treatment, to make a public health referral or send a packet of information.

GUIDELINES
Poison Prevention

- Assess possible contributing factors in occurrence of injury such as discipline, parent-child relationship, developmental ability, environmental factors, and behavior problems.
- Institute anticipatory guidance for possible future injuries based on child's age and developmental level.
- Provide assistance with environmental manipulation such as lead removal when necessary.
- Educate parents regarding safe storage of toxic substances.
- Advise parents to take drugs out of sight of children.
- Teach children the hazards of ingesting nonfood items.
- Advise parents against using plants for teas or medicine.
- Discuss problems of discipline and children's noncompliance, and offer strategies for effective discipline.
- Instruct parents regarding correct administration of drugs for therapeutic purposes and discontinuation of drug if there is evidence of mild toxicity.
- Advise parents to contact the poison control center or practitioner immediately when a poisoning occurs.
- Post the regional poison control center (800-222-1222) number with the emergency phone list by the telephone, or program the number in your cell phone.
- Include by the telephone the home address with nearest cross street in case an ambulance is needed. (In an emergency, family members may not remember the house address, and baby-sitters may not be aware of the information.)

injury-proofing measures. One method of identifying risk areas is to ask specific questions or have the parent complete a questionnaire designed to isolate factors that predispose children to poisoning. Another approach is to encourage parents to bend down to the child's eye level and survey the home environment for potential hazards. Have the parents try to open cabinets and reach shelves to access poisons.

Passive measures (those that do not require active participation) have been the most successful in preventing poisoning and include using child-resistant closures and limiting the number of tablets in one container. However, these measures alone are not sufficient to prevent poisoning because most toxic agents in the home do not have safety closures. Therefore active measures (those that require participation) are essential. See Guidelines box: Poison Prevention for guidelines on preventing the occurrence or recurrence of a poisoning.

HEAVY METAL POISONING

Heavy metal poisoning can occur from the ingestion of a variety of substances, the most common being lead. Other sources that are important in terms of children are iron and mercury. Mercury toxicity, a rare form of heavy metal poisoning, has occurred in children from a variety of sources such as predator fish (king mackerel, shark, swordfish, tile fish), broken thermometers or thermostats, broken fluorescent light bulbs, disk batteries, topical medications, gas regulators, cathartics, and interior latex house paint (Bose-O'Reilly, McCarthy, Steckling, et al., 2010). Elemental mercury (also called *metallic mercury* or *quicksilver*) is nontoxic if ingested and if the gastrointestinal tract is healthy (e.g., has no fistulas). However, mercury is volatile at room temperature and enters the bloodstream after it is inhaled, causing toxicity (tremors, memory loss, insomnia, gingivitis, diarrhea, anorexia, weight loss). The classic form of mercury poisoning is called *acrodynia* (or "painful extremities").

! NURSING ALERT

Mercury thermometers are no longer recommended because if they are broken the inhaled vapors can cause toxicity. To prevent inhalation, clean up spilled mercury quickly, using disposable towels and rubber gloves and washing the hands well afterward.

Heavy metals have an affinity for certain essential tissue chemicals, which must remain free for adequate cell functioning. When metals are bound to these substances, cellular enzyme systems are inactivated. Treatment involves *chelation,* use of a chemical compound that combines with the metal for rapid and safe excretion.

LEAD POISONING

Poisoning from lead has been a problem throughout history and throughout the world. In the United States the problem became apparent in the early 1900s when white lead was added to paints and tetraethyl lead was added to gasoline as an antiknock compound. Lead content in paint was decreased in 1950, and in 1978 the use of lead in household paint was banned. The use of lead in paint and leaded gasoline has been banned in the United States. After this change in policy, the average blood lead level (BLL) in the United States for people 1 to 74 years of age dropped from 12.8 mcg/dL in 1980 to 1.3 mcg/dL in 2010 (CDC, 2013). However, children continue to be exposed to lead; an estimated 0.8% of US children 1 to 5 years of age had BLLs of more than 10 mcg/dL in 2010, and more than 5% had BLLs of 5 mcg/dL (CDC, 2013).

Causes of Lead Poisoning

Although there are numerous sources of lead (Box 32.5), in most instances of acute childhood lead poisoning the source is nonintact lead-based paint in an older home or lead-contaminated bare soil in the yard. Microparticles of lead gain entrance into a child's body through ingestion or inhalation and, in the case of an exposed pregnant woman, by placental transfer. When measured, a mother's lead level is nearly the same as that of her unborn child. Although the level of lead may not be harmful to adult women, it can be harmful to fetuses.

Inhalation exposure usually occurs during renovation and remodeling activities in the home, but ingestion happens during normal day-to-day play and mouthing activities. Sometimes a child actually swallows loose chips of lead-based paint because it has a sweet taste. Water and food may also be contaminated with lead. A child does not need to eat loose paint chips to be exposed to the toxin; normal hand-to-mouth behavior,

BOX 32.5   Sources of Lead*

Lead-based paint in deteriorating condition
Lead solder
Lead crystal
Battery casings
Lead fishing sinkers
Lead curtain weights
Lead bullets
The following may contain lead:
- Ceramic ware
- Water
- Pottery
- Pewter
- Dyes
- Industrial factories
- Vinyl miniblinds
- Playground equipment
- Collectible toys
- Artists' paints
- Pool cue chalk
- Some imported toys or children's metal jewelry

Occupations and hobbies involving lead:
- Battery and aircraft manufacturing
- Lead smelting
- Brass foundry work
- Radiator repair
- Construction work
- Furniture refinishing
- Bridge repair work
- Painting contracting
- Mining
- Ceramics work
- Stained-glass making
- Jewelry making

*The US Consumer Product Safety Commission issues alerts and recalls for products that contain lead and that may unexpectedly pose a hazard to young children.

CULTURAL CONSIDERATIONS

Sources of Lead

In some cultures, the use of traditional ethnic remedies that contain lead may increase children's risk for lead poisoning. These remedies include the following:

Azarcon (Mexico): For digestive problems; a bright orange powder; often mixed with oil, milk, or sugar or sometimes given as a tea; sometimes a pinch is added to a baby bottle or tortilla dough for preventive purposes

Greta (Mexico): Yellow-orange powder used in the same way as azarcon

Paylooah (Southeast Asia): Used for rash or fever; an orange-red powder given straight or in a tea

Surma (India and Pakistan): Black powder used as a cosmetic and as teething powder

Unknown ayurvedic (Tibet): Small, gray-brown balls used to improve slow development; two balls are given orally 3 times per day

Tamarindo jellied fruit candy (Mexico): Fruit candy packaged in paper wrappers that contain high lead levels

Lozeena (Iraq): Bright orange powder used to color meat and rice

Litargirio (Dominican Republic): Yellow- or peach-colored powder used as a folk remedy and as an antiperspirant/deodorant

Ba-Baw-San (China): Herbal medicine used to treat colic pain

Adapted from Centers for Disease Control and Prevention. (1993). Lead poisoning associated with use of traditional ethnic remedies—California, 1991-1992. *Morbidity and Mortality Weekly Report, 42*(27), 521–524; Centers for Disease Control and Prevention. (1998). Lead poisoning associated with imported candy and powdered food coloring—California and Michigan. *Morbidity and Mortality Weekly Report, 47*(48), 1041–1043; Centers for Disease Control and Prevention. (2002). Childhood lead poisoning associated with tamarind candy and folk remedies—California, 1992-2000. *Morbidity and Mortality Weekly Report, 51*(31), 684–686; Centers for Disease Control and Prevention. (2005). Lead poisoning associated with use of litargirio—Rhode Island. *Morbidity and Mortality Weekly Report, 59*(9), 227–229.

coupled with the presence of lead dust in the environment that has settled over decades, is the usual method of poisoning (Campbell, Gracely, Tran, et al., 2012).

Because of family, cultural, or ethnic traditions, a source of lead may be a routine part of life for a child. Nurses must educate themselves about the practices of their patients and identify when such products may be a source of lead. The use of pottery or dishes containing lead may be an issue, as may be the use of folk remedies for stomachaches or the use of some cosmetics (see Cultural Considerations box: Sources of Lead). Children of immigrants and internationally adopted children may have been exposed to sources of lead before arrival in the United States and should also be carefully evaluated for lead exposure (Raymond, Kennedy, & Brown, 2013). Other risk factors for having an elevated BLL include living in poverty, being younger than 6 years of age, dwelling in urban areas, and living in older rental homes where lead decontamination may not be a priority. Nurses are often in a position to observe or elicit information about these practices and educate families about their potential harm.

Pathophysiology and Clinical Manifestations

Lead can affect any part of the body, including the renal, hematologic, and neurologic systems (Fig. 32.15). Of most concern for young children

is the developing brain and nervous system, which are more vulnerable than those of older children and adults. Lead in the body moves via an equilibration process between the blood, the soft tissues and organs, and the bones and teeth. It ultimately settles in the bones and teeth, where it remains inert and in storage. This makes up the largest portion of the body burden, approximately 75% to 90%. At the cellular level, it competes with molecules of calcium, interfering with the regulating action of calcium. In the brain, lead disrupts the biochemical processes and may have a direct effect on the release of neurotransmitters, may cause alterations in the blood-brain barrier, and may interfere with the regulation of synaptic activity (Cunningham, 2012).

There is a relationship between anemia and lead poisoning. Children who are iron deficient absorb lead more readily than those with sufficient iron stores. Lead can interfere with the binding of iron onto the heme molecule. This sometimes creates a picture of anemia even though the child is not iron deficient. Lead toxicity to the erythrocytes leads to the release of the enzyme erythrocyte protoporphyrin (EP). Because EP is not sensitive to BLLs of less than approximately 16 to 25 mcg/dL, it is no longer used as a screening test. Therefore the BLL test is currently used for screening and diagnosis. However, elevation of the EP level (>35 mcg/dL of whole blood) is a good indicator of toxicity from lead and reflects the length of exposure and body burden of lead in an individual child.

Although adults have been shown to experience adverse renal effects from occupational lead exposure, few studies document renal effects in children except at extremely high lead levels. One can hypothesize that lead can affect the renal integrity of both children and adults.

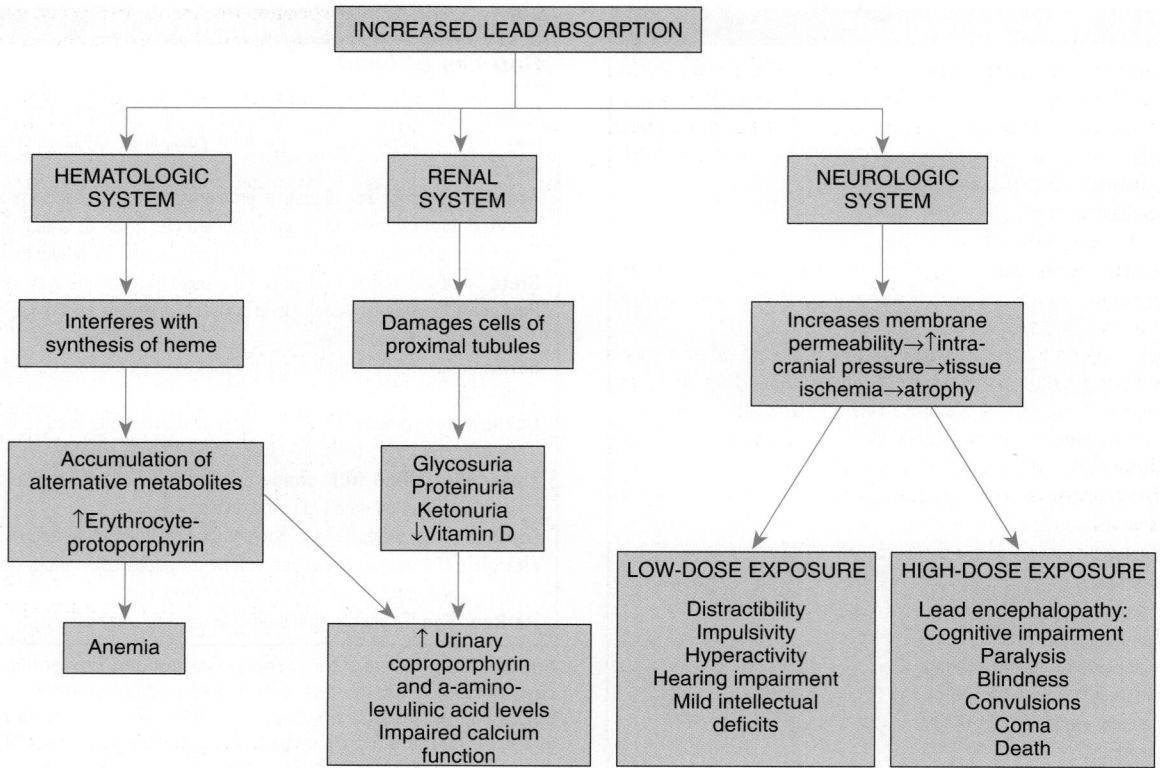

FIG 32.15 Main effects of lead on body systems.

Therefore the renal system of a child is still considered a potential target for the harmful effects of lead.

The lead levels identified in children have declined since the initiation of screening for children at risk for lead poisoning. With earlier intervention, the most prevalent effects have changed. Since the late 1960s, children have rarely died of lead poisoning, and seizures or cognitive impairment have become less likely. However, even mild and moderate lead poisoning can cause a number of cognitive and behavioral problems in young children, including aggression, hyperactivity, impulsivity, delinquency, disinterest, and withdrawal. Long-term neurocognitive signs of lead poisoning include developmental delays, lowered intelligence quotient (IQ), reading skill deficits, visual-spatial problems, visual-motor problems, learning disabilities, and lower academic success. Chronic lead toxicity may also affect physical growth and reproductive efficiency.

Diagnostic Evaluation

Children with lead poisoning rarely have symptoms, even at levels requiring chelation therapy. A diagnosis of lead poisoning is based only on the lead testing of a venous blood specimen from a venipuncture. The collection process is important. Blood must be collected carefully to avoid contamination by lead on the skin.

Anticipatory Guidance

The most effective prevention of lead exposure is ensuring that environmental exposures are reduced before children are exposed. The CDC (2012) recommends that the following information be made available to families beginning during prenatal and postnatal care:
- Hazards of lead-based paint in older housing
- Ways to control lead hazards safely
- How to choose safe toys
- Hazards accompanying repainting and renovating homes built before 1978

- Other exposure sources, such as traditional remedies, that might be relevant for a family

There has been recent concern regarding toys and other imported items with which children play that were found to contain lead. Parents should carefully evaluate the source of the toy (manufacturer) or item with which the child may play and not assume that it is safe because it is sold in a US market. The US Consumer Product Safety Commission (www.cpsc.gov) is an excellent resource for parents and caregivers concerned about the safety of a given toy or product that may be harmful.

Screening for Lead Poisoning

When primary prevention fails, secondary prevention screening efforts for elevated BLLs can identify children much earlier than in the past. This need is established using blood lead surveillance and other risk factor data collected over time to establish the status and risk of children throughout the state. Universal screening should be done at 1 and 2 years of age. Any child between 3 and 6 years of age who has not been previously screened should also be tested. All children with risk factors should be screened more often.

Targeted screening is acceptable when an area has been determined by existing data to have less risk. Children should be screened when they live in a high-risk geographic area or are members of a group determined to be at risk (e.g., Medicaid recipients) or if their family cannot answer "no" to the following personal risk questions:
- Does your child live in or regularly visit a house that was built before 1950?
- Does your child live in or regularly visit a house built before 1978 with recent or ongoing renovations or remodeling within the past 6 months?
- Does your child have a sibling or playmate who has or had lead poisoning?

Therapeutic Management

The degree of concern, urgency, and need for medical intervention change as the lead level increases. Education is one of the most important elements of the treatment process. Several areas that the nurse needs to discuss with the family of every child who has an elevated BLL (≥5 mcg/dL) include the following (CDC, 2012):

- The child's BLL and what it means
- Potential adverse health effects of an elevated BLL
- Sources of lead exposure and suggestions on how to reduce exposure such as the importance of wet cleaning to remove lead dust on floors, windowsills, and other surfaces
- Importance of good nutrition in reducing the absorption and effects of lead; for people with poor nutritional patterns, adequate intake of calcium and iron and importance of regular meals
- Need for follow-up testing to monitor the child's BLL
- Results of an environmental investigation if applicable
- Hazards of improper removal of lead paint (dry sanding, scraping, or open-flame burning)

Treatment actions vary, depending on the child's BLL. Based on a diagnosis from a venous BLL test, the CDC Advisory Committee on Childhood Lead Poisoning Prevention (2013) recommends that a BLL of 45 mcg/dL entails consideration of chelation therapy. Additional guidelines are expected to appear in publication in relation to the new recommendation that children 1 to 5 years of age with BLLs of 5 mcg/dL or more receive education and guidance for decreasing BLLs.

Chelation Therapy

Chelation is the term used for removing lead from circulating blood and theoretically some lead from organs and tissues. It is unclear whether chelation affects lead stores in bones. Although not an antidote in the truest sense, it does serve a similar purpose in that the toxic substance or poison is removed from the body. However, chelation does not counteract any effects of the lead.

Historically, three chelating agents have been used consistently: calcium disodium edetate (CaNa2EDTA, or calcium EDTA), British antilewisite (BAL, dimercaprol, dimercaptopropanol), and Meso-2,3-dimercaptosuccinic acid (DMSA, Chemet, Succimer). British antilewisite is used in conjunction with EDTA. All of the agents have potential toxic side effects and contraindications. Renal, hepatic, and hematologic parameters should be monitored.

Because of the equilibration process between blood, soft tissues, and other sites in the body, there is often a rebound of the BLL after chelation. After the body burden of lead is reduced enough to stabilize the BLL, rebound ceases. Multiple chelation treatments may be necessary. Adequate hydration is essential during therapy because the chelates are excreted via the kidneys.

Severe lead toxicity (lead level ≥70 mcg/dL) requires immediate inpatient treatment, whether symptoms are present or not. BAL is contraindicated in children with peanut allergies or hepatic insufficiency, nor should it be given in conjunction with iron. Also, use with caution in children with renal impairment or hypertension; monitor for hemolysis with presence of glucose 6-phosphate dehydrogenase deficiency. It must be given only at a deep intramuscular site, in repeated doses over several days. Calcium EDTA should be given intravenously or intramuscularly (in a different site from BAL). The intravenous route should not be used in children with cerebral edema.

For lead levels of 45 to 69 mcg/dL and an absence of symptoms, DMSA can be used. The capsule is opened and sprinkled on a small amount of food or may be swallowed whole. DMSA can be used in conjunction with iron. Adverse effects include nausea, vomiting, diarrhea, loss of appetite, rash, elevated liver function tests, and neutropenia. Because the chelates are excreted via the kidneys, adequate hydration is essential.

A less used oral chelating agent, d-penicillamine, is sometimes used to treat lead poisoning, but the medication is not approved by the Food and Drug Administration for use in the United States (Dapul & Laraque, 2014).

Prognosis

Although most of the pathophysiologic effects of lead are reversible, the most serious consequences of both high and low lead exposure are the effects on the CNS. In children with lead encephalopathy, permanent brain damage can result in cognitive impairment, behavior changes, possible paralysis, and seizures. However, low-dose exposure may also cause permanent neurologic deficits. Increased distractibility, short attention span, impulsivity, reading disabilities, and school failure have been associated with lead exposure (CDC, 2012).

Care Management

The primary nursing goal in lead poisoning is to prevent the child's initial or further exposure to lead. For children with low-level exposure, this requires identifying the sources of lead in the environment. Careful history taking is the most useful and most valuable tool and should concentrate on the personal risk questions. Suggestions for reducing lead in the child's environment are listed in the Community Focus box: Reducing Blood Lead Levels.

COMMUNITY FOCUS
Reducing Blood Lead Levels

- Make sure that child does not have access to peeling paint or chewable surfaces painted with lead-based paint, especially window sills and wells.
- If a house was built before 1978 and has hard-surface floors, wet mop them at least once per week. Wipe other hard surfaces (e.g., window sills, baseboards). If there are loose paint chips in an area, such as a window well, use a wet disposable cloth to pick up and discard them. Do not vacuum hard-surfaced floors or windowsills or wells because this spreads dust. Use vacuum cleaners with agitators to remove dust from rugs rather than vacuum cleaners with suction only. If a rug is known to contain lead dust and cannot be washed, it should be discarded.
- Wash and dry child's hands and face frequently, especially before eating.
- Wash toys and pacifiers frequently.

- Wipe your feet on mats before entering the home, especially if you work in occupations where lead is used. Removing your shoes when you are entering the home is a good practice to control lead.
- If soil around home is or is likely to be contaminated with lead (e.g., if home was built before 1978 or is near a major highway), plant grass or other ground cover; plant bushes around outside of house so child cannot play there.
- During remodeling of older homes, follow correct procedures. Be certain children and pregnant women are not in the home, day or night, until process is completed. After deleading, thoroughly clean house using cleaning solution to damp mop and dust before inhabitants return.
- In areas where the lead content of water exceeds the drinking water standard and a particular faucet has not been used for 6 hours or more, "flush" the

Continued

🏠 COMMUNITY FOCUS—cont'd

Reducing Blood Lead Levels

cold-water pipes by running the water until it becomes as cold as it will get (30 seconds to 2 minutes). The more time water has been sitting in pipes, the more lead it may contain.

- *Use only cold water* for consumption (drinking, cooking, and especially for reconstituting powder infant formula).
- Hot water dissolves lead more quickly than cold water and thus contains higher levels of lead. First-flush water may be used for nonconsumption uses (e.g., bathing).
- Have water tested by a competent laboratory. This action is especially important for apartment dwellers; flushing may not be effective in high-rise buildings or other buildings with lead-soldered central piping.
- Do not store food in open cans, particularly if cans are imported.
- Do not use pottery or ceramic ware that was inadequately fired or is meant for decorative use for food storage or service. Do not store drinks or food in lead crystal.

- Avoid folk remedies or cosmetics that contain lead.
- Avoid candy imported from Mexico (e.g., tamarind hard candy).
- Avoid imported toys and toy jewelry that may contain lead.
- Make sure that home exposure is not occurring from parental occupations or hobbies. Household members employed in occupations such as lead smelting should shower and change into clean clothing before leaving work. Construction and lead abatement workers may also bring home lead contaminants.
- Make sure that child eats regular meals because more lead is absorbed on an empty stomach.
- Make sure that child's diet contains sufficient iron and calcium and not excessive fat.
- Consider iron supplementation if the child does not regularly consume foods rich in iron.

The nurse prepares children who undergo chelation therapy for the injections and makes all efforts to reduce injection pain. Chelating agents are administered deeply into a large muscle mass. To lessen the pain from calcium EDTA, the local anesthetic procaine is injected with the drug. Rotation of sites is essential to prevent the formation of painful areas of fibrotic tissue. Because calcium EDTA and lead are toxic to the kidneys, keep records of fluid intake and output and assess the results of urinalysis to monitor renal functioning.

❗ NURSING ALERT

Use extreme caution with chelating agents. Incidences of child death from hypocalcemia have been recorded when Na2EDTA was substituted for CaNa2EDTA and used as a chelating agent (Fountain & Reith, 2014).

❗ NURSING ALERT

Calcium EDTA is only administered when there is adequate urinary output. Children receiving the drug intramuscularly must be able to maintain adequate oral intake of fluids.

Discharge planning for children with lead poisoning must include thorough education of families regarding safety from lead hazards, clear instructions regarding medication administration and follow-up, and confirmation that the child will be discharged to a home without lead hazards. Although the nurse must use caution to avoid alarming parents unnecessarily, it is important that they know the risk implications for their child's behavior and cognitive functions. Nurses should observe the development and behavior of children who are hospitalized. Thoroughly evaluate any concerns that are identified. Referral to a child development or speech and language specialist may be necessary.

As in any situational crisis, parents need support and understanding if their child is treated for lead poisoning. Many families at the highest risk for lead poisoning have the fewest resources to comply with measures such as relocation or removal of lead from the environment where the child experiences exposure.

▮ SAFETY PROMOTION AND INJURY PREVENTION

ASPIRATION AND SUFFOCATION

Suffocation death rates among infants younger than 1 year of age have dramatically increased in the last decade (Gilchrist et al., 2012).

Suffocation deaths usually occur in this age-group by wedging between a wall and mattress or crib side or collapse of a play yard wall (Theurer & Bhavsar, 2013).

Usually by 1 year of age children chew well, but they may have difficulty with large pieces of food (e.g., meat and whole hot dogs) and hard foods (e.g., nuts). Young children cannot discard pits from fruit or bones from fish. It takes practice to learn how to chew gum without swallowing it. Gel snacks that are sealed in plastic wrappers can also be difficult to manage, and the plastic wrapper can be aspirated. Therefore parents must implement the same precautions as discussed for infants regarding food selection (see Chapter 31).

Play objects for toddlers must still be chosen with an awareness of danger from small parts. Large, sturdy toys without sharp edges or removable parts are safest. Balloons, coins, paper clips, pins, bells, button batteries, pull-tabs on cans, thumbtacks, nails, screws, jewelry (especially pierced earrings), and all types of pins are common household objects that can cause significant harm if swallowed or aspirated. Because of the danger of aspiration, parents should be taught emergency procedures for choking.

Suffocation from causes seen during infancy is less frequent; but old refrigerators, ovens, and other large appliances are an ever-present threat. Toddlers can climb inside these appliances and, if they close the door behind them, can be trapped. Removing all doors before discarding or storing old appliances prevents such tragic deaths. Toddlers may also suffocate when unsafe toy box lids accidentally close on their heads or necks. Advise parents of this danger, and encourage them to buy storage chests with lightweight, removable covers.

FALLS

Falls are still a hazard to children in this age-group, although by the later part of early childhood gross and fine motor skills are well developed, decreasing the incidence of falls down stairs and from chairs. However, playground injuries are common. Children need to be taught safety at play areas such as no horseplay on high slides or jungle gyms, *sitting* on swings, and staying away from moving swings. Passive prevention includes placement of grass, sand, or wood chips under play equipment. Swing seats should be made of plastic, canvas, or rubber and have smooth or rounded edges. Slides should have inclines of no more than 30 degrees, and evenly spaced rungs for climbing.

The climbing and running of the typical toddler are complicated by the child's total disregard and lack of appreciation for danger, immature coordination, and a high center of gravity. Gates must be placed at both ends of stairs. Accessible windows must have window guards, not screens, to prevent falls to the ground below. Falling from furniture is a major cause of injury, with more children in this age-group sustaining head injuries than older children. Doors leading to stairwells or porches must be locked. A convenient type of lock is a sliding bar or hook that can be attached to the door and frame at a level higher than the child can reach; such locks also have safety clasps or devices that prevent children from being able to open them. Cribs and vehicles are other sources of falls. To avoid injury, crib rails should be fully raised, the mattress should be kept at the lowest position, and toys or bumper pads that may be used as steps to climb out should be removed. Ideally the floor under the crib should be carpeted or have a throw rug. Cribs, bassinets, and play yards are associated with a large number of accidental falls (66% of all fall injuries to children) (Yeh, Rochette, McKenzie, et al., 2011). The manufacture and sale of drop-side cribs has been banned by the Consumer Product Safety Commission (2010). When children reach a height of 89 cm (35 inches), they should sleep in a bed rather than a crib. If a bunk bed is selected, parents should be aware of possible dangers, including falls from the top bed and the ladder and head entrapment between the mattress and guardrail or between the supporting mattress slats.

Children can fall from high chairs, shopping carts, car seats, and strollers if not properly restrained or if balance changes by placing heavy objects. Therefore proper restraint and adequate supervision are essential. Children, especially older infants who are mobile, should not be placed in an infant seat on top of a shopping cart because the infant seat may fall off the cart; the safest place for an infant seat is inside the bed of the cart.

BODILY INJURY

Toddlers are still clumsy in many of their skills and can seriously harm themselves when walking while holding a sharp or pointed object or having food or objects, such as spoons, in their mouths. Preventing such occurrences is the best approach with toddlers. The child should be taught that, when walking with a pointed object such as a knife or scissors, the pointed end is held away from the face. Dangerous garden or workshop equipment and all firearms should be stored in locked cabinets. Power lawn mowers and weed eaters are especially dangerous because they can throw rocks and other solid items (projectiles), and young children should not be allowed in an area where such tools are in use; nor should they be taken for a ride on a mower or allowed to operate the device.

Safety education should include respect for firearms and their appropriate use, including nonpowder guns such as air guns, rifles (BB and pellet), and paintball guns, which can cause serious penetrating injuries. Firearm safety devices, such as trigger locks, gun safes, and personalized locks should be used to prevent unintentional firing of guns and subsequent injuries or fatalities. In addition, the child should be warned of and protected against potential danger from animals (see the "Animal Bites" section earlier in this chapter).

An additional safeguard for young children is the use of safety glass in doors, windows, and tabletops and the application of decals on glass doors and windows to reduce the likelihood of running through glass. In addition, children should not be allowed to run, jump, wrestle, or play ball near glass structures.

ANTICIPATORY GUIDANCE—CARE OF FAMILIES

Understanding toddlers is fundamental to successful child rearing. Nurses, particularly those in ambulatory or child health centers, are in a favorable position to help parents facilitate the tasks and meet the needs of children in this age-group. Prevention yields better results than treatment. Anticipatory guidance is paramount if one wishes to prevent future problems (see Family-Centered Care box: Guidance During Toddler Years).

FAMILY-CENTERED CARE
Guidance During Toddler Years

12 to 18 Months of Age
- Prepare parents for expected behavioral changes of toddler, especially negativism and ritualism.
- Assess present feeding habits, and encourage gradual weaning from bottle and increased intake of solid foods.
- Stress expected feeding changes of picky eating habits, food fads, and strong taste preferences; need for scheduled routine at mealtimes; inability to sit through an entire meal; and lack of table manners.
- Assess sleep patterns at night, particularly habit of a bedtime bottle, which is a major cause of early childhood caries (ECC), and procrastination behaviors that delay hour of sleep.
- Prepare parents for potential dangers of the home and motor vehicle environment, particularly motor vehicle injuries, drowning, accidental poisoning, and falling injuries; give appropriate suggestions for safety-proofing the home.
- Discuss need for firm but gentle discipline and ways to deal with negativism and temper tantrums; stress positive benefits of appropriate discipline.
- Emphasize importance for both child and parents of brief, periodic separations.
- Discuss toys that use developing gross and fine motor, language, cognitive, and social skills.

- Emphasize need for dental supervision, types of basic dental hygiene at home, and food habits that predispose to caries; stress importance of supplemental fluoride (according to age and fluoride content of local water supply).

18 to 24 Months of Age
- Stress importance of peer companionship in play.
- Explore need for preparation for additional sibling (as appropriate); stress importance of preparing child for new experiences.
- Discuss present discipline methods, their effectiveness, and parents' feelings about child's negativism; stress that negativism is an important aspect of developing self-assertion and independence and is not a sign of spoiling.
- Discuss signs of readiness for toilet training; emphasize importance of waiting for physical and psychologic readiness.
- Discuss development of fears such as darkness or loud noises and habits, such as security blanket or thumb sucking; stress normalcy of these transient behaviors.
- Prepare parents for signs of regression in time of stress.
- Assess child's ability to separate easily from parents for brief periods under familiar circumstances.

Continued

FAMILY-CENTERED CARE—cont'd

Guidance During Toddler Years

- Allow parents opportunity to express their feelings of weariness, frustration, and exasperation; be aware that it is often difficult to love toddlers when they are not asleep!
- Point out some of the expected changes of the next year such as longer attention span, somewhat less negativism, and increased concern for pleasing others.

24 to 36 Months of Age
- Discuss importance of imitation and domestic mimicry and need to include child in activities.

- Discuss approaches toward toilet training, particularly realistic expectations and attitude toward accidents.
- Stress uniqueness of toddlers' thought processes, especially through their use of language, poor understanding of time, causal relationships in terms of proximity of events, and inability to see events from another's perspective.
- Stress that discipline still must be structured and concrete and that relying solely on verbal reasoning and explanation leads to injuries, confusion, and misunderstanding.
- Discuss investigation of preschool or day care center toward completion of second year.

Advice is sometimes not the sole answer. Actual assistance such as being available for home visiting or telephone consulting, should be part of the nurse's flexible repertoire of interventions. Whether parents are experiencing the dilemmas of rearing a first or a subsequent child, they benefit from sharing their feelings, frustrations, and satisfactions. They need adult companionship, freedom from childrearing responsibilities, and periodic separations from their children. Part of a nurse's responsibility is to provide opportunities for parents to express their feelings and to meet their physical, mental, and spiritual needs.

REFERENCES

Abraham, V. M., Gaw, C. E., Chounthirath, T., et al. (2015). Toy-related injuries among children treated in US emergency departments, 1990-2011. *Clinical Pediatrics, 54*(2), 127–137.

Albertson, T. E., Owen, K. P., Sutter, M. E., et al. (2011). Gastrointestinal decontamination in the acutely poisoned patient. *International Journal of Emergency Medicine, 4*(1), 65.

American Academy of Pediatrics. (2015). *Car seats: Information for families for 2015.* Retrieved from http://www.healthychildren.org/English/safety-prevention/on-the-go/Pages/Car-Safety-Seats-Information-for-Families.aspx.

American Academy of Pediatrics, Committee on Infectious Diseases. (2015). L. Pickering (Ed.), *2015 Red book: report of the committee on infectious diseases* (30th ed.). Elk Grove Village, IL: Author.

American Academy of Pediatrics, Committee on Nutrition. (2014). *Pediatric nutrition handbook* (7th ed.). Elk Grove Village, IL: American Academy of Pediatrics.

American Academy of Pediatrics, Council on Communications and Media. (2016). *Media and Young minds.* Retrieved from http://dx.doi.org/10.1542/peds.2016-2591.

American Academy of Pediatric Dentistry. (2014a). *Guideline on infant oral health care.* Retrieved from http://www.aapd.org/media/Policies_Guidelines/G_InfantOralHealthCare.pdf.

American Academy of Pediatric Dentistry. (2014b). *Policy on early childhood caries (ECC): Classifications, consequences, and preventive strategies.* Retrieved from http://www.aapd.org/media/Policies_Guidelines/P_ECCClassifications.pdf.

American Academy of Pediatric Dentistry. (2014c). *Policy on use of fluoride.* Retrieved from http://www.aapd.org/media/Policies_Guidelines/P_FluorideUse.pdf.

American Academy of Pediatric Dentistry. (2014d). *Policy on dietary recommendations for infants, children, and adolescents.* Retrieved from http://www.aapd.org/media/Policies_Guidelines/P_DietaryRec.pdf.

Babcock, D. A. (2011). Evaluating sleep and sleep disorders in the pediatric primary care setting. *Pediatric Clinics of North America, 58*(3), 543–554.

Benson, B. E., Hoppu, K., Troutman, W. G., et al. (2013). Position paper update: gastric lavage for gastrointestinal decontamination. *Clinical Toxicology (Philadelphia), 51*(3), 140–146.

Berenbaum, S. A., & Beltz, A. M. (2011). Sexual differentiation of human behavior: effects of prenatal and pubertal organizational hormones. *Frontiers in Neuroendocrinology, 32*(2), 183–200.

Bhargava, S. (2011). Diagnosis and management of common sleep problems in children. *Pediatrics in Review, 32*(3), 91–98.

Bond, G. R., Woodward, R. W., & Ho, M. (2012). The growing impact of pediatric pharmaceutical poisoning. *Journal of Pediatrics, 160*(2), 265–279.

Bose-O'Reilly, S., McCarthy, K. M., Steckling, N., et al. (2010). Mercury exposure and children's health. *Current Problems in Pediatric and Adolescent Health Care, 40*(8), 186–215.

Brazelton, T. B. (1999). How to help parents of young children: The touchpoints model. *Journal of Perinatology, 19*(6 pt 2), S6–S7.

Bronstein, A. C., Spyker, D. A., Cantilena, L. R., Jr., et al. (2012). 2011 Annual report of the American Association of Poison Control Centers' National Poison Data System (NPDS): 29th annual report. *Clinical Toxicology (Philadelphia), 50*(10), 911–1161.

Brotanek, J. M., Schroer, D., Valentyn, L., et al. (2009). Reasons for prolonged bottle-feeding and iron deficiency among Mexican-American toddlers: An ethnographic study. *Academic Pediatrics, 9*(1), 17–25.

Buckley, N. A., Dawson, A. H., Juurlink, D. N., et al. (2016). Who gets antidotes? Choosing the chose few. *British Journal of Clinical Pharmacology, 81*(3), 402–407.

Butte, N. F., Fox, M. K., Briefel, R. R., et al. (2010). Nutrient intakes of US infants, toddlers, and preschoolers meet or exceed dietary reference intakes. *Journal of the American Dietetic Association, 110*(12 Suppl. 3), S27–S37.

Campbell, C., Gracely, E., Tran, M., et al. (2012). Primary prevention of lead exposure—Blood lead levels at age two years. *International Journal of Environmental Research and Public Health, 9,* 1216–1226.

Centers for Disease Control and Prevention. (2012). Injuries from batteries among children aged <13 years—United States, 1995-2010. *Morbidity and Mortality Weekly Report, 61*(34), 661–666.

Centers for Disease Control and Prevention. (2013). Blood lead levels in children aged 1-5years—United States, 1999-2010. *Morbidity and Mortality Weekly Report, 62*(13), 245–248.

Christakis, D. A. (2010). Infant media viewing: First, do no harm. *Pediatric Annals, 39*(9), 578–582.

Consumer Product Safety Commission. (2010). Full-size baby cribs and non–full-size baby cribs: Safety standards. *Federal Register, 75*(248), 81766–81788.

Craig, W. J., Mangels, A. R., & American Dietetic Association. (2009). Position of the American Dietetic Association: Vegetarian diets. *Journal of the American Dietetic Association, 109*(7), 1266–1282.

Cunningham, E. (2012). What role does nutrition play in the prevention or treatment of childhood lead poisoning? *Journal of the Academy of Nutrition and Dietetics, 112*(11), 1916.

Daniels, E., Mandleco, B., & Luthy, K. E. (2012). Assessment, management, and prevention of childhood temper tantrums. *Journal of the American Academy of Nurse Practitioners, 24*(10), 569–573.

Dapul, H., & Laraque, D. (2014). Lead poisoning in children. *Advances in Pediatrics, 61*, 313–333.

Durbin, D. R., & Committee on Injury, Violence, and Poison Prevention. (2011). Child passenger safety. *Pediatrics, 127*(4), e1050–e1066.

Duzinski, S. V., Barczyk, A. N., Wheeler, T. C., et al. (2014). Threat of paediatric hyperthermia in an enclosed vehicle: A year-round study. *Injury Prevention, 20*(4), 220–225.

Elder, J. S. (2016). Enuresis and voiding dysfunction. In R. M. Kliegman, B. F. Stanton, J. W. St. Geme, et al. (Eds.), *Nelson textbook of pediatrics* (20th ed.). Philadelphia, PA: Saunders/Elsevier.

Erikson, E. H. (1963). *Childhood and society* (2nd ed.). New York, NY: Norton.

Feigelman, S. (2016). The second year. In R. M. Kliegman, B. F. Stanton, J. W. St. Geme, & N. F. Schor (Eds.), *Nelson textbook of pediatrics* (20th ed.). Philadelphia, PA: Saunders/Elsevier.

Fountain, J. S., & Reith, D. M. (2014). Dangers of "EDTA. *New Zealand Medical Journal, 127*(1398), 126–127.

Fowler, J. W. (1981). *Stages of faith: the psychology of human development and the quest for meaning.* San Francisco, CA: Harper & Row.

Gilchrist, J., Ballesteros, M. F., & Parker, E. M. (2012). Vital signs: unintentional injury deaths among persons 0-19 years—United States, 2000-2009. *Morbidity and Mortality Weekly Report, 61*(15), 270–276.

Glenn, L. (2015). Pick your poison: What's new in poison control for the preschooler. *Journal of Pediatric Nursing, 30*(2), 395–401.

Hines, M. (2011). Gender development and the human brain. *Annual Review of Neuroscience, 34*, 69–88.

Huillet, A., Erdie-Lalena, C., Norvell, D., et al. (2011). Complementary and alternative medicine used by children in military pediatric clinics. *Journal of Alternative and Complementary Medicine, 17*(6), 531–537.

Institute of Medicine (IOM) (2005). *Dietary reference intakes for energy, carbohydrate, fiber, fat, fatty acids, cholesterol, protein, and amino acids.* Washington, DC: The Institute, National Academies Press.

Institute of Medicine (2010). *Dietary reference intakes for calcium and vitamin D.* Washington DC: The National Academies Press.

Jacob, S. E., Yang, A., Herro, E., & Zhang, C. (2010). Contact allergens in a pediatric population. *Journal of Clinical and Aesthetic Dermatology, 3*(101), 29–35.

Kemper, K. J., & Gardiner, P. M. (2016). Complementary therapies and integrative medicine. In R. M. Kliegman, B. F. Stanton, J. W. St. Geme, et al. (Eds.), *Nelson textbook of pediatrics* (20th ed.). Philadelphia, PA: Saunders/Elsevier.

Kendrick, D., Mulvaney, C. A., Ye, L., et al. (2013). Parenting interventions for the prevention of unintentional injuries in childhood. *Cochrane Database of Systematic Reviews, 2013*(3), CD006020.

Kendrick, D., Young, B., Mason-Jones, A. J., et al. (2012). Home safety education and provision of safety equipment for injury preventions. *Cochrane Database of Systematic Reviews, 2012*(9), CD005014.

Kiddoo, D. A. (2012). Toilet training children: When to start and how to train. *Canadian Medical Association Journal, 184*(5), 511–512.

Landier, W., & Tse, A. M. (2010). Use of complementary and alternative medical interventions for the management of procedural-related pain, anxiety, and distress in pediatric oncology: An integrative review. *Journal of Pediatric Nursing, 25*(6), 566–579.

Luangrath, A. (2011). Problem behavior in children: An approach for general practice. *Australian Family Physician, 40*(9), 678–681.

Meissner, W. W. (2009). The developmental progression from infancy to rapprochement. *Psychoanalytic Review, 96*(2), 219–259.

Mindell, J. A., Li, A. M., Sadeh, A., et al. (2015). Bedtime routines for young children: A dose-dependent association with sleep outcomes. *Sleep, 38*(5), 717–722.

Mindell, J. A., Sadeh, A., Kohyama, J., et al. (2010). Parental behaviors and sleep outcomes in infants and toddlers: A cross-cultural comparison. *Sleep Medicine, 11*(4), 393–399.

Mueller, C. R. (2010). Spirituality in children: Understanding and developing interventions. *Pediatric Nursing, 36*(4), 197–203, 208.

National Center for Complementary and Integrative Health. (2014). *What is complementary and alternative medicine?* Retrieved from http://nccam.nih.gov/health/whatiscam.

National Highway Traffic Safety Administration. (2010). *A parent's guide to booster seats (pamphlet).* Washington, DC: Author. Retrieved from nhtsa.gov.org.

Neuman, M. E. (2011). Addressing children's beliefs through Fowler's stages of faith. *Journal of Pediatric Nursing, 26*(1), 44–50.

Null, J. (2015). *Heatstroke deaths of children in vehicles.* Retrieved from http://noheatstroke.org/.

Owens, J. A. (2016). Sleep medicine. In R. M. Kliegman, B. F. Stanton, J. W. St. Geme, et al. (Eds.), *Nelson textbook of pediatrics* (20th ed.). Philadelphia, PA: Saunders/Elsevier.

Panella, N. J., Kirse, D. J., Pranikoff, T., et al. (2013). Disk battery ingestion: Case series with assessment of clinical and financial impact of a preventable disease. *Pediatric Emergency Care, 29*(2), 165–169.

Parks, E. P., Shaikhkhalil, A., Groleau, V., et al. (2016). Feeding healthy infants, children, and adolescents. In R. M. Kliegman, B. F. Stanton, J. W. St. Geme, et al. (Eds.), *Nelson textbook of pediatrics* (20th ed.). Philadelphia, PA: Saunders/Elsevier.

Raymond, J. S., Kennedy, C., & Brown, M. J. (2013). Blood lead level analysis among refugee children resettled in New Hampshire and Rhode Island. *Public Health Nursing, 30*(1), 70–79.

Rogers, J. (2013). Daytime wetting in children and acquisition of bladder control. *Nursing Children and Young People, 25*(6), 26–33.

Savic, I., Garcia-Falqueras, A., & Swaab, D. F. (2010). Sexual differentiation of the human brain in relation to gender identity and sexual orientation. *Progress in Brain Research, 186*, 41–62.

Schneider, L., Tilles, S., Lio, P., et al. (2013). Atopic dermatitis: A practice parameter update 2012. *Journal of Allergy and Clinical Immunology, 131*(2), 295–299.

Schwartz, S., & Benuck, I. (2013). Strategies and suggestions for a healthy toddler diet. *Pediatric Annals, 42*(9), 181–183.

Sharpe, S. J., Rochette, L. M., & Smith, G. A. (2012). Pediatric battery-related emergency department visits in the United States, 1990-2009. *Pediatrics, 129*(6), 1111–1117.

Steensma, T. D., Kreukels, B. P., de Vries, A. L., et al. (2013). Gender identity development in adolescence. *Hormones and Behavior, 64*(2), 288–297.

Theurer, W. M., & Bhavsar, A. K. (2013). Prevention of unintentional childhood injury. *American Family Physician, 87*(7), 502–509.

Ward, T. C., & Doering, J. J. (2014). Application of a socio-ecological model to mother-infant bed-sharing. *Health Education & Behavior, 41*(6), 577–589.

Weaver, N. L., Brixey, S. N., Williams, J., et al. (2013). Promoting correct car seat use in parents of young children: Challenges, recommendations, and implications for health communication. *Health Promotion Practice, 14*(2), 301–307.

Weiss, J., & American Academy of Pediatrics, Committee on Injury, Violence, and Poison Prevention. (2010). Technical report—Prevention of drowning. *Pediatrics, 126*(1), e253–e262.

Wolter, S., & Price, H. N. (2014). Atopic dermatitis. *Pediatric Clinics of North America, 61*(2), 241–260.

Wu, H. Y. (2010). Achieving urinary continence in children. *Nature Reviews Urology, 7*(7), 371–377.

Yeh, E. S., Rochette, L. M., McKenzie, L. B., et al. (2011). Injuries associated with cribs, playpens, and bassinets among young children in the US—1990-2008. *Pediatrics, 127*(3), 479–486.

Zimmerman, F. J., Gilkerson, J., Richards, J. A., et al. (2009). Teaching by listening: The importance of adult-child conversations to language development. *Pediatrics, 124*(1), 342–349.

Zuzak, T. J., Zuzak-Siegrist, I., Rist, L., et al. (2010). Medicinal systems of complementary and alternative medicine: A cross-sectional survey at a pediatric emergency department. *Journal of Alternative and Complementary Medicine, 16*(4), 473–479.

33

The Preschooler and Family

Cheryl C. Rodgers

ⓔ http://evolve.elsevier.com/Perry/maternal

PROMOTING OPTIMAL GROWTH AND DEVELOPMENT

BIOLOGIC DEVELOPMENT

The rate of physical growth slows and stabilizes during the preschool years. The average weight is 14.5 kg (32 pounds) at 3 years, 16.7 kg (36.8 pounds) at 4 years, and 18.7 kg (41.5 pounds) at 5 years. The average weight gain per year remains approximately 2 to 3 kg (4.5 to 6.5 pounds). Growth in height also remains steady, with an annual increase of 6.5 to 9 cm (2.5 to 3.5 inches), and generally occurs by elongation of the legs rather than the trunk. The average height is 95 cm (37.5 inches) at 3 years, 103 cm (40.5 inches) at 4 years, and 110 cm (43.5 inches) at 5 years.

Physical proportions no longer resemble those of the squat, pot-bellied toddler. The preschooler is slender but sturdy, graceful, agile, and postur-ally erect. There is little difference in physical characteristics according to gender, except as dictated by such factors as dress and hairstyle.

Most organ systems can adjust to moderate stress and change. During this period, most children are toilet trained. For the most part, motor development consists of increases in strength and refinement of previously learned skills such as walking, running, and jumping. However, muscle development and bone growth are still far from mature. Excessive activity and overexertion can injure delicate tissues. Good posture, appropriate exercise, and adequate nutrition and rest are essential for optimal development of the musculoskeletal system.

Gross and Fine Motor Skills

Walking, running, climbing, and jumping are well established by 36 months of age. Refinement in eye-hand and muscle coordination is evident in several areas. At 3 years of age, the preschooler rides a tricycle, walks on tiptoe, balances on one foot for a few seconds, and broad jumps. By 4 years of age, the child skips and hops proficiently on one foot (Fig. 33.1) and catches a ball reliably. By 5 years of age, he or she skips on alternate feet, jumps rope, and begins to skate and swim.

Fine motor development is evident in the child's increasingly skillful manipulation, such as in drawing and dressing. These skills provide readiness for learning and independence for entry into school.

PSYCHOSOCIAL DEVELOPMENT

Developing a Sense of Initiative (Erikson)

After preschoolers have mastered the tasks of the toddler period, they are ready to face the developmental endeavors of the preschool period. Erikson (1963) maintained that the chief psychosocial task of this period is acquiring a sense of *initiative*. Children are in a stage of energetic

🌐 CULTURAL CONSIDERATIONS
Learning Sociocultural Mores

Developing a conscience implies learning the sociocultural mores of the family's heritage. Depending on the type of attitudes conveyed, children learn not only appropriate behaviors but also tolerant, biased, or prejudicial values concerning their ethnic, religious, and social background and those of other groups. Much of this influence may remain dormant until they associate with children or adults of a different ethnic background. Then, depending on the particular group, they may be accepted or ostracized for their attitudes.

learning. They play, work, and live to the fullest and feel a real sense of accomplishment and satisfaction in their activities. Conflict arises when children overstep the limits of their ability and inquiry and experience a sense of *guilt* for not having behaved appropriately. Feelings of guilt, anxiety, and fear may also result from thoughts that differ from expected behavior.

A particularly stressful thought is wishing one's parent dead. As a sense of rivalry or competition develops between the child and same-sex parent, the child may think of ways to get rid of the interfering parent. In most situations, this rivalry is resolved when the child strongly identifies with the same-sex parent and peers during the school years. However, if that parent dies before the identification process is completed, the preschooler may be overwhelmed with guilt for having wished and therefore "caused" the death. Clarifying for children that wishes cannot and do not make events occur is essential in helping them overcome their guilt and anxiety.

Development of the *superego*, or *conscience*, begins toward the end of the toddler years and is a major task for preschoolers (see Cultural Considerations box: Learning Sociocultural Mores). Learning right from wrong and good from bad is the beginning of morality (see the "Moral Development" section later in this chapter).

COGNITIVE DEVELOPMENT

One of the tasks related to the preschool period is readiness for school and scholastic learning. Many of the thought processes of this period are crucial for achieving such readiness, and it is intentional that the child begins school between 5 and 6 years of age rather than at an earlier age.

Preoperational Phase (Piaget)

Piaget's cognitive theory does not include a period specifically for children who are 3 to 5 years of age. The *preoperational phase* covers the age span from 2 to 7 years and is divided into two stages: the *preconceptual*

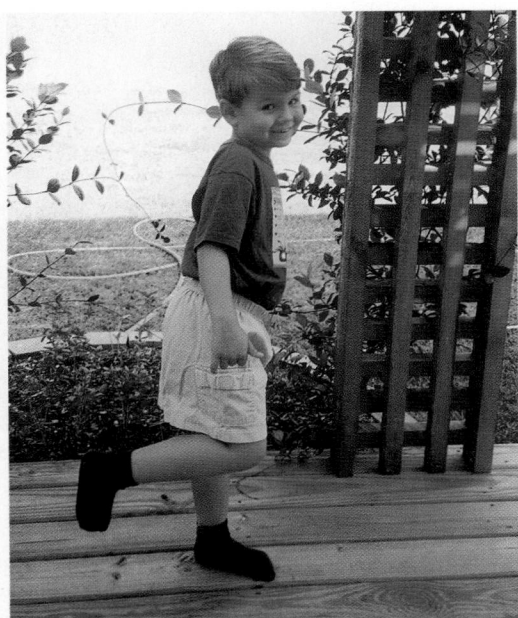

FIG 33.1 A 4-year-old child has sufficient balance to stand or hop on one foot.

phase, 2 to 4 years of age, and the phase of *intuitive thought,* 4 to 7 years of age. One of the main transitions during these two phases is the shift from totally egocentric thought to social awareness and the ability to consider other viewpoints. However, egocentricity is still evident.

Language continues to develop during the preschool period. Speech remains primarily a vehicle of egocentric communication. Preschoolers assume that everyone thinks as they do and that a brief explanation of their thinking makes the entire thought understood by others. Because of this self-referenced, egocentric verbal communication, it is often necessary to explore and understand the young child's thinking through other, nonverbal approaches. For children in this age group, the most enlightening and effective method is play, which becomes the child's way of understanding, adjusting to, and working out life's experiences.

Preschoolers increasingly use language without comprehending the meaning of words, particularly concepts of right and left, causality, and time. Children may use the concepts correctly but only in the circumstances in which they have learned them. For example, they may know how to put on shoes by remembering that the buckle is always on the outside of the foot. However, if different shoes have no buckles, they cannot reason which shoe fits which foot. In other words, they do not understand the concept of right and left.

Superficially, causality resembles logical thought. Preschoolers explain a concept as they heard it described by others, but their understanding is limited. An example is the concept of time. Because time is still incompletely understood, the child interprets it according to his or her own frame of reference, such as "A long time means until Christmas." Consequently time is best explained in relationship to an event such as, "Your mother will visit you after you finish your lunch." Avoiding words such as yesterday, tomorrow, next week, or Tuesday to express when an event is expected to occur and instead associating time with expected daily events help children learn about temporal relationships while increasing their trust in others' predictions.

Preschoolers' thinking is often described as *magical thinking.* Because of their egocentrism and transductive reasoning, they believe that thoughts are all-powerful. Such thinking places them in the vulnerable position of feeling guilty and responsible for bad thoughts, which may coincide with the occurrence of a wished event. Their inability to logically reason the cause and effect of an illness or injury makes it especially difficult for them to understand such events.

> **! NURSING ALERT**
>
> Counseling children whose parents are going through a divorce or separation should involve a discussion with the child about her or his role. Because of magical thinking the child may believe that she or he wished the other parent away. The child should be reassured that this is not the case.

Preschoolers believe in the power of words and accept their meaning literally. An example of this type of thinking is calling children "bad" because they did something wrong. In the preschooler's mind, calling them bad means that he or she is a bad person; thus it is better to say that the actions were bad (e.g., "That was a bad thing to do").

MORAL DEVELOPMENT

Preconventional or Premoral Level (Kohlberg)

Young children's development of moral judgment is at the most basic level. They have little, if any, concern about why something is wrong. They behave because of the freedom or restriction that is placed on actions. In the punishment and obedience orientation, children (from about 2 to 4 years of age) judge whether an action is good or bad depending on whether it results in reward or punishment. If children are punished for it, the action is bad. If they are not punished, the action is good regardless of the meaning of the act. For example, if parents allow hitting, the child perceives that hitting is good because it is not associated with punishment.

From approximately 4 to 7 years of age, children are in the stage of *naïve instrumental orientation,* in which actions are directed toward satisfying their needs and less frequently the needs of others. They have a concrete sense of justice and fairness during this period of development.

SPIRITUAL DEVELOPMENT

Children generally learn about faith and religion from significant others in their environment, usually from parents and their religious beliefs and practices. However, young children's understanding of spirituality is influenced by their cognitive level. Preschoolers have a concrete concept of a God with physical characteristics, often similar to an imaginary friend. They understand simple Bible stories, memorize short prayers, and imitate the religious practices of their parents without fully understanding the significance of these rituals. Preschoolers benefit from concrete representations of religious practices, such as picture Bible books and small statues, such as those of the Nativity scene.

Development of the conscience is strongly linked to spiritual development. At this age, children are learning right from wrong and behaving correctly to avoid punishment. Wrongdoing provokes feelings of guilt, and preschoolers often misinterpret illness as a punishment for real or imagined transgressions. Observing religious traditions and participating in a religious community can help children cope during stressful periods such as illness and hospitalization (Purow, Alisanski, Putnam, et al., 2011).

DEVELOPMENT OF BODY IMAGE

The preschool years play a significant role in the development of body image. With increasing comprehension of language, preschoolers recognize that individuals have desirable and undesirable appearances. They recognize differences in skin color and racial identity and are vulnerable to learning prejudices and biases. They are aware of the meaning of words such as *pretty* or *ugly*, and they reflect the opinions of others regarding their own appearance. By 5 years of age, children compare their size with that of their peers and can become conscious of being large or short, especially if others refer to them as "so big" or "so little" for their age. Research indicates that girls as young as preschool age already show concern about appearance and weight (Skouteris, McCabe, Swinburn, et al., 2010). Because these are formative years for both boys and girls, parents should make efforts to instill positive principles regarding body image, give their children encouraging feedback regarding their appearance, and emphasize the importance of accepting individuals no matter their differences in appearances. Children at this age should be educated regarding the benefits of physical activity and nutrition on health rather than focusing on weight.

Despite the advances in body-image development, preschoolers have poorly defined body boundaries and little knowledge of their internal anatomy. Intrusive experiences are frightening, especially those that disrupt the integrity of the skin, such as injections and surgery. They fear that, if their skin is "broken," all of their blood and "insides" can leak out. Therefore bandages are critical to "keep everything from coming out."

DEVELOPMENT OF SEXUALITY

Sexual development during these years is an important phase in a person's overall sexual identity and beliefs. Preschoolers are forming strong attachments to the opposite-sex parent while identifying with the same-sex parent. *Sex-typing,* or the process by which an individual develops the behavior, personality, attitudes, and beliefs appropriate for his or her culture and sex, occurs through several mechanisms during this period. Probably the most powerful mechanisms are childrearing practices and imitation. Gender identification is a result of complex prenatal and postnatal psychologic factors, as well as biologic, social, and genetic factors. Most children are aware of their gender and the expected sets of related behaviors by 1.5 to 2.5 years of age.

As sexual identity develops beyond gender recognition, modesty may become a concern. Sex-role imitation and dressing up like Mommy or Daddy are important activities. Attitudes and responses of others to role-playing can condition the child to accept the views of others. For example, comments such as "Boys shouldn't play with dolls" can influence a boy's self-concept of masculinity.

Sexual exploration may be more pronounced now than ever before, particularly in terms of exploring and manipulating the genitalia. Questions about sexual reproduction may come to the forefront in the preschooler's search for understanding (see the "Sex Education" section later in this chapter).

SOCIAL DEVELOPMENT

During the preschool period, the *separation*-individuation *process* is completed. Preschoolers have overcome much of the anxiety associated with strangers and the fear of separation of earlier years. They relate to unfamiliar people easily and tolerate brief separations from parents with little or no protest. However, they still need parental security, reassurance, guidance, and approval, especially when entering preschool or elementary school. Prolonged separation such as that imposed by illness and hospitalization is difficult, but preschoolers respond to anticipatory preparation and concrete explanation. Maintaining an established routine is still important in early preschoolers regardless of home, school, or hospital environment. They can cope with changes in daily routine much better than toddlers, although they may develop

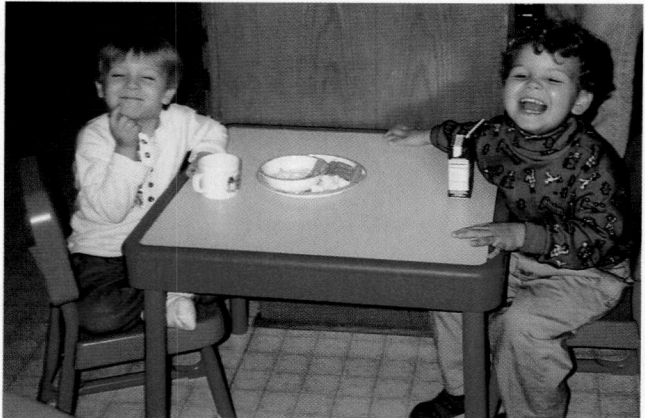

FIG 33.2 Preschool children enjoy friends and often use nonverbal messages to communicate.

more imaginary fears. Preschoolers gain security and comfort from familiar objects such as toys, dolls, or photographs of family members. They are able to work through many of their unresolved fears, fantasies, and anxieties through play, especially if guided with appropriate play objects (e.g., dolls, puppets) that represent family members, health care professionals, and other children.

Language

During the preschool years, language becomes more sophisticated and complex and the major mode of communication and social interaction (Fig. 33.2). Both cognitive ability and environment—particularly consistent role models—influence vocabulary, speech, and comprehension. Vocabulary increases dramatically, from 300 words at 2 years of age to more than 2100 words at the end of 5 years of age. Sentence structure, grammatical usage, and intelligibility also advance to a more adult level. Language development during these early years predicts school readiness (Harrison & McLeod, 2010) and sets the stage for later success in school (Reilly, Wake, Ukoumunne, et al., 2010).

Children between 3 and 4 years of age form sentences of about three or four words and include only the most essential words to convey a meaning. Such speech is often termed *telegraphic* for its brevity. Three-year-old children ask many questions and use plurals, correct pronouns, and the past tense of verbs. They name familiar objects, such as animals, parts of the body, relatives, and friends. They can give and follow simple commands. They talk incessantly regardless of whether anyone is listening or answering them. They enjoy musical or talking toys or dolls and imitate new words proficiently. Preschoolers also benefit from "reading" picture books with a parent or adult figure; this provides immediate feedback to the child and helps develop vocabulary as he or she hears the pronunciation of words from an adult (Feigelman, 2016).

From 4 to 5 years of age, preschoolers use longer sentences of four or five words and more words to convey a message (e.g., prepositions, adjectives, and a variety of verbs). They can follow simple directional commands such as, "Put the ball on the chair," but can carry out only one request at a time. They answer questions such as, "What do you do when you're hungry?" by describing the appropriate action. The pattern of asking questions is at its peak, and children usually repeat a question until they receive an answer. Preschoolers also are incapable of understanding figurative speech and are very literal in their understanding of the meaning of words (Feigelman, 2016). For example, saying that an IV cannula to be inserted for hydration is a straw is interpreted by the preschooler as literally a drinking straw because that is his or her common frame of reference for that object.

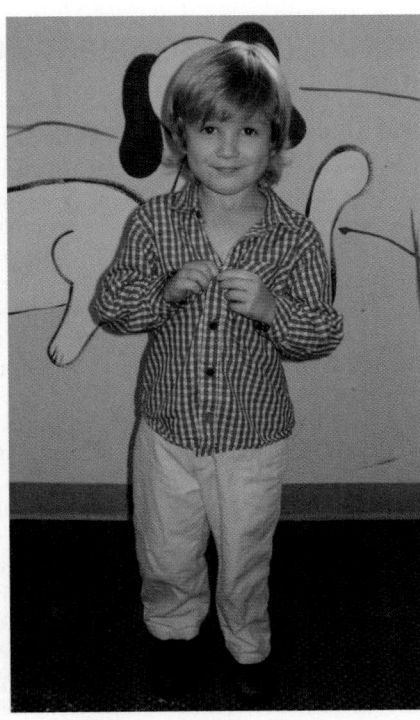

FIG 33.3 Most preschoolers are able to dress themselves but need help with more difficult items of clothing.

Personal-Social Behavior

The pervasive ritualism and negativism of toddlerhood gradually diminish during the preschool years. Although self-assertion is still a major theme, preschoolers demonstrate their sense of autonomy differently. They are able to verbalize their request for independence and perform independently because of their much-refined physical and cognitive development. By 4 or 5 years of age, they need little if any assistance with dressing, eating, or toileting (Fig. 33.3). They can be trusted to obey warnings of danger, although 3- or 4-year-old children may exceed their boundaries at times.

Preschoolers are also much more sociable and willing to please. They have internalized many of the standards and values of the family and culture. However, by the end of early childhood they begin to question parental values and compare them with those of their peer group and other authority figures. As a result, they may be less willing to abide by the family's code of conduct. Preschoolers become increasingly aware of their position and role within the family. Although this is a more secure age for experiencing the addition of another sibling, relinquishing the position of first or youngest is still difficult and requires appropriate preparation (see the "Sibling Rivalry" section in Chapter 32).

Play

Various types of play are typical of this period, but preschoolers especially enjoy *associative play* (i.e., group play in similar or identical activities but without rigid organization or rules). Play should provide for physical, social, and mental development.

Play activities for physical growth and refinement of motor skills include jumping, running, and climbing. Tricycles, wagons, gym and sports equipment, sandboxes, wading pools, and activities at water parks can help develop muscles and coordination (Fig. 33.4). Activities such as swimming and skating teach safety and muscle development and coordination. Children involved in the work of play do not require

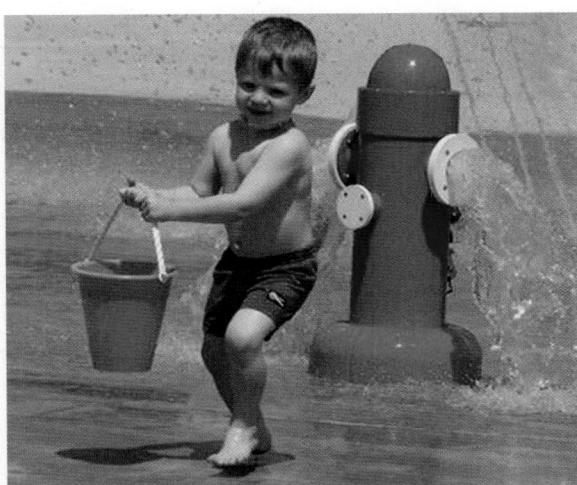

FIG 33.4 Preschoolers enjoy play activities that promote motor skills such as jumping and running. Water play is an exciting activity for preschoolers.

expensive toys and gadgets to keep them entertained but often enjoy playing with common household items such as a broom handle or even items that adults consider junk (boxes, sticks, rocks, and dirt).

Manipulative, constructive, creative, and educational toys provide for quiet activities, fine motor development, and self-expression. Easy construction sets, large blocks of various sizes and shapes, alphabet or number flash cards, paints, crayons, simple carpentry tools, musical toys, illustrated books, simple sewing or handicraft sets, large puzzles, and clay are suitable toys. Electronic games and computer programs are especially valuable in helping children learn basic skills such as letters and simple words.

Probably the most characteristic and pervasive preschool activity is imitative, imaginative, and dramatic play. Dress-up clothes, dolls, housekeeping toys, dollhouses, play store toys, farm animals and equipment, trains, trucks, cars, planes, hand puppets, and medical kits provide hours of self-expression (Fig. 33.5). Probably at no other time is the reproduction of adult behavior so faithful and absorbing as in 4- and 5-year-old children. Toward the end of the preschool period, children are less satisfied with make-believe or pretend objects and enjoy doing the actual activity such as cooking and carpentry.

Television and other media also have their place in children's play, although each should be only one part of children's total repertoire of social and recreational activities. Parents and other caregivers should supervise the selection of high-quality programs, and watch and discuss programs with their children (American Academy of Pediatrics, Council on Communications and Media, 2016). Considering the significant increase in media accessibility through various portable electronic devices and cell phones, parents need to be aware of the potential positive and negative effects of media exposure. Children enjoy and learn from educational programs; however, television viewing may limit time spent in other meaningful activities such as reading, physical activity, and socialization (American Academy of Pediatrics, Council on Communications and Media, 2016). Prolonged television viewing by young children has been linked to an increase in social-emotional delays and decreased time spent in active playing, which increases the risk for obesity among certain children (American Academy of Pediatrics, Council on Communications and Media, 2016).

Play is so much a part of young children's lives that reality and fantasy become blurred. Make-believe is reality during play and only becomes fantasy when the toys are put away or the dress-up clothes

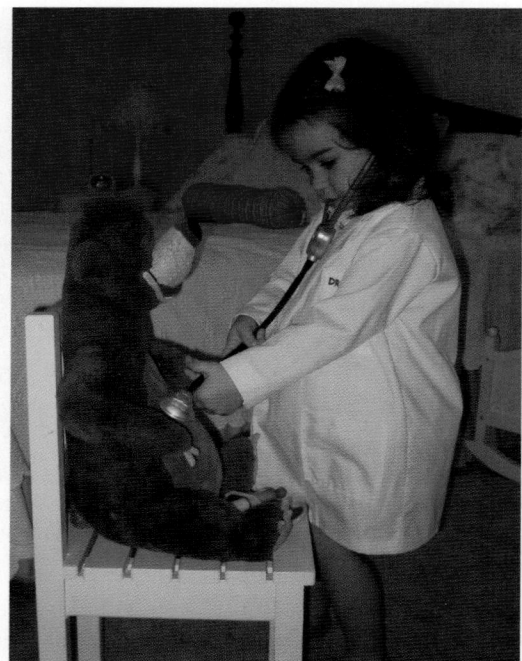

FIG 33.5 Imaginative and imitative play is typical of preschoolers.

are removed. It is no wonder that imaginary playmates are so much a part of this age period. The appearance of imaginary companions usually occurs between 2½ and 3 years of age, and for the most part, such playmates are relinquished when the child enters school. Differences in birth order and gender have been noted in studies of imaginary companion play. Firstborn children have a higher incidence of imaginary companions as do young girls; young boys more often tend to impersonate characters (Trionfi & Reese, 2009).

Imaginary companions serve many purposes: they become friends in times of loneliness, accomplish what the child is still attempting, and experience what the child wants to forget or remember. It is not unusual for the "friend" to have myriad vices and be blamed for wrongdoing. Sometimes the child hopes to escape punishment by saying, "My friend George broke the glass." At other times, the child may fantasize that the companion misbehaved and play the role of the parent. This becomes a way of assuming control and authority in a safe situation.

Parents often worry about the imaginary playmates, not realizing how normal and useful they are. They need to be reassured that the child's fantasy is a sign of health that helps differentiate make-believe and reality. Parents can acknowledge the presence of the imaginary companion by calling him or her by name and even agreeing to simple requests such as setting an extra place at the table, but they should not allow the child to use the playmate to avoid punishment or responsibility. For example, if the child blames the companion for messing up a room, parents need to state clearly that the child is the only one they see; therefore the child is responsible for cleaning up.

Children also benefit from play that occurs between them and a parent. Mutual play fosters development from birth through the school years and provides enriched opportunities for learning. Through mutual play, parents can provide tactile and kinesthetic experiences, maximize verbal and language abilities, and offer praise and encouragement for exploration of the world. In addition, mutual play encourages positive interactions between the parent and child, strengthening their relationship.

Table 33.1 summarizes the major developmental achievements for children 3, 4, and 5 years of age.

COPING WITH CONCERNS RELATED TO NORMAL GROWTH AND DEVELOPMENT

Preschool and Kindergarten Experience

Some children are home schooled, but many children attend some type of early childhood program, usually preschool or a day care center. Group care has become commonplace with the large number of parents currently employed outside the home (see the "Alternative Child Care Arrangements" section in Chapter 31). The effects of early education and stimulation on children have increasingly gained recognition. (For a discussion of the effects of day care on young children, see the "Working Mothers" section in Chapter 27.) Because social development widens to include age mates and other significant adults, preschool provides an excellent vehicle for expanding children's experiences with others. It is also excellent preparation for entrance into elementary school.

In preschool or day care centers, children are exposed to opportunities for learning group cooperation; adjusting to sociocultural differences; and coping with frustration, dissatisfaction, and anger. If activities are tailored to provide mastery and achievement, children increasingly have feelings of success, self-confidence, and personal competence. Whether structured learning is imposed is less important than the social climate, type of guidance, and attitude toward the children that is fostered by the teacher or leader. With a teacher who is aware of preschoolers' developmental abilities and needs, children learn from the activity that is provided. Most programs incorporate a daily schedule of quiet play, active outdoor activity, group activities such as games and projects, creative or free play, and snack and rest periods. Preschool is particularly beneficial for children who lack a peer-group experience such as only children and for children from impoverished homes.

One of the issues that parents face is their children's readiness for preschool or kindergarten. There are no absolute indicators for school readiness, but children's social and emotional maturity, especially attention span, are as important as their academic readiness. Using a developmental screening tool that addresses cognitive (especially language), social, and physical milestones can identify children who may benefit from diagnostic testing and early intervention programs before starting school. Parents should promote a positive attitude toward learning, read to their children, provide opportunities for social and emotional growth, and choose programs or schools that will partner with the family to foster learning (National Center on Parent, Family, and Community Engagement, 2014).

Nurses and other health care workers can guide parents in selecting enriched social and educational early intervention programs, schools, and child care centers. Careful selection of early childhood education is intrinsic to future learning and development. Licensed and regulated programs are mandated to abide by established standards, which represent minimum requirements and safeguards. Regulation is important to protect children from harm and promote the conditions essential for a child's healthy development and learning. The National Association for the Education of Young Children serves as the model for optimal care of small children.*

Areas for parents to evaluate include the facility's daily program, teacher qualifications, staff-to-student ratio, discipline policy, environmental safety precautions, provision of meals, sanitary conditions,

---

*Information about accreditation criteria and procedures of the National Association for the Education of Young Children Accreditation of Programs for Young Children is available from the National Association for the Education of Young Children, 1313 L Street NW, Suite 500, Washington, DC 20005, 800-424-2460 or 202-232-8777, http://www.naeyc.org. These criteria are excellent guidelines for evaluating preschools and day care centers.

TABLE 33.1 Growth and Development During Preschool Years

Physical	Gross Motor	Fine Motor	Language	Socialization	Cognition	Family Relationships
3 Years of Age						
Usual weight gain of 1.8 to 2.7 kg (4–6 lbs)	Rides tricycle	Builds tower of 9 to 10 cubes	Has vocabulary of about 900 words	Dresses self almost completely if helped with back buttons and told which shoe is right or left	Is in preconceptual phase	Attempts to please parents and conform to their expectations
Average weight of 14.5 kg (32 lbs)	Jumps off bottom step	Builds bridge with three cubes	Uses primarily telegraphic speech	Pulls on shoes	Is egocentric in thought and behavior	Is less jealous of younger sibling
Usual gain in height of 7.5 cm (3 inches) per year	Stands on one foot for a few seconds	Adeptly places small pellets in narrow-necked bottle	Uses complete sentences of three or four words	Has increased attention span	Has beginning understanding of time; uses many time-oriented expressions, talks about past and future as much as about present, pretends to tell time	Is aware of family relationships and sex-role functions
Average height of 95 cm (37.5 inches)	Goes up stairs using alternate feet; may still come down using both feet on step	In drawing, copies a circle, imitates a cross, names what has been drawn; cannot draw stick figure but may make circle with facial features	Talks incessantly regardless of whether anyone is paying attention	Feeds self completely	Has improved concept of space, as demonstrated by understanding of prepositions and ability to follow directional command	Boys tend to identify more with father or other male figure
May have achieved nighttime control of bowel and bladder	Broad jumps		Repeats sentence of six syllables	Can prepare simple meals such as cold cereal and milk	Has beginning ability to view concepts from another perspective	Has increased ability to separate easily and comfortably from parents for short periods
	May try to dance, but balance may not be adequate		Asks many questions	Can help set table; can dry dishes without breaking any		
				May have fears, especially of dark and going to bed		
				Knows own gender and gender of others		
				Play is parallel and associative; begins to learn simple games but often follows own rules; begins to share		
4 Years of Age						
Pulse and respiration rates decrease slightly	Skips and hops on one foot	Uses scissors successfully to cut out picture following outline	Has vocabulary of 1500 words or more	Very independent	Is in phase of intuitive thought	Rebels if parents expect too much, such as impeccable table manners
Growth rate is similar to that of previous year	Catches ball reliably	Can lace shoes but may not be able to tie bow	Uses sentences of four or five words	Tends to be selfish and impatient	Causality is still related to proximity of events	Takes aggression and frustration out on parents or siblings
Average weight of 16.5 kg (36.5 lbs)	Throws ball overhead	In drawing, copies a square, traces a cross and diamond, adds three parts to stick figure	Questioning is at peak	Aggressive physically and verbally	Understands time better, especially in terms of sequence of daily events	Do's and don'ts become important
Average height of 103 cm (40.5 inches)	Walks down stairs using alternate footing		Tells exaggerated stories	Takes pride in accomplishments	Unable to conserve matter	May have rivalry with older or younger siblings; may resent older sibling's privileges and younger sibling's invasion of privacy and possessions
Birth length has doubled			Knows simple songs	Has mood swings	Judges everything according to one dimension such as height, width, or order	May "run away" from home
Maximum potential for development of amblyopia			May be mildly profane if associates with older children	Shows off dramatically, enjoys entertaining others	Immediate perceptual clues dominate judgment	Identifies strongly with parent of opposite sex
			Obeys four prepositional phrases such as under, on top of, beside, in back of, or in front of	Tells family tales to others with no restraint	Is beginning to develop less egocentrism and more social awareness	Is able to run simple errands outside the home
			Names one or more colors	Still has many fears	May count correctly but has poor mathematical concept of numbers	
			Comprehends analogies such as, "If ice is cold, fire is _____."	Play is associative	Obeys because parents have set limits, not because of understanding of right or wrong	
				Imaginary playmates are common		
				Uses dramatic, imaginative, and imitative devices		
				Sexual exploration and curiosity demonstrated through play such as being "doctor" or "nurse"		

Continued

TABLE 33.1 Growth and Development During Preschool Years—cont'd

Physical	Gross Motor	Fine Motor	Language	Socialization	Cognition	Family Relationships
5 Years of Age						
Pulse and respiration rates decrease slightly	Skips and hops on alternate feet	Ties shoelaces	Has vocabulary of about 2100 words	Less rebellious and quarrelsome than at 4 years of age	Begins to question what parents think by comparing them with age-mates and other adults	Gets along well with parents
Average weight of 18.5 kg (41 lbs)	Throws and catches ball well	Uses scissors, simple tools, and pencil well	Uses sentences of six to eight words, with all parts of speech	More settled and eager to get down to business	May notice prejudice and bias in outside world	May seek out parent more often than at 4 years of age for reassurance and security, especially when entering school
Average height of 110 cm (43.5 inches)	Jumps rope	In drawing, copies a diamond and triangle; adds seven to nine parts to stick figure; prints a few letters, numbers, or words such as first name	Names coins (e.g., nickel, dime)	Not as open and accessible in thoughts and behavior as in earlier years	Is more able to view other's perspective but tolerates rather than understands them	Begins to question parents' thinking and principles
Eruption of permanent dentition may begin	Skates with good balance		Names four or more colors	Independent but trustworthy, not foolhardy; more responsible		Strongly identifies with parent of same sex, especially boys with their fathers
Handedness is established (about 90% are right-handed)	Walks backward with heel to toe		Describes drawing or pictures with much comment and elaboration	Has fewer fears; relies on outer authority to control world	May begin to show understanding of conservation of numbers through counting objects regardless of arrangement	Enjoys activities such as sports, cooking, and shopping with parent of same sex
	Jumps from height of 12 inches and lands on toes		Knows days of week, months, and other time-associated words	Eager to do things right and to please; tries to "live by the rules"	Uses time-oriented words with increased understanding	
	Balances on alternate feet with eyes closed		Knows composition of articles, such as "A shoe is made of ____"	Has better manners	Cautious about accepting or believing information	
			Can follow three commands in succession	Cares for self totally, occasionally needing supervision in dress or hygiene		
				Not ready for concentrated close work or small print because of slight farsightedness and still unrefined eye-hand coordination		
				Play is associative; tries to follow rules but may cheat to avoid losing		

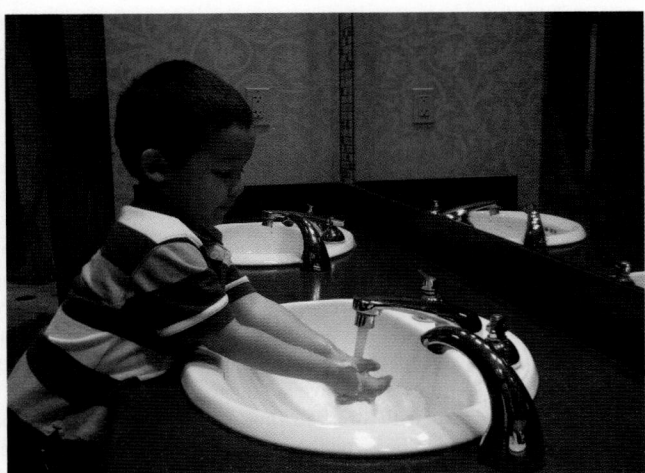

FIG 33.6 Thorough hand washing is the single most effective method of preventing infection.

adequate indoor and outdoor space per child, safety and injury prevention, and fee schedule. References from other parents help in evaluating a facility, but personal observation of the facility is recommended. Encourage parents to meet the director and some of the employees at a few facilities to make an informed choice.

Evaluation of the facility's health practices is extremely important. Preschoolers in child care centers have more illnesses than those not in child care centers, especially gastrointestinal tract and respiratory tract infections (Sacri, De Serres, Quach, Boulianne, Valiquette, & Skowronski, 2014). Nurses play an important role in infection control. Not only can they advise parents regarding the evaluation of the facility's sanitary practices, but they can also take an active part in educating staff in measures to minimize transmission of infection (Fig. 33.6). Parents should inquire about the policy of the center regarding the attendance and care of sick children.

Children need preparation for the preschool or kindergarten experience. For young children, it represents a change from their usual home environment and prolonged separation from their parents. Before children begin school, parents should present the idea as exciting and pleasurable. Talking to children about activities allows children to fantasize about the forthcoming event in a positive manner. When the first day of school arrives, parents should behave confidently. Such behavior requires them to have resolved their own feelings regarding the experience.

Parents should introduce their child to the teacher and the facility. In some instances, it is helpful for parents to remain with the child for at least part of the first day until the child is comfortable and at ease. Other specific actions that can help reduce separation anxiety include providing the school with detailed information about the child's home environment such as familiar routines, favorite activities, food preferences, names of siblings or pets, and personal habits. Such information helps the child feel familiar in the strange surroundings. When schools automatically request this information, the parent has a valuable clue to evaluating the quality of the program because the request represents the staff's awareness of each child's needs. Transitional objects such as a favorite toy may also help the child bridge the gap from home to school.

Sex Education

Preschoolers have assimilated a tremendous amount of information during their short lifetimes. Although their thinking may not be mature, they search constantly for explanations and reasons that are logical and reasonable to them. The word "why" seems to supplant the word "no,"

which was common in toddlerhood. It is only natural that, as they learn about "me," they will also want to know "why me" and "how me." Questions such as, "Where do babies come from?" are as casual as, "What makes it rain?" or "Who is that?" It is the way in which questions about procreation are answered that conditions children, even the youngest, to separate these questions from others about their world.

Two rules govern answering sensitive questions about topics such as sex. The first is to find out what children know and think. After investigating the theories children have produced as a reasonable explanation, parents can give correct information and help them understand why their explanation is inaccurate. Another reason for ascertaining what the child thinks before offering any information is that the "unasked for" answer may be given. For example, 4-year-old Emma asked her father, "Where did I come from?" Both parents quickly took this inquiry as a clue for offering sex education. After the explanation Emma exclaimed, "I don't know about all that! All I know is that Mary came from New York, and I want to know where I came from."

The second rule for giving information is to be honest. It is true that the preschooler will forget or misunderstand much of the correct information, but the correct information can be restated until the child absorbs and comprehends the facts. Even though the correct anatomic words may be hard to pronounce or even more difficult to remember, they become foundational content for explaining other concepts at a later time.

Honesty does not imply imparting to children every fact of life or allowing excessive permissiveness in sexual curiosity. When children ask one question, they are looking for one answer. When they are ready, they will ask about the other "unfinished" parts of the story. Sooner or later, they will wonder how the "sperm meets the egg" and "how the baby gets out," but during this period, it is best to wait until they ask.

Regardless of whether children are given sex education, they will engage in games of sexual curiosity and exploration. At about 3 years of age, children are aware of the anatomic differences between the sexes and concerned with how the other works. This is not really "sexual" curiosity because many children are still unaware of the reproductive function of the genitalia. Their curiosity is for the eliminative function of the anatomy. Little boys wonder how girls can urinate without a penis, so they watch girls go to the bathroom. Because they cannot see anything but the stream of urine coming out, they want to observe further. "Doctor play" is often a game invented for just such investigation. Little girls are no less curious about boys' anatomy. It is intriguing to closely inspect this "thing" that girls do not have.

One question that parents often have is how to handle such sexual curiosity. A positive approach is to neither condone nor condemn it but to express that if children have questions, they should ask the parents. Then parents can answer their questions and encourage them to engage in some other activity. In this way, children can be helped to understand that there are ways to satisfy their sexual curiosity other than through investigative games. This in no way condemns the act but stresses alternate methods to seek solutions and answers. Allowing children unrestricted permissiveness only intensifies their anxiety and concern because exploring and searching usually yield little evidence to satisfy their curiosity.

Many excellent books on sex education are available for preschool children at public libraries. The Sexuality Information and Education Council of the United States* and the American Academy of Pediatrics†

---

*Sexuality Information and Education Council of the United States (SIECUS), 1012 14th Street NW, Suite 1108, Washington, DC 20005, 202-265-2405, http://www.siecus.org.
†American Academy of Pediatrics, 141 Northwest Point Boulevard, Elk Grove Village, IL 60007, 847-434-4000, http://www.aap.org.

have bibliographies of suggested reading material. Parents should read the book themselves before giving or reading them to their children.

Another concern for some parents is masturbation, or self-stimulation of the genitalia. This occurs at any age for a variety of reasons and, if not excessive, is normal and healthy. It is most common at 4 years of age and during adolescence. For preschoolers, it is a part of sexual curiosity and exploration. If parents are concerned about their children masturbating, it is essential for nurses to investigate the circumstances associated with the activity because it may be an expression of anxiety, boredom, or unresolved conflicts. In the case of excessive masturbation, it may be associated with emotional or behavioral problems and physical or sexual abuse (Strachan & Staples, 2012). Management of normal childhood masturbation includes parent education and reassurance, redirection of the child to other activities, and discussion with the child regarding appropriate boundaries (Strachan & Staples, 2012). Parents should emphasize that masturbation is a private act, thus teaching children socially acceptable behavior.

Fears

A great number and variety of real and imagined fears are present during the preschool years, including fear of the dark, being left alone (especially at bedtime), animals (particularly large dogs), ghosts, sexual matters (castration), and objects or persons associated with pain. The exact cause of children's fears is often unknown. Parents often become perplexed about handling the fears because no amount of logical persuasion, coercion, or ridicule will send away the ghosts, boogeymen, monsters, and devils. Inappropriate television viewing by preschoolers may increase fears and anxieties because of the inability to separate reality-based experiences from fantasy portrayed on television.

The concept of animism (i.e., ascribing lifelike qualities to inanimate objects) helps explain why children fear objects. For example, a child may refuse to use the toilet after watching a television commercial in which the toilet bowel is portrayed as turning into a monster.

Preschoolers also experience fear of annihilation. Because of poorly defined body boundaries and improved cognitive abilities, young children develop concerns related to loss of body parts. They fear losing body parts with certain medical procedures, such as an intravenous insertion or cast application on a limb and may see these procedures as real threats to their existence. Preschoolers are often fearful when approaching the health care environment (office or hospital) and are especially fearful of pain. Because of their inability to sometimes discern reality from the imagined, a painful procedure such as a vaccination may be perceived as the end of existence (death) to the child; the preschooler is often unable to see beyond that experience. It is helpful to discuss the child's fears but maintain honesty and openness when working with preschoolers in the health care setting.

The best way to help children overcome their fears is by actively involving them in finding practical methods to deal with the frightening experience. This may be as simple as keeping a night light on in the child's bedroom for assurance that no monsters lurk in the dark. Exposing children to the feared object in a safe situation also provides a type of conditioning, or desensitization. For instance, children who are afraid of dogs should never be forced to approach or touch one, but they may be introduced gradually to the experience by watching other children play with the animal. This type of modeling, with others demonstrating fearlessness, can be effective if the child is allowed to progress at his or her own rate.

Usually by 5 or 6 years of age, children relinquish many of their fears. Explaining the developmental sequence of fears and their gradual disappearance may help parents feel more secure in handling preschoolers'

fears. Sometimes fears do not subside with simple measures or developmental maturation. When children experience severe fears that disrupt family life, professional help is required.

Stress

Although for parents the preschool years generally are less troublesome than toddlerhood, this period of life presents children with many unique stresses. Some such as fears are innate and stem from preschoolers' unique understanding of the world. Others are imposed, such as beginning school. Although minimal amounts of stress are beneficial during the early years to help children develop effective coping skills, excessive stress is harmful. Young children are especially vulnerable because of their limited capacity to cope. Expression of frustration, fear, or anxiety is hampered by inadequate expressive language.

To help parents deal with stress in their child's life, they must be aware of signs of stress and be helped to identify the source. Any number of stressors may be present such as the birth of a sibling, marital discord, separation and divorce, relocation, or illness.

The best approach to dealing with stress is prevention (i.e., monitoring the amount of stress in children's lives so levels do not exceed their coping ability and informing them of anticipated changes on a short-term basis). In many instances, structuring children's schedules to allow rest and preparing them for change, such as entering school, are sufficient measures.

Aggression

The term *aggression* refers to behavior that attempts to hurt a person or destroy property. Aggression differs from anger, which is a temporary emotional state, but anger may be expressed through aggression. Hyperaggressive behavior in preschoolers is characterized by unprovoked physical attacks on other children and adults, destruction of others' property, frequent intense temper tantrums, extreme impulsivity, disrespect, and noncompliance. Aggression is influenced by a complex set of biologic, sociocultural, and familial variables. Factors that tend to increase aggressive behavior are gender, frustration, modeling, and reinforcement.

Evidence indicates that types of aggression differ between genders. Boys exhibit more physical aggression than girls during preschool years (Lussier, Corrado, & Tzoumakis, 2012). Relational aggression is exhibited at similar rates in boys and girls of this age group; however, differences in the frequency of relational aggression between genders can vary depending upon peer interactions in various situations and settings (McEachern & Snyder, 2012).

Frustration, or the continual thwarting of self-satisfaction by disapproval, humiliation, punishment, or insults, can lead children to act out against others as a means of release. Especially if they fear their parents, these children displace their anger on others, particularly peers and other authority figures. This type of aggression often applies to children who are well-behaved at home but have a discipline problem at school or are bullies among their playmates.

Modeling, or imitating the behavior of significant others, is a powerful influencing force in preschoolers. Children who see their parents as physically abusive are observing behavior that they come to know as acceptable and therefore may exhibit this behavior with others (Knox, 2010). Another aspect of modeling is the "double standard" for acceptable conduct. For example, in some families aggression is synonymous with masculinity, and boys are encouraged to defend themselves. Media exposure is also a significant source for modeling at this impressionable age. Research indicates that there is a positive correlation between viewing violent programs and developing aggression; therefore, parents should be encouraged to supervise programming, especially for children with aggressive tendencies (Fitzpatrick, Barnett, & Pagani, 2012). The American

Academy of Pediatrics, Council on Communications and Media (2016) offers recommendations for media use for children 18 months to 5 years of age.

Reinforcement can also shape aggressive behavior. Sometimes the reward for aggression is negative (e.g., punishment) yet reinforcing because it brings attention. For example, children who are ignored by a parent until they hit a sibling or the parent learn that this act garners attention.

When children exhibit extreme behaviors such as aggression, parents may be concerned about the need for professional help. Generally the difference between normal and problematic behavior is not the behavior itself but its quantity (number of occurrences), severity (interference with social or cognitive functioning), distribution (different manifestations), onset (when behavior started), and duration (at least 4 weeks).*

Speech Problems

The most critical period for speech development occurs between 2 and 4 years of age. During this period, children are using their rapidly growing vocabulary faster than they can produce the words. Failure to master sensorimotor integrations results in stuttering or stammering as children try to say the word about which they are already thinking. This *dysfluency* in speech pattern is common during language development in children 2 to 5 years of age (Nelson, 2013). Stuttering affects boys more frequently than girls, has been shown to have a genetic link, and usually resolves during childhood (McQuiston & Kloczko, 2011). The National Institute on Deafness and Other Communication Disorders (2010) encourages parents and caregivers of children who stutter to speak slowly and relaxed, refrain from criticizing the child's speech, resist completing the child's sentences, and take time to listen attentively.

The best therapy for speech problems is prevention and early detection. Common causes of speech problems include hearing loss, developmental delay, autism, lack of environmental stimulation, and physical conditions that impede normal speech production (McLaughlin, 2011) Referral for further evaluation and treatment may be necessary to prevent a problem from interfering with learning. Anticipatory preparation of parents for expected developmental norms may allay caregiver concerns.

Children pressured into producing sounds ahead of their developmental level may develop *dyslalia* (articulation problems) or revert to using infantile speech. Prevention involves educating parents regarding the usual achievement of speech production during childhood. The *Denver Articulation Screening Examination* is an excellent tool for assessing articulation skills of a child and explaining to parents the expected progression of sounds.

PROMOTING OPTIMAL HEALTH DURING THE PRESCHOOL YEARS

NUTRITION

Healthy nutrition during childhood should include eating a variety of nutrient-dense foods, ensuring sufficient energy to promote growth and development, and balancing energy intake with energy expenditure to maintain a healthy weight (Kleinman & Greer, 2014). Nutritional

needs vary depending upon age, gender, activity level, and state of health. The estimated daily caloric requirement for preschoolers is 1000 to 1800 calories (Kleinman & Greer, 2014). Fluid requirements may decrease slightly to approximately 100 mL/kg/day, but requirements are affected by climatic conditions. Protein requirements increase during childhood, and the recommended intake for preschoolers is 13 to 19 g/day (0.45 to 0.67 oz/day) (US Department of Agriculture, 2011).

The American Academy of Pediatrics Committee on Nutrition recommends that the total fat intake over several days be 30% of total caloric intake for children 2 years of age and older (Kleinman & Greer, 2014). This recommendation is important in the prevention of childhood obesity and the development of other morbidities. Research has shown that the development of obesity, cardiovascular disease, diabetes, and cancer can be influenced by early eating patterns (Macaulay, Donovan, Leask, et al., 2014). While limiting fat consumption, it is also important to ensure that diets contain adequate nutrients. This can be done simultaneously as in the following example regarding calcium. The Recommended Dietary Allowance (RDA) of calcium intake for children 1 to 3 years of age is 700 mg/day, and the recommendation for children 4 to 8 years of age is 1000 mg/day (Institute of Medicine of the National Academies, 2011). Milk and dairy products are excellent sources of calcium. Low-fat and nonfat milk may be substituted for higher-fat choices, so the quantity of milk may remain the same while limiting fat intake overall.

Excessive consumption of fruit juices and other sugar-sweetened beverages has been associated with dental caries (Marshall, 2013) and adverse cardiometabolic effects (Kosova, Auinger, & Bremer, 2013). Parents should be educated regarding nonnutritious fruit drinks, which usually contain less than 10% fruit juice yet are often advertised as healthy and nutritious. When counseling parents regarding moderation in fruit juice consumption, providers should offer suggestions for more appropriate sources of nutrients such as ascorbic acid, folate, and potassium. In young children, intake of carbonated beverages that are acidic or contain high amounts of sugar is also known to contribute to dental caries; large amounts of nonnutritive calories in such beverages may also displace or preclude intake of nutrients necessary for growth.

An additional resource for dietary counseling includes MyPlate,* developed in 2011 by the U.S. Department of Agriculture. This colorful plate shows the five main food groups—fruits, grains, vegetable, protein, and dairy—with the intended purpose to involve children and their families in making appropriate food choices for meals. MyPlate provides an online interactive feature that allows the individual to select an individual food group and see choices for foods in that group. Approximate serving sizes are suggested, and vegetarian substitutions are also provided. This system is comprehensive and provides information for developing a healthy lifestyle at an early age. Parents can use this information to help their children make healthy lifestyle choices and prevent adverse health conditions secondary to poor nutrition. The importance of role modeling by parents cannot be overemphasized in regard to food intake and dietary habits; if parents will not eat a particular food or if their dietary habits are poor, children are likely to develop the same habits.

Some preschoolers still have food habits that are typical of toddlers such as food fads and strong taste preferences. When children reach 4 years of age, they enter another period of finicky eating, which is generally characteristic of the more rebellious behavior of children in this age group. As with toddlers, small portions of each item being served should be offered. The practice of having children remain at the

---

*Information on child development and behavior can be obtained through the American Academy of Pediatrics, Section on Developmental and Behavioral Pediatrics, http://www2.aap.org/sections/dbpeds.

*http://www.choosemyplate.gov/.

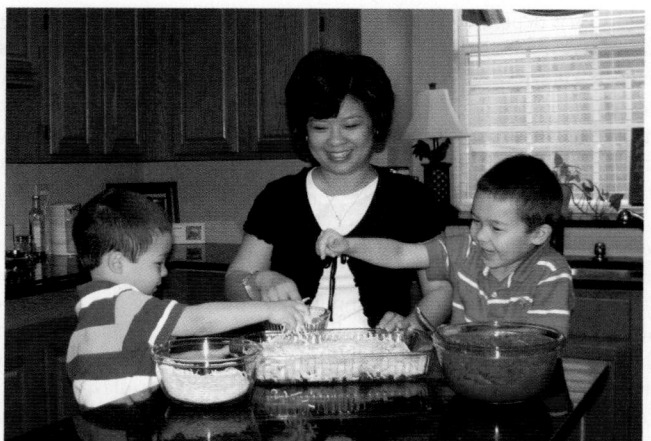

FIG 33.7 Preschool-age children enjoy helping adults and are more likely to try new foods if they can help in the preparation.

table until the plate is clean should be avoided because this may contribute to overeating and the development of poor eating habits that contribute to poor health later in life. By 5 years of age, children are more agreeable to trying new foods, especially if they are encouraged by an adult who allows them to help with food preparation or experiment with a new taste or different dish (Fig. 33.7). Mealtimes can become battlegrounds if parents expect perfect table manners.* Usually 5-year-old children are ready for the social aspects of eating, but 3- or 4-year-old children still have difficulty sitting quietly through long family meals.

The amount and variety of foods consumed by young children vary greatly from day to day. Consequently, parents sometimes worry about the quantity and quality of food that preschoolers consume. In general, the quality is much more important than the quantity, a fact that should be stressed during nutrition counseling. Eating habits are well established by 5 years of age, with the major contributing factor being the family, especially the parents.

> **! NURSING ALERT**
>
> Obesity has increased significantly over the past three decades in young children. Efforts to provide a healthy diet and encourage physical activity should begin early to help children achieve optimal health (Rogers, Hart, Motyka, et al., 2013).

In addition to unhealthy eating habits, experts recognize that a sedentary lifestyle contributes to cardiovascular disease and obesity. Therefore, experts recommend 60 minutes of physical activity per day for children 6 years of age and older (Centers for Disease Control and Prevention, 2015). One program recommends that preschoolers be encouraged to be involved in at least 2 hours of cumulative activity per 8-hour day in day care, including unstructured free playtime (Larson, Ward, Neelon, et al., 2011).

SLEEP AND ACTIVITY

Sleep patterns vary widely, but the average preschooler sleeps about 12 hours a night and infrequently takes daytime naps. Waking during the night is common throughout early childhood. An appropriate and consistent bedtime, nap schedule (as needed), and bedtime routine can help prevent and treat common sleep problems and night wakings experienced by young children (Honaker & Meltzer, 2014).

Motor activity levels continue to be high and allow preschoolers to explore their environment, begin learning physical games and sports, and interact with others. Sedentary activities such as television and video or computer games are increasingly appealing and can become unhealthy substitutes for active play.

Preschoolers' increased gross motor abilities and coordination allow them to engage in many physical activities, if only at a novice level. At this age, children benefit from free play and exposure to a variety of physical activities (Stricker, 2014). Whether young children should begin formalized training in an activity at this early age is controversial. The decision to participate should be based on the child's, not the parent's, motivation and enjoyment. Another key aspect of organized play for preschoolers is that the activity is developmentally appropriate and occurs in a nonthreatening, fun, and safe environment.

Sleep Problems

The preschool years are a prime time for sleep disturbances. Children may have trouble going to sleep, wake during the night, have difficulty resuming sleep after waking during the night, have nightmares or sleep terrors, or prolong the inevitable bedtime through elaborate rituals. Such sleep disturbances are typically related to increasing autonomy, negative sleep associations, nighttime fears, inconsistent bedtime routines, and lack of limit setting (Babcock, 2011).

Consequences of inadequate sleep include daytime tiredness, behavior changes, hyperactivity, difficulty concentrating, impaired learning ability, poor control of emotions and impulses, and strain on family relationships (Bhargava, 2011). Nurses should incorporate assessment of sleep patterns and education about the development of healthy sleep behaviors into every well-child visit. Recommendations for handling a sleep disturbance are offered only after a thorough assessment (Table 33.2). Cultural traditions may dictate sleep practices contrary to certain well-accepted professional recommendations. Thus, parents may not perceive particular sleep habits as problematic.

Interventions differ greatly; for example, *nightmares* and *sleep terrors* require different approaches (see Table 33.2). For children who delay going to bed, a recommended approach involves a consistent bedtime ritual and emphasizing the normalcy of this type of behavior in young children. Parents should ignore attention-seeking behavior and not take the child into the parents' bed or allow him or her to stay up past a reasonable hour. Other measures that may be helpful include keeping a light on in the room, providing transitional objects such as a favorite toy, or leaving a drink of water by the bed.

Helping children slow down before bedtime also reduces the resistance to going to bed. One strategy is to establish limited rituals that signal readiness for bed such as a bath or story. Parents can reinforce the pattern by stating, "After this story it's bedtime," and consistently carrying out the routine. If anticipated extra stimulation, such as having visitors arrive at bedtime, disrupts this routine, it is advisable to settle children in bed beforehand. Television viewing before bedtime may cause bedtime resistance and delay sleep.

---

*Excellent resources for parents related to mealtimes with toddlers and preschoolers include Jana, L.A., & Shu, J. (2012). *Food fights: winning the nutritional challenges of parenthood armed with insight, humor, and a bottle of ketchup* (2nd ed.). Elk Grove Village, IL: American Academy of Pediatrics, & Satter, E. (2005). *Your child's weight, helping without harming.* Madison, WI: Kelcy Press.

TABLE 33.2 Comparison of Nightmares to Sleep Terrors

Characteristics	Nightmares	Sleep Terrors
Description	A scary dream; takes place during REM sleep and is followed by full waking	A partial arousal from very deep sleep (state IV, non-REM) sleep
Time of distress	After dream is over, child wakes and cries or calls; not during nightmare itself	During terror itself, as child screams and thrashes; afterward is calm
Time of occurrence	In second half of night, when dreams are most intense	Usually 1 to 4 hours after falling asleep, when non-REM sleep is deepest
Child's behavior	Crying in younger children, fright in all; behaviors persistent even though child is awake	Initially may sit up, thrash, or run in bizarre manner; may cry, scream, talk, or moan; shows apparent fright, anger, or obvious confusion, which disappears when child is fully awake
Responsiveness to others	Is aware of and reassured by another's presence	Is not aware of another's presence, is not comforted, and may push person away and scream and thrash more if held or restrained
Return to sleep	May be considerably delayed because of persistent fear	Usually rapid; often difficult to keep child awake
Description of dream interventions	Accept dream as real fear	Requires little intervention
	Sit with child; offer comfort, assurance, and sense of protection	No memory of dream or of yelling or thrashing
	Avoid forcing child back to his or her own bed	Intervene only if necessary to protect child from injury
	Consider professional counseling for recurrent nightmares	Guide child back to bed if needed

Modified from Haupt, M., Sheldon, S.H., & Loghmanee, D. (2013). Just a scary dream? A brief review of sleep terrors, nightmares, and rapid eye movement sleep behavior disorder. *Pediatric Annals, 42*(10), 211–216.

DENTAL HEALTH

By the beginning of the preschool period, the eruption of the deciduous (primary) teeth is complete. Dental care is essential to preserve these temporary teeth and teach good dental habits (see Chapter 32). Although preschoolers' fine motor control is improved, they still require assistance and supervision with brushing, and flossing should be performed by parents. Professional care and prophylaxis, especially fluoride supplements (if needed), should be continued. The frequency of professional dental care should be based on a child's individual risk assessment, including family history, socioeconomic status, dental development, presence or absence of dental disease, special health care needs, and dietary habits (American Academy of Pediatric Dentistry, 2013). Trauma to teeth during this period is common, and prompt evaluation by a dentist is warranted if oral trauma occurs. Preservation of the space previously occupied by an avulsed tooth is necessary for proper eruption of the secondary tooth.

SAFETY PROMOTION AND INJURY PREVENTION

Because of improved gross and fine motor skills, coordination, and balance, preschoolers are less prone to falls than toddlers. They tend to be less reckless; listen more to parental rules; and are aware of potential dangers such as hot objects, sharp instruments, and dangerous heights. Putting objects in the mouth as part of exploration has all but ceased, although accidental poisoning is still a danger. Pedestrian motor vehicle injuries increase because of activities such as playing in the parking lot, driveway, or street; riding tricycles, bicycles, and other play vehicles; running after balls; or forgetting safety regulations when crossing streets.

In general, the guidelines suggested for injury prevention in Table 32.4 apply to children in this age-group as well. However, emphasis is now on education concerning safety and potential hazards in addition to appropriate protection. This is an excellent time to start enforcing the use of safety items such as bicycle helmets to prevent head trauma; children are less likely to warm to the idea later in life because of peer pressure. Because preschoolers are great imitators, it is essential that parents set a good example by "practicing what they preach." Children quickly observe discrepancies in what they are told to do and what they see others do. Establishing habits at this time, such as wearing protective equipment, can create long-term safety behaviors.

ANTICIPATORY GUIDANCE—CARE OF FAMILIES

The preschool years present fewer childrearing difficulties than do earlier years, and this stage of development is facilitated by appropriate anticipatory guidance in the areas already discussed (see Family-Centered Care box: Guidance During Preschool Years). There is a shift in childrearing practices from protection to education. Whereas injury prevention previously focused on safeguarding the immediate environment with less emphasis on reasoning, now the protective guardrails or electrical outlet caps may be replaced by verbal explanations of why danger exists and how to avoid it.

During this period, an emotional transition between parent and child occurs. Although children are still attached to their parents and accept all their values and beliefs, they are nearing the period of life when they will question previous teachings and prefer the companionship of peers. Entry into school marks a separation for parents and for children. Parents may need help in adjusting to this change, particularly if one parent has focused his or her daily activities primarily on home responsibilities. All family members must adjust to changes, which is part of the process of growth and development.

INFECTIOUS CONDITIONS: COMMUNICABLE DISEASES

The incidence of childhood communicable diseases has declined significantly since the advent of immunizations. Serious complications resulting from such infections have been reduced further with the use of antibiotics and antitoxins. However, infectious diseases do occur, and nurses must

FAMILY-CENTERED CARE

Guidance During Preschool Years

3 Years of Age
- Prepare parents for child's increasing interest in widening relationships.
- Encourage enrollment in preschool.
- Emphasize importance of setting limits.
- Prepare parents to expect exaggerated tension-reduction behaviors such as need for a "security blanket."
- Encourage parents to offer child choices.
- Prepare parents to expect marked changes at 3½ years, when child becomes insecure and exhibits emotional extremes.
- Prepare parents for normal dysfluency in speech, and advise them to avoid focusing on the pattern.
- Prepare parents to expect extra demands on their attention as a reflection of child's emotional insecurity and fear of loss of love.
- Warn parents that the equilibrium of a 3-year-old will change to the aggressive, out-of-bounds behavior of a 4-year-old.
- Inform parents to anticipate a more stable appetite with more food selections.
- Stress need for protection and education of child to prevent injury (see the "Safety Promotion and Injury Prevention" section later in this chapter.

4 Years of Age
- Prepare parents for more aggressive behavior, including motor activity and offensive language.
- Prepare parents to expect resistance to parental authority.
- Explore parental feelings regarding child's behavior.
- Suggest some type of respite for primary caregivers, such as placing child in preschool for part of the day.
- Prepare parents for child's increasing sexual curiosity.
- Emphasize importance of realistic limit setting on behavior and appropriate disciplinary techniques.
- Prepare parents for the highly imaginative 4-year-old who indulges in "tall tales" (to be differentiated from lies) and develops imaginary playmates.
- Prepare parents to expect nightmares or an increase in them.
- Provide reassurance that period of calmness begins at 5 years of age.

5 Years of Age
- Inform parents to expect tranquil period at 5 years of age.
- Help parents prepare children for entrance into school environment.
- Make certain that childhood immunizations are up to date before child enters school.
- Suggest that unemployed parental caregivers consider own activities when children begin school.

be familiar with the infectious agent to recognize the disease and institute appropriate preventive and supportive interventions (Table 33.3).

CARE MANAGEMENT

Table 33.3 describes the more common communicable diseases of childhood, their therapeutic management, and specific nursing care. The following is a general discussion of nursing care management for communicable diseases.

Identification of the infectious agent is of primary importance to prevent exposure of susceptible individuals. Nurses in ambulatory care settings, child care centers, and schools are often the first people to see signs of a communicable disease such as a rash or sore throat. The

nurse must operate under a high index of suspicion for common childhood diseases to identify potentially infectious cases and recognize diseases that require medical intervention. An example is the common complaint of sore throat. Although most often a symptom of a minor viral infection, it can signal an infection such as a streptococcal infection. Each of these bacterial conditions requires appropriate medical treatment to prevent serious sequelae.

When a communicable disease is suspected, it is important to assess the following:
- Recent exposure to a known case
- Prodromal symptoms (symptoms that occur between early manifestations of the disease and its overt clinical syndrome) or evidence of constitutional symptoms such as a fever or rash (see Table 33.3)
- Immunization history.
- History of having the disease

Immunizations are available for many diseases, and infection usually confers lifelong immunity; therefore the possibility of many infectious agents can be eliminated based on these criteria.

Prevent Spread

Prevention consists of two components: prevention of the disease and control of its spread to others. Primary prevention rests almost exclusively on immunizations.

Control measures to prevent spread of disease should include techniques to reduce risk of cross-transmission of infectious organisms between patients and protect health care workers from organisms harbored by patients. If a child is hospitalized, facility policies for infection control should be followed (see Chapter 39). The most important procedure is hand washing. People directly caring for children and handling contaminated articles must wash their hands and practice effective Standard Precautions in care of their patients.

Instruct children to practice good hand-washing technique before eating and after toileting. For diseases spread by droplets, instruct the parents in measures to reduce airborne transmission. Children who are old enough should use a tissue to cover their faces when coughing or sneezing; otherwise the parent should cover the child's mouth with a tissue and then discard it. Stress to the family the usual hygiene measures of not sharing eating and drinking utensils.

Prevent Complications

Although most children recover without difficulty, certain groups are at risk for serious, even fatal, complications from communicable diseases, especially the viral diseases chickenpox and erythema infectiosum (fifth disease) caused by human parvovirus B19.

Children with immunodeficiency (i.e., those receiving steroid or other immunosuppressive therapy, those with a generalized malignancy such as leukemia or lymphoma, and those with an immunologic disorder) are at risk for viremia from replication of the varicella-zoster virus* in the blood. Varicella occurs primarily in children younger than 15 years of age. However, it leaves the threat of herpes zoster, an intensely painful varicella that is localized to a single dermatome (body area innervated by a particular segment of the spinal cord). In children, the dermatomes most likely affected by herpes zoster are the cervical, lumbar, and thoracic dermatomes (Weinmann, Chun, Schmid, et al., 2013). Immunocompromised patients and healthy infants younger than 1 year of age (who also have reduced immunity) are at a higher risk for reactivation of varicella causing herpes zoster, probably as a result of a deficiency

---

*Educational materials may be obtained from the National Shingles Foundation, 603 West 115th Street, Suite 371, New York, NY 10025, 212-222-3390, www.vzvfoundation.org.

in cellular immunity (American Academy of Pediatrics, Committee on Infectious Diseases, 2015). Complications of herpes zoster virus in children include secondary bacterial infection, depigmentation, and rarely postherpetic neuralgia and scarring. The use of varicella-zoster immune globulin or intravenous immune globulin (IVIG) is recommended for children who are immunocompromised, who have no previous history of varicella, and who are likely to contract the disease and have complications as a result (American Academy of Pediatrics, Committee on Infectious Diseases, 2015). The antiviral agent acyclovir or valacyclovir may be used to treat varicella infections in susceptible immunocompromised people. It is effective in decreasing the number of lesions; shortening the duration of fever; and decreasing itching, lethargy, and anorexia.

Children with hemolytic disease, such as sickle cell disease, are at risk for aplastic anemia from erythema infectiosum. Human parvovirus B19 infects and lyses red blood cell precursors, thus interrupting the production of red blood cells. Therefore, the virus may precipitate a severe aplastic crisis in patients who need increased red blood cell production to maintain normal red blood cell volumes. Thrombocytopenia and neutropenia may also occur as a result of human parvovirus B19 infection. The fetus has a relatively high rate of red blood cell production and an immature immune system; the fetus may develop severe anemia and hydrops as a result of maternal human parvovirus infection. Fetal death rates as a result of human parvovirus B19 have been estimated to be between 2% and 6% (Koch, 2016; American Academy of Pediatrics, Committee on Infectious Diseases, 2015).

In the past decade, the incidence of pertussis has increased, particularly in infants younger than 6 months of age and children 10 to 14 years of age. Early clinical manifestations of pertussis in infants may include gagging, a dry, unproductive cough, nasal discharge, and low grade fever; the typical "whoop" associated with the disease is absent (Bentley, Pinfield, & Rouse, 2013). In older children, the disease may manifest as a common cold (see Table 33.3). It is now recommended that children 11 to 18 years of age receive a booster pertussis vaccine (tetanus and acellular pertussis [Tdap]) to prevent the disease. Because pertussis is contagious, especially among close household members, identify pertussis early and initiate treatment for the child and those who have been exposed. Azithromycin (for infants younger than 1 month of age) and erythromycin, clarithromycin, or azithromycin are administered to infants and children with pertussis (American Academy of Pediatrics, Committee on Infectious Diseases, 2015).

Prevention of complications from diseases such as diphtheria, pertussis, and scarlet fever requires compliance with antibiotic therapy. With oral preparations, stress the need to complete the entire course of therapy.

Provide Comfort

Many communicable diseases cause skin manifestations that are bothersome to children. The chief discomfort from most rashes is itching, and measures such as cool baths (usually without soap) and lotions (e.g., calamine) are helpful.

> **! NURSING ALERT**
>
> When lotions with active ingredients such as diphenhydramine in Caladryl are used, they are applied sparingly, especially over open lesions, where excessive absorption can lead to drug toxicity. Use these lotions with caution in children who are simultaneously receiving an oral antihistamine. Cooling the lotion in the refrigerator beforehand often makes it more soothing on the skin than at room temperature.

To avoid overheating, which increases itching, children should wear lightweight, loose, nonirritating clothing and keep out of the sun. If the child persists in scratching, keep the nails short and smooth, or use mittens and clothes with long sleeves or legs. For severe itching, antipruritic medication such as diphenhydramine (Benadryl) or hydroxyzine (Atarax) may be required, especially when the child has trouble sleeping because of itching. Loratadine, cetirizine, and fexofenadine do not cause drowsiness and may be preferred for urticaria during the day.

An elevated temperature is common, and both antipyretic medicine (acetaminophen or ibuprofen) and environmental manipulation are implemented (see the "Controlling Elevated Temperatures" section in Chapter 39). Acetaminophen is effective in lowering the fever but does not significantly reduce the symptoms of itching, anorexia, abdominal pain, fussiness, or vomiting.

A sore throat, another frequent symptom, is managed with lozenges, saline rinses (if the child is old enough to cooperate), and analgesics. Because most children are anorectic during an illness, bland foods and increased liquids are usually preferred. During the early stages of the disease, children voluntarily curtail their activity; and, although bed rest is beneficial, it should not be imposed unless specifically indicated. During periods of irritability quiet activity (e.g., reading, music, television, video games, puzzles, or coloring) helps distract children from the discomfort.

Support Child and Family

Most communicable diseases are benign, but may produce considerable concern and anxiety for parents. Often the occurrence of a disease, such as chickenpox, is the first time the child is acutely uncomfortable. Parents need assistance to cope with manifestations of the illness such as intense itching. The family and child need reassurance that generally recovery is rapid. However, visible signs of the dermatosis may be present for some time after the child is well enough to resume usual activities.

INTESTINAL PARASITIC DISEASES

Intestinal parasitic diseases, including helminths (worms) and protozoa, constitute the most frequent infections in the world. In the United States, the incidence of intestinal parasitic disease, especially giardiasis, has increased among young children who attend day care centers. Young children are especially at risk because of typical hand-mouth activity and uncontrolled fecal activity. Various infecting organisms cause intestinal parasitic diseases in humans. This discussion is limited to the two most common parasitic infections among children in the United States: giardiasis and pinworms.

GIARDIASIS

Giardiasis is caused by the protozoan *Giardia intestinalis* (formerly called *Giardia lamblia* and *Giardia duodenalis*). It is the most common intestinal parasitic pathogen in the United States. The potential for transmission is great because the cysts—the nonmotile stage of the protozoa—can survive in the environment for months. Chief modes of transmission are person to person, food, and animals, especially puppies. Contaminated water, especially in mountain lakes and streams, and swimming or wading pools frequented by diapered infants are common sources of transmission. In children, person-to-person transmission is the most likely cause. Child care centers and institutions providing care for persons with developmental disabilities are common sites for urban giardiasis, and the children may pass cysts for months. Although individuals infected with giardiasis may be asymptomatic, common symptoms include abdominal cramps and diarrhea (Box 33.1).

BOX 33.1 Clinical Manifestations of Giardiasis

Infants and young children:
 Diarrhea
 Vomiting
 Anorexia
 Growth failure (failure to thrive)—if chronic exposure
Children older than 5 years of age:
 Abdominal cramps
 Intermittent loose stools
 Constipation
Stools that are malodorous, watery, pale, and greasy
Spontaneous resolution of most infections in 4 to 6 weeks
Rare, chronic form:
 Intermittent loose, foul-smelling stools
 Possibility of abdominal bloating, flatulence, sulfur-tasting belches, epigastric
  pain, vomiting, headache, and weight loss

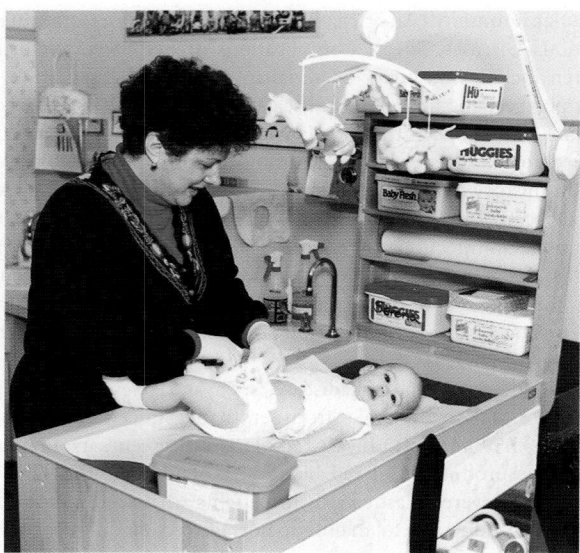

FIG 33.8 Prevention of giardiasis, especially in day care centers, requires sanitary practices during diaper changes, such as discarding paper diapers in a covered receptacle, changing paper covers on the diaper-changing surface, and having facilities for hand washing nearby. Note: Soiled cloth diapers and clothing should be stored in a plastic bag for transport home.

Diagnosis of giardiasis may be made by microscopic examination of stool specimens or duodenal fluid or by identification of *G. intestinalis* antigens in these specimens by techniques such as enzyme immunoassay (EIA) and direct fluorescent antibody (DFA) assays. Because the *Giardia* organisms live in the upper intestine and are excreted in a highly variable pattern, repeated microscopic examination of stool specimens may be required to identify trophozoites (active parasites) or cysts. Duodenal specimens are obtained by direct aspiration, biopsy, or the string test. In the string test, the child swallows a gelatin capsule with a nylon string attached. Several hours later, the string is withdrawn, and the contents are sent for laboratory analysis.

Therapeutic Management

The drugs of choice for treatment of giardiasis are metronidazole (Flagyl), tinidazole (Tindamax), and nitazoxanide (Alinia). Tinidazole is said to have an 80% to 100% cure rate after a single dose (American Academy of Pediatrics, Committee on Infectious Diseases, 2015). Metronidazole and tinidazole have a metallic taste and gastrointestinal side effects, including nausea and vomiting. Nitazoxanide does not have a bitter taste and should be taken with food to avoid gastrointestinal symptoms; it reportedly has very few adverse effects and is available in suspension form. Alternative drug therapy includes albendazole, furazolidone, and quinacrine (John, 2016). Quinacrine is only available from a compounding pharmacy.

Care Management

The most important nursing consideration is prevention of giardiasis and education of parents, child care center staff, and others who assume the daily care of small children. Attention to meticulous sanitary practices, especially during diaper changes, is essential (Fig. 33.8). Nurses can play an important role in educating parents of small children and day care staff regarding appropriate sanitation. In addition, discourage young children who are infected or who have diarrhea from swimming in community or private pools until they have been infection free for 2 weeks (American Academy of Pediatrics, Committee on Infectious Diseases, 2015). Lakes and streams may contain high numbers of Giardia spore cysts, which can be swallowed in the water. Discourage children from swimming in stagnant bodies of water and in water where there are known infected children swimming when there is a high chance of swallowing water. After children are infected, family education regarding drug administration is essential.

BOX 33.2 Clinical Manifestations of Pinworms

Intense perianal itching is the principal symptom. Evidence of itching in young
 children includes the following:
 General irritability
 Restlessness
 Poor sleep
 Bed-wetting
 Distractibility
 Short attention span
 Perianal dermatitis and excoriation secondary to itching
 If worms migrate, possible vaginal (vulvovaginitis) and urethral infection

ENTEROBIASIS (PINWORMS)

Enterobiasis, or pinworms, caused by the nematode *Enterobius vermicularis*, is the most common helminthic infection in the United States. It is universally present in temperate climatic zones and may infect more than 30% of all children at any one time. Crowded conditions, such as in classrooms and day care centers, favor transmission. Infection begins when the eggs are ingested or inhaled (the eggs float in the air). The eggs hatch in the upper intestine and then mature and migrate through the intestine. After mating, adult females migrate out the anus and lay eggs (American Academy of Pediatrics, Committee on Infectious Diseases, 2015). The movement of the worms on skin and mucous membrane surfaces causes intense itching. As the child scratches, eggs are deposited on the hands and underneath the fingernails. The typical hand-to-mouth activity of youngsters makes them especially prone to reinfection. Pinworm eggs persist in the indoor environment for 2 to 3 weeks, contaminating anything they contact, such as toilet seats, doorknobs, bed linen, underwear, and food. Except for the intense rectal itching associated with pinworms, the clinical manifestations are nonspecific (Box 33.2).

Text continued on p. 926

TABLE 33.3   Communicable Diseases of Childhood

Disease	Clinical Manifestations	Therapeutic Management and Complications	Care Management
Chickenpox (Varicella) (Fig. 33.9) **Agents:** Varicella-zoster virus (VZV) **Source:** Primary secretions of respiratory tract of infected people; to a lesser degree skin lesions (scabs not infectious) **Transmission:** Direct contact, droplet (airborne) spread, and contaminated objects **Incubation period:** 2 to 3 weeks, usually 14 to 16 days **Period of communicability:** Probably 1 day before eruption of lesions (prodromal period) until all lesions have crusted	**Prodromal stage:** Slight fever, malaise, and anorexia for first 24 hours; rash highly pruritic; begins as macule, rapidly progresses to papule and then vesicle (surrounded by erythematous base, becomes umbilicated and cloudy, breaks easily and forms crusts); all three stages (papule, vesicle, crust) present in varying degrees at one time **Distribution:** Centripetal, spreading to face and proximal extremities but sparse on distal limbs and less on areas not exposed to heat (i.e., from clothing or sun) **Constitutional signs and symptoms:** Elevated temperature from lymphadenopathy, irritability from pruritus	**Supportive:** Diphenhydramine hydrochloride or antihistamines to relieve itching; skin care to prevent secondary bacterial infection **Specific:** Antiviral agent acyclovir or valacyclovir for children at high risk (see text); varicella-zoster immunoglobulin or intravenous immunoglobulin (IVIG) after exposure in high-risk children only (see text) **Complications:** Secondary bacterial infections (abscesses, cellulitis, necrotizing fasciitis, pneumonia, sepsis) Encephalitis Varicella pneumonia (rare in healthy children) Hemorrhagic varicella (tiny hemorrhages in vesicles and numerous petechiae in skin) Chronic or transient thrombocytopenia **Preventive:** Childhood immunization	Maintain Standard, Airborne, and Contact Precautions if hospitalized until all lesions are crusted; for immunized child with mild breakthrough varicella, isolate until no new lesions are seen. Keep child in home away from susceptible individuals until vesicles have dried (usually 1 week after onset of disease), and isolate high-risk children from infected children. Provide skin care; give bath and change clothes and linens daily; administer topical calamine lotion; keep child's fingernails short and clean; apply mittens if child scratches. Keep child cool (may decrease number of lesions). Lessen pruritus; keep child occupied; use oatmeal or baking soda baths to minimize pruritus. Remove loose crusts that rub and irritate skin. Teach child to apply pressure to pruritic area rather than scratching it. *Avoid use of aspirin* (possible association with Reye syndrome).

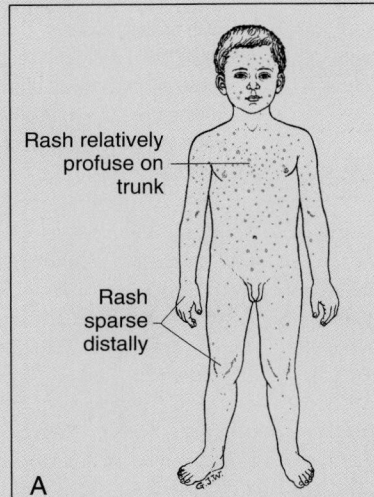
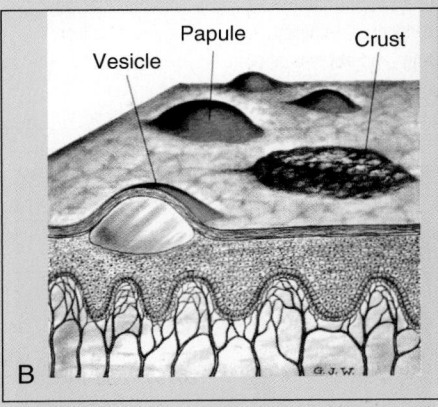
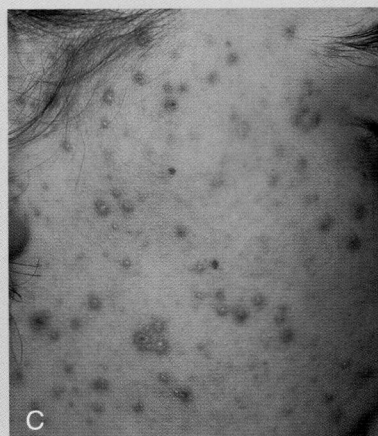

Rash relatively profuse on trunk

Rash sparse distally

Vesicle   Papule   Crust

A   B   C

FIG 33.9 Chickenpox (varicella). **A,** Progression of disease. **B,** Simultaneous stages of lesions. **C,** Clinical view. (C, From Habif, T.P. [2016]. *Clinical dermatology: A color guide to diagnosis and therapy* [6th ed.]. St. Louis, MO: Elsevier.)

Continued

TABLE 33.3 Communicable Diseases of Childhood—cont'd

Disease	Clinical Manifestations	Therapeutic Management and Complications	Care Management
Diphtheria			
Agent: *Corynebacterium diphtheriae* **Source:** Discharges from mucous membranes of nose and nasopharynx, skin, and other lesions of infected person **Transmission:** Direct contact with infected person, a carrier, or contaminated articles **Incubation period:** Usually 2 to 5 days, possibly longer **Period of communicability:** Varies; until virulent bacilli are no longer present (identified by three negative cultures); usually 2 weeks, but as long as 4 weeks	Vary according to anatomic location of pseudomembrane **Nasal:** Resembles common cold, serosanguineous mucopurulent nasal discharge without constitutional symptoms; may be frank epistaxis **Tonsillar/pharyngeal:** Malaise; anorexia; sore throat; low-grade fever; pulse increased above expected within 24 hours; smooth, adherent, white or gray membrane; lymphadenitis possibly pronounced ("bull's neck"); in severe cases, toxemia, septic shock, and death within 6 to 10 days **Laryngeal:** Fever, hoarseness, cough, with or without previous signs listed; potential airway obstruction, apprehensive, dyspneic retractions, cyanosis	Equine antitoxin (usually intravenously); preceded by skin or conjunctival test to rule out sensitivity to horse serum Antibiotics (penicillin G procaine or erythromycin) in addition to equine antitoxin Complete bed rest (prevention of myocarditis) Tracheostomy for airway obstruction Treatment of infected contacts and carriers **Complications:** Toxic cardiomyopathy (second to third week) Toxic neuropathy **Preventive:** Childhood immunization	Follow Standard and Droplet Precautions until two cultures are negative for *C. diphtheriae;* use Contact Precautions with cutaneous manifestations. Administer antibiotics in timely manner. Participate in sensitivity testing; have epinephrine available. Administer complete care to maintain bed rest. Use suctioning as needed. Observe respiration for signs of obstruction. Administer humidified oxygen as prescribed.
Erythema Infectiosum (Fifth Disease) (Fig. 33.10)			
Agent: Human parvovirus B19 **Source:** Infected persons, mainly school-age children **Transmission:** Respiratory secretions, blood, and blood products **Incubation period:** 4 to 14 days; may be as long as 21 days **Period of communicability:** Uncertain, but before onset of symptoms in children with aplastic crisis	Rash appearing in three stages: **I:** Erythema on face, chiefly on cheeks, "slapped face" appearance; disappears by 1 to 4 days **II:** About 1 day after rash appears on face, maculopapular red spots appear, symmetrically distributed on upper and lower extremities; rash progresses from proximal (trunk) to distal surfaces and may last more than 1 week. **III:** Rash subsides but reappears if skin is irritated or traumatized (sun, heat, cold, friction). In children with aplastic crisis, rash usually absent; prodromal illness includes fever, myalgia, lethargy, nausea, vomiting, and abdominal pain Child with sickle cell disease may have concurrent vaso-occlusive crisis.	**Supportive:** Antipyretics, analgesics, antiinflammatory drugs Possible blood transfusion for transient aplastic anemia **Complications:** Self-limited arthritis and arthralgia (arthritis may become chronic); more common in adult women May result in serious complications (anemia, hydrops) or fetal death if mother infected during pregnancy (primarily second trimester) Aplastic crisis in children with hemolytic disease or immunodeficiency Myocarditis (rare)	Isolation of child is not necessary, except hospitalized child (immunosuppressed or with aplastic crises) suspected of human parvovirus infection is placed on Droplet and Standard Precautions. Pregnant women need not be excluded from workplace where parvovirus infection is present; they should not care for patients with aplastic crises. Explain low risk of fetal death to those in contact with affected children; assist with routine fetal ultrasound for detection of fetal hydrops.

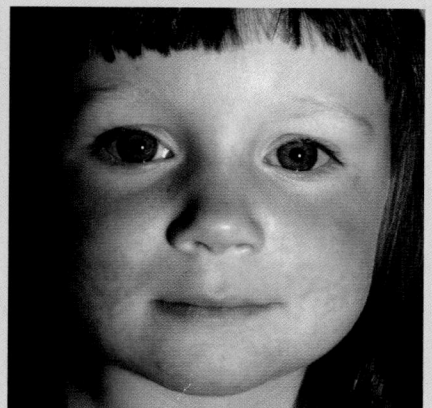

FIG 33.10 Erythema infectiosum. (From Habif, T.P. [2016]. *Clinical dermatology: A color guide to diagnosis and therapy* [6th ed.]. St. Louis, MO: Elsevier.)

TABLE 33.3 Communicable Diseases of Childhood—cont'd

Disease	Clinical Manifestations	Therapeutic Management and Complications	Care Management
Exanthem Subitum (Roseola Infantum; Sixth Disease) (Fig. 33.11)			
Agent: Human herpesvirus type 6 (HHV-6; rarely HHV-7) **Source:** Possibly acquired from saliva of healthy adult; entry via nasal, buccal, or conjunctival mucosa **Transmission:** Year-round; no reported contact with infected individual in most cases (virtually limited to children under 3 years of age, but peak age is between 6 and 15 months of age) **Incubation period:** Usually 5 to 15 days **Period of communicability:** Unknown	Persistent high fever for 3 to 7 days in child who appears well Precipitous drop in fever to normal with appearance of rash Bulging fontanel **Rash:** Discrete rose-pink macules or maculopapules appearing first on trunk, then spreading to neck, face, and extremities; nonpruritic, fades on pressure, lasts 1 to 2 days **Associated signs and symptoms:** Cervical/postauricular lymphadenopathy, inflamed pharynx, cough, coryza	Nonspecific Antipyretics to control fever **Complications:** Recurrent febrile seizures (possibly from latent infection of central nervous system that is reactivated by fever) Encephalitis Hepatitis (rare)	Use Standard Precautions Teach parents measures for lowering temperature (antipyretic drugs); ensure adequate parental understanding of specific antipyretic dosage to prevent accidental overdose. If child is prone to seizures, discuss appropriate precautions and possibility of recurrent febrile seizures. Ensure adequate oral fluid intake.

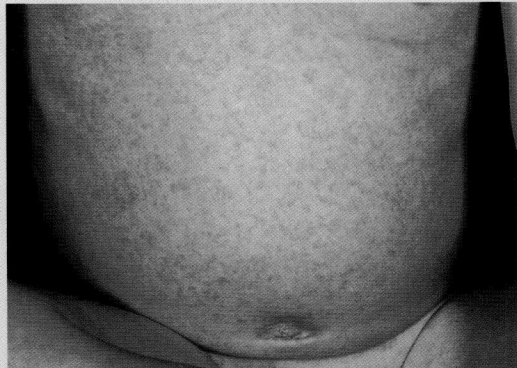

FIG 33.11 Roseola infantum. (From Habif, T.P. [2016]. *Clinical dermatology: A color guide to diagnosis and therapy* [6th ed.]. St. Louis, MO: Elsevier.)

Disease	Clinical Manifestations	Therapeutic Management and Complications	Care Management
Measles (Rubeola) (Fig. 33.12)			
Agent: Virus **Source:** Respiratory tract secretions, blood, and urine of infected person **Transmission:** Usually by direct contact with droplets of infected person; primarily in winter **Incubation period:** 10 to 20 days **Period of communicability:** From 4 days before to 5 days after rash appears but mainly during prodromal (catarrhal) stage	**Prodromal (catarrhal) stage:** Fever and malaise, followed in 24 hours by coryza, cough, conjunctivitis, Koplik spots (small, irregular red spots with a minute, bluish-white center first seen on buccal mucosa opposite molars 2 days before rash); symptoms gradually increasing in severity until second day after rash appears, when they begin to subside **Rash:** Appears 3 to 4 days after onset of prodromal stage; begins as erythematous maculopapular eruption on face and gradually spreads downward; more severe in earlier sites (appears confluent) and less intense in later sites (appears discrete); after 3 to 4 days, assumes brownish appearance, and fine desquamation occurs over area of extensive involvement **Constitutional signs and symptoms:** Anorexia, abdominal pain, malaise, generalized lymphadenopathy	Administer vitamin A for children with acute illness: 200,000 International units for children 12 months of age and older; 100,000 International units for children 6 to 11 months of age, 50,000 International units for infants younger than 6 months of age (American Academy of Pediatrics, Committee on Infectious Diseases, 2015) **Supportive:** Bed rest during febrile period; antipyretics Antibiotics to prevent secondary bacterial infection in high-risk children **Complications:** Otitis media Pneumonia (bacterial) Obstructive laryngitis and laryngotracheitis Encephalitis (rare but has high mortality) **Preventive:** Childhood immunization	Isolate until fifth day of rash; if hospitalized, institute Airborne Precautions. Encourage rest during prodromal stage; provide quiet activity. **Fever:** Instruct parents to administer antipyretics; avoid chilling; if child is prone to seizures, institute appropriate precautions. **Eye care:** Dim lights if photophobia present; clean eyelids with warm saline solution to remove secretions or crusts; keep child from rubbing eyes. **Coryza, cough:** Use cool-mist vaporizer; protect skin around nares with layer of petrolatum; encourage fluids and soft, bland foods. **Skin care:** Keep skin clean; use tepid baths as necessary.

Continued

TABLE 33.3   Communicable Diseases of Childhood—cont'd

Disease	Clinical Manifestations	Therapeutic Management and Complications	Care Management
Mumps **Agent:** Paramyxovirus **Source:** Saliva of infected persons **Transmission:** Direct contact with or droplet spread from an infected person **Incubation period:** 14 to 21 days **Period of communicability:** Most communicable immediately before and after swelling begins	**Prodromal stage:** Fever, headache, malaise, and anorexia for 24 hours, followed by "earache" that is aggravated by chewing **Parotitis:** By third day, parotid gland(s) (either unilateral or bilateral) enlarges and reaches maximum size in 1 to 3 days; accompanied by pain and tenderness; other exocrine glands (submandibular) may also be swollen	**Supportive:** Analgesics for pain and antipyretics for fever Intravenous fluid may be necessary for child refusing to drink or vomiting because of meningoencephalitis **Complications:** Sensorineural deafness Postinfectious encephalitis Myocarditis Arthritis Hepatitis Epididymo-orchitis Oophoritis Pancreatitis Sterility (extremely rare in adult males) Meningitis **Preventive:** Childhood immunization	Maintain isolation during period of communicability; institute Droplet and Contact Precautions during hospitalization. Encourage rest and decreased activity during prodromal phase until swelling subsides. Give analgesics for pain; if child is unable to swallow pills or tablets, use elixir form. Encourage fluids and soft, bland foods; avoid foods requiring chewing. Apply hot or cold compresses to neck, whichever is more comforting. To relieve orchitis, provide warmth and local support with tight-fitting underpants.

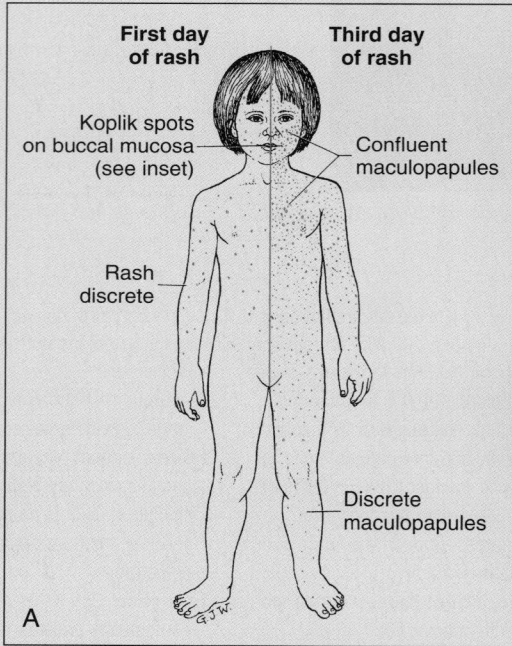

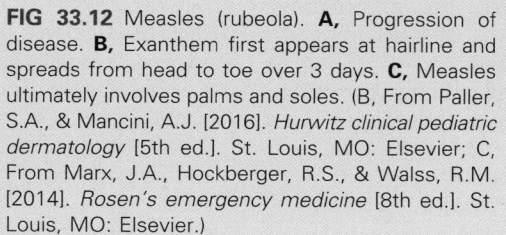

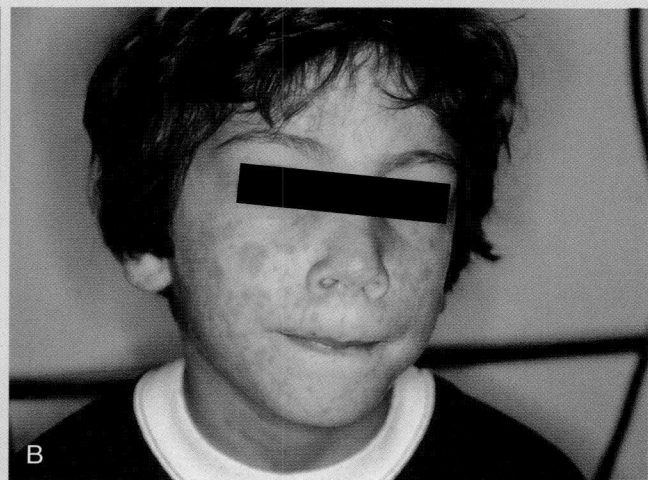

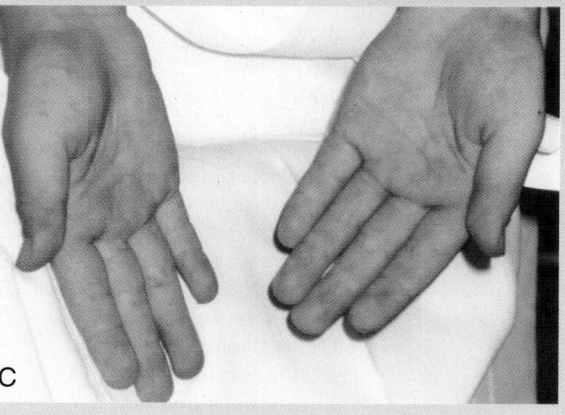

FIG 33.12 Measles (rubeola). **A,** Progression of disease. **B,** Exanthem first appears at hairline and spreads from head to toe over 3 days. **C,** Measles ultimately involves palms and soles. (B, From Paller, S.A., & Mancini, A.J. [2016]. *Hurwitz clinical pediatric dermatology* [5th ed.]. St. Louis, MO: Elsevier; C, From Marx, J.A., Hockberger, R.S., & Walss, R.M. [2014]. *Rosen's emergency medicine* [8th ed.]. St. Louis, MO: Elsevier.)

TABLE 33.3   Communicable Diseases of Childhood—cont'd

Disease	Clinical Manifestations	Therapeutic Management and Complications	Care Management
Pertussis (Whooping Cough) **Agent:** *Bordetella pertussis* **Source:** Discharge from respiratory tract of infected person **Transmission:** Direct contact or droplet spread from infected person; indirect contact with freshly contaminated articles **Incubation period:** 6 to 20 days; usually 7 to 10 days **Period of communicability:** Greatest during catarrhal stage before onset of paroxysms	**Catarrhal stage:** Begins with symptoms of upper respiratory tract infection, such as coryza, sneezing, lacrimation, cough, and low-grade fever; symptoms continue for 1 to 2 weeks when dry, hacking cough becomes more severe **Paroxysmal stage:** Cough most often occurs at night and consists of short, rapid coughs followed by sudden inspiration associated with a high-pitched crowing sound or "whoop"; during paroxysms, cheeks become flushed or cyanotic, eyes bulge, and tongue protrudes; paroxysm may continue until thick mucus plug is dislodged; vomiting frequently follows attack; stage generally lasts 4 to 6 weeks, followed by convalescent stage. Infants younger than 6 months of age may not have characteristic whoop cough but have difficulty maintaining adequate oxygenation with amount of secretions, frequent vomiting of mucus and formula or breast milk. Pertussis may occur in adolescents and adults with varying manifestations; cough and whoop may be absent, however, as many as 50% of adolescents may have a cough for up to 10 weeks (American Academy of Pediatrics, Committee on Infectious Diseases, 2015). Additional symptoms in adolescents include difficulty breathing and posttussive vomiting.	Antimicrobial therapy (e.g., erythromycin, clarithromycin, azithromycin) **Supportive:** Hospitalization sometimes required for infants, children who are dehydrated, or those who have complications Increased oxygen intake and humidity Adequate fluid intake Intensive care and mechanical ventilation may be necessary for infants younger than 6 months of age **Complications:** Pneumonia (usual cause of death in younger children) Atelectasis Otitis media Seizures Hemorrhage (scleral, conjunctival, epistaxis; pulmonary hemorrhage in neonate) Weight loss and dehydration Hernias (umbilical and inguinal) Prolapsed rectum Complications reported among adolescents include syncope, sleep disturbance, rib fractures, incontinence, and pneumonia (American Academy of Pediatrics, Committee on Infectious Diseases, 2015). **Preventive:** Immunization; childhood immunizations for pertussis does not confer lifelong immunity, so a pertussis booster is recommended for adolescents.	Maintain isolatation during catarrhal stage; if hospitalized, institute Droplet and Standard Precautions. Obtain nasopharyngeal culture for diagnosis. Encourage oral fluids; offer small amount of fluids frequently. Ensure adequate oxygenation during paroxysms; position infant on side to decrease chance of aspiration with vomiting. Provide humidified oxygen; suction as needed to prevent choking on secretions. Observe for signs of airway obstruction, such as increased restlessness, apprehension, retractions, cyanosis. Encourage compliance with antibiotic therapy for household contacts. Encourage adolescents to obtain pertussis booster (Tdap). Use Standard and Droplet Precautions in health care workers exposed to children with persistent cough and high suspicion of pertussis.
Poliomyelitis **Agent:** Enteroviruses, three types: type 1, most frequent cause of paralysis (paralytic form), both epidemic and endemic; type 2, least frequently associated with paralysis; type 3, second most frequently associated with paralysis **Source:** Feces and oropharyngeal secretions of infected persons, especially young children	May be manifested in three different forms: **Abortive or inapparent:** Fever, uneasiness, sore throat, headache, anorexia, vomiting, abdominal pain; lasts few hours to few days **Nonparalytic:** Same manifestations as abortive but more severe, with pain and stiffness in neck, back, and legs	**Supportive:** Complete bed rest during acute phase Mechanical or assisted ventilation in case of respiratory paralysis Physical therapy for muscles following acute stage	Institute Contact Precautions. Participate in physical therapy procedures (use of moist hot packs and range-of-motion exercises).

Continued

TABLE 33.3 Communicable Diseases of Childhood—cont'd

Disease	Clinical Manifestations	Therapeutic Management and Complications	Care Management
Transmission: Direct contact with persons with apparent or inapparent active infection; spread is via fecal-oral and pharyngeal-oropharyngeal routes Vaccine-acquired paralytic polio may occur as result of live oral polio vaccination (no longer available in the United States) **Incubation period:** Usually 7 to 14 days, with range of 5 to 35 days **Period of communicability:** Not exactly known; virus present in throat and feces shortly after infection and persists for about 1 week in throat and 4 to 6 weeks in feces	**Paralytic:** Initial course similar to nonparalytic type, followed by recovery and then signs of central nervous system paralysis	**Complications:** Permanent paralysis Respiratory arrest Hypertension Kidney stones from demineralization of bone during prolonged immobility **Preventive:** Childhood immunization	Position child to maintain body alignment and prevent contractures or skin breakdown; use footboard or appropriate orthoses to prevent footdrop; use pressure mattress for prolonged immobility. Encourage child to perform activities of daily living to capability, promote early ambulation with assistive devices; administer analgesics for maximum comfort during physical activity; give high-protein diet and bowel management for prolonged immobility. Observe for respiratory paralysis (difficulty in talking, ineffective cough, inability to hold breath, shallow and rapid respirations); report such signs and symptoms to practitioner.

Rubella (German Measles) (Fig. 33.13)

Agent: Rubella virus **Source:** Primarily nasopharyngeal secretions of person with apparent or inapparent infection; virus also present in blood, feces, and urine **Incubation period:** 14 to 21 days **Period of communicability:** 7 days before to about 5 days after appearance of rash **Constitutional signs and symptoms:** Occasionally low-grade fever, headache, malaise, and lymphadenopathy	**Prodromal stage:** Absent in children, present in adults and adolescents; consists of low-grade fever, headache, malaise, anorexia, mild conjunctivitis, coryza, sore throat, cough, and lymphadenopathy; lasts 1 to 5 days, subsides 1 day after appearance of rash **Rash:** First appears on face and rapidly spreads downward to neck, arms, trunk, and legs; by end of first day, body is covered with discrete, pinkish-red, maculopapular exanthema; disappears in same order as it began, and is usually gone by third day	No treatment necessary other than antipyretics for low-grade fever and analgesics for discomfort **Complications:** Rare (arthritis, encephalitis, or purpura); most benign of all childhood communicable diseases; greatest danger is teratogenic effect on fetus **Preventive:** Childhood immunization	Institute Droplet Precautions. Reassure parents of benign nature of illness in affected child. Use comfort measures as necessary. Avoid contact with pregnant woman. Monitor rubella titers in pregnant adolescent.

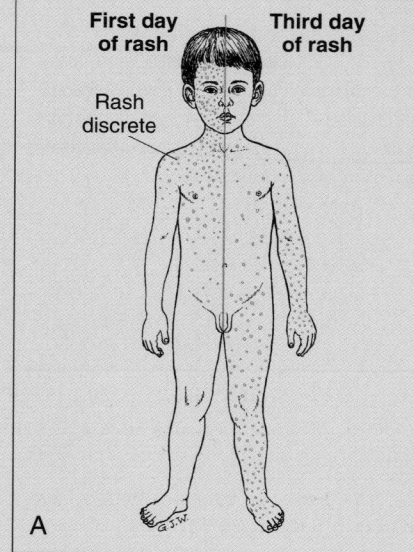

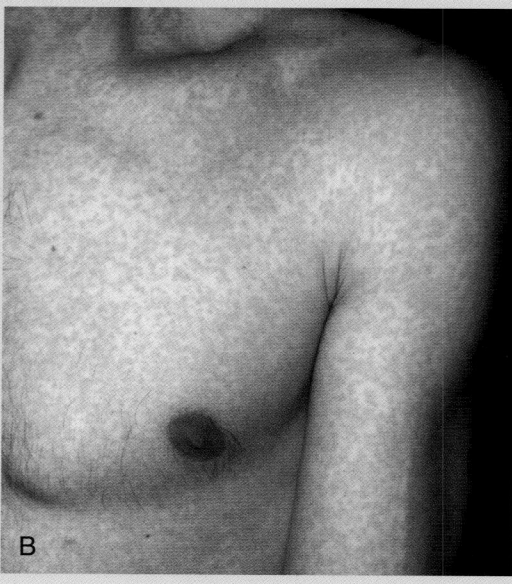

FIG 33.13 Rubella (German measles). **A,** Progression of rash. **B,** Clinical view. (B, From Habif, T.P. [2016]. *Clinical dermatology: A color guide to diagnosis and therapy* [6th ed.]. St. Louis, MO: Elsevier.)

TABLE 33.3   Communicable Diseases of Childhood—cont'd

Disease	Clinical Manifestations	Therapeutic Management and Complications	Care Management
Scarlet Fever* (Fig. 33.14) **Agent:** Group A β-hemolytic streptococci **Source:** Usually from nasopharyngeal secretions of infected persons and carriers **Transmission:** Direct contact with infected person or droplet spread; indirectly by contact with contaminated articles or ingestion of contaminated milk or other food **Incubation period:** 2 to 5 days, with range of 1 to 7 days **Period of communicability:** During incubation period and clinical illness, approximately 10 days; during first 2 weeks of carrier phase, although may persist for months	**Prodromal stage:** Abrupt high fever, pulse increased out of proportion to fever, vomiting, headache, chills, malaise, abdominal pain, halitosis **Enanthema:** Tonsils enlarged, edematous, reddened, and covered with patches of exudates; in severe cases, appearance resembles membrane seen in diphtheria; pharynx is edematous and beefy red; during first 1 to 2 days, tongue coated and papillae become red and swollen (white strawberry tongue); by fourth or fifth day, white coat sloughs off, leaving prominent papillae (red strawberry tongue); palate covered with erythematous punctate lesions **Exanthema:** Rash appears within 12 hours after prodromal signs; red pinhead-size punctate lesions rapidly become generalized but are absent on face, which becomes flushed with striking circumoral pallor; rash more intense in folds of joints; by end of first week, desquamation begins (fine, sandpaper-like on torso; sheetlike sloughing on palms and soles), which may be complete by 3 weeks or longer	Full course of penicillin (or erythromycin in penicillin-sensitive children), or oral cephalosporin Antibiotic therapy for newly diagnosed carriers (nose or throat cultures positive for streptococci) **Supportive:** Rest during febrile phase, analgesics for sore throat; antipruritics for rash if bothersome **Complications:** Peritonsillar and retropharyngeal abscess Sinusitis Otitis media Acute glomerulonephritis Acute rheumatic fever Polyarthritis (uncommon)	Institute Standard and Droplet Precautions until 24 hours after initiation of treatment. Ensure compliance with oral antibiotic therapy; intramuscular benzathine penicillin G (Bicillin) may be given. Encourage rest during febrile phase; provide quiet activity during convalescent period. Relieve discomfort of sore throat with analgesics, gargles, lozenges, antiseptic throat sprays, and inhalation of cool mist. Encourage oral fluids during febrile phase; avoid irritating liquids (certain citrus juices) or rough foods (chips); when child is able to eat, begin with soft diet. Advise parents to consult practitioner if fever persists after beginning therapy. Discuss procedures for preventing spread of infection; discard toothbrush; avoid sharing drinking and eating utensils.

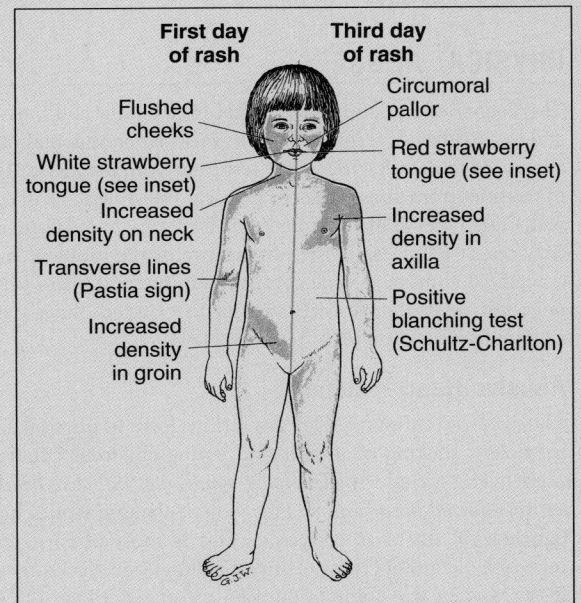

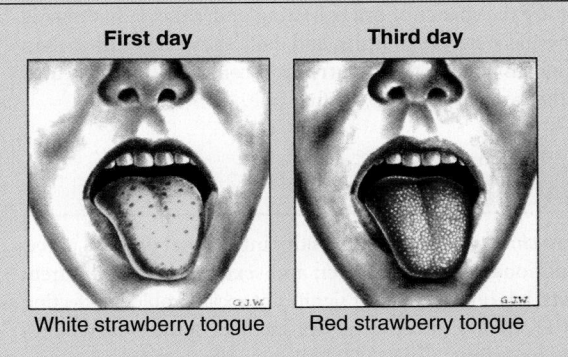

White strawberry tongue   Red strawberry tongue

FIG 33.14 Scarlet fever.

*Commonly called *streptococcal pharyngitis;* with the exception of the characteristic rash, scarlet fever and streptococcal pharyngitis have the same epidemiology, features, symptoms, signs, sequelae, and treatment (AAP, Committee on Infectious Diseases, 2015).

Diagnostic Evaluation

Diagnosis is most commonly made from the tape test (see the "Care Management" section). Repeated tests to collect eggs may be necessary (3 consecutive days in the early morning before the child washes are recommended for testing [American Academy of Pediatrics, Committee on Infectious Diseases, 2015]), and if there is a possibility that other family members may be infected, a tape test should be performed on them.

Therapeutic Management

The drugs available for treatment of pinworms include pyrantel pamoate (Pin-Rid, Antiminth) and albendazole. Mebendazole is no longer available in the United States, and it is not recommended for children younger than 2 years of age. If pyrvinium pamoate is prescribed, advise parents that the drug stains stool and vomitus bright red, as well as clothing or skin that comes in contact with the drug; it is available without prescription and should not be used in children younger than 2 years of age without consulting a primary practitioner. Because pinworms are easily transmitted, all household members should be treated. The dose of antiparasitic medication should be repeated in 2 weeks to completely eradicate the parasite and prevent reinfection.

Care Management

Direct nursing care at identifying the parasite, eradicating the organism, and preventing reinfection. Parents need clear, detailed instructions for the tape test. A loop of transparent (not "frosted" or "magic") tape, sticky side out, is placed around the end of a tongue depressor, which is then firmly pressed against the child's perianal area. A convenient, commercially prepared tape is also available for this purpose. Pinworm specimens are collected in the morning as soon as the child awakens and *before* the child has a bowel movement or bathes. The procedure may need to be performed on 3 or more consecutive days before eggs are collected. Parents are instructed to place the tongue blade in a glass jar or loosely in a plastic bag so that it can be brought in for microscopic examination. For specimens collected in the hospital, practitioner's office, or clinic, place the tape smoothly on a glass slide, sticky side down, for examination.

To prevent reinfection, washing all clothes and bed linens in hot water and vacuuming the house may be recommended. However, there is little documentation on the effectiveness of these measures because pinworms survive on many surfaces. Helpful suggestions include hand washing after toileting and before eating, keeping the child's fingernails short to minimize the chance of ova collecting under the nails, dressing children in one-piece sleeping outfits, and daily showering rather than tub bathing. Inform families that recurrence is common. Treat repeated infections in the same manner as the first one.

CHILD MALTREATMENT

The broad term *child maltreatment* includes intentional physical abuse or neglect; emotional abuse or neglect; and sexual abuse of children, usually by adults. It is one of the most significant social problems affecting children. In 2011, Child Protective Service agencies in the United States confirmed that an estimated 681,000 children were victims of one or more types of child maltreatment. Of the confirmed cases, approximately 18% suffered physical abuse, 9% sexual abuse, 79% neglect, and 8% psychologic maltreatment or emotional abuse. In 2011, there were an estimated 1570 child fatalities as a result of child abuse and neglect (US Department of Health and Human Services, 2012). Reported statistics only partially represent the actual incidence of child maltreatment because many cases are believed to be unreported.*

CHILD NEGLECT

Child neglect is the most common form of maltreatment. More than one-half of all reported cases are associated with deprivation of necessities, and 34% of deaths from maltreatment are in this group (US Department of Health and Human Services, 2012). *Neglect* is generally defined as the failure of a parent or other person legally responsible for the child's welfare to provide for her or his basic needs and an adequate level of care.

Important contributing factors for child neglect are lack of knowledge of the child's needs, lack of resources, and caregiver substance abuse. For example, neglectful parents often demonstrate poor parenting skills. They may be unaware that an infant needs to be fed every 3 to 4 hours, may not know what to feed the child, and may have insufficient funds to buy food. The most serious lack of knowledge is failure to recognize emotional nurturing as an essential need of children (see also the "Failure to Thrive" section in Chapter 31).

Types of Neglect

Neglect takes many forms and can be classified broadly as physical or emotional maltreatment. *Physical neglect* involves the deprivation of necessities such as food, clothing, shelter, supervision, medical care, and education. *Emotional neglect* generally refers to failure to meet the child's needs for affection, attention, and emotional nurturance.

Neglect may also include lack of intervention for or fostering of maladaptive behavior such as delinquency or substance abuse. *Emotional abuse* or *psychologic maltreatment,* an even more difficult aspect of maltreatment to define, refers to the deliberate attempt to destroy or significantly impair a child's self-esteem or competence. Emotional abuse may take the form of rejecting, isolating, terrorizing, ignoring, corrupting, verbally assaulting, or overpressuring the child (Hibbard, Barlow, MacMillian, et al., 2012).

PHYSICAL ABUSE

The deliberate infliction of physical injury on a child, usually by the child's caregiver, is termed *physical abuse.* Nonaccidental trauma is the term used to describe the injury resulting from the abuse. In 2011, 48% of fatalities from abuse suffered physical abuse alone or in combination with other types of maltreatment (US Department of Health and Human Services, 2012). Despite the importance of the problem, a universally accepted definition of what constitutes minor and major physical abuse does not exist. Rather each state in the United States defines abuse according to its individual reporting laws.

Abusive Head Trauma

Abusive head trauma (AHT) is a serious form of physical abuse caused by violent shaking of infants and young children. Other commonly used terms include *shaken baby syndrome, inflicted head injury,* or *neuro-inflicted brain injury.* This violent shaking would be easily recognized by others as dangerous and is most often a result of the inconsolable infant crying (Hinds, Shalaby-Rana, Jackson, et al., 2015). Every year in the United States an estimated 14 to 40 children per

---

*Additional information is available from the Children's Bureau, Administration for Children and Families, 370 L'Enfant Promenade SW, Washington, DC 20447, 800-422-4453, http://www.acf.hhs.gov/programs/cb.

100,000 children less than 1 year of age are shaken, and 6% to 36% of these victims die as a result of their injuries (Hinds et al.). Many have lifelong complications including neurologic, visual, cognitive, behavioral, and sleep abnormalities (Hinds et al.).

It is important to understand what happens in AHT. Infants have a large head-to-body ratio, weak neck muscles, and a large amount of water in the brain. Violent shaking causes the brain to rotate within the skull, resulting in shearing forces that tear blood vessels and neurons. The characteristic injuries that occur are intracranial bleeding (subdural hematoma) and in approximately 80% of cases retinal hemorrhages, which are classic results of repetitive acceleration-deceleration head trauma (Maguire, Watts, Shaw, et al., 2013). Injuries may also include fractures of the ribs and long bones; however, most often there are no signs of external injury. Practitioners base an abusive diagnosis on patterns of injuries to the infant, but this can be subjective. PredAHT, a prediction tool, assists clinicians with an AHT diagnosis by listing six key clinical features of AHT obtained from high-quality publications (Cowley, Morris, Maguire, et al., 2015). The PredAHT has high sensitivity and specificity in estimating the probability of AHT when three or more of the six features are present in the patient (Cowley et al.).

AHT is often not an isolated event. Victims of AHT can be seen with a variety of symptoms. Many of the presenting symptoms such as vomiting, irritability, poor feeding, and listlessness are often mistaken for common infant and childhood ailments. In more severe forms, presenting symptoms may include seizures, posturing, alterations in level of consciousness, apnea, bradycardia, or death. Nurses can take an active role in preventing AHT by teaching caregivers about care for infants and techniques to cope with inconsolable crying (Barr, 2012).

! NURSING ALERT

Stress to parents and caregivers the danger of shaking infants. Education must include coping mechanisms for caring for infants with inconsolable crying.

Munchausen Syndrome by Proxy

Munchausen syndrome by proxy (MSBP), also known as *medical child abuse* or *factitious disorder by proxy*, is a rare but serious form of child abuse in which caregivers deliberately exaggerate or fabricate histories and symptoms or induce symptoms. It is a form of child maltreatment that may include physical, emotional, and psychologic abuse for the gratification of the caregiver. In most cases, the perpetrator is the biologic mother with some degree of health care knowledge and training. Health care providers can become easily misled and unknowingly enable the perpetrator (Squires & Squires, 2013). Because of the history of symptoms provided by the caregiver, the child endures painful and unnecessary medical testing and procedures. Common symptoms presented are seizures, nausea and vomiting, diarrhea, and altered mental status; they are usually witnessed only by the perpetrator. The resolution of symptoms after separation from the perpetrator confirms the diagnosis.

Considerations when determining whether a child is a victim of MSBP include the following:

- Is the child's condition consistent with the reported history?
- Does diagnostic evidence support the reported history?
- Has anyone other than the caregiver witnessed the symptoms?
- Is treatment being provided primarily because of the caregiver's demands?

Factors Predisposing to Abuse

The causes of child abuse are multifaceted. Child maltreatment occurs across all socioeconomic, religious, cultural, racial, and ethnic groups (US Department of Health and Human Services, 2012). Three risk factors are commonly identified in child abuse: (1) parental characteristics, (2) characteristics of the child, and (3) environmental characteristics. However, no single factor or group of factors is predictive of abuse. Rather the interaction of these factors is thought to increase the risk for abuse occurring in a particular family.

Parental Characteristics

Some identified characteristics occur more frequently in parents who abuse their children and therefore are considered risk factors. Younger parents more often abuse their children. Single-parent families are at higher risk for abuse, and in single-parent families that include an unrelated partner, the partner is sometimes the abuser, although a biologic parent is most commonly the perpetrator (US Department of Health and Human Services, 2012).

Abusive families are often socially isolated and have few supportive relationships. They often have additional stressors, such as low-income circumstances with little education. Parents with substance-abuse problems pose a greater risk for abuse and neglect because of a variety of factors. The additional stressors of substance abuse with the demands of normal care of children create situations in which abuse and neglect can occur because these parents have impaired judgment and may react with violence while under the influence of drugs or alcohol (Lyden, 2011). With little or no available support system and concurrent stressors imposed by the child or environment, these parents are vulnerable to additional crises of any nature and may strike out at the child as a method of releasing their frustration and anxiety.

Other factors identified in abusive parents include low self-esteem and little knowledge of appropriate parenting skills. Parenting skills are learned behaviors, and parents who grew up with poor parental role models may have difficulty parenting their own children. Often, child abusers were abused or observed some types of abuse in their home (Lyden, 2011).

Characteristics of the Child

The onus for child abuse is always on the abuser. However, children who are abused do have some common characteristics. Children from birth to 1 year of age are at highest risk for being abused (U.S. Department of Health and Human Services, 2012). Infants and small children require constant attention and must have all their needs met by others. This can result in parental or caregiver fatigue that results in striking out at the child with physical force, shaking the child, or ignoring his or her needs.

The physical and emotional demands placed on the parents or caregiver of an unwanted, brain-damaged, hyperactive, or physically disabled child may overwhelm them, resulting in abuse. Children with disabilities may not understand that abusive behaviors are not appropriate; thus they may not tell others or defend themselves. Premature infants may be at risk for maltreatment because of failure of parent-child bonding during early infancy, increased physical care needs, or irritability. One child may be singled out in an abusive family. Removing that child from the home often places the other siblings at risk for abuse. Therefore no child is safe if left in the abusive environment unless the parents can be helped to learn new parenting skills, meet the children's needs, and release their frustration through alternatives other than attacking their children.

Environmental Characteristics

The environment is a significant part of the potentially abusive situation. A typical environment is one of chronic stress, including problems of divorce, poverty, unemployment, poor housing, frequent relocation, alcoholism, and drug addiction. Increased exposure between children and parents such as that which occurs in crowded living conditions also increases the likelihood of abuse.

Although most reporting of abuse has been from lower socioeconomic populations as stated previously, child abuse is not a problem of any one societal group. Stresses imposed by poverty predispose lower socioeconomic families to abusive situations, and abuse in these groups is more likely to be reported. However, concealed crises may also be present in upper-class families. Families who have substitute caregivers such as day care providers and babysitters may also be at risk for child abuse, especially if the family has not fully evaluated the caregiver. Nurses need to be aware of all these factors to identify the less obvious examples of child abuse and neglect.

SEXUAL ABUSE

Sexual abuse is one of the most devastating types of child maltreatment, and estimates indicate that it has increased significantly during the past decade (U.S. Department of Health and Human Services, 2012). Some of the apparent increase is because of increased awareness and increased reporting (Evans, 2011).

As with all forms of child maltreatment, no universal definition for sexual abuse exists. The Child Abuse and Prevention Act defines *sexual abuse* as "the employment, use, persuasion, inducement, enticement, or coercion of any child to engage in, or assist any other person to engage in, sexually explicit conduct or any simulation of such conduct; or rape, molestation, prostitution, or other form of sexual exploitation of children, or incest with children" (US Department of Health and Human Services, 2012).

Sexual abuse includes the following types of sexual maltreatment:

Incest: Any physical sexual activity between family members; blood relationship is not required (abusers can include stepparents, unrelated siblings, grandparents, uncles, and aunts); does not include sexual relations between legally sanctioned partners such as spouses

Molestation: A vague term that includes "indecent liberties" such as touching, fondling, kissing, single or mutual masturbation, or oral-genital contact

Exhibitionism: Indecent exposure, usually exposure of the genitalia by an adult man to children or women

Child pornography: Arranging and photographing, in any media, sexual acts involving children, alone or with adults or animals, regardless of consent by the child's legal guardian; also may denote distribution of such material in any form with or without profit

Child prostitution: Involving children in sex acts for profit and usually with changing partners

Pedophilia: Literally means "love of child" and does not denote a type of sexual activity but rather the preference of an adult for prepubertal children as the means of achieving sexual excitement

Human trafficking often involves some form of coerced sexual activity and thus sexual abuse that may also often involve physical and mental abuse. Many victims of human trafficking are females younger than 18 years of age who are forced to perform sexual acts for the monetary profit of the perpetrators. Nurses may encounter victims of sex trafficking and subsequent sexual and physical abuse who are seeking medical care in outpatient and emergent health care settings for a plethora of health problems (STIs, bruises, wound infections, PTSD, suicidal ideation, and addiction). However, nurses may not be aware of the victim's plight unless he or she delves further into the person's history and background (Sabella, 2011).

Characteristics of Abusers and Victims

Anyone, including siblings and mothers, can be sexual abusers; but a typical abuser is a man whom the victim knows. Offenders come from all levels of society; however, a higher risk for child abuse has been noted among families with incomes below the poverty level (Breyer &

MacPhee, 2015). In addition, parents with a high school education are more likely than parents with a college education to be abusers (Breyer & MacPhee). Many offenders hold full-time jobs, are active in community affairs, and may not have prior criminal records. Offenders often are employed (or volunteers) in positions such as teaching or coaching that bring them into contact with young girls and boys. Offenders may commit many assaults before being caught.

Incestuous relationships between father or stepfather and daughter are generally prolonged, and the victims are usually reluctant to report the situation because of fear of retaliation and fear that they will not be believed. Typically, incestuous relationships begin later than other forms of child abuse. The eldest daughter is usually abused, but in her absence another sister may be substituted. Sibling incest may also occur. Sexual abuse by relatives with a strong emotional bond with the victim such as a parent is often the most devastating to the child.

Boys are also victims of both intrafamilial and extrafamilial abuse. Compared with female victims, male victims are much less likely to report abuse, and they may suffer much greater emotional harm from incestuous relationships. Boys are likely to be subjected to anal penetration and oral-genital contact. They often have subtle physical findings and are abused by a father, stepfather, or mother's boyfriend.

Significant risk factors for child sexual abuse include parental unavailability, lack of emotional closeness and flexibility, social isolation, emotional deprivation, and communication difficulties. Most sexual abuse is committed by men and people known to the child, such as family members (Forsdike, Tarzia, Hindmarsh, et al., 2014).

Initiation and Perpetuation of Sexual Abuse

The cycle of sexual abuse often starts insidiously unless it involves an isolated attack, such as rape. Often offenders spend time with the victims to gain their trust before initiating any sexual contact. Most victims are then pressured into being an accessory to the sexual activity through various means (Box 33.3) and may be unaware that sexual activity is part of the offer. Children may not reveal the truth for fear that their parents would not believe them if they told, especially if the offender is a trusted member of the family. Some fear that they will be blamed for the situation; and many young children with limited vocabulary have difficulty describing the activity when they do have the courage or opportunity to reveal the abuse.

Incest most frequently occurs between siblings, but it may also be between fathers or stepfathers and daughters, or grandfather and granddaughter. Sibling incest has been found to have adverse outcomes during childhood that extend into adulthood and are just as damaging

---

BOX 33.3   Methods Used to Pressure Children Into Sexual Activity

- The child is offered gifts or privileges.
- The adult misrepresents moral standards by telling the child that it is "okay to do."
- Isolated and emotionally and socially impoverished children are enticed by adults who meet their needs for warmth and human contact.
- The offender asks the child for help in finding a favorite pet or object with which the child can easily identify.
- The successful sex offender pressures the victim into secrecy regarding the activity by describing it as a "secret between us" that other people may take away if they find out.
- The offender plays on the child's fears, including fear of punishment by the offender, fear of repercussions if the child tells, and fear of abandonment or rejection by the family.

GUIDELINES
Talking With Children Who Reveal Abuse

- Provide a private time and place to talk.
- Do not promise not to tell; tell them that you are required by law to report the abuse.
- Do not express shock or criticize their family.
- Use their vocabulary to discuss body parts.
- Avoid using any leading statements that can distort their report.
- Reassure them that they have done the right thing by telling.
- Tell them that the abuse is not their fault, that they are not bad or to blame.
- Determine their immediate need for safety.
- Let the child know what will happen when you report.

BOX 33.4 Warning Signs of Abuse

- Physical evidence of abuse or neglect, including previous injuries
- Conflicting stories about the "accident" or injury from the parents or others
- Cause of injury blamed on sibling or other party
- An injury inconsistent with the history such as a concussion and broken arm from falling off a bed
- History inconsistent with child's developmental level such as a 6-month-old turning on the hot water
- A complaint other than the one associated with signs of abuse (e.g., a chief complaint of a cold when there is evidence of first- and second-degree burns)
- Inappropriate response of caregiver such as an exaggerated or absent emotional response, refusal to sign for additional tests or agree to necessary treatment, excessive delay in seeking treatment, or absence of parents for questioning
- Inappropriate response of child such as little or no response to pain, fear of being touched, excessive or lack of separation anxiety, indiscriminate friendliness to strangers
- Child's report of physical or sexual abuse
- Previous reports of abuse in the family
- Repeated visits to emergency facilities with injuries
- Parent or caregiver report of being gone and finding the child unresponsive, indicating absence during the supposed event that resulted in harm

as father-daughter abuse (Krienert & Walsh, 2011). Victims may take years to disclose this abuse. However, not all incestuous relationships follow this pattern of silence. Reports of father-daughter incest during child custody conflicts have become more common and have raised serious concerns regarding the possibility of false accusation. Rather than tolerating or denying the child's sexual abuse, the other parent (usually the mother) is typically the chief accuser.

INTERPROFESSIONAL CARE OF THE MALTREATED CHILD

A critical responsibility of health care professionals is identifying abusive situations as early as possible. Nurses who increase their knowledge of the different types of abuse and neglect and underlying causes enhance their ability to identify, intervene, and prevent children from maltreatment and neglect (Lyden, 2011). The characteristics that may predispose members of some families to commit abuse can serve as a framework for assessing vulnerability but are never predictive of actual abuse. A careful, detailed history and interview combined with a thorough physical examination are the diagnostic tools needed to identify abuse. Nurses have a special role because they may be the first person to see the child and parent and are the consistent caregivers if the child is hospitalized (see Guidelines box: Talking With Children Who Reveal Abuse).

In interviewing the child and family, the nurse must be careful to avoid biasing the child's retelling of the events. Some experts suggest that health care professionals limit the interview to the child's physical and mental health concerns and leave topics of the family's social, legal, or other problems to law enforcement or Child Protective Services (Mollen, Goyal, & Frioux, 2012). If this is not possible, make an effort to coordinate the interview process so all pertinent health care professionals can be present for the interview.

Recognition of abuse or neglect necessitates a familiarity with both physical and behavioral signs that suggest maltreatment (Box 33.4). No one indicator can be used to diagnose maltreatment. It is a pattern or combination of indicators that should arouse suspicion and lead to further investigation. It is important to note that some situations, such as bleeding disorders, osteogenesis imperfecta, or sudden infant death syndrome, may be misinterpreted as abuse. In addition, some cultural practices such as cupping or coin rubbing (see the "Health Practices" section in Chapter 27), may mimic physical abuse. Unintentional injuries, such as burns from metal buckles on car seats, bruising from seat belts, or spiral fractures from a twist and fall injury, may also be wrongly diagnosed as abuse. Normal variants, such as mongolian spots and congenital anomalies of genitalia, can be mistaken for abuse.

Caregiver-Child Interaction

The initial contact with the family is used to assess the interaction between the caregiver and the child. Observations of the caregivers should include emotional support for the child, attentiveness to his or her needs, and concern for the child's injury. Although caregivers and children may vary in responses to a stressful event, note an unusual caregiver-child relationship and factor this into the overall evaluation of the child.

Certain behavioral responses of the parents to their child and to the interviewer should alert to the possibility of maltreatment. Abusive parents may have difficulty showing concern for their child. They may be unable or unwilling to comfort the child. Abusers may blame the child for the injuries or belittle her or him for being clumsy or stupid. When interacting with health care professionals, the parent may become hostile or uncooperative. During the child's hospitalization, they may not participate in her or his care and may show little concern for her or his progress, eventual discharge, or need for follow-up care.

Abused children's responses to their parents or the injury may also support the suspicion of abuse. Although no one pattern is typical, extremes of behavior may be observed. Children may be unresponsive to the parent or excessively clinging and intolerant of separation. They may be overly attached to the abusive parent, possibly in the hope of preventing any upset that may precipitate anger and another attack. During care of the injury, children may be passive and accepting of the discomfort or uncooperative and fearful of any physical contact. They may avoid eye contact. Some children maintain a wary watchfulness of all strangers; some shy away from strangers as if frightened; others are unusually affectionate and outgoing.

History and Interview
Child Physical Abuse

It is often difficult to distinguish child maltreatment from accidental injuries. Caregivers whose history of events may be deceptive or incomplete and children who are nonverbal may make the assessment more complex. A purposeful, skilled history and appropriate interview questions help ensure the right course of action. Knowledge of mechanism of injury and child development is essential. Cases of abuse are often detected when the child or caregiver history of events does not match with physical findings. Children who are verbal can often give a history of the injury. Separating the child from the caregiver may provide a more reliable history. It is important to ask nonleading, open-ended questions. The history should include a narrative of the injury from both caregiver and child (if verbal). Date, time, and location where the injury took place along with who was present at the time of the injury are essential questions. Family history for bleeding and bone disorders is important. Box 33.5 outlines areas of history that are concerning for abuse.

Neglect and Emotional Abuse

Each child may manifest different responses to neglect, depending on the situation and the child's developmental age. The goal of the interview is to determine whether the child is in a safe environment and whether the caregiver has the skills and resources to care for the child. It is often difficult to determine whether the circumstances constitute poor parenting skills or true neglect. Box 33.4 lists flags for behaviors to look for in neglected and abused children.

Sexual Abuse

An essential component to identifying sexual abuse is the interview. Several dynamics may impede the child's revelation of sexual abuse. Child sexual abuse is often perpetrated by someone known to the child, including family members. In some cases, the child may have been sworn to secrecy. The child may have been told that no one will believe the story or that the family would be harmed if he or she told someone about the abuse. Small children may imitate behaviors they have had perpetrated on themselves or have seen others do. Normal, age-related sexual curiosity and self-stimulating behaviors are distinguished. Typically children do not act out specific details of the sexual act or perform intrusive acts on others unless they have sexual knowledge beyond their normal age-related development (Dubowitz & Lane, 2016).

Children's reports of sexual abuse may vary from contradictory stories to unwavering versions of the experience. Stories that sound contradictory may reflect the child's experiences in several instances of abuse. In addition, children who repeatedly tell identical facts may have been prompted to do so.

Increasing evidence suggests that the types of interrogation to which children are exposed after reports of sexual abuse shape their thinking. To avoid biasing the interaction, nurses must be skillful interviewers when questioning children who may be victims of abuse. Medical records should include verbatim statements made by the child and interviewer that reflect appropriate nonleading questions and statements (Lyden, 2011). The child may not be emotionally ready to discuss the abuse. Establishing rapport with the child is essential to gaining his or her trust. Interviews should not be rushed. Engaging the child in play activities while encouraging conversation may help to the child discuss the abuse. It may take several interviews or psychologic counseling for the child to be forthcoming about the abuse. Information regarding the last sexual contact is important because it determines the need for a forensic evaluation. Children who have been sexually abused within the past 72 to 96 hours should be considered for forensic testing.

Unfortunately there is no typical profile of the victim, and the nurse must have a high index of suspicion to identify these children. Physical signs vary and may include any of those listed for sexual abuse. The victim may exhibit various behavioral manifestations, but none of these behaviors is diagnostic. When abused children exhibit these behaviors, the signs may be incorrectly attributed to the normal stresses of childhood, especially in older school-age children or adolescents. Even signs

considered most predictive of sexual abuse, such as certain genital findings, sexually inappropriate behavior for age, enactment of adult sexual activity, and intense focus on sexual activity (e.g., masturbation), do not always indicate that sexual abuse has occurred. Conversely abused children may not demonstrate more knowledge of sexual activity than non-abused children. However, one difference in the abused child's explanation of sexual activity may be unusual affective responses. For example, abused children may have an increased incidence of conduct disorders, aggressive behavior, and poor academic performance (Dubowitz & Lane, 2016).

> **! NURSING ALERT**
>
> When children report potentially sexually abusive experiences, their reports need to be taken seriously but also cautiously to avoid alarming the child or falsely accusing someone.

Physical Assessment
Child Physical Abuse

The goal of the physical assessment for child physical abuse is identification of all injuries. A systems approach ensures that the whole body is evaluated. In instances of severe abuse and injuries, the assessment should begin with a rapid assessment of airway, breathing, circulation, and neurologic systems. A systematic head-to-toe examination follows. Attention to areas often overlooked such as the scalp, behind the ears, and the frenulum is essential. The child's exterior genital area and posterior surface should be examined completely.

Record the location and a detailed description of all injuries. Note the color, size, and location of all bruising. Burn documentation should include the location, pattern, demarcation lines, and presence of eschar or blisters. Diagrams of the injuries using a body diagram form are helpful. If possible, obtain photographs of the injuries with a measurement tool.

Not all forms of physical abuse have obvious signs. Intraabdominal organ injury from blunt trauma to the abdomen can occur without signs of external abdominal bruising. Nurses should consider intraabdominal injury in infants and children who have any other signs of abuse.

All evidence collected must adhere to strict guidelines for legal purposes; the chain of custody must be appropriately maintained with local law enforcement personnel. Documentation on the chain of custody form should include the names of people collecting and receiving evidence (e.g., photographs and deoxyribonucleic acid [DNA] samples), types of evidence collected and received, and date of receipt (Lyden, 2011).

> **! NURSING ALERT**
>
> Incompatibility between the history and the injury is probably the most important criterion on which to base the decision to report suspected abuse.

Neglect and Emotional Abuse

Neglect from deprivation of necessities is easier to identify than emotional neglect or psychologic maltreatment because physical signs are usually evident. Assessment of the child's height, weight, nutritional status, hygiene, and age-appropriate interactions is important for the overall picture of potential neglect. Emotional maltreatment may be readily suspected, but it is difficult to substantiate. Physical signs are often nonspecific; and nurses must rely on behavioral indicators, which range from depression to acting-out behavior, to help identify a possibly abusive situation. Any persistent and unexplained change in the child's behavior is an important clue to possible emotional abuse.

BOX 33.5   Clinical Manifestations of Potential Child Maltreatment

Physical Neglect
Suggestive Physical Findings
- Failure to thrive (growth failure)
- Signs of undernutrition such as thin extremities, abdominal distention, lack of subcutaneous fat
- Poor personal hygiene
- Unclean or inappropriate dress
- Evidence of poor health care such as delayed immunizations, untreated infections, frequent colds
- Frequent injuries from lack of supervision

Suggestive Behaviors
- Dull and inactive affect; excessively passive or sleepy
- Self-stimulatory behaviors such as finger sucking or rocking
- Begging or stealing food
- Absenteeism from school
- Substance abuse
- Vandalism or shoplifting

Emotional Abuse and Neglect
Suggestive Physical Findings
- Failure to thrive (growth failure)
- Eating or feeding disorder
- Enuresis
- Sleep disorder

Suggestive Behaviors
- Self-stimulatory behaviors such as biting, rocking, sucking
- During infancy, lack of social smile and stranger anxiety
- Withdrawal from environment and people
- Unusual fearfulness
- Antisocial behavior such as destructiveness, stealing, cruelty to animals or people
- Extremes of behavior such as overcompliant and passive or aggressive and demanding
- Lag in emotional and intellectual development, especially language
- Suicide attempts or attempts to harm self

Physical Abuse
Suggestive Physical Findings
- Bruises and welts
  - On face, lips, mouth, back, buttocks, thighs, or areas of torso
  - Regular patterns descriptive of object used such as belt buckle, hand, wire hanger, chain, wooden spoon, squeeze or pinch marks
  - May be present in various stages of healing
- Burns
  - On soles of feet, palms of hands, back, or buttocks
  - Patterns descriptive of object used such as round cigar or cigarette burns; sharply demarcated areas from immersion in scalding water; rope burns on wrists or ankles from being bound; burns in the shape of an iron, radiator, or electric stove burner
  - Absence of "splash" marks and presence of symmetric burns
- Stun gun injury: lesions circular, fairly uniform (up to 0.5 cm), and paired about 5 cm (1¾ inches) apart
- Fractures and dislocations
  - Skull, nose, or facial structures
  - Injury denoting type of abuse such as spiral fracture or dislocation from twisting an extremity or whiplash from shaking child
  - Multiple new or old fractures in various stages of healing

- Lacerations and abrasions
  - On backs of arms, legs, torso, face, or external genitalia
  - Unusual symptoms such as abdominal swelling, pain, and vomiting from punching
  - Descriptive marks such as from human bites or pulling out of hair
- Chemical
  - Unexplained repeated poisoning, especially drug overdose
  - Unexplained sudden illness such as hypoglycemia from insulin administration

Suggestive Behaviors
- Wary of physical contact with adults
- Apparent fear of parents or going home
- Lying very still while surveying environment
- Inappropriate reaction to injury such as failure to cry from pain
- Lack of reaction to frightening events
- Apprehension when hearing other children cry
- Indiscriminate friendliness and displays of affection
- Superficial relationships
- Acting-out behavior such as aggression to seek attention
- Withdrawal behavior

Sexual Abuse
Suggestive Physical Findings
- Bruises, bleeding, lacerations, or irritation of external genitalia, anus, mouth, or throat
- Torn, stained, or bloody underclothing
- Pain on urination, or pain, swelling, and itching of genital area
- Penile discharge
- Sexually transmitted infection, nonspecific vaginitis, or venereal warts
- Difficulty in walking or sitting
- Unusual odor in genital area
- Recurrent urinary tract infections
- Presence of sperm
- Pregnancy in young adolescent

Suggestive Behaviors
- Sudden emergence of sexually related problems, including excessive or public masturbation, age-inappropriate sexual play, promiscuity, or overtly seductive behavior
- Withdrawn behavior, excessive daydreaming
- Preoccupation with fantasies, especially in play
- Poor relationships with peers
- Sudden changes such as anxiety, loss or gain of weight, clinging behavior
- In incestuous relationships, excessive anger at mother for not protecting daughter
- Regressive behavior such as bed-wetting or thumb-sucking
- Sudden onset of phobias or fears, particularly fears of dark, men, strangers, or particular settings or situations (e.g., undue fear of leaving house or staying at day care center or baby-sitter's house)
- Running away from home
- Substance abuse, particularly of alcohol or mood-elevating drugs
- Profound and rapid personality changes, especially extreme depression, hostility, and aggression (often accompanied by social withdrawal)
- Rapidly declining school performance
- Suicidal attempts or ideation

Sexual Abuse

Identifying instances of sexual abuse is particularly difficult because, often, few if any obvious physical indications of the activity exist. Physical signs vary and may include any of those listed in Box 33.5 for sexual abuse. The goal of the physical examination is to document genital findings. In most cases, the genital examination findings are normal, which does not mean that sexual abuse did not occur. Fondling or genital-to-genital contact without penetration may leave no physical findings. Forensic evidence obtained directly from a prepubertal victim's body diminishes greatly after 24 hours, with the best chance for evidence collection coming from bed linens or the child's underwear (Girardet, Bolton, Lohoti, et al., 2011). The female genital examination should include a description of the vulva, hymen, and surrounding tissue. Abnormal findings of concern are injuries to the posterior vulva or the lower half of the hymenal ring or abrasions, bruising, or bleeding of the genital or anal tissue. It is often helpful to use a magnifying instrument (colposcope) to detect subtle injuries. There are many variants of normal findings for female genital anatomy, so it is recommended that the examination be done by a practitioner experienced with these types of cases. Contrary to popular myth, the size of the hymenal opening does not predict the likelihood of sexual abuse (Adams, 2011). For male victims, swelling, abrasions, or bruising of the genital tissue raises concerns. Examine the anal area for symmetry, tone, fissures, or scars. Genital tissue heals very quickly and most often without scars. Therefore, unless the child is seen within a few days of injury, the genital tissue may appear normal. In addition, the vaginal and anal mucosa is elastic; therefore penetration without disruption of tissue is possible. This defies another myth that there is always evidence of female virginity. Consider the collection of specimens for determining the presence of sexually transmitted infections, which may have been contracted during the sexual contact.

Care Management
Protect Child From Further Abuse

Initially identification of instances of suspected abuse or neglect is essential. The nurse may come in contact with abused children in an emergency department, practitioner's office, home, day care center, or school.

> **! NURSING ALERT**
>
> The priority is to remove the child from the abusive situation to prevent further injury.

All states in North America have laws for mandatory reporting of child maltreatment. Suspected child abuse is reported to the local authorities.* Referrals usually come to the state child welfare department and are assigned to a caseworker in an agency such as Child Protective Services. After a referral has been made, a caseworker is assigned to investigate the report. Based on the findings, the child is left in the home or removed temporarily.

A court proceeding may be necessary before the child can be placed outside the home or when parental rights are to be terminated. When the courts are involved, they usually require firsthand testimony by the referring parties. Nurses may be subpoenaed to appear in court, or their notes may be introduced as evidence in court hearings. Accurate and factual documentation is essential. Behaviors are described, not interpreted, and are recorded daily to establish a progress record (see

---

*Telephone numbers are usually listed under "Child Abuse" in the business white pages of the local directory, or you can call the emergency child abuse hotline: 800-422-4453 (800-4-A-CHILD).

> ## 🗒 GUIDELINES
> ### *Recording Assessment Data in Suspected Abuse*
>
> **History of Injury**
> - Date, time, and place of occurrence
> - Sequence of events with recorded times
> - Presence of witnesses, especially person caring for child at time of incident
> - Time lapse between occurrence of injury and initiation of treatment
> - Interview with child when appropriate, including verbal quotations and information from drawing or other play activities
> - Interview with parent, witnesses, or other significant persons, including verbal quotations
> - Description of parent-child interactions (verbal interactions, eye contact, touching, parental concern)
> - Name, age, and condition of other children in home (if possible)
>
> **Physical Examination**
> - Location, size, shape, and color of bruises; approximate location, size, and shape on drawing of body outline
> - Distinguishing characteristics such as a bruise in the shape of a hand or a round burn (possibly caused by cigarette)
> - Symmetry or asymmetry of injury; presence of other injuries
> - Degree of pain; any bone tenderness
> - Evidence of past injuries; general state of health and hygiene
> - Developmental level of child; perform screening test (see the "Developmental Assessment" section in Chapter 28)

Guidelines box: Recording Assessment Data in Suspected Abuse). Conversations among the nurse, child, and parent are recorded verbatim as much as possible.

Support Child

Children suspected of being abused are often hospitalized for medical management of their injuries and to allow further assessment of their safety needs. The needs of these children are the same as those of any hospitalized child. The child should be treated as a child with the usual physical needs, developmental tasks, and play interests—not as a victim of abuse. The goal of the nurse-child relationship is to provide a role model for the parents in helping them relate positively and constructively to their child and to foster a therapeutic environment for the child in his or her reprieve from the abusing situation.

Support Family

The nurse also encourages the child's relationship with non-offending parents. The nurse does not become a substitute parent but rather acts as a role model for parents in helping them relate positively and constructively to their child. When parental ignorance of childrearing practices has played a part in the abuse, the nurse can educate the parent regarding children's physical and emotional needs. Because of the parents' own childrearing, they may not be aware of nonviolent methods of discipline, such as time-outs. They may also need help in dealing with their frustration so that they do not vent anger on the child. Because these parents may be sensitive to criticism or resistant to authority figures, teaching is implemented through demonstration and example rather than through lecturing. Praise any competent parenting abilities they demonstrate to promote their sense of parental adequacy.

Advise family members to encourage the child to resume normal activities and observe her or him for signs of distress (see the "Post-traumatic Stress Disorder" section in Chapter 34.) Children express their feelings primarily through behavior. Parents should be alert for changes in behavior that indicate distress resulting from the incident, such as remaining in the house, refusal to go to school, changes in sleeping patterns, and frequency of dreams and nightmares.

Referral to appropriate social service agencies is also essential. Many abusive parents live in poverty, and the daily stresses imposed by their circumstances are overwhelming. Seek resources for financial aid, improved housing, and child care. Self-help groups also provide important services. One such group is Parents Anonymous,* a group for parents who have abused or fear that they may abuse their child but only in terms of physical abuse, not sexual abuse.

Plan for Discharge

Discharge planning should begin as soon as the legal disposition for placement has been decided, which may be temporary foster home placement; return to the parents; or permanent termination of parental rights. Whenever children are sent to a foster home or juvenile institution, they must be allowed an opportunity to express their feelings. No matter how severe the abuse, they usually mourn the loss of their parents. They need help to understand why they must not return home and that this new home is in no way a punishment. Whenever possible, foster parents are encouraged to visit in the hospital, and the nurse should take an active role in helping the new parents understand the child and his or her health care needs. Studies have shown that the health care needs of children in foster care often go unmet (Schneiderman, Smith, & Palinkas, 2012).

Prevent Abuse

Prevention of child maltreatment has been an extremely difficult goal. However, nurses have played an important role in programs. The Nurse-Family Partnership is one program that has demonstrated evidence-based interventions resulting in the prevention of child maltreatment (Lane, 2014).

Nurses in a variety of settings can implement similar activities. For example, nurses in prenatal clinics can prepare expectant families for adjustment to parenthood. Nursery and postpartum nurses can foster the attachment process by encouraging parents to hold and look at their infant and by teaching coping mechanisms for prolonged crying. Nurses in neonatal intensive care units can minimize the effects of separation by encouraging parents to visit and can help parents become comfortable caring for their child. Nurses in ambulatory settings can teach parents appropriate methods of bathing, feeding, toileting, disciplining, and preventing injuries while stressing the normal needs and developmental characteristics of children. Nurses must be sensitive to parental needs for attention, reassurance, and reinforcement and should refer parents to community services and self-help groups.

Unlike preventive efforts for neglect and physical abuse, which have been aimed at the potential offender, prevention of child sexual abuse has centered on education of children to protect themselves. Materials are available for parents that describe sexual abuse and its prevention.[†] Helpful games such as, "What if the babysitter wants to wrestle and hug but tells you to keep it a secret?" can be used to explore dangerous situations in advance and help children learn the importance of saying "no." They need reassurance that, no matter what the other person says or does, the parents want to know about it and will not punish them. Even if children participate in the activity before telling their parents, they must be reassured that it was not their fault. It is equally important to teach children safety in terms of potential risk situations. Several suggestions for parents regarding protecting and educating children against possible molestation are presented in the Family-Centered Care box: Preventing or Dealing with Sexual Abuse of Children. The nurse is frequently in a position to discuss the topic of abuse with parents and provide guidelines. In addition, parents need to be made aware that "nice" people, including friends and relatives, can be offenders; they should carefully observe how others act toward the child. A sudden change in the child's behavior and a response such as, "I don't like Uncle Bob anymore" are clues to investigate the relationship. In the event of any doubt, prevent further solitary encounters between this person and the child. It is sometimes to the child's great misfortune that parents do not take certain comments seriously such as, "He hugs me too tight" or "I don't want to go with him." Casual parental statements such as, "He just loves you" or "You do whatever adults tell you to do" can place children in jeopardy. Health care professionals must alert parents to such dangers and guide them toward an appreciation of the problem, providing concrete guidelines toward child education and protection.

FAMILY-CENTERED CARE

Preventing or Dealing With Sexual Abuse of Children

Sexual assault of children is more common than most people realize. It may be preventable if children have proper preparation. *To provide protection and preparation:*

- Pay careful attention to who is around children. (Unwanted touch may come from someone liked and trusted.)
- Back up a child's right to say "no."
- Encourage communication by taking seriously what children say.
- Take a second look at signals of potential danger.
- Refuse to leave children in the company of those not trusted.
- Include information about sexual assault when teaching about safety.
- Provide specific definitions and examples of sexual assault.
- Remind children that even "nice" people sometimes do mean things.
- Urge children to tell about *anybody* who causes them to be uncomfortable.
- Prepare children to deal with bribes, threats, and possible physical force.
- Eliminate secrets between children and parents.
- Teach children how to say "no," ask for help, and control who touches them and how.
- Model self-protective and limit-setting behavior for children.

Should it ever become necessary to help a child recover from a sexual assault:
- Listen carefully to understand children.
- Support the child for telling through praise, belief, sympathy, and lack of blame.
- Know local resources, and choose help carefully.
- Provide opportunities to talk about the assault.
- Provide opportunities for entire family to go through recovery process.

Sexual assault affects everyone. To help deal with this social problem:
- Provide care and support to those who have been victimized.
- Recognize that offenders may not change behavior, even with an intervention.
- Organize neighborhood programs to support each other's efforts to protect children.
- Encourage schools to provide information about sexual assault as a problem of health and safety.
- Organize community groups to support educational-treatment and law-enforcement programs.

Modified from Adams, C., & Fay, J. (1981). *No more secrets: Protecting your child from sexual assault.* San Luis Obispo, CA: Impact.

---

*250 West First Street, Suite 250, Claremont, CA 91711; 909-621-6184; http://www.parentsanonymous.org.

[†]Sources of information are Prevent Child Abuse America, 228 S. Wabash Avenue, 10th Floor, Chicago, IL 60604, 312-663-3520 or 800-Children, www.preventchildabuse.org; and American Humane Association, 1400 16th Street NW, Suite 360, Washington, DC 20036; 800-227-4645, www.americanhumane.org.

REFERENCES

Adams, J. A. (2011). Medical evaluation of suspected child sexual abuse: 2011 update. *Journal of Child Sexual Abuse*, 20(5), 588–605.

American Academy of Pediatric Dentistry. (2013). *Guideline on periodicity of examination, preventive dental services, anticipatory guidance/counseling, and oral treatments for infants, children, and adolescents*. Retrieved from http://www.aapd.org/media/policies_guidelines/g_periodicity.pdf.

American Academy of Pediatrics, Committee on Infectious Diseases (2015). *Red book: 2015 report of the Committee on Infectious Diseases* (30th ed.). Elk Grove Village, IL: The Academy.

American Academy of Pediatrics, Council on Communications and Media. (2016). *Media and young minds*. Retrieved from http://dx.doi.org/10.1542/peds.2016-2591.

Babcock, D. A. (2011). Evaluating sleep and sleep disorders in the pediatric primary care setting. *Pediatric Clinics of North America*, 58(3), 543–554.

Barr, R. G. (2012). Preventing abusive head trauma resulting from a failure of normal interaction between infants and their caregivers. *Proceedings of the National Academy of Sciences of the United States of America*, 109(2 suppl), 17294–17301.

Bentley, J., Pinfield, J., & Rouse, J. (2013). Whooping cough: Identification, assessment, and management. *Nursing Standard*, 28(11), 50–57.

Bhargava, S. (2011). Diagnosis and management of common sleep problems in children. *Pediatrics in Review*, 32(3), 91–98.

Breyer, R. J., & MacPhee, D. (2015). Community characteristics, conservative ideology, and child abuse rates. *Child Abuse & Neglect*, 41, 126–135.

Centers for Disease Control and Prevention. (2015). *Youth physical activity guidelines toolkit*. Retrieved from http://www.cdc.gov/healthyschools/physicalactivity/guidelines.htm.

Cowley, L. E., Morris, C. B., Maguire, S. A., et al. (2015). Validation of a prediction tool for abusive head trauma. *Pediatrics*, 136(2), 290–298.

Dubowitz, H., & Lane, W. (2016). Abused and neglected children. In R. M. Kliegman, B. F. Stanton, J. W. St. Geme, et al. (Eds.), *Nelson textbook of pediatrics* (20th ed.). Philadelphia, PA: Saunders/Elsevier.

Erikson, E. (1963). *Childhood and society*. New York, NY: WW Norton.

Evans, H. (2011). Pediatrics tackles child sexual abuse. *Archives of Pediatrics and Adolescent Medicine*, 165(9), 783–784.

Feigelman, S. (2016). The preschool years. In R. M. Kliegman, B. F. Stanton, J. W. St. Geme, et al. (Eds.), *Nelson textbook of pediatrics* (20th ed.). Philadelphia, PA: Saunders/Elsevier.

Fitzpatrick, C., Barnett, T., & Pagani, L. S. (2012). Early exposure to media violence and later child adjustment. *Journal of Developmental and Behavioral Pediatrics*, 33(4), 291–297.

Forsdike, K., Tarzia, L., Hindmarsh, E., & Hegarty, K. (2014). Family violence across the life cycle. *Australian Family Physician*, 43(11), 768–774.

Girardet, R., Bolton, K., Lohoti, S., et al. (2011). Collection of forensic evidence from pediatric victims of sexual assault. *Pediatrics*, 128(2), 233–238.

Harrison, L. J., & McLeod, S. (2010). Risk and protective factors associated with speech and language impairment in a nationally representative sample of 4- to 5-year-old children. *Journal of Speech, Language and Hearing Research*, 53(2), 508–529.

Hibbard, R., Barlow, J., MacMillan, H., et al. (2012). Psychological maltreatment. *Pediatrics*, 130(2), 372–378.

Hinds, T., Shalaby-Rana, E., Jackson, A. M., et al. (2015). Aspects of abuse: Abusive head trauma. *Current Problems in Pediatric and Adolescent Health Care*, 45, 71–79.

Honaker, S. M., & Meltzer, L. J. (2014). Bedtime problems and night wakings in young children: An update of the evidence. *Paediatric Respiratory Reviews*, 15(4), 333–339.

Institute of Medicine of the National Academies. (2011). *Dietary reference intakes for calcium and vitamin D*. Retrieved from http://nationalacademies.org/hmd/reports/2010/dietary-reference-intakes-for-calcium-and-vitamin-d.aspx.

John, C. C. (2016). Giardia lamblia. In R. M. Kliegman, B. F. Stanton, J. W. St. Geme, et al. (Eds.), *Nelson textbook of pediatrics* (20th ed.). Philadelphia, PA: Saunders/Elsevier.

Kleinman, R. D., & Greer, F. R. (2014). *Pediatric nutrition* (7th ed.). Elk Grove Village, IL: American Academy of Pediatrics.

Knox, M. (2010). On hitting children: A review of corporal punishment in the United States. *Journal of Pediatric Health Care*, 24(2), 103–107.

Koch, W. C. (2016). Parvoviruses. In R. M. Kliegman, B. F. Stanton, J. W. St. Geme, et al. (Eds.), *Nelson textbook of pediatrics* (20th ed.). Philadelphia, PA: Saunders/Elsevier.

Kosova, E. C., Auinger, P., & Bremer, A. A. (2013). The relationships between sugar-sweetened beverage intake and cardiometabolic markers in young children. *Journal of the Academy of Nutrition and Dietetics*, 113(2), 219–227.

Krienert, J. L., & Walsh, J. A. (2011). Sibling sexual abuse: An empirical analysis of offender, victim, and event characteristics in National Incident-based Reporting System (NBRS) data, 2000-2007. *Journal of Child Sexual Abuse*, 20(4), 353–372.

Lane, W. G. (2014). Prevention of child maltreatment. *Pediatric Clinics of North America*, 61(5), 873–888.

Larson, N., Ward, D., Neelon, S. B., et al. (2011). *Preventing obesity among preschool children: how can child-care settings promote healthy eating and physical activity? Research synthesis*. Princeton, NJ: Robert Wood Johnson Foundation.

Lussier, P., Corrado, R., & Tzoumakis, S. (2012). Gender differences in physical aggression and associated developmental correlates in a sample of Canadian preschoolers. *Behavioral Sciences and the Law*, 30(5), 643–671.

Lyden, C. (2011). Uncovering child abuse. *Nursing Management*, 42(suppl), 1–5.

Macaulay, E. C., Donovan, E. L., Leask, M. P., et al. (2014). The importance of early life in childhood obesity and related diseases: A report from the 2014 Gravida Strategic Summit. *Journal of Developmental Origins of Health and Disease*, 5(6), 398–407.

Maguire, S. A., Watts, P. O., Shaw, A. D., et al. (2013). Retinal hemorrhages and related findings in abusive and non-abusive head trauma: A systematic review. *Eye*, 27(1), 28–36.

Marshall, T. A. (2013). Preventing dental caries associated with sugar-sweetened beverages. *Journal of the American Dental Association*, 144(10), 1148–1152.

McEachern, A. D., & Snyder, J. (2012). Gender differences in predicting antisocial behaviors: Developmental consequences of physical and relational aggression. *Journal of Abnormal Child Psychology*, 40(4), 501–512.

McLaughlin, M. R. (2011). Speech and language delay in children. *American Family Physician*, 83(10), 1183–1188.

McQuiston, S., & Kloczko, N. (2011). Speech and language development: Monitoring process and problems. *Pediatrics in Review*, 32(6), 230–238.

Mollen, C. J., Goyal, M. K., & Frioux, S. M. (2012). Acute sexual abuse. *Pediatric Emergency Care*, 28(6), 584–590.

National Center on Parent, Family, and Community Engagement. (2014). *Family engagement and school readiness*. Retrieved from http://eclkc.ohs.acf.hhs.gov/hslc/tta-system/family/docs/schoolreadiness-pfce-rtp.pdf.

National Institute on Deafness and Other Communication Disorders, National Institutes of Health. (2010). *Stuttering*. Retrieved from https://www.nidcd.nih.gov/health/stuttering.

Nelson, A. (2013). *Stuttering*. Retrieved from http://kidshealth.org/parent/emotions/behavior/stutter.html#.

Purow, B., Alisanski, S., Putnam, G., et al. (2011). Spirituality and pediatric cancer. *Southern Medical Journal*, 104(4), 299–302.

Reilly, S., Wake, M., Ukoumunne, O. C., et al. (2010). Predicting language outcomes at 4 years of age: Findings from Early Language in Victoria Study. *Pediatrics*, 126(6), 1530–1537.

Rogers, V. W., Hart, P. H., Motyka, E., et al. (2013). Impact of Let's Go! 5-2-1-0: A community-based, multisetting childhood obesity prevention program. *Journal of Pediatric Psychology*, 38(9), 1010–1020.

Sabella, D. (2011). The role of the nurse in combating human trafficking. *American Journal of Nursing*, 111(2), 28–37.

Sacri, A. S., De Serres, G., Quach, C., et al. (2014). Transmission of acute gastroenteritis and respiratory illness from children to parents. *Pediatric Infectious Disease Journal*, 33(6), 583–588.

Schneiderman, J. U., Smith, C., & Palinkas, L. A. (2012). The caregiver as gatekeeper for accessing health care for children in foster care: A qualitative study of kinship and unrelated caregivers. *Children and Youth Services Review, 34*(10), 2123–2130.

Skouteris, H., McCabe, M., Swinburn, B., et al. (2010). Healthy eating and obesity prevention for preschoolers: A randomized controlled trial. *BMC Public Health, 10*, 220.

Squires, J. E., & Squires, R. H. (2013). A review of Munchausen syndrome by proxy. *Pediatric Annals, 42*(4), 67–71.

Strachan, E., & Staples, B. (2012). Masturbation. *Pediatrics in Review, 33*(4), 190–191.

Stricker, P. R. (2014). *Sports goals and applications—Preschoolers.* Retrieved from www.healthychildren.org/English/ages-stages/preschool/nutrition-fitness/Pages/Sports-Goals-and-Applications-Preschoolers.aspx.

Trionfi, G., & Reese, E. (2009). Good story: Children with imaginary companions create richer narratives. *Child Development, 4*(80), 1301–1313.

US Department of Agriculture, Center for Nutrition Policy and Promotion. (2011). *A brief history of USDA food guides.* Retrieved from http://www.choosemyplate.gov/sites/default/files/printablematerials/ABrief HistoryOfUSDAFoodGuides.pdf.

US Department of Health and Human Services. (2012). *Child maltreatment 2011.* Washington, DC, U.S. Government Printing Office.

Weinmann, S., Chun, C., Schmid, D. S., et al. (2013). Incidence and clinical characteristics of herpes zoster among children in the varicella vaccine era, 2005-2009. *Journal of Infectious Diseases, 208*(11), 1859–1868.

34

The School-Age Child and Family

Cheryl C. Rodgers

(e) http://evolve.elsevier.com/Perry/maternal

PROMOTING OPTIMAL GROWTH AND DEVELOPMENT

The segment of the life span that extends from 6 years of age to approximately 12 years of age has a variety of labels, each of which describes an important characteristic of the period. These middle years are most often referred to as *school-age* or the *school years*. This period begins with entrance into the school environment, which has a significant impact on development and relationships.

Physiologically, the middle years begin with the shedding of the first deciduous tooth and end at puberty with the acquisition of the final permanent teeth (with the exception of the wisdom teeth). Before 5 or 6 years of age, children have progressed from helpless infants to sturdy, complicated individuals with an ability to communicate, conceptualize in a limited way, and become involved in complex social and motor behaviors. Physical growth is also rapid during the preschool-age years. In contrast, the period of middle childhood, between the rapid growth of early childhood and the prepubescent growth spurt, is a time of gradual growth and development with more even progress in both physical and emotional aspects.

BIOLOGIC DEVELOPMENT

During middle childhood, growth in height and weight assumes a slower but steady pace as compared with the earlier years. Between 6 and 12 years of age, children grow an average of 5 cm (2 inches) per year to gain 30 to 60 cm (1 to 2 feet) in height and almost double their weight, increasing 2 to 3 kg (4.4 to 6.6 pounds) per year. The average 6-year-old child is about 116 cm (46 inches) tall and weighs about 21 kg (46 pounds); the average 12-year-old child is about 150 cm (59 inches) tall and weighs approximately 40 kg (88 pounds). During this period, girls and boys differ little in size, although boys tend to be slightly taller and somewhat heavier than girls. Toward the end of the school-age years, both boys and girls begin to increase in size, although most girls begin to surpass boys in both height and weight, to the acute discomfort of both girls and boys.

Physical Changes

School-age children are more graceful than they were as preschoolers, and they are steadier on their feet. Their body proportions take on a slimmer look, with longer legs, varying body proportion, and a lower center of gravity. Posture improves over that of the preschool period to facilitate locomotion and efficiency in using the arms and trunk. These proportions make climbing, bicycle riding, and other activities easier. Fat gradually diminishes, and its distribution patterns change,

contributing to the thinner appearance of children during the middle years.

Accompanying the skeletal lengthening and fat diminution is an increase in the percentage of body weight represented by muscle tissue. By the end of this age period, both boys and girls double their strength and physical capabilities and their steady and relatively consistent development of coordination increases their poise and skill. However, this increased strength can be misleading. Although strength increases, muscles are still functionally immature when compared with those of adolescents, and they are more readily damaged by muscular injury caused by overuse.

The most pronounced changes that indicate increasing maturity in children are a decrease in head circumference in relation to standing height, a decrease in waist circumference in relation to height, and an increase in leg length in relation to height. These observations often provide a clue to a child's degree of physical maturity. Specific physiologic and anatomic characteristics are typical of school-age children. Facial proportions change as the face grows faster in relation to the remainder of the cranium. The skull and brain grow very slowly during this period and increase little in size. Because all of the primary (deciduous) teeth are lost during this age span, middle childhood is sometimes known as the age of the loose tooth (Fig. 34.1). The early years of middle childhood, when the new secondary (permanent) teeth appear too large for the face, are known as the ugly duckling stage.

Maturation of Systems

Maturity of the gastrointestinal system is reflected in fewer stomach upsets; better maintenance of blood glucose levels; and an increased stomach capacity, which permits retention of food for longer periods. School-age children do not need to be fed as promptly or as frequently as preschool-age children. Caloric needs (kcal/kg) are less than they were in the preschool years and lower than they will be during the coming adolescent growth spurt.

Physical maturation is evident in other body tissues and organs. Bladder capacity, although differing widely among individual children, is generally greater in girls than in boys. The heart grows more slowly during the middle years and is smaller in relation to the rest of the body than at any other period of life. Heart and respiratory rates steadily decrease, and blood pressure increases from 6 to 12 years of age.

The immune system becomes more competent in its ability to localize infections and to produce an antibody-antigen response. However, children have several infections in the first 1 to 2 years of school because of increased exposure to other children.

Bones continue to ossify throughout childhood but yield to pressure and muscle pulls more readily than with mature bones. Children need

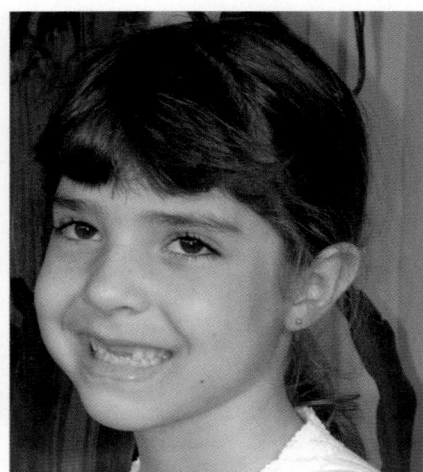

FIG 34.1 Middle childhood is the stage of development when deciduous teeth are shed.

ample opportunity to move around, but they should observe caution in carrying heavy loads. For example, they should shift books or tote bags from one arm to the other. Backpacks, when worn correctly, distribute weight more evenly than tote bags.

Wider differences between children are observed at the end of middle childhood than at the beginning. These differences become increasingly apparent and, if they are extreme or unique, may create emotional problems. The associated characteristics of height and weight relationships, rapid or slow growth, and other important features of development should be explained to children and their families. Physical maturity is not necessarily correlated with emotional and social maturity. Seven-year-old children who look like 10-year-old children will think and act like 7-year-old children. To expect behaviors appropriate for the older age is unrealistic and can be detrimental to their development of competence and self-esteem. Conversely, to treat 10-year-old children who look young physically as though they were younger is an equal disservice to them.

Prepubescence

Preadolescence is the period of approximately 2 years that begins at the end of middle childhood and ends with the thirteenth birthday. Because puberty signals the beginning of the development of secondary sex characteristics, prepubescence typically occurs during preadolescence.

Toward the end of middle childhood, the discrepancies in growth and maturation between boys and girls become apparent. On the average, there is a difference of approximately 2 years between girls and boys in the age of onset of pubescence. This is a period of rapid growth in height and weight, especially for girls.

There is no universal age at which children assume the characteristics of prepubescence. The first physiologic signs appear at about 9 years of age (particularly in girls) and are usually clearly evident in 11- to 12-year-old children. Although preadolescent children do not want to be different, variability in physical growth and physiologic changes among children of the same sex and between the two sexes is often striking at this time. This variability, especially in relation to the onset of secondary sexual characteristics, is of great concern to preadolescents. Either early or late appearance of these characteristics is a source of embarrassment and uneasiness to both sexes.

Preadolescence is a period of considerable overlapping of developmental characteristics of both middle childhood and early adolescence. However, several unique characteristics set this period apart from others. Generally, puberty begins at 10 years of age in girls and 12 years of age

in boys, but it can be normal for either sex after 8 years of age. Boys experience little visible sexual maturation during preadolescence.

PSYCHOSOCIAL DEVELOPMENT

Developing a Sense of Industry (Erikson)

Freud described middle childhood as the latency period, a time of tranquility between the Oedipal phase of early childhood and the eroticism of adolescence. During this time, children experience relationships with same-sex peers following the indifference of earlier years and preceding the heterosexual fascination that occurs for most boys and girls in puberty.

Successful mastery of Erikson's first three stages of psychosocial development is important in terms of development of a healthy personality. Successful completion of these stages requires a loving environment within a stable family unit. These experiences prepare the child to engage in experiences and relationships beyond the intimate family group.

A sense of industry or a stage of accomplishment is achieved somewhere between 6 years of age and adolescence. School-age children are eager to develop skills and participate in meaningful and socially useful work. They acquire a sense of personal and interpersonal competence; receive the systematic instruction prescribed by their individual cultures; and develop the skills needed to become useful, contributing members of their social communities. Failure to develop a sense of accomplishment may result in a sense of inferiority.

Interests expand in the middle years, and with a growing sense of independence, children want to engage in tasks that can be carried through to completion (Fig. 34.2). They gain satisfaction from independent behavior in exploring and manipulating their environment and from interaction with peers. Often the acquisition of skills provides a way to achieve success in social activities. Reinforcement in the form of grades, material rewards, additional privileges, and recognition provides encouragement and stimulation.

A sense of accomplishment also involves the ability to cooperate, to compete with others, and to cope effectively with people. Middle childhood is the time when children learn the value of doing things with others and the benefits derived from division of labor in the accomplishment of goals. Peer approval is a strong motivating power.

The danger inherent in this period of development is the occurrence of situations that might result in a sense of inferiority. This may happen if the previous stages have not been successfully mastered or if a child is incapable of or unprepared to assume responsibilities associated with developing sense of accomplishment. Children with physical and mental limitations may be at a disadvantage in the acquisition of certain skills. When the reward structure is based on evidence of mastery, children who are incapable of developing these skills risk feeling inadequate and inferior. Even children without chronic disabilities may experience feelings of inadequacy in some areas. No child is able to do everything well, and children must learn that they will not be able to master every skill that they attempt. All children, even children who usually have positive attitudes toward work and their own abilities, will feel some degree of inferiority when they encounter specific skills that they cannot master.

Children need and want real achievement. Children achieve a sense of industry when they have access to tasks that need to be done and they are able to complete the tasks well despite individual differences in their innate capacities and emotional development.

COGNITIVE DEVELOPMENT (PIAGET)

When children enter the school years, they begin to acquire the ability to relate a series of events to mental representations that can be expressed

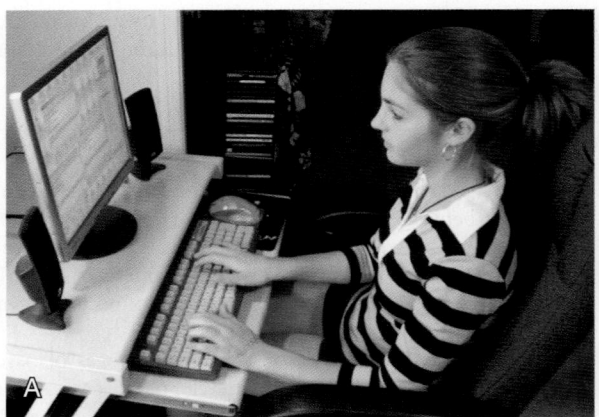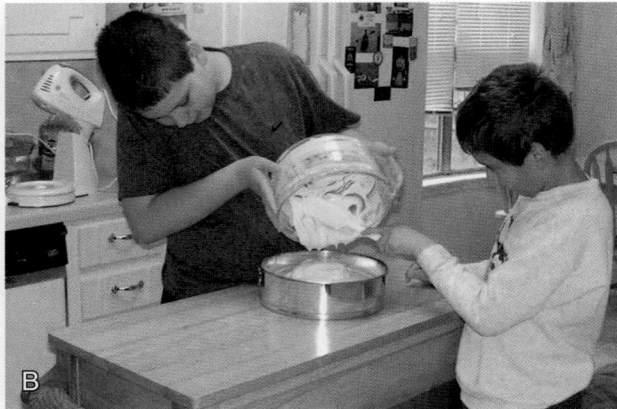

FIG 34.2 School-age children are motivated to complete tasks. **A,** Working alone. **B,** Working with others.

both verbally and symbolically. This is the stage Piaget describes as concrete operations, when children are able to use thought processes to experience events and actions. The rigid, egocentric view of the preschool years is replaced by mental processes that allow children to see things from another's point of view.

During this stage, children develop an understanding of relationships between things and ideas. They progress from making judgments based on what they see (perceptual thinking) to making judgments based on what they reason (conceptual thinking). They are increasingly able to master symbols and to use their memories of past experiences to evaluate and interpret the present.

One cognitive task of school-age children is mastering the concept of conservation (Fig. 34.3). There is a developmental sequence in children's capacity to understand conservation. At an early age (≈5 to 6 years of age), children grasp the concept of conservation of numbers. For example, they recognize that 5 remains 5 whether it is represented by 3+2, 4+1, five balls, or five buttons. Conservation of liquids, mass, and length usually is accomplished at about 6 to 7 years of age. They recognize that changing the shape of a substance such as a lump of clay does not alter its total mass. They learn conservation of weight sometime later (9 to 10 years of age) and conservation of volume or displacement last (9 to 12 years of age). For example, they no longer perceive a tall, thin glass of water as containing a greater volume than a short, wide glass; they can distinguish between the weight of items regardless of their size. School-age children also develop classification skills. They can group and sort objects according to the attributes that they share, place things in a sensible and logical order, and hold a concept in mind while making decisions based on that concept. Another characteristic of middle childhood is that children derive enjoyment from classifying and ordering their environment. They become occupied with collections of objects, such as stickers, shells, dolls, cars, cards, and stuffed animals. They may even begin to order friends and relationships (e.g., best friend, second-best friend).

They develop the ability to understand relational terms and concepts, such as bigger and smaller; darker and paler; heavier and lighter; to the right of and to the left of; and more than and less than. They view family relationships in terms of reciprocal roles (e.g., to be a brother, one must have a sibling).

School-age children learn the alphabet and the world of symbols called *words,* which can be arranged in terms of structure and their relationship to the alphabet. They learn to tell time, to see the relationship of events in time (history) and places in space (geography), and to combine time and space relationships (geology and astronomy).

The ability to read is acquired during the school years and becomes the most significant and valuable tool for independent inquiry. Children's capacity to explore, imagine, and expand their knowledge is enhanced by reading.

MORAL DEVELOPMENT (KOHLBERG)

As children move from egocentrism to more logical patterns of thought, they also move through stages in the development of conscience and moral standards. Young children do not believe that standards of behavior come from within themselves but that rules are established and set down by others. During the preschool years, children adopt and internalize the moral values of their parents. They learn standards for acceptable behavior, act according to these standards, and feel guilty when they violate them. Although children 6 or 7 years of age know the rules and behaviors expected of them, they do not understand the reasons behind them. Rewards and punishments guide their judgment; a "bad act" is one that breaks a rule or causes harm. Young children believe that what other people tell them to do is right and that what they themselves think is wrong. Consequently, children 6 or 7 years of age may interpret accidents or misfortunes as punishment for "bad" acts.

Older school-age children are able to judge an act by the intentions that prompted it rather than just its consequences. Rules and judgments become less absolute and authoritarian and begin to be founded on the needs and desires of others. For older children, a rule violation is likely to be viewed in relation to the total context in which it appears. The situation, as well as the morality of the rule itself, influences reactions. Although younger children judge an act only according to whether it is right or wrong, older children take into account different points of view. They are able to understand and accept the concept of treating others as they would like to be treated.

SPIRITUAL DEVELOPMENT

Children at this age think in concrete terms but are avid learners and have a great desire to learn about their God or deity. They picture God as human and use adjectives such as "loving" and "helping" to describe their deity. They are fascinated by the concepts of hell and heaven, with a developing conscience and concern about rules. They may fear going to hell for misbehavior. School-age children want and expect to be punished for misbehavior and, when given the option, tend to choose a punishment that "fits the crime." However, they may view illness or injury as a punishment for a real or imagined misdeed. The beliefs and

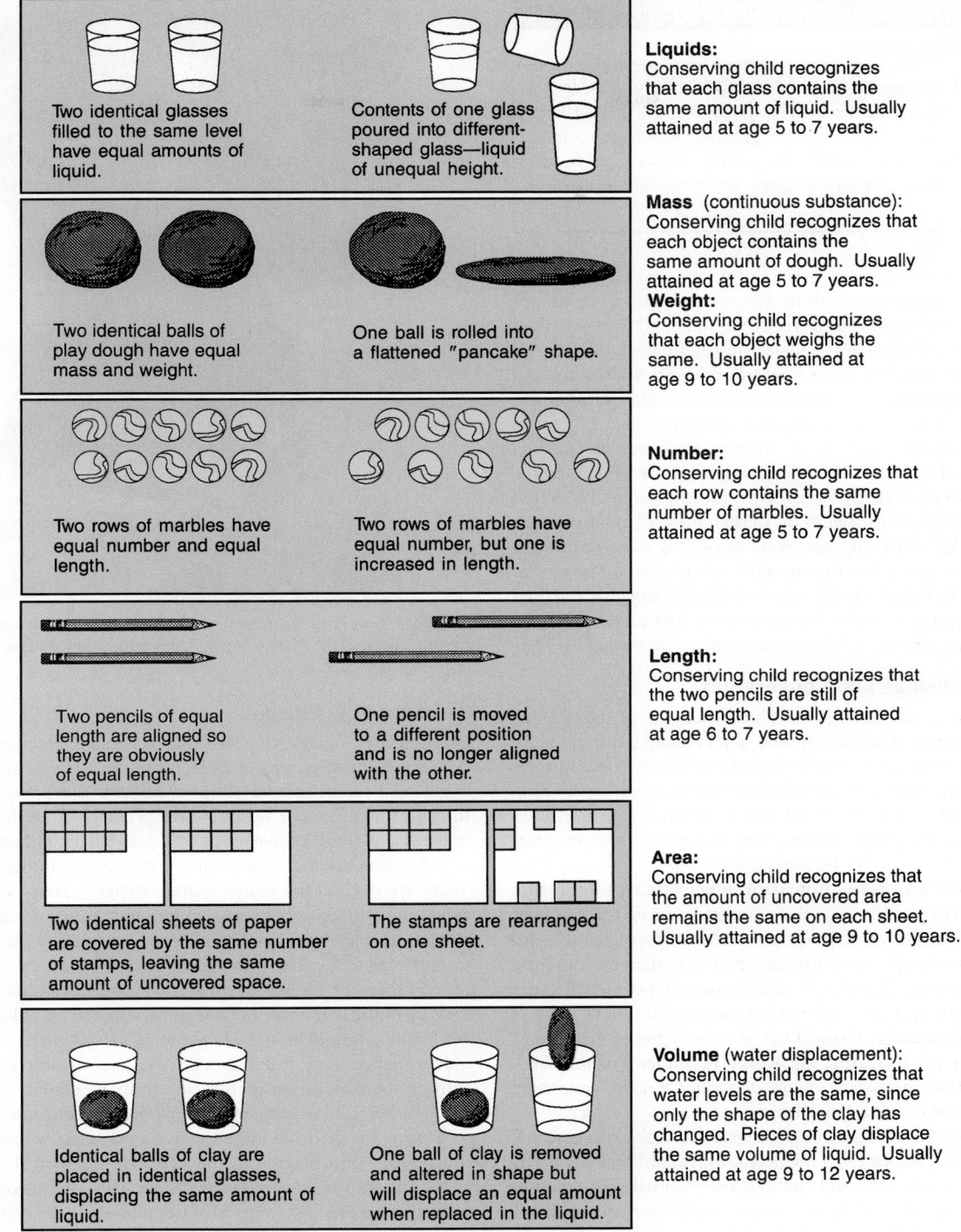

Liquids:
Conserving child recognizes that each glass contains the same amount of liquid. Usually attained at age 5 to 7 years.

Two identical glasses filled to the same level have equal amounts of liquid.

Contents of one glass poured into different-shaped glass—liquid of unequal height.

Mass (continuous substance): Conserving child recognizes that each object contains the same amount of dough. Usually attained at age 5 to 7 years.
Weight: Conserving child recognizes that each object weighs the same. Usually attained at age 9 to 10 years.

Two identical balls of play dough have equal mass and weight.

One ball is rolled into a flattened "pancake" shape.

Number: Conserving child recognizes that each row contains the same number of marbles. Usually attained at age 5 to 7 years.

Two rows of marbles have equal number and equal length.

Two rows of marbles have equal number, but one is increased in length.

Length: Conserving child recognizes that the two pencils are still of equal length. Usually attained at age 6 to 7 years.

Two pencils of equal length are aligned so they are obviously of equal length.

One pencil is moved to a different position and is no longer aligned with the other.

Area: Conserving child recognizes that the amount of uncovered area remains the same on each sheet. Usually attained at age 9 to 10 years.

Two identical sheets of paper are covered by the same number of stamps, leaving the same amount of uncovered space.

The stamps are rearranged on one sheet.

Volume (water displacement): Conserving child recognizes that water levels are the same, since only the shape of the clay has changed. Pieces of clay displace the same volume of liquid. Usually attained at age 9 to 12 years.

Identical balls of clay are placed in identical glasses, displacing the same amount of liquid.

One ball of clay is removed and altered in shape but will displace an equal amount when replaced in the liquid.

FIG 34.3 Common examples that demonstrate the child's ability to conserve (ages are only approximate).

ideals of family and religious people are more influential than those of their peers in matters of faith.

School-age children begin to learn the difference between the natural and the supernatural but have difficulty understanding symbols. Consequently, religious concepts must be presented to them in concrete terms. Prayer or other religious rituals comfort them, and if these activities are a part of their daily lives, they can help them cope with threatening situations. Their petitions to their God in prayers tend to be for tangible rewards. Although younger children expect their prayers to be answered, as they get older, they begin to recognize that this does not always occur and they become less concerned when their prayers are not answered. They are able to discuss their feelings about their faith and how it relates to their lives (see Cultural Considerations box: Religious Orientation).

SOCIAL DEVELOPMENT

One of the most important socializing agents in the school-age years is the peer group. In addition to parents and schools, the peer group

Religious Orientation

Many schools and communities have a Judeo-Christian orientation toward prayer, holidays, and values. This may result in conflict and discomfort for children of other religious or ethnic groups. Sensitivity must be exercised so as not to offend and confuse children from other religious backgrounds, such as the Buddhist, Hindu, and Muslim faiths, and those with no religious backgrounds.

conveys a substantial amount of information to its members. Peer groups have a culture of their own with secrets, traditions, and codes of ethics that promote feelings of solidarity and detachment from adults. Through peer relationships, children learn how to deal with dominance and hostility, how to relate to people in positions of leadership and authority, and how to explore ideas and the physical environment.

Peer-group identification is an important factor in gaining independence from parents. The aid and support of the group provide children with enough security to risk the moderate parental rejection brought about by small victories in the development of independence.

A child's concept of the appropriate gender role is acquired through relationships with peers. During the early school years, few gender differences exist in the play experiences of children. Both girls and boys share games and other activities. However, in the later school years, the differences in play of boys and girls become more marked.

Social Relationships and Cooperation

Daily relationships with peers provide important social interactions for school-age children. For the first time, children join group activities with unrestrained enthusiasm and steady participation. Previous interactions were limited to short periods under considerable adult supervision. With increased skills and wider opportunities, children become involved with one or more peer groups in which they can gain status as respected members.

Valuable lessons are learned from daily interaction with age mates. First, children learn to appreciate the numerous and varied points of view that are represented in the peer group. As children interact with peers who see the world in ways that are somewhat different from their own, they become aware of the limits of their own point of view. Because age mates are peers and are not forced to accept each other's ideas as they are expected to accept those of adults, other children have a significant influence on decreasing the egocentric outlook of the child. Consequently, children learn to argue, persuade, bargain, cooperate, and compromise to maintain friendships.

Second, children become increasingly sensitive to the social norms and pressures of the peer group. The peer group establishes standards for acceptance and rejection, and children are often willing to modify their behavior to be accepted by the group. The need for peer approval becomes a powerful influence toward conformity. Children learn to dress, talk, and behave in a manner acceptable to the group. A variety of roles, such as class joker or class hero, may be assumed by individual children to gain approval from the group.

Third, the interaction among peers leads to the formation of intimate friendships between same-sex peers. The school-age period is the time when children have "best friends" with whom they share secrets, private jokes, and adventures; they come to one another's aid in times of trouble. In the course of these friendships, children also fight, threaten each other, break up, and reunite. These relationships, in which the child experiences love and closeness with a peer, seem to be important as a foundation for relationships in adulthood (Fig. 34.4).

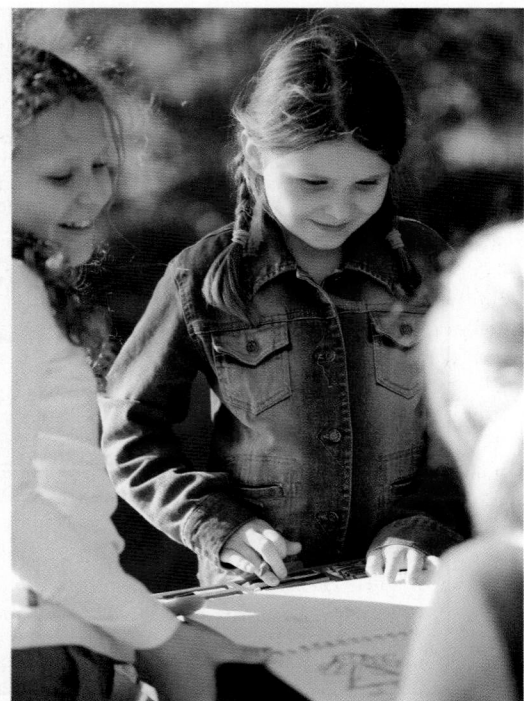

FIG 34.4 School-age children enjoy engaging in activities with a "best friend." (Copyright 2011 Photos.com, a division of Getty Images. All rights reserved.)

Clubs and Peer Groups

One of the outstanding characteristics of middle childhood is the formation of formalized groups, or clubs. A prominent feature of these groups is the rigid rules imposed on the members. There is exclusiveness in the selection of people who have the privilege of joining. Acceptance in the group is often determined on a pass-fail basis according to social or behavioral criteria. Conformity is the core of the group structure. There are often secret codes, shared interests, and special modes of dress, and special words that signify membership in the group. Each child must abide by a standard of behavior established by the members. Conforming to the rules provides children with feelings of security and relieves them of the responsibility of making decisions. By merging their identities with those of their peers, children are able to move from the family group to an outside group as a step toward seeking further independence. Peer groups and clubs allow children to substitute conformity to a peer group for conformity to a family at a time when children are still too insecure to function independently.

During the early school years, groups are usually small and loosely organized, with changing membership and no formal structure. The clubs and groups usually do not display elements of cooperation and order that are seen in groups of older children. In general, girls'; groups are less formalized than boys' groups, and although there may be a mixture of both sexes in the early school years, the groups of later school years are composed predominantly of children of the same sex. Common interests are the basis around which the group is structured.

Poor relationships with peers and a lack of group identification can contribute to bullying. Bullying is any recurring activity that intends to cause harm, distress, or control toward another in which there is a perceived imbalance of power between the aggressor(s) and the victim (Hensley, 2013). Although bullying can occur in any setting, it most often occurs at school where supervision is minimal but peers are present to witness the attack, such as playgrounds, hallways, bathrooms, or school buses (Carter & Wilson, 2015). Cyberbullying involves an electronic medium to harm or bother another individual and can be more harmful than traditional bullying, because the attack can instantly reach a wider audience, be available 24 hours a day, and allow the bully to remain anonymous (Carter & Wilson, 2015). Children who are targeted for bullying often have submissive characteristics such as those who are anxious, insecure, and sensitive, which make them an easy target for bullying (Juvonen & Graham, 2014). Bullies are generally defiant toward adults, antisocial, and likely to break school rules. They have aggressive attitudes, a positive view of violence, a lack of empathy, and may experience or witness violence or abuse at home (Hensley, 2013). Boys who bully tend to use physical force, referred to as *direct bullying,* but girls usually use *indirect bullying* methods, such as exclusion, gossip, or rumors (Shetgiri, 2013).

The long-term consequences of bullying are significant. Future problems of bullies include a higher risk for conduct problems, use of tobacco and illicit drugs, school dropout, unemployment, and participation in criminal behavior (Wolke & Lereya, 2015). Chronic bullies seem to continue their behaviors into adulthood, negatively influencing their ability to develop and maintain relationships. Victims of bullying are at increased risk for low self-esteem, self-harm, anxiety, depression, feelings of insecurity, loneliness, and psychosomatic complaints, such as headaches, stomach aches, or sleeping problems (Wolke & Lereya, 2015).

Because most bullying occurs in and around the school, there has been more emphasis on recognizing and dealing with the behaviors in schools.* Interventions should include recognizing the behavior in both the bully and the victim, protecting the victim, and stopping the behavior altogether. To be effective, behavioral changes from the bully and social changes in the school environment with the assistance of parents and adults in the school should occur. A recent meta-analysis on anti-bullying interventions including primarily school programs found positive effects for the interventions; however, further studies are needed (Langford, Bonell, Jones, et al., 2014).

There are also dangers in peer-group attachments that are too strong. Peer pressures force some children to take risks or engage in behaviors that are against their better judgment. Youth gang members continue to increase in the United States with the peak age of joining as 14 years (Pyrooz & Sweeten, 2015). A child's membership in a gang is associated with marked increases in serious delinquent behavior (Bradshaw, Waasdorp, Goldweber, et al., 2013). An integration of family-centered and school-based programs is needed to reduce the influences for children to become affiliated with gangs.

Relationships With Families

Although the peer group is influential and necessary for normal child development, parents are the primary influence in shaping their children's personalities, setting standards for behavior, and establishing value systems. Family values usually take precedence over peer value systems. Although children may appear to reject parental values while testing the new values of the peer group, ultimately they retain and incorporate into their own value systems the parental values they have found to be of worth.

In the middle school years, children want to spend more time in the company of peers, and they often prefer peer-group activities to family activities. This can be disturbing to parents. Children become intolerant and critical of their parents, especially when their parents' ways deviate from those of the group. They discover that parents can be wrong, and they begin to question the knowledge and authority of their parents, who were previously considered to be all-knowing and all-powerful. Parents can best serve the interests of their children through tolerant understanding and support.

Although increased independence is the goal of middle childhood, children are not prepared to abandon all parental control. They need and want restrictions placed on their behavior, and they are not prepared to cope with all of the problems of their expanding environment. They feel more secure knowing there is an authority figure to implement controls and restrictions. Children may complain loudly about restrictions and try to break down parental barriers, but they are uneasy if they succeed in doing so. They respect adults who prevent them from acting on every urge. Children view this behavior as an expression of love and concern for their welfare.

Children also need their parents to be adults, not friends. Sometimes parents, hurt by their children's rejection, attempt to maintain their love and gratitude by assuming the role of "pals." Children need the stable, secure strength provided by mature adults to whom they can turn during troubled relationships with peers or stressful changes in their world. With a secure base in a loving family, children are able to develop the self-confidence and maturity needed to break loose from the group and stand independently.

Play

Play takes on new dimensions that reflect a new stage of development in the school years. Play involves increased physical skill, intellectual ability, and fantasy. In addition, children develop a sense of belonging to a team or club by forming groups and cliques.

Rules and Rituals

The need for conformity in middle childhood is strongly manifested in the activities and games of school-age children. In the preschool years, children's games were either invented for them or played in the company of a friend or an adult. Now children begin to see the need for rules, and their games have fixed and unvarying rules that may be bizarre and extraordinarily rigid. Part of the enjoyment of the game is knowing the rules, because knowing means belonging. Conformity and ritual permeate their play and are also evident in their behavior and language. Childhood is full of chants and taunts, such as: "Eeny, meeny, miney, mo," "Last one is a rotten egg," and "Step on a crack, break your mother's back." Children derive a sense of pleasure and power from such sayings, which have been handed down with few changes through generations.

Team Play

A more complex form of play that evolves from the need for peer interaction is team games and sports. A referee, umpire, or person of authority may be required so that the rules can be followed more accurately. Team play teaches children to modify or exchange personal goals for goals of the group; it also teaches them that division of labor is an effective strategy for attaining a goal.

Team play can also contribute to children's social, intellectual, and skill growth (Eime, Young, Harvey, et al., 2013). Children work hard to develop the skills needed to become team members, to improve their contribution to the group, and to anticipate the consequences of their behavior for the group. Team play helps stimulate cognitive growth because children are called on to learn many complex rules, make judgments about those rules, plan strategies, and assess the strengths and weaknesses of members of their own team and members of the opposing team.

Quiet Games and Activities

Although play of school-age children is highly active, they also enjoy quiet and solitary activities. The middle years are the time for collections,

---

*Resources on bullying include: www.eyesonbullying.org and www.stopbullying.gov.

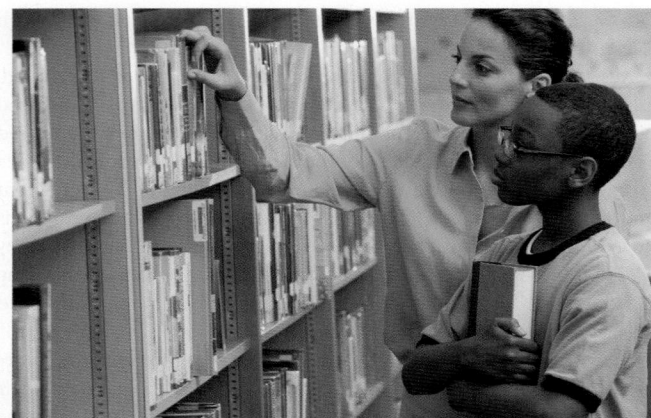

FIG 34.5 Selecting a book with the assistance of an adult. (Copyright 2011 by Photos.com, a division of Getty Images. All rights reserved.)

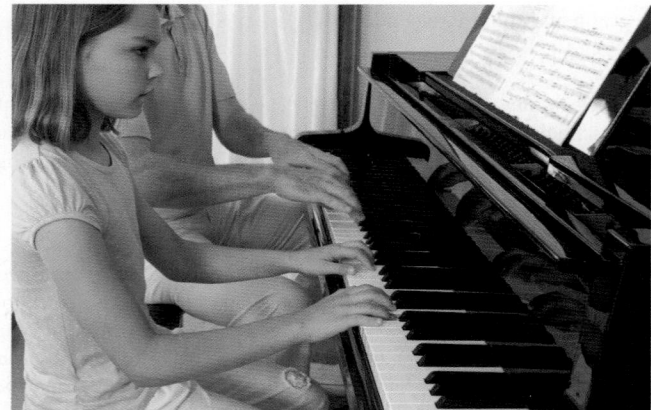

FIG 34.6 School-age children take pride in learning new skills. (Copyright 2011 by Photos.com, a division of Getty Images. All rights reserved.)

which constitute another ritual. Young school-age children's collections are an odd assortment of unrelated objects in messy, disorganized piles. Collections of later school years are more orderly, selective, and organized in scrapbooks, on shelves, or in boxes.

School-age children become fascinated with complex board, card, or computer games that they can play alone, with a best friend, or with a group. As in all games, adherence to the rules is fanatic. Disagreements over rules can cause much discussion and argument but are easily resolved by reading the rules of the game.

The newly acquired skill of reading becomes increasingly satisfying as school-age children expand their knowledge of the world through books (Fig. 34.5). School-age children never tire of stories and, as with preschool children, love to have stories read aloud. They also enjoy sewing, cooking, carpentry, gardening, and creative activities, such as painting. Many creative skills, such as music and art, as well as athletic skills such as swimming, karate, dancing, and skating, are learned during these years and continue to be enjoyed into adolescence and adulthood (Fig. 34.6).

DEVELOPMENT OF A SELF-CONCEPT

The term *self-concept* refers to a conscious awareness of self-perceptions, such as one's physical characteristics, abilities, values, self-ideals and expectancy, and idea of self in relation to others. It also includes one's

body image, sexuality, and self-esteem. Although primary caregivers continue to exert influence on children's self-evaluation, the opinions of peers and teachers provide valuable input during middle childhood. With the emphasis on skill building and broadened social relationships, children are continually engaged in the process of self-evaluation.

Body Image

School-age children have a relatively accurate and positive perception of their physical selves, but in general, they like their physical selves less as they grow older. The head appears to be the most important part of the school-age child's perceived image of self, with hair and eye color the characteristics used most frequently to describe the physical self.

Body image is influenced, but not solely determined, by significant others. The number of significant others who influence children's perception of themselves increases with age. Children are acutely aware of their own bodies, the bodies of their peers, and those of adults. They are also aware of deviations from the norm. Physical impairments, such as hearing or visual defects, ears that "stick out," or birthmarks, assume great importance. Increasing awareness of these differences, especially when accompanied by unkind comments and taunts from others, may cause a child to feel inferior and less desirable. This is especially true if the defect interferes with the child's ability to participate in games and activities.

Table 34.1 summarizes the major developmental achievements of the school-age years.

COPING WITH CONCERNS RELATED TO NORMAL GROWTH AND DEVELOPMENT

School Experience

School serves as the agent for transmitting the values of society to each succeeding generation of children. School is also the setting for relationships with peers. After the family, schools are the second most important socializing agent in the lives of children.

Entrance into school causes a sharp break in the structure of the child's world. For many children, it is their first experience in conforming to a group pattern imposed by an adult who is not a parent and who has responsibility for too many children to be constantly aware of each child as an individual. Children want to go to school and usually adapt to the new conditions with little difficulty. Successful adjustment is related to the child's physical and emotional maturity and the parent's readiness to accept the separation associated with school entrance. Unfortunately, some parents express their unconscious attempts to delay the child's maturity by clinging behavior, particularly with their youngest child.

By the time they enter school, most children have a fairly realistic concept of what school involves. They receive information regarding the role of a student from parents, siblings, playmates, and the media. In addition, most children have had some experience with day care, preschool, or kindergarten. Middle-class children have fewer adjustments to make and less to learn about expected behavior because schools tend to reflect dominant middle-class customs and values. If the child has attended a preschool program, the focus of the preschool program also affects the child's adjustment. Some preschool programs provide custodial care only, but others emphasize emotional, social, and intellectual development.

Role of Teachers

Children respond best to teachers who possess the characteristics of a warm, loving parent. Teachers in the early grades perform many of the activities formerly assumed by the parent, such as recognizing the child's personal needs (e.g., the need to go to the bathroom, need for help

TABLE 34.1 Growth and Development During the School-Age Years

Physical and Motor	Mental	Adaptive	Personal-Social
6 Years of Age			
Height and weight gain continues slowly	Develops concept of numbers	At table, uses knife to spread butter or jam on bread	Can share and cooperate better
Weight, 16 to 26.3 kg (35.5 to 58 pounds)	Can count 13 pennies	At play, cuts, folds, pastes paper; sews crudely if needle is threaded	Has great need for children of own age
Height, 106.7 to 123.5 cm (42 to 49 inches)	Knows whether it is morning or afternoon	Takes bath without supervision; performs bedtime activities alone	Will cheat to win
Central mandibular incisors erupt	Defines common objects such as fork and chair in terms of their use	Reads from memory; enjoys oral spelling game	Often engages in rough play
Loses first tooth	Obeys three commands in succession	Likes table games, checkers, simple card games	Often jealous of younger brother or sister
Gradual increase in dexterity	Knows right and left hands	Giggles a lot	Does what adults are seen doing
Active age; constant activity	Says which is pretty and which is ugly of a series of drawings of faces	Sometimes steals money or attractive items	May have occasional temper tantrums
Often returns to finger feeding	Describes the objects in a picture rather than simply enumerating them	Has difficulty owning up to misdeeds	Is a boaster
More aware of hand as a tool	Attends first grade	Tries out own abilities	Is more independent, probably an influence of school
Likes to draw, print, color			Has own way of doing things
Vision reaches maturity			Increases socialization
7 Years of Age			
Begins to grow at least 5 cm (2 inches) in height per year	Notices that certain items are missing from pictures	Uses table knife for cutting meat; may need help with tough or difficult pieces	Is becoming a real member of the family group
Weight, 17.7 to 30 kg (39 to 66 pounds)	Can copy a diamond	Brushes and combs hair acceptably without help	Takes part in group play
Height, 111.8 to 129.5 cm (44 to 51 inches)	Repeats three numbers backward	May steal	Boys prefer playing with boys; girls prefer playing with girls
Maxillary central incisors and lateral mandibular incisors erupt	Develops concept of time; reads ordinary clock or watch correctly to nearest quarter hour; uses clock for practical purposes	Likes to help and have a choice	Spends a lot of time alone; does not require a lot of companionship
More cautious in approaches to new performances	Attends second grade	Is less resistant and stubborn	
Repeats performances to master them	More mechanical in reading; often does not stop at the end of a sentence; skips words such as "it," "the," and "he"		
Jaw begins to expand to accommodate permanent teeth			
8 to 9 Years of Age			
Continues to gain 5 cm (2 inches) in height per year	Gives similarities and differences between two things from memory	Makes use of common tools such as hammer, saw, screwdriver	Is easy to get along with at home
Weight, 19.6 to 39.6 kg (43 to 87 pounds)	Counts backward from 20 to 1; understands concept of reversibility	Uses household and sewing utensils	Likes the reward system
Height, 116.8 to 141.8 cm (46 to 56 inches)	Repeats days of the week and months in order; knows the date	Helps with routine household tasks such as dusting, sweeping	Dramatizes
Lateral incisors (maxillary) and mandibular cuspids erupt	Describes common objects in detail, not merely their use	Assumes responsibility for share of household chores	Is more sociable
Movement fluid; often graceful and poised	Makes change out of a quarter	Looks after all of own needs at table	Is better behaved
Always on the go; jumps, chases, skips	Attends third and fourth grades	Buys useful articles; exercises some choice in making purchases	Is interested in boy-girl relationships but will not admit it
Increased smoothness and speed in fine motor control; uses cursive writing	Reads more; may plan to wake up early just to read	Runs useful errands	Goes about home and community freely, alone or with friends
Dresses self completely	Reads classic books but also enjoys comics	Likes pictorial magazines	Likes to compete and play games
Likely to overdo; hard to quiet down after recess	More aware of time; can be relied on to get to school on time	Likes school; wants to answer all the questions	Shows preference in friends and groups
More limber; bones grow faster than ligaments	Can grasp concepts of parts and whole (fractions)	Is afraid of failing a grade; is ashamed of bad grades	Plays mostly with groups of own sex, but is beginning to mix
	Understands concepts of space, cause and effect, nesting (puzzles), conservation (permanence of mass and volume)	Is more critical of self	Develops modesty
	Classifies objects by more than one quality; has collections	Takes music and sport lessons	Compares self with others
	Produces simple paintings or drawings		Enjoys organizations, clubs, and group sports

TABLE 34.1   Growth and Development During the School-Age Years—cont'd

Physical and Motor	Mental	Adaptive	Personal-Social
10 to 12 Years of Age			
Weight, 24.3 to 58 kg (54 to 128 pounds) Height, 127 to 162.5 cm (50 to 64 inches) Remainder of teeth will erupt and tend toward full development (except wisdom teeth) **Girls:** Pubescent changes may begin to appear; body lines soften and round out **Boys:** Slow growth in height and rapid weight gain; may become obese in this period	Writes brief stories Attends fifth to seventh grades Writes occasional short letters to friends or relatives on own initiative Uses telephone for practical purposes Responds to magazine, radio, or other advertising Reads for practical information or own enjoyment—stories or library books of adventure or romance, animal stories	Makes useful tools or does easy repair work Cooks or sews in small way Raises pets Washes and dries own hair; is responsible for a thorough job of cleaning hair, but may need reminding to do so Is sometimes left alone at home for an hour or so Is successful in looking after own needs or those of other children left in his or her care	Loves friends; talks about them constantly Chooses friends more selectively; may have a "best friend" Enjoys conversation Develops beginning interest in opposite sex Is more diplomatic Likes family; family really has meaning Likes mother and wants to please her in many ways Demonstrates affection Likes father, who is admired and may be idolized Respects parents

with clothing) and helping to develop their social behavior (e.g., manners).

Teachers, like parents, are concerned about the child's psychologic and emotional welfare. Although the functions of teachers and parents differ, both place constraints on behavior and both are in a position to enforce standards of conduct. However, the teacher's primary responsibility involves stimulating and guiding children's intellectual development, as opposed to providing for their physical welfare beyond the school setting.

Teachers serve as models that children try to emulate. Children seek their teachers' approval and avoid their disapproval. The teacher is a significant person in the life of the early school-age child, and hero worship of a teacher may extend into late childhood and preadolescence. Teachers who make supportive statements that reassure or commend children, use accepting and clarifying statements that help children refine ideas and feelings, and provide assistance that aids children with their own problem solving contribute to the development of a positive self-concept in the school-age child.

Role of Parents

Parents share responsibility for helping children achieve their maximal potential. Parents can supplement the school program in numerous ways (see Family-Centered Care box: Helping Children in School). Cultivating responsibility is the goal of parental assistance. Being responsible for schoolwork helps children learn to keep promises, meet deadlines, and succeed at their jobs as adults. Responsible children may occasionally ask for help (e.g., with a spelling list), but usually they prefer to think through their work by themselves. Excessive pressure or lack of encouragement from parents may inhibit the development of these desirable traits.

Latchkey Children

The term *latchkey children* is used to describe children who are left to care for themselves before or after school without the supervision of an adult. The large numbers of single-parent families and working parents, together with the lack of available child care, have created a stress-provoking situation for many school-age children. Some of these children may have a chronic illness as well.

Inadequate adult supervision after school leaves children at greater risk for injury and delinquent behavior. In some instances, outside activities are curtailed and relationships with peers may be significantly diminished. Latchkey children may feel more lonely, isolated, and fearful than children who have someone to care for them (Ruiz-Casares, Rousseau, Currie, et al., 2012). To cope with their fears and anxieties while alone, these children may devise strategies such as hiding, playing the television at a loud volume, or using pets for comfort.

Many communities and people concerned about the welfare of latchkey children are trying to help these children and their parents deal with this potentially serious problem. Some communities and employers have implemented after-school programs. Other types of programs include those designed to teach self-help skills to children, hotlines to provide telephone check-in and reassurance for children, and programs that link latchkey children with reassuring older people in their community. Nurses should be aware of these community services and encourage parents to teach self-help skills to these children.

Limit Setting and Discipline

Many factors influence the amount and manner of discipline and limit setting imposed on school-age children. Some of these factors are the parents' psychosocial maturity, the parents' childrearing experiences, the children's temperament, the context of the children's misconduct, and the children's response to rewards and punishments. Discipline serves many purposes: (1) to help the child interrupt or inhibit a forbidden action; (2) to point out a more acceptable form of behavior so that the child knows what is right in a future situation; (3) to provide some reason, understandable to the child, that explains why one action is inappropriate and another action is more desirable; and (4) to stimulate the child's ability to empathize with the victim of a misdeed.

To be effective, discipline should take place in a positive, supportive environment with the use of strategies to instruct and guide desired behaviors and eliminate undesired behaviors (Owen, Slep, & Heyman, 2012). Physically aggressive practices, such as spanking, are linked to children with poor internalizing behaviors, including depression, anxiety, hopelessness, and poor external behaviors, such as aggression and violence (Ferguson, 2013). Reasoning, on the other hand, is an effective technique for middle school–age children. With advancing cognitive skills, they

FAMILY-CENTERED CARE
Helping Children in School

General Guidelines

- Be supportive—provide companionship; share ideas and thoughts.
- Be positive—every child should experience some success each day.
- Share an interest in reading—use the library; discuss books they are reading.
- Support and encourage activity rather than passivity.
- Encourage originality—help children make their own projects from discarded articles or other available materials.
- Foster the development of hobbies and collections.
- Encourage children to wonder and reflect during free time.
- Encourage family experiences and trips to places of interest.
- Encourage questions—help children discover sources for information or places to explore and investigate.
- Stimulate creative thinking and problem solving—help children try out new solutions to problems without fear of making mistakes.
- Use rewards rather than punishment.

Specific Guidelines

- Meet the teacher at the beginning of school, and plan to visit the school to see what is taught and expected.
- Send the child to school every day. Teachers are concerned when parents make other plans for their children; it conveys the impression that school is unimportant.
- Demonstrate an interest in what the child is learning.
- Demonstrate an interest in content and growth more than in grades.
- Make it clear to the child that schoolwork is between the child and the teacher; the teacher and child should set goals for better school performance to allow the child to feel responsible for school successes and failures.
- Take advantage of situations that support and reinforce school learning.
- Share information with teachers that will help them understand the child better.
- Communicate with the teacher if there appears to be a problem; avoid waiting for a scheduled conference.
- Provide a quiet, well-lit area for study that is safe from interruption; do not allow television or music.
- Avoid dictating a study time, but do enforce rules, such as no video games until homework is done; accept the child's word that work is complete.
- Help with homework should focus on explaining the question, not giving the answer.
- Teach the child to break large tasks (e.g., a report) into smaller, manageable tasks spread over the allotted time rather than attempting the entire project the night before it is to be completed.
- Request special help for children with learning problems.
- Support the school staff by showing respect for both the school system and the teacher, at least in the child's presence.

are able to benefit from more complex disciplinary strategies. For example, withholding privileges, requiring compensation, imposing penalties, and contracting can be used with great success. Problem solving is the best approach to limit setting, and children themselves can be included in the process of determining appropriate disciplinary measures.

Dishonest Behavior

During middle childhood, children may engage in what is considered to be antisocial behavior. Previously well-behaved children may engage in lying, stealing, and cheating. Such behaviors are disturbing and challenging to parents.

Lying can occur for a number of reasons. By the time children enter school, they still "tell stories," often exaggerating a story or situation as a means of impressing their family or friends. However, during middle childhood, children become able to distinguish between fact and fantasy. If children do not develop this characteristic, parents need to teach them what is real and what is make-believe.

Young children may lie to escape punishment or to get out of some difficulty even when their misbehavior is evident. Older children may lie to meet expectations set by others to which they have been unable to measure up. However, most children know that lying and cheating are wrong, and they are concerned when it is observed in their friends. They are quick to tell on others when they detect cheating.

Parents need to be reassured that all children lie occasionally and that sometimes children may have difficulty separating fantasy from reality. Parents should be helped to understand the importance of being truthful in their relationships with children.

Cheating is most common in young children 5 to 6 years of age. They find it difficult to lose at a game or contest, so they may cheat to win. They have not yet realized that this behavior is wrong, and they do it almost automatically. This behavior usually disappears as they mature. However, because children model observed behaviors, parents need to be aware of their own behavior. When parents set examples of honesty, children are more likely to conform to these standards.

As with other ethically related behavior, stealing is not unexpected in younger children. Between 5 and 8 years of age, children's sense of property rights is limited and they tend to take things simply because they are attracted to them or to take money for what it will buy. They are equally likely to give away something valuable that belongs to them. When young children are caught and punished, they are penitent—they "didn't mean to" and "promise to never do it again"—but they are likely to repeat the performance the following day. Often they not only steal but also lie about their behavior or attempt to justify it with excuses. It is seldom helpful to trap children into admission by asking directly if they committed the offense. Children do not take responsibility for these behaviors until the end of middle childhood. Stealing can be an indication that something is seriously wrong or lacking in the child's life. For example, children may steal to make up for love or another satisfaction that they feel is lacking. In most situations, it is wise not to attempt to attach a hidden or deep meaning to the stealing. An admonition, together with an appropriate and reasonable punishment, such as having the older child pay back the money or return the stolen items, takes care of most cases. Most children can be taught to respect the property rights of others with little difficulty despite numerous temptations and opportunities. If children's personal rights are respected, they are likely to respect the rights of others. Some children simply need more time to learn the rules regarding private property.

Stress and Fear

Children today experience significant amounts of stress. Stress in childhood comes from a variety of sources, such as conflict within the family, interpersonal relationships, and low socioeconomic status (Riley, Scaramella, & McGoron, 2014). The school environment and participation in multiple organized activities can be additional sources of stress. The demands from teachers and parents with school work and standardized proficiency testing, in addition to peer pressure, can cause stress on school-age children (White, 2012). In addition, children in the middle school years are often overcommitted with activities such as dance, music, athletics, and other activities until the cumulative effect is overwhelming.

The increasing violence in society has infiltrated into the school setting. In the present information age in which tragedy is broadcast daily in the media, children come to school knowing more about the latest world events than any previous generation of children. Many children know other children who have been killed or children who have brought weapons to school. School-age children can be victims of bullying, verbal insults, unwanted sexual remarks, damaged or stolen property, and physical abuse in the school environment (King, 2014). Furthermore, children are stressed by conflict within the home, and the high number of single-parent families results in altered relationships and increasing responsibilities for children.

To help children cope with stress, parents, teachers, and health care providers must recognize signs that indicate a child is undergoing stress, identify the source of the stress promptly, and refer those children who need specialized treatment. They need to frequently reassure children that they are safe, have honest and open communication, encourage children to express their feelings, and provide time for unstructured play.

> ## ! NURSING ALERT
>
> The nurse who observes the following signs of stress in a child should explore the situation further:
> - Stomach pains or headache
> - Changes in sleep patterns or nightmares
> - Bed-wetting
> - Changes in eating habits
> - Aggressive or stubborn behavior
> - Withdrawal or reluctance to participate
> - Regression to earlier behaviors (e.g., thumb-sucking)
> - Trouble concentrating or changes in academic performance

Children 7 to 12 years of age are capable of identifying their own physiologic responses to stress including tight muscles, fast heartbeat, jitteriness, breathing difficulties, headache, or neck pain. Children should be taught to recognize these signs as indicators of stress and to use techniques to manage their stress. Children can learn relaxation techniques such as deep-breathing exercises, progressive relaxation of muscle groups, yoga, and positive imagery to reduce stress (Bothe, Grignon, & Olness, 2014; White, 2012). Encouraging them to "blow off steam" through physical activity reduces tension and anxiety. Children can be encouraged to observe effective coping strategies in others and adopt them for their own use. When an effective strategy has been developed for one situation, parents can show the child how to transfer the coping strategy or technique to other situations.

In addition to stress, school-age children experience a wide variety of fears, including fear of the dark, excessive worry about past behavior, self-consciousness, social withdrawal, and an excessive need for reassurance. These fears are considered normal for children this age. During the middle-school years, children become less fearful of body safety than they were as preschoolers but they still fear being hurt, being kidnapped, or having to undergo surgery. They also fear death and are fascinated by all the aspects of death and dying. The fears of noises, darkness, storms, and dogs lessen, but new fears related predominantly to school and family bother children during this time.

PROMOTING OPTIMAL HEALTH DURING THE SCHOOL YEARS

NUTRITION

Although caloric needs are diminished in relation to body size during middle childhood, resources are being laid down at this time for the increased growth needs of adolescence. Parents and children need to be aware of the value of a balanced diet to promote growth because children usually eat what their family members eat. The quality of the child's diet depends on the family's pattern of eating.

Likes and dislikes established at an early age continue in middle childhood, although preferences for single foods subside and children develop a taste for a variety of foods. However, the easy availability of fast-food restaurants, the influence of the mass media, and the temptation of "junk food" make it easy for children to fill up on empty calories. Foods that do not promote growth, such as sugars, starches, and excess fats, are common in school-age children's diets. The easy availability of high-calorie foods, combined with the tendency toward more sedentary activities, has also contributed to an epidemic of childhood obesity.

Parents are unable to monitor what their children eat when they are away from home. A parent may pack a lunch for school but is unaware of how much is eaten, traded, sold, or thrown away. Nutrition education can and should be integrated in the curriculum throughout the school years. Important aspects of nutrition education include the US Food and Drug Administration's MyPlate; elements of a wholesome diet; and how food products are grown, processed, and prepared. School cafeterias may not always provide healthy, nutritious meals; however, parents should advocate for the availability of nutritious food options and the elimination of unhealthy foods at schools.

SLEEP AND REST

The amount of sleep and rest required during middle childhood is highly individualized. The amount of sleep depends on the child's age, activity level, and state of health. The growth rate slows in the school-age years, and less energy is expended in growth than during preceding years.

School-age children usually do not require naps, but they do need to sleep approximately 11.5 hours at 5 years of age and 9 hours at 12 years of age each night (Galland, Taylor, Elder, & Herbison, 2012). Although fewer bedtime problems occur during these years, occasional difficulties are still associated with the bedtime ritual. Usually children 6 or 7 years of age exhibit few bedtime problems, and encouraging quiet activity before bedtime, such as coloring or reading, facilitates the task of going to bed. However, most children in middle childhood must be reminded frequently to go to bed; 8- to 9-year-old children and 11-year-old children are particularly resistant (Bhargava, 2011). Often these children are unaware that they are tired; if they are allowed to remain up later than usual, they are fatigued the following day. Sometimes bedtime resistance can be resolved by allowing a later bedtime as the child gets older. Twelve-year-old children usually offer no resistance at bedtime; some even retire early to read a book or listen to music.

EXERCISE AND ACTIVITY

The improved capabilities and adaptability of school-age children permit greater speed and effort in motor activities. Larger, stronger muscles permit longer and increasingly strenuous play without exhaustion. School-age children acquire the coordination, timing, and concentration that are required to participate in adult-type activities, but they may lack the strength, stamina, and control of adolescents and adults. They can engage in a greater amount of physical activity during the school years. However, parents, teachers, and coaches must remember that although children this age are large and appear strong, they may not be ready for strenuous competitive athletics.

All growing children need regular exercise and opportunities for satisfying experiences consistent with individual likes and dislikes. Appropriate activities during the school-age years include running, jumping rope, swimming, roller skating, ice skating, dancing, and bicycle riding. Positive reinforcement achieved by experiencing increasingly smooth, rhythmic, and efficient use of the body conditions the child toward regular physical activity. Exercise is essential for muscle development and tone, refinement of balance and coordination, increased strength and endurance, and stimulation of body functions and metabolic processes. Children need ample space to run, jump, skip, and climb in addition to safe indoor and outdoor facilities and equipment. Most children have abundant energy and need little encouragement to engage in physical activity. Children with disabling conditions or those who hesitate to become involved in active play (e.g., obese children) require special assessment and help so that activities appeal to them and are compatible with their limitations while also meeting their developmental needs.

Sports

Considerable controversy surrounds the trend toward early participation in competitive athletics and the amount and type of competitive sports that are appropriate for children in the elementary grades. The current view is that virtually every child is suited for some sport, and authorities do not discourage participation if children are matched to the type of sport appropriate to their abilities and to their physical and emotional constitution. School-age children enjoy competition (Fig. 34.7). However, teachers and coaches must understand the physical limitations of children this age and teach them the proper techniques and safety measures needed to avoid injuries. A safe and appropriate sport can be identified for even the most unskilled and uncompetitive child, including children

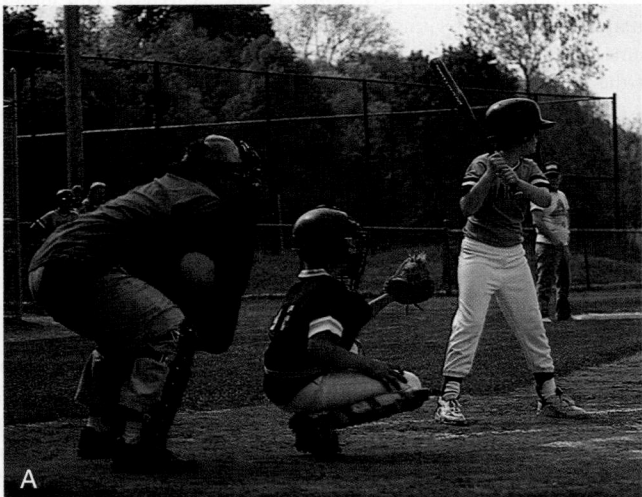

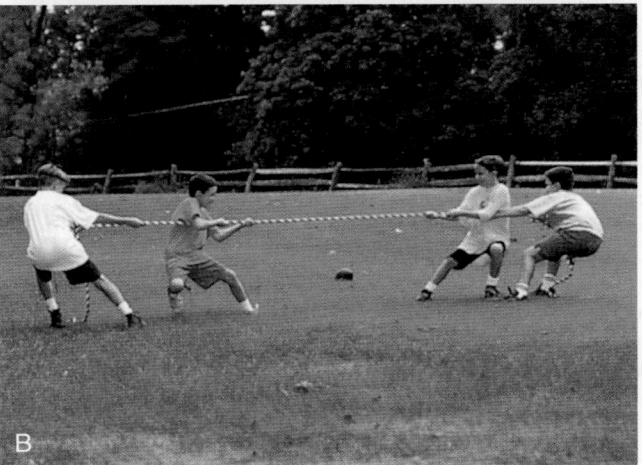

FIG 34.7 The activities engaged in by school-age children vary according to interest and opportunity. **A,** Little League competitors. **B,** Playing tug-of-war.

with chronic illnesses and intellectual disability. Common activities for school-age children include baseball, soccer, gymnastics, and swimming. Equipment must be maintained in safe condition, and protective apparatus should be worn to prevent serious injury.

During the school-age years, girls have the same basic body structure as boys and have a similar response to systematic exercise training. However, at puberty, boys become larger and have more muscle mass, and at this stage, it is usually recommended that girls compete only against other girls. Before puberty, there is no essential difference in strength and size between girls and boys, making these precautions unnecessary.

Preadolescence is a time to teach fundamental motor skills; develop fitness in a practical, safe, and gradual manner; and promote healthy attitudes and values. Activities should include both practice sessions and unstructured play; the actual game or event should be managed in a manner that stresses mastery of the sport and enhancement of self-image rather than winning or pleasing others. All children should have an opportunity to participate, and special ceremonies should recognize all participants, not just individuals who excel in sports or athletics.

Acquisition of Skills

School-age children demonstrate increasing fine motor abilities and complex artistic skills. Handedness is well established by the beginning of the school years, and children make great strides in writing and drawing during this period. It is a time of energetic and vibrant creative productivity. With the tools of language and reading, children create poems, stories, and plays. With more advanced fine motor skills, they are able to master an unlimited variety of handicrafts, such as ceramics, needlework, woodworking, and beadwork. They avidly pursue these skills in solitude, with a friend, or through organized groups such as boys' or girls' clubs or special interest groups that use crafts or other activities as a means to occupy, entertain, and educate children.

School-age children are capable of assuming responsibility for their own needs, although their distaste for soap and water and "dress" clothes is legendary. School-age children can and want to assume their share of household tasks, which usually are related to the male and female roles that have been defined by their culture. Many children also assume responsibility for tasks outside the home, such as baby-sitting, yard work, or paper routes.

TELEVISION, VIDEO GAMES, AND THE INTERNET

Children spend a significant amount of time each day involved in media-related activities, including the use of tablets, video games, and cell phones. Children 8 to 10 years of age spend at least 8 hours every day with various forms of media, and teenagers spend more than 11 hours per day (American Academy of Pediatrics, Council on Communications and Media, 2013). Because of the long periods of exposure, media has more time to develop children's attitudes than do parents and teachers.

There is no doubt that children learn from various forms of media, but the values and attitudes depicted on these forums are not always realistic and may conflict with previously taught values. Violence is common in various forms of media, and repeated exposure to violence can desensitize children to violence, convey a message that violence is acceptable, and teach children that initiating violent behavior is an appropriate form of protection (Brown & Tierney, 2011). Parents should make the ultimate decision about which programs, video games, and Internet sites they can access. These forms of media have valuable educational opportunities, but there are also risks that parents must acknowledge.

DENTAL HEALTH

The first permanent (secondary) teeth erupt at about 6 years of age, beginning with the 6-year molar, which erupts posterior to the deciduous molars. Other permanent teeth appear in approximately the same order as eruption of the primary teeth (see the "Teething" section in Chapter 31) and follow shedding of the deciduous teeth (Fig. 34.8). With the appearance of the second permanent (12-year) molar, most permanent teeth are present. Permanent dentition is more advanced in girls than in boys.

Because the permanent teeth erupt during the school-age years, dental hygiene and regular attention to dental caries are important parts of health supervision during this period (see the "Dental Health" section in Chapter 33). Correct brushing techniques should be taught or reinforced, and the role that fermentable carbohydrates play in production of dental caries should be emphasized. It is important to be alert to possible malocclusion problems that may result from irregular eruption of permanent teeth and that may impair function. Regular dental supervision and continued fluoride supplementation are integral parts of the health maintenance program.

The most effective means of preventing dental caries is proper oral hygiene. Children should be taught to perform their own dental care with the supervision and guidance of the parents. Parents should learn the correct brushing technique with their children, and they should monitor their child's efforts until the child can assume full responsibility.

Dental Problems

Limited or inadequate dental care results in the most common dental problems: dental caries, malocclusion, and periodontal disease. Trauma, especially tooth avulsion, is another important dental problem. All of these conditions benefit from early intervention to prevent tooth loss.

Dental caries (cavities) is the principal oral problem in children and adolescents. Reducing the incidence and consequences of dental caries is extremely important in childhood. If untreated, dental caries can result in total destruction of the involved teeth. The prevalence rate of caries increases steadily across the life span; whereas 25% of children younger than 5 years of age have caries, 68% of children have caries by 19 years of age (Mahat, Lyons, & Bowen, 2014).

Dental caries is a multifactorial disease involving susceptible teeth, cariogenic microflora, and an appropriate oral environment. The incidence of lesions and the likelihood of progressive invasion vary considerably and depend on a number of factors being present in the right combination. Because many children are exposed to health care but not dental care, oral inspection is an integral part of the physical assessment of every child. If there is any evidence of dental caries or other unhealthy dental state, the child should be referred for dental services. An alarming number of children do not receive regular dental supervision, and a significant number reach adulthood without dental examinations or treatment by a dentist.

Periodontal disease, an inflammatory and degenerative condition involving the gums and tissues supporting the teeth, often begins in childhood and accounts for a significant amount of tooth loss in adulthood. The more common periodontal problems are gingivitis (simple inflammation of the gums) and periodontitis (inflammation of the gums and loss of connective tissue and bone in the supporting structures of the teeth). Gingivitis, the most prevalent periodontal disease, is a reversible inflammatory disease that can begin in early childhood and is most often associated with the buildup of plaque on the teeth. Management is directed toward prevention by conscientious brushing and flossing, including the use of fluoride. Children should see a dentist at any signs of inflammation or irritation.

Malocclusion occurs when teeth of the upper and lower dental arches do not approximate in the proper relationships. As a result, the physiologic function of chewing is less effective and the cosmetic effect is displeasing. Teeth that are uneven, crowded, or overlapping are unable to meet their counterparts in the opposite jaw in the appropriate relationships and may be predisposed to disease in later years.

Orthodontic treatment is most successful when it is started in the late school-age or early teenage years after the last primary teeth have been shed and before growth ceases. However, referral should be made as soon as malocclusion is evident because some deformities can be corrected at an earlier age.

Dental injury may occur in childhood and includes fractures of varying degrees of severity, chipping, dislocation, or avulsion. All tooth injuries require prompt treatment by a competent dentist to prevent permanent displacement or loss. Delayed examination and diagnosis of tooth damage can result in infection or pulp involvement. Because it can affect the remaining teeth, replacement of the lost tooth is needed to maintain normal alignment and position of the other teeth.

A tooth that is avulsed (exarticulated, or "knocked out") should be replanted by the child, parent, or nurse and stabilized as soon as possible so that the blood supply to the tooth can be reestablished and the tooth kept alive (see Emergency Treatment box: Avulsed Permanent Tooth). A tooth that is replanted promptly has a good survival rate. Avulsed primary teeth are usually not reimplanted.

As with all injuries to the mouth, an avulsed tooth causes a large amount of bleeding, which is frightening to children and their families; therefore the nurse or anyone faced with dental trauma should be prepared to provide support and reassurance during the dental trauma.

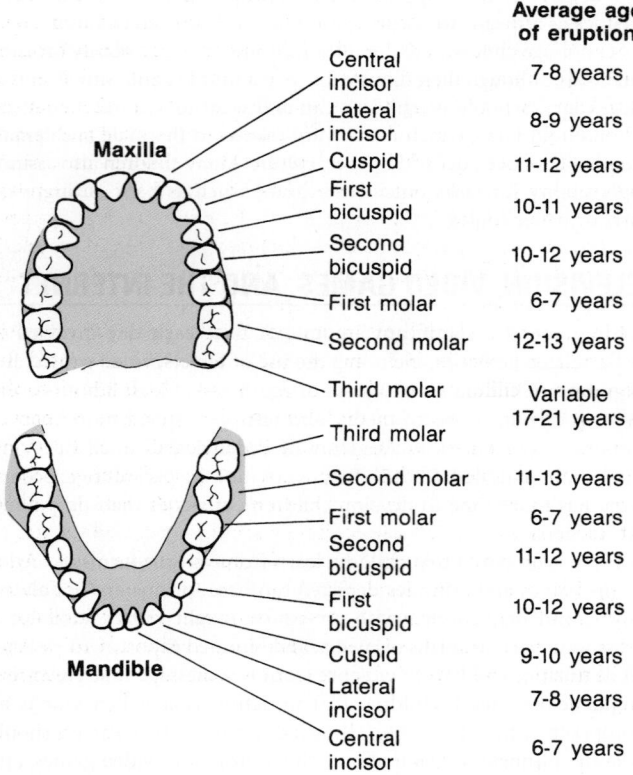

	Average age of eruption
Central incisor	7-8 years
Lateral incisor	8-9 years
Cuspid	11-12 years
First bicuspid	10-11 years
Second bicuspid	10-12 years
First molar	6-7 years
Second molar	12-13 years
Third molar	Variable 17-21 years
Third molar	
Second molar	11-13 years
First molar	6-7 years
Second bicuspid	11-12 years
First bicuspid	10-12 years
Cuspid	9-10 years
Lateral incisor	7-8 years
Central incisor	6-7 years

FIG 34.8 Sequence of eruption of the secondary teeth. (Data from Dean, J.A. [2016]. *McDonald and Avery's dentistry for the child and adolescent* [10th ed.]. St. Louis, MO: Elsevier.)

✚ EMERGENCY TREATMENT
Avulsed Permanent Tooth

- Recover tooth.
- Hold tooth by crown; avoid touching root area.
- If tooth is dirty, rinse it gently under running water or saline; be certain to insert stopper in sink or basin (to avoid tooth loss).

To Reimplant the Tooth
- Insert tooth into socket; be certain that the lip side (or convex surface) is facing front.
- Have child maintain tooth in place by slowly biting down on a piece of gauze.
- Transport child to dentist immediately.
- Avoid sudden stops or sharp turns to prevent dislodging tooth.

If Reluctant to Reimplant the Tooth
- Place avulsed tooth in suitable medium for transport:
  - Cold milk
  - Saliva—under child's or parent's tongue
- If child is holding tooth in the mouth, avoid sudden stops to prevent swallowing tooth.
- DO NOT FORGET TO TAKE THE TOOTH.

SEX EDUCATION

Many children experience some form of sex play during or before preadolescence as a response to normal curiosity, not as a result of love or sexual urges. Children are experimentalists by nature, and sex play is incidental and transitory. Any adverse emotional consequences or guilt feelings depend on how the behavior is managed by the parents if it is discovered or whether children view their actions as wrong in the eyes of significant people, particularly the parents.

An important component of ongoing sex education is effective communication. If parents either repress the child's sexual curiosity or avoid dealing with it, the sexual information that the child receives may be acquired almost entirely from peers. When peers are the primary source of sexual information, it is transmitted and exchanged in secret conversation and contains a large amount of misinformation.

Nurse's Role in Sex Education

No matter where nurses practice, they can provide information on human sexuality to both parents and children. To discuss the topic adequately, nurses must have an understanding of the physiologic aspects of sexuality; knowledge of the common myths and misconceptions associated with sex and the reproductive process; an understanding cultural and societal values; and an awareness of their own attitudes, feelings, and biases about sexuality.

When presenting sexual information to school-age children, nurses should treat sex as a normal part of growth and development. Questions should be answered honestly, in a matter-of- fact manner, and at the child's level of understanding. There may be times when boys and girls should be taught content separately; however each group needs information about both sexes.

Children need help to differentiate sex and sexuality. Exercises on clarifying values, identifying role models, engaging in problem-solving skills, and practicing responsibility are important to prepare children for early adolescence and puberty. In addition, children need explanations of sexual information that is provided via the media or jokes. Information concerning anatomy, pregnancy, contraceptives, and sexually transmitted diseases should be presented in simple, accurate terms. It is important to tell children what they want to know and what they can expect to happen as they become mature sexually.

During encounters with parents, nurses can be open and available for questions and discussion. They can set an example by the language they use in discussing body parts and their function and by the way in which they deal with problems that have emotional overtones, such as exploratory sex play and masturbation. Parents need help to understand normal behaviors and to view sexual curiosity in their children as a part of the developmental process. Assessing the parents' level of knowledge and understanding of sexuality provides cues to their need for supplemental information that will prepare them for the increasingly complex explanations they will need to provide as their children grow older.

SCHOOL HEALTH

Child health maintenance is ultimately the responsibility of the parents; however, the public schools and health departments in the United States have contributed to the improvement of child health by providing a healthful school environment, health services, and health education that emphasize sound health practices. Most of these functions constitute major components of community health services and involve large amounts of public funds and large numbers of health care professionals, including nurses.

A school health program is involved in ongoing health maintenance through assessment, screening, and referral activities. Routine health services provided by most schools include health appraisal, emergency care, safety education, communicable disease control, counseling, and follow-up care. Health education of school-age children is directed toward providing knowledge of health and influencing habits, attitudes, and conduct in relation to health and injury prevention.

Traditionally, school nurses were viewed as the individuals who detected diseases in the school, applied bandages, and cared for students who were ill or injured. Although these functions remain important parts of the school nurse's job, the role has acquired much broader dimensions. Today, school nurses develop, implement, and evaluate health care plans and programs. They manage and coordinate all the care required by regular students and students with special health care needs. In many settings, school health services have enlarged into family health centers that meet the needs of not only school-age children but also their families and the community. In these settings, school nurse practitioners provide health care that includes assessment of physical, psychomedical, psychoeducational, behavioral, and learning problems, as well as comprehensive well-child care.

The passage of the Education for All Handicapped Children Act and its amendments (Public Laws 94-142 and 99-457) mandated the integration of children with chronic illnesses and disabilities into the least restrictive environments, including regular classrooms whenever possible. School nurses are responsible for the medical and nursing needs of these children while they are in the school setting. School nurses develop, implement, and evaluate individualized health care plans for these children. Not all schools have a school nurse, and the use of unlicensed assistive personnel (UAP) is used in some cases. After appropriate training and supervision, UAP can provide standardized routine health care to students but must be overseen by a school nurse (Shannon & Kubelka, 2013). Delegation and supervision of UAP require skillful nursing assessment, effective communication, and professional judgment.

INJURY PREVENTION

Because school-age children have developed more refined muscular coordination and control and can apply their cognitive capacities to

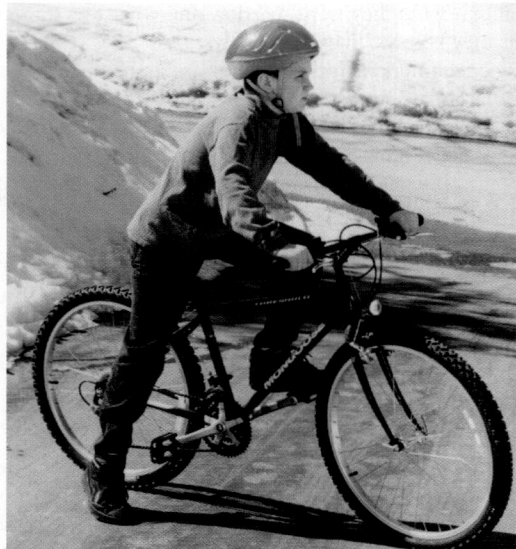

FIG 34.9 The right size bike is important; the child should be able to sit on the bike and place the balls of both feet on the ground. The foot should comfortably reach and manipulate the pedal in the down position. Wearing a protective helmet is mandatory. The helmet should be positioned so it sits low on the forehead and parallel to the ground when the head is held upright. It should not rock back and forth or shift from side to side. The strap should fasten securely under the chin.

their behavior, the number of injuries in middle childhood is diminished compared with the number in early childhood. The most common cause of severe injury and death in children older than 4 years of age is motor vehicle accidents—either as a pedestrian or passenger (National Highway Traffic Safety Administration, 2013). It is important that nurses continue to emphasize three automobile safety measures that have been found to reduce the severity of injuries: effective car restraint systems, door-lock mechanisms, and appropriate passenger seating locations in the motor vehicle (Table 34.2). The rear vehicle seat is the safest place for children younger than 13 years of age, and booster seats should be used until the child is 57 inches tall (Centers for Disease Control and Prevention, National Center for Injury Prevention and Control, 2015).

School-age children's desire for riding bicycles increases the risk for injury on streets. Other serious injuries include accidents on skateboards, roller skates, in-line skates, scooters, and other sports equipment. All-terrain vehicles (ATVs) are popular with children but are unstable, difficult to handle, and responsible for a large number of childhood injuries. Several organizations have developed policy and position statements to discourage the use of ATVs in any child younger than 16 years of age (Yanchar, 2012).

Most injuries occur in or near the home or school. The most effective means of prevention is education of the child and family regarding the hazards of risk taking and the improper use of equipment. Safety helmets, protective eye and mouth shields, and protective padding are strongly recommended for children engaging in active sports, even though they may not be required equipment. Falls from bicycles are the cause of a significant number of head injuries in school-age children, and the most important aspect of bicycle safety is to encourage children to wear protective helmets (Fig. 34.9) (Meehan, Lee, Fischer, et al., 2013). Family-Centered Care boxes provide guidelines for bicycle, skateboard, and in-line skate safety and guidance during the school years.

Physically active school-age children are also highly susceptible to cuts and abrasions, and the incidence of childhood fractures, strains, and sprains is high. Trampoline injuries are highest in children 5 to 14

FAMILY-CENTERED CARE
Bicycle Safety

- Always wear a properly fitted bicycle helmet that is approved by the US Consumer Product Safety Commission (CPSC); replace a damaged or outgrown helmet.
- Ride bicycles with traffic and away from parked cars.
- Ride single file.
- Walk bicycles through busy intersections only at crosswalks.
- Give hand signals well in advance of turning or stopping.
- Keep as close to the curb as practical.
- Watch for drain grates, potholes, soft shoulders, loose dirt, and gravel.
- Keep both hands on handlebars except with signaling.
- Never ride double on a bicycle.
- Do not carry packages that interfere with vision or control; do not drag objects behind a bike.
- Watch for and yield to pedestrians.
- Watch for cars backing up or pulling out of driveways; be especially careful at intersections.
- Look left, right, and then left before turning into traffic or roadway.
- Never hitch a ride on a truck or other vehicle.
- Learn rules of the road and respect for traffic officers.
- Obey all local ordinances.
- Wear shoes that fit securely while riding.
- Wear light colors at night, and attach fluorescent material to clothing and bicycle.
- Equip the bicycle with proper lights and reflectors.
- Be certain the bicycle is the correct size for rider (see Fig. 34.9).
- Have the bicycle inspected to ensure good mechanical condition.
- Children riding as passengers must wear appropriate-size helmets and sit in specially designed protective seats.

Adapted from American Academy of Pediatrics Committee on Injury and Poison Prevention. (2008). Bicycle helmets. *Pediatrics, 122*(2), 450.

FAMILY-CENTERED CARE
Skateboard, In-Line Skate, and Scooter Safety

- Children younger than 5 years of age should not use skateboards or in-line skates because they are not developmentally prepared to protect themselves from injury. Children 6 to 10 years of age should use these only with close adult supervision.
- The age when children are ready to use in-line skates safely is not known because of differences in the ability to acquire the skills needed to participate in the sport. Novice skaters should learn indoors on a flat, smooth surface. Children who ride skateboards, in-line skates, or scooters should wear helmets and other protective equipment, especially on their knees, wrists, and elbows, to prevent injury.
- Skateboards, in-line skates, and scooters should never be used near traffic or in streets. Their use should be prohibited on streets and highways. Activities that bring skateboards together (e.g., "catching a ride") are especially dangerous.
- Some types of use, such as riding homemade ramps on hard surfaces, may be particularly hazardous.

Data from Brudvik, C. (2006). Injuries caused by small wheel devices. *Prevention Science, 7,* 313–320; American Academy of Pediatrics, Committee on Injury and Poison Prevention. (2009). In-line skating injuries in children and adolescents. *Pediatrics, 123,* 1421–1422.

TABLE 34.2   Injury Prevention During the School-Age Years

Developmental Abilities Related to Risk for Injury	Injury Prevention
Motor Vehicle Accidents	
Is increasingly involved in activities away from home	Educate child regarding proper use of seat belts while a passenger in a vehicle.
Is excited by speed and motion	Maintain discipline while a passenger in a vehicle (e.g., keep arms inside, do not lean against doors, and do not interfere with driver).
Is easily distracted by environment	Remind parents and children that no one should ride in the bed of a pickup truck.
Can be reasoned with	Emphasize safe pedestrian behavior.
	Insist on child wearing safety apparel (e.g., helmet) when applicable, such as riding bicycle, motorcycle, moped, or all-terrain vehicle (see Family-Centered Care boxes).
Drowning	
Is apt to overdo	Teach child to swim.
May work hard to perfect a skill	Teach basic rules of water safety.
Has cautious, but not fearful, gross motor actions	Select safe and supervised places to swim.
Likes swimming	Check sufficient water depth for diving.
	Caution child to swim with a companion.
	Ensure that child uses an approved flotation device in water or boat.
	Advocate for legislation requiring fencing around pools.
	Learn cardiopulmonary resuscitation.
Burns	
Has increasing independence	Make certain home has smoke detectors.
Is adventurous	Set water heaters to 48.9°C (120°F) to avoid scald burns.
Enjoys trying new things	Instruct child regarding behavior in areas involving contact with potential burn hazards (e.g., gasoline, matches, bonfires or barbecues, lighter fluid, firecrackers, cigarette lighters, cooking utensils, chemistry sets).
	Instruct child to avoid climbing or flying kite around high-tension wires.
	Instruct child in proper behavior in the event of fire (e.g., fire drills at home and school).
	Teach child safe cooking (use low heat; avoid any frying; be careful of steam burns, scalds, or exploding foods, especially from microwaving).
Poisoning	
Adheres to group rules	Educate child regarding hazards of taking nonprescription drugs and chemicals, including aspirin and alcohol.
May be easily influenced by peers	Teach child to say "no" if offered illegal or dangerous drugs or alcohol.
Has strong allegiance to friends	Keep potentially dangerous products in properly labeled receptacles, preferably out of reach.
Bodily Damage	
Has increased physical skills	Help provide facilities for supervised activities.
Needs strenuous physical activity	Encourage playing in safe places.
Is interested in acquiring new skills and perfecting attained skills	Keep firearms safely locked up except under adult supervision.
	Teach proper care of, use of, and respect for potentially dangerous devices (e.g., power tools, firecrackers).
Is daring and adventurous, especially with peers	Teach children not to tease or surprise dogs, invade their territory, take dogs' toys, or interfere with dogs' feeding.
	Stress eye, ear, or mouth protection when using potentially hazardous objects or devices or when engaging in potentially hazardous sports.
Frequently plays in hazardous places	Teach safety regarding use of corrective devices (glasses); if child wears contact lenses, monitor duration of wear to prevent corneal damage.
Confidence often exceeds physical capacity	Stress careful selection, use, and maintenance of sports and recreation equipment, such as skateboards and in-line skates (see Family-Centered Care boxes).
Desires group loyalty and has strong need for friends' approval	Emphasize proper conditioning, safe practices, and use of safety equipment for sports or recreational activities.
	Do not permit use of trampolines except as part of supervised training. Use safety glass and decals on large glassed areas, such as sliding glass doors.
Delights in physical activity	Use window guards to prevent falls.
Attempts hazardous feats	Teach name, address, and phone number and emphasize that child should ask for help from appropriate people (e.g., cashier, security guard, police) if lost; have identification on child (e.g., sewn in clothes, inside shoe).
Accompanies friends to potentially hazardous facilities	Teach safety and stranger safety:
Is likely to overdo	Avoid clothing displaying the child's name or family name in public places.
Growth in height exceeds muscular growth and coordination	Caution child to never go with a stranger.
	Have child tell parents if anyone makes child feel uncomfortable in any way.
	Always listen to child's concerns regarding others' behavior.
	Teach child to say "no" when confronted by uncomfortable situations.

FAMILY-CENTERED CARE
Guidance During School Years

6 Years of Age
- Prepare parents to expect strong food preferences and frequent refusal of specific food items.
- Prepare parents to expect an increasingly ravenous appetite.
- Prepare parents for emotionality as child experiences erratic mood changes.
- Help parents anticipate continued susceptibility to illness.
- Teach injury prevention and safety, especially bicycle safety.
- Encourage parents to respect child's need for privacy and to provide a separate bedroom for child, if possible.
- Prepare parents for child's increasing interests outside the home.
- Help parents understand the need to encourage child's interactions with peers.

7 to 10 Years of Age
- Prepare parents to expect improvement in health with fewer illnesses, but warn them that allergies may increase or become apparent.
- Prepare parents to expect an increase in minor injuries.
- Emphasize caution in selecting and maintaining sports equipment, and reemphasize safety.
- Prepare parents to expect increased involvement with peers and interest in activities outside the home.
- Emphasize the need to encourage independence while maintaining limit setting and discipline.
- Prepare parents to expect more demands at 8 years of age.
- Prepare fathers to expect increasing admiration at 10 years; encourage father-child activities.
- Prepare parents for prepubescent changes in girls.

11 to 12 Years of Age
- Help parents prepare child for body changes of pubescence.
- Prepare parents to expect a growth spurt in girls.
- Make certain child's sex education is adequate with accurate information.
- Prepare parents to expect energetic but stormy behavior at 11 years of age, and becoming more even-tempered at 12 years of age.
- Encourage parents to support child's desire to "grow up" but to allow regressive behavior when needed.
- Prepare parents to expect an increase in child's masturbation.
- Instruct parents that the child may need more rest.
- Help parents educate child regarding experimentation with potentially harmful activities.

Health Guidance
- Help parents understand the importance of regular health and dental care for the child.
- Encourage parents to teach and model sound health practices, including diet, rest, activity, and exercise.
- Stress the need to encourage children to engage in appropriate physical activities.
- Emphasize providing a safe physical and emotional environment.
- Encourage parents to teach and model safety practices.

years of age and account for numerous fractures, sprains, and head injuries. Trampolines in the home environment, routine physical education classes, or outdoor playgrounds are not recommended for children younger than 6 years of age (American Academy of Pediatrics, Council on Sports Medicine and Fitness, 2012).

INFECTIONS OF THE SKIN

BACTERIAL INFECTIONS

Normally, the skin harbors a variety of bacterial flora, including the major pathogenic varieties of staphylococci and streptococci. The degree of their pathogenicity depends on the invasiveness and toxigenicity of the specific organism, the integrity of the skin (the host's barrier), and the host's immune and cellular defenses. Children with congenital or acquired immune disorders (e.g., acquired immunodeficiency syndrome [AIDS]), children receiving immunosuppressive therapy, and those with a malignancy such as leukemia or lymphoma) are at risk for developing bacterial infections.

Because of the characteristic "walling-off" process of the inflammatory reaction (abscess formation), staphylococci are more difficult to treat, and the local infected area is associated with an increase in bacteria all over the skin surface that serves as a source of continuing infection. Since the early 2000s, the number of methicillin-resistant *Staphylococcus aureus* (MRSA) community-acquired infections has risen dramatically (Skov, Christiansen, Dancer, et al., 2012). All of these factors underline the importance of careful hand washing and cleanliness when caring for infected children and their lesions to prevent the spread of infection and as an essential prophylactic measure when caring for infants and small children. Common bacterial skin disorders are outlined in Table 34.3.

VIRAL INFECTIONS

Viruses are intracellular parasites that produce their effect by using the intracellular substances of the host cells. Composed of only a deoxyribonucleic acid or ribonucleic acid core enclosed in an antigenic protein shell, viruses are unable to provide for their own metabolic needs or to reproduce themselves. After a virus penetrates a cell of the host organism, it sheds the outer shell and disappears within the cell, where the nucleic acid core stimulates the host cell to form more virus material from its intracellular substance. In a viral infection, the epidermal cells react with inflammation and vesiculation (as in herpes simplex) or by proliferating to form growths (warts).

Most of the communicable diseases of childhood are associated with rashes, and each rash is characteristic. Common viral disorders of the skin are in outlined in Table 34.4.

DERMATOPHYTOSES (FUNGAL INFECTIONS)

The dermatophytoses (ringworm) are infections caused by a group of closely related filamentous fungi that invade primarily the stratum corneum, hair, and nails. These are superficial infections by organisms that live on, not in, the skin. Dermatophytoses are designated by the Latin word *tinea*, with further designation relating to the area of the body where they are found (e.g., *tinea capitis* [ringworm of the scalp]). Table 34.5 outlines common dermatophytoses. Because of the infectious nature of the disease, affected children should not exchange grooming items, headgear, scarves, or other articles of apparel that have been in proximity to the infected area with other children. Because the infection can be acquired by animal-to-human transmission, all household pets should be examined for the disorder. Other sources of infection are seats with headrests (theater seats), seats in public transportation vehicles, helmets, and gymnasium mats.

SCABIES

Scabies is an endemic infestation caused by the scabies mite *Sarcoptes scabiei*. Lesions are created as the impregnated female scabies mite

TABLE 34.3 Bacterial Infections

Disorder and Organism	Manifestations	Management	Comments
Impetigo contagiosa: *Staphylococci*	Begins as a reddish macule then becomes vesicular Ruptures easily Exudate dries to form heavy, honey-colored crusts Pruritus common Systemic effects: Minimal or asymptomatic	Topical bactericidal ointment (mupirocin) or triple antibiotic ointment Oral or parenteral antibiotics (penicillin) in cases of severe or extensive lesions Vancomycin for methicillin-resistant *Staphylococcus aureus* (MRSA)	Tends to heal without scarring Autoinoculable and contagious May be superimposed on eczema
Pyoderma: *Staphylococci, streptococci*	Deeper extension of infection into dermis Tissue reaction more severe Systemic effects: Fever, lymphangitis, sepsis, heart disease	Soap and water cleansing Topical bactericidal ointment, such as mupirocin Antibiotics depending on causative organism	Autoinoculable and contagious May heal with or without scarring
Folliculitis (pimple), furuncle (boil), carbuncle (multiple boils): *Staphylococcus aureus*, methicillin-resistant *S. aureus* (MRSA)	Folliculitis: Infection of hair follicle Furuncle: Larger lesion with more redness and swelling at a single follicle Carbuncle: More extensive lesion with widespread inflammation and "pointing" at several follicular orifices Systemic effects: Malaise, if severe	Skin cleanliness Local warm, moist compresses Topical antibiotic agents Systemic antibiotics in severe cases Incision and drainage of severe lesions, followed by wound irrigations with antibiotics MRSA infections: • 5-inch soak of ½ cup bleach diluted in a standard 50-gallon tub one-fourth filled with water once or twice weekly • No sharing of towels or clothing • Disposal of razors after one use • Application of mupirocin to nares bid for 5 days	Autoinoculable and contagious Furuncle and carbuncle tend to heal with scar formation Lesion should never be squeezed
Cellulitis: *Streptococci, staphylococci, Haemophilus influenzae*	Inflammation of skin and subcutaneous tissues with intense redness, swelling, and firm infiltration; "streaking" often seen Involvement of regional lymph nodes May progress to abscess formation Systemic effects: Fever, malaise	Oral or parenteral antibiotics Rest and immobilization of both affected area and child	Hospitalization may be necessary for child with systemic symptoms

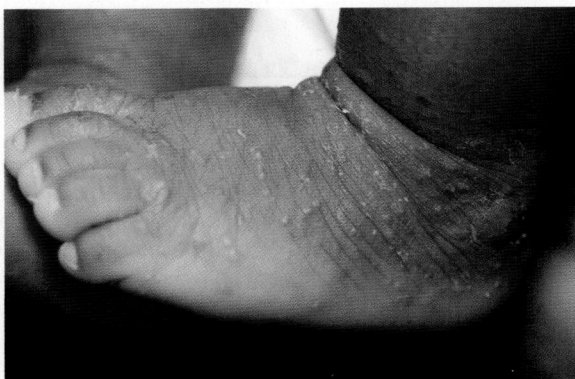

FIG 34.10 Scabies. (From Eichenfield, L.F., Frieden, I.J., Mathes, E.F., et al. [2015]. *Neonatal and infant dermatology* [3rd ed.]. Philadelphia, PA: Elsevier.)

burrows into the stratum corneum of the epidermis (never into living tissue), where she deposits her eggs and feces. The inflammatory response causes intense pruritus that leads to punctate discrete excoriations secondary to the itching. Maculopapular lesions are characteristically distributed in intertriginous areas: interdigital surfaces, the axillary-cubital area, popliteal folds, and the inguinal region. The observer must look for discrete papules, burrows, or vesicles (Fig. 34.10). Scabies is transmitted primarily through prolonged close personal contact, and it affects people regardless of age, sex, personal hygiene, and socioeconomic status.

Therapeutic Management

The treatment of scabies is the application of a scabicide. The drug of choice in children and infants older than 2 months of age is permethrin 5% cream (Elimite). Alternative drugs are 10% crotamiton (cream or lotion) or oral ivermectin. Lindane can be neurotoxic and is not recommended by the American Academy of Pediatrics (2015) for the treatment of scabies. Because of the length of time between infestation and physical symptoms (30 to 60 days), all people who were in close contact with the affected child need treatment.

PEDICULOSIS CAPITIS

Pediculosis capitis (head lice) is an infestation of the scalp by *Pediculus humanus capitis*, a common parasite in school-age children. These lice infestations create embarrassment and concern in the family and community. They can also cause a child to be ridiculed by other children. An important nursing role is education about pediculosis. Nurses should emphasize that anyone can get pediculosis; it has no respect for age, socioeconomic level, or cleanliness.

The louse is a blood-sucking organism that requires approximately five meals per day. The female louse lays her eggs at night at the junction

TABLE 34.4   Viral Skin Infection

Disorder and Organism	Manifestations	Management	Comments
Verruca (warts): Human papillomavirus (various types)	Usually well-circumscribed, gray or brown, elevated, firm papules with a roughened, finely papillomatous texture Occur anywhere, but usually appear on exposed areas, such as fingers, hands, face, and soles Asymptomatic	Local destructive therapy, individualized according to location, type, and number—surgical removal, electrocautery, curettage, cryotherapy (liquid nitrogen), caustic solutions (lactic acid and salicylic acid in flexible collodion, retinoic acid, salicylic acid plasters), laser ablation	Common in children Tend to disappear spontaneously Course unpredictable Most destructive techniques tend to leave scars Autoinoculable Repeated irritation will cause to enlarge
Verruca plantaris (plantar wart)	Located on plantar surface of feet and, because of pressure, are practically flat; may be surrounded by a collar of hyperkeratosis	Caustic chemical solution applied to wart, foam insole worn with hole cut to relieve pressure on wart; procedure repeated until wart comes out	Destructive techniques tend to leave scars, which may cause problems with walking
Cold sore, fever blister: Herpes simplex virus (HSV) type 1 Genital herpes: HSV type 2	Grouped burning and itching vesicles on inflammatory base, usually on or near mucocutaneous junctions (lips, nose, genitalia, buttocks) Vesicles dry, forming a crust, followed by exfoliation and spontaneous healing in 8 to 10 days May be accompanied by regional lymphadenopathy	Burrow solution compresses during weeping stages Oral antiviral (acyclovir [Zovirax]) for treatment or prophylaxis Oral antiviral (valacyclovir [Valtrex]) for episodic treatment; primarily recommended for immunocompromised patients	Heal without scarring unless secondary infection HSV-1 cold sores can be prevented by using sunscreens protecting against ultraviolet A and ultraviolet B light to prevent lip blisters Aggravated by corticosteroids May be fatal in children with depressed immunity
Herpes zoster, shingles: Varicella zoster virus	Caused by same virus that causes varicella (chickenpox) Crops of vesicles usually confined to dermatome following along course of affected nerve Usually preceded by neuralgic pain, hyperesthesias, and itching	Symptomatic treatment Analgesics for pain Ophthalmic variety: Systemic corticotropin or corticosteroids Acyclovir or valacyclovir Preventive vaccine is available for people >50 years of age	Isolate affected child from other children in a hospital or school May occur in children with depressed immunity Can be fatal
Molluscum contagiosum: Poxvirus	Flesh-colored papules (1 to 20) with a central caseous plug (umbilicated) that occur on trunk, face, and extremities; may be transmitted by sexual contact Usually asymptomatic	Cases in well children resolve spontaneously Treatment reserved for cosmetic purposes; alleviate discomfort; reduce autoinoculation; prevent secondary infection Numerous chemical agents including tretinoin gel 0.01% or cantharidin (Cantharone) liquid; podophyllin; imiquimod cream; these are painful treatments: use local anesthesia	Common in school-age children Spread by skin-to-skin contact, including autoinoculation and fomite-to-skin contact Outbreaks in child care centers have been reported

of a hair shaft and close to the skin because the eggs need a warm environment. The nits, or eggs, hatch in approximately 7 to 10 days. Itching, caused by the crawling insect and insect saliva on the skin, is usually the only symptom.

Common sites of involvement are the occipital area, behind the ears, and at the nape of the neck. Lice are small and grayish-tan, have no wings, and are visible to the naked eye. Observation of the white eggs (nits) firmly attached to the hair shafts confirms the diagnosis. The nits, or eggs, appear as tiny whitish oval specks adhering to the hair shaft about 6 mm (0.25 inch) from the scalp. The adherent nature of the nits distinguishes them from dandruff, which falls off readily. Empty nit cases, indicating hatched lice, are translucent rather than white and are located more than 6 mm from the scalp (Fig. 34.11).

Therapeutic Management

Treatment consists of the application of pediculicides and manual removal of nit cases. Because of its efficacy and lack of toxicity, the drug of choice for infants and children is permethrin 1% cream rinse (Nix), which kills adult lice and nits (Frankowski, Weiner, & American Academy of Pediatrics Committee on School Health, 2010). Most experts

advise a second treatment at 7 to 10 days to ensure a cure (American Academy of Pediatrics, 2015). Daily removal of nits from a child's hair with a metal nit or flea comb is an essential control measure following treatment with the pediculicide. The child's entire head should be completely combed every day until no more nits are found. Lice do not jump or fly, but they can be transmitted from one person to another on personal items. Children are cautioned against sharing combs, hair ornaments, hats, caps, scarves, coats, and other items used on or near the hair.

SCHOOL-AGE DISORDERS WITH BEHAVIORAL COMPONENTS

ATTENTION DEFICIT HYPERACTIVITY DISORDER AND LEARNING DISABILITY

Attention deficit hyperactivity disorder (ADHD) refers to developmentally inappropriate degrees of inattention, impulsiveness, and hyperactivity (American Psychiatric Association, 2013). Their behavior evokes negative responses from others, and repeated exposure to negative

TABLE 34.5 Dermatophytoses (Fungal Infections)

Disorder and Organism	Manifestations	Management	Comments
Tinea capitis: *Trichophyton tonsurans,* *Microsporum audouinii,* *Microsporum canis*	Lesions in scalp but may extend to hairline or neck Characteristic configuration of scaly, circumscribed patches or patchy areas of alopecia Pruritic Diagnosis: Microscopic examination of scales	Oral griseofulvin or terbinafine Oral ketoconazole for difficult cases Selenium sulfide shampoos, used twice a week	Person-to-person or animal-to-person transmission Rarely, permanent loss of hair Atopic individuals more susceptible
Tinea corporis: *Trichophyton rubrum,* *Trichophyton mentagrophytes, M. canis, Epidermophyton* organisms	Generally round or oval, erythematous scaling patch that spreads peripherally and clears centrally; may involve nails (tinea unguium) Usually unilateral Diagnosis: Direct microscopic examination of scales	Oral griseofulvin Local application of antifungal preparation, such as tolnaftate, naftifine, miconazole, terbinafine, clotrimazole; applied daily 2.5 cm (1 inch) beyond periphery of lesion; application continued 1 to 2 weeks after no sign of lesion	Usually of animal origin from infected pets but may occur from human transmission, soil, or fomites; commonly seen in wrestlers
Tinea cruris ("jock itch"): *Epidermophyton floccosum, T. rubrum, T. mentagrophytes*	Skin response similar to that in tinea corporis Localized to medial proximal aspect of thigh and crural fold; may involve scrotum in males Pruritic Diagnosis: Same as for tinea corporis	Local application of tolnaftate liquid; terbinafine, clotrimazole, ciclopirox	Rare in preadolescent children Health education regarding transmission via person-to-person (direct or indirect)
Tinea pedis ("athlete's foot"): *T. rubrum, Trichophyton interdigitale, E. floccosum* *Tinea unguium:* Nail infection	On intertriginous areas between toes or on plantar surface of feet Lesions vary: • Maceration and fissuring between toes • Patches with pinhead-sized vesicles on plantar surface Pruritic Diagnosis: Direct microscopic examination of scrapings	Local application of terbinafine, ciclopirox, clotrimazole, miconazole, or ketoconazole Oral itraconazole, terbinafine, or griseofulvin for severe infections or not responsive to topical Elimination of conditions of heat and perspiration by use of clean, light socks and well-ventilated shoes	Most frequent in adolescents and adults; rare in children, but common in locations such as showers, locker rooms and swimming pools where fungi proliferate
Candidiasis (moniliasis): *Candida albicans*	Grows in chronically moist areas Inflamed areas with white exudate, peeling, and easy bleeding Pruritic Diagnosis: Characteristic appearance; microscopic identification of scrapings Chronic or recurrent often seen with human immunodeficiency virus (HIV) infection and immunocompromised child	Oral: nystatin for neonates; clotrimazole troches for older children; fluconazole or itraconazole for immunocompromised children Esophagitis: oral or intravenous (IV) fluconazole; IV amphotericin, voriconazole, or micafungin Skin lesions: topical nystatin, miconazole, or clotrimazole Vulvovaginal: topical clotrimazole, miconazole, butoconazole, terconazole, or tioconazole	Common form of diaper dermatitis Oral form common in infants Disseminated disease in very low–birth weight infants and immunosuppressed children

feedback adversely affects their self-concept. Children with ADHD are at greater risk for conduct disorders, oppositional defiant disorders, depression, anxiety disorders, and developmental disorders (e.g., speech and language delays and learning disabilities) than are children without ADHD (American Academy of Pediatrics, 2011).

Clinical Manifestations

The behaviors exhibited by children with ADHD are not unusual aspects of child behavior. The difference lies in the quality of motor activity and the developmentally inappropriate inattention, impulsivity, and hyperactivity displayed by children with ADHD. The manifestations may be numerous or few and mild or severe, and vary with the child's developmental level (Minzenberg, 2012). Mild manifestations of symptoms are apparent in at least two settings, usually educational and

family environments. Every child with ADHD is different from all other children with ADHD.

Most behavioral manifestations of ADHD are apparent at an early age, but the learning disabilities may not become evident until the child enters school. A major clinical manifestation is distractibility. The stimuli may come from external sources or internal sources. Children often demonstrate immaturity relative to chronologic age. Selective attention is often seen, in which the child has difficulty attending to "non-preferred" tasks such as completing chores or finishing homework. The child may not consider the consequences of behavior, may take excessive physical risks (often beginning early in life), and may demonstrate inappropriate social skills.

Children with ADHD demonstrate one of three subtypes (American Psychiatric Association, 2013):

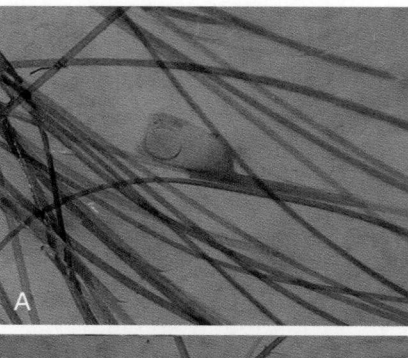
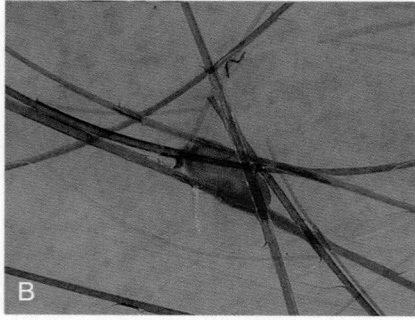

FIG 34.11 A, Empty nit case. **B,** Viable nits. (From Stefani, A.D., Hofmann-Wellenhof, R., Zalaudek, I. [2006]. Dermoscopy for diagnosis and treatment monitoring of pediculosis capitis. *Journal of the American Academy of Dermatology, 54*[5], 909–911.)

1. Combined type—Six (or more) symptoms of inattention and six (or more) symptoms of hyperactivity-impulsivity that persist for at least 6 months. Most children and adolescents with ADHD have the combined type.
2. Predominantly inattentive type—Six (or more) symptoms of inattention (but fewer than six symptoms of hyperactivity-impulsivity) that persist for at least 6 months.
3. Predominantly hyperactive-impulsive type—Six (or more) symptoms of hyperactivity-impulsivity (but fewer than six symptoms of inattention) that persist for at least 6 months. Inattention may often still be a significant clinical feature in such cases.

Diagnostic Evaluation

It is important to emphasize the need for a complete and thorough multidisciplinary evaluation of the child, incorporating the efforts of the primary pediatric health care provider and the family, as well as possible support from a psychologist, developmental pediatrician, neurologist, pediatric nurses, classroom teachers, and administrators. The clinicians and professionals must first determine whether the child's behavior is age appropriate or truly problematic.

Prior to diagnosis, a complete medical and developmental history is obtained. A description of the child's behavior in the home, school, and social situations are obtained from as many observers of the child as possible, especially the parents and teachers involved in the child's care. Behavioral checklists and adaptive scales should be completed by the child's caregivers and educators and scored by the primary care provider. A physical examination, including vision and hearing screening and a detailed neurologic evaluation, is completed. Psychologic testing, especially projective tests, is used to identify visual-perceptual difficulties, problems with spatial organization, and other phenomena that suggest cortical or diencephalic involvement, and it helps to identify the child's intelligence and achievement levels. Psychiatric disorders, medical problems, and traumatic experiences are ruled out, including lead poisoning, seizures, partial hearing loss, psychosis, and witnessing of sexual activity or violence.

Therapeutic Management

Management of the child with ADHD usually involves multiple approaches that include family education and counseling, medication, proper classroom placement, environmental manipulation, and behavioral therapy or psychotherapy.

Behavioral Therapy

Behavioral therapy focuses on the prevention of undesired behavior. Families are helped to identify new appropriate contingencies and reward systems to meet the child's developing needs. They may also receive instruction in effective parenting skills, such as delivering positive reinforcement, rewarding small increments of desired behaviors, and providing age-appropriate consequences (e.g., time-out, response cost). The use of organizational charts for completing self-care activities and the use of a word processor instead of manually writing assignments are emphasized. Through collaborative teamwork, parents learn techniques to help the child become more successful at home and in school.

Pharmacologic Therapy

The most commonly used medications are stimulants: methylphenidate hydrochloride and dextroamphetamine (Minzenberg, 2012). Non-stimulant medications, including norepinephrine reuptake inhibitors and adrenergic agonists, have also shown to be effective with fewer side effects in school-age and adolescent children (American Academy of Pediatrics, 2011). Children are given a small dosage initially, and the dosage is gradually increased until the desired response is achieved. Children who receive stimulants should be monitored carefully for side effects of the medication including appetite loss, abdominal pain, headaches, sleep disturbances, and growth velocity. Stimulants should be avoided in children who have a history of ticlike behaviors, a family history of Tourette syndrome (TS), or ADHD combined with TS because these medications may exaggerate tics.

Other medications, including tricyclic antidepressants and extended-release clonidine, may be used as adjunct therapy for ADHD, primarily for children with coexisting conditions, such as sleep disturbances (American Academy of Pediatrics, 2011). It is important to remember that these medications are not prescribed based on the child's weight (except atomoxetine) but on resolution of the symptoms; therefore, it is important to follow the child closely and evaluate for therapeutic effects and potential side effects. With all of these medications, regularly scheduled reevaluation of the child is essential to determine medication effectiveness, detect and evaluate any side effects, monitor development and health status (especially growth and blood pressure), and assess family interaction (see Clinical Reasoning Case Study).

Multimodal Treatment

The results of several studies suggest that multimodal treatment that involves the use of pharmacotherapy and behavioral intervention as well as close follow-up and feedback from school personnel is more effective than intensive behavioral treatment alone (Selekman, 2010).

Environmental Manipulation

Encourage families to modify the environment to allow the child to be more successful. Consistency is especially important for children with ADHD. Consistency between families and teachers in terms of reinforcing the same goals is essential. Fostering improved organizational skills requires a more highly structured environment than most children need. Children should be encouraged to make more appropriate choices and to take responsibility for their actions.

Attention Deficit Hyperactivity Disorder

Johnnie, 8 years of age, is a third grader who was recently diagnosed with ADHD. He has been taking methylphenidate (Ritalin) for about 1 month. In the short time that Johnnie has been taking this medication, his math teacher has noticed an improvement in his performance in math class. He is receiving a grade of B instead of his previous grades of D on most math quizzes. The math teacher has also noted that Johnnie is socializing more with his classmates and now has a "best friend" in math class. Johnnie usually receives his methylphenidate from the school nurse before lunch. Yesterday Johnnie's mother told the school nurse that he has not eaten his lunch for the past week and is not hungry.

What important issues regarding Johnnie's medication should the nurse consider in her discussions with Johnnie's mother?

Questions
1. Evidence—Is there sufficient evidence to draw conclusions about Johnnie's medication from his behavior?
2. Assumptions—Describe some underlying assumptions about the following:
   a. Pharmacologic action of methylphenidate in ADHD
   b. Side effects of methylphenidate
   c. Management of side effects
3. What implications for nursing care can be drawn at this time?
4. Does the evidence objectively support your conclusion?

ADHD, Attention deficit hyperactivity disorder.

Other helpful interventions include teaching parents how to make organizational charts (e.g., listing all activities that must be performed before leaving for school) and decrease distractions in the environment while the child is completing homework (e.g., turning off the television, having a consistent study area equipped with needed supplies), and helping parents understand ways to model positive behaviors and problem solving. The focus is on strategies to help the child succeed and cope with deficits while emphasizing strengths.

Appropriate Classroom Placement

Children with ADHD need an orderly, predictable, and consistent classroom environment with clear and consistent rules. Homework and classroom assignments may need to be reduced, and more time may need to be allotted for tests to allow the child to complete the task. Verbal instructions should be accompanied by visual references, such as written instructions on the blackboard. Schedules may need to be arranged so that academic subjects are taught in the morning when the child is experiencing the effects of the morning dose of medication. Low-interest and high-interest classroom activities should be intermingled to maintain the child's attention and interest. Regular and frequent breaks in activity are helpful because sitting in one place for an extended time may be difficult. Computers are helpful for children who have difficulty with writing (**dysgraphia**) and fine motor skills; in such children, handwriting will *not* improve. They need to find alternatives to physical competition that requires coordination of movement.

If the child has a learning disability, special training activities may be accomplished in self-contained classes limited to six to eight children, in special resource rooms with equipment and teaching teams, by mobile consultants who move from room to room to provide assistance to teachers and children, and in special first-grade programs in which high-risk children receive special attention to prevent or reduce the need for services as they progress. The purpose of programs for children with learning disabilities is to assist them toward more successful achievement, personal adjustment, and retention in the regular classroom.

A Child's Perception of Taking Ritalin at School

I feel embarrassed by having to leave class early to go take my medication. The other kids always ask where I'm going and why. It would be better if we could leave class at the same time as everyone else, go take the medication, and then just be a little late to the next class. Students don't ask why people are late for class, only why they leave early. It also bothers me when kids tell other kids, "Go take a pill" and other mean things just because someone is acting up.

What could nurses and teachers do to help? Most kids do not understand why other kids have to take medication. I think it would help if a nurse or teacher talked with the other kids and explained why some children take the medication and how ADHD affects people. That way there would be more understanding among all the kids.

Marissa White, Age 16 Years

ADHD, Attention deficit hyperactivity disorder.

Prognosis

With appropriate intervention, ADHD is relatively stable through early adolescence for most children. Some children experience decreased symptoms during late adolescence and adulthood, but a significant number of these children carry their symptoms into adulthood. The goal for children with ADHD is to help them identify their areas of weakness and learn to compensate for them.

Interprofessional Care Management of ADHD

Many health care professionals are active participants in the management of children with ADHD. Nurses and therapists in the community work with families and school personnel on a long-term basis to help plan and implement therapeutic regimens and to evaluate the effectiveness of therapy. They coordinate services and serve as a liaison between health and education professionals directly involved in the child's therapy program. School nurses understand the child's special needs and work with teachers (see Family-Centered Care box: A Child's Perception of Taking Ritalin at School). Nurses in any setting (community, school, hospital, practitioner's office) provide support and guidance to children and families during the difficult period of the child's growing up with a disabling condition.

Management begins with an explanation to the parents and the child about the diagnosis, including the nature of the problem and the practitioner's concept of the underlying CNS basis for the disorder. Parents need to be informed of the possible side effects of medications. If decreased appetite is a concern, parents can give the psychostimulants with or after meals rather than before, encourage consumption of nutritious snacks in the evening when the effects of the medication are decreasing, and serve frequent small meals with healthy "on-the-go" snacks. Sleeplessness is reduced by administering the medication early in the day.

Children taking tricyclic antidepressants display a dramatic increase in the incidence of dental caries. The marked anticholinergic action of the drugs increases saliva viscosity and produces a dry mouth. Emphasis on rigorous dental hygiene, conscientious home fluoride treatments, regular visits to the dentist, limited intake of refined carbohydrates, and use of artificial saliva is an important nursing function. The child should drink plenty of fluids and be well hydrated.

Parents often express concern that their children will become addicted to the psychostimulants or antidepressant drugs. Both types of drugs have the potential for abuse, and all children taking these drugs should be monitored closely for psychologic dependence, tolerance, depression, and other adverse behavior changes or idiosyncratic effects. Most children with ADHD are not interested in abusing their drugs because the effect of the drugs in these children is opposite that produced in normal individuals. However, caution parents to keep these drugs safely stored away from young children who may inadvertently ingest them and adolescents who may abuse them.

Parents need information about the prognosis and an understanding of the treatment plan. The greater their understanding of the disorder and its effects, the more likely they will be to carry out the recommended program of therapy. It is important that they understand that the therapy is not necessarily a panacea and that it will extend over a long period. This has particular significance for changes they need to make in environmental management. Reading material to help the child and family can be obtained from a variety of sources.

POSTTRAUMATIC STRESS DISORDER

Posttraumatic stress disorder (PTSD) refers to the development of characteristic symptoms after exposure to an extremely traumatic experience or catastrophic event. The traumatic experience is typically life-threatening to self or a significant other and may involve witnessing mutilation or death, experiencing or witnessing a serious injury, or physical coercion (e.g., an assault, a natural disaster, sexual abuse). It is important to note that PTSD is not limited to children who have lived in "war-torn" countries. Events such as automobile, school, or recreational accidents and bullying have also been identified as causes of PTSD.

The characteristic symptoms are persistent reexperiencing of the traumatic event, avoidance of stimuli associated with the event or trauma, numbing of general responsiveness, and persistent symptoms of increased arousal. The response to the event takes place in three stages. The initial response involves intense arousal, which usually lasts for a few minutes to 1 or 2 hours. The stress hormones are at the maximum as the individual prepares for "fight or flight." A prolonged arousal phase may indicate psychosis.

The second phase, which lasts approximately 2 weeks, is one in which defense mechanisms are mobilized. It is a period of calm in which the event appears to have produced no impression. The victim feels numb, and stress hormone secretion is absent. Defense mechanisms are less adaptive to specific situations and may not be what the situation demands. Denial that anything is wrong is a commonly observed defense mechanism.

The third phase is one of coping and consciously directed inquiry, which normally extends over 2 to 3 months. The victims want to know what happened and appear to be getting worse when actually they are getting better. Numerous psychologic symptoms such as depression, repetitive phenomena, phobic symptoms, anxiety, and conversion reactions may be present. Children often display repetitive actions. They play out the situation over and over again in an attempt to come to terms with their fear. Flashbacks are common. This phase can be self-perpetuating, and a prolonged reaction can develop into an obsession with the traumatic event.

Interprofessional Care Management of PTSD

Children need to deal with any traumatic events. Their reactions depend heavily on their social environment and the way in which their caregiving adults react to the event. In the second phase of PTSD, the appropriateness of the defense mechanism must be assessed, and children must be assisted in coping with their emotions.

Coping is a learned response, and children in the third phase of PTSD can be helped to deal with their fear. Children usually are willing

to accept reasoning. Those who are assisted in their catharsis and are allowed expression will survive without serious lasting effects. They should be encouraged to play out the stress and to discuss their feelings about the event. Children need professional help if any of the phases of PTSD are prolonged. Boys tend to have a prolonged defense phase more often than girls. Occasionally the event will be unrecognized, and the affected child will engage in what is considered to be unusual behavior. Children exhibiting any sudden change in behavior need to be assessed for exposure to a traumatic event. When the change in behavior is traced to a traumatic event, psychiatric services should be consulted to prevent or reduce the long-term emotional and psychologic effects of PTSD (Gerson & Rappaport, 2013).

SCHOOL REFUSAL

Children (other than beginning students) who resist going to school or who demonstrate extreme reluctance to attend school for a sustained period as a result of severe anxiety or fear of school-related experiences are said to have school refusal. The terms *school phobia* and *school avoidance* are also used to describe this behavior. School refusal occurs in children of all ages but is more common in children 10 years of age and older. School avoidance behaviors occur in both boys and girls and in children from all socioeconomic levels. Consequences of school refusal include poor academic performance, problems with peer relationships, employment difficulties, and increased risk for psychiatric illnesses (Lingenfelter & Hartung, 2015).

Anxiety that often verges on panic is a constant manifestation, and children can develop symptoms as a protective mechanism to keep them from facing the situation that distresses them. Physical symptoms are prominent and may affect any part of the body including anorexia, nausea, vomiting, diarrhea, dizziness, headache, leg pains, and abdominal pains. A striking feature of school refusal is the prompt subsiding of symptoms when it is evident that the child can remain at home. Another significant observation is an absence of symptoms on weekends and holidays unless they are related to other places such as Sunday school or parties.

Occasional mild reluctance to attend school is common among schoolchildren, but if the fear continues for longer than a few days, it must be considered a serious problem. The onset of school refusal is usually sudden and can be precipitated by a school-related incident including acts of violence, bullying, or pressure regarding academic achievement (Lingenfelter & Hartung, 2015). By taking a careful history, nurses determine the cause for the refusal.

Care Management

Treatment for school refusal depends on the cause. The primary goal is school attendance. The longer a child is permitted to stay out of school, the more difficult it is for the child to reenter. Parents must be convinced gently but firmly that an immediate return to school is essential and that it is their responsibility to insist on school attendance.

A school reentry protocol may be necessary for the child with severe symptoms. In reentry programs, the child role-plays routines that are involved in getting ready for school and occur at school. Relaxation techniques are also used. The child usually goes to school initially for a half day and then progresses to a full day. Often the school nurse is asked to provide support to the parents and the teacher during the reentry process. If the problem persists, professional help is recommended.

CONVERSION REACTION

A conversion reaction (also known as *hysteria, hysterical conversion reaction,* and *childhood hysteria*) is a sudden-onset psychophysiologic disorder that can usually be traced to a precipitating environmental event. The disorder is observed with equal frequency in both sexes in childhood, but affected girls outnumber affected boys during adolescence. Manifestations of conversion reaction involve primarily the voluntary musculature and special senses and include abdominal pain, fainting, pseudoseizures, paralysis, headaches, and visual field restriction. Once considered rare in childhood, this disorder occurs more frequently than has generally been acknowledged. The most commonly observed symptom is seizure activity that can be differentiated from symptoms of neurogenic origin by formal tests, the most useful of which is a normal electroencephalogram.

Many children with conversion reaction experienced a major family crisis before the onset of symptoms, such as the loss of a parent or other significant person through death, divorce, or moving. Children with conversion reaction characteristically come from families with communication problems or have a parent with depression or hypochondriasis.

Educating the child and family about the cause of emotional stresses or feelings and alternative approaches to coping with stress may alleviate the child's symptoms. If deep personality problems are evident, psychiatric consultation is indicated. Nursing care is similar to that for the child with recurrent abdominal pain.

CHILDHOOD DEPRESSION

Depression in childhood is often difficult to detect because children may be unable to express their feelings and tend to act out their problems and concerns rather than identifying them verbally. Some states of depression are temporary, such as acute depression precipitated by a traumatic event. The event might include a period of hospitalization, the loss of a parent through death or separation, or the loss of a significant relationship with something (a pet), a person (a friend, significant other, or family member), or a place (move from a familiar home, neighborhood, or city).

Manifestations are easily identifiable and include a sad face; tearfulness; irritability; and withdrawal from previously enjoyed activities and relationships. The child tends to spend more time in solitary activities and experiences hypersomnia, changes in appetite or weight (either increased or decreased), changes in school work, constipation, tiredness, and nonspecific complaints of not feeling well. Depressed children often exhibit a distinctive style of thinking characterized by low self-esteem, hopelessness, poor social engagement with peers, and a tendency to explain negative events in terms of personal shortcomings.

More serious and less common are the depressive responses to more chronic stress and loss. These are often observed in children with chronic illness or disability. Manifestations in the child are similar to those observed in acute reactions, but they occur more frequently and extend over a longer period.

Therapeutic Management

Depressed children are managed by a health care team that is specially trained in the care of children with mental disorders. Treatment is highly individualized and undertaken in the least restrictive environment. Suicidal children are admitted to the hospital for protection if the family is unable to provide constant monitoring. Most therapeutic regimens focus on various combinations of counseling, psychotherapy, family therapy, cognitive therapy, education (teaching social and life skills that facilitate coping), environmental improvement, and pharmacotherapy.

Pharmacotherapy may involve tricyclic antidepressants or selective serotonin reuptake inhibitors (SSRIs) such as sertraline (Zoloft), paroxetine (Paxil), bupropion (Wellbutrin), or venlafaxine (Effexor). There have been reports that antidepressant medications may cause increased suicidal thinking and behaviors in pediatric patients. This prompted the US Food and Drug Administration to require black box drug labeling detailing potential suicide-related risks for pediatric patients.

Interprofessional Care Management of Childhood Depression

Depression is a problem that can be easily overlooked in children and one that can interrupt normal growth and development. Recognizing depression and making appropriate referrals are important functions for all health care professionals. Identification of a depressed child requires a careful history (health, growth and development, social and family health), interviews with the child, and observations by the health care professional, parents, and teachers. If antidepressants are prescribed, the child and family need to know that antidepressants must be at a therapeutic level for 2 to 4 weeks to achieve a beneficial effect. The child and family also need to monitor the child for side effects of the specific drug prescribed and any interactions with other drugs.

CHILDHOOD SCHIZOPHRENIA

Childhood schizophrenia is a term that refers to severe deviations in ego functioning and is generally reserved for psychotic disorders that appear in children younger than 15 years of age. Childhood schizophrenia is a rare illness among children in the general population; only about 2 in every 1000 children with mental illness have childhood schizophrenia.

Childhood schizophrenia is characterized by symptoms that last for at least 6 months and seriously interfere with the child's functioning in school, at home, or in other social situations. The basic disturbance is a lack of contact with reality and the subsequent development of a world of the child's own. The most common manifestations involve language disturbances, impaired interpersonal relationships, and inappropriate affect (outward expression of emotion). Treatment involves management of the symptoms, prevention of relapse, and social and occupational rehabilitation. Antipsychotic drugs that may be used include haloperidol, clozapine, chlorpromazine, and risperidone. Family interventions and family therapy often result in improvements in psychotic symptoms, thought disorders, and social functioning among children with schizophrenia.

Interprofessional Care Management of Childhood Schizophrenia

Care of children with psychotic disorders is a highly specialized area. Health care professionals should be alert to the possibility that schizophrenia can occur in children and refer children to a psychiatrist for evaluation if they consistently demonstrate abnormal behavior. In addition, family members of children taking antipsychotic medications need to observe the child for possible side effects. Common side effects include dizziness, drowsiness, tachycardia, hypotension, and extrapyramidal effects such as abnormal movements and seizures.

REFERENCES

American Academy of Pediatrics. (2011). ADHD: Clinical practice guideline for the diagnosis, evaluation, and treatment of attention-deficit/hyperactivity disorder in children and adolescents. *Pediatrics, 128*(5), 1007–1022.

American Academy of Pediatrics, Committee on Infectious Diseases. (2015). L. Pickering (Ed.), *2015 Red book: Report of the Committee on Infectious Diseases* (30th ed.). Elk Grove Village, IL: The Academy.

American Academy of Pediatrics, Council on Communications and Media. (2013). Media education. *Pediatrics, 132*(5), 958–961.

American Academy of Pediatrics, Council on Sports Medicine and Fitness. (2012). Trampoline safety in childhood and adolescence. *Pediatrics, 130*(6), 1102–1109.

American Psychiatric Association. (2013). *Diagnostic and statistical manual of mental disorders* (5th ed.). Arlington, VA: Author.

Bhargava, S. (2011). Diagnosis and management of common sleep problems in children. *Pediatrics in Review, 32*(3), 91–98.

Bothe, D. A., Grignon, J. B., & Olness, K. N. (2014). The effects of a stress management intervention in elementary school children. *Journal of Developmental & Behavioral Pediatrics, 35*(1), 62–67.

Bradshaw, C. P., Waasdorp, T. E., Goldweber, A., et al. (2013). Bullies, gangs, drugs, and school: understanding the overlap and the role of ethnicity and urbanicity. *Journal of Youth and Adolescence, 42*(2), 220–234.

Brown, P., & Tierney, C. (2011). Media role in violence and the dynamics of bullying. *Pediatrics in Review, 32*(10), 453–454.

Carter, J. M., & Wilson, F. (2015). Cyberbullying: A 21st century health care phenomenon. *Pediatric Nursing, 41*(3), 115–125.

Centers for Disease Control and Prevention, National Center for Injury Prevention and Control. (2015). *Child passenger safety: Get the facts.* Retrieved from http://www.cdc.gov/MotorVehicleSafety/Child_Passenger _Safety/CPS-Factsheet.html.

Eime, R. M., Young, J. A., Harvey, J. T., et al. (2013). A systematic review of the psychological and social benefits of participation in sport for children and adolescents: Informing development of a conceptual model of health through sport. *International Journal of Behavioral Nutrition and Physical Activity, 10*, 98.

Ferguson, C. J. (2013). Spanking, corporal punishment and negative long-term outcomes: A meta-analytic review of longitudinal studies. *Clinical Psychology Review, 33*(1), 196–208.

Frankowski, B. L., Weiner, L. B., & American Academy of Pediatrics Committee on School Health. (2010). Clinical report: Guidance for the clinician in rendering pediatric care: head lice. *Pediatrics, 110*(3), 638–643.

Galland, B. C., Taylor, B. J., Elder, D. E., et al. (2012). Normal sleep patterns in infants and children: A systemic review of observational studies. *Sleep Medicine Reviews, 16*(3), 213–222.

Gerson, R., & Rappaport, N. (2013). Traumatic stress and posttraumatic stress disorder in youth: Recent research findings on clinical impact, assessment, and treatment. *Journal of Adolescent Health, 52*(2), 137–143.

Hensley, V. (2013). Childhood bullying: a review and implications for health care professionals. *Nursing Clinics of North America, 48*(2), 203–213.

Juvonen, J., & Graham, S. (2014). Bullying in schools: The power of bullies and the plight of victims. *Annual Review of Psychology, 65*, 159–185.

King, K. K. (2014). Violence in the school setting: A school nurse perspective. *Online Journal of Issues in Nursing.* Retrieved from http://www .nursingworld.org/MainMenuCategories/ANAMarketplace/ ANAPeriodicals/OJIN/TableofContents/Vol-19-2014/No1-Jan-2014/ Violence-in-School.html.

Langford, R., Bonell, C. P., Jones, H. E., et al. (2014). The WHO health promoting school framework for improving the health and well-being of students and their academic achievement. *Cochrane Database of Systematic Reviews, 2014*(4), CD008958.

Lingenfelter, N., & Hartung, S. (2015). School refusal behavior. *NASN School Nurse, 30*(5), 269–273.

Mahat, G., Lyons, R., & Bowen, F. (2014). Early childhood caries and the role of the pediatric nurse practitioner. *Journal for Nurse Practitioners, 10*(3), 189–193.

Meehan, 3rd, W. P., Lee, L. K., Fischer, C. M., et al. (2013). Bicycle helmet laws are associated with a lower fatality rate from bicycle-motor vehicle collisions. *Journal of Pediatrics, 163*(3), 726–729.

Minzenberg, M. J. (2012). Pharmacotherapy for attention-deficit/hyperactivity disorder: From cells to circuits. *Neurotherapeutics, 9*(3), 610–621.

National Highway Traffic Safety Administration. (2013). *Traffic safety facts 2011 data: Children.* Retrieved from http://www-nrd.nhtsa.dot.gov/pubs/ 811767.pdf.

Owen, D. J., Slep, A. M., & Heyman, R. E. (2012). The effect of praise, positive nonverbal response, reprimand, and negative nonverbal response on child compliance: A systematic review. *Clinical Child and Family Psychology Review, 15*(4), 364–385.

Pyrooz, D. C., & Sweeten, G. (2015). Gang membership between ages 5 and 17 years in the United States. *Journal of Adolescent Health, 56*(4), 414–419.

Riley, M. R., Scaramella, L. V., & McGoron, L. (2014). Disentangling the associations between contextual stress, sensitive parenting, and children's social development. *Family Relations, 63*, 287–299.

Ruiz-Casares, M., Rousseau, C., Currie, J. L., et al. (2012). 'I hold on to my teddy bear really tight': Children's experiences when they are home alone. *American Journal of Orthopsychiatry, 82*(1), 97–103.

Selekman, J. (2010). Attention-deficit/hyperactivity disorder. In P. Jackson, J. A. Vessey, & N. A. Schapiro (Eds.), *Primary care of children with chronic conditions* (5th ed.). St. Louis, MO: Mosby.

Shannon, R. A., & Kubelka, S. (2013). Reducing the risks of delegation: use of procedure skills checklists for unlicensed assistive personnel in schools, part 1. *NASN School Nurse, 28*(4), 178–181.

Shetgiri, R. (2013). Bullying and victimization among children. *Advances in Pediatrics, 60*(1), 33–51.

Skov, R., Christiansen, K., Dancer, S. J., et al. (2012). Update on the prevention and control of community-acquired methicillin-resistant *Staphylococcus aureus* (CA-MRSA). *International Journal of Antimicrobial Agents, 39*(3), 193–200.

White, L. S. (2012). Reducing stress in school-age girls through mindful yoga. *Journal of Pediatric Health Care, 26*(1), 45–56.

Wolke, D., & Lereya, S. T. (2015). Long-term effects of bullying. *Archives of Disease in Childhood, 100*(9), 879–885.

Yanchar, N. L. (2012). Preventing injuries from all-terrain vehicles. *Paediatrics & Child Health, 17*(9), 513–514.

35

The Adolescent and Family

Cheryl C. Rodgers

http://evolve.elsevier.com/Perry/maternal

PROMOTING OPTIMAL GROWTH AND DEVELOPMENT

Adolescence is a period of transition between childhood and adulthood—a time of rapid physical, cognitive, social, and emotional maturation.

Several terms are used to refer to this stage of growth and development. *Puberty* refers to the maturational, hormonal, and growth process that occurs when the reproductive organs begin to function and the secondary sex characteristics develop. This process is sometimes divided into three stages: *prepubescence*, the period of about 2 years immediately before puberty when the child is developing preliminary physical changes that herald sexual maturity; *puberty*, the point at which sexual maturity is achieved, marked by the first menstrual flow in girls but by less obvious indications in boys; and *postpubescence*, a 1- to 2-year period following puberty during which skeletal growth is completed and reproductive functions become fairly well established. *Adolescence*, which literally means "to grow into maturity," is generally regarded as the psychologic, social, and maturational process initiated by the pubertal changes. It involves three distinct subphases: *early adolescence* (11 to 14 years of age), *middle adolescence* (15 to 17 years of age), and *late adolescence* (18 to 20 years of age). The term *teenage years* is used synonymously with *adolescence* to describe 13 to 19 years of age. The changes that occur during the early, middle, and late phases of adolescence are summarized in Table 35.1.

BIOLOGIC DEVELOPMENT

The physical changes of puberty are primarily the result of hormonal activity and are controlled by the anterior pituitary gland in response to a stimulus from the hypothalamus. The obvious physical changes are noted in increased physical growth and in the appearance and development of secondary sex characteristics; less obvious are physiologic alterations and neurogonadal maturity, accompanied by the ability to procreate. Physical distinction between the sexes is made on the basis of distinguishing characteristics. Primary sex characteristics are the external and internal organs that carry out the reproductive functions (e.g., ovaries, uterus, breasts, penis). *Secondary sex characteristics* are the changes that occur throughout the body as a result of hormonal changes (e.g., voice alterations, development of facial and pubertal hair, fat deposits) but that play no direct part in reproduction.

Neuroendocrine Events of Puberty

The events of puberty are caused by a cluster or events that trigger the production of gonadotropin-releasing hormone (GnRH) by the hypothalamus. GnRH travels to the anterior pituitary gland, where is stimulates the production and secretion of follicle-stimulating hormone (FSH) and luteinizing hormone (LH). Increasing levels of FSH and LH stimulate a gonadal response, which for females consists of growth of ovarian follicles, production of estrogen, and initiation of ovulation, and for males consists of maturation of the testicles and testosterone and stimulation of sperm production.

The ovaries, testes, and adrenal glands secrete sex hormones. These hormones are produced in varying amounts by both sexes throughout the life span. The adrenal cortex is responsible for the small amounts secreted before the pubescent years, but the sex hormone production that accompanies maturation of the gonads is responsible for the biologic changes observed during puberty.

Estrogen, the feminizing hormone, is found in low quantities during childhood. Beginning in early puberty, FSH stimulates estrogen production by the ovaries; however, estrogen levels are not high enough to cause ovulation until mid-puberty. The increasing quantity of estrogen in early puberty causes a building of the endometrial lining of the uterus and first menstruation, or menarche. As puberty progresses, one ovarian follicle becomes dominant during each menstrual cycle and produces increasing amounts of estrogen that releases an ovum, a process called *ovulation*. After ovulation, the follicle involutes and estrogen production decreases. The pituitary gland responds to the decreased estrogen production by increasing production of FSH, which initiates a new menstrual cycle.

Androgens, the masculinizing hormones, are also secreted in small and gradually increasing amounts up to about 7 to 9 years of age, at which time there is a more rapid increase in both sexes, especially boys, until about 15 years of age. These hormones have tremendous growth-promoting properties that result in rapid increases of muscle mass, skeletal growth, and bone density. Androgens are responsible for the development of pubic, axillary, facial, and body hair; acne; body odor; and an increase in height. The capacity to ejaculate occurs approximately 1 year after initial testicular enlargement and pubic hair appearance. The production of viable sperm tends to follow boys' first ejaculation.

Sexual Maturation

The visible evidence of sexual maturation is achieved in an orderly sequence, and the state of maturity can be estimated on the basis of the appearance of these external manifestations. The age at which these changes are observed and the time required to progress from one stage to another may vary among children. The time from the appearance of breast buds to full maturity may be 1½ to 6 years for adolescent girls. It may take 2 to 5 years for male genitalia to reach adult size. The stages of development of secondary sex characteristics and genital development have been defined as a guide for estimating sexual maturity and are referred to as the *Tanner stages* (Box 35.1). The usual sequence of appearance of maturational changes is presented in Box 35.2.

TABLE 35.1   Growth and Development During Adolescence

Early Adolescence (11 to 14 Years of Age)	Middle Adolescence (15 to 17 Years of Age)	Late Adolescence (18 to 20 Years of Age)
Growth		
Rapidly accelerating growth	Growth decelerating in girls	Physically mature
Reaches peak velocity	Stature reaches 95% of adult height	Structure and reproductive growth almost complete
Secondary sex characteristics appear	Secondary sex characteristics well advanced	
Cognition		
Explores newfound ability for limited abstract thought	Developing capacity for abstract thinking	Established abstract thought
Clumsy groping for new values and energies	Enjoys intellectual powers, often in idealistic terms	Can perceive and act on long-range options
Comparison of "normality" with peers of same sex	Concern with philosophic, political, and social problems	Able to view problems comprehensively
		Intellectual and functional identity established
Identity		
Preoccupied with rapid body changes	Modifies body image	Body image and gender-role definition nearly secured
Trying out of various roles	Self-centered; increased narcissism	Mature sexual identity
Measurement of attractiveness by acceptance or rejection of peers	Tendency toward inner experience and self-discovery	Phase of consolidation of identity
Conformity to group norms	Has a rich fantasy life	Increase in self-esteem
Decline in self-esteem	Idealistic	Comfortable with physical growth
	Able to perceive future implications of current behavior and decisions; variable application	Social roles defined and articulated
Relationships With Parents		
Defining independence-dependence boundaries	Major conflicts over independence and control	Emotional and physical separation from parents completed
Strong desire to remain dependent on parents while trying to detach	Low point in parent-child relationship	Independence from family with less conflict
No major conflicts over parental control	Greatest push for emancipation; disengagement	Emancipation nearly secured
	Final and irreversible emotional detachment from parents; mourning	
Relationships With Peers		
Seeks peer affiliations to counter instability generated by rapid change	Strong need for identity to affirm self-image	Peer group recedes in importance in favor of individual friendship
Upsurge of close, idealized friendships with members of the same sex	Behavioral standards set by peer group	Testing of romantic relationships against possibility of permanent alliance
Struggle for mastery within peer group	Acceptance by peers extremely important—fear of rejection	Relationships characterized by giving and sharing
	Exploration of ability to attract opposite sex	
Sexuality		
Self-exploration and evaluation	Multiple plural relationships	Forms stable relationships and attachment to another
Limited dating, usually group	Internal identification of heterosexuality, homosexual, or bisexual attractions	Growing capacity for mutuality and reciprocity
Limited intimacy	Exploration of "self-appeal"	Dating as a romantic pair
	Feeling of "being in love"	May publicly identify as gay, lesbian, or bisexual
	Tentative establishment of relationships	Intimacy involves commitment rather than exploration and romanticism
Psychologic Health		
Wide mood swings	Tendency toward inner experiences; more introspective	More constancy of emotion
Intense daydreaming	Tendency to withdraw when upset or feelings are hurt	Anger more apt to be concealed
Anger outwardly expressed with moodiness, temper outbursts, and verbal insults and name-calling	Vacillation of emotions in time and range	
	Feelings of inadequacy common; difficulty in asking for help	

Sexual Maturation in Girls

In most girls, the initial indication of puberty is the appearance of breast buds, an event known as *thelarche*, which occurs between 8 and 13 years of age (Fig. 35.1). This is followed in approximately 2 to 6 months by growth of pubic hair on the mons pubis, known as *adrenarche* (Fig. 35.2). In a minority of normally developing girls, however, pubic hair may precede breast development. The average age of thelarche for Caucasian girls is 9.7 years of age, Hispanic girls is 9.3 years of age, and African-American girls is 8.8 years of age (Herman-Giddens, 2013).

BOX 35.1 Tanner Stages

The Tanner stages were developed by Dr. J.M. Tanner and colleagues. Tanner stages describe the stages of pubertal growth and are numbered from stage 1 (immature) to stage 5 (mature) for both males and females. In girls and young women, the Tanner stages describe pubertal development based on breast size and the shape and distribution of pubic hair. In boys and young men, the Tanner stages describe pubertal development based on the size and shape of the penis and scrotum and the shape and distribution of pubic hair.

Data from Tanner, J.M. (1962). *Growth of adolescents,* Oxford, UK: Blackwell Scientific Publications.

BOX 35.2 Usual Sequence of Maturational Changes

Girls
- Breast changes
- Rapid increase in height and weight
- Growth of pubic hair
- Appearance of axillary hair
- Menstruation (usually begins 2 years after first signs noted above)
- Abrupt deceleration of linear growth

Boys
- Enlargement of testicles
- Growth of pubic hair, axillary hair, hair on upper lip, hair on face and elsewhere on body (facial hair usually appears about 2 years after appearance of pubic hair)
- Rapid increase in height
- Changes in the larynx and consequently the voice (usually take place along with growth of penis)
- Nocturnal emissions
- Abrupt deceleration of linear growth

The initial appearance of menstruation, or menarche, occurs about 2 years after the appearance of the first pubescent changes, approximately 9 months after attainment of peak height velocity, and 3 months after attainment of peak weight velocity. There is evidence that girls are developing secondary sex characteristics at a younger age among various ethnicities. The explanation for this is not yet clear but appears to be influenced by being overweight as well as environmental influences (Currie, Ahluwalia, Godeau, et al., 2012). The normal age range of menarche ranges from $10\frac{1}{2}$ to 15 years, with the average age being 12 years, 8 months for Caucasian girls and 12 years 2 months for African-American girls (Cabrera, Bright, Frane, et al., 2014). Ovulation and regular menstrual periods usually occur 6 to 14 months after menarche. Girls may be considered to have pubertal delay if breast development has not occurred by 13 years of age (Villanueva & Argente, 2014).

Sexual Maturation in Boys

The first pubescent changes in boys are testicular enlargement accompanied by thinning, reddening, and increased looseness of the scrotum (Fig. 35.3). These events usually occur between $9\frac{1}{2}$ and 14 years of age. Early puberty is also characterized by the initial appearance of pubic hair. Penile enlargement begins, and testicular enlargement and pubic hair growth continue throughout mid-puberty. During this period, there is also increasing muscularity, early voice changes, and development of early facial hair. Temporary breast enlargement and tenderness,

gynecomastia, are common during early to mid-puberty, occurring in up to 70% of boys (Ali & Donohoue, 2016). The spurts in height and weight occur concurrently toward the end of mid-puberty. For most boys, breast enlargement disappears within 2 years; however, it may persist in obese individuals. By late puberty, there is a definite increase in the length and width of the penis, testicular enlargement continues, and the first ejaculation occurs. Axillary hair develops, and facial hair extends to cover the anterior neck. Final voice changes occur secondary to the growth of the larynx. Concerns about *pubertal delay* should be considered for boys who exhibit no enlargement of the testes or scrotal changes by 14 years of age (Villanueva & Argente, 2014).

Physical Growth During Puberty

A constant phenomenon associated with sexual maturation is a dramatic increase in growth. The final 20% to 25% of linear growth is achieved during puberty, and most of this growth occurs during a 24- to 36-month period—the adolescent growth spurt. This accelerated growth occurs in all children but, as in other areas of development, is highly variable in age of onset, duration, and extent. The growth spurt begins earlier in girls, usually between $9\frac{1}{2}$ and $14\frac{1}{2}$ years of age; on average, it begins between $10\frac{1}{2}$ and 16 years of age in boys. During this period, the average boy gains 10 to 30 cm (4 to 12 inches) in height and 7 to 30 kg (15.5 to 66 pounds) in weight. The average girl, in whom the growth spurt is slower and less extensive, gains 5 to 20 cm (2 to 8 inches) in height and 7 to 25 kg (15.5 to 55 pounds) in weight. Growth in height typically ceases 2 to $2\frac{1}{2}$ years after menarche in girls and at 18 to 20 years of age in boys.

This increase in size is acquired in a characteristic sequence. Growth in length of the extremities and neck precedes growth in other areas, and because these parts are the first to reach adult length, the hands and feet appear larger than normal during adolescence. Increases in hip and chest breadth take place in a few months, followed several months later by an increase in shoulder width. These changes are followed by increases in length of the trunk and depth of the chest. This sequence of changes is responsible for the characteristic long-legged, gawky appearance of early adolescent children.

Sex Differences in General Growth Patterns

Sex differences in general growth and distribution patterns are apparent in skeletal growth, muscle mass, adipose tissue, and skin. Skeletal growth differences between boys and girls are apparently a function of hormonal effects at puberty. The earlier cessation of growth in girls is caused by epiphyseal unity under the potent effect of estrogen secretion, and the hormonal effect on female bone growth is much stronger than the similar effect of testosterone in boys. In boys, the prolonged growth period before puberty and the less rapid epiphyseal closure are reflected in their greater overall height and longer arms and legs. Other skeletal differences are increased shoulder width in boys and broader hip development in girls.

Hypertrophy of the laryngeal mucosa and enlargement of the larynx and vocal cords occur in both boys and girls to produce voice changes. Girls' voices become slightly deeper and considerably fuller, but the effect in boys is striking. The change in the voice of adolescent boys occurs between Tanner stages 3 and 4, with the voice often shifting uncontrollably from deep to high tones in the middle of a sentence.

Growth of lean body mass, principally muscle, which tends to occur after the bone growth spurt, takes place steadily during adolescence. Lean body mass is both quantitatively and qualitatively greater in boys than in girls at comparable stages of pubertal development. Nonlean body mass, primarily fat, is also increased but follows a less orderly pattern. There may be a transient increase in subcutaneous fat just

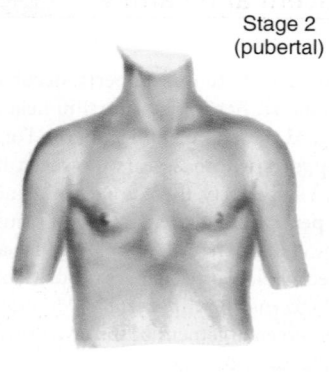
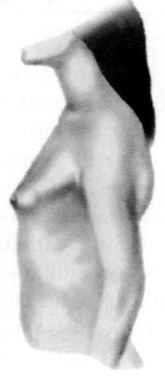

Stage 2
(pubertal)

Breast bud stage—small area of
elevation around papilla; enlargement
of areolar diameter

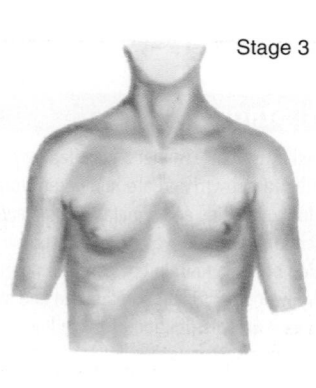
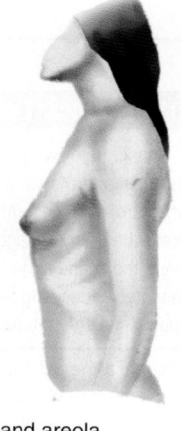

Stage 3

Further enlargement of breast and areola
with no separation of their contours

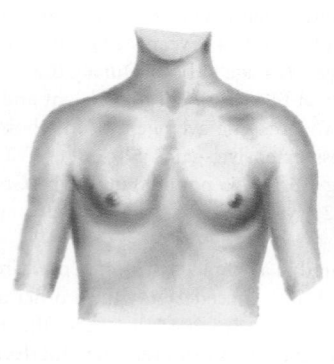
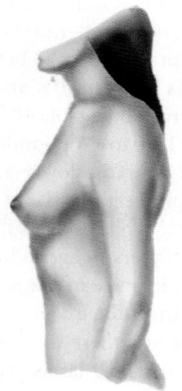

Stage 4

Projection of areola and papilla
to form a secondary mound (may
not occur in all girls)

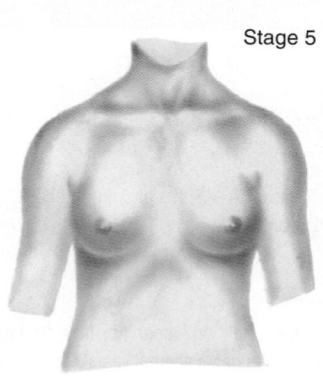
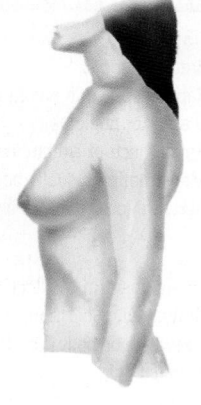

Stage 5

Mature configuration; projection of papilla
only caused by recession of areola
into general contour

FIG 35.1 Development of the breast in girls—average age span: 8 to 13 years. Stage 1 (prepubertal, elevation of papilla only) is not shown. (Adapted from Daniel, W.A., & Paulshock, B.Z. [1979]. A physician's guide to sexual maturity. *Patient Care, 13,* 122–124; Marshall, W.A., & Tanner, J.M. [1969]. Variations in pattern of pubertal changes in girls. *Archives of Disease in Childhood, 44*[235], 291.)

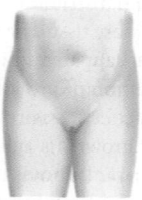

Stage 1
(prepubertal)

No pubic hair; essentially the same as
during childhood; no distinction between
hair on pubis and over the abdomen

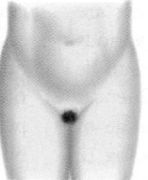

Stage 2

Sparse growth of long, straight, downy, and
slightly pigmented hair extending along labia;
between stages 2 and 3 begins to appear on pubis

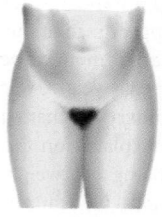

Stage 3

Hair darker, coarser, and curly and
spread sparsely over entire pubis in
the typical female triangle

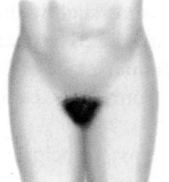

Stage 4

Pubic hair denser, curled, and adult in distribution
but less abundant and restricted to the pubic area

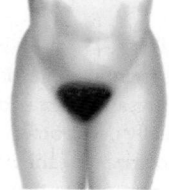

Stage 5

Hair adult in quantity, type, and pattern
with spread to inner aspect of thighs

FIG 35.2 Growth of pubic hair in girls—average age span for stages 2 to 5: 11 to 14 years. (Adapted from Daniel, W.A., & Paulshock, B.Z. [1979]. A physician's guide to sexual maturity. *Patient Care, 13,* 122–124; Marshall, W.A., & Tanner, J.M. [1969]. Variations in pattern of pubertal changes in girls. *Archives of Disease in Childhood, 44*[235], 291.)

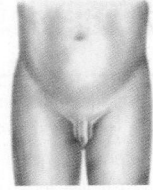

Stage 1
(prepubertal)

No pubic hair; essentially the same as
during childhood; no distinction between
hair on pubis and over the abdomen

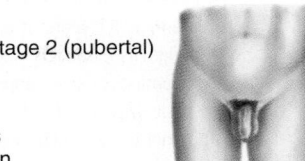

Stage 2 (pubertal)

Initial enlargement of scrotum and testes;
reddening and textural changes of scrotal skin;
sparse growth of long, straight, downy, and
slightly pigmented hair at base of penis

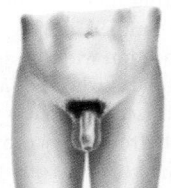

Stage 3

Initial enlargement of penis, mainly in
length; testes and scrotum further enlarged;
hair darker, coarser, and curly and spread
sparsely over entire pubis

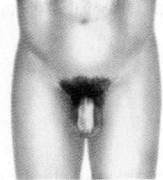

Stage 4

Increased size of penis with growth in diameter and
development of glans; glans larger and broader; scrotum
darker; pubic hair more abundant with curling but
restricted to pubic area

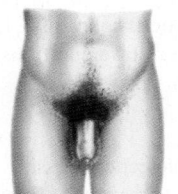

Stage 5

Testes, scrotum, and penis adult in size and shape;
hair adult in quantity and type with spread to inner
surface of thighs

FIG 35.3 Developmental stages of secondary sex characteristics and genital development in boys—average age span: 12½ to 16 years. (Adapted from Daniel, W.A., & Paulshock, B.Z. [1979]. A physician's guide to sexual maturity. *Patient Care, 13,* 122–124; Marshall, W.A., & Tanner, J.M. [1969]. Variations in pattern of pubertal changes in girls. *Archives of Disease in Childhood, 44*[235], 291.)

before the skeletal growth spurt, especially in boys. This is followed 1 to 2 years later by a modest to marked decrease, which is again more notable in boys. Later, variable amounts of fat are deposited to fill out and contour the mature physique in patterns characteristic of the adolescent's gender, particularly in the regions over the thighs, hips, and buttocks and around the breast tissue. It should be noted, however, that pediatric obesity is steadily on the increase in the United States, and obesity can change the timing of puberty. This may have long-term effects for increased risk for adult adiposity and obesity (Bralic, Tahirovic, Matanic, et al., 2012). An association is noted between obesity and onset of early puberty in girls rather than a causal relationship, and other factors such as hormones and insulin resistance may account for early-onset puberty; no correlations between body fat and earlier puberty in boys have been reported (Biro, Greenspan, & Galvez, 2012).

Other Physiologic Changes

A number of physiologic functions are altered in response to some of the pubertal changes. The size and strength of the heart, blood volume, and systolic blood pressure increase, whereas the heart rate decreases. Blood volume, which has increased steadily during childhood, reaches a higher value in boys than in girls, a fact that may be related to the increased muscle mass in pubertal boys. Adult values are reached for all formed elements of the blood. Respiratory rate and basal metabolic rate, decreasing steadily throughout childhood, reach the adult rate in adolescence. Respiratory volume and vital capacity are increased and to a far greater extent in males than in females. During this period, physiologic responses to exercise change drastically: performance improves, especially in boys, and the body is able to make the physiologic adjustments needed for normal functioning after exercise is completed. These capabilities are a result of the increased size and strength of muscles and the increased level of cardiac, respiratory, and metabolic functioning.

Responses to Puberty

The response to the physical changes of pubertal growth and development is manifested differently depending on the stage of development. During early adolescence, young adolescents become preoccupied with the rapid changes in their body and are interested in the anatomy, physiology, and function of their sexual organs. Boys must also confront the sexual feelings and tensions that accompany puberty, and the appearance of nocturnal emissions may be puzzling, troublesome, or embarrassing. Unless the boy has been prepared in advance, he may find it difficult to discuss his feelings with his parents and may turn to his friends for information and guidance. Many girls also find the rapid changes in their body to be sources of concern. Some girls perceive the increase in weight and associated fat deposition as evidence of obesity and may indulge in fad diets. Although many girls look forward to menstruation and take this event in stride, others may find the first menstrual period a distressing and frightening event. All teenagers, regardless of gender, are concerned with the question "Am I normal?" To answer this question, they compare their body with those of their peers and with images in the media. This leads to a great deal of uncertainty about their appearance and attractiveness. If an adolescent does not enter puberty at the same time as his or her peers, considerable inner conflict may occur. Nurses who work with adolescents must provide teaching and health care interventions that are appropriate for the adolescent's chronologic and cognitive development rather than the stage of physical maturation.

PSYCHOSOCIAL DEVELOPMENT

Developing a Sense of Identity (Erikson)

Traditional psychosocial theory holds that the developmental crisis of adolescence leads to the formation of a sense of identity (Erikson, 1963). Throughout childhood, individuals have been going through the process of identification as they concentrate on various parts of the body at specific times. During infancy, children identify themselves as being separate from the mother; during early childhood, they establish a gender-role identification with the appropriate-sex parent; and in later childhood, they establish who they are in relation to others. In adolescence, they come to see themselves as distinct individuals, somehow unique and separate from every other individual.

Adolescence begins with the onset of puberty and extends to relative physical and emotional stability at or near graduation from high school. During this time, the adolescent is faced with the crisis of *group identity versus alienation.* In the period that follows, the individual strives to attain autonomy from the family and develop a sense of *personal identity* as opposed to *role diffusion.* A sense of group identity appears to be essential to the development of a sense of personal identity. Young adolescents must resolve questions concerning relationships with a peer group before they are able to resolve questions about who they are in relation to family and society.

Group Identity

During the early stage of adolescence, pressure to belong to a group is intensified. Adolescents find it essential to have a group to which they feel they can belong and that provides them with status. Belonging to a crowd helps adolescents establish the differences between themselves and their parents. They dress as the group dresses and wear makeup and hairstyles according to group criteria, all of which are different from those of the parental generation. Language, music, and dancing reflect a culture that is exclusive to the adolescent. When adults begin to emulate these fashions and interests, their style changes immediately. The evidence of adolescent conformity to the peer group and nonconformity to the adult group provides adolescents with a frame of reference in which they can display their own self-assertion while they reject the identity of their parents' generation. To be different is to be unaccepted and alienated from the group.

Individual Identity

The quest for personal identity is part of the ongoing identification process. As adolescents establish identity within a group, they also attempt to incorporate multiple body changes into a concept of the self. Body awareness is part of self-awareness. In their search for identity, adolescents consider the relationships that have developed between themselves and others in the past, as well as the directions they hope to take in the future.

Significant others hold expectations for the adolescent's behavior. Often these expectations or demands are persistent enough to result in certain decisions that might be made differently or not at all if the individual could be solely responsible for identity formation. It is all too easy to slip into the roles that are expected by these external influences without incorporating personal goals or questioning these decisions. Thus individuals may become what parents or others wish them to be, based on these premature decisions. Adolescents might form a negative identity when society or their culture provides them with a self-image that is contrary to the values of the community. Labels such as "loser," "hoodlum," "troublemaker," or "failure" are applied to certain adolescents, who then accept and live up to these labels with behaviors that validate and strengthen them.

The process of evolving a personal identity is time-consuming and fraught with periods of confusion, depression, and discouragement. Determining an identity and a place in the world is a critical and perilous feature of adolescence (see Clinical Reasoning Case Study: Discussing the Future). However, as the pieces gradually shift and settle into place, a positive identity emerges. Role diffusion results when the individual is unable to formulate a satisfactory identity from the multiplicity of aspirations, roles, and identifications.

CLINICAL REASONING CASE STUDY
Discussing the Future

Jeremy is 17 years of age and will be graduating from high school in the spring. His mother, a single parent, tells you that she is concerned because graduation is quickly approaching and Jeremy has made no plans for what he will do with his life after graduation. Whenever Jeremy mentions the topic, his mother tells him "This is what you must do" and begins to outline the steps he must take. Jeremy just walks away. She asks, "What should I do?" What advice should you give Jeremy's mother?

1. Evidence—Is there sufficient evidence to draw any conclusions about what advice the nurse should give Jeremy's mother?
2. Assumptions—Describe an underlying assumption about each of the following issues:
   a. Adolescents and the search for personal identity
   b. The influence of others on the adolescent's search for personal identity
   c. Ways to communicate with adolescents
3. What implications and priorities for nursing care can be drawn at this time?
4. Does the evidence objectively support your argument (conclusion)?

Development of Self-Concept and Body Image

The sudden growth that takes place in early adolescence creates feelings of confusion for adolescents. They have lost the security of a familiar body and feel uncomfortable with their altered body. Consequently, they may try to either hide their body or advertise it or they may alternate between the two extremes. Teenagers are acutely aware of their appearance as they begin to acquire images of themselves as adults, but they see discrepancies between their ideal and actual skills and abilities.

Adolescents are continually comparing themselves with their peers and making judgments about their own normality based on these observations. Pubertal children feel most comfortable when they are just like their friends and age-mates. Perceived defects or deviations from the group average are threatening to their idealized image. Any blemish is likely to be magnified out of proportion, and any delay of the visible evidence of maturity is cause for worry. The diagnosis of chronic disease or a permanent physical disability has special significance during adolescence and creates additional stresses for both adolescents with the condition and health care providers.

Experts have determined that the body image established during adolescence is the one that individuals retain throughout life. Much of adolescents' search for identity takes place before a mirror as they try to read from the reflected features just who they are and what they look like to other people. Adolescents practice facial expressions and postures, try out hair arrangements, worry about a pimple, and in other ways attempt to assess the best means to achieve a maximum effect—to reveal the "true self." The self-concept becomes more differentiated as adolescents acquire a more complex picture of themselves, one that takes situational factors into account. The self-concept gradually becomes more individualized and more distinct from the concepts of others. By late adolescence, the heightened concern with body image has ended and is replaced by a general comfort with the body.

Sex-Role Identity

Adolescence is the time for consolidation of a sex-role identity. For young adolescents, the process of sexual identity development usually involves forming close friendships with same-sex peers. Many teenagers begin to make a shift from relationships with same-sex peers to intimate relationships with members of the opposite sex during middle adolescence (Fig. 35.4). The type and degree of seriousness of partner relationships

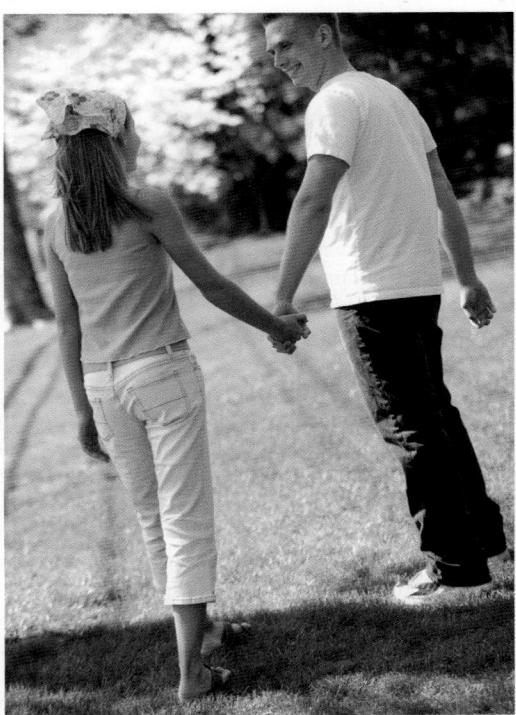

FIG 35.4 Relationships with peers of the opposite sex are an important part of adolescence. (Copyright 2011 by Photos.com, a division of Getty Images. All rights reserved.)

---

vary, but sexual activity is common by the late teen years, and 63% of 12th-grade students reported having sexual intercourse (Eaton, Kann, Kinchen, et al., 2012). An integrated sexual identity often emerges during late adolescence as individuals incorporate sexual experiences, feelings, and knowledge.

Sexual orientation is an important aspect of sexual identity. Sexual orientation is defined as a pattern of sexual arousal or romantic attraction toward people of the opposite gender (heterosexual), of the same gender (homosexual), or of both genders (bisexual). Sexual orientation encompasses several dimensions, including attraction, fantasy, actual sexual behavior, and self-labeling or group affiliation. Most adolescents identify themselves as being predominantly heterosexual; however, about 1% of high school students identify themselves as bisexual or homosexual, and 10% are unsure (Steever, Francis, Gordon, et al., 2014). For adolescents whose orientation encompasses any same-gender dimensions, the identity process during adolescence can be complicated, especially when community norms disapprove of orientations other than heterosexual. Adolescents who have witnessed harassment or violence may be reluctant to self-identify even when their attractions and behaviors are exclusively same-gender or bisexual.

The development of sexual orientation as part of sexual identity includes several developmental milestones during late childhood and throughout adolescence. These milestones do not necessarily occur in the same order for everyone, nor are they completed in the same amount of time. They include the following:

1. The realization of romantic or erotic attraction to people of one (or both) genders
2. Erotic daydreaming about one or both genders
3. Romantic partners or dates without sexual activity
4. Sexual activity with people of the preferred gender or genders (also, for some teens, sexual activity with a nonpreferred gender, out of curiosity or through social pressure)

CLINICAL REASONING CASE STUDY
Discussing Sexual Orientation With Adolescents

John, a 17-year-old adolescent, comes into the school-based clinic and tells the nurse practitioner that he thinks he is homosexual. Based on this information, answer the following questions:

1. Evidence—Is there sufficient evidence to draw any conclusions about John's sexual orientation at this time?
2. Assumptions—Describe an underlying assumption about each of the following issues:
   a. Sexual orientation in adolescents
   b. Society's reaction to homosexuality
   c. Health care professionals and sexuality
3. What is the most appropriate response by the nurse practitioner to John's statement?
4. Does the evidence objectively support your argument (conclusion)?

---

5. Self-identification of the orientation that best fits one's current circumstances and understanding
6. Publicly self-identifying that orientation, usually to intimate friends and family first and then the wider social group
7. An intimate, committed sexual relationship with a person of the gender appropriate to one's orientation

There is no evidence that homosexual or bisexual adults are more or less likely to create long-term, stable relationships than are heterosexual couples. It should be noted that bisexual adolescents and adults do not generally engage in sexual relationships with both genders concurrently; self-identification as bisexual usually refers to the ability to be attracted to either gender but does not imply that such a person requires partners of both genders or that one must be equally attracted to and have sexual experience with both genders to be bisexual.

Although the order of these milestones varies greatly among adolescents, adolescents who identify as gay, lesbian, or bisexual tend to publicly self-identify later than heterosexual peers. Without positive gay, lesbian, or bisexual role models or a supportive peer group, sexual-minority teens can feel isolated and they may not share their orientation with anyone for fear of rejection or violence (see Clinical Reasoning Case Study: Discussing Sexual Orientation With Adolescents).

COGNITIVE DEVELOPMENT (PIAGET)

Cognitive thinking culminates with the capacity for *abstract thinking*. This stage, the period of *formal operations*, is Piaget's fourth and last stage. Adolescents are no longer restricted to the real and actual, which was typical of the period of concrete thought; now they are also concerned with the possible. They now think beyond the present. Without having to center attention on the immediate situation, they can imagine a sequence of future events that might occur, such as college and occupational possibilities; how things might change in the future, such as relationships with parents; and the consequences of their actions, such as dropping out of school. At this time, their thoughts can be influenced by logical principles rather than just their own perceptions and experiences. They become increasingly capable of scientific reasoning and formal logic.

Adolescents are capable of mentally manipulating more than two categories of variables at the same time. For example, they can consider the relationship between speed, distance, and time in planning a trip. They can detect logical consistency or inconsistency in a set of statements and evaluate a system or set of values in a more analytic manner. For instance, they question the parent who insists on honesty in the teenager but at the same time cheats on an income tax report or expense account.

In adolescence, young people begin to think about both their own thinking and the thinking of others. They wonder what opinion others have of them, and they are able to imagine the thoughts of others. With this capacity comes the ability to differentiate between others' thoughts and their own and to interpret the thoughts of others more accurately. They are able to understand that few concepts are absolute or independent of other influencing factors. As they become aware that other cultures and communities have different norms and standards from their own, it becomes easier for them to accept members of these other cultures, and the decision to behave in their own culture in an accepted manner becomes a more conscious commitment.

MORAL DEVELOPMENT (KOHLBERG)

Although younger children merely accept the decisions or point of view of adults, adolescents question absolutes and rules, and they view moral standards as subjective and based on points of view that are subject to disagreement. When old principles are challenged but new independent values have not yet emerged to take their place, young people search for a moral code that preserves their personal integrity and guides their behavior. Their decisions involving moral dilemmas must be based on an *internalized set of moral principles* that provides them with the resources to evaluate the demands of the situation and to plan actions that are consistent with their ideals.

Late adolescence is characterized by serious questioning of existing moral values and their relevance to society and the individual. Adolescents can easily take the role of another. They understand duty and obligation based on reciprocal rights of others, as well as the concept of justice that is founded on making amends for misdeeds and repairing or replacing what has been spoiled by wrongdoing. However, they seriously question established moral codes, often as a result of observing that some adults verbally ascribe to a code but do not adhere to it.

SPIRITUAL DEVELOPMENT

Adolescents are capable of understanding abstract concepts and of interpreting analogies and symbols. They are able to empathize, philosophize, and think logically. Most adolescents search for ideals and speculate about illogical statements and conflicting ideologies. Their tendency toward introspection and emotional intensity often makes it difficult for others to know what they are thinking. However, they may reveal deep spiritual concerns. They need support and encouragement in their struggle for understanding and the freedom to question without censure.

Generally, the stated importance of participation in organized religion declines somewhat during the adolescent years. More high school students than post–secondary school young people attend religious services regularly, and, not surprisingly, the younger the adolescents, the more likely they are to view religion as being important to them. Among older adolescents, the importance of organized religion declines more among college students than among those not in college. Late adolescence appears to be a time when individuals reexamine and reevaluate many of the beliefs and values of their childhood. Consistent with developmental changes in value autonomy, the religious beliefs of young people are likely to become more personalized and less bound to the traditional religious practices they may have been exposed to when they were younger. As adolescents mature and form an identity, they may either reject their family's traditional beliefs or they may decide to conform to those beliefs (Neuman, 2011).

Greater levels of religiosity and spirituality are associated with fewer high-risk behaviors and more health-promoting behaviors (Michaelson,

Pickett, Robinson, et al., 2015). Nurses play an important role for teens by providing an opportunity to discuss issues regarding spirituality.

SOCIAL DEVELOPMENT

The biologic, cognitive, and social changes of adolescence are shaped by the social environment in which the changes take place. The social environment provides opportunities, barriers, role models, and support for individuals' development and health. Systems within the social environment, including family, peers, schools, community (including the Internet-based community), and the larger society, all contribute uniquely to an adolescent's development and health.

Relationships With Parents

During adolescence, the parent-child relationship changes from one of protection-dependency to one of mutual affection and equality. The process of achieving independence often involves turmoil and ambiguity as both parent and adolescent learn to play new roles and work toward establishing the ultimate relationship.

As teenagers assert their rights for grown-up privileges, they frequently create tensions within the home. They resist parental control, and conflicts can arise from almost any situation or any subject. Favorite topics of dispute include Internet and cell phone use, manners, dress, chores, homework, friendships, dating, money, automobiles, and time schedules. Adolescents' earliest attempts to achieve emancipation from parental controls are manifested in a period of rejection of the parents. They absent themselves from home and family activities and spend increasing time with the peer group. They confide less in their parents, but parents continue to play an important role in their personal and health-related decision making.

With advancing adolescence, teenagers become more competent and with this competence comes a need for more autonomy. Although they may be psychologically prepared for independence, they are often thwarted in their efforts by lack of money or other parental barriers. Conflict arises in relation to the teenagers' outside activities and the elements of privacy and trust. Parental monitoring remains important throughout adolescence and may have a direct influence on adolescent sexual and substance-use behavior. Parents should be guided toward an authoritative style of parenting in which authority is used to guide the adolescent while allowing developmentally appropriate levels of freedom and providing clear, consistent messages regarding expectations. However, to gain the trust of adolescents, parents must respect their adolescent's privacy and show an honest and sincere interest in what the adolescent believes and feels (see Family-Centered Care box: Communication With Adolescents: The Art of Listening).

Over the past several decades, changes have taken place within the family microsystem that have important implications for adolescent health. Changes in family structure and parent employment have resulted in adolescents having more time unsupervised by adults and increased time alone or with pers. Decreased adult supervision may result in more risk-taking behaviors, such as substance use and sexual intercourse, and decreased opportunities to develop a supportive relationship with parents. Adolescents who feel close to their parents show more positive psychosocial development and behavioral competence, less susceptibility to negative peer pressure, and lower tendencies to be involved in risk-taking behaviors (Smith, Stewart, Poon, et al., 2014).

Relationships With Peers

For the majority of teenagers, peers assume a more significant role in adolescence than they did during childhood. The peer group serves as a strong support to teenagers, individually and collectively, providing them with a sense of belonging and a feeling of strength and power.

FAMILY-CENTERED CARE

Communication With Adolescents: The Art of Listening

Conflicts between parents and their adolescents are often a result of a natural characteristic of parenthood: the desire to protect one's offspring from harm or from simply doing something "stupid" or embarrassing or something they may later regret. Teens sometimes "bounce" their thoughts and ideas off adults. At times, they really want some feedback; at other times, they simply want to elicit a reaction.

I found it easy to listen openly, thoughtfully, and without interrupting when my teenagers' friends discussed troublesome topics. However, one day, when one of my own teenagers had a similar conversation with me, the parent part kicked in. I felt responsible and spoke my piece on the spot. This brought communication to a halt and resulted in defensiveness. It was a long time before my child tried to talk to me about anything controversial again.

The next time one of my teenagers started a similar conversation, I decided to try to trick myself. Throughout the entire conversation, I told myself over and over again to act as if this were not my teenager but, rather, someone else's child. I found this actually worked quite well, and I was able to listen without interrupting. I continued to use the system, sometimes with more success than at other times.

Mother of Four

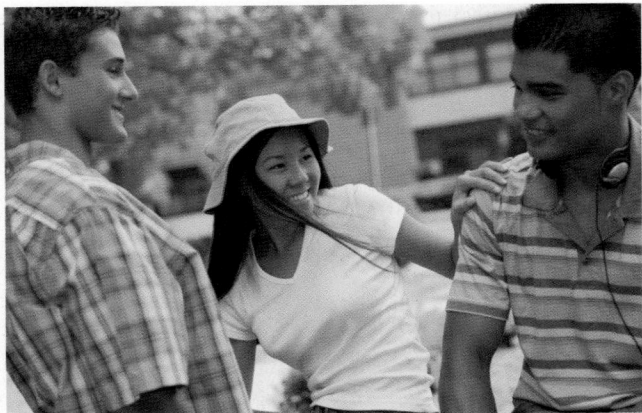

FIG 35.5 Teenagers like to gather in small groups. (Copyright 2011 by Photos.com, a division of Getty Images. All rights reserved.)

The peer group forms the transitional world between dependence and autonomy.

Adolescents are usually social, gregarious, and group-minded. Thus, the peer group has an intense influence on adolescents' self-evaluation and behavior. To gain acceptance by a group, younger adolescents tend to conform completely in such things as mode of dress, hairstyle, taste in music, and vocabulary. Peers can also be a positive force in health promotion by encouraging healthy behaviors, serving as role models, and promoting positive health norms. Adolescents use the peer group as a standard measure of what is normal.

School

In contemporary society, schools play an increasingly important role in preparing young people for adulthood. Schooling is essential for a successful future. Failure to complete high school reduces employment opportunities and the probability of earning an adequate income.

The school is psychologically important to adolescents as a focus of social life. Teenagers usually distribute themselves into a relatively predictable social hierarchy. They know to which groups they and others belong. A sense of school connectedness and optimal social connectedness is associated with positive outcomes for school completion, positive mood, and decreased high-risk behavior in adolescents (Chapman, Buckley, Reveruzzi, et al., 2014). School connectedness is correlated with caring teachers and the absence of prejudice or discrimination from peers. Within the larger groups are smaller, distinct, and rather exclusive crowds or cliques of selected close friends who are emotionally attached to each other. The selection is based on common interests, and background. Although cliques may become formalized, most remain informal and small. However, each has an identifying feature that proclaims its difference from others and its solidarity within itself, in much the same manner as the adolescent generation as a whole sets itself apart from the adult generation. Cliques are usually made up of one gender, and girls tend to be more cliquish than boys and to have a greater need for close friendships (Fig. 35.5). Within the intimacy of the group, adolescents gain support in learning about themselves,

consideration for the feelings of others, and increased ego development and self-reliance. To belong is of utmost importance; thus, adolescents behave in a way that will ensure their establishment in a group. Adolescents are highly susceptible to social approval, acceptance, and demands. To be ignored or criticized by peers creates feelings of inferiority, inadequacy, and incompetence.

Work

For the majority of young people in the United States, the workplace becomes another microsystem. Most adolescents are employed in an array of jobs as restaurant workers, cashiers, sales clerks, clerical assistants, and unskilled laborers. The jobs tend to require little initiative or decision making and rarely use skills learned in school. Adolescent work may negatively affect development as it fails to link adolescents to vocational mentors; is not intellectually stimulating; may take time away from other activities that could contribute to identity development; and can lead to fatigue, decreased interest in school, and poorer grades. These detrimental effects are likely to affect adolescents who work more than 20 hours per week.

Interests and Activities

Adolescents spend a large amount of time engaging in leisure-time activities. As teenagers progress through the developmental stages of adolescence, these leisure-time activities move from being family centered to being peer centered. In addition to providing teenagers with fun and enjoyment, leisure-time activities assist in the development of social, physical, and cognitive skills. Leisure-time activities also allow teenagers the opportunity to learn to set priorities and structure their time (Fig. 35.6).

The role of social media and advanced technology are nowhere more prominent than in the lives of today's adolescents. The widespread availability of the Internet and access to social networking websites such as Facebook, Snapchat, Instagram, e-mail, blogs, and Twitter have created "virtual" communities and ways for young people to interact with others; web cameras even allow those interactions to include real-time video communication. Cellular phones offer more mobile opportunities to talk on the phone, send text messages or instant messaging, send photos, or use video phone capabilities.

Social networking websites have created a more public arena for trying out identities and developing interpersonal skills with a wider network of people, occasionally with anonymity. This can create opportunities for young people who have a limited access to friends (because of rural location, shyness, or rare chronic conditions) to interact

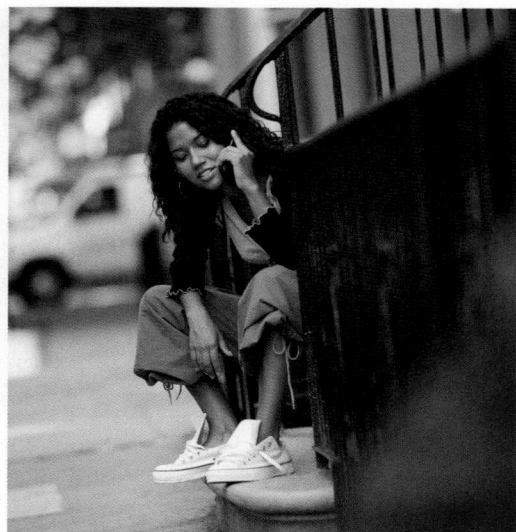

FIG 35.6 The cell phone allows adolescents to talk for hours with peers. (Copyright 2011 by Photos.com, a division of Getty Images. All rights reserved.)

CLINICAL REASONING CASE STUDY

Respecting Privacy

Jamie, a 17-year-old girl, arrives at the adolescent clinic with her mother, Mrs. S, for a routine history and physical examination with the nurse practitioner. As the nurse practitioner walks with Jamie to an examination room, Mrs. S whispers to the nurse practitioner, "I need to speak with you in private." How should the nurse practitioner respond to Mrs. S's request?

1. Evidence—Is there sufficient evidence to formulate a response to Mrs. S?
2. Assumptions—Describe an underlying assumption about each of the following topics:
   a. The role of the adolescent in health care
   b. The role of the parents in the health of their adolescent
   c. Adolescents and confidentiality
3. What implications for nursing care should be established at this time?
4. Does the evidence objectively support your argument (conclusion)?

with people like themselves. However, most adolescents appear to be using the online social environment to interact with the same peers that they spend their day with at school.

Text messaging has become a common activity and can sometimes be disruptive. In addition, both the online and text environment can create opportunities for cyberbullying, in which teens engage in insults, harassment, and publicly humiliating statements online or on cell phones.

Studies have noted that adolescents are not only enthusiastic technology users, but they frequently use multiple types of media at the same time. It is unclear how this multitasking and multiple media exposure will affect development of the brain and attention, but frequent media use has been associated with late nights and sleep deprivation (Owens & Adolescent Sleep Working Group Committee on Adolescence, 2014).

PROMOTING OPTIMAL HEALTH DURING ADOLESCENCE

For adolescents, health promotion involves helping youth acquire the power (including knowledge, attitudes, and skills), authority (permission to use their power), and opportunities to make choices that increase the likelihood of positive expressions of health for themselves. Adolescence provides an opportunity for teenagers to incorporate healthy lifestyle behaviors that will benefit them not only during the teenage years but also throughout the life span.

The rationale for focusing on health issues becomes obvious when one examines the major sources of mortality and morbidity during adolescence. The leading causes of mortality during adolescence in the United States are motor vehicle crashes, other accidental injuries, homicide, and suicide, which together are responsible for approximately 75% of all adolescent deaths (Blum & Qureshi, 2011; Eaton, et al., 2012). The sources of morbidity in adolescence include injury (primarily motor vehicle related), depression, eating disorders, substance use, sexually transmitted infections (STIs), and pregnancy; obesity may begin in childhood or adolescence, with secondary health consequences becoming evident in adolescence.

Effective health promotion for adolescents should incorporate a developmentally appropriate, multifaceted approach and incorporate

adolescents' perspectives on what health means. One strategy for health promotion used by nurses and other professionals in health care settings is the one-on-one health screening. Through a health screening interview, the health care professional can identify both assets and threats to an adolescent's health and well-being, and provides an opportunity to build a trusting relationship with the adolescent. As adolescents develop, they are able to assume additional responsibility for their own health, including maintaining health practices, taking prescribed medications, keeping appointments, and performing procedures when necessary. Health care professionals who work with adolescents should consider the adolescent's increasing independence and responsibility while maintaining privacy and ensuring confidentiality (see Guidelines box: Interviewing Adolescents and Clinical Reasoning Case Study: Respecting Privacy). Parents should also respect their teenager's independence and move toward the role of consultant about health issues while also maintaining some level of parental involvement throughout adolescence.

Several professional organizations have published guidelines aimed at improving and maintaining health care for adolescents and young adults. The American Academy of Pediatrics, American Academy of Family Physicians, American Medical Association, and US Preventive

Services Task Force have similar guidelines for health supervision of adolescents. These guidelines emphasize the need to provide health services to adolescents that meet their physical and emotional needs. They place great importance on the provision of health care by health care providers who are trained in meeting the adolescents' needs. Bright Futures (American Academy of Pediatrics, 2016) emphasizes that the following issues be addressed with adolescents over the course of multiple visits:

- Emotional well-being (coping, mood regulation, mental health, sexuality)
- Physical growth and development (physical and dental health, body image, healthy nutrition, physical activity)
- Social and academic competence (relationships with peers and family, school performance, interpersonal relationships)
- Risk reduction (tobacco, alcohol, other drugs, pregnancy, STIs)
- Violence and injury prevention (safety belt and helmet use, substance abuse and riding in a vehicle, guns, interpersonal violence, bullying)

Some practical suggestions for addressing the adolescent's individual health care needs are found in the following mnemonic*:

H—Home environment, belonging, decision making
E—Education/employment
E—Eating/nutrition
A—Activities, physical activities
D—Drugs (including smoking and alcohol use)
S—Sexuality
S—Suicide/depression
S—Safety

The following discussion of adolescent health will focus on some of the topics from this mnemonic as well as the Bright Futures topics listed earlier; other adolescent health issues are discussed later in this chapter.

EMOTIONAL WELL-BEING

Adolescents vacillate in their emotional states between considerable maturity and childlike behavior. One minute they are exuberant and enthusiastic; the next minute they are depressed and withdrawn. Unpredictable but essentially normal mood swings are common during this time. As the tension is relieved, emotion is brought under control and individuals retreat to review what has happened, to attempt to master their anger, and to increase their ability to control their emotions and gain from the new experience. Because of these mood swings, adolescents are frequently labeled as unstable, inconsistent, and unpredictable. Little things can cause an emotional upheaval and, depending on the teenager's interpretation, can mean a great deal.

Teenagers are better able to control their emotions in later adolescence. They can approach problems more calmly and rationally, and although they are still subject to periods of sadness, their feelings are less vulnerable, and they begin to demonstrate more mature emotions. Whereas early adolescents react immediately and emotionally, older adolescents can control their emotions until socially acceptable times and places for expression present themselves. They are still subject to heightened emotion, and when it is expressed, their behavior reflects feelings of insecurity, tension, and indecision.

As sources of credible information, support, and encouragement, nurses can help adolescents cope with the changes and challenges they face. To promote both emotional health and psychosocial adjustment, nurses and other health care professionals can encourage adolescents to develop (1) skills to cope with stress and change and (2) skills to become involved in personally meaningful activities.

NUTRITION

The rapid and extensive increase in height, weight, muscle mass, and sexual maturity of adolescence is accompanied by increased nutritional requirements. Because nutritional needs are closely related to the increase in body mass, the peak requirements occur in the years of maximum growth, during which the body mass almost doubles. The caloric and protein requirements during this time are higher than at almost any other time of life. As a result of this increased anabolic need, the adolescent is highly sensitive to caloric restrictions.

Current guidelines for caloric intake are provided by a number of sources. The Dietary Reference Intakes (DRIs) provide age-specific guidelines for nutrients (see Chapter 29). The 2015–2020 Dietary Guidelines for Americans* recommend specific caloric intakes for adolescents based on their levels of activity (sedentary, moderately active, and active) as well as recommendations to choose nutrient-dense foods and beverages across all food groups, limit calories from added sugars and saturated fats, and reduce sodium intake. MyPlate† is a scheme for eating a balanced diet of the five main food groups—fruits, grains, protein, vegetables, and dairy products. Adolescents usually have sufficient intake of protein to meet their needs except for those who limit their food intake because of economic problems or in an attempt to lose weight. There is a substantial increase in the need for the minerals such as *calcium, iron,* and *zinc* and vitamins during periods of rapid growth: calcium for skeletal growth, iron for expansion of muscle mass and blood volume, and zinc for the generation of both skeletal and bone tissue. The estimated average requirement (EAR) for calcium in adolescents 14 to 18 years of age is 1300 mg (Institute of Medicine, 2011). Calcium intake from food sources and supplements is essential during adolescence to assist in the prevention of osteoporosis. Eventual bone mass is a balance between the amount of bone laid down during adolescence and the amount later lost with aging. Overall, osteoporosis is a result of polygenic and multiple environmental factors such as nutrition, exercise, and chronic illness (Ma & Gordon, 2012). Girls with heavy or frequent menses may be especially susceptible to iron deficiency resulting from blood loss. Inadequate intake of certain vitamins (folic acid, vitamin B$_6$, vitamin A) is also evident, particularly among teenagers of low socioeconomic status. In combination with other factors, these dietary patterns could result in increased risk for obesity and chronic diseases such as heart disease, osteoporosis, and some types of cancer later in life. Dietary intervention should promote the regular consumption of breakfast and a balanced intake of a variety of foods.

Dietary Habits, Eating Disorders, and Obesity

Eating and attitudes toward food are primarily family centered during early and middle childhood, and food habits are largely related to cultural and individual family preferences and patterns. With adolescence and the move toward independence, family influences on the child diminish. Children's interests, attitudes, and routines are altered as an increasing number of meals are eaten away from home. These changes are largely a result of the high value that teenagers place on peer acceptability and sociability. Their peers easily influence their eating habits.

---

*From Duncan P, Pirretti AE: Bright futures for the busy clinical practice. American Academy of Pediatrics. *Adolescent Health Update, 22*(1), 1–10, 2009; Goldenring JM, & Rosen DS: Getting into adolescent heads: An essential update. *Contemporary Pediatrics, 21,* 64–90, 2004.

*Dietary Guidelines for Americans, http://health.gov/dietaryguidelines/2015/guidelines/.
†MyPlate, www.choosemyplate.gov.

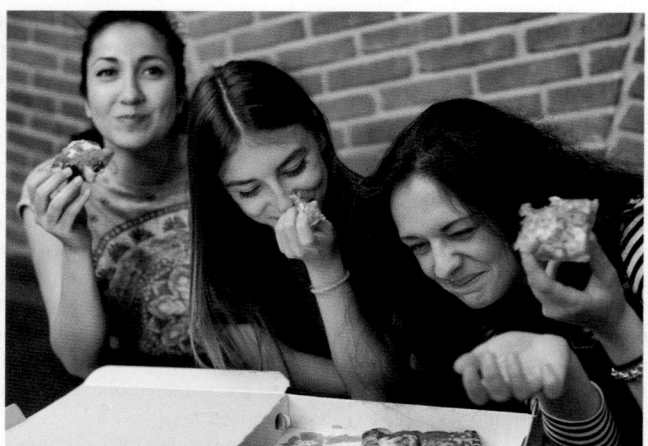

FIG 35.7 Snacking on empty calories is common among adolescents, especially during inactivity. (Copyright 2015 by iStock.com.)

Pressure for time and commitments to activities adversely affect teenagers' eating habits. Omitting breakfast or eating a breakfast that is nutritionally poor in quality is frequently a problem. Snacks, usually selected on the basis of accessibility rather than nutritional merit, become increasingly a part of the habitual eating pattern during adolescence (Fig. 35.7). Excess intake of calories, sugar, fat, cholesterol, and sodium is common among adolescents and is found in all income and racial or ethnic groups and both genders. Overeating or undereating during adolescence presents special problems. When they experience the normal increase in weight and fat deposition of the growth spurt, teenage girls often resort to dieting. The desire for a slim figure and a fear of becoming "fat" prompt teenage girls to embark on nutritionally inadequate reducing regimens that drain their energy and deprive their growing bodies of essential nutrients. They resort to diets on their own or with peers in an effort to conform. Many adopt current fad diets and are victims of food misinformation. Boys are less inclined to undereat. They are more concerned about gaining size and strength. However, they tend to eat foods high in calories but low in other essential nutrients.

Obesity is increasing among both children and adolescents in the United States. Poor dietary habits and increasingly sedentary lifestyles have caused this obesity epidemic. Currently 21% of children 2 to 19 years of age are obese (Centers for Disease Control and Prevention [CDC], 2015). The vast majority (90%) of obese adolescents remain obese into their 30s: 94% of women overall and 88% of men (Gordon-Larsen, The, & Adair, 2010).

Health problems traditionally thought of as adult comorbidities of obesity, including type 2 diabetes mellitus, obstructive sleep apnea, and nonalcoholic steatohepatitis, are occurring in adolescents. Routine nutrition screening for all adolescents should include questions about meal patterns, dieting behaviors, consumption of high-fat and high-salt foods, and recent changes in weight. Discuss healthy dietary habits with all adolescents, including the benefits of a healthy diet; ways to consume foods rich in calcium, iron, and other vitamins and minerals; and safe weight management. Lifestyle changes necessary for adolescents to lose weight require the involvement of family members who provide support and encourage active participation.

PHYSICAL FITNESS

Although today's youth are less fit than children 20 years ago, adolescents probably spend more time and energy practicing and participating in sports activities than members of any other age group. In 2011, nearly one half (49.5%) of all high school students reported that they participated in activities that made them "sweat and breathe hard for at least 20 minutes" three or more times in the past week (Eaton, et al., 2012). School-based, health-oriented physical education may provide both immediate effects of the activity and sustained effects through encouragement of lifelong activity patterns. Participation in school physical education classes declines with age, because schools often do not have mandatory requirements past grade 9 or 10. To improve health outcomes, the US Department of Health and Human Services recommended that school-age children and adolescents engage in a minimum of 60 minutes of moderate to vigorous physical activity daily and muscle-strengthening activity at least 3 days per week (Song, Carroll, & Fulton, 2013).

The practice of sports, games, and even dancing contributes significantly to growth and development, the education process, and better health. These activities provide exercise for growing muscles, interactions with peers, and a socially acceptable means of enjoying stimulation and conflict. In addition, competitive activities help teenagers in the process of self-appraisal and the development of self-respect and concern for others. Because physical fitness appears to be a major influence on one's lifelong health status, children should be encouraged to participate in activities that contribute to lifelong physical fitness. However, adolescents should not be encouraged to engage in physical activities that are beyond their physical or emotional capacity. Nurses can encourage participation as a way to promote health and build self-esteem.

HYPERTENSION

As adolescents experience sexual maturation, along with increases in height and weight, blood pressure increases from the onset of adolescence and continues to rise until the end of pubertal growth. This trend is especially apparent among males. Approximately 1% of adolescents have sustained hypertension, which is defined as a blood pressure greater than the 95th percentile of standards. The detection of hypertension during adolescence is important because hypertension is one of the major preventable risk factors for adult cardiovascular disease. With increasing levels of obesity, there have been reports of increasing incidence of hypertension among adolescents (Gurnani, Birken, & Hamilton, 2015). Screening for hypertension and associated risk factors should take place annually beginning at 3 years of age. Specific guidelines for monitoring and treatment of hypertension in adolescents are found in the 2011 National Heart Lung Blood Institute summary report (see Chapter 42).

HYPERLIPIDEMIA

Along with hypertension, smoking, and obesity, elevated serum cholesterol and triglyceride levels are major risk factors for the development of adult cardiovascular disease.

The National Heart Lung Blood Institute (2011) issued a recommendation for universal lipid (nonfasting or fasting) screening of all children and adolescents between 9 and 11 years of age and again between 17 and 21 years of age. Low-density lipoprotein (LDL) cholesterol–lowering drug therapy is recommended for children and adolescents 10 years of age and older whose LDL remains elevated after 6 months to 1 year on a restricted-fat diet, lifestyle modification (exercise), and weight management (National Heart Lung Blood Institute, 2011). Additional information and practice guidelines for monitoring cholesterol levels and initiation of LDL cholesterol–lowering medication as well as specific dietary modifications are found in the 2011 National Heart Lung Blood Institute summary report at http://www.nhlbi.nih.gov/health-pro/guidelines/current/cardiovascular-health-pediatric-guidelines/summary.

IMMUNIZATIONS

An immunization update is an important part of adolescent preventive care. Obtaining a record of the teenager's prior immunizations is important. The Tdap (tetanus, diphtheria, acellular pertussis) vaccine is recommended for adolescents 11 to 18 years of age who have not received a tetanus booster (Td) or Tdap dose and have completed the childhood DTaP/DTP series. When the Tdap is used as a booster dose, it may be administered earlier than the previous 5-year interval to provide adequate pertussis immunity (regardless of interval from the last Td dose) (CDC, 2016). Meningococcal vaccine (MenACWY-D [Menactra] or MenACWY-CRM [Menveo]) should be given to adolescents 11 to 12 years of age with a booster dose at 16 years of age. If not previously vaccinated, they should receive 1 dose between 13 and 18 years of age (CDC, 2016) (see the "Immunizations" section in Chapter 31).

The quadrivalent human papillomavirus (HPV) vaccine or the bivalent HPV vaccine is recommended for the prevention of cervical precancers and cancers for girls beginning at a minimum of 9 years of age. The HPV (Gardasil or Gardasil 9) vaccine is recommended for males 11 to 12 years of age but can be given at a minimum of 9 years of age (CDC, 2016). Each one of the HPV vaccines is administered in a three-dose series; it is important to follow the recommended dose intervals for optimal effectiveness.

All adolescents who have not previously received three doses of hepatitis B vaccine should be vaccinated against hepatitis B virus. The hepatitis A vaccine should be given to adolescents who live in areas where vaccination programs target older children or who are at increased risk for infection or for whom immunity against hepatitis A is desired (CDC, 2016). Annual influenza vaccination with either the live attenuated influenza vaccine or inactivated influenza vaccine is recommended for all children and adolescents. All adolescents should also be assessed for previous history of varicella infection or vaccination. Vaccination with the varicella vaccine is recommended for those with no previous history; for those with no previous infection or history, the varicella vaccine may be given in two doses 3 months apart to children 7 to 12 years of age and 4 weeks apart to adolescents 13 years of age and older (CDC, 2016). Adolescents should receive a tuberculin skin test if they have been exposed to active tuberculosis (TB), have lived in a homeless shelter, have been incarcerated, have lived in or come from an area with a high prevalence of TB, or currently work in a health care setting.

SLEEP AND REST

The changing social environment of adolescents can often change their sleep patterns at a time when their growth and development require additional sleep for health. Although adolescents should generally get around 9 hours of sleep each night, early morning school scheduling, extracurricular activities, homework, employment, and social time with peers can make it difficult to get sufficient sleep. Sleep deprivation can affect physical and mental health and has been associated with higher rates of overweight and obesity, depression, somatic complaints (e.g., headaches and stomachaches), fatigue, and difficulties with concentration. These physical and psychologic effects of inadequate sleep can also affect school performance and thus contribute to school problems. Health teaching and health promotion should include information to promote sufficient sleep.

DENTAL HEALTH

Dental health should not be neglected during adolescence, although the rate of caries formation is not as great as in childhood. Dental care is an aspect of preventive care that is not received by substantial proportions of children in the United States. It is recommended that an evaluation for caries takes place at a minimum of every year and optimally at 6-month intervals. Pit and fissure sealants are a safe and effective technique for dental caries prevention. Early adolescence is usually when corrective orthodontic appliances are worn, and these are frequently a source of embarrassment and concern to teens. Reassurance regarding the temporary nature of the annoyance and anticipation of an improved appearance help adolescents tolerate the inconvenience. It is also important to reinforce the orthodontist's directions regarding use and care of the appliances and to emphasize careful attention to toothbrushing during this time. During late adolescence, the third molars (wisdom teeth) should be evaluated to determine appropriate management (American Academy of Pediatric Dentistry, 2012).

PERSONAL CARE

Body-conscious teenagers are highly amenable to discussion and counseling about personal care and hygiene. Body changes associated with puberty bring special needs for cleanliness. The hyperactive sebaceous glands and newly functioning apocrine glands make frequent bathing or showering a necessity, and underarm deodorants assume an important place in personal care. Adolescents discover that hair requires more frequent shampooing, and girls often have questions about hair removal, use of cosmetics, and menstrual hygiene. Peer-group discussions center on the advantages of particular products or methods. Adolescents are continually bombarded with messages from the media regarding the best way to enhance their popularity and attractiveness. Nurses are in a position to help them evaluate the relative merits of commercial products.

POSTURE

Many adolescents demonstrate altered posture. Rapid skeletal growth is often associated with slower muscular growth, and as a result, some teenagers may appear awkward or slump and fail to stand or sit upright. However, some postural defects of adolescence require early medical intervention. Scoliosis is a defect of the spine that occurs frequently in adolescence and is more common in girls than in boys (see the "Idiopathic Scoliosis" section in Chapter 48). The majority of cases are idiopathic, and the defect manifests as a painless curvature of the spine. Fortunately, most of these spinal curvatures will not require treatment. However, because there is no way to predict which curvatures will progress, all curvatures of the spine should be referred for further evaluation.

BODY ART

Body art (piercing and tattooing) is an aspect of adolescent identity formation. The skin has become the latest source of parent-adolescent conflict. Adolescents often seek body art as an expression of their personal identity and style. Tattoos may mark significant life events such as new relationships, births, and deaths. Piercing the ear, nose, nipple, eyebrow, labia, navel, penis, or tongue may sometimes create a health problem. It is a nursing responsibility to caution girls and boys against having piercing performed by friends, parents, or themselves. Although in most cases piercings have few, if any, serious side effects, there is always a risk for complications such as infection, cyst or keloid formation, bleeding, dermatitis, or metal allergy. Using the same unsterilized needle to pierce body parts of multiple teenagers presents the same risk for human immunodeficiency virus (HIV), hepatitis C virus, and hepatitis B virus transmission as occurs with other needle-sharing activities.

A qualified operator using proper sterile technique should perform the procedure. This is especially important if an adolescent has a history of diabetes, allergies, or skin disorders. Adolescents should be informed about the approximate time for healing after body piercing and the care of the pierced area during and after healing. Some body sites need extra precautions. For example, cartilage (ear, nose) has a poor blood supply and heals slowly and scars easily; nipple piercing puts adolescents at risk for breast abscesses. Finally, migration of the piercing is common with naval and other flat skin surface piercing. Piercing guns should not be used for piercing anything other than the earlobe because guns place the piercing too deeply.

The presence of body art in the form of tattoos and branding is common among adolescents and young adults. Professionals as well as amateur artists administer tattoos. The risk to adolescents receiving tattoos is low. The greatest risk is for the tattoo artist, who comes in contact with the client's blood. Adolescents who are amateur tattoo artists benefit from discussions about Standard Precautions and the hepatitis B vaccination. Many states either have no regulations or do not enforce existing regulations of piercing and tattooing facilities. The local health department is a source of information about local regulatory requirements. The CDC has an excellent website that outlines safety concerns for people performing and receiving body art (http://www.cdc.gov/niosh/topics/body_art/).

TANNING

The quest for an attractive appearance leads many teenagers to excessive sunbathing and artificial means for tanning. However, this practice has serious long-term risks, and adolescents should be educated regarding the detrimental effects of sunlight on the skin (see discussion on sunburn in the "Burns" section in Chapter 32). Long-term effects include premature aging of the skin; increased risk for skin cancer; and, in susceptible individuals, phototoxic reactions.

The increasing popularity of artificial tanning has prompted concern from health care professionals regarding the use of sunlamps and tanning machines. The long-term effects of tanning machines are similar to those of the sun; dermatologists do not recommend tanning by this means. Those who insist on using tanning equipment should be warned that goggles must be worn in tanning booths to prevent serious corneal burning. Education on the use of sunscreens, including hypoallergenic products, with a sun protective factor (SPF) of at least 15 and a non-alcohol base without lanolin, parabens, or fragrance, is important. Broad-spectrum sunscreens that protect against both ultraviolet A and ultraviolet B (UVA and UVB) are the most effective. Self-tanning creams safely simulate the appearance of a tan; however, teens using these products should be cautioned that sun protection is still required. Targeting health education messages to adolescents and incorporating educational components relating to sun protection behaviors in school health curricula and in health care visits will increase adolescents' knowledge and awareness.

STRESS REDUCTION

The multiple changes occurring in adolescence can result in great stress (Fig. 35.8 and Box 35.3). Adolescents are faced with pressures from peers that often involve taking serious health risks, including pressures for sexual experimentation; use of drugs, alcohol, and cigarettes; and potentially dangerous physical activities.

Early-maturing girls and late-maturing children are especially sensitive to the stresses of being different from their peers. Many feel intense anxiety over their identity. Both early- and late-maturing children feel out of place among their classmates, but slow-maturing children appear

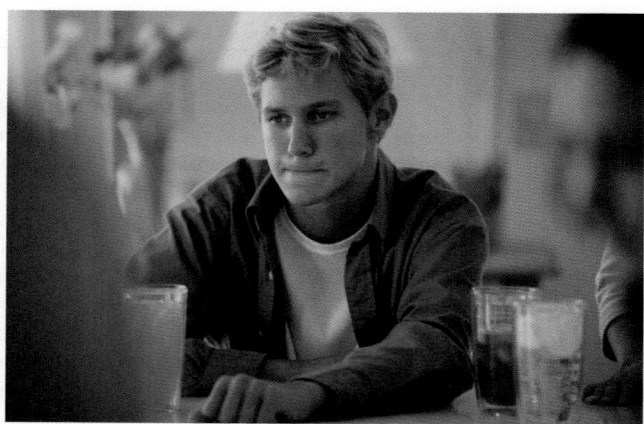

FIG 35.8 Adolescents use being alone as a method of coping with stress. Health care professionals need to assess whether this indicates clinical depression. (Copyright 2011 by Photos.com, a division of Getty Images. All rights reserved.)

BOX 35.3   Areas of Stress in Adolescence

- Body image
- Sexuality conflicts
- Academic pressures
- Competitive pressures
- Relationships with parents
- Relationships with siblings
- Relationships with peers
- Finances
- Decisions about present and future roles
- Career planning
- Ideologic conflicts

---

to experience the most pronounced inner turmoil and may be hesitant to voice their concerns. Slow-maturing adolescents need support and reassurance that they are not abnormal and need only be patient until the time comes when they, too, will mature physically.

SCHOOL AND LEARNING PROBLEMS

In 2011, 7% of American youth between 16 and 24 years of age old dropped out before completing high school (Davis & Bauman, 2013). Among in-school adolescents, a low grade point average has been associated with higher levels of emotional distress; cigarette, alcohol, and marijuana use; and earlier onset of sexual activity. School problems and dropping out of school can be markers for difficulties, such as learning disabilities, language barriers, family problems, lack of supportive relationships at school, and employment needs. In contemporary American society, education is critical to economic self-sufficiency. Adolescents who drop out of high school can expect to earn approximately $400,000 less over a lifetime than those who graduate (Center for Labor Market Studies, 2011).

Questions about recent grades, school absences, suspensions, and any history of repeating a grade in school can be used to screen for school-related problems. Specific management plans for youth who note school problems should be coordinated with school personnel and with the adolescent's parents or caregivers if possible.

SEXUALITY EDUCATION AND GUIDANCE

The average American teenager spends more than 11 hours every day in front of some type of medium (American Academy of Pediatrics, 2013). This potentially exposes them to unrealistic information and images, usually without adult supervision or interaction. In addition, social media use is a routine part of contemporary adolescents' daily lives, and there are many positive benefits including enhancing communication, social connection, and computer skills. However, there is increased danger of adolescents coming in contact and sharing personal information with sexual predators who pose as adolescents in an attempt to make personal contact with underage victims or engage them in sexting (sending sexually explicit or suggestive pictures or messages online) (Alexander, 2015). Adolescent sexting, rather than being an innocent anonymous activity, has been linked to risky sexual behaviors (Van Ouytsel, Walrave, Ponnet, et al., 2015).

The responsibility for providing sexuality education has been assumed by parents; schools; churches; community agencies such as Planned Parenthood Federation of America, Inc.;* and health care professionals, especially nurses. Many adolescents perceive nurses, especially school nurses, as individuals who possess important information and who are willing to discuss sex with them. To be able to discuss the topic adequately, nurses must have not only an understanding of the physiologic aspects of sexuality and a knowledge of cultural and societal values but also an awareness of their own attitudes, feelings, and biases about sexuality.

Comprehensive information about sexuality education is offered by the Sexuality Information and Education Council of the United States (SIECUS)† and the Sex Information and Education Council of Canada.‡ The SIECUS maintains that every sexuality education program should present the topic from six aspects, including biologic, social, health, personal adjustments and attitudes, interpersonal associations, and the establishment of values.

Sexuality education should consist of instruction concerning normal body functions and should be presented in a straightforward manner using correct terminology. When discussing sex and sexual activities, nurses should use simple but correct language—not street language, highly scientific terminology, or evasive jargon. After they understand the meaning of biologic terms such as uterus, testicles, and vagina, most teenagers prefer to use them in their discussions.

Teenagers need to discuss intercourse, alternative methods of sexual satisfaction, and how to resist peer pressure. With the increased incidence of sexually transmitted infections, the topic of "safe sex," especially abstinence or the use of condoms, is essential. Role-playing can help teenagers learn effective approaches to dealing with difficult situations. Sex and sexuality cannot be taught without discussions of mature decision making, sexual responsibility, and values clarification. Accurate and unbiased information regarding sexual practices should be provided in a setting wherein the adolescent feels comfortable asking questions without being degraded or made to feel uncomfortable for seeking information.

SAFETY PROMOTION AND INJURY PREVENTION

Injuries kill more adolescents in the United States than any other single cause, with unintentional injury accounting for 48% of deaths among

*434 West 33rd Street, New York, NY 10001; 800-230-PLAN (7526); www.plannedparenthood.org.
†90 John Street, Suite 402, New York, NY 10038; 212-819-9770; www.siecus.org.
‡850 Coxwell Avenue, Toronto, Ontario M4C 5R1; 416-466-5304; www.sieccan.org.

teens 12 to 19 years of age between 1996 and 2005 (Blum & Qureshi, 2011). Motor vehicle crashes are the single greatest source of unintentional injury and death in young people. Many factors contribute to the higher rate of crashes among teen drivers, including the lack of driving experience and maturity, driving too fast, using alcohol, and using cell phones to talk or text. Homicide, a form of intentional injury, is the second leading cause of death among all adolescents in the United States (CDC, 2012). Homicides among adolescents mostly involve firearms; many adolescents report easy access to a gun.

During adolescence, peak physical, sensory, and psychomotor function give teenagers a feeling of strength and confidence that they have never experienced before. One manifestation of this is an increase in energy that simply must be discharged through action, often at the expense of logical thinking and other control mechanisms. Their propensity for risk-taking behavior plus feelings of indestructibility make adolescents especially prone to injuries. Some of the developmental characteristics of teenagers and injury prevention suggestions are outlined in Box 35.4.

Motor Vehicle–Related Injuries

Adolescents' newly acquired ability to drive and the normal developmental need for independence and freedom make automobiles an attractive part of their lives. Motor vehicle crashes are the single greatest source of unintentional injury and death in young people in the United States. Many factors contribute to the higher rate of crashes among young drivers, including lacking driving experience and maturity, following too closely, driving too fast, having other teen passengers in the car, texting or answering a cell phone while driving, and driving under the influence of alcohol.

There has been recent attention on distracted teenage driving and cell phone talking or texting while driving. A recent survey found that 90% of college students use their cell phone to talk while driving, 50% text while on a freeway, 60% text in stop-and-go traffic, and 87% text at traffic lights (Hill, Rybar, Styer, et al., 2015). Many states have outlawed the use of handheld mobile devices while actively operating a vehicle, and all-driver texting bans have significantly lowered the odds of texting while driving (Qiao & Bell, 2016).

Nurses should educate teenagers and their parents about the risk of driving while drinking alcohol or of riding in an automobile with a drunk driver. Many families arrange a no-questions-asked ride home to prevent an adolescent from riding with a drunk driver. Families should also require adolescents to log several hours of supervised practice driving before taking the car out alone. Educational efforts should also discuss that the major risk for death in a motor vehicle accident is failure to use a safety restraint.

Other Vehicle Injuries

The increasing use of motorcycles, all-terrain vehicles, jet skis, and snowmobiles has caused an increase in injuries among young people who are below the legal age for driving automobiles. Many adolescents ride bicycles without helmets and without lights at night, and the overwhelming majority of deaths from bicycle injuries (primarily head injuries) involve teenagers. In-line skating and skateboarding without protective gear also contribute to a significant number of traumatic brain injuries in US adolescents and young people.

Firearms

Firearms are a major cause of intentional fatal injuries in the United States. Adolescence is the peak age for being either a victim or an offender in an injury involving a firearm. Gun carrying among adolescents is on the rise and is not limited to the stereotypic inner-city youth. Family members and acquaintances are a common source of guns for young people. Gun availability in the home is strongly linked to unintentional

BOX 35.4   Injury Prevention During Adolescence

Developmental Abilities Related to Risk for Injury
- Need for independence and freedom
- Testing independence
- Age permitted to drive a motor vehicle (varies from state to state)
- Inclination for risk-taking behaviors
- Feeling of indestructibility
- Need for discharging energy, often at expense of logical thinking and other control mechanisms
- Strong need for peer approval
- Attempting hazardous feats
- Peak incidence for practice and participation in sports
- Access to more complex tools, objects, and locations
- Can assume responsibility for own actions

Injury Prevention
Pedestrian
Emphasize and encourage safe pedestrian behavior:
- Use cross-walks.
- At night, walk with a friend.
- If someone is following you, go to nearest public place with people.
- Do not walk in secluded areas; take well-traveled walkways.

Motor or Nonmotor Vehicles
- Passenger—Promote appropriate behavior while riding in a motor vehicle. Refuse to ride with an impaired person or one who is driving recklessly.
- Driver—Provide competent driver education; encourage judicious use of vehicle; discourage drag racing or "playing chicken"; discourage text messaging; maintain vehicle in proper condition (e.g., brakes, tires).
- Teach and promote safety and maintenance of two- and three-wheeled vehicles.
- Promote and encourage wearing of safety apparel, such as helmet and long trousers.
- Discourage distractions while driving (e.g., cell phone talking or texting, eating, smoking, or reading).

Falls
- Teach and encourage general safety measures in all activities.

Submersion Injury
- Teach nonswimmer to swim.
- Teach basic rules of water safety:
  - Judicious selection of place to swim
  - Sufficient water depth for diving
  - Swimming with companion
  - Wearing life vest with water sports (e.g., boating, skiing)
  - Avoiding swimming, boating, or other water sports after or during alcohol consumption

Burns
- Reinforce proper behavior in areas involving contact with burn hazards (gasoline, electric wires, and fires).
- Advise regarding excessive exposure to natural or artificial sunlight (ultraviolet burn).
- Discourage smoking.
- Encourage use of sunscreen.

Poisoning
- Educate in hazards of drug use, including alcohol.

Bodily Damage
- Promote acquisition of proper instruction in sports and use of sports equipment.
- Instruct in safe use of and respect for firearms and other devices with potential danger (e.g., power tools, fireworks).
- Provide and encourage use of protective equipment when using potentially hazardous devices.
- Promote access to and/or provision of safe sports and recreational facilities.
- Be alert for signs of depression (potential suicide).
- Instruct regarding proper use of corrective devices (e.g., glasses, contact lenses, hearing aids).
- Encourage and foster judicious application of safety principles and prevention.

---

death and injury to children (Crossen, Lewis, & Hoffman, 2015). In addition, the presence of a gun in the home increases the risk for adolescent suicide and homicide. All families should be assessed for the presence of a gun in the home and informed of this risk. They must take preventive action to ensure that the guns are never loaded, that guns are locked up in a safe place, and that ammunition is stored and locked up separately in a location accessible only to appropriate adults.

Care Management

With continued increases in the numbers of adolescents in the United States and rising rates of health-related problems of youth, there is an unprecedented need for adolescent health promotion. Nursing professionals can make significant contributions to health promotion among adolescents and their families. Because nurses understand the biologic, cognitive, psychosocial, and social transitions of adolescence and their impact of health behavior, they can address adolescents' developmental and health needs. Working with colleagues from other disciplines, community members, parents, and adolescents themselves, nurses must become part of a comprehensive approach that delivers consistent messages across clinical, school, and community-based settings. Nurses

should be at the forefront of developing and disseminating culturally appropriate health-promotion interventions.

Both adolescents and their parents are often confused and perplexed about the changes and behavior of this stage of development. Parents need support and guidance to help them through this trying time. They need to understand the changes taking place and to accept the expected behaviors that accompany the process of detachment. Parents may need help to "let go" and to promote the changed relationship from one of dependence to one of mutuality. Suggestions for anticipatory guidance of parents of adolescents are listed in the Family-Centered Care box: Parent Strategies for Adolescent Support.

SPECIAL HEALTH PROBLEMS

DISORDERS OF THE FEMALE REPRODUCTIVE SYSTEM

Disorders related to the female reproductive system such as amenorrhea and dysmenorrhea are discussed in Chapter 4. Sexually transmitted infections are also discussed in Chapter 4.

FAMILY-CENTERED CARE
Parent Strategies for Adolescent Support

Encourage parents to do the following:
- Accept adolescent as a unique individual.
- Respect adolescent's ideas, likes and dislikes, and wishes
- Be involved with school functions, and attend adolescent's performances, whether it be a sporting event or a school play.
- Listen and try to be open to adolescent's views, even when they disagree with parental views.
- Avoid criticism about no-win topics.
- Provide opportunity for choosing options, and accept natural consequences of these choices.
- Allow young person to learn by doing, even when choices and methods differ from those of adults.
- Provide adolescent with clear, reasonable limits.
- Clarify house rules and consequences for breaking them. Let society's rules and consequences teach responsibility outside the home.
- Allow increasing independence within limitations of safety and well-being.
- Be available, but avoid pressing adolescent too far.
- Respect adolescent's privacy.
- Share adolescent's feelings of joy or sorrow.
- Respond to feelings, as well as words.
- Be available to answer questions, give information, and provide companionship.
- Make communication clear.
- Avoid comparisons with siblings.
- Assist adolescent in selecting appropriate career goals and preparing for adult role.
- Welcome adolescent's friends into the home, and treat them with respect.
- Provide unconditional love.
- Be willing to apologize when mistaken.

Be aware that adolescents:
- Are subject to turbulent, unpredictable behavior
- Are struggling for independence
- Are extremely sensitive to feelings and behavior that affect them
- May receive a different message from what was sent
- Consider friends extremely important
- Have a strong need to belong to a peer group of friends and not necessarily to family (except in certain circumstances)

DISORDERS OF THE MALE REPRODUCTIVE SYSTEM

Many obvious anomalies, such as hypospadias, hydrocele, phimosis, and cryptorchidism, are identified with corrective measures instituted during infancy or early childhood. Uncircumcised males may encounter problems related to a tight foreskin that cannot be retracted (phimosis) and are at a higher risk for infections, such as balanitis and prostatitis. The most frequent problems related to the reproductive organs in later childhood are as follows:
- Infections, such as urethritis (see the "Urinary Tract Infection" section in Chapter 45) or epididymitis
- Hematuria
- Penile problems, such as drug-induced priapism, carcinoma, and trauma
- Scrotal conditions, such as varicocele (elongation, dilation, and tortuosity of the veins superior to the testicle)

CLINICAL REASONING CASE STUDY
Testicular Self-Examination

At a recent faculty meeting, Paul, the pediatric nurse practitioner who runs the school-based health clinic, presented his plan for a class on testicular self-examination (TSE) to be delivered to the sophomore boys. Several teachers questioned the value of providing such a class when there is limited time to deliver content relating to "routine academic subjects." What important issues regarding testicular cancer and TSE should Paul use to justify providing this class to the sophomore boys?
1. Evidence—Is there sufficient evidence to justify teaching sophomore boys about TSE?
2. Assumptions—Describe the underlying assumption about each of the following:
   a. Detection of testicular cancers in adolescence
   b. Usual presenting symptom of testicular cancer
   c. Knowledge of genital anatomy among adolescent boys
   d. Ways to teach adolescent boys about their anatomy
3. What priorities and implications for nursing care can be drawn at this time?
4. Does the evidence objectively support your argument (conclusion)?

- Testicular torsion (a condition in which the testicle hangs free from its vascular structures, which can result in partial or complete venous occlusion with rotation)

Care Management

Adolescent boys are also self-conscious about their changing bodies and need preparation for a genital examination. The most successful approach is to assume a matter-of-fact attitude toward the examination, explain precisely what will take place, and maintain a continuous commentary about what is being done and the findings at each phase of the examination.

The routine health assessment of every adolescent boy should include teaching about testicular cancer and how to perform a testicular self-examination (TSE) every month. This rare malignancy is curable if detected early. Nurses are in an ideal position to teach TSE in a manner that is respectful of the adolescent boy's anxieties and that promotes early treatment (see Clinical Reasoning Case Study: Testicular Self-Examination).

In the TSE, each testicle is examined individually, preferably after a warm bath or shower when scrotal skin is more relaxed, using the thumbs and fingers of both hands and applying a small amount of firm, gentle pressure. The normal testicle is a firm organ with a smooth, egg-shaped contour; the epididymis is palpated as a raised swelling on the superior aspect of the testicle and should not be taken for an abnormality.

GYNECOMASTIA

Male breasts, although not strictly part of the male reproductive system, respond to hormonal changes. Some degree of bilateral or unilateral breast enlargement occurs frequently in boys during puberty. Approximately half of adolescent boys have transient gynecomastia, usually lasting less than 1 year, which subsides spontaneously with achievement of male development. A careful assessment of the pubertal stage at the onset of gynecomastia; medication history, including anabolic steroids; and the exclusion of renal, liver, thyroid, and endocrine disorders or dysfunction allow the examiner to reassure the adolescent that the changes are pubertal gynecomastia and that no further assessment is indicated. Gynecomastia may also be drug induced; calcium channel blockers, cancer chemotherapeutic agents, histamine$_2$-receptor antagonists, and oral ketoconazole medications have all been shown to cause the condition.

Care Management

Treatment of gynecomastia usually consists of assurance to the adolescent and his parents that this is a benign and temporary situation. A physical examination with palpation is necessary to differentiate gynecomastia from increased adiposity caused by being overweight. Adolescents who are distressed about physical integrity and masculinity may benefit from the knowledge that this condition occurs in more than 50% of all adolescent boys.

NUTRITIONAL AND EATING DISORDERS

OBESITY

Few problems in childhood and adolescence are so obvious to others, are so difficult to treat, and have such long-term effects on health as obesity. Several different definitions have been proposed for obesity and overweight. Obesity has been defined as an increase in body weight resulting from an excessive accumulation of body fat relative to lean body mass. Overweight refers to the state of weighing more than average for height and body build. Currently, the body mass index (BMI) measurement is recommended as the most accurate method for screening children and adolescents for obesity. It is highly specific for children with the greatest amount of body fat. Pediatric growth charts that include BMI for age and sex are available from the CDC.* Children with a BMI between the 85th and 95th percentiles are considered overweight, and obesity is defined by a BMI greater than or equal to the 95th percentile (Ogden, Carroll, Kit, et al., 2012). It is important to note that for children with high levels of muscle mass (e.g., athletes), the BMI measurement may misclassify these youth into overweight/obesity classifications. Clinical judgment is needed to understand if these youth are at risk for obesity.

Regardless of the definition used, the number of overweight children in the United States has reportedly reached epidemic status (Ogden, Carroll, Kit, et al., 2012). Approximately 12.7 million children are overweight or obese (CDC, 2014). Numerous studies dating back to the early 1960s have documented childhood overweight through comprehensive evaluations of dietary intake, physical activity, and anthropometric measures (CDC using the various National Health and Nutrition Examination Surveys [NHANES], I, II, III, and IV) (Ogden, Carroll, Kit, et al., 2012; Ogden, Carroll, & Flegal, 2008; Ogden, Kuczmarski, Flegal, et al., 2002; Ogden, Troiano, Briefel, et al., 1997). In the 1960s and 1970s, childhood overweight remained fairly constant at approximately 4% to 5.5%; however, surveys during the 1990s and early 2000s demonstrated a steady climb to reach 17% in both children and adolescents (Ogden, Carroll, Kit, et al., 2012; Flegal, Carroll, Kit, et al., 2012). This prevalence remains stable since 2003 but overall, the incidence remains high (Ogden, Carroll, Kit, et al., 2014). African-American and Hispanic children and youth are disproportionately represented by a higher prevalence of overweight/obesity (35% and 39%, respectively) compared with non-Hispanic white children (28.5%) (Ogden, Carroll, Kit, et al., 2012).

Because adult obesity is associated with increased mortality and morbidity from a variety of complications, both physical and psychologic, adolescent obesity is a serious condition. The probability that overweight school-age children will become obese adults is significant. In a large longitudinal study, overweight kindergartners were four times more likely to become obese by 14 years of age than normal weight kindergartners (Cunningham, Kramer, & Narayan, 2014). Furthermore, overweight adolescents are at risk for continuing to be obese as adults, thereby experiencing several health and social consequences (Van Cleave, Gortmaker, & Perrin, 2010).

Obesity in childhood and adolescence has been related to elevated blood cholesterol, high blood pressure, respiratory disorders, orthopedic conditions, cholelithiasis, some types of adult-onset cancer, nonalcoholic fatty liver disease (NAFLD), and type 2 diabetes mellitus. The incidence of metabolic syndrome was 30% in obese children (Kiess, Kratzsch, Sergeyev, et al., 2014). Common emotional consequences of obesity include low self-esteem, social isolation, anxiety, depression, and an increased risk for the development of eating disorders (Altman & Wilfley, 2015).

Etiology and Pathophysiology

Obesity results from a caloric intake that consistently exceeds caloric requirements and expenditure and may involve a variety of interrelated influences, including metabolic, hypothalamic, hereditary, social, cultural, and psychologic factors (Fig. 35.9). Because the etiology of obesity is multifactorial, the treatment requires multilevel interventions.

A balance between energy intake and energy expenditure is a critical factor in regulating body weight. For example, eating one small chocolate chip cookie (50 calories) is equivalent to walking briskly for 10 minutes. Factors that raise energy intake or decrease energy expenditure by even small amounts can have a long-term impact on the development of overweight and obesity. Physical inactivity has also been identified as

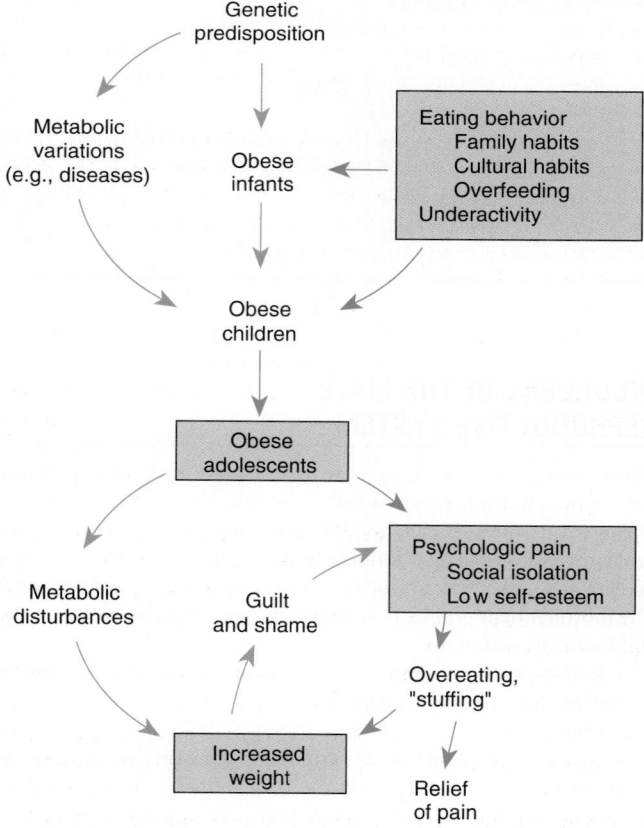

FIG 35.9 Complex relationships in obesity.

an important contributing factor in the development and maintenance of childhood overweight. There is little doubt that physical activity has decreased in elementary and secondary schools in the United States, and most of children's physical activity must occur within the family or outside of school. Decreased physical activity within the family is a powerful influence on children because children imitate their parents and other adults.

The growing attraction and availability of many sedentary activities, including television, video games, social media, and the Internet, have also greatly influenced the amount of time that children spend participating in sedentary behaviors. Studies have shown the association between screen time and obesity among children (De Jong, Visscher, Hirasing, et al., 2013; Thorn, DeLellis, Chandler, et al., 2013). A policy by the American Academy of Pediatrics (2013) encourages parents to limit total entertainment screen time in children to 2 hours or less per day. Genetic influence is an epidemiologic consideration in regard to children's weight. Genetic mutations, such as *FTO* (fat mass and obesity) and *INSIG2* (insulin-induced gene 2) are rare but can predispose individuals to becoming overweight or obese (Gahagan, 2016). Studies have also suggested a tendency for a combination of genetic and environmental factors. Parental BMI is a more potent predictor of obesity than genetics, suggesting that behaviors and environment play a greater role in obesity (Morandi, Meyre, Lobbens, et al., 2012). The increasing rates of obesity within genetically stable populations suggest that environmental and some perinatal factors (e.g., bottle feeding), and possible intrauterine factors (e.g., maternal gestational weight gain and stress) are contributors to the current increases in childhood obesity (Li, Magadia, Fein, et al., 2012). More research is needed to better understand the influences of family behavior and adolescent overweight.

Fewer than 5% of the cases of childhood obesity can be attributed to an underlying disease. Such diseases include hypothyroidism; adrenal hypercorticoidism; hyperinsulinism; and dysfunction or damage to the central nervous system as a result of tumor, injury, infection, or vascular accident. Obesity is a frequent complication of muscular dystrophy, paraplegia, Down syndrome, spina bifida, and other chronic illnesses that limit mobility.

There is little evidence to support a relationship between obesity and low metabolism. Small differences may exist in regulation of dietary intake or metabolic rate between obese and non-obese children that could lead to an energy imbalance and inappropriate weight gain, but these small differences are difficult to accurately quantify. Obese children tend to be less active than lean children, but it is uncertain whether inactivity creates the obesity or obesity is responsible for the inactivity. The tendency toward obesity is manifested whenever environmental conditions are favorable toward excessive caloric intake, such as an abundance of food, limited access to low-fat foods, reduced or minimum physical activity, and snacking combined with excessive screen time (computer, television, video games, cell phone). Family and cultural eating patterns, as well as psychologic factors, play important roles; many families and cultures consider fat to be an indication of good health. It is common for obese children to have families that emphasize large meals, admonish children for leaving food on their plates, or use food as a reward or punishment. Parents may have an exaggerated concept of the amount of food children require and expect them to eat more than they need.

Disparities in obesity rates exist among racial/ethnic minorities, immigrant and refugee communities, and socioeconomic status, with differences often becoming apparent before 6 years of age. Lower socioeconomic groups have a greater prevalence of obesity, especially in girls. Youth immigrating to the United States tend to have lower initial weight statuses, but on a population level, immigrant youth have higher BMIs than their native-born counterparts after one generation

of living in the United States. This is particularly true for Hispanic immigrants (Singh & Yu, 2012).

Some community factors that influence eating and activity patterns include a lack of built environment (food deserts, community gardens, farmers markets, sidewalks, parks, bike paths) or affordable and accessible facilities for low-income youth to be active, thus limiting their opportunities to participate in physical activities or healthful eating. Social policies also contribute to obesity. The increased availability of high-fat foods, pricing strategies that promote unhealthy food choices, and overzealous food advertising that targets children and adolescents with high-fat and high-sugar foods are some examples (Schwartz & Ustjanauskas, 2012).

Institutional factors also influence patterns of obesity and decreased physical activity. Many school policies allow students to leave school for lunch. Vending machines in school often are filled with high-fat and high-calorie foods and soft drinks. Although well-balanced, nutritious school lunches may be available to students, they often opt for less nutritious choices such as high-fat and high-sugar snacks.

Psychologic factors also affect eating patterns. In infancy, children experience relief from discomfort through feeding and learn to associate eating with a sense of well-being, security, and the comforting presence of a nurturing person. Eating is soon associated with the feeling of being loved. Many parents use food as a positive reward for desired behaviors. This practice may become a habit, and the child may continue to use food as a reward, a comfort, and a means of dealing with depression or hostility. Many individuals eat when they are not hungry or in response to boredom, loneliness, sadness, depression, or tiredness. Difficulty in determining feelings of satiety can lead to weight problems and may compound the factor of eating in response to emotional rather than physical hunger cues.

Frequency of family meals has consistently been shown to be a protective factor for obesity (Flattum, Draxten, Horning, et al., 2015). Family meals tend to provide access to a variety of nutrient-rich foods, particularly fruits and vegetables. This is also a time when parents can model healthy behaviors. Parental modeling of eating and physical activity and food availability in the home are predictors of excess weight gain during childhood and adolescence (Tandon, Zhou, Sallis, et al., 2012).

Diagnostic Evaluation

A careful history is obtained regarding the development of obesity, and a physical examination is performed to differentiate simple obesity from increased fat that results from organic causes. A family history of obesity, diabetes, coronary heart disease, and dyslipidemia should be obtained for all children who are overweight or at risk for being overweight. Specific information from the patient and family about the effects of obesity on daily functioning—for example, problems with nighttime breathing and sleep, daytime sleepiness, joint pain, inability to keep up with family activities and peers at school—is helpful. The physical examination should focus on identifying comorbid conditions and identifiable causes of obesity. For some, psychologic assessment by interviews and standardized personality tests may provide insight into the personality and emotional problems that contribute to obesity and that might interfere with therapy.

It is useful to estimate the degree of obesity to determine the component of body weight that can be modified. All of the following methods have been used to assess obesity: BMI, body weight, weight-height ratios, weight-age ratios, hydrostatic (underwater) weight, skinfold measurements, dual-energy x-ray absorptiometry (DXA) scan, bioelectrical analysis, computed tomography, magnetic resonance imaging, and neutron activation. Each of these methods has advantages and disadvantages. Hydrostatic, or underwater, weighing provides the most accurate measurement of lean body weight.

Body mass index is currently considered the best method to assess weight in children and adolescents. The calculation is based on the individual's height and weight. In adults, BMI definitions are fixed measures without regard for sex and age. The BMI in children and adolescents varies to accommodate age- and gender-specific changes in growth. The formula for BMI calculation is as follows:

$$\text{Weight in pounds} \div (\text{Height in inches})^2 \times 703$$

OR

$$\text{Weight in kilograms} \div (\text{Height in meters})^2$$

BMI measures in children and adolescents are plotted on growth charts that enable heath care professionals to determine BMI for age for the patient.

The initial assessment of obese children and adolescents should include screening to evaluate for comorbidities. The history is an important guide to determine the workup. A complete physical examination is important. Some areas to focus on include (1) skin for stretch markings and discolorations (e.g., acanthosis nigricans), (2) joints for swelling and evidence of pain, and (3) airway for evidence of obstruction and enlarged tonsils. Basic laboratory studies include a fasting lipid panel; fasting insulin level; fasting glucose hepatic enzymes, including γ-glutamyltransferase (GGT); and in some institutions, hemoglobin A1c. Other studies, such as a sleep study, metabolic studies, and radiographic evaluations, may be added based on the history and physical examination. These assessments may determine whether the patient needs a referral to specialty services for more focused evaluation and treatment, such as endocrinology (insulin resistance, diabetes), hepatology (elevated liver enzymes, NAFLD), orthopedics (Blount disease), or pulmonary medicine (sleep-disordered breathing, continuous positive airway pressure).

Therapeutic Management

The best approach to the management of obesity is a preventive one. Early recognition and control measures are essential before the child or adolescent reaches an obese state. Health care providers must educate families about the medical complications of obesity, and families are encouraged to be involved in the treatment plan.

Currently, the only treatments recommended for children are diet, exercise, behavior modification, and in some situations pharmacologic agents, such as orlistat. The treatment of obesity is difficult. Many approaches do not achieve long-term success. The average individual loses only about 5% to 10% of his or her weight with available therapies. Losing weight can have a significant positive effect on many comorbidities, but unfortunately, the lost weight is frequently regained in 1 or 2 years.

Diet modification is an essential part of weight-reduction programs. Dietary counseling is directed toward improving the nutritional quality of the diet rather than toward dietary restriction. Children and adolescents should avoid fad diets. Most dietitians and nutrition experts recommend a diet with no trans fats, low-saturated fat, moderate total fat (≤30%), low sodium, and at least nine servings of fruits and vegetables daily, consistent with the MyPlate* food guide for children. Also, promoting high-fiber foods and avoiding highly refined starches and sugars decrease caloric intake. Many programs recommend using a food diary as a helpful tool to increase awareness of food choices and eating behaviors. The goal is to encourage the individual to make healthy choices in food selection and discourage eating food by habit or to appease boredom. Box 35.5 contains helpful suggestions.

*www.choosemyplate.gov/index.html.

BOX 35.5   Recommended Behaviors for Preventing Obesity

In counseling adolescents whose body mass index (BMI) is between the 5th and 84th percentiles, physicians and health care providers should recommend the following steps to prevent obesity:

- Limit or avoid consumption of sugar-sweetened beverages.
- Consume recommended quantities of fiber, fruits, and vegetables.
- Limit screen time to no more than 2 hours per day, and remove television and computers from primary sleeping areas.
- Encourage 60 minutes of moderate to vigorous physical activity daily.
- Eat breakfast daily.
- Limit eating at fast food restaurants.
- Have frequent family meals in which parents and youth eat together.
- Recognize appropriate child-size portions.

Adapted from Daniels, S.R., Hassink, S.G. & American Academy of Pediatrics, Committee on Nutrition. (2015). The role of the pediatrician in primary prevention of obesity. *Pediatrics, 135*(1), e275-e292.

In patients with severe obesity, strict diets have been used, such as the protein-sparing modified fast, a hypocaloric diet, or a ketogenic diet that is designed to provide enough protein to minimize loss of lean body mass during weight loss. Such diets need to be closely monitored and should be used only with multidisciplinary teams that include a physician, nutritionist, and behavioral therapist. Generally, the diet consists of 1.5 to 2.5 g of protein per kilogram. The intake of carbohydrates is low enough to induce ketosis. The benefits of the diet are relatively rapid weight loss and anorexia induced by ketosis. Potential complications include protein losses, hypokalemia, hypoglycemia, inadequate calcium intake, orthostatic hypotension, and increased risk for osteoporosis. It is difficult to sustain such diets over the long term, and the long-term outcomes of using these diets have not been established.

Researchers continue searching for medications that will successfully treat obesity. Orlistat, a lipase inhibitor, has been approved for use in children 12 years of age and older; however, side effects of the drug include fatty or oily stools and possible malabsorption of fat-soluble vitamins (Kanekar & Sharma, 2010). There are currently no drugs approved for use in overweight or obese children younger than 12 years of age. Behavior modification approaches to weight loss are based on the observation that obese individuals have abnormal eating practices that can be altered. Attention is focused not on food but on the social and behavioral aspects surrounding food consumption. Combining behavior modification with pharmacologic therapy in children 12 years of age and older have produced mixed results referent to total weight loss maintained over a significant period of time (Barton & US Preventive Services Task Force, 2010). Programs including family-based behavior modification, dietary modification, and exercise have been shown to be successful in reducing obesity in some children (Altman & Wilfley, 2015).

Surgical techniques (bariatric surgery) that bypass portions of the intestine or occlude a segment of the stomach to produce a marked diet restriction and weight loss are hazardous and cause many metabolic complications. These complications include severe water and electrolyte depletion, persistent diarrhea, vitamin deficiency, internal herniation, and fatty infiltration and degeneration of the liver. Bariatric surgery may be the only practical alternative for increasing numbers of severely overweight adolescents who have failed organized attempts to lose or maintain weight loss through conventional nonoperative approaches and who have serious life-threatening conditions. Physicians must define clear, realistic, and restrictive guidelines to apply with younger patients when surgery is considered. Candidates for surgery should be referred to centers that offer a multidisciplinary team experienced in the management of childhood and adolescent obesity. The surgery should be performed by surgeons who have participated in subspecialty training in bariatric medical and surgical care as detailed by the American College of Surgeons and the American Society for Metabolic and Bariatric Surgery.

Care Management

Nurses play a key role in the adherence and maintenance phases of many weight-reduction programs. Nurses assess, manage, and evaluate the progress of many overweight adolescents. They also play an important role in recognizing potential weight problems and assisting parents and adolescents in preventing obesity.

The presence of obesity may not be obvious from appearance alone. Regular assessment of height and weight and computation of the BMI facilitate early recognition. Published guidelines and tools are available for childhood obesity prevention and treatment (Daniels, Hassink, & American Academy of Pediatrics, 2015; Avis, Komarnicki, Farmer, et al., 2016).

Before initiating a treatment plan, it is important to be certain that the family is ready for change. Lack of readiness may result in failure, frustration, and reluctance to address the problem in the future. The nurse should explore with adolescents the reasons behind the desire to lose weight because motivation to lose weight is the key to success. Adolescents need to take a personal responsibility for their dietary habits and physical activity. Young people who are forced by their parents to seek help are seldom motivated, become rebellious, and are unwilling to control their dietary intake.

Nutritional Counseling

Preventing an increase in body fat during growth is a realistic approach. This is often accomplished by adjusting four aspects of eating: (1) reducing the quantity eaten by purchasing, preparing, and serving smaller portions; (2) altering the quality consumed by substituting low-calorie, low-fat foods for high-calorie foods (especially for snacks); (3) eating regular meals and snacks, particularly breakfast; and (4) altering situations by severing associations between eating and other stimuli, such as eating while watching television. The most successful diets are those that use ordinary foods in controlled portions rather than diets that require the avoidance of specific foods. The emphasis of counseling should be on health outcomes, not weight. Studies have shown focusing on weight can be detrimental to therapies and may promote eating disorders (Altman & Wilfley, 2015).

Teach adolescents and parents how to incorporate favorite foods into their diet and to select satisfying substitutes. To maintain a healthy diet, it is necessary to encourage the consumption of high-nutrient foods such as fruits, vegetables, whole grains, and low-fat dairy protein products. Keep calories and fat to a healthy level without being significantly restricted. To be successful, a dietary program should be nutritionally sound with sufficient satiety value, produce the desired weight loss, and be accompanied by nutrition education and continued support. Children and adolescents should not initiate a reduction diet without health assessment and counseling. Davis and colleagues (2007) describe steps to approaching behavior change with youth (Box 35.6).

Behavioral Therapy

Altering eating behavior and eliminating inappropriate eating habits are essential to weight reduction, especially in maintaining long-term weight control. Most behavior modification programs include the following concepts:

- A description of the behavior to be controlled, such as eating habits
- Attempts to modify and control the stimuli that govern eating

---

BOX 35.6 Pediatric Obesity Prevention Protocol for Primary Care

Step 1: Assess
- Explain and conduct assessments of the following:
  - Weight, height, and body mass index percentile
  - Dietary intake (fruit, vegetables, sweetened beverages, and fast food)
  - Activity (screen time, moderate to vigorous activity)
  - Eating behaviors (breakfast, portion sizes, family meals)
- Provide and elicit feedback on body mass index and behaviors found to be inside and outside the optimal range.

Step 2: Set Agenda
- Explore interest in changing behaviors not in the optimal range.
- Agree on target behaviors with the patient and caregiver.

Step 3: Assess Motivation and Confidence
- With regard to interest in changing weight status or behaviors, assess the following:
  - Willingness
  - Perceived importance
  - Confidence in having success
- Probe the patient regarding ratings of willingness, perceived importance, and confidence to explore the advantages and disadvantages of changing.

Step 4: Summarize and Probe Possible Changes
- Summarize the advantages and disadvantages of change.
- Query possible next steps.
- Offer ideas for getting started in making a change as needed.
- Summarize the change plan.
- Provide positive feedback.

Step 5: Schedule Follow-Up Visit
- If a change plan is made, agree on a follow-up appointment within a specified number of weeks or months.
- If no change plan is made, agree to revisit the topic within a specific number of weeks or months.

Adapted from Davis, D.M., Gance-Cleveland, B., Hassink, S., et al. (2007). Recommendations for prevention of childhood obesity. *Pediatrics, 120*(suppl), S229–S253.

- Development of eating techniques designed to control speed of eating
- Positive reinforcement for these modifications through a suitable reward system that does not include food
- Creation of environments where the healthy choice is the easy choice

Box 35.5 includes specific strategies to modify eating habits.

Group Involvement

Commercial groups (e.g., Weight Watchers) and diet workshops composed primarily of adults may be helpful to some teenagers; however, a peer group is often more effective. Adolescent groups include summer camps designed for obese young people and conducted by health care professionals, school groups organized and led by a school nurse, and groups associated with special clinics.

These groups are concerned not only with weight loss but also with the development of a positive self-image and the encouragement of physical activity. Nutrition education, diet planning, and the improvement of social skills are essential components of these groups. Improvement is determined by positive changes in all aspects of behavior.

Family Involvement

There is a definite connection among family environment, interaction, and obesity. The nurse needs to educate parents in the purposes of the therapeutic measures and their role in management. The family needs nutrition education and counseling regarding the reinforcement plan, alterations in the food environment, and ways to maintain proper attitudes. They can support their child in efforts to change eating behaviors, food intake, and physical activity.

Physical Activity

The current recommendation for physical activity for children and adolescents is to participate in a combined total of 60 minutes of physical activity daily; this can be moderate to vigorous intensive exercise or activity (CDC, 2015). Regular physical activity is incorporated into all weight-reduction programs. Recommendations for physical activity need to consider the current health status and developmental level of the child or adolescent. The best choice for exercise is any form that is enjoyable and likely to be sustainable. Light exercises, such as walking, may provide an opportunity for the family to increase time together and increase caloric expenditure. Weight training can increase the basal metabolic rate and replace fat mass with muscle mass. However, weight training is not generally recommended for prepubertal children until they have reached physical and skeletal maturity. In prepubertal children, increasing outdoor playtime is likely to be beneficial. Limiting sedentary activities such as television viewing while eating snacks is very beneficial.

Prevention

Gradual accumulation of adipose tissue during childhood establishes a pattern of eating that is difficult to reverse in adolescence. Prevention of obesity should begin in early childhood with the development of healthy eating habits, regular exercise patterns, and a positive relationship between parents and children. Prevention of adolescent obesity is best accomplished by early identification of obesity in the preschool, school-age, and preadolescent periods. Health care professionals should encourage frequent health care visits for children who are overweight or obese and incorporate a dietary history and counseling into each well-infant, well-child, and well-adolescent visit.

ANOREXIA NERVOSA AND BULIMIA NERVOSA

Anorexia nervosa (AN) is an eating disorder characterized by a refusal to maintain a minimally normal body weight and by severe weight loss in the absence of obvious physical causes. It is a disorder with social, psychologic, behavioral, cultural, and physiologic components that result in significant morbidity and mortality. Individuals with AN are described as perfectionists, academically high achievers, conforming, and conscientious.

Bulimia (from the Greek meaning "ox hunger") refers to an eating disorder similar to AN. Bulimia nervosa (BN) is characterized by repeated episodes of binge eating followed by inappropriate compensatory behaviors, such as self-induced vomiting; misuse of laxatives, diuretics, or other medications; fasting; or excessive exercise (American Psychiatric Association, 2013). The binge behavior consists of secretive, frenzied consumption of large amounts of high-calorie (or "forbidden") foods during a brief time (usually about 2 hours). The binge is counteracted by a variety of weight-control methods (purging). These binge-purge cycles are followed by self-deprecating thoughts, a depressed mood, and an awareness that the eating pattern is abnormal. Although people with BN have many issues in common with those who have other eating disorders, impulse control and satiety regulation are important problems

in BN. Many individuals with BN begin with only occasional binges and purges "just for fun," enjoying the control over their weight while eating amounts of food that would normally produce obesity. As the condition progresses, the frequency of binges increases, the amount of food consumed increases, and they gradually lose control over the binge-purge cycle. The frequency of binging can be anywhere from once per week to 7 or 8 times per day. Because people with BN usually binge on high-calorie foods, especially sweets, ice cream, and pastries, insulin production is stimulated to cope with the added carbohydrates. When the food is vomited, the unused insulin stimulates hunger and the desire to eat.

A third eating disorder, identified as eating disorder not otherwise specified (EDNOS), has components of both AN and BN with varying degrees of symptomatology that are not always characteristic of the established diagnostic criteria for AN and BN. Binge eating disorder (BED) is a type of EDNOS. People with BED have recurrent episodes of eating large amounts of food in discrete periods of time with a feeling of loss of control over the situation (Lipsky & McGuinness, 2015).

The incidence of AN in adolescent females in the United States has been estimated at 0.5%, and between 1% and 5% meet the criteria for BN (Rosen, 2010). A nationally representative study found no differences in the prevalence of AN between adolescent boys and girls, but did find higher prevalences of BN among girls compared to boys (Swanson, Crow, Le Grange, et al., 2011). BED is more common among males (Smink, van Hoeken, & Hoek, 2012). People younger than 12 years of age are the fastest growing group of youth who report eating disorder tendencies (Funari, 2013).

Etiology and Pathophysiology

The etiology of these disorders remains unclear. A combination of genetic, neurochemical, psychodevelopmental, sociocultural, and environmental factors appear to cause the disorder (Stice, South, & Shaw, 2012). Dieting and body dissatisfaction appear to be common to the initiation of both AN and BN. Also characteristic is a childhood preoccupation with being thin reinforced by sociocultural and environmental factors, supporting the concepts of an ideal body shape. The dominant aspects of AN are a relentless pursuit of thinness and a fear of fatness, usually preceded by a period of mood disturbances and behavior changes.

Weight loss may be triggered by a typical adolescent crisis such as the onset of menstruation or a traumatic interpersonal incident that precipitates serious, out-of-control dieting. Situations of severe family stress (e.g., parental separation or divorce) or circumstances in which the adolescent perceives a lack of personal control (e.g., teasing at school, changing schools, or going to college) may precipitate a desire for control and the decision not to eat. Frequently, there is an exaggerated misinterpretation of the normal fat deposition characteristic of early adolescence or anxiety because of comments that the adolescent is putting on weight.

There are no strong empirical data to indicate that one particular family prototype is responsible for the development of an eating disorder. However, many experts have associated the development of an eating disorder with family characteristics such as an adolescent perception of high parental expectations for achievement and appearance, difficulty managing conflict and poor communication styles, enmeshment and occasionally estrangement among family members, devaluation of the mother or the maternal role, and marital tension. Families struggling with an eating disorder have been characterized as often having difficulties responding positively to the changing physical and emotional needs of the adolescent. Family stress of any kind may become a significant factor in the development of an eating disorder (Berge, Maclehose, Loth, et al., 2013).

Society's emphasis and the media's focus on tall, thin individuals may also play a role. Studies evaluating the possible association of eating disorders and sexual abuse have been conflicting. Childhood sexual abuse may be a factor in some cases of AN.

Individuals with eating disorders commonly have psychiatric problems, including affective disorder, anxiety disorder, obsessive-compulsive disorder (OCD), and personality disorder. Adult women with eating disorders were found to have higher rates of obsessive-compulsive behavior traits in their childhoods. Patients with eating disorders have also been found to have higher reported rates of substance abuse, with alcohol problems being more common in those with BN than AN (Wildes & Marcus, 2013). It is important to note that many of the clinical findings are directly related to the state of starvation and improve with weight gain. Research continues in an effort to better understand the etiology and pathogenesis of eating disorders.

Many sports and artistic endeavors that emphasize leanness (e.g., ballet and running) and sports in which the scoring is partly subjective (e.g., figure skating and gymnastics) or where weight class is prerequisite to participation (e.g., wrestling) have been associated with a higher incidence of eating disorders (Bratland-Sanda & Sundgot-Borgen, 2013). The term *female athlete triad*, characterized by an eating disorder, amenorrhea, and osteoporosis, has been applied to young women with restrictive eating disorders and amenorrhea (Deimel & Dunlap, 2012).

Diagnostic Evaluation

Diagnosis of AN is made on the basis of clinical manifestations (Box 35.7) and conformity to the criteria established by the American Psychiatric Association (2013). Characteristics of BN and AN are listed in Table 35.2.

A complete history and physical examination are important to rule out other causes of weight loss. The medical assessment of an eating disorder focuses on the complications of altered nutritional status and purging. A careful history assesses weight changes, dietary patterns, and the frequency and severity of purging and excessive exercise. Measure the patient's weight and height, and evaluate it for appropriateness according to standard weight for height, age, and sex determined according to the percentile of his or her expected body weight or BMI.

Particularly important parts of the physical examination are vital sign measurement (heart and blood pressure, both supine and standing, and temperature). Hypotension, bradycardia, and hypothermia are often seen in association with extremely low weight. Prolongation of the QT interval may be detected in some patients. Dry skin, lanugo, acrocyanosis, and breast atrophy are findings that have been associated with AN. Distinctive hand lesions (Russell sign) have been observed; the backs of the hands are often scarred and cut from repeated abrasion of the skin against the maxillary incisors during self-induced vomiting.

The diagnosis of eating disorder (ED) is made clinically, but additional laboratory diagnostic tests may be obtained to identify malnutrition or other associated complications. Laboratory assessment may include a complete blood count to evaluate for anemia and other hematologic abnormalities; erythrocyte sedimentation rate or C-reactive protein to detect evidence of inflammation; electrolytes as well as calcium, magnesium, phosphorus, blood urea nitrogen, and creatinine; and urinalysis, including specific gravity to detect water loading. In patients with prolonged amenorrhea, human chorionic gonadotropin is assessed to determine the presence of pregnancy. Other tests for patients with amenorrhea include thyroid function tests and measurement of serum prolactin and follicle-stimulating hormone to help rule out prolactinoma (hormone-secreting pituitary tumor), hyperthyroidism, hypothyroidism, or ovarian failure. In addition, a comprehensive cardiac evaluation is often recommended in those with AN. Further diagnostic tests may be required based on the history and findings from these diagnostic tests.

Screening Tools

All patients in high-risk categories for eating disorders should be screened during routine office visits. The medical history is most important for diagnosing eating disorders because the physical examination findings may be normal, especially early in the illness. A number of screening questionnaires are available to assist with the interview. For example, with the SCOFF questionnaire, 1 point is scored for every "yes." A score of 2 or more indicates a likely case of AN or BN. The questions related to the mnemonic SCOFF are (Trent, Moreira, Colwell, et al., 2013): (1) Do you make yourself *sick* because you feel uncomfortably full? (2) Do you worry that you have lost *control* over how much you eat? (3) Have you recently lost more than 6.4 kg (14 pounds or *one* stone) in a 3-month period? (4) Do you believe yourself to be *fat* when others say that you

---

BOX 35.7   Clinical Manifestations of Anorexia Nervosa

- Severe and profound weight loss
- Secondary amenorrhea (if menarche attained)
- Primary amenorrhea (if menarche not attained)
- Sinus bradycardia
- Lowered body temperature
- Hypotension
- Intolerance to cold
- Dry skin and brittle nails
- Appearance of lanugo hair
- Thinning hair
- Abdominal pain
- Bloating
- Constipation
- Fatigue
- Lightheadedness
- Evidence of muscle wasting (cachectic appearance)
- Bone pain with exercise

TABLE 35.2   Characteristics of Individuals With Eating Disorders

Factors	Anorexia Nervosa	Bulimia
Food	Turns away from food to cope	Turns to food to cope
Personality	Introverted	Extroverted
	Avoids intimacy	Seeks intimacy
	Negates feminine role	Aspires to feminine role
Behavior	"Model" child	Often acts out
	Obsessive-compulsive	Impulsive
School	High achiever	Variable school performance
Control	Maintains rigid control	Loses control
Body image	Body image distortion	Less frequent body image distortion
Health	Denies illness	Recognizes illness
		Health fluctuates
Weight	Body weight <85% of expected norm	Within 2.3 to 7 kg (5 to 15 lb) of normal body weight or may be overweight
Sexuality	Usually not sexually active	Often sexually active

are too thin? and (5) Do thoughts and *fears* about food and weight dominate your life?

Therapeutic Management

The treatment and management of AN involve three major goals: (1) reinstitution of normal nutrition or reversal of the severe state of malnutrition, (2) resolution of disturbed patterns of family interaction, and (3) individual psychotherapy to correct deficits and distortions in psychologic functioning. The treatment of eating disorders requires the cooperative efforts of an interdisciplinary team composed of a primary practitioner, nurse, dietitian, and mental health care provider with pediatric and adolescent health care experience. Because of the psychogenic nature of the disorder, the treatment may be long. Recent studies suggest that family-based therapy is more effective than individual cognitive behavioral therapy in reducing the maladaptive eating behaviors in adolescents with AN (Le Grange, Lock, Agras, et al., 2015).

Most adolescents are treated on an outpatient basis, but those with problems requiring immediate medical attention, such as severe malnutrition, electrolyte disturbances, vital sign abnormalities, or psychiatric disturbances (severe depression or suicidal ideation), may require hospitalization. People with BN may benefit from psychotherapy, antidepressant medications, or a combination of antidepressant medication and psychotherapy (Kreipe, 2016).

Nutrition Therapy

The most important goal is to treat any life-threatening malnutrition and to restore dietary stability and weight gain. This may require the administration of tube feedings or intravenous fluids if the malnutrition is severe. In most cases, it is best to reintroduce food and snacks slowly in a stepwise manner. A reasonable goal is to start caloric intake at 60% to 75% of estimated needs in undernourished patients (Agostino, Erdstein, & Di Meglio, 2013). When restoring nutrition, health care professionals must avoid the refeeding syndrome, which consists of cardiovascular, neurologic, and hematologic complications that occur when nutritional replacement is given too rapidly. This syndrome can be avoided with slow refeeding and the addition of phosphorus when total body phosphorus is depleted. Treatment goal weights are individualized and based on age, height, stage of puberty, premorbid weight, and previous growth charts. In young women who have reached menarche, resumption of menses is an objective measure of return to biologic health.

Dietary interventions are combined with behavioral therapy to improve the underlying psychologic misconceptions about weight loss. Another aspect of treatment is to relieve the anxiety related to eating and the depression that accompanies the disorder. Weight gain alone cannot be considered a cure for the disease and is an unreliable sign of progress. Relapses are frequent as the person may revert to previous eating patterns when removed from the therapeutic environment.

Cognitive Behavioral Therapy

Behavior modification, usually through cognitive behavioral therapy or motivational interviewing, has met varying degrees of success. The goal is to increase the patient's feelings of control and responsibility toward achieving recovery. Providing privileges or activities for weight gain or positive eating behaviors may be successful, but treatment should also address the conflict precipitating the disorder. Individual psychotherapy is aimed at helping the young person resolve the adolescent identity crisis, particularly as it relates to a distorted body image. If the disorder is related to a dysfunctional family situation, therapy is most successful when it is started soon after the onset of illness and directed toward disengagement and redirection of malfunctioning processes in the family.

Pharmacotherapy

Pharmacotherapy in the treatment of AN has been disappointing so far. Although some comorbidities have been shown to decrease, low recovery rates of the disorder are maintained (Flament, Bissada, & Spettigue, 2012). The few studies that have been done show a decrease of comorbid disorders such as OCD and depression. Anxiolytic medications may be helpful before meals to relieve some patients' anxiety.

Tricyclic antidepressants (TCAs) and fluoxetine belong to a group of medications known as *selective serotonin reuptake inhibitors (SSRIs)*, which have been more successful when used with BN. There is also some evidence that TCAs such as desipramine, imipramine, and amitriptyline; monoamine oxidase inhibitors; and buspirone are more effective compared with a placebo in decreasing binging and vomiting in patients with BN. Topiramate, an antiepileptic agent, and the selective serotonin antagonist *ondansetron* have demonstrated some benefit in treating patients with BN. The American Psychiatric Association's guidelines have discouraged using medication as the only therapy. Clearly more research is needed to clarify whether medications have a role in the treatment of eating disorders (Flament et al., 2012).

Psychotherapy

Psychotherapy is central to the treatment of eating disorders. Patients need to be active participants in the treatment process to better understand the impulses, feelings, and needs that have resulted in their eating disorder. The goal is to increase the patient's feelings of control and responsibility toward achieving recovery. Eating disorders are complex and multifaceted. If possible, treatment should match patients' readiness to change (Geller, Srikameswaran, Zelichowska, et al., 2012). It is important to treat eating disorder patients with respect and support preservation of their self-esteem to promote a successful recovery (Ozier & Henry, 2011).

Care Management

Nurses need to adopt and maintain a kind and supportive yet firm manner in managing the care of the adolescent with eating disorders without creating a passive-dependent attitude. The individual requires sustained support and reassurance to cope with ambivalent feelings related to body concept and the desire to be seen as cooperative, reliable, and worthy of receiving kindness. Encouraging the adolescent with education and activities that strengthen self-esteem facilitates the resocialization process and promotes social acceptance among peers.

It is important for nurses to be aware of the physical side effects of AN. Patients frequently limit their fluid intake. Urinary tract problems are common, and ketones and protein may be detected in the urine as a result of breakdown of fat and protein. Vital sign instability can be severe and can include orthostatic hypotension; the pulse becomes irregular, and the rate decreases markedly. Electrolyte imbalances can be life-threatening, and bradycardia and hypothermia can result in cardiac arrest (see Clinical Reasoning Case Study: Anorexia Nervosa).

Interprofessional Care Management of Anorexia Nervosa and Bulimia Nervosa

The team responsible for the management of young people with AN arranges a carefully structured environment. First, there must be consistency. The team decides on an approach and adheres to it. The plan is structured with reality testing regarding caloric intake and body image perception as an essential component. The team members provide a unified front to avoid any possibility of manipulation or inconsistency. Second, all team members are involved; responsibility for the program

CLINICAL REASONING CASE STUDY

Anorexia Nervosa

Jane is a 13-year-old girl whose grades have been excellent and whom the teachers describe as a "model student." Recently, Jane's teacher told the nurse practitioner that Jane's parents were in the middle of a "messy divorce." In addition, several of Jane's friends told the nurse practitioner that they are concerned about Jane because she runs every day at lunchtime and seldom eats lunch with them. Jane told her friends that she gained weight over the winter months and that she is running because she wants to qualify for the track team this spring. At the time of her routine health interview and sports physical examination, the nurse practitioner notes that Jane's oral temperature is 36° C (96.8° F) and that she weighs 34 kg (75 pounds). Jane has lost 9 kg (20 pounds) since her last sports physical. Jane tells the nurse practitioner that she has not had her menstrual period for 3 months.

1. Evidence—Is there sufficient evidence to draw any conclusions about Jane's behavior?
2. Assumptions—Describe some underlying assumptions about the following:
   a. Personality characteristics of individuals with anorexia nervosa (AN)
   b. Factors influencing the development of AN
   c. Clinical manifestations of AN
   d. Treatment of AN
3. What priorities for nursing care should be established for Jane at this time?
4. Does the evidence objectively support your argument (conclusion)?

cannot be left to one person. The role and boundaries of each member are clearly spelled out. Third, continuity of team members is important; it is helpful to have the same team members all the time. Fourth, communication among team members is essential. Communication with the patient regarding what is expected is also important. Fifth, the plan must provide for support of the adolescent, the family, and team members. The adolescent's efforts should be supported, and positive feedback should be provided for accomplishments made in normalizing eating habits. Meetings are held to discuss the feelings and concerns of the patient, immediate caregivers, and team members.

A behavioral contract, an agreement that the adolescent makes with others to change a maladaptive behavior, has proved to be effective in some cases. The written contract is constructed by the therapeutic team and approved and signed by the adolescent. Unless the adolescent agrees to its terms, the contract can become the source of a power struggle. However, it can be an effective tool that places the responsibility for weight gain or other behavioral change on the adolescent.

Family-based therapy is often used in the treatment of adolescent eating disorders. Encourage families to explore how it has become problematic to follow the normal developmental course of their family life cycle by looking at how the eating disorder and the interactional patterns in the family have become entangled.

Care of the adolescent with BN is similar to care of the patient with AN. Acute care involves careful monitoring of fluid and electrolyte alterations and observation for signs of cardiac complications. Nutritional consultation and follow-up care are essential. The adolescent and family members are encouraged to structure the environment to reduce the binging behavior. Avoiding and eliminating trigger foods that would result in binges; restricting eating to one room of the house; not engaging in other activities while eating; and substituting exercise, crafts, visualization, and relaxation techniques for binging are helpful interventions.

Patients and families can find assistance and information from several organizations. The National Association of Anorexia Nervosa and Associated Disorders* provides counseling, referral, and self-help programs for young people with AN. The National Eating Disorders Association† provides information and support services for both patients and families.

HEALTH PROBLEMS WITH A BEHAVIORAL COMPONENT

SUBSTANCE ABUSE

Although experimentation with drugs during childhood and adolescence is widespread, most children and teens do not become high-risk users. *Monitoring the Future* has been providing long-term research about the rates of substance use among adolescents, young adults, and adults since 1975 (Johnston, O'Malley, Miech, et al., 2016). The 2014 survey found that marijuana use and acceptance of marijuana use among 12th graders increased from 2006 to 2011 and then leveled from 2011 to 2013. Binge drinking (five or more alcoholic drinks at least once in the prior 2 weeks) has been on the decline since the early 1980s and reached historically low levels in 2014. Cigarette use was on a steady decline since the mid-1990s until 2004, which followed a leveling off through 2014. More teens used e-cigarettes in 2015 than any other tobacco product, with a prevalence of 16.2% among 12th graders (Johnston et al.). The use of illicit drugs other than marijuana has shown minimal change since 1992, with 21% of 12th graders in 2015 reporting use (Johnston et al.).

Drug abuse, misuse, and addiction are culturally defined and are voluntary behaviors. Drug tolerance and physical dependence are involuntary physiologic responses to the pharmacologic characteristics of drugs, such as opioids and alcohol. Consequently, an individual can be addicted to a narcotic with or without being physically dependent. A person can also be physically dependent on a narcotic without being addicted (e.g., patients who use opioids to control pain).

Motivation

Most drug use begins with experimentation. The drug may be used only once, may be used occasionally, or may become part of a drug-centered lifestyle. Children and adolescents initiate drug use out of curiosity. Adolescents who use drugs may fall into one of two broad categories—experimenters and compulsive users—or they may fall into a third category somewhere on the continuum between these extremes, referred to as *recreational users,* principally of drugs such as marijuana, cocaine, alcohol, and prescription drugs. For many, the goal is peer acceptance; these users fit more closely with the experimenting, intermittent users. For others, the goal is intoxication or the sustained intense effects from using a particular drug; these users resemble the compulsive users. These users may engage in periodic heavy use, or binges. The groups of greatest concern to health care workers are those whose patterns of use involve high doses or mixed drugs with the danger of overdose and compulsive users with the threat of dependence, withdrawal syndromes, and altered lifestyle.

Types of Drugs Abused

Any drug can be abused, and most are potentially harmful to adolescents still going through formative life experiences. Although rarely considered drugs by society, the chemically active substances frequently abused are

---

*Helpline 630-577-1330, available 9 AM to 5 PM Central, Monday through Friday; e-mail: anadhelp@anad.org; www.anad.org.
†603 Stewart Street, Suite 803, Seattle, WA 98101; 800-931-2237; www.nationaleatingdisorders.org/.

the xanthines and theobromines contained in chocolate, tea, coffee, and colas. Ethyl alcohol and nicotine are other drugs that are legal and socially sanctioned. Any of these substances can produce mild to moderate euphoric or stimulant effects and can lead to physical and psychologic dependence.

Drugs with mind-altering abilities that are available on the "street" and are of medical and legal concern are the hallucinogenic, narcotic, hypnotic, and stimulant drugs. In addition, health care professionals are concerned about the use of alcohol and volatile substances that are inhaled to achieve altered sensation (e.g., gasoline, antifreeze, plastic model airplane cement, organic solvents). Cough and cold preparations such as NyQuil, Coricidin, and Robitussin are common substances abused by adolescents and young adults. The abuse of prescription and synthetic drugs such as oxycodone, alprazolam (Xanax), dextromethorphan, and amphetamine-dextroamphetamine (Adderall) has been reported to have reached epidemic proportions among adolescents and young people (Maxwell, 2011). Many of the prescription drugs are available at a decreased cost compared with the more exotic drugs of abuse and are often found in the medicine or kitchen cabinet at home. Websites also promote the "safe use" of some psychoactive drugs and supply information on new "designer" drugs that are not detectable on a standard urine drug screening test.

Tobacco

Cigarette smoking has been on a slow decline since the peak in 1999 despite multiple efforts, including increased costs, changes in community attitudes about smoking among adults, media campaigns with counter-advertising, and tobacco-free environments. Use of all tobacco products among youth has not significantly changed between 2004 and 2015 (Johnston et al., 2016).

Cigarette smoking is still considered the chief avoidable cause of death. The hazards of smoking at any age are undisputed; however, a preventive approach to teenage smoking is especially important. Because of its addictive nature, smoking begun in childhood and adolescence can result in a lifetime habit, with increased morbidity and early mortality.

The effects of secondhand smoke exposure are also well known and include increased incidence of low birth weight and subsequent illness, increased incidence of sudden infant death syndrome (maternal smoking during and after pregnancy), increased incidence of lower respiratory tract infections and ear infections, exacerbation of asthma symptoms, sleep disturbances, and intellectual impairment (Homa, Neff, King, et al., 2015; Al-Sayed & Ibrahim, 2014).

Etiology. Teenagers begin smoking for a variety of reasons, including imitation of adult behavior; peer pressure; a desire to imitate behaviors and lifestyles portrayed in movies and advertisements; and a desire to control weight, especially among young women. Teenagers who do not smoke usually have family members and friends who do not smoke or who oppose smoking. Most teens who refrain from smoking have a desire to succeed in academics or athletics (particularly high-performance sports, such as basketball, swimming, and track) and plan to go to college (see Community Focus box: Early Sexual Maturation, Alcohol, and Cigarettes). Although smoking among college students has increased in recent years, rates of smoking are highest among adolescents who do not complete high school.

Smokeless tobacco. The term *smokeless tobacco* refers to tobacco products that are placed in the mouth but not ignited (e.g., snuff and chewing tobacco). This substitute for cigarettes continues to pose a hazard to adolescents, although use had steadily declined by about 50% since the peak prevalence in 1995. Children and adolescents continue to recognize the risk of smokeless tobacco and have expressed high rates of disapproval (Johnston et al., 2016). These products have also

COMMUNITY FOCUS
Early Sexual Maturation, Alcohol, and Cigarettes

Smoking cigarettes and drinking alcohol among adolescents are complex behaviors that are not explained by any one factor. Some theorists and investigators believe there is a relationship between biologic maturation and risk-taking behaviors. For example, young girls who are sexually mature at an earlier age than their peers are often attracted to older girls and boys who may engage in risk-taking behaviors. If older teens smoke, drink, and drive while under the influence of alcohol with no adverse consequences (e.g., no motor vehicle accidents), young girls may believe that they, too, will be safe while smoking, drinking, or riding in an automobile with friends who are drinking.

Although parents and nurses cannot influence the time of biologic maturation, they can identify young girls who are at risk for the initiation of risk-taking behaviors because of early puberty. Parents need to understand that an early-maturing daughter might be uncomfortable with her body, and they should take advantage of opportunities to build her self-esteem. Parental sensitivity to the importance of peer-group acceptance and parental support of a teenage daughter who feels left out or different are crucial. School nurses can provide anticipatory guidance to these girls and help them role-play coping strategies for situations that involve offers to smoke and drink. In addition, school nurses can provide information about physical development during puberty and emphasize that not all teenagers mature at the same time or rate.

Teachers, coaches, and community and church leaders can provide opportunities for these girls to "fit in" with their same-age peers through activities that stress mutual goals. For example, an early-maturing girl is typically taller than her age-mates and can be an asset in sports such as basketball and track-and-field events.

been proved to be carcinogenic, and regular use can cause dental problems, foul-smelling breath, and tooth erosion or loss.

Care Management

Prevention of regular smoking in teenagers is the most effective way to reduce the overall incidence of smoking. A variety of methods have been used. Posters, charts, displays, statistics, and the use of examples of actual damaged lungs to communicate the hazards of smoking all have their supporters and doubters. Some schools also use films and demonstrations in science classes.

For the most part, smoking prevention programs that focus on the negative, long-term effects of smoking on health have been ineffective. Youth-to-youth programs and those emphasizing the immediate effects are more effective but primarily in improving teenagers' attitudes toward not smoking. Because smoking and smoking-related behaviors are social symbols, antismoking campaigns must address the norms of potential smokers. Anything that ridicules or threatens the social norms of the peer group can be unproductive or counterproductive. Investigators have found that teaching resistance to peer pressure to smoke is effective in early adolescence. Although the effects of these programs may decrease with time, the effects can be enhanced in older adolescents by presenting information in class instead of simply handing out written material to the students.

Two areas of focus for antismoking programs are peer-led programs and use of media in smoking prevention (e.g., CDs, videos, and films). Peer-led programs emphasizing the social consequences of smoking have proved most successful. If a significant number of influential peers can "sell" their classmates on the idea that the habit is not popular, the followers will imitate their behavior. Such programs emphasize short-term rather than long-term consequences (e.g., the effects of smoking on

COMMUNITY FOCUS

Nonsmoking Strategies

Nurses who work in schools, hospitals, and community agencies can take advantage of all opportunities to provide education about the dangers of smoking, to discourage smoking initiation by children and adolescents, to encourage smoking cessation, and to promote smoke-free environments. In particular, school nurses must be alert to the vulnerability of young preteens when they enter junior high or middle school. These nurses are in an ideal position to assess stress, personal conflict, weight concerns, peer pressures, and other factors that place preteens at risk for smoking initiation. Nurses should serve as counselors to student, teacher, and parent groups and as advocates for antismoking legislative efforts. The following additional strategies are recommended:*

- Provide only brief information about long-term health consequences (e.g., cardiovascular and cancer risks).
- Discuss immediate physiologic consequences (e.g., changes in heart rate, blood pressure, respiratory symptoms, and blood carbon monoxide concentrations).
- Mention alternatives to smoking that also establish a self-image that appears independent, mature, or sophisticated (e.g., weight lifting; jogging; dancing; joining a boys' or girls' club; engaging in volunteer work for a hospital, political, religious, or community group).
- Mention the negative effects in detail (e.g., earlier wrinkling of skin; yellow stains on teeth and fingers; tobacco odor on breath, hair, and clothing).
- Mention the increasing ostracism of smokers by nonsmokers, both legal and informal, in the workplace and in public places.
- Mention the increasing evidence that secondhand smoke is injurious to the health of nonsmokers who are regularly exposed, especially small children.
- Acknowledge that many adults, who were enticed to start smoking as teenagers because of its social benefits, now wish they could stop smoking.
- Give cooperative adolescents effective arguments to deal with peer pressure (e.g., by not smoking, a teenager demonstrates independence and nonconformity, traits normally prized by youth).
- Request posters or pamphlets from local agencies (e.g., American Cancer Society, American Heart Association, and American Lung Association) to display in prominent places at school.

*The CDC has information on the effects of tobacco, smoking cessation, and tobacco control programs; 1600 Clifton Road, Atlanta, GA 30333; 800-232-4636; e-mail: tobaccoinfo@cdc.gov; www.cdc.gov/tobacco.

personal appearance, such as unattractive stains on teeth and hands and unpleasant odor of breath and clothing).

The impact of school-based antismoking programs can be strengthened by expanding these programs to include parents, mass media, youth groups, and community organizations. For example, mass media efforts that involve antismoking radio campaigns have been identified as the most cost-effective mass media intervention.

Smoking bans in schools also accomplish several goals: (1) they discourage students from starting to smoke; (2) they reinforce knowledge of the health hazards of cigarette smoking and exposure to environmental tobacco smoke; and (3) they promote a smoke-free environment as the norm (see Community Focus box: Nonsmoking Strategies).

Alcohol

Acute or chronic abuse of alcohol (ethanol) is responsible for many acts of violence, suicide, accidental injury, and death. Alcohol drinking is likely to begin in the middle-school years and increases with age. A national survey of high school students found that 75% of 12th-grade students have had at least one drink of alcohol in their life (CDC, 2014). Ethanol is a depressant that reduces inhibitions against aggressive and sexual acting out. Severe physical and psychologic symptoms accompany abrupt withdrawal, and long-term use leads to slow tissue destruction, especially of the brain and liver cells. The most noticeable effects of alcohol occur within the central nervous system and include changes in cognitive and autonomic functions such as judgment, memory, learning ability, and other intellectual capacities. Young people with alcoholism often drink alone and cannot control their use of alcohol. They often rely on the substance as a defense against depression, anxiety, fear, or anger. Not all of these characteristics are observed in adolescents who are abusing alcohol, but if several signs are evident, the child or adolescent should be considered at risk. Referral to a health care professional and detoxification therapy may be necessary. Information about alcohol and answers to questions are available through the Alcohol Hotline.* Other groups that provide support and counseling for families are Al-Anon, Alateen, Alatot, and Alcoholics Anonymous (an organization that has listings in all local directories).

Cocaine

Although cocaine is not pharmacologically considered a narcotic, it is legally categorized as such. Cocaine is available in two forms: water-soluble cocaine hydrochloride, which is administered by "snorting" or intravenous injection; and nonsoluble alkaloid (freebase) cocaine, which is used primarily for smoking. Crack, or "rock," is a purer, more menacing form of the drug. It can be produced cheaply and smoked in either water pipes or mentholated cigarettes.

Cocaine creates a sense of euphoria, or an indefinable high. Withdrawal does not produce the dramatic symptoms observed in withdrawal from other substances. The effects are those commonly seen in depression, including lack of energy and motivation, irritability, appetite changes, psychomotor delay, and irregular sleep patterns. More serious symptoms include cardiovascular manifestations and seizures. Physical withdrawal should not be confused with the so-called crash after a cocaine high, which consists of a long period of sleep. Answers to questions about the risks of using cocaine are available at the National Cocaine Hotline[†] which also provides referrals to support groups and treatment centers.

Narcotics

Narcotic drugs include opiates, such as heroin and morphine, and opioids (opiate-like drugs), such as hydromorphone (Dilaudid), hydrocodone, fentanyl, meperidine (Demerol), and codeine. These drugs produce a state of euphoria by removing painful feelings and creating a pleasurable experience and a sense of success accompanied by clouding of the consciousness and a dreamlike state. Physical signs of narcotic abuse include constricted pupils; respiratory depression; and, often, cyanosis. Needle marks may be visible on the arms or legs in chronic users. Physical withdrawal from opiates is extremely unpleasant unless controlled with supervised tapering doses of the opioid or substitution of methadone.

As important as the physical effects are the indirect consequences related to the illegal status of narcotic use and the problems associated with securing the drug (e.g., the time-consuming searches to obtain the drug and the often illegal methods used to meet the high cost of purchasing it). Health problems also result from self-neglect of physical needs (nutrition, cleanliness, dental care); overdose; contamination; and infection, including HIV and hepatitis B and hepatitis C infection.

*Toll-free 800-331-2900.
[†]800-COCAINE (800-262-2463).

Central Nervous System Depressants

Central nervous system depressants include a variety of hypnotic drugs that produce physical dependence and withdrawal symptoms on abrupt discontinuation. They create a feeling of relaxation and sleepiness but impair general functioning. Drugs in this category include barbiturates, nonbarbiturates, and alcohol. Barbiturates combined with alcohol produce a profound depressant effect. Flunitrazepam (Rohypnol), known as the "date rape drug," is a hypnotic drug abused by adolescents. Many women and men report being raped after unknowingly being given Rohypnol in a drink. Rohypnol is 10 times more powerful than diazepam (Valium). It produces prolonged sedation, a feeling of well-being, and short-term memory loss.

Central Nervous System Stimulants

Amphetamines and cocaine do not produce strong physical dependence and can be withdrawn without much danger. However, psychologic dependence is strong, and acute intoxication can lead to violent aggressive behavior or psychotic episodes characterized by paranoia, uncontrollable agitation, and restlessness. When combined with barbiturates, the euphoric effects are particularly addictive.

Methamphetamine can be snorted, injected, swallowed, or smoked and produces a burst of energy in its users, along with intense, alternating attacks of boldness and paranoia. It provokes excitement far more intense than that caused by cocaine. The drug, with the street names *crank,* *meth,* and *crystal,* is inexpensive and has a longer period of action than cocaine. Instead of a short (few minutes) high, as achieved with cocaine, a user can remain "up" for hours on a similar dose of crank.

Health care professionals are concerned about the use of various volatile substances, or inhalants such as gasoline, model airplane cement, and organic solvents; these substances are inhaled by the user to achieve an altered sensation, and the most recent surveillance has indicated a modest increase in use after nearly 1 decade of decline. Adolescents breathe or place these substances into paper or plastic bags or soda cans from which they rebreathe the fumes to produce a feeling of euphoria and altered consciousness. These substances contain chemical solvents and are extremely hazardous. Dusters contain Freon, a substance that can cause fatal cardiac dysrhythmias. Inhalants are the only substance that has a higher incidence of use among young adolescents. This is probably related to the fact that the products are readily available and may be the only substances available for young teens. Many young children are unaware of the dangers of "sniffing" or "huffing." In addition to rapid loss of consciousness and respiratory arrest, these substances may cause visual scanning problems, language deficiencies, motor instability, memory deficits, and attention and concentration problems.

Mind-Altering Drugs

Hallucinogens (psychedelics, psychotomimetics, psychotropics, or illusionogenics) are drugs that produce vivid hallucinations and euphoria. These drugs do not produce physical dependence, and they can be abruptly withdrawn without ill effect. However, the acute and long-term effects are variable, and in some individuals, the dissociative behavior may be prolonged. Cannabis (marijuana, hashish) and lysergic acid diethylamide (LSD) are also included in this category of drugs.

Care Management

Nurses who have contact with children and adolescents are in an excellent position to provide information about substance abuse and to serve as patient advocates. Nurses most often encounter young substance abusers when they are (1) experiencing overdose or withdrawal symptoms, (2) manifesting bizarre behavior or confusion secondary to drug ingestion,

---

CLINICAL REASONING CASE STUDY
Prescription Medication Abuse in Adolescence

An eighth-grade teacher calls the school nurse, Sally, to her classroom and reports that a girl is behaving "strangely"; the girl slept most of the period before lunch and has not participated in class discussions. Sally, RN, takes the girl to her office and performs an initial assessment. Upon assessment, the girl demonstrates short-term memory lapse and has slightly slurred speech and her pupillary reaction to light is delayed; her blood pressure is 112/68 mm Hg, respirations are 14 breaths/min and regular, and heart rate is 102 beats/min. She denies taking any pills or liquid initially but then states she had a migraine on arrival to school and a friend gave her two blue pills to help with the headache. She refuses to say who gave her the pills and does not know what they were but thought they were Tylenol. She states that she does not know where her mother or father are but thinks they are at work.

1. Evidence—Is there sufficient evidence for Sally to implement a plan of care for this adolescent?
2. What should Sally's next course of action involve? What is her professional responsibility in this case?
3. Assumptions—Describe some underlying assumptions about the following:
   a. The school nurse's physical assessment findings
   b. The misuse of prescription medications by adolescents
4. What nursing priorities and implications for care can be made at this time? What type of care should this eighth grader receive?

---

(3) worried that they are or will become addicted, or (4) worried about a friend or family member who is addicted.

In particular, nurses who care for hospitalized adolescents need to know if these youths use drugs compulsively. Drug withdrawal can seriously complicate other illnesses. Nurses should be alert for any physical or behavioral clues that indicate the onset of withdrawal or the effects of drugs. School nurses and nurses who work in the community play an essential role in identifying children, adolescents, and families with substance abuse problems. The school nurse may be the first to identify a child or adolescent who has ingested a particular drug by the child's erratic behavior in class or on the school grounds (see Clinical Reasoning Case Study: Prescription Medication Abuse in Adolescence). Early identification of those at risk for substance abuse problems is an essential aspect of prevention. Pediatric health care professionals also prevent substance abuse by creating trusting relationships so that children and adolescents feel comfortable asking questions about drugs, and health care professionals can alert them to websites and other aspects of society that discourage experimentation with drugs.

Interprofessional Care Management: Acute Care

Adolescents experiencing toxic drug effects or withdrawal symptoms are usually seen initially in the emergency department. Experienced emergency department personnel are familiar with the management of acute drug toxicity and the signs, symptoms, and behavioral characteristics associated with a variety of substances. When the drug is questionable or unknown, knowledge of these factors facilitates management and treatment. Often, observation or description of the child's or adolescent's behavior is more valuable than reports by patients or their friends.

The treatment for drug toxicity or withdrawal varies according to the drug and the method used. Every effort is made to determine the type, time of ingestion, amount of drug taken, mode of administration, and factors related to the onset of presenting symptoms. It is helpful to know the individual's pattern of use. For example, if two types of drugs are involved, they may require different treatments. Historically, gastric lavage has been used when the drug has been ingested recently and the cough reflex is intact, but it is of little value when the drug has been administered by the intravenous ("mainlined") or intranasal ("sniffed") route. More commonly, the administration of a drug antidote such as naloxone and the early (within 1 to 2 hours of ingestion) administration of activated charcoal may be used for opioid overdose. Because the actual content of most street drugs is highly questionable, other pharmaceutical agents are administered with caution, except perhaps the narcotic antagonists in cases of suspected opiate overdoses. It is also necessary to assess for possible trauma sustained while the patient was under the influence of the drug.

Interprofessional Care Management: Long-Term Management

A major factor in the treatment and rehabilitation of young drug users is careful assessment in the nonacute stage to determine the function that the drug plays in the adolescent's life. The motivation phase is directed toward exploring the factors that influence drug use. It also involves establishing a feeling of self-worth and a commitment to self-help in the teen.

Rehabilitation begins when adolescents decide that they can and are willing to change. Rehabilitation involves fostering healthy interdependent relationships with caring and supportive adults and exploring alternate mechanisms for problem solving while simultaneously reducing or eliminating drug use. People working with troubled youth must be prepared for recidivism, or the tendency to relapse, and maintain a plan for reentry into the treatment process.

Family Support

Most treatment programs for substance abusers are based on adult 12-step models such as Alcoholics Anonymous. Research is needed to determine whether these adult models are effective for adolescents. Tough Love* is one program that is based on the conviction that parents have the right and responsibility to be the policymakers in the family, to set limits on the behavior of their children, and to take control of the household from out-of-control adolescents. The premise is that allowing teenagers to experience the negative consequences of their behavior will bring them closer to accepting help or changing their behavior. Another group that provides support and counseling for families experiencing substance abuse and seeking strategies to cope with their children is Parents Anonymous.† Another source of information is the Substance Abuse and Mental Health Services Administration's National Clearinghouse for Alcohol and Drug Information.‡ The National Institute on Drug Abuse (NIDA)§ also contains an abundance of information for adolescents on the effects of abused substances, prevention, and treatment.

Prevention

Health care professionals play an important role in education efforts, as well as in individual observation, assessment, and therapy related to substance abuse. In recent years, a variety of educational programs have been applied with promising results. The most effective prevention strategies are those that are part of a broader, more general effort to promote overall health and success. Health-compromising behaviors are often interconnected and have common antecedents. Prevention efforts that focus on changing only one behavior (e.g., alcohol, other drug use) are less likely to be successful. Successful programs are those that promote parenting skills, social skills among distractible children, academic achievement, and skills to resist peer pressure.

Peer pressure is a powerful tool and can be used effectively in substance abuse prevention. A group that has had some success in reducing injury from drunk driving is Students Against Destructive Decisions (SADD).* Techniques used by this group include peer counseling, parental guidelines for teenage parties, and community awareness. Health care professionals should encourage the formation of SADD chapters in the high schools in their communities.

SUICIDE

Suicide is defined as the deliberate act of self-injury with the intent that the injury results in death. Most experts distinguish among suicidal ideation, suicide attempt (or parasuicide), and suicide.

Suicidal ideation involves a preoccupation with thoughts about committing suicide and may be a precursor to suicide. Although it is common for adolescents to experience occasional suicidal thoughts, expressions of preoccupation with suicide should be taken seriously and an assessment should be conducted for appropriate referral. A suicide attempt is intended to cause injury or death. The term *parasuicide* is used to refer to behaviors ranging from gestures to serious attempts to kill oneself. *Parasuicide* is a preferred term because it makes no reference to intent and because a person's motive may be too difficult or complex to determine. However, all parasuicidal activity should be taken seriously.

> **! NURSING ALERT**
>
> A history of a previous suicide attempt is a serious indicator for possible suicide completion in the future. Studies of adolescent suicides have found that as many as one-half of the adolescents had made previous attempts.

Results from the 2013 Youth Risk Behavior Surveillance indicated that 8% of students nationwide had attempted suicide at least once during the 12 months preceding the survey; the range of suicide attempts by adolescents across the states varied from 5.5% to 14.3% (CDC, 2014). The overall incidence of youth suicide has decreased since 1992, yet the CDC and other experts note that the incidence is still too high. Approximately 13.6% of the students in this survey reported that they had made a specific plan to attempt suicide in the 12 months preceding the survey. Suicide is currently the fourth leading cause of death during the teenage years, surpassed only by death from motor vehicle crashes, other unintentional injuries, and homicide (CDC, 2014).

Etiology

Individual, family, and social or environmental factors have all been implicated in suicide. The single most important individual factor is the presence of an active psychiatric disorder (depression, bipolar disorder, psychosis, substance abuse, or conduct disorder). Alcohol use in particular has been associated with a twofold increase in suicidal ideation (Nock, Green, Hwang, et al., 2013). For some teens, suicide becomes the final

---

*www.toughlove.com.
†250 West First Street, Suite 250, Claremont, CA 91711; 909-621-6184; www.parentsanonymous.org.
‡5600 Fishers Lane, Rockville, MD 20852; 877-SAMHSA-7; www.samhsa.gov.
§6001 Executive Boulevard, Room 5213, MSC 9561, Bethesda, MD 20892; 301-443-1124; www.drugabuse.gov/children-and-teens

*255 Main Street, Marlborough, MA 01752; 877-SADD-INC; www.sadd.org.

pathway for release from their psychiatric and social problems. Child and adolescent suicide victims are reported to have higher rates not only of depression but also of conduct disorders; bipolar disorders; substance abuse; interpersonal problems with parents; and a family history of depression, substance abuse, and suicidal behavior.

Gay, lesbian, and bisexual adolescents are at particularly high risk for suicide attempts, especially if raised in an environment where they are denied support systems (Lytle, De Luca, & Blosnich, 2014). Family factors influencing suicide include parental loss; family disruption; a family history of suicide, depression, substance abuse, or emotional disturbance; child abuse or neglect; unavailable parents; poor communication and isolation within the family; family conflict; and unrealistically high parental expectations or parental indifference with low expectations. Families who respect individuality, are cohesive and caring, balance discipline with a supportive and understanding relationship, have good systems of communication, and have at least one attentive and caring parent available to the child protect adolescents from suicidal outcomes. Social or environmental factors include incarceration, isolation, acute loss of a boyfriend or girlfriend, lack of future options, and availability of firearms in the home.

Methods

Firearms are by far the most commonly used instruments in completed suicides among males and females (Dowd, Sege, Council on Injury, Violence, and Poison Prevention Executive Committee & American Academy of Pediatrics, 2012). For adolescent males, the second and third most common means of suicide are hanging and overdose, respectively; for females, the second and third most common means are overdose and strangulation, respectively.

The most common method of suicide *attempt* is overdose or ingestion of a potentially toxic substance, such as drugs. The second most common method of suicide attempt is self-inflicted laceration.

! NURSING ALERT

Given what is known about youth suicide, nurses should ask parents, especially those with at-risk teenagers, if firearms are available in the house and, if so, recommend their removal. Parents must ensure that their children—especially those who are depressed, have poor problem-solving skills, or use drugs or alcohol—do not have access to firearms. Parents must also be educated on the warning signs of suicide (Box 35.8).

Motivation

Suicidal ideation is common in adolescents. It represents numerous fantasies, such as relief from suffering, a means of gaining comfort and sympathy, or a means of revenge against those who have hurt them. Adolescents have the erroneous perception that the act of suicide will evoke remorse and pity and that they will be able to return and witness the grief. Angry children or adolescents who are unable to directly punish those who have injured or insulted them may take revenge on those who love them through self-destruction ("They'll be sorry when they find me dead"; "They'll be sorry they were mean to me").

For adolescents who are severely depressed, suicide seems to be the only release from their despair. These adolescents rarely provide evidence of their intent and frequently conceal their suicidal thoughts. Many adolescents, however, tell their peers of their suicidal thoughts or plans but avoid telling adults. Social isolation is a significant factor in distinguishing adolescents who will kill themselves from those who will not. It is also more characteristic of those who complete suicide than of those who make attempts or threats.

BOX 35.8 Warning Signs of Suicide

- Preoccupation with themes of death—focuses on morbid thoughts
- Wants to give away cherished possessions
- Talks of own death, desire to die
- Loss of energy, loss of interest, listlessness
- Exhaustion without obvious cause
- Changes in sleep patterns—too much or too little
- Increased irritability, argumentativeness, or stubbornness
- Physical complaints—recurrent stomachaches, headaches
- Repeated visits to physician, nurse practitioner, or emergency department for treatment of injuries
- Reckless behavior
- Antisocial behavior—engages in drinking, uses drugs, fights, commits acts of vandalism, runs away from home, becomes sexually promiscuous
- Sudden change in school performance—lowered grades, cutting classes, dropping out of activities
- Resists or refuses to go to school
- Remains distant, sad, remote—flat affect, frozen facial expression
- Describes self as worthless
- Sudden cheerfulness after deep depression
- Social withdrawal from friends, activities, interests that were previously enjoyed
- Impaired concentration
- Dramatic change in appetite

The frequency of contagion or copycat suicides (i.e., an increase in youth suicide that occurs after the suicide of one teenager is publicized) is disturbing and may indicate that teenagers perceive suicide as glamorous. In addition, young people may not realize the finality of suicide because they have become desensitized from constantly viewing violence and death on television.

Diagnostic Evaluation

Depression is common among adolescents who attempt suicide. Depression is characterized by both subjective symptoms and objective signs that reflect the adolescent's sadness and despair. Adolescents describe feelings of sadness, despair, helplessness, hopelessness, boredom, loss of interest, and isolation. They may also feel self-reproach, self-deprecation, and guilt. Subjective symptoms of depression or specific changes in behavior place an adolescent at risk for suicide (Box 35.9).

Therapeutic Management

Threats of suicide should always be taken seriously. There has been a tendency to dismiss suicide attempts as impulsive acts resulting from temporary crises or depression. If a suicide attempt fails to draw attention to their problems or makes them worse, the child or adolescent may conclude that suicide is the only answer. Children and adolescents need to know that someone cares and must be provided with swift and efficient crisis intervention. Although ordinary practitioners can manage an acute depressive reaction without difficulty, the adolescent who has made a serious attempt or has a specific plan for suicide should receive immediate attention and competent psychiatric care.

Youths who are actively suicidal need inpatient care, monitoring, and treatment. Medications for depression and bipolar disorder often take several weeks to reach therapeutic levels. The time until medications and therapy begin to take effect can be trying for the adolescent and the family. It is important to encourage families to support their teen in adherence to the regimen prescribed. The SSRIs are often prescribed for depression, but teens who are taking such medications need careful, frequent monitoring.

BOX 35.9 Characteristics of Children or Adolescents With Depression

Behavior
- Predominantly sad facial expression with absence or diminished range of affective response (most of the day)
- Solitary play or work; tendency to be alone; lack of interest in play with friends
- Withdrawal from previously enjoyed activities and relationships
- Lowered grades in school; lack of interest in doing homework or achieving in school; refuses to wake up for school
- Diminished motor activity; tiredness
- Tearfulness or crying
- Inability to concentrate
- Dependent and clinging or aggressive and disruptive
- Recurrent suicidal thoughts or talk

Internal States
- Utterance of statements reflecting lowered self-esteem, sense of hopelessness, or guilt
- Suicidal ideation

Physiology
- Constipation
- Loss of energy; fatigue
- Nonspecific complaints of not feeling well
- Change in appetite resulting in weight loss or gain
- Alterations in sleeping pattern, sleeplessness, or hypersomnia

> **! NURSING ALERT**
>
> Adolescents who express suicidal feelings and have a specific plan should be monitored at all times. They should not have access to firearms, prescription or over-the-counter drugs, belts, scarves, shoestrings, sharp objects, matches, or lighters. If they are intoxicated, they must be restrained or placed in a protective environment until a psychiatrist or psychologist can assess them.

Interprofessional Care Management of Suicide

Health care professionals play a pivotal role in reducing adolescent suicide. They have the opportunity to provide anticipatory guidance to parents and adolescents. They can teach parents to be supportive and to develop positive communication patterns that help teens feel connected with and loved by their families. To foster healthy development, parents can be encouraged to provide teens with creative outlets and to assist young people in accepting strong emotions—pain, anger, and frustration—as a normal part of the human experience.

Care of suicidal adolescents includes early recognition, management, and prevention. The most important aspect of management is the recognition of warning signs that indicate that an adolescent is troubled and might attempt suicide. Any suicidal remarks are taken seriously, and the young person is not left alone until the degree of suicidality is assessed. A mnemonic for the assessment process is *SLAP*: specificity, lethality, accessibility, and proximity. The first step (specificity) is to ask adolescents whether they feel suicidal or as though they would like to take their own lives. If so, have they chosen a means of suicide, and do they have a specific plan? The second stage of assessment (lethality) involves determining the lethality of the methods available to them. Do they plan to use a gun or knife? Have they chosen highly lethal medications, hanging, or carbon monoxide poisoning? The third stage (accessibility) involves determining the availability of the means of

suicide, and the fourth stage (proximity) involves assessing whether they have determined a time to commit suicide and when.

Health care professionals must be alert to the signs of depression, and anyone who exhibits such behavior should be referred for thorough psychologic assessment. Depression is manifested differently in children and adolescents than in adults. In teens, it may be masked by impulsive aggressive behaviors. Defiance, disobedience, behavior problems, and psychosomatic disturbances can indicate underlying depression, suicidal ideation, and impending suicide attempts.

> **! NURSING ALERT**
>
> No threat of suicide should be ignored or challenged. Threats are a symptom that must be taken seriously. Too often, suicidal threats or minor attempts are confused with bids for attention. It is also a mistake to be lulled into a false sense of security when an adolescent's depression is apparently relieved. The improvement in attitude may mean that the adolescent has made the decision and found the means to carry out the threat.

Peers and other confidants are valuable observers and excellent sources of information about potential suicide attempts. They may not be able to diagnose depression, but they are able to sense when a friend has undergone a marked personality change. It is important to emphasize that the peer who detects any changes in a friend is a potential rescuer and should not remain silent about the observations. Friendship does not imply collusion. A peer who believes that a friend may be suicidal should alert someone who can help (e.g., a parent, teacher, guidance counselor, school nurse).

Routine health assessments of adolescents should include questions that assess the presence of suicidal ideation or intent. The following questions can be asked (Bono & Amendola, 2015):
1. How are things at home and school?
2. Have you ever felt that life is not worth living?
3. Do you have thoughts of death or wishing you were dead?
4. Have you ever felt like hurting yourself or wanting to kill yourself?
5. What suicide plans have you made in the last few days?
6. What suicide plans have you made and acted on in the last several months?

If adolescents answer "yes" to any of the questions 2, 3, or 4, they should be asked if they feel that way now to assess for current suicidality. If teens say they have attempted suicide in the past, assess the number of times, and ask them to describe what they were feeling, which method they used, what happened, if they would make a similar attempt, and how they would handle their despair now. Any previous suicide attempt indicates an increased risk for a future attempt. The risk for a suicide attempt in the near future increases as the frequency of suicidal ideation increases.

> **! NURSING ALERT**
>
> The National Suicide Prevention Lifeline (800-273-TALK [8255]; in Spanish, 888-628-9454) offers someone to talk to 24/7.

If children or adolescents express suicidal intent, nurses make a contract, asking them to sign an agreement that they will not attempt suicide during an agreed-on period and that they will call the 24-hour crisis line immediately if they feel that they cannot keep to their contract. The amount of time an adolescent feels comfortable contracting is usually an indication of his or her risk and stability.

Because a suicide attempt is frequently an outgrowth of family distress, it is essential to intervene with the family. It is important to assess family interactions and to recognize disturbed relationships. The most effective approach is recognition of susceptible adolescents during the early stages of family distress so that family counseling can be started. Prevention must be directed toward improving childrearing practices through support and education of parents and changing societal conditions that generate defeat, despair, and maladaptive behavior.

Although confidentiality is an essential part of adolescent counseling, in the case of self-destructive behaviors, confidentiality cannot be honored. Suicidal behavior is reported to the family and other professionals, and adolescents are informed that this will be done. Such action conveys an important message to the youth: that the professionals understand and care.

Many schools have instituted suicide prevention programs. These programs include services such as drop-in counseling and a peer counseling telephone line. Information can also be obtained from the American Association of Suicidology.*

REFERENCES

Agostino, H., Erdstein, J., & Di Meglio, G. (2013). Shifting paradigms: Continuous nasogastric feeding with high caloric intakes in anorexia nervosa. *Journal of Adolescent Health, 53*(3), 590–594.

Alexander, R. (2015). How to protect children from Internet predators: A phenomenological study. *Studies in Health Technology and Informatics, 219,* 82–88.

Ali, O., & Donohoue, P. A. (2016). Gynecomastia. In R. M. Kliegman, B. F. Stanton, J. W. St. Geme, et al. (Eds.), *Nelson textbook of pediatrics* (20th ed.). Philadelphia, PA: Saunders/Elsevier.

Al-Sayed, E. M., & Ibrahim, K. S. (2014). Second-hand tobacco smoke and children. *Toxicology and Industrial Health, 30*(7), 635–644.

Altman, M., & Wilfley, D. E. (2015). Evidence update on the treatment of overweight and obesity in children and adolescents. *Journal of Clinical Child & Adolescent Psychology, 44*(4), 521–537.

American Academy of Pediatric Dentistry. (2012). Guideline on periodicity of examination, preventive dental services, anticipatory guidance/counseling and oral treatment for infants, children, and adolescents. *AAPD Reference Manual 2011-2012, 33*(6), 103–108.

American Academy of Pediatrics. (2016). *Bright futures: Adolescence tools.* Retrieved from https://brightfutures.aap.org/materials-and-tools/tool-and-resource-kit/Pages/adolescence-tools.aspx.

American Academy of Pediatrics, Council on Communications and Media. (2013). Children, adolescents, and the media. *Pediatrics, 132*(5), 958–961.

American Psychiatric Association. (2013). *Diagnostic and statistical manual of mental disorders* (5th ed.). Arlington, VA: Author.

Avis, J. L., Komarnicki, A., Farmer, A. P., et al. (2016). Tools and resources for preventing childhood obesity in primary care: A method of evaluation and preliminary assessment. *Patient Education and Counseling, 99*(5), 769–775.

Barton, M., & US Preventive Services Task Force. (2010). Screening for obesity in children and adolescents: US Preventive Services Task Force recommendation statement. *Pediatrics, 125*(2), 361–367.

Berge, J. M., Maclehose, R., Loth, K. A., et al. (2013). Parent conversations about healthful eating and weight: Associations with adolescent disordered eating behaviors. *JAMA Pediatrics, 167*(8), 746–753.

Biro, F. M., Greenspan, L. C., & Galvez, M. P. (2012). Puberty in girls of the 21st century. *Journal of Pediatric & Adolescent Gynecology, 25*(5), 289–294.

Blum, R. W., & Qureshi, F. (2011). *Morbidity and mortality among adolescents and young adults in the United States.* Johns Hopkins Bloomberg School of Public Health. Retrieved from http://www.jhsph.edu/research/

centers-and-institutes/center-for-adolescent-health/_images/_pre-redesign/az/US%20Fact%20Sheet_FINAL.pdf.

Bono, V., & Amendola, C. L. (2015). Primary care assessment of patients at risk for suicide. *Journal of the American Academy of Physician Assistants, 28*(12), 35–39.

Bralic, I., Tahirovic, H., Matanic, D., et al. (2012). Association of early menarche age and overweight/obesity. *Journal of Pediatric Endocrinology and Metabolism, 25*(1-2), 57–62.

Bratland-Sanda, S., & Sundgot-Borgen, J. (2013). Eating disorders in athletes: Overview of prevalence, risk factors and recommendations for prevention and treatment. *European Journal of Sport Science, 13*(5), 499–508.

Cabrera, S. M., Bright, G. M., Frane, J. W., et al. (2014). Age of thelarche and menarche in contemporary US females: A cross-sectional analysis. *Journal of Pediatric Endocrinology and Metabolism, 27*(0), 47–51.

Center for Labor Market Studies. (2011). *High school dropouts in Chicago and Illinois: The growing labor market, income, civic, social and fiscal costs of dropping out of high school.* Retrieved from http://www.northeastern.edu/clms/wp-content/uploads/High-School-Dropouts-in-Chicago-and-Illinois.pdf.

Centers for Disease Control and Prevention. (2012). Vital signs: Unintentional injury deaths among persons aged 0-19 years—United States, 2000-2009. *Morbidity and Mortality Weekly Report, 61*(15), 270–276.

Centers for Disease Control and Prevention. (2014). Youth risk behavior surveillance—United States, 2013. *Morbidity and Mortality Weekly Report Supplement, 63*(4), 1–172.

Centers for Disease Control and Prevention. (2015). *How much physical activity do children need?* Retrieved from http://www.cdc.gov/physicalactivity/everyone/guidelines/children.html.

Centers for Disease Control and Prevention. (2016). *Recommended immunization schedules for persons aged 0 through 18 years, United States 2016.* Retrieved from http://www.cdc.gov/vaccines/schedules/downloads/child/0-18yrs-schedule.pdf.

Chapman, R. L., Buckley, L., Reveruzzi, B., et al. (2014). Injury prevention among friends: The benefits of school connectedness. *Journal of Adolescence, 37*(6), 937–944.

Crossen, E. J., Lewis, B., & Hoffman, B. D. (2015). Preventing gun injuries in children. *Pediatrics in Review, 36*(2), 43–50.

Cunningham, S. A., Kramer, M. R., & Narayan, K. M. (2014). Incidence of childhood obesity in the United States. *New England Journal of Medicine, 370*(5), 403–411.

Currie, C., Ahluwalia, N., Godeau, E., et al. (2012). Is obesity at individual and national level associated with lower age at menarche? Evidence from 34 countries in the health behavior in school-aged children study. *Journal of Adolescent Health, 50*(6), 621–626.

Daniels, S. R., Hassink, S. G., & American Academy of Pediatrics, Committee on Nutrition. (2015). The role of the pediatrician in primary prevention of obesity. *Pediatrics, 135*(1), e275–e292.

Davis, J., & Bauman, K. (2013). *School enrollment in the United States: 2011.* Retrieved from http://www.census.gov/prod/2013pubs/p20-571.pdf.

Davis, D. M., Gance-Cleveland, B., Hassink, S., et al. (2007). Recommendations for prevention of childhood obesity. *Pediatrics, 120*(suppl), S229–S253.

De Jong, E., Visscher, T., Hirasing, R., et al. (2013). Association between TV viewing, computer use and overweight, determinants and competing activities of screen time in 4- to 13-year-old children. *International Journal of Obesity, 37*(1), 47–53.

Deimel, J. F., & Dunlap, B. J. (2012). The female athlete triad. *Clinics in Sports Medicine, 31*(2), 247–254.

Dowd, M. D., Sege, R. D., & Council on Injury, Violence, and Poison Prevention Executive Committee & American Academy of Pediatrics. (2012). Firearm-related injuries affecting the pediatric population. *Pediatrics, 130*(5), e1416–e1423.

Eaton, D. K., Kann, L., Kinchen, S., et al. (2012). Youth risk behavior surveillance—United States, 2011. *Morbidity and Mortality Weekly Report Supplement, 61*(4), 1–162.

Erikson, E. H. (1963). *Childhood and society* (2nd ed.). New York, NY: WW Norton.

*5221 Wisconsin Avenue NW, Washington, DC 20015; 202-237-2280; www.suicidology.org.

Flament, M. F., Bissada, H., & Spettigue, W. (2012). Evidence-based pharmacotherapy of eating disorders. *International Journal of Neuropsychopharmacology, 15*(2), 189–207.

Flattum, C., Draxten, M., Horning, M., et al. (2015). HOME Plus: Program design and implementation of a family-focused, community-based intervention to promote the frequency and healthfulness of family meals, reduce children's sedentary behavior, and prevent obesity. *International Journal of Behavioral Nutrition and Physical Activity, 12*, 53.

Flegal, K. M., Carroll, M. D., Kit, B. K., et al. (2012). Prevalence of obesity and trends in the distribution of body mass index among US adults, 1999-2010. *Journal of the American Medical Association, 307*(5), 491–497.

Funari, M. (2013). Detecting symptoms, early intervention, and preventative education eating disorders and the school-age child. *NASN School Nurse, 28*(3), 162–166.

Gahagan, S. (2016). Overweight and obesity. In R. M. Kliegman, B. F. Stanton, J. W. St. Geme, et al. (Eds.), *Nelson textbook of pediatrics* (20th ed.). Philadelphia, PA: Saunders/Elsevier.

Geller, J., Srikameswaran, S., Zelichowska, J., et al. (2012). Working with severe and enduring eating disorders: enhancing engagement and matching treatment to client readiness. In J. R. E. Fox & K. P. Goss (Eds.), *Eating and its disorders.* Oxford: John Wiley & Sons.

Gordon-Larsen, P., The, N. S., & Adair, L. S. (2010). Longitudinal trends in obesity in the United States from adolescence to the third decade of life. *Obesity, 18*(9), 1801–1804.

Gurnani, M., Birken, C., & Hamilton, J. (2015). Childhood obesity: Causes, consequences, and management. *Pediatric Clinics of North America, 62*(4), 821–840.

Herman-Giddens, M. E. (2013). The enigmatic pursuit of puberty in girls. *Pediatrics, 132*(6), 1125–1126.

Hill, L., Rybar, J., Styer, T., et al. (2015). Prevalence of and attitudes about distracted driving in college students. *Traffic Injury Prevention, 16*(4), 362–367.

Homa, D. M., Neff, L. J., King, B. A., et al. (2015). Vital signs: Disparities in nonsmokers' exposure to secondhand smoke—United States, 1999-2012. *Morbidity and Mortality Weekly Report, 64*(4), 103–108.

Institute of Medicine. (2011). *Dietary reference intakes for calcium and vitamin D.* Washington DC: National Academies Press.

Johnston, L. D., O'Malley, P. M., Miech, R. A., et al. (2016). *Monitoring the future national results on drug use: 1975-2015: Overview, key findings on adolescent drug use.* Ann Arbor, MI: University of Michigan Institute for Social Research.

Kanekar, A., & Sharma, M. (2010). Pharmacological approaches for management of child and adolescent obesity. *Journal of Clinical Medicine Research, 2*(3), 105–111.

Kiess, W., Kratzsch, J., Sergeyev, E., et al. (2014). Metabolic syndrome in childhood and adolescence. *Clinical Biochemistry, 47*(9), 695.

Kreipe, R. E. (2016). Eating disorders. In R. M. Kliegman, B. F. Stanton, J. W. St. Geme, et al. (Eds.), *Nelson textbook of pediatrics* (20th ed.). Philadelphia, PA: Saunders/Elsevier.

Le Grange, D., Lock, J., Agras, W. S., et al. (2015). Randomized clinical trial of family-based treatment and cognitive-behavioral therapy for adolescent bulimia nervosa. *Journal of the American Academy of Child & Adolescent Psychiatry, 54*(11), 886–894.

Li, R., Magadia, J., Fein, S. B., et al. (2012). Risk of bottle-feeding for rapid weight gain during the first year of life. *Archives of Pediatrics and Adolescent Medicine, 166*(5), 431–436.

Lipsky, R. K., & McGuinness, T. M. (2015). Binge eating disorder and youth. *Journal of Psychosocial Nursing and Mental Health Services, 53*(8), 18–22.

Lytle, M. C., De Luca, S. M., & Blosnich, J. R. (2014). The influence of intersecting identities on self-harm, suicidal behaviors, and depression among lesbian, gay, and bisexual individuals. *Suicide and Life-Threatening Behavior, 44*(4), 384–391.

Ma, N. S., & Gordon, C. M. (2012). Pediatric osteoporosis: Where are we now? *Journal of Pediatrics, 161*(6), 983–990.

Maxwell, J. C. (2011). The prescription drug epidemic in the United States: A perfect storm. *Drug and Alcohol Review, 30*(3), 264–270.

Michaelson, V., Pickett, W., Robinson, P., et al. (2015). Participation in church or religious groups and its association with health, part 2: A qualitative, Canadian study. *Journal of Religion and Health, 54*(3), 1118–1133.

Morandi, A., Meyre, D., Lobbens, S., et al. (2012). Estimation of newborn risk for child or adolescent obesity: Lessons from longitudinal birth cohorts. *PLoS ONE, 7*(11), e49919.

National Heart Lung Blood Institute. (2011). *Expert panel on integrated guidelines for cardiovascular health and risk reduction in children and adolescents: summary report.* Retrieved from http://www.nhlbi.nih.gov/health-pro/guidelines/current/cardiovascular-health-pediatric-guidelines/summary.

Neuman, M. E. (2011). Addressing children's beliefs through Fowler's stages of faith. *Journal of Pediatric Nursing, 26*(1), 44–50.

Nock, M. K., Green, J. G., Hwang, I., et al. (2013). Prevalence, correlates, and treatment of lifetime suicidal behavior among adolescents. *JAMA Psychiatry, 70*(3), 300–310.

Ogden, C. L., Carroll, M. D., & Flegal, K. M. (2008). High body mass index for age among US children and adolescents, 2003-2006. *Journal of the American Medical Association, 299*(20), 2401–2405.

Ogden, C. L., Carroll, M. D., Kit, B. K., et al. (2012). Prevalence of obesity and trends in body mass index among US children and adolescents, 1999-2010. *Journal of the American Medical Association, 307*(5), 483–490.

Ogden, C. L., Kuczmarski, R. J., Flegal, K. M., et al. (2002). Centers for Disease Control and Prevention 2000 growth charts for the United States: Improvements to the 1977 National Center for Health Statistics version. *Pediatrics, 109*(1), 141–142.

Ogden, C. L., Troiano, R. P., Briefel, R. R., et al. (1997). Prevalence of overweight among preschool children in the United States, 1971 through 1994. *Pediatrics, 99*(4), e1.

Owens, J., & Adolescent Sleep Working Group, Committee on Adolescence. (2014). Insufficient sleep in adolescents and young adults: An update on causes and consequences. *Pediatrics, 134*(3), e921–e932.

Ozier, A. D., & Henry, B. W. (2011). American Dietetic Association: Position of the American Dietetic Association: Nutrition intervention in the treatment of eating disorders. *Journal of the American Dietetic Association, 111*(8), 1236–1241.

Qiao, N., & Bell, T. M. (2016). State all-driver distracted driving laws and high school students' texting while driving behavior. *Traffic Injury Prevention, 17*(1), 5–8.

Rosen, D. S. (2010). Identification and management of eating disorders in children and adolescents. *Pediatrics, 126*(6), 1240–1253.

Schwartz, M. B., & Ustjanauskas, A. (2012). Food marketing to youth: Current threats and opportunities. *Childhood Obesity, 8*(2), 85–88.

Singh, G. K., & Yu, S. M. (2012). The impact of ethnic-immigrant status and obesity-related risk factors on behavioral problems among US children and adolescents. *Scientifica (Cairo), 2012*, 648152.

Smith, A., Stewart, D., Poon, C., et al. (2014). *From Hasting Street to Haida Gwaii: Provincial results of the 2013 BC adolescent health survey.* Vancouver, Canada: McCreary Centre Society.

Smink, F. R., van Hoeken, D., & Hoek, H. W. (2012). Epidemiology of eating disorders: Incidence, prevalence and mortality rates. *Current Psychiatry Reports, 14*(4), 406–414.

Song, M., Carroll, D. D., & Fulton, J. E. (2013). Meeting the 2008 physical activity guidelines for Americans among US youth. *American Journal of Preventive Medicine, 44*(3), 216–222.

Steever, J., Francis, J., Gordon, L. P., et al. (2014). Sexual minority youth. *Primary Care, 41*(3), 651–669.

Stice, E., South, K., & Shaw, H. (2012). Future directions in etiologic, prevention, and treatment research for eating disorders. *Journal of Clinical Child & Adolescent Psychology, 41*(6), 845–855.

Swanson, S. A., Crow, S. J., Le Grange, D., et al. (2011). Prevalence and correlates of eating disorders in adolescents: Results from the national comorbidity survey replication adolescent supplement. *Archives of General Psychiatry, 68*(7), 714–723.

Tandon, P. S., Zhou, C., Sallis, J. F., et al. (2012). Home environment relationships with children's physical activity, sedentary time, and screen time by socioeconomic status. *International Journal of Behavioral Nutrition and Physical Activity, 9*, 88.

Thorn, J. E., DeLellis, N., Chandler, J. P., et al. (2013). Parent and child self-reports of dietary behaviors, physical activity, and screen time. *Journal of Pediatrics, 162*(3), 557–561.

Trent, S. A., Moreira, M. E., Colwell, C. B., et al. (2013). ED management of patients with eating disorders. *American Journal of Emergency Medicine, 31*(5), 859–865.

US Preventive Services Task Force. (2010). Screening for obesity in children and adolescents: US Preventive Services Task Force recommendation statement. *Pediatrics, 125*(2), 361–367.

Van Cleave, J., Gortmaker, S. L., & Perrin, J. M. (2010). Dynamics of obesity and chronic health conditions among children and youth. *Journal of the American Medical Association, 303*(7), 623–630.

Van Ouytsel, J., Walrave, M., Ponnet, K., et al. (2015). The association between adolescent sexting, psychosocial difficulties, and risk behavior: Integrative review. *Journal of School Nursing, 31*(1), 54–69.

Villanueva, C., & Argente, J. (2014). Pathology or normal variant: What constitutes a delay in puberty? *Hormone Research in Paediatrics, 82*(4), 213–221.

Wildes, J. E., & Marcus, M. D. (2013). Alternative methods of classifying eating disorders: Models incorporating comorbid psychopathology and associated features. *Clinical Psychology Review, 33*(3), 383–394.

36

Impact of Chronic Illness, Disability, or End-of-Life Care for the Child and Family

Marilyn J. Hockenberry

http://evolve.elsevier.com/Perry/maternal

CARE OF CHILDREN AND FAMILIES LIVING WITH OR DYING FROM CHRONIC OR COMPLEX DISEASES

SCOPE OF THE PROBLEM

Advances in medical and nursing care, such as the increasing viability of extremely preterm infants, the portability of life-sustaining technology (e.g., total parental nutrition, ventilatory support), and life-extending treatments for children with conditions that previously would have led to an early death (e.g., malignancies, genetic conditions), have led to an exponential rise in the prevalence of children with complex and chronic diseases (Burke & Alverson, 2010; Simon, Berry, Feudtner, et al., 2010). These children have complex conditions involving several organ systems and require multiple specialists, technologic supports, and community services to assist them to function to their healthiest potential. The complex, high level of skill required to meet their daily health care needs and the continuous nature and potential volatility of the condition sets this group apart from the broader population of children with special health care needs (Cohen, Kuo, Agrawal, et al., 2011; Simon et al.; Kuo, Cohen, Agrawal, et al., 2011). A range of terms, such as *complex chronic condition, medically complex, technology dependent,* and *multiply handicapped,* have been used to describe this vulnerable population of children (Carnevale, Rehm, Kirk, et al., 2008; Cohen, Friedman, Nicholas, et al., 2008; Cohen et al., 2011; Feudtner, Feinstein, Zhong, et al., 2014). Frequent and prolonged hospitalizations; complex and multisystem health and developmental needs; and reliance on technology and care that cross hospital, clinic, and home settings are the key characteristics that all of these terms seek to signify about the children they are used to represent (Berry, Hall, Hall, et al., 2013; Cohen et al., 2011; Feudtner et al., 2014).

The nature and severity of childhood chronic and complex conditions is widely heterogeneous. Table 36.1 is a nonexhaustive sampling of conditions organized by specialty. However, these children and families are similar in the vulnerability that they experience due to the health and developmental consequences of these diagnoses on the child, such as ongoing functional impairment, neurodevelopmental disability, dependence on medical technology, and the need for ongoing skilled, supportive care from health care providers and family members. Although many authors have described the rise in prevalence that has come about because of advances in medical care (Burns, Casey, Lyle, et al., 2010;

Council on Children with Disabilities, 2005; Simon et al., 2010), accurate estimates of the numbers of affected families are not known (Carnevale et al., 2008). However, the impact of chronic and complex illness in children is wide ranging. The family experiences significant challenges necessitated by the child's care requirements (Goudie, Narcisse, Hall, et al., 2014; Kratz, Uding, Trahms, et al., 2009; Kuo et al., 2011; MacDonald & Callery, 2008). A child's activity level and developmental opportunities can be affected. Days can be lost from school. Children with complex chronic conditions may be at increased risk for behavior or emotional problems. Parents may lose days from work, experience financial strain, and be challenged both emotionally and physically as they cope with care of the child.

Siblings are also affected by having a "different" brother or sister, and they may simultaneously feel guilt, anger, or jealousy toward their ill sibling. Clinicians need to know that siblings of children with chronic illnesses are at risk for negative psychologic effects (Hartling, Milne, Tjosvold, et al., 2014). Parents need encouragement and assistance with understanding the reactions of siblings to having a chronically ill family member (e.g., behavioral regression, anxiety, withdrawal, apathy). Additionally, secondary losses (e.g., the ability to participate in extracurricular activities or social events) occur because of routines imposed by the affected child's chronic condition.

TRENDS IN CARE

Developmental Focus

Focusing on the child's developmental level rather than chronologic age or diagnosis emphasizes the child's abilities and strengths rather than disabilities. Attention is directed to normalizing experiences, adapting the environment, and promoting coping skills. Nurses often are in vital positions to redirect attention from the pathologic model with its focus on weaknesses and problems to the developmental model to meet the unique needs of the child and family.

A developmental focus also considers family development. The life cycle of the family unit reflects changing ages and needs of family members, as well as changing external demands. A family member's serious illness can cause significant stress or crisis at any stage of the family life cycle. Just as with individual development, family development may be interrupted or even regress to an earlier level of functioning. Nurses can use the concept of family development to plan meaningful interventions and evaluate care.

TABLE 36.1	Chronic Conditions of Childhood
Specialty	**Examples of Chronic Conditions**
Cardiology	Complex congenital heart disease, congestive heart failure, cardiac dysrhythmias, Kawasaki disease, rheumatic fever, hyperlipidemia
Endocrinology	Diabetes, congenital adrenal hyperplasia, Cushing syndrome
Gastroenterology	Short bowel syndrome, biliary atresia, inflammatory bowel disease, hepatitis, cirrhosis, peptic ulcer disease, celiac disease
Hematology	Sickle cell anemia, thalassemia, aplastic anemia, hereditary anemias, hemophilia
Immunology	Immune deficiency, human immunodeficiency virus, Wiskott-Aldrich syndrome, severe combined immunodeficiency disease
Nephrology	Prune belly syndrome, renal disease
Neurology	Cerebral palsy, ataxia telangiectasia, muscular dystrophy, seizure disorder, spina bifida, traumatic brain injury
Oncology	Brain tumor, leukemia, lymphoma, solid tumors, bone tumors, rare tumors
Pulmonology	Asthma, chronic lung disease, cystic fibrosis, tuberculosis
Rheumatology	Systemic lupus erythematosus, juvenile rheumatoid arthritis, dermatomyositis

Family-Centered Care

Children's physical and emotional health, as well as their cognitive and social functioning, is strongly influenced by how well their families function (Dunst & Trivette, 2009; Treyvaud, 2014; Kuhlthau, Bloom, Van Cleave, et al., 2011). The importance of family-centered care—a philosophy that considers the family as the constant in the child's life—is especially evident in the care of children with special needs (see Family-Centered Care box: Using Defining Characteristics to Select an Appropriate Nursing Diagnosis in Chapter 26. As parents learn about the child's health care needs, they often become experts in delivering care. Health care providers, including nurses, are adjuncts to the child's care and need to form partnerships with parents. Effective communication and negotiation between parents and nurses are essential to forming trusting and effective partnerships and finding the best ways to meet the needs of the child and family (Corlett and Twycross, 2006; Kuo, Houtrow, Arango, et al., 2012). Collaborative relationships are characterized by communication, dialogue, active listening, awareness, and acceptance of others' differences (Kuhlthau et al.).

Family–Health Care Provider Communication

The disclosure of a serious chronic or complex condition of a child is one of the most stressful aspects of communication between families and health care professionals. Often, parents have suspected for some time that something is wrong with their child and believe that their concerns were minimized or ignored by health care professionals (Smaldone & Ritholz, 2011; Thomlinson, 2002; Whitehead & Gosling, 2003). After a diagnosis is made, factors that influence parent dissatisfaction with the way in which information is communicated include disrespectful attitudes, breaking bad news in an insensitive manner, withholding information, and changing a treatment course without preparing the child and family (Barnes, Gardiner, Gott, et al., 2012; Hsiao, Evan & Zeltzer, 2007). Conversely, parents report satisfaction

when they perceived health care providers to be available, demonstrate competence, and engage the child and parent in care decision making (Barnes et al.; Hsiao et al., 2007; Kuo, Sisterhen, Sigrest, et al., 2012). Similar factors are important in communication of changes in the child's condition throughout the course of the illness.

Providing information to families with a chronically ill child should be a process of repeated discussions to allow the family to process the information and their reactions to that information and allow them to ask for clarification and further information. Nurses play an important role in ensuring that families' needs are met during discussions related to the child's diagnosis, condition, and treatment (Kavanaugh, Moro, & Savage, 2010). This requires assessment regarding how much information the family is comfortable with, what they understand of the information already given to them, and how they are coping with the information both cognitively and emotionally. Nurses should ensure that the appropriate health care professionals address any concerns or further questions that families may have.

Establishing Therapeutic Relationships

Another important aspect of family-centered care of children with chronic and complex conditions is establishing a therapeutic relationship with the child and family, which has been shown to predict improved health-related outcomes (Kuhlthau et al., 2011). Families, most often the mother, take on enormous responsibility in providing technical care and symptom management of their child's condition outside of the health care institution (Goudie et al., 2014; Raina, O'Donnell, Rosenbaum, et al., 2005). To build successful therapeutic relationships with families, it is necessary for nurses to recognize parents' expertise with regard to their child's condition and needs. Health care environments for children with serious illnesses are fraught with obstacles that serve as barriers to successful therapeutic relationships with families. Individual discussions, especially with the case manager, primary nurse, clinical nurse specialist, or nurse practitioner, help establish a consistent and flexible care plan that can prevent conflicts or deal with these conflicts before they disrupt care.

The Role of Culture in Family-Centered Care

Issues of culture, ethnicity, and race affect access to services, utilization, and follow-through with referrals and recommendations (Coker, Rodriguez & Flores, 2010; Toomey, Chien, Elliott, et al., 2013). For some ethnic and minority populations, cultural understandings of illness, the structure of family life, social roles for individuals with disabilities, and other factors related to the perception of children may differ from those of mainstream American culture.

Although culture cannot completely explain how an individual will think and act, understanding cultural perspectives can help the nurse anticipate and understand why families may make certain decisions. Cultural attributes such as values and beliefs regarding an illness or chronic condition and its causation, social roles for people who are ill or disabled, family structure, the role of children, childrearing practices, self versus group orientation, spirituality, and time orientation also affect a family's response to an illness or chronic condition in a child (Carnevale, Alexander, Davis, et al., 2006; Dell'Api, Rennick & Rosmus, 2007; Wiener, McConnell, Latella, et al., 2013).

When parents are informed of their child's chronic illness, interpreters familiar with both culture and language should be used. Children, family members, and friends of the family should not be used as translators, because their presence may prevent parents from openly discussing the issues. When working with people of cultural backgrounds different from their own, nurses must listen carefully with an initial goal of understanding and articulating the family's perspective. The ability to interpret the mainstream medical culture to the family is also important.

Furthermore, every effort is made to incorporate traditional cultural beliefs of a family into treatment plans. It is important to keep in mind that "cultural norms" may not always apply to every family from a shared background. Developing a care plan in conjunction with the family, considering their preferences and priorities, is an important first step in formulating a plan that best meets the family's needs, no matter what their cultural background (Coker et al., 2010; Thibodeaux & Deatrick, 2007; Wiener et al., 2013).

Shared Decision Making

Shared decision making among the child, family, and health care team can result from open, honest, culturally sensitive communication and the establishment of a therapeutic relationship among the family and health care providers. In a shared decision-making model, the health care professionals provide honest, clear information regarding diagnosis, prognosis, treatment options, and risk-benefit assessment. The patient and family then share information with the health care team regarding important family values, acceptable levels of discomfort or inconvenience, and the ability to comply with recommended treatments (Kon, 2010; Wiener et al., 2013; Wyatt, List, Brinkman, et al., 2015). This process allows them to discuss all options in terms of the risks and benefits to the child and family, the prognosis or expected course of the illness, and the impact on the family's resources (Box 36.1). Together, the parents and health care team can make decisions that are best for the family and child at the time the decision is made (Kon, 2010).

Normalization

Normalization refers to the efforts family members make to create a normal family life, their perceptions of the consequences of these efforts, and the meanings they attribute to their management efforts (Knafl, Darney, Gallo, et al., 2010). For chronically ill children, such efforts may include attending school, pursuing hobbies and recreational interests, and achieving employment and a level of independence. For their families, it may entail adapting the family routine to accommodate the ill or disabled child's health and physical needs (Kratz et al., 2009; Kuo et al., 2011).

Children with chronic and complex conditions and their families face numerous challenges in achieving normalization. Families move between the "normal" of living with the experience of chronic childhood illness and the "normal" of the healthy outside world; they often redefine "normal" based on their particular experiences, needs, and circumstances (Knafl et al., 2010; Nelson, 2002). Normalization may be an important mediator of illness-related stressors (e.g., treatment demands, uncertainty) on family outcomes.

Nurses can assist families in normalizing their lives by assessing the family's everyday life, social support systems, coping strategies, family cohesiveness, and family and community resources. Interventions include encouraging families to reduce stress through delegation of care and family tasks, identifying ways to incorporate care into current routines, structuring the home environment to encourage the child's engagement in age-appropriate activities, and ensuring that families have access to appropriate community support services (Jokinen, 2004; Knafl & Santacroce, 2010). Being supportive of the child's illness and treatment and actively including the family in all aspects of care will improve their self-esteem and promote further development (Jones & Prinz, 2005; Knafl & Santacroce).

Home care represents the return to a system and set of priorities in which family values are as important in the care of a child with a chronic health problem as they are in the care of other children. Home care seeks to achieve goals that are consistent with the developmental model (Stein, 1985):

- Normalize the life of the child, including those with technologically complex care, in a family and community context and setting.
- Minimize the disruptive impact of the child's condition on the family.
- Foster the child's maximum growth and development.

With appropriate training and support, families provide complex procedures and treatments in the home. Parents are challenged to retain a homelike setting among monitors, ventilators, and other sophisticated equipment. Throughout the text, home care is discussed as appropriate for specific conditions. The process of transition from hospital to home is elaborated on in Chapter 38.

Paralleling normalization and home care is the process of **mainstreaming**, or integrating children with disabilities into regular classrooms. Children who attend school have the advantages of learning and socializing with a wide group of peers. There is an increased focus on individualization as plans are made to meet the academic needs of these children along with those of the rest of the students.

A variety of supplemental programs have been designed in the school system to accommodate special needs, both at school age and younger, through **early intervention**, which consists of any sustained and systematic effort to assist children from birth to 3 years of age with disabilities and who are developmentally vulnerable. This change and increasing opportunities for normalization for children with disabilities in large part have resulted from the passage of (1) the Education for All Handicapped Children Act of 1975 (Public Law 94-142) and its 1990 amendments (Public Law 101-476), which changed the name of the Act to the Individuals with Disabilities Education Act (IDEA); (2) the Education of the Handicapped Act Amendments of 1986 (Public Law 99-457), which directs states to develop and implement statewide comprehensive, coordinated, multidisciplinary interagency programs of early intervention services for infants and toddlers with disabilities, as well as support services for their families; and (3) the Americans with Disabilities Act of 1990. Nurses can provide parents with information about these laws and in some cases may participate in the development of individualized educational programs (IEPs) or individualized family service plans (IFSPs) for children with disabilities.

THE FAMILY OF THE CHILD WITH A CHRONIC OR COMPLEX CONDITION

A major goal in working with the family of a child with chronic or complex illness is to support the family's coping and promote their optimal functioning throughout the child's life. Long-term, comprehensive care involves forming parent-professional partnerships that can support a family's adaptation across the trajectory of the illness to the many changes that may be necessary in day-to-day life, determine expectations of and for the child, and provide a long-term perspective (Box 36.2).

Often the impact of a child's medical or developmental condition is first experienced as a crisis at the time of diagnosis, which may occur

---

BOX 36.1 Facilitating Shared Decision Making

- Continually assess the impact of the child's illness and treatment on the family.
- Provide honest, accurate information regarding the trajectory of the disease, anticipated complications, and prognostic information.
- Discuss what the family desires for the child's quality of life.
- Avoid personal opinion or judgment of the family's questions and decisions.
- Be aware of nurses' personal and cultural assumptions and the ways these assumptions impact communication, decision making, and judgment.

From Canam, C. (1993). Common adaptive tasks facing parents of children with chronic conditions. *Journal of Advanced Nursing, 18,* 46–53.

BOX 36.2   Adaptive Tasks of Parents Having Children With Chronic Conditions

1. Accept the child's condition.
2. Manage the child's condition on a day-to-day basis.
3. Meet the child's normal developmental needs.
4. Meet the developmental needs of other family members.
5. Cope with ongoing stress and periodic crises.
6. Assist family members to manage their feelings.
7. Educate others about the child's condition.
8. Establish a support system.

BOX 36.3   Anticipated Parental Stress Points

Diagnosis of the condition: Parents require considerable education while dealing with an emotional response.
Developmental milestones: Times that children normally achieve walking, talking, and self-care are delayed or impossible for the child.
Start of schooling: Particularly stressful are situations in which appropriate schooling will not be in a regular class placement.
Reaching the ultimate attainment: Parents must handle situations such as realizing that ambulation will be impossible or that the child will not learn to read.
Adolescence: Issues such as sexuality and independence become prominent.
Future placement: Decisions about placement must be made when the child becomes an adult or when the parents can no longer care for the child.
Death of the child

at birth, after a long period of diagnostic testing, or immediately after a tragic injury. But the impact may also be felt before the diagnosis is made, when parents are aware that something is wrong with their child but before medical confirmation (Smaldone & Ritholz, 2011; Thomlinson, 2002; Whitehead & Gosling, 2003).

The diagnosis and initial discharge home are critical times for parents (Coffey, 2006). Several factors can make this particularly difficult, including a long duration of uncertainty in the diagnostic process, negative perceptions of chronic illness, insufficient information, and lack of mutual trust between parents and their child's health care team (Huang, Kenzik, Sanjeev, et al., 2010; LeGrow, Hodnett, Stremler, et al., 2014; Monterosso, Kristjanson, Aoun, et al., 2007; Nuutila & Salanterä, 2006). Parental feelings of shock, helplessness, isolation, fear, and depression are common (Coffey, 2006; Nuutila & Salanterä, 2006). Throughout the first year, parents struggle to accept the child's diagnosis, care, and uncertainty of the future (Coffey, 2006). Optimal support at the time of diagnosis and initial discharge home can be encouraged by providing explicit and uncomplicated information to parents in an empathic way (Nuutila & Salanterä, 2006); assessing the family's daily routine, living conditions, background knowledge, skills and abilities, and coping behaviors; and evaluating the family's understanding of the information. It is also necessary to reassess parents' needs for information and support on a routine basis (Nuutila & Salanterä, 2006).

Other critical times include the exacerbation of the child's physical symptoms, which increases parental care. These crises often involve medical intervention and rehospitalization. Frequently, the child does not return to his or her precrisis level of functioning, and parents and family must adapt to new care needs and schedules. Instability may also follow transition points on the illness trajectory. Supporting parents, respecting their stress and emotions, and acknowledging their role as team members in the care of their child are important aspects of nursing care (Coffey, 2006; Nuutila & Salanterä, 2006; Panicker, 2013).

IMPACT OF THE CHILD'S CHRONIC ILLNESS

Each member in the family of a child with a chronic or complex illness is affected by the experience (Goudie et al., 2014; Kuo et al., 2011; Sullivan-Bolyai, Sadler, Knafl, et al., 2003). The effects on the parents and their responses may be so intense that they directly influence the other members' reactions and the child's own coping.

Parents

In addition to the stress of grieving for the loss of hope for a perfect child, parents are affected by whether or not they receive positive feedback from interactions with their child. Many parents feel satisfaction and fulfillment from the parenting role. For others, parenting may be a

series of unrewarding experiences that contribute to feelings of inadequacy and failure (Box 36.3). These responses may be most evident in parents who are responsible for the child's care. For example, parents may become preoccupied with their ability to carry out certain procedures, overlooking the child's personal comfort and satisfaction, or failing to offer praise for anything less than perfect cooperation or performance. They may pursue a frustrating activity until they achieve "success"—long after the child has become irritable and uncooperative. As a result, parents can become caught in a pattern of interaction that is mutually unrewarding and minimally productive. This situation may become exacerbated by disagreements or lack of support from other family members and judgment from caregivers and others in the community. For these parents, several strategies may be helpful, including education regarding what can reasonably be expected of their child, assistance in identifying the child's strengths, praise for a parental job well done, and respite care so that parents can renew their energies.

Parental Roles

Parenting a child with a complex chronic condition requires attending to the routine aspects of parenting with the added responsibility of performing complex technical care, symptom management, advocating for their child, and seeking and coordinating health and social services for their ill or disabled child (Kirk, Glendinning & Callery, 2005). These added responsibilities must then be balanced with the needs of other family members, extended family and friends, and personal health and obligations to minimize consequences to the overall functioning of the family (Coffey, 2006).

Often one parent or partner remains at home to manage existing family responsibilities, while the other remains with the ill child. The partner who is not included in the caregiving activities may feel neglected because all of the attention is directed toward the child and be resentful that he or she is not sufficiently informed to be competent in the care. Without active participation in the child's care, the parent has little appreciation of the time and energy involved in performing these activities. When this partner does attempt to participate, the other parent may criticize the less skillful efforts. As a result, communication and support for each other may be adversely affected.

The nurse can assist parents in avoiding role conflicts by providing anticipatory guidance early on. Teaching should address stressors often identified as having an impact on the marriage, including (1) the burden of care at home assumed by primarily one parent, (2) the financial burden, (3) the fear of the child dying, (4) pressure from relatives, (5) the hereditary nature of the disease (if applicable), and (6) fear of pregnancy. Other causes of tension may center on the inconveniences associated with care, such as long waits for an appointment, lack of parking near care facilities, or lack of overnight accommodations.

Mother-Father Differences

Mothers and fathers of a child with a complex condition often adjust and cope differently. Mothers are often the primary caregiver and are more likely than fathers to give up their jobs to care for their children, often resulting in social isolation (Coffey, 2006). Mothers often have greater needs for social support and positive appraisal of the situation than fathers.

Fathers of children with disabilities struggle with issues that may be distinct from those of the mothers (Swallow, Macfadyen, Santacroce, et al., 2012). Fathers may think that their role as protector is challenged, because they do not know how to help and cannot protect their family from the seemingly overwhelming recurring problems. The extensive stresses in the family can leave fathers feeling depressed, weak, guilty, powerless, isolated, embarrassed, and angry. Fearful that they will lose control or be viewed as weak or ineffectual, however, fathers often hide their feelings and display an outward confidence that may lead others to believe that everything is fine. Fathers worry about what the future holds for their children, their ability to manage the increasing financial burden, and the daily disruptions of the entire family (Davies, Gudmundsdottir, Worden, et al., 2004; Swallow et al.).

Single-Parent Families

Single-parent families are of special concern. As the only parent of a child who may require extensive, sophisticated, and lifelong care, the single parent may feel an enormous burden. Available financial and emotional resources may already be stretched to the limit. A special effort should be made to assist the single parent in finding financial and support services that can ease the burden of care. Nurses can also assist the single parent in identifying helping roles that may be acceptable to relatives and friends.

Siblings

Results of studies are less clear regarding the ways that siblings are affected by having a brother or sister with a complex condition (Anderson & Davis, 2011; Barlow & Ellard, 2006; Hartling et al., 2014; O'Brien, Duffy & Nicholl, 2009). Most evidence shows a negative effect on siblings of children with chronic illnesses compared with siblings of healthy children (Gold, Treadwell, Weissman, et al., 2011; Hartling et al.). Siblings of children with chronic illnesses report psychosocial problems more often than their peers (Gold et al.; O'Brien et al.). A number of factors increase the risk of negative effects for siblings of ill children. Responsibility for caregiving, differential treatment by parents, and limitations in family resources and recreational time are often the experiences of siblings of ill or disabled children (Lobato & Kao, 2002) (Box 36.4).

An important factor in sibling adjustment and coping is information and knowledge regarding their brother's or sister's illness or complex condition. What siblings piece together or overhear is often much worse than the truth. Often they imagine gruesome things regarding the experiences related to the illness, treatment, and hospitalization (Knafl & Santacroce, 2010). Latino siblings have reported less accurate information about their siblings' condition than non-Latino siblings (Lobato, Kao, & Plante, 2005). Parents are usually in the best position to impart information, although they are often overwhelmed with the medical crisis at hand (Fleitas, 2000). Nurses can encourage parents to talk with

---

BOX 36.4　Supporting Siblings of Children With Special Needs

Promote Healthy Sibling Relationships

Value each child individually, and avoid comparisons. Remind each child of his or her positive qualities and contribution to other family members.

Help siblings see the differences and similarities between themselves and the child with special needs. Create a climate in which children can achieve successes without feeling guilty.

Teach siblings ways to interact with the child.

Seek to be fair in terms of discipline, attention, and resources; require the affected child to do as much for himself or herself as possible.

Let siblings settle their own differences; intervene only to prevent siblings from hurting one another.

Legitimize reasonable anger. Even children with special needs behave badly sometimes.

Respect a sibling's reluctance to be with or to include the child with special needs in activities.

Help Siblings Cope

Listen to siblings to let them know that their thoughts and suggestions are valued.

Praise siblings when they have been patient, have sacrificed, or have been particularly helpful. Do not expect siblings to always act in this manner.

Acknowledge the personal strengths siblings have and their ability to cope with stress successfully.

Provide age-appropriate information about the child's condition, and update it when appropriate.

Let teachers know what is happening so that they can be understanding and helpful.

Recognize special stress times for siblings, and plan to minimize negative effects.

Schedule special time with siblings; have a friend or family member substitute when parent is unavailable.

Encourage siblings to join or help establish a sibling support group.

Use the services of professionals when needed. If parent feels that such a service is necessary, it should be provided in as vigorous a manner as a service for the child with special needs.

Involve Siblings

Seek out ways to realistically include siblings in the care and treatment of the child with special needs.

Limit caregiving responsibilities, and give recognition when siblings perform them.

Develop a library of children's books on special needs.

Invite siblings to attend meetings to develop plans for the child with special needs (e.g., individualized educational program [IEP], individualized family service plan [IFSP]).

Discuss future plans with siblings.

Solicit their ideas on treatment and service needs.

Have siblings visit professionals who work with the child.

Help siblings develop competencies to teach the child new skills.

Provide opportunities for siblings to advocate for the child.

Allow siblings to set their own pace for learning and involvement.

Data from Powell, T., & Ogle, P. (1985). *Brothers and sisters—A special part of exceptional families.* Baltimore, MD: Paul H Brooks; Spokane Washington Deaconess Medical Center, Pediatric Oncology Unit. (1987). Tips for dealing with siblings. *Candlelighters Childhood Cancer Foundation Quarterly Newsletter, 11*(3,4), 7; Carlson, J., Leviton, A., & Mueller, M. (1993). Services to siblings: An important component of family-centered practice. *ACCH Advocate, 1*(1), 53–56.

the siblings about how they perceive their sick brother or sister and to be accepting of the siblings' feelings. Nurses can be ideal educators and counselors of siblings during the course of their brother's or sister's illness.

COPING WITH ONGOING STRESS AND PERIODIC CRISES

Professionals can help families cope with stress by providing anticipatory guidance, providing emotional support, assisting the family in assessing and identifying specific stressors, aiding the family in developing coping mechanisms and problem-solving strategies, and working collaboratively with parents so that they become empowered in the process (Anderson & Davis, 2011).

Concurrent Stresses Within the Family

The ability to deal with the overwhelming stress of a chronic illness is challenged further when additional stresses are present. Stressors may be situational or developmental. They may be related to marital difficulties, sibling needs, homelessness, or social isolation. Some families may simultaneously be struggling with a family member's alcohol or other drug problem. Even relatively minor stressors, such as arranging care for siblings, managing the home, and traveling to distant treatment centers, can challenge a family's ability to cope successfully.

Most families, regardless of their income or insurance coverage, have financial concerns. The costs of caring for a child with a complex illness can be overwhelming. Nurses and social workers can help a family review various options for financial assistance, including insurance, managed care, or health maintenance organization policies; Medicaid; Supplemental Security Income; the Women, Infants, and Children program; the state Program for Children with Special Health Needs; disease-related associations; and local philanthropic organizations.

Coping Mechanisms

Coping mechanisms are behaviors aimed at reducing the tension caused by a crisis. Approach behaviors are coping mechanisms that result in movement toward adjustment and resolution of the crisis. Avoidance behaviors result in movement away from adjustment and represent maladaptation to the crisis. Several approach and avoidance behaviors used in coping with a chronic illness are listed in the Guidelines box: Assessing Coping Behaviors. Each behavior must be viewed in the context of all of the variables affecting the family. For example, the observation of several avoidance behaviors in an emotionally healthy family may denote significantly less risk to the successful resolution of the crisis than an equal number of avoidance behaviors in an individual who has few available supports.

Parental Empowerment

Empowerment can be seen as a process of recognizing, promoting, and enhancing competence. For parents of children with chronic conditions, empowerment may occur gradually as strength and capabilities are drawn on to master the child's care, manage family life, and plan for the future. Advocating for the child and developing parent-professional partnerships are part of taking charge (Panicker, 2013).

ASSISTING FAMILY MEMBERS IN MANAGING THEIR FEELINGS

Although some previous research has postulated stages of adaptation to a chronic illness, there is a great deal of individual variation in responses to the diagnosis, adjustments made, and time frames for coming to terms with a diagnosis. It is important that professionals

GUIDELINES

Assessing Coping Behaviors

Approach Behaviors

Asks for information regarding diagnosis and child's present condition

Seeks help and support from others

Anticipates future problems; actively seeks guidance and answers

Endows the chronic illness or complex condition with meaning

Shares burden of disorder with others

Plans realistically for the future

Acknowledges and accepts child's awareness of diagnosis and prognosis

Expresses feelings (e.g., sorrow, depression, and anger) and realizes reason for the emotional reaction

Realistically perceives child's condition; adjusts to changes

Recognizes own growth through passage of time, such as earlier denial and nonacceptance of diagnosis

Verbalizes possible loss of child

Avoidance Behaviors

Fails to recognize seriousness of child's condition despite physical evidence

Refuses to agree to treatment

Intellectualizes about the illness but in areas unrelated to child's condition

Is angry and hostile to members of the staff regardless of their attitude or behavior

Avoids staff, family members, or child

Entertains unrealistic future plans for child with little emphasis on the present

Is unable to adjust to or accept a change in progression of disease

Continually looks for new cures with no perspective toward possible benefit

Refuses to acknowledge child's understanding of disease and prognosis

Uses magical thinking and fantasy; may seek "occult" help

Places complete faith in religion to point of relinquishing own responsibility

Withdraws from outside world; refuses help

Punishes self because of guilt and blame

Makes no change in lifestyle to meet needs of other family members

Resorts to excessive use of alcohol or drugs to avoid problems

Verbalizes suicidal intent

Is unable to discuss possible loss of child or previous experiences with death

recognize and respect a wide range of reactions and coping mechanisms. In fact, members of the family of a child with a complex chronic condition may experience a number of difficult emotions, including fear, guilt, anger, resentment, and anxiety. Learning to manage these emotions promotes adaptive coping (see Guidelines box: Encouraging Expression of Emotion). Support from professionals, other family members, and friends can assist family members in managing their feelings. The following discussion examines some common phases of adjustment and emotional reactions.

Shock and Denial

The initial diagnosis of a chronic illness or complex condition is often met with intense emotion and is characterized by shock, disbelief, and sometimes denial. Denial as a defense mechanism is a necessary cushion to prevent disintegration and is a normal response to grieving for any type of loss. Probably all family members experience various degrees of adaptive denial as they learn of the impact that the diagnosis has on their lives.

Shock and denial can last from days to months, sometimes even longer. Examples of denial that may be exhibited at the time of diagnosis include the following:

- Physician shopping
- Attributing the symptoms of the actual illness to a minor condition

- Refusing to believe the diagnostic tests
- Delaying consent for treatment
- Acting happy and optimistic despite the revealed diagnosis
- Refusing to tell or talk to anyone about the condition
- Insisting that no one is telling the truth, regardless of others' attempts to do so
- Denying the reason for admission
- Asking no questions about the diagnosis, treatment, or prognosis

Generally, these mechanisms should be respected as short-term responses that allow individuals to distance themselves from the tremendous emotional impact and to collect and mobilize their energies toward goal-directed, problem-solving behaviors.

In children, the importance of denial has repeatedly been demonstrated as a factor in their positive coping with the diagnosis. Denial allows the child to maintain hope in the face of overwhelming odds and to function adaptively and productively. Similar to hope, denial may be an adaptive mechanism for dealing with loss that persists until a family or patient is ready or needs other responses.

Denial is probably the least understood and most poorly dealt-with reaction. If denial is labeled as maladaptive, it can lead to inappropriate attempts to strip away the reaction by repeated and sometimes blunt explanations of the prognosis. However, denial becomes maladaptive only when it prevents recognition of treatment or rehabilitative goals necessary for the child's optimal survival or development.

Adjustment

For most families, adjustment gradually follows shock and is usually characterized by an open admission that the condition exists. This stage may be accompanied by several responses, which are normal parts of the adaptation process. Probably the most universal of these feelings are guilt and self-accusation. Guilt is often greatest when the cause of the disorder is directly traceable to the parent, as in genetic diseases or accidental injury. However, it can occur even without any scientific or realistic basis for parental responsibility. Frequently, the guilt stems from a false assumption that the child's condition is a result of personal failure or wrongdoing, such as not doing something correctly during pregnancy or the birth. Guilt may also be associated with cultural or religious beliefs. Some parents are convinced that they are being punished for some previous misdeed. Others may see the illness as a trial sent by God to test their religious strength and faith. With correct information, support, and time, most parents master guilt and self-accusation.

Children, too, may interpret their serious illness as retribution for past misbehavior. The nurse should be particularly sensitive to the child who passively accepts all painful procedures. This child may believe that such acts are inflicted as deserved punishment. It is vital that parents and health care professionals reassure children that their illnesses are not their fault.

Other common and normal reactions to a diagnosis are bitterness and anger. Anger directed inward may be evident as self-reproaching or punitive behavior, such as neglecting one's health and verbally degrading oneself. Anger directed outward may be manifested in either open arguments or withdrawal from communication and may be evident in the person's relationship with any number of individuals, such as the spouse, the child, and siblings. Passive anger toward the ill child may be evident in decreased visiting, refusal to believe how sick the child is, or an inability to provide comfort. Health care providers are among the most common targets for parental anger. Parents may complain about the nursing care, the insufficient time physicians spend with them, or the lack of skill of those who draw blood or start intravenous infusions.

Children are apt to respond with anger as well, and this includes the affected child and the well siblings. Children are aware of the loss engendered by their illness or complex condition and may react angrily to the restrictions imposed or the feelings of being different. Siblings may also feel anger and resentment toward the ill child and parents for the loss of routine and parental attention. It is difficult for older children and almost impossible for younger children to comprehend the plight of the affected child. Their perception is of a brother or sister who has the undivided attention of their parents, is showered with cards and gifts, and is the focus of everyone's concern.

During the period of adjustment, four types of parental reactions to the child influence the child's eventual response to the disorder:

- **Overprotection:** The parents fear letting the child achieve any new skill, avoid all discipline, and cater to every desire to prevent frustration.
- **Rejection:** The parents detach themselves emotionally from the child but usually provide adequate physical care or constantly nag and scold the child.
- **Denial:** The parents act as if the disorder does not exist or attempt to have the child overcompensate for it.
- **Gradual acceptance:** The parents place necessary and realistic restrictions on the child, encourage self-care activities, and promote reasonable physical and social abilities.

Reintegration and Acknowledgment

For many families, the adjustment process culminates in the development of realistic expectations for the child and reintegration of family life with the illness or complex condition in a manageable perspective. Because a large portion of this phase is one of grief for a loss, total resolution is not possible until the child dies or leaves home as an independent adult. Therefore, one can regard adjustment as "increased comfort" with everyday living rather than a complete resolution.

This adjustment phase also involves social reintegration in which the family broadens its activities to include relationships outside of the home with the child as an acceptable and participating member of the group. This last criterion often differentiates the reaction of gradual acceptance during the adjustment period from total acceptance or perhaps is more descriptive of the acknowledgment process.

Many parents of children with chronic illnesses experience **chronic sorrow**, which are feelings of sorrow and loss that recur in waves over time. As the child's condition progresses, parents experience repeated losses that represent further declines and new caregiving demands. Consequently, families must be assessed on an ongoing basis and offered appropriate support and resources as their needs change over time (Bettle & Latimer, 2009; Gordon, 2009). This represents a critical period of time because the nursing and medical team approach and support provided during this period of time can directly impact the experience of complicated grief after the death of the child. Complicated grief, which is characterized as persistent distress and chronic stress response, may last 6 months or longer after the death of a child and has a significant impact on quality of life of the family left behind (Meert, Shear, Newth, et al., 2011). *Persistent complex bereavement disorder* is a new diagnostic entity included in the fifth edition of the *Diagnostic and Statistical Manual of Mental Disorders* (American Psychological Association, 2013).

ESTABLISHING A SUPPORT SYSTEM

The diagnosis of a child with a complex chronic condition is a major situational crisis that affects the entire family system. However, families can experience positive outcomes as they successfully deal with the many challenges that accompany a child with chronic illness (Hungerbuehler, Vollrath & Landolt, 2011).

One nursing goal is to assess which families are at risk for succumbing to the effects of the crisis. Several variables—available support system,

---

BOX 36.5   Concept of Functional Burden

Impact of the Child With Special Needs
The child's need for medical and nursing care
The child's fixed deficits
The child's age-appropriate dependency in activities of daily living
The disruptions in the family routine caused by the care
The psychologic burden of the prognosis on the family

Family Resources and Ability to Cope
The family's physical resources
The family's emotional resources
The family's educational resources
The family's social supports and available help
The competing demands for family members' time and energy

Data from Stein, R.E.K. (1985). Home care: A challenging opportunity. *Child Health Care, 14*(2), 90–95.

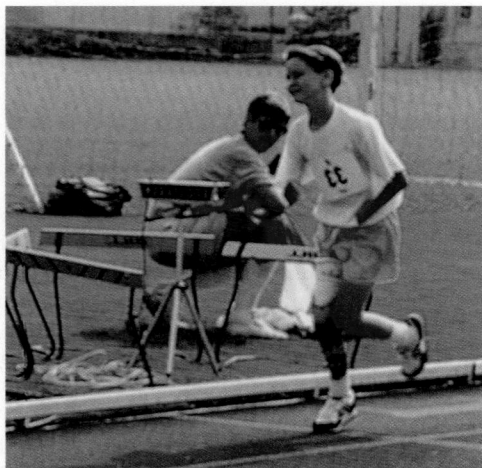

FIG 36.1 Children with any type of impairment should have the opportunity to develop their skills. (Courtesy of Poyo/Hinton Photography.)

---

perception of the event, coping mechanisms, reactions to the child, available resources, and concurrent stresses within the family—influence the resolution of a crisis. Although most families cope well, the needs of families at risk are great. If they receive emotional support and guidance early, there is an increased likelihood that they will also cope successfully.

Although it is easy to assume that families of children with the most severe illnesses or disabilities would have the poorest adjustment, the severity of the condition reflects only one part of the overall picture. The level of adjustment is significantly influenced by the **functional burden** on the family (Stein, 1985). This concept considers the issues related to caring for and living with the child in relation to the family's resources and ability to cope (Box 36.5). The family of a child with a high level of technology dependence demanding complex care yet having many resources and coping skills may adjust more successfully to the child's situation than the family of a child with a less serious condition and few resources to counterbalance.

Intrafamilial resources, social support from friends and relatives, parent-to-parent support, parent/professional partnerships, and community resources interweave to provide a flexible web of support for families of children with chronic conditions.

THE CHILD WITH A CHRONIC OR COMPLEX CONDITION

The child's reaction to chronic illness depends to a great extent on his or her developmental level, temperament, and available coping mechanisms; on the reactions of family members or significant others; and, to a lesser extent, on the condition itself. A child's conceptual understanding of his or her own illness is based not only on age and developmental level but also on the duration and type of experience accumulated with the disease. Knowledge of these variables is essential in providing the kind of information and support needed by these children to cope with an often overwhelming situation.

DEVELOPMENTAL ASPECTS

The impact of a complex chronic illness is influenced by the age at onset. Chronic illness affects children of all ages, but the developmental aspects of each age group dictate particular stresses and risks for the child. The nurse must also recognize that children need to redefine their condition and its implications as they develop and grow. For example, appearance, skills, and abilities are highly valued by peers

(Fig. 36.1). A teenager who is limited in any of these qualities is subject to rejection. This is especially marked when an illness interferes with sexual attractiveness. An understanding of these developmental factors facilitates planning care to support the child and minimize the risks. Developmental aspects of chronic illness on children are described in Table 36.2.

COPING MECHANISMS

Children with chronic conditions tend to use five distinct patterns of coping (Box 36.6). Children with more positive and accepting attitudes about their chronic illness use a more adaptive coping style characterized by optimism, competence, and compliance. They show fewer behavior problems at home and at school. The two maladaptive coping patterns— "Feels different and withdraws" and "Is irritable, is moody, and acts out"—are associated with poorer adaptation; children using these strategies have poorer self-concepts, more negative attitudes about their conditions, and more behavior problems at home and at school.

Well-adapted children gradually learn to accept their physical limitations and find achievement in a variety of compensatory motor and intellectual pursuits. They function well at home, at school, and with peers. They have an understanding of their disorder that allows them to accept their limitations, assume responsibility for their care, and assist in treatment and rehabilitation regimens. They express appropriate emotions, such as sadness, anxiety, and anger, at times of exacerbations but confidence and guarded optimism during periods of clinical stability (Fig. 36.2). They are able to identify with other similarly affected individuals, promoting positive self-images and displaying pride and self-confidence in their ability to master a productive, successful life despite their illnesses.

Hopefulness

Children, particularly adolescents, are sensitive to the presence or absence of hope. Hopefulness is an internal quality that mobilizes humans into goal-directed action that may be satisfying and life sustaining. A sense of hopefulness can produce increased participation in health-seeking behaviors and an improved sense of well-being (Ritchie, 2001).

Health Education and Self-Care

Health education is an intervention that promotes coping. Children need information about their condition, the therapeutic plan, and how

TABLE 36.2	Developmental Effects of Chronic Illness or Disability on Children	
Developmental Tasks	Potential Effects of Chronic Illness or Disability	Supportive Interventions
Infancy		
Develop a sense of trust	Multiple caregivers and frequent separations, especially if hospitalized	Encourage consistent caregivers in hospital or other care settings.
	Deprived of consistent nurturing	Encourage parental presence, "rooming in" during hospitalization, and participation in care.
Bond, or attach, to parent	Delayed because of separation; parental grief for loss of "dream" child; parental inability to accept the condition, especially a visible defect	Emphasize healthy, perfect qualities of infant. Help parents learn special care needs of infant for them to feel competent.
Learn through sensorimotor experiences	More exposure to painful experiences than pleasurable ones	Expose infant to pleasurable experiences through all senses (touch, hearing, sight, taste, movement).
	Limited contact with environment from restricted movement or confinement	Encourage age-appropriate developmental skills (e.g., holding bottle, finger feeding, crawling).
Begin to develop a sense of separateness from parent	Increased dependency on parent for care	Encourage all family members to participate in care to prevent overinvolvement of one member.
	Overinvolvement of parent in care	Encourage periodic respite from demands of care responsibilities.
Toddlerhood		
Develop autonomy	Increased dependency on parent	Encourage independence in as many areas as possible (e.g., toileting, dressing, feeding).
Master locomotor and language skills	Limited opportunity to test own abilities and limits	Provide gross motor skill activity and modification of toys or equipment, such as modified swing or rocking horse.
Learn through sensorimotor experience; beginning preoperational thought	Increased exposure to painful experiences	Give choices to allow simple feeling of control (e.g., choice of what book to look at, what kind of sandwich to eat). Institute age-appropriate discipline and limit setting. Recognize that negative and ritualistic behaviors are normal. Provide sensory experiences (e.g., water play, sandbox play, finger painting).
Preschool Age		
Develop initiative and purpose Master self-care skills	Limited opportunities for success in accomplishing simple tasks or mastering self-care skills	Encourage mastery of self-help skills. Provide devices that make tasks easier (e.g., self-dressing).
Begin to develop peer relationships	Limited opportunities for socialization with peers; may appear "like a baby" to age mates	Encourage socialization (e.g., inviting friends to play, day care experience, trips to park). Provide age-appropriate play, especially associative play opportunities. Emphasize child's abilities; dress appropriately to enhance desirable appearance.
	Protection within tolerant and secure family, causing child to fear criticism and withdraw	
Develop sense of body image and sexual identification	Awareness of body centering on pain, anxiety, and failure	Encourage relationships with same-sex and opposite-sex peers and adults.
	Sex-role identification focused primarily on mothering skills	
Learn through preoperational thought (magical thinking)	Guilt (thinking he or she caused the illness or disability or is being punished for wrongdoing)	Help child deal with criticisms; realize that too much protection prevents child from realities of world. Clarify that cause of child's illness or disability is not his or her fault or a punishment.
School Age		
Develop a sense of accomplishment	Limited opportunities to achieve and compete (e.g., many school absences, inability to join regular athletic activities)	Encourage school attendance; schedule medical visits at times other than school; encourage child to make up missed work.

Continued

TABLE 36.2   Developmental Effects of Chronic Illness or Disability on Children—cont'd

Developmental Tasks	Potential Effects of Chronic Illness or Disability	Supportive Interventions
Form peer relationships	Limited opportunities for socialization	Educate teachers and classmates about child's condition, abilities, and special needs. Encourage sports activities (e.g., Special Olympics). Encourage socialization (e.g., Girl Scouts, Campfire, Boy Scouts, 4-H Club; having a best friend or club membership).
Learn through concrete operations	Incomplete comprehension of the imposed physical limitations or treatment of the disorder	Provide child with information about his or her condition. Encourage creative activities (e.g., VSA Arts).
Adolescence		
Develop personal and sexual identity	Increased sense of feeling different from peers and reduced ability to compete with peers in appearance, abilities, special skills	Help child realize that many of the difficulties the teenager is experiencing are part of normal adolescence (rebelliousness, risk taking, lack of cooperation, hostility toward authority).
Achieve independence from family	Increased dependency on family; limited job or career opportunities	Provide instruction on interpersonal and coping skills. Encourage increased responsibility for care and management of the disease or condition (e.g., assuming responsibility for making and keeping appointment [ideally alone], sharing assessment and planning stages of health care delivery, contacting resources). Discuss planning for future and how condition can affect choices.
Form heterosexual relationships	Limited opportunities for heterosexual friendships; less opportunity to discuss sexual concerns with peers Increased concern with issues such as why did he or she get the disorder and whether he or she will marry and have a family	Encourage socialization with peers, including peers with special needs and those without special needs. Encourage activities appropriate for age (e.g., attending mixed-sex parties, sports activities, driving a car). Be alert to cues that signal readiness for information regarding implications of condition on sexuality and reproduction. Emphasize good appearance and wearing stylish clothes, use of makeup. Understand that adolescent has same sexual needs and concerns as any other teenager.
Learn through abstract thinking	Decreased opportunity for earlier stages of cognition impeding achievement of level of abstract thinking	Provide instruction on decision making, assertiveness, and other skills necessary to manage personal plans.

BOX 36.6   Coping Patterns Used by Children With Special Needs

Develops competence and optimism: Accentuates the positive aspects of the situation and concentrates more on what he or she has or can do than on what is missing or on what he or she cannot do; is as independent as possible

Feels different and withdraws: Sees self as being different from other children because of the chronic health condition; views being different as negative; sees self as less worthy than others; focuses on things he or she cannot do, and sometimes overrestricts activities needlessly

Is irritable, is moody, and acts out: Uses proactive and self-initiated coping behaviors, although usually counterproductive in that the behaviors are not ego enhancing or socially responsible and do not result in desired outcomes; acts out irritability, which may or may not be associated with condition's symptoms

Complies with treatment: Takes necessary medications, treatments; adheres to activity restrictions; also uses behaviors that indicate developing independence (e.g., assumes responsibility for taking medication)

Seeks support: Talks with adults, children, physicians, and nurses; develops plans to handle problems as they occur; uses downward comparison (i.e., realizes that others have it worse)

Modified from Austin, J., Patterson, J., & Huberty, T. (1991). Development of the coping health inventory for children. *Journal of Pediatric Nursing, 6*(3), 166–174.

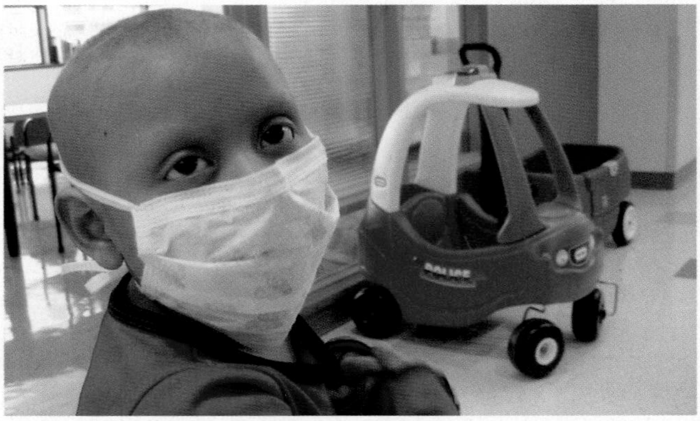

FIG 36.2 Periods of sadness and anger are appropriate in the child's adjustment to a chronic illness or disability, especially during exacerbations of the disorder.

the disease or the therapy might affect their particular situation. Children nearing puberty also need to understand the maturation process and how their chronic illness may alter this event. For example, a youngster with Crohn disease should understand that this disorder is associated with growth failure and delayed puberty, a child with diabetes needs to know that hormonal changes and increased growth needs will alter food and insulin requirements at this time, and a sexually active girl with sickle cell anemia or systemic lupus erythematosus needs to be aware of the risks of pregnancy. The information should not be given all at once but should be timed appropriately to meet their changing needs, and it should be described and repeated as often as the situation demands.

RESPONSES TO PARENTAL BEHAVIOR

Parental behavior toward the child is one of the most important factors influencing the child's adjustment. Children's perceptions of their mothers' support and maternal perceptions of the psychosocial impact of the child's chronic illness on the family were shown to be two of the greatest predictors of children's psychologic adjustment (Immelt, 2006). In addition, family organization, illness-related support, and involvement of the parents influence children's adjustment to chronic illness (Schor, 2003). They often display pride and confidence in their ability to cope successfully with the challenges imposed by their disorder. Anticipatory guidance by the nurse and encouragement of normalizing practices may assist parents in facilitating positive adjustment in their children.

TYPE OF ILLNESS OR CONDITION

The type of illness or condition also influences the child's emotional response. Interestingly, children with *more* severe disorders often cope better than those with milder conditions. However, the presence of multiple conditions may place a child at risk for more behavioral problems (Newacheck & Halfon, 1998). Because of children's cognitive ability and the timing of onset of abstract thinking in adolescence, an obvious condition may be easier for them to accept because its limitations are concrete.

The onset of a disabling condition may generate a state of confusion for children, who may have trouble differentiating between actual bodily functions and their image of their bodies. They may also experience problems in identifying themselves and those extensions of self (e.g., wheelchairs, braces, crutches, other mechanical or prosthetic devices) and may have difficulty in accepting functional aids.

NURSING CARE OF THE FAMILY AND CHILD WITH A CHRONIC OR COMPLEX CONDITION

ASSESSMENT

Because the nurse may meet a family during any phase of the adjustment process, several assessment areas are important. The family's ability to cope with previous stresses influences the current situation, and answers to questions about their usual coping skills are enlightening. Knowledge of concurrent stresses, such as financial, marital or nonmarital, and career or unemployment, helps identify families who may have fewer resources to cope with the child's needs.

Finally, awareness of the family members' reactions to the child and the illness or condition is important. Sample questions that the nurse and family can use to evaluate the support system, perception of the illness, coping mechanisms, resources, and concurrent stresses are listed in Table 36.3. Because factors affecting the family's response may change at any point during the illness, assessment must be a continuous process.

Special challenges exist in assessing the child's feelings about having a chronic condition. The nurse should use a variety of communication techniques, such as drawing and play, as assessment tools rather than relying solely on parental reports. Often, children are neglected partners in their care, and their unique needs are not identified (Dixon-Woods, Young & Heney, 1999; Young, Dixon-Woods, Windridge, et al., 2003).

The needs of working parents and siblings also should be assessed; this is a goal that requires flexibility in scheduling appointments. When working parents know that their input is valuable, they will often change their work schedule to meet with a health care professional. Because siblings can be of any age, the use of appropriate communication strategies for assessment must be considered. Nonverbal techniques should be considered for these children.

PROVIDE SUPPORT AT THE TIME OF DIAGNOSIS

The diagnosis is a critical time for parents and can influence how they perceive their health care providers across the trajectory of care. Although they may not hear or remember all that is said to them, they frequently sense a certain attitude of acceptance, rejection, hope, or despair that may influence their ability to absorb the shock and begin adapting to the family's altered future.

Parents may be encouraged to be together when they are informed of their child's condition, thus avoiding the problem of one parent having to interpret complex information and deal with the initial emotional reaction of the other. The informing session should take place in a private, comfortable setting free of distractions and interruptions in an atmosphere in which the parents feel free to express their emotions (Fig. 36.3). Their emotional needs are acknowledged by showing acceptance of expressions, such as crying, sadness, anger, and disappointment. Emotional support is offered by having tissues available if a family member cries and demonstrating through facial and body language that indeed this is a difficult and painful period. Although touching is a powerful expression of empathy, it must be used wisely. For example, it can prematurely terminate free expression of feelings, especially when combined with statements, such as "Everything will be all right." Nurses should also be aware of cultural issues regarding touching.

Parents should receive the kind of information they desire. This can be assessed by asking questions, such as "Do you prefer to hear detailed information?" Parents or other family members may have different

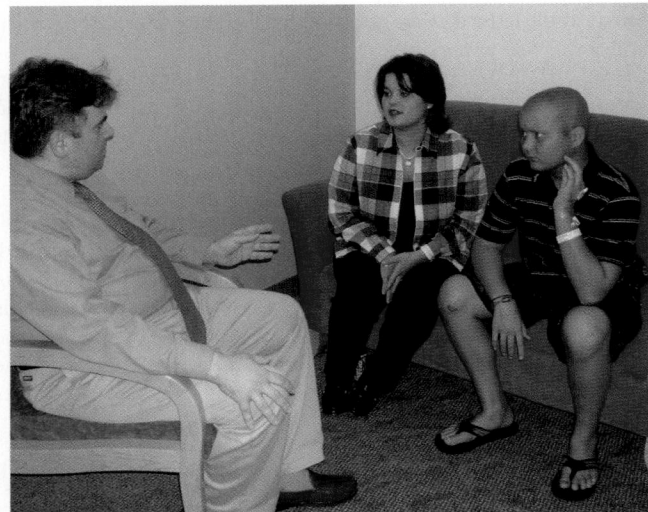

FIG 36.3 Information sessions should take place in a private, comfortable setting free of distractions and interruptions.

TABLE 36.3 Assessment of Factors Affecting Family Adjustment	
Factors Affecting Adjustment	**Assessment Questions**
Available Support System	
Status of marital relationship	To whom do you talk when you have something on your mind? (If answer is not the spouse, ask for the reason.)
Alternate support systems	When something is worrying you, what do you do?
	What helps you most when you are upset?
Ability to communicate	Does talking seem to help when you feel upset?
Perception of the Illness or Disability	
Previous knowledge of disorder	Have you ever heard the word (name of diagnosis) before? Tell me about it (if answer is yes).
Imagined cause of disorder	What are your thoughts about the causes of the disorder?
Effects of illness or disability on family	How has your child's illness or disability affected you and your family?
	How has your lifestyle changed?
Coping Mechanisms	
Reactions to previous crises	Tell me one time you've had another crisis (problem, bad time) in your family. How did you solve that problem?
Reactions to the child	Do you find yourself being a little more cautious with this child than with your other children?
Childrearing practices	Do you feel as comfortable disciplining this child as your other children?
Influence of religion	Has your religion or faith been of help to you? Tell me how (if answer is yes).
Attitudes	How is this child different from the siblings or other children of similar age?
	Describe your child's personality. Is it easy, difficult, or in between?
	When you think of your child's future, what thoughts come to mind?
Available Resources	
	What parts of your child's care are causing the most difficulty for you or your family?
	What services are available to help?
	What services do you need that currently are not available?
Concurrent Stresses	
	What other problems are you facing now? (Be specific; ask about financial, marital, sibling, and extended family or friends concerns.)

preferences regarding the amount of information that they wish to hear. Most parents want a clear, simple explanation of the diagnosis; a prediction of possible futures for the child; advice on what to do next; an opportunity to ask questions; a warm, sympathetic listener; and, most important, time. Understanding of explanations is elicited with questions, such as "Do you see what I mean?" or "Is this clear to you?" Technical terms are used with simple definitions. If the parents are unaware of the term, they are given written literature or at least a written summary of the diagnosis.

Finally, the informing conference does not end with the presentation of devastating news. Instead, the child's strengths, appealing behaviors, and potential for development are stressed, as are available rehabilitation efforts or treatments. Parents can be encouraged to view their experiences as a series of challenges that they are capable of handling, particularly with available professional feedback. The parents are assured that the nurse will be available to answer questions and to provide further assistance as needed.

The preceding discussion relates primarily to the initial informing interview. However, because of the need for long-term follow-up, it is only one in a series of continuing discussions. In all interactions, the family's input is solicited and incorporated into the care plan. Some situations require consideration of special problems (see Guidelines box: Situations Requiring Special Consideration).

SUPPORT THE FAMILY'S COPING METHODS

For the family to meet the stresses of optimally adjusting to the child's condition, each member must be individually supported so that the family system is strong. Although the family can indefinitely support a member who is in need of assistance, its greatest strength lies in every member supporting each other. The nurse should bear in mind that the family member in greatest need is not necessarily the affected child but may be a parent or sibling who is dealing with stresses that require intervention.

Parents

The nurse can provide support by being attentive to families' responses to their children. Mothers and fathers need to experience success, joy, and pride in their children to give the support they need. It is important for nurses to examine their attitudes to determine their ability to engage in parent-professional partnerships. An essential characteristic is the belief that parents are equal to professionals and are experts regarding their child (see Guidelines box: Developing Successful Parent-Professional Partnerships).

Parents can be encouraged to discuss their feelings toward the child, the impact of this event on their marriage, and associated stresses such as financial burdens. For most families, regardless of their income or insurance coverage, financial concerns exist. The costs of caring for a child with special needs can be overwhelming. In addition, one or both parents may have to sacrifice job opportunities to remain close to a medical facility or to avoid losing insurance benefits. Numerous volunteer and community resources are available that provide assistance, rehabilitation, equipment, and funding for a variety of health problems. National and local disease-oriented organizations may provide needed assistance and support to families that qualify. Many of these are discussed elsewhere

GUIDELINES
Situations Requiring Special Consideration

Congenital Anomaly

Tension in the delivery room conveys the sense that something is seriously wrong. Communication is often delayed while the physician is involved with the mother's care. The manner in which the infant is presented may well set the tone for the early parent-child relationship.

Clarify role with physician in regard to revealing information to enable immediate parental support.

Explain to parents briefly in simple language what the defect is and something concerning the immediate prognosis before showing them the infant. Later more information can be given when they are more ready to "hear" what is said.

Be aware of nonverbal communication. Parents watch facial expressions of others for signs of revulsion or rejection.

Present infant as something precious.

Emphasize well-formed aspects of infant's body.

Allow time and opportunity for parents to express their initial response.

Encourage parents to ask questions, and provide honest, straightforward answers without undue optimism or pessimism.

Cognitive Impairment

Unless cognitive impairment (or mental retardation) is associated with other physical problems, it is often easy for parents to miss clues to its presence or to make defensive excuses regarding the diagnosis.

Plan situations that help parents become aware of the problem.

Encourage parents to discuss their observations of child, but withhold diagnostic opinions.

Focus on what the child can do and appropriate interventions to promote progress (e.g., infant stimulation programs) to involve parents in their child's care while helping them gain an awareness of the child's condition.

Physical Disability

If loss of motor or sensory ability occurs during childhood, the diagnosis is readily apparent. The challenge lies in helping the child and parents over the period of shock and grief and toward the phase of acceptance and reintegration.

Institute early rehabilitation (e.g., using a prosthetic limb, learning to read braille, learning to read lips).

Be aware that physical rehabilitation usually precedes psychologic adjustment.

When the cause of the disability is accidental, avoid implying that parents or child was responsible for the injury, but allow them the opportunity to discuss feelings of blame.

Encourage expression of feelings (see the "Communication Techniques" section in Chapter 29).

Chronic Illness

Realization of the true impact may take months or years. Conflict over parents' versus child's concerns may result in serious problems. When condition is inherited, parents may blame themselves, or child may blame the parents.

Help each family member gain an appreciation of the others' concerns.

Discuss hereditary aspect of condition with parents at time of diagnosis to lessen guilt and accusatory feelings.

Encourage child to express feelings by using third-person technique (e.g., "Sometimes when a person has an illness that was passed on by the parents, that person feels angry or bitter toward them").

Multiple Disabilities

The child or parent may require additional time for the shock phase and may be able to attend to only one diagnosis before hearing significant information regarding other disorders.

Acknowledge parents' understanding and acceptance of all diagnoses, especially when an obvious and more hidden disability coexists.

Appreciate the devastating consequences of more than one disability for a child, especially if they interfere with expressive-receptive abilities.

Terminal Illness

Parents require much support to deal with their own feelings and guidance in how to tell the child the diagnosis. They may want to conceal the diagnosis from the child. They may believe that the child is too young to know, will not be able to cope with the information, or will lose hope and the will to live.

Approach the subject of disclosure in a positive way by asking, "How will you tell your child about the diagnosis?"

Help parents understand the disadvantages of not telling the child (e.g., deprives child of the opportunity to discuss feelings openly and ask questions, incurs the risk of child learning the truth from outside and sometimes less tactful sources, may lessen child's trust and confidence in the parents after learning the truth).

Guide parents to see the potential problems involved in fostering a conspiracy.

Offer parents guidelines for how and what to tell the child about the disease or the possibility of death. Explanations should be tailored to child's cognitive ability, be based on knowledge child already has, and be honest. Honesty must be tempered with concern for child's feelings.

Assure parents that telling a child the name of the illness and the reason for treatment instills hope, provides support from others, and serves as a foundation for explaining and understanding subsequent events.

Acknowledge that being honest is not always easy because the truth may prompt the child to ask other distressing questions, such as "Am I going to die?" However, even this difficult question must be answered.

---

in the text under the specific diagnosis. State and federal departments of health, mental health, social service, and labor may be able to help locate appropriate regional resources. For example, state programs for Children with Special Health Needs provide financial assistance for children with many disabling conditions. Local and national sources of respite care and medical day care may be useful to families. Nurses should become acquainted with those in their communities and with vocational programs for special groups.

Parent-to-Parent Support

Just being with another parent who has shared similar experiences is helpful. It may not need to be a parent of a child with the same diagnosis, because parents in the process of adjusting to a child with special needs—or finding respite services, educational or rehabilitative services, special equipment vendors, and financial counseling—tread a common path. If the agency does not have a parent staff position, the nurse can contact parent groups that will often send a representative. Another

GUIDELINES

Developing Successful Parent-Professional Partnerships

Promote primary nursing; in nonhospital settings, designate a case manager.

Acknowledge parents' overall competence and their unique expertise with their child.

Respect parents' time as having value equal to that of other members of child's health care team.

Explain or define any medical, technical, or discipline-specific terms.

Tell families, "I am not sure" or "I don't know" when appropriate.

Facilitate family's effectiveness in team meetings (e.g., provide parents with same information as other participants).

strategy is to ask another parent to talk to the parents. The nurse should seek out a parent who is a good listener, has a nonjudgmental approach to differences in families, and possesses good advocacy and problem-solving skills.

The parent self-help group can promote parent-to-parent support.* Group members feel less alone and have the opportunity to observe both coping and mastery role modeling from other members. Parent groups are rich resources for information. Even if parents are unable to attend meetings, they can still benefit from group newsletters and other literature that often accompany membership. Nurses can assist in starting a group by identifying one or two parents as leaders; sharing with them the names, telephone numbers, and addresses of other families who have expressed both an interest and a willingness to release their phone number and address; and guiding them in how to initiate a first meeting.

Advocate for Empowerment

Nurses can advocate for methods that foster opportunities for parent empowerment. For example, nurses can suggest reimbursement for travel and child care plus stipends to enable parents' voices to be heard at meetings and conferences. They can encourage parent membership on committees and advisory boards. They can keep parents informed of pending legislation on child health issues or take action when parents inform them.

The Child

Through ongoing contacts with the child, the nurse (1) observes the child's responses to the disorder, ability to function, and adaptive behaviors within the environment and with significant others; (2) explores the child's own understanding of his or her illness or condition; and (3) provides support while the child learns to cope with his or her feelings. Children are encouraged to express their concerns rather than allowing others to express them for them because open discussions may reduce anxiety (see Guidelines box: Encouraging Expression of Emotion).

One of the most important interventions is alleviating the child's feeling of being different and normalizing his or her life as much as possible (see Guidelines box: Promoting Normalization). Whenever possible, the nurse assists the family in assessing the child's daily routine for indications of a need for normalizing practices. For example,

---

*Information about self-help groups and books and pamphlets are available from the National Self-Help Clearinghouse, 365 Fifth Avenue, Suite 3300, New York, NY 10016; 217-817-1822; http://www.selfhelpweb.org.

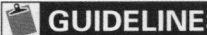

GUIDELINES

Encouraging Expression of Emotion

Describe the behavior: "You seem angry at everyone."
Give evidence of understanding: "Being angry is only natural."
Give evidence of caring: "It must be difficult to endure so many painful procedures."
Help focus on feelings: "Maybe you wonder why this happened to you."

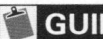

GUIDELINES

Promoting Normalization

Preparation: Prepare child in advance for changes that may occur from the chronic or complex condition.
 Example: Tell the child in advance the possible side effects of drug therapy.
Participation: Include child in as many decisions as possible, especially those relating to his or her care regimen.
 Example: The child is responsible for taking medications or scheduling home treatments.
Sharing: Allow both family members and child's peers to be a part of the care regimen whenever possible.
 Examples: Give the child his or her medication when the other siblings receive their vitamins.
 The parent cooks the same menu for the whole family.
 If the child is invited to another's home, the parent advises the family of the child's dietary restrictions.
Control: Identify areas where child can be in control so that feelings of uncertainty, passivity, and helplessness are decreased.
 Example: The child identifies activities that are appropriate to his or her energy level and chooses to rest when fatigued.
Expectation: Apply the same family rules to the child with a complex chronic illness as to the well siblings or peers.
 Example: The child is disciplined, is expected to fulfill household responsibilities, and attends school in accordance with abilities.

the child who remains in a bedroom all day requires a restructured daily routine to provide activities in different parts of the house, such as eating in the kitchen or dining room with the family. Such children may also be deprived of social, recreational, and academic activities that can be better accommodated by applying normalization practices. For example, home and out-of-home health-related treatments should be planned at times that least interfere with normal daily activities.

Children who are concerned that their condition detracts from their physical attractiveness need attention focused on the normal aspects of appearance and capabilities. Health care professionals help strengthen and consolidate the self-image by emphasizing the normal while allowing children to express anger, isolation, fear of rejection, feelings of sadness, and loneliness. The children need positive reinforcement for compliance and any evidence of improvement. Anything that might improve attractiveness and contribute to a positive self-image is used, such as makeup for a teenager with a scar, clothing that disguises a prosthesis, or a hairstyle or wig to cover a deformity or lost hair.

Siblings

The presence of a child with special needs in a family may result in parents paying less attention to the other children. Siblings may respond by developing negative attitudes toward the child or by expressing anger in different forms. The nurse can help by using anticipatory guidance, questioning the parents about what they believe is the best way to have siblings respond to the child, and guiding them through ways to meet their other children's needs for attention. This questioning should take place before serious negative effects occur.

Siblings may also experience embarrassment associated with having a brother or sister with a chronic or complex condition. Parents are then faced with the difficulty of responding to this embarrassment in an understanding and appropriate manner without punishing the siblings for how they feel. Parents are encouraged to talk with the siblings about how they view their affected sibling. For example, siblings of a child with developmental disabilities may express fears about their ability to bear normal children. Adolescents in particular may not be able to discuss these vital issues with their parents and may prefer to consult with the nurse. Many siblings benefit from sharing their concerns with other young people who are experiencing a similar situation. Support groups for siblings can help decrease isolation, promote expression of feelings, and provide examples of effective coping skills.

Many parents express concern about when and how to inform the other children in the family about a sibling's illness or disability. The answer depends on each child's level of sophistication and understanding. However, it is usually best to inform the siblings before a neighbor or other nonfamily member does so. Uninformed siblings may fantasize or develop apprehensions that are out of proportion to the child's actual condition. Furthermore, if parents choose to be silent or deceptive about the issue, they are setting a negative precedent for the siblings to follow rather than encouraging the siblings to cope with the experience in a healthy and nurturing way.

The nurse is sensitive to the reactions of siblings and whenever possible intervenes to promote more positive adjustment. For example, siblings often mention that they are expected to take on additional responsibilities to help the parents care for the child. It is not unusual for them to express a positive reaction to assuming the extra duties but a negative response to feeling unappreciated for doing so. Such feelings can often be minimized by encouraging siblings to discuss this with the parents and by suggesting to parents ways of showing gratitude, such as an increase in allowance; special privileges; and, most significantly, verbal praise.

EDUCATE ABOUT THE DISORDER AND GENERAL HEALTH CARE

Educating the family about the disorder is actually an extension of revealing the diagnosis. Education involves not only supplying technical information but also discussing how the condition will affect the child. Parents may only be able to process limited information at any one time. It may be helpful to provide essential information and then follow by asking, "What else would you like to know about your child's condition?" Responding to parents' questions and concerns ensures that their information needs are met.

Activities of Daily Living

Parents also need guidance in how the condition may interfere with or alter activities of daily living, such as eating, dressing, sleeping, and toileting. One area frequently affected is nutrition. Common problems are undernutrition resulting from food being inappropriately restricted or loss of appetite, vomiting, or motor deficits that interfere with feeding; overnutrition may also occur, usually because of a caloric intake in excess of energy expenditure because of boredom and lack of stimulation in other areas. Although the child requires the same basic nutrients as other children, the daily requirements may differ. Special nutritional considerations are discussed as appropriate throughout the text.

Safe Transportation

Modifications may also be needed regarding car safety. Children with conditions such as low birth weight or orthopedic, neuromuscular, or respiratory impairments often cannot safely use conventional car restraints. For example, children with hip spica casts cannot sit properly in child safety seats (see the "Developmental Dysplasia of the Hip" section in Chapter 48. Modifications can be made to some commercial models, and for older children, a special vest is available that secures the child to the back seat in a lying-down position.*

If a child requires a wheelchair, the family should consult the wheelchair manufacturer for specific instructions regarding safe car transportation. Considerations for wheelchairs used with vehicle transportation must address securing both the wheelchair and the occupant in the wheelchair. Wheelchairs should be secured facing forward with tie downs at four points. The tie-down system should be dynamically crash tested, as should the occupant securement system that secures the child in the wheelchair. For example, use of trays is not recommended for transportation. With children who must travel with additional medical equipment, this equipment (e.g., oxygen, monitors, or ventilators) should be anchored to the floor or underneath the vehicle seat or wheelchair. Soft padding should be added around the equipment to reduce movement. A second adult should be present to monitor the condition of a medically fragile child while traveling.

Primary Health Care

Children with special needs require all the usual health care recommended for any child. Attention to injury prevention, immunizations, dental health, and regular physical examinations is essential. Nurses can play an important role in reminding parents of these aspects of care that are so often neglected when the concern is focused on the child's chronic condition. Specific discussions of nutrition, sleep and activity, dental health, and injury prevention are presented in the chapters on health promotion for specific age groups. Immunizations are discussed in Chapter 31.

Parents also need to be aware of the importance of communicating the child's condition in the event of a medical emergency. Young children are unable to give information about their disorders, and although older children may be reliable sources, after an accident, they may be physically unable to speak. Therefore, all children with any type of chronic condition that may affect medical care should wear some type of identification, such as a MedicAlert bracelet,[†] or carry a card in their wallet that lists the medical condition and a phone number for emergency medical records and other personal information.

PROMOTE NORMAL DEVELOPMENT

Aside from knowledge of the condition and its effect on the child's abilities, the family must be guided toward fostering appropriate development in their child. Although each stage may take longer to achieve, parents are guided toward helping the child fully realize his or her potential in preparation for the next developmental stage. Table 36.2 outlines developmental aspects of complex conditions and supportive interventions. With appropriate planning and knowledge of strategies

---

*Information on car safety restraints for children with special needs is available from the Automotive Safety Program, 575 West Drive, Room 004, Indianapolis, IN 46202; 800-543-6227 or 317-274-2997; http://www.preventinjury.org.

[†]MedicAlert Foundation International, 2323 Colorado Avenue, Turlock, CA 95382; 888-633-4298; http://www.medicalert.org.

to improve the child's functional abilities, most children can live fulfilling and productive lives.

One important aspect of promoting normal development is to encourage the child's self-care abilities in both activities of daily living and the medical regimen. An assessment of the child's age and physical, emotional, and mental capacities, as well as the support and structure provided by the family, should be considered in determining the appropriate level of self-care in the medical regimen. Even toddlers can be involved in their own care by holding supplies for the parent during a procedure. Over time, children should be encouraged toward greater autonomy in the self-care arena.

Early Childhood

During infancy, the child is achieving basic trust through a satisfying, intimate, consistent relationship with his or her parents. However, affected children's early existence may be stressful, chaotic, and unsatisfying. Consequently, they may need more parental support and expressions of affection to achieve trust. Likewise, the parents require assistance in finding ways to meet the infant's needs, such as how to hold a rigid or flaccid infant, how to feed a child with tongue thrust or episodes of dyspnea, and how to stimulate a child who seems incapable of achieving any skills. If hospitalizations are frequent or prolonged, every effort is made to preserve the parent-child relationship.

During early childhood, the goal is to adapt to periods of separation from parents, autonomy, and initiative. However, the natural parental response to having a sick child is overprotection (Box 36.7). Parents need help in realizing the importance of brief separations of the child from them and from others involved in the child's care and of providing social experiences outside the home whenever possible. Respite care, which provides temporary relief for family members, can be essential in allowing caregivers time away from the daily burdens.

Young children also need the opportunity to develop independence. Frequently, the child is able to learn self-help skills, such as finger feeding, and removing simple articles of clothing, but the parent continues to perform the act. The nurse can provide parents with anticipatory guidance as to the usual milestones expected from the child. When a child is unable to perform a skill independently, functional aids should be used. With innovation, many adaptations can be implemented in children's environments to increase their mobility and independence and allow them to play like other children their age. For example, with slight modifications, a child with physical limitations may be able to ride a tricycle (Fig. 36.4).

Another critical component for normal child development is discipline. Discipline and guidance serve several purposes, such as providing children with boundaries on which to test out their behavior and teaching them socially acceptable behavior. Resentment and hostility can arise among siblings if different standards are applied to each child. The nurse's responsibility is to help parents learn successful methods of managing a child's behaviors before they become problems.

School Age

For school-age children, the major tasks are entry into school and achieving a sense of industry. Although the importance of school in the life of all children is well known, school absences are significantly higher among children with chronic illnesses than among their healthy peers. The more school absences the child experiences, the more difficult it is to resume attendance, and school phobia may result. The child should return to school as soon as possible after diagnosis or treatments.

Preparation for entry into or resumption of school is best accomplished through a team approach with the parents, child, teacher, school nurse, and primary nurse in the hospital. Ideally, this planning should begin before hospital discharge, provided that the child is well enough to resume usual activities. A structured plan should be developed, with attention to aspects of care that must be continued during school hours, such as administration of medication or other treatments.

Children also need preparation before entering or resuming school. Having a tutor in the hospital or home as soon as children are physically able helps them realize that school will continue and gives them time to consider this prospect (Fig. 36.5). They need to investigate possible answers to the many questions others will ask. One method of anticipatory preparation is to role-play, with the child as the "returned pupil" and the nurse or parent as "other schoolmates." If the child returns to school with some obvious physical change (such as, hair loss, amputation, or a visible scar), the nurse might also ask questions about these alterations to prompt preparatory responses from the child.

Classroom peers also need preparation, and a joint plan created by the teacher, nurse, and child is best. At a minimum, classmates should be given a description of the child's condition, prepared for any visible changes in the child, and allowed an opportunity to ask questions. The child should have the option of attending this session. As the child's

---

BOX 36.7 Characteristics of Parental Overprotection

Sacrifices self and rest of family for the child

Continually helps the child, even when the child is capable

Is inconsistent with regard to discipline or uses no discipline; frequently applies different rules to the siblings

Is dictatorial and arbitrary, making decisions without considering the child's wishes, such as keeping the child from attending school

Hovers and offers suggestions; calls attention to every activity; overdoes praise

Protects the child from every possible discomfort

Restricts play, often because of fear that the child will be injured

Denies the child opportunities for growing up and assuming responsibility, such as learning to give own medications or perform treatments

Does not understand the child's capabilities, and sets goals too high or too low

Monopolizes the child's time, such as sleeping with the child, permitting few friends, or refusing participation in social or educational activities

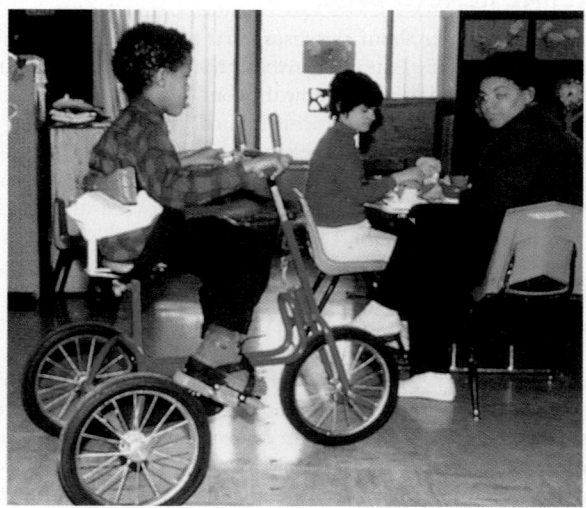

FIG 36.4 A modified tricycle with block pedals, self-adhesive straps for support, and a modified seat and handle bars can help a child with disabilities gain mobility.

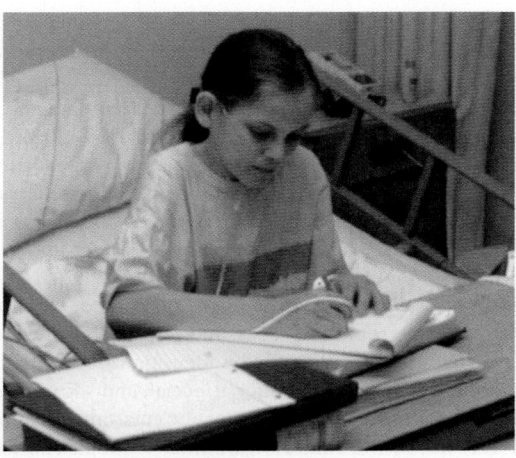

FIG 36.5 Children with disabilities should continue their schooling as soon as their condition permits.

condition changes, particularly if the illness is potentially fatal, school personnel, including the students, need periodic appraisal of the child's status and preparation for what to expect.

Children with special needs are encouraged to maintain or reestablish relationships with peers and to participate according to their capabilities in any age-appropriate activities. Alternative activities may be substituted for those that are impossible or that place a strain on the child's condition. Programs, such as the Special Olympics,* offer children an opportunity to compete with their peers and to achieve athletic skill. Summer camps† allow children to associate with peers and develop a wide variety of skills. Children with special needs can derive enormous benefits from expressive activities, such as art, music, poetry, dance, and drama. With adaptive equipment and imagination, children can participate in a variety of activities. Organizations such as VSA Arts allow children to celebrate and share their accomplishments.‡ Children need the opportunity to interact with healthy peers and to engage in activities with groups or clubs composed of similarly affected age-mates. Organizations such as ostomy clubs, diabetes clubs, and cerebral palsy groups share information and provide support related to the special problems the members face.

Adolescence

Adolescence can be a particularly difficult period for the teenager and family. All of the needs discussed previously apply to this age group as well. Developing independence or autonomy, however, is a major task for the adolescent as planning for the future becomes a prominent concern. Although the emphasis in the past has been on achieving

---

*1133 19th Street NW, Washington, DC 20036; 202-628-3630; www.specialolympics.org. Several pamphlets on sports and recreation for children with disabilities are available from Easter Seals and American Alliance for Health, Physical Education, Recreation and Dance, 1900 Association Drive, Reston, VA 20191; 703-476-3400 or 800-213-7193; www.shapeamerica.org.

†A directory of private and paying camps for children with a variety of chronic illnesses and general physical disabilities is available from the American Camp Association, 5000 State Road 67 North, Martinsville, IN 46151-7902; 765-342-8456; www.acacamps.org.

‡VSA Arts has affiliate chapters in all 50 states and in selected sites internationally; yearly festivals are held throughout the world. Information is available from the Department of VSA and Accessibility at the Kennedy Center 2700 F Street, NW Washington, DC 20566; 800-444-1324; http://www.kennedy-center.org/education/vsa.

independence from physical assistance, recent developments in the fields of special education, adolescent development, and family systems suggest redefining autonomy in terms of individuals' capacities to take responsibility for their own behavior, to make decisions regarding their own lives, and to maintain supportive social relationships. Given this understanding, even individuals with severe impairments can be viewed as autonomous if they perceive their own needs and take responsibility for meeting them, either directly or by engaging the assistance of others. As adolescents become more autonomous, the nurse can help them articulate their needs, participate in developing their own care plans, and discover and express how others can be of greatest assistance.

Physical symptoms are high on teenagers' list of health-related concerns. Because adolescence is a time of enormous physical and emotional changes, it is important for the nurse to distinguish between body changes that are related to the child's complex condition and those that are a result of normal body development. It can be a great comfort for teenagers with disabling conditions to know that many of the changes they experience are normal developmental outcomes.

A sense of feeling different from peers can lead to loneliness, isolation, and depression. Participation in groups of teenagers with chronic conditions or disabilities can alleviate feelings of isolation and smooth the transition to a meaningful relationship with one person in adulthood.

ESTABLISH REALISTIC FUTURE GOALS

One of the most difficult adjustments is setting realistic future goals for the child that are based on the child's own goals and values.

Planning for the future should be a gradual process. All along, the parents should cultivate realistic vocations for the child. For example, if children have physical disabilities, they can be directed toward intellectual, artistic, or musical pursuits. Children with developmental disabilities can be taught manual skills. In this way, the child's development proceeds in the direction of self-support through gainful employment.

With prolonged survival, young people with chronic illnesses must deal with new decisions and problems, such as marriage, employment, and insurance coverage. With appropriate guidance, individuals with disabilities can attain gainful employment, marriage, and a family. For those whose conditions are genetic, counseling is needed regarding future offspring. Prospective spouses often benefit from an opportunity to discuss their feelings regarding marriage to an individual with continued health needs and possibly a limited life span. Health insurance coverage is a critical issue for chronically ill children because of their enormous health care costs over time. The Affordable Care Act allows young adults to remain on their parents insurance until they are 26 years of age and prevents private insurance carriers from denying them coverage. Life insurance is another dilemma, especially when children have serious conditions, such as congenital heart anomalies.

PERSPECTIVES ON THE CARE OF CHILDREN AT THE END OF LIFE

Although most childhood illnesses and many injuries and other trauma respond favorably to treatment, some do not. When a child and family face a prolonged and life-limiting illness, health care professionals must confront the challenge of providing the best possible care to meet the physical, psychologic, spiritual, and emotional needs of the child and family during the uncertain course of the illness and at the time of death. When death is sudden and unexpected, nurses are challenged to respond to grief and shock in families and provide comfort and support in the absence of a prior relationship.

Many factors affect the causes of death that nurses are likely to encounter in children, including developmental factors, medical advances and technology, and changing social patterns. In infants, the leading causes of death are congenital anomalies, respiratory distress syndrome, disorders related to short gestation and low birth weight, and sudden infant death syndrome (Kochanek, Murphy, Xu, et al., 2014) (see Chapter 26). The leading causes of death in children 5 to 9 years of age include injuries (accidents), malignant neoplasms, congenital anomalies, assault (homicide), and heart disease. In children 10 to 14 years of age, suicide is the third leading cause of death after injuries (accidents) and malignant neoplasms. In youths 15 to 19 years of age, assault (homicide), suicide, malignant neoplasms, and heart disease follow accidents as the most prevalent causes of death (Anderson & Smith, 2005).

A child who is diagnosed with a life-threatening illness or who is suffering serious, life-threatening trauma needs medical diagnosis and intervention, as well as nursing assessment and care—sometimes for a short time and sometimes over a lengthy period. When cure is no longer possible and life-prolonging measures result in pain, suffering, and distress to the child, parents need information about care options that are available to assist them in deciding how they want the remaining time with their child to be managed by the health care team. It is important that families are reassured that although their child cannot be cured, active care will continue to be provided to maintain the child's comfort. Support is provided to assist the child and family during the dying process. As a result, nurses may care for children and families who are making the difficult transition from curative or restorative treatments to palliative care.

PRINCIPLES OF PALLIATIVE CARE

Palliative care involves a multidisciplinary approach to the care of children living with or dying from chronic, complex, or potentially life-limiting conditions with a primary focus on symptom control, supportive care, and quality of life rather than on cure or life prolongation in the absence of the possibility of a cure (Field & Behrman, 2004). The World Health Organization (1996) defines palliative care as the "active total care of patients whose disease is not responsive to curative treatment. Control of pain, of other symptoms, and of psychologic, social, and spiritual problems is paramount. The goal of palliative care is the achievement of the best possible quality of life for patients and their families." This goal is certainly compatible with care for patients who are pursuing curative or life-prolonging therapy. Therefore, there should be a distinction between palliative care and end-of-life care. End-of-life care is a part of palliative care, but the goals of palliative care extend to all aspects of a patient's quality of life and can be established early in the trajectory of a patient's disease. The World Health Organization (1998) amended the definition of palliative care for children to include the following:

- Palliative care for children is the active total care of the child's body, mind, and spirit and involves giving support to the family.
- It begins when illness is diagnosed and continues regardless of whether or not a child receives treatment directed at the disease.
- Health care providers must evaluate and alleviate the child's physical, psychologic, and social distress.
- Effective palliative care requires a broad multidisciplinary approach that includes the family and makes use of available community resources; it can be successfully implemented even if resources are limited.
- It can be provided in tertiary care facilities, in community health centers, and even in children's homes.

Palliative care interventions do not serve to hasten death. Rather, they provide pain and symptom management, attention to issues faced by the child and family with regard to death and dying, and promotion

of optimal functioning and quality of life during the time the child has remaining. The implementation of neonatal and pediatric palliative care consulting services within hospitals has led to enhanced quality of life and end-of-life care for children and their families and support for their care providers (Blume, Balkin, Aiyagari, et al., 2014; O'Quinn & Giambra, 2014). Several principles are hallmarks of palliative care.

The child and family are considered the unit of care. The death of a child is an extremely stressful event for a family, because it is out of the natural order of things. Children represent health and hope, and their death calls into question the understanding of life. A multidisciplinary team of health care professionals consisting of social workers, chaplains, nurses, personal care aides, and physicians skilled in caring for dying patients assist the family by focusing care on the complex interactions among physical, emotional, social, and spiritual issues.

Palliative care seeks to create a therapeutic environment as homelike as possible, if not in the child's own home. Through education and support of family members, an atmosphere of open communication is provided regarding the child's dying process and its impact on all members of the family (see Evidence-Based Practice box: Pediatric Pain and Symptom Management at the End of Life).

DECISION MAKING AT THE END OF LIFE

Discussions concerning the possibility that a child's illness or condition is not curable and that death is an inevitable outcome cause everyone involved a great deal of stress. Physicians, other members of the health care team, and families must consider all information regarding the child's situation and make decisions that all parties agree to and that will have a profound impact on the child and family.

Ethical Considerations in End-of-Life Decision Making

A number of ethical concerns arise when parents and health care professionals are deciding on the best course of care for the dying child. Many parents and health care providers are concerned that not offering treatment that would cause potential pain and suffering but might extend life would be considered euthanasia or assisted suicide. To eliminate such concerns, it is necessary to understand the various terms. Euthanasia involves an action carried out by a person other than the patient to end the life of the patient suffering from a terminal condition. The intent of this action is based on the belief that the act is "putting the person out of his or her misery." This action has also been called *mercy killing*. Assisted suicide occurs when someone provides the patient with the means to end his or her life and the patient uses that means to do so. The important distinction between these two actions involves who is actually acting to end the person's life.

The American Nurses Association *Code of Ethics for Nurses* (2015) does not support the active intent on the part of a nurse to end a person's life. However, it does permit the nurse to provide interventions to relieve symptoms in the dying patient even when the interventions involve substantial risks of hastening death. When the prognosis for a patient is poor and death is the expected outcome, it is ethically acceptable to withhold or withdraw treatments that may cause pain and suffering and provide interventions that promote comfort and quality of life.

Physician–Health Care Team Decision Making

Decisions by physicians regarding care are often made on the basis of the progression of the disease or amount of trauma, the availability of treatment options that would provide cure from disease or restoration of health, the impact of such treatments on the child, and the child's overall prognosis (Pousset, Bilsen, Cohen et al., 2010). Often the main determinants prompting physicians to discuss end-of-life issues and

EVIDENCE-BASED PRACTICE

Pediatric Pain and Symptom Management at the End of Life

Ask the Question

PICOT Question: In children, what is the pain and symptom experience at the end of life?

Search for the Evidence

Search Strategies

Published studies from using the subject terms *child, palliative care, pain,* and *symptoms* were identified and examined. Retrospective descriptive studies dominated the findings describing infants' and children's end-of-life experiences through the use of medical record reviews and provider and parental surveys.

Databases Used

PubMed, CINAHL

Critical Appraisal of the Evidence

Children experienced an average of 11 symptoms during their last week of life (Drake, Frost & Collins, 2003). Pain, dyspnea, and fatigue were the most frequently documented symptoms experienced by most children at the end of life (Bradshaw, Hinds, Lensing, et al., 2005; Carter, Howenstein, Gilmer, et al., 2004; Drake et al.; Hongo, Watanabe, Okada, et al., 2003). Children and their parents report high distress with pain and symptoms at the end of life. Parents reported pain and suffering as one of the most important factors in deciding to withhold or withdraw life support from their child in the pediatric intensive care unit (Meert, Thurston & Sarnaik, 2000).

Documentation was scarce related to symptom management. Morphine was the most commonly prescribed pain medication (Drake et al., 2003; Hongo et al., 2003). Parents reported their children as experiencing high levels of pain near the end of life (Contro, Larson, Scofield, et al., 2002). Physicians were more likely than nurses or parents to report that a child's pain and symptoms were well managed at the end of life, but the majority of both provider groups believed the child's physical management was difficult (Andresen, Seecharan, & Toce, 2004; Wolfe, Grier, Klar, et al., 2000).

Barriers to the adequate provision of pediatric palliative care include developmental issues specific to infants and children; symptoms, their causes, how they are related, and effective treatment strategies; lack of education; and reimbursement issues (Harris, 2004). Physicians report reliance on trial and error as they learn to care for children at the end of life and the need for specialty consults with palliative care service providers (Hilden, Emanuel, Fairclough, et al., 2001).

Apply the Evidence: Nursing Implications

There is **moderate-quality evidence** with a **strong recommendation** (Guyatt, Oxman, Vist, et al., 2008) for better pain management at the end of life. Although the philosophy of palliative care encompasses pain and symptom management for infants and children who may not outlive their disease, the provision of that care to ease suffering and provide comfort to those who will die continues to lag. Studies show that children experience significant pain and other distressing symptoms at the end of life that are not well managed. Discrepancies in perceptions of infants' and children's pain and suffering continue to exist between providers and parents. Barriers to the provision of pediatric palliative care exist. Improvements are needed in the management of pain and symptoms at the end of life for infants and children.

Quality and Safety Competencies: Evidence-Based Practice*

Knowledge

Differentiate clinical opinion from research and evidence-based summaries.

Describe common symptoms experienced at the end of life.

Skills

Base individualized care plan on patient values, clinical expertise, and evidence.

Integrate evidence into practice by carefully assessing pain and other symptoms in children at the end of life.

Attitudes

Value the concept of evidence-based practice as integral to determining best clinical practice.

Appreciate strengths and weakness of evidence for symptom assessment and management at the end of life.

References

Andresen, E. M., Seecharan, G. A., & Toce, S. S. (2004). Provider perceptions of child deaths. *Archives of Pediatrics and Adolescent Medicine, 158*(5), 430–435.

Bradshaw, G., Hinds, P. S., Lensing, S., et al. (2005). Cancer-related deaths in children and adolescents. *Journal of Palliative Medicine, 8*(1), 86–95.

Carter, B. S., Howenstein, B. S., Gilmer, M. J., et al. (2004). Circumstances surrounding the deaths of hospitalized children: Opportunities for pediatric palliative care. *Pediatrics, 114*(3), 361–366.

Contro, N., Larson, J., Scofield, S., et al. (2002). Family perspectives on the quality of pediatric palliative care. *Archives of Pediatrics and Adolescent Medicine, 156*(1), 14–19.

Drake, R., Frost, J., & Collins, J. J. (2003). The symptoms of dying children. *Journal of Pain and Symptom Management, 26*(1), 594–603.

Guyatt, G. H., Oxman, A. D., Vist, G. E., et al. (2008). GRADE: An emerging consensus on rating quality of evidence and strength of recommendations. *British Medical Journal, 336*(7650), 924–926.

Harris, M. B. (2004). Palliative care in children with cancer: which child and when? *Journal of the National Cancer Institute Monograph, 32*, 144–149.

Hilden, J. M., Emanuel, E. J., Fairclough, D. L., et al. (2001). Attitudes and practices among pediatric oncologists regarding end-of-life care: results of the 1998 American Society of Clinical Oncology Survey. *Journal of Clinical Oncology, 19*(1), 205–212.

Hongo, T., Watanabe, C., Okada, S., et al. (2003). Analysis of the circumstances at the end of life in children with cancer: Symptoms, suffering and acceptance. *Pediatrics International, 45*(1), 60–64.

Meert, K. L., Thurston, C. S., & Sarnaik, A. P. (2000). End-of-life decision-making and satisfaction with care: parental perspectives. *Pediatric Critical Care Medicine, 1*(2), 179–185.

Wolfe, J., Grier, H. E., Klar, N., et al. (2000). Symptoms and suffering at the end of life in children with cancer. *New England Journal of Medicine, 342*(5), 326–333.

*Adapted from the Quality and Safety Education for Nurses (QSEN) Institute.

options for children with critical illnesses include the child's age, premorbid cognitive condition and functional status, pain or discomfort, probability of survival, and quality of life (Pousset et al., 2010). When the physician discusses this information openly with families, a shared decision-making process can occur regarding do not attempt resuscitation (DNaR) orders and care that is focused on the comfort of the child and family during the dying process (Giannini, Messeri, Aprile, et al., 2008).

Unfortunately, many families are not given the option of terminating treatment and pursuing care that is focused on comfort and quality of life when cure is unlikely, and staff may be reluctant to raise the question of DNaR orders. This occurs for a number of reasons, including the belief that not being able to "save" a child is a "failure." Also, the physician and other members of the health care team may lack knowledge of and experience with the principles of palliative care (Baker, Torkildson, Baillargeon, et al., 2007; Price, Dornan & Quail, 2013).

FAMILY-CENTERED CARE
A Dying Child: A Nurse's Perspective

Claire was unresponsive with slow, gasping breathing. Her mother asked me what I thought was happening. I replied honestly, "Your baby is dying because of her brain tumor." The mother put her arms around me and cried. We arranged for Claire to be baptized.

Honesty. As painful as the loss of a child is, my job is to assist the family through this experience. Although I usually wait until a private moment, such as driving home, I found tears streaming down my face as family and friends gathered for Claire's baptism. I went into the kitchen to compose myself, only to find several of my colleagues crying as well. Saying good-bye to a dying child will always be a difficult but shared experience.

Jeanne O'Connor Egan, RN, MSN
Pediatric Clinical Specialist, Children's Hospital
Washington, DC

FAMILY-CENTERED CARE
Family of the Dying Child

As the group of health care professionals that is most involved with families, nurses are in an excellent position to ensure that families are presented with the options available to them. The nurse's first responsibility is to explore the family's wishes. This is best done in concert with the physician but at times may need to be initiated by the nurse. Statements such as, "Tell me about your thoughts for the type of care you want your child to receive when he is dying" or "Have you considered the types of interventions you would like us to use when your child is near death?" can begin discussion of this sensitive but critical aspect of terminal care.

Parental Decision Making

Rarely are families prepared to cope with the numerous decisions that must be made when a child is dying. When the death is unexpected, as in the case of an accident or trauma, the confusion of emergency services and possibly an intensive care setting presents challenges to parents as they are asked to make difficult choices. If the child has either experienced a life-threatening illness (e.g., cancer) or lived with a chronic illness that has now reached its terminal phase, parents are often unprepared for the reality of their child's impending death (see Family-Centered Care boxes: A Dying Child: A Nurse's Perspective and Family of the Dying Child). Numerous studies have found that families facing the impending death of a child depend on information provided to them by the health care team, particularly an honest appraisal of the child's prognosis, to make difficult decisions regarding care options for their children (Lipstein, Brinkman & Britto, 2012; Hinds, Oakes, Furman, et al., 2001; James & Johnson, 1997; Wolfe, Friebert & Hilden, 2002).

The Dying Child

Children need honest and accurate information about their illness, treatments, and prognosis. This information needs to be given in clear, simple language. In most situations, this best occurs as a gradual process over time that is characterized by increasingly open dialogue among parents, professionals, and the child (Barnes et al., 2012; Beale, Baile & Aaron, 2005; Young et al., 2003). Providing an atmosphere of open communication early in the course of an illness facilitates answering difficult questions as the child's condition worsens. Providing appropriate literature about the disease, as well as the experience of illness and possible death, is also helpful. Exactly how and when to involve children in decisions regarding care during their dying process and death is an

individual matter. The child's age or developmental level is an important consideration in the process (Table 36.4). In general, parents should be asked how they would like their child to be told of his or her prognosis, and they should be included in his or her care. Some parents may request that their child not be told that he or she is dying even if the child asks. This often places health care providers in a difficult situation. Children, even at a young age, are perceptive. Even if they are not told outright that they are dying, they realize that something is seriously wrong and that it involves them. Often, helping parents understand that honesty and shared decision making between them and their child are important to the child's and family's emotional health will encourage parents to allow discussion of dying with their child. Parents may require professional support and guidance in this process from a nurse, social worker, or child life specialist who has a good relationship with the child and family.

If given the opportunity, children will tell others how much they want to know. Nurses can help children set limits on how much truth they can accept and cope with by asking questions, such as "If the disease came back, would you want to know?" or "Do you want others to tell you everything even if the news isn't good?" or "If someone were not getting better [or more directly, were dying], do you think he would want to know?" Children need time to process feelings and information so that they can assimilate and ideally accept the reality of impending death.

Care of dying adolescents requires the nurse to become knowledgeable about any possible delays or alterations in normal growth and development. Legal and ethical issues also come to the forefront with respect to the age at which an adolescent should have autonomy in decision making with regard to care and treatment. Effective communication among the patient, family, and health care team is an important part of optimal care for dying adolescents (Barnes et al., 2012).

Treatment Options for Terminally Ill Children

Based on the child and family's decision regarding their wishes for terminal care, they have several options from which to choose.

Hospital

Families may choose to remain in the hospital to receive care if the child's illness or condition is unstable and home care is not an option or the family is uncomfortable with providing care at home. If a family chooses to remain at the hospital for terminal care, the setting should be made as homelike as possible. Families are encouraged to bring familiar items from the child's room at home. In addition, there should be a consistent and coordinated care plan for the comfort of the child and family.

Home Care

Some families prefer to take their child home and receive services from a home care agency. Generally, these services entail periodic nursing visits to administer a treatment or provide medications, equipment, or supplies. The child's care continues to be directed by the primary physician. Home care is often the option chosen by physicians and families because of the traditional view that a child must be considered to have a life expectancy of less than 6 months to be referred to hospice care. Fortunately, a number of hospice organizations are expanding their services to children based on the presence of a life-limiting disease process for which cure is not possible, rather than on the sole criteria of a limited time-projected prognosis.

Hospice Care

Parents should be offered the option of caring for their child at home during the final phases of an illness with the assistance of a hospice organization. Hospice* is a community health care organization that specializes in the care of dying patients by combining the hospice philosophy with the principles of palliative care. Hospice philosophy regards dying as a natural process and care of dying patients as including management of the physical, psychosocial, and spiritual needs of the patient and family. Care is provided by a multidisciplinary group of professionals in the patient's home or an inpatient facility that uses the hospice philosophy. Hospice care for children was introduced in the 1970s, and a number of community hospice organizations now accept children into their care (Keim-Malpass, Hart & Miller, 2013; Siden,

---

*For more information, contact National Hospice and Palliative Care Organization, 1700 Diagonal Road, Suite 625, Alexandria, VA 22314; 703-837-1500; fax: 703-837-1233; www.nhpco.org; and Children's Hospice International, 1101 King Street, Suite 360, Alexandria, VA 22314; 703-684-0330 or 800-24-CHILD; www.chionline.org.

Chavoshi, Harvey, et al., 2014). However, access to free-standing pediatric hospice services continues to be highly variable (Kassam & Wolfe, 2013). Collaboration between the child's primary treatment team and the hospice care team is essential to the success of hospice care. Families may continue to see their primary care physicians as they choose.

Hospice care is based on a number of important concepts that significantly set it apart from hospital care:
- Family members are usually the principal caregivers and are supported by a team of professional and volunteer staff.
- The priority of care is comfort. The child's physical, psychosocial, and spiritual needs are considered. Pain and symptom control are primary concerns, and no extraordinary efforts are used to attempt a cure or prolong life.
- The family's needs are considered to be as important as those of the patient.
- Hospice is concerned with the family's post-death adjustment, and care may continue for 1 year or longer.

TABLE 36.4 Children's Understanding of and Reactions to Death

Concepts of Death	Reactions to Death	Nursing Care Management
Infants and Toddlers		
Death has least significance to children younger than 6 months of age.	With the death of someone else, they may continue to act as though the person is alive.	Help parents deal with their feelings, allowing them greater emotional reserves to meet the needs of their children.
After parent-child attachment and trust are established, the loss, even if temporary, of the significant person is profound.	As children grow older, they will be increasingly able and willing to let go of the dead person.	Encourage parents to remain near child as much as possible, yet be sensitive to parents' needs.
Prolonged separation during the first several years is thought to be more significant in terms of future physical, social, and emotional growth than at any subsequent age.	Ritualism is important; a change in lifestyle could be anxiety producing.	Maintain as normal an environment as possible to retain ritualism.
Toddlers are egocentric and can only think about events in terms of their own frame of reference—living.	This age group reacts more to the pain and discomfort of a serious illness than to the probable fatal prognosis.	If a parent has died, encourage having a consistent caregiver for child.
Their egocentricity and vague separation of fact and fantasy make it impossible for them to comprehend absence of life.	This age group also reacts to parental anxiety and sadness.	Promote primary nursing.
Instead of understanding death, this age group is affected more by any change in lifestyle.		
Preschool Children		
Preschoolers believe their thoughts are sufficient to cause death; the consequence is the burden of guilt, shame, and punishment.	If they become seriously ill, they conceive of the illness as a punishment for their thoughts or actions.	Help parents deal with their feelings, allowing them greater emotional reserves to meet the needs of their children.
Their egocentricity implies a tremendous sense of self-power and omnipotence.	They may feel guilty and responsible for the death of a sibling.	Help parents understand behavioral reactions of their children.
They usually have some understanding of the meaning of death.	Greatest fear concerning death is separation from parents.	Encourage parents to remain near child as much as possible to minimize the child's great fear of separation from parents.
Death is seen as a departure, a kind of sleep.	They may engage in activities that seem strange or abnormal to adults.	If a parent has died, encourage having a consistent caregiver for child.
They may recognize the fact of physical death but do not separate it from living abilities.	Because they have fewer defense mechanisms to deal with loss, young children may react to a less significant loss with more outward grief than to the loss of a very significant person. The loss is so deep, painful, and threatening that the child must deny it for a time to survive its overwhelming impact.	Promote primary nursing.
Death is seen as temporary and gradual; life and death can change places with one another.	Behavior reactions such as giggling, joking, attracting attention, or regressing to earlier developmental skills indicate children's need to distance themselves from tremendous loss.	
They have no understanding of the universality and inevitability of death.		

Continued

TABLE 36.4 Children's Understanding of and Reactions to Death—cont'd

Concepts of Death	Reactions to Death	Nursing Care Management
School-Age Children		
Children still associate misdeeds or bad thoughts with causing death and feel intense guilt and responsibility for the event.	Because of their increased ability to comprehend, they may have more fears, for example:	Help parents deal with their feelings, allowing them greater emotional reserves to meet the needs of their children.

Because of their higher cognitive abilities, they respond well to logical explanations and comprehend the figurative meaning of words.	The reason for the illness
	  Communicability of the disease to themselves or others
	  Consequences of the disease
		Encourage parents to remain near child as much as possible, yet be sensitive to parents' needs.
		Because of children's fear of the unknown, anticipatory preparation is important.

They have a deeper understanding of death in a concrete sense.	The process of dying and death itself Their fear of the unknown is greater than their fear of the known.	Because the developmental task of this age is industry, interventions of helping children maintain control over their bodies and increasing
They particularly fear the mutilation and punishment that they associate with death.	The realization of impending death is a tremendous threat to their sense of security and ego strength.	their understanding allow them to achieve independence, self-worth, and self-esteem and avoid a sense of inferiority.
They personify death as the devil, a monster, or the bogeyman.	They are likely to exhibit fear through verbal uncooperativeness rather than actual physical aggression.	Encourage children to talk about their feelings, and provide aggressive outlets.
They may have naturalistic or physiologic explanations of death.	They are interested in post-death services.	Encourage parents to honestly answer questions about dying rather than avoiding the subject or fabricating euphemisms.
By 9 or 10 years of age, children have an adult concept of death, realizing that it is inevitable, universal, and irreversible.	They may be inquisitive about what happens to the body.	Encourage parents to share their moments of sorrow with their children. Provide preparation for post-death services.
Adolescents		
Adolescents have a mature understanding of death.	Adolescents straddle transition from childhood to adulthood.	Help parents deal with their feelings, allowing them greater emotional reserves to meet the needs of their children.
They are still influenced by remnants of magical thinking and are subject to guilt and shame.	They have the most difficulty in coping with death. They are least likely to accept cessation of life, particularly if it is their own.	Avoid alliances with either parent or child. Structure hospital admission to allow for maximum self-control and independence.
They are likely to see deviations from accepted behavior as reasons for their illness.	Concern is for the present much more than for the past or the future. They may consider themselves alienated from their peers and unable to communicate with their parents for emotional support, feeling alone in their struggle.	Answer adolescents' questions honestly, treating them as mature individuals and respecting their needs for privacy, solitude, and personal expressions of emotions.
	Adolescents' orientation to the present compels them to worry about physical changes even more than the prognosis.	Help parents understand their child's reactions to death and dying, especially that concern for present crises (e.g., loss of hair) may be much greater than for future ones, including possible death.
	Because of their idealistic view of the world, they may criticize funeral rites as barbaric, money making, and unnecessary.	

The goal of hospice care is for children to live life to the fullest without pain, with choices and dignity, in the familiar environment of their home, and with the support of their family. Hospice care is covered under state Medicaid programs and by most insurance plans. The service provides home visits from nurses, social workers, chaplains, and, in some cases, physicians. Medications, medical equipment, and any necessary medical supplies are all provided by the hospice organization providing care.

With children, the home has been the more common environment for implementing the hospice concept, and this benefits the family in a variety of ways. Children who are dying are allowed to remain with those they love and with whom they feel secure. Many children who were thought to be in imminent danger of death have gone home and lived longer than expected. Siblings can feel more involved in the care and often have more positive perceptions of the death. Parental adaptation is often more favorable, demonstrated by their perceptions of how the experience at home affected their marriage, social reorientation, religious beliefs, and views on the meaning of life and death.

If the home is chosen for hospice care, the child may or may not die in the home. Reasons for final admission to a hospital vary but may be related to the parents' or siblings' wish to have the child die outside the home, exhaustion on the part of the caregivers, and physical problems such as sudden, acute pain or respiratory distress.

NURSING CARE OF THE CHILD AND FAMILY AT THE END OF LIFE

Regardless of where the child is cared for during the terminal stage of illness, both the child and the family usually experience fear of (1) pain and suffering, (2) dying alone (child) or not being present when the child dies (parent), and (3) actual death. Nurses can help families by lessening their fears through attention to the care needs of the child and family.

FEAR OF PAIN AND SUFFERING

The presence of unrelieved pain in a terminally ill child can have detrimental effects on the quality of life experienced by the child and family. Parents feel that having their child in pain is unendurable and results in feelings of helplessness and a sense that they must be present and vigilant to get the necessary pain medications. Persistent pain also has an impact on the family as a whole. Nurses can alleviate the fear of pain and suffering by providing interventions aimed at treating the pain and symptoms associated with the terminal process in children.

Pain and Symptom Management

Pain control for children in the terminal stages of illness or injury must be given the highest priority. Despite ongoing efforts to educate physicians and nurses on pain management strategies in children, studies have reported that children continue to be undermedicated for their pain (Wolfe, Grier, Klar, et al., 2000). Nearly all children experience some amount of pain in the terminal phase of their illness. The current standard for treating children's pain follows the World Health Organization's (1996) analgesic stepladder, which promotes tailoring the pain interventions to the child's level of reported pain. Children's pain should be assessed frequently and medications adjusted as necessary. Pain medications should be given on a regular schedule, and extra doses for breakthrough pain should be available to maintain comfort. Opioid drugs such as morphine should be given for severe pain, and the dose should be increased as necessary to maintain optimal pain relief. Techniques, such as distraction, relaxation techniques, and guided imagery (Lambert, 1999), should be combined with drug therapy to provide the child and family strategies to control pain.

In addition to pain, children experience a variety of symptoms during their terminal course as a result of their disease process or as a side effect of medicines used to manage pain or other symptoms. These symptoms include fatigue, nausea and vomiting, constipation, anorexia, dyspnea, congestion, seizures, anxiety, depression, restlessness, agitation, and confusion (Hellsten, Hockenberry, Lamb, et al., 2000; von Lützau, Otto, Hechler, et al., 2012; Wolfe et al., 2002). Each of these symptoms should be aggressively managed with appropriate medications or treatments and with interventions such as repositioning, relaxation, massage, and other measures to maintain the child's comfort and quality of life.

Occasionally, children require very high doses of opioids to control pain. This may occur for several reasons. Children on long-term opioid pain management can become tolerant of the drug, meaning that it is necessary to give more drugs to maintain the same level of pain relief. This should not be confused with addiction, which is a psychologic dependence on the side effects of opioids. Addiction is not a factor in managing terminal pain in children. Other obvious reasons for requiring increased doses of opioids include progression of disease and other physiologic experiences of pain. It is important to understand that there is no maximum dose that can be given to control pain. However, nurses often express concern that administering doses of opioids that exceed what they are familiar with will hasten the child's death. The principle of double effect (Box 36.8) addresses such concerns. It provides an ethical standard that supports the use of interventions intended to relieve pain and suffering even though there is a foreseeable possibility that death may be hastened (Rousseau, 2001). In cases in which the child is terminally ill and in severe pain, using large doses of opioids and sedatives to manage pain is justified when no other treatment

---

> **BOX 36.8** **Ethical Principle of Double Effect**
>
> An action that has one good (intended) and one bad (unintended but foreseeable) effect is permissible if the following conditions are met:
> - The action itself must be good or indifferent. Only the good consequences of the action must be sincerely intended.
> - The good effect must not be produced by the bad effect.
> - There must be a compelling or proportionate reason for permitting the foreseeable bad effect to occur.

---

options are available that would relieve the pain but make the risk for death less likely (Hawryluck & Harvey, 2000; Jacobs, 2005).

Parents' and Siblings' Need for Education and Support

Parents are the primary caregivers when the child is at home, and nurses providing care to the child and family need to teach the family about the medications being given to the child, how to administer medications, and the use of nonpharmacologic techniques. This empowers parents and provides a sense of control over the child's comfort and well-being, reducing their fear that their child will be in pain or suffering as he or she is dying. Additionally, better bereavement outcomes (e.g., adaptive coping, family cohesion, and less anxiety, stress, and depression) have been reported by parents who were actively involved in the care of their child (Goodenough, Drew, Higgins, et al., 2004; Lauer, Mulhern, Schell, et al., 1989). The grief work of fathers in particular seems to be facilitated when their child dies in the home setting. This finding may be related to the increased opportunity of working fathers to provide care to and spend time with their child at home versus the hospital setting.

Siblings may feel isolated and displaced during the time that their brother or sister is dying. Parents devote the majority of their time to the care and comfort of the dying child, causing siblings to feel left out of the parent–sick child relationship. Siblings may become resentful of their sick sibling and begin to feel guilty or ashamed about such feelings (Murray, 1999). Nurses can assist the family by helping the parents identify ways to involve siblings in the caring process, perhaps by bringing some supplies or a favorite toy, game, or food item. Parents should also be encouraged to schedule time focusing on the siblings. Helping parents identify a trusted friend or family member who can sit with the ill child for a short period will allow them to attend to their own needs or those of their other children.

FEAR OF DYING ALONE OR OF NOT BEING PRESENT WHEN THE CHILD DIES

When a child is being cared for at home, the burden of care on parents and family members can be great. Often, as the child's condition declines, family members begin the "death vigil." Rarely is a child left alone for any length of time. This can be exhausting for family members, and nurses can assist the family by helping them arrange shifts so that friends or family members can be present with the child and allow others to rest. If the family has limited resources, community organizations, such as hospice or churches, often have volunteers who are willing to visit and sit with children. It is important that whoever is sitting with the child be aware of when the parent(s) would like to be notified to return to the child's bedside (Fig. 36.6).

When a child is dying in the hospital, the parents should be given full access to the child at all times. If the parents need to leave, they should be provided with a pager or other means of immediate communication and alerted if staff members note any change in the child that may indicate imminent death. Nurses should advocate for parents'

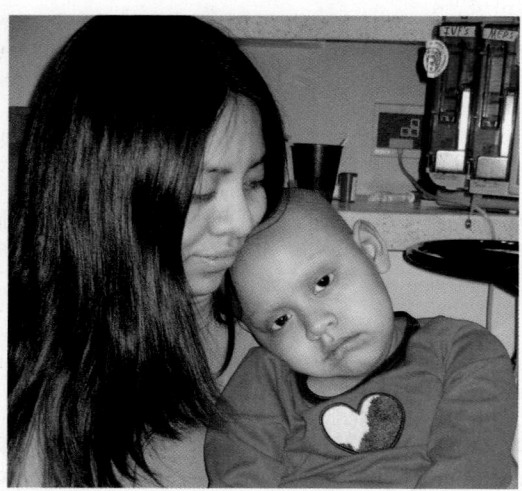

FIG 36.6 For a dying child, there is no greater comfort than the security and closeness of a parent.

BOX 36.9   **Physical Signs of Approaching Death**

Loss of sensation and movement in the lower extremities, progressing toward the upper body

Sensation of heat, although the body feels cool

Loss of senses:
- Tactile sensation decreasing
- Sensitivity to light
- Hearing the last sense to fail

Confusion, loss of consciousness, slurred speech

Muscle weakness

Loss of bowel and bladder control

Decreased appetite and thirst

Difficulty swallowing

Change in respiratory pattern:
- Cheyne-Stokes respirations (waxing and waning of depth of breathing with regular periods of apnea)
- "Death rattle" (noisy chest sounds from accumulation of pulmonary and pharyngeal secretions)

Weak, slow pulse; decreased blood pressure

---

presence in intensive care and emergency departments and attend to the parents' needs for food, drinks, comfortable chairs, blankets, and pillows.

FEAR OF ACTUAL DEATH

Home Deaths

The majority of children receiving hospice care die at home; they often die in their own room with family, pets, and loved possessions around them. The physical process of dying can be distressing to parents because often the child slowly becomes less alert in the days before the actual death. The nurse can assist the family by providing them with information about what changes will occur as the child progresses through the dying process (Box 36.9). During this time, nursing visits often become more frequent and longer in duration to provide the family with additional support as the death nears. The most distressing change for parents to observe is the change in the respiratory pattern. In the final hours of life, the dying patient's respirations may become labored, with deep breaths and long periods of apnea, referred to as *Cheyne-Stokes respirations*. Families should be reassured that this is not distressing to the child and that it is a normal part of the dying process. However, the use of opioids can slow the respirations to make the child breathe more easily, and scopolamine, usually applied as a topical patch, can help reduce noisy respirations known as the "death rattle." Noisy respirations are more likely to occur if the child is overhydrated.

All families have the option of admitting their child to the hospital if they feel unable to deal with the death. The child who dies at home must be pronounced dead. Hospice programs typically have provisions so that this proceeds smoothly. In some circumstances, the police may be notified, with an explanation of the circumstances to prevent unnecessary concern regarding abuse. Providing the police with the number of the responsible practitioner is usually all that is necessary to confirm the cause of death.

Hospital Deaths

Children dying in the hospital who are receiving supportive care interventions experience a similar process. Death resulting from accident or trauma or acute illness in settings such as the emergency department or intensive care unit, often requires the active withdrawal of some form of life-supporting intervention, such as a ventilator or bypass machine. These situations often raise difficult ethical issues (Sullivan, Monagle & Gillam, 2014), and parents are often less prepared for the actual moment of death. Nurses can assist these parents by providing detailed information about what will happen as supportive equipment is withdrawn, ensuring that appropriate pain medications are administered to prevent pain during the dying process and allowing the parents time before the start of the withdrawal to be with and speak to their child. It is important that the nurse attempt to control the environment around the family at this time by providing privacy, asking if they would like to play music, softening lights and monitor noises, and arranging for any religious or cultural rituals that the family may want performed.

After the child's death, the family should be allowed to remain with the body and hold or rock the child if they desire. After the nurse has removed all tubes and equipment from the body, the parents should be given the option of assisting with the preparation of the body, such as bathing and dressing. It is important for the nurse to determine whether the family has any specific needs because many cultures have adopted specific methods for coping with and mourning death, and impeding these practices may interfere with the grieving process (Clements, Vigil, Manno, et al., 2003).

At some point, the nurse discusses whether the family has made preparations for the burial service and whether the staff can help in any way. Parents often have concerns about the funeral, such as siblings' involvement in the death rituals. Although no absolute answers exist regarding the question of siblings attending the funeral or burial services, the consensus is that the surviving children benefit from being involved in these events. However, children need preparation for post-death services. They should be told what to expect, particularly how the deceased person will look if the coffin is open; allowed their private time to say good-bye; and permitted to stay as long as they wish. Ideally, the parents should prepare the siblings. If the parents' grief prevents this communication, a significant family member or friend should substitute.

ORGAN OR TISSUE DONATION AND AUTOPSY

For some families, organ or tissue donation may be a meaningful act—one that benefits another human being despite the loss of their child. Unfortunately, initiating a discussion about tissue donation is often stressful for staff, and there may be confusion regarding whose responsibility this is. In centers in which transplants are performed, a full-time transplant coordinator is usually available to inform the family about organ donation and to take care of details. If such services are not available, the staff needs to determine which members should discuss this topic with the family. Ideally, the person who knows the family best, knows when the death is expected, or has the opportunity to spend time with the family when the death is unexpected takes the role. Often nurses are in an optimal position to suggest tissue donation after consultation with the attending physician. When possible, the topic should be raised before death occurs. The request should be made in a private and quiet area of the hospital and should be simple and direct with questions, such as "Are you a donor family?" or "Have you ever considered organ donation?"

Many states have legislated a mandatory request for organ or tissue donation when a child dies, especially if the patient is brain dead. Written consent from the family is required before donation can proceed. When requests for organ donation are made, health care practitioners must address common misunderstandings families have about brain death and organ donation (Franz, DeJong, Wolfe, et al., 1997). Training health care professionals on sensitive approaches to requests for organ donation has been shown to increase families' willingness to consent to organ donation (Evanisko, Beasley, Brigham, et al., 1998; Workman, Myrick, Meyers, et al., 2013). The option to donate organs should always be separate from the communication of impending or actual death.

Nurses need to be aware of common questions about organ donation to help families make an informed decision. Healthy children who die unexpectedly are excellent candidates for organ donation. Children with cancer, chronic disease, or infection and those who have suffered prolonged cardiac arrest may not be suitable candidates, although this is individually determined. The nurse should ask whether organ donation was discussed with the child or whether the child ever expressed such a wish. Any number of body tissues or organs can be donated (skin, corneas, bone, kidney, heart, liver, pancreas), and their removal does not mutilate or desecrate the body or cause any suffering. The family may have an open casket, and there is no delay in the funeral. There is no cost to the donor family, but organ donation does not eliminate funeral or cremation responsibilities. With the exception of Orthodox Judaism, most religions permit organ donation as long as the recipient benefits from the transplant. In cases of unexplained death, violent death, or suspected suicide, autopsy is required by law. In other instances, it may be optional, and parents should be informed of this choice. The procedure, as well as forms that require signing, should be explained. The family should know that the child can be in an open casket after an autopsy.

GRIEF AND MOURNING

Grief is a process, not an event, of experiencing physiologic, psychologic, behavioral, social, and spiritual reactions to the loss of a child. Grief is highly individualized, encompassing a broad range of manifestations from person to person. It is a natural and expected reaction to loss. It is neither orderly nor predictable. Grieving in any form is necessary for healing to occur. When death is the expected or a possible outcome of a disorder, the child and family members may experience anticipatory grief. Anticipatory grief may be manifested in varying behaviors and intensities and may include denial, anger, depression, and other psychologic and physical symptoms.

Anticipatory guidance may assist grieving family members. Health care professionals should emphasize that grief reactions such as hearing the dead person's voice, feeling distant from others, or seeking reassurance that they did everything possible for the lost person are normal, necessary, and expected. They in no way signify poor coping, insanity, or an approaching mental breakdown. On the contrary, such behaviors signify that the survivor is working through the acute grief. Anticipatory guidance regarding the mourning process may help families recognize the normalcy of their experiences.

It is important to recognize that some family members may experience complicated grief. Complicated grief reactions (>1 year after the loss) include such symptoms as intense intrusive thoughts, pangs of severe emotion, distressing yearnings, feelings of excessive loneliness and emptiness, unusual sleep disturbance, and maladaptive levels of loss of interest in personal activities (Meert et al., 2011). Bereaved persons experiencing such prolonged and complicated grief should be referred to an expert in grief and bereavement counseling.

Another important aspect of grief is the individual nature of the grief experience. Each member of the family will experience the grief of the child's death in his or her own way based on the particular relationship with that child. This can create potential conflict for families, because each family member has expectations that the other family members should feel and grieve as they do. Nurses caring for families experiencing grief should be aware of the different grieving styles and help the family learn to recognize and support the uniqueness of each other's grief.

Parental Grief

Parental grief after the death of a child has been found to be the most intense, complex, long-lasting, and fluctuating grief experience compared with that of other bereaved individuals. Although parents experience the primary loss of their child, many secondary losses are felt, such as the loss of part of one's self, hopes and dreams for the child's future, the family unit, prior social and emotional community supports, and often spousal support. It is common for parents of the same child to experience different grief reactions.

Studies with bereaved parents have shown that grieving does not end with the severing of the bond with the deceased child but rather involves a continuing bond between the parent and the deceased child (Klass, 2001). Parental resolution of grief is a process of integrating the dead child into daily life in which the pain of losing a child is never completely gone but lessens. There are occasions of brief relapse, but not to the degree experienced when the loss initially occurred. Thus, parental grief work is never completed and is a timeless process of accommodating the new reality of being without a child as it changes over time (Davies, 2004). A child's death can also challenge the marital relationship in several ways. Maternal and paternal reactions often differ (Hendrickson, 2009; Moriarty, Carroll & Cotroneo, 1996; Scholtes & Browne, 2015; Vance, Najman, Thearle, et al., 1995). Different grieving styles between the couple may hinder communication and support for each other. Differing needs and expectations can place a strain on the marriage.

Sibling Grief

Each child grieves in his or her own way and on his or her own timeline. Children, even adolescents, grieve differently than adults. Adults and children differ more widely in their reactions to death than in their reactions to any other phenomenon. Children of all ages grieve the loss of a loved one, and their understanding and reactions to death depend on their age and developmental level. Children grieve for a longer duration, revisiting their grief as they grow and develop new understandings of death. However, they do not grieve 100% of the time. They grieve in spurts and can be emotional and sad in one instance and then, just as quickly, off and playing. Children express their grief through play and behavior. Children can be exquisitely attuned to their parents' grief and will try to protect them by not asking questions or by trying not to upset them. This can set the stage for the sibling to try to become the "perfect child." Children exhibit many of the grief reactions of adults, including physical sensations and illnesses, anger, guilt, sadness, loneliness, withdrawal, acting out, sleep disturbances, isolation, and search for meaning. Again, nurses should be attentive for signs that siblings are struggling with their grief and provide guidance to parents when possible.

At times, family members may need assistance in their grieving (see Guidelines box: Supporting Grieving Families). Communication with the bereaved family is essential, but often nurses do not know what to say and feel helpless in offering words of comfort. The most supportive approach is to avoid judging the family's reactions or offering advice or rationalizations and to focus on feelings. Perhaps the most valuable supportive measure the nurse can perform for families is to listen. Families understand that no words will relieve their pain; all they want is acceptance, understanding, and respect for their grief.

GUIDELINES

*Supporting Grieving Families**

General

Stay with the family; sit quietly if they prefer not to talk; cry with them if desired.

Accept the family's grief reactions; avoid judgmental statements (e.g., "You should be feeling better by now").

Avoid offering rationalizations for the child's death (e.g., "Your child isn't suffering anymore").

Avoid artificial consolation (e.g., "I know how you feel," or "You are still young enough to have another baby").

Deal openly with feelings such as guilt, anger, and loss of self-esteem.

Focus on feelings by using a feeling word in the statement (e.g., "You're still feeling all the pain of losing a child").

Refer the family to an appropriate self-help group or for professional help if needed.

At the Time of Death

Reassure the family that everything possible is being done for the child if they want lifesaving interventions.

Do everything possible to ensure the child's comfort, especially relieving pain.

Provide the child and family with the opportunity to review special experiences or memories in their lives.

Express personal feelings of loss or frustration (e.g., "We will miss him so much," "We tried everything; we feel so sorry that we couldn't save her").

Provide information that the family requests, and be honest.

Respect the emotional needs of family members, such as siblings, who may need brief respites from the dying child.

Make every effort to arrange for family members, especially the parents, to be with the child at the moment of death if they want to be present.

Allow the family to stay with the dead child for as long as they wish and to rock, hold, or bathe the child.

Provide practical help when possible, such as collecting the child's belongings.

Arrange for spiritual support based on the family's religious beliefs; pray with the family if no one else can stay with them.

Post Death

Attend the funeral or visitation if there was a special closeness with the family.

Initiate and maintain contact (e.g., sending cards, telephoning, inviting them back to the unit, making a home visit).

Refer to the dead child by name; discuss shared memories with the family.

Discourage the use of drugs and alcohol as a method of escaping grief.

Encourage all family members to communicate their feelings rather than remaining silent to avoid upsetting another member.

Emphasize that grieving is a painful process that often takes years to resolve.

*"Family" refers to all significant persons involved in the child's life, such as the parents, siblings, grandparents, and other close relatives or friends.

It is important for families to understand that mourning takes a long time. Whereas acute grief may last only weeks or months, resolving the loss is measured in years. Holidays and anniversaries can be particularly difficult, and people who previously had been supportive may now expect the family to have "adjusted." Consequently, prolonged mourning is often silent and lonely.

Many families never receive the support and guidance that could help them resolve the loss. A plan for regular follow-up with bereaved families can be beneficial. At minimum, one follow-up phone call or meeting with the family should be arranged. Families can also be referred to self-help groups. When such groups are not available, nurses can be instrumental in bringing families together or facilitating parent and sibling groups. Formal bereavement programs or bereavement counseling can be helpful as well.

NURSES' REACTIONS TO CARING FOR DYING CHILDREN

The death of a patient is one of the most stressful aspects of nursing.* Nurses experience reactions to the death of a patient that are very similar to the responses of family members, including denial, anger, depression, guilt, and ambivalent feelings.

Strategies that can assist nurses in maintaining the ability to work effectively in these settings include maintaining good general health, developing well-rounded interests, using distancing techniques such as taking time off when needed, developing and using professional and personal support systems, cultivating the capacity for empathy, focusing on the positive aspects of the caregiver role, and basing nursing interventions on sound theory and empiric observations. Attending shared-remembrance rituals assists some nurses in resolving grief (Davis and Eng, 1998). Similarly, attending the funeral services can be a supportive act for both the family and the nurse and in no way detracts from the professionalism of care.

REFERENCES

American Nurses Association (2015). *Code of ethics for nurses with interpretive statements.* Washington, DC: ANA Publishing.

American Psychological Association (2013). *Diagnostic and statistical manual of mental disorders (DSM-5)* (5th ed.). Arlington, VA: American Psychological Association.

Anderson, R. N., & Smith, B. L. (2005). Deaths: Leading causes for 2002. *National Vital Statistics Reports, 53*(17), 1–89.

Anderson, T., & Davis, C. (2011). Evidence-based practice with families of chronically ill children: A critical literature review. *Journal of Evidence-Based Social Work, 8*(4), 416–425.

Baker, J. N., Torkildson, C., Baillargeon, J. G., et al. (2007). National survey of pediatric residency program directors and residents regarding education in palliative medicine and end-of-life care. *Journal of Palliative Medicine, 10*(2), 420–429.

*Other sources of publications on life-threatening illness and death are: The Compassionate Friends, PO Box 3696, Oak Brook, IL 60522-3696; 630-990-0010 or 877-969-0010; https://www.compassionatefriends.org; Centering Corporation, 7230 Maple Street, Omaha, NE 68134; 866-218-0101; http://www.centering.org; Children's Hospice International, 1104 King Street, Suite 360, Alexandria, VA 22314; 800-24-CHILD or 703-684-0330; e-mail: info@chionline.org; www.chionline.org; and National Cancer Institute, Cancer Information Service, Building 21, Room 10A29, Bethesda, MD 20892-2580; 800-422-6237; https://www.cancer.gov.

Barlow, J. H., & Ellard, D. R. (2006). The psychosocial well-being of children with chronic disease, their parents and siblings: An overview of the research evidence base. *Child: Care, Health and Development, 32*(1), 19–31.

Barnes, S., Gardiner, C., Gott, M., et al. (2012). Enhancing patient-professional communication about end-of-life issues in life-limiting conditions: A critical review of the literature. *Journal of Pain and Symptom Management, 44*(6), 866–879.

Beale, E. A., Baile, W. F., & Aaron, J. (2005). Silence is not golden: Communicating with children dying from cancer. *Journal of Clinical Oncology, 23*(15), 3629–3631.

Berry, J. G., Hall, M., Hall, D. E., et al. (2013). Inpatient growth and resource use in 28 children's hospitals: A longitudinal, multi-institutional study. *JAMA Pediatrics, 167*(2), 170–177.

Bettle, A. M., & Latimer, M. A. (2009). Maternal coping and adaptation: A case study examination of chronic sorrow in caring for an adolescent with a progressive neurodegenerative disease. *Canadian Journal of Neuroscience Nursing, 31*(4), 15–21.

Blume, E. D., Balkin, E. M., Aiyagari, R., et al. (2014). Parental perspectives on suffering and quality of life at end-of-life in children with advanced heart disease: An exploratory study. *Pediatric Critical Care Medicine, 15*(4), 336–342.

Burke, R. T., & Alverson, B. (2010). Impact of children with medically complex conditions. *Pediatrics, 126*(4), 789–790.

Burns, K. H., Casey, P. H., Lyle, R. E., et al. (2010). Increasing prevalence of medically complex children in US hospitals. *Pediatrics, 126*(4), 638–646.

Carnevale, F. A., Alexander, E., Davis, M., et al. (2006). Daily living with distress and enrichment: The moral experience of families with ventilator-assisted children at home. *Pediatrics, 117*(1), e48–e60.

Carnevale, F. A., Rehm, R. S., Kirk, S., et al. (2008). What we know (and don't know) about raising children with complex continuing care needs. *Journal of Child Health Care, 12*(1), 4–6.

Clements, P. T., Vigil, G. J., Manno, M. S., et al. (2003). Cultural perspectives of death, grief, and bereavement. *Journal of Psychosocial Nursing and Mental Health Services, 41*(7), 18–26.

Coffey, J. S. (2006). Parenting a child with chronic illness: A metasynthesis. *Pediatric Nursing, 32*(1), 51–59.

Cohen, E., Friedman, J., Nicholas, D. B., et al. (2008). A home for medically complex children: The role of hospital programs. *Journal for Healthcare Quality, 30*(3), 7–15.

Cohen, E., Kuo, D. Z., Agrawal, R., et al. (2011). Children with medical complexity: An emerging population for clinical and research initiatives. *Pediatrics, 127*(3), 529–538.

Coker, T. R., Rodriguez, M. A., & Flores, G. (2010). Family-centered care for US children with special health care needs: Who gets it and why? *Pediatrics, 125*(6), 1159–1167.

Corlett, J., & Twycross, A. (2006). Negotiation of parental roles within family-centered care: A review of the research. *Journal of Clinical Nursing, 15*(10), 1308–1316.

Council on Children with Disabilities. (2005). Care coordination in the medical home: integrating health and related systems of care for children with special health care needs. *Pediatrics, 116*(5), 1238–1244.

Davies, B., Gudmundsdottir, M., Worden, B., et al. (2004). "Living in the dragon's shadow": Fathers' experiences of a child's life-limiting illness. *Death Studies, 28*(2), 111–135.

Davies, R. (2004). New understandings of parental grief: Literature review. *Journal of Advanced Nursing, 46*(5), 506–513.

Davis, B., & Eng, B. (1998). Special issues in bereavement and staff support. In D. Doyle, G. W. C. Hanks, & N. MacDonald (Eds.), *Oxford textbook of palliative medicine* (2nd ed.). Oxford, UK: Oxford University Press.

Dell'Api, M., Rennick, J. E., & Rosmus, C. (2007). Childhood chronic pain and health care professional interactions: Shaping the chronic pain experiences of children. *Journal of Child Health Care, 11*(4), 269–286.

Dixon-Woods, M., Young, B., & Heney, D. (1999). Partnerships with children. *British Medical Journal, 319*(7212), 778–780.

Dunst, C. J., & Trivette, C. M. (2009). Meta-analytic structural equation modeling of the influences of family-centered care on parent and child psychological health. *International Journal of Pediatrics, 2009*, 576840.

Evanisko, M. J., Beasley, C. L., Brigham, L. E., et al. (1998). Readiness of critical care physicians and nurses to handle requests for organ donation. *American Journal of Critical Care, 7*(1), 4–12.

Feudtner, C., Feinstein, J. A., Zhong, W., et al. (2014). Pediatric complex chronic conditions classification system version 2: Updated for ICD-10 and complex medical technology dependence and transplantation. *BMC Pediatrics, 14*, 199.

Field, M. J., & Behrman, R. E. (Eds.), (2004). *When children die: Improving palliative and end-of-life care for children and their families.* Washington, DC: National Academies Press.

Fleitas, J. (2000). When Jack fell down … Jill came tumbling after: Siblings in the web of illness and disability. *American Journal of Maternal/Child Nursing, 25*(5), 267–273.

Franz, H. G., DeJong, W., Wolfe, S. M., et al. (1997). Explaining brain death: A critical feature of the donation process. *Journal of Transplant Coordination, 7*(1), 14–21.

Giannini, A., Messeri, A., Aprile, A., et al. (2008). End-of-life decisions in pediatric intensive care: Recommendations of the Italian Society of Neonatal and Pediatric Anesthesia and Intensive Care (SARNePI). *Paediatric Anaesthesia, 18*(11), 1089–1095.

Gold, J. I., Treadwell, M., Weissman, L., et al. (2011). The mediating effects of family functioning on psychosocial outcomes in healthy siblings of children with sickle cell disease. *Pediatric Blood & Cancer, 57*(6), 1055–1061.

Goodenough, B., Drew, D., Higgins, S., et al. (2004). Bereavement outcomes for parents who lose a child to cancer: Are place of death and sex of parent associated with differences in psychological functioning? *Psycho-Oncology, 13*(11), 779–791.

Gordon, J. (2009). An evidence-based approach for supporting parents experiencing chronic sorrow. *Pediatric Nursing, 35*(2), 115–119.

Goudie, A., Narcisse, M. R., Hall, D. E., et al. (2014). Financial and psychological stressors associated with caring for children with disability. *Family, Systems, & Health, 32*(3), 280–290.

Hartling, L., Milne, A., Tjosvold, L., et al. (2014). A systematic review of interventions to support siblings of children with chronic illness or disability. *Journal of Paediatrics and Child Health, 50*(10), E26–E38.

Hawryluck, L. A., & Harvey, W. R. (2000). Analgesia, virtue, and the principle of double effect. *Journal of Palliative Care, 16*(suppl), S24–S30.

Hellsten, M. B., Hockenberry, M., Lamb, D., et al. (2000). *End-of-life care for children.* Austin, TX: Texas Cancer Council.

Hendrickson, K. C. (2009). Morbidity, mortality, and parental grief: A review of the literature on the relationship between the death of a child and the subsequent health of parents. *Palliative & Supportive Care, 7*(1), 109–119.

Hinds, P. S., Oakes, L., Furman, W., et al. (2001). End-of-life decision making by adolescents, parents, and healthcare providers in pediatric oncology: Research to evidence-based practice guidelines. *Cancer Nursing, 24*(2), 122–134.

Hsiao, J. L., Evan, E. E., & Zeltzer, L. K. (2007). Parent and child perspectives on physician communication in pediatric palliative care. *Palliative & Supportive Care, 5*(4), 355–365.

Huang, I. C., Kenzik, K. M., Sanjeev, T. Y., et al. (2010). Quality of life information and trust in physicians among families of children with life-limiting conditions. *Patient Related Outcome Measures, 2010*(1), 141–148.

Hungerbuehler, I., Vollrath, M. E., & Landolt, M. A. (2011). Posttraumatic growth in mothers and fathers of children with severe illnesses. *Journal of Health Psychology, 16*(8), 1259–1267.

Immelt, S. (2006). Psychological adjustment in young children with chronic medical conditions. *Journal of Pediatric Nursing, 21*(5), 362–377.

Jacobs, H. H. (2005). Ethics in pediatric end-of-life care: A nursing perspective. *Journal of Pediatric Nursing, 20*(5), 360–369.

James, L., & Johnson, B. (1997). The needs of parents of pediatric oncology patients during the palliative care phase. *Journal of Pediatric Oncology Nursing, 14*(2), 83–95.

Jokinen, P. (2004). The family life-path theory: A tool for nurses working in partnership with families. *Journal of Child Health Care, 8*(2), 124–133.

Jones, T. L., & Prinz, R. J. (2005). Potential roles of parental self-efficacy in parent and child adjustment: A review. *Clinical Psychology Review, 25*(3), 341–363.

Kassam, A., & Wolfe, J. (2013). The ambiguities of free-standing pediatric hospices. *Journal of Palliative Medicine, 16*(7), 716–717.

Kavanaugh, K., Moro, T. T., & Savage, T. A. (2010). How nurses assist parents regarding life support decisions for extremely premature infants. *Journal of Obstetric, Gynecologic, & Neonatal Nursing, 39*(2), 147–158.

Keim-Malpass, J., Hart, T. G., & Miller, J. R. (2013). Coverage of palliative and hospice care for pediatric patients with a life-limiting illness: A policy brief. *Journal of Pediatric Health Care, 27*(6), 511–516.

Kirk, S., Glendinning, C., & Callery, P. J. (2005). Parent or nurse? The experience of being the parent of a technology-dependent child. *Journal of Advanced Nursing, 51*(5), 456–464.

Klass, D. (2001). The inner representation of the dead child in the psychic and social narratives of bereaved parents. In R. A. Neimeyer (Ed.), *Meaning reconstruction and the experience of loss*. Washington, DC: American Psychological Association.

Knafl, K. A., Darney, B. G., Gallo, A. M., et al. (2010). Parental perceptions of the outcome and meaning of normalization. *Research in Nursing & Health, 33*(2), 87–98.

Knafl, K. A., & Santacroce, S. J. (2010). Chronic conditions and the family. In P. J. Allen, J. A. Vessey, & N. A. Schapiro (Eds.), *Primary care of the child with a chronic condition* (5th ed.). St Louis, MO: Mosby/Elsevier.

Kochanek, K. D., Murphy, S. L., Xu, J., et al. (2014). Mortality in the United States, 2013. *NCHS Data Brief, 178*, 1–8.

Kon, A. A. (2010). The shared decision-making continuum. *Journal of the American Medical Association, 304*(8), 903–904.

Kratz, L., Uding, N., Trahms, C. M., et al. (2009). Managing childhood chronic illness: Parent perspectives and implications for parent-provider relationships. *Families, Systems, & Health, 27*(4), 303–313.

Kuhlthau, K. A., Bloom, S., Van Cleave, J., et al. (2011). Evidence for family-centered care for children with special health care needs: A systematic review. *Academic Pediatrics, 11*(2), 136–143.

Kuo, D. Z., Cohen, E., Agrawal, R., et al. (2011). A national profile of caregiver challenges among more medically complex children with special health care needs. *Archives of Pediatrics and Adolescent Medicine, 165*(11), 1020–1026.

Kuo, D. Z., Houtrow, A. J., Arango, P., et al. (2012). Family-centered care: Current applications and future directions in pediatric health care. *Maternal and Child Health Journal, 16*(2), 297–305.

Kuo, D. Z., Sisterhen, L. L., Sigrest, T. E., et al. (2012). Family experiences and pediatric health services use associated with family-centered rounds. *Pediatrics, 130*(2), 299–305.

Lambert, S. (1999). Distraction, imagery, and hypnosis techniques for management of children's pain. *Journal of Child and Family Nursing, 2*(1), 5–15.

Lauer, M. E., Mulhern, R. K., Schell, M. J., et al. (1989). Long-term follow-up of parental adjustment following a child's death at home or hospital. *Cancer, 63*(5), 988–994.

LeGrow, K., Hodnett, E., Stremler, R., et al. (2014). Bourdieu at the bedside: Briefing parents in a pediatric hospital. *Nursing Inquiry, 21*(4), 327–335.

Lipstein, E. A., Brinkman, W. B., & Britto, M. T. (2012). What is known about parents' treatment decisions? A narrative review of pediatric decision making. *Medical Decision Making, 32*(2), 246–258.

Lobato, D. J., & Kao, B. T. (2002). Integrated sibling–parent group intervention to improve sibling knowledge and adjustment to chronic illness and disability. *Journal of Pediatric Psychology, 27*(8), 711–716.

Lobato, D. J., Kao, B. T., & Plante, W. (2005). Latino sibling knowledge and adjustment to chronic illness. *Journal of Family Psychology, 19*(4), 625–632.

MacDonald, H., & Callery, P. (2008). Parenting children requiring complex care: A journey through time. *Child: Care, Health and Development, 34*(2), 207–213.

Meert, K. L., Shear, K., Newth, C. J., et al. (2011). Follow-up study of complicated grief among parents eighteen months after a child's death in the pediatric intensive care unit. *Journal of Palliative Medicine, 14*(2), 207–214.

Monterosso, L., Kristjanson, L. J., Aoun, S., et al. (2007). Supportive and palliative care needs of families of children with life-threatening illnesses in Western Australia: Evidence to guide the development of a palliative care service. *Palliative Medicine, 1*(8), 689–696.

Moriarty, H., Carroll, R., & Cotroneo, M. (1996). Differences in bereavement reactions within couples following the death of a child. *Research in Nursing & Health, 19*(6), 461–469.

Murray, J. S. (1999). Siblings of children with cancer: A review of the literature. *Journal of Pediatric Oncology Nursing, 16*(1), 25–34.

Nelson, A. M. (2002). A metasynthesis: Mothering other-than-normal children. *Qualitative Health Research, 12*(4), 515–530.

Newacheck, P. W., & Halfon, N. (1998). Prevalence and impact of disabling chronic conditions in childhood. *American Journal of Public Health, 88*(4), 610–617.

Nuutila, L., & Salanterä, S. (2006). Children with a long-term illness: Parents' experiences of care. *Journal of Pediatric Nursing, 21*(2), 153–160.

O'Brien, I., Duffy, A., & Nicholl, H. (2009). Impact of childhood chronic illnesses on siblings: A literature review. *British Journal of Nursing, 18*(22), 1358, 1360-1365.

O'Quinn, L. P., & Giambra, B. K. (2014). Evidence of improved quality of life with pediatric palliative care. *Journal of Pediatric Nursing, 40*(6), 284–288, 296.

Panicker, L. (2013). Nurses' perceptions of parent empowerment in chronic illness. *Contemporary Nurse, 45*(2), 210–219.

Pousset, G., Bilsen, J., Cohen, J., et al. (2010). Medical end-of-life decisions in children in Flanders, Belgium: A population-based postmortem survey. *Archives of Pediatrics and Adolescent Medicine, 164*(6), 547–553.

Price, J., Dornan, J., & Quail, L. (2013). Seeing is believing—Reducing misconceptions about children's hospice care through effective teaching with undergraduate nursing students. *Nurse Education in Practice, 13*(5), 361–365.

Raina, P., O'Donnell, M., Rosenbaum, P., et al. (2005). The health and well-being of caregivers of children with cerebral palsy. *Pediatrics, 115*(6), e626–e636.

Ritchie, M. A. (2001). Self-esteem and hopefulness in adolescents with cancer. *Journal of Pediatric Nursing, 16*(1), 35–42.

Rousseau, P. (2001). Ethical and legal issues in palliative care. *Primary Care, 28*(2), 391–400.

Scholtes, D., & Browne, M. (2015). Internalized and externalized continuing bonds in bereaved parents: Their relationship with grief intensity and personal growth. *Death Studies, 39*(2), 75–83.

Schor, E. L., & American Academy of Pediatrics Task Force on the Family. (2003). Family pediatrics: Report of the Task Force on the Family. *Pediatrics, 111*(6 pt 2), 1541–1571.

Siden, H., Chavoshi, N., Harvey, B., et al. (2014). Characteristics of a pediatric hospice palliative care program over 15 years. *Pediatrics, 134*(3), e765–e772.

Simon, T. D., Berry, J., Feudtner, C., et al. (2010). Children with complex chronic conditions in inpatient hospital settings in the United States. *Pediatrics, 126*(4), 647–655.

Smaldone, A., & Ritholz, M. D. (2011). Perceptions of parenting children with type 1 diabetes diagnosed in early childhood. *Journal of Pediatric Health Care, 25*(2), 87–95.

Stein, R. E. K. (1985). Home care: A challenging opportunity. *Children's Health Care: Journal of the Association for the Care of Children's Health, 14*(2), 90–95.

Sullivan, J., Monagle, P., & Gillam, L. (2014). What parents want from doctors in end-of-life decision-making for children. *Archives of Disease in Childhood, 99*(3), 216–220.

Sullivan-Bolyai, S., Sadler, L., Knafl, K. A., et al. (2003). Great expectations: A position description for parents as caregivers, part I. *Journal of Pediatric Nursing, 29*(6), 52–56.

Swallow, V., Macfadyen, A., Santacroce, S. J., et al. (2012). Fathers' contributions to the management of their child's long-term medical condition: A narrative review of the literature. *Health Expectations, 15*(2), 157–175.

Thibodeaux, A. G., & Deatrick, J. A. (2007). Cultural influence on family management of children with cancer. *Journal of Pediatric Oncology Nursing, 24*(4), 227–233.

Thomlinson, E. H. (2002). The lived experience of families of children who are failing to thrive. *Journal of Advanced Nursing, 39*(6), 537–545.

Toomey, S. L., Chien, A. T., Elliott, M. N., et al. (2013). Disparities in unmet need for care coordination: The national survey of children's health. *Pediatrics*, *131*(2), 217–224.

Treyvaud, K. (2014). Parent and family outcomes following very preterm or very low birth weight birth: A review. *Seminars in Fetal and Neonatal Medicine*, *19*(2), 131–135.

Vance, J. C., Najman, J. M., Thearle, M. J., et al. (1995). Psychological changes in parents eight months after the loss of an infant from stillbirth, neonatal death, or sudden infant death syndrome—A longitudinal study. *Pediatrics*, *96*(5), 933–938.

von Lützau, P., Otto, M., Hechler, T., et al. (2012). Children dying from cancer: Parents' perspectives on symptoms, quality of life, characteristics of death, and end-of-life decisions. *Journal of Palliative Care*, *28*(4), 274–281.

Wiener, L., McConnell, D. G., Latella, L., et al. (2013). Cultural and religious considerations in pediatric palliative care. *Palliative & Supportive Care*, *11*(1), 47–67.

Whitehead, L. C., & Gosling, V. (2003). Parent's perceptions of interactions with health professionals in the pathway to gaining a diagnosis of tuberous sclerosis (TS) and beyond. *Research in Developmental Disabilities*, *24*(2), 109–119.

Wolfe, J., Friebert, S., & Hilden, J. (2002). Caring for children with advanced cancer integrating palliative care. *Pediatric Clinics of North America*, *49*(5), 1043–1062.

Wolfe, J., Grier, H. E., Klar, N., et al. (2000). Symptoms and suffering at the end of life in children with cancer. *New England Journal of Medicine*, *342*(5), 326–333.

Workman, J. K., Myrick, C. W., Meyers, R. L., et al. (2013). Pediatric organ donation and transplantation. *Pediatrics*, *131*(6), e1723–e1730.

World Health Organization (1996). *Cancer pain relief and palliative care.* Geneva, Switzerland: Author.

World Health Organization (1998). *Definition of palliative care for children.* Retrieved from http://www.who.int/cancer/palliative/definition/en.

Wyatt, K. D., List, B., Brinkman, W. B., et al. (2015). Shared decision making in pediatrics: A systematic review and meta-analysis. *Academic Pediatrics*, *15*(6), 573–583.

Young, B., Dixon-Woods, M., Windridge, K. C., et al. (2003). Managing communication with young people who have a potentially life threatening chronic illness: Qualitative study of patients and parents. *British Medical Journal*, *326*(7384), 305.

37

Impact of Cognitive or Sensory Impairment on the Child and Family

Marilyn J. Hockenberry

http://evolve.elsevier.com/Perry/maternal

COGNITIVE IMPAIRMENT

GENERAL CONCEPTS

Cognitive impairment (CI) is a general term that encompasses any type of intellectual disability. The term *intellectual disability* has widely replaced the term *mental retardation* as defined by the American Association on Intellectual and Developmental Disabilities (American Association on Intellectual and Developmental Disabilities, 2013; American Psychiatric Association, 2013). In this chapter, the term *CI* is used synonymously with *intellectual disability.*

Intellectual disability defined by the American Association on Intellectual and Developmental Disabilities in children consists of three components: (1) intellectual functioning, (2) functional strengths and weaknesses, and (3) age younger than 18 years at time of diagnosis. Intellectual functioning is measured by the intelligence quotient (IQ) test score of 70 and below or as high as 75. The child with an intellectual disability must demonstrate functional impairment in a number of different adaptive areas: communication, self-care, home living, social skills, leisure, health and safety, self-direction, functional academics, community use, and work (American Association on Intellectual and Developmental Disabilities, 2013). The American Psychiatric Association's *Diagnostic and Statistical Manual of Mental Disorders,* fifth edition (DSM-5), new criteria recommend moving away from exclusively relying on IQ testing toward using additional measures of adaptive functioning (American Psychiatric Association, 2013; Moran, 2013). The DSM-5 is the diagnostic standard and states that the child with CI must demonstrate deficits in adaptive functioning that result in failure to meet developmental and sociocultural standards for personal independence and social responsibility (Moran, 2013).

The American Psychiatric Association's DSM-5 terminology and diagnostic criteria are consistent with those terms established by American Association on Intellectual and Developmental Disabilities (Tassé, Luckasson, & Nygren, 2013). Careful evaluation to identify the needs of individuals with CI is focused on promoting habilitation for each person. It is anticipated that the functional capabilities of children with CI will improve over time when support is provided.

Diagnosis and Classification

The diagnosis of CI is usually made after professionals or the family suspects that the child's developmental progress is delayed. In some cases, it is confirmed at birth because of recognition of distinct syndromes, such as Down syndrome and fetal alcohol syndrome. At the other extreme, the diagnosis is made when problems such as speech delays or school problems arouse concern. In all cases, a high index of suspicion for developmental delay and behavioral signs is necessary for early diagnosis (Box 37.1); and routine developmental screening can assist in early identification. Delays are typically seen in gross and fine motor and speech development, although the latter is most predictive. *Developmental disability* can be described as any significant lag or delay in a child's physical, cognitive, behavioral, emotional, or social development when compared against developmental norms. CI is an impairment encompassing intellectual ability and adaptive behavior that are functioning significantly below average (see Box 37.1). In the absence of clear-cut evidence of CI, it is more appropriate to use a diagnosis of developmental disability.

Results of standardized tests are helpful in contributing to the diagnosis of CI. Tests for assessing adaptive behaviors include the Vineland Social Maturity Scale and the American Association on Mental Retardation Adaptive Behavior Scale. Informal appraisal of adaptive behavior may be made by those fully acquainted with the child (e.g., teachers, parents, other care providers). Frequently, these observations lead parents to seek evaluation of the child's development.

A more useful approach for clinical application is classification based on educational potential or symptom severity. For educational purposes, the mildly impaired group constitutes about 85% of all people with CI, and the group with moderate levels of CI accounts for about 10% of the intellectually disabled population (Shapiro & Batshaw, 2011; Shea, 2012).

Etiology

The causes of severe CI are primarily genetic, biochemical, and infectious. Although the etiology is unknown in the majority of cases, familial, social, environmental, and organic causes may predominate. Among individuals with CI, a sizable proportion of the cases are linked to Down syndrome, fragile X syndrome (FXS), or fetal alcohol syndrome. General categories of events that may lead to CI include the following (Katz & Lazcano-Ponce, 2008; Walker & Johnson, 2006):

- Infection and intoxication, such as congenital rubella, syphilis, maternal drug consumption (e.g., fetal alcohol syndrome), chronic lead ingestion, or kernicterus
- Trauma or physical agent (e.g., injury to the brain experienced during the prenatal, perinatal, or postnatal period)
- Inadequate nutrition and metabolic disorders, such as phenylketonuria or congenital hypothyroidism
- Gross postnatal brain disease, such as neurofibromatosis and tuberous sclerosis
- Unknown prenatal influence, including cerebral and cranial malformations, such as microcephaly and hydrocephalus

- Chromosomal abnormalities resulting from radiation; viruses; chemicals; parental age; and genetic mutations, such as Down syndrome and FXS
- Gestational disorders, including prematurity, low birth weight, and postmaturity
- Psychiatric disorders that have their onset during the child's developmental period up to 18 years of age, such as autism spectrum disorders (ASDs)
- Environmental influences, including evidence of a deprived environment associated with a history of intellectual disability among parents and siblings

NURSING CARE OF CHILDREN WITH IMPAIRED COGNITIVE FUNCTION

Nurses play a major role in identifying children with CI. In the newborn and early infancy periods, few signs are present, with the exception of Down syndrome (discussed later in this chapter). After this age, however, delayed developmental milestones are the major clues to CI. In addition, nurses must have a high index of suspicion for early behavior patterns that may suggest CI (see Box 37.1). Parental concerns, such as delayed development compared with siblings, need to be taken seriously. All children should receive regular developmental assessment, and the nurse is often the person responsible for performing such assessments. When delays are found, the nurse must use sensitivity and discretion in revealing this finding to parents.

Educate the Child and Family

To teach children with CI, one must investigate their learning abilities and deficits. This is important for the nurse who may be involved in a home care program or who may be caring for the child in a school or health care setting. The nurse who understands how these children learn can effectively teach them basic skills or prepare them for various health-related procedures.

Children with CI have a marked deficit in their ability to discriminate between two or more stimuli because of difficulty in recognizing the relevance of specific cues. However, these children can learn to discriminate if the cues are presented in an exaggerated, concrete form and if all extraneous stimuli are eliminated. For example, the use of colors to emphasize visual cues or the use of singing or rhymes to stress auditory cues can help them learn. Their deficit in discrimination also implies that concrete ideas are learned much more effectively than abstract ideas. Therefore, demonstration is preferable to verbal

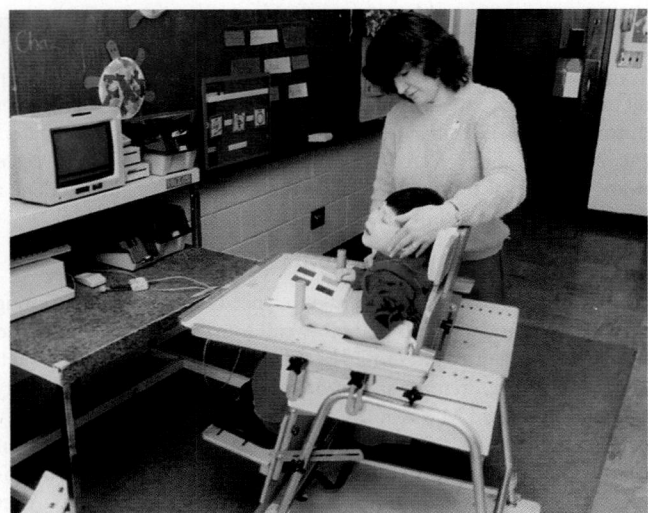

FIG 37.1 A push panel allows a child with cognitive impairment (CI) to turn a computer on and off.

explanation, and learning should be directed toward mastering a skill rather than understanding the scientific principles underlying a procedure.

Another cognitive deficit is in short-term memory. Whereas children of average intelligence can remember several words, numbers, or directions at one time, children with CI are less able to do so. Therefore, they need simple, one-step directions. Learning through a step-by-step process requires a task analysis in which each task is separated into its necessary components and each step is taught completely before proceeding to the next activity.

One critical area of learning that has had a tremendous impact on education for cognitively impaired individuals is motivation or the use of positive reinforcement to encourage the accomplishment of specific tasks or behaviors. Advances in technology have greatly aided in providing reinforcement, especially in children with severe disabilities and who may have physical disabilities that limit their range of capabilities. For example, with the use of specially designed switches, children are given control of some event in the environment, such as turning on the computer (Fig. 37.1). Activation of the computer becomes the reinforcement for pushing the switch. Repetitive use of these switches provides an early, simplistic association with a technical device that may progress to increasingly complex aids.

An early intervention program is a systematic program of therapy, exercises, and activities designed to address developmental delays in children with disabilities to help achieve their full potentials (Bull & Committee on Genetics, 2011; National Down Syndrome Society, 2012a; Weijerman & de Winter, 2010). Considerable evidence indicates that these programs are valuable for cognitively impaired children. Nurses working with these families need to be aware of the types of programs in their community. Under the Individuals with Disabilities Education Act (IDEA) of 1990 (Public Law 101-476), states are encouraged to provide full early intervention services and are required to provide educational opportunities for all children with disabilities from birth to 21 years of age. Services may be provided under state programs for Children with Special Health Care Needs (CSHCN) or Head Start, or by private organizations such as the National Down Syndrome Society,*

---

*Information on early intervention programs in each state is available from the National Down Syndrome Society, 666 Broadway, 8th Floor, New York, NY 10012-2317; 800-221-4602; email: info@ndss.org; www.ndss.org.

Easter Seals,* or The Arc of the United States.† Parents should inquire about these programs by contacting the appropriate agencies. The child's education should begin as soon as possible, because it has been shown that increased and early intervention exposure relates directly to greater improvements in cognitive development (Wallander, Biasini, Thorsten, et al., 2014). As children grow older, their education should be directed toward vocational training that prepares them for as independent a lifestyle as possible within their scope of abilities.

Teach the Child Self-Care Skills

When a child with CI is born, parents often need assistance in promoting normal developmental skills that other children learn easily. There is no way to predict when a child should be able to master self-care skills, such as feeding, toileting, dressing, and grooming, because a wide age variability exists in the CI child who is able to accomplish such functions.

Teaching self-care skills also necessitates a working knowledge of the individual steps needed to master a skill. For example, before beginning a self-feeding program, the nurse performs a task analysis. After a task analysis, the child is observed in a particular situation, such as eating, to determine what skills are possessed and the child's developmental readiness to learn the task. Family members are included in this process, because their "readiness" is as important as the child's. Numerous self-help aids are available to facilitate independence and can help eliminate some of the difficulties of learning, such as using a plate with suction cups to prevent accidental spills.‡

Promote the Child's Optimal Development

Optimal development involves more than achieving independence. It requires appropriate guidance for establishing acceptable social behavior and personal feelings of self-esteem, worth, and security. These attributes are not simply learned through a stimulation program. Rather, they must arise from the genuine love and caring that exist among family members. However, families need guidance in providing an environment that fosters optimal development. Often the nurse can provide assistance in these areas of childrearing.

Another important area for promoting optimal development and self-esteem is ensuring the child's physical well-being. Any congenital defects, such as cardiac, gastrointestinal, or orthopedic anomalies, should be repaired. Plastic surgery may be considered when the child's appearance can be substantially improved. Dental health is significant, and orthodontic and restorative procedures may improve facial appearance immensely.

Encourage Play and Exercise

Children who are cognitively impaired have the same need for play and exercise as any other child. However, because of the children's slower development, parents may be less aware of the need to provide such activities. Therefore, the nurse will need to guide parents toward selection

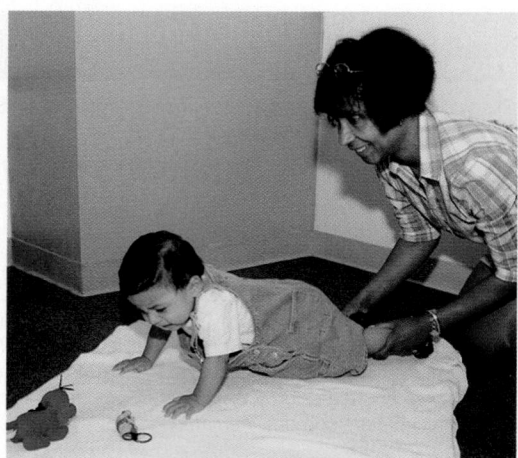

FIG 37.2 Placing an attractive object outside the child's reach encourages crawling movements. (Courtesy of James DeLeon, Texas Children's Hospital, Houston, TX.)

of suitable play and exercise activities. Because play has been discussed for children in each age group in earlier chapters, only the exceptions are presented here (Fig. 37.2).

The type of play is based on the child's developmental age, although the need for sensorimotor play may be prolonged. Parents should use every opportunity to expose the child to as many different sounds, sights, and sensations as possible. Appropriate toys include musical mobiles, stuffed toys, floating toys, a rocking chair or horse, a swing, bells, and rattles. The child should be taken on outings, such as trips to the grocery store or shopping center. Other people should be encouraged to visit in the home; and individuals should relate directly to the child through means such as cuddling, holding, rocking, and talking to the child in the face-to-face fashion.

Toys are selected for their recreational and educational value. For example, a large inflatable beach ball is a good water toy; it encourages interactive play and can be used to learn motor skills, such as balance, rocking, kicking, and throwing. Attractive toys encourage a child to reach, therefore assisting in the development of motor skills (see Fig. 37.2). Musical toys that mimic animal sounds or respond with social phrases are excellent ways of encouraging speech. A doll with removable clothes and different types of closures can help the child learn dressing skills. Toys should be simple in design so that the child can learn to manipulate them without help. For children with severe cognitive and physical impairment, electronic switches can be used to allow them to operate toys (Figs. 37.3 and 37.4).

Suitable activities for physical activity are based on the child's size, coordination, physical fitness and maturity, motivation, and health (see Fig. 37.4). Some children may have physical problems that prevent participation in certain sports, such as atlantoaxial instability in children with Down syndrome (later in this chapter). Children with CI often have greater success in individual and dual sports than in team sports and enjoy themselves most with children of the same developmental level. The Special Olympics* provides these children with a unique competitive opportunity.

*233 South Wacker Drive, Suite 2400, Chicago, IL 60606-4802; 800-221-6827; TTY: 312-726-4258; http://www.easterseals.com/; www.facebook.com/easterseals; twitter.com/EasterSealsON.
†1825 K Street NW, Suite 1200, Washington, DC 20006; 202-534-3700 or 800-433-5255; www.thearc.org; email: info@thearc.org; www.facebook.com/thearcus; twitter.com/thearcus; www.youtube.com/user/thearcoftheus.
‡A resource for a variety of self-help equipment is Performance Health, formerly known as Patterson Medical: Performance Health Corporate Headquarters, 28100 Torch Parkway, Suite 700, Warrenville, IL 60555-3938; Customer Service: 800-323-5547; www.performancehealth.com; www.facebook.com/Patterson-Medical. In Canada: 800-665-9200; www.performancehealth.ca; 905-858-6000.

*1133 19th Street NW, Washington, DC 20036; 800-700-8585 or 202-628-3630; www.specialolympics.org (Website includes listing of state offices.); info@specialolympics.org; twitter.com/mandynmurphy. In Canada: Special Olympics Canada, 21 St. Clair Avenue E, Suite 600, Toronto, ON M4T 1N5; 416-927-9050; 888-888-0608; www.specialolympics.ca.

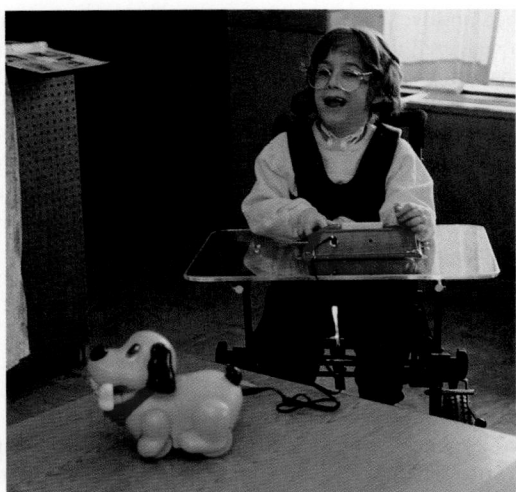

FIG 37.3 A manual switch allows a child with cognitive impairment (CI) to play with a battery-operated toy.

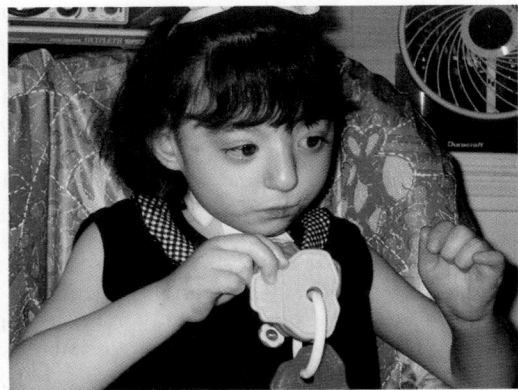

FIG 37.4 A favorite toy provides stimulation for a young child.

Safety is a major consideration in selecting recreational and exercise activities. For example, toys that may be appropriate developmentally may present dangers to a child who is strong enough to break them or use them incorrectly.

Provide Means of Communication

Verbal skills are typically delayed more than other physical skills. Speech requires adequate hearing and interpretation (receptive skills) and facial muscle coordination (expressive skills). Because both receptive and expressive skills may be impaired, children with CI need frequent audiometric testing and should be fitted with hearing aids if indicated. In addition, they may need help in learning to control their facial muscles. For example, some children may need tongue exercises to correct the tongue thrust or gentle reminders to keep the lips closed.

Nonverbal communication may be appropriate for some of these children, and various devices are available. For children with physical limitations, several adaptations or types of communication devices are available to facilitate selection of the appropriate picture or word (Fig. 37.5). Some children may be taught sign language or *Blissymbols*—a highly stylized system of graphic symbols representing words, ideas, and concepts. Although the symbols require education to learn their meaning, no reading skill is required. The symbols are typically arranged on a board, and the person points or uses some type of selector to convey a message.

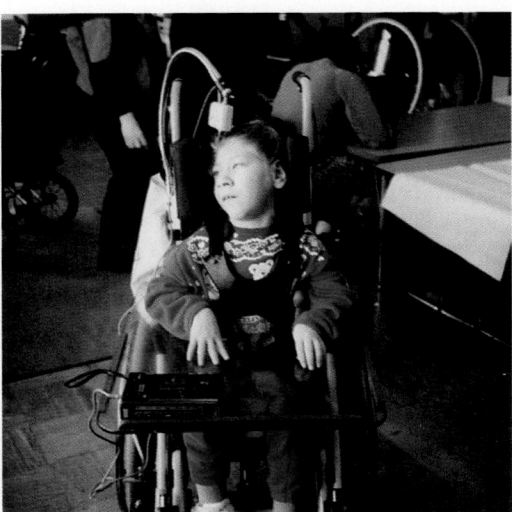

FIG 37.5 A child with cognitive and physical impairments can activate electronic and communication equipment by moving a device near her head.

Establish Discipline

Discipline must begin early. Limit-setting measures need to be simple, consistently applied, and appropriate for the child's mental age. Control measures are based primarily on teaching a specific behavior rather than on understanding the reasons behind it. Stressing moral lessons is of little value to a child who lacks the cognitive skills to learn from self-criticism or evaluation of previous mistakes. Behavior modification, especially reinforcement of desired actions, and use of time-out procedures are appropriate forms of behavior control.

Encourage Socialization

Acquiring social skills is a complex task, as is learning self-care procedures. Active rehearsals with role-playing and practice sessions and positive reinforcement for desired behavior have been the most successful approaches. Parents should be encouraged early to teach their child socially acceptable behavior: waving goodbye, saying "hello" and "thank you," responding to his or her name, greeting visitors, and sitting modestly. The teaching of socially acceptable sexual behavior is especially important to minimize sexual exploitation. Parents also need to expose the child to strangers so that he or she can practice manners, because there is no automatic transfer of learning from one situation to another.

Dressing and grooming are also important aspects of self-esteem and social acceptance. Clothes should be clean, age-appropriate, and well fitted with self-adhering fasteners and elastic openings to facilitate self-dressing.

Opportunities for social interaction and infant stimulation programs should began at an early age. As soon as possible, parents should enroll their child in early intervention or other appropriate preschool programs. Not only do these programs provide education and training, but they also offer an opportunity for social interaction with other children and adults. As children grow older, they should have peer experiences similar to those of other children, including group outings, sports, and organized activities, such as scouts and Special Olympics. Nurses should assess the child's abilities and encourage others (e.g., parents, teachers) to promote developmentally appropriate peer interaction, such as classroom and school activities, dance classes, clubs, vacations, and family outings (Bull & Committee on Genetics, 2011; National Down Syndrome Society, 2012b; Shapiro & Batshaw, 2011).

Provide Information on Sexuality

Adolescence may be a particularly difficult time for parents, especially in terms of the child's sexual behavior, possibility of pregnancy, future plans to marry, and ability to be independent. Frequently, minimal anticipatory guidance has been offered to parents to prepare the child for physical and sexual maturation. The nurse should help in this area by providing parents with information about sexuality education that is geared to the child's developmental level. For example, adolescent girls need a *simple* explanation of menstruation and instructions on personal hygiene during the menstrual cycle.

These adolescents also need practical sexual information regarding anatomy, physical development, and conception.* Because they are easy to persuade and lack judgment, they need a well-defined, concrete code of conduct with specific instructions for handling certain situations. The subtleties of social sexual behavior are less beneficial than specific instructions for handling certain situations. For example, an adolescent should be firmly told never to go alone anywhere with any person that he or she does not know well. To protect the child or adolescent from sexual abuse, parents must closely observe their child or adolescent's activities and associates. The question of contraceptive protection for these adolescents is often a parental concern.

Parents of these adolescents are often concerned about the advisability of marriage between two individuals with significant CI. There is no conclusive answer; each situation must be judged individually. In some instances, marriage is possible. The nurse should discuss this topic with parents and with the prospective couple, stressing suitable living accommodations and contraceptive methods to prevent pregnancy. If children are conceived, these parents require specialized assistance in learning to meet the needs of their offspring (Bull & Committee on Genetics, 2011; Shea, 2012).

Help the Family Adjust to Future Care

Not all families are able to cope with home care of children who are cognitively impaired, especially those who have severe or profound CI or multiple disabilities. Older parents may not be able to continue care responsibilities after they reach retirement or older age. The decision regarding residential placement is a difficult one for families, and the availability of such facilities varies widely. The nurse's role includes assisting parents in investigating and evaluating programs and helping parents adjust to the decision for placement.

Care for the Child During Hospitalization

Caring for the child during hospitalization can be a special challenge. Frequently, nurses are unfamiliar with children who are cognitively impaired, and they may cope with their feelings of insecurity and fear by ignoring or isolating the child. Not only is this approach nonsupportive, it may also be destructive to the child's sense of self-esteem and optimum development, and it may impair the parents' ability to cope with the stress of the experience. To prevent engaging in this nontherapeutic approach, nurses must use the mutual participation model in planning the child's care. Parents should stay with their child but not be made to feel as if the responsibility is totally theirs.

When the child is admitted, a detailed history is taken with special focus on all self-care abilities. Questions about the child's abilities are

approached positively. For example, rather than asking, "Is your child toilet trained yet?" the nurse may state, "Tell me about your child's toileting habits." The assessment should also focus on any special devices that the child uses, effective measures of limit setting, unusual or favorite routines, and any behaviors that may require intervention. If the parent states that the child engages in self-stimulatory or self-injurious activities (e.g., head banging, self-biting), the nurse should inquire about events that precipitate them and techniques (e.g., distraction, medication) that the parents use to manage them (Oliver & Richards, 2010).

The nurse also assesses the child's functional level of eating and playing; ability to express needs verbally; progress in toilet training; and relationship with objects, toys, and other children. The child is encouraged to be as independent as possible in the hospital.

Realizing that the child may be lonely in the hospital, the nurse makes certain that toys and other activities are provided. The child is placed in a room with other children of approximately the same developmental age, preferably a room with only two beds to avoid overstimulation. The nurse should treat the child with dignity and respect in a manner that promotes acceptance and understanding by other children, parents, and those with whom the child comes into contact in the hospital.

Explain procedures to the child using methods of communication that are at the appropriate cognitive level. Generally, explanations should be simple, short, and concrete, emphasizing what the child will physically experience. Demonstration either through actual practice or with visual aids is always preferable to verbal explanation. Include parents in preprocedural teaching to aid in the child's learning and to help the nurse learn effective methods of communicating with the child.

During hospitalization, the nurse should also focus on growth-promoting experiences for the child. For example, hospitalization may be an excellent opportunity to emphasize to parents abilities that the child does have but has not had the opportunity to practice, such as self-dressing. It may also be an opportunity for social experiences with peers, group play, or new educational and recreational activities. For example, one child who had the habit of screaming and kicking demonstrated a definite decrease in those behaviors after he learned to pound pegs and use a punching bag. Through social services, the parents may become aware of specialized programs for the child. Hospitalization may also offer parents a respite from everyday care responsibilities and an opportunity to discuss their feelings with a concerned professional.

Assist in Measures to Prevent Cognitive Impairment

Besides having a responsibility to families with a child with CI, nurses also need to be involved in programs aimed at preventing CI. Many of the familial, social, and environmental factors known to cause mild impairment are preventable. Counseling and education can reduce or eliminate such factors (e.g., poor nutrition, cigarette smoking, chemical abuse), which increase the risk for prematurity and intrauterine growth restriction. Interventions are directed toward improving maternal health by educating women regarding the dangers of chemicals, including prenatal alcohol exposure, which affects organogenesis, craniofacial development, and cognitive ability. Other preventive strategies that play an important role include adequate prenatal care; optimal medical care of high-risk newborns; rubella immunization; genetic counseling; and prenatal screening, especially in terms of Down syndrome or FXS. The use of folic acid supplements prevents neural tube defects during pregnancy and during the childbearing years; and the use of newborn screening for treatable inborn errors of metabolism (e.g., congenital hypothyroidism, phenylketonuria, and galactosemia) are early appropriate therapies to prevent developmental disabilities in children.

---

*Sources of information on sexuality and conception include Planned Parenthood Federation of America, 434 W. 33rd Street, New York, NY 10001; 212-541-7800 or 800-230-7526; www.plannedparenthood.org; www.facebook.com/PlannedParenthood/, and the ARC of the United States, www.thearc.org/.

DOWN SYNDROME

Down syndrome is the most common chromosomal abnormality of a generalized syndrome, occurring in 1 in 691 live births in the United States (National Down Syndrome Society, 2012c; Summar & Lee, 2011; Weijerman & de Winter, 2010). It occurs in people of all races and economic levels.

Etiology

The cause of Down syndrome is not known, but evidence from cytogenetic and epidemiologic studies supports the concept of multiple causality. Although the cause is unclear, the cytogenetics of the disorder are well established. Approximately 95% of all cases of Down syndrome are attributable to an extra chromosome 21 (group G), hence the name *nonfamilial trisomy 21.* Although children with trisomy 21 are born to parents of all ages, there is a statistically greater risk in older women, particularly those older than 35 years of age. For example, in women 35 years of age, the chance of conceiving a child with Down syndrome is about 1 in 350 live births; but in women 40 years of age, it is about 1 in 100. However, the majority (≈80%) of infants with Down syndrome are born to women younger than 35 years of age, because younger women have higher fertility rates (National Down Syndrome Society, 2012c; Summar & Lee, 2011). About 4% of the cases may be caused by *translocation* of chromosomes 15 and 21 or 22. This type of genetic aberration is usually hereditary and is not associated with advanced parental age. About 1% of affected people demonstrate *mosaicism,* which refers to a mixture of normal and abnormal chromosomes in the cells. The degree of cognitive and physical impairment is related to the percentage of cells with the abnormal chromosome makeup.

Diagnostic Evaluation

Down syndrome can usually be diagnosed by the clinical manifestations alone (Box 37.2 and Fig. 37.6), but a chromosome analysis should be done to confirm the genetic abnormality.

Several physical problems are associated with Down syndrome. Many of these children have congenital heart malformations, the most common being septal defects. Respiratory tract infections are prevalent and, when combined with cardiac anomalies, are the chief causes of death, particularly during the first year of life. Hypotonicity of chest and abdominal muscles and dysfunction of the immune system probably predispose the child to the development of respiratory tract infection. Other physical problems include thyroid dysfunction, especially congenital hypothyroidism, and an increased incidence of leukemia.

Therapeutic Management

Although no cure exists for Down syndrome, a number of therapies are advocated, such as surgery to correct serious congenital anomalies

---

BOX 37.2 Clinical Manifestations of Down Syndrome

Head and Eyes
Separated sagittal suture
Brachycephaly
Rounded and small skull
Flat occiput
Enlarged anterior fontanel
Oblique palpebral fissures (upward, outward slant)*
Inner epicanthal folds
Speckling of iris (Brushfield spots)

Nose and Ears
Small nose*
Depressed nasal bridge (saddle nose)*
Small ears and narrow canals
Short pinna (vertical ear length)
Overlapping upper helices
Conductive hearing loss

Mouth and Neck
High, arched, narrow palate*
Protruding tongue
Hypoplastic mandible
Delayed teeth eruption and microdontia
Abnormal teeth alignment common
Periodontal disease
Neck skin excess and laxity*
Short and broad neck

Chest and Heart
Shortened rib cage
Twelfth rib anomalies
Pectus excavatum or carinatum
Congenital heart defects common (e.g., atrial septal defect, ventricular septal defect)

Abdomen and Genitalia
Protruding, lax, and flabby abdominal muscles
Diastasis recti abdominis
Umbilical hernia
Small penis
Cryptorchidism
Bulbous vulva

Hands and Feet
Broad, short hands and stubby fingers
Incurved little finger (clinodactyly)
Transverse palmar crease
Wide space between big and second toes*
Plantar crease between big and second toes*
Broad, short feet and stubby toes

Musculoskeletal and Skin
Short stature
Hyperflexibility and muscle weakness*
Hypotonia
Atlantoaxial instability
Dry, cracked, and frequent fissuring
Cutis marmorata (mottling)

Other
Reduced birth weight
Learning difficulty (average intelligence quotient [IQ] of 50)
Hypothyroidism common
Impaired immune function
Increased risk for leukemia
Early-onset dementia (in one-third)

*Most common findings in modified chart (Pueschel, 1999).

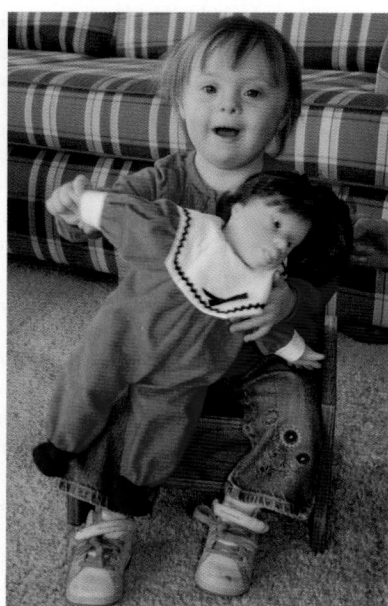

FIG 37.6 A young child with Down syndrome holding a doll with Down syndrome.

(e.g., heart defects, strabismus). These children also benefit from evaluative echocardiography soon after birth and regular medical care. Evaluation of sight and hearing is essential, and treatment of otitis media is required to prevent auditory loss, which can influence cognitive function. Periodic testing of thyroid function is recommended, especially if growth is severely delayed.

About 15% of children with Down syndrome have *atlantoaxial instability;* almost all of the children are asymptomatic. The American Academy of Pediatrics no longer recommends screening asymptomatic children with Down syndrome for atlantoaxial instability with cervical spine x-rays due to unproven value of detecting patients at risk for developing spinal cord compression injury (Bull & Committee on Genetics, 2011; National Down Syndrome Society, 2012d). However, the Special Olympics continues to require that all athletes with Down syndrome receive neck x-rays prior to sports participation, because neck x-ray is the only screen available (National Down Syndrome Society, 2012d).

> **! NURSING ALERT**
>
> Immediately report any child with the following signs of spinal cord compression:
> - Persistent neck pain
> - Loss of established motor skills and bladder or bowel control
> - Changes in sensation

Prognosis

Life expectancy for those with Down syndrome has improved in recent years but remains lower than for the general population. The majority of individuals with Down syndrome survive to 60 years of age and beyond (National Down Syndrome Society, 2012e; Weijerman & de Winter, 2010). As the prognosis continues to improve for these individuals, it will be important to provide for their long-term health care and social and leisure needs.

> **CLINICAL REASONING CASE STUDY**
> ### Diagnosis of Down Syndrome
>
> The parents of Melissa, a newborn diagnosed as having Down syndrome, ask the nurse, "What are we supposed to do with her?" They further state that they already have three other children at home.
>
> **Questions**
> 1. What evidence should you consider regarding this condition?
> 2. What additional information is required at this time?
> 3. List the nursing intervention(s) that have the highest priority.
> 4. Identify important patient-centered outcomes with reference to your nursing interventions.

Care Management
Support the Family at the Time of Diagnosis

Because of the unique physical characteristics, infants with Down syndrome are usually diagnosed at birth, and parents should be informed of the diagnosis at this time. Most parents usually prefer that both of them be present during the informing interview so that they can support one another emotionally. Parents appreciate receiving reading material about the syndrome* and being referred to parent groups and/or professional counseling.

Parental responses to the child may greatly influence decisions regarding future care. Whereas some families willingly take the child home, others consider foster care or adoption. The nurse must answer questions regarding developmental potential carefully, because the responses may influence the parents' decision. The nurse should share the available informative sources (e.g., parent groups, professional counseling, and literature) to help the family learn about Down syndrome (see Clinical Reasoning Case Study box: Diagnosis of Down Syndrome).

Assist the Family in Preventing Physical Problems

Many of the physical characteristics of infants with Down syndrome present challenges and nursing problems. The hypotonicity of muscles and hyperextensibility of joints complicate positioning. The limp, flaccid extremities resemble the posture of a rag doll; as a result, holding the infant is difficult and cumbersome. Sometimes parents perceive this lack of molding to their bodies as evidence of inadequate parenting. The extended body position promotes heat loss, because more surface area is exposed to the environment. Encourage the parents to swaddle or wrap the infant snugly in a blanket before picking up the child to provide security and warmth. The nurse also discusses with parents their feelings concerning attachment to the child, emphasizing that the child's lack of clinging or molding is a physical characteristic and not a sign of detachment or rejection.

Decreased muscle tone compromises respiratory expansion. In addition, the underdeveloped nasal bone causes a chronic problem of inadequate drainage of mucus. The constant stuffy nose forces the child to breathe by mouth, which dries the oropharyngeal membranes, increasing the susceptibility to upper respiratory tract infections. Measures to lessen these problems include clearing the nose with a bulb-type syringe, rinsing the mouth with water after feedings, increasing fluid intake, and using a cool-mist vaporizer to keep the mucous membranes moist and the secretions liquefied. Other helpful measures include changing the child's position frequently, practicing good hand washing,

---

*For the ARC and National Down Syndrome Society contact information, see the footnotes earlier in this chapter.

and properly disposing of soiled articles, such as tissues. If antibiotics are ordered, the nurse stresses the importance of completing the full course of therapy for successful eradication of the infection and prevention of growth of resistant organisms.

Inadequate drainage resulting in pooling of mucus in the nose also interferes with feeding. Because the child breathes by mouth, sucking for any length of time is difficult. When eating solids, the child may gag on the food because of mucus in the oropharynx. Parents are advised to clear the nose before each feeding; give small, frequent feedings; and allow opportunities for rest during mealtime.

The protruding tongue also interferes with feeding, especially of solid foods. Parents need to know that the tongue thrust is not an indication of refusal to feed but a physiologic response. Parents are advised to use a small but long, straight-handled spoon to push the food toward the back and side of the mouth. If food is thrust out, it should be refed.

Dietary intake needs supervision. Decreased muscle tone affects gastric motility, predisposing the child to constipation. Dietary measures, such as increased fiber and fluid, promote evacuation. The child's eating habits may need careful scrutiny to prevent obesity. Height and weight measurements should be obtained on a serial basis. The previously used Down syndrome–specific growth charts no longer reflect the current population styles and body proportions; and until new research quality standards are developed, National Center for Health Statistics or World Health Organization charts should be used (Bull & Committee on Genetics, 2011; Wyckoff, 2011).

During infancy, the child's skin is pliable and soft. However, it gradually becomes rough and dry and is prone to cracking and infection. Skin care involves the use of minimum soap and application of lubricants. Lip balm is applied to the lips, especially when the child is outdoors, to prevent excessive chapping.

Assist in Prenatal Diagnosis and Genetic Counseling

Prenatal diagnosis of Down syndrome is possible through chorionic villus sampling and amniocentesis, because chromosome analysis of fetal cells can detect the presence of trisomy or translocation. However, recent advances in development of noninvasive prenatal testing (NIPT) is a measurement of cell-free deoxyribonucleic acid (DNA) from the plasma of pregnant women, detecting nearly all cases of Down syndrome (Lewis, Hill, Silcock, et al., 2014; Liao, Chan, Jiang, et al., 2012; Huang, Zheng, Chen, et al., 2014; Palomaki, Kloza, Lambert-Messerlian, et al., 2011).

Offer prenatal testing and genetic counseling to women of advanced maternal age and those who have a family history of the disorder. If prenatal testing indicates that the fetus is affected, the nurse must allow the parents to express their feelings concerning elective abortion and support their decision to terminate or proceed with the pregnancy. It is important for nurses to be aware of their own attitudes regarding testing and related decisions.

FRAGILE X SYNDROME

FXS is the most common inherited cause of CI and the second most common genetic cause of CI or intellectual disability after Down syndrome. It has been described in all ethnic groups and races; the incidence of affected boys is 1 in 3600 to 4000, the incidence of affected girls is 1 in 4000 to 6000, the incidence of carrier girls is 1 in 151, and the incidence of carrier boys is 1 in 468 worldwide (National Fragile X Foundation, 2012a).

The syndrome is caused by an abnormal gene on the lower end of the long arm of the X chromosome. Chromosome analysis may demonstrate a *fragile site* (a region that fails to condense during mitosis and is characterized by a nonstaining gap or narrowing) in the cells of affected males and females and in carrier females. This fragile site is caused by a gene mutation that results in excessive repeats of nucleotide in a specific DNA segment of the X chromosome. The number of repeats in a normal individual is between 6 and 50. An individual with 50 to 200 base-pair repeats is said to have a *permutation* and is therefore a carrier. When passed from a parent to a child, these base-pair repeats can expand from 200 or more, which is termed a *full mutation*. This expansion occurs only when a carrier mother passes the mutation to her offspring; it does not occur when a carrier father passes the mutation to his daughters.

The inheritance pattern has been termed *X-linked dominant with reduced penetrance*. This is in distinct contrast to the classic X-linked recessive pattern in which all carrier females are normal, all affected males have symptoms of the disorder, and no males are carriers. Consequently, genetic counseling of affected families is more complex than that for families with a classic X-linked disorder, such as hemophilia. Both affected sexes are capable of transmitting the fragile X disorder. Prenatal diagnosis of the fragile X gene mutation is possible with direct DNA testing in a family with an established history using amniocentesis or chorionic villus sampling (National Fragile X Foundation, 2012b). The FMR1 mutation testing is highly accurate and is being researched regarding the incorporation into the newborn universal screening program (Abrams, Cronister, Brown, et al., 2012; Bagni, Tassone, Neri, et al., 2012; Finucane, Abrams, Cronister, et al., 2012; Hagerman, Berry-Kravis, Kaufmann, et al., 2009; Skinner, Choudhury, Sideris, et al., 2011).

Clinical Manifestations

The classic trend of physical findings in adult men with FXS consists of a long face with a prominent jaw (prognathism); large, protruding ears; and large testes (macroorchidism). In prepubertal children, however, these features may be less obvious, and behavioral manifestations may initially suggest the diagnosis (Box 37.3). In carrier females, the clinical manifestations are extremely varied.

Therapeutic Management

FXS has no cure. Medical treatment may include the use of serotonin agents, such as carbamazepine (Tegretol) or fluoxetine (Prozac), to control violent temper outbursts and the use of central nervous system stimulants or clonidine (Catapres) to improve attention span and decrease

---

BOX 37.3 Clinical Manifestations of Fragile X Syndrome

Physical Features
Increased head circumference
Long, wide, or protruding ears
Long, narrow face with prominent jaw
Strabismus
Mitral valve prolapse, aortic root dilation
Hypotonia
In postpubertal males, enlarged testicles

Behavioral Features
Mild to severe cognitive impairment (CI)
Speech delay; may be rapid speech with stuttering and word repetition
Short attention span, hyperactivity
Hypersensitivity to taste, sounds, touch
Intolerance to change in routine
Autistic-like behaviors, such as social anxiety and gaze aversion
Possible aggressive behavior

hyperactivity. Two possible treatments of FXS being investigated are reactivation of the affected gene and protein replacement (Bagni, Tassone, Neri, et al., 2012; Kuehn, 2011).

All affected children require referral to an early intervention program that requires interprofessional care (speech and language therapy, occupational therapy, and special education assistance) and interdisciplinary assessment, including cardiology, neurology, and orthopedic anomalies.

Prognosis

Individuals with FXS are expected to live a normal life span. Their CI may be improved by behavioral and educational interventions that usually begin in preschool-age children.

Care Management

Because CI is a fairly consistent finding in individuals with FXS, the care given to these families is the same as for any child with intellectual disability. Because the disorder is hereditary, genetic counseling is important to inform parents and siblings of the risks for transmission. In addition, any male or female with unexplained or nonspecific mental impairment should be referred for genetic testing and, if needed, counseling. Families with a member affected by the disorder should be referred to the National Fragile X Foundation.*

SENSORY IMPAIRMENT

HEARING IMPAIRMENT

Hearing impairment is one of the most common disabilities in the United States. An estimated 1 to 6 per 1000 well infants have hearing loss of varying degrees (Grindle, 2014). For infants admitted to neonatal intensive care units, the incidence rises sharply to approximately 2 to 4 per 100 neonates (American Academy of Pediatrics, Joint Committee on Infant Hearing, 2007; Almadhoob & Ohlsson, 2015; Colella-Santos, Hein, de Souza, et al., 2014). In the United States, there are about 1 million children with hearing impairment ranging from birth to 21 years of age, and almost one-third of these children have other disabilities, such as visual or cognitive deficits.

Definition and Classification

Hearing impairment is a general term indicating disability that may range in severity from slight to profound hearing loss. *Slight to moderately severe hearing loss* describes a person who has residual hearing sufficient to enable successful processing of linguistic information through audition, generally with the use of a hearing aid. *Severe to profound hearing loss* describes a person whose hearing disability precludes successful processing of linguistic information through audition with or without a hearing aid. Hearing-impaired people who are speech impaired tend not to have a physical speech defect other than that caused by the inability to hear.

Hearing defects may be classified according to etiology, pathology, or symptom severity. Each is important in terms of treatment, possible prevention, and rehabilitation.

Etiology

Hearing loss may be caused by a number of prenatal and postnatal conditions. These may include a family history of childhood hearing

impairment, anatomic malformations of the head or neck, low birth weight, severe perinatal asphyxia, perinatal infection (cytomegalovirus, rubella, herpes, syphilis, toxoplasmosis, bacterial meningitis), maternal prenatal substance abuse, chronic ear infection, cerebral palsy, Down syndrome, prolonged neonatal oxygen supplementation, or administration of ototoxic drugs (Colella-Santos, Hein, de Souza, et al., 2014; Grindle, 2014; Haddad, 2011; Jerry & Oghalai, 2011; Singh, 2015).

In addition, high-risk neonates who survive the once fatal prenatal or perinatal conditions may be susceptible to hearing loss from the disorder or its treatment. For example, sensorineural hearing loss may be a result of continuous humming noises or high noise levels associated with incubators, oxygen hoods, or intensive care units, especially when combined with the use of potentially ototoxic antibiotics.

Environmental noise is a special concern. Sounds loud enough to damage sensitive hair cells of the inner ear can produce irreversible hearing loss. Very loud, brief noise (e.g., gunfire) can cause immediate, severe, and permanent hearing loss. Longer exposure to less intense but still hazardous sounds (e.g., loud persistent music via headphones, sound systems, concerts, or industrial noises) may also produce hearing loss (Biassoni, Serra, Hinalaf, et al., 2014; Grindle, 2014; Harrison, 2012; Jerry & Oghalai, 2011; Serra, Biassoni, Hinalaf, et al., 2014). Loud noises combined with toxic substances (e.g., smoking or secondhand smoke) produce a synergistic effect on hearing that causes hearing loss (Fabry, Davila, Arheart, et al., 2011; Talaat, Metwaly, Khafagy, et al., 2014).

Pathology

Disorders of hearing are divided according to the location of the defect. *Conductive* or *middle-ear hearing loss* results from interference of transmission of sound to the middle ear. It is the most common of all types of hearing loss and most frequently a result of recurrent serous otitis media. Conductive hearing impairment involves mainly interference with loudness of sound.

Sensorineural hearing loss involves damage to the inner ear structures or the auditory nerve. The most common causes are congenital defects of inner ear structures or consequences of acquired conditions, such as kernicterus, infection, administration of ototoxic drugs, or exposure to excessive noise. Sensorineural hearing loss results in distortion of sound and problems in discrimination. Although the child hears some of everything going on around him or her, the sounds are distorted, severely affecting discrimination and comprehension.

Mixed conductive-sensorineural hearing loss results from interference with transmission of sound in the middle ear and along neural pathways. It frequently results from recurrent otitis media and its complications.

Central auditory imperception includes all hearing losses that are not linked to defects in the conductive or sensorineural structures. They are usually divided into organic or functional losses. In the organic type of central auditory imperception, the defect involves the reception of auditory stimuli along the central pathways and the expression of the message into meaningful communication. Examples are *aphasia*, the inability to express ideas in any form, either written or verbal; *agnosia*, the inability to interpret sound correctly; and *dysacusis*, difficulty in processing details or discriminating among sounds. In the *functional* type of hearing loss, no organic lesion exists to explain a central auditory loss. Examples of functional hearing loss are conversion hysteria (an unconscious withdrawal from hearing to block remembrance of a traumatic event), infantile autism, and childhood schizophrenia.

Symptom Severity

Hearing impairment is expressed in terms of a *decibel (dB)*, a unit of loudness (Table 37.1). Hearing is measured at various frequencies, such as 500, 1000, and 2000 cycles/second, the critical listening speech range.

---

*1615 Bonanza Street, Suite 202, Walnut Creek, CA 94597; 800-688-8765 or 925-938-9300; www.fragilex.org; email: natlfx@ fragilex.org; www .facebook.com/natlfragilex; twitter.com/FragileXnews.

TABLE 37.1 Intensity of Sounds Expressed in Decibels

Decibels	Representative Sound
0	Softest sound normal ear can hear
10	Heartbeat, rustling of leaves
20	Whisper at 1.5 m (5 feet)
30 to 45	Normal conversation
60	Noise in average restaurant
70 to 80	Street noises
80	Loud radio in home
90 to 100	Train
120	Thunder, loud music
140	Jet plane during departure
>140	Pain threshold

TABLE 37.2 Classification of Hearing Impairment Based on Symptom Severity

Hearing Level (dB)	Effect
Slight: 16 to 25	Has difficulty hearing faint or distant speech
	Usually is unaware of hearing difficulty
	Likely to achieve in school but may have problems
	No speech defects
Mild to moderate: 26 to 55	May have speech difficulties
	Understands face-to-face conversational speech at 0.9 to 1.5 m (3 to 5 ft)
Moderately severe: 56 to 70	Unable to understand conversational speech unless loud
	Considerable difficulty with group or classroom discussion
	Requires special speech training
Severe: 71 to 90	May hear a loud voice if nearby
	May be able to identify loud environmental noises
	Can distinguish vowels but not most consonants
	Requires speech training
Profound: 91	May hear only loud sounds
	Requires extensive speech training

dB, Decibels.

Hearing impairment can be classified according to *hearing threshold level* (the measurement of an individual's hearing threshold by means of an audiometer) and the degree of symptom severity as it affects speech (Table 37.2). These classifications offer only general guidelines regarding the effect of the impairment on any individual child, because children differ greatly in their ability to use residual hearing.

Therapeutic Management

Conductive Hearing Loss

Treatment of hearing loss depends on the cause and type of hearing impairment. Many conductive hearing defects respond to medical or surgical treatment, such as antibiotic therapy for acute otitis media or insertion of tympanostomy tubes for chronic otitis media. When the conductive loss is permanent, hearing can be improved with the use of a hearing aid to amplify sound.

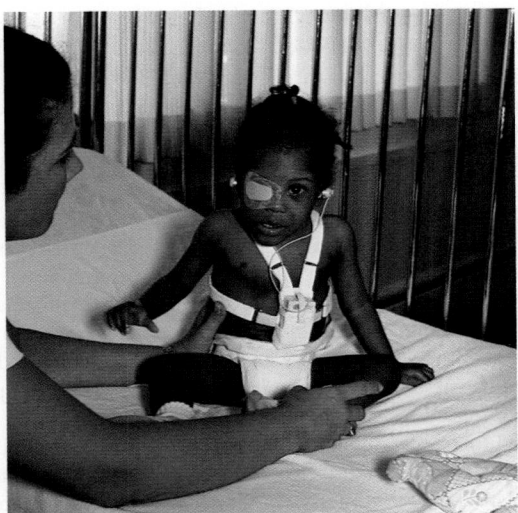

FIG 37.7 On-the-body hearing aids are convenient for young children, such as this child with severe bilateral hearing loss. Note eye patching for strabismus.

The nurse should be familiar with the types, basic care, and handling of hearing aids, especially when the child is hospitalized.* Types of aids include those worn in or behind the ear, models incorporated into an eyeglass frame, and types worn on the body with a wire connection to the ear (Fig. 37.7). One of the most common problems with a hearing aid is *acoustic feedback,* an annoying whistling sound usually caused by improper fit of the ear mold. Sometimes the whistling may be at a frequency that the child cannot hear but that is annoying to others. In this case, if children are old enough, they are told of the noise and asked to readjust the aid.

> **! NURSING ALERT**
>
> To reduce or eliminate whistling from a hearing aid, try removing and reinserting the aid, making certain that no hair is caught between the ear mold and the ear canal; cleaning the ear mold or ear; or lowering the volume of the aid.

As children grow older, they may be self-conscious about the device. Effort may be made to make the aid inconspicuous, such as styling the hair to cover behind-the-ear or in-the-ear models and encouraging the use of attractive frames for glasses with connected hearing aids. Give children responsibility for the care of the device as soon as they are able, because fostering independence is a primary goal of rehabilitation.

> **! NURSING ALERT**
>
> Stress to parents the importance of storing batteries for hearing aids in a safe location out of reach of children and teaching children not to remove the battery from the hearing aid (or supervising young children when they do so). Battery ingestion requires immediate emergency management.

---

*Information about hearing aids is available from the International Hearing Society, 16880 Middlebelt Road, Suite 4, Livonia, MI 48154; 800-521-5247 or 734-522-7200; www.ihsinfo.org; www.facebook.com/ihsinfo; twitter.com/IHSinfo.

Sensorineural Hearing Loss

Treatment for sensorineural hearing loss is much less satisfactory. Because the defect is not one of intensity of sound, hearing aids are of less value in this type of defect. The use of cochlear implants* (a surgically implanted prosthetic device) provides a sensation of hearing for individuals who have severe or profound hearing loss (Hayes, Geers, Trieman, et al., 2009; Lantos, 2012). Children with sensorineural hearing loss have lost or damaged some or all of their hair cells or auditory nerve fibers. Often these children cannot benefit from conventional hearing aids because they only amplify sound that cannot be processed by a damaged inner ear. A cochlear implant bypasses the hair cells to directly stimulate surviving auditory nerve fibers so that they can send signals to the brain. These signals can be interpreted by the brain to produce sound and sensations (Grindle, 2014; Lantos, 2012).

The multichannel implant is a sophisticated device that stimulates the auditory nerve at a number of locations with differently processed signals. This type of stimulation allows a person to use the pitch information present in speech signals, leading to better understanding of speech. The trend is toward early use of cochlear implants, usually by 12 months of age, to give the child maximum opportunity to develop listening, language, and speaking skills.

Care Management

Assessment of children for hearing impairment is a critical nursing responsibility. Identification of hearing loss before the first 3 months of age with intervention no later than 6 months of age is essential to improve the language and educational development for children with hearing impairments (Grindle, 2014; Lammers, Jansen, Grolman, et al., 2015; World Health Organization, 2012). The Joint Committee on Infant Hearing issued guidelines on auditory screening of newborns and infants to detect early hearing loss and implement intervention programs (American Academy of Pediatrics, Joint Committee on Infant Hearing, 2007; Joint Committee on Infant Hearing of the American Academy of Pediatrics, Muse, Harrison, et al., 2013).

At birth, the nurse can observe the neonate's response to auditory stimuli, as evidenced by the startle reflex, head turning, eye blinking, and cessation of body movement. The infant may vary in the intensity of the response, depending on the state of alertness. However, a consistent absence of a reaction should lead to suspicion of hearing loss. Box 37.4 summarizes other clinical manifestations of hearing impairment in infants.

Children who are profoundly hearing impaired are much more likely to be diagnosed during infancy than the child who is less severely affected. If the defect is not detected during early childhood, it likely will become evident during entry into school, when the child has difficulty learning. Unfortunately, some of these children are erroneously placed in special classes for students with learning disabilities or CI. Therefore, it is essential that the nurse suspect a hearing impairment in any child who demonstrates the behaviors listed in Box 37.4.

! NURSING ALERT

When parents express concern about their child's hearing and speech development, refer the child for a hearing evaluation. Absence of well-formed syllables (da, na, yaya) by 11 months of age should result in immediate referral.

---

*Hearing Enrichment Language Program of the Hough Ear Institute as part INTEGRIS Baptist Medical Center Cochlear Implant Clinic, 3300 N.W. Expressway, Oklahoma City, OK 73112; 405-949-3011 or 888-951-2277; http://integrisok.com/baptist-medical-center-oklahoma-city-ok-services-hearing; facebook.com/integrishealthOK.

BOX 37.4   Clinical Manifestations of Hearing Impairment

Infants

Lack of startle or blink reflex to a loud sound
Failure to be awakened by loud environmental noises
Failure to localize a source of sound by 6 months of age
Absence of babble or voice inflections by 7 months of age
General indifference to sound
Lack of response to the spoken word; failure to follow verbal directions
Response to loud noises as opposed to the voice

Children

Use of gestures rather than verbalization to express desires, especially after 15 months of age
Failure to develop intelligible speech by 24 months of age
Monotone and unintelligible speech; lessened laughter
Vocal play, head banging, or foot stamping for vibratory sensation
Yelling or screeching to express pleasure, needs, or annoyance
Asking to have statements repeated or answering them incorrectly
Greater response to facial expression and gestures than to verbal explanation
Avoidance of social interaction; prefer to play alone
Inquiring, sometimes confused facial expression
Suspicious alertness alternating with cooperation
Frequent stubbornness because of lack of comprehension
Irritability at not making themselves understood
Shy, timid, and withdrawn behavior
Frequent appearance of being "in a world of their own" or markedly inattentive

---

During early childhood, the primary importance of hearing impairment is the effect on speech development. A child with a mild conductive hearing loss may speak fairly clearly but in a loud, monotone voice. A child with a sensorineural defect usually has difficulty in articulation. Communication may be difficult, leading to frustration when words are not understood. For example, an inability to hear higher frequencies may result in the word *spoon* being pronounced "poon." Children with articulation problems need to have their hearing tested.

Lipreading

Although the child may become an expert at lipreading, only about 40% of the spoken word is understood, less if the speaker has an accent, mustache, or beard. Exaggerating pronunciation or speaking in an altered rhythm further lessens comprehension. Parents can help the child understand the spoken word by using the suggestions in the Guidelines box: Facilitating Lipreading. The child learns to supplement the spoken word with sensitivity to visual cues, primarily body language and facial expression (e.g., tightening the lips, muscle tension, eye contact).

Cued Speech

The cued speech method of communication is an adjunct to straight lipreading. It uses hand signals to help the hearing-impaired child to distinguish between words that look alike when formed by the lips (e.g., mat, bat). It is most commonly employed by hearing-impaired children who are using speech rather than those who are nonverbal.

Sign Language

Sign language, such as American Sign Language (ASL) or British Sign Language (BSL), is a visual-gestural language that uses hand signals that roughly correspond to specific words and concepts in the English language. Encourage family members to learn signing, because using

GUIDELINES

Facilitating Lipreading

Attract child's attention before speaking; use light touch to signal speaker's presence.

Stand close to child.

Face child directly, or move to a 45-degree angle.

Stand still; do not walk back and forth or turn away to point or look elsewhere.

Establish eye contact, and show interest.

Speak at eye level and with good lighting on speaker's face.

Be certain nothing interferes with speech patterns, such as chewing food or gum.

Speak clearly and at a slow and even rate.

Use facial expression to assist in conveying messages.

Keep sentences short.

Rephrase message if child does not understand the words.

or watching hands requires much less concentration than lipreading or talking. Also, a symbol method enables some hearing-impaired children to learn more and to learn faster.

Speech Language Therapy

The most formidable task in the education of a child who is profoundly hearing impaired is learning to speak. Speech is learned through a multisensory approach using visual, tactile, kinesthetic, and auditory stimulation. Encourage parents to participate fully in the learning process.

Additional Aids

Everyday activities present problems for older children with hearing impairment. For example, they may not be able to hear the telephone, doorbell, or alarm clock. Several commercial devices are available to help them adjust to these dilemmas. Flashing lights can be attached to a telephone or doorbell to signal its ringing. Trained hearing ear dogs can provide great assistance, because they alert the person to sounds, such as someone approaching, a moving car, a signal to wake up, or a child's cry. Special teletypewriters or telecommunications devices for the deaf (TDD or TTY) help hearing-impaired people to communicate with each other over the telephone; the typed message is conveyed via the telephone lines and displayed on a small screen.*

Any audiovisual medium presents dilemmas for these children, who can see the picture but cannot hear the message. However, with *closed captioning* a special decoding device is attached to the television, and the audio portion of a program is translated into subtitles that appear on the screen.†

Socialization

Socialization is extremely important to children's development. If children attend a special school for the hearing impaired, they are able to socialize

---

*Resources and support network information are provided by the Alexander Graham Bell Association for the Deaf and Hard of Hearing, 3417 Volta Place NW, Washington, DC 20007; voice: 202-337-5220; TTY: 202-337-5221; www.agbell.org; email: info@agbell.org; and Canadian Hearing Society, 271 Spadina Road, Toronto, ON M5R 2V3; voice: 416-928-2535 or 877-347-3427; TTY: 877-216-7310; www.chs.ca.

†Additional information is available from the National Captioning Institute, 3725 Concorde Parkway, Suite 100, Chantilly, VA 20151; voice/TTY: 703-917-7600; www.ncicap.org; email: mail@ncicap.org; https://www.facebook.com/National-Captioning-Institute-NCI-180151395413842/.

with peers in that setting. Classmates become a potential source of close friendships, because they communicate more easily among themselves. Encourage parents to promote these relationships whenever possible.

Children with a hearing impairment may need special help with school or social activities. For children wearing hearing aids, keep background noise to a minimum. Because many of these children are able to attend regular classes, the teacher may need assistance in adapting methods of teaching for the child's benefit. The school nurse is often in an optimal position to emphasize methods of facilitated communication, such as lipreading (see Guidelines box: Facilitating Lipreading). Because group projects and audiovisual teaching aids may hinder the hearing-impaired child's learning, carefully evaluate the use of these educational methods.

In a group setting, it is helpful for the other members to sit in a semicircle in front of the hearing-impaired child. Because one of the difficulties in following a group discussion is that the hearing-impaired child is unaware of who will speak next, someone should point out each speaker. Speakers can also be given numbers, or their names can be written down as each person talks. If one person writes down the main topic of the discussion, the child is able to follow lipreading more closely. Such practices can increase the child's ability to participate in sports, organizations such as Scouts, and group projects.

Support Child and Family

Once the diagnosis of hearing impairment is made, parents need extensive support to adjust to the shock of learning about their child's disability and an opportunity to realize the extent of the hearing loss. If the hearing loss occurs during childhood, the child also requires sensitive, supportive care during the long and often difficult adjustment to this sensory loss. Early rehabilitation is one of the best strategies for fostering adjustment. Progress in learning communication, however, may not always coincide with emotional adjustment. Depression or anger is common, and such feelings are a normal part of the grieving process.

Care for the Child During Hospitalization

The needs of the hospitalized child with impaired hearing are the same as those of any other child, but the disability presents special challenges to the nurse. For example, verbal explanations must be supplemented by tactile and visual aids, such as books or actual demonstration and practice. Children's understanding of the explanation needs to be constantly reassessed. If their verbal skills are poorly developed, they can answer questions through drawing, writing, or gesturing. For example, if the nurse is attempting to clarify where a spinal tap is done, ask the child to point to where the procedure will be done on the body. Because hearing-impaired children often need more time to grasp the full meaning of an explanation, the nurse needs to be patient, allowing ample time for understanding.

When communicating with the child, the nurse should use the same principles as those outlined for facilitating lipreading. Ideally, nurses without foreign accents should be assigned to the child. The child's hearing aid is checked to ensure that it is working properly. If it is necessary to awaken the child at night, the nurse should gently shake the child or turn on the hearing aid before arousing the child. The nurse should always make certain that the child can see him or her before any procedures, even routine ones such as changing a diaper or regulating an infusion. It is important to remember that the child may not be aware of the nurse's presence until alerted through visual or tactile cues.

Ideally, parents are encouraged to room with the child. However, the nurse must convey to them that this is not to serve as a convenience to the nurse but as a benefit to the child. Although the parents' aid can be enlisted in familiarizing the child with the hospital and explaining procedures, the nurse should also talk directly to the child, encouraging expression of feelings about the experience. If the child's speech is difficult to understand, try to become familiar with his or her pronunciation of words. Parents often can be helpful by explaining the child's usual speech habits. Nonverbal communication devices that use pictures or words that the child can point to are also available. The nurse can make boards by drawing pictures or writing the words on cardboard representing common needs, such as *parent, food, water,* or *toilet.*

The nurse has a special role as child advocate and is in a strategic position to alert other health team members and other patients to the child's special needs regarding communication. For example, the nurse should accompany other practitioners on visits to the child's room to ensure that they speak to the child and that the child understands what is said. Caregivers may forget that the child has the abilities to perceive and learn despite a hearing loss, and consequently they communicate only with the parents. As a result, the child's needs and feelings remain unrecognized and unaddressed.

Because children with impaired hearing may have difficulty forming social relationships with other children, introduce the child to roommates and encourage them to engage in play activities. The hospital setting can provide growth-promoting opportunities for social relationships. With the assistance of a child life specialist, the child can learn new recreational activities, experiment with group games, and engage in therapeutic play. Playing with puppets or dollhouses, role-playing with dress-up clothes, building with a hammer and nails, finger painting, and water play can help the child express feelings that previously were suppressed.

Assist in Measures to Prevent Hearing Impairment

A primary nursing role is prevention of hearing loss. Because the most common cause of impaired hearing is chronic otitis media, it is essential that appropriate measures be instituted to treat existing infections and prevent recurrences. Children with a history of ear or respiratory infections or any other condition known to increase the risk for hearing impairment should receive periodic auditory testing.

To prevent the causes of hearing loss that begin prenatally and perinatally, pregnant women need counseling regarding the necessity of early prenatal care, including genetic counseling for known familial disorders; avoidance of all ototoxic drugs, especially during the first trimester; tests to rule out syphilis, rubella, or blood incompatibility; medical management of maternal diabetes; strict control of alcohol intake; adequate dietary intake; and avoidance of smoke exposure. Stress the necessity of routine immunization during childhood to eliminate the possibility of acquired sensorineural hearing loss from rubella, mumps, or measles (encephalitis).

Exposure to excessive noise pollution is a well-established cause of sensorineural hearing loss. The nurse should routinely assess the possibility of environmental noise pollution and advise children and parents of the potential danger. When individuals engage in activities associated with high-intensity noise (e.g., flying model airplanes, target shooting, or snowmobiling), they should wear ear protection such as earmuffs or earplugs. Even common household equipment, such as lawn mowers, vacuum cleaners, and cordless telephones, can be harmful.

> **! NURSING ALERT**
>
> Suspect hazardous noise if the listener experiences (1) difficulty in communication while hearing the sound, (2) ringing in the ears (tinnitus) after exposure to the sound, or (3) muffled hearing after leaving the sound.

VISUAL IMPAIRMENT

Visual impairment is a common problem during childhood. In the United States, the prevalence of serious visual impairment in the pediatric population is estimated to be between 30 to 64 children per 100,000 population. Vision impairment such as refractive error, strabismus, and amblyopia occur in 5% to 10% of all preschoolers, who are usually identified through vision screening programs (Alley, 2013; Rahi, Cumberland, Peckham, et al., 2010; US Department of Health and Human Services, Office of Disease Prevention and Health Promotion, 2015; US Preventive Services Task Force, 2011). The nurse's role is one of assessment, detection, prevention, referral, and (in some instances) rehabilitation.

Definition and Classification

Visual impairment is a general term that encompasses both partial sight and legal blindness. *Partial sight* or *partial visual impairment* is defined as a visual acuity between 20/70 and 20/200. The child can generally use normal-sized print, because near vision is almost always better than distance vision. *Legal blindness* or *severe permanent visual impairment* is defined as a visual acuity of 20/200 or lower or a visual field of 20 degrees or less in the better eye. It is important to keep in mind that legal blindness is not a medical diagnosis but a legal definition. Educational and governmental agencies in the United States use the legal definition of blindness to determine tax status, eligibility for entrance into special schools, eligibility for financial aid, and other benefits.

Etiology

Visual impairment can be caused by a number of genetic and prenatal or postnatal conditions. These include perinatal infections (herpes, chlamydia, gonococci, rubella, syphilis, toxoplasmosis); retinopathy of prematurity; trauma; postnatal infections (meningitis); and disorders, such as sickle cell disease, juvenile rheumatoid arthritis, Tay-Sachs disease, albinism, and retinoblastoma. In many instances, such as with refractive errors, the cause of the defect is unknown.

Refractive errors are the most common types of visual disorders in children. The term *refraction* means bending and refers to the bending of light rays as they pass through the lens of the eye. Normally, light rays enter the lens and fall directly on the retina. However, in refractive disorders, the light rays either fall in front of the retina *(myopia)* or beyond it *(hyperopia)*. Other eye problems, such as strabismus, may or may not include refractive errors, but they are important because, if untreated, they result in severe permanent visual impairment from amblyopia. These, along with other less frequent visual disorders, are summarized in Box 37.5. In addition to these disorders, other visual problems can be a result of infection or trauma.

Trauma

Trauma is a common cause of visual impairment in children. Injuries to the eyeball and adnexa (supporting or accessory structures, such as eyelids, conjunctiva, or lacrimal glands) can be classified as penetrating or nonpenetrating. *Penetrating wounds* are most often a result of sharp instruments (e.g., sticks, knives, or scissors) or propulsive objects (e.g., firecrackers, guns, arrows, or slingshots). *Nonpenetrating injuries* may be a result of foreign objects in the eyes, lacerations, a blow from a blunt object such as a ball (baseball, softball, basketball, racquet sports) or fist, or thermal or chemical burns.

Treatment is aimed at preventing further ocular damage and is primarily the responsibility of the ophthalmologist. It involves adequate examination of the injured eye (with the child sedated or anesthetized in severe injuries); appropriate immediate intervention, such as removal of the foreign body or suturing of the laceration; and prevention of

BOX 37.5   Types of Visual Impairment

Refractive Errors

Myopia
Nearsightedness: Ability to see objects clearly at close range but not at a distance

Pathophysiology
Results from eyeball that is too long, causing images to fall in front of the retina

Clinical Manifestations
Headaches
Dizziness
Excessive eye rubbing
Head tilt or forward head thrusts
Difficulty in reading or doing other close work
Clumsiness; walking into objects
Blinking more than usual or irritability when doing close work
Inability to see objects clearly
Poor school performance, especially in subjects that require demonstration, such as arithmetic

Treatment
Corrected with biconcave lenses that focus rays on retina
May be corrected with laser surgery

Hyperopia
Farsightedness: Ability to see objects at a distance but not at close range

Pathophysiology
Results from eyeball that is too short, causing image to focus beyond retina

Clinical Manifestations
Because of accommodative ability, child can usually see objects at all ranges
Most children are normally hyperopic until about 7 years of age

Treatment
When required, corrected with convex lenses that focus rays on retina
May be corrected with laser surgery

Astigmatism
Unequal curvatures in refractive apparatus

Pathophysiology
Results from unequal curvatures in cornea or lens that cause light rays to bend in different directions

Clinical Manifestations
Depend on severity of refractive error in each eye
Possible clinical manifestations of myopia

Treatment
Corrected with special lenses that compensate for refractive errors
May be corrected with laser surgery

Anisometropia
Different refractive strength in each eye

Pathophysiology
May develop amblyopia because weaker eye is used less

Clinical Manifestations
Depend on severity of refractive error in each eye
Possible clinical manifestations of myopia

Treatment
Treated with corrective lenses, preferably contact lenses, to improve vision in each eye so that they work as a unit
May be corrected with laser surgery

Amblyopia
Lazy eye: Reduced visual acuity in one eye

Pathophysiology
Results when one eye does not receive sufficient stimulation
Each retina receives different images, resulting in diplopia (double vision)
Brain accommodates by suppressing less intense image
Visual cortex eventually does not respond to visual stimulation, with resultant loss of vision in that eye

Clinical Manifestations
Poor vision in affected eye

Treatment
Preventable if treatment of primary visual defect, such as anisometropia or strabismus, begins before 6 years of age

Strabismus
"Squint" or malalignment of eyes
Esotropia: Inward deviation of eye
Exotropia: Outward deviation of eye

Pathophysiology
May result from muscle imbalance or paralysis, poor vision, or congenital defect
Because visual axes are not parallel, brain receives two images, and amblyopia can result

Clinical Manifestations
Squints eyelids together or frowns
Difficulty in focusing from one distance to another
Inaccurate judgment in picking up objects
Inability to see print or moving objects clearly
Closing one eye to see
Tilting head to one side
If combined with refractive errors, may see any of the manifestations listed for refractive errors
Diplopia
Photophobia
Dizziness
Headaches

Treatment
Depends on cause of strabismus
May involve occlusion therapy (patching stronger eye) or surgery to increase visual stimulation to weaker eye
Early diagnosis essential to prevent vision loss

Cataracts
Opacity of crystalline lens

Pathophysiology
Prevents light rays from entering eye and refracting on retina

Clinical Manifestations
Gradual decrease in ability to see objects clearly
Possible loss of peripheral vision

Continued

BOX 37.5   Types of Visual Impairment—cont'd

Nystagmus (with permanent visual impairment)
Gray opacities of lens
Strabismus
Absence of red reflex

Treatment

Requires surgery to remove cloudy lens and replace lens (with intraocular lens implant, removable contact lens, prescription glasses)
Must be treated early to prevent permanent visual impairment from amblyopia

Glaucoma

Increased intraocular pressure

Pathophysiology

Congenital type results from defective development of some component related to flow of aqueous humor
Increased pressure on optic nerve causes eventual atrophy and severe permanent visual impairment

Clinical Manifestations

Loss of peripheral vision—mostly seen in acquired types
Possible bumping into objects
Perception of halos around objects
Possible complaint of pain or discomfort (severe pain, nausea, or vomiting if sudden rise in pressure)
Eye redness
Excessive tearing (epiphora)
Photophobia
Spasmodic winking (blepharospasm)
Corneal haziness
Enlargement of eyeball (buphthalmos)

Treatment

Requires surgical treatment (goniotomy) to open outflow tracts
May require more than one procedure

✚ EMERGENCY TREATMENT

Eye Injuries

Foreign Object

Examine eye for presence of a foreign body (evert upper eyelid to examine upper eye).
Remove a freely movable object with pointed corner of gauze pad lightly moistened with water.
Do not irrigate eye or attempt to remove a penetrating object (see Penetrating Injuries).
Caution child against rubbing eye.

Chemical Burns

Irrigate eye copiously with tap water for 20 minutes.
Evert upper eyelid to flush thoroughly.
Hold child's head with eye under a tap of running lukewarm water.
Take child to emergency department.
Have child rest with eyes closed.
Keep room darkened.

Ultraviolet Burns

If skin is burned, patch both eyes (make certain eyelids are completely closed); secure dressing with Kling bandages wrapped around head rather than with tape.
Have child rest with eyes closed.
Refer to an ophthalmologist.

Hematoma ("Black Eye")

Use a flashlight to check for gross hyphema (hemorrhage into anterior chamber; visible fluid meniscus across iris; more easily seen in light-colored than in brown eyes).
Apply ice for first 24 hours to reduce swelling if no hyphema is present.
Refer to an ophthalmologist immediately if hyphema is present.
Have child rest with eyes closed.

Penetrating Injuries

Take child to emergency department.
Never remove an object that has penetrated eye.
Follow strict aseptic technique in examining eye.
Observe for:
- Aqueous or vitreous leaks (fluid leaking from point of penetration)
- Hyphema
- Shape and equality of pupils, reaction to light, prolapsed iris (not perfectly circular)

Apply a Fox shield if available (not a regular eye patch), and apply patch over unaffected eye to prevent bilateral movement.
Maintain bed rest with child in a 30-degree Fowler's position.
Caution child against rubbing eye.
Refer to an ophthalmologist.

---

complications, such as administration of antibiotics or steroids and complete bed rest to allow the eye to heal and blood to reabsorb (see Emergency Treatment box: Eye Injuries). The prognosis varies according to the type of injury. It is usually guarded in all cases of penetrating wounds because of the high risk for serious complications.

Infections

Infections of the adnexa and structures of the eyeball or globe may occur in children. The most common eye infection is conjunctivitis. Treatment is usually with ophthalmic antibiotics. Severe infections may require systemic antibiotic therapy. Steroids are used cautiously because they exacerbate viral infections such as herpes simplex, increasing the risk for damage to the involved structures.

Care Management

Nursing care of the visually impaired child is a critical nursing responsibility. Discovery of a visual impairment as early as possible is essential to prevent social, physical, and psychologic damage to the child. Assessment involves (1) identifying those children who by virtue of their history are at risk, (2) observing for behaviors that indicate a vision loss, and (3) screening all children for visual acuity and signs of other ocular disorders such as strabismus. This discussion focuses on clinical manifestations of various types of visual problems (see Box 37.5). Vision testing is discussed in Chapter 29.

Infancy

At birth, the nurse should observe the neonate's response to visual stimuli, such as following a light or object and cessation of body movement. The infant may vary in the intensity of the response, depending on the state of alertness.

Of special importance in detecting visual impairment during infancy are the parents' concerns regarding visual responsiveness in their child. Their concerns, such as lack of eye contact from the infant, must be taken seriously. During infancy, the child should be tested for strabismus. Lack of binocularity after 2 to 4 months of age is considered abnormal and must be treated to prevent amblyopia (Rogers & Jordan, 2013).

> ### ! NURSING ALERT
>
> Suspect visual impairment in an infant who does not react to light and in a child of any age if the parents express concern.

Childhood

Because the most common visual impairment during childhood is refractive error, testing for visual acuity is essential. The school nurse usually assumes major responsibility for vision testing in schoolchildren. In addition to assessing for refractive errors, the nurse should be aware of signs and symptoms that indicate other ocular problems. If the family is given a referral requesting further eye testing, the nurse is responsible for follow-up concerning the recommendation.

Learning that their child is visually impaired precipitates an immense crisis for families. Encourage the family to investigate appropriate early intervention and educational programs for their child as soon as possible. Sources of information include state commissions for the visually impaired, local schools for children with visual impairments, the American Foundation for the Blind,* the National Federation of the Blind,† the National Association for Parents of Children with Visual Impairments,‡ the National Association for Visually Handicapped,§ the American Council of the Blind‖, and CNIB.¶

Promote Parent-Child Attachment

A crucial time in the life of visual impaired infants is when the infant and the parents are getting acquainted with each other. Pleasurable patterns of interaction between the infant and parents may be lacking if there is not enough reciprocity. For example, if the parent gazes fondly at the infant's face and seeks eye contact but the infant fails to respond because he or she cannot see the parent, a troubled cycle of responses may occur. The nurse can help parents learn to look for other

*2 Penn Plaza, Suite 1102, New York, NY 10021; 800-232-5463 or 212-502-7600; www.afb.org; email: afbinfo@afb.net.
†200 E. Wells Street at Jernigan Place, Baltimore, MD 21230; 410-659-9314; www.nfb.org; www.facebook.com/NationalFederationoftheBlind; twitter.com/NFB_voice.
‡PO Box 317, Watertown, MA 02471; 617-972-7441 or 800-562-6265; www.spedex.com.
§15 West 65th Street, New York, NY 10023/800-284-4422; www.lighthouseguild.org.
‖2200 Wilson Boulevard, Suite 650, Arlington, VA 22201; 800-424-8666; 202-467-5081; www.acb.org; www.facebook.com/AmericanCounciloftheBlindOfficial.
¶1929 Bayview Avenue, East York, ON M4G 0A1; Canada: 800-563-2642; www.cnib.ca; facebook.com/myCNIB; twitter.com/cnib.

cues that indicate the infant is responding to them, such as whether the eyelids blink; whether the activity level accelerates or slows; whether respiratory patterns change, such as faster or slower breathing, when the parents come near; and whether the infant makes throaty sounds when the parents speak to the infant. In time, parents learn that the infant has unique ways of relating to them. Encourage the parents to show affection using nonvisual methods, such as talking or reading, cuddling, and walking the child.

Promote the Child's Optimal Development

Promoting the child's optimum development requires rehabilitation in a number of important areas. These include learning self-help skills and appropriate communication techniques to become independent. Although nurses may not be directly involved in such programs, they can provide direction and guidance to families regarding the availability of programs and the need to promote these activities in their child.

Development and Independence

Motor development depends on sight almost as much as verbal communication depends on hearing. From earliest infancy, parents are encouraged to expose the infant to as many visual-motor experiences as possible, such as sitting supported in an infant seat or swing and being given opportunities for holding up the head, sitting unsupported, reaching for objects, and crawling.

Despite visual impairment, the child can become independent in all aspects of self-care. The same principles used for promoting independence in sighted children apply, with additional emphasis on nonvisual cues. For example, the child may need help in dressing, such as special arrangement of clothing for style coordination and braille tags to distinguish colors and prints.

The permanently visual impaired child also must learn to become independent in navigational skills. The two main techniques are the *tapping method* (use of a cane to survey the environment for direction and to avoid obstacles) and *guides,* such as a sighted human guide or a dog guide, such as a seeing eye dog. Children who are partially sighted may benefit from ocular aids, such as a monocular telescope.

Play and Socialization

Children with severe permanent visual impairments do not learn to play automatically. Because they cannot imitate others or actively explore the environment as sighted children do, they depend much more on others to stimulate and teach them how to play. Parents need help in selecting appropriate play materials, especially those that encourage fine and gross motor development and stimulate the senses of hearing, touch, and smell. Toys with educational value are especially useful, such as dolls with various clothing closures.

Children with severe permanent visual impairments have the same needs for socialization as sighted children. Because they have little difficulty in learning verbal skills, they are able to communicate with age mates and participate in suitable activities. The nurse should discuss with parents opportunities for socialization outside the home, especially regular preschools. The trend is to include these children with sighted children to help them adjust to the outside world for eventual independence.

To compensate for inadequate stimulation, these children may develop self-stimulatory activities, such as body rocking, finger flicking, or arm twirling. Discourage such habits because they delay the child's social acceptance. Behavior modification is often successful in reducing or eliminating self-stimulatory activities.

Education

The main obstacle to learning is the child's total dependence on nonvisual cues. Although the child can learn via verbal lecturing, he or she is unable to read the written word or to write without special education. Therefore, the child must rely on *braille*, a system that uses raised dots to represent letters and numbers. The child can then read braille with the fingers and can write messages using a braille writer. However, this system is not useful for communicating with others unless others read braille. A more portable system for written communication is the use of a braille slate and stylus or a microcassette tape recorder. A recorder is especially helpful for leaving messages for others and taking notes during classroom lectures. For mathematic calculations, portable calculators with voice synthesizers are available.*

Books on CDs and tapes are significant sources of reading material in addition to braille books, which are large and cumbersome. The Library of Congress† has talking books and braille books that are available at many local and state libraries and directly from the Library of Congress. The talking book machine and tape player are provided at no cost to families, and there is no postage fee for returning the materials. Learning Ally (formally known as Recording for the Blind and Dyslexic)‡ also provides texts and CDs and tapes of books, which are helpful for secondary and college students who are visually impaired. A means of writing is learning to use a home computer with a voice synthesizer that can be adapted to speak each letter or word typed.

Children with partial sight benefit from specialized visual aids that produce a magnified retinal image. The basic methods are accommodative techniques such as bringing the object closer; devices such as special plus lenses, handheld and stand magnifiers, telescopes, and video projection systems; and large print materials. Special equipment is available to enlarge print. Information about services for the partially sighted is available from the National Association for Visually Handicapped and American Foundation for the Blind. Children with diminished vision often prefer to do close work without their glasses and compensate by bringing the object very near to their eyes. This should be allowed. The exception is children with vision in only one eye, who should always wear glasses for protection.

Care for the Child During Hospitalization

Because nurses are more likely to care for children who are hospitalized for procedures that involve temporary loss of vision than for children who have severe permanent visual impairments, the following discussion concentrates primarily on the needs of such children. The nursing care objectives in either situation are to (1) reassure the child and family throughout every phase of treatment, (2) orient the child to the surroundings, (3) provide a safe environment, and (4) encourage independence. Whenever possible, the same nurse should care for the child to ensure consistency in the approach.

When sighted children temporarily lose their vision, almost every aspect of the environment becomes bewildering and frightening. They are forced to rely on nonvisual senses for help in adjusting to the visual impairment without the benefit of any special training. Nurses have a major role in minimizing the effects of temporary loss of vision. They need to talk to the child about everything that is occurring, emphasizing

---

*A catalog of numerous products for people with vision problems is available from Lighthouse Guild, 15 West 65th Street, New York, NY 10023; 800-284-4422

†National Library Service for the Blind and Physically Handicapped, Library of Congress, 1291 Taylor Street NW, Washington, DC 20011; 202-707-5100; 888-657-7323; TTD: 202-707-0744; www.loc.gov/nls. (State listings of libraries for visually impaired and physical handicapped readers, as well as other reference circulars, are available from this office.)

‡20 Roszel Road, Princeton, NJ 08540; 800-221-4792 or 866-RFBD-585; www.learningally.org; www.facebook.com/LearningAlly.org.

aspects of procedures that are felt or heard. They should always identify themselves as soon as they enter the room and before they approach the child. Because unfamiliar sounds are especially frightening, these are explained. Encourage the parents to room with their child and participate in the care. Familiar objects, such as a teddy bear or doll, should be brought from home to help lessen the strangeness of the hospital. As soon as the child is able to be out of bed, orient the child to the immediate surroundings. If the child is able to see on admission, this opportunity is taken to point out significant aspects of the room. Encourage the child to practice ambulating with the eyes closed to become accustomed to this experience.

The room is arranged with safety in mind. For example, a stool placed next to the bed will help the child climb in and out of bed. The furniture is always placed in the same position to prevent collisions. Remind cleaning personnel to keep the room in order. If the child has difficulty navigating by feeling the walls, a rope can be attached from the bed to the point of destination, such as the bathroom. Attention to details (such as, well-fitting slippers and robes that do not drag on the floor) is important in preventing tripping. Unlike the child who is visually impaired, these children are not familiar with navigating with a cane.

The child is encouraged to be independent in self-care activities, especially if the visual loss may be prolonged or potentially permanent. For example, during bathing, the nurse sets up all of the equipment and encourages the child to participate. At mealtimes, the nurse explains where each food item is on the tray, opens any special containers, prepares cereal or toast, and encourages the child in self-feeding. Favorite finger foods (e.g., sandwiches, hamburgers, hot dogs, or pizza) may be good selections. Praise the child for efforts at being cooperative and independent. Any improvements made in self-care, no matter how small, are stressed.

Appropriate recreational activities are provided, and if a child life specialist is available, such planning is done jointly. Because children with temporary visual impairment have a wide variety of play experiences to draw on, they are encouraged to select activities. For example, if they like to read, they may enjoy listening to books on CD or having someone to read to them. If they prefer manual activity, they may appreciate playing with clay or building blocks or feeling different textures and naming them. If they need an outlet for aggression, activities such as pounding or banging on a drum can be helpful. Simple board and card games can be played with a "seeing partner" or an opponent who helps with the game. They should have familiar toys from home to play with because familiar items are more easily manipulated than new ones. If parents want to bring presents, they should be objects that stimulate hearing and touch, such as a radio, music box, or stuffed animal.

Occasionally, children who are visually impaired come to the hospital for procedures to restore their vision. Although this is an extremely happy time, it also requires intervention to help them adjust to sight. They need an opportunity to take in all that they see. They should not be bombarded with visual stimuli. They may need to concentrate on people's faces or their own to become accustomed to this experience. They often need to talk about what they see and to compare the visual images with their mental ones. The children may also go through a period of depression, which must be respected and supported. Encourage the children to discuss how it feels to see, especially in terms of seeing themselves.

Newly sighted children also need time to adjust and engage in activities that were impossible before. For example, they may prefer to use braille to read rather than learning a new "visual approach" because of familiarity with the touch system. Eventually, as they learn to recognize letters and numbers, they will integrate these new skills into reading and writing. However, parents and teachers must be careful not to push them before they are ready. This applies to social relationships and physical activities as well as learning situations.

Assist in Measures to Prevent Visual Impairment

An essential nursing goal is to prevent visual impairment. This involves many of the same interventions discussed for hearing impairments:

- Prenatal screening for pregnant women at risk, such as those with rubella or syphilis infection and family histories of genetic disorders associated with visual loss
- Adequate prenatal and perinatal care to prevent prematurity
- Periodic screening of all children, especially newborns through preschoolers, for congenital and acquired visual impairments caused by refractive errors, strabismus, and other disorders
- Rubella immunization of all children
- Safety counseling regarding the common causes of ocular trauma, including safe practices when working with, playing with, and carrying objects such as scissors, knives, and balls

---

! NURSING ALERT

A helmet with a face mask should be required for children playing football, hockey, and baseball.

After detection of eye problems, the nurse should encourage the family to prevent further ocular damage by undertaking corrective treatment. For the child with strabismus, this often necessitates occlusion patching of the stronger eye. Compliance with the procedure is greatest during the early preschool years. It is more difficult to encourage school-age children to wear the occlusive patch because the poor visual acuity of the uncovered weaker eye interferes with school work and the patch sets them apart from their peers. In school, they benefit from being positioned favorably (closer to the white board or other visual media) and allowed extra time to read or complete an assignment. If treatment of the eye disorder requires instillation of ophthalmic medication, the family is taught the correct procedure.

Children who need glasses to correct refractive errors need time to adjust to wearing glasses. Young children who often pull off glasses benefit from temporal pieces that wrap around the ears or an elastic strap attached to the frames and around the back of the head to hold the glasses on securely. Once children appreciate the value of clear vision, they are more likely to wear the corrective lenses.

Glasses should not interfere with any activity. Special protective guards are available during contact sports to prevent accidental injury, and all corrective lenses should be made from safety glass, which is shatterproof. Often, corrective lenses improve visual acuity so dramatically that children are able to compete more effectively in sports. This in itself is a tremendous inducement to continue wearing glasses.

Contact lenses are a popular alternative to conventional glasses, especially for adolescents. Several types are available, such as hard lenses, including gas-permeable ones, and soft lenses, which may be designed for daily or extended wear. Contact lenses offer several advantages over glasses, such as greater visual acuity, total corrected field of vision, convenience (especially with the extended-wear type), and optimal cosmetic benefit. Unfortunately, they are usually more expensive and require much more care than glasses, including considerable practice to learn techniques for insertion and removal. If they are prescribed, the nurse can be helpful in teaching parents or older children how to care for the lenses.

Because trauma is the leading cause of visual impairment, the nurse has the major responsibility of preventing further eye injury until specific treatment is instituted. The major principles to follow when caring for

an eye injury are outlined in the Emergency Treatment box: Eye Injuries. Because patients with a serious eye injury fear visual impairment, the nurse should stay with the child and family to provide support and reassurance.

HEARING-VISUAL IMPAIRMENT

The most traumatic sensory impairment is loss of both vision and hearing, which may have profound effects on the child's development. These losses interfere with the normal sequence of physical, intellectual, and psychosocial growth. Although such children often achieve the usual motor milestones, their rate of development is slower. These children learn communication only with specialized training. *Finger spelling* is one desirable method often taught to these children. Words are spelled letter by letter into the hearing-visually impaired child's hand, and the child spells into the other person's hand. Some children with residual hearing or visual impairment can learn to speak. Whenever possible, encourage speech because it allows communication with other individuals.

The future prospects for hearing and visually impaired children are, at best, unpredictable. Congenital hearing and visual impairment are accompanied by other physical or neurologic problems, which further diminish the child's learning potential. The most favorable prognosis is for children who have acquired hearing and visual impairments with few, if any, associated disabilities. Their learning capacity is greatly potentiated by their developmental progress before the sensory impairments. Although total independence, including gainful vocational training, is the goal, some children with hearing-visual impairment are unable to develop to this level. They may require lifelong parental or residential care. The nurse working with such families helps them deal with future goals for the child, including possible alternatives to home care during the parents' advancing years.

COMMUNICATION IMPAIRMENT

AUTISM SPECTRUM DISORDERS

ASDs are complex neurodevelopmental disorders of unknown etiology. The American Psychiatric Association's *Diagnostic and Statistical Manual of Mental Disorders* (DSM-5) revised the definition for ASD based on two behavior domains that include difficulties in social communication and social interaction, and unusually restricted, repetitive behavior, interests, or activities (American Psychiatric Association, 2013; Brentani, dePaula, Bordini, et al., 2013; Lai, Lombardo, & Baron-Cohen, 2014).

ASD is now frequently diagnosed in toddlers because of their atypical development is being recognized early (Lai, Lombardo, & Baron-Cohen, 2014). It occurs in 1 in 68 children in the United States; is about four times more common in boys than in girls; and is not related to socioeconomic level, race, or parenting style (Centers for Disease Control and Prevention, 2014; National Autism Association, 2015a).

Etiology

The cause of ASD is unknown. Researchers are investigating a number of theories, including a link among hereditary causes, genetic factors, medical problems, immune dysregulation/neuroinflammation, oxidative stress (damage to cellular tissue), and environmental factors (Lai, Lombardo, & Baron-Cohen, 2014; Rossignol & Frye, 2012). Individuals with ASD may have abnormal electroencephalograms, epileptic seizures, delayed development of hand dominance, persistence of primitive reflexes, metabolic abnormalities (elevated blood serotonin), cerebellar vermis hypoplasia (part of the brain involved in regulating motion and some aspects of memory), and infantile abnormal head enlargement (Rutter, 2011).

The strong evidence for a genetic basis in twins is consistent with an autosomal recessive pattern of inheritance. Twin studies demonstrate a high concordance (60% to 96%) for monozygotic (identical) twins and less than 5% concordance for dizygotic (nonidentical) twins. In addition, between 5% and 16% of boys with ASD are positive for the fragile X chromosome (Clifford, Dissanayake, Bui, et al., 2007; Grafodatskaya, Chung, Szatmari, et al., 2010).

There is a relatively high risk for recurrence of ASD in families with one affected child (Chawarska, Shic, Macari, et al., 2014; Rutter, 2011; Yoder, Stone, & Walden, 2009). Several genes have been suggested as possible causative factors in ASD (Kolevzon, Gross, & Reichenberg, 2007; Talkowski, Minikel, & Gusella, 2014; Willsey & State, 2015).

The scientific evidence to date shows no link between measles, mumps, and rubella (MMR) and thimerosal-containing vaccines and ASDs (Barile,

Kuperminc, Weintraub, et al., 2012; Price, Thompson, Goodson, et al., 2010; Taylor, Swerdfeger, and Eslick, 2014; Uno, Uchiyama, Kurosawa, et al., 2015) (see Evidence-Based Practice box Thimerosal-Containing Vaccines and Autism Spectrum Disorders). ASD has been reported in association with a number of conditions, such as FXS, tuberous sclerosis, Prader-Willi syndrome, metabolic disorders, fetal rubella syndrome, *Haemophilus influenzae* meningitis, and structural brain anomalies (National Autism Association, 2015a; Peterson & Barbel, 2013). Recent reports have retrospectively tied ASD to prenatal and perinatal events, such as maternal and paternal ages over 40 years of age (for fathers, 1 in 116 births; for mothers, 1 in 123 births), uterine bleeding during pregnancy, low Apgar score, fetal distress, and neonatal hyperbilirubinemia (Amin, Smith, & Wang, 2011; Kolevzon, Gross & Reichenberg, 2007; Rutter, 2011). These same researchers, however, urge caution in interpreting these findings.

EVIDENCE-BASED PRACTICE

Thimerosal-Containing Vaccines and Autism Spectrum Disorders

Ask the Question

PICOT Question: Is the incidence of autism spectrum disorders (ASDs) increased in children receiving vaccines containing thimerosal?

Search for the Evidence

Search Strategies

Published studies from 2004 to 2015 focused on the pediatric population and restricted to the English language

Databases Used

PubMed, Cochrane Collaboration, MD Consult, Vaccine Adverse Events Reporting System (VAERS) database, American Academy of Pediatrics, Autism Research Institute

Critical Appraisal of the Evidence

Grade criteria: Moderate evidence with strong recommendations for practice (Balshem, Helfand, Schünemann, et al., 2011). Evidence does not support an association between the increased incidence of autism and mercury exposure from the pharmaceutical preservative thimerosal.

- A Cochrane systematic review of 64 studies assessing the effectiveness and adverse effects associated with the trivalent measles, mumps, and rubella (MMR) vaccine on healthy patients up to 15 years of age found no significant association between MMR with either autism or other conditions (Demicheli, Rivetti, Debalini, et al., 2012). Previously done studies supported the same conclusion, because the studies found no association between thimerosal-containing vaccines and ASD (Demicheli, Jefferson, Rivetti, et al., 2005; Hurley, Tadrous, & Miller, 2010; Parker, Schwartz, Todd, et al., 2004; Schultz, 2010; World Health Organization, 2012).
- Two large studies in Europe found no evidence that childhood vaccination with thimerosal-containing vaccines was associated with the development of ASDs. One longitudinal study evaluated more than 14,000 children in the United Kingdom. The mercury exposure from thimerosal-containing vaccines was recorded and calculated at 3, 4, and 6 months of age and compared with cognitive and behavioral-developmental assessments performed from 6 to 91 months of age (Heron, Golding, and ALSPAC Study Team, 2004). The second study, a cohort of 467,450 children in Denmark, compared the incidence of ASDs in children vaccinated with thimerosal-containing vaccines with the incidence of ASDs in children vaccinated with a thimerosal-free formulation of the same vaccine. Another study that evaluated 1047 children from early life to 7 to 10 years of age and their biologic mothers found no statistically significant associations between thimerosal exposure from vaccines early in life. It noted a small but statistically significant association between early

thimerosal exposure and the presence of tics in boys and recommended there be further research in this area (Barile, Kuperminc, Weintraub, et al., 2012).

- Case-control studies have also found no relationships between MMR vaccination and the increased risk for ASDs (Price, Thompson, Goodson, et al., 2010; Uno, Uchiyama, Kurosawa, et al., 2015). Another small case control study investigated the mercury level in maternal prenatal serum and early postnatal newborn serum of children with ASD (n = 84) compared to children with intellectual disability or developmental delay (n = 49) and the general population (n = 159) and found no significant association with the risk for ASD (Yau, Green, Alaimo, et al., 2014). A similar finding was concluded in a meta-analysis of evidence on impact of prenatal and early infancy exposures to mercury on autism and attention-deficit/hyperactivity disorder (ADHD) with the recommendation of further study to be conducted on effects of environmental perinatal mercury exposures and increase risk for developmental disorders (Yoshimasu, Kiyohara, Takemura, et al., 2014).
- Two review studies by the same first author reported new epidemiologic evidence of a significant relationship between increasing organic mercury exposure from thimerosal-containing vaccines and subsequent risk for neurodevelopmental disorders. Both case-control studies examined automated records updated through 2000 in the Vaccine Safety Datalink (VSD) for organic exposure to hepatitis B vaccine administered in the first 6 months of life and increased risk for neurodevelopmental disorder (Geier, Hooker, Kern, et al., 2014) and organic exposure from *Haemophilus influenzae* type b administered in first 15 months of life and increased risk for pervasive developmental disorder (Geier, Kern, King, et al., 2015). Conversely, the Global Advisory Committee on Vaccine Safety reviewed both animal and human toxicity studies in which the blood and brain did not attain toxic levels, making it biologically implausible for any relationship between thimerosal in vaccines and neurologic toxicity (World Health Organization, 2012). Another evidence-based meta-analysis of case-control studies and cohort studies supported the same conclusion; the findings suggest that vaccinations are not associated with the development of autism or ASD (Taylor, Swerdfeger, & Eslick, 2014).
- In 2013, the Institute of Medicine completed an update to the review of the evidence reported from January 1990 to May 2013 and concluded that the review did not reveal an evidence base, suggesting that the United States childhood immunization schedule is linked to learning or developmental disorders or attention deficit or disruptive disorders. Based on guidelines established by the US Food and Drug Administration (2014) and other government monitoring agencies, no children will be exposed to excessive mercury from childhood vaccines.

EVIDENCE-BASED PRACTICE—cont'd

Thimerosal-Containing Vaccines and Autism Spectrum Disorders

Apply the Evidence: Nursing Implications

There is moderate-quality evidence with a strong recommendation that there is no link between vaccines containing thimerosal and ASDs.

Quality and Safety Competencies: Evidence-Based Practice*

Knowledge

Differentiate clinical opinion from research and evidence-based summaries.

Compare research summaries that provide evidence of the lack of association between vaccines containing thimerosal and autism or other neurodevelopmental disorders.

Skills

Base individualized care plan on patient values, clinical expertise, and evidence.

Integrate evidence into practice by sharing results with parents regarding the benefits of vaccinating their children and the evidence regarding lack of association between immunizations and autism disorders.

Attitudes

Value the concept of evidence-based practice as integral to determining best clinical practice.

Appreciate strengths and weakness of the evidence that confirms the lack of a link between vaccines containing thimerosal and autism or other neurodevelopmental disorders.

References

Balshem, H., Helfand, M., Schünemann, H. J., et al. (2011). GRADE guidelines: 3. rating the quality of evidence. *Journal of Clinical Epidemiology, 64*(4), 401–406.

Barile, J. P., Kuperminc, G. P., Weintraub, E. S., et al. (2012). Thimerosal exposure in early life and neuropsychological outcomes 7-10 years later. *Journal of Pediatric Psychology, 37*(1), 106–118.

Demicheli, V., Jefferson, T., Rivetti, A., et al. (2005). Vaccines for measles, mumps and rubella in children. *Cochrane Database of Systematic Reviews, 2005*(4), CD004407.

Demicheli, V., Rivetti, A., Debalini, M. G., et al. (2012). Vaccines for measles, mumps and rubella in children. *Cochrane Database of Systematic Reviews, 2012*(2), CD004407.

Geier, D. A., Hooker, B. S., Kern, J. K., et al. (2014). A dose-response relationship between organic mercury exposure from thimerosal-containing vaccines and neurodevelopmental disorders. *International Journal of Environmental Research and Public Health, 11*(9), 9156–9170.

Geier, D. A., Kern, J. K., King, P. G., et al. (2015). A case-control study evaluating the relationship between thimerosal-containing *Haemophilus influenzae* type B vaccine administration and the risk for pervasive developmental disorder diagnosis in the United States. *Biological Trace Element Research, 163*(1-2), 28–38.

Heron, J., Golding, J., & ALSPAC Study Team. (2004). Thimerosal exposure in infants and developmental disorders: A prospective cohort study in the United Kingdom does not support a causal association. *Pediatrics, 114*(3), 577–583.

Hurley, A. M., Tadrous, M., & Miller, E. S. (2010). Thimerosal-containing vaccines and autism: Review of recent epidemiologic studies. *Journal of Pediatric Pharmacology and Therapeutics, 15*(3), 173–181.

Institute of Medicine. (2013). *The childhood immunization schedule and safety: stakeholders concerns, scientific evidence, and future studies.* Washington, DC: National Academies Press.

Parker, S. K., Schwartz, B., Todd, J., et al. (2004). Thimerosal-containing vaccines and autistic spectrum disorder: A critical review of published original data. *Pediatrics, 114*(3), 793–804.

Price, C. S., Thompson, W. W., Goodson, B., et al. (2010). Prenatal and infant exposure to thimerosal from vaccines and immunoglobulins and risk of autism. *Pediatrics, 126*(4), 656–664.

Schultz, S. T. (2010). Does thimerosal or other mercury exposure increase the risk for autism? A review of current literature. *Acta Neurobiologiae Experimentalis, 70*(2), 187–195.

Taylor, L. E., Swerdfeger, A. L., & Eslick, G. D. (2014). Vaccines are not associated with autism: An evidence-based meta-analysis of case-control and cohort studies. *Vaccine, 32*(29), 3623–3629.

Uno, Y., Uchiyama, T., Kurosawa, M., et al. (2015). Early exposure to the combined measles-mumps-rubella vaccine and thimerosal-containing vaccines and risk of autism spectrum disorder. *Vaccine, 33*(21), 2511–2516.

US Food and Drug Administration. (2014). *Thimerosal in vaccines.* Retrieved from http://www.fda.gov/BiologicsBloodVaccines/SafetyAvailability/vaccineSafety/UCM096228.

World Health Organization. (2012). *Global vaccine safety: Global Advisory Committee on Vaccine Safety, report of meeting held 6-7 June 2012.* Retrieved from http://www.who.int/vaccine_safety/committee/reports/Jun_2012/en/.

Yau, V. M., Green, P. G., Alaimo, C. P., et al. (2014). Prenatal and neonatal peripheral blood mercury levels and autism spectrum disorders. *Environmental Research, 133*, 294–303.

Yoshimasu, K., Kiyohara, C., Takemura, S., et al. (2014). A meta-analysis of the evidence on the impact of prenatal and early infancy exposures to mercury on autism and attention deficit/hyperactivity disorder in the childhood. *Neurotoxicology, 44*, 121–131.

Rosalind Bryant

*Adapted from the Quality and Safety Education for Nurses (QSEN) Institute.

Clinical Manifestations and Diagnostic Evaluation

Children with ASD demonstrate core deficits primarily in social interactions, communication, and behavior. Failure of social interaction and communication development is the one of the hallmarks of ASD. Parents of autistic children have reported their child showed less interest in social interaction (e.g., abnormal eye contact, decreased response to own name, decreased imitation, unusual repetitive behavior) and have verbal and motor delay (Bolton, Golding, Emond, et al., 2012; Golnik & Maccabee-Ryaboy, 2010; Kirchner, Hatre, Heekeren, et al., 2011; National Autism Association, 2015b). Children with ASD may have significant gastrointestinal symptoms. Constipation is a common symptom and can be associated with acquired megarectum in children with ASD (Buie, Campbell, Fuchs, et al., 2010; National Autism Association, 2015a).

Children with autism do not always have the same manifestations, from mild forms requiring minimal supervision to severe forms in which self-abusive behavior is common. The majority of children with autism have some degree of CI, with scores typically in the moderate to severe range. Despite their relatively moderate to severe disability, some children with autism (known as savants) excel in particular areas, such as art, music, memory, mathematics, or perceptual skills, such as puzzle building.

! NURSING ALERT

Claims of beneficial results from the use of secretin, a peptide hormone that stimulates pancreatic secretion, has been studied extensively in multiple randomized control trials, denoting clear evidence that it lacks any benefit (Krishnaswami, McPheeters, & Veenstra-Vanderweele, 2011; Williams, Wray, & Wheeler, 2012).*

*Additional information on secretin may be found by contacting the Autism Society, 4340 East-West Hwy., Suite 350, Bethesda, MD 20814-3067; 800-3AUTISM or 301-657-0881; http://www.autism-society.org.

Communication impairments are a common sign in children with ASD that may range from absent to delayed speech. Any child who does not display language skills such as babbling or gesturing by 12 months of age, single words by 16 months of age, and two-word phrases by 24 months of age is recommended for immediate hearing and language evaluation. Autism regression is when the child seems to develop normally then regresses suddenly; this is a red-flag event that has been frequently displayed in expressive language (Fernell, Ericksson, and Gillberg, 2013; National Autism Association, 2015b).

Early recognition, referral, diagnosis, and intensive early intervention tend to improve outcomes for children with ASD (Golnik & Maccabee-Ryaboy, 2010; Reichow, Barton, Boyd, et al., 2012; Peterson & Barbel, 2013; Zwaigenbaum, 2010). Unfortunately, diagnosis is often not made until 2 to 3 years after symptoms are first recognized. However, in a recent retrospective study, the majority of parents observed atypical development in their ASD children before 24 months of age (Lemcke, Juul, Parner, et al., 2013).

Prognosis

Even though ASD is usually a severely disabling condition, the symptoms associated with autism can be greatly improved with early and intensive interventions, and reported symptoms were completely overcome in some cases (National Autism Association, 2015a; Wodka, Mathy, & Kalb, 2013). Some ultimately achieve independence, but most require lifelong adult supervision. Aggravation of psychiatric symptoms occurs in about one-half of the children during adolescence, with girls having a tendency for continued deterioration.

Early recognition of behaviors associated with ASD is critical to implement appropriate interventions and family involvement. There is a growing body of evidence that parent-delivered interventions are associated with some improved outcomes, yet further research is needed in this area incorporating consistent measures (Bearss, Burrell, Stewart, et al., 2015; Brentani, de Paula, Bordini, et al., 2013; Oono, Honey, and McConachie, 2013). The prognosis is most favorable for children with higher intelligence, functional speech, and less behavioral impairment (Raviola, Gosselin, Walter, et al., 2011; Solomon, Buaminger, & Rogers, 2011).

Care Management

Therapeutic intervention for children with ASD is a specialized area involving professionals with advanced training emphasizing the importance of interprofessional care. Although there is no cure for ASD, numerous therapies have been used. The most promising results have been through highly structured and intensive behavior modification programs. In general, the objective in treatment is to promote positive reinforcement, increase social awareness of others, teach verbal communication skills, and decrease unacceptable behavior. Providing a structured routine for the child to follow is a key in the management of ASD.

When these children are hospitalized, the parents are essential to planning care and ideally should stay with the child as much as possible. Nurses should recognize that not all children with ASD are the same and that they require individual assessment and treatment. Decreasing stimulation by using a private room, avoiding extraneous auditory and visual distractions, and encouraging the parents to bring in possessions the child is attached to may lessen the disruptiveness of hospitalization. Because physical contact often upsets these children, minimal holding and eye contact may be necessary to avoid behavioral outbursts. Take care when performing procedures on, administering medicine to, and feeding these children because they may be either fussy eaters who willfully starve themselves or gag to prevent eating, or indiscriminate hoarders who swallow any available edible or inedible items, such as a thermometer. Eating habits of ASD children may be particularly problematic for families and may involve food refusal accompanied by mineral deficiencies, mouthing objects, eating nonedibles, and smelling and throwing food (Belschner, 2007; Herndon, DiGuiseppi, Johnson, et al., 2009).

Children with ASD need to be introduced slowly to new situations, with visits with staff caregivers kept short whenever possible. Because these children have difficulty organizing their behavior and redirecting their energy, they need to be told directly what to do. Communication should be at the child's developmental level, brief, and concrete.

Family Support

ASD, as with so many other chronic conditions, involves the entire family and often becomes "a family disease." Nurses can help alleviate the guilt and shame often associated with this disorder by stressing what is known from a biologic standpoint and by providing family support. It is imperative to help parents understand that they are not the cause of the child's condition.

Parents need expert counseling early in the course of the disorder and should be referred to the Autism Society website. The society provides information about education, treatment programs and techniques, and facilities such as camps and group homes. Other helpful resources for parents of children with ASD are the local and state departments of mental health and developmental disabilities; these organizations provide important programs and in-school programs throughout the United States for children with ASD.

As much as possible, the family is encouraged to care for the child in the home. With the help of family support programs in many states, families are often able to provide home care and assist with the educational services the child needs. As the child approaches adulthood and the parents become older, the family may require assistance in locating a long-term placement facility.

REFERENCES

Abrams, L., Cronister, A., Brown, W. T., et al. (2012). Newborn, carrier, and early childhood screening recommendations for fragile X. *Pediatrics*, *130*(6), 1126–1135.

Alley, C. L. (2013). Preschool vision screening: Update on guidelines and techniques. *Current Opinion in Ophthalmology*, *24*(5), 415–420.

Almadhoob, A., & Ohlsson, A. (2015). Sound reduction management in the neonatal intensive care unit for preterm or very low birth weight infants. *Cochrane Database of Systermatic Reviews*, *2015*(1), CD010333.

American Academy of Pediatrics, Joint Committee on Infant Hearing. (2007). Year 2007 position statement: Principles and guidelines for early hearing detection and intervention programs. *Pediatrics*, *120*(4), 898–921.

American Association on Intellectual and Developmental Disabilities. (2013). *Intellectual disability: definition, classification, and systems of supports* (11th ed.). Washington, DC: Author.

American Psychiatric Association (2013). *Diagnostic and statistical manual of mental disorders (DSM-V)* (5th ed.). Arlington, VA: American Psychiatric Association.

Amin, S. B., Smith, T., & Wang, H. (2011). Is neonatal jaundice associated with autism spectrum disorders: A systematic review. *Journal of Autism and Developmental Disorders*, *41*(11), 1455–1463.

Bagni, C., Tassone, F., Neri, G., et al. (2012). Fragile X syndrome: Causes, diagnosis, mechanisms, and therapeutics. *Journal of Clinical Investigation*, *122*(12), 4314–4322.

Barile, J. P., Kuperminc, G. P., Weintraub, E. S., et al. (2012). Thimerosal exposure in early life and neuropsychological outcomes 7-10 years later. *Journal of Pediatric Psychology*, *37*(1), 106–118.

Bearss, K., Burrell, T. L., Stewart, L., et al. (2015). Parent training in autism spectrum disorder: What's in a name? *Clinical Child and Family Psychology Review*, *18*(2), 170–182.

Belschner, R. A. (2007). Stop, assess and motivate: The SAM approach to autism spectrum disorder. *American Journal for Nurse Practitioners*, *11*(4), 43–50.

Biassoni, E. C., Serra, M. R., Hinalaf, M., et al. (2014). Hearing and loud music exposure in a group of adolescents at the ages of 14-15 and retested at 17-18. *Noise and Health*, *16*(72), 331–341.

Bolton, P. F., Golding, J., Emond, A., et al. (2012). Autism spectrum disorder and autistic traits in the Avon Longitudinal Study of Parents and Children: Precursors and early signs. *Journal of the American Academyy of Child and Adolescent Psychiatry, 51*(3), 249–260.

Brentani, H., Paula, C. S., Bordini, D., et al. (2013). Autism spectrum disorders: An overview on diagnosis and treatment. *Revista Brasileira de Psiquiatria, 35*(1 suppl), S62–S72.

Buie, T., Campbell, D. B., Fuchs, G. J., 3rd, et al. (2010). Evaluation, diagnosis, and treatment of gastrointestinal disorders in individuals with ASDs: A consensus report. *Pediatrics, 125*(1 suppl), S1–S18.

Bull, M. J., & Committee on Genetics. (2011). Health supervision for children with Down syndrome. *Pediatrics, 128*(2), 393–406.

Centers for Disease Control and Prevention. (2014). Prevalence of autism spectrum disorder among children aged 8 years—Autism and developmental disorders monitoring network, 11 sites, United States, 2010. *Morbidity and Mortality Weekly Report Surveillance Summaries, 63*(2), 1–21.

Chawarska, K., Shic, F., Macari, S., et al. (2014). 18-Month predictors of later outcomes in younger siblings of children with autism spectrum disorder: A baby siblings research consortium study. *Journal of the American Academyy of Child and Adolescent Psychiatry, 53*(12), 1317–1327.

Clifford, S., Dissanayake, C., Bui, Q. M., et al. (2007). Autism spectrum phenotype in males and females with fragile X full mutation and permutation. *Journal of Autism and Developmental Disorders, 37*(4), 738–747.

Colella-Santos, M. F., Hein, T. A., de Souza, G. L., et al. (2014). Newborn hearing screening and early diagnostic in the NICU. *BioMed Research International, 2014,* 845308.

Fabry, D. A., Davila, E. P., Arheart, K. L., et al. (2011). Secondhand smoke exposure and the risk of hearing loss. *Tobacco Control, 20*(1), 82–85.

Fernell, E., Eriksson, M. A., & Gillberg, C. (2013). Early diagnosis of autism and impact on prognosis: A narrative review. *Clinical Epidemiology, 5,* 33–43.

Finucane, B., Abrams, L., Cronister, A., et al. (2012). Genetic counseling and testing for FMRI gene mutations: Practice guidelines of the National Society of Genetic Counselors. *Journal of Genetic Counseling, 21*(6), 752–760.

Golnik, A., & Maccabee-Ryaboy, N. (2010). Autism: Clinical pearls for primary care. *Contemporary Pediatrics,* 42-60.

Grafodatskaya, D., Chung, B., Szatmari, P., et al. (2010). Autism spectrum disorders and epigenetics. *Journal of the American Academy of Child and Adolescent Psychiatry, 49*(8), 794–809.

Grindle, C. R. (2014). Pediatric hearing loss. *Pediatrics in Review, 35*(11), 456–463.

Haddad, J. (2011). Hearing loss. In R. M. Kliegman, R. F. Stanton, J. W. St. Geme III, et al. (Eds.), *Nelson textbook of pediatrics* (18th ed.). Philadelphia, PA: Elsevier/Saunders.

Hagerman, R. J., Berry-Kravis, E., Kaufmann, W. E., et al. (2009). Advances in the treatment of fragile X syndrome. *Pediatrics, 123*(1), 378–390.

Harrison, R. V. (2012). The prevention of noise induced hearing loss in children. *International Journal of Pediatrics, 2012,* 473541.

Hayes, H., Geers, A. E., Treiman, R., et al. (2009). Receptive vocabulary development in deaf children with cochlear implants: Achievement in an intensive auditory-oral educational setting. *Ear and Hearing, 30*(1), 128–135.

Herndon, A. C., DiGuiseppi, C., Johnson, S. L., et al. (2009). Does nutritional intake differ between children and autism spectrum disorders and children with typical development? *Journal of Autism and Developmental Disorders, 39*(2), 212–222.

Huang, X., Zheng, J., Chen, M., et al. (2014). Noninvasive prenatal testing of trisomies 21 and 18 by massively parallel sequencing of maternal plasma DNA in twin pregnancies. *Prenatal Diagnosis, 34*(4), 335–340.

Jerry, J., & Oghalai, J. S. (2011). Towards an etiologic diagnosis: Assessing the patient with hearing loss. *Advances in Oto-Rhino-Laryngology, 70,* 28–36.

Joint Committee on Infant Hearing of the American Academy of Pediatrics, Muse, C., Harrison, J., et al. (2013). Supplement to the JCIH 2007 position statement: Principles and guidelines for early intervention after confirmation that a child is deaf or hard of hearing. *Pediatrics, 131*(4), e1324–e1349.

Katz, G., & Lazcano-Ponce, E. (2008). Intellectual disability: Definition, etiological factors, classification, diagnosis, treatment and prognosis. *Salud Publica de Mexico, 50*(2 suppl), S132–S141.

Kirchner, J. C., Harte, A., Heekeren, H. R., et al. (2011). Autistic symptomatology, face processing abilities, and eye fixation patterns. *Journal of Autism and Developmental Disorders, 41*(2), 158–167.

Kolevzon, A., Gross, R., & Reichenberg, A. (2007). Prenatal and perinatal risk factors for autism: A review and integration of findings. *Archives of Pediatrics and Adolescent Medicine, 161*(4), 326–333.

Krishnaswami, S., McPheeters, M. L., & Veenstra-Vanderweele, J. (2011). A systematic review of secretin for children with autism spectrum disorders. *Pediatrics, 127*(5), e1322–e1325.

Kuehn, B. M. (2011). Scientists find promising therapies for fragile X and Down syndromes. *Journal of the American Medical Association, 305*(4), 344–346.

Lai, M. C., Lombardo, M. V., & Baron-Cohen, S. (2014). Autism. *Lancet, 383*(9920), 896–910.

Lammers, M. J., Jansen, T. T., Grolman, W., et al. (2015). The influence of newborn hearing screening on the age at cochlear implantation in children. *Laryngoscope, 125*(4), 985–990.

Lantos, J. D. (2012). Ethics for the pediatrician: The evolving risk of cochlear implants in children. *Pediatrics in Review, 33*(7), 323–326.

Lemcke, S., Juul, S., Parner, E. T., et al. (2013). Early signs of autism in toddlers: A follow-up study in the Danish National Birth Cohort. *Journal of Autism and Developmental Disorders, 43*(10), 2366–2375.

Lewis, C., Hill, M., Silcock, C., et al. (2014). Non-invasive prenatal testing for trisomy 21: A cross-sectional survey of service users' views and likely uptake. *International Journal of Obstetrics and Gynaecology, 121*(5), 582–594.

Liao, G. J., Chan, K. C., Jiang, P., et al. (2012). Noninvasive prenatal diagnosis of fetal trisomy 21 by allelic ratio analysis using targeted massively parallel sequencing of maternal plasma DNA. *PLoS ONE, 7*(5), e38154.

Moran, M. (2013). DSM-5 provides new take on neurodevelopment disorders. *Psychiatric News, 48*(2), 6–23.

National Autism Association. (2015a). *Autism fact sheet.* Retrieved from http://nationalautismassociation.org/resources/autism-fact-sheet/.

National Autism Association. (2015b). *Signs of autism.* Retrieved from http://nationalautismassociation.org/resources/signs-of-autism/.

National Down Syndrome Society. (2012a). *Early intervention.* Retrieved from http://www.ndss.org/Resources/Therapies-Development/Early-Intervention/.

National Down Syndrome Society. (2012b). *Recreation and friendship.* Retrieved from http://www.ndss.org/Resources/Wellness/Recreation-Friendship/.

National Down Syndrome Society. (2012c). *What is Down syndrome?* Retrieved from http://www.ndss.org/Down-Syndrome/What-Is-Down-Syndrome/.

National Down Syndrome Society. (2012d). *Atlantoaxial instability and Down syndrome.* Retrieved from http://www.ndss.org/Resources/Health-Care/Associated-Conditions/Atlantoaxial-Instability-Down-Syndrome/.

National Down Syndrome Society. (2012e). *Down syndrome facts.* Retrieved from http://www.ndss.org/Down-Syndrome/Down-Syndrome-Facts/.

National Fragile X Foundation. (2012a). *Prevalence.* Retrieved from https://fragilex.org/fragile-x-associated-disorders/prevalence/.

National Fragile X Foundation. (2012b). *Genetic counselor.* Retrieved from https://fragilex.org/treatment-intervention/genetic-counselor/.

Oliver, C., & Richards, C. (2010). Self-injurious behavior in people with intellectual disability. *Current Opinion in Psychiatry, 23*(5), 412–416.

Oono, I. P., Honey, E. J., & McConachie, H. (2013). Parent-mediated early intervention for young children with autism spectrum disorders (ASD). *Cochrane Database of Systematic Reviews, 2013*(4), CD009774.

Palomaki, G. E., Kloza, E. M., Lambert-Messerlian, G. M., et al. (2011). DNA sequencing of maternal plasma to detect Down syndrome: An international clinical validation study. *Genetics in Medicine, 13*(11), 913–920.

Peterson, K., & Barbel, P. (2013). On alert for autism spectrum disorders. *Nursing*, *43*(4), 28–34.

Price, C. S., Thompson, W. W., Goodson, B., et al. (2010). Prenatal and infant exposure to thimerosal from vaccines and immunoglobulins and risk of autism. *Pediatrics*, *126*(4), 656–664.

Pueschel, S. M. (1999). The child with Down syndrome. In M. D. Levine, W. B. Carey, & A. C. Crocker (Eds.), *Developmental-behavioral pediatrics* (3rd ed.). Philadelphia, PA: Saunders.

Rahi, J. S., Cumberland, P. M., Peckham, C. S., et al. (2010). Improving detection of blindness in childhood: The British Childhood Vision Impairment study. *Pediatrics*, *126*(4), e895–e903.

Raviola, G., Gosselin, G. J., Walter, H. J., et al. (2011). Pervasive developmental disorders and childhood psychosis. In R. M. Kliegman, B. F. Stanton, J. W. St. Geme III, et al. (Eds.), *Nelson textbook of pediatrics* (18th ed.). Philadelphia, PA: Elsevier/Saunders.

Reichow, B., Barton, E. E., Boyd, B. A., et al. (2012). Early intensive behavioral intervention (EIBI) for young children with autism spectrum disorders (ASD). *Cochrane Database of Systematic Reviews*, *2012*(10), CD009260.

Rogers, G. L., & Jordan, C. O. (2013). Pediatric vision screening. *Pediatrics in Review*, *34*(3), 126–133.

Rossignol, D. A., & Frye, R. E. (2012). A review of research trends in physiological abnormalities in autism spectrum disorders: Immune dysregulation, inflammation, oxidative stress, mitochondrial dysfunction and environmental toxicant exposures. *Molecular Psychiatry*, *17*(4), 389–401.

Rutter, M. L. (2011). Progress in understanding autism: 2007-2010. *Journal of Autism and Developmental Disorders*, *41*(4), 395–404.

Serra, M. R., Biassoni, E. C., Hinalaf, M., et al. (2014). Hearing and loud music exposure in 14-15 years old adolescents. *Noise and Health*, *16*(72), 320–330.

Shapiro, B. K., & Batshaw, M. L. (2011). Intellectual disability. In R. M. Kliegman, B. F. Stanton, J. W. St. Geme III, et al. (Eds.), *Nelson textbook of pediatrics* (18th ed.). Philadelphia: Elsevier/Saunders.

Shea, S. E. (2012). Intellectual disability (mental retardation). *Pediatrics in Review*, *33*(3), 110–121.

Singh, V. (2015). Newborn hearing screening: Present scenario. *Indian Journal of Community Medicine*, *40*(1), 62–65.

Skinner, D., Choudhury, S., Sideris, S., et al. (2011). Parents' decisions to screen newborns for FMR1 gene expansions in a pilot research project. *Pediatrics*, *127*(6), e1455–e1463.

Solomon, M., Buaminger, N., & Rogers, S. J. (2011). Abstract reasoning and friendship in high functioning preadolescents with autism spectrum disorders. *Journal of Autism and Developmental Disorders*, *41*(1), 32–43.

Summar, K., & Lee, B. (2011). Cytogenetics: Down syndrome and other abnormalities of chromosome number. In R. M. Kliegman, B. F. Stanton, J. W. St. Geme III, et al. (Eds.), *Nelson textbook of pediatrics* (18th ed.). Philadelphia, PA: Elsevier/Saunders.

Talaat, H. S., Metwaly, M. A., Khafagy, A. H., et al. (2014). Dose passive smoking induce sensorineural hearing loss in children? *International Journal of Pediatric Otorhinolaryngology*, *78*(1), 46–49.

Talkowski, M. E., Minikel, E. V., & Gusella, J. F. (2014). Autism spectrum disorder genetics: Diverse genes with diverse clinical outcomes. *Harvard Review of Psychiatry*, *22*(2), 65–75.

Tassé, M. J., Luckasson, R., & Nygren, M. (2013). AAIDD proposed recommendations for ICD-11 and the condition previously known as mental retardation. *Intellectual and Developmental Disabilities*, *51*(2), 127–131.

Taylor, L. E., Swerdfeger, A. L., & Eslick, G. D. (2014). Vaccines are not associated with autism: An evidence-based meta-analysis of case-control and cohort studies. *Vaccine*, *32*(29), 3623–3629.

Uno, Y., Uchiyama, T., Kurosawa, M., et al. (2015). Early exposure to the combined measles-mumps-rubella vaccine and thimerosal-containing vaccines and risk of autism spectrum disorder. *Vaccine*, *33*(21), 2511–2516.

US Department of Health and Human Services, Office of Disease Prevention and Health Promotion. (2015). *Healthy People 2020: Vision*. Retrieved from http://www.healthypeople.gov/2020/topics-objectives/topic/vision.

US Preventive Services Task Force. (2011). Vision screening for children 1 to 5 years of age: US Preventive Services Task Force Recommendation statement. *Pediatrics*, *127*(2), 340–346.

Walker, W. O., & Johnson, C. P. (2006). Mental retardation: Overview and diagnosis. *Pediatrics in Review*, *27*(6), 204–212.

Wallander, J. L., Biasini, F. J., Thorsten, V., et al. (2014). Dose of early intervention treatment during children's first 36 months of life is associated with developmental outcomes: An observational cohort study in three low/low-middle income countries. *BMC Pediatrics*, *14*, 281.

Weijerman, M. E., & de Winter, J. P. (2010). Clinical practice: The care of children with Down syndrome. *European Journal of Pediatrics*, *169*(12), 1445–1452.

Williams, K. J., Wray, J. J., & Wheeler, D. M. (2012). Intravenous secretin for autism spectrum disorder (ASD). *Cochrane Database of Systematic Reviews*, *2012*(4), CD003495.

Willsey, A. J., & State, M. W. (2015). Autism spectrum disorders: From genes to neurobiology. *Current Opinion in Neurobiology*, *30*, 92–99.

Wodka, E. L., Mathy, P., & Kalb, L. (2013). Predictors of phrase and fluent speech in children with autism and severe language delay. *Pediatrics*, *131*(4), e1128–e1134.

World Health Organization. (2012). *Deafness and hearing loss*. Retrieved from http://www.who.int/mediacentre/factsheets/fs300/en/.

Wyckoff, A. S. (2011). *AAP updates guidance on caring for children with Down syndrome*. Retrieved from http://aapnews.aappublications.org/content/early/2011/07/25/aapnews.20110725-3.full?rss=1.

Yoder, P., Stone, W. L., Walden, T., et al. (2009). Predicting social impairment and ASD diagnosis in younger siblings of children with autism spectrum disorder. *Journal of Autism and Developmental Disorders*, *39*(10), 1381–1391.

Zwaigenbaum, L. (2010). Advances in the early detection of autism. *Current Opinion in Neurology*, *23*(2), 97–102.

38

Family-Centered Care of the Child During Illness and Hospitalization

Marilyn J. Hockenberry

ℯ http://evolve.elsevier.com/Perry/maternal

STRESSORS OF HOSPITALIZATION AND CHILDREN'S REACTIONS

Often, illness and hospitalization are the first crises children must face. Especially during the early years, children are particularly vulnerable to these stressors because (1) stress represents a change from the usual state of health and environmental routine and (2) children have a limited number of coping mechanisms to resolve stressors. Major stressors of hospitalization include separation, loss of control, bodily injury, and pain. Children's reactions to these crises are influenced by their developmental age; their previous experience with illness, separation, or hospitalization; their innate and acquired coping skills; the seriousness of the diagnosis; and the support system available. Children also expressed fears caused by the unfamiliar environment or lack of information; child-staff relations; and the physical, social, and symbolic environment (Samela, Salanterä, & Aronen, 2009).

SEPARATION ANXIETY

The major stress from middle infancy throughout the preschool years, especially for children 6 to 30 months of age, is separation anxiety, also called *anaclitic depression*. The principal behavioral responses to this stressor during early childhood are summarized in Box 38.1. During the stage of protest, children react aggressively to the separation from the parent. They cry and scream for their parents, refuse the attention of anyone else, and are inconsolable in their grief (Fig. 38.1). In contrast, through the stage of despair, the crying stops, and depression is evident. The child is much less active, is uninterested in play or food, and withdraws from others (Fig. 38.2).

The third stage is detachment, also called *denial*. Superficially, it appears that the child has finally adjusted to the loss. The child becomes more interested in the surroundings, plays with others, and seems to form new relationships. However, this behavior is the result of resignation and is not a sign of contentment. The child detaches from the parent in an effort to escape the emotional pain of desiring the parent's presence and copes by forming shallow relationships with others, becoming increasingly self-centered, and attaching primary importance to material objects. This is the most serious stage in that reversal of the potential adverse effects is less likely to occur after detachment is established. However, in most situations, the temporary separations imposed by hospitalization do not cause such prolonged parental absences that the child enters into detachment. In addition, considerable evidence suggests that even with stressors (e.g., separation), children are remarkably adaptable, and permanent ill effects are rare.

Although progression to the stage of detachment is uncommon, the initial stages are frequently observed even with brief separations from either parent. Unless health team members understand the meaning of each stage of behavior, they may erroneously label the behaviors as positive or negative. For example, they may see the loud crying of the protest phase as "bad" behavior. Because the protests increase when a stranger approaches the child, they may interpret that reaction as meaning they should stay away. During the quiet, withdrawn phase of despair, health team members may think that the child is finally "settling in" to the new surroundings, and they may see the detachment behaviors as proof of a "good adjustment." The faster this stage is reached, the more likely it is that the child will be regarded as the "ideal patient."

Because children seem to react "negatively" to visits by their parents, uninformed observers feel justified in restricting parental visiting privileges. For example, during the protest stage, children outwardly do not appear happy to see their parents (Fig. 38.3). In fact, they may even cry louder. If they are depressed, they may reject their parents or begin to protest again. Often they cling to their parents in an effort to ensure their continued presence. Consequently, such reactions may be regarded as "disturbing" the child's adjustment to the new surroundings. If the separation has progressed to the phase of detachment, children will respond no differently to their parents than they would to any other person.

Such reactions are distressing to parents, who are unaware of their meaning. If parents are regarded as intruders, they will see their absence as "beneficial" to the child's adjustment and recovery. They may respond to the child's behavior by staying for only short periods, visiting less frequently, or deceiving the child when it is time to leave. The result is a destructive cycle of misunderstanding and unmet needs.

Early Childhood

Separation anxiety is the greatest stress imposed by hospitalization during early childhood. If separation is avoided, young children have a tremendous capacity to withstand any other stress. During this age period, the typical reactions just described are seen. However, children in the toddler stage demonstrate more goal-directed behaviors. For example, they may plead with the parents to stay and physically try to keep the parents with them or try to find parents who have left. They may demonstrate displeasure on the parents' return or departure by having temper tantrums; refusing to comply with the usual routines of mealtime, bedtime, or toileting; or regressing to more primitive levels of development. However, temper tantrums, bed-wetting, or other behaviors may also be expressions of anger, a physiologic response to stress, or symptoms of illness.

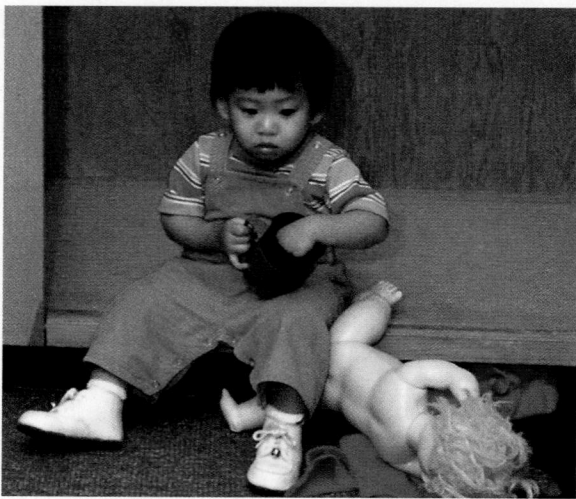

FIG 38.2 During the despair phase of separation anxiety, children are sad, lonely, and uninterested in food and play.

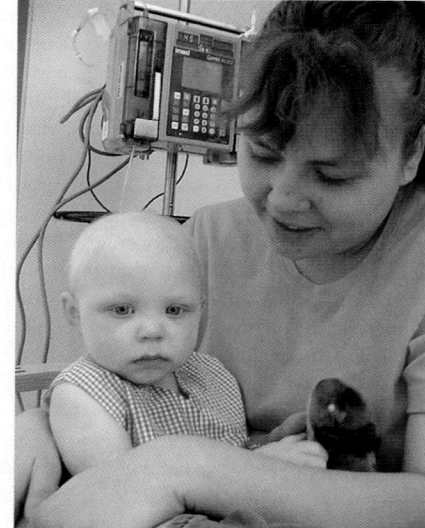

FIG 38.3 Young children may appear withdrawn and sad even in the presence of a parent. (Courtesy of E. Jacob, Texas Children's Hospital, Houston, TX.)

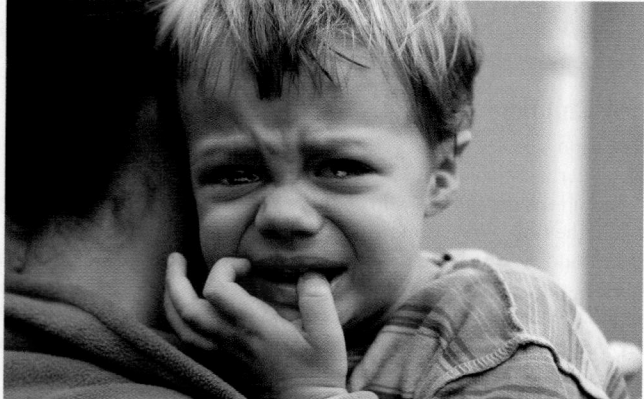

FIG 38.1 In the protest phase of separation anxiety, children cry loudly and are inconsolable in their grief for the parent. (Copyright 2015 iStock. com.)

Because preschoolers are more secure interpersonally than toddlers, they can tolerate brief periods of separation from their parents and are more inclined to develop substitute trust in other significant adults. However, the stress of illness usually renders preschoolers less able to cope with separation; as a result, they manifest many of the stage behaviors of separation anxiety, although in general, the protest behaviors are more subtle and passive than those seen in younger children. Preschoolers may demonstrate separation anxiety by refusing to eat, experiencing difficulty in sleeping, crying quietly for their parents, continually asking when the parents will visit, or withdrawing from others. They may express anger indirectly by breaking their toys, hitting other children, or refusing to cooperate during usual self-care activities. Nurses need to be sensitive to these less obvious signs of separation anxiety in order to intervene appropriately.

Later Childhood and Adolescence

Previous research, usually based on adult recollections, indicated that the family does not play as important a role for school-age children as it does during the toddler and preschool years. However, in a recent study that asked children about their fears when hospitalized, children listed their greatest fears regarding hospitalization as being separated from family and friends, being in an unfamiliar environment, receiving investigations or treatments, and losing self-determination or choices (Coyne, 2006). In a qualitative study of children 5 to 9 years of age, children described hospitalization in stories that focused on being alone and feeling scared, angry, or sad. These children also described the need for protection and companionship while hospitalized (Wilson, Megel, Enenbach, et al., 2010).

Although school-age children are better able to cope with separation in general, the stress and often accompanying regression imposed by illness or hospitalization may increase their need for parental security and guidance. This is particularly true for young school-age children who have only recently left the safety of the home and are struggling with the crisis of school adjustment. Middle and late school-age children may react more to the separation from their usual activities and peers than to the absence of their parents. These children have a high level of physical and mental activity that frequently finds no suitable outlets in the hospital environment, and even when they dislike school, they admit to missing its routine and worry that they will not be able to compete or "fit in" with their classmates when they return. Feelings of loneliness, boredom, isolation, and depression are common. Such reactions may occur more as a result of separation than of concern over the illness, treatment, or hospital setting.

School-age children may need and desire parental guidance or support from other adult figures but may be unable or unwilling to ask for it. Because the goal of attaining independence is so important to them, they are reluctant to seek help directly, fearing that they will appear weak, childish, or dependent. Cultural expectations to "act like a man" or to "be brave and strong" weigh heavily on these children, especially boys, who tend to react to stress with stoicism, withdrawal, or passive acceptance. Often the need to express hostile, angry, or other negative feelings finds outlets in alternate ways, such as irritability and aggression toward parents, withdrawal from hospital personnel, inability to relate to peers, rejection of siblings, or subsequent behavioral problems in school.

For adolescents, separation from home and parents may produce varied emotions, ranging from difficulty coping to welcoming the event. However, loss of peer-group contact may pose a severe emotional threat because of loss of group status, inability to exert group control or leadership, and loss of group acceptance. Deviations within peer groups are poorly tolerated, and although group members may express concern for the adolescent's illness or need for hospitalization, they continue their group activities, quickly filling the gap of the absent member. During the temporary separation from their usual group, ill adolescents may benefit from group associations with other hospitalized teens.

LOSS OF CONTROL

One of the factors influencing the amount of stress imposed by hospitalization is the amount of control that people perceive themselves as having. Lack of control increases the perception of threat and can affect children's coping skills. Many hospital situations decrease the amount of control a child feels. Although the usual sensory stimulations are lacking, the additional hospital stimuli of sight, sound, and smell may be overwhelming. Without an insight into the type of environment conducive to children's optimal growth, the hospital experience can at best temporarily slow development and at worst permanently restrict it. Because children's needs vary greatly depending on their age, the major areas of loss of control in terms of physical restriction, altered routine or rituals, and dependency are discussed for each age group.

EFFECTS OF HOSPITALIZATION ON THE CHILD

Children may react to the stresses of hospitalization before admission, during hospitalization, and after discharge. A child's concept of illness is even more important than age and intellectual maturity in predicting the level of anxiety before hospitalization (Clatworthy, Simon, & Tiedeman, 1999). This may or may not be affected by the duration of the condition or prior hospitalizations; therefore, nurses should avoid overestimating the illness concepts of children with prior medical experience (Box 38.2).

Individual Risk Factors

A number of risk factors make certain children more vulnerable than others to the stresses of hospitalization (Box 38.3). Rural children may exhibit significantly greater degrees of psychologic upset than urban children, possibly because urban children have opportunities to become familiar with a local hospital. Because separation is such an important issue surrounding hospitalization for young children, children who are active and strong-willed tend to fare better when hospitalized than those who are passive. Consequently, nurses should be alert to children

---

BOX 38.2   Post-Hospital Behaviors in Children

Young Children

They show initial aloofness toward parents; this may last from a few minutes (most common) to a few days.

This is frequently followed by dependency behaviors:
- Tendency to cling to parents
- Demands for parents' attention
- Vigorous opposition to any separation (e.g., staying at preschool or with a babysitter)

Other negative behaviors include the following:
- New fears (e.g., nightmares)
- Resistance to going to bed, night waking
- Withdrawal and shyness
- Hyperactivity
- Temper tantrums
- Food peculiarities
- Attachment to blanket or toy
- Regression in newly learned skills (e.g., self-toileting)

Older Children

Negative behaviors include the following:
- Emotional coldness followed by intense, demanding dependence on parents
- Anger toward parents
- Jealousy toward others (e.g., siblings)

BOX 38.3   Risk Factors That Increase Children's Vulnerability to the Stresses of Hospitalization

"Difficult" temperament

Lack of fit between child and parent

Age (especially between 6 months and 5 years of age)

Male gender

Below-average intelligence

Multiple and continuing stresses (e.g., frequent hospitalizations)

who passively accept all changes and requests; these children may need more support than "oppositional" children.

The stressors of hospitalization may cause young children to experience short- and long-term negative outcomes. Adverse outcomes may be related to the length and number of admissions, multiple invasive procedures, and the parents' anxiety. Common responses include regression, separation anxiety, apathy, fears, and sleeping disturbances, especially for children younger than 7 years of age (Melnyk, 2000). Supportive practices, such as family-centered care and frequent family visiting, may lessen the detrimental effects of such admissions. Nurses should attempt to identify children at risk for poor coping strategies (Small, 2002).

Changes in the Pediatric Population

The pediatric population in hospitals has changed dramatically over the past 2 decades. With a growing trend toward shortened hospital stays and outpatient surgery, a greater percentage of the children hospitalized today have more serious and complex problems than those hospitalized in the past. Many of these children are fragile newborns and children with severe injuries or disabilities who have survived because of major technologic advances, yet they have been left with chronic or disabling conditions that require frequent and lengthy hospital stays. The nature of their conditions increases the likelihood that they will experience more invasive and traumatic procedures while they are hospitalized. These factors make them more vulnerable to the emotional consequences of hospitalization and result in their needs being significantly different from those of the short-term patients of the past. The majority of these children are infants and toddlers, which is the age group most vulnerable to the effects of hospitalization.

Concern in recent years has focused on the increasing length of hospitalization because of complex medical and nursing care, elusive diagnoses, and complicated psychosocial issues. Without special attention devoted to meeting children's psychosocial and developmental needs in the hospital environment, the detrimental consequences of prolonged hospitalization may be severe.

Beneficial Effects of Hospitalization

Although hospitalization can be and usually is stressful for children, it can also be beneficial. The most obvious benefit is the recovery from illness, but hospitalization also can present an opportunity for children to master stress and feel competent in their coping abilities. The hospital environment can provide children with new socialization experiences that can broaden their interpersonal relationships. The psychologic benefits need to be considered and maximized during hospitalization. Appropriate nursing strategies to achieve this goal are presented later in this chapter.

STRESSORS AND REACTIONS OF THE FAMILY OF THE CHILD WHO IS HOSPITALIZED

PARENTAL REACTIONS

The crisis of childhood illness and hospitalization affects every member of the family. Parents' reactions to illness in their child depend on a variety of factors. Although one cannot predict which factors are most likely to influence their response, a number of variables have been identified (Box 38.4).

Recent research has identified common themes among parents whose children were hospitalized, including feeling an overall sense of helplessness, questioning the skills of staff, accepting the reality of hospitalization, needing to have information explained in simple language, dealing with fear, coping with uncertainty, and seeking reassurance from caregivers.

> **BOX 38.4   Factors Affecting Parents' Reactions to Their Child's Illness**
>
> Seriousness of the threat to the child
> Previous experience with illness or hospitalization
> Medical procedures involved in diagnosis and treatment
> Available support systems
> Personal ego strengths
> Previous coping abilities
> Additional stresses on the family system
> Cultural and religious beliefs
> Communication patterns among family members

Reassurance from the health care team can be in the form of collaboration, information sharing, preparation for procedures, ensuring formal and informal support for the family, and providing information in an unbiased and culturally sensitive manner (Eichner & Johnson, 2012).

SIBLING REACTIONS

Siblings' reactions to a sister's or brother's illness or hospitalization differ little when a child becomes temporarily ill. Siblings experience loneliness, fear, and worry, as well as anger, resentment, jealousy, and guilt. Illness may also result in children's loss of status within either their family or their social group. Various factors have been identified that influence the effects of the child's hospitalization on siblings. Recently, it has been found that parents of siblings of children with chronic illness tended to rate sibling health–related quality of life better than the siblings' self reports, and greater disease severity of affected child and older sibling age may be risk factors for impaired well-sibling quality of life (Limbers & Skipper, 2014). Although these factors are similar to those seen when a child has a chronic illness, Craft (1993) reported that the following factors regarding siblings are related specifically to the hospital experience and increase the effects on the sibling:

- Being younger and experiencing many changes
- Being cared for outside the home by care providers who are not relatives
- Receiving little information about their ill brother or sister
- Perceiving that their parents treat them differently compared with before their sibling's hospitalization

Parents are often unaware of the number of effects that siblings experience during the sick child's hospitalization and the benefit of simple interventions to minimize such effects, such as explicit explanations about the illness and provisions for the siblings to remain at home. Sibling visitation is usually beneficial to the patient, sibling, and parent but should be evaluated on an individual basis. Siblings should be prepared for the visit with developmentally appropriate information and be given the opportunity to ask questions.

NURSING CARE OF THE CHILD WHO IS HOSPITALIZED

PREPARATION FOR HOSPITALIZATION

Children and families require individualized care to minimize the potential negative effects of hospitalization. One method that can decrease negative feelings and fear in children is preparation for hospitalization. The rationale for preparing children for the hospital experience and related procedures is based on the principle that a fear of the unknown (fantasy) exceeds fear of the known. When children do not have paralyzing fear to cope with, they are able to direct their energies toward dealing with the other, unavoidable stresses of hospitalization.

Although preparation for hospitalization is a common practice, there is no universal standard or program for all settings. The preparation process may be elaborate with tours, puppet shows, and playtime with miniature hospital equipment; it may involve the use of books, videos, or films; or it may be limited to a brief description of the major aspects of any hospital stay. No consensus exists on the timing of preparation. Some authorities recommend preparing children 4 to 7 years of age about 1 week in advance so that they can assimilate the information and ask questions. For older children, the time may be longer. However, for young children, who may begin to fantasize about what they observed, 1 or 2 days before admission is sufficient time for anticipatory preparation. The length of the session should be tailored to the children's attention span—the younger the child, the shorter the program. The optimal approach is one that is individualized for each child and family.

Regardless of the specific type of program, all children, even those who have been hospitalized before, benefit from an introduction to the environment and routine of the unit. Sometimes it is not possible to prepare children and families for hospitalization, such as in the event of sudden, acute illness. However, care should be taken to orient the child and family to hospital routines, establish expectations, and allow for questions (Abraham & Moretz, 2012).

! NURSING ALERT

In many hospitals, child life specialists—health care professionals with extensive knowledge of child growth and development and of the special psychosocial needs of children who are hospitalized and their families—help prepare children for hospitalization, surgery, and procedures. Although the structure of a program may vary depending on the size of the pediatric facility, the patient population, and the availability of ancillary services, the two primary program objectives for child life are consistent: (1) to reduce the stress and anxiety related to the hospitalization or health care–related experiences and (2) to promote normal growth and development in the health care setting and at home (Thompson, 2009).

A collaborative effort between the nurse, child life specialist, and other members of the child's health care team helps ensure the best possible hospital experience for the child and family.

Admission Assessment

The nursing admission history refers to a systematic collection of data about the child and family that allows the nurse to plan individualized care. The nursing admission history presented in Box 38.5 is organized according to the Functional Health Patterns outlined by Gordon (2002) (see Nursing Diagnosis, Chapter 26. This assessment framework is a guideline for formulating nursing diagnoses. One of the main purposes of the history is to assess the child's usual health habits at home to promote a more normal environment in the hospital. Therefore, questions related to activities of daily living in the nutritional/metabolic, elimination, sleep/rest, and activity/exercise patterns are a major part of the assessment. The questions found under the health perception/health management pattern are directed toward evaluation of the child's preparation for hospitalization and are key factors in determining whether additional preparation is needed. The questions included in the self-perception/self-concept and role/relationship patterns offer insight into the child's potential reaction to hospitalization, especially in terms of separation.

The nurse should also inquire about the use of any medications at home, including complementary medicine practices (Box 38.6). In a study of children with cancer, 42% had used alternative or complementary

CLINICAL REASONING CASE STUDY
Complementary and Alternative Medicine

Maria, a 13-year-old Hispanic girl, has had severe nosebleeds. She is admitted to the hospital for a complete workup in an attempt to determine the cause. Her parents and grandparents have gathered around her bed. When you enter her room to begin admitting procedures, you notice an unusual scent. Maria's mother is rubbing the contents from an unfamiliar bottle of liquid on Maria. Meanwhile, the grandmother is rubbing Maria's head. She is startled at your entry and drops something on the floor near your feet. You bend over to pick it up and discover that it is a penny.

Questions
1. Evidence: Is there sufficient evidence to draw any conclusions?
2. Assumptions: What are some underlying assumptions that may be drawn from the data about the following:
   a. Complementary or alternative medical remedies
   b. The role of ethnic or folk remedies in modern health care practice
   c. The nurse's role in cases where alternative medicine is practiced (vs. traditional medicine)
3. What implications and priorities for nursing care can be drawn at this time?
4. Does the evidence objectively support your argument (conclusion)?

therapies simultaneously with or after conventional treatments (Fernandez, Pyesmany, & Stutzer, 1999). It is important that the use of any herbal or complementary therapy be noted in a preoperative assessment because of possible anesthesia or surgical complications related to herbal products (Flanagan, 2001) (see Clinical Reasoning Case Study box: Complementary and Alternative Medicine).

In addition to completing the nursing admission history, nurses should also perform a physical assessment before planning care. At the very least, the nurse's physical assessment of the child should include observation of the body for any bruises, rashes, signs of neglect, deformities, or physical limitations. The nurse should also listen to the heart and lungs to assess overall physical status. For example, it is impossible to evaluate improvement in respiratory function in a child admitted with pulmonary disease unless there are baseline data with which to compare subsequent findings.

Preparing the Child for Admission

The preparation that children require on the day of admission depends on the kind of prehospital counseling they have received. If they have been prepared in a formalized program, they usually know what to expect in terms of initial medical procedures, inpatient facilities, and nursing staff. However, prehospital counseling does not preclude the need for support during procedures, such as obtaining blood specimens, x-ray tests, or physical examination. For example, undressing young children before they feel comfortable in their new surroundings can be upsetting. Causing needless anxiety and fear during admission may adversely affect the nurse's establishment of trust with these children. Therefore, nursing assistance during the admission procedure is vital regardless of how well prepared any child is for the experience of hospitalization. In addition, spending this time with the child gives the nurse an opportunity to evaluate the child's understanding of subsequent procedures (Fig. 38.4). Ideally, a primary nurse is assigned whenever possible to allow for individualized care and to provide a substitute support person for the child.

When a child is admitted, nurses follow several fairly universal admission procedures (see Guidelines boxes: Hospital Admission and Special Hospital Admission). The minimum considerations for room

BOX 38.5 Nursing Admission History According to Functional Health Patterns*

Health Perception/Health Management Pattern

Why has your child been admitted?

How has your child's general health been?

What does your child know about this hospitalization?

- Ask the child why he or she came to the hospital.
- If the answer is "For an operation or for tests," ask the child to tell you about what will happen before, during, and after the operation or tests.

Has your child ever been in the hospital before?

- How was that hospital experience?
- What things were important to you and your child during that hospitalization? How can we be most helpful now?

What medications does your child take at home?

- Why are they given?
- When are they given?
- How are they given (if a liquid, with a spoon; if a tablet, swallowed with water; or other)?
- Does your child have any trouble taking medication? If so, what helps?
- Is your child allergic to any medications?

What, if any, forms of complementary medicine practices are being used?

Nutrition/Metabolic Pattern

What is the family's usual mealtime?

Do family members eat together or at separate times?

What are your child's favorite foods, beverages, and snacks?

- Average amounts consumed or usual size of portions
- Special cultural practices, such as family eats only ethnic food

What foods and beverages does your child dislike?

What are your child's feeding habits (bottle, cup, spoon, eats by self, needs assistance, any special devices)?

How does your child like the food served (warmed, cold, one item at a time)?

How would you describe your child's usual appetite (hearty eater, picky eater)?

- Has being sick affected your child's appetite? In what ways?

Are there any known or suspected food allergies?

Is your child on a special diet?

Are there any feeding problems (excessive fussiness, spitting up, colic); any dental or gum problems that affect feeding?

- What do you do for these problems?

Elimination Pattern

What are your child's toileting habits (diaper, toilet trained—day only or day and night, use of word to communicate urination or defecation, potty chair, regular toilet, other routines)?

What is your child's usual pattern of elimination (bowel movements)?

Do you have any concerns about elimination (bed-wetting, constipation, diarrhea)?

- What do you do for these problems?

Have you ever noticed that your child sweats a lot?

Sleep/Rest Pattern

What is your child's usual hour of sleep and awakening?

What is your child's schedule for naps; length of naps?

Is there a special routine before sleeping (bottle, drink of water, bedtime story, night light, favorite blanket or toy, prayers)?

Is there a special routine during sleep time, such as waking to go to the bathroom?

What type of bed does your child sleep in?

Does your child have a separate room or share a room; if shares, with whom?

Does your child sleep with someone or alone (e.g., sibling, parent, other person)?

What is your child's favorite sleeping position?

Are there any sleeping problems (falling asleep, waking during night, nightmares, sleep walking)?

Are there any problems in awakening and getting ready in the morning?

- What do you do for these problems?

Activity/Exercise Pattern

What is your child's schedule during the day (preschool, daycare center, regular school, extracurricular activities)?

What are your child's favorite activities or toys (both active and quiet interests)?

What is your child's usual television-viewing schedule at home?

What are your child's favorite programs?

Are there any television restrictions?

Does your child have any illness or disabilities that limit activity? If so, how?

What are your child's usual habits and schedule for bathing (bath in tub or shower, sponge bath, shampoo)?

What are your child's dental habits (brushing, flossing, fluoride supplements or rinses, favorite toothpaste); schedule of daily dental care?

Does your child need help with dressing or grooming, such as hair combing?

Are there any problems with these patterns (dislike of or refusal to bathe, shampoo hair, or brush teeth)?

- What do you do for these problems?

Are there special devices that your child requires help in managing (eyeglasses, contact lenses, hearing aid, orthodontic appliances, artificial elimination appliances, orthopedic devices)?

Note: Use the following code to assess functional self-care level for feeding, bathing and hygiene, dressing and grooming, toileting:

0: Full self-care

I: Requires use of equipment or device

II: Requires assistance or supervision from another person

III: Requires assistance or supervision from another person and equipment or device

IV: Is totally dependent and does not participate

Cognitive/Perceptual Pattern

Does your child have any hearing difficulty?

- Does the child use a hearing aid?
- Have "tubes" been placed in your child's ears?

Does your child have any vision problems?

- Does the child wear glasses or contact lenses?

Does your child have any learning difficulties?

What is the child's grade in school?

Self-Perception/Self-Concept Pattern

How would you describe your child (e.g., takes time to adjust, settles in easily, shy, friendly, quiet, talkative, serious, playful, stubborn, easygoing)?

What makes your child angry, annoyed, anxious, or sad? What helps?

How does your child act when annoyed or upset?

What have been your child's experiences with and reactions to temporary separation from you (parent)?

Does your child have any fears (places, objects, animals, people, situations)?

- How do you handle them?

Do you think your child's illness has changed the way he or she thinks about himself or herself (e.g., more shy, embarrassed about appearance, less competitive with friends, stays at home more)?

Role/Relationship Pattern

Does your child have a favorite nickname?

What are the names of other family members or others who live in the home (relatives, friends, pets)?

Who usually takes care of your child during the day and night (especially if other than parent, such as babysitter, relative)?

BOX 38.5   Nursing Admission History According to Functional Health Patterns*—cont'd

What are the parents' occupations and work schedules?

Are there any special family considerations (adoption, foster child, stepparent, divorce, single parent)?

Have any major changes in the family occurred lately (death, divorce, separation, birth of a sibling, loss of a job, financial strain, mother beginning a career, other)? Describe child's reaction.

Who are your child's play companions or social groups (peers, younger or older children, adults, or prefers to be alone)?

Do things generally go well for your child in school or with friends?

Does your child have "security" objects at home (pacifier, bottle, blanket, stuffed animal or doll)? Did you bring any of these to the hospital?

How do you handle discipline problems at home? Are these methods always effective?

Does your child have any condition that interferes with communication? If so, what are your suggestions for communicating with your child?

Will your child's hospitalization affect the family's financial support or care of other family members (e.g., other children)?

What concerns do you have about your child's illness and hospitalization?

Who will be staying with your child while hospitalized?

How can we contact you or another close family member outside of the hospital?

Sexuality/Reproductive Pattern

(Answer questions that apply to your child's age group.)

Has your child begun puberty (developing physical sexual characteristics, menstruation)? Have you or your child had any concerns?

Does your daughter know how to do breast self-examination?

Does your son know how to do testicular self-examination?

How have you approached topics of sexuality with your child?

Do you think you might need some help with some topics?

Has your child's illness affected the way he or she feels about being a boy or a girl? If so, how?

Do you have any concerns with behaviors in your child, such as masturbation, asking many questions or talking about sex, not respecting others' privacy, or wanting too much privacy?

Initiate a conversation about an adolescent's sexual concerns with open-ended to more direct questions and using the terms "friends" or "partners" rather than "girlfriend" or "boyfriend":

• Tell me about your social life.

• Who are your closest friends? (If one friend is identified, could ask more about that relationship, such as how much time they spend together, how serious they are about each other, if the relationship is going the way the teenager hoped.)

• Might ask about dating and sexual issues, such as the teenager's views on sexuality education, "going steady," "living together," or premarital sex.

• Which friends would you like to have visit in the hospital?

Coping/Stress Tolerance Pattern

(Answer questions that apply to your child's age group.)

What does your child do when tired or upset?

• If upset, does your child want a special person or object?

• If so, explain.

If your child has temper tantrums, what causes them, and how do you handle them?

Whom does your child talk to when worried about something?

How does your child usually handle problems or disappointments?

Have there been any big changes or problems in your family recently? If so, how have you handled them?

Has your child ever had a problem with drugs or alcohol or tried to commit suicide?

Do you think your child is "accident prone"? If so, explain.

Value/Belief Pattern

What is your religion?

How is religion or faith important in your child's life?

What religious practices would you like continued in the hospital (e.g., prayers before meals or bedtime; visit by minister, priest, or rabbi; prayer group)?

*The focus of the admission history is the child's psychosocial environment. Most of the questions are worded in terms of parental responses. Depending on the child's age, they should be addressed directly to the child when appropriate.

BOX 38.6   Complementary Medicine Practices and Examples

Nutrition, diet, and lifestyle or behavioral health changes: Macrobiotics, megavitamins, diets, lifestyle modification, health risk reduction and health education, wellness

Mind-body control therapies: Biofeedback, relaxation, prayer therapy, guided imagery, hypnotherapy, music or sound therapy, massage, aromatherapy, education therapy

Traditional and ethnomedicine therapies: Acupuncture, ayurvedic medicine, herbal medicine, homeopathic medicine, American Indian medicine, natural products, traditional Asian medicine

Structural manipulation and energetic therapies: Acupressure, chiropractic medicine, massage, reflexology, rolfing, therapeutic touch, Qi Gong

Pharmacologic and biologic therapies: Antioxidants, cell treatment, chelation therapy, metabolic therapy, oxidizing agents

Bioelectromagnetic therapies: Diagnostic and therapeutic application of electromagnetic fields (e.g., transcranial electrostimulation, neuromagnetic stimulation, electroacupuncture)

assignment are age, sex, and nature of the illness. No absolute rules govern room selection, but in general, placing children of the same age group and with similar types of illness in the same room is both psychologically and medically advantageous. However, there are many exceptions. For example, a child in traction may be therapeutic for another child confined to bed because of a serious illness. A child who is independent despite physical disabilities may help another child with similar or different limitations, and the parents of the child with disabilities may achieve deeper insight and acceptance of their child's disorder.

Age grouping is especially important for adolescents. Many hospitals make an effort to place teenagers on their own unit or in a separate designated section of the pediatric or general unit whenever possible.

NURSING INTERVENTIONS

Preventing or Minimizing Separation

A primary nursing goal is to prevent separation, particularly in children younger than 5 years of age. Many hospitals have developed a system of family-centered care. This philosophy of care recognizes the integral role of the family in a child's life and acknowledges the family as an essential part of the child's care and illness experience. The family is

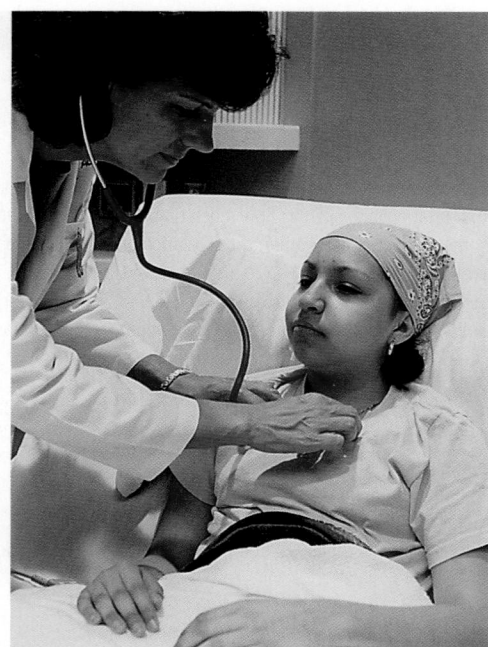

FIG 38.4 The initial admission procedures give the nurse an opportunity to get to know the child and to assess the child's understanding of the hospital experience.

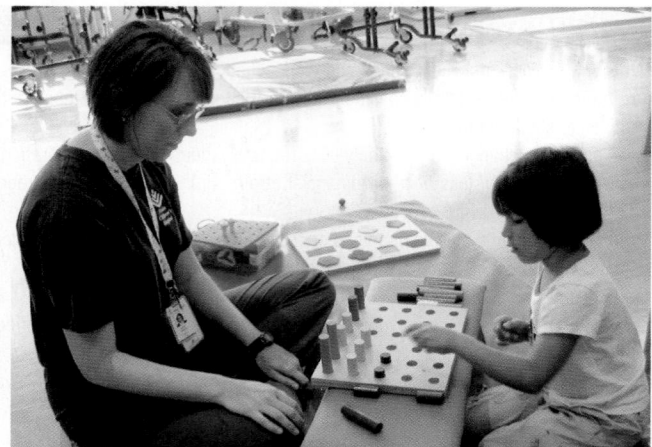

FIG 38.5 For extended hospitalizations, children enjoy doing projects to occupy time.

considered to be partners in the care of the child (Smith & Conant Rees, 2000). Family-centered care also supports the family by establishing priorities based on the needs and values of the family unit (Lewandowski & Tesler, 2003). Efforts to collaborate with families and encourage their involvement in the patient's care include optimizing family visitation, family-centered rounding, family presence during procedures or interventions, and opportunities for formal and informal family conferences (Meert, Clark, & Eggly, 2013). Historically hospitals have had restrictive visiting policies. Family-centered care started in pediatrics with the increased recognition of child and family separation trauma in the inpatient setting. Policies were adapted first in pediatrics to allow for rooming-in, longer visiting hours, sibling visits, and systems to allow families to accompany patients off the unit for procedures (Institute for Patient- and Family-Centered Care, 2010a, 2010b).

At the very least, most hospitals welcome parents at any time. Many provide facilities such as a chair or bed for at least one person per child, unit kitchen privileges, and other amenities that create a welcoming atmosphere for parents. However, not all hospitals provide such amenities, and parents' own schedules may prevent rooming-in. In such instances, strategies to minimize the effects of separation must be implemented.

Nurses must have an appreciation of the child's separation behaviors. As discussed earlier, the phases of protest and despair are normal. The child is allowed to cry. Even if the child rejects strangers, the nurse provides support through physical presence. *Presence* is defined as spending time being physically close to the child while using a quiet tone of voice, appropriate choice of words, eye contact, and touch in ways that establish rapport and communicate empathy. If behaviors of detachment are evident, the nurse maintains the child's contact with the parents by frequently talking about them; encouraging the child to remember them; and stressing the significance of their visits, telephone calls, or letters. The use of cellular phones can increase the contact between the hospitalized child and parents or other significant family members and friends. However, wireless technology devices may not be compatible with medical equipment, and use may be restricted in certain areas within the hospital.

Parental Absence During Infant Hospitalization

Familiar surroundings also increase the child's adjustment to separation. If the parents cannot stay with the child, they should leave favorite articles from home with the child, such as a blanket, toy, bottle, feeding utensil, or article of clothing. Because young children associate such inanimate objects with significant people, they gain comfort and reassurance from these possessions. They make the association that if the parents left this, the parents will surely return. Placing an identification band on the toy lessens the chances of its being misplaced and provides a symbol that the toy is experiencing the same needs as the child. Other reminders of home include photographs and recordings of family members reading a story, singing a song, saying prayers before bedtime, relating events at home, or taking a "talking walk" through the home. These reminders can be played at lonely times, such as on awakening or before sleeping. Some units allow pets to visit, which can have therapeutic benefits for a child. Older children also appreciate familiar articles from home, particularly photographs, a radio, a favorite toy or game, and their own pajamas. Often the importance of treasured objects to school-age children is overlooked or criticized. However, many school-age children have a special object to which they formed an attachment in early childhood. Therefore, such treasured or transitional objects can help even older children feel more comfortable in a strange environment.

The strange sights, smells, and sounds in the hospital that are commonplace for the nurse can be frightening and confusing for children. It is important for the nurse to try to evaluate stimuli in the environment from the child's point of view (considering also what the child may see or hear happening to other patients) and to make every effort to protect the child from frightening and unfamiliar sights, sounds, and equipment. The nurse should offer explanations or prepare the child for experiences that are unavoidable. Combining familiar or comforting sights with the unfamiliar can relieve much of the harshness of medical equipment.

Helping children maintain their usual contacts also minimizes the effects of separation imposed by hospitalization. This includes continuing school lessons during the illness and confinement, visiting with friends either directly or through letter writing or telephone calls, and participating in stimulating projects whenever possible (Fig. 38.5). For extended hospitalizations, youngsters enjoy personalizing the hospital room to make it "home" by decorating the walls with posters and cards, rearranging the furniture, and displaying a collection or hobby.

Minimizing Loss of Control

Feelings of loss of control result from separation, physical restriction, changed routines, enforced dependency, and magical thinking. Although

GUIDELINES

Hospital Admission

Preadmission

Assign a room based on developmental age, seriousness of diagnosis, communicability of illness, and projected length of stay.

Prepare roommate(s) for the arrival of a new patient; when children are too young to benefit from this consideration, prepare parents.

Prepare room for child and family, with admission forms and equipment nearby to eliminate need to leave child.

Admission

Introduce primary nurse to child and family.

Orient child and family to inpatient facilities, especially to assigned room and unit; emphasize positive areas of pediatric unit.

Room: Explain call light, bed controls, television, bathroom, telephone, and so on.

Unit: Direct to playroom, desk, dining area, or other areas.

Introduce family to roommate and his or her parents.

Apply identification band to child's wrist, ankle, or both (if not already done).

Explain hospital regulations and schedules (e.g., visiting hours, mealtimes, bedtime, limitations [give written information if available]).

Perform nursing admission history (see Box 38.5).

Take vital signs, blood pressure, height, and weight.

Obtain specimens as needed, and order needed laboratory work.

Support child and assist practitioner with physical examination (for purposes of nursing assessment).

GUIDELINES

Special Hospital Admission

Emergency Admission

Lengthy preparatory admission procedures are often impossible and inappropriate for emergency situations.

Focus assessment on airway, breathing, and circulation; weigh child whenever possible for calculation of drug dosages.

Unless an emergency is life-threatening, children need to participate in their care to maintain a sense of control.

Focus on essential components of admission counseling, including the following:
- Appropriate introduction to the family
- Use of child's name, not terms such as "honey" or "dear"
- Determination of child's age and some judgment about developmental age (If the child is of school age, asking about the grade level will offer some evidence of intellectual ability.)
- Information about child's general state of health, any problems that may interfere with medical treatment (e.g., allergies), and previous experience with hospital facilities
- Information about the chief complaint from both the parents and the child

Admission to Intensive Care Unit

Prepare child and parents for elective intensive care unit (ICU) admission, such as for postoperative care after cardiac surgery.

Prepare child and parents for unanticipated ICU admission by focusing primarily on the sensory aspects of the experience and on usual family concerns (e.g., people in charge of child's care, schedule for visiting, area where family can stay).

Prepare parents regarding child's appearance and behavior when they first visit child in ICU.

Accompany family to bedside to provide emotional support and answer questions.

Prepare siblings for their visit; plan length of time for sibling visitation; monitor siblings' reactions during visit to prevent them from becoming overwhelmed.

Encourage parents to stay with their child:
- If visiting hours are limited, allow flexibility in schedule to accommodate parental needs.
- Give family members a written schedule of visiting times.
- If visiting hours are liberal, be aware of family members' needs and suggest periodic respites.
- Assure family they can call the unit at any time.

Prepare parents for expected role changes, and identify ways for parents to participate in child's care without overwhelming them with responsibilities:
- Help with bath or feeding.
- Touch and talk to child.
- Help with procedures.

Provide information about child's condition in understandable language:
- Repeat information often.
- Seek clarification of understanding.
- During bedside conferences, interpret information for family members and child or, if appropriate, conduct report outside room.

Prepare child for procedures even if it involves explanation while procedure is performed.

Assess and manage pain; recognize that a child who cannot talk, such as an infant or child in a coma or on mechanical ventilation, can be in pain.

Establish a routine that maintains some similarity to daily events in child's life whenever possible:
- Organize care during normal waking hours.
- Keep regular bedtime schedules, including quiet times when television or radio is lowered or turned off.
- Provide uninterrupted sleep cycles (60 minutes for infants; 90 minutes for older children).
- Close and open drapes and dim lights to allow for day and night.
- Place curtain around bed for privacy.
- Orient child to day and time; have clocks or calendars in easy view for older children.

Schedule a time when child is left undisturbed (e.g., during naps, visit with family, playtime, or favorite program).

Provide opportunities for play.

Reduce stimulation in the environment:
- Refrain from loud talking or laughing.
- Keep equipment noise to a minimum.
- Turn alarms as low as safely possible.
- Perform treatments requiring equipment at one time.
- Turn off bedside equipment that is not in use, such as suction and oxygen.
- Avoid loud, abrupt noises.

some of these cannot be prevented, most can be minimized through individualized planning of nursing care.

Promoting Freedom of Movement

Younger children react most strenuously to any type of physical restriction or immobilization. Although temporary immobilization may be necessary for some interventions such as maintaining an intravenous line, most physical restriction can be prevented if the nurse gains the child's cooperation.

For young children, particularly infants and toddlers, preserving parent-child contact is the best means of decreasing the need for or stress of restraint. For example, almost the entire physical examination can be done in a parent's lap with the parent hugging the child for procedures, such as an otoscopic examination. For painful procedures, the nurse should assess the parents' preferences for assisting, observing, or waiting outside the room.

Environmental factors may also restrict movement. Keeping children in cribs or play yards may not represent immobilization in a concrete sense, but it certainly limits sensory stimulation. Increasing mobility by transporting children in carriages, wheelchairs, carts, or wagons provides them with a sense of freedom.

In some cases, physical restraint or isolation is necessary because of the child's medical diagnosis. In these cases, the environment can be altered to increase sensory freedom (e.g., moving the bed toward the window; opening window shades; providing musical, visual, or tactile activities).

Maintaining the Child's Routine

Altered daily schedules and loss of rituals are particularly stressful for toddlers and early preschoolers and may increase the stress of separation. The nursing admission history provides a baseline for planning care around the child's usual home activities. A frequently neglected aspect of altered routines is the change in the child's daily activities. A typical child's day, especially during the school years, is structured with specific times for eating, dressing, going to school, playing, and sleeping. However, this time structure vanishes when the child is hospitalized. Although nurses have a set schedule, the child is frequently unaware of it, and the new schedules that are imposed may be rigid. For example, some units have uniform nap times and bedtimes for all children, but others allow children to stay up late at night. Many children obtain significantly less sleep in the hospital than at home; the primary causes are a delay in sleep onset and early termination of sleep because of hospital routines. Not only are hours of sleep disrupted, but waking hours are spent in passive activities. For example, few institutions impose any limits on the amount of time the child spends watching television. This may lead to children's being less "tired" at bedtime and delay the onset of sleep.

One technique that can minimize the disruption in the child's routine is establishing a daily schedule. This approach is most suitable for non–critically ill school-age and adolescent children who have mastered the concept of time. It involves scheduling the child's day to include all those activities that are important to the child and nurse, such as treatment procedures, schoolwork, exercise, television, playroom, and hobbies. Together, the nurse, parent, and child then plan a daily schedule with times and activities written down (Fig. 38.6). This is left in the child's room, and a clock or watch is available for the child's use. Whenever possible, a calendar is also constructed with special events marked, such as favorite television programs, visits by friends or relatives, events in the playroom, and holidays or birthdays. If specific changes in treatment are expected (e.g., "beginning physical therapy in 2 days"), these are added.

Eric's Daily Schedule

7:30 AM – Breakfast, morning bath	3:00 PM – Tutor (M, W, F)
	– Study time (T, Th)
9:00 – Medications, dressing change	4:00 – Physical therapy
	5:30 – Dinner
11:00 – Physical therapy	9:00 – Medications, dressing change
12:00 PM – Lunch	9:15 – Bedtime

FIG 38.6 Time structuring is an effective strategy for normalizing the hospital environment and increasing the child's sense of control.

! NURSING ALERT

Ask the young child to select or draw pictures or symbols to represent daily or weekly fun activities (e.g., favorite television programs, family visits, and playroom times). Draw a clock face with the hands of the clock depicting the time each event will occur next to the child's representation. Have the child compare the clock on the schedule with a clock or watch in the room. When the two match, the child knows it is time for a favorite activity.

Encouraging Independence

The dependent role of the hospitalized patient imposes tremendous feelings of loss on older children. Principal interventions should focus on respect for individuality and the opportunity for decision making. Although these sound simple, their efficacy lies with nurses who are flexible and tolerant. It is also important for the nurse to empower the patient while not feeling threatened by a sense of lessened control.

Enabling children's control involves helping them maintain independence and promoting the concept of self-care. *Self-care* refers to the practice of activities that individuals personally initiate and perform on their own behalf in maintaining life, health, and well-being (Orem, 2001). Although self-care is limited by the child's age and physical condition, most children beyond infancy can perform some activities with little or no help. Whenever possible, these activities are encouraged in the hospital. Other approaches include jointly planning care, time structuring, wearing street clothes, making choices in food selections and bedtime, continuing school activities, and rooming with an appropriate age mate.

Promoting Understanding

Loss of control can occur from feelings of having too little influence on one's destiny or from sensing overwhelming control or power over fate. Although preschoolers' cognitive abilities predispose them most to magical thinking and delusions of power, all children are vulnerable to misinterpreting causes for stresses, such as illness and hospitalization.

Most children feel more in control when they know what to expect because the element of fear is reduced. Anticipatory preparation and provision of information help to lessen stress and increase understanding (see the "Preparation for Diagnostic and Therapeutic Procedures" section in Chapter 39).

Informing children of their rights while hospitalized fosters greater understanding and may relieve some of the feelings of powerlessness they typically experience. An increasing number of hospitals and organizations have developed a patient "bill of rights" that is prominently displayed throughout the hospital or is presented to children and their families on admission (Box 38.7).

Preventing or Minimizing Fear of Bodily Injury

Beyond early infancy, all children fear bodily injury from mutilation, bodily intrusion, body image change, disability, or death. In general, preparation of children for painful procedures decreases their fears and increases cooperation. Modifying procedural techniques for children in each age group also minimizes fear of bodily injury. For example, because toddlers and young preschoolers are traumatized by insertion of a rectal thermometer, axillary temperatures or temperatures taken with electronic or tympanic membrane devices can effectively be substituted. Whenever procedures are performed on young children, the most supportive intervention is to do the procedure as quickly as possible while maintaining parent-child contact.

Because of toddlers' and preschool children's poorly defined body boundaries, the use of bandages may be particularly helpful. For example, telling children that the bleeding will stop after the needle is removed does little to relieve their fears, but applying a small Band-Aid usually reassures them. The size of bandages is also significant to children in this age group; the larger the bandage, the more importance is attached to the wound. Watching their surgical dressings become successively smaller is one way young children can measure healing and improvement. Prematurely removing a dressing may cause these children considerable concern for their well-being.

For children who fear mutilation of body parts, it is essential that the nurse repeatedly stress the reason for a procedure and evaluate the child's understanding. For example, explaining cast removal to preschoolers may seem simple enough, but children's comprehension of the details may vary considerably from the explanation. Asking children to draw a picture of what they foresee happening presents substantial evidence of how they perceive events.

Children may fear bodily injury from a great variety of sources. Imaging machines, strange equipment used for examination, unfamiliar rooms, and awkward positions can be perceived as potentially hazardous. In addition, thoughts and actions can be imagined sources of bodily damage. Therefore, it is important to investigate imagined reasons, particularly of a sexual nature, for illness. Because children may fear revealing such thoughts, using techniques such as drawing or doll play may elicit previously undisclosed misconceptions.

Older children fear bodily injury of both internal and external origins. For example, school-age children are aware of the significance of the heart and may fear the actual operation as much as the pain, the stitches, and the possible scar. Adolescents may express concern about the actual procedure but be much more anxious over the resulting scar.

Children can grasp information only if it is presented on or close to their level of cognitive development. This necessitates an awareness of the words used to describe events or processes. For example, young children told that they are going to have a CAT (i.e., CT, computed tomography) scan may wonder, "Will there be cats or something that scratches?" It is clearer to describe the procedure in simple terms and explain what the letters of the common name stand for. Therefore, to prevent or alleviate fears, nurses must be keenly aware of the medical terminology and vocabulary that they use every day.

When children are upset about their illness, their perception can be changed by (1) providing a somewhat different and less negative account of the disease or (2) offering an explanation that is characteristic of the next stage of cognitive development. An example of the first strategy is reassuring a preschooler who fears that after a tonsillectomy, another sore throat means a second operation. Explaining that after tonsils are "fixed" they do not need fixing again can help relieve the fear. An example of the latter strategy is to explain that germs made the tonsils sick and even though germs can cause another sore throat, they cannot cause the tonsils to ever be sick again. This higher-level explanation is based on the school-age child's concept of germs as a cause of disease.

Providing Developmentally Appropriate Activities

A primary goal of nursing care for the child who is hospitalized is to minimize threats to the child's development. Many strategies (e.g., minimizing separation) have been discussed and may be all that the short-term patient requires. However, children who experience prolonged or repeated hospitalization are at greater risk for developmental delays or regression. The nurse who provides opportunities for the child to participate in developmentally appropriate activities further normalizes the child's environment and helps reduce interference with the child's ongoing development.

Interference with normal development may have long-term implications for developing infants and toddlers. The nurse plays a primary role in identifying children at risk and helping to plan, implement, and evaluate developmental intervention.

School is an integral part of the school-age child's and adolescent's development. Accreditation standards for hospitals serving children consider access to appropriate educational services a key factor in the accreditation decision process when a child's treatment requires a significant absence from school (The Joint Commission, 2011). The nurse can encourage children to resume schoolwork as quickly as their condition permits, help them schedule and protect a selected time for studies, and help the family coordinate hospital educational services with their children's schools. Children should have the opportunity to continue art and music classes, as well as their academic subjects.

To meet the unique developmental needs of adolescents, special units may be developed that provide privacy, increased socialization, and appropriate activities for these young people. Typically, these units can be set apart from the general pediatric facility so that the teenagers do not share space with younger children, who are often perceived as a threat to their maturity.

In caring for adolescent patients, it is essential to provide flexible routines and activities, such as more group activity, wearing of street clothes, and access to the items so critical to adolescents—wireless technology devices, MP3 players, DVD players, computers, email, electronic video game systems, and high-definition televisions. Because adolescents' food habits are rarely limited to the three traditional meals a day, a ready supply of snacks should be available. However, the most important benefit of these units is increased socialization with peers. In addition, staff members usually enjoy working with this age group and are able to establish the trust that is so essential for communication.

BOX 38.8 Functions of Play in the Hospital

Provides diversion and brings about relaxation
Helps the child feel more secure in a strange environment
Lessens the stress of separation and the feeling of homesickness
Provides a means for release of tension and expression of feelings
Encourages interaction and development of positive attitudes toward others
Provides an expressive outlet for creative ideas and interests
Provides a means for accomplishing therapeutic goals
Places the child in active role and provides opportunity to make choices and be in control

---

! NURSING ALERT

When adolescents must share a common activity room with younger patients, referring to the area as the "activity room" rather than the "playroom" may entice them to visit the room and participate in activities.

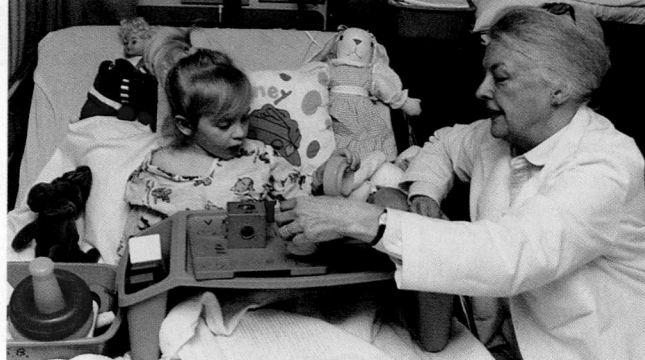

FIG 38.7 Play materials for children in the hospital need to be appropriate for their age, interests, and limitations.

Although regression is expected and normal for all age groups, nurses have the responsibility for fostering the child's growth and development. Hospitalization can become a significant opportunity for learning and advancing. Extended hospitalizations for long-term chronic illness or situations of failure to thrive, abuse, or neglect represent instances in which regression must be seen as an adjustment period to be followed by plans for promoting appropriate developmental skills.

Providing Opportunities for Play and Expressive Activities

Play is one of the most important aspects of a child's life and one of the most effective tools for managing stress. Because illness and hospitalization constitute crises in a child's life and often involve overwhelming stresses, children need to act out their fears and anxieties as a means of coping with these stresses. Play is essential to children's mental, emotional, and social well-being; however, play does not stop when children are ill or in the hospital. On the contrary, play in the hospital serves many functions (Box 38.8). Of all hospital facilities, no room probably alleviates the stressors of hospitalization more than the playroom (or activity room). In the playroom, children temporarily distance themselves from their illness, hospitalization, and the associated stressors. This room should be a safe haven for children, free from medical or nursing procedures (including medication administration), strange faces, and probing questions. The playroom then becomes a sanctuary in an otherwise frightening environment.

Engaging in play activities gives children a sense of control. In the hospital environment, most decisions are made for the child; play and other expressive activities offer the child much-needed opportunities to make choices for themselves. Even if a child chooses not to participate in a particular activity, the nurse has offered the child a choice, perhaps one of only a few real choices the child has had that day.

Hospitalized children typically have lower energy levels than healthy children of the same age. Therefore, children may not appear engaged and enthusiastic about an activity even though they are enjoying the experience. Activities may need to be adjusted or limited based on the child's age, endurance, and any special needs.

Diversional Activities

Almost any form of play can be used for diversion and recreation, but the activity should be selected on the basis of the child's age, interests, and limitations (Fig. 38.7). Children do not necessarily need special direction for using play materials. All they require is the raw materials with which to work and adult approval and supervision to help keep their natural enthusiasm or expression of feelings from getting out of control. Small children enjoy a variety of small, colorful toys that they can play with in bed or in their room or more elaborate play equipment, such as playhouses, sandboxes, rhythm instruments, or large boxes and blocks that may be a part of the hospital playroom.

Games that can be played alone or with another child or an adult are popular with older children, as are puzzles; reading material; quiet, individual activities, such as sewing, stringing beads, and weaving; and Lego blocks and other building materials. Assembling models is an excellent pastime, but one should make certain that all pieces and necessary materials are included in the package so that the child is not disappointed and frustrated.

Well-selected books are of infinite value to children. Children never tire of stories; having someone read aloud gives them endless hours of pleasure and is of special value to children who have limited energy to expend in play. A radio, DVD player, electronic games, and television, included among most hospital room equipment, are useful tools for entertaining children. Computers with access to the Internet can provide diversion, educational opportunities, and online support groups.

When supervising play for ill or convalescent children, it is best to select activities that are simpler than would normally be chosen for the child's specific developmental level. These children usually do not have the energy to cope with more challenging activities. Other limitations also influence the type of activities. Special consideration must be given to children who are confined in terms of movement, have a restricted extremity, or are isolated. Toys for isolated children must be disposable or need to be disinfected after every use.

Toys

Parents of hospitalized children often ask nurses about the types of toys that would be best to bring for their child. Although parents often want to buy new toys for the hospitalized child to offer cheer and comfort, it is often better to wait to bring new things, especially in the case of younger children. Small children need the comfort and reassurance of familiar things, such as the stuffed animal the child hugs for comfort and takes to bed at night. These familiar items are a link with home and the world outside the hospital. All toys brought into the hospital should be assessed for safety.

Large numbers of toys often confuse and frustrate small children. A few small, well-chosen toys are usually preferred to one large, expensive one. Children who are hospitalized for an extended time benefit from changes. Rather than a confusing accumulation of toys, older toys should be replaced periodically as interest wanes.

A highly successful diversion for a child who is hospitalized for a length of time and whose parents are unable to visit frequently is having the parents bring a box with several small, inexpensive, brightly wrapped items with a different day of the week printed on the outside of each package. The child will eagerly anticipate the time for opening each one. If the parents know when their next visit will be, they can provide the number of packages that corresponds to the time between visits. In this way, the child knows that the diminishing packages also represent the anticipated visit from the parent.

Expressive Activities

Play and other expressive activities provide one of the best opportunities for encouraging emotional expression, including the safe release of anger and hostility. Nondirective play that allows children freedom for expression can be tremendously therapeutic. Therapeutic play, however, should not be confused with play therapy, a psychologic technique reserved for use by trained and qualified therapists as an interpretative method with emotionally disturbed children. Therapeutic play, on the other hand, is an effective, nondirective modality for helping children deal with their concerns and fears, and at the same time, it often helps the nurse gain insights into children's needs and feelings.

Tension release can be facilitated through almost any activity; with younger ambulatory children, large-muscle activity such as use of tricycles and wagons is especially beneficial. Much aggression can be safely directed into pounding and throwing games or activities. Beanbags are often thrown at a target or open receptacle with surprising vigor and hostility. A pounding board is used with enthusiasm by young children; clay and play dough are beneficial for use at any age.

Creative Expression

Although all children derive physical, social, emotional, and cognitive benefits from engaging in art and other creative activities, children's need for such activities is intensified when they are hospitalized. Drawing and painting are excellent media for expression. Children are more at ease expressing their thoughts and feelings through art because humans think first in images and later learn to translate these images into words. Children need only to be supplied with the raw materials, such as crayons and paper, large brushes and an ample supply of newsprint supported on easels, or materials for finger painting (Fig. 38.8). Children can work individually or work together on a group project, such as a mural painted on a long piece of paper.

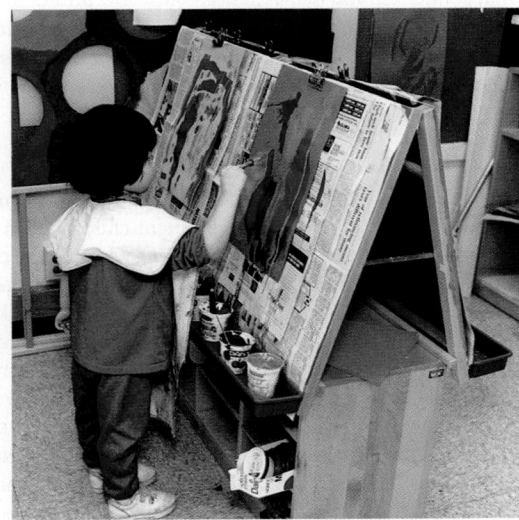

FIG 38.8 Drawing and painting are excellent media for expression.

Although interpretation of children's drawings requires special training, observing changes in a series of the child's drawings over time can be helpful in assessing psychosocial adjustment and coping. The nurse can use children's drawings, stories, poetry, and other products of creative expression as a springboard for discussion of thoughts, fears, and understanding of concepts or events. A child's drawing before surgery, for example, may reveal unvoiced concerns about mutilation, body changes, and loss of self-control.

Nurses can incorporate opportunities for musical expression into routine nursing care. For example, simple musical instruments, such as bracelets with bells, can be placed on infants' legs for them to shake to accompany mealtime music or dressing changes. Dance and movement suggestions may encourage a child to ambulate.

Holidays provide stimulus and direction for unlimited creative projects. Children can participate in decorating the pediatric unit; making pictures and decorations for their rooms gives the children a sense of pride and accomplishment. This is especially beneficial for children who are immobilized and isolated. Making gifts for someone at home helps to maintain interpersonal ties.

Dramatic Play

Dramatic play is a well-recognized technique for emotional release, allowing children to reenact frightening or puzzling hospital experiences. Through use of puppets, replicas of hospital equipment, or some actual hospital equipment, children can act out the situations that are a part of their hospital experience. Dramatic play enables children to learn about procedures and events that concern them and to assume the roles of the adults in the hospital environment.

Puppets are universally effective for communicating with children. Most children see them as peers and readily communicate with them. Children will tell the puppet feelings that they hesitate to express to adults. Puppets can share children's own experiences and help them to find solutions to their problems. Puppets dressed to represent figures in the child's environment—for example, a physician, nurse, child patient, therapist, and members of the child's own family—are especially useful. Small, appropriately attired dolls are equally effective in encouraging the child to play out situations, although puppets are usually best for direct conversation.

Play must consider medical needs, but at times, a procedure can be postponed briefly to allow the child to complete a special activity (see Clinical Reasoning Case Study box: Playroom and Hospital Procedures). Play must consider any limitations imposed by the child's condition. For example, small children may eat paste and other creative media; therefore, a child who is allergic to wheat should not be given finger paint made from wallpaper paste or modeling dough made with flour. A child on a restricted salt intake should not play with modeling dough because salt is one of its major constituents. At home, the play program can be planned around the therapy regimen. However, play can be satisfactorily incorporated into the child's care if the nurse and others involved allow some flexibility and use creativity in planning for play.

Maximizing Potential Benefits of Hospitalization

Although hospitalization generally represents a stressful time for children and families, it also represents an opportunity for facilitating positive change within the child and among family members. For some families, the stress of a child's illness, hospitalization, or both can lead to strengthening of family coping behaviors and the emergence of new coping strategies.

Fostering Parent-Child Relationships

The crisis of illness or hospitalization can mobilize parents into more acute awareness of their child's needs. For example, hospitalization

CLINICAL REASONING CASE STUDY
Playroom and Hospital Procedures

Joel, an 8-year-old with cystic fibrosis, has been hospitalized numerous times with complications from the condition. He is playing a board game with his brother, sister, and several other children in the playroom on the pediatric unit. A pediatric phlebotomist enters the playroom and says, "Joel, I need to take some blood. I can see that you are playing a game, so I'll just do it while you play. It will just take a minute." The playroom is usually off limits for invasive procedures. As Joel's nurse, you are aware that Dr. Lung wants the results of the laboratory studies as soon as possible to make a decision about the course of therapy.

Questions
1. Evidence: Is there sufficient evidence to draw any conclusions about this situation at this time?
2. Assumptions: What are some underlying assumptions about the following:
   a. Children and painful procedures, such as venipunctures
   b. The function of play in a hospitalized child
   c. The priority in performing the procedure
   d. Implications of performing the procedure in the playroom
3. What implications and priorities for nursing care can be drawn at this time (i.e., what will you do)?
4. Does the evidence objectively support your argument (conclusion)?

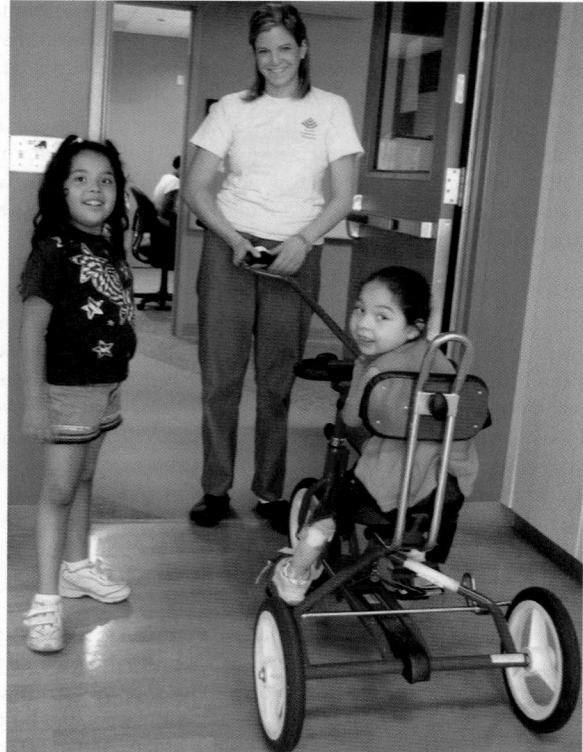

FIG 38.9 Placing children of the same age group with similar illnesses near each other on the unit is both psychologically and medically supportive. (Courtesy of E. Jacob, Texas Children's Hospital, Houston, TX.)

provides opportunities for parents to learn more about their children's growth and development. When parents are helped to understand children's usual reactions to stress, such as regression or aggression, they are not only better able to support the child through the hospital experience but also may extend their insights into childrearing practices after discharge.

Difficulties in parent-child relationships that existed before hospitalization that are characterized by feeding problems, negative behavior, and sleep disturbances may decrease during hospitalization. The temporary cessation of such problems sometimes alerts parents to the role they may be playing in propagating the negative behavior. With assistance from health care professionals, parents can restructure ways of relating to their children to foster more positive behavior.

Hospitalization may also represent a temporary reprieve or refuge from a disturbed home. Typically, abused or neglected children's dramatic physical and social improvement during hospitalization is proof of the benefits and potential growth that can occur during hospitalization. These children temporarily are able to seek support, reassurance, and security from new relationships, particularly with nurses and hospitalized peers.

Providing Educational Opportunities

Illness and hospitalization represent excellent opportunities for children and other family members to learn more about their bodies, each other, and the health care professionals. For example, during a hospital admission for a diabetic crisis, the child may learn about the disease; the parents may learn about the child's needs for independence, normalcy, and appropriate limits; and each of them may find a new support system in the hospital staff.

Illness or hospitalization can also help older children in choosing a career. Frequently, children have impressions of physicians or nurses that are disproportionately positive or negative. Actual experience with different health care professionals can influence their attitude about health care professionals and even a decision regarding a career in health care.

Promoting Self-Mastery

The experience of facing a crisis such as illness or hospitalization, coping successfully with it, and maturing as a result of it constitutes an opportunity for self-mastery. Younger children have the chance to test fantasy versus reality fears. They realize that they were not abandoned, mutilated, or punished. In fact, they were loved, cared for, and treated with respect for their individual concerns. It is not unusual for children who have undergone hospitalization or surgery to tell others that "it was nothing" or to display proudly their scars or bandages. For older children, hospitalization may represent an opportunity for decision making, independence, and self-reliance. They are proud of having survived the experience and may feel a genuine self-respect for their achievements. Nurses can facilitate such feelings of self-mastery by emphasizing aspects of personal competence in the child and not focusing on uncooperative or negative behavior.

Providing Socialization

Hospitalization may offer children a special opportunity for social acceptance. Lonely, asocial, and even delinquent children find a sympathetic environment in the hospital. Children who have a physical disability or are in some other way "different" from their age mates may find an accepting social peer group (Fig. 38.9). Although this does not always spontaneously occur, nurses can structure the environment to foster a supportive child group. For example, selection of a compatible roommate can help children gain a new friend and learn more about themselves. Forming relationships with significant members of the health care team, such as the physician, nurse, child life specialist, or social worker, can greatly enhance children's adjustment in many areas of life.

Parents may also encounter a new social group in other parents who have similar problems. The waiting room or hallway "self-help" groups are inherent to every institution. Parents meet while in the hospital or clinic and discuss their children's illnesses and treatments. Nurses can capitalize on this informal gathering by encouraging parents to discuss collectively their concerns and feelings. Nurses can also refer parents to organized parent groups or can use the help and support of parents of recovered hospitalized patients. It is important that nurses emphasize to families that each child responds differently to disease, treatments, and care. Any questions raised during group discussions should be clarified with a nurse or physician.

NURSING CARE OF THE FAMILY

Although it is not possible to predict exactly which factors are most likely to have an effect on a family's reactions, important variables are (1) the seriousness of the child's illness, (2) the family's previous experience with hospitalization, and (3) the medical procedures involved in the diagnosis and treatment. Important information is also obtained in the nursing admission history (see Box 38.5).

SUPPORTING FAMILY MEMBERS

Support involves the willingness to stay and listen to parents' verbal and nonverbal messages. Sometimes the nurse does not give this support directly. For example, the nurse may offer to stay with the child to allow the parents time alone or may discuss with other family members the parents' need for extra relief. Often relatives and friends want to help but do not know how. Suggesting ways, such as babysitting, preparing meals, doing laundry, or transporting the siblings to school, can prompt others to help reduce the responsibilities that burden parents.

Support may also be provided through the clergy. Parents with deep religious beliefs may appreciate the counsel of a clergy member, but because of their stress, they may not have sufficient energy to initiate the contact. Nurses can be supportive by arranging for clergy to visit, upholding parents' religious beliefs, and respecting the individual meaning and significance of those beliefs (Feudtner, Haney, & Dimmers, 2003).

Support involves accepting cultural, socioeconomic, and ethnic values. For example, health and illness are defined differently by various ethnic groups. For some, a disorder that has few outward manifestations of illness, such as diabetes, hypertension, or cardiac problems, is not a sickness. Consequently, following a prescribed treatment may be seen as unnecessary. Nurses who appreciate the influences of culture are more likely to intervene therapeutically.

Parents need help in accepting their own feelings toward the ill child. If given the opportunity, parents often disclose their feelings of loss of control, anger, and guilt. They often resist admitting to such feelings because they expect others to disapprove of behavior that is less than perfect. Unfortunately, health personnel, including nurses, sometimes do exercise little tolerance for deviation from the norm. This only increases the psychologic impact of a child's illness on family members. Helping parents identify the specific reason for such feelings and emphasizing that each is a normal, expected, and healthy response to stress may reduce the parents' emotional burden.

Family-centered care also addresses the needs of siblings. Support may involve preparing siblings for hospital visits, assessing their adjustment, and providing appropriate interventions or referrals when needed. The Family-Centered Care box: Supporting Siblings During Hospitalization suggests ways that parents can support siblings during hospitalization.

PROVIDING INFORMATION

One of the most important nursing interventions is providing information about (1) the disease, its treatment, prognosis, and home care; (2)

FAMILY-CENTERED CARE
Supporting Siblings During Hospitalization

Trade off staying at the hospital with spouse, or have a surrogate who knows the siblings well stay in the home.

Offer information about the child's condition to young siblings as well as older siblings; respect the sibling who avoids information as a means of coping with the situation.

Arrange for children to visit their brother or sister in the hospital if possible.

Encourage phone visits and mail between brothers and sisters; provide children with phone numbers, writing supplies, and stamps.

Help each sibling identify an extended family member or friend to be their support person and provide extra attention during parental absence.

Make or buy inexpensive toys or trinkets for siblings, one gift for each day the child will be hospitalized.

- Wrap each gift separately, and place them in a basket, box, or other container at the child's bedside.
- Instruct siblings to open one gift at bedtime and to remember that he or she is in their parent's thoughts.

If the child's condition is stable and distance is not prohibitive, plan a special time at home with the siblings or have spouse or another relative or friend bring the children to meet parent(s) at a restaurant or other location near the hospital.

- Have extended family members or friends schedule a visit to the child in the hospital during parental absence.
- Arrange a pass for the child to leave the hospital to join the family if the child's condition permits.

Adapted from Craft, M., & Craft, J. (1989). Perceived changes in siblings of hospitalized children: A comparison of sibling and parent reports. *Child Health Care, 10*(1), 42–48; Rollins, J. (1992). *Brothers and sisters: A discussion guide for families.* Landover, MD: Epilepsy Foundation of America.

---

the child's emotional and physical reactions to illness and hospitalization; and (3) the probable emotional reactions of family members to the crisis.

For many families, the child's illness is the first contact they have with the hospital experience. Often parents are not prepared for the child's behavioral reactions to hospitalization, such as separation behaviors, regression, aggression, and hostility. Providing the parents with information about these normal and expected behavioral responses can lessen the parents' anxiety during the hospital admission. The family is equally unfamiliar with hospital rules, which often compounds their confusion and anxiety. Therefore, the family needs clear explanations about what to expect and what is expected of them.

Parents also need to be aware of the effects of illness on the family and strategies that prevent negative changes. Specifically, parents should keep the family well informed and communicate with everyone as much as possible. They should treat all the children equally and as normally as before the illness occurred. Discipline, which initially may be lessened for the ill child, should be continued to provide a measure of security and predictability. When ill children know that their parents expect certain standards of conduct from them, they feel certain that they will recover. Conversely, when all limits are removed, they fear that something catastrophic will happen.

Helping parents understand the meaning of post-hospitalization behaviors in the sick child is necessary for them to tolerate and support such behaviors. In addition, parents should be forewarned of the common reactions after discharge (see Box 38.2). Parents who do not expect such reactions may misinterpret them as evidence of the child's "being spoiled" and demand perfect behavior at a time when the child is still reacting to the stress of illness and hospitalization. If the behaviors, especially the demand for attention, are dealt with in a supportive manner, most children are able to relinquish them and assume prior levels of functioning.

Nurses should also prepare parents for the reactions of siblings—particularly anger, jealousy, and resentment. Older siblings may deny such reactions because they provoke feelings of guilt. However, everyone needs outlets for emotions, and the repressed feelings may surface as problems in school or with age mates, as psychosomatic illnesses, or in delinquent behavior.

Probably one of the most neglected areas of communication involves giving information to siblings. Frequently, age becomes the only factor that leads to an awareness of this problem because older children may begin to ask questions or request explanations. Even in this situation, however, the information may be seriously inadequate. Children in every age group deserve some explanation of the sibling's illness or hospitalization. In addition, nurses can minimize a sibling's fear of also getting sick or having caused the illness.

ENCOURAGING PARENT PARTICIPATION

Preventing or minimizing separation is a key nursing goal with the child who is hospitalized, but maintaining parent-child contact is also beneficial for the family. One of the best approaches is encouraging parents to stay with their child and to participate in the care whenever possible. Although some health facilities provide special accommodations for parents, the concept of rooming in can be instituted anywhere. The first requirement is the staff's positive attitude toward parents. A negative attitude toward parent participation can create barriers to collaborative working relationships.

When hospital staff genuinely appreciate the importance of continued parent-child attachment, they foster an environment that encourages parents to stay. When parents are included in the care planning and understand that they are a contributing factor to the child's recovery, they are more inclined to remain with their child and have more emotional reserves to support themselves and the child through the crisis. An empowerment model of helping allows the nurse to focus on parents' strengths and seek ways to promote growth and family functioning so that the parents become empowered in caring for their child. Strategies such as bedside reporting that allow parents to be involved in the discussion of the child's current status are moving health care settings closer to family-centered care (Anderson & Mangino, 2006). Liaison nursing roles in tertiary care settings are also focused on improving communication between parents and health care providers (Caffin, Linton, & Pellegrini, 2007).

Because the mother tends to be the usual family caregiver, she usually spends more time in the hospital than the father. However, not all parents feel equally comfortable assuming responsibility for their child's care. Some may be under such great emotional stress that they need a temporary reprieve from total participation in caregiving activities. Others may feel insecure in participating in specialized areas of care, such as bathing the child after surgery. On the other hand, some mothers may feel a great need to control their child's care. This seems particularly true of young mothers, who have recently established their role as a parent; mothers of children too young to verbalize their needs; and ethnic minority mothers when the hospital setting is predominantly staffed by nonminority personnel. Individual assessment of each parent's preferred involvement is necessary to prevent the effects of separation while supporting parents in their needs as well.

With lifestyles and gender roles changing, fathers may assume all or some of the usual "mothering" roles in the household. In these cases, it may be the father-child relationship that requires preservation. Fathers need to be included in the care plan and respected for their parental role. For some fathers, the child's hospitalization may represent an opportunity to alter their usual caregiving role and increase their involvement. In single-parent families, the caregiver may not be a parent but an extended family member, such as a grandparent or aunt.

One of the potential problems with continuous parent involvement is neglect of the parent's need for sleep, nutrition, and relaxation. Often the sleeping accommodations are limited to a chair, and sleep is disrupted by nursing procedures. Encouraging the parents to leave for brief periods, arranging for sleeping quarters on the unit but outside the child's room, and planning a schedule of alternating visits with another family member can minimize the stresses for the parent.

All too often, nurses respond to parent participation by abandoning their patient responsibilities. Nurses need to restructure their roles to complement and augment the caregiving functions of parents (Hopia, Tomlinson, Paavilainen, et al., 2005). Even in units structured to provide care by parents, parents frequently feel anxiety in their caregiving responsibilities; those more involved in direct care may feel more anxiety than those less involved in direct care. Therefore, 24-hour responsibility may be too much for some parents. Assistance and relief by nursing personnel should always be available to these families, and nurses may need to work diligently to establish the strong bond of trust some parents need to take advantage of these opportunities.

PREPARING FOR DISCHARGE AND HOME CARE

Most hospitalizations necessitate some type of discharge preparation. Often this involves education of the family for continued care and follow-up in the home. Depending on the diagnosis, this may be relatively simple or highly complex. Preparing the family for home care demands a high degree of competence in planning and implementing discharge instructions.

Nurses are often key individuals in initiating and carrying out the discharge process. They collaborate with others in the planning and implementation phases to ensure appropriate care after hospitalization. Throughout the hospitalization, the nurse should be aware of the need for discharge planning and those assessment factors that affect the family's ability to provide home care. A thorough assessment of the family and home environment should be performed to ensure that the family's emotional and physical resources are sufficient to manage the tasks of home care. (For a discussion of family assessment strategies, see Chapter 29.) In addition to adequate family resources, an investigation of community services, including respite care, is needed to ensure that appropriate support agencies are available, such as emergency facilities, home health agencies, and equipment vendors. Financial resources are also a consideration. To coordinate the immense task of assessment and to plan implementation, a care coordinator or manager should be appointed early in the discharge process.

The preparation for hospital discharge and home care begins during the admission assessment. Short- and long-term goals are established to meet the child's physical and psychosocial needs. For children with complex care needs, discharge planning focuses on obtaining appropriate equipment and health care personnel for the home. Discharge planning is also concerned with treatments that parents or children are expected to continue at home. In planning appropriate teaching, nurses need to assess (1) the actual and perceived complexity of the skill, (2) the parents' or child's ability to learn the skill, and (3) the parents' or child's previous or present experience with such procedures.

The teaching plan incorporates levels of learning, such as observing, participating with assistance, and finally acting without help or guidance. The skill is divided into discrete steps, and each step is taught to the family member until it is learned. Return demonstration of the skill is requested before new skills are introduced. A record of teaching and performance provides an efficient checklist for evaluation. All families need to receive detailed *written* instructions about home care, with telephone numbers for assistance, before they leave the hospital. Communication between the nurse performing discharge planning and home health care is essential for ensuring a smooth transition for the child and family.

After the family is competent in performing the skill, they are given responsibility for the care. When possible, the family should have a transition or trial period to assume care with minimal health care supervision. This may be arranged on the unit; during a home pass; or in a facility, such as a motel, near the hospital. Such transitions provide a safe practice period for the family, with assistance readily available when needed, and are especially valuable when the family lives far from the hospital.

In many instances, parents need only simple instructions and understanding of follow-up care. However, the often overwhelming care assumed by some families, coupled with other stressors that they may be experiencing, necessitates continued professional support after discharge. A follow-up home visit or telephone call gives the nurse an opportunity to individualize care and provide information in perhaps a less stressful learning environment than the hospital. Appropriate referrals and resources may include visiting nurse or home health agencies, private nurse services, the school system, a physical therapist, a mental health counselor, a social worker, and any number of community agencies. Sharing the important issues surrounding the child's and family's needs is essential. Referral summaries should be concise, specific, and factual. When numerous support services are required, periodic collaboration among the professionals involved and the family is an excellent strategy to ensure efficient usage and comprehensive delivery of services.

CARE OF THE CHILD AND FAMILY IN SPECIAL HOSPITAL SITUATIONS

In addition to a general pediatric unit, children may be admitted to special facilities, such as an ambulatory or outpatient setting, an isolation room, or intensive care.

AMBULATORY OR OUTPATIENT SETTING

The ambulatory or outpatient setting provides needed medical services for the child while eliminating the necessity of overnight admission. The benefits of ambulatory care are (1) minimized stressors of hospitalization, especially separation from the family; (2) reduced chances of infection; and (3) increased cost savings. Admission to the ambulatory or outpatient hospital setting usually is for surgical or diagnostic procedures, such as insertion of tympanostomy tubes, hernia repair, adenoidectomy, tonsillectomy, cystoscopy, or bronchoscopy.

In the ambulatory or outpatient setting, adequate preparation is particularly challenging. Ideally, the child and parents should receive preadmission preparation, including a tour of the facility and a review of the day's events. Parents need information in advance to help prepare the child and themselves for surgery and enable them to care for the child at home after the procedure. Parents also appreciate suggestions for items to bring to the hospital, such as blankets or stuffed animals. When preadmission preparation is not possible, time should be allowed on the day of the procedure for children to become acquainted with their surroundings and for nurses to assess, plan, and implement appropriate teaching.

Explicit discharge instructions are important after outpatient surgery (see Family-Centered Care box: Discharge from Ambulatory Settings

---

👪 FAMILY-CENTERED CARE
Discharge From Ambulatory Settings

1. Before beginning, explain that all instructions will also be presented in writing for the family to refer to later.
2. Provide an overview of the typical trajectory (expected pattern) of recovery.
3. Discuss expected progression of the child's activity level during the postdischarge period (e.g., "Mary will probably sleep for the rest of the day and feel kind of tired most of tomorrow but will be back to her usual activities the next day").
4. Explain which activities the child is allowed and what is not permitted (e.g., bed rest, bathing).
5. Discuss dietary restrictions, being very specific and giving examples of "clear fluids" or what is meant by a "full liquid diet."
6. Discuss nausea and vomiting, if applicable, explaining how much is "normal" and what to do if more occurs (e.g., "Juan may be sick to his stomach and vomit. This is normal. However, if he vomits more than three times, please call us at this number right away").
7. Discuss fever and appropriate comfort measures, explaining how much fever is considered "normal," and specifically what to do if the child goes beyond the range.
8. Explain the amount, location, and kind of pain or discomfort the child may experience.
   - Give any prescribed medication before leaving the facility.
   - Send a pain scale home with the family.
   - Explain how much pain and discomfort is "normal" and what to do if the child surpasses that level or if pain management interventions are unsuccessful.
   - Discuss pain management, including dosage for pain medications and details on how to administer them.
   - Describe appropriate nonpharmacologic comfort measures, such as holding, rocking, or swaddling.
9. Provide information about each medication that the child will be taking at home.
   - Review the details, including dose and route.
   - Demonstrate how to administer medications, if necessary (e.g., how to take outer packaging off suppositories, how to insert).
   - Discuss guidelines for requesting other medications.
   - Request that all prescriptions be filled and given to the family before discharge.
10. Make certain the family has all of the equipment and supplies (e.g., gauze and tape for dressing changes) that they will need at home.
11. Discuss complications that may occur and the steps to take if they do.
12. Ensure that appropriate measures are in place for safe transport home.
   - Remind family to use a seat belt or car seat for the child.
   - Determine if there will be one person whose sole responsibility is helping ensure the child's safety and comfort during transport.
   - Discuss measures the driver may need to take if this is impossible (e.g., be certain a basin is within the child's reach in case vomiting occurs; take a route that permits slower traffic and has places along the roadside to stop if necessary).
   - Determine the availability of a blanket, pillow, and cup with a lid and straw for the child's use in the car.
13. Provide emergency phone numbers for the family to call with any concerns.
14. Explain that the family will be contacted (give an approximate time) to follow up on the child but that they should not hesitate to call if concerns arise before then.
15. Ask the family and child, if appropriate, if they have any questions, and problem solve with family members to meet their unique needs.

and the "Preparing for Discharge and Home Care" section earlier in this chapter). Parents need guidelines on when to call their practitioner regarding a change in the child's condition. A follow-up telephone call system allows for nurses to check on the child's progress within 48 to 72 hours after discharge. It also provides an opportunity for the nurse to review discharge information and answer questions.

> **! NURSING ALERT**
>
> Help the family prepare for the transportation home by offering the following suggestions:
> - Have a blanket and pillow in the car. (Always use the car safety restraint system.)
> - Take a basin or plastic bag in case of vomiting.
> - Use a cup with a cap and straw for the child to drink fluids (except in cases of oral facial surgery in which a straw may be contraindicated).
> - Give any prescribed pain medication before leaving the facility.
> - Provide parents verbal and written information regarding potential side effects of pain medication for which they should be vigilant after discharge.

ISOLATION

Admission to an isolation room increases all of the stressors typically associated with hospitalization. There is further separation from familiar people; additional loss of control; and added environmental changes, such as sensory deprivation and the strange appearance of visitors. Orientation to time and place is affected. These stressors are compounded by children's limited understanding of isolation. Preschool children have difficulty understanding the rationale for isolation, because they cannot comprehend the cause-and-effect relationship between germs and illness. They are likely to view isolation as punishment. Older children understand the causality better but still require information to decrease fantasizing or misinterpretation.

When a child is placed in isolation, preparation is essential for the child to feel in control. With young children, the best approach is a simple explanation, such as "You need to be in this room to help you get better. This is a special place to make all the germs go away. The germs made you sick, and you could not help that."

All children, but especially younger ones, need preparation in terms of what they will see, hear, and feel in isolation. Therefore, they are shown the mask, gloves, and gown and are encouraged to "dress up" in them. Playing with the strange apparel lessens the fear of seeing "ghostlike" people walk into the room. Before entering the room, nurses and other health personnel should introduce themselves and let the child see their faces before donning masks. In this way, the child associates them with significant experiences and gains a sense of familiarity in an otherwise strange and lonely environment.

When the child's condition improves, appropriate play activities are provided to minimize boredom, stimulate the senses, provide a real or perceived sense of movement, orient the child to time and place, provide social interaction, and reduce depersonalization. For example, the environment can be manipulated to increase sensory freedom by moving the bed toward the door or window. Opening window shades; providing musical, visual, or tactile toys; and increasing interpersonal contact can substitute mental mobility for the limitations of physical movement. Rather than dwelling on the negative aspects of isolation, the child can be encouraged to view this experience as challenging and positive. For example, the nurse can help the child look at isolation as a method of keeping others out and letting only special people in. Children often think of intriguing signs for their doors, such as "Enter at your own risk." These signs also encourage people "on the outside" to talk with the child about the ominous greeting.

> **! NURSING ALERT**
>
> Have the child select a place he or she would like to visit. Help the child decorate the bed and equipment to suit the theme (e.g., truck, circus tent, spaceship, sky). At a set time each day, pretend to go with the child to the special place. Consider including props such as a suitcase or picnic basket.

EMERGENCY ADMISSION

One of the most traumatic hospital experiences for the child and parents is an emergency admission. The sudden onset of an illness or the occurrence of an injury leaves little time for preparation and explanation. Sometimes the emergency admission is compounded by admission to an intensive care unit (ICU) or the need for immediate surgery. However, even in instances requiring only outpatient treatment, the child is exposed to a strange, frightening environment and to experiences that may elicit fear or cause pain.

There is a wide discrepancy between what constitutes a medically defined emergency and a patient-defined emergency. A growing concern is the use of major emergency departments for routine primary care health visits. To offset overcrowding in emergency departments, many facilities have minor emergency units or pediatric minor emergency units for after-hours health care. Telephone triage for minor illnesses for patients is also emerging as a health care delivery mode to differentiate illnesses such as a common cold from true life-threatening conditions that require immediate practitioner attention and intervention. Other factors contributing to the overuse of emergency departments (as opposed to the primary practitioner's office) include the increasing number of uninsured people and households where both parents work full time and cannot afford to take time off during the day to take the sick child to a practitioner.

In pediatric populations, most visits to the emergency department are for respiratory infections, skin conditions, gastrointestinal disorders, and trauma (e.g., poisoning). The most common reason parents give for bringing the child to the emergency department is concern about the illness worsening. However, practitioners may not think that the progressive symptoms necessitate immediate or emergency care. One of the nurse's primary goals is to assess the parents' perception of the event and their reasons for considering it serious or life-threatening.

Lengthy preparatory admission procedures are often inappropriate for emergency situations. In such instances, nurses must focus their nursing interventions on the essential components of admission counseling (see Guidelines boxes: Hospital Admission and Special Hospital Admission) and complete the process as soon as the child's condition has stabilized.

Unless an emergency is life-threatening, children need to participate in their care to maintain a sense of control. Because emergency departments are frequently hectic, there is a tendency to rush through procedures to save time. However, the extra few minutes needed to allow children to participate may save many more minutes of useless resistance and uncooperativeness during subsequent procedures. Other supportive measures include ensuring privacy, accepting various emotional responses to fear or pain, preserving parent-child contact, explaining all events before or as they occur, and personally remaining calm.

At times, because of the child's physical condition, little or no preparatory counseling for emergency hospitalization can be done. In such situations, counseling subsequent to the event has therapeutic value. The counseling should focus on evaluating children's thoughts regarding admission and related procedures. It is similar to precounseling techniques; however, instead of supplying information, the nurse listens to the explanations offered by the child. Projective techniques such as

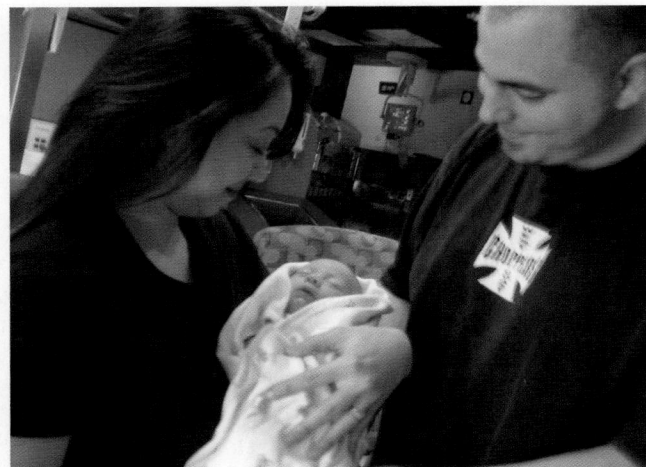

FIG 38.10 Parental presence during hospitalization provides emotional support for the child and increases the parent's sense of empowerment in the caregiver role. (Courtesy of E. Jacob, Texas Children's Hospital, Houston, TX.)

drawing, doll play, or storytelling are especially effective. The nurse then bases additional information on what has already been understood.

INTENSIVE CARE UNIT

Admission to an ICU can be traumatic for both the child and parents (Fig. 38.10). The nature and severity of the illness and the circumstances surrounding the admission are major factors, especially for parents. Parents experience significantly more stress when the admission is unexpected rather than expected. Stressors for the child and parent are described in Box 38.9. Although several studies have described what parents perceive as most stressful, the most effective strategy may be to simply ask parents what is stressful and implement interventions that will enhance their ability to cope (Board & Ryan-Wenger, 2003). Assessment should be repeated periodically to account for changes in perceptions over time. The use of daily patient goal sheets has been successful in improving communication among health care providers caring for children in the ICU (Agarwal, Frankel, Tourner, et al., 2008; Phipps & Thomas, 2007). By clearly defining daily patient care goals, health care providers believed that care was improved.

The family's emotional needs are paramount when a child is admitted to an ICU. A major stressor for parents of a child in the ICU is the child's appearance (Latour, van Goudoever, & Hazelzet, 2008). Although the same interventions discussed earlier for the stressors of separation and loss of control apply here, additional interventions may also benefit the family and child (see Box 38.9). In a qualitative study of 19 parents of 10 children in an ICU, parents reported that they simply wanted nurses to nurture the child in the same way the family would (Harbaugh, Tomlinson, & Kirschbaum, 2004). Nurse behaviors that exemplify caring and affection were perceived as helpful in decreasing stress. Behaviors perceived as not helpful included separating the child from the parents and communicating poorly with parents. Therefore, even critical care must be centered on the family. It is important that visiting hours be liberal and flexible enough to accommodate parental needs and involvement.

Critically ill children become the focus of the parents' lives, and parents' most pressing need is for information. They want to know if their child will live and, if so, whether the child will be the same as before. They need to know why various interventions are being done for the child, that the child is being treated for pain or is comfortable,

and that the child may be able to hear them even though not awake. When parents first visit the child in the ICU, they need preparation regarding the child's appearance. Ideally, the nurse should accompany the parents to the bedside to provide emotional support and answer any questions.

Despite the stresses normally associated with ICU admission, a special security develops from being carefully monitored and receiving individualized care. Therefore, planning for transition to the regular unit is essential and should include the following:

• Assignment of a primary nurse on the regular unit
• Continued visits by the ICU staff to assess the child's and parents' adjustment and to act as a temporary liaison with the nursing staff
• Explanation of the differences between the two units and the rationale for the change to less intense monitoring of the child's physical condition
• Selection of an appropriate room, such as one that is close to the nursing station, and a compatible roommate

REFERENCES

Abraham, M., & Moretz, J. G. (2012). Implementing patient- and family-centered care: Part I—Understanding the challenges. *Pediatric Nursing, 38*(1), 44–47.

Agarwal, S., Frankel, L., Tourner, S., et al. (2008). Improving communication in a pediatric intensive care unit using daily patient goal sheets. *Journal of Critical Care, 23*(2), 227–235.

Anderson, C. D., & Mangino, R. R. (2006). Nurse shift report: Who says you can't talk in front of the patient? *Nursing Administration Quarterly, 30*(2), 112–122.

Board, R., & Ryan-Wenger, N. (2003). Stressors and symptoms of mothers with children in the PICU. *Journal of Pediatric Nursing, 18*(3), 195–201.

Caffin, C. L., Linton, S., & Pellegrini, J. (2007). Introduction of a liaison nurse role in a tertiary paediatric ICU. *Intensive and Critical Care Nursing, 23*(4), 226–233.

Clatworthy, S., Simon, K., & Tiedeman, M. E. (1999). Child drawing: Hospital—an instrument designed to measure the emotional status of hospitalized school-aged children. *Journal of Pediatric Nursing, 14*(1), 2–9.

Coyne, I. (2006). Children's experiences of hospitalization. *Journal of Child Health Care, 10*(4), 326–336.

Craft, M. J. (1993). Siblings of hospitalized children: Assessment and intervention. *Journal of Pediatric Nursing, 8*(5), 289–297.

Eichner, J. M., & Johnson, B. H. (2012). Patient- and family-centered care and the pediatrician's role. *Pediatrics, 129*(2), 394–404.

Fernandez, C., Pyesmany, A., & Stutzer, C. (1999). Alternative therapies in childhood cancer. *New England Journal of Medicine, 340*(7), 569–570.

Feudtner, H. J., Haney, J., & Dimmers, M. A. (2003). Spiritual care needs of hospitalized children and their families: A national survey of pastoral care providers' perceptions. *Pediatrics, 111*(1), e67–e72.

Flanagan, K. (2001). Preoperative assessment: Safety considerations for patients taking herbal products. *Journal of Perianesthesia Nursing, 16*(1), 19–26.

Gordon, M. (2002). *Manual of nursing diagnosis* (10th ed.). St. Louis, MO: Mosby.

Harbaugh, B. L., Tomlinson, P. S., & Kirschbaum, M. (2004). Parents' perceptions of nurses' caregiving behaviors in the pediatric intensive care unit. *Issues in Comprehensive Pediatric Nursing, 27*(3), 163–178.

Hopia, H., Tomlinson, P. S., Paavilainen, E., et al. (2005). Child in hospital: Family experiences and expectations of how nurses can promote family health. *Journal of Clinical Nursing, 14*(2), 212–222.

Institute for Patient- and Family-Centered Care. (2010a). *Changing hospital "visiting" policies and practices: Supporting family presence and participation*. Retrieved from http://ipfcc.org/resources/visiting.pdf.

Institute for Patient- and Family-Centered Care. (2010b). *Advancing the practice of patient- and family-centered care in hospitals: How to get started....* Retrieved from http://www.ipfcc.org/resources/getting_started.pdf.

Latour, J. M., van Goudoever, J. B., & Hazelzet, J. A. (2008). Parent satisfaction in the pediatric ICU. *Pediatric Clinics of North America, 55*(3), 779–790.

Lewandowski, L. A., & Tesler, M. D. (2003). *Family centered care: Putting it into action*. Washington, DC: American Nurses Association.

Limbers, C., & Skipper, S. (2014). Health-related quality of life measurement in siblings of children with physical chronic illness: A systematic review. *Families, Systems & Health, 32*(4), 408–415.

Meert, K. L., Clark, J., & Eggly, S. (2013). Family-centered care in the pediatric intensive care unit. *Pediatric Clinics of North America, 60*(3), 761–772.

Melnyk, B. M. (2000). Intervention studies involving parents of hospitalized young children: An analysis of the past and future recommendations. *Journal of Pediatric Nursing, 15*(1), 4–13.

Orem, D. (2001). *Nursing: Concepts of practice* (5th ed.). New York, NY: Mosby.

Phipps, L. M., & Thomas, N. J. (2007). The use of a daily goals sheet to improve communication in the paediatric intensive care unit. *Intensive and Critical Care Nursing, 23*(5), 264–271.

Samela, M., Salanterä, S., & Aronen, E. (2009). Child-reported hospital fears in 4- to 6-year-old children. *Pediatric Nursing, 35*(5), 269–276, 303.

Small, L. (2002). Early predictors of poor coping outcomes in children following intensive care hospitalization and stressful medical encounters. *Pediatric Nursing, 28*(4), 393–401.

Smith, T., & Conant Rees, H. L. (2000). Making family-centered care a reality. *Seminars for Nurse Managers, 8*(3), 136–142.

The Joint Commission (2011). *Comprehensive accreditation manual for hospitals (CAMH)*. Oakbrook Terrace, IL: Author.

Thompson, R. (2009). *The handbook of child life: A guide for pediatric psychosocial care*. Springfield, IL: Charles C Thomas.

Wilson, M. E., Megel, M. E., Enenbach, L., et al. (2010). The voices of children: Stories about hospitalization. *Journal of Pediatric Health Care, 24*(2), 95–102.

39

Pediatric Variations of Nursing Interventions

Marilyn J. Hockenberry

ⓔ http://evolve.elsevier.com/Perry/maternal

GENERAL CONCEPTS RELATED TO PEDIATRIC PROCEDURES

INFORMED CONSENT

Before undergoing any invasive procedure, the patient or the patient's legal surrogate must receive sufficient information on which to make an informed health care decision. Informed consent should include the expected care or treatment; potential risks, benefits, and alternatives; and what might happen if the patient chooses not to consent. To obtain valid informed consent, health care providers must meet the following three conditions:

1. The person must be capable of giving consent; he or she must be over the age of majority (usually 18 years of age) and must be considered competent (i.e., possessing the mental capacity to make choices and understand their consequences).
2. The person must receive the information needed to make an intelligent decision.
3. The person must act voluntarily when exercising freedom of choice without force, fraud, deceit, duress, or other forms of constraint or coercion.

The patient has the right to accept or refuse any health care. If a patient is treated without consent, the hospital or health care provider may be charged with assault and held liable for damages.

Requirements for Obtaining Informed Consent

Written informed consent of the parent or legal guardian is usually required for medical or surgical treatment of a minor, including many diagnostic procedures. One universal consent is not sufficient. Separate informed permissions must be obtained for each surgical or diagnostic procedure, including the following:

- Major surgery
- Minor surgery (e.g., cutdown, biopsy, dental extraction, suturing a laceration [especially one that may have a cosmetic effect], removal of a cyst, closed reduction of a fracture)
- Diagnostic tests with an element of risk (e.g., bronchoscopy, angiography, lumbar puncture, cardiac catheterization, bone marrow aspiration)
- Medical treatments with an element of risk (e.g., blood transfusion, thoracentesis or paracentesis, radiotherapy)

Other situations that require patient or parental consent include the following:

- Photographs for medical, educational, or public use
- Removal of the child from the health care institution against medical advice

- Postmortem examination, except in unexplained deaths, such as sudden infant death, violent death, or suspected suicide
- Release of medical information

Decision making involving the care of older children and adolescents should include the patient's assent (if feasible), as well as the parent's consent. Assent means the child or adolescent has been informed about the proposed treatment, procedure, or research and is willing to permit a health care provider to perform it. Assent should include the following:

- Helping the patient achieve a developmentally appropriate awareness of the nature of his or her condition
- Telling the patient what he or she can expect
- Making a clinical assessment of the patient's understanding
- Soliciting an expression of the patient's willingness to accept the proposed procedure

Health care providers should use multiple methods to provide information, including age-appropriate methods (e.g., videos, peer discussion, diagrams, and written materials). The nurse should provide an assent form for the child to sign, and the child should keep a copy. By including the child in the decision-making process and gaining his or her acceptance, staff members demonstrate respect for the child. Assent is not a legal requirement but an ethical one to protect the rights of children.

Eligibility for Giving Informed Consent
Informed Consent of Parents or Legal Guardians

Parents have full responsibility for the care and rearing of their minor children, including legal control over them. As long as children are minors, their parents or legal guardians are required to give informed consent before medical treatment is rendered or any procedure is performed. If the parents are married to each other, consent from only one parent is required for nonurgent pediatric care. If the parents are divorced, consent usually rests with the parent who has legal custody (Berger & American Academy of Pediatrics Committee on Medical Liability, 2003). Parents also have a right to withdraw consent later.

Evidence of Consent

Regulations on obtaining informed consent vary from state to state, and policies differ at each health care facility. It is the physician's legal responsibility to explain the procedure, risks, benefits, and alternatives. The nurse witnesses the patient's, parent's, or legal guardian's signature on the consent form and may reinforce what the patient has been told. A signed consent form is the legal document that signifies that the process of informed consent has occurred. If parents are unavailable to sign consent forms, verbal consent may be obtained via the telephone in the presence of two witnesses. Both witnesses record that informed consent was given and by whom. Their signatures indicate that they witnessed the verbal consent.

Informed Consent of Mature and Emancipated Minors

State laws differ with regard to the age of majority, the age at which a person is considered to have all the legal rights and responsibilities of an adult. In most states, 18 years of age is the age of majority. Competent adults can give informed consent on their own behalf. An emancipated minor is one who is legally under the age of majority but is recognized as having the legal capacity of an adult under circumstances prescribed by state law, such as pregnancy, marriage, high school graduation, independent living, or military service. A mature minor exception to consent laws is recognized in a few states for children 14 years of age and older who can understand all elements of informed consent and make a choice based on the information; legal action may be required for designation as a mature minor.

Treatment Without Parental Consent

Exceptions to requiring parental consent before treating minor children occur in situations in which children need urgent medical or surgical treatment and a parent is not readily available to give consent or refuses to give consent. For example, a child may be brought to an emergency department accompanied by a grandparent, child care provider, teacher, or others. In the absence of parents or legal guardians, people in charge of the child may be given permission by the parents to give informed consent by proxy. A medical screening examination is required by federal law under the Emergency Medical Treatment and Active Labor Act (EMTALA) for all patients presenting to an emergency center. In emergencies, including danger to life or the possibility of permanent injury, appropriate care should not be withheld or delayed because of problems obtaining consent (American Academy of Pediatrics, Committee on Pediatric Emergency Medicine and Committee on Bioethics, 2011). The nurse should document any efforts made to obtain consent.

Parental refusal to give consent for life-saving treatment or to prevent serious harm can occur and requires notification to child protective services to render emergency treatment. Evaluation for child abuse or neglect can occur without parental consent and without notification to the state before evaluation in most states.

Adolescents, Consent, and Confidentiality

The Health Insurance Portability and Accountability Act of 1996 (HIPAA) was passed to help protect and safeguard the security and confidentiality of health information. Because adolescents are not yet adults, parents have the right to make most decisions on their behalf and receive information. Adolescents, however, are more likely to seek care in a setting in which they believe their privacy will be maintained. All 50 states have enacted legislation that entitles adolescents to consent to treatment without the parents' knowledge to one or more "medically emancipated" conditions, such as sexually transmitted infections, mental health services, alcohol and drug dependency, pregnancy, and contraceptive advice (American Academy of Pediatrics, Committee on Pediatric Emergency Medicine and Committee on Bioethics, 2011; Anderson, Schaechter, & Brosco, 2005; Tillett, 2005). Consent to abortion is controversial, and statutes vary widely by state. State law preempts HIPAA regardless of whether that law prohibits, mandates, or allows discretion about a disclosure.

Informed Consent and Parental Right to the Child's Medical Chart

Some state statutes give parents the unrestricted right to a copy of children's medical records. In states without statutes, the best practice is to allow parents to review or have a copy of minors' charts under reasonable circumstances. Practitioners should avoid restrictive requirements, such as review permitted only in the presence of a clinician. Rather, an appropriate practitioner should be available to answer any questions that parents may have during their reviews.

PREPARATION FOR DIAGNOSTIC AND THERAPEUTIC PROCEDURES

Technologic advances and changes in health care have resulted in more pediatric procedures being performed in a variety of settings. Many procedures are both stressful and painful experiences. For most procedures, the focus of care is psychologic preparation of the child and family. However, some procedures require the administration of sedatives and analgesics.

Psychologic Preparation

Preparing children for procedures decreases their anxiety, promotes their cooperation, supports their coping skills and may teach them new ones, and facilitates a feeling of mastery in experiencing a potentially stressful event. Many institutions have developed preadmission teaching programs designed to educate the pediatric patient and family by offering hands-on experience with hospital equipment, the procedure performed, and departments they will visit. Preparatory methods may be formal, such as group preparation for hospitalization. Most preparation strategies are informal, focus on providing information about the experience, and are directed at stressful or painful procedures. The most effective preparation includes the provision of sensory-procedural information and helping the child develop coping skills, such as imagery, distraction, or relaxation.

The Guidelines boxes describe general guidelines for preparing children for procedures along with age-specific guidelines that consider children's developmental needs and cognitive abilities. In addition to these suggestions, nurses should consider the child's temperament, existing coping strategies, and previous experiences in individualizing the preparatory process. Children who are distractible and highly active or those who are "slow to warm up" may need individualized sessions— shorter for active children and more slowly paced for shy children. Whereas children who tend to cope well may need more emphasis on using their present skills, those who appear to cope less adequately can benefit from more time devoted to simple coping strategies, such as relaxing, breathing, counting, squeezing a hand, or singing. Children with previous health-related experiences still need preparation for repeat or new procedures; however, the nurse must assess what they know, correct their misconceptions, supply new information, and introduce new coping skills as indicated by their previous reactions. Especially for painful procedures, the most effective preparation includes providing sensory-procedural information and helping the child develop coping skills, such as imagery or relaxation (see Guidelines box: Age-Specific Preparation of Children for Procedures Based on Developmental Characteristics).

> **! NURSING ALERT**
>
> Prepare a basket, toy chest, or cart to keep near the treatment area. Items ideal for the basket include a Slinky; a sparkling "magic" wand (sealed, acrylic tube partially filled with liquid and suspended metallic confetti); a soft foam ball; bubble solution; party blowers; pop-up books with foldout three-dimensional scenes; real medical equipment, such as a syringe, adhesive bandages, and alcohol packets; toy medical supplies or a toy medical kit; marking pens; a note pad; and stickers. Have the child choose an item to help distract and relax during the procedure. After the procedure, allow the child to choose a small gift, such as a sticker, or to play with items, such as medical equipment.

📋 GUIDELINES

Preparing Children for Procedures

- Determine details of exact procedure to be performed.
- Review parents' and child's present understanding.
- Base teaching on developmental age and existing knowledge.
- Incorporate parents in the teaching if they desire, especially if they plan to participate in care.
- Inform parents of their supportive role during procedure, such as standing near child's head or in child's line of vision and talking softly to child, as well as typical responses of children undergoing the procedure.
- Allow for ample discussion to prevent information overload and ensure adequate feedback.
- Use concrete, not abstract, terms and visual aids to describe procedure. For example, use a simple line drawing of a boy or girl, and mark the body part that will be involved in the procedure. Use nonthreatening but realistic models.*
- Emphasize that no other body part will be involved.
- If the body part is associated with a specific function, stress the change or noninvolvement of that ability (e.g., after tonsillectomy, child can still speak).
- Use words and sentence length appropriate to child's level of understanding (a rule of thumb for the number of words in a child's sentence is equal to his or her age in years plus 1).
- Avoid words and phrases with dual meanings (see Table 39.1) unless child understands such words.
- Clarify all unfamiliar words (e.g., "Anesthesia is a *special* sleep").
- Emphasize sensory aspects of procedure—what child will feel, see, hear, smell, and touch and what child can do during procedure (e.g., lie still, count out loud, squeeze a hand, hug a doll).
- Allow child to practice procedures that will require cooperation (e.g., turning, deep breathing, using incentive spirometry).
- Introduce anxiety-inducing information last (e.g., starting an intravenous [IV] line).
- Be honest with child about unpleasant aspects of a procedure, but avoid creating undue concern. When discussing that a procedure may be uncomfortable, state that it feels differently to different people.
- Emphasize end of procedure and any pleasurable events afterward (e.g., going home, seeing parents).
- Stress positive benefits of procedure (e.g., "After your tonsils are fixed, you won't have as many sore throats").
- Provide a positive ending, praising efforts at cooperation and coping.

*Soft-sculptured dolls and customized adapters and overlays for preparing children and families about procedures and as teaching models for technical care are available from Legacy Products, Inc., 508 S. Green Street, PO Box 267, Cambridge City, IN 47327; 800-238-7951; email: info@legacyproductsinc.com; http://www.legacyproductsinc.com.

Children differ in their "information-seeking dimension." Some actively ask for information about the intended procedure, but others characteristically avoid information. Parents can often guide nurses in deciding how much information is enough for the child, because parents know whether the child is typically inquisitive or satisfied with short answers. Asking older children their preferences about the amount of explanation is also important.

The exact timing of the preparation for a procedure varies with the child's age and the type of procedure. No exact guidelines govern timing, but in general, the younger the child, the closer the explanation should be to the actual procedure to prevent undue fantasizing and worrying. With complex procedures, more time may be needed for assimilation of information, especially with older children. For example,

the explanation for an injection can immediately precede the procedure for all ages, but preparation for surgery may begin the day before for young children and a few days before for older children, although the nurse should elicit older children's preferences.

Establish Trust and Provide Support

The nurse who has spent time with and established a positive relationship with a child usually finds it easier to gain cooperation. If the relationship is based on trust, the child will associate the nurse with caregiving activities that give comfort and pleasure most of the time rather than discomfort and stress. If the nurse does not know the child, it is best for the nurse to be introduced by another staff person whom the child trusts. The first visit with the child should not include any painful procedure and ideally should focus on the child first and then on an explanation of the procedure.

Parental Presence and Support

Children need support during procedures, and for young children, the greatest source of support is the parents. They represent security, protection, safety, and comfort. Several studies have reported a positive impact on parental distress and satisfaction and no difference in technical complications when parents remain with children (Piira, Sugiura, Champion, et al., 2005). Controversy exists regarding the role parents should assume during the procedure, especially if discomfort is involved. In 2006, 18 professional associations developed a consensus statement of support for the option of family presence during invasive procedures (Henderson & Knapp, 2006); several associations have published additional support (American Association of Critical Care Nurses, 2006; Emergency Nurses Association, 2005). The nurse should assess the parents' preferences for assisting, observing, or waiting outside the room, as well as the child's preference for parental presence. Respect the child's and parents' choices. Give parents who wish to stay appropriate explanation about the procedure, and coach them about where to sit or stand and what to say or do to help the child through the procedure. Support parents who do not want to be present in their decision, and encourage them to remain close by so that they can be available to support the child immediately after the procedure. Parents should also know that someone will be with their child to provide support. Ideally, this person should inform the parents after the procedure about how the child did.

Provide an Explanation

Age-appropriate explanations are one of the most widely used interventions for reducing anxiety in children undergoing procedures. Before performing a procedure, explain what is to be done and what is expected of the child. The explanation should be short, simple, and appropriate to the child's level of comprehension. Long explanations may increase anxiety in a young child. When explaining the procedure to parents with the child present, the nurse uses language appropriate to the child because unfamiliar words can be misunderstood (Table 39.1). If the parents need additional preparation, it is done in an area away from the child. Teaching sessions are planned at times most conducive to the child's learning (e.g., after a rest period) and for the usual span of attention.

Special equipment is not necessary for preparing a child, but for young children who cannot yet think conceptually, using objects to supplement verbal explanation is important. Allowing children to handle actual items that will be used in their care, such as a stethoscope, sphygmomanometer, or oxygen mask, helps them develop familiarity with these items and reduces the fear often associated with their use. Miniature versions of hospital items, such as gurneys and X-ray and intravenous (IV) equipment, can be used to explain what the children

GUIDELINES

Age-Specific Preparation of Children for Procedures Based on Developmental Characteristics

Infant: Developing Trust and Sensorimotor Thought

Attachment to Parent

Involve parent in procedure if desired.*

Keep parent in infant's line of vision.

If parent is unable to be with infant, place familiar object with infant (e.g., stuffed toy).

Stranger Anxiety

Have usual caregivers perform or assist with procedure.*

Make advances slowly and in a nonthreatening manner.

Limit number of strangers entering room during procedure.*

Sensorimotor Phase of Learning

During procedure, use sensory soothing measures (e.g., stroking skin, talking softly, giving pacifier).

Use analgesics (e.g., topical anesthetic, intravenous [IV] opioid) to control discomfort.*

Cuddle and hug infant after stressful procedure; encourage parent to comfort infant.

Increased Muscle Control

Expect older infants to resist.

Restrain adequately.

Keep harmful objects out of reach.

Memory for Past Experiences

Realize that older infants may associate objects, places, or people with prior painful experiences and will cry and resist at the sight of them.

Keep frightening objects out of view.*

Perform painful procedures in a separate room, not in crib (or bed).*

Use nonintrusive procedures whenever possible (e.g., axillary or tympanic temperatures, oral medications).*

Imitation of Gestures

Model desired behavior (e.g., opening mouth).

Toddler: Developing Autonomy and Sensorimotor to Preoperational Thought

Use same approaches as for infant plus the following.

Egocentric Thought

Explain procedure in relation to what child will see, hear, taste, smell, and feel.

Emphasize those aspects of procedure that require cooperation (e.g., lying still).

Tell child it is okay to cry, yell, or use other means to express discomfort verbally.

Designate one health care provider to speak during procedure. Hearing more than one can be confusing to a child*

Negative Behavior

Expect treatments to be resisted; child may try to run away.

Use firm, direct approach.

Ignore temper tantrums.

Use distraction techniques (e.g., singing a song with child).

Restrain adequately.

Animism

Keep frightening objects out of view (young children believe objects have lifelike qualities and can harm them).

Limited Language Skills

Communicate using gestures or demonstrations.

Use a few simple terms familiar to child.

Give child one direction at a time (e.g., "Lie down" and then "Hold my hand").

Use small replicas of equipment; allow child to handle equipment.

Use play; demonstrate on doll, but avoid child's favorite doll because child may think doll is really "feeling" procedure.

Prepare parents separately to avoid child's misinterpreting words.

Limited Concept of Time

Prepare child shortly or immediately before procedure.

Keep teaching sessions short (≈5 to 10 minutes).

Have preparations completed before involving child in procedure.

Have extra equipment nearby (e.g., alcohol swabs, new needle, adhesive bandages) to avoid delays.

Tell child when procedure is completed.

Striving for Independence

Allow choices whenever possible, but realize that child may still be resistant and negative.

Allow child to participate in care and to help whenever possible (e.g., drink medicine from a cup, hold a dressing).

Preschooler: Developing Initiative and Preoperational Thought

Egocentric

Explain procedure in simple terms and in relation to how it affects child (as with toddler, stress sensory aspects).

Demonstrate use of equipment.

Allow child to play with miniature or actual equipment.

Encourage "playing out" experience on a doll both before and after procedure to clarify misconceptions.

Use neutral words to describe the procedure (see Table 39.1).

Increased Language Skills

Use verbal explanation, but avoid overestimating child's comprehension of words.

Encourage child to verbalize ideas and feelings.

Limited Concept of Time and Frustration Tolerance

Implement same approaches as for toddler, but may plan longer teaching session (10 to 15 minutes); may divide information into more than one session.

Illness and Hospitalization Viewed as Punishment

Clarify why each procedure is performed; child will find it difficult to understand how medicine can make him or her feel better and can taste bad at the same time.

Ask child thoughts regarding why a procedure is performed.

State directly that procedures are never a form of punishment.

Animism

Keep equipment out of sight except when shown to or used on child.

*Applies to any age.

GUIDELINES

Age-Specific Preparation of Children for Procedures Based on Developmental Characteristics—cont'd

Fears of Bodily Harm, Intrusion, and Castration

Point out on drawing, doll, or child where procedure is performed.

Emphasize that no other body part will be involved.

Use nonintrusive procedures whenever possible (e.g., axillary temperatures, oral medication).

Apply an adhesive bandage over puncture site.

Encourage parental presence.

Realize that procedures involving genitalia provoke anxiety.

Allow child to wear underpants with gown.

Explain unfamiliar situations, especially noises or lights.

Striving for Initiative

Involve child in care whenever possible (e.g., hold equipment, remove dressing).

Give choices whenever possible, but avoid excessive delays.

Praise child for helping and attempting to cooperate; never shame child for lack of cooperation.

School-Age Child: Developing Industry and Concrete Thought

Increased Language Skills; Interest in Acquiring Knowledge

Explain procedure using correct scientific and medical terminology.

Explain procedure using simple diagrams and photographs.

Discuss why procedure is necessary; concepts of illness and bodily functions are often vague.

Explain function and operation of equipment in concrete terms.

Allow child to manipulate equipment; use doll or another person as model to practice using equipment whenever possible (doll play may be considered childish by older school-age child).

Allow time before and after procedure for questions and discussion.

Improved Concept of Time

Plan for longer teaching sessions (≈20 minutes).

Prepare up to 1 day in advance of procedure to allow for processing of information.

Increased Self-Control

Gain child's cooperation.

Tell child what is expected.

Suggest several ways of maintaining control the child may select from (e.g., deep breathing, relaxation, counting).

Striving for Industry

Allow responsibility for simple tasks (e.g., collecting specimens).

Include child in decision making (e.g., time of day to perform procedure, preferred site).

Encourage active participation (e.g., removing dressings, handling equipment, opening packages).

Developing Relationships With Peers

Prepare two or more children for same procedure, or encourage one to help prepare another.

Provide privacy from peers during procedure to maintain self-esteem.

Adolescent: Developing Identity and Abstract Thought

Increasing Abstract Thought and Reasoning

Discuss why procedure is necessary or beneficial.

Explain long-term consequences of procedures; include information about body systems working together.

Realize adolescent may fear death, disability, or other potential risks.

Encourage questioning regarding fears, options, and alternatives.

Consciousness of Appearance

Provide privacy; describe how the body will be covered and what will be exposed.

Discuss how procedure may affect appearance (e.g., scar) and what can be done to minimize it.

Emphasize any physical benefits of procedure.

Concern More With Present Than With Future

Realize that immediate effects of procedure are more significant than future benefits.

Striving for Independence

Involve adolescent in decision making and planning (e.g., time, place, individuals present during procedure, clothing, whether they will watch procedure).

Impose as few restrictions as possible.

Explore what coping strategies have worked in the past; they may need suggestions of various techniques.

Accept regression to more childish methods of coping.

Realize that adolescents may have difficulty accepting new authority figures and may resist complying with procedures.

Developing Peer Relationships and Group Identity

Same as for school-age child but assumes even greater significance.

Allow adolescents to talk with other adolescents who have had the same procedure.

---

can expect and permit them to safely experience situations that are unfamiliar and potentially frightening. Written and illustrated materials are also valuable aids to preparation.

 NURSING ALERT

Use photographs of children in different areas of the hospital (e.g., radiology department, operating room) to give children a more realistic idea of equipment they may encounter.

Physical Preparation

One area of special concern is the administration of appropriate sedation and analgesia before stressful procedures.

Performance of the Procedure

Supportive care continues during the procedure and can be a major factor in a child's ability to cooperate. Ideally, the same nurse who explains the procedure should perform or assist with the procedure. Before beginning, all equipment is assembled, and the room is readied to prevent unnecessary delays and interruptions that increase the child's anxiety. Minimizing the number of people present during the procedure also can decrease the child's anxiety.

 NURSING ALERT

To avoid a delay during a procedure, have extra supplies handy. For example, have tape, bandages, alcohol swabs, and an extra needle when performing an injection or venipuncture.

TABLE 39.1 Selecting Nonthreatening Words or Phrases

Words and Phrases to Avoid	Suggested Substitutions
Shot, bee sting, stick	Medicine under the skin
Organ	Special place in body
Test	To see how (specify body part) is working
Incision, cut	Special opening
Edema	Puffiness
Stretcher, gurney	Rolling bed, bed on wheels
Stool	Child's usual term
Dye	Special medicine
Pain	Hurt, discomfort, "owie," "boo-boo," sore, achy, scratchy
Deaden	Numb, make sleepy
Fix	Make better
Take (as in "take your temperature")	See how warm you are
Take (as in "take your blood pressure")	Check your pressure; hug your arm
Put to sleep, anesthesia	Special sleep so you won't feel anything
Catheter	Tube
Monitor	Television screen
Electrodes	Stickers, ticklers
Specimen	Sample

To promote long-term coping and adjustment, give special consideration to the patient's age, coping skills, and procedure to be performed in determining where a procedure will occur. Treatment rooms should be used for procedures requiring sedation, such as bone marrow aspirates and lumbar punctures in younger children. Traumatic procedures should never be performed in "safe" areas, such as the playroom. If the procedure is lengthy, avoid conversation that could be misinterpreted by the child. As the procedure is nearing completion, the nurse should inform the child that it is almost over in language the child understands.

Expect Success

Nurses who approach children with confidence and who convey the impression that they expect to be successful are less likely to encounter difficulty. It is best to approach a child as though cooperation is expected. Children sense anxiety and uncertainty in an adult and respond by striking out or actively resisting. Although it is not possible to eliminate such behavior in every child, a firm approach with a positive attitude tends to convey a feeling of security to most children.

Involve the Child

Involving children helps to gain their cooperation. Permitting choices gives them some measure of control. However, a choice is given only in situations in which one is available. Asking children, "Do you want to take your medicine now?" leads them to believe they have an option and provides them the opportunity to legitimately refuse or delay the medication. This places the nurse in an awkward, if not impossible, position. It is much better to state firmly, "It's time to drink your medicine now." Children usually like to make choices, but the choice must be one that they do indeed have (e.g., "It's time for your medicine. Do you want to drink it plain or with a little water?").

Many children respond to tactics that appeal to their maturity or courage. This also gives them a sense of participation and achievement. For example, preschool children will be proud that they can hold the dressing during the procedure or remove the tape. The same is true for school-age children, who often cooperate with minimal resistance.

Provide Distraction

Distraction is a powerful coping strategy during painful procedures (Uman, Chambers, McGrath, et al., 2006). It is accomplished by focusing the child's attention on something other than the procedure. Singing favorite songs, listening to music with a headset, counting aloud, or blowing bubbles to "blow the hurt away" are effective techniques.

> **! NURSING ALERT**
>
> Help the child select and practice a coping technique before the procedure. Consider having the parent or some other supportive person (such as, a child life specialist) "coach" the child in learning and using the coping skill.

Allow Expression of Feelings

The child should be allowed to express feelings of anger, anxiety, fear, frustration, or any other emotion. It is natural for children to strike out in frustration or to try to avoid stress-provoking situations. The child needs to know that it is all right to cry. Behavior is children's primary means of communication and coping and should be permitted unless it inflicts harm on them or those caring for them.

Postprocedural Support

After the procedure, the child continues to need reassurance that he or she performed well and is accepted and loved. If the parents did not participate, the child is united with them as soon as possible so that they can provide comfort.

Encourage Expression of Feelings

Planned activity after the procedure is helpful in encouraging constructive expression of feelings. For verbal children, reviewing the details of the procedure can clarify misconceptions and garner feedback for improving the nurse's preparatory strategies. Play is an excellent activity for all children. Infants and young children should have the opportunity for gross motor movement. Older children are able to vent their anger and frustration in acceptable pounding or throwing activities. Play-Doh is a remarkably versatile medium for pounding and shaping. Dramatic play provides an outlet for anger and places the child in a position of control, in contrast to the position of helplessness in the real situation. Puppets also allow the child to communicate feelings in a nonthreatening way. One of the most effective interventions is therapeutic play, which includes well-supervised activities, such as permitting the child to give an injection to a doll or stuffed toy to reduce the stress of injections (Fig. 39.1).

Positive Reinforcement

Children need to hear from adults that they did the best they could in the situation—no matter how they behaved. It is important for children to know that their worth is not being judged on the basis of their behavior in a stressful situation. Reward systems, such as earning stars, stickers, or a badge of courage, are appealing to children.

Returning to the child a short while after the procedure helps the nurse strengthen a supportive relationship. Relating with the child in a relaxed and nonstressful period allows him or her to see the nurse not only as someone associated with stressful situations but also as someone with whom to share pleasurable experiences.

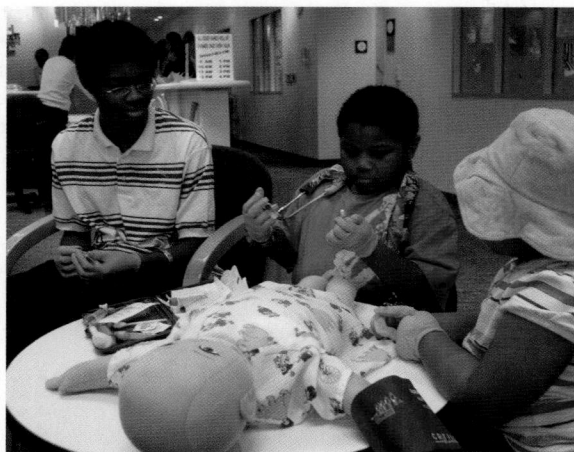

FIG 39.1 Playing with medical objects provides children with the opportunity to play out fears and concerns with supervision by a nurse or child life specialist.

Use of Play in Procedures

The use of play is an integral part of relationships with children. As such, its value in specific situations is discussed throughout this book, in relation to hospitalization. Many institutions have elaborate and well-organized play areas and programs under the direction of child life specialists. Other institutions have limited facilities. No matter what the institution provides for children, nurses can include play activities as part of nursing care. Play can be used to teach, express feelings, or achieve a therapeutic goal. Consequently, it should be included in preparing children for and encouraging their cooperation during procedures. Play sessions after procedures can be structured, such as directed toward needle play, or general, with a wide variety of equipment available for children to play with.

Routine procedures such as measuring blood pressure and oral administration of medication may be of concern to children. Box 39.1 describes suggestions for incorporating play into nursing procedures and activities for the hospitalized child that facilitate learning and adjustment to a new situation.

Preparing the Family

The process of patient education involves giving the family information about the child's condition, the regimen that must be followed and why, and other health teaching as indicated. The goal of this education is to enable the family to modify behaviors and adhere to the regimen that has been mutually established (see Guidelines box: General Principles of Family Education).

If equipment will be needed at home (e.g., suction machines, syringes), begin making the necessary arrangements in advance so that discharge can proceed smoothly. Whenever possible, make arrangements for the family to use the same equipment in the home that they are using in the hospital. This allows them to become familiar with the items. In addition, the staff can help troubleshoot the equipment in a controlled environment. Plan the teaching sessions well in advance of the time the family will be responsible for performing the care. The more complex the procedure, the more time is needed for training.

Review the instructions with family members (see Guidelines box: Family Preparation for Procedures). Encourage note taking if they desire. Allow ample practice time under supervision. At least one family member, but preferably two members, should demonstrate the procedure before they are expected to care for the child at home. Provide the family with

GUIDELINES
General Principles of Family Education

- Establish a rapport with the family.
- Avoid using any specialized terms or jargon. Clarify all terms with the family.
- When possible, allow family members to decide how they want to be taught (e.g., all at once or over 1 or 2 days). This gives the family a chance to incorporate the information at a rate that is comfortable.
- Provide accurate information to the family about the illness.
- Assist family members in identifying obstacles to their ability to comply with the regimen and in identifying the means to overcome those obstacles. Then help family members find ways to incorporate the plan into their daily lives.

GUIDELINES
Family Preparation for Procedures

Family education for specific procedures is included throughout this unit. General concepts applicable to most family education sessions include the following:
- Name of the procedure
- Purpose of the procedure
- Length of time anticipated to complete the procedure
- Anticipated effects
- Signs of adverse effects
- Assess the family's level of understanding
- Demonstrate and have family return demonstration (if appropriate)

the telephone numbers of resource individuals who are available to assist them in the event of a problem.

SURGICAL PROCEDURES

Preoperative Care

Children experiencing surgical procedures require both psychologic and physical preparation. An important concern is restriction of food and fluids before surgery to avoid aspiration during anesthesia. Infants require special attention to fluid needs. They should not be without oral fluids for an extended period preoperatively to avoid glycogen depletion and dehydration. Table 39.2 contains current preoperative fasting guidelines.

In general, psychologic preparation is similar to that discussed earlier for any procedure and uses many of the same techniques used in preparing a child for hospitalization, such as films, books, brochures, play, and tours. Stress points before and after surgery include the admission process, blood tests, injection of preoperative medication (if prescribed), transport to the operating room, the mask on the face during induction, and the stay in the postanesthesia care unit (PACU). Wearing a hospital gown without the security of underpants or pajama bottoms can also be traumatic. Therefore, these articles of clothing should be worn into the operating room and removed after induction of anesthesia. Children are at higher risk for ineffective response to anesthesia because of higher anxiety associated with stranger anxiety (infants), separation anxiety (toddlers and preschoolers), and fear of injury or death (adolescents) (Romino, Keatley, Secrest, et al., 2005).

Psychologic intervention consisting of systematic preparation, rehearsal of the forthcoming events, and supportive care at each of these points has shown to be more effective than a single-session

---

BOX 39.1   Play Activities for Specific Procedures

Fluid Intake

Make ice pops using child's favorite juice.

Cut gelatin into fun shapes.

Make a game out of taking a sip when turning page of a book or in games, such as Simon Says.

Use small medicine cups; decorate the cups.

Color water with food coloring or powdered drink mix.

Have a tea party; pour at a small table.

Let child fill a syringe and squirt it into mouth, or use it to fill small decorated cups.

Cut straws in half, and place in a small container (much easier for child to suck liquid).

Use a "crazy" straw.

Make a "progress poster;" give rewards for drinking a predetermined quantity.

Deep Breathing

Blow bubbles with a bubble blower.

Blow bubbles with a straw (no soap).

Blow on a pinwheel, feather, whistle, harmonica, balloon, or party blower.

Practice band instruments.

Have a blowing contest using balloons,* boats, cotton balls, feathers, marbles, ping-pong balls, or pieces of paper; blow such objects on a tabletop over a goal line, over water, through an obstacle course, up in the air, against an opponent, or up and down a string.

Suck paper or cloth from one container to another using a straw.

Dramatize stories, such as "I'll huff and puff and blow your house down" from the "Three Little Pigs."

Do straw-blowing painting.

Take a deep breath and "blow out the candles" on a birthday cake.

Use a little paint brush to "paint" nails with water and blow nails dry.

Range of Motion and Use of Extremities

Throw beanbags at a fixed or movable target, or throw wadded-up paper into a wastebasket.

Touch or kick Mylar balloons held or hung in different positions (if child is in traction, hang balloon from a trapeze).

Play "tickle toes;" have the child wiggle them on request.

Play Twister game or Simon Says.

Play pretend and guessing games (e.g., imitate a bird, butterfly, or horse).

Have tricycle or wheelchair races in a safe area.

Play kickball or throw ball with a soft foam ball in a safe area.

Position bed so that child must turn to view television or doorway.

Climb wall with fingers like a "spider."

Pretend to teach aerobic dancing or exercises; encourage parents to participate.

Encourage swimming if feasible.

Play video games or pinball (fine motor movement).

Play hide and seek: hide toy somewhere in bed (or room if ambulatory), and have child find it using specified hand or foot.

Provide clay to mold with fingers.

Paint or draw on large sheets of paper placed on floor or wall.

Encourage combing own hair; play "beauty shop" with "customer" in different positions.

Soaks

Play with small toys or objects (cups, syringes, soap dishes) in water.

Wash dolls or toys.

Pick up marbles or pennies* from bottom of bath container.

Make designs with coins on bottom of container.

Pretend a boat is a submarine by keeping it immersed.

Read to child during soaks; sing with child; or play game, such as cards, checkers, or other board game (if both hands are immersed, move board pieces for child).

Sitz bath: Give child something to listen to (music, stories) or look at (View-Master, book).

Punch holes in bottom of plastic cup, fill with water, and let it "rain" on child.

Injections

Let child handle syringe, vial, and alcohol swab and give an injection to doll or stuffed animal.

Draw a "magic circle" on area before injection; draw smiling face in circle after injection but avoid drawing on puncture site.

If multiple injections or venipunctures are planned, make a "progress poster;" give rewards for predetermined number of injections.

Have child count to 10 or 15 during injection.

Ambulation

Give child something to push:
- Toddler: Push-pull toy
- School-age child: Wagon or a doll in a stroller or wheelchair
- Adolescent: Decorated intravenous (IV) stand

Have a parade; make hats, drums, and so on.

Extending Environment (e.g., for Patients in Traction)

Make bed into a pirate ship or airplane with decorations.

Put up mirrors so that patient can see around room.

Move bed frequently to playroom, hallway, or outside.

*Small objects such as marbles and coins, as well as gloves and balloons, are unsafe for young children because of possible aspiration. Latex products also carry the risk for an allergic reaction.

---

preparation or consistent supportive care without systematic preparation and rehearsal (Kain, Caldwell-Andrews, Mayes, et al., 2007). A family-centered preoperative preparation program may consist of a tour of the perioperative areas with short explanations of the events 5 to 7 days before surgery, a video to take home and review a couple of times with additional explanations and demonstrations of perioperative processes, a mask to take home and practice with, pamphlets to guide parents on supporting children during induction, phone calls to coach parents on preparing children 1 or 2 days before surgery, and toys and supplies in the holding area. Therapeutic play is an effective strategy in preparing children, and increased familiarity with medical procedures decreases anxiety (Li, Lopez, & Lee, 2007).

Parental Presence

Some institutions support parental presence during induction of anesthesia. According to research conducted by Kain and colleagues (2007), benefits of well-prepared children and parents along with parental presence during induction of anesthesia include reduced anxiety for children and parents, lower doses of postoperative analgesia, lower incidence of severe emergence delirium symptoms, and shorter discharge time for short procedures. Other studies have not supported a reduction in children's anxiety (Yip, Middleton, Cyna, et al., 2009).

Concern exists regarding the appropriateness of parental presence during induction for all parents. Some parents may become upset by

TABLE 39.2 Fasting Recommendations to Reduce the Risk for Pulmonary Aspiration*

Ingested Material	Minimum Fasting Period (Hours)[†]
Clear liquids[‡]	>2
Breast milk	4
Infant formula	6
Nonhuman milk[§]	6
Light meal[‖]	6

From American Society of Anesthesiologists. (1999). Practice guidelines for preoperative fasting and the use of pharmacologic agents to reduce the risk of pulmonary aspiration: application to healthy patients undergoing elective procedures. *Anesthesiology, 90*(3), 896–905.

*These recommendations apply to healthy patients who are undergoing elective procedures. They are not intended for women in labor. Following the guidelines does not guarantee that complete gastric emptying has occurred.

[†]Fasting periods noted in chart apply to all ages.

[‡]Examples of clear liquids include water, fruit juices without pulp, carbonated beverages, clear tea, and black coffee.

[§]Because nonhuman milk is similar to solids in gastric emptying time, the amount ingested must be considered when determining appropriate fasting period.

[‖]A light meal typically consists of toast and clear liquids. Meals that include fried or fatty foods or meat may prolong gastric emptying time. Both the amount and type of foods ingested must be considered when determining an appropriate fasting period.

the rapid succession of induction events, by observing their child becoming limp, and by leaving the child in the care of strangers. Even though some parents may become anxious, most control their anxiety, do not disrupt the induction, and support the child. Whereas parents who are anxious before surgery tend to become even more anxious after the induction, the reverse is true of parents with little anxiety. Appropriate education is essential to help parents understand the stages of anesthesia, what to expect, and how to support their child.

Preoperative Sedation

The goals for using preoperative medications include anxiety reduction, amnesia, sedation, antiemetic effect, and reduction of secretions. When drugs are administered, they should be delivered atraumatically via oral, intranasal, or IV routes. Numerous preanesthetic drug regimens are used with children, and no consensus exists on the optimal method.

Postoperative Care

Various psychologic and physical interventions and observations help prevent or minimize possible unpleasant effects from anesthesia and the surgical procedure. Although the incidence of serious postoperative complications in healthy children undergoing surgery is less than 1% (Maxwell & Yaster, 2000), continuous monitoring of the child's cardiopulmonary status is essential during the immediate postoperative period. Postanesthesia complications such as airway obstruction, postextubation croup, laryngospasm, and bronchospasm make maintaining a patent airway and maximum ventilation critical.

Monitoring the patient's oxygen saturation and providing supplemental oxygen as needed, maintaining body temperature, and promoting fluid and electrolyte balance are important aspects of immediate postoperative care. Vital signs are continuously monitored, and each vital sign is evaluated in terms of side effects from anesthesia, shock, or respiratory compromise (Table 39.3).

A change in vital signs that demands immediate attention in the perioperative period is caused by malignant hyperthermia (MH), a potentially fatal pharmacogenetic disorder involving a defective calcium channel in the sarcoplasmic reticulum membrane. In susceptible children, inhaled anesthetics and the muscle relaxant succinylcholine trigger the disorder, producing hypermetabolism. Symptoms of MH include hypercarbia (increasing end-tidal carbon dioxide [$ETCO_2$]), elevated temperature, tachycardia, tachypnea, acidosis, muscle rigidity, and rhabdomyolysis (Rosenberg, Davis, & James, 2007). A family or previous history of sudden high fever associated with a surgical procedure and myotonia increase the risk for MH. Children who have successfully undergone prior surgery without adverse effects may still be considered susceptible.

Treatment of MH includes immediate discontinuation of the triggering agent, hyperventilation with 100% oxygen, and IV dantrolene sodium. If the child is hyperthermic, initiate cooling measures, such as ice packs to the groin, axillae, and neck and iced nasogastric (NG) lavage. The surgery may be discontinued or if it is emergent, it may be continued with a different anesthetic agent. The patient should be transferred to an intensive care unit for at least 36 hours and is closely monitored for stabilization of vital signs, metabolic state, and possible recurrence of symptoms.

Managing pain is a major nursing responsibility after surgery. The nurse should assess pain frequently and administers analgesics to provide comfort and facilitate cooperation with postoperative care, such as ambulation and deep breathing. Opioids are the most commonly used analgesics. Routinely scheduled IV analgesics, patient-controlled analgesia, and epidural infusions, rather than as-needed orders, provide excellent analgesia in postoperative pediatric patients.

Because respiratory tract infections are a potential complication of anesthesia, make every effort to aerate the lungs and remove secretions. The lungs are auscultated regularly to identify abnormal sounds or any areas of diminished or absent breath sounds. To prevent pneumonia, encourage respiratory movement with incentive spirometers or other motivating activities. If these measures are presented as games, the child is more likely to comply. The child's position is changed every 2 hours, and deep breathing is encouraged.

! NURSING ALERT

Because deep breathing is usually painful after surgery, be certain that the child has received analgesics. Have the child splint the operative site (depending on its location) by hugging a small pillow or a favorite stuffed animal.

During the recovery period, spend some time with the child to assess his or her perceptions of surgery. Play, drawing, and storytelling are excellent methods of discovering the child's thoughts. With such information, the nurse can support or correct the child's perceptions and boost his or her self-esteem for having endured a stressful procedure.

Many pediatric patients are discharged shortly after surgery. Preparation for discharge begins with the preadmission preparation visit. The nurse should discuss instructions for postoperative care and review them throughout the perioperative visit. After discharge, the nursing staff often makes phone calls to check the patient's status. Patient education and compliance with discharge instructions can also be assessed during these phone calls (see Guidelines box: Postoperative Care).

COMPLIANCE

Compliance, also termed *adherence,* refers to the extent to which the patient's behavior coincides with the prescribed regimen in terms of

TABLE 39.3 Potential Causes of Postoperative Vital Sign Alterations in Children

Alteration	Potential Cause	Comments
Heart Rate		
Increase	Decreased perfusion (shock)	Heart rate may increase to maintain cardiac output.
	Elevated temperature	
	Pain	
	Respiratory distress (early)	
	Medications (atropine, morphine, epinephrine)	
Decrease	Hypoxia	Bradycardia is of more concern in young child than tachycardia.
	Vagal stimulation	
	Increased intracranial pressure	
	Respiratory distress (late)	
	Medications (neostigmine [Prostigmin Bromide])	
Respiratory Rate		
Increase	Respiratory distress	Body responds to respiratory distress primarily by increasing rate.
	Fluid volume excess	
	Hypothermia	
	Elevated temperature	
	Pain	
Decrease	Anesthetics, opioids	Decreased respiratory rate from opioids may be compensated for
	Pain	by increased depth of respiration.
Blood Pressure		
Increase	Excess intravascular volume	This is serious in premature infants because it increases risk for
	Increased intracranial pressure	intraventricular hemorrhage.
	Carbon dioxide retention	
	Pain	
	Medication (ketamine, epinephrine)	
Decrease	Vasodilating anesthetic agents (halothane, isoflurane, enflurane)	Decreased blood pressure is late sign of shock because of
	Opioids (e.g., morphine)	elasticity and constriction of vessels to maintain cardiac output.
Temperature		
Increase	Shock (late sign)	Fever associated with infection usually occurs later than fever of
	Infection	noninfectious origin. Absence of fever does not rule out
	Environmental causes (warm room, excess coverings)	infection, especially in infants.
	Malignant hyperthermia	Malignant hyperthermia requires immediate treatment.
Decrease	Vasodilating anesthetic agents (halothane, isoflurane, enflurane)	Neonates are especially susceptible to hypothermia, with serious
	Muscle relaxants	or fatal consequences.
	Environmental causes (cool room)	
	Infusion of cool fluids or blood	

From Smith, D.P. (1991). *Comprehensive child and family nursing skills*. St. Louis, MO: Mosby.

taking medication, following diets, or executing other lifestyle changes. In developing strategies to improve compliance, the nurse must first assess level of compliance. Because many children are too young to assume partial or total responsibility for their care, parents are usually primarily responsible for home management.

Factors relating to the care setting are important in ensuring compliance and should be considered in planning strategies to improve compliance. Basically, any aspect of the health care setting that increases the family's satisfaction with the physical setting and the relationship with the practitioner positively influences adherence to the treatment regimen. However, the more complex, expensive, inconvenient, and disruptive the treatment protocol, the less likely the family is to comply. During long-term conditions that involve multiple treatments and considerable rearrangement of lifestyle, compliance is severely affected.

Although it is helpful to know those factors that influence compliance, assessment must include more direct measurement techniques. A number of methods exist, each with advantages and disadvantages. The most

successful approach includes a combination of at least two of the following methods:

Clinical judgment: This is subject to bias and inaccuracy unless the nurse carefully evaluates the criteria used in assessment.

Self-reporting: Most people overestimate their compliance by about 20% even when they admit to lapses.

Direct observation: This is difficult to use outside the health care setting, and awareness of being observed frequently affects performance.

Monitoring appointments: Keeping appointments indirectly indicates compliance with the prescribed care.

Monitoring therapeutic response: Few treatments yield directly measurable results (e.g., decreased blood pressure, weight loss); record on a graph or chart.

Pill counts: The nurse counts the number of pills remaining in the original container and compares the number missing with the number of times the medication should have been taken. Although this is a simple method, families may forget to bring the container or

GUIDELINES
Postoperative Care

- Ensure that preparations are made to receive child:
  - Bed or crib is ready.
  - Intravenous (IV) pumps and poles, suction apparatus, and oxygen flow meter are at bedside.
- Obtain baseline information:
  - Take vital signs, including blood pressure; keep blood pressure cuff in place and deflated to lessen disturbance to child.
  - Take and record vital signs more frequently if any value fluctuates.
  - Inspect operative area.
- Check dressing if present.
  - Outline any bleeding area on dressing or cast with pen.
  - Reinforce, but do not remove, loose dressing.
  - Observe areas below surgical site for blood that may have drained toward bed.
  - Assess for bleeding and other symptoms in areas not covered with a dressing, such as throat after tonsillectomy.
- Assess skin color and characteristics.
- Assess level of consciousness and activity.
- Notify primary care provider of any irregularities in child's condition.
- Assess for evidence of pain.
- Review surgeon's orders after completing initial assessment, and check that preoperative orders, such as seizure or cardiac medications, have been reordered and can be given by available routes (oral preparations may be contraindicated).
- Monitor vital signs as ordered and more often if indicated.
- Check dressings for bleeding or other abnormalities.
- Check bowel sounds.
- Observe for signs of shock, abdominal distention, and bleeding.
- Assess for bladder distention.
- Observe for signs of dehydration.
- Detect presence of infection:
  - Take vital signs every 2 to 4 hours as ordered.
  - Collect or request needed specimens.
  - Inspect wound for signs of infection: redness, swelling, heat, pain, and purulent drainage.

deliberately alter the number of pills to avoid detection. This method is also poorly suited to liquid medication. Another technique is the use of pill container caps that record every opening as a presumptive dose.

Chemical assay: For certain drugs, such as digoxin, measurement of plasma drug levels provides information on the amount of drug recently ingested. However, this method is expensive, indicates only short-term compliance, and requires precise timing of the assay for accurate results.

Compliance Strategies

Strategies to improve compliance involve interventions that encourage families to follow the prescribed treatment regimen. Some evidence suggests that higher levels of self-esteem and increased autonomy favorably affect adolescent compliance (KyngAs, Kroll, & Duffy, 2000). However, family factors are important, and characteristics associated with good compliance include family support, family reminders, good communication, and expectations for successful completion of the therapeutic regimen. No one approach is always successful, and the best results occur when at least two strategies are used.

Organizational **strategies** involve the care setting and the therapeutic plan. This may involve increasing the frequency of appointments, designating a primary practitioner, reducing the cost of medication by prescribing generic brands, reducing the treatment's disruption of the family's lifestyle, and using "cues" to minimize forgetting. Numerous devices are available commercially or can be improvised for cueing, such as pill dispensers, watches with alarms, charts to record completed therapy, messages on the refrigerator or morning coffee pot, and treatment schedules that incorporate the treatment plan into the daily routine (e.g., physical therapy after the evening bath).

The nurse instructs the family about the treatment plan. Although education is an important factor in enhancing compliance and patients who are more knowledgeable about their condition are more likely to comply, education alone does not ensure compliant behavior. The nurse should incorporate teaching principles known to enhance understanding and retention of material. Written materials are essential, especially in any regimen requiring multiple or complex treatments, and they need to be understandable to the average individual, who reads at about the fourth-grade level. Involvement of the immediate and extended family (e.g., grandparents) in education sessions may enhance compliance.

Treatment strategies relate to the child's refusal or inability to take the prescribed medication. The family may also have difficulty following a prescribed treatment regimen. They may remember and understand the instructions but may not be able to give the medicine as prescribed. Assess the reason for refusal. For example, the child may not be able to swallow pills. In this case, perhaps pills could be crushed or a liquid medication substituted (always review medication to ensure that crushing is acceptable before giving this instruction).

Assess the treatment and medication schedule to determine whether it is reasonable for a home situation. Although an every-6-hour or every-8-hour schedule is reasonable for hospitals, a parent would have difficulty getting up once or twice nightly. Instead the patient could take a medication during the day at times that would be easy to remember.

Behavioral strategies are designed to modify behavior directly. Nurses can use several effective strategies with children to encourage the desired behavior. Positive reinforcement is one strategy that strengthens the behavior. One example of this is the child earning stars or tokens, which can be exchanged for a special privilege or gift. At times, however, disciplinary techniques, such as time-out for young children or withholding privileges for older children, may be needed to improve compliance.

SKIN CARE AND GENERAL HYGIENE

MAINTAINING HEALTHY SKIN

Maintaining an IV line, removing a dressing, positioning a child in bed, changing a diaper, using electrodes, or using restraints have the potential to contribute to skin injury. General guidelines for skin care are listed in the Guidelines box: Skin Care.

Assessment of the skin is easiest to accomplish during the bath. Examine for early signs of injury. Risk factors include impaired mobility, protein malnutrition, edema, incontinence, sensory loss, anemia, infection, failure to turn the patient, and intubation. Critically ill children are at a higher risk for pressure ulcers and skin breakdown, because they often have several risk factors combined. The incidence in these children has been reported as high as 27% (Curley, Quigley, & Lin, 2003). Identification of risk factors helps to determine children who need a more thorough skin assessment. Several risk assessment scales are available for use in pediatrics, such as the Braden Q Scale (Curley, Razmus, Roberts, et al., 2003) and the Glamorgan Scale (Willock, Baharestani, & Anthony, 2009). Assessment should occur within 24 hours of admission to identify pressure ulcers and wounds that occurred before admission.

GUIDELINES

Skin Care

- Keep skin free of excess moisture (e.g., urine or fecal incontinence, wound drainage, excessive perspiration).
- Cleanse skin with mild nonalkaline soap or soap-free cleansing agents for routine bathing.
- Provide daily cleansing of eyes, oral and diaper or perineal areas, and any areas of skin breakdown.
- Apply non–alcohol-based moisturizing agents after cleansing to retain moisture and rehydrate skin.
- Use minimum amount of tape and adhesives. On very sensitive skin, use a protective, pectin-based or hydrocolloid skin barrier between skin and tape or adhesives.
- Place pectin-based or hydrocolloid skin barriers directly over excoriated skin. Leave barrier undisturbed until it begins to peel off or for 5 to 7 days. With wet, oozing excoriations, place a small amount of stoma powder on site, remove excess powder, and apply skin barrier. Hold barrier in place for several minutes to allow barrier to soften and mold to skin surface.
- Alternate electrode and probe placement sites, and thoroughly assess underlying skin typically every 8 to 24 hours.
- Eliminate pressure secondary to medical devices such as tracheostomy tubes, wheelchairs, braces, and gastrostomy tubes.
- Be certain fingers or toes are visible whenever extremity is used for intravenous (IV) or arterial line.
- Use a draw sheet to move child in bed or onto a stretcher; do not drag child from under the arms.
- Position in neutral alignment; pillows, cushions, or wedges may be needed to prevent hip abduction and pressure to bony prominences, such as heels, elbows, and sacral and occipital areas. When child is positioned laterally, pillows or cushions between the knees, under the head, and under the upper arm will help promote neutral body alignment. Avoid donut cushions because they can cause tissue ischemia. Elevate the head of the bed 30 degrees or less to reduce pressure unless contraindicated.
- Do not massage reddened bony prominences because this can cause deep tissue damage; provide pressure relief to those areas instead.
- Routinely assess the child's nutritional status. A child who is not permitted to take fluids by mouth (nothing by mouth [NPO]) for several days and is receiving only IV fluid is nutritionally at risk, which can also affect the skin's ability to maintain its integrity. Consider parenteral nutrition.

When capillary blood flow is interrupted by pressure, the blood flows back into the tissue when the pressure is relieved. As the body attempts to reoxygenate the area, a bright red flush appears. This *reactive hyperemia,* or flush, is the earliest sign of tissue compromise and pressure-related ischemia. If pressure is prolonged, reactive hyperemia will not be sufficient to revitalize ischemic tissue. Pressure ulcers can develop when the pressure on the skin and underlying tissues is greater than the capillary closing pressure, causing capillary occlusion. If the pressure remains unrelieved, vessels can collapse, resulting in tissue anoxia and cellular death. Pressure ulcers most often occur over bony prominences. These lesions are usually very deep (stage IV), extending into subcutaneous tissue or even more deeply into muscle, tendon, or bone.

Pressure ulcers are staged to classify the amount of tissue damage that has occurred.* Necrotic tissue must be removed so the tissue depth

---

*Staging of pressure ulcers and guidelines for prevention and management of pressure ulcers are available from the National Pressure Ulcer Advisory Panel, www.npuap.org.

can accurately be assessed. Accurate documentation of redness or obvious skin breakdown is essential. Color, size (diameter and depth), location, presence of sinus tracts, odor, exudate, and response to treatment are observed and recorded at least daily.

Pressure ulcers in children typically occur on the occiput, ears, sacrum, and scapula (Amlung, Miller, & Bosley, 2001); the heels and sacrum are common sites in adults. Critically ill children are at a higher risk for pressure ulcers and skin breakdown, because they often have several risk factors combined. Although pressure ulcers in hospitalized children are generally uncommon with reported rates of 1% to 13% (Noonan, Quigley, & Curley, 2006), the incidence in critically ill children has been reported as high as 27% (Curley, Quigley, & Lin, 2003). In a multisite study, risk factors associated with pressure ulcers in pediatric intensive care unit patients included 2 years of age and younger, length of stay 4 or more days, and ventilatory support (Schindler, Mikhailov, Kuhn, et al., 2011). Interventions found to prevent pressure ulcers in critically ill children include the following:

- Turning children every 2 hours
- Using pillows, blanket rolls, and positioning devices
- Draw sheets to minimize shear
- Utilization of pressure reduction surfaces (foam overlays, gel pads, specialty beds)
- Moisture reduction through the use of dry-weave diapers and disposable underpads
- Skin moisturizer
- Nutrition consults

Medical devices such as pulse oximeter probes, bilevel and continuous positive airway pressure masks, oxygen cannulas, orthotics, and casts can also cause pressure ulcers.

Friction and shear contribute to pressure ulcers. **Friction** occurs when the surface of the skin rubs against another surface, such as bed sheets. The skin may have the appearance of an abrasion. The skin damage is usually limited to the epidermal and upper layers. It most often occurs over the elbows, heels, or occiput. Prevention of friction injury includes the use of customized splinting over infants' heels; gel pillows under the heads of infants and toddlers; moisturizing agents; transparent dressings over susceptible areas; and soft, smooth bed linens and clothing (Baharestani & Ratliff, 2007). By itself, friction does not cause tissue necrosis, but when it acts with gravity, it results in shear injury.

Shear is the result of the force of gravity pushing down on the body and friction of the body against a surface, such as the bed or chair. For example, when a patient is in the semi-Fowler's position and begins to slide to the foot of the bed, the skin over the sacral area remains in the same place because of the resistance of the bed surface. The blood vessels in the area are stretched and may cause small-vessel thrombosis and tissue death. Prevention of shear injury includes using lift sheets when repositioning a patient, elevating the bed no more than 30 degrees for short periods, and using the knee gatch to interrupt the pull of gravity on the body toward the foot of the bed.

Epidermal stripping results when the epidermis is unintentionally removed when tape is removed. These lesions are usually shallow and irregularly shaped. Infants are at increased risk for epidermal injury. Prevention includes using no tape when possible and securing dressings with laced binders (Montgomery straps) or stretchy netting (Spandage or stockinette). Using porous or low-tack tapes (e.g., Medipore, paper, hydrogel), using alcohol-free skin sealants (No Sting Barrier Film), or picture framing wounds with hydrocolloid or wafer barriers (e.g., DuoDERM, Coloplast, Stomahesive) and then taping on top of the barrier also will reduce epidermal stripping.

Tape is placed so that there is no tension, traction, or wrinkles on the skin. To remove tape, slowly peel the tape away while stabilizing the underlying skin. Adhesive remover may be used to break the adhesive bond but may be drying to the skin. Avoid adhesive removers in preterm neonates because absorption rates vary and toxicity may occur. Remove the adhesive with water to prevent absorption and irritation. Wetting the tape with water or alcohol-based foam hand cleansers may facilitate removal.

Chemical factors can also lead to skin damage. Fecal incontinence, especially when mixed with urine; wound drainage; or gastric drainage around gastrostomy tubes can erode the epidermis. The skin can quickly progress from redness to denudement if exposure continues. Moisture barriers, gentle cleansing as soon after exposure as possible, and skin barriers can be used to prevent damage caused by chemical factors. In addition, foam dressings that wick moisture away from the skin are helpful around gastrostomy tubes and tracheostomy sites.

BATHING

Most infants and children can be bathed at the bedside or in a standard bathtub or shower. For infants and young children confined to bed, use commercially available bath cloths or the towel method. Immerse two towels in a dilute soap solution, and wring them damp. With the child lying supine on a dry towel, place one damp towel on top of the child and use it to gently clean the body. Discard the towel and dry the child and turn him or her prone. Repeat the procedure using the second damp towel. If bar soap is used, discard the basin and bar soap after a single bath (Marchaim, Taylor, Hayakawa, et al., 2012), because they can serve as a reservoir for pathogens in the hospital setting. Chlorhexidine is much less likely to harbor microbes (Powers, Peed, Burns, et al., 2012; Rupp, Huerta, Yu, et al., 2013), but it is generally not approved for use in infants younger than 2 months corrected gestational age.

Infants and small children are never left unattended in a bathtub, and infants who are unable to sit alone are securely held with one hand during the bath. The nurse securely supports the infant's head with one hand or grasps the infant's farther arm while the head rests comfortably on the nurse's arm. Children who are able to sit without assistance need only close supervision and a pad placed in the bottom of the tub to prevent slipping and loss of balance.

School-age children and adolescents may shower or bathe. Nurses need to use judgment regarding the amount of supervision the child requires. Some can assume this responsibility unaided, but others need someone in constant attendance. Children with cognitive impairments, physical limitations such as severe anemia or leg deformities, or suicidal or psychotic problems (who may commit bodily harm) require close supervision.

Areas that require special attention are the ears, between skinfolds, the neck, the back, and the genital area. The genital area should be carefully cleansed and dried, with particular care given to skinfolds. In uncircumcised boys, usually those older than 3 years of age, the foreskin should be gently retracted, the exposed surfaces cleansed, and the foreskin then replaced. If the condition of the glans indicates inadequate cleaning, such as accumulated smegma, inflammation, phimosis, or foreskin adhesions, teaching proper hygiene is indicated. In the Vietnamese and Cambodian cultures, the foreskin is traditionally not retracted until adulthood. Older children have a tendency to avoid cleaning the genitalia; therefore, they may need a gentle reminder.

ORAL HYGIENE

Mouth care is an integral part of daily hygiene and should be continued in the hospital. For some young children, this is their first introduction to the use of a toothbrush. Infants and debilitated children require the nurse or a family member to perform mouth care. Although young children can manage a toothbrush and are encouraged to use it, most need assistance to perform satisfactorily. Older children, although capable of brushing and flossing without assistance, sometimes need to be reminded.

HAIR CARE

Children should have their hair brushed and combed at least once daily. The hair is styled for comfort and in a manner pleasing to the child and parents. The hair should not be cut without parental permission, although clipping hair to provide access to a scalp vein for IV insertion may be necessary.

If children are hospitalized for more than a few days, the hair may need shampooing. With infants, the hair may be washed during the daily bath or less frequently. For most children, washing the hair and scalp once or twice weekly is sufficient unless there is an indication for more frequent washing, such as after a high fever and profuse sweating. Adolescents normally have increased oily sebaceous secretions that require frequent hair care and more frequent shampoos.

Almost any child can be transported to an accessible sink for shampooing. Those who are unable to be transported can receive a shampoo in their beds with adequate protection, specially adapted equipment or positioning, or dry shampoo caps. When necessary, a shampoo basin may be used or the child may be positioned near the edge of the bed, towels placed under the shoulders, a large plastic garbage bag draped at the edge of the bed with one open end under the shoulders, and the hair placed inside the opening. The other end is opened and placed in a collection container. Water can be transported in a basin.

For African-American children with curly hair, most standard combs are inadequate and may cause hair breakage and discomfort. Use a special comb with widely spaced teeth. It is also much easier to comb the hair after shampooing when it is wet. Use a special hair dressing or pomade, which usually has a coconut oil base. Rub the preparation on the hands, and then transfer it to the hair to make it more pliable and manageable. Consult the child's parents regarding the preparation to use on the child's hair, and ask if they can provide some for use during the child's hospitalization. Petroleum jelly should not be used. If braiding or plaiting the hair, weave it loosely while the hair is damp. The hair tightens as it dries, which could result in tension folliculitis.

FEEDING THE SICK CHILD

Loss of appetite is a symptom common to most childhood illnesses. Because an acute illness is usually short, the nutritional state is seldom compromised. Urging food on the sick child may precipitate nausea and vomiting. In most cases, children can usually determine their own need for food.

Refusing to eat may also be one way children can exert power and control in an otherwise helpless situation. For young children, loss of appetite may be related to depression caused by separation from their parents. Parents' concern with eating can intensify the problem. Forcing a child to eat meets with rebellion and reinforces the behavior as a control mechanism. Encourage parents to relax any pressure during an acute illness. Although it is best to provide high-quality nutritious foods, the child may desire foods and liquids that contain mostly empty or non-nutritional calories. Some well-tolerated foods include gelatin, diluted clear soups, carbonated drinks, flavored ice pops, dry toast, and crackers. Even though these substances are not nutritious, they can provide necessary fluid and calories.

Dehydration is always a hazard when children have a fever or anorexia, especially when accompanied by vomiting or diarrhea. Fluids should not be forced, and the child is not awakened to take fluids. Forcing

GUIDELINES
Feeding a Sick Child

Take a dietary history and use information to make eating time as similar to eating at home as possible.

Encourage parents or other family members to feed child or to be present at mealtimes.

Make mealtimes pleasant; avoid any procedures immediately before or after eating; make certain child is rested and pain free.

Serve small, frequent meals rather than three large meals, or serve three meals and nutritious between-meal snacks.

Provide finger foods for young children.

Involve children in food selection and preparation whenever possible.

Serve small portions, and serve each course separately, such as soup first followed by meat, potatoes, and vegetables and ending with dessert. With young children, camouflage size of food by cutting meat thicker so less appears on plate or by folding a cheese slice in half. Offer second helpings.

Ensure a variety of foods, textures, and colors.

Provide food selections that are favorites of most children, such as peanut butter and jelly sandwiches, hot dogs, hamburgers, macaroni and cheese, pizza, spaghetti, tacos, fried chicken, corn, and fruit yogurt.

Avoid foods that are highly seasoned, have strong odors, or are all mixed together unless typical of cultural practices.

Provide fluid selections that are favorites of most children, such as fruit punch, cola, ginger ale, sweetened tea, flavored ice pops, sherbet, ice cream, milk, milkshakes, pudding, gelatin, clear broth, or creamed soups.

Offer nutritious snacks, such as frozen yogurt or pudding, ice cream, oatmeal or peanut butter cookies, hot cocoa, cheese slices, pieces of raw vegetable or fruit, and dried fruit or cereal.

Make food attractive and different; for example:
- Serve a "picnic lunch" in a paper bag.
- Pack food in a Chinese take-out container; decorate container.
- Put a "face" or a "flower" on a hamburger or sandwich with pieces of vegetable.
- Use a cookie cutter to shape a sandwich.
- Serve pudding, yogurt, or juice frozen as an ice pop.
- Make Slurpies or snow cones by pouring flavored syrup on crushed ice.
- Add food coloring to water or milk.
- Serve fluids through brightly colored or unusually shaped straws.
- Make "bowtie" sandwiches by cutting them in triangles and placing two points together.
- Slice sandwiches into "fingers."
- Grate mounds of cheese.
- Cut apples horizontally to make circles.
- Put a banana on a hot dog bun, and spread with peanut butter.
- Break uncooked spaghetti into toothpick lengths, and skewer cheese, cold meat, vegetables, or fruit chunks.

Praise children for what they do eat.

Do not punish children for not eating by removing their dessert or putting them to bed.

fluids may create the same difficulties as urging the child to eat unwanted food. Gentle persuasion with preferred beverages will usually meet with success. Using play techniques can also be effective (see Guidelines box: Feeding a Sick Child).

An understanding of children's feeding habits can also increase food consumption. For example, if children are given all their food at one time, they generally eat the dessert first. Likewise, if they are presented with large portions, they often push the food away because the amount overwhelms them. If young children are not supervised during mealtime, they tend to play with the food rather than eat it. Therefore, nurses should present food in the usual order, such as soup first followed by small portions of meat, potatoes, and vegetables and ending with dessert.

When the child is feeling better, appetite usually begins to improve. It is best to take advantage of any hungry period by serving high-quality foods and snacks. If the child still refuses to eat, offer nutritious fluids, such as prepared breakfast drinks. Parents can help by bringing in food items from home; especially if the family's cultural eating habits differ from the hospital food. A clinical dietitian may be consulted for alternative food choices.

When children are placed on special diets, such as clear liquids after surgery or during episodes of diarrhea, assessment of their intake and readiness to advance to more complex foods is essential.

Regardless of the type of diet, charting the amount consumed is an important nursing responsibility. Descriptions need to be detailed and accurate, such as "4 ounces of orange juice, one pancake, and 8 ounces of milk." Comments such as "ate well" or "ate poorly" are inadequate. Charting the percentage of the meal eaten is also inadequate unless food is measured before serving.

If the parents are involved in the child's care, encourage them to keep a list of everything the child eats. Using a premeasured cup for fluids ensures a more accurate estimate of intake. A comparison of the intake at each meal can isolate food deficiencies, such as insufficient intake of meat or vegetables. Behaviors associated with mealtime also identify possible factors influencing appetite. For example, the observation, "child eats well when with other children but plays with food if left alone in room" helps the nurse plan mealtime activities that stimulate the child's appetite.

Although sick children's appetites may be poor and not characteristic of their home eating habits, the hospital stay provides numerous opportunities for nurses to assess the family's knowledge of good nutrition and to implement teaching as needed to improve nutritional intake.

CONTROLLING ELEVATED TEMPERATURES

An elevated temperature, most frequently from fever but occasionally caused by hyperthermia, is one of the most common symptoms of illness in children. This manifestation is a great concern to parents. To facilitate an understanding of fever, the following terms are defined:

Set point: The temperature around which body temperature is regulated by a thermostat-like mechanism in the hypothalamus

Fever (hyperpyrexia): An elevation in set point such that body temperature is regulated at a higher level; may be arbitrarily defined as temperature above 38° C (100.4° F)

Hyperthermia: Body temperature exceeding the set point, which usually results from the body or external conditions creating more heat than the body can eliminate, such as in heat stroke, aspirin toxicity, seizures, or hyperthyroidism

Body temperature is regulated by a thermostat-like mechanism in the hypothalamus. This mechanism receives input from centrally and peripherally located receptors. When temperature changes occur, these receptors relay the information to the thermostat, which either increases or decreases heat production to maintain a constant set point temperature. However, during an infection, pyrogenic substances cause an increase in the body's normal set point, a process that is mediated by prostaglandins. Consequently, the hypothalamus increases heat production until the core temperature reaches the new set point.

During the fever (febrile) state, shivering and vasoconstriction generate and conserve heat during the chill phase of fever, raising central temperatures to the level of the new set point. The temperature reaches a plateau when it stabilizes in the higher range. When the temperature is greater than the set point or when the pyrogen is no longer present, a crisis, or defervescence, of the temperature occurs.

Most fevers in children are of brief duration with limited consequences and are viral in origin. However, children who appear very ill and neonates are at high risk for serious bacterial illness, such as urinary tract infection or bacteremia, and will likely receive a sepsis workup, antibiotics, and hospitalization (Sahib El-Radhi, Carroll, & Klein, 2009).

Fever has physiologic benefits, including increased white blood cell activity, interferon production and effectiveness, and antibody production and enhancement of some antibiotic effects (Considine & Brennan, 2007). Contrary to popular belief, neither the rise in temperature nor its response to antipyretics indicates the severity or etiology of the infection, which casts doubt on the value of using fever as a diagnostic or prognostic indicator.

Therapeutic Management

Treatment of elevated temperature depends on whether it is attributable to a fever or hyperthermia. Because the set point is normal in hyperthermia but increased in fever, different approaches must be used to lower body temperature successfully.

Fever

The principal reason for treating fever is the relief of discomfort. Relief measures include pharmacologic and environmental intervention. The most effective intervention is the use of antipyretics to lower the set point.

Antipyretics include acetaminophen, aspirin, and nonsteroidal antiinflammatory drugs (NSAIDs). Acetaminophen is the preferred drug. Aspirin should not be given to children because of its association in children with influenza virus or chickenpox and Reye syndrome. One nonprescription NSAID, ibuprofen, is approved for fever reduction in children as young as 6 months of age. The dosage is based on the initial temperature level: 5 mg/kg of body weight for temperatures less than 39.2°C (102.6°F) or 10 mg/kg for temperatures greater than 39.2°C. The recommended dosage for pain is 10 mg/kg every 6 to 8 hours, and the recommended maximum daily dose for pain and fever is 40 mg/kg. The duration of fever reduction is generally 6 to 8 hours and is longer with the higher dose.

The recommended doses of acetaminophen should never be exceeded. Acetaminophen should be given every 4 hours but no more than five times in 24 hours. Because body temperature normally decreases at night, three or four doses in 24 hours will control most fevers. The temperature is usually retaken 30 minutes after the antipyretic is given to assess its effect but should not be repeatedly measured. The child's level of discomfort is the best indication for continued treatment.

The nurse can use environmental measures to reduce fever if they are tolerated by the child and if they do not induce shivering. Shivering is the body's way of maintaining the elevated set point by producing heat. Compensatory shivering greatly increases metabolic requirements above those already caused by the fever.

Traditional cooling measures, such as wearing minimum clothing; exposing the skin to air; reducing room temperature; increasing air circulation; and applying cool, moist compresses to the skin (e.g., the forehead), are effective if used approximately 1 hour after an antipyretic is given so that the set point is lowered. Cooling procedures (e.g., sponging or tepid baths) are ineffective in treating febrile children (these measures are effective for hyperthermia) either when used alone or in combination with antipyretics, and they cause considerable discomfort (Axelrod, 2000).

Seizures associated with a fever occur in 3% to 4% of all children, usually in those between 6 months and 6 years of age. About 30% of children have subsequent febrile seizures; a younger age at onset and a family history of febrile seizures are associated with increased incidence of recurring episodes. Evidence does not support the use of antipyretic

drugs (Rosenbloom, Finkelstein, Adams-Webber, et al., 2013) or anticonvulsants to prevent a second febrile seizure; nursing interventions should focus on ways to provide care and comfort during a febrile illness. Simple febrile seizures lasting less than 10 minutes do not cause brain damage or other debilitating effects (Jones & Jacobsen, 2007; Sadleir & Scheffer, 2007).

Hyperthermia

Unlike in fever, antipyretics are of no value in hyperthermia because the set point is already normal. Consequently, cooling measures are used. Cool applications to the skin help reduce the core temperature. Cooled blood from the skin surface is conducted to inner organs and tissues, and warm blood is circulated to the surface, where it is cooled and recirculated. The surface blood vessels dilate as the body attempts to dissipate heat to the environment and facilitate this cooling process.

Commercial cooling devices, such as cooling blankets or mattresses, are available to reduce body temperature. Place the patient on the bed, and cover with a sheet or lightweight blanket. Frequent temperature monitoring is essential to prevent excessive cooling of the body.

Traditionally, cool compresses decrease high temperature. For tepid tub baths, it is usually best to start with warm water and gradually add cool water until the desired water temperature of 37°C (98.6°F) is reached to acclimate the child to the lower water temperature. Generally, the temperature of the water only has to be 1°C (or 2°F) less than the child's temperature to be effective. The child is placed directly in the tub of tepid water for 15 to 20 minutes while water is gently squeezed from a washcloth over the back and chest or gently sprayed over the body from a sprayer. In the bed or crib, cool washcloths or towels are used, exposing only one area of the body at a time. Continue sponging for approximately 20 minutes.

After the tub or sponge bath, the child is dried and dressed in lightweight pajamas, a nightgown, or a diaper and placed in a dry bed. The child is dried by gently rubbing the skin surface with a towel to stimulate circulation. The temperature is retaken 30 minutes after the tub or sponge bath. The tub or sponge bath should not be continued or restarted until the skin surface is warm or if the child feels chilled. Chilling causes vasoconstriction, which defeats the purpose of the cool applications. In this condition, little blood is carried to the skin surface; the blood remains primarily in the viscera to become heated.

Whether a temperature elevation in the critically ill child is caused by fever or hyperthermia, it should be treated aggressively. The metabolic rate increases 10% for every 1°C increase in temperature and three to five times during shivering, thus increasing oxygen, fluid, and caloric requirements. If the child's cardiovascular or neurologic system is already compromised, these increased needs are especially hazardous. In all children with an elevated temperature, attention to adequate hydration is essential. Most children's needs can be met through additional oral fluids.

Family Teaching and Home Care

Fever is one of the most common problems for which parents seek health care. High levels of parental anxiety (fever phobia) surrounding potential complications of fever (e.g., seizures and dehydration) are prevalent and can result in overusing antipyretics (Purssell, 2009). Parents need to know that sponging is indicated for elevated temperatures from hyperthermia rather than fever and that ice water and alcohol are inappropriate, potentially dangerous solutions (Axelrod, 2000). Parents should know how to take the child's temperature, how to read the thermometer accurately, and when to seek professional care (see Family-Centered Care box: The Child with Fever). Some of the newer temperature-measuring devices, such as plastic strip or digital thermometers, may be better suited for home use. If the use of acetaminophen or ibuprofen is indicated,

The Child With Fever

Call Office Immediately If:

Your child is younger than 2 months of age.

The fever is over 40.6° C (105° F).

Your child looks or acts very sick, including a stiff neck, persistent vomiting, purplish spots on the skin, confusion, trouble breathing after you have cleansed his or her nose, or inability to be comforted.

Call Within 24 Hours If:

The fever is between 40° and 40.6° C (104° and 105° F), especially if your child is younger than 2 years of age.

Your child has had a fever for more than 24 hours without an obvious cause or location of infection.

Your child has had a fever for more than 3 days.

Your child has burning or pain with urination.

Your child has a history of febrile seizures.

The fever went away for more than 24 hours and then returned.

You have other concerns or questions.

Modified from Schmitt, B.D. (1999). *Instructions for pediatric patients* (2nd ed.). Philadelphia, PA: Saunders.

the parents need instructions in administering the drug. Emphasize accuracy in both the amount of drug given and the time intervals at which the drug is administered. Along with reduced activity, encourage small, frequent sips of clear liquids. Dress the child in light clothing; use a light blanket for children who are cold or shivering (Walsh & Edwards, 2006).

SAFETY

Safety is an essential component of any patient's care, but children have special characteristics that require an even greater concern for safety. Because small children in the hospital are separated from their usual environment and do not possess the capacity for abstract thinking and reasoning, it is the responsibility of everyone who comes in contact with them to maintain protective measures throughout their hospital stay. Nurses need to understand the age level at which each child is operating and plan for safety accordingly.

Identification (ID) bands are particularly important for children. Infants and unconscious patients are unable to tell or respond to their names. Toddlers may answer to any name or to a nickname only. Older children may exchange places, give an erroneous name, or choose not to respond to their own names as a joke, unaware of the hazards of such practices.

ENVIRONMENTAL FACTORS

All of the environmental safety measures for the protection of adults apply to children, including good illumination, floors that are clear of fluid and objects that might contribute to falls, and nonskid surfaces in showers and tubs. All staff members should be familiar with the area-specific fire plan. Elevators and stairways should be made safe.

All windows should be secured. Window blind and curtain cords should be out of reach with split cords to prevent strangulation. Pacifiers should not be tied around the neck or attached to an infant by string.

Electrical equipment should be in good working order and used only by personnel familiar with its use. It should not be in contact with moisture or situated near tubs. Electrical outlets should have covers to

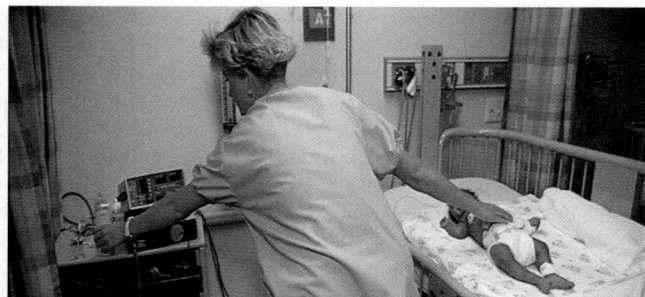

FIG 39.2 The nurse maintains hand contact when her back is turned.

prevent burns in small children, whose exploratory activities may extend to inserting objects into the small openings.

Staff members should practice proper care and disposal of small objects such as syringe caps, needle covers, and temperature probes. Staff also must carefully check bathwater before placing the child in it and never leave children alone in a bathtub. Infants are helpless in water, and small children (and some older ones) may turn on the hot water faucet and be severely burned.

Furniture is safest when it is scaled to the child's proportions, is sturdy, and is well balanced to prevent its being easily tipped over. A special hazard for children is the danger of entrapment under an electronically controlled bed when it is activated to descend. Infants and small children must be securely strapped into infant seats, feeding chairs, and strollers. Baby walkers should not be used because they provide access to hazards, resulting in burns, falls, and poisonings. Infants; young children; and children who are weak, paralyzed, agitated, confused, sedated, or cognitively impaired are never left unattended on treatment tables, on scales, or in treatment areas. Even premature infants are capable of surprising mobility; therefore, portholes in incubators must be securely fastened when not in use.

Crib sides up should always be raised and fastened securely. Use cribs that meet federal safety standards. Anyone attending an infant or small child on a stretcher or table should never turn away without maintaining hand contact with the child, that is, keeping one hand on the child's back or abdomen to prevent rolling, crawling, or jumping from the open crib (Fig. 39.2). A child who is likely to climb over the sides of the crib is safest when placed in a specially constructed crib with a cover over the top. Never tie nets to the movable crib sides or use knots that do not permit quick release.

The safest sleeping position to prevent sudden infant death syndrome is wholly supine (American Academy of Pediatrics, Task Force on Sudden Infant Death Syndrome, 2011). No pillows should be placed in a young infant's crib while the infant is sleeping. A firm sleep surface without soft bedding in a shared room (not a shared bed), and the avoidance of overheating, exposure to tobacco smoke, alcohol, and illicit drugs further increase the safety of an infant's sleeping environment.

Toys

Toys play a vital role in the everyday lives of children, and they are no less important in the hospital setting. Nurses are responsible for assessing the safety of toys brought to the hospital by well-meaning parents and friends. Toys should be appropriate to the child's age, condition, and treatment. For example, if the child is receiving oxygen, electrical or friction toys or equipment are not safe because sparks can cause oxygen to ignite. Inspect toys to ensure they are nonallergenic, washable, and unbreakable and that they have no small, removable parts that can be aspirated or swallowed or can otherwise inflict injury on a child. All objects within reach of children younger than 3 years of age should pass the choke tube test. A toilet paper roll is a handy guide. If a toy or object fits into the cylinder (items <1¼ inches across or balls <1¾ inches in diameter), it is a potential choking danger to the child. Latex balloons pose a serious threat to children of all ages. If the balloon breaks, a child may put a piece of the latex in his or her mouth. If it is aspirated or swallowed, the latex piece is difficult to remove, resulting in choking. Latex balloons should never be permitted in the hospital setting.

Preventing Falls

Falls prevention begins with identification of children most at risk for falls. Pediatric hospitals use various methods to identify a child's risk for falls (Child Health Corporation of America Nursing Falls Study Task Force, 2009). After a risk assessment is performed, multiple interventions are needed to minimize pediatric patients' risk for falling, including education of patient, family, and staff.

To identify children at risk for falling, perform a fall risk assessment on patients on admission and throughout hospitalization. Risk factors for hospitalized children include the following:

- Medication effects: Postanesthesia or sedation; analgesics or narcotics, especially in those who have never had narcotics in the past and in whom effects are unknown
- Altered mental status: Secondary to seizures, brain tumors, or medications
- Altered or limited mobility: Reduced skill at ambulation secondary to developmental age, disease process, tubes, drains, casts, splints, or other appliances; new to ambulation with assistive devices such as walkers or crutches
- Postoperative children: Risk for hypotension or syncope secondary to large blood loss, a heart condition, or extended bed rest
- History of falls
- Infants or toddlers in cribs with side rails down or on the daybed with family members
- Once children at risk for falls have been identified, alert other staff members by posting signs on the door and at the bedside, applying a special colored armband labeled "Fall Precautions," labeling the chart with a sticker, or documenting information on the chart.

Prevention of falls requires alterations in the environment, including the following:

- Keep the bed in the lowest position with the brakes locked and the side rails up.
- Place the call bell within reach.
- Ensure that all necessary and desired items are within reach (e.g., water, glasses, tissues, snacks).
- Offer toileting on a regular basis, especially if the patient is taking diuretics or laxatives.
- Keep lights on at all times, including dim lights while sleeping.
- Lock wheelchairs before transferring patients.
- Ensure that the patient has an appropriate size gown and nonskid footwear. Do not allow gowns or ties to drag on the floor during ambulation.
- Keep the floor clean and free of clutter. Post a "wet floor" sign if the floor is wet.
- Ensure that the patient has glasses on if he or she normally wears them.
- Preventing falls also relies on age-appropriate education of patients. Assist the child with ambulation even though he or she may have ambulated well before hospitalization. Patients who have been lying in bed need to get up slowly, sitting on the side of the bed before standing.

The nurse also needs to educate family members:

- Call the nursing staff for assistance, and do not allow patients to get up independently.

- Keep the side rails of the crib or bed up whenever the patient is in the crib or bed.
- Do not leave infants on the daybed; put them in the crib with the side rails up.
- When all family members need to leave the bedside, notify the staff and ensure that the patient is in the bed or crib with the side rails up and call bell within reach (if appropriate).

INFECTION CONTROL

According to the Centers for Disease Control and Prevention, approximately 2 million patients each year develop nosocomial (hospital-acquired) infections. These infections occur when there is interaction among patients, health care personnel, equipment, and bacteria (Collins, 2008). Nosocomial infections are preventable if caregivers practice meticulous cleaning and disposal techniques.

Standard Precautions synthesize the major features of Universal (blood and body fluid) Precautions (designed to reduce the risk for transmission of bloodborne pathogens) and body substance isolation (designed to reduce the risk for transmission of pathogens from moist body substances). Standard Precautions involve the use of barrier protection, such as gloves, goggles, gown, or mask, to prevent contamination from (1) blood; (2) all body fluids, secretions, and excretions except sweat, regardless of whether they contain visible blood; (3) nonintact skin; and (4) mucous membranes. Standard Precautions are designed for the care of all patients to reduce the risk for transmission of microorganisms from both recognized and unrecognized sources of infection. Respiratory hygiene/cough etiquette was added to Standard Precautions in 2007 by the Centers for Disease Control and Prevention, along with safe injection practices. Anyone with cough, congestion, runny nose, or secretions should cover their mouth and nose when coughing; a mask should be worn by the coughing person when tolerated (usually not suitable for young children). Safe injection practices include the use of a new sterile needle or cannula each time medication or fluid is withdrawn from a vial or bag and for each injection. Reuse of needles/cannulas in multidose vials and IV bags has resulted in transmission of hepatitis and other infections.

Transmission-Based Precautions are designed for patients with documented or suspected infection or colonization (presence of microorganisms in or on patient but without clinical signs and symptoms of infection) with highly transmissible or epidemiologically important pathogens for which additional precautions beyond Standard Precautions are needed to interrupt transmission in hospitals. There are three types of transmission-based precautions: Airborne Precautions, Droplet Precautions, and Contact Precautions. They may be combined for diseases that have multiple routes of transmission (Box 39.2). They are to be used in addition to Standard Precautions.

Airborne Precautions reduce the risk for airborne transmission of infectious agents. Airborne transmission occurs by dissemination of either airborne droplet nuclei (small-particle residue [<5 mm] of evaporated droplets that may remain suspended in the air for long periods) or dust particles containing the infectious agent. Microorganisms carried in this manner can be dispersed widely by air currents and may become inhaled by or deposited on a susceptible host within the same room or over a longer distance from the source patient, depending on environmental factors. Special air handling and ventilation are required to prevent airborne transmission. Airborne precautions apply to patients with known or suspected infection with pathogens transmitted by the airborne route, such as measles, varicella, and tuberculosis.

Droplet Precautions reduce the risk for droplet transmission of infectious agents. Droplet transmission involves contact of the conjunctivae or the mucous membranes of the nose or mouth of a susceptible

Standard Precautions for Prevention of Transmission of Pathogens
Use Standard Precautions for the care of all patients.

Airborne Precautions
In addition to Standard Precautions, use Airborne Precautions for patients known or suspected to have serious illnesses transmitted by airborne droplet nuclei. Examples of such illnesses include measles, varicella (including disseminated zoster), and tuberculosis.

Droplet Precautions
In addition to Standard Precautions, use Droplet Precautions for patients known or suspected to have serious illnesses transmitted by large-particle droplets. Examples of such illnesses include the following:
- Invasive *Haemophilus influenzae* type b disease, including meningitis, pneumonia, epiglottitis, and sepsis
- Invasive *Neisseria meningitidis* disease, including meningitis, pneumonia, and sepsis
- Other serious bacterial respiratory tract infections spread by droplet transmission, including diphtheria (pharyngeal), mycoplasmal pneumonia, pertussis, pneumonic plague, streptococcal pharyngitis, pneumonia, and scarlet fever in infants and young children
- Serious viral infections spread by droplet transmission, including adenovirus, influenza, mumps, parvovirus B19, and rubella

Contact Precautions
In addition to Standard Precautions, use Contact Precautions for patients known or suspected to have serious illnesses easily transmitted by direct patient contact or by contact with items in the patient's environment. Examples of such illnesses include the following:
- Gastrointestinal, respiratory, skin, or wound infections or colonization with multidrug-resistant bacteria judged by the infection control program based on current state, regional, or national recommendations, to be of special clinical and epidemiologic significance
- Enteric infections with a low infectious dose or prolonged environmental survival, including *Clostridium difficile;* for diapered or incontinent patients: enterohemorrhagic *Escherichia coli* O157:H7, *Shigella* organisms, hepatitis A, or rotavirus
- Respiratory syncytial virus (RSV), parainfluenza virus, or enteroviral infections in infants and young children
- Skin infections that are highly contagious or that may occur on dry skin, including diphtheria (cutaneous), herpes simplex virus (neonatal or mucocutaneous), impetigo, major (noncontained) abscesses, cellulitis or decubitus, pediculosis, scabies, staphylococcal furunculosis in infants and young children, zoster (disseminated or in the immunocompromised host)
- Viral or hemorrhagic conjunctivitis
- Viral hemorrhagic infections (Ebola, Lassa, or Marburg)

person with large-particle droplets (>5 mm) containing microorganisms generated from a person who has a clinical disease or who is a carrier of the microorganism. Droplets are generated from the source person primarily during coughing, sneezing, or talking and during procedures such as suctioning and bronchoscopy. Transmission requires close contact between source and recipient individuals because droplets do not remain suspended in the air and generally travel only short distances, usually 3 feet or less, through the air. Because droplets do not remain suspended in the air, special air handling and ventilation are not required to prevent droplet transmission. Droplet precautions apply to any patient with known or suspected infection with pathogens that can be transmitted by infectious droplets (see Box 39.2).

Contact Precautions reduce the risk for transmission of microorganisms by direct or indirect contact. Direct-contact transmission involves skin-to-skin contact and physical transfer of microorganisms to a susceptible host from an infected or colonized person, such as occurs when turning or bathing patients. Direct-contact transmission also can occur between two patients (e.g., by hand contact). Indirect contact transmission involves contact of a susceptible host with a contaminated intermediate object, usually inanimate, in the patient's environment. Contact Precautions apply to specified patients known or suspected to be infected or colonized with microorganisms that can be transmitted by direct or indirect contact.

> **! NURSING ALERT**
>
> The most common piece of medical equipment, the stethoscope, can be a potent source of harmful microorganisms and nosocomial infections.

Nurses caring for young children are frequently in contact with body substances, especially urine, feces, and vomitus. Nurses need to exercise judgment concerning situations when gloves, gowns, or masks are necessary. For example, nurses should wear gloves and possibly gowns for changing diapers when there are loose or explosive stools. Otherwise, the plastic lining of disposable diapers provides a sufficient barrier between the hands and body substances.

During feedings, wear gowns if the child is likely to vomit or spit up, which often occurs during burping. When wearing gloves, wash the hands thoroughly after removing the gloves because gloves fail to provide complete protection. The absence of visible leaks does not indicate that the gloves are intact.

Another essential practice of infection control is that all needles (uncapped and unbroken) are disposed of in a rigid, puncture-resistant container located near the site of use. Consequently, these containers are installed in patients' rooms. Because children are naturally curious, extra attention is needed in selecting a suitable type of container and a location that prevents access to the discarded needles. The use of needleless systems allows secure syringe or IV tubing attachment to vascular access devices without the risk for needlestick injury to the child or nurse.

TRANSPORTING INFANTS AND CHILDREN

Infants and children need to be transported within the unit and to areas outside the pediatric unit. Infants and small children can be carried for short distances within the unit, but for more extended trips, the child should be securely transported in a suitable conveyance.

Small infants can be held or carried in the horizontal position with the back supported and the thigh grasped firmly by the carrying arm (Fig. 39.3, *A*). In the football hold, the infant is carried on the nurse's arm with the head supported by the hand and the body held securely between the nurse's body and elbow (see Fig. 39.3, *B*). Both of these holds leave the nurse's other arm free for activity. The infant also can be held in the upright position with the buttocks on the nurse's forearm and the front of the body resting against the nurse's chest. The infant's head and shoulders are supported by the nurse's other arm in case the infant moves suddenly (see Fig. 39.3, *C*). Older infants are able to hold their heads erect but are still subject to sudden movements.

The method of transporting children depends on their age, condition, and destination. Older children are safe in wheelchairs or on stretchers. Younger children can be transported in a crib, on a stretcher, in a wagon

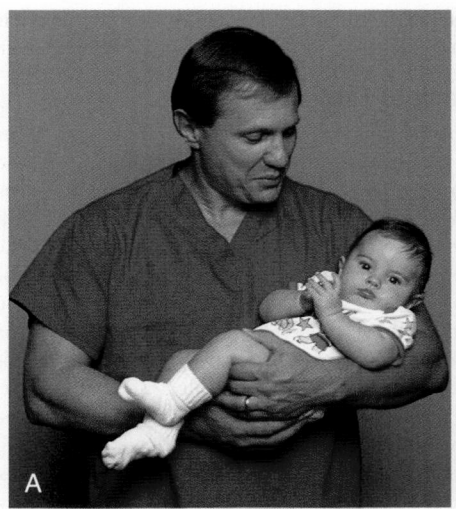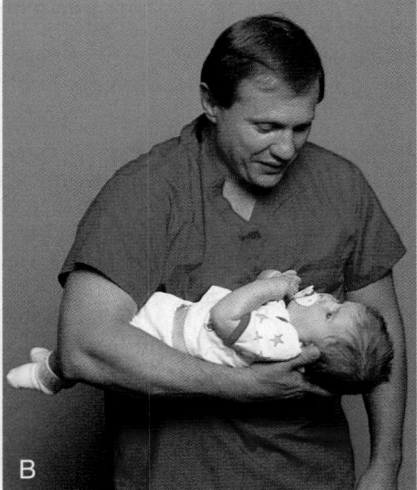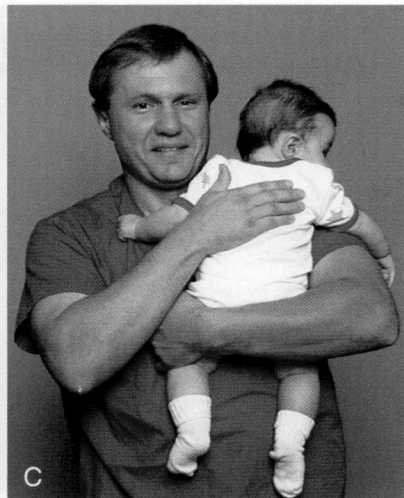

FIG 39.3 Transporting infants. **A,** The infant's thigh firmly grasped in the nurse's hand. **B,** Football hold. **C,** Back supported.

with raised sides, or in a wheelchair with a safety belt. Stretchers should be equipped with high sides and a safety belt, both of which are secured during transport.

Special care is needed in transporting critically ill patients in the hospital. Critically ill children should always be transported on a stretcher or bed (rather than carried) by at least two staff members with monitoring continued during transport. A blood pressure monitor (or standard blood pressure cuff), pulse oximeter, and cardiac monitor/defibrillator should accompany every patient (Warren, Fromm, Orr, et al., 2004). Airway equipment and emergency medications should accompany the patient.

RESTRAINING METHODS

The Centers for Medicare and Medicaid Services have established regulations to minimize the use and ensure safety of patients in restraints. The Centers for Medicare and Medicaid Services (2013) defines restraint as "any manual method, physical or mechanical device, material, or equipment that immobilizes or reduces the ability of a patient to move his or her arms, legs, body, or head freely…or a drug or medication when it is used as a restriction to manage the patient's behavior or restrict the patient's freedom of movement and is not a standard treatment or dosage for the patient's condition." The physical force may be human, mechanical devices, or a combination of the two. Examples of restraints include limb restraints, elbow restraints, vest restraints, and tight tucking of sheets to prevent movement in bed.

The use of mechanical supports such as immobilizers for fractures, orthopedic devices to maintain proper body alignment, leg braces, protective helmets, and surgical dressings are not considered restraints. An armboard to secure a peripheral intravenous (PIV) line is not considered a restraint, unless it is pinned to the bed or immobilizes the entire limb. Hand mitts are not considered a restraint, unless pinned to the bed or used in conjunction with a wrist restraint. Developmentally age-appropriate safety interventions for infants, toddlers, and preschoolers (e.g., net enclosures on beds, crib domes, crib side rails, and high chair lap safety belts) are generally not considered a restraint. Picking up, redirecting, or holding an infant, toddler, or preschooler is not considered restraint. Interventions that would typically be employed by a child care provider outside of a health care environment to ensure safety in young children are not considered to be restraints.

Before initiating restraints, the nurse completes a comprehensive assessment of the patient to determine whether the need for a restraint outweighs the risk of not using one. Restraints can result in loss of dignity, violation of patient rights, psychologic harm, physical harm, and even death. Consider alternative methods first, and document them in the patient's record. Some examples of alternative measures include bringing a child to the nurses' station for continuous observation, providing diversional activities such as music, and encouraging participation of the parents. The use of restraints can often be avoided with adequate preparation of the child; parental or staff supervision of the child; or adequate protection of a vulnerable site, such as an infusion device.

The nurse needs to assess the child's development, mental status, potential to hurt others or self, and safety. The nurse is responsible for selecting the least restrictive type of restraint. Using less restrictive restraints is often possible by gaining the cooperation of the child and parents. Examples of less restrictive restraints are provided in Table 39.4. An order must be obtained as soon as possible (during application or within a few minutes) after the initiation of restraints and specify the time frame they can be used, the reason they are being used, and reasons for discontinuation. Discontinuation of restraints should occur as soon as safe, even if the order time frame has not expired.

Restraints for violent, self-destructive behavior are limited to situations with a significant risk for patients physically harming themselves or others because of behavioral reasons and when nonphysical interventions are not effective. Before initiating a behavioral restraint, the nurse should assess the patient's mental, behavioral, and physical status to determine the cause for the child's potentially harmful behavior. If behavioral restraints are indicated, a collaborative approach involving the patient (if appropriate), the family, and the health care team should be used.

Unless state law is more restrictive, behavioral restraints for children must be reordered every 1 hour for children younger than 9 years of age and every 2 hours for children 9 to 17 years of age; orders for adults 18 years of age and older are required every 4 hours. A licensed independent practitioner or specially trained nurse must conduct an in-person evaluation within 1 hour and at least every 24 hours to continue restraints.

Children in behavioral restraints must be observed and assessed according to facility policy, typically continuously, every 15 minutes, or every 2 hours. Assessment components include signs of injury associated with applying restraint, nutrition and hydration, circulation

TABLE 39.4   Restraining Children: Less Restrictive to More Restrictive Techniques

Technique or Device	Less Restrictive to More Restrictive				
Extremities					
Sleeves	X				
Hand mitts, mittens	X				
Stockinette		X			
Elbows (no-no's)			X		
Arm board				X	
One or two limbs					X
Three or four limbs					X
Chest and Body					
Belts, safety belts	X				
Posey vest, safety jacket			X		
Mummy restraint					X
Papoose board					X
Environment					
Side rails		X			
Crib tops		X			
Seclusion					X
Other					
Chemical					X

Adapted from Selekman, J., & Snyder, B. (1996). Uses of and alternatives to restraints in pediatric settings. *AACN Clinical Issues,* *7*(4), 603–610.

and range-of-motion of extremities, vital signs, hygiene and elimination, physical and psychologic status and comfort, and readiness for discontinuation of restraint. The nurse must use clinical judgment in setting a schedule within the facility's policy for when each of these parameters needs to be evaluated.

Nonviolent/non–self-destructive patients may also require restraints. Examples of nonbehavioral restraints include removal of an artificial airway or airway adjunct for delivery of oxygen, indwelling catheters, tubes, drains, lines, pacemaker wires, or disruption of suture sites. The medical-surgical restraint is used to ensure that safe care is given to the patient. Patient confusion, agitation, unconsciousness, or developmental inability to understand direct requests or instructions also are examples of when nonbehavioral restraints may be required to maintain patient safety. The potential risks of the restraint are offset by the potential benefit of providing safer care.

Nonbehavioral restraints can be initiated by an individual order or by protocol; the use of the protocol must be authorized by an individual order. The order for continued use of restraints must be renewed each day. Patients are monitored per facility policy, typically at least every 2 hours.

Restraints with ties must be secured to the bed or crib frame, not the side rails. Suggestions for increasing safety and comfort while the child is in a restraint include leaving one finger breadth between skin and the device and tying knots that allow for quick release. The nurse can also increase safety by ensuring the restraint does not tighten as the child moves and decreasing wrinkles or bulges in the restraint. Placing jacket restraints over an article of clothing; placing limb restraints below waist level, below knee level, or distal to the IV; and tucking in dangling straps also increase safety and comfort. Do not place objects over the patient's face to protect staff from being spit upon or bitten. Masks and face shields should be readily available for staff to wear; some facilities also provide bite gloves and arm/hand wraps made of

strong barrier materials (e.g., Kevlar) for staff to wear to prevent injury from bites and scratches.

Mummy Restraint or Swaddle

When an infant or small child requires short-term restraint for examination or treatment that involves the head and neck (e.g., venipuncture, throat examination, gavage feeding), a papoose board with straps or a mummy wrap effectively controls the child's movements. A blanket or sheet is opened on the bed or crib with one corner folded to the center. The infant is placed on the blanket with the shoulders at the fold and feet toward the opposite corner. With the infant's right arm straight down against the body, the right side of the blanket is pulled firmly across the infant's right shoulder and chest and secured beneath the left side of the body. The left arm is placed straight against the infant's side, and the left side of the blanket is brought across the shoulder and chest and locked beneath the body on the right side. The lower corner is folded and brought over the body and tucked or fastened securely with safety pins. Safety pins can be used to fasten the blanket in place at any step in the process. To modify the mummy restraint for chest examination, bring the folded edge of the blanket over each arm and under the back, and then fold the loose edge over and secure it at a point below the chest to allow visualization and access to the chest (Fig. 39.4, *A*).

Jacket Restraint

A jacket restraint is sometimes used to keep the child safe in various chairs. The jacket is put on the child with the ties in back so the child is unable to manipulate them. The jacket restraint is also useful as a means for maintaining the child in a desired horizontal position. The long tapes, secured to the understructure of the crib, keep the child inside the crib.

Arm and Leg Restraints

Occasionally, the nurse needs to restrain one or more extremities or limit their motion. Several commercial restraining devices are available, including disposable wrist and ankle restraints (see Fig. 39.4, *B*). Restraints must be appropriate to the child's size and padded to prevent undue pressure, constriction, or tissue injury; and the extremity must be observed frequently for signs of irritation or impaired circulation. The ends of the restraints are never tied to the side rails because lowering the rail will disturb the extremity, frequently with a jerk that may hurt or injure the child.

Elbow Restraint

Sometimes it is important to prevent the child from reaching the head or face (e.g., after cleft lip or palate surgery, when a scalp vein infusion is in place, or to prevent scratching in skin disorders). Elbow restraints fashioned from a variety of materials function well (see Fig. 39.4, *C*). Commercial elbow restraints are available. They extend from just below the axilla to the wrist and are sometimes referred to as "no-no's." A shoulder strap to prevent slipping may be used in an awake, active older infant or toddler to prevent slippage, but should not be used when sleeping.

POSITIONING FOR PROCEDURES

Infants and small children are unable to cooperate for many procedures. Therefore, the nurse is responsible for minimizing their movement and discomfort with proper positioning. Older children usually need only minimal, if any, restraint. Careful explanation and preparation beforehand and support and simple guidance during the procedure are usually sufficient. For painful procedures, the child should receive adequate analgesia and sedation to minimize pain and the need for excessive

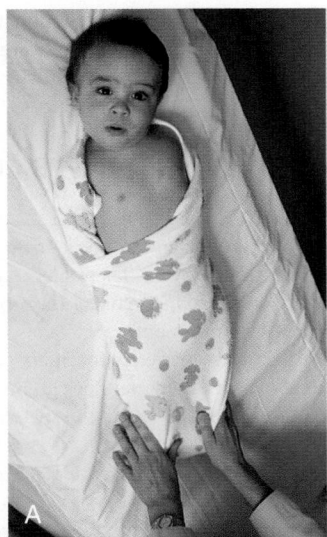

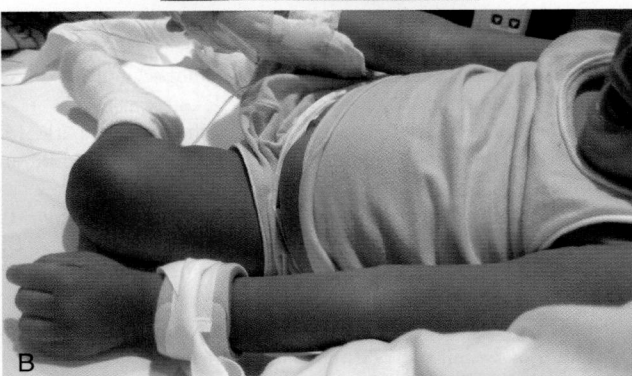

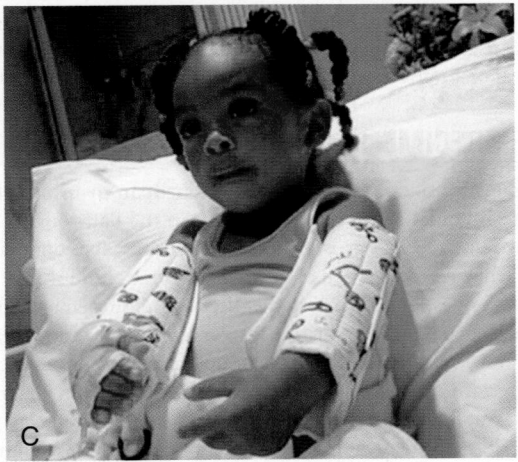

FIG 39.4 Restraint examples from most restrictive to least restrictive. **A,** Mummy restraint. **B,** Wrist restraints. **C,** Elbow restraints.

restraint. For local anesthesia, use buffered lidocaine to reduce the stinging sensation or a topical anesthetic.

FEMORAL VENIPUNCTURE

The nurse places the child supine with the legs in a frog position to provide extensive exposure of the groin area. The infant's legs can be effectively controlled by the nurse's forearms and hands (Fig. 39.5). Only the side used for the venipuncture is uncovered so that the

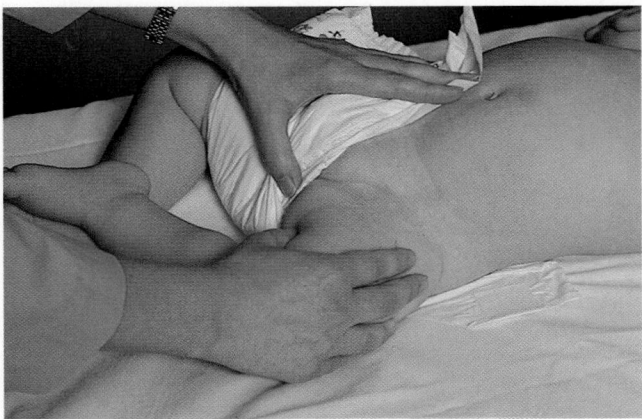

FIG 39.5 Positioning infant for femoral venipuncture.

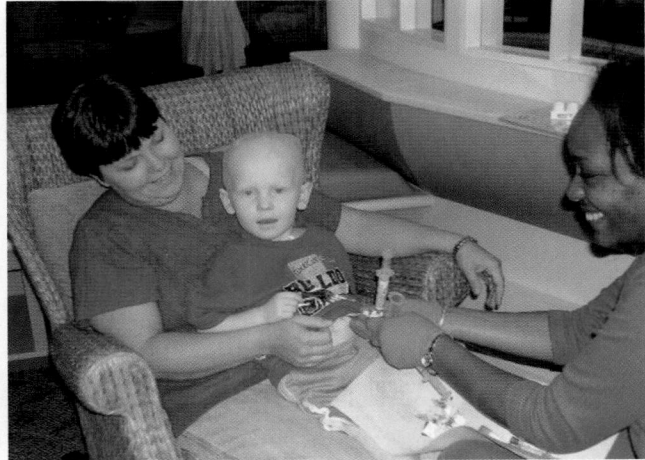

FIG 39.6 Therapeutic holding of child for extremity venipuncture with parental assistance.

practitioner is protected if the child urinates during the procedure. Apply pressure to the site to prevent oozing from the site.

EXTREMITY VENIPUNCTURE OR INJECTION

The most common sites of venipuncture are the veins of the extremities, especially the arm and hand. A convenient position is to place the child in the parent's (or assistant's) lap with the child facing the parent and in the straddle position. Next, place the child's arm for venipuncture on a firm surface, such as a treatment table. The nurse can partially stabilize the child's outstretched arm and have the parent hug the child's upper body, preventing movement; the nurse can then use the parent's arm to immobilize the venipuncture site. This type of restraint also comforts the child because of the close body contact and allows each person to maintain eye contact (Fig. 39.6).

LUMBAR PUNCTURE

Pediatric lumbar puncture sets contain smaller spinal needles, but sometimes the practitioner will specify a different size or type of needle. The technique for lumbar puncture in infants and children is similar to that in adults, although modifications are suggested in neonates, who have less distress in a side-lying position with modified neck extension than in flexion or a sitting position.

Children are usually easiest to control in the side-lying position, with the head flexed and the knees drawn up toward the chest. Even

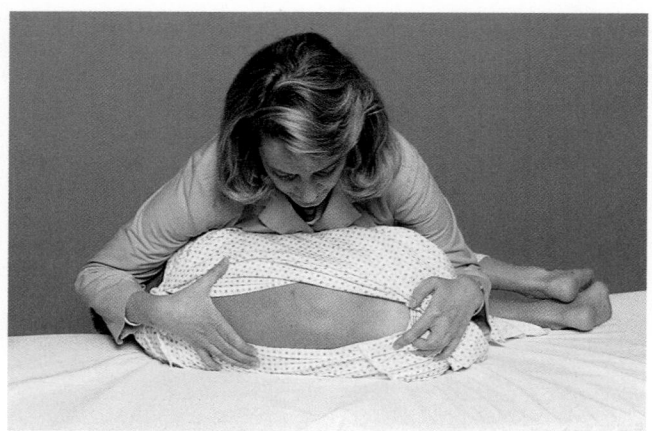

FIG 39.7 Side-lying position for lumbar puncture.

cooperative children need to be held gently to prevent possible trauma from unexpected, involuntary movement. They can be reassured that, although they are trusted, holding will serve as a reminder to maintain the desired position. It also provides a measure of support and reassurance to them.

A flexed sitting or side-lying position may be used, depending on the child's ability to cooperate and whether sedation will be used. In the sitting position with the hips flexed, the interspinous space is maximized (Abo, Chen, Johnston, et al., 2010). The child is placed with the buttocks at the edge of the table. The nurse's hands immobilize the infant's arms and legs. Neck flexion is not necessary (Fig. 39.7).

> **! NURSING ALERT**
>
> The sitting position may interfere with chest expansion and diaphragm excursion, and in infants the soft, pliable trachea may collapse. Therefore, observe the child for difficulty with breathing.

Specimens and spinal fluid pressure are obtained, measured, and sent for analysis in the same manner as for adult patients. Take vital signs as ordered, and observe the child for any changes in level of consciousness, motor activity, and other neurologic signs. Post–lumbar puncture headache may occur and is related to postural changes; this is less severe when the child lies flat. Headache is seen much less frequently in young children than in adolescents.

BONE MARROW ASPIRATION OR BIOPSY

The position for a bone marrow aspiration or biopsy depends on the chosen site. In children, the posterior or anterior iliac crest is most frequently used, but in infants, the tibia may be selected because it is easy to access the site and hold the child.

If the posterior iliac crest is used, the child is positioned prone. Sometimes a small pillow or folded blanket is placed under the hips to facilitate obtaining the bone marrow specimen. Children should receive adequate analgesia or anesthesia to relieve pain. If the child might awaken, he or she may need to be held, preferably by two people—one person to immobilize the upper body and a second person to immobilize the lower extremities.

COLLECTION OF SPECIMENS

Many of the specimens needed for diagnostic examination of children are collected in much the same way as they are for adults. Older children

are able to cooperate if given proper instruction regarding what is expected of them. Infants and small children, however, are unable to follow directions or control body functions sufficiently to help in collecting some specimens.

FUNDAMENTAL PROCEDURE STEPS COMMON TO ALL PROCEDURES

The following steps are very important for every procedure and should be considered fundamental aspects of care. These steps, although important, are not listed in each of the specimen collection procedures.

1. Assemble the necessary equipment.
2. Identify the child using two patient identifiers (e.g., patient name and medical record or birth date; neither can be a room number). Compare the same two identifiers with the specimen container and order.
3. Perform hand hygiene, maintain aseptic technique, and follow Standard Precautions.
4. Explain the procedure to parents and child according to the developmental level of the child; reassure the child that the procedure is not a punishment.
5. Provide atraumatic care, and position the child securely.
6. Prepare area with antiseptic agent.
7. Place specimens in appropriate containers, and apply a patient ID label to the specimen container in the presence of the child and family.
8. Discard puncture device in puncture-resistant container near the site of use.
9. Wash the procedural preparation agent off if povidone/iodine is used, if skin is sensitive, and for infants.
10. Remove gloves, and perform hand hygiene after the procedure. Have children wash their hands if they have helped.
11. Praise the child for helping.
12. Document pertinent aspects of the procedure, such as number of attempts, site and amount of blood or urine withdrawn, as well as type of test performed.

URINE SPECIMENS

Older children and adolescents can use a bedpan or urinal or can be trusted to follow directions for collection in the bathroom. However, they may have special needs. School-age children are cooperative but curious. They are concerned about the reasons behind things and are likely to ask questions regarding the disposition of their specimen and what one expects to discover from it. Self-conscious adolescents may be reluctant to carry a specimen through a hallway or waiting room and appreciate a paper bag for disguising the container. The presence of menses may be an embarrassment or a concern to teenage girls; therefore, it is a good idea to ask them about this and make adjustments as necessary. The specimen can be delayed or a notation made on the laboratory slip to explain the presence of red blood cells.

Preschoolers and toddlers are usually unable to void on request. It is often best to offer them water or other liquids that they enjoy and wait about 30 minutes until they are ready to void voluntarily.

> **! NURSING ALERT**
>
> In infants, wipe the abdomen with an alcohol pad and fan it dry; the cooling effect often causes voiding within 2 minutes. Apply pressure over the suprapubic area, or stroke the paraspinal muscles (along the spine) to elicit the Perez reflex; in infants 4 to 6 months of age, this reflex causes crying, extension of the back, flexion of the extremities, and urination.

Children will better understand what is expected if the nurse uses familiar terms, such as "pee-pee," "wee-wee," or "tinkle." Some have difficulty voiding in an unfamiliar receptacle. Potty chairs or a potty hat placed on the toilet is usually satisfactory. Toddlers who have recently acquired bladder control may be especially reluctant, because they undoubtedly have been admonished for "going" in places other than those approved by parents. Enlisting the parents' help usually leads to success.

At times, parents may be asked to bring a urine sample to a health care facility for examination, especially when infants are unable to void during an outpatient visit. In these instances, parents need instructions on applying the collection device and storing the specimen. Ideally, the specimen should be brought to the designated place as soon as possible. If there is a delay, the sample should be refrigerated and the lapsed time reported to the examiner.

For some types of urine testing (e.g., specific gravity, ketones, glucose, and protein), the nurse can aspirate urine directly from the diaper. If the urine is not tested within 30 minutes, the specimen is refrigerated or placed in a sterile container with a preservative. Superabsorbent gel disposable diapers may absorb all urine and may also produce a false crystalluria. Specific gravity measurements are accurate for up to 4 hours provided that the disposable diapers are kept folded. Urine samples collected by the cotton ball method were accurate for pH and specific gravity and were atraumatic to the skin of newborns (Kennedy, Griffin, Su, et al., 2009).

Urine Collection Bags

For infants and toddlers who are not toilet trained, special urine collection bags with self-adhering material around the opening at the point of attachment may be used. To prepare the infant, the genitalia, perineum, and surrounding skin are washed and dried thoroughly because the adhesive will not stick to a moist, powdered, or oily skin surface. The collection bag is easiest to apply if attached first to the perineum, progressing to the symphysis pubis (Fig. 39.8). With girls, the perineum is stretched taut during application to ensure a leak-proof fit. With boys, the penis and sometimes the scrotum are placed inside the bag. The adhesive portion of the bag must be firmly applied to the skin all around the genital area to avoid leakage. The bag is checked frequently and removed as soon as the specimen is available, because the moist bag may become loosened on an active child.

The American Academy of Pediatrics guidelines (American Academy of Pediatrics, Subcommittee on Urinary Tract Infections, Steering Committee on Quality Improvement and Management, & Roberts, 2011) for diagnosis and management of urinary tract infections in infants 2 to 24 months of age recommend a positive screen obtained from a bag specimen be confirmed by culture via bladder catheterization or suprapubic aspiration due to an unacceptably high rate of false-positives. Although

the bag specimen collection method is less invasive and traumatic to an infant, some families and clinicians may prefer to collect only one definitive specimen and avoid additional delay in a obtaining a second specimen.

> ### ! NURSING ALERT
>
> When using a urine collection bag, cut a small slit in the diaper and pull the bag through to allow room for urine to collect and to facilitate checking on the contents. To obtain small amounts of urine, use a syringe without a needle to aspirate urine directly from the diaper. If diapers with absorbent gelling material that trap urine are used, place a small gauze dressing, some cotton balls, or a urine collection device inside the diaper to collect urine and aspirate the urine with a syringe.

Clean-Catch Specimens

Clean-catch specimen traditionally refers to a urine sample obtained for culture after the urethral meatus is cleansed and the first few milliliters of urine are voided (midstream specimen). In girls, the perineum is wiped with an antiseptic pad from front to back. In boys, the tip of the penis is cleansed.

Twenty-Four–Hour Collection

For a 24-hour collection, collection bags are required in infants and small children. Older children require special instruction about notifying someone when they need to void or have a bowel movement so that urine can be collected separately and is not discarded. Some older school-age children and adolescents can take responsibility for collection of their own 24-hour specimens and can keep output records and transfer each voiding to the 24-hour collection container.

The collection period always starts and ends with an empty bladder. At the time the collection begins, instruct the child to void and discard the specimen. All urine voided in the subsequent 24 hours is saved in a container with a preservative or is placed on ice. Twenty-four hours from the time the precollection specimen was discarded, the child is again instructed to void, the specimen is added to the container, and the entire collection is taken to the laboratory.

Infants and small children who are bagged for 24-hour urine collection require a special collection bag. Frequent removal and replacement of adhesive collection devices can produce skin irritation. A thin coating of sealant, such as Skin-Prep, applied to the skin helps to protect it and aids adhesion (unless its use is contraindicated, such as in premature infants or children with irritated skin). Plastic collection bags with collection tubes attached are ideal when the container must be left in place for a time. These can be connected to a collecting device or emptied periodically by aspiration with a syringe. When such devices are not

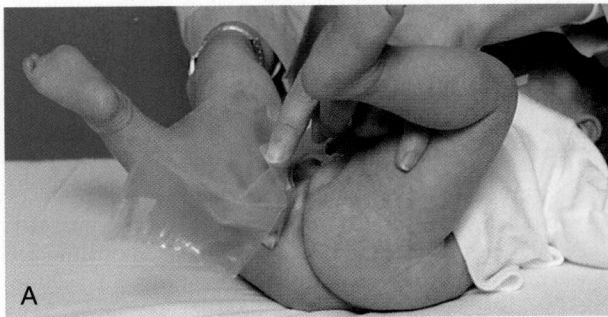
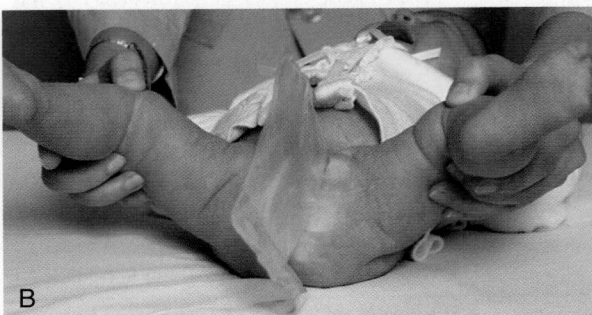

FIG 39.8 Application of urine collection bag. **A,** On female infants, the adhesive portion is applied to the exposed and dried perineum first. **B,** The bag adheres firmly around the perineal area to prevent urine leakage.

available, a regular bag with a feeding tube inserted through a puncture hole at the top of the bag serves as a satisfactory substitute. However, take care to empty the bag as soon as the infant urinates to prevent leakage and loss of contents. An indwelling catheter may also be placed for the collection period.

Bladder Catheterization and Other Techniques

Bladder catheterization or suprapubic aspiration is used when a specimen is urgently needed or a child is unable to void or otherwise provide an adequate specimen. The American Academy of Pediatrics recommends that a urine specimen be obtained by bladder catheterization or suprapubic aspiration in ill-appearing febrile infants with no apparent source of infection prior to antimicrobial administration and to confirm a positive screen for infection (American Academy of Pediatrics, Subcommittee on Urinary Tract Infections, Steering Committee on Quality Improvement and Management, & Roberts, 2011).

Preparation for catheterization includes instruction on pelvic muscle relaxation whenever possible. The toddler, preschooler, or younger child should blow on a pinwheel and press the hips against the bed or procedure table during catheterization to relax the pelvic and periurethral muscles. The nurse describes the location and function of the pelvic muscles briefly to the older child or adolescent. The patient then contracts and relaxes the pelvic muscles, and the relaxation procedure is repeated during catheter insertion. If the patient vigorously contracts the pelvic muscles when the catheter reaches the striated sphincter (proximal urethra in boys and midurethra in girls), catheter insertion is temporarily stopped. The catheter is neither removed nor advanced; instead, the child is helped to press the hips against the bed or examining table and relax the pelvic muscles. The catheter is then gently advanced into the bladder (Gray, 1996).

Catheterization is a sterile procedure, and Standard Precautions for body substance protection should be followed. If the catheter is to remain in place, a Foley catheter is used. Table 39.5 gives guidelines for choosing the appropriate-size catheter and length of insertion. The supplies needed for this procedure include sterile gloves, sterile lubricant anesthetic, the appropriate-size catheter, povidone/iodine (Betadine) swabs or an alternative cleansing agent and 4 × 4-inch gauze squares, a sterile drape, and a syringe with sterile water if a Foley catheter is used. Test the balloon of the Foley catheter by injecting sterile water before catheter insertion.

Adolescent boys and children with a history of urethral surgery may be catheterized with a coudé-tipped catheter. Children with myelodysplasia and those who have been identified as being sensitive or allergic to latex are catheterized with catheters manufactured from an alternative material. When an indwelling catheter is indicated for urinary drainage, a lubricious-coated or silicone catheter is selected, because these materials produce less irritation of the urethral mucosa compared with Silastic or latex catheters when left in place for more than 72 hours.

A 2% lidocaine lubricant with applicator is assembled according to the manufacturer's instructions, and several drops of the lubricant are placed at the meatus. The child is advised that the lubricant is used to reduce any discomfort associated with inserting the catheter and that introduction of the catheter into the urethra will produce a sensation of pressure and a desire to urinate (Gray, 1996) (see Evidence-Based Practice box: The Use of Lidocaine Lubricant for Urethral Catheterization).

In male patients, grasp the penis with the nondominant hand and retract the foreskin. In uncircumcised newborns and infants, the foreskin may be adhered to the shaft; use care when retracting. If the penis is pendulous, place a sterile drape under the penis. Using the sterile hand, swab the glans and meatus three times with povidone/iodine. Gently introduce the tip of the lidocaine jelly applicator into the urethra 1 to 2 cm (0.4 to 0.8 inch) so that the lubricant flows only into the urethra; insert 5 to 10 mL 2% lidocaine lubricant into the urethra, and hold it in place for 2 to 3 minutes by gently squeezing the distal penis. Lubricate the catheter, and insert it into the urethra while gently stretching the penis and lifting it to a 90-degree angle to the body. Resistance may occur when the catheter meets the urethral sphincter. Ask the patient to inhale deeply, and advance the catheter. Do not force a catheter that does not easily enter the meatus, particularly if the child has had corrective surgery. For indwelling catheters, after urine is obtained, advance the catheter to the hub, inflate the balloon with sterile water, pull it back gently to test inflation, and connect it to the closed drainage system. Cleanse the glans and meatus, and replace retracted foreskin. If blood is seen at any time during the procedure, discontinue the procedure and notify the primary care provider.

In female patients, place a sterile drape under the buttocks. Use the nondominant hand to gently separate and pull up the labia minora to visualize the meatus. Swab the meatus from front to back three times using a different povidone/iodine swab each time. Place 1 to 2 mL 2% lidocaine lubricant on the periurethral mucosa, and insert the lubricant 1 to 2 mL into the urethral meatus. Delay catheterization for 2 to 3 minutes to maximize absorption of the anesthetic into the periurethral and intraurethral mucosa. Add lubricant to the catheter, and gently insert it into the urethra until urine returns; then advance the catheter an additional 2.5 to 5 cm (1 to 2 inches). When using an indwelling Foley catheter, inflate the balloon with sterile water and gently pull back; then connect to a closed drainage system. Cleanse the meatus and labia (see Cultural Considerations box: Bladder Catheterization). Because the use of lidocaine jelly can increase the volume of intraurethral lubricant, urine return may not be as rapid as when minimal lubrication is used.

TABLE 39.5 Straight Catheter or Foley Catheter*

	Size (Length of Insertion [cm]) for Girls	Size (Length of Insertion [cm]) for Boys
Term neonate	5 to 6 (5)	5 to 6 (6)
Infant to 3 years of age	5 to 8 (5)	5 to 8 (6)
4 to 8 years of age	8 (5 to 6)	8 (6 to 9)
8 years of age to prepubertal	10 to 12 (6 to 8)	8 to 10 (10 to 15)
Pubertal	12 to 14 (6 to 8)	12 to 14 (13 to 18)

*Foley catheters are approximately 1 Fr size larger because of the circumference of the balloon (for example, 10-Fr Foley catheter = ≈12-Fr calibration).

⚡ SAFETY ALERT

Do not advance the catheter too far into the bladder. Knotting of catheters and tubes within the bladder has been reported in several case studies. Feeding tubes should not be used for urinary catheterization because they are more flexible, longer, and prone to knotting compared with commercially designed urinary catheters (Kilbane, 2009; Levison & Wojtulewicz, 2004; Lodha, Ly, Brindle, et al., 2005; Turner, 2004).

Suprapubic aspiration is mainly used when the bladder cannot be accessed through the urethra (e.g., with some congenital urologic birth defects) or to reduce the risk for contamination that may be present when passing a catheter. With the advent of small catheters (5- and 6-French straight catheters), the need for suprapubic aspiration has decreased. Access to the bladder via the urethra has a much higher success rate than suprapubic aspiration, in which success depends on

EVIDENCE-BASED PRACTICE

The Use of Lidocaine Lubricant for Urethral Catheterization

Ask the Question

PICOT Question: In children, does a lidocaine lubricant decrease the pain associated with urethral catheterization?

Search for the Evidence
Search Strategies

Search selection criteria included English-language publications, research-based studies, and review articles on use of the lidocaine lubricant before urethral catheterization.

Databases Used

Cochrane Collaboration, PubMed, MD Consult, BestBETs, American Academy of Pediatrics

Critical Appraisal of the Evidence

Gray (1996) published a review of strategies to minimize distress associated with urethral catheterization in children and supported intraurethral instillation of a local anesthetic that contains 2% lidocaine before catheter insertion.

One prospective, double-blind, placebo-controlled trial evaluated the use of lidocaine lubricant for discomfort in 20 children before urethral catheterization. Two doses of lidocaine lubricant instilled into the urethra 5 minutes apart significantly reduced pain and distress during urethral catheterization (Gerard, Cooper, Duethman, et al., 2003).

Boots and Edmundson (2010) conducted a randomized controlled trial in 200 children in a follow-up to the study by Gerard and colleagues. Conclusions were that a topical application of 2% lidocaine gel followed by urethral instillation of lidocaine gel is effective in reducing discomfort prior to urinary catheterization, and two urethral instillations offered no significant difference over a single instillation.

Mularoni, Cohen, DeGuzman, and colleagues (2009) found in a three-armed placebo-controlled, double-blind, randomized, controlled trial of 43 children younger than 2 years of age that topical and intraurethral lidocaine lubricant were superior to the placebos of topical aqueous lubricant alone and topical and intraurethral aqueous lubricant in lowering distress, but did not fully alleviate pain.

A placebo-controlled, double-blind, randomized, controlled trial of 115 children younger than 2 years of age found no significant difference when 2% lidocaine gel was compared with a nonanesthetic lubricant. The lubricant was applied to the genital mucosa for 2 to 3 minutes and liberally applied to the catheter but not instilled into the urethra (Vaughn, Paton, Bush, et al., 2005).

Apply the Evidence: Nursing Implications

There is **moderate-quality evidence** with a **strong recommendation** (Guyatt, Oxman, Vist, et al., 2008) for using a lidocaine lubricant to decrease pain associated with urethral catheterization.

Three published research studies were found to support the use of anesthetic before urethral catheterization, and one found topical application alone insufficient to reduce pain. Several publications support its effectiveness in clinical practice. Topical application followed by one or two transurethral instillations of 2% lidocaine gel before urethral catheterization minimizes distress and reduces pain prior to urinary catheterization.

Quality and Safety Competencies: Evidence-Based Practice*
Knowledge

Differentiate clinical opinion from research and evidence-based summaries.

Describe use of lidocaine gel for pain reduction during urethral catheterization.

Skills

Base individualized care plan on patient values, clinical expertise, and evidence.

Integrate evidence into practice by using lidocaine gel for pain reduction during urethral catheterization in children.

Attitudes

Value the concept of evidence-based practice as integral to determining best clinical practice.

Appreciate the strengths and weakness of evidence for using lidocaine gel for pain reduction during urethral catheterization in children.

References

Boots, B. K., & Edmundson, E. E. (2010). A controlled, randomised trial comparing single to multiple application lidocaine analgesia in paediatric patients undergoing urethral catheterisation procedures. *Journal of Clinical Nursing, 19*(5-6), 744–748.

Gerard, L. L., Cooper, C. S., Duethman, K. S., et al. (2003). Effectiveness of lidocaine lubricant for discomfort during pediatric urethral catheterization. *Journal of Urology, 170*(2 Pt. 1), 564–567.

Gray, M. (1996). Atraumatic urethral catheterization of children. *Pediatric Nursing, 22*(4), 306–310.

Guyatt, G. H., Oxman, A. D., Vist, G. E., et al. (2008). GRADE: An emerging consensus on rating quality of evidence and strength of recommendations. *British Medical Journal, 336*(7650), 924–926.

Mularoni, P. P., Cohen, L. L., DeGuzman, M., et al. (2009). A randomized clinical trial of lidocaine gel for reducing infant distress during urethral catheterization. *Pediatric Emergency Care, 25*(7), 439–443.

Vaughn, H., Paton, E. A., Bush, A., et al. (2005). Does lidocaine gel alleviate the pain of bladder catheterization in young children? A randomized, controlled trial. *Pediatrics, 116*(4), 917–920.

*Adapted from the Quality and Safety Education for Nurses (QSEN) Institute.

🌐 CULTURAL CONSIDERATIONS

Bladder Catheterization

Parents may be upset when their child is catheterized. Aside from the trauma the child experiences, some parents may fear that the procedure affects the daughter's virginity. To correct this misconception, the family may benefit from a detailed explanation of the genitourinary anatomy, preferably with a model that shows the separate vaginal and urethral openings. The nurse can also indicate that catheterization has no effect on virginity.

the practitioner's skill at assessing the location of the bladder and the amount of urine in the bladder.

Suprapubic aspiration involves aspirating bladder contents by inserting a 20- or 21-gauge needle in the midline approximately 1 cm (0.4 inch) above the symphysis pubis and directed vertically downward. The nurse prepares the skin as for any needle insertion, and the bladder should contain an adequate volume of urine. This can be assumed if the infant has not voided for at least 1 hour or the bladder can be palpated above the symphysis pubis. This technique is useful for obtaining sterile specimens from young infants because the bladder is an abdominal

ATRAUMATIC CARE

Bladder Catheterization or Suprapubic Aspiration

- Use distraction to help the child relax (e.g., blowing bubbles, deep breathing, singing a song).
- Use lidocaine jelly to anesthetize the area before insertion of the catheter. EMLA cream (a eutectic mixture of lidocaine and prilocaine) or LMX cream may lessen an infant's discomfort as the needle passes through the skin for suprapubic aspiration, but care should be taken that the site is thoroughly cleansed and prepped before the procedure.
- Children often become agitated at being restrained for either procedure. Use comfort measures through touch and voice, both during and after the procedure, to help reduce the child's distress.

EMLA, Eutectic mixture of local anesthetics; *LMX,* lidocaine.

organ and is easily accessed. Suprapubic aspiration is painful; therefore, pain management during the procedure is important (see Atraumatic Care box: Bladder Catheterization or Suprapubic Aspiration).

STOOL SPECIMENS

Stool specimens are frequently collected from children to identify parasites and other organisms that cause diarrhea, assess gastrointestinal function, and check for occult (hidden) blood. Ideally, stool should be collected without contamination with urine, but in children wearing diapers, this is difficult unless a urine bag is applied. Children who are toilet trained should urinate first, flush the toilet, and then defecate into the toilet or a bedpan (preferably one that is placed on the toilet to avoid embarrassment) or a commercial potty hat.

! NURSING ALERT

To obtain a stool specimen, place plastic wrap over the toilet bowl before defecation. Use a tongue depressor or disposable spoon or knife to collect the stool.

Stool specimens should be large enough to obtain an ample sampling, not merely a fecal fragment. Specimens are placed in an appropriate container, which is covered and labeled. If several specimens are needed, mark the containers with the date and time and keep them in a specimen refrigerator. Exercise care in handling the specimen because of the risk for contamination.

BLOOD SPECIMENS

Whether the specimen is collected by the nurse or by others, the nurse is responsible for making certain that specimens, such as serial examinations and fasting specimens, are collected on time and that the proper equipment is available. Collecting, transporting, and storing specimens can have a major impact on laboratory results.

Venous blood samples can be obtained by venipuncture or by aspiration from a peripheral or central access device. Benefits of sampling blood from an indwelling catheter include decreased anxiety, discomfort, and dissatisfaction associated with venipuncture samples (Infusion Nurses Society, 2011). Withdrawing blood specimens through peripheral lock devices in small peripheral veins has varying degrees of success. Although it avoids an additional venipuncture for the child, attempting to aspirate blood from the peripheral lock may shorten the life of the device. When using an IV infusion site for specimen collection, consider the type of fluid being infused. For example, a specimen collected for glucose determination would be inaccurate if removed from a catheter through which glucose-containing solution was being administered.

Although central lines can also be used to withdraw blood specimens, risks include catheter-associated bloodstream infection and occlusion. A common technique is to withdraw and discard 0.5 to 10 mL of blood. The Infusion Nurses Society (2011) recommends withdrawing and discarding 1.5 to 2 times the fill volume of the central vascular access device (CVAD). Limited research supports using the initial volume obtained as a blood culture specimen. Some facilities allow reinfusion of the blood initially withdrawn from the CVAD, especially when blood conservation is essential. Another technique that conserves blood is the push-pull method in which blood is withdrawn into a syringe and reinfused three times back into the CVAD. A new sterile syringe is then attached and the specimen is withdrawn; no blood is discarded.

When venipuncture is performed, the needed specimens are quickly collected, and pressure is applied to the puncture site with dry gauze until bleeding stops (see Atraumatic Care box: Guidelines for Skin and Vessel Punctures). The arm should be extended, not flexed, while pressure is applied for a few minutes after venipuncture in the antecubital fossa to reduce bruising. The nurse then covers the site with an adhesive bandage. In young children, adhesive bandages pose an aspiration hazard, so avoid using them or remove the adhesive bandage as soon as the bleeding stops. Applying warm compresses to ecchymotic areas increases circulation, helps remove extravasated blood, and decreases pain.

Arterial blood samples are sometimes needed for blood gas measurement, although noninvasive techniques, such as transcutaneous oxygen monitoring and pulse oximetry, are used frequently. Arterial samples may be obtained by arterial puncture using the radial, brachial, or femoral arteries or from indwelling arterial catheters. Assess adequate circulation before arterial puncture by observing capillary refill or performing the **Allen test**, a procedure that assesses the circulation of the radial, ulnar, or brachial arteries. Because unclotted blood is required, use only heparinized collection tubes or syringes. In addition, no air bubbles should enter the tube because they can alter blood gas concentration. Crying, fear, and agitation affect blood gas values; therefore, make every effort to comfort the child. Pack the blood samples in ice to reduce blood cell metabolism, and take it to the laboratory immediately.

Take capillary blood samples from children by finger stick. A common method for taking peripheral blood samples from infants younger than 6 months of age is by a heel stick. Before the blood sample is taken, warm the heel for 3 minutes and cleanse the area with alcohol. Holding the infant's foot firmly with the free hand, the nurse then punctures the heel with an automatic lancet device. An automatic device delivers a more precise puncture depth and is less painful than using a lance (Vertanen, Fellman, Brommels, et al., 2001). A surgical blade of any kind is contraindicated. An example of a safe device is the BD Quickheel Safety Lancet. The Tenderfoot Preemie device was compared with the Monolet lancet and was found to be safer than the lancet and required fewer heel punctures, less collection time, and lower recollection rates (Kellam, Sacks, Wailer, et al., 2001). Shepherd, Glenesk, Niven, and colleagues (2005) reported that the Tenderfoot device was more effective and safer than a lancet for newborn screening tests. Although obtaining capillary blood gases is a common practice, these measures may not accurately reflect arterial values.

The most serious complications of infant heel puncture are necrotizing osteochondritis from lancet penetration of the underlying calcaneus bone, infection, and abscess of the heel. To avoid osteochondritis, the puncture should be no deeper than 2 mm and should be made at the outer aspect of the heel. The boundaries of the calcaneus can be marked by an imaginary line extending posteriorly from a point between the fourth and fifth toes and running parallel with the lateral aspect of the heel and another line extending posteriorly from the middle of the

ATRAUMATIC CARE

Guidelines for Skin and Vessel Punctures

To reduce the pain associated with heel, finger, venous, or arterial punctures:

- Apply EMLA topically over the site if time permits (>60 minutes). LMX cream also may be used and requires a shorter application time (30 minutes). To remove the transparent dressing atraumatically, grasp opposite sides of the film and pull the sides away from each other to stretch and loosen the film. After the film begins to loosen, grasp the other two sides of the film and pull. Use a vapo-coolant spray or buffered lidocaine (injected intradermally near the vein with a 30-gauge needle) to numb the skin.
- Use nonpharmacologic methods of pain and anxiety control (e.g., ask the child to take a deep breath when the needle is inserted and again when the needle is withdrawn, to exhale a large breath or blow bubbles to "blow hurt away," or to count slowly and then faster and louder if pain is felt).
- Keep all equipment out of sight until used.
- Enlist parents' presence or assistance if they wish.
- Restrain child only as needed to perform the procedure safely; use therapeutic holding (see Fig. 39.6).
- Allow the skin preparation to dry completely before penetrating the skin.
- Use the smallest-gauge needle (e.g., 25 gauge) that permits free flow of blood; a 27-gauge needle can be used for obtaining 1 to 1.5 mL of blood and for prominent veins (needle length is only 1.25 cm [0.5 inch]).
- If possible, avoid putting an IV line in the dominant hand or the hand the child uses to suck the thumb.
- Use an automatic lancet device for precise puncture depth of the finger or heel; press the device lightly against the skin; avoid steadying the finger against a hard surface.
- Have a "two-try" only policy to reduce excessive insertion attempts—two operators each have two insertion attempts. If insertion is not successful after four punctures, consider alternative venous access, such as a PICC; have a policy for identifying children with difficult access and appropriate interventions (e.g., most experienced operator for the first attempt, use transilluminator or ultrasonography for insertion guidance).

For Multiple Blood Samples

- Use an intermittent infusion device (saline lock) to collect additional samples from an existing IV line; consider PICC lines early, not as a last resort.
- Coordinate care to allow several tests to be performed on one blood sample using micromethods of testing.
- Anticipate tests (e.g., drug levels, chemistry, immunoglobulin levels), and ask the laboratory to save blood for additional testing.

For Heel Lancing in Newborns

- Heel lancing has shown to be more painful than venipuncture (Shah & Ohlsson, 2007).
- Kangaroo care (placing the diapered newborn against the parent's bare chest in skin-to-skin contact) 10 to 15 minutes before and during heel lance reduces pain. In two studies, mothers were slightly more effective than fathers in decreasing pain (Shah & Jefferies, 2012; Johnston, Campbell-Yeo, & Filion, 2011; Gray, Watt, & Blass, 2000).
- Breastfeeding during a neonatal heel lance is effective in reducing pain and has been found to be more effective than sucrose in some studies (Shah, Herbozo, Aliwalas, et al., 2012; Shah & Jefferies, 2012)
- If breast milk is unavailable, administer sucrose and encourage the newborn to suck a pacifier. When commercially manufactured 24% sucrose solution is unavailable, add 1 tsp of table sugar to 4 tsp of sterile water. Use this solution to coat the pacifier or administer 2 mL to the tongue 2 minutes before the procedure (see Evidence-Based Practice box: Reduction of Minor Procedural Pain in Infants, Chapter 30.
- Although safe for use in preterm infants when applied correctly, EMLA has been found to be no more effective than placebo in preventing pain during heel lancing (Anand & Hall, 2006; Stevens, Johnston, Taddio, et al., 1999; Essink-Tebbes, Wuis, Liem, et al., 1999).

EMLA, Eutectic mixture of local anesthetics; *IV,* Intravenous; *LMX,* lidocaine; *PICC,* peripherally inserted central catheter.

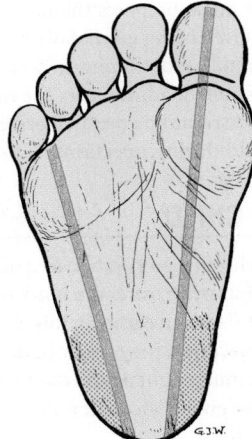

FIG 39.9 Puncture site (colored stippled area) on the sole of an infant's foot.

great toe and running parallel with the medial aspect of the heel (Fig. 39.9). Repeated trauma to the walking surface of the heel can cause fibrosis and scarring that may interfere with locomotion.

No matter how or by whom the specimen is collected, children (even some older ones) fear the loss of their blood. This is particularly true for children whose condition requires frequent blood specimens. They mistakenly believe that blood removed from their body is a threat to their lives. Explaining to them that their body continuously produces blood provides them a measure of reassurance. When the blood is drawn, a comment such as, "Just look how red it is. You're really making a lot of nice red blood," confirms this information and affords them an opportunity to express their concern. An adhesive bandage gives them added assurance that the vital fluids will not leak out through the puncture site.

Children also dislike the discomfort associated with venous, arterial, and capillary punctures. Children have identified these procedures as the ones most frequently causing pain during hospitalization, and an arterial puncture as being one of the most painful of all procedures experienced. Toddlers are most distressed by venipuncture followed by school-age children and then adolescents. Consequently, nurses need to institute pain reduction techniques to lessen the discomfort of these procedures.

RESPIRATORY SECRETION SPECIMENS

Collection of sputum or nasal discharge is sometimes required for the diagnosis of respiratory infections, especially tuberculosis and respiratory syncytial virus (RSV). Older children and adolescents are able to cough as directed and supply sputum specimens when given proper directions.

The nurse must make it clear to them that a coughed specimen, not mucus cleared from the throat, is needed. It is helpful to demonstrate a deep cough. Infants and small children are unable to follow directions to cough and will swallow any sputum produced; therefore, gastric washings (lavage) may be used to collect a sputum specimen. Sometimes a satisfactory specimen can be obtained using a suction device (e.g., a mucus trap) if the catheter is inserted into the trachea and the cough reflex elicited. A catheter inserted into the back of the throat is not sufficient. For children with a tracheostomy, a specimen is easily aspirated from the trachea or major bronchi by attaching a collecting device to the suction apparatus.

Nasal washings are usually obtained to diagnose an infection of RSV. The child is placed supine, and 1 to 3 mL of sterile normal saline is instilled with a sterile syringe (without needle) into one nostril. The contents are aspirated using a small, sterile bulb syringe and are placed in a sterile container. Another method uses a syringe with 5 cm (2 inches) of 18- to 20-gauge tubing. The saline is quickly instilled and then aspirated to recover the nasal specimen. To prevent any additional discomfort, all of the equipment should be ready before beginning the procedure.

Other respiratory secretion collection methods include nasopharyngeal swabs to diagnose *Bordetella* pertussis and throat cultures. The nurse swabs both the tonsils and the posterior pharynx when obtaining a throat culture. The swab stick is inserted into the culture tube. Some culture kits require squeezing an ampule to release the culture medium.

ADMINISTRATION OF MEDICATION

DETERMINATION OF DRUG DOSAGE

Nurses must have an understanding of the safe dosages of medications that they administer to children, as well as the expected actions, possible side effects, and signs of toxicity. Unlike with adult medications, there are few standardized pediatric dosage ranges, and with a few exceptions, drugs are prepared and packaged in average adult-dosage strengths.

Factors related to growth and maturation significantly alter an individual's capacity to metabolize and excrete drugs. Immaturity or defects in any of the important processes of absorption, distribution, biotransformation, or excretion can significantly alter the effects of a drug. Newborn and premature infants with immature enzyme systems in the liver (where most drugs are broken down and detoxified), lower plasma concentrations of protein for binding with drugs, and immaturely functioning kidneys (where most drugs are excreted) are particularly vulnerable to the harmful effects of drugs. Beyond the newborn period, many drugs are metabolized more rapidly by the liver, necessitating larger doses or more frequent administration. This is particularly important in pain control, when the dosage of analgesics may need to be increased or the interval between doses decreased.

Various formulas involving age, weight, and body surface area (BSA) as the basis for calculations have been devised to determine children's drug dosages. Because the administration of medication is a nursing responsibility, nurses need to have not only knowledge of drug action and patient responses but also resources for estimating safe dosages for children. Children's dosages are most often expressed in units of measure per body weight (mg/kg). Some medications, such as chemotherapy, are more precisely dosed using BSA. The ratio of BSA to weight varies inversely with length; therefore, an infant who is shorter and weighs less than an older child or adult has relatively more BSA than would be expected from the weight. BSA is based on the West nomogram and is easily determined using conversion programs widely available on the Internet.

CHECKING DOSAGE

Administering the correct dosage of a drug is a shared responsibility between the practitioner who orders the drug and the nurse who carries out that order. Children react with unexpected severity to some drugs, and ill children may be especially sensitive to drugs. When a dose is ordered that is outside the usual range or when there is some question regarding the preparation or the route of administration, the nurse should check with the prescribing practitioner before proceeding with the administration, because the nurse is legally liable for any drug administered.

Even when it has been determined that the dosage is correct for a particular child, many drugs are potentially hazardous or lethal. Most facilities have regulations requiring specified drugs to be double-checked by another nurse before giving them to the child. Among drugs that require such safeguards are antiarrhythmics, anticoagulants, chemotherapeutic agents, and insulin. Others frequently included are epinephrine, opioids, and sedatives. Even if this precaution is not mandatory, nurses are wise to take such precautions. Errors in decimal point placement may occur and may result in a tenfold or greater dosage error.

IDENTIFICATION

Before the administration of any medication, the child must be correctly identified using two identifiers (e.g., name and medical record number or birth date). With an infant, young child, or nonverbal child, the parent or guardian (if present) can verify the child's identity. After verbal verification of the child's identity (by the parent, guardian, or child), the ID band should be verified using two identifiers. Bedside computers to scan the ID bracelet for electronic record updating may also be used.

PREPARING THE PARENTS

Nearly all parents have given some type of medication to their child and can describe the approaches that they have found successful. In some cases, it is less traumatic for the child if a parent gives the medication, provided that the nurse prepares the medication and supervises its administration. Children being given daily medications at home are accustomed to the parent's functioning in this capacity and are less likely to fuss than if a stranger administers the medication. Individual decisions need to be made regarding parental presence and participation, such as holding the child during injections.

PREPARING THE CHILD

Every child requires psychologic preparation for parenteral administration of medication and supportive care during the procedure (see the "Psychologic Preparation" section earlier in this chapter). Even if children have received several injections, they rarely become accustomed to the discomfort and have as much right as any other child to understanding and patience from those giving the injection.

ORAL ADMINISTRATION

The oral route is preferred for administering medications to children because of the ease of administration. Most medications are dissolved or suspended in liquid preparations. Although some children are able to swallow or chew solid medications at an early age, solid preparations are not recommended for young children because of the danger of aspiration.

ATRAUMATIC CARE

Encouraging a Child's Acceptance of Oral Medication

- Give the child a flavored ice pop or small ice cube to suck to numb the tongue before giving the drug.
- Mix the drug with a small amount (≈1 tsp) of sweet-tasting substance, such as honey (except in infants because of the risk for botulism), flavored syrups, jam, fruit purees, sherbet, or ice cream; avoid essential food items because the child may later refuse to eat them.
- Give a "chaser" of water, juice, soft drink, or ice pop or frozen juice bar after the drug.
- If nausea is a problem, give a carbonated beverage poured over finely crushed ice before or immediately after the medication.
- When medication has an unpleasant taste, have the child pinch the nose and drink the medicine through a straw. Much of what we taste is associated with smell.
- Flavorings, such as apple, banana, and bubble gum (e.g., FLAVORx), can be added at many pharmacies at nominal additional cost. An alternative is to have the pharmacist prepare the drug in a flavored, chewable troche or lozenge.*

*Infants will suck medicine from a needleless syringe or dropper in small increments (0.25 to 0.5 mL) at a time. Use a nipple or special pacifier with a reservoir for the drug.

Most pediatric medications come in palatable and colorful preparations for added ease of administration. Some have a slightly unpleasant aftertaste, but most children swallow these liquids with little, if any, resistance. Complaints of dislike from the child can be accepted, and the taste can be camouflaged whenever possible. Most pediatric units have preparations available for this purpose (see Atraumatic Care box: Encouraging a Child's Acceptance of Oral Medication).

Preparation

The devices available to measure medicines are not always sufficiently accurate for measuring the small amounts needed in pediatric nursing practice. The most accurate means for measuring small amounts of medication is the plastic disposable calibrated oral syringe. Not only does the syringe provide a reliable measure, but it also serves as a convenient means for transporting and administering the medication. The medication can be placed directly into the child's mouth from the syringe.

A device called the Rx Medibottle (The Medicine Bottle Company, Hinsdale, IL) has shown to be more effective in delivering unpleasant tasting oral medication to infants than an oral syringe (Purswani, Radhakrishnan, Irfan, et al., 2009; Kraus, Stohlmeyer, Hannon, et al., 2001). This device allows an infant to suck juice or other liquids from a nipple attached to a specially designed bottle while receiving undiluted medication dispensed in spurts from a syringe inserted into a central sleeve of the bottle.

Paper cups are totally unsuitable for liquid medications because they collapse easily, are likely to have irregularly shaped or crumpled bottoms, and retain considerable amounts of thick medication. Molded plastic cups have measuring lines and are often supplied with over-the-counter medications for cough and fever, but the vast majority of families in one study could not measure a 5-mL dose within 0.5 mL (Sobhani, Christopherson, Ambrose, et al., 2008). Measures less than 1 tsp are impossible to determine accurately with a medicine cup.

The teaspoon is also an inaccurate measuring device and is subject to error. Teaspoons vary greatly in capacity, and different people using the same spoon will pour different amounts. Therefore, measure a drug ordered in teaspoons in milliliters; the established standard is 5 mL/tsp. A convenient hollow-handled medicine spoon is available to accurately measure and administer the drug. Household measuring spoons can also be used when other devices are not available.

Another unreliable device for measuring liquids is the dropper, which varies to a greater extent than the teaspoon or measuring cup. The volume of a drop varies according to the viscosity (thickness) of the liquid measured (Peacock, Parnapy, Raynor, et al., 2010). Viscous fluids produce much larger drops than thin liquids. Many medications are supplied with caps or droppers designed for measuring each specific preparation. These are accurate when used to measure that specific medication but are not reliable for measuring other liquids. Emptying dropper contents into a medicine cup invites additional error. Because some of the liquid clings to the sides of the cup, a significant amount of the drug can be lost.

Young children and some older children have difficulty swallowing tablets or pills. Because a number of drugs are not available in pediatric preparations, tablets need to be crushed before being given to these children. Commercial devices* are available, or simple methods can be used for crushing tablets. Not all drugs can be crushed (e.g., medication with an enteric or protective coating or formulated for slow release).

The nurse can teach children who must take solid oral medication for an extended period to swallow tablets or capsules. Training sessions include using verbal instruction, demonstration, reinforcement for swallowing progressively larger candy or capsules, no attention for inappropriate behavior, and gradual withdrawal of guidance after children can swallow their medication.

Because pediatric doses often require dividing adult preparations of medication, the nurse may be faced with the dilemma of accurate dosage. With tablets, only those that are scored can be halved or quartered accurately. If the medication is soluble, the tablet or contents of a capsule can be mixed in a small premeasured amount of liquid and the appropriate portion given. For example, if half a dose is required, the tablet is dissolved in 5 mL of water, and 2.5 mL is given.

Administration

Although administering liquids to infants is relatively easy, the nurse must take care to prevent aspiration. While holding the infant in a semireclining position, place the medication in the mouth from a spoon, plastic cup, dropper, or syringe (without a needle). It is best to place the dropper or syringe along the side of the infant's tongue and administer the liquid slowly in small amounts, waiting for the child to swallow between deposits.

> **! NURSING ALERT**
>
> In infants up to 11 months of age and children with neurologic impairments, blowing a small puff of air in the face frequently elicits a swallow reflex.

Medicine cups can be used effectively for older infants who are able to drink from a cup. Because of the natural outward tongue thrust in infancy, medications may need to be retrieved from the lips or chin and refed. Allowing the infant to suck the medication that has been placed in an empty nipple or inserting the syringe or dropper into the side of the mouth, parallel to the nipple, while the infant nurses is another convenient method for giving liquid medications to infants. Medication is not added to the infant's formula feeding because the

---

*Several styles of pill crushers are available from Trademark Medical, 449 Sovereign Court, St Louis, MO 63011; 800-325-9044; http://www.trademarkmedical.com.

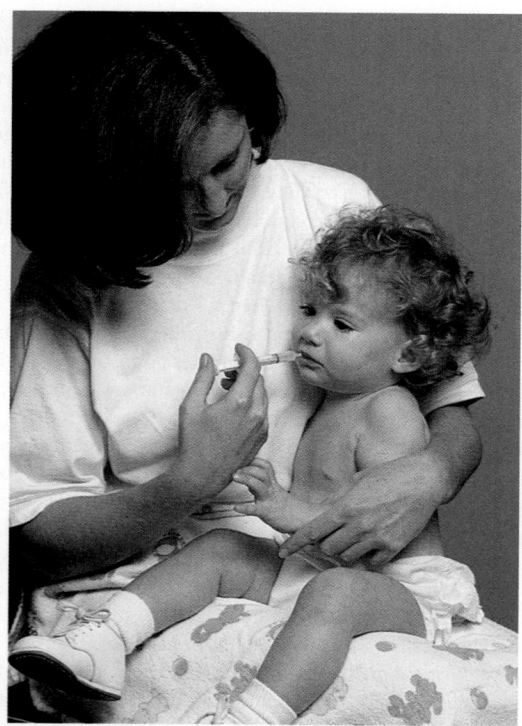

FIG 39.10 A nurse partially restrains a child for easy and comfortable administration of oral medication.

child may subsequently refuse the formula. Dispose of any plastic covers that may be on the ends of syringes because these covers are choking hazards.

Young children who refuse to cooperate or resist consistently despite explanation and encouragement may require mild physical coercion. If so, it is carried out quickly and carefully. Make every effort to determine why the child resists, and explain the reasons for the coercion in such a way that the child knows it is being carried out for his or her well-being and is not a form of punishment. There is always a risk in using even mild forceful techniques. A crying child can aspirate a medication, particularly when lying on the back. If the nurse holds the child in the lap with the child's right arm behind the nurse, the left hand firmly grasped by the nurse's left hand, and the head securely cradled between the nurse's arm and body, the medication can be slowly poured into the mouth (Fig. 39.10).

INTRAMUSCULAR ADMINISTRATION

Selecting the Syringe and Needle

The volume of medication prescribed for small children and the small amount of tissue available for injection necessitate selection of a syringe that can measure small amounts of solution. For volumes less than 1 mL, the tuberculin syringe, calibrated in 0.01-mL increments, is appropriate. Minute doses may require the use of a 0.5-mL, low-dose syringe. These syringes, along with specially constructed needles, minimize the possibility of inadvertently administering incorrect amounts of a drug because of dead space, which allows fluid to remain in the syringe and needle after the plunger is pushed completely forward. A minimum of 0.2 mL of solution remains in a standard needle hub; therefore, when very small amounts of two drugs are combined in the syringe, such as mixtures of insulin, the ratio of the two drugs can be altered significantly. Measures that minimize the effect of dead space are (1) when two drugs are combined in the syringe, always draw them

up in the same order to maintain a consistent ratio between the drugs, (2) use the same brand of syringe (dead space may vary between brands), and (3) use one-piece syringe units (needle permanently attached to the syringe).

Dead space is also an important factor to consider when injecting medication because flushing the syringe with an air bubble adds an additional amount of medication to the prescribed dose. This can be hazardous when very small amounts of a drug are given. Consequently, flushing is not recommended, especially when less than 1 mL of medication is given. Syringes are calibrated to deliver a prescribed drug dose, and the amount of medication left in the hub and needle is not part of the syringe barrel calibrations. Certain drugs (e.g., iron dextran and diphtheria and tetanus toxoid) may cause irritation when tracked into the subcutaneous tissue. The Z-track method is recommended for use in infants and children rather than an air bubble. Changing the needle after withdrawing the fluid from the vial is another technique to minimize tracking.

The needle length must be sufficient to penetrate the subcutaneous tissue and deposit the medication into the body of the muscle. The needle gauge should be as small as possible to deliver the fluid safely. Smaller-diameter (25- to 30-gauge) needles cause the least discomfort, but larger gauges are needed for viscous medication and prevention of accidental bending of longer needles.

Determining the Site

Factors to consider when selecting a site for an intramuscular (IM) injection on an infant or child include the following:

- The amount and character of the medication to be injected
- The amount and general condition of the muscle mass
- The frequency or number of injections to be given during the course of treatment
- The type of medication being given
- Factors that may impede access to or cause contamination of the site
- The child's ability to assume the required position safely

Older children and adolescents usually pose few problems in selecting a suitable site for IM injections, but infants, with their small and underdeveloped muscles, have fewer available sites. It is sometimes difficult to assess the amount of fluid that can be safely injected into a single site. Usually 1 mL is the maximum volume that should be administered in a single site to small children and older infants. The muscles of small infants may not tolerate more than 0.5 mL. As the child approaches adult size, the nurse can use volumes approaching those given to adults. However, the larger the amount of solution, the larger the muscle at the injection site must be.

Injections must be placed in muscles large enough to accommodate the medication, while avoiding major nerves and blood vessels. The IM immunization site recommended for infants by the Centers for Disease Control and Prevention, World Health Organization, and American Academy of Pediatrics is the anterolateral thigh or vastus lateralis (Table 39.6). However, in two studies, immunizations at the ventrogluteal site have been found to have fewer local reactions and fever (Cook & Murtagh, 2003; Junqueira, Tavares, Martins, et al., 2010). Cook and Murtagh (2003) also found fewer systemic reactions (irritability and persistent crying or screaming) and greater parental acceptance for the ventrogluteal site. The ventrogluteal site is relatively free of major nerves and blood vessels, is a relatively large muscle with less subcutaneous tissue than the dorsal site, has well-defined landmarks for safe site location, and is easily accessible in several positions. Distraction and prevention of unexpected movement may be more easily achieved by placing the child supine on a parent's lap for ventrogluteal site use (Cook & Murtagh, 2006).

TABLE 39.6 Intramuscular Injection Sites in Children

Site	Discussion
Vastus Lateralis 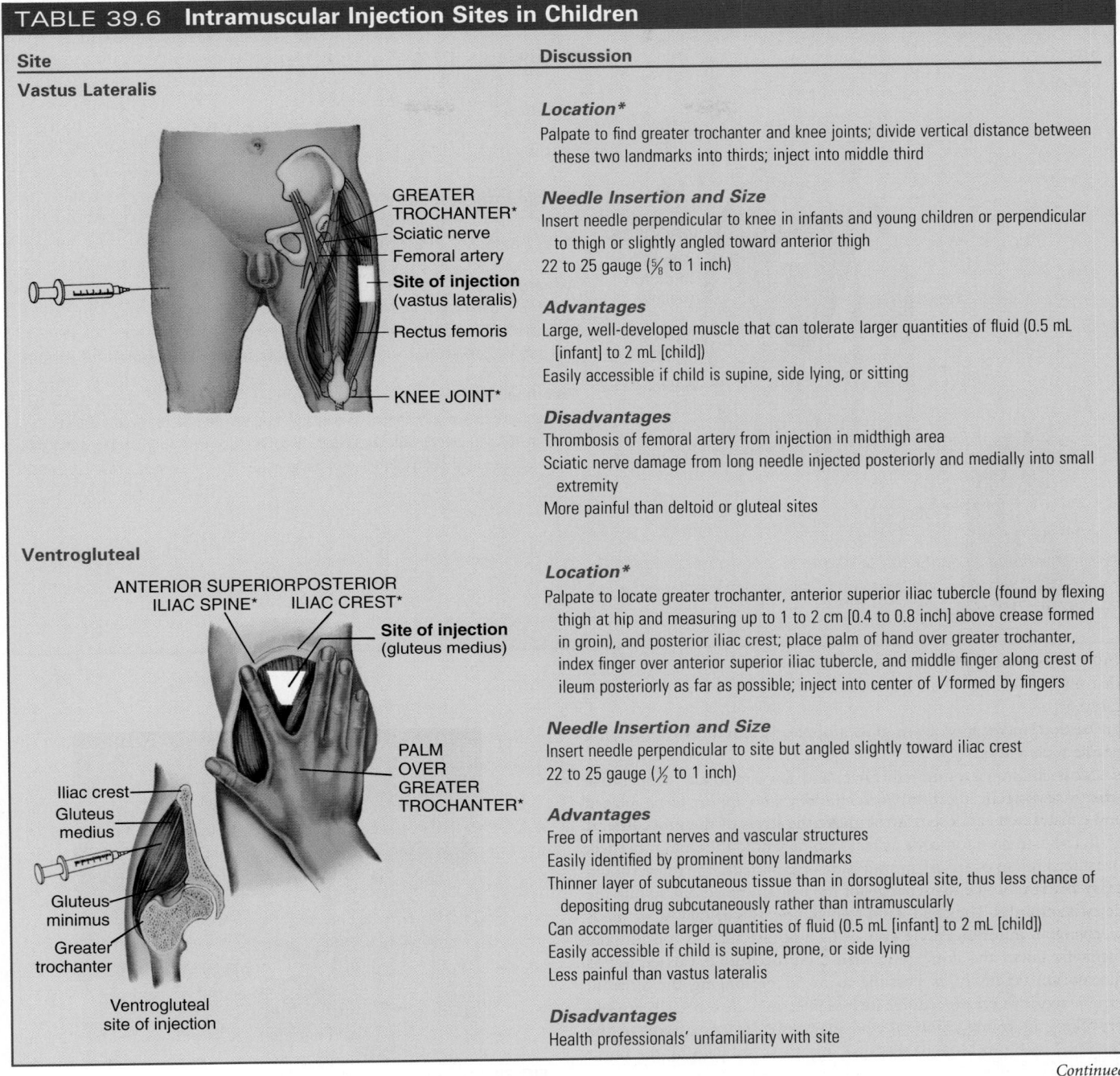	**Location*** Palpate to find greater trochanter and knee joints; divide vertical distance between these two landmarks into thirds; inject into middle third **Needle Insertion and Size** Insert needle perpendicular to knee in infants and young children or perpendicular to thigh or slightly angled toward anterior thigh 22 to 25 gauge (⅝ to 1 inch) **Advantages** Large, well-developed muscle that can tolerate larger quantities of fluid (0.5 mL [infant] to 2 mL [child]) Easily accessible if child is supine, side lying, or sitting **Disadvantages** Thrombosis of femoral artery from injection in midthigh area Sciatic nerve damage from long needle injected posteriorly and medially into small extremity More painful than deltoid or gluteal sites
Ventrogluteal	**Location*** Palpate to locate greater trochanter, anterior superior iliac tubercle (found by flexing thigh at hip and measuring up to 1 to 2 cm [0.4 to 0.8 inch] above crease formed in groin), and posterior iliac crest; place palm of hand over greater trochanter, index finger over anterior superior iliac tubercle, and middle finger along crest of ileum posteriorly as far as possible; inject into center of *V* formed by fingers **Needle Insertion and Size** Insert needle perpendicular to site but angled slightly toward iliac crest 22 to 25 gauge (½ to 1 inch) **Advantages** Free of important nerves and vascular structures Easily identified by prominent bony landmarks Thinner layer of subcutaneous tissue than in dorsogluteal site, thus less chance of depositing drug subcutaneously rather than intramuscularly Can accommodate larger quantities of fluid (0.5 mL [infant] to 2 mL [child]) Easily accessible if child is supine, prone, or side lying Less painful than vastus lateralis **Disadvantages** Health professionals' unfamiliarity with site

Labels in Vastus Lateralis figure: GREATER TROCHANTER*, Sciatic nerve, Femoral artery, Site of injection (vastus lateralis), Rectus femoris, KNEE JOINT*

Labels in Ventrogluteal figure: ANTERIOR SUPERIOR ILIAC SPINE*, POSTERIOR ILIAC CREST*, Site of injection (gluteus medius), PALM OVER GREATER TROCHANTER*, Iliac crest, Gluteus medius, Gluteus minimus, Greater trochanter, Ventrogluteal site of injection

Continued

The deltoid muscle, a small muscle near the axillary and radial nerves, can be used for small volumes of fluid in children as young as 18 months of age. Its advantages are less pain and fewer side effects from the injectate (as observed with immunizations), compared with the vastus lateralis. Table 39.6 summarizes the three major injection sites and illustrates the location of the preferred IM injection sites for children.

Administration

Although injections that are executed with care seldom cause trauma to children, there have been reports of serious disability related to IM injections in children. Repeated use of a single site has been associated with fibrosis of the muscle with subsequent muscle contracture. Injections close to large nerves, such as the sciatic nerve, have been responsible for permanent disability, especially when potentially neurotoxic drugs are administered. When such drugs are injected, use great care in locating the correct site. Aspiration during IM vaccine administration is no longer recommended by the Centers for Disease Control and Prevention, World Health Organization, American Academy of Pediatrics, or the Immunization Action Coalition (Petousis-Harris, 2008). One classic study of IM injection techniques revealed that the straighter the path of needle insertion (e.g., 90-degree angle), the less displacement and shear to tissue, causing less discomfort (Katsma & Smith, 1997).

A reported potential hazard with medication in glass ampules is the presence of glass particles in the ampule after the container is broken. When the medication is withdrawn into the syringe, the glass particles are also withdrawn and subsequently injected into the patient. As a

TABLE 39.6   Intramuscular Injection Sites in Children—cont'd

Site	Discussion
Deltoid 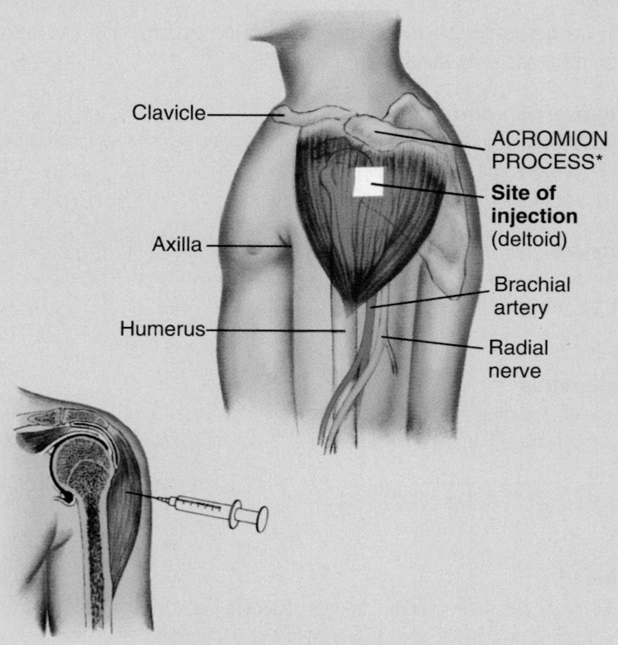 Clavicle ACROMION PROCESS* Site of injection (deltoid) Axilla Brachial artery Humerus Radial nerve	**Location*** Locate acromion process; inject only into upper third of muscle that begins about two finger breadths below acromion **Needle Insertion and Size** Insert needle perpendicular to site but angled slightly toward shoulder 22 to 25 gauge ($\frac{1}{2}$ to 1 inch) **Advantages** Faster absorption rates than gluteal sites Easily accessible with minimal removal of clothing Less pain and fewer local side effects from vaccines compared with vastus lateralis **Disadvantages** Small muscle mass; only limited amounts of drug can be injected (0.5 to 1 mL) Small margins of safety with possible damage to radial nerve and axillary nerve (not shown; lies under deltoid at head of humerus)

*Locations are indicated by asterisks on illustrations.

precaution, medication from glass ampules is only drawn through a needle with a filter.

Most children are unpredictable, and few are totally cooperative when receiving an injection. Even children who appear to be relaxed and constrained can lose control under the stress of the procedure. It is advisable to have someone available to help hold the child if needed. Because children often jerk or pull away unexpectedly, the nurse should carry an extra needle to exchange for the contaminated one so that the delay is minimal. The child, even a small one, is told that he or she is receiving an injection (preferably using a phrase such as "putting the medicine under the skin"), and then the procedure is carried out as quickly and skillfully as possible to avoid prolonging the stressful experience. Invasive procedures such as injections are especially anxiety provoking in young children, who may associate any assault to the "behind" with punishment. Because injections are painful, the nurse should use excellent injection techniques and effective pain reduction measures to reduce discomfort (see Guidelines box: Intramuscular Administration of Medication).

Small infants offer little resistance to injections. Although they squirm and may be difficult to hold in position, they can usually be restrained without assistance. A larger infant's body can be securely restrained between the nurse's arm and body. To inject into the body of a muscle, the nurse firmly grasps the muscle mass between the thumb and fingers to isolate and stabilize the site (Fig. 39.11). However, in obese children, it is preferable to first spread the skin with the thumb and index finger to displace subcutaneous tissue and then grasp the muscle deeply on each side.

If medication is given around the clock, the nurse must wake the child. Although it may seem easier to surprise the sleeping child and do it quickly, this can cause the child to fear going back to sleep. When

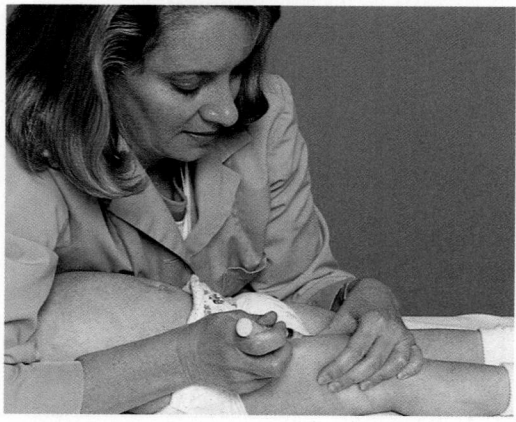

FIG 39.11 Holding a small child for intramuscular (IM) injection. Note how the nurse isolates and stabilizes the muscle.

awakened first, children will know that nothing will be done to them unless they are forewarned. The Guidelines box: Intramuscular Administration of Medication summarizes administration techniques that maximize safety and minimize the discomfort often associated with injections.

A needleless injection system (e.g., Biojector) delivers IM or subcutaneous injections without the use of a needle and eliminates the risk for accidental needle puncture. This needle-free injection system uses a carbon dioxide cartridge to power the delivery of medication through the skin. Although it is not painless, it may reduce pain and the anxiety of seeing the needle.

GUIDELINES

Intramuscular Administration of Medication

Apply EMLA (a eutectic mix of lidocaine and prilocaine) or LMX cream (lidocaine) topically over site if time permits. (See Pain Management, Chapter 30)

Prepare medication.

- Select appropriately sized needle and syringe.
- If withdrawing medication from an ampule, use a needle equipped with a filter that removes glass particles; then use a new, nonfilter needle for injection.
- The maximum volume to be administered in a single site is 1 mL for older infants and small children.
- Have medication at room temperature before injection.

Determine site of injection (see Table 39.6); make certain that muscle is large enough to accommodate volume and type of medication.

- For infants and small or debilitated children, use the vastus lateralis or ventrogluteal muscles; the dorsogluteal muscle is insufficiently developed to be a safe site for infants and small children.

Obtain sufficient help in restraining child.

Explain briefly what is to be done and, if appropriate, what child can do to help.

Expose injection area for unobstructed view of landmarks.

Select a site where skin is free of irritation and danger of infection; palpate for and avoid sensitive or hardened areas.

With multiple injections, rotate sites.

Place child in a lying or sitting position; child is not allowed to stand because landmarks are more difficult to assess, restraint is more difficult, and the child may faint and fall.

- *Ventrogluteal:* On side with upper leg flexed and placed in front of lower leg
- *Vastus lateralis:* Supine, lying on side, or sitting

Use a new, sharp needle (not one that has pierced rubber stopper on vial) with smallest diameter that permits free flow of the medication.

Grasp muscle firmly between thumb and fingers to isolate and stabilize muscle for deposition of drug in its deepest part; in obese children, spread skin with thumb and index finger to displace subcutaneous tissue, and grasp muscle deeply on each side.

Allow skin preparation to dry completely before penetrating skin.

Decrease perception of pain.

- Distract child with conversation.
- Give child something on which to concentrate (e.g., squeezing a hand or side rail, pinching own nose, humming, counting, yelling "Ouch!").
- Spray vapo-coolant (e.g., ethyl chloride or fluoromethane) on site before injection, place a cold compress or wrapped ice cube on site about 1 minute before injection, or apply cold to contralateral site.
- Have child hold a small adhesive bandage and place it on puncture site after IM injection is given.

Insert needle quickly using a dartlike motion at a 90-degree angle unless contraindicated.

Avoid tracking any medication through superficial tissues:

- Replace needle after withdrawing medication.
- Use the Z-track or air-bubble technique as indicated.
- Avoid any depression of the plunger during insertion of the needle.

Remove needle quickly; hold gauze firmly against skin near needle when removing it to avoid pulling on tissue.

Apply firm pressure to site after injection; massage site to hasten absorption unless contraindicated, as with irritating drugs.

Place a small adhesive bandage on puncture site; with young children, decorate it by drawing a smiling face or other symbol of acceptance.

Hold and cuddle young child, and encourage parents to comfort child; praise older child.

Allow expression of feelings.

Discard syringe and uncapped, uncut needle in puncture-resistant container located near site of use.

Record time of injection, drug, dose, and injection site.

EMLA, Eutectic mixture of local anesthetics; *IM,* intramuscular; *LMX,* lidocaine.

SUBCUTANEOUS AND INTRADERMAL ADMINISTRATION

Subcutaneous and intradermal injections are frequently administered to children, but the technique differs little from the method used with adults. Examples of subcutaneous injections include insulin, hormone replacement, allergy desensitization, and some vaccines. Tuberculin testing, local anesthesia, and allergy testing are examples of frequently administered intradermal injections.

Techniques to minimize the pain associated with these injections include changing the needle if it pierced a rubber stopper on a vial, using 26- to 30-gauge needles (only to inject the solution), and injecting small volumes (≤0.5 mL). The angle of the needle for the subcutaneous injection is typically 90 degrees. In children with little subcutaneous tissue, some practitioners insert the needle at a 45-degree angle. However, the benefit of using the 45-degree angle rather than the 90-degree angle remains controversial.

Although subcutaneous injections can be given anywhere there is subcutaneous tissue, common sites include the center third of the lateral aspect of the upper arm, the abdomen, and the center third of the anterior thigh. Some practitioners believe it is not necessary to aspirate before injecting subcutaneously; for example, this is an accepted practice in the administration of insulin. Automatic injector devices do not aspirate before injecting.

When giving an intradermal injection into the volar surface of the forearm, the nurse should avoid the medial side of the arm, where the skin is more sensitive.

 NURSING ALERT

Families often need to learn injection techniques to administer medications, such as insulin, at home. Begin teaching as early as possible to allow the family the maximum amount of practice time.

INTRAVENOUS ADMINISTRATION

The IV route for administering medications is frequently used in pediatric therapy. For some drugs, it is the only effective route. This method is used for giving drugs to children who:

- Have poor absorption as a result of diarrhea, vomiting, or dehydration
- Need a high serum concentration of a drug
- Have resistant infections that require parenteral medication over an extended time
- Need continuous pain relief
- Require emergency treatment

Intravenous Line Placement

The nurse needs to consider several factors in relation to IV medication. When a drug is administered intravenously, the effect is almost instantaneous and further control is limited. Most drugs for IV administration require a specified minimum dilution, rate of flow, or both, and many drugs are highly irritating or toxic to tissues outside the vascular system. In addition to the precautions and nursing observations commonly related to IV therapy, factors to consider when preparing and administering drugs to infants and children by the IV route include the following:

- Amount of drug to be administered
- Minimum dilution of drug and whether child is fluid restricted
- Type of solution in which drug can be diluted
- Length of time over which drug can be safely administered
- Rate limitations of child, vascular system, and infusion equipment
- Time that this or another drug is to be administered
- Compatibility of all drugs that child is receiving intravenously
- Compatibility with infusion fluids

Before any IV infusion, check the site of insertion for patency. Never administer medications with blood products. Only one antibiotic should be administered at a time. Extra fluids needed to administer IV medications can be problematic for infants and fluid-restricted children. Syringe pumps are often used to deliver IV medication, because they minimize fluid requirements and more precisely deliver small volumes of medication compared with large-volume infusion pumps. Regardless of the technique, the nurse must know the minimum dilutions for safe administration of IV medications to infants and children.

Peripheral Intermittent Infusion Device

The *peripheral lock*, also known as an *intermittent infusion device* or *saline* or *heparin lock*, is an alternative to a keep-open infusion when extended access to a vein is required without the need for continuous fluid. It is most frequently used for intermittent infusion of medication into a peripheral venous route. A short, flexible catheter is used as the lock device, and a site is selected where there will be minimal movement, such as the forearm. The catheter is inserted and secured in the same manner as for any IV infusion device, but the hub is occluded with a stopper or injection cap.

The type of device used may vary, and the care and use of the peripheral lock are carried out according to the protocol of the institution or unit. However, the general concept is the same. The catheter remains in place and is flushed with saline after infusion of the medication. See the Evidence-Based Practice box: Normal Saline or Heparinized Saline Flush Solution in Pediatric Intravenous Lines and Table 39.7 on flushing with normal saline or heparin.

Children may be discharged with a peripheral lock in place to continue receiving medications without hospitalization; this is usually reserved

EVIDENCE-BASED PRACTICE

Normal Saline or Heparinized Saline Flush Solution in Pediatric Intravenous Lines

Ask the Question

PICOT Question: Is there a significant difference in the longevity of intravenous (IV) intermittent infusion locks in children when normal saline (NS) is used as a flush instead a heparinized saline (HS) solution?

Search for the Evidence
Search Strategies
Selection criteria included evidence during the years 1992 to 2013 with the following terms: *saline versus heparin intermittent flush, children's heparin lock flush, heparin lock patency, peripheral venous catheter in children*.

Databases Used
CINAHL, PubMed

Critical Appraisal of the Evidence

- In trials of HS administration versus NS, placebo, or no treatment in neonates, no strong evidence regarding the effectiveness and safety of heparin in prolonging catheter life was found (Shah, Ng, & Sinha, 2005). No differences in patency were established in a double-blind prospective, randomized study in neonates. Saline flush was deemed preferable to heparin in peripheral intravenous (PIV) locks in neonates, in consideration of complications associated with heparin (Arnts, Heijnen, Wilbers, et al., 2011).
- No significant statistical difference was found between HS and NS flushes for maintaining catheter patency in children (Hanrahan, Kleiber, & Berends, 2000; Hanrahan, Kleiber, & Fagan, 1994; Heilskov, Kleiber, Johnson, et al., 1998; Kotter, 1996; Mok, Kwong, & Chan, 2007; Schultz, Drew, & Hewitt, 2002).
- Increased incidence of pain or erythema was associated with HS flushing of infusion devices (Hanrahan, Kleiber, & Fagan, 1994; McMullen, Fioravanti, Pollack, et al., 1993; Nelson & Graves, 1998; Robertson, 1994).
- Increased patency or longer dwell times were found with HS solutions versus NS in 24-gauge catheters (Beecroft, Bossert, Chung, et al., 1997; Danek & Noris, 1992; Gyr, Burroughs, Smith, et al., 1995; Hanrahan, Kleiber, & Berends, 2000; Mudge, Forcier, & Slattery, 1998; Tripathi, Kaushik & Singh, 2008).

- Younger children and preterm neonates with lower gestational ages were associated with shorter patency of IV catheters (McMullen, Fioravanti, Pollack, et al., 1993; Paisley, Stamper, Brown, et al., 1997; Robertson, 1994; Tripathi, Kaushik, & Singh, 2008).
- Infusion devices flushed with NS lasted longer than those flushed with HS (Goldberg, Sankaran, Givelichian, et al., 1999; Le Duc, 1997; Nelson & Graves, 1998).
- When measured and reported, the length of time between flushing peripheral devices affected the dwell time (Crews, Gnann, Rice, et al., 1997; Gyr, Burroughs, Smith, et al., 1995).
- Preterm neonates are at higher risk for development of clotting problems as a result of heparin; none of the studies cited anticoagulation-associated complications with HS (Klenner, Fusch, Rakow, et al., 2003).
- 0.9% sodium chloride injection is safe for maintaining patency of peripheral locks in adults and children older than 12 years of age (American Society of Hospital Pharmacists Commission on Therapeutics, 2006).
- Either preservative-free heparin or preservative-free 0.9% sodium chloride may be used to flush a PIV line; however, catheter patency may be maintained by flushing with saline when converting from continuous to intermittent use (Infusion Nurses Society, 2011).
- After each catheter use, peripheral catheters should be locked with preservative-free 0.9% sodium chloride (Infusion Nurses Society, 2011).

Apply the Evidence: Nursing Implications
There is **low-quality evidence with a weak recommendation (**Guyatt, Oxman, Vist, et al., 2008) for using NS versus HS flush solution in pediatric IV lines. Further research is still needed with larger samples of children, especially preterm neonates, using small-gauge catheters (24 gauge) and other gauge catheters flushed with NS and HS as intermittent infusion devices only (no continuous infusions). Variables to be considered include catheter dwell time; medications administered; period between regular flushing and flushing associated with medication administration; pain, erythema, and other localized complications; concentration and amount of HS used; flush method (positive-pressure technique

Normal Saline or Heparinized Saline Flush Solution in Pediatric Intravenous Lines—cont'd

vs. no specific technique); reason for IV device removal; and complications associated with either solution. NS is a safe alternative to HS flush in infants and children with intermittent IV locks larger than 24 gauge; smaller neonates may benefit from HS flush (longer dwell time), but the evidence is inconclusive for all weight ranges and gestational ages.

Quality and Safety Competencies: Evidence-Based Practice*
Knowledge

Differentiate clinical opinion from research and evidence-based summaries.

Describe methods for using NS or HS flush solution in pediatric IV lines.

Skills

Base individualized care plan on patient values, clinical expertise, and evidence.

Integrate evidence into practice on NS or HS flush solution in pediatric IV lines.

Attitudes

Value the concept of evidence-based practice as integral to determining best clinical practice.

Appreciate the strengths and weakness of evidence for NS or HS flush solution in pediatric IV lines.

References

American Society of Hospital Pharmacists Commission on Therapeutics. (2006). ASHP therapeutic position statement on the institutional use of 0.9% sodium chloride injection to maintain patency of peripheral indwelling intermittent infusion devices. *American Journal of Health-System Pharmacy, 63*(13), 1273–1275.

Arnts, I. J., Heijnen, J. A., Wilbers, H. T., et al. (2011). Effectiveness of heparin solution versus normal saline in maintaining patency of intravenous locks in neonates: A double blind randomized controlled study. *Journal of Advanced Nursing, 67*(12), 2677–2685.

Beecroft, P. C., Bossert, E., Chung, K., et al. (1997). Intravenous lock patency in children: Dilute heparin versus saline. *Journal of Pediatric Pharmacy Practice, 2*(4), 211–203.

Crews, B. E., Gnann, K. K., Rice, M. H., et al. (1997). Effects of varying intervals between heparin flushes on pediatric catheter longevity. *Pediatric Nursing, 23*(1), 87–91.

Danek, G. D., & Noris, E. M. (1992). Pediatric IV catheters: efficacy of saline flush. *Pediatric Nursing, 18*(2), 111–113.

Goldberg, M., Sankaran, R., Givelichian, L., et al. (1999). Maintaining patency of peripheral intermittent infusion devices with heparinized saline and saline: A randomized double blind controlled trial in neonatal intensive care and a review of literature. *Neonatal Intensive Care: Journal of Perinatology-Neonatology, 12*(1), 18–22.

Guyatt, G. H., Oxman, A. D., Vist, G. E., et al. (2008). GRADE: An emerging consensus on rating quality of evidence and strength of recommendations. *British Medical Journal, 336*(7650), 924–926.

Gyr, P., Burroughs, T., Smith, K., et al. (1995). Double blind comparison of heparin and saline flush solutions in maintenance of peripheral infusion devices. *Pediatric Nursing, 21*(4), 383–389.

Hanrahan, K. S., Kleiber, C., & Berends, S. (2000). Saline for peripheral intravenous locks in neonates: Evaluating a change in practice. *Neonatal Network, 19*(2), 19–24.

Hanrahan, K. S., Kleiber, C., & Fagan, C. (1994). Evaluation of saline for IV locks in children. *Pediatric Nursing, 20*(6), 549–552.

Heilskov, J., Kleiber, C., Johnson, K., et al. (1998). A randomized trial of heparin and saline for maintaining intravenous locks in neonates. *Journal of the Socety of Pediatric Nurses, 3*(3), 111–116.

Infusion Nurses Society. (2011). Infusion nursing standards of practice. *Journal of Infusion Nursing, 34*(1S), S63–S64.

Klenner, A. F., Fusch, C., Rakow, A., et al. (2003). Benefit and risk of heparin for maintaining peripheral venous catheters in neonates: A placebo-controlled trial. *Journal of Pediatrics, 143*(6), 741–745.

Kotter, R. W. (1996). Heparin vs. saline for intermittent intravenous device maintenance in neonates. *Neonatal Network, 15*(6), 43–47.

Le Duc, K. (1997). Efficacy of normal saline solution versus heparin solution for maintaining patency of peripheral intravenous catheters in children. *Journal of Emergency Nursing, 23*(4), 306–309.

McMullen, A., Fioravanti, I. D., Pollack, D., et al. (1993). Heparinized saline or normal saline as a flush solution in intermittent intravenous lines in infants and children. *American Journal of Maternal/Child Nursing, 18*(2), 78–85.

Mok, E., Kwong, T. K., & Chan, M. E. (2007). A randomized controlled trial for maintaining peripheral intravenous lock in children. *International Journal of Nursing Practice, 13*(1), 33–45.

Mudge, B., Forcier, D., & Slattery, M. J. (1998). Patency of 24-gauge peripheral intermittent infusion devices: A comparison of heparin and saline flush solutions. *Pediatric Nursing, 24*(2), 142–149.

Nelson, T. J., & Graves, S. M. (1998). 0.9% Sodium chloride injection with and without heparin for maintaining peripheral indwelling intermittent infusion devices in infants. *American Journal of Heath-System Pharmacy, 55*(6), 570–573.

Paisley, M. K., Stamper, M., Brown, T., et al. (1997). The use of heparin and normal saline flushes in neonatal intravenous catheters. *Journal of Pediatric Nursing, 23*(5), 521–527.

Robertson, J. (1994). Intermittent intravenous therapy: A comparison of two flushing solutions. *Contemporary Nursing, 3*(4), 174–179.

Schultz, A. A., Drew, D., & Hewitt, H. (2002). Comparison of normal saline and heparinized saline for patency of IV locks in neonates. *Applied Nursing Research, 15*(1), 28–34.

Shah, P. S., Ng, E., & Sinha, A. K. (2005). Heparin for prolonging peripheral intravenous catheter use in neonates. *Cochrane Database of Systematic Reviews, 2002*(4), CD002774.

Tripathi, S., Kaushik, V., & Singh, V. (2008). Peripheral IVs: factors affecting complications and patency—A randomized controlled trial. *Journal of Infusion Nursing, 31*(3), 182–188.

*Adapted from the Quality and Safety Education for Nurses (QSEN) Institute.

for children who require medications on a short-term basis and are referred to a home-based infusion company. Those with chronic illnesses who require repeated blood sampling or medications, long-term chemotherapy, or frequent hyperalimentation or antibiotic therapy are best managed with a central venous catheter.

Central Venous Access Device

Central venous access devices (CVADs) have several different characteristics. Factors that can influence the type of CVAD include the reason for placement of the catheter (diagnosis), length of therapy, risk to the patient in placement of the catheter, and availability of resources to assist the family in maintaining the catheter.

Short-term or nontunneled catheters are used in acute care, emergency, and intensive care units. These catheters are made of polyurethane and are placed in large veins, such as the subclavian, femoral, or jugular. Insertion is by surgical incision or large percutaneous threading. A chest X-ray should be taken to verify placement of the catheter tip before administration of fluids or medications.

Peripherally inserted central catheters (PICCs) can be used for short-term to moderate-length therapy. These catheters consist of silicone or polymer material and are placed by specially trained nurses, physicians, or interventional radiologists (Gamulka, Mendoza, & Connolly, 2005). The most common insertion site is above the antecubital area using the median, cephalic, or basilic vein. The catheter is threaded either with or without a guidewire into the superior vena cava. PICCs can be trimmed before insertion, and the decision can be made to insert the catheter midline, which is considered between the insertion site and the axilla. If the catheter is threaded midline, total parenteral nutrition (TPN) or any other drug known to irritate a peripheral vein (e.g., chemotherapy drugs) should not be administered. The high concentration

TABLE 39.7   Intravenous Catheter Flushes for Lines Without Continuous Fluid Infusions

Peripheral lines (Hep-Lock or saline locks)	NS* after medications or every 8 hours for dormant lines; instill 2½ times tubing volume 24-g catheters: NS* or heparin 2 units/mL 2 mL
Midline	Heparin 10 units/mL; 3 mL in a 10-mL syringe† after medications or every 8 hours if dormant Newborns: Heparin 1 to 2 units/mL to run continuously at ordered rate
External central line (nonimplanted, nontunneled, tunneled, or PICC)	Heparin 10 units/mL; 3 mL in a 10-mL syringe† after medications or once daily if dormant Newborns: Heparin 2 units/mL; 2 to 3 mL after medications or to check line patency *or* heparin 1 to 2 units/mL to run continuously at ordered rate
Totally implanted central line (TIVAS, implanted port)	Heparin 10 units/mL; 5 mL after medications or once daily if dormant and accessed; if not accessed, heparin 100 units/mL; 5 mL every month
Arterial and central venous pressure continuous monitored lines	Heparin 2 units/mL in 55-mL syringe to run continuously at 1 mL/hour

NS, Normal saline; *PICC*, peripherally inserted central catheter; *TIVAS*, totally implantable venous access device.
*Use 5% dextrose in water when medication is incompatible with saline.
†Smaller syringes may be used when flush is delivered by a pump.

of glucose in TPN makes it irritating to the vessel; it should be infused through a central catheter.

The decision to insert a PICC needs to be made before several attempts at IV insertion are done. When the antecubital veins have been punctured repeatedly, they are not considered candidates for this type of catheter. Because this catheter is the least costly and has less chance of complications than other CVADs, it is an excellent choice for many pediatric patients.

> **! NURSING ALERT**
>
> Most peripherally inserted central catheter (PICC) lines are not sutured into place, so care is needed when changing the dressing.

Long-term CVADs include tunneled catheters and implanted infusion ports (Table 39.8 and Fig. 39.12). They may have single, double, or triple lumens. Multilumen (several lumens) catheters allow more than one therapy to be administered at the same time. Reasons to use multilumen catheters include repeated blood sampling, TPN, administration of blood products or infusion of large quantities or concentrations of fluids, administration of incompatible drugs or fluids at the same time (through different lumens), and central venous pressure monitoring.

With any of the central venous catheters, medication is easily instilled through the injection cap. Maintenance of the catheter includes dressing changes, flushing to maintain patency, and prevention of occlusion or dislodgment.

> **! NURSING ALERT**
>
> When working with tunneled catheters, peripherally inserted central catheters (PICCs), and peripheral intravenous (PIV) lines, avoid the use of any scissors around the tubing or dressing. Removal is best accomplished using fingers and much patience. In the event that a tunneled catheter is cut, use a padded clamp to clamp the catheter proximal to the exit site to avoid blood loss. Repair kits are available, which may save the catheter and avoid surgery to replace a cut catheter.

With the implanted device, the port must be palpated for placement and stabilized, the overlying skin cleansed, and only special noncoring Huber needles used to pierce the port's diaphragm on the top or side, depending on the style. To avoid repeated skin punctures, a special infusion set with a Huber needle and extension tubing with a Luer connection can be used (see Fig. 39.12). With this attached, the injection procedure is the same as for an intermittent infusion device or a central venous catheter. To prevent infection, meticulous aseptic technique must be used any time the devices are entered, including instillation of heparin or saline to prevent clotting. There should be a protocol stating that the Huber needle needs to be changed at established intervals, usually 5 to 7 days.

The children and parents are taught the procedure for care of the CVAD before discharge from the hospital, including preparation and injection of the prescribed medication, the flush, and dressing changes. A protective device may be recommended for some active children to prevent their accidentally dislodging the needle. Many children take responsibility for preparing and administering medications. Both verbal and written step-by-step instructions are provided for the learners.

> **! NURSING ALERT**
>
> A pocket sewn on the inside of a T-shirt provides a place in which to coil the catheter line while the child is at play if a dressing is not used.

Infection and catheter occlusion are two of the most common complications of central venous catheters. They require treatment with antibiotics for infection and a fibrinolytic agent, such as alteplase, for thrombus formation (Blaney, Shen, Kerner, et al., 2006; Fisher, Deffenbaugh, Poole, et al., 2004; Kerner, Garcia-Careaga, Fisher, et al., 2006; Shen, Li, Murdock, et al., 2003). Uncapping can be prevented by taping the cap securely to the catheter and the clamped line to the dressing. Leaks can be prevented by using a smooth-edged clamp only. The parents are cautioned to keep scissors away from the child to prevent accidental cutting of the catheter. If the catheter leaks, the parents are instructed to tape it above the leak and then clamp the catheter at the taped site. The child should be taken to the practitioner as soon as possible to prevent infection or clotting after a catheter leak.

> **! NURSING ALERT**
>
> If a central venous catheter is accidentally removed, apply pressure to the entry site to the vein, not the exit site on the skin.

INTRAOSSEOUS INFUSION

Situations may occur in which rapid establishment of systemic access is vital, and venous access may be hampered by peripheral circulatory collapse, hypovolemic shock (secondary to vomiting or diarrhea, burns, or trauma), cardiopulmonary arrest, or other conditions. It is recommended that intraosseous access be obtained if venous access cannot

TABLE 39.8   Comparison of Long-Term Central Venous Access Devices

Description	Benefits	Care Considerations
Tunneled Catheter (e.g., Hickman or Broviac Catheter)		
Silicone, radiopaque, flexible catheter with open ends or VitaCuffs (biosynthetic material impregnated with silver ions) on catheter(s) enhances tissue ingrowth May have more than one lumen	Reduced risk for bacterial migration after tissue adheres to cuff Easy to use for self-administered infusions Removal requires pulling catheter from site (nonsurgical procedure)	Requires daily heparin flushes Must be clamped or have clamp nearby at all times Must keep exit site dry Heavy activity restricted until tissue adheres to cuff Water sports may be restricted (risk for infection) Risk for infection still present Protrudes outside body; susceptible to damage from sharp instruments and may be pulled out; may affect body image More difficult to repair Patient or family must learn catheter care
Groshong Catheter		
Clear, flexible, silicone, radiopaque catheter with closed tip and two-way valve at proximal end Dacron cuff or VitaCuff on catheter enhances tissue ingrowth May have more than one lumen	Reduced time and cost for maintenance care; no heparin flushes needed Reduced catheter damage; no clamping needed because of two-way valve Increased patient safety because of minimal potential for blood backflow or air embolism Reduced risk for bacterial migration after tissue adheres to cuff Easily repaired Easy to use for self-administered IV infusions	Requires weekly irrigation with normal saline Must keep exit site dry Heavy activity restricted until tissue adheres to cuff Water sports may be restricted (risk for infection) Risk for infection still present Protrudes outside body; susceptible to damage from sharp instruments and may be pulled out; can affect body image Patient or family must learn catheter care
Implanted Ports (e.g., Port-A-Cath, Infus-A-Port, Mediport, Norport, Groshong Port)		
Totally implantable metal or plastic device that consists of self-sealing injection port with top or side access with preconnected or attachable silicone catheter that is placed in large blood vessel	Reduced risk for infection Placed completely under the skin and therefore much less likely to be pulled out or damaged No maintenance care and reduced cost for family Heparinized monthly and after each infusion to maintain patency (only Groshong port requires saline) No limitations on regular physical activity, including swimming Dressing needed only when port accessed with Huber needle that is not removed No or only slight change in body appearance (slight bulge on chest)	Must pierce skin for access; pain with insertion of needle; can use local anesthetic (EMLA, LMX) or intradermal buffered lidocaine before accessing port Special noncoring needle (Huber) with straight or angled design must be used to inject into port Skin preparation needed before injection Difficult to manipulate for self-administered infusions Catheter may dislodge from port, especially if child "plays" with port site (twiddler syndrome) Vigorous contact sports generally not allowed Removal requires surgical procedure

EMLA, Eutectic mixture of local anesthetics; *IV,* intravenous; *LMX,* lidocaine.

be readily achieved in a pediatric resuscitation (Kleinman, Chameides, Schexnayder, et al., 2010; Tobias & Ross, 2010). Intraosseous infusion provides a rapid, safe, and lifesaving alternate route for administration of fluids and medications until intravascular access is possible.

A large-bore needle, such as a bone marrow aspiration needle (e.g., Jamshidi) or an intraosseous needle (e.g., Cook), is inserted into the medullary cavity of a long bone, most often the proximal tibia. This procedure is usually reserved for children who are unconscious or for those who are receiving analgesia because the procedure is painful. Local anesthesia should be used for semiconscious patients. A battery-powered (EZ-IO) intraosseous needle driver is also available for use in prehospital and hospital settings and has a high rate of success in pediatric resuscitation and stabilization (Greene, Bhananker, & Ramaiah, 2012).

Once the bone marrow needle is in place, the needle should stand alone and feel secure. Tape and gauze are used to secure the needle to the leg. Gauze should be built up around the needle to provide support and prevent trauma or dislodgment. Drugs may be pushed and fluids delivered via an infusion pump. Observe the dependent tissue closely for swelling because extravasation may be hidden under the leg, and compartment syndrome may result. Other complications, although rare,

include fractures, skin necrosis, osteomyelitis, and cellulitis (Tobias & Ross, 2010). The intraosseous line may be discontinued after IV access has been achieved.

MAINTAINING FLUID BALANCE

MEASUREMENT OF INTAKE AND OUTPUT

Accurate measurements of fluid intake and output (I&O) are essential to the assessment of fluid balance. Measurements from all sources—including gastrointestinal and parenteral I&O from urine, stools, vomitus, fistulas, NG suction, sweat, and drainage from wounds—must be taken and considered. Although the practitioner usually indicates when I&O measurements are to be recorded, it is a nursing responsibility to keep an accurate I&O record on certain children, including those:

- Receiving IV therapy
- Who underwent major surgery
- Receiving diuretic or corticosteroid therapy
- With severe thermal burns or injuries
- With renal disease or damage

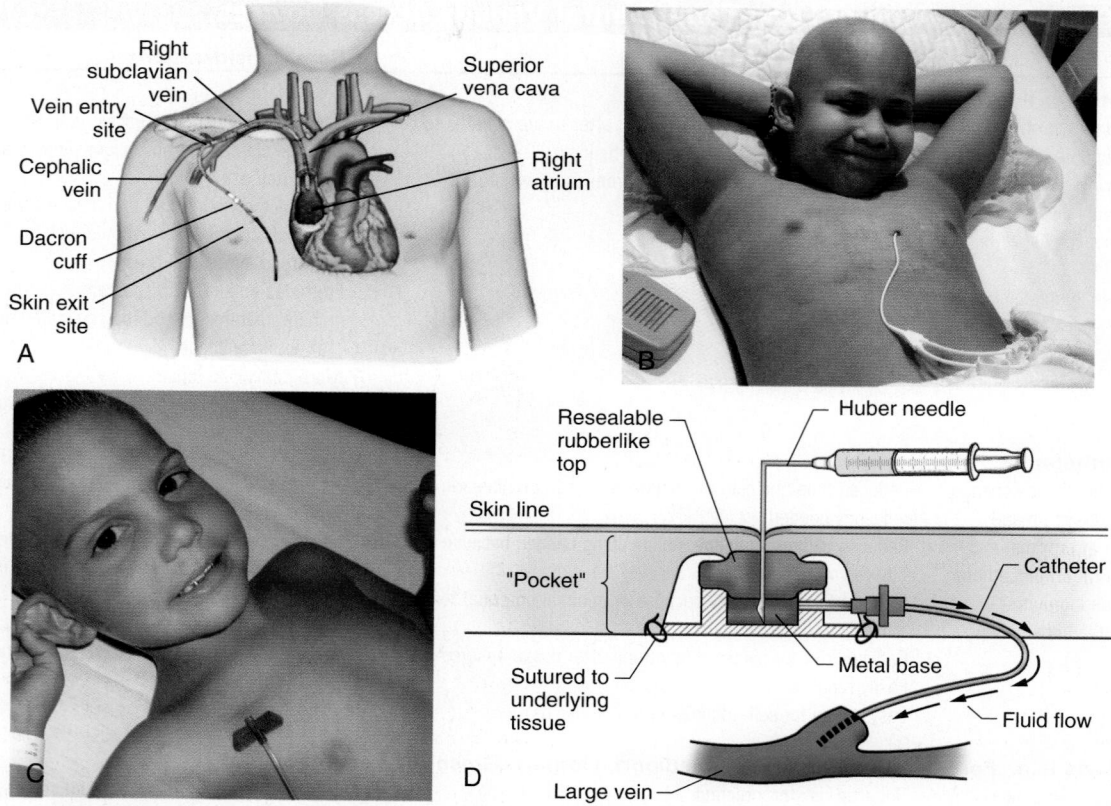

FIG 39.12 Venous access devices. **A,** External central venous catheter insertion and exit site. **B,** Child with an external central venous catheter (dressing removed for photo). **C,** Child with an implanted port with a Huber needle in place (dressing removed for photo). **D,** Side view of an implanted port.

- With congestive heart failure
- With dehydration
- With diabetes mellitus
- With oliguria
- In respiratory distress
- With chronic lung disease

Infants and small children who are unable to use a bedpan and those who have bowel movements with every voiding require the application of a collecting device. If collecting bags are not used, wet diapers or pads are carefully weighed to ascertain the amount of fluid lost. This includes liquid stool, vomitus, and other losses. The volume of fluid in milliliters is equivalent to the weight of the fluid measured in grams. The specific gravity as a measure of osmolality assists in assessing the degree of hydration.

> ⚠ **NURSING ALERT**
>
> 1 g of wet diaper weight = 1 mL of urine

In infants with diapers, weigh all dry diapers to be used and note in an indelible marker the dry weight of the diaper; when there is fluid (urine or liquid stool) in the diaper, the amount of output can be approximated by subtracting the weight of the dry diaper from the weighed amount of the wet diaper.

Disadvantages of the weighed-diaper method of fluid measurement include (1) an inability to differentiate one type of loss from another because of admixture, (2) loss of urine or liquid stool from leakage or evaporation (especially if the infant is under a radiant warmer), and (3) additional fluid in the diaper (superabsorbent disposable type) from absorption of atmospheric moisture (in high-humidity incubators).

SPECIAL NEEDS WHEN THE CHILD IS NOT PERMITTED TO TAKE FLUIDS BY MOUTH

Infants or children who are unable or not permitted to take fluids by mouth (nothing by mouth [NPO]) have special needs. To ensure that they do not receive fluids, a sign can be placed in some obvious place, such as over their beds or on their shirts, to alert others to the NPO status. To prevent the temptation to drink, fluids should not be left at the bedside.

Oral hygiene, a part of routine hygienic care, is especially important when fluids are restricted or withheld. For young children who cannot brush their teeth or rinse their mouth without swallowing fluid, the mouth and teeth can be cleansed and kept moist by swabbing with saline-moistened gauze.

> ⚠ **NURSING ALERT**
>
> To keep the mouth feeling moist when the child is not permitted to take fluids by mouth, give ice chips (if this is permitted by the practitioner) or spray the mouth from an atomizer. To meet the need to suck, infants are provided with a safe commercial pacifier.

The child who is fluid restricted presents an equal challenge. Limiting fluids is often more difficult for the child than being NPO, especially when IV fluids are also eliminated. To make certain the child does not

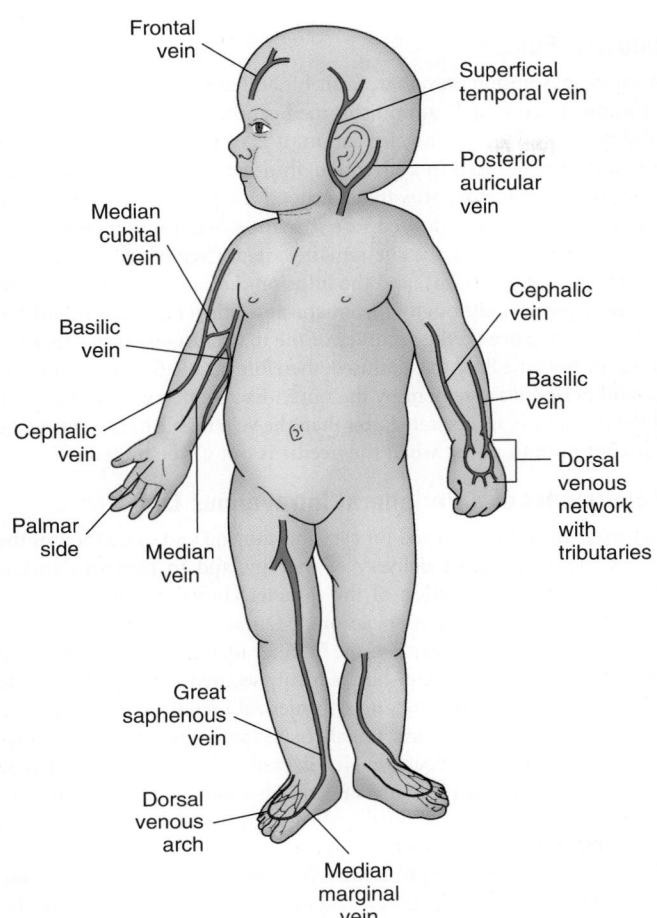

FIG 39.13 Preferred sites for venous access in infants.

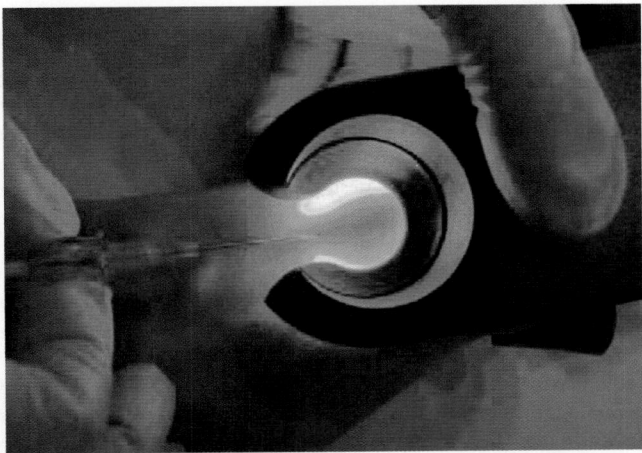

FIG 39.14 Transilluminator: Low-heat light-emitting diode (LED) light placed on the skin to illuminate veins; an opening allows cannulation of vein. (Courtesy of Professor Mark Waltzman, Children's Hospital, Boston MA.)

drink the entire amount allowed early in the day, the daily allotment is calculated to provide fluids at periodic intervals throughout the child's waking hours. Serving the fluids in small containers gives the illusion of larger servings. No extra liquid is left at the bedside.

PARENTERAL FLUID THERAPY

Site and Equipment

The site selected for PIV infusion depends on accessibility and convenience. Although it is possible to use any accessible site in older children, the child's developmental, cognitive, and mobility needs must be considered when selecting a site. Ideally, in older children, the superficial veins of the forearm should be used, leaving the hands free. An older child can help select the site and thereby maintain some measure of control. For veins in the extremities, it is best to start with the most distal site and avoid the child's favored hand to reduce the disability related to the procedure. Restrict the child's movements as little as possible—avoid a site over a joint in an extremity, such as the antecubital space. In small infants, a superficial vein of the hand, wrist, forearm, foot, or ankle is usually most convenient and most easily stabilized (Fig. 39.13). Foot veins should be avoided in children learning to walk and in children already walking. Superficial veins of the scalp have no valves, insertion is easy, and they can be used in infants up to about 9 months of age, but they should be used only when other site attempts have failed.

A transilluminator (Fig. 39.14) aids in finding and evaluating veins for access. Although not as powerful as ultrasound, a transilluminator

requires minimal training and experience to use. Small veins that may not be visible or palpable (especially in infants and toddlers) are often more readily visualized using a transilluminator and more often result in successful cannulation on the first or second attempt. Some devices require assistance to hold in place. Commercial devices have not caused burns in infants or children. Because veins stand out so clearly with transillumination, they appear more superficial than they are. Practice in this technique is necessary for optimal outcomes.

Selection of a scalp vein may require clipping the area around the site to better visualize the vein and provide a smoother surface on which to tape the catheter hub and tubing. Clipping a portion of the infant's hair is upsetting to parents; therefore, they should be told what to expect and reassured that the hair will grow in again rapidly (save the hair because parents often wish to keep it). Remove as little as possible directly over the insertion site and taping surface. A rubber band slipped onto the head from brow to occiput will usually suffice as a tourniquet, although if the vessel is visible, a tourniquet may not be necessary.

> **! NURSING ALERT**
>
> A tab of tape should be placed on the rubber band to help grasp it when removing it from the infant's head. The rubber band should be cut to avoid accidentally dislodging the catheter when moving the rubber band over the IV insertion site. The tape tab will lift the rubber band and allow it to be cut. Hold the rubber band in two places, and cut between these areas to prevent the rubber band from snapping on the head.

For most IV infusions in children, a 20- to 24-gauge catheter may be used if therapy is expected to last less than 5 days. The smallest gauge and shortest length catheter that will accommodate the prescribed therapy should be chosen. The length of the catheter may be directly related to infection or embolus formation—the shorter the catheter, the fewer the complications. The gauge of the catheter should maintain adequate flow of the infusate into the cannulated vein while allowing adequate blood flow around the catheter walls to promote proper hemodilution of the infusate.

Determining the best catheter for the patient early in the therapy provides the best chance of avoiding catheter-related complications. As the length of therapy increases, decisions regarding the type of infusion device (short peripheral, midline, PICC, or central venous catheter) should be explored. Guidelines such as flow charts and algorithms are available to help in these decisions.

Safety Catheters and Needleless Systems

Over-the-needle IV catheters with hollow-bore needles carry a high risk for transmission of bloodborne pathogens from needlestick injuries. Safety catheters prevent accidental needlesticks with the use of over-the-needle IV catheters.

Needleless IV systems are designed to prevent needlestick injuries during administration of IV push medications and IV piggyback medications. Some needleless devices can be used with any tubing, but others require use of the entire IV delivery system for compatibility. Needleless IV systems rely on pre-pierced septa that are accessed by blunted plastic cannulas or systems that use valves that open and close a fluid path when activated by insertion of a syringe.

Blunt plastic cannulas and pre-slit injection port sites (Fig. 39.15) eliminate the need for steel needles and conventional injection port sites but remain accessible via hypodermic needles, a drawback except in emergent situations. Systems that do not permit needled access enhance safety by preventing health care workers from attempting to use needles. A syringe with a blue spike is available to access a single-dose vial (see Fig. 39.15, A). The pre-slit injection port sites are identified by a white ring surrounding the port; this ring alerts users that the system is needleless (see Fig. 39.15, B). Syringes are available with the blunt plastic cannula for accessing these sites (see Fig. 39.15, C). A lever lock (see Fig. 39.15, D) or threaded lock cannula (see Fig. 39.15, E) attaches to an IV line, IV Y site, or peripheral intermittent infusion device. A pre-slit universal vial adapter (not pictured) provides access to standard multiple-dose vials, and syringe cannulas are then used to access the adapter. Valve technology allows syringes and IV tubing to connect directly in-line without the use of an adapter.

> **! NURSING ALERT**
>
> Misconnections of tubing have occurred, resulting in patient deaths. Many needleless IV systems allow other types of tubing such as blood pressure and oxygen tubing to connect and instill air directly into the IV line. Before tubing is connected or reconnected to a patient, trace it completely from the patient to the point of origin for verification.

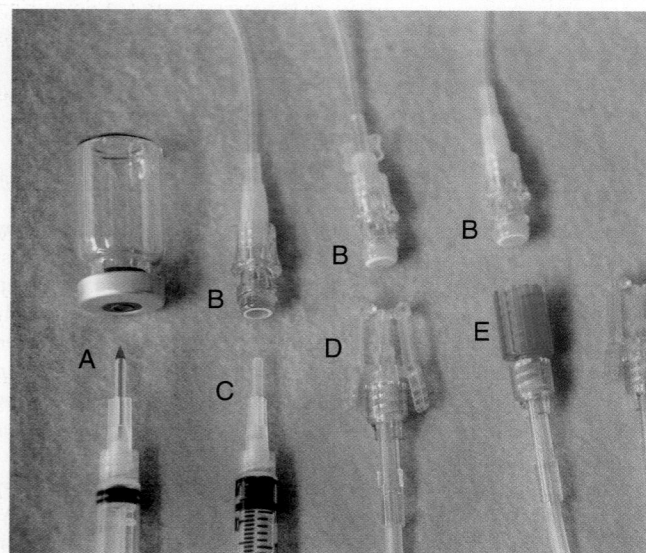

FIG 39.15 Interlink intravenous (IV) access systems. **A,** Blue spike syringe. **B,** Pre-slit injection port (needleless). **C,** Blunt plastic cannula syringe. **D,** Lever lock cannula. **E,** Threaded lock cannula.

Infusion Pumps

A variety of infusion pumps are available and used in nearly all pediatric infusions to accurately administer medication and minimize the possibility of overloading the circulation. It is important to calculate the amount to be infused in a given length of time, set the infusion rate, and monitor the apparatus frequently (at least every 1 to 2 hours) to make certain that the desired rate is maintained, the integrity of the system remains intact, the site remains intact (free of redness, edema, infiltration, or irritation), and the infusion does not stop. Continuous infusion pumps, although convenient and efficient, are not without risks. Overreliance on the accuracy of the machine can cause either too much or too little fluid to be infused; therefore, its use does not eliminate careful periodic assessment by the nurse. Excess pressure can build up if the machine is set at a rate faster than the vein is able to accommodate (or continues to pump when the needle is out of the lumen).

Securement of a Peripheral Intravenous Line

Catheters must be stabilized for easy monitoring and evaluation of the access site, to promote delivery of therapy, and to prevent damage, dislodgement, or migration of the catheter (Infusion Nurses Society, 2011; Registered Nurses' Association of Ontario, 2008).

To maintain the integrity of the IV line, adequate protection of the site is required. The catheter hub is firmly secured at the puncture site with a transparent dressing and commercial securement device (e.g., StatLock) (Fig. 39.16) or clear nonallergenic tape. Transparent dressings are ideal because the insertion site is easily observed. Minimal tape should be used at the puncture site and on about 1 to 2 inches of skin beyond the site to avoid obscuring the insertion site for early detection of infiltration.

A protective cover is applied directly over the catheter insertion site to protect the infusion site. Easy access to the IV site for frequent (hourly) assessments must be considered (Infusion Nurses Society, 2011). Improvised plastic cups that are cut in half with the ridged edges covered with tape should not be used because they have injured patients. A commercial site protector, I.V. House, is available in different sizes (Fig. 39.17). Its ventilation holes prevent moisture from accumulating under the dome. This device is designed to protect the IV site and allows for visibility of the site. The device also minimizes use of padded boards, splints, or other restraints and tape and maintains skin integrity. The connector tubing or extension tubing can be looped to make it small enough to fit under the protective cover to prevent accidental snagging of the catheter. It is important to safely secure the IV tubing to prevent

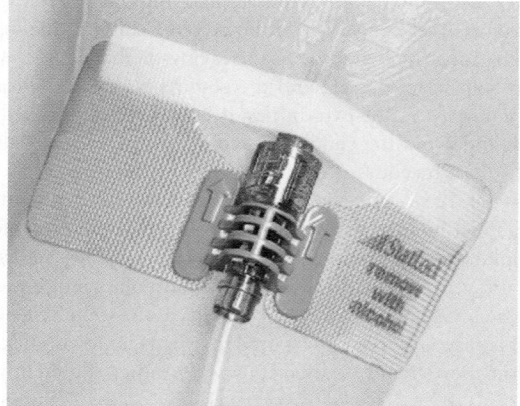

FIG 39.16 StatLock securement devices enhance peripheral intravenous (PIV) line dwell time and decrease phlebitis.

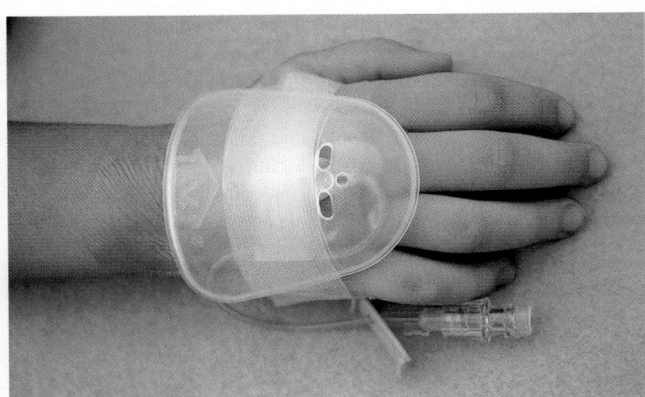

FIG 39.17 I.V. House used to protect the intravenous (IV) site.

infants and children from becoming entangled in the tubing and from accidentally pulling the catheter or needle out. Securing the tubing in this manner also eliminates movement of the catheter hub at the insertion site (mechanical manipulation). A colorful and interesting sticker can be applied to the protecting device to add a positive note to the procedure.

Finger and toe areas are left unoccluded by dressings or tape to allow for assessment of circulation. The thumb is never immobilized because of the danger of contractures with limited movement later on. An extremity should never be encircled with tape. The use of roll gauze, self-adhering stretch bandages (Coban), and ACE bandages can cause the same constriction and hide signs of infiltration.

> **⚠ NURSING ALERT**
>
> Opaque covering should be avoided; however, if any type of opaque covering is used to secure the IV line, the insertion site and extremity distal to the site should be visible to detect an infiltration. If these sites are not visible, they must be checked frequently to detect problems early.

Traditionally, padded boards and splints have been used to partially immobilize the IV site. Padded boards and splints and restraints were appropriate when metal needles were inserted into the vein to prevent the sharp end from puncturing the vessel, especially at a joint. With the more recent use of soft, pliable catheters, arm or leg boards may not be necessary and have several disadvantages. They obscure the IV site, can constrict the extremity, may excoriate the underlying tissue and promote infection, can cause a contracture of a joint, restrict useful movement of the extremity, and are uncomfortable. Unfortunately, no research has been conducted to demonstrate their proposed benefit of increasing dwell time (patency of the IV line). Adequate securement should eliminate the need for padded boards in most circumstances. Older children who are alert and cooperative can usually be trusted to protect the IV site.

Removal of a Peripheral Intravenous Line

When it comes time to discontinue an IV infusion, many children are distressed by the thought of catheter removal. Therefore, they need a careful explanation of the process and suggestions for helping. Encouraging children to remove or help remove the tape from the site provides them with a measure of control and often fosters their cooperation. The procedure consists of turning off any pump apparatus, occluding the IV tubing, removing the tape, pulling the catheter out of the vessel in the opposite direction of insertion, and exerting firm pressure at the site. A dry dressing (adhesive bandage strip) is placed over the puncture

site. The use of adhesive-removal pads can decrease the pain of tape removal, but the skin should be washed after use to avoid irritation. To remove transparent dressings (e.g., OpSite, Tegaderm), pull the opposing edges parallel to the skin to loosen the bond. Inspect the catheter tip to ensure the catheter is intact and that no portion remains in the vein.

> **⚠ NURSING ALERT**
>
> Consider the child's age, development, and neurologic status, as well as the predictability of the child (how the child responds to painful treatments), when determining the need for assistance to maintain safety. Manual removal of tape is the preferred method. Only if absolutely necessary should a small cut be made in the tape, using bandage scissors, to facilitate its removal. Before cutting the tape:
> - Ensure that all digits are visible.
> - Remove any barrier that hinders visibility, such as a protective covering.
> - Protect the child's skin and digits by sliding own finger(s) between the tape and the child's skin so that the scissors do not touch the patient.
> - Cut on the tape on the medial aspect (thumb side) of the extremity.

Maintenance

In a consensus guideline of 16 organizations and professional associations, the following maintenance recommendations were made (O'Grady, Alexander, Burns, et al., 2011):

- Use transparent dressings to allow site visualization. If diaphoresis, bleeding, or oozing prevents adequate adhesion, gauze dressings can be used.
- Replace any dressing when damp, visibly soiled, or loose. Routinely replace transparent dressings every 7 days and gauze dressings every 2 days unless the risk for central catheter dislodgement outweighs the benefits of the dressing change.
- During dressing changes, use chlorhexidine to cleanse skin surrounding central lines and either chlorhexidine, tincture of iodine, an iodophor, or alcohol surrounding PIV lines. No recommendations can be made for the use of chlorhexidine in infants younger than 2 months of age.
- Chlorhexidine-impregnated sponge dressings should be used for short-term central catheters in patients older than 2 months of age when central line–associated bloodstream rates are not decreasing with other efforts, such as chlorhexidine skin cleansing, maximum sterile barrier precautions during insertion, and staff education.
- Do not apply ointments to the insertion site; they promote fungal growth and antimicrobial resistance.
- Replace IV administration sets at the following frequencies:
  - Continuous infusions of crystalloids at no less than 96-hour intervals, but at least every 7 days.
  - Blood products or lipid emulsions sets within 24 hours of starting the infusion.
  - Propofol sets every 6 to 12 hours and when the vial is changed.
  - No recommendation was made on the frequency of intermittent set changes.
  - Include all needleless components (including injection caps at the catheter hub) in administration set changes.
- In pediatric patients, PIV catheters may remain in place until a complication occurs or the therapy is complete.
- Promptly remove temporary central catheters or PIV catheters as soon as they are no longer needed.

Complications

The same precautions regarding maintenance of asepsis, prevention of infection, and observation for infiltration are carried out with patients of any age. However, infiltration is more difficult to detect in infants and small children than in adults. The increased amount of subcutaneous fat and the amount of tape used to secure the catheter often obscure the early signs of infiltration. When the fluid appears to be infusing too slowly or ceases, the usual assessment for obstruction within the apparatus—kinks, screw clamps, shutoff valve, and positioning interference (e.g., a bent elbow)—often locates the difficulty. When these actions fail to detect the problem, it may be necessary to carefully remove some of the dressing to obtain a clear view of the venipuncture site. Dependent areas, such as the palm and undersides of the extremity or the occiput and behind the ears, are examined.

Whenever possible, the IV infusion should be placed in an extremity to which the ID band (or bracelet) is not attached. Serious circulatory impairment can result from infiltrated solution distal to the band, which acts as a tourniquet, preventing adequate venous return. To check for return blood flow through the catheter, the tubing is removed from the infusion pump, and the bag is lowered below the level of the infusion site. Resistance during flushing or aspiration for blood return also indicates that the IV infusion may have infiltrated surrounding tissue. A good blood return, or lack thereof, is not always an indicator of infiltration in small infants. Flushing the catheter and observing for edema, redness, or streaking along the vein are appropriate for assessment of the IV.

IV therapy in pediatrics tends to be difficult to maintain because of mechanical factors such as vascular trauma resulting from the catheter, the insertion site, vessel size, vessel fragility, pump pressure, the patient's activity level, operator skill and insertion technique, forceful administration of boluses of fluid, and infusion of irritants or vesicants through a small vessel. These factors cause infiltration and extravasation injuries. Infiltration is defined as inadvertent administration of a nonvesicant solution or medication into surrounding tissue. Extravasation is defined as inadvertent administration of vesicant solution or medication into surrounding tissue (Infusion Nurses Society, 2011). A vesicant or sclerosing agent causes varying degrees of cellular damage when even minute amounts escape into surrounding tissue. Guidelines are available for determining the severity of tissue injury by staging characteristics, such as the amount of redness, blanching, the amount of swelling, pain, the quality of pulses below infiltration, capillary refill, and warmth or coolness of the area (Infusion Nurses Society, 2011).*

Treatment of infiltration or extravasation varies according to the type of vesicant. Guidelines are available outlining the sequence of interventions and specific treatment of infiltration or extravasation with antidotes.

> ### ! NURSING ALERT
>
> When infiltration or extravasation is observed (signs include erythema, pain, edema, blanching, streaking on the skin along the vein, and darkened area at the insertion site), immediately stop the infusion, elevate the extremity, notify the primary care provider, and initiate the ordered treatment as soon as possible. Remove the IV line when it is no longer needed (e.g., after infusing an antidote).

Phlebitis, or inflammation of the vessel wall, may also develop in children who require IV therapy. Lamagna and MacPhee (2004) describe three types of phlebitis: mechanical (caused by rapid infusion rate, manipulation of the IV), chemical (caused by medications), and bacterial (caused by staphylococcal organisms). The initial sign of phlebitis is erythema (redness) at the insertion site. Pain may or may not be present.

PIV catheters are the most commonly used intravascular device. Heavy cutaneous colonization of the insertion site is the single most important predictor of catheter-related infection with all types of short-term, percutaneously inserted catheters. Phlebitis, largely a mechanical rather than infectious process, remains the most important complication associated with the use of peripheral venous catheters.*

> ### ! NURSING ALERT
>
> The most effective ways to prevent infection of an IV site are to cleanse hands between each patient, wear gloves when inserting a catheter, and closely inspect the insertion site and physical condition of the dressing. Proper education of the patient and family regarding signs and symptoms of an infected site can help prevent infections from going unnoticed.

RECTAL ADMINISTRATION

The rectal route for administration is less reliable but is sometimes used when the oral route is difficult or contraindicated. It is also used when oral preparations are unsuitable to control vomiting. Some of the drugs available in suppository form are acetaminophen, aspirin, sedatives, analgesics (morphine), and antiemetics. The difficulty in using the rectal route is that unless the rectum is empty at the time of insertion, the absorption of the drug may be delayed, diminished, or prevented by the presence of feces. Sometimes the drug is later evacuated, securely surrounded by stool.

Remove the wrapping on the suppository, and lubricate the suppository with warm water (water-soluble jelly may affect medication absorption). Rectal suppositories are traditionally inserted with the apex (pointed end) foremost. Reverse contractions or the pressure gradient of the anal canal may help the suppository slip higher into the canal. Using a glove or finger cot, quickly but gently insert the suppository into the rectum beyond both of the rectal sphincters. Then hold the buttocks together firmly to relieve pressure on the anal sphincter until the urge to expel the suppository has passed, which occurs within 5 to 10 minutes. Sometimes the amount of drug ordered is less than the dose available. The irregular shape of most suppositories makes the process of dividing them into a desired dose difficult if not dangerous. If it must be halved, it should be cut lengthwise. However, there is no guarantee that the drug is evenly dispersed throughout the petrolatum base.

If medication is administered via a retention enema, the same procedure is used. Drugs given by enema are diluted in the smallest amount of solution possible to minimize the likelihood of being evacuated.

OPTIC, OTIC, AND NASAL ADMINISTRATION

There are few differences in administering eye, ear, and nose medication to children and to adults. The major difficulty is in gaining children's cooperation. Older children need only an explanation and direction. Although the administration of optic, otic, and nasal medication is not painful, these drugs can cause unpleasant sensations, which can be eliminated with various techniques.

---

*Guidelines for determining tissue injury severity are available from the Infusion Nurses Society, 315 Norwood Park South, Norwood, MA 02062; 781-440-9408; http://www.ins1.org.

*Guidelines for prevention of intravascular device–related infections are available from the Centers for Disease Control and Prevention, 1600 Clifton Road, Atlanta, GA 30333; 404-639-1515; http://www.cdc.gov/hai/.

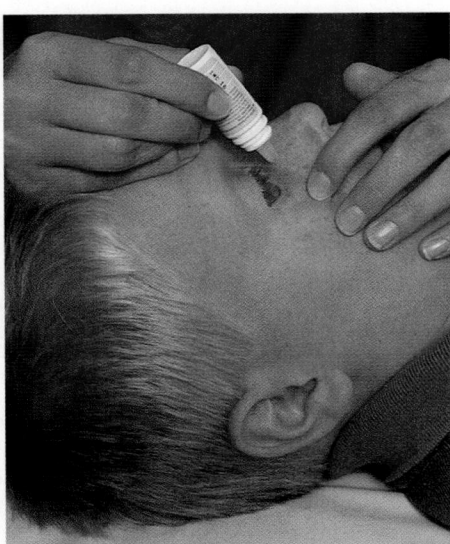

FIG 39.18 Administering eye drops.

To instill eye medication, place the child supine or sitting with the head extended and ask the child to look up. Use one hand to pull the lower eyelid downward; the hand that holds the dropper rests on the head so that it may move synchronously with the child's head, thus reducing the possibility of trauma to a struggling child or dropping medication on the face (Fig. 39.18). When the lower eyelid is pulled down, a small conjunctival sac is formed; apply the solution or ointment to this area rather than directly on the eyeball. Another effective technique is to pull the lower eyelid down and out to form a cup effect, into which the medication is dropped. Gently close the eyelids to prevent expression of the medication. Wipe excess medication from the inner canthus outward to prevent contamination to the contralateral eye.

> ## ! NURSING ALERT
>
> To reduce unpleasant sensations when administering medications:
> - Eye: Apply finger pressure to the lacrimal punctum at the inner aspect of the eyelid for 1 minute to prevent drainage of medication to the nasopharynx and the unpleasant "tasting" of the drug.
> - Ear: Allow medications stored in the refrigerator to warm to room temperature before instillation.
> - Nose: Position the child with the head hyperextended to prevent strangling sensations caused by medication trickling into the throat rather than up into the nasal passages.

Instilling eye drops in infants can be difficult because they often clench the eyelids tightly closed. One approach is to place the drops in the nasal corner where the eyelids meet. The medication pools in this area, and when the child opens the eyelids, the medication flows onto the conjunctiva. For young children, playing a game can be helpful, such as instructing the child to keep the eyes closed to the count of three and then open them, at which time the drops are quickly instilled. Ointment can be applied by gently pulling down the lower eyelid and placing the ointment in the lower conjunctival sac.

> ## ⬮ MEDICATION ALERT
>
> If both eye ointment and drops are ordered, give drops first, wait 3 minutes, and then apply the ointment to allow each drug to work. When possible, administer eye ointments before bedtime or naptime because the child's vision will be blurred temporarily.

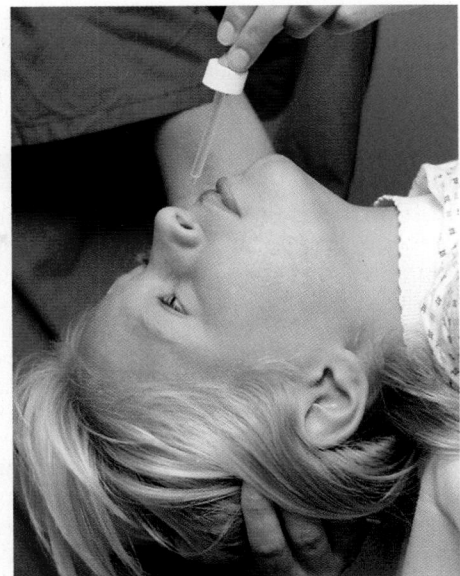

FIG 39.19 Proper position for instilling nose drops.

Ear drops are instilled with the child in the prone or supine position and the head turned to the appropriate side. For children younger than 3 years of age, the external auditory canal is straightened by gently pulling the pinna downward and straight back. The pinna is pulled upward and back in children older than 3 years of age. To place the drops deep into the ear canal without contaminating the tip of the dropper, place a disposable ear speculum in the canal and administer the drops through the speculum. Position the bottle so that the drops fall against the side of the ear canal. After instillation, the child should remain lying on the unaffected side for a few minutes. Gentle massage of the area immediately anterior to the ear facilitates the entry of drops into the ear canal. The use of cotton pledgets prevents medication from flowing out of the external canal. However, they should be loose enough to allow any discharge to exit from the ear. Premoistening the cotton with a few drops of medication prevents the wicking action from absorbing the medication instilled in the ear.

Nose drops are instilled in the same manner as in the adult patient. Remove mucus from the nose with a clean tissue or a washcloth. Unpleasant sensations associated with medicated nose drops are minimized when care is taken to position the child with the head extended well over the edge of the bed or pillow (Fig. 39.19). Depending on size, infants can be positioned in the football hold (see Fig. 39.3, *B*), in the nurse's arm with the head extended and stabilized between the nurse's body and elbow and the arms and hands immobilized with the nurse's hands, or with the head extended over the edge of the bed or a pillow. After instillation of the drops, the child should remain in position for 1 minute to allow the drops to come in contact with the nasal surfaces. Insert nasal spray dispensers into the naris vertically, and then angle them to avoid trauma to the septum and to direct medication toward the inferior turbinate.

AEROSOL THERAPY

Aerosol therapy can be effective in depositing medication directly into the airway. The value of aerosolized water, or "mist therapy," is controversial. This route of administration can be useful in avoiding the systemic side effects of certain drugs and in reducing the amount of drug necessary to achieve the desired effect. Bronchodilators, steroids, mucolytics, and antibiotics, suspended in particulate form, can be inhaled so that the medication reaches the small airways. Aerosol therapy is particularly challenging in children who are too young to cooperate with controlling the rate and depth of breathing. Administration of this therapy requires skill, patience, and creativity.

> ### 💊 MEDICATION ALERT
>
> Medications can be aerosolized or nebulized with air or with oxygen-enriched gas. The metered-dose inhaler (MDI) is a self-contained, handheld device that allows for intermittent delivery of a specified amount of medication. Many bronchodilators are available in this form and are successfully used by children with asthma. A spacer device attached to the MDI can help with coordination of breathing and aerosol delivery. It also allows the aerosolized particles to remain in suspension longer. Handheld nebulizers discharge a medicated mist into a small plastic mask, which the child holds over the nose and mouth. To avoid particle deposition in the nose and pharynx, the child is instructed to take slow, deep breaths through an open mouth during the treatment. For home use, an air compressor is necessary to force air through the liquid medication to form the aerosol. Compact, portable units can be obtained from health equipment companies.

Assessment of breath sounds and work of breathing should be done before and after treatments. Young children who become upset by having a mask held close to the face may become fatigued with fighting the procedure and may actually appear worse during and immediately after the therapy. It may be necessary to spend a few minutes calming the child after the procedure and allowing the vital signs to return to baseline to accurately assess changes in breath sounds and work of breathing.

FAMILY TEACHING AND HOME CARE

The nurse usually assumes responsibility for preparing families to administer medications at home. The family should understand why the child is receiving the medication and the effects that might be expected, as well as the amount, frequency, and length of time the drug is to be administered. Instruction should be carried out in an unhurried, relaxed manner, preferably in an area away from a busy ward or office.

Instruct the caregiver carefully regarding the correct dosage. Some people have difficulty understanding medical terminology, and just because they nod or otherwise indicate they understand, the nurse should not assume that the message is clear. It is important to ascertain their interpretation of a teaspoon, for example, and to be certain they have acceptable devices for measuring the drug. If the drug is packaged with a dropper, syringe, or plastic cup, the nurse should show or mark the point on the device that indicates the prescribed dose and demonstrate how the dose is drawn up into a dropper or syringe, measured, and the bubbles eliminated. If the nurse has any doubts about the parent's ability to administer the correct dose, the parent should give a return demonstration. This is essential when the drug has potentially serious consequences from incorrect dosage, such as insulin or digoxin, or when more complex administration is required, such as parenteral injections. When teaching a parent to give an injection, the nurse must allot adequate time for instruction and practice.

Home modifications are often necessary because the availability of equipment or assistance can differ from the hospital setting. For example, the parent may need guidance in devising methods that allow one person to hold the child and safely give the drug.

> ### ❗ NURSING ALERT
>
> To administer oral, nasal, or optic medication when only one person is available to hold the child, use the following procedure:
> - Place child supine on a flat surface (bed, couch, floor).
> - Sit facing child so child's head is between operator's thighs, and child's arms are under operator's legs.
> - Place lower legs over child's legs to restrain lower body, if necessary.
> - To administer oral medication, place a small pillow under child's head to reduce risk for aspiration.
> - To administer nasal medication, place a small pillow under child's shoulders to aid flow of liquid through nasal passages.

The nurse should clarify with parents the time that the drug is to be administered. For instance, when a drug is prescribed in association with meals, the number of meals that the family is accustomed to eating influences the amount of drug the child receives. Does the family have meals twice per day or five times per day? When a drug is to be given several times during the day, together the nurse and parents can work out a schedule that accommodates the family's routine. This is particularly significant if a drug must be given at equal intervals throughout a 24-hour period. For example, telling parents that the child needs 1 tsp of medicine four times a day is subject to misinterpretation, because the parents may routinely schedule the doses at incorrect times. Instead, a preplanned schedule based on 6-hour intervals should be set up with the number of days required for the therapeutic dosage listed. Modification should also be made to accommodate sleep schedules. Written instructions should accompany all drug prescriptions.

> ### ❗ NURSING ALERT
>
> If parents have difficulty reading or understanding English, use colors to convey instructions. For example, mark each drug with a color and place the appropriate color on a calendar chart or on a drawing of a clock to identify when the drug needs to be given. If a liquid medication and syringe are used, also mark the syringe at the place the plunger needs to be with color-coded tape.

NASOGASTRIC, OROGASTRIC, AND GASTROSTOMY ADMINISTRATION

When a child has an indwelling feeding tube or a gastrostomy, oral medications are usually given via that route. An advantage of this method is the ability to administer oral medications around the clock without disturbing the child. A disadvantage is the risk for occluding, or clogging, the tube, especially when giving viscous solutions through small-bore feeding tubes. The most important preventive measure is adequate flushing after the medication is instilled (see Guidelines box: Nasogastric, Orogastric, or Gastrostomy Medication Administration in Children).

ALTERNATIVE FEEDING TECHNIQUES

Some children are unable to take nourishment by mouth because of anomalies of the throat, esophagus, or bowel; impaired swallowing capacity; severe debilitation; respiratory distress; or unconsciousness. These children are frequently fed by way of a tube inserted orally or nasally into the stomach (orogastric [OG] or NG gavage) or duodenum-jejunum (enteral gavage) or by a tube inserted directly into the stomach (gastrostomy) or jejunum (jejunostomy). Such feedings may be

GUIDELINES

Nasogastric, Orogastric, or Gastrostomy Medication Administration in Children

Use elixir or suspension (rather than tablet) preparations of medication whenever possible.

Dilute viscous medication or syrup with a small amount of water if possible.

If administering tablets, crush tablet to a fine powder and dissolve drug in a small amount of warm water.

Never crush enteric-coated or sustained-release tablets or capsules.

Avoid oily medications because they tend to cling to side of tube.

Do not mix medication with enteral formula unless fluid is restricted. If adding a drug:

- Check with pharmacist for compatibility.
- Shake formula well, and observe for any physical reaction (e.g., separation, precipitation).
- Label formula container with name of medication, dosage, date, and time infusion started.

Check for correct placement of nasogastric (NG) or orogastric (OG) tube (see Evidence-Based Practice box: Confirming Nasogastric Tube Placement in Pediatric Patients).

Attach syringe (with adaptable tip but without plunger) to tube.

Pour medication into syringe.

Unclamp tube, and allow medication to flow by gravity.

Adjust height of container to achieve desired flow rate (e.g., increase height for faster flow).

As soon as syringe is empty, pour in water to flush tubing.

- Amount of water depends on length and gauge of tubing.
- Determine amount before administering any medication by using a syringe to fill completely an unused NG or OG tube with water. Amount of flush solution is usually 1.5 times this volume.
- With certain drug preparations (e.g., suspensions), more fluid may be needed.

If administering more than one drug at the same time, flush tube between each medication with clear water.

Clamp tube after flushing unless tube is left open.

---

intermittent or by continuous drip. During gavage or gastrostomy feedings, infants are given a pacifier. Nonnutritive sucking has several advantages, such as increased weight gain and decreased crying. However, only pacifiers with a safe design can be used to prevent the possibility of aspiration. Using improvised pacifiers made from bottle nipples is not a safe practice.

When a child is concurrently receiving continuous-drip gastric or enteral feedings and parenteral (IV) therapy, the potential exists for inadvertent administration of the enteral formula through the circulatory system. The possibility for error increases when the parenteral solution is a fat emulsion, a milky-appearing substance. Safeguards to prevent this potentially serious error include the following:

- Use a separate, specifically designed enteral feeding pump mounted on a separate pole for continuous-feeding solutions.
- Label all tubing of continuous enteral feeding with brightly colored tape or labels.
- Use specifically designed continuous-feeding bags to contain the solutions instead of parenteral equipment, such as a burette.
- Whenever access or connections are made, trace the tubing all the way from the patient to the bag to ensure that the correct tubing source is selected.

GAVAGE FEEDING

Infants and children can be fed simply and safely by a tube passed into the stomach through either the nares or the mouth. The tube can be left in place or inserted and removed with each feeding. In older children, it is usually less traumatic to tape the tube securely in place between feedings. When this alternative is used, the tube should be removed and replaced with a new tube according to facility policy, specific orders, and the type of tube used. Meticulous hand washing is practiced during the procedure to prevent bacterial contamination of the feeding, especially during continuous-drip feedings.

Preparations

The equipment needed for gavage feeding includes the following:

- A suitable tube selected according to the child's size, the viscosity of the solution being fed, and anticipated duration of treatment
- A receptacle for the fluid; for small amounts, a 10- to 30-mL syringe barrel or Asepto syringe is satisfactory; for larger amounts, a 60-mL syringe with a catheter tip is more convenient
- A 10-mL barrel syringe to aspirate stomach contents after the tube has been placed
- Water or water-soluble lubricant to lubricate the tube; sterile water is used for infants
- Paper or nonallergenic tape to mark the tube and to attach the tube to the infant's or child's cheek (and nose if placed through the nares)
- pH paper to determine the correct placement in the stomach
- The solution for feeding

Not all feeding tubes are the same. Polyethylene and polyvinylchloride types lose their flexibility and need to be replaced frequently, usually every 3 or 4 days. Polyurethane and silicone tubes remain flexible, so they can remain in place up to 30 days. Advantages of small-bore tubes include a reduced incidence of pharyngitis, otitis media, aspiration, and discomfort. Disadvantages include difficulty during insertion (may require a stylet or metal guide wire), collapse of the tube during aspiration of gastric contents to test for correct placement, dislodgment during forceful coughing, migration out of position, knotting, occlusion, and unsuitability for thick feedings.

Procedure

Infants are easier to control if they are first wrapped in a mummy restraint (see Fig. 39.4, *A*). Even tiny infants with random movements can grasp and dislodge the tube. Preterm infants do not ordinarily require restraint, but if they do, a small blanket folded across the chest and secured beneath the shoulders is usually sufficient. Be careful so that breathing is not compromised.

Whenever possible, the infant should be held and provided with a means for nonnutritive sucking during the procedure to associate the comfort of physical contact with the feeding. When this is not possible, gavage feeding is carried out with the infant or child on the back or toward the right side and the head and chest elevated. Feeding the child in a sitting position helps maintain placement of the tube in the lowest position, thus increasing the likelihood of correct placement in the stomach.

Although the most accurate method for testing tube placement is radiography, this practice is not always possible before each feeding. Research indicates that bedside assessment of gastrointestinal aspirate color and pH is useful in predicting feeding tube placement (see Evidence-Based Practice box: Nasogastric Tube Placement in Pediatric Patients). If doubt exists regarding correct placement, consult the practitioner. The Guidelines box: Nasogastric Tube Feedings in Children describes the procedure for gavage feeding.

EVIDENCE-BASED PRACTICE
Confirming Nasogastric Tube Placement in Pediatric Patients

Ask the Question
PICOT Question: In children, how should correct placement of nasogastric (NG) tubes be assessed during hospitalization?

Search for the Evidence
Search Strategies
Search selection criteria included English-language, research-based articles, and children and adolescents requiring NG tube placement. Search areas included aspirate, auscultation and radiology methods, NG tube–length prediction methods, age-related height-based methods, and accurate NG tube placement. Searches excluded newborns and preterm infants.

Databases Used
PubMed, Cochrane Collaboration, MDConsult, Joanna Briggs Institute, AHRQ-National Guideline Clearinghouse, TRIP database Plus, PedsCCM, BestBETS

Critical Appraisal of the Evidence
Studies compared various methods used to evaluate correct placement of the NG tube.

Accurate Nasogastric Tube Length Measurement
- Children 8 years, 4 months of age or younger: Use age-related height-based equation for NG length predictions.
- Children older than 8 years, 4 months of age, short stature, or when you cannot obtain accurate height: Use nose-ear-midxiphoid-umbilicus (NEMU) (Beckstrand, Ellet, Welch, et al., 1990; Beckstrand, Cirgin-Ellett, & McDaniel, 2007; Ellett, Beckstrand, Welch, et al., 1992; Strobel, Byrne, Ament, et al., 1979).

Nonradiologic Verification Methods
- A pH of 5 or less supports that the tip of the tube is in the gastric location (Ellett, Croffie, Cohen, et al., 2005; Huffman, Pieper, Jarczyk, et al., 2004; Metheny & Stewart, 2002; Metheny, Reed, Wiersema, et al., 1993; Metheny, Stewart, Smith, et al., 1997, 1999; Neumann, Meyer, Dutton, et al., 1995; Nyqvist, Sorell, & Ewald, 2005; Phang, Marsh, Barlows, et al., 2004; Westhus, 2004; Society of Pediatric Nurses, 2011).
- A pH greater than 5 does not reliably predict correct distal tip location. This may indicate respiratory or esophageal placement or the presence of medications to suppress acid secretion. Gastric aspirate pH means are statistically significantly lower compared with means from intestinal and respiratory pH aspirates (Ellett, Croffie, Cohen, et al., 2005; Metheny & Stewart, 2002; Metheny, Stewart, Smith, et al., 1997, 1999; Phang, Marsh, Barlows, et al., 2004; Westhus, 2004; Society of Pediatric Nurses, 2011).

Visual Inspection of Aspirate
- Visual inspection is less accurate than pH to confirm placement. Aspirate colors are specific to the intended placement location. Gastric contents are clear, off-white, or tan or may be brown-tinged if blood is present. Respiratory secretions may look the same. Intestinal contents are often bile stained, light to dark yellow, or greenish-brown (Metheny, Reed, Berglund, et al., 1994; Metheny & Stewart, 2002; Metheny, Stewart, Smith, et al., 1999; Phang, Marsh, Barlows, et al., 2004; Westhus, 2004; Society of Pediatric Nurses, 2011).

Enzyme Testing
- Aspirate testing of enzyme levels for bilirubin, pepsin, and trypsin is highly accurate but limited to laboratory assessment (Ellett, Croffie, Cohen, et al.,

2005; Metheny & Stewart, 2002; Metheny, Stewart, Smith, et al., 1999; Westhus, 2004).

Carbon Dioxide Monitoring
- CO_2 monitoring is a reliable method to determine incorrect tube placement in the respiratory tract; it requires a capnograph monitor (Ellett, Croffie, Cohen, et al., 2005; Metheny & Stewart, 2002; Metheny, Stewart, Smith, et al., 1999).

Gastric Auscultation
- Auscultation as a verification tool is reliable only 60% to 80% of the time and should not be used without additional methods (Metheny, McSweeney, Wehrle, et al., 1990; Neumann, Meyer, Dutton, et al., 1995).
- Using aspirate and nonaspirate NG tube placement verification methods in combination increases the likelihood for accurate NG tube placement to 97% to 99%, similar to the radiologic chest radiography gold standard of 99% (Ellett, Croffie, Cohen, et al., 2005; Metheny & Stewart, 2002; Metheny, Reed, Berglund, et al., 1994; Metheny, Reed, Wiersema, et al., 1993; Metheny, Stewart, Smith, et al., 1999; Neumann, Meyer, Dutton, et al., 1995; Phang, Marsh, Barlows, et al., 2004; Westhus, 2004; Society of Pediatric Nurses, 2011).

Apply the Evidence: Nursing Implications
There is **good evidence** with **strong recommendations** that a combination of verification methods to confirm NG tube placement will reduce the required number of x-rays in children (Guyatt, Oxman, Vist, et al., 2008; Society of Pediatric Nurses, 2011). These methods include pH testing and visual inspection of the pH aspirate. There is also good evidence that improving the accuracy of predicting NG tube length before insertion will enhance the precision of successful NG tube placement. Auscultation is used in combination with other NG tube verification methods.

Quality and Safety Competencies: Evidence-Based Practice*
Knowledge
Differentiate clinical opinion from research and evidence-based summaries.
Describe the various verification methods to confirm NG tube placement.

Skills
Base individualized care plan on patient values, clinical expertise, and evidence.
Integrate evidence into practice by using the techniques for NG tube placement verification in clinical care.

Attitudes
Value the concept of evidence-based practice as integral to determining best clinical practice.
Appreciate the strengths and weakness of evidence for confirming NG tube placement.

References
Beckstrand, J., Cirgin-Ellett, M. L., & McDaniel, A. (2007). Predicting internal distance to the stomach for positioning nasogastric and orogastric feeding tubes in children. *Journal of Advanced Nursing, 59*(3), 274–289.

Beckstrand, J., Ellet, M., Welch, J., et al. (1990). The distance to the stomach for feeding tube placement in children predicted from regression on height. *Research in Nursing & Health, 13*(6), 411–420.

Ellett, M., Beckstrand, J., Welch, J., et al. (1992). Predicting the distance for gavage tube placement in children. *Pediatric Nursing, 18*(2), 119–121.

Ellett, M. L., Croffie, J. M., Cohen, M. D., et al. (2005). Gastric tube placement in young children. *Clinical Nursing Research, 14*(3), 238–252.

EVIDENCE-BASED PRACTICE

Confirming Nasogastric Tube Placement in Pediatric Patients—cont'd

Guyatt, G. H., Oxman, A. D., Vist, G. E., et al. (2008). GRADE: An emerging consensus on rating quality of evidence and strength of recommendations. *British Medical Journal, 336*(7650), 924–926.

Huffman, S., Pieper, P., Jarczyk, K. S., et al. (2004). Methods to confirm feeding tube placement: Application of research in practice. *Pediatric Nursing, 30*(1), 10–13.

Metheny, N., McSweeney, M., Wehrle, M. A., et al. (1990). Effectiveness of the auscultatory method in predicting feeding tube location. *Nursing Research, 39*(5), 262–267.

Metheny, N., Reed, L., Berglund, B., et al. (1994). Visual characteristics of aspirates from feeding tubes as a method for predicting tube location. *Nursing Research, 43*(5), 282–287.

Metheny, N., Reed, L., Wiersema, L., et al. (1993). Effectiveness of pH measurements in predicting feeding tube placement: an update. *Nursing Research, 42*(6), 324–331.

Metheny, N. A., & Stewart, B. J. (2002). Testing feeding tube placement during continuous tube feedings. *Appl Nursing Research, 15*(4), 254–258.

Metheny, N. A., Stewart, B. J., Smith, L., et al. (1997). pH and concentrations of pepsin and trypsin in feeding tube aspirates as predictors of tube placement. *Journal of Parenteral and Enteral Nutrition, 21*(5), 279–285.

Metheny, N. A., Stewart, B. J., Smith, L., et al. (1999). pH and concentration of bilirubin in feeding tube aspirates as predictors of tube placement. *Nursing Research, 48*(4), 189–197.

Neumann, M. J., Meyer, C. T., Dutton, J. L., et al. (1995). Hold that x-ray: Aspirate pH and auscultation prove tube placement. *Journal of Clinical Gastroenterology, 20*(4), 293–295.

Nyqvist, K. H., Sorell, A., & Ewald, U. (2005). Litmus tests for verification of feeding tube location in infants: Evaluation of their clinical use. *Journal of Clinical Nursing, 14*(4), 486–495.

Phang, J. S., Marsh, W. A., Barlows, T. G., et al. (2004). Determining feeding tube location by gastric and intestinal pH values. *Nutrition in Clinical Practice, 19*(6), 640–644.

Society of Pediatric Nurses Clinical Practice Committee, SPN Research Committee, & Longo, M. A. (2011). Best evidence: Nasogastric tube placement verification. *Journal of Pediatric Nursing, 26*(4), 373–376.

Strobel, C. T., Byrne, W. J., Ament, M. E., et al. (1979). Correlation of esophageal lengths in children with height: Application to the Tuttle test without prior esophageal manometry. *Journal of Pediatrics, 94*(1), 81–84.

Westhus, N. (2004). Methods to test feeding tube placement in children. *American Journal of Maternal/Child Nursing, 29*(5), 282–291.

*Adapted from the Quality and Safety Education for Nurses (QSEN) Institute.

Studies evaluating NG and OG tube length in infants and children found that age-specific methods for predicting the distance based on height is a more accurate estimate of internal distance to the stomach (Beckstrand, Ellett, & McDaniel, 2007; Klasner, Luke, & Scalzo, 2002). The morphologic measure most commonly used by clinicians, nose-ear-xiphoid distance, is often too short to locate the entire tube pore span in the stomach. However, the nose-ear-midxiphoid umbilicus span approached the accuracy of the age-specific prediction equations and is easier to use in a clinical setting. The best option is to adapt the nose-ear-midxiphoid umbilicus measurement for NG or OG tube length (Fig. 39.20, *A*) (see Guidelines box: Nasogastric Tube Feedings in Children).

Ellett and Beckstrand (1999) found significant tube placement errors (43.5%) in a study of 39 hospitalized children. Children who were comatose or semicomatose, were inactive, had swallowing difficulty, or had Argyle tubes experienced increased tube placement errors. Findings supported the effectiveness of radiographs in documenting tube placement.

GASTROSTOMY FEEDING

Feeding by way of gastrostomy, or G tube, is often used for children in whom passage of a tube through the mouth, pharynx, esophagus, and cardiac sphincter of the stomach is contraindicated or impossible. It is also used to avoid the constant irritation of an NG tube in children who require tube feeding over an extended period. A gastrostomy tube may be placed with the child under general anesthesia or percutaneously using an endoscope with the patient sedated and under local anesthesia (percutaneous endoscopic gastrostomy [PEG]). The tube is inserted through the abdominal wall into the stomach about midway along the greater curvature and secured by a purse-string suture. The stomach is anchored to the peritoneum at the operative site. The tube used can be a Foley, wing-tip, or mushroom catheter. Immediately after surgery, the catheter may be left open and attached to gravity drainage for 24 hours or more.

Direct postoperative care of the wound site toward prevention of infection and irritation. Cleanse the area with soap and water at least daily or as often as needed to keep the area free of drainage. After healing, meticulous care is needed to keep the area surrounding the

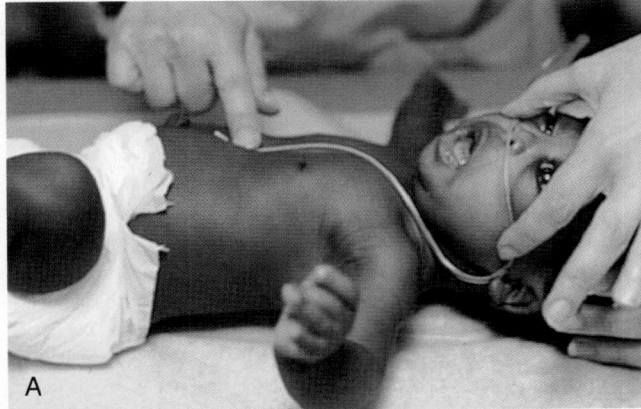

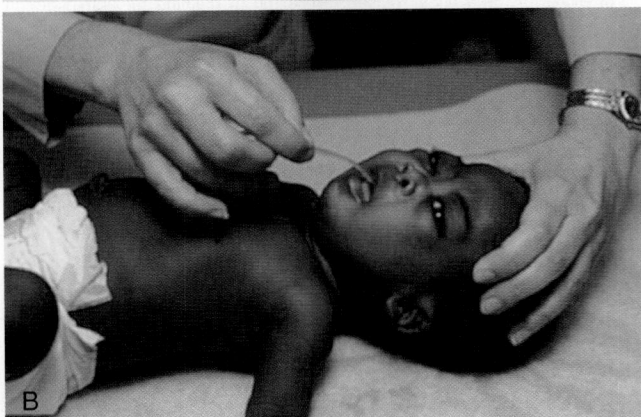

FIG 39.20 Gavage feeding. **A,** Measuring the tube for orogastric (OG) feeding from the tip of the nose to the earlobe and to the midpoint between the end of the xiphoid process and the umbilicus. **B,** Inserting the tube.

tube clean and dry to prevent excoriation and infection. Exercise care to prevent excessive pull on the catheter that might cause widening of the opening and subsequent leakage of highly irritating gastric juices. Use barrier ointments such as zinc oxide, petrolatum-based ointment, and nonalcohol skin barrier film to control leakage; add absorptive

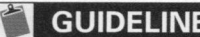

GUIDELINES

Nasogastric Tube Feedings in Children

Place child supine with head slightly hyperflexed or in a sniffing position (nose pointed toward ceiling).

Measure the tube for approximate length of insertion, and mark the point with a small piece of tape.

Insert a tube that has been lubricated with sterile water or water-soluble lubricant through either the mouth or one of the nares to the predetermined mark. Because most young infants are obligatory nose breathers, insertion through the mouth causes less distress and helps stimulate sucking. In older infants and children, the tube is passed through the nose and alternated between nostrils. An indwelling tube is almost always placed through the nose.

- When using the nose, slip the tube along the base of the nose, and direct it straight back toward the occiput.
- When entering through the mouth, direct the tube toward the back of the throat (see Fig. 39.20, *B*).
- If the child is able to swallow on command, synchronize passing the tube with swallowing.

Confirm placement (see Evidence-Based Practice box: Confirming Nasogastric Tube Placement in Pediatric Patients).

Stabilize the tube by holding or taping it to the cheek, not to the forehead, because of possible damage to the nostril. To maintain correct placement, measure and record the amount of tubing extending from the nose or mouth to the distal port when the tube is first positioned. Recheck this measurement before each feeding.

Warm the formula to room temperature. Do not microwave! Pour formula into the barrel of the syringe attached to the feeding tube. To start the flow, give a gentle push with the plunger, but then remove the plunger and allow the fluid to flow into the stomach by gravity. The rate of flow should not exceed 5 mL every 5 to 10 minutes in premature and very small infants and 10 mL/min in older infants and children to prevent nausea and regurgitation. The rate is determined by the diameter of the tubing and the height of the reservoir containing the feeding and is regulated by adjusting the height of the syringe. A usual feeding may take 15 to 30 minutes to complete.

Flush the tube with sterile water (1 or 2 mL for small tubes to 5 to 15 mL or more for large ones), or see discussion of flushing for administering medication through nasogastric (NG) tubes in the Guidelines box: Nasogastric, Orogastric, or Gastrostomy Medication Administration in Children to clear it of formula.

Cap or clamp indwelling tubes to prevent loss of feeding.

- If the tube is to be removed, first pinch it firmly to prevent escape of fluid as the tube is withdrawn. Withdraw the tube quickly.

Position the child with the head elevated 30 to 45 degrees or on the right side for 30 to 60 minutes in the same manner as after any infant feeding to minimize the possibility of regurgitation and aspiration. If the child's condition permits, burp the child after the feeding.

Record the feeding, including the type and amount of residual, the type and amount of formula, and how it was tolerated.

- For most infant feedings, any amount of residual fluid aspirated from the stomach is refed to prevent electrolyte imbalance, and the amount is subtracted from the prescribed amount of feeding. For example, if the infant is to receive 30 mL and 10 mL is aspirated from the stomach before the feeding, the 10 mL of aspirated stomach contents is refed along with 20 mL of feeding. Another method can be used in children. If residual fluid is more than one-fourth of the last feeding, return the aspirate and recheck in 30 to 60 minutes. When residual fluid is less than one-fourth of the last feeding, give the scheduled feeding. If large amounts of aspirated fluid persist and the child is due for another feeding, notify the primary care provider.

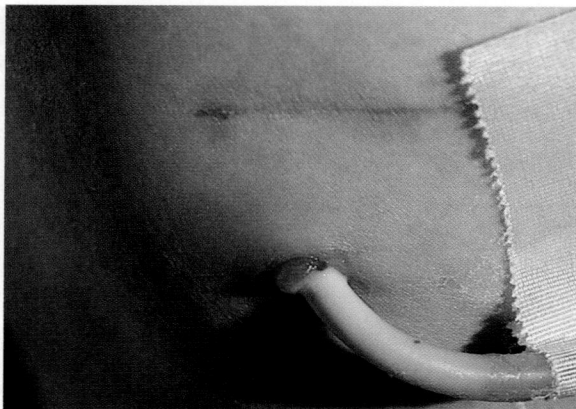

FIG 39.21 Appearance of healthy granulation tissue around a stoma.

powders and pectin-based skin barrier wafers if skin irritation is present (Wound Ostomy and Continence Nurses Society, 2008). Secure the tube to the abdomen using a commercial stabilizer, polyurethane foam, or the H tape method, and leave a small loop of tubing at the exit site to prevent tension on the site.

Granulation tissue may grow around a gastrostomy site (Fig. 39.21). This moist, beefy red tissue is not a sign of infection. However, if it continues to grow, the excess moisture can irritate the surrounding skin. The use of hydrogen peroxide for routine site cleansing has been identified as one of the possible causes of hypergranulation tissue (Wound Ostomy and Continence Nurses Society, 2008), corrosion and excessive drying of the tissue (McClave & Neff, 2006), and disruption of wound healing (Borkowski & Rogers, 2004; Borkowski, 2005). Clinical guidelines issued by the Wound Ostomy and Continence Nurses Society (2008) recommend managing hypergranulation by stabilizing the tube, keeping the peristomal area dry by applying polyurethane foam, and using triamcinolone (0.5%) three times a day. Silver nitrate may also be used for hypergranulation.

For children receiving long-term gastrostomy feeding, a skin-level device (e.g., MIC-KEY, Bard Button) offers several advantages. The small, flexible silicone device protrudes slightly from the abdomen, is cosmetically pleasing, affords increased comfort and mobility to the child, is easy to care for, and is fully immersible in water. The one-way valve at the proximal end minimizes reflux and eliminates the need for clamping. However, the skin-level device requires a well-established gastrostomy site and is more expensive than the conventional tube. In addition, the valve may become clogged. When functioning, the valve prevents air from escaping; therefore, the child may require frequent bubbling. With some devices, during feedings, the child must remain fairly still, because the tubing easily disconnects from the opening if the child moves. With other devices, extension tubing can be securely attached to the opening (Fig. 39.22). The feeding is instilled at the other end of the tubing in a manner similar to that for a regular gastrostomy. The extension tubing may also have a separate medication port. Both the feeding and the medication ports have plugs attached. Some skin-level devices require a special tube to be able to decompress the stomach (to check residual or decompress air).

Feeding of water, formula, or pureed foods is carried out in the same manner and rate as for gavage feeding. A mechanical pump may be used to regulate the volume and rate of feeding. After feedings, the infant or child is positioned on the right side or in the Fowler position, and the tube may be clamped or left open and suspended between feedings, depending on the child's condition. A clamped tube allows more mobility but is only appropriate if the child can tolerate intermittent feedings without vomiting or prolonged backup of feeding into the tube.

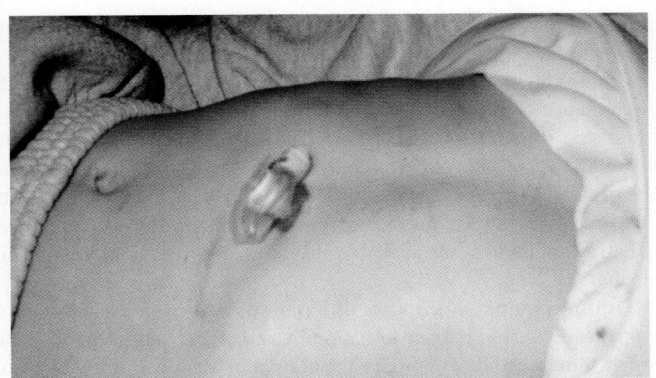

FIG 39.22 Child with a skin-level gastrostomy device (MIC-KEY), which provides for secure attachment of extension tubing to the gastrostomy opening.

Sometimes a Y tube is used to allow for simultaneous decompression during feeding. If a Foley catheter is used as the gastrostomy tube, apply very slight tension. The tube is securely taped to maintain the balloon at the gastrostomy opening and prevent leakage of gastric contents and the tube's progression toward the pyloric sphincter, where it may occlude the stomach outlet. As a precaution, the length of the tube is measured postoperatively and then remeasured each shift to be certain it has not slipped. The nurse can make a mark above the skin level to further ensure its placement. When the gastrostomy tube is no longer needed, it is removed; the skin opening usually closes spontaneously by contracture.

NASODUODENAL AND NASOJEJUNAL TUBES

Children at high risk for regurgitation or aspiration such as those with gastroparesis, mechanical ventilation, or brain injuries may require placement of a postpyloric feeding tube. A trained practitioner inserts the nasoduodenal or nasojejunal tube because of the risk for misplacement and potential for perforation in tubes requiring a stylet. Accurate placement is verified by radiography. Small-bore tubes may easily clog. Flush the tube when feeding is interrupted, before and after medication administration, and routinely every 4 hours or as directed by facility policy. Tube replacement should be considered monthly to ensure optimal tube patency. Continuous feedings are delivered by a mechanical pump to regulate their volume and rate. Bolus feeds are contraindicated. Tube displacement is suspected in children showing signs of feeding intolerance, such as vomiting. In these cases, stop the feedings and notify the primary care provider.

TOTAL PARENTERAL NUTRITION

TPN provides for the total nutritional needs of infants and children whose lives are threatened because feeding by way of the gastrointestinal tract is impossible, inadequate, or hazardous.

TPN therapy involves IV infusion of highly concentrated solutions of protein, glucose, and other nutrients. The solution is infused through conventional tubing with a special filter attached to remove particulate matter or microorganisms that may have contaminated the solution. The highly concentrated solutions require infusion into a vessel with sufficient volume and turbulence to allow for rapid dilution. The wide-diameter vessels selected are the superior vena cava and innominate or intrathoracic subclavian veins approached by way of the external or internal jugular veins. The highly irritating nature of concentrated glucose precludes the use of the small peripheral veins in most instances.

However, dilute glucose-protein hydrolysates that are appropriate for infusing into peripheral veins are being used with increasing frequency. When peripheral veins are used, soybean oil (Intralipid) becomes the major calorie source. For long-term alimentation, central venous catheters are usually used.

The major nursing responsibilities are the same as for any IV therapy and include control of sepsis, monitoring of the infusion rate, and assessment of the patient. The TPN solution must be prepared under rigid aseptic conditions, which is best accomplished by specially trained technicians. Specially trained nurses should change the solution and tubing and redress the infusion using meticulous aseptic precautions. In some institutions, this may be a nursing responsibility. If so, the procedure is carried out according to hospital protocol.

The infusion is maintained at a constant rate by means of an infusion pump to ensure the proper concentrations of glucose and amino acids. Accurate calculation of the rate is required to deliver a measured amount in a given length of time. Because alterations in flow rate are relatively common, the drip should be checked frequently to ensure an even, continuous infusion. The TPN infusion rate should not be increased or decreased without the practitioner being informed because alterations can cause hyperglycemia or hypoglycemia.

General assessments, such as vital signs, input and output measurements, and checking results of laboratory tests, facilitate early detection of infection or fluid and electrolyte imbalance. Additional amounts of potassium and sodium chloride are often required in hyperalimentation; therefore, observation for signs of potassium or sodium deficit or excess is part of nursing care. This is rarely a problem except in children with reduced renal function or metabolic defects. Hyperglycemia may occur during the first day or two as the child adapts to the high-glucose load of the hyperalimentation solution. Although hyperglycemia occurs infrequently, insulin may be required to help the body adjust. When this occurs, nursing responsibilities include blood glucose testing. To prevent hypoglycemia when the hyperalimentation is disconnected, the rate of the infusion and the amount of insulin are decreased gradually.

FAMILY TEACHING AND HOME CARE

When alternative feedings are needed for an extended period, the family needs to learn how to feed the child with an NG, gastrostomy, or TPN feeding regimen. Plan ample time for the family to learn and perform the procedures under supervision before they assume full responsibility for the child's care. Refer the family to community agencies that provide support and practical assistance. The Oley Foundation* is a nonprofit research and education organization that assists people receiving enteral nutrition and home TPN.

PROCEDURES RELATED TO ELIMINATION

ENEMA

The procedure for giving an enema to an infant or child does not differ essentially from that for an adult except for the type and amount of fluid administered and the distance for inserting the tube into the rectum (Table 39.9). Depending on the volume, use a syringe with rubber tubing, an enema bottle, or an enema bag.

An isotonic solution is used in children. Plain water is not used because, being hypotonic, it can cause rapid fluid shift and fluid overload. The Fleet enema (pediatric or adult sized) is not advised for children

---

*214 Hun Memorial, MC-28, Albany Medical Center, Albany, NY 12208; 800-776-OLEY; http://www.oley.org.

TABLE 39.9	Administration of Enemas to Children	
Age	**Amount (mL)**	**Insertion Distance**
Infant	120 to 240	2.5 cm (1 inch)
2 to 4 years of age	240 to 360	5 cm (2 inches)
4 to 10 years of age	360 to 480	7.5 cm (3 inches)
11 years of age	480 to 720	10 cm (4 inches)

because of the harsh action of its ingredients (sodium biphosphate and sodium phosphate). Commercial enemas can be dangerous to patients with megacolon and to dehydrated or azotemic children. The osmotic effect of the Fleet enema may produce diarrhea, which can lead to metabolic acidosis. Other potential complications are extreme hyperphosphatemia, hypernatremia, and hypocalcemia, which may lead to neuromuscular irritability and coma.

> **! NURSING ALERT**
>
> If prepared saline is not available, the nurse can make some by adding 1 tsp of table salt to 500 mL (1 pint) of tap water.

Because infants and young children are unable to retain the solution after it is administered, the buttocks must be held together for a short time to retain the fluid. The enema is administered and expelled while the child is lying with the buttocks over the bedpan and with the head and back supported by pillows. Older children are ordinarily able to hold the solution if they understand what to do and if they are not expected to hold it for too long. The nurse should have the bedpan handy or, for ambulatory children, ensure that the bathroom is available before beginning the procedure. An enema is an intrusive procedure and thus threatening to preschool children; therefore, a careful explanation is especially important to ease possible fear.

A preoperative bowel preparation solution given orally or through an NG tube is increasingly being used instead of an enema. The polyethylene glycol–electrolyte lavage solution (GoLYTELY) mechanically flushes the bowel without significant absorption, thereby avoiding potential fluid and electrolyte imbalances. NuLYTELY, a modification of GoLYTELY, has the same therapeutic advantages as GoLYTELY and was developed to improve on the taste. Another effective oral cathartic is magnesium citrate solution.

OSTOMIES

Children may require stomas for various health problems. The most frequent causes in infants are necrotizing enterocolitis and imperforate anus and, less often, Hirschsprung disease. In older children, the most frequent causes are inflammatory bowel disease, especially Crohn disease (regional enteritis), and ureterostomies for distal ureter or bladder defects.

Care and management of ostomies in older children differ little from the care of ostomies in adult patients. The major emphasis in pediatric care is preparing the child for the procedure and teaching care of the ostomy to the child and family. The basic principles of preparation are the same as for any procedure. Simple, straightforward language is most effective together with the use of illustrations and a replica model (e.g., drawing a picture of a child with a stoma on the abdomen and explaining it as "another opening where bowel movements [or any other term the child uses] will come out"). At another time, the nurse can draw a pouch over the opening to demonstrate how the

contents are collected. Using a doll to demonstrate the process is an excellent teaching strategy, and special books are available.

Children with ileostomies are fitted immediately after surgery with an appliance to protect the skin from the proteolytic enzymes in the liquid stool. Infants may not be fitted with a pouch in the immediate postoperative period. When stomal drainage is minimal, as is often the case in small or preterm infants, gauze dressing will suffice. Give parents a choice of caring for the colostomy with or without an appliance. Pediatric appliances are available in a variety of sizes to ensure an adequate fit.*

Ostomy equipment consists of a one- or two-piece system with a hypoallergenic skin barrier to maintain peristomal skin integrity. The pouch should be large enough to contain a moderate amount of stool and flatus but not so large as to overwhelm the infant or child. A backing helps minimize the risk for skin breakdown from moisture trapped between the skin and pouch. Avoid small clips and rubber bands to prevent choking in young children.

Protection of the peristomal skin is a major aspect of stoma care. Well-fitting appliances are important to prevent leakage of contents. Before applying the appliance, prepare the skin with a skin sealant that is allowed to dry. Then apply stoma paste around the base of the stoma or to the back of the wafer. The sealant and paste work together to prevent peristomal skin breakdown.

In infants with a colostomy left unpouched, skin care is similar to that of any diapered child. However, protect the peristomal skin with a barrier substance (e.g., zinc oxide ointment [Sensi-Care] or a mixture of zinc oxide ointment and stoma powder [Stomahesive]). A diaper larger than the one usually worn may be needed to extend upward over the stoma and absorb drainage. If the skin becomes inflamed, denuded, or infected, the care is similar to the interventions used for diaper dermatitis. A zinc-based product helps protect healthy skin, heal excoriated skin, and minimize pain associated with skin breakdown. The skin protectant adheres to denuded, weeping skin. The nurse can apply zinc-based products over topical antifungal and antibacterial agents if infection is present. No-sting barrier film is a skin sealant that has no alcohol base and can be used on open skin without stinging.

With young children, preventing them from pulling off the pouch is also an important consideration. One-piece outfits keep exploring hands from reaching the pouch, and the loose waist avoids any pressure on the appliance. Keeping the child occupied with toys during the pouch change is also helpful. As children mature, encourage their participation in ostomy care. Even preschoolers can assist by holding supplies, pulling paper backings from the appliance, and helping clean the stoma area. Toilet training for bladder control needs to begin at the appropriate time as for any other child.

Older children and adolescents should eventually have total responsibility for ostomy care just as they would for usual bowel function. During adolescence, concerns for body image and the ostomy's impact on intimacy and sexuality emerge. The nurse should stress to teenagers that the presence of a stoma need not interfere with their activities. These youngsters can choose which ostomy equipment is best suited to their needs. Attractively designed and decorated pouch covers are well liked by teenagers.

Children with familial adenomatous polyposis may require a colectomy with ileoanal reservoir to prevent or treat carcinoma of the colon. Peristomal skin care for these children is particularly challenging because of increased liquid stools, increased digestive enzymes that may cause skin breakdown, and the stoma being at skin level rather than raised.

---

*Parents may find helpful information at the ConvaTec website: http://www.convatec.com.

Additional care with this condition includes close monitoring of fluid and electrolyte status and increased incidence of bowel obstruction.

An enterostomal therapy nurse specialist is an important member of the health care team and will have additional suggestions and assistance with skin care information and ostomy pouching options. The nurse can obtain further information by contacting the Wound, Ostomy and Continence Nurses Society.*

Family Teaching and Home Care

Because these children are almost always discharged with a functioning colostomy, preparation of the family should begin as early as possible in the hospital. The nurse instructs the family in the application of the device (if used), care of the skin, and appropriate action in case skin problems develop. Early evidence of skin breakdown or stomal complications (e.g., ribbonlike stools, excessive diarrhea, bleeding, prolapse, or failure to pass flatus or stool) is brought to the attention of the physician, nurse, or stoma specialist.

PROCEDURES FOR MAINTAINING RESPIRATORY FUNCTION

INHALATION THERAPY

Oxygen Therapy

Oxygen is administered for hypoxemia and may be delivered by mask, nasal cannula, face tent, hood, face mask, or ventilator. The mode of delivery is selected on the basis of the concentration needed and the child's ability to cooperate in its use. Oxygen therapy is frequently administered in the hospital, although increasing numbers of children are receiving oxygen in the home. Oxygen is dry and therefore must be humidified.

Oxygen delivered to infants is well tolerated by using a plastic hood (Fig. 39.23). At least 7 L/min of flow is necessary to maintain oxygen concentrations and remove the exhaled carbon dioxide. The humidified oxygen should not be blown directly into the infant's face. Older, cooperative infants and children can use a nasal cannula or prongs, which can supply a concentration of oxygen of about 50%. A high-flow nasal cannula (5 to 8 L/min using pediatric tubing) may be used to avoid intubation, postextubation, in palliative care, and as a mode of

---

*1120 Route 73, Suite 200, Mount Laurel, NJ 08054; 888-224-9626; http://www.wocn.org.

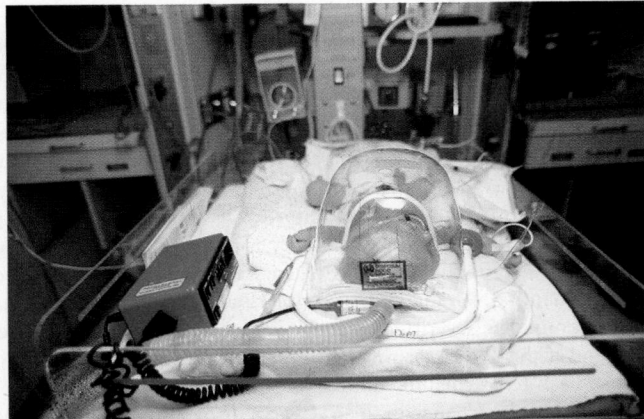

FIG 39.23 Oxygen administered to an infant by means of a plastic hood. Note the oxygen analyzer (blue machine).

ventilatory support in very low–birthweight infants. Care with prong size, placement, and maintenance is important to prevent breakdown of the nasal alae.

Oxygen masks are available in pediatric sizes but may not be well tolerated in children, because a snug fit is required to ensure adequate oxygen delivery. A face tent or bucket is often better tolerated because this soft piece of plastic sits beneath the child's chin and allows oxygen to be directed to the mouth and nose without enclosure (Curley & Moloney-Harmon, 2001). Oxygen tents (croup tents) are rarely used today in developed countries. Oxygen concentration is difficult to control, and the child's clothing can become saturated with water from the humidification and cause hypothermia.

> ### 💊 MEDICATION ALERT
>
> Prolonged exposure to high oxygen tensions can damage some body tissues and functions. This is called *oxygen toxicity*. The organs most vulnerable to the adverse effects of excessive oxygenation are the retinas of extremely preterm infants and the lungs of people at any age.

> ### ❗ NURSING ALERT
>
> Inspect all toys for safety and suitability (e.g., vinyl or plastic, not stuffed items that absorb moisture and are difficult to keep dry). The high-level oxygen environment makes any source of sparks (e.g., mechanical or electrical toys) a potential fire hazard.

Oxygen-induced carbon dioxide narcosis is a physiologic hazard of oxygen therapy that may occur in people with chronic pulmonary disease, such as cystic fibrosis. In these patients, the respiratory center has adapted to the continuously higher arterial carbon dioxide ($PaCO_2$) tension levels, and therefore hypoxia becomes the more powerful stimulus for respiration. When the arterial oxygen (PaO_2) tension level is elevated during oxygen administration, the hypoxic drive is removed, causing progressive hypoventilation and increased $PaCO_2$ levels, and the child rapidly becomes unconscious. Carbon dioxide narcosis can also be induced by the administration of sedation in these patients.

Monitoring Oxygen Therapy

Pulse oximetry is a continuous, noninvasive method of determining arterial oxygen saturation (SaO_2) to guide oxygen therapy. A sensor composed of a light-emitting diode (LED) and a photodetector is placed in opposition around a foot, hand, finger, toe, or earlobe, with the LED placed on top of the nail when digits are used (Fig. 39.24). The diode emits red and infrared lights that pass through the skin to the photodetector. The photodetector measures the amount of each type of light absorbed by functional hemoglobins. Hemoglobin saturated with oxygen (oxyhemoglobin) absorbs more infrared light than does hemoglobin not saturated with oxygen (deoxyhemoglobin). Pulsatile blood flow is the primary physiologic factor that influences accuracy of the pulse oximeter. In infants, reposition the probe at least every 4 to 8 hours to prevent pressure necrosis; poor perfusion and very sensitive skin may necessitate more frequent repositioning.

Another noninvasive method is transcutaneous monitoring (TCM), which provides continuous monitoring of transcutaneous partial pressure of oxygen in arterial blood ($tcPaO_2$) and, with some devices, of transcutaneous partial pressure of carbon dioxide in arterial blood ($tcPaCO_2$). An electrode is attached to the warmed skin to facilitate arterialization of cutaneous capillaries. The site of the electrode must be changed

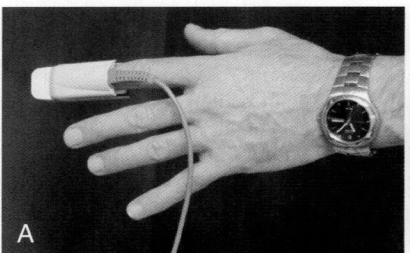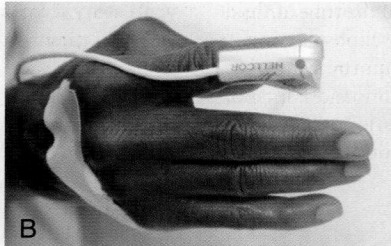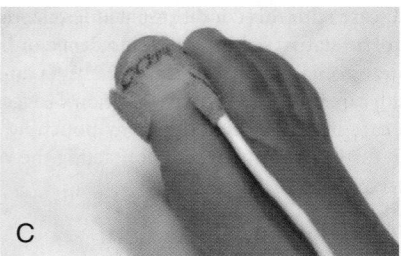

FIG 39.24 Oximeter sensor on the great toe. Note that the sensor is positioned with a light-emitting diode (LED) opposite the photodetector. (From Roberts, J.R. [2014]. *Roberts and Hedges' clinical procedures in emergency medicine* [6th ed.]. Philadelphia, PA: Elsevier.)

every 3 to 4 hours to avoid burning the skin, and the machine must be calibrated with every site change. TCM is used frequently in neonatal intensive care units, but it may not reflect PaO_2 in infants with impaired local circulation.

Oximetry is insensitive to hyperoxia, because hemoglobin approaches 100% saturation for all PaO_2 readings greater than approximately 100 mm Hg, which is a dangerous situation for preterm infants at risk for developing retinopathy of prematurity (see Chapter 25). Therefore, preterm infants being monitored with oximetry should have their upper limits identified, such as 90% to 95%, and a protocol should be established for decreasing oxygen when saturations are high.

Oximetry offers several advantages over TCM. Oximetry (1) does not require heating the skin, thus reducing the risk for burns; (2) eliminates a delay period for transducer equilibration; and (3) maintains an accurate measurement regardless of the patient's age or skin characteristics or the presence of lung disease.

> **! NURSING ALERT**
>
> It is important to make certain that sensor connectors and oximeters are compatible. Wiring that is incompatible can generate considerable heat at the tip of the sensor, causing second- and third-degree burns under the sensors. Pressure necrosis can also occur from sensors attached too tightly. Therefore, inspect the skin under the sensor frequently.

Applying the sensor correctly is essential for accurate SaO_2 measurements. Because the sensor must identify every pulse beat to calculate the SaO_2, movement can interfere with sensing. Some devices synchronize the SaO_2 reading with the heartbeat, thereby reducing the interference caused by motion. Sensors are not placed on extremities used for blood pressure monitoring or with indwelling arterial catheters because pulsatile blood flow may be affected.

> **! NURSING ALERT**
>
> **Infant:** Secure the sensor to the great toe, and tape the wire to the sole of the foot (or use a commercial holder that fastens with a self-adhering closure). Place a snug-fitting sock over the foot, but check the site frequently for color, temperature, and pulse.
> **Child:** Secure the sensor securely to the index finger, and tape the wire to the back of the hand.

Ambient light from ceiling lights and phototherapy, as well as high-intensity heat and light from radiant warmers, can interfere with readings. Therefore, the sensor should be covered to block these light sources. IV dyes; green, purple, or black nail polish; nonopaque synthetic nails; and possibly ink used for footprinting can also cause inaccurate SaO_2 measurements. The dyes should be removed or, in the case of porcelain nails, a different area used for the sensor. Skin color, thickness, and edema do not affect the readings.

Blood gas measurements are sensitive indicators of change in respiratory status in acutely ill patients. They provide valuable information regarding lung function, lung adequacy, and tissue perfusion. The pH, $PaCO_2$, bicarbonate (HCO_3), and PaO_2 levels can provide information about whether the child is compensating and guide critical treatment decisions.

END-TIDAL CARBON DIOXIDE MONITORING

End-tidal carbon dioxide ($ETCO_2$) monitoring measures exhaled carbon dioxide noninvasively. Capnometry provides a numeric display, and capnography provides a graph over time. Continuous capnometry is available in many bedside physiologic monitors, as well as stand-alone monitors. $ETCO_2$ differs from pulse oximetry in that it is more sensitive to the mechanics of ventilation rather than oxygenation. Hypoxic episodes can be prevented through the early detection of hypoventilation, apnea, or airway obstruction.

Children who are experiencing an asthma exacerbation, receiving procedural sedation, or who are mechanically ventilated may have $ETCO_2$ monitoring. Special sampling cannulas are used for nonintubated patients, and a small device is placed between the endotracheal (ET) tube and the ventilator tubing in intubated patients. Although $ETCO_2$ monitoring is not a substitute for arterial blood gases, it does have the information of providing ventilation information continuously and noninvasively. Normal $ETCO_2$ values are 30 to 43 mm Hg, which is slightly lower than normal PCO_2 of 35 to 45 mm Hg. During cardiopulmonary resuscitation (CPR), $ETCO_2$ values consistently below 15 mm Hg indicate ineffective compressions or excessive ventilation. Changes in waveform and numeric display follow changes in ventilation by a very few seconds and precede changes in respiratory rate, skin color, and pulse oximetry values.

For years, disposable colorimetric $ETCO_2$ detectors have been used to assess ET tube placement. A color change with each exhaled breath when there is adequate systemic perfusion indicates that the tube is in the lungs. These devices do not provide numbers or graphic representation and do not provide the same early detection of hypoventilation as the continuous quantitative monitors.

Additional uses of $ETCO_2$ monitoring have limited supporting research. Although waveform analysis does not yet have standardized nomenclature, some clinicians use the angles of the waveform coupled with the quantitative value of $ETCO_2$ to classify the severity of asthma exacerbations. The severity of diabetic ketoacidosis (Fearon & Steele, 2002) and acidosis from gastroenteritis (Nagler, Wright, & Krauss, 2006) has also been researched in children and is used in some facilities.

When there is a change in the $ETCO_2$ value or waveform, assess the patient quickly for adequate airway, breathing, and circulation. Sedated patients may be hypoventilating and need stimulation. Intubated patients may need suctioning, have self-extubated or dislodged the tube, or have equipment failure or disconnection. Patients with asthma may have a worsening condition. Problems with the $ETCO_2$ monitoring system can include a kink in the sample line or disconnection. In general, check the patient first and then the equipment.

BRONCHIAL (POSTURAL) DRAINAGE

Bronchial drainage is indicated whenever excessive fluid or mucus in the bronchi is not being removed by normal ciliary activity and cough. Positioning the child to take maximum advantage of gravity facilitates removal of secretions. Postural drainage can be effective in children with chronic lung disease characterized by thick mucus, such as cystic fibrosis.

Postural drainage is carried out three or four times daily and is more effective when it follows other respiratory therapy, such as bronchodilator or nebulization medication. Bronchial drainage is generally performed before meals (or 1 to $1\frac{1}{2}$ hours after meals) to minimize the chance of vomiting and is repeated at bedtime. The duration of treatment depends on the child's condition and tolerance; it usually lasts 20 to 30 minutes. Several positions facilitate drainage from all major lung segments.

CHEST PHYSICAL THERAPY

Chest physical therapy (CPT) usually refers to the use of postural drainage in combination with adjunctive techniques that are thought to enhance the clearance of mucus from the airway. These techniques include manual percussion, vibration, and squeezing of the chest; cough; forceful expiration; and breathing exercises. Special mechanical devices are also currently used to perform CPT (e.g., vest-type percussors). Postural drainage in combination with forced expiration has been shown to be beneficial.

Common techniques used in association with postural drainage include manual percussion of the chest wall and percussion with mechanical devices, such as a high-frequency handheld chest compression device. A "popping," hollow sound, not a slapping sound, should be the result. The procedure should be done over the rib cage only and should be painless. Percussion can be performed with a soft circular mask (adapted to maintain air trapping) or a percussion cup marketed especially for the purpose of aiding in loosening secretions. CPT is contraindicated when patients have pulmonary hemorrhage, pulmonary embolism, end-stage renal disease, increased intracranial pressure, osteogenesis imperfecta, or minimal cardiac reserves.

INTUBATION

Rapid-sequence intubation (RSI) is commonly performed in pediatric (and some neonatal) patients to induce an unconscious, neuromuscular blocked condition to avoid the use of positive-pressure ventilation and the risk for possible aspiration (Bottor, 2009). Atropine, fentanyl, and vecuronium or rocuronium are drugs commonly used during RSI. In neonates, ET tube intubation is often a stressful event, and hypoxia and pain are commonly associated with routine intubation; RSI in neonates may serve to prevent such adverse events (Bottor).

Indications for intubation include the following:
- Respiratory failure or arrest, agonal or gasping respirations, apnea
- Upper airway obstruction
- Significant increase in work of breathing, use of accessory muscles
- Potential for developing partial or complete airway obstruction—respiratory effort with no breath sounds, facial trauma, and inhalation injuries
- Potential for or actual loss of airway protection, increased risk for aspiration
- Anticipated need for mechanical ventilation related to chest trauma, shock, increased intracranial pressure
- Hypoxemia despite supplemental oxygen
- Inadequate ventilation

In preparation for intubation, the child should be preoxygenated with 100% oxygen using an appropriately sized bag and mask. Historically, uncuffed ET tubes were used in children younger than 8 years of age, but there is evidence that the use of these tubes in small children does not produce a higher incidence of complications; newer cuff designs are reported to decrease complications, such as stridor and tracheal mucosal injury (Kuch, 2013; Taylor, Subaiya, & Corsino, 2011). Air or gas delivered directly to the trachea must be humidified. During intubation, the cardiac rhythm, heart rate, and oxygen saturation should be monitored continuously with audible tones. ET tube placement should be verified by at least one clinical sign and at least one confirmatory technology:
- Visualization of bilateral chest expansion
- Auscultation over the epigastrium (breath sounds should not be heard) and the lung fields bilaterally in the axillary region (breath sounds should be equal and adequate)
- Color change on $ETCO_2$ detector during exhalation after at least 3 to 6 breaths or waveform/value verification with continuous capnography
- Chest radiography

Apply a protective skin barrier, and secure the ET tube with tape or a securement device. An NG tube is typically inserted after intubation.

MECHANICAL VENTILATION

ET intubation can be accomplished by the nasal (nasotracheal), oral (orotracheal), or direct tracheal (tracheostomy) routes. Although it is more difficult to place, nasotracheal intubation is preferred to orotracheal intubation because it facilitates oral hygiene and provides more stable fixation, which reduces the complication of tracheal erosion and the danger of accidental extubation.

Basic ongoing assessment of the mechanically ventilated patient includes observing the chest rise and fall for symmetry, bilateral breath sounds equal or unchanged from last assessment, level of consciousness, capillary refill and skin color, and vital signs. A heart rate that is too fast or too slow is a possible indication of hypoxemia, air leak, or low cardiac output. Pulse oximetry and $ETCO_2$ monitoring is also routine along with periodic arterial blood gas analysis. If sudden deterioration of an intubated patient occurs, consider the following etiologies:
- DOPE*
  - **D**isplacement: The tube is not in the trachea or has moved into a bronchus (right mainstream most common).
  - **O**bstruction: Secretions or kinking of the tube.
  - **P**neumothorax: Chest trauma, barotraumas, or noncompliant lung disease.
  - **E**quipment failure: Check the oxygen source, Ambu bag, and ventilator.
- Verify placement again during each transport and when patients are moved to different beds.

To maintain skin integrity in the mechanically ventilated patient, reposition the patient at least every 2 hours as the patient's condition tolerates. Apply a hydrocolloid barrier to protect the facial cheeks. Place gel pillows under pressure points, such as occiput, heels, elbows, and shoulders. Allow no tubes, lines, wires, or wrinkles in bedding under the patient. Provide meticulous skin care.

*American Heart Association, 2015.

Provide analgesia and sedation as needed. Use a system for communication that includes sign boards, pointing, and opening and closing eyes. To maintain safety, use soft restraints if necessary to maintain a critical airway.

Ventilator-associated pneumonia (VAP) is a complication that can be prevented through the use of aggressive hand hygiene, wearing gloves to handle respiratory secretions or contaminated objects, use of closed suctioning systems, routine oral care, and elevation of the head of the bed between 30 and 45 degrees (unless contraindicated) (Centers for Disease Control and Prevention, 2012). Enteral nutrition is often provided to decrease the risk for bacterial translocation. Routinely assess the patient's intestinal motility (e.g., by auscultating for bowel sounds and measuring residual gastric volume or abdominal girth), and adjust the rate and volume of enteral feeding to avoid regurgitation. In high-risk patients (decreased gag reflex, delayed gastric emptying, gastroesophageal reflux, severe bronchospasm), postpyloric (duodenal or jejunal) feeding tubes are often used. To prevent the aspiration of pooled secretions, suction the hypopharynx before suctioning the ET tube, before repositioning the ET tube, and before repositioning the patient. Prevent ventilator circuits' condensate from entering ET tube or in-line medication nebulizers. Additional measures to prevent VAP include oral intubation and changing ventilator circuits only when they are visibly soiled (Kline-Tilford, Sorce, Levin, et al., 2013).

Assess readiness to extubate daily. Indications that a child is ready to be extubated include an improvement in underlying condition, hemodynamic stability, and mechanical support no longer being necessary. Assess level of consciousness and ability to maintain a patent airway by mobilizing pulmonary secretions through effective coughing. Maintain NPO status 4 hours before extubation. After extubation, monitor for respiratory distress, which may develop within minutes or hours. Signs of postintubation respiratory distress include stridor, hoarseness, increased work of breathing, unstable vital signs, and desaturations.

TRACHEOSTOMY

A tracheostomy is a surgical opening in the trachea; the procedure may be done on an emergency basis or may be an elective one, and it may be combined with mechanical ventilation. Pediatric tracheostomy tubes are usually made of plastic or Silastic (Fig. 39.25). The most common types are the Bivona, Shiley, Tracoe, Arcadia, and Hollinger tubes. These tubes are constructed with a more acute angle than adult tubes, and they soften at body temperature, conforming to the contours of the trachea. Because these materials resist the formation of crusted respiratory secretions, they are made without an inner cannula. On occasion, tracheostomy tubes with inner cannulas are used (Portex).

Children who have undergone a tracheostomy must be closely monitored for complications, such as hemorrhage, edema, aspiration, accidental decannulation, tube obstruction, and the entrance of free air into the pleural cavity. The focuses of nursing care are maintaining a patent airway, facilitating the removal of pulmonary secretions, providing humidified air or oxygen, cleansing the stoma, monitoring the child's ability to swallow, and teaching while simultaneously preventing complications.

Because the child may be unable to signal for help, direct observation and use of respiratory and cardiac monitors are essential in the early postoperative period. Respiratory assessments include breath sounds and work of breathing, vital signs, tightness of the tracheostomy ties, and the type and amount of secretions. Large amounts of bloody secretions are uncommon and should be considered a sign of hemorrhage. The practitioner should be notified immediately if this occurs.

The child is positioned with the head of the bed raised or in the position most comfortable to the child with the call light easily available. Suction catheters, suction source, gloves, sterile saline, sterile gauze for wiping away secretions, scissors, an extra tracheostomy tube of the same size with ties already attached, another tracheostomy tube one size smaller, and the obturator are kept at the bedside. A source of humidification is provided because the normal humidification and filtering functions of the airway have been bypassed. IV fluids ensure adequate hydration until the child is able to swallow sufficient amounts of fluids.

Suctioning

The airway must remain patent and may require frequent suctioning during the first few hours after a tracheostomy to remove mucous plugs and excessive secretions. Proper vacuum pressure and suction catheter size are important to prevent atelectasis and decrease hypoxia from the suctioning procedure. Vacuum pressure should range from 60 to 100 mm Hg for infants and children and from 40 to 60 mm Hg for preterm infants. Unless secretions are thick and tenacious, the lower range of negative pressure is recommended. Tracheal suction catheters are available in a variety of sizes. The catheter selected should have a diameter that is one-half the diameter of the tracheostomy tube. If the catheter is too large, it can block the airway. The catheter is constructed with a side port so that the catheter is introduced without suction and removed while simultaneous intermittent suction is applied by covering the port with the thumb (Fig. 39.26). The catheter is inserted just to the end of the tracheostomy tube. The practice of instilling sterile saline in the tracheostomy tube before suctioning is not supported by research and is no longer recommended (see Evidence-Based Practice box: Normal Saline Instillation Before Endotracheal or Tracheostomy Suctioning: Helpful or Harmful?).

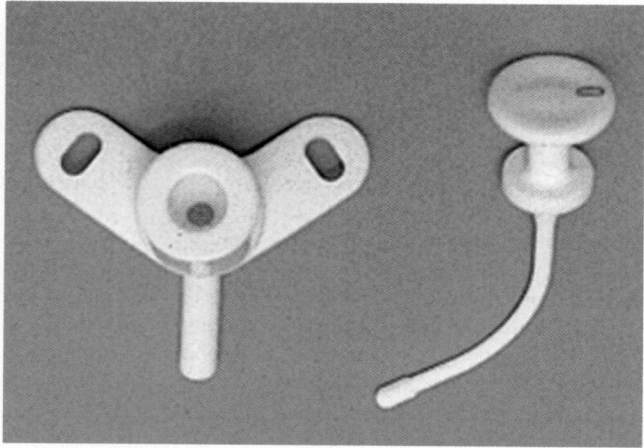

FIG 39.25 Silastic pediatric tracheostomy tube and obturator.

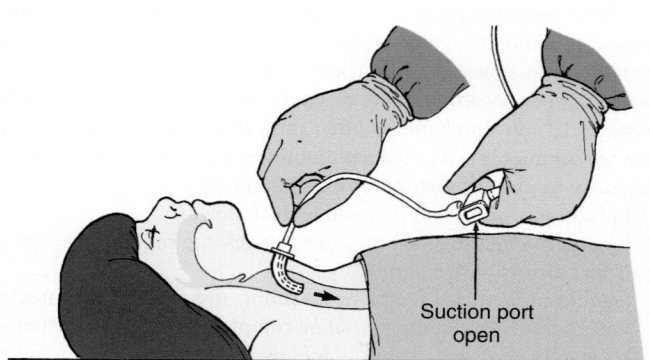

Suction port open

FIG 39.26 Tracheostomy suction catheter insertion. Note that the catheter is inserted just to the end of the tracheostomy tube.

EVIDENCE-BASED PRACTICE

Normal Saline Instillation Before Endotracheal or Tracheostomy Suctioning: Helpful or Harmful?

Ask the Question

PICOT Question: In intubated children and those with tracheostomy, is normal saline (NS) instillation before suctioning helpful or harmful?

Search for the Evidence

Search Strategies

All English-language literature from 1980 to 2013 was searched.

Databases Used

PubMed, Cochrane Collaboration, MDConsult, BestBETs, PedsCCM

Critical Appraisal of the Evidence

GRADE criteria: Evidence quality moderate; recommendation strong (Balshem, Helfand, Schunemann, et al., 2011)

- Instillation of NS before endotracheal (ET) tube suctioning has been used for years to loosen and dilute secretions, lubricate the suction catheter, and promote cough. In recent years, the possible adverse effects of this procedure have been explored. Adult studies have found decreased oxygen saturation, increased frequency of nosocomial pneumonia, and increased intracranial pressure after instillation of NS before suctioning (Ackerman, 1993; Ackerman & Gugerty, 1990; Bostick & Wendelgass, 1987; Hagler & Traver, 1994; Kinlock, 1999; O'Neal, Grap, Thompson, et al., 2001; Reynolds, Hoffman, Schlichtig, et al., 1990).

- Two of the first research studies evaluating the effect of NS instillation before suctioning in neonates found no deleterious effects. Shorten, Byrne, and Jones (1991) found no significant differences in oxygenation, heart rate, or blood pressure before or after suctioning in a group of 27 intubated neonates.

- In a second study of nine neonates acting as their own controls, no adverse effects on lung mechanics were found after NS instillation and suctioning (Beeram & Dhanireddy, 1992).

- A study evaluating the effects of NS instillation before suctioning in children found results similar to those in the previously published adult studies. Ridling, Martin, and Bratton (2003) evaluated the effects of NS instillation before suctioning in a group of 24 critically ill children, 10 weeks to 14 years of age (level 1 evidence). A total of 104 suctioning episodes were analyzed. Children experienced significantly greater oxygen desaturation after suctioning if NS was instilled. Sedigheh and Hossein (2011) also found that instillation of NS before suctioning can cause an adverse effect on oxygen saturation. Another study by Zahran and Abd El-Razik (2011) found a significant increase in arterial carbon dioxide ($PaCO_2$) after suctioning and a reduction in oxygen tension and arterial oxygen saturation (SaO_2) 5 minutes after suctioning. The authors advocate to educate caregivers to avoid using saline to liquefy secretions before suctioning and recommend adequate hydration and humidification, as well as the use of mucolytics.

- Gardner and Shirland (2009) evaluated 10 studies on the effects of instilling NS in intubated neonates and concluded that the evidence does not support routine instillation of NS; however, the evidence indicating adverse effect of NS instillation is abundant. Morrow and Argent (2008) suggest that despite evidence indicating the detriment of the use of saline for suctioning in adults, evidence is lacking in the pediatric population. They conclude, however, that saline should not be routinely used for suctioning infants and children.

Apply the Evidence: Nursing Implications

Studies support the contention that the adverse effects of NS instillation before suctioning in children are similar to those found for adults. This technique causes a significant reduction in oxygen saturation that can last up to 2 minutes after suctioning. The evidence does not support the use of NS instillation before ET suctioning in children.

References

Ackerman, M. H. (1993). The effect of saline lavage prior to suctioning. *American Journal of Critical Care, 2*(4), 326–330.

Ackerman, M. H., & Gugerty, B. (1990). The effect of normal saline bolus instillation in artificial airways. *Journal of the Society of Otorhinolaryngology and Head-Neck Nurses, 8,* 14–17.

Balshem, H., Helfand, M., Schunemann, H. J., et al. (2011). GRADE Guidelines: Rating the quality of evidence. *Journal of Clinical Epidemiology, 64*(4), 401–406.

Beeram, M. R., & Dhanireddy, R. (1992). Effects of saline instillation during tracheal suction on lung mechanics in newborn infants. *Journal of Perinatology, 12*(2), 120–123.

Bostick, J., & Wendelgass, S. T. (1987). Normal saline instillation as part of the suctioning procedure: Effects of PaO_2 and amount of secretions. *Heart and Lung: Journal of Critical Care, 16*(5), 532–537.

Gardner, D. L., & Shirland, L. (2009). Evidence-based guideline for suctioning the intubated neonate and infant. *Neonatal Network, 28*(5), 281–302.

Hagler, D. A., & Traver, G. A. (1994). Endotracheal saline and suction catheters: Sources of lower airway contamination. *American Journal of Critical Care, 3*(6), 444–447.

Kinlock, D. (1999). Instillation of normal saline during endotracheal suctioning: Effects on mixed venous oxygen saturation. *American Journal of Critical Care, 8*(4), 231–240.

Morrow, B. M., & Argent, A. C. (2008). A comprehensive review of pediatric endotracheal suctioning: Effects, indications, and clinical practice. *Pediatric Critical Care Medicine, 9*(5), 465–477.

O'Neal, P. V., Grap, M. J., Thompson, C., et al. (2001). Level of dyspnoea experienced in mechanically ventilated adults with and without saline instillation prior to endotracheal suctioning. *Intensive and Critical Care Nursing, 17*(6), 356–363.

Reynolds, P., Hoffman, L. A., Schlichtig, R., et al. (1990). Effects of normal saline instillation on secretion volume, dynamic compliance, and oxygen saturation (abstract). *American Review of Respiratory Disease, 141,* A574.

Ridling, D. A., Martin, L. D., & Bratton, S. L. (2003). Endotracheal suctioning with or without instillation of isotonic sodium chloride in critically ill children. *American Journal of Critical Care, 12*(3), 212–219.

Sedigheh, I., & Hossein, R. (2011). Normal saline instillation with suctioning and its effect on oxygen saturation, heart rate, and cardiac rhythm. *International Journal of Nursing Education, 3*(1), 42.

Shorten, D. R., Byrne, P. J., & Jones, R. L. (1991). Infant responses to saline instillations and endotracheal suctioning. *Journal of Obstetric, Gynecologic, & Neonatal Nursing, 20*(6), 464–469.

Zahran, E. M., & Abd El-Razik, A. A. (2011). Tracheal suctioning with versus without saline instillation. *Journal of American Science, 7*(8), 23–32.

! NURSING ALERT

In a closed suction system, a suction catheter is directly attached to the ventilator tubing. This system has several advantages. First, there is no need to disconnect the patient from the ventilator, which allows for better oxygenation. Second, the suction catheter is enclosed in a plastic sheath, which reduces the risk that the nurse will be exposed to the patient's secretions.

! NURSING ALERT

Suctioning should require no more than 5 seconds for infants and 10 seconds for children (Ireton, 2007). Counting—one one-thousand, two one-thousand, three one-thousand, and so on—while suctioning is a simple means for monitoring the time. Without a safeguard, the airway may be obstructed for too long. Hyperventilating the child with 100% oxygen before and after suctioning (using a bag-valve-mask or increasing the fraction of inspired oxygen concentration [FiO_2] ventilator setting) may be performed to prevent hypoxia. Closed tracheal suctioning systems that allow for uninterrupted oxygen delivery may also be used.

The child is allowed to rest for 30 to 60 seconds after each aspiration to allow oxygen saturation to return to normal; then the process is repeated until the trachea is clear. Suctioning should be limited to about three aspirations in one period. Oximetry is used to monitor suctioning and prevent hypoxia.

> **! NURSING ALERT**
>
> Suctioning is carried out only as often as needed to keep the tube patent. Signs of mucus partially occluding the airway include an increased heart rate, a rise in respiratory effort, a drop in arterial oxygen saturation (SaO_2), cyanosis, and an increase in the positive inspiratory pressure on the ventilator.

In the acute care setting, aseptic technique is used during care of the tracheostomy. Secondary infection is a major concern because the air entering the lower airway bypasses the natural defenses of the upper airway. Gloves are worn during the aspiration procedure, although a sterile glove is needed only on the hand touching the catheter. A new tube, gloves, and sterile saline solution are used each time.

Routine Care

The tracheostomy stoma requires daily care. Assessments of the stoma area include observations for signs of infection and breakdown of the skin. The skin is kept clean and dry, and crusted secretions around the stoma may be gently removed with half-strength hydrogen peroxide. Hydrogen peroxide should not be used with sterling silver tracheostomy tubes, because it tends to pit and stain the silver surface. The nurse should be aware of wet tracheostomy dressings, which can predispose the peristomal area to skin breakdown. Several products are available to prevent or treat excoriation. The Allevyn tracheostomy dressing is a hydrophilic sponge with a polyurethane back that is highly absorptive. Other possible barriers to help maintain skin integrity include the use of hydrocolloid wafers (e.g., DuoDERM CGF, Hollister Restore, Mepilex Lite) under the tracheostomy flanges, as well as extra-thin hydrocolloid wafers under the chin.

The tracheostomy tube is held in place with tracheostomy ties made of a durable, nonfraying material. The ties are changed daily and when soiled. A self-adhering Velcro collar is commonly used. The collar or ties should be tight enough to allow just a fingertip to be inserted between the ties and the neck (Fig. 39.27). It is easier to ensure a snug fit if the child's head is flexed rather than extended while the ties are being secured.

Routine tracheostomy tube changes are usually carried out weekly after a tract has been formed to minimize the formation of granulation tissue. The first change is usually performed by the surgeon; subsequent

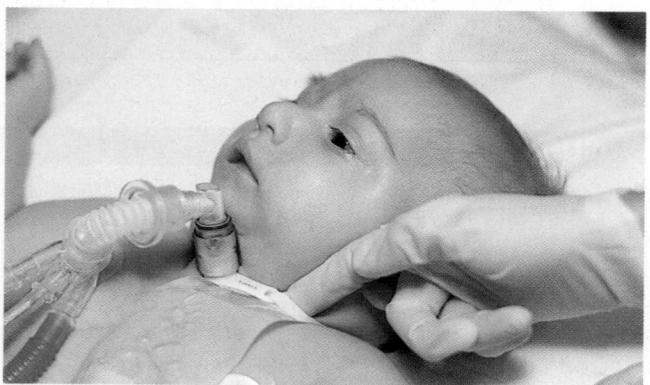

FIG 39.27 Tracheostomy ties are snug but allow one finger to be inserted.

changes are performed by the nurse and, if the child is discharged home with the tracheostomy, by either a parent or a visiting nurse. Ideally, two caregivers participate in the procedure to assist with positioning the child.

Changing the tracheostomy tube is accomplished using strict aseptic technique. A gown and eye protection should be worn to change the tracheostomy. Sterile gloves may be worn for insertion of the sterile tracheostomy tube, but clean gloves may be used for tubes that are cleaned and reused. Tube changes should occur before meals or 2 hours after the last meal. Continuous feedings should be turned off at least 1 hour before a tube change. The new sterile tube is prepared by inserting the obturator and attaching new ties. The child may be suctioned if necessary before the procedure and then restrained and positioned with the neck slightly extended. One caregiver removes the old ties and removes the tube from the stoma. The new tube is inserted gently into the stoma (using a downward and forward motion that follows the curve of the trachea), the obturator is removed, and the ties are secured. The adequacy of ventilation must be assessed after a tube change because the tube can be inserted into the soft tissue surrounding the trachea; therefore, breath sounds and respiratory effort are carefully monitored.

Supplemental oxygen is always delivered with a humidification system to prevent drying of the respiratory mucosa. Humidification of room air for an established tracheostomy can be intermittent if secretions remain thin enough to be coughed or suctioned from the tracheostomy. Direct humidification via a tracheostomy mask can be provided during naps and at night so that the child is able to be up and around unencumbered during much of the day. Room humidifiers are also used successfully.

The inner cannula, if used, should be removed with each suctioning, cleaned with sterile saline and pipe cleaners to remove crusted material, dried thoroughly, and reinserted.

Emergency Care: Tube Occlusion and Accidental Decannulation.

Occlusion of the tracheostomy tube is life-threatening, and infants and children are at greater risk than adults because of the smaller diameter of the tube. Maintaining patency of the tube is accomplished with suctioning and routine tube changes to prevent the formation of crusts that can occlude the tube.

> **! NURSING ALERT**
>
> Suctioning is carried out only as often as needed to keep the tube patent. Signs of mucus partially occluding the airway include an increased heart rate, a rise in respiratory effort, a drop in oxygen saturation, cyanosis, or an increase in the positive inspiratory pressure on the ventilator.

Accidental decannulation also requires immediate tube replacement. Some children have a fairly rigid trachea, so the airway remains partially open when the tube is removed. However, others have malformed or flexible tracheal cartilage, which causes the airway to collapse when the tube is removed or dislodged. Because many infants and children with upper airway problems have little airway reserve, if replacement of the dislodged tube is impossible, a smaller-sized tube should be inserted. If the stoma cannot be cannulated with another tracheostomy tube, oral intubation should be performed.

CHEST TUBE PROCEDURES

A chest tube is placed to remove fluid or air from the pleural or pericardial space. Chest tube drainage systems collect air and fluid while inhibiting backflow into the pleural or pericardial space. Indications for chest tube placement include pneumothorax, hemothorax, chylothorax, empyema, pleural or pericardial effusion, and prevention of accumulation of fluid in the pleural and pericardial space after cardiothoracic surgery. Nursing responsibilities include assisting with chest tube placement, managing chest tubes, and assisting with chest tube removal.

Before chest tube insertion, assess hematologic and coagulation studies for any risk for bleeding during the procedure. Notify the physician of abnormal findings. Prepare the drainage system with sterile water as described in the package insert (some systems may not require this step). Administer pain and sedation medications as ordered. Monitor airway, breathing, circulation, and pulse oximetry throughout the procedure.

After the tube has been inserted and connected to the chest drainage system, secure the tubing so that it does not become disconnected. If suction is required, use connection tubing to join the drainage system to a wall suction adapter and adjust suction on the drainage system as ordered (usually −10 to −20 cm H_2O). There should be gentle, continuous bubbling in the suction control chamber. Place an occlusive dressing over the chest tube insertion site per facility policy. Note the date, time, and your initials on the dressing. If gauze is used, use presplit gauze; "homemade" split gauze may leave loose threads in the wound. Ensure that the drainage system is positioned below the patient's chest and secured to the floor or bed. Keep the drainage tubing free of dependent loops. Obtain a chest radiograph to confirm placement of the chest tube. Ensure that daily chest x-rays are scheduled to monitor placement of the chest tube as well as resolution of the pneumothorax or effusion.

Disposable chest drainage systems typically consist of three chambers next to one another in one drainage unit (Fig. 39.28). The fluid collection chamber collects drainage from the patient's pleural or pericardial space. The water seal chamber is directly connected to the fluid collection chamber and acts as a one-way valve, protecting patients from air returning to the pleural or pericardial space. The suction chamber may be a dry suction or calibrated water chamber. It is connected to external vacuum suction set to the amount of suction ordered and controls the amount of suction that patients experience.

Assess for blood clots and fibrin strands in tubes with sanguinous or serosanguineous drainage, and ensure that there are no obstructions to drainage in the tube. Maintain chest tube clearance per facility policy. Milking or stripping of chest tubes is not recommended for chest tube clearance because of the high negative intrathoracic pressure that is created. However, some special circumstances warrant chest tube clearance with these methods, such as maintaining chest tube patency while a patient is bleeding. Notify the physician immediately if chest tube obstruction is suspected. Generally, chest tubes should not be clamped. However, it may be necessary to clamp a chest tube when exchanging the collection chamber or to determine the site of an air leak (see Guidelines box: Ongoing Patient and Chest Drainage System Assessment).

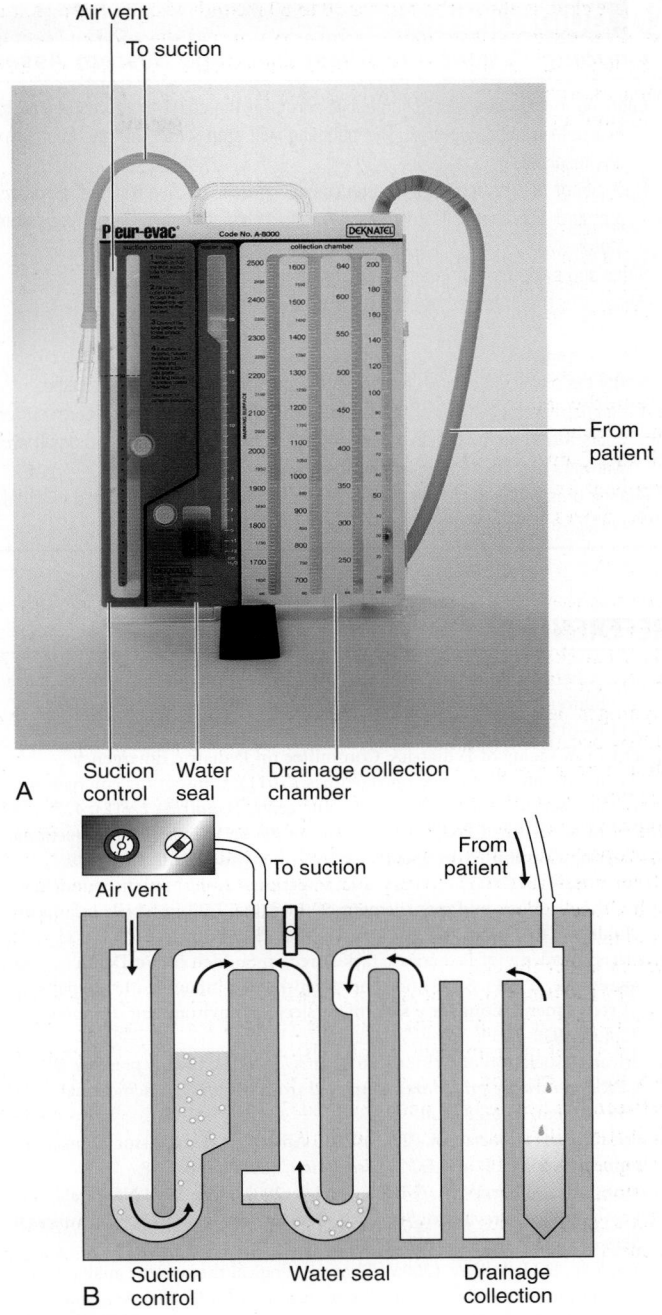

FIG 39.28 A, The Pleur-Evac drainage system, a commercial three-bottle chest drainage device. **B,** Schematic of the drainage device. (From Igna-tavicius, D.D., Workman, L.M. [2013]. *Medical-surgical nursing: Patient-centered collaborative care* [7th ed.]. Philadelphia, PA: Saunders/Elsevier.)

GUIDELINES

Ongoing Patient and Chest Drainage System Assessment

Drainage type (sanguinous, serosanguineous, serous, chylous, empyemic), color, amount, consistency. If there is a marked decrease in the amount of drainage, assess for drainage around the chest tube insertion site. Dressing is clean, dry, and intact.	Chest tube sutures are intact. Prescribed amount of suction is applied. Water level is at 2 cm. If the water column is too high, the flow of air from the chest may be impeded.

Continued

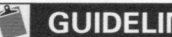
GUIDELINES

Ongoing Patient and Chest Drainage System Assessment—cont'd

Bubbling in the water seal chamber is normal if the chest tube was placed to evacuate a pneumothorax. The bubbling will stop when the pneumothorax has resolved.

Fluctuations may be seen in the water column because of changes in intrathoracic pressure. Substantial fluctuations may reflect changes in a patient's respiratory status.

Signs and symptoms of infection or skin breakdown.

Palpate for the presence of subcutaneous air.

Interventions

Notify the physician of any changes in the quantity or quality of drainage.

If 3 mL/kg/hour or greater of sanguinous drainage occurs for 2 to 3 consecutive hours after cardiothoracic surgery, it may indicate active hemorrhaging and warrants immediate attention of the physician.

Change dressing, and perform site care per facility policy. Typically, a minimal, occlusive dressing is applied.

When the collection chamber is almost full, exchange existing drainage system with a new one per manufacturer's instructions using sterile technique.

To lower the water column, depress the manual vent on the back of the unit until the water level reaches 2 cm. Do not depress the filtered manual vent when the suction is not functioning or connected.

If evacuation of a pneumothorax was not the indication for placement of the chest tube, bubbling in the water seal chamber may be the result of a break in the chest drainage system. Identify the break in the system by briefly clamping the system between the drainage unit and the patient. When the clamp is placed between the unit and the break in the system, the bubbling will stop. Tighten any loose connections. If the air leak is suspected to be at the patient's chest wall, notify the primary care provider.

Encourage patient ambulation. Secure chest tube drainage system to prevent chest tube dislodgment from patient or disconnection from drainage system.

REFERENCES

Abo, A., Chen, L., Johnston, P., et al. (2010). Positioning for lumbar puncture in children evaluated by bedside ultrasound. *Pediatrics, 125*(5), e1149–e1153.

American Academy of Pediatrics, Committee on Pediatric Emergency Medicine and Committee on Bioethics. (2011). Consent for emergency medical services for children and adolescents. *Pediatrics, 128*(2), 427–433.

American Academy of Pediatrics, Subcommittee on Urinary Tract Infections, Steering Committee on Quality Improvement and Management, & Roberts, K. B. (2011). Urinary tract infection: Clinical practice guideline for the diagnosis and management of the initial UTI in febrile infants and children 2 to 24 months. *Pediatrics, 128*(3), 595–610.

American Academy of Pediatrics, Task Force on Sudden Infant Death Syndrome. (2011). SIDS and other sleep-related infant deaths: Expansion of recommendations for a safe infant sleeping environment. *Pediatrics, 128*(5), 1030–1039.

American Association of Critical Care Nurses. (2006). *Family presence during CPR and invasive procedures.* Retrieved from http://ajcc.aacnjournals .org/content/16/3/283.full.

American Heart Association. (2015). 2015 American Heart Association guidelines for CPR and ECC. *Circulation, 132*(2 suppl), 18.

Amlung, S. R., Miller, W. L., & Bosley, L. M. (2001). The 1999 National Pressure Ulcer Prevalence Survey: A benchmarking approach. *Advances in Skin & Wound Care, 14*(6), 297–301.

Anand, K. J., & Hall, R. W. (2006). Pharmacological therapy for analgesia and sedation in the newborn. *Archives of Disease in Childhood. Fetal and Neonatal Edition, 91*(6), 448–453.

Anderson, S. L., Schaechter, J., & Brosco, J. P. (2005). Adolescent patients and their confidentiality: Staying within legal bounds. *Contemporary Pediatrics, 22*(7), 54.

Axelrod, P. (2000). External cooling in the management of fever. *Clinical Infectious Diseases, 31*(5 suppl), S224–S229.

Baharestani, M. M., & Ratliff, C. R. (2007). Pressure ulcers in neonates and children: An NPUAP white paper. *Advances in Skin & Wound Care, 20*(4), 208–220.

Beckstrand, J., Cirgin-Ellett, M. L., & McDaniel, A. (2007). Predicting internal distance to the stomach for positioning nasogastric and orogastric feeding tubes in children. *Journal of Advanced Nursing, 59*(3), 274–289.

Berger, J. E., American Academy of Pediatrics Committee on Medical Liability. (2003). Consent by proxy for nonurgent pediatric care. *Pediatrics, 112*(5), 1186–1195.

Blaney, M., Shen, V., Kerner, J. A., et al. (2006). Alteplase for the treatment of central venous catheter occlusion in children: Results of a prospective, open-label, single-arm study (The Cathflo Activase Pediatric Study). *Journal of Vascular and Interventional Radiology, 17*(11 pt 1), 1745–1751.

Borkowski, S. (2005). G tube care: Managing hypergranulation tissue. *Nursing, 35*(8), 24.

Borkowski, S., & Rogers, V. E. (2004). Similar gastrostomy peristomal skin irritations in three pediatric patients. *Journal of Wound Ostomy & Continence Nursing, 31*(4), 201–206.

Bottor, L. T. (2009). Rapid sequence intubation in the neonate. *Advances in Neonatal Care, 9*(3), 111–117.

Centers for Disease Control and Prevention. (2012). *Healthcare-associated infections (HAIs): Ventilator-associated pneumonia (VAP).* Retrieved from http://www.cdc.gov/HAI/vap/vap.html.

Centers for Medicare and Medicaid Services. (2013). *State operations manual: Appendix A—Survey protocol, regulations and interpretive guidelines for hospitals.* Retrieved from http://www.cms.gov/Regulations-and -Guidance/Guidance/Manuals/downloads/som107ap_a_hospitals.pdf.

Child Health Corporation of America Nursing Falls Study Task Force. (2009). Pediatric falls: State of the science. *Pediatric Nursing, 35*(4), 227–231.

Collins, A. S. (2008). Preventing health care-associated infections. In R. G. Hughes (Ed.), *Patient safety and quality: An evidence-based handbook for nurses.* Rockville, MD: Agency for Healthcare Research and Quality.

Considine, J., & Brennan, D. (2007). Effect of an evidence-based education programme on ED discharge advice for febrile children. *Journal of Clinical Nursing, 16*(9), 1687–1694.

Cook, I. F., & Murtagh, J. (2003). Comparative reactogenicity and parental acceptability of pertussis vaccines administered into the ventrogluteal area and anterolateral thigh in children aged 2, 4, 6, and 18 months. *Vaccine, 21*(23), 3330–3334.

Cook, I. F., & Murtagh, J. (2006). Ventrogluteal area—A suitable site for intramuscular vaccination of infants and toddlers. *Vaccine, 24*(13), 2403–2408.

Curley, M. A. Q., & Moloney-Harmon, P. A. (2001). *Critical care nursing of infants and children* (2nd ed.). Philadelphia, PA: Saunders/Elsevier.

Curley, M. A., Quigley, S. M., & Lin, M. (2003). Pressure ulcers in pediatric intensive care: Incidence and associated factors. *Pediatric Critical Care Medicine, 4*(3), 284–290.

Curley, M. A., Razmus, I. S., Roberts, K. E., et al. (2003). Predicting pressure ulcer risk in pediatric patients: The Braden Q Scale. *Nursing Research, 52*(1), 22–33.

Ellett, M. L., & Beckstrand, J. (1999). Examination of gavage tube placement in children. *Journal of the Society of Pediatric Nurses, 4*(2), 51–60.

Emergency Nurses Association. (2005). *Family presence at the bedside during invasive procedures and resuscitation.* Retrieved from https://www.ena.org/ practice-research/research/CPG/Documents/FamilyPresenceCPG.pdf.

Essink-Tebbes, C. M., Wuis, E. W., Liem, K. D., et al. (1999). Safety of lidocaine-prilocaine cream application four times a day in premature neonates: A pilot study. *European Journal of Pediatrics, 158*(5), 421–423.

Fearon, D. M., & Steele, D. W. (2002). End-tidal carbon dioxide predicts the presence and severity of acidosis in children with diabetes. *Academic Emergency Medicine, 9*(12), 1373–1378.

Fisher, A. A., Deffenbaugh, C., Poole, R. L., et al. (2004). The use of alteplase for restoring patency to occluded central venous access devices in infants and children. *Journal of Infusion Nursing, 27*(3), 171–174.

Gamulka, B., Mendoza, C., & Connolly, B. (2005). Evaluation of a unique, nurse-inserted, peripherally inserted central catheter program. *Pediatrics, 115*(6), 1602–1606.

Gray, L., Watt, L., & Blass, E. M. (2000). Skin-to-skin contact is analgesic in healthy newborns. *Pediatrics, 105*(1), e14.

Gray, M. (1996). Atraumatic urethral catheterization of children. *Pediatric Nursing, 22*(4), 306–310.

Greene, N., Bhananker, S., & Ramaiah, R. (2012). Vascular access, fluid resuscitation, and blood transfusion in pediatric trauma. *International Journal of Critical Illness and Injury Science, 2*(3), 135–142.

Henderson, D. P., & Knapp, J. F. (2006). Report of the National Consensus Conference on Family Presence During Pediatric Cardiopulmonary Resuscitation and Procedures. *Journal of Emergency Nursing, 33*(1), 23–29.

Infusion Nurses Society. (2011). Infusion nursing standards of practice. *Journal of Infusion Nursing, 34*(1 suppl), S63–S64.

Ireton, J. (2007). Tracheostomy suction: A protocol for practice. *Paediatric Nursing, 19*(10), 14–18.

Johnston, C. C., Campbell-Yeo, M., & Filion, F. (2011). Paternal vs maternal kangaroo care for procedural pain in preterm neonates: A randomized crossover trial. *Archives of Pediatrics and Adolescent Medicine, 165*(9), 792–796.

Jones, T., & Jacobsen, S. J. (2007). Childhood febrile seizures: Overview and implications. *International Journal of Medical Sciences, 4*(2), 110–114.

Junqueira, A. L., Tavares, V. R., Martins, R. M., et al. (2010). Safety and immunogenicity of hepatitis B vaccine administered into ventrogluteal vs. anterolateral thigh sites in infants: A randomized controlled trial. *International Journal of Nursing Studies, 47*(9), 1074–1079.

Kain, Z. N., Caldwell-Andrews, A. A., Mayes, L. C., et al. (2007). Family-centered preparation for surgery improves perioperative outcomes in children. *Anesthesiology, 106*(1), 65–74.

Katsma, D., & Smith, G. (1997). Analysis of needle path during intramuscular injection. *Nursing Research, 46*(5), 288–292.

Kellam, B., Sacks, L. M., Wailer, J. L., et al. (2001). Tenderfoot Preemie vs a manual lancet: A clinical evaluation. *Neonatal Network, 20*(7), 31–36.

Kennedy, M. J., Griffin, A., Su, R., et al. (2009). Urine collected from diapers can be used for 2-D PAGE in infants and young children. *Proteomics. Clinical Applications, 3*(8), 989–999.

Kerner, J. A., Jr., Garcia-Careaga, M. G., Fisher, A. A., et al. (2006). Treatment of catheter occlusion in pediatric patients. *Journal of Parenteral and Enteral Nutrition, 30*(1 suppl), S73–S81.

Kilbane, B. J. (2009). Images in emergency medicine: Knotting of a urinary catheter. *Annals of Emergency Medicine, 53*(5), e3–e4.

Klasner, A. E., Luke, D. A., & Scalzo, A. J. (2002). Pediatric orogastric and nasogastric tubes: A new formula evaluated. *Annals of Emergency Medicine, 39*(3), 268–272.

Kleinman, M. E., Chameides, L., Schexnayder, S. M., et al. (2010). Pediatric advance life support: 2010 American Heart Association guidelines for cardiopulmonary resuscitation and emergency cardiovascular care. *Pediatrics, 126*(5), e1361–e1399.

Kline-Tilford, A. M., Sorce, L. R., Levin, D. L., et al. (2013). Pulmonary disorders. In M. F. Hazinski (Ed.), *Nursing care of the critically ill child* (3rd ed.). St. Louis, MO: Elsevier.

Kraus, D. M., Stohlmeyer, L. A., Hannon, D. R., et al. (2001). Effectiveness and infant acceptance of the Rx Medibottle versus the oral syringe. *Pharmacotherapy, 21*(4), 416–423.

Kuch, B. A. (2013). Respiratory monitoring and support. In M. F. Hazinski (Ed.), *Nursing care of the critically ill child* (3rd ed.). St. Louis, MO: Elsevier.

KyngAs, H. A., Kroll, T., & Duffy, M. E. (2000). Compliance in adolescents with chronic diseases: A review. *Journal of Adolescent Health, 26*(6), 379–388.

Lamagna, P., & MacPhee, M. (2004). Phlebitis and infiltration: Troubleshooting pediatric peripheral IVs. *Nurse Week (Heartland), 5*(4), 20, 26, 28.

Levison, J., & Wojtulewicz, J. (2004). Adventitious knot formation complicating catheterization of the infant bladder. *Journal of Paediatrics and Child Health, 40*(8), 493–494.

Li, H. C., Lopez, V., & Lee, T. L. (2007). Psychoeducational preparation of children for surgery: The importance of parental involvement. *Patient Education and Counseling, 65*(1), 34–41.

Lodha, A., Ly, L., Brindle, M., et al. (2005). Intraurethral knot in a very-low-birth-weight infant: Radiological recognition, surgical management and prevention. *Pediatric Radiology, 35*(7), 713–716.

Marchaim, D., Taylor, A. R., Hayakawa, K., et al. (2012). Hospital bath basins are frequently contaminated with multidrug-resistant human pathogens. *American Journal of Infection Control, 40*(6), 562–564.

Maxwell, L. G., & Yaster, M. (2000). Perioperative management issues in pediatric patients. *Anesthesiology Clinics of North America, 18*(3), 601–632.

McClave, S. A., & Neff, R. L. (2006). Care and long-term maintenance of percutaneous endoscopic gastrostomy tubes. *Journal of Parenteral and Enteral Nutrition, 30*(1 suppl), S27–S38.

Nagler, J., Wright, R. O., & Krauss, B. (2006). End-tidal carbon dioxide as a measure of acidosis among children with gastroenteritis. *Pediatrics, 118*(1), 260–267.

Noonan, C., Quigley, S., & Curley, M. A. (2006). Skin integrity in hospitalized infants and children: A prevalence survey. *Journal of Pediatric Nursing, 21*(6), 445–453.

O'Grady, N. P., Alexander, M., Burns, L. A., et al. (2011). Guidelines for the prevention of intravascular catheter-related infections. *Clinical Infectious Diseases, 52*(9), e162–e193.

Peacock, G., Parnapy, S., Raynor, S., et al. (2010). Accuracy and precision of manufacturer-supplied liquid medication administration devices before and after patient education. *Journal of the American Pharmacists Association, 50*(1), 84–86.

Petousis-Harris, H. (2008). Vaccine injection technique and reactogenicity—Evidence for practice. *Vaccine, 26*(50), 6299–6304.

Piira, T., Sugiura, T., Champion, G. D., et al. (2005). The role of parental presence in the context of children's medical procedures: A systematic review. *Child: Care, Health and Development, 31*(2), 233–243.

Powers, J., Peed, J., Burns, L., et al. (2012). Chlorhexidine bathing and microbial contamination in patients' bath basins. *American Journal of Critical Care, 21*(5), 338–342.

Purssell, E. (2009). Parental fever phobia and its evolutionary correlates. *Journal of Clinical Nursing, 18*(2), 210–218.

Purswani, M. U., Radhakrishnan, J., Irfan, K. R., et al. (2009). Infant acceptance of a bitter-tasting liquid medication: A randomized controlled trial comparing the Rx Medibottle with an oral syringe. *Archives of Pediatrics and Adolescent Medicine, 163*(2), 186–188.

Registered Nurses' Association of Ontario (2008). *Care and maintenance to reduce vascular access complications, guideline supplement.* Toronto, ON: Author.

Romino, S. L., Keatley, V. M., Secrest, J., et al. (2005). Parental presence during anesthesia induction in children. *AORN Journal, 81*(4), 780–792.

Rosenberg, H., Davis, M., & James, D. (2007). Malignant hyperthermia. *Orphanet Journal of Rare Diseases, 2,* 21.

Rosenbloom, E., Finkelstein, Y., Adams-Webber, T., et al. (2013). Do antipyretics prevent the recurrence of febrile seizures in children? A systematic review of randomized controlled trials and meta-analysis. *European Journal of Paediatric Neurology, 17*(6), 585–588.

Rupp, M. E., Huerta, T., Yu, S., et al. (2013). Hospital basins used to administer chlorhexidine baths are unlikely microbial reservoirs. *Infection Control & Hospital Epidemiology, 34*(6), 643–645.

Sadleir, L. G., & Scheffer, I. E. (2007). Febrile seizures. *British Medical Journal, 334*(7588), 307–311.

Sahib El-Radhi, A., Carroll, J., & Klein, N. (Eds.), (2009). *Clinical manual of fever in children.* Berlin, Germany: Springer-Verlag.

Shah, P. S., Herbozo, C., Aliwalas, L. L., et al. (2012). Breastfeeding or breast milk for procedural pain in neonates. *Cochrane Database of Systematic Reviews, 2012*(12), CD004950.

Schindler, C. A., Mikhailov, T. A., Kuhn, E. M., et al. (2011). Protecting fragile skin: Nursing interventions to decrease development of pressure ulcers in pediatric intensive care. *American Journal of Critical Care, 20*(1), 26–35.

Shah, V., & Jefferies, A. (2012). Preterm infants receiving heel lance procedures have slightly lower pain scores and quicker time to return to baseline heart rate when held in kangaroo care by the mother than by the father. *Journal of Evidence-Based Medicine, 17*(5), 153–154.

Shah, V., & Ohlsson, A. (2007). Venepuncture versus heel lance for blood sampling in term neonates. *Cochrane Database of Systematic Reviews, 2007*(4), CD001452.

Shen, V., Li, X., Murdock, M., et al. (2003). Recombinant tissue plasminogen activator (alteplase) for restoration of function to occluded central venous catheters in pediatric patients. *Journal of Pediatric Hematology/Oncology, 25*(1), 38–45.

Shepherd, A. J., Glenesk, A., Niven, C. A., et al. (2005). A Scottish study of heel-prick blood sampling in newborn babies. *Midwifery, 22*(2), 158–168.

Sobhani, P., Christopherson, J., Ambrose, P. J., et al. (2008). Accuracy of oral liquid measuring devices: Comparison of dosing cup and oral dosing syringe. *Annals of Pharmacotherapy, 42*(1), 46–52.

Stevens, B., Johnston, C., Taddio, A., et al. (1999). Management of pain from heel lance with lidocaine-prilocaine (EMLA) cream: Is it safe and efficacious in preterm infants? *Journal of Developmental and Behavioral Pediatrics, 20*(4), 216–221.

Taylor, C., Subaiya, L., & Corsino, D. (2011). Pediatric cuffed endotracheal tubes: an evolution of care. *Ochsner Journal, 11*(1), 52–56.

Tillett, J. (2005). Adolescents and informed consent: Ethical and legal issues. *Journal of Perinatal & Neonatal Nursing, 19*(2), 112–121.

Tobias, J. D., & Ross, A. K. (2010). Intraosseous infusion: A review for the anesthesiologist with a focus on pediatric use. *Anesthesia & Analgesia, 110*(2), 391–401.

Turner, T. W. (2004). Intravesical catheter knotting: An uncommon complication of urinary catheterization. *Pediatric Emergency Care, 20*(2), 115–117.

Uman, L. S., Chambers, C. T., McGrath, P. J., et al. (2006). Psychological interventions for needle-related procedural pain and distress in children and adolescents. *Cochrane Database of Systematic Reviews, 2006*(4), CD005179.

Vertanen, H., Fellman, V., Brommels, M., et al. (2001). An automatic incision device for obtaining blood samples from the heels of preterm infants causes less damage than a conventional manual lancet. *Archives of Disease in Childhood: Fetal and Neonatal Edition, 84*(1), F53–F55.

Walsh, A., & Edwards, H. (2006). Management of childhood fever by parents: Literature review. *Journal of Advanced Nursing, 54*(2), 217–222.

Warren, J., Fromm, R. E., Jr., Orr, R. A., et al. (2004). Guidelines for the inter- and intrahospital transport of critically ill patients. *Critical Care Medicine, 32*(1), 256–262.

Willock, J., Baharestani, M. M., & Anthony, D. (2009). The development of the Glamorgan paediatric pressure ulcer risk assessment scale. *Journal of Wound Care, 18*(1), 17–21.

Wound Ostomy and Continence Nurses Society. (2008). *Management of gastrostomy tube complications for the pediatric and adult patient.* Retrieved from http://c.ymcdn.com/sites/www.wocn.org/resource/resmgr/Publications/Mgmt_of_G-Tube_Complications.pdf.

Yip, P., Middleton, P., Cyna, A. M., et al. (2009). Non-pharmacological interventions for assisting the induction of anaesthesia in children. *Cochrane Database of Systematic Reviews, 2009*(3), CD006447.

40

The Child With Respiratory Dysfunction

Cheryl C. Rodgers

ⓔ http://evolve.elsevier.com/Perry/maternal

RESPIRATORY INFECTION

GENERAL ASPECTS OF RESPIRATORY INFECTIONS

Infections of the respiratory tract are described according to the anatomic area of involvement. The *upper respiratory tract,* or *upper airway,* consists of the oronasopharynx, pharynx, larynx, and upper part of the trachea. The *lower respiratory tract* consists of the lower trachea, mainstem bronchi, segmental bronchi, subsegmental bronchioles, terminal bronchioles, and alveoli. In this discussion, the trachea is considered with lower tract disorders, and infections of the epiglottis and larynx are categorized as croup syndromes. However, respiratory infections seldom fall into discrete anatomic areas. Infections often spread from one structure to another because of the contiguous nature of the mucous membrane lining the entire tract. Consequently, respiratory tract infections involve several areas rather than a single structure, although the effect on one area may predominate in any given illness.

Etiology and Characteristics

Respiratory infections account for the majority of acute illnesses in children. The etiology and course of these infections are influenced by the age of the child, the season, living conditions, and preexisting medical problems.

Infectious Agents

The respiratory tract is subject to a wide variety of infective organisms. Most infections are caused by viruses, particularly respiratory syncytial virus (RSV), rhinovirus, nonpolio enteroviruses (coxsackieviruses A and B), adenovirus, parainfluenza virus, influenza virus, and human metapneumovirus. Other agents involved in primary or secondary invasion include group A beta-hemolytic streptococci (GABHS), staphylococci, *Haemophilus influenzae, Bordetella pertussis, Chlamydia trachomatis, Mycoplasma* organisms, and pneumococci.

Age

Healthy full-term infants younger than 3 months of age are presumed to have a lower infection rate than older infants because of the protective function of maternal antibodies; however, infants may be susceptible to specific respiratory tract infections, namely pertussis, during this period. The infection rate increases from 3 to 6 months of age—the time between the disappearance of maternal antibodies and the infant's own antibody production. The viral infection rate remains high during the toddler and preschool years. By 5 years of age, viral respiratory tract infections are less frequent, but the incidence of *Mycoplasma pneumoniae* and GABHS infections increases. The amount of lymphoid tissue increases throughout middle childhood, and repeated exposure to organisms confers increasing immunity as children grow older.

Some viral or bacterial agents produce a mild illness in older children but severe lower respiratory tract illness or croup in infants. For example, pertussis causes a relatively harmless tracheobronchitis in childhood but is a serious disease in infancy.

Size

Anatomic differences influence the response to respiratory tract infections. The diameter of the airways is smaller in young children and subject to considerable narrowing from edematous mucous membranes and increased production of secretions. The distance between structures within the respiratory tract is also shorter in the young child, and organisms may move rapidly down the respiratory tract, causing more extensive involvement. The relatively short and open eustachian tube in infants and young children allows pathogens easy access to the middle ear.

Resistance

The ability to resist invading organisms depends on several factors. Deficiencies of the immune system place the child at risk for infection. Other conditions that decrease resistance are malnutrition, anemia, and fatigue. Conditions that weaken defenses of the respiratory tract and predispose children to infection also include allergies (e.g., allergic rhinitis), preterm birth, bronchopulmonary dysplasia (BPD), asthma, history of RSV infection, cardiac anomalies that cause pulmonary congestion, and cystic fibrosis (CF). Day care attendance and exposure to secondhand smoke increase the likelihood of infection.

Seasonal Variations

The most common respiratory pathogens appear in epidemics during the winter and spring months. However, mycoplasmal infections occur more often in autumn and early winter. Infection-related asthma occurs more frequently during cold weather, whereas winter and spring are typically the "RSV seasons."

BOX 40.1 Signs and Symptoms Associated With Respiratory Infections in Infants and Small Children

Fever
- May be absent in neonates (<28 days of age)
- Greatest at 6 months to 3 years of age
- Temperature may reach 39.5° to 40.5°C (103° to 105°F) even with mild infections
- Often appears as first sign of infection
- May lead to listlessness and irritability, with altered activity pattern
- Tendency to develop high temperatures with infection in certain families
- May precipitate febrile seizures (see Chapter 46)

Poor Feeding and Anorexia
- Common with most childhood illnesses
- Frequently the initial evidence of illness
- Persists to a greater or lesser degree throughout febrile stage of illness; often extends into convalescence

Vomiting
- Common in small children with illness
- A clue to onset of infection
- May precede other signs by several hours
- Usually short-lived, but may persist during the illness
- Is frequent cause of dehydration

Diarrhea
- Usually mild, transient diarrhea but may become severe
- Often accompanies viral respiratory infections
- Frequent cause of dehydration

Abdominal Pain
- Common complaint
- Sometimes indistinguishable from pain of appendicitis
- May represent referred pain (e.g., chest pain associated with pneumonia)
- May be caused by mesenteric lymphadenitis
- May be linked to muscle spasms from vomiting, especially in nervous, tense child

Nasal Blockage
- Small nasal passages of infants easily blocked by mucosal swelling and exudation
- Can interfere with respiration and feeding in infants
- May contribute to the development of otitis media (OM) and sinusitis

Nasal Discharge
- Frequent occurrence
- May be thin and watery (rhinorrhea) or thick and purulent
- Depends on the type or stage of infection
- Associated with itching
- May irritate upper lip and skin surrounding the nose

Cough
- Common feature
- May be evident only during acute phase
- May persist several months after a disease

Respiratory Sounds
- Sounds associated with respiratory disease:
  - Cough
  - Hoarseness
  - Grunting
  - Stridor
  - Wheezing
- Findings on auscultation:
  - Wheezing
  - Crackles
  - Absence of breath sounds (air movement)

Sore Throat
- Frequent complaint of older children
- Young children (unable to describe symptoms) may not complain even when highly inflamed
- Often accompanied by refusal to take oral fluids or solids

Meningismus
- Meningeal signs without infection of the meninges
- Occurs with abrupt onset of fever, accompanied by:
  - Headache
  - Pain and stiffness in the back and neck
  - Presence of Kernig and Brudzinski signs
- Signs subside as the temperature decreases

Clinical Manifestations

Infants and young children, especially those between 6 months and 3 years of age, react more severely to acute respiratory tract infection than do older children. Young children display a number of generalized signs and symptoms and local manifestations (Box 40.1).

Care Management

Assessment of the respiratory system follows the guidelines described in Chapter 29 (for assessment of the ears, nose, mouth and throat, chest, and lungs). The assessment should include respiratory rate, depth, and rhythm; heart rate; oxygenation; hydration status; body temperature; activity level; level of consciousness; and level of comfort. Special attention should also be given to the components and observations listed in Box 40.2. A noninvasive pulse oximeter (oxygen saturation [SaO_2]) measurement should be performed on *all* children with a respiratory condition as part of the routine physical assessment. The nursing process in the care of the child with acute respiratory tract infection is outlined in the Nursing Care Plan box: The Child with Acute Respiratory Tract Infection.

Ease Respiratory Efforts

Many acute respiratory tract infections are mild and cause few symptoms. Although children may feel uncomfortable and have a "stuffy" nose and some mucosal swelling, acute respiratory distress occurs infrequently. Interventions delivered at home are usually sufficient to relieve minor discomfort and ease respiratory efforts. However, in some cases, the infant or child may require close observation by health care professionals.

Warm or cool mist is a common therapeutic measure for symptomatic relief of respiratory discomfort. The moisture soothes inflamed membranes and is beneficial when there is hoarseness or laryngeal involvement. Mist tents have been used in the hospital for humidifying the air and relieving discomfort. The use of steam vaporizers in the

BOX 40.2 Components for Assessing Respiratory Function

Pattern of Respirations

- Rate: Rapid *(tachypnea)*, normal, or slow for the particular child
- Depth: Normal depth, too shallow *(hypopnea)*, too deep *(hyperpnea)*; usually estimated from the amplitude of thoracic and abdominal excursion
- Ease: Effortless, labored *(dyspnea)*, difficult breathing except in upright position *(orthopnea)*; associated with intercostal or substernal retractions (inspiratory "sinking in" of soft tissues in relation to the cartilaginous and bony thorax); pulsus paradoxus (blood pressure falling with inspiration and rising with expiration); flaring nares; head bobbing (head of sleeping child with suboccipital area supported on caregiver's forearm bobs forward in synchrony with each inspiration); grunting, wheezing, or stridor
- Labored breathing: Continuous, intermittent, becoming steadily worse, sudden onset, at rest or on exertion, associated with wheezing, grunting, or chest pain
- Rhythm: Variation in rate and depth of respirations

Other Observations

In addition to respirations, particular attention is addressed to the following:

- Evidence of infection: Check for elevated temperature; enlarged cervical lymph nodes; inflamed mucous membranes; and purulent discharges from the nose, ears, or lungs (sputum).
- Cough: Observe characteristics of cough (if present); under what circumstances cough is heard (e.g., night only, on arising); nature of cough (paroxysmal with or without wheeze; "croupy" or "brassy"); frequency of cough; associated with swallowing or other activity; character of cough (moist and dry); productivity.
- Wheeze: Note if it occurs with expiration or inspiration, high-pitched or musical, prolonged, slowly progressive or sudden, associated with labored breathing.
- Cyanosis: Note distribution (peripheral, perioral, facial, trunk, and face), degree, duration, associated with activity.
- Chest pain: May be a complaint of older children; note location and circumstances: localized or generalized, referred to base of neck or abdomen, dull or sharp, deep or superficial, associated with rapid, shallow respirations or grunting.
- Sputum: Older children may provide sputum sample by coughing, whereas young children may need use of bulb or wall suction to provide a sample; note volume, color, viscosity, and odor.
- Bad breath (halitosis): May be associated with some lung infections.

---

home is often discouraged because of the hazards related to their use and limited evidence to support their efficacy (Himdani, Javed, Hughes, et al., 2016).

A time-honored method (albeit not evidence based) of producing steam is the shower. Running a shower of hot water into the empty bathtub or open shower stall with the bathroom door closed produces a quick source of steam. Keeping a child in this environment for approximately 10 to 15 minutes humidifies inspired air and can help relieve symptoms. A small child can be held on the lap of a parent or other adult. Older children can sit in the bathroom under the supervision of an adult. The use of kettles or bowls of boiling water are strongly discouraged due to the risk for accidental scalding.

Promote Rest

Children who have an acute febrile illness usually have limited activity. One of the cardinal signs that the child is feeling better is the increase in activity; this may, however, be temporary if a high fever returns after

a few hours of increased activity. Children should be encouraged to rest or play quietly to avoid exacerbating symptoms.

Promote Comfort

Older children are usually able to manage nasal secretions with little difficulty. For very young infants, who normally breathe through their noses, an infant nasal aspirator or a bulb syringe is helpful in removing nasal secretions, especially before being put to bed to sleep and before feeding. This practice, preceded by instillation of saline nose drops as needed, may clear nasal passages and promote feeding. Saline nose drops can be prepared at home by dissolving 1 tsp of salt in 1 pint of warm water. Two to three drops of saline can be put into the nostril, and a bulb syringe can be used to suction it out.

For children older than 2 years of age who can tolerate decongestants, vasoconstrictive nose drops may be administered every 4 hours as needed. Phenylephrine 0.25% (for children older than 2 years of age) or oxymetazoline 0.05% (for children older than 6 years of age) is sometimes prescribed. Bottles of nose drops should be used for only one child and one illness because they are easily contaminated with bacteria and viruses.

> ### ! NURSING ALERT
> To avoid rebound congestion, vasoconstrictive nose drops or sprays should not be administered for more than 3 days.

Topical vapor rubs could be considered for children older than 2 years of age to ease nasal congestion, lessen cough severity, and improve sleep quality (Fashner, Ericson, & Werner, 2012). However, some children may not tolerate the strong smell. These vapor rubs should never be given orally or placed directly beneath the nose.

Hot or cold applications sometimes provide relief for children with painful cervical adenitis. An ice bag or heating pad applied to the neck may decrease the discomfort, but safety precautions must be observed to prevent burns. The ice bag or heating device must be covered, and the heating pad should not be set at high settings.

Prevent Spread of Infection

Careful hand washing is important when caring for children with respiratory tract infections. Older children should use a tissue or their arm to cover their nose and mouth when they cough or sneeze, dispose of the tissue properly, and wash their hands. Remembering to cover the nose or mouth is often difficult for small children. Used tissues should be immediately thrown into the wastebasket and not allowed to accumulate in a pile. Children with respiratory tract infections should not share drinking cups, eating utensils, washcloths, or towels. To decrease contamination, wash hands frequently, and do not touch eyes or noses with hands. Parents should try to remove affected children from contact with other children. Parents should also keep affected children out of school or day care settings to prevent the spread of infection. An effort should be made to teach well children to stay away from ill children, to wash their hands frequently, and to avoid eating and drinking from the same utensils or cups.

Reduce Temperature

If the child has a significantly elevated body temperature, controlling the fever is important. Parents should know how to take a child's temperature and read a thermometer accurately. Nurses should not assume that all parents can read a thermometer and should provide education when needed.

If the practitioner prescribes an antipyretic such as acetaminophen or ibuprofen (for infants and children 6 months of age and older), parents may need instruction on how to administer it. Most parents

⊚ NURSING CARE PLAN

The Child With Acute Respiratory Tract Infection

Case Study

Sarah is a 7-month-old patient who is being evaluated in the emergency room for fever and cough. Sara's mother reports that Sarah has not been as active as usual and has been eating less over the past 2 days. She started coughing during the night and upon awakening was noted to have a temperature of 103°F.

Assessment

Based on these events, what are the most important subjective and objective data that should be assessed?

Defining Characteristics

Usually high fever, tachypnea, tachycardia
Retractions
Nasal flaring
Dyspnea (reported by older children)
Breath sounds (usually rhonci or fine crackles)
Cough (productive or nonproductive)
Skin color (pallor or cyanosis depending on severity)
Irritable, restless, or lethargic

Nursing Diagnoses

Ineffective Breathing Pattern
Ineffective Airway Clearance
Hyperthermia
Infection
Risk for Fluid Volume Deficit

Nursing Interventions and Rationales

What are the most appropriate nursing interventions for this infant with acute respiratory tract infection?

Nursing Interventions	Rationales
Position Sarah for maximum ventilation and airway patency.	To allow for increased chest expansion
Monitor vital signs including respiratory and oxygen status.	To quickly identify alterations in temperature, respiratory status, or circulation and determine the need for additional interventions
Provide humidified oxygen as indicated.	To improve oxygenation
Suction airway (nose, mouth) as necessary.	To remove secretions and maintain airway patency
Provide gentle chest percussion and postural drainage (CPT) as indicated.	To facilitate secretion removal
Administer antipyretics as indicated.	To reduce fever and promote comfort
Administer bronchodilators as indicated.	To promote bronchodilation and improve ventilation
Administer antibiotics as indicated	To treat infection source
Obtain specimens (i.e., secretions, blood) as indicated.	To identify infective organisms
Maintain appropriate precautions such as Standard Precautions, aseptic suction, and frequent hand washing.	To prevent spread of infection
Monitor hydration status through strict intake and output and daily weights.	To prevent dehydration or fluid overload
Implement comfort measures such as allowing parent presence, parent holding infant, and comfort item such as favorite blanket or stuffed animal.	To reduce anxiety and promote comfort

Expected Outcomes

Respiration rate will be in an acceptable range and nonlabored.
Airway will remain patent.
Body temperature will remain in acceptable range.
Infection will resolve.
Adequate hydration status will be maintained.

Case Study (Continued)

Sarah's parents are anxious and upset about their daughter's condition and hospitalization. You want to educate them on what is happening to their daughter.

Assessment

What are the most important aspects of care to discuss with her parents at this time?

Defining Characteristics

Understanding of acute respiratory tract infection
Description of treatment regimen including rationale for medications
Expression of fears and concerns
Display of appropriate reactions to child's condition

Nursing Diagnosis

Readiness for Enhanced Knowledge related to parents' interest in Sarah's health status.

Nursing Interventions and Rationales

What are the most appropriate nursing interventions for this diagnosis?

Nursing Interventions	Rationales
Educate family about characteristics of acute respiratory tract infection.	To promote understanding of etiology and symptoms of respiratory infections
Educate family about strategies to facilitate ventilation (i.e., sitting up) and encourage secretion clearance (i.e., CPT, nasal suctioning).	To promote understanding of measures to enhance ventilation and airway clearance
Educate family about Sarah's hospital and discharge medications, including antipyretics, bronchodilators, and antibiotics.	To promote understanding of treatment regimen
Allow family to remain with Sarah, and encourage family's involvement in the Sarah's care.	To decrease effects of separation and promote family sense of control and involvement in care
Arrange for social worker to meet with family to assess emotional and financial needs.	To identify and modify stressors associated with hospitalization

Expected Outcomes

Parents will verbalize understanding of acute respiratory tract infection.
Parents will verbalize understanding of treatment including medication and strategies to promote ventilation and airway clearance.
Parents will verbalize understanding of medications including antipyretics, bronchodilators, and antibiotics.
Parents will remain involved in Sarah's care.
Parents will verbalize resources available for emotional and financial support as indicated.

can read the label and calculate the desired dosage, but parents of infants and toddlers require detailed instruction and dosing parameters. It is important to emphasize accuracy in determining both the amount of drug to be given and the time intervals for administration.

Cool liquids are encouraged to reduce the temperature and minimize the chances of dehydration (see the "Controlling Elevated Temperatures" section in Chapter 39).

> ## ! NURSING ALERT
>
> Caution parents about the use of over-the-counter combination "cold" remedies, since these often include acetaminophen. Careful calculation of both the acetaminophen given separately and the acetaminophen in combination medications is necessary to avoid an overdose.

Promote Hydration

Dehydration is a potential complication when children have respiratory tract infections and are febrile or anorectic, especially when vomiting or diarrhea is present. Infants are especially prone to fluid and electrolyte deficits when they have a respiratory illness because a rapid respiratory rate that accompanies such illnesses precludes adequate oral fluid intake. In addition, the presence of fever increases the total body fluid turnover in infants. If the infant has nasal secretions, this further prevents adequate respiratory effort by blocking the narrow nasal passages when the infant reclines to bottle feed or breastfeed and ceases the compensatory mouth breathing effort, thus causing the child to limit intake of fluids. Adequate fluid intake is encouraged by offering small amounts of favorite fluids (clear liquids if vomiting) at frequent intervals. Oral rehydration solutions, such as Infalyte or Pedialyte, should be considered for infants, and water or a low-carbohydrate (≤5 g per 8 oz) flavored drink should be considered for older children. Fluids with caffeine (tea, coffee) are avoided because these may act as diuretics and promote fluid loss. Sports drinks and energy drinks are not recommended for oral rehydration (American Academy of Pediatrics, 2011). Breastfeeding infants should continue to be breastfed because human milk confers some degree of protection from infection (see Chapter 24). Fluids should not be forced, because this creates the same problem as urging unwanted food. Gentle persuasion with preferred beverages or sugar-free popsicles is usually more successful. Younger children may like to drink smaller amounts from a plastic medicine cup or syringe.

To assess their child's level of hydration (see Chapter 41), parents are advised to observe the frequency of voiding and to notify the nurse or practitioner if there is insufficient voiding. Counting the number of wet diapers in a 24-hour period is a satisfactory method to assess output in infants and toddlers. In the hospital, diapers are weighed to assess output, which should be at least 1 mL/kg/hr in a child who weighs less than 30 kg. Urinary output should be at least 30 mL per hour in patients weighing more than 30 kg. The practitioner should be notified if the urine output is low.

Provide Nutrition

Loss of appetite is characteristic of children with acute infections. In most cases, children can be permitted to determine their own need for food. Many children show no decrease in appetite, and others respond well to foods such as gelatin, soup, and puddings (see the "Feeding the Sick Child" section in Chapter 39). Urging foods for children who are sick may precipitate nausea and vomiting and cause an aversion to feeding that may extend into the convalescent period and beyond.

Provide Family Support and Home Care

Young children with respiratory tract infections may be irritable and difficult to comfort; therefore the family needs support, encouragement, and practical suggestions concerning comfort measures and administration of medication. In addition to antipyretics and nose drops, the child may require antibiotic therapy. Parents of children receiving oral antibiotics must understand the importance of regular administration and continuing the drug for the prescribed length of time, regardless of whether the child appears ill. Parents are cautioned against giving their child any medications that are not approved by the practitioner and to avoid giving antibiotics left over from a previous illness or prescribed for another child. Administering unprescribed antibiotics can produce serious side effects and adverse reactions (see Chapter 39 for administration of medications and family teaching).

UPPER RESPIRATORY TRACT INFECTIONS

ACUTE VIRAL NASOPHARYNGITIS

Acute nasopharyngitis, or the equivalent of the "common cold," is caused by rhinoviruses, RSV, adenoviruses, enteroviruses, influenza virus, and parainfluenza virus. Symptoms are more severe in infants and children than in adults. Fever is common in young children, and older children have low-grade fevers, which appear early in the course of the illness. Other clinical manifestations are listed in Box 40.3. Symptoms may last up to 14 days.

Therapeutic Management

Children with nasopharyngitis are managed at home. There is no specific treatment, and effective vaccines are not available. Antipyretics may be indicated for fever and discomfort (see Chapter 39 for management of

---

> ### BOX 40.3   Clinical Manifestations of Nasopharyngitis and Pharyngitis
>
> | Nasopharyngitis | Pharyngitis |
> |---|---|
> | **Younger Child** | **Younger Child** |
> | • Fever | • Fever |
> | • Irritability, restlessness | • General malaise |
> | • Poor feeding and decreased fluid intake | • Anorexia |
> | • Sneezing | • Moderate sore throat |
> | • Nasal mucus (abundant) causing mouth breathing | • Headache |
> | • Vomiting or diarrhea | **Older Child** |
> | | • Fever (may reach 40° C [104° F]) |
> | **Older Child** | • Headache |
> | • Dryness and irritation of nose and throat initially | • Anorexia |
> | • Nasal discharge causing mouth breathing | • Dysphagia |
> | • Sneezing, chilling | • Abdominal pain |
> | • Muscular aches | • Vomiting |
> | • Cough, sometimes | **Physical Signs** |
> | **Physical Signs** | *Younger Child* |
> | • Edema and vasodilation of mucosa | • Mild to moderate hyperemia |
> | | *Older Child* |
> | | • Mild to bright red, edematous pharynx |
> | | • Hyperemia of tonsils and pharynx; may extend to soft palate and uvula |
> | | • Often abundant follicular exudate that spreads and coalesces to form pseudomembrane on tonsils |
> | | • Cervical glands enlarged and tender |

fever). Fluids and rest are recommended. The provision of a humidified environment and increasing oral fluids may be beneficial to some children with a cold.

Cough suppressants containing dextromethorphan should be used with caution (cough is a protective way of clearing secretions) but may be prescribed every 6 to 8 hours for a dry, hacking cough, especially at night. However, some preparations contain 22% alcohol and can cause adverse effects such as confusion, hyperexcitability, dizziness, nausea, and sedation. Parents should monitor the child carefully for potential adverse effects. Recent concerns regarding serious side effects of cough and cold preparations in young children, particularly infants, and lack of convincing evidence that such medications are effective in reducing symptoms have prompted recommendations by health care experts to carefully evaluate the benefits and risks of recommending such preparations for children younger than 6 years of age (Yang & So, 2014). Over-the-counter cold preparations such as pseudoephedrine and some antihistamines are not appropriate for the treatment of the common cold in infants and toddlers; these may cause serious side effects in such children and have been associated with death in infants (Hampton, Nguyen, Edwards, et al., 2013). Over-the-counter cough and cold medications do not work for children younger than 4 years of age and in some cases may pose a health risk (Hampton et al.).

Antihistamines are largely ineffective in treatment of nasopharyngitis. These drugs have a weak atropine-like effect that dries secretions, but they can cause drowsiness or, paradoxically, have a stimulatory effect on children. There is no support for the usefulness of expectorants, and antibiotics are usually not indicated because most infections are viral.

Prevention

Nasopharyngitis is so widespread in the general population that it is impossible to prevent. The best methods for preventing transmission of these viruses are frequent hand washing and avoiding touching one's eyes, nose, and mouth. Children are more susceptible because they have not yet developed resistance to many viruses. Young infants are subject to serious complications, so they should be protected from exposure.

Care Management

A cold is often the parents' first introduction to an illness in their infant. Most discomfort of nasopharyngitis is related to the nasal obstruction, especially in small infants. Elevating the head of the bed or crib mattress assists with drainage of secretions. Suctioning and vaporization may also provide relief. Saline nose drops and gentle suction with a bulb syringe before feeding and sleep time may be useful.

Maintaining adequate fluid intake is essential. Although a child's appetite for solid foods is usually diminished for several days, it is important to offer appropriate fluids to prevent dehydration.

Because nasopharyngitis is spread from secretions, the best means for prevention is avoiding contact with affected people. This goal is difficult to accomplish in family settings, classrooms, and day care centers. Family members with a cold should carefully dispose of tissues; not share towels, glasses, or eating utensils; cover the mouth and nose with tissues when coughing or sneezing; and wash hands thoroughly after nose blowing or sneezing. The most frequent carriers of infection are the human hands, which deposit viruses on doorknobs, faucets, and other everyday objects. Children should be taught to wash their hands thoroughly and avoid touching their eyes, nose, and mouth.

Family Support

Support and reassurance are important elements of care for families of young children with recurrent upper respiratory infections (URIs). Because URIs are frequent in children younger than 3 years of age,

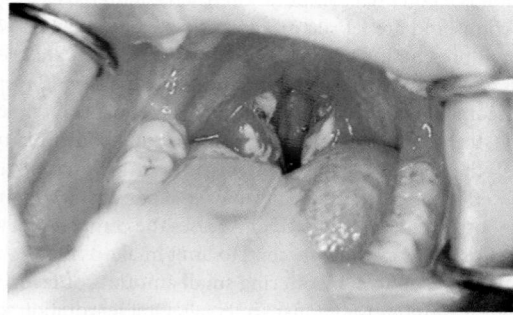

FIG 40.1 Tonsillitis and pharyngitis. (Courtesy of Dr. Edward L. Applebaum, Head, Department of Otolaryngology, University of Illinois Medical Center, Chicago, IL.)

families may feel they are on an endless roller coaster of illness. They need reassurance that frequent colds are a normal part of childhood and that by 5 years of age, their children will have developed immunity to many viruses. When children spend time in day care centers, their infection rate is higher than if they are cared for in the home because of increased exposure. Likewise, for children who were cared for at home before starting school, their infection rate increases when exposed to more children at school.

Parents should know the signs of respiratory complications and should notify a health care professional if complications occur or the child does not improve within 2 to 3 days (Box 40.4).

ACUTE INFECTIOUS PHARYNGITIS

Acute infectious pharyngitis can be caused by many bacteria or viruses. GABHS infection is the most common causative organism for this infection. Children who experience GABHS infection of the upper airway (strep throat) are at risk for rheumatic fever (RF), an inflammatory disease of the heart, joints, and central nervous system (CNS) (see Chapter 42), and acute glomerulonephritis (AGN), an acute kidney infection (see Chapter 44). Permanent damage can result from these sequelae, especially RF. GABHS may also cause skin manifestations, including impetigo and pyoderma.

Clinical Manifestations

GABHS infection is generally a relatively brief illness that varies in severity from subclinical (no symptoms) to severe toxicity. The onset is often abrupt and characterized by pharyngitis, headache, fever, and abdominal pain. The tonsils and pharynx may be inflamed and covered with exudate (Fig. 40.1), which usually appears by the second day of illness. However, streptococcal infections should be suspected in children older than 2 years of age who have pharyngitis without exudate or nasal symptoms. The tongue may appear edematous and red (strawberry tongue), and the child may have a fine sandpaper rash on the trunk, axillae, elbows, and groin seen in scarlet fever (caused by a strain of group A streptococcus). The uvula is edematous and red. Anterior cervical lymphadenopathy (in 30% to 50% of cases) usually occurs early, and the nodes are often tender. Pain can be relatively mild to severe enough to make swallowing difficult. Clinical manifestations usually subside in 3 to 5 days unless complicated by sinusitis or parapharyngeal, peritonsillar, or retropharyngeal abscess. Nonsuppurative complications may appear after the onset of GABHS—AGN in about 10 days and RF in an average of 18 days.

Children who are GABHS carriers may have a positive throat culture but often experience a coincidental viral illness.

Diagnostic Evaluation

Although 80% to 90% of all cases of acute pharyngitis are viral, a throat culture or rapid streptococcal antigen testing should be performed to rule out GABHS. Most streptococcal infections are short-term illnesses, and antibody responses (e.g., antistreptolysin-O titer) appear later than symptoms and are useful only for retrospective diagnosis.

Rapid identification of GABHS with diagnostic test kits (rapid antigen detection test) is possible in the office or clinic setting. Because of the high specificity of these rapid tests, a positive test result does not require throat culture confirmation. However, the sensitivities of these kits vary considerably and a confirmatory throat culture is recommended in patients who have a negative test result (American Academy of Pediatrics Committee on Infectious Diseases & Pickering, 2012).

Therapeutic Management

If streptococcal sore throat infection is present, oral penicillin V or amoxicillin is prescribed for 10 days to eliminate any organisms that might remain to initiate RF symptoms. Penicillin does not prevent the development of AGN in susceptible children; however, it may prevent the spread of a nephrogenic strain of GABHS to others in the family. Penicillin usually produces a prompt response within 24 hours. Patients who have a history of RF or who remain symptomatic after a full course of antibiotics may require a follow-up throat swab.

Intramuscular (IM) benzathine penicillin G is an appropriate therapy, but it is painful and is not the first choice for children. An oral macrolide (erythromycin, azithromycin, clarithromycin) is indicated for children who are allergic to penicillin. Other antibiotics used to treat GABHS are oral cephalosporins, clindamycin, and amoxicillin with clavulanic acid (American Academy of Pediatrics Committee on Infectious Diseases & Pickering, 2012).

Care Management

The nurse often obtains a throat swab for culture or rapid antigen testing and instructs the parents about administering oral antibiotics and analgesics as prescribed. Cold or warm compresses to the neck may provide relief. In children who can cooperate, warm saline gargles may offer relief of throat discomfort. Acetaminophen and ibuprofen may be effective in decreasing the throat pain; liquid preparations or chewable forms may be preferable because of the pain associated with swallowing. Pain may interfere with oral intake, and children should not be forced to eat, but fluid intake is essential. Cool liquids, ice chips, or flavored ice pops may be tolerated better than solid foods.

Special emphasis is placed on correct administration of oral medication and completion of the course of antibiotic therapy (see the "Administration of Medication" and "Compliance" sections in Chapter 39). If an injection of penicillin is required, it must be administered deep into a large muscle mass (e.g., vastus lateralis or ventrogluteal muscle). To prevent pain, application of a topical anesthetic cream, such as LMX4 (4% lidocaine) or eutectic mixture of lidocaine and prilocaine (EMLA) over the injection site before the injection is helpful (see Guidelines box: Intramuscular Administration of Medication in Chapter 39). The injection site may be tender for 1 to 2 days.

Children are considered infectious to others at the onset of symptoms and up to 24 hours after initiation of antibiotic therapy, but they should not return to school or day care until they have been taking antibiotics for a full 24-hour period. Nurses should remind the children to discard their toothbrushes and replace them with new ones after they have been taking antibiotics for 24 hours. Orthodontic appliances should be washed thoroughly because they may harbor the organisms. Parents are cautioned to prevent other household members, especially if immunocompromised, from having close contact with the sick child and avoid sharing drinking or eating items.

If the child continues to have a high fever that does not respond to antipyretics, has an extremely sore throat, refuses liquids, and appears toxic 24 to 48 hours after starting antibiotics, further evaluation by a practitioner is recommended.

TONSILLITIS

The tonsils are masses of lymphoid tissue located in the pharyngeal cavity. They filter and protect the respiratory and alimentary tracts from invasion by pathogenic organisms and play a role in antibody formation. Although tonsil size varies, children generally have much larger tonsils than do adolescents or adults. This difference is thought to be a protective mechanism because young children are especially susceptible to URIs.

Pathophysiology

Several pairs of tonsils are part of a mass of lymphoid tissue encircling the nasal and oral pharynx, known as the Waldeyer *tonsillar ring* (Fig. 40.2). The palatine, or faucial, tonsils are located on either side of the oropharynx behind and below the pillars of the fauces (opening from the mouth). A surface of the palatine tonsils is usually visible during oral examination. The palatine tonsils are those removed during tonsillectomy. The pharyngeal tonsils, also known as the adenoids, are located above the palatine tonsils on the posterior wall of the nasopharynx.

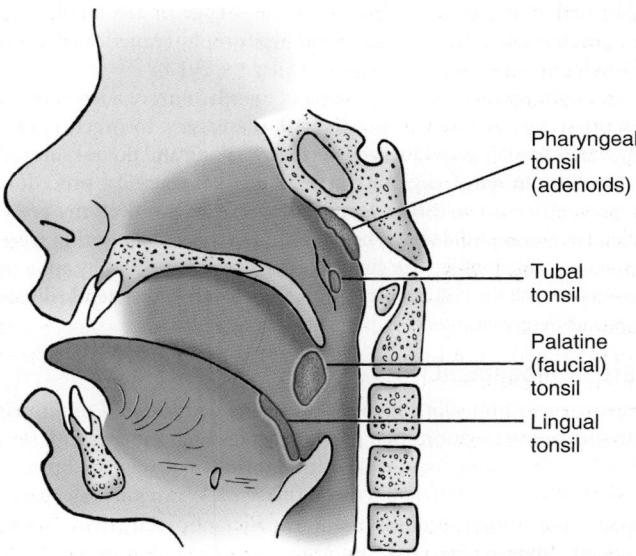

FIG 40.2 Location of various tonsillar masses.

Their proximity to the nares and eustachian tubes causes difficulties in instances of inflammation.

Etiology

Tonsillitis often occurs with pharyngitis. Because of the abundant lymphoid tissue and the frequency of URIs, tonsillitis is a common cause of illness in young children. The causative agent may be viral or bacterial.

Clinical Manifestations

The manifestations of tonsillitis are caused by inflammation. As the palatine tonsils enlarge from edema, they may meet in the midline (kissing tonsils), obstructing the passage of air or food. The child has difficulty swallowing and breathing. When enlargement of the adenoids occurs, the space behind the posterior nares becomes blocked, making it difficult or impossible for air to pass from the nose to the throat. As a result, the child breathes through the mouth.

Therapeutic Management

Because tonsillitis is self-limiting, treatment of viral pharyngitis is symptomatic. Throat cultures positive for GABHS infection warrant antibiotic treatment. It is important to differentiate between viral and streptococcal infection in febrile exudative tonsillitis. Because most infections are of viral origin, early rapid tests can eliminate unnecessary antibiotic administration.

Tonsillectomy is the surgical removal of the palatine tonsils. Absolute indications for a tonsillectomy are recurrent throat infections (seven or more episodes in the preceding year, five or more episodes in each of the preceding 2 years, or three or more episodes in each of the preceding 3 years) and sleep-disordered breathing (Baugh, Archer, Mitchell, et al., 2011).

Adenoidectomy (the surgical removal of the adenoids) is recommended for children who have a history of four or greater episodes of recurrent purulent rhinorrhea in the previous 12 months in a child younger than 12 years of age (one episode should be documented by intranasal examination or imaging (American Academy of Otolaryngology—Head and Neck Surgery, 2012). Other indications include persisting symptoms of adenoiditis after two courses of antibiotics, sleep disturbance with nasal obstruction for more than 3 months, hyponasal speech, otitis media with effusion (OME) for more than 3 months, dental malocclusion or orofacial growth disturbance as validated by an orthodontist/dentist, OME with effusion in a child at least 4 years of age, or cardiopulmonary complications associated with adenoid hypertrophy (American Academy of Otolaryngology—Head and Neck Surgery, 2012).

For some children, the effectiveness of tonsillectomy or adenoidectomy is modest and may not justify the risk of surgery. In practice, many physicians rely on individualized decision making and do not subscribe to an absolute set of eligibility criteria for these surgical procedures. Contraindications to either tonsillectomy or adenoidectomy are (1) cleft palate because the tonsils help minimize escape of air during speech; (2) acute infections at the time of surgery because locally inflamed tissues increase the risk for bleeding; (3) uncontrolled systemic diseases or blood dyscrasias; and (4) poor anesthetic risk.

Care Management

Nursing care of tonsillitis involves providing comfort and minimizing activities or interventions that precipitate bleeding. Patients with sleep-disordered breathing require close monitoring of airway and breathing postoperatively. A soft to liquid diet is preferred. Warm salt-water gargles, warm fluids, throat lozenges, and analgesic/antipyretic drugs such as acetaminophen are used to promote comfort. Opioids are often needed to reduce pain so the child can drink. Combination non-opioid and opioid elixirs such as acetaminophen with codeine or with hydrocodone (Lortab) relieve pain and should be given regularly as prescribed.

If surgery is required, the child requires the same psychologic preparation and physical care as for any other surgical procedure. Most tonsillectomy and adenoidectomy surgeries now take place in outpatient settings; however, the priorities of preoperative and postoperative care remain the same. The following discussion focuses on postoperative nursing care for tonsillectomy and adenoidectomy, although both procedures may not be performed.

Until fully awake, the child is placed on his or her abdomen or side to facilitate drainage of secretions. Routine suctioning is avoided, but when performed, it is done carefully to avoid trauma to the oropharynx. When alert, the child may prefer sitting up. The child is discouraged from coughing frequently, clearing the throat, blowing the nose, and any other activity that may aggravate the operative site.

Some secretions are common, particularly dried blood from surgery. All secretions and vomitus are inspected for evidence of fresh bleeding (some blood-tinged mucus is expected). Dark brown (old) blood is usually present in the emesis, in the nose, and between the teeth. If parents do not expect this, they often become frightened at a time when they need to be calm and reassuring.

The throat is sore after surgery. An ice collar may provide relief, but many children find it bothersome and refuse to use it. Most children experience moderate pain after a tonsillectomy and adenoidectomy and need pain medication regularly for at least the first few days. Analgesics may be given rectally or intravenously to avoid the oral route. Because the pain is continuous, analgesics should be administered at regular intervals, even at night (see the "Pain Management" section in Chapter 30). An antiemetic such as ondansetron (Zofran) may be administered postoperatively if nausea or vomiting is present.

Food and fluids are restricted until the child is fully alert and there are no signs of hemorrhage. Cool water, crushed ice, flavored ice pops, or diluted fruit juice may be given, but fluids with a red or brown color are avoided to distinguish fresh or old blood in emesis from the ingested liquid. Citrus juice may cause discomfort and is poorly tolerated. Soft foods, particularly gelatin, cooked fruits, sherbet, soup, and mashed potatoes, are started on the first or second postoperative day or as the child tolerates feeding. The pain from surgery often inhibits fluid intake, reinforcing the need for adequate and regular administration of analgesics. Milk, ice cream, and pudding are usually not offered because milk products coat the mouth and throat and may cause the child to clear the throat, which can initiate bleeding.

Postoperative hemorrhage is uncommon but can occur in up to 5% of patients up to 14 days after surgery. The nurse observes the throat directly for evidence of bleeding—using a good source of light and, if necessary, carefully inserting a tongue depressor. Other signs of hemorrhage are tachycardia, pallor, frequent clearing of the throat or swallowing by a younger child, and vomiting of bright red blood. Restlessness, an indication of hemorrhage, may be difficult to differentiate from general discomfort after surgery. Decreasing blood pressure is a late sign of shock.

Surgery may be required to ligate a bleeding vessel. Airway obstruction may also occur as a result of edema or accumulated secretions and is indicated by signs of respiratory distress, such as stridor, drooling, restlessness, agitation, increasing respiratory rate, and progressive cyanosis. Suction equipment and oxygen should be available after tonsillectomy.

! NURSING ALERT

The most obvious early sign of bleeding is the child's continuous swallowing of the trickling blood. While the child is sleeping, note the frequency of swallowing. If continuous bleeding is suspected, notify the surgeon immediately.

Family Support and Home Care

Discharge instructions include (1) avoiding irritating and highly seasoned foods, (2) avoiding gargles or vigorous toothbrushing, (3) avoiding coughing or clearing of the throat or putting objects in the mouth (e.g., a straw), (4) using analgesics or an ice collar for pain, and (5) limiting activity to decrease the potential for bleeding. Chewing gum may prevent throat and ear pain in older children. Objectionable mouth odor and slight ear pain with a low-grade fever are common for 5 to 10 days postoperatively. However, persistent severe earache, fever, or cough requires medical evaluation. Most children are ready to resume normal activity within 1 to 2 weeks after the operation. The child's voice may sound different postoperatively, especially if the tonsils were large.

INFLUENZA

Influenza, or the "flu," is caused by three orthomyxoviruses, which are antigenically distinct: types A and B, which cause epidemic disease; and type C, which is antigenically stable and causes milder disease. Influenza is spread from one individual to another by direct contact (large-droplet infection) or by articles recently contaminated by nasopharyngeal secretions. Attack rates are highest in young children who have had no previous contact with a strain. Influenza is frequently most severe in infants. During epidemics, infection among school-age children is believed to be a major source of transmission in a community. The disease is more common during the winter months and has a 1- to 3-day incubation period. Affected people are most infectious for 24 hours before and after the onset of symptoms. The virus has a peculiar affinity for epithelial cells of the respiratory tract mucosa, where it destroys ciliated epithelium with metaplastic hyperplasia of the tracheal and bronchial epithelium with associated edema. The alveoli may also become distended with a hyaline-like material. The viruses can be isolated from nasopharyngeal secretions early after the onset of infection, and serologic tests identify the type by complement fixation or the subgroups by hemagglutination inhibition.

Clinical Manifestations

The manifestations of influenza may be subclinical, mild, moderate, or severe. Most patients have a dry throat and nasal mucosa, a dry cough, and a tendency toward hoarseness. A flushed face, photophobia, myalgia, hyperesthesia, and sometimes exhaustion and lack of energy accompany a sudden onset of fever and chills. Subglottal croup is common, especially in infants. The symptoms of influenza last for 4 to 5 days. Complications include severe viral pneumonia (often hemorrhagic); encephalitis; and secondary bacterial infections such as otitis media, sinusitis, or pneumonia.

Therapeutic Management

Uncomplicated influenza in children usually requires only symptomatic treatment, including acetaminophen or ibuprofen for fever and sufficient fluids to maintain hydration. There are four influenza antiviral drugs approved by the US Food and Drug Administration (FDA) for use in the United States, but only oseltamivir (Tamiflu) and zanamivir (Relenza) are recommended because of widespread resistance to amantadine (Symmetrel) and rimantadine (Flumadine) (American Academy of Pediatrics Committee on Infectious Diseases & American Academy of Pediatrics Bronchiolitis Guidelines Committee, 2014).

Oseltamivir is a neuraminidase inhibitor that may be administered orally for 5 days to children older than 1 year of age (and adults) to decrease the flu symptoms; this drug must be taken within 2 days of the onset of symptoms. It is reported to be effective for types A and B influenza (American Academy of Pediatrics Committee on Infectious Diseases & Pickering, 2012).

Zanamivir can be used for treatment of influenza in patients 7 years of age and older and for prophylaxis of influenza in patients 5 years of age and older. It must be started within 48 hours of the onset of symptoms. Zanamivir is an inhaled medication effective for type A and B influenza. The drug is taken twice daily for 5 days and is administered by a specially designed oral inhaler (Diskhaler). Bronchospasm and a decline in lung function can occur when zanamivir is used in patients with underlying airway disease, such as asthma or chronic obstructive pulmonary disease (COPD).

Prevention

The influenza vaccine is now recommended annually for children older than 6 months of age. Influenza vaccine (trivalent inactivated influenza vaccine [TIV]) may be given to healthy children 6 months of age and older. The TIVs are safe and effective provided the antigens in the vaccine correlate with the circulating influenza viruses (see the "Immunizations" section in Chapter 31). Patients who have a hypersensitivity to eggs with a history of hives after exposure, may receive the trivalent recombinant influenza vaccine in a setting with readily available personnel and equipment.

The live-attenuated influenza vaccine (LAIV) is a nasal spray flu vaccine approved by the FDA that is licensed for administration to people 2 to 49 years of age. However, this preparation contains a live virus and should not be used in individuals who are immunocompromised or receiving immunosuppressants, have reactive airway disease, have a febrile illness, are receiving aspirin therapy, have a chronic respiratory condition, have received a live vaccine in the previous 28 days, are or could be pregnant, or have a history of Guillain-Barré syndrome (Centers for Disease Control and Prevention, 2012). Patients who have had anaphylactic reactions to egg protein should receive a risk-assessment evaluation by a physician with expertise in the management of allergic conditions (Centers for Disease Control and Prevention, 2012).

Care Management

Nursing care for influenza is the same as for any child with a URI, including implementing measures to relieve symptoms. The greatest danger to affected children is development of a secondary infection. Prolonged fever or the appearance of fever during early convalescence is a sign of secondary bacterial infection and should be reported to the health care provider for antibiotic therapy. Children with influenza (or other similar viruses) should not receive aspirin because of its possible link with Reye syndrome.

OTITIS MEDIA

OM is the presence of fluid in the middle ear along with acute signs of illness and symptoms of middle ear inflammation (Klein & Pelton, 2013). The standard terminology used to define OM is outlined in Box 40.5. OM is one of the most prevalent diseases of early childhood. Its incidence is highest in winter months. Many cases of bacterial OM are preceded by a viral respiratory infection. The two viruses most likely to precipitate OM are RSV and influenza. Most episodes of acute otitis media (AOM) occur in the first 24 months of life, but the incidence decreases with age except for a small increase at 5 or 6 years of age when children enter school. OM occurs infrequently in children older than 7 years of age. Preschool-age boys are affected more frequently than preschool-age girls. Children who have siblings or parents with a history of chronic OM have a higher incidence of OM. Children living in households with many members (especially smokers) are more likely to have OM than those living with fewer people. Passive smoking increases the risk for persistent middle ear effusion by enhancing attachment of the pathogens that cause OM to the respiratory epithelium in the middle ear space, by prolonging the inflammatory response, and by impeding drainage through the eustachian tube (Lieberthal, Carroll, Chonmaitree, et al., 2013). Family socioeconomic status and extent of exposure to other children are the two most important identifiable risk factors for the occurrence of OM (Lieberthal et al.).

Etiology

Streptococcus pneumoniae, H. influenzae, and *Moraxella catarrhalis* are the three most common bacteria causing acute otitis media (AOM). The etiology of noninfectious OM is unknown, but OM may occur because of blocked eustachian tubes, which results in negative ear pressure. Fluid is pulled from the mucosal lining, which accumulates and becomes colonized by infectious organisms. Predisposing factors include URIs, allergic rhinitis, Down syndrome, cleft palate, day care attendance, exposure to secondhand smoke, and bottle propping during feeding. Breastfed infants have a lower incidence of OM than formula-fed infants (Bowatte, Tham, Allen, et al., 2015). Breastfeeding may protect infants against respiratory viruses and allergy because it contains secretory immunoglobulin A, which limits the exposure of the eustachian tube and middle ear mucosa to microbial pathogens and foreign proteins. Reflux of milk up the eustachian tubes is less likely in breastfed infants because of the semivertical positioning during breastfeeding compared with bottle feeding.

Pathophysiology

OM is primarily a result of malfunctioning eustachian tubes. Mechanical or functional obstruction of the eustachian tube causes accumulation of secretions in the middle ear. Intrinsic obstruction can be caused by infection or allergy; extrinsic obstruction is usually a result of enlarged adenoids or nasopharyngeal tumors. When the passage is not totally obstructed, contamination of the middle ear can take place by reflux, aspiration, or insufflation during crying, sneezing, nose blowing, and swallowing when the nose is obstructed.

Diagnostic Evaluation

Careful assessment of tympanic membrane mobility with a pneumatic otoscope is essential to differentiate AOM from OM with effusion (OME) (Lieberthal et al., 2013). A diagnosis of AOM is made if visual inspection of the tympanic membrane reveals a purulent discolored effusion and a bulging or full, opacified, or reddened immobile membrane, (Lieberthal et al.). An immobile tympanic membrane or an orange, discolored membrane indicates OME. Clinical symptoms of OM are also helpful in making the diagnosis (Box 40.6). In AOM, symptoms such as acute onset of ear pain, fever, and a bulging yellow or red tympanic membrane are usually present.

Therapeutic Management

Treatment for AOM is one of the most common reasons for antibiotic use in the ambulatory setting. Recently, however, concerns about drug-resistant *S. pneumoniae* and other drug resistances have led infectious disease authorities to recommend careful and judicious use of antibiotics for the treatment of this illness. Current literature indicates that waiting up to 72 hours for spontaneous resolution is safe and appropriate management of AOM without severe signs and symptoms in healthy infants older than 6 months of age (Lieberthal et al., 2013). Furthermore, there is no clear evidence that antibiotics improve outcomes in children younger than 2 years of age with uncomplicated AOM. However, the watchful waiting approach is not recommended for children younger than 2 years of age who have persistent acute symptoms of fever and severe ear pain (Kerschner & Preciado, 2016). In addition, all cases of AOM in infants younger than 6 months of age should be treated with antibiotics because of their immature immune systems and the potential for infection with bacteria.

When antibiotics are warranted, oral amoxicillin in high doses (80 to 90 mg/kg/day divided twice daily) is the treatment of choice for initial episodes of AOM in children who have not received amoxicillin within the past month (Lieberthal et al., 2013). The recommendation for the duration of antibiotic therapy in severe AOM is 10 days. A 5- to 7-day course may be sufficient in children 6 years of age and older with uncomplicated AOM or a moderate or mild infection (American Academy of Pediatrics Committee on Infectious Diseases & Pickering, 2012).

Second-line antibiotics used to treat OM include amoxicillin-clavulanate and cephalosporins (e.g., cefdinir, cefuroxime, and cefpodoxime). IM ceftriaxone is used if the causative organism is a highly resistant pneumococcus or if the parents are noncompliant with the therapy. An important consideration with the use of single-dose IM injections is the pain involved in this therapy. One strategy to minimize pain at the injection site is to reconstitute the cephalosporin with 1% lidocaine. A topical analgesic cream such as EMLA or LMX4 can also be applied to the site beforehand to reduce pain. *Myringotomy,* a surgical incision of the eardrum, may be necessary to alleviate the severe pain of AOM or OME. Myringotomy is also performed to drain infected middle ear fluid in the presence of complications (mastoiditis, labyrinthitis, or facial paralysis) or to allow purulent middle ear fluid to drain into the ear canal for culture. A minimally invasive laser-assisted myringotomy procedure may be performed in outpatient settings. These procedures should be performed only by ear, nose, and throat (ENT) specialists (Yousaf, Malik, & Zada, 2014).

Tympanostomy tube placement and adenoidectomy are surgical procedures that may be done to treat recurrent chronic OM (defined as three bouts in 6 months, six in 12 months, or six by 6 years of age). Tympanostomy tubes are pressure-equalizer tubes or grommets that facilitate continued drainage of fluid and allow ventilation of the middle ear. They are inserted to treat severe eustachian tube dysfunction, OME, or complications of OM (mastoiditis, facial nerve paralysis, brain abscess, labyrinthitis). Adenoidectomy is not recommended for treatment of AOM and is performed only in children with recurrent AOM or chronic OME with postnasal obstruction, adenoiditis, or chronic sinusitis.

In some children, residual middle ear effusions remain after episodes of AOM. Some children have fluid that persists in the middle ear for weeks or months. Antibiotics are not required for initial treatment of OME but may be indicated for children with persistent effusion for more than 3 months (van Zon, van der Heijden, van Dongen, et al., 2012). Placement of tympanostomy tubes is recommended after a total of 4 to 6 months of bilateral effusion with a bilateral hearing deficit (Zakrzewski & Lee, 2013). This therapy allows for mechanical drainage of the fluid, which promotes healing of the membrane and prevents scar formation and loss of elasticity. Myringotomy with or without insertion of pressure-equalizer tubes should not be performed for initial management of OME but may be recommended for children who have recurrent episodes of OME with a long cumulative duration (Zakrzewski & Lee).

OME is frequently associated with mild to moderate impairment of hearing; therefore a hearing test should also be performed if OME persists for 3 months or more or if there is evidence of language or learning delays. Follow-up examinations of children with chronic OME should be maintained on a 3- to 6-month basis until the OME is resolved, a significant hearing loss is identified, or structural defect of the tympanic membrane or middle ear is identified (Rosenfeld, Schwartz, Pynnonen, et al., 2013). Children with hearing loss should be referred to a pediatric otolaryngologist and should receive a speech and language evaluation as necessary.

Prevention

Routine immunization with the pneumococcal conjugate vaccine PCV7 (Prevnar 7) has reduced the incidence of AOM in many infants and children (American Academy of Pediatrics Committee on Infectious Diseases & Pickering, 2012). In February 2010, a 13-valent pneumococcal conjugate vaccine (PCV13) was approved for use in children 6 weeks to 71 months of age to protect against 13 pneumococcal serotypes. The vaccine is administered as a four-dose series beginning at 2 months of age; infants and children who have started the series with Prevnar 7 may complete the series with Prevnar 13 (Centers for Disease Control and Prevention, 2010). The latest AAP clinical guidelines also recommend an annual influenza vaccination as a prevention for AOM (Lieberthal et al., 2013).

Parents are encouraged to reduce risk factors for AOM by breastfeeding infants for at least the first 6 months of life, avoiding propping the formula bottle, and preventing exposure to tobacco smoke (Lieberthal et al., 2013).

Care Management

Nursing objectives for children with AOM include (1) relieving pain, (2) facilitating drainage when possible, (3) preventing complications or recurrence, (4) educating the family in care of the child, and (5) providing emotional support to the child and family.

Analgesic drugs such as acetaminophen (all ages) and ibuprofen (6 months of age and older) are used to treat mild pain.

If the ear is draining, the external canal may be cleaned with sterile cotton swabs or pledgets coupled with topical antibiotic treatment. If ear wicks or lightly rolled sterile gauze packs are placed in the ear after surgical treatment, they should be loose enough to allow accumulated drainage to flow out of the ear; otherwise, infection may be transferred to the mastoid process. The wicks need to stay dry during shampoos or baths. Occasionally, drainage is so profuse that the auricle and the skin surrounding the ear become excoriated from the exudate. This is prevented by frequent cleansing and application of various moisture barriers (e.g., Proshield Plus), zinc oxide–based products, or petrolatum jelly (e.g., Vaseline).

Tympanostomy tubes may allow water to enter the middle ear, but recommendations for earplugs are inconsistent. However, lake and river water are potentially contaminated and wearing earplugs while swimming in a lake or non-chlorinated pool prevents total flooding of the external canal and possible infections (Rosenfeld et al., 2013). Bathwater and shampoo water should be kept out of the ear, if possible, because soap reduces the surface tension of water and facilitates entry through the tube (Rosenfeld et al.). Parents should be aware of the appearance of a grommet (usually a tiny, white, plastic spool-shaped tube) so that they can recognize it if it falls out. They are reassured that this is normal and requires no immediate intervention, although they should notify the practitioner.

Prevention of recurrence requires adequate education regarding antibiotic therapy. The symptoms of pain and fever usually subside within 24 to 48 hours, but nurses must emphasize that all of the prescribed medication should be taken. Parents should be aware that potential complications of OM, such as hearing loss, can be prevented with adequate treatment and follow-up care.

Parents also need anticipatory guidance regarding methods to reduce the risks of OM, especially in children younger than 2 years of age. Reducing the chances of OM is possible with simple measures, such as sitting or holding an infant upright for feedings, maintaining routine childhood immunizations, and exclusively breastfeeding until at least 6 months of age. Propping bottles is discouraged to avoid pooling of milk while the child is in the supine position and to encourage human contact during feeding. Eliminating tobacco smoke and known allergens is also recommended. Early detection of middle ear effusion is essential to prevent complications. Infants and preschool children should be screened for effusion, and all schoolchildren, especially those with learning disabilities, should be tested for hearing deficits related to a middle ear effusion.

INFECTIOUS MONONUCLEOSIS

Infectious mononucleosis is an acute, self-limiting infectious disease that is common among people younger than 25 years of age. Symptoms include fever, exudative pharyngitis, lymphadenopathy, hepatosplenomegaly, and an increase in atypical lymphocytes. The course is usually mild but occasionally can be severe or, rarely, accompanied by serious complications.

Etiology and Pathophysiology

The Epstein-Barr virus (EBV) is the principal cause of infectious mononucleosis. It appears in both sporadic and epidemic forms, but the sporadic cases are more common. The mechanism of spread has not been proven, but it is believed to be transmitted in saliva by direct intimate contact, although it survives in saliva for many hours outside of the body. The incubation period after exposure is approximately 30 to 50 days (American Academy of Pediatrics Committee on Infectious Diseases & Pickering, 2012).

BOX 40.7 Clinical Manifestations of Infectious Mononucleosis

Early Signs
- Headache
- Malaise
- Fatigue
- Chills
- Low-grade fever
- Loss of appetite
- Puffy eyes

Acute Disease
Cardinal Features
- Fever
- Sore throat
- Cervical adenopathy

Common Features
- Splenomegaly (may persist for several months)
- Palatine petechiae
- Macular eruption (especially on trunk)
- Exudative pharyngitis or tonsillitis
- Hepatic involvement to some degree, often associated with jaundice

Diagnostic Tests

The onset of symptoms may be acute or insidious and may appear anywhere from 10 days to 6 weeks after exposure. The presenting symptoms vary greatly in type, severity, and duration (Box 40.7). The clinical manifestations of infectious mononucleosis are usually less severe (often subclinical or unapparent), and the convalescent phase is shorter in younger children than in older children and young adults. Heterophil antibody tests (Paul-Bunnell or Monospot) determine the extent to which the patient's serum will agglutinate sheep red blood cells; the response in these tests is primarily to immunoglobulin M (IgM), which is present in the first 2 weeks of the illness and may last up to 1 year (American Academy of Pediatrics Committee on Infectious Diseases & Pickering, 2012). The spot test (Monospot) is a slide test of venous blood that has high specificity. It is rapid, sensitive, inexpensive, and easy to perform and has the advantage over the Paul-Bunnell test in that it can detect significant agglutinins at lower levels, thus allowing earlier diagnosis. Blood is usually obtained for the test by finger puncture or venous sampling and is placed on special paper. If the blood agglutinates, forming fragments or clumps, the test result is positive for the infection.

Therapeutic Management

No specific treatment exists for infectious mononucleosis. A mild analgesic is often sufficient to relieve the headache, fever, and malaise. Rest is encouraged for fatigue but is not imposed for any specific period. Affected people are instructed to regulate activities according to their own tolerance unless complicating factors are present. Contact sports are discouraged in the presence of splenomegaly.

Antibiotics are contraindicated unless beta-hemolytic streptococci are present (amoxicillin or ampicillin can cause a rash in patients with EBV infection). If sore throat is severe, effective therapies include gargles; warm drinks; anesthetic troches; or analgesics, including opioids. Corticosteroids have been used to treat respiratory distress from significant tonsillar inflammation, myocarditis, hemolytic anemia, thrombocytopenia, and neurologic complications; however, routine use of steroids is not recommended (American Academy of Pediatrics Committee on Infectious Diseases & Pickering, 2012).

Prognosis

The course of this disease is usually self-limiting and uncomplicated. Acute symptoms often disappear within 7 to 10 days, and persistent fatigue subsides within 2 to 4 weeks. Some adolescents may need to restrict their activities for 2 to 3 months, but the disease rarely extends

for longer periods. The adolescent is encouraged to maintain limited exercise to prevent deconditioning.

Care Management

Nursing responsibilities are directed toward providing comfort measures to relieve symptoms. The child is advised to limit exposure to people outside the family, especially during the acute phase of illness. Throat pain may be severe enough to require an analgesic, such as acetaminophen or ibuprofen. Careful nursing assessment of swallowing ability is essential to detect serious airway edema and airway compromise.

! NURSING ALERT

Advise the family to seek medical evaluation of the child or adolescent if the following occurs:
- Breathing becomes difficult.
- Severe abdominal pain develops.
- Sore throat pain is so severe that the child is unable to eat or drink.
- Respiratory stridor is observed.

CROUP SYNDROMES

Croup is a general term applied to a symptom complex characterized by hoarseness, a resonant cough described as "barking" or "brassy" (croupy), varying degrees of inspiratory stridor, and varying degrees of respiratory distress resulting from swelling or obstruction in the region of the larynx. Acute infections of the larynx are important in infants and small children because of their increased incidence in these age groups and because the small diameter of the airway in infants and children places them at risk for significant narrowing with inflammation.

Croup syndromes can affect the larynx, trachea, and bronchi. However, laryngeal involvement often dominates the clinical picture because of the severe effects on the voice and breathing. Croup syndromes are described according to the primary anatomic area affected (i.e., epiglottitis [or supraglottitis], laryngitis, laryngotracheobronchitis [LTB], and tracheitis). In general, LTB occurs in very young children, and epiglottitis is more common in older children. A comparison of croup syndromes is provided in Table 40.1.

With widespread immunization programs aimed at preventing *H. influenzae* type b, the cause of most cases of croup in the United States is attributed to viruses, namely parainfluenza virus, human metapneumovirus, influenza types A and B, adenovirus, and measles.

ACUTE EPIGLOTTITIS

A presumptive diagnosis of acute epiglottitis, or acute supraglottitis, is a medical emergency. It is a serious obstructive inflammatory process that occurs predominantly in children 2 to 5 years of age but can occur from infancy to adulthood. The obstruction is supraglottic as opposed to the subglottic obstruction of laryngitis. The responsible organism is usually *H. influenzae*. LTB and epiglottitis do not occur together.

Clinical Manifestations

The onset of epiglottitis is abrupt, and it can rapidly progress to severe respiratory distress. The child usually goes to bed asymptomatic to awaken later, complaining of sore throat and pain on swallowing. The child has a fever; appears sicker than clinical findings suggest; and insists on sitting upright and leaning forward with the chin thrust out, mouth open, and tongue protruding *(tripod position)*. Drooling of saliva is common because of the difficulty or pain on swallowing and excessive secretions.

TABLE 40.1   Comparison of Croup Syndromes

	Acute Epiglottitis	Acute Laryngotracheobronchitis (Ltb)	Acute Spasmodic Laryngitis	Acute Tracheitis
Age-group affected	2 to 5 years of age, but varies	Infant or child younger than 5 years of age	1 to 3 years of age	1 month to 6 years of age
Etiologic agent	Bacterial	Viral	Viral with allergic component	Viral or bacterial with allergic component
Onset	Rapidly progressive	Slowly progressive	Sudden; at night	Moderately progressive
Major symptoms	Dysphagia	URI	URI	URI
	Stridor aggravated when supine	Stridor	Croupy cough	Croupy cough
	Drooling	Brassy cough	Stridor	Purulent secretions
	High fever	Hoarseness	Hoarseness	High fever
	Toxic appearance	Dyspnea	Dyspnea	No response to LTB therapy
	Rapid pulse and respirations	Restlessness	Restlessness	
		Irritability	Symptoms awakening child but disappearing during day	
		Low-grade fever	Tendency to recur	
		Nontoxic appearance		
Treatment	Airway protection	Humidified oxygen if needed	Cool mist	Antibiotics
	Corticosteroids	Corticosteroids	Reassurance	Fluids
	Fluids	Fluids		
	Antibiotics	Reassurance		
	Reassurance			

LTB, Laryngotracheobronchitis; *URI,* upper respiratory infection.

❗ NURSING ALERT

Three clinical observations that are predictive of epiglottitis are absence of spontaneous cough, presence of drooling, and agitation.

The child is irritable; extremely restless; and has an anxious, apprehensive, and frightened expression. The voice is thick and muffled, with a froglike croaking sound on inspiration, but the child is not hoarse. Suprasternal and substernal retractions may be evident. The child seldom struggles to breathe, and slow, quiet breathing provides better air exchange. The throat is red and inflamed, and a distinctive large, cherry red, edematous epiglottis is visible on careful throat inspection.

❗ NURSING ALERT

Throat inspection should be attempted only by experienced personnel when equipment is available to proceed with immediate intubation or tracheostomy.

Therapeutic Management

The course of epiglottitis may be fulminant, with respiratory obstruction appearing suddenly. Progressive obstruction leads to hypoxia, hypercapnia, and acidosis followed by decreased muscular tone; reduced level of consciousness; and, when obstruction becomes more or less complete, a rather sudden death.

The child who is suspected of having epiglottitis should be examined in a setting where emergency airway equipment is readily available. Examination of the throat with a tongue depressor is contraindicated until experienced personnel and equipment are available to proceed with immediate intubation or tracheostomy in the event that the examination precipitates further or complete obstruction (see Clinical Reasoning Case Study: Croup Syndrome).

Nasotracheal intubation or tracheostomy is usually considered for the child with epiglottitis with severe respiratory distress. It is recommended

CLINICAL REASONING CASE STUDY

Croup Syndrome

Kim, a 5-year-old patient, is admitted to the emergency department in the early evening hours with a sore throat, pain on swallowing, drooling, and a fever of 39°C (102.2°F). She looks ill; her skin is flushed; she is agitated; and she prefers to sit up leaning on her arms. According to Kim's mother, she has not had anything to eat or drink since this morning. What nursing interventions should the nurse implement in this situation?

1. Evidence—Is there sufficient evidence to draw any conclusions about Kim's condition at this time?
2. Assumptions—Describe some underlying assumptions about each of the following:
   a. Epiglottitis in children
   b. Symptoms of epiglottitis
   c. Precautions to be taken when a child has suspected epiglottitis
   d. Immediate nursing interventions when caring for a child with epiglottitis
3. What priorities for nursing care can be drawn at this time?
4. Does the evidence objectively support your argument (conclusion)?

that the intubation or tracheostomy and any invasive procedure, such as starting an intravenous (IV) infusion, be performed in an area where emergency airway maintenance can be easily and quickly accomplished. Humidified oxygen is administered as necessary either via mask in older children or blow-by in younger children to avoid further agitation. Whether or not there is an artificial airway, the child requires intensive observation by experienced personnel. The epiglottal swelling usually decreases after 24 hours of antibiotic therapy (ceftriaxone sodium or alternate cephalosporin), and the epiglottis is near normal by the third day. Intubated children are generally extubated at this time. The use of corticosteroids for reducing edema may be beneficial during the early treatment phase.

Children with suspected bacterial epiglottitis are given antibiotics intravenously followed by oral administration to complete a 7- to 10-day course. Family contacts with children younger than 4 years of age and any contacts younger than 4 years of age are treated with rifampin for 4 days (American Academy of Pediatrics Committee on Infectious Diseases & Pickering, 2012).

Care Management

Epiglottitis is a serious and frightening disease for the child and family. It is important to act quickly but calmly and to provide support without increasing anxiety. The child is allowed to remain in the position that provides the most comfort and security, and the parents are reassured that everything possible is being done to obtain relief for their child.

> **! NURSING ALERT**
>
> When epiglottitis is suspected, the nurse should not attempt to visualize the epiglottis directly with a tongue depressor or take a throat culture but should refer the child for medical evaluation immediately.

Acute care of the child is the same as that described later for the child with LTB. Continuous monitoring of respiratory status, including pulse oximetry (and blood gases if the patient is intubated), is an important part of nursing observations, and the IV infusion is maintained as described in Chapter 39.

ACUTE LARYNGOTRACHEOBRONCHITIS

Acute LTB is the most common croup syndrome. It affects primarily children 6 months to 3 years of age, and the causative organisms are viral agents, particularly the parainfluenza virus types 1, 2 and 3, adenovirus, enterovirus, RSV, rhinovirus, and influenza A and B (Zoorob, Sidani, & Murray, 2011). Bacterial organisms are rarely a causative organism but can include *M. pneumonia* and diphtheria (Zoorob et al). The disease is usually preceded by a URI, which gradually descends to adjacent structures. It is characterized by a gradual onset of low-grade fever, and the parents often report that the child went to bed and later awoke with a barky, brassy cough. Inflammation of the mucosa lining the larynx and trachea causes a narrowing of the airway. When the airway is significantly narrowed, the child struggles to inhale air past the obstruction and into the lungs, producing the characteristic inspiratory stridor and suprasternal retractions. Other classic manifestations include cough and hoarseness. Respiratory distress in infants and toddlers may be manifested by nasal flaring, intercostal retractions, tachypnea, and continuous stridor. The typical child with LTB develops the classic barking or seal-like cough and acute stridor after several days of rhinitis. When the child is unable to inhale a sufficient volume of air, symptoms of hypoxia become evident. Obstruction that is severe enough to prevent adequate ventilation and exhalation of carbon dioxide can cause respiratory acidosis and eventually respiratory failure.

Therapeutic Management

The major objective in medical management is maintaining the airway and providing adequate respiratory exchange. Children with mild croup (no stridor at rest) can be managed at home. Parents are taught the signs of respiratory distress and instructed to obtain professional help early if needed. Children with labored respirations and stridor or other respiratory symptoms should receive medical attention.

The application of humidity with cool mist provides some relief for most children with mild croup. A cool-air vaporizer can be used at home. In the hospital, a nebulized mist for older infants and toddlers may be used to provide increased humidity and supplemental oxygen.

However, controversy surrounds the use of mist therapy to treat croup. The cool temperature therapy modalities assist by constricting edematous blood vessels. A ride in the car with the windows down may help relieve symptoms.

Nebulized epinephrine (racemic epinephrine) is often used in children with severe disease, stridor at rest, retractions, or difficulty breathing. The beta-adrenergic effects cause mucosal vasoconstriction and subsequently decrease subglottic edema. The onset of action is rapid, and the peak effect is observed in 2 hours. Children may be discharged home following racemic epinephrine after a 2- to 3-hour period of observation for return of acute symptoms.

Oral steroids (dexamethasone) have proven effective in the treatment of croup (often as a single dose); IM dexamethasone may be given to children who are unable to tolerate oral dosing. Nebulized budesonide may be administered in conjunction with IM dexamethasone. Antibiotics are only used to treat specific complications of croup.

In severe cases of LTB, the administration of heliox (a mixture of 70% to 80% helium and 20% to 30% oxygen) may be used to reduce the work of breathing and relieve airway obstruction. It reduces airway turbulence but is not recommended as a standard treatment of croup (Moraa, Sturman, McGuire, et al., 2013). On occasion, intubation and ventilation may be required when airway obstruction becomes more severe.

Care Management

The most important nursing function in the care of children with LTB is continuous, vigilant observation and accurate assessment of respiratory status. Cardiac, respiratory, and pulse oximetry monitoring supplement visual observation. Changes in therapy are frequently based on the nurses' observations and assessments, the child's response to therapy, and tolerance of procedures. The trend away from early intubation of children with LTB emphasizes the importance of nursing observations and the ability to recognize impending respiratory failure so that intubation can be implemented without delay.

> **! NURSING ALERT**
>
> Early signs of impending airway obstruction include increased pulse and respiratory rate; substernal, suprasternal, and intercostal retractions; flaring nares; and increased restlessness.

In most acute care facilities, the infant is allowed to be held by the parent. If cool mist is used in the treatment, it can be administered through a tube held in front of the patient while the child is held on the parent's lap. Children need the security of the parent's presence, because crying increases respiratory distress and hypoxia.

The rapid progression of croup, the alarming sound of the cough and stridor, and the child's apprehensive behavior and ill appearance combine to create a frightening experience for the parents and family. The family should be allowed to remain with their child as much as possible. Parents need frequent reassurance provided in a calm, quiet manner and education regarding what they can do to make their child more comfortable. Fortunately, as the crisis subsides and the child responds to therapy, breathing becomes easier and the recovery is generally prompt. Home care includes monitoring for worsening symptoms, continued humidity, adequate hydration, and nourishment.

ACUTE SPASMODIC LARYNGITIS

Acute spasmodic laryngitis (spasmodic croup) is distinct from laryngitis and LTB and is characterized by recurrent paroxysmal attacks of laryngeal obstruction that occur chiefly at night. Signs of inflammation are absent or mild, and it is followed by an uneventful recovery. The child feels well the next day. Some children appear to be predisposed to the condition; allergies or hypersensitivities may be implicated in some cases. Management is the same as for infectious croup.

BACTERIAL TRACHEITIS

Bacterial tracheitis, an infection of the mucosa and soft tissues of the upper trachea, is a distinct entity with features of both croup and epiglottitis. The disease occurs typically at a mean age between 5 and 7 years of age and may cause severe airway obstruction (Roosevelt, 2016). It is believed to be a complication of LTB, and although *Staphylococcus aureus* is the most frequent organism responsible, *M. catarrhalis, S. pneumonia,* and *H. influenzae* have also been implicated.

Many of the manifestations of bacterial tracheitis are similar to those of LTB but are unresponsive to LTB therapy. The child has a history of previous URI with croupy cough, stridor unaffected by position, toxicity, absence of drooling, absence of dysphagia, and high fever. Thick, purulent tracheal secretions are common, and respiratory difficulties are secondary to these copious secretions. The child's white blood cell count will be elevated.

Therapeutic Management and Care Management

Bacterial tracheitis requires vigorous management with oxygen therapy, antipyretics, and antibiotics. Many younger children require endotracheal intubation and mechanical ventilation; patients are closely monitored for impending respiratory failure if not intubated. Early recognition to prevent life-threatening airway obstruction is essential.

INFECTIONS OF THE LOWER AIRWAYS

The reactive portion of the lower respiratory tract includes the bronchi and bronchioles in children. The smooth muscle in these structures represents a major factor in the constriction of the airway, particularly in the bronchioles—the portion that extends from the bronchi to the alveoli. Table 40.2 compares some of the major features of bronchial and bronchiolar infections.

BRONCHITIS

Bronchitis (sometimes referred to as *tracheobronchitis*) is an inflammation of the large airways (trachea and bronchi), which is frequently associated with URIs. Viral agents are the primary cause of the disease, although *M. pneumoniae* is a common cause in children older than 6 years of age. A dry, hacking, nonproductive cough that worsens at night and becomes productive in 2 to 3 days characterizes this condition.

Bronchitis is a mild, self-limiting disease that requires only symptomatic treatment, including analgesics, antipyretics, and humidity. Cough suppressants may be useful to allow rest but can interfere with clearance of secretions. Most patients recover uneventfully in 5 to 10 days. It can be associated with other underlying conditions (such as CF and bronchiectasis) and can become chronic in nature (cough >3 months). Adolescents with bronchitis (>3 months) should be screened for tobacco or marijuana use.

RESPIRATORY SYNCYTIAL VIRUS AND BRONCHIOLITIS

Bronchiolitis is a common, acute viral infection with upper respiratory symptoms and lower respiratory infection of the bronchioles due to inflammation. The infection occurs primarily in winter and early spring. By 3 years of age, most children have been infected at least once. RSV infection is the most frequent cause of hospitalization in children younger than 1 year of age. In addition, severe RSV infections in the first year of life represent a significant risk factor for the development of asthma up to 13 years of age (Knudson & Varga, 2015). RSV infection may also

TABLE 40.2	Comparison of Conditions Affecting the Bronchi		
	Asthma	**Bronchitis**	**Bronchiolitis**
Description	Exaggerated response of bronchi to a trigger such as URI, animal dander, cold air, exercise Bronchospasm, exudation, and edema of bronchi, airway obstruction Inflammatory response	Usually occurs in association with URI Seldom an isolated entity	Most common infectious disease of lower airways Maximum obstructive impact at bronchiolar level
Age-group affected	Infancy to adolescence	First 4 years of life	Usually children 2 to 12 months of age Peak incidence approximately 6 months of age
Etiologic agents	Most often viruses such as RSV in infants, but may be any of a variety of URI pathogens	Usually viral Other agents (e.g., bacteria, fungi, allergic disorders, airborne irritants) can trigger symptoms	Viruses, predominantly RSV; also adenoviruses, parainfluenza viruses, human metapneumovirus, and *Mycoplasma pneumoniae*
Predominant characteristics	Wheezing, cough, labored respirations	Persistent dry, hacking cough (worse at night) becoming productive in 2 to 3 days	Labored respirations, poor feeding, cough, tachypnea, retractions, nasal flaring, emphysema, increased nasal mucus, wheezing, may have fever
Treatment	Inhaled corticosteroids, bronchodilators, leukotriene modifiers, allergen and "triggers" control, long-term antiinflammatory medications	Cough suppressants if needed	Supplemental oxygen if saturations ≤90%; bronchodilators (optional) Suctioning nasopharynx Ensuring adequate fluid intake Maintaining adequate oxygenation

RSV, Respiratory syncytial virus; *URI,* upper respiratory infection.

occur in children older than 1 year of age who have a chronic or serious disabling illness. Although most cases of bronchiolitis are caused by RSV, adenoviruses and parainfluenza viruses are also implicated; human metapneumovirus has also been associated with bronchiolitis in children. It can also rarely be caused by *M. pneumoniae*.

RSV is transmitted from exposure to contaminated secretions. RSV can live on fomites for several hours and on hands for 30 minutes (American Academy of Pediatrics Committee on Infectious Diseases & Pickering, 2012).

Pathophysiology

RSV affects the epithelial cells of the respiratory tract. The ciliated cells swell, protrude into the lumen, and lose their cilia. The walls of the bronchi and bronchioles are infiltrated with inflammatory cells, and varying degrees of intraluminal obstruction lead to hyperinflation, obstructive emphysema resulting from partial obstruction, and patchy areas of atelectasis. Dilation of bronchial passages on inspiration allows sufficient space for intake of air, but narrowing of the passages on expiration prevents air from leaving the lungs. Thus air is trapped distal to the obstruction and causes progressive overinflation (emphysema).

Clinical Manifestations

The illness usually begins with a URI after an incubation of about 5 to 8 days. Symptoms such as rhinorrhea and low-grade fever often appear first. OM and conjunctivitis may also be present. In time, a cough may develop. If the disease progresses, it becomes a lower respiratory tract infection and manifests typical symptoms (Box 40.8). Infants may have several days of URI symptoms or no symptoms except slight lethargy, poor feeding, or irritability. Children who are infected with RSV are usually contagious for 3 to 8 days, but some infants and patients with weakened immune systems can be contagious for as long as 4 weeks (Centers for Disease Control and Prevention, 2014).

When the lower airway is involved, classic manifestations include signs of altered air exchange, such as wheezing, retractions, crackles, dyspnea, tachypnea, and diminished breath sounds. Apnea may be the first recognized indicator of RSV infection in very young infants (younger than 1 month of age).

Diagnostic Evaluation

Identification has been simplified by the development of tests done on nasopharyngeal secretions, using either a rapid immunofluorescent antibody–direct fluorescent antibody (DFA) staining or an enzyme-linked immunosorbent assay (ELISA) for RSV antigen detection (see the "Respiratory Secretion Specimens" section in Chapter 39). Hyperinflation of the lungs is generally seen on the chest radiograph.

BOX 40.8   Signs and Symptoms of Respiratory Syncytial Virus

Initial
- Rhinorrhea
- Pharyngitis
- Coughing/sneezing
- Wheezing
- Possible ear or eye drainage
- Intermittent fever

With Progression of Illness
- Increased coughing and wheezing
- Tachypnea and retractions
- Cyanosis

Severe Illness
- Tachypnea, >70 breaths/min
- Listlessness
- Apneic spells
- Poor air exchange; decreased breath sounds

Therapeutic Management

Children with bronchiolitis are treated at home if they are maintaining hydration, do not have respiratory distress, and do not need oxygen therapy. Hospitalization is recommended for children with respiratory distress and those who cannot maintain adequate hydration. Other reasons for hospitalization include complicating conditions, such as underlying lung or heart disease or associated debilitated states, or a home environment where adequate management is questionable. An infant who is tachypneic or apneic, has marked retractions, appears listless, has a history of poor fluid intake, or is dehydrated should be closely observed for respiratory failure.

Humidified oxygen is administered in concentrations sufficient to maintain adequate oxygenation (Spo_2) at or above 90% as measured by pulse oximetry. Routine chest percussion and postural drainage (formerly chest physiotherapy [CPT]) are not recommended for children who have bronchiolitis. Infants with abundant nasal secretions benefit from regular suctioning, especially for feeding.

Fluids by mouth may be contraindicated because of tachypnea, weakness, and fatigue; therefore IV fluids may be used until the acute stage of the disease has passed. Nasogastric fluids may be required if the infant is unable to tolerate oral fluids and a peripheral IV is difficult to establish.

Clinical assessments, noninvasive oxygen monitoring, and blood gas values may guide therapy. Medical therapy for bronchiolitis is primarily supportive and aimed at decreasing airway hyperresonance and inflammation and promoting adequate fluid intake. Racemic epinephrine has been shown to produce modest improvement in ventilation status. The use of systemic corticosteroids is controversial but may be used in some centers. A recent Cochrane Review found no evidence to support the use of antibiotics for bronchiolitis; therefore, antibiotics should not be part of the treatment of bronchiolitis unless there is a coexisting bacterial infection, such as OM or pneumonia (Farley, Spurling, Eriksson, et al., 2014). Additional recommendations from the American Academy of Pediatrics clinical practice guideline are to encourage breastfeeding, avoid passive tobacco smoke exposure, and promote preventive measures, including hand washing and the administration of palivizumab (Synagis) to high-risk infants (Ralston, Lieberthal, Meissner, et al., 2014). The American Academy of Pediatrics no longer recommends a trial dose of a bronchodilator to be used for patient with bronchiolitis (Ralston et al.). They also specify that testing for specific viruses is unnecessary because bronchiolitis may be caused by multiple viruses, although some institutions continue to test to detect RSV.

Ribavirin, an antiviral agent (synthetic nucleoside analog), is the only specific therapy approved for hospitalized children. Due to potential toxic effects of the medication to exposed health care staff and conflicting results of efficacy, the American Academy of Pediatrics recommends against routine use of ribavirin to treat RSV. Based on current literature, ribavirin should be reserved for treatment in patients at high risk for mortality related to the infection, such as infants and transplant recipients (Turner, Kopp, Paul, et al., 2014).

Prevention of Respiratory Syncytial Virus Infection

The only product available in the United States for prevention of RSV infection is palivizumab (Synagis), a monoclonal antibody, which is given monthly in an IM injection to prevent hospitalization associated with RSV. According to the American Academy of Pediatrics (2014), candidates for palivizumab include infants in their first year of life born before 29 weeks of gestation and infants in their first year of life with chronic lung disease of prematurity (<32 weeks, 0 days of gestation) who needed less than 21% oxygen for at least 28 days after birth.

Additional age and condition recommendations are outlined in the American Academy of Pediatrics policy statement (American Academy of Pediatrics Committee on Infectious Diseases & American Academy of Pediatrics Bronchiolitis Guidelines Committee, 2014).

> ### ! NURSING ALERT
>
> The lyophilized powder form of palivizumab should be administered within 6 hours of being reconstituted with sterile water because it is preservative free.

Care Management

Children admitted to the hospital with suspected RSV infection are usually assigned separate rooms or grouped with other RSV-infected children. Droplet and Standard Precautions are used, including hand washing, not touching the nasal mucosa or conjunctiva, and using gloves and gowns when entering the patient's room; Contact Precautions are also recommended. Other isolation procedures of potential benefit are those aimed at limiting the number of hospital personnel, visitors, and uninfected children in contact with the child. Another measure is to make patient assignments so that nurses assigned to children with RSV infection are not caring for other patients who are considered high risk.

Infants with RSV infection often have copious nasal secretions, making breathing and breastfeeding or bottle feeding difficult. This engenders concerns that the child will lose weight or stop breastfeeding altogether. Breastfeeding mothers are encouraged to continue feeding the infant or, if feedings are contraindicated because of the acuity of the illness, mothers should pump their milk and store it appropriately for later use (see Chapter 24). Parents are taught how to instill normal saline drops into the nares and suction the mucus before feedings and before bedtime so the child may eat and rest better. A bulb syringe can be used for suctioning in the home setting.

To address the issue of decreased fluid intake, parents may offer small amounts of fluids frequently to maintain adequate hydration. Infants may cough or vomit as the secretions settle in the stomach and make them prone to emesis of such secretions.

Additional nursing care is aimed at monitoring oxygenation with pulse oximetry, ensuring any bronchodilator therapy is optimized by using a small mask for delivery, monitoring IV fluids and nasogastric (NG) fluids, and providing information for the parent and family regarding the infant's status. For the most part, infants recover quickly from the disease and resume normal daily activities, including fluid intake. Such infants are at risk for further episodes of wheezing that may or may not involve another RSV infection; parents, however, may be concerned that the infant has another serious case of RSV infection. More severe cases of RSV require the administration of positive airway pressure via a mask or ventilation.

PNEUMONIAS

Pneumonia, inflammation of the pulmonary parenchyma, is common in childhood but occurs more frequently in early childhood. Clinically, pneumonia may occur either as a primary disease or as a complication of another illness. The causative agent is either inhaled into the lungs directly or comes from the bloodstream.

The most useful classification of pneumonia is based on the etiologic agent (e.g., viral, bacterial, mycoplasmal, or aspiration of foreign substances) (see the "Aspiration Pneumonia" section later in this chapter). Many organisms can cause pneumonia, and these vary according to the child's age (Ho, 2013):

- **Neonates**—Group B streptococci, gram-negative enteric bacteria, cytomegalovirus, *S. aureus*, *S. pyogenes*, *Listeria monocytogenes*, *C. trachomatis*

> ### BOX 40.9   General Signs of Pneumonia
>
> Fever: Usually high (≥39.5° C [103° F])
> Respiratory:
> - Cough: Nonproductive to productive with whitish sputum
> - Tachypnea
> - Breath sounds: Crackles, decreased breath sounds
> - Dullness with percussion
> - Chest pain
> - Retractions
> - Nasal flaring
> - Pallor to cyanosis (depends on severity)
>
> Chest x-ray: Diffuse or patchy infiltration with peribronchial distribution
> Behavior: Irritability, restlessness, malaise, lethargy
> Gastrointestinal: Anorexia, vomiting, diarrhea, abdominal pain

- **Infants**—RSV and other respiratory viruses, *S. pneumoniae*, *S. aureus*, *H. influenzae*, *M. pneumoniae*, *Mycobacterium tuberculosis*
- **Preschool-age children**—RSV and other respiratory viruses, *S. pneumoniae*, *H. influenzae*, *M. pneumoniae*, *M. tuberculosis*
- **School-age children**—*S. pneumoniae*, *M. pneumoniae*, *Chlamydophila pneumoniae*, *M. tuberculosis*, influenza and other respiratory viruses

Histomycosis, coccidioidomycosis, and other fungi also cause pneumonia. *Pneumonitis* is a localized acute inflammation of the lung without the toxemia associated with lobar pneumonia.

The clinical manifestations of pneumonia vary depending on the etiologic agent, the child's age, the child's systemic reaction to the infection, the extent of the lesions, and the degree of bronchial and bronchiolar obstruction. The causative agent is identified from the clinical history, the child's age, the general health history, the physical examination, radiography, and the laboratory examination.

Viral Pneumonia

Viral pneumonias, which occur more frequently than bacterial pneumonias, are seen in children of all ages and are often associated with viral URIs. Viruses that cause pneumonia include RSV in infants and parainfluenza, influenza, human metapneumovirus, enterovirus, and adenovirus in older children. Differentiation among viruses is usually made by clinical features such as the child's age, medical history, season of the year, and radiographic and laboratory examination (Box 40.9).

Viral infections of the respiratory tract render the affected child more susceptible to secondary bacterial infection, especially when there is denuded bronchial mucosa. Treatment is symptomatic and includes measures to promote oxygenation and comfort, such as oxygen administration with cool mist, postural drainage, antipyretics for fever management, monitoring fluid intake, and family support. Antimicrobial therapy is usually reserved for children in whom a bacterial infection is demonstrated by appropriate cultures.

Primary Atypical Pneumonia

Atypical pneumonia refers to pneumonia that is caused by pathogens other than the traditionally most common and readily cultured bacteria (e.g., *S. pneumoniae*). In the category of atypical pneumonias, *M. pneumoniae* is the most common cause of community-acquired pneumonia in children 5 to 15 years of age (Cardinale, Cappiello, Mastrototaro, et al., 2013). It occurs primarily in the fall and winter months and is more prevalent in crowded living conditions. Most affected people recover from acute illness at home in 7 to 10 days with symptomatic treatment followed by 1 week of convalescence. The incubation period is 2 to 3 weeks, but the cough may last several weeks.

Chlamydial pneumonia, caused by *C. trachomatis,* can occur in infants and generally appears between 1 and 3 months of age (Workowski, Bolan, & Centers for Disease Control and Prevention, 2015). The infant contracts this from the infected genital tract of the mother at birth. Chlamydial pneumonia is characterized by a persistent cough, tachypnea, and sometimes rales. Oral erythromycin or ethylsuccinate is the treatment of choice; alternatively, azithromycin can be given (Workowski, et al.).

Bacterial Pneumonia

S. pneumoniae is the most common bacterial pathogen responsible for community-acquired pneumonia in both children and adults (Cardinale et al., 2013). Other bacteria that cause pneumonia in children are pneumococcus, group A streptococcus, *S. aureus, M. catarrhalis, M. pneumonia,* and *C. pneumoniae.*

Beyond the neonatal period, bacterial pneumonias display distinct clinical patterns that facilitate their differentiation from other forms of pneumonia. The onset of illness is abrupt and generally follows a viral infection that disturbs the natural defense mechanisms of the upper respiratory tract.

The child with bacterial pneumonia usually appears ill. Symptoms include fever, malaise, rapid and shallow respirations, cough, and chest pain. The associated cough may persist for several weeks or months. The pain of pneumonia may be referred to the abdomen in young children. Chills and meningeal symptoms (meningism) without meningitis are common.

Most older children with pneumonia can be treated at home if the condition is recognized and treatment is initiated early. Antibiotic therapy, rest, liberal oral intake of fluid, and administration of an antipyretic for fever are the principal therapeutic measures. Chest percussion and postural drainage may be indicated; however, there is a lack of evidence to show that they have benefit to children with pneumonia.

Follow-up examination is recommended for small infants and toddlers. Hospitalization is indicated when pleural effusion or empyema accompanies the disease, when moderate or severe respiratory distress or deoxygenation occurs, in situations in which compliance with therapy is estimated to be poor, in infants younger than 6 months of age, and when there are chronic illnesses such as congenital heart disease or BPD (Barson, 2014). IV fluids may be necessary to ensure adequate hydration, and oxygen is required if the child is in respiratory distress; some children may require initial therapy with parenteral antibiotics because of the severity of illness.

Complications

At present, the classic features and clinical course of pneumonia are seen infrequently because of early and vigorous antibiotic and supportive therapy. However, some children, especially infants, with staphylococcal pneumonia develop empyema, pyopneumothorax, or tension pneumothorax. AOM and pleural effusion are common in children with pneumococcal pneumonia (Box 40.10) (see Evidence-Based Practice box: Nursing Interventions for Prevention of Ventilator-Associated Pneumonia in Children).

Continuous closed chest drainage may be instituted when purulent fluid is aspirated. If a large amount of purulent drainage is obtained, an appropriate antibiotic may be instilled into the chest cavity, and chest drainage is discontinued for approximately 1 hour after the instillation. Closed drainage via a chest tube is continued until drainage fluid is minimal, which rarely requires more than 5 to 7 days. Sometimes repeated pleural taps are sufficient to remove fluid; however, if the purulent drainage accumulates rapidly and is highly viscous, continuous drainage is preferred. Rarely thoracotomy with open debridement of the infected lung tissue may be required. If empyema and pneumothorax

---

BOX 40.10 Pneumothorax

Pneumothorax occurs when there is an accumulation of air in the pleural space; this air increases intrapleural pressure, making it more difficult to expand the affected lung. This leads to the clinical manifestations of dyspnea, chest pain and often back pain, labored respirations, tachycardia, and decreased oxygen saturation. In neonates and infants on mechanical ventilation, the first clinical signs of pneumothorax are oxygen desaturation and hypotension. The three major types of pneumothorax are tension, spontaneous, and traumatic. The definitive diagnosis of pneumothorax is a chest radiograph. The emergent treatment involves needle aspiration of the air within the pleural space; subsequently a chest tube to closed drainage is usually inserted to prevent the reaccumulation of air. *Pleural effusion* occurs when there is an excessive accumulation of fluid in the pleural space. The diagnosis is made by chest radiography, and the treatment involves evacuation of the fluid by needle aspiration followed by insertion of a chest tube to closed drainage.

---

tend to recur, a partial thoracoscopic lobectomy may be performed. Alternatively, video-assisted thoracoscopy (VATS) and intrapleural fibrinolytic therapy may preclude the use of open debridement and thoracotomy (Winnie & Lossef, 2016).

Interprofessional Care Management

Care of the child with pneumonia is primarily supportive and symptomatic but necessitates thorough respiratory assessment and administration of fluids and antibiotics. The respiratory therapist is involved in the child's care if supplemental oxygen is needed. For some children, a pulmonologist may be consulted. The child's respiratory rate, rhythm, and depth, oxygenation, general disposition, and level of activity are frequently assessed. To prevent dehydration, fluids are frequently administered intravenously during the acute phase. If the child is ill, solid foods may be rejected; fluid intake is encouraged until the child feels well enough to eat solids. Dieticians can perform a nutritional assessment and provide nutritional interventions if indicated.

Nursing care of the child with a chest tube requires close attention to respiratory status, as noted previously; the chest tube and drainage device used are monitored for proper function (i.e., drainage is not impeded, vacuum setting is correct, tubing is free of kinks, dressing covering chest tube insertion site is intact, water seal is maintained [if used], and chest tube remains in place). Movement in bed and ambulation with a chest tube are encouraged according to the child's respiratory status, but children require frequent doses of an analgesic. Supplemental oxygen may be required in the acute phase of the illness and may be administered by nasal cannula, face mask, or flow-by. Children are usually more comfortable in a semi-erect position (Fig. 40.3) but should be allowed to determine the position of comfort. Lying on the affected side if the pneumonia is unilateral ("good lung up") splints the chest on that side and reduces the pleural rubbing that often causes discomfort. Fever is controlled by the cool environment and administration of antipyretic drugs. Children, especially infants, with ineffectual cough or difficulty handling secretions may require suctioning to maintain a patent airway. A simple bulb suction syringe is usually sufficient for clearing the nares and nasopharynx of infants, but mechanical suction should be readily available if needed. A noninvasive suction device (nasal aspirator) may be used to suction the infant's nares without the danger of causing nasal trauma; the device may be connected to mechanical suction for best results. Older children can usually handle secretions without assistance. Chest percussion, postural drainage, and nebulized bronchodilator treatments may be prescribed depending on the child's condition. Chest percussion and postural drainage currently lack

EVIDENCE-BASED PRACTICE

Nursing Interventions for Prevention of Ventilator-Associated Pneumonia in Children

Ask the Question
PICOT Question: What nursing interventions prevent VAP in children?

Search for the Evidence
Search Strategies
Search selection included English publications on nursing interventions for prevention of VAP in children and adolescents.

Databases Used
PubMed, AHRQ

Critical Appraisal of the Evidence
- Implementation of VAP bundle resulted in a decreased VAP rate from 5.6 infections per 1000 ventilator days at baseline to 0.3 per 1000 ventilator days (Bigham, Amato, Bondurrant, et al, 2009).
- Common VAP prevention interventions include the following (Bigham et al, 2009; Garland, 2010; Morrow, Argent, Jeena, et al., 2009; Norris, Barnes, & Roberts, 2009):
  - Change ventilator circuits and in-line suction catheters only when soiled.
  - Every 2 to 4 hours, drain condensate from ventilator circuit (use heated wire circuits to reduce rainout).
  - Rinse oral suction devices after use, and store in a nonsealed plastic bag at the bedside.
  - Perform hand hygiene before and after contact with ventilator circuit.
  - Wear PPE before providing care to patients when soiling from respiratory secretions is anticipated.
  - Follow unit mouth care policy every 2 to 4 hours.
  - Unless contraindicated, elevate head of bed to 30 to 45 degrees.
  - Before repositioning patient, always drain ventilator circuit.
  - For patients older than 12 years of age, when possible, use ET tube with dorsal lumen above ET tube cuff to help suction secretions above the cuff.
  - Evaluate daily for possible extubation.
  - Avoid reintubation.
- Infants in supine position (infant lying on back with ET tube held upright in the vertical position) had increased colony counts or new organisms in tracheal aspirate compared to infants in the lateral position (infant lying on side with ET tube at same level as trachea) (Aly, Badawy, El-Kholy, et al., 2008).
- Staff education on VAP and improvements to practice changes can have a substantial impact on reducing VAP (Garland, 2010; Richardson, Hines, Dixon, et al., 2010; Turton, 2008).
- A 7-day versus 3-day ventilator circuit change was not associated with increased VAP rates (Samransamruajkit, Jirapaiboonsuk, Siritantiwat, et al, 2010).
- Use of low-sodium solution for airway care was associated with a decrease in VAP as well as chronic lung disease (Christensen, Henry, Baer, et al, 2010).

- In bronchoalveolar lavage fluid, PAI-1 levels can aid in early diagnosis of VAP (Srinivasan, Song, Wiener-Kronish, et al., 2011).
- Reduced mortality rates were observed in patients with VAP when a silver-coated ET tube was used versus an uncoated ET tube (Afessa, Shorr, Anzueto, et al, 2010).

Apply the Evidence: Nursing Implications
There is moderate evidence with strong recommendations (Guyatt, Oxman, Vist, et al, 2008) for use of interventions to prevent VAP in children. Some of the prevention methods included in VAP bundles are hand hygiene, oral hygiene, use of PPE, and elevation of head of bed 30 to 45 degrees. Staff education and engagement in VAP prevention initiatives are important.

References
Afessa, B., Shorr, A. F., Anzueto, A. R., et al. (2010). Association between a silver-coated endotracheal tube and reduced mortality in patients with ventilator-associated pneumonia. *Chest, 137*(5), 1015–1021.

Aly, H., Badawy, M., El-Kholy, A., et al. (2008). Randomized, controlled trial on tracheal colonization of ventilated infants: can gravity prevent ventilator-associated pneumonia? *Pediatrics, 122*, 770–774.

Bigham, M. T., Amato, R., Bondurrant, P., et al. (2009). Ventilator-associated pneumonia in the pediatric intensive care unit: Characterizing the problem and implementing a sustainable solution. *Journal of Pediatrics, 154*, 582–587.

Christensen, R. D., Henry, E., Baer, V. L., et al. (2010). A low-sodium solution for airway care: results of a multicenter trial. *Respiratory Care, 55*(12), 1680–1685.

Garland, J. S. (2010). Strategies to prevent ventilator-associated pneumonia in neonates. *Clinics in Perinatology, 37*, 629–643.

Guyatt, G. H., Oxman, A. D., Vist, G. E., et al. (2008). GRADE: An emerging consensus on rating quality of evidence and strength of recommendations. *British Medical Journal, 336*, 924–926.

Morrow, B. M., Argent, A. C., Jeena, P. M., et al. (2009). Guideline for the diagnosis, prevention and treatment of paediatric ventilator-associated pneumonia. *South African Medical Journal, 99*(4), 255–267.

Norris, S. C., Barnes, A. K., & Roberts, T. D. (2009). When ventilator-associated pneumonias haunt your NICU: One unit's story. *Neonatal Network, 28*(1), 59–66.

Richardson, M., Hines, S., Dixon, G., et al. (2010). Establishing nurse-led ventilator-associated pneumonia surveillance in paediatric intensive care. *Journal of Hospital Infection, 75*(3), 220–224.

Samransamruajkit, R., Jirapaiboonsuk, S., Siritantiwat, S., et al. (2010). Effect of frequency of ventilator circuit changes (3 vs 7 days) on the rate of ventilator-associated pneumonia in PICU. *Journal of Critical Care, 25*(1), 56–61.

Srinivasan, R., Song, Y., Wiener-Kronish, J., et al. (2011). Plasminogen activation inhibitor concentrations in bronchoalveolar lavage fluid distinguishes ventilator-associated pneumonia from colonization in mechanically ventilated pediatric patients. *Pediatric Critical Care Medicine, 12*(1), 21–27.

Turton, P. (2008). Ventilator-associated pneumonia in paediatric intensive care: A literature review. *Nursing in Critical Care, 13*(5), 241–248.

ET, Endotracheal; *PAI,* plasminogen activator inhibitor; *PPE,* personal protective equipment; *VAP,* ventilator-associated pneumonia.

empirical support for improving the child's condition or decreasing the length of stay in children with community-acquired pneumonia. For the child being cared for at home, the nurse educates the parent regarding observation for worsening symptoms, antibiotic and antipyretic administration, and encouragement of oral fluid intake. Return to school or day care is usually permitted according to the type of pneumonia, severity of illness, and health care provider recommendation. It should be emphasized that the infection may be transmitted to other children with close contact.

OTHER RESPIRATORY TRACT INFECTIONS

PERTUSSIS (WHOOPING COUGH)

Pertussis, or whooping cough, is an acute respiratory tract infection caused by *B. pertussis,* which in the past occurred primarily in children younger than 4 years of age who were not immunized. It is highly contagious and is particularly threatening in young infants, who have a higher morbidity and mortality rate. Complications in adolescents

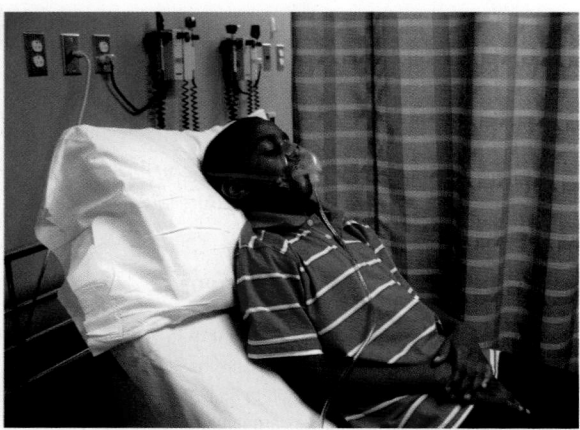

FIG 40.3 Child placed in semi-erect position is often more comfortable, and this position enhances diaphragmatic expansion.

commonly include syncope, rib fractures, insomnia, and weight loss, whereas in younger children, seizures, pneumonia, and conjunctival bleeding can occur (Kilgore, Salim, Zervos, et al., 2016). Infants younger than 6 months of age may not come to the health care provider with the typical cough; in this age-group, apnea is a common presenting manifestation (American Academy of Pediatrics Committee on Infectious Diseases & Pickering, 2012). Likewise, older children are known to manifest the disease with a persistent cough and the absence of the characteristic whoop (see Table 33.3 for signs, symptoms, and management of pertussis). The incidence is highest in the spring and summer months, and a single attack confers lifetime immunity.

The resurgence of pertussis in the United States, particularly among children 10 years of age and older, has prompted concerns of the long-term effects of the pertussis vaccine. Consequently, two acellular pertussis booster vaccines have been approved for children: tetanus, diphtheria, acellular pertussis vaccine (Boostrix) for people 10 to 64 years of age and Adacel for those 10 to 64 years of age (see the "Immunizations" section in Chapter 31).

Most children with pertussis can be managed at home; care is supportive in nature, including encouraging adequate hydration and administering antipyretics. When coughing spasms occur in small children, they can be frightening for the parent and family. Admission to the hospital occurs if respiratory symptoms are severe or if apnea occurs. Diagnosis is obtained via culture or *B. pertussis* polymerase chain reaction (PCR) test on specimens obtained with a nasopharyngeal swab. Treatment with antibiotics (erythromycin, clarithromycin, or azithromycin) in the catarrhal stage may result in a milder form of the infection, but treatment also prevents spread to others (Kilgore et al., 2016). Patients are considered infectious until at least 5 days of antibiotics have been completed or for 3 weeks if no antibiotics have been administered. Family and other contacts, such as children in child care or school, may also be treated. Symptoms can develop up to 3 weeks after exposure to pertussis. Inpatients must be placed on droplet precautions. Symptoms usually last for 6 to 10 weeks but may persist for longer.

TUBERCULOSIS

Tuberculosis (TB) along with human immunodeficiency virus is the leading cause of death from a single infectious disease (World Health Organization, 2016). Nine million people worldwide are infected with TB (Longo, Horsburgh, Barry, et al., 2015). Case rates of TB for all ages are higher in urban, low-income areas and among nonwhite racial and ethnic groups (Hartman-Adams, Clark, & Juckett, 2014). The following groups have the greatest rates of latent TB infection: recent immigrants, health care professionals, refugees from or travelers to high-prevalence regions (Asia, Africa, Eastern Europe, Central America, and South America), homeless individuals, and people living or working in institutional settings (Hartman-Adams et al). Children with human immunodeficiency virus (HIV) infection have an increased incidence of TB disease, and all children with TB disease should be tested for HIV (Marais, 2014).

TB is caused by *M. tuberculosis*, an acid-fast bacillus. Children are susceptible to the human *(M. tuberculosis)* and the bovine *(Mycobacterium bovis)* organisms. In parts of the world where TB in cattle is not controlled or milk is not pasteurized, the bovine type is a common source of infection.

The source of TB infection in children is usually an infected member of the household or a frequent visitor to the home, such as a babysitter or domestic worker. The airway is the usual portal of entry for the organism. In the lungs, a proliferation of epithelial cells surrounds and encapsulates the multiplying bacilli in an attempt to wall it off, thus forming the typical tubercle. Extension of the primary lesion at the original site causes progressive tissue destruction as it spreads within the lung, discharges material from foci to other areas of the lungs (e.g., bronchi, pleura), or produces pneumonia. Erosion of blood vessels by the primary lesion can cause widespread dissemination of the tubercle bacillus to near and distant sites (miliary TB). Extrapulmonary (miliary) TB may be manifested as malaise, fever, weight loss, superior lymphadenitis, meningitis, hepatomegaly, splenomegaly, and osteoarthritis (American Academy of Pediatrics Committee on Infectious Diseases & Pickering, 2012). With the exception of meningitis, the treatment for extrapulmonary TB may be the same drug regimen as for pulmonary TB. Infants and children younger than 3 years of age are more likely to develop miliary TB.

Diagnostic Evaluation

Diagnosis of TB is based on information derived from physical examination, history, tuberculin skin testing, radiographic examinations, and cultures of the organism. The clinical manifestations of the disease are extremely variable (Box 40.11).

The tuberculin skin test (TST) is the most important indicator of whether a child has been infected with the tubercle bacillus. Universal testing of all children for TB is no longer recommended. A targeted testing method is employed wherein only children and adolescents at high risk for contracting the disease, in addition to patients at risk for progression to TB disease, are screened. A risk factor questionnaire

(Box 40.12) has been developed to facilitate screening pediatric populations at high risk.

Skin tests must be carried out correctly to obtain accurate results. The standard dose of purified protein derivative (PPD) is 5 units, which is administered using a 27-gauge needle and a 1-mL syringe intradermally into the volar aspect of the forearm. Creation of a visible wheal is crucial to accurate testing. If the wheal is not formed, the procedure is repeated. The reaction to the skin test is determined in 48 to 72 hours by a health care professional. The size of the transverse diameter of induration, not the erythema, is measured. Administration of the TST and interpretation of the results must be performed and read only by specially educated health care professionals (Hartman-Adams et al., 2014).

A positive reaction indicates that the individual has been infected and has developed sensitivity to the protein of the tubercle bacillus. It does not, however, confirm the presence of active disease. Once an individual reacts positively, he or she will always react positively. Prompt radiographic evaluation of all children with a positive TST reaction is recommended.

The term *latent tuberculosis infection (LTBI)* is used to indicate infection in a person who has a positive TST, no physical findings of disease, and normal chest radiograph findings. The majority of children are asymptomatic when a positive skin test result is found, and most of them do not go on to develop the disease.

The term *TB disease* or *clinically active TB* is used when a child has clinical symptoms or radiographic manifestations caused by the *M. tuberculosis* organism. A diagnosis of TB disease represents recent transmission of the *M. tuberculosis* organism and is an urgent event for public health. Prompt evaluation, treatment, and identification and treatment of contacts are key components to managing TB.

Therapeutic Management

Medical management of TB disease in children consists of adequate nutrition, pharmacotherapy, prevention of unnecessary exposure to other infections that further compromise the body's defenses, prevention of reinfection, and sometimes surgical procedures. Family members and other contacts should also be assessed for symptoms by public health practitioners and treated accordingly.

Isoniazid (INH), pyrazinamide (PZA), and rifampin are common medications used to treat TB in children; ethambutol is added if drug resistance is speculated and can be discontinued when susceptibility to the initial three drugs have been confirmed (Longo et al., 2015). They are prescribed daily or twice weekly with direct observation of therapy (DOT) if daily treatment is not possible. *DOT* means that a health care worker or other responsible, mutually agreed-on individual is present when medications are administered to the patient. The duration of treatment depends on the medication, presence of disease versus LTBI, whether or not multidrug-resistant TB is present, and the patient's immune status.

For the child with clinically active TB disease, the goal is to achieve sterilization of the tuberculous lesion. Recommended drug therapy for treating TB disease includes combinations of INH, rifampin, and PZA. The AAP recommends a 6-month regimen consisting of INH, rifampin, and PZA given daily for the first 2 months followed by INH and rifampin given 2 or 3 times per week by DOT for the remaining 4 months (American Academy of Pediatrics Committee on Infectious Diseases & Pickering, 2012). DOT decreases the rates of relapse, treatment failures, and drug resistance and is recommended for treatment of children and adolescents with TB in the United States. Optimal therapy for TB in children with HIV infection has not been established, and consultation with a specialist is advised.

Surgical procedures may be required to remove the source of infection in tissues that are inaccessible to pharmacotherapy or that are destroyed by the disease. Orthopedic procedures may be performed for correction of bone deformities, and bronchoscopy may be done for removal of a tuberculous granulomatous polyp.

Prognosis

Most children recover from primary TB infection and are often unaware of its presence. However, very young children have a higher incidence of disseminated disease. TB is a serious disease during the first 2 years of life, during adolescence, and in children who are HIV positive. Except in cases of tuberculous meningitis, death seldom occurs in treated children. Antibiotic therapy has decreased the death rate and the hematogenous spread from primary lesions.

Prevention

The only definite means to prevent TB is to avoid contact with the tubercle bacillus. Maintaining an optimal state of health with adequate nutrition and avoiding fatigue and debilitating infections promote natural resistance but do not prevent infection. Pasteurization and routine testing of milk and elimination of diseased cattle have reduced the incidence of bovine TB.

Limited immunity can be produced by administration of bacille Calmette-Guérin (BCG), a live vaccine containing bovine bacilli with reduced virulence (attenuated). In most instances, positive tuberculin reactions develop after inoculation with BCG. The distribution of BCG is controlled by local or state health departments, and the vaccine is not used extensively, even in areas with a high prevalence of disease. BCG vaccination is not generally recommended for use in the United States. However, it may be recommended for long-term protection of infants and children with negative TST results who are not infected with HIV and who (1) are at high risk for continuing exposure to people with infectious pulmonary TB or (2) are continuously exposed to people with TB who have bacilli resistance to both INH and rifampin (American Academy of Pediatrics Committee on Infectious Diseases & Pickering, 2012).

Care Management

Children with TB receive their care in ambulatory settings, outpatient departments, schools, and public health settings. Most children are not contagious and require only standard precautions. Children with no cough and negative sputum smears can be hospitalized in a regular patient room. However, Airborne Precautions and a negative-pressure room are required for children who are contagious and hospitalized with active TB disease. Infection control for hospital personnel in contagious cases should include the use of a personally fitted air-purifying

N95 or N100 respirator (powered air-purifying respirator [PAPR]) for all patient contacts.

Asymptomatic children with TB can attend school or day care facilities if they are receiving pharmacotherapy. They can return to regular activities as soon as effective therapy has been instituted, adherence to therapy has been documented, and clinical symptoms have diminished. Children receiving pharmacotherapy for TB can receive measles and other age-appropriate live virus vaccines unless they are receiving high-dose corticosteroids, are severely ill, or have specific contraindications to immunization.

Because the success of therapy depends on compliance with the drug regimen, parents are instructed about the importance and rationale for DOT. Case finding in the community and follow-up of known contacts—individuals from whom the affected child may have acquired the disease and people who may have been exposed to the child with the disease—are essential control measures.

PULMONARY DYSFUNCTION CAUSED BY NONINFECTIOUS IRRITANTS

FOREIGN BODY ASPIRATION

Small children characteristically explore matter with their mouth and are prone to aspirate foreign bodies (FBs). Small children also place objects such as beads, paper clips, small magnets, or food items in the nose, which can easily be aspirated into the trachea. FB aspiration can occur at any age but is most common in children 1 to 3 years of age. Severity is determined by the location, type of object aspirated, and extent of obstruction. For example, dry vegetable matter (e.g., a seed, nut, or piece of carrot or popcorn) that does not dissolve and that may swell when wet creates a particularly difficult problem. The high fat content of potato chips and peanuts may cause the added risk for lipoid pneumonia. "Fun foods" are the worst offenders in terms of potential for choking. Offending foods in the order of frequency of choking are hot dogs, round candies, peanuts or other nuts, grapes, cookies or biscuits, pieces of meats, caramels, carrots, apples, peas, celery, popcorn, fruit and vegetable seeds, cherry pits, gum, and peanut butter. Other items include burst latex balloons, plastic or glass beads, marbles, pen or marker caps, button or disc batteries, and coins. Objects such as small lithium or cadmium batteries may cause esophageal or tracheal corrosion.

Diagnostic Evaluation

The diagnosis of FB aspiration is suspected on the basis of the history and physical signs. Initially, a FB in the air passages produces choking, gagging, wheezing, or coughing. Laryngotracheal obstruction most commonly causes dyspnea, cough, stridor, and hoarseness because of decreased air entry. Up to one-half of all children with FB ingestion may be asymptomatic. Cyanosis may occur if the obstruction becomes worse. Bronchial obstruction usually produces cough (frequently paroxysmal), wheezing, asymmetric breath sounds, decreased airway entry, and dyspnea. When an object is lodged in the larynx, the child is unable to speak or breathe. If the obstruction progresses, the child's face may become livid, and if the obstruction is total, the child can become unconscious and die of asphyxiation. If obstruction is partial, hours, days, or even weeks may pass without symptoms after the initial period. Secondary symptoms are related to the anatomic area in which the object is lodged and are usually caused by a persistent respiratory tract infection distal to the obstruction. FB aspiration should also be suspected in the presence of acute or chronic pulmonary lesions. Often, by the time secondary symptoms appear, the parents have forgotten the initial episode of coughing and gagging. Nasal FBs

often manifest by unilateral purulent drainage that does not improve with time.

Radiographic examination reveals opaque FBs but is of limited use in localizing nonradiographic matter. Bronchoscopy is required for a definitive diagnosis of objects in the larynx and trachea. Fluoroscopic examination is valuable in detecting FBs in the bronchi. The mainstay of diagnosis and management of FBs is endoscopy. If there is doubt about the presence of an FB, endoscopy can be diagnostic and therapeutic.

Therapeutic Management

FB aspiration may result in life-threatening airway obstruction, especially in infants because of the small diameters of their airways. Current recommendations for the emergency treatment of the choking child include the use of abdominal thrusts for children older than 1 year of age and back blows and chest thrusts for children younger than 1 year of age.

A FB is rarely coughed up spontaneously. Most frequently, it must be removed instrumentally by bronchoscopy. This procedure usually requires sedation with an agent (such as IV propofol or midazolam) and is carried out as quickly as possible because the progressive local inflammatory process triggered by the foreign material hampers removal. A chemical pneumonia soon develops, and vegetable matter begins to macerate within a few days, making it even more difficult to remove. After removal of the FB, the child is usually observed for any complications such as laryngeal edema and then discharged home within a matter of hours if vital signs are stable and recovery is satisfactory.

Prevention

Nurses are in a position to teach prevention in a variety of settings. They can educate parents singly or in groups about hazards of aspiration in relation to the developmental level of their children and encourage them to teach their children safety. Parents should be cautioned about behaviors that their children might imitate (e.g., holding foreign objects, such as pins, nails, and toothpicks, in their lips or mouth). Parents should be educated on access to age-appropriate toys and how older siblings' toys could be hazardous for younger siblings. Magnets must be kept away from younger children.

Care Management

A major role of nurses caring for a child who has aspirated an FB is to recognize the signs of FB aspiration, observe for worsening of respiratory symptoms, and implement immediate measures to relieve an emergency obstruction. Choking on food or other material should not be fatal. To aid a child who is choking, nurses must recognize the signs of distress. A blind sweep of the child's mouth should never be performed because it may lodge the agent farther into the airway. Not every child who gags or coughs while eating is truly choking.

> ### ! NURSING ALERT
>
> The child in severe distress (1) cannot speak, (2) becomes cyanotic, and (3) collapses. These three signs indicate that the child is truly choking and requires immediate action. The child can die within 4 minutes.

ASPIRATION PNEUMONIA

Aspiration pneumonia occurs when food, secretions, inert materials, volatile compounds, or liquids enter the lung and cause inflammation and a chemical pneumonitis. Aspiration of fluid or foods is a particular hazard in the child who has difficulty with swallowing or is unable to swallow because of paralysis, weakness, debility, congenital anomalies, or absent cough reflex or in the child who is force-fed, especially while crying or breathing rapidly.

Clinical signs of the aspiration of oral secretions may not be distinguishable from those of other forms of acute bacterial pneumonia. For example, if vegetable matter has been aspirated, manifestations may not appear for several weeks after the event. Classic symptoms include an increasing cough or fever with foul-smelling sputum, deteriorating oxygenation, evidence of infiltrates on chest radiographs, and other signs of lower airway involvement. These deviations may persist for weeks, even while the child starts to feel better. Rarely, aspiration causes immediate death from asphyxia; more often, the irritated mucous membrane becomes a site for secondary bacterial infection. In addition to fluids, food, vomitus, and nasopharyngeal secretions, other substances that may cause pneumonia are hydrocarbons, lipids, powder, and contrast dye or barium. The severity of the lung injury depends on the pH of the aspirated material.

Interprofessional Care Management

Care of the child with aspiration pneumonia is the same as that described for the child with pneumonia from other causes. However, the major focus of care is on prevention of aspiration. Proper feeding techniques should be carried out, and preventive measures should be used to prevent aspiration of any material that might enter the nasopharynx. The presence of an NG feeding tube or a history of gastroesophageal reflux disease places the child at risk for aspiration. NG tubes used for feedings should be checked before the initiation of bolus feedings; continuous NG tube feedings should also be evaluated periodically for proper tube placement.

Children who are at risk for swallowing difficulties as a result of illness, physical debilitation, anesthesia, or sedation are kept on nothing by mouth (NPO) status until they can properly swallow fluids effectively. A formal evaluation by an occupational therapist of a child's ability to swallow is recommended with patients who are at risk for aspiration. The child may receive nutrition by alternate means (such as an enteral feeding tube), and a dietician can determine the best nutrition. The child who is at risk for vomiting and incapable of protecting the airway should be positioned in a side-lying recovery position. Educating parents on its prevention is important.

PULMONARY EDEMA

Pulmonary edema (PE) is the movement of fluid into the alveoli and interstitium of the lungs caused by extravasation of fluid from the pulmonary vasculature (Mazor & Green, 2016). There are two main types of PE: cardiogenic and noncardiogenic.

Cardiogenic (hydrostatic, hemodynamic) PE is caused by an increase in pulmonary capillary pressure because of an increase in pulmonary venous pressure. It can be caused by excessive IV fluid administration, left ventricular failure, heart valve disorder (aortic regurgitation, aortic stenosis, mitral regurgitation), severe hypertension, renal artery stenosis, or severe renal disease (Pinto & Kociol, 2014).

Noncardiogenic PE is caused by various conditions that result in increased pulmonary capillary permeability. Some subtypes of noncardiogenic PE include permeability PE (caused by acute respiratory distress syndrome [ARDS] or acute lung injury [ALI]), high-altitude PE (caused by rapid ascension to heights above 12,000 feet), or neurogenic PE (after CNS insult such as seizures, head injury, or cerebral hemorrhage). Some less common forms of PE are reperfusion PE (after removal of thromboemboli from the lung or a lung transplant), reexpansion PE (caused by rapid reexpansion of a collapsed lung), or PE that results from opiate overdose (methadone or heroin), salicylate toxicity (chronic), aspiration (FB inhalation), inhalation injuries, near drowning, pulmonary

embolism, viral infections, or pulmonary venoocclusive disease. Other causes include traumatic injury, organ dysfunction caused by sepsis, multiorgan failure, alcoholism or substance abuse, pregnancy (eclampsia), chronic renal impairment, malnutrition, hypertension, or a blood transfusion (transfusion-related ALI).

Pathophysiology

Fluid flows from the pulmonary vasculature into the alveolar interstitial space and then returns to the systemic circulation in a normal lung. Movement of this fluid is controlled by the net difference between hydrostatic and osmotic pressures and the permeability of the capillary membrane. Increased pulmonary hydrostatic pressure or increased permeability of the vascular membrane results in movement of fluid into the alveoli and interstitium of the lung. The pulmonary lymph system normally drains away any fluid from the alveoli, but when the amount of fluid present in the alveoli exceeds lymph drainage, PE occurs.

Symptoms include extreme shortness of breath, cyanosis, tachypnea, diminished breath sounds, anxiety, agitation, confusion, diaphoresis, orthopnea, respiratory crackles, expiratory wheezing (in young infants), heart murmur, third heart sound (S3) gallop, cool extremities, jugular venous distention, nocturnal dyspnea, cough, pink frothy sputum (if severe), tachycardia, hypertension, or hypotension (if caused by left ventricle dysfunction).

Therapeutic Management

Management of PE depends on the cause but can include oxygen therapy, positive end-expiratory pressure (PEEP) via continuous positive airway pressure (CPAP), and intubation with ventilatory support if respiratory failure occurs. If ventricular failure is the cause, medications such as diuretics, digoxin, positive inotropes, and vasodilators (nitroglycerin) may be started and the child may be placed on a fluid and sodium restriction. Morphine may be prescribed to relieve dyspnea. The primary goal of management is to determine why PE occurred and treat the underlying condition.

Care Management

Nursing care of the child with PE is similar to that for any other acute respiratory condition. Pulse oximetry is monitored, and vital signs are observed closely for any deterioration. The nurse should note changes in oxygen saturation (SaO_2), end-tidal carbon dioxide ($ETCO_2$), and arterial blood gas (ABG) values. An ongoing assessment of the child's cardiopulmonary status is needed by checking lung sounds and observing respiratory rate, rhythm, depth, and effort. Oxygen, medications, and other respiratory treatments are administered as prescribed. Close monitoring of intake and output, electrolytes, and comfort is important. The child should be monitored for restlessness, anxiety, and air hunger. Placing the child in a high Fowler position may help with lung expansion. Because this position places pressure on bony prominences in the sacrum and hips, pressure areas must be relieved at intervals. Most of the care of PE occurs in the intensive care unit, which is anxiety provoking for the child and family. They should be given the opportunity to express their fears and anxieties and to ask questions. (For other nursing care activities, see the following section on ARDS.)

ACUTE RESPIRATORY DISTRESS SYNDROME

ARDS is a potentially life-threatening inflammatory lung condition that may occur in both children and adults. This syndrome may be caused by direct injury to the lungs or by systemic insults that lead indirectly to lung injury with subsequent hypoxemia and respiratory failure due to non-cardiogenic PE. Sepsis, trauma, viral pneumonia, aspiration, fat emboli, drug overdose, reperfusion injury after lung transplantation, smoke inhalation, and near-drowning, among others, have been associated with ARDS.

Pathologically, the hallmark of ARDS is increased permeability of the alveolar-capillary membrane that results in PE. During the acute phase of ARDS, inflammatory mediators damage the alveolocapillary membrane, with an increasing pulmonary capillary permeability with resulting interstitial edema. Later stages are characterized by pneumocyte and fibrin infiltration of the alveoli, with the start of either the healing process or fibrosis. When fibrosis occurs, the child may demonstrate respiratory distress and the need for mechanical ventilation. In ARDS, the lungs become stiff as a result of surfactant inactivation; gas diffusion is impaired; and eventually, bronchiolar mucosal swelling and congestive atelectasis occur. The net effect is decreased functional residual capacity, pulmonary hypertension, and increased intrapulmonary right-to-left shunting of pulmonary blood flow. Surfactant secretion is reduced, and the atelectasis and fluid-filled alveoli provide an excellent medium for bacterial growth. Hypoxemia or increased work of breathing may require ventilatory support.

Diagnostic Evaluation

Diagnostic criteria were established by the American European Consensus Conference (Bernard, Artigas, Brigham, et al, 1994) and have been superseded by the Berlin definition of ARDS (ARDS Definition Task Force, Ranieri, Rubenfeld, et al., 2012). According to the Berlin definition, ARDS occurs within 1 week of a known clinical insult or new or worsening respiratory symptoms; is characterized by bilateral opacities on chest imaging not fully explained by effusions, lobar/lung collapse, or nodules; and manifests as respiratory failure not fully explained by cardiac failure or fluid overload (ARDS Definition Task Force et al). Hypoxemia is expressed in terms of the ratio of partial pressure of oxygen (PaO_2) to the fraction of inspired oxygen (FiO_2), or P/F ratio.

Therapeutic Management

The child with ARDS may first demonstrate only symptoms caused by an injury or infection, but as the condition deteriorates, hyperventilation, tachypnea, increasing respiratory effort, cyanosis, and decreasing oxygen saturation occur. At times, the developing hypoxemia is not responsive to oxygen administration.

Treatment involves supportive measures to maintain adequate oxygenation and pulmonary perfusion, treatment of infection (or the precipitating cause), and maintenance of adequate cardiac output and vascular volume. After the underlying cause has been identified, specific treatment (e.g., antibiotics for infection) is initiated. Many patients require mechanical ventilatory support. This is usually achieved invasively (i.e., after endotracheal intubation), but occasionally noninvasive ventilation is used in milder cases. Patients requiring invasive mechanical ventilation usually require sedation, at least initially, to allow for ventilatory synchrony. Fluid administration to maintain adequate intravascular volume and end-organ perfusion must be balanced against the desire to decrease lung fluid to improve oxygenation. The provision of adequate nutrition, maintenance of patient comfort, and prevention of complications such as gastrointestinal ulceration are essential. Psychologic support of the patient and family is also important.

It has been demonstrated that inappropriate use of mechanical ventilatory support may worsen the lung injury by causing volutrauma, barotrauma, atelectrauma, and biotrauma to the injured lungs. Protective ventilatory strategies using low tidal volumes (6 mL/kg ideal body weight) have been demonstrated to improve outcomes in adults and theoretically are also appropriate in children. PEEP is applied to decrease atelectasis and maintain an "open" lung. Permissive hypercapnia may also be used.

Other strategies used in the support of patients with ARDS include use of the prone position, inhaled nitric oxide, inhaled prostaglandins, high-frequency oscillatory ventilation (HFOV), and extracorporeal membrane oxygenation (ECMO), although evidence to support these therapies is scant.

Prognosis

The prognosis for patients with ARDS is improving. Nonetheless, the mortality rate remains high, and in children, it ranges from 14% to 45% (Lopez-Fernandez, Azagra, de la Oliva, et al., 2012). The precipitating disorder influences the outcome; the worst prognosis is associated with profound hypoxemia, uncontrolled sepsis, bone marrow transplantation, cancer, and multisystem involvement with hepatic failure. Children who recover may have persistent cough and exertional dyspnea.

Interprofessional Care Management

The child with ARDS is cared for in the intensive care unit during the acute stages of illness and involves professionals from a variety of disciplines. Care of the patient involves close monitoring of oxygenation and respiratory status as well as assessment of cardiac output, perfusion, fluid and electrolyte balance, and renal function (urinary output). Blood gas analysis, acid-base status, and pulse oximetry are important evaluation tools. Diuretics may be administered to reduce pulmonary fluid, and vasodilators may be administered to decrease pulmonary vascular pressure. Nutritional support is often required because of the prolonged acute phase of the illness. Intensivists, pulmonologists, dieticians, respiratory therapists, and oftentimes cardiologists and nephrologists are involved in the child's care.

Management also includes monitoring the effects of the numerous parenteral fluids and drugs used to stabilize the child and monitoring for changes in the child's hemodynamic status. Most children with ARDS require invasive monitoring via a central venous catheter. Care of the child with ARDS also involves close observance of skin condition, prevention of skin breakdown by pressure area relief, and passive range of motion. Physical therapists can assist with care to prevent muscle atrophy and contractures.

Respiratory distress is a frightening situation for both the child and the parents, and attention to their psychologic needs is a major element in the care of these children. The child is often sedated during the acute phase of the illness, and weaning from sedation requires close monitoring for anxiety reduction and comfort. Social workers and child life specialists can assist the patient and family with coping.

SMOKE INHALATION INJURY

A number of noxious substances that may be inhaled are toxic to humans. They are primarily products of incomplete combustion and cause more deaths from fires than flame injuries. The severity of the injury depends on the nature of the substances generated by the material burned, whether the victim is confined in a closed space, and the duration of contact with the smoke.

Three distinct syndromes of pulmonary complications may occur in children with inhalation injury: (1) early carbon monoxide (CO) poisoning, airway obstruction, and PE; (2) ARDS occurring at 24 to 48 hours or later in some cases; and (3) late complications of bronchopneumonia and pulmonary emboli (Antoon & Donovan, 2016). Smoke inhalation results in three types of injury: heat, chemical, and systemic.

Heat injury involves thermal injury to the upper airway. Air has low specific heat; therefore the injury goes no farther than the upper airway. Reflex closure of the glottis prevents injury to the lower airway.

Chemical injury involves gases that may be generated during the combustion of materials such as clothing, furniture, and floor coverings. Acids, alkalis, and their precursors in smoke can produce chemical burns. These substances can be carried deep into the respiratory tract, including the lower respiratory tract, in the form of insoluble gases. Soluble gases tend to dissolve in the upper respiratory tract. Chemical burns to the airways are similar to burns on the skin, except they are painless because the tracheobronchial tree is relatively insensitive to pain.

Inhalation of small amounts of noxious irritants produces alveolar and bronchiolar damage that can lead to obstructive bronchiolitis. Severe exposure causes further injury, including alveolocapillary damage with hemorrhage, necrotizing bronchiolitis, inhibited secretion of surfactant, and formation of hyaline membranes, which are all manifestations of ARDS.

Systemic injury occurs from gases that are nontoxic to the airways (e.g., CO, hydrogen cyanide). However, these gases cause injury and death by interfering with or inhibiting cellular respiration. CO is responsible for more than one-half of all fatal inhalation poisonings in the United States. CO is a colorless, odorless gas with an affinity for hemoglobin 230 times greater than that of oxygen. When CO enters the bloodstream, it binds readily with hemoglobin to form carboxyhemoglobin (COHb). Because it is released less readily than oxygen, tissue hypoxia reaches dangerous levels before oxygen is available to meet tissue needs.

> **! NURSING ALERT**
>
> With carbon monoxide (CO) poisoning, the oxygen saturation (SaO_2) obtained by pulse oximetry will be normal because the device measures only oxygenated and deoxygenated hemoglobin; it does not measure dysfunctional hemoglobin, such as carboxyhemoglobin (COHb).

Accidental CO poisoning is usually a result of exposure to fumes of heaters or smoke from structural fires, although poorly ventilated recreational vehicles with improperly operated or maintained gas lamps or stoves and cooking in underventilated areas with charcoal grills are also frequent causes. CO is produced by incomplete combustion of carbon or carbonaceous material such as wood or charcoal.

The signs and symptoms of CO poisoning are secondary to tissue hypoxia and vary with the level of COHb. Mild manifestations include headache, visual disturbances, irritability, and nausea; more severe intoxication causes confusion, hallucinations, ataxia, and coma. The bright, cherry-red lips and skin often described are less common than pallor and cyanosis.

Therapeutic Management

Treatment of children with smoke inhalation injury is largely symptomatic. The most widely accepted treatment is placing the child on humidified 100% oxygen as quickly as possible (assuming no previous medical conditions exist contraindicating this) to rapidly reverse tissue hypoxia and to displace CO and cyanide from protein binding sites. The child is monitored for signs of respiratory distress and impending failure, and intubation may be required. A laryngoscopy or bronchoscopy evaluation may be done to assess for airway damage. Baseline ABGs and COHb levels are obtained. PaO_2 may be within normal limits unless there is marked respiratory depression. If CO poisoning is confirmed, 100% oxygen is continued until COHb levels fall to the nontoxic range of about 10%. If CO poisoning is severe, the patient may benefit from hyperbaric oxygen therapy. Hyperbaric oxygen therapy may be useful in the treatment of neurologic complications related to CO poisoning.

Pulmonary care may be facilitated by bronchodilators, humidification, chest percussion, and postural drainage to enhance the removal of necrotic material, minimize bronchoconstriction, and avoid atelectasis. Bronchoscopy may be needed to clear heavy secretions.

Respiratory distress may occur early in the course of smoke inhalation as a result of hypoxia, or patients who are breathing well on admission may suddenly develop respiratory distress. Therefore, endotracheal intubation equipment should be readily available. Transient edema of the airways can occur at any level in the tracheobronchial tree. Assessment and localization of the obstruction should be accomplished before severe swelling of the head, neck, or oropharynx occurs. Intubation is often necessary when (1) severe burns in the area of the nose, mouth, and face increase the likelihood of developing oropharyngeal edema and obstruction; (2) vocal cord edema causes obstruction; (3) the patient has difficulty handling secretions; and (4) progressive respiratory distress requires artificial ventilation. Controversy surrounds tracheostomy, but many prefer this procedure when the obstruction is proximal to the larynx and reserve nasotracheal intubation for lower tract involvement.

Care Management

Care of the child with inhalation injury is the same as that for any child with respiratory distress. The initial goal is to maintain a patent airway and effective ventilation status. Vital signs and other respiratory assessments (oxygenation, work of breathing, acid-base status) are performed frequently, and the pulmonary status is carefully observed and maintained. The administration of nebulized bronchodilators, humidified oxygen, and inhaled corticosteroids is often part of the child's care. Chest percussion and postural drainage are often part of the therapy, as well as mechanical ventilation if needed. Fluid requirements for children experiencing inhalation injury are greater than for those with surface burns alone; however, one concern is the development of PE. Therefore accurate monitoring of fluid intake and output is essential.

In addition to observation and management of the physical aspects of inhalation injury, the nurse also deals with the psychologic needs of a frightened child and distraught parents. As with any accidental injury, the parents may feel overwhelming guilt even when the injury occurred through no fault of their own. Parents need support, reassurance, and information regarding the child's condition, treatment, and progress. The nurse can provide anticipatory guidance and educate families on prevention of inhalation injuries and the importance of CO detectors in the home.

ENVIRONMENTAL TOBACCO SMOKE EXPOSURE

Numerous investigations indicate that parental or family smoking is an important cause of morbidity in children. Children exposed to (secondhand) passive or environmental tobacco smoke have an increased number of respiratory illnesses, increased respiratory symptoms (i.e., cough, sputum, and wheezing), and reduced performance on pulmonary function tests (PFTs). AOM and OME are also increased in children who have smoking parents. Indoor exposure to tobacco smoke has been linked to asthma in children (Sheikh, Pitts, Ryan-Wenger, et al., 2016). Among children with asthma, there is an association between parental cigarette smoking and asthma exacerbations, trips to the emergency department (ED), medication use, and impaired recovery after hospitalization for acute asthma. Maternal cigarette smoking is associated with a significant risk factor for sudden infant death syndrome (SIDS) (Mitchell & Krous, 2015). The risk for diagnosis of early-onset asthma in the first 6 years of life is associated with in utero exposure to maternal smoking (Neuman, Hohmann, Orsini, et al., 2012). Exposure to tobacco smoke during childhood may also contribute to the development of chronic lung disease in the adult.

FAMILY-CENTERED CARE

Decreasing Childhood Exposure to Environmental Tobacco Smoke*

- Do not smoke around infants and children.
- Maintain a smoke-free home. Do not allow visitors to smoke in the home.
- Encourage exclusive breastfeeding for the first 6 months.
- Change clothing after smoking and before holding an infant in close proximity.
- Restrict smoking to outside the house where the children do not play.
- Do not smoke in motor vehicles with children.

*For further information on the effects of secondhand smoke on child health, go to http://www.surgeongeneral.gov/library/reports/secondhandsmoke/secondhandsmoke.pdf.

The use of electronic cigarettes (e-cigarettes) has become more prevalent with adolescents and adults in recent years. The National Youth Tobacco Survey, 2011-2013 reported a three-fold increase in the use of e-cigarettes among adolescents who had never smoked cigarettes (Bunnell, Agaku, Arrazola, et al., 2014). Further studies are needed on the impact of e-cigarette emissions on air quality and on nicotine deposition on surfaces. E-cigarettes may be a source of nicotine exposure to bystanders (Czogala, Goniewicz, Fidelus, et al., 2014), and children may be at risk for poisoning due to ingestion of the nicotine liquid in cartridges.

Care Management

Nurses must provide information about the hazards of environmental smoke exposure in all of their interactions with children and their family members. This information is especially important for children with respiratory and allergic illnesses. In families in which smokers refuse to quit, appropriate guidance is provided for reducing smoke in the child's environment (see Family-Centered Care box: Decreasing Childhood Exposure to Environmental Tobacco Smoke). Nurses should set an example for children and families and become advocates for "no smoking" ordinances in public places, prohibition of advertising tobacco products in the media, and inclusion of health warnings of sidestream smoke on tobacco products.* Nurses have an important role in providing parents with affordable smoking-cessation education resources, including the appropriate use of smoking-cessation pharmacologic aids. Nurses also have a role in educating adolescents about avoiding using tobacco products or smoking marijuana.

LONG-TERM RESPIRATORY DYSFUNCTION

ASTHMA

Asthma is a chronic inflammatory disorder of the airways characterized by recurring symptoms, airway obstruction, bronchial hyperresponsiveness, and an underlying inflammation process (Trent, Zimbro, & Rutledge, 2015). In susceptible children, inflammation causes recurrent episodes of wheezing, breathlessness, chest tightness, and cough, especially at night or in the early morning. The airflow limitation or obstruction is reversible either spontaneously or with treatment. Inflammation causes an increase in bronchial hyperresponsiveness to a variety of stimuli (Liu, Covar, Spahn, et al., 2016). Recognition of the key role of inflammation

*For further information on the effects of secondhand smoke on child health, go to http://www.surgeongeneral.gov/library/reports/secondhandsmoke/secondhandsmoke.pdf.

BOX 40.13   Asthma Severity Classification in Children 0 to 11 Years of Age*

Step 5 or 6: Severe Asthma
- Continual symptoms throughout the day
- Frequent nighttime symptoms (>1 time per week (0 to 4 years of age), 7 nights per week (5 years of age and older)
- Pulmonary expiratory flow (PEF): <60%
- Forced expiratory volume in 1 second (FEV_1): <75% of predicted value
- Interference with normal activity: extremely limited
- Use of short-acting β agonist for symptom control: several times per day

Step 3 or 4: Moderate Asthma
- Daily symptoms
- Nighttime symptoms: 3 to 4 times per month (0 to 4 years of age), >1 per week but not nightly (5 to 11 years of age)
- PEF: 60% to 80% of predicted value (5 years of age and older)
- FEV_1: 75% to 80% (5 years of age and older)
- PEF variability: >30%
- Interference with normal activity: some limitation
- Use of short-acting β agonist for symptom control: daily

Step 2: Mild Asthma
- Symptoms >2 times per week but <1 time per day
- Nighttime symptoms: 1 to 2 times per month (0 to 4 years of age), 3 to 4 times per month (5 to 11 years of age)
- PEF or FEV_1: ≥80% of predicted value
- PEF variability: 20% to 30%
- Interference with normal activity: minor limitation
- Use of short-acting β agonist for symptom control: >2 days per week, but not daily

Step 1: Intermittent Asthma
- Symptoms ≤2 days per week
- Nighttime symptoms (awakenings): None (0 to 4 years of age); ≤2 nights per month (5 to 11 years of age)
- PEF or FEV_1: ≥80% of predicted value
- PEF variability: <20%
- Interference with normal activity: none
- Use of short-acting β agonist for symptom control: <2 days per week

FEV_1, Forced expiratory volume in 1 second; *PEF,* peak expiratory flow.

*The presence of one clinical feature of severity is sufficient to place a patient in that category. An individual should be assigned to the most severe grade in which any feature occurs. The characteristics in this box are general and may overlap because asthma is highly variable. An individual's classification may change over time. Risk factors for each category are not presented in this box. See original reference for additional classification data. Asthma treatment should not be based on this box.

From National Asthma Education and Prevention Program. (2007). *Guidelines for the diagnosis and management of asthma: Summary report 2007.* Retrieved from www.nhlbi.nih.gov/guidelines/asthma/index.htm.

---

has made the use of antiinflammatory agents, especially inhaled steroids, a major component in the treatment of asthma.

Asthma is classified into four categories based on the symptom indicators of disease severity. These categories are *intermittent, mild, moderate,* and *severe.* Symptoms increase in frequency or intensity until the last category of severe persistent asthma (Box 40.13). These categories provide a stepwise approach to the pharmacologic management, environmental control, and educational interventions needed for each category (Liu et al., 2016). These categories emphasize the multifaceted aspect of the disease for consideration of effects on present quality of life and functional capacity and the future risk for adverse events.

Asthma is the most common chronic disease of childhood, the primary cause of school absences, and the third leading cause of hospitalizations in children younger than 15 years of age (Trent et al., 2015). Although the onset of asthma may occur at any age, 80% to 90% of children have their first symptoms before 4 or 5 years of age. Boys are affected more frequently than girls until adolescence, when the trend reverses. Asthma prevalence, morbidity, and mortality are increasing in the United States, especially among non-Hispanic black children (Akinbami, Simon, & Rossen, 2016). Morbidity and mortality increases may result from worsening air pollution, more premature infants with chronic lung disease, poor access to medical care, underdiagnosis, and undertreatment.

Etiology

Studies of children with asthma indicate that allergies influence both the persistence and the severity of the disease. In fact, *atopy*, or the genetic predisposition for the development of an immunoglobulin E (IgE)–mediated response to common aeroallergens, is the strongest identifiable predisposing factor for developing asthma (Loutsios, Farahi, Porter, et al., 2014). However, 20% to 40% of children with asthma have no evidence of allergic disease. In addition to allergens, other substances and conditions can serve as triggers that may exacerbate asthma (Box 40.14). Evidence shows that viral respiratory infections, including RSV infection, may also have a significant role in the development and expression of asthma (Knudson & Varga, 2015).

Pathophysiology

There is general agreement that inflammation contributes to heightened airway reactivity in asthma. It is unlikely that asthma is caused by either a single cell or a single inflammatory mediator; rather, it appears that asthma results from complex interactions among inflammatory cells, mediators, and the cells and tissues present in the airways (Liu et al., 2016). However, recognition of the importance of inflammation has made the use of antiinflammatory agents a key component of asthma therapy.

Another important component of asthma is bronchospasm and airflow obstruction. The mechanisms responsible for the obstructive symptoms in asthma include (1) inflammatory response to stimuli; (2) airway edema and accumulation and secretion of mucus; (3) spasm of the smooth muscle of the bronchi and bronchioles, which decreases the caliber of the bronchioles; and (4) airway remodeling, which causes permanent cellular changes (Liu et al., 2016) (Fig. 40.4).

Airflow is determined by the size of the airway lumen, degree of bronchial wall edema, mucus production, smooth muscle contraction, and muscle hypertrophy. Bronchial constriction is a normal reaction to foreign stimuli; however, with asthma, it is abnormally severe, producing impaired respiratory function. Because the bronchi normally dilate and elongate during inspiration and contract and shorten on expiration, the respiratory difficulty is more pronounced during the expiratory phase of respiration.

BOX 40.14   Triggers Tending to Precipitate or Aggravate Asthmatic Exacerbations

Allergens
- Outdoor: Trees, shrubs, weeds, grasses, molds, pollens, air pollution, spores
- Indoor: Dust or dust mites, mold, cockroach antigen

Irritants: Tobacco smoke, wood smoke, odors, sprays
Exposure to occupational chemicals
Exercise
Cold air
Changes in weather or temperature
Environmental change (e.g., moving to a new home, starting a new school)
Colds and infections
Animals: Cats, dogs, rodents, horses
Medications: Aspirin, NSAIDs, antibiotics, β blockers
Strong emotions: Fear, anger, laughing, crying
Conditions: Gastroesophageal reflux, tracheoesophageal fistula
Food additives: Sulfite preservatives
Foods: Nuts, milk/dairy products
Endocrine factors: Menses, pregnancy, thyroid disease

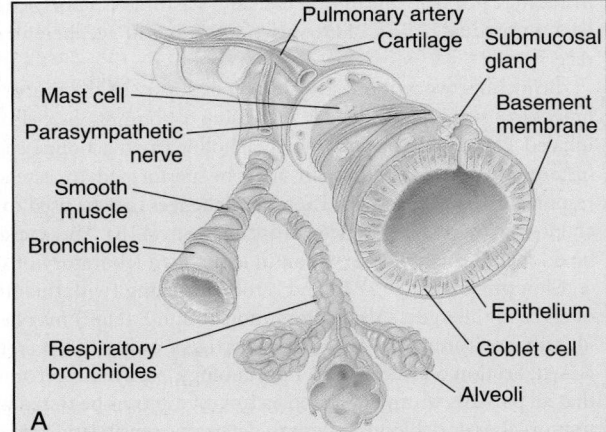
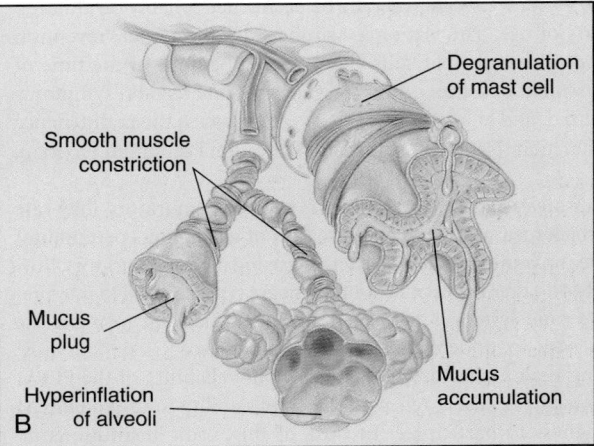

FIG 40.4 Airway obstruction caused by asthma. **A,** A normal lung. **B,** Bronchial asthma: thick mucus, mucosal edema, and smooth muscle spasm causing obstruction of small airways; breathing becomes labored, and expiration is difficult. (Adapted from Des Jardins, T., & Burton, G.G. [1995]. *Clinical manifestations and assessment of respiratory disease* [3rd ed.]. St. Louis, MO: Mosby.)

Increased resistance in the airway causes forced expiration through the narrowed lumen. The volume of air trapped in the lungs increases as airways are functionally closed at a point between the alveoli and the lobar bronchi. This trapping of gas forces the individual to breathe at higher and higher lung volumes. Consequently, the person with asthma fights to inspire sufficient air. This expenditure of effort for breathing causes fatigue, decreased respiratory effectiveness, and increased oxygen consumption. The inspiration occurring at higher lung volumes hyperinflates the alveoli and reduces the effectiveness of the cough. As the severity of obstruction increases, there is a reduced alveolar ventilation with carbon dioxide retention; hypoxemia; respiratory acidosis; and, eventually, respiratory failure.

Chronic inflammation may also cause permanent damage (airway remodeling) to airway structures, which cannot be prevented by and is not responsive to current treatments (Sferrazza Papa, Pellegrino, & Pellegrino, 2014).

Diagnostic Evaluation

The classic manifestations of asthma are dyspnea, wheezing, and coughing. An attack may develop gradually or appear abruptly and may be preceded by a URI. The age of the child is often a significant factor because the first attack frequently occurs before 5 years of age, with some children manifesting clinical signs and symptoms in infancy. In infancy, an attack usually follows a respiratory infection. Some children may experience a prodromal itching at the front of the neck or over the upper part of the back just before an attack, especially if the attack is related to allergies (Box 40.15).

> **! NURSING ALERT**
>
> Shortness of breath with air movement in the chest restricted to the point of absent breath sounds (silent chest) accompanied by a sudden rise in respiratory rate is an ominous sign indicating ventilatory failure and imminent respiratory arrest.

The diagnosis is determined primarily on the basis of clinical manifestations, history, physical examination, and, to a lesser extent, laboratory tests. Generally, chronic cough in the absence of infection or diffuse wheezing during the expiratory phase of respiration is sufficient to establish a diagnosis.

Pulmonary function tests (PFTs) provide an objective method of evaluating the presence and degree of lung disease, as well as the response to therapy. Spirometry can generally be performed reliably on children 5 or 6 years of age. The National Asthma Education and Prevention Program recommends that spirometry testing be done at the time of initial assessment of asthma, after treatment is initiated and symptoms have stabilized, and at least every 1 to 2 years to assess the maintenance of airway function (National Asthma and Education Prevention Program, 2012).

Another measurement to consider is the peak expiratory flow rate (PEFR), which measures the maximum flow of air (in liters per minute) that can be forcefully exhaled in 1 second using a peak expiratory flow meter (PEFM). Three zones of measurement are typically used to interpret PEFR. The zone system is patterned after a traffic light to make the categories easy to understand and remember (see Guidelines box: Interpreting Peak Expiratory Flow Rates). The reliability of the PEFM is controversial, because it relies on the child's ability to use the PEFM and willingness to participate. Because of this, some institutions no longer rely on the PEFR results to guide asthma management. The child's technique on doing the PEFR should be examined on an ongoing basis and reeducation provided when needed. Families are encouraged to record PEFM at regular intervals and to bring a record of this to any

---

BOX 40.15 Clinical Manifestations of Asthma

Cough
- Hacking, paroxysmal, irritative, and nonproductive
- Becomes rattling and productive of frothy, clear, gelatinous sputum

Respiratory-Related Signs
- Shortness of breath
- Prolonged expiratory phase
- Audible wheeze
- May have a malar flush and red ears
- Lips deep dark red color
- Possible progression to cyanosis of nail beds or circumoral cyanosis
- Restlessness
- Apprehension
- Prominent sweating as the attack progresses
- Older children sit upright with shoulders in a hunched-over position, hands on the bed or chair, and arms braced (tripod position)
- Speech: May speak in short, panting, broken phrases

Chest
- Hyperresonance on percussion
- Coarse, loud breath sounds
- Wheezes throughout the lung fields
- Prolonged expiration
- Crackles
- Generalized inspiratory and expiratory wheezing; increasingly high pitched

With Repeated Episodes
- Barrel chest
- Elevated shoulders
- Use of accessory muscles of respiration
- Facial appearance: flattened malar bones, circles beneath the eyes, narrow nose, prominent upper teeth

---

medical appointments for health care providers to review trends. Each child needs to establish his or her personal best value during a 2- to 3-week period when the child's asthma is stable. After the personal best value has been established, the child's current PEFR on any occasion can be compared with the personal best value. In some cases, a low PEFR may not truly mean that the child's asthma is poorly controlled. Each individual child's PEFR varies according to age, height, sex, and race.

Bronchoprovocation testing, direct exposure of the mucous membranes to a suspected antigen in increasing concentrations, helps identify inhaled allergens. Exposure to methacholine (methacholine challenge), histamine, or cold or dry air may be performed to assess airway responsiveness or reactivity. Exercise challenges may be used to identify children with exercise-induced bronchospasm (EIB). These tests should be done under close observation in a qualified laboratory or clinic.

Skin prick testing (SPT) and serologic testing (with quantification of sIgE) for allergen-specific immunoglobulin E (sIgE) may be used to identify environmental allergens that trigger asthma (Sicherer, Wood, & AAP Section on Allergy and Immunology, 2012). It is recommended that all patients with year-round asthma symptoms be tested with skin tests or laboratory blood analysis to determine sensitization to perennial allergens (e.g., house dust mites, cats, dogs, cockroaches, molds, and fungi) (Liu et al., 2016).

In addition to these tests, other tests may be performed, including laboratory tests (complete blood count [CBC] with differential) and

GUIDELINES

*Interpreting Peak Expiratory Flow Rates**

Green (80% to 100% of personal best) signals *all clear*. Asthma is under reasonably good control. No symptoms are present, and the routine treatment plan for maintaining control can be followed.

Yellow (50% to 79% of personal best) signals *caution*. Asthma is not well controlled. An acute exacerbation may be present. Maintenance therapy may need to be increased. Call the health care provider if the child stays in this zone.

Red (below 50% of personal best) signals a *medical alert*. Severe airway narrowing may be occurring. A short-acting bronchodilator should be administered. Notify the health care provider if the peak expiratory flow rate does not return immediately and stay in yellow or green zones.

*These zones are guidelines only. Specific zones and management should be individualized for each child.

chest radiographs. The presence of eosinophilia of greater than 500/mm^3 suggests the presence of an allergic or inflammatory disorder. Frontal and lateral radiographs may show infiltrates and hyperexpansion of the airways, with the anteroposterior diameter on physical examination indicating an increased diameter (suggestive of barrel chest). Radiography may assist in ruling out a respiratory tract infection or other conditions, such as CF.

Therapeutic Management

The overall goals of asthma management are to maintain normal activity levels, maintain normal pulmonary function, prevent chronic symptoms and recurrent exacerbations, provide optimal drug therapy with minimal or no adverse effects, and assist the child in living as normal and happy a life as possible. This includes facilitating the child's social adjustments in the family, school, and community and normal participation in recreational activities and sports. To accomplish these goals, several treatment principles need to be followed (Brown, Gallagher, Fowler, et al., 2010):

- Regular visits to the health care provider are necessary to evaluate therapeutic response and revise the plan of care if needed.
- Prevention of exacerbations includes avoiding triggers, avoiding allergens, and using medications as needed.
- Therapy includes efforts to reduce underlying inflammation and relieve or prevent symptomatic airway narrowing.
- Therapy includes education, environmental control, pharmacologic management, and the use of objective measures to monitor the severity of disease and guide the course of therapy.
- Managing asthma should be fostered in the child as the child increases in age and maturity.

Allergen Control

Nonpharmacologic therapy is aimed at the prevention and reduction of exposure to airborne allergens and irritants. House dust mites and other components of house dust are frequent agents identified in children who are allergic to inhalants. The cockroach, another common household inhabitant, is an important allergen in many locations. Exterminating live cockroaches, carefully cleaning kitchen floors and cabinets, putting food away after eating, and taking trash out in the evening are essential measures to control cockroaches. The mouse allergen is the most recent allergen to be identified in the homes of inner-city children with asthma. The role of cat and dog dander in allergen-induced asthma has also been studied. Studies suggest that exposure to pets at a young age has no effect on the development of asthma, but continuing pet exposure can increase the risk for asthma development later in life (Ownby &

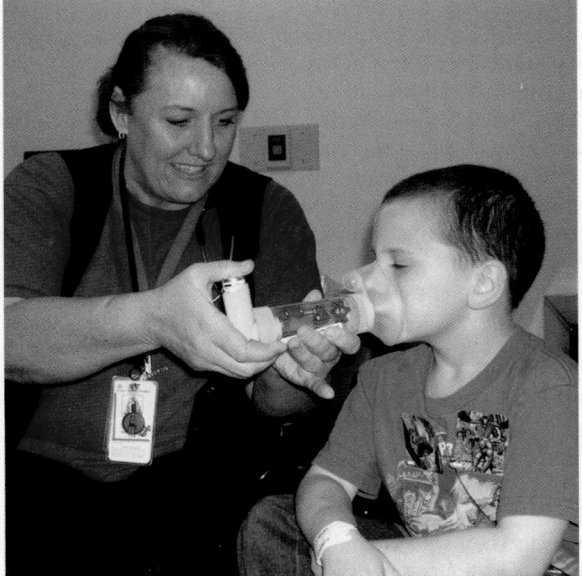

FIG 40.5 Child using metered-dose inhaler with spacer and face mask.

Johnson, 2016). Additional sources of pollutants include ozone, particulate matter produced by tobacco smoke, wood-burning stoves, cleaning products, pesticides, mold spores, nitrogen dioxide, and sulfur dioxide; these are believed to contribute to asthma morbidity in children and should be avoided or minimized (Liu et al., 2016). Living in homes close to busy roads, living in damp homes with mold, and exposure to tobacco smoke are significant contributing factors in the development of asthma in infants and small children (Heinrich, 2011).

Skin testing identifies specific allergens so steps can be taken to eliminate or avoid them. Often, simply removing the offending environmental allergens or irritants (e.g., removing carpeting from the home of a child sensitive to mold and dust particles) will decrease the frequency of asthma episodes. Dehumidifiers or air conditioners may control nonspecific factors that trigger an episode, such as extremes of temperature.

Drug Therapy

Pharmacologic therapy is used to prevent and control asthma symptoms, reduce the frequency and severity of asthma exacerbations, and reverse airflow obstruction. A stepwise approach is recommended based on the severity of the child's asthma. Because inflammation is considered an early and persistent feature of asthma, therapy is directed toward long-term suppression of inflammation.

Asthma medications are categorized into two general classes: long-term control medications (preventive medications) to achieve and maintain control of inflammation; and quick-relief medications (rescue medications) to treat symptoms and exacerbations.

Quick-relief and long-term medications are often used in combination. Inhaled corticosteroids, cromolyn sodium, long-acting β_2 agonists (LABAs), methylxanthines, and leukotriene modifiers are used as long-term control medications. Short-acting β_2 agonists, anticholinergics, and systemic corticosteroids are used as quick-relief or rescue medications.

Many asthma medications are given by inhalation with a nebulizer or a metered-dose inhaler (MDI). The MDI is always attached to a spacer, which can be equipped with a mask or a mouthpiece (Fig. 40.5). Pharmaceutical companies are currently mandated to produce inhalers that do not contain chlorofluorocarbons (CFCs) as the propellant because CFCs have been linked to damage and depletion of the earth's ozone layer. Several currently available CFC-free MDI devices use dry powder (and are called dry-powder inhalers); these include the Diskus inhaler and the Turbuhaler. These devices are breath activated, and the child needs to inhale as quickly and deeply as possible to use them effectively. The Diskhaler and Aerosolizer are similar, but with the Aerosolizer, the medication must be loaded into the inhaler before use. Children who have difficulty using MDIs or other inhalers can receive their asthma medications via a nebulizer, which administers the medication via compressed air or oxygen. Children are instructed to breathe normally with the mouth open to provide a direct route to the trachea.

Corticosteroids are antiinflammatory drugs used to treat reversible airflow obstruction, control symptoms, and reduce bronchial hyper-responsiveness in chronic asthma. Inhaled corticosteroids are used as first-line therapy in children older than 5 years of age. Clinical studies of corticosteroids have indicated significant improvement of all asthma parameters, including decreases in symptoms, ED visits, and medication requirements (Bekmezian, Fee, & Weber, 2015).

Corticosteroids may be administered parenterally, orally, or by inhalation. Oral medications are metabolized slowly, with an onset of action up to 3 hours after administration and peak effectiveness occurring within 6 to 12 hours. Oral systemic steroids may be given for short periods (e.g., 3- or 10-day "bursts") to gain prompt control of inadequately controlled persistent asthma or to manage severe persistent asthma. These drugs should be given in the lowest effective dose. These medications have few side effects (cough, dysphonia, and oral thrush), and strong evidence indicates that they improve the long-term outcomes for children of all ages with mild or moderate persistent asthma. Some studies have monitored children for 6 years after starting inhaled corticosteroids, and they indicate that when used at recommended doses, they do not have long-term significant effects on growth, bone mineral density, or suppression of the adrenal-pituitary axis (Liu et al., 2016). However, primary care providers should frequently monitor (at least every 3 to 6 months) the growth of children and adolescents taking corticosteroids to assess the systemic effects of these drugs and make appropriate reductions in dosages or changes to other types of asthma therapy when necessary. Inhaled corticosteroids include budesonide and fluticasone.

β-Adrenergic agonists (short-acting) (primarily albuterol, levalbuterol [Xopenex], and terbutaline) are used for treatment of acute exacerbations and for the prevention of EIB. These drugs bind with the β receptors on the smooth muscle of airways, where they activate adenylate cyclase and convert adenosine monophosphate (AMP) to cyclic AMP (cAMP). The increased cAMP enhances binding of intracellular calcium to the cell membrane, reducing the availability of calcium and thus allowing smooth muscle to relax. Other effects of the drug help stabilize mast cells to prevent release of mediators. Most β-adrenergics used in asthma therapy affect predominantly the β_2-receptors, which help eliminate bronchospasm. β_1-receptor effects, such as increased heart rate and gastrointestinal disturbances, have been minimized. Albuterol is given orally (liquid or pill) or via nebulizer or inhaler. Levalbuterol is given via nebulizer or MDI. Terbutaline is given orally, via nebulizer, subcutaneously, or intravenously. The inhaled drugs have a more rapid onset of action than oral forms. Inhalation also reduces troublesome systemic side effects, including irritability, tremor, nervousness, and insomnia.

Salmeterol (Serevent) is a LABA (bronchodilator) that is used twice a day (no more frequently than every 12 hours). This drug is added to antiinflammatory therapy and used for long-term prevention of symptoms, especially nighttime symptoms, and EIB. Salmeterol can be used in children 4 years of age and older, and it is not used to treat acute symptoms or exacerbations. LABA (e.g., salmeterol) should be added to a low- or medium-dosage inhaled corticosteroid among children with persistent asthma not controlled with inhaled corticosteroid

treatment alone, in order to decrease asthma symptoms and the need for a short-acting β_2 agonist (Miraglia del Giudice, Matera, Capristo, et al., 2013). LABAs can only be used as an adjuvant therapy in patients who are currently receiving but are not adequately controlled on a long-term asthma-control medication. LABAs can increase the risk for severely worsening asthma symptoms, potentially leading to hospitalizations and death (US Food and Drug Administration, 2011).

Theophylline is a methylxanthine drug used for decades to relieve symptoms and prevent asthma attacks; however, it is now used primarily in the ICU when the child is not responding to maximal therapy (Dalabih, Harris, Bondi, et al., 2013). Adding theophylline to inhaled glucocorticoids can be more effective than increasing the steroid dose alone. Therapeutic levels should be obtained with this drug because it has a narrow therapeutic window.

Cromolyn sodium is a medication used in maintenance therapy for asthma in children older than 2 years of age. It stabilizes mast cell membranes; inhibits activation and release of mediators from eosinophil and epithelial cells; and inhibits the acute airway narrowing after exposure to exercise, cold dry air, and sulfur dioxide. It does not result in immediate relief of symptoms and has minimal side effects (occasional coughing on inhalation of the powder formulation). It is now available as an oral preparation or via nebulizer. *Nedocromil sodium* inhibits the bronchoconstrictor response to inhaled antigens and inhibits the activity of and release of inflammatory cell types, such as histamine, leukotrienes, and prostaglandins. The drug has few side effects and is used for maintenance therapy in asthma; it is not effective for reversal of acute exacerbations and is not used in children younger than 5 years of age.

Leukotrienes are mediators of inflammation that cause increases in airway hyperresponsiveness. Leukotriene modifiers (e.g., zafirlukast [Accolate] and montelukast sodium [Singulair]) block inflammatory and bronchospasm effects. These drugs are not used to treat acute episodes but are given orally in combination with β_2 agonists and steroids to provide long-term control and prevent symptoms in mild persistent asthma. Montelukast is approved for children 12 months of age and older, and zafirlukast is approved for children 5 years of age and older.

Anticholinergics (atropine and ipratropium [Atrovent]) may relieve acute bronchospasm. However, these drugs have adverse side effects that include drying of respiratory secretions, blurred vision, and cardiac and CNS stimulation. The primary anticholinergic drug used is ipratropium, which does not cross the blood-brain barrier and therefore elicits no CNS effects. Ipratropium, when used in combination with albuterol, can be effective during acute severe asthma in improving lung function in children coming to the ED (Liu et al., 2016).

Omalizumab (Xolair) is a *monoclonal antibody* that blocks the binding of IgE to mast cells. Blocking this interaction inhibits the inflammation that is associated with asthma. It is used in patients with moderate to persistent asthma who have confirmed perennial aeroallergen sensitivity, have total serum IgE levels between 30 and 700 international units/mL, and have had poor control of symptoms on inhaled steroids. Many patients with asthma are atopic and possess specific IgE antibodies to allergens responsible for airway inflammation. Xolair has been approved for use in children 12 years of age and older in the United States. The drug is administered once or twice per month by subcutaneous injection. Efficacy of omalizumab is not immediate and can take up to 16 weeks (Humbert, Busse, & Hanania, 2014). In early 2007, the FDA added a "black box warning" to the drug, which highlights the risk for anaphylaxis. Since that time, the US Food and Drug Administration reported an increase in cardiovascular and cerebrovascular adverse events related to its use. Some children with severe asthma and a history of severe life-threatening episodes may need a prescription for an EpiPen (subcutaneous injectable epinephrine).

Exercise

Exercise-induced bronchospasm (EIB) is an acute, reversible, usually self-terminating airway obstruction that develops during or after vigorous activity, reaches its peak 5 to 10 minutes after stopping the activity, and usually stops in another 20 to 30 minutes. Patients with EIB have cough, shortness of breath, chest pain or tightness, wheezing, and endurance problems during exercise, but an exercise challenge test in a laboratory is necessary to make the diagnosis.

The problem is rare in activities that require short bursts of energy (e.g., baseball, sprints, gymnastics, skiing) and more common in those that involve endurance exercise (e.g., soccer, basketball, distance running). Swimming is well tolerated by children with EIB because they are breathing air fully saturated with moisture and because of the type of breathing required in swimming.

Children with asthma are often excluded from exercise by parents, teachers, and practitioners, as well as by the children themselves because they are reluctant to provoke an attack. However, this practice can seriously hamper peer interaction and physical health. Exercise is advantageous for children with asthma, and most children can participate in activities at school and in sports with minimal difficulty, provided their asthma is under control. Appropriate prophylactic treatment with β-adrenergic agents or cromolyn sodium before exercise usually permits full participation in strenuous exertion.

Breathing Exercises

Breathing exercises and physical training help produce physical and mental relaxation, improve posture, strengthen respiratory musculature, and develop more efficient patterns of breathing. For motivated children, breathing exercises and controlled breathing are of value in preventing overinflation and improving efficiency of the cough. However, these exercises are not recommended during acute, uncomplicated exacerbation of asthma.

Hyposensitization

The role of hyposensitization in childhood asthma has become controversial. In the past, immunotherapy was used for seasonal allergies and when single substances were identified as the offending allergen. It is not recommended for allergens that can be eliminated, such as foods, drugs, and animal dander. Immunotherapy is considered for asthma patients in the following situations (Kwong & Leibel, 2013):

- Patient's preference
- Poor adherence to therapy
- Incomplete response to allergen avoidance
- Significant medication side effects or adverse effects
- Multiple- and/or high-dose medication requirements

Injection therapy is usually limited to clinically significant allergens. The initial dose of the offending allergen(s), based on the size of the skin reaction, is injected subcutaneously. The amount is increased at weekly intervals until a maximum tolerance is reached, after which a maintenance dose is given at 4-week intervals. This may be extended to 5- or 6-week intervals during the off-season for seasonal allergens. Successful treatment is continued for a minimum of 3 years and then stopped. If no symptoms appear, acquired immunity is assumed; if symptoms recur, treatment is reinstituted. Hyposensitization injections should be administered only with emergency equipment and medications readily available in the event of an anaphylactic reaction.

Status Asthmaticus

Status asthmaticus is a medical emergency that can result in respiratory failure and death if untreated. Children who continue to display respiratory distress despite vigorous therapeutic measures, especially the use of sympathomimetics (e.g., albuterol, epinephrine), are in status asthmaticus. The condition may develop gradually or rapidly, often coincident with complicating conditions, such as pneumonia or a respiratory virus, that can influence the duration and treatment of the exacerbation.

! NURSING ALERT

A child with asthma who sweats profusely, remains sitting upright, and refuses to lie down is in severe respiratory distress. Also, a child who suddenly becomes agitated or an agitated child who suddenly becomes quiet may have serious hypoxia and requires immediate intervention.

Therapy for status asthmaticus is aimed at improving ventilation, decreasing airway resistance, relieving bronchospasm, correcting dehydration and acidosis, allaying child and parent anxiety related to the severity of the event, and treating any concurrent infection. Humidified oxygen is recommended and should be given to maintain an oxygen saturation greater than 90%. Inhaled aerosolized short-acting β_2 agonists are recommended for all patients. Three treatments of β_2 agonists spaced 20 to 30 minutes apart are usually given as initial therapy, and continuous administration of β_2 agonists via nebulizer may be initiated. A systemic corticosteroid (oral, IV, or IM) is given to decrease the effects of inflammation. An anticholinergic agent, such as ipratropium bromide, may be added to the aerosolized solution of the β_2 agonist. Anticholinergics have been shown to result in additional bronchodilation in patients with severe airflow obstruction. An IV infusion is often initiated to provide a means for hydration and to administer medications. Correction of dehydration, acidosis, hypoxia, and electrolyte disturbance is guided by frequent determination of arterial pH, blood gases, and serum electrolytes.

Additional therapies in acute asthma attacks include the use of IV magnesium sulfate, a potent muscle relaxant that acts to decrease inflammation and improves pulmonary function and peak flow rate among pediatric patients with moderate to severe asthma when treated in the ED. Heliox may be administered to decrease airway resistance and thereby decrease the work of breathing; heliox can be delivered via a nonrebreathing face mask from premixed tanks, which may be blended in a stand-alone unit or within a ventilator. Heliox may be used in acute exacerbations as an adjunct to β_2-agonist and IV corticosteroid therapy to improve pulmonary function until the two latter medications have time to take full effect in decreasing bronchospasm; whereas the effects of heliox are usually seen within 20 minutes of administration, other drugs may take longer to exert the desired effect. Ketamine, a dissociative anesthetic, is believed to cause smooth muscle relaxation and decrease airway resistance caused by severe bronchospasm in acute asthma; it may be administered as an adjunct to other therapies mentioned previously, although evidence on the use of this in asthma is limited. Antibiotics should not be used to treat acute asthma attacks except when a bacterial infection resulting from another condition such as pneumonia or sinusitis is present.

A child suspected of having status asthmaticus is usually seen in the ED and is often admitted to a pediatric ICU for close observation and continuous cardiorespiratory monitoring. A key component in the prevention of morbidity is helping the child, parents, teachers, coaches, and other adults recognize features of deteriorating respiratory status, use the correct rescue drugs effectively, and immediately place the child with deteriorating respiratory status into the care of health care professionals instead of waiting to see if the asthma improves on its own. For the child going into early status asthmaticus, immediate medical care is required to prevent irreversible respiratory failure and possible death (see Nursing Care Plan box: The Child with Acute Respiratory Tract Infection).

Prognosis

Although deaths from asthma have been relatively uncommon since the 1980s, the rate of death from asthma increased steadily in the United States until it peaked in the mid-1990s. Asthma-related deaths decreased from 2000 to 2009; 84 deaths were noted among children in the United States in 2000 compared to 33 deaths among children in the United States in 2009 (Hasegawa, Tsugawa, Brown, et al., 2013). The rate of hospitalization due to asthma decreased significantly from 2000 to 2009 in children younger than 18 years of age; however, the use of invasive and noninvasive mechanical ventilation significantly increased during that time (Hasegawa et al). African-American children have 2 to 7 times more hospitalizations, ED visits, and deaths than those of white and Hispanic children (Liu et al., 2016). Most asthma deaths in children occur in the home, school, or community before lifesaving medical care can be administered.

Some children's asthma symptoms may improve at puberty, but up to two thirds of children with asthma continue to have symptoms through puberty and into adulthood. The prognosis for control or disappearance of symptoms varies in children from those who have rare and infrequent attacks to those who are constantly wheezing or are subject to status asthmaticus. Risk factors that may predict the persistence of symptoms into childhood (from infancy) include atopy, male gender, exposure to environmental tobacco, and maternal history of asthma. Many children who outgrow their exacerbations continue to have airway hyperresponsiveness and cough as adults.

The younger child and adolescent age group appear to be the most vulnerable, with the greatest increase occurring in children younger than 4 years of age and 12 to 17 years of age (Hasegawa et al., 2013). No reliable data exist to explain this increase. Factors that have been postulated include exposure of atopic individuals to more allergens (particularly in large urban centers), change in severity of the disease, abuse of drug therapy (toxicity), failure of families and practitioners to recognize the severity of asthma, and psychologic factors, such as denial and refusal to accept the disease. On the other hand, studies have shown that children living in rural areas and farming communities have a decreased incidence of asthma and allergy (Liu et al, 2016).

Risk factors for asthma deaths include early onset, frequent attacks, difficult-to-manage disease, adolescence, history of respiratory failure, psychologic problems (refusal to take medications), dependency on or misuse of asthma drugs (high use), presence of physical stigmata (barrel chest, intercostal retractions), and abnormal PFT results.

Interprofessional Care Management

Acute Asthma Care

Children who are admitted to the hospital with acute asthma are ill, anxious, and uncomfortable. The importance of continual observation and assessment cannot be overemphasized.

When β_2 agonists, supplemental oxygen, and corticosteroids are given, the child is monitored closely and continuously for relief of respiratory distress and signs of side effects or toxicity. Pulse oximetry is monitored along with rate and depth of breathing, auscultation of air movement, adventitious sounds, and any signs of respiratory distress (e.g., nasal flaring, tachypnea, retractions). The child on supplemental oxygen requires intermittent or continuous oxygenation monitoring depending on severity of respiratory compromise and initial oxygenation status. The child in status asthmaticus should be placed on continuous cardiorespiratory (including blood pressure) and pulse oximetry monitoring. Oral fluid intake may be limited during the acute phase; IV fluid replacement may be required to provide adequate tissue hydration.

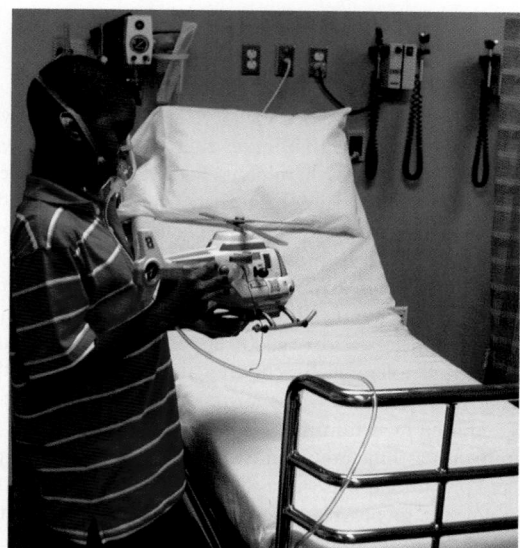

FIG 40.6 Child with asthma is allowed play activity as tolerated.

Older children may be more comfortable standing (Fig. 40.6), sitting upright, or leaning slightly forward (Fig. 40.7). Shortness of breath makes talking difficult. The calm, efficient presence of a care provider helps reassure children that they are safe and will be cared for during this stressful period. It is important to assure children that they will not be left alone and that their parents are allowed to remain with them. Parents want to be informed of their child's condition and therapies. They may believe that they have in some way contributed to the child's condition or could have prevented the episode. Reassurance regarding their efforts expended on the child's behalf and their parenting capabilities can help alleviate their stress. Efforts to reduce parental apprehension will also reduce the child's distress. Some institutions use an asthma scoring tool assessing the child's respiratory rate, oxygen requirements, auscultation findings, retractions, and degree of dyspnea to evaluate asthma severity. Members of the health care team can use this tool to evaluate how the child is responding to the medications and other therapies.

Long-Term Asthma Care

Care of children with asthma involves helping children and their families learn to live with the condition. The disease can be managed so that it does not require hospitalization or interfere with family life, physical activity, or school attendance. The nursing process in the care of the child with asthma is outlined in the Nursing Care Plan box: The Child with Asthma.

Nurses may perform a variety of functions in asthma care. These may include asthma education in the primary care setting and in schools and other community settings, care of the child with asthma in the acute care setting, ambulatory care, care coordination, and intensive care. Nurses also obtain information on how asthma affects the child's everyday activities and self-concept, the child's and family's adherence to the prescribed therapy, and their personal treatment goals. Every effort is made to build a partnership between the child and family and the health care team, and effective communication is an essential part of this partnership. In particular, the child and family's satisfaction with asthma control and with the quality of care should be assessed. The nurse should also assess the child and family's perception of the severity of the disease and their level of social support.

One of the major emphases is outpatient management by the family. Parents are taught how to prevent exacerbations, to recognize and respond

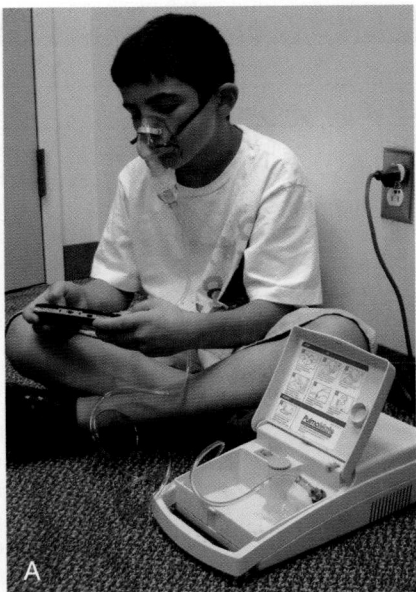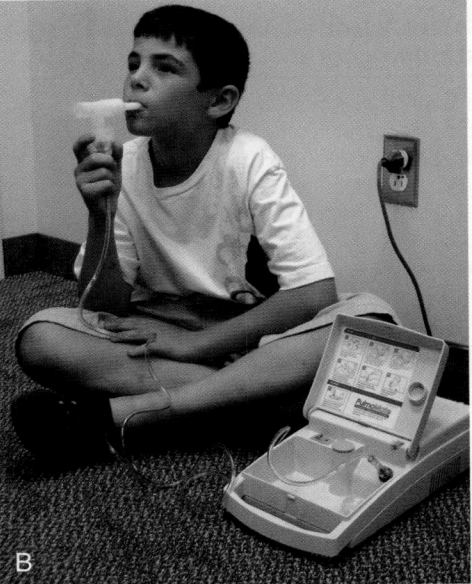

FIG 40.7 Children with asthma may take a nebulized aerosol treatment with a mask **(A)** or mouthpiece **(B).** (Courtesy of Texas Children's Hospital, Houston, TX.)

◎ NURSING CARE PLAN

The Child With Asthma

Case Study

Jeremy is a 17-year-old patient with a history of asthma. His asthma symptoms have been controlled with use of a long-acting inhaler twice daily, but an increase in seasonal allergies and a recent upper respiratory infection has caused an exacerbation of his symptoms. Jeremy rarely uses his peak expiratory flow meter, instead he waits until his symptoms become severe before starting to use his rescue medications. He now presents to his primary care provider with his mother to seek further treatment as his symptoms are not resolving with his current treatment.

Assessment

Based on these events, what are the most important subjective and objective data that should be assessed?

Defining Characteristics

Dyspnea
Shortness of breath
Diminished breath sounds and/or adventitious breath sounds (wheezing)
Increased respiratory rate
Use of accessory muscles (retractions)
Dry cough
Chest tightness or chest pain

Nursing Diagnoses

Impaired Breathing Pattern
Ineffective Airway Clearance
Ineffective Health Management

Nursing Interventions and Rationales

What are the most appropriate nursing interventions for a child with acute respiratory tract infection?

Nursing Interventions	Rationales
Monitor airway, breathing, and circulation (ABCs) closely.	To provide supportive measures as needed to maintain airway, breathing, and circulation
Allow Jeremy to assume position of comfort.	To promote maximum ventilator function
Administer humidified oxygen to maintain oxygen saturation above 90%.	To enhance oxygenation of tissues
Administer rescue medications (as prescribed) that can include inhalers, nebulizer, and/or oral or intravenous steroids.	To open constricted airways and allow air exchange and to enhance tissue oxygenation
Assess patient's response to rescue medications.	To determine need for more aggressive interventions
Assist Jeremy in recognizing factors that trigger asthma symptoms.	To avoid factors that exacerbate asthma
Assist Jeremy to understand the purpose and use of peak expiratory flow meter (PEFM).	To allow early recognition of asthma symptoms before acute exacerbation
Observe technique for use of PEFM, inhaler, and/or nebulizer.	To ensure appropriate technique to maximize accuracy and effectiveness

Expected Outcomes

Adolescent will breathe easily with nonlabored respirations at a rate within normal limits for age.
Adolescent will maintain patent airway.
Adolescent will verbalize understanding of health maintenance measures (i.e., avoiding triggers, use of peak flow meter, use of inhalers).

Case Study (Continued)

Jeremy had no improvement with the nebulized treatment provided in the primary care office, and his symptoms worsened. He was transferred to a nearby hospital

Continued

◎ NURSING CARE PLAN

The Child With Asthma—cont'd

for further evaluation. Upon arrival to the emergency department (ED), Jeremy is unable to answer questions, refuses to lie down, and displays short rapid breaths with significant retractions. His mother is concerned about what is happening to him.

Assessment

What are the most important signs and symptoms based on this scenario?

Defining Characteristics

Inability to speak in full sentences
Agitation, confusion
Rapidly progressive shortness of breath
Tachypnea and tachycardia
Chest tightness
Retractions
Cyanosis

Nursing Diagnoses

Impaired Breathing Pattern
Ineffective Airway Clearance
Impaired Gas Exchange
Readiness for Enhanced Knowledge (family)

Nursing Interventions and Rationales

What are the most appropriate nursing interventions for this child?

Nursing Interventions	Rationales
Monitor airway, breathing, and circulation (ABCs) closely.	To provide supportive measures as needed to maintain airway, breathing, and circulation
Allow Jeremy to assume position of comfort.	To promote maximum ventilator function

Nursing Interventions	Rationales
Administer humidified oxygen to maintain oxygen saturation above 90%.	To enhance oxygenation of tissues
Administer short-acting beta agonists continuously via nebulizer (as prescribed).	To open constricted airways and allow air exchange and to enhance tissue oxygenation
Obtain blood specimen for electrolytes, complete blood count, renal function tests, and arterial blood gases (ABGs).	To determine current status of patient and institute therapy based on results
Obtain intravenous (IV) access and administer corticosteroid, hydration, and electrolytes as prescribed.	To decrease inflammation and correct dehydration, acidosis, and electrolyte disturbances
Educate family about status asthmaticus and treatment underway to resolve condition.	To promote understanding of characteristics and treatment for status asthmaticus
Arrange for social worker to meet with family to assess emotional and financial needs.	To identify and modify stressors associated with acute exacerbation of illness and sudden hospitalization
Transfer Jeremy from the emergency department (ED) to the pediatric intensive care unit (PICU).	To allow for continuous cardiorespiratory monitoring and further treatment

Expected Outcomes

Respirations will be nonlabored at a rate within normal limits for age.
Airway will be patent
Adequate gas exchange will be maintained.
Family will verbalize understanding of condition and treatment.

---

to bronchospasm, to maintain health and prevent complications, and to promote normal activities. Cultural or ethnic beliefs or practices may influence management and necessitate modifications in approaches to meet the family's needs. Inconsistent home care, on the part of either the child or the parents, often leads to unnecessary ED visits for management.

Avoid Allergens

One goal of asthma management is avoidance of an exacerbation. Children and parents need to know how to avoid allergens that precipitate asthma episodes. The nurse and social worker assist the parent in modifying the environment to reduce contact with the offending allergen(s). Parents are cautioned to avoid exposing a sensitive child to excessive cold, wind, and other extremes of weather; smoke (open fire or tobacco); sprays; scents; and other irritants. Foods known to provoke symptoms should be eliminated from the diet.

Approximately 2% to 6% of children with asthma are sensitive to aspirin; therefore, nurses should caution parents to use other analgesic and antipyretic drugs for discomfort or fever and to read package labeling. Although aspirin is rarely given to children in the United States, salicylate compounds are in other common medicines such as Pepto-Bismol. Children with aspirin-induced asthma may also be sensitive to nonsteroidal antiinflammatory drugs (NSAIDs) and tartrazine (yellow dye number 5, a common food coloring).

❗ NURSING ALERT

Parents are encouraged to avoid administering aspirin to any child due to the risk for Reye syndrome, unless specifically recommended by and under the supervision of a health care provider. Acetaminophen is safe for children and is the analgesic of choice.

Relieve Bronchospasm

Teach parents and older children to recognize early signs and symptoms of an impending attack so that it can be controlled before symptoms become distressing. Most children can recognize prodromal symptoms well before an attack (about 6 hours) and implement preventive therapy. Objective signs that parents may observe include rhinorrhea, cough, low-grade fever, irritability, itching (especially in front of the neck and chest), apathy, anxiety, sleep disturbance, abdominal discomfort, and loss of appetite.

Children who use a nebulizer, MDI, Diskus, or Turbuhaler to deliver drugs need to learn how to use the device correctly. The MDI device delivers medication directly to the airways; therefore the child needs to learn to breathe slowly and deeply for better distribution to narrowed airways (see Patient Teaching box: Use of a Metered-Dose Inhaler).

PATIENT TEACHING

*Use of a Metered-Dose Inhaler**

Steps for Using the Inhaler With a Mouthpiece

1. Remove the cap, and hold the inhaler upright.
2. Shake the inhaler.
3. Attach a spacer, as appropriate.
4. Tilt the head back slightly, and breathe out slowly.
5. With the inhaler in an upright position, insert the mouthpiece:
   a. About 3 to 4 cm (1 to 1½ inches) from the mouth *or*
   b. Into the mouth, forming an airtight seal between the lips and the mouthpiece
6. At the end of a normal expiration, depress the top of the inhaler canister firmly to release the medication (into the mouth), and breathe in slowly (about 3 to 5 seconds). Relax the pressure on the top of the canister.
7. Hold the breath for at least 5 to 10 seconds to allow the aerosol medication to reach deeply into the lungs.
8. Remove the inhaler, and breathe out slowly through the nose.
9. Wait 1 minute between puffs (if an additional puff is needed) when using a bronchodilator.

Steps for Using the Inhaler With an AeroChamber (See Fig. 40.5)

1. Remove the cap, and hold the inhaler upright.
2. Shake the inhaler.
3. Attach the AeroChamber.
4. With the inhaler in an upright position, insert the mouthpiece into the back of the AeroChamber.
5. Apply the AeroChamber mask to the child's face, and make sure there is a good seal.
6. Have the child breathe slow, regular breaths. Depress the top of the inhaler canister firmly to release the medication (into the AeroChamber) as the child breathes slowly in and out. Relax the pressure on the top of the canister.
7. Hold the AeroChamber in place over the child's face until six breaths have been taken. Give one puff at a time.
8. Remove the inhaler and AeroChamber.
9. Wait 1 minute between puffs (if an additional puff is needed) when using a bronchodilator.

*Inhaled dry powder such as budesonide (Pulmicort) requires a different inhalation technique. To use a dry-powder inhaler, the base of the device is turned until a click is heard. It is important to close the mouth tightly around the mouthpiece of the inhaler and inhale rapidly.

A spacer or AeroChamber device should be used with MDI inhalers. These devices allow the parent or child to deliver the medication from the MDI and slowly inhale it. Spacers also help prevent yeast infections in the mouth when corticosteroids are inhaled via an MDI (see Fig. 40.5).

The child and parents also need to be cautioned about the adverse effects of prescribed drugs and the dangers of overuse of β_2 agonists. They should know that it is important to use these drugs when needed but not indiscriminately or as a substitute for avoiding the symptom-provoking allergen.

! NURSING ALERT

Long-acting β2-agonist inhalers (salmeterol) should be used only as directed (usually every 12 hours) and not more frequently. They are not intended to relieve acute asthmatic symptoms.

The family may be asked to obtain a PEFM and learn to use this device to monitor the child's asthma if the child is 5 years of age and older. A written asthma action plan that includes the three peak flow meter zones and the child's asthma medications may be obtained from the child's primary care provider. A home asthma action plan may reduce the risk for asthma death by 70% (Liu et al., 2016). Medications used for asthma exacerbations are also included in the asthma plan. This action plan should be used to make decisions about asthma management at home and at school. The nurse may assist the child and family in understanding the written action plan, emphasizing that the child and family determine the success of the plan, not the health professionals. Teach parents how to read labels on prepared foods and snacks to determine the presence of allergens.

The child should be protected from a respiratory tract infection that can trigger an attack or aggravate the asthmatic state, especially in young children whose airways are mechanically smaller and more reactive. Annual influenza vaccinations are recommended for all children older than 6 months of age. Pneumococcal vaccines should also be maintained. Equipment used for the child, such as nebulizers, must be kept absolutely clean to decrease the chances of contamination with bacteria and fungi.

Teach breathing exercises and controlled breathing, and the nurse should provide information concerning activities that promote diaphragmatic breathing, side expansion, and improved mobility of the chest wall. Play techniques that can be used for younger children to extend their expiratory time and increase expiratory pressure include blowing cotton balls or a Ping-Pong ball on a table, blowing a pinwheel, blowing bubbles, or preventing a tissue from falling by blowing it against the wall.

Self-care and asthma self-management programs are important in helping the child and family cope with asthma. Self-contained programs and brochures for patient education are available from the Asthma and Allergy Foundation of America* and the American Lung Association.[†] The National Heart, Lung, and Blood Institute[‡] provides fact sheets and educational materials for asthma education in the school setting. Practice parameters and guidelines can be obtained from the American Academy of Allergy Asthma & Immunology.[§]

Support Child or Adolescent and Family

The nurse working with children with asthma can provide support in a number of ways. Many children voice frustration because their exacerbations interfere with their daily activities and social lives. Children need education on their condition and reassurance from the health care team that they can learn to control and cope with their asthma and live a normal life.

Children in disruptive family situations (divorce, separation, violence, custodial battles) may disregard their daily asthma medication regimen or may be at higher risk as a result of neglect by adults who are in charge of their care. Adolescents struggling with a sense of identity and body image often regard asthma as a condition that will "go away," especially if there is a time lapse between symptoms, and may abandon the therapeutic regimen. Referral for counseling and guidance is appropriate when the child's or adolescent's life is potentially in harm's

---

*8201 Corporate Drive, Suite 1000, Landover, MD 20785; 800-7-Asthma; www.aafa.org.

[†]1301 Pennsylvania Avenue NW, Suite 800, Washington, DC 20004; 800-548-8252; national headquarters: 202-785-3385; www.lungusa.org.

[‡]NHLBI Health Information Center, PO Box 30105, Bethesda, MD 20824-0105; 301-592-8573; www.nhlbi.nih.gov.

[§]555 E. Wells Street, Suite 1100, Milwaukee, WI 53202; 414-272-6071; http://aaaai.org.

way and the therapeutic regimen for asthma is abandoned because of personal or family crises.

CYSTIC FIBROSIS

Cystic fibrosis (CF) is inherited as an autosomal recessive trait; the affected child inherits the defective gene from both parents, with an overall risk of 1 in 4 if both parents carry the gene. The mutated gene responsible for CF is located on the long arm of chromosome 7. This gene codes a protein of 1480 amino acids called *the cystic fibrosis transmembrane conductance regulator (CFTR)*. The CFTR protein is related to a family of membrane-bound glycoproteins. The glycoproteins constitute a cAMP-activated chloride channel and regulate other chloride and sodium channels at the surfaces of the epithelial cells.

Pathophysiology

CF is characterized by several clinical features, which are increased viscosity of mucous gland secretions, a striking elevation of sweat electrolytes, an increase in several organic and enzymatic constituents of saliva, and abnormalities in autonomic nervous system function. Although both sodium and chloride are affected, the defect appears to be primarily a result of abnormal chloride movement; the CFTR appears to function as a chloride channel. Children with CF demonstrate an increase in sodium and chloride in both saliva and sweat. This characteristic is the basis for the sweat chloride diagnostic test. The sweat electrolyte abnormality is present from birth, continues throughout life, and is unrelated to the severity of the disease or the extent to which other organs are involved.

The primary factor, and the one that is responsible for many of the clinical manifestations of the disease, is mechanical obstruction caused by the increased viscosity of mucous gland secretions (Fig. 40.8). Instead of forming a thin, freely flowing secretion, the mucous glands produce a thick mucoprotein that accumulates and dilates them. Small passages in organs, such as the pancreas and bronchioles, become obstructed as secretions precipitate or coagulate to form concretions in glands and ducts. The earliest postnatal manifestation of CF is often *meconium ileus* in the newborn, in which the small intestine is blocked with thick, puttylike, tenacious, mucilaginous meconium.

In the pancreas, the thick secretions block the ducts, eventually causing pancreatic fibrosis. This blockage prevents essential pancreatic enzymes from reaching the duodenum, which causes marked impairment in the digestion and absorption of nutrients. The disturbed function is reflected in bulky stools that are frothy from undigested fat (steatorrhea) and foul smelling from putrefied protein (azotorrhea).

Because of the changes in pancreatic architecture and diminished blood supply over time in children with CF, the incidence of diabetes mellitus (DM) (cystic fibrosis–related diabetes [CFRD]) is greater in children with CF than in the general population. Prevalence is estimated at 18% of adolescents with CF that increases to 30% by 30 years of age (Dashiff, Suzui-Crumly, Krace, Britton, & Moreland, 2013). CFRD is reported to be the most common complication associated with CF. The primary characteristic of CFRD is severe insulin deficiency as a result of β-cell dysfunction; however, CFRD also may demonstrate fluctuating insulin resistance, especially during acute illness. Thus, CFRD has characteristics of both type 1 DM and type 2 DM but is considered to be its own entity (Moran, Pillay, Becker, et al., 2014). The positive

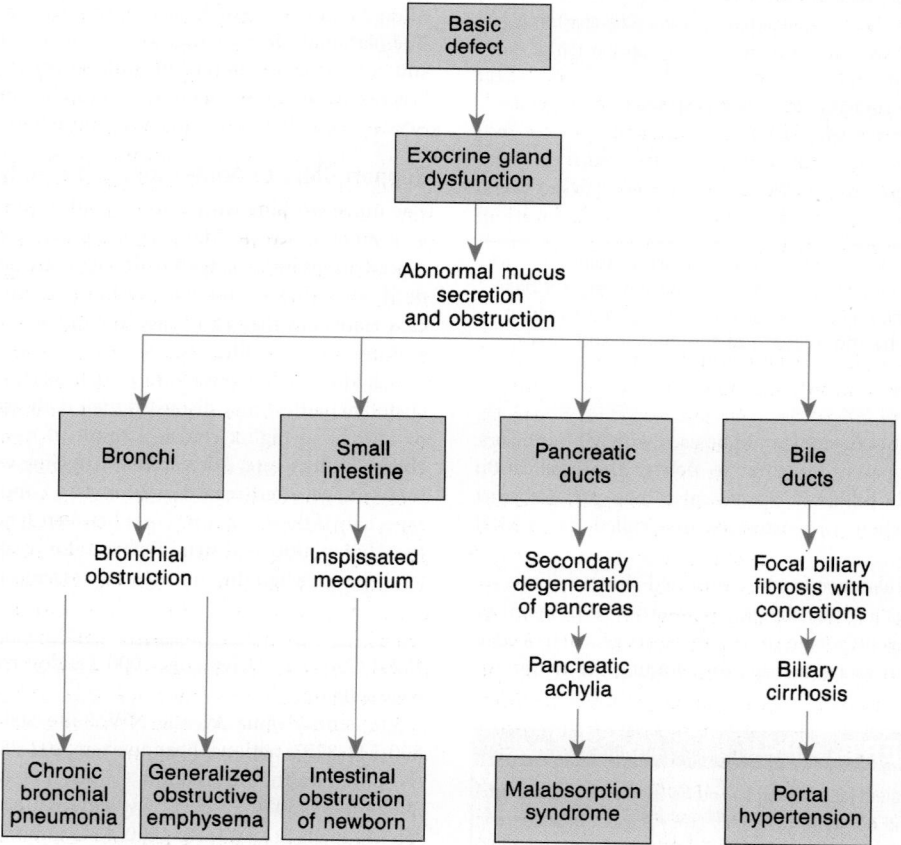

FIG 40.8 Various effects of exocrine gland dysfunction in cystic fibrosis.

correlation between nutritional status and optimal pulmonary function in patients with CF has been described; the presence of adequate insulin appears to be a key factor in maintaining an adequate nutritional status. Experts continue to recommend a high-fat, high-calorie diet in CF patients, and at this time there is no evidence to support a change in this diet for patients with CFRD (Ode & Moran, 2013).

A common gastrointestinal complication associated with CF is *prolapse of the rectum*, which occurs in infancy and childhood and is related to large, bulky stools; malabsorption; and increased intra-abdominal pressure secondary to paroxysmal cough. Affected children of all ages are subject to intestinal obstruction from heavy or impacted feces. Gum-like masses in the cecum can obstruct the bowel and produce a partial or complete obstruction, a condition that is referred to as *distal intestinal obstruction syndrome*.

Pulmonary complications are present in almost all children with CF, but the onset and extent of involvement are variable. Symptoms are produced by stagnation of mucus in the airways, with eventual bacterial colonization leading to destruction of lung tissue. The abnormally viscous and tenacious secretions are difficult to expectorate and gradually obstruct the bronchi and bronchioles, causing scattered areas of bronchiectasis, atelectasis, and hyperinflation. The stagnant mucus also offers a favorable environment for bacterial growth. The reproductive systems of both males and females with CF are affected. Fertility can be inhibited by highly viscous cervical secretions, which act as a plug, blocking sperm entry. Women with CF who become pregnant have an increased incidence of premature labor and birth and infant low birth weight. Favorable nutritional status and pulmonary function are positively correlated with favorable pregnancy outcomes. Most men (95%) with CF are sterile, which may be caused by blockage of the vas deferens with abnormal secretions or by failure of normal development of the wolffian duct structures (vas deferens, epididymis, and seminal vesicles), resulting in decreased or absent sperm production.

Growth and development are often affected in children with moderate to severe forms of CF. Physical growth may be restricted as a result of decreased absorption of nutrients, including vitamins and fat; increased oxygen demands for pulmonary function; and delayed bone growth. The usual pattern is one of growth failure (failure to thrive) with increased weight loss despite an increased appetite and gradual deterioration of the respiratory system. Clinical manifestations of CF are listed in Box 40.16.

Diagnostic Evaluation

Traditionally, the diagnosis of CF was based on the presence of one or more characteristic features (chronic sinopulmonary disease, gastrointestinal or nutritional abnormalities, salt loss syndromes, genital abnormalities in males), a history of CF in a sibling, or a positive newborn screen plus laboratory confirmation of an abnormality in the *CFTR* gene or protein. However, more than 2000 mutations have now been identified in the *CFTR* gene, not all of which result in CF (Barrio, 2015).

Newer diagnostic methods make it possible to screen newborns for CF. Universal newborn screening for CF is now required by law in all states in the United States. The newborn screening test consists of an immunoreactive trypsinogen (IRT) analysis performed on a dried spot of blood, which may be followed by direct analysis of DNA for the presence of the ΔF508 mutation or other mutations on the same dried blood spot. A positive screen indicates persistent hypertrypsinogenemia and does not diagnose CF but identifies infants at risk for CF. Further testing is needed to confirm or rule out CF. Benefits of early screening and detection include preventing undernutrition of identified infants to optimize lung function and improve height and weight. A disadvantage of newborn screening is parental anxiety associated with a false-positive

---

BOX 40.16 Clinical Manifestations of Cystic Fibrosis

Meconium Ileus*
- Abdominal distention
- Vomiting
- Failure to pass stools
- Rapid development of dehydration

Gastrointestinal Manifestations
- Large, bulky, loose, frothy, extremely foul-smelling stools
- Voracious appetite (early in disease)
- Loss of appetite (later in disease)
- Weight loss
- Marked tissue wasting
- Growth failure
- Distended abdomen
- Thin extremities
- Sallow skin
- Evidence of deficiency of fat-soluble vitamins A, D, E, and K
- Anemia

Pulmonary Manifestations
Initial Signs
- Wheezing respirations
- Dry, nonproductive cough

Eventually
- Increased dyspnea
- Paroxysmal cough
- Evidence of obstructive emphysema and patchy areas of atelectasis

Progressive Involvement
- Overinflated, barrel-shaped chest
- Cyanosis
- Clubbing of fingers and toes
- Repeated episodes of bronchitis and bronchopneumonia

*In about 10% of cases.

---

result. An in utero diagnosis of CF is also possible based on detection of two CF mutations in the fetus.

The consistent finding of abnormally high sodium and chloride concentrations in the sweat is a unique characteristic of CF. Parents may report that their infant tastes "salty" when they kiss him or her. The quantitative sweat chloride test (pilocarpine iontophoresis) involves stimulating the production of sweat with a special device (involves stimulation with 3-mA electric current), collecting the sweat on filter paper, and measuring the sweat electrolytes. The quantitative analysis requires a sufficient volume of sweat (>75 mg). Two separate samples are collected to ensure the reliability of the test for any individual. Normally, sweat chloride content is less than 40 mEq/L, with a mean of 18 mEq/L. A chloride concentration greater than 60 mEq/L in a child 6 months of age or older is diagnostic of CF; a concentration between 40 and 59 mmol/L is indeterminate, and a repeat test should be performed in 1 to 2 months (Nicholson, 2013). In some situations, DNA testing may be substituted for the sweat test. The presence of a mutation known to cause CF on each *CFTR* gene predicts with a high degree of certainty that the individual has CF; however, multiple CFTR mutations may also be present and detected with DNA assay.

Chest radiography reveals characteristic patchy atelectasis and obstructive emphysema. PFTs are sensitive indexes of lung function, providing evidence of abnormal small airway function in CF. Other diagnostic tools that may aid in diagnosis include stool fat or enzyme analysis. Stool analysis requires a 72-hour sample with accurate recording of food intake during that time. Radiographs, including a contrast enema, are used for diagnosis of meconium ileus.

Therapeutic Management

Improved survival among patients with CF during the past 2 decades is attributable largely to antibiotic therapy and improved nutritional and respiratory management. Goals of CF therapy are to (1) prevent or minimize pulmonary complications, (2) prevent chronic pseudomonas infection, (3) ensure adequate nutrition for growth, and (4) encourage appropriate physical activity. A multidisciplinary approach to treatment is needed to accomplish these goals.

Management of Pulmonary Problems

Management of pulmonary problems is directed toward prevention and treatment of pulmonary infection by improving ventilation, removing mucopurulent secretions, and administering antimicrobial agents. Many children develop respiratory symptoms by 3 years of age. The large amounts and viscosity of respiratory secretions in children with CF contribute to the likelihood of respiratory tract infections. Recurrent pulmonary infections in children with CF result in greater damage to the airways; small airways are destroyed, causing bronchiectasis.

The most common pathogens responsible for pulmonary infections are *Pseudomonas aeruginosa, Burkholderia cepacia, S. aureus, H. influenzae, Escherichia coli,* and *Klebsiella pneumoniae. P. aeruginosa,* and *B. cepacia* are particularly pathogenic for children with CF, and infections with these organisms are difficult to eradicate. In addition, children with CF who are chronically colonized with these organisms have poorer survival rates than children who are not colonized. Colonization and infection with methicillin-resistant *Staphylococcus aureus* (MRSA) has emerged as a critical factor in lung infection and pulmonary function in patients with CF, especially in patients 11 to 24 years of age (Zobell, Epps, Young, et al., 2015). Depending on the severity of the infection, patients with MRSA can be treated with oral antibiotics as an outpatient or may require IV antibiotics as an inpatient. Fungal colonization with *Candida* or *Aspergillus* organisms in the respiratory tract is also common in patients with CF.

Airway clearance therapies (ACTs) are an essential part of CF management and include percussion and postural drainage, positive expiratory pressure (PEP), active-cycle-of-breathing technique, autogenic drainage, oscillatory PEP, high-frequency chest compressions (HFCCs), and exercise. Studies have demonstrated that no particular ACT has any advantage over the other in relation to outcomes of sputum production; however, it is recommended that individualized assessment occur to determine the best ACT for each patient. *Airway clearance therapies* such as percussion and postural drainage are usually performed on average twice daily (on rising and in the evening) and more frequently if needed, especially during pulmonary infection. The Flutter mucus clearance device is a small handheld plastic pipe with a stainless-steel ball on the inside that facilitates removal of mucus. It has the advantage of increasing sputum expectoration and being used without an assistant. Handheld percussors may be used to loosen secretions. Another method to clear mucus is hHFCC in which the child temporarily wears a mechanical vest device that provides high-frequency chest wall oscillation.

The active cycle of breathing technique is a series of breathing techniques to help clear secretions. Forced expiration, or "huffing," with the glottis partially closed helps move secretions from the small airways so that subsequent coughing can move secretions forcefully from the large airways. Another mucus-clearing technique involves use of a PEP mask; this technique involves breathing into a mask attached to a one-way valve, which creates resistance; as the patient exhales, the airway is kept open by the pressure, and mucus is forced into the upper airway for expulsion.

Bronchodilator medication delivered in an aerosol opens bronchi for easier expectoration and is administered before percussion and postural drainage when the patient exhibits evidence of reactive airway disease or wheezing. Another aerosolized medication is recombinant human deoxyribonuclease (DNase, known generically as dornase alfa [Pulmozyme]), which decreases the viscosity of mucus. It is well tolerated

and has no major adverse effects; minor reactions are voice alterations and laryngitis. This medication, given daily via nebulization generally before or with percussion and postural drainage, has resulted in improvements in spirometry, PFTs, dyspnea scores, and perceptions of well-being and has reduced the viscosity of sputum.

Nebulized hypertonic saline (7%) has been shown to be effective in improving airway hydration and increases mucus clearance in patients with CF. However, this treatment causes bronchospasm and may not be recommended for patients with severe disease (Furnari, Termini, Traverso, et al., 2012).

Physical exercise is an important adjunct to daily ACT. Exercise stimulates mucus excretion and provides a sense of well-being and increased self-esteem. Any aerobic exercise that the patient enjoys should be encouraged. The ultimate aim of exercise is to increase lung vital capacity, remove secretions, increase pulmonary blood flow, and maintain healthy lung tissue for effective ventilation.

Pulmonary infections are treated as soon as they are recognized. In patients with CF, characteristic signs of pulmonary infection—fever, tachypnea, and chest pain—may be absent. Therefore, a careful history and physical examination are essential. The presence of anorexia, weight loss, and decreased activity alerts the practitioner to pulmonary infection and the need for an antibiotic regimen. Aerosolized antibiotics, such as tobramycin, aztreonam, and colistin, are beneficial for patients with frequent pulmonary exacerbations and are administered in 2- to 4-week cycles.

IV antibiotics may be administered at home as an alternative to hospitalization. The use of peripherally inserted central catheters (PICCs) for the administration of antibiotics in children with CF is a viable option with limited complications and fewer needle punctures to obtain blood specimens and to maintain often lengthy treatment with parenteral antibiotics. Alternatively, an implanted vascular access device offers the advantage of access for blood draws and antibiotic infusion. When pulmonary function does not improve with outpatient management, hospitalization may be recommended for continued antibiotic therapy and vigorous ACT. Periodic hospitalizations for preventive IV antibiotic therapy and percussion and postural drainage occur less frequently than in the past due to limited evidence to support this practice and concern about making organisms more multidrug resistant. Oxygen administration is used for children with acute episodes but must be used cautiously because many children with CF have chronic carbon dioxide retention, and the unsupervised use of oxygen can be harmful. With repeated infection and inflammation, bronchial cysts and emphysema may develop. These cysts may rupture, resulting in pneumothorax.

> **! NURSING ALERT**
>
> Signs of pneumothorax are usually nonspecific and include tachypnea, tachycardia, dyspnea, pallor, and cyanosis. A subtle drop in oxygen saturation (measured by pulse oximetry) may be an early sign of pneumothorax.

Blood streaking of the sputum is usually associated with increased pulmonary infection and often requires no specific treatment. Hemoptysis indicates a potentially life-threatening event and needs to be treated immediately. Sometimes bleeding can be controlled with bed rest, IV antibiotics, replacement of acute blood loss, IV conjugated estrogens (Premarin) or vasopressin (Pitressin), and correction of any coagulation defects with vitamin K or fresh-frozen plasma. If hemoptysis persists, the site of bleeding should be localized via bronchoscopy and cauterized or embolized. In severe cases, a lung resection may be required.

Nasal polyps can develop in two thirds of patients with CF and occur due to chronic inflammation. Treatment of nasal polyps includes intranasal corticosteroids, decongestants, and mucolytics. If these measures are ineffective, surgical interventions may be necessary. Saline irrigations are often prescribed to remove thick nasal secretions and to treat chronic sinusitis associated with CF.

Because pulmonary damage in patients with CF is believed to be caused by the inflammatory process that occurs with frequent infections, the use of corticosteroids has been studied; however, treatment with corticosteroids for prolonged periods found only a modest effect and numerous side effects including linear growth restriction, glucose tolerance abnormalities, and cataract formation. Antiinflammatory medications such as ibuprofen are becoming more important in the treatment of CF, but careful monitoring for adverse effects (gastrointestinal bleeding) is essential.

Management of Gastrointestinal Problems

The principal treatment for pancreatic insufficiency is replacement of pancreatic enzymes, which are administered with meals and snacks to ensure that digestive enzymes are mixed with food in the duodenum. Enteric-coated products prevent the neutralization of enzymes by gastric acids, thus allowing activation to occur in the alkaline environment of the small bowel. The amount of enzymes depends on the severity of the insufficiency, the child's response to enzyme replacement, and the practitioner's philosophy. Usually one to five capsules are administered with a meal, and a smaller amount is taken with snacks. The amount of enzyme is adjusted to achieve normal growth and a decrease in the number of stools to one or two per day. Capsules can be swallowed whole or taken apart and the contents (enteric-coated beads) sprinkled on a small amount of food to be taken at the beginning of the meal or within 30 minutes of eating. The enteric-coated beads should not be chewed or crushed because destroying the enteric coating can lead to inactivation of the enzymes and excoriation of oral mucosa. The powder form is used with infants and young children but should be used cautiously because inhalation of the powder may precipitate acute bronchospasm and, if mixed with food, predigests the food, making it unpalatable. The mouth must be rinsed after enzymes are administered to avoid breakdown of the oral mucosa or a breastfeeding mother's nipples.

Children with CF require a well-balanced, high-protein, high-caloric diet (because of their impaired intestinal absorption). In fact, they often require up to 150% of the recommended daily allowances to meet their needs for growth. Breastfeeding with enzyme supplementation should be continued as long as possible and, when necessary, supplemented with a higher-calorie-per-ounce formula. For formula-fed infants, commercial cow's milk–based formulas are usually adequate, although frequently a partial hydrolysate formula with medium-chain triglycerides (e.g., Pregestimil or Alimentum) may be recommended. Enzymes are mixed into cereal or fruit, such as applesauce. Because the uptake of fat-soluble vitamins is decreased, water-miscible forms of these vitamins (A, D, E, and K) are given along with multivitamins and the enzymes. When high-fat foods are eaten, the child is encouraged to add extra enzymes.

Growth failure despite adequate nutritional support may indicate deterioration of pulmonary status. Patients with CF may experience frequent anorexia as a result of the copious amounts of mucus produced and expectorated, persistent cough, effect of medications, fatigue, and sleep disruption. They may be placed on oral nutritional supplements, nighttime supplemental gastrostomy or NG tube feedings, or, rarely, parenteral alimentation in an effort to build up nutritional reserves if there has been a history of inability to maintain weight.

Meconium ileus and meconium ileus equivalent, or total or partial intestinal obstruction, can occur at any age. Constipation is often the result of a combination of malabsorption (either from inadequate pancreatic enzyme dosage or a failure to take the enzymes), decreased intestinal motility, and abnormally viscous intestinal secretions. These problems usually do not require surgical intervention and may be treated with MiraLAX or Colyte (osmotic solutions given orally or by NG tube), other laxatives, stool softeners, or rectal administration of meglumine diatrizoate (Gastrografin).

Rectal prolapse occurs in a small number of infants with CF, due to steatorrhea, malnutrition, and repetitive coughing (Egan, Green, & Voynow, 2016). The first episode of rectal prolapse is frightening to both the parents and child. Its reduction usually requires immediate guidance and intervention, which is managed by simply guiding the rectum back into place with a gloved, lubricated finger. Further management usually involves attempting to decrease the bulk of daily stools through enzyme replacement.

Children with CF often experience transient or chronic gastroesophageal reflux, which should be treated with the appropriate histamine-receptor antagonist and gastrointestinal motility drug, dietary modifications, and an upright position after feedings and meals.

Management of Endocrine Problems

The management of CFRD is critical in the therapeutic treatment of the child with CF. CFRD presents a combination of insulin resistance and insulin deficiency, with unstable glucose homeostasis in the presence of acute lung infection and treatment. Children with CFRD require close monitoring of blood glucose, administration of oral glucose-lowering agents or insulin injections, diet and exercise management, and quarterly glycosylated hemoglobin (HgA1c) measurements. Children with CF may be at increased risk for glucose management problems as a result of decreased nutrient absorption, anorexia, and severity of pulmonary illness. The prevalence of CFRD increases with age, and there is increased morbidity and mortality among children with CFRD compared with those without. Microvascular complications such as retinopathy and nephropathy may occur in children and adolescents with CFRD (Siwamogsatham, Alvarez, & Tangpricha, 2014). However, ketoacidosis is reported to be rare in individuals with CFRD (Egan et al., 2016). Children with CFRD should perform *self–blood glucose monitoring (SBGM)* three times daily and should be on an insulin regimen. Target glucose levels should be the same as for any other patient with diabetes. There is no evidence that oral glycemic agents are effective. During acute CF exacerbations, the nondiabetic child should be monitored closely for hyperglycemia. Although HgA1c may be low in patients with CF, the HgA1c trend may be useful to identify overall blood sugar control (Siwamogsatham et al., 2014).

Bone health is of concern in children and adults with CF. The pancreatic insufficiency of CF and chronic steroid use present potential risks for less-than-optimum bone growth in such children. Assessment of bone health by history and bone mass density evaluation should be considered in assessing the child's (8 years of age and older) health status to detect and prevent osteoporosis and osteopenia.

Prognosis

The median survival age for the CF patient is 40 years, and approximately 50% of patients are 18 years of age and older (Cystic Fibrosis Foundation, 2015). Lung, heart, pancreas, and liver transplantation have increased survival rates among some patients with CF. Heart/lung and double-lung transplants have been successfully performed in children with advanced pulmonary vascular disease and hypoxia. The obstacles surrounding this technique are availability of donated organs; complications from surgery; pulmonary infections; and recurrence of obstructive bronchiolitis, which decreases transplanted lung function.

Interprofessional Care Management

Assessment of the child with CF involves comprehensive assessment of all affected systems with special focus on the pulmonary and gastrointestinal systems. Pulmonary assessment is the same as that described for asthma, with special attention to lung sounds, observation of cough, and evidence of decreased activity or fatigue. Gastrointestinal assessment primarily involves observing the frequency and nature of the stools and abdominal distention. The observer is also alert to evidence of growth failure (e.g., weight loss, muscle wasting, pallor, anorexia, decreased activity [from baseline norm]). Family members are interviewed to determine the child or adolescent's eating and eliminating habits and to confirm a history of frequent respiratory tract infections or bowel obstruction in infancy.

The nurse assesses the newborn for feeding and stooling patterns, which may indicate a potential problem, such as meconium ileus. The dietician is consulted to assist in maximizing caloric intake.

The uncertainty, fear, and initial shock associated with the diagnosis are overwhelming to parents. They must face the impact of the chronic, life-threatening nature of the disease and the prospect of intensive treatment, for which they must assume a major part of the responsibility and for which they may be ill prepared. They often fear that they will be unable to provide the care the child needs. One of the most difficult aspects of the diagnosis is the implications inherent in its etiology (i.e., the recognition that each parent contributed the gene responsible for the defect).

Hospital Care

Most patients with CF require hospitalization only for treatment of pulmonary infection, uncontrolled diabetes, or a coexisting medical problem that cannot be treated on an outpatient basis. Therefore, when patients with CF are hospitalized, implement Standard Precautions with meticulous hand washing to decrease the nosocomial spread of organisms to the CF patient and among other hospitalized CF patients (especially when MRSA is prevalent). Contact Precautions may be required for specific infections. Some institutions issue Contact Precautions on all patients admitted with CF for their protection.

When the child with CF is hospitalized for diagnosis or treatment of pulmonary complications, aerosol therapy, percussion, and postural drainage are instituted or continued. Respiratory therapists often initiate, supervise, and provide these treatments; however, it is the nurse's responsibility to monitor the patient's tolerance to the procedure and evaluate the effectiveness of the procedure in relation to treatment goals. The nurse may at times administer aerosol therapy, perform chest percussion and postural drainage, assist with ACTs such as the mechanical vest, and teach breathing exercises. Chest percussion and postural drainage should not be performed before or immediately after meals. Planning percussion and postural drainage so it does not coincide with meals is essential to the effectiveness of this treatment.

Assessments, including observation of respiratory pattern, work of breathing, and lung auscultation, are vital assessments. Noninvasive pulse oximetry provides valuable data about the patient's oxygenation status. Supplemental oxygen therapy is administered to the child with mild or moderate respiratory distress, and the child requires frequent assessment of the tolerance to the procedure.

One of the challenges in the care of the child with CF is encouraging compliance with the therapeutic medication regimen, which often involves a significant number of medications—pancreatic enzymes; vitamins A, D, E, and K; oral antifungals for Candida infection; antihistamines; antiinflammatory agents; and oral antibiotics. This may be overwhelming to the child. Factor in multiple inhaled bronchodilators, ACTs and postural and aerosol treatments, blood glucose monitoring and insulin administration, various other medications, and increased mucus production during the acute phase, and it is common for the child with CF to rebel and be reluctant to adhere to the prescribed regimen. Education, positive reinforcement, and frank negotiation may be required to enlist cooperation for effective medication compliance.

The diet for the child with CF represents another challenge; careful planning with a pediatric dietitian and the child's input may help decrease the loss of appetite and weight loss that are often part of the condition. Children in the early stages of CF often have a good appetite. With infection and increased lung involvement, the child's appetite diminishes, and eventually it becomes a challenge to provide appropriate nutrition. When dietary intake fails to meet the child's needs for growth, enteral feedings or supplements may be considered. These feedings may be administered via a gastrostomy tube during the night to minimize the disruption of daily activities, including school. A low-profile gastrostomy affords the child few activity restrictions and minimal disruption of body image compared with a NG tube or conventional gastrostomy tube. The child and parents are encouraged to not perceive this therapy as a last-ditch effort but as an adjunct therapy to maintain optimum growth and prevent excessive weight loss. Depression, anxiety, and disturbed self-image may occur in children and adolescents with CF. Older adolescents and young adults with severe symptoms may be especially prone to depression as a result of the realization of the poor prognosis and the reality of unmet life expectations and goals.

Providing support to both the child and the family is essential. Skilled nursing care and sympathetic attention to the emotional needs of the child and family help them cope with the stresses associated with repeated respiratory tract infections and hospitalizations. The use of support groups or counseling may also be beneficial to the child.

Home Care

Most children and adolescents with CF can be managed at home. The goals of care include normalization and daily activities, including school and peer involvement. The care plan should be flexible so that family activities are disrupted as little as possible. Parents may initially require assistance finding and contacting durable medical equipment companies that will provide home care equipment. They also need opportunities to learn how to use the equipment and to solve problems that they may encounter while delivering therapy at home. A home health care provider may be required for initial assistance.

Patients and family members need education about the preferred diet of nutritious meals with tolerated fat, increased protein and carbohydrate, and the administration of pancreatic enzymes and nutritional supplements. It is important to stress to parents that the enzymes, in the amount regulated to the child's needs, should be administered at the beginning of all meals and snacks. For enteral feeds administered overnight, enzymes are generally administered at the start and finish of the feeds.

One of the most important aspects of educating parents for home care is teaching techniques for the removal of mucus (ACT, vest, forced expiration) and breathing exercises. The success of a therapy program depends on conscientious performance of these treatments regularly as prescribed. The number of times these therapies are performed each day is determined on an individual basis, and often parents readily learn to adjust the number and intensity of the treatments to the child's needs. For pulmonary infection, home IV antibiotics may be prescribed pending verification of insurance coverage and availability of an agency with adequate staff to perform multiple daily home antibiotic infusions. With use of the venous access devices, such as PICC lines and implanted ports, the parents and child can be taught the technique of direct administration into the IV line.

Families also need information about medications and possible side effects. Children receiving multiple antibiotics may require serum drug levels to ensure therapeutic dosing as well as other laboratory testing.

If the child has CFRD, education on blood glucose monitoring, insulin therapy, diet control, and possible complications related to this is needed. Follow-up with a pediatric endocrinologist is recommended.

Children and adolescents with CF should receive routine primary care with special attention to diet, growth and development, and immunizations. Care providers should be alert to any weight loss or flattening in the growth curve associated with loss of appetite, which could indicate a pulmonary exacerbation in children with CF. Anticipatory guidance concerning issues of discipline, how to incorporate aspects of the treatment regimen into the school environment, and delayed pubertal development are also important considerations for the primary care provider.

Home palliative care for the child or adolescent with CF who is in the terminal stages may be carried out with the assistance of palliative care or hospice as appropriate (see Chapter 36).

The nurse can assist the family in contacting resources that provide help to families with affected children. Various special child health services, many local clinics, private agencies, service clubs, and other community groups often offer equipment and medications either free or at reduced rates. The Cystic Fibrosis Foundation* has chapters throughout the United States that provide education and services to families and professionals.

Family Support

One of the most challenging aspects of providing care for the family of a child or adolescent with CF is meeting the emotional needs of the child and family. The diagnosis, treatment, and prognosis for CF are often associated with many problems and frustrations. The diagnosis can evoke feelings of guilt and self-recrimination in parents.

The long-range problems for an infant, child, or adolescent with CF are those encountered in any chronic illness (see Chapter 36). Both the child and the family must make many adjustments, the success of which depends on their ability to cope and on the quality and quantity of support they receive from outside sources. It is often the nurse who assesses the home situation, organizes and coordinates these services, and collects the data needed to evaluate the effectiveness of the services.

The persistent need for treatment several times per day places tremendous strain on the family. When the child is young, a family member must perform postural drainage and other ACTs. Children can balk at these treatments, and the parents are placed in the position of insisting on adherence. The stress and anxiety related to this routine may produce feelings of resentment in both the child and the family members. When possible, occasional trusted respite care should be available to allow parents to leave the situation for short periods without undue anxiety about the child's welfare.

The affected child or adolescent may become resentful about the disease, its relentless routine of therapy, and the necessary curtailment it places on activities and relationships. The child's activities are interrupted or built around treatments, medications, and diet. This imposes hardships and influences the child's quality of life. The child should be encouraged to attend school, seek employment when old enough, and join age-appropriate peer groups to foster a life that is as normal and productive as possible. Sports are often an important part of the child's and adolescent's life; interaction with peers includes valuable life experiences, especially to adolescents. Children and adolescents with CF should be encouraged to participate in sports activities to the extent that their physical and pulmonary health allows. Exercise is encouraged to increase pulmonary vital capacity, promote muscle development, and enhance cardiovascular function.

As the disease progresses, however, family stress should be expected and the patient may become angry and may resist medical therapy. It is important for care providers to recognize the family's changing needs and the grief they may experience as the CF worsens. Families should be made aware of resources for counseling. Patients need to be guided into activities that enable them to express anger, sorrow, and fear without guilt.

Transition to Adulthood

As life expectancy continues to rise for children and adolescents with CF, issues related to marriage, sexuality, childbearing, and career choice become more pressing. Male patients must be informed at some point that they will often be unable to produce offspring. It is important that the distinction be made between sterility and impotence. Normal sexual relationships can be expected. Female patients may be able to bear children but should be informed of the possible deleterious effects on the respiratory system created by the burden of pregnancy. They also need to know that their children will be carriers of the *CFTR* gene. Adolescent females may need counseling concerning the use of oral contraceptives and other contraceptive options (Roe, Traxler, & Schreiber, 2016).

Adolescents with CF are encouraged to take personal ownership and management of the illness to maximize their life's potential. Many adolescents and young people with the illness enroll in college or vocational and technical training school and complete degrees either by distance learning or by attending a local school. Young people are encouraged to set life goals and live normal lives to the extent that their illness allows.

It is important to prepare the child and family members for end-of-life decisions and care when appropriate. Anticipatory grieving and other aspects related to care of a child with a terminal illness are an important part of nursing care.

OBSTRUCTIVE SLEEP-DISORDERED BREATHING

Pediatric obstructive sleep-disordered breathing reportedly affects approximately 600,000 children 5 to 19 years of age in the United States (Weiss & Owens, 2014). Obstructive sleep-disordered breathing is an abnormal respiratory pattern or abnormal deoxygenation associated with hypoventilation that results in repetitive partial or complete airway obstruction of the upper airway during sleep. The most severe form of this condition is obstructive sleep apnea syndrome (OSAS). Common symptoms include nightly snoring, labored breathing during sleep, interrupted or disturbed sleep patterns, sleep enuresis, and daytime neurobehavioral problems (Marcus, Brooks, Draper, et al., 2012). OSAS is to be distinguished from primary snoring, which is snoring without obstructive apnea, frequent sleep arousals, or abnormalities in gas exchange. Children with OSAS usually do not exhibit daytime sleepiness as do adults, with the possible exception of obese children. If left untreated, obstructive sleep-disordered breathing may result in complications such as growth failure, cor pulmonale, hypertension, poor learning, behavioral problems, attention deficit hyperactivity disorder, and death.

The diagnosis of obstructive sleep-disordered breathing is made by a sleep study (polysomnography), which provides evidence of sleep disturbance, respiratory pauses, and changes in oxygenation. The six-channel polysomnography can be performed in children of all ages

---

*6931 Arlington Road, Bethesda, MD 20814-3205; 301-951-4422 or 800-FIGHT CF; www.cff.org. In Canada: Canadian Cystic Fibrosis Foundation, 2221 Yonge Street, Suite 601, Toronto, Ontario, Canada M4S 2B4; 800-378-2233 (toll free in Canada only); www.cysticfibrosis. ca. For information about specialized medications and equipment for CF and other pulmonary diseases, contact the Cystic Fibrosis Services Pharmacy, 6931 Arlington Road, 2nd floor, Bethesda, MD; 800-541-4959; www.cfservicespharmacy.com.

with videotaping or audiotaping, and abbreviated (vs. full night sleep study) polysomnography may be useful; however, these latter methods do not predict the severity of OSAS (Marcus et al., 2012). Polysomnography can distinguish between OSAS and primary snoring (Owens, 2016).

Obstructive sleep-disordered breathing in children has been associated with enlarged tonsils, obesity, chronic nasal congestion, asthma, prematurity, cerebral palsy, muscular dystrophy, Down syndrome, craniofacial anomalies, and nasal septal deviation (Weiss & Owens, 2014). A common treatment is adenotonsillectomy, provided there is evidence of adenotonsillar hypertrophy (Marcus et al., 2012). However, evidence indicates that this procedure may not be as successful in children with obesity (Lee, Hsu, Chang, et al., 2015). CPAP and bilevel (cycles between high and low pressure) positive airway pressure (BiPAP) may be helpful in older children with sleep-disordered breathing whose condition persists after surgical intervention. CPAP or BiPAP is a long-term therapy that requires frequent assessments to evaluate the required amount of pressure and the overall effectiveness of the intervention. For obese children with OSAS, a weight management plan is implemented. Care of the child with sleep-disordered breathing involves early detection by observation of the infant's or child's sleep patterns, active participation in the diagnostic polysomnography, observation of oxygenation and vital signs, application of CPAP when indicated, and monitoring the patient's response to diagnostic therapy. Counseling families of children with sleep-disordered breathing may involve dietary counseling for exercise programs and weight management, use of the CPAP or BiPAP equipment, and direct postoperative care after the surgical intervention of tonsillectomy or adenoidectomy. Some children may resist wearing CPAP or BiPAP devices and will need encouragement to do this. The nurse can help identify the most appropriate mask that can be tolerated by the child and can provide education about use of the CPAP or BiPAP at home.

RESPIRATORY EMERGENCY

RESPIRATORY FAILURE

Effective pulmonary gas exchange requires clear airways, normal lungs and chest wall, and adequate pulmonary circulation. Anything that affects these functions or their relationships can compromise respiration. In general, the term *respiratory insufficiency* is applied to two situations: (1) when there is increased work of breathing but gas exchange function is near normal; and (2) when normal blood gas tensions cannot be maintained and hypoxemia and acidosis develop secondary to carbon dioxide retention.

Respiratory failure is defined as the inability of the respiratory system to maintain adequate oxygenation of the blood with or without carbon dioxide retention. This process involves pulmonary dysfunction that generally results in impaired alveolar gas exchange, which can lead to hypoxemia or hypercapnia. Respiratory failure is the most common cause of cardiopulmonary arrest in children. *Respiratory arrest* is the complete cessation of respiration. *Apnea* is the cessation of breathing for more than 20 seconds or for a shorter period when associated with cyanosis, pallor, or bradycardia (Eichenwald & American Academy of Pediatrics Committee on Fetus and Newborn, 2016). Apnea can be (1) central, in which both airflow and chest wall movement are absent; (2) obstructive, in which airflow is absent but chest wall motion is present; and (3) mixed, in which both central and obstructive components are present.

Respiratory dysfunction may have an abrupt or an insidious onset. Respiratory failure can occur as an emergency situation or may be preceded by gradual and progressive deterioration of respiratory function.

Most clinical manifestations are nonspecific and are affected by variations among individual patients and differences in the severity and duration of inadequate gas exchange.

Diagnostic Evaluation

The diagnosis of respiratory failure is determined by the combined application of three sources of information:
1. Presence or history of a condition that might predispose the patient to respiratory failure
2. Observation of respiratory failure
3. Measurement of ABGs, including pH

Nursing observation and judgment are vital to the recognition and early management of respiratory failure. Nurses must be able to assess a situation and initiate appropriate action within moments. Signs of respiratory failure are listed in Box 40.17.

Therapeutic Management

The interventions used in the management of respiratory failure are often dramatic, requiring special skills and emergency procedures. If respiratory arrest occurs, the primary objectives are to recognize the situation and immediately initiate resuscitative measures, such as opening the airway, positioning, administration of supplemental oxygen, and cardiopulmonary resuscitation (CPR). When the situation is not an arrest, the suspicion of respiratory failure is confirmed by assessment; the severity may be defined by ABG analysis. Interventions such as administering supplemental oxygen, positioning, stimulation, suctioning,

---

BOX 40.17 Clinical Manifestations of Respiratory Failure

Cardinal Signs
- Restlessness
- Tachypnea
- Tachycardia
- Diaphoresis

Early but Less Obvious Signs
- Mood changes such as euphoria or depression
- Headache
- Altered depth and pattern of respirations
- Hypertension
- Exertional dyspnea
- Anorexia
- Increased cardiac output and renal output
- Central nervous system symptoms (decreased efficiency, impaired judgment, anxiety, confusion, restlessness, irritability, depressed level of consciousness)
- Nasal flaring
- Chest wall retractions
- Expiratory grunt
- Wheezing or prolonged expiration

Signs of More Severe Hypoxia
- Hypotension or hypertension
- Altered vision
- Somnolence
- Stupor
- Coma
- Dyspnea
- Depressed respirations
- Bradycardia
- Cyanosis, peripheral or central

and CPAP, BiPAP, or early intubation may avert an arrest. When the severity is established, an attempt is made to determine the underlying cause by thorough evaluation.

The principles of management are to (1) maintain ventilation and maximize oxygen delivery, (2) correct hypoxemia and hypercapnia, (3) treat the underlying cause, (4) minimize extrapulmonary organ failure, (5) apply specific and nonspecific therapy to control oxygen demands, and (6) anticipate complications. Monitoring the patient's condition closely is critical.

Care Management

For families whose child has a respiratory arrest, support is aimed at keeping the family informed of the child's status and helping them cope with a near-death experience or an actual death (see Chapter 36). Knowing that their child requires CPR is a frightening and often overwhelming experience for parents. Uncertainty regarding the outcome is a primary concern. Traditionally, family members are not allowed to be present during resuscitation efforts. However, studies indicate that family presence during emergencies alleviates the family's anger about being separated from the patient during a crisis, reduces their anxiety, eliminates doubts about what was done to help the patient, and facilitates the grieving process if the patient dies (Meert, Clark, & Eggly, 2013).

Regardless of whether an institution permits parental presence during CPR, nurses must consider the needs, fears, and concerns of family members during this situation. If family presence is not permitted, nurses should arrange for someone to remain with the family. After the child's recovery or death, the family will continue to need support and thorough medical information regarding lifesaving measures, the prognosis if the child survives, and the cause of death if the child dies.

REFERENCES

Akinbami, L. J., Simon, A. E., & Rossen, L. M. (2016). Changing trends in asthma prevalence among children. *Pediatrics, 137*(1). [Epub ahead of print.]

American Academy of Otolaryngology—Head and Neck Surgery. (2012). *Clinical indicators: Adenoidectomy.* Retrieved from http://www.entnet.org/content/clinical-indicators-adenoidectomy.

American Academy of Pediatrics Committee on Infectious Diseases & American Academy of Pediatrics Bronchiolitis Guidelines Committee. (2014). Updated guidance for palivizumab prophylaxis among infants and young children at increased risk of hospitalization for respiratory syncytial virus infection. *Pediatrics, 134*(2), 415–420.

American Academy of Pediatrics Committee on Infectious Diseases, & Pickering, L. (2012). *Red book: 2012 report of the Committee on Infectious Diseases* (29th ed.). Elk Grove Village, IL: Author.

American Academy of Pediatrics Committee on Nutrition and the Council on Sports Medicine and Fitness. (2011). Clinical report—Sports drinks and energy drinks for children and adolescents: Are they appropriate? *Pediatrics, 127*(6), 1182–1189.

Antoon, A. Y., & Donovan, M. K. (2016). Burn injuries. In R. M. Kliegman, B. F. Stanton, J. W. St. Geme, et al. (Eds.), *Nelson textbook of pediatrics* (20th ed.). Philadelphia, PA: Elsevier/Saunders.

ARDS Definition Task Force, Ranieri, V. M., Rubenfeld, G. D., et al. (2012). Acute respiratory distress syndrome: The Berlin definition. *Journal of the American Medical Association, 307*(23), 2526–2533.

Barson, W. J. (2014). ED evaluation and management of pediatric community-acquired pneumonia. *Pediatric Emergency Medicine Reports.* Retrieved from https://www.ahcmedia.com/articles/118868-ed-evaluation-and-management-of-pediatric-community-acquired-pneumonia.

Barrio, R. (2015). Management of endocrine disease: Cystic fibrosis–related diabetes: novel pathogenic insights opening new therapeutic avenues. *European Journal of Endocrinology, 172*(4), R131–R141.

Baugh, R. F., Archer, S. M., Mitchell, R. B., et al. (2011). Clinical practice guideline: Tonsillectomy in children. *Otolaryngology-Head and Neck Surgery, 144*(1 suppl), S1–S30.

Bekmezian, A., Fee, C., & Weber, E. (2015). Clinical pathway improves pediatric asthma management in the emergency department and reduces admissions. *Journal of Asthma, 52*(8), 806–814.

Bernard, G. R., Artigas, A., Brigham, K. L., et al. (1994). Report of the American-European consensus conference on ARDS: Definitions, mechanisms, relevant outcomes and clinical trial coordination. The Consensus Committee. *Intensive Care Medicine, 20*(3), 225–232.

Bowatte, G., Tham, R., Allen, K. J., et al. (2015). Breastfeeding and childhood acute otitis media: A systematic review and meta-analysis. *Acta Paediatrica, 104*, 85–95.

Brown, N., Gallagher, R., Fowler, C., et al. (2010). The role of parents in managing asthma in middle childhood: An important consideration in chronic care. *Collegian (Royal College of Nursing, Australia), 17*(2), 71–76.

Bunnell, R. E., Agaku, I. T., Arrazola, R., et al. (2014). *Intentions to smoke cigarettes among never-smoking US middle and high school electronic cigarette users, National Youth Tobacco Survey, 2011-2013.* Retrieved from http://www.cdc.gov/tobacco/basic_information/e-cigarettes/youth-intentions/index.htm.

Cardinale, F., Cappiello, A. R., Mastrototaro, M. F., et al. (2013). Community-acquired pneumonia in children. *Early Human Development, 89*, S49–S52.

Centers for Disease Control and Prevention. (2010). Licensure of a 13-valent pneumococcal conjugate vaccine (PCV13) and recommendations for use among children—Advisory Committee on Immunization Practices (ACIP), 2010. *Morbidity and Mortality Weekly Report, 59*(9), 258–261.

Centers for Disease Control and Prevention. (2012). Prevention and control of influenza with vaccines: Recommendations of the Advisory Committee on Immunization Practices (ACIP)—United States, 2012–2013 influenza season. *Morbidity and Mortality Weekly Report, 61*(32), 613–618.

Centers for Disease Control and Prevention. (2014). *Respiratory syncytial virus infection (RSV): Transmission and prevention.* Retrieved from http://www.cdc.gov/rsv/about/transmission.html.

Cystic Fibrosis Foundation. (2015). *About cystic fibrosis.* Retrieved from http://www.cff.org/AboutCF/Faqs/.

Czogala, J., Goniewicz, M. L., Fidelus, B., et al. (2014). Secondhand exposure to vapors from electronic cigarettes. *Nicotine & Tobacco Research, 16*(6), 655–662.

Dalabih, A., Harris, Z. L., Bondi, S. A., et al. (2013). Contemporary aminophylline use for status asthmaticus in pediatric ICUs. *Chest, 141*(4), 1122–1123.

Dashiff, C., Suzuki-Crumly, J., Kracke, B., et al. (2013). Cystic fibrosis-related diabetes in older adolescents: Parental support and self-management. *Journal for Specialists in Pediatric Nursing, 18*(1), 42–53.

Egan, M., Green, D. M., & Voynow, J. A. (2016). Cystic fibrosis. In R. M. Kliegman, B. F. Stanton, J. W. St. Geme, et al. (Eds.), *Nelson textbook of pediatrics* (20th ed.). Philadelphia, PA: Elsevier/Saunders.

Eichenwald, E. C., & American Academy of Pediatrics Committee on Fetus and Newborn. (2016). Apnea of prematurity. *Pediatrics, 137*(1). [Epub ahead of print.]

Farley, R., Spurling, G. K., Eriksson, L., et al. (2014). Antibiotics for bronchiolitis in children under two years of age. *Cochrane Database of Systematic Reviews, 2014*(10), CD005189.

Fashner, J., Ericson, K., & Werner, S. (2012). Treatment of the common cold in children and adults. *American Family Physician, 86*(2), 153–159.

Furnari, M. L., Termini, L., Traverso, G., et al. (2012). Nebulized hypertonic saline containing hyaluronic acid improves tolerability in patients with cystic fibrosis and lung disease compared with nebulized hypertonic saline alone: A prospective, randomized, double-blind, controlled study. *Therapeutic Advances in Respiratory Disease, 6*(6), 315–322.

Hampton, L. M., Nguyen, D. B., Edwards, J. R., et al. (2013). Cough and cold medication adverse events after market withdrawal and labeling revision. *Pediatrics, 132*(6), 1047–1054.

Hartman-Adams, H., Clark, K., & Juckett, G. (2014). Update on latent tuberculosis infection. *American Family Physician, 89*(11), 889–896.

Hasegawa, K., Tsugawa, Y., Brown, D. F., et al. (2013). Childhood asthma hospitalization in the United States, 2000-2009. *Journal of Pediatrics, 163*(4), 1127–1133.

Heinrich, J. (2011). Influence of indoor factors in dwellings on the development of childhood asthma. *International Journal of Hygiene and Environmental Health, 214*(1), 1–25.

Himdani, S. A., Javed, M. U., Hughes, J., et al. (2016). Home remedy or hazard? Management and costs of paediatric steam inhalation therapy burn injuries. *British Journal of General Practice, 66*, e193–e199.

Ho, E. (2013). Community-acquired pneumonia in adults and children. *Primary Care, 40*(3), 655–669.

Humbert, M., Busse, W., & Hanania, N. A. (2014). Omalizumab in asthma: An update on recent developments. *Journal of Allergy and Clinical Immunology: In Practice, 2*(5), 525–536.

Kerschner, J. E., & Preciado, D. (2016). Otitis media. In R. M. Kliegman, B. F. Stanton, J. W. St. Geme, et al. (Eds.), *Nelson textbook of pediatrics* (20th ed.). Philadelphia, PA: Saunders/Elsevier.

Kilgore, P. E., Salim, A. M., Zervos, M. J., et al. (2016). Pertussis: Microbiology, disease, treatment, and prevention. *Clinical Microbiology Reviews, 29*(3), 449–486.

Klein, J. O., & Pelton, S. (2013). *Acute otitis media in children: Epidemiology, microbiology, clinical manifestations and complications.* Retrieved from http://www.uptodate.com/contents/acute-otitis-media-in-children-epidemiology-microbiology-clinical-manifestations-and-complications.

Knudson, C. J., & Varga, S. M. (2015). The relationship between respiratory syncytial virus and asthma. *Veterinary Pathology, 52*(1), 97–106.

Kwong, K. Y., & Leibel, S. (2013). Update on allergen immunotherapy for treatment of allergic disease. *Advances in Pediatrics, 60*(1), 141–165.

Lee, C. H., Hsu, W. C., Chang, W. H., et al. (2015). Polysomnographic findings after adenotonsillectomy for obstructive sleep apnea in obese and non-obese children: A systematic review and meta-analysis. *Clinical Otolaryngology, 41*(5), 498–510.

Lieberthal, A. S., Carroll, A. E., Chonmaitree, T., et al. (2013). The diagnosis and management of acute otitis media. *Pediatrics, 131*(3), e964–e994.

Liu, A. H., Covar, R. A., Spahn, J. D., et al. (2016). Childhood asthma. In R. M. Kliegman, B. F. Stanton, J. W. St. Geme, et al. (Eds.), *Nelson textbook of pediatrics* (20th ed.). Philadelphia, PA: Elsevier/Saunders.

Longo, D. L., Horsburgh, C. R., Barry, C. E., et al. (2015). Treatment of tuberculosis. *New England Journal of Medicine, 373*, 2149–2160.

Lopez-Fernandez, Y., Azagra, A. M., de la Oliva, P., et al. (2012). Pediatric acute lung injury epidemiology and natural history study: Incidence and outcome of the acute respiratory distress syndrome in children. *Critical Care Medicine, 40*(12), 3238–3245.

Loutsios, C., Farahi, N., Porter, L., et al. (2014). Biomarkers of eosinophilic inflammation in asthma. *Expert Review of Respiratory Medicine, 8*(2), 143–150.

Marais, B. J. (2014). Tuberculosis in children. *Journal of Paediatrics and Child Health, 50*(10), 759–767.

Marcus, C. L., Brooks, L. J., Draper, K. A., et al. (2012). Diagnosis and management of childhood obstructive sleep apnea syndrome. *Pediatrics, 130*(3), 576–584.

Mazor, R., & Green, T. P. (2016). Pulmonary edema. In R. M. Kliegman, B. F. Stanton, J. W. St. Geme, et al. (Eds.), *Nelson textbook of pediatrics* (20th ed.). Philadelphia, PA: Elsevier/Saunders.

Meert, K. L., Clark, J., & Eggly, S. (2013). Family-centered care in the pediatric intensive care unit. *Pediatric Clinics of North America, 60*(3), 761–772.

Miraglia del Giudice, M., Matera, M. G., Capristo, C., et al. (2013). LABAs in asthmatic children: Highlights and new inside. *Pulmonary Pharmacology & Therapeutics, 26*(5), 540–543.

Mitchell, E. A., & Krous, H. F. (2015). Sudden unexpected death in infancy: A historical perspective. *Journal of Paediatrics and Child Health, 51*(1), 108–112.

Moraa, I., Sturman, N., McGuire, T., et al. (2013). Heliox for croup in children. *Cochrane Database of Systematic Reviews, 2013*(12), CD006822.

Moran, A., Pillay, K., Becker, D. J., et al. (2014). ISPAD clinical practice consensus guidelines 2014, management of cystic fibrosis-related diabetes in children and adolescents. *Pediatric Diabetes, 15*(20 suppl), 65–76.

National Asthma Education and Prevention Program. (2012). *Asthma care quick reference: Diagnosing and managing asthma.* Retrieved from https://www.nhlbi.nih.gov/files/docs/guidelines/asthma_qrg.pdf.

Neuman, A., Hohmann, C., Orsini, N., et al. (2012). Maternal smoking in pregnancy and asthma in preschool children. *American Journal of Respiratory and Critical Care Medicine, 186*(10), 1037–1043.

Nicholson, K. N. (2013). Screening for cystic fibrosis. *Journal for Nurse Practitioners, 38*(9), 24–32.

Ode, K. L., & Moran, A. (2013). New insights into cystic fibrosis–related diabetes in children. *The Lancet Diabetes & Endocrinology, 1*(1), 52–58.

Owens, J. A. (2016). Sleep medicine. In R. M. Kliegman, B. F. Stanton, J. W. St. Geme, et al. (Eds.), *Nelson textbook of pediatrics* (20th ed.). Philadelphia, PA: Elsevier/Saunders.

Ownby, D., & Johnson, C. C. (2016). Recent understandings of pet allergies. *F1000Research, 5*.

Pinto, D. S., & Kociol, R. D. (2014). *Pathophysiology of cardiogenic pulmonary edema.* Retrieved from http://www.uptodate.com/contents/pathophysiology-of-cardiogenic-pulmonary-edema.

Ralston, S. L., Lieberthal, A. S., Meissner, H. C., et al. (2014). Clinical practice guideline: The diagnosis, management, and prevention of bronchiolitis. *Pediatrics, 134*(5), e1474–e1502.

Roe, A. H., Traxler, S., & Schreiber, C. A. (2016). Contraception in women with cystic fibrosis: A systematic review of the literature. *Contraception, 93*(1), 3–10.

Roosevelt, G. E. (2016). Acute inflammatory upper airway obstruction. In R. M. Kliegman, B. F. Stanton, J. W. St. Geme, et al. (Eds.), *Nelson textbook of pediatrics* (20th ed.). Philadelphia, PA: Elsevier/Saunders.

Rosenfeld, R. M., Schwartz, S. R., Pynnonen, M. A., et al. (2013). Clinical practice guideline: Tympanostomy tubes in children. *Otolaryngology–Head and Neck Surgery, 149*(1 suppl), S1–S35.

Sferrazza Papa, G. F., Pellegrino, G. M., & Pellegrino, R. (2014). Asthma and respiratory physiology: Putting lung function into perspective. *Respirology (Carlton, Vic.), 19*(7), 960–969.

Sheikh, S., Pitts, J., Ryan-Wenger, N. A., et al. (2016). Environmental exposures and family history of asthma. *Journal of Asthma, 53*(5), 465–470.

Sicherer, S. H., Wood, R. A., & AAP Section on Allergy and Immunology. (2012). Allergy testing in childhood: Using allergen-specific IgE tests. *Pediatrics, 129*(1), 193–197.

Siwamogsatham, O., Alvarez, J. A., & Tangpricha, V. (2014). Diagnosis and treatment of endocrine comorbidities in patients with cystic fibrosis. *Current Opinion in Endocrinology, Diabetes, and Obesity, 21*(5), 422–429.

Trent, C. A., Zimbro, K. S., & Rutledge, C. M. (2015). Barriers in asthma care for pediatric patients in primary care. *Journal of Pediatric Health Care, 29*(1), 70–79.

Turner, T. L., Kopp, B. T., Paul, G., et al. (2014). Respiratory syncytial virus: Current and emerging treatment options. *ClinicoEconomics and Outcomes Research, 6*, 217–225.

US Food and Drug Administration. (2011). *FDA requires post-market safety trials for long-acting beta-agonists (LABAs).* Retrieved from http://www.fda.gov/Drugs/DrugSafety/ucm251512.htm.

van Zon, A., van der Heijden, G. J., van Dongen, T. M., et al. (2012). Antibiotics for otitis media with effusion in children. *Cochrane Database of Systematic Reviews, 2012*(9), CD009163.

Weiss, M., & Owens, J. (2014). Recognizing pediatric sleep apnea. *Journal for Nurse Practitioners, 39*(8), 43–49.

Winnie, G. B., & Lossef, S. V. (2016). Pneumothorax. In R. M. Kliegman, B. F. Stanton, J. W. St. Geme, et al. (Eds.), *Nelson textbook of pediatrics* (20th ed.). Philadelphia, PA: Elsevier/Saunders.

Workowski, K. A., Bolan, G. A., & Centers for Disease Control and Prevention. (2015). Sexually transmitted diseases treatment guidelines, 2015. *Morbidity and Mortality Weekly Report Recommendations and Reports, 64*(RR03), 1–137.

World Health Organization. (2016). *Tuberculosis: WHO global tuberculosis report*. Retrieved from: http://www.who.int/tb/publications/global_report/en/.

Yang, M., & So, T. Y. (2014). Revisiting the safety of over-the-counter cough and cold medications in the pediatric population. *Clinical Pediatrics, 53*(4), 326–330.

Yousaf, M., Malik, S. A., & Zada, B. (2014). Laser and incisional myringotomy in otitis media with effusion—A comparative study. *Journal of Ayub Medical College, Abbottabad, 26*(4), 441–443.

Zakrzewski, L., & Lee, D. T. (2013). An algorithmic approach to otitis media with effusion. *Journal of Family Practice, 62*(12), 700–706.

Zobell, J. T., Epps, K. L., Young, D. C., et al. (2015). Utilization of antibiotics for methicillin-resistant *Staphylococcus aureus* infection in cystic fibrosis. *Pediatric Pulmonology, 50*(6), 552–559.

Zoorob, R., Sidani, M., & Murray, J. (2011). Croup: An overview. *American Family Physician, 83*(9), 1067–1073.

41

The Child With Gastrointestinal Dysfunction

Cheryl C. Rodgers

http://evolve.elsevier.com/Perry/maternal

DISTRIBUTION OF BODY FLUIDS

The distribution of body fluids, or total body water (TBW), involves the presence of intracellular fluid (ICF) and extracellular fluid (ECF). Water is the major constituent of body tissues, and the TBW in an individual ranges from 75% (in term newborns) to 45% (in late adolescence) of total body weight.

The ICF refers to the fluid contained within the cells, whereas the ECF is the fluid outside the cells. The ECF is further broken down into several components: intravascular (contained within the blood vessels), interstitial (surrounding the cell; the location of most ECF), and transcellular (contained within specialized body cavities, such as cerebrospinal, synovial, and pleural fluid). In the newborn, about 50% of the body fluid is contained within the ECF, whereas 30% of a toddler's body fluid is contained within the ECF.

Under normal conditions, the amount of water ingested closely approximates the amount of urine excreted in a 24-hour period. Maintenance water requirement is the volume of water needed to replace obligatory fluid loss, such as that from insensible water loss (IWL) through the skin and respiratory tract, evaporative water loss, and losses through urine and stool formation. The amount and type of these losses may be altered by disease states such as fever (with increased sweating), diarrhea, gastric suction, and pooling of body fluids in a body space (often referred to as *third spacing*).

Nurses should be alert for altered fluid requirements in various conditions:

Increased requirements:
- Fever (add 12% per rise of 1° C)
- Vomiting, diarrhea
- High-output kidney failure
- Diabetes insipidus
- Diabetic ketoacidosis
- Burns
- Shock
- Tachypnea
- Radiant warmer (preterm infant)
- Phototherapy (infants)
- Postoperative bowel surgery (e.g., gastroschisis)

Decreased requirements:
- Heart failure
- Syndrome of inappropriate antidiuretic hormone (SIADH)
- Mechanical ventilation
- After surgery
- Oliguric renal failure
- Increased intracranial pressure

Basal maintenance calculations for required body water are based on the body's requirements for water in a normometabolic state at rest; estimated fluid requirements are then increased or decreased from these parameters based on increased or decreased water losses, such as with elevated body temperature (increased) or heart failure (decreased). Daily maintenance fluid requirements for infants, toddlers, and older children are listed in Table 41.1.

Maintenance fluids contain both water and electrolytes and can be estimated from the child's age, body weight, degree of activity, and body temperature. Basal metabolic rate (BMR) is derived from standard tables and adjusted for the child's activity, temperature, and disease state. For example, for afebrile patients at rest, the maintenance water requirement is approximately 100 mL for each 100 kcal expended. Children with fluid losses or other alterations require adjustment of these basic needs to accommodate abnormal losses of both water and electrolytes as a result of a disease state. For example, insensible losses increase when basal expenditure increases by fever or hypermetabolic states. Hypometabolic states, such as hypothyroidism and hypothermia, decrease the BMR.

The percentage of TBW varies among individuals and in adults and older children; it is related primarily to the amount of body fat. Consequently, females, who have more body fat than males, and obese people tend to have less water content in relation to weight.

GASTROINTESTINAL DYSFUNCTION

The extensive surface area of the gastrointestinal (GI) tract and its digestive function represent the major means of exchange between the human organism and the environment. Disorders that impair the functional integrity of the GI system have the potential to cause serious alterations in fluid and electrolyte balance. Disorders that involve GI losses of large amounts of fluid, absorption disorders, inflammatory disorders, and decreased or excessive water intake have the potential to cause fluid and electrolyte imbalance in infants and children. In any disorder that involves GI losses of large amounts of fluid, dehydration poses a serious threat to life and demands immediate attention.

DEHYDRATION

Dehydration is a common body fluid disturbance in infants and children and occurs whenever the total output of fluid exceeds the total intake, regardless of the underlying cause. Although dehydration can result from impaired oral intake, it is often a result of abnormal losses such as those that occur in vomiting or diarrhea, when oral intake only

TABLE 41.1 Daily Maintenance Fluid Requirements*	
Body Weight	**Amount of Fluid per Day**
1 to 10 kg	100 mL/kg
11 to 20 kg	1000 mL plus 50 mL/kg for each kg >10 kg
>20 kg	1500 mL plus 20 mL/kg for each kg >20 kg

*Not appropriate for neonatal use.

partially compensates for the abnormal losses. Other significant causes of dehydration include diabetic ketoacidosis and extensive burns.

Types of Dehydration

Sodium is the chief solute in ECF and the primary determinant of ECF volume. It is considered a unique electrolyte in that water balance determines sodium concentration; when water is lost and sodium concentration becomes elevated, compensatory mechanisms in the kidney stop ADH secretion so water is retained. The thirst mechanism (not fully functional in infants) is also stimulated so water is replaced, thus increasing the total body water content and returning sodium to a normal level (Greenbaum, 2016). Potassium is found primarily inside the cell (intracellular), but small amounts are also found in ECF. Sodium depletion in diarrhea occurs in two ways: out of the body in stool and into the ICF compartment to replace potassium to maintain electrolyte equilibrium.

Dehydration is classified into three categories on the basis of osmolality and depends primarily on the serum sodium concentration: (1) isotonic, (2) hypotonic, and (3) hypertonic.

Hypotonic (hyposmotic or hyponatremic) dehydration occurs in conditions in which electrolyte and water deficits are present in approximately balanced proportions. This is the primary form of dehydration in children. Water and sodium are lost in approximately equal amounts. The observable fluid losses are not necessarily isotonic because losses from other avenues make adjustments, so the sum of all losses, or the net loss, is isotonic. There is no osmotic force between the ICF and the ECF; thus the major loss is sustained from the ECF compartment. This significantly reduces the plasma volume and the circulating blood volume, which affects the skin, muscles, and kidneys. Shock is the greatest threat to life, and the child with isotonic dehydration displays symptoms characteristic of hypovolemic shock. Plasma sodium remains within normal limits, between 130 and 150 mEq/L.

Hypotonic (hyposmotic or hyponatremic) dehydration occurs when the electrolyte deficit exceeds the water deficit, leaving the serum hypotonic. Because ICF is more concentrated than ECF in hypotonic dehydration, water moves from the ECF to the ICF to establish osmotic equilibrium. This movement further increases the ECF volume loss, and shock is a frequent finding. Because there is a greater proportional loss of ECF in hypotonic dehydration, the physical signs tend to be more severe with smaller fluid losses than with isotonic or hypertonic dehydration. Serum sodium concentration is typically less than 130 mEq/L.

Hypertonic (hyperosmotic or hypernatremic) dehydration results from water loss in excess of electrolyte loss and is usually caused by a proportionately larger loss of water or a larger intake of electrolytes. This type of dehydration is the most dangerous and requires more specific fluid therapy. Hypertonic dehydration may occur in infants with diarrhea who are given fluids by mouth that contain large amounts of solute or in children who receive high-protein nasogastric (NG) tube feedings that place an excessive solute load on the kidneys. In hypertonic dehydration, fluid shifts from the lesser concentration of the ICF to the ECF. Plasma sodium concentration is greater than 150 mEq/L.

Because the ECF volume is proportionately larger, hypertonic dehydration consists of a greater degree of water loss for the same intensity of physical signs. However, central nervous system (CNS) disturbances, such as seizures, are more likely to occur. Cerebral changes are serious and may result in permanent damage. These include disturbances of consciousness, poor ability to focus attention, lethargy, increased muscle tone with hyperreflexia, and hyperirritability to stimuli (tactile, auditory, bright lights).

Degree of Dehydration

Diagnosis of the type and degree of dehydration is necessary to develop an effective plan of therapy. The degree of dehydration has been described as a percentage of body weight dehydrated: mild—less than 5% in infants or less than 3% in older children; moderate—5% to 10% in infants and 3% to 6% in older children; and severe—more than 10% in infants and more than 6% in older children (Greenbaum, 2016). Water constitutes only 60% to 70% of an infant's weight. However, adipose tissue contains little water and is highly variable in individual infants and children. A more accurate means of describing dehydration is to reflect acute loss (time frame of ≤48 hours) in milliliters per kilogram of body weight. For example, a loss of 50 mL/kg is considered to be a mild fluid loss, but a loss of 100 mL/kg produces severe dehydration.

A detailed history is the first step when assessing for dehydration. Parent reports of fluid intake, urine output, diarrhea, and emesis can aid in the identification of dehydration. In addition, parents are asked about tears; a child who is able to produce tears is less likely to have moderate or severe dehydration (Churgay & Aftab, 2012a). Clinical signs provide clues to the extent of dehydration (Table 41.2). Weight is the most important determinant of the percent of total body fluid loss in infants and younger children. Other predictors of fluid loss include a changing level of consciousness (irritability to lethargy), altered response to stimuli, decreased skin elasticity and turgor, prolonged capillary refill (>2 seconds), increased heart rate, and sunken eyes and fontanels. The earliest detectable sign is usually tachycardia followed by dry skin and mucous membranes, sunken fontanels, signs of circulatory failure (coolness and mottling of extremities), loss of skin elasticity, and prolonged capillary filling time (see Table 41.2).

Compensatory mechanisms attempt to maintain fluid volume by adjusting to these losses. Interstitial fluid moves into the vascular compartment to maintain the blood volume in response to hemoconcentration and hypovolemia, and vasoconstriction of peripheral arterioles helps maintain pumping pressure. When fluid losses exceed the ability of the body to sustain blood volume and blood pressure, circulation is seriously compromised, and the blood pressure falls. This results in tissue hypoxia with accumulation of lactic acid, pyruvate, and other acid metabolites, which contribute to the development of metabolic acidosis.

Renal compensation is impaired by reduced blood flow through the kidneys, and little urine is formed. Increased serum osmolality stimulates the secretion of antidiuretic hormone (ADH) to conserve fluid and initiates the renin/angiotensin mechanisms in the kidney, causing further vasoconstriction. Aldosterone is released to promote sodium retention and conserve water in the kidneys. If dehydration increases in severity, urine formation is greatly diminished, and metabolites and hydrogen ions that are normally excreted by this route are retained.

Shock, a common manifestation of severe depletion of ECF volume, is preceded by tachycardia and signs of poor perfusion and tissue oxygenation (e.g., low pulse oximeter readings). Peripheral circulation is poor as a result of reduced blood volume; therefore the skin is cool and mottled, with decreased capillary filling. Impaired kidney circulation often leads to oliguria and azotemia. Although low blood pressure may

TABLE 41.2   Evaluating Extent of Dehydration

| Clinical Signs | LEVEL OF DEHYDRATION | | |
	Mild	Moderate	Severe
Weight loss—infants	3% to 5%	6% to 9%	≥10%
Weight loss—children	3% to 4%	6% to 8%	10%
Pulse	Normal	Slightly increased	Very increased
Respiratory rate	Normal	Slight tachypnea (rapid)	Hyperpnea (deep and rapid)
Blood pressure	Normal	Normal to orthostatic (>10 mm Hg change)	Orthostatic to shock
Behavior	Normal	Irritable, more thirsty	Hyperirritable to lethargic
Thirst	Slight	Moderate	Intense
Mucous membranes*	Normal (moist)	Dry	Parched
Tears	Present	Decreased	Absent, sunken eyes
Anterior fontanel	Normal	Normal to sunken	Sunken
External jugular vein	Visible when supine	Not visible except with supraclavicular pressure	Not visible even with supraclavicular pressure
Skin*	Capillary refill >2 seconds	Slowed capillary refill (2 to 4 seconds [decreased turgor])	Very delayed capillary refill (>4 seconds) and tenting; skin cool, acrocyanotic or mottled
Urine	Decreased	Oliguria	Oliguria or anuria

*These signs are less prominent in patients who have hypernatremia.
Data from Jospe, N., & Forbes, G (1996). Fluids and electrolytes—clinical aspects, *Pediatrics in Review, 17*(11), 395–403; Steiner, M.J., DeWalt, D.A., & Byerly, J.S. (2004). Is this child dehydrated? *Journal of the American Medical Association, 291*(22), 2746–2754.

accompany other symptoms of shock, in infants and young children it is usually a late sign and may herald the onset of cardiovascular collapse.

Diagnostic Evaluation

To initiate a therapeutic plan, several factors must be determined:

- The degree of dehydration based on physical assessment
- The type of dehydration based on the pathophysiology of the specific illness responsible for the dehydrated state
- Specific physical signs other than general signs
- Initial plasma sodium concentrations
- Serum bicarbonate concentration
- Any associated electrolyte (especially serum potassium) and acid-base imbalances (as indicated)

Initial and regular ongoing evaluations assess the patient's progress toward equilibrium and the effectiveness of therapy.

In the examination of an infant or younger child, one of the most important determinants of the extent of dehydration is body weight because this can help to determine the percentage of total body fluid lost; however, because the pre-illness weight is often unknown, clinical manifestations must be evaluated. Clinical signs of abnormal capillary refill, abnormal skin turgor, and abnormal respiratory pattern are the most useful in predicting dehydration in children (Churgay & Aftab, 2012a). Objective signs of dehydration are present at a fluid deficit of less than 5%.

Laboratory data are useful only when results are significantly abnormal. Urine specific gravity and blood urea nitrogen (BUN) measurements are unreliable assessments for determining dehydration in children (Churgay & Aftab, 2012a). However, a serum bicarbonate level greater than 17 mEq/L reduces the chances of dehydration, whereas a bicarbonate level less than 13 mEq/L increases the chance of dehydration requiring IV intervention (Churgay & Aftab). Shock, tachycardia, and very low blood pressure are common features of severe depletion of ECF volume (see the "Shock" section in Chapter 42).

Therapeutic Management

Medical management is directed at correcting the fluid imbalance and treating the underlying cause. When the child is alert, awake, and not in danger, correction of dehydration may be attempted with oral fluid administration. Mild cases of dehydration can be managed at home by this method. Several commercial rehydration fluids are available for use (Table 41.3). Oral rehydration management consists of replacement of fluid loss over 4 to 6 hours, replacement of continuing losses, and provision for maintenance fluid requirements. In general, a mildly dehydrated child may be given 50 mL/kg of oral rehydration solution (ORS), and a child with moderate dehydration may be given 100 mL/kg of ORS. A child with fluid losses from diarrhea or vomiting may be given 10 mL/kg for each stool or emesis (Churgay & Aftab, 2012b). Amounts and rates are determined from body weight and the severity of dehydration and are increased if rehydration is incomplete or if excess losses continue until the child is well hydrated and the basic problem is under control.

Enhance the flavor of an ORS such as Pedialyte (unflavored) by adding 1 tsp of unsweetened flavored drink mix, such as Kool-Aid, to each 60 to 90 mL of ORS. Older children may take a small popsicle orally instead of fluids that require drinking. Many commercially available popsicles are relatively inexpensive and contain small amounts of sucrose and approximately 40 to 50 mL of fluid. Frozen oral hydration may be accepted by some children when conventional ORS is rejected.

The child may not be thirsty even though dehydrated and may refuse oral fluids initially for fear of continued emesis (if occurring) or because of decreased strength, oral stomatitis, or thrush. In such children, rehydration may proceed by administering 2 to 5 mL of ORS by a syringe or small medication cup every 2 to 3 minutes until the child is able to tolerate larger amounts; if the child has emesis, administering small amounts (5 to 10 mL) of ORS after 10 minutes and administering every 5 minutes may help overcome fluid deficit, and the emesis often lessens over time (Churgay & Aftab, 2012b). Oral rehydration therapy (ORT) is effective for treating mild or moderate dehydration in children, is less expensive, and involves fewer complications than parenteral therapy (American Academy of Pediatrics, Committee on Nutrition, 2014). ORSs are available in the United States as commercially prepared solutions and are successful in treating the majority of infants and children with dehydration.

TABLE 41.3	Clinical Manifestations of Dehydration		
Manifestation	**Isotonic (Loss of Water and Sodium)**	**Hypotonic (Loss of Sodium in Excess of Water)**	**Hypertonic (Loss of Water in Excess of Sodium)**
Skin			
Color	Gray	Gray	Gray
Temperature	Cold	Cold	Cold or hot
Turgor	Poor	Very poor	Fair
Feel	Dry	Clammy	Thickened, doughy
Mucous membranes	Dry	Slightly moist	Parched
Tearing and salivation	Absent	Absent	Absent
Eyeball	Sunken	Sunken	Sunken
Fontanel	Sunken	Sunken	Sunken
Body temperature	Subnormal or elevated	Subnormal or elevated	Subnormal or elevated
Pulse	Rapid	Very rapid	Moderately rapid
Respirations	Rapid	Rapid	Rapid
Behavior	Irritable to lethargic	Lethargic or comatose; seizures	Marked lethargy with extreme hyperirritability on stimulation

Parenteral Fluid Therapy

Parenteral fluid therapy is initiated whenever the child is unable to ingest sufficient amounts of fluid and electrolytes to (1) meet ongoing daily physiologic losses, (2) replace previous deficits, and (3) replace ongoing abnormal losses. Patients who usually require IV fluids are those with severe dehydration, uncontrollable vomiting, inability to drink for any reason (e.g., extreme fatigue, coma), and severe gastric distention.

Because dehydration (volume depletion) constitutes a great threat to life, the first priority is the restoration of circulation by rapid expansion of the ECF volume to treat or prevent shock. IV administration of fluid begins immediately, although the exact nature of the dehydration and the serum electrolyte values may not initially be known. The solution selected is based on what is known regarding the probable type and cause of the dehydration. This usually involves an isotonic solution such as 0.9% sodium chloride or lactated Ringer's solution, both of which are close to the body's serum osmolality of 285 to 300 mOsm/kg and do not contain dextrose (which is contraindicated in the early treatment stages of diabetic ketoacidosis).

Parenteral rehydration therapy has three phases. The initial therapy is used to expand volume quickly to ensure tissue perfusion (Greenbaum, 2016). During initial therapy, an isotonic electrolyte solution is used at a rate of 20 mL/kg given as an IV bolus over 5 to 20 minutes and repeated as necessary after assessment of the child's response to therapy (Friedman, 2010). Subsequent therapy is used to replace deficits, meet maintenance water and electrolyte requirements, and catch up with ongoing losses. Water and sodium requirements for the deficit, maintenance, and ongoing losses are calculated at 8-hour intervals, taking into consideration the amount of fluids given with the initial boluses and the amount administered during the first 24-hour period. With improved circulation during this phase, water and electrolyte deficits can be evaluated, and acid-base status can be corrected either directly through the administration of fluids or indirectly through improved renal function. Potassium is withheld until kidney function is restored and assessed and circulation has improved.

The final phase of therapy allows the patient to return to normal and begin oral feedings, with a gradual correction of total body deficits. The potassium loss in ICF is replaced slowly by way of the ECF. The body fat and protein stores are replaced through diet. If the child is unable to eat or if feeding aggravates a chronic condition, IV maintenance fluids are provided.

Although the initial phase of fluid replacement is rapid in both isotonic and hypotonic dehydration, it is contraindicated in hypertonic dehydration because of the risk for water intoxication, especially in the brain cells, specifically the central pontine cells. Central pontine myelinolysis may occur with an overcorrection of fluid deficit and an overly rapid correction of serum sodium concentration (Alleman, 2014). There is an apparent lag time for sodium to reach a steady state when diffusing in and out of brain cells, but water diffuses almost instantaneously. Consequently, rapid administration of fluid causes equally rapid diffusion of water into the dehydrated brain cells, causing marked cerebral edema. Because ECF volume is maintained relatively well in hypertonic as opposed to the other types of dehydration, shock is not a usual manifestation.

Care Management

Nursing observation and intervention are essential for detection and therapeutic management of dehydration. A variety of circumstances cause fluid losses in infants and small children, and changes can take place quickly. An important nursing responsibility is observing for signs of dehydration. Nursing assessment should begin with observing general appearance and proceed to more specific observations. Ill children usually have drawn expressions, have dry mucous membranes and lips, and "look sick." Loss of appetite is one of the first behaviors observed in most childhood illnesses, and the infant's or child's activity level is diminished from baseline or usual activities. The cry of an ill infant is less vigorous, often whining, and higher pitched than usual. The child is irritable, seeks the parent's comfort and attention, and displays purposeless movements and inappropriate responses to people and familiar objects. In some cases, the child may not protest advances by the health care worker and procedures such as taking vital signs or starting an IV infusion. These are signs that the child truly feels bad and that the condition is serious and immediate intervention is necessary. As the child's illness and level of dehydration become more severe, irritability progresses to lethargy and even unconsciousness.

Assess capillary filling time by pinching the abdominal skin, chest, arm, or leg and estimating the time it takes for the blood to return. Capillary filling time in mild dehydration is less than 2 seconds, increasing to more than 4 seconds in severe dehydration. The technique is effective in children of all ages. However, it can be altered in the presence of heart failure, which affects circulation time, and hypertonic dehydration, in which fluid loss is primarily intracellular. Additional clinical signs observed in children with dehydration include cool mottled extremities, sunken eyes, tachypnea, and changes in sensorium.

When caring for the ill child, assess the vital signs as often as every 15 to 30 minutes, and record fluid intake and output and body weight frequently during the initial phase of therapy. It is important to use the same scale each time the child is weighed and predetermine the weight of any equipment or devices that must remain attached during the weighing process, including elbow restraints, and any clothing the child might be wearing. Obtain routine weights at the same time each day using the same scales. Accurate intake and output are vital to the assessment of fluid balance. This includes oral and parenteral intake and losses from urine, stools, vomiting, fistulas, NG suction, sweat, and wound drainage:

Urine—Frequency, color, consistency, and volume (when weighing diapers, ≈1 g of wet diaper weight equals 1 mL of urine)

Stools—Frequency, volume, and consistency

Vomitus—Volume, frequency, and type

Sweating—Can only be estimated from frequency of clothing and linen changes

In addition to fluid intake and output, the following observations help to assess dehydration:

Vital signs—Temperature (normal, elevated, or lowered depending on degree of dehydration), pulse (tachycardia), respirations (hyperpnea), and blood pressure (hypotension)

Skin—Color, temperature, turgor, presence or absence of edema, and capillary refill

Mucous membranes—Moisture, color, and presence and consistency of secretions

Body weight—Decreased in relation to degree of dehydration

Fontanel (infants)—Sunken, soft, or normal

Sensory alterations—Presence of thirst (only in older child)

It is important to measure and record all intake, oral and parenteral, and output from all sources, including urine, stool, emesis, drainage tubes, fistulas, and wounds from which appreciable amounts of fluid are lost. Advise parents to observe the number of times and how much the child voids at home. For nursing interventions, see discussion under specific disorders in this chapter.

EDEMA

Edema represents an abnormal accumulation of fluid within the interstitial tissue and subsequent tissue and develops when there is a defect in the normal cardiovascular circulation or a failure in the lymphatic drainage systems. Edema results from anything that (1) alters the retention of sodium, such as renal disease or hormonal influences; (2) affects the formation or destruction of plasma proteins, such as starvation or liver disease; or (3) alters membrane permeability, such as nephrotic syndrome or trauma.

Edema may be localized to a small or large area, or it can be generalized. Several types of edema include the following:

- Peripheral edema, or localized or generalized palpable swelling of the interstitial space
- Ascites, or the accumulation of fluid in the abdominal cavity (usually associated with renal or liver abnormalities)
- Pulmonary edema, which occurs when interstitial volume increases
- Cerebral edema, which is a particularly threatening form of edema caused by trauma, infection, or other etiologic factors, including vascular overload or injudicious IV administration of hypotonic solutions
- Overall fluid gain, which is especially seen in patients with kidney disease

Assessment

Generalized edema resulting from any of the above types is manifested by swelling in the extremities, face, perineum, and torso. Loss of normal skin creases may be assessed. Daily weights are more sensitive indicators of water gain or loss and should be obtained. Abdominal girth measurement changes may also be an indicator of edema in children. Pitting edema may occur and can be assessed by pressing the fingertip against a bony prominence for 5 seconds. If the tissue rebounds immediately on removing the finger, the patient does not have pitting edema.

Therapeutic Management

The primary goal in the management of edema is treatment of the underlying disease process, which is discussed elsewhere in relation to the specific disorder. However, an essential aspect in the management of any fluid overload is early recognition in which nurses play a vital role. The management of edema is discussed throughout the text with specific conditions.

DISORDERS OF MOTILITY

DIARRHEA

Diarrhea is a symptom that results from disorders involving digestive, absorptive, and secretory functions. It is caused by abnormal intestinal water and electrolyte transport. Worldwide there are an estimated 1.7 billion episodes of diarrhea each year (Walker, Rudan, Liu, et al., 2013). The incidence and morbidity of diarrhea are more prominent in low-income countries, such as areas of Asia and Africa (Walker et al., 2013), and among children younger than 5 years of age (Liu , Johnson, Cousens, et al., 2012). In the United States, approximately 370 children younger than 5 years of age die of diarrhea and dehydration each year (Esposito, Holman, Haberling, et al., 2011).

Diarrheal disturbances involve the stomach and intestines (gastroenteritis), the small intestine (enteritis), the colon (colitis), or the colon and intestines (enterocolitis). Diarrhea is classified as acute or chronic.

Acute diarrhea is defined as a sudden increase in frequency and a change in consistency of stools, often caused by an infectious agent in the GI tract. It may be associated with upper respiratory or urinary tract infections, antibiotic therapy, or laxative use. Acute diarrhea is usually self-limited (<14 days' duration) and subsides without specific treatment if dehydration does not occur. Acute infectious diarrhea (infectious gastroenteritis) is caused by a variety of viral, bacterial, and parasitic pathogens (Table 41.4).

Chronic diarrhea is an increase in stool frequency and increased water content with a duration of more than 14 days. It is often caused by chronic conditions such as malabsorption syndromes, inflammatory bowel disease (IBD), immunodeficiency, food allergy, lactose intolerance, or chronic nonspecific diarrhea or as a result of inadequate management of acute diarrhea.

Intractable diarrhea of infancy is a syndrome that occurs in the first few months of life, persists for more than 2 weeks with no recognized pathogens, and is refractory to treatment. The most common cause is inadequately managed acute infectious diarrhea.

Chronic nonspecific diarrhea (CNSD), also known as *irritable colon of childhood* and *toddlers' diarrhea*, is a common cause of chronic diarrhea in children 6 to 54 months of age. These children have loose stools, often with undigested food particles, and diarrhea lasting more than 2 weeks. Children with CNSD grow normally and have no evidence of malnutrition, no blood in their stool, and no enteric infection. Poor dietary habits and food sensitivities have been linked to chronic diarrhea.

TABLE 41.4 Infectious Causes of Acute Diarrhea

Organism	Pathology	Characteristics	Comments
Viral Agents			
Rotavirus Incubation: 48 hours Diagnosis: enzyme immunoassay (EIA)	Fecal-oral transmission Seven groups (A to G): Most group A viruses replicate in mature villous epithelial cells of small intestine; leads to (1) imbalance in ratio of intestinal fluid absorption to secretion, and (2) malabsorption of complex carbohydrates	Mild-to-moderate fever Vomiting followed by the onset of watery stools Fever and vomiting generally abate in approximately 2 days, but diarrhea persists for 5 to 7 days	Most common cause of diarrhea in children younger than 5 years of age; Infants 6 to 12 months of age are most vulnerable Affects all ages; usually milder in children older 3 years of age; immunocompromised children at greater risk for complications Peak occurrences in winter months Important cause of nosocomial infections Two vaccines available
Noroviruses (formerly Norwalk-like) Also called *caliciviruses* Incubation: 12 to 48 hours Diagnosis: EIA,	Fecal-oral transmission; contaminated water Pathology similar to rotavirus; affects villous epithelial cells of small intestine leading to (1) imbalance in ratio of intestinal fluid absorption to secretion, and (2) malabsorption of complex carbohydrates	Abdominal cramps; nausea, vomiting, malaise, low-grade fever, watery diarrhea without blood; duration 2 to 3 days; tends to resemble so-called *food poisoning* symptoms with nausea predominating	Affects all ages Multiple strains often named for location of outbreak (e.g., Norwalk, Sapporo, Snow Mountain, Montgomery)
Bacterial Agents			
Escherichia coli Incubation: 3 to 4 days; variable depending on strain Diagnosis: sorbitol MacConkey agar positive for blood, but fecal leukocytes absent or rare	*E. coli* strains produce diarrhea as a result of enterotoxin production, adherence, or invasion: enterotoxigenic-producing *E.coli,* enterohemorrhagic *E.coli,* enteroaggregative *E.coli*	Watery diarrhea 1 to 2 days; then severe abdominal cramping and bloody diarrhea Can progress to hemolytic uremic syndrome	Foodborne pathogen Traveler's diarrhea Highest incidence in summer Cause of nursery epidemics Symptomatic treatment Antibiotics may worsen course Avoid antimotility agents and opioids
***Salmonella* groups (nontyphoidal)** Gram-negative rods, nonencapsulated, nonsporulating Incubation 6 to 72 hours Diagnosis: Gram-stain, stool culture	Invasion of mucosa in small and large intestine; edema of lamina propria; focal acute inflammation with disruption of mucosa and microabscesses	Nausea, vomiting, colicky abdominal pain, bloody diarrhea, fever; symptoms variable (mild to severe) May have headache, and cerebral manifestations (e.g., drowsiness, confusion, meningismus, seizures) Infants may be afebrile and nontoxic May result in life-threatening septicemia and meningitis Nausea/vomiting typically short duration; diarrhea may persist as long as 2 to 3 weeks Typically shed virus for average of 5 weeks; cases reported up to 1 year	Incidence highest in summer months; foodborne outbreaks common Usually transmitted person to person, but may transmit via undercooked meats or poultry Poultry and poultry products cause about one-half of the cases In children, related to pets (e.g., dogs, cats, hamsters, turtles) Communicable as long as organisms are excreted Antibiotics not recommended in uncomplicated cases Antimotility agents also not recommended—prolong transit time and carrier state Incidence decreasing over past 10 years
Salmonella typhi Produces enteric fever–systemic syndrome Incubation: Usually 7 to 14 days but could be 3 to 30 days depending on size of inoculum Diagnosis: positive blood cultures; also sometimes positive stool and urine cultures Late stage: positive bone marrow culture	Bloodstream invasion; after ingestion, organism attaches to microvilli of ileal brush borders, and bacteria invade intestinal epithelium via Peyer's patches Next, organism is transported to intestinal lymph nodes and enters bloodstream via thoracic ducts; circulating organisms reach reticuloendothelial cells, causing bacteremia	Manifestations depend on age Abdominal pain; diarrhea; nausea, vomiting, high fever, lethargy Must be treated with antibiotics	Incidence is much lower in developed countries; about 400 cases per year in the United States; 65% of US cases acquired via international cases Ingestion of foods and water contaminated with human feces is most common mode of transmission Congenital and intrapartum transmission possible Three vaccines available

Continued

TABLE 41.4	Infectious Causes of Acute Diarrhea—cont'd		
Organism	**Pathology**	**Characteristics**	**Comments**
***Shigella* species** Gram-negative nonmotile anaerobic bacilli Incubation: 1 to 7 days Diagnosis: stool culture loaded with polymorphonuclear leukocytes	Enterotoxins: invade epithelium with superficial mucosal ulcerations	Children appear sick Symptoms begin with fever, fatigue, anorexia Crampy abdominal pain precedes watery or bloody diarrhea Symptoms usually subside in 5 to 10 days	Most cases in children younger than 9 years of age, with about one-third of cases in children 1 to 4 weeks of age Antibiotics shorten illness and lower mortality All patients at risk for dehydration Acute symptoms may persist for 1 week or more Antidiarrheal medications not recommended; may predispose patient to toxic megacolon
Yersinia enterocolitica Incubation: dose dependent, 1 to 3 weeks Diagnosis: stool culture, ELISA Patients have leukocytosis; elevated sedimentation rate	Pathology poorly understood; possible production of enterotoxin	Mucoid diarrhea, sometimes bloody; abdominal pain suggestive of appendicitis; fever, vomiting	Seen more frequently in winter months Transmitted by pets and contaminated food Antibiotics usually do not alter clinical course in uncomplicated cases; should be used in complicated infections and compromised hosts
Campylobacter jejuni Microaerophilic, motile, gram-negative bacilli Incubation: 1 to 7 days Ability to cause illness appears dose related Diagnosis: stool culture, sometimes in blood culture Commonly found in GI tract of wild or domestic animals	Not fully understood; possibly (1) adherence to intestinal mucosa by toxin; (2) invasion of mucosa in terminal ileum and colon; (3) translocation, in which organisms penetrate mucosa and replicate in lamina propria	Fever, abdominal pain, vomiting, diarrhea that can be bloody Watery, profuse, foul-smelling diarrhea Clinically similar to infection by *Salmonella* or *Shigella* organisms Fecal-oral transmission	Most infections in humans relate to consumption of contaminated foods or water, such as undercooked meats, particularly chicken Also acquired from contaminated household pets (e.g., dogs, cats, hamsters) Bimodal peaks in infants younger than 1 year of age and again at 15 to 29 years of age Antibiotics do not prolong carriage of bacteria and may eliminate organism more quickly Erythromycin is the drug of choice Antimotility agents are not recommended and tend to prolong symptoms
Vibrio cholerae Gram-negative, motile, curved bacillus living in bodies of salt water Incubation: 1 to 3 days Diagnosis; stool culture	Enters via oral route in contaminated food or water; if survives acid stomach environment, travels to small intestine, adheres to mucosa, and produces toxin	Onset abrupt; vomiting, watery diarrhea without cramping or tenesmus Dehydration can occur quickly	More prevalent in developing countries Rehydration most important treatment Antibiotics can shorten diarrhea Despite continued efforts, no vaccine available
Clostridium difficile Gram-positive anaerobic bacillus with the ability to produce spores Diagnosis: by detecting *C. difficile* toxin in stool culture	Produces two important toxins (A and B) Toxin binds to enterocyte surface receptor, resulting in altered permeability, protein synthesis, and direct cytotoxicity	Mostly mild, watery diarrhea lasting a few days Some prolonged diarrhea and illness May cause pseudomembranous colitis Some individuals are extremely ill with high fever, leukocytosis, hypoalbuminemia	Associated with alteration of normal intestinal flora by antibiotics Adults tend to have more severe symptoms than children Treatment with antibiotics (metronidazole) in mildly to moderately symptomatic patients; for nonresponders, give vancomycin Resistant strains have developed Relapse common
Clostridium perfringens Anaerobic, gram-positive, spore-producing bacilli Incubation: 8 to 24 hours	Toxins produced in intestine after ingestion of organism	Acute onset: watery diarrhea, crampy abdominal pain Fever, nausea and vomiting rare Duration of illness usually 24 hours	Transmitted by contaminated food products, most often meats and poultry Usually self-limiting, and medical intervention not needed Oral rehydration usually sufficient Antibiotics serve no purpose and should not be used

TABLE 41.4 Infectious Causes of Acute Diarrhea—cont'd

Organism	Pathology	Characteristics	Comments
Clostridium botulinum Gram-positive, anaerobic, spore-producing bacilli Incubation: 12 to 26 hours (range, 6 hours to 8 days) Diagnosis: Blood and stool culture sent to special laboratory (usually state health department) to detect toxin	Botulism caused by binding of toxin to neuromuscular junction	Clinical presentation related to age and strain of botulism Abdominal pain, cramping, and diarrhea Other strains: respiratory compromise, central nervous system symptoms	Transmitted in contaminated food products Treatment is supportive care and neutralization of toxin
Staphylococcus Gram-positive, nonmotile, aerobic, or facultative anaerobic bacteria Incubation: generally short, 1 to 8 hours Diagnosis: identify organism in food, blood, pus, aspirate	Direct tissue invasion and production of toxin	Clinical presentation depends on site of entry In food poisoning: profuse diarrhea, nausea and vomiting	Transmitted in inadequately cooked or refrigerated foods Self-limiting Symptomatic treatment

CNS, Central nervous system; *EIA,* enzyme immunoassay; *ELISA,* enzyme-linked immunosorbent assay; *GI,* gastrointestinal.

The excessive intake of juices and artificial sweeteners such as sorbitol, which is a substance found in many commercially prepared beverages and foods, may be a factor.

Etiology

Most pathogens that cause diarrhea are spread by the fecal-oral route through contaminated food or water or are from person to person where there is close contact (e.g., day care centers). Lack of clean water, crowding, poor hygiene, nutritional deficiency, and poor sanitation are major risk factors, especially for bacterial or parasitic pathogens. Infants are often more susceptible to frequent and severe bouts of diarrhea because their immune system has not been exposed to many pathogens and has not acquired protective antibodies. Worldwide the most common causes of acute gastroenteritis are infectious agents, viruses, bacteria, and parasites.

Rotavirus is the most important cause of serious gastroenteritis among children, with 28% of all cases causing fatality (Walker et al., 2013). The virus is spread through the fecal-oral route or through contaminated food or water, and almost all children are infected with rotavirus at least once by 5 years of age (Esona & Gautam, 2015). Rotavirus is the most common cause of diarrhea-associated hospitalization, with an estimated 20 to 60 deaths per year in the United States (Esona & Gautam, 2015).

Salmonella, Shigella, and *Campylobacter* organisms are the most frequently isolated bacterial pathogens in the United States (Scallan, Mahon, Hoekstra, et al., 2013). These organisms are gram-negative bacteria and can be contracted through raw or undercooked food, contaminated food or water, or through the fecal-oral route. Among children younger than 5 years of age, *Salmonella* occurs in approximately 617 out of 100,000 children; *Campylobacter* occurs in 409 out of 100,000 children; and *Shigella* occurs in 312 out of 100,000 children (Scallan et al.) (see the "Intestinal Parasitic Diseases" section in Chapter 33).

Antibiotic administration is frequently associated with diarrhea because antibiotics alter the normal intestinal flora, resulting in an overgrowth of other bacteria such as *Clostridium difficile*. *Clostridium difficile* is the most common bacterial overgrowth and accounts for approximately 20% of all antibiotic-associated diarrhea (Barakat, El-Kady,

Mostafa, et al., 2011). Antibiotic-associated diarrhea can also be caused by *Klebsiella oxytoca* organisms, *Clostridium porringers,* and *Staphylococcus aureus* pathogens (Barakat et al.).

Pathophysiology

Invasion of the GI tract by pathogens results in increased intestinal secretion as a result of enterotoxins, cytotoxic mediators, or decreased intestinal absorption secondary to intestinal damage or inflammation. Enteric pathogens attach to the mucosal cells and form a cuplike pedestal on which the bacteria rest. The pathogenesis of the diarrhea depends on whether the organism remains attached to the cell surface, resulting in a secretory toxin (noninvasive, toxin-producing, noninflammatory type diarrhea) or penetrates the mucosa (systemic diarrhea). Noninflammatory diarrhea is the most common diarrheal illness, resulting from the action of enterotoxin that is released after attachment to the mucosa. The most serious and immediate physiologic disturbances associated with severe diarrheal disease are (1) dehydration, (2) acid-base imbalance with acidosis, and (3) shock that occurs when dehydration progresses to the point that circulatory status is seriously impaired.

Diagnostic Evaluation

Evaluation of a child with acute gastroenteritis begins with a careful history that seeks to discover the possible cause of diarrhea, assess the severity of symptoms and the risk for complications, and elicit information about current symptoms indicating other treatable illnesses that could be causing the diarrhea. The history should include questions about recent travel, exposure to untreated drinking or washing water sources, contact with animals or birds, day care center attendance, recent treatment with antibiotics, or recent diet changes. History questions should also explore the presence or absence of other symptoms such as fever and vomiting, frequency and character of stools (e.g., watery, bloody), urinary output, dietary habits, and recent food intake.

Extensive laboratory evaluation is not indicated in children who have uncomplicated diarrhea and no evidence of dehydration because most diarrheal illnesses are self-limiting. Laboratory tests are indicated for children who are severely dehydrated and receiving IV therapy. Watery, explosive stools suggest glucose intolerance; foul-smelling, greasy,

TABLE 41.5   Treatment of Acute Diarrhea

Degree of Dehydration	Signs and Symptoms	Rehydration Therapy*	Replacement of Stool Losses	Maintenance Therapy†
Mild (5% to 6%)	Increased thirst Slightly dry buccal mucous membranes	ORS, 50 mL/kg within 4 hours	ORS, 10 mL/kg (for infants) or 150 to 250 mL at a time (for older children) for each diarrheal stool	Breastfeeding, if established, should continue; give regular infant formula if tolerated.
Moderate (7% to 9%)	Loss of skin turgor, dry buccal mucous membranes, sunken eyes, sunken fontanel	ORS, 100 mL/kg within 4 hours	Same as above	If lactose intolerance suspected, give undiluted lactose-free formula (or half-strength lactose-containing formula for brief period only);
Severe (>9%)	Signs of moderate dehydration plus one of following: rapid, thready pulse; cyanosis; rapid breathing; lethargy; or coma	IV fluids (lactated Ringer's solution), 40 mL/kg until pulse and state of consciousness return to normal; then 50 to 100 mL/kg or ORS	Same as above	infants and children who receive solid food should continue their usual diet.

IV, Intravenous; *NS*, normal saline; *ORS*, oral rehydration solution.
*If no signs of dehydration are present, rehydration therapy is not necessary. Proceed with maintenance therapy and replacement of stool losses.
†Maintenance therapy applies to all degrees of dehydration.
Modified from King, C.K., Glass, R., Bresee, J.S., et al. (2003). Managing acute gastroenteritis among children: Oral rehydration, maintenance, and nutritional therapy. *Morbidity and Mortality Weekly Report Recommendations and Reports, 52*(RR-16), 1–16.

bulky stools suggest fat malabsorption. Diarrhea that develops after the introduction of cow's milk, fruits, or cereal may be related to enzyme deficiency or protein intolerance. Neutrophils or red blood cells in the stool indicate bacterial gastroenteritis or IBD. The presence of eosinophils suggests protein intolerance or parasitic infection. Stool cultures should be performed only when blood, mucus, or polymorphonuclear leukocytes are present in the stool; when symptoms are severe; when there is a history of travel to a developing country; and when a specific pathogen is suspected. Gross or occult blood may indicate pathogens such as *Shigella, Campylobacter,* or hemorrhagic *Escherichia coli* strains. An enzyme-linked immunosorbent assay (ELISA) may be used to confirm the presence of rotavirus or *Giardia* organisms. If there is a history of recent antibiotic use, the stool should be tested for *C. difficile* toxin. When bacterial and viral culture results are negative and diarrhea persists for more than a few days, examine stools for ova and parasites. A stool specimen with a pH of less than 6.0 and the presence of reducing substances may indicate carbohydrate malabsorption or secondary lactase deficiency. Stool electrolyte measurements may help identify children with secretory diarrhea.

The serum bicarbonate (HCO_3) may be useful when combined with other clinical signs. In the presence of metabolic acidosis, an anion gap may be helpful to distinguish between types of metabolic imbalance. Obtain a complete blood count (CBC), serum electrolytes, creatinine, and BUN in the child who has moderate-to-severe dehydration or who requires hospitalization. The hemoglobin, hematocrit, creatinine, and BUN levels are usually elevated in acute diarrhea and should normalize with rehydration.

Therapeutic Management

The major goals in the management of acute diarrhea include (1) assessment of fluid and electrolyte imbalance, (2) rehydration, (3) maintenance fluid therapy, and (4) reintroduction of an adequate diet. Treat infants and children with acute diarrhea and dehydration first with *oral rehydration therapy (ORT)*. ORT is one of the major worldwide health care advances. It is more effective, safer, less painful, and less costly than IV rehydration. The American Academy of Pediatrics, World Health Organization, and Centers for Disease Control recommend ORT as the treatment of choice for most cases of dehydration caused by diarrhea (Churgay & Aftab, 2012b). *Oral rehydration solutions (ORSs)*

enhance and promote the resorption of sodium and water; these solutions greatly reduce vomiting, volume loss from diarrhea, and the duration of the illness. ORSs are available in the United States as commercially prepared solutions and are successful in treating the majority of infants with dehydration. Guidelines for rehydration recommended by the American Academy of Pediatrics are included in Table 41.5.

After rehydration, ORS may be used during maintenance fluid therapy by alternating the solution with a low-sodium fluid such as breast milk, lactose-free formula, or half-strength lactose-containing formula. In older children, ORS can be given, and a regular diet continued. Ongoing stool losses should be replaced on a 1:1 basis with ORS. If the stool volume is not known, approximately 10 mL/kg of ORS should be given for each diarrheal stool.

Solutions for oral hydration are useful in most cases of dehydration, and vomiting is not a contraindication. Give a child who is vomiting an ORS at frequent intervals and in small amounts. For young children, the caregiver may give the fluid with a spoon or small syringe in 5- to 10-mL increments every 1 to 5 minutes. An ORS may also be given via NG or gastrostomy tube infusion. Infants without clinical signs of dehydration do not need ORT. However, they should receive the same fluids recommended for infants with signs of dehydration in the maintenance phase and for ongoing stool losses. The use of probiotics in tandem with rehydration therapy reduces the duration of antibiotic-associated diarrhea in children (Churgay & Aftab, 2012b).

> **! NURSING ALERT**
>
> Diarrhea is not managed by encouraging intake of clear fluids by mouth such as fruit juices, carbonated soft drinks, and gelatin. These fluids usually have high carbohydrate content, very low electrolyte content, and high osmolality. Avoid caffeinated soda because caffeine is a mild diuretic and may lead to increased loss of water and sodium. Chicken or beef broth is not given because it contains excessive sodium and inadequate carbohydrate. A BRAT diet (bananas, rice, applesauce, and toast or tea) is contraindicated for children and especially for infants with acute diarrhea because it has little nutritional value (low in energy and protein), is high in carbohydrates, and is low in electrolytes (Churgay & Aftab, 2012b).

Early reintroduction of nutrients is desirable and has gained more widespread acceptance. Continued feeding or early reintroduction of a normal diet after rehydration has no adverse effects and actually lessens the severity and duration of the illness and improves weight gain compared with the gradual reintroduction of foods (Churgay & Aftab, 2012b; Bhutta, 2016). Infants who are breastfeeding should continue to do so, and ORS should be used to replace ongoing losses in these infants. Formula-fed infants should resume their formula; if it is not tolerated, a lactose-free formula may be used for a few days. In toddlers, there is no contraindication to continuing soft or pureed foods. In older children, a regular diet, including milk, generally can be offered after rehydration has been achieved. In cases of severe dehydration and shock, IV fluids are initiated whenever the child is unable to ingest sufficient amounts of fluid and electrolytes to (1) meet ongoing daily physiologic losses, (2) replace previous deficits, and (3) replace ongoing abnormal losses. Select the IV solution for fluid replacement based on what is known regarding the probable type and cause of the dehydration. The type of fluid normally used is a saline solution containing 5% dextrose in water. Although the initial phase of fluid replacement is rapid in both isotonic and hypotonic dehydration, rapid replacement is contraindicated in hypertonic dehydration because of the risk for water intoxication.

After the severe effects of dehydration are under control, specific diagnostic and therapeutic measures are begun to detect and treat the cause of the diarrhea. The use of antibiotic therapy in children with acute gastroenteritis is controversial. Antibiotics may shorten the course of some diarrheal illnesses (e.g., those caused by *Shigella* organisms). However, most bacterial diarrheas are self-limiting, and the diarrhea often resolves before the causative organism can be determined. Antibiotics may prolong the carrier period for bacteria such as *Salmonella* spp. However, they may be considered in patients who are younger than 3 months of age, on immunosuppressive medication, or who have clinical signs of shock, severe malnutrition, dysentery, suspected cholera, or suspected giardiasis (Dekate, Jayashree, & Singhi, 2013). Antimotility drugs such as loperamide are not recommended in children. Because of the self-limiting nature of vomiting and its tendency to improve when dehydration is corrected, the use of antiemetic agents historically has not been recommended; however, ondansetron has few side effects and may be administered if vomiting persists and interferes with ORT (Bhutta, 2016).

Care Management

The management of most cases of acute diarrhea takes place in the home with education of the caregiver. Teach caregivers to monitor for signs of dehydration (especially the number of wet diapers or voidings) and the amount of fluids taken by mouth and to assess the frequency and amount of stool losses. Education relating to ORT, including the administration of maintenance fluids and replacement of ongoing losses, is important (see Clinical Reasoning Case Study: Diarrhea). ORS should be administered in small quantities at frequent intervals. Vomiting is not a contraindication to ORT unless it is severe. Information concerning the introduction of a normal diet is essential. Parents need to know that a slightly higher stool output initially occurs with continuation of a normal diet and with ongoing replacement of stool losses. The benefits of a better nutritional outcome with fewer complications and a shorter duration of illness outweigh the potential increase in stool frequency. Parents' concerns should be addressed to ensure adherence to the treatment plan.

If the child with acute diarrhea and dehydration is hospitalized, an accurate weight must be obtained, and fluid intake and output carefully monitored. The child may be placed on parenteral fluid therapy with nothing by mouth (NPO) for 12 to 48 hours, but small amounts of

---

CLINICAL REASONING CASE STUDY
Diarrhea

A mother brings her 8-month-old infant, Mary, to the primary care clinic. The mother reports that Mary has had a "cold" for about 2 days, and this morning she began to vomit and has had diarrhea for the past 8 hours. The mother states that Mary is still breastfeeding, but she is not taking as much fluid as usual and she is having three times as many stools as usual (the stools are watery in consistency). When the nurse practitioner examines Mary, she notes that her temperature is 38° C (100.4° F), her pulse and blood pressure are in the normal range, her mucous membranes are moist, and she has tears when she cries. The nurse practitioner also notes that Mary's weight has not changed from what it was when she was seen in the clinic 2 weeks ago for her well-child visit.

1. Evidence—Is there sufficient evidence for the nurse and nurse practitioner to draw any conclusions for her initial plan of management?
2. Assumptions—Describe some underlying assumptions about the following:
   a. Clinical manifestations of various levels of dehydration
   b. Management of acute diarrhea
   c. Breastfeeding and the management of acute diarrhea
   d. Use of antidiarrheal medications for acute diarrhea
3. Which nursing interventions should the nurse and nurse practitioner implement at this time?
4. Does the evidence support the nurse and nurse practitioner's conclusion?

---

oral fluids may be started unless there are other illness factors that preclude ORT. Monitoring the IV infusion is an important nursing function. The nurse must ensure that the correct fluid and electrolyte concentration is infused, the flow rate is adjusted to deliver the desired volume in a given time, and the IV site is maintained.

Accurate measurement of output is essential to determine whether renal blood flow is sufficient to permit the addition of potassium to the IV fluids. The nurse is responsible for examination of stools and collection of specimens for laboratory examination (see the "Collection of Specimens" section in Chapter 39). Take care when obtaining and transporting stools to prevent possible spread of infection. Transport stool specimens to the laboratory in appropriate containers and media according to hospital policy.

Diarrheal stools are highly irritating to the perianal skin, and extra care is needed to protect the skin of the diaper region from excoriation (see the "Diaper Dermatitis" section in Chapter 31). Avoid taking the temperature rectally because it stimulates the bowel, increasing the passage of stool.

Support for the child and family involves the same care and consideration given to all hospitalized children (see Chapter 38). Keep parents informed of the child's progress and instructed in the use of frequent and proper hand washing and the disposal of soiled diapers, clothes, and bed linens. Everyone caring for the child must be aware of "clean" and "dirty" areas, especially in the hospital, where the sink in the child's room is used for many purposes. Discard soiled diapers and linens in receptacles close to the bedside.

Prevention

The best intervention for diarrhea is prevention. The fecal-oral route spreads most infections, and parents need information about preventive measures such as personal hygiene, protection of the water supply from contamination, and careful food preparation. Meticulous attention to perianal hygiene, disposal of soiled diapers, proper hand washing, and isolation of infected people also minimize the transmission of infection (see the "Infection Control" section in Chapter 39).

Parents need information about preventing diarrhea while traveling. They are cautioned against giving their children adult medications that are used to prevent traveler's diarrhea. The best measure during travel to areas where water may be contaminated is to allow children to drink only bottled water and carbonated beverages. Tap water, ice, unpasteurized dairy products, raw vegetables, unpeeled fruits, meats, and seafood should also be avoided.

Two rotavirus vaccines are now available for children. Human-bovine reassortant rotavirus vaccine (RotaTeq), which became available in 2006, and live-attenuated human rotavirus vaccine (Rotarix) may be used to prevent this infectious diarrheal disease (see the "Immunizations" section in Chapter 31). Population-based studies show a reduction of diarrhea-associated hospitalizations by as much as 87% in the years after rotavirus vaccination (Esona & Gautam, 2015).

CONSTIPATION

Constipation is an alteration in the frequency, consistency, or ease of passing stool. It is defined as a decrease in bowel movement frequency or trouble defecating for more than 2 weeks (Agarwal, 2013). The frequency of bowel movements varies by age, but most children have an average of 1.7 stools per day at 2 years of age and an average of 1.2 stools per day at 4 years of age or older (Petersen, 2014). Constipation is often associated with painful bowel movements, blood-streaked or retained stool, abdominal pain, lack of appetite, and stool incontinence (i.e., soiling) (Rogers, 2012). The frequency of bowel movements is not considered a diagnostic criterion because it varies widely among children. Having extremely long intervals between defecation is *obstipation*. Constipation with fecal soiling is *encopresis*.

Constipation may arise secondary to a variety of organic disorders or in association with a wide range of systemic disorders. Structural disorders of the intestine, such as strictures, ectopic anus, and Hirschsprung disease, may be associated with constipation. Systemic disorders associated with constipation include hypothyroidism, hypercalcemia resulting from hyperparathyroidism or vitamin D excess, and chronic lead poisoning. Constipation is also associated with use of drugs such as antacids, diuretics, antiepileptics, antihistamines, opioids, and iron supplementation. Spinal cord lesions may be associated with loss of rectal tone and sensation. Affected children are prone to chronic fecal retention and overflow incontinence.

The majority of children have *idiopathic* or *functional constipation* because no underlying cause can be identified. Chronic constipation may occur as a result of environmental or psychosocial factors, or a combination of both. Transient illness, withholding and avoidance secondary to painful or negative experiences with stooling, and dietary

intake with decreased fluid and fiber all play a role in the etiology of constipation.

Newborn Period

Normally, newborn infants pass a first meconium stool within 24 to 36 hours of birth. Any newborn that does not do so should be assessed for evidence of intestinal atresia or stenosis, Hirschsprung disease, hypothyroidism, meconium plug, or meconium ileus. *Meconium plug* is caused by meconium that has reduced water content and is usually evacuated after digital examination but may require irrigations with a hypertonic solution or contrast medium. *Meconium ileus,* the initial manifestation of cystic fibrosis, is the luminal obstruction of the distal small intestine by abnormal meconium. Treatment is the same as for a meconium plug; early surgical intervention may be needed to evacuate the small intestine.

Infancy

The onset of constipation frequently occurs during infancy and may result from organic causes such as Hirschsprung disease, hypothyroidism, and strictures. It is important to differentiate these conditions from functional constipation. Constipation in infancy is often related to dietary practices. It is less common in breastfed infants, who have softer stools than bottle-fed infants. Breastfed infants may also have decreased stools because of more complete digestion of breast milk with little residue. When constipation occurs with a change from human milk or modified cow's milk to whole cow's milk, simple measures such as adding or increasing the amount of vegetables and fruit in the infant's diet and increasing fluids usually corrects the problem. When a bottle-fed infant passes a hard stool that results in an anal fissure, stool-withholding behaviors may develop in response to pain on defecation (see Clinical Reasoning Case Study: Constipation).

Childhood

Most constipation in early childhood is attributable to environmental changes or normal development when a child begins to attain control over bodily functions. A child who has experienced discomfort during bowel movements may deliberately try to withhold stool. Over time, the rectum accommodates to the accumulation of stool, and the urge to defecate passes. When the bowel contents ultimately are evacuated, the accumulated feces are passed with pain, thus reinforcing the desire to withhold stool.

Constipation in school-age children may represent an ongoing problem or a first-time event. The onset of constipation at this age is often the result of environmental changes, stresses, and changes in toileting patterns. A common cause of new-onset constipation at school entry is fear of using the school bathrooms, which are noted for their lack of privacy. Early and hurried departure for school immediately after breakfast may also impede bathroom use.

Therapeutic Management

Treatment of constipation depends on the cause and duration of symptoms. A complete history and physical examination are essential to determine appropriate management. The management of simple constipation consists of a plan to promote regular bowel movements. Often this is as simple as changing the diet to provide more fiber and fluids, eliminating foods known to be constipating, and establishing a bowel routine that allows for regular passage of stool. An increase in dietary fiber is recommended as a treatment for constipation in the healthy child. The amount of fiber for children for different ages varies by authorities, but the formula of "age + 5 g" daily intake of fiber is recommended for children 3 years of age and older (Kranz, Brauchla, Slavin, et al., 2012). Stool-softening agents such as docusate or lactulose may also be helpful. Polyethylene glycol (PEG) 3350 without electrolytes (MiraLAX) is a chemically inert polymer that has been introduced as a new laxative in recent years. It is usually tolerated well by children because it can be mixed in a beverage of choice. If other symptoms such as vomiting, abdominal distention, or pain and evidence of growth failure are associated with the constipation, the condition should be investigated further.

Care Management

Constipation tends to be self-perpetuating. A child who has difficulty or discomfort when attempting to evacuate the bowels has a tendency to retain the bowel contents, and this may initiate a vicious cycle. Nursing assessment begins with an accurate history of bowel habits; diet; events associated with the onset of constipation; drugs or other substances that the child may be taking; and the consistency, color, frequency, and other characteristics of the stool. If there is no evidence of a pathologic condition, the major task is to educate the parents regarding normal stool patterns and participate in the education and treatment of the child.

Dietary modifications are essential in preventing constipation. Fiber is an important part of the diet. Parents benefit from guidance in selecting foods high in fiber (Table 41.6). They need reassurance concerning the prognosis for establishing normal bowel habits. It is also important to discuss their attitudes and expectations regarding toilet habits.

HIRSCHSPRUNG DISEASE

Hirschsprung disease is a congenital anomaly that results in mechanical obstruction from inadequate motility of part of the intestine. It accounts for about one-fourth of all cases of neonatal intestinal obstruction. The incidence is 1 in 5000 live births (Liang, Ji, Yuan, et al., 2014). It is four times more common in males than in females and follows a familial pattern in a small number of cases. A recent meta-analysis of mutations in the *RET* protooncogene confirmed a significant association between *RET* polymorphisms and Hirschsprung disease (Liang et al., 2014).

Pathophysiology

The pathology of Hirschsprung disease relates to the absence of ganglion cells in the affected areas of the intestine, resulting in a loss of the

TABLE 41.6 Fiber Content of Select Foods

Food	Serving Size	Grams of Fiber
Apple, raw, with skin	1 apple	3.3
Bananas, ripe, raw	1 small-size banana	3.1
Beans, baked, canned	1 cup	10.4
Beans, pinto, mature seeds*	1 cup	15.4
Beets*	1 cup	3.4
Blackberries, raw	1 cup	7.6
Blueberries, raw	1 cup	3.5
Bread, mixed grain (includes whole grain)	1 slice	1.6
Broccoli*	1 cup	5.1
Brussel sprouts*	1 cup	4.1
Carrots*	1 cup	4.7
Cereals, ready-to-eat, General Mills, Cheerios	1 cup	3.6
Cereals, ready-to-eat, General Mills, Raisin Nut Bran	1 cup	5.1
Cereals, ready-to-eat, Kellogg's All Bran, Original	½ cup	8.8
Cereals, ready-to-eat, Kellogg's Raisin Bran	1 cup	7.3
Collards*	1 cup	5.3
Dates, deglet noor	1 cup	14.2
Lentils, mature seeds*	1 cup	15.6
Lima beans, large, mature*	1 cup	13.2
Oat bran, cooked	1 cup	5.7
Pears, raw	1 pear	5.1
Peas, green, frozen*	1 cup	8.8
Raisins, seedless	1 cup	5.4
Spinach*	1 cup	4.3
Vegetables, mixed, frozen*	1 cup	8.0
Wheat flour, whole grain	1 cup	14.6
Wheat flour, white, all-purpose, enriched	1 cup	3.5

*Cooked, boiled, drained, no salt.
Modified from USDA National Nutrient Database for Standard Reference, Release 27. Retrieved from http://ndb.nal.usda.gov/ndb/nutrients/index.

rectosphincteric reflex and an abnormal microenvironment of the cells of the affected intestine. The term *congenital aganglionic megacolon* describes the primary defect, which is the absence of ganglion cells in the myenteric plexus of Auerbach and the submucosal plexus of Meissner (Fig. 41.1).

The absence of ganglion cells in the affected bowel results in a lack of enteric nervous system stimulation, which decreases the ability of the internal sphincter to relax. Unopposed sympathetic stimulation of the intestine results in increased intestinal tone. In addition to the contraction of the abnormal bowel and the resulting lack of peristalsis, there is a loss of the rectosphincteric reflex. Normally, when a stool bolus enters the rectum, the internal sphincter relaxes, and the stool is evacuated. In Hirschsprung disease, the internal sphincter does not relax. In most cases, the aganglionic segment includes the rectum and some portion of the distal colon. In 80% of cases, the aganglionosis is restricted to the internal sphincter, rectum, and a few centimeters of the sigmoid colon and is termed *short-segment disease* (Liang et al., 2014). However, the entire colon or part of the small intestine may be involved; this is considered *long-segment disease*. Occasionally, skip

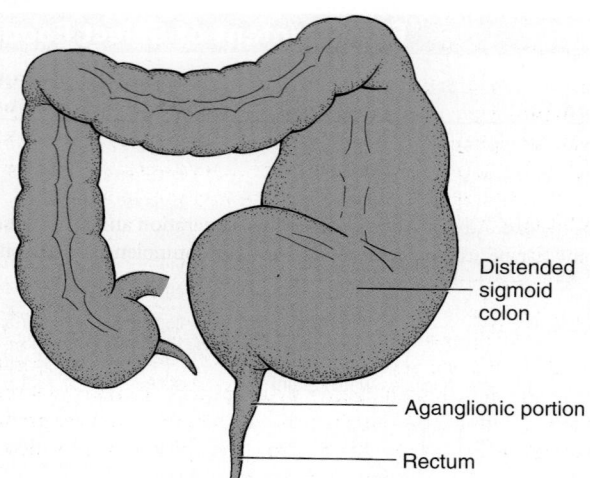

Distended
sigmoid
colon

Aganglionic portion

Rectum

FIG 41.1 Hirschsprung disease.

BOX 41.1 Clinical Manifestations of Hirschsprung Disease

Newborn Period
- Failure to pass meconium within 24 to 48 hours after birth
- Refusal to feed
- Bilious vomiting
- Abdominal distention

Infancy
- Failure to thrive
- Constipation
- Abdominal distention
- Episodes of diarrhea and vomiting
- Signs of enterocolitis: explosive, watery diarrhea; fever; appears significantly ill

Childhood (Symptoms Appear More Chronic)
- Constipation
- Ribbonlike, foul-smelling stools
- Abdominal distention
- Visible peristalsis
- Easily palpable fecal mass
- Undernourished, anemic appearance

---

segments or total intestinal aganglionosis may occur. Rarely, total colonic aganglionosis, in which there is no innervation of the large and small intestine from the anus to the ileocecal valve, may occur.

Diagnostic Evaluation

Most children with Hirschsprung disease are diagnosed in the first few months of life. Clinical manifestations vary according to the age when symptoms are recognized and the presence of complications, such as enterocolitis (Box 41.1). A neonate usually is seen with distended abdomen, feeding intolerance with bilious vomiting, and delay in the passage of meconium. Typically 99% of normal term infants pass meconium in the first 48 hours of life, but fewer than 10% of infants with Hirschsprung disease do so (Gourlay, 2013).

The history is an important part of diagnosis and typically includes a chronic pattern of constipation. On examination, the rectum is empty

---

of feces, the internal sphincter is tight, and leakage of stool and accumulated gas may occur if the aganglionic segment is short. To confirm the diagnosis, rectal biopsy is performed either surgically to obtain a full-thickness biopsy specimen or by suction biopsy for histologic evidence of the absence of ganglion cells.

Therapeutic Management

The majority of children with Hirschsprung disease require surgery rather than medical therapy with frequent enemas (Gourlay, 2013). After the child is stabilized with fluid and electrolyte replacement if needed, surgery is performed with a high rate of success. Surgical management consists primarily of the removal of the aganglionic portion of the bowel to relieve obstruction, restore normal motility, and preserve the function of the external anal sphincter. With earlier diagnosis, the proximal bowel may not be extremely distended, thus allowing for a primary pull-through or one-stage procedure and eliminating the need for a temporary colostomy. The transanal Soave endorectal pull-through procedure is often performed and consists of pulling the end of the normal bowel through the muscular sleeve of the rectum, from which the aganglionic mucosa has been removed. Simpler operations such as an anorectal myomectomy may be indicated in very short–segment disease.

Prognosis

After the pull-through procedure, the majority of children achieve fecal continence. However, some children may experience anal stricture, recurrent enterocolitis, prolapse, perianal abscess, and incontinence may occur and require further therapy, including dilations or bowel retraining therapy (Fiorino & Liacouras, 2016).

Care Management

The nursing concerns depend on the child's age and the type of treatment. If the disorder is diagnosed during the neonatal period, the main objectives are to (1) help the parents adjust to a congenital defect in their child, (2) foster infant-parent bonding, (3) prepare them for the medical-surgical intervention, and (4) assist them to assume care of the child after surgery.

Preoperative Care

The child's preoperative care depends on age and clinical condition. A child who is malnourished may not be able to withstand surgery until his or her physical status improves. Often this involves symptomatic treatment with enemas; and a low-fiber, high-calorie, high-protein diet.

Physical preoperative preparation includes the same measures that are common to any surgery (see the "Surgical Procedures" section in Chapter 39). In newborns whose bowels are relatively sterile, no additional preparation may be necessary. However, in older children preparation for the pull-through procedure involves emptying the bowels with saline enemas and decreasing bacterial flora with oral or systemic antibiotics and colonic irrigations using antibiotic solution. Enterocolitis is the most serious complication of Hirschsprung disease. Emergency preoperative care includes frequent monitoring of vital signs and blood pressure for signs of shock; monitoring fluid and electrolyte replacements and plasma or other blood derivatives; and observing for symptoms of bowel perforation such as fever, increasing abdominal distention, vomiting, increased tenderness, irritability, dyspnea, and cyanosis.

Because progressive distention of the abdomen is a serious sign, the nurse measures abdominal circumference with a paper tape measure, usually at the level of the umbilicus or at the widest part of the abdomen. The point of measurement is marked with a pen to ensure reliability of subsequent measurements. Abdominal measurement can be obtained with the vital sign measurements and is recorded in serial order so that any change is obvious. To reduce stress to the acutely ill child when frequent measurements of abdominal circumference are needed, the tape measure can be left in place beneath the child rather than removed each time.

The child's age dictates the type and extent of psychologic preparation. When a colostomy is performed, the child who is of preschool age is told about the procedure in concrete terms with the use of visual aids (see Chapter 39). It is important to time explanations appropriately to prevent the anxiety and confusion that could result from too much information. It is also important to stress to parents and older children that a colostomy for Hirschsprung disease is temporary unless so much bowel is involved that a permanent ileostomy must be performed. In most instances, the extent of bowel resection is known before surgery, although the nurse should be aware of cases when doubt exists concerning repair. Although a temporary colostomy is favorable in terms of future health and adjustment, it requires additional surgery, which may be stressful to parents and children.

Postoperative Care

Postoperative care is the same as that for any child or infant with abdominal surgery (see the "Surgical Procedures" section in Chapter 39). The nurse involves the parents in the care of the child, allowing them to help with feedings and observe for signs of wound infection or irregular passage of stool. Some children will require daily anal dilations in the postoperative period to avoid anastomotic strictures; parents are often taught to perform the procedure in the home (Temple, Shawyer, & Langer, 2012). When a colostomy is part of the corrective procedure, skin and stomal care is a major nursing task (see the "Ostomies" section in Chapter 39). Parents are taught how to care for the colostomy and how to provide skin care to prevent skin breakdown.

VOMITING

Vomiting is the forceful ejection of gastric contents through the mouth. It is a well-defined, complex, coordinated process that is under CNS control and is often accompanied by nausea and retching. Vomiting has many causes including acute infectious diseases, increased intracranial pressure, toxic ingestions, food intolerances and allergies, mechanical obstruction of the GI tract, metabolic disorders, nephrologic disease, and psychogenic problems (Singhi, Shah, Bansal, et al., 2013). Vomiting is common in childhood, is usually self-limiting, and requires no specific treatment. However, complications may occur, including acute fluid volume loss (dehydration) and electrolyte disturbances, malnutrition, aspiration, and Mallory-Weiss syndrome (small tears in the distal esophageal mucosa).

Characteristics of the emesis and pattern of vomiting help determine the cause. The color and consistency of the emesis vary according to the cause. Green bilious vomiting suggests bowel obstruction. Curdled stomach contents, mucus, or fatty foods that are vomited several hours after ingestion suggest poor gastric emptying or high intestinal obstruction. Gastric irritation by certain medicines, foods, or toxic substances may cause vomiting. Vomiting is also a response to psychologic stress due to a rise in adrenaline levels that stimulates the chemoreceptor trigger zone. Forceful vomiting is associated with pyloric stenosis. Cyclic vomiting is a rare disorder characterized by bouts of vomiting that can last from hours to several days but between bouts, the child appears healthy and participates in normal activities (Tarbell & Li, 2015).

Associated symptoms also help identify the cause. Fever and diarrhea accompanying vomiting suggest an infection. Constipation associated with vomiting suggests an anatomic or functional obstruction. Localized abdominal pain and vomiting often occur with appendicitis, pancreatitis, or peptic ulcer disease (PUD).

Therapeutic Management

Management is directed toward detection and treatment of the cause of the vomiting and prevention of complications, such as dehydration and malnutrition. Fluids are administered in the same manner and in an electrolyte composition similar to those administered for diarrhea. Although most children respond to these measures, antiemetic drugs may be needed. Adverse effects with earlier-generation antiemetics (such as promethazine and metoclopramide) include somnolence, nervousness, irritability, and dystonic reactions and should not be routinely administered to children (Singhi et al., 2013). Ondansetron (Zofran) is an antiemetic with limited adverse effects and is beneficial when the child is not able to tolerate anything orally or in the case of postoperative vomiting, chemotherapy-induced vomiting, cyclic vomiting syndrome, or acute motion sickness (Singhi et al.). For children who are prone to motion sickness, it is helpful to administer an appropriate dose of dimenhydrinate (Dramamine) before a trip.

Care Management

The major focus of nursing care of the vomiting infant and child is observing and reporting vomiting behavior and associated symptoms and implementing measures to reduce the vomiting. Accurate assessment of the type of vomiting, appearance of the emesis, and the child's behavior in association with the vomiting helps to establish a diagnosis.

The cause of the vomiting determines the nursing interventions. When it is a manifestation of improper feeding methods, establishing proper techniques through teaching and example usually corrects the situation. If vomiting is believed to be an indication of obstruction, food is usually withheld or special feeding techniques are implemented. In situations in which vomiting is related to concurrent infection, efforts are directed toward maintaining hydration or preventing dehydration.

The thirst mechanism is the most sensitive guide to fluid needs, and *ad libitum* administration of an oral rehydration solution to an alert child restores water and electrolytes satisfactorily. It is important to include carbohydrate to spare body protein and avoid ketosis resulting from exhaustion of glycogen stores. Small, frequent feedings of fluids or foods are preferred. After vomiting has stopped, offer more liberal amounts of fluids followed by gradual resumption of the regular diet.

Position the vomiting infant or child on the side or semi-reclining to prevent aspiration, and observe for evidence of dehydration. It is important to emphasize the need for the child to brush the teeth or rinse the mouth after vomiting to dilute hydrochloric acid that comes in contact with the teeth. Careful monitoring of fluid and electrolyte status is necessary to prevent an electrolyte disturbance.

GASTROESOPHAGEAL REFLUX

Gastroesophageal reflux (GER) is defined as the transfer of gastric contents into the esophagus. This phenomenon is physiologic, occurring throughout the day, most frequently after meals and at night; therefore it is important to differentiate GER from *gastroesophageal reflux disease (GERD)*. GERD represents symptoms or tissue damage that result from GER. The peak incidence of GER occurs at 4 months of age and generally resolves spontaneously in most infants before 12 months of age (Khan & Orenstein, 2016a). GER becomes a disease when complications (e.g., failure to thrive, respiratory problems, or dysphagia) develop.

Certain conditions predispose children to a high prevalence of GERD, including neurologic impairment, hiatal hernia, and morbid obesity (Singhal & Khaitan, 2014). Sandifer syndrome is an uncommon condition, usually occurring in young children and characterized by repetitive stretching and arching of the head and neck that can be mistaken for a seizure. This maneuver likely represents a physiologic neuromuscular

BOX 41.2 Clinical Manifestations of Gastroesophageal Reflux

Infants
- Spitting up, regurgitation, vomiting (may be forceful)
- Excessive crying, irritability, arching of the back with neck extension, stiffening
- Weight loss, failure to grow (thrive)
- Respiratory problems (cough, wheeze, stridor, gagging, choking with feedings)
- Hematemesis
- Apnea or apparent life-threatening event

Children
- Heartburn
- Abdominal pain
- Noncardiac chest pain
- Chronic cough
- Dysphagia
- Nocturnal asthma
- Recurrent pneumonia

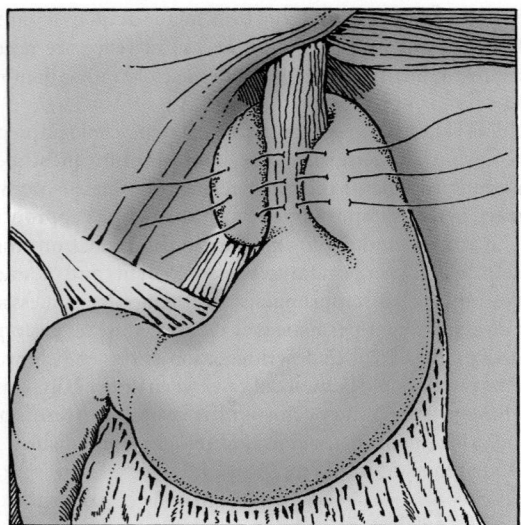

FIG 41.2 Nissen fundoplication sutures passing through esophageal musculature. (Redrawn from Campbell, A., & Ferrara, B. [1993]. *AORN Journal, 57*, 671–679.)

response attempting to prevent acid refluxate from reaching the upper portion of the esophagus (Goldani, Nunes & Ferreira, 2012).

Infants who are prone to develop GER include preterm infants and those with bronchopulmonary dysplasia. Children who have had tracheoesophageal or esophageal atresia repairs, neurologic disorders, scoliosis, asthma, cystic fibrosis, or cerebral palsy are also prone to developing GER. The clinical manifestations of GER are listed in Box 41.2.

Pathophysiology

Although the pathogenesis of GER is multifactorial, its primary causative mechanism likely involves inappropriate transient relaxation of the lower esophageal sphincter (LES). Factors that increase abdominal pressure such as coughing and sneezing, scoliosis, and overeating may contribute to GER. Esophageal symptoms are caused by inflammation from the acid in the gastric refluxate, whereas reactive airway disease may result from stimulation of airway reflexes by the acid refluxate.

Diagnostic Evaluation

The history and physical examination are usually sufficiently reliable to help establish the diagnosis of GER. However, the upper GI series is helpful in evaluating the presence of anatomic abnormalities (e.g., pyloric stenosis, malrotation, annular pancreas, hiatal hernia, esophageal stricture). The 24-hour intraesophageal pH monitoring study is the gold standard in the diagnosis of GER (Wilshire & Watson, 2013). Endoscopy with biopsy may be helpful to assess the presence and severity of esophagitis, strictures, and Barrett esophagus and to exclude other disorders such as Crohn's disease. *Scintigraphy* detects radioactive substances in the esophagus after a feeding of the compound and assesses gastric emptying. It can differentiate between aspiration of gastric contents from reflux versus aspiration from poor oropharyngeal muscle coordination.

Therapeutic Management

Therapeutic management of GER depends on its severity. No therapy is needed for the infant who is growing and has no respiratory complications. Avoidance of certain foods that exacerbate acid reflux (e.g., caffeine, citrus, tomatoes, alcohol, peppermint, and spicy or fried foods), lifestyle modifications in older children (e.g., weight control if indicated; small, more frequent meals), and feeding maneuvers in infants (e.g., thickened feedings) can improve mild GER symptoms.

Feedings thickened with 1 teaspoon to 1 tablespoon of rice cereal per ounce of formula may be recommended. This may benefit infants who are underweight as a result of GERD. This may benefit infants who are underweight as a result of GERD; however, the additional calories are not beneficial among infants who are overweight. These infants may benefit from pre-thickened formulas that are now commercially available. NG feedings may be necessary for infants with severe reflux and growth failure until surgery can be performed. Elevating the head of the bed or placing the infant in an infant seat for 1 hour after feedings may decrease GER. Prone positioning of infants also decreases episodes of GER, but due to the risk for sudden infant death syndrome, all infants should sleep in the supine position (Khan & Orenstein, 2016a). The American Academy of Pediatrics continues to recommend supine positioning for sleep (see Chapter 31). A weight loss program may be necessary for children with GERD symptoms that occur as a result of obesity.

Pharmacologic therapy may be used to treat infants and children with GERD. Both H_2-receptor antagonists (cimetidine [Tagamet], ranitidine [Zantac], or famotidine [Pepcid]) and proton pump inhibitors (PPIs; esomeprazole [Nexium], lansoprazole [Prevacid], omeprazole [Prilosec], pantoprazole [Protonix], and rabeprazole [Aciphex]) reduce gastric hydrochloric acid secretion and may stimulate some increase in LES tone. Use of metoclopramide remains controversial; there is no sufficient evidence to support the effectiveness with GER, and several side effects have been noted among infants; however, the medication is still commonly prescribed.

Surgical management of GER is reserved for children with severe complications such as recurrent aspiration pneumonia, apnea, severe esophagitis, or failure to thrive and for children who have failed to respond to medical therapy. The *Nissen fundoplication* (Fig. 41.2) is the most common surgical procedure (Wilshire & Watson, 2013). This surgery involves passage of the gastric fundus behind the esophagus to encircle the distal esophagus. Complications from fundoplication include breakdown of the wrap, small bowel obstruction, gas-bloat syndrome, infection, retching, and dumping syndrome (Wilshire & Watson, 2013).

Care Management

Nursing care is directed at (1) identifying children with symptoms suggestive of GER; (2) educating parents regarding home care, including feeding, positioning, and medications when indicated; and (3) caring for the child undergoing surgical intervention. For the majority of infants, parental reassurance of the benign nature of the condition and its relationship to physiologic maturity is the most important intervention. To help parents cope with the inconvenience of dealing with a child who spits up or regurgitates frequently, simple tips such as using bibs and protective clothes during feeding and prone positioning when holding the infant after feeding are beneficial.

It is important to educate and reassure parents about positioning. In the past, recommendations encouraged upright positioning during sleeping for both infants and older children. The supine position for sleeping continues to be the recommended infant sleeping position. Parents should not place infants on their sides as an alternative to fully supine sleeping, and avoiding soft bedding and soft objects in the bed is important. Rescheduling of the family's routine may be required to accommodate more frequent feeding times. If parents thicken formula, they should also enlarge the nipple opening for easier sucking. Usually breastfeeding may continue, and the mother may provide more frequent feeding times or express the milk for thickening with rice cereal. Parents should avoid feeding the child spicy foods or any foods that they find aggravate symptoms in general and avoid caffeine, chocolate, tobacco smoke, and alcohol when breastfeeding. Other practical advice includes advising the parents to avoid vigorous play after feedings and feeding just before bedtime.

When regurgitation is severe and growth is restricted, continuous NG tube or gastrostomy feedings may decrease the amount of emesis and provide constant buffering of gastric acid. Special preparation of caregivers is required when this type of nutritional therapy is indicated.

The nurse can support the family by providing information about all aspects of treatment. Parents often require specific information about the medications given for GER. PPIs are most effective when administered 30 minutes before breakfast so the peak plasma concentrations occur with mealtime. If they are given twice per day, the second best time for administration is 30 minutes before the evening meal. Parents need to be reassured that they may not see results right away because it takes several days of administration to achieve a steady state of acid suppression. A number of new formulations available in PPIs allow for more efficient administration. Some preparations are available in dissolvable pills. Powder and granule preparations are available as well. Many pharmacies compound the medication in a liquid form for administration. Postoperative nursing care after the Nissen fundoplication is similar to that for other types of laparoscopic or open abdominal surgery.

NUTRITIONAL DISORDERS

Reports of severe nutritional disorders in childhood in most developed countries are uncommon, yet there exist small numbers of children who may experience a nutritional deficiency of some type. The 2008 Feeding Infants and Toddlers Study (FITS) found that usual nutrient intake of infants, toddlers, and preschoolers (0 to 47 months of age) met or exceeded energy and protein requirements based on the Dietary Reference Intakes (DRIs) and the 2005 Dietary Guidelines for Americans (Butte, Fox, Briefel, et al., 2010). According to the study, a small but significant number of infants were at risk for inadequate intake of iron and zinc. Dietary fiber intakes in toddlers and preschoolers were low, and saturated fat intakes exceeded recommendations for the majority of preschoolers (Butte et al.). Nutritional requirements should be met through a wide variety of fruits, vegetables, and whole grains rather than an increased dependence on processed foods (Solomons & Vossenaar, 2013).

The findings of these studies and other similar reports are important for nurses who work with infants and children. Nurses must work to promote healthy nutrition habits early in children's lives through proper education of families and children about healthy lifestyle habits, including diet and exercise for health promotion and prevention of morbidities associated with poor micronutrient intake and sedentary lifestyle.

VITAMIN IMBALANCES

Although true vitamin deficiencies are rare in the United States, subclinical deficiencies are commonly seen in population subgroups in which either maternal or child dietary intake is imbalanced and contains inadequate amounts of vitamins. *Vitamin D–deficiency rickets,* once rarely seen because of the widespread commercial availability of vitamin D–fortified milk, increased before the turn of the century. Populations at risk include the following:

- Children who are breastfed exclusively by mothers with an inadequate intake of vitamin D or breastfed exclusively longer than 6 months without adequate maternal vitamin D intake or supplementation
- Children with dark skin pigmentation who are exposed to minimal sunlight because of socioeconomic, religious, or cultural beliefs or housing in urban areas with high levels of pollution or who live above or below a latitude of 33 degrees north and south where sunlight does not produce vitamin D (Wacker & Holick, 2013)
- Children with diets that are low in sources of vitamin D and calcium
- Individuals who use milk products not supplemented with vitamin D (e.g., yogurt* raw cow's milk) as the primary source of milk
- Children who are overweight or obese (Turer, Lin, & Flores, 2013)

The American Academy of Pediatrics (2008) recommends that infants who are breastfed exclusively receive 400 IU of vitamin D beginning shortly after birth to prevent rickets and vitamin D deficiency. Vitamin D supplementation should continue until the infant is consuming at least 1 L/day (or 1 quart/day) of vitamin D–fortified formula (American Academy of Pediatrics, 2008). Nonbreastfed infants who are taking less than 1 L/day of vitamin D–fortified formula should also receive a daily vitamin D supplement of 400 IU. Inadequate maternal ingestion of cobalamin (vitamin B_{12}) may contribute to infant neurologic impairment when exclusive breastfeeding (past 6 months) is the only source of the infant's nutrition. A correlation between the incidence of childhood upper respiratory infections and vitamin D deficiency has been found, but the implications of the findings have yet to be completely understood (Xiao, Xing, Yang, et al., 2015).

Children may also be at risk for vitamin deficiencies secondary to disorders or their treatment. For example, vitamin deficiencies of the fat-soluble vitamins A and D may occur in malabsorptive disorders such as cystic fibrosis and short bowel syndrome. Preterm infants may develop rickets in the second month of life as a result of inadequate intake of vitamin D, calcium, and phosphorus. Children receiving high doses of salicylates may have impaired vitamin C storage. Environmental tobacco smoke exposure has been implicated in decreased concentrations of of vitamin A and E in newborn infants (Titova, Ayvazova, Bichkaeva, et al., 2012). Children with chronic illnesses resulting in anorexia, decreased food intake, or possible nutrient malabsorption as a result of multiple medications should be evaluated carefully for adequate vitamin and mineral intake in some form (parenteral or enteral).

Children with thalassemia are reported to have suboptimal intakes (according to DRI recommendations) of vitamins A, D, E, and K, folate, calcium, and magnesium, and the inadequacies continue to increase

---

*Yogurt does not contain adequate amounts of vitamins A and D (unless specifically fortified with these vitamins) but is an acceptable source of calcium and phosphorus.

with advanced age (Fung, Xu, Trachtenberg, et al., 2012). One study found that children with intestinal failure who were being transitioned from parenteral to enteral nutrition had at least one vitamin and mineral deficiency; vitamin D was the most common deficiency identified, and zinc and iron were the most common minerals identified as being deficient (Yang, Duro, Zurakowski, et al., 2011).

Vitamin A deficiency has been reported with increased risk for blindness in children with measles. However, a Cochrane review of studies assessing the efficacy of vitamin A in children with measles found no information specifically related to ocular morbidities (Bello, Meremikwu, Ejemot-Nwadiaro, et al., 2014). Despite the lack of evidence, vitamin A supplementation has minimal side effects and should be administered to children with measles (Bello et al.). Complications from diarrhea and infections are often increased in infants and children with vitamin A deficiency. Although scurvy (caused by a deficiency of vitamin C) is rare in developed countries, cases have been reported in infants and children with malnutrition but can also be found in patients with eating disorders and after gastric surgery (Wijkmans & Talsma, 2016).

An excessive dose of a vitamin is generally defined as 10 or more times the Recommended Dietary Allowance (RDA), although the fat-soluble vitamins, especially vitamins A and D, tend to cause toxic reactions at lower doses. With the addition of vitamins to commercially prepared foods, the potential for *hypervitaminosis* has increased, especially when combined with the excessive use of vitamin supplements. Hypervitaminosis of vitamins A and D presents the greatest problems because these fat-soluble vitamins are stored in the body. High intakes of vitamin A present with dry, scaly skin that progresses to desquamation and fissures, and include anorexia, vomiting, and bulging fontanelle (Hayman & Dalziel, 2012). Vitamin D is the most likely of all vitamins to cause toxic reactions in relatively small overdoses. The water-soluble vitamins, primarily niacin, B_6, and C, can also cause toxicity. Poor outcomes in infants (e.g., fatal hypermagnesemia) have been associated with mega-vitamin therapy with high doses of magnesium oxide.

One vitamin supplement that is recommended for all women of childbearing age is a daily dose of 0.4 mg of folic acid, the usual RDA. Folic acid taken before conception and during early pregnancy can reduce the risk for neural tube defects such as spina bifida by as much as 70% (Czeizel, Dudás, Paput, et al., 2011). Drugs such as oral contraceptives and antidepressants may decrease folic acid absorption; thus adolescent girls taking such medications should consider supplementation (see Chapter 49).

MINERAL IMBALANCES

A number of minerals are essential nutrients. The *macrominerals* refer to those with daily requirements greater than 100 mg and include calcium, phosphorus, magnesium, sodium, potassium, chloride, and sulfur. *Microminerals,* or *trace elements,* have daily requirements of less than 100 mg and include several essential minerals and those in which the exact role in nutrition is still unclear. The greatest concern with minerals is deficiency, especially iron deficiency anemia (see Chapter 43). However, other minerals that may be inadequate in children's diets, even with supplementation, include calcium, phosphorus, magnesium, and zinc. Low levels of zinc can cause nutritional failure to thrive. Some of the macrominerals may be overlooked inadvertently when a child with intestinal failure or recent surgery is making the transition from total parenteral to enteral intake.

An imbalance in the intake of calcium and phosphorous may occur in infants who are given whole cow's milk instead of infant formula; neonatal tetany may be observed in such cases. Whole cow's milk is also a poor source of iron, and inadequate intake of iron from other food sources, such as iron-fortified cereal, may cause iron deficiency anemia.

The regulation of mineral balance in the body is a complex process. Dietary extremes of mineral intake can cause a number of mineral-mineral interactions that could result in unexpected deficiencies or excesses. For example, excessive amounts of one mineral such as zinc can result in a deficiency of another mineral, such as copper, even if sufficient amounts of copper are ingested. Thus, megadose intake of one mineral may cause an inadvertent deficiency of another essential mineral by blocking its absorption in the blood or intestinal wall or competing with binding sites on protein carriers needed for metabolism.

Deficiencies can also occur when various substances in the diet interact with minerals. For example, iron, zinc, and calcium can form insoluble complexes with phytates or oxalates (substances found in plant proteins), which impair the bioavailability of the mineral. This type of interaction is important in vegetarian diets because plant foods, such as soy, are high in phytates. Contrary to popular opinion, spinach is not an ideal source of iron or calcium because of its high oxalate content. Children with certain illnesses are at greater risk for growth failure, especially in relation to bone mineral deficiency as a result of the treatment of the disease, decreased nutrient intake, or decreased absorption of necessary minerals. Those at risk for such deficiencies include children who are receiving or have received radiation and chemotherapy for cancer; children with human immunodeficiency virus (HIV), sickle cell disease, cystic fibrosis, gastrointestinal (GI) malabsorption, or nephrosis; and extremely low–birth weight (ELBW) and very low–birth weight (VLBW) preterm infants.

Care Management

Identification of adequacy of nutrient intake is the initial nursing goal and requires assessment based on a dietary history and physical examination for signs of deficiency or excess (see the "Nutrition" section in Chapter 32 and the "Nutritional Assessment" section in Chapter 29). After assessment data are collected, this information is evaluated against standard intakes to identify areas of concern. DRIs are one source of standard nutrient intakes (see the "Dietary Guidelines" section in Chapter 32).

Standardized growth reference charts should be used in infants, children, and adolescents to compare and assess growth parameters such as height and head circumference with the percentile distribution of other children at the same ages. The World Health Organization growth chart is a standardized growth reference recommended for infants and toddlers up to 24 months of age. This growth chart includes head circumference, height, and weight references that were derived from healthy children in six different countries around the world. These growth standards are based on the growth of healthy breastfed infants throughout the first year of life. The Centers for Disease Control and Prevention (CDC) growth charts are also recommended for children 2 to 19 years of age.

Infants should be breastfed for the first 6 months and preferably for 1 year, be introduced to some solid foods after about 4 to 6 months, and receive iron-fortified cereal for at least 18 months (see Chapter 31). Vitamin B_{12} supplementation is recommended if the breastfeeding mother's intake of the vitamin is inadequate or if she is not taking vitamin supplements (Roumeliotis, Dix, & Lipson, 2012). If the infant is being breastfed exclusively after 4 months (when fetal iron stores are depleted), iron supplementation (1 mg/kg/day) is recommended until appropriate iron-containing complementary foods, such as iron-fortified cereal, are introduced (Baker, Greer, & American Academy of Pediatrics Committee on Nutrition, 2010). The introduction of solids for vegetarian infants may occur using the same guidelines as for other children (see

Chapter 32). A variety of foods should be introduced during the early years to ensure a well-balanced intake. Infants who are identified as having particular nutritional deficits should be identified; a multidisciplinary approach should be taken for identifying the deficit and the etiology, and a plan established with the caregiver to promote adequate growth and development.

SEVERE ACUTE MALNUTRITION (PROTEIN-ENERGY MALNUTRITION)

Malnutrition continues to be a major health problem in the world today, particularly in children younger than 5 years of age. However, lack of food is not always the primary cause of malnutrition. In many developing and underdeveloped nations, diarrhea (gastroenteritis) is a major factor. Additional factors are bottle-feeding (in poor sanitary conditions), inadequate knowledge of proper child care practices, parental illiteracy, economic and political factors, climate conditions, and cultural and religious food preferences. Poverty is an underlying cause of malnutrition due to the association of poor environmental conditions and lack of adequate food (Imdad, Sadiq, & Bhutta, 2011). The most extreme forms, or protein-energy malnutrition (PEM), are kwashiorkor and marasmus. Some authorities, including the World Health Organization, suggest that severe malnutrition encompasses more than protein-energy deficits and thus prefer the term *severe acute malnutrition (SAM)*. SAM may also be subdivided into edematous (kwashiorkor), severe wasting (marasmus) types, or marasmic kwashiorkor, which has features of both marasmus and kwashiorkor (Ashworth, 2016).

In the United States, milder forms of PEM are seen as a result of primary malnutrition, although the classic cases of marasmus and kwashiorkor may also occur. Unlike in developing countries, where the main reason for SAM is inadequate food, in the United States SAM occurs despite ample dietary supplies (see the "Failure to Thrive [Growth Failure]" section in Chapter 31). SAM may also be seen in people with chronic health problems such as cystic fibrosis, renal dialysis, cancer, chronic diarrhea syndromes, burns, inborn errors of metabolism, and GI malabsorption. Kwashiorkor has been reported in the United States in children fed only a rice beverage diet and in infants who were fed nonstandard infant diets such as flour water, corn porridge, molasses, and nondairy creamer (Tierney, Sage, & Shwayder, 2010). Other reported cases of kwashiorkor in developed countries involved infants who were fed extremely restricted diets due to perceived or actual reactions to foods or food allergies (Tierney et al., 2010). Kwashiorkor has also been reported in the United States when infants have been fed inappropriate food as a result of parental (caretaker) nutritional ignorance, a perceived cow's milk–based formula intolerance, family social chaos, or cow's milk intolerance. Therefore it is important that health care workers not assume that SAM cannot occur in developed countries; a comprehensive dietary history should be obtained in any child with clinical features resembling SAM.

Kwashiorkor

Kwashiorkor has been defined primarily as a deficiency of protein with an adequate supply of calories. A diet consisting mainly of starch grains or tubers provides adequate calories in the form of carbohydrates but an inadequate amount of high-quality proteins. However, some evidence supports a multifactorial etiology, including cultural, psychologic, and infective factors that may interact to place the child at risk for kwashiorkor. Kwashiorkor may result from the interplay of nutrient deprivation and infectious or environmental stresses, which produces an imbalanced response to such insults (Trehan & Manary, 2015). Kwashiorkor often occurs subsequent to an infectious outbreak of measles and dysentery. There is further evidence that oxidative stress occurs in children with

kwashiorkor, resulting in free radical damage, which may precipitate cellular changes, resulting in edema and muscle wasting (Bandsma, Spoelstra, Mari, et al., 2011).

Taken from the Ga language (Ghana), the word *kwashiorkor* means "the sickness the older child gets when the next baby is born" and aptly describes the syndrome that develops in the first child, usually between 1 and 4 years of age, when weaned from the breast after the second child is born.

The child with kwashiorkor has thin, wasted extremities and a prominent abdomen from edema (ascites). The edema often masks severe muscular atrophy, making the child appear less debilitated than he or she actually is. The skin is scaly and dry and has areas of depigmentation. Several dermatoses may be evident, partly resulting from the vitamin deficiencies. Permanent blindness often results from the severe lack of vitamin A. Mineral deficiencies are common, especially iron, calcium, and zinc. Acute zinc deficiency is a common complication of severe SAM and results in skin rashes, loss of hair, impaired immune response and susceptibility to infections, digestive problems, night blindness, changes in affective behavior, defective wound healing, and impaired growth. Its depressant effect on appetite further limits food intake. The hair is thin, dry, coarse, and dull. Depigmentation is common, and patchy alopecia may occur.

Diarrhea (persistent diarrhea malnutrition syndrome) commonly occurs from a lowered resistance to infection and further complicates the electrolyte imbalance. Low levels of cytokines (protein cells involved in the primary response to infection) have been reported in children with kwashiorkor, suggesting that such children have a blunted immune response to infection. A large number of deaths in children with kwashiorkor occur in those who develop HIV infection. GI disturbances such as fatty infiltration of the liver and atrophy of the acini cells of the pancreas occur. Anemia is also a common finding in malnourished children. Protein deficiency increases the child's susceptibility to infection, which eventually results in death. Fatal deterioration may be caused by diarrhea and infection or by circulatory failure.

Marasmus

Marasmus results from general malnutrition of both calories and protein. It is common in underdeveloped countries during times of drought, especially in cultures where adults eat first; the remaining food is often insufficient in quality and quantity for the children.

Marasmus is usually a syndrome of physical and emotional deprivation and is not confined to geographic areas where food supplies are inadequate. It may be seen in children with growth failure in whom the cause is not solely nutritional but primarily emotional. Marasmus may be seen in infants as young as 3 months of age if breastfeeding is not successful and there are no suitable alternatives. *Marasmic kwashiorkor* is a form of SAM in which clinical findings of both kwashiorkor and marasmus are evident; the child has edema, severe wasting, and stunted growth. In marasmic kwashiorkor, the child has inadequate nutrient intake and superimposed infection. Fluid and electrolyte disturbances, hypothermia, and hypoglycemia are associated with a poor prognosis.

Marasmus is characterized by gradual wasting and atrophy of body tissues, especially of subcutaneous fat. The child appears to be very old, with loose and wrinkled skin, unlike the child with kwashiorkor, who appears more rounded from the edema. Fat metabolism is less impaired than in kwashiorkor; thus deficiency of fat-soluble vitamins is usually minimal or absent. In general, the clinical manifestations of marasmus are similar to those seen in kwashiorkor, except with marasmus, there is no edema from hypoalbuminemia or sodium retention, which contributes to a severely emaciated appearance; no dermatoses caused by vitamin deficiencies; little or no depigmentation of hair or skin;

moderately normal fat metabolism and lipid absorption; and a smaller head size and slower recovery after treatment.

The child is fretful, apathetic, withdrawn, and so lethargic that prostration frequently occurs. Intercurrent infection with debilitating diseases such as tuberculosis, parasitosis, HIV, and dysentery is common.

Therapeutic Management

The treatment of SAM includes providing a diet with high-quality proteins, carbohydrates, vitamins, and minerals. When SAM occurs as a result of persistent diarrhea, three management goals are identified:

1. Rehydration with an oral rehydration solution (ORS) that also replaces electrolytes
2. Administration of antibiotics to prevent intercurrent infections
3. Provision of adequate (energy intake) nutrition by either breastfeeding or a proper weaning diet

Local protocols are used in developing countries to deal with SAM. Experts recommend a three-phase treatment protocol: (1) acute or initial phase in the first 2 to 10 days involving initiation of treatment for oral rehydration, diarrhea, and intestinal parasites; prevention of hypoglycemia and hypothermia; and subsequent dietary management; (2) recovery or rehabilitation (2 to 6 weeks) focusing on increasing dietary intake and weight gain; and (3) follow-up phase, focusing on care after discharge in an outpatient setting to prevent relapse and promote weight gain, provide developmental stimulation, and evaluate cognitive and motor deficits. In the acute phase, care is taken to prevent fluid overload; the child is observed closely for signs of food or fluid intolerance. Refeeding syndrome may occur when carbohydrates are administered too rapidly causing severe hypophosphatemia that may cause sudden death in a child who has been malnourished (Kliegman, 2016). Vitamin and mineral supplementation is required in most cases of SAM. Vitamin A, zinc, and copper are recommended; iron supplementation is not recommended until the child is able to tolerate a steady food source. In addition, the child is observed for signs of skin breakdown, which should be treated to prevent infection. Breastfeeding is encouraged if the mother and child are able to do so effectively; in some cases, partial supplementation with a modified cow's milk–based formula may be necessary.

The World Health Organization issued a statement recognizing the importance of breastfeeding for the first 6 months in developing countries where HIV is prevalent among childbearing women and children (Lawrence, 2013). The World Health Organization recognizes that appropriate sources of food and water for infants may not be available after the 6 months are concluded and that the risk for malnutrition is greater among such children than the theoretic risk for HIV. Furthermore, the organization recommends that breastfeeding continue after 6 months with the introduction of complementary foods, provided they are safe for child consumption. In severely malnourished children, a modest energy food source is given initially, followed by a high-protein and high-energy food source; severely malnourished children do not tolerate a high-energy and high-protein source initially. A number of food sources may be provided to treat SAM. They include oral rehydration solutions (ReSoMal), amino acid–based elemental food, and ready-to-feed foods that do not require the addition of water (to minimize contaminated water consumption); parenteral and oral antibiotics are often part of the standard treatment for SAM (Jones & Berkley, 2014).

Interprofessional Care Management

Because SAM appears early in childhood, primarily in children 6 months to 2 years of age, and is associated with early weaning, a low-protein diet, delayed introduction of complementary foods, and frequent infections (Grover & Ee, 2009), it is essential that care focus on *prevention*

of SAM. Parent education should address feeding practices during this crucial period. Prevention among health care providers should also focus on the nutritional health of pregnant women because this directly impacts the health of their unborn children. Breastfeeding is the optimal method of feeding for the first 6 months. The immune properties naturally found in breast milk not only nourish infants but also help prevent opportunistic infections, which may contribute to SAM. Providing for essential physiologic needs such as appropriate nutrient intake, protection from infection, adequate hydration, skin care, and restoration of physiologic integrity is paramount. Additional care focuses on education about and administration of childhood vaccinations to prevent illness, promotion of nutrition and well-being for the lactating mother, encouragement and participation in well-child visits for infants and toddlers, appropriate food sources for children being weaned from breastfeeding, and education regarding sanitation practices to prevent childhood GI diseases.

Poor skin integrity further increases the chance of infections, hypothermia, water loss, and skin breakdown. Tube feedings may be required for infants too weak to breastfeed or bottle-feed. Oral rehydration with an approved oral rehydration solution is commonly used in cases of SAM in which diarrhea and infection are not immediately life-threatening.

One approach that has gained acceptance for treating childhood malnutrition in developing countries is the use of ready-to-use therapeutic food (RUTF). RUTF is a paste based on peanuts, powdered milk, sugar, and vegetable oil; it requires no mixing with water or milk (Ashworth, 2016). The packaged RUTF can be stored without refrigeration. Studies have demonstrated improved survival rates in malnourished children (Amthor, Cole, & Manary, 2009; Park, Kim, Ouma, et al., 2012). Some of the reported advantages of home-based (community-based) treatment include that children are not exposed to hospital-acquired infections and may receive the RUTF from village health aides (Park et al., 2012).

It is imperative that nurses be at the forefront in educating, reinforcing healthy nutrition habits in parents of small children to prevent malnutrition, and eliciting consults from other health care providers when indicated. Because children with marasmus may experience emotional starvation as well, care should be consistent with that for children with FTT.

The World Health Organization has published a guideline for the dietary treatment and management of children with severe acute malnutrition (http://apps.who.int/iris/bitstream/10665/95584/1/9789241506328_eng.pdf?ua=1). This guideline provides a summary of the evidence along with specific recommendations regarding the care of infants and children with SAM.

FOOD SENSITIVITY

In 2010, the National Institute of Allergy and Infectious Diseases, working with 34 other professional organizations, published new evidence-based guidelines for the diagnosis and management of food allergy. A *food allergy* is defined by the National Institute of Allergy and Infectious Diseases as "an adverse health effect arising from a specific immune response that occurs reproducibly on exposure to a given food" (Boyce, Assa'ad, Burks, et al., 2011, p. 64). *Food allergens* are defined as specific components of food or ingredients in food, such as a protein, that are recognized by allergen-specific immune cells eliciting an immune reaction that results in the characteristic symptoms (Boyce et al.). *Food intolerance* is said to exist when a food or food component elicits a reproducible adverse reaction but does not have an established or likely immunologic mechanism (Boyce et al.). For example, a person may have an immune-mediated allergy to cow's milk protein, but the person who is unable to digest the lactose in cow's milk is considered to be intolerant, not allergic to it. The National Institute of Allergy and Infectious Diseases guidelines classify food allergy according to the following: food-induced anaphylaxis, GI food allergies, and specific syndromes; cutaneous reactions to foods; respiratory manifestation; and Heiner syndrome (Boyce et al.). The exact prevalence of food allergies in children is reported to be much lower than that which parents report. Approximately 6% of children may experience food allergic reactions in the first 2 to 3 years of life; 1.5% will have an allergy to eggs, 2.5% to cow's milk, and 1% to peanuts (Nowak-Wegrzyn, Sampson, & Sicherer, 2016). Seafood allergies in children are reported to be low in the United States: 0.2% for fish and 0.5% for crustaceans (Boyce et al.). Most children will eventually be able to tolerate milk, eggs, soy, and wheat; far fewer will ever tolerate tree nuts and peanuts (Boyce et al.). The National Institute of Allergy and Infectious Diseases guidelines also recommend the following (Boyce et al.; Burks, Jones, Boyce, et al., 2011):

- Infants should be breastfed exclusively until 4 to 6 months of age.
- Soy formula is not recommended to prevent the development of food allergy.
- Introduction of complementary foods should not be delayed beyond 6 months of age.
- Hydrolyzed formula (versus cow's milk) may be used in at-risk infants to prevent or modify food allergy.
- Maternal diet during pregnancy or lactation should not be restricted to prevent food allergy.
- Children should be vaccinated with the measles, mumps, and rubella (MMR) and measles, mumps, rubella, and varicella (MMRV) vaccines (even with egg allergy [unless severe reaction occurred]).
- Patients with severe egg allergy reactions should not receive the influenza vaccine without consulting the primary care provider for an analysis of the risks versus benefits (see Chapter 31).

A summary of the National Institute of Allergy and Infectious Diseases guidelines is provided by McBride (2011) and Burks and colleagues (2011).

The clinical manifestations of food allergy may be divided as follows (American Academy of Pediatrics, 2014):

Systemic—Anaphylactic, growth failure
GI—Abdominal pain, vomiting, cramping, diarrhea
Respiratory—Cough, wheezing, rhinitis, infiltrates
Cutaneous—Urticaria, rash, atopic dermatitis

Food allergies usually occur either as an immunoglobulin E (IgE)–mediated or non–IgE-mediated immune response; some toxic reactions may occur as a result of a toxin found within the food. Food allergy is caused by exposure to allergens, usually proteins (but not the smaller amino acids), that are capable of inducing IgE antibody formation (sensitization) when ingested. *Sensitization* refers to the initial exposure of an individual to an allergen, resulting in an immune response; subsequent exposure induces a much stronger response that is clinically apparent. Consequently, food allergy typically occurs after the food has been ingested one or more times. The National Institute of Allergy and Infectious Diseases indicate that sensitization alone is not sufficient to classify as a food allergy; rather an immune-mediated response and manifestation of specific signs and symptoms are necessary to categorize an individual as having a food allergy (Boyce et al., 2011). The most common food allergens are listed in Box 41.3.

Oral allergy syndrome occurs when a food allergen (commonly fruits and vegetables) is ingested and there is subsequent edema and pruritus involving the lips, tongue, palate, and throat. Recovery from symptoms is usually rapid. *Immediate GI hypersensitivity* is an IgE-mediated reaction to a food allergen; reactions include nausea, abdominal pain, cramping, diarrhea, vomiting, anaphylaxis, or all of these. Additional food allergies seen in young children include allergic eosinophilic

---

BOX 41.3   Common Allergenic Foods and Sources

Nuts*—Some chocolates, candy, baked goods, cherry soda (may be flavored with a nut extract), walnut oil

Eggs*—Mayonnaise, creamy salad dressing, baked goods, egg noodles, some cake icing, meringue, custard, pancakes, French toast, root beer

Wheat*—Almost all baked goods, wieners, bologna, pressed or chopped cold cuts, gravy, pasta, some canned soups

Legumes—Peanuts,* peanut butter or oil, beans, peas, lentils

Fish or shellfish*—Cod liver oil, pizza with anchovies, Caesar salad dressing, any food fried in same oil as fish

Soy*—Soy sauce, teriyaki or Worcestershire sauce, tofu, baked goods using soy flour or oil, soy nuts, soy infant formulas or milk, soybean paste, tuna packed in vegetable oil, many margarines

Chocolate—Cola beverages, cocoa, chocolate-flavored drinks

Milk—Ice cream, butter, margarine (if it contains dairy products), yogurt, cheese, pudding, baked goods, wieners, bologna, canned creamed soups, instant breakfast drinks, powdered milk drinks, milk chocolate

Buckwheat—Some cereals, pancakes

Pork, chicken—Bacon, wieners, sausage, pork fat, chicken broth

Strawberries, melon, pineapple—Gelatin, syrups

Corn—Popcorn, cereal, muffins, cornstarch, corn meal, corn bread, corn tortillas, corn syrup

Citrus fruits—Orange, lemon, lime, grapefruit; any of these in drinks, gelatin, juice, or medicines

Tomatoes—Juice, some vegetable soups, spaghetti, pizza sauce, catsup

Spices—Chili, pepper, vinegar, cinnamon

*Most common allergens.

---

esophagitis, allergic eosinophilic gastroenteritis, food protein–induced proctocolitis, and food protein–induced enterocolitis.

Food allergy or hypersensitivity may also be classified according to the interval between ingestion and the manifestation of symptoms: immediate (within minutes to hours) or delayed (2 to 48 hours) (American Academy of Pediatrics, 2014).

Food allergies can occur at any time but are common during infancy because the immature intestinal tract is more permeable to proteins than the mature intestinal tract, thus increasing the likelihood of an immune response. Allergies in general demonstrate a genetic component: children who have one parent with an allergy have a 50% or greater risk for developing allergy; children who have both parents with an allergy have up to a 100% risk for developing allergy. Allergy with a hereditary tendency is referred to as *atopy*. Some infants with atopy can be identified at birth from elevated levels of IgE in umbilical cord blood.

Deaths have been reported in children who experienced an anaphylactic reaction to food. Onset of the reactions occurred shortly after ingestion (5 to 30 minutes). In most of the children, the reactions did not begin with skin signs such as hives, red rash, and flushing but rather mimicked an acute asthma attack (wheezing, decreased air movement in airways, dyspnea). Watch children with food anaphylaxis closely because a biphasic response has been recorded in a number of cases in which there is an immediate response, apparent recovery, and acute recurrence of symptoms (Alqurashi, Stiell, Chan, et al., 2015). Children with extremely sensitive food allergies should wear a medical alert identification bracelet and have an injectable epinephrine cartridge (EpiPen) readily available (see the "Anaphylaxis" section in Chapter 42). Any child with a history of food allergy or previous severe reaction to food should have a written emergency treatment plan and an EpiPen (see Emergency Treatment box: Management of Anaphylaxis). Note

---

✚ EMERGENCY TREATMENT
Management of Anaphylaxis

Drug—Epinephrine 0.01 mg/kg up to maximum of 0.5 mg
Dosage—EpiPen Jr 0.15 mg intramuscularly (IM) for child weighing 8 to 25 kg (17.5 to 55 pounds) or EpiPen (0.3 mg) IM for child weighing more than 25 kg (55 pounds)
Monitor—for adverse reactions, such as tachycardia, hypertension, irritability, headache, nausea, and tremors.

Data from Sampson, H.A., Wang, J., & Sicherer, S.H. (2016). Anaphylaxis. In R.M. Kliegman, B.F. Stanton, J.W. St. Geme, et al. (Eds), *Nelson textbook of pediatrics* (20th ed.). Philadelphia, PA: Saunders/Elsevier.

that diphenhydramine and cetirizine are effective for cutaneous and nasal manifestations but not for airway manifestations (Keet, 2011).

Although the reason is unknown, many children "outgrow" their food allergies (Nowak-Wegrzyn et al., 2016). Children who are allergic to more than one food may develop tolerance to each food at a different time. The most common allergens such as peanuts are outgrown less readily than other food allergens. Because of the tendency to lose the hypersensitivity, allergenic foods should be reintroduced into the diet after a period of abstinence (usually ≥1 year) to evaluate whether the food can safely be added to the diet. However, foods that are associated with severe anaphylactic reactions continue to present a lifelong risk and must be avoided.

❗ NURSING ALERT

Indications for the administration of intramuscular epinephrine in a child with a life-threatening anaphylactic reaction or one who is experiencing severe symptoms include any one of the following (Simons, Ardusso, Biló, et al., 2012):

- Itching sensation or tightness in throat; hoarseness
- "Barky" cough
- Difficulty swallowing; dyspnea
- Wheezing or stridor
- Itching, flushing, urticaria, angioedema
- Anxiety, confusion, sense of impending doom
- Syncope, bradycardia, dysrhythmia, or hypotension

Diagnosis and Therapeutic Management

The diagnosis of food allergy is made based on a number of factors, including the occurrence of anaphylaxis or any combination of 37 symptoms listed in the National Institute of Allergy and Infectious Diseases guidelines within minutes to hours of ingesting food or if such symptoms have occurred after the ingestion of a specific food on one or more occasions. The gold standard is the double-blind, placebo-controlled food challenge; the skin prick test and serum IgE measurements may be used as an adjunct to diagnose food allergy but singly should not be used for the diagnosis. The atopy patch test, intradermal test, and serum IgE test are not recommended for establishing a diagnosis. A single oral food challenge may be used in certain circumstances (Boyce et al., 2011). The traditional management of food allergy consists of avoiding the specific food or ingredient that causes the manifestations. Because children with food allergies (usually two or more) are at risk for inadequate nutrient intake and growth failure, it is recommended that they have an annual nutritional assessment to prevent such problems.

CLINICAL REASONING CASE STUDY
Food Allergy Anaphylaxis

A group of nursing students is holding a health promotion fair at a local elementary school for first, second, and third graders. The nursing students have several booths set up in the school cafeteria. Three second-grade boys are engaging in horseplay in front of one of the booths when one of the boys, Jason, an 8-year-old child, suddenly starts coughing and clutching his throat. The students also observe that he is developing red splotches on his face, neck, and throat and that he is scratching. Jason says, "I'm having trouble breathing!" The school nurse is nearby and comes over to see what the commotion is about. One of the boys with Jason says, "We didn't mean any harm! We were just goofing around when we put peanuts in his trail mix." One of the student nurses says, "He's in obvious distress. What should we do?"

1. Evidence—Is there sufficient evidence to draw any conclusions at this time about Jason's condition?
2. Assumptions—Describe some underlying assumptions about the following:
   a. Clinical manifestations of food allergy
   b. The emergency treatment of a food allergy "reaction," or anaphylaxis
   c. Which one of the following interventions would have highest immediate priority?
      (1) Call Jason's parents, and ask them to come pick him up from school.
      (2) Call Jason's family practitioner to obtain orders for medication.
      (3) Promptly administer an intramuscular dose of epinephrine.
      (4) Call 911, and wait for the emergency response personnel to arrive.
3. What implication for nursing care exists in this situation after an intervention in the previous question has been chosen and implemented?
4. Describe the potential results of taking a "let's observe Jason for a few minutes before we do anything" stance in this scenario.
5. Is there evidence to support your immediate and secondary nursing interventions? Provide objective evidence to support your decisions for action.

Care Management

Nursing care of children with potential food allergy consists of assisting in collecting vital health assessment data for the establishment of a diagnosis and assisting with diagnostic tests. It is important for nurses to be informed about food allergy and provide parents, caregivers, and older children with accurate information regarding food allergy.

Educate parents, teachers, and day care workers regarding signs and symptoms of food allergy and reactions. Children with a history of food allergy may spend a considerable amount of time in day care; therefore people working in day care centers and other children's settings need to be educated properly regarding recognition and management of severe anaphylactic reactions (see Clinical Reasoning Case Study: Food Allergy Anaphylaxis). People with food allergy should avoid unfamiliar foods and restaurants that do not disclose food ingredients. New labeling guidelines require that food additives, such as spices and flavoring, be labeled clearly on commercially sold, store-bought foods. Hidden ingredients in prepared foods are also potential sources of food allergy.

Breastfeeding is a primary strategy for avoiding atopy in families with known food allergies; however, there is no evidence that maternal avoidance (during pregnancy or lactation) of cow's milk protein or other dietary products known to cause food allergy prevents food allergy in children (American Academy of Pediatrics, 2014; Boyce et al., 2011). Researchers indicate that delaying the introduction of highly allergenic foods past 4 to 6 months of age may not be as protective for food allergy as previously believed (Fleischer, Spergel, Assa'ad, et al., 2013). Likewise

BOX 41.4   Common Clinical Manifestations of Cow's Milk Allergy

Gastrointestinal
- Diarrhea
- Vomiting
- Colic
- Abdominal pain
- Gastroesophageal reflux
- Blood streaked mucous, loose stools

Respiratory
- Rhinitis
- Bronchitis
- Wheezing
- Sneezing
- Coughing
- Chronic nasal discharge
- Asthma exacerbation

Cutaneous
- Urticaria
- Atopic dermatitis

Systemic
- Anaphylaxis

Other Signs and Symptoms
- Eczema
- Excessive crying
- Pallor (from anemia secondary to chronic blood loss in gastrointestinal tract)
- Fussiness, irritability

studies have shown that soy formula does not prevent allergic disease in infants and children (Fleischer et al., 2013).*

Cow's Milk Allergy

Cow's milk allergy (CMA) is a multifaceted disorder representing adverse systemic and local GI reactions to cow's milk protein. Approximately 2.5% of infants develop cow's milk hypersensitivity, with 60% of these being IgE mediated. Some studies suggest that milk allergy may persist, and some children may not be able to tolerate milk until they are 16 years of age (American Academy of Pediatrics, 2014). (This discussion centers on cow's milk protein contained in commercial infant formulas; whole milk is not recommended for infants younger than 12 months of age.) The allergy may be manifested within the first 4 months of life through a variety of signs and symptoms that may appear within 45 minutes of milk ingestion or after several days (Box 41.4). The diagnosis initially may be made from the history, although the history alone is not diagnostic. The timing and diversity of clinical manifestations vary greatly. For example, CMA may be manifested as colic (see Chapter

---

*Additional information for parents of infants with food allergies is available from the American Academy of Allergy, Asthma and Immunology, 555 E. Wells Street, Suite 1100, Milwaukee, WI 53202, 414-272-6071, www.aaaai.org. Additional helpful websites for information on food allergy include MedlinePlus (sponsored by the US National Library of Medicine and National Institutes of Health), www.nlm.nih.gov/medlineplus; Food Allergy and Anaphylaxis Network, 800-929-4040, www.foodallergy.org; and National Institute of Allergy and Infectious Diseases, www.niaid.nih.gov and Allergic Child, www.allergicchild.com.

31), diarrhea, vomiting, GI bleeding, gastroesophageal reflux, chronic constipation, or sleeplessness in an otherwise healthy infant.

Diagnostic Evaluation

A number of diagnostic tests may be performed, including stool analysis for blood, eosinophils, and leukocytes (both frank and occult bleeding can occur from the colitis); serum IgE levels; skin-prick or scratch testing; and radioallergosorbent test (RAST) (measures IgE antibodies to specific allergens in serum by radioimmunoassay). Both skin testing and RAST may help identify the offending food, but the results are not always conclusive. No single diagnostic test is considered definitive for the diagnosis (American Academy of Pediatrics, 2014).

The most definitive diagnostic strategy is elimination of milk in the diet followed by challenge testing after improvement of symptoms. A clinical diagnosis is made when symptoms improve after removal of milk from the diet and two or more challenge tests produce symptoms (Kattan, Cocco, & Järvinen, 2011). *Challenge testing* involves reintroducing small quantities of milk in the diet to detect resurgence of symptoms; at times it involves the use of a placebo so the parent is unaware of (or "blind" to) the timing of allergen ingestion. A double-blind, placebo-controlled food challenge is the gold standard for diagnosing food allergies such as CMA, yet it may not be used often for diagnosing CMA because of the expense, time involved, and risk for further exposure and anaphylactic reaction (Dupont, 2014). Careful observation of the child is required during a challenge test because of the possibility of anaphylactic reaction.

Therapeutic Management

Treatment of CMA is elimination of cow's milk–based formula and all other dairy products. For infants fed cow's milk–based formula, this primarily involves changing the formula to a casein hydrolysate milk formula (Pregestimil, Nutramigen, or Alimentum) in which the protein has been broken down into its amino acids through enzymatic hydrolysis. Although the American Academy of Pediatrics (2014) recommends the use of extensively hydrolyzed formulas for CMA, many health care providers may start a soy formula instead because of the expense of the hydrolyzed formulas. Approximately 50% of infants who are sensitive to cow's milk protein also demonstrate sensitivity to soy, but soy is less expensive than protein hydrolysate formula. Other choices for children who are intolerant to cow's milk–based formula are the amino acid–based formulas Neocate or EleCare, but their cost is a major consideration. Goat's milk (raw) is not an acceptable substitute because it cross-reacts with cow's milk protein, is deficient in folic acid, has a high sodium and protein content, and is unsuitable as the only source of calories. Some suggest that goat's milk infant formula may be a suitable substitute for cow's milk formula; however, anaphylactic reaction to goat's milk has been noted in infants who are also allergic to cow's milk (Ehlayel, Bener, Hazeima, et al., 2011). Infants usually remain on the milk-free diet for 12 months, after which time small quantities of milk are reintroduced.

Children who have CMA may tolerate extensively heated cow's milk (Dupont, 2014). One study reports that these children became tolerant to uncooked milk products over time after consuming baked milk products (Kim, Nowak-Wegrzyn, Sicherer, et al., 2011).

Care Management

The principal nursing objectives are identification of potential CMA and appropriate counseling of parents regarding substitute formulas. Parents often interpret GI symptoms such as spitting up and loose stools or fussiness as indications that the infant is allergic to cow's milk and switch the infant to a variety of formulas in an attempt to resolve the problem.

Parents need much reassurance regarding the needs of nonverbal infants with such an array of symptoms. Endless nights of lost sleep and a crying infant may promote feelings of parenting inadequacy and role conflict, thus aggravating the situation. Nurses can reassure parents that many of these symptoms are common and the reasons are often never found, yet the child does achieve appropriate growth and development. Report acute symptoms to the practitioner for further evaluation. Parents need reassurance that the infant will receive complete nutrition from the new formula and will have no ill effects from the absence of cow's milk.

When solid foods are started, parents need guidance in avoiding milk products. Carefully reading all food labels helps avoid exposure to prepared foods containing milk products. Although labeled as nondairy, milk, cream, and butter substitutes may contain cow's milk protein (Kattan et al., 2011).

RECURRENT AND FUNCTIONAL ABDOMINAL PAIN

Recurrent abdominal pain (RAP) is a complaint of childhood that is often attributed to psychogenic causes, although it can be a symptom of either psychosomatic or organic disease. RAP is characterized by three or more separate episodes of abdominal pain at least 3 months before diagnosis that interferes with daily activities (El-Radhi, 2015). The disorder affects school-age children 4 to 18 years of age but is more common in children approximately 11 years of age, and it occurs more often in girls than in boys (Chiou, How, & Ong, 2013). The most common causes of RAP in childhood are: (1) functional abdominal pain, (2) irritable bowel syndrome (IBS), (3) abdominal migraine, and (4) food intolerance/allergy (El-Radhi, 2015). Most children with RAP suffer from functional abdominal pain (FAP).

ETIOLOGY AND PATHOPHYSIOLOGY

Only a minority of children and adolescents with RAP have an organic basis for their pain. Organic causes include IBD, PUD, lactose intolerance, pelvic inflammatory disease, urinary tract infection, and pancreatitis. Psychogenic causes of abdominal pain, such as school phobia, depression, acute reactive anxiety, and conversion reaction, account for a small number of cases.

In cases in which no organic disorder is identifiable, the abdominal pain of RAP has been attributed to dysfunction. Dysfunctional conditions causing RAP include constipation, chronic stool retention, overeating, irritable colon, and intestinal gas with heightened awareness of intestinal motility or dysmotility. The symptoms of RAP may result from multiple causes, and it is important to assess a number of factors that could place a child at risk for this condition. These include (1) somatic predisposition, dysfunction, or disorder; (2) lifestyle and habit, including routines, diet, and life tempo; (3) temperament and learned response patterns, such as the child's behavior style, personality, and learned coping skills; and (4) milieu and critical events (i.e., the child's intimate surroundings [familial, social, and cultural norms] and unexpected sources of stress or gratification).

DIAGNOSTIC EVALUATION

Diagnosis is based on a complete family history, the child's health history, physical examination, and laboratory tests. The family history may provide evidence of a hereditary disorder or mimicry of adult symptoms. The child is evaluated for evidence of an organic basis for symptoms, such as pain that radiates to the back, pain that awakens the child from sleep, persistent right upper or right lower quadrant pain, unexplained or recurrent fever, weight loss, GI blood loss, significant vomiting, chronic severe diarrhea, or family history of IBD. Pain is assessed for location, quality, frequency, duration, any associated symptoms, alleviating factors, and exacerbating factors.

THERAPEUTIC MANAGEMENT

Treatment involves providing reassurance and reducing or eliminating symptoms. Initial efforts are directed toward ruling out organic causes of the pain, relieving discomfort, and attempting to determine the situations that precipitate attacks.

Emphasize a high-fiber diet, psyllium bulk agents, lubricants, such as mineral oil, and bowel training for pain associated with bowel patterns. Treatment may also include acid-reduction therapy for pain associated with dyspepsia; antispasmodic agents, smooth muscle relaxants, or low doses of psychotropic agents for pain. Dietary modifications may include removal of dairy products, fructose, and gluten for 2 to 3 weeks to rule out lactose intolerance, sensitivity to high sugar content, and celiac disease. Other treatments include cognitive-behavioral therapy and biofeedback.

CARE MANAGEMENT

The nurse can be instrumental in assessment and management of RAP in children. Evaluate the child's social and psychologic adjustment, and obtain the details of the pain directly from the child. Questions that provide clues to parent-child relationships and the way that the family deals with angry feelings provide information for diagnosis and management. Relationships with peers, school problems, and other concerns of the child need to be explored. Note any evidence of depression.

Once the diagnosis has been established, the parents and the child need an explanation of the pain, which can be compared to a skeletal muscle cramp, "charley horse," or headache for easier comprehension. Reassurance that the symptoms are not unique to their child and that the pain is rarely associated with a severe disease can help relieve parental fears and anxieties. After the parents are reassured that there is no organic cause for the pain, they need guidance on what to do during a pain episode. Often they feel helpless and anxious, which tends to compound the child's distress. The simple measure of having the child rest in a peaceful, quiet environment and providing comfort will often relieve the symptoms in a short time. Application of a heating pad may also ease the discomfort. If pain is not relieved by these simple measures, teach parents how to administer antispasmodics, if prescribed.

Discuss a high-fiber diet with the child and family, and emphasize bowel training. The child is encouraged to establish a pattern of sitting on the toilet for 10 to 15 minutes immediately after breakfast to take advantage of the increased colonic activity following meals. If necessary, have the child use stimulatory suppositories to induce early morning defecation.

The most valuable assistance that the nurse can provide is support and reassurance to the family. When open communication is established and families are able to see a relationship between stress-provoking situations and the child's symptoms, the chance for remedial action is enhanced. Follow-up care and continued support are essential because the symptoms tend to remit and exacerbate; therefore, the availability of a supportive health professional can be a source of comfort to the child and family.

IRRITABLE BOWEL SYNDROME

Irritable bowel syndrome (IBS) is classified as a functional GI disorder. Children with IBS often have alternating diarrhea and constipation, flatulence, bloating or a feeling of abdominal distention, lower abdominal pain, a feeling of urgency when needed to defecate, and a feeling of incomplete evacuation of the bowel. These symptoms should be present for 6 months or longer and present for at least 3 days per month over the last 3 months (Wadlund, 2012). IBS has been identified as a cause of RAP in 21% to 45% of school-age children (Rajindrajith & Devanarayana, 2012). Typically there are no abnormal physical findings on examination. Many children with symptoms appear active and healthy and have normal growth.

The cause of IBS is not clear, but it is believed to involve a combination of autonomic and psychologic factors. Children with IBS are evaluated to rule out organic causes of their symptoms, such as inflammatory bowel disease (IBD), lactose intolerance, and parasitic infections. The long-range goal of treatment is development of regular bowel habits and relief of symptoms.

Care Management

The disorder is stressful to children and parents, and the primary nursing goal is family support and education. The nurse provides support and reassurance that, although the symptoms are difficult to deal with, the disorder is not generally a threat to the child's health.

ACUTE APPENDICITIS

Appendicitis, inflammation of the *vermiform appendix* (blind sac at the end of the cecum), is the most common cause of emergency abdominal surgery in childhood. In the United States, 70,000 cases are diagnosed each year (Pepper, Stanfill, & Pearl, 2012). The average age of children with appendicitis is 10 years of age, with boys and girls equally affected before puberty (Pepper et al., 2012). Classically the first symptom of appendicitis is periumbilical pain followed by nausea, right lower quadrant pain, and later vomiting with fever (Balachandran, Singhi, & Lal, 2013). Perforation of the appendix can occur within approximately 48 hours of the initial complaint of pain and occurs in 20% to 40% of children with appendicitis (Wheeler, 2011). Complications from appendiceal perforation include major abscess, phlegmon, enterocutaneous fistula, peritonitis, and partial bowel obstruction (Pepper et al.). A *phlegmon* is an acute suppurative inflammation of subcutaneous connective tissue that spreads.

Etiology

The cause of appendicitis is obstruction of the lumen of the appendix, usually by hardened fecal material *(fecalith)*. Swollen lymphoid tissue, frequently occurring after a viral infection, can also obstruct the appendix. Another rare cause of obstruction is a parasite such as *Enterobius vermicularis*, or pinworms, which can obstruct the appendiceal lumen.

Pathophysiology

With acute obstruction, the outflow of mucus secretions is blocked, and pressure builds within the lumen, resulting in compression of blood vessels. The resulting ischemia is followed by ulceration of the epithelial lining and bacterial invasion. Subsequent necrosis causes perforation or rupture with fecal and bacterial contamination of the peritoneal cavity. The resulting inflammation spreads rapidly throughout the abdomen *(peritonitis)*, especially in young children who are unable to localize infection. Progressive peritoneal inflammation results in functional intestinal obstruction of the small bowel *(ileus)* because intense GI reflexes severely inhibit bowel motility. Because the peritoneum represents a major portion of total body surface, the loss of ECF to the peritoneal cavity leads to electrolyte imbalance and hypovolemic shock.

Diagnostic Evaluation

Diagnosis is not always straightforward. Fever, vomiting, abdominal pain, and an elevated white blood cell (WBC) count are associated with

BOX 41.5 Clinical Manifestations of Appendicitis

- Right lower quadrant abdominal pain
- Fever
- Rigid abdomen
- Decreased or absent bowel sounds
- Vomiting (typically follows onset of pain)
- Constipation or diarrhea may be present
- Anorexia
- Tachycardia
- Rapid, shallow breathing
- Pallor
- Lethargy
- Irritability
- Stooped posture (guarding)

appendicitis but are also seen in IBD, pelvic inflammatory disease, gastroenteritis, urinary tract infection, right lower lobe pneumonia, mesenteric adenitis, Meckel diverticulum, and intussusception. Prolonged symptoms and delayed diagnosis often occur in younger children, in whom the risk for perforation is greatest because of their inability to verbalize their complaints.

The diagnosis is based primarily on the history and physical examination (Box 41.5). Pain, the cardinal feature, initially is generalized (usually periumbilical); however, it usually descends to the lower right quadrant. The most intense site of pain may be at McBurney point, located at a point midway between the anterior superior iliac crest and the umbilicus. Rebound tenderness is extremely painful to the child but not a reliable sign. Referred pain, elicited by light percussion around the perimeter of the abdomen, indicates peritoneal irritation. Movement, such as riding over bumps in an automobile or wheelchair, aggravates the pain. In addition to pain, significant clinical manifestations include fever, a change in behavior, anorexia, and vomiting.

Laboratory studies usually include a CBC, urinalysis (to rule out a urinary tract infection), and in adolescent females serum human chorionic gonadotropin (to rule out an ectopic pregnancy). A WBC count greater than 10,000/mm^3 and an elevated C-reactive protein (CRP) are common but not necessarily specific for appendicitis. An elevated percentage of bands (often referred to as *a shift to the left*) may indicate an inflammatory process. CRP is an acute-phase reactant that rises within 12 hours of the onset of infection.

Computed tomography (CT) has become the imaging technique of choice, although ultrasonography may also be helpful in diagnosing appendicitis. A CT scan result is considered positive in the presence of enlarged appendiceal diameter; appendiceal wall thickening; and periappendiceal inflammatory changes, including fat streaks, phlegmon, fluid collection, and extraluminal gas (Balachandran et al., 2013). The accuracy of CT scan is 96% for diagnosing appendicitis (Pepper et al., 2012).

! NURSING ALERT

Signs of peritonitis, in addition to fever, include sudden relief from pain after perforation; subsequent increase in pain (usually diffuse and accompanied by rigid guarding of the abdomen); progressive abdominal distention; tachycardia; rapid, shallow breathing; pallor; chills; irritability; and restlessness.

Therapeutic Management

Treatment of appendicitis before perforation is surgical removal of the appendix *(appendectomy)*. Usually antibiotics are administered preoperatively. IV fluids and electrolytes are often required before surgery, especially if the child is dehydrated as a result of the marked anorexia characteristic of appendicitis.

The operation is usually performed through a right lower quadrant incision (open appendectomy). Laparoscopic surgery is now commonly used to treat nonperforated acute appendicitis. Advantages of laparoscopic appendectomy include reduced time in surgery and anesthesia, and reduced risk for postoperative wound infection (Wray, Kao, Millas, et al., 2013).

Ruptured Appendix

Management of the child diagnosed with peritonitis caused by a ruptured appendix often begins preoperatively with IV administration of fluid and electrolytes, systemic antibiotics, and NG decompression. Postoperative management includes IV fluids, continued administration of antibiotics, and NG suction for abdominal decompression until intestinal activity returns. Sometimes surgeons close the wound after irrigation of the peritoneal cavity. At other times, the wound is left open (delayed closure) to prevent wound infection. A Penrose drain may be used to permit transperitoneal drainage.

Prognosis

Complications are uncommon after a simple appendectomy, and recovery is usually rapid and complete. The mortality rate for perforating appendicitis has improved from nearly certain death a century ago to 1% or less at the present time (Wray et al., 2013). Early recognition of the illness is essential to prevent complications.

Care Management

Because abdominal pain is the most common childhood complaint with appendicitis, it is important to assess the severity of pain (see the "Pain Assessment" section in Chapter 30). One of the most reliable estimates is the degree of change in behavior. Younger, nonverbal children assume a rigid, motionless, side-lying posture with the knees flexed on the abdomen, and there is decreased range of motion of the right hip. Older children may exhibit all of these behaviors while complaining of abdominal pain.

> **! NURSING ALERT**
>
> In any instance in which severe abdominal pain is observed, be aware of the danger of administering laxatives or enemas. Such measures stimulate bowel motility and increase the risk for perforation.

Postoperative Care

Postoperative care for the nonperforated appendix is the same as for most abdominal procedures. Care of the child with a ruptured appendix and peritonitis involves more complex care, and the course of recovery is considerably longer. The child is maintained on IV fluids, is kept NPO, and the NG tube is kept on low continuous gastric decompression until there is evidence of intestinal activity. Listening for bowel sounds and observing for other signs of bowel activity (e.g., passage of flatus or stool) are part of the routine assessment. A drain may be placed in the wound during surgery, and frequent dressing changes with meticulous skin care are essential to prevent excoriation of the area surrounding the surgical site. Wound care includes irrigation with antibacterial solution or saline.

Management of pain from the incision and repeated dressing changes and irrigations are an essential part of the child's care. Because pain is continuous during the first few postoperative days, analgesics are given regularly to control pain. Procedures are performed when the analgesics are at peak effect. Psychologic care of the child and parents is similar to that used in other emergency situations. Parents and older children need to express their feelings and concerns regarding the events surrounding the illness and hospitalization. The nurse can provide education and psychosocial support to promote adequate coping and alleviate anxiety for both the child and the family (see Nursing Care Plan: The Child with Appendicitis).

MECKEL DIVERTICULUM

Meckel diverticulum is a remnant of the fetal omphalomesenteric duct, which connects the yolk sac with the primitive midgut during fetal life (Kotecha, Bellah, Pena, Jaimes & Mattei, 2012). Normally the structure is obliterated between the fifth ad ninth week of gestation, when the placenta replaces the yolk sac as the source of nutrition for the fetus. Failure of obliteration may result in an omphalomesenteric fistula (a fibrous band connecting the small intestine to the umbilicus), referred to as Meckel diverticulum.

Meckel diverticulum is a true diverticulum because it arises from the antimesenteric border of the small intestine and includes all layers of the intestinal wall. The position of the diverticulum varies, but it is usually found within 40 to 50 cm (16 to 20 inches) of the ileocecal valve. Meckel diverticulum is often referred to by the "rule of twos" because it occurs in 2% of the population, has a 2:1 male-to-female ratio, is located within 2 feet of the ileocecal valve, is commonly 2 cm in diameter and 2 inches in length, contains two types of ectopic tissue (pancreatic and gastric), and is more common before 2 years of age (Pepper et al., 2012).

Pathophysiology

Bleeding, obstruction, or inflammation causes the symptomatic complications of Meckel diverticulum. Bleeding, which is the most common problem in children, is caused by peptic ulceration or perforation because of the unbuffered acidic secretion. Several mechanisms may cause obstruction such as intussusception or entanglement of the small intestine (Pepper et al., 2012).

Diagnostic Evaluation

Diagnosis is usually based on the history, physical examination, and radiographic studies. Meckel diverticulum is often a diagnostic challenge. A technetium-99 pertechnetate scan (Meckel scan) is the most effective diagnostic testing, especially for a bleeding diverticulum, with sensitivity ranging from 65% to 85% (Pepper et al., 2012). CT, magnetic resonance imaging (MRI), and mesenteric angiography may be used to investigate complications of Meckel diverticulum, but each test has associated risks, such as the use of contrast for CT scans, exposure to radiation for MRI scans, and the blood loss for tagged red blood cells with mesenteric angiography (Pepper et al.). Laboratory studies are usually part of the general workup to rule out any bleeding disorder and evaluate the severity of the anemia.

The most common clinical presentation in children includes painless rectal bleeding, abdominal pain, or signs of intestinal obstruction (Box 41.6). Bleeding, which may be mild or profuse, often appears as dark red or "currant jelly" stools; it may be significant enough to cause hypotension.

Therapeutic Management

The standard treatment for symptomatic Meckel diverticulum is surgical removal of the diverticulum. When severe hemorrhage increases the surgical risk, interventions to correct hypovolemic shock such as blood replacement, IV fluids, and oxygen may be necessary. Antibiotics may be used before surgery to control infection. If intestinal obstruction

NURSING CARE PLAN
The Child With Appendicitis

Case Study

Lisa is a 10-year-old girl who has a 2-day history of generalized periumbilical pain and anorexia. Today she developed a fever and vomiting, so her parents took her to her pediatrician. On examination, Lisa was febrile with abdominal pain midway between the anterior superior iliac crest and umbilicus. The pain intensifies with any activity or deep breathing. Blood work was performed, and a complete blood count with differential shows a white blood cell count of 21,000/mm³, 79% bands, 14% lymphocytes, 6% eosinophils, and a normal hemoglobin and platelet count. With Lisa's history and physical findings, she was referred to a local emergency department.

Assessment

Based on Lisa's history, what are the most important signs and symptoms that you need to be aware of?

Defining Characteristics

A 2-day history of abdominal pain that started around the umbilicus and has now progressed to the lower-right abdomen (McBurney's point)
Fever
Anorexia
Nausea and vomiting
Elevated white blood cell count (>10,000/mm³) along with a high percentage of bands (left shift)
Elevated C-reactive protein

Nursing Diagnoses

Pain, Acute
Body Temperature, Imbalanced
Infection
Nausea
Risk for Electrolyte Imbalance
Risk for Fluid Volume Deficit
Knowledge Deficit

Nursing Interventions and Rationales

What are the most appropriate nursing interventions for a child with appendicitis?

Nursing Interventions	Rationales
Close monitoring of Lisa's status. Follow clinical and laboratory findings. Blood studies included CBC, CRP, and electrolytes	To identify infection, signs of inflammation, changes in fluid and electrolyte status, which require additional treatment
Close monitoring of diagnostic evaluation studies (i.e., CT scan and/or ultrasound).	To confirm diagnosis of appendicitis
Administer IV fluids.	To correct fluid deficit and electrolyte imbalances
Administer analgesics as ordered.	To reduce pain
Administer antiemetics as ordered.	To reduce nausea and alleviate vomiting
Monitor temperature and vital signs.	To observe for signs of infection
Administer antipyretic medication as indicated.	To reduce fever
Administer antibiotics as ordered.	To treat infection
Maintain NPO status.	To keep stomach empty in anticipation of possible surgery

Nursing Interventions	Rationales
Identify patient and family stressors that may accompany a diagnosis of appendicitis.	Providing financial and emotion support for family can help decrease some of the stressors associated with this condition.
Review disease, medication, dietary restrictions.	Understanding the medical condition and therapies allows family to make informed decisions about care

Expected Outcomes

Lisa will exhibit decreased pain
Lisa will exhibit no evidence of nausea or vomiting
Lisa's body temperature is within normal limits
Sufficient fluid and electrolytes are maintained
Lisa and her family indicate understanding of appendicitis and treatment

Case Study (Continued)

Results of the CT scan demonstrate a ruptured appendix. Lisa is now being prepared for surgery. The nurse performing the assessment finds Lisa's temperature to be elevated. Lisa reports the pain had initially resolved but she now reports increasing pain (rated 9 out of 10) and nausea.

Assessment

What concerns you most based on the scenario?
 Lisa's appendix has ruptured, and the recurrence of pain and fever is likely related to an infection or possible abscess.
 What immediate steps should be taken to further evaluate Lisa's status?
Check CBC and differential.
Document temperature and vital signs (pulse, respirations, blood pressure).
Assess and document location and rating of pain.
Administer antipyretic agent, analgesic, antiemetic, and intravenous fluids.
 The following laboratory results have returned from Lisa's blood work:
CBC: WBC 26,000/mm³, bands 81%, lymphocytes 12%, eosinophils 5%, normal hemoglobin and normal platelets
Electrolytes and kidney function: potassium 3.4, sodium 135, BUN 25, serum creatinine 1.2

Nursing Diagnoses

Pain, Acute
Body Temperature, Imbalanced
Infection
Nausea
Risk for Electrolyte Imbalance
Risk for Fluid Volume Deficit

Nursing Interventions and Rationales

What are the most appropriate nursing interventions for Lisa before and after surgery?

Nursing Interventions	Rationales
Administer antibiotics as ordered. Intravenous antibiotics are given for a minimum of 3 days postoperatively in children with complicated appendicitis and are transitioned to oral antibiotics at discharge.	To treat infection

Continued

◎ NURSING CARE PLAN

The Child With Appendicitis—cont'd

Nursing Interventions	Rationales
Administer analgesics as ordered.	To reduce pain
Administer antiemetics as ordered.	To reduce nausea and alleviate vomiting
Monitor temperature and vital signs.	To observe for signs of infection and shock
Administer IV fluids, and monitor electrolytes.	To correct fluid deficit and electrolyte imbalances
Follow laboratory findings. Blood studies including CBC, CRP, and intraoperative cultures if obtained.	To identify infection, and signs of inflammation
Advance diet as tolerated postoperatively.	To maintain nutritional status

Expected Outcomes

Lisa will exhibit no signs of infection.

Lisa's pain will be controlled initially with intravenous analgesics, and then Lisa will transition to oral analgesics.

Lisa will exhibit no evidence of nausea or vomiting.

Lisa will tolerate a regular diet.

Lisa's body temperature is within normal limits.

Sufficient fluid and electrolytes are maintained.

Case Study (Continued)

Lisa's parents are anxious and upset with the urgent need for surgery and hospitalization. You are concerned that they do not understand what is happening to their daughter.

Assessment

What are the most important aspects of Lisa's care to discuss with her parents at this time?

Defining Characteristics

- Understands definition of appendicitis and ruptured appendix
- Describes rationale for urgent surgery
- Describes rationale for subsequent hospitalization and need for intravenous antibiotics
- Expresses fears and concerns
- Shows appropriate reactions to child's illness

Nursing Diagnosis

Readiness for Enhanced Knowledge related to parents' interest in Lisa's health status.

Nursing Interventions and Rationales

What are the most appropriate nursing interventions for this diagnosis?

Nursing Interventions	Rationales
Review disease and treatment prior to surgery.	Understanding the medical condition and therapies allow families to make informed decisions about care.
Review disease and treatment after surgery.	To increase knowledge and compliance with treatment plan to control pain, treat infection, maintain adequate fluid and electrolyte balance, and maximize nutrition
Arrange for social worker to meet with family to assess emotional and financial needs.	To identify and modify stressors associated with urgent and prolonged hospitalization
As child nears discharge, arrange for discussions with parents to discuss home care.	Family must be aware of necessary treatment and monitoring in order to be compliant with care.

Expected Outcomes

Parents will indicate understanding of appendicitis and treatment.

Parents will verbalize understanding the signs and symptoms of infection and understand the actions to treat infection.

Parents will verbalize understanding of the plan for managing postsurgical treatment at home.

BOX 41.6   Clinical Manifestations of Meckel Diverticulum

Abdominal Pain
- Similar to appendicitis
- May be vague and recurrent

Bloody Stools
- Painless
- Bright or dark red with mucus (currant jelly–like stools)
- In infants, bleeding sometimes accompanied by pain

Sometimes
- Severe anemia
- Shock

---

has occurred, appropriate preoperative measures are used to reverse electrolyte imbalances and prevent abdominal distention.

Prognosis

If symptomatic Meckel diverticulum is diagnosed and treated early, full recovery is likely. The mortality rate of untreated Meckel diverticulum is approximately 6% (Caracappa, Gullá, Lombardo, Burini, Castellani et al., 2014). Because of the potential for surgical complications, resection of asymptomatic Meckel diverticulum remains controversial.

Care Management

Nursing care is the same as for any child undergoing abdominal surgery (see Chapter 38). When intestinal bleeding is present, specific preoperative considerations include frequent monitoring of vital signs, including blood pressure and recording the approximate amount of blood lost in stools. Pain management is essential to preoperative and postoperative care of the child with this condition.

Postoperatively, the child requires IV fluids and an NG tube for decompression and evacuation of gastric secretions; laparoscopic surgery may avoid the necessity for an NG tube. Signs of return of normal bowel function should be monitored in the postoperative period. Because the onset of illness is usually rapid, psychologic support is important, as in other acute conditions, such as appendicitis. It is important to remember that rectal bleeding is usually traumatic to both the child and the parents and may significantly affect their emotional reaction to hospitalization and surgery.

INFLAMMATORY BOWEL DISEASE

Inflammatory bowel disease (IBD) should not be confused with IBS. IBD is a term used to refer to two major forms of chronic intestinal

TABLE 41.7 Clinical Manifestations of Inflammatory Bowel Diseases

Characteristics	Ulcerative Colitis	Crohn Disease
Rectal bleeding	Common	Uncommon
Diarrhea	Often severe	Moderate to severe
Pain	Less frequent	Common
Anorexia	Mild or moderate	May be severe
Weight loss	Moderate	May be severe
Growth delay	Usually mild	May be severe
Anal and perianal lesions	Rare	Common
Fistulas and strictures	Rare	Common
Rashes	Mild	Mild
Joint pain	Mild to moderate	Mild to moderate

inflammation: Crohn disease (CD) and ulcerative colitis (UC). Crohn disease and ulcerative colitis have similar epidemiologic, immunologic, and clinical features, but they are distinct disorders (Table 41.7). Approximately 1 million people in the United States have IBD, with 10% of these being children (D'Auria & Kelly, 2013). Over the past 30 years, the incidence of Crohn disease has risen, but the incidence of ulcerative colitis in children has remained stable (Aloi, D'Arcangelo, Pofi, et al., 2013). Both Crohn disease and ulcerative colitis have been noted to be more aggressive if the onset occurs in childhood (Aloi et al.).

Etiology

Despite decades of research, the etiology of IBD is not completely understood, and there is no known cure. There is evidence to indicate a multifactorial etiology. Research is focused on theories of defective immunoregulation of the inflammatory response to bacteria or viruses in the GI tract in individuals with a genetic predisposition (Szigethy, McLafferty, & Goyal, 2011). In Crohn disease, the chronic immune process is characterized by a T-helper 1 cytokine profile, whereas in ulcerative colitis the response is more humoral and mediated by T-helper 2 cells; however, recent studies have shown a subset of T cells (Th17) that are critical in inflammation for both forms of IBD (Szigethy et al., 2011). Development of IBD also may have a genetic influence. Family-based genetic studies have linked chromosome 6 in ulcerative colitis with the *NOD2* gene in Crohn disease (Szigethy et al.).

Pathophysiology

The inflammation found with ulcerative colitis is limited to the colon and rectum, with the distal colon and rectum the most severely affected. Inflammation affects the mucosa and submucosa and involves continuous segments along the length of the bowel with varying degrees of ulceration, bleeding, and edema. Thickening of the bowel wall and fibrosis are unusual, but long-standing disease can result in shortening of the colon and strictures. Extraintestinal manifestations are less common in ulcerative colitis than in Crohn disease. Toxic megacolon is the most dangerous form of severe colitis.

The chronic inflammatory process of Crohn disease involves any part of the GI tract from the mouth to the anus but most often affects the terminal ileum. The disease involves all layers of the bowel wall (transmural) in a discontinuous fashion, meaning that between areas of intact mucosa, there are areas of affected mucosa (skip lesions). The inflammation may result in ulcerations; fibrosis; adhesions; stiffening of the bowel wall; stricture formation; and fistulas to other loops of bowel, bladder, vagina, or skin.

Diagnostic Evaluation

The diagnosis of ulcerative colitis and Crohn disease comes from the history, physical examination, laboratory evaluation, and other diagnostic procedures. Laboratory tests include a CBC to detect anemia and an erythrocyte sedimentation rate (ESR) or CRP to assess the systemic reaction to the inflammatory process. Levels of total protein, albumin, iron, zinc, magnesium, vitamin B_{12}, and fat-soluble vitamins may be low in children with Crohn disease. Stools are examined for blood, leukocytes, and infectious organisms. A serologic panel is often used in combination with clinical findings to diagnose IBD and differentiate between Crohn disease and ulcerative colitis.

In patients with Crohn disease, an upper GI series with small-bowel follow-through assists in assessing the existence, location, and extent of disease. Upper endoscopy and colonoscopy with biopsies are an integral part of diagnosing IBD (Ellis & Cole, 2011). Endoscopy allows direct visualization of the surface of the GI tract so the extent of inflammation and narrowing can be evaluated. CT and ultrasonography also may be used to identify bowel wall inflammation, intraabdominal abscesses, and fistulas. Colonoscopy can confirm the diagnosis and evaluate the extent of the disease. Discrete ulcers are commonly seen in patients with Crohn disease, whereas microulcers and diffuse abnormalities and inflammation are seen in patients with ulcerative colitis (Grossman & Baldassano, 2016). Crohn disease lesions may pierce the walls of the small intestine and colon, creating tracts called *fistulas* between the intestine and adjacent structures such as the bladder, anus, vagina, or skin.

Therapeutic Management

The natural history of the disease continues to be unpredictable and characterized by recurrent flare-ups that can severely impair patients' physical and social functioning (D'Auria & Kelly, 2013). The goals of therapy are to (1) control the inflammatory process to reduce or eliminate the symptoms, (2) obtain long-term remission, (3) promote normal growth and development, and (4) allow as normal a lifestyle as possible. Treatment is individualized and managed according to the type and the severity of the disease, its location, and the response to therapy. Crohn disease is more disabling, has more serious complications, and is often less amenable to medical and surgical treatment than is ulcerative colitis. Because ulcerative colitis is confined to the colon, a colectomy may cure ulcerative colitis.

Medical Treatment

The goal of any treatment regimen is first to induce remission of acute symptoms and then to maintain remission over time. 5-Aminosalicylates (5-ASAs) are effective in the induction and maintenance of remission in mild-to-moderate ulcerative colitis. Mesalamine, olsalazine, and balsalazide are now preferred over sulfasalazine because of reduced side effects (headache, nausea, vomiting, neutropenia, and oligospermia). Suppository and enema preparations of mesalamine are used to treat left-sided colitis. These drugs decrease inflammation by inhibiting prostaglandin synthesis. 5-ASAs can be used to induce remission in mild Crohn disease.

Corticosteroids such as prednisone and prednisolone are indicated in induction therapy in children with moderate-to-severe ulcerative colitis and Crohn disease. These drugs inhibit the production of adhesion molecules, cytokines, and leukotrienes. Although these drugs reduce the acute symptoms of IBD, they have side effects that relate to long-term use, including growth suppression (adrenal suppression), weight gain, and decreased bone density. High doses of IV corticosteroids may be administered in acute episodes and tapered according to clinical response. Budesonide, a synthetic corticosteroid, is designed for controlled release in the ileum and indicated for ileal and right-sided colitis; budesonide has fewer side effects than prednisone and prednisolone (Szigethy et al., 2011). Rectal steroid therapy (enemas and foam-based preparations) are available for both induction and maintenance therapy in left-sided colitis (Szigethy et al.).

Immunomodulators such as azathioprine and its metabolite 6-mercaptopurine (6-MP) are used to induce and maintain remission in children with IBD who are steroid resistant or steroid dependent and to treat chronic draining fistulas. They block the synthesis of purine, thus inhibiting the ability of deoxyribonucleic acid (DNA) and ribonucleic acid (RNA) to hinder lymphocyte function, especially that of T-cells. Side effects include infection, pancreatitis, hepatitis, bone marrow toxicity, arthralgia, and malignancy. Methotrexate is also useful in inducing and maintaining remission in Crohn disease patients who are unresponsive to standard therapies. Cyclosporine and tacrolimus have both been effective in inducing remission in severe steroid-dependent ulcerative colitis. 6-MP or azathioprine is then used to maintain remission. Patients taking immunomodulating medications require regular monitoring of their CBC and differential to assess for changes that reflect suppression of the immune system because many of the side effects can be prevented or managed by dose reduction or discontinuation of medication.

Antibiotics, such as metronidazole and ciprofloxacin, may be used as an adjunctive therapy to treat complications, such as perianal disease or small-bowel bacterial overgrowth in Crohn disease. Side effects of these drugs are peripheral neuropathy, nausea, and a metallic taste.

Biologic therapies act to regulate inflammatory and antiinflammatory cytokines. With the emergence of the biologic agents, specifically the use of tumor necrosis factor-alpha (TNF-α) agents, progress has been made in targeting specific pathogenetic mechanisms and achieving a more prolonged clinical response (Bradley & Oliva-Hemker, 2012; Szigethy et al., 2011). TNF-α is believed to influence active inflammation.

Nutritional Support

Nutritional support is important in the treatment of patients with IBD. Growth failure is a common serious complication, especially in Crohn disease. Growth failure is characterized by weight loss, alteration in body composition, restricted height, and delayed sexual maturation. Malnutrition causes the growth failure, and its etiology is multifactorial. Malnutrition occurs as a result of inadequate dietary intake, excessive GI losses, malabsorption, drug-nutrient interaction, and increased nutritional requirements. Inadequate dietary intake occurs with anorexia and episodes of increased disease activity. Excessive loss of nutrients (protein, blood, electrolytes, and minerals) occurs secondary to intestinal inflammation and diarrhea. Carbohydrate, lactose, fat, vitamin, and mineral malabsorption as well as vitamin B_{12} and folic acid deficiencies occur with disease episodes, with drug administration, and when the terminal ileum is resected. Finally, nutritional requirements are increased with inflammation, fever, fistulas, and periods of rapid growth (e.g., adolescence).

The goals of nutritional support include (1) correction of nutrient deficits and replacement of ongoing losses, (2) provision of adequate energy and protein for healing, and (3) provision of adequate nutrients to promote normal growth. Nutritional support includes both enteral nutrition and parenteral nutrition (PN). A well-balanced, high-protein, high-calorie diet is recommended for children whose symptoms do not prohibit an adequate oral intake. There is little evidence that avoiding specific foods influences the severity of the disease. Supplementation with multivitamins, iron, and folic acid is recommended.

Special enteral formulas given either by mouth or continuous NG infusion (often at night) may be required. Elemental formulas are completely absorbed in the small intestine with almost no residue. A diet consisting only of elemental formula not only improves nutritional status but also induces disease remission, either without steroids or with a diminished dosage of steroids required. An elemental diet is a safe and potentially effective primary therapy for patients with Crohn disease. Unfortunately, remission is not sustained when NG feedings are discontinued unless maintenance medications are added to the treatment regimen.

Total parenteral nutrition (TPN) has also improved nutritional status in patients with IBD. Short-term remissions have been achieved after TPN, although complete bowel rest has not reduced inflammation or added to the benefits of improved nutrition by TPN. Nutritional support is less likely to induce a remission in ulcerative colitis than in Crohn disease. However, improvement of nutritional status is important in preventing deterioration of the patient's health status and preparing the patient for surgery.

Surgical Treatment

Surgery is indicated for ulcerative colitis when medical and nutritional therapies fail to prevent complications. Surgical options include a subtotal colectomy and ileostomy that leaves a rectal stump as a blind pouch. A reservoir pouch is created in the configuration of a J or S to help improve continence after surgery. An ileoanal pull-through preserves the normal pathway for defecation. *Pouchitis*, an inflammation of the surgically created pouch, is the most common late complication of this procedure. In many cases, ulcerative colitis can be cured with a total colectomy.

Surgery may be required in children with Crohn disease when complications cannot be controlled by medical and nutritional therapy. Segmental intestinal resections are performed for small-bowel obstructions, strictures, or fistulas. Partial colonic resection is not curative, and the disease often recurs (Ellis & Cole, 2011).

Prognosis

IBD is a chronic disease. Relatively long periods of quiescent disease may follow exacerbations. The outcome is influenced by the regions and severity of involvement and appropriate therapeutic management. Malnutrition, growth failure, and bleeding are serious complications. The overall prognosis for ulcerative colitis is good.

The development of colorectal cancer (CRC) is a long-term complication of IBD. In ulcerative colitis, the median duration of a CRC diagnosis was 23.5 years with a range of 11 to 48 years (Latella, 2012). Because the risk for CRC occurs 10 years after diagnosis, surveillance colonoscopy with multiple biopsies should begin approximately 10 years after diagnosis of ulcerative colitis or Crohn disease (Latella, 2012). In Crohn disease, however, surgical removal of the affected colon does not prevent cancer from developing elsewhere in the GI tract.

Interprofessional Care Management

The nursing considerations in the management of patients with IBD extend beyond the immediate period of hospitalization. These interventions involve continued guidance of families in terms of (1) managing diet; (2) coping with factors that increase stress and emotional lability; (3) adjusting to a disease of remissions and exacerbations; and (4) when indicated, preparing the child and parents for the possibility of diversionary bowel surgery.

Because nutritional support is an essential part of therapy, encouraging the anorexic child to consume enough food is often a challenge. Successful interventions include involving the child in meal planning; encouraging small, frequent meals or snacks rather than three large meals per day; serving meals around medication schedules when diarrhea, mouth pain, and intestinal spasm are controlled; and preparing high-protein, high-calorie foods such as eggnog, milkshakes, cream soups, puddings, or custard (if lactose is tolerated). Using bran or a high-fiber

CLINICAL REASONING CASE STUDY
Inflammatory Bowel Disease

Susan, a 13-year-old girl, was admitted to the hospital because of bloody diarrhea, abdominal pain, and weight loss. After a thorough evaluation, including laboratory tests, radiographic studies, and GI endoscopy procedures, the diagnosis of Crohn disease was made. Medical treatment, including corticosteroid drugs and nutritional support, was implemented during this hospitalization.

Susan has improved considerably and is to be discharged home this week. Enteral formula administered by continuous nighttime nasogastric (NG) tube infusion will be continued at home, and both Susan and her family are eager to learn how to perform these feedings. You are the nurse who is responsible for Susan's discharge planning.

1. Evidence—Are there sufficient data to formulate any specific interventions for discharge?
2. Assumptions—Describe some underlying assumptions about the following:
   a. The goals of nutritional support for children with Crohn disease
   b. Teaching required by an adolescent or family member who is administering NG tube feedings at home
   c. Psychosocial issues related to Crohn disease
3. What are the priorities for discharge planning at this time?
4. Does the evidence support your conclusion?

diet for active IBD is questionable. Bran, even in small amounts, has been shown to worsen the condition. Occasionally the occurrence of aphthous stomatitis further complicates adherence to dietary management. Mouth care before eating and the selection of bland foods help relieve the discomfort of mouth sores.

When NG feedings or TPN is indicated, dieticians determine the best formula. Nurses play an important role in explaining the purpose and expected outcomes of this therapy. The nurse should acknowledge the anxieties of the child and family members and give them adequate time to demonstrate the skills necessary to continue the therapy at home if needed (see Clinical Reasoning Case Study: Inflammatory Bowel Disease).

The importance of continued drug therapy despite remission of symptoms must be stressed to the child and family members by all health care providers. Failure to adhere to the pharmacologic regimen can result in exacerbation of the disease (see the "Compliance" section in Chapter 39). Unfortunately, exacerbation of IBD can occur even if the child and family are compliant with the treatment regimen; this is difficult for the child and family to cope with.

Emotional Support

The nurse should attend to the emotional components of the disease and assess any sources of stress. Frequently she or he can help children adjust to problems of growth restriction, delayed sexual maturation, dietary restrictions, feelings of being "different" or "sickly," inability to compete with peers, and necessary absence from school during exacerbations of the illness (see the "Impact of the Child's Chronic Illness" section in Chapter 36).

If a permanent colectomy-ileostomy is required, the nurse teaches the child and family how to care for the ileostomy. The nurse emphasizes the positive aspects of the surgery, particularly accelerated growth and sexual development, permanent recovery, the eliminated risk for colonic cancer in ulcerative colitis, and the normality of life despite bowel diversion. Introducing the child and parents to other ostomy patients, especially those who are the same age, can be effective in fostering eventual acceptance. Whenever possible, offer continent ostomies as options to the child, although they are not performed in all centers in the United States.

Because of the chronic and often lifelong nature of the disease, families benefit from the educational services provided by organizations such as the Crohn's and Colitis Foundation of America.* If diversionary bowel surgery is indicated, the United Ostomy Associations of America† and the Wound, Ostomy and Continence Nurses Society‡ are available to assist with ileostomy care and provide important psychologic support through their self-help groups. Adolescents often benefit by participating in peer-support groups, which are sponsored by the Crohn's and Colitis Foundation of America.

PEPTIC ULCER DISEASE

Peptic ulcer disease (PUD) is a chronic condition that affects the stomach or duodenum. Ulcers are described as gastric or duodenal and as primary or secondary. A *gastric ulcer* involves the mucosa of the stomach; a *duodenal ulcer* involves the pylorus or duodenum. Most primary ulcers are idiopathic or associated with *Helicobacter pylori* infection and tend to be chronic, occurring more frequently in the duodenum (Blanchard & Czinn, 2016). *Secondary ulcers* result from the stress of a severe underlying disease or injury (e.g., severe burns, sepsis, increased intracranial pressure, severe trauma, multisystem organ failure) and are more frequently gastric with an acute onset (Blanchard & Czinn, 2016). About 1.8% to 5% of children in North America are diagnosed with PUD (Sullivan, 2010). Primary ulcers are more common in children older than 10 years of age, and secondary ulcers are more common in infants and children with underlying disease, and children taking nonsteroidal antiinflammatory drugs (NSAIDs), corticosteroids, or sodium valproate medications (Sullivan, 2010).

Etiology

The exact cause of PUD is unknown, although infectious, genetic, and environmental factors are important. There is a significant relationship between the bacterium *Helicobacter pylori* and ulcers. *H. pylori* is a microaerophilic, gram-negative, slow-growing, spiral-shaped, and flagellated bacterium known to colonize the gastric mucosa in about one-half of the population of the world (Ertem, 2012). *H. pylori* synthesizes the enzyme urease, which hydrolyses urea to form ammonia and carbon dioxide. Ammonia then absorbs acid to form ammonium, thus raising the gastric pH. *H. pylori* may cause ulcers by weakening the gastric mucosal barrier and allowing acid to damage the mucosa. It is believed that it is acquired via the fecal-oral route, and this hypothesis is supported by finding viable *H. pylori* in feces.

In addition to ulcerogenic drugs, both alcohol and smoking contribute to ulcer formation. There is no conclusive evidence to implicate particular foods such as caffeine-containing beverages or spicy foods, but polyunsaturated fats and fiber may play a role in ulcer formation. Psychologic factors may play a role in the development of PUD, and stressful life events, dependency, passiveness, and hostility have all been implicated as contributing factors.

---

*386 Park Avenue South, 17th Floor, New York, NY 10016, 800-932-2423, www.ccfa.org. In Canada: Crohn's and Colitis Foundation of Canada, www.ccfc.ca.

†P.O. Box 512, Northfield, MN 55057-0512, 800-826-0826, www.ostomy.org. In Canada: United Ostomy Association of Canada, 344 Bloor Street West, Suite 501, Toronto, ON M5S 3A7, 416-595-5452, www.ostomycanada.ca.

‡15000 Commerce Parkway, Suite C, Mt. Laurel, NJ, 888-224-9626, www.wocn.org.

Pathophysiology

Most likely the pathology is caused by an imbalance between the destructive (cytotoxic) factors and defensive (cytoprotective) factors in the GI tract. The toxic mechanisms include acid, pepsin, medications such as aspirin and NSAIDs, bile acids, and infection with *H. pylori*. The defensive factors include the mucus layer, local bicarbonate secretion, epithelial cell renewal, and mucosal blood flow. Prostaglandins play a role in mucosal defense because they stimulate both mucus and alkali secretion. The primary mechanism that prevents the development of peptic ulcer is the secretion of mucus by the epithelial and mucous glands throughout the stomach. The thick mucus layer acts to diffuse acid from the lumen to the gastric mucosal surface, thus protecting the gastric epithelium. The stomach and the duodenum produce bicarbonate, decreasing acidity on the epithelial cells and thereby minimizing the effects of the low pH. When abnormalities in the protective barrier exist, the mucosa is vulnerable to damage by acid and pepsin. Exogenous factors such as aspirin and NSAIDs cause gastric ulcers by inhibition of prostaglandin synthesis.

Zollinger-Ellison syndrome may occur in children who have multiple, large, or recurrent ulcers. This syndrome is characterized by hypersecretion of gastric acid, intractable ulcer disease, and intestinal malabsorption caused by a gastrin-secreting tumor of the pancreas.

Diagnostic Evaluation

Diagnosis is based on the history of symptoms, physical examination, and diagnostic testing. The focus is on symptoms such as epigastric abdominal pain, nocturnal pain, oral regurgitation, heartburn, weight loss, hematemesis, and melena (Box 41.7). History should include questions relating to the use of potentially causative substances such as NSAIDs, corticosteroids, alcohol, and tobacco. Frequently a history

of epigastric and periumbilical pain accompanies PUD. However, children often find it difficult to describe the location of their pain and often indicate the location by moving their hand in circular movement all around the stomach area. Asking the child to take one finger and point to the area where it hurts the most often helps to identify the location of the pain. Pain may also be elicited during the examination with palpation. Laboratory tests include a CBC to detect anemia; stool analysis for occult blood; liver function tests (LFTs); ESR or CRP to evaluate inflammation; amylase and lipase to evaluate pancreatitis; and gastric acid measurements to identify hypersecretion. A lactose breath test may be performed to detect lactose intolerance.

Radiographic studies such as an upper GI series may be performed to evaluate obstruction or malrotation, although they are rarely helpful in identifying ulcers in children. Fiber-optic endoscopy is the most reliable procedure to detect PUD in children. A biopsy can determine the presence of *H. pylori*. A blood test can also identify the presence of the antigen to this organism. The C^{13} urea breath test measures bacterial colonization in the gastric mucosa. This test may be used to screen for *H. pylori* in adults and children. Polyclonal and monoclonal stool antigen tests are an accurate, noninvasive method for both the initial diagnosis of *H. pylori* and the confirmation of its eradication after treatment (Ertem, 2012). In children, an initial upper endoscopy is recommended to evaluate and confirm *H. pylori* disease (Blanchard & Czinn, 2016).

Therapeutic Management

The major goals of therapy for children with PUD are to relieve discomfort, promote healing, prevent complications, and prevent recurrence. Management is primarily medical and consists of administration of medications to treat the infection and reduce or neutralize gastric acid secretion. Antacids are beneficial medications to neutralize gastric acid. Histamine (H_2) receptor antagonists (antisecretory drugs) act to suppress gastric acid production. Cimetidine (Tagamet), ranitidine (Zantac), and famotidine (Pepcid) are examples of these medications. These medications have few side effects.

PPIs, such as omeprazole, lansoprazole, pantoprazole, and esomepraole, act to inhibit the hydrogen ion pump in the parietal cells, thus blocking the production of acid. These agents have been shown to be effective in children and adolescents but not in infants (van der Pol, Smits, van Wijk, et al., 2011).

Mucosal protective agents, such as sucralfate and bismuth-containing preparations, may be prescribed for PUD. Sucralfate is an aluminum-containing agent that forms a protective barrier over ulcerated mucosa to protect against acid and pepsin. Bismuth compounds are sometimes prescribed for the relief of ulcers, but they are used less frequently than PPIs. Although these compounds inhibit the growth of microorganisms, the mechanism of their activity is poorly understood. In combination with antibiotics, bismuth is effective against *H. pylori*. Although concern has been expressed about the use of bismuth salts in children because of potential side effects, none of these side effects has been reported when these compounds have been used in the treatment of *H. pylori* infection. These agents are available in both pill and liquid forms. Because they block the absorption of other medications, they should be given separately from other medications.

Triple-drug therapy is the standard first-line treatment regimen for *H. pylori* (Ertem, 2012). Examples of drug combinations used in triple therapy are (1) bismuth, clarithromycin, and metronidazole; (2) lansoprazole, amoxicillin, and clarithromycin; and (3) metronidazole, clarithromycin, and omeprazole. Common side effects of medications include diarrhea and nausea and vomiting. In addition to medications, children with PUD should have a nutritious diet and avoid caffeine. Warn adolescents about gastric irritation associated with alcohol use and smoking.

BOX 41.7 Characteristics of Peptic Ulcer

Neonates
- Usually gastric and secondary ulcers
- Commonly has a history of preterm birth, respiratory distress, sepsis, hypoglycemia, or an intraventricular hemorrhage
- Perforation may lead to massive bleeding

Infants to Children 2 Years of Age
- Most likely to have a secondary ulcer located equally in the stomach or duodenum
- Primary ulcers less common and usually located in the stomach
- Likely to occur in relation to illness, surgery, or trauma
- Hematemesis, melena, or perforation

Children 2 to 6 Years of Age
- Primary or secondary ulcers
- Located equally in the stomach or duodenum
- Perforation more likely in secondary ulcers
- Periumbilical pain, poor eating, vomiting, irritability, nighttime waking, hematemesis, melena

Children Older Than 6 Years of Age
- Usually primary and most often duodenal ulcers
- More typical of adult type
- Chance of recurrence greater
- Often associated with *Helicobacter pylori*
- Epigastric pain or vague abdominal pain
- Nighttime waking, hematemesis, melena, and anemia possible

Children with an acute ulcer who have developed complications, such as massive hemorrhage, require emergency care. The administration of IV fluids, blood, or plasma depends on the amount of blood loss. Replacement with whole blood or packed cells may be necessary for significant loss.

Surgical intervention may be required for complications, such as hemorrhage, perforation, or gastric outlet obstruction. Ligation of the source of bleeding or closure of a perforation is performed. A vagotomy and pyloroplasty may be indicated in children with recurring ulcers despite aggressive medical treatment (Sullivan, 2010).

Prognosis

The long-term prognosis for PUD is variable. Many ulcers are successfully treated with medical therapy; however, primary duodenal peptic ulcers often recur. Complications such as GI bleeding can occur and extend into adult life. The effect of maintenance drug therapy on long-term morbidity remains to be established with further studies.

Care Management

The primary nursing goal is to promote healing of the ulcer through compliance with the medication regimen. If an analgesic or antipyretic is needed, acetaminophen, not aspirin or NSAIDs, is used. Critically ill neonates, infants, and children in intensive care units should receive H_2 blockers to prevent stress ulcers.

> **! NURSING ALERT**
>
> Critically ill children receiving IV H_2 blockers should have their gastric pH values checked at frequent intervals.

For nonhospitalized children with chronic illnesses, consider the role stress plays. In children, many ulcers occur secondary to other conditions, and the nurse should be aware of family and environmental conditions that may aggravate or precipitate ulcers. Children may benefit from psychologic counseling and from learning how to cope constructively with stress.

HEPATIC DISORDERS

ACUTE HEPATITIS

Etiology

Hepatitis is an acute or chronic inflammation of the liver that can result from infectious or noninfectious reasons. Many types of hepatitis are caused by viruses such as the hepatitis viruses, Epstein-Barr virus (EBV), and cytomegalovirus (CMV). Other causes of hepatitis are nonviral (abscess, amebiasis), autoimmune, metabolic, chemical, anatomic (choledochal duct cyst and biliary atresia [BA]), hemodynamic (shock, congestive heart failure), and idiopathic (sclerosing cholangitis and Reye syndrome). Determining the cause of acute or chronic hepatitis is important in determining the treatment and prognosis for the child. Table 41.8 compares the features of hepatitis A virus (HAV), hepatitis B virus (HBV), and hepatitis C virus (HCV).

Hepatitis A

Hepatitis A incidence in the United States has declined 92% since the introduction of a vaccine in 1995, with approximately 21,000 cases annually in the United States (Matheny & Kingery, 2012). The virus is spread directly or indirectly by the fecal-oral route by ingestion of contaminated foods, direct exposure to infected fecal material, or close contact with an infected person. The virus is particularly prevalent in developing countries with poor living conditions, inadequate sanitation,

crowding, and poor personal hygiene practices. The spread of HAV has been associated with improper food handling and high-risk areas such as households with infected people, residential centers for people with disabilities, and day care centers. The average incubation period is about 28 days, with a range of 15 to 50 days (Matheny & Kingery, 2012). Fecal shedding of the virus can occur for 2 weeks before and for 1 week after the onset of jaundice. During this time, although the individual is asymptomatic, the virus is most likely to be transmitted. Infants with HAV infection are likely to be asymptomatic (anicteric hepatitis). Children often have diarrhea, and their symptoms are frequently attributed to gastroenteritis. Younger children rarely develop jaundice; however, 70% of older children and adults infected with HAV develop clinical signs with icteric hepatitis (Matheny & Kingery). The prognosis of HAV infection is usually good, and complications are rare.

Hepatitis B

Although the incidence of HBV is declining after the introduction of a universal immunization program, approximately 1.25 million people in the United States are infected with HBV (Jensen & Balistereri, 2016). Hepatitis B can be an acute or chronic infection, ranging from an asymptomatic, limited infection to fatal, fulminant (rapid and severe) hepatitis. There are no environmental or animal reservoirs for HBV. Humans are the main source of infection. HBV may be transmitted parenterally, percutaneously, or transmucosally. Hepatitis B surface antigen (HBsAg) has been found in all body fluids, including feces, bile, breast milk, sweat, tears, vaginal secretions, and urine; but only blood, semen, and saliva have been found to contain infectious HBV particles. HBV infection from human bites has been documented, but transmission from feces has not. HBV has been acquired after blood transfusion, but the likelihood of this has been reduced through blood product screening procedures. Adults whose occupations are associated with considerable exposure to blood or blood products such as health care workers are at an increased risk for contracting HBV.

Most HBV infection in children is acquired perinatally. Transmission from mother to infant during the perinatal period (e.g., blood exposure during delivery) results in chronic infection in 90% of infants if the mother is positive for HBsAg and HBeAg (Paganelli, Stephenne, & Sokal, 2012). HBsAg has been inconsistently detected in breast milk, but no increased risk for transmission has been found, and breastfeeding is currently recommended after infant immunization (Clemente & Schwarz, 2011). Infants and children who are not infected during the perinatal period remain at high risk for acquiring person-to-person transmission from their mother, with a 30% incidence of transmission during the first 5 years of life (Clemente & Schwarz). HBV infection occurs in children and adolescents in specific high-risk groups, which are (1) individuals with hemophilia or other disorders who have received multiple transfusions, (2) children and adolescents involved in IV drug abuse, (3) institutionalized children, (4) preschool children in endemic areas, and (5) individuals engaged in sexual activity with an infected partner. The incubation period for HBV infection ranges from 45 to 160 days, with an average of 120 days (Jensen & Balistereri, 2016). HBV infection can cause a carrier state and lead to chronic hepatitis with eventual cirrhosis or hepatocellular carcinoma in adulthood.

Hepatitis C

HCV is the most common cause of chronic liver disease, with an estimated 4 million affected people in the United States (Jensen & Balistereri, 2016). HCV is transmitted parenterally through exposure to blood and blood products from HCV-infected people, whereas perinatal transmission is the most common mode of transmission in children (Jensen & Balistereri, 2016). Recent improvements in donor screening and inactivation procedures for blood products, such as the factor concentrates

TABLE 41.8   Comparison of Types A, B, and C Hepatitis

Characteristics	Type A	Type B	Type C
Incubation period	15 to 50 days; average 28 days	45 to 160 days; average 120 days	2 to 24 weeks; average 7 to 9 weeks
Period of communicability	Believed to be latter half of incubation period to first week after onset of clinical illness	Variable Virus in blood or other body fluids during late incubation period and acute stage of disease; may persist in carrier state for years to lifetime	Begins before onset of symptoms May persist in carrier state for years
Mode of transmission	Principal route—fecal-oral Rarely—parenteral	Principal route—parenteral Less frequent route—oral, sexual, any body fluid Perinatal transfer—transplacental blood (last trimester); at delivery; or during breastfeeding, especially if mother has cracked nipples	Principal route—parenteral Nonparenteral spread possible
Clinical features			
Onset	Usually rapid, acute	More insidious	Usually insidious
Fever	Common and early	Less frequent	Less frequent
Anorexia	Common	Mild to moderate	Mild to moderate
Nausea and vomiting	Common	Sometimes present	Mild to moderate
Rash	Rare	Common	Sometimes present
Arthralgia	Rare	Common	Rare
Pruritus	Rare	Sometimes present	Sometimes present
Jaundice	Present (many cases anicteric)	Present	Present
Immunity	Present after one attack; no crossover to type B or C	Present after one attack; no crossover to type A or C	Present after one attack; no crossover to type A or B
Carrier state	No	Yes	Yes
Chronic infection	No	Yes	Yes
Prophylaxis			
IG	Passive immunity Successful, especially in early incubation period and preexposure prophylaxis	Passive immunity Inconsistent benefits; probably of no use	Not currently recommended by CDC
HAV vaccine	Two inactivated vaccines approved for children 12 months to 18 years of age: Havrix and Vaqta; given in a two-dose schedule (6 to 12 months between doses)		
HBV immunoglobulin (HBIG)	No benefit	Postexposure protection possible if given immediately after definite exposure	No benefit
HBV vaccine	No benefit	Provides active immunity Universal vaccination recommended for all newborns	No benefit
Mortality rate	0.1% to 0.2%	0.5% to 2% in uncomplicated cases; may be higher in complicated cases	1% to 2% in uncomplicated cases; may be higher in complicated cases

CDC, Centers for Disease Control and Prevention; *HAV,* hepatitis A virus; *HBIG,* hepatitis B immunoglobulin; *HBV,* hepatitis B virus; *IG,* immunoglobulin.

used for patients with hemophilia, have significantly reduced the risk for transmission through blood products.

The clinical course varies. The incubation period for HCV ranges from 2 to 24 weeks, with an average of 7 to 9 weeks (Jensen & Balistereri, 2016). The natural history of the disease in children is not well defined. Some children may be asymptomatic, but hepatitis C can become a chronic condition and can cause cirrhosis and hepatocellular carcinoma. About 85% of individuals infected with HCV develop chronic disease (Jensen & Balistereri).

Hepatitis D

Hepatitis D occurs rarely in children and must occur in individuals already infected with HBV (Clemente & Schwarz, 2011). HDV is a defective RNA virus that requires the helper function of HBV. The

incubation period is from 2 to 8 weeks, but with co-infection of HBV, the incubation period is similar to an HBV infection (Jensen & Balistereri, 2016). HDV infection occurs through blood and sexual contact and commonly occurs among drug abusers, individuals with hemophilia, and people immigrating from endemic areas.

Hepatitis E

Hepatitis E was formerly known as non-A, non-B hepatitis. Transmission may occur through the fecal-oral route or from contaminated water. The incubation period ranges from 15 to 60 days, with an average of 40 days (Jensen & Balistereri, 2016). This illness is uncommon in children, does not cause chronic liver disease, is not a chronic condition, and has no carrier state. However, it can be a devastating disease among pregnant women, with an unusually high case-fatality rate.

Pathophysiology

Pathologic changes occur primarily in the parenchymal cells of the liver and result in variable degrees of swelling; infiltration of liver cells by mononuclear cells; and subsequent degeneration, necrosis, and fibrosis. Structural changes within the hepatocyte account for altered liver functions such as impaired bile excretion, elevated transaminase levels, and decreased albumin synthesis. The disorder may be self-limiting with regeneration of liver cells without scarring, leading to complete recovery. However, some forms of hepatitis do not result in complete return of liver function. These include fulminant hepatitis, which is characterized by a severe, acute course with massive destruction of the liver tissue causing liver failure and high mortality within 1 to 2 weeks, and subacute or chronic active hepatitis, which is characterized by progressive liver destruction, uncertain regeneration, scarring, and potential cirrhosis.

The progression of liver disease is characterized pathologically by four stages: (1) stage one is characterized by mononuclear inflammatory cells surrounding small bile ducts; (2) in stage two, there is proliferation of small bile ductules; (3) stage three is characterized by fibrosis or scarring; and (4) stage four is cirrhosis (Angulo & Lindor, 2010).

Clinical Manifestations

The clinical manifestations and course of uncomplicated acute viral hepatitis are similar for most of the hepatitis viruses. Usually the prodromal, or anicteric, phase (absence of jaundice) lasts from 5 to 7 days. Anorexia, malaise, lethargy, and easy fatigability are the most common symptoms. Fever may be present, especially in adolescents. Nausea, vomiting, and epigastric or right upper quadrant abdominal pain or tenderness may occur. Arthralgia and skin rashes may occur and are more likely in children with hepatitis B than those with hepatitis A. The transaminases rather than bilirubin are often elevated in acute hepatitis, and hepatomegaly may be present. Some mild cases of acute viral hepatitis do not cause symptoms or can be mistaken for influenza.

In young children, most of the prodromal symptoms disappear with the onset of jaundice, or the icteric phase. However, many children with acute viral hepatitis never develop jaundice. If jaundice occurs, it is often accompanied by dark urine and pale stools. Pruritus may accompany jaundice and can be bothersome for children.

Children with chronic active hepatitis may be asymptomatic but more commonly have nonspecific symptoms of malaise, fatigue, lethargy, weight loss, or vague abdominal pain. Hepatomegaly may be present, and the transaminases are often very high, with mild-to-severe hyperbilirubinemia.

Fulminant hepatitis is due primarily to HBV or HCV. Many children with fulminant hepatitis develop characteristic clinical symptoms and rapidly develop manifestations of liver failure, including encephalopathy, coagulation defects, ascites, deepening jaundice, and an increasing WBC count. Changes in mental status or personality indicate impending liver failure. Although children with acute hepatitis may have hepatomegaly, a rapid decrease in the size of the liver (indicating loss of tissue caused by necrosis) is a serious sign of fulminant hepatitis. Complications of fulminant hepatitis include GI bleeding, sepsis, renal failure, and disseminated coagulopathy.

Diagnostic Evaluation

Diagnosis is based on the history; physical examination; and serologic markers for hepatitis A, B, and C. No LFT is specific for hepatitis, but serum aspartate aminotransferase (AST) and serum alanine aminotransferase (ALT) levels are markedly elevated. Serum bilirubin levels peak 5 to 10 days after clinical jaundice appears. Histologic evidence from liver biopsy may be required to establish the diagnosis

and assess the severity of the liver disease. Serologic markers indicate the antibodies or antigens formed in response to the specific virus and confirm the diagnosis. Serum immunologic tests are not available to detect HAV antigen, but there are two HAV antibody tests: anti-HAV immunoglobulin G (IgG) and immunoglobulin M (IgM). Anti-HAV antibodies are present at the onset of the disease and persist for life. A positive anti-HAV antibody test can indicate acute infection, immunity from past infection, passive antibody acquisition (e.g., from transfusion, serum immunoglobulin infusion), or immunization. To diagnose an acute or recent HAV infection, a positive anti-HAV IgM test result that is present with the onset of the disease and that persists for only 2 or 3 days is required.

Diagnosis of hepatitis B is confirmed by the detection of various hepatitis virus antigens and the antibodies that are produced in response to the infection. These antibodies and antigens and their significance include the following:

HBsAg: Hepatitis B surface antigen (found on the surface of the virus), indicating ongoing infection or carrier state

Anti-HBs: Antibody to surface antigen HBsAg, indicating resolving or past infection

HBcAg: Hepatitis B core antigen (found on the inner core of the virus), detected only in the liver

Anti-HBc: Antibody to core antigen HBcAg, indicating ongoing or past infection

HBeAg: Hepatitis Be antigen (another component of the HBV core), indicating active infection

Anti-HBe: Antibody to HBeAg, indicating resolving or past infection

IgM anti-HBc: IgM antibody to core antigen

Tests are available for detection of all the HBV antigens and antibodies except HBcAg. HBsAg is detectable during acute infection. Presence of HBsAg indicates that the individual has been infected with the hepatitis virus. If the infection is self-limiting, HBsAg disappears in most patients before serum anti-HBs can be detected (termed the *window phase of infection*). IgM anti-HBc is highly specific in establishing the diagnosis of acute infection and during the window phase in older children and adults. However, IgM anti-HBc usually is not present in perinatal HBV infection. Clinical improvement is usually associated with a decrease in or disappearance of these antigens followed by the appearance of their antibodies. For example, anti-HBc of the IgM class often occurs early in the disease followed by a rise in anti-HBc of the IgG class. Because the antibodies persist indefinitely, they are used to identify the carrier state (individuals with HBV who have no clinical disease but are able to transmit the organism). People with chronic HBV infection have circulating HBsAg and anti-HBc, and on rare occasions, anti-HBsAg is present. Both anti-HBs and anti-HBc are detected in people with resolved infection, but anti-HBs alone is present in individuals who have been immunized with the HBV vaccine.

HCV RNA is the earliest serologic marker for HCV. HCV-RNA can be detected during the incubation period before symptoms of HCV disease are expressed. A positive HCV-RNA result indicates active infection, and persistence of HCV-RNA indicates chronic infection. A negative test result correlates with resolution of the disease. HCV-RNA is also used to determine patient response to antiviral therapy for HCV.

The history of all patients should include questions to seek evidence of (1) contact with a person known to have hepatitis, especially a family member; (2) unsafe sanitation practices such as contaminated drinking water; (3) ingestion of certain foods such as clams or oysters (especially from polluted water); (4) multiple blood transfusions; (5) ingestion of hepatotoxic drugs such as salicylates, sulfonamides, antineoplastic agents, acetaminophen, and anticonvulsants; and (6) parenteral administration of illicit drugs or sexual contact with a person who uses these drugs.

Therapeutic Management

The goals of management include early detection, support and monitoring of the disease, recognition of chronic liver disease, and prevention of spread of the disease. Special high-protein, high-carbohydrate, low-fat diets are generally not of value. The use of corticosteroids alone or with immunosuppressive drugs is not advocated in the treatment of chronic viral hepatitis. However, steroids have been used to treat chronic autoimmune hepatitis. Hospitalization is required in the event of coagulopathy or fulminant hepatitis.

Therapy for hepatitis depends on the severity of inflammation and the cause of the disorder. HAV is treated primarily with supportive care. The US Food and Drug Administration approved several medications for treatment of children with HBV and HCV. Human interferon-α has been used successfully in the treatment of chronic hepatitis B and C in children. A number of antiviral medications are being used currently to treat HBV and HCV. Lamivudine is used for the treatment of HBV. It is well tolerated with no significant side effects and is approved for children older than 3 years of age (Paganelli et al., 2012). Combined therapy with lamivudine and interferon-α reduces the rate of antiviral resistance compared with lamivudine monotherapy (Paganelli et al.). Adefovir is used to treat HBV in children older than 12 years of age, and entecavir is a recently approved treatment for HBV in adolescents 16 years of age and older (Paganelli et al.). Pegylated interferon, interferon alpha-2b, and ribavirin have been approved for use in the treatment of HCV infections in children 3 years of age and older (Jensen & Balistereri, 2016). Products such as telbivudine and tenofovir are under current investigation in clinical trials, largely with adult patients.

Prevention

Proper hand washing and Standard Precautions prevent the spread of viral hepatitis. Prophylactic use of standard immunoglobulin is effective in preventing hepatitis A in situations of preexposure (e.g., anticipated travel to areas where HAV is prevalent) or within 2 weeks of exposure.

Hepatitis B immunoglobulin (HBIG) is effective in preventing HBV infection after one-time exposures, such as accidental needle punctures or other contact of contaminated material with mucous membranes, and should be given to newborns whose mothers are HBsAg positive. HBIG is prepared from plasma that contains high titers of antibodies against HBV. HBIG should be given within 72 hours of exposure.

Vaccines have been developed to prevent HAV and HBV infection (see Table 41.8). HBV vaccination is recommended for all newborns and children who did not receive the vaccination as a newborn (see the "Immunizations" section in Chapter 31). Because HDV cannot be transmitted in the absence of HBV infection, it is possible to prevent HDV infection by preventing HBV infection. Routine serologic testing for anti-HCV of children born to women previously identified as being infected with HCV is also recommended (Jensen & Balistereri, 2016).

Prognosis

The prognosis for children with hepatitis varies and depends on the type of virus and the child's age and immunocompetency. Hepatitis A and E are usually mild, brief illnesses with no carrier state. Hepatitis B can cause a wide spectrum of acute and chronic illness. Infants are more likely than older children to develop chronic hepatitis. Hepatocellular carcinoma during adulthood is a potentially fatal complication of chronic HBV infection. Hepatitis C frequently becomes chronic, and cirrhosis may develop in these children.

Interprofessional Care Management

Care depends largely on the severity of the hepatitis, the medical treatment, and factors influencing the control and transmission of the disease.

Because children with mild viral hepatitis are frequently cared for at home, it is often the nurse's responsibility to explain any medical therapies and infection control measures. When further assistance is needed for parents to comply with instructions, a public health nursing referral is necessary.

Encourage a well-balanced diet and a schedule of rest and activity adjusted to the child's condition. Because the child with HAV is not infectious within 1 week after the onset of jaundice, the child may feel well enough to resume school shortly thereafter. Caution parents about administering any medication to the child because normal doses of many drugs may become dangerous due to the inability of the liver to detoxify and excrete them.

Standard precautions are followed when children are hospitalized. However, these children are not usually isolated in a separate room unless they are fecally incontinent or their toys and other personal items are likely to become contaminated with feces. Discourage children from sharing their toys.

Hand washing is the single most effective measure in prevention and control of hepatitis in any setting. Parents and children need an explanation of the usual ways in which hepatitis is spread (fecal-oral route and parenteral route). Parents should also be aware of the recommendation for universal vaccination against HBV for newborns and adolescents (see Chapter 31).

Health care providers have the responsibility of helping young people with HBV infection who have a known or suspected history of illicit drug use to realize the associated dangers of drug abuse, stressing the parenteral mode of transmission of hepatitis, and encouraging them to seek counseling through a drug program.

CIRRHOSIS

Cirrhosis occurs at the end stage of many chronic liver diseases, including BA and chronic hepatitis. It can also result from infectious diseases, autoimmune disorders, toxic injury, and chronic diseases such as hemophilia and cystic fibrosis. A cirrhotic liver is irreversibly damaged.

Clinical manifestations of cirrhosis include jaundice, poor growth, anorexia, muscle weakness, and lethargy. Ascites, edema, GI bleeding, anemia, and abdominal pain may be present in children with impaired intrahepatic blood flow. Pulmonary function may be impaired because of pressure against the diaphragm caused by hepatosplenomegaly and ascites. Dyspnea and cyanosis may occur, especially on exertion. Intrapulmonary arteriovenous shunts may develop, which can also cause hypoxemia. Spider angiomas and prominent blood vessels on the upper torso are often present.

Diagnostic Evaluation

The diagnosis of cirrhosis is based on (1) the history, especially in regard to prior liver disease, such as hepatitis; (2) physical examination, particularly hepatosplenomegaly; (3) laboratory evaluation, especially LFTs, ammonia, albumin, cholesterol, and prothrombin time; and (4) liver biopsy for characteristic changes. Doppler ultrasonography of the liver and spleen is useful to confirm ascites, to evaluate blood flow through the liver and spleen, and to determine patency and size of the portal vein if liver transplantation is considered.

Therapeutic Management

Unfortunately, there is no successful treatment to arrest the progression of cirrhosis. The goals of management include monitoring liver function and managing specific complications such as esophageal varices and malnutrition. Assessment of the child's degree of liver dysfunction is important so that the child can be evaluated for transplantation at the appropriate time.

Liver transplantation has improved the prognosis substantially for many children with cirrhosis. The combination of new immunosuppressive medications and new surgical techniques has resulted in 83% to 91% 1-year survival rates in many large hospital centers (Kamath & Olthoff, 2010). The policy governing the allocation of livers for transplantation by the United Network for Organ Sharing allows patients with acute fulminant liver failure or those with chronic liver disease to be placed at the top of the network's transplantation lists. Although this change has benefited many pediatric patients, the shortage of available donors for children continues to dictate transplantation decisions, and many children continue to die while waiting for a suitable donor.

Nutritional support is an important therapy for children with cirrhosis and malnutrition. Supplements of fat-soluble vitamins are often required, and mineral supplements may be indicated. In some instances, aggressive nutritional support in the form of enteral feedings or PN may be necessary.

Esophageal and gastric varices are life-threatening complications of portal hypertension. Acute hemorrhage is managed with IV fluids, blood products, vitamin K if needed to correct coagulopathy, vasopressin or somatostatin, and gastric lavage. If acute hemorrhage persists, the most common secondary approach is endoscopic sclerotherapy or endoscopic banding ligation (El-Tawil, 2012). Balloon tamponade with a Sengstaken-Blakemore tube may be indicated for the unstable patient with acute hemorrhage (El-Tawil). Ascites can be managed by sodium restriction and diuretics. Severe ascites with respiratory compromise can be managed with administration of albumin or by paracentesis.

Although the full mechanism of hepatic encephalopathy is unknown, failure of the damaged liver to remove endogenous toxins such as ammonia plays a role. Treatment is directed at limiting the ammonia formation and absorption that occur in the bowel, especially with the drugs neomycin and lactulose. Because ammonia is formed in the bowel by the action of bacteria on ingested protein, neomycin reduces the number of intestinal bacteria so that less ammonia is produced. The fermentation of lactulose by colonic bacteria produces short-chain fatty acids that lower the colonic pH, thereby inhibiting bacterial metabolism. This decreases the formation of ammonia from bacterial metabolism of protein.

Prognosis

The success of liver transplantation has revolutionized the approach to liver cirrhosis. Liver failure and cirrhosis are indications for transplantation. Careful monitoring of the child's condition and quality of life is necessary to evaluate the need for and timing of transplantation.

Care Management

Several factors influence nursing care of the child with cirrhosis, including the cause of the cirrhosis, the severity of complications, and the prognosis. The prognosis is often poor unless successful liver transplantation occurs. Therefore nursing care of the child is similar to that for any child with a life-threatening illness (see Chapter 36). Hospitalization is required when complications such as hemorrhage, severe malnutrition, or hepatic failure occur. Nursing assessments are directed at monitoring the child's condition, and interventions are aimed at treatment of specific complications. If liver transplantation is an option, the family needs support and assistance to cope.

BILIARY ATRESIA

Biliary atresia, or extrahepatic biliary atresia (EHBA), is a progressive inflammatory process that causes both intrahepatic and extrahepatic bile duct fibrosis, resulting in eventual ductal obstruction. The incidence of BA is approximately 1 in 10,000 to 15,000 live births (Hassan &

Balistreri, 2016). Associated malformations include polysplenia, intestinal atresia, and malrotation of the intestine. If untreated, BA usually leads to cirrhosis, liver failure, and death in the first 2 years of life.

Etiology and Pathophysiology

The exact cause of BA is unknown, although immune mechanisms or viral injury may be responsible for the progressive process that results in complete obliteration of the bile ducts. BA is not seen in fetuses or stillborn or newborn infants. This suggests that BA is acquired late in gestation or in the perinatal period and is manifested a few weeks after birth. The majority of cases of BA (85%) have a complete obliteration of the extrahepatic biliary tree at or above the porta hepatitis (Hassan & Balistreri, 2016).

Many infants with BA are full term and appear healthy at birth. If jaundice persists beyond 2 weeks of age, especially if the direct (conjugated) serum bilirubin is elevated, the nurse should suspect BA. The urine may be dark, and the stools often become progressively acholic or gray, indicating absence of bile pigment. Hepatomegaly is present early in the course of the disease, and the liver is firm on palpation.

Diagnostic Evaluation

Early diagnosis is critical to the survival of children with BA. Infants who undergo surgery in the first 60 days of life have more favorable outcomes than patients with delayed treatment. The diagnosis of BA is suspected on the basis of the history, physical findings, and laboratory studies (Box 41.8). Laboratory tests should include a CBC, electrolytes, bilirubin, and liver function studies. Additional laboratory analyses, including α_1-antitrypsin level, TORCH titers (see the "Maternal Infections" section in Chapter 25), hepatitis serology, and urine CMV may be indicated to rule out other conditions that cause persistent cholestasis and jaundice. Abdominal ultrasonography allows inspection of the liver and biliary system. The patency of the extrahepatic biliary system will be demonstrated by a nuclear scintiscan using technetium-99m iminodiacetic acid (^{99m}Tc IDA) or hepatobiliary iminodiacetic acid (HIDA) scan. If there is no evidence of radioactive material excreted into the duodenum, BA is the most probable diagnosis. Because the nuclear scan may take up to 5 days for the results, a percutaneous liver biopsy is probably the most useful method of diagnosing BA (Hassan & Balistreri, 2016). The definitive diagnosis of BA is further established during an exploratory laparotomy and an intraoperative cholangiogram that demonstrates complete obstruction at some level of the biliary tree.

BOX 41.8   Clinical Manifestations of Biliary Atresia

Jaundice
- Earliest manifestation and most striking feature of disorder
- First observed in sclera
- Usually not apparent until 2 to 3 weeks of age, after resolution of neonatal jaundice

Dark yellow urine

Stools lighter than expected or white or tan

Hepatomegaly and abdominal distention common

Splenomegaly occurs later

Poor fat metabolism results in:
- Poor weight gain
- Failure to thrive

Pruritus

Irritability; difficulty comforting infant

Therapeutic Management

The primary treatment of BA is *hepatic portoenterostomy* (Kasai procedure) in which a segment of intestine is anastomosed to the resected porta hepatis to attempt bile drainage. A Roux-en-Y jejunal limb is then anastomosed to the porta hepatis (a *Y*-shaped anastomosis performed to provide bile drainage without reflux). After the Kasai procedure, approximately one-third of infants become jaundice free and regain normal liver function. Another one-third of infants demonstrate liver damage; however, they may be supported by medical and nutritional interventions. A final one-third require liver transplantation.

Medical management of BA is primarily supportive. It includes nutritional support with infant formulas that contain medium-chain triglycerides and essential fatty acids. Supplementation with fat-soluble vitamins (A, D, E, and K); a multivitamin; and minerals, including iron, zinc, and selenium, is usually required. Aggressive nutritional support in the form of continuous gastrostomy feedings or TPN may be indicated for moderate to severe growth failure; the enteral solution should be low in sodium. Phenobarbital may be prescribed after hepatic portoenterostomy to stimulate bile flow, and ursodeoxycholic acid may be used to decrease cholestasis and the intense pruritus from jaundice. In cases of advanced liver dysfunction, management is the same as in infants with cirrhosis.

Prognosis

Untreated BA results in progressive cirrhosis and death in most children by 10 years of age (Baumann & Ure, 2012). The Kasai procedure improves the prognosis but is not a cure. Biliary drainage can often be achieved if the surgery is done before the intrahepatic bile ducts are destroyed, and the success rate decreases to 20% if surgery is performed in an infant older than 3 months of age (Baumann & Ure). Long-term survival of 75% to 90% has been reported in children who receive the Kasai procedure (Baumann & Ure). However, even with successful bile drainage, many children ultimately develop liver failure and require liver transplantation.

Advances in surgical techniques and the use of immunosuppressive and antifungal drugs have improved the success of transplantation to survival rates of 80% to 90% (Baumann & Ure, 2012). The major obstacle continues to be a shortage of donor livers.

Interprofessional Care Management

Interventions for the child with BA include support of the family before, during, and after surgical procedures and education regarding the treatment plan. In the postoperative period of a portoenterostomy, care is similar to that after major abdominal surgery. Teaching includes the proper administration of medications. Administration of nutritional therapy, including special formulas, vitamin and mineral supplements, gastrostomy feedings, or PN, is an essential nursing responsibility. Growth failure in such infants is common, and increased metabolic needs combined with ascites, pruritus, and nutritional anorexia constitute a challenge for care. Teaching includes how to monitor and administer nutritional therapy in the home, and a home care agency may be consulted for continued teaching in the home. Pruritus may be a significant problem that is addressed by drug therapy and comfort measures such as baths in colloidal oatmeal compounds and trimming of fingernails. The risk for complications of BA, such as cholangitis, portal hypertension, GI bleeding, and ascites, should be explained to caregivers.

Children and their families also need psychosocial support. The uncertain prognosis, discomfort, and waiting for transplantation produce considerable stress. In addition, extended hospitalizations, pharmacologic therapy, and nutritional therapy can impose significant financial burdens on the family, as with any chronic condition. Families can receive help from psychosocial services and from support groups, such as the Children's Liver Association for Support Services* and the American Liver Foundation[†].

STRUCTURAL DEFECTS

CLEFT LIP AND CLEFT PALATE

Clefts of the lip (CL) and palate (CP) are facial malformations that occur during embryonic development and are the most common congenital deformities in the United States. They may appear separately or more often together.

The palate can be divided into the primary and secondary palates. The primary palate consists of the medial portion of the upper lip and the portion of the alveolar ridge that contains the central and lateral incisors. The secondary palate consists of the remaining portion of the hard palate and all of the soft palate. CL may vary from a small notch in the upper lip to a complete cleft extending into the base of the nose, including the lip and the alveolar ridge (Fig. 41.3). CL can be unilateral or bilateral. Deformed dental structures are associated with CL. Isolated CP occurs in the midline of the secondary palate and may also vary from a bifid uvula (the mildest form of CP) to a complete cleft extending from the soft to the hard palate.

Cleft lip and palate (CL/P) is more common than CP alone and varies by ethnicity. The occurrence is 1 in 750 births in Caucasians, 1 in 500 births in Asians, 1 in 300 births in Native Americans, and 1 in 2500 births in African-Americans (Tinanoff, 2016). CL/P tends to be more common in males, and isolated CP occurs more frequently in females.

Etiology

Cleft deformities may be an isolated anomaly, or they may occur with a recognized syndrome. Clefts of the secondary palate alone are more likely to be associated with syndromes than are isolated CL or CL/P.

Most cases of CL and CP have multifactorial inheritance, which is generally caused by a combination of genetic and environmental factors. Researchers do not yet know which gene(s) are responsible for clefting or to what extent environmental factors impact the developing structures. Exposure to teratogens such as alcohol, cigarette smoking, anticonvulsants, steroids, and retinoids are associated with higher rates of oral clefting. Folate deficiency is also a risk factor for clefting.

Pathophysiology

Cleft deformities represent a defect in cell migration that results in a failure of the maxillary and premaxillary processes to come together between the fourth and tenth weeks of embryonic development. Although often appearing together, CL and CP are distinct malformations embryologically, occurring at different times during the developmental process. Merging of the primary palate (upper lip and alveolus bilaterally) is completed by the seventh week of gestation. Fusion of the secondary palate (hard and soft palate) takes place later, between the seventh and tenth weeks of gestation. In the process of migrating to a horizontal position, the palates are separated by the tongue for a short time. If there is delay in this movement or if the tongue fails to descend soon enough, the remainder of development proceeds, but the palate never fuses.

---

*25379 Wayne Mills Place, Suite 143, Valencia, CA 91355, 877-679-8256, www.classkids.org.
[†]39 Broadway, Suite 2700, New York, NY 10006, 212-668-1000, www.liverfoundation.org/about/education/.

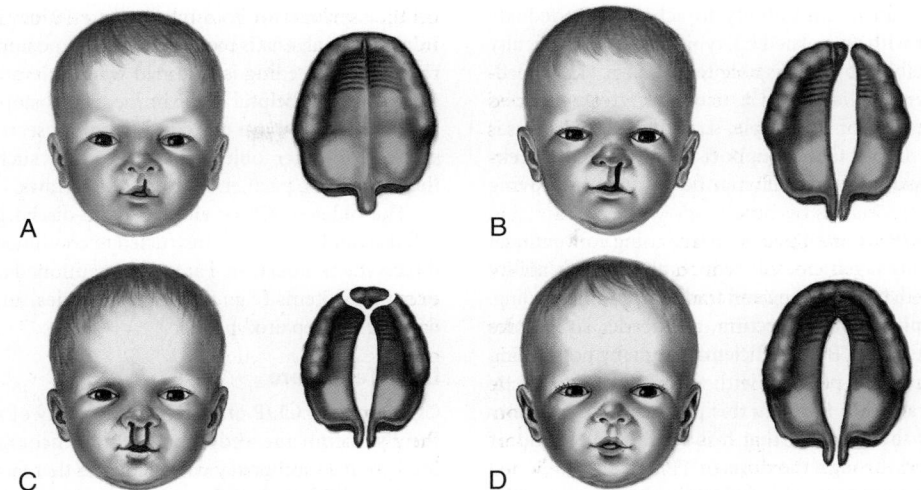

FIG 41.3 Variations in clefts of lip and palate at birth. **A,** Notch in vermilion border. **B,** Unilateral cleft lip and cleft palate. **C,** Bilateral cleft lip and cleft palate. **D,** Cleft palate.

Diagnostic Evaluation

CL and CL/P are apparent at birth. CP is less obvious than CL and may not be detected immediately without a thorough assessment of the mouth. CP is identified through visual examination of the oral cavity or when the examiner places a gloved finger directly on the palate. Clefts of the hard and soft palate form a continuous opening between the mouth and the nasal cavity. The severity of the CP has an impact on feeding; the infant is unable to create suction in the oral cavity that is necessary for feeding. However, in most cases the infant's ability to swallow is normal.

Prenatal diagnosis with fetal ultrasonography is not reliable until the soft tissues of the fetal face can be visualized at 13 to 14 weeks. About 20% to 30% of infants with CL and CL/P are prenatally diagnosed through ultrasonography (Robbins, Damiano, Druschel, et al., 2010), although infants with CP only are rarely diagnosed prenatally.

Interprofessional Management

Treatment of the child with CL and CP involves the cooperative efforts of a multidisciplinary health care team, including pediatrics, plastic surgery, orthodontics, otolaryngology, speech/language pathology, audiology, nursing, and social work. Management is directed toward closure of the cleft(s), prevention of complications, and facilitation of normal growth and development in the child.

Surgical Correction of Cleft Lip

CL repair typically occurs at most centers between 2 and 3 months of age. The two most common procedures for repair of CL are the Fisher technique and the Millard rotational advancement technique. Improved surgical techniques have minimized scar retraction, and in the absence of infection or trauma healing occurs with little scar formation. Nasoalveolar molding may also be used to bring the cleft segments closer together before definitive CL repair, reducing the need for CL revision. However, optimal cosmetic results may be difficult to obtain in severe defects. Additional revisions may be necessary at a later age.

Surgical Correction of Cleft Palate

CP repair typically occurs before 12 months of age to enhance normal speech development (Tinanoff, 2016). The most common techniques to repair CP include the Veau-Wardill-Kilner V-Y pushback procedure

and the Furlow double-opposing Z-plasty. Approximately 20% to 30% of children with repaired CP need a secondary surgery to improve velopharyngeal closure for speech. Secondary procedures may include palatal lengthening, pharyngeal flap, sphincter pharyngoplasty, or posterior pharyngeal wall augmentation. If the child is not a candidate for surgical revision to improve velopharyngeal function, prosthetic management should be considered.

Prognosis

Children with CL may require multiple surgeries to achieve optimal aesthetic outcomes but are not at risk for increased speech problems. Although some children with CP and CL/P do not require speech therapy, many have some degree of speech impairment that requires speech therapy at some point throughout childhood. Articulation errors result from a history of velopharyngeal dysfunction, incorrect articulatory placement, improper tooth alignment, and varying degrees of hearing loss. Improper drainage of the middle ear as a result of inefficient function of the eustachian tube relating to the history of CP contributes to recurrent otitis media, which leads to conductive hearing loss in many children with CP. As a prophylactic measure, many children with palatal clefts have pressure-equalization tubes placed. Extensive orthodontics and prosthodontics may be needed to correct malposition of the teeth and maxillary arches. Academic achievement, social adjustment, and behavior should be monitored, particularly in children with syndromic cleft conditions.

Interprofessional Care Management

The immediate nursing problems for an infant with CL/P deformities are related to feeding. Parents of newborns with clefts place high priority on learning how to feed their infants and identify when they are sick, but they also express interest in learning about the infant's "normal" features. Whenever possible, they should be referred to a comprehensive CP team.

Feeding

Feeding the infant with CL/P deformities presents a challenge. Growth failure in infants with CL/P or CP has been attributed to preoperative feeding difficulties. After surgical repair, most infants who have isolated CL, CP, or CL/P with no associated syndromes gain weight or achieve adequate weight and height for age.

CL may interfere with an infant's ability to achieve an adequate anterior lip seal. An infant with an isolated CL typically has no difficulty breastfeeding because the breast tissue is able to conform to the cleft. If bottle-fed, an infant with an isolated CL may have greater success using bottles with a wide base of the nipple, such as a Playtex nurser or a NUK (orthodontic) nipple. Cheek support (squeezing the cheeks together to decrease the width of the cleft) may be useful in improving lip seal during feeding.

Infants with CP and CL/P are often unable to feed using conventional methods before surgical management. CP reduces the infant's ability to suck, which interferes with breastfeeding and traditional bottle-feeding. Modifications to positioning, bottle selection, and feeder supportive techniques can help infants with CP feed efficiently. Begin by positioning an infant with CP in an upright position with the head supported by the caregiver's hand or cradled in the arm; this position allows gravity to assist with the flow of the liquid so that it is swallowed instead of resulting in a loss of liquid through the nose.

Suction is almost certainly impaired in infants with CP because the velum is unable to elevate and separate the oral nasal cavities while generating adequate negative intraoral pressure. Several types of bottles work well with infants unable to generate adequate suction, including the Special Needs Feeder (formerly Haberman), the Pigeon bottle, and the Mead-Johnson Cleft Palate Nurser. The Special Needs Feeder and the Pigeon bottles use a one-way flow valve that allows the infant to feed successfully by compressing the nipple with the intact segments of the palate and the mandible or tongue. With the one-way flow valve in place, the liquid flows into the oral cavity rather than back into the bottle chamber when the nipple is compressed. The Special Needs Feeder also has a large nipple chamber that allows the feeder to provide extra assistance by squeezing the chamber if needed. The tip of the Special Needs Feeder has a slit cut, which allows the feeder to control the flow of liquid by positioning the slit vertically or horizontally within the mouth, which can reduce choking and gagging. The Pigeon bottle comes with two nipple sizes, standard and small, each with a Y-cut nipple that increases the flow of liquid. The third bottle, the Mead Johnson Cleft Palate Nurser, is a squeezable bottle with a long, thin X-cut nipple; this bottle requires the feeder to rhythmically squeeze the bottle throughout the feeding and does not require the infant to actively compress the nipple during the feeding.

Infants with clefts tend to swallow excessive air during feedings; thus it is important to pause during feedings and burp the infant. Some CP specialists advocate for the use of feeding obturators to assist with feeding; these devices may increase compression surfaces within the oral cavity but do not improve feeding efficiency or growth within the first year of life (Jindal & Khan, 2013).

Regardless of the feeding method used, the mother should begin feeding the infant as soon as possible, preferably after the initial nursery feeding. When maternal feeding is initiated early, the mother can help to determine the method best suited to her, and the infant and can become adept in the technique before discharge from the hospital.

Preoperative Care

In preparation for surgical repair, parents may be taught to use alternative feeding systems (e.g., syringes) several days before surgery.

Postoperative Care

The major efforts in the postoperative period are directed toward protecting the operative site. For CL, parents may be advised to apply petroleum jelly to the operative site for several days after surgery. For CL, CP, or CL/P, elbow immobilizers may be used to prevent the infant from rubbing or disturbing the suture line; they are applied immediately after surgery and may be used for 7 to 10 days. Some centers advocate

using a syringe for feeding for 7 to 10 days after CL or CP repair. Adequate analgesia is required to relieve postoperative pain and prevent restlessness. Feeding is resumed when tolerated. An upright or infant seat position is helpful in the immediate postoperative period (especially for infants who have difficulty handling secretions). Avoid the use of suction or other objects in the mouth such as tongue depressors, thermometers, pacifiers, spoons, and straws.

The older infant or child may be discharged on a blenderized or soft diet, and parents are instructed to continue the diet until the surgeon directs them otherwise. Parents are cautioned against allowing the child to eat hard items (e.g., toast, hard cookies, and potato chips) that can damage the repaired palate.

Long-Term Care

Children with CL/P often require a variety of services during recovery. Family members need support and encouragement by health care professionals and guidance in activities that facilitate a normal outcome for their child. Parents frequently cite financial stress as a difficult issue. With the combined efforts of the family and the health care team, most children achieve a satisfactory outcome. Many children with CL/P have surgical correction that creates a near normal–appearing lip and permits good function of the palate for speech and feeding. Parents need to understand the function of speech therapy and the purpose and care of all orthodontic appliances, as well as the importance of establishing good mouth care and proper brushing habits.

Throughout the child's development, an important goal is the development of a healthy personality and self-esteem. Many communities have CP parents' groups that offer help and support to families. Agencies that provide services and information for children with CL/P and their families include the American Cleft Palate–Craniofacial Association (www.acpa-cpf.org), the Cleft Palate Foundation (www.cleftline.org), Cleft Advocate (www.cleftadvocate.org), the March of Dimes (www.marchforbabies.org), and various state children's medical services.

ESOPHAGEAL ATRESIA AND TRACHEOESOPHAGEAL FISTULA

Congenital esophageal atresia (EA) and tracheoesophageal fistula (TEF) are rare malformations that represent a failure of the esophagus to develop as a continuous passage and a failure of the trachea and esophagus to separate into distinct structures. These defects may occur as separate entities or in combination, and without early diagnosis and treatment they pose a serious threat to the infant's well-being.

The incidence of EA is estimated to be approximately 1 in 4000 live births (Kunisaki & Foker, 2012). There appears to be a slightly higher incidence in males, and the birth weight of most affected infants is significantly lower than average, with an unusually high incidence of preterm birth with EA and a subsequent increase in mortality. A history of maternal polyhydramnios is present in approximately 50% of infants with the defect.

Approximately 50% of the cases of EA/TEF are a component of VATER or VACTERL association, which are acronyms used to describe associated anomalies (VATER for vertebral defects, imperforate anus, tracheoesophageal fistula, and radial and renal dysplasia; and VACTERL for vertebral, anal, cardiac, tracheal, esophageal, renal, and limb) (Khan & Orenstein, 2016b). Cardiac anomalies may also occur with EA/TEF; therefore, all patients should undergo a workup for associated anomalies.

Pathophysiology

Anomalies involving the trachea and esophagus are caused by defective separation, incomplete fusion of the tracheal folds after this separation, or altered cellular growth during embryonic development. In the most frequently encountered form of EA and TEF (80% to 90% of cases), the proximal esophageal segment terminates in a blind pouch, and the distal segment is connected to the trachea or primary bronchus by a short fistula at or near the bifurcation. The second most common variety (7% to 8%) consists of a blind pouch at each end, widely separated and with no communication to the trachea. An H-type EA refers to an otherwise normal trachea and esophagus connected by a fistula (4% to 5%). Extremely rare anomalies involve a fistula from the trachea to the upper esophageal segment (0.8%) or to both the upper and lower segments (0.7% to 6%).

Diagnostic Evaluation

Although the diagnosis is established on the basis of clinical signs and symptoms (Box 41.9), the exact type of anomaly is determined by radiographic studies. A radiopaque catheter is inserted into the hypopharynx and advanced until it encounters an obstruction. Chest radiographs are taken to ascertain esophageal patency or the presence and level of a blind pouch. Occasionally fistulas are not patent, which makes them more difficult to diagnose. A careful bronchoscopic examination may be performed in an attempt to visualize the fistula.

The presence of polyhydramnios (accumulation of 2000 mL of amniotic fluid) prenatally is a clue to the possibility of EA in the unborn infant, especially with defect type A, B, or C. With these types of EA/TEF, amniotic fluid normally swallowed by the fetus is unable to reach the GI tract to be absorbed and excreted by the kidneys. The result is an abnormal accumulation of amniotic fluid, or polyhydramnios.

Therapeutic Management

The treatment of patients with EA and TEF includes maintenance of a patent airway, prevention of pneumonia, gastric or blind pouch decompression, supportive therapy, and surgical repair of the anomaly.

When EA with a TEF is suspected, the infant is immediately deprived of oral intake, IV fluids are initiated, and the infant is positioned to facilitate drainage of secretions and decrease the likelihood of aspiration. Accumulated secretions are suctioned frequently from the mouth and pharynx. A double-lumen catheter should be placed into the upper esophageal pouch and attached to intermittent or continuous low suction. The infant's head is kept upright to facilitate removal of fluid collected in the pouch and prevent aspiration of gastric contents. Broad-spectrum antibiotic therapy is often instituted if there is a concern about aspiration of gastric contents.

The surgery consists of a thoracotomy with division and ligation of the TEF and an end-to-end or end-to-side anastomosis of the esophagus. A chest tube may be inserted to drain intrapleural air and fluid. For infants who are not stable enough to undergo definitive repair or those with a lengthy gap (>3 to 4 cm) between the proximal and distal esophagus, a staged operation is preferred that involves gastrostomy, ligation of the TEF, and constant drainage of the esophageal pouch. A

delayed esophageal anastomosis is usually attempted after several weeks to months. Thoracoscopic repair of EA/TEF is being used successfully, thus negating the need for a thoracotomy and minimizing associated postoperative complications and morbidities (Guidry & McGahren, 2012; Kunisaki & Foker, 2012).

If an esophageal anastomosis cannot be accomplished, a gastrostomy is recommended; a cervical esophagostomy (to allow drainage of saliva through a stoma in the neck) is performed in cases of a long gap atresia, but this is no longer recommended because it makes subsequent surgical repair more difficult (Kunisaki & Foker, 2012).

A primary anastomosis may be impossible because of insufficient length of the two segments of esophagus. This occurs if the distance between the two segments is 3 to 4 cm (1.2 to 1.6 inches) (Khan & Orenstein, 2016b). In these cases, an esophageal replacement procedure using a part of the colon or gastric tube interposition may be necessary to bridge the missing esophageal segment. Further surgical techniques may be performed later to facilitate esophageal lengthening. Tracheomalacia may occur as a result of weakness in the tracheal wall that exists when a dilated proximal pouch compresses the trachea early in fetal life. It may also occur as a result of inadequate intratracheal pressure causing abnormal tracheal development. Clinical signs of tracheomalacia include a barking cough, stridor, wheezing, recurrent respiratory tract infections, cyanosis, and sometimes apnea.

Prognosis

The survival rate is nearly 100% in otherwise healthy children. Most deaths are the result of extreme prematurity or other lethal associated anomalies. Potential complications after the surgical repair of EA and TEF depend on the type of defect and surgical correction. Complications of repair include an anastomotic leak, strictures caused by tension or ischemia, esophageal motility disorders causing dysphagia, respiratory compromise, and GER. Anastomotic esophageal strictures may cause dysphagia, choking, and respiratory distress. The strictures are often treated with routine esophageal dilation. Feeding difficulties are often present for months or years after surgery, and the infant must be monitored closely to ensure adequate weight gain, growth, and development. In some cases, laparoscopic fundoplication may be required. At times, the infant must be fed via gastrostomy or jejunostomy to provide adequate caloric intake.

Care Management

Nursing responsibility for detection of this serious malformation begins immediately after birth. For an infant with the classic signs and symptoms of EA, the major concern is the establishment of a patent airway and prevention of further respiratory compromise. Cyanosis is usually a result of laryngeal spasm caused by overflow of saliva into the larynx from the proximal esophageal pouch or aspiration; it normally resolves after removal of the secretions from the oropharynx by suctioning. The passage of a small-gauge orogastric feeding tube via the mouth into the stomach during the initial nursing physical assessment is helpful to rule out EA or other obstructive defects.

> **! NURSING ALERT**
>
> Any infant who has an excessive amount of frothy saliva in the mouth or difficulty with secretions and unexplained episodes of apnea, cyanosis, or oxygen desaturation should be suspected of having an EA or TEF and referred immediately for medical evaluation.

Preoperative Care

The nurse carefully suctions the mouth and nasopharynx and places the infant in an optimum position to facilitate drainage and avoid aspiration. The most desirable position for a newborn who is suspected of having the typical EA with a TEF (e.g., type C) is supine (or sometimes prone) with the head elevated on an inclined plane of at least 30 degrees. This positioning minimizes the reflux of gastric secretions at the distal esophagus into the trachea and bronchi, especially when intraabdominal pressure is elevated.

It is imperative to immediately remove any secretions that can be aspirated. Until surgery, the blind pouch is kept empty by intermittent or continuous suction through an indwelling double-lumen catheter passed orally or nasally to the end of the pouch. In some cases, a percutaneous gastrostomy tube is inserted and left open so any air entering the stomach through the fistula can escape, thus minimizing the danger of gastric contents being regurgitated into the trachea. The gastrostomy tube is emptied by gravity drainage. Feedings through the gastrostomy tube and irrigations with fluid are contraindicated before surgery in an infant with a distal TEF.

Nursing interventions include respiratory assessment, airway management, thermoregulation, fluid and electrolyte management, and PN support.

Often the infant must be transferred to a hospital with a specialized care unit and pediatric surgical team. The nurse advises the parents of the infant's condition and provides them with necessary support and information.

Postoperative Care

Postoperative care for these infants is the same as for any high-risk newborn. Adequate thermoregulation is provided, the double-lumen NG catheter is attached to low-suction or gravity drainage, PN is provided, and the gastrostomy tube (if applicable) is returned to gravity drainage until feedings are tolerated. If a thoracotomy is performed and a chest tube is inserted, attention to the appropriate function of the closed drainage system is imperative. Pain management in the postoperative period is important even if only a thoracoscopic approach is used. In the first 24 to 36 hours, the nurse should provide pain management for the neonate. Tracheal suction should only be done using a premeasured catheter and with extreme caution to avoid injury to the suture line.

If tolerated, gastrostomy feedings may be initiated and continued until the esophageal anastomosis is healed. Before oral feedings are initiated and the chest tube (if applicable) is removed, a contrast study or esophagram will verify the integrity of the esophageal anastomosis.

The nurse must carefully observe the initial attempt at oral feeding carefully to make certain the infant is able to swallow without choking. Until the infant is able to take a sufficient amount by mouth, oral intake may need to be supplemented by bolus or continuous gastrostomy feedings. Ordinarily infants are not discharged until they can take oral fluids well. The gastrostomy tube may be removed before discharge or maintained for supplemental feedings at home.

Special Problems

Upper respiratory tract complications are a threat to life in both the preoperative and postoperative periods. In addition to pneumonia, there is a constant danger of respiratory distress resulting from atelectasis, pneumothorax, and laryngeal edema. Any persistent respiratory difficulty after removal of secretions is reported to the surgeon immediately. The infant is monitored for anastomotic leaks, as evidenced by purulent chest tube drainage, increased WBC count, and temperature instability.

For an infant who requires esophageal replacement, nonnutritive sucking is provided by a pacifier. Sometimes small amounts of water or formula are given orally, and although the liquid drains from the esophagostomy, this process allows the infant to develop mature sucking patterns. Other appropriate oral stimulation prevents feeding aversion.

Infants who remain NPO for an extended period or who have not received oral stimulation have difficulty eating by mouth after corrective surgery and may develop oral hypersensitivity and food aversion. They require patient, firm guidance to learn how to take food into the mouth and swallow after repair. A referral to a multidisciplinary feeding behavior program is recommended.

Some infants with EA/TEF may require periodic esophageal dilations on an outpatient basis. Discharge education should include instructions about feeding techniques in the infant with a repaired esophagus, including a semi-upright feeding position, small feedings, and observation for adequacy of swallowing (regurgitation, cyanosis, choking). Tracheomalacia is often a complication, and parents are educated regarding the signs and symptoms of this condition. GER may also occur when feedings resume and may contribute to reactive airway disease with wheezing and labored respirations as the prominent clinical manifestations. Problems with thriving and gaining weight may occur in the first 5 years of life in the child with EA/TEF, especially if the infant is born preterm, and the nurse should be alert to the achievement of developmental milestones that indicate a need for early intervention and multidisciplinary referral.

Preparing parents for discharge involves teaching them skills they will need at home. Parents are taught to observe for behaviors that indicate the need for suctioning and signs of respiratory distress and constriction of the esophagus (e.g., poor feeding, choking, dysphagia, drooling, regurgitation of undigested food). Discharge planning also includes obtaining the necessary equipment and home nursing services to provide home care.

HERNIAS

A hernia is a protrusion of a portion of an organ or organs through an abnormal opening. The danger from herniation arises when the organ protruding through the opening is constricted to the extent that circulation is impaired or when the protruding organs encroach on and impair the function of other structures.

The umbilical hernia is a common hernia observed in infants. An umbilical hernia usually is an isolated defect, but it may be associated with other congenital anomalies, such as Down syndrome (trisomy 21) and trisomies 13 and 18. Inguinal hernias account for approximately 80% of all childhood hernias and occur more frequently in boys than in girls. An inguinal hernia that cannot be reduced easily is called an *incarcerated hernia*. A *strangulated inguinal hernia* is one in which the blood supply to the herniated organ is impaired. If left untreated, both incarcerated and strangulated hernias will progress to necrotic bowel. The herniations of concern are those that protrude through the diaphragm, the abdominal wall, or the inguinal canal. The abdominal wall defects gastroschisis and omphalocele are considered separately in Table 41.9.

OBSTRUCTIVE DISORDERS

Obstruction in the GI tract occurs when the passage of nutrients and secretions is impeded by a constricted or occluded lumen or when there is impaired motility *(paralytic ileus)*. Obstructions may be congenital or acquired. Congenital obstructions, such as atresia, imperforate anus, meconium plug, and meconium ileus, usually appear in the neonatal period. Other obstructions of congenital etiology, such as malrotation, Hirschsprung disease, pyloric stenosis, volvulus, incarcerated hernia, and Meckel diverticulum, appear after the first few weeks of life. Intestinal obstruction from acquired causes such as intussusception and tumors may occur in infancy or childhood. Intestinal obstructions from any cause are characterized by similar signs and symptoms (Box 41.10).

TABLE 41.9   Abdominal Wall Defects

Defect	Symptoms	Nursing Management
Omphalocele—Protrusion of intraabdominal viscera into base of umbilical cord; sac covered with a translucent peritoneal sac	Usually obvious on inspection; however, small omphalocele may appear to be a hematoma in umbilical cord Observe for associated malformations	**Therapeutic:** Surgical repair of defect. **Nursing:** *Preoperative:* Protect defect from trauma or drying. Keep sac or viscera moist with a bowel bag or moist dressings. Maintain thermoregulation. Administer prophylactic antibiotics and IV fluids as prescribed. Provide nasogastric suction for gastric decompression. Keep patient NPO. Assess for associated birth defects. *Postoperative:* Monitor vital signs. Assess for and manage pain. Provide nasogastric suction for bowel decompression. Administer IV fluids and parenteral nutrition. Keep NPO until return of bowel function, then feedings may resume.
Gastroschisis—Protrusion of intraabdominal contents through defect in abdominal wall lateral to umbilical ring; no peritoneal sac covering the exposed bowel	Defect obvious at delivery if not detected prenatally by ultrasonography	**Therapeutic:** Surgical repair of defect. For large lesions, provide gradual reduction of abdominal contents via Silastic silo before surgical closure. **Nursing:** *Preoperative:* Keep sac covered with a bowel bag to prevent trauma and drying. Provide nasogastric suction for bowel decompression. Maintain thermoregulation. Administer antibiotics and IV fluids. Observe exposed bowel for signs of necrosis or constriction at exit site. *Postoperative:* Monitor vital signs and BP. Assess for and manage pain. Provide nasogastric suction for bowel decompression. Administer IV fluids and parenteral nutrition. Monitor surgical closure site for infection. Monitor lower extremities for pulses and circulation (in case of vena cava compression by large bowel in small abdominal cavity). Monitor for return of bowel function and peristalsis. In event of Silastic silo, nursing care should also include monitoring vital signs, keeping pouch clean, and aseptic technique with dressing changes (if not done by surgeon). Provide emotional support for parents. Long-term problems associated with feeding and weight gain.

IV, Intravenous; *NG,* nasogastric; *NPO,* nothing by mouth.

HYPERTROPHIC PYLORIC STENOSIS

Hypertrophic pyloric stenosis (HPS) occurs when the circumferential muscle of the pyloric sphincter becomes thickened, resulting in elongation and narrowing of the pyloric channel. This produces an outlet obstruction and compensatory dilation, hypertrophy, and hyperperistalsis of the stomach. This condition usually develops in the first few weeks of life, causing nonbilious vomiting, which occurs after a feeding. If the condition is not diagnosed early, dehydration, metabolic alkalosis, and failure to thrive may occur. The precise etiology is unknown. Boys are affected four to six times more frequently than girls (Hunter & Liacouras, 2016). It is more common in white infants and is seen less frequently in African-American and Asian infants (Hunter & Liacouras, 2016).

Pathophysiology

The circular muscle of the pylorus thickens as a result of hypertrophy. This produces severe narrowing of the pyloric canal between the stomach and the duodenum, causing partial obstruction of the lumen (Fig. 41.4, *A*). Over time, inflammation and edema further reduce the size of the opening, resulting in complete obstruction. The hypertrophied pylorus may be palpable as an olive-like mass in the upper abdomen.

Pyloric stenosis is not a congenital disorder. It is believed that local innervation may be involved in the pathogenesis. In most cases, HPS is an isolated lesion; however, it may be associated with intestinal malrotation, esophageal and duodenal atresia, and anorectal anomalies.

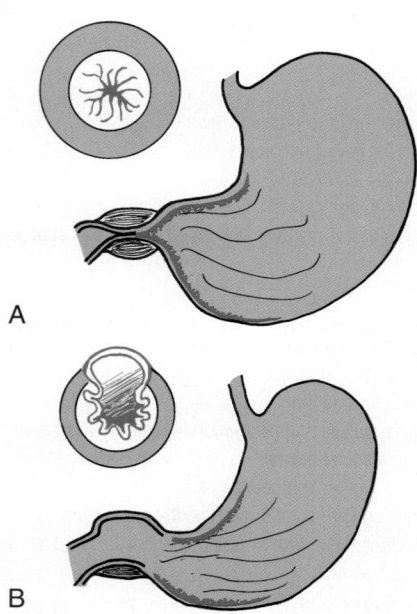

FIG 41.4 Hypertrophic pyloric stenosis. **A,** Enlarged muscular area nearly obliterates pyloric channel. **B,** Longitudinal surgical division of muscle down to submucosa establishes adequate passageway.

Diagnostic Evaluation

The diagnosis of HPS is often made after the history and physical examination. The olive-like mass is easily palpated when the stomach is empty, the infant is quiet, and the abdominal muscles are relaxed. Vomiting usually occurs 30 to 60 minutes after feeding and becomes projectile as the obstruction progresses. Emesis is nonbilious in the early stages. These infants may become dehydrated and appear malnourished if an early diagnosis is not established.

If the diagnosis is inconclusive from the history and physical signs (Box 41.11), ultrasonography demonstrates an elongated, sausage-shaped mass with an elongated pyloric channel. If ultrasonography fails to demonstrate a hypertrophied pylorus, an upper GI radiography should

be done to rule out other causes of vomiting. If the condition is not diagnosed early, laboratory findings reflect the metabolic alterations (hypochloremic metabolic alkalosis) created by severe depletion of both fluid and electrolytes from extensive and prolonged vomiting.

Therapeutic Management

Surgical relief of the pyloric obstruction by *pyloromyotomy* is the standard therapy for this disorder. Preoperatively, the infant must be rehydrated and metabolic alkalosis corrected with parenteral fluid and electrolyte administration. Replacement fluid therapy may delay surgery for 24 to 48 hours. The stomach is decompressed with an NG tube if the infant continues with vomiting. In infants with no evidence of fluid and electrolyte imbalance, surgery is performed without delay.

The surgical procedure is often performed by laparoscope and consists of a longitudinal incision through the circular muscle fibers of the pylorus down to, but not including, the submucosa (pyloromyotomy, or the Fredet-Ramstedt procedure) (see Fig. 41.4, *B*). The procedure has a high success rate. Laparoscopic surgery through a single small incision often results in a shorter surgical time, more rapid postoperative feeding, and shorter hospital stay (Hunter & Liacouras, 2016).

Feedings are usually begun 4 to 6 hours postoperatively, beginning with small, frequent feedings of an electrolyte solution such as Pedialyte or water. If clear fluids are retained, formula or breast feedings are initiated about 24 hours after surgery to the infant's tolerance. The amount and the interval between feedings are gradually increased until a full feeding schedule is reinstated, which usually takes about 48 hours.

Prognosis

The prognosis for infants and small children with HPS is excellent when the diagnosis is confirmed early. Most infants recover completely and rapidly after pyloromyotomy. Postoperative complications include persistent pyloric obstruction and rarely wound dehiscence.

Care Management

Nursing care involves primarily observation for clinical features that help establish the diagnosis, careful regulation of fluid therapy, and reestablishment of normal feeding patterns. Assessment is based on observation of eating behaviors and evidence of other characteristic clinical manifestations.

Preoperatively, the emphasis is placed on restoring hydration and electrolyte balance. Infants are usually given no oral feedings and receive IV fluids with dextrose and electrolyte replacement based on laboratory serum electrolyte values and clinical appearance.

Observations also include assessment of vital signs, particularly those that might indicate fluid or electrolyte imbalances. These infants are prone to metabolic alkalosis from loss of hydrogen ions and to potassium, sodium, and chloride depletion. Assess the skin, mucous membranes, and daily weight for alterations in hydration status.

If stomach decompression is used preoperatively, the nurse is responsible for ensuring that the tube is patent and functioning properly and for measuring and recording the type and amount of drainage. Parental involvement is encouraged and promoted.

Postoperative vomiting is common, and even with successful surgery most infants exhibit some vomiting during the first 24 to 48 hours. IV fluids are administered until the infant is taking and retaining adequate amounts by mouth. Much of the same care that was instituted before surgery is continued postoperatively, including observation of vital signs, monitoring of IV fluids, and careful monitoring of fluid intake and output. In addition, the infant is observed for responses to the stress of surgery and evidence of pain. Appropriate analgesics should be given around the clock because pain is continuous. The surgical incision(s) is inspected for drainage or erythema, and any signs of infection are reported to the surgeon. A surgical adhesive may be used for incision closure, and parents are instructed regarding the care of the incision and any dressings before discharge.

Feedings are usually instituted within 12 to 24 hours postoperatively, beginning with clear liquids and advancing to formula or breast milk as tolerated. Observation and recording of feedings and the infant's responses to feedings are a vital part of postoperative care. Care of the operative site consists of observation for any drainage or signs of inflammation and care of the incision.

INTUSSUSCEPTION

Intussusception is the most common cause of intestinal obstruction in children between 5 months and 3 years of age (Kennedy & Liacouras, 2016). Intussusception is more common in males than in females and is more common in children younger than 2 years of age. Although specific intestinal lesions occur in a small percentage of the children, generally the cause is not known. More than 90% of intussusceptions do not have a pathologic lead point such as a polyp, lymphoma, or Meckel diverticulum. The idiopathic cases may be caused by hypertrophy of intestinal lymphoid tissue secondary to viral infection.

Pathophysiology

Intussusception occurs when a proximal segment of the bowel telescopes into a more distal segment, pulling the mesentery with it. The mesentery is compressed and angled, resulting in lymphatic and venous obstruction. As the edema from the obstruction increases, pressure within the area of intussusception increases. When the pressure equals the arterial pressure, arterial blood flow stops, resulting in ischemia and the pouring of mucus into the intestine. Venous engorgement also leads to leaking of blood and mucus into the intestinal lumen, forming the classic currant jelly–like stools. The most common site is the ileocecal valve (ileocolic), where the ileum invaginates into the cecum and then further into the colon (Fig. 41.5). Other forms include *ileoileal* (one part of the ileum invaginates into another section of the ileum) and *colocolic* (one part of the colon invaginates into another area of the colon) intussusceptions, usually in the area of the hepatic or splenic flexure or at some point along the transverse colon.

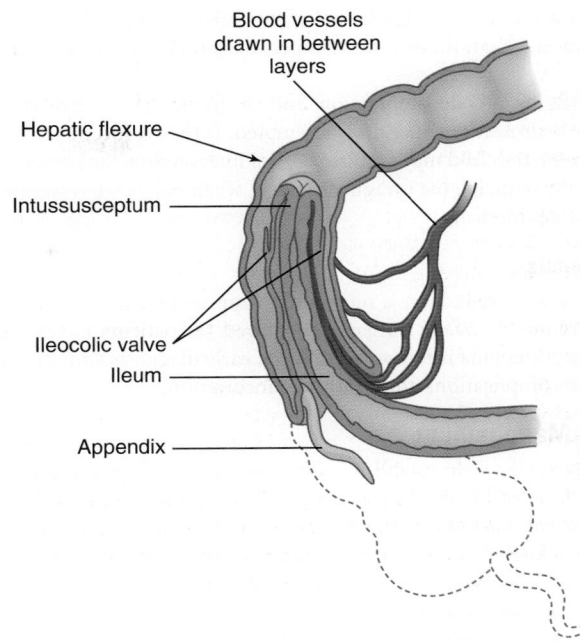

FIG 41.5 Ileocecal intussusception.

Labels: Blood vessels drawn in between layers; Hepatic flexure; Intussusceptum; Ileocolic valve; Ileum; Appendix

BOX 41.12   Clinical Manifestations of Intussusception

- Sudden acute abdominal pain
- Child screaming and drawing the knees toward the chest
- Child appearing comfortable during intervals between episodes of pain
- Vomiting
- Lethargy
- Passage of red, currant jelly–like stools (stool mixed with blood and mucus)
- Tender, distended abdomen
- Palpable sausage-shaped mass in upper right quadrant
- Empty lower right quadrant (Dance sign)
- Eventual fever, prostration, and other signs of peritonitis

! NURSING ALERT

The classic triad of intussusception symptoms (abdominal pain, abdominal mass, bloody stools) is present in fewer than 30% of children (Kennedy & Liacouras, 2016). A more chronic case may be presented, characterized by diarrhea, anorexia, weight loss, occasional vomiting, and periodic pain. Because intussusception is potentially life-threatening, be aware of such signs, and closely observe and refer these children for further medical evaluation.

Diagnostic Evaluation

Frequently subjective findings lead to the diagnosis (Box 41.12), which can be confirmed by ultrasonography. A rectal examination reveals mucus, blood, and occasionally a low intussusception itself.

Therapeutic Management

Conservative treatment consists of radiologist-guided pneumoenema (air enema) with or without water-soluble contrast or ultrasound-guided hydrostatic (saline) enema; the advantage of the latter is that no ionizing radiation is needed (Kennedy & Liacouras, 2016). Recurrence of intussusception after conservative treatment is rare; however, this procedure should not be attempted with prolonged intussusception, signs of shock, peritoneal irritation, or intestinal perforation (Kennedy & Liacouras, 2016).

IV fluids, NG decompression, and antibiotic therapy may be used before hydrostatic reduction is attempted. If these procedures are not successful, the child may require surgical intervention. Surgery involves manually reducing the invagination and, when indicated, resecting any nonviable intestine.

Prognosis

Nonoperative reduction is successful in approximately 65% to 75% of cases (Gourlay, 2013). Surgery is required for patients in whom the hydrostatic enema is unsuccessful. With early diagnosis and treatment, serious complications and death are uncommon.

Care Management

The nurse can help establish a diagnosis by listening to the parent's description of the child's physical and behavioral symptoms. It is not unusual for parents to state that they thought something was seriously wrong before others shared their concerns. The description of the child's severe colicky abdominal pain combined with vomiting is a significant sign of intussusception.

As soon as a possible diagnosis of intussusception is made, the nurse prepares the parents for the immediate need for hospitalization, the nonsurgical technique of hydrostatic reduction, and the possibility of surgery. It is important to explain the basic defect of intussusception. A model of the defect is easily demonstrated by pushing the end of a finger on a rubber glove back into itself or using the example of a telescoping rod. The principle of reduction by hydrostatic pressure can be simulated by filling the glove with water, which pushes the "finger" into a fully extended position.

Physical care of the child does not differ from that for any child undergoing abdominal surgery. Even though nonsurgical intervention may be successful, the usual preoperative procedures such as maintenance of NPO status, routine laboratory testing (CBC and urinalysis), signed parental consent, and preanesthetic sedation, are performed. Before surgery, the nurse monitors all stools. Children with perforation will require IV fluids, systemic antibiotics, and bowel decompression before undergoing surgery. Fluid volume replacement and restoration of electrolytes may be required in such children before surgery.

> **! NURSING ALERT**
>
> Passage of a normal brown stool usually indicates that the intussusception has reduced itself. This is reported to the health care provider immediately, who may choose to alter the diagnostic and therapeutic care plan.

Postprocedural care includes observations of vital signs, blood pressure, intact sutures and dressing, and the return of bowel sounds. After spontaneous or hydrostatic reduction, the nurse observes for passage of water-soluble contrast material (if used) and the stool patterns because the intussusception may recur. Children may be admitted to the hospital or monitored on an outpatient basis. A recurrence of intussusception is treated with the conservative reduction techniques described earlier, but a laparotomy is considered for multiple recurrences.

MALROTATION AND VOLVULUS

Malrotation of the intestine is caused by the abnormal rotation of the intestine around the superior mesenteric artery during embryologic development. Malrotation may manifest in utero or may be asymptomatic throughout life. Infants may have intermittent bilious vomiting, recurrent

abdominal pain, distention, or lower GI bleeding. Malrotation is the most serious type of intestinal obstruction because if the intestine undergoes complete volvulus (the intestine twisting around itself), compromise of the blood supply results in intestinal necrosis, peritonitis, perforation, and death.

Diagnostic Evaluation

It is imperative that malrotation and volvulus be diagnosed promptly and surgical treatment instituted quickly. In addition to a history and physical examination, a plain abdominal radiograph and lateral decubitus view are obtained; bowel distention will be present proximal to the distention on plain radiograph, and a lateral view will demonstrate air-fluid levels in the distended bowel (Bales & Liacouras, 2016). An upper GI series is the definitive procedure to diagnose this condition.

Therapeutic Management

Surgery is indicated to remove the affected area. Because of the extensive nature of some lesions, short-bowel syndrome is a postoperative complication.

Care Management

Preoperatively, the nursing care is the same as that provided to an infant or child with intestinal obstruction. IV fluids, NG decompression, and systemic antibiotics are implemented; in the rapidly deteriorating infant, fluid volume resuscitation and vasopressors may be required for preoperative stabilization. Postoperatively, the nursing care is similar to that provided to the infant or child who has undergone abdominal surgery.

ANORECTAL MALFORMATIONS

Anorectal malformations are among the more common congenital malformations caused by abnormal development, with an incidence of approximately 1 in 5000 births (Herman & Teitelbaum, 2012). These malformations may range from simple imperforate anus to include other associated complex anomalies of genitourinary (GU) and pelvic organs, which may require extensive treatment for fecal, urinary, and sexual function. Anorectal malformations may occur in isolation or as a part of the VACTERL association (see earlier in this chapter). These anomalies are classified according to the newborn's gender and abnormal anatomic features, including GU defects.

Rectal atresia and stenosis occur when the anal opening appears normal, there is a midline intergluteal groove, and usually no fistula exists between the rectum and urinary tract. *Rectal atresia* is a complete obstruction (inability to pass stool) and requires immediate surgical intervention. *Rectal stenosis* may not become apparent until later in infancy when the infant has a history of difficult stooling, abdominal distention, and ribbonlike stools.

The anus and rectum originate from an embryologic structure called the *cloaca*. Lateral growth of the cloaca forms the urorectal septum that separates the rectum dorsally from the urinary tract ventrally. The rectum and urinary tract separate completely by the seventh week of gestation. A *persistent cloaca* is a complex anorectal malformation in which the rectum, vagina, and urethra drain into a common channel opening into the perineum (Fig. 41.6, *A*).

Imperforate anus includes several forms of malformation without an obvious opening (see Fig. 41.6, *B*). Frequently a *fistula* (an abnormal communication) leads from the distal rectum to the perineum or GU system (see Fig. 41.6, *B*). The fistula may be evidenced when meconium is evacuated through the vaginal opening, the perineum below the vagina, the male urethra, or the perineum under the scrotum. The presence of meconium on the perineum does not indicate anal patency. A fistula may not be apparent at birth, but as peristalsis increases,

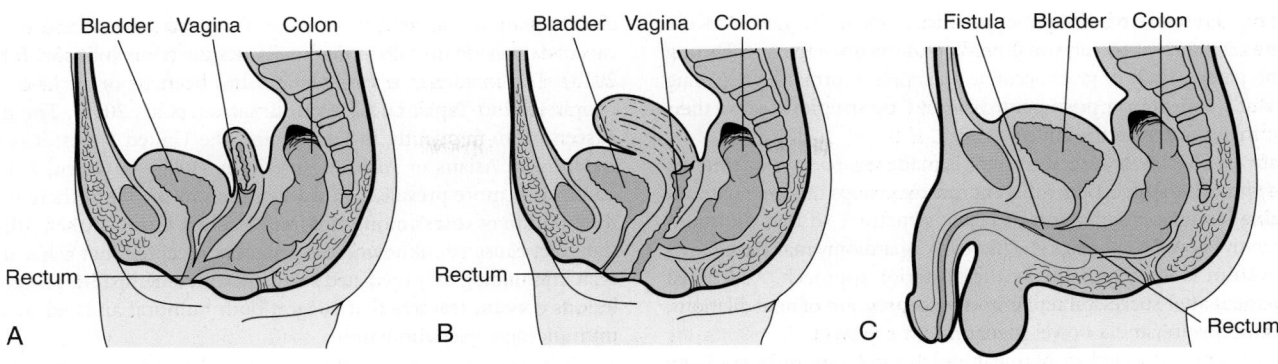

FIG 41.6 Anorectal malformations. **A,** Typical cloaca (female). **B,** Low rectovaginal fistula (female). **C,** Rectourethral bulbar fistula (male).

BOX 41.13 Classification of Anorectal Malformations

Male Defects	Female Defects
• Perineal fistula	• Perineal fistula
• Rectourethral bulbar fistula	• Retrovestibular fistula
• Rectourethral prostatic fistula	• Imperforate anus without fistula
• Rectovesicular (bladder neck) fistula	• Rectal atresia and stenosis
• Imperforate anus without fistula	• Cloaca
• Rectal atresia and stenosis	

From Peña, A., & Hong, A. (2000). Advances in the management of anorectal malformations. *American Journal of Surgery, 180*(5), 370–376.

---

meconium is forced through the fistula into the urethra or onto the newborn's perineum. Anorectal anomalies are classified according to gender and abnormal anatomic features, including GU and associated pelvic anomalies (Box 41.13).

Diagnostic Evaluation

The diagnosis of an anorectal malformation is based on the physical finding of an absent anal opening. Other symptoms may include abdominal distention, vomiting, absence of meconium passage, or presence of meconium in the urine. Additional physical findings with an anorectal malformation are a flat perineum and the absence of a midline intergluteal groove. The appearance of the perineum alone does not predict the extent of the defect and associated anomalies accurately. GU and spinal-vertebral anomalies associated with anorectal malformations should be considered when an anomaly is noted. EA with or without TEF, cardiac defects, and neural tube defects or vertebral anomalies may occur in association with anorectal malformations, and the infant should be carefully evaluated for the presence of these and other anomalies.

A perineal fistula may be diagnosed by clinical observation. Abdominal and pelvic ultrasonography is performed to further evaluate the infant's anatomic malformation. An IV pyelogram and a voiding cystourethrogram are performed to evaluate associated anomalies involving the urinary tract. Other diagnostic examinations that may be performed include pelvic MRI, radiography, ultrasonography, and fluoroscopic examination of pelvic anatomic contents and lower spinal anatomy.

Therapeutic Management

The primary management of anorectal malformations is surgical. Once the defect has been identified, take steps to rule out associated life-threatening defects, which need immediate surgical intervention. Provided no immediate life-threatening problems exist, the newborn is stabilized and kept NPO for further evaluation. IV fluids are provided to maintain glucose and fluid and electrolyte balance. The current recommendation is that surgery be delayed at least 24 hours to evaluate for the presence of a fistula and possibly other anomalies (Herman & Teitelabum, 2012).

The surgical treatment of anorectal malformations varies according to the defect but usually involves one or possibly a combination of several of the following procedures: anoplasty, colostomy, *posterior sagittal anorectoplasty* (PSARP) or other pull-through with colostomy, and colostomy (take-down) closure. The "Care Management" section that follows outlines some aspects of preoperative and postoperative care.

A primary laparoscopic repair (without colostomy) of anorectal malformations is being performed successfully in some centers. This minimizes surgical risks, associated morbidity, and postoperative pain management.

Care Management

The first nursing responsibility is assisting to identify anorectal malformations. A newborn who does not pass stool within 24 hours after birth or has meconium that appears at a location other than the anal opening requires further assessment. Preoperative care includes diagnostic evaluation, GI decompression, bowel preparation, and IV fluids.

For the newborn with a perineal fistula, an *anoplasty* is performed, which involves moving the fistula opening to the center of the sphincter and enlarging the rectal opening. Postoperative nursing care after anoplasty is primarily directed toward healing the surgical site without other complications. A program of anal dilations is usually initiated when the child returns for the 2-week checkup. Feedings are started soon after surgical repair, and breastfeeding is encouraged because it causes less constipation.

In neonates with anomalies such as cloaca (females), rectourethral prostatic fistula (males), and vestibular fistula (females), a descending colostomy may be performed to allow fecal elimination and avoid fecal contamination of the distal imperforate section and subsequent urinary tract infection in infants with urorectal fistulas. With a colostomy, postoperative nursing care is directed toward maintaining appropriate skin care at the stoma sites (both distal and proximal), managing postoperative pain, and administering IV fluids and antibiotics. Postoperative NG decompression may be required with laparotomy, and nursing care focuses on maintenance of appropriate drainage (see the "Ostomies" section in Chapter 39 for colostomy care).

The PSARP is a common surgical procedure for the repair of anorectal malformations in infants approximately 1 to 2 months after the initial colostomy. Preoperative PSARP care often involves irrigation of the distal stoma to prevent fecal contamination of the operative site. During this time, parents must be given accurate yet simple information regarding the infant's appearance postoperatively and expectations as to their level of involvement in the child's care.

In the PSARP procedure, the repair is made via a posterior midline sacral approach to dissect the different muscle groups involved without damaging strategic innervation of pelvic structures so that optimum postoperative bowel continence is achieved. A laparotomy may be required if the rectum is unidentifiable by the posterior approach. Additional management after successful repair involves a program of anal dilations, colostomy closure, and a bowel management program.

Parents are instructed in perineal and wound care or care of the colostomy as needed. Anal dilations may be necessary for some infants. Parents should observe stooling patterns and signs of anal stricture or complications. Information about dietary modifications and administration of medications is included in counseling. Nurses have a vital role in helping families of a child with anorectal malformations provide optimum care so bowel management is successful and quality of life enhanced for the child and family.

Family Support, Discharge Planning, and Home Care

Long-term follow-up is important for children with complex malformations. After the definitive pull-through procedure, toilet training is delayed, and complete continence is seldom achieved at the usual age of 2 to 3 years. Bowel habit training, bowel management irrigation programs, diet modification, and administration of stool softeners or fiber help children improve bowel function and social continence. Some children never achieve bowel continence and must rely on daily bowel irrigations. Support and reassurance are important during the slow progression to socially acceptable function.

MALABSORPTION SYNDROMES

Chronic diarrhea and malabsorption of nutrients characterize malabsorption syndromes. An important complication of malabsorption syndromes in children is failure to thrive. Most cases are classified according to the location of the supposed anatomic or biochemical defect. The term *celiac disease* is often used to describe a symptom complex with four characteristics: (1) steatorrhea (fatty, foul, frothy, bulky stools), (2) general malnutrition, (3) abdominal distention, and (4) secondary vitamin deficiencies.

Digestive defects are conditions in which the enzymes necessary for digestion are diminished or absent, such as (1) cystic fibrosis, in which pancreatic enzymes are absent; (2) biliary or liver disease, in which bile flow is affected; or (3) lactase deficiency, in which there is congenital or secondary lactose intolerance.

Absorptive defects are conditions in which the intestinal mucosal transport system is impaired. This may occur because of a primary defect (e.g., celiac disease) or secondary to inflammatory disease of the bowel that results in impaired absorption because bowel motility is accelerated (e.g., ulcerative colitis). Obstructive disorders (e.g., Hirschsprung disease) also cause secondary malabsorption from enterocolitis.

Anatomic defects such as extensive resection of the bowel or SBS affect digestion by decreasing the transit time of substances and affect absorption by severely compromising the absorptive surface.

CELIAC DISEASE (GLUTEN-SENSITIVE ENTEROPATHY)

Celiac disease, also known as *gluten-induced enteropathy, gluten-sensitive enteropathy,* and *celiac sprue,* is a permanent intestinal intolerance to dietary gluten, a protein present in wheat, barley, rye, and oats that causes damage to the villi in the small intestine (Paul, Johnson, & Speed, 2013). The incidence is variable and has been reported in 1 in 141 people (Rubio-Tapia, Ludvigsson, Brantner, et al., 2012). The disease is seen more frequently in Europe and the United States; it is rarely reported in Asians or African-Americans (Reilly & Green, 2012). As adults, it is more prevalent in women than in men, but there is equal distribution of cases among children (Reilly & Green, 2012). Although the exact cause is unknown, it is generally accepted that celiac disease is an immunologically mediated small intestine enteropathy. The mucosal lesions contain features that suggest both humoral and cell-mediated immunologic overstimulation.

Pathophysiology

Celiac disease is characterized by villous atrophy in the small bowel in response to the protein gluten. When individuals are unable to digest the gliadin component of gluten, an accumulation of a toxic substance that is damaging to the mucosal cells, damage to the mucosa of the small intestine leads to villous atrophy, hyperplasia of the crypts, and infiltration of the epithelial cells with lymphocytes. Villous atrophy leads to malabsorption caused by the reduced absorptive surface area.

Genetic predisposition is an essential factor in the development of celiac disease. Membrane receptors involved in preferential antigen presentation to CD4+ T-cells play a crucial role in the immune response characteristic of celiac disease. Children with genetic susceptibilities, namely *HLA-DQ2* or *HLA-DQ8,* are more susceptible to being diagnosed with celiac disease (Paul et al., 2013). Symptoms of celiac disease appear when solid foods such as beans and pasta are introduced into the child's diet, typically between 1 and 5 years of age (Box 41.14). Other symptoms include failure to thrive, chronic diarrhea, abdominal distention and pain, muscle wasting, aphthous ulcers, and fatigue. These clinical manifestations are usually insidious and chronic.

Diagnostic Evaluation

Gluten should not be excluded from the diet until the diagnostic evaluation is complete so that proper identification can occur. The first step

---

BOX 41.14   Clinical Manifestations of Celiac Disease

Impaired Fat Absorption
Steatorrhea (excessively large, pale, oily, frothy stools)
Exceedingly foul-smelling stools

Impaired Nutrient Absorption
Malnutrition
Muscle wasting (especially prominent in legs and buttocks)
Anemia
Anorexia
Abdominal distention

Behavioral Changes
Irritability
Uncooperativeness
Apathy

Celiac Crisis
Acute, severe episodes of profuse watery diarrhea and vomiting
May be precipitated by:
- Infections (especially gastrointestinal)
- Prolonged fluid and electrolyte depletion
- Emotional disturbance

is a serologic blood test for tissue transglutaminase and antiendomysial antibodies in children 18 months of age and older (Paul et al., 2013). Positive serologic markers should be followed by an upper GI endoscopy with biopsy. The diagnosis of celiac disease is based on a biopsy of the small intestine demonstrating the characteristic changes of mucosal inflammation, crypt hyperplasia, and villous atrophy (Paul et al.).

Therapeutic Management

Treatment of celiac disease is primarily dietary management. Although the diet is called "gluten free," it is actually *low* in gluten because it is impossible to remove every source of this protein. Because gluten is found primarily in the grains of wheat and rye but also in smaller quantities in barley and oats, these four foods are eliminated. Corn and rice become substitute grain foods.

Children with untreated celiac disease may have lactose intolerance, especially if their mucosal lesions are extensive. Lactose intolerance usually improves as the mucosa heals with gluten withdrawal. Specific nutritional deficiencies such as iron, folic acid, and fat-soluble vitamin deficiencies are treated with appropriate supplements.

Prognosis

Celiac disease is regarded as a chronic disease; its severity varies greatly among children. The most severe symptoms usually occur in early childhood and again in adult life. Most children who comply with dietary management are healthy and remain free from symptoms and complications; however, children should be evaluated annually for nutritional deficiencies, impaired growth, delayed puberty, and reduced bone mineral density (Paul et al., 2013).

Care Management

The main nursing consideration is helping the child adhere to the dietary regimen. Considerable time is involved in explaining the disease process to the child and parents, the specific role of gluten in aggravating the disorder, and the foods that must be restricted. It is difficult to maintain a diet indefinitely when the child has no symptoms and temporary transgressions result in no difficulties. However, most individuals who relax their diet experience a relapse of their disease.

Although the chief sources of gluten are cereal and baked goods, grains are frequently added to processed foods as thickeners or fillers. To compound the difficulty, gluten is added to many foods as hydrolyzed vegetable protein, which is derived from cereal grains. The nurse must advise parents of the necessity of reading all label ingredients carefully to avoid hidden sources of gluten.

Many of children's favorite foods contain gluten, including bread, cake, cookies, crackers, donuts, pies, spaghetti, pizza, prepared soups, some processed ice cream, many types of chocolate candy, milk preparations such as malts, hot dogs, luncheon meats, meat gravy, and some prepared hamburgers. Many of these products can be eliminated from an infant's or young child's diet fairly easily, but monitoring the diet of a school-age child or adolescent is more difficult. Luncheon preparation away from home is particularly difficult because bread, luncheon meats, and instant soups are not allowed. For families on restricted food budgets, the diet adds an additional financial burden because many inexpensive and convenient foods cannot be used.

In addition to restricting gluten, other dietary alterations may be necessary. For example, in some children who have more severe mucosal damage, the digestion of disaccharides is impaired, especially in relation to lactose. Therefore these children often need a temporarily lactose-free diet, which necessitates eliminating all milk products. In general, dietary management includes a diet high in calories and proteins with simple carbohydrates such as fruits and vegetables but low in fats. Because the bowel is inflamed as a result of the pathologic processes in absorption, the child must avoid high-fiber foods such as nuts, raisins, raw vegetables, and raw fruits with skin, until inflammation has subsided.

It is important to stress long-range complications and remind parents of the child's physical status before dietary treatment and the dramatic improvement after treatment. The nurse can be instrumental in allowing the child to express concerns and frustration while focusing on ways in which the child can still feel normal. Encourage the child and parents to find new recipes using suitable ingredients such as Mexican or Chinese dishes that use corn or rice. Consult a registered dietician to provide children and their families with detailed dietary instructions and education.

Several resources are available to help children and parents in all aspects of coping with celiac disease. The Celiac Sprue Association* provides support and guidance to families and supplies educational materials concerning a gluten-free diet, food sources, recipes, and travel information.

LACTOSE INTOLERANCE

Lactose intolerance refers to the inability to digest lactose, a sugar found in milk and dairy products. It involves a deficiency of the enzyme *lactase*, which is needed for the hydrolysis or digestion of lactose in the small intestine; lactose is hydrolyzed into glucose and galactose.

There are at least four types of lactase deficiency that leads to lactose intolerance. *Congenital lactase deficiency* occurs soon after birth after the newborn has consumed lactose-containing milk (human milk or commercial formula). This inborn error of metabolism involves the complete absence or severely reduced presence of lactase, is extremely rare, and requires a lifelong lactose-free or extremely reduced lactose diet. *Developmental lactase deficiency* refers to the relative lactase deficiency observed in preterm infants younger than 34 weeks of gestation and is usually reversible with time. *Primary lactase deficiency* is the most common type of lactose intolerance and is manifested usually by 2 years of age, although the time of onset is variable. Ethnic groups with a high incidence of lactase deficiency include Asians, American Indians, and African-Americans; individuals of northern Europe descent tend to have the lowest incidence (Carter & Attel, 2013). *Secondary lactase deficiency* may occur secondary to damage of the intestinal lumen, which decreases or destroys the enzyme lactase. Cystic fibrosis, sprue, celiac disease, kwashiorkor, and infections such as giardiasis or rotavirus may cause a temporary or permanent lactose intolerance.

The primary symptoms of lactose intolerance include abdominal pain, abdominal bloating, flatulence, diarrhea, and nausea after the ingestion of lactose. The onset of symptoms occurs within 30 minutes to several hours of lactose consumption. Lactose intolerance is often perceived as an allergy or irritable bowel syndrome; however, a dairy allergy is often immediate and accompanied by a skin rash or hives, and IBS is triggered by ingestion of fat, caffeine, sorbitol, and fructose in addition to lactose (Carter & Attel, 2013).

Lactose intolerance may be diagnosed on the basis of the history and improvement with a lactose-reduced diet. The breath hydrogen test is used to positively diagnose the condition. After ingesting 50 grams of a lactose solution, breath samples in lactose-deficient individuals will yield a higher percentage of hydrogen (≥ 20 ppm [parts per million] above baseline). In infants, lactose malabsorption may be diagnosed

---

*PO Box 31700, Omaha, NE 68131-0700, 877-CSA-4CSA or 402-558-0600, www.csaceliacs.org. In Canada: Canadian Celiac Association, 5025 Orbitor Drive, Suite 400, Mississauga, ON L4W 4Y5, 800-363-7296, 905-507-6208, www.celiac.ca.

by evaluating fecal pH and reducing substances after ingesting a lactose load; however, fructose, gastric motility, and water excretion can alter the sensitivity of the test (Carter & Attel, 2013).

Treatment of lactose intolerance is elimination of offending dairy products; however, some advocate decreasing amounts of dairy products rather than total elimination. Most individuals with lactose intolerance can tolerate a single serving of lactose (12 grams) per day, especially when consumed with food (Carter & Attel, 2013). The enzyme, lactase, can be added to foods or beverages to promote the breakdown of lactose. One concern is that dairy avoidance in children and adolescents with lactose intolerance will contribute to reduced bone mineral density (Setty-Shah, Maranda, Candela, et al., 2013). It is recommended that individuals with lactose maldigestion who do not experience lactose intolerance symptoms continue to consume small amounts of dairy products with meals to prevent reduced bone mass density and subsequent osteoporosis. A systematic review of interventions to reduce lactose intolerance symptoms found insufficient evidence on the use of probiotics (Shaukat, Levitt, Taylor, et al., 2010). Because dairy products are a major source of calcium and vitamin D, supplementation of these nutrients is needed to prevent deficiency. Yogurt contains inactive lactase enzyme, which is activated by the temperature and pH of the duodenum; this lactase activity substitutes for the lack of endogenous lactase. Fresh, plain yogurt may be tolerated better than frozen or flavored yogurt; hard cheeses, lactase-treated dairy products, and lactase tablets taken with dairy products are also viable options.

Care Management

Nursing care is similar to the interventions discussed for CMA in this chapter and includes explaining the dietary restrictions to the family; identifying alternate sources of calcium such as yogurt and calcium supplementation; explaining the importance of supplementation; and discussing sources of lactose, especially hidden sources such as its use as a bulk agent in certain medications, and ways of controlling the symptoms. Parents are advised to check with the pharmacist regarding this possibility when obtaining medication.

SHORT-BOWEL SYNDROME

SBS is a malabsorptive disorder that occurs as a result of decreased mucosal surface area, usually because of extensive resection of the small intestine. Malabsorption may be exacerbated by other factors such as bacterial overgrowth and dysmotility. The most common causes of SBS in children are necrotizing enterocolitis, volvulus, and intestinal malformations (Pironi, 2016). Less frequent causes include trauma to the GI tract and total colonic aganglionosis with extension into the small bowel (Soden, 2010).

The definition of SBS includes two important findings: (1) decreased intestinal surface area that is less than 25% of expected length for gestational age; and (2) a need for PN (Pironi, 2016). The prognosis for infants with SBS has improved dramatically with survival rates between 73% and 89%; however, children on PN have a lower survival rate at approximately 60% (Soden, 2010).

Therapeutic Management

The goals of therapy for infants and children with SBS include: (1) preserve as much length of bowel as possible during surgery; (2) maintain optimum nutritional status, growth, and development while intestinal adaptation occurs; (3) stimulate intestinal adaptation with enteral feeding; and (4) minimize complications related to the disease process and therapy (Uko, Radhakrishnan, & Alkhouri, 2012).

Nutritional support is the long-term focus of care for children with SBS (Uko et al., 2012). The initial phase of therapy includes PN as the primary source of nutrition. The second phase is the introduction of enteral feeding, which usually begins as soon as possible after surgery. Elemental formulas containing glucose, sucrose and glucose polymers, hydrolyzed proteins, and medium-chain triglycerides facilitate absorption. Usually these formulas are given by continuous infusion through an NG or gastrostomy tube. As the enteral feedings are advanced, the PN solution is decreased in terms of calories, amount of fluid, and total hours of infusion per day. If enteral feedings are tolerated, oral feedings should be attempted to minimize oral aversion and preserve oral skills (Goulet, Olieman, Ksiazyk, et al., 2013).

The final phase of nutritional support occurs when growth and development are sustained. When PN is discontinued, there is a risk for nutritional deficiency secondary to malabsorption of fat-soluble vitamins (A, D, E, and K) and trace minerals (iron, selenium, and zinc). Monitor serum vitamin and mineral levels closely, and provide enteral supplementation of vitamins and minerals if needed. Pharmacologic agents have been used to reduce secretory losses. H_2 blockers, PPIs, and octreotide inhibit gastric or pancreatic secretion. Cholestyramine is often prescribed to improve diarrhea that is associated with bile salt malabsorption. Growth factors have also been used to hasten adaptation and enhance mucosal growth, but these uses are still experimental and results are controversial (Uko et al., 2012).

Numerous complications are associated with SBS and long-term PN. Infectious, metabolic, and technical complications can occur. Sepsis can occur after improper care of the catheter. The GI tract can also be a source of microbial seeding of the catheter. Bowel atrophy may foster increased intestinal permeability of bacteria. A lack of adequate sites for central lines may become a significant problem for the child in need of long-term PN. Hepatic dysfunction, cholestasis, and chronic renal failure may also occur (Pironi, 2016).

Bacterial overgrowth is likely to occur when the ileocecal valve is absent or when stasis exists as a result of a partial obstruction or a dilated segment of bowel with poor motility. Alternating cycles of broad-spectrum antibiotics are used to reduce bacterial overgrowth. This treatment may also decrease the risk for bacterial translocation and subsequent central venous catheter infections. Other complications of bacterial overgrowth and malabsorption include metabolic acidosis and gastric hypersecretion.

Many surgical interventions, including intestinal valves, tapering enteroplasty or stricturoplasty, intestinal lengthening, and interposed segments, have been used to slow intestinal transit, reduce bacterial overgrowth, or increase mucosal surface area. Intestinal transplantation has been performed successfully in children. Only children with a permanent dependence on PN or severe complications of long-term PN are candidates for transplantation.

Prognosis

The prognosis for infants with SBS has improved with advances in PN and with the understanding of the importance of intraluminal nutrition. Improved supportive care for the management of therapy-related problems and the development of more specific immunosuppressive medications for transplantation have all contributed to improved management. The prognosis depends in part on the length of the residual small intestine. An intact ileocecal valve also improves the prognosis. Infants and children with SBS die from PN-related problems such as fulminant sepsis or severe PN cholestasis.

Interprofessional Care Management

The most important components of care are administering and monitoring of nutritional therapy. During PN therapy, care must be taken to minimize the risk for complications related to the central venous access device (i.e., catheter infections, occlusions, dislodgment, or accidental removal). Care of enteral feeding tubes and monitoring of enteral feeding tolerance are also important nursing responsibilities.

When long-term PN is required, preparing the family for home care is a major nursing responsibility. Many infants and children can be cared for at home successfully with enteral nutrition and PN when the family is prepared and provided with adequate support services. Most families benefit from home nursing care to assist with and supervise therapy. Home infusion companies provide portable infusion equipment, which enables the child and family to maintain a more normal lifestyle. Follow-up by a multidisciplinary nutritional support team is essential.

Many infants with SBS have an intestinal ostomy performed at the time of the initial bowel resection. Routine ostomy care is another important nursing responsibility. Because infants and children with SBS have chronic diarrhea, perineal skin irritation is often a problem after ostomy closure. Frequent diaper changes, gentle perineal cleansing, and protective skin barriers help prevent skin breakdown.

When hospitalization is prolonged, the child's developmental and emotional needs must be met. This often requires special planning to promote normal family adjustment and adaptation of the hospital routines. Care of hospitalized children is discussed in Chapter 38.

REFERENCES

Agarwal, J. (2013). Chronic constipation. *Indian Journal of Pediatrics, 80*(12), 1021–1025.

Alleman, A. M. (2014). Osmotic demyelination syndrome: Central pontine myelinolysis and extrapontine myelinolysis. *Seminars in Ultrasound, CT, and MRI, 35*(2), 153–159.

Aloi, M., D'Arcangelo, G., Pofi, F., et al. (2013). Presenting features and disease course of pediatric ulcerative colitis. *Journal of Crohn's and Colitis, 7*(11), e509–e515.

Alqurashi, W., Stiell, I., Chan, K., et al. (2015). Epidemiology and clinical predictors of biphasic reactions in children with anaphylaxis. *Annals of Allergy, Asthma & Immunology, 115*(3), 217–223.

American Academy of Pediatrics (AAP). (2008). Prevention of rickets and vitamin D deficiency in infants, children, and adolescents. *Pediatrics, 122*(5), 1142–1148.

American Academy of Pediatrics, Committee on Nutrition, Kleinman, R. E., & Greer, F. R. (Eds.), 2014). *Pediatric nutrition handbook* (7th ed.). Elk Grove Village, IL: American Academy of Pediatrics.

Amthor, R. E., Cole, S. M., & Manary, M. J. (2009). The use of home-based therapy with ready-to-use therapeutic food to treat malnutrition in a rural area during a food crisis. *Journal of the American Dietetic Association, 109*(3), 464–467.

Angulo, P., & Lindor, K. D. (2010). Primary biliary cirrhosis. In M. Feldman, L. S. Friedman & L. J. Brandt (Eds.), *Sleisenger and Fordtran's gastrointestinal and liver disease* (9th ed.). Philadelphia, PA: Saunders.

Ashworth, A. (2016). Nutrition, food security, and health. In R. M. Kliegman, B. F. Stanton, J. W. St. Geme, et al. (Eds.), *Nelson textbook of pediatrics* (20th ed.). Philadelphia, PA: Saunders/Elsevier.

Baker, R. D., Greer, F. R., & American Academy of Pediatrics Committee on Nutrition. (2010). Clinical report—Diagnosis and prevention of iron deficiency and iron-deficiency anemia in infants and young children (0–3 years of age). *Pediatrics, 126*(5), 1040–1050.

Balachandran, B., Singhi, S., & Lal, S. (2013). Emergency management of acute abdomen in children. *Indian Journal of Pediatrics, 80*(3), 226–234.

Bales, C., & Liacouras, C. A. (2016). Intestinal atresia, stenosis, and malrotation. In R. M. Kliegman, B. F. Stanton, J. W. St Geme, et al. (Eds.), *Nelson textbook of pediatrics* (20th ed.). Philadelphia, PA: Saunders/Elsevier.

Bandsma, R. H., Spoelstra, M. N., Mari, A., et al. (2011). Impaired glucose absorption in children with severe malnutrition. *Journal of Pediatrics, 158*(2), 282–287.

Barakat, M., El-Kady, Z., Mostafa, M., et al. (2011). Antibiotic-associated bloody diarrhea in infants: Clinical, endoscopic, and histopathologic profiles. *Journal of Pediatric Gastroenterology and Nutrition, 52*(1), 60–64.

Baumann, U., & Ure, B. (2012). Biliary atresia. *Clinics and Research in Hepatology and Gastroenterology, 36*(3), 257–259.

Bello, S., Meremikwu, M. M., Ejemot-Nwadiaro, R. I., et al. (2014). Routine vitamin A supplementation for the prevention of blindness due to measles infection in children. *Cochrane Database of Systematic Reviews, 2014*(8), CD007719.

Bhutta, Z. A. (2016). Acute gastroenteritis in children. In R. M. Kliegman, B. F. Stanton, J. W. St Geme, et al. (Eds.), *Nelson textbook of pediatrics* (20th ed.). Philadelphia, PA: Saunders/Elsevier.

Blanchard, S. S., & Czinn, S. J. (2016). Peptic ulcer disease in children. In R. M. Kliegman, B. F. Stanton, J. W. St Geme, et al. (Eds.), *Nelson textbook of pediatrics* (20th ed.). Philadelphia, PA: Saunders/Elsevier.

Boyce, J. A., Assa'ad, A., Burks, A. W., et al. (2011). Guideline for the diagnosis and management of food allergy in the United States: Summary of the NIAID-sponsored expert panel report. *Nutrition Research, 31*(1), 61–75.

Bradley, G. M., & Oliva-Hemker, M. (2012). Infliximab for the treatment of pediatric ulcerative colitis. *Expert Review of Gastroenterology & Hepatology, 6*(6), 659–665.

Burks, A. W., Jones, S. M., Boyce, J. A., et al. (2011). NAID-sponsored 2010 guidelines for managing food allergy: Applications in the pediatric population. *Pediatrics, 128*(5), 955–965.

Butte, N. F., Fox, M. K., Briefel, R. R., et al. (2010). Nutrient intakes of US infants, toddlers, and preschoolers meet or exceed dietary reference intakes. *Journal of the American Dietetic Association, 110*(12 suppl), S27–S37.

Caracappa, D., Gullá, N., Lombardo, F., et al. (2014). Incidental finding of carcinoid tumor on Meckel's diverticulum: Case report and literature review, should prophylactic resection be recommended? *World Journal of Surgical Oncology, 12*, 144.

Carter, S. L., & Attel, S. (2013). The diagnosis and management of patients with lactose-intolerance. *Journal for Nurse Practitioners, 38*(7), 23–28.

Chiou, F. K., How, C. H., & Ong, C. (2013). Recurrent abdominal pain in childhood. *Singapore Medical Journal, 54*(4), 195–200.

Churgay, C. A., & Aftab, Z. (2012a). Gastroenteritis in children: Part I Diagnosis. *American Family Physician, 85*(11), 1059–1062.

Churgay, C. A., & Aftab, Z. (2012b). Gastroenteritis in children: Part II Prevention and management. *American Family Physician, 85*(11), 1066–1070.

Clemente, M. G., & Schwarz, K. (2011). Hepatitis: general principles. *Pediatrics in Review, 32*(8), 333–340.

Czeizel, A. E., Dudás, I., Paput, L., et al. (2011). Prevention of neural-tube defects with periconceptional folic acid, methylfolate, or multivitamins? *Annals of Nutrition and Metabolism, 58*(4), 263–271.

D'Auria, J. P., & Kelly, M. (2013). Inflammatory bowel disease: Top resources for children, adolescents, and their families. *Journal of Pediatric Health Care, 27*(2), e25–e28.

Dekate, P., Jayashree, M., & Singhi, S. C. (2013). Management of acute diarrhea in emergency room. *Indian Journal of Pediatrics, 80*(3), 235–246.

Dupont, C. (2014). Diagnosis of cow's milk allergy in children: Determining the gold standard? *Expert Review of Clinical Immunology, 10*(2), 257–267.

Ehlayel, M., Bener, A., Hazeima, K., et al. (2011). Camel milk is a safer choice than goat milk for feeding children with cow milk allergy. *ISRN Allergy, 391641*, 1–5.

El-Radhi, A. S. (2015). Management of abdominal pain in children. *British Journal of Nursing, 24*(1), 44–47.

Ellis, M., & Cole, A. (2011). Crohn's disease in children and adolescents. *Gastrointestinal Nursing, 9*(1), 41–46.

El-Tawil, A. M. (2012). Trends on gastrointestinal bleeding and mortality: Where are we standing? *World Journal of Gastroenterology, 18*(11), 1154–1158.

Ertem, D. (2012). Clinical practice: *Helicobacter pylori* infection in childhood. *European Journal of Pediatrics, 171*(9), 1–8.

Esona, M. D., & Gautam, R. (2015). Rotavirus. *Clinics in Laboratory Medicine, 35*(2), 363–391.

Esposito, D. H., Holman, R. C., Haberling, D. L., et al. (2011). Baseline estimates of diarrhea-associated mortality among United States children before rotavirus vaccine introduction. *Pediatric Infectious Disease Journal, 30*(11), 942–947.

Fiorino, K., & Liacouras, C. A. (2016). Congenital aganglionic megacolon (Hirschsprung disease). In R. M. Kliegman, B. F. Stanton, J. W. St Geme, et al. (Eds.), *Nelson textbook of pediatrics* (20th ed.). Philadelphia, PA: Saunders/Elsevier.

Fleischer, D. M., Spergel, J. M., Assa'ad, A. H., & Pongracic, J. A. (2013). Primary prevention of allergic disease through nutritional interventions. *Journal of Allergy and Clinical Immunology: In Practice, 1*(1), 29–36.

Friedman, A. (2010). Fluid and electrolyte therapy: A primer. *Pediatric Nephrology, 25*(5), 843–846.

Fung, E. B., Xu, Y., Trachtenberg, F., et al. (2012). Inadequate dietary intake in patients with thalassemia. *Journal of the Academy of Nutrition and Dietetics, 112*(7), 980–990.

Goldani, H. A., Nunes, D. L., & Ferreira, C. T. (2012). Managing gastroesophageal reflux disease in children: The role of endoscopy. *World Journal of Gastrointestinal Endoscopy, 4*(8), 339–346.

Goulet, O., Olieman, J., Ksiazyk, J., et al. (2013). Neonatal short bowel syndrome as a model of intestinal failure: Physiological background for enteral feeding. *Clinical Nutrition, 32*(2), 162–171.

Gourlay, D. M. (2013). Colorectal considerations in pediatric patients. *Surgical Clinics of North America, 93*(2), 251–272.

Greenbaum, L. A. (2016). Electrolyte and acid-base disorders. In R. M. Kliegman, B. F. Stanton, J. W. St Geme, et al. (Eds.), *Nelson textbook of pediatrics* (20th ed.). Philadelphia, PA: Saunders/Elsevier.

Grossman, A. B., & Baldassano, R. N. (2016). Chronic ulcerative colitis. In R. M. Kliegman, B. F. Stanton, J. W. St Geme, et al. (Eds.), *Nelson textbook of pediatrics* (20th ed.). Philadelphia, PA: Saunders/Elsevier.

Grover, Z., & Ee, L. C. (2009). Protein energy malnutrition. *Pediatric Clinics of North America, 56*(5), 1055–1068.

Guidry, C., & McGahren, E. D. (2012). Pediatric chest I: Developmental and physiologic conditions for the surgeon. *Surgical Clinics of North America, 92*(3), 615–643.

Hassan, H. H., & Balistreri, W. F. (2016). Cholestasis. In R. M. Kliegman, B. F. Stanton, J. W. St Geme, et al. (Eds.), *Nelson textbook of pediatrics* (20th ed.). Philadelphia, PA: Saunders/Elsevier.

Hayman, R. M., & Dalziel, S. R. (2012). Acute vitamin A toxicity: A report of three paediatric cases. *Journal of Paediatrics and Child Health, 48*(3), e98–e100.

Herman, R. S., & Teitelbaum, D. H. (2012). Anorectal malformations. *Clinics in Perinatology, 39*(2), 403–422.

Hunter, A. K., & Liacouras, C. A. (2016). Pyloric stenosis and other congenital anomalies of the stomach. In R. M. Kliegman, B. F. Stanton, J. W. St Geme, et al. (Eds.), *Nelson textbook of pediatrics* (20th ed.). Philadelphia, PA: Saunders/Elsevier.

Imdad, A., Sadiq, K., & Bhutta, Z. A. (2011). Evidence-based prevention of childhood malnutrition. *Current Opinion in Clinical Nutrition and Metabolic Care, 14*(3), 276–285.

Jensen, M. K., & Balistreri, W. F. (2016). Viral hepatitis. In R. M. Kliegman, B. F. Stanton, J. W. St Geme, et al. (Eds.), *Nelson textbook of pediatrics* (20th ed.). Philadelphia, PA: Saunders/Elsevier.

Jindal, M. K., & Khan, S. Y. (2013). How to feed cleft patient? *International Journal of Clinical Pediatric Dentistry, 6*(2), 100–103.

Jones, K. D., & Berkley, J. A. (2014). Severe acute malnutrition and infection. *Paediatrics and International Child Health, 34*(1 suppl), S1–S29.

Kamath, B. M., & Olthoff, K. M. (2010). Liver transplantation in children: Update 2010. *Pediatric Clinics of North America, 57*(2), 401–414.

Kattan, J. D., Cocco, R. R., & Järvinen, K. M. (2011). Milk and soy allergy. *Pediatric Clinics of North America, 58*(2), 407–426.

Keet, C. (2011). Recognition and management of food-induced anaphylaxis. *Pediatric Clinics of North America, 58*(2), 377–388.

Kennedy, M., & Liacouras, C. A. (2016). Intussusception. In R. M. Kliegman, B. F. Stanton, J. W. St Geme, et al. (Eds.), *Nelson textbook of pediatrics* (20th ed.). Philadelphia, PA: Saunders/Elsevier.

Khan, S., & Orenstein, S. R. (2016a). Gastroesophageal reflux disease. In R. M. Kliegman, B. F. Stanton, J. W. St Geme, et al. (Eds.), *Nelson textbook of pediatrics* (20th ed.). Philadelphia, PA: Saunders/Elsevier.

Khan, S., & Orenstein, S. R. (2016b). Esophageal atresia and tracheoesophageal fistula. In R. M. Kliegman, B. F. Stanton, J. W. St Geme, et al. (Eds.), *Nelson textbook of pediatrics* (20th ed.). Philadelphia, PA: Saunders/Elsevier.

Kim, J. S., Nowak-Wegrzyn, A., Sichere, S. H., et al. (2011). Dietary baked milk accelerates the resolution of cow's milk allergy in children. *Journal of Allergy and Clinical Immunology, 128*(1), 125–131.

Kliegman, R. M. (2016). Refeeding syndrome. In R. M. Kliegman, B. F. Stanton, J. W. St. Geme, et al. (Eds.), *Nelson textbook of pediatrics* (20th ed.). Philadelphia, PA: Saunders/Elsevier.

Kotecha, M., Bellah, R., Pena, A. H., et al. (2012). Multimodality imaging manifestations of the Meckel diverticulum in children. *Pediatric Radiology, 41*, 95–103.

Kranz, S., Brauchla, M., Slavin, J. L., et al. (2012). What do we know about dietary fiber intake in children and health? The effects of fiber intake on constipation, obesity, and diabetes in children. *Advances in Nutrition, 3*(1), 47–53.

Kunisaki, S. M., & Foker, J. E. (2012). Surgical advances in the fetus and neonate: Esophageal atresia. *Clinics in Perinatology, 39*(2), 349–361.

Latella, G. (2012). Colorectal cancer in inflammatory bowel disease: What is the real magnitude of the risk? *World Journal of Gastroenterology, 18*(29), 3839–3848.

Lawrence, R. M. (2013). Circumstances when breastfeeding is contraindicated. *Pediatric Clinics of North America, 60*(1), 295–318.

Liang, C. M., Ji, D. M., Yuan, X., et al. (2014). RET and PHOX2B genetic polymorphisms and Hirschsprung's disease susceptibility: A meta-analysis. *PLoS ONE, 9*(3), e90091.

Liu, L., Johnson, H. L., Cousens, S., et al. (2012). Global, regional, and national causes of child mortality: An updated systematic analysis for 2010 with time trends since 2000. *Lancet, 379*(9832), 2151–2161.

Matheny, S. C., & Kingery, J. E. (2012). Hepatitis A. *American Family Physician, 86*(11), 1027–1034.

McBride, D. L. (2011). New food allergy guidelines. *Journal of Pediatric Nursing, 26*(3), 262–263.

Nowak-Wegrzyn, A., Sampson, H. A., & Sicherer, S. H. (2016). Food allergy and adverse reactions to foods. In R. M. Kliegman, B. F. Stanton, J. W. St. Geme, et al. (Eds.), *Nelson textbook of pediatrics* (20th ed.). Philadelphia, PA: Saunders/Elsevier.

Paganelli, M., Stephenne, X., & Sokal, E. M. (2012). Chronic hepatitis B in children and adolescents. *Journal of Hepatology, 57*(4), 885–896.

Park, S. E., Kim, S., Ouma, C., et al. (2012). Community management of acute malnutrition in the developing world. *Pediatric Gastroenterology, Hepatology & Nutrition, 15*(4), 210–219.

Paul, S. P., Johnson, J., & Speed, H. R. (2013). Clinical update: Coeliac disease in children. *Community Practitioner, 86*(1), 35–37.

Pepper, V. K., Stanfill, A. B., & Pearl, R. H. (2012). Diagnosis and management of pediatric appendicitis, intussusceptions, and Meckel's diverticulum. *Surgical Clinics of North America, 92*(3), 505–526.

Petersen, B. (2014). Diagnosis and management of functional constipation: A common pediatric problem. *Journal for Nurse Practitioners, 39*(8), 1–6.

Pironi, L. (2016). Definitions of intestinal failure and the short bowel syndrome. *Best Practice & Research: Clinical Gastroenterology, 30*(2), 173–185.

Rajindrajith, S., & Devanarayana, N. M. (2012). Subtypes and symptomatology of irritable bowel syndrome in children and adolescents: A school-based survey using Rome III criteria. *Journal of Neurogastroenterology and Motility, 18*(3), 298–304.

Reilly, N. R., & Green, P. H. (2012). Epidemiology and clinical presentations of celiac disease. *Seminars in Immunopathology, 34*(4), 473–478.

Robbins, J. M., Damiano, P., Druschel, C. M., et al. (2010). Prenatal diagnosis of orofacial clefts: Association with maternal satisfaction, team care, and treatment outcomes. *Cleft Palate–Craniofacial Journal, 47*(5), 476–481.

Rogers, J. (2012). Assessment, prevention and treatment of constipation in children. *Nursing Standard, 26*(29), 46–52.

Roumeliotis, N., Dix, D., & Lipson, A. (2012). Vitamin B(12) deficiency in infants secondary to maternal causes. *Canadian Medical Association Journal, 184*(14), 1593–1598.

Rubio-Tapia, A., Ludvigsson, J. F., Brantner, T. L., et al. (2012). The prevalence of celiac disease in the United States. *American Journal of Gastroenterology, 107*(10), 1538–1544.

Scallan, E., Mahon, B. E., Hoekstra, R. M., et al. (2013). Estimates of illnesses, hospitalizations and deaths caused by major bacterial enteric pathogens in young children in the United States. *Pediatric Infectious Disease Journal, 32*(3), 217–221.

Setty-Shah, N., Maranda, L., Candela, N., et al. (2013). Lactose intolerance: Lack of evidence for short stature or vitamin D deficiency in prepubertal children. *PLoS ONE, 8*(10), e78653.

Shaukat, A., Levitt, M. D., Taylor, B. C., et al. (2010). Systematic review: Effective management strategies for lactose intolerance. *Annals of Internal Medicine, 152*(12), 797–803.

Simons, F. E., Ardusso, L. R., Biló, M. B., et al. (2012). 2012 Update: World Allergy Organization guidelines for the assessment and management of anaphylaxis. *Current Opinion in Allergy and Clinical Immunology, 12*(4), 389–399.

Singhal, V., & Khaitan, L. (2014). Gastroesophageal reflux disease: Diagnosis and patient selection. *Indian Journal of Surgery, 76*(6), 453–560.

Singhi, S. C., Shah, R., Bansal, A., et al. (2013). Management of a child with vomiting. *Indian Journal of Pediatrics, 80*(4), 318–325.

Soden, J. S. (2010). Clinical assessment of the child with intestinal failure. *Seminars in Pediatric Surgery, 19*(1), 10–19.

Solomons, N. W., & Vossenaar, M. (2013). Nutrient density in complementary feedings of infants and toddlers. *European Journal of Clinical Nutrition, 67*(5), 501–506.

Sullivan, P. (2010). Peptic ulcer disease in children. *Paediatrics and Child Health, 20*(10), 462–464.

Szigethy, E., McLafferty, I., & Goyal, A. (2011). Inflammatory bowel disease. *Pediatric Clinics of North America, 58*(4), 903–920.

Tarbell, S. E., & Li, B. U. (2015). Anxiety measures predict health-related quality of life in children and adolescents with cyclic vomiting syndrome. *Journal of Pediatrics, 167*(3), 633–638.

Temple, S. J., Shawyer, A., & Langer, J. C. (2012). Is daily dilatation by parents necessary after surgery for Hirschsprung disease and anorectal malformations? *Journal of Pediatric Surgery, 47*(1), 209–212.

Tierney, E. P., Sage, R. J., & Shwayder, T. (2010). Kwashiorkor from a severe dietary restriction in an 8-month infant in suburban Detroit, Michigan: Case report and review of the literature. *International Journal of Dermatology, 49*(5), 500–506.

Tinanoff, N. (2016). Cleft lip and palate. In R. M. Kliegman, B. F. Stanton, J. W. St Geme, et al. (Eds.), *Nelson textbook of pediatrics* (20th ed.). Philadelphia, PA: Saunders/Elsevier.

Titova, O. E., Ayvazova, E. A., Bichkaeva, F. A., et al. (2012). The influence of active and passive smoking during pregnancy on umbilical cord blood levels of vitamins A and E and neonatal anthropometric indices. *British Journal of Nutrition, 108*(8), 1241–1345.

Trehan, I., & Manary, M. J. (2015). Management of severe acute malnutrition in low-income and middle-income countries. *Archives of Disease in Childhood, 100*(3), 283–287.

Turer, C. B., Lin, H., & Flores, G. (2013). Prevalence of vitamin D deficiency among overweight and obese US children. *Pediatrics, 131*(1), e152–e161.

Uko, V., Radhakrishnan, K., & Alkhouri, N. (2012). Short bowel syndrome in children: Current and potential therapies. *Pediatric Drugs, 14*(3), 179–188.

van der Pol, R. J., Smits, M. J., van Wijk, M. P., et al. (2011). Efficacy of proton pump inhibitors in children with gastroesophageal reflux disease: A systematic review. *Pediatrics, 127*(5), 925–935.

Wacker, M., & Holick, M. F. (2013). Vitamin D—Effects on skeletal and extraskeletal health and the need for supplementation. *Nutrients, 5*(1), 11–148.

Wadlund, D. L. (2012). Meeting the challenge of IBS. *Journal for Nurse Practitioners, 37*(5), 22–30.

Walker, C. L., Rudan, I., Liu, L., et al. (2013). Global burden of childhood pneumonia and diarrhea. *Lancet, 381*(9875), 1405–1416.

Wheeler, R. A. (2011). Appendicitis in children and young people. *Clinical Risk, 17*, 126–129.

Wijkmans, R. A., & Talsma, K. (2016). Modern scurvy. *Journal of Surgical Case Reports, 2016*, 1.

Wilshire, C. L., & Watson, T. J. (2013). Surgical management of gastroesophageal reflux disease. *Gastroenterology Clinics of North America, 42*(1), 119–131.

Wray, C. J., Kao, L. S., Millas, S. G., et al. (2013). Acute appendicitis: Controversies in diagnosis and management. *Current Problems in Surgery, 50*(2), 54–86.

Xiao, L., Xing, C., Yang, Z., et al. (2015). Vitamin D supplementation for the prevention of childhood acute respiratory infections: A systematic review of randomised controlled trials. *British Journal of Nutrition, 114*(7), 1026–1034.

Yang, C. F., Duro, D., Zurakowski, D., et al. (2011). High prevalence of multiple micronutrient deficiencies in children with intestinal failure: A longitudinal study. *Journal of Pediatrics, 159*(1), 39–44.

42

The Child With Cardiovascular Dysfunction

Marilyn J. Hockenberry

ⓔ http://evolve.elsevier.com/Perry/maternal

CARDIOVASCULAR DYSFUNCTION

Cardiovascular disorders in children are divided into two major groups, congenital heart disease and acquired heart disorders. *Congenital heart disease (CHD)* includes primarily anatomic abnormalities present at birth that result in abnormal cardiac function. The clinical consequences of congenital heart defects fall into two broad categories, heart failure (HF) and hypoxemia. *Acquired cardiac disorders* are disease processes or abnormalities that occur after birth and can be seen in the normal heart or in the presence of congenital heart defects. They result from various factors, including infection, autoimmune responses, environmental factors, and familial tendencies. The pathophysiology review found in Fig. 42.1 describes the flow of blood through the heart.

HISTORY AND PHYSICAL EXAMINATION

Taking an accurate health history is an important first step in assessing an infant or child for possible heart disease. Parents may have specific concerns, such as an infant with poor feeding or fast breathing, or a 7-year-old who can no longer keep up with friends on the soccer field. Others may not realize that their child has a medical problem because their baby has always been pale and fussy.

Asking details about the mother's health history, pregnancy, and birth history is important in assessing infants. Mothers with chronic health conditions, such as diabetes or lupus, are more likely to have infants with heart disease. Some medications, such as phenytoin (Dilantin), are teratogenic to fetuses. Maternal alcohol use or illicit drug use increases the risk for congenital heart defects. Exposures to infections, such as rubella, early in pregnancy may result in congenital anomalies. Infants with low birth weight resulting from intrauterine growth restriction are more likely to have congenital anomalies. High–birth weight infants have an increased incidence of heart disease.

A detailed family history is also important. There is an increased incidence of congenital cardiac defects if either parent or a sibling has a heart defect. Some diseases, such as Marfan syndrome, and some cardiomyopathies are hereditary. A family history of frequent fetal loss, sudden infant death, and sudden death in adults may indicate heart disease. Congenital heart defects are seen in many syndromes such as Down and Turner syndromes.

The physical assessment of suspected cardiac disease begins with observation of general appearance and then proceeds with more specific observations. The following lists are supplementary to the general assessment techniques described for physical examination of the chest and heart in Chapter 29.

Inspection

Nutritional state: Failure to thrive or poor weight gain is associated with heart disease.

Color: Cyanosis is a common feature of CHD, and pallor is associated with poor perfusion.

Chest deformities: An enlarged heart sometimes distorts the chest configuration.

Unusual pulsations: Visible pulsations of the neck veins are seen in some patients.

Respiratory excursion: This refers to the ease or difficulty of respiration (e.g., tachypnea, dyspnea, expiratory grunt).

Clubbing of fingers: This is associated with cyanosis.

Palpation and Percussion

Chest: These maneuvers help discern heart size and other characteristics (e.g., thrills) associated with heart disease.

Abdomen: Hepatomegaly or splenomegaly may be evident.

Peripheral pulses: Rate, regularity, and amplitude (strength) may reveal discrepancies.

Auscultation

Heart rate and rhythm: Listen for fast heart rates (tachycardia), slow heart rates (bradycardia), and irregular rhythms.

Character of heart sounds: Listen for distinct or muffled sounds, murmurs, and additional heart sounds.

DIAGNOSTIC EVALUATION

A variety of invasive and noninvasive tests may be used in the diagnosis of heart disease (Table 42.1). Some of the more common diagnostic tools that require nursing assessment and intervention are described in the following sections.

Electrocardiogram

Electrocardiography (ECG or EKG) measures the electrical activity of the heart, provides a graphic display, and supplies information on heart rate and rhythm, abnormal rhythms or conduction, ischemic changes, and other information. A standard ECG uses 12 leads to get different views of the heart. An ECG takes about 15 minutes to perform; infants and young children may be fussy with lead placement.

Bedside cardiac monitoring with a single lead of the ECG is commonly used in pediatrics, especially in the care of children with heart disease. An alarm can be set with parameters for individual patient requirements and will sound if the heart rate is above or below the set parameters.

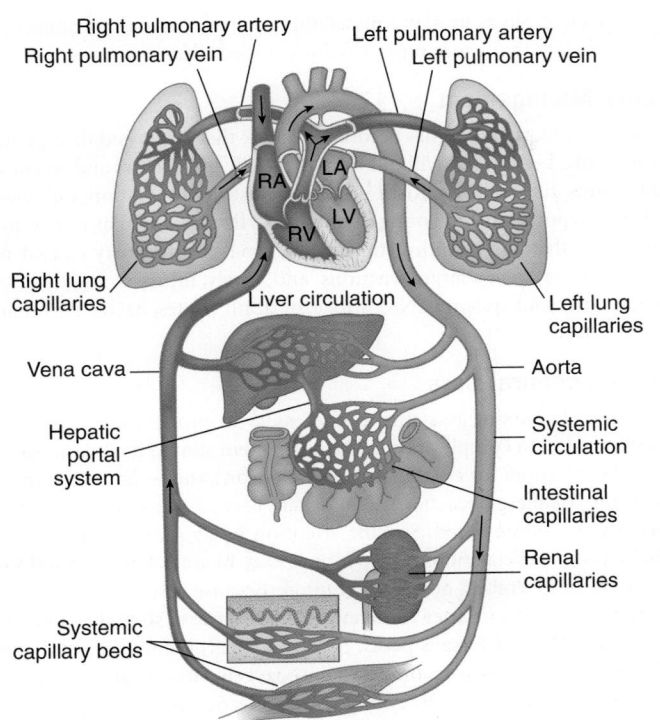

FIG 42.1 Diagram showing serially connected pulmonary and systemic circulatory systems and how to trace the flow of blood. Right heart chambers propel unoxygenated blood through the systemic circulation. *LA,* Left atrium; *LV,* left ventricle; *RA,* right atrium; *RV,* right ventricle. (From McCance, K.L., & Heuther, S.E. [2010]. *Pathophysiology: The biological basis for disease in adults and children* [6th ed.]. St. Louis, MO: Mosby.)

Gelfoam electrodes are commonly used and placed on the right side of the chest (above the level of the heart) and on the left side of the chest, and a ground electrode is placed on the abdomen. Bedside monitors are an adjunct to patient care and should never be substituted for direct assessment and auscultation of heart sounds. The nurse should assess the patient, not the monitor.

> **! NURSING ALERT**
>
> Electrodes for cardiac monitoring are often color coded: white for right, green (or red) for ground, and black for left. Always check to ensure that these colors are placed correctly.

Echocardiography

Echocardiography involves the use of ultra-high–frequency sound waves to produce an image of the heart's structure. A transducer placed directly on the chest wall delivers repetitive pulses of ultrasound and processes the returned signals (echoes). It is the most frequently used test for describing cardiac anatomy and detecting cardiac dysfunction in children. In many cases, a prenatal diagnosis of CHD can be made by fetal echocardiography.

Although the test is noninvasive, painless, and associated with no known side effects, it can be stressful for children. A full echocardiogram can take 1 hour, and the child must lie quietly in the standard echocardiographic positions. Therefore, infants and young children may need a mild sedative; older children benefit from preparation for the test. The distraction of a video or movie is often helpful.

Cardiac Magnetic Resonance Imaging

Cardiac magnetic resonance imaging (MRI) is often used to define unresolved anatomic pathways when a child may have poor acoustic windows or a complex structure that is difficult to visualize by ultrasound

TABLE 42.1	Procedures for Cardiac Diagnosis
Procedure	**Description**
Chest radiography (x-ray)	Provides information on heart size and pulmonary blood flow patterns
ECG	Graphic measure of electrical activity of heart
Holter monitor	24-hour continuous ECG recording used to assess dysrhythmias
Echocardiography	Use of high-frequency sound waves obtained by a transducer to produce an image of cardiac structures
Transthoracic	Done with transducer on chest
M-mode	One-dimensional graphic view used to estimate ventricular size and function
Two-dimensional	Real-time, cross-sectional views of heart used to identify cardiac structures and cardiac anatomy
Doppler	Identifies blood flow patterns and pressure gradients across structures
Fetal	Imaging fetal heart in utero
TEE	Transducer placed in esophagus behind heart to obtain images of posterior heart structures or in patients with poor images from chest approach
Cardiac catheterization	Imaging study using radiopaque catheters placed in a peripheral blood vessel and advanced into heart to measure pressures and oxygen levels in heart chambers and visualize heart structures and blood flow patterns
Hemodynamics	Measures pressures and oxygen saturations in heart chambers
Angiography	Use of contrast material to illuminate heart structures and blood flow patterns
Biopsy	Use of special catheter to remove tiny samples of heart muscle for microscopic evaluation; used in assessing infection, inflammation, or muscle dysfunction disorders; also used to evaluate for rejection after heart transplant
EPS	Special catheters with electrodes employed to record electrical activity from within heart; used to diagnose rhythm disturbances
Exercise stress test	Monitoring of heart rate, BP, ECG, and oxygen consumption at rest and during progressive exercise on a treadmill or bicycle
Cardiac MRI	Noninvasive imaging technique; used in evaluation of vascular anatomy outside of heart (e.g., COA, vascular rings), estimates of ventricular mass and volume; uses for MRI are expanding

BP, Blood pressure; *COA,* coarctation of the aorta; *ECG,* electrocardiography; *EPS,* electrophysiology; *MRI,* magnetic resonance imaging; *TEE,* transesophageal echocardiography.

alone. In today's practices, cardiac MRI is increasingly used in conjunction with other imaging modalities for assessment of blood flow, and evaluation of myocardial perfusion and viability (Prakash, Powell, Krishnamurthy, et al., 2004).

Cardiac catheterization is an invasive diagnostic procedure in which a radiopaque catheter is introduced through a large bore needle into a peripheral vessel (usually the femoral artery or vein in children) and then guided into the heart with the aid of fluoroscopy. After the tip of the catheter is within a heart chamber, measurements of pressures and saturations in the different cardiac chambers are obtained. Contrast material is injected, and images are taken of the circulation inside the heart (angiography). Types of cardiac catheterizations include the following:

Diagnostic catheterizations: These studies are used to diagnose congenital cardiac defects, particularly in symptomatic infants and before surgical repair. They can include right-sided catheterizations, in which the catheter is introduced through a vein (usually the femoral vein) and threaded to the right atrium, and left-sided catheterizations, in which the catheter is threaded through an artery into the aorta and into the heart.

Interventional catheterizations (therapeutic catheterizations): A balloon catheter or other device is used to alter the cardiac anatomy. Examples include dilating stenotic valves or vessels or closing abnormal connections (Table 42.2).

Electrophysiology studies: Catheters with tiny electrodes that record the impulses of the heart directly from the conduction system are used to evaluate dysrhythmias. Other catheters can destroy abnormal pathways that cause rapid rhythms (called *ablation*).

Care Management

Cardiac catheterization has become a routine diagnostic and therapeutic procedure, but it is not without risks, especially in neonates and seriously ill infants and children. Risks include exposure to radiation and anesthesia, hypothermia in young infants, arrhythmias, vascular injury and bleeding that may require transfusion, renal insufficiency caused by contrast material, allergic reactions, and, rarely, injury to the heart or central nervous system (CNS), stroke, or death (Feltes, Bacha, Beekman, et al., 2011).

Preprocedural Care

A complete nursing assessment is necessary to ensure a safe procedure with minimum complications. This assessment should include accurate height (essential for correct catheter selection) and weight. Obtaining a history of allergic reactions is important because some of the contrast agents are iodine based. Specific attention to signs and symptoms of infection is crucial. Severe diaper rash may be a reason to cancel the procedure if femoral access is required. Because assessment of pedal pulses is important after catheterization, the nurse should assess and mark the pulses (dorsalis pedis, posterior tibial) before the child goes to the catheterization room. Baseline oxygen saturation using pulse oximetry in children with cyanosis is also recorded.

Preparing the child and family for the procedure is the joint responsibility of the patient care team. School-age children and adolescents benefit from a description of the catheterization laboratory and a chronologic explanation of the procedure, emphasizing what they will see, feel, and hear. Older children and adolescents may bring earphones and favorite music so that they can listen to music during the catheterization procedure. Preparation materials such as picture books, videos, or tours of the catheterization laboratory may be helpful. Preparation should be geared to the child's developmental level. The child's caregivers often benefit from the same explanations. Additional information, such as the expected length of the catheterization, description of the child's appearance after catheterization, and usual postprocedure care, should be outlined (see the "Prepare the Child and Family for Invasive Procedures" section later in this chapter).

Methods of sedation vary among institutions and may include oral or intravenous (IV) medications (see Chapter 39). The child's age, heart defect, clinical status, and type of catheterization procedure planned are considered when sedation is determined. General anesthesia is needed for most interventional procedures. Children are allowed nothing by mouth (NPO) for 6 to 8 hours or more before the procedure. Infants and patients with polycythemia may need IV fluids to prevent dehydration and hypoglycemia.

Post-Procedural Care

Post catheterization care may occur in a recovery unit, hospital room, or intensive care unit (ICU) depending on the patient's acuity and care needs. Some catheterizations may be done as outpatient procedures, but most patients having interventional procedures are observed overnight in the hospital. Patients are placed on a cardiac monitor and a pulse oximeter for the first few hours of recovery. The most important nursing responsibility is observation of the following for signs of complications:

- **Pulses,** especially below the catheterization site, for equality and symmetry (Pulse distal to the site may be weaker for the first few hours after catheterization but should gradually increase in strength.)
- **Temperature and color of the affected extremity** because coolness or blanching may indicate arterial obstruction

TABLE 42.2 Current Interventional Cardiac Catheterization Procedures in Children

Intervention	Diagnosis
Balloon atrioseptostomy: Use well established in newborns; may also be done under echocardiographic guidance	Transposition of great arteries Some complex single-ventricle defects

Balloon dilation: Treatment of choice	Valvular pulmonic stenosis
	Branch pulmonary artery stenosis
	Congenital valvular aortic stenosis
	Rheumatic mitral stenosis
	Recurrent coarctation of aorta
	Further follow-up required in:
	    Native coarctation of aorta in patients older than 7 months
	    Congenital mitral stenosis

Coil occlusion: Accepted alternative to surgery	PDA (<4 mm)
Transcatheter device closure: Several devices used in clinical trials	ASD
Amplatzer septal occluder: Approved for ASD closure	ASD
VSD devices: Used in clinical trials	VSD
Stent placement	Pulmonary artery stenosis Coarctation of the aorta in adolescents Use to treat other lesions investigational
RF ablation	Some tachydysrhythmias

ASD, Atrial septal defect; *PDA,* patent ductus arteriosus; *RF,* radiofrequency; *VSD,* ventricular septal defect.

After Cardiac Catheterization

Cover catheter insertion site with an adhesive bandage strip, and change daily for 2 days.

Keep site clean and dry. Avoid tub baths and swimming for several days; patient may shower or have a sponge bath.

Observe site for redness, swelling, drainage, and bleeding. Monitor for fever. Notify practitioner if these occur.

Encourage rest and quiet activities for the first 3 days, and avoid strenuous exercise.

Discuss returning to school and resuming other activities with the practitioner.

Resume regular diet without restrictions.

Use acetaminophen for pain.

Keep follow-up appointments per practitioner's instruction.

Modified from Children's Hospital (Boston) Cardiovascular Program, 2012.

CLINICAL REASONING CASE STUDY
Cardiac Catheterization

Tommy, a 3-year-old patient with tetralogy of Fallot, has just returned to his hospital room from the cardiac catheterization recovery room. His mother calls you to the bedside to tell you that he is vomiting and bleeding. You arrive to find Tommy anxious, pale, crying, and sitting in a puddle of blood.

Questions
1. Evidence: Is there sufficient evidence to draw conclusions about Tommy's situation?
2. Assumptions: Describe an underlying assumption about each of the following:
   a. Risks of cardiac catheterization
   b. Association between vomiting and bleeding after cardiac catheterization
   c. Concerns related to acute blood loss
3. What priorities for nursing care should be established for Tommy?
4. Does the evidence support your nursing interventions?

- **Vital signs,** which are taken as frequently as every 15 minutes, with special emphasis on heart rate, which is counted for 1 full minute for evidence of dysrhythmias or bradycardia
- **Blood pressure (BP),** especially for hypotension, which may indicate hemorrhage from cardiac perforation or bleeding at the site of initial catheterization
- **Dressing,** for evidence of bleeding or hematoma formation in the femoral or antecubital area
- **Fluid intake,** both IV and oral, to ensure adequate hydration (Blood loss in the catheterization laboratory, the child's NPO status, and diuretic actions of dyes used during the procedure put children at risk for hypovolemia and dehydration.)
- **Blood glucose levels** for hypoglycemia, especially in infants, who should receive dextrose-containing IV fluids

> ❗ **NURSING ALERT**
>
> If bleeding occurs, direct continuous pressure is applied 2.5 cm (1 inch) above the percutaneous skin site to localize pressure over the vessel puncture.

Depending on hospital policy, the child may be kept in bed with the affected extremity maintained straight for 4 to 6 hours after venous catheterization and 6 to 8 hours after arterial catheterization to facilitate healing of the cannulated vessel. If younger children have difficulty complying, they can be held in the parent's lap with the leg maintained in the correct position. The child's usual diet can be resumed as soon as tolerated, beginning with sips of clear liquids and advancing as the condition allows. The child is encouraged to void to clear the contrast material from the blood. Generally, there is only slight discomfort at the percutaneous site. To prevent infection, the catheterization area is protected from possible contamination. If the child wears diapers, the dressing can be kept dry by covering it with a piece of plastic film and sealing the edges of the film to the skin with tape. However, the nurse must be careful to continue observing the site for any evidence of bleeding (see Family-Centered Care box: After Cardiac Catheterization and Clinical Reasoning Case Study box: Cardiac Catheterization).

CONGENITAL HEART DISEASE

The incidence of CHD in children is approximately 8 to 12 per 1000 live births (Park, 2014). CHD is the major cause of death (other than prematurity) in the first year of life. Although there are more than 35 well-recognized cardiac defects, the most common heart anomaly is ventricular septal defect (VSD).

The exact cause of most congenital cardiac defects is unknown. Most are thought to be a result of multiple factors, including a complex interaction of genetic and environmental influences. Some risk factors are known to be associated with increased incidence of congenital heart defects. Maternal risk factors include chronic illnesses (e.g., diabetes or poorly controlled phenylketonuria), alcohol consumption, and exposure to environmental toxins and infections. Family history of a cardiac defect in a parent or sibling increases the likelihood of a cardiac anomaly. In general, when one child is affected, the risk for recurrence in siblings is about 3%, and for those who have a child with hypoplastic left heart syndrome (HLHS) the risk for CHD in subsequent children is reported to be 10% (Park, 2014).

Congenital heart anomalies are often associated with chromosomal abnormalities, specific syndromes, or congenital defects in other body systems. Down syndrome (trisomy 21) and trisomies 13 and 18 are highly correlated with congenital heart defects. Syndromes associated with heart defects include DiGeorge syndrome, a syndrome characterized by deletion of part of chromosome 22q11 (interrupted aortic arch, truncus arteriosus, tetralogy of Fallot, and posterior malaligned VSDs); Noonan syndrome (pulmonic valve anomalies and cardiomyopathy); Williams syndrome (aortic and pulmonic stenosis); and Holt-Oram syndrome (upper limb anomalies and atrial septal defect [ASD]). Extracardiac defects (e.g., tracheoesophageal fistula, renal abnormalities, and diaphragmatic hernia) are seen in association with heart anomalies.

CIRCULATORY CHANGES AT BIRTH

Blood carrying oxygen and nutritive materials from the placenta enters the fetal system through the umbilicus via the large umbilical vein. The blood then travels to the liver, where it divides. Part of the blood enters the portal and hepatic circulation of the liver, and the remainder travels directly to the inferior vena cava (IVC) by way of the ductus venosus. Oxygenated blood enters the heart by way of the IVC. Because of the higher pressure of blood entering the right atrium, it is directed posteriorly in a straight pathway across the right atrium and through the foramen ovale to the left atrium. In this way, the better-oxygenated blood enters the left atrium and ventricle to be pumped through the aorta to the head and upper extremities. Blood from the head and upper extremities entering the right atrium from the superior vena cava is directed downward through the tricuspid valve into the right

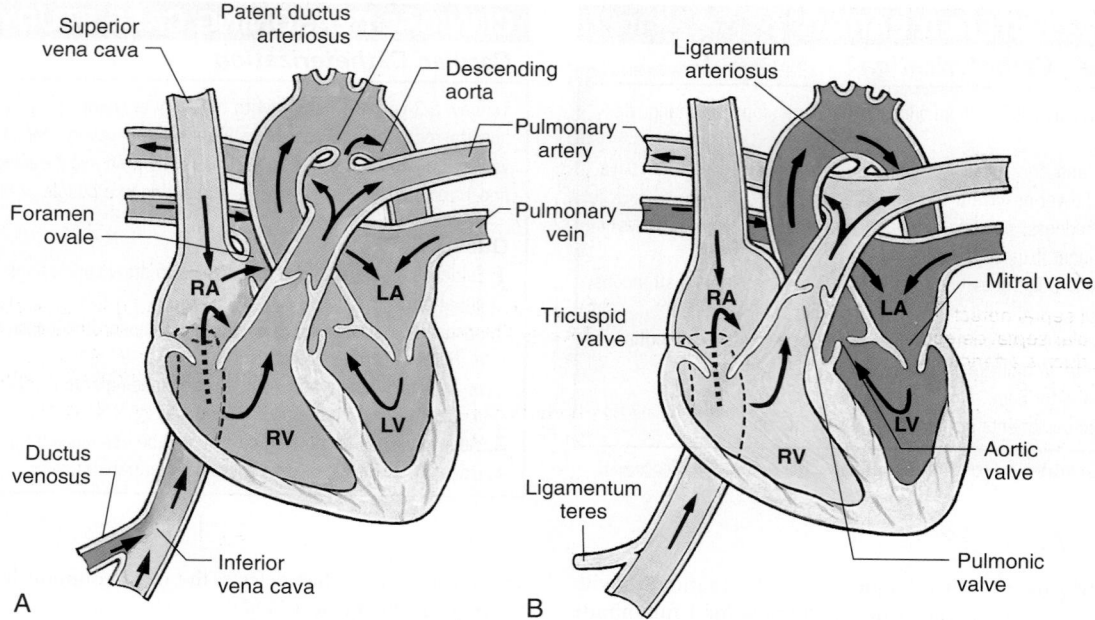

FIG 42.2 Changes in circulation at birth. *A,* Prenatal circulation. *B,* Postnatal circulation. *Arrows* indicate direction of blood flow. Although four pulmonary veins enter the left atrium (LA), for simplicity, this diagram shows only two. *LV,* Left ventricle; *RA,* right atrium; *RV,* right ventricle.

ventricle. From there it is pumped through the pulmonary artery, where the major portion is shunted to the descending aorta via the ductus arteriosus. Only a small amount flows to and from the nonfunctioning fetal lungs (Fig. 42.2, *A*).

Before birth, the high pulmonary vascular resistance created by the collapsed fetal lung causes greater pressures in the right side of the heart and the pulmonary arteries. At the same time, the free-flowing placental circulation and the ductus arteriosus produce a low vascular resistance in the remainder of the fetal vascular system. With the cessation of placental blood flow from clamping of the umbilical cord and the expansion of the lungs at birth, the hemodynamics of the fetal vascular system undergo pronounced and abrupt changes (see Fig. 42.2, *B*).

With the first breath, the lungs are expanded, and increased oxygen causes pulmonary vasodilation. Pulmonary pressures start to fall as systemic pressures, given the removal of the placenta, start to rise. Normally, the foramen ovale closes as the pressure in the left atrium exceeds the pressure in the right atrium. The ductus arteriosus starts to close in the presence of increased oxygen concentration in the blood and other factors.

ALTERED HEMODYNAMICS

To appreciate the physiology of heart defects, it is necessary to understand the role of pressure gradients, flow, and resistance within the circulation. As blood is pumped through the heart, it (1) flows from an area of high pressure to one of low pressure and (2) takes the path of least resistance. In general, the higher the pressure gradient, the faster the rate of flow; and the higher the resistance, the slower the rate of flow.

Normally, the pressure on the right side of the heart is lower than that on the left side, and the resistance in the pulmonary circulation is less than that in the systemic circulation. Vessels entering or exiting these chambers have corresponding pressures. Therefore, if an abnormal connection exists between the heart chambers (e.g., a septal defect), blood will necessarily flow from an area of higher pressure (left side) to one of lower pressure (right side). Such a flow of blood is termed a

left-to-right shunt. Anomalies resulting in cyanosis may result from a change in pressure so that the blood is shunted from the right to the left side of the heart *(right-to-left shunt)* because of either increased pulmonary vascular resistance or obstruction to blood flow through the pulmonic valve and artery. Cyanosis may also result from a defect that allows mixing of oxygenated and deoxygenated blood within the heart chambers or great arteries, such as occurs in truncus arteriosus.

CLASSIFICATION OF DEFECTS

There are typically two classification systems used to categorize congenital heart defects. Traditionally, cyanosis, a physical characteristic, has been used as the distinguishing feature, dividing anomalies into acyanotic defects and cyanotic defects. In clinical practice, this system is problematic because children with acyanotic defects may develop cyanosis. Also, more often, those with cyanotic defects may appear pink and have more clinical signs of HF.

A more useful classification system is based on hemodynamic characteristics (blood flow patterns within the heart). These blood flow patterns are (1) increased pulmonary blood flow; (2) decreased pulmonary blood flow; (3) obstruction to blood flow out of the heart; and (4) mixed blood flow, in which saturated and desaturated blood mix within the heart or great arteries. As a comparison, Fig. 42.3 outlines both classification systems. With the hemodynamic classification system, the clinical manifestations of each group are more uniform and predictable. Defects that allow blood flow from the higher-pressure left side of the heart to the lower-pressure right side (left-to-right shunt) result in increased pulmonary blood flow and cause HF. Obstructive defects impede blood flow out of the ventricles; whereas obstruction on the left side of the heart results in HF, severe obstruction on the right side causes cyanosis. Defects that cause decreased pulmonary blood flow result in cyanosis. Mixed lesions present a variable clinical picture based on the degree of mixing and amount of pulmonary blood flow; hypoxemia (with or without cyanosis) and HF usually occur together. Using this classification system, the clinical presentation and management

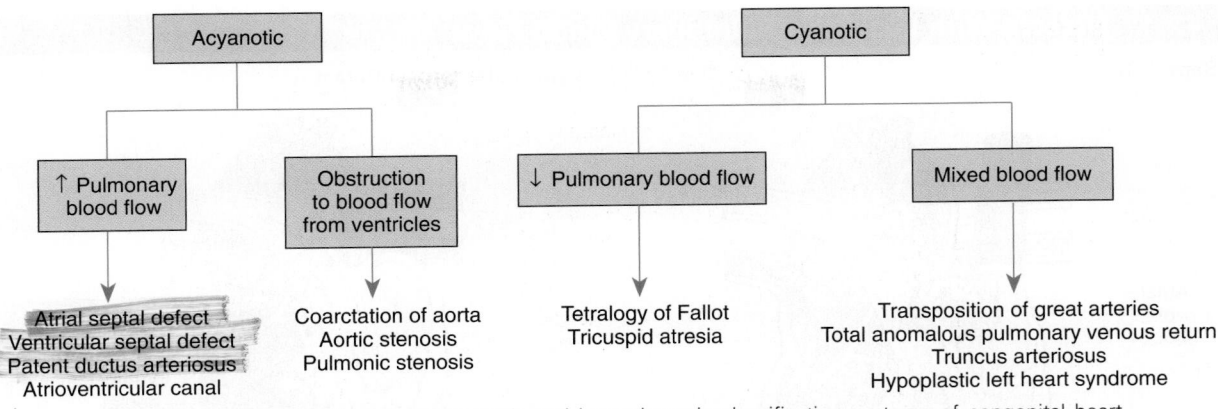

FIG 42.3 Comparison of acyanotic-cyanotic and hemodynamic classification systems of congenital heart disease (CHD).

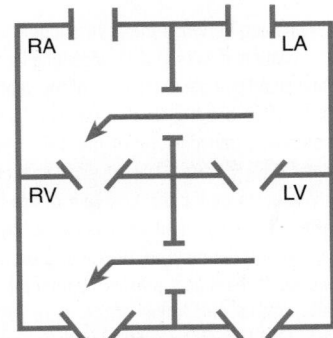

FIG 42.4 Hemodynamics in defects with increased pulmonary blood flow. *LA,* Left atrium; *LV,* left ventricle; *RA,* right atrium; *RV,* right ventricle.

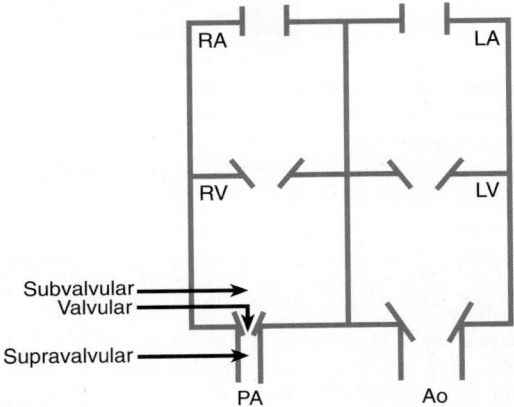

FIG 42.5 Obstruction to ventricular ejection can occur at the valvular level *(shown),* below the valve (subvalvular), or above the valve (supravalvular). Pulmonary stenosis is shown here. *Ao,* Aorta; *LA,* left atrium; *LV,* left ventricle; *PA,* pulmonary artery; *RA,* right atrium; *RV,* right ventricle.

of the most common defects are outlined in the following sections and Box 42.1.

The outcomes of surgical treatment for patients with moderate to severe disease are variable. Patient risk factors for increased morbidity and mortality include prematurity or low birth weight, a genetic syndrome, multiple cardiac defects, a noncardiac congenital anomaly, and age at time of surgery (neonates are a higher-risk group). For example, aortic stenosis or coarctation manifesting in the first week of life is more severe and carries a higher mortality than if it becomes apparent at 1 year of age. Outcomes for surgical repair of similar congenital heart defects also vary among treatment centers. In general, the outcomes of surgical procedures have steadily improved in the past decade, with mortality rates for many severe defects below 10% and a decrease in the incidence of complications and length of hospital stay.

Defects With Increased Pulmonary Blood Flow

In this group of cardiac defects, intracardiac communications along the septum or an abnormal connection between the great arteries allows blood to flow from the higher-pressure left side of the heart to the lower-pressure right side of the heart (Fig. 42.4). Increased blood volume on the right side of the heart increases pulmonary blood flow at the expense of systemic blood flow. Clinically, patients demonstrate signs and symptoms of HF. ASD, VSD, and patent ductus arteriosus are typical anomalies in this group (see Box 42.1).

Obstructive Defects

Obstructive defects are those in which blood exiting the heart meets an area of anatomic narrowing *(stenosis),* causing obstruction to blood flow. The pressure in the ventricle and in the great artery before the obstruction is increased, and the pressure in the area beyond the obstruction is decreased. The location of the narrowing is usually near the valve (Fig. 42.5), as follows:

Valvular: At the site of the valve itself

Subvalvular: Narrowing in the ventricle below the valve (also referred to as the *ventricular outflow tract*)

Supravalvular: Narrowing in the great artery above the valve

Coarctation of the aorta (narrowing of the aortic arch), aortic stenosis, and pulmonic stenosis are typical defects in this group (Box 42.2). Hemodynamically, there is a pressure load on the ventricle and decreased cardiac output. Clinically, infants and children exhibit signs of HF. Children with mild obstruction may be asymptomatic. Rarely, as in severe pulmonic stenosis, hypoxemia may be seen.

Defects With Decreased Pulmonary Blood Flow

In this group of defects, there is obstruction of pulmonary blood flow and an anatomic defect (ASD or VSD) between the right and left sides of the heart (Fig. 42.6). Because blood has difficulty exiting the right side of the heart via the pulmonary artery, pressure on the right side increases, exceeding left-sided pressure. This allows desaturated blood to shunt right to left, causing desaturation in the left side of the heart and in the systemic circulation. Clinically, these patients have hypoxemia

BOX 42.1 Defects With Increased Pulmonary Blood Flow

Atrial Septal Defect

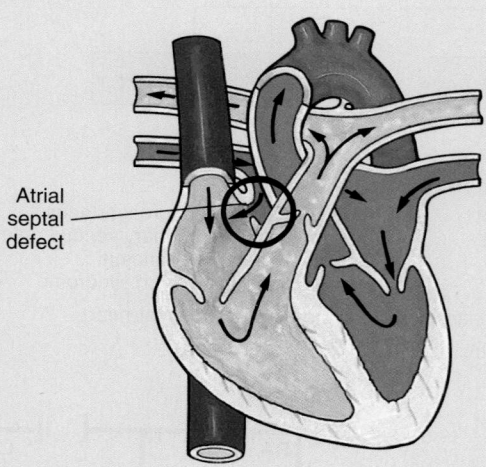

Atrial septal defect

Description: Abnormal opening between the atria, allowing blood from the higher-pressure left atrium to flow into the lower-pressure right atrium. There are three types of ASD:

Ostium primum (ASD 1): Opening at lower end of septum; may be associated with mitral valve abnormalities

Ostium secundum (ASD 2): Opening near center of septum

Sinus venosus defect: Opening near junction of superior vena cava and right atrium; may be associated with partial anomalous pulmonary venous connection

Pathophysiology: Because left atrial pressure slightly exceeds right atrial pressure, blood flows from the left to the right atrium, causing an increased flow of oxygenated blood into the right side of the heart. Despite the low pressure difference, a high rate of flow can still occur because of low pulmonary vascular resistance and the greater distensibility of the right atrium, which further reduces flow resistance. This volume is well tolerated by the right ventricle because it is delivered under much lower pressure than with a VSD. Although there is right atrial and ventricular enlargement, cardiac failure is unusual in an uncomplicated ASD. Pulmonary vascular changes usually occur only after several decades if the defect is left unrepaired.

Clinical manifestations: Patients may be asymptomatic. They may develop HF. There is a characteristic systolic murmur with a fixed split second heart sound. There may also be a diastolic murmur. Patients are at risk for atrial dysrhythmias (probably caused by atrial enlargement and stretching of conduction fibers) and pulmonary vascular obstructive disease and emboli formation later in life from chronically increased pulmonary blood flow.

Surgical treatment: Surgical patch closure (pericardial patch or Dacron patch) is done for moderate to large defects. Open repair with cardiopulmonary bypass is usually performed before school age. In addition, the sinus venosus defect requires patch placement, so the anomalous right pulmonary venous return is directed to the left atrium with a baffle. ASD 1 type may require mitral valve repair or, rarely, replacement of the mitral valve.

Nonsurgical treatment: ASD 2 closure with a device during cardiac catheterization is becoming commonplace and can be done as an outpatient procedure. The Amplatzer Septal Occluder is most commonly used. Smaller defects that have a rim around them for attachment of the device can be closed with a device; large, irregular defects without a rim require surgical closure. Successful closure in appropriately selected patients yields results similar to those from surgery but involves shorter hospital stays and fewer complications. Patients receive low-dose aspirin for 6 months (Park, 2014).

Prognosis: Operative mortality is very low (<0.5%).

Ventricular Septal Defect

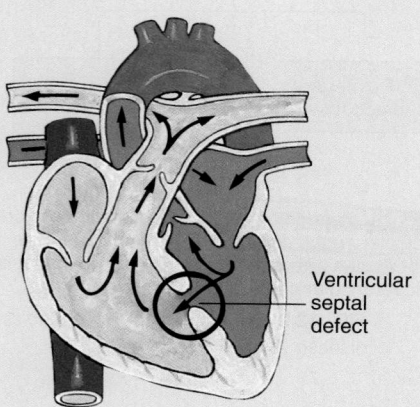

Ventricular septal defect

Description: Abnormal opening between the right and left ventricles. May be classified according to location: membranous (accounting for 80%) or muscular. May vary in size from a small pinhole to absence of the septum, which results in a common ventricle. VSDs are frequently associated with other defects, such as pulmonary stenosis, transposition of the great vessels, PDA, atrial defects, and COA. Many VSDs (20% to 60%) close spontaneously. Spontaneous closure is most likely to occur during the first year of life in children having small or moderate defects. A left-to-right shunt is caused by the flow of blood from the higher-pressure left ventricle to the lower-pressure right ventricle.

Pathophysiology: Because of the higher pressure within the left ventricle and because the systemic arterial circulation offers more resistance than the pulmonary circulation, blood flows through the defect into the pulmonary artery. The increased blood volume is pumped into the lungs, which may eventually result in increased pulmonary vascular resistance. Increased pressure in the right ventricle as a result of left-to-right shunting and pulmonary resistance causes the muscle to hypertrophy. If the right ventricle is unable to accommodate the increased workload, the right atrium may also enlarge as it attempts to overcome the resistance offered by incomplete right ventricular emptying.

Clinical manifestations: HF is common. There is a characteristic loud holosystolic murmur heard best at the left sternal border. Patients are at risk for BE and pulmonary vascular obstructive disease.

Surgical treatment:

Palliative: Pulmonary artery banding (placement of a band around the main pulmonary artery to decrease pulmonary blood flow) may be done in infants with multiple muscular VSDs or complex anatomy. Improvements in surgical techniques and postoperative care make complete repair in infancy the preferred approach.

Complete repair (procedure of choice): Small defects are repaired with sutures. Large defects usually require that a knitted Dacron patch be sewn over the opening. CPB is used for both procedures. The approach for the repair is generally through the right atrium and the tricuspid valve. Postoperative complications include residual VSD and conduction disturbances.

Prognosis: Risks depend on the location of the defect, the number of defects, and the presence of other associated cardiac defects. Single-membranous defects are associated with low mortality (<1%); multiple muscular defects can carry a higher risk for infants, especially infants younger than 2 months of age (Park, 2014).

BOX 42.1   Defects With Increased Pulmonary Blood Flow—cont'd

Atrioventricular Canal Defect

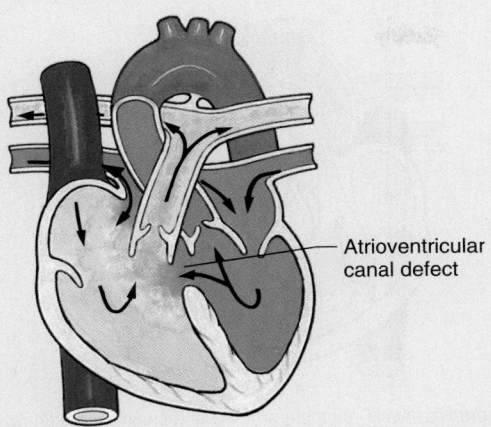

Atrioventricular canal defect

Patent Ductus Arteriosus

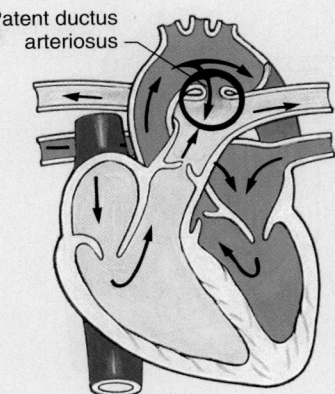

Patent ductus arteriosus

Description: Incomplete fusion of the endocardial cushions. Consists of a low ASD that is continuous with a high VSD and clefts of the mitral and tricuspid valves, which create a large central AV valve that allows blood to flow between all four chambers of the heart. The directions and pathways of flow are determined by pulmonary and systemic resistance, left and right ventricular pressures, and the compliance of each chamber, although flow is generally from left to right. It is the most common cardiac defect in children with Down syndrome.

Pathophysiology: The alterations in hemodynamics depend on the severity of the defect and the child's pulmonary vascular resistance. Immediately after birth, while the newborn's pulmonary vascular resistance is high, there is minimum shunting of blood through the defect. When this resistance falls, left-to-right shunting occurs, and pulmonary blood flow increases. The resultant pulmonary vascular engorgement predisposes the child to development of HF.

Clinical manifestations: Patients usually have moderate to severe HF. There is a loud systolic murmur. There may be mild cyanosis that increases with crying. Patients are at high risk for developing pulmonary vascular obstructive disease.

Surgical treatment:

Palliative: Pulmonary artery banding is occasionally done in small infants with severe symptoms. Complete repair in infancy is most common.

Complete repair: Surgical repair consists of patch closure of the septal defects and reconstruction of the AV valve tissue (either repair of the mitral valve cleft or fashioning of two AV valves). Postoperative complications include heart block, HF, mitral regurgitation, dysrhythmias, and pulmonary hypertension.

Prognosis: Operative mortality has been 3% to 10%. Factors that increase surgical risk are younger age, severe AV valve regurgitation, hypoplasia of the left ventricle and severe failure preoperatively, as well as other heart defects (Park, 2014). A potential later problem is mitral regurgitation, which may require valve replacement.

Description: Failure of the fetal ductus arteriosus (artery connecting the aorta and pulmonary artery) to close within the first weeks of life. The continued patency of this vessel allows blood to flow from the higher-pressure aorta to the lower-pressure pulmonary artery, which causes a left-to-right shunt.

Pathophysiology: The hemodynamic consequences of PDA depend on the size of the ductus and the pulmonary vascular resistance. At birth, the resistance in the pulmonary and systemic circulations is almost identical so that the resistance in the aorta and pulmonary artery is equalized. As the systemic pressure comes to exceed the pulmonary pressure, blood begins to shunt from the aorta across the duct to the pulmonary artery (left-to-right shunt). The additional blood is recirculated through the lungs and returned to the left atrium and left ventricle. The effects of this altered circulation are increased workload on the left side of the heart, increased pulmonary vascular congestion and possibly resistance, and potentially increased right ventricular pressure and hypertrophy.

Clinical manifestations: Patients may be asymptomatic or show signs of HF. There is a characteristic machinery-like murmur. A widened pulse pressure and bounding pulses result from runoff of blood from the aorta to the pulmonary artery. Patients are at risk for BE and pulmonary vascular obstructive disease in later life from chronic excessive pulmonary blood flow.

Medical management: Administration of indomethacin (a prostaglandin inhibitor) has proved successful in closing a PDA in preterm infants and some newborns.

Surgical treatment: Surgical division or ligation of the patent vessel is performed via a left thoracotomy. In a newer technique, video-assisted thoracoscopic surgery, a thoracoscope and instruments are inserted through three small incisions on the left side of the chest to place a clip on the ductus. The technique is used in some centers and eliminates the need for a thoracotomy, thereby speeding postoperative recovery.

Nonsurgical treatment: Coils to occlude the PDA are placed in the catheterization laboratory in many centers. Preterm or small infants (with small-diameter femoral arteries) and patients with large or unusual PDAs may require surgery.

Prognosis: Both surgical procedures can be done at low risk with zero percent mortality. PDA closure in very preterm infants has a higher mortality rate because of the additional significant medical problems. Complications are rare, but can include injury to the laryngeal nerve, paralysis of the left hemidiaphragm, or injury to the thoracic duct (Park, 2014).

ASD, Atrial septal defect; *AV,* atrioventricular; *BE,* bacterial endocarditis; *COA,* coarctation of the aorta; *CPB,* cardiopulmonary bypass; *HF,* heart failure; *PDA,* patent ductus arteriosus; *VSD,* ventricular septal defect.

BOX 42.2 Obstructive Defects

Coarctation of the Aorta

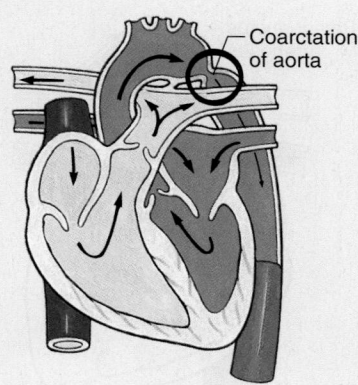

Coarctation of aorta

Description: Localized narrowing near the insertion of the ductus arteriosus, which results in increased pressure proximal to the defect (head and upper extremities) and decreased pressure distal to the obstruction (body and lower extremities).

Pathophysiology: The effect of a narrowing within the aorta is increased pressure proximal to the defect (upper extremities) and decreased pressure distal to it (lower extremities).

Clinical manifestations: The patient may have high BP and bounding pulses in the arms, weak or absent femoral pulses, and cool lower extremities with lower BP. There are signs of HF in infants. In infants with critical coarctation, the hemodynamic condition may deteriorate rapidly with severe acidosis and hypotension. Mechanical ventilation and inotropic support are often necessary before surgery. Older children may experience dizziness, headaches, fainting, and epistaxis resulting from hypertension. Patients are at risk for hypertension, ruptured aorta, aortic aneurysm, and stroke.

Surgical treatment: Surgical repair is the treatment of choice for infants younger than 6 months of age and for patients with long-segment stenosis or complex anatomy; it may be performed for all patients with coarctation. Repair is by resection of the coarcted portion with an end-to-end anastomosis of the aorta or enlargement of the constricted section using a graft of prosthetic material or a portion of the left subclavian artery. Because this defect is outside the heart and pericardium, cardiopulmonary bypass is not required, and a thoracotomy incision is used. Postoperative hypertension is treated with IV sodium nitroprusside, esmolol, or milrinone followed by oral medications, such as ACE inhibitors or beta blockers. Residual permanent hypertension after repair of COA seems to be related to age and time of repair. To prevent both hypertension at rest and exercise-provoked systemic hypertension after repair, elective surgery for COA is advised within the first 2 years of life. There is a 15% to 30% risk for recurrence in patients who underwent surgical repair as infants (Beekman, 2001). Percutaneous balloon angioplasty techniques have proved to be effective in relieving residual postoperative coarctation gradients.

Nonsurgical treatment: Balloon angioplasty is being performed as a primary intervention for COA in older infants and children, Balloon angioplasty has a higher associated rate of recoarctation than surgical repair, and the rate of complication, particularly femoral artery injury, is high during infancy.

Prognosis: Mortality is less than 5% in patients with isolated coarctation; the risk is increased in infants with other complex cardiac defects (Park, 2014).

Aortic Stenosis

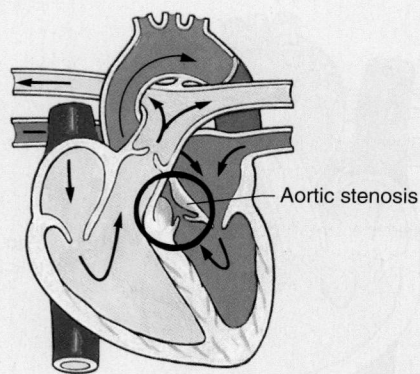

Aortic stenosis

Description: Narrowing or stricture of the aortic valve, causing resistance to blood flow in the left ventricle, decreased cardiac output, left ventricular hypertrophy, and pulmonary vascular congestion. The prominent anatomic consequence of AS is the hypertrophy of the left ventricular wall, which eventually leads to increased end-diastolic pressure, resulting in pulmonary venous and pulmonary arterial hypertension. Left ventricular hypertrophy also interferes with coronary artery perfusion and may result in myocardial infarction or scarring of the papillary muscles of the left ventricle, which causes mitral insufficiency. Valvular stenosis, the most common type, is usually caused by malformed cusps that result in a bicuspid rather than tricuspid valve or fusion of the cusps. Subvalvular stenosis is a stricture caused by a fibrous ring below a normal valve; supravalvular stenosis occurs infrequently. Valvular AS is a serious defect for the following reasons: (1) the obstruction tends to be progressive; (2) sudden episodes of myocardial ischemia, or low cardiac output, can result in sudden death; and (3) surgical repair rarely results in a normal valve. This is one of the rare instances in which strenuous physical activity may be curtailed because of the cardiac condition.

Pathophysiology: A stricture in the aortic outflow tract causes resistance to ejection of blood from the left ventricle. The extra workload on the left ventricle causes hypertrophy. If left ventricular failure develops, left atrial pressure will increase; this causes increased pressure in the pulmonary veins, which results in pulmonary vascular congestion (pulmonary edema).

Clinical manifestations: Newborns with critical AS demonstrate signs of decreased cardiac output with faint pulses, hypotension, tachycardia, and poor feeding. Children show signs of exercise intolerance, chest pain, and dizziness when standing for a long period. A systolic ejection murmur may or may not be present. Patients are at risk for BE, coronary insufficiency, and ventricular dysfunction.

Valvular Aortic Stenosis

Surgical treatment: Aortic valvotomy is performed under inflow occlusion. Used rarely because balloon dilation in the catheterization laboratory is the first-line procedure. Newborns with critical AS and small left-sided structures may undergo a stage 1 Norwood procedure (see Hypoplastic Left Heart Syndrome in Box 42.4).

Prognosis: Aortic valve replacement offers a good treatment option and may lead to normalization of left ventricular size and function (Arnold, Ley-Zaporozhan, Ley, et al., 2008). Aortic valvotomy remains a palliative procedure, and approximately 25% of patients require additional surgery within 10 years for recurrent stenosis. A valve replacement may be required at the second procedure. An aortic homograft with a valve may also be used (extended aortic root replacement), or the pulmonary valve may be moved to the aortic position and replaced with a homograft valve (Ross procedure).

BOX 42.2 Obstructive Defects—cont'd

Nonsurgical treatment: The narrowed valve is dilated using balloon angioplasty in the catheterization laboratory. This procedure is usually the first intervention.

Prognosis: Complications include aortic insufficiency or valvular regurgitation, tearing of the valve leaflets, and loss of pulse in the catheterized limb.

Subvalvular Aortic Stenosis

Surgical treatment: Procedure may involve incising a membrane if one exists or cutting the fibromuscular ring. If the obstruction results from narrowing of the left ventricular outflow tract and a small aortic valve annulus, a patch may be required to enlarge the entire left ventricular outflow tract and annulus and replace the aortic valve; this is known as the *Konno procedure.*

Prognosis: Mortality from surgical repairs of subvalvular AS is less than 5% in major centers. About 20% of these patients will develop recurrent subaortic stenosis and will require additional surgery (Schneider & Moore, 2008).

Pulmonic Stenosis

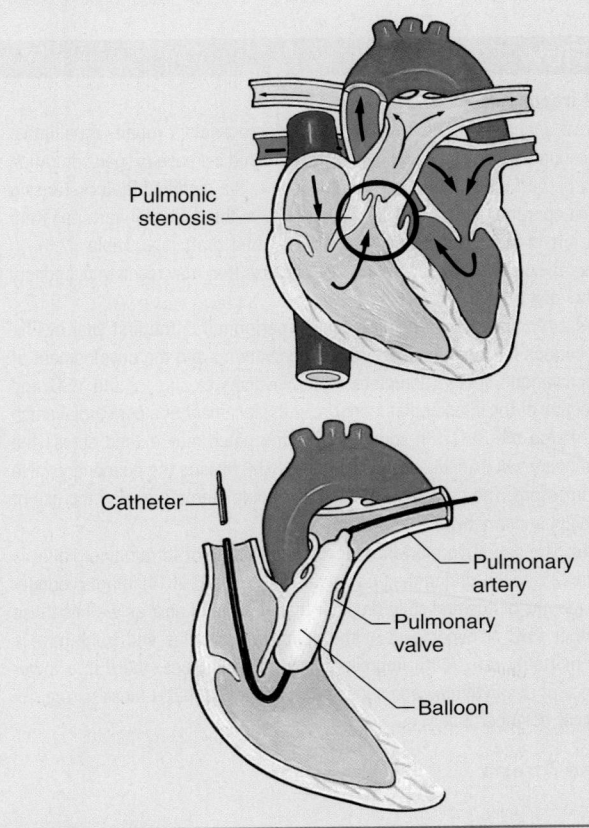

Description: Narrowing at the entrance to the pulmonary artery. Resistance to blood flow causes right ventricular hypertrophy and decreased pulmonary blood flow. Pulmonary atresia is the extreme form of PS in that there is total fusion of the commissures and no blood flows to the lungs. The right ventricle may be hypoplastic.

Pathophysiology: When PS is present, resistance to blood flow causes right ventricular hypertrophy. If right ventricular failure develops, right atrial pressure will increase, and this may result in reopening of the foramen ovale, shunting of unoxygenated blood into the left atrium, and systemic cyanosis. If PS is severe, HF occurs, and systemic venous engorgement will be noted. An associated defect such as a PDA partially compensates for the obstruction by shunting blood from the aorta to the pulmonary artery and into the lungs.

Clinical manifestations: Patients may be asymptomatic; some have mild cyanosis or HF. Progressive narrowing causes increased symptoms. Newborns with severe narrowing are cyanotic. A loud systolic ejection murmur at the upper-left sternal border may be present. However, in severely ill patients, the murmur may be much softer because of decreased cardiac output and shunting of blood. Cardiomegaly is evident on chest radiography. Patients are at risk for BE.

Surgical treatment: In infants, transventricular (closed) valvotomy (Brock procedure) is the surgical treatment. In children, pulmonary valvotomy with CPB is the surgical treatment. Need for surgical treatment is rare with widespread use of balloon angioplasty techniques.

Nonsurgical treatment: Balloon angioplasty in the cardiac catheterization laboratory to dilate the valve. A catheter is inserted across the stenotic pulmonic valve into the pulmonary artery, and a balloon at the end of the catheter is inflated and rapidly passed through the narrowed opening (see figure at left). The procedure is associated with few complications and has proved to be highly effective. It is the treatment of choice for discrete PS in most centers and can be done safely in neonates.

Prognosis: The risk is low for both surgical and nonsurgical procedures; mortality is lower than 1% and slightly higher in neonates (Park, 2014). Both balloon dilation and surgical valvotomy leave the pulmonic valve incompetent because they involve opening the fused valve leaflets; however, these patients are clinically asymptomatic. Long-term problems with restenosis or valve incompetence may occur.

ACE, Angiotensin-converting enzyme; *AS*, aortic stenosis; *BE*, bacterial endocarditis; *BP*, blood pressure; *COA*, coarctation of the aorta; *CPB*, cardiopulmonary bypass; *HF*, heart failure; *IV*, intravenous; *PDA*, patent ductus arteriosus; *PS*, pulmonic stenosis.

and usually appear cyanotic. Tetralogy of Fallot and tricuspid atresia are the most common defects in this group (Box 42.3).

Mixed Defects

Many complex cardiac anomalies are classified together in the mixed category (Box 42.4), because survival in the postnatal period depends on mixing of blood from the pulmonary and systemic circulations within the heart chambers. Hemodynamically, fully saturated systemic blood flow mixes with the desaturated pulmonary blood flow, causing a relative desaturation of the systemic blood flow. Pulmonary congestion occurs because the differences in pulmonary artery pressure and aortic pressure favor pulmonary blood flow. Cardiac output decreases because of a volume load on the ventricle. Clinically, these patients have a variable picture that combines some degree of desaturation (although cyanosis is not always visible) and signs of HF. Some defects, such as transposition of the great arteries, cause severe cyanosis in the first days of life and later cause HF. Others, such as truncus arteriosus, cause severe HF in the first weeks of life and mild desaturation.

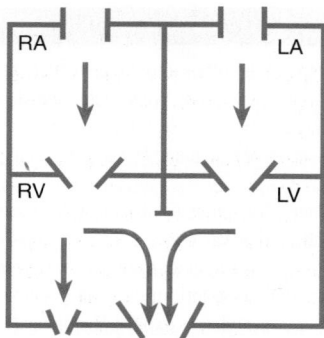

FIG 42.6 Hemodynamic defects with decreased pulmonary blood flow. *LA,* Left atrium; *LV,* left ventricle; *RA,* right atrium; *RV,* right ventricle.

CLINICAL CONSEQUENCES OF CONGENITAL HEART DISEASE

HEART FAILURE

HF is the inability of the heart to pump an adequate amount of blood to the systemic circulation at normal filling pressures to meet the body's metabolic demands. In children, HF most frequently occurs secondary to structural abnormalities (e.g., septal defects) that result in increased blood volume and pressure within the heart. It can also result from myocardial failure in which the contractility or relaxation of the ventricle is impaired. This can occur with cardiomyopathy, dysrhythmias, or severe electrolyte disturbances. HF can also occur because of excessive demands on a normal heart muscle, such as sepsis or severe anemia.

Pathophysiology

HF is often separated into two categories, right-sided and left-sided failure. In right-sided failure, the right ventricle is unable to pump

---

BOX 42.3 Defects With Decreased Pulmonary Blood Flow

Tetralogy of Fallot

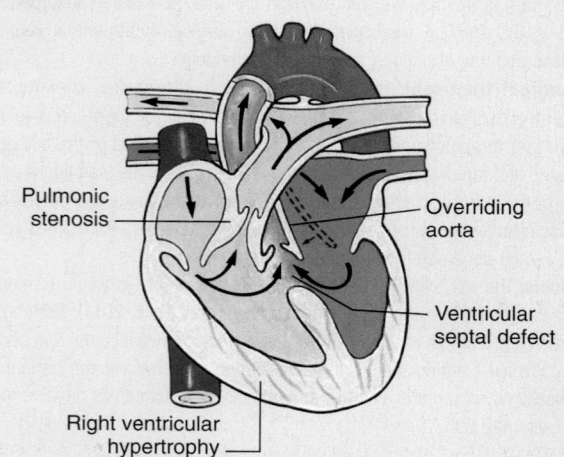

Description: The classic form includes four defects: (1) VSD, (2) PS, (3) overriding aorta, and (4) right ventricular hypertrophy. Tetralogy of Fallot occurs in 5% to 10% of all CHDs and is the most common cyanotic lesion (Park, 2014).

Pathophysiology: The alteration in hemodynamics varies widely, depending primarily on the degree of PS but also on the size of the VSD and the pulmonary and systemic resistance to flow. Because the VSD is usually large, pressures may be equal in the right and left ventricles. Therefore, the shunt direction depends on the difference between pulmonary and systemic vascular resistance. If pulmonary vascular resistance is higher than systemic resistance, the shunt is from right to left. If systemic resistance is higher than pulmonary resistance, the shunt is from left to right. PS decreases blood flow to the lungs and consequently the amount of oxygenated blood that returns to the left side of the heart. Depending on the position of the aorta, blood from both ventricles may be distributed systemically.

Clinical manifestations: Some infants may be acutely cyanotic at birth; others have mild cyanosis that progresses over the first year of life as the PS worsens. There is a characteristic systolic murmur that is often moderate in intensity. There may be acute episodes of cyanosis and hypoxia, called *blue spells* or *tet spells.* Anoxic spells occur when the infant's oxygen requirements exceed the blood supply, usually during crying or after feeding. Patients are at risk for emboli, seizures, and loss of consciousness or sudden death after an anoxic spell.

Surgical treatment:

Palliative shunt: In infants who cannot undergo primary repair, a palliative procedure to increase pulmonary blood flow and increase oxygen saturation may be performed. The preferred procedure is a modified Blalock-Taussig shunt operation, which provides blood flow to the pulmonary arteries from the left or right subclavian artery via a tube graft (see Table 42.4). In general, however, shunts are avoided because they may result in pulmonary artery distortion.

Complete repair: Elective repair is usually performed in the first year of life. Indications for repair include increasing cyanosis and the development of hypercyanotic spells. Complete repair involves closure of the VSD and resection of the infundibular stenosis, with placement of a pericardial patch to enlarge the RVOT. In some repairs, the patch may extend across the pulmonary valve annulus (transannular patch), making the pulmonary valve incompetent. The procedure requires a median sternotomy and the use of cardiopulmonary bypass.

Prognosis: The operative mortality for total correction of tetralogy of Fallot is less than 2% to 3% during the first 2 years of life (Park, 2014) Infants younger than 3 months of age and children older than 4 years of age, as well as those with other CHD or hypoplasia of the pulmonary annulus and trunk have a higher mortality rate. With improved surgical techniques, there is a lower incidence of dysrhythmias and sudden death; surgical heart block is rare. HF may occur postoperatively.

Tricuspid Atresia

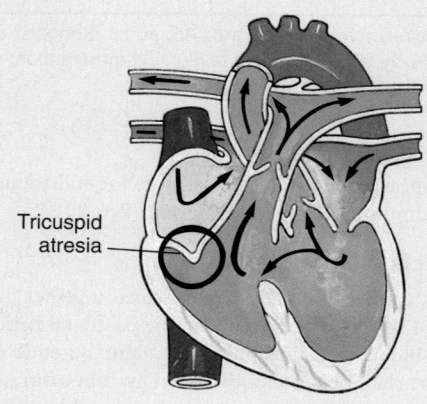

BOX 42.3   Defects With Decreased Pulmonary Blood Flow—cont'd

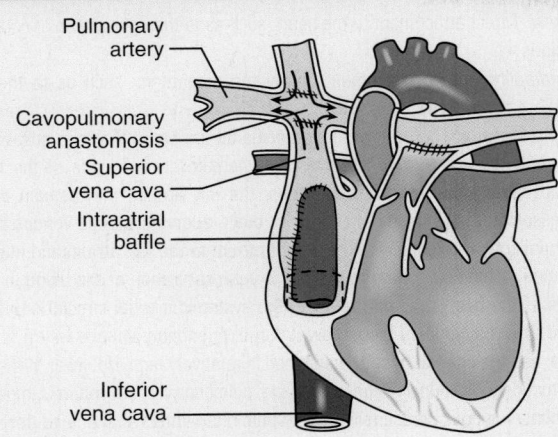

Pulmonary artery

Cavopulmonary anastomosis

Superior vena cava

Intraatrial baffle

Inferior vena cava

Description: The tricuspid valve fails to develop; consequently there is no communication from the right atrium to the right ventricle. Blood flows through an ASD or a patent foramen ovale to the left side of the heart and through a VSD to the right ventricle and out to the lungs. The condition is often associated with PS and TGA. There is complete mixing of unoxygenated and oxygenated blood in the left side of the heart, which results in systemic desaturation, and varying amounts of pulmonary obstruction, which causes decreased pulmonary blood flow.

Pathophysiology: At birth, the presence of a patent foramen ovale (or other atrial septal opening) is required to permit blood flow across the septum into the left atrium; the PDA allows blood flow to the pulmonary artery into the lungs for oxygenation. A VSD allows a modest amount of blood to enter the right ventricle and pulmonary artery for oxygenation. Pulmonary blood flow usually is diminished.

Clinical manifestations: Cyanosis is usually seen in the newborn period. There may be tachycardia and dyspnea. Older children have signs of chronic hypoxemia with clubbing.

Therapeutic management: For neonates whose pulmonary blood flow depends on the patency of the ductus arteriosus, a continuous infusion of prostaglandin E_1 is started at 0.1 mcg/kg/min until surgical intervention can be arranged.

Surgical treatment: Palliative treatment is the placement of a shunt (pulmonary–to–systemic artery anastomosis) to increase blood flow to the lungs. If the ASD is small, an atrial septostomy is performed during cardiac catheterization. Some children have increased pulmonary blood flow and require pulmonary artery banding to lessen the volume of blood to the lungs. A bidirectional Glenn shunt (cavopulmonary anastomosis) may be performed at 4 to 9 months of age as a second stage.

Modified Fontan procedure: Systemic venous return is directed to the lungs without a ventricular pump through surgical connections between the right atrium and the pulmonary artery. A fenestration (opening) is sometimes made in the right atrial baffle to relieve pressure. The patient must have normal ventricular function and a low pulmonary vascular resistance for the procedure to be successful. The modified Fontan procedure separates oxygenated and unoxygenated blood inside the heart and eliminates the excess volume load on the ventricle but does not restore normal anatomy or hemodynamics. This operation is also the final stage in the correction of many complex defects with a functional single ventricle, including HLHS.

Prognosis: Surgical mortality following the Fontan procedure is less than 3% (Park, 2014). The overall survival rate after the Fontan operation was above 95% at follow up of 50 months (Hirsch, Goldberg, Bove, et al., 2008). Postoperative complications include dysrhythmias, systemic venous hypertension, pleural and pericardial effusions, and ventricular dysfunction. Long-term concerns are the development of protein-losing enteropathy, atrial dysrhythmias, late ventricular dysfunction, and developmental delays.

ASD, Atrial septal defect; *CHD,* congenital heart disease; *HF,* heart failure; *HLHS,* hypoplastic left heart syndrome; *PDA,* patent ductus arteriosus; *PS,* pulmonic stenosis; *RVOT,* right ventricular outflow tract; *TGA,* transposition of the great arteries; *VSD,* ventricular septal defect.

BOX 42.4   Mixed Defects

Transposition of the Great Arteries, or Transposition of the Great Vessels

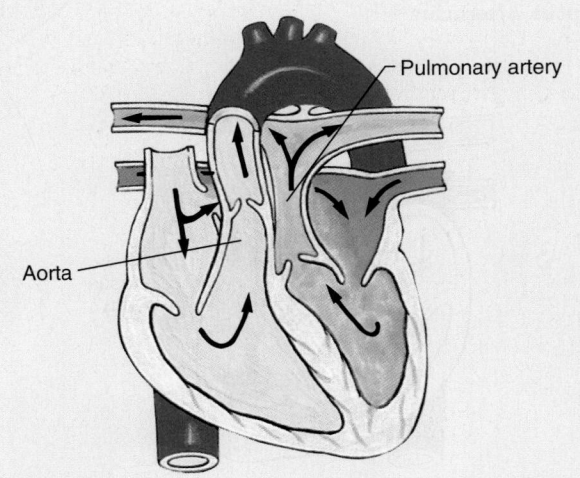

Pulmonary artery

Aorta

Description: The pulmonary artery leaves the left ventricle, and the aorta exits from the right ventricle with no communication between the systemic and pulmonary circulations.

Pathophysiology: Associated defects, such as septal defects or PDA, must be present to permit blood to enter the systemic circulation or the pulmonary circulation for mixing of saturated and desaturated blood. The most common defect associated with TGA is a patent foramen ovale. At birth, there is also a PDA, although in most instances this closes after the neonatal period. Another associated defect may be a VSD. The presence of a VSD increases the risk for HF because it permits blood to flow from the right to the left ventricle, into the pulmonary artery, and finally to the lungs. However, it also produces high pulmonary blood flow under high pressure, which can result in high pulmonary vascular resistance.

Clinical manifestations: These depend on the type and size of the associated defects. Newborns with minimum communication are severely cyanotic and have depressed function at birth. Those with large septal defects or a PDA may be less cyanotic but have symptoms of HF. Heart sounds vary according to the type of defect present. Cardiomegaly is usually evident a few weeks after birth.

Therapeutic management (to provide intracardiac mixing): The administration of IV prostaglandin E_1 may be initiated to keep the ductus arteriosus open to temporarily increase blood mixing and provide an oxygen saturation of 75% or to maintain cardiac output. During cardiac catheterization or under echocardiographic guidance, a balloon atrial septostomy (Rashkind procedure) may also be performed to increase mixing by opening the atrial septum.

Continued

BOX 42.4   Mixed Defects—cont'd

Surgical treatment: An arterial switch procedure is the procedure of choice performed in the first weeks of life. It involves transecting the great arteries and anastomosing the main pulmonary artery to the proximal aorta (just above the aortic valve) and anastomosing the ascending aorta to the proximal pulmonary artery. The coronary arteries are switched from the proximal aorta to the proximal pulmonary artery to create a new aorta. Reimplantation of the coronary arteries is critical to the infant's survival, and they must be reattached without torsion or kinking to provide the heart with its supply of oxygen. The advantage of the arterial switch procedure is the reestablishment of normal circulation, with the left ventricle acting as the systemic pump. Potential complications of the arterial switch include narrowing at the great artery anastomoses and coronary artery insufficiency.

Intraatrial baffle repairs: Intraatrial baffle repairs are rarely performed, although many adolescents and adults survive today with repairs that were done more than 15 years ago. An intraatrial baffle is created to divert venous blood to the mitral valve and pulmonary venous blood to the tricuspid valve using the patient's atrial septum (Senning procedure) or a prosthetic material (Mustard procedure). A disadvantage is the continuing role of the right ventricle as the systemic pump and the late development of right ventricular failure and rhythm disturbances. Other potential postoperative complications include loss of normal sinus rhythm, baffle leaks, and ventricular dysfunction.

Rastelli procedure: This procedure is the operative choice in infants with TGA, VSD, and severe PS. It involves closure of the VSD with a baffle so that left ventricular blood is directed through the VSD into the aorta. The pulmonic valve is then closed, and a conduit is placed from the right ventricle to the pulmonary artery to create a physiologically normal circulation. Unfortunately, this procedure requires multiple conduit replacements as the child grows.

Prognosis: Mortality rate varies dependent upon the anatomy and procedure performed. The operative mortality rate for neonates with TGA and intact ventricular septum is at 6% (Park, 2014). Potential long-term problems include suprapulmonic stenosis and neoaortic dilation and regurgitation, as well as coronary artery obstruction.

Total Anomalous Pulmonary Venous Connection

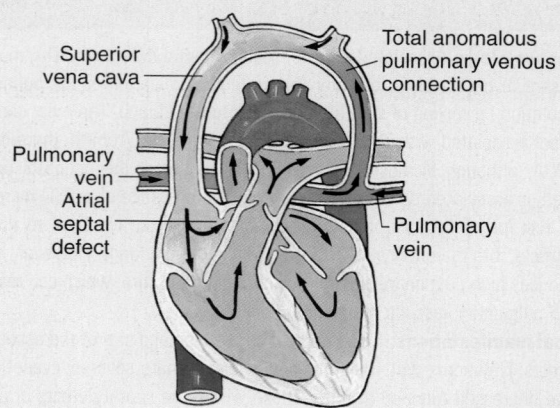

Description: Rare defect characterized by failure of the pulmonary veins to join the left atrium. Instead, the pulmonary veins are abnormally connected to the systemic venous circuit via the right atrium or various veins draining toward the right atrium, such as the SVC. The abnormal attachment results in mixed blood being returned to the right atrium and shunted from the right to the left through an ASD. TAPVC (also called *total anomalous pulmonary venous return* or *total anomalous pulmonary venous drainage*) is classified according to the pulmonary venous point of attachment as follows:

Supracardiac: Attachment above the diaphragm, such as to the SVC (most common form) (see Fig. 42.9)

Cardiac: Direct attachment to the heart, such as to the right atrium or coronary sinus

Infradiaphragmatic: Attachment below the diaphragm, such as to the IVC (most severe form)

Pathophysiology: The right atrium receives all the blood that normally would flow into the left atrium. As a result, whereas the right side of the heart hypertrophies, the left side, especially the left atrium, may remain small. An associated ASD or patent foramen ovale allows systemic venous blood to shunt from the higher-pressure right atrium to the left atrium and into the left side of the heart. As a result, the oxygen saturation of the blood in both sides of the heart (and ultimately in the systemic arterial circulation) is the same. If the pulmonary blood flow is large, pulmonary venous return is also large, and the amount of saturated blood is relatively high. However, if there is obstruction to pulmonary venous drainage, pulmonary venous return is impeded, pulmonary venous pressure rises, and pulmonary interstitial edema develops and eventually contributes to HF. Infradiaphragmatic TAPVC is often associated with obstruction to pulmonary venous drainage and is a surgical emergency.

Clinical manifestations: Most infants develop cyanosis early in life. The degree of cyanosis is inversely related to the amount of pulmonary blood flow—the more pulmonary blood, the less cyanosis. Children with unobstructed TAPVC may be asymptomatic until pulmonary vascular resistance decreases during infancy, increasing pulmonary blood flow with resulting signs of HF. Cyanosis becomes worse with pulmonary vein obstruction; when obstruction occurs, the infant's condition usually deteriorates rapidly. Without intervention, cardiac failure will progress to death.

Surgical treatment: Corrective repair is performed in early infancy. The surgical approach varies with the anatomic defect. In general, however, the common pulmonary vein is anastomosed to the back of the left atrium, the ASD is closed, and the anomalous pulmonary venous connection is ligated. The cardiac type is most easily repaired; the infradiaphragmatic type carries the highest morbidity and mortality because of the higher incidence of pulmonary vein obstruction. Potential postoperative complications include reobstruction; bleeding; dysrhythmias, particularly heart block; PAH; and persistent heart failure.

Prognosis: Mortality is between 5% and 10% for infants without obstruction, and it can be as high as 20% for infants with infradiaphragmatic type (Park, 2014).

Truncus Arteriosus

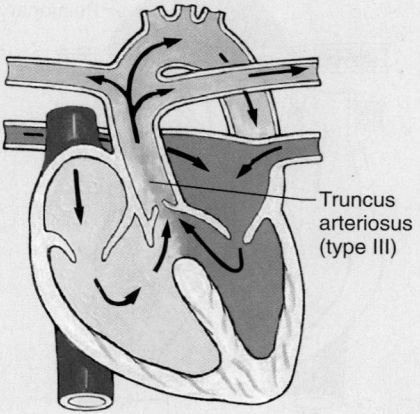

Description: Failure of normal septation and division of the embryonic bulbar trunk into the pulmonary artery and the aorta, which results in development of a single vessel that overrides both ventricles. Blood from both ventricles mixes in the common great artery, which leads to desaturation and hypoxemia.

BOX 42.4   Mixed Defects—cont'd

Blood ejected from the heart flows preferentially to the lower-pressure pulmonary arteries so that pulmonary blood flow is increased and systemic blood flow is reduced. There are three types:

Type I: A single pulmonary trunk arises near the base of the truncus and divides into the left and right pulmonary arteries.

Type II: The left and right pulmonary arteries arise separately but in close proximity and at the same level from the back of the truncus.

Type III: The pulmonary arteries arise independently from the sides of the truncus.

Pathophysiology: Blood ejected from the left and right ventricles enters the common trunk so that pulmonary and systemic circulations are mixed. Blood flow is distributed to the pulmonary and systemic circulations according to the relative resistances of each system. The amount of pulmonary blood flow depends on the size of the pulmonary arteries and the pulmonary vascular resistance. Generally, resistance to pulmonary blood flow is less than systemic vascular resistance, which results in preferential blood flow to the lungs. Pulmonary vascular disease develops at an early age in patients with truncus arteriosus.

Clinical manifestations: Most infants are symptomatic with moderate to severe HF and variable cyanosis, poor growth, and activity intolerance. There is a holosystolic murmur at the left sternal murmur with a diastolic murmur present if truncal regurgitation is present. Thirty-five percent of patients have 22q11 deletions (Goldmuntz, Clark, Mitchell, et al., 1998).

Surgical treatment: Early repair is performed in the first month of life. It involves closing the VSD so that the truncus arteriosus receives the outflow from the left ventricle and excising the pulmonary arteries from the aorta and attaching them to the right ventricle by means of a homograft. Currently, homografts (segments of cadaver aorta and pulmonary artery that are treated with antibiotics and cryopreserved) are preferred over synthetic conduits to establish continuity between the right ventricle and pulmonary artery. Homografts are more flexible and easier to use during the procedure and appear less prone to obstruction. Postoperative complications include persistent heart failure, bleeding, PAH, dysrhythmias, and residual VSD. Because conduits are not living tissue, they will not grow along with the child and may also become narrowed with calcifications. One or more conduit replacements will be needed in childhood.

Prognosis: Mortality is greater than 10%; future operations are required to replace the conduits.

Hypoplastic Left Heart Syndrome

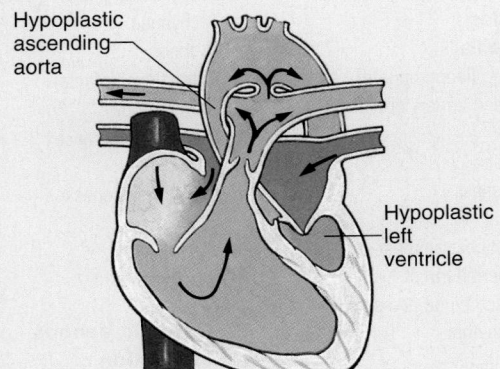

Description: Underdevelopment of the left side of the heart, resulting in a hypoplastic left ventricle and aortic atresia. Most blood from the left atrium flows across the patent foramen ovale to the right atrium, to the right ventricle, and out the pulmonary artery. The descending aorta receives blood from the PDA supplying systemic blood flow.

Pathophysiology: An ASD or patent foramen ovale allows saturated blood from the left atrium to mix with desaturated blood from the right atrium and to flow through the right ventricle and out into the pulmonary artery. From the pulmonary artery, the blood flows both to the lungs and through the ductus arteriosus into the aorta and out to the body. The amount of blood flow to the pulmonary and systemic circulations depends on the relationship between the pulmonary and systemic vascular resistances. The coronary and cerebral vessels receive blood by retrograde flow through the hypoplastic ascending aorta.

Clinical manifestations: The patient has mild cyanosis and signs of HF until the PDA closes and then progressive deterioration with cyanosis and decreased cardiac output, leading to cardiovascular collapse. The condition is usually fatal in the first months of life without intervention.

Therapeutic management: Neonates require stabilization with mechanical ventilation and inotropic support preoperatively. A prostaglandin E_1 infusion is needed to maintain ductal patency and ensure adequate systemic blood flow.

Surgical treatment: A multiple-stage approach is used. The first stage is a Norwood procedure, which involves an anastomosis of the main pulmonary artery to the aorta to create a new aorta, shunting to provide pulmonary blood flow (usually with a modified Blalock-Taussig shunt), and creation of a large ASD. Postoperative complications include imbalance of systemic and pulmonary blood flow, bleeding, low cardiac output, and persistent heart failure. A new modification of the first-stage repair is the use of a right ventricle–to–pulmonary artery homograft conduit instead of a shunt to supply pulmonary blood flow (Sano procedure). The second stage is often a bidirectional Glenn shunt procedure (see Fig. 42.9) or a hemi-Fontan operation. Both involve anastomosing the SVC to the right pulmonary artery so that SVC flow bypasses the right atrium and flows directly to the lungs. The procedure is usually done at 3 to 6 months of age to relieve cyanosis and reduce the volume load on the right ventricle. The final repair is a modified Fontan procedure (see Tricuspid Atresia in Box 42.3).

Transplantation: Heart transplantation in the newborn period is another option for these infants. Problems include the shortage of newborn organ donors, risk for rejection, long-term problems with chronic immunosuppression, and infection (see the "Heart Transplantation" section earlier in this chapter).

Prognosis: For the first-stage repair, survival rates vary widely in different centers. Much progress has been made, and some experienced centers are reporting mortality rates of about 10% (Tweddell, Hoffman, Mussatto, et al., 2002). Long-term problems with repair include worsening ventricular function, tricuspid regurgitation, recurrent aortic arch narrowing, dysrhythmias, and developmental delays. There is a risk for mortality between surgical procedures. The mortality for the later two operations is less than 5%.

ASD, Atrial septal defect; *HF,* heart failure; *IV,* intravenous; *IVC,* inferior vena cava; *PAH,* pulmonary artery hypertension; *PDA,* patent ductus arteriosus; *PS,* pulmonic stenosis; *SVC,* superior vena cava; *TAPVC,* total anomalous pulmonary venous connection; *TGA,* transposition of the great arteries; *VSD,* ventricular septal defect.

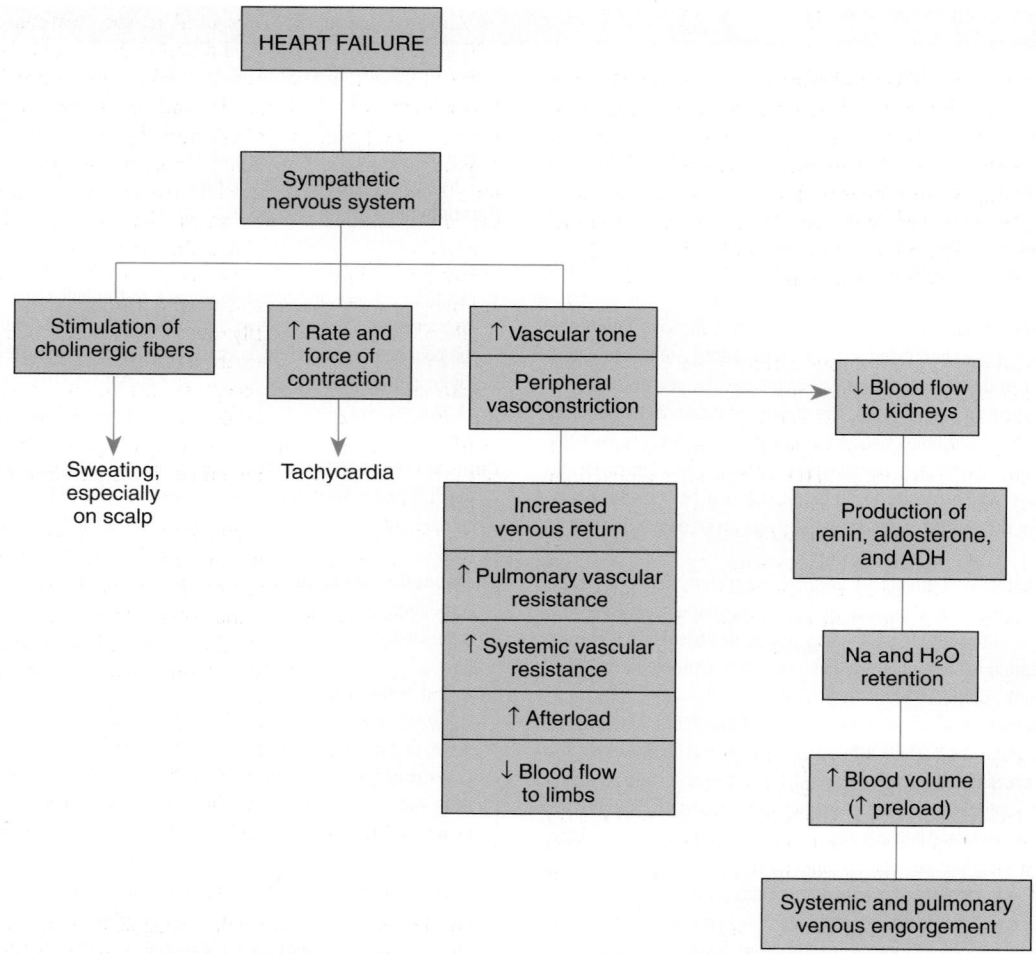

FIG 42.7 Pathophysiology of heart failure. *ADH,* Antidiuretic hormone.

blood effectively into the pulmonary artery, resulting in increased pressure in the right atrium and systemic venous circulation. Systemic venous hypertension causes hepatosplenomegaly and occasionally edema. In left-sided failure, the left ventricle is unable to pump blood into the systemic circulation, resulting in increased pressure in the left atrium and pulmonary veins. The lungs become congested with blood, causing elevated pulmonary pressures and pulmonary edema.

Although each type of HF produces different signs and symptoms, clinically, it is unusual to observe solely right- or left-sided failure in children. Because each side of the heart depends on adequate function of the other side, failure of one chamber causes a reciprocal change in the opposite chamber.

If the abnormalities precipitating HF are not corrected, the heart muscle becomes damaged. Despite compensatory mechanisms, the heart is unable to maintain an adequate cardiac output. Decreased blood flow to the kidneys continues to stimulate sodium and water reabsorption, leading to fluid overload, increased workload on the heart, and congestion in the pulmonary and systemic circulations (Fig. 42.7).

Clinical Manifestations

The signs and symptoms of HF can be divided into three groups: (1) impaired myocardial function, (2) pulmonary congestion, and (3) systemic venous congestion (Box 42.5). Because these hemodynamic changes occur from different causes and at differing times, the clinical presentation may vary among children.

BOX 42.5   Clinical Manifestations of Heart Failure

Impaired Myocardial Function
Tachycardia
Sweating (inappropriate)
Decreased urinary output
Fatigue
Weakness
Restlessness
Anorexia
Pale, cool extremities
Weak peripheral pulses
Decreased blood pressure (BP)
Gallop rhythm
Cardiomegaly

Pulmonary Congestion
Tachypnea
Dyspnea
Retractions (infants)
Flaring nares
Exercise intolerance
Orthopnea
Cough, hoarseness
Cyanosis
Wheezing
Grunting

Systemic Venous Congestion
Weight gain
Hepatomegaly
Peripheral edema, especially periorbital
Ascites
Neck vein distention (children)

Diagnostic Evaluation

Diagnosis is made on the basis of clinical symptoms, such as tachypnea and tachycardia at rest, dyspnea, retractions, activity intolerance (especially during feeding in infants), feeding intolerance, weight gain caused by fluid retention, and hepatomegaly. Chest radiography demonstrates cardiomegaly and increased pulmonary blood flow. Ventricular hypertrophy, abnormal rhythm, or decreased voltages appear on the ECG. An echocardiogram is done to determine the cause of HF, such as a congenital heart defect or poor ventricular function.

Therapeutic Management

The goals of treatment are to (1) improve cardiac function (increase contractility and decrease afterload), (2) remove accumulated fluid and sodium (decrease preload), (3) decrease cardiac demands, and (4) improve tissue oxygenation and decrease oxygen consumption. For most infants diagnosed with HF, the cause is CHD. Infants are stabilized on medical therapy and then referred for surgical repair. Today many children are being surgically repaired in the neonatal and early infancy stages before the onset of HF symptoms (Margossian, 2008). For children newly diagnosed with HF, the cause may be worsening ventricular function following a previous cardiac repair, cardiomyopathy, arrhythmia, or other conditions. In addition to management of HF, the underlying cause is treated if possible.

Improve Cardiac Function

Three groups of drugs are used to enhance myocardial function in HF: (1) digitalis glycosides (digoxin), which improve contractility, (2) angiotensin-converting enzyme (ACE) inhibitors, which reduce the afterload on the heart and thus make it easier for the heart to pump, and (3) beta blockers. Myocardial efficiency is improved through administration of digitalis glycosides. The beneficial effects are increased cardiac output, decreased heart size, decreased venous pressure, and relief of edema. In children, digoxin (Lanoxin) is used almost exclusively because of its more rapid onset. Note the dose is calculated in micrograms (1000 mcg = 1 mg). During initiation, the child is monitored by means of an ECG to observe for the desired effects (prolonged PR interval and reduced ventricular rate) and detect side effects, especially dysrhythmias.

Another group of drugs used in the treatment of HF, the ACE inhibitors, inhibit the normal function of the renin/angiotensin system in the kidney. The ACE inhibitors block the conversion of angiotensin I to angiotensin II so that, instead of vasoconstriction, vasodilation occurs. Vasodilation results in decreased pulmonary and systemic vascular resistance, decreased BP, and a reduction in afterload. It also reduces the secretion of aldosterone, which reduces preload by preventing volume expansion from fluid retention and decreases the risk for hypokalemia. Common medications used in children are captopril (Capoten), enalapril (Vasotec), and lisinopril. The principal side effects of ACE inhibitors are hypotension, cough, and renal dysfunction.

Beta blockers, specifically carvedilol (Coreg), are the newest medications to be added to the treatment of some children with chronic HF. The α- and β-adrenergic receptors are blocked, causing decreased heart rate, decreased BP, and vasodilation. It has been shown to decrease morbidity and mortality in some adults with HF and is being used selectively in children. Side effects included dizziness, headache, and hypotension.

Cardiac resynchronization therapy (CRT) using biventricular pacing is an effective treatment in adult patients with HF and is beginning to be applied in the pediatric population. With pharmacologic therapies described earlier, CRT has the potential to improve cardiac function in this group of patients, including those with a single ventricle (Cecchin, Frangini, Brown, et al., 2009; Dubin, Janousek, Rhee, et al., 2005).

> **! NURSING ALERT**
>
> Because ACE inhibitors also block the action of aldosterone, the addition of potassium supplements or spironolactone (Aldactone) to the drug regimen of patients taking diuretics is usually not needed and may cause hyperkalemia.

Remove Accumulated Fluid and Sodium

Treatment consists of diuretics, possible fluid restriction, and possible sodium restriction. Diuretics are the mainstay of therapy to eliminate excess water and salt to prevent reaccumulation. The most frequently used agents are listed in Table 42.3. Because furosemide and the thiazides are potassium-losing diuretics, potassium supplements may be prescribed, and rich dietary sources of the electrolyte are encouraged.

TABLE 42.3 Diuretics Used in Heart Failure

Actions	Comments	Care Management
Furosemide (Lasix): Blocks reabsorption of sodium and water in proximal renal tubule and interferes with reabsorption of sodium	Drug of choice in severe HF Causes excretion of chloride and potassium (hypokalemia may precipitate digitalis toxicity)	Begin to record output as soon as drug is given. Observe for dehydration caused by profound diuresis. Observe for side effects (nausea and vomiting, diarrhea, ototoxicity, hypokalemia, dermatitis, postural hypotension). Encourage foods high in potassium, or give potassium supplements. Monitor chloride and acid-base balance with long-term therapy. Observe for signs of digoxin toxicity.
Chlorothiazide (Diuril): Acts directly on distal tubules to decrease sodium, water, potassium, chloride, and bicarbonate absorption	Less frequently used drug Causes hypokalemia, acidosis from large doses	Observe for side effects (nausea, weakness, dizziness, paresthesia, muscle cramps, skin eruptions, hypokalemia, acidosis). Encourage foods high in potassium, or give potassium supplements.
Spironolactone (Aldactone): Blocks action of aldosterone, which promotes retention of sodium and excretion of potassium	Weak diuretic Has potassium-sparing effect; frequently used with thiazides, furosemide Poorly absorbed from GI tract Takes several days to achieve maximum actions	Observe for side effects (skin rash, drowsiness, ataxia, hyperkalemia). Do not administer potassium supplements.

GI, Gastrointestinal; *HF,* heart failure.

Fluid restriction may be required in the acute stages of HF and must be carefully calculated to avoid dehydrating the child, especially if cyanotic CHD and significant polycythemia are present. Infants rarely need fluid restrictions because HF makes feeding so difficult that they struggle to take maintenance fluids.

Sodium-restricted diets are used less often in children than in adults to control HF because of their potential negative effects on the child's appetite and ultimate growth. If salt intake is restricted, additional table salt and highly salted foods are avoided.

Decrease Cardiac Demands

To lessen the workload on the heart, metabolic needs are minimized by (1) providing a neutral thermal environment to prevent cold stress in infants, (2) treating any existing infections, (3) reducing the effort of breathing (by placement in the semi-Fowler's position), (4) using medication to sedate an irritable child, and (5) providing for rest and decreasing environmental stimuli.

Improve Tissue Oxygenation

The preceding measures serve to increase tissue oxygenation, either by improving myocardial function or by lessening tissue oxygen demands. In addition, supplemental cool humidified oxygen may be administered to increase the amount of available oxygen during inspiration. Oxygen administration is especially helpful in patients with pulmonary edema, intercurrent respiratory tract infections, and increased pulmonary vascular resistance (oxygen is a vasodilator that decreases pulmonary vascular resistance).

An oxygen hood, nasal cannula, or face tent is used to deliver oxygen. Nasal cannulas are ideal for long-term oxygen administration because the child can be ambulatory and can easily eat and drink. Cool humidification is necessary to counteract the drying effect of oxygen. The amount of cool humidity is carefully regulated to prevent chilling.

QUALITY PATIENT OUTCOMES: Heart Failure
- Adequate cardiac output
- Decreased cardiac demands
- Improved respiratory function
- No evidence of fluid excess
- Adequate support and education

Care Management

The infant or child with HF may be acutely ill, and some may require intensive care until the symptoms improve. Expert nursing care is essential to reduce the cardiac demands that strain the failing heart muscle. During this time, the child and family require emotional support. Although the objectives of nursing care are the same, interventions

BOX 42.6 Common Signs of Digoxin Toxicity in Children

Gastrointestinal	Cardiac
Nausea	Bradycardia
Vomiting	Dysrhythmias
Anorexia	

differ depending on the child's age (see Nursing Care Plan box: The Child with Heart Failure).

Assist in Measures to Improve Cardiac Function

The nurse's responsibility in administering digoxin includes calculating and administering the correct dosage, observing for signs of toxicity, and instituting parental teaching regarding drug administration at home. The child's apical pulse is always checked before administering digoxin. As a general rule, the drug is not given if the pulse is below 90 to 110 beats/min in infants and young children or below 70 beats/min in older children (the cutoff point for adults is 60 beats/min). However, because the pulse rate varies in children in different age groups, the written drug order should specify at what heart rate the drug is withheld. The nurse should also use judgment in evaluating the pulse rate. If it is significantly lower than the previous recording, the dose should be withheld until the practitioner is notified.

The apical rate is taken because a pulse deficit (radial pulse rate lower than apical) may be present with decreased cardiac output. It is auscultated for 1 full minute to evaluate alterations in rhythm. If the child is monitored by means of an ECG, a rhythm strip is obtained and attached to the chart for rate and rhythm analysis, such as abnormal lengthening of the PR interval (>50% increase over predigitalization interval) and dysrhythmias.

Digoxin is a potentially dangerous drug because of its narrow margin of safety of therapeutic, toxic, and lethal doses. Many toxic responses are extensions of its therapeutic effects. Therefore, the nurse must maintain a high index of suspicion for signs of toxicity when administering digoxin (Box 42.6).

Because digoxin toxicity can occur from accidental overdose, great care must be taken in properly calculating and measuring the dosage. When converting milligrams to micrograms to milliliters, the nurse carefully checks the placement of the decimal point, because an error causes a significant change in dosage. For example, 0.1 mg is 10 times the dosage of 0.01 mg.

These same principles are taught to parents in preparation for discharge, although the correct dose in milliliters is usually specified on the container, thus reducing potential errors in calculation. The nurse watches the parent measure the elixir in the dropper and stresses the level mark as the meniscus of the fluid that is observed at eye level.

Parents are also advised of the signs of toxicity. According to the practitioner's preference, they may be taught to take the pulse before giving the drug. A return demonstration of the procedure from the parents or another principal caregiver is included as part of the teaching plan. Their level of anxiety in counting the pulse is assessed because

NURSING CARE PLAN

The Child With Heart Failure

Case Study

George is a 2-week-old patient with congenital heart disease (CHD). At birth he initially showed no signs or symptoms, but within the first week he developed symptoms of heart failure (HF). He was found to have coarctation of the aorta and is now under the care of the cardiology team and scheduled for surgery. George is experiencing more signs of HF, and the care is now focused on preventing further symptoms before he goes to surgery.

Assessment

What are the most important signs of HF that you need to look for in a young infant?

Heart Failure: Defining Characteristics

Tachycardia
Tachypnea
Ineffective peripheral circulation, cool extremities
Hypotension
Rapid, weak peripheral pulses
Prolonged capillary refill, longer than 2 or 3 seconds
Narrow pulse pressure
Distended neck veins in older children
Cardiomegaly revealed on chest radiograph
Gallop rhythm
Edema
Rapid weight gain
Feeding difficulty
Irritability

Nursing Diagnosis

Decreased Cardiac Output related to inadequate volume of blood pumped by the heart per minute to meet the metabolic demands of the body.

Nursing Interventions and Rationales

What are the most appropriate nursing interventions for an infant in heart failure?

Nursing Interventions	Rationales
Assess and record heart rate, respiratory rate, blood pressure (BP), and any signs or symptoms of decreased cardiac output every 2 to 4 hours and as necessary.	To detect change in vital signs and infant's physical status that reflect altered cardiac output and cardiogenic shock
Administer cardiac drugs on schedule. Assess and record any side effects or any signs and symptoms of toxicity. Follow hospital protocol for administration.	To avoid dangers inherent in failure to administer cardiac drugs as prescribed and to perform careful assessment before administration
Keep accurate record of intake and output.	To detect HF, which causes decreased urinary output
Weigh George on same scale at same time of day as previously. Document results, and compare to previous weight.	To monitor for weight increases, which may indicate excess fluid accumulation
Administer diuretics on schedule. Assess and record effectiveness and any side effects noted.	To eliminate excess water and salt because fluid retention commonly occurs with HF
Offer small, frequent feedings to George's tolerance.	To increase caloric intake and compensate for fatigue during feeding and increased metabolic rate because of poor cardiac function
Organize nursing care to allow George uninterrupted rest.	To allow adequate rest because poor cardiac output decreases energy level and lowers tolerance to activity

Expected Outcomes

George's cardiac function will be protected by decreasing cardiac demands, improving respiratory function, and preventing fluid excess.

George will have adequate cardiac output as evidenced by:
- Heart rate within acceptable range (state specific range)
- Respiratory rate within acceptable range (state specific range)
- Skin warm to touch
- Strong and equal peripheral pulses
- BP normal for age
- Brisk capillary refill within 2 or 3 seconds
- Lack of distended neck veins
- Normal sinus rhythm
- Lack of edema
- Adequate urinary output (1 to 2 mL/kg/hour)
- Age-appropriate weight gain on standardized growth curve
- Successful feeding

Case Study (Continued)

George's BP is increased, and the pulses in his arms are bounding. You find weak femoral pulses, and his extremities are cool to touch. George's breathing appears labored, and you note nasal flaring but no intercostal retractions at this time. His color is pale and slightly mottled.

Assessment

What are the most important signs and symptoms of impaired breathing in this infant?

Defining Characteristics

Tachypnea
Dyspnea
Retractions
Crackles
Shortness of breath
Cyanosis
Pallor
Mottling
Nasal flaring
Grunting
Head bobbing
Cough
Use of accessory muscles
Activity intolerance

Case Study (Continued)

Do the findings described in the case study concern you?

The effect of the coarctation of the aorta causes a narrowing within the aorta that increases pressure proximal to the defect (upper extremities) and a decreased pressure distal to it (lower extremities). It is not surprising to find high BP, bounding upper extremity pulses, and weak or even absent femoral pulses and cool extremities in these infants. You should follow his breathing patterns closely and observe for breathing changes.

Continued

NURSING CARE PLAN

The Child With Heart Failure—cont'd

How would you assess the effectiveness of these interventions?
Evaluate for changes in breathing patterns, respiratory rate, and labored breath sounds; observe for nasal flaring or change in color to dusky or blue.
Why are breathing pattern changes a concern?
Coarctation of the aorta can cause pulmonary congestion as a result of decreased cardiac output. Breathing difficulties can be a sign of progression of heart failure.

Nursing Diagnosis
Impaired Breathing Pattern related to pulmonary congestion, decreased cardiac output.

Nursing Interventions and Rationales
What are the most appropriate nursing interventions for this diagnosis?

Nursing Interventions	Rationales
Assess and record oxygen saturation every 2 to 4 hours or more often as needed.	To evaluate pulmonary effectiveness
Elevate head of bed at a 30- to 45-degree angle.	To promote maximum chest expansion
Assess and record respiratory rate, breath sounds, and any signs or symptoms of ineffective pattern every 2 to 4 hours and as needed.	To detect indicators of worsening HF
Administer humidified oxygen in correct amount and route of delivery. Record percent of oxygen and route of delivery. Assess and record George's response to therapy.	To reduce respiratory distress by easing respiratory effort
Suction if George has ineffective cough or is unable to manage secretions. Assess and record amount and characteristics of secretions.	To maintain patent airway to promote respiratory expansion

Expected Outcomes
George will have an effective breathing pattern and maintain stable respiratory pattern until surgery as evidenced by respiratory rate within acceptable limits for age.
Infant will have effective breathing pattern as evidenced by:
- Respiratory rate within acceptable range (state specific range)
- Clear and equal breath sounds bilaterally anteriorly and posteriorly
- Pink or tan color
- Absence of nasal flaring, retractions, cough, and head bobbing

- Unlabored breath sounds
- Tolerance of activities appropriate for age

Case Study (Continued)
George's parents ask you what you have found in your initial assessment. They ask about why he seems to be having problems breathing. What should you say to his parents?

Assessment
What are the most important aspects of George's care to discuss with his parents at this time?

Family's Knowledge of Illness-Defining Characteristics
Understands definition of heart failure
States four characteristics of signs of heart failure
Describes medications the infant is taking
Expresses fears and concerns
Shows appropriate reactions to infant's illness

Nursing Diagnosis
Readiness for Enhanced Knowledge related to parents' interest in George's health status.

Nursing Interventions and Rationales
What are the most appropriate nursing interventions for this diagnosis?

Nursing Interventions	Rationales
Educate family about characteristics of HF. Assess and record effectiveness of teaching session.	To promote understanding of measures to improve cardiac function and decrease demands
Educate family about George's daily care, such as medication administration. Assess and record results and family's participation in care.	To promote understanding of disease and medication side effects
Educate family regarding illness factors that should prompt them to take George to the primary care provider (fever, blue skin color, poor eating).	To prevent further compromise of cardiac and respiratory status.

Expected Outcomes
George's parents will understand the signs and symptoms of HF and will understand the actions being taken by the health care team.

overconcern about the heart rate may result in excessive withholding of the drug.

Monitor Afterload Reduction
For patients receiving ACE inhibitors for afterload reduction, the nurse should carefully monitor BP before and after dose administration, observe for symptoms of hypotension, and notify the practitioner if BP is low. Numerous medications affecting the kidney can potentiate renal dysfunction, so children taking multiple diuretics and an ACE inhibitor require careful assessment of serum electrolytes and renal function.

Decrease Cardiac Demands
The infant requires rest and conservation of energy for feeding. Every effort is made to organize nursing activities to allow for uninterrupted periods of sleep. Whenever possible, parents are encouraged to stay with their infant to provide the holding, rocking, and cuddling that help children sleep more soundly. To minimize disturbing the infant, changing bed linens and complete bathing are done only when necessary. Feeding is planned to accommodate the infant's sleep and wake patterns. The child is fed at the first sign of hunger, such as when sucking on fists, rather than waiting until he or she cries for a bottle because the stress of crying exhausts the limited energy supply. Because infants with HF tire easily and may sleep through feedings, smaller feedings every 3 hours may be helpful. Gavage feedings may be instituted to provide adequate nutrition and allow the infant to rest.

Every effort is made to minimize unnecessary stress. Older children need an explanation of what is happening to them to decrease anxiety about their illness and necessary treatments, such as cardiac monitoring, oxygen administration, and medications. Outlining a plan for the day, preparing the child for tests and procedures, providing quiet activities, and providing adequate rest periods are all helpful interventions with older children. Some infants and children require sedation during the acute phase of illness to allow them to rest.

Temperature is carefully monitored because hyperthermia or hypothermia increases the need for oxygen. Febrile states are reported to the physician because infection must be promptly treated. Maintaining body temperature is of special importance in children who are receiving cool, humidified oxygen and in infants, who tend to be diaphoretic and lose heat by way of evaporation.

Skin breakdown from edema is prevented with a change of position every 2 hours (from side to side while in the semi-Fowler's position) and use of a pressure-relieving mattress or bed. The skin, especially over the sacrum, is checked for evidence of redness from pressure.

Reduce Respiratory Distress

Careful assessment, positioning, and oxygen administration can reduce respiratory distress. Respirations are counted for 1 full minute during a resting state. Any evidence of increased respiratory distress is reported, because this may indicate worsening HF.

Infants are positioned to encourage maximum chest expansion, with the head of the bed elevated; they should sit up in an infant seat or be held at a 45-degree angle. Children prefer to sleep on several pillows and remain in the semi-Fowler's or high-Fowler's position during waking hours. Safety restraints, such as those used with infant seats, are applied low on the abdomen and loosely enough to provide both safety and maximum expansion.

The infant or child is often given humidified supplemental oxygen via oxygen hood or tent, nasal cannula, or mask. The child's response to oxygen therapy is carefully evaluated by noting respiratory rate, ease of respiration, color, and especially oxygen saturation as measured by oximetry.

Respiratory tract infections can exacerbate HF and should be appropriately treated and prevented if possible. The child should be protected from persons with respiratory tract infections and have a noninfectious roommate. Good hand washing is practiced before and after caring for any hospitalized child. Antibiotics may be given to combat respiratory tract infection. The nurse ensures that the drug is given at equally divided times over a 24-hour schedule to maintain high blood levels of the antibiotic.

Maintain Nutritional Status

Meeting the nutritional needs of infants with HF or serious cardiac defects is a nursing challenge. The metabolic rate of these infants is greater because of poor cardiac function and increased heart and respiratory rates. Their caloric needs are greater than those of the average infant because of their increased metabolic rate, yet their ability to take in adequate calories is hampered by their fatigue. Feeding for a fragile infant with serious CHD is similar to exercising for an adult, and these infants often do not have the energy or cardiac reserve to do extra work. The nurse seeks measures to enable the infant to feed easily without excess fatigue and to increase the caloric density of the formula.

The infant should be well rested before feeding and fed soon after awakening so as not to expend energy on crying. A 3-hour feeding schedule works well for many infants. (Feeding every 2 hours does not provide enough rest between feedings, and a 4-hour schedule requires an increased volume of feeding, which many infants are unable to take.) The feeding schedule should be individualized to the infant's needs. A feeding goal of 150 mL/kg/day and at least 120 kcal/kg/day is common for newborns with significant heart disease (Steltzer, Rudd, & Pick, 2005). A soft preemie nipple or a slit in a regular nipple to enlarge the

opening decreases the infant's energy expenditure while sucking. Infants should be well supported and fed in a semiupright position. Infants may need to rest frequently and may need to have the jaw and cheeks stroked to encourage sucking. Generally, giving an infant about a half hour to complete a feeding is reasonable. Prolonging the feeding time can exhaust the infant and decrease the rest period between feedings.

Infants with feeding difficulties are often gavage fed using a nasogastric tube to supplement their oral intake and ensure adequate calories. If they are very stressed and fatigued, experiencing signs of respiratory distress, or tachypneic to 80 to 100 breaths/min, oral feedings may be withheld and all nutrition given by gavage feedings. Gavage feedings are usually a temporary measure until the infant's medical status improves and nutritional needs can be met through oral feedings. Some infants with severe HF, neurologic deficits, or significant gastroesophageal reflux may need placement of a gastrostomy tube to allow adequate nutrition.

The caloric density of formulas is frequently increased by concentration and then adding Polycose, medium-chain triglyceride oil, or corn oil. Infant formulas provide 20 kcal/oz, and the use of additives can increase the calories to 30 kcal/oz or more. This allows the infant to obtain more calories despite a smaller volume intake of formula. The caloric density of the formula needs to be increased slowly (by 2 kcal/oz/day) to prevent diarrhea or formula intolerance. Breastfeeding mothers are encouraged to provide the infant with alternating feedings of breast milk and high-calorie formulas. Some lactating mothers prefer to feed the child expressed breast milk that has been fortified with Similac or Enfamil powder, Polycose, or corn oil to increase caloric intake. A diet plan specific to the individual infant's needs is calculated and prescribed by the nutritionist in collaboration with the other health personnel. The nurse needs to reinforce this information with the parents as necessary.

Assist in Measures to Promote Fluid Loss

When diuretics are given, the nurse records fluid intake and output and monitors body weight at the same time each day to evaluate benefit from the drug. Because profound diuresis may cause dehydration and electrolyte imbalance (loss of sodium, potassium, chloride, bicarbonate), the nurse observes for signs indicating either complication, as well as signs and symptoms suggesting reactions to the drugs. Diuretics should be given early in the day to children who are toilet trained to avoid the need to urinate at night. If potassium-losing diuretics are given, the nurse encourages foods high in potassium, such as bananas, oranges, whole grains, legumes, and leafy vegetables and administers prescribed supplements. Serum potassium levels are checked frequently.

> **! NURSING ALERT**
>
> Mix the elixir with fruit juice (red punch or grape juice works well) to disguise the bitter taste and to prevent intestinal irritation from a concentrated solution.

Fluid restriction is rarely necessary in infants because of their difficulty in feeding. However, if fluids are restricted, the nurse plans fluid intake schedules for a 24-hour period, allowing for most fluids during waking hours. Toddlers and preschoolers should be given small amounts of liquid in small cups so the containers appear full. Older children's cooperation is gained by placing them in charge of recording their fluid intake.

If salt is limited, the nurse discusses food sources of sodium with the family and discourages their bringing salt-containing treats to the child. At mealtimes, the child's tray is checked to make sure the appropriate diet is given.

FAMILY-CENTERED CARE

Diagnosis of Heart Disease

Remember, we don't have your experience. We don't see children every day who have heart disease. We would have been upset finding out our child had to have his tonsils out. How could we ever be prepared for this? Please remember, we only know people who have trivial heart murmurs. How could we ever expect this to happen? And to us, this is the worst problem we've ever heard of.

We still fear most what we don't know and understand. Be honest with us. If you don't know either, tell us. But at least don't leave us wondering about what you know and we don't. Not knowing anything really can be worse than knowing something bad. Be honest but don't strip us of hope.

Please, remember we are trying to learn complex information in a moment of time. And trying to learn it in a context of great pain and emotional investment. This is our lives you're talking about. Please be thorough but keep it simple. Tell us again, maybe even again and again, when we can hear better.

From Schrey, C., Schrey, M. (1994). A parent's perspective: our needs and our message. *Critical Care Nursing Clinics of North America, 6*(1), 113–119.

Support Child and Family

HF is a serious complication of heart disease. Parents and older children are usually acutely aware of the critical nature of the condition. Because stress places additional demands on cardiac function, the nurse should focus on reducing anxiety through anticipatory preparation, frequent communication with the parent regarding the child's progress, and constant reassurance that everything possible is being done.

Home care involves many of the same interventions discussed in the Plan for Discharge and Home Care section. The nurse teaches the family about the medications that need to be administered and alerts them to the signs of worsening HF that require medical attention, such as increased sweating, decreased urinary output (noted in fewer wet diapers or infrequent use of the toilet), or poor feeding. Every effort is made to improve the family's adherence to the medication schedule by adapting the schedule to their usual home routines, avoiding medications during the night, making it as simple as possible, and using charts or visual aids to remember when to give medications (see Chapter 39). Written instructions regarding correct administration of digoxin are essential (see Family-Centered Care box: Diagnosis of Heart Disease), including an explanation regarding signs of toxicity.

If HF is the end stage of a severe heart defect, the nurse cares for this child as for any child who is terminally ill, using the principles discussed in Chapter 36.

HYPOXEMIA

Hypoxemia refers to an arterial oxygen tension (or pressure, PaO_2) that is less than normal and can be identified by a decreased arterial saturation or a decreased PaO_2. *Hypoxia* is a reduction in tissue oxygenation that results from low oxygen saturations and PaO_2 and results in impaired cellular processes. *Cyanosis* is a blue discoloration in the mucous membranes, skin, and nail beds of the child with reduced oxygen saturation. It results from the presence of deoxygenated hemoglobin (hemoglobin not bound to oxygen) in a concentration of 5 g/dL of blood. Cyanosis is usually apparent when arterial oxygen saturations are 80% to 85%. Determination of cyanosis is subjective. It can vary depending on skin pigment, quality of light, color of the room, or clothing worn by the child. The presence of cyanosis may not accurately reflect arterial hypoxemia because both oxygen saturation and the amount of circulating

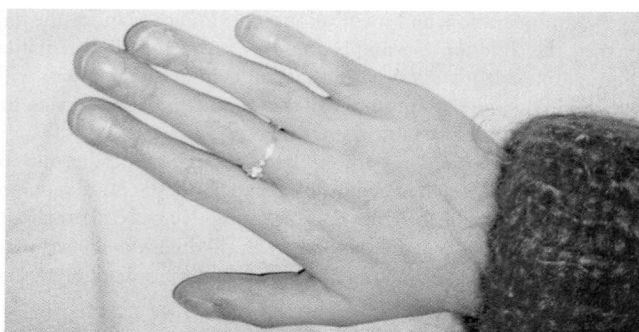

FIG 42.8 Clubbing of the fingers.

hemoglobin are involved. Children with severe anemia may not be cyanotic despite severe hypoxemia because the hemoglobin level may be too low to produce the characteristic blue color. Conversely, patients with polycythemia may appear cyanotic despite a near-normal PaO_2. Heart defects that cause hypoxemia and cyanosis result from desaturated venous blood (blue blood) entering the systemic circulation without passing through the lungs.

Clinical Manifestations

Over time, two physiologic changes occur in the body in response to chronic hypoxemia: polycythemia and clubbing. Polycythemia, an increased number of red blood cells, increases the oxygen-carrying capacity of the blood. However, anemia may result if iron is not readily available for the formation of hemoglobin. Polycythemia increases the viscosity of the blood and crowds out clotting factors. *Clubbing*, a thickening and flattening of the tips of the fingers and toes, is thought to occur because of chronic tissue hypoxemia and polycythemia (Fig. 42.8). Infants with mild hypoxemia may be asymptomatic except for cyanosis and exhibit near-normal growth and development. Those with more severe hypoxemia may exhibit fatigue with feeding, poor weight gain, tachypnea, and dyspnea. Severe hypoxemia resulting in tissue hypoxia is manifested by clinical deterioration and signs of poor perfusion.

Hypercyanotic spells, also referred to as *blue spells* or *tet spells* because they are often seen in infants with tetralogy of Fallot, may occur in any child whose heart defect includes obstruction to pulmonary blood flow and communication between the ventricles. The infant becomes acutely cyanotic and hyperpneic because sudden infundibular spasm decreases pulmonary blood flow and increases right-to-left shunting (the proposed mechanism in tetralogy of Fallot). Spells, rarely seen before 2 months of age, occur most frequently in the first year of life. They occur more often in the morning and may be preceded by feeding, crying, defecation, or stressful procedures. Because profound hypoxemia causes cerebral hypoxia, hypercyanotic spells require prompt assessment and treatment to prevent brain damage or possibly death.

Persistent cyanosis as a result of cyanotic heart defects places the child at risk for significant neurologic complications. Cerebrovascular accident (CVA; stroke), brain abscess, and developmental delays (especially in motor and cognitive development) may result from chronic hypoxia.

Diagnostic Evaluation

Cyanosis in a newborn can be the result of cardiac, pulmonary, metabolic, or hematologic disease, although cardiac and pulmonary causes occur most often. To distinguish between the two, a hyperoxia test is helpful. The infant is placed in a 100% oxygen environment, and blood parameters are monitored. A PaO_2 of 100 mm Hg or higher suggests lung disease,

GUIDELINES

Treating Hypercyanotic Spells

Place infant in knee/chest position (Fig. 42.10).
Use a calm, comforting approach.
Administer 100% "blow-by" oxygen.
Give morphine subcutaneously or through an existing IV line.
Begin IV fluid replacement and volume expansion if needed.
Repeat morphine administration.

IV, Intravenous.

and a PaO$_2$ lower than 100 mm Hg suggests cardiac disease (Park, 2014). An accurate history, a chest radiograph, and especially an echocardiogram contribute to the diagnosis of cyanotic heart disease.

Therapeutic Management

Newborns generally exhibit cyanosis within the first few days of life as the ductus arteriosus, which provided pulmonary blood flow, begins to close. Prostaglandin E$_1$, which causes vasodilation and smooth muscle relaxation, thus increasing dilation and patency of the ductus arteriosus, is administered intravenously to reestablish pulmonary blood flow. The use of prostaglandins has been lifesaving for infants with ductus-dependent cardiac defects. The increase in oxygenation allows the infant to be stabilized and have a complete diagnostic evaluation performed before further treatment is needed.

Hypercyanotic spells occur suddenly, and prompt recognition and treatment are essential. In the hospital setting, spells are often seen during blood drawing or IV insertion, when the child is highly agitated, or after cardiac catheterization. Treatment of a hypercyanotic spell is outlined in the Guidelines box: Treating Hypercyanotic Spells. Morphine, administered subcutaneously or through an existing IV line, helps reduce infundibular spasm. A spell indicates the need for prompt surgical treatment if possible. In infants with defects not amenable to surgical repair, a shunt may be created surgically to increase blood flow to the lungs. Several commonly used shunt procedures are described in Table 42.4 and Fig. 42.9.

The cyanotic infant and child are well hydrated to keep the hematocrit and blood viscosity within acceptable limits to reduce the risk for CVAs. The infant is monitored closely for anemia because of the risk for CVAs and the reduced arterial oxygen-carrying capacity that occurs. Iron supplementation and possibly blood transfusion are used as needed.

Respiratory tract infections or reduced pulmonary function from any cause can worsen hypoxemia in the cyanotic child. Aggressive pulmonary hygiene, chest physical therapy, administration of antibiotics, and use of oxygen to improve arterial saturations are important interventions.

Care Management

The general appearance of infants and children with significant cyanosis poses unique concerns. Blue lips and fingernails are obvious signs of their hidden cardiac defect. Clubbing and small, thin stature in older children further indicate severe heart disease. Adolescents are especially concerned about their body image; children with cyanosis are often teased about their appearance and singled out as different. Many children, when asked what surgery will do, reply, "Make me pink." Their joy and excitement after surgery are evident when they see their pink fingers. Parents are often fearful of their child's bluish color because cyanosis is usually associated with lack of oxygen and severe illness. They also must deal with comments from relatives, friends, and strangers about their child's abnormal color. They need a simple explanation of hypoxemia

TABLE 42.4 Selected Shunt Procedures for Children With Cardiac Defects

Shunt Type	Comments
Modified Blalock-Taussig shunt: Subclavian artery to pulmonary artery using Gore-Tex or Impra tube graft	Shunt flow sometimes excessive, requiring use of diuretics Possibility of thrombosis; aspirin usually prescribed postoperatively Easy to ligate at time of definitive correction Shunt size fixed and may become too small as child grows
Sano modification: Right ventricular to pulmonary artery using Gore-Tex graft	Prevents diastolic runoff of systemic blood into the pulmonary arteries Provides a higher diastolic BP and seemingly better coronary perfusion Used in place of the Modified Blalock-Taussig shunt in the Norwood procedure
Central shunt: Ascending aorta to main pulmonary artery using Gore-Tex graft	Length of shunt acts to restrict blood flow; possibility of symptoms of HF; diuretic therapy sometimes required Uncommon; used when modified Blalock-Taussig shunt cannot be used Easy to insert and remove at time of repair Possibility of thrombosis; aspirin usually prescribed postoperatively
Bidirectional Glenn shunt (cavopulmonary anastomosis): SVC to side of right pulmonary artery; blood flow to both lungs	Done as a second shunt; often used as a staging step to a Fontan procedure Can be incorporated into eventual modified Fontan procedure Relieves severe cyanosis and decreases volume overload on ventricle Carries risk for embolic events (mixing defect); aspirin often prescribed Pulmonary arteriovenous fistulas may occur months or years later, causing desaturation (uncommon finding)

BP, Blood pressure; *HF*, heart failure; *SVC*, superior vena cava.

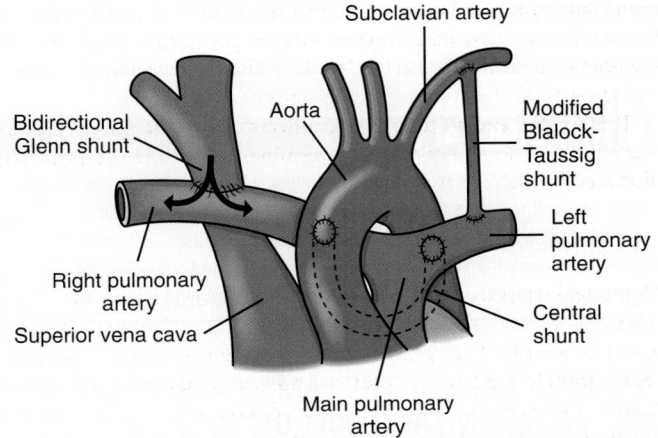

FIG 42.9 Schematic diagram of cardiac shunts.

and cyanosis and reassurance that cyanosis does not imply a lack of oxygen to the brain. Their questions and fears need to be addressed in a calm, supportive manner, and positive aspects of their child's growth and development are emphasized. They are taught the treatment for hypercyanotic spells (see Guidelines box: Treating Hypercyanotic Spells).

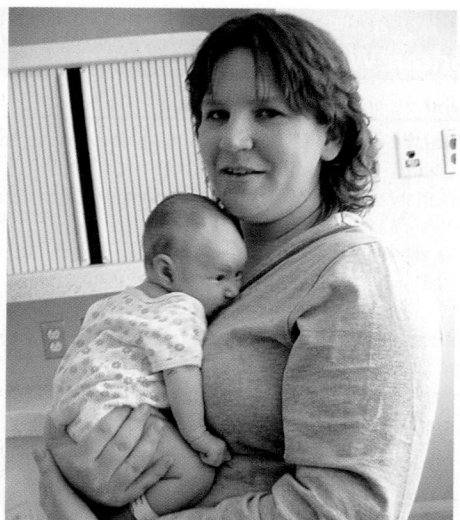

FIG 42.10 Infant held in a knee/chest position.

Dehydration must be prevented in children with hypoxemia because it potentiates the risk for CVAs. Fluid status is carefully monitored, with accurate intake and output and daily weight measurements. Maintenance fluid therapy is the minimum requirement, supplemental fluids should be readily available, and gavage feeding or IV hydration is given to children unable to take adequate oral fluids. Fever, vomiting, and diarrhea can cause dehydration and require prompt treatment. Parents are instructed in the importance of adequate fluid intake and measures to prevent dehydration. An oral electrolyte solution should be available at home in the event that the infant is unable to tolerate the usual formula. The practitioner should be notified of fever, vomiting, diarrhea, or other problems.

Preventive measures and accurate assessment of respiratory infection are important nursing considerations. Any compromise in pulmonary function will increase the infant's hypoxemia. Good hand washing and protection from individuals with an obvious respiratory tract infection are important. Aggressive pulmonary hygiene, treatment with antibiotics or antiviral agents as indicated, and supplemental oxygen to decrease hypoxemia are necessary measures. Infants may need to be gavage fed or given parenteral hydration if respiratory distress prevents oral feeding.

> **! NURSING ALERT**
>
> Intracardiac shunting of blood from the right side (desaturated) to the left side of the heart allows air in the venous system to go directly to the brain, resulting in an air embolism. Therefore, all IV lines should have filters in place to prevent air from entering the system, the entire tubing should be checked for air, all connections should be taped securely, and any air should be removed.

NURSING CARE OF THE FAMILY AND CHILD WITH CONGENITAL HEART DISEASE

When a child is born with a severe cardiac anomaly, the parents are faced with the immense psychologic and physical tasks of adjusting to the birth of a child with special needs. The following discussion is primarily directed toward (1) the family of the infant who has a serious heart defect and requires home care before definitive repair and (2) the preparation and care of the child and family when invasive procedures (catheterization and surgery) are performed. For nursing care related to the child with hypoxemia and HF, the reader should refer to earlier discussions of these topics.

Nursing care of the child with a congenital heart defect begins as soon as the diagnosis is suspected. Prenatal diagnosis of congenital heart defects is becoming increasingly frequent. New demands are being placed on nurses to counsel and support families as they prepare for the birth of these infants.

HELP THE FAMILY ADJUST TO THE DISORDER

When parents learn of the heart defect, they are initially in a period of shock followed by high anxiety and fear that the child will die. The family needs time to grieve before they can assimilate the meaning of the defect. Unfortunately, the demands for medical treatment may not allow this, instead necessitating that the parents immediately give informed consent for diagnostic-therapeutic procedures. The nurse can be instrumental in supporting parents in their loss, assessing their level of understanding, supplying information as needed, and helping other members of the health care team understand the parents' reactions (see Family-Centered Care box: Diagnosis of Heart Disease).

Severely ill newborns usually remain in the hospital. Parent-infant attachment is supported by encouraging parents to hold, touch, and look at their child and providing time and privacy for the parents to spend with their newborn.

The effect of a child with a serious heart defect on the family is complex. No member, regardless of the degree of positive adjustment, is unaffected. Mothers frequently feel inadequate in their mothering ability because of the more complex care infants with congenital heart defects require. They often feel exhausted from the pressures of caring for these children and the other family members. Fathers and siblings may feel neglected and resentful, which is a reaction similar to the feelings toward family members with other chronic conditions (see Chapter 36). Often, parents do not feel confident leaving the child in another person's care. This often sets up a trap for parents, especially mothers, who become locked into the child's care with no relief. Although the fears are justified, they can be minimized by gradually teaching someone (a reliable relative or neighbor) how to care for the child.

The need to maintain discipline and set consistent limits can be difficult for parents. Using behavior modification techniques, in the form of either concrete awards (e.g., a favorite activity) or social reinforcement (e.g., approval), can be effective. However, it is most beneficial if used *before* the child learns to control the family. To prevent later problems, it is necessary to begin discussions with parents while the child is in infancy regarding the need for discipline as the child gets older.

Another issue that may develop within family relationships is the child's overdependency. This is often the result of parental fear that the child may die. Parents need guidance to recognize the eventual hazards of continuing dependency and protectiveness as the child grows older, and the nurse can assist parents in learning ways to foster optimum development. Unless parents are shown what activities the child can do, they may focus on physical limitations and encourage dependency.

The child also needs opportunities for normal social interaction with peers. These children do not need to be prevented from playing with other children because of concern regarding overexertion. Children usually limit their activities if allowed to set their own pace. A child with CHD may constitute a long-term family crisis. Frequently, the continuing unremitting stresses of care—physical exhaustion, financial costs, emotional upset, fear of death, and concern for the child's future—are not fully appreciated by those caring for the family. Even when the child's condition is stabilized or corrected, the family may need to make adjustments in their lifestyle. Introducing them to other families with similarly affected children can help them adjust to the daily stresses.

EDUCATE THE FAMILY ABOUT THE DISORDER

When parents are ready to hear about the heart condition, they require a clear explanation based on their level of understanding. A review of the basic structure and function of the heart is helpful before describing the defect. A simple diagram, pictures, or a model of the heart can help parents visualize the heart and the congenital defect. Parents appreciate receiving written information about the specific condition.* Health care professionals should take advantage of subsequent encounters to assess parental understanding of the condition and clarify information as needed.

Increasingly, families are using the Internet as a source of information about heart disease in children. They are also finding support through contacts with other parents and parent groups.† It is important for parents to realize that not all websites offer medically accurate information and that information from other parents might not be applicable to their own situation. Some children with rare, complex heart defects require individualized treatment plans, and general information on the Internet or in books may not apply to their child. Parents should use their health care team, in particular their cardiologist, to discuss information they have received from other sources.

Information given to the child must be tailored to the child's developmental age. As the child matures, the level of information is revised to meet the child's new cognitive level. Preschoolers need basic information about what they will experience more than what is actually occurring physiologically. School-age children benefit from a concrete explanation of the defect. Including the child at this age early in their own health care and education about their condition will improve self-care and their own accountability (Mickley, Burkhart, & Sigler, 2013). Preadolescents and adolescents often appreciate a more detailed description of how the defect affects their heart. Children of all ages need to express their feelings concerning the diagnosis.

HELP THE FAMILY MANAGE THE ILLNESS AT HOME

Parents are the child's principal caregivers and need to develop a positive, supportive working relationship with the health care team. Because most children spend the majority of their time at home with episodic trips to the hospital, parents manage their child's illness on a daily basis. They monitor for signs of illness, give medications and treatments, bring their child to appointments, work with a variety of caregivers, and alert the team about problems. Successful relationships are partnerships between parents and caregivers that are built on mutual trust and respect. Good communication among the family, the cardiology

specialists, and the primary care provider is essential. As children reach adolescence, they begin to take a larger role in managing their illness and making decisions about their care.

Parents should be aware of the symptoms of their child's cardiac condition and signs of worsening clinical status. Parents of children who may develop HF should be familiar with the symptoms (see Box 42.5) and know when to contact the practitioner. Parents of children with cyanosis should be informed about fluid management and hypercyanotic spells (see earlier in this chapter). Parents should have an information sheet with their child's diagnosis, significant treatments such as surgical procedures, allergies, other health care problems, current medications, and health care providers' contact numbers available in case of emergencies and to share with other caregivers such as teachers, babysitters, and day care providers.

The family also needs to be knowledgeable regarding the therapeutic management of the disorder and the role that surgery, other procedures, medications, and a healthy lifestyle play in maintaining good health. Medications play a critical role in managing some cardiac conditions, such as dysrhythmias, severe HF, anticoagulation for artificial valves, and antirejection medications after heart transplantation. Some patients must take multiple medications daily for their lifetime. Many medications can be dangerous if taken incorrectly and require close monitoring. Parents are taught the correct procedure for giving medications and cautioned to keep them in a safe area to prevent accidental ingestion.

Another area of parental concern is the child's level of physical activity. Most children do not need to restrict activity, and the best approach is to treat the child normally and allow self-limited activity. Exceptions to self-determined activity primarily involve strenuous recreational and competitive sports in children with specific cardiac problems. Activities and exercise restrictions should be discussed with the child's cardiologist. In 2013, the American Heart Association published guidelines for promotion of physical activity in children and adults with CHD. Regular exercise can assist the child with CHD in maintaining a healthy weight, foster normal development, help with self-esteem, and help with acceptance into peer groups (Longmuir, Brothers, de Ferranti, et al., 2013).

Infants and children with CHD require good nutrition. Breastfeeding should be possible for many infants with CHD. Providing adequate nutrition to infants with HF or complex congenital defects is especially difficult due to their high caloric requirements and inability to suck effectively because of fatigue and tachypnea. Instructing parents in feeding methods that decrease the infant's work and giving high-calorie formula are important interventions (see the "Maintain Nutritional Status" section earlier in this chapter for a discussion on feeding the infant with HF). Children with severe cardiac defects are often anorexic. Encouraging them to eat can be a tremendous challenge. Consultation with a dietitian is often helpful. The child should be given a choice of available high-nutrient foods.

Infants with heart disease should be immunized according to the current guidelines. Immunization schedules may need to be modified around times of acute illness or surgical procedures. Infants and children younger than 12 months of age with hemodynamically significant CHD or those younger than 24 months of age undergoing cardiac transplantation during RSV season should receive the vaccine for respiratory syncytial virus (RSV) monthly during RSV season (November to April in North America) for a total of five doses (American Academy of Pediatrics Committee on Infectious Diseases & American Academy of Pediatrics Bronchiolitis Guidelines Committee, 2014).

Infants and children who have serious heart disease are at risk for developmental delays. Multiple factors can influence neurodevelopmental outcomes, including genetics (chromosomal abnormalities and microdeletions), family background (parental intelligence quotient [IQ] and

---

*American Heart Association, 7272 Greenville Avenue, Dallas, TX 75231; 800-242-8721; http://www.heart.org; Kids with Heart National Association for Children's Heart Disorders, PO Box 12504, Green Bay, WI 54307; 800-538-5390; http://kidswithheart.org; Little Hearts, Inc., PO Box 171 Cromwell, CT 06416; 860-635-0006, 866-435-4673; http://www.littlehearts.org.

†The Congenital Heart Information Network, http://tchin.org; Heart Rhythm Society (information on arrhythmias), http://www.hrsonline.org; Adult Congenital Heart Association, http://www.achaheart.org; Children's Heart Foundation, http://www.childrensheartfoundation.org. Many major medical centers that perform pediatric heart surgery also have information on their websites.

socioeconomic status), preoperative factors (including prematurity, cyanosis, shock), intraoperative factors (use of cardiopulmonary bypass, deep hypothermic circulatory arrest), and postoperative factors (hemo-dynamic instability, hypoxia, acidosis, cardiac arrest, stroke, ischemic events).

Research in the past decade has begun to identify specific risk factors and common developmental concerns for CHD. In complex CHD, altered flow of oxygen to the brain, both in utero and postnatally may impact brain development. One study demonstrated that the brain in utero of infants with complex CHD is delayed, thus the brain is less mature than it is by gestational age in a certain population (Licht, Shera, Clancy, et al., 2009). The American Heart Association's 2012 Scientific Statement reinforces that children with CHD are at increased risk for developmental disorder or disabilities or developmental delay. The American Heart Association recommends that all children with CHD be developmentally screened, evaluated, and reevaluated, because this may identify deficits and allow therapies and education to assist academic, behavioral, and psychosocial functioning.

Recent efforts to limit the time of deep hypothermic circulatory arrest and provide better neuroprotection during infant surgery may improve outcomes in the future. Although most children with serious heart disease are within the normal range for IQ, there is a higher incidence of neurodevelopmental deficits in children after heart surgery than in the normal population, specifically in speech and language, fine motor skills, and cognitive processes (Majnemer & Limperopoulos, 1999). Severe neurologic problems such as cerebral palsy, epilepsy, and mental retardation are uncommon.

PREPARE THE CHILD AND FAMILY FOR INVASIVE PROCEDURES

Chapter 39 provides an extensive discussion of the principles for preparing children for invasive procedures. The American Heart Association published a scientific statement, "Recommendations for Preparing Children and Adolescents for Invasive Cardiac Procedures" (LeRoy, Elixson, O'Brien, et al., 2003), which addresses issues specific to the child with heart disease. The following discussion highlights some important aspects of preparation for cardiac catheterization and cardiac surgery.

The expected outcomes for preprocedure preparation include reducing anxiety, improving patient cooperation with procedures, enhancing recovery, developing trust with caregivers, and improving long-term emotional and behavioral adjustments after procedures (LeRoy et al., 2003). Important factors to consider in planning preparation strategies are the child's cognitive development, previous hospital experiences, the child's temperament and coping style, the timing of preparation, and the involvement of the parents. The most beneficial preparation strategies usually combine information giving and coping skills training, such as conscious breathing exercises, distraction techniques, guided imagery, or other behavioral interventions.

Outpatient preoperative and precatheterization workups are common for most elective procedures. Children are then admitted on the morning of the procedure. Preprocedure teaching is often done in the clinic setting or at home and may include a tour of the ICU and inpatient facilities. Children of different ages and developmental levels require different amounts of information and different approaches. Whereas young children should be prepared close in time to the event, older children and adolescents may benefit from teaching several weeks in advance. Parents should be included in the preparation session to support their child and learn about upcoming events.

Topics to include in preoperative or precatheterization preparation include information on the environment, equipment, and procedures that the child will encounter during and after the procedure. Many information-giving techniques can be used, such as verbal and written information, hospital tours, preoperative classes, picture books, or videos. Information about what the child will see, hear, and feel should be included, especially for older children and adolescents. Some of the sensory experiences of being in an ICU or catheterization laboratory include sights (monitors, many people, a lot of equipment), sounds (beeping noises, alarms, voices), and sensations (lines and dressings, tape, discomfort, thirst). Familiar aspects of the environment, such as BP cuffs, stethoscopes, or oximeter probes, are reviewed, and new equipment, such as monitors, IV lines, and oxygen masks, are described. Comforting aspects of the environment, such as play areas, chairs for parents, and televisions, are emphasized. Many patients who will be sedated during catheterization or receive narcotic pain relievers after surgery will have minimal recall of that period and will not need detailed information about the equipment or procedures used. Information should be specific to the planned procedure for each patient.

A discussion of ways the child can cope with the experience should be included. For a young child, bringing a familiar stuffed animal or comfort object will help relieve anxiety, and advising an older child to bring headphones and favorite music to the catheterization laboratory will help distract him or her during the procedure. Recovery topics after catheterization include lying still to prevent bleeding at the catheter site, advancing diet, controlling pain, and monitoring. After surgery, the nurse reviews the importance of ambulation, coughing, deep breathing, drinking, and eating and describes pain management and monitoring routines. Simple coping strategies for use during painful procedures should be reviewed; these include distraction techniques such as counting, blowing, singing, and telling stories.

Children and their families should have a choice about an ICU tour. Exposure to the ICU environment can actually increase anxiety in some children, particularly young children, those with previous hospital experiences, and those who are highly anxious (LeRoy et al., 2003). Usually the day before the procedure is ample time to allow the child to ask questions and to prevent undue fantasizing about the experience. The child should be protected from the frightening sights in the unit; equipment not in view postoperatively, such as equipment located behind or below the bed, needs less attention. The child and parents are encouraged to ask questions or to explore further any equipment in the room, but they should not be pushed to assimilate more information than they are able.

Preoperative physical care differs little, if any, from that for any other surgery and is discussed in Chapter 39. The child should be assured that the parents will be there when the child wakes up; they should be allowed to accompany their child as far as possible to the operating suite (see the "Surgical Procedures" section in Chapter 39). After all of the equipment and procedures have been explained, it is important to talk about "getting well" and going home.

PROVIDE POSTOPERATIVE CARE

Immediate postoperative care is usually provided by specially trained nurses in ICUs. Many of the procedures, such as arterial pressure and central venous pressure (CVP) monitoring, and the observations related to vital functions require advanced educational training (readers should refer to critical care texts for further information). However, nurses caring for the child before surgery and during the convalescent period need to be familiar with the major principles of care. Selected complications that may occur postoperatively are described in Box 42.7.

Observe Vital Signs

Vital signs and BP are recorded frequently until stable. Heart rate and respirations are counted for 1 full minute, compared with the ECG

BOX 42.7   Selected Complications After Cardiac Surgery and Treatment Approaches

Cardiac

Heart failure: Digoxin, diuretics

Low cardiac output: Intravenous (IV) inotropes

Dysrhythmias: Identification, drug treatment, possible pacing, cardioversion

Tamponade (blood or fluid in the pericardial space constricting the heart): Prompt removal of fluid by pericardiocentesis

Respiratory

Atelectasis: Chest physical therapy, coughing, deep breathing, ambulation

Pulmonary edema: Diuretics

Pleural effusions: Diuretics, possible chest tube drainage

Pneumothorax: Possible chest tube drainage

Neurologic

Seizures: Assessment, antiepileptic drugs

Cerebrovascular accident (CVA; stroke), cerebral edema, neurologic deficits: Assessment and treatment

Infectious Disease

Infections (especially wound, pneumonia, otitis media, and sepsis): Antibiotics

Hematologic

Anemia: Iron supplementation, possible transfusion

Postoperative bleeding: Initially, clotting factors, blood products; may need repeat surgery to locate and ligate source of bleeding

Other

Postpericardiotomy syndrome (syndrome of fever, leukocytosis, friction rub, pericardial and pleural effusions, and lethargy seen about 7 to 21 days after cardiac surgery; possible viral or autoimmune etiologies): Antipyretics, diuretics, antiinflammatory medications

---

monitor, and recorded with activity. The heart rate is normally increased after surgery. The nurse observes cardiac rhythm and notifies the practitioner of any changes in regularity. Dysrhythmias may occur postoperatively secondary to anesthetics, acid-base and electrolyte imbalance, hypoxia, surgical intervention, or trauma to conduction pathways.

At least hourly, the lungs are auscultated for breath sounds. Diminished or absent sounds may indicate an area of atelectasis or a pleural effusion or pneumothorax, which necessitates further medical assessment. Temperature changes are typical during the early postoperative period. Hypothermia is expected immediately after surgery from hypothermia procedures, effects of anesthesia, and loss of body heat to the cool environment. During this period, the child is kept warm to prevent additional heat loss. Infants may be placed under radiant heat warmers. During the next 24 to 48 hours, the body temperature may rise to 37.7° C (100° F) or slightly higher as part of the inflammatory response to tissue trauma. After this period, an elevated temperature is most likely a sign of infection and warrants immediate investigation for probable cause.

Intraarterial monitoring of BP is commonly done after open-heart surgery. A catheter is passed into the radial artery or other artery, and the other end is attached to an electronic monitoring system, which provides a continuous recording of the BP. The intraarterial line is maintained with a low-rate, constant infusion of heparinized saline to prevent clotting.

Several IV lines are inserted preoperatively, including a peripheral IV to give fluids and medications and a central venous line that is placed in a large vessel to measure CVP. Additional, intracardiac monitoring lines are sometimes placed intraoperatively in the right atrium, left atrium, or pulmonary artery. Intracardiac lines allow assessment of pressures inside the cardiac chambers, providing vital information about volume status, cardiac output, and ventricular function. All lines must be cared for using strict aseptic technique, and patients must be carefully assessed for bleeding at the time of line removal.

Maintain Respiratory Status

Infants usually require mechanical ventilation in the immediate postoperative period. Early extubation in the operating room or early postoperative period is becoming more common. Children, especially those not requiring cardiopulmonary bypass, may be extubated in the operating room or in the first few postoperative hours. Suctioning is performed only as needed and performed carefully to avoid vagal stimulation (which can trigger cardiac dysrhythmias) and laryngospasm, especially in infants. Suctioning is intermittent and maintained for no more than 5 seconds at a time to avoid depleting the oxygen supply. Supplemental oxygen is administered with a manual resuscitation bag before and after the procedure to prevent hypoxia. The heart rate is monitored after suctioning to detect changes in rhythm or rate, especially bradycardia. The child should always be positioned facing the nurse to permit assessment of the child's color and tolerance of the procedure.

When weaning and extubation are completed, humidified oxygen is delivered by mask, hood, or nasal cannula to prevent drying of mucosa. The child is encouraged to turn and deep breathe at least hourly. Incentive spirometer use should be encouraged. Measures are used to enhance ventilation and decrease pain, such as splinting of the operative site and use of analgesics. Chest tubes are inserted into the pleural or mediastinal space during surgery or in the immediate postoperative period to remove secretions and air to allow reexpansion of the lung. Drainage is checked hourly for color and quantity. Immediately after surgery the drainage may be bright red, but afterward it should be serous. The largest volume of drainage occurs in the first 12 to 24 hours and is greater in extensive heart surgery.

> **! NURSING ALERT**
>
> Chest tube drainage greater than 3 mL/kg/hour for more than 3 consecutive hours or 5 to 10 mL/kg in any 1 hour is excessive and may indicate postoperative hemorrhage. The surgeon should be notified immediately because cardiac tamponade can develop rapidly and is life-threatening.

Chest tubes are usually removed on the first to third postoperative day. Removal of chest tubes is a painful, frightening experience. Analgesics such as morphine sulfate, often combined with midazolam (Versed), should be given before the procedure. Older children are forewarned that they will feel a sharp, momentary pain. After the suture is cut, the tubes are quickly pulled out at the end of full inspiration in the extubated patient to prevent intake of air into the pleural cavity. (In the intubated patient, the tubes are pulled out on inspiration because the lungs are stented open with the positive pressure ventilation). A purse-string suture (placed when the tubes were inserted) is pulled tight to close the opening. A petrolatum-covered gauze dressing is immediately applied over the wound and securely taped on all four sides to the skin so that an airtight seal is formed. It is left on for 1 or 2 days. Breath sounds are checked to assess for pneumothorax, a possible complication of chest tube removal. A chest radiograph is usually obtained after removal to evaluate for possible pneumothorax or pleural effusion.

Monitor Fluids

Intake and output of all fluids must be accurately calculated. Intake is primarily IV fluids; however, a record of fluid used to flush the arterial and CVP lines or to dilute medications is also kept. Output includes hourly recordings of urine (usually a Foley catheter is inserted and attached to a closed collecting device), drainage from chest and nasogastric tubes, and blood drawn for analysis. Renal failure is a potential risk from a transient period of low cardiac output.

> ### ! NURSING ALERT
>
> The signs of renal failure are decreased urinary output (<1 mL/kg/hour) and elevated levels of blood urea nitrogen and serum creatinine.

Fluids are restricted during the immediate postoperative period to prevent hypervolemia, which places additional demands on the myocardium, predisposing the patient to cardiac failure. If the child is to be extubated within the first 24 to 48 hours, fluids are provided primarily intravenously. If the child is to be intubated longer, fluids may be given via a nasogastric or nasojejunal tube to optimize nutrition and gut motility. Approximately 4 hours after extubation, enteral fluids may be reinitiated in the setting of a stable hemodynamic and respiratory status. To monitor fluid retention, the child is weighed daily, and the same scale is used at approximately the same time each day to avoid errors in measurement. Fluid restriction may be imposed even when oral fluids are given. The nurse calculates the distribution over a 24-hour period based on the child's preoperative weight and drinking habits. The distribution should allow for most fluid to be given during the child's most wakeful and active periods.

Provide Rest and Progressive Activity

After heart surgery, rest should be provided to decrease the workload of the heart and promote healing. The simplest way to ensure individualized, efficient, high-quality care is to plan at the beginning of the shift the nursing procedures to be done, with periods of rest identified. The schedule should be shared with parents to allow them to visit at the most advantageous times, such as after a rest period when no special treatments are anticipated.

A progressive schedule of ambulation and activity is planned, based on the child's preoperative activity patterns and postoperative cardiovascular and pulmonary function. Ambulation is initiated early, usually by the second postoperative day, when chest tubes, arterial lines, and assisted ventilatory equipment have been removed. Activity progresses from sitting on the edge of the bed and dangling the legs to standing up and sitting in a chair. Heart rate and respirations are carefully monitored to assess the degree of cardiac demand imposed by each activity. Tachycardia, dyspnea, cyanosis, desaturation, progressive fatigue, and dysrhythmias indicate the need to limit further energy expenditure.

Provide Comfort and Emotional Support

Heart surgery is both painful and frightening for children, and comfort is a primary nursing concern. Several types of incisions are used by the cardiac surgeon. A median sternotomy is most common, following the sternum down the center of the chest. A ministernotomy opens the lower sternum. A thoracotomy incision is most uncomfortable because it goes through muscle tissue. It allows access to the side of the chest through an incision from under the arm around the back to the scapula.

Most patients need IV analgesics for pain control during the immediate postoperative period. Patient-controlled analgesia may be used with children old enough to understand the concept. Nonsteroidal antiinflammatory drugs (NSAIDs) such as ketorolac (Toradol) may be used

intravenously. Paralyzing agents may also be used with the analgesics for children who are hemodynamically unstable.

After extubation and removal of lines and tubes, pain can be satisfactorily controlled with oral medications such as ibuprofen, codeine with acetaminophen (Tylenol No. 3), or oxycodone and acetaminophen. Acetaminophen alone provides adequate pain relief for most children at discharge. Sternotomy incisions are usually well tolerated, with some discomfort when walking and coughing. Thoracotomy incisions are usually more painful because the incision is through muscle; a more aggressive pain management plan with around-the-clock medications for several days is often necessary to allow for adequate rest, ambulation, and pulmonary hygiene.

In addition to pharmacologic pain control, every effort is made to minimize the discomfort of procedures, such as using a firm pillow or favorite stuffed animal placed against the chest incision during movement and performing treatments *after* pain medication is given, preferably at a time that coincides with the drug's peak effect. Nonpharmacologic measures are used to lessen the perception of pain, and parents are encouraged to comfort their child as much as possible (see the "Pain Management" and "Pain Assessment" sections in Chapter 30).

Children may become depressed after surgery. This is thought to be caused by preoperative anxiety, postoperative psychologic and physiologic stress, and sensory overstimulation. Typically, the child's disposition improves on leaving the ICU.

Children may also be angry and uncooperative after surgery as a response to the physical pain and to the loss of control imposed by the surgery and treatments. They need an opportunity to express feelings, either verbally or through activity. Children often regress in their behavior during the stress of surgery and hospitalization. They also may express feelings of anger or rejection toward their parents. The nurse can support the parents by being available for information and explaining all of the procedures to them. The first few postoperative days are particularly difficult because parents see their child in pain and realize the potential risks from surgery. They often are overwhelmed by the physical environment of the ICU and feel useless because they can do so little for their child. The nurse can minimize such feelings by including parents in caregiving activities and comfort and play activities, providing information about the child's condition, and being sensitive to their emotional and physical needs. The importance of their presence in making the child feel more secure is stressed even if they do not provide physical care.

> **QUALITY PATIENT OUTCOMES:** **Congenital Heart Disease**
> - Improved cardiac function
> - Prevention of fluid and sodium overload
> - Decreased cardiac demands
> - Improved oxygenation
> - Reduced respiratory distress

PLAN FOR DISCHARGE AND HOME CARE

Ideally, discharge planning begins on admission for cardiac surgery and includes an assessment of the parents' adjustment to the child's altered state of health. Neonates need additional screening tests (e.g., newborn metabolic screen and hearing tests) and may need immunizations, as well as a car seat test before discharge (American Academy of Pediatrics, 2012). The family will need both verbal and written instructions on medication, nutrition, activity restrictions, return to school, wound care, and signs and symptoms of infection or complications (see Family-Centered Care box: Topics to Include in Discharge Teaching After Cardiac Surgery). Referrals to community agencies may be warranted to assist parents in the transition from the hospital to home and to reinforce the teaching.

FAMILY-CENTERED CARE

Topics to Include in Discharge Teaching After Cardiac Surgery

- Medication teaching
- Activity restrictions
- Diet and nutrition
- Wound care (including dressings, if any; suture removal; bathing)
- Bacterial (infective) endocarditis prophylaxis (see Box 42.9)
- Follow-up appointments (cardiologist, primary care provider)
- Community agencies as needed (visiting nurse service, early developmental intervention)
- When to call practitioner; signs and symptoms of postoperative problems
- Review of cardiac defect and surgical repair

The parents will also need clear instructions on when to seek medical care for complications and how to contact the health care provider. Follow-up with the cardiologist and primary care provider is also arranged before discharge. Parents should have a summary, including their child's medical condition, medications, and health care providers available for emergencies. Appropriate identification, such as a MedicAlert device, is indicated for children with a pacemaker or a heart transplant and for those receiving anticoagulation therapy or antidysrhythmic medication.

Although surgical correction of heart defects has improved dramatically, it is still not possible to completely repair many of the complex anomalies. For many children, repeat procedures are required to replace conduits or grafts or to manage complications, such as restenosis. Consequently, the long-term prognosis is uncertain, and full recovery is not always possible. For these families, medical follow-up and continued emotional support are essential. The nurse can often serve as an important primary health care professional and as a resource for referrals when needed.

ACQUIRED CARDIOVASCULAR DISORDERS

INFECTIVE ENDOCARDITIS

Infective endocarditis (IE) (previously called *bacterial endocarditis* or *subacute bacterial endocarditis [SBE]*) is an infection of the inner lining of the heart (endocardium), generally involving the valves. Though rare in children, it carries a mortality rate of 20% to 25% (Bragg & Alvarez, 2014). It is most often a sequela of bacteremia in children with acquired or congenital anomalies of the heart or great vessels, particularly those with valvular abnormalities, prosthetic valves, shunts, recent cardiac surgery with invasive lines, and rheumatic heart disease (RHD) with valve involvement. There is an increased incidence of IE in children without cardiac abnormalities, likely related to the increased use of indwelling central lines to treat other serious diseases (Bragg & Alvarez).

Pathophysiology

Organisms may enter the bloodstream from any site of localized infection. Endocarditis may occur from routine exposure to bacteremia associated with usual daily activities such as brushing teeth, although it can also occur after procedures such as dental work; invasive procedures involving the gastrointestinal and genitourinary tracts; cardiac surgery, especially if synthetic material is used (valves, patches, conduits); or from long-term indwelling catheters. The most common causative agents are *Staphylococcus aureus* and *Streptococcus viridans;* other causative agents include gram-negative bacteria and fungi such as *Candida albicans.* The microorganisms grow on the endocardium, forming vegetations

BOX 42.8 Clinical Manifestations of Infective Endocarditis

Onset usually insidious
Unexplained fever (low grade and intermittent)
Anorexia
Malaise
Weight loss
Characteristic findings caused by extracardiac emboli formation:
- Splinter hemorrhages (thin black lines) under the nails
- Osler nodes (red, painful intradermal nodes found on pads of phalanges)
- Janeway lesions (painless hemorrhagic areas on palms and soles)
- Petechiae on oral mucous membranes
May be present:
- Heart failure
- Cardiac dysrhythmias
- New murmur or change in previously existing one

(verrucae), deposits of fibrin, and platelet thrombi. The lesion may invade adjacent tissues, such as the aortic and mitral valves, and may break off and embolize elsewhere, especially in the spleen, kidney, and CNS.

Diagnostic Evaluation

The diagnosis of IE is suspected on the basis of clinical manifestations (Box 42.8). The most commonly used diagnostic guidelines are the revised Duke criteria, which outline major and minor criteria consistent with IE (Li, Sexton, Mick, et al., 2000). Definitive diagnosis rests on growth and identification of the causative agent in the blood. At least three blood cultures are drawn at different times to aid in diagnosis. Vegetations on the valve and abnormal valve function can often be visualized by echocardiography. A diagnosis of culture-negative IE is made when the patient has echocardiographic or clinical evidence of IE but no organism can be cultured. Several laboratory findings may suggest IE including anemia, elevated erythrocyte sedimentation rate [ESR], leukocytosis, and microscopic hematuria.

Therapeutic Management

Treatment should be instituted immediately and consists of administration of high doses of appropriate antibiotics intravenously for 2 to 8 weeks. Blood cultures are taken periodically to evaluate the response to antibiotic therapy. Cardiac function is monitored by echocardiograms. Heart surgery to repair or replace the affected valve may be necessary.

Prevention involves administration of prophylactic antibiotic therapy to high-risk patients prior to dental procedures that are associated with the risk for entry of organisms (Box 42.9). Drugs of choice for prophylaxis, given 1 hour prior to the procedure, include amoxicillin, ampicillin, and clindamycin in penicillin-allergic patients (Wilson, Taubert, Gewitz, et al., 2007).

QUALITY PATIENT OUTCOMES: Bacterial (Infective) Endocarditis
- Prevention in high-risk patients with antibiotic prophylaxis
- Early recognition and treatment

Care Management

Nurses counsel parents of high-risk children concerning the signs and symptoms of endocarditis and the need for prophylactic antibiotic therapy before dental work. The family's dentist should be advised of the child's cardiac diagnosis as an added precaution to ensure preventive treatment. It is important that all children with congenital or acquired heart disease maintain the highest level of oral health to reduce the chance of bacteremia from oral infections.

Parents should also have a high index of suspicion regarding potential infections. Without unduly alarming them, the nurse stresses that any unexplained fever, weight loss, or change in behavior (lethargy, malaise, anorexia) must be brought to the practitioner's attention. Early diagnosis and treatment are important in preventing further cardiac damage, embolic complications, and growth of resistant organisms.

Treatment of endocarditis requires long-term parenteral drug therapy. In many cases, IV antibiotics may be administered at home with nursing supervision. Nursing goals during this period are (1) preparation of the child for IV infusion, usually with an intermittent-infusion device and several venipunctures for blood cultures; (2) observation for side effects of antibiotics, especially inflammation along venipuncture sites; (3) observation for complications, including embolism and HF; and (4) education regarding the importance of follow-up visits for cardiac evaluation, echocardiographic monitoring, and blood cultures. Some children may need preparation for surgery and later, postoperative care.

ACUTE RHEUMATIC FEVER AND RHEUMATIC HEART DISEASE

Acute rheumatic fever (ARF) is a result of an abnormal immune response to a group A strep (GAS) infection, usually pharyngitis, in a genetically susceptible host (Marijon, Mirabel, Celermajer, et al., 2012; Mirabel, Narayanan, Jouven, et.al., 2014). It occurs most often in late school-age children and adolescents and is rare in adults. ARF is a self-limited illness that involves the joints, skin, brain, and heart, but cardiac valve damage, which is referred to as *rheumatic heart disease (RHD)*, the most significant complication of ARF, occurs in more than one-half of the cases. The mitral valve is most often affected. In developed countries, ARF and RHD have become uncommon. However, in developing countries, because of overcrowded living conditions and poor access to medical care, ARF and resulting RHD is the leading cause of HF in young people (Remenyi, Carapetis, Wyber, et al., 2013).

Etiology

Strong evidence supports a relationship between upper respiratory tract infection with GAS and subsequent development of ARF (usually within 2 to 6 weeks). Prevention or treatment of GAS infection prevents ARF. If the GAS infection is untreated, antibodies are produced to fight the infection, which can also act against the heart valves causing damage. If children have one strep infection, they are at greater risk for repeated infections, and recurrent infections cause the cumulative valve damage of RHD.

Diagnostic Evaluation

Diagnosis is based on a set of guidelines, and later revisions, known as the *modified Jones criteria* (Special Writing Group of the Committee on Rheumatic Fever, Endocarditis, and Kawasaki Disease of the Council on Cardiovascular Disease in the Young of the American Heart Association, 1992; Ferrieri & Jones Criteria Working Group, 2002). The updated Jones criteria suggest that the presence of two major manifestations or one major and two minor manifestations, with supportive evidence of recent GAS infection, indicates a high probability of ARF (see Guidelines box: Diagnosis of Initial Attack of Rheumatic Fever).

Children suspected of having ARF are tested for streptococcal antibodies. The most reliable and best standardized test is an elevated or rising antistreptolysin O (ASO or ASLO) titer, which occurs in 80% of children with ARF. Additional antistreptococcal antibody titers may be sent if ASO titers are negative. Acute-phase reactants, ESR, and C-reactive protein (CRP) are usually elevated as well. Echocardiograms play an important role in diagnosing RHD and monitoring deteriorating valve function.

Therapeutic Management

Primary prevention involves prompt diagnosis and treatment of strep throat infections so that ARF does not occur. Penicillin is the drug of choice or an alternative in penicillin-sensitive children (Gerber, Baltimore, Eaton, et al., 2009).

If children have ARF, antibiotics are given to treat the GAS infection and salicylates are used to control the inflammatory process, especially in the joints, and reduce the fever and discomfort. Supportive care involves bed rest initially and then quiet activities as symptoms subside. Good nutrition is important. Children who have had ARF are susceptible to recurrent infections that are likely to result in RHD and further damage to the heart valves. Prophylactic treatment against recurrence of ARF (secondary prevention) is started after the acute therapy. The treatment of choice is intramuscular injections of benzathine penicillin G every 28 days because it is most effective. Alternative therapy includes oral doses of penicillin or erythromycin twice a day, or one daily dose of sulfadiazine. The duration of secondary prophylaxis is based on the presence of residual heart disease. If ARF occurs without carditis, then prophylaxis is recommended for 5 years or until 21 years of age, whichever is longer. In patients with carditis, 10 years is recommended or until 21 years of age. In patients with RHD, prophylaxis can continue until 40 years of age and may be indicated indefinitely depending on the individual's risk (Gerber et al., 2009).

Management of RHD may require surgical valve repair or replacement. Valve replacement with a mechanical valve requires lifelong anticoagulation with warfarin.

QUALITY PATIENT OUTCOMES: Acute Rheumatic Fever
- Group A strep (GAS) tonsillopharyngitis identified and treated
- Early recognition and treatment to prevent cardiac valve damage
- Recurrence prevented with prophylaxis compliance

Care Management

The objective of nursing care is, first, prevention. For the child with ARF, nursing care (1) encourages compliance with drug regimens, (2) facilitates recovery from the illness, and (3) provides emotional support. Nurses play an important role in prevention by educating parents about

GUIDELINES

Diagnosis of Initial Attack of Rheumatic Fever (Jones Criteria, 1992 Update)*

Major Manifestations
Carditis
Tachycardia out of proportion to degree of fever
Cardiomegaly
New murmurs or change in preexisting murmurs
Muffled heart sounds
Pericardial friction rub
Chest pain
Changes in ECG (especially prolonged PR interval)

Polyarthritis
Swollen, hot, red, painful joint(s)
After 1 to 2 days, different joint(s) affected
Favors large joints: Knees, elbows, hips, shoulders, wrists

Erythema Marginatum
Erythematous macules with clear center and wavy, well-demarcated border
Transitory
Nonpruritic
Primarily affects trunk and extremities (inner surfaces)

Chorea (St. Vitus Dance, Sydenham Chorea)
Sudden aimless, irregular movements of extremities
Involuntary facial grimaces
Speech disturbances

Emotional lability
Muscle weakness (can be profound)
Muscle movements exaggerated by anxiety and attempts at fine motor activity; relieved by rest

Subcutaneous Nodes
Nontender swelling
Located over bony prominences
May persist for some time and then gradually resolve

Minor Manifestations
Clinical Findings
Arthralgia
Fever

Laboratory Findings
Elevated acute-phase reactants
- ESR
- CRP
- Prolonged PR interval

Supporting Evidence of Antecedent Group A Streptococcal Infection
Positive throat culture or rapid streptococcal antigen test result
Elevated or rising streptococcal antibody titer

From Special Writing Group of the Committee on Rheumatic Fever, Endocarditis, and Kawasaki Disease of the Council on Cardiovascular Disease in the Young of the American Heart Association. (1992). Guidelines for the diagnosis of rheumatic fever, Jones criteria, 1992 update. *Journal of the American Medical Association, 268*(15), 2069–2073.
CRP, C-reactive protein; *ECG,* electrocardiogram; *ESR,* erythrocyte sedimentation rate.
*If supported by evidence of preceding group A streptococcal infection, the presence of two major manifestations or of one major and two minor manifestations indicates a high probability of acute rheumatic fever.

the complications of strep infections and working with patients and families to ensure follow up with antibiotic prophylaxis. Because compliance is a major concern in long-term drug therapy, every effort is made to encourage adherence to the therapeutic plan (see the "Compliance" section in Chapter 39). When compliance is poor, monthly injections may be substituted for daily oral administration of antibiotics, and children need preparation for this often-dreaded procedure.

Interventions for ARF are primarily concerned with providing rest, adequate nutrition, and management of cardiac symptoms or chorea. One of the most disturbing manifestations of ARF is chorea. The onset is gradual and may occur weeks to months after the illness. Sometimes mistaken for nervousness, clumsiness, or inattentiveness, it is usually a source of great frustration to the child because the movements, incoordination, and weakness severely limit physical ability. It is important that parents and teachers are aware of the involuntary, sudden nature of the movements and that the movements are transitory and will eventually disappear.

Children with RHD will need lifelong follow-up, education, and management of HF and monitoring for progressive valve disease. If surgery is required, preparation for the procedure is provided. An important aspect of postoperative care is education about anticoagulation medications and follow-up.

HYPERLIPIDEMIA (HYPERCHOLESTEROLEMIA)

Hyperlipidemia is a general term for excessive lipids (fat and fatlike substances); *hypercholesterolemia* refers to excessive cholesterol in the

blood. *Dyslipidemia* is a term used to describe all abnormalities in lipid metabolism, including low levels of high-density lipoprotein (HDL) or "good" cholesterol, high low-density lipoprotein (LDL) or "lousy" cholesterol, or high triglycerides. Abnormal lipid or cholesterol levels play an important role in producing atherosclerosis (fatty plaque on the arteries), which eventually can lead to coronary artery disease, which is a primary cause of morbidity and mortality in the adult population. A presymptomatic phase of atherosclerosis begins in childhood/adolescence, providing the template for later clinical disease. Preventive cardiology focuses on the identification of high-risk patients and management of lipid levels in childhood/adolescence.

Cholesterol is part of the lipoprotein complex in plasma that is essential for cellular metabolism. Triglycerides, natural fats synthesized from carbohydrates, are used for energy. Both are major lipids transported on *lipoproteins,* a combination of lipids and proteins, which include the following:

Low-density lipoproteins (LDLs): LDL is the major carrier of cholesterol to the cells. Cells use cholesterol for synthesis of membranes and steroid production. Elevated circulating LDL is a strong risk factor in cardiovascular disease. In addition, particle size and density of LDL may affect overall risk, with small, dense particles associated with increased atherosclerosis.

High-density lipoproteins (HDLs): HDL cholesterol contains very low concentrations of triglycerides, relatively little cholesterol, and high levels of protein. They transport free cholesterol to the liver for excretion in the bile. High levels of HDL are thought to be protective against cardiovascular disease.

Very-low-density lipoproteins (VLDLs): Contain high concentration of triglycerides, some cholesterol, and a little protein. Triglycerides are the main storage form of fuel or energy for the body.

Diagnostic Evaluation

Hyperlipidemia can have a genetic basis (familial homozygous or heterozygous), and/or a lifestyle component, or can be caused by secondary problems, such as hypothyroidism. Hyperlipidemia is diagnosed on the basis of analysis of blood. A complete lipid profile should be drawn after a 12-hour fast. In children with elevated cholesterol levels, a screening thyroid-stimulating hormone is measured at diagnosis in order to rule out hypothyroidism as a cause of secondary hypercholesterolemia. Additional blood work is individualized based on other risk factors. Lipid values may be affected by recent high fevers, and therefore cholesterol values should not be drawn if a child has had a fever within the past 3 weeks. Diagnostic values for acceptable, borderline, and high total cholesterol and LDL cholesterol levels are listed in Table 42.5.

The National Heart, Lung, and Blood Institute published comprehensive guidelines for cardiovascular health and risk reduction in children and adolescents in 2012. In contrast to prior guidelines, the National Heart, Lung, and Blood Institute guidelines now recommend universal screening for all children between 9 and 11 years of age and again between 17 and 21 years of age. In addition, selective lipid screening continues to be recommended for children older than 2 years of age who have a family history of dyslipidemia or early heart disease in a first- or second-degree relative, as well as for those children who have individual coronary risk factors (Expert Panel on Integrated Guidelines for Cardiovascular Health and Risk Reduction in Children and Adolescents, & National Heart, Lung, and Blood Institute, 2012) (see Evidence-Based Practice box: Rationale for Universal Cholesterol Screening for Children). Although not without controversy, the goal of this new approach is to identify children earlier in order decrease coronary risk factors, particularly in the current era of an increased prevalence of obesity in young people (Daniels, 2012; de Ferranti, Daniels, Gillman, et al., 2012; McCrindle, Kwiterovich, McBride, et al., 2012). In addition to abnormal cholesterol levels, known risk factors that correlate with the development CHD include the following:

- Positive family history of elevated cholesterol and/or early heart disease
- Cigarette smoking
- Obesity
- Sedentary lifestyle
- Nutritional factors
- Older age
- Male gender
- Hypertension
- Type 1 or type 2 diabetes

In addition to the risk factors noted earlier, the American Heart Association and National Heart, Lung, and Blood Institute have identified children who are considered to be at higher risk for atherosclerosis because of coexisting health problems including the following:
- Chronic inflammatory diseases
- Cancer survivors
- Transplant patients
- CHD
- A history of Kawasaki disease with coronary artery aneurysms

Therapeutic Management

The first step in the treatment of high cholesterol is focused on lifestyle modification. The National Heart, Lung, and Blood Institute guidelines advocate the benefits of a heart-healthy diet for all children (Box 42.10). In addition, children with known elevated cholesterol should have

---

TABLE 42.5   Classification of Cholesterol Levels in Children

Category	Normal mg/dL	Borderline High mg/dL	Elevated g/dL
Triglycerides	<170	170–199	≥200
Low-density lipoprotein (LDL)	<110	110–120	≥130
Non–high-density lipoprotein (HDL)	<120	120–144	≥145
High-density lipoprotein (HDL)*	>45	N/A	N/A

Data adapted from the Expert Panel on Integrated Guidelines for Cardiovascular Health and Risk Reduction in Children and Adolescents, Daniels, S.R., Benuck, I., et al. (2012). Expert Panel on Integrated Guidelines for Cardiovascular Health and Risk Reduction in Children and Adolescents: Summary report. Bethesda, MD: US Department of Health and Human Services, National Heart, Lung, and Blood Institute, National Institutes of Health.
N/A, Not applicable.
*Borderline low HDL 40–45; Low HDL <40.

BOX 42.10   Recommendations for Dietary/Lifestyle Management of Dyslipidemia for Children/Adolescents Older Than 2 Years of Age

For All Children/Adolescents
- Obtain 1 hour of moderate or vigorous physical activity at least 5 days per week
- Less than 2 hours per day of sedentary screen time
- Avoid firsthand and secondhand smoke exposure
- Eat a diverse diet rich in fruits, vegetables, whole grains, lean meats, and fish
- Refer to a registered dietician for individual nutritional counseling

Elevated Low-Density Lipoprotein Cholesterol
- 25% to 30% of calories from fat
- Less than 7% from saturated fats (approximately 12 to 15 g/day)
- Avoid trans fats
- Favor monounsaturated fats
- Less than 200 mg/day of dietary cholesterol

Elevated Triglycerides or Non–High-Density Lipoprotein Cholesterol
- Decrease intake of simple sugars
  - Avoid white bread, white pasta, white potatoes, white rice, sugary cereals, cookies, cakes, candy
  - No sugar-sweetened beverages
  - Replace simple sugars with complex carbohydrates
- 25% to 30% of calories from fat
- Less than 7% from saturated fat
- Favor monounsaturated fats (beneficial effects on high-density lipoprotein [HDL] cholesterol)
  - Use olive oil, canola oil, avocados, nuts, and fish
- Avoid trans fats
- Increase dietary fish intake for omega-3 fatty acids

Adapted from Expert Panel on Integrated Guidelines for Cardiovascular Health and Risk Reduction in Children and Adolescents, & National Heart, Lung, and Blood Institute. (2011). Expert Panel on Integrated Guidelines for Cardiovascular Health and Risk Reduction in Children and Adolescents: Summary report. *Pediatrics, 128*(Suppl 5), S213–S256.

EVIDENCE-BASED PRACTICE
Rationale for Universal Cholesterol Screening for Children

Ask the Question
PICOT Question: Should cholesterol screening be performed in children?

Search for the Evidence
Search Strategies
The literature was searched to locate clinical research studies related to this issue. Selection criteria included English-language publications within the past 10 years, research-based articles (level 3 or lower), and infant and child populations.

Databases Used
PubMed, Cochrane Collaboration, MD Consult, Joanna Briggs Institute, National Guidelines Clearinghouse (AHRQ), TRIP Database Plus, PedsCCM, BestBETs

Critical Appraisal of the Evidence
- In late 2011, an expert panel of the National Heart, Lung, and Blood Institute made a recommendation that lipid screening be performed on all children 9 to 11 years of age; this recommendation was based on evidence that as many as 30% to 60% of children with dyslipidemia might be missed when screening is performed by family history alone (National Heart, Lung, and Blood Institute, 2011). The expert panel's guidelines also include comprehensive screening and treatment guidelines for children with cardiovascular disease risk factors.
- Diagnosis of obesity is paramount in enhancing care of obese pediatric patients. Current laboratory (cholesterol or glucose) screening rates (10%) are inadequate in the outpatient setting (Patel, Madsen, Maselli, et al., 2010).
- Testing for cardiovascular risk factors: HDL cholesterol, LDL cholesterol, fasting glucose, HgA1c, BP, thyroid-stimulating hormone, and ALT should be considered in pediatric patients with increased waist circumference and even normal BMI (l'Allemand-Jander, 2010).
- In obese children, LDL cholesterol, HDL cholesterol, total cholesterol, and triglycerides are significantly different from subjects who are not obese (Simsek, Balta, Balta, et al., 2010).
- Serum triglyceride levels are a predictive risk factor of carotid intima-media thickness (Simsek et al., 2010).
- In children and adolescents (12 to 19 years of age) fasting non-HDL cholesterol levels were strongly associated with metabolic syndrome. A non-HDL cholesterol threshold of 120 mg/dL indicated borderline risk for metabolic syndrome, and a threshold of 145 mg/dL indicated high metabolic syndrome risk (Li, Ford, McBride, et al., 2011).
- Cholesterol levels in childhood are a major population predictor for adult cholesterol levels (Daniels, Greer, & Committee on Nutrition, 2008).
- Precursors of atherosclerosis are present in young people. The atherosclerotic process begins early in life with early phases characterized by the development of fatty streaks in the vessels (PDAY study) (Enos, Holmes, & Beyer, 1953; Strong, Malcom, McMahan, et al., 1999).
- Atherosclerosis is related to the presence and degree of cardiovascular risk factors in adults (Berenson, Srinivasan, Bao, et al., 1998).
- Most severely affected children come from families with a high incidence of early heart disease. Children whose genetic family history is unknown should also be screened (National Heart, Lung, and Blood Institute, 2011).
- Universal cholesterol screening in children would identify all individuals with dyslipidemia. Using solely the family history to identify subjects for cholesterol screening missed individuals with moderate dyslipidemia and those with potentially genetic dyslipidemia (Ritchie, Murphy, Ice, et al., 2010).

Apply the Evidence: Nursing Implications
There are strong recommendations (Guyatt, Oxman, Vist, et al., 2008) that lipid screening should be performed on all children 9 to 11 years of age and again between 17 and 21 years of age. Selective screening is still recommended for children older than 2 years of age with affected first- or second-degree relatives or those with individual cardiac risk factors. The National Heart, Lung, and Blood Institute guidelines have been endorsed by the American Academy of Pediatrics (National Heart, Lung, and Blood Institute, 2011).

Quality and Safety Competencies: Evidence-Based Practice*
Knowledge
Differentiate clinical opinion from research and evidence-based summaries.
Describe use of cholesterol screening in children.

Skills
Base individualized care plan on patient values, clinical expertise, and evidence.
Integrate evidence into practice by using cholesterol screening in children.

Attitudes
Value the concept of evidence-based practice as integral to determining best clinical practice.
Appreciate strengths and weakness of evidence for using cholesterol screening in children.

References
Berenson, G. S., Srinivasan, S. R., Bao, W., et al. (1998). Association between multiple cardiovascular risk factors and atherosclerosis in children and young adults: The Bogalusa Heart Study. *New England Journal of Medicine, 338*(23), 1650–1656.

Daniels, S. R., Greer, F. R., & Committee on Nutrition. (2008). Lipid screening and cardiovascular health in childhood. *Pediatrics, 122*(1), 198–208.

Enos, W. F., Holmes, R. H., & Beyer, J. (1953). Coronary disease among United States soldiers killed in action in Korea; Preliminary report. *Journal of the American Medical Association, 152*(12), 1090–1093.

Expert Panel on Integrated Guidelines for Cardiovascular Health and Risk Reduction in Children and Adolescents, & National Heart, Lung, and Blood Institute. (2011). Expert panel on integrated guidelines for cardiovascular health and risk reduction in children and adolescents: Summary report. *Pediatrics, 128*(Suppl. 5):S213–S256.

Guyatt, G. H., Oxman, A. D., Vist, G. E., et al. (2008). GRADE: An emerging consensus on rating quality of evidence and strength of recommendations. *British Medical Journal, 336*(7650), 924–926.

l'Allemand-Jander, D. (2010). Clinical diagnosis of metabolic and cardiovascular risk in overweight children: Early development of chronic diseases in the obese child. *International Journal of Obesity, 34*(2 suppl), S32–S36.

Li, C., Ford, E. S., McBride, P. E., et al. (2011). Non-high-density lipoprotein cholesterol concentration is associated with the metabolic syndrome among US youth aged 12-19 years. *Journal of Pediatrics, 158*(2), 201–207.

Patel, A. I., Madsen, K. A., Maselli, J. H., et al. (2010). Underdiagnosis of pediatric obesity during outpatient preventive care visits. *Academic Pediatrics, 10*(6), 405–409.

Ritchie, S. K., Murphy, E. C., Ice, C., et al. (2010). Universal versus targeted blood cholesterol screening among youth: The CARDIAC project. *Pediatrics, 126*(2), 260–265.

Simsek, E., Balta, H., Balta, Z., et al. (2010). Childhood obesity-related cardiovascular risk factors and carotid intima-media thickness. *Turkish Journal of Pediatrics, 52*(6), 602–611.

Strong, J. P., Malcom, G. T., McMahan, C. A., et al. (1999). Prevalence and extent of atherosclerosis in adolescents and young adults: Implications for prevention from the Pathobiological Determinants of Atherosclerosis in Youth Study. *Journal of the American Medical Association, 281*(8), 727–735.

Updated by Olga A. Taylor

ALT, Alanine aminotransferase; *BMI,* body mass index; *BP,* blood pressure; *HDL,* high-density lipoprotein; *HgA1c,* hemoglobin A1c test; *LDL,* low-density lipoprotein.
*Adapted from the Quality and Safety Education for Nurses (QSEN) Institute.

individual nutritional counseling, ideally by a dietician with expertise in pediatric lipids.

Research continues to support the benefit of diets low in saturated fats. Current thinking favors a "Mediterranean"-type diet. Whole grains, fruits, and vegetables form the foundation of this diet. In addition, this diet recommends the use of monounsaturated fats, such as olive oil, canola oil, nuts, avocados, and fish, which have beneficial effects on HDL cholesterol values. Patients who have elevated triglycerides, particularly those with an elevated body mass index (BMI), should receive targeted counseling aimed at a low glycemic diet. Daily aerobic exercise of at least 60 minutes per day 5 days per week is also recommended for children. In addition, patients and parents should be counseled regarding the negative effects of smoking (both firsthand and secondhand).

For children with severe hypercholesterolemia who fail to respond to dietary modifications, drug therapy may be necessary. Pharmacologic therapy is recommended for children older than 10 years of age who have LDL cholesterol greater than 190 mg/dL without other risk factors or greater than 160 mg/dL in patients with two or more other risk factors or with a family history of early heart disease in a first-degree relative. In young people who are considered to have individual risk conditions (e.g., diabetes, chronic kidney disease, Kawasaki disease with aneurysms, or heart transplant recipients), the threshold for medication is lower and may be considered when LDL values are greater than 130 mg/dL.

The use of medication in a child/adolescent needs to be a cooperative decision with the parents. Parents and patients should understand the available data related to statin use in young people particularly because prospective, long-term evidence-based practice is not practical or available for this population. Options for lipid-lowering medications include bile acid–binding resins, 3-hydroxy-3-methylglutaryl coenzyme A (HMG-CoA) reductase inhibitors (statins), ezetimibe, and fibrates. Nicotinic acid is generally not used in children or adolescents.

The most recent guidelines on lipid abnormalities in children recommend treatment with statins if pharmacologic therapy is indicated after lifestyle modification has been attempted (Expert Panel on Integrated Guidelines for Cardiovascular Health and Risk Reduction in Children and Adolescents & National Heart, Lung, and Blood Institute, 2012). Statins are effective in lowering LDL cholesterol. To a lesser degree, they also help lower triglyceride levels and can raise HDL cholesterol somewhat. Statins work by inhibiting the enzyme necessary for cholesterol synthesis. Statins are most effective when taken in the evening and are started at the lowest possible dose in young people. Blood work should be followed closely in children and adolescents and usually includes a fasting lipid profile, liver function tests, and creatinine kinase repeated 1 month or so after initiation, and then twice yearly as well as with any dosage changes.

Patients beginning therapy with a statin should be counseled regarding rare but potentially serious side effects (e.g., rhabdomyolysis) as well as more minor potential side effects. Patients should discontinue their medication and contact their practitioner if they develop dark urine or new muscle aches. Statin medications are not safe during pregnancy; therefore, sexually active adolescents need to take adequate birth control measures. Very long–term studies are unlikely to be available over decades; however, in the shorter-term studies that have been completed, statins seem to have a similar safety profile for children as they do for adults (McCrindle, Urbina, Dennison, et al., 2007). Ezetimibe is sometimes given in combination with statins to further reduce LDL cholesterol, which it accomplishes by decreasing reabsorption of cholesterol from the gut. Another class of lipid-lowering drugs includes bile acid–binding resins. Bile acid– binding resins act by binding bile acids in the intestinal lumen. Because the intestine does not absorb them, resin binders do not produce systemic toxicity and are safe for children. Cholestyramine (Questran) and colestipol (Colestid) are both powders that are mixed with water or juice just before ingestion. Unfortunately, the vast majority of patients do not get adequate reduction in LDL cholesterol from bile acid–binding resins alone. Many cannot tolerate the medication because of the taste; gritty texture; and side effects, the most significant being constipation, abdominal pain, gastrointestinal bloating, flatulence, and nausea. Lastly, it is not common to use medications to lower triglyceride values unless they are significantly elevated (>500 mg/dL), in which case fibrates, which decrease the production of triglycerides, may be considered.

Care Management

Nurses play an important role in the screening, education, and support of children with lipid abnormalities and their families. When a child is referred to a preventive cardiology clinic, it is essential that the family be adequately prepared for the first visit. Generally, the parents will be asked to keep a dietary history of the child before this visit. Sometimes they will need to complete a questionnaire regarding the child's normal dietary habits. Families should be instructed to keep their child fasting for at least 12 hours before lab work. In addition, parents should be aware that lipids should not be drawn within 3 weeks of a febrile illness because doing so can affect cholesterol values. It is important to schedule the blood test early in the morning and to arrange for nourishment immediately thereafter. At the visit, a full family history should be taken, including the health of both parents and all first-degree relatives. Specific questions should be asked regarding early heart disease, hypertension, strokes (CVAs), sudden death, hyperlipidemia, diabetes, and endocrine abnormalities.

Patients and parents should be educated about cholesterol and lipid abnormalities. This should include a brief introduction of the different lipoprotein categories, including an explanation of the components of the lipid profile. Also, lifestyle risk factors for heart disease, such as smoking and exercise, should be reviewed. For management to be effective, parents and patients need to understand that the rationale for dietary or pharmacologic intervention is prevention of future cardiovascular disease and is part of any treatment plan for lipid abnormalities.

A child with a lipid disorder should not be viewed as having a disease, and stringent dietary guidelines may become an issue of control and a source of great stress for many families. Rather, the positive aspects of healthy eating, regularly exercising, and avoiding smoking should be emphasized. Basic dietary changes should be encouraged for the whole family so that the affected child is not singled out. Cultural differences must be considered and recommendations individualized. Substitution rather than elimination needs to be emphasized. Visual aids (e.g., test tubes depicting the amount of fat in a hot dog or the number or packs of sugar in a glass of juice) are often helpful, especially for children. Diets should be flexible and individually tailored by a nutritionist who is experienced in lipid disorders. Dietary recommendations need to meet the nutritional demands of growing children while providing benefit to the overall profile. Parents and patients are encouraged to participate in dietary and educational sessions, ask questions, and share ideas and experiences.

Parents often feel guilty about the hereditary component of hyperlipidemia. Many also believe they have failed if the diet alone is not making a significant difference in their child's lipid profile. They need to be reassured that a dietary approach alone is often not sufficient, especially for children with genetically elevated values.

Parents of children who require pharmacologic therapy need to understand the purpose, dosage, and possible side effects of the various drugs. Medication schedules should remain flexible and should not interfere with the child's daily activities. Follow-up phone calls by the nurse between visits allow parents to discuss their concerns and ask any questions that have arisen.

CARDIAC DYSRHYTHMIAS

Dysrhythmias, or abnormal heart rhythms, can occur in children with structurally normal hearts, as features of some congenital heart defects, and in patients after surgical repair of congenital heart defects. They are also seen in patients with cardiomyopathy and with cardiac tumors. They can occur secondary to metabolic and electrolyte imbalances. They can be classified in several ways, including by heart rate characteristics (bradycardia and tachycardia) and by the origin of the dysrhythmia in the atria or ventricles. Some dysrhythmias are well tolerated and self-limiting. Others may cause decreased cardiac output with associated symptoms. Some dysrhythmias can cause sudden death. Treatment depends on the cause of the dysrhythmia and its severity.

Many advances have been made in the diagnosis and treatment of pediatric dysrhythmias in the past decade. Improvements in technology have allowed better diagnosis, the development of ablation techniques, and the expansion of pacemaker capabilities. New antidysrhythmic medications have proven safe and effective in children. Radiofrequency ablation has offered a cure for some dysrhythmias. Pediatric electrophysiology has become a highly specialized field, and students should consult more detailed sources for an in-depth discussion. The following sections address diagnostic studies and provide a general discussion of the most common tachycardia (supraventricular tachycardia [SVT]) and the most common bradycardia (complete heart block) that require treatment in the pediatric population.

Diagnostic Evaluation

Nurses must be familiar with the standards of normal heart rate for the particular age group. An initial nursing responsibility is recognition of an abnormal heartbeat, either in rate or rhythm. When a dysrhythmia is suspected, the apical rate is counted for 1 full minute and compared with the radial rate, which may be lower because not all of the apical beats are felt. Consistently, high or low heart rates should be regarded as suspicious. The patient should be placed on a cardiac monitor with recording capabilities. A 12-lead ECG yields more information than the monitor recording and should be done as soon as possible.

The basic diagnostic procedure is the ECG, including 24-hour Holter monitoring. Electrophysiologic cardiac catheterization allows for identification of the conduction disturbance and immediate investigation of drugs that may control the dysrhythmia. Another procedure that may be used is transesophageal recording. An electrode catheter is passed to the lower esophagus and, when in position at a point proximal to the heart, is used to stimulate and record dysrhythmias.

Dysrhythmias can be classified according to various criteria, such as effect on heart rate and rhythm, as follows:

Bradydysrhythmias: Abnormally slow rate
Tachydysrhythmias: Abnormally rapid rate
Conduction disturbances: Irregular heart rate

Bradydysrhythmias

Sinus bradycardia (slower than normal rate) in children can be attributed to the influence of the autonomic nervous system, as with hypervagal tone, or in response to hypoxia and hypotension. Sinus bradycardias are also known to develop after some complex cardiac surgical repairs involving extensive atrial suture lines, such as atrial baffle repairs (Mustard and Senning repairs) and the Fontan procedure.

Complete atrioventricular (AV) block is also referred to as *complete heart block.* This can be either congenital (occurring in children with structurally normal hearts) or acquired after surgery to repair cardiac defects. AV blocks are most often related to edema around the conduction system and resolve without treatment. Temporary epicardial wires are placed in most patients at surgery; if a rhythm disturbance occurs,

temporary pacing can be used. Several days after surgery, the health practitioner removes the wires by pulling slowly and deliberately down on them from the site of insertion.

Some children may need a permanent pacemaker. The pacemaker takes over or assists in the heart's conduction function. The implantation of a pacemaker, in the operating room or possibly the catheterization laboratory, is usually a low-risk procedure. The pacemaker is made up of two basic parts, the pulse generator and the lead. The pulse generator is composed of the battery and the electronic circuitry. The lead is an insulated, flexible wire that conducts the electrical impulse from the pulse generator to the heart. Two types of leads are available, transvenous and epicardial. After the lead has been attached to the heart, a small incision is made, and a pocket is formed under the muscle to house and protect the generator. Continuous ECG monitoring is necessary during the recovery phase to assess pacemaker function. The nurse should be aware of the programmed rate and expected individual generator variations. The pacemaker insertion site is monitored for signs of infection. Analgesics are given for pain.

Pacemaker functions have become more sophisticated, and some models can adjust the heart rate to activity demands or be programmed for overdrive pacing or cardioversion.

Discharge teaching includes information about the signs and symptoms of infection, general wound care, and activity restrictions. Parents, and patients if they are old enough, should be taught to take a pulse and know the settings of the pacemaker. If the patient's low rate is set at 80 beats/min and the heart rate is only 68 beats/min, there is a possible problem with the pacemaker that needs to be investigated. Instructions for telephone transmission of ECG readings are also given. Telephone transmission can be used to transmit ECG strips and to monitor battery life and pacemaker function. The pacemaker generator will have to be replaced periodically because of battery depletion. Children with pacemakers should wear a MedicAlert device, and their parents should have a paper identification card with specific pacer data in case of an emergency. Cardiopulmonary resuscitation (CPR) instruction is suggested for parents.

Tachydysrhythmias

Sinus tachycardia (an abnormally fast heart rate) secondary to fever, anxiety, pain, anemia, dehydration, or any other etiologic factor requiring increased cardiac output should be ruled out before diagnosing an increased heart rate as pathologic. SVT is the most common tachydysrhythmia found in children and refers to a rapid regular heart rate of 200 to 300 beats/min. As many as 1 in 250 children experience SVT (Schlechte, Boramanand & Funk, 2008). The onset of SVT is often sudden, the duration is variable, and the rhythm may end abruptly and convert back to a normal sinus rhythm. Clinical signs in infants and young children are poor feeding, extreme irritability, and pallor. Children may experience palpitations, dizziness, chest pain, and diaphoresis. If SVT is sustained, signs of HF may be seen.

The treatment of SVT depends on the degree of compromise imposed by the dysrhythmia (see Clinical Reasoning Case Study: Supraventricular Tachycardia). In some cases, vagal maneuvers, such as applying ice to the face, massaging the carotid artery (on one side of the neck only), or having an older child perform a Valsalva maneuver (e.g., exhaling against a closed glottis, blowing on a thumb as if it were a trumpet for 30 to 60 seconds), have terminated SVT. If vagal maneuvers fail or the child is hemodynamically unstable, adenosine (a drug that impairs AV conduction) may be used. Adenosine is given by rapid IV push with a saline bolus immediately after the drug because of its very short half-life. If this is unsuccessful or cardiac output is compromised, esophageal overdrive pacing or synchronized cardioversion (delivering an electrical shock to the heart) can be used in the intensive care setting. Sedation

CLINICAL REASONING CASE STUDY
Supraventricular Tachycardia

You are working in the emergency department when a father comes through the doors, crying, carrying his 1-month-old infant. The infant is awake and very irritable. The father reports that the infant has not been feeding well for the past 6 hours, and the father has noticed sweating (diaphoresis) with attempted feeds. No history of fever is noted. Further assessment reveals a diaphoretic, crying infant with a respiratory rate of 60 breaths/min, blood pressure of 60/40 mm Hg, and heart rate that is too fast to count by auscultation. When the infant is attached to the cardiorespiratory monitor, the heart rate is 220 beats/min, nonvariable, with an oxygen saturation of 97%. Capillary refill time is slightly prolonged at 3 seconds, and femoral pulses are palpable but weak.

Questions
1. Evidence: Is there sufficient evidence to draw conclusions about this infant?
2. Assumptions: Describe an underlying assumption about each of the following:
   a. Symptoms associated with heart failure
   b. An infant younger than 3 months of age with poor feeding
   c. Tachyarrhythmias in infants
3. What priorities for nursing care should be established?
4. Does the evidence support your nursing interventions?

is needed for both procedures. Cardioversion should never be done in a conscious patient. More long-term pharmacologic treatment includes digoxin or possibly propranolol (Inderal) or amiodarone for severe or recurrent SVT.

A primary focus of nursing care is education of the family regarding the symptoms of SVT and its treatment. SVT may occur again despite therapy. Parents should be taught to take a radial pulse for 1 full minute. If medication is prescribed, instructions regarding accurate dosage and the importance of administering the correct dose at specified intervals are stressed.

Radiofrequency ablation has become first-line therapy for some types of SVT. The procedure is done in the cardiac catheterization laboratory and begins with mapping of the conduction system to identify the dysrhythmia focus. A catheter delivering radiofrequency current is directed at the site, and the area is heated to destroy the tissue in the area. These are lengthy procedures, often lasting 6 to 8 hours, and sedation or general anesthesia is required. Preparation is similar to that for cardiac catheterization. Another procedure, cryoablation, is also used in treatment of SVT. Liquid nitrous oxide is used to cool a catheter to subfreezing temperatures, which then destroys the tissue of target by freezing.

PULMONARY ARTERY HYPERTENSION

Pulmonary artery hypertension (PAH) is a disease of the entire pulmonary circulation. The pulmonary arteries are described as having vascular narrowing due to decreased vascular growth and surface area, as well as structure remodeling of the vessel wall (Abman & Ivy, 2011). This leads to an increase in pulmonary vascular resistance. These disorders are poorly understood, and until recently, there was no treatment beyond supportive care. PAH is a progressive, eventually fatal disease for which there is no known cure. It can be difficult to diagnose in the early stages. Often when patients become symptomatic and a diagnosis is made, their disease is rapidly progressing, treatment is unsuccessful, and death occurs within several years. There is also evidence of a genetic basis for some PAH (Newman, Phillips, & Loyd, 2008).

There are many possible causes of PAH. Cardiac causes occur primarily in patients with a large left-to-right shunt producing increased pulmonary blood flow. If these defects are not repaired early, the high pulmonary flow will cause changes in the pulmonary artery vessels, and the vessels will lose their elasticity. Other causes of PAH include hypoxic lung diseases, thromboembolic diseases causing pulmonary vascular obstruction, collagen vascular diseases, exposure to toxic substances, and congenital heart defects with a large left-to-right shunt, from increased pulmonary blood flow. Many of the patients have no identifiable cause for PAH and have primary or idiopathic PAH.

Clinical Manifestations

Clinical manifestations include dyspnea with exercise, chest pain, and syncope. Dyspnea is the most common symptom and is caused by impaired oxygen delivery. Chest pain is the result of coronary ischemia in the right ventricle from severe hypertrophy. Syncope reflects a limited cardiac output leading to decreased cerebral blood flow. Right-sided heart dysfunction is steadily progressive, and when symptoms of venous congestion and edema are present, the prognosis is poor.

Therapeutic Management

Although no cure is known, several therapies have shown promise in slowing the progression of the disease and improving quality of life. In general, situations that may exacerbate the disease and cause hypoxia, such as exercise and high altitudes, are avoided. Supplemental oxygen, especially at night while sleeping, is commonly used to relieve hypoxia. Patients are at risk for thromboembolic events leading to pulmonary emboli, so anticoagulation with warfarin (Coumadin) is often prescribed.

A number of new drug therapies have been used in this patient population and have promise in improving quality of life and survival. Several studies and newer approaches in treatment emphasize combined therapy that targets each of the major pathways of the disease process rather than monotherapy approaches.

Vasodilator therapy (which relaxes vascular smooth muscle and reduces pulmonary artery pressure) can prolong survival of patients with PAH. Oral calcium channel blockers have been successful in some children. For patients who are nonresponders in vasodilator testing, a new oral drug, bosentan (an endothelin-receptor antagonist), is now available that reduces pulmonary artery pressure and resistance and is safe and well tolerated in children (Barst, Ivy, Dingemanse, et al., 2003). It has been used in combination with IV prostacyclin.

Lung transplantation may be another treatment option for those with severe disease. Patients with pulmonary hypertension have had a higher mortality rate than after lung transplantation than other lung transplant patients. The management of PAH continues to evolve as new information is learned and new combination therapies are tested and evaluated.

QUALITY PATIENT OUTCOMES: Hypertension
- Underlying cause of hypertension identified
- Blood pressure (BP) control maintained
- Dietary practices and lifestyle changes effectively used to control hypertension
- Compliance with medication regimen, if prescribed

CARDIOMYOPATHY

Cardiomyopathy refers to abnormalities of the myocardium in which the cardiac muscles' ability to contract is impaired. Cardiomyopathies are relatively rare in children. Possible etiologic factors include familial or genetic causes, infection, deficiency states, metabolic abnormalities, and collagen vascular diseases. Most cardiomyopathies in children are considered primary or idiopathic, in which the cause is unknown and the cardiac dysfunction is not associated with systemic disease. Some of the known causes of secondary cardiomyopathy are anthracycline toxicity (the antineoplastic agents, doxorubicin [Adriamycin] and daunomycin), hemochromatosis (from excessive iron storage), Duchenne muscular dystrophy, Kawasaki disease, collagen diseases, and thyroid dysfunction.

Cardiomyopathies can be divided into three broad clinical categories according to the type of abnormal structure and dysfunction present: (1) dilated cardiomyopathy, (2) hypertrophic cardiomyopathy, and (3) restrictive cardiomyopathy.

Dilated cardiomyopathy is characterized by ventricular dilation and greatly decreased contractility, resulting in symptoms of HF. This is the most common type of cardiomyopathy in children. Its cause is often unknown. The clinical findings are HF with tachycardia, dyspnea, hepatosplenomegaly, fatigue, and poor growth. Dysrhythmias may be present and may be more difficult to control with worsening HF.

Hypertrophic cardiomyopathy is characterized by an increase in heart muscle mass without an increase in cavity size, usually occurring in the left ventricle and associated with abnormal diastolic filling. It is a familial autosomal dominant genetic abnormality in most cases and is probably the most common genetically transmitted cardiovascular disease (Maron, 2001). The expression of clinical disease varies greatly among patients. Clinical symptoms usually appear during the school-age period or adolescence and may include anginal chest pain, dysrhythmias, and syncope. One recent study confirmed that unexplained syncope in the childhood age group (younger than 18 years of age) with known hypertrophic cardiomyopathy had a 60% cumulative risk for sudden death within 5 years of the syncopal event (Spirito, Autore, Rapezzi, et al., 2009). Presentation in infancy includes signs of HF and has a poor prognosis. The ECG demonstrates left ventricular hypertrophy, often with ST-T changes. The echocardiogram is most helpful and demonstrates asymmetric septal hypertrophy and an increase in left ventricular wall thickness, with a small left ventricle cavity.

Restrictive cardiomyopathy, which is rare in children, describes a restriction to ventricular filling caused by endocardial or myocardial disease or both. It is characterized by diastolic dysfunction and absence of ventricular dilation or hypertrophy. Symptoms are similar to those of HF (see earlier in this chapter).

Therapeutic Management

Treatment is directed toward correcting the underlying cause whenever feasible. However, in most affected children, this is not possible, and treatment is aimed at managing HF (see earlier in this chapter) and dysrhythmias. Digoxin, diuretics, and aggressive use of afterload reduction agents have been found to be helpful in managing symptoms in those with dilated cardiomyopathy. Practice guidelines for the management of HF in children have been outlined and provide an in-depth review of available therapies (Rosenthal, Chrisant, Edens, et al., 2004; Rossano & Shaddy, 2014). Digoxin and inotropic agents are usually not helpful in the other forms of cardiomyopathy because increasing the force of contraction may exacerbate the muscular obstruction and actually impair ventricular ejection. Beta blockers (e.g., propranolol) and calcium channel blockers (e.g., verapamil) have been used to reduce left ventricular outflow obstruction and improve diastolic filling in those with hypertrophic cardiomyopathy.

Careful monitoring and treatment of dysrhythmias are essential. The placement of an automatic implantable cardioverter defibrillator (AICD) should be considered for patients at high risk for sudden death because of ventricular dysrhythmias. Anticoagulants may be given to reduce the risk for thromboemboli, a complication of the sluggish circulation through the heart. For worsening HF and signs of poor perfusion, IV inotropic or vasodilating drugs may be needed. Severely ill children may require mechanical ventilation, oxygen administration, and IV medications. Heart transplantation may be a treatment option for patients who have worsening symptoms despite maximum medical therapy.

Care Management

Because of the poor prognosis in many children with cardiomyopathy, nursing care is consistent with that for any child with a life-threatening disorder (see Chapter 36). One of the most difficult adjustments for the child may be the realization of failing health and the need for restricted activity. The child should be included in decisions regarding activity and allowed to discuss feelings, particularly if the disease follows a progressively fatal course. After symptoms of HF or dysrhythmias develop, the same nursing interventions are implemented as discussed earlier in this chapter. If heart transplantation is considered, the needs of the child and family are great in terms of psychologic preparation and postoperative care. The nurse plays an important role in assessing the family's understanding of the procedure and long-term consequences. Children of school age and older should be fully informed to give their assent to the procedure (see the "Informed Consent" section in Chapter 39).

HEART TRANSPLANTATION

Heart transplantation has become a treatment option for infants and children with worsening HF and a limited life expectancy despite maximum medical and surgical management. Indications for heart transplantation in children are cardiomyopathy and end-stage CHD. It is also an option for patients with some forms of complex congenital cardiac defects, such as HLHS, for whom conventional surgical approaches have a high mortality rate.

The heart transplant procedure may be orthotopic or heterotopic. *Orthotopic heart transplantation* refers to removing the recipient's own heart and implanting a new heart from a donor who has had brain death but a healthy heart. The donor and recipient are matched by weight and blood type. *Heterotopic heart transplantation* refers to leaving the recipient's own heart in place and implanting a new heart to act as an additional pump, or "piggyback" heart; this type of transplant is rarely done in children.

Before transplantation, potential recipients undergo a careful cardiac evaluation to determine if there are any other medical or surgical options to improve the patient's cardiac status. Other organ systems are assessed to identify problems that might increase the risk of or preclude transplantation. A psychosocial evaluation of the patient and family is done to assess family function, support systems, and ability to comply with the complex medical regimen after the transplant. Support services to help the family successfully care for their child are provided when possible. Parents and older adolescents need extensive education about the risks and benefits of transplantation so that they can make an informed decision. Patients are listed on a national computer network organized by the United Network for Organ Sharing to match donors and recipients (see the "Organ or Tissue Donation and Autopsy" section in Chapter 36).

The total number of pediatric heart transplants has increased from 274 in 1998 to 372 in 2012 (Scientific Registry of Transplant Recipients, 2012). Primary diagnosis for the majority of candidates continues to be complex CHD, and most (87.9%) candidates are status 1A at the time of transplant (Scientific Registry of Transplant Recipients). The 1-year graft survival rate for pediatric heart transplants performed in 2012 was 87.5% (Scientific Registry of Transplant Recipients).

Waiting list mortality remains high, particularly in the smallest children. Recent progress in suitable ventricular assist devices for use in children as a bridge to transplantation has made outcomes to survival for cardiac transplantation more successful (Blume, Naftel, Bastardi, et al., 2006). A multicenter study using the US Scientific Registry of Transplant Recipients was recently conducted (Almond, Thiagarajian, Piercy, et al., 2009). Among 3098 children listed for a heart transplant between 1999 and 2006, the median age was 2 years. Sixty percent of patients were listed as a top status (30% ventilated and 18% on supportive measures), and of those children, 17% died, 63% received transplants, 8% recovered, and 12% remained listed. These numbers concluded that waiting time in the United States remains high in the current era, and high-risk groups in these categories could benefit from emerging cardiac assist devices, such as extracorporeal membrane oxygenation and ventricular assist devices.

The posttransplant course is complex. Although heart function is greatly improved or normal after transplantation, the risk for rejection is serious. The leading cause of death in the first 3 years after heart transplantation is rejection, with the greatest risk in the first 6 months (Blume, 2003). Rejection of the heart is diagnosed primarily by endomyocardial biopsy in older children. Serial echocardiograms are often used in infants and young children to reduce the need for invasive biopsies. Immunosuppressants must be taken for life and have many systemic side effects. Triple-drug therapy for immunosuppression with a calcineurin inhibitor (cyclosporine or tacrolimus), steroids, and mycophenolate mofetil or azathioprine is most commonly used in pediatric patients. Steroids are weaned in the first year and may be discontinued in some patients; many pediatric centers are avoiding long-term steroids by utilizing induction therapy protocols of high-dose steroids and thymoglobulin at the time of transplant (Thrush & Hoffman, 2014).

Infection is always a risk. Potential long-term problems that may limit survival include chronic rejection, causing coronary artery disease; renal dysfunction and hypertension resulting from cyclosporine administration; lymphoma; and infection. Coronary artery disease is the leading cause of death among late survivors of heart transplantation (Boucek, Aurora, Edwards, et al., 2007). In the short term, after successful transplantation, children are able to return to full participation in age-appropriate activities and appear to adapt well to their new lifestyle. Transplantation is not a cure because patients must live with the lifetime consequences of chronic immunosuppression.

Care Management

Successfully caring for a child after a heart transplant requires the expertise and dedication of many members of the health care team. Nurses play vital roles in assessment, coordination of care, psychosocial support, and patient and family education. The heart transplant recipient must be carefully monitored for signs of rejection, infection, and the side effects of the immunosuppressant medications. The patient's and family's psychosocial well-being also needs to be assessed to identify issues such as increased family stress, depression, substance abuse, and school problems. Noncompliance with an intense medication regimen, especially during adolescence, can lead to serious medical problems and can be fatal. Immunosuppressants and nursing implications are discussed in Chapter 44 in relation to renal transplantation. Care of the immunosuppressed child is reviewed in Chapter 43. Psychosocial concerns and appropriate interventions for the child with a life-threatening disorder are presented in Chapter 36.

The first 6 months to 1 year after the transplant are most intense because the risk for complications is greatest and the patient and family are adjusting to a new lifestyle. Patients are monitored closely by the health care team, with frequent visits and laboratory tests. Care is usually shared between local health care providers and the transplant center. Many patients are able to return to school and other age-appropriate activities within 2 to 3 months after the transplant.

VASCULAR DYSFUNCTION

SYSTEMIC HYPERTENSION

Hypertension is defined as the consistent elevation of BP beyond values considered to be the upper limits of normal. The two major categories are *essential hypertension* (no identifiable cause) and *secondary hypertension* (subsequent to an identifiable cause). In recent years, there has been increasing incidence in this disorder in adolescents and children, which is most likely related to the obesity epidemic. Hypertension in children and adolescents is defined as having a systolic or diastolic BP that consistently falls at or over the 95th percentile. This group is further delineated as follows:

Stage 1 hypertension includes patients who have BP readings between the 95th and 99th percentiles.

Stage 2 hypertension includes patients with BP readings over the 99th percentile plus 5 mm Hg.

An additional group includes children and adolescents who have prehypertension (or high-normal BP). This prehypertensive group includes those with BP readings that fall consistently between the 90th and 95th percentiles. *The Fourth Report on the Diagnosis, Evaluation, and Treatment of High Blood Pressure in Children and Adolescents* outlines in detail the identification, testing, and treatment recommendations for young people with high BP (National High Blood Pressure Education Program Working Group on High Blood Pressure in Children and Adolescents, 2004). These recommendations were reiterated in the more recent Expert Panel on Integrated Guidelines for Cardiovascular Health and Risk Reduction (Expert Panel on Integrated Guidelines for Cardiovascular Health and Risk Reduction in Children and Adolescents, & National Heart, Lung, and Blood Institute, 2011).

Etiology

Most instances of hypertension in young children occur secondary to a structural abnormality or an underlying pathologic process, although this is being challenged by screening programs of relatively healthy children. The most common cause of secondary hypertension is renal disease followed by cardiovascular, endocrine, and some neurologic disorders. As a rule, the younger the child and the more severe the hypertension, the more likely it is to be secondary.

The causes of essential hypertension are undetermined, but evidence indicates that both genetic and environmental factors play a role. The incidence of hypertension has been shown to be higher in children whose parents are hypertensive. African-Americans have a higher incidence of hypertension than whites, and in African-Americans it develops earlier, is frequently more severe, and results in death at an earlier age. Environmental factors that contribute to the risk for developing hypertension include obesity, salt ingestion, smoking, and stress.

Diagnostic Evaluation

BP assessment should be a routine part of annual assessment in healthy children older than 3 years of age. BP readings should also be done in those children younger than 3 years of age who have high-risk family histories or those with individual risk factors, including CHD, kidney disease, malignancy, transplant, certain neurologic problems, or systemic illnesses known to cause hypertension. Although clinical manifestations associated with hypertension depend largely on the underlying cause, some observations can provide clues to the examiner that an elevated BP may be a factor (Box 42.11). In infants and very young children who cannot communicate symptoms, observation of behavior may provide clues, although gross behavioral changes may not be apparent until complications are present.

No definitive cutoff values are used in the diagnosis of hypertension in the pediatric patient. The Expert Panel on Integrated Guidelines for Cardiovascular Health and Risk Reduction in Children and Adolescents (National Heart, Lung, and Blood Institute, 2012) endorsed the National Heart, Lung, and Blood Institute's *Fourth Report on the Diagnosis, Evaluation, and Treatment of High Blood Pressure in Children and Adolescents* (National High Blood Pressure Education Program Working Group on High Blood Pressure in Children and Adolescents, 2004). Both documents provide normative data for children. BP tables include the 50th, 90th, 95th, and 99th percentiles for BP readings based on age, gender, and height percentiles. These guidelines are based on auscultatory readings, and therefore this is currently the preferred method of assessment. These charts take into account differences in body height but not weight or BMI. It is therefore important to note that a child who is large for his or her age may normally have a higher BP than a child of average size. Before a diagnosis is made, BP should be measured on at least three separate occasions. An ambulatory BP monitor may be ordered if "white-coat hypertension" is suspected. These are useful in that they provide BP readings over a 24-hour period. There are different normative values for ambulatory BP readings (Urbina, Alpert, Flynn, et al., 2008).

A careful medical history and family history should be obtained to screen for other relatives with hypertension or other cardiovascular risk factors. In children with suspected hypertension, initial laboratory data include a urinalysis, renal function studies (e.g., creatinine and blood urea nitrogen), a lipid profile, complete blood count, and electrolytes. Depending on the severity of hypertension, additional testing may be indicated. Testing may include a retinal examination, renal ultrasonography to measure kidney size, and Doppler flow to detect the likelihood of a renal etiology. In addition, an ECG and an echocardiogram help to evaluate the presence of end-organ involvement, such as left ventricular hypertrophy. Further testing for a secondary cause of hypertension may be indicated in children with significant hypertension and normal initial screening test findings.

Oral contraceptives can be a cause of hypertension because of their pressor effects. A trial off of oral contraceptives may be indicated; however, other contraceptive options should be discussed before this decision is made.

Therapeutic Management

Therapy for secondary hypertension involves diagnosis and treatment of the underlying cause. Children and adolescents with consistently elevated BP readings from no known cause or those with secondary hypertension not amenable to surgical correction may be treated with a combination of lifestyle and pharmacologic interventions. Dietary practices and lifestyle changes are important in the control of hypertension both for children and for adults. Nonpharmacologic measures, such as weight control in overweight patients, increased exercise, limited salt intake (such as recommended in the Dietary Approaches to Stop Hypertension [DASH] diet), and avoidance of stress and smoking, carry no risk and should be instituted as first-line therapy except in severe cases in which pharmacologic therapy may be indicated as well.

Drug therapy is instituted with caution in children with significant elevations of BP despite lifestyle modification. The treatment should begin with one drug with additional drug added if control is not obtained. The classes of oral antihypertensive drugs used in children include the β blockers, ACE inhibitors, calcium channel blockers, angiotensin-receptor blockers, and diuretics. The goal is to achieve a normotensive state without accompanying drug side effects.

Care Management

BP measurement should be a part of the routine assessment of children older than 3 years of age and patients younger than 3 years of age who are considered to be at high risk for hypertension. To obtain an accurate reading, care is taken to quiet the child or relax the adolescent while the measurement is recorded to avoid false readings caused by excitement. BP should be measured in the sitting position with the arm at the level of the heart. Initial evaluation should also include four extremity pressures (in the supine position) to rule out coarctation of the aorta. The chief cause of falsely elevated BP readings is the use of improperly fitting, narrow cuffs. Therefore, attention to correct measurement technique is essential (see the "Blood Pressure" section in Chapter 29).

Education aimed at understanding hypertension and its implication over the life span is essential in promoting patient and family compliance with both non-pharmacologic and pharmacologic therapies (see the "Compliance" section in Chapter 39).

Ambulatory/home BP measurements can facilitate surveillance in patients being assessed for hypertension or can document the effectiveness of therapy for those being treated for chronic hypertension. In addition, a family member can be instructed in how to take and record accurate BP measurements, thus decreasing the number of trips to a health care facility. This individual needs to have parameters, above which they should contact the practitioner. In addition, the school nurse can often be a valuable resource in monitoring BP. The nurse plays an important role in assessing individual families and providing targeted information regarding nonpharmacologic modes of intervention, such as diet, weight loss, smoking cessation, and exercise programs. A DASH diet—low in sodium, red meats, and sugar, and high in fruits, vegetables, whole grains, beans, nuts, low-fat dairy, fish, and poultry—is recommended for children/adolescents with elevated BP/hypertension. The child should be referred to a nutritionist with expertise in working with children and adolescents with hypertension. Exercise regimens should be individualized but should emphasize the benefits of regular aerobic exercise (ideally 300 minutes of aerobic exercise weekly). School-age children and young adolescents generally prefer team sports rather than individual training, which they may view as a burden rather than an enjoyable activity. If peers and family members can be encouraged to participate in any of the management strategies, the child's compliance is likely to be greater.

If drug therapy is prescribed, the nurse needs to provide information to the family regarding the reasons for it, how the drug works, and possible side effects. General instructions for antihypertensive drugs include the following:

- Rise slowly from a horizontal position, and avoid sudden position changes.
- Take drugs as prescribed.
- Maintain adequate hydration.
- Notify the practitioner if unpleasant side effects occur, but do not discontinue the drug.
- Avoid alcohol, and stay on the prescribed diet.

The need for regular follow-up is stressed, especially because antihypertensive therapy can sometimes be safely discontinued if BP remains under control over time.

KAWASAKI DISEASE

Kawasaki disease is an acute systemic vasculitis of unknown cause. It is seen in every racial group, with 75% of the cases occurring in children younger than 5 years of age. The peak incidence is in the toddler age group. The acute disease is self-limited; however, without treatment, approximately 20% to 25% of children develop coronary artery dilation or aneurysm formation. Infants younger than 1 year of age are at the greatest risk for heart involvement, although an increased incidence has also been reported in older children, perhaps because of later diagnosis in many.

The etiology of Kawasaki disease is unknown. The illness is not spread by person-to-person contact; however, several factors support an infectious etiologic trigger, possible in a genetically susceptible host. It is often seen in geographic and seasonal outbreaks, with an increased incidence reported in the late winter and early spring (Newburger, de Ferranti, Fulton, et al., 2015; Newburger, Takahashi, Gerber, et al., 2004).

Pathophysiology

The principal area of concern in Kawasaki disease is the cardiovascular system. During the initial stage of the illness, extensive inflammation of the arterioles, venules, and capillaries is evident, resulting in many of the clinical symptoms. In addition, segmental damage to the medium-sized muscular arteries, mainly the coronary arteries, can occur, resulting in the formation of coronary artery aneurysms in some children. Death is very rare in Kawasaki disease (<0.17% of cases) and is usually the result of myocardial ischemia from coronary thrombosis during the first few months of illness or years later from severe scar formation and stenosis in coronary aneurysms (Wilder, Palinkas, Kao, et al., 2007).

Clinical Manifestations

Because no specific diagnostic test exists for Kawasaki disease, the diagnosis is established on the basis of clinical findings and associated laboratory results (Box 42.12). These criteria should be used as guidelines. It is important to note that many children with Kawasaki disease do not fulfill standard diagnostic criteria, and infants in particular often have an incomplete presentation. It is therefore important to consider

BOX 42.12   Diagnostic Criteria for Kawasaki Disease

Child must have fever for more than 5 days along with four of five clinical criteria* (diagnosis may be made on day 4 by an experienced practitioner if child has all the clinical criteria):
1. Changes in the extremities: In the acute-phase edema, erythema of the palms and soles; in the subacute phase, periungual desquamation (peeling) of the hands and feet
2. Bilateral conjunctival injection (inflammation) without exudation
3. Changes in the oral mucous membranes, such as erythema of the lips, oropharyngeal reddening; or "strawberry tongue" (large papillae are exposed)
4. Polymorphous rash
5. Cervical lymphadenopathy (one lymph node >1.5 cm)

*Incomplete Kawasaki disease should be considered in the situation of prolonged fever (see algorithm for incomplete Kawasaki disease from American Heart Association guidelines). Kawasaki disease can be diagnosed with fewer clinical criteria when coronary artery changes are noted.

Kawasaki disease as a possible diagnosis in any infant or child with prolonged fever that is unresponsive to antibiotics and is not attributable to another cause.

Kawasaki disease manifests in three phases: acute, subacute, and convalescent. The acute phase begins with an abrupt onset of a high fever that is unresponsive to antibiotics and antipyretics. The remaining diagnostic symptoms evolve over the next week or so. Symptoms may come and go and do not need to be present simultaneously for diagnosis, although the fever is generally persistent throughout. During this stage, the child is typically very irritable. The subacute phase begins with resolution of the fever and lasts until all clinical signs of Kawasaki disease have disappeared. During this phase, coronary artery aneurysms may be noticed or previously dilated vessels may continue to increase in size. Irritability persists during this phase. In the convalescent phase, all of the clinical signs of Kawasaki disease have resolved, but the laboratory values have not returned to normal. This phase is complete when all blood values are normal (6 to 8 weeks after onset). At the end of this stage, the child has regained his or her usual temperament, energy, and appetite.

Cardiac Involvement

Long-term complications of Kawasaki disease include the development of coronary artery aneurysms, potentially disrupting blood flow. Children with large (giant) aneurysms have the potential for myocardial infarction, which can result from thrombotic occlusion of a coronary aneurysm or late-stenosis of the same vessel.

Affected coronary arteries dilate progressively, reaching their maximal diameter approximately 1 month from the onset of fever. Over time, as the damaged vessel tries to heal, stenosis of the aneurysm may develop and may lead to myocardial ischemia. Most of the morbidity and mortality occur in children affected with the largest aneurysms (giant aneurysms >8 mm or z-score >10). Symptoms of acute myocardial infarction in young children can be confusing and may include abdominal pain, vomiting, restlessness, inconsolable crying, pallor, and shock, as well as chest pain or pressure (noted more in older children). In the initial phase of the illness, children with Kawasaki disease may have signs or symptoms related to inflammation of the myocardium, including myocarditis, valvulitis, or arrhythmias.

Echocardiograms are accurate in assessing coronary artery dilation and are used to monitor coronary artery dimensions, myocardial function, and valvar function. A baseline echocardiogram should be obtained at the time of diagnosis and is used for comparison with future studies, which are obtained at 1 week after the initial diagnosis and again at 4 to 6 weeks later. Additional echocardiograms should be done (often as frequently as twice per week) in situations where a child has coronary artery dilation or obvious aneurysm formation or when response to treatment is incomplete.

Therapeutic Management

The current treatment of children with Kawasaki disease includes high-dose intravenous immunoglobulin (IVIG) along with salicylate therapy. IVIG has been demonstrated to be effective at reducing the incidence of coronary artery abnormalities when given within the first 10 days of the illness and ideally in the first 7 days of illness. A single, large infusion of 2 g/kg over 10 to 12 hours is recommended. Retreatment with IVIG and/or other antiinflammatory drugs may be given to patients with an incomplete response to the initial IVIG (continued or recrudescent fever) or those with coronary artery dilation.

Aspirin is used in an antiinflammatory dose (80 to 100 mg/kg/day in divided doses every 6 hours) to control fever and symptoms of inflammation. However, after the fever has subsided, aspirin can be reduced to an antiplatelet dose (3 to 5 mg/kg/day). Low-dose aspirin is continued in patients without echocardiographic evidence of coronary abnormalities until the platelet count has returned to normal (6 to 8 weeks). If the child develops coronary abnormalities, salicylate therapy is continued indefinitely. Additional anticoagulation (e.g., clopidogrel [Plavix], enoxaparin [Lovenox], or warfarin) may be indicated in children who have medium-sized or giant coronary artery aneurysms.

Prognosis

Most children with Kawasaki disease recover fully after treatment. However, when cardiovascular complications occur, serious morbidity may result. The prognosis for patients is strongly related to the extent of coronary damage, with patients who have giant aneurysms being at the highest risk for complications and those with normal coronary dimensions having an excellent long-term prognosis.

QUALITY PATIENT OUTCOMES: Kawasaki Disease
- Early diagnosis and treatment
- Prevention of cardiovascular complications

Care Management

In the initial phase, the nurse must monitor the child's cardiac status carefully. Intake and output and daily weight measurements are recorded. Although the child may be reluctant to eat and therefore may be partially dehydrated, fluids need to be administered with care because of the usual finding of myocarditis. The child should be assessed frequently for signs of HF, including decreased urinary output, gallop rhythm (an additional heart sound), tachycardia, and respiratory distress.

Administration of IVIG should follow the same guidelines as for any blood product, with frequent monitoring of vital signs. Patients must be watched for allergic reactions. Cardiac status must be monitored because of the large volume being administered to patients who may have diminished left ventricular function.

The majority of nursing care in the hospital focuses on symptomatic relief. To minimize skin discomfort, cool cloths; unscented lotions; and soft, loose clothing are helpful. During the acute phase, mouth care, including lubricating ointment to the lips, is important for mucosal inflammation. Clear liquids and soft foods can be offered.

Patient irritability is perhaps the most challenging problem. These children need a quiet environment that promotes adequate rest. Their parents need to be supported in their efforts to comfort an often inconsolable child. They may need time away from their child, and nurses can often provide respite care for the family. Parents need to understand that irritability is a hallmark of Kawasaki disease and that it will resolve. They need not feel guilty or embarrassed about their child's behavior.

Discharge Teaching

Parents need accurate information about the course of the illness, including the importance of follow-up monitoring and when they should contact their practitioner. Irritability is likely to persist for up to 2 months after the onset of symptoms. Periungual desquamation (peeling of the hands and feet) begins in the second and third weeks. Usually the fingertips peel first followed by the feet. The peeling is painless, but the new skin may be tender. Arthritis is always temporary but may involve the larger weight-bearing joints and may persist for several weeks. Affected children are typically most stiff in the mornings, during cold weather, and after naps. Passive range-of-motion exercises in the bathtub are often helpful in increasing flexibility. Any live immunizations (e.g., measles, mumps, and rubella; varicella) should be deferred for 11 months after the administration of IVIG because the body might not produce the appropriate amount of antibodies to provide lifelong immunity. The decision to give the varicella (chickenpox) vaccine while the child is receiving aspirin therapy is made individually by the practitioner. Daily temperatures should be recorded in the first week or two after discharge, and the occurrence of fever should be communicated to the health care provider.

At discharge, the ultimate cardiac sequelae is generally not fully known yet because vessels may be evolving. Parents of children with large aneurysms should be educated as to the unlikely but real possibility of myocardial infarction, as well as the signs and symptoms of cardiac ischemia in a child. CPR should be taught to parents of children with severe coronary artery aneurysms.

Long-Term Follow-Up

The frequency and type of follow-up is based on the presence or absence of coronary damage. The long-term outlook for children without aneurysms is excellent. Increased incidence of early heart disease in this population has not been observed with over 40 years of follow-up. In order to keep the coronary arteries as healthy as possible, it is recommended that these children follow the national guidelines, which recommend screening for the presence of coronary risk factors as they grow older. They should have a cholesterol screen performed at routine physical examinations; routine BP monitoring; and education recommending a heart-healthy lifestyle, including exercise, a heart-healthy diet, and avoidance of smoking.

In patients with aneurysms, follow-up focuses on the prevention and early detection of coronary ischemia. Noninvasive modalities of coronary imaging (e.g., echocardiography, EKGs, and stress testing to assess for reversible ischemia) are used as much as possible with other forms of imaging such as cardiac computed tomography angiography, MRI, and cardiac catheterization recommended based on the individual situation.

In addition to regular monitoring, patients with coronary aneurysms may require long-term antiplatelet or anticoagulation and possibly β-blocker therapy or other therapies, depending on the severity of coronary involvement.

SHOCK

Shock, or *circulatory failure*, is a complex clinical syndrome characterized by inadequate tissue perfusion to meet the metabolic demands of the body, resulting in cellular dysfunction and eventual organ failure. Although the causes are different, the physiologic consequences are the same and include hypotension, tissue hypoxia, and metabolic acidosis. Circulatory failure in children is a result of hypovolemia, altered peripheral vascular resistance, or pump failure. Types of shock are listed in Box 42.13.

Pathophysiology

A healthy child's circulatory system is able to transport oxygen and metabolic substrates to body tissues, which require a constant source for these essential needs. The cardiac output and distribution to the various body tissues can change rapidly in response to intrinsic (myocardial and intravascular) or extrinsic (neuronal) control mechanisms. In shock states, these mechanisms are altered or challenged.

Reduced blood flow, as in hypovolemic shock, causes diminished venous return to the heart, low CVP, low cardiac output, and hypotension. Vasomotor centers in the medulla are signaled, causing a compensatory increase in the force and rate of cardiac contraction and constriction of arterioles and veins, thereby increasing peripheral vascular resistance. Simultaneously, the lowered blood volume leads to the release of large amounts of catecholamines, antidiuretic hormone, adrenocorticosteroids, and aldosterone in an effort to conserve body fluids. This causes reduced

BOX 42.13   Types of Shock

Hypovolemic
Characteristics
Reduction in size of vascular compartment
Falling BP
Poor capillary filling
Low CVP

Most Frequent Causes
Blood loss (hemorrhagic shock): Trauma, gastrointestinal bleeding, intracranial hemorrhage
Plasma loss: Increased capillary permeability associated with sepsis and acidosis, hypoproteinemia, burns, peritonitis
Extracellular fluid loss: Vomiting, diarrhea, glycosuric diuresis, sunstroke

Distributive
Characteristics
Reduction in peripheral vascular resistance
Profound inadequacies in tissue perfusion
Increased venous capacity and pooling
Acute reduction in return blood flow to the heart
Diminished cardiac output

Most Frequent Causes
Anaphylaxis (anaphylactic shock): Extreme allergy or hypersensitivity to a foreign substance
Sepsis (septic shock, bacteremic shock, endotoxic shock): Overwhelming sepsis and circulating bacterial toxins
Loss of neuronal control (neurogenic shock): Interruption of neuronal transmission (spinal cord injury)
Myocardial depression and peripheral dilation: Exposure to anesthesia or ingestion of barbiturates, tranquilizers, opioids, antihypertensive agents, or ganglionic blocking agents

Cardiogenic
Characteristic
Decreased cardiac output

Most Frequent Causes
After surgery for CHD
Primary pump failure: Myocarditis, myocardial trauma, biochemical derangements, heart failure
Dysrhythmias: SVT, AV block, and ventricular dysrhythmias; secondary to myocarditis or biochemical abnormalities (occasionally)

AV, Atrioventricular; *BP,* blood pressure; *CHD,* congenital heart disease; *CVP,* central venous pressure; *SVT,* supraventricular tachycardia.

BOX 42.14   Clinical Manifestations of Shock

Compensated	**Decompensated**
Apprehensiveness	Confusion and somnolence
Irritability	Tachypnea
Unexplained tachycardia	Moderate metabolic acidosis
Normal blood pressure (BP)	Oliguria
Narrowing pulse pressure	Cool, pale extremities
Thirst	Decreased skin turgor
Pallor	Poor capillary filling
Diminished urinary output	
Reduced perfusion of extremities	**Irreversible**
	Thready, weak pulse
	Hypotension
	Periodic breathing or apnea
	Anuria
	Stupor or coma

Complications of shock create further hazards. CNS hypoperfusion may eventually lead to cerebral edema, cortical infarction, or intraventricular hemorrhage. Renal hypoperfusion causes renal ischemia with possible tubular or glomerular necrosis and renal vein thrombosis. Reduced blood flow to the lungs can interfere with surfactant secretion and result in acute respiratory distress syndrome, which is characterized by sudden pulmonary congestion and atelectasis with formation of a hyaline membrane. Gastrointestinal tract bleeding and perforation are always possibilities after splanchnic ischemia and necrosis of intestinal mucosa. Metabolic complications of shock may include hypoglycemia, hypocalcemia, and other electrolyte disturbances.

Diagnostic Evaluation

The etiology of shock can be discerned from the history and the physical examination. The severity of the shock is determined by measurements of vital signs, including CVP and capillary filling (Box 42.14). Shock can be regarded as a form of compensation for circulatory failure. Because of the progressive nature of shock, it can be divided into the following three stages or phases:

1. **Compensated shock:** Vital organ function is maintained by intrinsic compensatory mechanisms; blood flow is usually normal or increased but generally uneven or maldistributed in the microcirculation.
2. **Decompensated shock:** Efficiency of the cardiovascular system gradually diminishes until perfusion in the microcirculation becomes marginal despite compensatory adjustments. The outcomes of circulatory failure that progress beyond the limits of compensation are tissue hypoxia, metabolic acidosis, and eventual dysfunction of all organ systems.
3. **Irreversible, or terminal, shock:** Damage to vital organs, such as the heart or brain, is of such magnitude that the entire organism will be disrupted regardless of therapeutic intervention. Death occurs even if cardiovascular measurements return to normal levels with therapy.

At all stages, the principal differentiating signs are observed in the (1) degree of tachycardia and perfusion to the extremities, (2) level of consciousness, and (3) BP. Additional signs or modifications of these more universal signs may be present depending on the type and cause of the shock. Initially, the child's ability to compensate is effective; therefore, early signs are subtle. As the shock state advances, signs are more obvious and indicate early decompensation.

Additional signs may be present, depending on the type and cause of the shock. In early septic shock, there are chills, fever, and vasodilation,

blood flow to the skin, kidneys, muscles, and viscera to shunt the available blood to the brain and heart. Consequently, the skin feels cold and clammy, there is poor capillary filling, and glomerular filtration rate and urinary output are significantly reduced.

As a result of impaired perfusion, oxygen is depleted in the tissue cells, causing them to revert to anaerobic metabolism, producing lactic acidosis. The acidosis places an extra burden on the lungs as they attempt to compensate for the metabolic acidosis by increasing the respiratory rate to remove excess carbon dioxide. Prolonged vasoconstriction results in fatigue and atony of the peripheral arterioles, which leads to vessel dilation. Venules, which are less sensitive to vasodilator substances, remain constricted for a time, causing massive pooling in the capillary and venular beds, which further depletes blood volume.

with increased cardiac output that results in warm, flushed skin (hyperdynamic, or "hot," shock). A later and ominous development is disseminated intravascular coagulation (DIC) (see Chapter 43), the major hematologic complication of septic shock. Anaphylactic shock is frequently accompanied by urticaria and angioneurotic edema, which is life-threatening when it involves the respiratory passages (see the "Anaphylaxis" section later in this chapter).

Laboratory tests that assist in assessment are: blood gas measurements, pH, and sometimes liver function tests. Coagulation tests are evaluated when there is evidence of bleeding, such as oozing from a venipuncture site, bleeding from any orifice, or petechiae. Cultures of blood and other sites are indicated when there is a high suspicion of sepsis. Renal function tests are performed when impaired renal function is evident.

Therapeutic Management

Treatment of shock consists of three major interventions: (1) ventilation, (2) fluid administration, and (3) improvement of the pumping action of the heart (vasopressor support). The first priority is to establish an airway and administer oxygen. After the airway is ensured, circulatory stabilization is the major concern. Establishment of adequate IV access, ideally with multilumen central lines, is essential to deliver fluids and medications.

Ventilatory Support

The lung is the organ that is most sensitive to shock. Decreased distribution or redistribution of blood flow to respiratory muscles plus the increased work of breathing can rapidly lead to respiratory failure. Critically ill patients are unable to maintain an adequate airway. To place the lung at rest and improve ventilation, tracheal intubation is initiated early with positive-pressure ventilation. Supplemental oxygen is always given as soon as possible. Blood gases and pH are monitored frequently.

Increased extravascular lung water caused by edema contributes to the development of respiratory complications. Therapy is directed toward maintaining normal arterial blood gas measurements, normal acid-base balance, and circulation. Efforts are made to remove fluid and prevent its accumulation with the use of diuretics.

Cardiovascular Support

In most cases, rapid restoration of blood volume is all that is needed for resuscitation of the child in shock. An isotonic crystalloid solution (normal saline or lactated Ringer's solution) is the fluid of choice; colloids (e.g., albumin) are also used. Successful resuscitation is reflected by an increase in BP and a reduction in heart rate; increased cardiac output results in improved capillary circulation and skin color. CVP measurements of right atrial pressure help guide fluid therapy, and urinary output measurement is an important indicator of adequacy of circulation. Correction of acidosis, hypoxemia, hypoglycemia, hypothermia, and any metabolic derangements is mandatory.

Temporary pharmacologic support may be required to enhance myocardial contractility, reverse metabolic or respiratory acidosis, and maintain arterial pressure. The principal agents used to improve cardiac output and circulation are catecholamines, such as dopamine (Intropin) and epinephrine (Adrenalin). Vasodilators that are sometimes used include nitroprusside (Nipride) and milrinone.

QUALITY PATIENT OUTCOMES: Shock
- Oxygen content of blood optimized
- Cardiac output improved
- Oxygen demand reduced
- Metabolic abnormalities corrected
- Type of shock identified and treated

✚ EMERGENCY TREATMENT
Shock

Ventilation
Establish airway; be prepared for intubation.
Administer oxygen, usually 100% by mask.

Fluid Administration
Restore fluid volume as ordered.

Cardiovascular Support
Administer vasopressors (epinephrine 1:1000, 0.01 mg/kg subcutaneously; maximum dose of 0.5 mg; may repeat if needed).

General Support
Keep child flat with legs raised above level of heart.
Keep child warm and calm.

Care Management

The child who is in shock requires intensive observation and care. *The initial action is to ensure adequate tissue oxygenation.* The nurse should be prepared to administer oxygen by the appropriate route and to assist with any intubation and ventilatory procedures indicated. Other procedures and activities that require immediate attention are establishing an IV line, weighing the child, obtaining baseline vital signs, placing an indwelling catheter, obtaining blood gases and other measurements, and administering medications as indicated. The child is best positioned flat with the legs elevated.

❗ NURSING ALERT

Early clinical signs of shock include apprehension, irritability, normal BP, narrowing pulse pressure (difference between diastolic and systolic BP), thirst, pallor, diminished urinary output, unexplained mild tachycardia, and decreased perfusion of the hands and feet.

The nurse's responsibilities are to monitor the IV infusion, intake and output, vital signs (including CVP), and general systems assessments on a routine basis. IV medications are titrated according to patient responses, and vital signs are taken every 15 minutes during the critical periods and thereafter as needed. Urinary output is measured hourly; blood gases, hematocrit, pH, and electrolytes are monitored frequently to assess the child's status and the efficacy of therapy. An apnea and cardiac monitor is attached and monitored continuously. In the initial stages of acute shock, more than one nurse is often needed to manage all of the necessary activities that must be carried out simultaneously (see Emergency Treatment box: Shock).

Throughout the intense activity, support for the family must not be overlooked. Someone should contact family members at frequent intervals to inform them about what is being done and whether there is any progress. Ideally, someone should remain with the parents to serve as a liaison between them and the intensive care team. However, this is not always feasible in such a critical situation. As soon as possible, the family should be allowed to see the child. A member of the clergy or a social worker may be called to help provide comfort and support.

ANAPHYLAXIS

Anaphylaxis is the acute clinical syndrome resulting from the interaction of an allergen and a patient who is hypersensitive to that allergen. When the antigen enters the circulatory system, a generalized reaction rapidly takes place. Vasoactive amines (principally histamine or a histamine-like substance) are released and cause vasodilation, bronchoconstriction, and increased capillary permeability.

Severe reactions are immediate in onset; are often life-threatening; and frequently involve multiple systems, primarily the cardiovascular, respiratory, gastrointestinal, and integumentary systems. Exposure to the antigen can be by ingestion, inhalation, skin contact, or injection. Examples of common allergens associated with anaphylaxis include drugs (e.g., antibiotics, chemotherapeutic agents, radiologic contrast media), latex, foods, venom from bees or snakes, and biologic agents (antisera, enzymes, hormones, blood products).

! NURSING ALERT

Penicillin allergy is associated with immediate onset (within 1 hour of administration) or accelerated onset (1 to 72 hours after administration) of skin eruption, especially an urticarial rash, or more serious symptoms such as laryngeal edema or anaphylactic shock.

Clinical Manifestations

The onset of clinical symptoms usually occurs within seconds or minutes of exposure to the antigen, and the rapidity of the reaction is directly related to its intensity: the sooner the onset, the more severe the reaction. The reaction may be preceded by symptoms of uneasiness, restlessness, irritability, severe anxiety, headache, dizziness, paresthesia, and disorientation. The patient may lose consciousness. Cutaneous signs of flushing and urticaria are common early signs followed by angioedema, most notable in the eyelids, lips, tongue, hands, feet, and genitalia.

Bronchiolar constriction may follow, causing narrowing of the airway; pulmonary edema and hemorrhage also may occur. Laryngeal edema with severe acute upper airway obstruction may be life-threatening and requires rapid intervention. Shock occurs as a result of mediator-induced vasodilation, which causes capillary permeability and loss of intravascular fluid into the interstitial space. Sudden hypotension and impaired cardiac output with poor perfusion are seen.

Therapeutic Management

Successful outcome of anaphylactic reactions depends on rapid recognition and institution of treatment. The goals of treatment are to provide ventilation, restore adequate circulation, and prevent further exposure by identifying and removing the cause when possible.

A mild reaction with no evidence of respiratory distress or cardiovascular compromise can be managed with subcutaneous administration of antihistamines, such as diphenhydramine (Benadryl) and epinephrine.

Moderate or severe distress presents a potentially life-threatening emergency. Establishing an airway is the first concern, as with all shock states. Epinephrine is given subcutaneously or intravenously as an antihistamine and to support the cardiovascular system and increase BP. Other routes for giving epinephrine are intramuscular and via the airway, either nebulized or injected through an endotracheal tube. In severe anaphylaxis, epinephrine by any route is better than none. Fluids are given to restore blood volume. Additional vasopressors may be given to improve cardiac output.

Prevention of a reaction is preferable. Preventing exposure is more easily accomplished in children known to be at risk, including those with (1) a history of previous allergic reaction to a specific antigen; (2) a history of atopy; (3) a history of severe reactions in immediate family members; and (4) a reaction to a skin test, although skin tests are not available for all allergens. Desensitization may be recommended in certain cases.

QUALITY PATIENT OUTCOMES: Anaphylaxis
- Early recognition of symptoms
- Airway patency maintained
- Adequate circulation restored and maintained
- Further exposure to allergic agent prevented

Care Management

When an anaphylactic reaction is suspected, both immediate intervention and preparation for medical therapy are nursing responsibilities. Placing the child in a head-elevated position ensures ventilation, unless contraindicated by hypotension, to facilitate breathing and administer oxygen. If the child is not breathing, CPR is initiated and emergency medical services are summoned.

If the cause can be determined, measures are implemented to slow the spread of the offending substance. An IV infusion is established immediately. Emergency medications are given intravenously whenever possible; however, epinephrine may be given subcutaneously (see Emergency Treatment box: Shock). Vital signs and urinary output are monitored frequently. Medications are administered as prescribed, with regular assessment to monitor effectiveness and to detect signs of side effects of medication and fluid overload.

To prevent an anaphylactic reaction, parents are always asked about possible allergic responses to foods, latex, medications, and environmental conditions. These are displayed prominently on the patient's chart. The specific allergen is noted, as are the type and severity of the reaction. Parents are excellent historians, especially when the child has displayed a pronounced reaction to a substance. Drugs, including related drugs (e.g., penicillin, nafcillin), and other items (e.g., latex) that have produced a reaction previously are *never* used. If the child is allergic to insect venom, the family is instructed to purchase an emergency kit to be kept with the child at all times. Both the family and the child, if the child is old enough, are taught how to use the equipment. The patient should carry medical identification at all times.

SEPTIC SHOCK

Sepsis and septic shock are caused by infectious organisms. Normally, an infection triggers an inflammatory response in a local area, which results in vasodilation, increased capillary permeability, and eventually elimination of the infectious agent. The widespread activation and systemic release of inflammatory mediators is called the *systemic inflammatory response syndrome (SIRS)*. Box 42.15 provides the exact definitions for SIRS, infection, sepsis, and severe sepsis. SIRS can occur in response to both infectious and noninfectious (e.g., trauma, burns) causes. When caused by infection, it is called *sepsis*. Septic shock is defined as sepsis with organ dysfunction and hypotension.

Most of the physiologic effects of shock occur because the exaggerated immune response triggers more than 30 different mediators that result in diffuse vasodilation, increased capillary permeability, and maldistribution of blood flow. This impairs oxygen and nutrient delivery to the cells, resulting in cellular dysfunction. If the process continues, multiple-organ dysfunction occurs and may result in death. Table 42.6 includes the age-specific vital signs and laboratory values reflective of septic shock in children. Although the incidence of shock continues to be on the increase, survival rate due to early detection and treatment improves (Martin, 2012).

Three stages have been identified in septic shock. In early septic shock, the patient has chills, fever, and vasodilation with increased cardiac output, which results in warm, flushed skin that reflects vascular tone abnormalities and hyperdynamic, warm, or hyperdynamic-compensated responses. BP and urinary output are normal. The patient has the best chance for survival in this stage. The second stage—the normodynamic, cool, or hyperdynamic-decompensated stage—lasts only a few hours. The skin is cool, but pulses and BP are still normal. Urinary output diminishes, and the mental state becomes depressed. With advancing

---

BOX 42.15 Definitions of Systemic Inflammatory Response Syndrome, Infection, Sepsis, and Severe Sepsis

Systemic inflammatory response syndrome (SIRS): The presence of at least two of the following four criteria, one of which must be abnormal temperature or leukocyte count:

1. Core temperature of more than 38.5° C (101.3° F) or less than 36° C (96.8° F)
2. Tachycardia, defined as a mean heart rate more than two standard deviations above normal for age in the absence of external stimulus, chronic drugs, or painful stimuli; or otherwise unexplained persistent elevation over a 0.5- to 4-hour period; or, for children younger than 1 year of age: bradycardia, defined as a mean heart rate less than the 10th percentile for age in the absence of external vagal stimulus, β-blocker drugs, or CHD; or otherwise unexplained persistent depression over a 0.5-hour period
3. Mean respiratory rate more than two standard deviations above normal for age or mechanical ventilation for an acute process not related to underlying neuromuscular disease or the receipt of general anesthesia
4. Leukocyte count elevated or depressed for age (not secondary to chemotherapy-induced leukopenia) or more than 10% immature neutrophils

Infection: A suspected or proven (by positive culture, tissue stain, or PCR test) infection caused by any pathogen; or a clinical syndrome associated with a high probability of infection. Evidence of infection includes positive findings on clinical examination, imaging, or laboratory tests (e.g., white blood cells in a normally sterile body fluid, perforated viscus, chest radiograph consistent with pneumonia, petechial or purpuric rash, or purpura fulminans).

Sepsis: SIRS in the presence of or as a result of suspected or proven infection.

Severe sepsis: Sepsis plus cardiovascular organ dysfunction or ARDS or two or more other organ dysfunctions.

From Goldstein, B., Giroir, B., Randolph, A., et al. (2005). International Pediatric Sepsis Consensus Conference: Definitions for sepsis and organ dysfunction in pediatrics. *Pediatric Critical Care Medicine* 6(1), 2–8; used with permission.
ARDS, Acute respiratory distress syndrome; *CHD,* congenital heart disease; *PCR,* polymerase chain reaction.

---

disease, certain signs of circulatory decompensation that deteriorate to signs of circulatory collapse are indistinguishable from late shock of any cause. In the hypodynamic, or cold, stage of shock, cardiovascular function progressively deteriorates even with aggressive therapy. The patient has hypothermia, cold extremities, weak pulses, hypotension, and oliguria or anuria. Patients are severely lethargic or comatose. Multiorgan failure is common. This is the most dangerous stage of shock.

Management of septic shock involves measures to provide hemodynamic stability and adequate oxygenation to the tissues and the use of antimicrobials to treat the infectious organism. As with other forms of shock, hemodynamic stability is achieved with fluid volume resuscitation and inotropic agents as needed. Providing adequate oxygenation often requires intubation and mechanical ventilation, supplemental oxygen, sedation, and paralysis to decrease the work of breathing. Septic shock involves activation of complement proteins that promote clumping of the granulocytes in the lung. The granulocytes can release chemicals that can cause direct lung injury to the pulmonary capillary endothelium. This causes a fluid leak into the alveoli, which causes stiff, noncompliant lungs. DIC and multiorgan dysfunction may also occur and require prompt assessment and management.

Newer therapies are being developed to modify the host immune response by attempting to block various mediators, thereby interrupting the inflammatory cascade.

Early identification of the symptoms of septic shock is critical to patient survival. A high index of suspicion is required in all critically ill patients who are at greater risk for sepsis because of multiple invasive lines and devices, poor nutrition, and impaired immune function. Subtle alterations in tissue perfusion and unexplained tachypnea and tachycardia often are early warning signs. Identification of the infectious agent and prompt treatment are also critical to patient survival. Broad-spectrum antibiotics should be given, and the site of infection should be removed if possible (e.g., drain abscesses, remove indwelling lines). Patients should be managed in an ICU in which continuous monitoring and sophisticated cardiac and respiratory support are available. Multidisciplinary collaboration is essential in managing these critically ill patients.

TOXIC SHOCK SYNDROME

Toxic shock syndrome (TSS) is a relatively rare condition caused by the toxins produced by the *Staphylococcus* bacteria. First described in 1978, TSS can cause acute multisystem organ failure and a clinical picture that resembles septic shock. TSS became well known in 1980 because of the striking relationship between the disease and tampon use (Nakase, 2000). An aggressive health education campaign about

---

TABLE 42.6 Age-Specific Vital Signs and Laboratory Variables in Septic Shock*

Age Group	HEART RATE (beats/min) Tachycardia	Bradycardia	Respiratory Rate (breaths/min)	Leukocyte Count (Leukocytes × 10³/mm³)	Systolic Blood Pressure (mm Hg)
0 days to 1 week of age	>180	<100	>50	>34	<65
1 week to 1 month of age	>180	<100	>40	>19.5 or <5	<75
1 month to 1 year of age	>180	<90	>34	>17.5 or <5	<100
2 to 5 years of age	>140	N/A	>22	>15.5 or <6	<94
6 to 12 years of age	>130	N/A	>8	>13.50 or <4.5	<105
13 to <18 years of age	>110	N/A	>4	>11 or <4.5	<117

From Goldstein, B., Giroir, B., Randolph, A., et al. (2005). International Pediatric Sepsis Consensus Conference: Definitions for sepsis and organ dysfunction in pediatrics. *Pediatric Critical Care Medicine,* 6(1), 2–8; used with permission.
N/A, Not applicable.
*Lower values for heart rate, leukocyte count, and systolic blood pressure are for fifth percentile, and upper values for heart rate, respiratory rate, or leukocyte count are for 95th percentile.

BOX 42.16   Criteria for Definition of Toxic Shock Syndrome

Toxic Shock Syndrome (Other Than Streptococcal)
2011 Case Definition

Clinical Criteria
An illness with the following clinical manifestations:
- Fever: Temperature ≥102° F (≥38.9° C)
- Rash: Diffuse macular erythroderma
- Desquamation: 1 to 2 weeks after onset of rash
- Hypotension: Systolic blood pressure (BP) ≤90 mm Hg for adults or less than fifth percentile by age for children younger than 16 years of age
- Multisystem involvement (three or more of the following organ systems):
  - Gastrointestinal: Vomiting or diarrhea at onset of illness
  - Muscular: Severe myalgia or creatine phosphokinase level at least twice the upper limit of normal
  - Mucous membrane: Vaginal, oropharyngeal, or conjunctival hyperemia
  - Renal: Blood urea nitrogen or creatinine at least twice the upper limit of normal for laboratory or urinary sediment with pyuria (≥5 leukocytes per high-power field) in the absence of urinary tract infection
  - Hepatic: Total bilirubin, alanine aminotransferase enzyme, or aspartate aminotransferase enzyme levels at least twice the upper limit of normal for laboratory
  - Hematologic: Platelets <100,000/mm^3
  - Central nervous system (CNS): disorientation or alterations in consciousness without focal neurologic signs when fever and hypotension are absent

Laboratory Criteria for Diagnosis
Negative results on the following tests, if obtained:

- Blood or cerebrospinal fluid (CSF) culture may be positive for *Staphylococcus aureus*
- Negative serologies for Rocky Mountain spotted fever, leptospirosis, or measles

Case Classification
Probable
A case that meets the laboratory criteria and in which four of the five clinical criteria described in the following section are present

Confirmed
A case that meets the laboratory criteria and in which all five of the clinical criteria described below are present, including desquamation, unless the patient dies before desquamation occurs:
1. Fever of 38.9° C (102° F) or higher
2. Presence of diffuse macular erythroderma
3. Desquamation, particularly of palms and soles, 1 to 2 weeks after onset of illness
4. Hypotension, defined as a systolic BP of 90 mm Hg or less for adults and below the fifth percentile for children younger than 16 years of age; or an orthostatic drop in diastolic BP of 15 mm Hg or more with a change from lying to sitting; or orthostatic syncope; or orthostatic dizziness
5. Involvement of three or more of the following organ systems: Gastrointestinal (GI), muscular, mucous membrane, renal, hepatic, hematologic, or CNS

Toxic shock syndrome (TSS) is probable when four of the five major criteria are fulfilled. In addition, if blood and CSF cultures are obtained, they must be negative for any organisms other than *S. aureus*. Serologic tests for Rocky Mountain spotted fever, leptospirosis, and measles also must be negative.

Modified From Centers for Disease Control and Prevention: National Notifiable Diseases Surveillance System (NNDSS). (2011). *Toxic shock syndrome (other than streptococcal) (TSS) 2011 case definition.* Retrieved from http://wwwn.cdc.gov/nndss/script/casedef.aspx?CondYrID=869&DatePub=1/1/2011.

the dangers of prolonged tampon use and a change in the chemical composition of tampons have markedly reduced the incidence of TSS in menstruating women. Cases of TSS have also been reported in men, older women, and children.

Diagnostic Evaluation

Diagnosis is established on the basis of the criteria established by the Centers for Disease Control and Prevention's toxic case definition (Box 42.16). A history of tampon use contributes to the diagnosis. Additional laboratory tests include cultures from blood, the vagina, the cervix, and any discharge. Other laboratory tests are those that facilitate the management of shock.

Therapeutic Management

The management of patients with TSS is the same as management of shock of any cause and may range from supportive care in mild cases to hospitalization and intensive care in severe cases. Appropriate parenteral antibiotics are usually administered after cultures are obtained.

Care Management

Because the disease is relatively rare, the major efforts of nursing are directed toward prevention. The association between the disease and the use of tampons provides some direction for education. Avoiding the use of tampons offers the most certain preventive measure, although this approach is probably unacceptable to most adolescent girls, who prefer the freedom, comfort, and inconspicuousness that tampons afford.

Adolescent girls who use tampons can be taught general hygiene measures, such as good hand washing and careful insertion to avoid vaginal abrasion. It is wise to modify their use, alternating with sanitary napkins—perhaps using the napkins during the night, when at home during the day, and when flow is slight. Young girls are advised not to use super-absorbent tampons and not to leave any tampon in the body for more than 4 to 6 hours.

REFERENCES

Abman, S. H., & Ivy, D. D. (2011). Recent progress in understanding pediatric pulmonary hypertension. *Current Opinion in Pediatrics, 23*(2), 298–304.

Almond, C., Thiagarajian, R. R., Piercy, G. E., et al. (2009). Waiting list mortality among children listed for heart transplantation in the United States. *Circulation, 119*(5), 717–727.

American Academy of Pediatrics. (2012). *Car seat checkup.* Retrieved from http://www.healthychildren.org/English/safety-prevention/on-the-go/Pages/Car-Safety-Seat-Checkup.aspx.

American Academy of Pediatrics Committee on Infectious Diseases, American Academy of Pediatrics Bronchiolitis Guidelines Committee. (2014). Updated guidance for palivizumab prophylaxis among infants and young children at increased risk of hospitalization for respiratory syncytial virus infection. *Pediatrics, 134*(2), 415–420.

Arnold, R., Ley-Zaporozhan, J., Ley, S., et al. (2008). Outcome after mechanical aortic valve replacement in children and young adults. *Annals of Thoracic Surgery, 85*(2), 604–610.

Barst, R. J., Ivy, D., Dingemanse, J., et al. (2003). Pharmacokinetics, safety, and efficacy of bosentan in pediatric patients with pulmonary artery hypertension. *Clinical Pharmacology and Therapeutics, 73*(4), 372–382.

Beekman, R. H. (2001). Coarctation of the aorta. In H. D. Allen, D. J. Driscoll, R. E. Shaddy, et al. (Eds.), *Moss and Adams' heart disease in infants, children and adolescents* (6th ed.). Philadelphia, PA: Lippincott.

Blume, E. D. (2003). Current status of heart transplantation in children: Update 2003. *Pediatric Clinics of North America, 50*(6), 1375–1391.

Blume, E. D., Naftel, D. C., Bastardi, H. J., et al. (2006). Outcomes of children bridged to heart transplantation with ventricular assist devices: A multi-institutional study. *Circulation, 113*(19), 2313–2319.

Boucek, M. M., Aurora, P., Edwards, L. B., et al. (2007). The Registry of the International Society for Heart and Lung Transplantation: Tenth official pediatric heart transplantation report—2007. *Journal of Heart and Lung Transplantation, 26*(8), 796–807.

Bragg, L., & Alvarez, A. (2014). Endocarditis. *Pediatrics in Review, 35*(4), 162–167.

Cecchin, F., Frangini, P. A., Brown, D. W., et al. (2009). Cardiac resynchronization therapy (and multisite pacing) in pediatrics and congenital heart disease: Five years experience in a single institution. *Journal of Cardiovascular Electrophysiology, 20*(1), 58–65.

Daniels, S. R. (2012). Management of hyperlipidemia in pediatrics. *Current Opinion in Cardiology, 27*(2), 92–97.

de Ferranti, S. D., Daniels, S. R., Gillman, M., et al. (2012). NHLBI Integrated Guidelines on Cardiovascular Disease Risk Reduction: Can we clarify the controversy about cholesterol screening and treatment in childhood? *Clinical Chemistry, 58*(12), 1626–1630.

Dubin, A. M., Janousek, J., Rhee, E., et al. (2005). Resynchronization therapy in pediatric and congenital heart disease patients. *Journal of the American College of Cardiology, 46*(12), 2277–2283.

Expert Panel on Integrated Guidelines for Cardiovascular Health and Risk Reduction in Children and Adolescents, & National Heart, Lung, and Blood Institute. (2011). Expert panel on integrated guidelines for cardiovascular health and risk reduction in children and adolescents: Summary report. *Pediatrics, 128*(5 suppl):S213–S256.

Feltes, T. F., Bacha, E., Beekman, R. H., 3rd, et al. (2011). Indications for cardiac catheterization and intervention in pediatric heart disease: A scientific statement from the American Heart Association. *Circulation, 123*(22), 2607–2652.

Ferrieri, P., & Jones Criteria Working Group. (2002). Proceedings of the Jones Criteria Workshop. *Circulation, 106*(19), 2521–2523.

Gerber, M. A., Baltimore, R. S., Eaton, C. B., et al. (2009). Prevention of rheumatic fever and diagnosis and treatment of acute Streptococcal pharyngitis: A scientific statement from the American Heart Association. *Circulation, 119*(11), 1541–1551.

Goldmuntz, E., Clark, B. J., Mitchell, L. E., et al. (1998). Frequency of 22q11 deletion in patients with conotruncal defects. *Journal of the American College of Cardiology, 32*(2), 492–498.

Hirsch, J. C., Goldberg, C., Bove, E. L., et al. (2008). Fontan operation in the current era: A 15-year single institute experience. *Annals of Surgery, 248*(3), 402–410.

LeRoy, S., Elixson, E. M., O'Brien, P., et al. (2003). Recommendations for preparing children and adolescents for invasive cardiac procedures: A statement from the American Heart Association Pediatric Nursing Subcommittee of the Council on Cardiovascular Nursing in collaboration with the Council on Cardiovascular Diseases of the Young. *Circulation, 108*(20), 2550–2564.

Li, J. S., Sexton, D. J., Mick, N., et al. (2000). Proposed modifications to the Duke criteria for the diagnosis of infective endocarditis. *Clinical Infectious Diseases, 30*(4), 633–638.

Licht, D. J., Shera, D. M., Clancy, R. R., et al. (2009). Brain maturation is delayed in infants with complex congenital heart defects. *Journal of Thoracic and Cardiovascular Surgery, 137*(3), 529–536.

Longmuir, P. E., Brothers, J. A., de Ferranti, S. D., et al. (2013). Promotion of physical activity for children and adults with congenital heart disease: A scientific statement from the American Heart Association. *Circulation, 127*(21), 2147–2159.

Majnemer, A., & Limperopoulos, C. (1999). Developmental progress of children with congenital heart defects requiring open heart surgery. *Seminars in Pediatric Neurology, 6*(1), 12–19.

Margossian, R. (2008). Contemporary management of pediatric heart failure. *Expert Review of Cardiovascular Therapy, 6*(2), 187–197.

Marijon, E., Mirabel, M., Celermajer, D. S., et al. (2012). Rheumatic heart disease. *Lancet, 379*(9819), 953–964.

Maron, B. J. (2001). Hypertrophic cardiomyopathy. In H. D. Allen, D. J. Driscoll, R. E. Shaddy, et al. (Eds.), *Moss and Adams' heart disease in infants, children, and adolescents* (6th ed.). Philadelphia, PA: Lippincott.

Martin, G. S. (2012). Sepsis, severe sepsis and septic shock: Changes in incidence, pathogens, and outcomes. *Expert Review of Anti-infective Therapy, 10*(6), 701–706.

McCrindle, B. W., Kwiterovich, P. O., McBride, P. E., et al. (2012). Guidelines for lipid screening in children and adolescents: Bringing evidence to the debate. *Pediatrics, 130*(2), 353–356.

McCrindle, B. W., Urbina, E. M., Dennison, B. A., et al. (2007). Drug therapy of high-risk lipid abnormalities in children and adolescents: A scientific statement from the American Heart Association Atherosclerosis, Hypertension, and Obesity in Youth Committee, Council of Cardiovascular Disease in the Young, with the Council on Cardiovascular Nursing. *Circulation, 115*(14), 1948–1967.

Mickley, K. L., Burkhart, P. V., & Sigler, A. N. (2013). Promoting normal development and self-efficacy in the school-age children managing chronic conditions. *Nursing Clinics of North America, 48*(2), 319–328.

Mirabel, M., Narayanan, K., Jouven, X., et al. (2014). Cardiology patient page: Prevention of acute rheumatic fever and rheumatic heart disease. *Circulation, 130*(5), e35–e37.

Nakase, J. Y. (2000). Update on emerging infections from the Centers for Disease Control and Prevention. *Annals of Emergency Medicine, 36*(3), 268–270.

National Heart, Lung, and Blood Institute. (2012). *Expert panel on integrated guidelines for cardiovascular health and risk reduction in children and adolescents: Summary report.* Bethesda, MD: US Department of Health and Human Services, National Heart, Lung, and Blood Institute, National Institutes of Health.

National High Blood Pressure Education Program Working Group on High Blood Pressure in Children and Adolescents. (2004). The fourth report on the diagnosis, evaluation, and treatment of high blood pressure in children and adolescents. *Pediatrics, 114*(2 suppl), 555–576.

Newburger, J. W., de Ferranti, S. D., & Fulton, D. R. (2015). *Cardiovascular sequelae of Kawasaki disease.* Retrieved from http://www.uptodate.com/contents/cardiovascular-sequelae-of-kawasaki-disease.

Newburger, J. W., Takahashi, M., Gerber, M. A., et al. (2004). Diagnosis, treatment, and long-term management of Kawasaki disease: A statement for health professionals from the Committee on Rheumatic Fever, Endocarditis and Kawasaki Disease, Council on Cardiovascular Disease in the Young, American Heart Association. *Circulation, 110*(17), 2747–2771.

Newman, J. H., Phillips, J. A., 3rd, & Loyd, J. E. (2008). The enigma of pulmonary arterial hypertension: New insights from genetic studies. *Annals of Internal Medicine, 148*(4), 278–283.

Park, M. K. (2014). *Park's pediatric cardiology for practitioners* (6th ed.). Philadelphia, PA: Elsevier/Saunders.

Prakash, A., Powell, A. J., Krishnamurthy, R., et al. (2004). Magnetic resonance imaging evaluation of myocardial perfusion and viability in congenital and acquired pediatric heart disease. *American Journal of Cardiology, 93*(5), 657–661.

Remenyi, B., Carapetis, J., Wyber, R., et al. (2013). Position statement of the World Heart Federation on the prevention and control of rheumatic heart disease. *Nature Reviews Cardiology, 10*(5), 284–292.

Rosenthal, D., Chrisant, M. R., Edens, E., et al. (2004). International Society for Heart and Lung Transplantation: Practice guidelines for management of heart failure in children. *Journal of Heart and Lung Transplantation, 23*(12), 1313–1333.

Rossano, J. W., & Shaddy, R. E. (2014). Heart failure in children: Etiology and treatment. *Journal of Pediatrics, 165*(2), 228–233.

Schlechte, E. A., Boramanand, N., & Funk, M. (2008). Supraventricular tachycardia in the pediatric primary care setting: Age-related presentation, diagnosis, and management. *Journal of Pediatric Health Care, 22*(5), 289–299.

Schneider, D. J., & Moore, J. W. (2008). Aortic stenosis. In H. D. Allen, D. J. Driscoll, R. E. Shaddy, et al. (Eds.), *Moss and Adams' heart disease in infants, children, and adolescents* (7th ed.). Philadelphia, PA: Lippincott.

Scientific Registry of Transplant Recipients. (2012). *OPTN/SRTR 2012 annual data report.* Rockville, MD: Department of Health and Human Services,

Health Resources and Services Administration, Healthcare Systems Bureau, Division of Transplantation.

Special Writing Group of the Committee on Rheumatic Fever, Endocarditis, and Kawasaki Disease of the Council on Cardiovascular Disease in the Young of the American Heart Association. (1992). Guidelines for the diagnosis of rheumatic fever, Jones criteria, 1992 update. *Journal of the American Medical Association, 268*(15), 2069–2073.

Spirito, P., Autore, C., Rapezzi, C., et al. (2009). Syncope and risk of sudden death in hypertrophic cardiomyopathy. *Circulation, 119*(13), 1703–1710.

Steltzer, M., Rudd, N., & Pick, B. (2005). Nutrition care for newborns with congenital heart disease. *Clinics in Perinatology, 32*(4), 1017–1030.

Thrush, P. T., & Hoffman, T. M. (2014). Pediatric heart transplantation— Indications and outcomes in the current era. *Journal of Thoracic Disease, 6*(8), 1080–1096.

Tweddell, J. S., Hoffman, G. M., Mussatto, K. A., et al. (2002). Improved survival of patients undergoing palliation of hypoplastic left heart syndrome: Lessons learned from 115 consecutive patients. *Circulation, 106*(12 suppl 1), 182–189.

Urbina, E., Alpert, B., Flynn, J., et al. (2008). Ambulatory blood pressure monitoring in children and adolescents: Recommendations for standard assessment: A scientific statement from the American Heart Association Atherosclerosis, Hypertension, and Obesity in Youth Committee of the Council on Cardiovascular Disease in the Young and the Council for High Blood Pressure Research. *Hypertension, 52*(3), 433–451.

Wilder, M. S., Palinkas, L. A., Kao, A. S., et al. (2007). Delayed diagnosis by physicians contributes to the development of coronary artery aneurysms in children with Kawasaki syndrome. *Pediatric Infectious Disease, 26*(3), 256–260.

Wilson, W., Taubert, K. A., Gewitz, M., et al. (2007). Prevention of infective endocarditis: Guidelines from the American Heart Association. *Circulation, 116*(15), 1736–1754.

43

The Child With Hematologic or Immunologic Dysfunction

Marilyn J. Hockenberry

http://evolve.elsevier.com/Perry/maternal

HEMATOLOGIC AND IMMUNOLOGIC DYSFUNCTION

Several tests can be performed to assess hematologic function, including additional procedures to identify the cause of the dysfunction. The following discussion is limited to a description of the most common and one of the most valuable tests, the complete blood count (CBC). Other procedures, such as those related to iron, coagulation, and immune status, are discussed throughout the chapter as appropriate. The nurse should be familiar with the significance of the findings from the CBC (Table 43.1).

As with any disorder, the history and physical examination are essential to identify hematologic dysfunction, and the nurse is often the first person to suspect a problem based on information from these sources. Comments by the parent regarding the child's lack of energy, food diary of poor sources of iron, frequent infections, and bleeding that is difficult to control offer clues to the more common disorders affecting the blood. A careful physical appraisal, especially of the skin, can reveal findings (e.g., pallor, petechiae, bruising) that may indicate minor or serious hematologic conditions. Nurses need to be aware of the clinical manifestations of blood diseases to assist in recognizing symptoms and establishing a diagnosis.

> **! NURSING ALERT**
>
> A common term used in describing an abnormal complete blood count (CBC) is *shift to the left*, which refers to the presence of immature neutrophils in the peripheral blood from hyperfunction of the bone marrow, as seen during a bacterial infection.

RED BLOOD CELL DISORDERS

ANEMIA

The term *anemia* describes a condition in which the number of red blood cells (RBCs) or the hemoglobin (Hgb or Hb) concentration is reduced below normal values for age. This diminishes the oxygen-carrying capacity of the blood, causing a reduction in the oxygen available to the tissues. The anemias are the most common hematologic disorder of infancy and childhood and are not diseases but an indication or manifestation of an underlying pathologic process.

Classification

Anemias can be classified using two basic approaches: *etiology or physiology*, manifested by erythrocyte or Hgb depletion, and *morphology,*

the characteristic changes in RBC size, shape, or color (Box 43.1). Although the morphologic classification is useful in terms of laboratory evaluation of anemia, the etiology provides direction for planning nursing care. For example, anemia with reduced Hgb concentration may be caused by a dietary depletion of iron, and the principal intervention is replenishing iron stores. The classification of anemias is found in Fig. 43.1.

Consequences of Anemia

The basic physiologic defect caused by anemia is a decrease in the oxygen-carrying capacity of blood and consequently a reduction in the amount of oxygen available to the cells. When the anemia has developed slowly, the child usually adapts to the declining Hgb level.

The effects of anemia on the circulatory system can be profound. Because the viscosity of blood depends almost entirely on the concentration of RBCs, the resulting hemodilution of severe anemia decreases peripheral resistance, causing greater quantities of blood to return to the heart. The increased circulation and turbulence within the heart may produce a murmur. Because the cardiac workload is greatly increased, especially during exercise, infection, or emotional stress, cardiac failure may ensue.

Children seem to have a remarkable ability to function well despite low levels of Hgb. Cyanosis, which results from an increased quantity of deoxygenated Hgb in arterial blood, is typically not evident. Growth restriction, resulting from decreased cellular metabolism, and coexisting anorexia is a common finding in chronic severe anemia. It is frequently accompanied by delayed sexual maturation in the older child.

Diagnostic Evaluation

In general, anemia may be suspected based on findings in the history and physical examination, such as a lack of energy, easy fatigability, and pallor. Unless the anemia is severe, one of the first clues to the disorder may be alterations in the CBC, such as decreased RBCs, and decreased Hgb and hematocrit (Hct) levels (see Fig. 43.1). Although anemia is sometimes defined as an Hgb level below 10 or 11 g/dL, this arbitrary cutoff is inappropriate for all children, since Hgb levels normally vary with age (see Table 43.1).

Other tests specific to a particular type of anemia are used to determine the underlying cause of anemia. These are discussed in relation to the particular disorder.

Therapeutic Management

The objective of medical management is to reverse the anemia by treating the underlying cause. In nutritional anemias, the specific deficiency is replaced. In blood loss from acute hemorrhage, RBC transfusion may be given. In patients with severe anemia, supportive medical care may

TABLE 43.1   Tests Performed as Part of a Complete Blood Count

Test (Average Value)	Description, Comments
RBC count (4.5 to 5.5 million/mm³)	Number of RBCs/mm³ of blood Indirectly estimates Hgb content of blood Reflects function of bone marrow
Hgb determination (11.5 to 15.5 g/dL)	Amount of Hgb (g)/dL of whole blood Total blood Hgb primarily depends on number of circulating RBCs but also on amount of Hgb in each cell
Hct (35% to 45%)	Percent volume of packed RBCs in whole blood Indirectly measures Hgb content Is approximately three times Hgb content
RBC indices	
MCV (77 to 95 fL)	Average or mean volume (size) of a single RBC MCV value is expressed as femtoliter (fL) or cubic micron (mm³)
MCH (25 to 33 pg/cell)	Average or mean quantity (weight) of Hgb in a single RBC MCH value is expressed as picogram (pg) or micromicrogram (mmcg) Whereas MCV and MCH depend on accurate counts of RBCs, MCHC does not; therefore, MCHC is often more reliable All indices depend on average cell measurements and do not show individual RBC variations (anisocytosis)
MCHC (31% to 37% Hgb [g]/dL RBC)	Average concentration of Hgb in a single RBC MCHC values are expressed as percent Hgb (g)/cell or Hgb (g)/dL RBC
RBC volume distribution width (13.4% ± 1.2%)	Average size of RBCs Differentiates some types of anemia
Reticulocyte count (0.5% to 1.5% erythrocytes)	Percent reticulocytes in RBCs Index of production of mature RBCs by bone marrow Decreased count indicates depressed bone marrow function Increased count indicates erythrogenesis in response to some stimulus When reticulocyte count is extremely high, other forms of immature RBCs (normoblasts, even erythroblasts) may be present Indirectly estimates hypochromic anemia Usually elevated in patients with chronic hemolytic anemia
WBC count (4.5 to 13.5 × 10³ cells/mm³)	Number of WBCs/mm³ of blood Total number of WBCs less important than differential count
Differential WBC count	Inspection and quantification of WBC types present in peripheral blood Values are expressed as percentages; to obtain absolute number of any type of WBC, multiply its respective percentage by total number of WBCs
Neutrophils (polys) (54% to 62%) (3 to 5.8 × 10³ cells/mm³)	Primary defense in bacterial infection; capable of phagocytizing and killing bacteria
Bands (3% to 5%) (0.15–0.4 × 10³ cells/mm³)	Immature neutrophil Increased numbers in bacterial infection Also capable of phagocytosis and killing
Eosinophils (1% to 3%) (0.05 to 0.25 × 10³ cells/mm³)	Named for their staining characteristics with eosin dye Increased in allergic disorders, parasitic diseases, certain neoplasms, and other diseases
Basophils (0.075%) (0.015 to 0.03 × 10³ cells/mm³)	Named for their characteristic basophilic stippling Contain histamine, heparin, and serotonin; believed to cause increased blood flow to injured tissues while preventing excessive clotting
Lymphocytes (25% to 33%) (1.5 to 3 × 10³ cells/mm³)	Involved in development of antibody and delayed hypersensitivity
Monocytes (3% to 7%)	Large phagocytic cells that are involved in early stage of inflammatory reaction
ANC (>1000/mm³)	Percent neutrophils/bands times WBC count Indicates body's capability to handle bacterial infections
Platelet count (150 to 400 × 10³/mm³)	Number of platelets/mm³ of blood Cellular fragments that are necessary for clotting to occur
Stained peripheral blood smear	Visual estimation of amount of Hgb in RBCs and overall size, shape, and structure of RBCs Various staining properties of RBC structures may be evidence of immature forms of erythrocytes Shows variation in size and shape of RBCs: microcytic, macrocytic, poikilocytic (variable shapes)

ANC, Absolute neutrophil count; *Hct,* hematocrit; *Hgb,* hemoglobin; *MCH,* mean corpuscular hemoglobin; *MCHC,* mean corpuscular hemoglobin concentration; *MCV,* mean corpuscular volume; *RBC,* red blood cell; *WBC,* white blood cell.

include oxygen therapy, bed rest, and replacement of intravascular volume with intravenous (IV) fluids. In addition to these general measures, the nurse may implement more specific interventions, depending upon the cause. The next sections will discuss these interventions.

Care Management

The assessment of anemia includes the basic techniques that are applicable to any condition. The age of the infant or child provides some clues regarding the possible etiology of the anemia. For example, iron deficiency anemia occurs more frequently in toddlers between 12 and 36 months of age and during the growth spurt of adolescence.

Racial or ethnic background is significant. For example, the anemias related to abnormal Hgb levels are found in Southeast Asians and people of African or Mediterranean ancestry. These same groups may be genetically deficient in the enzyme lactase after the period of infancy.

Affected individuals are unable to tolerate lactose in the diet, with consequent intestinal irritation and chronic blood loss.

Special emphasis is placed on a careful history to elicit any information that might help identify the cause of the anemia. For example, a statement such as "My child drinks lots of milk" is a frequent finding in toddlers with iron deficiency anemia. An episode of diarrhea may have precipitated temporary lactose intolerance in a young child.

Stool examination for occult (microscopic) blood (Hemoccult test) can identify chronic intestinal bleeding that results from primary or secondary lactase deficiency. It is also important to understand the significance of various blood tests (see Table 43.1).

Prepare the Child and Family for Laboratory Tests

Usually, several blood tests are ordered, but because they are generally done sequentially rather than at one time, the child is subjected to multiple finger or heel punctures or venipunctures. Laboratory technicians frequently are not aware of the trauma that repeated punctures represent to a child. These invasive procedures need not be painful (see the "Blood Specimens" section in Chapter 39) with the topical application of an eutectic mixture of local anesthetics (EMLA; lidocaine and prilocaine) or 4% lidocaine (ELA-Max or LMX) before needle punctures (see the "Pain Management" section in Chapter 30). Therefore, the nurse's responsibilities for preparing the child and family for the tests include the following:

- Explaining the significance of each test, particularly why the tests are not all done at one time
- Encouraging parents or another supportive person to be with the child during the procedure
- Allowing the child to play with the equipment on a doll or participate in the actual procedure (e.g., by holding the Band-Aid)

Older children may appreciate the opportunity to observe the blood cells under a microscope or in photographs. This experience is especially important if a serious blood disorder, such as aplastic anemia, is suspected because it serves as a foundation for explaining the pathophysiology of the disorder.

Bone marrow aspiration is not a routine hematologic test but is essential for definitive diagnosis of the certain anemias such as severe aplastic anemia.

BOX 43.1   Red Blood Cell Morphology

Size (Cell Size)
Variation in RBC sizes (anisocytosis)
- Normocytes (normal cell size)
- Microcytes (smaller than normal cell size)
- Macrocytes (larger than normal cell size)

Shape (Cell Shape)
Variation in RBC shapes (poikilocytosis)
- Spherocytes (globular cells)
- Drepanocytes (sickle-shaped cells)
- Numerous other irregularly shaped cells

Color (Cell Staining Characteristics)
Variation in hemoglobin concentration in the RBC
- Normochromic (sufficient or normal amount of hemoglobin per RBC)
- Hypochromic (reduced amount of hemoglobin per RBC)
- Hyperchromic (increased amount of hemoglobin per RBC)

RBC, Red blood cell.

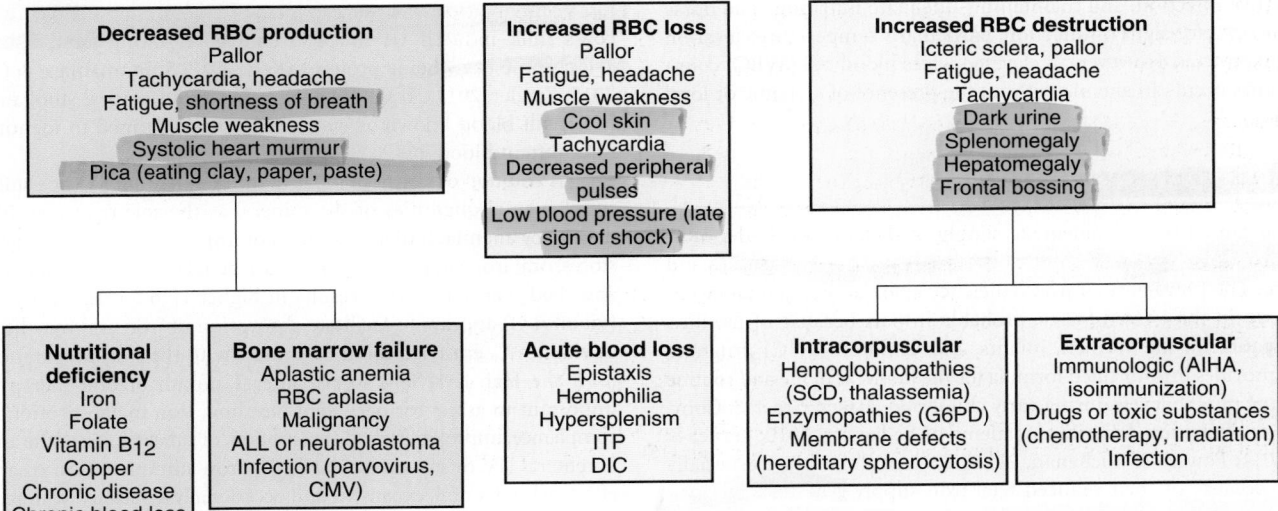

FIG 43.1 Classifications of anemias. *AIHA,* Autoimmune hemolytic anemia; *ALL,* acute lymphoid leukemia; *CMV,* cytomegalovirus; *DIC,* disseminated intravascular coagulation; *G6PD,* glucose-6-phosphate dehydrogenase; *ITP,* idiopathic thrombocytopenic purpura; *RBC,* red blood cell; *SCD,* sickle cell disease.

Decrease Tissue Oxygen Needs

Because the basic pathologic process in anemia is a decrease in oxygen-carrying capacity, an important nursing responsibility is to minimize tissue oxygen needs by continual assessment of the child's energy level. Assess the child's level of tolerance for activities of daily living and play, and make adjustments to allow as much self-care as possible without undue exertion. During periods of rest, the nurse measures vital signs and observes behavior to establish a baseline of nonexertion energy expenditure. During periods of activity, the nurse repeats these measurements and observations to compare them with resting values.

Prevent Complications

Children with anemia are prone to infection because tissue hypoxia causes cellular dysfunction that weakens the body's defense against infectious agents. Take all of the usual precautions to prevent infection, such as practicing thorough hand washing, selecting an appropriate room in a noninfectious area, restricting visitors or hospital personnel with active infection, and maintaining adequate nutrition. The nurse also observes for signs of infection, particularly temperature elevation and leukocytosis. However, an elevated white blood cell (WBC) count sometimes occurs in anemia without the presence of systemic or local infection.

IRON DEFICIENCY ANEMIA

Anemia caused by an inadequate supply of dietary iron is the most prevalent and preventable nutritional disorder in the United States and globally. The prevalence of iron deficiency anemia during infancy has decreased in the United States, probably in part because of families' participation in the Women, Infants, and Children (WIC) program, which provides iron-fortified formula for the first year of life and routine screening of Hgb levels during early childhood (Baker, Greer, & Committee on Nutrition American Academy of Pediatrics, 2010; Lerner & Sills, 2011; Powers & Buchanan, 2014). Preterm infants are especially at risk because of their reduced fetal iron supply. Children 12 to 36 months of age are at risk for anemia as a result of primarily cow's milk intake and not eating an adequate amount of iron-containing food (Baker et al.; Eussen, Alles, Uijterschout, et al., 2015; Paoletti, Bogen, & Ritchey, 2014). Adolescents are also at risk because of their rapid growth rate combined with poor eating habits, menses, obesity, or strenuous activities.

Pathophysiology

Iron deficiency anemia can be caused by any number of factors that decrease the supply of iron, impair its absorption, increase the body's need for iron, or affect the synthesis of Hgb. Although the clinical manifestations and diagnostic evaluation are similar regardless of the cause, the therapeutic and nursing care management depends on the specific reason for the iron deficiency. The following discussion is limited to iron deficiency anemia resulting from inadequate iron in the diet.

During the last trimester of pregnancy, iron is transferred from the mother to the fetus. Most of the iron is stored in the circulating erythrocytes of the fetus, with the remainder stored in the fetal liver, spleen, and bone marrow. These iron stores are usually adequate for the first 5 to 6 months in a full-term infant but for only 2 to 3 months in preterm infants and multiple births. If dietary iron is not supplied to meet the infant's growth demands after the fetal iron stores are depleted, iron deficiency anemia results. Physiologic anemia should not be confused with iron deficiency anemia resulting from nutritional causes.

Although infants with iron deficiency anemia are underweight, many are overweight because of excessive milk ingestion (known as *milk babies*). These children become anemic for two reasons: (1) milk, a poor source of iron, is given almost to the exclusion of solid foods, and (2) increased fecal loss of blood occurs in 50% of iron-deficient infants fed cow's milk.

Therapeutic Management

After the diagnosis of iron deficiency anemia is made, therapeutic management focuses on increasing the amount of supplemental iron the child receives. This is usually done through dietary counseling and the administration of oral iron supplements.

In formula-fed infants, the most convenient and best sources of supplemental iron are iron-fortified commercial formula and iron-fortified infant cereal. Iron-fortified formula provides a relatively constant and predictable amount of iron and is not associated with an increased incidence of gastrointestinal (GI) symptoms, such as colic, diarrhea, or constipation. Infants younger than 12 months of age should *not* be given fresh cow's milk because it may increase the risk for GI blood loss occurring from exposure to a heat-labile protein in cow's milk or cow's milk–induced GI mucosal damage resulting from a lack of cytochrome iron (heme protein) (Kett, 2012; Subramaniam & Girish, 2015; Ziegler, 2011). If GI bleeding is suspected, several stool analyses for occult blood known as *guaiac tests* are performed to identify any intermittent blood loss.

The addition of iron-rich foods to the diet may not provide sufficient supplemental quantities of the mineral as the sole treatment of iron deficiency anemia. If dietary sources of iron cannot replenish the body stores, oral iron supplements are prescribed. Ferrous iron, more readily absorbed than ferric iron, results in higher Hgb levels. Ascorbic acid (vitamin C) appears to facilitate absorption of iron and may be given as vitamin C–enriched foods and juices with the iron preparation.

If the Hgb level fails to rise after 1 month of oral therapy, it is important to assess for persistent bleeding, iron malabsorption, noncompliance, improper iron administration, or other causes of the anemia. Parenteral (IV or intramuscular [IM]) iron administration is safe and effective but painful, expensive, and occasionally associated with regional lymphadenopathy, transient arthralgias, or serious allergic reaction (Andrews, Ullrich, & Fleming, 2009; Bregman & Goodnough, 2014; Lerner & Sills, 2011). Therefore, parenteral iron is reserved for children who have iron malabsorption, chronic hemoglobinuria, or intolerance to oral preparations. Transfusions are indicated for the most severe anemia and in cases of serious infection, cardiac dysfunction, or surgical emergency when anesthesia is required. Packed RBCs (2 to 3 mL/kg), not whole blood, are used to minimize the chance of circulatory overload. Supplemental oxygen is administered when tissue hypoxia is severe.

Prognosis

The prognosis for a child with iron deficiency anemia is very good. However, evidence indicates that if the iron deficiency anemia is severe and longstanding, cognitive, behavioral, and motor impairment and even death may result (Andrews et al., 2009; Jauregui-Lobera, 2014; Lokeshwar, Mehta, Mehta, et al., 2011; Scott, Chen-Edinboro, Caulfield, et al., 2014). However, there is lack of convincing evidence that iron treatment of young children with iron deficiency anemia has an effect on psychomotor development or cognitive function (McDonagh, Blazina, Dana, et al., 2015; Thompson, Biggs, & Pasricha, 2013; Wang, Zhan, Gong, et al., 2013). Therefore, there is need for further large long-term follow-up randomized interventional studies to be conducted in this area.

> **QUALITY PATIENT OUTCOMES: Iron Deficiency Anemia**
> - Early recognition of signs and symptoms of iron deficiency anemia
> - Appropriate quantity of milk, use of iron-fortified infant formula, and introduction of solid foods
> - Adherence to oral iron supplement with appropriate administration
> - Hemoglobin increased within 1 month and anemia resolved within 6 months

Care Management

An essential nursing responsibility is instructing parents in the administration of iron. Oral iron should be given as prescribed in two divided doses between meals, when the presence of free hydrochloric acid is greatest, because more iron is absorbed in the acidic environment of the upper GI tract. A citrus fruit or juice taken with the medication aids in absorption.

> **◉ MEDICATION ALERT**
>
> Cow's milk contains substances that bind the iron and interfere with absorption. Iron supplements should not be administered with milk or milk products (Carley, 2003; Powers & Buchanan, 2014).

An adequate dosage of oral iron turns the stools a tarry green or black color. The nurse advises parents of this normally expected change and inquires about its occurrence on follow-up visits. Absence of the greenish black stool may be a clue to poor compliance (e.g., in schedule, in dosage, in administration, in side effects). If compliance is an issue, make every effort to institute strategies to improve adherence to the medication regimen, such as changing the schedule to more convenient times.

> **◉ MEDICATION ALERT**
>
> Liquid preparations of iron may temporarily stain the teeth. If possible, the medication should be taken through a straw or given through a syringe or medicine dropper placed toward the back of the mouth. Brushing the teeth after administration of the drug lessens the discoloration.

> **❗ NURSING ALERT**
>
> Because iron ingestion in excessive quantities is toxic or even fatal, parents should be instructed to keep no more than 1 month's supply in the home and store it safely away from the reach of children.

If parenteral iron preparations are prescribed, iron dextran must be injected deeply into a large muscle mass using the Z-track method. The injection site is *not* massaged after injection to minimize skin staining and irritation. Because no more than 1 mL should be given in one injection site, the IV route should be considered to avoid multiple injections. Careful observation with IV iron administration is required because of the risk for anaphylaxis, so a test dose is recommended before use. Several IV iron preparations (e.g., ferumoxytol, ferric carboxymaltose, iron sucrose complex, iron isomaltoside) show promise in complete replacement of iron with little toxicity (Auerbach, 2011; Bregman & Goodnough, 2014; Smith, 2012).

Diet

A primary nursing objective is to prevent nutritional anemia through family education. The nurse must reinforce the importance of administering iron supplementation to exclusively breastfed infants by 4 months of age because breast milk is a low iron source (Baker et al., 2010; Lokeshwar et al., 2011; Ziegler, Nelson, & Jeter, 2011). The American Academy of Pediatrics recommends that preterm, marginally low– and low–birth weight infants, or infants with inadequate iron stores at birth receive iron supplements at approximately 2 months of age (Berglund, Westrup, & Domellof, 2010).

In formula-fed infants, the nurse discusses with parents the importance of using iron-fortified formula and of introducing solid foods at the appropriate age during the first year of life. Traditionally, cereals are one of the first semisolid foods to be introduced into the infant's diet at approximately 6 months of age (Baker et al., 2010; Lerner & Sills, 2011; Lokeshwar et al., 2011). The best solid-food source of iron is commercial iron-fortified cereals. It may be difficult at first to teach the infant to accept foods other than milk. The same principles are applied as those for introducing new foods, especially feeding the solid food before the milk. Predominantly milk-fed infants rebel against solid foods, and parents are cautioned about this and the need to be firm in not relinquishing control to the child. It may require intense problem solving on the part of both the family and the nurse to overcome the child's resistance.

A difficulty encountered in discouraging the parents from feeding milk to the exclusion of other foods is dispelling the popular myth that milk is a "perfect food." Many parents believe that milk is best for infants and equate weight gain with "healthiness." Although milk is an excellent food, it is deficient in iron, vitamin C, zinc, and fluoride. Sources of each of these nutrients and the role they play in preventing deficiencies need to be discussed with the family, especially the person responsible for feeding the infant. Also stress that overweight is not synonymous with good health.

Diet education of teenagers is difficult, especially because teenage girls are particularly prone to following weight-reduction diets. Emphasizing the effect of anemia on appearance (pallor) and energy level (difficulty maintaining popular activities) may be useful.

SICKLE CELL ANEMIA

Sickle cell anemia (SCA) is one of a group of diseases collectively termed *hemoglobinopathies* in which normal adult Hgb (Hgb A [HbA]) is partly or completely replaced by abnormal sickle Hgb (HbS). Sickle cell disease (SCD) refers to a group of hereditary disorders, all of which are related to the presence of HbS. Although the term *SCD* is sometimes used to refer to SCA, this use is incorrect. The correct terms for SCA are *homozygous sickle cell disease* (HgbSS) and *homozygous SCD*.

The following are the most common forms of SCD in the United States:

- **SCA,** the homozygous form of the disease (HbgSS), in which valine, an amino acid, is substituted for glutamic acid at the sixth position of the β chain
- **Sickle cell–C disease,** a heterozygous variant of SCD (HgbSC) is characterized by the presence of both HgbS and HgbC, in which lysine is substituted for glutamic acid at the sixth position of the β chain
- **Sickle thalassemia disease,** a combination of sickle cell trait and β-thalassemia trait (Sβthal). In the β⁺ (beta plus) form, some normal HbA can be produced. In the β⁰ (beta zero) form, there is no ability to produce HbA.

Of the SCDs, SCA is the most common form in African Americans followed by sickle cell–C disease and sickle thalassemia disease. Numerous other sickle syndromes exist in which HbS is paired with other mutant globin.

SCD is one of the most common genetic diseases worldwide, affecting approximately 100,000 Americans, including other nationalities, such as Africans; Hispanics; Italians; Greeks; Iranians; Turks; individuals of Arab, Caribbean, and Asian Indian descent; and other ethnic groups. The incidence of the disease varies in different geographic locations. Among African Americans, the incidence of sickle cell trait is about 8%, whereas among inhabitants of West Africa, the incidence is reported to be as high as 40%. The high incidence of sickle cell trait in West Africans is believed by some to be the result of selective protection afforded trait carriers against one type of malaria.

The gene that determines the production of HbS is situated on an autosome and, when present, is always detectable and therefore dominant. Heterozygous individuals who have both normal HbA and abnormal

HbS are said to have sickle cell trait. Homozygous individuals have predominantly HbS and have SCA. The inheritance pattern is essentially that of an autosomal recessive disorder. Therefore, when both parents have sickle cell trait, there is a 25% chance with each pregnancy of producing an offspring with SCA.

Although the defect is inherited, the sickling phenomenon is usually not apparent until later in infancy because of the presence of fetal Hgb (HbF). As long as the child has predominantly HbF, sickling does not occur because there is less HbS. Newborns with SCA are generally asymptomatic because of the protective effect of HbF (60% to 80% HbF), but this rapidly decreases during the first year, so these children are at risk for sickle cell–related complications (Driscoll, 2007; Ellison, 2012; Heeney & Dover, 2009; Meier & Miller, 2012).

Pathophysiology

The clinical features of SCA are primarily the result of (1) obstruction caused by the sickled RBCs with other cells, (2) vascular inflammation, and (3) increased RBC destruction (Fig. 43.2). The abnormal adhesion, entanglement, and enmeshing of rigid sickle-shaped cells accompanied by the inflammatory process intermittently blocks the microcirculation causing vaso-occlusion (Fig. 43.3). The resultant absence of blood flow to adjacent tissues causes local hypoxia, leading to tissue ischemia and infarction (cellular death). Most of the complications seen in SCA can be traced to this process and its impact on various organs of the body (Box 43.2).

The clinical manifestations of SCA vary greatly in severity and frequency. The most acute symptoms of the disease occur during periods of exacerbation called *crises*. There are several types of episodic crises,

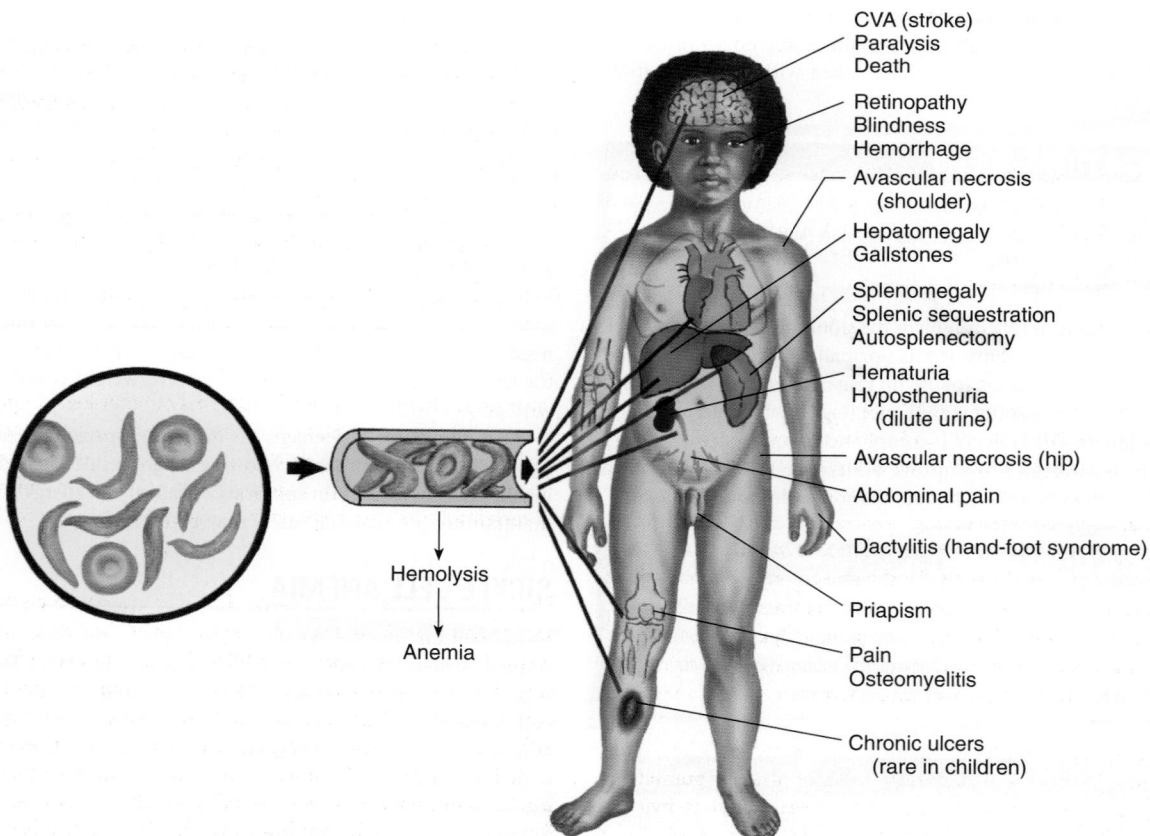

FIG 43.2 Clinical features of sickle cell anemia (SCA) from red blood cell (RBC) obstruction and destruction. *CVA,* Cerebrovascular accident.

Normal red blood cells

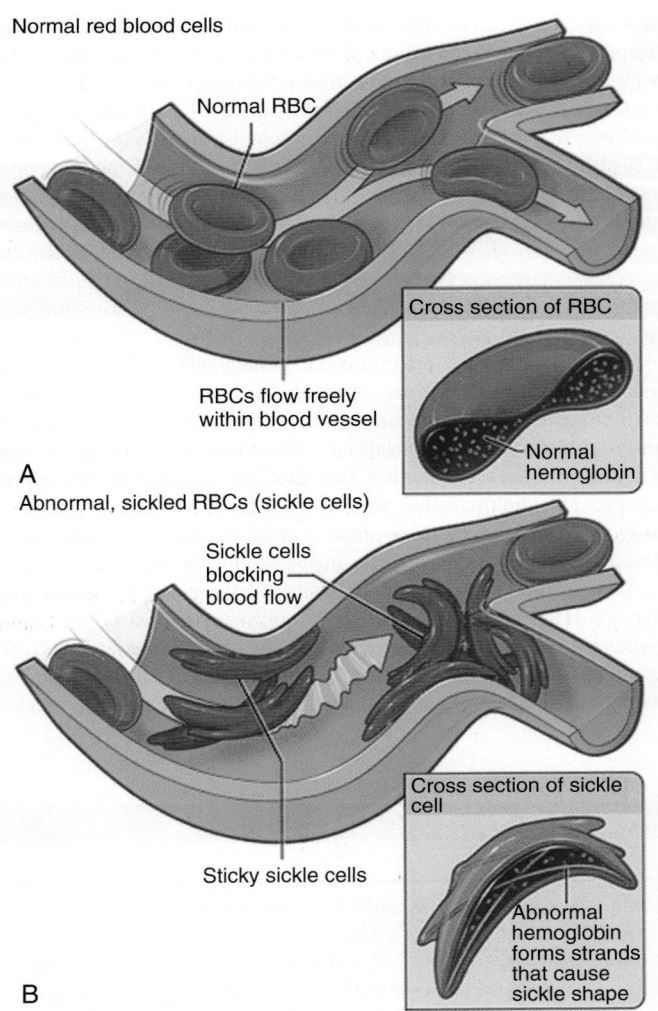

Normal RBC

RBCs flow freely
within blood vessel

Cross section of RBC

Normal
hemoglobin

A
Abnormal, sickled RBCs (sickle cells)

Sickle cells
blocking
blood flow

Cross section of sickle
cell

Sticky sickle cells

Abnormal
hemoglobin
forms strands
that cause
sickle shape

B

FIG 43.3 A, Normal red blood cells (RBCs) flowing freely in a blood vessel. The inset shows a cross-section of a normal RBC with normal hemoglobin. **B,** Abnormal, sickled RBCs clumping and blocking blood flow in a blood vessel. (Other cells also may play a role in this clumping process.) The inset shows a cross-section of a sickle cell with abnormal hemoglobin. (From National Heart, Lung, and Blood Institute. [2008]. *What is sickle cell anemia?* Bethesda, MD: Author.)

BOX 43.2 Clinical Manifestations of Sickle Cell Anemia

General
Possible growth restriction
Chronic anemia (hemoglobin level of 6 to 9 g/dL)
Possible delayed sexual maturation
Marked susceptibility to sepsis

Vaso-Occlusive Crisis
Pain in area(s) of involvement
Manifestations related to ischemia of involved areas
  Extremities: Painful swelling of hands and feet (sickle cell dactylitis, or hand/foot syndrome), painful joints
  Abdomen: Severe pain resembling acute surgical condition
  Cerebrum: Stroke, visual disturbances
  Chest: Symptoms resembling pneumonia, protracted episodes of pulmonary disease
  Liver: Obstructive jaundice, hepatic coma
  Kidney: Hematuria
  Genitalia: Priapism (painful penile erection)

Sequestration Crisis
Pooling of large amounts of blood
  Hepatomegaly
  Splenomegaly
  Circulatory collapse

Effects of Chronic Vaso-Occlusive Phenomena
  Heart: Cardiomegaly, systolic murmurs
  Lungs: Altered pulmonary function, susceptibility to infections, pulmonary insufficiency
  Kidneys: Inability to concentrate urine, enuresis, progressive renal failure
  Liver: Hepatomegaly, cirrhosis, intrahepatic cholestasis
  Spleen: Splenomegaly, susceptibility to infection, functional reduction in splenic activity progressing to autosplenectomy
  Eyes: Intraocular abnormalities with visual disturbances; sometimes progressive retinal detachment and blindness
  Extremities: Avascular necrosis of hip or shoulder; skeletal deformities, especially lordosis and kyphosis; chronic leg ulcers; susceptibility to osteomyelitis
  Central nervous system (CNS): Hemiparesis, seizures

including vaso-occlusive, acute splenic sequestration, aplastic, hyperhemolytic, cerebrovascular accident (CVA), chest syndrome, and infection. The crises may occur individually or concomitantly with one or more other crises. The *vaso-occlusive crisis (VOC)*, preferably called a "painful episode," is characterized by ischemia causing mild to severe pain that may last from minutes to days or longer. *Sequestration crisis* is a pooling of a large amount of blood usually in the spleen and infrequently in the liver that causes a decreased blood volume and ultimately shock. *Aplastic crisis* is diminished RBC production, usually triggered by viral infection that may result in profound anemia. *Hyperhemolytic crisis* is an accelerated rate of RBC destruction characterized by anemia, jaundice, and reticulocytosis.

Another serious complication is *acute chest syndrome* (ACS), which is clinically similar to pneumonia. It is the presence of a new pulmonary infiltrate and may be associated with chest pain, fever, cough, tachypnea, wheezing, and hypoxia. A *cerebrovascular accident* (CVA, stroke) is a sudden and severe complication, often with no related illnesses. Sickled cells block the major blood vessels in the brain, resulting in cerebral

infarction, which causes variable degrees of neurologic impairment. The current treatment for SCD children who have experienced a stroke is chronic transfusion therapy. Repeat CVAs causing progressively greater brain damage occur in approximately 70% of untreated children who have experienced one stroke (Heeney & Dover, 2009; Wang & Dwan, 2013).

Diagnostic Evaluation

Universal screening of newborns for SCD has become standard in the United States in all 50 states and the territories (McCavit, 2012; McGann, Nero, & Ware, 2013; Meier & Miller, 2012). However, global newborn screening varies by country and is not a common practice in most countries where SCD is a public health concern (Aygun & Odame, 2012; Huttle, Maestre, Lantigua, et al., 2015). The screening provides early identification of these children before complications develop. At birth, infants have up to 80% of HbF, which does not carry the defect. Because levels of HbS are low at birth, Hgb electrophoresis or other tests that measure Hgb concentrations are indicated. Early diagnosis (before 3 months of age) enables initiation of appropriate interventions to minimize complications. The family is taught to administer prophylactic antibiotics and identify early signs of infection to seek medical therapy as soon as possible.

Although SCD is usually reported during the prenatal or neonatal periods, it may not be recognized until the toddler and preschool period during a crisis precipitated by an acute respiratory tract or GI infection. However, early diagnosis (before 2 months of age) facilitates initiation of appropriate interventions to minimize complications. There are several specific tests that detect the presence of the abnormal Hgb in the heterozygous or the homozygous form of SCD. For screening purposes, the sickle-turbidity test (Sickledex) is used because it can be performed on blood from a finger or heel stick and yields accurate results in 3 minutes. If the test result is positive, however, Hgb electrophoresis is necessary to distinguish between children with the trait and those with the disease. *Hemoglobin electrophoresis* (referred to as "fingerprinting" of the protein) is a specially prepared blood test that separates various hemoglobins by high voltage. The blood test is accurate, rapid, and specific for detecting the homozygous and heterozygous forms of the disease, as well as the percentages of the various types of Hgb. The hemoglobin electrophoresis is increasingly used as the initial screening test in centers within the United States.

Therapeutic Management

The aims of therapy are to prevent the sickling phenomena, which are responsible for the pathologic sequelae, and treat the medical emergencies

of sickle cell crisis. The successful achievement of the aims depends on prompt nursing interventions, medical therapies, patient and family preventive measures, and use of innovative treatments.

Medical management of a crisis is directed by an interprofessional care team that provides supportive, symptomatic, and specific treatments. The main objectives are to provide (1) rest to minimize energy expenditure and to improve oxygen utilization; (2) hydration through oral and IV therapy; (3) electrolyte replacement because hypoxia results in metabolic acidosis, which also promotes sickling; (4) analgesia for the severe pain from vaso-occlusion; (5) blood replacement to treat anemia and to reduce the viscosity of the sickled blood; and (6) antibiotics to treat any existing infection.

Administration of pneumococcal, *Haemophilus influenza,* and meningococcal vaccines is recommended for these children because of their susceptibility to infection as a result of functional asplenia. In addition to routine immunizations, children with SCD should receive a yearly influenza vaccination (see the "Immunizations" section in Chapter 31). Oral penicillin prophylaxis is recommended by 2 months of age to reduce the chance of pneumococcal sepsis (see Evidence-Based Practice box: Sickle Cell Anemia and Penicillin Prophylaxis).

Oxygen therapy is of little therapeutic value unless the patient has hypoxia (Heeney & Dover, 2009). Severe hypoxia must be prevented because it causes massive systemic sickling that can be fatal. Oxygen administration is usually not effective in reversing sickling or reducing pain because the oxygen is unable to reach the enmeshed sickled

---

EVIDENCE-BASED PRACTICE

Sickle Cell Anemia and Penicillin Prophylaxis

Ask the Question
PICOT Question: In children with sickle cell anemia (SCA), does prophylaxis with penicillin reduce the risk for pneumococcal infection?

Search for the Evidence
Search Strategies
Search selection criteria included English-language publications within the past 25 years, research-based articles (level 3 or lower), and child populations.

Databases Used
PubMed, Cochrane Collaboration, MD Consult

Critical Appraisal of the Evidence
- Hirst and Owusu-Ofori (2014) conducted an updated systematic Cochrane review of three trials that showed a reduced rate of infection in children with homozygous sickle cell disease (SCD) (HgbSS or HgbSβ0Thal) receiving prophylactic penicillin. Two trials looked at whether treatment was effective. The third trial followed from one of the early trials and looked at when it was safe to stop treatment. Adverse drug effects were rare and minor. Penicillin given prophylactically significantly reduces the risk for pneumococcal infection in children with SCD younger than 5 years of age and is associated with minimal adverse reactions. Supporting the same conclusion that there is strong evidence that daily oral penicillin prophylaxis greatly reduces the risk for pneumococcal infection in children with SCA younger than 3 years of age was reported in a systematic review (Gwaram & Gwaram, 2014).
- Researchers combined the clinical experiences of three sickle cell programs in the eastern United States in an attempt to determine the age and disease-specific risk for *Streptococcus pneumoniae* bacteremia and meningitis in children with SCD at a time when penicillin prophylaxis was routine. Forty-seven pneumococcal infections (44 bacteremia; 3 meningitis) among 40 patients

with SCD were observed. Most children in whom infections developed were taking prophylactic penicillin and received Pneumovax at 24 months of age. The observed severe pneumococcal infection rate in HgbSS children younger than 5 years of age was less than that reported before penicillin prophylaxis in this specific population (Hord, Byrd, Stowe, et al., 2002).
- Administration of oral prophylactic penicillin was compared with the 14-valent pneumococcal vaccine in preventing pneumococcal infection in 242 children between 6 months and 3 years of age with HgbSS. In the first 5 years of the trial, there were 11 pneumococcal infections in the pneumococcal vaccine group and higher infection rates in those given the vaccine before 1 year of age. No pneumococcal isolates were found in the group receiving penicillin, although four pneumococcal isolates were found in this group within 1 year of stopping the penicillin prophylaxis at 3 years of age. This study supported the use of penicillin prophylaxis to prevent pneumococcal infection in children younger than 3 years of age (John, Ramlal, Jackson, et al., 1984).
- In a multicenter, randomized, double-blind, placebo-controlled clinical trial, 105 children received penicillin twice daily; a control group of 110 children received a placebo twice daily. The trial was terminated 8 months early when an 84% reduction in the incidence of pneumococcal infections was observed in the group treated with penicillin compared with the placebo group. There were no deaths in the penicillin group, but three deaths from infection occurred in the placebo group. Researchers stressed the importance of screening children during the neonatal period and prescribing prophylactic penicillin to decrease the morbidity and mortality associated with pneumococcal infection (Gaston, Verter, Woods, et al., 1986).
- Zarkowsky, Gallagher, Gill, et al. (1986) conducted a retrospective analysis of 178 episodes of bacteremia in children with sickle hemoglobinopathies that occurred during 13,771 patient-years of follow-up (n = 3451). The predominant pathogen in patients younger than 6 years of age was *S. pneumoniae* (66%), and gram-negative organisms were responsible for 50% of the

EVIDENCE-BASED PRACTICE

Sickle Cell Anemia and Penicillin Prophylaxis—cont'd

bacteremias in patients 6 years of age and older. The incidence of pneumococcal bacteremia in children with SCA younger than 3 years of age was 6.1 events per 100 patient-years. The results of this study supported prophylactic administration of penicillin for prevention of pneumococcal bacteremia in children younger than 3 years of age.

- A cohort study of 315 patients with HgbSS who lived in Jamaica was conducted between June 1973 and December 1981. The patients were divided into three groups to determine whether interventions such as penicillin prophylaxis, parental education in early diagnosis of acute splenic sequestration, and close monitoring in a sickle cell clinic improved survival. A significant decline in deaths from acute splenic sequestration and pneumococcal septicemia and meningitis was found. The research indicated that early detection of SCD and prophylactic measures could significantly reduce deaths associated with HgbSS (Lee, Thomas, Cupidore, et al., 1995).

- Riddington and Owusu-Ofori (2002) conducted a systematic review of randomized, controlled trials evaluating the effectiveness of prophylactic antibiotic administration in preventing pneumococcal infection in children with SCD. The review of published research found that penicillin prophylaxis significantly reduced the risk for pneumococcal infection in children with HgbSS with minimal adverse reactions.

- McCavit, Gilbert, & Buchanan (2013) conducted a cross-sectional electronic survey of 106 pediatric hematologists with expertise in SCD regarding their practices related to penicillin prophylaxis in children with SCD after 5 years of age. Eighty-four percent of pediatric hematologists from 76 centers completed the survey, and 76% routinely recommended cessation of penicillin prophylaxis after 5 years of age.

Apply the Evidence: Nursing Implications

There is good evidence with a strong recommendation (Guyatt, Oxman, Vist, et al., 2008) that penicillin prophylaxis significantly reduces the risk for pneumococcal infection in children with SCA. The epidemiologic studies strongly suggest that all children with SCA should be started on prophylactic penicillin at 2 months of age. Parents and children with SCA should be instructed in the importance of taking the prophylactic penicillin twice daily and seeking medical attention immediately for acute illness, especially if the temperature exceeds 38.3° C (101° F), regardless of the use of prophylaxis.

Quality and Safety Competencies: Evidence-Based Practice*

Knowledge

Differentiate clinical opinion from research and evidence-based summaries.

Summarize the epidemiologic studies that strongly suggest that children with SCA should be started on prophylactic penicillin.

Skills

Base individualized care plan on patient values, clinical expertise, and evidence.

Integrate evidence into practice by making sure infants with SCD are started on penicillin at 2 months of age.

Attitudes

Value the concept of evidence-based practice as integral to determining best clinical practice.

Appreciate strengths and weaknesses of evidence for preventing pneumococcal infection in children with SCD.

References

Gaston, M. H., Verter, J. I., Woods, G., et al. (1986). Prophylaxis with oral penicillin in children with sickle cell anemia: A randomized trial. *New England Journal of Medicine*, *314*(25), 1593–1599.

Guyatt, G. H., Oxman, A. D., Vist, G. E., et al. (2008). GRADE: An emerging consensus on rating quality of evidence and strength of recommendations. *British Medical Journal*, *336*(7650), 924–926.

Gwaram, H. A., & Gwaram, B. A. (2014). A systematic review of effectiveness of daily oral penicillin v prophylaxis in the prevention of pneumococcal infection in children with sickle cell anaemia. *Nigerian Journal of Medicine*, *23*(2), 118–129.

Hirst, C., & Owusu-Ofori, S. (2014). Prophylactic antibiotics for preventing pneumococcal infection in children with sickle cell disease. *Cochrane Database of Systematic Reviews*, *2014*(11), CD003427.

Hord, J., Byrd, R., Stowe, L., et al. (2002). Streptococcus pneumoniae sepsis and meningitis during the penicillin prophylaxis era in children with sickle cell disease. *Journal of Pediatric Hematology/Oncology*, *24*(6), 470–472.

John, A. B., Ramlal, A., Jackson, H., et al. (1984). Prevention of pneumococcal infection in children with homozygous sickle cell disease. *British Medical Journal*, *288*(6430), 1567–1570.

Lee, A., Thomas, P., Cupidore, L., et al. (1995). Improved survival in homozygous sickle cell disease: Lessons from a cohort study. *British Medical Journal*, *311*(7020), 1600–1602.

McCavit, T. L., Gilbert, M., & Buchanan, G. R. (2013). Prophylactic penicillin after 5 years of age in patients with sickle cell disease: A survey of sickle cell disease experts. *Pediatric Blood & Cancer*, *60*(6), 935–939.

Riddington, C., & Owusu-Ofori, S. (2002). Prophylactic antibiotics for preventing pneumococcal infection in children with sickle cell disease. *Cochrane Database of Systematic Reviews*, *2002*(3), CD003427.

Zarkowsky, H. S., Gallagher, D., Gill, F. M., et al. (1986). Bacteremia in sickle hemoglobinopathies. *Journal of Pediatrics*, *109*(4), 579–585.

*Adapted from the Quality and Safety Education for Nurses (QSEN) Institute.

erythrocytes in clogged vessels. In addition, prolonged administration of oxygen can depress bone marrow, further aggravating the anemia.

Another important component of care is the use of blood transfusions. Exchange RBC transfusion (erythrocytapheresis) is the replacement of sickle cells with normal RBCs. Exchange transfusion is a successful, rapid method of reducing the number of circulating sickle cells and therefore slowing down the vicious circle of hypoxia, thrombosis, tissue ischemia, and injury. Therapy including simple and exchange transfusions are used in life-threatening ACS and after acute overt stroke to prevent recurrence and further tissue damage (Velasquez, Mariscalco, Goldstein, et al., 2009; Meier & Miller, 2012; Wang & Dwan, 2013). A transcranial Doppler (TCD) test identifies the child with SCA or HgbS-β⁰ thalassemia who is at high risk for developing a CVA by monitoring the intracranial vascular flow (Driscoll, 2007; Kwiatkowski, Yim, Miller, et al., 2011;

Meier & Miller, 2012). The TCD is performed yearly for children from 2 to 16 years of age. The recommended treatment for children with confirmed abnormal TCD is chronic transfusion therapy (Armstrong-Wells, Grimes, Sidney, et al., 2009; Kwiatkowski, Yim, Miller, et al., 2011; Wang & Dwan, 2013). The duration of transfusion is indefinite, although current studies are addressing whether patients may be transitioned safely to hydroxyurea to prevent stroke (McCavit, 2012). Multiple transfusions carry the risk for transmission of viral infection, hyperviscosity, transfusion reactions, alloimmunization, and hemosiderosis (Driscoll, 2007; Heeney & Dover, 2009; Jordan, Casella, & DeBaun, 2012; Yawn, Buchanan, Afenyi-Annan, et al., 2014). After a CVA, blood transfusions are usually given every 3 to 4 weeks to help prevent a repeat stroke. To reduce iron overload from chronic transfusion therapy, chelation therapy may be started (see later in this chapter).

In children with recurrent life-threatening splenic sequestration, splenectomy may be a lifesaving measure. However, the spleen usually atrophies on its own through progressive fibrotic changes (functional asplenia) by 6 years of age in children with SCA. Prophylactic penicillin and pneumococcal vaccines have decreased the incidence of pneumococcal sepsis in children with SCD. Packed RBC transfusions are recommended not only for treatment of splenic sequestration but also stroke and used preoperatively accompanied with maintenance IV hydration for most surgical procedures in children with SCD.

VOC, the most common, severe, painful episode, is considered the clinical hallmark of SCD that is usually accompanied by increasing health care cost because of prolonged hospitalization (Ballas, 2011; McCavit, 2012; Raphael, Mei, Mueller, et al., 2012; Yawn et al., 2014). The chronic nature of this pain can greatly affect the child's development. A multidisciplinary team (e.g., physician, psychologist, child life specialist, family, nurse, social worker) approach is best for vaso-occlusive pain management that includes pharmacologic treatments, hydration, physical therapy, and nonpharmacologic and complementary treatment (e.g., prayer, spiritual healing, massage, heating pads, herbs, relaxation, breathing exercises, distraction, music, guided imagery, self-motivation, acupuncture, and biofeedback) (Ballas, 2011; Brandow, Weisman, & Panepinto, 2011; Meier & Miller, 2012; Redding-Lallinger & Knoll, 2006). When mild to moderate VOC is reported, nonsteroidal antiinflammatory medication (e.g., ibuprofen, ketorolac) or nonopioids (e.g., acetaminophen) are used initially. If these drugs are not effective alone, an opioid may be added. The dosages of both drugs are titrated (adjusted) to a therapeutic level. Opioids such as immediate- and sustained-release morphine, oxycodone, hydrocodone, hydromorphone (Dilaudid), and methadone are administered intravenously or orally for severe pain and are given around the clock. In conjunction with the opioid, IV ketorolac for a maximum of a 5-day course is commonly used to enhance the pain management effect. Patient-controlled analgesia (PCA) has been used successfully for sickle cell–related pain. PCA reinforces the patient's role and responsibility in managing the pain and provides flexibility in dealing with pain, which may vary in severity over time (see the "Pain Management" section in Chapter 30).

MEDICATION ALERT

Meperidine (Demerol) is not recommended. Normeperidine, a metabolite of meperidine, is a central nervous system (CNS) stimulant that produces anxiety, tremors, myoclonus, and generalized seizures when it accumulates with repetitive dosing. Patients with SCD are particularly at risk for normeperidine-induced seizures (Ellison, 2012; Howard & Davies, 2007; National Institutes of Health & National Heart, Lung, and Blood Institute, Division of Blood Disease and Resources, 2002).

Prognosis

The prognosis varies, but most patients live into the fifth decade. The greatest risk is usually in children younger than 5 years of age, and the majority of deaths in these children are caused by overwhelming infection. Consequently, SCA is a chronic illness with a potentially terminal outcome. Physical and sexual maturation are delayed in adolescents with SCA. Although adults achieve normal height, weight, and sexual function, the delay may present problems to adolescents (Heeney & Dover, 2009; Redding-Lallinger & Knoll, 2006).

Individuals with SCD who have higher levels of HbF tend to have a milder disease with fewer complications than those with lower levels (Driscoll, 2007; Meier & Miller, 2012). Hydroxyurea is a US Food and Drug Administration–approved medication that increases the production

of HbF, reduces endothelial adhesion of sickle cells, improves the sickle cell hydration and cell size, increases nitric oxide production (a vasodilator), and lowers leukocyte and reticulocyte counts (McGann & Ware, 2011; National Institutes of Health, National Heart, Lung, and Blood Institute, Division of Blood Disease and Resources, 2002; Yawn et al., 2014). Long-term follow-up of patients taking hydroxyurea alone revealed a 40% reduction in mortality and decreased frequency of VOC, ACS, hospital admissions, and need for transfusions, thus making SCD crises milder (Anderson, 2006; Strouse, Lanzkron, Beach, et al., 2008; Voskaridou, Christoulas, Bilalis, et al., 2010). Pediatric studies have shown that hydroxyurea can be safely used in children (Wang, Ware, Miller, et al., 2011; Zimmerman, Schultz, Davis, et al., 2004).

Allogeneic hematopoietic stem cell transplantation (HSCT) offers a curative treatment for children with SCD, with an overall survival of 92% to 95% and an event-free survival of 82% to 86% (Bernaudin, Socie, Kuentz, et al., 2007; Haining, Duncan, & Lehmann, 2009; Hsieh, Fitzhugh, Weitzel, et al., 2014; Locatelli & Pagliara, 2012).

Since SCD is an autosomal recessive disorder, curative strategies for correction, replacement, addition, or modulation of the globin gene continue to evolve in the basic and clinical research settings (Meier & Miller, 2012).

QUALITY PATIENT OUTCOMES: Sickle Cell Disease

- Early recognition of signs and symptoms of sickle cell anemia (SCA)
- Tissue deoxygenation minimized
- Sickle cell crisis prevented or quickly managed
- Pain appropriately managed
- Stroke prevented
- Prophylactic penicillin regimen followed
- Hypoxia prevented when surgery is necessary
- Pneumococcal, *H. influenzae* type b, and meningococcal vaccines administered

Care Management
Educate the Family and Child

Family education begins with an explanation of the disease and its consequences (see Nursing Care Plan box: The Child with Sickle Cell Anemia). After this explanation, the most important issues to teach the family are to (1) seek early intervention for problems, such as fever of 38.5° C (101.3° F) or greater; (2) give penicillin as ordered; (3) recognize signs and symptoms of stroke, splenic sequestration, as well as respiratory problems that can lead to hypoxia; and (4) treat the child normally. The nurse tells the family that the child is normal but can get sick in ways that other children cannot.

! NURSING ALERT

One simple yet graphic way to demonstrate the effect of sickling is to roll rounded objects, such as marbles or beads, through a tube to simulate normal circulation and then roll pointed objects, such as screws or jacks, through the tube. The effect of sickling and clumping of the pointed objects is especially noticeable at a bend or slight narrowing of the tube.

The nurse emphasizes the importance of adequate hydration to prevent sickling and delay the vaso-occlusion and hypoxia-ischemia cycle. It is not sufficient to advise parents to "force fluids" or "encourage drinking." They need specific instructions on how many daily glasses or bottles of fluid are required. Many foods are also a source of fluid, particularly soups, flavored ice pops, ice cream, sherbet, gelatin, and puddings.

Increased fluids combined with impaired kidney function result in the problem of enuresis. Parents who are unaware of this fact frequently

◎ NURSING CARE PLAN
The Child With Sickle Cell Anemia

Case Study

Donny is a 2-year-old male with sickle cell anemia (HgbSS). He returns to the hematology clinic this morning after being seen last night in the emergency department (ED) for pain. His mother states he is having more pain in his feet over the past several hours, and he no longer wants to walk. The mother has been giving Donny the pain medications as prescribed by the ED physician, but she feels his pain is getting worse. On examination, you find that his feet and hands are swollen, and he cries out when you touch them.

Assessment

What are the most important signs of acute pain that you need to look for in a young child with sickle cell disease (SCD)?

Sickle Cell Vaso-Occlusive Pain: Defining Characteristics

Pain can be in any location in the body; can be rapid in onset and severe, may be localized or generalized

Low-grade fever may be present

Localized swelling over joints with arthralgia can occur

Nursing Diagnosis

Acute Pain related to tissue anoxia (vaso-occlusive episode or crisis)

Nursing Interventions and Rationales

What are the most appropriate nursing interventions for a child with SCD experiencing pain?

Nursing Interventions	Rationales
Discuss schedule of medication around the clock with parents.	To control pain
Encourage high level of fluid intake.	To ensure hydration
Recognize that various analgesics, including opioids and medication schedules, may need to be tried.	To ensure satisfactory pain relief
Reassure Donny and family that analgesics, including opioids, are medically indicated, that high doses may be needed, and that children rarely become addicted.	To avoid needless suffering because of unfounded fears
Apply heat application or massage to affected area. Avoid applying cold compresses.	To prevent vasoconstriction that may enhance sickling

Case Study (Continued)

Donny's pain is not being controlled by oral pain medications, and the plan is to begin intravenous (IV) pain medications to control his pain. What is the most appropriate IV medication for Donny at this time?

A dose of morphine (0.1 to 0.2 mg/kg/dose) is given every 10 minutes for three doses.

What important nursing interventions should be implemented at this time?

Give both the morphine and ketorolac. If pain is still not relieved after three doses of morphine, then switch to patient-controlled analgesia (PCA) and admit. Give ketorolac 1 mg/kg for first dose, and then 0.5 mg/kg /dose IV every 6 hours; not to exceed 5 days (maximum of 30 mg/dose).

Nursing Interventions	Rationales
Administer morphine and ketorolac safely.	To prevent adverse effects and overdose
Monitor for side effects of morphine; assess respiratory status closely, and prevent constipation.	To prevent discomfort and adverse effects following administration
Monitor for side effects of ketorolac; assess for bleeding (gastrointestinal [GI] or renal) closely.	

Nursing Interventions	Rationales
Educate parents on the safety and effectiveness of morphine and ketorolac as pain-relieving medications.	To reduce unfounded fears
Reassess the child's pain level after administering morphine and ketorolac; continue to assess frequently.	To ensure satisfactory pain relief
Recognize that various analgesics and doses may need to be tried.	To assure optimal pain relief

Case Study (Continued)

Because Donny is only 2 years of age, what kind of pain assessment tool is most appropriate for a child this age?

Because Donny is in a great deal of pain, the FLACC Behavioral Pain Assessment Scale is an appropriate observational tool to use at this time. The FLACC tool is an interval scale that includes the five categories of behavior: facial expression (F), leg movement (L), activity (A), cry (C), and consolability (C). See Chapter 5 for more discussion of this tool.

How frequently should Donny's pain be assessed?

Donny's pain should be assessed frequently to determine whether the IV morphine is providing enough pain relief. Morphine (0.1 to 0.2 mg/kg/dose) is given every 10 minutes for three doses. After this initial intervention, pain assessment will help determine what to do next. Donny may require additional medications to control his pain. If the IV morphine provided relief, then discharge on oral morphine (0.2 to 0.5 mg/kg) or convert to home opioid equivalent with ibuprofen every 6 hours. Instruct to continue around-the-clock medications at home, emphasize increased fluid intake, and start bowel regimen to prevent constipation. If his pain is still not under control after three doses of IV morphine, then initiate morphine PCA and admit to hospital.

PCA: Loading dose of 0.1 mg/kg (maximum 8 mg); basal rate of 0.01 mg/kg and intermittent dose 0.035 mg/kg (maximum 8 mg) with the interval lockout ≈10 minutes. A 4-hour limit 0.5 to 0.75 mg/kg with IV fluids at 1½ maintenance rate is administered unless history of acute chest syndrome *(ACS), then IV is at maintenance rate.*

Once the pain is controlled (e.g., decreased swelling, using extremities, no crying when touch extremities), then gradually decrease IV analgesic. If drinking orally, at least maintenance and half fluids daily, and then may convert to home oral opioid equivalent with ibuprofen every 6 hours and discharge home. If pain remains under control and Donny is drinking fluids adequately at home, instruct parents to continue home oral opioid every 24 hours, then stop opioid and continue to observe for any signs of pain. Continue ibuprofen for 24 hours after stopping the opioid, and then stop ibuprofen with no signs of pain observed.

Expected Outcomes

Donny's pain will be controlled in a timely manner.

Case Study (Continued)

Donny is not eating or drinking this morning and appears lethargic in the examination room. When you question his mother regarding the last time he drank something, she remembers it was over 12 hours ago.

Assessment

What are the most important signs and symptoms of dehydration in a child with SCD?

Defining Characteristics

Dry mucous membranes

Loss of skin turgor

Continued

◎ NURSING CARE PLAN

The Child With Sickle Cell Anemia—cont'd

Sunken eyes
No or diminished tears
Sunken fontanel
Dark urine
Rapid, thready pulse
Rapid breathing

Nursing Diagnosis
Deficient Fluid Volume

Nursing Interventions and Rationales
What are the most appropriate nursing interventions for dehydration in a young child with sickle cell anemia (SCA) who is experiencing a vaso-occlusive crisis (VOC)?

Nursing Interventions	Rationales
Calculate recommended daily fluid intake (1600 mL/m²/day), and base Donny's fluid requirements on this amount.	To ensure adequate hydration
Increase fluid intake above minimum requirements during physical exercise or emotional stress and during a crisis.	To compensate for additional fluid needs
Give parents written instructions regarding specific quantity of fluid required daily.	To encourage compliance
Encourage child to drink.	To ensure adequate hydration
Increase fluid intake above minimum requirements during physical exercise or emotional stress and during a crisis.	To compensate for additional fluid needs

Expected Outcomes
Donny will receive appropriate hydration and will demonstrate electrolyte and fluid stability.
Donny's parents ask you what you have found in your initial assessment. They ask about why he has swollen hands and feet and how that causes pain from SCD. They are very worried and think it is their fault that this happened.

Assessment
What are the most important aspects of Donny's care to discuss with his parents at this time? What should be included regarding SCD in a young child?

Defining Characteristics
Lack of understanding
Inability to identify signs and symptoms of painful crises
Inability to follow disease management guidelines
Difficulty describing treatment plan

Nursing Diagnosis
Readiness for Enhanced Knowledge related to parents' interest in Donny's health status.

Nursing Interventions and Rationales
What are the most appropriate nursing interventions to help a family manage a young child with SCD?

Nursing Interventions	Rationales
Explain signs of developing complications, such as fever, pallor, respiratory distress, persistent headaches, and pain. Discuss dactylitis in the young child.	To ensure prompt and appropriate treatment
Reinforce basic information regarding trait transmission, and refer to genetic counseling services if appropriate.	To allow for informed decision making
Provide information on what to do when complications occur, such as fever, pallor, respiratory distress, persistent headaches, and pain.	To ensure prompt and appropriate treatment
Stress importance of adequate nutrition; routine immunizations, including pneumococcal and meningococcal vaccinations; protection from known sources of infection; and frequent health evaluation and regularly scheduled comprehensive evaluation.	To encourage preventive measures and decrease risk for infection exposure

Expected Outcomes
Parents will understand the signs and symptoms of SCD and will understand the actions being taken by the health care team.
Parents will be prepared to manage his disease at home.

---

use the usual measures to discourage bedwetting, such as limiting fluids at night, and may resort to punishment and shame to force bladder control. The nurse should discuss this problem with the parents, stressing that the child's ability to concentrate urine is impaired. Reminding the child to urinate frequently during the day and prior to bedtime may be helpful, and waking the child during the night may help if the child's sleep pattern is not disturbed. Enuresis is treated as a complication of the disease, such as joint pain or some other symptom, to alleviate parental pressure on the child.

Promote Supportive Therapies During Crises

The success of many of the medical therapies relies heavily on nursing implementation. Management of pain is an especially difficult problem and often involves experimenting with various analgesics, including opioids, and schedules before relief is achieved. Unfortunately, these children tend to be undermedicated, resulting in "clock watching" and demands for additional doses sooner than might be expected. Often

this incorrectly raises suspicions of drug addiction, when in fact the problem is one of improper dosage (see Family-Centered Care box: Fear of Addiction). In choosing and scheduling analgesics, the goal should be *prevention* of pain.

! NURSING ALERT

Advise parents to be particularly alert to situations in which dehydration may be a possibility (e.g., hot weather, playing sports) and to recognize early signs of reduced fluid intake, such as decreased urinary output (e.g., fewer wet diapers) and increased thirst.

Any pain program should be combined with psychologic support to help the child deal with the depression, anxiety, and fear that may accompany the disease. This includes regular visits with the child to discuss any concerns during the hospitalization and positive reinforcement of coping skills, such as successful methods of dealing with the

FAMILY-CENTERED CARE
Fear of Addiction

Although the pain during a sickle cell crisis is usually severe and opioids are needed, many families fear that their child will become addicted to the narcotic. Unfortunately, misinformed health care professionals may foster this unfounded fear, which results in needless suffering. Extremely few children who receive opioids for severe pain become behaviorally addicted to the drug (American Pain Society, 2015; Howard & Davies, 2007; National Institutes of Health & National Heart, Lung, and Blood Institute, Division of Blood Disease and Resources, 2002). Families and older children, especially adolescents, need to be reassured that opioids are medically indicated, high doses may be needed, and children rarely become addicted.

pain and compliance with treatment prescriptions. To reduce the negative connotation associated with the term *crisis,* it is best to say *pain episode.*

If blood transfusions or exchange transfusions are given, the nurse has the responsibility of observing for signs of transfusion reaction (see Table 43.3 later in this chapter). Because hypervolemia from too-rapid transfusion can increase the workload of the heart, the nurse also must be alert to signs of cardiac failure.

In splenic sequestration, gently measure the size of the spleen, because increasing splenomegaly is an ominous sign (see the "Abdomen" section in Chapter 29). A decrease in spleen size denotes response to therapy. The nurse also closely monitors vital signs and blood pressure to detect impending shock. Anemia is typically not a presenting complication in VOC but is a critical problem in other types of crises. The nurse monitors for evidence of increasing anemia and institutes appropriate nursing interventions (see earlier in this chapter). Oxygen is not beneficial in vaso-occlusive episodes unless hypoxemia is present (Heeney & Dover, 2009). It does not reverse sickled RBCs, and if used in a nonhypoxic patient, it will decrease erythropoiesis (Vichinsky & Styles, 1996). Because prolonged use of oxygen can aggravate the anemia, report any signs of lack of therapeutic benefit, such as restlessness, increased pallor, and continued pain.

Record intake, especially of IV fluids, and output. The child's weight should be taken on admission, because it serves as a baseline for evaluating hydration. Because diuresis can result in electrolyte loss, the nurse observes for signs of hypokalemia and should be familiar with normal serum electrolyte values to report changes.

Recognize Other Complications

Nurses also need to be aware of the signs of ACS and CVA, which are both potentially fatal complications.

! NURSING ALERT

Report signs of the following immediately:

Acute chest syndrome (ACS)
- Severe chest, back, or abdominal pain
- Fever of 38.5° C (101.3° F) or higher
- Cough
- Dyspnea, tachypnea
- Retractions
- Declining oxygen saturation (oximetry)

Cerebrovascular accident (CVA):
- Severe, unrelieved headaches
- Severe vomiting
- Jerking or twitching of the face, legs, or arms
- Seizures
- Strange, abnormal behavior
- Inability to move an arm or leg
- Stagger or an unsteady walk
- Stutter or slurred speech
- Weakness in the hand, foot, or leg
- Changes in vision

Support the Family

Families need the opportunity to discuss their feelings regarding transmitting a potentially fatal, chronic illness to their child. Because of the widely publicized prognosis for children with SCA, many parents express their fear of the child's death. Three manifestations of SCD that may appear in the first 2 years of life (dactylitis, severe anemia, leukocytosis) can be predictors of disease severity (Miller, Sleeper, Pegelow, et al., 2000). The nurse should care for the family as for any family with a child who has a chronic and life-threatening illness and give consideration to the siblings' reactions, the stress on the marital relationship, and the childrearing attitudes displayed toward the child. Several resources are available to families with a sickling disorder.*

The nurse advises parents to inform all treating personnel of the child's condition. The use of medical identification, such as a bracelet, is another way of ensuring awareness of the disease.

If family members have the SCD trait or SCA, genetic counseling is necessary. A primary consideration in genetic counseling is informing parents of the 25% chance with each pregnancy of having a child with the disease when both parents carry the trait.

BETA-THALASSEMIA (COOLEY ANEMIA)

Worldwide, thalassemia is a common genetic disorder, affecting as many as 15 million people (Yaish, 2015). The term *thalassemia,* which is derived from the Greek word *thalassa,* meaning "sea," is applied to a variety of inherited blood disorders characterized by deficiencies in the rate of production of specific globin chains in Hgb. The name appropriately refers to people living near the Mediterranean Sea, namely Italians, Greeks, Syrians, Asians, Africans, and their descendants. Evidence suggests that the high incidence of the disorders among these groups is a result of the selective advantage of the trait in protecting against malaria, as is postulated in SCD. The disorder has a wide geographic distribution, probably as a result of genetic migration through intermarriage or possibly as a result of spontaneous mutation.

Beta-thalassemia is the most common of the thalassemias and occurs in four forms:
- Two heterozygous forms, *thalassemia minor,* an asymptomatic silent carrier, and *thalassemia trait,* which produces a mild microcytic anemia
- *Thalassemia intermedia,* which may involve either homozygous or heterozygous abnormalities and is manifested as splenomegaly and moderate to severe anemia
- A homozygous form, *thalassemia major* (also known as *Cooley anemia*), which results in a severe anemia that would lead to cardiac failure and death in early childhood without transfusion support

*Sickle Cell Disease Association of America, Inc., 231 E. Baltimore Street, Suite 800, Baltimore, MD 21202; 410-528-1555, 800-421-8453; email: scdaa@sicklecelldisease.org; www.sicklecelldisease.org; www.facebook.com/sicklecellcampaign; Sickle Cell Information Center, PO Box 109, Grady Memorial Hospital, 80 Jesse Hill Jr Drive SE, Atlanta, GA 30303; 404-616-3572; email: aplatt@emory.edu; www.scinfo.org; National Heart, Lung, and Blood Institute Health Information Center, PO Box 30105, Bethesda, MD 20824-0105; 301-592-8573; http://www.nhlbi.nih.gov; http://www.ahcpr.gov. Guideline for the management of acute and chronic pain in sickle-cell disease is available from the American Pain Society, 4700 W. Lake Avenue, Glenview, IL 60025-1485; 847-375-4715; email: info@ampainsoc.org; www.americanpainsociety.org; www.facebook.com/americanpainsociety.

Pathophysiology

Normal postnatal Hgb is composed of two α- and two β-polypeptide chains. In β-thalassemia, there is a partial or complete deficiency in the synthesis of the β-chain of the Hgb molecule. Consequently, there is a compensatory increase in the synthesis of α-chains, and γ-chain production remains activated, resulting in defective Hgb formation. This unbalanced polypeptide unit is very unstable; when it disintegrates, it damages RBCs, causing severe anemia.

To compensate for the hemolytic process, an overabundance of erythrocytes is formed unless the bone marrow is suppressed by transfusion therapy. Excess iron from packed RBC transfusions and from the rapid destruction of defective cells is stored in various organs (*hemosiderosis*).

Diagnostic Evaluation

The onset of clinical manifestations in thalassemia major may be insidious and not recognized until late infancy or early toddlerhood. The clinical effects of thalassemia major are primarily attributable to defective synthesis of HbA, structurally impaired RBCs, and shortened life span of erythrocytes (Box 43.3).

Hematologic studies reveal the characteristic changes in RBCs (e.g., microcytosis, hypochromia, anisocytosis, poikilocytosis, target cells, and basophilic stippling of various stages). Low Hgb and Hct levels are seen in severe anemia, although they are typically lower than the reduction in RBC count because of the proliferation of immature erythrocytes. Hgb electrophoresis confirms the diagnosis and is helpful in distinguishing the type of thalassemia because it analyzes the quantity and kind of hemoglobin variants found in the blood.

Therapeutic Management

The objectives of supportive therapy are to maintain sufficient Hgb levels to prevent bone marrow expansion and bony deformities and to provide sufficient RBCs to support normal growth and normal physical activity. Transfusions are the foundation of medical management with the goal of maintaining the Hgb level above 9.5 g/dL, an aim that may require transfusions as often as every 3 to 5 weeks. The advantages of this therapy include (1) improved physical and psychologic well-being because of the ability to participate in normal activities, (2) decreased cardiomegaly and hepatosplenomegaly, (3) fewer bone changes, (4) normal or near-normal growth and development until puberty, and (5) fewer infections.

One of the potential complications of frequent blood transfusions is iron overload (hemosiderosis). Because the body has no effective means of eliminating the excess iron, the mineral is deposited in body tissues. To minimize the development of hemosiderosis, oral iron chelators (deferasirox, deferiprone) have shown in short-term studies to be a safe equivalent to deferoxamine (Desferal), a parenteral iron-chelating agent, and more tolerable by patients and families (Bakai & Pennell, 2014; Cappellini, Porter, El-Beshlawy, et al., 2010; Meerpohl, Schell, Rucker, et al., 2014; Vichinsky, Bernaudin, Forni, et al., 2011).

In some children with severe splenomegaly who require repeated transfusions, a splenectomy may be necessary to decrease the disabling effects of abdominal pressure and to increase the life span of supplemental RBCs. Over time, the spleen may accelerate the rate of RBC destruction and thus increase transfusion requirements. After a splenectomy, children generally require fewer transfusions, although the basic defect in Hgb synthesis remains unaffected. A major postsplenectomy complication is severe and overwhelming infection. Therefore, these children are often on prophylactic antibiotics with close medical supervision for many years and should receive the pneumococcal and meningococcal vaccines in addition to the regularly scheduled immunizations (see the "Immunizations" section in Chapter 31).

> ### ! NURSING ALERT
>
> Ensure that the family and patient understand the need to notify the health professional of all fevers of 38.5° C (101.3° F) or greater because of the risk for sepsis in a child with asplenia.

Prognosis

Most children treated with blood transfusion and early chelation therapy survive well into adulthood. The most common causes of death are heart disease, postsplenectomy sepsis, and multiple-organ failure secondary to hemochromatosis (Cunningham, Sankaran, Nathan, et al., 2009; Yaish, 2015). A curative treatment for some children is HSCT. Children younger than 16 years of age who undergo allogeneic HSCT have a high rate of complication-free survival; approximately 80% to 97% of these children are cured (Isgro, Gaziev, Sodani, et al., 2010; Lucarelli, Isgro, Sodani, et al., 2012).

Care Management

The objectives of nursing care are to (1) promote compliance with transfusion and chelation therapy, (2) assist the child in coping with the anxiety-provoking treatments and the effects of the illness, (3) foster the child's and family's adjustment to a chronic illness, and (4) observe for complications of multiple blood transfusions. Basic to each of these goals is explaining to parents and older children the defect responsible for the disorder, its effect on RBCs, and the potential effects of untreated iron overload (e.g., delayed growth and maturation, heart disease). Because this condition is prevalent among families of Mediterranean descent, the nurse also inquires about the family's previous knowledge about thalassemia. All families with a child with thalassemia should be tested for the trait and referred for genetic counseling.

As with any chronic illness, the family's needs must be met for optimal adjustment to the stresses imposed by the disorder (see Chapter 36). Sources of information for the family include the Cooley's Anemia Foundation* and the Northern California Comprehensive Thalassemia

---

*330 Seventh Avenue, No. 200, New York, NY 10001; 800-522-7222; http://www.thalassemia.org; www.facebook.com/pages/Thalassemia-org/162500870481012.

BOX 43.3 Clinical Manifestations of Beta-Thalassemia

Anemia (Before Diagnosis)
Pallor
Unexplained fever
Poor feeding
Enlarged spleen or liver

Progressive Anemia
Signs of chronic hypoxia
  Headache
  Precordial and bone pain
  Decreased exercise tolerance
  Listlessness
  Anorexia

Other Features
Small stature
Delayed sexual maturation
Bronzed, freckled complexion (if not receiving chelation therapy)

Bone Changes (Older Children if Untreated)
Enlarged head
Prominent frontal and parietal bossing
Prominent malar eminences
Flat or depressed bridge of the nose
Enlarged maxilla
Protrusion of the lip and upper central incisors and eventual malocclusion
Generalized osteoporosis

Center. Genetic counseling for the parents and fertile offspring is mandatory, and both prenatal diagnosis using amniocentesis or fetal blood sampling and screening for thalassemia trait are available.

APLASTIC ANEMIA

Aplastic anemia (AA) is a rare and life-threatening disorder that can be satisfactorily treated in about 90% of cases (Miano & Dufour, 2015). It refers to a bone marrow failure condition in which the formed elements of the blood are simultaneously depressed. To diagnose AA, the peripheral blood smear demonstrates pancytopenia with at least two of the following present: profound anemia, leukopenia, and thrombocytopenia, whereas hypoplastic anemia is characterized by a profound depression of RBCs but normal or slightly decreased WBCs and platelets.

Etiology

AA can be primary (congenital, or present at birth) or secondary (acquired). The best-known congenital disorder of which AA is an outstanding feature is *Fanconi syndrome,* a rare hereditary disorder characterized by pancytopenia, hypoplasia of the bone marrow, and patchy brown discoloration of the skin resulting from the deposit of melanin. It is associated with multiple congenital anomalies of the musculoskeletal and genitourinary systems. The syndrome appears to be inherited as an autosomal recessive trait with varying penetrance; therefore, affected siblings may demonstrate several different combinations of defects.

Several etiologic factors contribute to the development of acquired AA; however, most of the cases are considered idiopathic (Box 43.4). The following discussion focuses on severe acquired AA, which carries a poorer prognosis and follows a more rapidly fatal course than the primary types.

Diagnostic Evaluation

The onset of clinical manifestations, which include anemia, leukopenia, and decreased platelet count, is usually insidious. Definitive diagnosis is determined from bone marrow examination, which demonstrates the conversion of red bone marrow to yellow, fatty bone marrow. Severe AA is based on Camitta's criteria that include less than 25% bone marrow cellularity with at least two of the following findings: absolute granulocyte count less than 500/mm^3, platelet count less than 20,000/mm^3, and absolute reticulocyte count less than 40,000/mm^3 (Miano & Dufour, 2015; Passweg & Marsh, 2010). Moderate AA is defined as more than 25% bone marrow cellularity with the presence of mild or moderate cytopenia (Miano & Dufour, 2015; Shimamura & Guinan, 2009).

Therapeutic Management

The objectives of treatment established by the interprofessional care team are based on the recognition that the underlying disease process

---

BOX 43.4 Common Causes of Acquired Aplastic Anemia

- Human parvovirus infection, hepatitis, or overwhelming infection
- Irradiation
- Immune disorders, such as eosinophilic fasciitis and hypoimmunoglobulinemia
- Drugs, such as certain chemotherapeutic agents, anticonvulsants, and antibiotics
- Industrial and household chemicals, including benzene and its derivatives, which are found in petroleum products, dyes, paint remover, shellac, and lacquers
- Infiltration and replacement of myeloid elements, such as in leukemia or the lymphomas
- Idiopathic (In most cases, no identifiable precipitating cause can be found.)

---

is failure of the bone marrow to carry out its hematopoietic functions. Therefore, therapy is directed at restoring function to the marrow and involves two main approaches: (1) immunosuppressive therapy (IST) to remove the presumed immunologic functions that prolong aplasia or (2) replacement of the bone marrow through transplantation. Bone marrow transplantation is the treatment of choice for severe AA when a suitable donor exists (see later in this chapter).

Antilymphocyte globulin (ALG) or *antithymocyte globulin (ATG)* is the principal drug treatment used for AA. The rationale for using ATG is based on the theory that AA may be a result of autoimmunity. IST is a combination of ATG and cyclosporine that suppress T cell–dependent autoimmune responses by recognizing human lymphocyte cell surface antigen and decreasing the lymphocytes without causing bone marrow suppression (Peinemann & Labeit, 2014). Cyclosporine is administered orally for several weeks to months. ATG usually is administered intravenously over 12 to 16 hours for 4 days after a test dose to check for hypersensitivity. Response to IST is typically delayed, and responses generally do not start before 3 to 4 months (Samarasinghe & Webb, 2012). An IST course may be repeated, depending on the reduction in circulating lymphocytes and the patient's response. Because of the hypersensitivity response associated with ATG (i.e., fever, chills, myalgias), methylprednisolone is given intravenously to prevent these side effects. Growth factors, given parenterally, may be used to prevent neutropenic infection and enhance bone marrow production (Passweg & Marsh, 2010). Androgens may be used with ATG to stimulate erythropoiesis if the AA is unresponsive to initial therapies.

HSCT should be considered early in the course of the disease if a compatible donor can be found. Transplantation is more successful when performed before multiple transfusions have sensitized the child to leukocyte and *human leukocyte antigens* (HLAs). HSCT is associated with an approximately 90% survival rate in patients who receive a bone marrow transplant from an HLA-identical sibling (Hord, 2011; Scheinberg, 2012).

Care Management

The care of the child with AA is similar to that of the child with leukemia (see Chapter 44) and includes preparing the child and family for the diagnostic and therapeutic procedures, preventing complications from the severe pancytopenia, and emotionally supporting them in the face of a potentially fatal outcome. Information and support are available from the Aplastic Anemia and MDS International Foundation, Inc.*

The aspects of nursing care are discussed in the "Leukemias" section in Chapter 44, therefore only interventions specific to AA are presented here. The drug ATG is usually administered by way of a central vein. If not, vigilant care must be directed to the IV infusion to prevent extravasation. Meticulous care of the venous access is essential because of the child's susceptibility to infection. Chemotherapeutic agents have been used in the treatment of relapsed patients with AA after unresponsive IST. Many of the side effects associated with chemotherapy such as nausea and vomiting, alopecia, and mucositis are experienced by children receiving treatment for AA. Specialized care is required for AA children who have HSCT; this is discussed in Chapter 44.

DEFECTS IN HEMOSTASIS

Hemostasis is the process that stops bleeding when a blood vessel is injured. Vascular and plasma clotting factors, as well as platelets, are required. A complex system of clotting, anticlotting, and clot breakdown

---

*100 Park Avenue, Suite 108, Rockville, MD 20850; 800-747-2820, 301-279-7202; email: help@aamds.org; http://www.aamds.org; www.facebook.com/aamds.

(fibrinolysis) mechanisms exists in equilibrium to ensure clot formation only in the presence of blood vessel injury and to limit the clotting process to the site of vessel wall injury. Dysfunction in these systems leads to bleeding or abnormal clotting. Although the coagulation process is complex, clotting depends on three factors: (1) vascular influence, (2) platelet role, and (3) clotting factors.

HEMOPHILIA

The term *hemophilia* refers to a group of bleeding disorders resulting from congenital deficiency, dysfunction, or absence of specific coagulation proteins or factors (Montgomery, Gill, & DiPaola, 2009; Sharathkumar and Pipe, 2008). Although the symptomatology is similar regardless of which clotting factor is deficient, the identification of specific factor deficiencies allows definitive treatment with replacement agents.

In about 80% of all cases of hemophilia, the inheritance pattern is demonstrated as X-linked recessive. The two most common forms of the disorder are *factor VIII deficiency* (hemophilia A, or classic hemophilia) and *factor IX deficiency* (hemophilia B, or Christmas disease), with a prevalence of approximately 1 in 5000 and 1 in 20,000 to 30,000 live births, respectively (McLean, Fiebelkorn, Temte, et al., 2013; Sharathkumar & Carcao, 2011; Zimmerman & Valentino, 2013). *Von Willebrand disease* (vWD) is another hereditary bleeding disorder characterized by a deficiency, abnormality, or absence of the protein called *von Willebrand factor (vWF)*. The following discussion is primarily concerned with factor VIII deficiency, which accounts for 80% of all hemophilia cases.

Pathophysiology

The basic defect of hemophilia A is a deficiency of factor VIII (antihemophilic factor [AHF]). Factor VIII is produced by the liver and is necessary for the formation of thromboplastin in phase I of blood coagulation (Fig. 43.4). The less factor VIII that is found in the blood, the more severe the disease. Individuals with hemophilia have two of the three factors required for coagulation: vascular influence and platelets. Therefore, they may bleed for longer periods but not at a faster rate.

Subcutaneous and IM hemorrhages are common. Hemarthrosis, which refers to bleeding into joint cavities, especially the knees, elbows, and ankles, is the most frequent form of internal bleeding. Bony changes and crippling deformities occur after repeated bleeding episodes over several years. Early signs of hemarthrosis are a feeling of stiffness, tingling or achiness in the affected joint, followed by decrease in joint movement. Obvious affected joint signs and symptoms are increased warmth, redness, and swelling and severe pain with loss of movement. Bleeding in the neck, mouth, or thorax is serious because the airway can become obstructed. Intracranial hemorrhage can have fatal consequences and is one of the major causes of death. Hemorrhage anywhere along the GI tract can lead to anemia, and bleeding into the retroperitoneal cavity is especially hazardous because of the large space for blood to accumulate. Hematomas in the spinal cord can cause paralysis.

Diagnostic Evaluation

The diagnosis is usually made from a history of bleeding episodes, evidence of X-linked inheritance (only one-third of the cases are new mutations), and laboratory findings. To understand the significance of various tests of hemostasis, it is helpful to recall the usual mechanism to control bleeding (e.g., the function of platelets and clotting factors). The test specific for hemophilia plasma includes factor VIII and factor IX assay, procedures normally performed in specialized laboratories. Other tests are those that depend on specific factors for a reaction to occur, especially the partial thromboplastin time (PTT). Carrier detection is possible in classic hemophilia using deoxyribonucleic acid (DNA) testing and is an important consideration in families in which female offspring may have inherited the trait.

Therapeutic Management

The primary therapy for hemophilia is replacement of the missing clotting factor. The products available are factor VIII concentrates, either produced through genetic engineering (recombinant form) or derived from pooled plasma, which are reconstituted with sterile water immediately before use. A synthetic form of vasopressin, 1-deamino-8-d-arginine vasopressin (DDAVP), increases plasma factor VIII activity and is the treatment of choice in mild hemophilia and vWD types I and IIA only if the child shows an appropriate response. After DDAVP administration, a threefold to fourfold rise in factor VIII–level activity

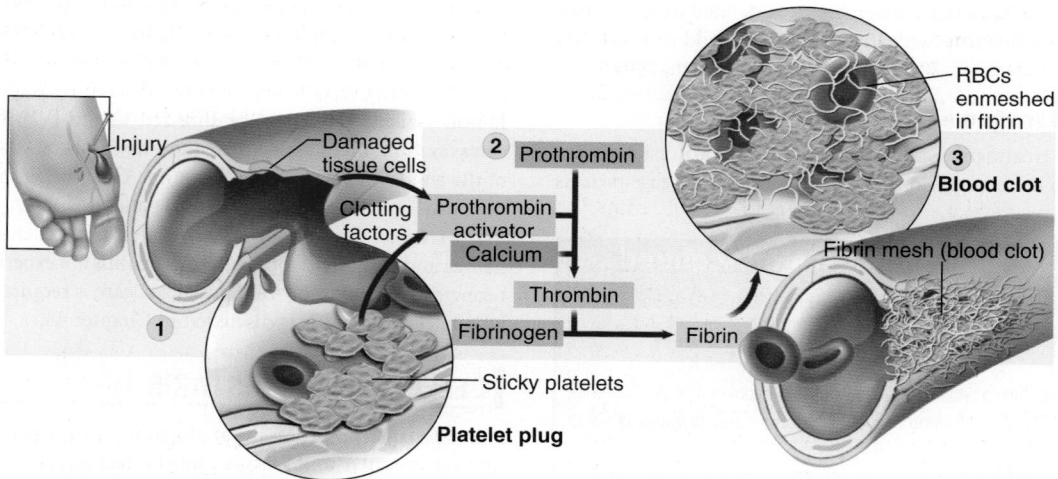

FIG 43.4 Blood clotting. The extremely complex clotting mechanism can be distilled into three basic steps: (1) release of clotting factors from both injured tissue cells and sticky platelets at the injury site (which form a temporary platelet plug); (2) a series of chemical reactions that eventually result in the formation of thrombin; and (3) formation of fibrin and trapping of red blood cells (RBCs) to form a clot. (From Patton, T., & Thibodeau, G.A. [2016]. *Anatomy & physiology* [9th ed.]. St. Louis, MO: Elsevier.)

should occur. It is not effective in the treatment of severe hemophilia A, severe vWD, or any form of hemophilia B. Aggressive factor concentrate replacement therapy is initiated to prevent chronic crippling effects from joint bleeding.

Other drugs may be included in the therapy plan, depending on the source of the hemorrhage. Corticosteroids are given for hematuria, acute hemarthrosis, and chronic synovitis. Nonsteroidal antiinflammatory drugs (NSAIDs), such as ibuprofen, are effective in relieving pain caused by synovitis; however, they are occasionally used with caution because they inhibit platelet function (Curry, 2004; Hermans, De Moerloose, Fischer, et al., 2011). Oral administration of ε-aminocaproic acid (Amicar) prevents clot destruction. Its use is limited to mouth trauma or surgery with a dose of factor concentrate given first.

The interprofessional care team will recommend a regular program of exercise, and physical therapy is an important aspect of management. Physical activity within reasonable limits strengthens muscles around joints and may decrease the number of spontaneous bleeding episodes.

Treatment without delay results in more rapid recovery and a decreased likelihood of complications; therefore, most children are treated at home. The family is taught the technique of venipuncture and to administer the AHF to children older than 2 to 3 years of age. The child learns the procedure for self-administration at 8 to 12 years of age. Home treatment is highly successful, and the rewards, in addition to the immediacy, are less disruption of family life, fewer school or work days missed, and enhancement of the child's self-esteem and independence.

Prophylactic therapy is periodic factor replacement for children with severe hemophilia to prevent bleeding complications, including arthropathy and spontaneous life-threatening bleeding events (Coppola, Tagliaferri, Di Capua, et al., 2012; Montgomery et al., 2009; Scott & Montgomery, 2011; Zimmerman & Valentino, 2013). Primary prophylaxis involves the infusion of factor VIII concentrate on a regular basis before the onset of joint damage. Secondary prophylaxis involves the infusion of factor VIII concentrate on a regular basis after the child experiences his or her first joint bleed. The administration of infusions differs among treatment centers and may range from every other day to three times per week for several weeks to promote healing. On-demand factor replacement may be a cost-effective alternative to primary prophylaxis, but prophylaxis decreases the development of joint disease and preserves joint function compared with on-demand factor replacement treatment (Iorio, Marchesini, Marcucci, et al., 2011; Manco-Johnson, Abshire, Shapiro, et al., 2007). Prompt appropriate treatment of hemorrhage and prophylactic therapy are key to excellent care and prevention of long-term morbidity in patients with hemophilia (Lillicrap, 2013; Montgomery et al., 2009).

Prognosis

Although there is no cure for hemophilia, its symptoms can be controlled and its potentially crippling deformities greatly reduced or even avoided. Today many children with hemophilia function with minimal or no joint damage. They have an average life expectancy and are normal in every respect but one—they have a tendency to bleed, which is a significant inconvenience but not necessarily a life-threatening event.

Gene therapy may prove to be a treatment option in the future. Techniques are under development to introduce factor VIII and factor IX genes into hepatocytes, fibroblasts, and endothelial cells using adeno-associated viral vectors, and other novel ideas for genetic correction (Branchford, Monahan, & Di Paola, 2013; Nienhuis, 2008; Walsh & Batt, 2013). Problems exist with appropriate selection of the vector, identification of the cell for gene expression, and control of side effects (Mátrai, Chuah, & VandenDriessche, 2010; Montgomery et al., 2009; Sharathkumar & Carcao, 2011).

QUALITY PATIENT OUTCOMES Hemophilia
- Early recognition of signs and symptoms of hemophilia
- Bleeding episodes prevented
- Bleeding episodes treated early with factor replacement
- Adherence to prophylactic factor replacement program when indicated
- Hemarthrosis prevented when possible with limited joint damage
- Exercise program and physical therapy ongoing

Care Management

The earlier a bleeding episode is recognized, the more effectively it can be treated. Signs that indicate internal bleeding are especially important to recognize. Children are aware of internal bleeding and are reliable in telling the examiner the location of an internal bleed. In addition to the manifestations described (Box 43.5), the nurse maintains a high level of suspicion when a child with hemophilia shows signs such as headache, slurred speech, loss of consciousness (from cerebral bleeding), and black, tarry stools (from GI bleeding).

Prevent Bleeding

The goal of prevention of bleeding episodes is directed toward decreasing the risk for injury. Prevention of bleeding episodes is geared mostly toward appropriate exercises to strengthen muscles and joints and to allow age-appropriate activity. During infancy and toddlerhood, the normal acquisition of motor skills creates innumerable opportunities for falls, bruises, and minor wounds. Restraining the child from mastering motor development can bring more serious long-term problems than allowing the behavior. However, the environment should be made as safe as possible, with close supervision during playtime to minimize incidental injuries.

For older children, the family usually needs assistance in preparing for school. A nurse who knows the family can be instrumental in discussing the situation with the school nurse and in jointly planning an appropriate activity schedule. Because almost all individuals with hemophilia are boys, the physical limitations in regard to active sports may be a difficult adjustment, and activity restrictions must be tempered with sensitivity to the child's emotional and physical needs. Use of protective equipment, such as helmets, face masks, shin/wrist/forearm guards, kneepads, and other equipment appropriate for the type of athletic activity, is encouraged to prevent injury. Children and adolescents with severe hemophilia may participate in noncontact sports, such as aerobic exercise, stretching exercises, swimming, walking, jogging, tennis, golf, fishing, and bowling (Blaney, Forsyth, Zourikian, et al., 2010). However, the use of prophylaxis to prevent joint hemorrhage or use of exercise during low-impact athletic participation remains unknown (Broderick, Herbert, Latimer, et al., 2012; Michael, Mulder & Strike, 2014; Ross, Goldenberg, Hund, et al., 2009).

BOX 43.5   Clinical Manifestations of Hemophilia

- Prolonged bleeding anywhere from or in the body
- Hemorrhage from any trauma: Loss of deciduous teeth, circumcision, cuts, epistaxis, injections
- Excessive bruising, even from a slight injury, such as a fall
- Subcutaneous and intramuscular (IM) hemorrhages
- Hemarthrosis (bleeding into the joint cavities), especially the knees, ankles, and elbows
- Hematomas: Pain, swelling, and limited motion
- Spontaneous hematuria

To prevent oral bleeding, some readjustment in terms of dental hygiene may be needed to minimize trauma to the gums, such as use of a water irrigating device, softening the toothbrush in warm water before brushing, or using a sponge-tipped disposable toothbrush. A regular toothbrush should be soft-bristled and small.

Because any trauma can lead to a bleeding episode, all people caring for these children must be aware of their disorder. These children should wear a medical alert identification bracelet, and older children should be encouraged to recognize situations in which disclosing their condition is important, such as during dental extraction or injections. Health personnel need to take special precautions to prevent the use of procedures that may cause bleeding, such as IM injections. The subcutaneous route is substituted for IM injections whenever possible. Venipunctures for blood samples are usually preferred for these children. There is usually less bleeding after the venipuncture than after finger or heel punctures. Neither aspirin nor any aspirin-containing compound should be used. Acetaminophen is a suitable aspirin substitute, especially for controlling pain at home.

Recognize and Control Bleeding

As noted, the earlier a bleeding episode is recognized, the more effectively it can be treated. Factor replacement therapy should be instituted according to established medical protocol, and supportive measures may be implemented, such as RICE, which stands for *rest*, *ice*, *compression*, and *elevation*. When parents and older children are taught such measures beforehand, they can be prepared to initiate immediate treatment. Plastic bags of ice or cold packs should be kept in the freezer for such emergencies. However, such measures do not take the place of factor replacement.

Prevent Crippling Effects of Bleeding

As a result of repeated episodes of hemarthrosis, incompletely absorbed blood in the joints, and limitation of motion, bone and muscle changes occur that result in flexion contractures and joint fixation. During bleeding episodes, the joint is elevated and immobilized. Active range-of-motion exercises are usually instituted after the acute phase. This allows the child to control the degree of exercise according to the level of discomfort. If an exercise program is instituted in the home, a physical therapist or public health nurse may need to supervise compliance with the regimen. Rarely, orthopedic intervention (e.g., casting, application of traction, or aspiration of blood) may be necessary to preserve joint function. Diet is also an important consideration because excessive body weight can increase the strain on affected joints, especially the knees, and predispose the child to hemarthrosis. Consequently, calories need to be supplied in accordance with energy requirements.

Support the Family and Prepare for Home Care

Genetic counseling is essential, and the interprofessional care team recommends this to occur as soon as possible after diagnosis. Unlike many other disorders in which both parents carry the trait, the feeling of responsibility for this condition usually rests with the mother. Unless she has an opportunity to discuss her feelings, the couple's relationship can suffer. Technology is now available to identify classic hemophilia carriers using DNA testing and may reduce the anxiety regarding childbearing in women who may be at risk for carrying the defective gene. Factor concentrates have greatly changed the outlook for these children by minimizing bleeding and allowing the child to live a normal, unrestricted life. Children are taught to take responsibility for their disease at an early age. They learn their limitations, preventive measures, and self-administration of the prophylactic AHF.

The needs of families who have children with hemophilia are best met through a comprehensive team approach of physicians (pediatrician,

hematologist, orthopedist), nurse practitioner, nurse, social worker, and physical and psychologic therapist. Parent-group discussions are beneficial in meeting the needs that are often best met by similarly affected families. For example, with the improved prognosis for these children, parents and adolescents with hemophilia face vocational and financial problems in addition to concern over future childbearing. This can be disastrous in terms of the cost of treatment, which can exceed $100,000 per year. Financial support is particularly important. The National Hemophilia Foundation* and the Canadian Hemophilia Society† provide numerous services and publications for both health care providers and families.

Children who have become infected with human immunodeficiency virus (HIV) through transfusions and factor replacement products are faced with the consequences of this dreaded disease. Consequently, they need the support of health care professionals, especially in the areas of safe sexual practices to avoid disease transmission and public education regarding acquired immune deficiency syndrome (AIDS) and ways to deal with public reactions to people who have AIDS.

IMMUNE THROMBOCYTOPENIA (IDIOPATHIC THROMBOCYTOPENIC PURPURA)

Idiopathic thrombocytopenic purpura (ITP), the formerly used term because purpura is an infrequent sign at presentation, is now referred to as *immune thrombocytopenia* (Rodeghiero, Stasi, Gernsheimer, et al., 2009). ITP is an acquired hemorrhagic disorder characterized by (1) thrombocytopenia, (2) absence or minimal signs of bleeding (easy bruising, mucosal bleeding, petechiae) in most childhood cases, and (3) normal bone marrow with a normal or increased number of immature platelets (megakaryocytes) and eosinophils. Although all causes of ITP are not known, it is understood that ITP involves the evolution of antibodies against multiple platelet antigens, leading to reduced platelet survival and impaired platelet production (Consolini, 2011; McCrae, 2011). ITP is the most common thrombocytopenia of childhood, with the majority of cases in children younger than 10 years of age and a peak incidence between 1 and 5 years of age (Consolini, 2011; McCrae, 2011; Montgomery & Scott, 2011).

The disease occurs in one of two forms: (1) an acute, self-limiting course or (2) a chronic condition (>12 months' duration). The acute form occurs most commonly after upper respiratory tract infections; after the childhood diseases measles, rubella, mumps, and chickenpox; or after infection with human parvovirus.

Diagnostic Evaluation

The diagnosis is suspected on the basis of clinical manifestations (Box 43.6). In ITP, the platelet count is reduced to less than 20,000/mm³; therefore, tests that depend on platelet function, such as the tourniquet test, bleeding time, and clot retraction, are abnormal. There is no definitive test that establishes a diagnosis of ITP; several tests are usually performed to rule out other disorders in which thrombocytopenia is a manifestation, such as systemic lupus erythematosus, lymphoma, or leukemia.

Therapeutic Management

Interprofessional care management of ITP is primarily supportive, because the disease is self-limiting in the majority of cases. Activity is

---

*116 W. 32nd Street, 11th Floor, New York, NY 10001; 800-42-HANDI, 212-328-3700; email: handi@hemophilia.org; https://www.hemophilia.org; www.facebook.com/NationalHemophiliaFoundation.
†400-1255 University Street, Montreal, Quebec, Canada H3B 3B6; 800-668-2686, 514-848-0503; email: chs@hemophilia.ca; www.hemophilia.ca.

BOX 43.6   Clinical Manifestations of Immune Thrombocytopenia (Idiopathic Thrombocytopenic Purpura)

Easy Bruising
- Petechiae
- Ecchymoses
- Most often over bony prominences

Bleeding From Mucous Membranes
- Epistaxis
- Bleeding gums
- Internal hemorrhage evidenced by the following:
  - Hematuria
  - Hematemesis
  - Melena
  - Hemarthrosis
  - Menorrhagia
  - Hematomas over lower extremities

BOX 43.7   Criteria for Anti-D Antibody Therapy

- Age between 1 and 19 years of age; Rh(D)-positive blood type
- Normal WBC count and hemoglobin level for age; platelet count of 20,000/mm^3
- No active mucosal bleeding
- No history of reaction to plasma products
- No known immunoglobulin A deficiency
- No concurrent infection
- Absence of Evans syndrome (characterized by the combination of ITP and autoimmune hemolytic anemia)
- No suspicion of lupus erythematosus or other collagen vascular disorder
- No splenectomy

ITP, Idiopathic thrombocytopenic purpura; *WBC,* white blood cell.

restricted at the onset while the platelet count is low and while active bleeding or progression of lesions is occurring. Treatment for acute presentation is symptomatic and has included prednisone, intravenous immunoglobulin (IVIG), and anti-D antibody. These are not curative therapies. *Anti-D antibody* is a plasma-derived immunoglobulin that causes a transient hemolytic anemia in Rh (D)-positive patients with ITP. With the clearance of antibody-coated RBCs, there is prolonged survival of platelets resulting from the blockade of the Fc receptors of the reticuloendothelial cells. The platelet count usually increases approximately 48 hours after an infusion of anti-D antibody; therefore, it is not appropriate therapy for patients who are actively bleeding. The benefits of choosing anti-D antibody IV therapy over prednisone or IVIG are that anti-D antibody can be given in one dose over 5 to 10 minutes and is significantly less expensive than IVIG. Historically, patients who are treated with prednisone may first undergo a bone marrow examination to rule out leukemia, which is controversial because leukemia rarely manifests with low platelet count alone (Montgomery & Scott, 2011; Wilson, 2009). Therefore, the use of anti-D antibody and IVIG alleviates the need for a bone marrow examination. Before receiving the initial dose of anti-D antibody, patients must meet certain criteria (Box 43.7). Premedication with acetaminophen 5 to 10 minutes before the infusion is recommended.

! NURSING ALERT

After administration of anti-D antibody, observe the child for a minimum of 1 hour and maintain a patent IV line. Obtain baseline vital signs measurements before the infusion and again 5, 20, and 60 minutes after beginning the infusion. If fever, chills, and headache occur during or shortly after the infusion, the nurse should administer acetaminophen, diphenhydramine (Benadryl), and/or hydrocortisone (Solu-Cortef) as ordered and observe the patient for an additional hour after the reaction.

Splenectomy is for patients who have chronic ITP that is not responsive to pharmacologic management and have increased risk for severe hemorrhage. It is an option associated with long-term remission for these children and reduces the risk for hemorrhage (McCrae, 2011; Montgomery & Scott, 2011; Wilson, 2009). Before splenectomy is considered, it is recommended to wait until the child is older than 5 years of age because of the increased risk for bacterial infection. Administration of pneumococcal, meningococcal, and *H. influenzae* vaccines are recommended before splenectomy (see the "Immunizations" section in Chapter 31). The child also receives penicillin prophylaxis after splenectomy. The length of prophylactic therapy is controversial, but in general, a minimum of 3 years of therapy is recommended.

Prognosis

The majority of children have a self-limited course without major complications. Some children may develop chronic ITP and require ongoing therapy. A splenectomy may modify the disease process, and the child may be asymptomatic.

QUALITY PATIENT OUTCOMES: Idiopathic Thrombocytopenic Purpura

- Serious bleeding episode prevented
- Activities that increase risk for serious bleeding avoided
- Treatment administered without serious side effects

Care Management

Nursing care is largely supportive and should include teaching regarding possible side effects of therapy and limitation in activities while the child's platelet count is less than 50,000/mm^3 (Consolini, 2011). Children with ITP should not participate in *any* contact sports, bike riding, skateboarding, in-line skating, gymnastics, climbing, or running. Parents are encouraged to engage their children in quiet activities and to prevent any injuries, especially to the child's head. Instruct the parents to obtain prompt medical evaluation if the child sustains head or abdominal trauma. As in any condition with an uncertain outcome, the family needs emotional support.

DISSEMINATED INTRAVASCULAR COAGULATION

Disseminated intravascular coagulation (DIC), also known as *consumption coagulopathy,* is characterized by diffuse fibrin deposition in the microvasculature, consumption of coagulation factors, and endogenous generation of thrombin and plasmin. DIC is a secondary disorder of coagulation that occurs as a complication of a number of pathologic processes, such as hypoxia, acidosis, shock, endothelial damage (e.g., burns), and many severe systemic diseases (e.g., congenital heart disease, necrotizing enterocolitis, gram-negative bacterial sepsis, rickettsial infections, and some severe viral infections). The hallmarks of this disorder are bleeding and clotting that occurs simultaneously.

BOX 43.8   Clinical Manifestations of Disseminated Intravascular Coagulation

Petechiae
Purpura
Bleeding from openings in the skin
- Venipuncture site
- Surgical incision

Bleeding from umbilicus, trachea (newborn)
Evidence of gastrointestinal (GI) bleeding
Hypotension
Organ dysfunction from infarction and ischemia

✚ EMERGENCY TREATMENT
Epistaxis

- Have child sit up and lean forward (not lie down).
- Apply continuous pressure to nose with thumb and forefinger for at least 10 minutes.
- Insert cotton or wadded tissue into each nostril, and apply ice or cold cloth to bridge of nose if bleeding persists.
- Keep child calm and quiet.

Pathophysiology

DIC occurs when the first stage of the coagulation process is abnormally stimulated. Although no well-defined sequence of events occurs, two distinct phases can be identified. First, when the clotting mechanism is triggered in the circulation, thrombin is generated in greater amounts than can be neutralized by the body. Consequently, there is rapid conversion of fibrinogen to fibrin, with aggregation and destruction of platelets. Local and widespread fibrin deposition occurs in blood vessels that causes obstruction of blood flow with eventual necrosis of tissues. Concurrently, the fibrinolytic mechanism is activated, which causes extensive destruction of clotting factors. With a deficiency of clotting factors, the child is vulnerable to uncontrollable hemorrhage into vital organs. An additional complication is damage and hemolysis of RBCs.

Diagnostic Evaluation

DIC is suspected when the patient has an increased tendency to bleed (Box 43.8). Hematologic findings include prolonged prothrombin time, PTT, thrombin time, and increased D-dimer antigen (byproduct of fibrinolytic process). There is a profoundly depressed platelet count, fragmented RBCs, and depleted fibrinogen.

Therapeutic Management

Treatment of DIC is directed toward control of the underlying or initiating cause, which in most instances stops the coagulation problem spontaneously. Platelets and fresh-frozen plasma may be needed to replace lost plasma components, especially in children whose underlying disease remains uncontrolled. Extremely ill newborn infants may require exchange transfusion with fresh blood. The administration of IV heparin to inhibit thrombin formation is most often restricted to patients who have no response to treatment of the underlying disease or replacement of coagulation factors and platelets.

Care Management

The goals of nursing care are to be aware of the possibility of DIC in severely ill children and to recognize signs that might indicate its presence. The skills needed to monitor IV infusion and blood transfusions and to administer heparin are the same as for any child receiving these therapies.

EPISTAXIS (NOSE BLEEDING)

Isolated and transient episodes of epistaxis, or nose bleeding, are common in childhood. The nose, especially the septum, is a highly vascular structure, and bleeding usually results from direct trauma, including blows to the nose, foreign bodies, and nose picking, or from mucosal inflammation associated with allergic rhinitis and upper respiratory tract infections. The bleeding usually stops with minimal pressure and requires no medical evaluation or therapy.

Recurrent epistaxis and severe bleeding may indicate an underlying disease, particularly vascular abnormalities, leukemia, thrombocytopenia, and clotting factor deficiency diseases (e.g., hemophilia, vWD). Nosebleeds are sometimes associated with administration of aspirin, even in normal amounts. Persistent episodes of epistaxis require medical evaluation.

Care Management

In the event of a nosebleed, an essential intervention is to remain calm. Otherwise, the child will become more agitated, the blood pressure will increase, and the child will not cooperate. Although in most instances a nosebleed is not serious, it can be upsetting to family members as well. They need reassurance that the loss of blood is not serious and that the bleeding usually stops in less than 10 minutes with nasal pressure.

To control the bleeding, the child is instructed to sit up and lean forward (not to lie down or hold head backwards) to avoid aspiration of blood. Most of the nose bleeding originates in the anterior part of the nasal septum and can be controlled by applying pressure to the soft lower portion of the nose with the thumb and forefinger (see the Emergency Treatment box: Epistaxis). During this time, the child breathes through the mouth.

In the event that hemorrhage continues, the child should be evaluated by a practitioner who may pack the nose with epinephrine-soaked gauze. After a nosebleed, a water-soluble jelly can be inserted into each nostril to prevent crusting of old blood and to lessen the likelihood of the child's picking at the nose and restarting the hemorrhage. If a child has numerous nosebleeds, factors believed to increase the likelihood of bleeds are eliminated, such as discouraging nose picking or altering the household humidity by placing a cool-mist humidifier in the child's room. Repeated bleeding episodes lasting longer than 30 minutes may be an indication to refer the child for evaluation for the possibility of a bleeding disorder.

▌IMMUNOLOGIC DEFICIENCY DISORDERS

A number of disorders can cause profound, often life-threatening alterations within the body's immune system. The most serious are those conditions that completely depress immunity, such as severe combined immunodeficiency disease (SCID). However, the one disorder that generates the most anxiety, within both the family and the community at large, is HIV infection and the subsequent development of AIDS.

Several classifications of immune dysfunction exist. AIDS, SCID, and Wiskott-Aldrich syndrome (WAS) are syndromes wherein the body is unable to mount an immune response. The immune response can also be misdirected. In autoimmune disorders, antibodies, macrophages, and lymphocytes attack healthy cells.

HUMAN IMMUNODEFICIENCY VIRUS INFECTION AND ACQUIRED IMMUNE DEFICIENCY SYNDROME

HIV infection and AIDS have generated intense medical investigation and constitute one of world's most serious medical, public health, and social challenges of our time (Ezekowitz, 2009; Joint United Nations Programme on HIV/AIDS [UNAIDS], 2013). Research has led to early diagnosis and improved medical treatments for HIV infection, changing this disease from a rapidly fatal one to a chronic disease.

Epidemiology

The first AIDS cases in the pediatric population in the United States were identified in children born to HIV-infected mothers and in children who received blood products. More than 90% of these children acquired the disease perinatally from their mothers. Smaller numbers of children were infected through the transfusion of contaminated blood or blood products before establishment of screening blood products routinely for HIV. Currently, the principal modes of HIV transmission to the pediatric population are mother-to-child transmission and adolescent risky behaviors, such as sexual activity and IV drug use (Siberry, 2014; Simpkins, Siberry, & Hutton, 2009; Joint United Nations Programme on HIV/AIDS [UNAIDS], 2013).

The estimated number of children with perinatally acquired AIDS peaked in 1992; subsequent years have seen significant declines. This trend is a result of implementation of recommended HIV counseling and voluntary testing practices and the use of highly active antiretroviral therapy (HAART) to prevent perinatal transmission. HAART (combination of two nucleoside analog reverse transcriptase inhibitors and a non-nucleoside reverse transcriptase inhibitor protease inhibitor or integrase inhibitor), is the current standard in the United States for the treatment of HIV-infected pregnant women, and it has significantly reduced the transmission of HIV (Hayden, 2013; Siberry, 2014; Siegfried, van der Merwe, Brocklehurst, et al., 2011; Simpkins et al., 2009). Routine HIV counseling and voluntary testing using the opt-in (must agree) or opt-out approach (right of refusal) is the recommended standard of care for pregnant women in the United States (Centers for Disease Control and Prevention, 2006; 2014b; American Academy of Pediatrics Committee on Pediatric AIDS, 2008; Siberry, 2014; Simpkins et al., 2009).

Etiology

HIV is a retrovirus that is transmitted by lymphocytes and monocytes. It is found in blood, semen, vaginal secretions, and breast milk. It has an incubation or latency period of months to years (Yogev & Chadwick, 2011). There are different strains of HIV. Whereas HIV-2 is prevalent in Africa, HIV-1 is the dominant strain in the United States and elsewhere. Horizontal transmission of HIV occurs through intimate sexual contact or parenteral exposure to blood or body fluids containing visible blood. Perinatal (vertical) transmission occurs when an HIV-infected pregnant woman passes the infection to her infant. There is no evidence that *casual* contact between infected and uninfected individuals can spread the virus.

Pathophysiology

The HIV virus primarily infects a specific subset of T lymphocytes, the CD_4^+ T cells, but it can also invade cells of the monocyte-macrophage lineage. The virus takes over the machinery of the CD_4^+ lymphocyte, using it to replicate itself, rendering the CD_4^+ cell dysfunctional. The $CD4^+$ lymphocyte count gradually decreases over time, and physical symptoms appear at some point. The count eventually reaches a critical level below which there is substantial risk for opportunistic illnesses, followed by death.

Clinical Manifestations

Common clinical manifestations of HIV infection in children are varied (Box 43.9). The diagnosis of AIDS is associated with certain illnesses or conditions. The most common AIDS-defining conditions observed

> **BOX 43.9 Common Clinical Manifestations of Human Immunodeficiency Virus Infection in Children**
>
> - Lymphadenopathy
> - Hepatosplenomegaly
> - Oral candidiasis
> - Chronic or recurrent diarrhea
> - Failure to thrive
> - Developmental delay
> - Parotitis

> **BOX 43.10 Common Defining Conditions for Acquired Immune Deficiency Syndrome in Children**
>
> - *Pneumocystis carinii* pneumonia (PCP)
> - Lymphoid interstitial pneumonitis (LIP)
> - Recurrent bacterial infections
> - Wasting syndrome
> - Candidal esophagitis
> - Human immunodeficiency virus (HIV) encephalopathy
> - Cytomegalovirus disease
> - *Mycobacterium avium-intracellulare* complex infection
> - Pulmonary candidiasis
> - Herpes simplex disease
> - Cryptosporidiosis

among children in the United States are listed in Box 43.10. Other problems in these children may include short stature, malnutrition, and cardiomyopathy. CNS abnormalities resulting from HIV infection may include neuropsychologic deficits; developmental disabilities; and deficits in motor skills, communication, and behavioral functioning.

Diagnostic Evaluation

For children 18 months of age and older, the HIV enzyme-linked immunosorbent assay (ELISA) and Western blot immunoassay are performed to determine HIV infection. In infants born to HIV-infected mothers, results of these assays are positive because of the presence of maternal antibodies derived transplacentally. Maternal antibodies may persist in the infant up to 18 months of age. Therefore, other diagnostic tests are used—most commonly the HIV polymerase chain reaction (PCR) for detection of proviral DNA. A controlled-center study tested recombinase polymerase amplification (RPA) as a novel technology that is ideal for early infant diagnosis of HIV-1, because it amplifies target DNA in less than 20 minutes at a constant temperature without the need for complex thermocycling equipment needed for the PCR assay (Boyde, Lehman, Lillis, et al., 2013). RPA may become a beneficial yet inexpensive test for early diagnosis of HIV-infected individuals worldwide. There is a need for further research to compare the RPA assay to the gold standard PCR-based assay in a real-world setting. With these techniques, almost all infected infants can be diagnosed between 1 and 6 months of age (Siberry, 2014; Yogev & Chadwick, 2011).

HIV testing is entering a new era in the United States because of Food and Drug Administration approval of (1) combination tests that detect both HIV antigen and antibody, and (2) tests that accurately differentiate HIV-1 from HIV-2 antibodies (Centers for Disease Control and Prevention, 2014a). With the identification of HIV antigen, individuals may be diagnosed with HIV infection prior to development of symptoms.

The Centers for Disease Control and Prevention (1994) has developed a classification system to describe the spectrum of HIV disease in children (Table 43.2). The system indicates the severity of clinical signs and symptoms and the degree of immunosuppression. The nonsymptomatic

TABLE 43.2 **Pediatric Human Immunodeficiency Virus Infection Classification***

Immunologic Category	N: No Signs or Symptoms	A: Mild Signs or Symptoms	B: Moderate Signs or Symptoms[†]	C: Severe Signs or Symptoms[†]
No evidence of suppression	N1	A1	B1	C1
Evidence of moderate suppression	N2	A2	B2	C2
Severe suppression	N3	A3	B3	C3

From Centers for Disease Control and Prevention. (1994). 1994 Revised classification system for human immunodeficiency virus infection in children less than 13 years of age. *Morbidity and Mortality Weekly Report Recommendations and Reports, 43*(RR-12), 1–10.
*Children whose human immunodeficiency virus (HIV) infection status is not confirmed are classified by using this table with the letter *E* (for perinatally exposed) placed before the appropriate classification code (e.g., *EN2*).
[†]Both category C and lymphoid interstitial pneumonitis (LIP) in category B are reportable to state and local health departments as acquired immune deficiency syndrome (AIDS).

category includes either no signs and symptoms or one of the conditions listed in the mildly symptomatic category. The mildly symptomatic category includes signs and symptoms, such as lymphadenopathy, parotitis, hepatosplenomegaly, dermatitis, and recurrent or persistent sinusitis or otitis media. The moderately symptomatic category includes signs and symptoms such as lymphoid interstitial pneumonitis (LIP) and a variety of organ-specific dysfunctions or infections. The severely symptomatic category includes signs and symptoms, such as AIDS-defining illnesses with the exception of LIP. Children with LIP have a better prognosis than those with other AIDS-defining illnesses. In children whose HIV infection is not yet confirmed, the letter *E* (vertically exposed) is placed in front of the classification. The immune categories are based on CD_4^+ lymphocyte counts and percentages. Age adjustment of these numbers is necessary because normal counts, which are relatively high in infants, decline steadily until 6 years of age, which is when they reach adult norms.

Therapeutic Management

The interprofessional care team establishes goals of therapy for HIV infection that include slowing the growth of the virus, preventing and treating opportunistic infections, and providing nutritional support and symptomatic treatment. Antiretroviral drugs work at various stages of the HIV life cycle to prevent reproduction of functional new virus particles. Although not a cure, these drugs can suppress viral replication, prevent further deterioration of the immune system, and delay disease progression. Classes of antiretroviral agents include nucleoside reverse transcriptase inhibitors (e.g., zidovudine, didanosine, stavudine, lamivudine, abacavir), nonnucleoside reverse transcriptase inhibitors (e.g., nevirapine, delavirdine, efavirenz), nucleotide reverse transcriptase inhibitors (e.g., adefovir), and protease inhibitors (e.g., indinavir, saquinavir, ritonavir, nelfinavir, amprenavir). Combinations of antiretroviral drugs are used to stall the emergence of drug resistance. Antiretroviral therapy regimens and guidelines are continually evolving. Therapy is lifelong, making adherence difficult. Laboratory markers (CD_4^+ lymphocyte count, viral load) assist in monitoring both disease progression and response to therapy.

Pneumocystis carinii pneumonia (PCP) is the most common opportunistic infection of children infected with HIV. It occurs most frequently between 3 and 6 months of age. All infants born to HIV-infected women should receive prophylaxis by 6 weeks of age until HIV infection is reasonably excluded (Siberry, 2014; Simpkins et al., 2009). Trimethoprim/sulfamethoxazole (TMP-SMZ) is the agent of choice. If adverse effects are experienced with TMP-SMZ, dapsone or pentamidine can be used. Prophylaxis is often employed for other opportunistic infections, such as disseminated *Mycobacterium avium-intracellulare* complex, candidiasis, or herpes simplex. Intravenous gamma globulin (IVGG) has been helpful in preventing recurrent or serious bacterial infections in some HIV-infected children.

Immunization against common childhood illnesses, including the pneumococcal and influenza vaccines, is recommended for all children exposed to and infected with HIV (American Academy of Pediatrics Committee on Pediatric AIDS, 2000b; Leggat, Iyer, Ohtola, et al., 2015; Simpkins et al., 2009). Varicella (chickenpox) vaccine and measles, mumps, and rubella (MMR) vaccine can be administered if there is no evidence of severe immunocompromise. Because antibody production to vaccines may be poor or decrease over time, immediate prophylaxis after exposure to several vaccine-preventable diseases (e.g., measles, varicella) is warranted. It should be recognized that children receiving IVGG prophylaxis may not respond to the MMR vaccine if given in close proximity to the IVGG dose (McLean, Fiebelkorn, Temte, et al., 2013).

HIV infection often leads to marked failure to thrive and multiple nutritional deficiencies. Nutritional management may be difficult because of recurrent illness, diarrhea, and other physical problems. The nurse should implement intensive nutritional interventions if the child's growth begins to slow or weight begins to decrease.

Prognosis

Early recognition and improved medical care have changed HIV disease from a rapidly fatal illness to a chronic disease. After the introduction of combination antiretroviral therapy, the number of new AIDS cases and deaths declined substantially. In the United States, from 2009 to 2013, the annual estimated number and rate of deaths of HIV-infected children younger than 13 years of age has remained stable (Centers for Disease Control and Prevention, 2015; Simpkins et al., 2009). In contrast, adolescents and young adults (13 to 24 years of age) with AIDS that represent a minority of cases in the United States (≈5%) constitute one of the fastest growing groups of newly infected people in the country (Simpkins et al.; Yogev & Chadwick, 2011).

QUALITY PATIENT OUTCOMES: **Human Immunodeficiency Virus**

- Early recognition of human immunodeficiency virus (HIV) infection
- HIV infection slowed or maintained
- Growth and development promoted
- No infectious complications or cancer development
- Adherence to antiretroviral therapy
- Prolonged survival
- Quality of life supported

Care Management

Education concerning transmission and control of infectious diseases, including HIV infection, is essential for children with HIV infection and anyone involved in their care. The basic tenets of Standard

Precautions should be presented in an age-appropriate manner, with careful consideration of the educational levels of the individuals (see the "Infection Control" section in Chapter 39. Safety issues, including appropriate storage of special medications and equipment (e.g., needles and syringes), are emphasized.

Unfortunately, relatives, friends, and others in the general public may be fearful of contracting HIV infection, and criticism and ostracism of the child and family may occur. In an effort to protect the child and deal with fears of the community, the family may limit the child's activities outside the home. Although certain precautions are justified in limiting exposure to sources of infections, they must be tempered with concern for the child's normal developmental needs. Both the family and the community need ongoing education about HIV to dispel many of the myths that have been perpetuated by uninformed people.*

Prevention is a key component of HIV education. Educating adolescents about HIV is essential in preventing HIV infection in this age group. Education should include the routes of transmission, the hazards of IV and other recreational drug use, and the value of sexual abstinence and safe sex practices. Such education should be a part of anticipatory guidance provided to all adolescent patients. Nurses should also encourage adolescents at risk to undergo HIV counseling and testing. In addition to identifying infected teenagers and getting them into care, such counseling affords adolescents an opportunity to learn about, and possibly change, their risky behaviors.

Because approximately 20% to 25% of individuals living with HIV infection are unaware of their positive status, the US Preventive Services Task Force recommended clinicians screen for HIV infection in individuals 15 to 64 years of age and all individuals who are at increased risk regardless of age (Moyer & US Preventive Services Task Force, 2013). The US Preventive Services Task Force's recommendation was supported by a report on two health care settings that screened 32,534 individuals from 2011 to 2013 of which 148 tested HIV-positive with 120 (81%) linked to HIV medical care (Lin, Dietz, Rodriguez, et al., 2014c). Early detection of HIV-infected individuals and linking them to medical care and counseling through screening programs in the health care setting provides effective treatment and decreases the transmission of HIV (Suthar, Ford, Bachanas, et al., 2013).

The multiple complications associated with HIV disease are potentially painful (Ezekowitz, 2009). Aggressive pain management is essential for these children to have an acceptable quality of life. Their pain may be caused by infections (e.g., otitis media, dental abscess), encephalopathy (e.g., spasticity), adverse effects of medications (e.g., peripheral neuropathy), or an unknown source (e.g., deep musculoskeletal pain). Pain is not only related to the disease processes but also to various treatments these children often undergo, including venipunctures, lumbar punctures, biopsies, and endoscopies. Ongoing assessment of pain is crucial and is most easily accomplished in older children who are able to communicate. Nonverbal and developmentally delayed children are more difficult to assess. The nurse should be alert for signs of pain, such as emotional detachment, lack of interactive play, irritability, and depression. Effective pain management depends on the appropriate use of pharmacologic agents, including EMLA or LMX cream, acetaminophen, NSAIDs, muscle relaxants, and opioids. Tolerance to opioids may indicate increased dosing; monitored use ensures safety. Nonpharmacologic interventions (e.g., guided imagery, hypnosis, relaxation, and distraction techniques) are useful adjuncts.

Common psychosocial concerns include disclosing the diagnosis to the child, making custody plans when the parent is infected, and anticipating the loss of a family member. Other stressors may include financial difficulties, HIV-associated stigma, attempts to keep the diagnosis secret, infection of other family members, and any losses associated with HIV. Most mothers of these children are single mothers who are also HIV infected. As primary caretakers, they often attend to the needs of their child first, neglecting their own health in the process. The nurse should encourage the mother to receive regular health care. As an integral part of the multidisciplinary team, the nurse is necessary for the successful management of the complex medical and social problems of these families.

Children with HIV infection attend day care centers and schools. It is well established that the risk for HIV transmission in these settings is minimal. These institutions are required to follow Centers for Disease Control and Prevention and Occupational Safety and Health Administration guidelines for infection control measures. Standard Precautions describing proper management of blood and body fluids should also be followed. It is recommended that school personnel receive current HIV information and include it in the health education curriculum for kindergarten through twelfth grade (American Academy of Pediatrics Committee on Pediatric AIDS and Committee on Infectious Diseases, 1999; American Academy of Pediatrics Committee on Pediatric AIDS, 2000a). School nurses play a vital role in educating the school staff, students, and parents. They are also invaluable in monitoring the needs of known affected children.

Confidentiality is another major issue in day care or school attendance. Parents and legal guardians have the right to decide whether they inform the day care or school of their child's HIV diagnosis. Unfortunately, myths about HIV infection continue to exist, and the family often wishes to avoid any potential criticism or ostracism of the child.

SEVERE COMBINED IMMUNODEFICIENCY DISEASE

SCID is a defect characterized by absence of both humoral and cell-mediated immunity. The terms *Swiss-type lymphopenic agammaglobulinemia,* which refers to the autosomal recessive form of the disease, and *X-linked lymphopenic agammaglobulinemia* have been used to describe this disorder, which, as the names imply, can follow either mode of inheritance.

The most common manifestation is susceptibility to infection early in life, most often in the first month. The disorder in children is characterized by chronic infections, failure to completely recover from infections, frequent reinfection, and infection with unusual agents. Failure to thrive is a consequence of the persistent illnesses.

Diagnosis is usually based on a history of recurrent, severe infections from early infancy; a familial history of the disorder; and specific laboratory findings, which include lymphopenia, lack of lymphocyte response to antigens, and absence of plasma cells in the bone marrow. Documentation of immunoglobulin deficiency is difficult during infancy because of the normally delayed response of infants in producing their own immunoglobulins and maternal transfer of immunoglobulin G (IgG).

Therapeutic Management

The definitive treatment for SCID is HSCT. If the condition is diagnosed at birth or within the first 3 months of life, more than 95% of cases can be treated successfully with an HLA-identical or T-cell–depleted haploidentical donor (usually a parent), or a matched unrelated donor bone marrow stem cell transplant (Bonilla & Geha, 2009; Buckley, 2011). Other approaches to management of SCID include providing passive immunity with IVIG infusions and maintaining the child in a sterile environment. PCP prophylaxis is used to augment the humoral immunity until the transplant is performed. Several investigators are attempting gene therapy with some success, offering hope that gene therapy may

*Additional information is available from the National HIV/AIDS Hotline: 800-448-0440; outside of the United States: 301-315-2816.

eventually be the treatment of choice for cases of SCID (Bonilla & Geha, 2009; Buckley, 2011).

Care Management

Nursing care focuses on preventing infection and supporting the child and family. The care is consistent with that needed for HSCT for any condition (see earlier in this chapter). Because the prognosis for SCID is very poor if a compatible bone marrow donor is not available, nursing care is directed at supporting the family in caring for a child with a life-threatening illness (see Chapter 36). Genetic counseling is essential because of the modes of transmission in either form of the disorder.

WISKOTT-ALDRICH SYNDROME

WAS is a congenital X-linked recessive disorder characterized by a triad of abnormalities: thrombocytopenia, eczema, and immunodeficiency of selective functions of B lymphocytes and T lymphocytes. An abnormal gene has been identified on the proximal arm of the X chromosome and designated the WAS protein (Bonilla & Geha, 2009; Buckley, 2011). At birth, the presenting feature may be increased bleeding at the circumcision site or bloody diarrhea as a result of thrombocytopenia. As the child grows older, recurrent infection and eczema become more severe, and the bleeding becomes less frequent.

Eczema is typical of the allergic type and readily becomes superinfected. Chronic infection with herpes simplex is a frequent problem and may lead to chronic keratitis of the eye with loss of vision. Chronic pulmonary disease, sinusitis, and otitis media result from repeated infections. In children who survive the bleeding episodes and overwhelming infections, malignancy presents an additional risk to survival. Medical treatment involves the following:

- Counteracting the bleeding tendencies with platelet transfusions
- Administering IVIG to provide passive immunity
- Administering prophylactic antibiotics to prevent and control infection
- Providing aggressive local therapy for the eczema

WAS is usually cured with HSCT and should be performed as early as possible (Albert, Notarangelo, & Ochs, 2011; Buckley, 2011; Mahlaoui, Pellier, Mignot, et al., 2013). Several clinical trials focused on replacing the WAS gene are being conducted to determine the most effective vector (Albert, Notarangelo, & Ochs, 2011).

Care Management

Because of the poor prognosis for these children, the main nursing consideration is supporting the family in the care of a terminally ill child (see Chapter 36). Physical care should be directed at controlling the problems imposed by the disorder. The measures used to control bleeding are similar to those for hemophilia and vWD (see previous discussions). Another major goal is prevention or control of infection. Because eczema is a troublesome problem, nursing measures specific to this condition are especially important. The genetic implications of this X-linked recessive disorder differ little from those of any other X-linked disease.

TECHNOLOGIC MANAGEMENT OF HEMATOLOGIC AND IMMUNOLOGIC DISORDERS

BLOOD TRANSFUSION THERAPY

Technologic advances in blood banking and transfusion medicine enable the administration of only the blood component needed by the child, such as packed RBCs in anemia or platelets for bleeding disorders. Regardless of the blood component administered, the nurse must be aware of the possible transfusion reactions. Table 43.3 summarizes the major complications of transfusions, the signs and symptoms typically associated with each, and nursing responsibilities. General guidelines that apply to all transfusions include the following:

- Take vital signs, including blood pressure, *before* administering blood to establish baseline data for pretransfusion and posttransfusion comparison; 15 minutes after initiation; hourly while blood is infusing; and on completion of transfusion.
- Check the identification of the recipient along with his or her blood type and group against the donor, regardless of the blood product being used.
- Administer the first 50 mL of blood or initial 20% of the volume (whichever is smaller) *slowly,* and stay with the child.
- Administer with normal saline on a piggyback setup, or have normal saline available.
- Administer blood through an appropriate filter to eliminate particles in the blood and prevent the precipitation of formed elements; gently shake the container frequently.
- Use blood within 30 minutes of its arrival from the blood bank; if it is not used, return it to the blood bank—do not store it in the regular unit refrigerator.
- Infuse a unit of blood (or the specified amount) within 4 hours. If the infusion will exceed this time, the blood should be divided into appropriately sized quantities by the blood bank and the unused portion refrigerated under controlled conditions.
- If a reaction of any type is suspected, stop the transfusion, take vital signs, maintain a patent IV line with normal saline and new tubing, notify the primary care provider, and do not restart the transfusion until the child's condition has been medically evaluated.

Although hemolytic reactions are rare, ABO incompatibility remains the most common cause of death from blood transfusion, and human error (e.g., administration of the wrong type to the patient or mislabeling of the blood product) is usually responsible (Lavoie, 2011; Tondon, Pandey, Mickey, et al., 2010). Hemolysis can also cause the release of large quantities of phospholipids, which are capable of stimulating DIC. Acute kidney shutdown and eventual renal failure are a result of renal vasoconstriction from antigen-antibody complexes derived from the RBC surface.

Blood is usually administered to children by infusion pump; therefore, the usual precautions and management related to pumps apply. When the blood infusion begins with a standard transfusion set, the filter chamber is filled to allow the total filter to be used. The drip chamber is partially filled with blood to permit counting of the drops. In adjusting the flow rate, it is important to remember that blood administration sets do not use microdrops (60 drops/mL) but regular drops (usually 10 to 15 drops/mL). The nurse must consider this when calculating the flow rate.

APHERESIS

Apheresis is the removal of blood from an individual, separation of the blood into its components, retention of one or more of these components, and reinfusion of the remainder of the blood into the individual. Apheresis is most often used to remove large quantities of platelets from healthy adult donors. These transfusion products have greatly prolonged the survival of patients with hematologic and oncologic diseases.

TABLE 43.3   Nursing Care of the Child Receiving Blood Transfusions

Complication	Signs and Symptoms	Precautions and Nursing Responsibilities
Immediate Reactions		

Hemolytic reactions
Most severe type but rare
Incompatible blood
Incompatibility in multiple
  transfusions
	Sudden, severe headache
	Chills
	Shaking
	Fever
	Pain at needle site and along
	  venous tract
	Nausea and vomiting
	Sensation of tightness in chest
	Red or black urine
	Flank pain
	Progressive signs of shock or
	  renal failure
		Identify donor and recipient blood types and groups before transfusion is begun; verify
		  with another nurse or practitioner.
		Transfuse blood slowly for the first 15 to 20 minutes or initial 20% of blood volume;
		  remain with patient.
		Stop transfusion immediately in event signs or symptoms occur, maintain patent IV line,
		  and notify primary care provider.
		Save donor blood to re-crossmatch with patient's blood.
		Monitor for evidence of shock.
		Insert urinary catheter, and monitor hourly outputs.
		Send samples of patient's blood and urine to laboratory for presence of hemoglobin
		  (indicates intravascular hemolysis).
		Observe for signs of hemorrhage resulting from DIC.
		Support medical therapies to reverse shock.

Febrile reactions Leukocyte or platelet antibodies Plasma protein antibodies	Fever Chills	May give acetaminophen for prophylaxis. Leukocyte-poor RBCs are less likely to cause reaction. Stop transfusion immediately; report to primary care provider for evaluation.
Allergic reactions Recipient reaction to allergens in donor's blood	Urticaria Pruritus Flushing Asthmatic wheezing Laryngeal edema	Give antihistamines for prophylaxis to children with tendency to allergic reactions. Stop transfusion immediately. Administer epinephrine for wheezing or anaphylactic reaction.

Circulatory overload
Too rapid transfusion (even a
  small quantity)
Transfusion of excessive
  quantity of blood (even
  slowly)
	Precordial pain
	Dyspnea
	Rales
	Cyanosis
	Dry cough
	Distended neck veins
	Hypertension
		Transfuse blood slowly.
		Prevent overload by using packed RBCs or administering divided amounts of blood.
		Use infusion pump to regulate and maintain flow rate.
		Stop transfusion immediately if there are signs of overload.
		Place child upright with feet in dependent position to increase venous resistance.

Air emboli
May occur when blood is
  transfused under pressure
	Sudden difficulty in breathing
	Sharp pain in chest
	Apprehension
		Normalize pressure before container is empty when infusing blood under pressure.
		Clear tubing of air by aspirating air with syringe at nearest Y connector if air is
		  observed in tubing; disconnect tubing and allow blood to flow until air has escaped
		  only if a Y connector is not available.

Hypothermia	Chills Low temperature Irregular heart rate Possible cardiac arrest	Allow blood to warm at room temperature (<1 hour). Use approved mechanical blood warmer or electric warming coil to warm blood rapidly; never use microwave oven. Take temperature if patient complains of chills; if subnormal, stop transfusion.

Electrolyte disturbances
Hyperkalemia (in massive
  transfusions or in patients
  with renal problems)
	Nausea, diarrhea
	Muscular weakness
	Flaccid paralysis
	Paresthesia of extremities
	Bradycardia
	Apprehension
	Cardiac arrest
		Use washed RBCs or fresh blood if patient is at risk.

Delayed Reactions		

Transmission of infection
Hepatitis
HIV infection
Malaria
Syphilis
Other bacterial or viral infection
	Signs of infection (e.g., jaundice)
	Toxic reaction: High fever, severe
	  headache or substernal pain,
	  hypotension, intense flushing,
	  vomiting or diarrhea
		Blood is tested for antibodies to HIV, hepatitis C virus, and hepatitis B core antigen; in
		  addition, blood is tested for hepatitis B surface antigen and alanine aminotransferase,
		  and a serologic test is performed for syphilis. Units that test positive are destroyed.
		  Individuals at risk for carrying certain viruses are deterred from donation.
		Report any sign of infection, and if it occurs during transfusion, stop transfusion
		  immediately, send sample for culture and sensitivity testing, and notify primary care
		  provider.

Alloimmunization
Antibody formation
Occurs in patients receiving
  multiple transfusions
	Increased risk for hemolytic,
	  febrile, and allergic reactions
		Use limited number of donors.
		Observe carefully for signs of reactions.

Delayed hemolytic reaction	Destruction of RBCs and fever 5 to 10 days after transfusion	Observe for posttransfusion anemia and decreasing benefit from successive transfusion.

DIC, Disseminated intravascular coagulation; *HIV,* human immunodeficiency virus; *RBC,* red blood cell.

REFERENCES

Albert, M. H., Notarangelo, L. D., & Ochs, H. D. (2011). Clinical spectrum, pathophysiology and treatment of Wiskott-Aldrich syndrome. *Current Opinion in Hematology*, 18(1), 42–48.

American Academy of Pediatrics Committee on Pediatric AIDS. (2000a). Identification and care of HIV-exposed and HIV-infected infants, children, and adolescents in foster care. *Pediatrics*, 106(1), 149–153.

American Academy of Pediatrics Committee on Pediatric AIDS. (2000b). Technical report: Perinatal human immunodeficiency virus testing and prevention of transmission. *Pediatrics*, 106(6), 1–12.

American Academy of Pediatrics Committee on Pediatric AIDS. (2008). HIV testing and prophylaxis to prevent mother-to-child transmission in the United States. *Pediatrics*, 122(5), 1127–1134.

American Academy of Pediatrics Committee on Pediatric AIDS and Committee on Infectious Diseases. (1999). Issues related to human immunodeficiency virus transmission in schools, child care, medical settings, the home, and community. *Pediatrics*, 104(2), 318–324.

American Pain Society. (2015). *Guidelines for the management of acute and chronic pain in sickle-cell disease*. Glenview, IL: Author.

Anderson, N. (2006). Hydroxyurea therapy: Improving the lives of patients with sickle cell disease. *Pediatric Nursing*, 32(6), 541–543.

Andrews, N. C., Ullrich, C. K., & Fleming, M. D. (2009). Disorders of iron metabolism and sideroblastic anemia. In S. H. Orkin, D. Nathan, D. Ginsburg, et al. (Eds.), *Nathan and Oski's hematology of infancy and childhood* (7th ed.). Philadelphia, PA: Saunders/Elsevier.

Armstrong-Wells, J., Grimes, B., Sidney, S., et al. (2009). Utilization of TCD screening for primary stroke prevention in children with sickle cell disease. *Neurology*, 72(15), 1316–1321.

Auerbach, M. (2011). Should intravenous iron be upfront therapy for iron deficiency anemia? *Pediatric Blood & Cancer*, 56(4), 511–512.

Aygun, B., & Odame, I. (2012). A global perspective on sickle cell disease. *Pediatric Blood & Cancer*, 59(2), 386–390.

Bakai, A. J., & Pennell, D. J. (2014). Randomized controlled trials of iron chelators for the treatment of cardiac siderosis in thalassaemia major. *Frontiers in Pharmacology*, 5, 217.

Baker, R. D., Greer, F. R., & Committee on Nutrition American Academy of Pediatrics. (2010). Diagnosis and prevention of iron deficiency and iron-deficiency anemia in infants and young children (0-3 years of age). *Pediatrics*, 126(5), 1040–1050.

Ballas, S. K. (2011). Update on pain management in sickle cell disease. *Hemoglobin*, 35(5-6), 520–529.

Berglund, S., Westrup, B., & Domellof, M. (2010). Iron supplements reduce the risk of iron deficiency anemia in marginally low birth weight infants. *Pediatrics*, 126(4), e874–e883.

Bernaudin, F., Socie, G., Kuentz, M., et al. (2007). Long-term results of related myeloablative stem-cell transplantation to cure sickle cell disease. *Blood*, 110(7), 2749–2756.

Blaney, G., Forsyth, A., Zourikian, N., et al. (2010). Comprehensive elements of physiotherapy exercise programme in hemophilia—A global perspective. *Haemophilia*, 16(5 suppl), 136–145.

Bonilla, F. A., & Geha, R. S. (2009). Primary immunodeficiency diseases. In S. H. Orkin, D. Nathan, D. Ginsburg, et al. (Eds.), *Nathan and Oski's hematology of infancy and childhood* (7th ed.). Philadelphia, PA: Saunders/Elsevier.

Boyde, D. S., Lehman, D. A., Lillis, L., et al. (2013). Rapid detection of HIV-1 proviral DNA for early infant diagnosis using recombinase polymerase amplification. *mBio*, 4(2), e00135–13.

Branchford, B. R., Monahan, P. E., & Di Paola, J. (2013). New developments in the treatment of pediatric hemophilia and bleeding disorders. *Current Opinion in Pediatrics*, 25(1), 23–30.

Brandow, A. M., Weisman, S. J., & Panepinto, J. A. (2011). The impact of a multidisciplinary pain management model on sickle cell disease pain hospitalizations. *Pediatric Blood & Cancer*, 56(5), 789–793.

Bregman, D. B., & Goodnough, L. T. (2014). Experience with intravenous ferric carboxymaltose in patients with iron deficiency anemia. *Therapeutic Advances in Hematology*, 5(2), 48–60.

Broderick, C. R., Herbert, R. D., Latimer, J., et al. (2012). Association between physical activity and risk of bleeding in children with hemophilia. *Journal of the American Medical Association*, 308(14), 1452–1459.

Buckley, R. H. (2011). Primary combined antibody and cellular immunodeficiencies. In R. M. Kliegman, H. Jenson, R. E. Behrman, et al. (Eds.), *Nelson textbook of pediatrics* (19th ed.). Philadelphia, PA: Saunders/Elsevier.

Cappellini, M. D., Porter, J. B., El-Beshlawy, A., et al. (2010). Tailoring iron chelation by iron intake and serum ferritin trends: The prospective multicenter EPIC study of deferasirox in 1744 patients with various transfusion-dependent anemias. *Haematologica*, 95(4), 557–566.

Carley, A. (2003). Anemia: When is it iron deficiency? *Journal of Pediatric Nursing*, 29(2), 127–133.

Centers for Disease Control and Prevention. (1994). 1994 Revised classified system for human immunodeficiency virus infection in children less than 13 years of age. *Morbidity and Mortality Weekly Report Recommendations and Reports*, 43(RR-12), 1–10.

Centers for Disease Control and Prevention. (2006). Revised recommendations for HIV testing of adults, adolescents, and pregnant women in health-care settings. *Morbidity and Mortality Weekly Report Recommendations and Reports*, 55(RR-14), 1–17.

Centers for Disease Control and Prevention. (2014a). National HIV Testing Day and new testing recommendations. *Morbidity and Mortality Weekly Report*, 63(25), 537.

Centers for Disease Control and Prevention. (2014b). *Reducing HIV transmission from mother-to-child: An opt-out approach to HIV screening*. Retrieved from http://www.cdc.gov/hiv/group/gender/pregnantwomen/opt-out.html.

Centers for Disease Control and Prevention. (2015). *HIV surveillance report, 2013* (vol 25). Retrieved from http://www.cdc.gov/hiv/library/reports/surveillance.

Consolini, D. M. (2011). Thrombocytopenia in infants and children. *Pediatrics in Review*, 32(4), 135–151.

Coppola, A., Tagliaferri, A., Di Capua, M., et al. (2012). Prophylaxis in children with hemophilia: Evidence-based achievements, old and new challenges. *Seminars in Thrombosis and Hemostasis*, 38(1), 79–94.

Cunningham, M. J., Sankaran, V. G., Nathan, D. G., et al. (2009). The thalassemias. In S. H. Orkin, D. G. Nathan, D. Ginsburg, et al. (Eds.), *Nathan and Oski's hematology of infancy and childhood* (7th ed.). Philadelphia, PA: Saunders/Elsevier.

Curry, H. (2004). Bleeding disorder basics. *Pediatric Nursing*, 30(5), 402–405.

Driscoll, M. C. (2007). Sickle cell disease. *Pediatrics in Review*, 28(7), 259–267.

Ellison, A. M. (2012). *About sickle cell disease: Advice on handling emergencies*. Retrieved from http://contemporarypediatrics.modernmedicine.com/contemporary-pediatrics/news/modernmedicine/modern-medicine-feature-articles/about-sickle-cell-disea?page=full.

Eussen, S., Alles, M., Uijterschout, L., et al. (2015). Iron intake and status of children aged 6-36 months in Europe: A systematic review. *Annals of Nutrition and Metabolism*, 66(2-3), 80–92.

Ezekowitz, R. A. B. (2009). Hematologic manifestations of systemic diseases. In S. H. Orkin, D. G. Nathan, D. Ginsburg, et al. (Eds.), *Nathan and Oski's hematology of infancy and childhood* (7th ed.). Philadelphia, PA: Saunders/Elsevier.

Haining, W. N., Duncan, C., & Lehmann, L. E. (2009). Principles of bone marrow and stem cell transplantation. In S. H. Orkin, D. G. Nathan, D. Ginsburg, et al. (Eds.), *Nathan and Oski's hematology of infancy and childhood* (7th ed.). Philadelphia, PA: Saunders/Elsevier.

Hayden, E. C. (2013). Bid to cure HIV ramps up. *Nature*, 498(7455), 417–418.

Heeney, M., & Dover, G. J. (2009). Sickle cell disease. In S. H. Orkin, D. G. Nathan, D. Ginsburg, et al. (Eds.), *Nathan and Oski's hematology of infancy and childhood* (7th ed.). Philadelphia, PA: Saunders/Elsevier.

Hermans, C., De Moerloose, P., Fischer, K., et al. (2011). Management of acute haemarthrosis in haemophilia A without inhibitors: Literature review, European survey and recommendations. *Haemophilia*, 17(3), 383–392.

Hord, J. D. (2011). The acquired pancytopenia. In R. M. Kliegman, H. T. S. Jenson, R. E. Behrman, et al. (Eds.), *Nelson textbook of pediatrics* (19th ed.). Philadelphia, PA: Saunders/Elsevier.

Howard, J., & Davies, S. C. (2007). Sickle cell disease in North Europe. *Scandinavian Journal of Clinical and Laboratory Investigation, 67*(1), 27–38.

Hsieh, M. M., Fitzhugh, C. D., Weitzel, R. P., et al. (2014). Nonmyeloablative HLA-matched sibling allogeneic hematopoietic stem cell transplantation for severe sickle cell phenotype. *Journal of the American Medical Association, 312*(1), 48–56.

Huttle, A., Maestre, G. E., Lantigua, R., et al. (2015). Sickle cell in Latin America and the United States. *Pediatric Blood & Cancer, 62*(7), 1131–1136.

Iorio, A., Marchesini, E., Marcucci, M., et al. (2011). Clotting factor concentrates given to prevent bleeding and bleeding-related complications in people with hemophilia A or B. *Cochrane Database of Systematic Reviews, 2011*(9), CD003429.

Isgro, A., Gaziev, J., Sodani, P., et al. (2010). Progress in hematopoietic stem cell transplantation as allogeneic cellular gene therapy in thalassemia. *Annals of the New York Academy of Sciences, 1202*, 149–154.

Jauregui-Lobera, I. (2014). Iron deficiency and cognitive functions. *Neuropsychiatric Disease and Treatment, 10*, 2087–2095.

Joint United Nations Programme on HIV/AIDS (UNAIDS). (2013). *Global report: UNAIDS report on the global AIDS epidemic 2013*. Retrieved from http://www.unaids.org/sites/default/files/media_asset/UNAIDS_Global_Report_2013_en_1.pdf.

Jordan, L. C., Casella, J. F., & DeBaun, M. R. (2012). Prospects for primary stroke prevention in children with sickle cell anaemia. *British Journal of Haematology, 157*(1), 14–25.

Kett, J. C. (2012). Anemia in infancy. *Pediatrics in Review, 33*(4), 186–187.

Kwiatkowski, J. L., Yim, E., Miller, S., et al. (2011). Effect of transfusion therapy on transcranial Doppler ultrasonography velocities in children with sickle cell disease. *Pediatric Blood & Cancer, 56*(5), 777–782.

Lavoie, J. (2011). Blood transfusion risks and alternate strategies in pediatric patients. *Pediatric Anaesthesia, 21*(1), 14–24.

Leggat, D. J., Iyer, A. S., Ohtola, J. A., et al. (2015). Response to pneumococcal polysaccharide vaccination in newly diagnosed HIV-positive individuals. *Journal of AIDS and Clinical Research, 6*(2).

Lerner, N., & Sills, R. (2011). Iron-deficiency anemia. In R. M. Kliegman, H. B. Jenson, R. E. Behrman, et al. (Eds.), *Nelson textbook of pediatrics* (19th ed.). Philadelphia, PA: Elsevier.

Lillicrap, D. (2013). The future of hemostasis management. *Pediatric Blood & Cancer, 60*(1 suppl), S44–S47.

Lin, X., Dietz, P. M., Rodriguez, V., et al. (2014c). Routine HIV screening in two health-care settings—New York City and New Orleans, 2011-2013. *Morbidity and Mortality Weekly Report, 63*(25), 537–541.

Locatelli, F., & Pagliara, D. (2012). Allogeneic hematopoietic stem cell transplantation in children with sickle cell disease. *Pediatric Blood & Cancer, 59*(2), 372–376.

Lokeshwar, H. R., Mehta, M., Mehta, N., et al. (2011). Prevention of iron deficiency anemia (IDA): How far have we reached? *Indian Journal of Pediatrics, 78*(5), 593–602.

Lucarelli, G., Isgro, A., Sodani, P., et al. (2012). Hematopoietic stem cell transplantation in thalassemia and sickle cell anemia. *Cold Spring Harbor Perspectives in Medicine, 2*(5), a011825.

Mahlaoui, N., Pellier, I., Mignot, C., et al. (2013). Characteristics and outcome of early-onset, severe forms of Wiskott-Aldrich syndrome. *Blood, 121*(9), 1510–1516.

Manco-Johnson, M. J., Abshire, T. C., Shapiro, A. D., et al. (2007). Prophylaxis versus episodic treatment to prevent joint disease in boys with severe hemophilia. *New England Journal of Medicine, 357*(6), 535–544.

Mátrai, J., Chuah, M. K., & VandenDriessche, T. (2010). Preclinical and clinical progress in hemophilia gene therapy. *Current Opinion in Hematology, 17*(5), 387–392.

McCavit, T. L. (2012). Sickle cell disease. *Pediatrics in Review, 33*(5), 195–206.

McCrae, K. (2011). Immune thrombocytopenia: No longer "idiopathic." *Cleveland Clinic Journal of Medicine, 78*(6), 358–373.

McDonagh, M. S., Blazina, I., Dana, T., et al. (2015). Screening and routine supplementation for iron deficiency anemia: A systematic review. *Pediatrics, 135*(4), 723–733.

McGann, P. T., Nero, A. C., & Ware, R. E. (2013). Current management of sickle cell anemia. *Cold Spring Harbor Perspectives in Medicine, 3*(8).

McGann, P. T., & Ware, R. E. (2011). Hydroxyurea for sickle cell anemia: What have we learned and what questions remain? *Current Opinion in Hematology, 18*(3), 158–165.

McLean, H. Q., Fiebelkorn, A. P., Temte, J. L., et al. (2013). Prevention of measles, rubella, congenital rubella syndrome, and mumps, 2013: Summary recommendations of the Advisory Committee on Immunization Practices (ACIP). *Morbidity and Mortality Weekly Report Recommendations and Reports, 62*(RR-04), 1–34.

Meerpohl, J. J., Schell, L. K., Rucker, G., et al. (2014). Deferasirox for managing transfusional iron overload in people with sickle cell disease. *Cochrane Database of Systematic Reviews, 2014*(5), CD007477.

Meier, E. R., & Miller, J. L. (2012). Sickle cell disease in children. *Drugs, 72*(7), 895–906.

Miano, M., & Dufour, C. (2015). The diagnosis and treatment of aplastic anemia: A review. *International Journal of Hematology, 101*(6), 527–535.

Michael, R., Mulder, K., & Strike, K. (2014). Exercise for hemophilia. *Cochrane Database of Systematic Reviews, 2014*(12), CD011180.

Miller, S. T., Sleeper, L. A., Pegelow, C. H., et al. (2000). Prediction of adverse outcomes in children with sickle cell disease. *New England Journal of Medicine, 342*(2), 83–89.

Montgomery, R. R., Gill, J. C., & DiPaola, J. (2009). Hemophilia and von Willebrand disease. In S. H. Orkin, D. Nathan, D. Ginsburg, et al. (Eds.), *Nathan and Oski's hematology of infancy and childhood* (7th ed.). Philadelphia, PA: Saunders/Elsevier.

Montgomery, R. R., & Scott, J. P. (2011). Platelet and blood vessel disorders. In R. M. Kliegman, H. T. S. Jenson, R. E. Behrman, et al. (Eds.), *Nelson textbook of pediatrics* (19th ed.). Philadelphia, PA: Saunders/Elsevier.

Moyer, V. A., & US Preventive Services Task Force. (2013). Screening for HIV. US Preventive Services Task Force recommendation statement. *Annals of Internal Medicine, 159*(1), 51–60.

National Institutes of Health, & National Heart, Lung, and Blood Institute, Division of Blood Disease and Resources. (2002). *The management of sickle cell disease*, NIH Pub No 02-2117. Bethesda, MD: NHLBI Health Information Network.

Nienhuis, A. W. (2008). Development of gene therapy for blood disorders. *Blood, 111*(9), 4431–4444.

Paoletti, G., Bogen, D. L., & Ritchey, A. K. (2014). Severe iron-deficiency anemia still an issue in toddlers. *Clinical Pediatrics, 53*(14), 1352–1358.

Passweg, J. R., & Marsh, J. C. (2010). Aplastic anemia: First-line treatment by immunosuppression and sibling marrow transplantation. *Hematology: American Society of Hematology, Education Program, 2010*, 36–42.

Peinemann, F., & Labeit, A. M. (2014). Stem cell transplantation of matched sibling donors compared with immunosuppressive therapy for acquired severe aplastic anaemia: A Cochrane systematic review. *BMJ Open, 4*(7), e005039.

Powers, J. M., & Buchanan, G. R. (2014). Diagnosis and management of iron deficiency anemia. *Hematology/Oncology Clinics of North America, 28*(4), 729–745.

Raphael, J. L., Mei, M., Mueller, B. U., et al. (2012). High resource hospitalizations among children with vaso-occlusive crises in sickle cell disease. *Pediatric Blood & Cancer, 58*(4), 584–590.

Redding-Lallinger, R., & Knoll, C. (2006). Sickle cell disease—Pathophysiology and treatment. *Current Problems in Pediatric and Adolescent Health Care, 36*(10), 346–376.

Rodeghiero, F., Stasi, R., Gernsheimer, T., et al. (2009). Standardization of terminology, definitions, and outcome criteria in immune thrombocytopenic purpura of adults and children: Report from an international working group. *Blood, 113*(11), 2386–2393.

Ross, C., Goldenberg, N. A., Hund, D., et al. (2009). Athletic participation in severe hemophilia: Bleeding and joint outcomes in children on prophylaxis. *Pediatrics, 124*(5), 1267–1272.

Samarasinghe, S., & Webb, D. K. (2012). How I manage aplastic anaemia in children. *British Journal of Haematology, 157*(1), 26–40.

Scheinberg, P. (2012). Aplastic anemia: Therapeutic updates in immunosuppression and transplantation. *Hematology: American Society of Hematology, Education Program, 2012*, 292–300.

Scott, S. P., Chen-Edinboro, L. P., Caulfield, L. E., et al. (2014). The impact of anemia on child mortality: An updated review. *Nutrients, 6*(12), 5915–5932.

Scott, J. P., & Montgomery, R. R. (2011). Hereditary clotting factor deficiencies. In R. M. Kliegman, H. T. S. Jenson, R. E. Behrman, et al. (Eds.), *Nelson textbook of pediatrics* (19th ed.). Philadelphia, PA: Saunders/Elsevier.

Sharathkumar, A. A., & Carcao, M. (2011). Clinical advances in hemophilia management. *Pediatric Blood & Cancer, 57*(6), 910–920.

Sharathkumar, A. A., & Pipe, S. W. (2008). Post-thrombotic syndrome in children: A single center experience. *Journal of Pediatric Hematology/Oncology, 30*(4), 261–266.

Shimamura, A., & Guinan, E. C. (2009). Acquired aplastic anemia. In S. H. Orkin, D. Nathan, D. Ginsburg, et al. (Eds.), *Nathan and Oski's hematology of infancy and childhood* (7th ed.). Philadelphia, PA: Saunders.

Siberry, G. K. (2014). Preventing and managing HIV infection in infants, children, and adolescents in the United States. *Pediatrics in Review, 35*(7), 268–286.

Siegfried, N., van der Merwe, L., Brocklehurst, P., et al. (2011). Antiretrovirals for reducing the risk of mother-to-child transmission of HIV infection. *Cochrane Database of Systematic Reviews, 2011*(7), CD003510.

Simpkins, E. P., Siberry, G. K., & Hutton, N. (2009). Thinking about HIV infection. *Pediatrics in Review, 30*(9), 337–349.

Smith, A. (2012). Guide to evaluation and treatment of anaemia in general practice. *Prescriber, 23*(21), 25–42.

Strouse, J. J., Lanzkron, S., Beach, M. C., et al. (2008). Hydroxyurea for sickle cell disease: A systematic review for efficacy and toxicity in children. *Pediatrics, 122*(6), 1332–1342.

Subramaniam, G., & Girish, M. (2015). Iron deficiency anemia in children. *Indian Journal of Pediatrics, 82*(6), 558–564.

Suthar, A. B., Ford, N., Bachanas, P. J., et al. (2013). Towards universal voluntary HIV testing and counseling: A systematic review and meta-analysis of community-based approaches. *PLoS Medicine, 10*(8), e1001496.

Thompson, J., Biggs, B. A., & Pasricha, S. R. (2013). Effects of daily iron supplementation in 2- to 5-year-old children: Systematic review and meta-analysis. *Pediatrics, 131*(4), 739–753.

Tondon, R., Pandey, P., Mickey, K. B., et al. (2010). Errors reported in cross match laboratory: A prospective data analysis. *Transfusion and Apheresis Science, 43*(3), 309–314.

Velasquez, M. P., Mariscalco, M. M., Goldstein, S. L., et al. (2009). Erythrocytapheresis in children with sickle cell disease and acute chest syndrome. *Pediatric Blood & Cancer, 53*(6), 1060–1063.

Vichinsky, E., Bernaudin, F., Forni, G. L., et al. (2011). Long-term safety and efficacy of deferasirox (Exjade) for up to 5 years in transfusional iron-overloaded patients with sickle cell disease. *British Journal of Haematology, 154*(3), 387–397.

Vichinsky, E., & Styles, L. (1996). Pulmonary complications. *Hematology/Oncology Clinics of North America, 10*(6), 1275–1286.

Voskaridou, E., Christoulas, D., Bilalis, A., et al. (2010). The effect of prolong administration of hydroxyurea on morbidity and mortality in adult patients with sickle cell syndromes: Results of a 17-year single-center trial (LaSHS). *Blood, 115*(12), 2354–2363.

Walsh, C. E., & Batt, K. M. (2013). Hemophilia clinical gene therapy: Brief review. *Translational Research, 161*(4), 307–312.

Wang, W. C., & Dwan, K. (2013). Blood transfusion for preventing primary and secondary stroke in people with sickle cell disease. *Cochrane Database of Systematic Reviews, 2013*(11), CD003146.

Wang, W. C., Ware, R. E., Miller, S. T., et al. (2011). Hydroxycarbamide in very young children with sickle-cell anaemia: A multicenter, randomised, controlled trial (BABY HUG). *Lancet, 377*(9778), 1663–1672.

Wang, B., Zhan, S., Gong, T., et al. (2013). Iron therapy for improving psychomotor development and cognitive function in children under the age of three with iron deficiency anemia. *Cochrane Database of Systematic Reviews, 2013*(6), CD001444.

Wilson, D. B. (2009). Acquired platelet defects. In S. H. Orkin, D. G. Nathan, D. Ginsburg, et al. (Eds.), *Nathan and Oski's hematology of infancy and childhood* (7th ed.). Philadelphia, PA: Saunders.

Yaish, H. M. (2015). *Pediatric thalassemia.* Retrieved from http://emedicine.medscape.com/article/958850-overview.

Yawn, B. P., Buchanan, G. R., Afenyi-Annan, A. N., et al. (2014). Management of sickle cell disease summary of the 2014 evidence-based report by expert panel members. *Journal of the American Medical Association, 312*(10), 1033–1048.

Yogev, R., & Chadwick, E. G. (2011). Acquired immunodeficiency syndrome (human immunodeficiency virus). In R. M. Kliegman, H. B. Jenson, R. E. Behrman, et al. (Eds.), *Nelson textbook of pediatrics* (19th ed.). Philadelphia, PA: Saunders/Elsevier.

Ziegler, E. E. (2011). Consumption of cow's milk as a cause of iron deficiency in infants and toddlers. *Nutrition Reviews, 69*(1 suppl), S37–S42.

Ziegler, E. E., Nelson, S. E., & Jeter, J. M. (2011). Iron supplementation of breastfed infants. *Nutrition Reviews, 69*(1 suppl), S71–S77.

Zimmerman, S. A., Schultz, W. H., Davis, J. S., et al. (2004). Sustained long-term hematologic efficacy of hydroxyurea at maximum tolerated dose in children with sickle cell disease. *Blood, 103*(6), 2039–2045.

Zimmerman, B., & Valentino, L. A. (2013). Hemophilia: In review. *Pediatrics in Review, 34*(7), 289–295.

44

The Child With Cancer

Cheryl C. Rodgers

http://evolve.elsevier.com/wong/essentials

CANCER IN CHILDREN

Few situations in nursing exceed the challenges of caring for a child with cancer. Despite the dramatic improvements in survival rates for these children, the family's needs are tremendous as they cope with a serious physical illness and the fear that the child will not be cured. Nurses should base support of patients and their families on the premise that communication promotes understanding and clarity. With understanding, fear diminishes and hope emerges, and in the presence of hope, anything is possible.

EPIDEMIOLOGY

Childhood cancer is rare; approximately 16,400 cases of cancer are diagnosed in children younger than 20 years of age in the United States each year (Scheurer, Lupo, & Bondy, 2016). Despite the relatively low incidence, approximately 1300 children younger than 15 years of age die from their disease each year, making cancer the leading cause of death from disease in this age group (Scheurer et al.). The incidence of cancer in children and adolescents is approximately 18 cases per 100,000 children (Henley, Singh, King, et al., 2015).

The incidence of specific subtypes of childhood cancer can vary according to age, sex, and race. For example, males have a higher overall incidence of cancer compared with females, with a ratio of 1.1:1 (Scheurer et al., 2016). This is due to the higher incidence of acute lymphoblastic leukemia (ALL), non-Hodgkin lymphoma (NHL), and central nervous system (CNS) tumors—the most common types of childhood cancer—in young boys. Unlike adults, Caucasian children have an overall higher incidence of cancer compared to African-American children. This is accounted for by the higher incidence in ALL, Ewing sarcoma, and melanoma in Caucasian children. The incidence of childhood cancer is more pronounced in children 0 to 4 years of age and adolescents 15 to 19 years of age; however, the types of cancers among these two groups are very distinct, with neuroblastoma and retinoblastoma occurring more commonly in young children and lymphoma and sarcoma occurring more commonly in adolescents (Scheurer et al.).

ETIOLOGY

Often the first questions parents of newly diagnosed children with cancer ask is "How did my child get this, and did I do something to cause it?" Parents are also understandably concerned with the question of the likelihood that their other children will get cancer. Although there are numerous hypotheses concerning the origin of cancer, the most enduring theory is that some genetic alteration results in the unregulated proliferation of cells. Significant advances have been made in our understanding of cell proliferation, programmed cell death (apoptosis), genes that activate tumor growth (oncogenes), and genes that keep tumor growth in check (tumor suppressor genes). Cancer is the result of multiple genetic events but is not necessarily hereditary. Overall, the incidence of cancers caused by direct inheritance is low.

In the early 1970s, Alfred Knudson described the "two-hit hypothesis." This explanation of cancer inheritance is best described in retinoblastoma. Like most genes, the retinoblastoma gene *(Rb)* is present in two copies on each cell. It is a tumor suppressor gene, responsible for controlling cell growth. When just one of these copies is lost—the "first hit," the cell remains normal. However, when the second copy is lost—the "second hit," abnormal cell proliferation occurs and retinoblastoma develops (Knudson, Hethcote & Brown, 1975). A child can inherit one altered copy of the retinoblastoma gene from a mother or father. Therefore, it takes only one more hit for retinoblastoma to develop. Perhaps the most well-known inherited cancer predisposition syndrome is Li-Fraumeni syndrome, which is mainly due to constitutional (in all cells) mutation in the tumor suppressor gene, *p53*. This syndrome is characterized by early incidence brain tumors, premenopausal breast cancer, soft-tissue and bone sarcoma, leukemias, and lymphomas (Plon & Malkin, 2016).

Chromosome abnormalities have been identified in many childhood malignancies and are important in the development of various types of cancer. Chromosome abnormalities can be confined to the tumor or can be present in all cells; the latter are called *germ-line mutations*. Chromosome abnormalities can be due to translocations (a rearrangement of information between two chromosomes) or abnormal numbers of chromosomes. Many well-established chromosome translocations have been identified in childhood leukemia and some solid tumors.

Other genetic syndromes that can affect genes or chromosomes and are associated with a predisposition to cancer include Fanconi anemia, Bloom syndrome, Beckwith-Weidemann syndrome, neurofibromatosis type 1, ataxia-telangiectasia, and Klinefelter syndrome.

Children with immunodeficiencies, such as Wiskott-Aldrich syndrome or acquired immunodeficiency syndrome, or children whose immune system has been suppressed, such as following transplant procedures, are at a greater risk for developing various cancers. Of major concern is the increased risk for secondary cancers in some children successfully treated for their primary malignancy.

Risk Factors

Lifestyle-related behaviors are the main factors that increase the risk for cancer in adults, but they have little to no effect on childhood cancer. There is relatively little information to support a strong environmental role in the development of childhood cancer. However, some risk factors are well established. Known risk factors include exposure to ionizing radiation, carcinogenic drugs, immunosuppressive therapy, infections (e.g., Epstein Barr virus), race, and genetic conditions (Scheurer et al., 2016).

Prevention

Knowledge of the risk factors that increase the likelihood of cancer holds the promise of prevention. Unfortunately, the known carcinogens are limited in children. Therefore, at present there is really no known prevention.

Health care professionals, however, have two roles. One is aimed at preventing adult type of cancers by educating parents and children about the hazards of known carcinogens, particularly the effects of cigarette smoking and excessive exposure to sunlight. Lung cancer is the leading cause of death from cancer in adults, and malignant melanoma is the leading cause of death from diseases of the skin. In addition, to provide early detection of other types of cancer, males should learn testicular self-examination, and female adolescents should learn breast self-examination and seek periodic health examinations, including a Papanicolaou smear.

Second, health care professionals need to be aware of the cardinal symptoms of childhood cancer (Box 44.1). Unfortunately, fever and pain are manifestations of common childhood disorders and, without a high index of suspicion, may be attributed to minor ailments. The other signs are subtle and easily missed. If parents suspect an abnormality, their concerns must be taken seriously. The greatest weapons against all forms of cancer are early detection and treatment.

DIAGNOSTIC EVALUATION

The evaluation of a child suspected of having cancer may take several days to complete. Specific signs and symptoms depend on the type of cancer and its location. The essential components of a comprehensive evaluation for childhood cancer include complete history and review of symptoms, physical examination, laboratory tests, diagnostic imaging, diagnostic procedures (e.g., lumbar puncture [LP], bone marrow aspirate, and biopsy), and surgical pathology.

Laboratory Tests

Several laboratory tests must be performed to accurately diagnose and treat children with cancer. The majority of patients have a complete blood count, serum chemistries, liver function tests, coagulation studies, and urinalysis done on initial presentation. Frequent complete blood counts are necessary to monitor effects of therapy and in some

hematologic malignancies, response to therapy. Blood chemistry yields important information with regard to kidney, liver, bone function, and electrolyte balance. These tests are important to help detect the extent of disease and also to monitor for side effects during therapy.

Diagnostic Procedures

LP is a routine test employed in leukemia, brain tumors, and other cancers that may metastasize to the CNS. LPs are also used to administer intrathecal drugs in patients with various malignancies, such as leukemia.

A bone marrow aspirate test is performed by aspirating marrow with a large- or fine-bore needle. A bone marrow biopsy is performed by obtaining a piece of bone through a special type of needle. These tests are performed to determine the presence or absence of tumor or response to therapy in this specific location.

Diagnostic Imaging

Modern-day diagnostic imaging has greatly improved our ability to accurately diagnose childhood cancers. The most commonly employed modes of imaging include chest X-rays, computed tomography (CT), magnetic resonance imaging (MRI), positron emission tomography (PET), and metaiodobenzylguanidine (MIBG) scan, which is being used increasingly in certain types of pediatric malignancies, such as neuroblastoma and soft-tissue tumors. Interventional radiology is playing an increasing role in the diagnosis and management of pediatric malignancies.

Pathologic Evaluation

A biopsy is necessary to establish the diagnosis of a malignancy. Besides determining what type of cancer the patient has, this tissue sample can also be sent for various biologic studies that define the patient's prognosis and allow health care providers to tailor therapy according to the risk group. For example, a bone marrow biopsy determines whether the patient has acute lymphocytic leukemia or acute myelocytic leukemia and also tells what specific subtype of leukemia the patient has and how aggressively it should be treated. Similarly, patients with neuroblastoma undergo a biopsy of the tumor to establish the diagnosis and to evaluate the tumor for *N-myc* amplification, which determines the type of treatment they receive.

TREATMENT MODALITIES

The use of multimodal therapy consisting of surgery, chemotherapy, and radiotherapy; enrollment of large numbers of children in cooperative group clinical trials or protocols; and improvements in supportive care have greatly increased the survival of children with cancer. Eighty percent of these patients are now expected to be cured of their disease.

Current efforts are aimed at increasing the survival of patients with high-risk tumors, decreasing the acute and long-term side effects of treatment, and studying the biology of the diseases to better identify patients who are at different risk levels for disease recurrence and can therefore benefit from risk-adapted therapies.

Surgery

The main goal of surgery, besides obtaining biopsies, is to remove all traces of the tumor and restore normal body functioning. Surgery is most successful when the tumor is encapsulated and localized (confined to the site of origin). It may be used for palliative care when the cancer is regional (metastasized to an area adjacent to the original site) or advanced (widespread throughout the body). Obviously the best prognosis is directly related to early detection of the tumor.

Because the majority of pediatric cancers respond well to chemotherapy, more conservative surgical excision is increasingly used in a variety of tumors in an attempt to preserve function and cosmesis. For example, in some types of bone cancer, such as osteosarcoma, patients are successfully treated with resection of the diseased portion of the bone rather than amputation. There is an increasing emphasis on the use of combination drug therapy and radiotherapy after limited surgical intervention.

Chemotherapy

Chemotherapy may be the primary form of treatment, or it may be an adjunct to surgery or radiotherapy. The majority of chemotherapy agents work by interfering with the function or production of nucleic acids, deoxyribonucleic acid (DNA), or ribonucleic acid (RNA). Although several drugs with antineoplastic capabilities have been effective in treating different forms of cancer, the remarkable survival rates have been the result of improved combination drug regimens. Combining drugs allows for optimum cell cycle destruction with minimum toxic effects and decreased resistance by the cancer cells to the agent.

In addition to more effective combinations of drugs, several advances in the administration of chemotherapy have permitted continuous or intermittent intravenous (IV) administration without multiple venipunctures. The use of venous access devices (e.g., catheters and implantable infusion ports) has greatly facilitated safe and effective drug administration with minimum discomfort for the child. Continuous infusions over an extended period using syringe pumps have made possible the administration of certain drugs (e.g., cytosine arabinoside) in higher doses with less toxicity than when the drug is administered intermittently.

Chemotherapeutic agents can be classified according to their primary mechanism of action. Alkylating agents replace a hydrogen atom of a molecule by an alkyl group. The irreversible combination of alkyl groups with nucleotide chains, particularly DNA, causes unbalanced growth of unaffected cell constituents so that the cell eventually dies. These agents have a steep dose-response curve and, for this reason, can be used in high-dose therapy regimens. Examples of alkylating agents include cyclophosphamide, ifosfamide, cisplatin (Platinol), and dacarbazine. Antimetabolites resemble essential metabolic elements needed for cell growth but are sufficiently altered in molecular structure to inhibit further synthesis of DNA or RNA; their maximum effect occurs in cells that are actively producing DNA. Examples of antimetabolites include methotrexate and mercaptopurine. Plant alkaloids arrest cells in metaphase (a phase of mitosis) by binding to microtubular protein needed for spindle formation. Examples include vincristine and vinblastine. Antitumor antibiotics are natural products that interfere with cell division by reacting with DNA in such a way as to prevent further replication of DNA and transcription of RNA. Examples include doxorubicin and daunomycin.

A number of agents are not categorized according to the preceding classifications. For example, L-asparaginase is an enzyme isolated from extracts of bacterial cultures of *Escherichia coli* or *Erwinia carotovora*. It hydrolyzes L-asparagine, an amino acid, to L-aspartic acid, which prevents the cell from synthesizing protein needed for DNA and RNA synthesis. Because L-asparagine is synthesized by normal cells but must be exogenously supplied to certain leukemia and lymphoma cells, administration of the enzyme destroys the essential exogenous supply while sparing normal cells of untoward effects.

An understanding of the actions and side effects of these drugs is essential to nursing care of children with cancer. Unfortunately, almost all drugs are not selectively cytotoxic for malignant cells, and other cells with a high rate of proliferation (e.g., the bone marrow elements, hair, skin, and epithelial cells of the gastrointestinal tract) are also affected. Frequently the problems related to the destruction of these normal cells require more nursing care than the disease itself.

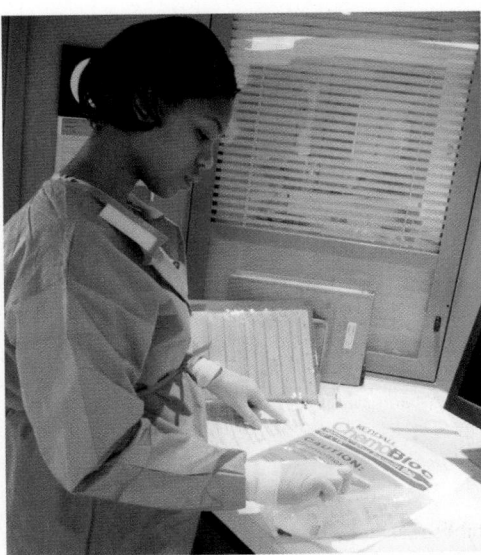

FIG 44.1 Nurses caring for children with cancer require expertise in the safe administration of chemotherapy.

A number of targeted agents called *tyrosine kinase inhibitors* have been developed and are being used in a variety of pediatric and adult malignancies. Examples of some of these agents include imatinib, sunitinib, and sorafenib.

Precautions in Administering and Handling Chemotherapeutic Agents

Many chemotherapeutic agents are *vesicants* (sclerosing agents) that can cause severe cellular damage if even minute amounts of the drug infiltrate surrounding tissue. Only nurses experienced with chemotherapeutic agents should administer vesicants (Fig. 44.1). Guidelines are available* and must be followed meticulously to prevent tissue damage to patients.

In addition to extravasation, a potentially fatal complication is anaphylaxis, especially from L-asparaginase, bleomycin, cisplatin, and etoposide (VP-16). Hypersensitivity reactions to these chemotherapeutic agents are characterized by urticaria, angioedema, flushing, rashes, difficulty breathing, hypotension, and nausea or vomiting. Nursing responsibilities include prevention, recognition, and preparation for serious reactions. If a reaction is suspected, the nurse discontinues the drug, flushes and maintains the IV line with saline, and monitors the child's vital signs and subsequent responses.

> **! NURSING ALERT**
>
> When chemotherapeutic and immunologic agents with known anaphylactic potential are given, it is standard practice to observe the child for at least 1 hour after the infusion for signs of anaphylaxis (e.g., rash, urticaria, hypotension, wheezing, nausea, vomiting). Emergency equipment (especially blood pressure monitor, bag and valve mask, and suction) and emergency drugs (especially oxygen, epinephrine, antihistamines, aminophylline, corticosteroids, and vasopressors) must be readily available.

ASCO/ONS Chemotherapy Safety Standards is available from the Oncology Nursing Society, 125 Enterprise Drive, Pittsburgh, PA 15275; 412-859-6100 or 866-257-4667; https://www.ons.org/practice-resources/standards-reports/chemotherapy.

TABLE 44.1 Early Side Effects of Radiotherapy

Site	Effects	Nursing Interventions
Gastrointestinal tract	Nausea and vomiting	Give antiemetic on schedule around the clock.
		Measure amount of emesis to assess for dehydration.
	Anorexia	Encourage fluids and foods best tolerated, usually light, soft diet and small, frequent meals.
		Monitor weight.
	Mucosal ulceration	Use frequent mouth rinses and oral hygiene to prevent mucositis.
	Diarrhea	Control with antispasmodics and kaolin pectin preparations.
		Observe for signs of dehydration.
Skin	Alopecia (within 2 weeks; hair may regrow by 3 to 6 months)	Introduce idea of wig.
		Stress necessity of scalp hygiene and need for head covering in sun and cold weather.
	Dry or moist desquamation	Do not refer to skin change as a "burn" (implies use of too much radiation).
		Avoid lotions and other creams to skin.
		Wash daily, using soap (e.g., Dove) sparingly.
		Do not remove skin marking for radiation fields.
		Avoid exposure to sun.
		For desquamation, consult health care provider for skin hygiene and care.
Head	Nausea and vomiting (from stimulation of vomiting center in brain)	Same as for gastrointestinal tract.
	Alopecia	Same as for skin.
	Mucositis	Encourage regular dental care, fluoride treatments.
	Potential effects: • Parotitis • Sore throat • Loss of taste	Provide analgesics as needed to relieve discomfort.
	Xerostomia (dry mouth)	Combat severe dryness of mouth with oral hygiene and liquid diet.
Urinary bladder	Rarely cystitis	Encourage liberal fluid intake and frequent voiding.
		Evaluate for hematuria.
Bone marrow	Myelosuppression	Observe for fever (temperature >101° F [38.3° C]).
		Initiate workup for sepsis as ordered.
		Administer antibiotics as prescribed.
		Avoid use of suppositories, rectal temperatures.
		Institute bleeding precautions.
		Observe for signs of anemia.

In addition to the many responsibilities during chemotherapy administration, nurses must also use safeguards to protect themselves. Handling chemotherapeutic agents may present risks to handlers and to their offspring, although the exact degree of risk is not known. The Oncology Nursing Society has published comprehensive guidelines for safe practice issues related to administration of chemotherapy.* They have also established safe management procedures for chemotherapy administered in the home.

Radiotherapy

Radiotherapy is frequently used in the treatment of childhood cancer, usually in conjunction with chemotherapy or surgery. It can be used for curative purposes or for palliation to relieve symptoms by shrinking the size of the tumor. Recent advances in radiotherapy have optimized its beneficial effects and minimized many of the undesirable side effects, although high-dose irradiation is associated with many serious late effects.

Ionizing radiation is cytotoxic in at least three different ways: (1) damaging the pyrimidine bases cytosine, thymine, and uracil needed

for the synthesis of nucleic acids; (2) causing single-strand breaks in the DNA or RNA molecule; or (3) causing double helical–strand breaks in these molecules. The effect of disturbing cellular metabolic and reproductive functions is either sublethal or lethal damage. *Lethal damage* refers to the death of the cell. *Sublethal damage* refers to injured cells that may subsequently be repaired. Many of the acute side effects are the result of lethal damage to radiosensitive tissue, particularly proliferating cells such as those of the bone marrow, gastrointestinal tract, and hair follicles. Late effects are usually the result of cell death.

The acute untoward reactions from radiotherapy depend primarily on the area to be irradiated. Total-body irradiation is associated with the most severe reactions and is employed to prepare the immune system for blood or marrow transplantation (BMT). Table 44.1 summarizes the acute effects of radiotherapy and nursing interventions that may be helpful in mitigating or preventing them. In limited areas of the country, proton beam radiation is available. Protons are positively charged subatomic particles that deposit energy differently than x-ray beams. There is no "exit dose" beyond the tumor involved in proton radiotherapy; therefore, the local control of the therapy is a huge benefit with no long-term effects to organs surrounding the target area (Hill-Kayser, Tochner, Both, et al., 2013). For example, some brain tumor patients receive radiation to the spine. With traditional forms of radiotherapy, long-term effects to nearby vital organs like the heart and lungs are possible; however,

*Chemotherapy and Biotherapy Guidelines and Recommendations for Practice can be purchased from the Oncology Nursing Society, 125 Enterprise Drive, Pittsburgh, PA 15275; 866-257-4667, 412-859-6100; www.ons.org.

with proton therapy the heart and lungs would not be affected, greatly reducing long-term effects.

Biologic Response Modifiers

Biologic response modifiers (BRMs) alter the relationship between tumor and host by therapeutically changing the host's biologic response to tumor cells. These agents or interventions may affect the host's immunologic mechanisms (immunotherapy); have direct antitumor activity; or stimulate cell growth, reducing the hematologic toxicity associated with chemotherapy (Fry, Sondel, & Mackall, 2016). Much of the current work in biotherapy is directed toward the use of monoclonal antibodies in the diagnosis and treatment of cancers. Through a complex process, special cells are fused to form a hybrid clone, or hybridoma, that produces antibodies that recognize a single specific antigen—hence the term *monoclonal antibody* (*mono* meaning "one" and *clone* meaning "exact duplicate"). These clones are then frozen, maintained in culture, or grown as tumors in mice to produce large quantities of the antibody. Monoclonal antibodies have several mechanisms of cytotoxic action, but their main effect is exerted on the small molecule inhibitors of the cell surface proteins (Fry et al.). A commonly used monoclonal antibody is rituximab, which directs its effect on the B-cell surface protein CD20 and is used for the treatment of NHL (Fry et al.).

Blood or Marrow Transplantation

Another approach to the treatment of childhood cancer is BMT. Candidates for transplantation are children who have diseases that require high doses of chemotherapy and/or replacement of dysfunctional bone marrow. The conditioning regimen consists of radiotherapy and/or high-dose chemotherapy to rid the body of malignant cells and suppress the immune system to prevent rejection of the transplanted marrow. Next, the marrow, stem cells, or cord blood obtained from a family member or volunteer donor (allogeneic) or the cells previously stored from the patient (autologous) are given to the patient by IV infusion. The newly transfused marrow or stem cells begin to produce functioning nonmalignant blood cells. In essence, the recipient accepts a new blood-forming organ.

The selection process for a suitable donor and the potential complications in transplantation are related to the human leukocyte antigen (HLA) system complex. There is a wide diversity for each of these HLA loci. The genes are inherited as a single unit, or *haplotype*. A child inherits one unit from each parent; thus a child and each parent have one identical and one nonidentical haplotype. Because the possible haplotype combinations among siblings follow the laws of Mendelian genetics, there is a one in four chance that two siblings have two identical haplotypes and are perfectly matched at the HLA loci.

The importance of HLA matching is to prevent the serious complication of graft-versus-host disease (GVHD). Because the child's immune system is essentially rendered nonfunctional, the recipient is unlikely to reject the bone marrow. However, the donor's marrow may contain antigens not matched to the recipient's antigens, which begin attacking body cells. The more closely the HLA systems match, the less likely GVHD is to develop. However, GVHD can occur even with a perfect HLA match because of unidentified and thus unmatched histocompatibility antigens (Gottschalk, Naik, Hegde, et al., 2016).

COMPLICATIONS OF THERAPY

Although tremendous advances have been achieved through current modes of cancer therapy, the successes are not without consequences. Numerous side effects are expected with chemotherapy and radiotherapy. Other complications that are less common but generally more serious are described here.

Pediatric Oncologic Emergencies

Tumor Lysis Syndrome

Life-threatening conditions may develop in children with cancer as a result of the malignancy and/or aggressive treatment modalities. Acute tumor lysis syndrome has hallmark metabolic abnormalities that are the direct result of rapid release of intracellular contents during the lysis of malignant cells. This typically occurs in patients with ALL or Burkitt lymphoma during the initial treatment period but may occur spontaneously before onset of therapy. Tumor lysis syndrome may also occur in other malignancies that have a large tumor burden, are very sensitive to chemotherapy, or have a rapid proliferative rate. The hallmark metabolic abnormalities of tumor lysis syndrome include hyperuricemia, hypocalcemia, hyperphosphatemia, and hyperkalemia. The crystallization of uric acid that can occur in cases of hyperuricemia can lead to obstructive nephropathy, tubular injury, acute renal failure, and death (McCurdy & Shanholtz, 2012).

Risk factors for development of tumor lysis syndrome include high white blood cell count at diagnosis, large tumor burden, sensitivity to chemotherapy, and high proliferative rate. In addition to the described metabolic abnormalities, children may develop a spectrum of clinical symptoms, including flank pain, lethargy, nausea and vomiting, muscle cramps, pruritus, tetany, and seizures.

Management of tumor lysis syndrome consists of early identification of patients at risk, prophylactic measures, and early interventions. Patients at risk for tumor lysis syndrome should have serum chemistries and urine pH monitored frequently, strict record of intake and output, and aggressive IV fluids. Medications to reduce uric acid formation and promote excretion of byproducts of purine metabolism, such as allopurinol, are often used. If tumor lysis syndrome occurs, IV hydration continues and the specific metabolic abnormalities are treated. Hyperuricemia is now effectively treated with recombinant urate oxidase, or rasburicase. This medication converts uric acid to allantoin, which is more soluble in urine. Exchange transfusions are sometimes necessary to reduce the metabolic consequences of massive tumor lysis, especially in children with a high tumor burden.

Hyperleukocytosis

Hyperleukocytosis, which is defined as a peripheral white blood cell count greater than $100,000/mm^3$, can lead to capillary obstruction, microinfarction, and organ dysfunction. Children often experience respiratory distress and cyanosis. They also experience neurologic changes, including altered level of consciousness, visual disturbances, agitation, confusion, ataxia, and delirium. Management consists of rapid cytoreduction by chemotherapy, hydration, urinary alkalinization, and allopurinol. Leukapheresis or exchange transfusion may be necessary.

Superior Vena Cava Syndrome

Space-occupying lesions located in the chest, especially from Hodgkin disease and NHL, may cause superior vena cava syndrome (SVCS), leading to airway compromise and potentially to respiratory failure. Children are initially seen with cyanosis of the face, neck, and upper chest; facial and upper extremity edema; and distended neck and chest veins. They may be anxious and have dyspnea, wheezing, or a frequent cough from airway obstruction. Management consists of airway protection and alleviation of respiratory distress. Rapid treatment is initiated, and symptoms typically improve as the disease is effectively treated.

Spinal Cord Compression

Different malignancies can invade or impinge on the spinal cord, causing acute symptoms of cord compression. Children with primary CNS tumors can have tumors that originate or spread to the spinal cord.

Other solid tumors, like neuroblastoma or rhabdomyosarcoma, can metastasize to the spinal cord and cause compression. Back pain is a common initial manifestation, but other symptoms can include sensation change, extremity weakness, loss of bowel and bladder function, and respiratory insufficiency. Careful physical examination is essential in early detection of symptoms, and MRI is the gold standard for diagnosis (McCurdy & Shanholtz, 2012). Treatment may include high-dose steroids to reduce associated edema and alleviate symptoms and rapid initiation of treatment such as emergent radiation or laminectomy if indicated.

CARE MANAGEMENT

This section presents an overview of general nursing concepts that apply to most childhood cancers. Specific nursing care for children with a particular type of cancer is discussed under each disease section later in this chapter. This discussion focuses on the physical aspects of care. Chapter 36 presents the emotional aspects.

QUALITY PATIENT OUTCOMES: The Child With Cancer
- Child and family educated on disease and treatment
- Treatment administered on schedule with appropriate drug doses
- Side effects of treatment managed
- Treatment complications prevented
- Child and family coping skills supported
- Quality of life during treatment maintained
- Child and family adjusted to chronic illness
- Growth and development maintained during treatment

SIGNS AND SYMPTOMS OF CANCER IN CHILDREN

Early detection is critical to early treatment and eventual cure. Cancers in children are often difficult to recognize. Therefore, being alert to the persistence of unusual symptoms is essential (see Box 44.1). This section discusses some of the more significant clues to pediatric cancer.

Pain may be an early or late initial sign of cancer and requires a careful history of its onset, characteristics, location, intensity, and alleviating factors. Pain may be generalized or present at a specific location. For example, bone pain occurs in approximately 20% of children with leukemia. Pain, swelling, and tenderness at the tumor site may be the initial sign in solid tumors. In addition, a mass is a typical finding in children with solid tumors. An abdominal mass in a child must be evaluated for a malignancy, such as Wilms tumor or neuroblastoma.

Fever is a frequent occurrence during childhood and is caused by numerous illnesses, including cancer. The cause of fever in cancer patients is infection or the malignant process itself. A careful skin assessment will reveal signs and symptoms of a low platelet count. Ecchymosis and petechiae are most commonly found on the child's extremities and under constricting parts of clothing like waistbands. Spontaneous gum or nose bleeding may occur when the platelet count falls below 20,000/mm³.

The child with malignant invasion of the bone marrow often appears pale, with symptoms of lethargy, weight loss, and generalized malaise. These symptoms may be attributed to anemia caused by the replacement of normal cells with malignant cells in the bone marrow. The nurse should assess for signs and symptoms of anemia (see Chapter 43).

Swollen lymph glands are another common finding in children. However, enlarged, firm lymph nodes in a child with fever for more than 1 week, a recent history of weight loss, or an abnormal chest X-ray may indicate a serious disease and should be evaluated further.

The presence of a white reflection as opposed to the normal red pupillary reflex in the pupil of a child's eye is the classic sign of retinoblastoma. Squinting, strabismus, or swelling can indicate other solid tumors of the eye.

The child with a brain tumor develops signs and symptoms according to the exact area of the brain involved. The nurse must perform a thorough neurologic assessment to identify the specific area of tumor involvement.

MANAGING SIDE EFFECTS OF TREATMENT

Cancer care encompasses more than treatments aimed at eliminating the malignant cells. Because of the delicate balance between killing malignant cells and preserving functional cells, supportive therapy is frequently needed during those times that serious damage occurs to normal body tissues. A major concern for the child receiving treatment for cancer is the risk for the development of complications secondary to the treatment.

Infection

The nurse caring for the child with fever must be aware of the signs and symptoms of septic shock, as discussed in Chapter 42. The child with fever who has an absolute neutrophil count (ANC) lower than 500/mm³ is at risk for the following (see Guidelines box: Calculating the Absolute Neutrophil Count):
- Overwhelming infection
- General malaise
- Invasion of organisms producing secondary infections

The child with fever is evaluated for potential sites of infection, such as from a needle puncture, mucosal ulceration, minor abrasion, or skin tear (e.g., a hangnail). Although the body may not be able to produce an adequate inflammatory response to the infection and the usual clinical signs of infection may be partially expressed or absent, fever will occur. Therefore, monitor the temperature closely. To identify the source of infection, the health care team takes blood, stool, urine, and nasopharyngeal cultures and chest X-ray.

Once infection is suspected, broad-spectrum IV antibiotic therapy is begun before the organism is identified and may be continued for 7 to 10 days. If the child does not have a venous access device, a peripheral IV should be inserted to prevent the inconvenience of multiple venipunctures in administering antibiotic therapy.

The organisms most lethal to these children are (1) viruses, particularly varicella (chickenpox), herpes zoster, herpes simplex, respiratory syncytial virus, influenza, and cytomegalovirus; (2) protozoa and *Toxoplasma gondii*; (3) fungi, especially *Pneumocystis jiroveci* (formally known as *P. carinii*) and *Candida albicans*; (4) gram-negative bacteria, such as *Pseudomonas aeruginosa, E. coli,* and *Klebsiella* organisms; and (5) gram-positive bacteria, especially *Staphylococcus* and *Enterococcus* species (Ardura & Koh, 2016). Prophylaxis against *Pneumocystis*

GUIDELINES

Calculating the Absolute Neutrophil Count

1. Determine the total percentage of neutrophils ("polys" or "segs," and "bands").
2. Multiply white blood cell (WBC) count by percentage of neutrophils.

Example

WBC = 1000/mm³, neutrophils = 7%, nonsegmented neutrophils (bands) = 7%

Step 1: 7% + 7% = 14%

Step 2: 0.14 × 1000 = 140/mm³ ANC

ANC, Absolute neutrophil count.

Fever and Neutropenia

Billy, 9 years of age, is undergoing chemotherapy for high-risk acute lymphoblastic leukemia (ALL) but has recently been hospitalized with a fever of 103° F (39.5° C). He last received chemotherapy 10 days ago with vincristine, doxorubicin, and PEG-L-asparaginase and is currently taking oral dexamethasone for 21 days. His current white blood cell count is 0.1/mm³, with an absolute neutrophil count (ANC) of 0. His platelet count is 31,000/mm³, and his hemoglobin is 8.1 g/dL. He has noticeable petechiae on his arms and legs with multiple bruises in various stages of healing.

After your morning report, you visit Billy, start your assessment, and note the following: Billy is an alert and oriented 9-year-old Caucasian boy. His tongue and oral mucosa are covered with a white plaque. Vital signs are as follows: Temperature, 102.6° F (39.2° C), axial; respiratory rate, 24 breaths/min; heart rate, 140 beats/min; and blood pressure, 100/56 mm Hg. Further observation of the patient and his surroundings reveals (1) a sign over his bed that reads "no needle punctures;" (2) he is currently getting 6 liters of oxygen via nasal cannula; (3) the Port-A-Cath is accessed with intravenous (IV) fluids infusing, and the dressing is clean and dry; and (4) a tympanic thermometer is in the room.

1. What evidence should you consider regarding this condition?
2. What additional information is required at this time?
3. List the nursing intervention(s) that have the highest priority.
4. Identify important patient-centered outcomes with reference to your nursing interventions.

Bleeding

Paul, 14 years of age, is undergoing chemotherapy for non-Hodgkin lymphoma (NHL) but has recently been hospitalized with an infection. He last received chemotherapy 12 days ago. His current platelet count is 28,000/mm³. He has noticeable petechiae on his arms and legs with multiple bruises in various stages of healing. After your morning report, you visit Paul, start your assessment, and note the following: Paul is an alert and oriented 14-year-old Caucasian boy. The right sclera has a hemorrhage, and multiple petechiae and bruises are on his arms and legs. Petechiae are noted on the buccal mucosa and palate. Further observation of the patient and his surroundings reveals (1) a sign over his bed that reads "no needle punctures;" (2) he is currently getting 6 liters of oxygen via nasal cannula; (3) the Port-A-Cath is accessed with intravenous (IV) fluids infusing, and the dressing is clean and dry; and (4) a tympanic thermometer is in the room.

1. What evidence should you consider regarding this condition?
2. What additional information is required at this time?
3. List the nursing intervention(s) that have the highest priority.
4. Identify important patient-centered outcomes with reference to your nursing interventions.

pneumonia, such as trimethoprim-sulfamethoxazole, is routinely given to most children during treatment for cancer (Ardura & Koh, 2016).

Colony-stimulating factors (CSFs), a family of glycoprotein hormones that regulate the reproduction, maturation, and function of blood cells, are now routinely used as supportive measures to prevent the side effects caused by low blood counts. CSFs promote stem cell proliferation and stimulate a more rapid maturation of the cells, allowing them to enter the bloodstream earlier. G-CSF (filgrastim [Neupogen], pegfilgrastim [Neulasta]) directs granulocyte development and can decrease the duration of neutropenia. This reduces the incidence and duration of infection in children receiving treatment for cancer. G-CSF is also being used to decrease the bone marrow recovery time after BMT (Ardura & Koh, 2016). Prevention of infection continues as a priority after discharge from the hospital. Some institutions allow the child to return to school when the ANC is above 500/mm³. Other institutions place no restrictions on the child, regardless of the blood count. If the level falls below this value, cautious isolation from crowded areas, such as shopping centers or subways, is advisable. At all times, encourage family members to practice good hand washing to avoid introducing pathogens into the home (see Clinical Reasoning Case Study box: Fever and Neutropenia).

Hemorrhage

Before the use of transfused platelets, hemorrhage was a leading cause of death in children with some types of cancer. Now most bleeding episodes can be prevented or controlled with judicious administration of platelet concentrates or platelet-rich plasma. Severe spontaneous internal hemorrhage varies but usually does not occur until the platelet count is 20,000/mm³ or less (Hockenberry, Kline, & Rodgers, 2016).

Platelet transfusions are generally reserved for active bleeding episodes that do not respond to local treatment, and that may occur during induction or relapse therapy. Epistaxis and gingival bleeding are the most common. The nurse teaches parents and other children measures to control nose bleeding. Applying pressure at the site without disturbing clot formation is the general rule. Platelet concentrates normally do not have to be cross-matched for blood group or type. However, because platelets contain specific antigen components similar to blood group factors, children who receive multiple transfusions may become sensitized to a platelet group other than their own. Therefore, platelets are cross-matched with the donor's blood components whenever possible.

During bleeding episodes, the parents and child need much emotional support (see Clinical Reasoning Case Study box: Bleeding). The sight of oozing blood is upsetting. Often parents request a platelet transfusion, unaware of the necessity of trying local measures first. The nurse can help calm their anxiety by explaining the reason for delaying a platelet transfusion until absolutely necessary. Because compatible donors decrease the risk for antigen formation in the recipient, the nurse should encourage parents to locate suitable donors for eventual blood use.

Children at home who have low platelet counts (usually <100,000/mm³) should avoid activities that might cause injury or bleeding, such as riding bicycles or skateboards, roller skating or in-line skating, climbing trees or playground equipment, and contact sports such as football or soccer. Once the platelet count rises, these restrictions are not necessary. In addition, aspirin and aspirin-containing products are not used; for mild pain or significantly elevated temperature, acetaminophen is substituted.

Anemia

Initially anemia may be profound from replacement of the healthy bone marrow by cancer cells. During induction therapy, blood transfusions with packed red blood cells may be necessary to raise the hemoglobin to levels approaching 10 g/dL. The usual precautions in caring for the child are instituted (see Chapter 43).

Anemia is also a consequence of drug-induced myelosuppression. Although not as severely affected as the white blood cells, erythrocyte production may be delayed. Because children have an amazing capacity to withstand low hemoglobin levels, the best approach is to allow the child to regulate activity with reasonable adult supervision. It may be necessary for the parents to alert the teacher to the child's physical limitations, particularly in terms of strenuous activity.

Nausea and Vomiting

The nausea and vomiting that occur shortly after administration of chemotherapy and as a result of cranial or abdominal irradiation can be profound. 5-Hydroxytryptamine-3 receptor antagonists are the antiemetics of choice to manage nausea and vomiting caused by chemotherapy and radiotherapy (Dupuis, Boodhan, Holdsworth, et al., 2013). The advantage of these agents over conventional drugs is that they produce no extrapyramidal side effects. Multiple studies have shown ondansetron (Zofran) to be effective for patients receiving moderate to highly emetic chemotherapy, and ondansetron in combination with dexamethasone has been more effective than ondansetron alone (Dupuis et al.).

Other agents for mild to moderate vomiting include phenothiazine-type drugs. In addition, synthetic cannabinoids are used in children undergoing chemotherapy, such as dronabinol. Dronabinol helps control nausea and vomiting and also is an effective appetite stimulant (Feyer & Jordan, 2011).

The most beneficial regimen for antiemetic control has been the administration of the antiemetic before the chemotherapy begins (30 minutes to 1 hour before) and regular (not as-needed) administration for at least 24 hours after chemotherapy. The goal is to prevent the child from ever experiencing nausea or vomiting, because this can prevent the development of anticipatory symptoms (the conditioned response of developing nausea and vomiting before receiving the drug). Giving the antineoplastic drug with a mild sedative at bedtime is also helpful for some children, and there is evidence that nighttime administration of drugs such as methotrexate and 6-mercaptopurine may be more effective cytotoxically than morning administration.

Altered Nutrition

Altered nutrition is a common side effect of treatment. Continued assessment of the child's nutritional status, child's intake, and energy expenditure must occur throughout treatment. The child's height, weight, and head circumference (for children younger than 3 years of age) must be measured routinely during visits to the hospital or clinic. Energy reserves should be evaluated with routine skinfold measurements. Biochemical assays such as serum prealbumin, transferrin, and albumin may be helpful to evaluate nutritional status in some children, but a single assay should not be used alone for a nutritional evaluation (Lawson, Daley, Sams, et al., 2013). There are no specific criteria that mandate nutritional interventions in children undergoing cancer treatment. Instead each child should have an individualized nutritional care plan based on routine assessments.

Nutritional status is important to maintain because a compromised nutritional status can contribute to reduced tolerance to treatment, altered metabolism of chemotherapy drugs, prolonged episodes of neutropenia, and increased risk for infection.

Supportive nutrition measures include oral supplements with high-protein and high-calorie foods. Ways to increase calories include using whole milk, adding tofu (high in protein) to meals, and serving full-fat instead on nonfat or low-fat items. Cooking with butter; adding sugar or cheese on foods; and making high-calorie snacks such as trail mix, peanut butter, or dried fruit readily available for the child are other ways to increase calories. Enteral feeding or parenteral hyperalimentation may be necessary when children are unable to maintain the necessary calories to prevent weight loss. Chapter 39 discusses these interventions in more detail.

Mucosal Ulceration

One of the most distressing side effects of several chemotherapy drugs is gastrointestinal mucosal cell damage, which results in ulcers anywhere along the alimentary tract. Oral ulcers (stomatitis) are red, eroded, painful areas in the mouth or pharynx. Similar lesions may extend along the esophagus and occur in the rectal area. They greatly compound anorexia because eating is extremely uncomfortable.

> **! NURSING ALERT**
>
> Viscous lidocaine is not recommended for young children. If applied to the pharynx, it may depress the gag reflex, increasing the risk for aspiration. Seizures have also been associated with the use of oral viscous lidocaine, most likely as a result of the rapid absorption into the bloodstream via the oral lesions (Lutwak, Howland, Gambetta, et al., 2013).

Some interventions that are helpful when oral ulcers develop are feeding a bland, moist, soft diet; using a soft sponge toothbrush (Toothette) instead of a toothbrush; frequently rinsing the mouth with chlorhexidine mouthwash or sodium bicarbonate and salt mouth rinses (using a solution of 1 tsp of baking soda and $\frac{1}{2}$ tsp of table salt in 1 quart of water); using sucralfate; and administering local anesthetics without alcohol, such as a solution of diphenhydramine and Maalox (aluminum and magnesium hydroxide) (Miller, Donald, & Hagemann, 2012). Although local anesthetics are effective in temporarily relieving the pain, many children dislike the taste and numb feeling they produce.

> **! NURSING ALERT**
>
> Avoid agents such as lemon glycerin swabs and hydrogen peroxide because of the drying effects on the mucosa. In addition, lemon may be very irritating, especially on eroded tissue.

Administering mouth care is particularly difficult in infants and toddlers. A satisfactory method of cleaning the gums is to wrap a piece of gauze around a finger; soak it in saline or plain water; and swab the gums, palate, and inner cheek surfaces with the finger. Children should perform mouth care routinely before and after any feeding and as often as every 2 to 4 hours to rid mucosal surfaces of debris, which becomes an excellent medium for bacterial and fungal growth.

Difficulty eating is a major problem with stomatitis and may warrant hospitalization if the child refuses fluids. The child usually chooses the foods that are best tolerated. Drinking can usually be encouraged if a straw is used to bypass the ulcerated oral mucosa. The nurse should encourage parents to relax any eating pressures because the anorexia accompanying stomatitis is well justified and usually temporary. Ordinarily, severe mucosal ulceration indicates a need for decreased chemotherapy until complete healing takes place. Analgesics, including opioids, may be needed when treatment cannot be altered, such as during BMT.

If rectal ulcers develop, meticulous toilet hygiene, warm sitz baths after each bowel movement, and an occlusive ointment applied to the ulcerated area promote healing; the use of stool softeners is necessary to prevent further discomfort. Parents should record bowel movements because the child may voluntarily avoid defecation to prevent discomfort. Rectal temperatures and suppositories are always avoided because they may traumatize the area.

Neurologic Problems

Vincristine, and to a lesser extent vinblastine, can cause various neurotoxic effects. One of the more common neurotoxic effects is severe constipation caused from decreased bowel innervation. Administration of opioids can further aggravate constipation. The nurse advises parents to record bowel movements and to notify the health care provider of a change in stool habits. Physical activity and stool softeners are helpful in preventing the problem, but laxatives, such as polyethylene glycol, are often necessary to stimulate evacuation. Dietary changes such as increased fiber may not be effective, because the increased bulk tends to increase fecal distention and discomfort without producing the necessary mechanical stimulation.

Footdrop and weakness and numbness of the extremities are another common neurotoxic effect and may cause difficulty in walking or fine hand movement. The nurse should look for these problems and warn parents of these side effects, which are reversible once the drug is stopped. Wearing high-top tennis shoes or using a footboard in bed is used to preserve proper alignment. If weakness occurs while the child is attending school, temporary alteration of activity may be necessary. Parents should inform the teacher of the situation to avoid unrealistic expectations of the child's abilities.

Another neurotoxic effect is severe jaw pain. Analgesics may help relieve the discomfort. Children may avoid movement by not talking or chewing, although continuous chewing, such as with gum, may actually reduce the pain. A neurologic syndrome, postirradiation somnolence, may develop 5 to 8 weeks after CNS irradiation and last for 4 to 15 days. It is characterized by somnolence with or without fever, anorexia, and nausea and vomiting. Parents should be warned of the possibility of such symptoms and encouraged to seek medical evaluation, because somnolence may be an early indicator of long-term neurologic sequelae after cranial irradiation.

Hemorrhagic Cystitis

Sterile hemorrhagic cystitis is a side effect of chemical irritation to the bladder from chemotherapy or radiotherapy. It can be prevented by (1) a liberal oral or parenteral fluid intake (at least one and a half times the recommended daily fluid requirement [2 L/m^2/day]); (2) frequent voiding immediately after feeling the urge, including immediately before bed, one nighttime void, and upon arising; (3) administration of the drug early in the day to allow for sufficient fluids and frequent voiding; and (4) administration of mesna, a drug that inhibits the urotoxicity of cyclophosphamide and ifosfamide.

> **! NURSING ALERT**
>
> If signs of cystitis such as dysuria or hematuria occur, prompt medical evaluation is needed. Hemorrhagic cystitis warrants a full workup and prompt intervention.

In most cases, IV fluids are given before, during, and after the drug to ensure adequate hydration, thereby eliminating the need for the child's drinking large amounts of fluid. If oral home administration is prescribed, the family needs specific instructions on exactly how much fluid the child must have.

Alopecia

Hair loss is a side effect of several chemotherapeutic drugs and cranial irradiation. Not all children lose their hair during drug therapy, and some children may experience thinning of the hair rather than baldness. However, retaining hair is the exception rather than the rule. It is better to warn children and parents of this side effect to allow time to adapt to the side effect.

The family should know that the hair falls out in clumps, causing patchy baldness. To lessen the trauma of seeing large amounts of hair on bed linen or clothing, the child can wear a disposable surgical cap to collect the shed hair during the period of greatest hair loss, or the hair can be cut short or shaved. Families should also be aware that wigs are tax deductible and that hair typically regrows in 3 to 6 months. The hair is often a different color and texture than before cancer treatment.

> **! NURSING ALERT**
>
> Encouraging children to choose a wig similar to their own hairstyle and color before the hair falls out is helpful in fostering later adjustment to hair loss.

If the child chooses not to wear a wig, attention to some type of head covering is important, especially in cold or sunny climates. Scalp hygiene is also important. The scalp should be washed regularly as with any other body part.

Steroid Effects

Short-term steroid therapy produces physical changes and alterations in body image, which, although not clinically significant, can be extremely distressing to older children. One of these is cushingoid appearance. The child's face becomes rounded and puffy. Unlike hair loss, little can be done to camouflage this obvious change, although careful avoidance of salt and salt-containing foods can help reduce fluid accumulation. It is not unusual for other children to tease the child. It is helpful to reassure the child that, after cessation of the drug, the facial contours will return to normal. The use of loose-fitting clothes, such as warm-up outfits, can help camouflage the change in weight.

Children receiving steroid therapy look healthy. The moon face, red cheeks, supraclavicular fat pads, protuberant abdomen, and fluid retention indicate weight gain. However, the actual weight gain resulting from increased muscle mass and subcutaneous tissue may be small. Therefore, the nurse should evaluate weight gain by observing the extremities and measuring skinfold thickness and arm circumference during steroid therapy to determine whether the weight gain is a result of increased dietary intake.

Shortly after beginning steroid therapy, children may experience a number of mood changes, which range from feelings of well-being and euphoria to depression and irritability. If parents are unaware of these drug-induced changes, they may become unduly concerned. Therefore, the nurse should warn them of the reactions and encourage them to discuss the behavioral changes with each other and the child.

NURSING CARE DURING BLOOD OR MARROW TRANSPLANTATION

Because of the aggressive preconditioning therapy used to remove the marrow and the potential for complications while waiting for engraftment of transplanted stem cells, children undergoing BMT are hospitalized for several weeks. BMT patients must have numerous procedures performed, such as the insertion of a venous access device, administration of intensive chemotherapy and irradiation, and strict infectious precautions. During the period after transplantation and before the new marrow begins adequately replacing granulocytes, the child is extremely susceptible to infection, and any infection can be life-threatening. In addition, many of the side effects previously discussed occur in the child undergoing BMT.

The most common complication in allogeneic transplants is acute GVHD, which can affect the skin, gastrointestinal tract, and liver. The characteristics and severity of the manifestations vary according to the severity and area affected. Emphasis is now placed on the prevention of GVHD, using various agents such as a calcineurin inhibitor in conjunction with mycophenolate mofetil, methotrexate, or sirolimus (Gottschalk et al., 2016). Treatment involves the use of steroids or other immunosuppressive medications. However, this treatment further increases the risk for infection in the already susceptible patient. All blood products should be irradiated to minimize the introduction of additional antigens.

Throughout this long ordeal, the family is worried about successful engraftment and fatal complications. An unfortunate posttransplant possibility is recurrence of the disease after engraftment. Consequently, nurses need to provide sensitive care and maintain a supportive attitude during the many crises that may arise. If the procedure is not successful, the care needed by these families is consistent with that required by the family of any child with a life-threatening disorder (see Chapter 36).

PREPARATION FOR PROCEDURES

Children in particular need psychologic preparation for the various treatment modalities, which often involve surgery, IV injections, bone marrow aspiration, and LP. The diagnostic procedures initially employed to confirm the diagnosis and those that are repeated to monitor treatment can be a source of discomfort and stress to the child and family. Even noninvasive procedures such as imaging and radiologic tests are frightening to a young child. Many of these tests require the child to lie absolutely motionless for a prolonged time in a confined space with little or no communication with a supportive adult. Consequently, infants and young children are usually sedated, and older children need an explanation of what to expect and reminders during the test of how much longer they must remain still. The same principles for preparing children for procedures that are discussed in Chapter 39 apply here, including the option of having parents stay with the child whenever possible. Children who undergo repeated tests need additional preparation and emotional support to decrease their stress.

Two procedures, bone marrow studies and LP, are so commonly performed in many types of childhood cancer that they deserve special consideration in preparing children (Fig. 44.2). Professionals caring for children with cancer recommend the use of developmentally appropriate support using both pharmacologic and nonpharmacologic approaches and sedation if required (see Chapter 30).

Topical anesthetics such as eutectic mixture of local anesthetics (EMLA) and LMX4 creams are used as a local anesthetic before intrusive procedures, including venipunctures, implanted port access, LPs, and subcutaneous or intramuscular injections (Hockenberry et al., 2016). Local intradermal anesthesia of lidocaine is frequently used for LP and bone marrow examination. To reduce the stinging sensation from lidocaine, sodium bicarbonate should be added (see the "Pain Management" section in Chapter 30). Deeper infiltration of the muscle and periosteum of the bone with buffered lidocaine further reduces the pain from the large-bore aspiration or biopsy needle entering the bone. For bone marrow studies, LPs, and other procedures, children of preschool

age and beyond should be prepared beforehand. Physical care after the procedures is minimal. A small pressure bandage is applied to the bone marrow puncture site, and an adhesive bandage is applied to the LP site. No activity restriction is necessary after the bone marrow test, although the site is usually sore and the child may prefer to remain quiet. Recommendations after LP vary.

PAIN MANAGEMENT

Nurses must be knowledgeable about the basic pathophysiology of cancer pain and treatment-related side effects. The World Health Organization's three-step analgesic pain ladder should be incorporated into the approach to pain management for every child with cancer (Wong, Lau, Palozzi, et al., 2012). Nurses must acquire extensive knowledge of nonopioid and opioid analgesics used in pediatric pain management. Interdisciplinary pain management teams are used in many pediatric cancer centers. These teams serve as consultants and provide expertise in the assessment and management of pain. The nurse often serves as the coordinator of care, playing a key role in cancer pain management.

Chapter 30 discusses pharmacologic management of disease-related pain, which involves a variety of methods. It may take more than a trial of one type of medication to find the appropriate agent to manage a patient's pain. Nonsteroidal antiinflammatory drugs (NSAIDs), acetaminophen with codeine, oxycodone, and morphine are commonly used agents in the management of disease-related pain (Wong et al., 2012). Appropriate dosing is imperative. Doses are titrated to increase the amount of analgesia and minimize side effects.

HEALTH PROMOTION

Children with cancer require the same basic health supervision as any child. Sometimes the overwhelming needs and demands placed on the family, coupled with the singular concern focused on the cancer by both family and practitioners, result in a lack of attention to normal health care needs. Nurses should monitor the type of primary care the child receives, using as a guideline recommendations for health supervision. Areas of particular concern are growth, physical and cognitive development, and neurologic status. Two other areas are also important: (1) dental care, because of potential side effects from treatment, and (2) immunizations, because of concern with live virus vaccines and immunosuppression.

Dental Care

Irradiation to the head and neck can cause a number of late complications (Landier, Armenian, Meadows, et al., 2016). Some are irreversible, such as facial asymmetry, but those affecting the teeth and gums (e.g., caries, periodontal disease) benefit from excellent oral hygiene, including regular use of systemic and topical fluoride and regular dental examinations and cleaning (see the "Dental Health" section in Chapter 34). There is evidence of delayed or absent development of the permanent teeth (Effinger et al., 2014). Children need to be aware of this possibility and need help to explain the delay to peers.

Immunizations

Viral replication after the administration of live vaccine for polio, measles, rubella, and mumps can cause serious disease in immunocompromised children. The child receiving chemotherapy for cancer should not receive live, attenuated vaccines. Inactivated vaccines can be given to immunosuppressed children. Siblings and other family members can receive the live measles, mumps, and rubella vaccine and the varicella vaccine without risk to the child who is immunosuppressed.

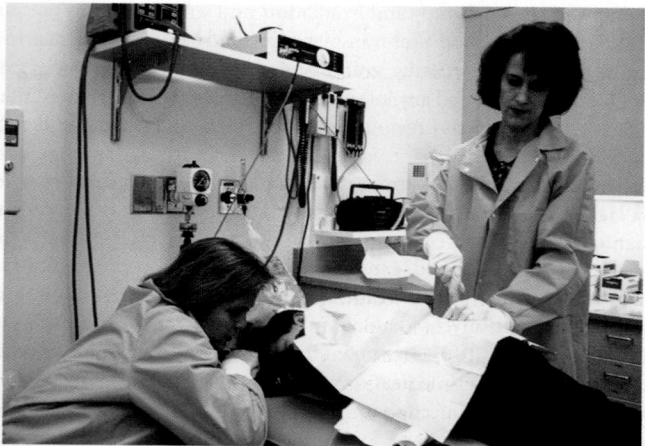

FIG 44.2 Child with leukemia undergoing bone marrow aspiration.

An important indication for isolation is an outbreak of childhood disease, especially chickenpox. If the child has been exposed to the varicella virus, varicella-zoster immune globulin given within 96 hours may favorably alter the course of the disease. Antiviral agents, such as acyclovir, should be given if the child develops varicella. Without treatment, death from disseminated varicella occurs in 7% to 20% of patients, due to disseminated disease in the liver, lung, and CNS (Ardura & Koh, 2016) (see the "Immunizations" section in Chapter 31.)

> **! NURSING ALERT**
>
> Children vaccinated 2 weeks before or during chemotherapy should be considered unimmunized and should be revaccinated or receive live virus vaccines 6 months after chemotherapy has stopped (Ruggiero, Battista, Coccia, et al., 2011). Most institutions have individual guidelines regarding vaccinations in a child undergoing immunosuppressive therapy. The nurse should be aware of these guidelines and educate patients and families.

FAMILY EDUCATION

Nurses working with children who have cancer have a significant supportive role in helping the family understand the various therapies, preventing or managing expected side effects or toxicities, and observing for late effects of treatment. Education is a constant feature of the nursing role, especially in terms of new treatments, clinical trials, and home care. Because of the anxiety generated by the diagnosis of cancer, some families may resort to unproven methods of treatment. Nurses are instrumental in helping families avoid seeking unproven and potentially unsafe "remedies" by encouraging the families to discuss concerns and questions openly with their health care provider. The American Cancer Society and local and state medical societies are reliable sources of information concerning research on investigational versus quack methods of cancer therapy. The Association of Pediatric Hematology/Oncology Nurses* has developed numerous educational materials for family and child teaching. The American Childhood Cancer Organization† is an international organization providing support, education, and advocacy programs for children with cancer and their families.

Instruction regarding home care frequently involves teaching about medication schedules, observing for side effects or toxicities that require further evaluation, taking measures to prevent or manage these problems, and caring for special devices such as central venous catheters.‡ Compliance is an important issue, because poor adherence to regimens can result in disease relapse or serious medical complications. Every effort must be made to ensure that the family understands the importance of adhering to the prescribed treatment schedule and measures to improve compliance (see Chapter 39).

CESSATION OF THERAPY

Care does not end when the child completes therapy. With the increasing awareness of late effects, nurses play an important role in the assessment

*8735 W. Higgins Road, Suite 300, Chicago, IL 60631; 847-375-4724; www.aphon.org.
†PO Box 498, Kensington, MD 20895; 855-858-2226 or 301-962-3520; www.acco.org.
‡Home care instructions for giving medications to children and caring for a central venous catheter are available in Wilson, D., & Hockenberry, M.J. (2008). *Wong's clinical manual of pediatric nursing* (7th ed.). St. Louis, MO: Mosby/

of the child for problems, such as delayed growth, secondary malignancies, and disturbances in any body system. The family needs to be aware of the importance of continued medical supervision. Other health care professionals caring for the child (e.g., school nurses, family physicians, and dentists) should be informed of the child's cancer diagnosis. As children reach adulthood, they may benefit from genetic counseling regarding cancers that are likely to be inherited. If the possibility of infertility exists, fertility options should be discussed for pubertal males and females prior to the start of treatment. The Children's Oncology Group (2014) has developed guidelines for long-term follow-up care for pediatric cancer survivors. Nurses involved with these children should be familiar with these guidelines and use all opportunities to teach patients and families regarding needed continued care.

CANCERS OF BLOOD AND LYMPH SYSTEMS

LEUKEMIAS

Acute Leukemias

Leukemia is a broad term given to a group of malignant diseases of the bone marrow and lymphatic system. It is a complex disease of varying heterogeneity. Consequently, classification has become increasingly complex, sophisticated, and essential because identification of the subtype of leukemia has therapeutic and prognostic implications. The following is an overview of the major classification systems currently used.

Morphology

In children, two forms are generally recognized: ALL and acute myelogenous leukemia (AML). Synonyms for ALL include lymphatic, lymphocytic, lymphoid, and lymphoblastic leukemia. ALL is the most common form of childhood cancer, with an annual incidence of 2 to 5 cases per 100,000 children (Rabin, Gramatges, Margolin, et al., 2016). It occurs more frequently in boys than in girls and in Caucasians than in African-Americans (Rabin et al.). The peak onset is between 2 and 5 years of age. It is one of the forms of pediatric cancer that has demonstrated dramatic improvements in survival rates. Before the use of antileukemic agents in 1948, a child with ALL lived 2 to 3 months. Current long-term disease-free survival rates for children with ALL approach 80% in major research centers.

AML accounts for 20% of all cases of childhood leukemia and has an annual incidence of 8 cases per 1 million children (Arceci & Meshinchi, 2016). The incidence is similar for males and females, and higher rates are seen during the first year of life. Overall survival rates vary dramatically according to sex, race, and constitutional characteristics of the disease (Arceci & Meshinchi, 2016).

Pathologic and Related Clinical Manifestations

Leukemia is an unrestricted proliferation of immature white blood cells in the blood-forming tissues of the body. Although not a "tumor" as such, the leukemic cells demonstrate the neoplastic properties of solid cancers. Thus the resultant pathologic and clinical manifestations of the disease are caused by infiltration and replacement of any tissue of the body with nonfunctional leukemic cells. Highly vascular organs, such as the spleen and liver, are most severely affected.

To understand the pathophysiology of the leukemic process, it is important to clarify two common misconceptions. First, although leukemia is an overproduction of white blood cells, most often the leukocyte count is low. Instead, the peripheral blood smear and, more definitively, the bone marrow examination reveal greatly elevated counts of immature cells, or blasts. Second, these immature cells do not deliberately attack and destroy the normal blood cells or vascular tissues. Cellular destruction occurs through the process of infiltration and

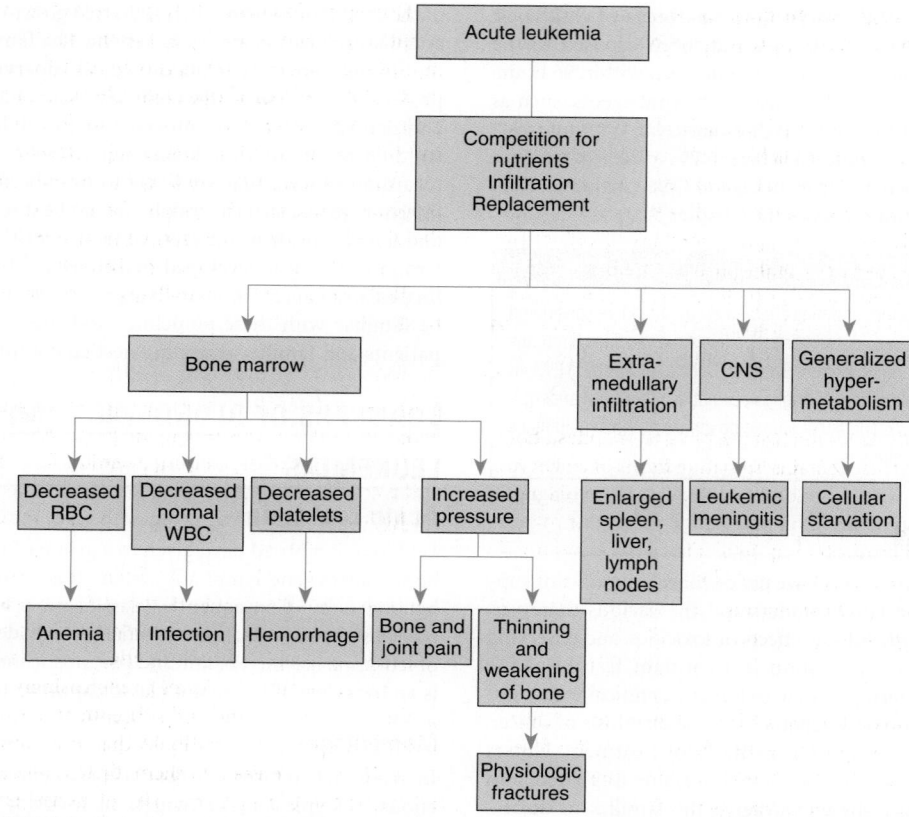

FIG 44.3 Principal sites of tissue involvement in leukemia. *CNS,* Central nervous system; *RBC,* red blood cell; *WBC,* white blood cell.

subsequent competition for metabolic elements. The following discussion elaborates on the pathologic process and related clinical manifestations in the most susceptible organs of the body (Fig. 44.3).

Bone Marrow Dysfunction

In all types of leukemia, the proliferating cells depress bone marrow production of the formed elements of the blood by competing for and depriving the normal cells of the essential nutrients for metabolism. The three main consequences are (1) anemia from decreased erythrocytes, (2) infection from neutropenia, and (3) bleeding from decreased platelet production.

The invasion of the bone marrow with leukemic cells gradually causes a weakening of the bone and a tendency toward fractures. As leukemic cells invade the periosteum, increasing pressure causes severe pain. The most frequent presenting signs and symptoms of leukemia are a result of infiltration of the bone marrow. These include fever, pallor, fatigue, anorexia, hemorrhage (usually petechiae), and bone and joint pain. In the presence of neutropenia, the body's normal bacterial flora can become aggressive pathogens. Any break in the skin is a potential site of infection. Frequently, vague abdominal pain is caused by areas of inflammation from normal flora within the intestinal tract.

Disturbance of Involved Organs

The spleen, liver, and lymph glands demonstrate marked infiltration, enlargement, and eventually fibrosis. Hepatosplenomegaly is typically more common than lymphadenopathy.

The next most important site of involvement is the CNS. Less than 5% of patients with CNS involvement have B-cell ALL, and 10% to 20% of patients with CNS involvement have T-cell ALL (Rabin et al.,

2016). The use of prophylactic CNS intrathecal therapy has dramatically decreased the incidence of CNS relapse in these patients.

Additional sites of involvement may be the cranial nerves (most often cranial nerve VII, or the facial nerve) and spinal nerves, particularly of the lumbosacral plexus, hypothalamus, and cerebellum. Clinical manifestations for these sites are directly related to the area involved. For example, with lumbosacral invasion, the patient has weakness in the lower extremities, pain radiating down the legs to the feet, and difficulty in voiding. Although such signs may suggest a brain tumor, the absence of localized signs often leads to the discovery of CNS involvement in leukemia. Other sites that may become invaded with leukemic cells include the kidneys, testes, prostate, ovaries, gastrointestinal tract, and lungs.

Onset

The onset of leukemia varies from acute to insidious. In most instances, the child displays remarkably few symptoms. For example, leukemia may be diagnosed when a minor infection, such as a cold, fails to completely disappear. The child is pale, listless, irritable, febrile, and anorexic. Parents often suspect some underlying problem when they observe the weight loss, petechiae, bruising without cause, and continued complaints of bone and joint pain.

At other times leukemia is diagnosed after an extended history of signs and symptoms mimicking such conditions as rheumatoid arthritis or mononucleosis. In some cases, the diagnosis of leukemia accompanies some totally unrelated event, such as a routine physical examination or injury.

The history not only yields valuable medical information regarding the subsequent course of the illness but also bears heavily on the parents' emotional reaction to the diagnosis. In most instances, the diagnosis is an unexpected revelation of catastrophic proportion.

Prognostic Factors

The most important prognostic factors in determining long-term survival for children with ALL are the initial white blood cell count, the patient's age at diagnosis, cytogenetics, the immunologic subtype, and the child's sex. Favorable indicators include a white blood cell count <50,000/mm^3, 2 to 10 years of age, hyperdiploid cytogenetics, early pre–B cell immunologic subtype, and female sex. For children with AML, prognostic factors associated with a poorer prognosis include certain chromosome abnormalities (monosomy 5 or 7), chromosome rearrangements, and a poor initial response to therapy (Arceci & Meshinchi, 2016).

Diagnostic Evaluation

Leukemia is usually suspected from the history, physical manifestations, and a peripheral blood smear that contains immature forms of leukocytes, frequently in combination with low blood counts. Definitive diagnosis is based on bone marrow aspiration or biopsy. Typically the bone marrow shows a monotonous infiltrate of blast cells. Once the diagnosis is confirmed, a LP is performed to determine whether there is any CNS involvement. Although only a small number of children have CNS involvement, they are usually asymptomatic.

Therapeutic Management

Treatment of leukemia involves the use of IV and intrathecal chemotherapeutic agents. Radiation is sometimes used for resistant CNS disease or testicular relapse. Typically leukemia treatment is divided into phases: (1) induction therapy, which achieves a complete remission or clinical disappearance of leukemic cells; (2) intensification (or consolidation) therapy, which further decreases the total tumor burden; and (3) maintenance therapy, which consists of further chemotherapy to ensure the disease stays in remission. Although the combination of drugs and possibility of irradiation may vary according to the institution, the patient's prognostic or risk characteristics, and the type of leukemia being treated, the following general principles for each phase are consistently employed.

Induction Therapy

Almost immediately after confirmation of the diagnosis, induction therapy is begun and lasts for 4 to 5 weeks. A complete remission is determined by the absence of clinical signs or symptoms of the disease and the presence of less than 5% blast cells in the bone marrow (Rabin et al., 2016).

Because many of the chemotherapy drugs also cause myelosuppression of normal blood elements, the period immediately after a remission can be critical. The body is defenseless against invading organisms (especially normal bacterial flora) and susceptible to spontaneous hemorrhage. Consequently, supportive therapy during this time is essential.

Intensification or Consolidation Therapy

Intensification or consolidation therapy is used to further decrease the number of leukemic cells in the child's body. The intensification phase consists of pulses of chemotherapy medications given periodically during the first 6 months of treatment. The specific agents used for intensification therapy depend on the type of leukemia and the child's risk factors.

Maintenance Therapy

The goal of maintenance therapy is to preserve remission and further reduce the number of leukemic cells. Combined drug regimens have been more successful in maintaining remissions and preventing drug resistance.

During maintenance therapy, weekly or monthly complete blood counts are taken to evaluate the marrow's response to the drugs. If myelosuppression becomes severe (usually indicated by an ANC less than 1000/mm^3) or if toxic side effects occur, therapy is temporarily stopped or the dose decreased. Duration of therapy has been based on clinical experience comparing survival rates for various time intervals and is concerned with preventing deleterious effects of excessive treatment. Although the optimum time for discontinuing therapy is not known, current practice is to continue treatment for 2 to 3 years. After cessation of therapy, all children require regular medical evaluation for surveillance of relapse and long-term sequelae of treatment.

Central Nervous System Prophylactic Therapy

Children with leukemia are at risk for invasion of the CNS by the leukemic cells. For this reason, many children receive CNS prophylactic therapy. Because of the concern regarding late effects of cranial irradiation and secondary malignancies, this mode of therapy is generally reserved for high-risk patients or those with resistant CNS disease.

Reinduction Therapy After Relapse

For many children, additional therapy becomes necessary when a relapse occurs, as evidenced by the presence of leukemic cells within the bone marrow. Although remissions may be achieved after more than one relapse, each relapse indicates an increasingly poor prognosis. However, more long-term second and subsequent remissions are occurring, and these may have better outlooks than previously thought.

A site that is resistant to chemotherapy and is responsible for leukemic relapse is the testes. A minority of males experience relapses during maintenance therapy or have occult disease after cessation of therapy. Treatment for testicular disease includes bilateral testicular irradiation, and intensive systemic chemotherapy (Rabin et al., 2016).

Blood or Marrow Transplantation

BMT has been used successfully in treating some children with ALL and AML. In general, BMT is not recommended for children with ALL during the first remission because of the excellent results possible with chemotherapy. The indication for BMT are those with ALL who are stratified as high risk or have a poor early therapy response (Gottschalk et al., 2016). Because of the poorer prognosis in children with AML, transplantation may be considered during the first remission when a suitable donor is available (Gottschalk et al., 2016).

Care Management

Nursing care of the child with leukemia is directly related to the regimen of therapy. Myelosuppression, drug toxicity, and leukemic infiltration cause secondary complications that necessitate supportive physical care. This discussion focuses on supportive interventions for the child with leukemia and the family. General aspects of care appropriate for the child with leukemia are discussed in the "Care Management" section earlier in this chapter.

Prepare the Family for Diagnostic and Therapeutic Procedures

From the time before diagnosis to cessation of therapy, children must undergo several tests, the most traumatic of which are bone marrow aspiration or biopsy and LP. Multiple finger sticks and venipunctures for blood analysis and drug infusion are common occurrences for several years after the diagnosis. Therefore, the child needs an explanation of the rationale for each procedure and what can be expected (see the "Preparation for Diagnostic and Therapeutic Procedures" section in Chapter 39).

Provide Continued Emotional Support

Nursing care of the child with leukemia is based on typical problems the family confronts during the treatment phases. The nurse's role is one of continual support, guidance, clarification, and judgment. Parents need to know how to recognize symptoms that demand medical attention. Although some of the reactions discussed are expected, parents should still report them to their health care provider. Warning parents of their possible occurrence beforehand also allows them to prepare. At the same time, it reassures them that these reactions are not caused by a return of leukemic cells.

Another aspect of continued emotional support involves prognosis. Leukemia is not invariably fatal, but present statistics must be correctly interpreted. Although almost 80% of children with ALL live 5 years or longer, these are average estimates that apply to those children treated with the most successful protocols since diagnosis. For the high-risk child with ALL, the prognosis may be significantly poorer, and a portion of patients will relapse. The nurse must realize that parents' understanding of the chances for survival requires an adjustment period. During the initial diagnosis or when a relapse occurs, parents may find it difficult to "hear" the facts. An understanding of each member's emotional needs, as well as competent care of physical ones, is essential to the positive, growth-promoting support of the family. Comprehensive emotional support for the family of a child with a chronic illness and the child at end of life is discussed in Chapter 36.

LYMPHOMAS

The lymphomas, a group of neoplastic diseases that arise from the lymphoid and hematopoietic systems, are divided into Hodgkin disease and NHL. These diseases are further subdivided according to tissue type and extent of disease (staging). In children, NHL is more common than Hodgkin disease. Although Hodgkin disease is extremely rare before 5 years of age, there is a striking increase in children 15 to 19 years of age, when it occurs with almost the same frequency as leukemia.

Hodgkin Disease

Hodgkin disease affects about 29 in 1 million children, mostly adolescents (National Cancer Institute, 2015a). The malignancy originates in the lymphoid system and primarily involves the lymph nodes. It predictably metastasizes to non-nodal or extralymphatic sites, especially the spleen, liver, bone marrow, lungs, and mediastinum (i.e., mass of tissues and organs separating the lungs, including the heart and its vessels, trachea, esophagus, thymus, and lymph nodes), although no tissue is exempt from involvement (Fig. 44.4). It is classified according to four histologic types: (1) lymphocytic predominance, (2) nodular sclerosis, (3) mixed cellularity, and (4) lymphocytic depletion. With present treatment protocols, the histologic stage of the disease has less prognostic significance.

Staging and Prognosis

Accurate staging of the extent of disease is the basis for treatment protocols and expected prognosis. More than one staging system exists; Box 44.2 shows the Ann Arbor Staging Classification.

Each stage is further subdivided into A, B, E, or S. Stage A denotes absence of associated general symptoms. Stage B indicates presence of symptoms, such as night sweats, fever (100.4°F [38°C]), or weight loss of 10% or more during the preceding 6 months. Stage E represents extralymphatic disease beyond the contiguous nodal disease. Stage S is used when the disease involves the spleen. Subtype B has a significantly poorer prognosis than others (Metzger, Krasin, Choi, et al., 2016).

The prognosis for patients with Hodgkin disease has improved dramatically, largely as a result of the systematic staging procedure and

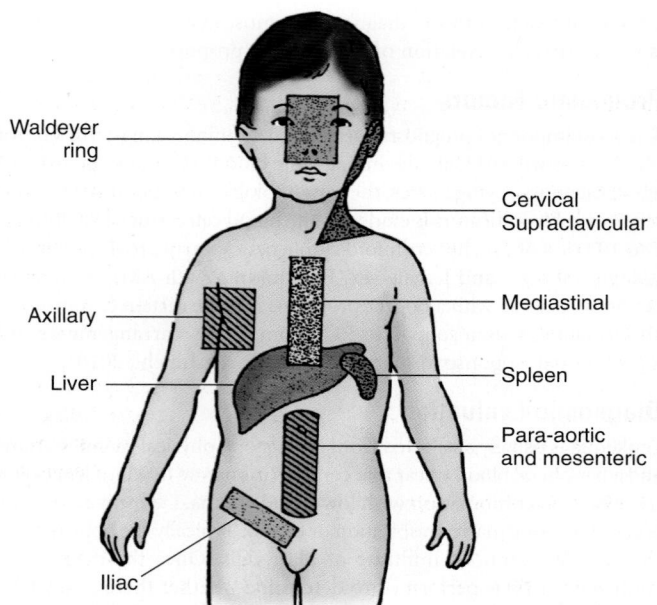

FIG 44.4 Main areas of lymphadenopathy and organ involvement in Hodgkin disease.

BOX 44.2   Staging of Hodgkin Disease

Stage I: Disease limited to one lymph node area or only one additional extralymphatic site (I-E), such as the liver, lungs, kidney, or intestines

Stage II: Two or more lymph node regions on the same side of the diaphragm or one additional extralymphatic site or organ (II-E) on the same side of the diaphragm

Stage III: Lymph node regions on both sides of the diaphragm and has spread to one extralymphatic site (III-E), spleen (III-S), or both (III-SE)

Stage IV: Disease has metastasized diffusely throughout the body to one or more extralymphatic sites with or without involvement of associated lymph nodes

---

improved treatment protocols. Overall the survival rate for patients with Hodgkin disease is as high as 95%; however, the survival rate is dependent on histology and staging (Frew, Lewis, & Lucraft, 2013). Even in those with disseminated disease, long-term remissions are possible in more than one-half of patients. For relapses, complete remission may occur in 30% to 60% of patients undergoing autologous BMT (Metzger et al., 2016).

Clinical Manifestations

Hodgkin disease is characterized by painless enlargement of lymph nodes. The most common finding is enlarged, firm, nontender, movable nodes in the supraclavicular or cervical area. In children, the sentinel node located near the left clavicle may be the first enlarged node. Enlargement of axillary and inguinal lymph nodes is less frequent (see Fig. 44.4).

Other signs and symptoms depend on the extent and location of involvement. Mediastinal lymphadenopathy may cause a persistent, nonproductive cough. Enlarged retroperitoneal nodes may produce unexplained abdominal pain. Systemic symptoms include low-grade or intermittent fever (Pel-Ebstein disease), anorexia, nausea, weight loss, night sweats, and pruritus. Generally, such symptoms indicate advanced lymph node and extralymphatic involvement.

their child's behavior. For example, they should know that it is not unusual for the child to be lethargic for a few days after surgery.

The nurse should participate in preoperative conferences with the physician and parents. By attending the conference, the nurse knows what information the parents have been given in order to provide further explanations or emotional support when necessary.

> **! NURSING ALERT**
>
> Report sluggish, dilated, or unequal pupils immediately because they may indicate increased ICP and potential brainstem herniation—a medical emergency.

Prevent Postoperative Complications

After surgery, the surgeon prescribes specific orders for taking vital signs, positioning, regulating fluids, and administering medication. These vary somewhat, depending on the location of the craniotomy. The following are general principles of care for infratentorial or supratentorial surgery. Chapter 46 discusses additional aspects of care, such as care of the child with seizures and care of the unconscious child in terms of respiratory status and neurologic assessment.

Assessment

Vital signs are taken as often as every 15 to 30 minutes until the patient is stable. Temperature measurement is particularly important because of hyperthermia resulting from surgical intervention in the hypothalamus or brainstem and from some types of general anesthesia.

> **! NURSING ALERT**
>
> To keep an accurate account of drainage, circle the soiled area with a pen and monitor for signs of continuous bleeding.

The presence of colorless drainage is reported immediately because it most likely is cerebrospinal fluid leaking from the incisional area. A foul odor from the dressing may indicate an infection. Such a finding is reported, and a culture is taken. The most likely types of infection are meningitis and respiratory tract infection. The probable cause of meningitis is wound contamination. The risk for respiratory tract infections is high because of the imposed immobility, danger of aspiration, and possible depression from the brainstem. The usual precautions of deep breathing and turning as allowed are instituted. Regular pulmonary assessments are performed to identify adventitious sounds or any areas of diminished or absent breath sounds.

As soon as possible, the nurse should begin testing reflexes, hand grip, and functioning of the cranial nerves. Muscle strength is usually less after surgery because of general weakness but should improve daily. Ataxia may be significantly worse with cerebellar intervention, but it slowly improves. Edema near the cranial nerves may depress important functions, such as the gag, blink, or swallowing reflex.

Neurologic checks are an essential aspect of care and include pupillary reaction to light, level of consciousness, sleep patterns, and response to stimuli. Although children may be comatose for a few days, once they regain consciousness, there should be a steady increase in alertness. Regression to a lethargic, irritable state indicates increasing pressure, possibly caused by meningitis, hemorrhage, or edema.

Once the younger child is alert, the arms may need to be restrained to preserve the dressing. Even a child who has been cooperative before surgery must be closely supervised during the initial stages of regaining consciousness, which is when disorientation and restlessness are common. Elbow restraints are satisfactory to prevent the hands from reaching the head.

Positioning

Correct positioning after surgery is critical to prevent pressure against the operative site, reduce ICP, and avoid the danger of aspiration. If a large tumor was removed, the child is not placed on the operative side, because the brain may suddenly shift to that cavity, causing trauma to the blood vessels, linings, and the brain itself. The nurse confers with the surgeon to be certain of the correct position, including the degree of neck flexion. The first 24 to 48 hours after brain surgery are critical. If positioning is restricted, notice of this is posted above the head of the bed. When the child is turned, every precaution is used to prevent jarring or misalignment to prevent undue strain on the sutures. Two nurses, one supporting the head and the other the body, are needed. The use of a turning sheet may facilitate turning a heavy child.

> **! NURSING ALERT**
>
> The Trendelenburg position is contraindicated in both infratentorial and supratentorial surgeries because it increases ICP and the risk for hemorrhage. If shock is impending, the health care provider is notified immediately, before the head is lowered.

Fluid Regulation

With an infratentorial craniotomy, the child is allowed nothing by mouth for at least 24 hours or longer if the gag and swallowing reflexes are depressed or the child is comatose. With a supratentorial procedure, feeding may be resumed soon after the child is alert, sometimes within 24 hours. Clear water is always started first because of the danger of aspiration. If the child vomits, stop oral liquids. Vomiting not only predisposes the child to aspiration but also increases ICP and the risk for incisional rupture.

IV fluids are continued until fluids are well tolerated. Because of the cerebral edema postoperatively and the danger of increased ICP, fluids are carefully monitored and usually infused less than the maintenance rate. A hypertonic solution such as mannitol may be necessary to remove excess fluid. These drugs cause rapid diuresis. Urinary output is monitored after administration of these drugs to evaluate their effectiveness.

Comfort Measures

Headache may be severe and is largely the result of cerebral edema. Measures to relieve some of the discomfort include providing a quiet, dimly lit environment; restricting visitors; preventing any sudden jarring movement, such as banging into the bed; and preventing an increase in ICP. The last is most effectively achieved by proper positioning and prevention of straining, such as during coughing, vomiting, or defecating. The use of opioids, such as morphine, to relieve pain is controversial because it is thought that they may mask signs of altered consciousness or depress respirations. However, opioids are considered safe because naloxone can be used to reverse opioid effects, such as sedation or respiratory depression. Acetaminophen and codeine are also effective analgesics. Regardless of the drugs used, adequate dosage and regular administration are essential to provide optimum pain relief (see the "Pain Assessment" and "Pain Management" sections in Chapter 30).

Brain edema may severely depress the gag reflex, necessitating suctioning of oral secretions. Facial edema may also be present, necessitating eye care if the lids remain partially open. Ice compresses applied to the eyes for short periods help relieve the edema. A depressed blink reflex also predisposes the corneas to ulceration. Irrigating the eyes with saline drops and covering them with eye dressings are important steps in preventing this complication.

Support the Family

The family's emotional needs are great when the diagnosis is a brain tumor, and the extent of surgery, any neurologic deficits, the prognosis, and additional therapy influence these feelings. Because few definitive answers can be given before surgery, the surgeon's report is a significant finding that can vary from a completely benign, resected neoplasm to a highly malignant, invasive, and only partially removed tumor. Although parents try to prepare themselves for a potentially fatal diagnosis, it is understandably a shock for them.

Ideally, a nurse who will be involved in the continuing care of this child should be with the family when the physician discusses the prognosis and plan of therapy. Regardless of the future prospects, direct the parents' thinking toward helping the child recover and resume a normal life to his or her fullest potential. Provide an opportunity for the family to share their concerns and questions, and encourage parents to verbalize their feelings about the diagnosis.*

During this period, the nurse should also discuss with parents what they plan to tell the child. If the child was prepared honestly, as described previously, the diagnosis can be expressed in a similar manner, such as "The surgeon removed most of the tumor, and the rest will be treated with special drugs and x-ray treatments." During recovery, the child needs additional explanation about the treatment and the reason for residual neurologic effects, such as ataxia or blindness. Hair loss is a normal concern for the child, and its regrowth will be delayed, depending on the length of therapy. At this point, it is advisable to reintroduce the idea of a wig.

Promote Return to Optimum Functioning

The ultimate goal is a cured child who has optimum functioning. As soon as possible, the child should resume usual activities within tolerable limits, especially returning to school.[†] Until the skull is completely healed, the child may need to wear a helmet when engaging in any active sport. This decision is made by the child's neurosurgeon. The school nurse and teacher should confer with the parents on activity restrictions, such as physical education, and the reactions of schoolmates to the child's appearance.

The vast realm of possible consequences after the diagnosis of a brain tumor is not discussed here. Rather, the reader is referred to other sections of the text that deal with possible outcomes, such as the paralyzed, visually impaired, or unconscious child or the child with a ventricular shunt, seizure disorder, or meningitis. Numerous physical problems can occur with progression of the tumor that may necessitate additional procedures. For example, frequent vomiting, anorexia, and nausea may require nonoral routes of feeding, such as gastrostomy or parenteral alimentation. Whenever these procedures are instituted, the nurse may be responsible for teaching the family appropriate home care to allow the child the highest quality of life (see the discussion of discharge planning and home care in Chapter 38).

NEUROBLASTOMA

Neuroblastoma is the most common extracranial solid tumor of childhood and the most common cancer diagnosed in infancy. Approximately 650 new cases of neuroblastoma are diagnosed every year in the United

---

*Information about support groups is available from the National Brain Tumor Society, 55 Chapel Street, Suite 200, Newton MA 02458; 617-924-9997; www.braintumor.org.

[†]Information on returning to school is available from the American Brain Tumor Association, 8550 W. Bryn Mawr Avenue, Suite 550, Chicago, IL 60631; 1-800-886-2282; www.abta.org.

States (National Cancer Institute, 2015c). The median age at diagnosis is 19 months (National Cancer Institute). These tumors originate from embryonic neural crest cells that normally give rise to the adrenal medulla and the sympathetic nervous system. Consequently, the majority of the tumors arise from the adrenal gland or from the retroperitoneal sympathetic chain. The primary site is within the abdomen; other sites include the head and neck region, chest, and pelvis.

Clinical Manifestations

The signs and symptoms of neuroblastoma depend on the location and stage of the disease. With abdominal tumors, the most common presenting sign is a firm, nontender, irregular mass in the abdomen that crosses the midline (in contrast to Wilms tumor, which is usually confined to one side). Other primary tumor sites may cause significant clinical effects such as neurologic impairment, respiratory obstruction from a thoracic mass, or varying degrees of paralysis from compression of the spinal cord.

Distant metastasis frequently causes supraorbital ecchymosis, periorbital edema, and proptosis (exophthalmos) from invasion of retrobulbar soft tissue. Lymphadenopathy, hepatomegaly, and skeletal pain are also present in patients with disseminated disease. Vague symptoms of widespread metastasis include pallor, weakness, irritability, anorexia, and weight loss.

Diagnostic Evaluation

Diagnostic evaluation is aimed at locating the primary site and areas of metastasis. A CT scan of the abdomen, pelvis, or chest is the preferred imaging modality to locate the primary tumor. A bone scan and MIBG (iodine-131 metaiodobenzylguanidine) scan should be performed to evaluate for the presence of skeletal metastases. Examination of the bone marrow with bilateral aspirates and biopsies should be performed in all patients. Neuroblastomas, particularly those arising in the adrenal glands or from a sympathetic chain, excrete the catecholamines epinephrine and norepinephrine. Urinary excretion of catecholamines is detected in approximately 95% of children with adrenal or sympathetic tumors.

Staging and Prognosis

Neuroblastoma is a "silent" tumor. In more than 70% of cases, diagnosis is made after metastasis occurs, with the first signs caused by involvement in the nonprimary site, usually the lymph nodes, bone marrow, skeletal system, or liver. Because of the frequency of invasiveness, the prognosis for neuroblastoma is generally poor.

The child's age and the stage of the disease (Box 44.4) at diagnosis are important prognostic factors. Survival is inversely correlated with age. If all stages are grouped together, the survival rates are approximately 80% for children younger than 1 year of age and less than 50% for children older than 1 year of age (Brodeur, Hogarty, Bagatell, et al., 2016). This marked difference in survival rates by age is partly accounted for by the larger proportion of very young children with stage I, II, or IV-S disease and the absence of the *MYC-N* gene amplification.

Infants who remain free from disease for 1 year after treatment are usually cured, but older children have experienced relapses several years after cessation of treatment. Surgical resection of the tumor in stage I appears to be greater than 90% curative (Brodeur et al., 2016). Stage IV-S neuroblastoma is one of the few tumors that demonstrate spontaneous regression, possibly as a result of maturity of the embryonic cell or development of an active immune system.

Therapeutic Management

Accurate clinical staging is important for establishing initial treatment. Therefore, the purpose of surgery is both to remove as much of the tumor as possible and to obtain biopsies. In stages I and II, complete surgical removal of the tumor is the treatment of choice. If the tumors are large, partial resection is attempted, with a course of irradiation postoperatively to shrink the tumor in the hope of complete removal at a later date. Surgery is usually limited to biopsy in stages III and IV because of the extensive metastasis.

The precise role of radiotherapy is unclear. It does not appear to be of any benefit in children with stage I and II disease. It is can be used with stage III disease, although it may not improve survival expectancy. Radiotherapy for paraspinal neuroblastoma is no longer recommended because the radiation therapy has long-term morbidity, and chemotherapy is a safe and effective initial treatment modality (Brodeur et al., 2016).

Chemotherapy is the mainstay of therapy for extensive local or disseminated disease. The drugs are administered in a variety of combinations according to specific protocols. In addition, the use of consolidative myeloablative therapy using autologous marrow or peripheral stem cells followed by 13-*cis*-retinoic acid has improved the outcome of patients with high-risk disease.

Care Management

Care management is similar to that discussed in the "Care Management" section earlier in this chapter, including psychologic and physical preparation for diagnostic and operative procedures; prevention of postoperative complications for abdominal, thoracic, or cranial surgery; and explanation of chemotherapy and radiotherapy and their side effects (see Tables 44.1 and 44.3).

Because this tumor carries a poor prognosis for many children, evaluate and address the needs of the family in terms of coping with a life-threatening illness (see Chapter 36). Because of the high degree of metastasis at the time of diagnosis, many parents suffer guilt for not having recognized signs earlier. Parents need much support in dealing with these feelings and expressing them to the appropriate people.

▍BONE TUMORS

GENERAL CONSIDERATIONS

Bone tumors consist of osteosarcoma and Ewing sarcoma and account for about 6% of all malignant neoplasms in children in the United States (Scheurer et al., 2016). Osteosarcoma is the most common bone tumor, with approximately 4.4 cases per 1 million children annually in the United States, whereas Ewing sarcoma occurs in 1 case per 1 million annually among children younger than 20 years of age (National Cancer Institute, 2015d). The peak age for pediatric bone tumors is 15 years of age, and they occur more often in males.

Clinical Manifestations

Most malignant bone tumors produce localized pain in the affected site, which may be severe or dull and may be attributed to trauma or the vague complaint of "growing pains." The pain is often relieved by a flexed position, which relaxes the muscles overlying the stretched periosteum. Frequently it draws attention when the child limps, curtails physical activity, or is unable to hold heavy objects. A palpable mass is also a common manifestation of bone tumors, but systemic symptoms (e.g., fever) and other clinical symptoms (e.g., spinal cord compression and respiratory distress) are more frequent in patients with Ewing sarcoma.

Diagnostic Evaluation

Diagnosis begins with a thorough history and physical examination. A primary objective is to rule out causes such as trauma or infection. Careful questioning regarding pain is essential in attempting to determine the duration and rate of tumor growth. Physical assessment focuses on functional status of the affected area; signs of inflammation; size of the mass; and any systemic indication of generalized malignancy, such as anemia, weight loss, and frequent infection.

Definitive diagnosis is based on radiologic studies, such as plain films and CT or MRI scan of the primary site, CT scan of the chest, and radioisotope bone scans to evaluate metastasis, and bone marrow examination in patients with Ewing sarcoma. A needle or surgical biopsy is necessary to establish the diagnosis. Ewing sarcoma most commonly involves the pelvis, long bones of the lower extremities, and chest wall and radiographically involves the diaphysis with detachment of the periosteum from the bone (Codman triangle). In osteosarcoma, lesions are most commonly located in the metaphyseal region of the bone, often involving the long bones. Radial ossification in the soft tissue gives the tumor a "sunburst" appearance on plain radiograph.

Prognosis

A better understanding of the biology of neoplastic growth has resulted in more aggressive treatment and an improved prognosis. The natural history of osteogenic sarcoma and Ewing sarcoma suggests that multiple submicroscopic foci of metastatic disease are present at the time of diagnosis despite clinical evidence of localized involvement. The lungs, distant bones, and bone marrow are the most common sites for metastatic bone tumor disease. With current therapies that include surgery and chemotherapy for osteosarcoma and surgery, radiotherapy, and chemotherapy for Ewing sarcoma, the majority of patients with localized disease can be cured.

OSTEOSARCOMA

Osteosarcoma (osteogenic sarcoma) presumably arises from bone-forming mesenchyme, which gives rise to malignant osteoid tissue. Most primary tumor sites are in the diaphyseal and metaphyseal region (wider part of the shaft, adjacent to the epiphyseal growth plate) of long bones, especially in the lower extremities. More than one-half occur in the femur, particularly the distal portion, with the rest involving the humerus, tibia, pelvis, jaw, and phalanges.

Therapeutic Management

Optimum treatment of osteosarcoma includes surgery and chemotherapy. The surgical approach consists of surgical biopsy followed by either limb salvage or amputation. To ensure local control, all gross and microscopic tumors must be resected. A limb salvage procedure has become the standard approach to surgical intervention and involves resection of the primary tumor with prosthetic replacement of the involved bone (Gorlick, Janeway, & Marina, 2016). Frequently children undergoing a limb salvage procedure receive preoperative chemotherapy in an attempt to decrease the tumor size and make surgery more manageable (Arndt, Rose, Folpe, et al., 2012).

Chemotherapy plays a vital role in treatment of osteosarcoma. Antineoplastic drugs may be administered singly or in combination and may be employed both before and after surgical resection of the tumor. When pulmonary metastases are found, thoracotomy and chemotherapy have resulted in prolonged survival and potential cure. These combined-modality approaches have significantly improved the prognosis in osteosarcoma to approximately 75% for nonmetastatic patients (Arndt et al., 2012).

Care Management

Nursing care depends on the type of surgical approach. The family may have more difficulty adjusting to an amputation than a limb salvage procedure. In either instance, preparation of the child and family is critical. Straightforward honesty is essential in gaining the child's cooperation and trust. The diagnosis of cancer should not be disguised with falsehoods such as "infection." To accept the need for surgery, the child should be told a few days before surgery to allow him or her time to think about the diagnosis and consequent treatment and to ask questions.

Sometimes children have many questions about the prosthesis, limitations on physical ability, and prognosis in terms of cure. At other times they react with silence or with a calm manner that belies their concern and fear. Either response must be accepted, since it is part of the grieving process of a loss. For those who desire information, it may be helpful to introduce them to another amputee before surgery or to show them pictures of the prosthesis.* However, the nurse must be careful not to overwhelm children with information. A sound approach is to answer questions without offering additional information. For those who do not pursue additional information, the nurse expresses a willingness to talk.

The child is also informed of the need for chemotherapy and its side effects before surgery. Exercise caution about offering too much information at one time. When discussing hair loss, emphasize coping strategies, such as wearing a wig. Because bone tumors affect adolescents and young adults, it is not unusual for them to become angry over all the radical body alterations.

The child requires stump care, which is the same as for any amputee. If an amputation is performed, the child is usually fitted with a temporary prosthesis immediately after surgery, which permits early functioning and fosters psychologic adjustment. A permanent prosthesis is usually fitted within 6 to 8 weeks. During hospitalization, the child begins physical therapy to become proficient in the use and care of the device.

Phantom limb pain may develop in 60% to 80% of patients after amputation and is caused by interruption of sensory nerve impulses (Wolff, Vanduynhoven, van Kleef, et al, 2011). This symptom is characterized by sensations such as tingling, itching, and, more frequently, pain felt in the amputated limb. The child and family need to know that the sensations are real, not imagined. A recent Cochrane Review reported that various medications such as morphine, gabapentin, and ketamine

have been used for phantom limb pain, but complete pain relief has been unsuccessful (Alviar, Hale & Dungca, 2011).

Discharge planning must begin early in the postoperative period. Once the child has begun physical therapy, the nurse should consult with the therapist and health care provider to evaluate the child's physical and emotional readiness to reenter school. It is an opportune time to involve a community nurse in the child's home care. Every effort is made to promote normalcy and gradual resumption of realistic pre-amputation activities.* Role playing in anticipation of such experiences is beneficial in preparing the child for the inevitable confrontation by others. Environmental barriers, such as stairs, are assessed in terms of accessibility in the school and home, especially because the child may need to use crutches or a wheelchair before complete healing and prosthetic competency are achieved. The nurse encourages the child to select clothing that best camouflages the prosthesis, such as pants or long-sleeved shirts. Well-fitted prostheses are so natural looking that girls can usually wear sheer stockings without revealing the device. Encouraging the child to wear jeans and a T-shirt may distract attention from the deformity and focus on familiar aspects of appearance.

The family and child need much support in adjusting not only to a life-threatening diagnosis but also to alteration in body form and function. Because loss of a limb entails a grieving process, those caring for the child need to recognize that the reactions of anger and depression are normal and necessary. Often parents view the anger as a direct affront to them for allowing the amputation to occur, or they see the depression as rejection. These are not personal attacks but the child's attempts to cope with a loss.

EWING SARCOMA (PRIMITIVE NEUROECTODERMAL TUMOR OF THE BONE)

Ewing sarcomas, which includes primitive neuroectodermal tumor of the bone, arise in the marrow spaces of the bone rather than from osseous tissue. The tumor originates in the shaft of long and trunk bones, most often affecting the pelvis, femur, tibia, fibula, humerus, ulna, vertebra, scapula, ribs, and skull. It occurs almost exclusively in individuals younger than 30 years of age and affects Caucasians much more often than other races (National Cancer Institute, 2015d).

Therapeutic Management

Limb salvage procedures might be feasible in extremity lesions, and amputation may be considered if the results of radiotherapy render the extremity useless or deformed (e.g., from retarded growth in young children). The treatment of choice for the majority of lesions is involved field radiotherapy and chemotherapy.

Care Management

The psychologic adjustment to Ewing sarcoma is typically less traumatic than it is to osteosarcoma when there is preservation of the affected limb. Many families accept the diagnosis with a sense of relief in knowing that this type of bone cancer does not necessitate amputation. Consequently, they need preparation for the various diagnostic tests, including bone marrow aspiration and surgical biopsy, and adequate explanation of the treatment regimen. Radiotherapy often causes a skin reaction of dry or moist desquamation followed by hyperpigmentation. The child should wear loose-fitting clothes over the irradiated area to minimize additional skin irritation. Because of increased sensitivity, protect the area from sunlight and sudden changes in temperature. Encourage the child to use the extremity as tolerated.

The child needs the same considerations for adjusting to the effects of chemotherapy as any other patient with cancer. The drug regimen usually results in hair loss, severe nausea and vomiting, peripheral

---

*Information about prostheses can be obtained from the National Amputation Foundation, 40 Church Street, Malverne, NY 11565; 516-887-3600; www.nationalamputation.org.

neuropathy, and possible cardiotoxicity. Make every effort to outline a treatment plan that allows the child maximum resumption of a normal lifestyle and activities.

OTHER SOLID TUMORS

In addition to the cancers already discussed, several other types of solid tumors may occur in children. Wilms tumor, rhabdomyosarcoma, and retinoblastoma are unique in that they tend to be diagnosed early, typically before 5 years of age. Wilms tumor and retinoblastoma are also unusual in that they are among the few types of cancer that may occur in both hereditary and nonhereditary forms.

WILMS TUMOR

Wilms tumor, or nephroblastoma, is the most common kidney tumor of childhood (Davidoff, 2012). Its frequency is estimated to be 8 cases per 1 million children younger than 15 years of age, with approximately 650 new cases per year (Davidoff). Seventy-five percent of patients with Wilms' tumor are diagnosed when they are younger than 5 years of age, and it has a peak incidence between 2 and 3 years of age (Davidoff). About 5% of Wilms tumors are familial (Davidoff).

Clinical Manifestations

The most common presenting sign is painless swelling or mass within the abdomen. The mass is characteristically firm, nontender, confined to one side, and deep within the flank. If it is on the right side, it may be difficult to distinguish from the liver, although, unlike that organ, it does not move with respiration. Parents usually discover the mass during routine bathing or dressing of the child.

Other clinical manifestations are the result of compression from the tumor mass, metabolic alterations secondary to the tumor, or metastasis. Hematuria occurs in less than one-fourth of children with Wilms tumor. Anemia, usually secondary to hemorrhage within the tumor, results in pallor, anorexia, and lethargy. Hypertension, caused by secretion of excess amounts of renin by the tumor, occurs occasionally. Other effects of malignancy include weight loss and fever. If metastasis has occurred, symptoms of lung involvement (e.g., dyspnea, cough, shortness of breath, and chest pain) may be evident.

Diagnostic Evaluation

In a child suspected of having Wilms tumor, special emphasis is placed on the history and physical examination for the presence of congenital anomalies; a family history of cancer; and signs of malignancy, such as weight loss, enlarged liver and spleen, indications of anemia, and lymphadenopathy. Specific tests include radiographic studies, such as abdominal ultrasound, CT, and MRI of the abdomen; CT of the chest to evaluate for the presence of metastases in the lung; and Doppler ultrasound of the inferior vena cava. Laboratory studies should include a complete blood count (polycythemia is sometimes present if the tumor secretes excess erythropoietin), biochemical studies, and urinalysis. Studies to demonstrate the relationship of the tumor to the ipsilateral kidney and the presence of a normally functioning kidney on the contralateral side are essential.

Staging and Prognosis

Wilms tumor arises from a malignant, undifferentiated metanephrogenic blastoma (a cluster of primordial cells capable of initiating the regeneration of an abnormal structure). Its occurrence slightly favors the left kidney, which is advantageous because surgically this kidney is easier to manipulate and remove. Although the tumor may become large, it remains encapsulated for an extended period.

The histology of the tumor cells is identified and classified according to two groups: favorable histology (FH) and unfavorable histology (UH). Only about 10% of Wilms tumors demonstrate UH, which is associated with a poorer prognosis and demands a more aggressive treatment protocol, regardless of the clinical stage (Davenport, Blanco, & Sandler, 2012).

Survival rates for Wilms tumor are one of the highest among all childhood cancers. Children with localized tumor have a 90% chance of cure with multimodal therapy (Davenport et al., 2012). For those children who relapse, a better expectancy of disease-free survival is associated with FH of the tumor; time to recurrence and site of recurrence are no longer considered prognostic indicators (Davidoff, 2012).

Therapeutic Management

Combined treatment with surgery and chemotherapy, with or without irradiation, is based on the clinical stage and histologic pattern. In unilateral disease, a large transabdominal incision is performed for optimum visualization of the abdominal cavity. The tumor, affected kidney, and adjacent adrenal gland are removed. Great care is taken to keep the encapsulated tumor intact because rupture can seed cancer cells throughout the abdomen, lymph channel, and bloodstream. The contralateral kidney is carefully inspected for evidence of disease or dysfunction. Regional lymph nodes are inspected, and a biopsy is performed when indicated. Any involved structures (e.g., part of the colon, diaphragm, or vena cava) are removed. Metal clips are placed around the tumor site for exact marking during radiotherapy.

If both kidneys are involved, the child may be treated with chemotherapy preoperatively to shrink the tumor, allowing more successful surgery (Davenport et al., 2012). In some cases, a partial nephrectomy is performed, followed with additional administration of chemotherapy. When additional therapy is not effective, bilateral nephrectomy is performed with obligatory dialysis and a renal transplant is pursued (Davenport et al.).

Postoperative radiotherapy is indicated for children with metastatic disease (Davenport et al., 2012). Chemotherapy is indicated for all children. The duration of therapy ranges from 6 to 15 months.

Care Management

The nursing care of the child with Wilms tumor is similar to that of other cancers treated with surgery, irradiation, and chemotherapy. However, some significant differences are discussed for each phase of nursing intervention.

Preoperative Care

As with many of the other cancers, the diagnosis of Wilms tumor is a shock. Frequently the child has no physical indication of the seriousness of the disorder other than a palpable abdominal mass. Because the parents usually discover the mass, the nurse needs to take into account their feelings regarding the diagnosis. Whereas some parents are grateful for their detection of the tumor, others feel guilty for not finding it sooner or anger toward the health care provider for missing it on earlier examinations.

The preoperative period is one of swift diagnosis. Typically, surgery is scheduled within 24 to 48 hours of admission. The nurse is faced with the challenge of preparing the child and parents for all laboratory and operative procedures. Because of the little time available, keep explanations simple and repeat them often, with attention to what the child will experience. In addition to usual preoperative observations, monitor blood pressure, because hypertension from excess renin production is a possibility.

There are several special preoperative concerns, the most important of which is not to palpate the tumor unless absolutely necessary because manipulation of the mass may cause dissemination of cancer cells to adjacent and distant sites.

> ## ! NURSING ALERT
>
> To reinforce the need for caution, it may be necessary to post a sign on the bed that reads "Do not palpate abdomen." Careful bathing and handling are also important in preventing trauma to the tumor site.

Because radiotherapy and chemotherapy are usually begun immediately after surgery, parents need an explanation of what to expect, such as major benefits and side effects, although the timing of the information should be considered to avoid overwhelming the family. Ideally the nurse should be present during physician-parent conferences to answer questions as they arise.

Postoperative Care

Despite the extensive surgical intervention necessary in many children with Wilms tumor, the recovery period is usually rapid. The major nursing responsibilities are those following any abdominal surgery. Because these children are at risk for intestinal obstruction from postsurgical adhesion formation or side effects from the chemotherapy and radiation, the nurse monitors gastrointestinal activity, such as bowel movements, bowel sounds, distention, and vomiting. Other considerations are frequent evaluation of blood pressure and observation for signs of infection, especially during chemotherapy.

Support the Family

The postoperative period is frequently difficult for parents. The shock of seeing their child immediately after surgery may be the first realization of the seriousness of the diagnosis. From surgery, the stage and pathology of the tumor are determined. The physician discusses this information with the parents. The nurse's presence during this conversation is important to provide additional support and assess the parents' understanding of this information.

Older children need an opportunity to deal with their feelings concerning the many procedures to which they have been subjected in rapid succession. Therapeutic play can be beneficial in helping children of any age understand what they have undergone and express their feelings.

RHABDOMYOSARCOMA

Rhabdomyosarcoma (*rhabdo* means striated) is the most common soft-tissue sarcoma in children. Striated (skeletal) muscle is found almost anywhere in the body, so these tumors occur in many sites—the most common of which are the head and neck, especially the orbit. The disease occurs in children in all age-groups but is most common in children 9 years of age or younger and is slightly more common in males (Wexler, Skapek, & Helman, 2016). Its incidence is approximately 4.5 cases per 1 million children annually (National Cancer Institute, 2015e).

Rhabdomyosarcoma arises from embryonic mesenchyme with three recognized subtypes (Box 44.5). These malignant neoplasms originate from undifferentiated mesenchymal cells in muscles, tendons, bursae, and fascia, or in fibrous, connective, lymphatic, or vascular tissue. They derive their name from the specific tissue(s) of origin, such as myosarcoma (*myo* means muscle).

Clinical Manifestations

The initial signs and symptoms are related to the site of the tumor and compression of adjacent organs. Some tumor locations, such as the

> ### BOX 44.5 Subtypes of Rhabdomyosarcoma
>
> **Embryonal:** Most common type; most frequently found in the head, neck, abdomen, and genitourinary tract
> **Alveolar:** Second most common type; most often seen in deep tissues of the extremities and trunk
> **Pleomorphic:** Rare in children; most often occurs in soft parts of extremities and trunk

orbit, manifest early in the course of the illness. Other tumors, such as those of the retroperitoneal area, only produce symptoms when they are relatively big and compress adjacent organs. Unfortunately, many of the signs and symptoms attributable to rhabdomyosarcoma are vague and frequently suggest a common childhood illness, such as "earache" or "runny nose." Often the primary tumor site is never identified.

Diagnostic Evaluation

Diagnosis begins with a careful history and physical examination. Radiographic studies to delineate the primary tumor site should include PET/CT or MRI scans. Metastatic evaluation should include a CT of the chest, bone scan, and bilateral bone marrow aspirates and biopsies. For patients with tumors in the parameningeal area, a LP is performed to examine the spinal fluid. An excisional biopsy or surgical resection of the tumor, when possible, is done to confirm the diagnosis.

Staging and Prognosis

Careful staging is extremely important for planning treatment and determining the prognosis. The Intergroup Rhabdomyosarcoma Study has developed a surgicopathologic staging system, which includes four stage classifications depending on disease involvement.

With the use of contemporary multimodal therapy, more than 60% of patients with nonmetastatic disease are expected to survive, and if diagnosed in the early stage, the survival rate increases to 80% (Davenport et al., 2012). If relapse occurs, the prognosis for long-term survival is poor.

Therapeutic Management

All rhabdomyosarcomas are high-grade tumors with the potential for metastases. Therefore, multimodal therapy is recommended for all patients. Complete removal of the primary tumor is advocated whenever possible. However, because the tumor is chemosensitive, radical procedures with high morbidity should be avoided. In the majority of cases, a biopsy is followed by chemotherapy, irradiation, or both.

Care Management

The nursing responsibilities are similar to those for other types of cancer, especially the solid tumors when surgery is employed. Specific objectives include careful assessment for signs of the tumor, especially during well-child examinations; preparation of the child and family for the multiple diagnostic tests; and supportive care during each stage of multimodal therapy. The reader is urged to review Chapter 36 for information on emotional support of the family in the event of a poor prognosis.

RETINOBLASTOMA

Retinoblastoma, which arises from the retina, is the most common intraocular malignancy of childhood (Dimaras, Kimani, Dimba, et al., 2012). Approximately 4 cases per 1 million children occur annually in the United States (National Cancer Institute, 2015f). The average age of the child at the time of diagnosis is 2 years of age, and bilateral and hereditary disease is diagnosed earlier than unilateral and nonhereditary disease (Hurwitz, Shields, Shields, et al, 2016). Of all cases of retinoblastoma, 60% are unilateral and nonhereditary, 25% are bilateral and hereditary, and 15% are unilateral and hereditary (National Cancer Institute, 2015f).

Retinoblastoma may be caused by various genetic alterations of the *Rb* gene, including a somatic mutation in nonhereditary cases, a germ-line mutation in hereditary cases, or a chromosome 13 deletion. A "two-hit hypothesis" was developed to explain genetic and sporadic cases and states that as few as two mutational events are required for tumor initiation. Children who have chromosome aberrations and retinoblastoma also often have an increased incidence of cognitive impairment and congenital malformations, although the vast majority of children with retinoblastomas apparently have normal chromosomes and intelligence.

Clinical Manifestations

Retinoblastoma has few grossly obvious signs. Typically the parents are the ones who first observe a whitish "glow" in the pupil, known as the *cat's eye reflex,* or *leukocoria* (Fig. 44.6). The reflex represents visualization of the tumor as the light momentarily falls on the mass. When a tumor arises in the macular region (which is the area directly at the back of the retina when the eye is focused straight ahead), a white reflex may be visible when the tumor is small. It is best observed when a bright light is shining toward the child as the child looks forward. Sometimes parents accidentally discover it when taking a photograph of their child using a flash attachment.

When the tumor arises in the periphery of the retina, it must grow to a considerable size before light can strike it sufficiently to produce the cat's eye reflex. In this situation, it is visible only when the child looks in certain directions (sideways) or if the observer stands at an oblique angle to the child's face as the child looks straight ahead. The fleeting nature of the reflex often results in a delayed diagnosis because health care professionals fail to appreciate the ominous significance of the parents' findings.

The next most common sign is strabismus resulting from poor fixation of the visually impaired eye, particularly if the tumor develops in the macula, the area of sharpest visual acuity. Blindness is usually a late sign, but it frequently is not obvious unless the parent consciously observes for behaviors indicating loss of sight, such as bumping into objects, slowed motor development, or turning of the head to see objects

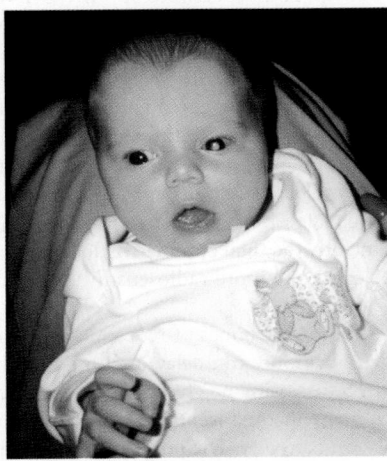

FIG 44.6 Cat's eye reflex. Whitish appearance of lens is produced as light falls on tumor mass in left eye.

lateral to the affected eye. Other signs and symptoms include heterochromia (different color of the iris), glaucoma, and pain.

Diagnostic Evaluation

A detailed family history and recording of eye symptoms are essential. Children suspected of having this disorder are referred to an ophthalmologist; the diagnosis is usually based on indirect ophthalmoscopy, ultrasound, CT, and MRI scans.

Metastatic disease at the time of retinoblastoma diagnosis is rare (Hurwitz et al, 2016); therefore, staging procedures such as bone marrow aspiration, bone scan, and LP are not routinely performed.

Staging and Prognosis

Staging of retinoblastomas is done under indirect ophthalmoscopy before surgery to accurately determine the tumor size (measured in disc diameters [DDs]) and location (according to an imaginary line called the *equator* drawn on the midplane of the eye) (Hurwitz et al, 2016).

Various classification systems have been used to stage retinoblastoma, including the Reese-Ellsworth system and the International Classification of Retinoblastoma. The overall 10-year survival rate is nearly 90% for unilateral and bilateral tumors (Hurwitz et al, 2016). Retinoblastoma is one of the tumors that may spontaneously regress.

Of major concern in long-term survivors is the development of secondary tumors. Children with bilateral disease (hereditary form) are more likely to develop secondary cancers than are children with unilateral disease. Currently providers believe these individuals are predisposed to developing cancer and that radiation increases their risk.

Therapeutic Management

Treatment of retinoblastoma is complex. Enucleation may be used to treat advanced disease with optic nerve invasion in which there is no hope for salvage of vision. Irradiation can be used when there is vitreous seeding. Chemotherapy has been used to decrease the tumor size to allow treatment with local therapies, such as plaque brachytherapy (surgical implantation of an iodine-125 applicator on the sclera until the maximum radiation dose has been delivered to the tumor), photocoagulation (use of a laser beam to destroy retinal blood vessels that supply nutrition to the tumor), and cryotherapy (freezing of the tumor, which destroys the microcirculation to the tumor and the cells themselves through microcrystal formation). The use of chemotherapy along with radiation or high-dose chemotherapy with autologous stem cell rescue is used to treat metastatic disease (Hurwitz et al, 2016).

Care Management
Prepare the Family for Diagnostic and Therapeutic Procedures and Home Care

Because the tumor is usually diagnosed in infants or very young children, most of the preparation for diagnostic tests and treatment involves parents. Once the disease is staged, the physician confers with the parents regarding treatment. In most cases, enucleation can be avoided. In the event that an enucleation is performed, tell parents about the procedure and the benefits of a prosthesis. Showing parents pictures of another child with an artificial eye may help them adjust to the procedure. Although the loss of vision is distressing, most parents realize that there is no alternative. Emphasizing that the unaffected eye retains normal vision and that the affected eye is probably already blind is particularly helpful in promoting acceptance of the imposed impairment.

After surgery, the parents need to be prepared for the child's facial appearance. An eye patch is in place, and the child's face may be edematous and ecchymotic. Parents often fear seeing the surgical site because they imagine a cavity in the skull. On the contrary, the lids are usually closed, and the area does not appear sunken because a surgically implanted sphere maintains the shape of the eyeball. The implant is covered with conjunctiva, and when the lids are open, the exposed area resembles the mucosal lining of the mouth. Once the child is fitted for a prosthesis, usually within 3 weeks, the facial appearance returns to normal.

After an uneventful recovery from enucleation, plans can be made for discharge from the hospital, usually within 3 to 4 days postoperatively. Parents need instruction regarding care of the surgical site and preparation for any additional therapy. They should be given the opportunity to see the socket as soon after surgery as possible. A good time to do this without unduly pressuring them is during dressing changes. They should then be encouraged to participate in the dressing changes.

Care of the socket is minimal and easily accomplished. The wound itself is clean and has little or no drainage. If an antibiotic ointment is prescribed, it is applied in a thin line on the surface of the tissues of the socket. The dressing consists of an eye pad changed daily. Once the socket has healed completely, a dressing is no longer necessary, although there are several reasons for having the child continue to wear an eye patch. Infants and toddlers explore their environment with their hands, and without an eye patch in place, the socket is available to exploring fingers. Although there is little danger of the child injuring the socket, parents may feel more secure with the socket covered. This also helps prevent infection.

The ocularist, who fits and manufactures the prosthesis, gives initial instructions for care of the device. Once in place, the prosthesis need not be removed unless cleaning is necessary, in which case it is taken out by gently pulling down on the lower lid, which frees the lower edge of the prosthesis, and applying pressure to the upper lid. The prosthesis is cleaned by placing it in hot water and soaking it for several minutes. Reinsertion is easier if the prosthesis remains wet. To reinsert the prosthesis, the lids are separated; and with the prosthesis held in the correct position (it should be marked to indicate the nasal side); it is pushed up under the upper lid, allowing the lower lid to cover its lower edge.

Safety is a major concern to prevent damage to the unaffected eye. Safety measures should be practiced at all times, and children should avoid rough contact sports or wear protective eyewear.

Support the Family

The diagnosis of retinoblastoma presents some special concerns in addition to those raised by any type of cancer. Families with a history of the disorder may feel guilt for transmitting the defect to their offspring, especially if they knowingly "played the odds" and parented an affected child. In families with no history of retinoblastoma, the diagnosis is a shock, frequently complicated by guilt for not having discovered it sooner. Consider each of these variables while offering supportive care to the family.

Other concerns also relate to the hereditary aspects of the disease. Of great importance to parents is the risk for retinoblastoma in their subsequent offspring and in the offspring of the surviving affected child. With improving prognoses for these children, genetic counseling to prevent transmission of the disease is assuming greater importance. Encourage these families to seek regular follow-up care for the affected child to detect secondary tumors, and all subsequent offspring of unaffected parents and survivors should undergo regular ophthalmoscopy to detect retinoblastoma at its earliest stage.

GERM CELL TUMORS

Germ cell tumors account for about 2% of all tumors in children younger than 15 years of age but account for 14% of all tumors in children 15

to 19 years of age (Frazier, Olson, Schneider, et al., 2016). Teratoma is the most common subtype of germ cell tumor in childhood (Frazier et al). The most common ovarian tumors are the mature cystic teratomas, followed by dysgerminomas and yolk sac tumors. The most common testicular tumors are yolk sac tumors, followed by teratomas. In general, most teratomas and localized gonadal tumors that are surgically resected can be observed without the need for further therapy. For patients with more advanced disease, the use of chemotherapy has produced excellent results.

Care Management

To supplement routine health assessment, every adolescent male should know how to perform frequent testicular self-examination to familiarize himself with his own anatomy and to ensure early detection of any abnormality. Ideally self-examination should be performed once a month beginning when physical development reaches Tanner stage 3, usually about 13 or 14 years of age (see Fig. 35.3). Each testicle is examined individually, preferably after a warm bath or shower (when scrotal skin is more relaxed), using the thumbs and fingers of both hands and applying a small amount of firm, gentle pressure. The normal testicle is a firm organ with a smooth egg-shaped contour. The epididymis can be palpated as a raised swelling on the superior aspect of the testicle and should not be confused with an abnormality.

LIVER TUMORS

Liver tumors account for 1% of all childhood cancers; the most common histologic subtype is hepatoblastoma (Agarwala, 2012). Surgical resection is the treatment of choice for these tumors but is usually performed after the administration of chemotherapy to make the tumor resection more successful (Meyers, Trobaugh-Lotrario, Malogolowkin, et al., 2016). Liver transplantation is often used in unresectable tumors. Survival rates for patients with hepatoblastoma can be as high as 85% with current therapies (Agarwala, 2012).

THE CHILDHOOD CANCER SURVIVOR

Survival for children with cancer has greatly improved over the past 20 years. The overall 5-year survival rate is 80% (Scheurer et al., 2016). Vigorous treatment of childhood cancers has resulted in dramatically improved survival rates. However, treatment programs combining surgery, irradiation, and chemotherapy are not without their complications. Some may occur immediately, such as loss of a limb from surgical amputation. However, current concern is with late effects—adverse changes related to treatment modalities, interactions between modes of treatment, individual characteristics of the child, and the disease process that may appear months to years after lifesaving treatment. Because more children are being cured and surviving into adulthood, increasing documentation of late effects is emerging (Table 44.3). Almost no organ is exempt, and almost every antineoplastic agent (especially irradiation) is responsible for some adverse effect. Many factors influence the development of late effects from irradiation; some of the more important ones include the total cumulative dose given, the child's age (the younger the child, the more radiosensitive the body organs are), and the tumor's location.

Radiotherapy to growing bones or reproductive glands responsible for growth-related hormones can delay or stunt growth. Nurses must document growth by assessing height and weight at each visit. Radiotherapy and some chemotherapy agents can cause hormonal dysfunction, decreased fertility, and sterility. The potential for gonadal dysfunction depends on the child's age and sex, the type of treatment, and the duration and total doses of treatment. Nursing assessment must begin

TABLE 44.3 Late Effects of Cancer Treatment

Systemic Effects and Clinical Manifestations	Associated Mode of Treatment
Central Nervous System	
Leukoencephalopathy (syndrome ranging from lethargy, dementia, and seizures to quadriplegia and death)	Methotrexate, intrathecal chemotherapy, or CNS irradiation
Mineralizing microangiopathy (headaches, focal seizures, incoordination, gait abnormalities)	Methotrexate or CNS irradiation
Peripheral neuropathy (footdrop, tingling sensation in hands and/or feet, incoordination)	Vincristine
Cognitive deficits (decline with intelligence, memory, attention, nonlanguage skills)	Intrathecal chemotherapy or cranial irradiation (especially before 3 years of age)
Cardiovascular	
Cardiomyopathy (tachycardia, tachypnea, dyspnea, shortness of breath, edema, palpitations)	Anthracyclines (doxorubicin and daunorubicin) or irradiation to heart High-dose cyclophosphamide
Pericardial damage (pleural effusion, cardiomegaly)	Mediastinal irradiation
Respiratory	
Pneumonitis (dyspnea, nonproductive cough, fever)	Lung irradiation, alkylating agents, possibly bleomycin, vinblastine, cisplatin
Pulmonary fibrosis (dyspnea, restrictive ventilation, decreased exercise tolerance)	
Gastrointestinal	
Chronic enteritis (colic, abdominal pain, vomiting, diarrhea, obstipation, bleeding)	Abdominal irradiation, methotrexate, cytosine arabinoside
Hepatic fibrosis (jaundice, hepatomegaly)	Methotrexate, 6-mercaptopurine
Urinary	
Hemorrhagic cystitis (microscopic hematuria to gross hemorrhage)	Cyclophosphamide; ifosfamide; irradiation
Bladder fibrosis (decreased bladder capacity, ureteral reflux)	Cisplatin
Tubular necrosis (decreased creatinine clearance)	
Endocrine	
Thyroid dysfunction (see Chapter 47)	Irradiation to thyroid gland, pituitary gland, testes, ovaries
Reproductive	
Possible gonadal damage, both sexes (delayed puberty, amenorrhea, decreased sperm count, increased follicle-stimulating and luteinizing hormones, decreased testosterone or estrogen)	Alkylating agents Irradiation to pituitary gland, testes, ovaries
Skeletal	
Growth retardation (short stature)	Irradiation, long-term steroids
Spinal deformities, scoliosis, kyphosis, asymmetric growth, pathologic fractures	Irradiation
Immune	
Asplenia (overwhelming infection, fever)	Splenectomy
Sensory Organs	
Cataracts (opacity over pupil)	Cranial irradiation, high-dose steroids
Hearing (decreased hearing, especially with high-frequency loss)	Cisplatin
Additional Effects	
Dental Problems	
Increased caries, periodontal disease, hypoplastic teeth, hypodontia (delayed or absent tooth development)	Irradiation to maxilla and mandible
Second Malignancies	
Bone and soft-tissue tumors	Irradiation, alkylating agents
Leukemia (ALL or AML)	

ALL, Acute lymphoblastic leukemia; *AML,* acute myelogenous leukemia; *CNS,* central nervous system.

with careful documentation of the child's sexual development using the Tanner staging scale (see the "Sexual Maturation" section in Chapter 35).

Irradiation to developing bone and cartilage may cause numerous abnormalities. Assessment includes close observation of the irradiated bone for defects, such as spinal kyphoscoliosis, functional limitations, and osteoporosis. Children who have received irradiation to the mandibular area are at risk for dental caries, arrested tooth development, and incomplete dental calcification. A careful assessment in children who have received irradiation is performed at each clinic visit.

REFERENCES

Agarwala, S. (2012). Primary malignant liver tumors in children. *Indian Journal of Pediatrics, 79*(6), 793–800.

Allen, C. E., Kamdar, K. Y., Bollard, C. M., et al. (2016). Malignant non-Hodgkin lymphomas in children. In P. A. Pizzo & D. G. Poplack (Eds.), *Principles and practices of pediatric oncology* (7th ed.). Philadelphia, PA: Lippincott.

Alviar, M. J., Hale, T., & Dungca, M. (2011). Pharmacologic interventions for treating phantom limb pain. *Cochrane Database of Systematic Reviews, 2011*(12), CD006380.

Arceci, R. J., & Meshinchi, A. (2016). Acute myeloid leukemia and myelodysplastic disorders. In P. A. Pizzo & D. G. Poplack (Eds.), *Principles and practices of pediatric oncology* (7th ed.). Philadelphia, PA: Lippincott.

Ardura, M. I., & Koh, A. Y. (2016). Infectious complications in pediatric cancer patients. In P. A. Pizzo & D. G. Poplack (Eds.), *Principles and practices of pediatric oncology* (7th ed.). Philadelphia, PA: Lippincott.

Arndt, C. A., Rose, P. S., Folpe, A. L., et al. (2012). Common musculoskeletal tumors of childhood and adolescence. *Mayo Clinic Proceedings, 87*(5), 475–487.

Brodeur, G. M., Hogarty, M. D., Bagatell, R., et al. (2016). Neuroblastoma. In P. A. Pizzo & D. G. Poplack (Eds.), *Principles and practices of pediatric oncology* (7th ed.). Philadelphia, PA: Lippincott.

Children's Oncology Group. (2014). *Long-term follow-up guidelines for survivors of childhood, adolescent, and young adult cancers.* Retrieved from http://www.survivorshipguidelines.org/.

Crawford, J. (2013). Childhood brain tumors. *Pediatrics in Review, 34*(2), 63–78.

Davenport, K. P., Blanco, F. C., & Sandler, A. D. (2012). Pediatric malignancies, neuroblastoma, Wilm's tumor, hepatoblastoma, rhabdomyosarcoma, and sacrococcygeal teratoma. *Surgical Clinics of North America, 92*(3), 745–767.

Davidoff, A. M. (2012). Wilms tumor. *Advances in Pediatrics, 59*(1), 247–267.

Dimaras, H., Kimani, K., Dimba, E. A., et al. (2012). Retinoblastoma. *Lancet, 379*(9824), 1436–1446.

Dupuis, L. L., Boodhan, S., Holdsworth, M., et al. (2013). Guideline for the prevention of acute nausea and vomiting due to antineoplastic medication in pediatric cancer patients. *Pediatric Blood & Cancer, 60*(7), 1073–1082.

Effinger, K. E., Migliorati, C. A., Hudson, M. M., et al. (2014). Oral and dental late effects in survivors of childhood cancer: A Children's Oncology Group report. *Supportive Care in Cancer, 22*(7), 2009–2019.

Feyer, P., & Jordan, K. (2011). Update and new trends in antiemetic therapy: The continuing need for novel therapies. *Annals of Oncology, 22*(1), 30–38.

Fleming, A. J., & Chi, S. N. (2012). Brain tumors in children. *Current Problems in Pediatric and Adolescent Health Care, 42*(4), 80–103.

Frazier, A. L., Olson, T. A., Schneider, D. T., et al. (2016). Germ cell tumors. In P. A. Pizzo & D. G. Poplack (Eds.), *Principles and practices of pediatric oncology* (7th ed.). Philadelphia, PA: Lippincott.

Frew, J. A., Lewis, J., & Lucraft, H. H. (2013). The management of children with lymphomas. *Clinical Oncology, 25*(1), 11–18.

Fry, T. J., Sondel, P. M., & Mackall, C. L. (2016). Tumor immunology and pediatric cancer. In P. A. Pizzo & D. G. Poplack (Eds.), *Principles and practices of pediatric oncology* (7th ed.). Philadelphia, PA: Lippincott.

Gorlick, R., Janeway, K., & Marina, N. (2016). Osteosarcoma. In P. A. Pizzo & D. G. Poplack (Eds.), *Principles and practices of pediatric oncology* (7th ed.). Philadelphia, PA: Lippincott.

Gottschalk, S., Naik, S., Hegde, M., et al. (2016). Hematopoietic stem cell transplantation in pediatric oncology. In P. A. Pizzo & D. G. Poplack (Eds.), *Principles and practices of pediatric oncology* (7th ed.). Philadelphia, PA: Lippincott.

Henley, S. J., Singh, S. D., King, J., et al. (2015). Invasive cancer incidence and survival—United States, 2011. *Morbidity and Mortality Weekly Report, 64*(9), 237–242.

Hill-Kayser, C., Tochner, Z., Both, S., et al. (2013). Proton versus photon radiation therapy for patients with high-risk neuroblastoma: The need for a customized approach. *Pediatric Blood & Cancer, 60*(10), 1606–1611.

Hockenberry, M. J., Kline, N. E., & Rodgers, C. (2016). Nursing support of the child with cancer. In P. A. Pizzo & D. G. Poplack (Eds.), *Principles and practices of pediatric oncology* (7th ed.). Philadelphia, PA: Lippincott.

Hurwitz, R. L., Shields, C. L., Shields, J. A., et al. (2016). Retinoblastoma. In P. A. Pizzo & D. G. Poplack (Eds.), *Principles and practices of pediatric oncology* (7th ed.). Philadelphia, PA: Lippincott.

Knudson, A. G., Jr., Hethcote, H. W., & Brown, B. W. (1975). Mutation and childhood cancer: A probabilistic model for the incidence of retinoblastoma. *Proceedings of the National Academy of Sciences of the United States of America, 72*(12), 5116–5120.

Landier, W., Armenian, S. H., Meadows, A. T., et al. (2016). Late effects of childhood cancer and its treatment. In P. A. Pizzo & D. G. Poplack (Eds.), *Principles and practices of pediatric oncology* (7th ed.). Philadelphia, PA: Lippincott.

Lawson, C. M., Daley, B. J., Sams, V. G., Martindale, R., Kudsk, K. A., et al. (2013). Factors that impact patient outcome: Nutrition assessment. *Journal of Parenteral and Enteral Nutrition, 37*(5 suppl), 30S–38S.

Lutwak, N., Howland, M. A., Gambetta, R., et al. (2013). Even "safe" medications need to be administered with care. *BMJ Case Reports, 2013*.

McCurdy, M. T., & Shanholtz, C. B. (2012). Oncologic emergencies. *Critical Care Medicine, 40*(7), 2212–2222.

Metzger, M., Krasin, M. J., Choi, J. K., et al. (2016). Hodgkin lymphoma. In P. A. Pizzo & D. G. Poplack (Eds.), *Principles and practices of pediatric oncology* (7th ed.). Philadelphia, PA: Lippincott.

Meyers, R. L., Trobaugh-Lotrario, A. D., Malogolowkin, M. H., Katzenstein, H. M., López-Terrada, D. H., et al. (2016). Liver tumors. In P. A. Pizzo & D. G. Poplack (Eds.), *Principles and practices of pediatric oncology* (7th ed.). Philadelphia, PA: Lippincott.

Miller, M. M., Donald, D. V., & Hagemann, T. M. (2012). Prevention and treatment of oral mucositis in children with cancer. *Journal of Pediatric Pharmacology and Therapeutics, 174*, 340–350.

National Cancer Institute. (2015a). *Childhood Hodgkin lymphoma treatment— For health professionals.* Retrieved from http://www.cancer.gov/types/lymphoma/hp/child-hodgkin-treatment-pdq.

National Cancer Institute. (2015b). *Childhood non-Hodgkin lymphoma treatment.* Retrieved from http://www.cancer.gov/types/lymphoma/hp/child-nhl-treatment-pdq#link/_536_toc.

National Cancer Institute. (2015c). *Neuroblastoma treatment—For health professionals.* Retrieved from http://www.cancer.gov/types/neuroblastoma/hp/neuroblastoma-treatment-pdq.

National Cancer Institute. (2015d). *Ewing sarcoma treatment—For health professionals.* Retrieved from http://www.cancer.gov/types/bone/hp/ewing-treatment-pdq.

National Cancer Institute. (2015e). *Childhood rhabdomyosarcoma treatment— For health professionals.* Retrieved from http://www.cancer.gov/types/soft-tissue-sarcoma/hp/rhabdomyosarcoma-treatment-pdq.

National Cancer Institute. (2015f). *Retinoblastoma treatment—For health professionals.* Retrieved from http://www.cancer.gov/types/retinoblastoma/hp/retinoblastoma-treatment-pdq.

Parsons, D. W., Pollack, I. F., Haas-Kogan, D. A., et al. (2016). Gliomas, ependymomas, and other nonembryonal tumors of the central nervous system. In P. A. Pizzo & D. G. Poplack (Eds.), *Principles and practices of pediatric oncology* (7th ed.). Philadelphia, PA: Lippincott.

Plon, S. E., & Malkin, D. (2016). Childhood cancer and heredity. In P. A. Pizzo & D. G. Poplack (Eds.), *Principles and practices of pediatric oncology* (7th ed.). Philadelphia, PA: Lippincott.

Rabin, K. R., Gramatges, M. M., Margolin, J. F., et al. (2016). Acute lymphoblastic leukemia. In P. A. Pizzo & D. G. Poplack (Eds.), *Principles and practices of pediatric oncology* (7th ed.). Philadelphia, PA: Lippincott.

Ruggiero, A., Battista, A., Coccia, P., et al. (2011). How to manage vaccinations in children with cancer. *Pediatric Blood & Cancer, 57*(7), 1104–1108.

Scheurer, M. E., Lupo, P. J., & Bondy, M. L. (2016). Epidemiology of childhood cancer. In P. A. Pizzo & D. G. Poplack (Eds.), *Principles and practices of pediatric oncology* (7th ed.). Philadelphia, PA: Lippincott.

Wexler, L. H., Skapek, S. X., & Helman, L. J. (2016). Rhabdomyosarcoma. In P. A. Pizzo & D. G. Poplack (Eds.), *Principles and practices of pediatric oncology* (7th ed.). Philadelphia, PA: Lippincott.

Wolff, A., Vanduynhoven, E., van Kleef, M., et al. (2011). Phantom pain. *Pain Practice, 11*(4), 403–413.

Wong, C., Lau, E., Palozzi, L., et al. (2012). Pain management in children: Part I—Pain assessment tools and a brief review of nonpharmacological and pharmacological treatment options. *Canadian Pharmacists Journal, 145*(5), 222–225.

45

The Child With Genitourinary Dysfunction

Marilyn J. Hockenberry

GENITOURINARY DYSFUNCTION

Assessment of kidney and urinary tract integrity and diagnosis of renal or urinary tract disease are based on several evaluative tools. Physical examination, history taking, and observation of symptoms are the initial procedures. In suspected urinary tract diseases or disorders, further assessment by laboratory, radiologic, and other evaluative methods is carried out. Fig. 45.1 provides a review of the kidney and nephron structures.

CLINICAL MANIFESTATIONS

As in most disorders of childhood, the incidence and type of kidney or urinary tract dysfunction change with the age and maturation of the child. In addition, the presenting complaints and the significance of these complaints vary with age. For example, a complaint of enuresis has greater significance at 8 years of age than at 4 years of age. In newborns, renal abnormalities may be associated with a number of other malformations, for example, obvious neural tube defects to the subtle abnormal shape or position of the outer ear. Failure to thrive in children may be a sign of impaired renal function.

Many of the clinical manifestations of renal disease are common to a variety of childhood disorders, but their presence is an indication to obtain further information from the child's history, family history, and laboratory studies as part of a complete physical examination. Suspected renal disease can be further evaluated by means of radiographic studies and renal biopsy (Table 45.1).

LABORATORY TESTS

Both urine and blood studies contribute vital information for detection of renal problems. The single most important test is probably routine urinalysis. Specific urine and blood tests provide additional information. Because nurses are usually the persons who collect the specimens for examination and who often perform many of the screening tests, they should be familiar with the test, its function, and factors that can alter or distort the results of the test. The major urine tests and blood tests are outlined in Tables 45.2 and 45.3, respectively.

CARE MANAGEMENT

Interprofessional care responsibilities in the assessment of genitourinary disorders or diseases begin with observation of the child for any manifestations that might indicate dysfunction. Many conditions have specific characteristics that distinguish them from other disorders. These are discussed as appropriate throughout the chapter.

The nurse is generally the one who is responsible for preparing infants, children, and parents for tests and for collection of urine and (sometimes) blood specimens for observation and laboratory analysis (see the "Preparation for Diagnostic and Therapeutic Procedures" and "Collection of Specimens" sections in Chapter 39). An important nursing responsibility is to maintain careful intake and output measurements and blood pressure for most children with genitourinary dysfunction and those who might be at risk for developing renal complications (e.g., children in shock, postoperative patients). For example, any significant degree of renal disease can diminish the glomerular filtration rate (GFR), a measure of the amount of plasma from which a given substance is totally cleared in 1 minute. A number of substances can be used, but the most useful clinical estimation of glomerular filtration is the clearance of *creatinine,* an end product of protein metabolism in muscle and a substance that is freely filtered by the glomerulus and secreted by renal tubular cells. The nurse's responsibility in this test is collection of urine, usually a 12- or 24-hour specimen.

GENITOURINARY TRACT DISORDERS AND DEFECTS

Urinary Tract Infection

Urinary tract infection (UTI) is a common and potentially serious problem in children. The overall prevalence is approximately 7% in infants and young children, although there is some variability based on age, gender, race, and circumcision status (Shaikh, Morone, Bost, et al., 2008). Caucasians, females, and uncircumcised boys have the highest rates. Specifically, girls have a twofold to fourfold higher prevalence than do circumcised boys. Uncircumcised males younger than 3 months of age and females younger than 12 months of age have the highest baseline prevalence of UTI (Shaikh et al.). UTI may involve the urethra and bladder (lower urinary tract) or the ureters, renal pelvis, calyces, and renal parenchyma (upper urinary tract). Because of the difficulty in distinguishing upper from lower tract infection, particularly in young children, UTI is often broadly defined. Upper UTIs or kidney infections tend to present with fever and may lead to renal scarring that may be associated with decreased kidney function, hypertension, and renal disease over time. Diagnosis of UTI is made based on the presence of both pyuria and at least 50,000 colonies per mL of a single uropathic organism in an appropriately collected specimen (American Academy of Pediatrics Subcommittee on Urinary Tract Infection, Steering Committee on Quality Improvement and Management, & Roberts, 2011).

Classification

Infection of the urinary tract may be present with or without clinical symptoms. As a result, the site of infection is often difficult to pinpoint

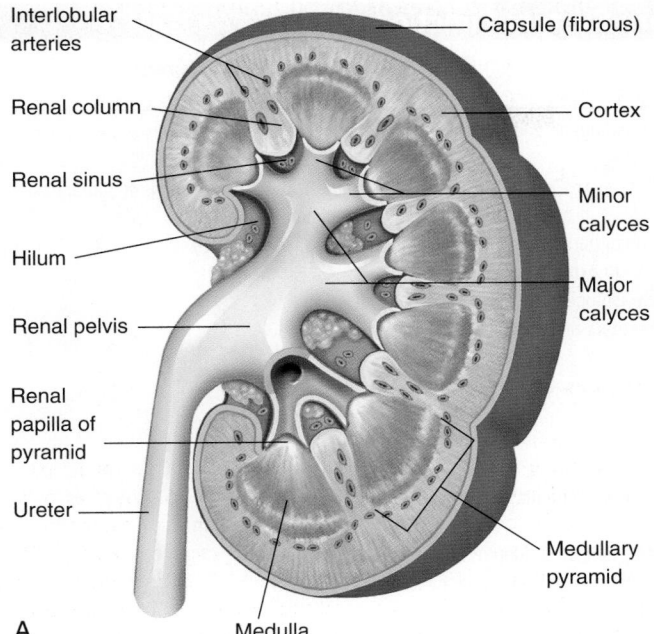

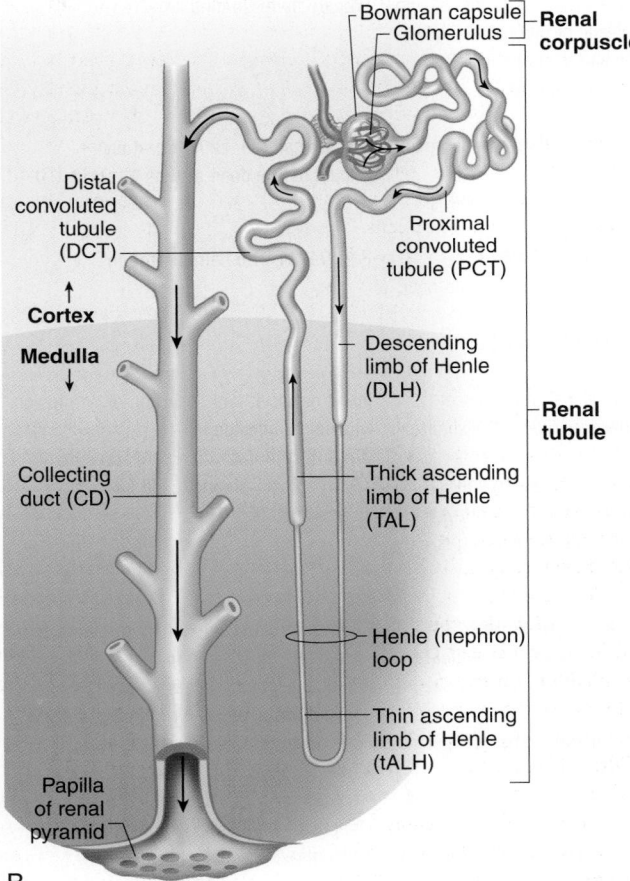

FIG 45.1 A, Kidney structure. **B,** Components of the nephron. (From Patton K.T., & Thibodeau, G.A. [2016]. *Anatomy and physiology* [9th ed.]. St. Louis, MO: Elsevier.)

with any degree of accuracy. Various terms used to describe urinary tract disorders include the following:

Bacteriuria: Presence of bacteria in the urine

Pyuria: Presence of white blood cells in the urine

Asymptomatic bacteriuria: Significant bacteriuria (usually defined as >100,000 colony-forming units [CFUs]) with no evidence of clinical infection

Symptomatic bacteriuria: Bacteriuria accompanied by physical signs of UTI (dysuria, suprapubic discomfort, hematuria, fever)

Recurrent UTI: Repeated episode of bacteriuria or symptomatic UTI

Persistent UTI: Persistence of bacteriuria despite antibiotic treatment

Febrile UTI: Bacteriuria accompanied by fever and other physical signs of UTI; presence of a fever typically implies pyelonephritis

Cystitis: Inflammation of the bladder

Urethritis: Inflammation of the urethra

Pyelonephritis: Inflammation of the upper urinary tract and kidneys

Urosepsis: Febrile UTI coexisting with systemic signs of bacterial illness; blood culture reveals presence of urinary pathogen

Etiology

A variety of organisms can be responsible for UTI. *Escherichia coli* remains the most common uropathogen overall, but the prevalence is higher in females (83%) than males (50%) (Edlin, Shapiro, Hersh, et al., 2013). Other gram-negative organisms associated with UTI include *Proteus mirabilis, Pseudomonas aeruginosa, Klebsiella,* and *Enterobacter.* Gram-positive bacterial pathogens include *Enterococcus, Staphylococcus saprophyticus,* and, rarely, *Staphylococcus aureus.* Viruses and fungi are uncommon causes of UTI in children. Most uropathogens originate in the gastrointestinal tract, migrate to the periurethral area, and ascend to the bladder. A number of factors contribute to the development of UTI, including anatomic, physical, and chemical conditions or properties of the host's urinary tract.

Anatomic and Physical Factors

The structure of the lower urinary tract has traditionally been thought to account for the increased incidence of bacteriuria in females. The short urethra, which measures about 2 cm (0.75 inch) in young girls and 4 cm (1.6 inches) in mature women, provides a ready pathway for invasion of organisms. In addition, the closure of the urethra at the end of micturition may return contaminated bacteria to the bladder. The longer male urethra (as long as 20 cm [8 inches] in an adult) and the antibacterial properties of prostatic secretions inhibit the entry and growth of pathogens. The importance of the length of the urethra in the pathogenesis of UTI has been questioned because of the high incidence of UTI in male neonates. The presence or absence of the foreskin has been shown to be a significant factor, with prevalence of UTI in infant males younger than 3 months of age being 2.4% in circumcised males and 20.1% in uncircumcised males (Shaikh et al., 2008). The presence of a foreskin is associated with a preputial colonization of uropathic bacteria that can ascend the urethra easily (Balat, Karakok, Guler, et al., 2008). Virulence factors are important in the pathogenesis; and these, coupled with the propensity of bacteria to adhere to the female periurethral mucosa may explain the increased incidence of UTI in females.

> **! NURSING ALERT**
>
> Considerable evidence shows significant reduction in the risk for urinary tract infection (UTI) in the first year of life in circumcised male infants. Current evidence indicates the health benefits of circumcision outweigh the risks and the benefits of the procedure justify access for families who choose it, but are not sufficient to recommend routine circumcision for all male newborns (American Academy of Pediatrics Task Force on Circumcision, 2012).

TABLE 45.1	**Radiologic and Other Tests of Urinary System Function**		
Test	**Procedure**	**Purpose**	**Comments and Nursing Responsibilities**
Urine culture and sensitivity	Collection of sterile specimen	Determines presence of pathogens and the drugs to which they are sensitive	Send specimen to laboratory immediately after collection Catheterization, clean-catch, or suprapubic specimen
Renal and bladder ultrasonography	Transmission of ultrasonic waves through renal parenchyma, along ureteral course, and over bladder	Allows visualization of renal parenchyma and renal pelvis without exposure to external-beam radiation or radioactive isotopes Visualization of dilated ureters and bladder wall also possible Can show renal cysts and stones, though less sensitive than CT Doppler ultrasonography can be used to evaluate renal vascular flow	Noninvasive procedure
Testicular (scrotal) ultrasonography	Transmission of ultrasonic waves through scrotal contents and testis	Allows visualization of scrotal contents, including testis Testicular ultrasonography is used to identify masses, and Doppler-enhanced ultrasonography is used to differentiate hyperemia of epididymo-orchitis from ischemia or torsion	Noninvasive procedure
Plain film of the abdomen	Flat plate radiograph of abdomen and pelvis for KUB	Can identify certain types of stones that are calcium containing as well as calculi or opaque foreign bodies in bladder (diagnostic test of choice for nephrolithiasis is noncontrast helical CT) Assess stool burden	Prepare as for routine x-ray
Voiding cystourethrography	Contrast medium injected into bladder through urethral catheter until bladder is full; films taken before, during, and after voiding	Visualizes bladder outline and urethra, reveals reflux of urine into ureters Provides information on bladder emptying and is also used to diagnosis PUV	Prepare child for catheterization Should not be done at time of active UTI
Radionuclide (nuclear) cystogram	Radionuclide-containing fluid injected through urethral catheter until bladder is full; images generated before, during, and after voiding	Alternative to voiding cystourethrography to evaluate reflux, although visualization of anatomic details is relatively poor Used in some institutions for follow up if initial VCUG due to less radiation	Prepare child for catheterization
Radioisotope imaging studies (renal scans)	Contrast medium injected intravenously; computer analysis to measure uptake or washout (excretion) for analysis of organ function	DMSA radioisotope used to visualize renal scars and differential renal function; does not visualize ureters and bladder MAG3 radioisotope assesses obstruction and differential function between the two kidneys DTPA is an alternative to MAG3, but imaging is limited because it is only filtered at the glomerulus	Insert or assist with insertion of IV infusion Monitor IV infusion Urethral catheterization may accompany MAG3 scan; prepare child for catheterization when indicated
MRI	Uses strong magnetic fields and radio waves to form images	MRI of kidneys used to evaluate renal mass Magnetic resonance angiography used to evaluate renovascular hypertension and has reduced need for renal angiography Magnetic resonance urogram used to detect specific urologic abnormalities, such as ectopic ureter	MRI often requires sedation in infants and children due to need to stay still, typically in an enclosed space; follow NPO guidelines depending on timing of study Assist with IV access if indicated Magnetic devices or implants may be unsafe for MRI, including cochlear implants and permanent pacemakers
CT	Narrow-beam x-rays and computer analysis provide precise reconstruction of area	Visualizes vertical or horizontal cross-section of kidney Especially valuable to distinguish tumors, cysts, and stones Noncontrast helical CT is gold standard for radiologic diagnosis of renal stone disease Renal CT angiogram used to evaluate blood flow in hypertensive patients and is now used more commonly than renal arteriography	Noncontrast scan is noninvasive Contrast-enhanced CT scan preparation may require child to be NPO for a few hours With speed of newer scans, the need for sedation is decreased but if required will also require NPO Assist with IV access if needed Used selectively due to higher radiation exposure

TABLE 45.1	Radiologic and Other Tests of Urinary System Function—cont'd		
Test	**Procedure**	**Purpose**	**Comments and Nursing Responsibilities**
Cystoscopy	Direct visualization of bladder and lower urinary tract through small scope inserted via urethra	Investigation of bladder and lower tract lesions; visualizes ureteral openings, bladder wall, trigone, and urethra	NPO orders per protocol, typically no solid food after midnight, liquids until 4 to 6 hours before procedure Carry out preoperative preparations; cystoscopy is done under anesthesia in children
Renal biopsy	Removal of kidney tissue by open or percutaneous technique for study by light, electron, or immunofluorescent microscopy	Yields histologic and microscopic information about glomeruli and tubules; helps distinguish among types of nephritic syndromes Distinguishes other renal disorders	Nothing orally 4 to 6 hours before test Premedicate as ordered Prepare setup for procedure Assist with procedure Take vital signs Apply pressure to area with pressure dressing and, if feasible, a sandbag Bed rest for 24 hours Observe for abdominal pain, tenderness Monitor input and output Surgical incision may be required in infants
Urodynamics	Set of tests designed to measure bladder filling, storage, and evacuation functions: **Uroflowmetry:** Test to determine efficiency of urination **Cystometrography:** Graphic comparison of bladder pressure as a function of volume **Voiding pressure study:** Comparison of detrusor contraction pressure, sphincter electromyelogram, and urinary flow	Determine characteristic of voiding dysfunction. Used to identify type (cause) of incontinence or urinary retention Especially valuable for voiding dysfunction complicated by urinary infection, urinary retention, or neurogenic bladder dysfunction	Prepare child for urinary catheterization The bladder will be filled with contrast, sterile water, or saline solution, and filling pressures will be recorded; the child may experience fullness, coolness from the fluid, and urine leakage during the study Insertion of needles may be required for sphincter EMG (institution-specific, often use electrode patches)

CT, Computed tomography; *DMSA,* dimercaptosuccinic acid; *DTPA,* diethylenetriamine pentaacetic acid; *EMG,* electromyography; *IV,* intravenous; *KUB,* kidney, ureters, and bladder; *MAG3,* mercaptoacetyltriglycine; *MRI,* magnetic resonance imaging; *NPO,* nothing by mouth; *PUV,* posterior urethral valve; *UTI,* urinary tract infection; *VCUG,* voiding cystourethrogram.

The single most important host factor influencing the occurrence of UTI is *urinary stasis.* Ordinarily, urine is sterile, but at 37° C (98.6° F), it provides an excellent culture medium. Under normal conditions, the act of completely and repeatedly emptying the bladder flushes away any organisms before they have an opportunity to multiply and invade surrounding tissue. However, urine that remains in the bladder allows bacteria from the urethra to rapidly become established in the rich medium. Incomplete bladder emptying (stasis) may result from *reflux* (see the "Vesicoureteral Reflux" section later in this chapter), anatomic abnormalities, neurogenic bladder, voiding dysfunction, or extrinsic ureteral or bladder compression that may be caused by constipation. Overdistention of the bladder may increase the risk for infection by decreasing host resistance, probably as a result of decreased blood flow to the mucosa. This occurs more often in a neurogenic bladder with increased bladder pressure, but it can be the result of voluntarily holding back urine (Vasudeva & Madersbacher, 2014).

Altered Urine and Bladder Chemistry

Several mechanical and chemical characteristics of the urine and bladder mucosa help maintain urinary sterility. Increased fluid intake promotes flushing of the normal bladder and lowers the concentration of organisms in the infected bladder. Diuresis also seems to enhance the antibacterial properties of the renal medulla.

Most pathogens favor an alkaline medium. Normally, urine is slightly acidic with a median pH of 6. A urine pH of 5 hampers but does not eliminate bacterial multiplication. Much has been reported about the use of cranberry products for prevention of UTI. Initially it was thought to alter the urine acidity, but studies have not shown that ingestion results in a lower pH; but instead it appeared to decrease the adherence of certain bacteria to the bladder wall. Recent review of the literature showed that cranberry products did not significantly reduce the occurrence of symptomatic UTI overall or in any of the subgroups, including children. Because the benefit is small, cranberry juice cannot currently be recommended for prevention of UTIs. Other cranberry preparations need to be quantified using standardized methods to ensure the potency before being evaluated in clinical studies or recommended for use (Jepson, Williams & Craig, 2012).

Diagnostic Evaluation

The clinical manifestations of UTI depend on the child's age (Box 45.1). Diagnosis of UTI is confirmed by detection of bacteria in urine culture, but urine collection is often difficult, especially in infants and very

TABLE 45.2   Urine Tests of Renal Function

Test	Normal Range	Deviations	Significance of Deviations
Physical Tests			
Volume	Age related	Polyuria	Osmotic factors (urinary glucose level in diabetes mellitus)
	Newborn: 30 to 60 mL	Oliguria	Retention caused by obstructive disease
	Children: Bladder capacity		Inadequate bladder emptying caused by neurogenic bladder or obstructive disorder
	(oz) = Age (years) + 2	Anuria	Obstruction of urinary tract; AKI
Specific gravity	With normal fluid intake:	High	Dehydration
	1.016 to 1.022		Presence of protein or glucose
	Newborn: 1.001 to 1.020		Presence of radiopaque contrast medium after radiologic examinations
	Others: 1.001 to 1.030	Low	Excessive fluid intake
			Distal tubular dysfunction
			Insufficient ADH
			Diuresis
Osmolality	Newborn: 50 to 600 mOsm/L	Fixed at 1.01	Chronic glomerular disease
	Thereafter: 50 to	High or low	Same as for specific gravity
	1400 mOsm/L		More sensitive index than specific gravity
Appearance	Clear pale yellow to deep	Cloudy	Contains sediment
	gold	Cloudy reddish pink to	Blood from trauma or disease
		reddish brown	Myoglobin after severe muscle destruction
		Light	Dilute
		Dark	Concentrated
		Red	Trauma
Chemical Tests			
pH	Newborn: 5 to 7	Weak acid or neutral	If associated with metabolic acidosis, suggests tubular acidosis
	Thereafter: 4.8 to 7.8	Alkaline	If associated with metabolic alkalosis, suggests potassium deficiency
	Average: 6		Urinary infection
			Metabolic alkalosis
Protein level	Absent	Present	Abnormal glomerular permeability (e.g., glomerular disease, changes in blood pressure)
			Most kidney disease
			Orthostatic in some individuals
Glucose level	Absent	Present	Diabetes mellitus
			Infusion of concentrated glucose-containing fluids
			Glomerulonephritis
			Impaired tubular reabsorption
Ketone levels	Absent	Present	Conditions of acute metabolic demand (stress)
			Diabetic ketoacidosis
Leukocyte esterase	Absent	Present	Can identify both lysed and intact WBCs via enzyme detection
Nitrites	Absent	Present	Most species of bacteria convert nitrates to nitrites in the urine
Microscopic Tests			
WBC count	<1 or 2	>5 polymorphonuclear leukocytes/field	Urinary tract inflammatory process
		Lymphocytes	Allograft rejection
			Malignancy
RBC count	<1 or 2	4 to 6/field in centrifuged specimen	Trauma
			Stones
			Glomerular injury
			Infection
			Neoplasms
Presence of bacteria	Absent to a few	>100,000 organisms/mL in centrifuged specimen	UTI
Presence of casts	Occasional	Granular casts	Tubular or glomerular disorders
		Cellular casts	Degenerative process in advanced renal disease
		WBC	Pyelonephritis
		RBC	Glomerulonephritis
		Hyaline casts	Proteinuria; usually transient

ADH, Antidiuretic hormone; *AKI,* acute kidney injury; *RBC,* red blood cell; *UTI,* urinary tract infection; *WBC,* white blood cell.

TABLE 45.3 Blood Tests of Renal Function

Test	Normal Range (mg/dL)	Deviations	Significance of Deviations
BUN	Newborn: 4 to 18 Infant, child: 5 to 18	Elevated	Renal disease: Acute or chronic (the higher the BUN, the more severe the disease) Increased protein catabolism Dehydration Hemorrhage High protein intake Corticosteroid therapy
Uric acid	Child: 2 to 5.5	Increased	Severe renal disease
Creatinine	Infant: 0.2 to 0.4 Child: 0.3 to 0.7 Adolescent: 0.5 to 1	Increased	Renal impairment

BUN, Blood urea nitrogen.

BOX 45.1 Clinical Manifestations of Urinary Tract Disorders or Disease

Neonatal Period (Birth to 1 Month of Age)
Poor feeding
Vomiting
Failure to gain weight
Rapid respiration (acidosis)
Respiratory distress
Spontaneous pneumothorax or pneumomediastinum
Frequent urination
Screaming on urination
Poor urine stream
Jaundice
Seizures
Dehydration
Other anomalies or stigmata
Enlarged kidneys or bladder

Infancy (1 to 24 Months of Age)
Poor feeding
Vomiting
Failure to gain weight
Excessive thirst
Frequent urination
Straining or screaming on urination
Foul-smelling urine
Pallor
Fever
Persistent diaper rash
Seizures (with or without fever)
Dehydration
Enlarged kidneys or bladder

Childhood (2 to 14 Years of Age)
Poor appetite
Vomiting
Growth failure
Excessive thirst
Enuresis, incontinence, frequent urination
Painful urination
Swelling of face
Seizures
Pallor
Fatigue
Blood in urine
Abdominal or back pain
Edema
Hypertension
Tetany

small children. Several factors may alter a urine specimen, and contamination of a specimen by organisms from sources other than the urine, such as perineal and perianal flora in bag specimens, is the most frequent cause of false-positive results. Unless the specimen is a first morning sample, a recent high fluid intake may indicate a falsely low organism count. Therefore, children should not be encouraged to drink large volumes of water in an attempt to obtain a specimen quickly.

> **! NURSING ALERT**
>
> A child who exhibits the following should be evaluated for UTI:
> - Incontinence in a toilet-trained child
> - Strong-smelling urine in association with other symptoms
> - Frequency or urgency
> - Pain with urination

The most accurate tests of bacterial content are suprapubic aspiration (for children younger than 2 years of age) and properly performed bladder catheterization (as long as the first few milliliters are excluded from collection). The specimen must be fresh (<1 hour with storage at room temperature or <4 hours with refrigeration) to ensure sensitivity and specificity of the urinalysis and to prevent growth of organisms (American Academy of Pediatrics Subcommittee on Urinary Tract Infection, et al., 2011). Clean catch and specimens collected by urine bags are prone to contamination, given the difficulty of obtaining a true mid-stream specimen with wiping of the meatus and retraction of the labia or foreskin or cleaning the perineum. In these instances, a negative specimen excludes infection, and a positive culture is not necessarily diagnostic.

Predictive tests are utilized to direct therapy when UTI is suspected. Urine dipsticks indicate the presence of leukocyte esterase and nitrites and are quick and inexpensive. Leukocyte esterase is a surrogate marker for pyuria, and nitrite is converted from dietary nitrates in the presence of most gram-negative enteric bacteria in the urine. Because the conversion takes 4 hours in the bladder, it is not a sensitive marker for infants or children who empty their bladder frequently. Also, not all urinary pathogens reduce nitrate to nitrite (American Academy of Pediatrics Subcommittee on Urinary Tract Infection, et al., 2011).

Further radiographic evaluation, such as ultrasonography, voiding cystourethrogram (VCUG), and renal scans such as a dimercaptosuccinic acid (DMSA) scan, may be performed after the infection subsides to identify anatomic abnormalities contributing to the development of infection and existing kidney changes from recurrent infection.

Therapeutic Management

The objectives of treatment of children with UTI are to (1) eliminate current infection, (2) identify contributing factors to reduce the risk for recurrence, (3) prevent systemic spread of the infection, and (4) preserve renal function. Antibiotic therapy should be initiated on the basis of identification of the pathogen, the child's history of antibiotic use, and the location of the infection. Several antimicrobial drugs are available for treating UTI, but all of them can occasionally be ineffective because of resistance of organisms. Common antiinfective agents used for UTI include the penicillins, sulfonamide (including trimethoprim-sulfamethoxazole), the cephalosporins, and nitrofurantoin.

If anatomic defects such as primary reflux or bladder neck obstruction are present, surgical correction or urinary prophylaxis may be necessary to prevent recurrent infection. The aim of therapy and careful follow-up is to reduce the chance of renal scarring.

Vesicoureteral Reflux

Vesicoureteral reflux (VUR) refers to the retrograde flow of urine from the bladder into the upper urinary tract. *Primary reflux* results from congenitally abnormal insertion of ureters into the bladder; *secondary reflux* occurs as a result of an acquired condition.

Reflux increases the chance for febrile UTI but does not cause it. When bladder pressure is high enough, refluxing urine can fill the ureter and the renal pelvis. The International Reflux Study Group developed a classification system that describes the degree of reflux, ranging from Grade I to V, which is important because higher grades are associated with renal abnormalities and renal damage. Reflux with infection is the most common cause of pyelonephritis in children. These children are usually very symptomatic with high fevers, vomiting, and chills. In most cases, conservative therapy is sufficient with a high rate of spontaneous resolution of VUR over time: 51% at a mean duration of 2 years for all grades of VUR (Estrada, Passerotti, Graham, et al., 2009). Prevention of infection has been the goal with use of continuous antibiotic prophylaxis (CAP) common practice until resolution or correction of VUR. This practice was reviewed in a recent multisite trial and found to be associated with a substantially decreased risk for recurrence of UTI but not of renal scarring, leaving the use of CAP controversial (Hoberman, Chesney, & RIVUR Trial Investigators, 2014). Urine cultures are not recommended routinely but should be obtained if there are symptoms or unexplained fever, because breakthrough infections can occur despite CAP.

Surgical management of VUR corrects the anatomy at the insertion of the refluxing ureter into the bladder and consists of open or laparoscopic and robotic techniques or endoscopic correction. Surgical intervention is indicated in patients who are unlikely to resolve their VUR and are at risk for renal scarring, including those with Grade V reflux with scarring, Grade V reflux over 6 years of age, and children who fail medical therapy.

Prognosis

With prompt and adequate treatment at the time of diagnosis, the long-term prognosis for UTI is usually excellent. However, the risk for progressive renal injury due to scarring from a first UTI has been found to be highest in children with an abnormal renal bladder ultrasound or with a combination of high fever (≥39° C or 102° F) and an etiologic organism other than *E. coli* (Shaikh, Craig, Rovers, et al., 2014). The presence of VUR, particularly high grade (IV to V) is an important risk factor for the development of renal scarring.

QUALITY PATIENT OUTCOMES: Urinary Tract Infections
- Treatment based on culture and sensitivity
- Renal function maintained
- Appropriate diagnosis of renal abnormalities

Care Management

Nurses should instruct parents to observe for signs and symptoms suggestive of UTI. These are not always obvious, particularly in an infant, young child, or developmentally delayed child. A high fever without obvious cause should be a signal to check the urine. Because infants and young children often are unable to express their feelings and sensations verbally, it is difficult to detect discomfort they may be experiencing from dysuria. A careful history regarding voiding habits, stooling pattern, feeding tolerance, and episodes of unexplained irritability may assist in detecting less obvious cases of UTI.

!　NURSING ALERT

Another strategy for obtaining a daily urine protein is to place cotton balls in the diaper at night before bedtime and then squeeze them out in the morning.

When infection is suspected, collecting an appropriate specimen is essential. It is the nurse's responsibility to take every precaution to obtain acceptable clean-voided specimens in a child who is able to void volitionally, taking care to cleanse the meatus and retract the foreskin in uncircumcised males or keep the labia separated in females. Having a young girl sit backwards on the toilet can facilitate this process, particularly the ability to obtain urine midstream, decreasing the risk for contamination. Because of the unreliability of a specimen obtained via a urine collection bag, suprapubic aspiration of urine or sterile catheterization should be done in infants and young children whose illness warrants immediate antibiotic therapy, such as high fever, vomiting, and lethargy.

Frequently, additional tests are performed to detect anatomic defects. Children are prepared for these tests as appropriate for their age. This includes an explanation of the procedure, its purpose, and what the children will experience (see the "Preparation for Diagnostic and Therapeutic Procedures" section in Chapter 39). Sometimes a simple description of the urinary system is helpful. For children younger than 3 to 4 years of age, the procedure can be explained on a doll. For those who are older, a simple drawing of the bladder, urethra, ureters, and kidneys makes the procedure more understandable.

Handling actual equipment when feasible can be helpful in allaying anxiety in children of all ages. Anticipatory instruction on distraction techniques such as deep breathing, storytelling, and imagery may help the child relax and be more cooperative during the actual procedures.

Because antibacterial drugs are indicated in UTI, the nurse advises parents of proper dosage and administration. When used in low dose for prevention of UTI, parents need an explanation of the drug's continued necessity when no signs of infection are present. For all children, adequate fluid intake is encouraged.

Prevention

Prevention is the most important goal in both primary and recurrent infection, and many preventive measures are simple hygienic habits that should be a routine part of daily care (see Guidelines box: Prevention of Urinary Tract Infection). For example, parents are taught to cleanse their infant's genital areas from front to back to avoid contaminating the urethral area with fecal organisms. Girls are taught to wipe from front to back after voiding and defecating. Children should void as soon as they feel the urge.

Sexually active female adolescents are advised to urinate as soon as possible after they have intercourse to flush out any bacteria introduced. Children who have recurrent UTIs or neurogenic bladder are sometimes maintained on daily low-dose antibiotics. Giving the dose at bedtime in children who stay dry through the night allows the drug to remain in the bladder longer. The nurse should reinforce the importance of compliance to parents and older children.

Obstructive Uropathy

Structural or functional abnormalities of the urinary system that obstruct the normal flow of urine can result in renal dysfunction. The area above the obstruction may demonstrate increased pressure, dilation, and urinary stasis. If the blockage is low in the urinary tract, both ureters and kidneys may be affected; if one kidney or ureter is affected, the other may be normal. The renal pelvis and calyces typically show dilation

Prevention of Urinary Tract Infection

Factors Predisposing to Development
Short female urethra close to vagina and anus
Incomplete emptying and overdistention of bladder
Concentrated urine
Constipation

Measures of Prevention
Practice perineal hygiene; wipe from front to back.
Avoid tight clothing or diapers; wear cotton panties rather than nylon.
Avoid "holding" urine; encourage child to void frequently.
Take time to empty bladder completely. This may be helped by relaxed toilet posture for girls, with feet supported on a stool and knees apart. Some children benefit from "double voiding" (void, wait a few minutes, and void again).
Avoid constipation.
Encourage adequate fluid intake.

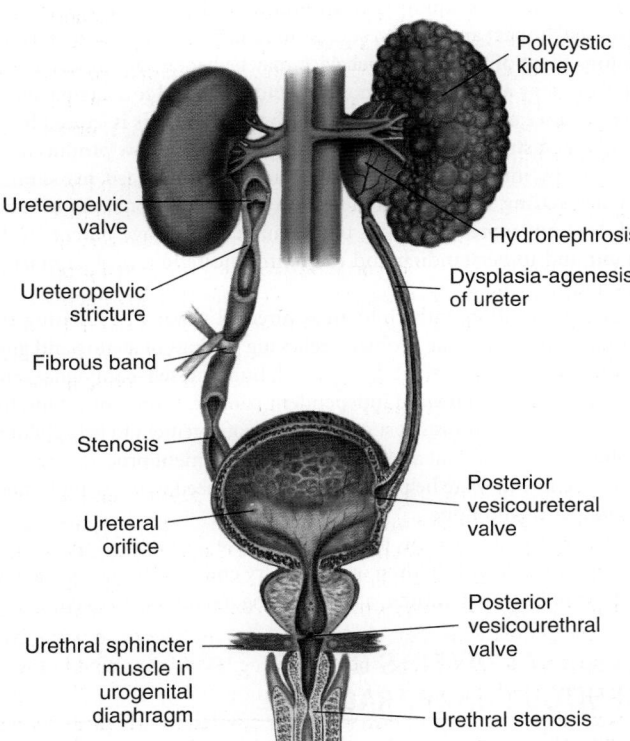

FIG 45.2 Major sites of urinary tract obstruction.

termed *hydronephrosis* from obstruction, although a kidney may have hydronephrosis and not be obstructed.

Obstruction may be congenital or acquired, unilateral or bilateral, and complete or incomplete with acute or chronic manifestations. The obstruction can occur at any level of the upper or lower urinary tract (Fig. 45.2). Partial obstruction may not be symptomatic, and changes caused may be partially or completely reversible if there is early intervention. Boys are affected more frequently than girls, and malformations should be suspected when patients have associated congenital defects (e.g., prune belly syndrome, chromosomal anomalies, anorectal malformations,

neural tube defects). Prenatal diagnosis with ultrasonography has been a factor leading to early diagnosis and intervention with subsequent decrease in renal impairment.

Causes of obstructive uropathy include congenital problems, such as posterior urethral valves (PUVs), ureteropelvic junction (UPJ) and ureterovesical junction (UVJ) obstruction, and ureterocele. Acquired causes include renal or bladder stones, tumor, and trauma. PUVs are obstructing membranous folds within the lumen of the posterior urethra and are the most common cause of obstruction of the urinary tract in newborn males, as well as the most common cause of chronic renal injury from obstructive uropathy (Khan, Fahim, & Mansoor, 2012). Because the obstruction occurs in the urethra, the bladder and upper urinary tract is affected. Damage to distal nephrons in chronic uropathy may cause decreased glomerular filtration, which can lead to renal insufficiency. Damage to smooth muscle of the bladder and upper urinary tract also may occur with obstruction and can contribute to bladder dysfunction. Because stasis of urine serves as a medium for bacterial growth, infection can magnify destructive changes of obstruction and cause increased renal damage as well as increased morbidity.

Early diagnosis and surgical correction or procedures that divert the flow of urine to bypass the obstruction may prevent progressive renal damage. Medical complications of acute or chronic renal failure (CRF) or infection are managed as described for those disorders.

Care Management

Interprofessional care goals in urinary tract obstruction include helping to identify cases, assisting with diagnostic procedures, and caring for children with complications (described elsewhere). Preparing parents and children for procedures is a major nursing responsibility (see the "Preparation for Diagnostic and Therapeutic Procedures" section in Chapter 39).

Parents and children need emotional support and counseling during the potentially lengthy management of these disorders. Children may be discharged with urinary drainage systems that require nursing education of the parents and older child to provide care and to recognize problems, such as obstruction of urine flow or infection. Drainage tubes should be observed for obstruction resulting from sediment, small blood clots, or kinking. If indicated, instructions on site care and drainage tube irrigation need to be provided, including observation for signs of infection or dislodgement.

Children with external diversional systems need psychologic support and guidance, especially as they reach adolescence and body image concerns assume more prominence. Those with progressive renal deterioration may face the prospect of dialysis or transplantation and the physical and psychologic challenges that accompany these procedures.

PROBLEMS RELATED TO ELIMINATION

ENURESIS

Enuresis (bedwetting), or nocturnal enuresis, is a common and troublesome disorder that is defined as the intentional or involuntary passage of urine into the bed (usually at night) in children who are beyond the age when voluntary bladder control should normally have been acquired. The inappropriate voiding of urine must occur at least twice per week for at least 3 months, and the chronologic or developmental age of the child must be at least 5 years. The predominant symptom is urgency that is immediate and is accompanied by acute discomfort, restlessness, and urinary frequency. In addition, the urinary incontinence must not be related to the direct physiologic effects of a substance (e.g., diuretics) or a general medical condition (e.g., diabetes mellitus or diabetes insipidus, spina bifida, seizure disorder, or sickle cell disease).

Enuresis is more common in boys; nocturnal bedwetting usually ceases between 6 and 8 years of age. Enuresis can also be defined as primary (bedwetting in children who have never been dry for extended periods) or secondary (the onset of wetting after a period of established urinary continence). The passage of urine may be monosymptomatic and occur only during nighttime sleep, with the child remaining dry during the day; or it may be polysymptomatic, in which the child has daytime urinary urgency and an occasional daytime accident in conjunction with other conditions such as sleep apnea, urinary tract infection, neurologic impairment, constipation, or emotional stressors. The nocturnal, monosymptomatic type is most common. The condition may be particularly distressing to adolescents, who may refuse therapy (Wolfe-Christensen, Kovacevic, Mirkovic, et al., 2013). Although enuresis may occur during the daytime, the following discussion primarily focuses on nocturnal enuresis.

Before psychogenic factors are considered, organic causes that may be related to enuresis should be ruled out. These include structural disorders of the urinary tract; urinary tract infection; neurologic deficits; disorders that increase the normal output of urine, such as diabetes; and disorders that impair the concentrating ability of the kidneys, such as chronic renal failure or sickle cell disease. A bladder volume of 300 to 350 mL (10 to 12 oz) is sufficient to hold a night's urine. Normal bladder capacity (in ounces) is the child's age plus 2 (up to 14 years of age). In other cases, enuresis is influenced by emotional factors, although it is doubtful that they are causative factors. Nocturnal enuresis has a strong familial tendency. Age, male gender, parents' history of enuresis, and siblings' history of enuresis are significant predictive factors for nocturnal enuresis (Sarici, Telli, Ozgur, et al., 2016).

Therapeutic techniques used to manage nocturnal enuresis include medications, complementary and alternative medicine techniques (e.g., hypnotherapy), restriction or elimination of fluids after the evening meal, avoidance of caffeinated and sugar-containing beverages after 4 PM, purposeful interruption of sleep to void, motivational therapy, and various devices designed to establish a conditioned reflex response to waken the child at the initiation of voiding (alarms).

Drug therapy is increasingly being prescribed to treat enuresis. Three types of drugs are used: tricyclic antidepressants (TCAs), antidiuretics, and antispasmodics. The drug used depends on the interpretation of the cause. The most commonly used drug is the TCA imipramine (Tofranil), which exerts an anticholinergic action in the bladder to inhibit urination. The dosage and time of administration are individualized, and the drug is given in amounts sufficient to lighten sleep but not to cause wakefulness. Some practitioners prescribe low doses, which reduces bedwetting in two-thirds of children. However, it is important to note that almost all children relapse when the medication is stopped. The suggested length of treatment is 6 to 8 weeks followed by gradual withdrawal over 4 weeks. Because overdosage of this drug is especially dangerous, caution parents about the safe use of this drug and the need to keep supplies of the drug out of the reach of children.

Anticholinergic drugs, especially oxybutynin, reduce uninhibited bladder contractions and may be helpful for children with daytime urinary frequency (Kinlaw, Jonsson Funk, Steiner, et al., 2016). Success has also been achieved with desmopressin acetate (DDAVP) nasal spray, an analog of vasopressin, which reduces nighttime urinary output to a volume less than functional bladder capacity. Typically, the child receives two sprays before bedtime. The medication is generally well tolerated but may cause nasal irritation or, rarely, headache or nausea. A preparation of desmopressin acetate is also available in tablet form. This preparation is as effective and safe as the nasal spray but avoids the problem of nasal irritation.

These drugs are considered second-line management, and parents should be cautioned not to think these agents will cure the condition; parents are also advised of the side effects of these drugs.

Care Management

No matter which techniques are used, the nurse can help both children and parents understand the problem of enuresis, the treatment plan, and the difficulties they may encounter in the process. Essential to the success of any method is the supportive management of parents and their children. Both need encouragement and patience. The problem is discussed with both the parent and the child because all treatments involve and require the child's active participation. In some treatment interventions, the child is in charge of the intervention; therefore parents must learn to support the child rather than intervene themselves. For example, children can strip their wet covers, limit fluids, and use the toilet before bedtime. Parents should encourage the child to maintain a regular bowel evacuation regimen; constipation can contribute to nocturnal enuresis. A calendar with wet and dry nights may be helpful to motivate the child to stay dry and maintain a positive perspective on the problem; positive rewards are also helpful.

Parents need to understand that punishment such as scolding, shaming, and threatening is contraindicated because of its negative emotional impact and limited success in reducing the behavior. Positive reinforcement of the desired behavior may be beneficial. Children need to believe they are helping themselves, and they need to sustain feelings of confidence and hope. Many parents believe enuresis is caused by an emotional disturbance and fear that they have somehow produced the situation by improper childrearing practices. They need reassurance that bedwetting is not a manifestation of an emotional disturbance and does not represent willful misbehavior. Encourage parents to be patient and understanding and to communicate love and support to the child.

Communication with children is directed toward eliminating the emotional impact of the problem, relieving feelings of shame and guilt and the burden of parental disapproval, building self-confidence, and motivating children toward independent control. More important, the nurse can provide consistent support and encouragement to help children through the inconsistent and unpredictable treatment process. Children need to believe they are helping themselves and need to maintain feelings of confidence and hope.

Parents should also be taught to observe for side effects of any medications used. All children with primary enuresis should be encouraged to void before bedtime, and diapering should be avoided.

EXTERNAL DEFECTS OF THE GENITOURINARY TRACT

Defects of the external genitourinary tract have the potential to cause distortions of body image. Satisfactory surgical repair is successful for the more common disorders and is carried out or initiated as early as possible. The major anomalies of the lower genitourinary tract, their description, and their management are outlined in Table 45.4.

PHIMOSIS

Phimosis is a narrowing or stenosis of the preputial opening of the foreskin that prevents retraction of the foreskin over the glans penis. It is a normal finding in infants and young boys and usually resolves as the child grows and the distal prepuce dilates. Occasionally the narrowing obstructs the flow of urine, resulting in a dribbling stream or even ballooning of the foreskin with accumulated urine during voiding.

TABLE 45.4 Defects of the Genitourinary Tract

Defect	Therapeutic Management
Inguinal hernia: Protrusion of abdominal contents through inguinal canal into scrotum	Detected as painless inguinal swelling of variable size Surgical closure of inguinal defect
Hydrocele: Fluid in scrotum	Surgical repair indicated if persists past 1 year of age
Phimosis: Narrowing or stenosis of preputial opening of foreskin	**Mild cases:** May not require therapy if urine flow not obstructed; steroid cream may be prescribed, typically twice a day for 1 month **Severe cases:** Circumcision or dorsal slit in severe, rare cases
Hypospadias: Urethral opening located behind glans penis or anywhere along ventral surface of penile shaft	Objectives of surgical correction: • Enable child to void in standing position and direct stream voluntarily in usual manner • Improve physical appearance of genitalia • Produce a sexually adequate organ
Chordee: Ventral curvature of penis, often associated with hypospadias	Surgical release of fibrous band causing the deformity
Epispadias: Meatal opening located on dorsal surface of penis	Surgical correction, usually including penile and urethral lengthening and bladder neck reconstruction (if necessary)
Cryptorchidism: Failure of one or both testes to descend normally through inguinal canal	Detected by inability to palpate testes within scrotum **Medical:** Administration of hormonal therapy has historically been used in some institutions to induce testicular descent but is controversial and not currently recommended **Surgical:** Orchiopexy Objectives of therapy: Place and fix viable undescended testes in a normal scrotal position, or remove nonviable testicular remnants Allows for easier examination of the testis because there is an increased risk for testicular cancer in undescended testes; early surgical correction may reduce the risk for cancer as well as infertility Decrease risk for trauma and torsion Decrease risk for inguinal hernia by closing the inguinal canal Potential improved body satisfaction
Exstrophy of bladder: Eversion of posterior bladder through anterior bladder wall and lower abdominal wall; associated with open pubic arch (a severe defect)	Potential objectives of surgical correction: • Preserve renal function • Attain urinary control • Provide adequate reconstructive repair • Improve sexual function

Balanitis is an inflammation or infection of the phimotic foreskin, which occurs occasionally and is managed as any other inflammation or infection. Phimosis is often treated effectively by application of steroid cream twice a day for 1 month, with the option for surgical treatment with circumcision in severe cases.

Care Management

Proper hygiene of the phimotic foreskin in infants and young boys consists of external cleansing during routine bathing. The foreskin should not be forcibly retracted, because it may create scarring that can prevent future retraction. Furthermore, retraction of the tight foreskin can result in paraphimosis, a condition in which the retracted foreskin cannot be replaced in its normal position over the glans. This causes edema and venous congestion created by constriction by the tight band of foreskin—a urologic emergency that requires immediate evaluation.

HYDROCELE

A *hydrocele* is the presence of peritoneal fluid in the scrotum between the parietal and visceral layers of the tunica vaginalis and is the most common cause of painless scrotal swelling in children and adolescents, along with nonincarcerated inguinal hernia. Hydroceles may be communicating or noncommunicating. A communicating hydrocele usually develops when the processus vaginalis does not close during development, allowing for communication with the peritoneum. Noncommunicating hydroceles have no connection to the peritoneum with fluid coming from the mesothelial lining of the tunica vaginalis. Hydroceles are common in newborns and often resolve spontaneously, usually by 12 months of age. In older children, noncommunicating hydroceles may be idiopathic or a result of trauma, epididymitis, orchitis, testicular torsion, torsion of the appendix testis or appendix epididymis, or tumor.

Communicating hydroceles may change in size during the day or with straining, whereas noncommunicating hydroceles are not reducible and do not change size with crying or straining. Surgical repair is indicated for communicating hydroceles persisting past 1 year of age, because there is a risk for development of incarcerated inguinal hernia. Idiopathic hydroceles are repaired if symptomatic, and reactive hydroceles usually resolve with treatment of underlying cause, such as epididymitis.

Care Management

Surgical correction is an outpatient procedure. Advise parents that there may be temporary swelling and discoloration of the scrotum that resolves spontaneously. Straddle toys are avoided for 2 to 4 weeks, and strenuous activities in older boys may be avoided for 1 month. If a dressing is used, it is removed in 2 to 3 days, and typically the child can bathe in 3 days.

CRYPTORCHIDISM (CRYPTORCHISM)

Cryptorchidism is failure of one or both testes to descend normally through the inguinal canal into the scrotum. Absence of testes within the scrotum can be a result of undescended (cryptorchid) testes, retractile testes, or anorchism (absence of testes). Undescended testes can be categorized further according to location:

Abdominal: Proximal to the internal inguinal ring

Canalicular: Between the internal and external inguinal rings

Ectopic: Outside the normal pathways of descent between the abdominal cavity and the scrotum

The incidence of cryptorchidism is reported to be as high as 45% in preterm boys and less than 5% in full-term boys; by 1 year of age, the incidence decreases to less than 2% and does not change thereafter (Sijstermans, Hack, Meijer, et al., 2008).

Pathophysiology

Cryptorchidism occurs when one or both testes fail to descend through the inguinal canal and into the scrotum. Several processes may slow or arrest testicular descent, including endocrinologic abnormalities affecting the hypothalamic-pituitary-testicular axis, denervation of the genitofemoral nerve, traction of the gubernaculum, abnormal development of the epididymis, or preterm birth. Congenital hernias and abnormal testes often accompany cryptorchid testes, and they are at risk for subsequent torsion.

Anorchism is the complete absence of a testis. Anorchism is suspected whenever one or both testes cannot be palpated in the patient with apparent cryptorchidism. In some cases, bilateral anorchism is associated with disorders of sex development with genotypic and phenotypic abnormalities, specifically congenital adrenal hyperplasia (CAH). Although it is commonly associated with a normal karyotype (46,XY) and normal genital development, it is critical to rule out the possibility of CAH in the newborn because of the potential for serious harm due to inability to regulate electrolyte levels (Kolon, Herndon, Baker, et al., 2014). An absent testis may be due to atrophy from prenatal testicular torsion, also known as *vanishing testes* or *testicular regression syndrome.*

The cryptorchid or ectopic testis must be differentiated from anorchism because of the risk for malignant degeneration and subfertility when the testis is left in an extrascrotal location. This differentiation requires laparoscopic or direct surgical exploration (Kolon et al., 2014).

Retractile testes can be found at any level within the path of testicular descent, but they are most commonly identified in the groin. Fortunately, they are not truly cryptorchid. Instead, they are introverted to an inguinal or abdominal position because of an overactive cremasteric reflex. The cremasteric reflex, observed as withdrawal of the testis above the scrotum and into the inguinal canal in response to various stimuli, including exposure to cool temperatures, is active during infancy and peaks around 4 to 5 years of age. Unlike the cryptorchid testis, the retractile testis can be gently moved into the scrotum without residual tension and does not require treatment. Retractile testes can become ascending testes and require annual monitoring.

Clinical Manifestations

A nonpalpable testis is typically observed by the parent or detected during routine physical examination by a health care provider. If one testis is not palpable, the affected hemiscrotum will appear smaller than the other. With bilateral nonpalpable testes, both hemiscrota appear small. In the case of retractile testes, the parents may report intermittently observing the testes in the scrotum, interspersed with periods when they cannot be visualized or palpated. Frequently, the retractile testis will be observed in the scrotum when the child is being bathed in warm water.

Diagnostic Evaluation

It is important to differentiate the true undescended testis from the more common retractile testis. Retractile testes can be "milked" or pushed back into the scrotum, but truly undescended ones cannot. For examination, the nurse can obviate the cremasteric reflex by placing the child in a squatting or cross-legged sitting position prior to checking the position of the testes.

Therapeutic Management

Although primary hormonal therapy with luteinizing hormone–releasing hormone (nasal spray) and human chorionic gonadotropin (injection) has been used more commonly in Europe, it is no longer recommended to induce testicular descent. Evidence shows low response rates and lack of long-term efficacy (Kolon et al., 2014). *Orchiopexy*, or surgical repositioning of the testis, is performed on palpable testes. Exploratory surgery may be required if the testis is not palpable. The goal of surgery is to place and fix viable undescended testes to a normal scrotal position or to remove nonviable testicular remnants. Scrotal positioning reduces the risk for torsion and trauma and permits easier examination of the testis, because there is an increased risk for testicular cancer despite treatment of undescended testes. In the routine surgical procedure for undescended testes, the testes are brought down into the scrotum and secured in that position without tension or torsion. A simple orchiopexy for a palpable testis can usually be performed as an outpatient. If exploratory surgery is needed to determine if a testis is present, an examination under anesthesia is the initial step. Depending on findings, a diagnostic laparoscopic procedure or an open inguinal approach may be performed. If an intraabdominal testis is identified, this permits planning for a definitive procedure, which may be open or laparoscopic. Approximately 10% of boys with nonpalpable testes are found to have an absent testicle at the time of surgery.

Care Management

Postoperative nursing care is directed toward preventing infection and instructing parents in home care of the child, including pain control. Observation of the wound for complications and activity restrictions are discussed. The child should avoid vigorous sports activities and use of straddle toys for 2 to 4 weeks postoperatively. General care is similar to that described for hydrocele repair.

Parents may be concerned about the child's future fertility, and recent studies show some decreased fertility in bilateral cryptorchism, but in unilateral patients the fertility rate approximates that found in the general population. The risk for testicular cancer is a concern that is decreased if surgery is done before puberty, but all boys with cryptorchidism should be taught testicular self-examination at puberty to potentially facilitate early detection (Kolon et al., 2014). Surgical treatment is indicated as soon as possible after 6 months of age and definitely should be completed by 2 years of age because spontaneous descent rarely occurs after 6 months of age, and treatment by 1 to 2 years of age is associated with improved fertility and testicular growth.

HYPOSPADIAS

Hypospadias is a congenital anomaly of the male urethra that results in abnormal ventral placement of the urethral opening on the underside of the penis, ranging from the glans to the perineum (Fig. 45.3). It is one of the most common congenital anomalies with an incidence reported to be 1 per 250 to 300 live births, with 10% to 15% having a first-degree male relative (sibling or father) with the same condition (Bukowski & Zeman, 2001; Gray & Moore, 2009). Both genetic and environmental factors have been associated with hypospadias. Severity of hypospadias is based on the position of the urethral opening and the degree of *chordee,* or ventral curvature of the penis. The more distant the opening from the normal position at the tip of the glans and the more marked curvature increases the severity and the need for more extensive surgical

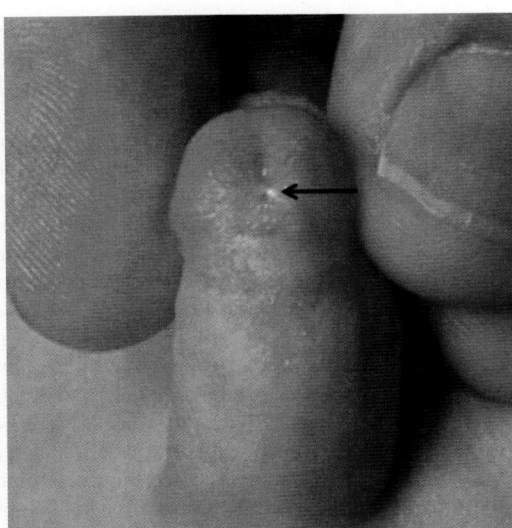

FIG 45.3 Distal hypospadias with a stenotic meatus (arrow) located on the glans with no chordee. (From Holcomb, G.W., Murphy, J.P., & Ostlie, D.J. [2014]. *Ashcraft's pediatric surgery* [6th ed.]. Philadelphia, PA: Elsevier.)

correction. In mild cases, the meatus is just below the tip of the penis. In the most severe malformation, the meatus is on the perineum between the halves of the bifid scrotum. In addition, the foreskin is usually absent ventrally and, when combined with chordee, gives the organ a hooded and crooked appearance. In severe cases, the altered appearance may leave the infant's gender in doubt at birth because of the perineal position of the meatus and small penis. In any case of ambiguous genitalia, additional evaluation is essential. Cryptorchidism is present in about 10% of infants with hypospadias and increases with more proximal hypospadias with the meatus at the scrotum or perineum. There is an increased risk for disorders of sex development in patients with severe hypospadias, both with and without cryptorchidism.

Surgical Correction

The principal objectives of surgical correction are (1) to enhance the child's ability to void in the standing position with a straight stream, (2) to improve the physical appearance of the genitalia for psychologic reasons, and (3) to preserve a sexually adequate organ. The choice of surgical procedure is affected primarily by the severity of the defect and the presence of associated anomalies. Numerous techniques are utilized in repair of hypospadias and are performed under general anesthesia and typically as an outpatient procedure.

Hypospadias repair may be done by primary tubularization for milder forms in which a new urethra is made by rolling a ventral strip of penile shaft skin that normally would have formed the urethra. For more severe hypospadias, an onlay island flap is used to create the urethra, transferring a strip of inner foreskin onto the ventral urethral plate. In severe forms of hypospadias, including those with significant chordee, a two-stage repair is used to straighten the penis and create a new urethra. These are typically performed at least 6 months apart. There is no consensus on the best surgical approach for correcting severe hypospadias, and complication rates are high, specifically development of urethrocutaneous fistula, urethral stricture or meatal stenosis, and urethral diverticulum (Prat, Natasha, Polak, et al., 2012).

The preferred time for surgical repair is 6 to 12 months of age, before the child has developed body image. Occasionally a short course of testosterone is administered preoperatively to achieve additional penile size to facilitate the surgery.

Care Management

Neonatal circumcision should be avoided in hypospadias where there is incomplete foreskin, because this is not conductive to a safe clamp or Plastibell circumcision. In severe cases, the foreskin may be used in reconstruction. In mild hypospadias, the foreskin is not incomplete and the abnormality may not be noted until after circumcision. This does not affect future successful reconstruction if it is needed. In most cases, the appearance after reconstruction will be of a circumcised normal penis. Preparation of parents for the type of procedure to be done and the expected cosmetic result helps avert problems.

Frequently parents are informed of what is to be surgically corrected but are not advised of what to expect as a reasonable consequence. More refined surgical techniques performed by surgeons specializing in pediatric urologic conditions have improved cosmetic and functional outcomes in these boys. If children are old enough to understand what is occurring, the nurse also prepares them for the operation and the expected outcome.

Hypospadias repair may require some type of urinary diversion with a silicone stent or feeding tube to promote optimum healing and to maintain the position and patency of the newly formed urethra. This is left in the bladder to drain urine for 5 to 10 days. In most infants and children who are not toilet trained, the catheter drains directly into the diaper. In older children, the catheter is connected to a leg bag or a larger bedside bag at night. Drainage bags should always be positioned below the bladder level for proper drainage. Tub baths are avoided until the catheter is removed. Most children will have a caudal or penile nerve block in addition to general anesthesia, which lasts 6 to 8 hours. Appropriate administration of prescribed pain medication for 48 to 72 hours after surgery will help control discomfort. When a catheter is left in place, bladder spasms are common and are very uncomfortable. Anticholinergic medications, such as oxybutynin, are typically used to prevent spasms. Parents should be advised that bladder spasms, which are usually brief and intense, may occur, and that the child may arch his back, bring his knees up to his chest, and leak urine around the catheter with a spasm. Oxybutynin is given every 8 hours typically and may require dosing adjustment, such as increasing frequency to every 6 hours to control spasms. Once the catheter is removed, the medication is no longer needed. Often a prophylactic antibiotic is given until shortly after catheter removal. Anticholinergic medication is constipating; this problem is common in the postoperative period and may be avoided with preventative measures, such as giving adequate fluid and a stool softener or laxative if needed. Preparing parents for these potential problems is an important nursing responsibility. Patients usually go home with a dressing that often comes off in 1 to 2 days and typically is removed in the bath in 3 days if there is no stent in place. If the dressing is soiled, it can be cleaned gently and removed once the parent is prepared that the appearance of the penis is often swollen, discolored, and/or bruised, and this is expected and will resolve with time. While healing, applying petroleum jelly or KY jelly to the diaper to prevent the penis from sticking can help prevent bleeding and increase comfort.

EXSTROPHY-EPISPADIAS COMPLEX

Bladder exstrophy is a severe defect involving the musculoskeletal system and the urinary, reproductive, and intestinal tracts. It is one of three anomalies that define the exstrophy-epispadias complex (EEC). *Epispadias* is an exposed or open dorsal urethra. Bladder exstrophy is a more severe defect characterized by an open, inside-out bladder with the inner surface exposed and the dorsal urethra on the lower abdominal wall (Figs. 45.4 and 45.5). The third disorder, *cloacal exstrophy,* is the most severe, and includes bladder exstrophy as well as exstrophy of the large intestine

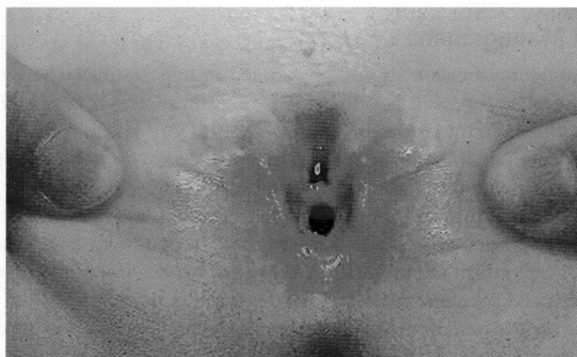

FIG 45.4 Epispadias. (From Gearhart, J.P. Rink, R.C., & Mouriquand, P.D.E. [2010]. *Pediatric urology* [2nd ed.]. Philadelphia, PA: Saunders.)

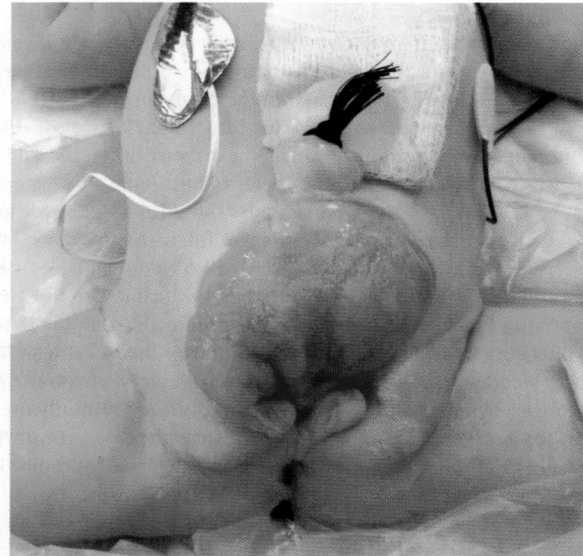

FIG 45.5 Exstrophy of bladder. (From Sirisreetreerux, P., Lue, K.M., Michaud, J.E., et al. [2016]. Duplicated renal collecting system with ectopic ureter in female bladder exstrophy: A case report. *Urology, 89,* 129–131.)

(hindgut) through an abdominal wall defect. In addition, there is anal atresia, omphalocele, hypoplasia of the colon, anomalous genitalia, and often spinal dysraphism. Fortunately, incidence of cloacal exstrophy is low—less than 1 per 100,000 live births (Feldkamp, Botto, Amar, et al., 2011). Classic bladder exstrophy typically includes findings of diastasis (separation) of the symphysis pubis (pelvic bone), low-set umbilicus, anteriorly displaced anus, defects of the genitalia, and inguinal hernia. The incidence of bladder exstrophy ranges from 3.3 to 5 per 100,000 live births and is more common in males than in females (Jayachandran, Bythell, Platt, et al., 2011).

Pathophysiology

Exstrophy results from failure of the abdominal wall and underlying structures, including the ventral wall of the bladder, to fuse in utero. As a result, the lower urinary tract is exposed, and the everted bladder appears bright red through the abdominal opening. This is accompanied by a constant seepage of urine from the exposed ureteral orifices, making the area malodorous and susceptible to infection. The constant accumulation of urine on the surrounding skin produces tissue ulceration and

further infection. Progressive renal damage from infection and obstruction may cause renal failure if left untreated.

In males with bladder exstrophy, the defect of the genitalia includes epispadias and upward curvature of a shortened penis and may include other problems, such as undescended testes and inguinal hernias. In females, there is epispadias, a bifid clitoris, and small labia minora. The vagina is shortened compared with normal appearance, and vaginal dilation may be needed to allow for sexual intercourse. In cloacal exstrophy patients, there are often more severe anomalies, such as bifid or duplicated uterus, split clitoris, completely separated labia, and a duplicate or absent vagina in females. Males may have a split penis and scrotum or a short, flat penis with hypospadias. In either sex, separation of the pubic bones is generally corrected by pelvic osteotomy, particularly if there is extreme diastasis to increase the likelihood of successful bladder closure. In bladder exstrophy patients, the upper urinary tract is usually normal. Fertility is possible in females but decreased in males, possibly because of semen abnormalities, abnormal ejaculation, or a combination of both. Assisted reproductive techniques remain a viable option for patients with infertility. Recent studies indicate good long-term outcomes on erectile and general sexual function in both men and women with epispadias and bladder exstrophy (Suominen, Santtila & Taskinen, 2015).

Therapeutic Management

The objectives of treatment are (1) preservation of renal function, (2) attainment of urinary control, (3) adequate reconstructive repair for acceptable appearance, (4) prevention of UTIs, and (5) preservation of optimum external genitalia with continence and sexual function. There are two surgical approaches currently utilized to correct bladder exstrophy. One is termed *modern staged repair of exstrophy (MSRE)*, typically involving three surgeries beginning with closure of the bladder and abdominal wall. Complete primary repair of bladder exstrophy (CPRE) is a single-stage surgical closure combining closure of the bladder, abdominal wall, partial tightening of the bladder neck, and bilateral ureteral reimplantation to correct reflux. Often, pelvic osteotomies are performed at the time of primary closure to deepen the flattened pelvis, close the pubic diastasis, and release tension on the abdominal wall to improve success of primary closure (Inouye, Tourchi, & Di Carlo, 2014).

For the child with bladder exstrophy, CPRE may be performed within the first 72 hours of life or as a delayed procedure at about 2 months of age. For the child with cloacal exstrophy, pelvic osteotomies are needed because of the wide pelvic diastasis, and surgery is done within 48 to 72 hours of life to close the bladder and omphalocele and perform intestinal diversion (Inouye et al., 2014).

In some children, reconstruction (tightening) of the bladder neck may not provide sufficient resistance to achieve urinary continence. In these cases, suburethral collagen injections or implantation of an artificial urinary sphincter may be performed. Occasionally, the bladder fails to achieve an adequate functional capacity, and augmentation enterocystoplasty is required. This procedure is typically combined with the creation of a Mitrofanoff appendiceal stoma, because catheterization is difficult after reconstruction of the proximal urethra. Abnormalities of the genitalia are addressed to ensure optimal sexual function. In boys, the testes are typically cryptorchid, and bilateral orchiopexy is combined with reconstruction of the bifid scrotum to preserve testicular function. In girls, surgical enlargement of the vaginal introitus may be needed to permit intercourse. In both genders, plastic surgery to reduce scarring of the genital area or to create an umbilicus may significantly improve the child's body image and emerging sexual identity.

Care Management

It is important to limit trauma to the exposed bladder mucosa, and the bladder is covered with a nonadherent film of plastic wrap or transparent dressing that will not stick to the bladder but can adhere to the surrounding skin. After bladder closure, the neonate is monitored for urinary output and for signs of urinary tract or wound infection. At the time of closure, the pelvic diastasis may be corrected with an osteotomy, but even if that is not performed, patients typically require immobilization of the pelvis with traction for 2 to 4 weeks. A common form of traction for newborns is the modified Bryant's traction, but spica casting and other alternatives are used. Monitoring of skin condition and circulation is critical as well as monitoring the incision for wound dehiscence. The focus of nursing care is pain management and maintenance of immobilization. Pain management may be achieved with continuous epidural therapy or patient/parent/nurse-controlled intravenous analgesia (PCA) and may involve the acute pain service working with the bedside nurse to provide optimal pain control (Kozlowski, 2008). Postoperative nursing care also includes monitoring of hemodynamic stability, maintaining patency and stability of tubes and drains, provision of intravenous (IV) fluids and nutrition, and inclusion of the family in care.

Postoperative nursing care after bladder neck reconstruction and antireflux surgery (ureteral reimplantation) includes routine wound care and careful monitoring of urinary output from the bladder and ureteral drainage tubes. Care after a penile lengthening, chordee release, and urethral reconstruction is similar to care after hypospadias repair.

Children who fail to attain urinary continence after bladder neck reconstruction are offered a continent diversion. In addition to routine postoperative care, nursing care after a continent diversion includes wound care, observation of nasogastric (NG) suction (surgery requires bowel resection), and measurement and observation of urinary output. Clean intermittent catheterization (CIC) is used to regularly empty the urinary reservoir. Most children are able to learn self-catheterization by 6 or 7 years of age. Adult supervision is needed to ensure the child is compliant.

Family Support and Home Care

Bladder exstrophy and the other disorders of the EEC are significant congenital abnormalities that require lifelong care by a team of specialists. Improvement in surgical techniques has helped achieve better outcomes, specifically that of the goal of continence. Parental stress is significant, and support services may be helpful for positive adaptation. Patients may also benefit from psychologic support as adjustment problems are common, particularly in adolescents. Parents should receive teaching and practice on care of the infant or child at home and have access to resources to call if there are questions. Allowing time for parents to voice concerns can facilitate evaluation of their understanding and help direct discharge needs. When the infant is discharged with an unrepaired defect, plastic wrap is placed over the defect, and diapers are changed frequently to prevent infection, ulceration, and odor. Parents are taught to recognize the signs of UTI and to report a suspected infection to the patient care provider. General infant care remains unchanged—except for sponge baths rather than immersion in water.

DISORDERS OF SEX DEVELOPMENT

The term *disorders of sex development (DSD)* has a comprehensive definition that includes any problem noted at birth in which the genitalia are atypical in relation to the chromosomes or gonads (Lee, Houk, Ahmed, et al., 2006). The presentation at birth may be a genital appearance that does not permit gender declaration, and this is termed *ambiguous genitalia.* These may include bilateral cryptorchidism, perineal hypospadias with bifid scrotum, clitoromegaly, posterior labial fusion, phenotypic female appearance with a palpable gonad, and hypospadias and unilateral nonpalpable gonad. Also included in the DSD category

are infants with discordant genitalia and sex chromosomes. Turner syndrome (45, XO) and Klinefelter syndrome (47, XXY) are also DSDs that do not present with ambiguous genitalia.

Pathophysiology

Normal sexual differentiation starts at 7 weeks of gestation when fetuses with a Y chromosome begin developing testes. Early on, both female (XX) and male (XY) fetuses have a similar reproductive structure. Multiple genes contribute to this process, and mutations in these genes can lead to various DSDs. Congenital malformation of the genitalia are most frequently because of androgen deficiency in XY individuals and androgen excess in XX patients, though in many cases no endocrine etiology can be found (Grinspon & Rey, 2014).

Initial evaluation includes karyotype and assessment of adrenal and gonadal function, and this information can be used to categorize the infant into one of three categories:
- Virilized XX (XX DSD)
- Undervirilized XY (XY DSD)
- Mixed sex chromosome pattern

Therapeutic Management

The most common cause of ambiguous genitalia is congenital adrenal hyperplasia (CAH), which can lead to life-threatening salt-wasting adrenal insufficiency in the first weeks of life. Though now a part of neonatal screening in the United States, any infant with genital ambiguity should be evaluated urgently. Laboratory testing includes a measurement of 17-hydroxyprogesterone in addition to karyotype with immediate probe for SRY (sex-determining region on the Y chromosome). Serum electrolytes are monitored, as signs and symptoms of adrenal insufficiency may include hypoglycemia, hypovolemia, hyponatremia, hyperkalemia, vomiting, and diarrhea. Fluids and electrolytes need to be replaced urgently, and the nurse plays a key role in assessing the infant and providing prescribed therapy. Additional laboratory testing may be indicated, as well as pelvic and abdominal ultrasonography to evaluate for gonads, uterus, and vagina.

Family Support

The birth of a child with ambiguous genitalia has been termed a *psychosocial emergency for the family.* They require support because the answers to a seemingly simple question as to what sex is their child requires evaluation and time. Involvement in a multidisciplinary team that may include endocrinology, urology, genetics, surgeons, in addition to nurses and social workers can make clear communication challenging, and the nurse may be instrumental in coordinating family meetings with the team.

The infant and child with DSD pose very complex and controversial management questions, including sex assignment and potential genital surgery. Traditional approaches are being questioned and continue to evolve. Referral to a specialized center for children with DSD is recommended.

Psychologic Problems Related to Genital Surgery

Improved understanding of the psychologic implications of genitourinary surgery in children, improvements in technical aspects of surgery, and advances in pediatric anesthesia have resulted in modifications of the surgical approach to children requiring genitourinary surgery. Some of the problems of hospitalization, separation, and anxiety can be eased by hospital practices that are sensitive to the child's needs (see Chapter 38).

A child's body image is largely derived as a result of feedback from primary caregivers and peers; and parental anxiety regarding an acceptable physical appearance is readily communicated to an affected child. This subtle communication increases the risk for development of a distorted body image, and early repair may facilitate a positive body image. Sexual body image is another area that has been thought to be largely a function of socialization. In terms of disorders of sex development, this becomes a much more complex and multifaceted area.

The child's reaction to surgery is related to emotional and cognitive development. Separation of parent and child is important to minimize, particularly in the first 1 to 2 years of life. From about 3 to 6 years of age, children are frightened of what they perceive to be threats to their body and bodily function. They are egocentric in their view of the world and may perceive surgery as punishment for real or imagined wrongdoing and require reassurance that they are not to blame. By 7 years of age, they have more ability to understand but may still associate surgery with punishment. Surgical repair is ideally performed before these fears and anxieties develop. In terms of anesthesia risk, elective procedures are generally performed after 6 months of age. It is thought that children do not have memory of procedures performed by 18 to 24 months of age. Age 24 to 36 months may be a time when trauma of surgery is relatively less, but in the case of an external defect this prolongs correction. The American Academy of Pediatrics Action Committee on Surgery first published recommendations in terms of timing of elective surgery on the genitalia of male children as a review in 1996.

Care Management

Preparing children and their families for diagnostic and surgical procedures (see the "Preparation for Diagnostic and Therapeutic Procedures" section in Chapter 39) and for home care is a major nursing function. Most postoperative care involves care of the surgical site. Tub baths may be discouraged for a few days or longer, depending on procedure, if a stent or catheter is left in place, and surgeon preference. It is common practice to leave a urethral stent or catheter in place to drain directly into the diaper after some reconstructive procedures, such as hypospadias repair. The surgical site is kept clean and is inspected for signs of infection or bleeding. More complex surgeries require additional care and observation, such as drainage tube care and irrigation, dressing changes, and monitoring of collection devices.

Postoperative activity restrictions vary with age and type of surgery. Activity of infants and toddlers is not typically limited with the exception of avoiding straddle toys following penile or scrotal surgery. Older children may need more restriction from strenuous activity for 1 month after these type procedures. In the case of more extensive abdominal surgery, there may be restrictions on lifting and strenuous activity for a longer period. Swimming may be restricted especially when any drains are still in place or until incisions are healed. Precise restrictions depend on the specific type of surgery and surgeon preference.

In most cases, the results of surgery are satisfactory. However, in some of the more severe defects, such as exstrophy and severe hypospadias, additional psychologic support may be needed to help adjust to concerns about penis size, appearance of the genitalia, potential ability to procreate, and rejection by peers (especially the opposite sex). Ongoing open discussion and support groups for parents and children are useful in promoting optimum emotional adjustment, particularly during adolescence.

GLOMERULAR DISEASE

NEPHROTIC SYNDROME

Nephrotic syndrome is a clinical state that includes massive proteinuria, hypoalbuminemia, hyperlipidemia, and edema. The disorder can occur as (1) a primary disease known as *idiopathic nephrosis, childhood nephrosis,*

or *minimal-change nephrotic syndrome (MCNS);* (2) a secondary disorder that occurs as a clinical manifestation after or in association with glomerular damage that has a known or presumed cause; or (3) a congenital form inherited as an autosomal recessive disorder. The disorder is characterized by increased glomerular permeability to plasma protein, which results in massive urinary protein loss. This discussion is devoted to MCNS because it constitutes 80% of nephrotic syndrome cases.

Pathophysiology

The onset of MCNS can occur at any age but predominantly occurs in children between 2 and 7 years of age. It is rare in children younger than 6 months of age, uncommon in infants younger than 1 year of age, and unusual after 8 years of age. Patients with MCNS are twice as likely to be male.

The pathogenesis of MCNS is not fully understood. There may be a metabolic, biochemical, physiochemical, or immune-mediated disturbance that causes the basement membrane of the glomeruli to become increasingly permeable to protein, but the cause and mechanisms are only speculative.

The glomerular membrane, normally impermeable to albumin and other proteins, becomes permeable to proteins, especially albumin, that leak through the membrane and are lost in urine (*hyperalbuminuria*). This reduces the serum albumin level (*hypoalbuminemia*), decreasing the colloidal osmotic pressure in the capillaries. As a result, the vascular hydrostatic pressure exceeds the pull of the colloidal osmotic pressure, causing fluid to accumulate in the interstitial spaces (*edema*) and body cavities, particularly in the abdominal cavity (*ascites*). The shift of fluid from the plasma to the interstitial spaces reduces the vascular fluid volume (*hypovolemia*), which in turn stimulates the renin-angiotensin system and the secretion of antidiuretic hormone and aldosterone. Tubular reabsorption of sodium and water is increased in an attempt to increase intravascular volume. The elevation of serum lipids is not fully understood. The sequence of events in nephrotic syndrome is diagrammed in Fig. 45.6.

Diagnostic Evaluation

The disease is suspected on the basis of clinical manifestations (Box 45.2). The generalized edema may develop rapidly or gradually but eventually prompts the family to seek medical attention. Parents usually give a history of the child being well but steadily gaining weight; appearing edematous; and then becoming anorexic, irritable, and less active.

The diagnosis of MCNS is suspected on the basis of the history and clinical manifestations (edema, proteinuria, hypoalbuminemia, and

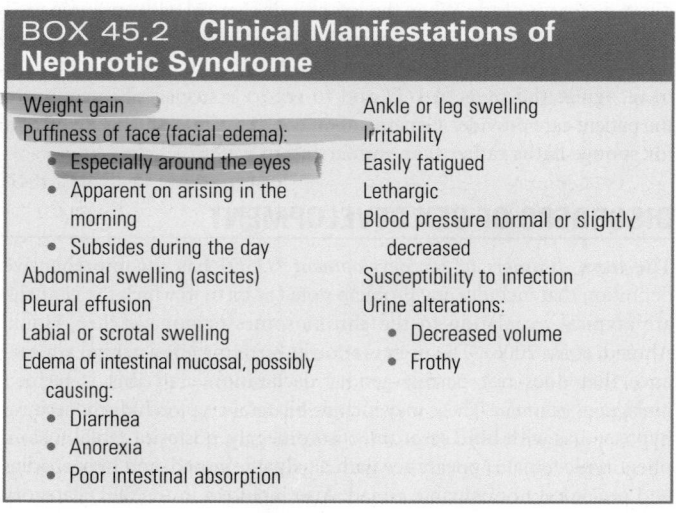

BOX 45.2   Clinical Manifestations of Nephrotic Syndrome

Weight gain	Ankle or leg swelling
Puffiness of face (facial edema):	Irritability
• Especially around the eyes	Easily fatigued
• Apparent on arising in the morning	Lethargic
• Subsides during the day	Blood pressure normal or slightly decreased
Abdominal swelling (ascites)	Susceptibility to infection
Pleural effusion	Urine alterations:
Labial or scrotal swelling	• Decreased volume
Edema of intestinal mucosal, possibly causing:	• Frothy
• Diarrhea	
• Anorexia	
• Poor intestinal absorption	

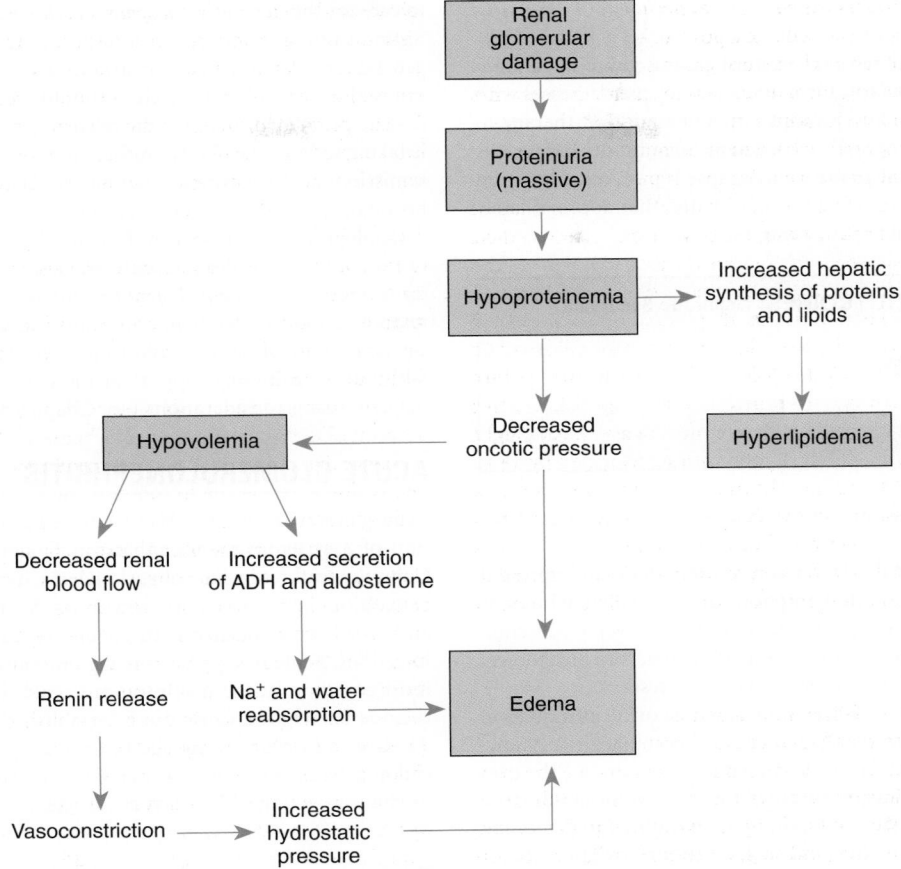

FIG 45.6 Sequence of events in nephrotic syndrome. *ADH,* Antidiuretic hormone.

hypercholesterolemia in the absence of hematuria and hypertension) in children between 2 and 8 years of age. The hallmark of MCNS is massive proteinuria (higher than 2+ on urine dipstick). Hyaline casts, oval fat bodies, and a few red blood cells (RBCs) can be found in the urine of some affected children, although there is seldom gross hematuria. The GFR is usually normal or high. Kidney function must be monitored, however, because acute kidney injury (AKI) may occur due to intravascular volume depletion, interstitial nephritis, acute tubular necrosis, or other factors (Rheault, Wei, Hains, et al., 2014).

Total serum protein concentration is low, with the serum albumin significantly reduced and plasma lipids elevated. Hemoglobin and hematocrit are usually normal or elevated as a result of hemoconcentration. The platelet count may be elevated. Serum sodium concentration may be low. If the patient does not respond to an 8-week course of daily steroids, a renal biopsy may be needed to distinguish among other types of nephrotic syndrome. The biopsy results of children with MCNS are remarkable for effacement of the foot processes of the epithelial cells lining the basement membrane, but otherwise the kidney tissue is normal.

Therapeutic Management

Objectives of therapeutic management include (1) reducing excretion of urinary protein, (2) reducing fluid retention in the tissues, (3) preventing infection, and (4) minimizing complications related to therapies. Dietary restrictions include a low-salt diet and, in more severe cases, fluid restriction. If complications of edema develop, diuretic therapy may be initiated to provide temporary relief from edema. Sometimes

infusions of 25% albumin are used. Acute infections are treated with appropriate antibiotics.

Corticosteroids are the first line of therapy for MCNS. The starting dosage for prednisone is usually 2 mg/kg body weight/day for 6 weeks followed by 1.5 mg/kg every other day for 6 weeks (Lombel, Gipson & Hodson, 2013). About two-thirds of children with MCNS have a relapse, heralded first by increased urine protein. Relapses can be diagnosed early if parents are taught routine home monitoring of urine protein by dipstick. Relapses are treated with a repeated, but usually shorter, course of high-dose steroid therapy. Side effects of the steroids include increased appetite, weight gain, rounding of the face, and behavior changes. Long-term therapy may result in hirsutism, growth retardation, cataracts, hypertension, gastrointestinal bleeding, bone demineralization, infection, and hyperglycemia. Children who do not respond to steroid therapy, those who have frequent relapses, and those in whom the side effects threaten their growth and general health may be considered for a course of therapy using other immunosuppressant medications (cyclophosphamide, chlorambucil, or cyclosporine).

Episodes of MCNS, both the first episode and relapse, often happen in conjunction with a viral or bacterial infection. Relapses can also be triggered by allergies and immunizations. Relapses in children with MCNS may continue over many years.

Complications of nephrotic syndrome include infection, circulatory insufficiency secondary to hypovolemia, and thromboembolism. Infections that may be seen in children with nephrotic syndrome include peritonitis, cellulitis, and pneumonia and require prompt recognition and vigorous treatment with appropriate antibiotic therapy.

Prognosis

The prognosis for ultimate recovery in most cases is good. In children who respond to steroid therapy, the tendency to relapse decreases with time. With early detection and prompt implementation of therapy to eradicate proteinuria, progressive basement membrane damage is minimized so that when the tendency to relapse is past, renal function is usually normal or near normal. It is estimated that approximately 80% of affected children have this favorable prognosis.

> **QUALITY PATIENT OUTCOMES: Nephrotic Syndrome**
> * Protein-free urine
> * Acute infections prevented
> * Edema absent or minimal
> * Nutrition maintained
> * Metabolic abnormalities controlled

Care Management

Continuous monitoring of fluid retention or excretion is an important nursing function. Strict intake and output records are essential but may be difficult to obtain from very young children. Application of collection bags is irritating to edematous skin that is readily subject to breakdown. Applying diapers or weighing wet pads may be necessary.

Other methods of monitoring progress include urine examination for albumin, daily weight, and measurement of abdominal girth. Assessment of edema (e.g., increased or decreased swelling around the eyes and dependent areas), the degree of pitting, and the color and texture of skin are part of nursing care. Vital signs are monitored to detect any early signs of complications, such as shock or an infective process.

Infection is a constant source of danger to edematous children and those receiving corticosteroid therapy. These children are particularly vulnerable to upper respiratory tract infection; therefore, they must be kept warm and dry, active, and protected from contact with infected individuals (e.g., roommates, visitors, and personnel). The pneumococcal conjugate vaccine (13-valent) and pneumococcal polysaccharide vaccine (PPSV, 23-valent) are recommended for children with nephrotic syndrome (Centers for Disease Control and Prevention, 2014).

Loss of appetite accompanying relapse creates a perplexing problem for nurses. The combined efforts of nurse, dietitian, parents, and child are needed to formulate a nutritionally adequate and attractive diet. Salt is restricted (but not eliminated) during the edema phase and while the child is on steroid therapy. Fluid restriction (if prescribed) is limited to short-term use during massive edema. Every effort should be made to serve attractive meals with preferred foods and a minimum of fuss, but it usually requires considerable ingenuity to entice the child to eat (see the "Feeding the Sick Child" section in Chapter 39). Once the child feels better, the appetite (enhanced by steroids) returns. At this point, care must be taken to prevent excessive caloric intake and weight gain.

Children usually adjust activities according to their tolerance level. However, they may require guidance in selecting play activities. Suitable recreational and diversional activities are an important part of their care. Irritability and mood swings that accompany steroid therapy are not unusual in these children and may create an additional challenge for the nurse and family.

Family Support and Home Care

Continuous support of the child and family is one of the major nursing considerations. Parents are taught to detect signs of relapse and to call for changes in treatment at the earliest indication. Unless the edema and proteinuria are severe or the parents, for some reason, are unable to care for the ill child, *home care is preferred*. Parents are instructed in testing urine for albumin, administering medications, and providing general care. Parents are also instructed regarding avoiding contact with infected playmates, but the child should attend school.

The prolonged course of the relapsing form of nephrotic syndrome is taxing to both the child and the family. The up-and-down course of remissions and exacerbations with periodic disruption of family life by hospitalization places a severe strain on the child and the family, both psychologically and financially. Reassurance regarding this characteristic of the course of the disease, with emphasis on the importance of long-term care, needs to be provided to parents and children. A satisfactory response is more likely when relapses are detected and therapy is instituted early, and remissions are prolonged when instructions are carried out faithfully. Continuous support of the child and family is one of the major nursing considerations (see Chapter 36).

ACUTE GLOMERULONEPHRITIS

Acute glomerulonephritis (AGN) may be a primary event or a manifestation of a systemic disorder that can range from minimal to severe. Common features include oliguria, edema, hypertension and circulatory congestion, hematuria, and proteinuria. Most cases are postinfectious and have been associated with pneumococcal, streptococcal, and viral infections. Acute poststreptococcal glomerulonephritis (APSGN) is the most common of the postinfectious renal diseases in childhood and the one for which a cause can be established in the majority of cases. APSGN can occur at any age but affects primarily early school-age children, with a peak age of onset of 6 to 7 years of age. It is uncommon in children younger than 2 years of age, and boys outnumber girls 2 to 1.

Etiology

APSGN is an immune-complex disease that occurs after an antecedent streptococcal infection with certain strains of the group A beta-hemolytic streptococci (GABHS). Most streptococcal infections do not cause APSGN. A latent period of 10 to 21 days occurs between the streptococcal infection and the onset of clinical manifestations. Disease secondary to streptococcal pharyngitis is more common in the winter or spring, but when APSGN is associated with pyoderma (principally impetigo), it may be more prevalent in late summer or early fall, especially in warmer climates. Second episodes of APSGN are rare.

Pathophysiology

The pathophysiology of APSGN is still uncertain. Immune complexes are deposited in the glomerular basement membrane. The glomeruli become edematous and infiltrated with polymorphonuclear leukocytes, which occlude the capillary lumen. The resulting decrease in plasma filtration results in an excessive accumulation of water and retention of sodium that expands plasma and interstitial fluid volumes, leading to circulatory congestion and edema. The cause of the hypertension associated with AGN cannot be completely explained by fluid retention. Excess renin may also be produced.

Diagnostic Evaluation

Typically, affected children are in good health until they experience a streptococcal infection. In some instances, they have a history of only a mild cold or no previous infection at all. The onset of nephritis appears after an average latency period of about 1 to 3 weeks (Box 45.3). Because the child appears to be well during the latency period, parents may not recognize the association. The edema is usually relatively moderate and may not be appreciated by someone unfamiliar with the child's normal appearance.

Urinalysis during the acute phase characteristically shows hematuria and proteinuria. Proteinuria generally parallels the hematuria and may be 3+ or 4+ in the presence of gross hematuria. Gross discoloration of the urine reflects RBC and hemoglobin content. Microscopic examination of the sediment shows many RBCs, leukocytes, epithelial cells, and granular and RBC casts. Bacteria are not seen.

Azotemia that results from impaired glomerular filtration is reflected in elevated blood urea nitrogen (BUN) and creatinine levels in at least 50% of cases. Occasionally, proteinuria is excessive, and the patient may have nephrotic syndrome (i.e., hypoproteinemia and hyperlipidemia).

Cultures of the pharynx are rarely positive for streptococci because the renal disease occurs weeks after the infection.

Some serologic tests are necessary to make the diagnosis of APSGN. Circulating serum antibodies to streptococci indicate the presence of a previous infection. The antistreptolysin O (ASO) titer is the most familiar and readily available test for streptococcal infection. Other antibodies that may aid in diagnosis are elevated antihyaluronidase (AHase), anti-deoxyribonuclease B (ADNase-B), and streptozyme. All patients with APSGN have reduced serum complement 3 (C3) activity in the early stages of the disease. Rising C3 levels are used as a guide to indicate improvement of the disease and should be normal in almost all patients 8 weeks after the disease onset.

Studies that may be useful include chest x-ray, which generally shows cardiac enlargement, pulmonary congestion, or pleural effusion during the edematous phase of acute disease. Renal biopsy for diagnostic purposes is seldom required but may be useful in the diagnosis of atypical cases.

Therapeutic Management

Management consists of the interprofessional care team providing general supportive measures and early recognition and treatment of complications. Children who have normal blood pressure and a satisfactory urinary output can generally be treated at home. Those with substantial edema, hypertension, gross hematuria, or significant oliguria should be hospitalized because of the unpredictability of complications.

Dietary restrictions depend on the stage and severity of the disease, especially the extent of edema. Moderate sodium restriction and even fluid restriction may be instituted for children with hypertension and edema. Foods with substantial amounts of potassium are generally restricted during the period of oliguria.

Regular measurement of vital signs, body weight, and intake and output is essential to monitor the progress of the disease and to detect complications that may appear at any time during the course of the disease. A record of daily weight is the most useful means for assessing fluid balance. Rarely, children with APSGN will develop AKI with oliguria that significantly alters the fluid and electrolyte balance (resulting in hyperkalemia, acidosis, hypocalcemia, or hyperphosphatemia). These children require careful management. Peritoneal dialysis or hemodialysis is seldom needed.

Acute, sometimes severe, hypertension must be anticipated and identified early. Blood pressure measurements are taken every 4 to 6 hours. A variety of antihypertensive medications and diuretics are used to control hypertension. Antibiotic therapy is indicated only for children with evidence of persistent streptococcal infections. It is used to prevent transmission of nephritogenic streptococci to other family members.

Prognosis

Almost all children correctly diagnosed as having APSGN recover completely, and specific immunity is conferred, so subsequent recurrences are uncommon. Less than 1% of children will go on to develop end-stage renal disease (ESRD), although abnormal urinalysis and renal function may persist for decades (Nast, 2012).

Care Management

Interprofessional care of the child with glomerulonephritis involves careful assessment of the disease status, with regular monitoring of vital signs (including frequent measurement of blood pressure), fluid balance, and behavior.

Vital signs provide clues to the severity of the disease and early signs of complications. They are carefully measured, and any deviations are reported and recorded. The volume and character of urine are noted, and the child is weighed daily. Children with restricted fluid intake, especially those who are not severely edematous or those who have lost weight, are observed for signs of dehydration.

Assessment of the child for signs of cerebral complications is an important nursing function, because the severity of the acute phase is variable and unpredictable. The child with edema, hypertension, and gross hematuria may be subject to complications, and anticipatory preparations such as seizure precautions and IV equipment are included in the nursing care plan (see the Nursing Care Plan box: The Child with Chronic Kidney Disease later in this chapter).

For most children, a regular diet is allowed, but it should contain no added salt. Foods high in sodium and salted treats are eliminated, and parents and friends are advised not to bring snacks, such as potato chips or pretzels. Fluid restriction, if prescribed, is more difficult, and the amount permitted should be evenly divided throughout the waking hours. Meal preparation and service require special attention because the child is indifferent to meals during the acute phase. Again, collaboration with parents and the dietitian and special consideration for food preferences facilitate meal planning.

During the acute phase, children are generally content to lie in bed. As they begin to feel better and their symptoms subside, they will want to be up and about. Activities should be planned to allow for frequent rest periods and avoidance of fatigue. Children who have mild edema and no hypertension, as well as convalescent children who are being treated at home, need follow-up care. Parent education and support in preparation for discharge and home care include education in home management, dietary restrictions, infection prevention, and the need for follow-up care and health supervision. Health supervision is continued with weekly followed by monthly visits for evaluation and urinalysis.

MISCELLANEOUS RENAL DISORDERS

HEMOLYTIC UREMIC SYNDROME

Hemolytic uremic syndrome (HUS) is an uncommon, acute renal disease that occurs primarily in infants and small children between 6 months and 5 years of age. HUS is one of the most frequent causes of acquired AKI in children (Grisaru, 2014). The clinical features of the disease include acquired hemolytic anemia, thrombocytopenia, renal injury, and central nervous system (CNS) symptoms. The etiology of HUS is thought to be associated with bacterial toxins, chemicals, and viruses. The appearance of the disease has been associated with *Rickettsia* organisms, viruses (especially coxsackievirus, echovirus, and adenovirus), *E. coli,* pneumococci, shigellae, and salmonellae and may represent an unusual response to these infections. Multiple cases of HUS caused by enteric infection of the *E. coli* O157:H7 serotype have been traced to undercooked meat, especially ground beef. Other sources are unpasteurized milk or fruit juice, especially apple; alfalfa sprouts; lettuce; and salami. Drinking or swimming in sewage-contaminated water can also cause infection. The clinical presentation is usually a history of a prodromal illness (most often gastroenteritis or an upper respiratory tract infection) followed by the sudden onset of hemolysis and renal failure.

Pathophysiology

The primary site of injury appears to be the endothelial lining of the small glomerular arterioles, which become swollen and occluded with deposits of platelets and fibrin clots (intravascular coagulation). RBCs are damaged as they attempt to move through the partially occluded blood vessels. These damaged cells are removed by the spleen, causing acute hemolytic anemia. The platelet aggregation within the damaged blood vessels or the damage and removal of platelets produce the characteristic thrombocytopenia.

Diagnostic Evaluation

The triad of anemia, thrombocytopenia, and renal failure is sufficient for diagnosis (Box 45.4). Renal involvement is evidenced by proteinuria, hematuria, and urinary casts; BUN and serum creatinine levels are elevated. A low hemoglobin and hematocrit and a high reticulocyte count confirm the hemolytic nature of the anemia.

Therapeutic Management

The goals of therapy are early diagnosis and aggressive, supportive care of the AKI and hemolytic anemia. Hemodialysis or peritoneal dialysis is instituted in any child who has been anuric for 24 hours or who demonstrates oliguria with uremia or hypertension and seizures. Other treatments include use of pharmacologic agents, fresh-frozen plasma,

---

and plasmapheresis. Blood transfusions with fresh, washed packed cells are administered for severe anemia but are used with caution to prevent circulatory overload from added volume.

Prognosis

With prompt treatment, the recovery rate is about 95%, but residual renal impairment ranges from 10% to 50%. Long-term complications include chronic kidney disease (CKD), hypertension, and CNS disorders. Death is usually caused by residual renal impairment or CNS injury.

Care Management

Interprofessional care is the same as that provided in AKI and, for children with continued impairment, includes management of chronic disease. Because of the sudden and life-threatening nature of the disorder in a previously well child, parents are often ill prepared for the impact of hospitalization and treatment. Therefore, support and understanding are especially important aspects of care.

RENAL FAILURE

Renal failure is the inability of the kidneys to excrete waste material, concentrate urine, and conserve electrolytes. It can occur suddenly (e.g., AKI) in response to inadequate perfusion, kidney disease, or urinary tract obstruction, or it can develop slowly (e.g., CKD) as a result of long-standing kidney disease or an anomaly.

Azotemia and *uremia* are terms often used in relation to renal failure. Azotemia is the accumulation of nitrogenous waste within the blood. Uremia is a more advanced condition in which retention of nitrogenous products produces toxic symptoms. Whereas azotemia is not life-threatening, uremia is a serious condition that often involves other body systems.

ACUTE KIDNEY INJURY

AKI is said to exist when the kidneys suddenly are unable to regulate the volume and composition of urine appropriately in response to food and fluid intake and the needs of the organism. The principal feature of AKI is oliguria* associated with azotemia, metabolic acidosis, and diverse electrolyte disturbances. AKI is not common in childhood, and the outcome depends on the cause, associated findings, and prompt recognition and treatment.

The pathologic conditions that produce AKI caused by glomerulonephritis and HUS are discussed in relation to those disorders. AKI can also develop as a result of a large number of related or unrelated clinical conditions: poor renal perfusion; urinary tract obstruction; acute renal injury; cardiac surgery (Susantitaphong, Cruz, Cerda, et al., 2013), or the final expression of chronic, irreversible renal disease. The most common cause in children is transient renal failure resulting from severe dehydration or other causes of poor perfusion that may respond to restoration of fluid volume.

Pathophysiology

AKI is usually reversible, but the deviations of physiologic function can be extreme, and mortality in the pediatric age group remains high. There is severe reduction in the GFR, an elevated BUN level, and a significant reduction in renal blood flow.

The clinical course is variable and depends on the cause. In reversible AKI, there is a period of severe oliguria, or a low-output phase, followed

---

BOX 45.4   Clinical Manifestations of Hemolytic Uremic Syndrome

Vomiting	Oliguria or anuria
Irritability	Central nervous system (CNS)
Lethargy	involvement:
Marked pallor	• Seizures
Hemorrhagic manifestations:	• Stupor or coma
• Bruising	Signs of acute heart failure
• Petechiae	(sometimes)
• Jaundice	
• Bloody diarrhea	

---

*The definition of *oliguria* varies extensively in the literature, from 1.8 to 4 dL/m^2 every 24 hours.

by an abrupt onset of diuresis, or a high-output phase, and then a gradual return to (or toward) normal urine volumes.

In many instances of AKI, the infant or child is already critically ill with the precipitating disorder, and the explanation for development of oliguria may or may not be readily apparent (Box 45.5). When a previously well child develops AKI without an obvious cause, a careful history is taken to reveal symptoms that may be related to glomerulonephritis, obstructive uropathy, or exposure to nephrotoxic chemicals (e.g., ingestion of heavy metals, inhalation of organic solvents, or medications such as vancomycin, aminoglycosides, or nonsteroidal antiinflammatory drugs) (Blatt & Liebman, 2013). Significant laboratory measurements during renal failure that serve as a guide for therapy are BUN, serum creatinine, pH, sodium, potassium, and calcium.

Diminished urinary output and lethargy in a child who is dehydrated, is in shock, or has recently undergone surgery should be evaluated for possible AKI.

Therapeutic Management

Treatment of AKI is directed toward (1) treatment of the underlying cause, (2) management of the complications of renal failure, and (3) provision of supportive therapy within the constraints imposed by the renal failure.

Treatment of poor perfusion resulting from dehydration consists of volume restoration, as described in Chapter 41, in treatment of dehydration. If oliguria persists after restoration of fluid volume or if the renal failure is caused by intrinsic renal damage, the physiologic and biochemical abnormalities that have resulted from kidney dysfunction must be corrected or controlled. Initially, a Foley catheter is inserted to rule out urine retention, to collect available urine for analysis, and to monitor results of diuretic administration. The catheter may or may not be removed during the oliguric phase.

The amount of exogenous water provided should not exceed the amount needed to maintain zero water balance. It is calculated on the basis of estimated endogenous water formation and losses from sensible (primarily gastrointestinal) and insensible sources. No allotment is calculated for urine as long as oliguria persists.

When the output begins to increase, either spontaneously or in response to diuretic therapy, the intake of fluid, potassium, and sodium must be monitored and adequate replacement provided to prevent depletion and its consequences. Some patients pass enormous amounts of electrolyte-rich urine.

Complications

The child with AKI has a tendency to develop water intoxication and hyponatremia, which makes it difficult to provide calories in sufficient amounts to meet the child's needs and reduce tissue catabolism, metabolic acidosis, hyperkalemia, and uremia. If the child is able to tolerate oral foods, food sources high in concentrated carbohydrate and fat but low in protein, potassium, and sodium may be provided. However, many children have functional disturbances of the gastrointestinal tract, such as nausea and vomiting; therefore, the IV route is generally preferred and usually consists of essential amino acids or a combination of essential and nonessential amino acids administered by the central venous route.

Control of water balance in these patients requires careful monitoring of feedback information, such as accurate intake and output, body weight, and electrolyte measurements. In general, during the oliguric phase, no sodium, chloride, or potassium is given unless there are other large, ongoing losses. Regular measurement of plasma electrolyte, pH, BUN, and creatinine levels is required to assess the adequacy of fluid therapy and to anticipate complications that require specific treatment.

Hyperkalemia is the most immediate threat to the life of the child with AKI. Hyperkalemia can be minimized and sometimes avoided by eliminating potassium from all food and fluid, reducing tissue catabolism, and correcting acidosis. Measures used for the reduction of serum potassium levels are oral or rectal administration of an ion-exchange resin, such as sodium polystyrene sulfonate (Kayexalate) and peritoneal dialysis or hemodialysis (see later in this chapter). The resin produces its effect by exchange of its sodium for the potassium, thus binding potassium for removal from the body. This increased sodium concentration may contribute to fluid overload, hypertension, and cardiac failure. Dialysis removes potassium and other waste products from the serum by diffusion through a semipermeable membrane.

Hypertension is a frequent and serious complication of AKI, and to detect it early, blood pressure measurements are made every 4 to 6 hours. The most common cause of hypertension in AKI is overexpansion of extracellular fluid and plasma volume together with activation of the renin-angiotensin system. Hypertension is controlled with antihypertensive drugs. Other measures that may be used include limiting fluids and salt.

Anemia is frequently associated with AKI, but transfusion is not recommended unless the hemoglobin drops below 6 g/dL. Transfusions, if used, consist of fresh, packed RBCs given slowly to reduce the likelihood of increasing blood volume, hypertension, and hyperkalemia.

Seizures may occur when renal failure progresses to uremia and are also related to hypertension, hyponatremia, and hypocalcemia. Treatment is directed to the specific cause when known. More obscure causes are managed with antiepileptic drugs.

Cardiac failure with pulmonary edema is almost always associated with hypervolemia. Treatment is directed toward reduction of fluid volume, with water and sodium restriction and administration of diuretics.

Prognosis

The prognosis of AKI depends largely on the nature and severity of the causative factor or precipitating event and the promptness and competence of management. The outcome is least favorable in children with rapidly progressive nephritis and cortical necrosis. Children in whom AKI is a result of HUS or AGN may recover completely, but residual renal impairment or hypertension is more often seen. Complete recovery is usually expected in children whose renal failure is a result of dehydration, nephrotoxins, or ischemia. AKI after cardiac surgery is less favorable. It is often impossible to assess the extent of recovery for several months.

QUALITY PATIENT OUTCOMES: Acute Kidney Injury
- Underlying cause of acute kidney injury (AKI) identified and treated
- Water balance maintained
- Hypertension controlled
- Electrolyte balance maintained
- Diet maintains calories while minimizing tissue catabolism, metabolic acidosis, hyperkalemia, and uremia

---

Care Management

Meticulous attention to fluid intake and output is mandatory and includes all of the physical measurements discussed previously in relation to problems of fluid balance. Monitoring fluid balance and vital signs is a continuous process, and observers are constantly on the alert for signs of complications so that appropriate interventions can be implemented. Because these children require intensive observation and often specialized treatment (e.g., dialysis), they are usually admitted to an intensive care unit in which needed equipment and trained personnel are available (see the Nursing Care Plan box: The Child with Chronic Kidney Disease later in this chapter).

Limiting fluid intake requires ingenuity on the part of caregivers to cope with the child who is thirsty. Rationing the daily intake in small amounts of fluid served in containers that give the impression of larger volumes is one strategy. Older children who understand the rationale of fluid limits can help determine how their daily ration should be distributed.

Meeting nutritional needs is sometimes a problem; the child may be nauseated, and encouraging concentrated foods without fluids may be difficult. When nourishment is provided by the IV route, careful monitoring is essential to prevent fluid overload. In addition, nursing measures such as maintaining an optimal thermal environment, reducing any elevation of body temperature, and reducing restlessness and anxiety are used to decrease the rate of tissue catabolism.

The nurse must be continually alert for changes in behavior that indicate the onset of complications. Infection from reduced resistance, anemia, and general morbidity is a constant threat. Fluid overload and electrolyte disturbances can precipitate cardiovascular complications, such as hypertension and cardiac failure. Fluid and electrolyte imbalances, acidosis, and accumulation of nitrogenous waste products can produce neurologic involvement manifested by coma, seizures, or alterations in sensorium.

Although children with AKI are usually quite ill and voluntarily diminish their activity, infants may become restless and irritable, and children are often anxious and frightened. Frequent, painful, and stress-producing treatments and tests must be performed. A supportive, empathetic nurse can provide comfort and stability in a threatening and unnatural environment.

Family Support

Providing support and reassurance to parents is among the major nursing responsibilities. The seriousness of AKI and its emergency nature are stressful to parents, and most feel some degree of guilt regarding the child's condition, especially when the illness is a result of ingestion of a toxic substance, dehydration, or a genetic disease. They also need to be kept informed of the child's progress and provided explanations regarding the therapeutic regimen. The equipment and the child's behavior are sometimes frightening and anxiety provoking. Nurses can do much to help parents comprehend and deal with the stresses of the situation.

CHRONIC KIDNEY DISEASE

The kidneys are able to maintain the chemical composition of fluids within normal limits until more than 50% of functional renal capacity is destroyed by disease or injury. Chronic renal insufficiency or failure begins when the diseased kidneys can no longer maintain the normal chemical structure of body fluids under normal conditions. Progressive deterioration over months or years produces a variety of clinical and biochemical disturbances that eventually culminate in the clinical syndrome known as *uremia*.

A variety of diseases and disorders can result in CKD. The most frequent causes are congenital renal and urinary tract malformations, VUR associated with recurrent UTI, chronic pyelonephritis, hereditary disorders, chronic glomerulonephritis, and glomerulonephropathy associated with systemic diseases, such as anaphylactoid purpura and lupus erythematosus (see the Nursing Care Plan box: The Child with Chronic Kidney Disease).

Pathophysiology

Early in the course of progressive renal failure, the child remains asymptomatic with only minimal biochemical abnormalities. Unless the presence of CKD is detected in the process of routine assessment, signs and symptoms that indicate advanced renal damage frequently emerge only late in the course of the disease. Midway in the disease process, as increasing numbers of nephrons are totally destroyed and most others are damaged to varying degrees, the few that remain intact are hypertrophied but functional. These few normal nephrons are able to make sufficient adjustments to stresses to maintain reasonable degrees of fluid and electrolyte balance. Definitive biochemical examination at this time will reveal restricted tolerance to excesses or restrictions. As the disease progresses to the end stage, because of a severe reduction in the number of functioning nephrons, the kidneys are no longer able to maintain fluid and electrolyte balance, and the features of uremic syndrome appear.

The accumulation of various biochemical substances in the blood resulting from diminished renal function produces complications such as the following:

Retention of waste products, especially BUN and creatinine

Water and sodium retention, which contributes to edema and vascular congestion

Hyperkalemia of dangerous levels

Metabolic acidosis of a sustained nature because of continual hydrogen ion retention and bicarbonate loss

Calcium and phosphorus disturbances, resulting in altered bone metabolism, which in turn causes growth arrest or retardation, bone pain, and deformities known as *renal osteodystrophy*

Anemia caused by hematologic dysfunction, including a shortened life span of RBCs, impaired RBC production related to decreased production of erythropoietin, prolonged bleeding time, and nutritional anemia

Growth disturbance, probably caused by such factors as renal osteodystrophy, poor nutrition associated with dietary restrictions and loss of appetite, and biochemical abnormalities

Children with CKD seem to be more susceptible to infection, especially pneumonia, UTI, and septicemia, although the reason for this is unclear. These children become extraordinarily sensitive to changes in vascular volume that may cause pulmonary overload, CNS symptoms, hypertension, and cardiac failure.

◎ NURSING CARE PLAN
The Child With Chronic Kidney Disease

Case Study

Susie is a 9-year-old girl who has a history of chronic pyelonephritis. Over the past several months, she has experienced increased fatigue and lack of appetite, was unable to participate in physical activities, and appeared pale and listless. Her parents took her to her pediatrician who on examination, found signs and symptoms of weight loss, facial puffiness, bone and joint pain, and dryness of the skin. Susie told her pediatrician that she was having headaches and nausea. With Susie's history of chronic pyelonephritis, she was immediately referred to a pediatric nephrologist.

Assessment

Based on Susie's history, what are the most important signs and symptoms that you need to be aware of?

Defining Characteristics

Elevated serum creatinine
Evidence of hyperkalemia, hyperphosphatemia, hypernatremia, and uremia
Anemia
Oliguria
Anuria uncommon (except in obstructive disorders)
Nonspecific (may develop):
  Nausea
  Vomiting
  Headaches
  Drowsiness
  Edema
  Dryness and itchiness of the skin
  Hypertension
  Inadequate growth
  Poor nutritional intake

Nursing Diagnoses

Risk for Electrolyte Imbalance
Risk for Ineffective Renal Perfusion
Risk for Poor Growth
Risk for Anemia
Risk for Cardiovascular Complications
Risk for Renal Bone Disease
Knowledge Deficit regarding chronic kidney disease (CKD) and treatments

Nursing Interventions and Rationales

What are the most appropriate nursing interventions for a child with CKD?

Nursing Interventions	Rationales
Close monitoring of Susie's status. Follow clinical and laboratory findings. Blood studies include complete blood count (CBC), electrolyte and kidney status.	To identify changes in kidney status that require additional treatment
Observe for evidence of accumulated waste products.	To ensure prompt treatment
Provide dietary instructions for foods that reduce excretory demands on kidneys and provide sufficient calories and protein for growth.	To encourage appropriate diet, which can reduce kidney demands
Limit phosphorus, salt, and potassium as prescribed.	To prevent mineral excess

Nursing Interventions	Rationales
Monitor growth closely since short stature is a significant side effect.	To provide early detection of growth failure and, if appropriate, treatment with growth hormone
Monitor cardiovascular status including blood pressure measurement.	Early identification and treatment of hypertension decreases the risk for end organ damage such as left ventricular hypertrophy and further kidney damage
Minimize renal bone disease by maintaining optimal calcium, phosphorus, and intact parathyroid hormone levels, and acid base balance.	Prevention and early treatment of renal bone disease optimizes growth
Monitor for anemia. Susie may require school accommodations and rest periods due to fatigue.	Early identification of anemia allows for treatment with iron supplement and erythropoiesis-stimulating medication maximizing energy level
Identify patient and family stressors that may accompany a diagnosis of CKD.	To provide financial and emotional support for family to help decrease some of the stressors associated with this condition
Review disease, medication, dietary, and other information at every encounter.	Understanding the medical condition and therapies allows family to make informed decisions about care

Expected Outcomes

Susie will exhibit no evidence of waste product accumulation.
Sufficient calories and protein for growth will be maintained.
Excretory demands made on the kidney will be limited.
Metabolic bone disease (osteodystrophy) will be minimal.
Fluid and electrolyte disturbances will be managed.
Hypertension will be managed.
Patient/family will indicate understanding of CKD and treatments.

Case Study (Continued)

Susie is now being followed by a nephrology specialty team and has returned to the clinic for her monthly evaluation. The nurse performing the assessment finds Susie's blood pressure to be elevated, and she notices that her skin appears pale and sallow in appearance. Susie tells her nurse that she has been really tired lately and her headaches have returned.

Assessment

What concerns you most based on the scenario?
  Susie's kidney status may be deteriorating based on the history and examination. See the defining characteristics of CKD listed earlier.
What immediate steps should be taken to further evaluate Susie's kidney status?
  Check CBC, electrolyte status, and kidney function tests.
  Document weight, height, and blood pressure; compare to previous visit.
  Evaluate patient adherence to medication and dietary recommendations.
The following laboratory results have returned from Susie's blood work:
  CBC: Hemoglobin, 9.1; hematocrit (Hct), 27; white blood cells (WBCs), 8500; platelets, normal
  Urinalysis: Elevated protein
  Electrolytes and kidney function: Potassium, 5.9; sodium, 138; phosphate, 6; calcium, 9.1; magnesium, 2.5; blood urea nitrogen (BUN), 25; serum creatinine, 1.8

Continued

NURSING CARE PLAN

The Child With Chronic Kidney Disease—cont'd

Glomerular filtration rate (GFR), 30 mL/min/1.73 m^2 (The GFR shows how well the kidneys are working to pass liquid and waste from the bloodstream to the kidneys.)

Nursing Diagnoses

Risk for Electrolyte Imbalance (hyperkalemia)
Risk for Ineffective Renal Perfusion

Nursing Interventions and Rationales

What are the most appropriate nursing interventions for Susie at this time?

Nursing Interventions	Rationales
Treat hyperkalemia with dietary restrictions and perhaps medication, such as Kayexalate.	To prevent cardiac arrhythmias and other symptoms associated with elevated potassium levels
Observe for evidence of accumulated waste products.	To ensure prompt treatment
Provide dietary instructions for foods that reduce excretory demands on kidneys and provide sufficient calories and protein for growth. This may include restriction of potassium, sodium, and/or phosphorus intake.	To encourage appropriate diet, which can reduce kidney demands
Treat anemia with adequate rest periods and possibly iron and erythropoiesis-stimulating medications.	To maximize energy level

Expected Outcomes

Susie will be managed to minimize further kidney function deterioration.

Case Study (Continued)

Susie's parents are anxious and upset with the new problems she is now having. They are concerned that she will need kidney transplantation in the near future. You are concerned that they are not adhering to the management plan that was designed for the parents to follow at home.

Assessment

What are the most important aspects of Susie's care to discuss with her parents at this time?

Defining Characteristics

Understands definition of CKD
States four signs of kidney failure
Describes medications the child is taking and rationale for use
Describes dietary modifications and rationale for use
Expresses fears and concerns
Shows appropriate reactions to child's illness

Nursing Diagnosis

Readiness for Enhanced Knowledge related to parents' interest in Susie's health status.

Nursing Interventions and Rationales

What are the most appropriate nursing interventions for this diagnosis?

Nursing Interventions	Rationales
Review disease, medication, dietary, and other information at every encounter.	Understanding the medical condition and therapies allows families to make informed decisions about care. Optimal consistency with treatment maximizes renal function.
Arrange for renal dietitian to meet with family to review allowable foods and assist in dietary planning.	Improved understanding of the child's dietary needs increases ability to adhere to modifications.
Arrange for social worker to meet with family to assess emotional and financial needs.	This assistance is to identify and modify stressors associated with CKD.
As Susie nears end-stage kidney failure, arrange for discussions with a kidney transplant coordinator and/or dialysis nurse to discuss renal replacement therapies.	Family must be aware of positive and negative aspects of each therapy in order to make informed decisions.

Expected Outcomes

Susie's parents will understand the signs and symptoms of CKD and will understand the actions being taken by the health care team.
Susie and her parents will follow the plan designed for managing her chronic kidney failure at home.

Diagnostic Evaluation

The diagnosis of CKD is usually suspected on the basis of any number of clinical manifestations, a history of prior renal disease, or biochemical findings. The onset is usually gradual, and the initial signs and symptoms are vague and nonspecific (Box 45.6).

Laboratory and other diagnostic tools and tests are of value in assessing the extent of renal damage, biochemical disturbances, and related physical dysfunction (see Tables 45.1 to 45.3). Often they can help establish the nature of the underlying disease and differentiate among other disease processes and the pathologic consequences of renal dysfunction.

Therapeutic Management

In irreversible renal failure, the goals of medical management are to (1) promote maximum renal function, (2) maintain body fluid and electrolyte balance within safe biochemical limits, (3) treat systemic complications, and (4) promote as active and normal a life as possible for the child for as long as possible. The child is allowed unrestricted activity and is allowed to set his or her own limits regarding rest and extent of exertion. School attendance is encouraged as long as the child is able. When the effort is too great, home tutoring is arranged.

Diet regulation is the most effective means, short of dialysis, of reducing the quantity of materials that require renal excretion. The goal of diet management in renal failure is to provide sufficient calories and protein for growth while limiting the excretory demands made on the kidneys, to minimize metabolic bone disease (osteodystrophy), and to minimize fluid and electrolyte disturbances. Dietary protein intake is limited only to the reference daily intake (Recommended Dietary Allowance [RDA]) for the child's age. Restriction of protein intake below the RDA is believed to negatively affect growth and neurodevelopment. Malnutrition due to factors including anorexia, dietary restrictions, metabolic acidosis, and increased energy expenditure is common in these children (Carrero, Stenvinkel, Cuppari, et al., 2013).

BOX 45.6 Clinical Manifestations of Chronic Renal Failure

Early signs:
- Loss of normal energy
- Increased fatigue on exertion
- Pallor, subtle (may not be noticed)
- Elevated blood pressure (sometimes)

As the disease progresses:
- Decreased appetite (especially at breakfast)
- Less interest in normal activities
- Increased or decreased urinary output with compensatory intake of fluid
- Pallor more evident
- Sallow, muddy appearance of skin

Child may complain of:
- Headache
- Muscle cramps
- Nausea

Other signs and symptoms:
- Weight loss
- Facial edema
- Malaise
- Bone or joint pain
- Growth retardation
- Dryness or itching of the skin
- Bruised skin

- Sensory or motor loss (sometimes)
- Amenorrhea (common in adolescent girls)

Uremic syndrome (untreated):
- Gastrointestinal symptoms
  - Anorexia
  - Nausea and vomiting
- Bleeding tendencies
  - Bruises
  - Bloody diarrheal stools
  - Stomatitis
  - Bleeding from lips and mouth
- Intractable itching
- Uremic frost (deposits of urea crystals on skin)
- Unpleasant "uremic" breath odor
- Deep respirations
- Hypertension
- Congestive heart failure
- Pulmonary edema
- Neurologic involvement
  - Progressive confusion
  - Dulled sensorium
  - Coma (ultimately)
  - Tremors
  - Muscle twitching
  - Seizures

Sodium and water are not usually limited unless there is evidence of edema or hypertension, and potassium is not usually restricted. However, restrictions of any or all three may be imposed in later stages or at any time that abnormal serum concentrations are evident.

Dietary phosphorus is controlled through reduction of protein and milk intake to prevent or correct the calcium-phosphorus imbalance. Phosphorus levels can be further reduced by oral administration of calcium carbonate preparations or other phosphate-binding agents that combine with the phosphorus to decrease gastrointestinal absorption and thus the serum levels of phosphate. Treatment with (inactive) 25-OH vitamin D and/or (active) 1, 25-dihydroxy vitamin D is begun to increase calcium absorption and suppress elevated parathyroid hormone levels (Wesseling-Perry & Salusky, 2013).

Metabolic acidosis is alleviated through administration of alkalizing agents, such as sodium bicarbonate or a combination of sodium and potassium citrate.

Growth failure is one major consequence of CKD, especially in preadolescents. These children grow poorly both before and after the initiation of hemodialysis. The use of recombinant human growth hormone to accelerate growth in children with growth retardation secondary to CKD has been successful (Gupta & Lee, 2012). Osseous deformities that result from renal osteodystrophy, especially those related to ambulation, are troublesome and require correction if they occur. Dental defects are common in children with CKD, and the earlier the onset of the disease, the more severe are the dental manifestations (including hypoplasia, hypomineralization, tooth discoloration, alteration

in size and shape of teeth, malocclusion, and ulcerative stomatitis). Therefore, regular dental care is important in these children.

Anemia in children with CKD is related to decreased production of erythropoietin. Recombinant human erythropoietin (rHuEPO) is being offered to these children as thrice-weekly or weekly subcutaneous injections and is replacing the need for frequent blood transfusions. The drug corrects the anemia that in turn increases appetite, activity, and general well-being in the children who receive it.

Hypertension may be managed initially by cautious use of a low-sodium diet, fluid restriction, and perhaps diuretics, such as hydrochlorothiazide or furosemide. Severe hypertension requires the use of other antihypertensive agents, singly or in combination.

Intercurrent infections are treated with appropriate antimicrobials at the first sign of infection; however, any drug eliminated through the kidneys is administered with caution. Other complications are treated symptomatically (e.g., central-acting antiemetics for nausea, antiepileptics for seizures, and diphenhydramine [Benadryl] for pruritus).

When the child reaches end-stage kidney failure, death will eventually occur unless waste products and toxins are removed from body fluids by dialysis or kidney transplantation. These techniques have been adapted for infants and small children and are implemented in most cases of renal failure after conservative management is no longer effective (see the "Technologic Management of Renal Failure" section later in this chapter).

Prognosis

Dialysis and transplantation are the only treatments currently available for children with ESRD. Although children may survive on dialysis, it is not an ideal long-term modality. Complications include infection of access sites, growth failure, and disruption of normal socialization. Many pediatric centers encourage families of children with ESRD to consider kidney transplantation. The North American Pediatric Renal Trials and Collaborative Studies' (2010) annual transplant report documents graft survival of 96% at 1 year and 84% at 5 years for living donor kidneys and 95% at 1 year and 78% at 5 years for deceased donor kidneys.

Posttransplant complications include infection, hypertension, steroid toxicity, hyperlipidemia, aseptic necrosis, malignancy, and growth retardation (Sharma, Ramanathan, Posner, et al., 2013). Long-term graft survival is not guaranteed, and many children require a second or third transplant. Successful kidney transplantation does improve rehabilitation of children with CKD, both educationally and psychologically. Increasing use of primary or preemptive kidney transplants is becoming the optimal form of renal replacement therapy, leading to substantial improvement in quality of life (Goldstein, Rosburg, Warady, et al., 2009).

QUALITY PATIENT OUTCOMES: Chronic Kidney Disease
- Sufficient calories and protein for growth maintained
- Excretory demands made on the kidney are limited
- Metabolic bone disease (osteodystrophy) minimal
- Fluid and electrolyte disturbances managed
- Hypertension managed
- Growth retardation treated

Care Management

The multiple complications of ESRD are managed according to medical protocols, such as the National Kidney Foundation Kidney Disease Outcomes Quality Initiative's evidence-based clinical practice guidelines (http://www.kidney.org/professionals/KDOQI). However, progressive disease places a number of stresses on the child and family, including those of a potentially fatal illness (see Chapter 36). There is a continuing need for repeated examinations that often entail painful procedures, side effects, and frequent hospitalizations. Diet therapy becomes progressively more restricted and intense, and the child is required to take a variety of medications. Ever present in all aspects of the treatment regimen is the realization that without treatment, death is inevitable.

Some specific stresses related to ESRD and its treatment are predictable. When it first becomes apparent that ESRD is inevitable, both parents and child experience depression and anxiety. Acceptance is particularly difficult if renal failure progresses rapidly after diagnosis. Denial and disbelief are usually pronounced. After renal failure is established and symptoms become progressively more distressing, the initiation of dialysis is usually perceived as a positive experience, and after experiencing initial concerns regarding the treatment, the child begins to feel better, and parental anxiety is relieved for a time.

For children, however, initiating a dialysis regimen is a traumatic and anxiety-provoking experience, because it involves surgery for implantation of a graft, fistula, or peritoneal catheter. The initial experience with the dialysis procedure is frightening to most children. They need reassurance about the nature of the preparations for dialysis and the conduct of the treatment.

Adolescents, with their increased need for independence and their urge for rebellion, usually adapt less well than younger children. They resent the control and enforced dependence imposed by the rigorous and unrelenting therapy program. They resent being dependent on hemodialysis technology, their parents, and the professional staff. Depression or hostility is common in adolescents undergoing hemodialysis.

Both the graft and the fistula require needle insertions at each dialysis. The goal is to perform pain-free venipuncture. Using buffered lidocaine with a small-gauge needle (30-gauge) to anesthetize the area before venipuncture of the graft or fistula is one method. Using an anesthetizing topical preparation, such as eutectic mixture of local anesthetics (EMLA; lidocaine and prilocaine) 1 hour before venipuncture is another approach (see the "Pain Management" section in Chapter 30). External dual-lumen venous access devices eliminate the need for needles but are more prone to infection and other central line complications.

The availability of home peritoneal dialysis has offered a greater degree of freedom for persons undergoing long-term dialysis. The nurse is responsible for teaching the family about (1) the disease, its implications, and the therapeutic plan; (2) the possible psychologic effects of the disease and the treatment; and (3) the technical aspects of the procedure. The family learns to manage the various aspects of the dialysis procedure, how to maintain accurate records, and how to observe for signs of complications that need to be reported to the proper people.

Body changes related to the disease process (such as, pale or ashen skin color, growth retardation, and lack of sexual maturation) are stress provoking. Dietary restrictions are particularly burdensome for both children and parents. Children feel deprived when they are unable to eat foods previously enjoyed and that are unrestricted for other family members. Consequently, they may fail to cooperate. Diet restrictions may be interpreted as punishment. Some children, unable to understand fully the purpose of restrictions, will sneak forbidden food items at every opportunity. Allowing children, especially adolescents, maximum participation in and responsibility for their own treatment program is helpful.

After months or years of dialysis, the parents and child feel anxiety associated with the prognosis and continued pressures of the treatment. The continuous need for treatment interferes with family plans. The time spent in transportation to and from the dialysis unit and the time spent undergoing dialysis treatments cut into time for outside activities, including school. Graft and fistula problems, as well as peritoneal catheter exit site infections, may develop and present a common source of aggravation (see Family-Centered Care box: Family Priorities).

FAMILY-CENTERED CARE
Family Priorities

Families that have children with long-term chronic illnesses, such as end-stage renal disease (ESRD), spend much time in hospitals, outpatient clinics, and primary health care facilities. When they miss appointments or respond less quickly than anticipated, sometimes they are quickly labeled "noncompliant." It is important to remember that families have to develop priorities for the unit as a whole. Sometimes the family may decide that it is more important for the parent to go to work or to attend a sibling's school performance than to attend an appointment scheduled for them by health care personnel. The chronically ill child cannot and should not always be the number-one priority for the family. The professional staff who works with the family can help the parents prioritize the needs of the ill child within the needs of the family constellation.

Teresa Hall, MS, RN
Hathaway Children's Services
Sylmar, CA

The possibility of kidney transplantation often provides hope for relief from the rigors of hemodialysis and peritoneal dialysis. Most children and families respond well to a kidney transplant, and most children can be successfully rehabilitated.

The National Kidney Foundation* and other agencies provide a number of services and information for families of children with renal disease.

TECHNOLOGIC MANAGEMENT OF RENAL FAILURE

DIALYSIS

Dialysis is the process of separating colloids and crystalline substances in solution by the difference in their rate of diffusion through a semipermeable membrane. Methods of dialysis currently available for clinical management of renal failure are *peritoneal dialysis*, wherein the abdominal cavity acts as a semipermeable membrane through which water and solutes of small molecular size move by osmosis and diffusion according to their respective concentrations on either side of the membrane, and *hemodialysis*, in which blood is circulated outside the body through artificial membranes that permit a similar passage of water and solutes. A third type of dialysis is *hemofiltration*, in which blood filtrate is circulated outside the body by hydrostatic pressure exerted across a semipermeable membrane with simultaneous infusion of a replacement solution. Types of hemofiltration include continuous venovenous hemofiltration, continuous venovenous hemodialysis, and continuous venovenous hemofiltration. These continuous renal replacement therapies are used in AKI, severe fluid overload, and inborn errors of metabolism or after bone marrow transplant.

Peritoneal dialysis is the preferred form of dialysis for infants, children, and parents who wish to remain independent, families who live a long distance from the medical center, and children who prefer fewer dietary restrictions and a gentler form of dialysis. Chronic peritoneal dialysis is most often performed at home. The two types of peritoneal dialysis are *continuous ambulatory peritoneal dialysis* and *continuous cycling peritoneal dialysis*. In both methods, commercially available sterile dialysis

---

*30 E. 33rd Street, New York, NY 10016; 212-889-2210, 800-622-9010; http://www.kidney.org. In Canada: Kidney Foundation of Canada, 300–5165 Sherbrooke Street W, Montreal, QC H4A 1T6; 514-369-4806, 800-361-7494; http://www.kidney.ca.

solution is instilled into the peritoneal cavity through a surgically implanted indwelling catheter tunneled subcutaneously and sutured into place. The warmed solution is allowed to enter the peritoneal cavity by gravity and remains a variable length of time according to the rate of solute removal and glucose absorption in individual patients. The care and management of the procedure are the responsibility of the parents of young children. Some centers have initiated use of home health nurses to give parents respite from care. Older children and adolescents can carry out the procedure themselves, which provides them with some control and less dependency. This is especially important for adolescents.

> ## ! NURSING ALERT
> Observe for changes in the color of the dialysate draining from the child. The spent solution should be clear. If the color is cloudy, notify the patient care provider immediately.

Hemodialysis requires the creation of a vascular access and the use of special dialysis equipment—the hemodialyzer, or so-called *artificial kidney*. Vascular access may be one of three types: fistulas, grafts, or external vascular access devices. An *arteriovenous fistula* is an access in which a vein and artery are connected surgically. The preferred site is the radial artery and a forearm vein that produces dilation and thickening of the superficial vessels of the forearm to provide easy access for repeated venipuncture. An alternative is the creation of a subcutaneous (internal) arteriovenous graft by anastomosing artery and vein, with a synthetic prosthetic graft for circulatory access. The most commonly used material is expanded polytetrafluoroethylene (ePTFE). Both the graft and the fistula require needle insertions with each dialysis treatment.

For external vascular access devices, percutaneous catheters are inserted in the femoral, subclavian, or internal jugular veins, even in very small children. A more permanent form of external access is available via a central catheter inserted surgically into the internal jugular vein. This catheter has a dual lumen, which allows a larger volume of blood flow with minimum recirculation. Catheters eliminate the need for skin punctures but require some home care.

Hemodialysis is best suited to children who do not have someone in the family who is able to perform home peritoneal dialysis and to those who live close to a dialysis center. The procedure is usually performed three times per week for 4 to 6 hours, depending on the child's size. Studies suggest that intensified hemodialysis (shorter sessions done 5 to 7 days weekly or longer sessions done overnight three to seven times weekly) may improve outcomes (Thumfart, Pommer, Querfeld, et al., 2014). Hemodialysis achieves rapid correction of fluid and electrolyte abnormalities but can cause problems in association with this rapid change, such as muscle cramping and hypotension. Disadvantages include school absence during dialysis and strict fluid and dietary restrictions between dialysis sessions. Boredom for the child and family is often a problem during dialysis, and planned activities should be introduced (Fig. 45.7).

Most children show rapid clinical improvement with the implementation of dialysis, although it is directly related to the duration of uremia before dialysis and good nutrition. Growth rate and skeletal maturation improve, but recovery of normal growth is infrequent. In many cases, sexual development, although delayed, progresses to completion.

TRANSPLANTATION

Kidney transplantation is an acceptable and effective means of therapy in the pediatric age group. Although peritoneal dialysis and hemodialysis are life-preserving, both require major alterations in lifestyle. Transplantation

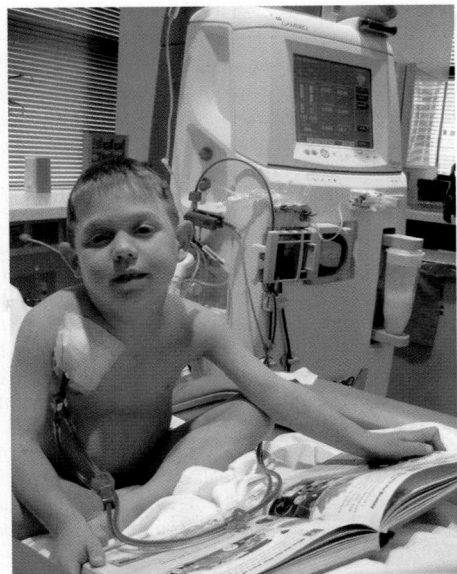

FIG 45.7 Diversional activities help lessen the boredom children can experience during hemodialysis.

offers the opportunity for a relatively normal life and is the preferred form of treatment for children with ESRD.

Kidneys for transplant are available from two sources: a **living related donor**, usually a parent or a sibling, or a **cadaver donor**, wherein the family of a dead or brain-dead patient consents to donation of a healthy kidney. Retransplantation may be required if rejection occurs.

The primary goal in transplantation is the long-term survival of grafted tissue by securing tissue that is antigenically similar to that of the recipient and by suppressing the recipient's immune mechanism. The immunosuppressant therapy of choice has been corticosteroids (prednisone) in conjunction with cyclosporine or tacrolimus and mycophenolate mofetil. Other therapies include antilymphoblast globulin or monoclonal antibodies. New immunosuppressant medications and early withdrawal of steroids or steroid-free protocols are rapidly coming into clinical trials and use in large transplant centers (Kim, Webster, & Craig, 2013). It is important for the nurse to learn about the medications used in the antirejection protocol(s) and their side effects. Because the immunosuppressant medications are taken indefinitely, transplant patients experience many side effects of the drugs, including hypertension, growth retardation, cataracts, risk for infection, obesity, characteristics of Cushing syndrome, and hirsutism.

> ## ! NURSING ALERT
> The child with a kidney transplant who exhibits any of the following should be evaluated immediately for possible rejection:
> * Fever
> * Swelling and tenderness over graft area
> * Diminished urinary output
> * Elevated blood pressure
> * Elevated serum creatinine

Rejection of the transplanted kidney is the most common cause of transplant failure. Rejection is treated aggressively with immunosuppressant medications and can often be reversed. Some patients do not respond to treatment of acute rejection or develop chronic rejection and must eventually return to dialysis or undergo another kidney transplant.

REFERENCES

American Academy of Pediatrics Subcommittee on Urinary Tract Infection, Steering Committee on Quality Improvement and Management, & Roberts, K. B. (2011). Urinary tract infection: Clinical practice guideline for the diagnosis and management of the initial UTI in febrile infants and children 2 to 24 months. *Pediatrics, 128*(3), 595–610.

American Academy of Pediatrics Task Force on Circumcision. (2012). Circumcision policy statement. *Pediatrics, 130*(3), 585–586.

Balat, A., Karakok, M., Guler, E., et al. (2008). Local defense systems in the prepuce. *Scandinavian Journal of Urology and Nephrology, 42*(1), 63–65.

Blatt, A. E., & Liebman, S. E. (2013). Drug induced acute kidney injury. *Hospital Medicine Clinics, 2*(4), e525–e541.

Bukowski, T. P., & Zeman, P. A. (2001). Hypospadias: Of concern but correctable. *Contemporary Pediatrics, 18*(2), 89–109.

Carrero, J. J., Stenvinkel, P., Cuppari, L., et al. (2013). Etiology of the protein-energy wasting syndrome in chronic kidney disease: A consensus statement from the International Society of Renal Nutrition and Metabolism (ISRNM). *Journal of Renal Nutrition, 23*(2), 77–90.

Centers for Disease Control and Prevention. (2014). *Recommended immunization schedules for persons aged 0 through 18 years—United States.* Retrieved from http://www.cdc.gov/vaccines/schedules.

Edlin, R. S., Shapiro, D. J., Hersh, A. L., et al. (2013). Antibiotic resistance patterns of outpatient pediatric urinary tract infections. *Journal of Urology, 190*(1), 222–227.

Estrada, C. R., Passerotti, C. C., Graham, D. A., et al. (2009). Nomograms for predicting annual resolution rate of primary vesicoureteral reflux: Results from 2,462 children. *Journal of Urology, 185*(4), 1535–1541.

Feldkamp, M. L., Botto, L. D., Amar, E., et al. (2011). Cloacal exstrophy: An epidemiological study from the International Clearinghouse for Birth Defects Surveillance and Research. *American Journal of Medical Genetics. Part C, Seminars in Medical Genetics, 157C*(4), 333–343.

Goldstein, S. L., Rosburg, N. M., Warady, B. A., et al. (2009). Pediatric end stage renal disease health-related quality of life differs by modality: A PedsQL ESRD analysis. *Pediatric Nephrology, 24*(8), 1553–1560.

Gray, M., & Moore, K. N. (2009). Atlas of genitourinary anatomy and physiology. In *Urologic disorders: Adult and pediatric care.* St. Louis, MO: Mosby/Elsevier.

Grinspon, R. P., & Rey, R. A. (2014). When hormone defects cannot explain it: Malformative disorders of sex development. *Birth Defects Research Part C: Embryo Today, 102*(4), 359–373.

Grisaru, S. (2014). Management of hemolytic-uremic syndrome in children. *International Journal of Nephrology and Renovascular Disease, 7*, 231–239.

Gupta, V., & Lee, M. (2012). Growth hormone in chronic renal disease. *Indian Journal of Endocrinology and Metabolism, 16*(2), 195–203.

Hoberman, A., Chesney, R. W., & RIVUR Trial Investigators. (2014). Antimicrobial prophylaxis for children with vesicoureteral reflux. *New England Journal of Medicine, 371*(11), 1072–1073.

Inouye, B. M., Tourchi, A., Di Carlo, H. N., et al. (2014). Modern management of the exstrophy-epispadias complex. *Surgery Research and Practice, 2014*, 58764.

Jayachandran, D., Bythell, M., Platt, M. W., et al. (2011). Register based study of bladder exstrophy-epispadias complex: Prevalence, associated anomalies, prenatal diagnosis and survival. *Journal of Urology, 186*(5), 2056–2060.

Jepson, R. G., Williams, G., & Craig, J. C. (2012). Cranberries for preventing urinary tract infections. *Cochrane Database of Systematic Reviews, 2012*(10), CD001321.

Khan, S. Z., Fahim, F., & Mansoor, K. (2012). Obstructive uropathy: Causes and outcome in pediatric patients. *Journal of Postgraduate Medical Institute, 26*(2), 176–182.

Kim, S., Webster, A. C., & Craig, J. C. (2013). Current trends in immunosuppression following organ transplantation in children. *Current Opinion in Organ Transplantation, 18*(5), 537–542.

Kinlaw, A. C., Jonsson Funk, M., Steiner, M. J., et al. (2016). Trends in pharmacotherapy for bladder dysfunction among children in the United States, 2000 to 2013. *Clinical Pediatrics (Philadelphia).* [Epub ahead of print.]

Kolon, T. F., Herndon, C. D., Baker, L. A., et al. (2014). Evaluation and treatment of cryptorchidism: AUA guideline. *Journal of Urology, 192*(2), 337–345.

Kozlowski, L. J. (2008). The acute pain service nurse practitioner: A case study in the postoperative care of the child with bladder exstrophy. *Journal of Pediatric Health Care, 22*(6), 351–359.

Lee, P. A., Houk, C. P., Ahmed, S. F., et al. (2006). Consensus statement on management of intersex disorders. International Consensus Conference on Intersex. *Pediatrics, 118*(2), e488–e500.

Lombel, R. M., Gipson, D. S., Hodson, E. M., et al. (2013). Treatment of steroid-sensitive nephrotic syndrome: New guidelines from KDIGO. *Pediatric Nephrology, 28*(3), 415–426.

Nast, C. C. (2012). Infection-related glomerulonephritis: Changing demographics and outcomes. *Advances in Chronic Kidney Disease, 19*(2), 68–75.

North American Pediatric Renal Trials and Collaborative Studies. (2010). *NAPRTCS 2010 annual transplant report.* Retrieved from https://web.emmes.com/study/ped/annlrept/2010_Report.pdf.

Prat, D., Natasha, A., Polak, A., et al. (2012). Surgical outcome of different types of primary hypospadias repair during three decades in a single center. *Urology, 79*(6), 1350–1353.

Rheault, M. N., Wei, C. C., Hains, D. S., et al. (2014). Increasing frequency of acute kidney injury amongst children hospitalized with nephrotic syndrome. *Pediatric Nephrology, 29*(1), 139–147.

Sarici, H., Telli, O., Ozgur, B. C., et al. (2016). Prevalence of nocturnal enuresis and its influence on quality of life in school-aged children. *Journal of Pediatric Urology, 12*(3), 159.e1–159.e6.

Shaikh, N., Craig, J. C., Rovers, M. M., et al. (2014). Identification of children and adolescents at risk for renal scarring after a first urinary tract infection: A meta-analysis with individual patient data. *JAMA Pediatrics, 168*(10), 893–900.

Shaikh, N., Morone, N. E., Bost, J. E., et al. (2008). Prevalence of urinary tract infection in childhood: A meta-analysis. *Pediatric Infectious Disease Journal, 27*(4), 302–308.

Sharma, A., Ramanathan, R., Posner, M., et al. (2013). Pediatric kidney transplantation: A review. *Transplant Research and Risk Management, 5*, 21–31.

Sijstermans, K., Hack, W. W., Meijer, R. W., et al. (2008). The frequency of undescended testis from birth to adulthood: A review. *International Journal of Andrology, 31*(1), 1–11.

Suominen, J. S., Santtila, P., & Taskinen, S. (2015). Sexual function in patients operated for bladder exstrophy and epispadias. *Journal of Urology, 194*(1), 195–199.

Susantitaphong, P., Cruz, D. N., Cerda, J., et al. (2013). World incidence of AKI: A meta-analysis. *Clinical Journal of the American Society of Nephrology, 8*(9), 1482–1493.

Thumfart, J., Pommer, W., Querfeld, U., et al. (2014). Intensified hemodialysis in adults, and in children and adolescents. *Deutsches Ärzteblatt International, 111*(14), 237–243.

Vasudeva, P., & Madersbacher, H. (2014). Factors implicated in pathogenesis of urinary tract infections in neurogenic bladders: Some revered, few forgotten, others ignored. *Neurourology and Urodynamics, 33*(1), 95–100.

Wesseling-Perry, K., & Salusky, I. B. (2013). Phosphate binders, vitamin D and calcimimetics in the management of chronic kidney disease-mineral bone disorders (CKD-MBD) in children. *Pediatric Nephrology, 28*(4), 617–625.

Wolfe-Christensen, C., Kovacevic, L. G., Mirkovic, J., et al. (2013). Lower health related quality of life and psychosocial difficulties in children with monosymptomatic nocturnal enuresis—Is snoring a marker of severity? *Journal of Urology, 190*(4 suppl), 1501–1504.

46

The Child With Cerebral Dysfunction

Cheryl C. Rodgers

ⓔ http://evolve.elsevier.com/Perry/maternal

CEREBRAL DYSFUNCTION

Most of the information about the status of the brain is obtained by indirect measurements. Some of these measurements are discussed elsewhere in relation to numerous aspects of child care (e.g., as part of assessments of health [Chapter 29], newborn status [Chapter 22], intellectual disability [Chapter 37], hypoxic injury [cerebral palsy, Chapter 49], and attainment of developmental milestones at each stage of development). Because increased intracranial pressure (ICP) and altered states of consciousness have such prominent places in neurologic dysfunction, they are described here, followed by techniques for neurologic assessment and diagnostic tests.

INCREASED INTRACRANIAL PRESSURE

The brain, tightly enclosed in the solid bony cranium, is well protected but highly vulnerable to pressure that may accumulate within the enclosure (Fig. 46.1). The total volume of the cranium—brain (80%), cerebrospinal fluid (CSF) (10%), and blood (10%)—must remain approximately the same at all times. A change in the proportional volume of one of these components (e.g., increase or decrease in intracranial blood) must be accompanied by a compensatory change in another. In this way, the volume and pressure normally remain constant. Examples of compensatory changes are reduction in blood volume, decrease in CSF production, increase in CSF absorption, or shrinkage of brain mass by displacement of intracellular and extracellular fluid.

Children with open fontanels compensate for increased volume by skull expansion and widened sutures. However, at any age the capacity for spatial compensation is limited. An increase in ICP may be caused by tumors or other space-occupying lesions, accumulation of fluid within the ventricular system, bleeding, or edema of cerebral tissues. When compensation is exhausted, any further increase in the volume of the cranium results in a rapid rise in ICP.

Early signs and symptoms of increased ICP are often subtle and assume many patterns (Box 46.1). As pressure increases, signs and symptoms become more pronounced, and the level of consciousness (LOC) deteriorates.

ALTERED STATES OF CONSCIOUSNESS

Consciousness implies awareness (i.e., the ability to respond to sensory stimuli and have subjective experiences). There are two components of consciousness: *alertness,* an arousal-waking state, including the ability to respond to stimuli; and *cognitive power,* including the ability to process stimuli and produce verbal and motor responses.

An altered state of consciousness usually refers to varying states of unconsciousness that may be momentary or extend for hours, for days, or indefinitely. *Unconsciousness* is depressed cerebral function (i.e., the inability to respond to sensory stimuli and have subjective experiences). *Coma* is defined as a state of unconsciousness from which the patient cannot be aroused even with powerful stimuli.

Levels of Consciousness

Assessment of LOC remains the earliest indicator of improvement or deterioration in neurologic status. LOC is determined by observations of the child's responses to the environment. When LOC is being assessed in young children, it is often useful to have a parent present to help elicit a desired response. An infant or child may not respond in an unfamiliar environment or to unfamiliar voices. Children older than 3 years of age should be able to give their name, although they may not be cognizant of place or time. Other diagnostic tests such as motor activity, reflexes, and vital signs vary more and do not necessarily directly parallel the depth of the comatose state. The most consistently used terms are described in Box 46.2.

Coma Assessment

Several scales have been devised in an attempt to standardize the description and interpretation of the degree of depressed consciousness. The most popular of these is the Glasgow Coma Scale (GCS), which consists of a three-part assessment: eye opening, verbal response, and motor response (Fig. 46.2). Numeric values of 1 to 5 are assigned to the levels of response in each category. The sum of these numeric values provides an objective measure of the patient's LOC. A person with an unaltered LOC would score the highest, 15; a score of 8 or below is generally accepted as a definition of coma; and the lowest score, 3, indicates deep coma. A decrease in the GCS score indicates a deterioration of the patient's condition. The pronouncement of brain death requires two conditions: (1) complete cessation of clinical evidence of brain function (as evidenced by lack of activity on flow study) and (2) irreversibility of the condition.

NEUROLOGIC EXAMINATION

GENERAL ASPECTS

Children younger than 2 years of age require special evaluation because they are unable to respond to directions designed to elicit specific neurologic responses. Early neurologic responses in infants are primarily reflexive; these responses are gradually replaced by meaningful movement in the characteristic cephalocaudal direction of development. This

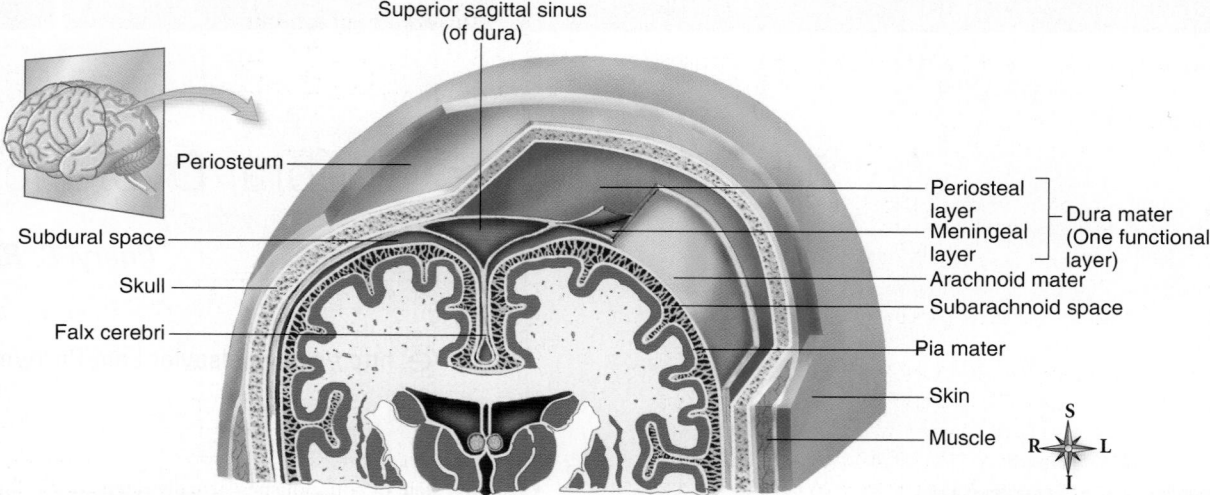

FIG 46.1 Coronal section of the top of the head showing meningeal layers. (From Patton, K.T., Thibodeau, G.A. [2016]. *Anatomy and physiology* [7th ed.]. St, Louis, MO: Elsevier.)

BOX 46.1 Clinical Manifestations of Increased Intracranial Pressure in Infants and Children

Infants
- Tense, bulging fontanel
- Separated cranial sutures
- Macewen (cracked-pot) sign
- Irritability and restlessness
- Drowsiness
- Increased sleeping
- High-pitched cry
- Increased frontooccipital circumference
- Distended scalp veins
- Poor feeding
- Crying when disturbed
- Setting-sun sign

Children
- Headache
- Nausea
- Forceful vomiting
- Diplopia, blurred vision

- Seizures
- Indifference, drowsiness
- Decline in school performance
- Diminished physical activity and motor performance
- Increased sleeping
- Inability to follow simple commands
- Lethargy

Late Signs in Infants and Children
- Bradycardia
- Decreased motor response to command
- Decreased sensory response to painful stimuli
- Alterations in pupil size and reactivity
- Extension or flexion posturing
- Cheyne-Stokes respirations
- Papilledema
- Decreased consciousness
- Coma

---

evidence of progressive maturation reflects more extensive myelinization and changes in neurochemical and electrophysiologic properties.

Most information about infants and small children is gained by observing their spontaneous and elicited reflex responses. As they develop increasingly complex motor skills and communicative skills, more sophisticated techniques are used to assess acquisition of developmental milestones. Delay or deviation from expected milestones helps identify high-risk children. Persistence or reappearance of reflexes that normally disappear indicates a pathologic condition. In evaluating an infant or young child, it is also important to obtain the pregnancy and delivery history to determine the possible impact of intrauterine environmental influences known to affect the orderly maturation of the central nervous system (CNS). These influences include maternal infections, chemicals, medications, illicit drug use, trauma, and metabolic insults.

General aspects of assessment that provide clues to the etiology of dysfunction include the following:

Family history: Sometimes offers clues regarding possible genetic disorders with neurologic manifestations.

Health history: May provide valuable clues regarding the cause of dysfunction. Information should include Apgar scores, age of developmental milestones, trauma or injuries, acute and chronic illnesses, encounters with animals or insects, and ingestion or inhalation of neurotoxic substances.

Physical examination of infants, including assessment of the following:
- Level of alertness
- Size and shape of the head, including presence of fontanels
- Sensory responses
- Motor function, including posture, tone, and muscle strength
- Motility, including symmetry of movements and involuntary movements
- Respirations, including signs of prolonged apnea, ataxic breathing, paradoxical chest movement, or hyperventilation

BOX 46.2 Levels of Consciousness

Full consciousness: Awake and alert, orientated to time, place, and person; behavior appropriate for age

Confusion: Impaired decision making

Disorientation: Confusion regarding time, place; decreased level of consciousness (LOC)

Lethargy: Limited spontaneous movement, sluggish speech, drowsy

Obtundation: Arousable with stimulation

Stupor: Remaining in a deep sleep, responsive only to vigorous and repeated stimulation

Coma: No motor or verbal response or extension posturing to noxious (painful) stimuli

Persistent vegetative state: Permanently lost function of the cerebral cortex; eyes follow objects only by reflex or when attracted to the direction of loud sounds; all four limbs are spastic but can withdraw from painful stimuli; hands show reflexive grasping and groping; the face can grimace, some food may be swallowed, and the child may groan or cry but utter no words.

- Dysmorphic facial features
- Behavioral cues, including consolability and habituation
- Primitive and deep tendon reflexes
- Cranial nerves

NEUROLOGIC EXAMINATION

The purpose of the neurologic examination is to establish an accurate, objective baseline of neurologic information. It is essential that the neurologic examination be documented in a descriptive and detailed fashion. This allows for a comparison of the findings so the observer can detect subtle changes in the neurologic status that might not otherwise be evident. Descriptions of behaviors should be simple, objective, and easily interpreted, for example: "Drowsy but awake and conversationally oriented to person, place, and time"; "Arousable only with vigorous physical stimuli. Pressure to nail base of right hand results in upper-extremity flexion/lower-extremity extension."

Vital Signs

Pulse, respiration, and blood pressure provide information regarding the adequacy of circulation and the possible underlying cause of altered consciousness. Autonomic activity is most intensively disturbed in cases of deep coma or brainstem lesions.

Body temperature is often elevated, and sometimes the elevation may be extreme. High temperature is most frequently a sign of an acute infectious process or heat stroke but may also be caused by ingestion of some drugs (especially salicylates, alcohol, and barbiturates) or intracranial bleeding, especially subarachnoid hemorrhage. Hypothalamic involvement may cause elevated or decreased temperature. Some infection may produce hypothermia.

The pulse varies and may be rapid, slow and bounding, or feeble. Blood pressure may be normal, elevated, or very low. The Cushing reflex, or pressor response, causes a slowing of the pulse and an increase in blood pressure and is uncommon in children; when it occurs it is a very late sign of ICP. Medications may affect the vital signs. For assessment purposes, actual changes in pulse and blood pressure are more important than the direction of the change.

Respirations are often slow, deep, and irregular. Slow, deep breathing is often seen in heavy sleep caused by sedatives, after seizures, or in cerebral infections. Slow, shallow breathing may result from sedatives or opioids. Hyperventilation (deep and rapid respirations) is usually a result of metabolic acidosis or abnormal stimulation of the respiratory

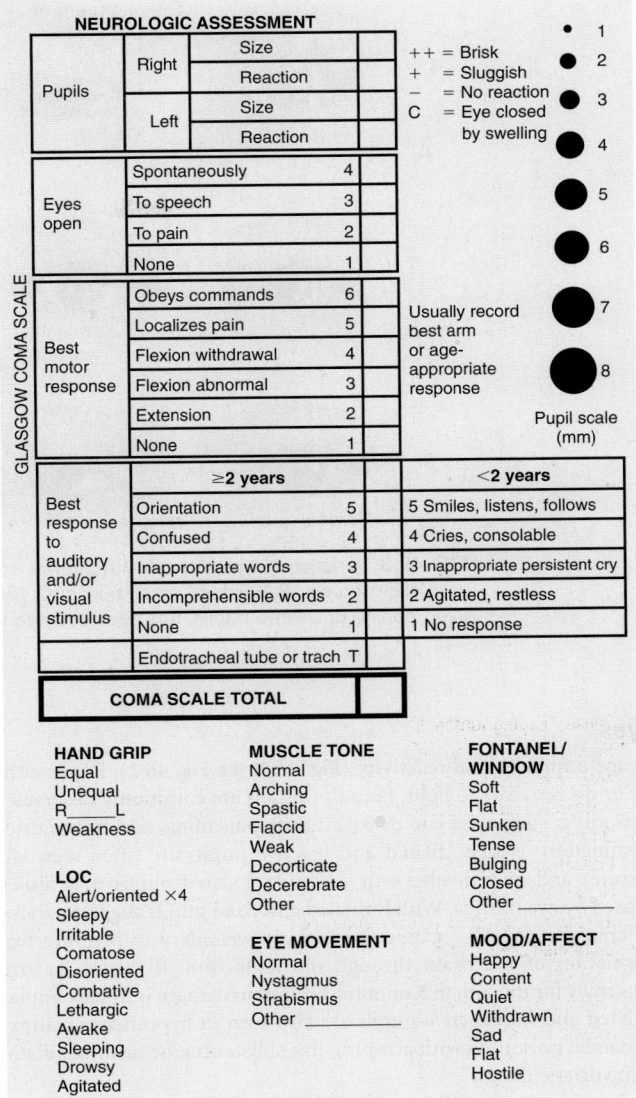

FIG 46.2 Pediatric coma scale.

center in the medulla caused by salicylate poisoning, hepatic coma, or Reye's syndrome (RS).

Breathing patterns have been described with a number of terms (e.g., *apneustic, cluster, ataxic, Cheyne-Stokes*). However, it is better to describe what is being observed rather than placing a label on it because the traditional terms are often used and interpreted incorrectly. Periodic or irregular breathing is an ominous sign of brainstem (especially medullary) dysfunction that often precedes complete apnea. The odor of the breath may provide additional clues (e.g., the fruity, acetone odor of ketosis; the foul odor of uremia; the fetid odor of hepatic failure; or the odor of alcohol).

Skin

The skin should be evaluated for color (such as pallor, cyanosis, erythema, or jaundice), temperature, and turgor. In addition, the skin may offer clues to the cause of unconsciousness. The body surface should be examined for signs of injury, needle marks, petechiae, bites, and ticks. Evidence of toxic substances may be found on the hands, face, mouth, and clothing, especially in small children.

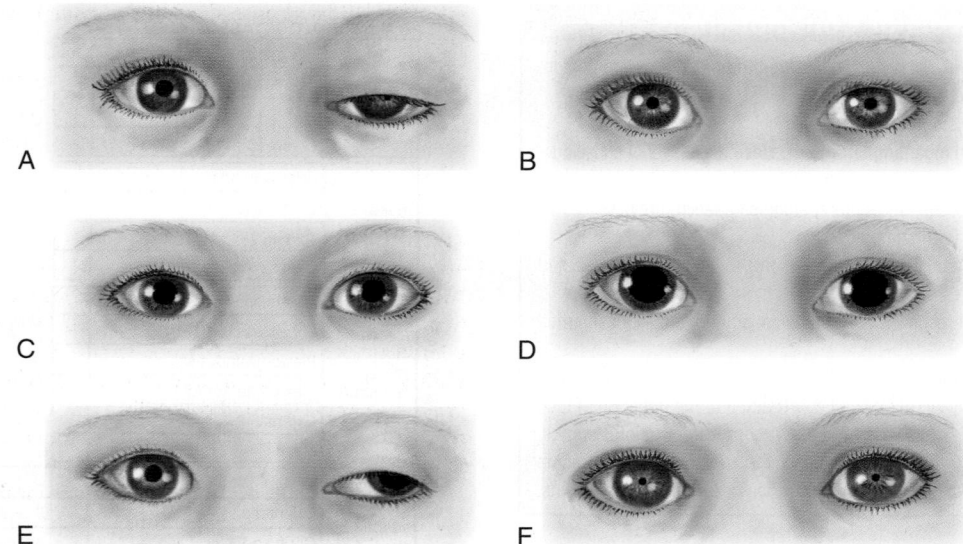

FIG 46.3 Variations in pupil size with altered states of consciousness. **A,** Ipsilateral pupillary constriction with slight ptosis. **B,** Bilateral small pupils. **C,** Midposition, light fixed to all stimuli. **D,** Bilateral dilated and fixed pupils. **E,** Dilated pupils, left eye abducted with ptosis. **F,** Pinpoint pupils.

Eyes

Assess pupil size and reactivity (Fig. 46.3; see Fig. 46.2). Pupils either do or do not react to light. Pinpoint pupils are commonly observed in poisoning, such as opiate or barbiturate poisoning, and in brainstem dysfunction. Widely dilated and reactive pupils are often seen after seizures and may involve only one side. Dilated pupils may also be caused by eye trauma. Widely dilated and fixed pupils suggest paralysis of cranial nerve III (oculomotor nerve) secondary to pressure from herniation of the brain through the tentorium. If pupils are fixed bilaterally for more than 5 minutes, brainstem damage is usually implied. Dilated and nonreactive pupils are also seen in hypothermia, anoxia, ischemia, poisoning with atropine-like substances, or prior instillation of mydriatic drugs.

Special tests, usually performed by qualified persons, include the following:

- Doll's head maneuver: Elicited by rotating the child's head quickly to one side and then to the other. Conjugate (paired or working together) movement of the eyes in the direction opposite to the head rotation is normal. Absence of this response suggests dysfunction of the brainstem or oculomotor nerve (cranial nerve III).
- Caloric test, or oculovestibular response (RS): Elicited with the child's head up (head of bed is elevated 30 degrees) by irrigating the external auditory canal with 10 mL of ice water for 20 seconds, which normally causes conjugate movement of the eyes toward the side of stimulation. This response is lost when the pontine centers are impaired, thus providing important information in assessment of the comatose patient.
- Funduscopic examination: Reveals additional clues. *Papilledema* is not evident early in the course of unconsciousness because if it develops, it takes 24 to 48 hours. Papilledema is characterized by optic disc swelling, indistinct optic disc margins, hemorrhage, tortuosity of vessels, and absence of venous pulsations. The presence of preretinal (subhyaloid) hemorrhages in children is almost invariably a result of acute trauma with intracranial bleeding, usually subarachnoid or subdural hemorrhage.

> ⚠ **NURSING ALERT**
>
> Any tests that require head movement are not attempted until after cervical spine injury has been ruled out.

> ⚠ **NURSING ALERT**
>
> The caloric test is painful and is never performed on a child who is awake or an individual with a ruptured tympanic membrane.

> ⚠ **NURSING ALERT**
>
> The sudden appearance of a fixed and dilated pupil(s) is a neurologic emergency.

Motor Function

Observation of spontaneous activity, gait, and response to painful stimuli provides clues to the location and extent of cerebral dysfunction. Asymmetric movements of the limbs or absence of movement suggests paralysis. In hemiplegia, the affected limb lies in external rotation and falls uncontrollably when lifted and allowed to drop. All motor functions should be described rather than labeled.

In the deeper comatose states, there is little or no spontaneous movement, and the musculature tends to be flaccid. There is considerable variability in the motor behavior in lesser degrees of coma. For example, the child may be relatively immobile or restless and hyperkinetic; muscle tone may be increased or decreased. Tremors, twitching, and spasms of muscles are common observations. The patient may display purposeless movements. Combative or negativistic behavior is common. Hyperactivity is more common in acute febrile and toxic states than in cases of increased ICP. Seizures are common in children and may be

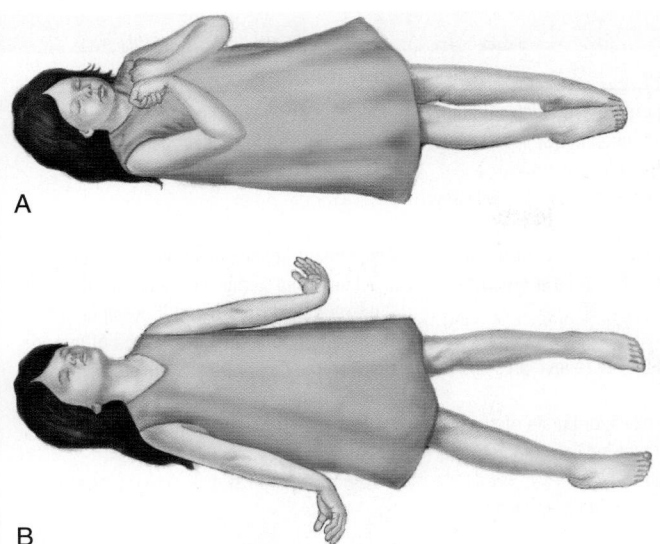

FIG 46.4 A, Flexion posturing. **B,** Extension posturing.

present from any cause. Any repetitive or seizure movements should be described precisely.

Posturing

Primitive postural reflexes emerge as cortical control over motor function is lost in brain dysfunction. These reflexes are evident in posturing and motor movements directly related to the area of the brain involved. Posturing reflects a balance between the lower exciting and the higher inhibiting influences and strong muscles overcoming weaker ones. *Decorticate* or *flexion posturing* (Fig. 46.4, *A*) is seen with severe dysfunction of the cerebral cortex or lesions to corticospinal tracts above the brainstem. Typical posturing includes rigid flexion with the arms held tightly to the body; flexed elbows, wrists, and fingers; plantar flexed feet; legs extended and internally rotated; and possibly the presence of fine tremors or intense stiffness. *Decerebrate posture* or *extension posturing* (see Fig. 46.4, *B*) is a sign of dysfunction at the level of the midbrain or lesions to the brainstem. It is characterized by rigid extension and pronation of the arms and legs, flexed wrists and fingers, a clenched jaw, an extended neck, and possibly an arched back. Unilateral decerebrate posture is often caused by tentorial herniation.

Posturing may not be evident when the child is quiet but can usually be elicited by applying painful stimuli such as a blunt object pressed on the base of the nail. Nurses should avoid applying thumb pressure to the supraorbital region of the frontal bone (risk for orbital damage). Noxious stimuli (e.g., suctioning) elicits a response, as may turning or touching. When the nurse is describing posturing, the stimulus needed to provoke the response is as important as the reaction.

Reflexes

Testing of some reflexes may be of limited value. In general the corneal, pupillary, muscle-stretch, superficial, and plantar reflexes tend to be absent in deep coma. The state of reflexes varies in lighter grades of unconsciousness and depends on the underlying pathologic process and the location of the lesion. Absence of corneal reflexes and presence of a tonic neck reflex are associated with severe brain damage. The Babinski reflex, in which the lateral portion of the foot is stroked, may be of value if it is found to be present consistently in children older than 1 year of age. A positive Babinski reflex is significant in assessment of pyramidal tract lesions when it is unilateral and associated with

other pyramidal signs. A fluctuating Babinski reflex is often observed with seizures.

> **❗ NURSING ALERT**
>
> Three key reflexes that demonstrate neurologic health in young infants are the Moro, tonic neck, and withdrawal reflexes.

SPECIAL DIAGNOSTIC PROCEDURES

Numerous diagnostic procedures are used for the assessment of cerebral function. Laboratory tests that may help delineate the cause of unconsciousness include blood glucose, urea nitrogen, and electrolyte (pH, sodium, potassium, chloride, calcium, and bicarbonate) tests; clotting studies; a complete blood count; liver function tests; blood cultures if there is fever; and toxicology screen and blood lead levels if clinically indicated.

An electroencephalogram (EEG) may provide important information. For example, generalized random, slow activity suggests suppressed cortical function, and localized slow activity suggests a space-occupying issue. A flat tracing is one of the criteria used as evidence of brain death. Examination of spinal fluid is performed when toxic encephalopathy or infection is suspected. Lumbar puncture ordinarily is delayed if intracranial hemorrhage is suspected and is contraindicated in the presence of ICP because of the potential for brainstem herniation.

Auditory and visual evoked potentials are sometimes used in neurologic evaluation of infants and young children. Brainstem auditory evoked potentials are useful for assessing brainstem function and are particularly useful for detecting demyelinating disease and neoplasms.

Highly sophisticated tests are carried out with specialized equipment. Two imaging techniques, computed tomography (CT) and magnetic resonance imaging (MRI), assist in diagnosis by scanning both soft tissues and solid matter. Most of these tests are outlined in Table 46.1. Because such tests can be threatening to children, the nurse needs to prepare patients for the tests and provide support and reassurance during the tests (see the "Preparation for Diagnostic and Therapeutic Procedures" section in Chapter 39). Children who are old enough to understand require careful explanation of the procedure, reason for the procedure, what they will experience, and how they can help. School-age children usually appreciate a more detailed description of why contrast material is injected.

The importance of lying still for tests needs to be stressed. Children unfamiliar with the machines can be shown a picture beforehand. Although radiographic examinations are not painful, the appearance of the machinery is often so frightening that the child protests because of anxiety. This is especially true of CT and MRI, both of which require that the child's head be placed within a special immobilizing device. Chin and cheek pads are sometimes used to prevent the slightest head movement, and straps are applied to the body to prevent a slight change in body position. The nurse can explain these events to a child by comparing them to an astronaut's preparation for a space flight. It is important to emphasize to the child that at no time is the procedure painful.

The nurse should not expect cooperation from a young child. Sedation may be required. If so, children should be helped through the preparation and administration and assured that someone will remain with them (if possible). Many different agents are currently used for sedation of children undergoing neurologic diagnostic procedures. Chloral hydrate or benzodiazepines have been used for decades as short-term sedative agents and remain safe methods of pediatric sedation (Arlachov & Ganatra, 2012). Other sedative agents have been used safely, alone and

TABLE 46.1	**Neurologic Diagnostic Procedures**		
Test	**Description**	**Purpose**	**Comments**
Lumbar puncture (LP)	Spinal needle is inserted between L3 and L4 or L4 and L5 vertebral spaces into subarachnoid space; CSF pressure is measured, and sample is collected for examination.	Diagnostic—Measures spinal fluid pressure, obtains CSF for laboratory analysis Therapeutic—Injection of medication	Contraindicated in patients with increased ICP or infected skin over puncture site.
Subdural tap	Needle is inserted into anterior fontanel or coronal suture (midline to pupil).	Helps rule out subdural effusions Removes CSF to relieve pressure	Place infant in semi-erect position after subdural tap to minimize leakage from site; prevent child from crying if possible. Check site frequently for evidence of leakage.
Ventricular puncture	Needle is inserted into lateral ventricle via coronal suture (midline to pupil).	Removes CSF to relieve pressure	Risk for intracerebral or ventricular hemorrhage.
Electroencephalography (EEG)	EEG records changes in electrical potential of brain. Electrodes are placed at various points to assess electrical function in a particular area. Impulses are recorded by electromagnetic pen or digitally.	Detects spikes, or bursts of electrical activity that indicate the potential for seizures Used to determine brain death	Patient should remain quiet during procedure; may require sedation. Minimize external stimuli during procedure.
Nuclear brain scan	Radioisotope is injected intravenously and then counted and recorded after fixed time intervals. Radioisotope accumulates in areas where blood-brain barrier is defective.	Identifies focal brain lesions (e.g., tumors, abscesses) Positive uptake of material with encephalitis and subdural hematoma Visualizes CSF pathways	Requires IV access; patient may require sedation. In normal children or noncommunicating hydrocephalus, no retrograde filling of ventricles occurs. Areas of concentrated uptake of material are termed *hot spots*.
Encephalography	Pulses of ultrasonic waves are beamed through head; echoes from reflecting surfaces are recorded graphically.	Identifies shifts in midline structures from their normal positions as a result of intracranial lesions May show ventricular dilation	Simple, safe, rapid procedure.
Real-time ultrasonography (RTUS)	Similar to CT but uses ultrasound instead of ionizing radiation.	Allows high-resolution anatomic visualization in variety of imaging planes	Produces images similar to CT scan. Especially useful in neonatal CNS problems.
Radiography	Skull X-rays are taken from different views—lateral, posterolateral, axial (submentoventricular), half-axial.	Shows fractures, dislocations, spreading suture lines, craniosynostosis Shows degenerative changes, bone erosion, calcifications	Simple, noninvasive procedure.
Computed tomography (CT) scan	Pinpoint X-ray beam is directed on horizontal or vertical plane to provide series of images that are fed into computer and assembled in image displayed on video screen. CT uses ionizing radiation.	Visualizes horizontal and vertical cross-section of brain in three planes (axial, coronal, sagittal) Distinguishes density of various intracranial tissues and structures—congenital abnormalities, hemorrhage, tumors, demyelinating and inflammatory processes, calcification	Requires IV access if contrast agent is used. Patient may require sedation.
Magnetic resonance imaging (MRI)	MRI produces radiofrequency emissions from elements (e.g., hydrogen, phosphorus), which are converted to visual images by computer.	Permits visualization of morphologic feature of target structures Permits tissue discrimination unavailable with many techniques	MRI is noninvasive procedure except when IV contrast agent is used. No exposure to radiation occurs. Patient may require sedation. Parent or attendant can remain in room with child. MRI does not visualize bone detail or calcifications. No metal can be present in scanner.
Positron emission tomography (PET)	PET involves IV injection of positron-emitting radionucleotide; local concentrations are detected and transformed into visual display by computer.	Detects and measures blood volume and flow in brain, metabolic activity, and biochemical changes within tissue	Requires lengthy period of immobility. Minimum exposure to radiation occurs. Patient may require sedation.

TABLE 46.1   Neurologic Diagnostic Procedures—cont'd

Test	Description	Purpose	Comments
Digital subtraction angiography (DSA)	Contrast dye is injected intravenously; computer "subtracts" all tissues without contrast medium, leaving clear image of contrast medium in vessels studied.	Visualizes vasculature of target tissue Visualizes finite vascular abnormalities	Safe alternative to angiography. Patient must remain still during procedure; may require sedation.
Single-photon emission computed tomography (SPECT)	Involves IV injection of photon-emitting radionuclide; radionuclides are absorbed by healthy tissue at different rate than by diseased or necrotic tissue; data are transferred to computer that converts image to film.	Provides information regarding blood flow to tissues; analyzing blood flow to organ may help determine how well it is functioning	Requires lengthy period of immobility. Minimum exposure to radiation occurs. Patient may require sedation.

CNS, Central nervous system; *CSF*, cerebrospinal fluid; *ICP*, intracranial pressure; *IV*, intravenous.

in combination, for children and include intravenous (IV) sodium pentobarbital (Nembutal), IV fentanyl (Sublimaze), IV midazolam (Versed), and intranasal midazolam (Arlachov & Ganatra). Propofol is a good sedation agent for diagnostic procedures because of its short induction and recovery time, but this medication should be used with caution because it can cause respiratory depression and apnea with little warning (Arlachov & Ganatra) (see the "Pain Management" section in Chapter 30).

Children need continual support and reinforcement during procedures in which they remain conscious. Vital signs and physiologic responses to the procedure are monitored throughout. The nurse should review written instructions with parents if the child is discharged after a procedure. Children who have undergone a procedure with a general anesthetic require postanesthesia care, including positioning, to prevent aspiration of secretions and frequent assessment of the vital signs and LOC. In addition, other neurologic functions such as pupillary responses, motor strength, and movement are tested at regular intervals. Any surgical wound resulting from the test is checked for bleeding, CSF leakage, and other complications. Children who undergo repeated subdural taps should have their hematocrit monitored to detect excessive blood loss from the procedure.

NURSING CARE OF THE UNCONSCIOUS CHILD

The unconscious child requires nursing attention, with observation, recording, and evaluation of changes in objective signs. These observations provide valuable information regarding the patient's progress and often serve as a guide to diagnosis and treatment. Therefore careful and detailed observations are essential for the patient's welfare. In addition, vital functions must be maintained, and complications prevented through conscientious and meticulous nursing care. The outcome of unconsciousness is variable and ranges from early and complete recovery, to death within a few hours or days, or persistent and permanent unconsciousness, or recovery with varying degrees of residual mental or physical disability. The outcome and recovery of the unconscious child may depend on the level of nursing care and observational skills.

Direct emergency measures toward ensuring circulation, a patent airway, and breathing (CAB); stabilizing the spine when indicated; treating shock; and reducing ICP if present. Delayed treatment often leads to increased damage. As soon as emergency measures have been implemented, and in many cases concurrently, therapies for specific causes are begun. Because nursing care is closely related to medical management, both are considered here.

Continual observation of LOC, pupillary reaction, and vital signs is essential to manage CNS disorders. Regular assessment of neurologic status is an intergral part of nursing care of unconscious children. The assessment frequency depends on the cause of unconsciousness, the LOC, and the progression of cerebral involvement. Intervals between observations may be as short as every 15 minutes or as long as every 2 hours. Significant alterations must be reported immediately.

Vital signs provide important information about the status of the unconscious child. The temperature is taken every 2 to 4 hours. Fevers can indicate an infective process, heat stroke, or hypothalamic regulatory abnormalities (Sharma, Kochar, Sankhyan, et al., 2010). Tachycardia is common with fevers, hypovolemic shock, or heart failure, whereas increased ICP or myocardial injury can cause bradycardia (Sharma et al). Tachypnea is associated with lung pathology, but quiet tachypnea indicates acidosis that can be associated with diabetic ketoacidosis or some poisonings (Sharma et al). The LOC is assessed periodically and includes evaluating pupillary size, equality, and reaction to light. Signs of meningeal irritation such as nuchal rigidity are assessed. Assessment of LOC includes response to vocal commands, spontaneous behavior, resistance to care, and response to painful stimuli. Note any abnormal movement, changes in muscle tone or strength, and body position. Seizure activity is described according to the duration and body areas involved.

Pain management for the unconscious child requires astute nursing observation and management. Responses to pain include motor reactions such as increased agitation or posturing; and alterations in vital signs such as tachycardia, tachypnea, or hypertension. Because these findings may not be specific for pain, the nurse should observe for their appearance during times of induced or suspected pain and their disappearance after the inciting procedure or the administration of analgesia. A pain assessment record should be used to document indications of pain and the effectiveness of interventions (see the "Pain Assessment" section in Chapter 30).

The use of opioids such as morphine to relieve pain is controversial because they may mask signs of altered consciousness or depress respirations. However, unrelieved pain activates the stress response, which can elevate ICP. To block the stress response, some authorities advocate the use of analgesics, sedatives, and in some cases paralyzing agents via continuous IV infusion. A frequently used combination is fentanyl, midazolam, and vecuronium (Norcuron). If there are concerns about assessing the LOC or respiratory depression, naloxone (Narcan) can be used to reverse the opioid effects. Regardless of which drugs are used, adequate dosage and regular administration are essential to provide optimal pain relief (see the "Pain Management" section in Chapter 30).

Other measures to relieve discomfort include providing a quiet, dimly lit environment; limiting visitors; preventing any sudden, jarring movement such as banging into the bed; and preventing an increase in ICP. The last is most effectively achieved by proper positioning and prevention of straining such as during coughing, vomiting, suctioning, and defecating. Antiepileptic drugs may be ordered for control of seizure activity.

 MEDICATION ALERT

When opioids are used, bowel elimination must be monitored closely because of the potential constipating effect. Stool softeners should be given regularly with laxatives as needed to prevent constipation.

RESPIRATORY MANAGEMENT

Respiratory effectiveness is the primary concern in the care of the unconscious child, and establishing an adequate airway is *always* the first priority. Carbon dioxide has a potent vasodilating effect and increases cerebral blood flow (CBF) and ICP. Cerebral hypoxia at a normal body temperature that lasts longer than 4 minutes nearly always causes irreversible brain damage.

Children in lighter states of coma may be able to cough and swallow, but those in deeper states are unable to manage secretions, which tend to pool in the throat and pharynx. Dysfunction of CN IX and CN X places the child at risk for aspiration and cardiac arrest. Therefore, position the child with the head and body to the side to prevent aspiration of secretions, and empty the stomach to reduce the likelihood of vomiting. In infants, blockage of air passages from secretions can happen in seconds. In addition, upper airway obstruction from laryngospasm is a frequent complication in comatose children.

An oral airway can be used for children who have a temporary loss of consciousness, such as after a contusion, seizure, or anesthesia. For children who remain unconscious for a longer time, a nasotracheal or orotracheal tube is inserted to maintain the open airway and facilitate removal of secretions. A tracheostomy is performed in cases in which laryngoscopy for introduction of an endotracheal tube would be difficult or dangerous or for a child who needs long-term ventilatory support. Suctioning is used only as needed to clear the airway, exerting care to prevent increasing ICP. Respiratory status is observed and evaluated regularly. Signs of respiratory distress may be an indication for ventilatory assistance.

When the respiratory center is involved, mechanical ventilation is usually indicated (see Chapter 39). Blood gas analysis is performed regularly, and oxygen is administered as indicated. Moderately severe hypoxia and respiratory acidosis are often present but not always evident from clinical manifestations. Hyperventilation frequently accompanies unconsciousness and may lead to respiratory alkalosis, or it may represent the attempt by the body to compensate for metabolic acidosis. Therefore, blood gas and pH determinations are essential guides for therapy. Chest physiotherapy is carried out on a regular basis, and the child's position is changed at least every 2 hours to prevent pulmonary complications.

INTRACRANIAL PRESSURE MONITORING

Management of the child with increased ICP is a complex and important task. ICP monitoring is used to guide therapy to reduce ICP and provides information on intracranial compliance, cerebrovascular status, and cerebral perfusion (Sankhyan, Raju, Sharma, et al., 2010). Indications for inserting an ICP monitor are as follows (Singhi & Tiwari, 2009):
- GCS evaluation of less than or equal to 8
- GCS evaluation greater than 8 with respiratory assistance
- Deterioration of condition
- Subjective judgment regarding clinical appearance and response
  Four major types of ICP monitors are as follows:

1. Intraventricular catheter with fibroscopic sensors attached to a monitoring system
2. Subarachnoid bolt (Richmond screw)
3. Epidural sensor
4. Anterior fontanel pressure monitor

Direct ventricular pressure measurement remains the gold standard of ICP monitoring (Walker, Stone, Jacobson, et al., 2012). The catheter method involves introduction of a catheter into the lateral ventricle on the nondominant side, if known, or placement in the subdural space. The catheter has the advantage of providing a means of extraventricular (or continuous) drainage of CSF to reduce pressure. A drainage bag attached to the system is kept at the level of the ventricles and can be lowered to decrease ICP (see Clinical Reasoning Case Study box: Hydrocephalus). This device requires full penetration of the brain, requires skill and experience with placement, and carries the risk for infection. An epidural sensor can be placed between the dura and the skull through a burr hole and connected to a stopcock assembly and transducer, which provides a readout of the pressure. Although less invasive, ICP measurements may be inconsistent. In infants, a fontanel transducer can be used to detect impulses from a pressure sensor and convert them to electrical energy. The electrical energy is then converted to visible waves or numeric readings on an oscilloscope. ICP measurement from the anterior fontanel is noninvasive but may prove to be inaccurate if the equipment is poorly placed or inconsistently recalibrated.

⚠ NURSING ALERT

If the external ventricular drain is unclamped for CSF drainage, carefully monitor the level of the collection container. If the container is too low, improper CSF decompression could lower ICP too rapidly, causing bleeding and pain.

⚠ NURSING ALERT

The bolt is stabilized with dressings, and these are not changed or disturbed, even to check the site.

Placement of the subarachnoid bolt is not adjusted by anyone except the neurosurgeon who placed the device. The neurosurgeon is notified if a satisfactory waveform on the ICP monitoring is not observed.

An epidural sensor provides a readout of the ICP with a stopcock assembly and transducer. Although less invasive, ICP measurements may be inconsistent. In infants, a fontanel transducer can be used to detect impulses from a pressure sensor and convert them to electrical energy. The electrical energy is then converted to visible waves or numeric readings on an oscilloscope. ICP measurement from the anterior fontanel is noninvasive but may prove to be inaccurate if the equipment is poorly placed or recalibrated inconsistently.

ICP can be increased by instilling solutions; therefore antibiotics are administered systemically if a positive CSF culture is obtained. CSF is a body fluid; therefore standard precautions are implemented according to institutional policy (see Chapter 39).

Nurses caring for patients with intracranial monitoring devices must be acquainted with the system, assist with insertion, interpret the monitor readings, and be able to distinguish between danger signals and mechanical dysfunction. Because systematic blood pressure, ICP, and therefore cerebral perfusion pressure (CPP) are normally lower in children, the child's age must be taken into account when deciding what constitutes abnormally high ICP or abnormally low CPP.

Several medical measures are available to treat increased ICP resulting from cerebral edema. Osmotic diuretics may provide rapid relief of increased ICP in emergency situations. Although their effect is transient, lasting only about 6 hours, they can be lifesaving in emergencies. These substances are rapidly excreted by the kidneys and carry with them large quantities of sodium and water. Mannitol (or sometimes urea) administered intravenously is the drug most frequently used for rapid reduction. The infusion is generally given slowly but may be pushed rapidly in cases of herniation or impending herniation. Adrenocorticosteroids are not recommended for cerebral edema secondary to head trauma. Arterial carbon dioxide ($Paco_2$) should be maintained at approximately 30 mm Hg to produce vasoconstriction, which reduces CBF, thereby decreasing ICP.

Activities

In cases of high levels of increased ICP, procedures tend to trigger reactive pressure waves in many patients. For example, increased intrathoracic or abdominal pressure is transmitted to the cranium. Particular care is taken in positioning these patients to avoid neck vein compression, which may further increase ICP by interfering with venous return.

> **! NURSING ALERT**
>
> The head of the bed is elevated 15 to 30 degrees, and the child is positioned so the head is maintained in midline to facilitate venous drainage and avoid jugular compression. Turning side to side is contraindicated because of the risk for jugular compression.

It is important to avoid activities that may increase ICP by causing pain or emotional stress. Clustering nursing activities together and minimizing environmental stimuli by decreasing noxious procedures help to control ICP. Gentle range-of-motion exercises can be carried out but should not be performed vigorously. Nontherapeutic touch can cause an increase in ICP. Any disturbing procedures to be performed should be scheduled to take advantage of therapies such as osmotherapy and sedation that reduce ICP. Take efforts to minimize or eliminate environmental noise. Assessment and intervention to relieve pain are important nursing functions to decrease ICP.

Suctioning and percussion are poorly tolerated; therefore, these procedures are contraindicated unless concurrent respiratory problems exist. Hypoxia and the Valsalva maneuver associated with cough acutely elevate ICP. Vibration, which does not increase ICP, accomplishes excellent results and should be tried first if treatment is needed. If suctioning is necessary, it should be used judiciously and preceded by hyperventilation with 100% oxygen, which can be monitored during suctioning with a pulse oxygen sensor reading to determine oxygen saturation.

NUTRITION AND HYDRATION

In the unconscious child, fluids and calories are supplied initially by the IV route (see Chapter 39). An IV infusion is started early, and the type of fluid administered is determined by the patient's general condition. Fluid therapy requires careful monitoring and adjustment based on neurologic signs and electrolyte determinations. The goal of fluid therapy is euvolemia. Often unconscious children cannot tolerate the same amounts of fluid as when they are healthy. Overhydration must be avoided to prevent fatal cerebral edema. When cerebral edema is a threat, fluids may be restricted to reduce the chance of fluid overload. Examine skin and mucous membranes for signs of dehydration. Adjustments to fluid administration are based on urinary output, serum electrolytes and osmolarity, blood pressure, and arterial filling pressure. Observation for signs of altered fluid balance related to abnormal pituitary secretions is a part of nursing care.

Provide long-term nutrition with a balanced formula via a nasogastric or gastrostomy tube. Most children have continuous feedings, but if bolus feedings are used, the tube is rinsed with water after each feeding. Avoid overfeeding to prevent vomiting and the risk for aspiration.

Altered Pituitary Secretion

An altered ability to handle fluid loads is attributed in part to the syndrome of inappropriate antidiuretic hormone secretion (SIADH) and diabetes insipidus (DI) resulting from hypothalamic dysfunction (see Chapter 47). SIADH frequently accompanies CNS diseases such as head injury, meningitis, encephalitis, brain abscess, brain tumor, and subarachnoid hemorrhage. In patients with SIADH, scant quantities of urine are excreted, electrolyte analysis reveals hyponatremia and hyposmolality, and manifestations of overhydration are evident. It is important to evaluate all parameters because the reduced urinary output might be erroneously interpreted as a sign of dehydration. The treatment of SIADH consists of fluid restriction until serum electrolytes and osmolality return to normal levels.

DI may occur after intracranial trauma. In DI, there is increased urinary volume and the accompanying danger of dehydration. Adequate replacement of fluids is essential, and observation of electrolyte balance is necessary to detect signs of hypernatremia and hyperosmolality. Exogenous vasopressin may be administered.

MEDICATIONS

The cause of unconsciousness determines specific drug therapies. Children with infectious processes are given antibiotics appropriate to the disease and the infecting organism. Corticosteroids are prescribed for inflammatory conditions and edema. Cerebral edema is an indication for osmotic diuretics. Sedatives or antiepileptics are prescribed for seizure activity. Sedation in the combative child provides amnesic and anxiolytic properties in conjunction with a paralytic agent. The combination decreases ICP and allows treatment of cerebral edema. Usual drugs include morphine and midazolam. Midazolam is attractive because of its short half-life.

Deep coma induced by administration of barbiturates is controversial in the management of ICP. Barbiturates are currently reserved for the reduction of increased ICP when all else has failed. Barbiturates decrease the cerebral metabolic rate for oxygen and protect the brain during times of reduced CPP. Barbiturate coma requires extensive monitoring, cardiovascular and respiratory support, and ICP monitoring to assess response to therapy. Paralyzing agents such as vecuronium may be needed to aid in performing diagnostic tests, improving effectiveness of therapy, and reducing the risk for secondary complications. Elevation of ICP or heart rate of patients who are being given paralyzing agents or are under sedation may indicate the need for another dose of either or both medications.

THERMOREGULATION

Hyperthermia often accompanies cerebral dysfunction; if it is present, measures are implemented to reduce the temperature to prevent brain damage and reduce metabolic demands generated by the increased body temperature. Antipyretic agents are the method of choice for fever reduction; cooling devices should be used for hyperthermia. Laboratory tests and other methods are used in an attempt to determine the cause of the hyperthermia.

ELIMINATION

A urinary catheter is usually inserted in the acute phase, although diapers may be used and weighed to record urinary output. The child who formerly had bowel and bladder control is generally incontinent. If the child remains unconscious for a long period, the indwelling catheter may be removed, and periodic bladder emptying can be accomplished by intermittent catheterization. Stool softeners are usually sufficient to maintain bowel function, but suppositories or enemas may be needed occasionally for adequate elimination and to prevent fecal impaction. The passage of liquid stool after a period of no bowel activity is usually a sign of an impaction. To avoid this preventable problem, daily recording of bowel activity is essential.

HYGIENIC CARE

Routine measures for cleansing and maintaining skin integrity are an integral part of nursing care of the unconscious child. Unconscious children undergo numerous invasive procedures, and the skin sites used for these procedures require special assessment and intervention to promote healing and prevent infection. Skinfolds also require special attention to prevent excoriation.

Mouth care is performed at least twice daily because the mouth tends to become dry or coated with mucus. The teeth are brushed carefully with a soft toothbrush or cleaned with gauze saturated with saline. Commercially prepared cleansing devices such as Toothettes are convenient for cleansing the mouth and teeth. Lips are coated with ointment or other preparations to protect them from drying, cracking, or blistering.

Unconscious children are susceptible to eye irritation. The corneal reflexes are absent; therefore the eyes are easily irritated or damaged by linen, dust, or other substances that may come in contact with them. Excessive dryness results from incomplete closure of the eyelids, especially if the child is undergoing osmotherapy to reduce or prevent cerebral edema.

> **! NURSING ALERT**
>
> The eyes should be examined regularly and carefully for early signs of irritation or inflammation. Artificial tears are placed in the eyes every 1 to 2 hours. Eye patches may be necessary to protect the eyes from possible damage.

POSITIONING AND EXERCISE

The unconscious child is positioned to minimize ICP and prevent aspiration of saliva, nasogastric secretions, and vomitus. The head of the bed is elevated, and the child is placed in a side-lying or semi-prone position. A small, firm pillow is placed under the head, and the uppermost limbs are flexed and supported with pillows. The weight of the body should not rest on the dependent arm. In the semi-prone position, the child lies with the dependent arm at the side behind the body, the opposite side supported on pillows, and the uppermost arm and leg flexed and resting on the pillows. This position prevents undue pressure on the dependent extremities. The dependent position of the face encourages drainage of secretions and prevents the flaccid tongue from obstructing the airway.

Normal range-of-motion exercises help maintain function and minimize contractures of joints and prevent skin breakdown. Perform exercises gently to minimize increasing ICP. Place a small rolled pad in the palms to help maintain proper position of fingers. Footboards or high-top shoes can help prevent footdrop; and in some cases, splinting is needed to prevent severe contractures of the wrist, knee, or ankle in children.

STIMULATION

Sensory stimulation is important in the care of the unconscious child. It helps arouse a temporarily unconscious or semiconscious child to the conscious state and orient the child to time and place. Auditory and tactile stimulation are especially valuable. Tactile stimulation is not appropriate for children in whom it may elicit an undesirable response. However, for other children, tactile contact often has a relaxing and calming effect. When the child's condition permits, holding or rocking has a soothing effect and provides the body contact needed by young children.

The auditory sense is often intact in a state of coma. Hearing is the last sense to be lost and the first one to be regained; therefore, speak to the child as any other child. Conversation around the child should not include thoughtless or derogatory remarks. Soft music is used frequently to provide auditory stimulation. Singing the child's favorite songs or reading a favorite story is a tactic used to maintain the child's contact with a familiar world. Playing songs or favorite stories recorded in the parents' voices can provide a continuous source of familiar stimulation.

REGAINING CONSCIOUSNESS

Awakening from a coma is a gradual process; however, sometimes children regain consciousness within a short time. Regaining orientation involves knowing person, place, and time in that order.

Certain behaviors have been observed when children awaken from the unconscious state. The stress and anxiety they appear to feel in a strange and unfamiliar environment can be expressed in silent, withdrawn behavior. Children respond to basic questioning but usually do not display their prehospitalization personality and social behavior until they are transferred from the critical care area.

FAMILY SUPPORT

Helping the parents of an unconscious child cope with the situation is especially difficult. They may demonstrate all of the guilt, fear, hostility, and anxiety of any parent of a seriously ill child (see Chapter 38). In addition, these parents face the uncertain outcome of the cerebral dysfunction. The fear of death, cognitive impairment, or other permanent disability is present. Nursing intervention with parents depends on the nature of the pathologic condition, the parents' personality, and the parent-child relationship before the injury or illness.

Probably the most difficult situations involve children who never regain consciousness. Unlike losing a child through death, these situations lack finality, which often leaves the parents in a state of suspended grief. An awareness of these behaviors and coping mechanisms provides nurses with the understanding that helps them support the parents in their grief process.

Superimposed on the process of grieving for the "lost" child, parents may be faced with difficult decisions. When the child's brain is so severely damaged that vital functions must be maintained by artificial means, the parents must make the final decision of whether to remove life-support systems. Nurses continue to provide specialty care during this time that maintains the patient's physiologic status while addressing the informational and psychologic needs of the family. This decision is difficult for parents, but having an open and honest dialog about the child's medical condition and prognosis can help make patient-centered conclusions (de Vos, Bos, Plötz, et al., 2015). Parents' cultural, religious, and language needs along with their intellectual level, decision-making preferences, and emotional state are considered during the discussions (Allen, 2014). Sometimes parents may choose to refuse or not initiate treatment if they believe it to be best for the child and the family (informed dissent). At other times they request that "everything possible" be done for the child.

When the child has survived the cerebral insult but physical or mental capacity is limited either minimally or severely, families must cope with the long and tedious rehabilitation process and the uncertain outcome. The drain on financial, emotional, and social resources can be enormous. For parents who choose to care for their child at home, planning begins early in the recovery process. The family should become involved with the child's care as soon as they indicate an interest and ability to do so. They need education and support in learning to care for the child, regular follow-up observation and assessment of the home management, and planning for respite care. Parents need to understand that it is important to plan for periodic relief from the continual care of the child (see the "Preparing for Discharge and Home Care" section in Chapter 38).

CEREBRAL TRAUMA

HEAD INJURY

Head injury is a pathologic process involving the scalp, skull, meninges, or brain as a result of trauma. According to the Centers for Disease Control and Prevention (2012) and Safe Kids Worldwide,[*] unintentional injuries are the number-one health risk for children and the leading cause of death in children 1 to 19 years of age. Tragically, 12,175 children 0 to 19 years of age are killed every year by unintentional injuries (Centers for Disease Control and Prevention, 2012). It has been estimated that each year approximately 511,000 children 0 to 14 years of age sustain a traumatic brain injury and that 2174 children die as a result of the brain injury (Faul, Xu, Wald, et al., 2010).

Etiology

The three major causes of brain damage in childhood, in order of importance, are falls, motor vehicle injuries, and bicycle or sports-related injuries. Neurologic injury accounts for the highest mortality rate, with

---

[*]1301 Pennsylvania Avenue NW, Suite 1000, Washington, DC 20004-1707, 202-662-0600, www.safekids.org.

boys affected twice as often as girls. Falls are the major source of all head injuries in children between 0 and 14 years of age (Faul et al., 2010). In motor vehicle accidents, children younger than 2 years of age are almost exclusively injured as passengers, but older children may also be injured as pedestrians or cyclists. The majority of deaths from brain trauma caused by bicycle injuries occur between 5 and 19 years of age. Bicycle helmet laws have been effective in reducing the risk for head injury by 85% and brain injury by 88% (Rivara & Grossman, 2016).

Many of the physical characteristics of children predispose them to craniocerebral trauma. For example, infants can be left unattended on beds, in high chairs, and in other places from which they can fall. Because the head of an infant or toddler is proportionately larger and heavier in relation to other body parts, it is the most likely to be injured. Incomplete motor development contributes to falls at young ages, and the natural curiosity and exuberance of children also increase their risk for injury.

Pathophysiology

The pathology of brain injury is directly related to the force of impact. Intracranial contents (brain, blood, CSF) are damaged because the force is too great to be absorbed by the skull and musculoligamentous support of the head. Although nervous tissue is delicate, it usually requires a severe blow to cause significant damage.

Primary head injuries are those that occur at the time of trauma and include skull fracture, contusions, intracranial hematoma, and diffuse injury. Subsequent complications include hypoxic brain damage, increased ICP, infection, and cerebral edema. The predominant feature of a child's brain injury is the amount of diffuse swelling that occurs. Hypoxia and hypercapnia threaten the energy requirements of the brain and increase CBF. The added volume across the blood-brain barrier, along with the loss of autoregulation, exacerbates cerebral edema. Pressure inside the skull that is greater than arterial pressure results in inadequate perfusion.

A child's response to head injury is different from that of an adult. The larger head size and insufficient musculoskeletal support render the very young child particularly vulnerable to head injuries. Physical forces act on the head through acceleration, deceleration, or deformation. Acceleration or deceleration is responsible for most head injuries. When the stationary head receives a blow, the sudden acceleration causes deformation of the skull and mass movement of the brain. Continued movement of the intracranial contents allows the brain to strike parts of the skull (e.g., the sharp edges of the sphenoid or the irregular surface of the anterior fossa) or the edges of the tentorium. Sudden deceleration such as takes place during a fall causes the greatest cerebral injury at the point of impact.

Although the brain volume remains unchanged, significant distortion takes place as the brain changes shape in response to the force of impact to the skull. This deformation can cause bruising at the point of impact (coup) or at a distance as the brain collides with the unyielding surfaces far removed from the point of impact (contrecoup) (Fig. 46.5). Thus, a blow to the occipital region can cause severe injury to the frontal and temporal areas of the brain. Children with an acceleration-deceleration injury demonstrate diffuse generalized cerebral swelling produced by increased blood volume or a redistribution of cerebral blood volume (cerebral hyperemia) rather than by increased water content (edema).

Another effect of brain movement is shearing stresses, which may tear small arteries and cause subdural hemorrhages. Although shearing forces are maximum at the cerebral surface and extend toward the center of rotation within the brain, the most serious effects are often in the area of the brainstem. Damage can also occur when severe compression of the skull causes the brain to be forced through the

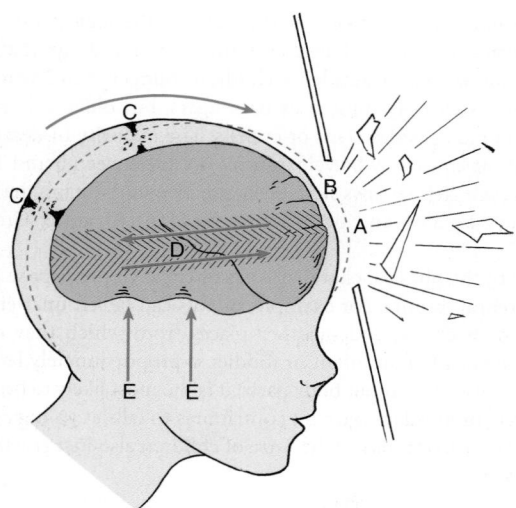

FIG 46.5 Mechanical distortion of the cranium during a closed head injury. **A,** Preinjury contour of the skull. **B,** Immediate postinjury contour of the skull. **C,** Torn subdural vessels. **D,** Shearing forces. **E,** Trauma from contact with the floor of the cranium. (Redrawn from Grubb, R.L., & Coxe, W.S. [1974]. Central nervous system trauma: cranial. In Eliasson, Presky, & Hardin Jr. *Neurological pathophysiology.* New York, NY: Oxford University Press.)

tentorial opening. This can produce irreparable damage to the brainstem (see Fig. 46.6).

Concussion

The most common head injury is *concussion,* a transient disturbance of brain function often traumatically induced that involves a complex pathophysiologic process (Liebig & Congeni, 2016). Confusion and amnesia after head injury are the hallmarks of concussion; however, loss of consciousness is not an accurate indicator for the presence of a concussion. Concussions usually resolve in 1 to 3 weeks without complications, but the child should rest until symptoms resolve, and then resume activities gradually (Liebig & Congeni).

The pathogenesis of concussion is still unclear but may be a result of shearing forces that cause stretching, compression, and tearing of nerve fibers, particularly in the area of the central brainstem, which is the seat of the reticular activating system. It has also been suggested that the anatomic alterations of nerve fibers cause the release of large quantities of acetylcholine into the CSF and a reduction in oxygen consumption with increased lactate production.

Contusion and Laceration

The terms *contusion* and *laceration* are used to describe visible bruising and tearing of cerebral tissue. Contusions represent petechial hemorrhages or localized bruising along the superficial aspects of the brain at the site of impact (coup injury) or a lesion remote from the site of direct trauma (contrecoup injury). In serious accidents, there may be multiple sites of injury.

The major areas of the brain susceptible to contusion or laceration are the occipital, frontal, and temporal lobes. In addition, the irregular surfaces of the anterior and middle fossae at the base of the skull are capable of producing bruises or lacerations on forceful impact. Contusions may cause focal disturbances in strength, sensation, or visual awareness. The degree of brain damage in the contused areas varies according to the extent of vascular injury. Signs vary from mild, transient weakness of a limb to prolonged unconsciousness and paralysis. However,

the signs and symptoms may be clinically indistinguishable from those of concussion.

Infants who are shaken roughly (referred to as *shaken baby syndrome* or *abusive head trauma*) can sustain profound neurologic impairment, seizures, retinal hemorrhages (usually bilateral), and intracranial subarachnoid or subdural hemorrhages (Sieswerda-Hoogendoorn, Boos, Spivack, et al., 2012).

Cerebral lacerations are generally associated with penetrating or depressed skull fractures. However, they may occur without fracture in small children. When brain tissue is actually torn, with bleeding into and around the tear, more severe and prolonged unconsciousness and paralysis occur, leaving permanent scarring and some degree of disability.

Fractures

Skull fractures result from a direct blow or injury to the skull and are often associated with intracranial injury. Falls are the most common cause of head injury. Many of the falls that resulted in a skull fracture in children younger than 2 years of age involved short distances less than 3 feet, such as falls from a caregiver's arms (Ibrahim, Wood, Margulies, et al., 2012).

The types of skull fractures that occur are *linear, depressed, comminuted, basilar, open,* and *growing.* As a rule, the faster the blow, the greater the likelihood of a depressed fracture; a low-velocity impact tends to produce a linear fracture.

Linear skull fractures are a single fracture line that starts at the point of maximum impact but does not cross suture lines. Linear fractures constitute the majority of childhood skull fractures. Most linear skull fractures are associated with an overlying scalp hematoma, particularly in infants younger than 1 year of age and in the parietal or temporal region (Erlichman, Blumfield, Rajpathak, et al., 2010).

Depressed fractures are those in which the bone is broken locally, usually into several irregular fragments that are pushed inward. Depressed skull fractures may be associated with direct underlying parenchymal damage and should be suspected when a child's head appears misshapen. Surgery may be needed to elevate the depressed bone fragment if there is an associated intracranial hematoma and if the depression is greater than 1 cm (0.4 inch).

Comminuted fractures consist of multiple associated linear fractures. They usually result from intense impact. These fractures often result from repeated blows against an object or ejection from a car at a high rate of speed. They may suggest child abuse.

Basilar fractures involve the bones at the base of the skull in either the posterior or anterior region. The bones involved are the ethmoid, sphenoid, temporal, or occipital bones and usually result in a dural tear. Because of the proximity of the fracture line to structures surrounding the brainstem, a basal skull fracture is a serious head injury. Approximately 80% of the cases may include clinical features such as subcutaneous bleeding over the mastoid process *(battle sign),* bleeding around the orbit (raccoon eyes), bleeding behind the tympanic membrane *(hemotympanum),* or CSF leakage from the nose or ear (Perheentupa, Kinnunen, Grénman, et al., 2010).

Open fractures cause communication between the skull and the scalp or the mucosa of the upper respiratory tract. Open fractures increase the risk for CNS infection when the fracture creates an opening in the paranasal sinuses or middle ear that causes CSF leakage. They may have a skin laceration overlying the bone fracture called a *compound fracture.* Antibiotics are recommended to prevent osteomyelitis.

Growing fractures are skull fractures associated with an underlying dura tear that fails to heal properly. The enlargement may be caused by a leptomeningeal cyst, dilated ventricles, or a herniated brain. The majority of growing skull fractures occur before 3 years of age (Liu,

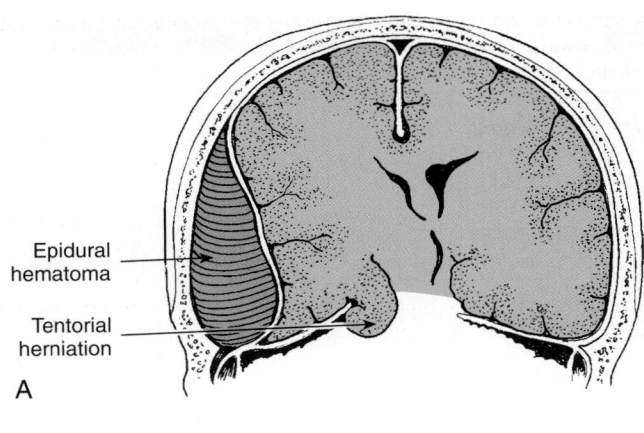

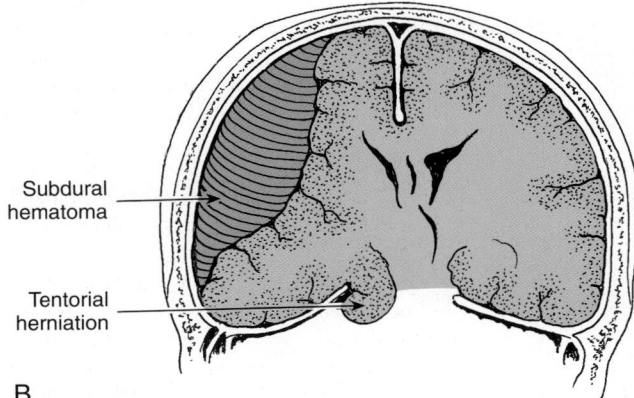

FIG 46.6 A, Epidural (extradural) hematoma and compression of temporal lobe through tentorial hiatus. **B,** Subdural hematoma.

You, & Lu, 2012). Physical examination reveals a pulsatile mass or enlarging and sunken skull defect.

Complications

The major complications of trauma to the head are hemorrhage, infection, edema, and herniation through the brainstem. Infection is always a hazard in open injuries, and edema is related to tissue trauma. Vascular rupture may occur even in minor head injuries, causing hemorrhage between the skull and cerebral surfaces. Compression of the underlying brain produces effects that can be rapidly fatal or insidiously progressive.

Epidural Hemorrhage

An epidural hemorrhage is bleeding into the space between the dura and the skull that forms a hematoma. As the hematoma enlarges, the dura is stripped from the skull, forcing the underlying brain contents downward and inward as the brain expands (Fig. 46.6, *A*). Because bleeding is generally arterial, brain compression occurs rapidly. Most often the expanding hematoma is located in the parietal and temporal regions (Teichert, Rosales, Lopes, et al., 2012). The lower incidence of epidural hematoma in childhood has been attributed to the fact that the middle meningeal artery is not embedded in the bone surface of the skull until approximately 2 years of age. Therefore a fracture of the temporal bone is less likely to lacerate the artery.

The classic clinical picture of epidural hemorrhage consists of momentary unconsciousness, followed by a normal period, and then followed with lethargy and coma due to blood accumulation in the epidural space and compression of the brain (see Box 46.3 for clinical manifestations). The period of impaired consciousness is lacking, and

common symptoms are irritability, pallor with anemia, and cephalhematoma. Infants may have hypotonia, seizures, a bulging fontanel, and lethargy. An epidural hematoma can be detected by a CT scan. If the severity of the child's signs and symptoms is not recognized, herniation and death will occur.

Subdural Hemorrhage

A subdural hemorrhage is bleeding between the dura and the arachnoid membrane, usually as a result of rupture of cortical veins that bridge the subdural space (see Fig. 46.6, *B*). Subdural hematomas are more common than epidural hematomas, occurring most often in infancy, frequently as a result of birth trauma, falls, assaults, or violent shaking.

Unlike epidural hemorrhage, which develops inwardly against the less resistant brain tissue, subdural hemorrhage tends to develop more slowly and spreads thinly and widely, crossing cranial sutures, until it is limited by the dural barriers (i.e., the falx and tentorium). The small subdural space and the dura, which is firmly attached to the skull in this area, are highly vulnerable to increased ICP.

Presenting signs can include irritability, vomiting, increased head circumference, bulging fontanels in infants, lethargy, coma, or seizures. In infants with open fontanels, large amounts of intracranial blood may accumulate, causing hemorrhagic shock or fever before there are any changes in the neurologic examination. Hemiparesis, hemiplegia, and unequal pupils are signs of brainstem compression and increased ICP. A child with a GCS of 12 or less requires emergency consultation with the neurosurgeon.

> ! **NURSING ALERT**
>
> Children with a subdural hematoma and retinal hemorrhages should be evaluated for the possibility of child abuse, especially shaken baby syndrome.

The need for surgical evacuation of the hematoma depends on the physical examination, size of the hematoma, and CT scan abnormalities. Various surgical options to treat subdural hematomas include transfontanel percutaneous aspiration, subdural drains, placement of a burr hole, or craniotomy (Klimo, Matthews, Lew, et al., 2011).

Cerebral Edema

Some degree of brain edema is expected after craniocerebral trauma. Cerebral edema peaks at 24 to 72 hours after injury and may account for changes in a child's neurologic status. Cerebral edema associated with traumatic brain injury may be caused by cytotoxic edema or vasogenic edema. Either mechanism can result in increased ICP as a result of the increased intracranial volume and changes in CBF as a result of loss of autoregulation and/or hypercapnia or hypoxia.

Diagnostic Evaluation

A detailed health history, both past and present, is essential in evaluating the child with craniocerebral trauma. Certain disorders, such as drug allergies, hemophilia, diabetes mellitus, or epilepsy, may produce similar symptoms. Even minor traumatic injury can aggravate a preexisting disease process, thereby producing neurologic signs out of proportion to the injury.

After a minor injury, initial unconsciousness (if present) is brief, and the child ordinarily exhibits a transient period of confusion, somnolence, and listlessness; this period is most often accompanied by irritability, pallor, and one episode of vomiting. Because head injuries are frequently accompanied by injuries in other areas, the examination is performed with care to avoid further damage.

> **! NURSING ALERT**
>
> Stabilize a child's spine after head injury until a spinal cord injury is ruled out.

Initial Assessment

Priorities in the initial stabilization phase of a child with a head injury include assessment of the CAB (circulation, airway, breathing); neurologic examination focusing on mental status, pupillary responses, and motor responses; and assessment for spinal cord injury. The assessment is carried out quickly in relation to vital signs (see Emergency Treatment box: Head Injury).

> **! NURSING ALERT**
>
> Deep, rapid, periodic, or intermittent and gasping respirations; wide fluctuations or noticeable slowing of the pulse; and widening pulse pressure or extreme fluctuations in blood pressure are signs of brainstem involvement. Marked hypotension may represent internal injuries.

Ocular signs such as fixed, dilated, and unequal pupils; fixed and constricted pupils; and pupils that are poorly reactive or nonreactive to light and accommodation indicate increased ICP or brainstem involvement. It is important to remain with the child who demonstrates fixed and dilated pupils because these are ominous signs with a high probability of respiratory arrest. Dilated, nonpulsating blood vessels indicate increased ICP before the appearance of papilledema. Retinal hemorrhages are seen in acute head injuries, including shaken baby syndrome.

> **! NURSING ALERT**
>
> Observation of asymmetric pupils or one dilated, nonreactive pupil in a comatose child is a neurologic emergency.

Less urgent but important additional assessments include examination of the scalp for lacerations, widely separated sutures, and the size and tension of fontanels, which indicate intracranial hemorrhage or rapidly

> **✚ EMERGENCY TREATMENT**
>
> ### Head Injury
>
> 1. Assess child:
>   - **C**—Circulation
>   - **A**—Airway
>   - **B**—Bleeding
>   - Neurologic and thermoregulatory status
> 2. Stabilize neck and spine immediately. Use jaw thrust, not chin lift, to open airway.
> 3. Clean any abrasions with soap and water.
>   - Apply clean dressing.
>   - If bleeding, apply pressure and then ice to relieve pain and swelling.
> 4. Keep NPO until instructed otherwise.
> 5. Assess pain, but do not give analgesics or sedatives.
> 6. Check pupil reaction every 4 hours (including twice during the night) for 48 hours.
> 7. Awaken twice during the night to check LOC.
> 8. Seek medical attention if any of the following apply:
>   - Injury sustained:
>   - At high speed (e.g., automobile)
>   - From fall from a significant distance (e.g., height greater than that of the child)
>   - From great force (e.g., baseball bat)
>   - Under suspicious circumstances
>   - Loss of consciousness
>   - Amnesia
>   - Discomfort (crying) more than 10 minutes after injury
>   - Headache that is severe, worsening, interferes with sleep, or lasts more than 24 hours
>   - Fluid leak from ears or nose; blackened eyes
>   - Vomiting three or more times, beginning after injury, or continuing 4 to 6 hours after injury
>   - Swelling in front of or above earlobe or swelling that increases in size
>   - Confusion or abnormal behavior
>   - Difficulty arousing child from sleep
>   - Difficulty speaking
>   - Blurred vision or diplopia
>   - Unsteady gait
>   - Difficulty using extremities, weakness, or incoordination
>   - Neck pain or stiffness
>   - Pupils dilated, unequal, or fixed
>   - Infant with bulging fontanel
>   - Seizures

LOC, Level of consciousness; *NPO,* nothing by mouth.

developing cerebral edema. A significant amount of blood loss can occur from scalp lacerations. An underlying skull fracture should be ruled out by CT scan.

> **! NURSING ALERT**
>
> Bleeding from the nose or ears needs further evaluation, and a watery discharge from the nose (rhinorrhea) that is positive for glucose (as tested with Dextrostix) suggests leaking of CSF from a skull fracture.

An accurate assessment of clinical signs provides baseline information. Serial evaluations, preferably by a single observer, help to detect changes in the neurologic status. Alterations in mental status, evidenced by increased difficulty in rousing the child, mounting agitation, development of focal lateral neurologic signs, or marked changes in vital signs, usually indicate extension or progression of the basic pathologic process.

Special Tests

After a thorough clinical examination, a variety of diagnostic tests are helpful in providing a more definitive diagnosis of the type and extent of the trauma. The severity of a head injury may not be apparent on clinical examination of a child but is detectable on a CT scan. Whenever the child has a history consistent with a serious head injury (unrestrained occupant in a severe motor vehicle accident or a fall from a significant height), it is important to perform a diagnostic scan, even if the child initially appears alert and oriented. All children with head injuries who have any alteration of consciousness, headache, vomiting, skull fracture, seizure, or a predisposing medical condition should undergo a diagnostic evaluation that includes CT scanning.

MRI may be useful in evaluating cerebral edema or structural brain abnormalities. A neurobehavioral assessment may be useful in documenting cognitive impairments. Other radiographic tests may be indicated, depending on the severity or cause of the trauma. EEG is not helpful for diagnosis of head injury but is useful for defining seizure activity. Lumbar puncture is rarely used in craniocerebral trauma and is contraindicated in the presence of increased ICP because of the possibility of herniation.

Posttraumatic Syndromes

Posttraumatic syndromes include postconcussion syndrome, posttraumatic seizures, and structural complications after a head injury.

Postconcussion syndrome is a common sequela to brain injury with or without loss of consciousness. Symptoms can develop within hours to days after a mild head injury but can also occur after moderate to severe head injury. The manifestations vary with the child's age and include nausea, dizziness, headache, photophobia, fatigue, irritability, restlessness, difficulty concentrating, and memory impairment (Babcock, Byczkowski, Wade, et al., 2013). The duration of manifestations can vary from several days to several months.

Posttraumatic seizures occur in a number of children who survive a head injury, often within 24 hours after the injury but can occur up to 1 week after the trauma (Christensen, 2012). In comparison to children with no brain injury, seizures are two times more likely to occur in children with mild traumatic brain injury and seven times more likely to occur in children with severe head injury (Christensen).

Structural complications (e.g., hydrocephalus) may occur as a result of head injuries. Clinical sequelae include cognitive deterioration, gait changes, optic atrophy, cranial nerve palsies, or aphasia. The type of residual effect depends on the location and nature of the trauma.

Therapeutic Management

The majority of children with mild traumatic brain injury who have not lost consciousness can be cared for and observed at home after a careful examination reveals no serious intracranial injury. Nurses should provide parents with verbal and written instructions of signs and symptoms that warrant concern and the need for medical reevaluation (see Family-Centered Care box: Maintaining Contact).

Parents are instructed to check the child every 2 hours to determine any changes in responsiveness. The sleeping child should be awakened to see if he or she can be roused normally. Parents are advised to maintain contact with the health care provider, who typically examines the child again in 1 or 2 days. The manifestations of epidural hematoma in children do not generally appear until 24 hours or more after injury.

Children with severe injuries, those who have lost consciousness for more than a few minutes, and those with prolonged and continued seizures or other focal or diffuse neurologic signs must be hospitalized

until their condition is stable and their neurologic signs have diminished. The child is maintained on NPO (nothing by mouth) status or restricted to clear liquids until it is determined that vomiting will not occur. IV fluids are indicated in the child who is comatose, displays dulled sensorium, or is vomiting persistently. The volume of IV fluid is carefully monitored to minimize the possibility of overhydration in cases of SIADH and cerebral edema. However, damage to the hypothalamus or pituitary gland may produce DI with its accompanying hypertonicity and dehydration. Fluid balance is monitored closely by daily weights; accurate intake and output measurements; and serum osmolality to detect early signs of water retention.

Sedating drugs are commonly withheld in the acute phase. Headaches are usually controlled with acetaminophen, although opioids may be needed. Antiepileptics are used for seizure control. Antibiotics may be administered if lacerations or penetrating injuries are present. Cerebral edema is managed as described for the unconscious child. Hyperthermia is controlled with tepid sponges or a hypothermia blanket.

Surgical Therapy

Scalp lacerations are sutured after the underlying bone is carefully examined. Depressed fractures require surgical reduction and removal of bone fragments. Torn dura is sutured. Ping-pong ball skull fractures in very young infants ordinarily correct themselves within a few weeks; however, depressions larger than 5 mm may require surgical intervention (López-Elizalde, Leyva-Mastrapa, Muñoz-Serrano, Godínez-Rubí, Preciado-Barón et al., 2013).

Prognosis

The outcome of craniocerebral trauma depends on the extent of injury and complications. In general, the prognosis is more favorable for children than for adults. More than 90% of children with concussions or simple linear fractures recover without symptoms after the initial period. Outcomes in children with brain injuries are focused increasingly on long-term cognitive, emotional, and mental problems.

True coma (not obeying commands, eyes closed, and not speaking) usually does not last more than 2 weeks. A child's eventual outcome can range from brain death to a persistent vegetative state to complete recovery. However, even the best recovery may be associated with personality changes, including mood lability and loss of confidence, impaired short-term memory, headaches, and subtle cognitive impairments. Many children are left with significant disabilities after head injury that appear months later as learning difficulties, behavioral changes, or emotional disturbances (Anderson, Le Brocque, Iselin, et al., 2012).

Interprofessional Care Management

The hospitalized child requires careful neurologic assessment and evaluation that are repeated at frequent intervals to establish a correct diagnosis, identify signs and symptoms of increased ICP, determine clinical management, and prevent many complications.

The child is placed on bed rest, usually with the head of the bed elevated slightly and the head in midline position. Appropriate safety measures, such as side rails kept up and seizure precautions, are implemented. Children may be restless and irritable, but often their reaction is to fall asleep when left undisturbed. A quiet environment helps reduce restlessness and irritability. For extremely restless children, hard surfaces may need to be padded and restraint used to prevent the possibility of further injury. Care is individualized according to the child's specific needs. Shining bright lights directly into the child's face is irritating and makes assessment of ocular responses difficult.

Frequent examinations of vital signs, neurologic signs, and LOC are extremely important observations. When possible, they should be performed by a single observer to better detect subtle changes that may indicate worsening neurologic status. Pupils are checked for size, equality, reaction to light, and accommodation. After the initial changes are seen after injury, the vital signs generally return to normal unless there is brainstem involvement.

The most important observation is assessment of the child's LOC. Alterations in consciousness appear earlier in the progression of an injury than alterations of vital signs or focal neurologic signs. Frequent examinations of alertness are fatiguing to the child. The child often desires to fall asleep, which may be confused with depressed consciousness. It is common to observe ocular divergence through the partially closed eyelids.

An important consideration is to provide sedation and analgesia for the child. The conflict between the need to promote comfort and relieve anxiety in the child versus the need to assess for neurologic changes presents a dilemma. Both goals can be achieved with close observation of the child's LOC and response to analgesics (using of a pain assessment record), and effective communication with the health care provider. Decreasing restlessness after administration of an analgesic most likely reflects pain control rather than a declining LOC.

Observations of position and movement provide additional information. Note any abnormal posturing and whether it occurs continuously or intermittently. Questions nurses might consider include the following:
- Are the child's handgrips strong and equal in strength?
- Are there any signs of flexion or extension posturing?
- What is the child's response to stimulation?
- Is movement purposeful, random, or absent?
- Are movement and sensation equal on both sides or restricted to one side only?

The child may complain of headache or other discomfort. A child who is too young to describe a headache may be fussy and resist being handled. A child who has vertigo often assumes a position of comfort. Forcible movement causes the child to vomit and display spontaneous nystagmus. Seizures are relatively common in children with head trauma and may be of any type. Carefully observe, record, and report in detail any seizure activity. Children in postictal (postseizure) states are lethargic with sluggish pupils.

Document drainage from any orifice. Bleeding from the ear suggests the possibility of a basal skull fracture. Clear nasal drainage suggests an anterior basal skull fracture. The amount and characteristics of the drainage is observed, recorded, and reported.

Head trauma is frequently accompanied by other undetected injuries; therefore any bruises, lacerations, or evidence of internal injuries or fractures of the extremities are noted and reported. Associated injuries are evaluated and treated appropriately.

The child with normal LOC is usually allowed clear liquids unless fluid is restricted. If the child has an IV infusion, it is maintained as prescribed. The diet is advanced to that appropriate for the child's age as soon as the condition permits. Intake and output are measured and recorded, and any incontinence of bowel or bladder is noted if the child has been toilet trained.

Observe the child for any unusual behavior, but behavior should be interpreted in relation to the child's normal behavior. For example, urinary incontinence during sleep would be of no consequence in a child who routinely wets the bed but would be highly significant for one who is always dry. Parents are valuable resources in evaluating objective behavior of their child. Information obtained from parents at or shortly after admission is essential in evaluating the child's behavior (e.g., the ease with which the child is roused normally, the usual sleeping position and patterns, motor activities [rolling over, sitting up, climbing], hearing and visual acuity, appetite, and manner of eating [spoon, bottle, cup]).

Family Support

The emotional and educational support of the family presents a challenging aspect to nursing care. Witnessing the parents' grief and helplessness on seeing their child in an altered state, connected to monitoring equipment, and in an intensive care unit evokes empathy. The nurse can encourage the family to be involved in the child's care, bring in familiar belongings, or make a tape recording of familiar voices and sounds. Parents may need a demonstration on how to touch or cuddle their child and may want to talk about their grief. The nurse listens attentively, reinforces what is being done to assist the child, and directs parents toward signs and symptoms of recovery to instill hope without promises. Honesty and kindness, along with competent care, can help families through this difficult time.

Rehabilitation

Rehabilitation and management of the child with permanent brain injury are essential aspects of care. Rehabilitation begins as soon as feasible and usually involves the family and a rehabilitation team. Careful assessment of the child's capabilities, limitations, and probable potential is made as early as possible, and appropriate interventions are implemented to maximize the residual capacities. The Brain Injury Association of America* provides information and listings of rehabilitation services and support groups throughout the country.

Pediatric trauma rehabilitation is a national concern. Coordinating care and services for early rehabilitation involves identifying the child's and family's response to the traumatic injury and disability, securing available resources, and recognizing the parental role in the process.

Children with disabilities resulting from head trauma require assessment on a physical, cognitive, emotional, and social level. These children have experienced separation, pain, sensory deprivation and overload, changes in circadian cycle, and fear of the unknown. Recovery and transition require new coping strategies at the same time that regressive and acting-out behavior may start. Parents and children need honest communication for decision making. Rehabilitation is recommended when the child has progressed beyond what can be provided in a hospital setting. The Rancho Los Amigos Scale provides a systematic assessment

---

! NURSING ALERT

Suctioning through the nares is contraindicated because of the risk of the catheter entering the brain parenchyma through a fracture in the skull.

---

*1608 Spring Hill Road, Suite 110, Vienna, VA 22182, 703-761-0750, www.biausa.org.

of the possible progress that a child may achieve after a severe head injury.

Prevention

Tremendous strides have been taken to prevent cerebral damage after head injury in children. New developments are directed toward the prevention of cellular injury or the primary insult. Education can exert a valuable influence on prevention of children's head injuries. Preventable head injuries occur because unnecessary risks go unchecked. Inadequate supervision combined with children's natural sense of curiosity and exploration can lead to lethal results. Nurses are in the unique position of influencing caregivers in terms of growth and development risks. Banning the use of infant walkers is an example. This equipment does not help develop motor skills and places infants at risk for head and neck injuries from falls, especially down steps. Public education coupled with legislative support can prevent childhood injuries.

SUBMERSION INJURY

Submersion injury is a major cause of unintentional injury related death in children 1 to 19 years of age, with the highest rate occurring in children 1 to 4 years of age (Mott & Latimer, 2016). The term *submersion injury* has replaced *near-drowning* to include any person who experiences distress from submersion or immersion in liquid that results either in death (drowning) or survival at least 24 hours after submersion (near-drowning) (Mott & Latimer). Most cases of submersion are accidental, usually involving children who are helpless in water, such as inadequately attended children in or near swimming pools or infants in bathtubs; small children who fall into ponds, streams, and flooded excavations; occupants of pleasure boats who fail to wear life preservers; children who have diving accidents; and children who are able to swim but overestimate their endurance. Accidental drowning occurs more commonly in toddlers, boys, and African-Americans (Nasrullah & Muazzam, 2011).

Submersion injury can take place in any body of liquid, and sites of drowning are important to consider for preventive education. Children younger than 1 year of age are most likely to have a submersion injury in a bathtub, whereas top-heavy toddlers fall head first into a pail of liquid and are unable to free themselves (Caglar & Quan, 2016). Preschoolers are at risk for injury in swimming pools, and school-age children and adolescents are most commonly at risk in natural bodies of water, such as lakes, ponds, and rivers (Caglar & Quan). The suction created at the outlet of pools, hot tubs, or whirlpool spas is strong enough to trap any child, even larger children, underwater. Submersion injury as a form of fatal child abuse has also been recognized as a problem.

Pathophysiology

Physiologically most organ systems are affected, especially pulmonary, cardiovascular, and neurologic systems. Cerebral hypoxia is the major component of morbidity and mortality with submersion events. Within minutes of a submersion, a lack of oxygen leads to loss of consciousness and progressive decreased cardiac output and ultimately apnea and cardiac arrest (Caglar & Quan, 2016). Recovery depends on the timeliness and effectiveness of initial resuscitation and subsequent supportive care measures.

Physiologic features in submersion injuries are hypoxia, aspiration, and hypothermia.

Hypoxia is related to the duration of anoxia and asphyxia. Different cells tolerate variable lengths of anoxia, causing variations of cell damage. Neurons, especially cerebral cells, sustain irreversible damage after 4 to 6 minutes of submersion; but the heart and lungs can survive up to 30 minutes. Regardless of the amount of liquid aspirated, there is arterial hypoxemia (resulting from atelectasis with shunting of blood through the nonventilated alveoli) and a combined respiratory acidosis (resulting from retained carbon dioxide) and metabolic acidosis (caused by buildup of acid metabolites from anaerobic metabolism). Approximately 10% of submersion injury victims die without aspirating fluid but succumb from acute asphyxia as a result of prolonged reflex laryngospasm.

Aspiration of fluid occurs in the majority of submersion injuries. The aspirated fluid results in pulmonary edema, atelectasis, airway spasm, and pneumonitis, which aggravates the hypoxia. *Hypothermia* is common after submersion; children are at an increased risk for hypothermia because of their large surface area relative to body mass, decreased subcutaneous fat, and limited thermoregulation (Caglar & Quan, 2016). The temperature of the liquid plays an important role in developing hypoxemia. Cold water decreases metabolic demands and activates the diving reflex, which causes blood to be shunted away from the periphery to vital organs (i.e., the brain and heart). However, prolonged submersion in cold liquids can impair cognition, coordination, and muscle strength, ultimately resulting in a loss of consciousness, decreased cardiac output, and cardiac arrest (Caglar & Quan).

Therapeutic Management

With rapid treatment, some children can be saved. Resuscitative measures should begin at the scene, and the victim should be transported to the hospital with maximum ventilatory and circulatory support. In the hospital, intensive care is implemented and continued according to the patient's needs.

In general, the management of the victims with submersion injuries is based on the degree of cerebral insult. The first priority is to restore oxygen delivery to the cells and prevent further hypoxic damage. A spontaneously breathing child does well in an oxygen-enriched atmosphere; a more severely affected child requires endotracheal intubation and mechanical ventilation. Blood gases and pH are monitored frequently as a guide to oxygen, fluid, and electrolyte therapies. Seizures may occur due to hypoxia and cerebral edema.

All children who have a submersion injury should be observed for at least 6 to 8 hours. Almost one-half of asymptomatic or minimally symptomatic alert children experience complications (e.g., respiratory compromise, cerebral edema) during the first 4 to 8 hours after the incident (Caglar & Quan, 2016). Aspiration pneumonia is a frequent complication that occurs about 48 to 72 hours after the episode. Bronchospasm, alveolocapillary membrane damage, atelectasis, abscess formation, and acute respiratory distress syndrome are other complications that occur after aspiration of fluid.

Prognosis

The best predictors of a good outcome are length of submersion less than 5 minutes and the presence of sinus rhythm, reactive pupils, and neurologic responsiveness at the scene. The worst prognoses—for death or severe neurologic impairment—are for children submerged for more than 10 minutes and not responding to advanced life support within 25 minutes. Most children without spontaneous purposeful movement and normal brainstem function 24 hours after a submersion injury have sustained severe neurologic deficits or death (Caglar & Quan, 2016) (see Guidelines box: Establishing Brain Death in Children).

Care Management

Nursing care depends on the child's condition. A child who survives may need intensive respiratory nursing care with attention to vital signs, mechanical ventilation, or tracheostomy, blood gas determination, chest physiotherapy, and IV infusion. A child who has sustained a submersion

GUIDELINES

Establishing Brain Death in Children

1. Coma and apnea must coexist. Child must exhibit complete loss of consciousness, vocalization, and volitional activity.
2. Brainstem function must be absent, as defined by the following:
   a. Midposition or fully dilated pupils in both eyes that do not respond to light. Drugs may influence and invalidate pupillary assessment.
   b. Absence of spontaneous eye movements and those induced by oculocephalic and caloric (oculovestibular) testing.
   c. Absence of movement of bulbar musculature, including facial and oropharyngeal muscles.
   d. Absence of the corneal, gag, cough, sucking, and rooting reflexes.
   e. Absence of respiratory movements when child is removed from the respirator. Apnea testing using standardized methods can be performed but is done after other criteria are met.
3. Child must not be significantly hypothermic or hypotensive for age.
4. Flaccid tone and absence of spontaneous or induced movements, including spinal cord events such as reflex withdrawal or spinal myoclonus, should exist.
5. Examination should remain consistent with brain death throughout the observation and testing period.
6. Observation periods according to age:
   37 weeks gestation to term infant 30 days of age—Two separate examinations and two EEGs separated by at least 24 hours
   Older than 30 days to 18 years of age—Two separate examinations and two EEGs separated by at least 12 hours

EEG, Electroencephalogram.
Adapted from Nakagawa, T.A., Ashwal, S., Mathur, M., et al. (2011). Guidelines for the determination of brain death in infants and children: An update of the 1987 task force recommendations. *Pediatrics, 128,* e720–e740.

injury requires the same care as an unconscious child. A difficult aspect in the care of the child victim of submersion injury is helping the parents cope with severe guilt reactions. Given the magnitude of the event, parents need repeated assurance that everything possible is being done to treat the child.

The parents of the child who is saved from death face the anxiety of not knowing the final outcome. The situation generates such intense feelings of loneliness and guilt that it is important for families to know that they are not alone. They should be reminded frequently that people are available to assist them through the crisis. Additional sources of support include psychiatric and social work consultants, community services, and religious support. Self-help groups may be beneficial if available in the community.

Nurses often have difficulty relating to the parents if obvious neglect has precipitated the accident and subsequent problems; therefore it is important for those who care for these children and their families to assess their own feelings about the situation, in addition to assessing the family's coping abilities and resources. Caring for victims of a submersion injury and their families requires nurses to be sensitive to the needs of the child and family and recognize their own reactions and emotions.

Prevention

Most submersion injuries are preventable. The most common cause of submersion injury of infants and young children is inadequate adult supervision, including a momentary lapse of supervision (Weiss & American Academy of Pediatrics Committee on Injury, Violence, and Poison Prevention, 2010). Close adult supervision of infants and children

around any body of water is essential and should include the adult not engaging in any distracting activities. Other strategies include environmental prevention strategies, such as pool fencing, pool covers, water-entry alarms, and lifeguard and individual prevention such as swimming and survival skills, cardiopulmonary resuscitation training, and the use of personal flotation devices (Mott & Latimer, 2016).

INTRACRANIAL INFECTIONS

The nervous system is subject to infection by the same organisms that affect other organs of the body. However, the nervous system is limited in the ways in which it responds to injury. Laboratory studies are needed to identify the causative agent. The inflammatory process can affect the meninges (meningitis) or brain (encephalitis).

Meningitis can be caused by a variety of organisms, but the three main types are (1) bacterial, or pyogenic, caused by pus-forming bacteria, especially meningococci and pneumococci organisms; (2) viral, or aseptic, caused by a wide variety of viral agents; and (3) tuberculous, caused by the tuberculin bacillus. The majority of children with acute febrile encephalopathy have either bacterial meningitis or viral meningitis as the underlying cause.

BACTERIAL MENINGITIS

Bacterial meningitis is an acute inflammation of the meninges and CSF. Suspected bacterial meningitis is a medical emergency, and immediate action must be taken to identify the causative organism and to initiate prompt treatment.

The advent of antimicrobial therapy has had a significant effect on the overall clinical course and prognosis of children with bacterial meningitis. The introduction of the *Haemophilus* influenza type b (Hib) vaccine in 1990 and *Streptococcus pneumoniae* (pneumococcus) in 2000 has led to dramatic changes in the epidemiology of bacterial meningitis. Currently *S. pneumoniae* is the leading cause of bacterial meningitis in children 3 months to 11 years of age, whereas *Neisseria meningitidis* is the leading cause in children 11 to 17 years of age (Thigpen, Whitney, Messonnier, et al., 2011). The leading causes of neonatal meningitis are group b streptococci (Thigpen et al). Meningococcal meningitis occurs in epidemic form and is the only type readily transmitted by droplet infection from nasopharyngeal secretions. Although this condition may develop at any age, the risk for meningococcal infection increases with the number of contacts; therefore it occurs predominantly in school-age children and adolescents. College students, especially those living in dormitory residences, are at moderately increased risk for meningococcal disease compared with other people their age. There appear to be some seasonal variations with the organisms. Pneumococcal and meningococcal infections can occur at any time but are more common in later winter and early spring.

Pathophysiology

The most common route of infection is vascular dissemination from a focus of infection elsewhere. For example, organisms from the nasopharynx invade the underlying blood vessels, cross the blood-brain barrier, and multiply in the CSF. Invasion by direct extension from infections in the paranasal and mastoid sinuses is less common. Organisms also gain entry by direct implantation after penetrating wounds, skull fractures that provide an opening into the skin or sinuses, lumbar puncture or surgical procedures, anatomic abnormalities such as spina bifida, or foreign bodies such as an internal ventricular shunt or an external ventricular device. Once implanted, the organisms spread into the CSF, by which the infection spreads throughout the subarachnoid space.

The infective process is similar to that seen in any bacterial infection and includes inflammation, exudation, white blood cell accumulation, and varying degrees of tissue damage. The brain becomes hyperemic and edematous, and the entire surface of the brain is covered by a layer of purulent exudate that varies with the type of organism. For example, meningococcal exudate is most evident over the parietal, occipital, and cerebellar regions; the thick, fibrinous exudate of pneumococcal infection is confined chiefly to the surface of the brain, particularly the anterior lobes; and the exudate of streptococcal infections is similar to that of pneumococcal infections but thinner. As infection extends to the ventricles, thick pus, fibrin, or adhesions may occlude the narrow passages and obstruct the flow of CSF.

Clinical Manifestations

The onset of illness may be abrupt and rapid, or develop progressively over 1 day or several days, and may be preceded by a febrile illness. Most children with meningitis present with fever, chills, headache, and vomiting that are quickly followed by alterations in the sensorium; however, some may present only with lethargy and irritability. The child is extremely irritable and agitated and may develop seizures, photophobia, confusion, hallucinations, drowsiness, stupor, or coma. See Box 46.4 for clinical manifestations of bacterial meningitis. Nuchal rigidity is manifested by inability to flex neck and place chin on chest and presence of Kernig and Brudzinski signs. The Kernig sign is present if the patient, in the supine position with the hip and knee flexed at 90 degrees, cannot extend the knee more than 135 degrees and pain is felt in the hamstrings. Flexion of the opposite knee may also occur. The Brudzinski sign is present if the patient, while in the supine position, flexes the lower extremities if passive flexion of the neck is attempted.

> **! NURSING ALERT**
>
> Any child who is ill and develops a purpuric or petechial rash may have meningococcemia and must receive medical attention immediately.

Diagnostic Evaluation

A lumbar puncture is the definitive diagnostic test for meningitis. The fluid pressure is measured; and samples are obtained for culture, Gram stain, blood cell count, and determination of glucose and protein content. These findings are usually diagnostic. Culture and sensitivity testing are needed to identify the causative organism. Spinal fluid pressure is usually elevated, but interpretation is often difficult when the child is crying. Sedation with fentanyl and midazolam can alleviate the child's pain and fear associated with this procedure. If there is evidence or suspicion of increased ICP (papilledema, focal neurologic deficits, bulging fontanel), a CT scan of the head is warranted before the procedure. Lumbar puncture is contraindicated in any patient with imaging to suggest that the procedure is not safe (e.g., midline shift, mass effect, transependymal migration of CSF).

The patient with meningitis generally has an elevated white blood cell count, often predominantly polymorphonuclear leukocytes. Typically, in bacterial meningitis the CSF glucose level is reduced, generally in proportion to the duration and severity of the infection. The protein concentration is usually increased.

BOX 46.4   Clinical Manifestations of Bacterial Meningitis

Children and Adolescents
- Usually abrupt onset
- Fever
- Chills
- Headache
- Vomiting
- Alterations in sensorium
- Seizures (often the initial sign)
- Irritability
- Agitation
- May develop:
  - Photophobia
  - Delirium
  - Hallucinations
  - Aggressive behavior
  - Drowsiness
  - Stupor
  - Coma
- Nuchal rigidity; may progress to opisthotonos
- Positive Kernig and Brudzinski signs
- Hyperactivity but variable reflex responses
- Signs and symptoms peculiar to individual organisms:
  - Petechial or purpuric rashes (meningococcal infection), especially when associated with a shocklike state
  - Joint involvement (meningococcal and *Haemophilus influenzae* infection)
  - Chronically draining ear (pneumococcal meningitis)

Infants and Young Children
- Classic presentation in children (above) is rarely seen in children between 3 months and 2 years of age
- Fever
- Poor feeding
- Vomiting
- Marked irritability
- Frequent seizures (often accompanied by a high-pitched cry)
- Bulging fontanel
- Nuchal rigidity possible
- Brudzinski and Kernig signs not helpful in diagnosis
- Difficult to elicit and evaluate in this age-group
- Subdural empyema (*H. influenzae* infection)

Neonates
Specific Signs
- Child well at birth but within a few days begins to look and behave poorly
- Refuses feedings
- Poor sucking ability
- Vomiting or diarrhea
- Poor tone
- Lack of movement
- Weak cry
- Full, tense, and bulging fontanel may appear late in course of illness
- Neck usually supple

Nonspecific Signs That May Be Present
- Hypothermia or fever (depending on infant's maturity)
- Jaundice
- Irritability
- Drowsiness
- Seizures
- Respiratory irregularities or apnea
- Cyanosis
- Weight loss

A blood culture is advisable for all children suspected of having meningitis and occasionally is positive when CSF culture is negative. Nose and throat cultures may provide helpful information in some cases.

Therapeutic Management

Acute bacterial meningitis is a medical emergency that requires early recognition and immediate institution of therapy to prevent death or residual disabilities. The initial therapeutic management includes the following:

- Isolation precautions
- Initiation of antimicrobial therapy
- Maintenance of hydration
- Maintenance of ventilation
- Reduction of increased ICP
- Management of systemic shock
- Control of seizures
- Control of temperature
- Treatment of complications

The child is isolated from other children, usually in an intensive care unit for close observation. An IV infusion is started to facilitate the administration of antimicrobial agents, fluids, antiepileptic drugs, and blood, if needed. The child is placed in respiratory isolation.

Drugs

Until the causative organism is identified, empirical therapy is administered. After identification of the organism, antimicrobial agents are adjusted accordingly.

> ### 💊 MEDICATION ALERT
>
> Dexamethasone may play a role in the initial management of symptoms occurring from a cytokine-mediated inflammatory response after treatment has begun. Evidence indicates that dexamethasone therapy decreases the risk for neurologic sequelae in children with *H. influenza* type b meningitis, but data regarding the benefits in other types of bacterial meningitis are inconclusive (Prober & Matthew, 2016).

Signs of gastrointestinal hemorrhage or secondary infection may complicate steroid administration. Antibiotic treatment with cephalosporins demonstrates superiority for promptly sterilizing the CSF and reducing the incidence of severe hearing impairment.

Nonspecific Measures

Maintaining hydration is a prime concern, and the type and amount of IV fluids are determined by the patient's condition. The optimum hydration involves correction of any fluid deficits and electrolyte abnormalities followed by fluid restriction until normal serum sodium levels and no signs of increased ICP are present. If needed, measures to decrease ICP are implemented (see earlier in this chapter). Long-term fluid restriction is not the standard of care because a lack of adequate fluid volume can reduce blood pressure and CPP, causing CNS ischemia (Prober & Matthew, 2016).

Complications such as aspiration of subdural effusion in infants and treatment for disseminated intravascular coagulation syndrome are treated appropriately. Shock is managed by restoration of circulating blood volume and maintenance of electrolyte balance. Seizures can occur during the first few days of treatment. These are controlled with the appropriate antiepileptic drug. Hearing loss is common. The patient should undergo auditory evaluation 6 months after the illness has resolved.

Lumbar puncture is carried out as needed to determine the effectiveness of therapy. The patient is evaluated neurologically during the convalescent period.

Prognosis

Less than 10% of cases of bacterial meningitis are fatal (Thigpen et al, 2011). The child's age, duration of illness before antibiotic therapy, rapidity of diagnosis after onset, type of organism, and adequacy of therapy are important in the prognosis of bacterial meningitis. Survivors can experience significant physical and neurologic sequelae, including hearing loss, learning disabilities, and seizure disorder (Chandran, Herbert, Misurski, et al., 2011).

Clinical features that are associated with an increased risk for developing neurologic complications include young age, infection with *S. pneumoniae,* CSF with more than 10^7 colony-forming units/mL or low CSF glucose content, delay in antimicrobial therapy for longer than 2 days, prolonged or complicated seizures, focal neurologic deficits, and adequacy of response to infection (Chandran et al., 2011). The residual deficits in infants are primarily a result of communicating hydrocephalus and the greater effects of cerebritis on the immature brain. In older children, they are related to the inflammatory process itself or result from vasculitis associated with the disease.

Prevention

Vaccines are available for types A, C, Y, and W-135 meningococci and Hib. Meningococcal polysaccharide vaccination is given routinely to children 11 to 12 years of age with a booster at 16 years of age; however, children 2 to 10 years of age may be given the vaccine if they are at increased risk for meningococcal disease (Prober & Matthew, 2016). Routine vaccinations for Hib and pneumococcal conjugate vaccines are recommended for all children beginning at 2 months of age (see Evidence-Based Practice box: Children with Bacterial Meningitis and Preventive Vaccines).

> ### ❗ NURSING ALERT
>
> A major priority of nursing care of a child suspected of having meningitis is to administer antibiotics as soon as they are ordered. The child is placed on respiratory isolation for at least 24 hours after initiation of antimicrobial therapy.

Care Management

Keep the room as quiet as possible, and keep environmental stimuli at a minimum because most children with meningitis are sensitive to noise, bright lights, and other external stimuli. Most children are more comfortable without a pillow and with the head of the bed slightly elevated. A side-lying position is more often assumed because of nuchal rigidity. The nurse should avoid actions that cause pain or increase discomfort such as lifting the child's head. Evaluating the child for pain and implementing appropriate relief measures are important during the initial 24 to 72 hours. Acetaminophen with codeine is often used. The nurse should be cautious to evaluate if a patient is febrile before giving acetaminophen or ibuprofen because either of these medications may mask a fever, which is an important clinical indication of infection.

The nursing care of the child with meningitis is determined by the child's symptoms and treatment. Observation of vital signs, neurologic signs, LOC, urinary output, and other pertinent data is carried out at frequent intervals. The child who is unconscious is managed as described earlier in this chapter, and all children are observed carefully for signs of the complications just described, especially increased ICP, shock, or respiratory distress. Frequent assessment of the open fontanels is needed in the infant because subdural effusions and obstructive hydrocephalus can develop as a complication of meningitis.

Administration of fluids and nourishment are determined by the child's status. The child with dulled sensorium is usually kept NPO. Other children are allowed clear liquids initially and, if these are tolerated,

---

EVIDENCE-BASED PRACTICE
Children With Bacterial Meningitis and Preventive Vaccines

Ask the Question

PICOT Question: In children and adolescents with bacterial meningitis, has the administration of *Haemophilus influenzae* type B (Hib), pneumococcal, and meningococcal preventive vaccines reduced the incidence and mortality associated with bacterial meningitis?

Search for the Evidence
Search Strategies

Search selection criteria included English language, publications within the past 10 years, research-based articles, and children populations.

Databases Used

PubMed and Cochrane Collaboration

Critical Appraisal of the Evidence

- Haddy, Perry, Chacko, and colleagues (2005) compared the incidence of *Streptococcus pneumoniae* disease before and after the introduction of conjugated pneumococcal vaccine from 1999 to 2002. The trend in the rates of invasive pneumococcal disease cases showed significant declines during the study period for all ages after the introduction of the heptavalent *S. pneumoniae* protein conjugate vaccine.
- Watt, Wolfson, O'Brien, and colleagues (2009) performed a literature review with studies evaluating Hib disease incidence, fatality ratios, and the effect of Hib vaccine. In 2000, there were 173,000 cases of Hib meningitis and 78,300 deaths among children younger than 5 years of age worldwide. Expanded use of Hib vaccine can reduce the incidence and mortality of Hib-related disease.
- A Cochrane review determined the effect, duration of protection, and age-specific effects of polysaccharide serogroup A vaccine (SgAV) to prevent meningococcal meningitis in children. The vaccine had a 95% protective effect during the first year in children older than 5 years of age, but its efficacy after the first year could not be determined. Children 1 to 5 years of age in low-income countries were also protected, but the exact efficacy could not be determined (Patel & Lee, 2005).
- A systematic review assessed the impact of the 7-valent pneumococcal vaccination on morbidity and mortality from invasive pneumococcal diseases. The six studies from North America consistently reported a decline in invasive pneumococcal disease mortality after the introduction of the pneumococcal

vaccine, with reductions ranging from 57% to 62% among children and 37% to 76% among all age groups (Myint, Madhava, Balmer, et al., 2013).
- Comparing invasive pneumococcal disease (IPD) in children from the pre–PCV 13 (2007–2009) to the post–PCV 13 (2010–2012) eras, Iroh Tam, Madoff, and colleagues (2014) found a significant decline in incidence rates among the two groups (46/100,000 pre–PCV 13 and 23/100,000 post–PCV 13, p <0.00001) but no difference in mortality (3.6% pre–PCV13 and 3.5% post–PCV 13).
- Using laboratory-based and population-based data, IPD was compared to actual incidence versus expected incidence if PCV 13 had not replaced PCV 7. Moore, Link-Gelles, Schaffner, and colleagues (2015) estimated that 10,000 IPD cases and 90 deaths among children were prevented in the first 3 years after the introduction of PCV 13.

Apply the Evidence: Nursing Implications

The evidence strongly suggests that all children should be immunized against the most common organisms responsible for bacterial meningitis (i.e., Hib, *S. pneumoniae,* and *Neisseria meningitidis*) as preventive vaccines to decrease the incidence of bacterial meningitis. Nurses should stress to parents, children, adolescents, and young adults the importance of adhering to the immunization schedule to protect the child against serious childhood diseases.

References

Haddy, R. I., Perry, K., Chacko, C. E., et1 al. (2005). Comparison of incidence in invasive *Streptococcus pneumoniae* disease among children before and after introduction of conjugated pneumococcal vaccine. *Pediatric Infectious Disease Journal, 24*(4), 320–330.

Iroh Tam, P. Y., Madoff, L. C., Coombes, B., et al. (2014). Invasive pneumococcal disease after implementation of 13-valent conjugate vaccine. *Pediatrics, 134*(2), 210–217.

Moore, M. R., Link-Gelles, R., Schaffner, W., et al. (2015). Effect of use of 13-valent pneumococcal conjugate vaccine in children on invasive pneumococcal disease in children and adults in the USA: Analysis of multisite, population-based surveillance. *Lancet Infectious Diseases, 15*(3), 301–309.

Myint, T., Madhava, H., Balmer, P., et al. (2013). The impact of 7-valent pneumococcal conjugate vaccine on invasive pneumococcal disease: A literature review. *Advances in Therapy, 30*(2), 127–151.

Patel, M., & Lee, C. K. (2005). Polysaccharide vaccines for preventing serogroup A meningococcal meningitis. *Cochrane Database of Systematic Reviews, 2005*(1), CD001093.

Watt, J. P., Wolfson, L. J., O'Brien, K. L., et al. (2009). Burden of disease caused by Haemophilus influenzae type b in children younger than 5 years: Global estimates. *Lancet, 374*, 903–911.

---

progress to a diet suitable for their age. Careful monitoring and recording of intake and output are needed to determine deviations that might indicate impending shock or increasing fluid accumulation such as cerebral edema or subdural effusion.

One of the most difficult problems in the nursing care of children with meningitis is maintaining IV infusion for the length of time needed to provide adequate antimicrobial therapy (usually 10 days). Because continuous IV fluids are usually not necessary, an intermittent infusion device is used. In some cases, children who are recovering uneventfully are sent home with the device, and the parents are taught IV drug administration.

Family Support

The sudden nature of the illness makes emotional support of the child and parents extremely important. Parents are upset and concerned about their child's condition and often feel guilty for not having suspected the seriousness of the illness sooner. They need much reassurance that

the natural onset of meningitis is sudden and that they acted responsibly in seeking medical assistance when they did. The nurse encourages the parents to openly discuss their feelings to minimize blame and guilt. They also are kept informed of the child's progress and of all procedures, results, and treatments. In the event that the child's condition worsens, they need the same psychologic supportive care as parents who face the possible death of their child (see Chapter 36).

NONBACTERIAL (ASEPTIC) MENINGITIS

The term *aseptic meningitis* refers to the onset of meningeal symptoms, fever, and pleocytosis without bacterial growth from CSF cultures. Aseptic meningitis is caused by many different viruses, including arbovirus, herpes simplex virus (HSV), cytomegalovirus, adenovirus, and human immunodeficiency virus (HIV). Enteroviruses are the most common cause of aseptic meningitis (Prober & Matthew, 2016). The onset may be abrupt or gradual, and many of the presenting signs and symptoms

TABLE 46.2   Variation of Cerebrospinal Fluid Analysis in Bacterial and Viral Meningitis

Manifestations	Bacterial*	Viral
White blood cell count	Elevated; increased neutrophils	Slightly elevated; increased lymphocytes
Protein content	Elevated	Normal or slightly increased
Glucose content	Decreased	Normal
Gram stain; bacteria culture	Positive	Negative
Color	Turbid or cloudy	Clear or slightly cloudy

*Results may vary in the neonate.

BOX 46.5   Clinical Manifestations of Encephalitis

Onset: Sudden or Gradual
- Malaise
- Fever
- Headache
- Dizziness
- Apathy
- Lethargy
- Nuchal rigidity
- Ataxia
- Tremors
- Hyperactivity
- Speech difficulties: mutism
- Altered mental status

Severe Cases
- High fever
- Stupor
- Seizures
- Disorientation
- Spasticity
- Coma (may proceed to death)
- Ocular palsies
- Paralysis

are the same as bacterial meningitis, including headache, fever, photophobia, and nuchal rigidity.

Diagnosis is based on clinical features and CSF findings. Variations in CSF values in bacterial and viral meningitis are listed in Table 46.2. It is important to differentiate this self-limiting disorder from the more serious forms of meningitis.

Treatment is primarily symptomatic, such as acetaminophen for headache and muscle pain, maintenance of hydration, and positioning for comfort. Until a definitive diagnosis is made, antimicrobial agents may be administered, and isolation enforced as a precaution against the possibility that the disease might be of bacterial origin. Nursing care is similar to the care of the child with bacterial meningitis. The clinical course of viral meningitis is much shorter and typically without any significant complications.

ENCEPHALITIS

Encephalitis can occur as a result of (1) direct invasion of the CNS by a virus or (2) postinfectious involvement of the CNS after a viral disease. Often the specific type of encephalitis may not be identified. The cause of more than one-half of the cases reported in the United States is unknown. The majority of cases of known etiology are associated with the childhood diseases of measles, mumps, varicella, and rubella and, less often, with the enteroviruses, herpesviruses, and West Nile virus.

Herpes simplex encephalitis is an uncommon disease, but 30% of cases involve children. The initial clinical findings are nonspecific (fever, altered mental status), but most cases evolve to demonstrate focal neurologic signs and symptoms. Children may experience focal seizures. The CSF is abnormal in most cases. Because of a rise in the number of children with herpes simplex encephalitis, suspected cases require prompt attention, especially because the diagnosis can be difficult. CSF polymerase chain reaction (PCR) testing can confirm the clinical diagnosis rapidly. The early use of IV acyclovir reduces mortality and morbidity. Empiric therapy with acyclovir is given before precise virologic diagnosis has been established. The multiplicity of causes of viral encephalitis makes diagnosis difficult. Most are those involved with arthropod vectors (togaviruses and bunyaviruses) and those associated with hemorrhagic fevers (arenaviruses, filoviruses, and hantaviruses). In the United States, the vector reservoir for most agents pathogenic for humans is the mosquito (St Louis or West Nile encephalitis); therefore most cases of encephalitis appear during the hot summer months and subside during the autumn.

The clinical features of encephalitis are similar regardless of the agent involved. Manifestations can range from a mild benign form that resembles aseptic meningitis, lasts a few days, and is followed by rapid and complete recovery, to fulminating encephalitis with severe CNS involvement. The onset may be sudden or gradual with malaise, fever, headache, dizziness, apathy, nuchal rigidity, nausea and vomiting, ataxia, tremors, hyperactivity, and speech difficulties (Box 46.5). In severe cases, the patient has a high fever, stupor, seizures, disorientation, spasticity, and coma that may proceed to death. Ocular palsies and paralysis also may occur.

Diagnostic Evaluation

The diagnosis is made on the basis of clinical findings and, when possible, identification of the specific virus. Early in the course of encephalitis, CT scan results may be normal. Later hemorrhagic areas in the frontotemporal region may be seen. Togaviruses (some of which were formerly labeled *arboviruses*) are rarely detected in the blood or spinal fluid, but viruses of herpes, mumps, measles, and enteroviruses may be found in the CSF. Serologic testing may be required. The first blood sample should be drawn as soon as possible after onset, with the second sample drawn 2 or 3 weeks later.

Therapeutic Management

Patients suspected of having encephalitis are hospitalized promptly for observation, including ICP monitoring. Only herpes simplex encephalitis has specific treatment available. In other cases, treatment is primarily supportive and includes conscientious nursing care, control of cerebral manifestations, and adequate nutrition and hydration, with observation and management as for other cerebral disorders. Viral encephalitis can cause devastating neurologic injury.

The prognosis for the child with encephalitis depends on the child's age, the type of organism, and residual neurologic damage. Very young children (younger than 2 years of age) may exhibit increased neurologic disabilities, including learning difficulties and epilepsy. Follow-up care with periodic reevaluation is important because symptoms are often subtle, and rehabilitation is essential for patients who develop residual effects of the disease.

Care Management

Nursing care of the child with encephalitis is the same as for any unconscious child and for children with meningitis. Additional nursing interventions include observation for deterioration in consciousness. Isolation of the child is not necessary; however, follow good hand washing technique. A main focus of nursing management is the control of rapidly rising ICP. Neurologic monitoring, administration of medications, and support of the child and parents are the major aspects of care.

RABIES

Rabies is an acute infection of the nervous system caused by a virus that is almost invariably fatal if left untreated. It is transmitted to humans by the saliva of an infected mammal and is introduced through a bite or skin abrasion. After entry into a new host, the virus multiplies in muscle cells and is spread through neural pathways without stimulating a protective host immune response.

Approximately 91% of rabies cases are transmitted by wild animals, and 9% from domestic animals (Weant & Baker, 2013). Carnivorous wild animals such as skunks, raccoons, foxes, and bats are the animals most often infected with rabies and the cause of most indigenous cases of human rabies in the United States (Weant & Baker, 2013). The circumstances of a biting incident are important. An unprovoked attack is more likely than a provoked attack to indicate a rabid animal. Bites inflicted on a child attempting to feed or handle an apparently healthy animal can generally be regarded as provoked. Any child bitten by a wild animal is assumed to be exposed to rabies.

Although rabies is common among wildlife species, human rabies is rarely acquired. The highest incidence occurs in children younger than 15 years of age. The incubation period usually ranges from 1 to 3 months but may be as short as 5 days or longer than 6 months (Willoughby, 2016). Modern-day prophylaxis is nearly 100% successful. Only 10% to 15% of people bitten develop the disease, but when symptoms are present, rabies progresses to a fatal outcome. In the United States, human fatalities associated with rabies occur in people who fail to seek medical attention, usually because they are unaware of their exposure.

The disease is characterized by a period of nonspecific symptoms, including general malaise, fever, headache, and weakness, followed by typical symptoms of severe encephalitis, including agitation, changes in LOC, and seizures. Attempts at swallowing may cause such severe spasm of the pharynx, neck, and diaphragm muscles that apnea, cyanosis, and anoxia (i.e., the characteristics from which the term *hydrophobia* was derived) are produced.

Diagnosis is made on the basis of history and clinical features. Hydrophobia is a cardinal sign of a rabies diagnosis. The diagnosis is confirmed by skin biopsy, and antibodies may be detected 7 to 8 days after the onset of clinical symptoms (Crowcroft & Thampi, 2015).

Therapeutic Management

Treatment is of little avail after symptoms appear, but the long incubation period allows time for the induction of active and passive immunity before the onset of illness. The current therapy for a rabid animal bite consists of three steps: (1) thoroughly cleansing the wound with soap and water, and avoiding suturing the wound whenever possible; (2) administering rabies vaccine; and (3) administering rabies immunoglobulin. The rabies vaccine consists of four doses administered intramuscularly at days 0, 3, 7, and 14 but can be stopped if the animal remains healthy throughout the 10-day observation period or is proved to be negative for rabies by a reliable laboratory (Crowcroft & Thampi, 2015). Rabies immunoglobulin is administered locally at the wound and provides passive antibodies at the site of exposure. Rabies immunoglobulin is given once within 7 days after the first vaccine dose before the child develops an active immune response (Crowcroft & Thampi).

Care Management

Parents and children are frightened by the urgency and seriousness of the situation. They need anticipatory guidance for the therapy and support and reassurance regarding the efficacy of the preventive measures for this dreaded disease. The vaccine is well tolerated by children, although they need preparation for the series of injections. Mass immunization is unnecessary and unlikely to be implemented. In areas where rabies is rare, the schedule given is sufficient. However, certain circumstances may warrant pre-exposure vaccination, such as when a child is being taken to an area of the world where rabies in stray dogs is still a problem.

REYE'S SYNDROME

RS is a disorder defined as metabolic encephalopathy associated with other characteristic organ involvement. It is characterized by fever, profoundly impaired consciousness, and disordered hepatic function.

The etiology of RS is not well understood, but most cases follow a common viral illness, typically influenza or varicella. RS is a condition characterized pathologically by cerebral edema and fatty changes of the liver. The onset is notable for profuse effortless vomiting and lethargy that quickly progresses to neurologic impairment, including delirium, seizures, and coma, that ultimately lead to increased ICP, herniation, and death (Ibrahim & Balistreri, 2016). The cause of RS is a mitochondrial insult induced by various viruses, drugs, exogenous toxins, and genetic factors. Elevated serum ammonia levels tend to correlate with the clinical manifestations and prognosis.

Definitive diagnosis is established by liver biopsy. The staging criteria for RS are based on liver dysfunction and neurologic signs that range from lethargy to coma. As a result of improved diagnostic techniques, children who would have been diagnosed with RS in the past are now diagnosed with other illnesses, such as viral or inborn metabolic errors affecting organic acid, ammonia, and carbohydrate metabolism. Cases of unrecognized, drug-induced encephalopathy by antiemetics given to children during viral illnesses have symptoms similar to those of RS.

The potential association between aspirin therapy for the treatment of fever in children with varicella or influenza and the development of RS precludes its use in these patients. However, by the time the US Food and Drug Administration required aspirin product labeling in 1986, most of the decline in RS incidence had already occurred.

Care Management

The most important aspect of successful management of a child with RS is early diagnosis and aggressive supportive therapy. Rapid progression to coma and high peak ammonia concentrations are associated with a more serious prognosis. Cerebral edema with increased ICP represents the most immediate threat to life.

Care and observations are implemented as for any child with an altered state of consciousness (see earlier in this chapter) and increasing ICP. Accurate and frequent monitoring of intake and output is essential for adjusting fluid volumes to prevent both dehydration and cerebral edema. Because of related liver dysfunction, monitor laboratory studies to determine impaired coagulation such as prolonged bleeding time.

Keep parents of children with RS informed of the child's progress, and explain diagnostic procedures and therapeutic management. Families need to be aware that salicylate, the alleged offending ingredient in aspirin, is contained in other products (e.g., Pepto-Bismol). They should refrain from administering any product for influenza-like symptoms without first checking the label for "hidden" salicylates.

Prognosis

Recovery from RS is rapid and usually without sequelae if the diagnosis is determined early and therapy is initiated promptly. Patients who survive have full liver function recovery (Ibrahim & Balistreri, 2016).

SEIZURE DISORDERS

A seizure is a "transient occurrence of signs and/or symptoms due to abnormal excessive and synchronous neuronal activity in the brain" (Fisher, Acevedo, Arzimanoglou, et al., 2014). Seizures are the most common pediatric neurologic disorder. About 4% to 10% of children will have at least one seizure by 16 years of age (Mikati & Hani, 2016). Seizures are caused by excessive and disorderly neuronal discharges in the brain. The manifestation of seizures depends on the region of the brain in which they originate and may include unconsciousness or altered consciousness, involuntary movements, and changes in perception, behaviors, sensations, and/or posture.

Seizures are a symptom of an underlying disease process. Potential causes include infectious, intracranial lesions or hemorrhage, metabolic disorders, trauma, brain malformations, genetic disorders, or toxic ingestion. *Epilepsy* is a condition characterized by two or more unprovoked seizures more than 24 hours apart and can be caused by a variety of pathologic processes in the brain. A single seizure event is not classified as epilepsy and is generally not treated with long-term antiepileptic drugs. Some seizures may result from an acute medical or neurologic illness and cease after the illness is treated. In other cases, children may have one or more seizures without the cause ever being known.

After it is determined that the child has had a seizure, it is important to classify it according to the International Classification of Epileptic Seizures. Optimum treatment and prognosis require an accurate diagnosis and a determination of the cause whenever possible.

Etiology

Seizures in children have many different causes. They are classified not only according to type but also according to etiology. Acute symptomatic seizures are associated with an acute insult, such as head trauma or meningitis. Remote symptomatic seizures are those without an immediate cause but with an identifiable prior brain injury such as major head trauma, meningitis or encephalitis, hypoxia, stroke, or a static encephalopathy such as cognitive impairment or cerebral palsy. Cryptogenic seizures are those occurring with no clear cause. Idiopathic seizures are genetic in origin. A partial list of causative factors is presented in Box 46.6.

Pathophysiology

Regardless of the etiologic factor or type of seizure, the basic mechanism is the same. Abnormal electrical discharges (1) may arise from the simultaneous activation of neurons in both hemispheres of the brain (generalized seizures); (2) may be restricted to one area of the cerebral cortex, producing manifestations characteristic of that particular anatomic focus (partial seizure); or (3) may begin in a localized area of the cortex as a partial seizure and spread to other portions of the brain and, if sufficiently extensive, produce generalized seizure activity.

A seizure occurs when there is sudden excessive excitation and loss of inhibition within neuronal circuits, allowing the circuits to amplify their discharges simultaneously. These discharges occur in response to the activity of sodium, potassium, calcium, and chloride ion channels. Normally these discharges are restrained by inhibitory mechanisms. In response to physiologic stimuli, such as brain injury or infection, genetic abnormalities, cellular dehydration, severe hypoglycemia, electrolyte imbalance, sleep deprivation, emotional stress, and toxic exposures, these abnormal neuronal discharges can spread to nearby cortex and subcortical structures. Primary generalized seizures begin with abnormal discharges in both hemispheres, which can involve connections between the thalamus and neocortex. On the basis of these characteristic neuronal discharges (manifested as stereotypic symptoms observed and reported during seizures and/or as recorded by the EEG), seizures are designated as *partial, generalized,* and *unclassified* epileptic seizures.

Seizure Classification and Clinical Manifestations

There are many different types of seizures, and each has unique clinical manifestations (Box 46.7 and Table 46.3). Seizures are classified into two major categories:

BOX 46.6 Etiology of Seizures in Children

Nonrecurrent (Acute)	Recurrent (Chronic)
• Febrile episodes	• Idiopathic epilepsy
• Intracranial infection	• Epilepsy secondary to:
• Intracranial hemorrhage	• Trauma
• Space-occupying lesions (cyst, tumor)	• Hemorrhage
• Acute cerebral edema	• Anoxia
• Anoxia	• Infections
• Toxins	• Toxins
• Drugs	• Degenerative phenomena
• Tetanus	• Congenital defects
• Lead encephalopathy	• Parasitic brain disease
• *Shigella* or *Salmonella* organisms	• Hypoglycemia injury
• Metabolic alterations:	• Epilepsy—sensory stimulus
• Hypocalcemia	• Epilepsy-stimulating states
• Hypoglycemia	• Narcolepsy and catalepsy
• Hyponatremia or hypernatremia	• Psychogenic
• Hypomagnesemia	• Tetany from hypocalcemia, alkalosis
• Alkalosis	• Hypoglycemic states
• Disorders of amino acid metabolism	• Hyperinsulinism
• Deficiency states	• Hypopituitarism
• Hyperbilirubinemia	• Adrenocortical insufficiency
	• Hepatic disorders
	• Uremia
	• Allergy
	• Cardiovascular dysfunction or syncopal episodes
	• Migraine

- Partial seizures, which have a local onset and involve a relatively small location in the brain
- Generalized seizures, which involve both hemispheres of the brain from onset or secondarily generalize from partial seizures

Diagnostic Evaluation

Establishing a diagnosis is critical for establishing a prognosis and planning appropriate treatment. The process of diagnosis in a child suspected of having had a seizure(s) or having epilepsy includes (1) determining whether the events thought to be seizures are epileptic seizures or non-epileptic events (NEEs), and (2) identifying the underlying cause, if possible. The assessment and diagnosis rely heavily on a thorough history, skilled observation, and several diagnostic tests.

It is important to differentiate epilepsy from other brief alterations in consciousness or behavior. Clinical entities that mimic seizures include staring, migraine headaches, toxic effects of drugs, syncope (fainting), breath-holding spells in infants and young children, movement disorders (tics, tremor, chorea), prolonged QT syndrome and other cardiac arrhythmias, sleep disturbances (night terrors), psychogenic seizures, rage attacks, and transient ischemic attacks (rare in children). The toxic effects of maternal drug use and withdrawal from these drugs should be considered in the differential diagnosis of new-onset seizure activity in a newborn.

A detailed description of the seizure should be obtained from the caregiver(s) who witnessed it. Ask questions about the child's behavior during the event, especially at the onset, and the time at which the seizure occurred (e.g., early morning, while awake, or during sleep). Any factors that may have precipitated the seizure are important, including fever, infection, head trauma, anxiety, fatigue, sleep deprivation, menstrual cycle, alcohol, and activity (e.g., hyperventilation or exposure

BOX 46.7 Classification and Clinical Manifestations of Seizures

Partial Seizures

Simple Partial Seizures With Motor Signs

Characterized by:

- Localized motor symptoms
- Somatosensory, psychic, autonomic symptoms
- Combination of these
- Abnormal discharges remaining unilateral

Manifestations

- Aversive seizure (most common motor seizure in children)—eye or eyes and head turn away from the side of the focus; awareness of movement or loss of consciousness
- Rolandic (Sylvan) seizure—tonic-clonic movements involving the face, salivation, arrested speech; most common during sleep
- Jacksonian march (rare in children)—orderly, sequential progression of clonic movements beginning in a foot, hand, or face and moving, or "marching," to adjacent body parts

Simple Partial Seizures With Sensory Signs

Uncommon in children younger than 8 years of age

Characterized by various sensations, including:

- Numbness, tingling, prickling, paresthesia, or pain originating in one area (e.g., face or extremities) and spreading to other parts of the body
- Visual sensations or formed images
- Motor phenomena such as posturing or hypertonia

Complex Partial Seizures (Psychomotor Seizures)

Observed more often in children from 3 years of age through adolescence

Characterized by:

- Period of altered behavior
- Amnesia for event (no recollection of behavior)
- Inability to respond to environment
- Impaired consciousness during event
- Drowsiness or sleep usually following seizure
- Confusion and amnesia possibly prolonged
- Complex sensory phenomena (aura)—most frequent sensation is strange feeling in the pit of the stomach that rises toward the throat and is often accompanied by odd or unpleasant odors or tastes; complex auditory or visual hallucinations; ill-defined feelings of elation or strangeness (e.g., déjà vu, a feeling of familiarity in a strange environment); strong feelings of fear and anxiety; a distorted sense of time and self; and in small children emission of a cry or attempt to run for help

Patterns of motor behavior:

- Stereotypic
- Similar with each subsequent seizure
- May suddenly cease activity, appear dazed, stare into space, become confused and apathetic, and become limp or stiff or display some form of posturing
- May be confused
- May perform purposeless, complicated activities in a repetitive manner (automatisms) such as walking, running, kicking, laughing, or speaking incoherently, most often followed by postictal confusion or sleep; may exhibit oropharyngeal activities such as smacking, chewing, drooling, swallowing, and nausea or abdominal pain followed by stiffness, a fall, and postictal sleep; rarely manifests actions such as rage or temper tantrums; aggressive acts uncommon during seizure

Generalized Seizures

Tonic-Clonic Seizures (Formerly Known as Grand Mal)

Most common and dramatic of all seizure manifestations

- Occur without warning
- Tonic phase lasts approximately 10 to 20 seconds

Manifestations

- Eyes roll upward
- Immediate loss of consciousness
- If standing, falls to floor or ground
- Stiffens in generalized, symmetric tonic contraction of entire body musculature
- Arms usually flexed
- Legs, head, and neck extended
- May utter a peculiar piercing cry
- Apneic, may become cyanotic
- Increased salivation and loss of swallowing reflex

  Clonic phase: lasts about 30 seconds but can vary from only a few seconds to a half hour or longer

Manifestations

- Violent jerking movements as the trunk and extremities undergo rhythmic contraction and relaxation
- May foam at the mouth
- May be incontinent of urine and feces
- As event ends, movements less intense, occurring at longer intervals and then ceasing entirely

Status epilepticus—series of seizures at intervals too brief to allow the child to regain consciousness between the time one event ends and the next begins

- Requires emergency intervention
- Can lead to exhaustion, respiratory failure, and death

  Postictal state:

- Appears to relax
- May remain semiconscious and difficult to arouse
- May awaken in a few minutes
- Remains confused for several hours
- Poor coordination
- Mild impairment of fine motor movements
- May have visual and speech difficulties
- May vomit
- When left alone, usually sleeps for several hours
- On awakening is fully conscious
- Usually feels tired and complains of sore muscles and headache
- No recollection of entire event

Absence Seizures (Formerly Called Petit Mal or Lapses)

Characterized by:

- Onset usually between 4 and 12 years of age
- More common in girls than in boys
- Usually cease at puberty
- Brief loss of consciousness
- Minimum or no alteration in muscle tone
- May go unrecognized because of little change in child's behavior
- Abrupt onset; suddenly develops 20 or more attacks daily
- Event often mistaken for inattentiveness or daydreaming

Continued

BOX 46.7   Classification and Clinical Manifestations of Seizures—cont'd

- Events possibly precipitated by hyperventilation, hypoglycemia, stresses (emotional and physiologic), fatigue, or sleeplessness

Manifestations
- Brief loss of consciousness
- Appear without warning or aura
- Usually last about 5 to 10 seconds
- Slight loss of muscle tone may cause child to drop objects
- Ability to maintain postural control; seldom falls
- Minor movements such as lip smacking, twitching of eyelids or face, or slight hand movements
- Not accompanied by incontinence
- Amnesia for episode
- May need to reorient self to previous activity

Atonic and Akinetic Seizures (Also Known as Drop Attacks)
Characterized by:
- Onset usually between 2 and 5 years of age
- Sudden, momentary loss of muscle tone and postural control
- Events recurring frequently during the day, particularly in the morning hours and shortly after awakening

Manifestations
- Loss of tone causing child to fall to the floor violently
- Unable to break fall by putting out hand
- May incur serious injury to face, head, or shoulder
- Loss of consciousness only momentary

Myoclonic Seizures
- Variety of seizure episodes
- May be isolated as benign essential myoclonus

- May occur in association with other seizure forms
Characterized by:
- Sudden, brief contractures of a muscle or group of muscles
- Occur singly or repetitively
- No postictal state
- May or may not be symmetric
- May or may not include loss of consciousness

Infantile Spasms
Also called *infantile myoclonus, massive spasms, hypsarrhythmia, salaam episodes,* or *infantile myoclonic spasms*
- Most commonly occur during the first 6 to 8 months of life
- Twice as common in boys than in girls
- Numerous seizures during the day without postictal drowsiness or sleep
- Poor outlook for normal intelligence

Manifestations
- Possible series of sudden, brief, symmetric, muscular contractions
- Head flexed, arms extended, and legs drawn up
- Eyes sometimes rolling upward or inward
- May be preceded or followed by a cry or giggling
- May or may not include loss of consciousness
- Sometimes flushing, pallor, or cyanosis
Infants who are able to sit but not stand:
- Sudden dropping forward of head and neck with trunk flexed forward and knees drawn up—the *salaam* or *jackknife* seizure
Less often: alternate clinical forms
- Extensor spasms rather than flexion of arms, legs, and trunk, and head nodding
- Lightning events involving a single, momentary, shocklike contraction of the entire body

TABLE 46.3   Comparison of Simple Partial, Complex Partial, and Absence Seizures

Clinical Manifestations	Simple Partial	Complex Partial	Absence
Age of onset	Any age	Uncommon before 3 years of age	Uncommon before 3 years of age
Frequency (per day)	Variable	Rarely over one or two times	Multiple
Duration	Usually <30 seconds	Usually >60 seconds, rarely <10 seconds	Usually <10 seconds, rarely >30 seconds
Aura	May be sole manifestation of seizure	Frequent	Never
Impaired consciousness	Never	Always	Always; brief loss of consciousness
Automatisms	Never	Frequent	Frequent
Clonic movements	Frequent	Occasional	Occasional
Postictal impairment	Rare	Frequent	Never
Mental disorientation	Rare	Common	Unusual

to strong stimuli such as bright flashing light or loud noises). Record any sensory phenomena that the child can describe and if the child was able to hear during the seizure. The duration and progression of the seizure (if any) and the postictal feelings and behavior (e.g., confusion, inability to speak, amnesia, headache, and sleep) should also be noted. For children who have epilepsy, document how often they have seizures: daily, weekly, or monthly. Knowing the age of the child when they had their first seizure is important. It is important to determine whether more than one seizure type exists. It is often more informative to ask the parents to show you what the seizure looked like rather than relying on their verbal description. Demonstrating a seizure often reveals features, such as head turning, that would otherwise go unrecognized. Some

seizures are overlooked by parents. For example, some parents may not identify brief head nods or brief single jerks as seizures unless specifically asked whether their child has these symptoms.

A thorough medical history must be obtained beginning with conception. Questions to consider include: Was the mother's pregnancy complicated by illness and drug use, either prescribed or recreational? How old was the baby when discharged from the hospital after birth? Has the child had any overnight hospitalizations or surgeries? A complete history is designed to uncover possible risk factors for the development of seizures or epilepsy.

The family history should include whether other family members have ever had a seizure of any kind, cognitive impairments, cerebral palsy, autism, or other neurologic disorders. Ask if there is a family history of sudden, unexpected deaths. A family history can offer clues to paroxysmal disorders, such as migraine headaches, breath-holding spells, febrile seizures, or neurologic diseases.

A complete physical and neurologic examination, including developmental assessment of language, learning, behavior, and motor abilities, may provide clues to the cause of the seizures. A number of laboratory and neuroimaging tests may be ordered, depending on the child's age, whether it is a new-onset seizure, characteristics of the seizure, and the history. Laboratory studies that may prove valuable include a white blood cell count (for signs of infection) and blood glucose measurements that may indicate hypoglycemic episodes. Serum electrolytes, blood urea nitrogen, calcium, serum amino acids, lactate, ammonia, and urine organic acids may indicate metabolic disturbances. Blood for chromosomal analysis may also be tested if a genetic etiology is suspected. A toxic screen should be performed if alcohol or drug ingestion is suspected. Lumbar puncture can confirm a suspected diagnosis of meningitis. CT may be done to detect a cerebral hemorrhage, infarctions, and gross malformations. MRI provides greater anatomic detail and is used to detect developmental malformations, tumors, and cortical dysplasias.

An EEG is obtained for most children with seizures. The EEG is the most useful tool for evaluating the child's risk for recurrent seizures, helping to determine the type of seizure the child had, and diagnosing the type of epilepsy. It confirms the presence of abnormal electrical discharges and provides information on the seizure type and the focus. The EEG is carried out under varying conditions (e.g., with the child asleep, awake, awake with provocative stimulation [flashing lights, noise], and hyperventilation). Stimulation may elicit abnormal electrical activity, which is recorded on the EEG. Various seizure types produce characteristic EEG patterns: high-voltage spike discharges are seen in tonic-clonic seizures, with abnormal patterns in the intervals between seizures; a three-per-second spike and wave pattern is observed in an absence seizure; and absence of electrical activity in an area suggests a large lesion such as an abscess or subdural collection of fluid.

A normal EEG does not rule out seizures because the EEG is only a surface recording. It only represents approximately 1 hour of time and therefore may show normal interictal activity. If there is concern about whether a child has seizures or the seizure type cannot be determined, then a long-term video EEG may be done to record the child during wakefulness and sleep. The full-body image is recorded on video, with selected EEG channels displayed on the same screen for simultaneous recording and viewing. Although the EEG is very valuable, it should not be used alone to determine the type of seizure. Rather, the EEG interpretation along with a thorough clinical description of the child's behavior during the seizure episode guides to the correct classification of the seizure and the appropriate treatment choice.

Therapeutic Management

The goal of treatment of seizures and epilepsy is to control the seizures or reduce their frequency and severity so that the child may live as normal a life as possible. Discovering and, when possible, correcting the underlying cause of the seizures can lead to complete control of all seizures. If the seizure activity is a manifestation of an infectious, traumatic, or metabolic process, the seizure therapy is instituted as part of the general therapeutic regimen. Management of epilepsy has four treatment options: drug therapy, the ketogenic diet, vagus nerve stimulation (VNS), and epilepsy surgery.

Drug Therapy

It is known that people predisposed to epilepsy have seizures when their basal level of neuronal excitability exceeds a critical point; no event occurs if the excitability is maintained below this threshold. The administration of antiepileptic drugs serves to raise this threshold and prevent seizures. Consequently, the primary therapy for seizure disorders is the administration of the appropriate antiepileptic drug or combination of drugs in a dosage that provides the desired effect without causing undesirable side effects or toxicity. Antiepileptic drugs are believed to exert their effect primarily by reducing the responsiveness of normal neurons to the sudden, high-frequency nerve impulses that arise in the epileptogenic focus. Thus the seizure is effectively suppressed; however, the abnormal brain waves may or may not be altered. The chance of total control of seizures depends on the underlying cause of the seizures.

The initiation of anticonvulsant therapy is based on several factors, including the child's age, type of seizure, risk for recurrence, and other comorbid or predisposing medical issues. For children who develop recurrent seizures or epilepsy, treatment is begun with a single drug known to be effective and have the lowest toxicity (i.e., the safest side-effect profile for the child's particular type of seizure). The dosage is gradually increased until the seizures are controlled or the maximum recommended dose has been reached and seizures are still not controlled. If a child develops intolerable side effects, the medication is stopped and another one is tried. If the drug reduces but does stop all the seizures, a second drug is added in gradually increasing doses. When seizures are controlled, the first drug may be tapered to reduce the potential adverse effects and drug interactions of polytherapy. Mono-therapy remains the treatment method of choice for epilepsy, but a combination of medications may be a viable alternative for children who cannot attain seizure control with only one medication (Mikati & Hani, 2016).

Sleepiness, changes in mood or behavior, vision changes, and ataxia are some of the potential side effects of antiepileptic medications. These are very distressing to both children and families. They often disappear over time or when drug dosages are reduced. Blood cell counts, urinalysis, and liver function tests are obtained at regular intervals in children receiving particular antiepileptic medications that can affect organ function. If complete seizure control is maintained on an anticonvulsant drug for 2 years, it may be safe to slowly discontinue the drug for patients with no risk factors. When seizure medications are discontinued, the dosage is decreased gradually over weeks or months. Sudden withdrawal of a drug is not recommended because it can cause seizures, which may be longer and more intense than previously, to recur. Risk factors for recurrence of seizures include older age at onset, numerous seizures before control is achieved, presence of a neurologic dysfunction (e.g., motor or cognitive impairment), and the characteristics of epilepsy syndrome (Verrotti, D'Egidio, Agostinelli, et al., 2012). Recurrence occurs most frequently within the first year of discontinuation (Braun & Schmidt, 2014).

💊 MEDICATION ALERT

Intravenous (IV) fosphenytoin is often used to treat seizures instead of IV phenytoin because of possible complications and drug interactions associated with IV phenytoin. If IV phenytoin is used, it should be administered via slow IV push at a rate that does not exceed 50 mg/min. Because phenytoin precipitates when mixed with glucose, only normal saline is used to flush the tubing or catheter. Fosphenytoin may be given in saline or glucose solutions at a rate of up to 150 mg phenytoin equivalent (PE)/min, and it may be given intramuscularly if necessary.

Ketogenic Diet

The ketogenic diet is a high-fat, low-carbohydrate, and adequate protein diet (Kossoff, 2013). Consumption of the ketogenic diet forces the body to shift from using glucose as the primary energy source to using fat, and the individual develops a state of ketosis. Ketones can be measured in both the child's urine and blood. The mechanism(s) of action remain unclear. The diet is rigorous. All foods and liquids that the child consumes must be carefully weighed and measured. The diet is deficient in vitamins and minerals; therefore vitamin and mineral supplementation is necessary. Early side effects of the diet are diarrhea, hypoglycemia, dehydration, acidosis, and lethargy; long-term side effects include dyslipidemia, kidney stones, and poor growth (Kossoff, 2013).

The ketogenic diet has been shown to be an efficacious and tolerable treatment for medically refractory seizures, with seizure control comparable to antiepileptic drugs in some children. In a meta-analysis of the ketogenic diet, at least 38% of children had a 50% reduction in seizures for at least 1 year (Levy, Cooper & Giri, 2012).

Vagus Nerve Stimulation

VNS was developed as a palliative treatment for patients with seizures not controlled by drugs and who are not candidates for diet or surgical therapy (Moshé, Perucca, Ryvlin, et al., 2015). It is currently indicated as adjunct therapy in patients 12 years of age and older with partial-onset seizures (with or without secondary generalization) who are refractory to antiepileptic drugs (Elliott, Rodgers, Bassani, et al., 2011). A programmable signal generator is implanted subcutaneously in the chest. Electrodes tunneled beneath the skin deliver electrical impulses to the left vagus nerve (cranial nerve X). The device is programmed noninvasively to deliver a precise pattern of stimulation to the left vagus nerve. The patient or caregiver can activate the device using a magnet at the onset of a seizure. No long-term adverse effects have been reported with VNS, but dysphonia, throat or neck pain, and cough can occur during stimulation. Studies show that approximately one-third to one-half of patients have a reduction in seizures after 1 year of therapy (Elliott et al, 2011).

Surgical Therapy

When seizures are determined to be caused by a hematoma, vascular malformation, or tumor, surgical removal is usually recommended. Epilepsy surgery is the most effective treatment for children with medically refractory epilepsy due to focal cortical dysplasia and mesial temporal sclerosis. About 80% of these patients will be seizure-free 4 years after surgery (Moosa & Gupta, 2014). Refractory seizures are usually defined as the persistence of seizures despite adequate trials of three antiepileptic medications, alone or in combination (Téllez-Zenteno, Hernández-Ronquillo, Buckley, et al., 2014). Epilepsy surgery does not always eliminate the need for antiepileptic drug therapy. The goal is to improve seizure control without worsening or producing serious deficits. Some children will see improvements in their cognition, behavior, and quality of life (Ryvlin, Cross, & Rheims, 2014). Types of surgeries include focal resection of the epileptogenic focus, functional hemispherectomy, and corpus callosotomy, which severs the connection between the hemispheres.

Status Epilepticus

Status epilepticus is a continuous seizure that lasts more than 30 minutes or a series of seizures from which the child does not regain a premorbid LOC (Huff & Fountain, 2011). It has been suggested that the term *impending status epilepticus* be used for a continuous seizure or series of seizures lasting between 5 and 30 minutes with the designation of *impending status* indicating that treatment should begin after 5 minutes of seizure activity (Freilich, Schreiber, Zelleke, et al., 2014). The initial treatment is directed toward support of vital functions (i.e., the CABs of life support, administering oxygen, and gaining IV access) immediately followed by IV administration of antiepileptic agents (Dulac & Takahashi,

2013). Simultaneously with life support measures and emergency medications, the underlying cause of the status epilepticus is identified and corrected (Abend & Loddenkemper, 2014).

 MEDICATION ALERT

Buccal midazolam and rectal diazepam are quick, effective, and safe treatments for home or prehospital treatment of status epilepticus (Shorvon, 2011). Cessation of seizure occurred in 8 minutes with buccal midazolam and 15 minutes with rectal diazepam (Shorvon, 2011). Respiratory depression is a potential side effect when more than two doses are given (Abend & Loddenkemper, 2014), and patients should be monitored closely after administration. Intranasal midazolam is safe and effective for stopping seizures and also easier to administer than rectal diazepam or buccal lorazepam.

For in-hospital management of status epilepticus, IV diazepam or lorazepam (Ativan) is the first-line drug of choice (Abend & Loddenkemper, 2014). Lorazepam is the preferred agent because of its rapid onset (2 to 5 minutes) and long half-life (12 to 24 hours). The child must be monitored closely during administration to detect early alterations in vital signs that may indicate impending respiratory depression. When a benzodiazepine (diazepam or lorazepam) is ineffective, IV phenytoin or IV fosphenytoin or IV phenobarbital is given as the next line of treatment. This combination of therapy places the child at high risk for apnea; therefore respiratory support is generally necessary. Children may also receive an antiepileptic medication, IV valproate or levetiracetam. Children who continue to have seizures despite this drug treatment may require general anesthesia with a continuous infusion of midazolam, propofol, or pentobarbital (Abend & Loddenkemper, 2014). In this situation, the child will need to be intubated, and continuous EEG monitoring begun to monitor for and treat electrographic seizures (Abend & Loddenkemper).

Nursing care of a child with status epilepticus includes, in addition to the CABs of life support, monitoring blood pressure and body temperature. During the first 30 to 45 minutes of the seizure, the blood pressure may be elevated. Thereafter, the blood pressure typically returns to normal but may be decreased, depending on the medications being administered for seizure control. Hyperthermia requiring treatment may occur as a result of increased motor activity. Status epilepticus is a medical emergency that requires immediate intervention to prevent possible brain injury and death. Diagnosis and correction of the underlying cause of the status epilepticus is essential.

Prognosis

Only about one-half of children who experience a first seizure will experience additional seizures (El-Radhi, 2015). Therefore, children who have had a single seizure are rarely started on anti-epileptic drugs. Prognosis for eventual remission of childhood epilepsy depends on the etiology and epilepsy syndrome diagnosis. Some seizures almost always remit, whereas others almost never do (Camfield & Camfield, 2014). Intractable seizures are failure to control seizures after two appropriately selected antiepileptic medications are trialed (Wassenaar, Leijten, Egberts, et al., 2013). Most mortality in children with epilepsy is due to factors associated with a child's coexisting neurologic conditions and poorly controlled seizures (Berg & Rychlik, 2015). Deaths from epilepsy in children who have no other neurologic conditions occur at the same rate as childhood deaths from other causes, such as accidents (Nickels, Grosshardt, & Wirrell, 2012).

Interprofessional Care Management

An important responsibility among all health care providers is to observe the seizure episode and accurately document the events. Any alterations

BOX 46.8   General Observations: The Child During a Seizure

Observations During Seizure

Describe

Order of events (before, during, and after)

Duration of seizure

- Tonic-clonic—from first signs of event until jerking stops
- Absence—from loss of consciousness until consciousness is regained
- Complex partial—from first sign of unresponsiveness, motor activity, and automatisms until there are signs of responsiveness to environment

Onset

Time of onset

Significant precipitating events—missed medication dosage, illness, stress, sleep deprivation, menses

Behavior

Change in facial expression

Cry or other sound

Stereotypic or automatous movements

Random activity (wandering)

Position of eyes, head, body, extremities

Unilateral or bilateral posturing of one or more extremities

Movement

Change of position, if any

Site of commencement—hand, thumb, mouth, generalized

- Tonic phase—length, parts of body involved
- Clonic phase—twitching or jerking movements, parts of body involved, sequence of parts involved, generalized, change in character of movements
- Lack of movement or muscle tone of body part or entire body

Face

- Color change—pallor, cyanosis, flushing
- Perspiration

- Mouth—position, deviating to one side, teeth clenched, tongue bitten, frothing at mouth, flecks of blood or bleeding
- Lack of expression
- Asymmetric expression

Eyes

- Position—straight ahead, deviation upward or outward, conjugate or divergent gaze
- Pupils—change in size, equality, reaction to light

Respiratory Effort

- Presence and length of apnea

Other

- Incontinence

Postictal Observations

- Duration of postictal period
- State of consciousness
- Orientation
- Arousability
- Motor ability
- Any change in motor function
- Ability to move all extremities
- Paresis or weakness
- Speech
- Sensations
- Complaint of discomfort or pain
- Any sensory impairment
- Recollection of preseizure sensations or aura

---

in behavior preceding the seizure and the characteristics of the episode, such as sensory-hallucinatory phenomena (e.g., an aura), motor effects (e.g., eye movements, muscular contractions), alterations in consciousness, and postictal state (e.g., behavior after the seizure) are noted and recorded (Box 46.8). Health care providers should describe only what is observed rather than trying to label a seizure type. Note the duration of the seizure with start and stop times.

Based on a thorough assessment, several nursing diagnoses are identified. The more common diagnoses for the child with a seizure disorder are included in the Nursing Care Plan: The Child with Seizures.

The child must be protected from injury during the seizure. Nursing observations made during the event provide valuable information for diagnosis and management of the disorder (see Emergency Treatment box: Seizures).

It is impossible to physically stop a seizure once it has begun, and no attempt should be made to do so. Health care providers must remain calm, stay with the child, and prevent the child from sustaining any harm during the seizure. If possible, isolate the child from the view of others by closing a door or curtain. If other people are present, they should be assured that everything is being done for the child. After the seizure, they can be given a simple explanation about the event as needed.

If the health care provider is able to reach the child in time, a child who is standing or seated in a chair is eased to the floor immediately.

Do not remove a child from a wheelchair as the wheelchair provides support and padding. During (and sometimes after) the tonic-clonic seizure, the swallowing reflex is lost, salivation increases, and the tongue is hypotonic. Therefore, the child is at risk for aspiration and airway occlusion. Placing the child on the side facilitates drainage and helps maintain a patent airway. Suctioning the oral cavity and posterior oropharynx may be necessary. Take vital signs, and allow the child to rest if at school or away from home. When feasible, the child is integrated back into the environment. Sending a child with a chronic seizure disorder home from school is not necessary unless requested by the parents.

Seizure precautions are required for children who have a history of seizures (Box 46.9).

Long-Term Care

Care of the child with epilepsy involves physical care and instruction regarding the importance of adherence to the treatment plan. Probably more significant is education and support regarding the potential for the development of psychosocial, educational, and emotional problems in children with epilepsy and their families. Few diseases generate as much anxiety among families, friends, and school personnel as epilepsy. Fears and misconceptions about the disease and its treatment are common. For many it represents the archetype of severe hereditary affliction. Care is directed toward educating the child and family about epilepsy, helping them develop strategies for coping with the psychosocial

NURSING CARE PLAN
The Child With Seizures

Case Study
Jacob is a 7-year-old male who was playing during physical education class at school when he suddenly stopped his activity, stared into space, repetitively moved his left arm up and down, and smacked his lips. After approximately 1 minute, he stopped the behavior and was drowsy but responsive to his environment. Jacob had no memory of the event. Jacob was accompanied to the school nurse by his teacher for further assessment.

Assessment
Based on these events, what are the most important subjective and objective data that should be assessed?

Defining Characteristics
From patient:
> Aura
> Sensory phenomena that the child can describe during the event (i.e., ability to hear)
> Postictal feelings (i.e., confusion, inability to speak, amnesia, headache, sleepiness)

From person who observed the seizure:
> Time of onset of seizure
> Duration of seizure
> Change in level of consciousness (LOC) before, during, and after the seizure
> Movements (ask for demonstration of the seizure rather than relying on verbal description)

From parent or primary caregiver:
> Previous seizures
> Family history of seizures
> Recent illness
> Current medications

Nursing Diagnoses
Risk for Injury
Risk for Aspiration
Risk for Ineffective Coping

Nursing Interventions and Rationales
What are the most appropriate nursing interventions for a child with seizures?

Nursing Interventions	Rationales
Monitor time (onset and duration), movements, and LOC during seizure.	To provide an accurate description of the seizure, including the order of events before, during, and after the seizure
If Jacob is at risk for falling, ease him to floor. Prevent Jacob from hitting head on objects. Do not attempt to restrain him or use force.	To prevent physical harm
During seizure, place Jacob in a side-lying position on a flat surface such as floor. Do not put anything in his mouth.	To prevent possible aspiration
Stay with Jacob, and reassure him when awakening from seizure.	To decrease Jacob's anxiety and fear
Evaluate postictal feelings.	To provide accurate description of the postictal state

Nursing Interventions	Rationales
Ensure antiepileptic drugs are being administered as directed.	To prevent further seizure activity
Involve Jacob and parents in discussion of fears, anxieties, and resources and support options available to them.	To promote coping by discussing fear and anxieties and encouraging participation in support resources

Expected Outcomes
Jacob will not experience physical injury as a result of seizure activity.
Jacob's airway will remain patent.
Jacob and his parents will cope with the condition and receive adequate support.

Case Study (Continued)
The following week, Jacob had another seizure while playing with his siblings in the backyard. His brother ran inside to get help, and Jacob's mother ran outside to see Jacob staring into space with his head turned to the side and his left arm moving rhythmically up and down. This activity stopped for a few seconds then started back again. Jacob did not regain consciousness in between the episodes and was unable to speak. Jacob's mother called for emergency assistance (911), and Jacob was transported to a nearby hospital. Jacob had not regained consciousness during the transport.

Assessment
What are the most important signs and symptoms based in this child?

Defining Characteristics
Series of seizure activity
Lack of consciousness between seizures
Do the findings described in the case study concern you?
The fact that the child is not regaining a premorbid LOC between seizures is concerning and meets criteria for a diagnosis of status epilepticus. The child's circulation, airway, breathing (CABs) should be monitored closely and supportive measures initiated (i.e., cardiopulmonary resuscitation) when indicated.

Nursing Diagnoses
Risk for Impaired Breathing Pattern
Risk for Aspiration
Risk for Injury
Risk for Imbalanced Body Temperature
Risk for Impaired Cardiovascular Function

Nursing Interventions and Rationales
What are the most appropriate nursing interventions for Jacob?

Nursing Interventions	Rationales
Monitor airway, breathing, and circulation (CABs) closely.	To provide supportive measures as needed to maintain airway, breathing, and circulation
Monitor and record characteristics, onset, and duration of each episode including motor effects, alterations in consciousness, and postictal state.	To accurately describe the seizure activity and postictal state

NURSING CARE PLAN
The Child With Seizures—cont'd

Nursing Interventions	Rationales
Do not attempt to stop the seizure; ease Jacob to the floor if upright. A child in a wheelchair usually has adequate support and padding and does not need to be removed. Side rails should be padded for a child on a stretcher.	To prevent injury during seizure
Place Jacob in a side-lying position; suction the oral cavity and posterior oropharynx as needed.	During seizures, the swallowing reflex may be lost, salivation may increase, and the tongue is hypotonic, which causes the child to be at risk for aspiration and airway occlusion.
Administration of antiepileptic medications • During transport: buccal or intranasal midazolam, buccal lorazepam, rectal diazepam • Upon arrival to the hospital: Intravenous (IV) lorazepam, valproate, or levetiracetam	To decrease or stop the seizure activity
Closely monitor vital signs including temperature, respirations, heart rate, and blood pressure.	Hyperthermia and hypertension are a common result of increased motor activity. In addition, side effects from the medications may cause respiratory depression.
If possible, isolate Jacob from view of others by closing door or curtain.	To maintain privacy for Jacob and family and to minimize distress to the family, and other visitors
Perform diagnostic testing as indicated.	To determine the underlying cause of status epilepticus

Expected Outcomes
Jacob will have effective ventilation.
Jacob's airway will remain patent.
Jacob will not experience physical injury as a result of seizure activity.
Jacob's body temperature will remain in acceptable range
Jacob's blood pressure will remain normal for age

Case Study (Continued)
Jacob's parents are anxious and upset with the seizures. You are concerned that they do not understand what is happening to their son.

Assessment
What are the most important aspects of care to discuss with her parents at this time?

Defining Characteristics of Family's Knowledge
Understands definition of seizure and status epilepticus
Describes measures implemented to prevent harm during seizure

Describes treatment regimen including rationale for medications
Expresses fears and concerns
Shows appropriate reactions to child's condition

Nursing Diagnosis
Readiness for Enhanced Knowledge related to parents' interest in Jacob's health status.

Nursing Interventions and Rationales
What are the most appropriate nursing interventions for this diagnosis?

Nursing Interventions	Rationales
Educate family about characteristics of seizures including aura, seizure activity, and postictal state.	To promote understanding of seizures, including signs of impending seizure and characteristics to monitor during and after seizure
Educate family about safety precautions before and during a seizure including side-lying positioning, padding area if needed, and not placing items in mouth or attempting to stop the seizure.	To promote understanding of measures needed to protect Jacob from harm
Educate family about Jacob's medication administration including scheduled and as necessary (prn) medications and potential side effects of medications.	To promote understanding of medications including monitoring for side effects
Arrange for social worker to meet with family to assess emotional and financial needs. Consider consultation with child life specialist to assist with education of school personnel and classmates.	To identify and modify stressors associated with chronic illnesses and to assist with re-entry into school
Education family about Jacob's daily care including the following: • Have Jacob wear medical identification. • Always swim with a companion. • Shower preferred, and bathe only with close supervision. • Use protective helmet and padding during bicycle riding, skateboarding, and in-line skating.	To promote understanding of safety measures for daily life

Expected Outcomes
Parents will verbalize understanding of seizure and status epilepticus and necessary monitoring.
Parents will verbalize safety measures for daily living and during seizure activity.
Parents will verbalize understanding of medications, including schedule, route, and potential side effects.
Parents will verbalize resources available for emotional, financial, and school support as indicated.

problems related to epilepsy, and directing them to resources for children and families living with epilepsy.

Children with epilepsy are prescribed antiepileptic medications. These medications are administered at regular intervals to maintain adequate levels in the blood. It is sometimes easy to skip doses or omit them for a variety of reasons, especially when the child is free from seizures most of the time. This is particularly so when the child is older and assumes responsibility for his or her medication. It is important to impress on the family and child, the importance of giving the antiepileptic medication as scheduled to prevent recurrent seizures. In general, antiepileptic medications are continued until the child has been seizure free for 2 years (Braun & Schmidt, 2014). The medication

✚ EMERGENCY TREATMENT

Seizures

Tonic-Clonic Seizure

During the Seizure
- Remain calm.
- Time seizure episode.
- If child is standing or seated, ease child down to floor.
- Turn child to one side.
- Place pillow or folded blanket under child's head.
- Loosen restrictive clothing.
- Remove eyeglasses.
- Clear area of any hazards or hard objects.
- Allow seizure to end without interference.
- Do not:
  - Attempt to restrain child or use force to control his or her movements.
  - Put anything in child's mouth.
  - Give any food or liquids.

After the Seizure
- Time postictal period.
- Check for breathing. Check position of head and tongue.
- Reposition if head is hyperextended. If child is not breathing, give rescue breathing and call EMS.
- Keep child on side.
- Remain with child.
- Do not give food or liquids until child is fully alert and swallowing reflex has returned.
- Look for medical identification, and determine which factors occurred before onset of seizure that may have been triggering factors.
- Check head and body for possible injuries.
- Check inside of mouth to see if tongue or lips have been bitten.

Complex Partial Seizure

During the Seizure
- Do not restrain child's movements.
- Remove harmful objects from area.
- Redirect to safe area.
- Talk in calm, reassuring manner.
- Do not expect child to follow instructions.
- Watch to see if seizure generalizes.

After the Seizure
- Stay with child, and reassure until fully conscious.

Call EMS if:
- Child stops breathing.
- There is evidence of injury, or child has diabetes or is pregnant.
- Seizure lasts for more than 5 minutes (unless duration of seizure is typically longer than 5 minutes), and written medical order is present.
- Seizures continue for more than 10 minutes after administration of rescue medication.
- Status epilepticus occurs.
- Pupils are not equal after seizure.
- Child vomits continuously 30 minutes after seizure has ended (sign of possible acute problem).
- Child cannot be awakened and is unresponsive to pain after seizure has ended.
- Seizure occurs in water.
- This is child's first seizure.

EMS, Emergency medical services.

Modified from Epilepsy Foundation. (2013). *Seizure recognition and first aid*. Retrieved from http://www.epilepsynw.org/wp-content/themes/epilepsy/brochures/First-Aid-and-Seizure-Response/Seizure-Recognition-and-First-Aid.pdf .

BOX 46.9   Seizure Precautions

The extent of precautions depends on type, severity, and frequency of seizures. They may include the following:
- Side rails raised when child is sleeping or resting
- Side rails and other hard objects padded
- Waterproof mattress or pad on bed or crib

Appropriate precautions during potentially hazardous activities may include the following:
- Swimming with a companion
- Showers preferred; bathing only with close supervision
- Use of protective helmet and padding during bicycle riding, skateboarding, and in-line skating
- Supervision during use of hazardous machinery or equipment
  Have child carry or wear medical identification.
  Alert other caregivers to need for any special precautions.
  Child may not drive or operate hazardous machinery or equipment unless seizure free for designated period (varies by state).

is then slowly tapered over a period of weeks to decrease the possibility of precipitating a seizure. The seizure threshold may be lowered during any illness but particularly with fever. Therefore parents should be aware that, if their child has an illness, he or she is at increased risk for seizures. They should contact their health care provider if the child misses medications during an illness because of vomiting.

Rectal preparations of some antiepileptic medications are highly effective when a child is unable to take oral medications because of repeated vomiting, surgery, or status epilepticus. Parents can learn to administer rectal antiepileptic medication for home treatment. Buccal and intranasal midazolam or rectal diazepam are useful adjunctive home treatment for children at risk for prolonged seizures or clusters of seizures and can minimize the need for hospitalization while enhancing parental confidence.

💊 MEDICATION ALERT

Children taking phenobarbital or phenytoin should receive adequate vitamin D and folic acid because deficiencies of both have been associated with these drugs. Phenytoin should not be taken with milk.

Nurses should educate the child and parents about the possible adverse reactions to the medications used to treat seizures. Parents must understand the rare but potentially serious side effect of allergic reaction to the medication. They must immediately report rashes to the child's health care provider. More common but less serious potential side effects include excessive sleepiness, changes in appetite, and worsening behavior and mood. Parents should be encouraged to share their observations with their child's health care provider. Parents should understand that the child needs periodic physical assessment. Depending on the medication prescribed, some children will need regular testing of their complete blood count and liver functions. Possible adverse effects on the hematopoietic system, liver, and kidneys may be reflected in symptoms, such as fever, sore throat, enlarged lymph nodes, jaundice, and bleeding (e.g., easy bruising, petechiae, ecchymosis, and epistaxis). Children with epilepsy are not at increased risk for injury with the exception of head injury (Baca, Vickrey, Vassar, et al., 2013). The degree to which activities are restricted is individualized for each child and depends on the type, frequency, and severity of the seizures; the child's response to therapy; and the length of time the seizures have been controlled. To prevent head injuries, children should always wear helmets and other safety devices when participating in sports, such as biking, skiing, skateboarding, horseback riding, and in-line skating. Only children with frequent seizures must avoid these activities. Children with epilepsy should avoid activities involving heights, such as climbing on play structures taller than they are. Submersion injuries are a serious risk for children with a history of seizures. Children should never be left alone in the bathtub, even for a few seconds. Older children and adolescents should be encouraged to use a shower and reminded not to lock the bathroom door when showering. They must have eyes-on supervision at all times when swimming. Because the child is encouraged to attend school, camp, and other normal activities, the school nurse and teachers should be made aware of the child's condition and therapy. They can help ensure regularity of medication administration and provision of any special care the child might need. Teachers, child care providers, camp counselors, youth organization leaders, coaches, and other adults who assume responsibility for children should be instructed regarding care of the child during a seizure so that they can react calmly, provide for the child's safety, and influence the attitude of the child's peers.

Triggering Factors

Careful and detailed documentation of seizures over time may indicate a pattern of seizures. About one-half of the people 12 years of age and older with epilepsy can recognize at least one trigger for their seizures (Wassenaar, Kasteleijn-Nolst Trenité, de Haan, et al., 2014). When this occurs, the child, nurse, or responsible adult can intervene to make changes in the lifestyle or environment that may prevent seizures or decrease their frequency. Often the necessary changes are simple but can make an enormous difference in the lives of the child and family.

The most common factors that may trigger seizures in children include emotional stress, sleep deprivation, fatigue, fever, and illness (Novakova, Harris, Ponnusamy, et al., 2013). Other precipitating factors include flickering lights, menstrual cycle, and alcohol (Wassenaar et al., 2014). Some individuals have pattern- or photo-sensitive epilepsy (i.e., seizures precipitated by changes in dark-light patterns such as those that occur with a flash on a camera, automobile headlights, reflections of light on snow or water, or rotating blades on a fan). Most of these individuals have absence, myoclonic, or generalized tonic-clonic seizures. A small minority of children have seizures while playing video games. Only these children need to be restricted from playing video games.

FEBRILE SEIZURES

A febrile seizure is a seizure associated with a febrile illness in a child who does not have a CNS infection. By definition, children who have a febrile seizure cannot have a history of neonatal or unprovoked seizures (Syndi Seinfeld & Pellock, 2013). Febrile seizures are the single most common seizure type, occurring in 2% to 5% of children between 1 month and 5 years of age (Syndi Seinfeld & Pellock).

There is evidence for both genetic and environmental causes for febrile seizures. Children with a family history of febrile seizures are at increased risk for both a single febrile seizure (10% to 46%) and for recurrent febrile seizures (Saghazadeh, Mastrangelo, & Rezaei, 2014). Environmental factors that have been implicated include a viral illness and an age younger than 18 months (Mewasingh, 2014).

Most febrile seizures have stopped by the time the child is taken to a medical facility and require no treatment. If the seizure continues for more than 5 minutes, it is likely that it will continue for some time (Seinfeld, Shinnar, Sun, et al., 2014). Initial treatment consists of administering a benzodiazepine: IV lorazepam; IV or rectal diazepam; or IV, buccal, or intranasal midazolam. The majority of children with febrile status epilepticus will require administration of multiple anti-epileptic medications for seizure control (Seinfeld et al). Antipyretic therapies will not prevent a seizure and are ineffective at lowering the temperature of a fever that leads to a febrile seizure (Rosenbloom, Finkelstein, Adams-Webber, et al., 2013). Tepid sponge baths are not recommended for several reasons: they are ineffective in significantly lowering the temperature, the shivering effect further increases metabolic output, and cooling causes discomfort to the child. Parental education and emotional support are important interventions. Information may need to be repeated depending on the parents' anxiety and education level. Parents need reassurance that children who have had febrile seizures but do not have underlying developmental problems will perform as well as other children academically and behaviorally.

There is no indication for the use of daily prophylactic antiepileptic medication for febrile seizures because the risk for adverse side effects outweighs any potential benefit (Offringa & Newton, 2013). Children who have had four or more febrile seizures, have a family history of epilepsy, and have complex febrile seizures have an increased risk but still a low rate of 2% to 7%, for developing epilepsy throughout the life span (Pavlidou & Panteliadis, 2013). The mechanism is unknown but is thought to be primarily genetic.

> **! NURSING ALERT**
>
> If a febrile seizure lasts more than 5 minutes, parents should seek medical attention right away. They should call for emergency assistance (911) and not place the child who is actively having a seizure in the car.

CEREBRAL MALFORMATIONS

CRANIAL DEFORMITIES

Hydrocephalus

Hydrocephalus is a condition caused by an imbalance in the production and absorption of CSF in the ventricular system. When production is greater than absorption, CSF accumulates within the ventricular system, usually under increased pressure, producing passive dilation of the ventricles.

Pathophysiology

The causes of hydrocephalus are varied, but the result is either (1) impaired absorption of CSF fluid within the subarachnoid space, obliteration of the subarachnoid cisterns, or malfunction of the arachnoid villi (*nonobstructive* or *communicating hydrocephalus*); or (2) obstruction to the flow of CSF through the ventricular system (*obstructive* or *noncommunicating hydrocephalus*) (Kinsman & Johnston, 2016). Any imbalance of secretion and absorption causes an increased accumulation of CSF in the ventricles, which become dilated (ventriculomegaly) and compress the brain substance against the surrounding rigid bony cranium. When this occurs before fusion of the cranial sutures, it causes enlargement of the skull and dilation of the ventricles (Fig. 46.7). In children younger than 12 years of age, previously closed suture lines, especially the sagittal

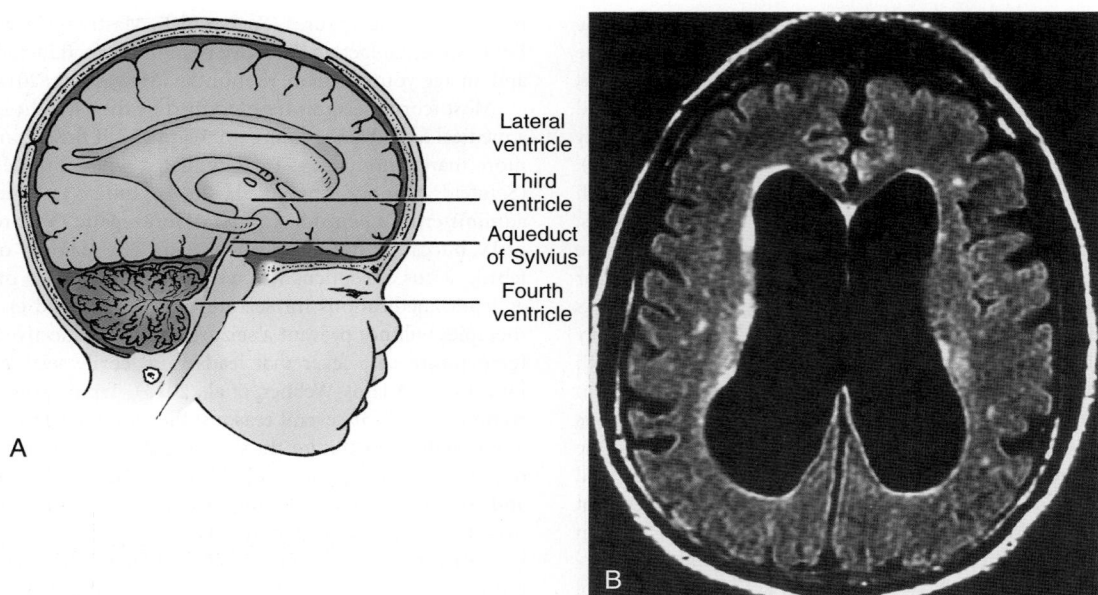

FIG 46.7 Hydrocephalus: a block in flow of cerebrospinal fluid (CSF). **A,** Patent CSF circulation. **B,** Normal-pressure hydrocephalus. (B, From Nadgir, R., Yousem, D.M. [2017]. *Neuroradiology: The prerequisites* [2nd ed.]. St. Louis, MO: Elsevier.)

suture, may become diastatic or opened. After 12 years of age, the sutures are fused and will not open.

Most cases of hydrocephalus are a result of developmental malformations. Although the defect usually is apparent in early infancy, it may become evident at any time from the prenatal period to late childhood or early adulthood. Other causes include neoplasms, CNS infections, and trauma. An obstruction to the normal flow can occur at any point in the CSF pathway to produce increased pressure and dilation of the pathways proximal to the site of obstruction.

Developmental defects (e.g., Chiari malformations, aqueduct stenosis, aqueduct gliosis, and atresia of the foramina of Luschka and Magendie [Dandy-Walker syndrome]) account for most cases of hydrocephalus from birth to 2 years of age. Hydrocephalus is so often associated with myelomeningocele that all such infants should be observed for its development. In the remainder of cases, there is a history of intrauterine infection, hemorrhage, and neonatal meningoencephalitis. In older children, hydrocephalus is most often a result of intracranial masses, intracranial infections, hemorrhage, preexisting developmental defects (e.g., aqueduct stenosis, Chiari malformation), or trauma.

Clinical Manifestations

The factors that influence the clinical picture in hydrocephalus are the time of onset, acuity of onset, and associated structural malformations. In infancy, before closure of the cranial sutures, head enlargement (increasing occipitofrontal circumference) is the predominant sign, but in older infants and children, the lesions responsible for hydrocephalus produce other neurologic signs through pressure on adjacent structures (Box 46.10).

In infants with hydrocephalus, the head grows at an abnormal rate, although the first signs may be bulging fontanels. The anterior fontanel is tense, often bulging and nonpulsatile. Scalp veins are dilated, especially when the infant cries. With the increase in intracranial volume, skull bones become thin and the sutures become palpably separated to produce a cracked-pot sound (Macewen sign) on percussion of the skull. In severe cases, infants display frontal protrusion (frontal bossing), eyes depressed and rotated downward (setting-sun sign), and sluggish pupils.

The signs and symptoms in early-to-late childhood are caused by increased ICP, and specific manifestations are related to the focal lesion. Most commonly resulting from posterior fossa neoplasms and aqueduct stenosis, the clinical manifestations are primarily those associated with space-occupying lesions (e.g., headaches on awakening with improvement after emesis or being in an upright position, strabismus, ataxia).

Diagnostic Evaluation

Hydrocephalus in infants is based on head circumference that crosses one or more percentile line on the head measurement chart within 2 to 4 weeks. In evaluation of a preterm infant, specially adapted head circumference charts are consulted to distinguish abnormal head growth from normal rapid head growth. The primary diagnostic tools to detect hydrocephalus in older infants and children are CT and MRI. Diagnostic evaluation of children who have symptoms of hydrocephalus after infancy is similar to that used in those with suspected intracranial tumor. In neonates, echoencephalography is useful in comparing the ratio of lateral ventricle to cortex.

Therapeutic Management

The treatment of hydrocephalus is directed toward relief of ventricular pressure, treatment of the cause, treatment of associated complications, and management of problems related to the effect of the disorder on psychomotor development. With few exceptions, the treatment is surgical. This is accomplished by direct removal of an obstruction (e.g., a tumor or hematoma). Most children require placement of a shunt that provides primary drainage of the CSF from the ventricles to an extracranial compartment, usually the peritoneum (*ventriculoperitoneal [VP] shunt*) (Fig. 46.8).

Most shunt systems consist of a ventricular catheter, a flush pump, a unidirectional flow valve, and a distal catheter. In all models, the valves are designed to open at a predetermined intraventricular pressure and close when the pressure falls below that level, thus preventing backflow of secretions.

The major complications of VP shunts are malfunction and infection. All shunts are subject to mechanical difficulties, such as kinking, plugging,

BOX 46.10 Clinical Manifestations of Hydrocephalus

Infancy (Early)
- Abnormally rapid head growth
- Bulging fontanels (especially anterior) sometimes without head enlargement:
  - Tense
  - Nonpulsatile
- Dilated scalp veins
- Separated sutures
- Macewen sign (cracked-pot sound on percussion)
- Thinning of skull bones

Infancy (Later)
- Frontal enlargement, or bossing
- Depressed eyes
- Setting-sun sign (sclera visible above iris)
- Pupils sluggish with unequal response to light

Infancy (General)
- Irritability
- Lethargy
- Infant cries when picked up or rocked and quiets when allowed to lie still
- Early infantile reflex acts may persist
- Normally expected responses fail to appear
- May display:
  - Change in level of consciousness (LOC)
  - Opisthotonos (often extreme)
  - Lower-extremity spasticity
  - Vomiting
- Advanced cases:
- Difficulty in sucking and feeding
- Shrill, brief, high-pitched cry
- Cardiopulmonary embarrassment

Childhood
- Headache on awakening; improvement after emesis or upright posture
- Papilledema
- Strabismus
- Extrapyramidal tract signs (e.g., ataxia)
- Irritability
- Lethargy
- Apathy
- Confusion
- Incoherence
- Vomiting

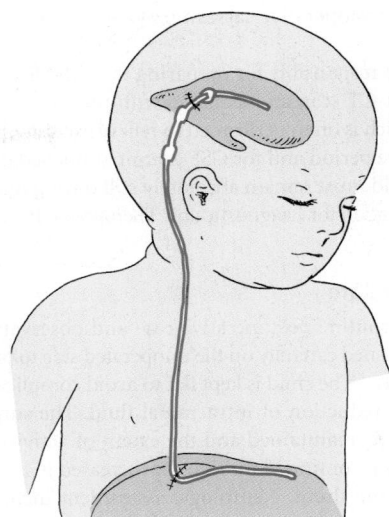

FIG 46.8 Ventriculoperitoneal shunt. The catheter is threaded beneath the skin.

wound infection, shunt nephritis, meningitis, and ventriculitis. Meningitis and ventriculitis are of greatest concern because any complicating CNS infection is a significant predictor of subnormal intellectual outcome. Infection is treated with antibiotics administered intravenously or intrathecally for a minimum of 7 to 10 days. A persistent infection requires removal of the shunt until the infection is controlled. External ventricular drainage (EVD) is used until CSF is sterile. The EVD allows for removal of CSF through a tube that is placed in the child's ventricle and flows by gravity into a collection device.

Prognosis

The prognosis for children with treated hydrocephalus depends largely on the cause of the dilated ventricles before shunt placement and the amount of irreversible brain damage before shunting (Kinsman & Johnston, 2016). For example, children with malignant tumors may have a high mortality rate regardless of other complicating factors.

Surgically treated hydrocephalus in patients with little or no evidence of irreversible brain damage has a survival rate of about 80%, with the highest incidence of mortality occurring within the first year of treatment (Paulsen, Lundar, & Lindegaard, 2010). Those with poor outcomes include children shunted for posthemorrhagic hydrocephalus or meningitis. Most children who require shunting must depend on the shunt for the remainder of their life.

Interprofessional Care Management

An infant with diagnosed or suspected hydrocephalus is observed carefully for signs of increasing ventricular size and increasing ICP. In infants, the head is measured daily at the largest measurement, the frontooccipital circumference (see the "Head Circumference" section in Chapter 29 for technique). Fontanels and suture lines are palpated for size, signs of bulging, tenseness, and separation. Irritability, lethargy, or seizure activity and altered vital signs and feeding behavior may indicate an advancing pathologic condition.

In older children, the most valuable indicators of increasing ICP are alterations in the child's LOC, headaches, and changes in interactions with the environment. Changes are identified by observation and comparison of present behavior with customary behavior, sleep patterns, developmental capabilities, and habits obtained through a detailed history and a baseline assessment. This baseline information serves as

or separation or migration of the tubing. Malfunction is most often caused by mechanical obstruction either within the ventricles from particulate matter (tissue or exudate) or at the distal end from thrombosis or displacement as a result of growth. Functional obstruction of a shunt's anti-siphon device remains a common complication. Revisions are needed when signs of malfunction appear. The child with a shunt obstruction is often first seen in an emergency department with clinical manifestations of increased ICP, which is frequently accompanied by worsening neurologic status.

The most serious complication, shunt infection, can occur at any time, but the period of greatest risk is within the first 6 months after placement (Sivaganesan, Krishnamurthy, Sahni & Viswanathan, 2012). The infection is generally a result of intercurrent infections at the time of shunt placement. Infections include sepsis, bacterial endocarditis,

a guide for postoperative assessment and evaluation of shunt function.

The nurse is responsible for preparing the child for diagnostic tests such as MRI or CT scan and assisting with procedures such as a ventricular tap, which is often performed to relieve excessive pressure during the preoperative period and for CSF examination. Sedation is required because the child must remain absolutely still during diagnostic testing (see the "Preparation for Diagnostic and Therapeutic Procedures" section in Chapter 39).

Postoperative Care

In addition to routine postoperative care and observation, the infant or child is positioned carefully on the unoperated side to prevent pressure on the shunt valve. The child is kept flat to avoid complications resulting from too rapid reduction of intracranial fluid. The surgeon indicates the position to be maintained and the extent of activity allowed.

Observation is continued for signs of increased ICP, which indicates obstruction of the shunt. Neurologic assessment includes evaluation of pupillary dilation (pressure causes compression or stretching of the oculomotor nerve, producing dilation on the same side as the pressure) and blood pressure (hypoxia to the brainstem causes variability in these vital signs).

> **!** **NURSING ALERT**
>
> Arbitrary pumping of the shunt may cause obstruction or other problems and should not be performed unless indicated by a neurosurgeon.

Because infection is the greatest hazard of the postoperative period, nurses are continually on the alert for the usual manifestations of CSF infection such as elevated temperature, poor feeding, vomiting, decreased responsiveness, and seizure activity. There may be signs of local inflammation at the operative sites and along the shunt tract. The child is also observed for abdominal distention because CSF may cause peritonitis or a postoperative ileus as a complication of distal catheter placement. Antibiotics are administered by the IV route as ordered, and the nurse may also need to assist with intraventricular instillation. Inspect the incision site for leakage, and test any suspected drainage for glucose, an indication of CSF.

Family Support

Specific needs and concerns of parents during periods of hospitalization are related to the reason for the child's hospitalization (shunt revision, infection, diagnosis) and the diagnostic and surgical procedures to which the child is subjected. Parents may have little understanding of anatomy; therefore they need further exploration and reinforcement of information that was given to them by the physician and neurosurgeon, including information about what to expect. They are especially frightened of any procedure that involves the brain, and the fear of disability or brain damage is real and pervasive. Nurses can calm their anxiety with explanations of the rationale underlying the various nursing and medical activities, such as positioning or testing, and by simply being available and willing to listen to their concerns.

To prepare for the child's discharge and home care, the parents are instructed on how to recognize signs that indicate shunt malfunction or infection. Active children may have injuries, such as a fall that can damage the shunt, and the tubing may pull out of the distal insertion site or become disconnected during normal growth. Contact sports should be avoided, and a helmet should be worn when outside play is vigorous. It is also important for the nurse to encourage families to enroll infants and toddlers with hydrocephalus into an early childhood development program.

The management of hydrocephalus in a child is a demanding task for both family and health care providers, and helping a family cope with the child's difficulties is an important nursing responsibility. Children with hydrocephalus have lifelong special health care needs and require evaluation on a regular basis. The overall aim is to establish realistic goals and an appropriate educational program that will help the child to achieve his or her optimal potential. Families can be referred to community agencies for support and guidance. The National Hydrocephalus Foundation* and the Hydrocephalus Association† provide information on the condition for families and help interested groups establish local organizations.

REFERENCES

Abend, N. S., & Loddenkemper, T. (2014). Pediatric status epilepticus management. *Current Opinion in Pediatrics, 26*(6), 668–674.

Allen, K. A. (2014). Parental decision-making for medically complex infants and children: An integrated literature review. *International Journal of Nursing Studies, 51*(9), 1289–1304.

Anderson, V., Le Brocque, R., Iselin, G., et al. (2012). Adaptive ability, behavior and quality of life pre- and posttraumatic brain injury in childhood. *Disability and Rehabilitation, 34*(19), 1639–1647.

Arlachov, Y., & Ganatra, R. H. (2012). Sedation/anaesthesia in paediatric radiology. *British Journal of Radiology, 85*(1019), e1018–e1031.

Babcock, L., Byczkowski, T., Wade, S. L., et al. (2013). Predicting postconcussion syndrome after mild traumatic brain injury in children and adolescents who present to the emergency department. *JAMA Pediatrics, 167*(2), 156–161.

Baca, C. B., Vickrey, B. G., Vassar, S. D., et al. (2013). Injuries in adolescents with childhood-onset epilepsy compared with sibling controls. *Journal of Pediatrics, 163*(6), 1684–1691.

Berg, A. T., & Rychlik, K. (2015). The course of childhood-onset epilepsy over the first two decades: A prospective, longitudinal study. *Epilepsia, 56*(1), 40–48.

Braun, K. P., & Schmidt, D. (2014). Stopping antiepileptic drugs in seizure-free patients. *Current Opinion in Neurology, 27*(2), 219–226.

Caglar, D., & Quan, L. (2016). Drowning and submersion injury. In R. M. Kliegman, B. F. Stanton, J. W. St. Geme, et al. (Eds.), *Nelson textbook of pediatrics* (20th ed.). Philadelphia, PA: Elsevier/Saunders.

Camfield, C., & Camfield, P. (2014). Most adults with childhood-onset epilepsy and their parents have incorrect knowledge of the cause 20-30 years later: A population-based study. *Epilepsy & Behavior, 37,* 100–103.

Centers for Disease Control and Prevention. (2012). *Protect the ones you love: child injuries are preventable.* Retrieved from https://www.cdc.gov/safechild/.

Chandran, A., Herbert, H., Misurski, D., & Santosham, M. (2011). Long-term sequelae of childhood bacterial meningitis: An underappreciated problem. *Pediatric Infectious Disease Journal, 30*(1), 3–6.

Christensen, J. (2012). Traumatic brain injury: Risks of epilepsy and implications for medicolegal assessment. *Epilepsia, 53*(4 suppl), 43–47.

Crowcroft, N. S., & Thampi, N. (2015). The prevention and management of rabies. *British Medical Journal, 350,* 7827.

de Vos, M. A., Bos, A. P., Plötz, F., et al. (2015). Talking with parents about end-of-life decisions for their children. *Pediatrics, 135*(2), e465–e476.

Dulac, O., & Takahashi, T. (2013). Status epilepticus. *Handbook of clinical neurology, 111,* 681–689.

---

*12413 Centralia Road, Lakewood, CA 90715-1653, 562-924-6666, 888-857-3434, http://www.nhfonline.org.
†4340 East West Highway, Suite 905, Bethesda, MD 20814, 888-598-3789, http://www.hydroassoc.org.

Erlichman, D. B., Blumfield, E., Rajpathak, S., et al. (2010). Association between linear skull fractures and intracranial hemorrhage in children with minor head trauma. *Pediatric Radiology, 40,* 1375–1379.

Elliott, R. E., Rodgers, S. D., Bassani, L., et al. (2011). Vagus nerve stimulation for children with treatment resistant epilepsy. *Journal of Neurosurgery. Pediatrics, 7,* 491–500.

El-Radhi, A. S. (2015). Management of seizures in children. *British Journal of Nursing, 24*(3), 152–155.

Faul, M., Xu, L., Wald, M. M., et al. (2010). *Traumatic brain injury in the United States.* Retrieved from www.cdc.gov/traumaticbraininjury/pdf/tbi_blue_book_age.pdf.

Fisher, R. S., Acevedo, C., Arzimanoglou, A., et al. (2014). A practical clinical definition of epilepsy. *Epilepsia, 55*(4), 475–482.

Freilich, E. R., Schreiber, J. M., Zelleke, T., et al. (2014). Pediatric status epilepticus: Identification and evaluation. *Current Opinion in Pediatrics, 26*(6), 655–661.

Huff, J. S., & Fountain, N. B. (2011). Pathophysiology and definitions of seizures and status epilepticus. *Emergency Medicine Clinics of North America, 29*(1), 1–13.

Ibrahim, S. H., & Balistreri, W. F. (2016). Mitochondrial hepatopathies. In R. M. Kliegman, B. F. Stanton, J. W. St. Geme, et al. (Eds.), *Nelson textbook of pediatrics* (20th ed.). Philadelphia, PA: Elsevier/Saunders.

Ibrahim, N. G., Wood, J., Margulies, S. S., et al. (2012). Influence of age and fall type on head injuries in infants and toddlers. *International Journal of Developmental Neuroscience, 30*(3), 201–206.

Kinsman, S. L., & Johnston, M. V. (2016). Hydrocephalus. In R. M. Kliegman, B. F. Stanton, J. W. St. Geme, et al. (Eds.), *Nelson textbook of pediatrics* (20th ed.). Philadelphia, PA: Elsevier/Saunders.

Klimo, P., Jr., Matthews, A., Lew, S. M., et al. (2011). Minicraniotomy versus bur holes for evacuation of chronic subdural collections in infants—A preliminary single-institution experience. *Journal of Neurosurgery. Pediatrics, 8*(5), 423–429.

Kossoff, E. H. (2013). Nonpharmacological approaches: Diet and neurostimulation. *Handbook of Clinical Neurology, 111,* 803–808.

Levy, R. G., Cooper, P. N., & Giri, P. (2012). Ketogenic diet and other dietary treatments for epilepsy. *Cochrane Database of Systematic Reviews, 2012*(3), CD001903.

Liebig, C. W., & Congeni, J. A. (2016). Sports-related traumatic brain injury (concussion). In R. M. Kliegman, B. F. Stanton, J. W. St. Geme, et al. (Eds.), *Nelson textbook of pediatrics* (20th ed.). Philadelphia, PA: Elsevier/Saunders.

Liu, X. S., You, C., & Lu, M. (2012). Growing skull fracture stages and treatment strategy. *Journal of Neurosurgery. Pediatrics, 9*(6), 670–675.

López-Elizalde, R., Leyva-Mastrapa, T., Muñoz-Serrano, J. A., et al. (2013). Ping-pong fractures: Treatment using a new medical device. *Child's Nervous System, 29*(4), 679–683.

Mewasingh, L. D. (2014). Febrile seizures. *BMJ Clinical Evidence, 324.*

Mikati, M. A., & Hani, A. J. (2016). Seizures in childhood. In R. M. Kliegman, B. F. Stanton, J. W. St. Geme, et al. (Eds.), *Nelson textbook of pediatrics* (20th ed.). Philadelphia, PA: Elsevier/Saunders.

Moosa, A. N., & Gupta, A. (2014). Outcome after epilepsy surgery for cortical dysplasia in children. *Child's Nervous System, 30*(11), 1905–1911.

Moshé, S. L., Perucca, E., Ryvlin, P., et al. (2015). Epilepsy: New advances. *Lancet, 385*(9971), 884–898.

Mott, T. F., & Latimer, K. M. (2016). Prevention and treatment of drowning. *American Family Physician, 93*(7), 576–582.

Nasrullah, M., & Muazzam, S. (2011). Drowning mortality in the United States 1999–2006. *Journal of Community Health, 36,* 69–75.

Nickels, K. C., Grossardt, B. R., & Wirrell, E. C. (2012). Epilepsy-related mortality is low in children: A 30-year population-based study in Olmstead County, MN. *Epilepsia, 53*(12), 2164–2171.

Novakova, B., Harris, P. R., Ponnusamy, A., et al. (2013). The role of stress as a trigger for epileptic seizures: A narrative review of evidence from human and animal studies. *Epilepsia, 54*(11), 1866–1876.

Offringa, M., & Newton, R. (2013). Prophylactic drug management for febrile seizures in children (review). *Evidence-Based Child Health, 8*(4), 1376–1485.

Paulsen, A. H., Lundar, T., & Lindegaard, K. F. (2010). Twenty-year outcome in young adults with childhood hydrocephalus: Assessment of surgical outcome, work participation, and health-related quality of life. *Journal of Neurosurgery. Pediatrics, 6,* 527–535.

Pavlidou, E., & Panteliadis, C. (2013). Prognostic factors for subsequent epilepsy in children with febrile seizures. *Epilepsia, 54*(12), 2101–2107.

Perheentupa, U., Kinnunen, I., Grénman, R., et al. (2010). Management and outcome of pediatric skull base fractures. *International Journal of Pediatric Otorhinolaryngology, 74,* 1245–1250.

Prober, C. G., & Matthew, R. (2016). Acute bacterial meningitis beyond the neonatal period. In R. M. Kliegman, B. F. Stanton, J. W. St. Geme, et al. (Eds.), *Nelson textbook of pediatrics* (20th ed.). Philadelphia, PA: Elsevier/Saunders.

Rivara, F. P., & Grossman, D. C. (2016). Injury control. In R. M. Kliegman, B. F. Stanton, J. W. St. Geme, et al. (Eds.), *Nelson textbook of pediatrics* (20th ed.). Philadelphia, PA: Elsevier/Saunders.

Rosenbloom, E., Finkelstein, Y., Adams-Webber, T., et al. (2013). Do antipyretics prevent the recurrence of febrile seizures in children? A systematic review of randomized controlled trials and meta-analysis. *European Journal of Paediatric Neurology, 17*(6), 585–588.

Ryvlin, P., Cross, J. H., & Rheims, S. (2014). Epilepsy surgery in children and adults. *Lancet Neurology, 13*(11), 1114–1126.

Safe Kids. (2008). *Report to the nation: Trends in unintentional childhood injury mortality and parental views on child safety.* Retrieved from www.safekids.org/research-report/report-nation-trends-unintentional-childhood-injury-mortality-and-parental-views.

Saghazadeh, A., Mastrangelo, M., & Rezaei, N. (2014). Genetic background of febrile seizures. *Reviews in the Neurosciences, 25*(1), 129–161.

Sankhyan, N., Raju, K. N., Sharma, S., et al. (2010). Management of raised intracranial pressure. *Indian Journal of Pediatrics, 77,* 1409–1416.

Seinfeld, S., Shinnar, S., Sun, S., et al. (2014). Emergency management of febrile status epilepticus: Results of the FEBSTAT study. *Epilepsia, 55*(3), 388–395.

Sharma, S., Kochar, G. S., Sankhyan, N., et al. (2010). Approach to the child with coma. *Indian Journal of Pediatrics, 77*(11), 1279–1287.

Shorvon, S. (2011). The treatment of status epilepticus. *Current Opinion in Neurology, 24,* 165–170.

Sieswerda-Hoogendoorn, T., Boos, S., Spivak, B., et al. (2012). Abusive head trauma part I: Clinical aspects. *European Journal of Pediatrics, 171*(3), 415–423.

Sivaganesan, A., Krishnamurthy, R., Sahni, D., et al. (2012). Neuroimaging of ventriculoperitoneal shunt complications in children. *Pediatric Radiology, 42*(9), 1029–1046.

Singhi, S. C., & Tiwari, L. (2009). Management of intracranial hypertension. *Indian Journal of Pediatrics, 76,* 519–529.

Syndi Seinfeld, D., & Pellock, J. M. (2013). Recent research on febrile seizures: A review. *Journal of Neurology & Neurophysiology, 4,* 165–171.

Teichert, J. H., Rosales Jr., P. R., Lopes, P. B., et al. (2012). Extradural hematoma in children: Case series of 33 patients. *Pediatric Neurosurgery, 48*(4), 216–220.

Téllez-Zenteno, J. F., Hernández-Ronquillo, L., Buckley, S., et al. (2014). A validation of the new definition of drug-resistant epilepsy by the International League Against Epilepsy. *Epilepsia, 55*(6), 829–834.

Thigpen, M. C., Whitney, C. G., Messonnier, N. E., et al. (2011). Bacterial meningitis in the United States 1998–2007. *New England Journal of Medicine, 364*(21), 2016–2025.

Verrotti, A., D'Egidio, C., Agostinelli, S., et al. (2012). Antiepileptic drug withdrawal in childhood epilepsy: What are the risk factors associated with seizure relapse? *European Journal of Paediatric Neurology, 16*(6), 599–604.

Walker, C. T., Stone, J. J., Jacobson, M., et al. (2012). Indications for pediatric external ventricular drain placement and risk factors for conversion to a ventriculoperitoneal shunt. *Pediatric Neurosurgery, 48*(6), 342–347.

Wassenaar, M., Kasteleijn-Nolst Trenité, D. G., de Haan, G. J., et al. (2014). Seizure precipitants in a community-based epilepsy cohort. *Journal of Neurology, 261*(4), 717–724.

Wassenaar, M., Leijten, F. S., Egberts, T. C., et al. (2013). Prognostic factors for medically intractable epilepsy: A systematic review. *Epilepsy Research*, *106*(3), 301–310.

Weant, K. A., & Baker, S. N. (2013). Review of human rabies prophylaxis and treatment. *Critical Care Nursing Clinics of North America*, *25*(2), 225–242.

Weiss, J., & American Academy of Pediatrics Committee on Injury, Violence, and Poison Prevention. (2010). Prevention of drowning. *Pediatrics*, *126*, e253–e262.

Willoughby, R. E., Jr. (2016). Rabies. In R. M. Kliegman, B. F. Stanton, J. W. St. Geme, et al. (Eds.), *Nelson textbook of pediatrics* (20th ed.). Philadelphia, PA: Elsevier/Saunders.

47

The Child With Endocrine Dysfunction

Cheryl C. Rodgers

http://evolve.elsevier.com/Perry/maternal

THE ENDOCRINE SYSTEM

The endocrine system controls and regulates metabolism; this includes energy production, growth, fluid and electrolyte balance, response to stress, and sexual development (Gardner & Shoback, 2011). The endocrine system consists of three components: (1) the cells, which send chemical messages by means of hormones; (2) the target cells or organs, which receive chemical messages; and (3) the environment through which the chemicals are transported (blood, lymph, extracellular fluids) from the sites of synthesis to the sites of cellular action. The pathophysiology review in Fig. 47.1 provides a summary of the principal pituitary hormones and their target organs.

HORMONES

A hormone is a complex chemical substance produced and secreted into body fluids by a cell or group of cells that exerts a physiologic controlling effect on other cells. These effects may be local or distant and may affect either most cells of the body or specific "target" tissues. Most hormones are released by the endocrine glands into the bloodstream, and production is regulated by a feedback mechanism. The master gland of the endocrine system is the anterior pituitary gland, which is responsible for stimulation and inhibition of tropic hormones. However, some hormones, such as insulin, are regulated by other mechanisms.

DISORDERS OF PITUITARY FUNCTION

The pituitary gland is divided into two lobes—the anterior (adenohypophysis) and the posterior (neurohypophysis) lobe. Each lobe is responsible for secreting different hormones. Disorders of the anterior pituitary hormones may be attributable to organic defects or have an idiopathic etiology and may occur as a single hormonal problem or in combination with other hormonal disorders. The clinical manifestations of pituitary dysfunction depend on the hormones involved and the age of the patient. *Panhypopituitarism* is defined clinically as the loss of all anterior pituitary hormones, leaving only posterior function intact (Lang, Mead, & Sykes, 2015).

> **! NURSING ALERT**
>
> Children with panhypopituitarism should wear a medical alert identification, such as a bracelet or necklace.

HYPOPITUITARISM

Hypopituitarism is diminished secretion of one or more pituitary hormones. The consequences of the condition depend on the degree of dysfunction. It often leads to: gonadotropin deficiency with absence or regression of secondary sex characteristics; growth hormone (GH) deficiency, in which children display stunted somatic growth; thyroid-stimulating hormone (TSH) deficiency, which produces hypothyroidism; and adrenocorticotropic hormone (ACTH) deficiency, which results in adrenal hypofunction.

Hypopituitarism can result from any of the conditions listed in Box 47.1. The most common organic cause of pituitary undersecretion is a tumor in the pituitary or hypothalamic region, especially the craniopharyngiomas. Congenital hypopituitarism can be seen in newborn infants and can run in families, suggesting a genetic cause (Alatzoglou & Dattani, 2010). Symptoms of apnea, cyanosis, or severe hypoglycemia with or without seizure often manifest in infants with congenital hypopituitarism (Parks & Felner, 2016).

Idiopathic hypopituitarism, or idiopathic pituitary growth failure, is usually related to GH deficiency, which inhibits somatic growth in all cells of the body (Amin, Mushtaq, & Alvi, 2015). Growth failure is defined as an absolute height of less than −2 standard deviation (SD) for age or a linear growth velocity consistently less than −1 SD for age. When this occurs without the presence of hypothyroidism, systemic disease, or malnutrition, rather than abnormality of the GH–insulin-like growth factor (IGF-I) axis should be considered (Richmond & Rogol, 2008).

Not all children with short stature have GH deficiency. In most instances, the cause is considered idiopathic. Most children with idiopathic short stature (ISS) have either familial short stature or constitutional growth delay. *Familial short stature* refers to otherwise healthy children who have ancestors with adult height in the lower percentiles. *Constitutional growth* delay refers to individuals (usually boys) with delayed linear growth, generally beginning as a toddler, and skeletal and sexual maturation that is behind that of age mates (Amin et al., 2015). GH therapy in children with ISS continues to be debated frequently by pediatric endocrinologists.

Clinical Manifestations

Children with GH deficiency generally grow normally during the first year and then follow a slowed growth curve that is below the third percentile. These children may appear overweight or obese due to stunted height in combination with good nutrition. A nourished appearance is an important diagnostic clue that may differentiate patients with GH

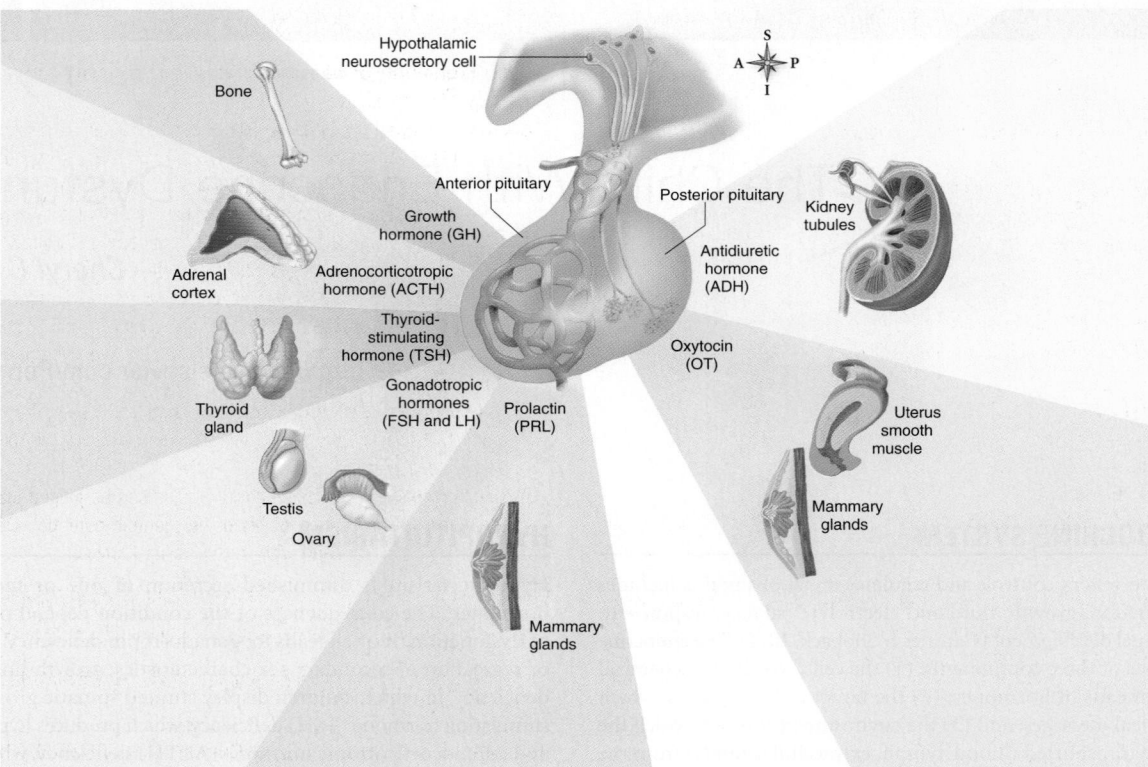

FIG 47.1 Principal anterior and posterior pituitary hormones and their target organs. *FSH,* Follicle-stimulating hormone; *LH,* luteinizing hormone. (From Patton K.T., & Thibodeau, G.A. [2016]. *Anatomy and physiology* [9th ed.]. St. Louis, MO: Elsevier.)

deficiency from patients with failure to thrive. Sexual development is usually delayed but is otherwise normal unless the gonadotropin hormones are deficient. Growth may extend into the third or fourth decade of life, but permanent height is usually diminished if the disorder is left untreated. Because of an underdeveloped jaw, teeth may be crowded or malpositioned. Clinical manifestations of panhypopituitarism are listed in Box 47.1.

Diagnostic Evaluation

Only a small number of children with delayed growth or short stature have hypopituitary dysfunction. Diagnostic evaluation is aimed at isolating organic causes, which, in addition to GH deficiency, may include tumor growth, hypothyroidism, oversecretion of cortisol, gonadal aplasia, chronic illness, nutritional inadequacy, Russell-Silver dwarfism, or hypochondroplasia.

A complete diagnostic evaluation should include a family history, a history of the child's growth patterns and previous health status, physical examination, and psychosocial evaluation. Specific radiographic imaging, including magnetic resonance imaging (MRI), endocrine studies, and genetic testing may be warranted (Stanley, 2012). Accurate measurement of height and weight, and comparison with standard growth charts are essential. Multiple height measures reflect a more accurate assessment of abnormal growth patterns (Box 47.2). Parental height and familial patterns of growth are important clues to diagnosis. A skeletal survey in children younger than 3 years of age and radiographic examination of the hand-wrist for centers of ossification (bone age) (Box 47.3) in older children are important in evaluating growth.

Definitive diagnosis of GH deficiency is based on absent or subnormal reserves of pituitary GH. Because GH levels are variable in children, GH stimulation testing is usually required for diagnosis. It is recommended that GH stimulation tests be reserved for children with low serum IGF-I and insulin-like growth factor binding protein 3 (IGFBP3) levels and poor growth who do not have other causes for short stature (Hokken-Koelega, 2011). GH stimulation testing involves the use of pharmacologic agents such as levodopa, clonidine, arginine, insulin, propranolol, or glucagon followed by the measurement of GH blood levels (Parks & Felner, 2016). Children with poor linear growth, delayed bone age, and abnormal GH stimulation tests are considered GH deficient.

Therapeutic Management

Treatment of GH deficiency caused by organic lesions is directed toward correction of the underlying disease process (e.g., surgical removal or irradiation of a tumor). The definitive treatment of GH deficiency is replacement of GH, which is successful in 80% of affected children. Biosynthetic GH is administered subcutaneously on a daily basis. Growth velocity increases in the first year of treatment and then declines in subsequent years. Final height is likely to remain less than normal (Deodati & Cianfarani, 2011), and early diagnosis and intervention are essential.

The decision to stop GH therapy is made jointly by the child, family, and health care team. Growth rates of less than 1 inch per year and a bone age of more than 14 years in girls and more than 16 years in boys are often used as criteria to stop GH therapy (Parks & Felner, 2016).

BOX 47.1 Clinical Manifestations of Panhypopituitarism

Growth Hormone
- Short stature but proportional height and weight
- Delayed epiphyseal closure
- Delayed bone age proportional to height
- Premature aging common in later life
- Increased insulin sensitivity

Thyroid-Stimulating Hormone
- Short stature with infantile proportions
- Dry, coarse skin; yellow discoloration, pallor
- Cold intolerance
- Constipation
- Somnolence
- Bradycardia
- Dyspnea on exertion
- Delayed dentition, loss of teeth

Gonadotropins
- Absence of sexual maturation or loss of secondary sexual characteristics
- Atrophy of genitalia, prostate gland, breasts
- Amenorrhea without menopausal symptoms
- Decreased spermatogenesis

Adrenocorticotropic Hormone
- Severe anorexia, weight loss
- Hypoglycemia
- Hypotension
- Hyponatremia, hyperkalemia
- Adrenal apoplexy, especially in response to stress
- Circulatory collapse

Antidiuretic Hormone
- Polyuria
- Polydipsia
- Dehydration

Melanocyte-Stimulating Hormone
- Decreased pigmentation

BOX 47.2 Evaluating the Growth Curve

Ensure reliability of measurements: Accurately obtain and plot height and weight measurements.

Determine absolute height: The child's absolute height bears some relationship to the likelihood of a pathologic condition. However, the majority of children who have a height below the lowest percentile (either the third or fifth percentile on the height curve) do not have a pathologic growth problem.

Assess height velocity: The most important aspect of a growth evaluation is the observation of a child's height over time, or height velocity. Accurate determination of height velocity requires at least 4 and preferably 6 months of observation. A substantial deceleration in height velocity (crossing several percentiles) between 3 and 12 or 13 years of age indicates a pathologic condition until proven otherwise.

Determine weight-to-height relationship: Determination of the weight-to-height ratio has some diagnostic value in ascertaining the cause of growth delay in a short child.

Project target height: The height of a child can be judged inappropriately short only in the context of his or her genetic potential. Determine the target height of the child with the following formula:

[father's height (cm) + mother's height (cm)] + 13/2 for boys

[father's height (cm) + mother's height (cm)] − 13/2 for girls

Most children achieve an adult stature within approximately 10 cm (4 inches) of the target height.

Adapted from Vogiatzi, M.G., & Copeland, K.C. (1998). The short child. *Pediatrics in Review, 19*(3), 92–99.

BOX 47.3 Bone Age for Evaluating Growth Disorders

Bone age refers to a method of assessing skeletal maturity by comparing the appearance of representative epiphyseal centers obtained on x-ray examination with age-appropriate published standards.

Most conditions that cause poor linear growth also cause a delay in skeletal maturation and a delayed bone age. Observation of even a profoundly delayed bone age is never diagnostic or even indicative of a specific diagnosis. A delayed bone age merely indicates that the associated short stature is to some extent "partially reversible" because linear growth will continue until epiphyseal fusion is complete. In comparison, a bone age that is not delayed in a short child is of much greater concern and may, in fact, be of some diagnostic value under certain circumstances.

Adapted from Vogiatzi, M.G., & Copeland, K.C. (1998). The short child. *Pediatrics in Review, 19*(3), 92–99.

Children with other hormone deficiencies require replacement therapy to correct the specific disorders.

Care Management

The principal nursing consideration is identifying children with growth problems. Even though the majority of growth problems are not a result of organic causes, any delay in normal growth and sexual development poses special emotional adjustments for these children.

The nurse may be a key person in helping establish a diagnosis. For example, if serial height and weight records are not available, the nurse can question parents about the child's growth compared with that of siblings, peers, or relatives. Preparation of the child and family for diagnostic testing is especially important if a number of tests are being performed, and the child requires particular attention during provocative testing. Blood samples are usually taken every 30 minutes for a 3-hour period. Children also have difficulty overcoming hypoglycemia generated by tests with insulin, so they must be observed carefully for signs of

hypoglycemia. Those receiving glucagon are at risk for nausea and vomiting. Clonidine may cause hypotension, requiring administration of intravenous (IV) fluids.

Child and Family Support

Children undergoing hormone replacement require additional support. The nurse should provide education for patient self-management during the school-age years. Nursing functions include family education concerning medication preparation and storage, injection sites, injection technique, and syringe disposal (see Chapter 39). Administration of GH is facilitated by family routines that include a specific time of day for the injection.

Even when hormone replacement is successful, these children attain their eventual adult height at a slower rate than their peers; therefore, they need assistance in setting realistic expectations regarding improvement. Because these children appear younger than their chronologic age, others may relate to them in infantile or childish ways. Parents and teachers benefit from guidance directed toward setting realistic expectations for the child based on age and abilities. For example, in the home, such children should have the same age-appropriate responsibilities as their siblings. As they approach adolescence, they should be encouraged to participate in group activities with peers. If abilities and strengths are emphasized rather than physical size, such children are more likely to develop a positive self-image.

Professionals and families can find resources for research, education, support, and advocacy from the Human Growth Foundation.* Treatment is expensive, but the cost is often partially covered by insurance if the child has a documented deficiency.

PITUITARY HYPERFUNCTION

Excess GH before closure of the epiphyseal shafts results in proportional overgrowth of the long bones until the individual reaches a height of 2.4 m (8 ft) or more. Vertical growth is accompanied by rapid and increased development of muscles and viscera. Weight is increased but is usually in proportion to height. Proportional enlargement of head circumference also occurs and may result in delayed closure of the fontanels in young children. Children with a pituitary-secreting tumor may also demonstrate signs of increasing intracranial pressure, especially headache.

If oversecretion of GH occurs after epiphyseal closure (growth plate), growth is in the transverse direction, producing a condition known as *acromegaly*. Typical facial features include overgrowth of the head, lips, nose, tongue, jaw, and paranasal and mastoid sinuses; separation and malocclusion of the teeth in the enlarged jaw; disproportion of the face to the cerebral division of the skull; increased facial hair; thickened, deeply creased skin; and an increased tendency toward hyperglycemia and diabetes mellitus (DM). Acromegaly can develop slowly, leading to delays in diagnosis and treatment.

Diagnostic Evaluation

Excessive secretion of GH by a pituitary adenoma causes most cases of acromegaly. Diagnosis is based on a history of excessive growth during childhood and evidence of increased levels of GH. MRI may reveal a tumor or an enlarged sella turcica, normal bone age, enlargement of bones (e.g., the paranasal sinuses), and evidence of joint changes. Endocrine studies to confirm excess of other hormones, specifically thyroid, cortisol, and sex hormones, should also be included in the differential diagnosis.

*997 Glen Cove Avenue, Suite 5, Glen Head, NY 11545; 800-451-6434; www.hgfound.org.

Therapeutic Management

If a lesion is present, surgery is performed to remove the tumor when feasible. Other therapies aimed at destroying pituitary tissue include external irradiation and radioactive implants. Several pharmacologic agents have evolved and may be used in combination with other therapies (Muhammad, van der Lely, & Neggers, 2015). Depending on the extent of surgical extirpation and degree of pituitary insufficiency, hormone replacement with thyroid extract, cortisone, and sex hormones may be necessary.

Care Management

The primary nursing consideration is early identification of children with excessive growth rates. Although medical management cannot reduce growth already attained, further growth can be retarded. The earlier the treatment, the more control there is in predetermining a normal adult height. Nurses should also observe for signs of a tumor, especially headache, and evidence of concurrent hormonal excesses, particularly the gonadotropins, which cause sexual precocity. Children with excessive growth rates require as much emotional support as those with short stature.

PRECOCIOUS PUBERTY

Manifestations of sexual development before 9 years of age in boys or 8 years of age in girls have traditionally been considered precocious development, and these children were recommended for further evaluation (Brito, Spinola-Castro, Kochi, et al., 2016). However, recent examination of the age limit for defining when puberty is precocious reveals that the onset of puberty in girls is occurring earlier than previous studies have documented. The mean onset of puberty is 10.2 years of age in Caucasian girls and 9.6 years of age in African-American girls. Based on these findings, precocious puberty evaluation for a pathologic cause should be performed for Caucasian girls younger than 7 years of age or for African-American girls younger than 6 years of age (Latronico, Brito, & Carel, 2016). No change in the guidelines for evaluation of precocious puberty in boys is recommended.

Normally, the hypothalamic-releasing factors stimulate secretion of the gonadotropic hormones from the anterior pituitary gland at the time of puberty. In boys, interstitial cell–stimulating hormone stimulates Leydig cells of the testes to secrete testosterone; in girls, FSH and LH stimulate the ovarian follicles to secrete estrogens. This sequence of events is known as the *hypothalamic-pituitary-gonadal axis*. If for some reason the cycle undergoes premature activation, the child will display evidence of advanced or precocious puberty. Causes of precocious puberty are found in Box 47.4.

Isosexual precocious puberty is more common in girls than in boys. Approximately 1 in 5000 to 10,000 girls with precocious puberty in the United States have *central precocious puberty (CPP)*, in which pubertal development is activated by the hypothalamic gonadotropin-releasing hormone (GnRH) (Latronico et al., 2016). This produces early maturation and development of the gonads with secretion of sex hormones, development of secondary sex characteristics, and sometimes production of mature sperm and ova (Li, Li, & Yang, 2014). CPP may be the result of congenital anomalies; infectious, neoplastic, or traumatic insults to the central nervous system (CNS); or treatment of long-standing sex hormone exposure (Latronico et al., 2016). CPP occurs more frequently in girls and is usually idiopathic, with 90% demonstrating no causative factor (Latronico et al., 2016). *Peripheral precocious puberty (PPP)* includes early puberty resulting from hormone stimulation other than the hypothalamic GnRH–stimulated pituitary gonadotropin release. Isolated manifestations that are usually associated with puberty may be seen as

BOX 47.4   Causes of Precocious Puberty

Central Precocious Puberty

Idiopathic, with or without hypothalamic hamartoma

Secondary:
- Congenital anomalies
- Postinflammatory: Encephalitis, meningitis, abscess, granulomatous disease
- Radiotherapy
- Trauma
- Neoplasms

After effective treatment of long-standing pseudosexual precocity

Peripheral Precocious Puberty

Familial male-limited precocious puberty

Albright syndrome

Gonadal or extragonadal tumors

Adrenal:
- Congenital adrenal hyperplasia (CAH)
- Adenoma, carcinoma
- Glucocorticoid resistance

Exogenous sex hormones

Primary hypothyroidism

Incomplete Precocious Puberty

Premature thelarche

Premature menarche

Premature pubarche or adrenarche

Adapted from Root, A.W. (2000).: Precocious puberty. *Pediatrics in Review* 21(1):10–19.

variations in normal sexual development. They appear without other signs of pubescence and are caused by excess secretion of sex hormones through the gonads or adrenal glands and may be isosexual or contrasexual. Included are premature thelarche (development of breasts in prepubertal girls), premature pubarche (premature adrenarche, early development of sexual hair), and premature menarche (isolated menses without other evidence of sexual development).

Therapeutic Management

Treatment of precocious puberty is directed toward the specific cause when known. In 50% of cases, precocious pubertal development regresses or stops advancing without any treatment (Carel & Leger, 2008). If needed, precocious puberty of central (hypothalamic-pituitary) origin is managed with monthly injections of a synthetic analog of luteinizing hormone–releasing hormone, which regulates pituitary secretions (Latronico et al., 2016). The available preparation, leuprolide acetate (Lupron Depot), is given once every 4 to 12 weeks depending on the preparation. With the initiation of treatment, breast development regresses or does not advance, and growth returns to normal rates. Studies suggest that not all patients attain adult targeted heights, and the addition of GH therapy may be warranted (Menon & Vijayakumar, 2014). Treatment is discontinued at a chronologically appropriate time, allowing pubertal changes to resume.

Interprofessional Care Management

Both parents and the affected child should be taught the injection procedure. Psychologic support and guidance of the child and family are the most important aspects of management. Parents need anticipatory guidance, support and information resources, and reassurance of the benign nature of the condition. Dress and activities for the physically precocious child should be appropriate to the chronologic age. Sexual interest is not usually advanced beyond the child's chronologic age, and

parents need to understand that the child's mental age is congruent with the chronologic age.

DIABETES INSIPIDUS

The principal disorder of posterior pituitary hypofunction is diabetes insipidus (DI), also known as *neurogenic DI*, resulting from undersecretion of antidiuretic hormone (ADH) or vasopressin, producing a state of uncontrolled diuresis (Di Iorgi, Morana, Napoli, et al., 2015). This disorder is not to be confused with nephrogenic DI, a rare hereditary disorder affecting primarily males and caused by unresponsiveness of the renal tubules to the hormone.

Neurogenic DI may result from a number of different causes. Primary causes are familial or idiopathic; of the total cases, approximately 20% to 50% are idiopathic (Di Iorgi, Allegri, Napoli, et al., 2014). Secondary causes include trauma (accidental or surgical), tumors, granulomatous disease, infections (meningitis or encephalitis), and vascular anomalies (aneurysm). Certain drugs, such as alcohol and phenytoin (diphenylhydantoin), can cause a transient polyuria. DI may be an early sign of an evolving cerebral process (Di Iorgi et al., 2015).

The cardinal signs of DI are polyuria and polydipsia. In older children, signs such as excessive urination accompanied by a compensatory insatiable thirst may be so intense that the child does little more than go to the toilet and drink fluids. Frequently, the first sign is enuresis. In infants, the initial symptom is irritability that is relieved with feedings of water but not milk. These infants are also prone to dehydration, electrolyte imbalance, hyperthermia, azotemia, and potential circulatory collapse.

Dehydration is usually not a serious problem in older children, who are able to drink larger quantities of water. However, any period of unconsciousness, such as after trauma or anesthesia, may be life-threatening because the voluntary demand for fluid is absent. During such instances, careful monitoring of urine volumes, blood concentration, and IV fluid replacement is essential to prevent dehydration.

> **! NURSING ALERT**
>
> Children with diabetes insipidus (DI) complicated by congenital absence of the thirst center must be encouraged to drink sufficient quantities of liquid to prevent electrolyte imbalance.

Diagnostic Evaluation

The simplest test used to diagnose this condition is restriction of oral fluids and observation of consequent changes in urine volume and concentration. Normally, reducing fluids results in concentrated urine and diminished volume. In DI, fluid restriction has little or no effect on urine formation but causes weight loss from dehydration. Accurate results from this procedure require strict monitoring of fluid intake and urinary output, measurement of urine concentration (specific gravity or osmolality), and frequent weight checks. A weight loss between 3% and 5% indicates significant dehydration and requires termination of the fluid restriction.

> **! NURSING ALERT**
>
> Small children require close observation during fluid deprivation to prevent them from drinking, even from toilet bowls, flower vases, and other unlikely sources of fluid.

If this test result is positive, the child should be given a test dose of injected aqueous vasopressin, which should alleviate the polyuria and polydipsia. Unresponsiveness to exogenous vasopressin usually indicates nephrogenic DI. An important diagnostic consideration is to differentiate DI from other causes of polyuria and polydipsia, especially DM.

Therapeutic Management

The usual treatment is intranasal, oral, or parenteral desmopressin (DDAVP), a synthetic hormone replacement of aqueous lysine vasopressin (Di lorgi et al., 2015). The injectable form has the advantage of lasting 48 to 72 hours; however, it has the disadvantage of requiring frequent injections and proper preparation of the drug.

> **! NURSING ALERT**
>
> To be effective, injectable vasopressin must be thoroughly resuspended before administration. If this is not done, the oil may be injected minus the antidiuretic hormone (ADH). Small brown particles, which indicate drug dispersion, must be seen in the suspension.

Interprofessional Care Management

An early sign of DI may be sudden enuresis in a child who is toilet trained. Excessive thirst with bed-wetting is an indication for further investigation. Another clue is persistent irritability and crying in an infant who is relieved only by bottle feedings of water. After head trauma or certain neurosurgical procedures, the development of DI can be anticipated; therefore, these patients must be closely monitored.

Assessment includes frequent measurement of the patient's weight, serum electrolytes, blood urea nitrogen (BUN), hematocrit, and urine specific gravity. Fluid intake and output should be carefully measured and recorded. Alert patients are able to adjust intake to urine losses, but unconscious or very young patients require closer fluid observation. In children who are not toilet trained, collection of urine specimens may require application of a urine-collecting device.

After confirmation of DI, parents need comprehensive teaching. Specific clarification that DI is a different condition from DM should be reinforced. Parents and children must realize that treatment is lifelong. Caregivers should be taught the correct procedure for preparation and administration of the drug. When children are old enough, they should be encouraged to assume full responsibility for their care.

For emergency purposes, children with DI should wear medical alert identification. Older children should carry the nasal spray with them for temporary relief of symptoms. School personnel need to be aware of the problem so they can grant children unrestricted use of the lavatory.

SYNDROME OF INAPPROPRIATE ANTIDIURETIC HORMONE SECRETION

The disorder that results from hypersecretion of ADH from the posterior pituitary hormone is known as *syndrome of inappropriate antidiuretic hormone secretion (SIADH)*. It is observed with increased frequency in a variety of conditions, especially those involving infections, tumors, or other CNS disease or trauma, and it is the most common cause of hyponatremia in the pediatric population (Reid-Adam, 2013).

The manifestations are directly related to fluid retention and hypotonicity. Excess ADH causes most of the filtered water to be reabsorbed from the kidneys back into central circulation. Serum osmolality is low, and urine osmolality is inappropriately elevated. When serum sodium levels are diminished to 120 mEq/L, affected children may display anorexia, nausea (and sometimes vomiting), stomach cramps, irritability, and personality changes. With progressive reduction in sodium, other neurologic signs, stupor, and seizures may occur. The symptoms usually disappear when the underlying disorder is corrected.

The immediate management consists of restricting fluids. Subsequent management depends on the cause and severity. Fluids continue to be restricted to one-fourth to one-half maintenance. When there are no fluid abnormalities but SIADH can be anticipated, fluids are often restricted expectantly at two-thirds to three-fourths maintenance.

Care Management

The first goal of management is recognizing the presence of SIADH from symptoms described in patients at risk.

> **! NURSING ALERT**
>
> Nausea, vomiting, and malaise may precede the onset of more severe stages, such as disorientation, confusion, coma, and seizures (Gardner & Shoback, 2011).

Accurately measuring intake and output, noting daily weight, and observing for signs of fluid overload are primary nursing functions, especially in children receiving IV fluids. Seizure precautions are implemented. Patients and families need education regarding the rationale for fluid restrictions. The rare child with chronic SIADH will be placed on long-term ADH-antagonizing medication, and the child and family will require instructions for its administration.

DISORDERS OF THYROID FUNCTION

The thyroid gland secretes two types of hormones: *thyroid hormone (TH)*, which consists of the hormones *thyroxine (T_4)* and *triiodothyronine (T_3)*, and *calcitonin*. The secretion of THs is controlled by TSH from the anterior pituitary gland, which in turn is regulated by thyrotropin-releasing factor (TRF) from the hypothalamus as a negative feedback response. Consequently, hypothyroidism or hyperthyroidism may result from a defect in the target gland or from a disturbance in the secretion of TSH or TRF. Because the functions of T_3 and T_4 are qualitatively the same, the term *thyroid hormone* is used throughout the discussion.

The synthesis of TH depends on available sources of dietary iodine and tyrosine. The thyroid is the only endocrine gland capable of storing excess amounts of hormones for release as needed. During circulation in the bloodstream, T_4 and T_3 are bound to carrier proteins (T_4-binding globulin). They must be unbound before they are able to exert their metabolic effect.

The main physiologic action of TH is to regulate the basal metabolic rate and thereby control the processes of growth and tissue differentiation. Unlike GH, TH is involved in many more diverse activities that influence the growth and development of body tissues. Therefore, a deficiency of TH exerts a more profound effect on growth than that seen in GH deficiency.

Calcitonin helps maintain blood calcium levels by decreasing the calcium concentration. Its effect is the opposite of parathyroid hormone (PTH) in that it inhibits skeletal demineralization and promotes calcium deposition in the bone.

JUVENILE HYPOTHYROIDISM

Hypothyroidism is one of the most common endocrine problems of childhood. It may be either congenital or acquired and represents a deficiency in secretion of TH (Parks & Felner, 2016).

Beyond infancy, primary hypothyroidism may be caused by a number of defects. For example, a congenital hypoplastic thyroid gland may provide sufficient amounts of TH during the first 1 or 2 years but be inadequate when rapid body growth increases demands on the gland. A partial or complete thyroidectomy for cancer or thyrotoxicosis can

Decelerated growth:
• Less when acquired at later age
Myxedematous skin changes:
• Dry skin
• Puffiness around eyes
• Sparse hair
• Constipation
• Sleepiness
• Mental decline

Enlarged Thyroid Gland
• Usually symmetric
• Firm
• Freely movable
• Nontender

Tracheal Compression
• Sense of fullness
• Hoarseness
• Dysphagia

Hyperthyroidism (Possible)
• Nervousness
• Irritability
• Increased sweating
• Hyperactivity

leave insufficient thyroid tissue to furnish hormones for body requirements. Radiotherapy for Hodgkin disease or other malignancies may lead to hypothyroidism (Pizzo & Poplack, 2016). Infectious processes may cause hypothyroidism. It can also occur when dietary iodine is deficient, although it is now rare in the United States because iodized salt is a readily available source of the nutrient.

Clinical manifestations depend on the extent of dysfunction and the child's age at onset. Primary congenital hypothyroidism is characterized by low levels of circulating THs and raised levels of TSH at birth (Rastogi & LaFranchi, 2010). If left untreated, congenital hypothyroidism causes decreased mental capacity. Improvements in newborn screening have led to earlier detection and prevention of complications. The presenting symptoms are decelerated growth from chronic deprivation of TH or thyromegaly. Impaired growth and development are less severe when hypothyroidism is acquired at a later age, and because brain growth is nearly complete by 2 to 3 years of age, intellectual disability and neurologic sequelae are not associated with juvenile hypothyroidism. Other manifestations are myxedematous skin changes (dry skin, puffiness around the eyes, sparse hair), constipation, lethargy, and mental decline (Box 47.5).

Therapy is TH replacement, the same as for hypothyroidism in infants, although the prompt treatment needed in infants is not required in children. Levothyroxine is administered over a period of 4 to 8 weeks to avoid symptoms of hyperthyroidism. Children treated early continue to have mild delays in reading, comprehension, and arithmetic but catch up. However, adolescents may demonstrate problems with memory, attention, and visuospatial processing.

Care Management

Growth cessation in a child whose growth has previously been normal should alert the health care provider to the possibility of hypothyroidism. Treatment is daily oral TH replacement. The importance of daily compliance and the need for periodic monitoring of serum thyroid level should be stressed to parents. Children should learn to take responsibility for their own health as soon as they are old enough.

GOITER

A *goiter* is an enlargement or hypertrophy of the thyroid gland. It may occur with deficient (hypothyroid), excessive (hyperthyroid), or normal (euthyroid) TH secretion. It can be congenital or acquired. Congenital disease occurs as a result of maternal administration of antithyroid drugs or iodides during pregnancy or as an inborn error of TH production. Acquired disease can result from increased secretion of pituitary TSH in response to decreased circulating levels of TH or from infiltrative neoplastic or inflammatory processes. In areas where dietary iodine (essential for TH production) is deficient, goiter can be endemic.

Enlargement of the thyroid gland may be mild and noticeable only when there is an increased demand for TH (e.g., during periods of rapid growth). Enlargement of the thyroid gland at birth can be sufficient to cause severe respiratory distress. TH replacement is necessary to treat the hypothyroidism and reverse the TSH effect on the gland.

Interprofessional Care Management

Large goiters are identified by their obvious appearance. Smaller nodules may be evident only on palpation. Benign enlargement of the thyroid gland may occur during adolescence and should not be confused with pathologic states. Nodules rarely are caused by a cancerous tumor but always require evaluation. Questions regarding exposure to radiation should be included in patient assessments.

Immediate surgery to remove part of the gland may be lifesaving in infants born with a goiter. When thyroid replacement is necessary, parents have the same needs regarding its administration as discussed for the parents of children who have hypothyroidism.

LYMPHOCYTIC THYROIDITIS

Lymphocytic thyroiditis (*Hashimoto disease, chronic autoimmune thyroiditis*) is the most common cause of thyroid disease in children and adolescents and accounts for the largest percentage of juvenile hypothyroidism. It accounts for many of the enlarged thyroid glands formerly designated *thyroid hyperplasia of adolescence* or *adolescent goiter*. Although lymphocytic thyroiditis can occur during the first 3 years of life, it occurs more frequently after 6 years of age, with peak incidence occurring during adolescence. The presence of a goiter and elevated antithyroglobulin antibody with progressive increase in both thyroid peroxidase antibody and TSH may be predictive factors for future development of hypothyroidism (Kim, Lee, Jung, et al., 2016).

An enlarged thyroid gland is often detected during a routine examination, although it may be noted by parents when the child swallows. In most children, the entire gland is enlarged symmetrically (although it may be asymmetric) and is firm, freely movable, and nontender. There may be manifestations of moderate tracheal compression (sense of fullness, hoarseness, and dysphagia), but it is extremely rare for a nontoxic diffuse goiter to cause airway obstruction. Most children are euthyroid, but some display symptoms of hypothyroidism, including delayed growth and puberty and declining school performance. Other signs suggestive of thyroiditis are found in Box 47.6.

Diagnostic Evaluation

Thyroid function test results are usually normal, although TSH levels may be slightly or moderately elevated. With progressive disease, the T$_4$ decreases followed by a decrease in T$_3$ levels and an increase in TSH. The majority of children have antithyroid antibody titers. However, levels in children are lower than in adults; therefore, repeated measurements may be needed in doubtful cases because titers may increase later in the disease.

Therapeutic Management

In many cases, the goiter is transient, asymptomatic, and regresses spontaneously within 1 or 2 years. Therapy of a nontoxic diffuse goiter is usually simple, uncomplicated, and effective. Oral administration of TH provides the feedback needed to suppress TSH stimulation and decrease the size of the thyroid gland. TSH levels should be monitored, with the goal of restoring normal growth and development. Surgery is contraindicated in this disorder. Untreated patients should be evaluated periodically.

Interprofessional Care Management

Care consists of identifying the child with thyroid enlargement, and providing reassurance and education regarding therapy and positive outcome.

HYPERTHYROIDISM

Graves' disease is the most common cause of hyperthyroidism in children. This disease often runs in families. Graves' disease–associated hyperthyroidism is caused by autoantibodies to the TSH receptor causing excess secretion of TH. Most cases of Graves' disease in children occur in adolescence, with a peak incidence between 12 and 14 years of age. Transient Graves' disease may be present at birth in children of thyrotoxic mothers. The incidence is higher in girls than in boys (Léger & Carel, 2013). There is no cure for Graves' disease, and treatment options continue to be debated among pediatric endocrinologists (Léger & Carel, 2013).

Signs and symptoms of Graves' disease develop gradually, with an interval between onset and diagnosis of approximately 6 to 12 months. Clinical features include irritability, hyperactivity, short attention span, tremors, insomnia, and emotional lability. Clinical manifestations are presented in Box 47.7.

Exophthalmos (protruding eyeballs), which is observed in many children, is accompanied by a wide-eyed staring expression, increased blinking, eyelid lag, lack of convergence, and absence of wrinkling of the forehead when looking upward. As exophthalmos increases, the eyelid may not completely cover the cornea. Visual disturbances may include blurred vision and loss of visual acuity. Eye disease associated with hyperthyroidism can develop long before or after the clinical diagnosis.

Diagnostic Evaluation

Graves' disease is established on the basis of increased levels of T_4 and T_3. TSH is suppressed to unmeasurable levels (Ma, Kuang, Xie, et al., 2008). Other tests are rarely indicated.

Therapeutic Management

Therapy for hyperthyroidism is controversial, but all methods are directed toward slowing the rate of hormone secretion. The three acceptable modes available are antithyroid drugs; subtotal thyroidectomy; and ablation with radioiodine (^{131}I iodide) (Lee & Hwang, 2014; Léger & Carel, 2013). Each is effective, but each has advantages and disadvantages. Pharmacologic therapy may induce a remission, and treatment may be discontinued. However, relapse may occur. Radioactive iodine ablation is usually effective but response may be slower, and there have been concerns about a possible link to thyroid cancer in younger children. Surgery is often used when other treatments are not effective. These children require lifelong monitoring.

BOX 47.7   Clinical Manifestations of Hyperthyroidism (Graves' Disease)

Cardinal Signs
- Emotional lability
- Physical restlessness, characteristically at rest
- Decelerated school performance
- Voracious appetite with weight loss in 50% of cases
- Fatigue

Physical Signs
- Tachycardia
- Widened pulse pressure
- Dyspnea on exertion
- Exophthalmos (protruding eyeballs)
- Wide-eyed, staring expression with eyelid lag
- Tremor
- Goiter (hypertrophy and hyperplasia)
- Warm, moist skin
- Accelerated linear growth
- Heat intolerance (may be severe)
- Hair fine and unable to hold a curl
- Systolic murmurs

Thyroid Storm
Acute onset:
- Severe irritability and restlessness
- Vomiting
- Diarrhea
- Hyperthermia
- Hypertension
- Severe tachycardia
- Prostration

May progress rapidly to:
- Delirium
- Coma
- Death

When affected children exhibit signs and symptoms of hyperthyroidism (e.g., increased weight loss, pulse, pulse pressure, and blood pressure), their activity should be limited to classwork only. Vigorous exercise is restricted until thyroid levels are decreased to normal or near-normal values.

Thyrotoxicosis (thyroid "crisis" or thyroid "storm") may occur from sudden release of TH. Although thyrotoxicosis is unusual in children, a crisis can be life-threatening. These "storms" are evidenced by the acute onset of severe irritability and restlessness, vomiting, diarrhea, hyperthermia, hypertension, severe tachycardia, and prostration. There may be rapid progression to delirium, coma, and even death. A crisis may be precipitated by acute infection, surgical emergencies, or discontinuation of antithyroid therapy. In addition to antithyroid drugs, beta blockers are used to control symptoms until normal thyroid function is achieved (Léger & Carel, 2013). Therapy is usually required for 2 to 3 weeks.

The American Thyroid Association* has an extensive website with information related to prevention, treatment, and cure of thyroid disease.

---

*6066 Leesburg Pike, Suite 550, Falls Church, VA 22041; 800-THYROID; www.thyroid.org.

Interprofessional Care Management

Because the clinical manifestations often appear gradually, the goiter and ophthalmic changes may not be noticed, and the excessive activity may be attributed to behavioral problems. Health care providers in all settings, particularly schools, need to be alert to signs that suggest this disorder, especially weight loss despite an excellent appetite, academic difficulties resulting from a short attention span, inability to sit still, unexplained fatigue and sleeplessness, and difficulty with fine motor skills such as writing. Exophthalmos may develop long before the onset of signs and symptoms of hyperthyroidism and may be the only presenting sign.

Much of these children's care is related to treating physical symptoms before a response to drug therapy is achieved. Children with hyperthyroidism need a quiet, unstimulating environment that is conducive to rest. Increased metabolic rate may cause heat intolerance and increased food intake in these patients. Mood swings and irritability can disrupt relationships, creating difficulties within and outside the home. A school consultation is important to provide education and suggest ways to assist a child after diagnosis. The child and parents should be encouraged to express feelings about the behavior and its effect on others. Heat intolerance may be minimized by the use of light cotton clothing, good ventilation, air conditioning or fans, frequent baths, and adequate hydration. Dietary requirements should be adjusted to meet the child's increased metabolic rate. Rather than three large meals, the child's appetite may be better satisfied by five or six moderate meals throughout the day.

> ## ! NURSING ALERT
>
> Children being treated with propylthiouracil or methimazole must be carefully monitored for side effects of the drug. Because sore throat and fever accompany the grave complication of leukopenia, these children should be seen by a health care provider if such symptoms occur. Parents and children should be taught to recognize and report symptoms immediately.

> ## ! NURSING ALERT
>
> The earliest indication of hypoparathyroidism may be anxiety and mental depression followed by paresthesia and evidence of heightened neuromuscular excitability, such as the following:
> - Chvostek sign: Facial muscle spasm elicited by tapping the facial nerve in the region of the parotid gland
> - Trousseau sign: Carpal spasm elicited by pressure applied to nerves of the upper arm
> - Tetany: Carpopedal spasm (sharp flexion of wrist and ankle joints), muscle twitching, cramps, seizures, and stridor

DISORDERS OF PARATHYROID FUNCTION

The parathyroid glands secrete *parathyroid hormone (PTH)*. Along with vitamin D and calcitonin, PTH regulates the homeostasis of serum calcium concentration (Gardner & Shoback, 2011). The effect of PTH on calcium is opposite that of calcitonin. PTH and vitamin D work together to maintain serum calcium levels within a narrow normal range. They are required for bone mineralization. Secretion of PTH is controlled by a negative feedback system involving the serum calcium ion concentration. Low ionized calcium levels stimulate PTH secretion, causing absorption of calcium by the target tissues; high ionized calcium concentrations suppress PTH.

HYPOPARATHYROIDISM

Hypoparathyroidism is a spectrum of disorders that result in deficient PTH. *Congenital hypoparathyroidism* may be caused by a specific defect in the synthesis or cellular processing of PTH or by aplasia or hypoplasia of the gland (Gardner & Shoback, 2011).

Other causes, including infection and autoimmune syndromes, may cause hypoparathyroidism. Postoperative hypoparathyroidism may follow thyroidectomy. Two forms of transient hypoparathyroidism may be present in newborns, both of which are the result of a relative PTH deficiency. One type is caused by maternal hyperparathyroidism. A more common form appears almost exclusively in infants fed a milk formula with a high phosphate-to-calcium ratio.

Pseudohypoparathyroidism occurs when there is a genetic defect in the cellular receptors to PTH. The result is normal parathyroid gland and elevated PTH levels. Abnormal calcium and phosphorus levels are not affected by administration of PTH. These children typically have a short, stocky build; a round face; and abnormally shaped hands and fingers. They have an increased risk for neuropsychiatric disorders, cataracts, and seizures (Underbjerg, Sikjaer, Mosekilde, et al., 2016).

Clinical signs of hypoparathyroidism are found in Box 47.8. Muscle cramps are an early symptom, progressing to numbness, stiffness, and tingling in the hands and feet. A positive Chvostek or Trousseau sign or laryngeal spasms may be present. Convulsions with loss of consciousness may occur. These episodes may be preceded by abdominal discomfort, tonic rigidity, head retraction, and cyanosis. Headaches and vomiting with increased intracranial pressure and papilledema may occur and may suggest a brain tumor (Doyle, 2016).

Diagnostic Evaluation

The diagnosis of hypoparathyroidism is made on the basis of clinical manifestations associated with decreased serum calcium and increased serum phosphorus. Levels of plasma PTH are low in idiopathic hypoparathyroidism but high in pseudohypoparathyroidism. End-organ responsiveness is tested by the administration of PTH with measurement of urinary cyclic adenosine monophosphate (cAMP). Kidney function tests are included in the differential diagnosis to rule out renal insufficiency. Magnesium levels should also be tested. Although bone radiograph findings are usually normal, they may demonstrate increased bone density and suppressed growth.

Therapeutic Management

The objective of treatment is to maintain normal serum calcium and phosphate levels with minimal complications. Acute or severe tetany is corrected immediately by IV and oral administration of calcium gluconate and follow-up daily doses to achieve normal levels. Twice-daily serum calcium measurements are taken to monitor the efficacy of therapy and prevent hypercalcemia. When diagnosis is confirmed, vitamin D therapy is begun. Vitamin D therapy is somewhat difficult to regulate because the drug has a prolonged onset and a long half-life. Some advocate beginning with a lower dose with stepwise increases and careful monitoring of serum calcium until stable levels are achieved. Others prefer rapid induction with higher doses and rapid reduction to lower maintenance levels (Doyle, 2016).

Long-term management usually consists of vitamin D and oral calcium supplementation. Blood calcium and phosphorus are monitored frequently until the levels have stabilized. Renal function, blood pressure, and serum vitamin D levels are measured every 6 months. Serum magnesium levels are measured to permit detection of hypomagnesemia, which may raise the requirement for vitamin D.

BOX 47.8 Clinical Manifestations of Hypoparathyroidism

Pseudohypoparathyroidism
- Short stature
- Round face
- Short, thick neck
- Short, stubby fingers and toes
- Dimpling of skin over knuckles
- Subcutaneous soft-tissue calcifications
- Intellectual disability a prominent feature

Idiopathic Hypoparathyroidism
- None of the above physical characteristics observed
- May include papilledema
- May have intellectual disability

Both Types
- Dry, scaly, coarse skin with eruptions
- Hair often brittle
- Nails thin and brittle with characteristic transverse grooves
- Dental and enamel hypoplasia
- Muscle contractions:
  - Tetany
  - Carpopedal spasm
  - Laryngospasm (laryngeal stridor)
  - Muscle cramps and twitching
  - Positive Chvostek sign or Trousseau sign
  - Paresthesias, tingling
- Neurologic:
  - Headache
  - Seizures (generalized, absence, or focal)
  - Swings of emotion
  - Loss of memory
  - Depression
  - Confusion possible
- Gastrointestinal:
  - Muscle cramps
  - Diarrhea
  - Vomiting
- Delayed skeletal growth

BOX 47.9 Clinical Manifestations of Hyperparathyroidism

Gastrointestinal
- Nausea
- Vomiting
- Abdominal discomfort
- Constipation

Central Nervous System
- Delusions
- Confusion
- Hallucinations
- Impaired memory
- Lack of interest and initiative
- Depression
- Varying levels of consciousness

Neuromuscular
- Weakness
- Easy fatigability
- Muscle atrophy (especially proximal muscles of lower limbs)
- Tongue twitching
- Paresthesias in extremities

Skeletal
- Vague bone pain
- Subperiosteal resorption of phalanges
- Spontaneous fractures
- Absence of lamina dura around teeth

Renal
- Polyuria
- Polydipsia
- Renal colic
- Hypertension

Interprofessional Care Management

The initial objective is recognition of hypocalcemia. Unexplained convulsions, irritability (especially to external stimuli), gastrointestinal symptoms (diarrhea, vomiting, cramping), and positive signs of tetany are signs of hypocalcemia related to hypoparathyroidism. Care includes institution of seizure and safety precautions; reduction of environmental stimuli; and observation for signs of laryngospasm such as stridor, hoarseness, and a feeling of tightness in the throat. A tracheostomy set and injectable calcium gluconate should be available for emergency use. The administration of calcium gluconate requires precautions against extravasation of the drug and tissue destruction.

The family is educated about daily administration of calcium and vitamin D. Because vitamin D toxicity can be a serious consequence of therapy, parents are advised to watch for signs that include weakness, fatigue, lassitude, headache, nausea, vomiting, and diarrhea. Early renal impairment is manifested by polyuria, polydipsia, and nocturia.

HYPERPARATHYROIDISM

Hyperparathyroidism is rare in childhood but can be primary or secondary. The most common cause of primary hyperparathyroidism is adenoma of the gland (Doyle, 2016). The most common causes of secondary hyperparathyroidism are chronic renal disease, renal osteodystrophy, and congenital anomalies of the urinary tract. The common factor is hypercalcemia. The clinical signs of hyperparathyroidism are listed in Box 47.9.

Diagnostic Evaluation

Blood studies to identify elevated calcium and decreased phosphorus levels are routinely performed. Measurement of PTH and tests to isolate the cause of hypercalcemia, such as renal function studies, should be included. If parathyroid adenoma is suspected, imaging using ultrasound and a sestamibi nuclear subtraction study are recommended (Iqbal & Wahoff, 2009). Other procedures used to substantiate the physiologic consequences of the disorder include electrocardiography and radiographic bone surveys.

Therapeutic Management

Treatment depends on the cause of hyperparathyroidism. The treatment of primary hyperparathyroidism is surgical removal of the tumor or hyperplastic tissue. Treatment of secondary hyperparathyroidism is directed at the underlying contributing cause, which subsequently restores the serum calcium balance. However, in some instances, such as in chronic renal failure, the underlying disorder is irreversible. In this case, treatment is aimed at raising serum calcium levels to inhibit the stimulatory effect of low levels on the parathyroid glands. This includes oral administration of calcium salts, high doses of vitamin D to enhance calcium absorption, a low-phosphorus diet, and administration of a phosphorus-mobilizing aluminum hydroxide to reduce phosphate absorption.

Interprofessional Care Management

The initial objective is recognition of the disorder. Because secondary hyperparathyroidism is a consequence of chronic renal failure, the health care provider is always alert to signs that suggest this complication, especially bone pain and fractures. Because urinary symptoms are the earliest indication, assessment of other body systems for evidence of high calcium levels is indicated when polyuria and polydipsia coexist. Clues to the possibility of hyperparathyroidism include change in behavior, especially inactivity; unexplained gastrointestinal symptoms; and cardiac irregularities.

DISORDERS OF ADRENAL FUNCTION

The *adrenal cortex* secretes three main groups of hormones collectively called *steroids* and classified according to their biologic activity: (1) glucocorticoids (cortisol, corticosterone); (2) mineralocorticoids (aldosterone); and (3) sex steroids (androgens, estrogens, and progestins). The glucocorticoids and mineralocorticoids affect metabolism and stress. The sex steroids influence sexual development but are not essential because the gonads secrete the major supply of these hormones.

The *adrenal medulla* secretes the *catecholamines epinephrine* and *nor-epinephrine*. Both hormones have essentially the same effects on various organs as those caused by direct sympathetic stimulation except that the hormonal effects last several times longer. Catecholamine-secreting tumors are the primary cause of adrenal medullary hyperfunction.

ACUTE ADRENOCORTICAL INSUFFICIENCY

The acute form of adrenocortical insufficiency (*adrenal crisis*) may have a number of causes during childhood. Although a rare disorder, some of the more common etiologic factors include hemorrhage into the gland from trauma, which may be caused by difficult labor; fulminating infections, such as meningococcemia, which result in hemorrhage and necrosis (Waterhouse-Friderichsen syndrome); abrupt withdrawal of exogenous sources of cortisone or failure to increase exogenous supplies during stress; or congenital adrenogenital hyperplasia of the salt-wasting type.

Early symptoms of adrenocortical insufficiency include increased irritability, headache, diffuse abdominal pain, weakness, nausea and vomiting, and diarrhea. Other clinical signs are found in Box 47.10. In newborns, adrenal crisis is accompanied by high fever, tachypnea, cyanosis, and seizures. Usually there is no evidence of infection or clinical signs of bleeding. However, hemorrhage into the adrenal gland may be evident as a palpable retroperitoneal mass.

Diagnostic Evaluation

There is no rapid, definitive test to confirm acute adrenocortical insufficiency. Diagnosis is usually made based on clinical presentation, especially when a fulminating sepsis is accompanied by hemorrhagic manifestations and signs of circulatory collapse despite adequate antibiotic therapy. Because there is no real danger in administering a cortisol preparation for a short period, treatment should be instituted immediately. Improvement with cortisol therapy confirms the diagnosis.

Therapeutic Management

Treatment involves replacement of cortisol, replacement of body fluids to combat dehydration and hypovolemia, administration of glucose solutions to correct hypoglycemia, and specific antibiotic therapy in the presence of infection. Initially, IV hydrocortisone (Solu-Cortef) is administered. Normal saline containing 5% glucose is given parenterally

| BOX 47.10 | Clinical Manifestations of Acute Adrenocortical Insufficiency |

Early Symptoms
- Increased irritability
- Headache
- Diffuse abdominal pain
- Weakness
- Nausea and vomiting
- Diarrhea

Generalized Hemorrhagic Manifestations (Waterhouse-Friderichsen Syndrome)
- Fever (increases as condition worsens)
- Central nervous system signs:
  - Nuchal rigidity
  - Seizures
  - Stupor
  - Coma

Shocklike State
- Weak, rapid pulse
- Decreased blood pressure
- Shallow respirations
- Cold, clammy skin
- Cyanosis
- Circulatory collapse (terminal event)

Newborn
- Hyperpyrexia
- Tachypnea
- Cyanosis
- Seizures
- Gland evident as palpable retroperitoneal mass (hemorrhagic)

to replace lost fluid, electrolytes, and glucose. If hemorrhage has been severe, whole blood may be replaced. In the event that these measures do not reverse the circulatory collapse, vasopressors are used for immediate vasoconstriction and elevation of blood pressure.

After the child's condition has been stabilized, oral doses of cortisone, fluids, and salt are given, similar to the regimen used for chronic adrenocortical insufficiency described later in this chapter. To maintain sodium retention, aldosterone is replaced by synthetic salt-retaining steroids.

Interprofessional Care Management

Because of the abrupt onset and potentially fatal outcome of this condition, prompt recognition is essential. Vital signs, including blood pressure, are taken every 15 minutes. Seizure precautions are instituted. The health care provider should monitor the child's response to fluid and cortisol replacement. Rapid administration of fluids can precipitate cardiac failure, and overdosage with cortisol may cause hypotension and a sudden fall in temperature.

When the acute phase is over and the hypovolemia has been corrected, the child is given oral fluids in small quantities. Rapid ingestion of oral fluids may induce vomiting, which increases dehydration. Therefore, a gradual schedule for reintroducing liquids is planned.

> **! NURSING ALERT**
>
> Monitor serum electrolyte levels, and observe for signs of hypokalemia or hyperkalemia (e.g., weakness, poor muscle control, paralysis, cardiac dysrhythmias, and apnea). The condition is rapidly corrected with IV or oral potassium replacement.

> **! NURSING ALERT**
>
> When an oral potassium preparation is given, it should be mixed with a small amount of strongly flavored fruit juice to disguise its bitter taste.

The sudden, severe nature of this disorder necessitates a great deal of emotional support for the child and family. The child may be placed in an intensive care unit where the surroundings are strange and frightening. Despite the need for emergency intervention, health care providers must be sensitive to the family's psychologic needs and prepare them for each procedure, even if this is a brief statement, such as "The IV infusion is necessary to replace fluid that your child is losing." Because recovery within 24 hours is often dramatic, health care providers should keep the parents apprised of the child's condition, emphasizing signs of improvement such as a lowered temperature and improved blood pressure.

CHRONIC ADRENOCORTICAL INSUFFICIENCY (ADDISON DISEASE)

Chronic adrenocortical insufficiency is rare in children. Causes include infections, destructive lesion of the adrenal gland or neoplasms, and autoimmune processes, but they may also be idiopathic. Because 90% of adrenal tissue must be nonfunctional before signs of insufficiency are manifested, onset of symptoms is often gradual. However, during periods of stress, when demands for additional cortisol are increased, symptoms of acute insufficiency may appear in a previously well child (Box 47.11).

Definitive diagnosis is based on measurements of functional cortisol reserve. The fasting serum cortisol and urinary 17-hydroxycorticosteroid levels are low and fail to rise, and plasma *adrenocorticotropic hormone (ACTH)* levels are elevated with corticotropin (ACTH) stimulation, the definitive test for the disease.

Therapeutic Management

Treatment involves replacement of *glucocorticoids (cortisol)* and *mineralocorticoids (aldosterone)*. Some children are able to be maintained solely on oral supplements of cortisol (cortisone or hydrocortisone preparations) with a liberal intake of salt. During stressful situations, such as fever, infection, emotional upset, or surgery, the dosage must

be tripled to accommodate the body's increased need for glucocorticoids. Failure to meet this requirement will precipitate an acute crisis. Overdosage produces appearance of cushingoid signs.

Children with more severe states of chronic adrenocortical insufficiency require mineralocorticoid replacement to maintain fluid and electrolyte balance. Other forms of therapy include monthly injections of desoxycorticosterone acetate or implantation of desoxycorticosterone acetate pellets subcutaneously every 9 to 12 months.

Interprofessional Care Management

After the disorder is diagnosed, parents need guidance concerning drug therapy. They must be aware of the continuous need for cortisol replacement. Sudden termination of the drug because of inadequate supplies or inability to ingest the oral form because of vomiting, places the child in danger of an acute adrenal crisis. Therefore, parents should always have a spare supply of the medication in the home. Ideally, families will have a prefilled syringe of hydrocortisone and be instructed in proper technique for intramuscular administration of the drug during a crisis. Unnecessary administration of cortisone will not harm the child, but if it is needed, it may be lifesaving. Any evidence of acute insufficiency should be reported to the health care provider immediately.

Undesirable side effects of cortisone include gastric irritation, which is minimized by ingestion with food or the use of an antacid; increased excitability and sleeplessness; weight gain, which may require dietary management to prevent obesity; and, occasionally, behavioral changes, including depression or euphoria. Parents should be aware of signs of overdose and report these to the health care provider. In addition, the drug has a bitter taste, which creates a challenge in its administration.

Because the body cannot supply endogenous sources of cortical hormones during times of stress, the home environment should be stable and relatively free of stress. Parents need to be aware that during periods of emotional or physical crisis, the child requires additional hormone replacement. The child should wear medical alert identification to notify medical personnel to adjust requirements during emergency care.

CUSHING SYNDROME

Cushing syndrome is a characteristic group of manifestations caused by excessive circulating free cortisol. It can result from a variety of causes, which generally fall into one of five categories (Box 47.12).

Cushing syndrome is uncommon in children. When seen, it is often caused by excessive or prolonged steroid therapy that produces a

---

BOX 47.11 Clinical Manifestations of Chronic Adrenocortical Insufficiency

Neurologic Symptoms
- Muscle weakness
- Mental fatigue
- Irritability, apathy, and negativism
- Increased sleeping, listlessness

Pigmentary Changes
- Previous scars
- Palmar creases
- Mucous membranes
- Hair
- Hyperpigmentation over pressure points (elbows, knees, or waist)
- Less frequently, vitiligo (loss of pigmentation)

Gastrointestinal Symptoms
- Dehydration
- Anorexia
- Weight loss

Circulatory Symptoms
- Hypotension
- Small heart size
- Dizziness
- Syncopal (fainting) attacks

Hypoglycemia
- Headache
- Hunger
- Weakness
- Trembling
- Sweating

Other Signs (Seen in Some Children)
- Recurrent, unexplained seizures
- Intense craving for salt
- Acute abdominal pain
- Electrolyte imbalances

BOX 47.12 Etiology of Cushing Syndrome

Pituitary: Cushing syndrome with adrenal hyperplasia, usually attributed to an excess of ACTH
Adrenal: Cushing syndrome with hypersecretion of glucocorticoids, generally a result of adrenocortical neoplasms
Ectopic: Cushing syndrome with autonomous secretion of ACTH, most often caused by extrapituitary neoplasms
Iatrogenic: Cushing syndrome frequently a result of administration of large amounts of exogenous corticosteroids
Food dependent: Inappropriate sensitivity of adrenal glands to normal postprandial increases in secretion of gastric inhibitory polypeptide

ACTH, Adrenocorticotropic hormone.
Adapted from Magiakou, M.A., Mastorakos, G., Oldfield, E.H., et al. (1994). Cushing's syndrome in children and adolescents: Presentation, diagnosis, and therapy. *New England Journal of Medicine, 331*(10), 629–636.

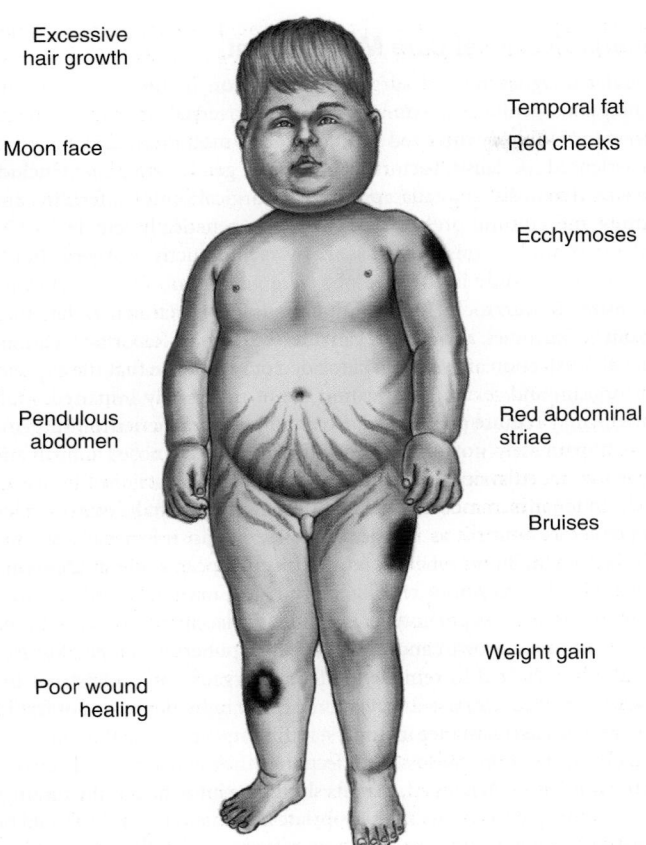

Excessive hair growth

Moon face

Temporal fat

Red cheeks

Ecchymoses

Pendulous abdomen

Red abdominal striae

Bruises

Weight gain

Poor wound healing

FIG 47.2 Characteristics of Cushing syndrome.

cushingoid appearance (Fig. 47.2). This condition is reversible after the steroids are gradually discontinued. Abrupt withdrawal will precipitate acute adrenal insufficiency. Gradual withdrawal of exogenous supplies is necessary to allow the anterior pituitary gland an opportunity to secrete increasing amounts of ACTH to stimulate the adrenal glands to produce cortisol.

Clinical Manifestations

Because the actions of cortisol are widespread, clinical manifestations are equally profound and diverse. The symptoms that produce changes in physical appearance occur early in the disorder and are of considerable concern to school-age and older children. The physiologic disturbances, such as hyperglycemia, susceptibility to infection, hypertension, and hypokalemia, may have life-threatening consequences unless recognized early and treated successfully. Children with short stature may be responding to increased cortisol levels, resulting in Cushing syndrome. Cortisol inhibits the action of GH.

Diagnostic Evaluation

Several tests are helpful in confirming Cushing syndrome. Serum cortisol levels should be measured at midnight and in the morning along with corticotropin hormone, urinary free cortisol, fasting blood glucose levels for hyperglycemia, serum electrolyte levels for hypokalemia and alkalosis, and 24-hour urinary levels of elevated 17-hydroxycorticoids and 17-ketosteroids (Lowitz & Keil, 2015). Imaging of the pituitary and adrenal glands to assess for tumors, bone density studies for evidence of osteoporosis, and skull radiographs to determine enlargement of the sella turcica may also aid in the diagnosis. Another procedure used to establish a more definitive diagnosis is the dexamethasone (cortisone)

suppression test (Ceccato & Boscaro, 2016). Administration of an exogenous supply of cortisone normally suppresses ACTH production. However, in individuals with Cushing syndrome, cortisol levels remain elevated. This test is helpful in differentiating between children who are obese and those who appear to have cushingoid features.

Therapeutic Management

Treatment depends on the cause. In most cases, surgical intervention involves bilateral adrenalectomy and postoperative replacement of the cortical hormones (interventions are the same as those discussed earlier for chronic adrenocortical insufficiency). If a pituitary tumor is found, surgical extirpation or irradiation may be chosen. In either of these instances, treatment of panhypopituitarism with replacement of GH, TH, ADH, gonadotropins, and steroids may be necessary for an indefinite period (Lau, Rutledge, & Aghi, 2015).

Interprofessional Care Management

Care depends on the cause. When cushingoid features are caused by steroid therapy, the effects may be lessened with administration of the drug early in the morning and on an alternate-day basis. Giving the drug early in the day maintains the normal diurnal pattern of cortisol secretion. If given during the evening, it is more likely to produce symptoms because endogenous cortisol levels are already low and the additional supply exerts more pronounced effects. An alternate-day schedule allows the anterior pituitary gland an opportunity to maintain more normal hypothalamic-pituitary-adrenal control mechanisms.

If an organic cause is found, care is related to the treatment regimen. Although a bilateral adrenalectomy permanently solves one condition, it reciprocally produces another syndrome. Before surgery, parents need to be adequately informed of the operative benefits and disadvantages. Postoperative teaching regarding drug replacement is the same as discussed in the previous section.

> **! NURSING ALERT**
>
> Postoperative complications of adrenalectomy are related to the sudden withdrawal of cortisol. Observe for shocklike symptoms (e.g., hypotension, hyperpyrexia).

Anorexia and nausea and vomiting are common and may be improved with the use of nasogastric decompression. Muscle and joint pain may be severe, requiring use of analgesics. The psychologic depression can be profound and may not improve for months. Parents should be aware of the physiologic reasons behind these symptoms in order to be supportive of the child.

CONGENITAL ADRENAL HYPERPLASIA

Congenital adrenal hyperplasia (CAH) is a family of disorders caused by decreased enzyme activity required for cortisol production in the adrenal cortex. The adrenal gland produces excessive amounts of cortisol precursors and androgens to compensate. The most common defect is *21-hydroxylase deficiency*, which constitutes more than 90% of all cases of CAH (Yau, Khattab, & New, 2016). This deficiency is an autosomal recessive disorder that results in improper steroid hormone synthesis (Mendes, Vaz Matos, Ribeiro, et al., 2015).

Excessive androgens cause masculinization of the urogenital system at approximately the tenth week of fetal development. The most pronounced abnormalities occur in girls, who are born with varying degrees of ambiguous genitalia. Masculinization of external genitalia causes the clitoris to enlarge so that it appears as a small phallus. Fusion of the labia produces a saclike structure resembling the scrotum without testes.

However, no abnormal changes occur in the internal sexual organs, although the vaginal orifice is usually closed by the fused labia. The label *ambiguous genitalia* should be applied to any infant with hypospadias or micropenis and no palpable gonads, and a diagnostic evaluation for CAH should be contemplated (Gardner & Shoback, 2011).

Increased pigmentation of skin creases and genitalia caused by increased ACTH may be a subtle sign of adrenal insufficiency. A salt-wasting crisis frequently occurs, usually within the first few weeks of life (White, 2016a). Infants fail to gain weight, and hyponatremia and hyperkalemia may be significant. Cardiac arrest can occur.

Untreated CAH results in early sexual maturation, with enlargement of the external sexual organs; development of axillary, pubic, and facial hair; deepening of the voice; acne; and a marked increase in musculature with changes toward an adult male physique. However, in contrast to precocious puberty, breasts do not develop in girls and they remain amenorrheic and infertile. In boys, the testes remain small and spermatogenesis does not occur. In both sexes, linear growth is accelerated and epiphyseal closure is premature, resulting in short stature by the end of puberty.

Diagnostic Evaluation

Clinical diagnosis is initially based on congenital abnormalities that lead to difficulty in assigning sex to the newborn and on signs and symptoms of adrenal insufficiency. Newborn screening is currently done in all 50 states by measurement of the cortisol precursor 17-hydroxyprogesterone. Definitive diagnosis is confirmed by evidence of increased 17-ketosteroid levels in most types of CAH (Yau et al., 2016). In complete 21-hydroxylase deficiency, blood electrolytes demonstrate loss of sodium and chloride and elevation of potassium. In older children, bone age is advanced and linear growth is increased. DNA analysis for positive sex determination and to rule out any other genetic abnormality (e.g., Turner syndrome) is always done in any case of ambiguous genitalia.

Another test that can be used to visualize the presence of pelvic structures is ultrasonography, a noninvasive, painless imaging technique that does not require anesthesia or sedation. It is especially useful in CAH because it readily identifies the absence or presence of female reproductive organs or male testes in a newborn or child with ambiguous genitalia. Because ultrasonography yields immediate results, it has the advantage of determining the child's sex long before the more complex laboratory results for chromosome analysis or steroid levels are available.

Therapeutic Management

After diagnosis is confirmed, medical management includes administration of glucocorticoids to suppress the abnormally high secretions of ACTH and adrenal androgens. If cortisone is begun early enough, it is very effective. Cortisone depresses the secretion of ACTH by the anterior pituitary gland, which in turn inhibits the secretion of adrenocorticosteroids, which stems the progressive virilization. The signs and symptoms of masculinization in girls gradually disappear, and excessive early linear growth is slowed. Puberty occurs normally at the appropriate age.

The recommended oral dosage is divided to simulate the normal diurnal pattern of ACTH secretion. Because these children are unable to produce cortisol in response to stress, it is necessary to increase the dosage during episodes of infection, fever, surgery, or other stresses. Acute emergencies require immediate IV or intramuscular administration. Children with the salt-wasting type of CAH require aldosterone replacement, as discussed earlier for chronic adrenocortical insufficiency, and supplementary dietary salt. Frequent laboratory tests are conducted to assess the effects on electrolytes, hormonal profiles, and renin levels. The frequency of testing is individualized to the child.

Interprofessional Care Management

Gender assignment and surgical intervention in the newborn with ambiguous genitalia is complex and controversial. It is a significant stress for families, who need support from a multidisciplinary team of experienced specialists. Factors that influence gender assignment include genetic diagnosis, genitalia appearance, surgical options, fertility, and family and cultural preferences. Generally, genetically female (46XX) infants should be raised as girls. Early reconstructive surgery should be considered only in the case of severe virilization (Sturm, Durbin-Johnson, & Kurzrock, 2015). Emphasis is on functional rather than cosmetic outcomes, and surgery can often be delayed. Reports concerning sexual satisfaction after partial clitoridectomy indicate that the capacity for orgasm and sexual gratification is not necessarily impaired. Male infants may require phallic reconstruction by an experienced surgeon.

Unfortunately, not all children with CAH are diagnosed at birth and raised in accordance with their genetic sex. Particularly in the case of affected females, masculinization of the external genitalia may have led to gender assignment as a male. In males, diagnosis is usually delayed until early childhood, when signs of virilism appear. In these situations, it is advisable to continue rearing the child as a male in accordance with assigned gender and phenotype. Hormone replacement may be required to permit linear growth and to initiate male pubertal changes. Surgery is usually indicated to remove the female organs and reconstruct the phallus for satisfactory sexual relations. These individuals are not fertile.

Parents need assistance in understanding and accepting the condition and time to grieve for the loss of perfection in their newborn child. As soon as the gender is determined, parents should be informed of the findings and encouraged to choose an appropriate name, and the child should be identified as a male or female with no reference to ambiguous gender.

In general, rearing a genetically female child as a girl is preferred because of the success of surgical intervention and the satisfactory results with hormones in reversing virilism and providing a prospect of normal puberty and the ability to conceive. This is in contrast to the choice of rearing the child as a boy, in which case the child is sterile and may never be able to function satisfactorily in heterosexual relationships. If the parents persist in their decision to assign a male gender to a genetically female child, a psychologic consultation should be requested to explore their motivations and ensure their understanding of the future consequences for the child.

Interventions regarding cortisol and aldosterone replacement are the same as those discussed earlier for chronic adrenocortical insufficiency. Because infants are especially prone to dehydration and salt-wasting crises, parents need to be aware of signs of dehydration and the urgency of immediate medical intervention to stabilize the child's condition. Parents should have injectable hydrocortisone available and know how to prepare and administer the intramuscular injection (see Chapter 39).

In the unfortunate situation in which the gender is erroneously assigned and the correct gender determined later, parents need a great deal of help in understanding the reason for the incorrect gender identification and the options for gender reassignment or medical-surgical intervention.

Parents should be referred for genetic counseling before they conceive another child because CAH is an autosomal recessive disorder. Prenatal diagnosis and treatment are available.

> **! NURSING ALERT**
>
> Parents should be advised that there is no physical harm in treating for suspected adrenal insufficiency that is not present, but the consequence of not treating acute adrenal insufficiency can be fatal.

PHEOCHROMOCYTOMA

Pheochromocytoma is a rare tumor characterized by secretion of catecholamines. The tumor most commonly arises from the chromaffin cells of the adrenal medulla but may occur wherever these cells are found, such as along the paraganglia of the aorta or thoracolumbar sympathetic chain. In children, they are frequently bilateral or multiple and are generally benign. Often there is a familial transmission of the condition as an autosomal dominant trait (White, 2016b).

The clinical manifestations of pheochromocytoma are caused by an increased production of catecholamines, producing hypertension, tachycardia, headache, decreased gastrointestinal activity with resultant constipation, increased metabolism with anorexia, weight loss, hyperglycemia, polyuria, polydipsia, hyperventilation, nervousness, heat intolerance, and diaphoresis. In severe cases, signs of congestive heart failure are evident.

Diagnostic Evaluation

The clinical manifestations mimic those of other disorders, such as hyperthyroidism or DM. Usually the tumor is identified by computed tomography (CT) or magnetic resonance imaging (MRI). Definitive tests include 24-hour measurement of urinary levels of the catecholamine metabolites, histamine stimulation, and α-adrenergic blocking agents.

Therapeutic Management

Definitive treatment consists of surgical removal of the tumor. In children, the tumors may be bilateral, requiring a bilateral adrenalectomy and lifelong glucocorticoid and mineralocorticoid therapy. The major complications that can occur during surgery are severe hypertension, tachydysrhythmias, and hypotension. The first two are caused by excessive release of catecholamines during manipulation of the tumor, and the latter results from catecholamine withdrawal and hypovolemic shock.

Preoperative medication to inhibit the effects of catecholamines is begun 1 to 3 weeks before surgery to prevent these complications. The major group of drugs used is the α-adrenergic blocking agents. To control catecholamine release when α-adrenergic blocking agents are inadequate, the child is given β-adrenergic blocking agents. Success of therapy is judged by lowering of blood pressure to normal, absence of hypertensive attacks (flushing or blanching, fainting, headache, palpitations, tachycardia, nausea and vomiting, profuse sweating), heat tolerance, a decrease in perspiration, and disappearance of hyperglycemia. A disadvantage of these drugs is their inability to block the effects of catecholamines on beta receptors.

Interprofessional Care Management

Children with hypertension and hypertensive attacks should be assessed for pheochromocytoma. Because of behavioral changes (nervousness, excitability, overactivity, and even psychosis), increased cardiac and respiratory activity may appear to be related to an acute anxiety attack. Therefore a careful history of the onset of symptoms and association with stressful events is helpful in distinguishing between an organic and a psychologic cause for the symptoms.

Preoperative care involves frequent monitoring of vital signs and observation for evidence of hypertensive attacks and congestive heart failure. Therapeutic effects are evidenced by normal vital signs and absence of glycosuria. Daily blood glucose levels, urine acetone, and any signs of hyperglycemia are closely monitored.

! NURSING ALERT

Do not palpate the mass. Preoperative palpation of the mass releases catecholamines, which can stimulate severe hypertension and tachydysrhythmias.

The environment is made conducive to rest and free of emotional stress. This requires adequate preparation during hospital admission and before surgery. Parents are encouraged to room-in with their child and to participate in care. Play activities need to be tailored to the child's energy level without being overly strenuous or challenging because these can increase metabolic rate and promote frustration and anxiety.

After surgery, the child is observed for signs of shock from removal of excess catecholamines. If a bilateral adrenalectomy was performed, the interventions are the same as those discussed earlier for chronic adrenocortical insufficiency.

DISORDERS OF PANCREATIC HORMONE SECRETION

DIABETES MELLITUS

DM is a chronic disorder of metabolism characterized by hyperglycemia and insulin resistance. It is the most common metabolic disease, resulting in metabolic adjustment or physiologic change in almost all areas of the body. In the United States, approximately 215,000 individuals younger than 20 years of age have either type 1 or type 2 diabetes (Centers for Disease Control and Prevention [CDC], 2012). The odds are higher for African-American and Hispanic children—nearly 50% of them will develop diabetes (CDC, 2012). DM in children can occur at any age, but 40% of children diagnosed are between 10 and 14 years of age, and 60% are between 15 and 19 years of age. Girls are 1.3 to 1.7 times more likely to develop type 2 diabetes than boys (Laffel & Svoren, 2015).

Traditionally, DM had been classified according to the type of treatment needed. The former categories were insulin-dependent diabetes mellitus (IDDM), or type I, and non–insulin-dependent diabetes mellitus (NIDDM), or type II. In 1997, these terms were eliminated because treatment can vary (some people with NIDDM require insulin) and because the terms do not indicate the underlying problem. The new terms are *type 1* and *type 2*, using Arabic symbols to avoid confusion (e.g., *type II* could be read as *type eleven*) (American Diabetes Association, 2001). The characteristics of type 1 DM and type 2 DM are outlined in Table 47.1.

In the age-group younger than 10 years of age, most diabetes cases are type 1 and occur most frequently in non-Hispanic whites. In the age-group 10 to 19 years of age, type 1 diabetes is more prominent in non-Hispanic whites followed by African-Americans and then Hispanics; the lowest prevalence is among Native Americans. In type 2 diabetes, Native Americans have the highest incidence followed by African-Americans, Asian Pacific individuals, and Hispanics; the lowest prevalence is in non-Hispanic whites (CDC, 2011). Type 1 diabetes is characterized by destruction of the pancreatic beta cells, which produce insulin; this usually leads to absolute insulin deficiency. Type 1 diabetes has two forms. Immune-mediated DM results from an autoimmune destruction of the beta cells; it typically starts in children or young adults who are slim, but it can arise in adults of any age. Idiopathic type 1 refers to rare forms of the disease that have no known cause.

Type 2 diabetes usually arises because of insulin resistance in which the body fails to use insulin properly combined with relative (rather than absolute) insulin deficiency. People with type 2 can range from predominantly insulin resistant with relative insulin deficiency to predominantly deficient in insulin secretion with some insulin resistance. It typically occurs in those who are older than 45 years of age, are overweight and sedentary, and have a family history of diabetes.

The symptomatology of diabetes is more readily recognizable in children than in adults, so it is surprising that the diagnosis may sometimes be missed or delayed. Diabetes is a great imitator; influenza,

TABLE 47.1   Characteristics of Type 1 and Type 2 Diabetes Mellitus

Characteristic	Type 1	Type 2
Age at onset	<20 years	Increasingly occurring in younger children
Type of onset	Abrupt	Gradual
Sex ratio	Affects males slightly more than females	Females outnumber males
Percentage of diabetic population	5% to 8%	85% to 90%
Heredity:		
Family history	Sometimes	Frequently
Human leukocyte antigen	Associations	No association
Twin concordance	25% to 50%	90% to 100%
Ethnic distribution	Primarily whites	Increased incidence in Native Americans, Hispanics, African-Americans
Presenting symptoms	3 *P*s common: polyuria, polydipsia, polyphagia	May be related to long-term complications
Nutritional status	Underweight	Overweight
Insulin (natural):		
Pancreatic content	Usually none	>50% normal
Serum insulin	Low to absent	High or low
Primary resistance	Minimum	Marked
Islet cell antibodies	80% to 85%	<5%
Therapy:		
Insulin	Always	20% to 30% of patients
Oral agents	Ineffective	Often effective
Diet only	Ineffective	Often effective
Chronic complications	>80%	Variable
Ketoacidosis	Common	Infrequent

BOX 47.13   Clinical Manifestations of Type 1 Diabetes Mellitus

- Polyphagia
- Polyuria
- Polydipsia
- Weight loss
- Enuresis or nocturia
- Irritability; "not himself" or "herself"
- Shortened attention span
- Lowered frustration tolerance
- Dry skin
- Blurred vision
- Poor wound healing
- Fatigue
- Flushed skin
- Headache
- Frequent infections
- Hyperglycemia:
  - Elevated blood glucose levels
  - Glucosuria
- Diabetic ketosis:
  - Ketones and glucose in urine
  - Dehydration in some cases
- Diabetic ketoacidosis (DKA):
  - Dehydration
  - Electrolyte imbalance
  - Acidosis
  - Deep, rapid breathing (Kussmaul respirations)

gastroenteritis, and appendicitis are the conditions most often diagnosed when it turns out that the disease is really diabetes (Box 47.13).

Pathophysiology

Insulin is needed to support the metabolism of carbohydrates, fats, and proteins, primarily by facilitating the entry of these substances into the cells. Insulin is needed for the entry of glucose into the muscle and fat cells, prevention of mobilization of fats from fat cells, and storage of glucose as glycogen in the cells of liver and muscle. Insulin is not needed for the entry of glucose into nerve cells or vascular tissue. The chemical composition and molecular structure of insulin are such that it fits into receptor sites on the cell membrane. Here it initiates a sequence of poorly defined chemical reactions that alter the cell membrane to facilitate the entry of glucose into the cell and stimulate enzymatic systems outside the cell that metabolize the glucose for energy production.

With a deficiency of insulin, glucose is unable to enter the cells and its concentration in the bloodstream increases. The increased concentration of glucose (hyperglycemia) produces an osmotic gradient that causes the movement of body fluid from the intracellular space to the interstitial space and then to the extracellular space and into the glomerular filtrate to "dilute" the hyperosmolar filtrate. Normally, the renal tubular capacity to transport glucose is adequate to reabsorb all the glucose in the glomerular filtrate. When the glucose concentration in the glomerular filtrate exceeds the renal threshold (180 mg/dL), glucose spills into the urine (glycosuria) along with an osmotic diversion of water (polyuria), a cardinal sign of diabetes. The urinary fluid losses cause the excessive thirst (polydipsia) observed in diabetes. This water "washout" results in a depletion of other essential chemicals, especially potassium.

Protein is also wasted during insulin deficiency. Because glucose is unable to enter the cells, protein is broken down and converted to glucose by the liver (glucogenesis); this glucose then contributes to the hyperglycemia. These mechanisms are similar to those seen in starvation when substrate (glucose) is absent. The body is actually in a state of starvation during insulin deficiency. Without the use of carbohydrates for energy, fat and protein stores are depleted as the body attempts to meet its energy needs. The hunger mechanism is triggered, but increased food intake (polyphagia) enhances the problem by further elevating blood glucose.

Ketoacidosis

When insulin is absent or insulin sensitivity is altered, glucose is unavailable for cellular metabolism and the body chooses alternate sources of energy, principally fat. Consequently, fats break down into fatty acids, and glycerol in the fat cells is converted by the liver to ketone bodies (β-hydroxybutyric acid, acetoacetic acid, acetone). Any excess is eliminated in the urine (ketonuria) or the lungs (acetone breath). The ketone bodies in the blood (ketonemia) are strong acids that lower serum pH, producing ketoacidosis.

Ketones are organic acids that readily produce excessive quantities of free hydrogen ions, causing a fall in plasma pH. Then chemical buffers in the plasma, principally bicarbonate, combine with the hydrogen ions to form carbonic acid, which readily dissociates into water and carbon dioxide. The respiratory system attempts to eliminate the excess carbon dioxide by increased depth and rate (Kussmaul respirations, or the hyperventilation characteristic of metabolic acidosis). The ketones are buffered by sodium and potassium in the plasma. The kidneys attempt to compensate for the increased pH by increasing tubular secretion of hydrogen and ammonium ions in exchange for fixed base, thus depleting the base buffer concentration.

With cellular death, potassium is released from the cells (intracellular fluid) into the bloodstream (extracellular fluid) and excreted by the kidneys, where the loss is accelerated by osmotic diuresis. The total body potassium is then decreased even though the serum potassium level may be elevated as a result of the decreased fluid volume in which it circulates. Alteration in serum and tissue potassium can lead to cardiac arrest.

If these conditions are not reversed by insulin therapy in combination with correction of the fluid deficiency and electrolyte imbalance, progressive deterioration occurs, with dehydration, electrolyte imbalance, acidosis, coma, and death. *Diabetic ketoacidosis (DKA)* should be diagnosed promptly in a seriously ill patient and therapy instituted in an intensive care unit.

Long-Term Complications

Long-term complications of diabetes involve both the microvasculature and the macrovasculature. The principal microvascular complications are nephropathy, retinopathy, and neuropathy. Microvascular disease develops during the first 30 years of diabetes, beginning in the first 10 to 15 years after puberty, with renal involvement evidenced by proteinuria and clinically apparent retinopathy. Macrovascular disease develops after 25 years of diabetes and creates the predominant problems in patients with type 2 DM. The process appears to be one of glycosylation, wherein proteins from the blood become deposited in the walls of small vessels (e.g., glomeruli), where they become trapped by "sticky" glucose compounds (glycosyl radicals). The buildup of these substances over time causes narrowing of the vessels, with subsequent interference with microcirculation to the affected areas (Dominqueti, Dusse, Carvalho, et al., 2016).

With poor diabetic control, vascular changes can appear as early as $2\frac{1}{2}$ to 3 years after diagnosis; however, with good to excellent control, changes can be postponed for 20 or more years. Intensive insulin therapy appears to delay the onset and slow the progression of retinopathy, nephropathy, and neuropathy. Hypertension and atherosclerotic cardiovascular disease are also major causes of morbidity and mortality in patients with DM (Mays, 2015).

Other complications have been observed in children with type 1 DM. Hyperglycemia appears to influence thyroid function, and altered function is frequently observed at the time of diagnosis and in poorly controlled diabetes. Limited mobility of small joints of the hand occurs in 30% of 7- to 18-year-old children with type 1 DM and appears to be related to changes in the skin and soft tissues surrounding the joint as a result of glycosylation.

> **! NURSING ALERT**
>
> Recurrent vaginal and urinary tract infections, especially with *Candida albicans*, are often an early sign of type 2 DM, especially in adolescents.

Diagnostic Evaluation

Three groups of children who should be considered as candidates for diabetes are (1) children who have glycosuria, polyuria, and a history of weight loss or failure to gain despite a voracious appetite; (2) those with transient or persistent glycosuria; and (3) those who display manifestations of metabolic acidosis, with or without stupor or coma. In every case, diabetes must be considered if there is glycosuria, with or without ketonuria, and unexplained hyperglycemia.

Glycosuria by itself is not diagnostic of diabetes. Other sugars, such as galactose, can produce a positive result with certain test strips, and a mild degree of glycosuria can be caused by other conditions, such as infection, trauma, emotional or physical stress, hyperalimentation, and some renal or endocrine diseases.

DM is diagnosed based upon any of the following four abnormal glucose metabolites: (1) an 8-hour fasting blood glucose level of 126 mg/dL or more, (2) a random blood glucose value of 200 mg/dL or more accompanied by classic signs of diabetes, (3) an oral glucose tolerance test (OGTT) finding of 200 mg/dL or more in the 2-hour sample, and (4) a hemoglobin A1c of 6.5% or more is almost certain to indicate diabetes (Laffel & Svoren, 2015). Postprandial blood glucose determinations and the traditional OGTTs have yielded low detection rates in

children and are not usually necessary for establishing a diagnosis. Serum insulin levels may be normal or moderately elevated at the onset of diabetes; delayed insulin response to glucose indicates impaired glucose tolerance.

Ketoacidosis must be differentiated from other causes of acidosis or coma, including hypoglycemia, uremia, gastroenteritis with metabolic acidosis, salicylate intoxication encephalitis, and other intracranial lesions. DKA is a state of relative insulin insufficiency and may include the presence of hyperglycemia (blood glucose level ≥200 mg/dL), ketonemia (strongly positive), acidosis (pH <7.30 and bicarbonate <15 mmol/L), glycosuria, and ketonuria (Wolsdorf, Craig, Daneman, et al., 2009). Tests used to determine glycosuria and ketonuria are the glucose oxidase tapes (Keto-Diastix).

Therapeutic Management

The definitive treatment is replacement of insulin that the child is unable to produce. However, insulin needs are also affected by emotions, nutritional intake, activity, and other life events such as illnesses and puberty. The complexity of the disease and its management require that the child and family incorporate diabetes needs into their lifestyle. Medical and nutritional guidance are primary, but management also includes continuing diabetes education, family guidance, and emotional support.

Insulin Therapy

Insulin replacement is the cornerstone of management of type 1 DM. Insulin dosage is tailored to each child based on home blood glucose monitoring. The goal of insulin therapy is maintaining near-normal blood glucose values while avoiding too frequent episodes of hypoglycemia. Insulin is administered as two or more injections per day or as continuous subcutaneous infusion using a portable insulin pump.

Healthy pancreatic cells secrete insulin at a low but steady basal rate with superimposed bursts of increased secretion that coincide with intake of nutrients. Consequently, insulin levels in the blood increase and decrease coincidentally with the rise and fall in blood glucose levels. In addition, insulin is secreted directly into the portal circulation; therefore the liver, which is the major site of glucose disposal, receives the largest concentration of insulin. No matter which method of insulin replacement is used, this normal pattern cannot be duplicated. Subcutaneous injection results in absorption of the drug into the general circulation, thus reducing the concentrations of insulin to which the liver is exposed.

Insulin Preparations

Insulin is available in highly purified pork preparations and in human insulin biosynthesized by and extracted from bacterial or yeast cultures. Most health care providers suggest human insulin as the treatment of choice. Insulin is available in rapid-, intermediate-, and long-acting preparations, and all are packaged in the strength of 100 units/mL. Some insulins are available as premixed insulins, such as 70/30 and 50/50 ratios, the first number indicating the percentage of intermediate-acting insulin and the second number the percentage of rapid-acting insulin. The different types of insulin are found in Box 47.14.

> **! NURSING ALERT**
>
> The human insulins from various manufacturers may be interchangeable, but human insulin and pork insulin or pure pork insulin should never be substituted for one another.

Dosage. Conventional management has consisted of a twice-daily insulin regimen of a combination of *rapid-acting* and *intermediate-acting* insulin drawn up into the same syringe and injected before breakfast and before the evening meal. The amount of morning regular insulin is determined by patterns in the late morning and lunchtime blood glucose values. The morning intermediate-acting dosage is determined by patterns in the late afternoon and dinner blood glucose values. Fasting blood glucose patterns at breakfast help determine the evening dose of intermediate-acting insulin, and the blood glucose patterns at bedtime help determine the evening dose of rapid-acting (regular) insulin. For some children, better morning glucose control is achieved by a later (bedtime) injection of intermediate-acting insulin.

Regular insulin is best administered at least 30 minutes before meals. This allows sufficient time for absorption and results in a significantly greater reduction in the postprandial rise in blood glucose than if the meal were eaten immediately after the insulin injection. Intensive therapy consists of multiple injections throughout the day with a once- or twice-daily dose of long-acting (Ultralente) insulin to simulate the basal insulin secretion and injections of rapid-acting insulin before each meal. A multiple daily injection program reduces microvascular complications of diabetes in young, healthy patients who have type 1 DM.

BOX 47.14   Types of Insulin

There are four types of insulin, based on the following criteria:
- How soon the insulin starts working (onset)
- When the insulin works the hardest (peak time)
- How long the insulin lasts in the body (duration)

However, each person responds to insulin in his or her own way. That is why onset, peak time, and duration are given as ranges.

Rapid-acting insulin (e.g., NovoLog) reaches the blood within 15 minutes after injection. The insulin peaks 30 to 90 minutes later and may last as long as 5 hours.

Short-acting (regular) insulin (e.g., Novolin R) usually reaches the blood within 30 minutes after injection. The insulin peaks 2 to 4 hours later and stays in the blood for about 4 to 8 hours.

Intermediate-acting insulins (e.g., Novolin N) reach the blood 2 to 6 hours after injection. The insulins peak 4 to 14 hours later and stay in the blood for about 14 to 20 hours.

Long-acting insulin (e.g., Lantus) takes 6 to 14 hours to start working. It has no peak or a very small peak 10 to 16 hours after injection. The insulin stays in the blood between 20 and 24 hours.

Some insulins come mixed together (e.g., Novolin 70/30). For example, you can buy regular insulin and NPH insulins already mixed in one bottle, which makes it easier to inject two kinds of insulin at the same time. However, you cannot adjust the amount of one insulin without also changing how much you get of the other insulin.

NPH, Neutral Protamine Hagedorn.

The precise dose of insulin needed cannot be predicted. Therefore the total dosage and percentage of regular- to intermediate-acting insulin should be determined empirically for each child. Usually 60% to 75% of the total daily dose is given before breakfast, and the remainder is given before the evening meal. Furthermore, insulin requirements do not remain constant but change continuously during growth and development; the need varies according to the child's activity level and pubertal status. For example, less insulin is required during spring and summer months when children are more active. Illness also alters insulin requirements. Some children require more frequent insulin administration. This includes children with difficult-to-control diabetes and children during the adolescent growth spurt.

Methods of administration. Daily insulin is administered subcutaneously by twice-daily injections, by multiple-dose injections, or by means of an insulin infusion pump. The insulin pump is an electromechanical device designed to deliver fixed amounts of regular or lispro insulin continuously (basal rate), thereby more closely imitating the release of the hormone by the islet cells. Although the pump delivers a programmed amount of basal insulin, the child or parent must program a dose for the pump to deliver before each meal.

The system consists of a syringe to hold the insulin, a plunger, and a computerized mechanism to drive the plunger. The insulin flows from the syringe through a catheter to a needle inserted into subcutaneous tissue (the abdomen or thigh), and the lightweight device is worn on a belt or a shoulder holster. The needle and catheter are changed every 48 to 72 hours by the child or parent using aseptic technique and then taped in place.

Although the pump provides more consistent insulin delivery, it has certain disadvantages. Pump therapy is expensive and requires commitment from the parent and child. A certain level of mathematical skills is required to calculate infusion rates. It should also not be removed for more than 1 hour at a time, which may limit some activities. Skin infections are common, and as with any other mechanical device, it is subject to malfunction. However, the pumps are equipped with alarms that signal problems, such as a depleted battery, an occluded needle or tubing, or a microprocessor malfunction.

Monitoring

Daily monitoring of blood glucose levels is an essential aspect of appropriate DM management. Plasma blood glucose and hemoglobin A1c goal ranges are found in Table 47.2.

Blood glucose. *Self-monitoring of blood glucose (SMBG)* has improved diabetes management and is used successfully by children from the onset of their diabetes. By testing their own blood, children are able to change their insulin regimen to maintain their glucose level in the euglycemic (normal) range of 80 to 120 mg/dL. Diabetes management

TABLE 47.2   Plasma Blood Glucose and Hemoglobin A1c Goals for Type 1 Diabetes Mellitus by Age-Group

Age	Value* Before Meals (Mg/dL)	Value* at Bedtime/ Overnight (Mg/dL)	Hemoglobin A1c (%)	Implications
Toddlers and preschoolers (<6 years)	100 to 180	110 to 200	≤8.5% (but ≥7.5%)	High risk and vulnerability to hypoglycemia
School age (6 to 12 years)	90 to 180	100 to 180	<8%	Risks for hypoglycemia and relatively low risk for complications before puberty
Adolescents (>12 years) and young adults	90 to 130	90 to 150	<7.5%	Risk for hypoglycemia Developmental and psychologic issues

*Plasma blood glucose goal range.
Adapted from American Diabetes Association. (2005). Standards of medical care in diabetes. *Diabetes Care* 28(Suppl):S4–36.

depends to a great extent on SMBG. In general, children tolerate the testing well.

Glycosylated hemoglobin. The measurement of glycosylated hemoglobin (hemoglobin A1c) levels is a satisfactory method for assessing control of the diabetes. As red blood cells circulate in the bloodstream, glucose molecules gradually attach to the hemoglobin A molecules and remain there for the lifetime of the red blood cell, approximately 120 days. The attachment is not reversible; therefore this glycosylated hemoglobin reflects the average blood glucose levels over the previous 2 to 3 months. The test is a satisfactory method for assessing control, detecting incorrect testing, monitoring the effectiveness of changes in treatment, defining patients' goals, and detecting nonadherence. Nondiabetic hemoglobin A1c values are generally between 4% and 6% but can vary by laboratory. Diabetes control depends on comorbidities, but hemoglobin A1c levels less than 7% indicate an acceptable level for most individuals (Mays, 2015).

Urine. Urine testing for glucose is no longer used for diabetes management; there is poor correlation between simultaneous glycosuria and blood glucose concentrations. However, urine testing can be carried out to detect evidence of ketonuria.

> **! NURSING ALERT**
>
> It is recommended that urine be tested for ketones every 3 hours during an illness or whenever the blood glucose level is over 240 mg/dL when illness is not present.

Nutrition

Essentially, the nutritional needs of children with diabetes are no different from those of healthy children. Children with diabetes need no special foods or supplements. They need sufficient calories to balance daily expenditure for energy and to satisfy the requirement for growth and development. Unlike children without diabetes, whose insulin is secreted in response to food intake, insulin injected subcutaneously has a relatively predictable time of onset, peak effect, duration of action, and absorption rate depending on the type of insulin used. Consequently, the timing of food consumption must be regulated to correspond to the timing and action of the insulin prescribed.

Meals and snacks must be eaten according to peak insulin action, and the total number of calories and proportions of basic nutrients must be consistent from day to day. The constant release of insulin into the circulation makes the child prone to hypoglycemia between the three daily meals unless a snack is provided between meals and at bedtime. The distribution of calories should be calculated to fit the activity pattern of each child. For example, a child who is more active in the afternoon will need a larger snack at that time. This larger snack might also be split to allow some food at school and some food after school. Food intake should be altered to balance food, insulin, and exercise. Extra food is needed for increased activity.

Concentrated sweets are discouraged, and because of the increased risk for atherosclerosis in persons with DM, fat is reduced to 30% or less of the total caloric requirement. Dietary fiber has become increasingly important in dietary planning because of its influence on digestion, absorption, and metabolism of many nutrients. It has been found to diminish the rise in blood glucose after meals.

For growing children, food restriction should never be used for diabetes control, although caloric restrictions may be imposed for weight control if the child is overweight. In general, the child's appetite should be the guide for the amount of calories needed, with the total caloric intake adjusted to appetite and activity.

Exercise

Exercise is encouraged and never restricted unless indicated by other health conditions. Exercise lowers blood glucose levels, depending on the intensity and duration of the activity. Consequently, exercise should be included as part of diabetes management, and the type and amount of exercise should be planned around the child's interests and capabilities. However, in most instances, children's activities are unplanned, and the resulting decrease in blood glucose can be compensated for by providing extra snacks before and, if the exercise is prolonged, during the activity. In addition to a feeling of well-being, regular exercise aids in utilization of food and often results in a reduction of insulin requirements.

Hypoglycemia

Occasional episodes of hypoglycemia are an integral part of insulin therapy, and an objective of diabetes management is to achieve the best possible glycemic control while minimizing the frequency and severity of hypoglycemia. Even with good control, a child may frequently experience mild symptoms of hypoglycemia. If the signs and symptoms are recognized early and promptly relieved by appropriate therapy, the child's activity should be interrupted for no more than a few minutes.

> **! NURSING ALERT**
>
> Hypoglycemic episodes most commonly occur before meals or when the insulin effect is peaking.

The signs and symptoms of hypoglycemia are caused by both increased adrenergic activity and impaired brain function. The increased adrenergic nervous system activity plus increased secretion of catecholamines produce tremulousness, sweating, hunger, and behavioral changes (Mays, 2015). Weakness, dizziness, headache, drowsiness, irritability, loss of coordination, seizures, and coma are more severe responses and reflect CNS glucose deprivation and the body's attempts to elevate the serum glucose levels.

It is often difficult to distinguish between hyperglycemia and a hypoglycemic reaction (Table 47.3). Because the symptoms are similar and usually begin with changes in behavior, the simplest way to differentiate between the two is to test the blood glucose level. The blood glucose level is low in hypoglycemia, but in hyperglycemia, the glucose level is significantly elevated. Urinary ketones may be present after hypoglycemia as a result of starvation. In doubtful situations, it is safer to give the child some simple carbohydrate. This will help alleviate the symptoms in the case of hypoglycemia but will do little harm if the child is hyperglycemic.

Children are usually able to detect the onset of hypoglycemia, but some are too young to implement treatment. Parents should become adept at recognizing the onset of symptoms—for example, a change in a child's behavior, such as tearfulness or euphoria. In the majority of cases, 10 to 15 g of simple carbohydrate, such as 1 Tbsp of table sugar, will elevate the blood glucose level and alleviate the symptoms. The simpler the carbohydrate, the more rapidly it will be absorbed (8 oz of milk equals 15 g of carbohydrate). The rapidly releasing sugar is followed by a complex carbohydrate, such as a slice of bread or a cracker, and by a protein, such as peanut butter or milk.

For a mild reaction, milk or fruit juice is a good food to use in children. Milk supplies them with lactose or milk sugar, as well as a more prolonged action from the protein and fat (aids in decreased absorption). Other glucose sources include Insta-Glucose (cherry-flavored glucose), carbonated drinks (not sugarless), sherbet, gelatin, or cake icing. All children with diabetes should carry with them glucose tabs,

TABLE 47.3   Comparison of Manifestations of Hypoglycemia and Hyperglycemia

Variable	Hypoglycemia	Hyperglycemia
Onset	Rapid (minutes)	Gradual (days)
Mood	Labile, irritable, nervous, weepy	Lethargic
Mental status	Difficulty concentrating, speaking, focusing, coordinating Nightmares	Dulled sensorium Confusion
Inward feeling	Shaky feeling Hunger Headache Dizziness	Thirst Weakness Nausea and vomiting Abdominal pain
Skin	Pallor Sweating	Flushed Signs of dehydration
Mucous membranes	Normal	Dry, crusty
Respirations	Shallow, normal	Deep, rapid (Kussmaul)
Pulse	Tachycardia, palpitations	Less rapid, weak
Breath odor	Normal	Fruity, acetone
Neurologic	Tremors	Diminished reflexes Paresthesia
Ominous signs	Late: Hyperreflexia, dilated pupils, seizure Shock, coma	Acidosis, coma
Blood:		
Glucose	Low: <60 mg/dL	High: ≥250 mg/dL
Ketones	Negative	High, large
Osmolarity	Normal	High
pH	Normal	Low (≤7.25)
Hematocrit	Normal	High
Bicarbonate	Normal	<20 mEq/L
Urine:		
Output	Normal	Polyuria (early) to oliguria (late)
Glucose	Negative	Enuresis, nocturia
Ketones	Negative or trace	High
Vision	Diplopia	Blurred vision

Insta-Glucose, sugar cubes, or sugar-containing candy such as LifeSavers. A difficulty with candies or icing is that the child may learn to fake a reaction to get the sweets; therefore, commercial treatment products such as Insta-Glucose or glucose tabs may be preferred.

Glucagon is sometimes prescribed for home treatment of hypoglycemia. It is available as an emergency kit that must be mixed at the time of use and is administered intramuscularly or subcutaneously. Glucagon functions by releasing stored glycogen from the liver and requires about 15 to 20 minutes to elevate the blood glucose level.

❗ NURSING ALERT

Vomiting may occur after administration of glucagon; therefore precautions against aspiration must be taken (e.g., placing the child on the side) because the child often becomes unconscious.

Morning hyperglycemia. The management of elevated morning blood glucose levels depends on whether the increase is a true dawn phenomenon *(insulin waning)*, or a rebound hyperglycemia *(the Somogyi*

effect). Insulin waning is a progressive rise in blood glucose levels from bedtime to morning. It is treated by increasing the nocturnal insulin dose. The true dawn phenomenon shows a relatively normal blood glucose level until about 3 AM, when the level begins to rise. The Somogyi effect may occur at any time but often entails an elevated blood glucose level at bedtime and a drop at 2 AM with a rebound rise following. The treatment for this phenomenon is decreasing the nocturnal insulin dose to prevent the 2 AM hypoglycemia. The rebound rise in the blood glucose level is a result of counterregulatory hormones (epinephrine, GH, and corticosteroids), which are stimulated by hypoglycemia. More frequent blood monitoring (especially at times of anticipated peak insulin action) will usually identify these conditions. Trace amounts of urinary ketones aid in identifying undetected hypoglycemia.

Illness Management

Illness alters diabetes management, and maintaining control is usually related to the seriousness of the illness. In a well-controlled child, an illness will run its course as it does in unaffected children. The goals during an illness are to restore euglycemia, treat urinary ketones, and maintain hydration. Blood glucose levels and urinary ketones should be monitored every 3 hours. Some hyperglycemia and ketonuria are expected in most illnesses, even with diminished food intake, and are an indication for increased insulin. Insulin should never be omitted during an illness, although dosage requirements may increase, decrease, or remain unchanged, depending on the severity of the illness and the child's appetite. Often the child will need supplemental insulin between usual dose times. If the child vomits more than once, if blood glucose levels remain above 240 mg/dL, or if urinary ketones remain high, the health care provider should be notified. Simple carbohydrates may be substituted for carbohydrate-containing exchanges in the meal plan. Although insulin and diet are important tools in sick-day care, fluids are the most important intervention. Fluids must be encouraged to prevent dehydration and to flush out ketones.

Therapeutic Management of Diabetic Ketoacidosis

DKA, the most complete state of insulin deficiency, is a life-threatening situation. Management consists of rapid assessment, adequate insulin to reduce the elevated blood glucose level, fluids to overcome dehydration, and electrolyte replacement (especially potassium).

DKA constitutes an emergency situation, thus a child should be admitted to an intensive care facility for management. The priority is to obtain a venous access for administration of fluids, electrolytes, and insulin. The child should be weighed, measured, and placed on a cardiac monitor. Blood glucose and ketone levels are determined at the bedside, and samples are obtained for laboratory measurement of glucose, electrolytes, BUN, arterial pH, Po_2, Pco_2, hemoglobin, hematocrit, white blood cell count and differential, calcium, and phosphorus.

Oxygen may be administered to patients who are cyanotic and in whom arterial oxygen is less than 80%. Gastric suction is applied to unconscious children to avoid the possibility of pulmonary aspiration. Antibiotics may be administered to febrile children after appropriate specimens are obtained for culture. A Foley catheter may or may not be inserted for urine samples and measurement. Unless the child is unconscious, a collection bag is usually sufficient for accurate assessments.

Fluid and Electrolyte Therapy

All patients with DKA experience dehydration (10% of total body weight in severe ketoacidosis) because of the osmotic diuresis, accompanied by depletion of electrolytes, sodium, potassium, chloride, phosphate, and magnesium. Serum pH and bicarbonate reflect the degree of acidosis. Prompt and adequate fluid therapy restores tissue perfusion and suppresses the elevated levels of stress hormones.

The initial hydrating solution is 0.9% saline solution. A fluid bolus of 10 to 20 mL/kg can be given over 1 to 2 hours if the patient is hemodynamically unstable; however, total resuscitation volumes should not exceed 40 to 50 mL/kg during the first 4 hours of treatment to avoid the risk for cerebral edema (Olivieri & Chasm, 2013). After the initial bolus, the goal for rehydration is to replace fluids evenly over a period of 24 to 48 hours (Olivieri & Chasm, 2013).

> **! NURSING ALERT**
>
> Potassium must never be given until the serum potassium level is known to be normal or low and urinary voiding is observed. All maintenance IV fluids should include 30 to 40 mEq/L of potassium. Never give potassium as a rapid IV bolus, or cardiac arrest may result.

Serum potassium levels may be normal on admission, but after fluid and insulin administration, the rapid return of potassium to the cells can seriously deplete serum levels, with the attendant risk for cardiac dysrhythmias. As soon as the child has established renal function (is voiding at least 25 mL/hour) and insulin has been given, vigorous potassium replacement is implemented. The cardiac monitor is used as a guide to therapy, and configuration of T waves should be observed every 30 to 60 minutes to determine changes that might indicate alterations in potassium concentration (widening of the QT interval and the appearance of a U wave following a flattened T wave indicate hypokalemia; an elevated and spreading T wave and shortening of the QT interval indicate hyperkalemia).

Insulin should not be given until urinary ketones and a blood glucose level have been obtained. Continuous IV regular insulin is given at a dosage of 0.1 units/kg/hour. Insulin therapy should be started after the initial rehydration bolus because serum glucose levels fall rapidly after volume expansion. Blood glucose levels should decrease by 50 to 100 mg/dL/hour. When blood glucose levels fall to 250 to 300 mg/dL, dextrose is added to the IV solution. The goal is to maintain blood glucose levels between 120 and 240 mg/dL by adding 5% to 10% dextrose. Sodium bicarbonate is not recommended for use in children with DKA and has been associated with the development of cerebral edema (Olivieri & Chasm, 2013).

When the critical period is over, the task of regulating the insulin dosage in relation to diet and activity is started. Children should be actively involved in their own care and are given responsibility according to their ability and the guidance of the nurse.

> **! NURSING ALERT**
>
> Because insulin can chemically bind to plastic tubing and in-line filters, thereby reducing the amount of medication reaching the systemic circulation, an insulin mixture is run through the tubing to saturate the insulin-binding sites before the infusion is started.

Interprofessional Care Management

The management of the child with type 1 DM consists of a multidisciplinary approach involving the family; the child (when appropriate); and professionals, including a pediatric endocrinologist, diabetes nurse educator, nutritionist, and exercise physiologist. Often psychologic support from a mental health professional is also needed. Communication among the team members is essential and extends to other individuals in the child's life, such as teachers, school nurse, school guidance counselor, and coach.

Children with DM may be admitted to the hospital at the time of their initial diagnosis; during illness or surgery; or for episodes of ketoacidosis, which may be precipitated by any of a variety of factors. Many children are able to keep the disease under control with periodic assessment and adjustment of insulin, diet, and activity as needed under the supervision of a health care provider. Under most circumstances, these children can be managed well at home and require hospitalization only for serious illnesses or upsets.

However, a small number of children with diabetes exhibit a degree of metabolic lability and have repeated episodes of DKA that require hospitalization, which interferes with their education and social development. These children appear to display a characteristic personality structure. They tend to be unusually passive and nonassertive and to come from families that are inclined to smooth over conflicts without resolution. Children in this type of setting experience emotional arousal with little, if any, opportunity or ability to resolve it. Other children from psychosocially dysfunctional families display behavioral and personality problems. This emotional stress causes an increased production of endogenous catecholamines, which stimulate fat breakdown, leading to ketonemia and ketonuria.

Hospital Management

Children with DKA require intensive nursing care. Vital signs should be observed and recorded frequently. Hypotension caused by the contracted blood volume of the dehydrated state may cause decreased peripheral blood flow, which can be particularly hazardous to the heart, lungs, and kidneys. An elevated temperature may indicate infection and should be reported so that treatment can be implemented immediately.

Careful and accurate records should be maintained, including vital signs (pulse, respiration, temperature, and blood pressure), weight, IV fluids, electrolytes, insulin, blood glucose level, and intake and output. A urine collection device or retention catheter is used to obtain the urine measurements, which include volume, specific gravity, and glucose and ketone values. The volume relative to the glucose content is important because 5% glucose in a 300-mL sample is a significantly greater amount than a similar reading from a 75-mL sample. A diabetic flow sheet maintained at the bedside provides an ongoing record of the vital signs, urine and blood tests, amount of insulin given, and intake and output. The level of consciousness is assessed and recorded at frequent intervals. The comatose child generally regains consciousness fairly soon after initiation of therapy but is managed like any unconscious child until then.

When the critical period is over, the task of regulating insulin dosage to diet and activity is begun. The same meticulous records of intake and output, urine glucose and acetone levels, and insulin administration are maintained. Capable children should be actively involved in their own care and are given responsibility for keeping the intake and output record; testing the blood and urine; and, when appropriate, administering their own insulin—all under the supervision and guidance of the nurse (see Nursing Care Plan: The Child With Diabetes Mellitus).

Child and Family Education

Several organizations are prepared to assist with education and dissemination of knowledge about diabetes. The American Diabetes Association,* Diabetes Canada,† Juvenile Diabetes Research Foundation International,‡ and American Association of Diabetes Educators§ are

---

*1701 N. Beauregard Street, Alexandria, VA 22311; 800-342-2383; www.diabetes.org.

†1400-522 University Avenue, Toronto, ON M5G 2R5; 800-226-8464; www.diabetes.ca.

‡26 Broadway, 14th Floor, New York, NY 10004; 800-533-CURE; www.jdrf.org.

§200 W. Madison Street, Suite 800, Chicago, IL 60606; 800-338-3633; www.diabeteseducator.org.

NURSING CARE PLAN

The Child With Diabetes Mellitus

Case Study

Tommy is an 8-year-old who has been healthy all his life. Recently his mother noticed that he has lost weight and that he is getting up several times during the night to go to the bathroom. He was drinking a great deal more during the past week, and she thought that was the reason for being awakened at night to use the bathroom. However, today Tommy says he is too tired to go to school and when she goes into his bedroom she notices that he has wet the bed during the night. She becomes alarmed and calls the pediatrician for an appointment the next day. Tommy's mother has a brother with diabetes and thinks that Tommy's symptoms are similar to her brother's problems when he was first diagnosed as a child.

Assessment

What are the most important signs of type 1 diabetes mellitus (DM) that you need to look for in a child?

Defining Characteristics

Polyphagia
Polyuria
Polydipsia
Weight loss
Enuresis or nocturia
Irritability; "not himself" or "herself"
Shortened attention span
Lowered frustration tolerance
Fatigue
Dry skin
Blurred vision
Poor wound healing
Flushed skin
Headache
Frequent infections

Nursing Diagnosis

Risk for Injury related to insulin deficiency

Case Study (Continued)

At the pediatrician's office, several tests are completed to evaluate Tommy. His blood glucose level is 220 mg/dL, and his hemoglobin (Hgb) A1c level is 10.5%. Tommy provides a urine specimen, and the urine dip test is positive for glucose and ketones. Tommy is admitted to the hospital for further evaluation to establish a diagnosis.

Tommy has met the criteria for new-onset diabetes that will require insulin injections to help manage. Initially Tommy will start with a twice-daily insulin regimen combining a rapid-acting (regular) insulin with an intermediate-acting insulin (neutral protamine Hagedorn [NPH]/Lente) drawn up in the same syringe. One injection will be given at least 30 minutes before breakfast. The second one will be given 30 minutes before dinner. Tommy will learn how to self-monitor his blood glucose. Even though he will start off only administering insulin twice daily, he will still need to check his blood glucose before meals and at bedtime. Based on Tommy's age, his glucose goal range should be 90 to 180 mg/dL before meals and 100 to 180 mg/dL at bedtime.

Nursing Interventions and Rationales

What are the most appropriate nursing interventions for administering insulin in a child newly diagnosed with type 1 DM?

Nursing Interventions	Rationales
Obtain blood glucose level before administering insulin.	To determine most appropriate dose of insulin

Nursing Interventions	Rationales
Administer insulin as prescribed.	To maintain normal blood glucose level
Understand the action of insulin: differences in composition, time of onset, and duration of action for the various preparations.	To ensure accurate insulin administration
Employ aseptic techniques when preparing and administering insulin.	To prevent infection
Rotate insulin injection sites.	To enhance absorption of insulin

Expected Outcomes

Tommy's glucose levels will be maintained within the targeted range.
Diabetic ketoacidosis (DKA) will be prevented.
HgA1c levels will range from 6.5% to 8%.

Case Study (Continued)

Tommy's parents are in shock and are asking lots of questions related to diabetes and the care Tommy will require. Tommy is quiet and listens as his parents talk with you and express their fear and concern.

Nursing Interventions and Rationales

What are the most important interventions to focus on with Tommy and his family regarding his diagnosis? Where would you start to teach him and his family regarding diabetes management?

Treatment consists of glucose monitoring, insulin therapy, observing for common problems, encouraging healthy eating, and physical activity. Focus on these four major categories for beginning your education with Tommy and his family.

Nursing Interventions	Rationales
Discuss glucose monitoring.	To determine most appropriate dose of insulin
Teach how to administer insulin.	To maintain normal blood glucose level
Discuss signs and symptoms to look for.	To prevent complications
Promote healthy eating patterns.	To ensure accurate insulin administration
Encourage physical activity.	To enhance absorption of insulin

Expected Outcomes

Parents and Tommy demonstrate an understanding of the following:
- What diabetes is
- The need to administer insulin
- How to administer insulin
- How to monitor glucose
- Signs and symptoms to observe when glucose is low or high
- How to promote healthy eating
- How to remain physically active

Case Study (Continued)

Tommy is expecting to be discharged today. After the morning dose of insulin when the nurse is preparing the family for discharge, Tommy tells her that he feels funny and his head hurts. He is dizzy when he stands, and his hands are shaking. In questioning Tommy's mother about the morning, you are told that he did not eat breakfast because he wanted to eat on the way home.

Assessment

What are the most important signs and symptoms of hypoglycemia?

Defining Characteristics

Hypoglycemia
Shaky feeling

◎ **NURSING CARE PLAN**
The Child With Diabetes Mellitus—cont'd

Hunger
Headache
Dizziness
Difficulty concentrating, speaking, and focusing
Tremors
Tachycardia
Shallow respirations
Can lead to convulsion, shock, and coma

Nursing Diagnosis
Risk for Injury related to hypoglycemia

Nursing Interventions and Rationales
What are the most appropriate nursing interventions for a child newly diagnosed with diabetes who is experiencing hypoglycemia?

Nursing Interventions	Rationales
Immediately administer ½ cup of fruit juice or a glass of nonfat or 1% milk.	To increase blood sugar
Check blood glucose after 15 minutes.	To check blood sugar
Give a starch-protein snack.	To stabilize blood sugar
Give parents instructions regarding signs and symptoms of hypoglycemia versus hyperglycemia.	To promote maintaining blood sugar within an acceptable range
Teach parents how to administer intramuscular (IM) glucagon if unresponsive, unconscious, or seizing.	To increase blood sugar

Expected Outcomes
Tommy's blood sugar will return to the targeted range.

Case Study (Continued)
After 15 minutes, Tommy is feeling better and his blood sugar is within an acceptable range. Tommy's mother is quite concerned and is worried that she will not be able to identify whether his blood sugar level is too high or too low. She is quite worried about Tommy being discharged today.

Assessment
What are some key points that you can review with Tommy's mother about the signs and symptoms of low and high blood sugar?

Defining Characteristics
Hypoglycemia (see earlier)
Hyperglycemia
   Thirst
   Weakness
   Fatigue
   Nausea and vomiting
   Abdominal pain
   Frequent urination
   Confusion
   Flushed
   Rapid respirations
   Breath odor (fruity)

Nursing Diagnosis
Knowledge Deficit related to signs and symptoms of hypoglycemia and hyperglycemia.

Nursing Interventions and Rationales
What should you focus on regarding the family's education needs at this time to ensure Tommy's blood glucose is kept within the targeted range?

Nursing Interventions	Rationales
Review how to recognize high and low blood sugar levels to prevent glucose levels that lead to medical emergencies.	To ensure prompt and appropriate treatment
Reinforce the importance of keeping the blood sugar within a target range.	To keep blood glucose levels stable
Discuss when to contact the health care provider, including fever, vomiting and diarrhea, inability to keep fluids down, and glucose levels above target range.	To ensure prompt and appropriate treatment
Discuss that exercise and increased activity will affect blood glucose levels, so increased monitoring will be necessary.	To keep blood glucose levels stable

Expected Outcomes
Tommy and his parents will understand the signs and symptoms of high or low blood sugar levels and will understand the actions needed when this occurs. His parents will be prepared to help Tommy manage his disease at home.

---

valuable resources for a wide variety of educational materials. The National Institute of Diabetes and Digestive and Kidney Diseases* publishes a number of comprehensive annotated bibliographies, a compilation of resource materials for children, siblings, parents, teachers, and health care professionals, including *What I Need to Know About Physical Activity and Diabetes.*

Medical Identification

One of the first things the nurse should call to the parents' attention is the need for the child to wear some means of medical identification. Usually recommended is the Medic-Alert identification, a stainless steel or silver- or gold-plated identification bracelet that is visible and

immediately recognizable. It contains a telephone number that medical personnel can call around the clock for medical records and personal information.

Nature of Diabetes

The better the parents understand the pathophysiology of diabetes and the function and action of insulin and glucagon in relation to caloric intake and exercise, the better they will understand the disease and its effects on the child. Parents need answers to a number of questions (voiced or unvoiced) to increase their confidence in coping with the disease. For example, they may want to know about the various procedures performed on their child and treatment rationale, such as what is being put in the IV fluid and the expected effect.

Meal Planning

Normal nutrition is a major aspect of the family education program. Diet instruction is usually conducted by the nutritionist, with reinforcement

*Office of Communications and Public Liaison, NIDDK, NIH, Building 31, Room 9A06, 31 Center Drive, MSC 2560, Bethesda, MD 20892-2560; 301-496-3583; www.niddk.nih.gov.

and guidance from the nurse. The emphasis is on adequate intake for age, consistent menus, complex carbohydrates, and consistent eating times. The family is taught how the meal plan relates to the requirements of growth and development, the disease process, and the insulin regimen. Meals and snacks are modified based on the child's preferences and current menu, preserving cultural patterns and preferences as much as possible. Extensive exchange lists are available that include foods compatible with most lifestyles.

Learning about foods within specific food groups helps in making choices. Weights and measures of foods are used as eye-training devices for defining serving sizes and should be practiced for about 3 months, with gradual progression to estimation of food portions. Even when the child and family become competent in estimating portion sizes, reassessment should take place weekly or monthly and when there is any change of brands.

Family members should also be guided in reading labels for the nutritional value of foods and food content. They need to become familiar with the carbohydrate content of food groups. Substitution with foods of equal carbohydrate content is the skill needed for successful carbohydrate counting. Substitution might be necessary if a food is not available in sufficient quantity or for the teenager who wishes to eat fast food with peers. The use of a multiple daily injection program lends flexibility to the timing of meals.

Lists of popular fast-food items and items served at the major fast-food chains can be obtained from the restaurants to help guide food selections. It is important that the child know the nutritional value of these items (the major chains are remarkably uniform), but the child should be cautioned to avoid high-fat and high-sugar/high-carbohydrate items; for example, the child could choose a plain hamburger instead of a double cheeseburger.

Children should use sugar substitutes in moderation in items such as soft drinks. Artificial sweeteners have been shown to be safe, but if there is any question about amounts, the health care provider such as the physician, dietitian, or nurse can provide guidelines on consumption based on body weight. Sugar-free chewing gum and candies made with sorbitol may be used in moderation by children with DM. Although sorbitol is less cariogenic than other varieties of sugar substitutes, it is an alcohol sugar that is metabolized to fructose and then to glucose. Furthermore, large amounts can cause osmotic diarrhea. Most dietetic foods contain sorbitol. They are more expensive than regular foods. Also, although a product may be sugar free, it is not necessarily carbohydrate free.

Traveling

Traveling requires planning, especially when a trip involves crossing time zones. A number of tips are included in pamphlets available free of charge. Suggestions for traveling encompass what will be needed from the health care provider before leaving, what and how much to take along, needs in transit, what to consider at the destination, and planning for when the child returns home. Planning is needed no matter what type of travel is considered—automobile, plane, bus, or train.

Insulin

Families need to understand the treatment method and the insulin prescribed, including the effective duration, onset, and peak action. They also need to know the characteristics of the various types of insulins, the proper mixing and dilution of insulins, and how to substitute another type when their usual brand is not available (insulin is a nonprescription drug). Insulin need not be refrigerated but should be maintained at a temperature between 15° and 29.4° C (59° and 85° F). Freezing renders insulin inactive.

Insulin bottles that have been "opened" (i.e., the stopper has been punctured) should be stored at room temperature or refrigerated for up to 28 to 30 days. After 1 month, these vials should be discarded. Unopened vials should be refrigerated and are good until the expiration date on the label. Diabetic supplies should not be left in a hot environment.

Injection procedure. Learning to give insulin injections is a source of anxiety for both parents and children. It is helpful for the learner to know that this important aspect of care will become as routine as brushing the teeth. First, the basic injection technique is taught using an orange or similar item and sterile normal saline for practice. To gain children's confidence, the nurse can demonstrate the technique by giving a skillful injection to the parent and then having the parent return the demonstration by giving the nurse an injection. With practice and confidence, the parents will soon be able to give the insulin injection to their children and their children will trust them. Another effective strategy is to instruct the children and then have them teach the technique to the parents while the nurse observes. Both parents should participate, and as little time as possible should elapse between instruction and the actual injection, especially with parents and teenage learners.

Insulin can be injected into any area in which there is adipose (fat) tissue over muscle; the drug is injected at a 90-degree angle. Newly diagnosed children may have lost adipose tissue, and care should be exerted not to inject intramuscularly. The pinch technique is the most effective method for tenting the skin to allow easy entrance of the needle to subcutaneous tissues in children. The site selected will sometimes depend on whether children or parents administer the insulin. The arms, thighs, hips, and abdomen are usual injection sites for insulin. The children can reach the thighs, abdomen, and part of the hip and arm easily but may require help to inject other sites. For example, a parent can pinch a loose fold of skin of the arm while the child injects the insulin.

The parents and child are helped to work out a rotation pattern to various areas of the body to enhance absorption because insulin absorption is slowed by fat pads that develop in overused injection areas. The most efficient rotation plan involves giving about four to six injections in one area (each injection about 2.5 cm [1 inch] apart, or the diameter of the insulin vial from the previous injection) and then moving to another area.

Remember that the absorption rate varies in different parts of the body (Table 47.4). The methodical use of one anatomic area and then movement to another (as described in the previous paragraph) minimizes variations in absorption rates. However, absorption is also altered by vigorous exercise, which enhances absorption from exercised muscles; therefore, it is recommended that a site be chosen other than the exercising extremity (e.g., avoiding legs and arms when playing in a tennis tournament).

Injection sites for an entire month can be determined in advance on a simple chart. For example, a "paper doll" (body outline) can be constructed and insulin sites marked by the child. After injection, the child places the date on the appropriate site. To keep in practice, it is

TABLE 47.4 Onset and Duration of Action Related to Injection Site

	SITE OF INJECTION			
	Abdomen	**Arm**	**Leg**	**Buttock**
Rate	Very fast	Fast	Slow	Very slow
Duration	Very short	Short	Long	Very long

From Albisser, A.M., & Sperlich, M. (1992). Adjusting insulins. *Diabetes Educator, 18*(3), 211–218.

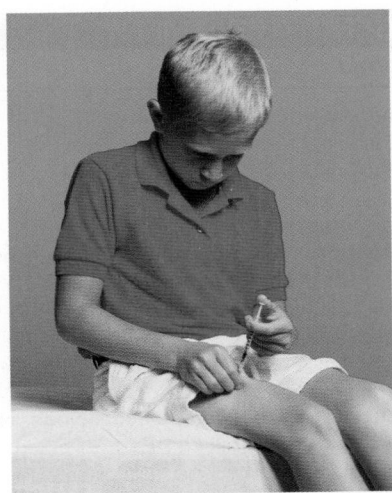

FIG 47.3 School-age children are able to administer their own insulin.

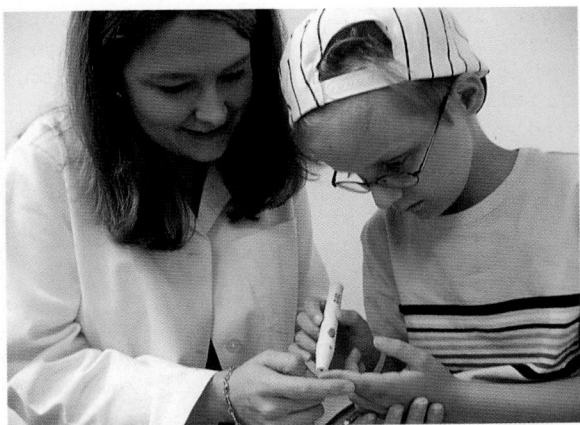

FIG 47.4 Child using a fingerstick device to obtain a blood sample.

a good idea for the parent to give two or three injections per week in areas that are difficult for the child to reach. The same basic methodology is used when teaching children to give their own insulin injections (Fig. 47.3). They should practice first on an orange or a doll, building courage gradually. Other devices are available for insulin injection and may offer advantages to some children. Children who do not wish to give themselves injections can be taught to use a syringe-loaded injector (Inject-Ease). With the device, puncture is always automatic. Adolescents respond well to a self-contained and compact device resembling a fountain pen (NovoPen), which eliminates conventional vials and syringes. Preloaded pens may also cause less pain because the needle is not blunted by piercing the rubber top of the insulin vial.

Continuous subcutaneous insulin infusion. Some children are considered candidates for use of a portable insulin pump, and even some young children with unsatisfactory metabolic control can benefit from its use. The child and the parents are taught to operate the device, including the mechanics of the pump, battery changes, and alarm systems. A number of devices are on the market that vary in the basal rates they are able to deliver and in the cost of the equipment. Families can investigate the various devices and select the model that best suits their needs. Product information is available from pump manufacturers and distributors.*

Parents and children learn (1) the technical aspects of the pump and SMBG; (2) prevention and treatment for hyperglycemia, sick-day management, and meal planning; (3) the effects of exercise, stress, and diet on blood glucose levels; and (4) decision-making strategies to evaluate blood glucose patterns and make adjustments in all aspects of the regimen.

Numerous blood glucose measurements (at least 4 times per day) are an essential part of infusion pump use. Intensive education and supervision are critical to obtaining maximum efficiency and control. This is particularly important if the family has been accustomed to a conventional insulin regimen. They must realize that simply wearing the pump will not normalize blood glucose. The pump is merely an insulin delivery device, and frequent, routine blood glucose determinations are necessary to adjust the insulin delivery rate.

The major problems with use of the insulin pump are inflammation from irritation and infection at the insertion site. The site should be cleansed thoroughly before the needle is inserted and then covered with

*Medtronic, www.medtronicdiabetes.com; Accu-Chek, www.accu-chek. com; Animas, www.animas.com.

ATRAUMATIC CARE
Minimizing Pain of Blood Glucose Monitoring

- To enhance blood flow to the finger, hold it under warm water for a few seconds before the puncture.
- When obtaining blood samples, use the ring finger or thumb (blood flows more easily to these areas) and puncture the finger just to the side of the finger pad (more blood vessels and fewer nerve endings).
- To prevent a deep puncture, press the platform of the lancet device lightly against the skin and avoid steadying the finger against a hard surface.
- Use lancet devices with adjustable-depth tips. Begin with the shallowest setting.
- Use glucose monitors that require small blood samples (e.g., Ascensia Elite) to avoid repeated punctures.

a transparent dressing. The site is changed and rotated every 48 to 72 hours (this may vary) or at the first sign of inflammation. Nurses working where pumps are part of the therapeutic regimen should become familiar with the operation of the specific device being used and the protocol of disease management. Others should be aware of this management technique and be prepared to assist patients using the pump.

Monitoring

Nurses should also be prepared to teach and supervise blood glucose monitoring. SMBG is associated with few complications, and although it does not necessarily lead to improved metabolic control, it provides a more accurate assessment of blood glucose levels than can be obtained with the historical urine testing. Blood glucose monitoring has the added advantage that it can be performed anywhere (see Atraumatic Care box: Minimizing Pain of Blood Glucose Monitoring).

Blood for testing can be obtained by two different methods: manually or with a mechanical bloodletting device. A mechanical device is recommended for children, although the child and family should learn to use both methods in the event of mechanical failure. Several lancet devices are available, and each provides a means for obtaining a large drop of blood for testing (Fig. 47.4).

! NURSING ALERT

Caution children not to allow anyone else to use their lancet because of the risk for contracting hepatitis B virus or human immunodeficiency virus infection.

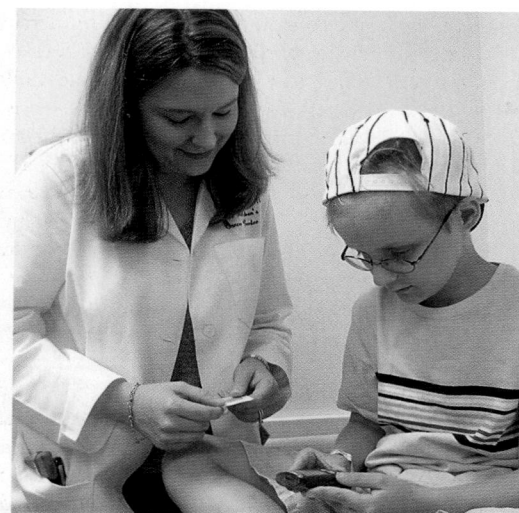

FIG 47.5 Child using a blood glucose monitor and reagent strips to test his blood for glucose.

The blood sample may be obtained from fingertips or alternate sites such as the forearm. Alternate site testing requires a meter that can test a small volume of blood. Not all meters are capable of this.

Signs of redness and soreness at the site of finger puncture should be examined by the health care provider. It may be evidence of poor technique, poor hygiene, or poor skin healing relative to poor control. Many types of blood-testing meters are available for home use. Newer technology has brought about improvements in meter size and ease of use. The family should be shown features of several meters, including advantages and disadvantages, and allowed to choose equipment that best meets their needs.

The least expensive testing method uses a reagent strip to which blood is applied (Fig. 47.5). After blotting, the color change is compared against a color scale for an estimation of the blood glucose level. The strips can be cut in half (although not all professionals recommend this) to obtain two readings per strip. This method is not accepted practice but may be necessary for some families or situations.

Urine testing. Testing for urinary ketones is recommended during times of illness and when blood glucose values are elevated. Information on a specific ketone-testing product should include correct procedure, storage, and product expiration. Families need a clear understanding of home management of ketones (fluids and additional insulin as directed by the health care team).

Signs of Hyperglycemia

Severe hyperglycemia is most often caused by illness, growth, emotional upset, or missed insulin doses. Emotional stress from school finals or examinations and physical response to immunizations are examples of causes of hyperglycemia. With careful glucose monitoring, any elevation can be managed by adjustment of insulin or food intake. Parents should understand how to adjust food, activity, and insulin at the time of illness or when the child is treated for an illness with a medication known to raise the blood glucose level (e.g., steroids). Hyperglycemia is managed by increasing insulin soon after the increased glucose level is noted. Health care professionals should be aware that adolescent girls often become hyperglycemic around the time of their menses and should be advised to increase insulin dosages if necessary.

Signs of Hypoglycemia

Hypoglycemia is caused by imbalances of food intake, insulin, and activity. Ideally, hypoglycemia should be prevented, and parents need

to be prepared to prevent, recognize, and treat the problem. They should be familiar with the signs of hypoglycemia and instructed in treatment, including care of the child with seizures. Early signs are adrenergic, including sweating and trembling, which help raise the blood glucose level, similar to the reaction when an individual is startled or anxious. The second set of symptoms that follow an untreated adrenergic reaction is neuroglycopenic (also called *brain hypoglycemia*). These symptoms typically include difficulty with balance, memory, attention, or concentration; dizziness or lightheadedness; and slurred speech. Severe and prolonged hypoglycemia leads to seizures, coma, and possible death (Mays, 2015). Hypoglycemia can be managed effectively as outlined in the Emergency Treatment box: Hypoglycemia.

It is advisable for parents to plan for anticipated excitement or exercise. In addition, gastroenteritis may decrease insulin needs slightly as a result of poor appetite, vomiting, or diarrhea. If the blood glucose level is low but urinary ketones are present, the family should be aware of the increased need for simple carbohydrates and liquids.

Hygiene

All aspects of personal hygiene should be emphasized for children with diabetes. Children should be cautioned against wearing shoes without socks, wearing sandals, and walking barefoot. Correct nail and extremity care tailored to the individual child (with the guidance of a podiatrist) can begin health practices that last a lifetime. These children's eyes should be checked once per year unless the child wears glasses and then as directed by the ophthalmologist. Regular dental care is emphasized, and cuts and scratches should be treated with plain soap and water unless otherwise indicated. Diaper rash in infants and candida infections in adolescents may indicate poor diabetes control.

Exercise

Exercise is an important component of the treatment plan. If the child is more active at one time of the day than at another time, food or insulin can be altered to meet that activity pattern. Food should be increased in the summer, when children tend to be more active. Decreased activity on return to school may require a decrease in food intake or insulin dosage. Children who are active in team sports will need a snack about a half hour before the anticipated activity. Races or other competition may call for a slightly higher food intake than at practice times.

Food intake will usually need to be repeated for prolonged activity periods, often as frequently as every 45 minutes to 1 hour. Families should be informed that if increased food is not tolerated, decreased insulin is the next course of action. If the timing of the exercise is changed so that the dinner meal is delayed, the insulin in the second or third dose of the day may be moved back to precede the mealtime. Sugar may sometimes be needed during exercise periods for quick response. Elevated blood glucose levels after extreme activity may represent the body's adrenergic response to exercise. If the blood glucose level is elevated (>240 mg/dL) before planned exercise, urinary ketones should be checked and the activity may need be postponed until the blood glucose is controlled.

> ## ! NURSING ALERT
>
> Ketonuria in the presence of hyperglycemia is an early sign of ketoacidosis and a contraindication to exercise.

Record Keeping

Home records are an invaluable aid to diabetes self-management. The nurse and family devise a method to chart insulin administered, blood glucose values, urine ketone results, and other factors and events that affect diabetes control. The child and family are encouraged to observe for patterns of blood glucose responses to events such as exercise. If lapses in management occur (e.g., eating a candy bar), the child should be encouraged to note this and not be criticized for the transgression.

Self-Management

Self-management is the key to close control. Being able to make changes when they are needed rather than waiting until the next contact with health care professionals is important for self-management and gives the individual and family the feeling that they have control over the disease. Psychologically, this helps family members believe they are useful and participating members of the team. Allowing the child to learn to look at records objectively promotes independence in self-management support. As children grow and assume more responsibility for self-management, they develop confidence in their ability to manage their disease and confidence in themselves as people. They learn to respond to the disease and to make more accurate interpretations and changes in treatment when they become adults.

Puberty is associated with decreased sensitivity to insulin that normally would be compensated for by an increased insulin secretion. Health care professionals should anticipate that pubertal patients will have more difficulty maintaining glycemic control. Patients should be taught to give themselves additional doses of rapid-acting insulin (5% to 10% of their daily dose) when their blood glucose levels are increased. The use of supplemental rapid-acting insulin is preferred to withholding food in adolescents.

Child or Adolescent and Family Support

Just as the physiologic responses affect the child, the parents and other family members of the child with newly diagnosed DM experience various emotional responses to the crisis. Care in the acute setting is short but may create fears and frustrations. The prospect of a chronic illness in their child engenders all the feelings and concerns that are faced by parents of children with other chronic illnesses (see Chapter 36). The threat of complications and death is always present, as well as the continuing drain on emotional and financial resources.

Certain fears may develop as a result of past experiences with the disease. A severe insulin reaction with seizures can contribute to fear of repetition. If parents observe a seizure or the adolescent has one

in a public place, the desire to maintain better control is reinforced. They must understand how to prevent problems and how to handle problems calmly and coolly if they occur, and they must understand the complexities of the body, the disease, and its complications. Young children usually adjust well to problems related to the disease. With toddlers and preschoolers, insulin injections and glucose testing may be difficult at first. However, they usually accept the procedures when the parents use a matter-of-fact approach, without calling attention to a "hurt," and treat the procedure like any other routine part of the child's life. After the injection, time with some special and positive attention, such as reading, talking, or another pleasant activity, is one way to convert children who initially refuse injections to those who accept them.

In the years before adolescence, children probably accept their condition most easily. They are able to understand the basic concepts related to their disease and its treatment. They are able to test blood glucose and urine, recognize food groups, give injections, keep records, and distinguish fear or excitement from hypoglycemia. They understand how to recognize, prevent, and treat hypoglycemia. However, they still need considerable parental involvement.

> ## ! NURSING ALERT
>
> Ongoing motivation to adhere to a regimen is difficult. An older child and parent (or another caregiver) may enjoy negotiating a day off when the responsibility for testing and recording blood glucose is delegated from the child to the caregiver (or vice versa).

Adolescents appear to have the most difficulty adjusting. Adolescence is a time of stress in trying to be perfect and similar to one's peers, and no matter what others say, having diabetes is being different. Some adolescents are more upset about not being able to have a candy bar than about injections, diet, and other aspects of management. If children can accept the difference as a part of life—in other words, that each person is different in some way—then, with adequate parental support, they should be able to adjust well (see Clinical Reasoning Case Study: Type 1 Diabetes Mellitus).

CLINICAL REASONING CASE STUDY

Type 1 Diabetes Mellitus

Shelly, a 14-year-old adolescent with a 3-year history of type 1 DM, has been admitted to the pediatric intensive care unit for treatment of DKA. This is her fifth hospital admission for DKA in the past year. Shelly's parents are divorced, and she has four younger siblings, none of whom has diabetes. Shelly's mother has maintained two jobs for the past 5 years and frequently leaves Shelly in charge of the household. In anticipation of her discharge, you are planning a patient education program for Shelly and her mother. What important issues regarding Shelly's unstable diabetes management must you consider to plan the education program?

1. Evidence: Is there sufficient evidence to draw conclusions about Shelly's recurrent episodes of DKA?
2. Assumptions: Describe an underlying assumption about each of the following:
   a. Type 1 DM in adolescence
   b. Type 1 DM and menses
   c. Emotional stress and elevated blood glucose levels
   d. Blood glucose monitoring for insulin management
3. What priorities for nursing care should be established for Shelly?
4. Does the evidence support your nursing intervention?

DKA, Diabetic ketoacidosis; *DM*, diabetes mellitus.

Camping and other special group activities are useful. At diabetes camp, children learn that they are not alone. As a result, they become more independent and resourceful in other settings. Useful information about such camps and organizations can be obtained from the American Diabetes Association. A list of accredited camps specifically for children and teenagers with diabetes is also available from the American Camping Association.*

REFERENCES

Alatzoglou, K. S., & Dattani, M. T. (2010). Genetic causes and treatment of isolated growth hormone deficiency—An update. *Nature Reviews. Endocrinology, 6*(10), 562–576.

American Diabetes Association. (2001). Report of the Expert Committee on the Diagnosis and Classification of Diabetes Mellitus. *Diabetes Care, 24* (1 suppl), S5–S20.

Amin, N., Mushtaq, T., & Alvi, S. (2015). Fifteen-minute consultation: The child with short stature. *Archives of Disease in Childhood. Education and Practice Edition, 100*(4), 180–184.

Brito, V. N., Spinola-Castro, A. M., Kochi, C., et al. (2016). Central precocious puberty: Revisiting the diagnosis and therapeutic management. *Archives of Endocrinology and Metabolism, 60*(2), 163–172.

Carel, J. C., & Léger, J. (2008). Clinical practice. Precocious puberty. *New England Journal of Medicine, 358*(22), 2366–2377.

Ceccato, F., & Boscaro, M. (2016). Cushing syndrome: Screening and diagnosis. *High Blood Pressure & Cardiovascular Prevention, 23*(3), 209–215.

Centers for Disease Control and Prevention (2011). *National diabetes fact sheet 2011: National estimates and general information on diabetes and prediabetes in the US.* Atlanta, GA: Author.

Centers for Disease Control and Prevention (2012). *Diabetes report card.* Atlanta, GA: Centers for Disease Control and Prevention, US Department of Health and Human Services.

Deodati, A., & Cianfarani, S. (2011). Impact of growth hormone therapy on adult height of children with idiopathic short stature: Systematic review. *British Medical Journal, 342*, c7157.

Di Iorgi, N., Allegri, A. E., Napoli, F., et al. (2014). Central diabetes insipidus in children and young adults: Etiological diagnosis and long-term outcome of idiopathic cases. *Journal of Clinical Endocrinology and Metabolism, 99*(4), 1264–1272.

Di Iorgi, N., Morana, G., Napoli, F., et al. (2015). Management of diabetes insipidus and adipsia in the child. *Best Practice & Research: Clinical Endocrinology & Metabolism, 29*(3), 415–436.

Dominqueti, C. P., Dusse, L. M., Carvalho, M., et al. (2016). Diabetes mellitus: The linkage between oxidative stress, inflammation, hypercoagulability and vascular complications. *Journal of Diabetes and Its Complications, 30*(4), 738–745.

Doyle, D. A. (2016). Hypoparathyroidism. In R. M. Kliegman, B. Stanton, J. W. St. Geme, et al. (Eds.), *Nelson textbook of pediatrics* (20th ed.). Philadelphia, PA: Elsevier/Saunders.

Gardner, D., & Shoback, D. (2011). *Greenspan's basic and clinical endocrinology* (9th ed.). New York, NY: Lange Medical Books/McGraw-Hill.

Hokken-Koelega, A. C. (2011). Diagnostic workup of the short child. *Hormone Research in Paediatrics, 76*(3 suppl), 6–9.

Igbal, C. W., & Wahoff, D. C. (2009). Diagnosis and management of pediatric endocrine neoplasms. *Current Opinion in Pediatrics, 21*(3), 379–385.

Kim, S. Y., Lee, Y. A., Jung, H. W., et al. (2016). Pediatric goiter: Can thyroid disorders be predicted at diagnosis and in follow-up? *Journal of Pediatrics, 170*, 253–259.e1-e2.

Laffel, L., & Svoren, B. (2015). *Epidemiology, presentation, and diagnosis of type 2 diabetes mellitus in children and adolescents.* Retrieved from http://

www.uptodate.com/contents/epidemiology-presentation-and-diagnosis-of-type-2-diabetes-mellitus-in-children-and-adolescents.

Lang, D., Mead, J. S., & Sykes, D. B. (2015). Hormones and the bone marrow: Panhypopituitarism and pancytopenia in a man with a pituitary adenoma. *Journal of General Internal Medicine, 30*(5), 692–696.

Latronico, A. C., Brito, V. N., & Carel, J. C. (2016). Causes, diagnosis, and treatment of central precocious puberty. *Lancet Diabetes & Endocrinology, 4*(3), 265–274.

Lau, D., Rutledge, C., & Aghi, M. K. (2015). Cushing's disease: Current medical therapies and molecular insights guiding future therapies. *Neurosurgical Focus, 38*(2), E11.

Lee, H. S., & Hwang, J. S. (2014). The treatment of Graves' disease in children and adolescents. *Annals of Pediatric Endocrinology & Metabolism, 19*(3), 122–126.

Léger, J., & Carel, J. C. (2013). Hyperthyroidism in childhood: Causes, when and how to treat. *Journal of Clinical Research in Pediatric Endocrinology, 5*(1 suppl), 50–56.

Li, P., Li, Y., & Yang, C. L. (2014). Gonadotropin releasing hormone agonist treatment to increase final status in children with precocious puberty: A meta-analysis. *Medicine, 93*(27), e260.

Lowitz, J., & Keil, M. F. (2015). Cushing syndrome: Establishing a timely diagnosis. *Journal of Pediatric Nursing, 30*(3), 528–530.

Ma, C., Kuang, A., Xie, J., et al. (2008). Radioiodine treatment for pediatric Grave's disease (protocol). *Cochrane Database of Systematic Reviews, 2008*(3), CD006294.

Mays, L. (2015). Diabetes mellitus standards of care. *Nursing Clinics of North America, 50*(4), 703–711.

Mendes, C., Vaz Matos, I., Ribeiro, L., et al. (2015). Congenital adrenal hyperplasia due to 21-hydroxylase deficiency: Genotype-phenotype correlation. *Acta Medica Portuguesa, 28*(1), 56–62.

Menon, P. S., & Vijayakumar, M. (2014). Precocious puberty—Perspectives on diagnosis and management. *Indian Journal of Pediatrics, 81*(1), 76–83.

Muhammad, A., van der Lely, A. J., & Neggers, S. J. (2015). Review of current and emerging treatment options in acromegaly. *Netherlands Journal of Medicine, 73*(8), 362–367.

Olivieri, L., & Chasm, R. (2013). Diabetic ketoacidosis in the pediatric emergency department. *Emergency Medicine Clinics of North America, 31*(3), 755–773.

Parks, J. S., & Felner, E. I. (2016). Hypopituitarism. In R. M. Kliegman, B. Stanton, J. St. Geme, et al. (Eds.), *Nelson textbook of pediatrics* (20th ed.). Philadelphia, PA: Elsevier/Saunders.

Pizzo, P. A., & Poplack, D. G. (2016). *Principles and theories of pediatric oncology.* Philadelphia, PA: Lippincott.

Rastogi, M. V., & LaFranchi, S. H. (2010). Congenital hypothyroidism. *Orphanet Journal of Rare Diseases, 5*, 17.

Reid-Adam, J. (2013). Hyponatremia. *Pediatrics in Review, 24*(9), 417–419.

Richmond, E. J., & Rogol, A. D. (2008). Growth hormone deficiency in children. *Pituitary, 71*, 115–120.

Stanley, T. (2012). Diagnosis of growth hormone deficiency in childhood. *Current Opinion in Endocrinology, Diabetes and Obesity, 19*(1), 47–52.

Sturm, R. M., Durbin-Johnson, B., & Kurzrock, E. A. (2015). Congenital adrenal hyperplasia: Current surgical management at academic medical centers in the United States. *Journal of Urology, 193*(5 suppl), 1796–1801.

Underbjerg, L., Sikjaer, T., Mosekilde, L., et al. (2016). Pseudohypoparathyroidism—Epidemiology, mortality and risk of complications. *Clinical Endocrinology (Oxford), 84*(6), 904–911.

White, P. C. (2016a). Congenital adrenal hyperplasia and related disorders. In R. M. Kliegman, B. Stanton, J. W. St. Geme, et al. (Eds.), *Nelson textbook of pediatrics* (20th ed.). Philadelphia, PA: Elsevier/Saunders.

White, P. C. (2016b). Pheochromocytoma. In R. M. Kliegman, B. Stanton, J. W. St. Geme, et al. (Eds.), *Nelson textbook of pediatrics* (20th ed.). Philadelphia, PA: Elsevier/Saunders.

Wolsdorf, J., Craig, M. E., Daneman, D., et al. (2009). Diabetic ketoacidosis in children and adolescents with diabetes. *Pediatric Diabetes, 10*(12 suppl), 118–133.

Yau, M., Khattab, A., & New, M. I. (2016). Prenatal diagnosis of congenital adrenal hyperplasia. *Endocrinology Metabolism Clinics of North America, 45*(2), 267–281.

*5000 State Road 67 N, Martinsville, IN 46151; 800-428-2267; http://www.acacamps.org.

48

The Child With Musculoskeletal or Articular Dysfunction

Marilyn J. Hockenberry

http://evolve.elsevier.com/Perry/maternal

THE IMMOBILIZED CHILD

IMMOBILIZATION

One of the most difficult aspects of illness in children is the immobility it often imposes on a child. Children's natural tendency to be active influences all aspects of their growth and development. Impaired mobility presents a challenge to children, their families, and their caregivers.

PHYSIOLOGIC EFFECTS OF IMMOBILIZATION

Many clinical studies, including space program research, have documented predictable consequences that occur after immobilization and the absence of gravitational force. Functional and metabolic responses to restricted movement can be noted in most of the body systems. Each has a direct influence on the child's growth and development because of homeostatic mechanisms that thrive on normal use and feedback to maintain dynamic equilibrium. Inactivity leads to a decrease in the functional capabilities of the whole body as dramatically as the lack of physical exercise leads to muscle weakness.

Disuse from illness, injury, or a sedentary lifestyle can limit function and potentially delay age-appropriate milestones. Most of the pathologic changes that occur during immobilization arise from decreased muscle strength and mass, decreased metabolism, and bone demineralization, which are closely interrelated, with one change leading to or affecting the others.

The major effects of immobilization are outlined briefly in Table 48.1 and are related directly or indirectly to decreased muscle activity, which produces numerous primary changes in the musculoskeletal system with secondary alterations in the cardiovascular, respiratory, skeletal, metabolic, and renal systems. The musculoskeletal changes that occur during disuse are a result of alterations in the effect of gravity and stress on the muscles, joints, and bones. Muscle disuse leads to tissue breakdown and loss of muscle mass (atrophy). Muscle atrophy causes decreased strength and endurance, which may take weeks or months to restore.

The daily stresses on bone created by motion and weight bearing maintain the balance between bone formation (osteoblastic activity) and bone resorption (osteoclastic activity). During immobilization, increased calcium leaves the bone, causing osteopenia (demineralization of the bones), which may predispose bone to pathologic fractures. A joint contracture begins when the arrangement of collagen, the main structural protein of connective tissues, is altered, resulting in a denser tissue that does not glide as easily. Eventually, muscles, tendons, and ligaments can shorten and reduce joint movement, ultimately producing contractures that restrict function. The major musculoskeletal consequences of immobilization are as follows:

- Significant decrease in muscle size, strength, and endurance
- Bone demineralization leading to osteoporosis
- Contractures and decreased joint mobility

Circulatory stasis combined with hypercoagulability of the blood, which results from factors such as damage to the endothelium of blood vessels (Virchow triad), can lead to thrombus and embolus formation. Deep vein thrombosis (DVT) involves the formation of a thrombus in a deep vein, such as the iliac and femoral veins, and can cause significant morbidity if it remains undetected and untreated. The larger the portion of the body immobilized and the longer the immobilization, the greater the risks of immobility.

PSYCHOLOGIC EFFECTS OF IMMOBILIZATION

For children, one of the most difficult aspects of illness is immobilization. Throughout childhood, physical activity is an integral part of daily life and is essential for physical growth and development. It also serves children as an instrument for communication and expression and as a means for learning about and understanding their world. Activity helps them deal with a variety of feelings and impulses and provides a mechanism by which they can exert control over inner tensions. Children respond to anxiety with increased activity. Removal of this power deprives them of necessary input and a natural outlet for their feelings and fantasies. Through movement, children also gain sensory input, which provides an essential element for developing and maintaining body image.

When children are immobilized by disease or as part of a treatment regimen, they experience diminished environmental stimuli with a loss of tactile input and an altered perception of themselves and their environment. Sudden or gradual immobilization narrows the amount and variety of environmental stimuli children receive by means of all their senses: touch, sight, hearing, taste, smell, and proprioception (a feeling of where they are in their environment). This sensory deprivation frequently leads to feelings of isolation and boredom and of being forgotten, especially by peers.

The quest for mastery at every stage of development is related to mobility. Even speech and language skills require sensorimotor activity and experience. For toddlers, exploration and imitative behaviors are essential to developing a sense of autonomy. Preschoolers' expression of initiative is evidenced by the need for vigorous physical activity. School-age children's development is strongly influenced by physical achievement and competition. Adolescents rely on mobility to achieve independence.

TABLE 48.1 Summary of Physical Effects of Immobilization With Nursing Interventions*

Primary Effects	Secondary Effects	Nursing Considerations
Muscular System		
Decreased muscle strength, tone, and endurance	Decreased venous return and decreased cardiac output	Use antiembolism stockings or intermittent compression devices to promote venous return (monitor circulatory and neurovascular status of extremities when such devices are used).
	Decreased metabolism and need for oxygen	
	Decreased exercise tolerance	Plan play activities to use uninvolved extremities.
	Bone demineralization	Place in upright posture when possible.
Disuse atrophy and loss of muscle mass	Catabolism	Have patient perform range-of-motion, active, passive, and stretching exercises.
	Loss of strength	
Loss of joint mobility	Contractures, ankylosis of joints	Maintain correct body alignment.
		Use joint splints as indicated to prevent further deformity.
		Maintain range of motion.
Weak back muscles	Secondary spinal deformities	Maintain body alignment.
Weak abdominal muscles	Impaired respiration	See nursing considerations for respiratory system.
Skeletal System		
Bone demineralization— osteoporosis, hypercalcemia	Negative bone calcium uptake	With paralysis, use upright posture on tilt table.
	Pathologic fractures	Handle extremities carefully when turning and positioning.
	Calcium deposits	Administer calcium-mobilizing drugs (diphosphonates) and normal saline infusions if ordered.
	Extraosseous bone formation, especially at hip, knee, elbow, and shoulder	Ensure adequate intake of fluid; monitor output.
		Acidify urine.
	Renal calculi	Promptly treat urinary tract infections.
Negative bone calcium uptake	Life-threatening electrolyte imbalance	Monitor serum calcium levels.
		Provide electrolyte replacement as indicated.
Metabolism		
Decreased metabolic rate	Slowing of all systems	Mobilize as soon as possible.
	Decreased food intake	Have patient perform active and passive resistance exercises and deep-breathing exercises.
		Ensure adequate food intake.
		Provide a high-protein, high-fiber diet.
Negative nitrogen balance	Decline in nutritional state	Encourage small, frequent feedings with protein and preferred foods.
	Impaired healing	Prevent pressure areas.
Hypercalcemia	Electrolyte imbalance	See nursing consideration for skeletal system.
Decreased production of stress hormones	Decreased physical and emotional coping capacity	Identify causes of stress.
		Implement appropriate interventions to lower physical and psychosocial stresses.
Cardiovascular System		
Decreased efficiency of orthostatic neurovascular reflexes	Inability to adapt readily to upright position (orthostatic intolerance)	Monitor peripheral pulses and skin temperature changes.
	Pooling of blood in extremities in upright posture	Use antiembolism stockings or intermittent compression devices to decrease pooling when upright.
Diminished vasopressor mechanism	Orthostatic intolerance with syncope, hypertension, deceased cerebral blood flow, tachycardia	Provide abdominal support.
		In severe cases, use antigravitational pants.
		Position horizontally.
Altered distribution of blood volume	Increased cardiac workload	Monitor hydration, blood pressure, and urinary output.
	Decreased exercise tolerance	
Venous stasis	Pulmonary emboli or thrombi	Encourage and assist with frequent position changes.
		Elevate extremities without knee flexion.
		Ensure adequate fluid intake.
		Have patient perform active or passive exercises or movement as needed.
		Prescribe routine wearing of antiembolism stockings or intermittent compression devices.
		Monitor for signs of pulmonary embolism: sudden dyspnea, chest pain, respiratory arrest.
		Promptly intervene to maintain adequate oxygenation if signs and symptoms of pulmonary emboli are noted.
		Measure circumference of extremities periodically.
		Give anticoagulant drugs as prescribed.

TABLE 48.1   Summary of Physical Effects of Immobilization With Nursing Interventions*—cont'd

Primary Effects	Secondary Effects	Nursing Considerations
Dependent edema	Tissue breakdown and susceptibility to infection	Administer skin care. Turn every 2 to 4 hours. Monitor skin color, temperature, and integrity. Use pressure-reduction surface as necessary to prevent skin breakdown (see Chapter 39).
Respiratory System		
Decreased need for oxygen	Altered oxygen/carbon dioxide exchange and metabolism	Promote exercise as tolerated. Encourage deep-breathing exercises.
Decreased chest expansion and diminished vital capacity	Diminished oxygen intake Dyspnea and inadequate arterial oxygen saturation; acidosis	Position for optimum chest expansion. Semi-Fowler position may assist in lung expansion if patient can tolerate. Use prone positioning without pressure on abdomen to allow gravity to aid in diaphragmatic excursion. Ensure that patient maintains proper alignment when sitting to prevent pressure on respiratory mechanism.
Poor abdominal tone and distention	Interference with diaphragmatic excursion	Avoid restriction of chest and abdominal musculature. Supply torso support to promote chest expansion.
Mechanical or biochemical secretion retention	Hypostatic pneumonia Bacterial and viral pneumonia Atelectasis	Change position frequently. Carry out chest percussion, vibration, and drainage (or suctioning) as necessary. Use incentive spirometer Monitor breath sounds.
Loss of respiratory muscle strength	Poor cough	Encourage coughing and deep breathing. Support chest wall by splinting with pillow when patient coughs. Use incentive spirometer. Observe for signs of respiratory distress with pulse oximetry or blood gas measurement as necessary.
	Upper respiratory tract infection	Prevent contact with infected people. Provide adequate hydration. Administer immunizations as necessary (pneumococcal, meningococcal).
Gastrointestinal System		
Distention caused by poor abdominal muscle tone	Interference with respiratory movements Difficulty in feeding in prone position	Monitor bowel sounds. Encourage small, frequent feedings.
No specific primary effect	Possible constipation caused by gravitational effect on feces through ascending colon or weakened smooth muscle tone Anorexia	Have patient sit in upright position in bedside chair if possible. Carry out bowel training program with hydration, stool softeners, increased fiber intake, and mild laxatives if necessary. Stimulate appetite with favored foods.
Urinary System		
Alteration of gravitational force	Difficulty in voiding in prone position	Position as upright as possible to void.
Impaired ureteral peristalsis	Urinary retention in calyces and bladder Infection Renal calculi	Hydrate to ensure adequate urinary output for age. Stimulate bladder emptying with warm running water, as necessary. Catheterize only for severe urinary retention. Administer antibiotics as indicated.
Integumentary System		
Altered tissue integrity	Decreased circulation and pressure leading to tissue injury	Turn and reposition at least every 2 to 4 hours. Frequently inspect total skin surface. Eliminate mechanical factors causing pressure, friction, moisture, or irritation. Place on pressure-reduction mattress.
	Difficulty with personal hygiene	Assess ability to perform self-care and assist with bathing, grooming, and toileting as needed. Encourage self-care to potential ability. Ensure adequate intake of protein, vitamins, and minerals.

*Individualize care according to a child's needs; interventions may vary in different institutions.

The monotony of immobilization may lead to sluggish intellectual and psychomotor responses; decreased communication skills; increased fantasizing; and rarely, hallucinations and disorientation. Children are likely to become depressed over loss of ability to function or the marked changes in body image. Physical interference with the activity of infants and young children gives them a feeling of helplessness. They may regress to earlier developmental behaviors, such as wanting to be fed, bedwetting, and baby talk.

Children may react to immobility by active protest, anger, and aggressive behavior, or they may become quiet, passive, and submissive. They may believe the immobilization is a justified punishment for misbehavior. Children should be allowed to display their anger, but it should be within the limits of safety to their self-esteem and not damaging to the integrity of others (see the "Providing Opportunities for Play and Expressive Activities" section in Chapter 38). When children are unable to express anger, aggression is often displayed inappropriately through regressive behavior and outbursts of crying or temper tantrums.

EFFECT ON FAMILIES

Even brief periods of immobilization may disrupt family function, and catastrophic illness or disability may severely tax a family's resources and coping abilities. The family's needs often must be met by the services of a multidisciplinary team, and nurses play a key role in anticipating the services that they will need and in coordinating conferences to plan care. Home management is frequently planned prior to discharge, including special considerations for addressing cultural, economic, physical, and psychologic needs. A child with a severe disability is very dependent, and caregivers need respite to revitalize themselves. Individual and group counseling is beneficial for solving problems in advance and provides an emotional support system. Parent groups are also helpful and often allow nonthreatening social contact. The families of children with permanent disabilities need long-term resources because some of the most difficult problems arise as they try to sustain high-quality care for many years (see Chapter 36).

Care Management

Physical assessment of the child who is immobilized for any number of reasons (e.g., injury or illness) includes a focus not only on the injured part (e.g., fracture) but also on the functioning of other systems that may be affected secondarily—the circulatory, renal, respiratory, muscular, and gastrointestinal systems. With long-term immobilization, there may also be neurologic impairment and changes in electrolytes (especially calcium), nitrogen balance, and the general metabolic rate. The psychologic impact of immobilization should also be assessed.

Children who require prolonged total immobility and are unable to move themselves in bed should be placed on a pressure-reduction mattress to prevent skin breakdown. Frequent position changes also help prevent dependent edema and stimulate circulation, respiratory function, gastrointestinal motility, and neurologic sensation. Children at greater risk for skin breakdown include those with prolonged immobilization, mechanical ventilation, casts, and assistive devices including orthotics, prosthetics, and wheelchairs. Additional risk factors include poor nutrition, friction (from bed linen with traction), and moist skin (from urine or perspiration). Nursing care of children at risk includes strategies for preventing skin breakdown when such conditions are present. The Braden Q Scale is a reliable, objective tool that may be used in the assessment for pressure ulcer development in children who are acutely ill or who are at risk for skin breakdown from neurologic conditions and immobilization (Noonan, Quigley & Curley, 2011).

The use of antiembolism stockings or intermittent compression devices prevents circulatory stasis and dependent edema in the lower extremities and the development of DVT. Anticoagulant therapy may also be implemented with low-molecular-weight heparin, unfractionated heparin, or vitamin K antagonists. The child should be allowed as much activity as possible within the limitations of the illness or treatment. Any functional mobility, however minimal, is preferred to total immobility.

High-protein, high-calorie foods are encouraged to prevent negative nitrogen balance, which may be difficult to correct by diet, especially if there is anorexia as a result of immobility and decreased gastrointestinal function (decreased motility and possibly constipation). Stimulating the appetite with small servings of attractively arranged, preferred foods may be sufficient. At times, supplementary nasogastric or gastrostomy feedings or intravenous (IV) nutrition or fluids may be needed, but these are reserved for serious disability in which oral intake is impossible. Adequate hydration and, when possible, an upright position and remobilization promote bowel and kidney function and help prevent complications in these systems.

Children are encouraged to be as active as their condition and restrictive devices allow. This poses few problems for children, whose innate ingenuity and natural inclination toward mobility provide them with the impetus for physical activity. They need the opportunity, the materials and objects to stimulate activity, and the encouragement and participation of others. Those who are unable to move may benefit from passive exercise and movement in consultation with a physical therapist.

Using dolls, stuffed animals, or puppets to illustrate and explain the immobilization method (e.g., traction, cast) is a valuable tool for small children. Placing a cast, tubing, or other restraining equipment on the doll offers the child a nonthreatening opportunity to express, through the doll, feelings concerning the restrictions and feelings toward the nurse and other health care providers. The doll or puppet may also be used for teaching the child and family procedures, such as IV therapy, procedural sedation, and general anesthesia.

Whenever possible, transporting the child outside the confines of the room increases environmental stimuli and allows social contact with others. Specially designed wheelchairs or carts for increased mobility and independence are available. While hospitalized, children benefit from visitors, computers, books, interactive video games, and other items brought from their own room at home. An activity center or slanting tray can be helpful for the child with limited mobility to use for drawing, coloring, writing, and playing with small toys, such as trucks and cars. Accessibility to clocks, calendars, and a program of diversional therapy are also beneficial. All these interventions help children to function in a more typical way while hospitalized. Children are able to express frustration, displeasure, and anger through play activities (see Chapter 38), which is helpful in their recovery. A child life specialist should be consulted for recreational planning.

All efforts should be made to minimize family disruption resulting from the hospitalization. Children should be allowed to wear their own clothes (street clothes, especially for preadolescent and adolescent girls) and resume school and preinjury activities if able. A parent or sibling should be allowed to stay overnight and room in with the hospitalized child to prevent the effects of family disruption. Visits from significant persons, such as family members and friends, offer occasions for emotional support and also provide opportunities for learning how to care for the child. Privacy is necessary, especially for adolescents.

One of the most useful interventions to help children cope with immobility is participation in their own care. Self-care to the maximum extent is usually well received by children. They can help plan their daily routine; select their diet; and choose "street clothes," including innovative adornment, such as a baseball cap or brightly colored stockings to express their autonomy and individuality. They are encouraged to do as much for themselves as they are able to keep their muscles active and their interest alive.

Although most of the suggestions discussed relate to hospital care, the same consultations (physical therapist, occupational therapist, child life specialist, speech therapist) and environment may be considered in the home as well to help the child and family achieve independence and normalization (see Chapter 36). For a child with greatly restricted movement (e.g., child with a bilateral hip spica cast or confined to bed rest), care is often a challenge. These situations require long-term management either in the hospital or at home. Wherever the care occurs, consistent planning and coordination of activities with other health care workers and caregivers are vital nursing functions.

Family Support and Home Care

The needs of a child with severe disabilities can be complex, and family members require time to assimilate the teachings and demonstrations needed to understand the child's situation and care. Even a child who is confined on a short-term basis can be a challenge for the family, which is usually unprepared for the problems imposed by the child's special needs. Home modification is usually needed for facilitating care, especially when it involves traction, a large cast, or extended confinement. Suitable child care may be needed for times when all family members work.

Just as in the hospital, the child at home is encouraged to be as independent as possible and to follow a schedule that approximates his or her normal lifestyle as nearly as possible, such as continuing school lessons, regular bedtime, and suitable recreational activities.

TRAUMATIC INJURY

SOFT-TISSUE INJURY

Injuries to the muscles, ligaments, and tendons are common in children (Fig. 48.1). In young children, soft-tissue injury usually results from mishaps during play. In older children and adolescents, participation in sports is a common cause of such injuries.

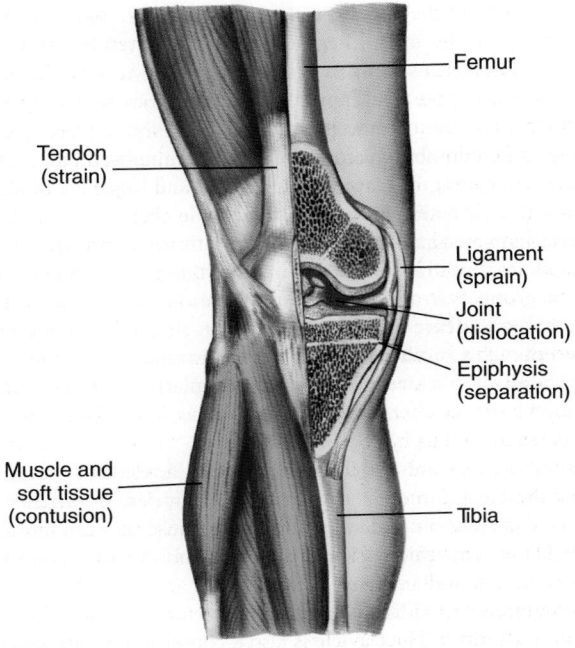

Femur

Tendon (strain)

Ligament (sprain)

Joint (dislocation)

Epiphysis (separation)

Muscle and soft tissue (contusion)

Tibia

FIG 48.1 Sites of injuries to bones, joints, and soft tissues.

Contusions

A contusion (bruise) is damage to the soft tissue, subcutaneous structures, and muscle. The tearing of these tissues and small blood vessels and the inflammatory response lead to hemorrhage, edema, and associated pain when the child attempts to move the injured part. The escape of blood into the tissues is observed as *ecchymosis*, a black-and-blue discoloration.

Large contusions cause gross swelling, pain, and disability and usually receive immediate attention from health care personnel. Smaller injuries may go unnoticed, allowing continued participation. However, they can become disabling after rest because of pain and muscle spasm. Immediate treatment consists of cold application, as in the treatment of sprains described later. Return to participation is allowed when the strength and range of motion of the affected extremity are equal to those of the opposite extremity or are demonstrated under conditions, such as sport-specific tests. Myositis ossificans may occur from deep contusions to the biceps or quadriceps muscles; this condition may result in a restriction of flexibility of the affected limb.

Crush injuries occur when children's extremities or digits are crushed (e.g., fingers slammed in doors, folding chairs, or equipment) or hit (as when hammering a nail). A severe crush injury involves the bone, with swelling and bleeding beneath the nail (subungual) and sometimes laceration of the pulp of the nail. The subungual hematoma can be released by creating a hole at the proximal end of the nail with a special cautery device or a heated sterile 18-gauge needle.

Dislocations

Long bones are held in approximation to one another at the joint by ligaments. A dislocation occurs when the force of stress on the ligament is so great as to displace the normal position of the opposing bone ends or the bone end to its socket. The predominant symptom is pain that increases with attempted passive or active movement of the extremity. In dislocations, there may be an obvious deformity and inability to move the joint. Children with naturally lax joints are more prone to dislocation of joints. Dislocation of the phalanges is the most common type seen in children, followed by elbow dislocation. In the adolescent population, shoulder dislocations are more common, and dislocation unaccompanied by fracture is rare.

A common injury in young children is subluxation, or partial dislocation, of the radial head, also called *pulled elbow* or *nursemaid's elbow*. In the majority of cases, the injury occurs in a child younger than 5 years of age who receives a sudden longitudinal pull or traction at the wrist while the arm is fully extended and the forearm pronated. It usually occurs when an individual who is holding the child by the hand or wrist gives a sudden pull or jerk to prevent a fall or attempts to lift the child by pulling the wrist or when the child pulls away by dropping to the floor or ground. The child often cries, appears anxious, complains of pain in the elbow or wrist, and refuses to use the affected limb. The practitioner manipulates the arm by applying firm finger pressure to the head of the radius and then supinates and flexes the forearm to return the bone structure to normal alignment. A click may be heard or felt, and functional use of the arm returns within minutes. Immobilization is not required. However, the longer the subluxation is present, the longer it takes for the child to recover mobility after treatment. No anesthetic is usually required, but a mild pain reliever such as acetaminophen or ibuprofen may be administered. In an older child, severe elbow injury or dislocation should be immediately evaluated by a practitioner. If a traumatic elbow injury in a younger child is not a subluxation or if attempts at reduction are unsuccessful, the child should be carefully evaluated, with the consideration of radiographs.

In children younger than 5 years of age, the hip can be dislocated by a fall. The greatest risk after this injury is the potential loss of blood supply to the head of the femur. Relocation of the hip within 60 minutes after the injury provides the best chance for prevention of damage to the femoral head.

Shoulder dislocations and separations occur most often in older adolescents and are often sports related. Temporary restriction of the joint, with a sling or bandage that secures the arm to the chest in a shoulder dislocation, can provide sufficient comfort and immobilization until medical attention is received.

Simple dislocations should be reduced as soon as possible with the child under procedural sedation combined with local anesthesia. An unreduced dislocation may be complicated by increased swelling, making reduction difficult and increasing the risk for neurovascular problems. Treatment is determined by the severity of the injury.

Sprains

A sprain occurs when trauma to a joint is so severe that a ligament is partially or completely torn or stretched by the force created as a joint is twisted or wrenched, often accompanied by damage to associated blood vessels, muscles, tendons, and nerves. Common sprain sites include ankles and knees.

The presence of joint laxity is the most valid indicator of the severity of a sprain. In a severe injury, the child complains of the joint "feeling loose" or as if "something is coming apart" and may describe hearing a "snap," "pop," or "tearing." Pain may or may not be the principal subjective symptom, and in some children, it may prevent optimal examination of ligamentous instability. There is a rapid onset of swelling, often diffuse, accompanied by immediate disability and appreciable reluctance to use the injured joint.

Strains

A strain is a microscopic tear to the musculotendinous unit and has features in common with sprains. The area is painful to touch and swollen. Most strains are incurred over time rather than suddenly, and the rapidity of the appearance provides clues regarding severity. In general, the more rapidly the strain occurs, the more severe the injury. When the strain involves the muscular portion, there is more bleeding, often palpable soon after injury and before edema obscures the hematoma.

Therapeutic Management

The first 12 to 24 hours are the most critical period for virtually all soft-tissue injuries. Basic principles of managing sprains and other soft-tissue injuries are summarized in the acronyms RICE and ICES.

Rest	**I**ce
Ice	**C**ompression
Compression	**E**levation
Elevation	**S**upport

Soft-tissue injuries should be iced immediately. This is best accomplished with crushed ice wrapped in a towel, a screw-top ice bag, or a resealable plastic storage bag. Chemical-activated ice packs are also effective for immediate treatment but are not reusable and must be closely monitored for leakage. A wet elastic wrap, which transfers cold better than dry wrap, is applied to provide compression and to keep the ice pack in place. A cloth barrier should be used between the ice container and the skin to prevent trauma to the tissues. Ice has a rapid cooling effect on tissues that reduces edema and pain. Ice should never be applied for more than 30 minutes at a time.

> **! NURSING ALERT**
>
> A plastic bag of frozen vegetables, such as peas, serves as a convenient ice pack for soft-tissue injuries. It is clean, watertight, and easily molded to the injured part. When available, snow placed in a plastic bag may serve as an ice bag.

Elevating the extremity uses gravity to facilitate venous return and reduce edema formation in the damaged area. The point of injury should be kept several inches above the level of the heart for therapy to be effective. Several pillows can be used for elevation. Allowing the extremity to be dependent causes excessive fluid accumulation in the area of injury, delaying healing and causing painful swelling.

Torn ligaments, especially those in the knee, are usually treated by immobilization with a knee immobilizer or a knee brace that allows flexion and extension until the child is able to walk without a limp. Crutches are used for mobility to rest the affected extremity. Passive leg exercises, gradually increased to active ones, are begun as soon as sufficient healing has taken place. Parents and children are cautioned against using any form of liniment or other heat-producing preparation before examination. If the injury requires casting or splinting, the heat generated in the enclosed space can cause extreme discomfort and even tissue damage. In some cases, torn knee ligaments are managed with arthroscopy and ligament repair or reconstruction as necessary depending on the extent of the tear, ligaments involved, and child's age. Surgical reconstruction of the anterior cruciate ligament may be performed in young athletes who wish to continue in active sports.

FRACTURES

Bone fractures occur when the resistance of bone against the stress being exerted yields to the stress force. Fractures are a common injury at any age but are more likely to occur in children and older adults. Because childhood is a time of rapid bone growth, the pattern of fractures, problems of diagnosis, and methods of treatment differ in children compared with adults. In children, fractures heal much faster than in adults. Consequently, children may not require as long a period of immobilization of the affected extremity as an adult with a fracture.

Fracture injuries in children are most often a result of traumatic incidents at home, at school, in a motor vehicle, or in association with recreational activities. Children's everyday activities include vigorous play that predisposes them to injury, including climbing, falling down, running into immovable objects, skateboarding, jumping on trampolines, skiing, participating in playground activities, and receiving blows to any part of their bodies by a solid, immovable object.

Aside from automobile accidents or falls from heights, true injuries that cause fractures rarely occur in infancy. Bone injury in children of this age group warrants further investigation. In any small child, radiographic evidence of fractures at various stages of healing is, with few exceptions, a result of nonaccidental trauma (child abuse). Any investigation of fractures in infants, particularly multiple fractures, should include consideration of osteogenesis imperfecta (OI) after nonaccidental trauma has been ruled out.

Fractures in school-age children are often a result of playground falls or bicycle/automobile or skateboard injuries. Adolescents are vulnerable to multiple and severe trauma because they are mobile on bicycles, all-terrain vehicles, skateboards, skis, snowboards, trampolines, and motorcycles and are active in sports.

A distal forearm (radius, ulna, or both) fracture is the most common fracture in children. The clavicle is also a common fracture sustained in childhood, with approximately one-half of clavicle fractures occurring

---

BOX 48.1 **Types of Fractures in Children**

Plastic deformation: Occurs when the bone is bent but not broken. A child's flexible bone can be bent 45 degrees or more before breaking. However, if bent, the bone will straighten slowly but not completely, producing some deformity but without the angulation seen when the bone breaks. Bends occur most commonly in the ulna and fibula, often in association with fractures of the radius and tibia.

Buckle, or torus, fracture: Produced by compression of the porous bone; appears as a raised or bulging projection at the fracture site. These fractures occur in the most porous portion of the bone near the metaphysis (the portion of the bone shaft adjacent to the epiphysis) and are more common in young children.

Greenstick fracture: Occurs when a bone is angulated beyond the limits of bending. The compressed side bends, and the tension side fails, causing an incomplete fracture similar to the break observed when a green stick is broken.

Complete fracture: Divides the bone fragments. These fragments often remain attached by a **periosteal hinge**, which can aid or hinder reduction.

---

in children younger than 10 years of age. Common mechanisms of injury include a fall with an outstretched hand or direct trauma to the bone. In neonates, a fractured clavicle may occur with a large newborn and a small maternal pelvis. This may be noted in the first few days after birth by a unilateral Moro reflex or at the 2-week well-child check, when a fracture callus is palpated on the infant's healing clavicle.

Types of Fractures

A fractured bone consists of fragments: the fragment closer to the midline, or the proximal fragment, and the fragment farther from the midline, or the distal fragment. When fracture fragments are separated, the fracture is *complete*; when fragments remain attached, the fracture is *incomplete*. The fracture line can be any of the following:

Transverse: Crosswise at right angles to the long axis of the bone

Oblique: Slanting but straight between a horizontal and a perpendicular direction

Spiral: Slanting and circular, twisting around the bone shaft

The twisting of an extremity while the bone is breaking results in a spiral break. If the fracture does not produce a break in the skin, it is a *simple*, or *closed*, fracture. *Open*, or *compound*, fractures are those with an open wound through which the bone protrudes. If the bone fragments cause damage to other organs or tissues (e.g., lung, liver), the injury is said to be a *complicated fracture*. When small fragments of bone are broken from the fractured shaft and lie in the surrounding tissue, the injury is a *comminuted fracture*. This type of fracture is rare in children. The types of fractures that are seen most often in children are described in Box 48.1 and Fig. 48.2.

Growth Plate (Physeal) Injuries

The weakest point of long bones is the cartilage growth plate, or the *physis*. Consequently, this is a frequent site of damage of childhood trauma. Growth plate fractures are classified with the Salter-Harris classification system (Fig. 48.3). Detection of physeal injuries is sometimes difficult but critical. Close monitoring and early treatment, if indicated, is essential to prevent longitudinal or angular growth deformities (or both). Treatment of these fractures may include surgical open reduction and internal fixation to prevent or reduce growth disturbances.

Immediately after a fracture occurs, the muscles contract and physiologically splint the injured area. This phenomenon accounts for the muscle tightness observed over a fracture site and the deformity that is produced as the muscles pull the bone ends out of alignment. This

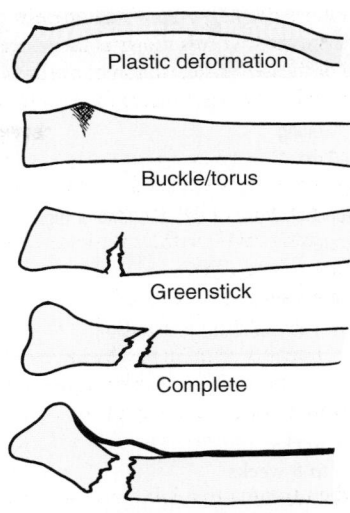

FIG 48.2 Types of fractures in children.

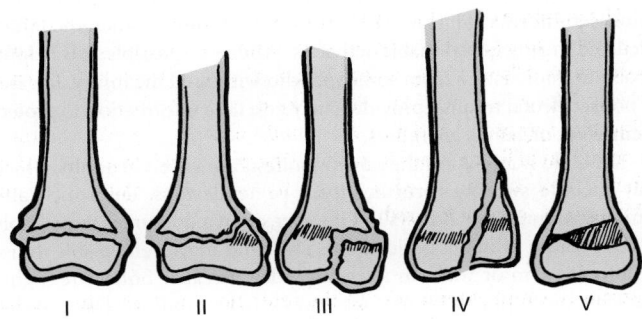

FIG 48.3 Salter-Harris fracture classification. Types of epiphyseal injury in order of increasing risk. The injuries are classified as follows: Type I, separation or slip of growth plate without fracture of the bone; type II, separation of growth plate and breaking off of section of metaphysis; type III, fracture of epiphysis extending through joint surface; type IV, fracture of growth plate, epiphysis, and metaphysis; and type V, crushing injury of epiphysis (can be diagnosed only in retrospect). This classification of epiphyseal injuries was developed by orthopedists R.B. Salter and W.R. Harris. (First published in Salter, R.B., & Harris, W.R. [1963]. Injuries involving the physeal plate. *Journal of Bone and Joint Surgery, 45*([3], 587–622.)

muscle response must be overcome by traction or complete muscle relaxation (e.g., anesthesia) to realign the distal bone fragment to the proximal bone fragment.

Bone Healing and Remodeling

Bone healing is rapid in growing children because of the thickened periosteum and generous blood supply. When there is a break in the continuity of bone, the osteoblasts are stimulated to maximal activity. New bone cells are formed in immense numbers almost immediately after the injury and, in time, are evidenced by a bulging growth of new bone tissue between the fractured bone fragments. This is followed by deposition of calcium salts to form a callus. Remodeling is a process that occurs in the healing of long bone fractures in growing children. The irregularities produced by the fracture become indistinct as the angles and bone overgrowth are smoothed out, giving the bone a straighter appearance.

Fractures heal in less time in children than in adults. The approximate healing times for a femoral shaft are as follows:

BOX 48.2   Clinical Manifestations of a Fracture

Signs of injury:
- Generalized swelling
- Pain or tenderness
- Deformity
- Diminished functional use of affected limb or digit

May also demonstrate:
- Bruising
- Severe muscular rigidity
- Crepitus (grating sensation at fracture site)

Neonatal period: 2 to 3 weeks
Early childhood: 4 weeks
Later childhood: 6 to 8 weeks
Adolescence: 8 to 12 weeks

Diagnostic Evaluation

A history of the injury may be lacking in childhood injuries. Infants and toddlers are unable to communicate, and older children may not volunteer information (even under direct questioning) when the injury occurred during questionable activities. Whenever possible, it is helpful to obtain information from someone who witnessed the injury. In cases of nonaccidental trauma, providers may give false information to protect themselves or family members.

The child may exhibit the same manifestations seen in adults, which may include swelling, bruising, pain or tenderness, deformity, and diminished function (Box 48.2). However, often a fracture is remarkably stable because of intact periosteum. The child may even be able to use an affected arm or walk on a fractured leg. Because bones are highly vascular, a soft, pliable hematoma may be felt around the fracture site.

! NURSING ALERT

A fracture should be strongly suspected in a small child who refuses to walk or crawl.

Radiographic examination is the most useful diagnostic tool for assessing skeletal trauma. The calcium deposits in bone make the entire structure radiopaque. Radiographic films are taken after fracture reduction and, in some cases, may be taken during the healing process to determine satisfactory progress.

Therapeutic Management

The goals of fracture management are as follows:
- To regain alignment and length of the bony fragments (reduction)
- To retain alignment and length (immobilization)
- To restore function to the injured parts
- To prevent further injury and deformity

The majority of children's fractures heal well, and nonunion is rare. Fractures are splinted or casted to immobilize and protect the injured extremity. Children with displaced fractures may have immediate surgical reduction and fixation (internal or external) rather than being immobilized by traction (Fig. 48.4). This practice is more common and holds true for all types of fractures, including femur fractures, although there is variation based on provider preference and institutional practice. Some conditions require immediate medical attention, including open fractures, compartment syndrome, fractures associated with vascular or nerve injury, and joint dislocations that are unresponsive to reduction maneuvers.

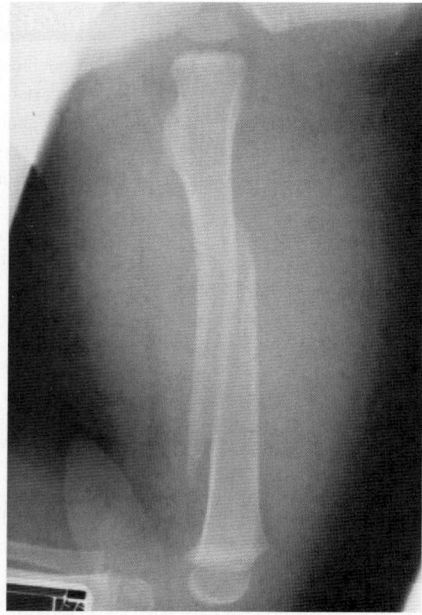

FIG 48.4 Fractured femur. Most fractured femurs in childhood are of the spiral type shown here. (From Mark, J.A., Hockberger, R.S., & Walls, R.M. [2014]. *Rosen's emergency medicine: Concepts and clinical practice* [8th ed.]. St. Louis, MO: Elsevier.)

In children, immobilization is used until adequate callus is formed. The position of the bone fragments in relation to one another influences the rapidity of healing and residual deformity. Weight bearing and active movement for the purpose of regaining function may begin after the fracture site is determined to be stable by the health care provider. The child's natural tendency to be active is usually sufficient to restore normal mobility, and physical or occupational therapy is rarely indicated.

Children are most frequently hospitalized for fractures of the femur and supracondylar area of the distal humerus. If simple reduction cannot be achieved or a neurovascular problem is detected after the injury, observation in a hospital setting may be indicated. The trend is to avoid hospitalization. The major methods for immobilizing a fracture, casting and traction, are described later in this chapter.

Care Management

Nurses are frequently the people who make the initial assessment of a child with a suspected fracture (see Emergency Treatment box: Fracture). The child and parents may be frightened and upset, and the child is often in pain. Therefore, if the child is alert and there is no evidence of hemorrhage, the initial nursing interventions are directed toward calming and reassuring the child and parents so that a more extensive assessment can be more easily accomplished.

While remaining calm and speaking in a quiet voice, the nurse can ask the parents and older child to describe what happened. The child may arrive with the limb supported in some manner; if not, careful support or immobilization may be provided to the affected site. In the event that the limb is supported or immobilized, it may be best not to touch the child but to ask him or her to point to the painful area and to wiggle the fingers or toes. By this time the child may feel relatively safe and will allow someone to gently touch the area just enough to feel the pulses and test for sensation. A child's anxiety is greatly influenced by previous experiences with injury and with health care professionals. However, he or she needs to be told what will happen and what to do to help. The affected limb need not be palpated, and it should not be moved unless properly splinted. If the child is at home or if the

✚ EMERGENCY TREATMENT

Fracture

Determine the mechanism of injury.

Assess the 6 *P*s.

Move the injured part as little as possible.

Cover open wounds with a sterile or clean dressing.

Immobilize the limb, including joints above and below the fracture site; do not attempt to reduce the fracture or push protruding bone under the skin.

Use a soft splint (pillow or folded towel) or rigid splint (rolled newspaper or magazine).

The uninjured leg can serve as a splint for a leg fracture if no splint is available.

Reassess neurovascular status.

Apply traction if circulatory compromise is present.

Elevate the injured limb if possible.

Apply cold to the injured area.

Call emergency medical services, or transport to a medical facility.

BOX 48.3   Compartment Syndrome Evaluation

Assess the extent of injury—"the 6 *P*s":

1. **Pain:** Severe pain that is not relieved by analgesics or elevation of the limb, movement that increases pain
2. **Pulselessness:** Inability to palpate a pulse distal to the fracture or compartment
3. **Pallor:** Pale appearing skin, poor perfusion, capillary refill greater than 3 seconds
4. **Paresthesia:** Tingling or burning sensations
5. **Paralysis:** Inability to move extremity or digits
6. **Pressure:** Involved limb or digits may feel tense and warm; skin is tight, shiny; pressure within the compartment is elevated

---

practitioner is not present to examine the child, some type of splint is applied carefully for transport to the medical facility. Parental anxiety may be heightened by the child's pain reaction and fear and possibly by other events surrounding the accident. It is important to communicate to the parent that the child will receive the necessary care, including pain management.

❗ NURSING ALERT

Compartment syndrome is a serious complication that results from compression of nerves, blood vessels, and muscle inside a closed space. This injury may be devastating, resulting in tissue death, and thus requires emergency treatment (fasciotomy). The six *P*s of ischemia from a vascular, soft-tissue, nerve, or bone injury should be included in an assessment of any injury:

1. Pain
2. Pulselessness
3. Pallor
4. Paresthesia
5. Paralysis
6. Pressure (Box 48.3)

THE CHILD IN A CAST

The completeness of the fracture, the type of bone involved, and the amount of weight bearing influence how much of the extremity must be included in the cast to immobilize the fracture site completely. In

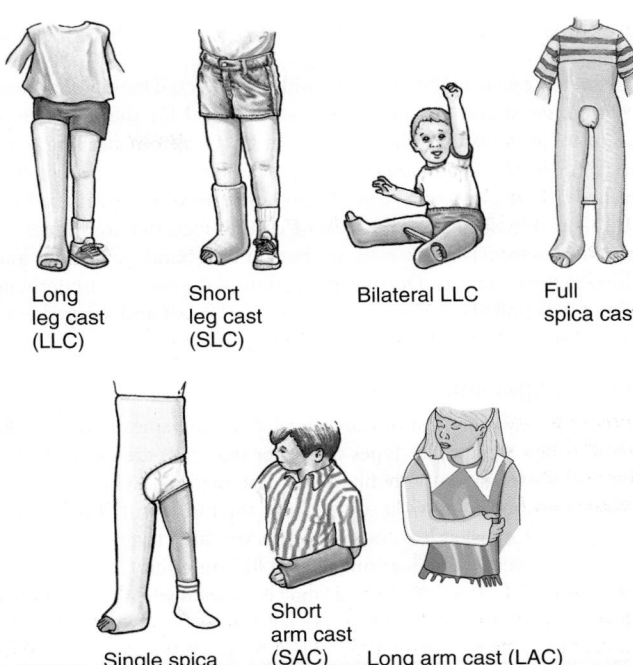

Long leg cast (LLC)   Short leg cast (SLC)   Bilateral LLC   Full spica cast

Single spica   Short arm cast (SAC)   Long arm cast (LAC)

FIG 48.5 Types of casts.

most cases, the joints above and below the fracture are immobilized to eliminate the possibility of movement that might cause displacement at the fracture site. Four major categories of casts are used for fractures: upper extremity to immobilize the wrist or elbow, lower extremity to immobilize the ankle or knee, spinal and cervical to immobilize the spine, and spica casts to immobilize the hip and knee (Fig. 48.5).

The Cast

Casts are constructed from gauze strips and bandages impregnated with plaster of Paris or, more commonly, from synthetic lighter weight and water-resistant materials (e.g., waterproof liners, fiberglass and polyurethane resin).

Both types of casting produce heat from chemical reaction activated by water immediately after application. Plaster casts mold closely to the body part, take 10 to 72 hours to dry, have a smooth exterior, and are inexpensive. The newer synthetic casting material is lightweight, dries in 5 to 20 minutes, permits earlier weight bearing, and is water resistant when applied with a waterproof liner. It is always desirable to give children choices, and synthetic casting materials come in a variety of colors. The disadvantages of synthetic casting are its inability to mold closely to body parts and its rough exterior, which may scratch surfaces. Synthetic casts are also difficult to write on; a waterproof marker or color markers may be used.

Cast Application

The child's developmental age should be considered before the cast is applied. For preschoolers who fear bodily harm and fantasize about the loss of an extremity, it may be helpful to use a plastic doll or stuffed animal to explain the procedure beforehand. Toddlers and preschoolers do not have easily defined body boundaries; if an extremity is wrapped in a bandage, cast, or splint, to the young child the extremity ceases to function or exist. It is also helpful to explain that some synthetic cast material will become warm during application but will not burn. During the application of the cast, various distraction methods can be used, including discussing favorite pets or activities at school, blowing bubbles, and so forth. In this age group, explanations, such as "This will help your arm get better," are futile because the child has no concept of causality.

Before the cast is applied, the extremities are checked for any abrasions, cuts, or other alterations in the skin surface and for the presence of rings or other items that might cause constriction from swelling; such objects are removed. A tube of cloth stockinette or Gore-Tex liner is stretched over the area to be casted, and bony prominences are padded with soft cotton sheeting. Dry rolls of casting material are immersed in a pail of water. The wet rolls are put on in a bandage fashion and molded to the extremity. During application of the cast, the underlying stockinette is pulled over the rough edges of the cast and secured with casting material to form a padded edge to protect the skin.

Care Management

The complete evaporation of the water from a hip spica cast can take 24 to 48 hours when older types of plaster materials are used. Drying occurs within minutes with fiberglass cast material. The cast must remain uncovered to allow it to dry from the inside out. Turning the child in a plaster cast at least every 2 hours will help to dry a body cast evenly and prevent complications related to immobility. A regular fan or cool-air hair dryer to circulate air may be helpful when the humidity is high.

> ! **NURSING ALERT**
>
> Heated fans or dryers are not used because they cause the cast to dry on the outside and remain wet beneath or cause burns from heat conduction by way of the cast to the underlying tissue.

A wet plaster cast should be supported by a pillow that is covered with plastic and handled by the palms of the hands to prevent indenting the cast, which can create pressure areas. A dry plaster-of-Paris cast produces a hollow sound when it is tapped with the finger. After it has dried, "hot spots" felt on the cast surface or a foul-smelling odor may indicate an infection. This should be reported for further evaluation, and if concern continues, an opening, or a "window," may be exposed over the area of concern to evaluate the site.

During the first few hours after a cast is applied, the chief concern is that the extremity may continue to swell to the extent that the cast becomes a tourniquet, shutting off circulation and producing neurovascular complications (compartment syndrome) (see Box 48.3). To reduce the likelihood of this potential problem, the body part can be elevated, thereby increasing venous return. If edema is excessive, casts are bivalved (i.e., cut to make anterior and posterior halves that are held together with an elastic bandage). The cast and the involved extremity are observed frequently for neurovascular integrity and any signs of compromise. Permanent muscle and tissue damage can occur within a few hours.

> ! **NURSING ALERT**
>
> Observations such as pain (unrelieved by pain medication 1 hour after administration, especially with passive range of motion), swelling, discoloration (pallor or cyanosis) of the exposed portions, decreased pulses, decreased temperature, paresthesia, or the inability to move the distal exposed part(s) should be reported immediately. Pallor, paralysis, and pulselessness are late signs (see Box 48.3).

When an extremity that has sustained an open fracture is casted, a window is often left over the wound area to allow for observation and dressing of the wound. For the first few hours after surgery, substantial bleeding may soak through the cast. Periodically, the circumscribed bloodstained area should be outlined with a waterproof marker and

FAMILY-CENTERED CARE
Cast Care

Keep the casted extremity elevated on pillows or similar support for the first day or as directed by the health care professional.

Avoid denting the plaster cast with fingertips (use palms of hand to handle) while it is still wet to avoid creating pressure points.

Expose the plaster cast to air until dry.

Observe the extremities (fingers or toes) for any evidence of swelling or discoloration (darker or lighter than a comparable extremity), and contact the health care professional if noted.

Check movement and sensation of the visible extremities frequently.

Follow health care professionals orders regarding any restriction of activities.

Restrict strenuous activities for the first few days:
- Engage in quiet activities, but encourage use of muscles.
- Move the joints above and below the cast on the affected extremity.

Encourage frequent rest for a few days, keeping the injured extremity elevated while resting.

Avoid allowing the affected limb to hang in a dependent position for any length of time:
- Keep an injured upper extremity elevated (e.g., in a sling) while upright.
- Elevate a lower limb when sitting, and avoid standing for too long.

Do not allow the child to put anything inside the cast. Keep small items that might be placed inside the cast away from small children.

Keep a clear path for ambulation. Remove toys, hazardous floor rugs, pets, and other items over which the child might stumble.

Use crutches appropriately if lower limb fracture requires non–weight bearing on affected extremity.

The crutches should fit properly, have a soft rubber tip to prevent slipping, and be well padded at the axilla.

With crutch walking, the child's body weight is supported on the hand grips, not the axilla.

the time indicated to provide a guide for assessing the amount of bleeding.

Appropriate cast care guidelines for the child's caregiver are necessary before discharge. Instructions are also given for checking for signs and symptoms that indicate that the cast is too tight (see Family-Centered Care box: Cast Care). Parents should also be told to take the child to the health care professional for attention if the cast becomes too loose because a loose cast no longer serves its purpose.

Nurses can help families adapt the child's home environment to meet the temporary encumbrance of a large cast or one that restricts the child's mobility (e.g., a long-leg or spica cast [Fig. 48.6]). Commonplace situations become problematic (e.g., transporting a child safely and comfortably in a car). Standard seat belts and car seats may not be readily adapted for use by children in some casts. Specially designed car seats and restraints are available that meet safety requirements.* Alterations to standard car seats to accommodate the cast are not recommended because the structure may be adversely altered and

*For information on specially adapted molded-plastic chairs for children who have spica casts, contact R82 at 844 US MOBILITY; http://www.r82.com. The E-Z-On vest is a special safety harness for larger children with poor trunk control. Additional safety restraints and a listing of distributors are available from SafetyBeltSafe U.S.A., http://www.carseat.org. Another resource is the National Center for the Safe Transportation of Children with Special Health Care Needs; 800-543-6227; http://www.preventinjury.org/Special-Needs-Transportation/Child-Seats-for-Children-with-Special-Needs.

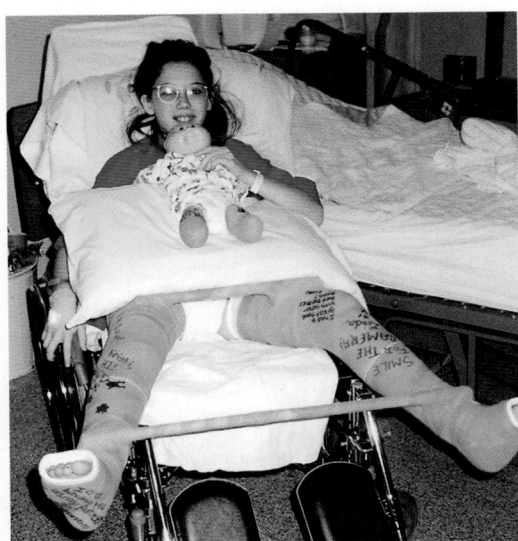

FIG 48.6 Spica cast with hip abductor. Note casts on doll as well.

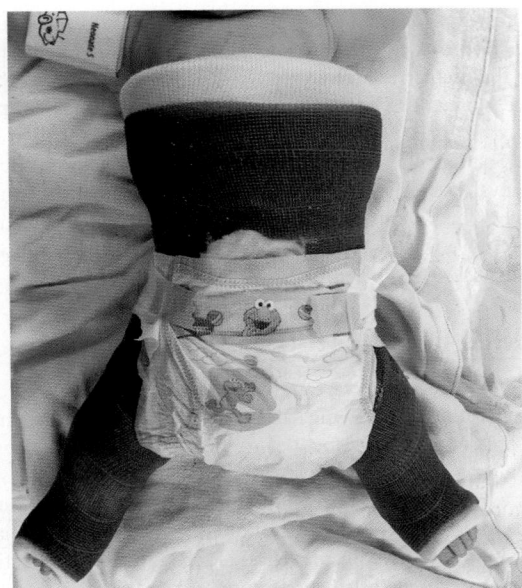

FIG 48.7 Spica cast. Note diaper to maintain dryness. (From Arlen, A.M., & Smith, E.A. [2014]. Disorders of the bladder and cloacal anomaly. *Clinics in Perinatology, 41*[3], 695-707.)

fail to properly restrain the child. A bedside commode or rental wheelchair maybe be necessary equipment for a child who is nonambulatory.

Parents are taught the proper care of the cast or brace and are helped to devise means for maintaining cleanliness. A superabsorbent disposable diaper is tucked beneath the entire perineal opening of the cast. A larger diaper can be applied and fastened over the small diaper and cast to hold the smaller diaper in place. In the event that the larger diaper becomes wet or soiled, it is likely the cast is as well.

For tightly fitting casts, transparent film dressings can be cut into strips as for petaling with one edge applied to the cast edge and the other directly to the perineum; this forms a continuous, waterproof bridge between the perineum and the cast to prevent leakage. An additional advantage to the use of this transparent dressing is that it keeps both the skin and the cast dry while allowing for observation of skin beneath the dressing.

Older infants and small children may stuff bits of food, small toys, or other items under the cast; parents should be alerted to this possibility so they can initiate suitable preventive measures.

Feeding an infant in a hip spica cast offers problems in positioning. Very young infants can be fed in the supine position with the head elevated. With the infant's hips and legs supported on a pillow at the side, the parent can cuddle the infant in his or her arms during feeding. A somewhat similar position can be used for breastfeeding (i.e., with the infant supported on pillows or held in a "football" hold facing the mother with the legs behind her). An alternate position is to hold the infant upright on the caregiver's lap with the legs of the infant astride the adult's leg.

Children in spica casts usually find the prone position easier for self-feeding from a small table placed next to the dining table; alternatively, they may manage a semi-sitting position in bed or in a wheelchair (Fig. 48.7). The use of a conventional toilet is almost impossible. A bedside toilet can be adapted for use. Small bedpans or other containers offer alternatives for elimination. The nurse may suggest waterproofing methods by devising plastic wraps for elimination and showers. Baths are possible only if the plaster cast is kept out of the water and covered to prevent it from becoming wet.

Cast Removal

Cutting the cast to remove it or to relieve tightness is frequently a frightening experience for children. They fear the sound of the cast

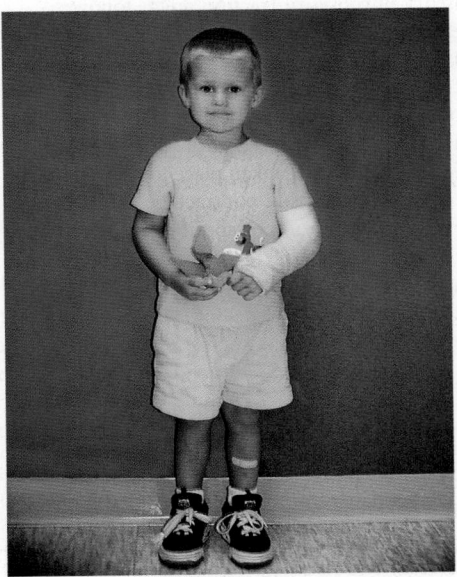

FIG 48.8 Young children come to regard a cast as part of their body.

cutter and are terrified that their flesh, as well as the cast, will be cut. The oscillating blade vibrates rapidly back and forth and will not cut when placed *lightly* on the skin. Children have described it as producing a "tickly" sensation. The vibration also generates heat that may be felt by the child. Both of these feelings should be explained.

Preparation for the procedure will help reduce anxiety, especially if a trusting relationship has been established between the child and the nurse. Many young children come to regard the cast as part of themselves, which intensifies their fear of removal (Fig. 48.8). They need continual reassurance that all is going well and that their behavior is accepted. After the cast is removed, the parents and child should be given the option of keeping the cast. If the cast has been in place for a lengthy period, decreased muscle mass will be noted. The child should be reassured that resuming exercise and routine activities will return function and appearance (provided there was no significant trauma beforehand).

After the cast is removed, the skin surface will be caked with desquamated skin and sebaceous secretions. Application of mineral oil (e.g., baby oil) or lotion may remove the particles as well as provide comfort. Soaking the extremity in a bathtub is usually sufficient for their removal, but it may take several days to eliminate the accumulation completely. The parents and child should be instructed not to pull or forcibly remove this material with vigorous scrubbing because it may cause excoriation and bleeding.

THE CHILD IN TRACTION

The ever-changing health care arena has witnessed the demise of many long-term treatments involving lengthy hospitalization; one such change is in the area of traction. Most balanced skeletal traction is applied in children after a severe or complex injury to allow physiologic stability, align bone fragments, and permit closer evaluation of the injured site. Newer technology has produced orthopedic fixation devices that allow partial or full mobility, thus preventing long-term immobilization and its consequences. In many situations, surgical intervention may be carried out within a matter of days; therefore, skeletal traction devices described herein may be used infrequently in pediatrics.

Purposes of Traction

The six primary purposes of traction are as follows:
1. To fatigue the involved muscles and reduce muscle spasm so that bones can be realigned
2. To position the distal and proximal bone ends in desired realignment to promote satisfactory bone healing
3. To immobilize the fracture site until realignment has been achieved and sufficient healing has taken place to permit casting or splinting
4. To help prevent or improve contracture deformity
5. To provide immobilization of specific areas of the body
6. To reduce muscle spasms (rare in children)

The three essential components of traction management are *traction, counter traction,* and *friction* (Fig. 48.9). To reduce or realign a fracture site, traction (forward force) is produced by attaching weight to the distal bone fragment. Body weight provides counter traction (backward force), and the patient's contact with the bed constitutes the frictional force. These forces are used to align the distal and proximal bone fragments by adjusting the line of pull upward or downward and adducting or abducting the extremity.

To attain equilibrium, the amount of forward force is adjusted by adding weight to or subtracting weight from the traction, or counter traction can be increased by elevating the foot of the bed to create a greater gravitational pull to the backward force.

The *all-or-none law,* characteristic of muscle contractibility, influences the complete relaxation. When muscles are stretched, muscle spasm ceases, which permits the realignment of the bone ends. The continuous maintenance of traction is important during this phase because releasing the traction allows the muscle's normal contracting ability to again cause a malpositioning of the bone ends.

Realignment of the fragments is a gradual process that is achieved more rapidly in infants, who have limited muscle tone, than in muscular teenagers. The desired vector force and callus formation are checked periodically by radiographic examination. The traction pull to some degree immobilizes the fracture site; however, adjunctive immobilizing devices such as splints or casts are sometimes used with skeletal traction. Immobilization with traction is maintained until the bone ends are in satisfactory realignment after which a less confining type of immobilization—a cast, pins, or external stabilization device—is applied.

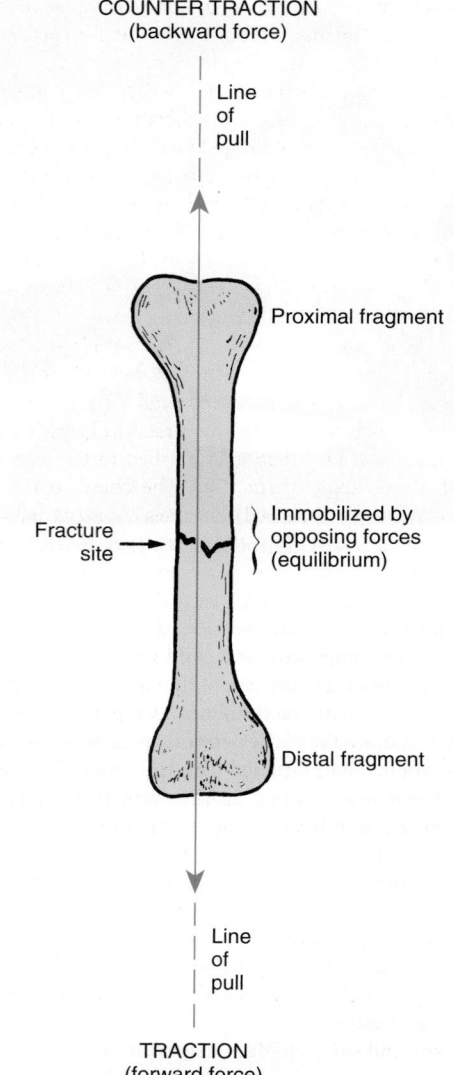

FIG 48.9 Application of traction for maintaining equilibrium.

BOX 48.4   Types of Traction

Manual traction: Applied to the body part by the hand placed distal to the fracture site. Manual traction may be provided during application of a cast but more commonly when a closed reduction is performed.

Skin traction: Applied directly to the skin surface and indirectly to the skeletal structures. The pulling mechanism is attached to the skin with adhesive material or an elastic bandage. Both types are applied over soft, foam-backed traction straps to distribute the traction pull.

Skeletal traction: Applied directly to the skeletal structure by a pin, wire, or tongs inserted into or through the diameter of the bone distal to the fracture.

Types of Traction

The pull needed for traction can be applied to the distal bone fragment in several ways (Box 48.4). The type of traction applied is determined primarily by the child's age, the condition of the soft tissues, and the type and degree of displacement of the fracture. Fractures most commonly treated by application of traction are those involving the femur and vertebrae. The major types of traction for specific fractures are briefly discussed in the following paragraphs.

The use of upper extremity traction in children is uncommon. Newer surgical techniques allow for early mobilization and optimal results without traction. Nursing care of the child with upper extremity traction is the same as that for lower extremity traction, which is discussed later.

The frequent site for a femoral fracture is in the middle third of the shaft. With this fracture, there may be significant overriding but minimal displacement. In a fracture in the lower third of the shaft, the pull of the gastrocnemius muscle causes the distal fragment to become downwardly displaced.

Fractures of the femur can often be reduced with immediate application of a hip spica cast in young children. When traction is required, several types may be used based on the initial assessment.

Bryant traction is a type of running traction in which the pull is in only one direction. Skin traction is applied to the legs, which are flexed at a 90-degree angle at the hips. The child's trunk (with the buttocks raised slightly off the bed) provides counter traction.

Buck extension traction (Fig. 48.10) is a type of traction with the legs in an extended position. Except for fracture cases, turning from side to side with care is permitted to maintain the involved leg in alignment. Buck extension traction is used primarily for short-term immobilization, such as preoperative management of a child with a dislocated hip, or for correction of contractures or bone deformities, such as in Legg-Calvé-Perthes disease. Buck traction may be accomplished with either skin straps or a special foam boot designed for traction.

Russell traction uses skin traction on the lower leg and a padded sling under the knee. Two lines of pull, one along the longitudinal line of the lower leg and one perpendicular to the leg, are produced. This

combination of pulls allows realignment of the lower extremity and immobilizes the hip and knee in a flexed position. The hip flexion must be kept at the prescribed angle to prevent fracture malalignment because there is no direct support under the fracture and the skin traction may slip. Special nursing measures include carefully checking the position of the traction so that the amount of desired hip flexion is maintained and damage to the common peroneal nerve under the knee does not produce footdrop.

A common skeletal traction is 90-degree–90-degree traction (90-90 traction). The lower leg is supported by a boot cast or a calf sling, and a skeletal Steinmann pin or Kirschner wire is placed in the distal fragment of the femur, resulting in a 90-degree angle at both the hip and the knee. From a nursing standpoint, this traction facilitates position changes, toileting, and prevention of complications related to traction.

Balanced suspension traction may be used with or without skin or skeletal traction. Unless used with another traction, the balanced suspension merely suspends the leg in a desired flexed position to relax the hip and hamstring muscles and does not exert any traction directly on a body part. A *Thomas splint* extends from the groin to midair above the foot, and a *Pearson attachment* supports the lower leg. Towels or pieces of felt covered with stockinette are clipped or pinned to the splints for leg support. When the child is lifted off the bed, the traction lifts with the child without loss of alignment. This traction requires careful checking of splints and ropes to make certain that no slippage or fraying has occurred. The traction is of great value in an older and heavier child when it is essential to lift the patient for care.

The cervical area is a vulnerable site for flexion or extension injuries to muscle, vertebrae, or the spinal cord. Cervical muscle trauma without other complications is treated with a cervical hard collar to relieve the weight of the head from the fracture site. When a child displaces or fractures a cervical vertebra, it may be necessary to reduce and immobilize the site with cervical skeletal traction. The spinal cord runs through the intravertebral canal, and dislocation or fracture of the vertebrae can also cause spinal cord injury. Nursing assessment of neurologic function is essential to prevent further injury during the application and use of cervical skeletal traction.

Most cervical traction is accomplished with the use of a halo brace or halo vest (Fig. 48.11, A). This device consists of a steel halo attached to the head by four screws inserted into the outer skull; several rigid bars connect the halo to a vest that is worn around the chest, thus providing greater mobility of the rest of the body while avoiding cervical spinal motion altogether. If the injury has been limited to a vertebral

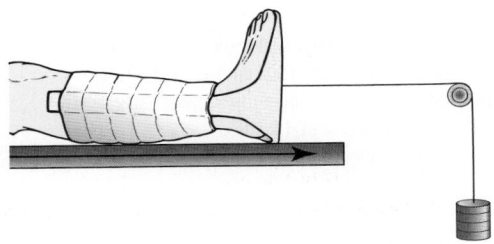

FIG 48.10 Buck extension traction.

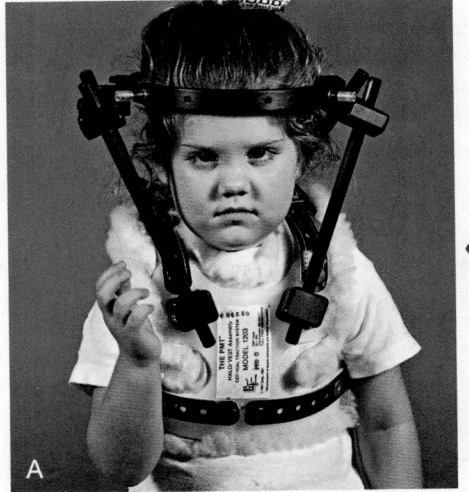
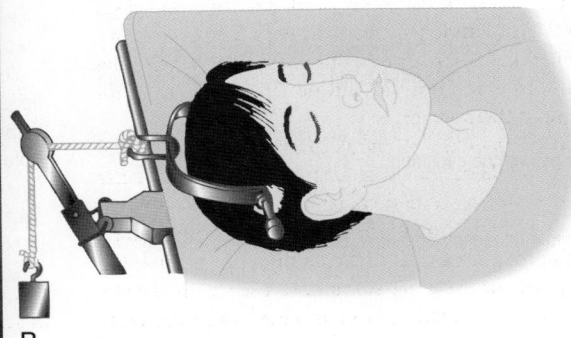

FIG 48.11 **A,** Halo vest. **B,** Cervical traction with Gardner-Wells tong.

fracture without neurologic deficit, a halo brace can be applied to permit earlier ambulation. Gardner-Wells tongs may be used with cervical traction to immobilize the cervical spine (see Fig. 48.11, *B*). Gardner-Wells tongs are spring loaded, so making burr holes and shaving hair are not required; a local anesthetic may be used during application. As the neck muscles fatigue with constant traction pull, the vertebral bodies gradually separate so that the cord is no longer pinched between the vertebrae. Immobilization until fracture healing or surgical fixation can occur is an essential goal of cervical traction. If immobilization is required in an infant or young child, a special cervical spine cast (Minerva cast) is applied.

Care Management

To assess the child in traction, it is essential to know the purpose for which the traction is applied and to understand the basic principles of traction. Regular assessment of both the child and the traction apparatus is required (see Guidelines box: Traction Care). Many of the nursing problems associated with a child in traction are related to

immobility. Modifying the child's diet, encouraging fluids, increasing fiber, and offering a mild stool softener may be necessary to prevent constipation.

> **! NURSING ALERT**
>
> Skeletal traction is never released by the nurse (except under direct supervision by the practitioner). This precaution includes not lifting the weights that are applying traction (e.g., for moving the child in bed, for repositioning).

In addition to routine skin observation and care, the child in skeletal traction will need special skin care at the pin sites according to hospital policy or practitioner preference. Pin sites should be frequently assessed and cleaned to prevent infection; after the first 48 to 72 hours, pin site care may be performed once daily or weekly for mechanically stable pins (Holmes, Brown & Pin Site Care Expert Panel, 2005). Use of a 2-mg/mL chlorhexidine solution has been proposed as best practice care for skeletal pin sites by the National Association of Orthopaedic

---

 GUIDELINES

Traction Care

Understand Therapy
Understand purpose of traction.
Understand function of traction in each specific situation.

Maintain Traction
Check desired line of pull and relationship of distal fragment to proximal fragment.
  Check whether fragment is being directed upward, adducted, or abducted.
Check function of each component:
  • Position of bandages, frames, splints, specialized boot
  • Ropes: In center track of pulley, taut, no fraying, knots tied securely
  • Pulleys: In original position on attachment bar; have not slid from original site; wheels freely movable
  • Weights: Correct amount of weight, hanging freely, in safe location
Check bed position: Head or foot elevated as directed for desired amount of pull and counter traction.
Do not remove skeletal traction or adhesive traction straps on skin traction.

Maintain Alignment
Observe for correct body alignment with emphasis on alignment of shoulder, hip, and leg.
Check after child has moved.
Maintain correct angles at joints.

Skin Traction
Replace nonadhesive straps or elastic bandage on skin traction when permitted or absolutely necessary, but make certain that traction on limb is maintained by someone during procedure.
Assess straps or bandages to ascertain if they are correctly applied (diagonal or spiral) and not too loose or too tight, which could cause slippage and malalignment of traction.
Assess traction boot to ensure it has not slipped and is not causing compression of the foot, thus impairing the circulation.

Skeletal Traction
Check pin sites frequently for signs of bleeding, inflammation, or infection.
Cleanse and dress pin sites per institutional protocol or as ordered.
Apply topical antiseptic or antibiotic to pin sites daily as ordered.
Cover ends of pins with protective rubber or padding to prevent child being scratched by pin.

Note pull of traction on pin; pull should be even.
Check pin screws to be certain that screws are tight in metal clamp that attaches traction apparatus to pin.

Prevent Skin Breakdown
Provide alternating-pressure mattress underneath hips and back.
Make total-body skin checks for redness or breakdown, especially over areas that receive greatest pressure.
Wash and dry skin at least daily.
Inspect pressure points daily or more often if risk for breakdown is observed.
Use a skin breakdown assessment scale, such as Braden Q.
Stimulate circulation with gentle massage over pressure areas.
Change position at least every 2 hours to relieve pressure.
Encourage increase in intake of oral fluids.
Provide and encourage patient to eat a balanced diet, including vegetables and fruits.

Prevent Complications
Check pulses in affected area, and compare with pulses in contralateral site.
Assess circular dressings for excessive tightness.
Assess restrictive bandages or devices used to maintain traction on affected limb:
  1. Make certain that they are not too loose or too tight.
  2. Remove periodically, and check for skin breakdown or pressure areas.
Encourage deep breathing or use of incentive spirometry:
  • Monitor the 6 *P*s (see Box 48.3).
Take immediate action to correct problem or report to practitioner if neurovascular changes are present.
Record findings of neurovascular changes.
Carry out passive, active, or active-with-resistance exercises of uninvolved joints.
Note if any tightness, weakness, edema, or contractures are developing in uninvolved joints and muscles.
Take measures to correct or prevent further development of weakness, such as applying footboard or foot orthoses to prevent footdrop.
When indicated by the attending practitioner, the nurse may remove nonadhesive skin traction. In these cases, intermittent traction is periodically released and reapplied as ordered. A child may have several types of traction at one time, and each one must be assessed separately to avoid problems.

Nurses (Holmes et al.). A pressure-reduction device, such as a pressure-reduction mattress, decreases the chance of skin breakdown.

> **! NURSING ALERT**
>
> A small hand mirror facilitates visualization of inaccessible skin areas.

When the child is first placed in traction, increased discomfort is common as a result of the traction pull fatiguing the muscle. It has been determined that orthopedic conditions are associated with a higher-than-average number of painful events and a higher percentage of bodily symptoms than other common conditions. Analgesics, including IV opioids, and muscle relaxants, help during this phase of care and should be administered liberally.

> **! NURSING ALERT**
>
> For skeletal traction to be effective, ensure that the weights are hanging freely at all times.

The specific nursing responsibilities for the patient in traction are outlined earlier in this chapter in the Guidelines box: Traction Care.

DISTRACTION

Unlike traction, which helps bones realign and fuse properly, *distraction* is the process of separating opposing bone to encourage regeneration of new bone in the created space. Distraction can also be used when limbs are of unequal lengths and new bone is needed to elongate the shorter limb.

External Fixation

Monolateral, Taylor Spatial Frame, and Ilizarov external fixators (IEFs) are common external fixation devices. The IEF uses a system of wires, rings, and telescoping rods that permits limb lengthening to occur by manual distraction (Fig. 48.12). In addition to lengthening bones, the

device can be used to correct angular or rotational defects or to immobilize fractures. The device is attached surgically by securing a series of external full or half rings to the bone with wires. External telescoping rods connect the rings to each other. Manual distraction is accomplished by manipulating the rods to increase the distance between the rings. A percutaneous osteotomy is performed when the device is applied to create a "false" growth plate. A special osteotomy or corticotomy involves cutting only the cortex of the bone while preserving its blood supply, bone marrow, endosteum, and periosteum. Capillary blood flow to the transected area is essential for proper bone growth. Cut bone ends typically grow at a rate of 1 cm (0.4 inches) per month. The IEF can result in up to a 15-cm (6-inch) gain in length.

Care Management

Success of the fixation devices depends on the child's and family's cooperation; therefore, before surgery, they must be fully informed of the appearance of the device, how it accomplishes bone growth and limits bone mobility, alterations in activities, and home and follow-up care. Children are involved in learning to adjust the device to accomplish distraction. Children and parents should be instructed in pin care, including observation for infection and loosening of the pins. Cleaning routines for the pin sites vary among practitioners but should not traumatize the skin.

Children who participate actively in their care report less discomfort. Because the device is external, the child and family need to be prepared for the reactions of others and assisted in camouflaging the device with appropriate apparel, such as wide-legged pants that close with self-adhering fasteners around the device. A loose sock or stockinette may also be used over the device to decrease public awareness. Partial weight bearing is allowed, and the child learns to walk with crutches. Alterations in activity include modifications at school and in physical education (PE). Full weight bearing is not allowed until the distraction is completed and bone consolidation has occurred. Follow-up care is essential to maintain appropriate distraction until the desired limb length is achieved. The device is removed surgically after the bone has consolidated, and the child may need to use crutches or have a cast for 4 to 6 weeks after removal to reduce the risk for fracture.

AMPUTATION

A child may be born with the congenital absence of an extremity, have a traumatic loss of an extremity, or need a surgical amputation for a pathologic condition such as osteosarcoma. With today's surgical technology and the quick thinking of bystanders who save a traumatically amputated body part, some children have had fingers and arms sewn back on with variable degrees of functional use regained.

> **! NURSING ALERT**
>
> For an amputated limb or body part that may be reattached, do the following:
> 1. Rinse the limb gently with normal saline.
> 2. Loosely wrap the limb in sterile gauze.
> 3. Place the wrapped limb in a watertight bag.
> 4. Cool (without freezing) the bag in ice water (do not pack in ice because this may harm tissue).
> 5. Label with the child's name, date, and time, and transport with the child to the hospital.

Surgical amputation or the surgical repair of a permanently severed limb focuses on constructing an adequately nourished residual limb. A smooth, healthy, padded stump, free of nerve endings, is important in prosthesis fitting and subsequent ambulation. In some situations in

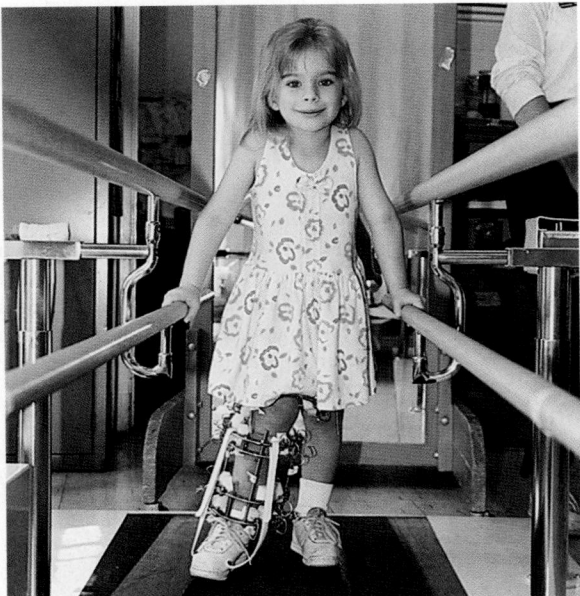

FIG 48.12 Child with Ilizarov external fixator (IEF; on right leg) during physical therapy on parallel bars.

which there is no vascular or neurologic deficit, a cast is applied to the stump immediately after the procedure, and a pylon, metal extension, and artificial foot are attached so the patient can walk on the temporary prosthesis within a few hours.

Care Management

Stump shaping is done postoperatively with special elastic bandaging using a figure-eight bandage, which applies pressure in a cone-shaped fashion. This technique decreases stump edema, controls hemorrhage, and aids in developing desired contours so the child will bear weight on the posterior aspect of the skin flap rather than on the end of the stump. Stump elevation may be used during the first 24 hours, but after this time, the extremity should not be left in this position because contractures in the proximal joint will develop and seriously hamper ambulation. Monitoring proper body alignment will further decrease the risk for flexion contractures.

For older children and adolescents, arm exercises, bed pushups, and prosthesis-training programs using parallel bars help build up the arm muscles necessary for walking with crutches. Full range-of-motion exercises of joints above the amputation must be performed several times daily using active and isotonic exercises. Young children are often spontaneously active and require little encouragement.

Depending on the child's age, children or their parents will need to learn hygiene, including carefully washing with soap and water every day and checking for skin irritation, breakdown, and infection. A tube of stockinette or powder is used to slide the prosthesis on more easily. Skin must be checked carefully every time the prosthesis is removed, and prosthesis tolerance time must be adjusted to prevent skin breakdown.

For children who have had an amputation, phantom limb sensation is an expected experience because the nerve-brain connections are still present. Gradually, these sensations fade, although in many people who have had amputations, they persist for years. Preoperative discussion of this phenomenon will aid a child in understanding these "unusual feelings" and not hiding the experiences from others. Limb pain, especially pain that increases with ambulation, should be evaluated for the possibility of a neuroma at the free nerve endings in the stump or other problems such as a poorly fitting prosthesis or joint instability.

SPORTS PARTICIPATION AND INJURY

Every sport has the potential for injury to participants—whether an adolescent engages in serious competition or participates for enjoyment. Serious injury occurs most often during rough contact sports or to people who are not physically prepared for the activity. Injuries also occur when the children's or adolescents' bodies are not suited to the sport, when their muscles and body systems (respiratory and cardiovascular) are not conditioned to endure physical stress, or when they lack the insight and judgment to recognize that an activity exceeds their physical abilities. Rapidly growing bones, muscles, joints, and tendons are especially vulnerable to unusual strain. In general, more injuries occur during recreational sports participation than during organized athletic competition.

The environment and the sports or recreational equipment can also present risks (Fig. 48.13). Children and adolescents who participate in physical activity or sports do so in many different environments, including indoors and outdoors, on floors, on the ground and snow, on or beneath water surfaces, and sometimes in free air space. Most of these activities also involve equipment, which children and adolescents may not be physically mature enough to manage safely. A common example is skateboarding when the child or adolescent does not take safety precautions and perceives increased risk taking as a part of the sport.

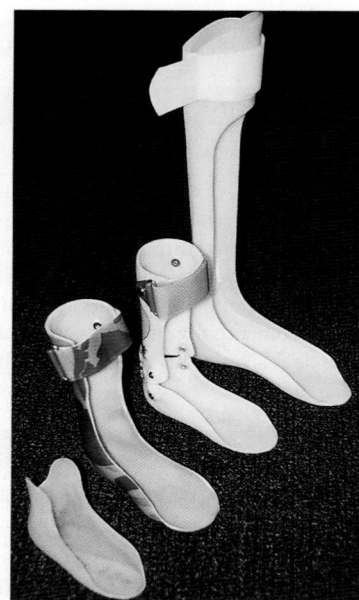

FIG 48.13 Left to right: Supramalleolar orthosis (SMO), solid ankle-foot orthosis (AFO), articulating AFO, and floor reaction AFO.

Acute overload injuries are those that occur suddenly during an activity and produce immediate symptoms. A blow or overstretching, twisting, or sudden stress to tissues can cause these injuries. For descriptions and management of traumatic injuries, see the "Traumatic Injuries" section earlier in this chapter.

OVERUSE SYNDROMES

To excel in sports, young athletes are forced to train longer, harder, and earlier in life than previously. The rewards are an increased level of fitness, better performance, faster times, and the satisfaction of attaining a personal goal. However, risks are associated when young people overtrain; these risks include recurrent upper respiratory infections, sleep and mood disturbances, loss of appetite, decreased interest in training and competition, and inability to concentrate (Winsley & Matos, 2011). Growing numbers of young people participate in organized sports, resulting in an increase in overuse injuries. Nearly one-half of all injuries evaluated in pediatric sports medicine are overuse injuries (Biber & Gregory, 2010).

The risk for overuse injury is always present and can be related to several factors, including training errors, muscle/tendon imbalance, anatomic malalignment (e.g., femoral anteversion, excessive lumbar lordosis, tibial torsion), incorrect footwear or playing surface, an associated disease state, and growth (growth cartilage is less resistant to microtrauma). Chronic pain in athletes is often associated with overuse injury, which can occur at any level of athletic participation. The common feature in overuse injuries is the repetitive microtrauma that occurs to a particular anatomic structure. Performing the same movements repeatedly can cause several types of injury:

1. **Frictional**, or rubbing of one structure against another
2. **Tractional**, or repeated pull on a ligament or tendon
3. **Cyclic**, or repetitive loading of impact forces (stress fractures)

The end result is inflammation of the involved structure with complaints of pain, tenderness, swelling, and disability.

Stress Fractures

Stress fractures are a consequence of repetitive, excessive stress on the bone that causes microfractures within the bone. Continued stress to the bone can lead to spread of the microfracture and eventual macrofracture. The pathogenesis of stress injury to the bone is multifactorial and includes everything from the footwear to the fitness level of the athlete. Stress fractures occur most commonly in the lower extremities, particularly the tibia. Track and field athletes have the highest incidence of stress fractures (Patel, Roth, & Kapil, 2011).

The most common symptom of stress fracture is a sharp, persistent, progressive pain or a deep, persistent dull ache located over the bone. Sometimes there is pain on impact (heel strike), but the most important clinical sign is pain over the involved bony surface. Diagnosis is based on clinical observation and history. Plain radiographs are rarely diagnostic of stress fractures during the initial few weeks because callus formation is not yet evident. Magnetic resonance imaging (MRI) is used when other causes of pain must be ruled out.

Therapeutic Management

Development of inflammation is common to all overuse syndromes; therefore, management involves rest or alteration of activities, physical therapy, and medication. Rest is the primary therapy, usually interpreted as reduced activity and the use of alternative exercise—not bed rest or immobilization with an orthosis. The main purpose is to alleviate the repetitive stress that initiated the symptoms. It is important to keep the adolescent mobile, and training can be continued. Alternative exercise is selected that maintains conditioning without aggravating the injury. For example, pool running (treading water in the deep end of a pool) can use the same movements as running but without the weight bearing; bicycling, swimming, and rowing are viable alternatives.

Other modalities include cryotherapy and cold whirlpool baths. Sometimes taping, bracing, splinting, and other orthoses are used, depending on the injury. Nonsteroidal antiinflammatory drugs (NSAIDs) are often prescribed to reduce inflammation and pain. Topical medications are of questionable value.

NURSE'S ROLE IN SPORTS FOR CHILDREN AND ADOLESCENTS

Nurses are often involved in sports activities in the areas of preparation and evaluation for activities, prevention of injury, treatment of injuries, and rehabilitation after injury. Selecting an appropriate sport for both recreation and competition is a joint effort of the adolescent, parents, and the interprofessional care team. The best approach to counseling children, adolescents, and parents regarding sports participation is to encourage activities that are most likely to provide pleasure and physical benefits throughout childhood and into adulthood. Exposure to a variety of activities is better for young children than limiting them to one sport. Parents should be cautioned against overcommitting children to sports activities so they have time for other activities.

When children sustain athletic injuries, nurses are often responsible for instructions regarding care. Instructions (e.g., schedule for appointments, application of ice, any restrictions in activity) should be clear and accompanied by written directions. The importance of taking medications as prescribed is emphasized, especially if medications are needed for an extended period and if adherence is an issue. Antiinflammatory medications given 1 hour before practice or competition may help children continue their activities.

Prevention of sports injuries is the most important aspect of athletic programs. Children should be suited to the activity, and the environment and the equipment must be safe. Children should be prepared for the sport, especially if it requires strenuous or continuous physical exertion. Nurses, coaches, and athletic trainers must collaborate to ensure that safety measures are implemented. Stretching exercises, warm-up and cool-down activities, and appropriate training are requirements for safe participation. Protective measures such as pads, taping, and wrapping are also important to prevent injury. Finally, nurses must be aware of environmental safety risks (see the "Head Injury" section in Chapter 46).

BIRTH AND DEVELOPMENTAL DEFECTS

Some skeletal defects may be diagnosed at birth or within days, weeks, or months after birth. In other cases, the deviation may be difficult to detect without careful inspection. Therefore, it is imperative that nurses become acquainted with signs of these defects and understand the principles of therapy in order to direct families in the care and management of these children.

DEVELOPMENTAL DYSPLASIA OF THE HIP

The broad term *developmental dysplasia of the hip (DDH)* describes a spectrum of disorders related to abnormal development of the hip that may occur at any time during fetal life, infancy, or childhood. A change in terminology from *congenital hip dysplasia* and *congenital dislocation of the hip* to *DDH* more properly reflects a variety of hip abnormalities in which there is a shallow acetabulum, subluxation, or dislocation.

The incidence of hip dysplasia varies depending on ethnicity/race but is approximately 1 to 2 infants per 1000 live births in the United States. Girls are affected more commonly than boys, and a positive family history increases a child's risk for having DDH. Approximately 7% to 40% of infants with DDH have a breech intrauterine position (Loder & Skopelja, 2011a).

Pathophysiology

The cause of DDH is unclear but is likely multifactorial. Certain factors such as gender, birth order, family history, intrauterine position, joint laxity, and postnatal positioning are believed to affect the risk for DDH. Predisposing factors associated with DDH may be divided into three broad categories: (1) physiologic factors, which include maternal hormone secretion and intrauterine positioning; (2) mechanical factors, which involve breech presentation, multiple fetus, oligohydramnios, and large infant size, as well as swaddling, where the hips are maintained in adduction and extension, which in time may cause a dislocation; and (3) genetic factors, which entail a higher incidence of DDH in siblings of affected infants and an even greater incidence of recurrence if a sibling and one parent were affected.

Some experts categorize DDH into two major groups: (1) *idiopathic*, in which the infant is neurologically intact, and (2) *teratologic*, which involves a neuromuscular defect, such as arthrogryposis or myelodysplasia. The teratologic forms usually occur in utero and are much less common.

Three degrees of DDH are illustrated in Fig. 48.14.

1. **Acetabular dysplasia:** This is the mildest form of DDH, in which there is a delay in acetabular development evidenced by osseous hypoplasia of the acetabular roof that is oblique and shallow, although the cartilaginous roof is comparatively intact. The femoral head remains in the acetabulum.
2. **Subluxation:** The largest percentage of DDH, subluxation, implies incomplete dislocation of the hip. The femoral head remains in contact with the acetabulum, but a stretched capsule and ligamentum teres cause the head of the femur to be partially displaced. Pressure on the cartilaginous roof inhibits ossification and produces a flattening of the socket.
3. **Dislocation:** The femoral head loses contact with the acetabulum and is displaced posteriorly and superiorly over the fibrocartilaginous rim. The ligamentum teres is elongated and taut.

Factors related to infant handling are indicated in the Cultural Considerations box: Developmental Dysplasia of the Hip.

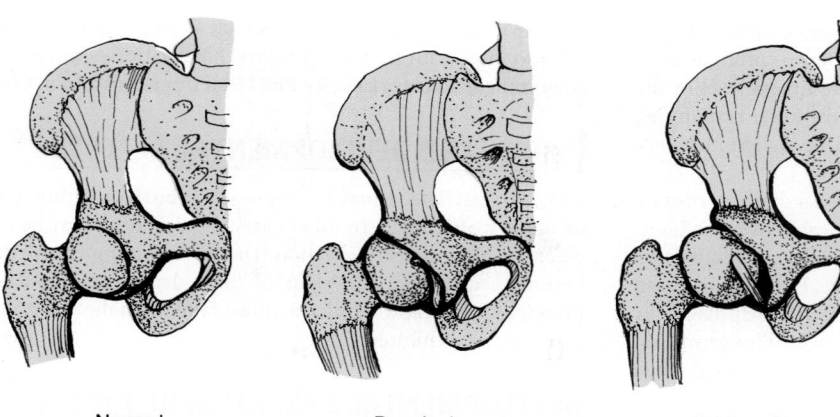

Normal   Dysplasia   Subluxation   Dislocation

FIG 48.14 Configuration and relationship of structures in developmental dysplasia of the hip (DDH).

🌐 CULTURAL CONSIDERATIONS
Developmental Dysplasia of the Hip

A striking relationship exists between the development of hip dislocation and methods of swaddling the hips. Among the cultures with the highest incidence of dislocation (Navajo Indians and Canadian Natives), newly born infants are tightly wrapped with the hips adducted and extended in blankets or other swaddling material or are strapped to cradle boards. In cultures such as those in Central and South America, Asia, and Africa, where mothers traditionally carry infants on their backs with the infants' hips in the abducted and flexed hip position, hip dysplasia is much less common.

Recently, several prominent orthopedic specialty organizations recommended that infants' hips be placed in slight flexion and abduction during swaddling. It was further recommended that infants' knees be maintained in slight flexion and that forced or sustained passive hip extension in the first few months should be avoided (Price & Schwend, 2011). These recommendations were supported by evidence that demonstrated a significant relationship between tight swaddling and hip dysplasia and are aimed at decreasing the incidence of hip dysplasia in infants.

Diagnostic Evaluation

DDH is often not detected at the initial examination after birth; thus, all infants should be carefully monitored for hip dysplasia at follow-up visits throughout the first year of life at routine well-child checks. In the newborn period, hip dysplasia usually appears as hip joint laxity rather than as outright dislocation. Subluxation and the tendency to dislocate can be demonstrated by the Ortolani or Barlow maneuvers (Fig. 48.15, *D*). The Ortolani and Barlow tests are most reliable from birth to 4 weeks of age. With the Barlow test, the thigh is adducted and light pressure is applied to see if the femoral head can be felt to slip posteriorly out of the acetabulum. The Ortolani test involves abducting the thighs and placing anterior pressure at the hip to see if the femoral head slips forward into the acetabulum. Other signs of DDH are shortening of the limb on the affected side (see Fig. 48.15, *C*), asymmetric thigh and gluteal folds (see Fig. 48.15, *A*), and decreased hip abduction on the affected side (see Fig. 48.15, *B*). See Box 48.5.

❗ NURSING ALERT

These tests must be performed by an experienced clinician to prevent an injury to the infant's hip.

BOX 48.5 Clinical Manifestations of Developmental Dysplasia of the Hip

Infants
Shortening of limb on affected side (Galeazzi sign)
Restricted abduction of hip on affected side
Unequal gluteal folds (best visualized with infant prone)
Positive Ortolani test (hip is reduced by abduction)
Positive Barlow test (hip is dislocated by adduction)

Older Infants and Children
Affected leg appears shorter than the other
Telescoping or piston mobility of joint: Head of femur felt to move up and down in buttock when extended thigh is pushed first toward child's head and then pulled distally
Trendelenburg sign: When child stands first on one foot and then on the other (holding onto a chair, rail, or someone's hands) bearing weight on affected hip, pelvis tilts downward on normal side instead of upward, as it would with normal stability
Greater trochanter prominent and appearing above a line from anterosuperior iliac spine to tuberosity of ischium
Marked lordosis and waddling gait (bilateral hip dislocation)

Radiographic examination in early infancy is not reliable because ossification of the femoral head does not normally take place until the fourth to sixth month of life. However, the cartilaginous head can be visualized directly by ultrasonography. Universal newborn screening with ultrasonography has been proposed; however, numerous studies reveal that this approach has a high rate of false-positive results and subsequent overtreatment. Therefore, ultrasonography is recommended as an adjunct to the physical examination (American Academy of Pediatrics, 2000). In infants older than 6 months of age and in children, radiographic examination is useful in confirming the diagnosis. An upward slope in the roof of the acetabulum (acetabular angle) greater than 30 degrees with upward and outward displacement of the femoral head is seen in a child with hip dysplasia. The American Academy of Pediatrics (2000) has published extensive clinical guidelines for screening and early detection of DDH.

Therapeutic Management

Treatment is begun as soon as the condition is recognized because early intervention is more favorable to the restoration of normal bony architecture and function. The longer treatment is delayed, the more

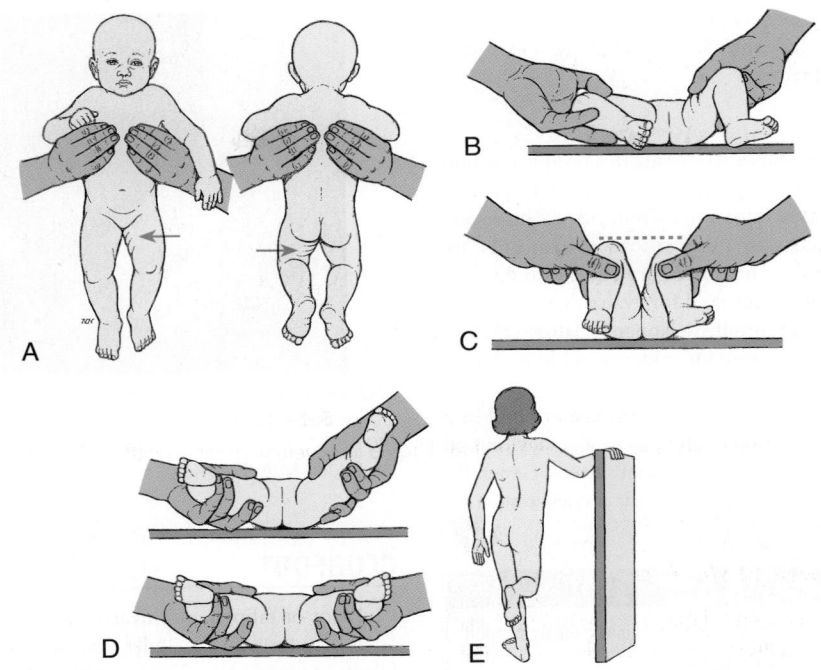

FIG 48.15 Signs of developmental dysplasia of the hip (DDH). **A,** Asymmetry of gluteal and thigh folds. **B,** Limited hip abduction, as seen in flexion. **C,** Apparent shortening of the femur, as indicated by the level of the knees in flexion (Galeazzi sign). **D,** Ortolani maneuver with clunk elicited. **E,** Positive Trendelenburg sign (if child is weight bearing).

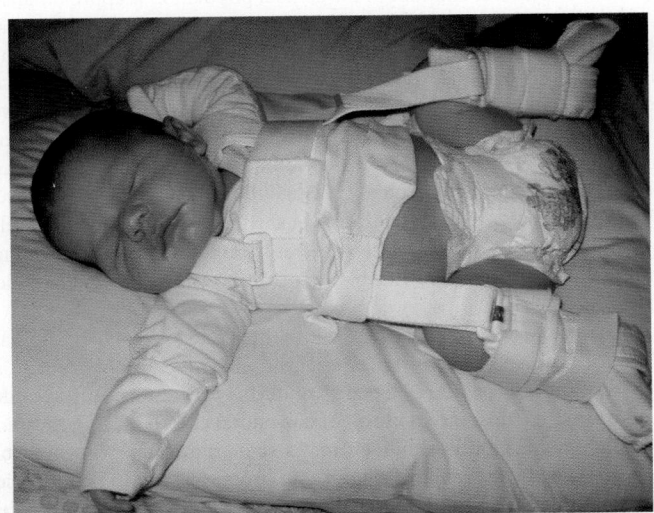

FIG 48.16 Child in Pavlik harness. (Courtesy of Amanda Politte, St. Louis, MO.)

severe the deformity, the more difficult the treatment, and the less favorable the prognosis. The treatment varies with the child's age and the extent of the dysplasia. The goal of treatment is to obtain and maintain a safe, congruent position of the hip joint to promote normal hip joint development.

Newborn to 6 Months of Age

The hip joint is maintained, by dynamic splinting, in a safe position with the proximal femur centered in the acetabulum in a degree of flexion. Of the numerous devices available, the Pavlik harness is the most widely used, and with time, motion, and gravity, the hip works into a more abducted, reduced position (Fig. 48.16). The harness is worn continuously until the hip is proved stable on both clinical and ultrasound examination, usually within 6 to 12 weeks.

When there is difficulty in maintaining stable reduction of the femoral head, a surgical closed reduction of the hip and application of a hip spica cast is performed. The cast is changed periodically to accommodate the child's growth. Once sufficient stability is acquired, after approximately 3 months, the child is transitioned to a removable hip abduction orthosis. The duration of treatment in the orthosis depends on development of the acetabulum.

6 to 24 Months of Age

In this age group, the dislocation is often not recognized until the child begins to stand and walk, when shortening of the limb and contractures of hip adductor and flexor muscles become apparent. In less severe DDH or acetabular dysplasia, use of a hip abduction orthosis may be initiated. Duration of treatment depends on development of the acetabulum. When adduction contracture is present, devices such as traction may be used to slowly and gently stretch the hip to full abduction, after which wide abduction is maintained until stability is attained. A surgical closed reduction of the hip is performed in cases of hip subluxation or dislocation, and in the event that the hip remains unstable, an open reduction may be necessary. The child is placed in a spica cast for approximately 12 weeks, and a hip abduction orthosis may be used following casting.

Older Children

Correction of the hip deformity in older children is inherently more difficult than in the preceding age groups because secondary adaptive changes and other etiologic factors (e.g., juvenile arthritis and cerebral palsy) complicate the condition. Operative reduction, which may involve preoperative traction, lengthening of contracted muscles, and pelvic osteotomy procedures designed to construct an acetabular roof, often combined with proximal femoral osteotomy, are usually required. After cast removal, range-of-motion exercises help restore movement. Other rehabilitation measures may include muscle strengthening, a period of crutch or walker use, and gait training.

Care Management

Nurses as part of the interprofessional care team are in a unique position to detect DDH in early infancy. During the infant assessment process and routine nurturing activities, the hips and extremities are inspected for any deviations from normal. Any observations or concerns are reported to the attending provider. An ambulatory child who displays a limp or an unusual gait should be referred for evaluation. This may indicate an orthopedic or neurologic problem. Nonambulatory children with cerebral palsy should also be assessed for evidence of hip problems throughout their growing years.

The major nursing problems in the care of an infant or child in a cast or other device are related to maintenance of the device and adaptation of nurturing activities to meet the patient's needs. Generally, treatment and follow-up care of these children are carried out in an outpatient setting.

> **! NURSING ALERT**
>
> The former practice of double or triple diapering for DDH is not recommended because there is no evidence to support its efficacy.

The primary nursing goal is teaching parents to apply and maintain the reduction device. The Pavlik harness allows for easy handling of the infant and usually produces less apprehension in the parent than heavy braces and casts. It is important that parents understand the correct use of the harness, which may or may not allow for its removal during bathing. Removing the harness is determined individually on the basis of the health care provider's recommendation, the degree of hip instability, and the family's level of understanding. Parents are instructed to not adjust the harness. The child should be examined by the health care provider before any adjustment is attempted to make certain the hips are in correct placement.

Skin care is an important aspect of care of an infant in a harness. The following instructions for preventing skin breakdown are stressed:

- Check frequently (at least two or three times per day) for red areas or skin irritation in skin folds or under the straps.
- Gently massage healthy skin under the straps once per day to stimulate circulation. In general, avoid lotions and powders because they can cake and irritate the skin.
- Always place the diaper under the straps.

Parents are encouraged to hold the infant with a harness and continue care and nurturing activities. The nurse can assist by being available for parents' questions about the necessary adaptations to daily care to decrease the parents' anxiety and possible feelings about the child being hurt by routine care.

Casts and orthotic devices (braces) offer more challenging nursing and caregiver problems because they cannot be removed for routine care, although sometimes a brace may be removed for bathing. Care of an infant or small child with a cast requires nursing innovation to reduce irritation and to maintain cleanliness of both the child and the cast, particularly in the diaper area (see the "Care of the Child in a Cast" section earlier in this chapter).

It is important for nurses, parents, and other caregivers to understand that children in corrective devices need to be involved in all typical age-appropriate activities. Confinement in a cast or appliance should not exclude children from family (or unit) activities. They can be held astride the lap for comfort and transported to areas of activity. An adapted wheelchair, stroller, or wagon can offer mobility to an older infant or child.

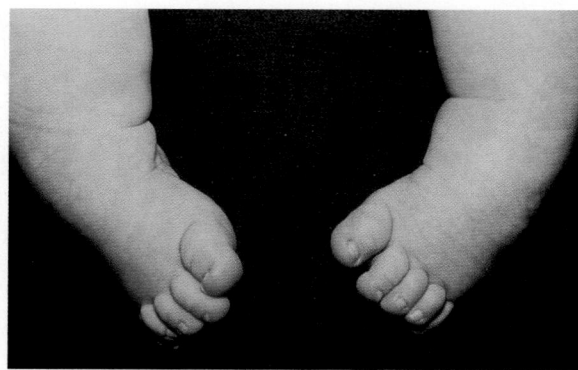

FIG 48.17 Bilateral congenital talipes equinovarus (TEV; clubfoot) in a 2-month-old infant. (From Zitelli, B.J., McIntire, S.C., & Nowalk, A.J. [2012]. *Zitelli and Davis' atlas of pediatric physical diagnosis* [6th ed.]. St. Louis, MO: Elsevier.)

CLUBFOOT

Clubfoot or talipes equinovarus (TEV) is a complex deformity of the ankle and foot that includes forefoot adduction, midfoot supination, hindfoot varus, and ankle equinus. The foot is pointed downward (plantarflexed) and inward in varying degrees of severity (Fig. 48.17). Clubfoot may occur as an isolated deformity or in association with other disorders or syndromes, such as chromosomal abnormalities, arthrogryposis, or spina bifida.

The incidence of clubfoot in the general population is approximately 1 per 1000 live births, with boys affected twice as often as girls. Bilateral clubfeet occur in 50% of the cases (Winell & Davidson, 2016). The precise cause of clubfoot is unknown. However, there is a strong familial tendency, with a 1 in 10 chance that a parent with clubfoot will have an affected offspring. Other possible theories as to the cause of clubfoot include arrested or abnormal fetal development or abnormal positioning and restricted movement in utero, although the evidence is not conclusive. Whereas arrested development during this early stage tends to result in a rigid deformity, mechanical pressures from intrauterine positioning are likely causes of more flexible deformities (Shyy, Wang, Sheffield et al., 2010).

Clubfoot may be further divided into three categories: (1) positional clubfoot (also called *transitional, mild,* or *postural* clubfoot), which is believed to occur primarily from intrauterine crowding and responds to simple stretching and casting; (2) congenital clubfoot (also referred to as *idiopathic* clubfoot), which may occur in an otherwise normal child and has a wide range of rigidity and prognosis; and (3) syndromic (or teratologic) clubfoot, which is associated with other congenital anomalies (e.g., myelomeningocele or arthrogryposis) and is a more severe form of clubfoot that is often resistant to typical treatment.

Classification

The mild, or postural, clubfoot may correct spontaneously or may require passive exercise or serial casting. There is no bony abnormality, but there may be tightness and shortening of the soft tissues medially and posteriorly. The teratologic clubfoot usually requires surgical correction and has a high incidence of recurrence. The congenital idiopathic clubfoot, or "true clubfoot," almost always requires surgical intervention because there is bony abnormality.

Diagnostic Evaluation

The deformity is readily apparent at birth if it has not been detected prenatally through ultrasonography. However, it must be differentiated from some positional deformities that can be passively corrected. Once it is detected, a careful yet comprehensive physical assessment of the affected foot (or feet) should be completed to allow for appropriate decision making regarding treatment plans and prognosis. The affected foot (or feet) is usually smaller and shorter with an empty heel pad midfoot medial crease. When the deformity is unilateral, the affected limb may be shorter and calf atrophy is present. Radiographs of the feet are generally not necessary. A thorough hip examination should be performed for all infants with clubfoot; an increased risk for hip dysplasia is associated with clubfoot deformities.

Therapeutic Management

The goal of treatment for clubfoot is to achieve a painless, plantigrade, and functional foot. Treatment of clubfoot involves three stages: (1) correction of the deformity, (2) maintenance of the correction until normal muscle balance is regained, and (3) follow-up observation to avert possible recurrence of the deformity. Some feet respond to treatment readily; some respond only to prolonged, vigorous, and sustained efforts; and the improvement in others remains disappointing even with maximal effort.

Recommended treatment of clubfoot is with the use of the Ponseti method. Serial casting is begun shortly after birth. Weekly gentle manipulation and stretching of the foot along with placement of serial long-leg casts allow for gradual improvement in the alignment of the foot (Fig. 48.18). The extremity or extremities are casted until maximum correction is achieved, usually within 6 to 10 weeks. The majority of the time, a percutaneous heel-cord tenotomy is performed at the end of casting to correct the equinus deformity. After the tenotomy, a long-leg cast is applied and left in place for 3 weeks. After casting is completed, children are transitioned to utilizing Ponseti sandals with a bar set in abduction to help maintain the correction and prevent a recurrence of the foot deformity. Inability to achieve normal foot alignment after casting and tenotomy indicates the need for surgical intervention (Ponseti, 1996).

Care Management

Nursing care of the child with clubfoot is the same as for any child who has a cast (see the "Care of the Child in a Cast" section earlier in this chapter). Because the child will spend considerable time in a corrective device, nursing care plans include both long- and short-term goals. Careful observation of the skin and circulation is particularly important in young infants because of their rapid growth rate.

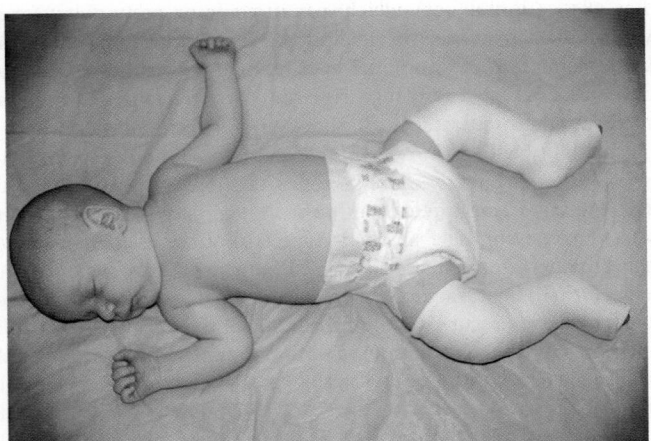

FIG 48.18 Feet casted for correction of bilateral talipes equinovarus (TEV).

Because treatment and follow-up care are handled in the orthopedic clinic or outpatient department, parent education and support are important in nursing care of these children. It is important for parents to understand the diagnosis, overall treatment program, the importance of regular cast changes, and the role they play in the long-term effectiveness of the therapy. Reinforcing and clarifying the orthopedic provider's explanations and instructions, teaching parents about care of the cast or bracing (including vigilant observation for potential problems), and encouraging parents to facilitate normal development within the limitations imposed by the treatment are all part of nursing responsibilities.

METATARSUS ADDUCTUS (VARUS)

Metatarsus adductus, or metatarsus varus, is probably the most common congenital foot deformity. In most instances, it is a result of abnormal intrauterine positioning, particularly in a firstborn child, and is usually detected at birth. The deformity is characterized by medial adduction of the toes and forefoot, frequently in association with inversion and convexity of the lateral border of the foot (kidney shaped). Metatarsus adductus may be divided into three categories:

- Type I: The forefoot is flexible and corrects easily with manipulation.
- Type II: The forefoot is only partially flexible and corrects passively past neutral position, but only to neutral position with active manipulation.
- Type III: The forefoot is rigid and will not stretch to neutral position with manipulation.

Unlike a clubfoot, with which it is often confused, the angulation occurs at the tarsometatarsal joint while the heel and ankle remain in a neutral position. Ankle range of motion is normal. This deformity may cause a pigeon-toed or intoeing gait in the child. A thorough hip examination should be performed for all infants with metatarsus adductus as an increased risk for hip dysplasia is associated with foot deformities.

Management depends on the rigidity and type of the deformity. With types I and II, correction can usually be accomplished by gentle manipulation and passive stretching of the foot, which the parent is taught to perform. Repeated and consistent stretching is continued for the first 6 weeks, after which the treatment is based on the flexibility of the foot. With type III, the child usually requires serial manipulation and casting to correct the deformity, after which a corrective shoe or orthosis may be used. Surgical correction is rarely required for the condition but may be performed in children older than 4 to 6 years of age who have considerable pain on ambulation or functional difficulties as a result of the deformity (Winell & Davidson, 2016).

Care Management

The nursing role primarily involves identifying the defect so that early therapy and instruction of the parents can be initiated. The nurse teaches the parents how to hold the heel firmly and to stretch only the forefoot; otherwise, undue force on the heel may produce a valgus deformity. If casting or an orthosis is required, the nurse instructs the parents in cast care and use of the brace.

SKELETAL LIMB DEFICIENCY

Congenital limb deficiencies, or reduction malformations, are manifested by a variety of degrees of loss of functional capacity. They are characterized by underdevelopment of skeletal elements of the extremities. The range of malformation can extend from minor defects of the digits to serious abnormalities, such as *amelia,* absence of an entire extremity, or *meromelia,* partial absence of an extremity, which includes *phocomelia* (seal limbs), an interposed deficiency of long bones with relatively good development of hands and feet attached at or near the shoulder or the hips. Most reduction defects are primary defects of development of the limb, but prenatal destruction of the limb can occur, such as full or partial amputation of a limb in utero from constriction of an amniotic band (amniotic band syndrome). Neonates with congenital limb deficiencies often have associated malformations and should be thoroughly assessed for cardiovascular, central nervous system, renal, and digestive abnormalities (Stoll, Alembik, Dott et al., 2010).

Pathophysiology

Limb deficiencies can be attributed to both heredity and environment and can originate at any stage of limb development. Formation of limbs may be suppressed at the time of limb bud formation, or there may be interference in later stages of differentiation and growth. Heredity appears to play a prominent role, and prenatal environmental insults have been implicated in a number of cases, such as the well-publicized thalidomide tragedy of the 1950s and early 1960s, which demonstrated a clear relationship between the time of exposure of the pregnant woman to the antiemetic drug and the presence and type of limb deformity in the newborn. There are still drugs that may have similar teratogenic effects in the first trimester of pregnancy. Therefore, medication administration during this period should be carefully evaluated by the provider.

Therapeutic Management

The child with a limb deficiency should be fitted with prosthetic devices, and the devices should be applied at the earliest possible stage of development in an attempt to match the infant's motor readiness. This favors natural progression of prosthetic use. For example, an infant with an upper extremity deficiency is fitted with a simple passive device between 3 and 6 months of age to encourage limb exploration, sitting (with the extremities needed for support), and bilateral hand activities. Lower limb prostheses are applied when the infant is ready to pull to a standing position.

In preparation for prosthetic devices, surgical modification of the residual limb may be necessary to ensure the most effective use of the device or prosthetic. Phocomelic digits are preserved for controlling switches of externally powered appliances in the upper extremities. Digits (in both the upper and lower extremities) provide the child with surfaces for tactile exploration and stimulation. Prostheses are replaced to accommodate the child's growth and increasing capabilities.

Care Management

Prosthetic application, training, and use are most successfully carried out in an institution that specializes in meeting the special needs of these children, especially very young children and those with multiple amputations or missing limbs. Management involves a prosthetist, who as a member of the interprofessional care team, specializes in the development, fitting, and maintenance of prosthetic limbs, and other health care providers, such as physical and occupational therapists. Parents need support and are encouraged to assist the child in making age-appropriate adjustments to the environment. Although these children need assistance, overprotection may produce overdependence, with later maladjustment to school and other situations.

OSTEOGENESIS IMPERFECTA

OI is a rare genetic disorder characterized by bones that fracture easily. Although inheritance follows an autosomal dominant pattern in most cases, rare autosomal recessive inheritance exists. Most types of OI have defects in the *COL1A1* or *COL1A2* genes, which code for polypeptide chains in type 1 procollagen, a precursor of type 1 collagen, which is a major structural component of bone. The error results in faulty bone

---

> ## BOX 48.6 **Classification of Osteogenesis Imperfecta***
>
> **Type I***[†]
> **A:** Mild bone fragility; blue sclerae; normal teeth; hearing loss (occurs between 20 and 30 years of age); autosomal dominant inheritance
> **B:** Same as A except dentinogenesis imperfecta instead of normal teeth
> **C:** Same as B but no bone fragility
> **Type II:** Lethal; stillborn or die in early infancy; severe bone fragility, multiple fractures at birth; 10% of cases of OI; autosomal recessive inheritance
> **Type III:** Severe bone fragility leading to severe progressive deformities; normal sclerae; marked growth failure; most autosomal recessive inheritance; few autosomal dominant inheritance
> **Type IV**
> **A:** Mild to moderate bone fragility; normal sclerae; normal teeth; short stature; variable deformity; autosomal dominant inheritance
> **B:** Same as A except dentinogenesis imperfecta instead of normal teeth; approximately 6% of cases of OI
> **Type V:** Clinically similar to type IV; hyperplastic callus; collagen mutation negative
> **Type VI:** Sclerae and dentition normal; moderate to severe bone fragility; diagnosis by bone biopsy because of similarities to other types
> **Types VII and VIII (recessive form):** Clinically overlap types II and III but have white sclerae, rhizomelia, and small to normal head circumference; severe osteochondroplastica and short stature in survivors. Type VII is associated with *CRTAP* gene, and type VIII is associated with the *LEPRE1* genetic mutation.

OI, Osteogenesis imperfecta.
*Two-thirds of cases are type I.
†This classification is based on that proposed by Sillence, D.O., Senn, A., & Danks, D.M. (1979). Genetic heterogeneity in osteogenesis imperfecta. *Journal of Medical Genetics*, *16*[2], 101–116, which originally included OI types I to IV. Additional types have been described but are not included herein.

---

mineralization, abnormal bone architecture, and increased susceptibility to fracture. There are at least 12 described types of OI, which accounts for significant disease variability. Clinical features may include varying degrees of bone fragility and deformity, short stature, blue sclerae, hearing loss, and dentinogenesis imperfecta (hypoplastic discolored teeth) (Marini & Blissett, 2013).

Classification is based on clinical features and patterns of inheritance (Box 48.6). Clinically, type I is the most common and mildest form, with most fractures occurring before puberty. Stature is near normal, and bone deformity is minimal or absent. Type II is the most severe and considered lethal in infancy. Type III OI is characterized by multiple fractures often present at birth, short stature, severe bone deformity, and disability with a shortened life expectancy. Type IV is similar to type I although slightly more severe, with short stature and mild to moderate bone deformities. Types V and VI do not have a type 1 collagen defect and are clinically similar to type IV. Both types demonstrate a unique pattern to their bone. Affected individuals have hypertrophic callus formation at fracture sites, a radiodense metaphyseal band, and calcification of the interosseous membrane of the forearm. In type VI, bone has a characteristic mineralization defect or microscopic "fish scale" appearance with elevated alkaline phosphatase activity. Types VII through XII are rare, recessive forms of OI with different genetic defects being found. Clinical severity is variable and overlaps types II and III in relation to clinical features. Those who survive have white sclerae, short stature, and rhizomelia (Marini & Blissett, 2013).

Therapeutic Management

The treatment for OI has historically been primarily supportive; although patients and families are optimistic about new research advances. The use of bisphosphonate therapy with IV pamidronate to promote increased bone density and prevent fractures has become standard therapy for many children with OI. However, bisphosphonate therapy is reportedly more beneficial for increasing vertebral bone density and less effective for long bones (Marini, 2016).

The goals of a rehabilitative approach to management are directed toward preventing (1) positional contractures and deformities, (2) muscle weakness and osteoporosis, and (3) malalignment of lower extremity joints prohibiting weight bearing. Lightweight braces and splints help support limbs, prevent fractures, and aid in ambulation. Physical therapy helps prevent disuse osteoporosis and strengthens muscles, which in turn improves bone density. Surgery is sometimes used to help treat the manifestations of the disease. Surgical techniques are used to prevent or correct deformities that interfere with bracing, standing, or walking. The placement of intramedullary rods into the long bones can provide stability to bone, as well as prevent or correct deformities.

Care Management

Infants and children with this disorder require careful handling to prevent fractures. They must be supported when they are being turned, positioned, moved, and held. Even changing a diaper may cause a fracture in severely affected infants. These children should never be held by the ankles when being diapered but should be gently lifted by the buttocks or supported with pillows. However, nurses should not be afraid to touch or handle the infant or child with OI. Such children need compassionate handling and care as much as any other patient.

Both parents and the affected child need education regarding the child's limitations and guidelines in planning suitable activities that promote optimal development and protect the child from harm. Realistic occupational planning and genetic counseling are part of the long-term goals of care. Educational materials and information can be obtained from the Osteogenesis Imperfecta Foundation,* which also has a network that places families in contact with other families with a similar condition.

Children with current fractures or healing fractures should be screened for OI; the assumption that abuse or neglect is the cause of fractures in children must be carefully evaluated by a multidisciplinary team. A detailed history, no evidence of associated soft-tissue injury, and the presence of other symptoms related to OI help to determine the diagnosis.

ACQUIRED DEFECTS

LEGG-CALVÉ-PERTHES DISEASE

Legg-Calvé-Perthes disease is a self-limiting disorder in which there is avascular necrosis of the femoral head. The disease affects children 2 to 12 years of age, but most cases occur as an isolated event in boys between 4 and 8 years of age, with a male-to-female ratio of 4:1. In approximately 10% of cases, the involvement is bilateral; most affected children have a skeletal age significantly below their chronologic age. Caucasian children are affected 10 times more frequently than African-American children (Loder & Skopelja, 2011b).

*804 W. Diamond Avenue, Suite 210, Gaithersburg, MD 20878; 800-981-2663; http://www.oif.org.

> ### BOX 48.7   Radiographic Stages of Legg-Calvé-Perthes Disease
>
> **Stage I:** Initial, or avascular, stage: Avascular necrosis or infarction of the proximal femoral epiphysis with degenerative changes producing flattening of the upper surface of the femoral head or a decrease in femoral head height.
>
> **Stage II:** Fragmentation, or resorptive, stage: Femoral head resorption and revascularization produces collapse of the femoral head and fragmentation that gives a mottled appearance on radiographs.
>
> **Stage III:** Reossification stage: New bone formation, which is represented on radiographs as calcification and ossification or increased density in the areas of radiolucency; this filling-in process appears to begin in the periphery of the femoral head and progress centrally.
>
> **Stage IV:** Healing, or remodeling, stage: Gradual reformation of the head of the femur without radiolucency; this occurs until skeletal maturity.

Pathophysiology

The cause of the disease is unknown, but a temporary disturbance of circulation or vascular supply to the femoral capital epiphysis produces an ischemic avascular necrosis of the femoral head. During middle childhood, circulation to the femoral epiphysis is more tenuous than at other ages and can become obstructed by trauma, inflammation, coagulation defects, and a variety of other causes. The pathologic events seem to take place in four stages (Box 48.7). The entire disease process may encompass as little as 18 months or continue for several years. The reformed femoral head may be severely altered or minimally impacted.

Clinical Manifestations and Diagnostic Evaluation

The onset of Legg-Calvé-Perthes disease is usually insidious, and the history may reveal only intermittent appearance of a limp on the affected side or a symptom complex, including hip soreness, ache, or stiffness, which can be constant or intermittent. The parents may report seeing the child limping, and the limp becomes more pronounced with increased activity. The pain may be experienced in the hip, along the entire thigh, or in the vicinity of the knee joint. The pain and limp are usually most evident on arising and at the end of a long day of activities. The pain is usually accompanied by joint dysfunction and limited range of motion at the hip. There may be a vague history of trauma but not necessarily. The diagnosis is established by characteristic radiographic findings including medial joint space widening, flattening of the femoral head with irregular ossification, and possible subchondral fracture. A perfusion MRI of the hip may be obtained to assess the blood flow to the femoral head.

Therapeutic Management

Because deformity occurs early in the disease process, the aims of treatment are to restore and maintain adequate hip range of motion; prevent femoral head collapse, extrusion, or subluxation; and preserve as well-rounded femoral head as possible at the time of healing. Treatment varies according to the child's age at the time of diagnosis and the appearance of the femoral head and position within the acetabulum. Activity causes microfractures of the soft ischemic epiphysis, which tend to induce synovitis, stiffness, and adductor contracture.

The initial therapy is rest or activity restrictions and limited weight bearing, which helps reduce inflammation and irritability of the hip. The use of NSAIDs can provide relief of pain or discomfort; physical therapy or range-of-motion exercises help restore hip motion. In some cases, traction is applied to stretch tight adductor muscles and improve containment of the femoral head. Abduction braces or casting may also

Legg-Calvé-Perthes Disease

A family with five healthy children was startled one day to learn that their 2-year-old son could no longer walk. He was diagnosed with Legg-Calvé-Perthes disease. Through several years of prosthetic devices and numerous physician visits, hospitalizations, and surgeries, this family turned a potentially devastating experience into one with cherished memories.

Today, the parents reflect on how their family coped with the reality of a debilitating disease. It was difficult for the parents to observe an eager, energetic child watch other children riding bicycles, running, or playing outdoor games. They are warmed by memories of watching their other children make the difference for their sibling. They all developed a strong bond through caring and sharing with one another. Coping as a family was an easy adjustment and, most of all, therapeutic. Today, more than 20 years later, the parents believe that each family member has grown with feelings of faith and trust. The experience proved to them that life will go on and that life is what you make it!

Shona Swenson Lenss, MS, RN, FNP
Cheyenne, WY

---

be utilized for containment of the femoral head. If nonsurgical or conservative management is unsuccessful, surgical reconstruction or containment procedures such as a pelvic or proximal femoral osteotomy may be necessary.

The disease is self-limiting, but the ultimate outcome of therapy depends on early and efficient treatment. Children 5 years of age and younger, whose epiphyses are more cartilaginous, tend to have the best prognosis or outcome. Children older than 8 years of age have a significant risk for degenerative arthritis, especially if they have femoral head deformity at the time of diagnosis. The later the diagnosis is made, the more femoral damage will have occurred before treatment is implemented (Herring, 2011).

Care Management

Because these children are largely cared for on an outpatient basis, the major emphasis of nursing care is teaching the family the required care and management. The family needs to comprehend the diagnosis and understand the purpose and function of activity restrictions and limitations in achieving the desired outcome. The child and family may rely on the nurse to help them understand and adjust to therapeutic measures (see Family-Centered Care box: Legg-Calvé-Perthes Disease).

One of the most difficult aspects associated with the disorder is the need to cope with a normally active child who feels well but must remain relatively inactive. It is important to emphasize that children should continue to attend school and engage in activities that can be adapted to the prescribed regimen. Suitable activities must be devised to meet the needs of a child in the process of developing a sense of initiative or industry. Activities that fulfill creative urges are well received.

SLIPPED CAPITAL FEMORAL EPIPHYSIS

Slipped capital femoral epiphysis (SCFE) refers to the spontaneous displacement of the proximal femoral epiphysis in a posterior and inferior direction. It develops most frequently shortly before or during accelerated growth and the onset of puberty (children between 8 and 15 years of age; median age of 12 years of age for boys and 11 years of age for girls) and is seen more often in boys and obese children. The incidence is 0.3 to 24 cases per 100,000 children. Bilateral involvement occurs in up to 50% of cases (Loder & Skopelja, 2011c).

BOX 48.8 **Clinical Manifestations of Slipped Capital Femoral Epiphysis**

Very often obese (body mass index >95%)
Limp on affected side
Possible inability to bear weight because of severe pain
Pain in groin, thigh, or knee
- May be acute, chronic, or acute-on-chronic
- Continuous or intermittent
Affected leg is externally rotated
Loss of hip flexion, abduction, and internal rotation as severity increases
Affected leg may appear shorter

Pathophysiology

In a hip with SCFE, the capital femoral epiphysis remains in the acetabulum, but the femoral neck slips, deforming the femoral head and stretching blood vessels to the epiphysis. Most cases of SCFE are idiopathic, although it can be associated with endocrine disorders, such as hypothyroidism, low growth hormone levels, pituitary tumors, and renal osteodystrophy. The cause of idiopathic SCFE is multifactorial and includes obesity, physeal architecture and orientation, and pubertal hormone changes that affect physeal strength. Although obesity stresses the physeal plate, SCFE can also occur in children who are not obese.

Diagnostic Evaluation

SCFE is suspected when an adolescent or preadolescent displays clinical signs of a limp or complains of hip, groin, thigh, or knee pain. See Box 48.8 for additional clinical manifestations. The diagnosis is confirmed by anteroposterior and frog-leg hip radiographs that reflect a change in position of the proximal femoral epiphysis. Radiographs show medial displacement of the epiphysis and uncovered upper portion of the femoral neck adjacent to the physis. There is a widened growth plate and irregular metaphysis.

Therapeutic Management

The treatment goals of SCFE are to prevent further slipping of the femoral epiphysis until physeal closure, avoid further complication such as avascular necrosis, and maintain adequate hip function (Peck & Herrara-Soto, 2014). If the diagnosis is suspected or has been established, the child should be non–weight bearing to prevent further slippage. Surgical intervention is necessary and most often occurs within 24 hours to avoid further slippage and potential complications such as avascular necrosis.

Currently, in situ pinning using a single screw or alternatively multiple screws through the femoral neck into the proximal femoral epiphysis is the treatment of choice. For moderate to severe SCFE, an experienced surgeon may choose to perform a surgical hip dislocation to improve the anatomy at the site of the deformity (Tibor & Sink, 2013). Postsurgical care includes non–weight bearing or limited weight bearing with use of crutches for ambulation for weeks to months. Children may be restricted from certain sports or activities until fusion or closure of the proximal femoral physis has occurred in order to prevent further slippage.

Care Management

Nursing care involves preparing the child and family for the surgical procedure and recovery. Postoperative care involves hemodynamic stabilization, pain management, and assessment for complications. The adolescent is taught the proper use of crutches and the importance of avoiding weight bearing on the affected hip. Self-care and performance

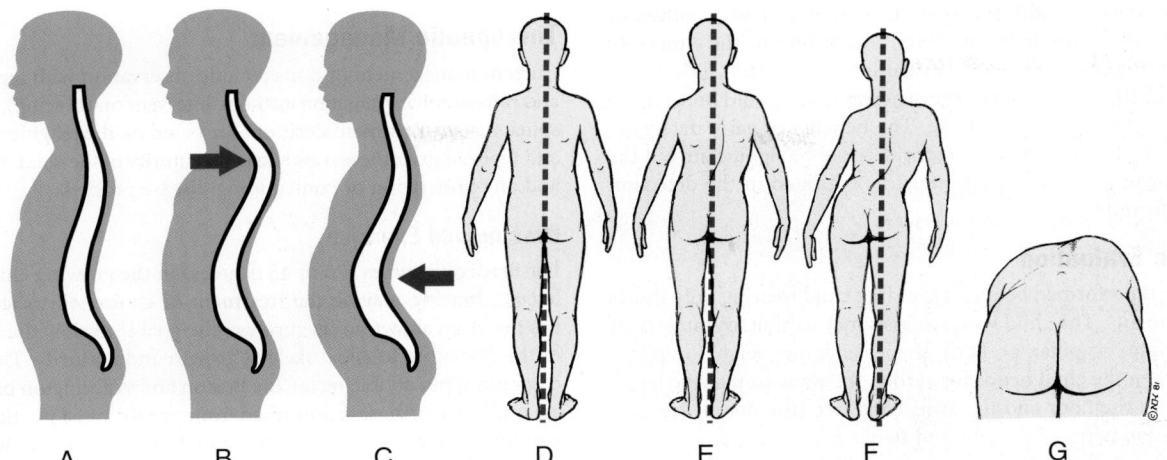

FIG 48.19 Defects of spinal column. **A,** Normal spine. **B,** Kyphosis. **C,** Lordosis. **D,** Normal spine in balance. **E,** Mild scoliosis in balance. **F,** Severe scoliosis not in balance. **G,** Rib hump and flank asymmetry seen in flexion caused by rotary component. (Redrawn from Hilt, N.E., & Schmitt, E.W. [1975]. *Pediatric orthopedic nursing.* St. Louis, MO: Mosby.)

of activities of daily living to capability are encouraged to promote confidence and decrease a sense of helplessness.

> ⚠ **NURSING ALERT**
>
> Children with hip issues, such as Legg-Calvé-Perthes disease or slipped capital femoral epiphysis (SCFE), often present with groin, thigh, or knee pain. This is often because of referred pain and is anatomically related to the obturator nerve. Any time a child presents with groin, thigh, or knee pain, a complete hip examination is paramount to rule out underlying hip pathology.

KYPHOSIS AND LORDOSIS

The spine, which consists of numerous segments, can acquire deformity curves of three types: kyphosis, lordosis, and scoliosis (Fig. 48.19). *Kyphosis* is the lateral convex angulation in the curvature of the thoracic spine (see Fig. 48.19, *B*). If it is increased (greater than 45 degrees), it may occur secondary to disease processes, such as tuberculosis (TB), chronic arthritis, osteodystrophy, or compression fractures of the thoracic spine. The most common form of hyperkyphosis is posture-related. Children, especially during the time when skeletal growth outpaces growth of muscle, are prone to exaggeration of a normal kyphosis. This is particularly common in self-conscious adolescent girls who assume a round-shouldered slouching posture in an attempt to hide their developing breasts and increasing height. *Scheuermann kyphosis* is a thoracic curve greater than 45 degrees with wedging of more than 5 degrees of at least three adjacent vertebral bodies and vertebral irregularity.

Postural (flexible) hyperkyphosis is almost always accompanied by a compensatory postural lordosis, an abnormally exaggerated concave lumbar curvature. Treatment of kyphosis consists of exercises to strengthen shoulder and abdominal muscles and bracing for more marked deformity. With adolescents who are significantly self-conscious about their appearance, the best approach is to emphasize the cosmetic value of corrective therapy and to place the responsibility on the adolescent for carrying out an exercise program at home with regular visits to and assessments by a physical therapist. Treatment with a brace may be indicated until skeletal maturity, and surgical fusion may be considered for severe, painful, or progressive thoracic curves, such as Scheuermann kyphosis.

Lordosis is the lateral inward curve of the cervical or lumbar curvature (see Fig. 48.19, *C*). Hyperlordosis may be a secondary complication of a disease process, a result of trauma, or idiopathic. Hyperlordosis is a normal observation in toddlers and, in older children, is often seen in association with flexion contractures of the hip, obesity, DDH, and SCFE. During the pubertal growth spurt, lordosis of varying degrees is observed in teenagers, especially girls. In obese children, the weight of the abdominal fat alters the center of gravity, causing a compensatory lordosis. Unlike kyphosis, severe lordosis is usually accompanied by pain.

Treatment involves management of the predisposing cause when possible, such as weight loss and correction of deformities. Postural exercises or support garments are helpful in relieving symptoms in some cases; however, these do not usually provide a permanent cure.

IDIOPATHIC SCOLIOSIS

Scoliosis is a complex spinal deformity in three planes, usually involving lateral curvature, spinal rotation causing rib asymmetry, and when in the thoracic spine, often thoracic hypokyphosis (see Fig. 48.19, *E* to *G*). It is the most common spinal deformity and is classified according to age of onset: *congenital* occurs in fetal development; *infantile* occurs at birth up to 3 years of age; *juvenile* occurs in children 3 to 10 years of age; and *adolescent* occurs at 10 years of age or older.

Scoliosis can be caused by a number of conditions and may occur alone or in association with other diseases, particularly neuromuscular conditions (neuromuscular scoliosis). In most cases, however, there is no apparent cause, hence the name *idiopathic scoliosis*. There appears to be a genetic component to the etiology of idiopathic scoliosis; however, the exact relationship has yet to be established. The following section is limited to a discussion of adolescent idiopathic scoliosis.

Clinical Manifestations

Idiopathic scoliosis is most commonly identified during the preadolescent growth spurt. Parents frequently bring a child for follow-up on an abnormal school scoliosis screening or because of ill-fitting clothes, such as poorly fitting jeans. School screening is controversial because there are no controlled studies to demonstrated improved outcomes and a reported number of false-positive results lead to referrals. The American Academy of Orthopaedic Surgeons and the American Academy of Pediatrics published a joint statement favoring scoliosis screening for preadolescents and adolescents in the school, provider's office, or nurses' clinic (Richards & Vitale, 2008). According to the American Academy of Orthopaedic Surgeons (Richards & Vitale, 2008), girls should be screened at 10 and 12 years of age, whereas boys should be screened once either at 13 or 14 years of age. The benefits of early detection, referral, and medical treatment are considered to be significant, but the people performing the screenings must be educated in the detection of spinal deformity.

Diagnostic Evaluation

Observation is performed behind a standing child wearing only shorts or undergarments. The child with scoliosis may exhibit asymmetry of shoulder height, scapular or flank shape, and hip height or pelvic obliquity. When the child bends forward at the waist so that the trunk is parallel with the floor and the arms hang free (the Adams forward bend test), asymmetry of the ribs and flanks may be appreciated (see Fig. 48.19, G). A scoliometer is used in the initial screening to measure truncal rotation. Often a primary curve and a compensatory curve will place the head in alignment with the gluteal cleft. However, with an uncompensated curve, the head and hips are not aligned (see Fig. 48.19, E and F).

Definitive diagnosis is made by radiographs of the child in the standing position and use of the Cobb technique, a standard measurement of angle curvature. The Risser scale is used to evaluate skeletal maturity on the radiograph. This scale assists in making a determination of the likely progression of the spinal curvature based on growth potential. The sexual maturity rating is also used to evaluate the risk for curve progression in adolescents. Not all spinal curvatures are scoliosis. A curve of less than 10 degrees is considered a postural variation. Curves measured between 10 and 25 degrees are mild and, if nonprogressive, do not require treatment (Hresko, 2013).

Intraspinal conditions or other disease processes that can cause scoliosis must be ruled out. The presence of pain, sacral dimpling or hairy patches, cutaneous vascular changes, absent or abnormal reflexes, bowel or bladder incontinence, or a left thoracic curve may indicate an intraspinal abnormality, such as syringomyelia, diastematomyelia, or tethered cord syndrome. An MRI scan of the spine is usually obtained for evaluation.

Therapeutic Management

Current management options include observation with regular clinical and radiographic evaluation, orthotic intervention (bracing), and surgical spinal fusion. Treatment decisions are based on the magnitude, location, and type of curve; the age and skeletal maturity of the child or adolescent; and any underlying or contributing disease process.

Bracing and Exercise

For moderate curves (25 to 45 degrees) in the growing child and adolescent, bracing may be the treatment of choice. Historically bracing has not been shown to be curative; the goal is to slow the progression of the curvature to allow skeletal growth and maturity. The two most common types of bracing are the Boston and Wilmington braces, which are underarm orthoses customized from prefabricated plastic shells, with corrective forces using lateral pads and decreasing lumbar lordosis, and a thoracolumbosacral orthosis (TLSO), which is an underarm orthosis made of plastic that is custom molded to the body and then shaped to correct or hold the deformity (Fig. 48.20). The Milwaukee brace, which is an individually adapted brace that includes a neck ring, is rarely used in scoliosis but is sometimes used in the treatment of kyphosis. The Charleston nighttime bending brace is worn only when the child is in bed, because it prevents walking because of the severity of the trunk bend. Wearing the brace is challenging due to the child's age and preoccupation with body image and appearance. Bracing, although used as the gold standard treatment for moderate curves in a growing child, has not proved to be entirely effective in the treatment of idiopathic scoliosis.

There is very limited evidence regarding the effect of exercises and chiropractic treatment in the prevention of curve progression in scoliosis. Transcutaneous electrical nerve stimulation has proved to be an ineffective treatment. Exercises are of benefit when used in conjunction with bracing to maintain and increase the strength and range of motion of the spine.

Operative Management

Surgical intervention may be required for treatment of severe curves, which are typically greater than 45 degrees (Mistovich & Spiegel, 2016). The child's age, location of the curvature, and curve magnitude influence the decision for surgery. Any progressive or severe curve that does not

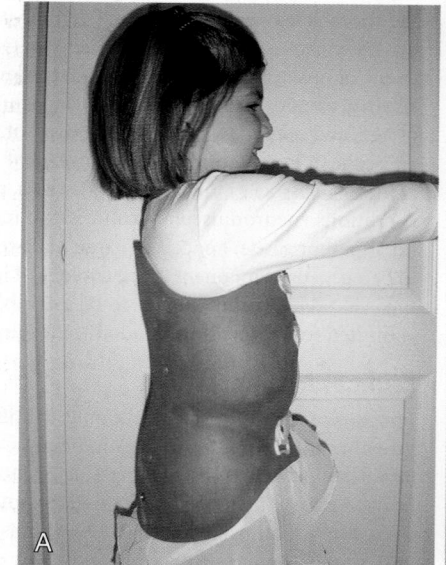
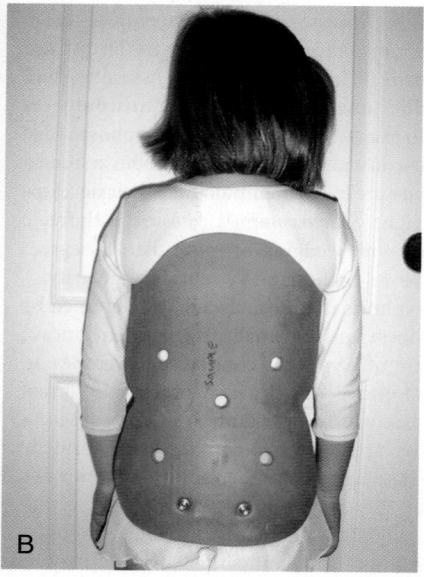

FIG 48.20 A, Standard thoracolumbosacral orthotic (TLSO) brace for idiopathic scoliosis. The brace may be decorated to make it more acceptable to adolescents. **B,** Posterior view of the same brace.

respond to conservative orthotic measures (e.g., bracing) requires surgical correction. Bracing and exercise have been found to be ineffective in managing curves greater than 45 degrees. Neuromuscular, dysplastic and congenital curves, which eventually progress, are best treated with surgical stabilization. Difficulties with balance or seating, respiratory compromise, or pain are also considered.

There are a number of surgical techniques for severe scoliosis. A spinal fusion consists of realignment and straightening of the spine with internal fixation and instrumentation combined with bony fusion (arthrodesis). Posterior and/or anterior surgical approaches may be implemented. The goals of surgical intervention are to improve the curvatures on the sagittal and coronal planes and to provide a solid, pain-free fusion in a well-balanced torso, with maximum mobility of the remaining spinal segments.

Advances in surgical technology currently being evaluated include thoracoscopic spinal fusion and placement of implants; metallic staples may also be placed into the vertebral bodies to achieve spinal fusion and to correct the deformity (Mistovich & Spiegel, 2016). The use of minimally invasive surgery techniques has gained acceptance for its small incisions, decreased blood loss, decreased recovery time, earlier mobilization, and decreased pain and need for pain medications (Sarwahi, Wollowick, Sugarman et al., 2011).

Care Management

Treatment for scoliosis extends over a significant portion of the affected child's period of growth. In adolescents, this period is the one in which their identity, both physical and psychologic, is formed. The identification of scoliosis as a "deformity," in combination with unattractive braces and a significant surgical procedure, can have a negative effect on the already fragile adolescent body image. The adolescent and family require excellent nursing care to meet not only physical needs but also psychologic needs associated with the diagnosis, surgery, postoperative recovery, and eventual rehabilitation.

Although adolescents with scoliosis are encouraged to participate in most peer activities, necessary therapeutic modifications are likely to make them feel different and isolated. Nursing care of the adolescent who is facing scoliosis surgery, potential social isolation, pain, and uncertainty, not to mention misunderstood emotions and body image issues, must be evaluated from the adolescent's perspective to be successful in meeting the individual's needs.

When a child or adolescent first faces the prospect of a prolonged period in a brace or other device, the therapy program and the nature of the device must be explained thoroughly to both the child and the parents so they will understand the anticipated results, how the appliance corrects the defect, the freedoms and constraints imposed by the device, and what they can do to help achieve the desired goal. Management involves the skills and services of a team of specialists, including the orthopedist, physical therapist, orthotist (a specialist in fitting orthopedic braces), nurse, social worker, and sometimes a thoracic or pulmonary specialist.

It is difficult for a child to be restricted at any phase of development, but adolescents need continual positive reinforcement, encouragement, and as much independence as can be safely assumed during this time. Adolescents appreciate guidance and assistance by the interprofessional care team regarding anticipated problems, such as selection of clothing and participation in social activities. Socialization with peers is strongly encouraged, and every effort is expended to help the adolescent feel attractive and worthwhile.

Preoperative Care

The preoperative workup usually involves a radiographic series, including bending or traction spine films, pulmonary function studies, and serologic laboratory studies (including prothrombin, partial thromboplastin, and platelet function test; blood count; electrolyte levels; urinalysis and urine culture; and blood levels of any medications). Spinal surgery typically results in considerable blood loss, so several options are considered preoperatively to maintain or replace blood volume. These options include autologous blood donations obtained from the patient before the surgery; intraoperative blood salvage; intraoperative hemodilution; erythropoietin administration; and controlled induced hypotension, which must be carefully monitored at all times to prevent physiologic instability.

Surgery for spinal fusion is complex, and often adolescents who require the procedure due to idiopathic scoliosis are not familiar with medical terms or procedures. Preoperative teaching is critical for the adolescent to be able to cooperate and participate in his or her treatment and recovery. Because the surgery is extensive, the patient is taught how to manage his or her own patient-controlled analgesia (PCA) pump; how to log roll; and the use and function of other equipment, such as a chest tube (for anterior repair) and Foley urinary catheter. It is recommended that the child or adolescent bring a favorite toy (age dependent) or personal items such as a favorite stuffed animal, laptop computer, cell phone, MP3 player, or movie player for postoperative use. Meeting with a peer who has undergone a similar surgery may also be valuable.

Postoperative Care

Following surgery, patients are monitored in an acute care setting and log rolled when changing position to prevent damage to the fusion and instrumentation. In some cases, an immobilization brace or cast is used postoperatively depending on the type of surgical intervention. Skin care is important, and pressure-relieving mattresses or beds may be needed to prevent pressure wounds (see the "Maintaining Healthy Skin" section in Chapter 39).

In addition to the usual postoperative assessments of wound, circulation, and vital signs, the neurologic status of the patient's extremities requires special attention. Prompt recognition of any neurologic impairment is imperative because delayed paralysis may develop that requires surgical intervention. Common postoperative problems after spinal fusion include neurologic injury or spinal cord injury, hypotension from acute blood loss, wound infection, syndrome of inappropriate antidiuretic hormone, atelectasis, pneumothorax, ileus, delayed neurologic injury, and implanted hardware complications (Freeman, 2013). Superior mesenteric artery syndrome may occur several days after spinal surgery; this involves duodenal compression by the aorta and superior mesenteric artery and may result in acute partial or complete duodenal obstruction. Clinical manifestations include epigastric pain, nausea, copious vomiting, and eructation; symptoms are aggravated in the supine position and often relieved with the patient in a left lateral decubitus or prone position.

The adolescent usually has considerable pain for the first few days after surgery and requires frequent administration of pain medication, preferably opioids administered intravenously on a regular schedule. For children able to understand the concept, PCA is recommended (see the "Pain Assessment" and "Pain Management" sections in Chapter 30). In addition to pain management, the patient is evaluated for skin integrity, adequate urinary output, fluid and electrolyte balance, and ileus. Discharge planning should include a timetable for follow-up with the provider and resumption of regular activities.

In most cases, the patient begins ambulation as soon as possible. Depending on the instrumentation used and the surgical approach, most patients are walking by the second or third postoperative day and discharged within 5 to 7 days. The patient may start physical therapy as soon as he or she is able, beginning with range-of-motion exercises on the first postoperative day and many of the activities of daily living in the following days. Self-care, such as washing and eating, is always encouraged. Throughout the hospitalization, age-appropriate activities and contact with family and friends are important parts of nursing care and planning (see the "Immobilization" section earlier in this chapter). The family is encouraged to become involved in the patient's care to facilitate the transition from hospital to home management. An organization that provides education and services to both families and professionals is the National Scoliosis Foundation.*

INFECTIONS OF BONES AND JOINTS

OSTEOMYELITIS

Osteomyelitis, an infectious process in the bone, can occur at any age but most frequently is seen in children 10 years of age or younger. Boys are more commonly affected than girls, and the median age of diagnosis is 5 to 6 years of age. The limbs most commonly affected include the foot, femur, tibia, and pelvis. *Staphylococcus aureus* is the most common causative organism. Neonates are also likely to have osteomyelitis caused by group B streptococci. Children with sickle cell disease may develop osteomyelitis from *Salmonella* organisms as well as *S. aureus*. *Neisseria gonorrhoeae* is a potential causative organism in sexually active adolescents. *Kingella kingae* has been reported as one of the most causative organisms in children younger than 5 years of age (Kaplan, 2016a).

Acute hematogenous osteomyelitis results when a bloodborne bacterium causes an infection in the bone. Common foci include infected lesions, upper respiratory tract infections, otitis media, tonsillitis, abscessed teeth, pyelonephritis, and infected burns. Exogenous osteomyelitis is acquired from direct inoculation of the bone from a puncture wound, open fracture, surgical contamination, or adjacent tissue infection. Subacute osteomyelitis has a longer course and may be caused by less virulent microbes with a walled-off abscess or Brodie abscess, typically in the proximal or distal tibia. Chronic osteomyelitis is a progression of acute osteomyelitis and is characterized by dead bone, bone loss, and drainage and sinus tracts.

Generally, healthy bone is not likely to become infected. Factors that contribute to infection include inoculation with a large number of organisms, presence of a foreign body, bone injury, high virulence of an organism, immunosuppression, and malnutrition; certain types and locations of bone are also more vulnerable to infection.

Typically, children with acute hematogenous osteomyelitis are seen with a 2- to 7-day history of pain, warmth, tenderness, and decreased range of motion in the affected limb along with systemic symptoms of fever, irritability, and lethargy (Box 48.9). Infants may have an adjacent joint effusion as well. Symptoms often resemble those observed in other conditions involving bones, such as arthritis, leukemia, or sarcoma.

Pathophysiology

In acute osteomyelitis, bacteria adhere to bone, causing a suppurative infection with inflammatory cells, edema, vascular congestion, and small-vessel thrombosis; the result is bone destruction, abscess formation, and dead bone (sequestra). Infection within the bone can rupture through the cortex into the subperiosteal space, stripping loose periosteum and forming an abscess. As dead bone is resorbed, new bone is formed along the live bone and infection borders. This surrounding sheath of live bone is called an *involucrum*. Sinus tracts from perforations in the involucrum may drain pus through soft tissue to the skin.

---

*5 Cabot Place, Stoughton, MA 02072; 800-673-6922; http://www.scoliosis.org.

BOX 48.9 Causative Microorganisms of Osteomyelitis According to Age

Newborns
Staphylococcus aureus
Group B streptococcus
Gram-negative enteric rods

Infants
S. aureus (methicillin-sensitive *S. aureus*, methicillin-resistant *S. aureus* [MRSA])
Haemophilus influenzae

Older Children
S. aureus
Pseudomonas organisms
Salmonella organisms
Neisseria gonorrhoeae

Adolescents and Adults
Pseudomonas organisms
Mycobacterium tuberculosis

From McCance, K.L., & Huether, S.E. (2010). *Pathophysiology: The biological basis for disease in adults and children* [6th ed.]. St. Louis, MO: Mosby/Elsevier.

The pathology of osteomyelitis is different in infants, children older than 1 year of age, and adults. In infants, blood vessels cross the growth plate into the epiphysis and joint space, which allows infection to spread into the joint. In children, the infection is contained by the growth plate, and joint infection is less likely (unless the infection is intracapsular). In older adolescents (with a closed growth plate), the infection is poorly contained and the joint is compromised. Adult periosteum is attached to bone; consequently, rupture through the periosteum and sinus drainage is more common in adults.

Diagnostic Evaluation

Organism identification and antibiotic susceptibility testing are essential for effective therapy. Cultures of aspirated purulent drainage along with cultures of blood, joint fluid, and infected skin samples should be obtained. Bone biopsy is indicated if blood culture results and radiographic findings are not consistent with osteomyelitis. Supporting evidence for osteomyelitis includes leukocytosis and elevated erythrocyte sedimentation rate (ESR) and C-reactive protein (CRP). Radiographic signs, except for soft-tissue swelling, are evident only after 2 to 3 weeks. A three-phase technetium bone scan can show areas of increased blood flow, such as occurs in early stages in infected bone, and is useful in locating multiple sites; however, it is not a diagnostic test. CT can detect bone destruction, and MRI provides anatomic details useful in delineating the area of involvement, especially if surgical intervention is planned. MRI is reported to be the most sensitive diagnostic radiologic tool for diagnosing osteomyelitis (Kaplan, 2016a). Sometimes the osteomyelitis may be unrecognized if it occurs as a complication of a severe toxic and debilitating disease. Neonates may not present with clinical manifestations other than limited mobility of the affected extremity; fever may or may not be present, and the neonate may not appear to be sick (Kaplan, 2016a).

Therapeutic Management

After culture specimens are obtained, empiric therapy is started with IV antibiotics covering the mostly likely organisms. For *S. aureus*, nafcillin or clindamycin is generally used. Consideration should be given to the increased rates of community-acquired methicillin-resistant *S. aureus* (MRSA) in the selection of first-line antibiotic therapy; MRSA may require vancomycin, or in some cases, clindamycin may be appropriate. When the infectious agent is identified, administration of the appropriate antibiotic is initiated and continued for at least 3 to 4 weeks, but the length of therapy is determined by the duration of the symptoms, the response to treatment, and the sensitivity of the organism; 6 weeks to 4 months may be required in some cases (Kaplan, 2016a). In selected cases, oral antibiotic therapy may follow the IV treatment. Because of the prolonged duration of high-dose antibiotic therapy, it is important to monitor for hematologic, renal, hepatic, ototoxic, and other potential side effects. To prevent antibiotic-associated diarrhea in some children, administration of a probiotic may be considered.

Surgery may be indicated if there is no response to specific antibiotic therapy, there is a penetrating injury, a persistent soft-tissue abscess is seen, or the infection has spread to the joint. Opinions differ regarding surgical intervention, but many advocate sequestrectomy and surgical drainage to decompress the metaphyseal space before purulent fluid erupts and spreads to the subperiosteal space, forming abscesses that strip the periosteum from bone or form draining sinuses. When these complications occur, a chronic infection usually persists, which may require antibiotic therapy for several months.

Care Management

During the acute phase of illness, movement of the affected limb will cause discomfort; therefore, the child is positioned comfortably with the affected limb supported. A temporary splint or cast may be applied. Weight bearing is avoided in the acute phase, and moving and turning are carried out carefully to minimize pain. The child may require long-term pain medication to deal with the bone pain. Postoperatively, pain medication should be considered as with any other surgical procedure.

Antibiotic therapy requires careful observation and monitoring of the IV equipment and site. A peripherally inserted central catheter (PICC) may be inserted for long-term antibiotic therapy. Antibiotic therapy is often continued at home or through an outpatient infusion clinic.

Standard precautions are implemented by the interprofessional care team for all children with osteomyelitis. If there is an open wound, it is managed according to standard wound care precautions. If a PICC line or central venous catheter (CVC) is inserted, meticulous care should be taken to prevent catheter-related infection.

Provision of diversional and constructive activities becomes an important nursing intervention. Children are usually confined to bed for some time during the acute phase but may be allowed to move about on a stretcher or in a wheelchair if isolation is not necessary.

As the infection subsides, physical therapy is instituted to ensure restoration of optimum function. The child may eventually be transitioned to a regimen of oral antibiotics, and progress is followed closely for some time.

SEPTIC ARTHRITIS

Septic arthritis is a bacterial infection in the joint. It usually results from hematogenous spread or from direct extension of an adjacent cellulitis or osteomyelitis. Direct inoculation from trauma accounts for 15% to 20% of septic arthritis cases. The most common causative organism is *S. aureus*. Community-acquired MRSA is commonly a cause of septic arthritis. In addition to *S. aureus*, pathogens seen in neonates include group B streptococci, *Escherichia coli*, and *Candida albicans*. In children 2 months to 5 years of age, *S. aureus*, *Streptococcus pyogenes*, *Streptococcus pneumoniae*, and *K. kingae* are the primary organisms causing infection. Children older than 5 years of age are more likely to be infected by *S. aureus* and *S. pyogenes*, and sexually active adolescents may be infected by *N. gonorrhoeae* (Gutierrez, 2005; Kaplan, 2016b).

The knees, hips, ankles, and elbows are the most common joints affected. Clinical manifestations include severe joint pain, swelling, warmth of overlying tissue, and occasional erythema. An infection involving the hip, however, is considered a surgical emergency to prevent compromised blood supply to the head of the femur (Kaplan, 2016b).

The child is resistant to any joint movement. Features of systemic illness such as fever, malaise, headache, nausea, vomiting, and irritability may also be present.

Therapeutic Management and Care Management

The affected joint is aspirated and the specimen evaluated by Gram stain, cultures (including separate cultures for *H. influenzae* and *N. gonorrhoeae*), and determination of leukocyte count. In addition, perform blood cultures and obtain complete blood count with differential and ESR or CRP level. Early radiographic findings are limited to soft-tissue swelling but may reveal a foreign body, and such films always provide a baseline for comparison. Technetium scans reveal areas of increased blood flow but will not differentiate between sites. MRI and CT scans provide more detailed images of cartilage loss, joint narrowing, erosions, and ankylosis of progressive disease. Ultrasonography is helpful in the detection of joint effusions and fluid in the soft tissue and subperiosteum (Kaplan, 2016b).

Treatment is IV antibiotic therapy based on Gram stain results and the clinical presentation. The benefits of serial aspirations to demonstrate sterility of synovium fluid and reduce pressure or pain are controversial. Pain management is an important aspect of nursing care, particularly with involvement of a large joint such as the hip. Surgical intervention may also be required if there was a penetrating wound or a foreign object was possibly involved. Physical therapy may be initiated for the child who is immobilized to prevent flexion contractures. Additional nursing care is the same as for osteomyelitis.

SKELETAL TUBERCULOSIS

In children, tubercular infection of the bones and joints is acquired by lymphohematogenous spread at the time of primary infection. Occasionally, it is from chronic pulmonary TB. Skeletal tubercular infection is not common in the United States but should be considered in communities with high TB case rates. The condition is a late manifestation of TB and is most likely to involve the vertebrae, causing tubercular spondylitis. If the infection is progressive, it causes Pott disease with destruction of the vertebral bodies and results in kyphosis and spinal malalignment. Symptoms are insidious. The child may report persistent or intermittent pain. Other findings include joint swelling and stiffness; fever and weight loss are not common. Tubercular arthritis can also affect single joints (e.g., a knee or hip) and tends to cause severe destruction of adjacent bone. Infection in the fingers causes spina ventosa, a tuberculous dactylitis.

As with pulmonary TB, the index case should be located. A family and environmental history needs to be obtained and tuberculin skin tests (TSTs) performed. Results of TSTs are positive for the majority of children with tuberculous arthritis; however, the results are not diagnostic, and the clinical and laboratory features do not differentiate tubercular arthritis from a nontubercular septic arthritis. Diagnosis requires isolation of *Mycobacterium tuberculosis* from the site. Patients with the susceptible organism start treatment with combined antituberculosis chemotherapy (isoniazid, rifampin, and pyrazinamide); directly observed therapy (DOT) is preferred.

Care Management

Nursing care depends on the site and extent of infection. Tuberculous spondylitis and hip infection may require immobilization, casting, and surgical fusion. Nursing care is individualized but is generally the same as for osteomyelitis and septic arthritis.

DISORDERS OF JOINTS

JUVENILE IDIOPATHIC ARTHRITIS

Juvenile idiopathic arthritis (JIA) refers to chronic childhood arthritis. A group of heterogeneous autoimmune diseases, JIA causes inflammation in the joint synovium and surrounding tissue. The cause of JIA is unknown. JIA starts before 16 years of age, with a peak onset between 1 and 3 years of age. Twice as many girls as boys are affected. The reported incidence of chronic childhood arthritis varies from 1 to 20 cases per 100,000 children, with a prevalence of 10 to 400 cases per 100,000 children (Cassidy & Petty, 2011). Genetic factors and environmental triggers (e.g., rubella, Epstein-Barr virus, parvovirus B19) have been associated with the onset of JIA, but the etiology remains unclear.

Pathophysiology

The disease process is characterized by chronic inflammation of the synovium with joint effusion and eventual erosion, destruction, and fibrosis of the articular cartilage. Adhesions between joint surfaces and ankylosis of joints may occur if the inflammatory process persists.

Clinical Manifestations

Whether single or multiple joints are involved, swelling and loss of motion develop in the affected joint. The swollen joint may be slightly warm and mildly tender to touch, but it is not uncommon for pain not to be reported despite a large joint effusion. Loss of motion in the joint from joint inflammation and muscle spasm may be exacerbated by inactivity. Morning stiffness of the joints(s) is characteristic of JIA and may be present on arising or inactivity. Functional change may be an obvious limp or subtle limitations in joint motion, such as fisting to avoid wrist extension with pressure. Growth disturbances (either overgrowth or undergrowth) may occur, such as bony enlargement of the adjacent femoral or tibial condyles with a knee effusion or a receding chin from temporomandibular arthritis.

Classification of Juvenile Idiopathic Arthritis

JIA is not a single disease but a heterogeneous group of diseases. The universal Durban classification of JIA, developed in 1997 and revised in 1998 and 2001, lists several disease categories, each with its own set of criteria and exclusions, which continue to be revised (Petty, Southwood, Manners et al., 2004).

- Systemic arthritis is arthritis in one or more joints associated with at least 2 weeks of quotidian fever and daily for at least 3 days and one or more of the following: rash, lymphadenopathy, hepatosplenomegaly, and serositis. *Exclusions: a, b, c, d*
- Oligoarthritis is arthritis in one to four joints for the first 6 months of disease. It is subdivided to persistent oligoarthritis if it remains in four joints or fewer, or it becomes extended oligoarthritis if it involves more than four joints after 6 months. *Exclusions: a, b, c, d, e*
- Polyarthritis rheumatoid factor (RF) negative affects five or more joints in the first 6 months with a negative RF. *Exclusions: a, b, c, e*
- Polyarthritis RF positive also affects five or more joints in the first 6 months, but these children have a positive RF. *Exclusions: a, b, c, e*
- Psoriatic arthritis is arthritis with psoriasis or an associated dactylitis, nail pitting, or onycholysis or psoriasis in a first-degree relative. *Exclusions: b, c, d, e*
- Enthesitis-related arthritis is arthritis or enthesitis associated with at least two of the following: sacroiliac or lumbosacral pain, HLA-B27 antigen, arthritis in a boy older than 6 years of age, acute anterior uveitis, inflammatory bowel disease, Reiter syndrome, or acute anterior uveitis in a first-degree relative. *Exclusions: a, d, e*
- Undifferentiated arthritis fits no other category above or fits more than one category.

Diagnostic Evaluation

JIA is a diagnosis of exclusion; there are no definitive tests. Classifications are based on the clinical criteria of age of onset before 16 years of age, arthritis in one or more joints for 6 weeks or longer, and exclusion of other causes. Laboratory tests may provide supporting evidence of disease. The ESR/CRP may or may not be elevated. Leukocytosis is frequently present during exacerbations of systemic JIA. Antinuclear antibodies are common in JIA but are not specific for arthritis; however, they help identify children who are at greater risk for uveitis. Plain radiographs are the best initial imaging studies and may show soft-tissue swelling and joint space widening from increased synovial fluid in the joint. Later films can reveal osteoporosis, narrow joint space, erosions, subluxation, and ankylosis. A slit lamp eye examination is necessary to diagnosis uveitis, inflammation in the anterior chamber of the eye, which is most common in antinuclear antibody–positive young girls with oligoarthritis. Routine examinations are necessary for early diagnosis and treatment to avoid or minimize sight-threatening disease (Qian & Acharya, 2010).

Therapeutic Management

There is no cure for JIA. The major goals of therapy are to control pain, preserve joint range of motion and function, minimize effects of inflammation such as joint deformity, and promote normal growth and development. Outpatient care is the mainstay of therapy; lengthy hospitalizations are infrequent in this era of managed care. The treatment plan can be exhaustive and intrusive for the child and family, including medications, physical and occupational therapy, ophthalmologic slit lamp examinations, splints, comfort measures, dietary management, school modifications, and psychosocial support.

Medications

In 2011, the American College of Rheumatology published recommendations for the treatment of JIA intended to lend guidance to the provider. The guidelines are divided into four groups: (1) children with four or fewer affected joints, (2) five or more affected joints, (3) systemic arthritis and active systemic features, and (4) systemic arthritis with active arthritis. Each path provides recommendations for a stepwise escalation of the medication and therapy (Beukelman, Patkar, Saag et al., 2011). All tracks consider poor prognostic indicators, such as erosions on radiograph; arthritis of the hip, cervical spine, ankle, or wrist; and a positive RF. Additionally, each track takes into account disease activity levels that include elevated acute phase reactants and global assessments of both the provider and the patient/parent.

Medications contained in the guidelines include those described in the following sections.

Nonsteroidal Antiinflammatory Drugs

NSAIDs (e.g., naproxen and ibuprofen) are used alone or in combination with other drugs depending on the amount of disease activity and poor prognostic features. NSAIDs offer an analgesic effect but may require higher dosing for an antiinflammatory effect. Patient/parent education

---

*Exclusion: (a) Psoriasis/history of psoriasis in the patient or first-degree relative; (b) arthritis in an HLA-B27–positive male beginning after the sixth birthday; (c) ankylosing spondylitis, enthesitis-related arthritis, sacroiliitis with inflammatory bowel disease, Reiter syndrome, or symptomatic anterior uveitis, or a history of one of these disorders in a first-degree relative; (d) the presence of immunoglobulin M rheumatoid factor (RF) on at least two occasions at least 3 months apart; (e) the presence of systemic JIA in the patient.

is important and should include potential side effects of gastrointestinal, renal, hepatic, and prolonged coagulation.

Disease-Modifying Antirheumatic Drugs

Disease-modifying antirheumatic drugs (DMARDs) include nonbiologic drugs, methotrexate and sulfasalazine. The decision to use a DMARD at initiation of therapy or later in the escalation of therapy is guided by the amount of disease activity and poor prognostic features. Effective against arthritis and uveitis, antirheumatic low-dose methotrexate has a time-proven safety profile, but parents may be overwhelmed with the potential adverse effects of liver disease, infections, bone marrow suppression, gastrointestinal disturbance, teratogenic effects, and alarming but unconfirmed risk for cancer. Patient/parent education includes frank discussion about sexual activity and birth defects. Sexually active teenagers need effective birth control. As a precaution, pregnant caregivers or those trying to conceive need to avoid contact with methotrexate. Instructions about avoiding live immunizations and alchohol are essential during patient education. Sulfasalazine may be used in children with axial arthritis, a positive test result for HLA-B27, or symptoms of inflammatory bowel disease, given this drug's success in these select groups of patients.

Biologic Disease-Modifying Antirheumatic Drugs

Biologic DMARDs are initiated when there is significant disease activity and/or poor prognostic indicators after unsuccessful treatment with methotrexate. Tumor necrosis factor–alpha (TNF-α) inhibitors are the most frequently used biologic DMARDs and include etanercept, infliximab, and adalimumab. All three reduce the proinflammatory response that promotes arthritis. Anakinra (interleukin-1 receptor antagonist), tocilizumab (interleukin-6 receptor antagonist), and abatacept (selective T-cell costimulation blocker) are also biologics that may be selected for use in systemic JIA (tocilizumab and off-label anakinra) or in children with JIA and limited response to other biologics (tocilizumab and abatacept). Patient education focuses on the increased risk for infection, holding the scheduled dose if the child has fever or symptoms of infection, and seeking medical attention at early onset of illness. All patients starting biologic DMARDs need a negative TST prior to starting. Although biologic DMARDs have been found safe and effective, the potential for malignancy needs to be addressed and patients need routine safety monitoring (Tarkiainen, Tynjälä, Vähäsalo et al., 2015; Ruperto & Martini, 2011).

Glucocorticoids

Glucocorticoids are potent antiinflammatory agents; however the significant adverse effects of long-term systemic steroids are undesirable. Consequently, they are used in conjunction with other medications to provide a prompt antiinflammatory response with acute arthritis, and then they are tapered and discontinued. High-dose IV steroids may be used with acutely active arthritis or systemic features (fevers, rash, and pericarditis). Intraarticular long-acting steroid injections are effective in treating individual joint effusions with minimal adverse effects and frequently provide sustained control. Glucocorticoid education is extensive and includes discussion of potential risk for infection, adrenal insufficiency, cushingoid features, weight gain, mood/sleep changes, hypertension, diabetes, osteoporosis, and avascular necrosis. Simultaneous dietary changes (low calorie and low salt) and, if possible, an active exercise program should be considered when steroids are initiated.

Physical and Occupational Therapy

Physical therapy programs are individualized for each child and designed to reach the ultimate goal—preserving function or preventing deformity. Physical therapy is directed toward specific joints, focusing on strengthening muscles, mobilizing restricted joint motion, and preventing or correcting deformities. Occupational therapists are responsible for evaluating and improving performance of activities of daily living.

Treatment or maintenance programs vary; a child may be seen a couple times per week, or monthly, but the mainstay of any program is the child doing his or her daily home exercise program, which is demonstrated and revised at each therapy session.

Exercising in a pool is excellent therapy, because it allows an almost weightless freedom of movement against gentle resistance of water. If there is pain on motion, a hot pack or warm bath before therapy may help.

Providers may recommend nighttime splinting to help minimize pain and reduce flexion deformity. Joints most frequently splinted are the knees, wrists, and hands. Loss of extension in the knee, hip, and wrist causes special problems and requires vigilance to detect the earliest signs of involvement and vigorous attention to prevent deformity with specialized passive stretching, positioning, and resting splints.

Care Management

Interprofessional care of the child with JIA involves assessment of the child's general health, the status of involved joints, and the child's emotional response to all ramifications of the disease—discomfort, physical restrictions, therapies, and self-concept.

The effects of JIA are manifest in every aspect of the child's life, including physical activities, social experiences, and personality development. Nursing interventions to support the parents may foster successful adaptation for the entire family. Parental concerns about the disease prognosis, financial and insurance issues, spouse and sibling relationships, and job and schedule conflicts must all be addressed. Referral to social workers, counselors, or support groups may be needed.

Relieve Pain

The pain of JIA is related to several aspects of the disease, including disease severity, functional status, individual pain threshold, family variables, and psychologic adjustment. The aim is to provide as much relief as possible with medication and other therapies to help children tolerate the pain and cope as effectively as possible. Nonpharmacologic modalities, such as behavioral therapy and relaxation techniques, have proved effective in modifying pain perception (see the "Pain Management" section in Chapter 30) and activities that aggravate pain. Opioid analgesics are typically avoided in juvenile arthritis; however, for children immobilized with refractory pain, short-term opioid analgesics can be part of a comprehensive plan that uses multiple pain relief techniques (Connelly & Schanberg, 2006).

Promote General Health

The child's general health must be considered. A well-balanced diet with sufficient calories to maintain growth is essential. If the child is relatively inactive, caloric intake needs to match energy needs to avoid excessive weight gain, which places additional stress on affected joints. Sleep and rest are essential for children with JIA. Some children require rest during the day; however, daytime napping that interferes with nighttime sleepiness should be avoided. A bedtime routine that involves comfort measures can help induce sleep. A firm mattress, electric blanket, or sleeping bag helps provide warmth, comfort, and rest. Nighttime splints needed to maintain range of motion might initially be a source of bedtime conflict. The family needs to be instructed on how to use the splint appropriately; the splint should not be painful or impede sleep. Behavior modification programs that reward splint and exercise compliance may be helpful in reducing adherence barriers. Well-child care to assess growth, development, and immunization requirements needs to be coordinated between the primary care provider and the rheumatologist. Common childhood illnesses, such as upper respiratory tract infections, may cause arthritis to worsen; consequently, medical attention must be sought quickly for relatively minor illness to prevent arthritis flares. Effective communication among the family, the primary care provider, and the rheumatology team is essential for care coordination.

Children are encouraged to attend school even on days when they have some pain or discomfort. The school nurse's assistance is enlisted so that the child is permitted to take the prescribed medication at school and to arrange for rest in the nurse's office during the day. Split days or half days may help the child remain involved in school. Permitting the child to come to school late allows time to gain joint movement and reduces the time at school to avoid exhaustion. It is important that the child attend school to learn skills and engage in social interaction, especially if the JIA continues to limit physical skills. Arranging for two sets of textbooks—one for home and one for school—eliminates heavy backpacks, or rolling backpacks may be used. Additionally, extra time to take tests, allowing the child to stand and stretch, participation in PE as tolerated or in a modified PE program, an elevator pass, and extra time to change classes can all reduce barriers and maximize the child's attendance and participation in school. A formal school hearing may be necessary to obtain an individualized education program (IEP), ensured by public law, which includes intensive school modifications.

Facilitate Adherence

The child and family need to be actively involved in the treatment plan to commit to it. They need to know the purpose and correct use of any splints, exercise programs, and medications prescribed. Pillboxes can help foster adherence, although parents should continue to monitor adherence of the older child who is able to safely take medications independently. Nurses can facilitate adherence by demonstrating and providing written instructions on proper techniques for pill crushing or pill swallowing. Teaching parents and patients how to give subcutaneous injections lays the groundwork for future adherence by identifying and addressing potential barriers. Shots are never a pleasant activity; but if available, enlist a child life specialist as a resource in providing the child skills to cope and better understand and accept unpleasant but necessary medical treatments.

Comfort Measures and Exercise

Heat has been shown to be beneficial to children with arthritis. Moist heat is best for relieving pain and stiffness, and the most efficient and practical method is in the bathtub with warm water. In some cases, a daily whirlpool bath, paraffin bath, or hot packs may be used as needed for temporary relief of acute swelling and pain. Hot packs are easily applied using a damp hand towel wrung out after being immersed in hot water or heated in a microwave oven; after testing for heat, hot packs are applied to the area, and covered with plastic to retain heat. Commercial pads that warm in only a few seconds in the microwave are also available. Painful hands or feet can be immersed in a pan of warm water or a paraffin unit.

Pool therapy is the easiest method for exercising a large number of joints. Swimming activities strengthen muscles and maintain mobility in larger joints. Very small children who are frightened of the water can carry out their exercises in the bathtub. Small children love to splash, kick, and throw things in the water. Remember, adult supervision is necessary for all water activities.

Activities of daily living provide satisfactory exercise for older children to maintain maximal mobility with minimal pain. These children are encouraged in their efforts to be independent and patiently allowed to dress and groom themselves, to assume daily tasks, and to care for their belongings. It is often difficult for children to manipulate buttons, comb or brush their hair, and turn faucets, but unless there is an acute flare

with significant loss of motion and pain, parents and other caregivers should not offer assistance but extra time and encouragement to proceed independently. In turn, children should learn and understand why others do not help them. Many helpful devices, such as self-adhering fasteners, tongs for manipulating difficult items, and grab bars installed in bathrooms for safety, can be used to facilitate tasks. A raised (higher) toilet seat often makes the difference between dependent and independent toileting because weak quadriceps muscles and sore knees inhibit the ability to raise the body from a low sitting position.

A child's natural affinity for play offers many opportunities for incorporating therapeutic exercises. Throwing or kicking a ball and riding a tricycle (with the seat raised to achieve maximum leg extension) are excellent moving and stretching exercises for a young child whose daily living activities are physically limited.

An effective approach to beginning the day's activities is to awaken children early to give them their medication and then to allow them to sleep for 1 hour. On arising, children take a hot bath (or shower) and perform a simple ritual of limbering-up exercises, after which they commence the activities of the day, such as going to school. Exercise, heat, and rest are spaced throughout the remainder of the day according to the child's individual needs and schedules. Parents are instructed in exercises that meet the child's needs.

The Arthritis Foundation and the American Juvenile Arthritis Alliance (an organization within the Arthritis Foundation) provide information and services for both parents and professionals, and nurses can refer families to these agencies as an added resource.

Support the Child and Family

JIA affects every aspect of life for the child and family. Physical limitations may interfere with self-care, school participation, and recreational activities. The intensive treatment plan, including multiple medications, physical therapy, comfort measures, and medical appointments, is intrusive and disruptive to the parents' work schedule and the family routine. To prevent isolation and foster independence, the family is encouraged to pursue their normal activities. Unfortunately, the adaptations necessary to make that occur take resourcefulness and commitment from all family members. At diagnosis and throughout the span of JIA, it is essential to recognize signs of stress and counterproductive coping and provide the necessary support to maximize adaptation. The problems and needs of these families are discussed in Chapter 36, and readers are directed to that chapter for guidance in planning care.

SYSTEMIC LUPUS ERYTHEMATOSUS

Systemic lupus erythematosus (SLE) is a severe chronic autoimmune disease that results in inflammation and multiorgan system damage. Other forms of lupus include discoid lupus, which is limited to the skin, and neonatal lupus, which occurs when maternal autoantibodies cause a transient lupus-like syndrome in a newborn with the potential serious complication of heart block. The remaining discussion focuses on SLE.

The Lupus Foundation of America (2015) estimates that 1.5 million individuals have lupus, and 10% to 15% of these adults were diagnosed with SLE as children or adolescents. SLE in children tends to be more severe at onset and has more aggressive clinical course than the adult-onset type (Mina & Brunner, 2013).

SLE is more common in girls, with an approximate 4:3 female-to-male predominance before 10 years of age and a 4:1 female-to-male predominance in the second decade, indicating a potential hormonal trigger with maturation. There is a familial tendency, although many newly diagnosed patients are unaware of other affected family members. SLE has been reported in all cultures, but within the United States, there has been a disproportionately higher incidence in African-American, Asian, and Hispanic children.

The cause of SLE is not known. It appears to result from a complex interaction of genetics with an unidentified trigger that activates the disease. Suspected triggers include exposure to ultraviolet (UV) light, estrogen, pregnancy, infections, and drugs. Genetic predisposition to SLE is evidenced in an increased concordance rate in twins (tenfold), increased incidence within family members (10% to 16%), and increased frequency of certain gene alleles in population-based studies.

Clinical Manifestations and Diagnostic Evaluation

The child with SLE may have any clinical manifestation with mild to life-threatening severity (Box 48.10). The diagnosis is established when 4 of the 11 diagnostic criteria are met (Box 48.11). Kidney involvement heralds progressive disease and the need for rigorous therapeutic management.

BOX 48.10   Manifestations of Systemic Lupus Erythematosus

Constitutional: Fever, fatigue, weight loss, anorexia
Cutaneous: Erythematosus butterfly rash over bridge of nose and across cheeks, discoid rash, photosensitivity, mucocutaneous ulceration, alopecia, periungual telangiectasias
Musculoskeletal: Arthritis, arthralgia, myositis, myalgia, tenosynovitis
Neurologic: Headache, seizure, forgetfulness, behavior change, change in school performance, psychosis, chorea, stroke, cranial and peripheral neuropathy, pseudotumor cerebri
Pulmonary and cardiac: Pleuritis, basilar pneumonitis, atelectasis, pericarditis, myocarditis, and endocarditis
Renal: Glomerulonephritis, nephrotic syndrome, hypertension
Gastrointestinal: Abdominal pain, nausea, vomiting, blood in stool, abdominal crisis, esophageal dysfunction, colitis
Hepatic, splenic, and nodal: Hepatomegaly, splenomegaly, lymphadenopathy
Hematologic: Anemia, cytopenia
Ophthalmologic: Cotton wool spots, papilledema, retinopathy
Vascular: Raynaud phenomenon, thrombophlebitis, livedo reticularis

BOX 48.11   Classification Criteria for Systemic Lupus Erythematosus*

Malar rash: Fixed malar erythema
Discoid rash: Patchy erythematous lesions
Photosensitivity: Rash with sunlight exposure
Oronasal ulcers: Painless ulcers in mouth and nose
Arthritis: Swelling, tenderness, or effusion in two or more peripheral joints (nonerosive)
Serositis: Pleuritis, pericarditis
Renal disorder: Proteinuria, casts in urine
Neurologic disorder: Psychosis, seizures
Hematologic disorder: Hemolytic anemia, thrombocytopenia, leukopenia, lymphopenia
Immunologic disorder: Anti–double-stranded deoxyribonucleic acid, anti-Sm, antiphospholipid antibodies; lupus anticoagulant; false-positive result on syphilis test (rapid plasma reagin)
Antinuclear antibodies: Presence of antinuclear antibody by immunofluorescence or an equivalent assay

*The presence of four criteria is required for classification as systemic lupus erythematosus (SLE).

Therapeutic Management

The goal of treatment by the interprofessional care team is to ensure the child's health by balancing the medications necessary to avoid exacerbation and complications while preventing or minimizing treatment-associated morbidity. Therapy involves the use of specific medications and general supportive care. The drugs used to control inflammation are corticosteroids administered in doses sufficient to control inflammation and then tapered to the lowest suppressive dose or given intravenously during acute flares. Hydroxychloroquine, an antimalarial, is a useful medication for inflammatory control, rash, and arthritis; NSAIDs are used to relieve muscle and joint inflammation; and immunosuppressive agents, such as cyclophosphamide are used for renal and CNS disease. Mycophenolate, azathioprine, and methotrexate are effective immunosuppressive drugs that may be used to control SLE and allow steroids to be reduced. Rituximab is a monoclonal antibody that results in decreased antibody formation and has been used off-label in pediatric lupus patients who have not responded to standard therapy (Nwobi, Abitbol, Chandar et al., 2008). Antihypertensives, low-dose aspirin (as a blood thinner), and calcium and vitamin D supplements are just a few of the additional remedies that may be necessary to treat or avoid complications.

General supportive care includes sufficient nutrition, sleep and rest, and exercise. Exposure to the sun and ultraviolet B (UVB) light is limited because of its association with SLE exacerbation.

Care Management

The principal nursing goal is to help the child and family positively adjust to the disease and therapy. The child and family must learn to recognize subtle signs of disease exacerbation and potential complications of medication therapy and to communicate these concerns to their health care provider. Consequently, patient and family education is an ongoing process initiated at diagnosis and tailored to the patient's individual needs. Referral to other members of the interprofessional care team such as the social worker, psychologist, or support group may help the child and family make a successful adjustment. Support groups are associated with the Lupus Foundation of America and the Arthritis Foundation.

Key issues include therapy compliance; body-image problems associated with rash, hair loss, and steroid therapy; school attendance; vocational activities; social relationships; sexual activity; and pregnancy (see Chapter 36 for a discussion on adjusting to a chronic illness). Specific instructions for avoiding exposure to the sun and UVB light, such as using sunscreens, wearing sun-resistant clothing, and altering outdoor activities, must be provided with great sensitivity to ensure compliance while minimizing the associated feeling of being different from peers. Patients need to be instructed to maintain regular medical supervision and seek attention quickly during illness or before elective surgical procedures, such as dental extraction, because of potential needs for increased steroids or prophylactic antibiotics. People with SLE should carry medical alert identification for their disease and steroid dependence.

REFERENCES

American Academy of Pediatrics. (2000). Clinical practice guideline: Early detection of developmental dysplasia of the hip. *Pediatrics, 105*(4pt 1), 896–905.

Beukelman, T., Patkar, N. M., Saag, K. G., et al. (2011). 2011 American College of Rheumatology recommendations for the treatment of juvenile idiopathic arthritis: initiation and safety monitoring of therapeutic agents for the treatment of arthritis and systemic features. *Arthritis Care & Research, 63*(4), 465–482.

Biber, R., & Gregory, A. (2010). Overuse injuries in youth sports: Is there such a thing as too much sports? *Pediatric Annals, 39*(5), 286–292.

Cassidy, J. T., & Petty, R. E. (2011). Chronic arthritis in childhood. In J. T. Cassidy, R. E. Petty, R. M. Laxer, et al. (Eds.), *Textbook of pediatric rheumatology* (6th ed.). Philadelphia, PA: Elsevier/Saunders.

Connelly, M., & Schanberg, L. (2006). Opioid therapy for the treatment of refractory pain in children with juvenile rheumatoid arthritis. *Nature Clinical Practice. Rheumatology, 2*(12), 636–637.

Freeman, B. L., III (2013). Scoliosis and kyphosis. In S. T. Canale & J. H. Beaty (Eds.), *Campbell's operative orthopaedics* (12th ed.). Philadelphia, PA: Mosby.

Gutierrez, K. (2005). Bone and joint infections in children. *Pediatric Clinics of North America, 52*(3), 779–794.

Herring, J. A. (2011). Legg-Calvé-Perthes disease at 100: A review of evidence-based treatment. *Journal of Pediatric Orthopaedics, 31*(2 suppl), S137–S140.

Holmes, S. B., Brown, S. J., & Pin Site Care Expert Panel. (2005). Skeletal pin site care: National Association of Orthopaedic Nurses guidelines for orthopedic nursing. *Orthopaedic Nursing, 24*(2), 99–107.

Hresko, M. T. (2013). Idiopathic scoliosis in adolescents. *New England Journal of Medicine, 368*(9), 834–841.

Kaplan, S. L. (2016a). Osteomyeltitis. In R. M. Kliegman, B. F. Stanton, J. W. St. Geme, et al. (Eds.), *Nelson textbook of pediatrics* (20th ed.). Philadelphia, PA: Saunders/Elsevier.

Kaplan, S. L. (2016b). Septic arthrisits. In R. M. Kliegman, B. F. Stanton, J. W. St. Geme, et al. (Eds.), *Nelson textbook of pediatrics* (20th ed.). Philadelphia, PA: Saunders/Elsevier.

Loder, R. T., & Skopelja, E. N. (2011a). *The epidemiology and demographics of hip dysplasia.* ISRN Orthopedics, 238607.

Loder, R. T., & Skopelja, E. N. (2011b). *The epidemiology and demographics of Legg-Calvé-Perthes disease.* ISRN Orthopedics, 504393.

Loder, R. T., & Skopelja, E. N. (2011c). *The epidemiology and demographics of slipped capital femoral epiphysis.* ISRN Orthopedics, 486512.

Lupus Foundation of America. (2015). *Understanding lupus: What is lupus?* Retrieved from http://www.lupus.org/answers/entry/what-is-lupus.

Marini, J. C., & Blissett, A. R. (2013). New genes in bone development: What's new in osteogenesis imperfecta. *Journal of Clinical Endocrinology and Metabolism, 98*(8), 3095–3103.

Marini, J. C. (2016). Osteogenesis imperfecta. In R. M. Kliegman, B. F. Stanton, J. W. St. Geme, et al. (Eds.), *Nelson textbook of pediatrics* (20th ed.). Philadelphia, PA: Saunders/Elsevier.

Mina, R., & Brunner, H. I. (2013). Update on differences between childhood-onset and adult-onset systemic lupus erythematosus. *Arthritis Research & Therapy, 15*(4), 218.

Mistovich, R. J., & Spiegel, D. A. (2016). Idiopathic scoliosis. In R. M. Kliegman, B. F. Stanton, J. W. St. Geme, et al. (Eds.), *Nelson textbook of pediatrics* (20th ed.). Philadelphia, PA: Saunders/Elsevier.

Noonan, C., Quigley, S., & Curley, M. A. (2011). Using the Braden Q Scale to predict pressure ulcer risk in pediatric patients. *Journal of Pediatric Nursing, 26*(6), 566–575.

Nwobi, O., Abitbol, C. L., Chandar, J., et al. (2008). Rituximab therapy for juvenile-onset systemic lupus erythematosus. *Pediatric Nephrology, 23*(3), 413–419.

Patel, D. S., Roth, M., & Kapil, N. (2011). Stress fractures: Diagnosis, treatment, and prevention. *American Family Physician, 83*(1), 39–46.

Peck, K., & Herrara-Soto, J. (2014). Slipped capital femoral epiphysis: What's new? *Orthopedic Clinics of North America, 45*(1), 77–86.

Petty, R. E., Southwood, T. R., Manners, P., et al. (2004). International League of Associations for Rheumatology classification of juvenile idiopathic arthritis: Second revision, Edmonton, 2001. *Journal of Rheumatology, 31*(2), 390–392.

Ponseti, I. V. (1996). *Congenital clubfoot: Fundamentals of treatment.* Oxford, UK: Oxford University Press.

Price, C. T., & Schwend, R. M. (2011). Improper swaddling A risk factor for developmental dysplasia of hip. *AAP News, 32*(9), 11–12.

Qian, Y., & Acharya, N. R. (2010). Juvenile idiopathic arthritis-associated uveitis. *Current Opinion in Ophthalmology, 21*(6), 468–472.

Richards, B. S., & Vitale, M. G. (2008). Screening for idiopathic scoliosis in adolescents: An information statement. *Journal of Bone and Joint Surgery. American Volume, 90*(1), 195–198.

Ruperto, N., & Martini, A. (2011). Pediatric rheumatology: JIA, treatment and possible risk of malignancies. *Nature Reviews Rheumatology, 7*(1), 6–7.

Sarwahi, V., Wollowick, A. L., Sugarman, E. P., et al. (2011). Minimally invasive scoliosis surgery: An innovative technique in patients with adolescent idiopathic scoliosis. *Scoliosis, 6,* 16.

Shyy, W., Wang, K., Sheffield, V. C., et al. (2010). Evaluation of embryonic and perinatal myosin gene mutations and the etiology of congenital idiopathic clubfoot. *Journal of Pediatric Orthopaedics, 30*(3), 231–234.

Stoll, C., Alembik, Y., Dott, B., et al. (2010). Associated malformations in patients with limb reduction deficiencies. *European Journal of Medical Genetics, 53*(5), 286–290.

Tarkiainen, M., Tynjälä, P., Vähäsalo, P., et al. (2015). Occurrence of adverse events in patients with JIA receiving biologic agents: Long-term follow-up in a real-life setting. *Rheumatology, 54*(7), 1170–1176.

Tibor, L. M., & Sink, E. L. (2013). Risks and benefits of the modified Dunn approach for treatment of moderate or severe slipped capital femoral epiphysis. *Journal of Pediatric Orthopaedics, 33*(1 suppl), S99–S102.

Winell, J. J., & Davidson, R. S. (2016). Talipes equinovarus (clubfoot). In R. M. Kliegman, B. F. Stanton, J. W. St. Geme, et al. (Eds.), *Nelson textbook of pediatrics* (20th ed.). Philadelphia, PA: Saunders/Elsevier.

Winsley, R., & Matos, N. (2011). Overtraining and elite young athletes. *Medicine and Sport Science, 56,* 97–105.

49

The Child With Neuromuscular or Muscular Dysfunction

Marilyn J. Hockenberry

ⓔ http://evolve.elsevier.com/Perry/maternal

CONGENITAL NEUROMUSCULAR OR MUSCULAR DISORDERS

CEREBRAL PALSY

A new definition proposed in 2006 describes cerebral palsy (CP) as a "group of permanent disorders of the development of movement and posture, causing activity limitation, that are attributed to nonprogressive disturbances that occurred in the developing fetal or infant brain" (Rosenbaum, Paneth, Leviton et al., 2007). In addition to motor disorders, the condition often involves disturbances of sensation, perception, communication, cognition, and behavior; secondary musculoskeletal problems; and epilepsy (Rosenbaum et al.). The etiology, clinical features, and course vary and are characterized by abnormal muscle tone and coordination as the primary disturbances. CP is the most common permanent physical disability of childhood, and the incidence is reported to be between 2.4 to 3.6 per every 1000 live births in the United States (Hirtz, Thurman, Gwinn-Hardy et al., 2007; Yeargin-Allsopp, Van Naarden Braun, Doernberg et al., 2008).

One systematic review and meta-analysis indicated a prevalence of 2.11 per 1000 live births, with the highest prevalence among infants born weighing 1000 grams to 1499 grams at birth; the prevalence of CP was higher among infants born prior to completion of 28 weeks of gestation (Oskoui, Coutinho, Dykeman et al., 2013). Since the 1960s, the prevalence of CP has risen approximately 20%, which most likely reflects the improved survival of extremely low birth weight (ELBW) and very low birth weight (VLBW) infants.

However, in the past 2 decades, there has been a decrease in the incidence of CP in ELBW and VLBW infants (Hack & Costello, 2008). The incidence is higher in males than in females and is more likely to occur in African-American children than in Caucasian or Hispanic children (Centers for Disease Control and Prevention [CDC], 2013).

Although the prevalent traditional hypothesis has been that CP results from perinatal problems, especially birth asphyxia, it is now believed that CP results more often from existing prenatal brain abnormalities; the exact cause of these abnormalities remains elusive but may include genetic factors, including clotting disorders as well as brain malformations. It has been estimated that as many as 70% to 80% of the cases of CP are caused by unknown prenatal factors (Johnston, 2016; Krigger, 2006). Intrauterine exposure to maternal chorioamnionitis is associated with an increased risk for CP in infants of normal birth weight and preterm infants (Hermansen & Hermansen, 2006; Shatrov, Birch, Lam et al., 2010); however, not all term infants exposed to chorioamnionitis develop CP.

In general, infants exposed to maternal and perinatal infections are at increased risk for the development of CP as a result of the effects on the developing brain. Although CP occurs in term births, preterm birth of ELBW and VLBW infants continues to be the single most important risk factor for CP. Still, in some cases no identifiable cause is determined. Periventricular leukomalacia and intracerebral hemorrhage in low–birth weight (LBW) infants are significant risk factors in the development of CP. Perinatal ischemic stroke is also associated with a later diagnosis of CP (Golomb, Saha, Garg et al., 2007).

Additional factors that may contribute to the development of CP postnatally include bacterial meningitis, multiple births, viral encephalitis, motor vehicle crashes, and child abuse (shaken baby syndrome [traumatic brain injury]) (Krigger, 2006). One study found a higher risk for CP occurring among infants born at 42 weeks of gestation or later than among those born at 37 or 38 weeks of gestation (Moster, Wilcox, Vollset et al., 2010). One study found that 10% to 15% of children with CP acquired the condition after birth from causes such as falls, motor vehicle crashes, and infections, such as meningitis (CDC, 2013). A significant percentage (15% to 60%) of children with CP also have epilepsy. In summary, as many as 80% of the total cases of CP may be linked to a perinatal or neonatal brain lesion or brain maldevelopment, regardless of the cause (Krageloh-Mann & Cans, 2009). A number of biochemical disorders may cause motor abnormalities often seen in CP and may be initially misdiagnosed as CP (Nehring, 2010).

Pathophysiology

It is difficult to establish a precise location of neurologic lesions on the basis of etiology or clinical signs, because there is no characteristic pathologic picture. In some cases, there are gross malformations of the brain. In others, there may be evidence of vascular occlusion, atrophy, loss of neurons, and laminar degeneration that produce narrower gyri, wider sulci, and low brain weight. Anoxia appears to play the most significant role in the pathologic state of brain damage, which is often secondary to other causative mechanisms.

There are a few exceptions. In some cases, the manifestation or etiology is related to anatomic areas. For example, CP associated with preterm birth is usually spastic diplegia caused by hypoxic infarction or hemorrhage with periventricular leukomalacia in the area adjacent to the lateral ventricles. The athetoid (extrapyramidal) type of CP is most likely to be associated with birth asphyxia but can also be caused by kernicterus and metabolic genetic disorders, such as mitochondrial disorders and glutaric aciduria (Johnston, 2016). Hemiplegic (hemiparetic) CP is often associated with a focal cerebral infarction (stroke) secondary to an intrauterine or perinatal thromboembolism, usually a result of maternal thrombosis or a hereditary clotting disorder (Johnston, 2016). Cerebral hypoplasia and sometimes severe neonatal hypoglycemia are related to ataxic CP. Generalized cortical and cerebral

BOX 49.1 Clinical Classification of Cerebral Palsy

Spastic (Pyramidal)

Characterized by persistent primitive reflexes, positive Babinski reflex, ankle clonus, exaggerated stretch reflexes, eventual development of contractures

- 70% to 80% of all cases of cerebral palsy (CP)
- Diplegia: All extremities affected; lower more than upper (30% to 40% of spastic CP)
- Tetraplegia: All four extremities involved—legs and trunk, mouth, pharynx, and tongue (10% to 15% of spastic CP)
- Triplegia: Three limbs involved
- Monoplegia: Only one limb involved
- Hemiplegia: Motor dysfunction on one side of the body; upper extremity more affected than lower extremity (20% to 30% of spastic CP)

Other features:
- Hypertonicity with poor control of posture, balance, and coordinated motion
- Impairment of fine and gross motor skills

Dyskinetic (Nonspastic, Extrapyramidal)

Athetoid: Chorea (involuntary, irregular, jerking movements); characterized by slow, wormlike, writhing movements that usually involve the extremities, trunk, neck, facial muscles, and tongue

Dystonic: Slow, twisting movements of the trunk or extremities; abnormal posture

Involvement of the pharyngeal, laryngeal, and oral muscles causing drooling and dysarthria (imperfect speech articulation)

Ataxic (Nonspastic, Extrapyramidal)

Wide-based gait

Rapid, repetitive movements performed poorly

Disintegration of movements of the upper extremities when the child reaches for objects

Mixed Type

Combination of spastic CP and dyskinetic CP

May be labeled *mixed* when no specific motor pattern is dominant; however, this term is losing favor to more precise descriptions of motor function and affected area of brain involved (Rosenbaum, Paneth, Leviton et al., 2007)

Data from Nehring, W. (2010). Cerebral palsy. In Allen, P.J., Vessey, J.A., & Schapiro, N.A. (Eds), *Primary care of the child with a chronic condition* [5th ed.]. St. Louis, MO: Mosby/Elsevier; Jones, M.W., Morgan, E., Shelton, J.E., et al. (2007). Cerebral palsy: Introduction and diagnosis, part 1. *Journal of Pediatric Health Care, 21*(3), 146–152; and National Institute of Neurologic Disorders and Stroke. [2015]. *Cerebral palsy: Hope through research.* Retrieved from https://www.ninds.nih.gov/Disorders/Patient-Caregiver-Education/Hope-Through-Research/Cerebral-Palsy-Hope-Through-Research.

atrophy often cause severe quadriparesis with cognitive impairment and microcephaly.

Clinical Classification

A revision of the Winter classification was proposed in 2005 to reflect the child's actual clinical problems and their severity, an assessment of the child's physical and quality-of-life status across time, and long-term support needs (Bax, Goldstein, Rosenbaum et al., 2005; Nehring, 2010). The proposed new definition has four major dimensions of classification (Bax, Goldstein, Rosenbaum et al., 2005):

Motor abnormalities: Nature and typology of the motor disorder; functional motor abilities

Associated impairments: Seizures; hearing or vision impairment; attentional, behavioral, communicative, or cognitive deficits; oral motor and speech function

Anatomic and radiologic findings: Anatomic distribution or parts of the body affected by motor impairments or limitations; radiologic findings sometimes including white matter lesions or brain anomaly noted on computed tomography (CT) or magnetic resonance imaging (MRI)

Causation and timing: Identification of a clearly identified cause such as a postnatal event (e.g., meningitis, traumatic brain injury).

CP has four primary types of movement disorders: spastic, dyskinetic, ataxic, and mixed (Nehring, 2010). The most common clinical type, spastic CP (77.4% reported by the CDC [2013]), represents an upper motor neuron muscular weakness (Box 49.1). The reflex arc is intact, and the characteristic physical signs are increased stretch reflexes, increased muscle tone, and (often) weakness. Early neurologic manifestations are usually generalized hypotonia or decreased tone that lasts for a few weeks or may extend for months or even as long as 1 year.

Diagnostic Evaluation

Infants at risk according to known etiologic factors associated with CP warrant careful assessment during early infancy to identify the signs of neuromotor dysfunction as early as possible. The neurologic examination and history are the primary modalities for diagnosis. Neuroimaging of the child with suspected brain abnormality and CP is now recommended for diagnostic assessment, with MRI being a strong predictor of CP when performed at term (corrected age); general movements assessment (GMA) also had a strong predictive value in children older than 2 years of age and younger than 5 years of age (Bosanquet, Copeland, Ware et al., 2013). Metabolic and genetic testing is recommended if no structural abnormality is identified by neuroimaging; routine laboratory tests are no longer recommended in the diagnostic process for CP.

Early recognition is made more difficult by the lack of reliable neonatal neurologic signs. However, nurses should monitor infants with known etiologic risk factors and evaluate them closely in the first 2 years of life. Because cortical control of movement does not occur until later in infancy, motor impairment associated with voluntary control is usually not apparent until after 2 to 4 months of age at the earliest. More often the diagnosis cannot be confirmed until 2 years of age, because motor tone abnormalities may be indicative of another neuromuscular condition. In addition, some children who show signs consistent with CP before 2 years of age do not demonstrate such signs after 2 years of age (Nehring, 2010). However, there is no consensus regarding an age cutoff for the onset of symptoms. Clinical manifestations of CP at the time of diagnosis are listed in Box 49.2; early warning signs are listed in Box 49.3, but these are not considered diagnostic.

Establishing a diagnosis may be facilitated by the persistence of primitive reflexes: (1) either the asymmetric tonic neck reflex or the persistent Moro reflex (beyond 4 months of age) and (2) the crossed extensor reflex. The tonic neck reflex normally disappears between 4 and 6 months of age. An obligatory response is considered abnormal. This is elicited by turning the infant's head to one side and holding it there for 20 seconds. When a crying infant is unable to move from the asymmetric posturing of the tonic neck reflex, it is considered obligatory and an abnormal response. The crossed extensor reflex, which normally disappears by 4 months of age, is elicited by applying a noxious stimulus to the sole of one foot with the knee extended. Normally, the contralateral foot responds with extensor, abduction, and then adduction movements. The possibility of CP is suggested if these reflexes persist after 4 months of age.

BOX 49.2 Clinical Manifestations of Cerebral Palsy (at Time of Diagnosis)

Delayed Gross Motor Development
- A universal manifestation
- Delay in all motor accomplishments
- Increases as growth advances
- Delays more obvious as growth advances

Abnormal Motor Performance
- Very early preferential unilateral hand preference
- Abnormal and asymmetric crawl
- Standing or walking on toes
- Uncoordinated or involuntary movements
- Poor sucking
- Feeding difficulties
- Persistent tongue thrust

Alterations of Muscle Tone
- Increased or decreased resistance to passive movements
- Opisthotonic posturing (arching of back)
- Feels stiff on handling or dressing
- Difficulty in diapering
- Rigid and unbending at the hip and knee joints when pulled to sitting position (early sign)

Abnormal Postures
- Maintains hips higher than trunk in prone position with legs and arms flexed or drawn under the body
- Scissoring and extension of legs with feet plantarflexed in supine position
- Persistent infantile resting and sleeping position
- Arms abducted at shoulders
- Elbows flexed
- Hands fisted

Reflex Abnormalities
- Persistence of primitive infantile reflexes
- Obligatory tonic neck reflex at any age
- Nonpersistence beyond 6 months of age
- Persistence or hyperactivity of the Moro, plantar, and palmar grasp reflexes
- Hyperreflexia, ankle clonus, and stretch reflexes elicited in many muscle groups on fast, passive movements

Associated Disabilities*
- Altered learning and reasoning
- Seizures
- Impaired behavioral and interpersonal relationships
- Sensory impairment (vision, hearing)

From Nehring, W.M. (2010). Cerebral palsy. In Allen, P.J., Vessey, J.A., & Schapiro, N.A. (Eds), *Primary care of the child with a chronic condition* [5th ed.]. St. Louis, MO: Mosby/Elsevier. Adapted from Jones, M.W., Morgan, E., & Shelton, J.E. (2007). Primary care of the child with cerebral palsy: A review of systems (part II). *Journal of Pediatric Health Care, 21*, 226–237.
*May or may not be present.

A number of assessment instruments are now available to evaluate muscle spasticity; functional independence in self-care, mobility, and cognition; self-initiated movements over time; and capability and performance of functional activities in self-care, mobility, and social function (Krigger, 2006).

BOX 49.3 Early Signs of Cerebral Palsy

- Failure to meet any developmental milestones, such as rolling over, raising head, sitting up, crawling
- Persistent primitive reflexes, such as Moro, atonic neck
- Poor head control (head lag) and clenched fists after 3 months of age
- Stiff or rigid arms or legs; scissoring legs
- Pushing away or arching back; stiff posture
- Floppy or limp body posture, especially while sleeping
- Inability to sit up without support by 8 months of age
- Using only one side of the body or only the arms to crawl
- Feeding difficulties
- Persistent gagging or choking when fed
- After 6 months of age, tongue pushing soft food out of the mouth
- Extreme irritability or crying
- Failure to smile by 3 months of age
- Lack of interest in surroundings

Data from Pathways Awareness Foundation. (1991). *Parents if you see any of these warning signs don't delay,* Chicago: Author; Nehring, W. (2004). Cerebral palsy. In Allen, P.J., & Vessey, J.A. (Eds), *Primary care of the child with a chronic condition.* St. Louis, MO: Mosby/Elsevier; Jones, M.W., Morgan, E., Shelton, J.E., et al. (2007). Cerebral palsy: Introduction and diagnosis, part 1. *Journal of Pediatric Health Care, 21*(3), 146–152.

Therapeutic Management

The interprofessional care team's goals of therapy for children with CP are early recognition and promotion of optimal development to enable affected children to attain normalization and realize their potential within the limits of the existing health problems. The disorder is permanent, and therapy is primarily preventive and symptomatic.

Therapy has five broad goals:
1. To establish locomotion, communication, and self-help skills
2. To gain optimal appearance and integration of motor functions
3. To correct associated defects as early and effectively as possible
4. To provide educational opportunities adapted to the child's needs and capabilities
5. To promote socialization experiences with other affected and unaffected children

Each child is evaluated and managed on an individual basis. The plan of therapy may involve a variety of settings, facilities, and specially trained people. The scope of the child's needs requires multidisciplinary planning and care coordination among professionals and the child's family. The outcome for the child and family with CP is normalization and promotion of self-care activities that empower the child and family to achieve maximum potential.

Ankle-foot orthoses (AFOs, braces) are worn by many of these children and are used to help prevent or reduce deformity, increase the energy efficiency of gait, and control alignment. Wheeled scooter boards allow children to propel themselves while on the abdomen, or the total body is supported while the legs are positioned with wedges to prevent scissoring. Wheeled go-carts provide sitting balance that may serve as early "wheelchair" experience for young children. Manual or powered wheelchairs allow for more independent mobility (Figs. 49.1 and 49.2). Strollers can be equipped with custom seats for dependent mobilization. A number of wheelchairs can be customized to meet the needs and preferences of older children.

Orthopedic surgery may be required to correct contracture or spastic deformities, to provide stability for an unstable joint, and to provide balanced muscle power. This includes tendon-lengthening procedures, release of spastic muscles, and correction of hip and adductor muscle

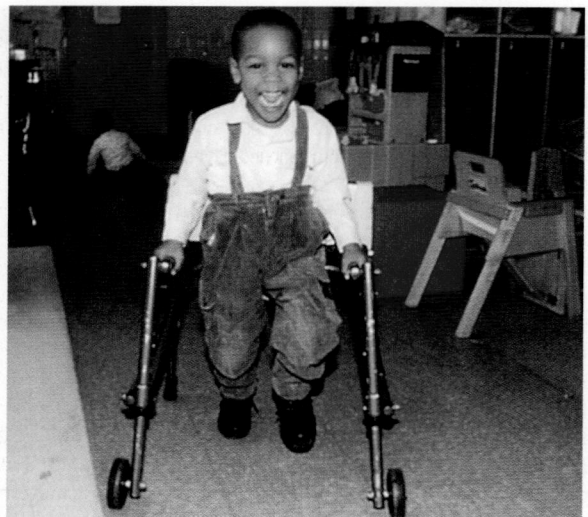

FIG 49.1 Mobilization device for a child.

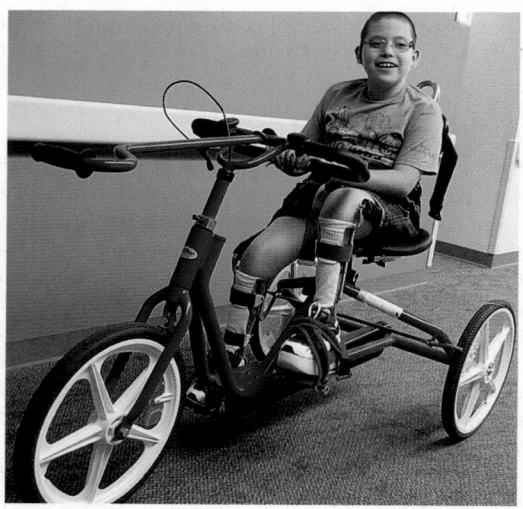

FIG 49.2 Bike walker used to provide mobility and to enhance leg muscle strength. (Courtesy of Texas Children's Hospital, Houston, TX.)

spasticity or contracture to improve locomotion. Hip dislocation often occurs in children with CP, so hip surveillance may be routine care for a child with CP. Spinal fusion may be required for scoliosis. Computerized motion analysis, radiographs, and clinical findings are used to make decisions about orthopedic surgery. Selective dorsal rhizotomy may provide marked improvement in some children with CP (Nordmark, Josenby, Lagergren et al., 2008). The procedure involves selectively cutting dorsal column sensory rootlets that have an abnormal response to electrical stimulation. Achieving the benefits from the surgery requires intensive physical therapy and family commitment. Because the procedure results in flaccid muscles, the child must be retaught to sit, stand, and walk.

Surgical intervention is usually reserved for children who do not respond to more conservative measures, but it is also indicated for children whose spasticity causes progressive deformities. Orthopedic surgery is generally not performed until after the child is 6 years of age (Nehring, 2010). Surgery is primarily used to improve function rather than for cosmetic purposes and is followed by physical therapy. Surgery

may also be performed to improve caloric intake, correct gastroesophageal reflux disease, prevent aspiration, and correct associated dental problems (Nehring, 2010).

Intense pain may occur with muscle spasms in patients with CP. Pharmacologic agents given orally (dantrolene sodium, baclofen [Lioresal], and diazepam [Valium]) have had limited effectiveness in improving muscle coordination in children with CP; however, they are effective in decreasing overall spasticity. The most common side effects of these agents include hepatotoxicity (dantrolene), drowsiness, fatigue, and muscle weakness; less commonly, central nervous system (CNS) depression, hypotension, diaphoresis, and constipation may be seen with baclofen. Diazepam is used frequently but should be restricted to older children and adolescents.

Botulinum toxin A (Botox) is also used to reduce spasticity in targeted muscles. Botulinum toxin A is injected into a selected muscle (commonly the quadriceps, gastrocnemius, or medial hamstrings) after a topical anesthetic is applied. The drug inhibits the release of acetylcholine into a specific muscle group, thereby reducing spasticity. When administered early in the course of the condition, affected muscle contractures may be minimized, particularly in the lower extremities, thus avoiding surgical procedures with possible adverse effects. The goal is to allow stretching of the muscle as it relaxes and permit ambulation with an AFO. The major reported adverse effects of botulinum toxin A injection are pain at the injection site and temporary weakness (Lukban, Rosales, & Dressler, 2009). Prime candidates for botulinum toxin A injections are children with spasticity confined to the lower extremities; the drug reduces spasticity so that the muscles can be stretched and the child may walk with or without orthoses. The onset of action occurs within 24 to 72 hours, with a peak effect observed at 2 weeks and a duration of action of 3 to 6 months.

Children with CP may also experience pain as a result of surgical procedures intended to reduce contracture deformities, body position, gastroesophageal reflux, and physical therapy (McKearnan, Kieckhefer, Engel et al., 2004). Therefore, pain management is an important aspect of the care of children with CP. Decreasing spasticity with botulinum toxin A may also result in less pain from spasms (Lundy, Lumsden & Fairhurst, 2009).

The neurosurgical and pharmacologic approach to managing the spasticity associated with CP involves the implantation of a pump to infuse baclofen directly into the intrathecal space surrounding the spinal cord to provide relief of spasticity. Intrathecal baclofen therapy is best suited for children with severe spasticity that interferes with activities of daily living (ADLs) and ambulation. High doses of oral baclofen are associated with significant side effects, including drowsiness and confusion, yet are often unable to provide adequate relief of spasticity. Direct infusion of baclofen into the intrathecal space provides relief without as many side effects (Motta, Antonello, & Stignani, 2011). Intrathecal baclofen is especially helpful in improving comfort (Morton, Gray, & Vloeberghs, 2011). Oral tizanidine given in conjunction with botulinum toxin A has been reported to be more effective than oral baclofen and botulinum toxin A in one study of children with CP (Dai, Wasay, & Awan, 2008).

Patients may be screened before pump placement by the infusion of a "test dose" of intrathecal baclofen delivered via lumbar puncture. Close monitoring for side effects (hypotonia, somnolence, seizures, nausea, vomiting, headache) is necessary. Relief of spasticity occurs for several hours after infusion. If a favorable response is noted, the patient is considered a candidate for pump placement. The implantation procedure is done in the operating room by a neurosurgeon. The pump, which is approximately the size of a hockey puck, is placed in the subcutaneous space of the midabdomen. An intrathecal catheter is tunneled from the lumbar area to the abdomen and connected to the pump. The pump is filled with baclofen and programmed to provide a set dose using a telemetry wand and a computer. Benefits of intrathecal baclofen include fewer systemic side effects than oral baclofen, dosage titration for maximizing effects, and reversibility of therapy with removal of the pump if so desired. The patient may remain hospitalized for 3 to 7 days to adjust the dosage and ensure proper healing. Outpatient visits to refill the pump and make dosage adjustments are scheduled about every 3 to 6 months depending on the patient's response to the treatment. This procedure is most suited for a multidisciplinary setting where rehabilitation specialists are readily available and consistently involved in the patient's ongoing care. Abrupt withdrawal of intrathecal baclofen may result in adverse effects, such as rebound spasticity, pruritus, hyperthermia, rhabdomyolysis, disseminated intravascular coagulation, multiorgan failure, and death; in some cases, intrathecal baclofen withdrawal may mimic sepsis. Treatment of withdrawal centers on reestablishing the medication dosage, with improvements observed within 1 to 2 hours. Hospitalization and surgery may be required for withdrawal as a result of pump or catheter failure.

Antiepileptic drugs (AEDs) such as carbamazepine (Tegretol), divalproex (valproate sodium and valproic acid; Depakote), lacosamide (Vimpat), levetiracetam (Keppra), oxcarbazepine (Trileptal), and lamotrigine (Lamictal) are prescribed routinely for children who have seizures. Other medications include levodopa for treating dystonia; trihexyphenidyl (Artane) for treating dystonia, and for increasing the use of upper extremities and vocalizations; and reserpine for hyperkinetic movement disorders, such as chorea or athetosis (Johnston, 2016). Gabapentin (Neurontin) has been used for decreasing spasticity pain in children with CP successfully (National Institute of Neurologic Disorders and Stroke, 2015). All medications should be weighed for risk/benefit ratio and monitored for maintenance of therapeutic levels and avoidance of subtherapeutic or toxic levels.

Dental hygiene is essential in the care of children with CP. Regular visits to the dentist and prophylaxis, including brushing, fluoride, and flossing, should be started as soon as the teeth erupt. Dental care is especially important for children given phenytoin because they often develop gum hyperplasia. Decreased oral intake can lead to more tartar buildup. Additional problems common among children with CP include constipation caused by neurologic deficits and lack of exercise; poor bladder control and urinary retention; osteopenia (related to decreased bone density from immobility); chronic respiratory tract infections; problems with airway clearance; and aspiration pneumonia, which may be a consequence of gastroesophageal reflux, abnormal muscle tone, immobility, and altered positioning. Skin problems may result from pressure areas, malalignment, poor bracing, nutrition, and immobility. Latex allergy has also been reported in children with CP (Nehring, 2010).

A wide variety of technical aids are available to improve the function of children with CP. Airway clearance devices help mobilize secretions (e.g., therapy vest that essentially performs what was done formerly by clap pulmonary therapy, or physiotherapy). Eye/hand coordination can be enhanced by computerized toys and games. Toys may be operated by a head or hand switch. Microcomputers combined with voice synthesizers aid children with speech difficulties to "speak." Smart phones with speech applications are appropriate for some children.

Many other electronic devices allow independent functioning. Sensors can be activated and deactivated by using a head stick or tongue or other voluntary muscle movement over which the child has control. Voice-activated computer technology may also allow increased mobility and ambulation with specially designed devices, such as wheelchairs. The application of this technology makes it possible for people with CP to function in their own residences and can be extended into the workplace.

There is some evidence that neuromuscular electrical stimulation (NMES) in addition to dynamic splinting may result in increased muscle strength, range of motion, and function of upper limbs in children with CP. Further studies are needed in children with CP to support the use of botulinum toxin A in conjunction with NMES to decrease muscle spasticity and improve function (Wright, Durham, Ewins et al., 2012).

Behavior problems are common and often interfere with the child's development. Attention-deficit/hyperactivity disorder and other learning problems require professional attention. In addition, children with CP may have vision difficulties, such as strabismus, nystagmus, and optic atrophy (Johnston, 2016). Speech-language therapy involves the services of a speech-language pathologist who may also assist with feeding problems.

Physical therapy is one of the most frequently used conservative treatment modalities. This requires the specialized skills of a qualified therapist with an extensive repertoire of exercise methods that can design a program to stimulate and guide each child to achieve his or her functional goals.

An active therapy program involves the family; the physical therapist; and often other members of the health care team, including the nurse. The most common approach uses traditional types of therapeutic exercises that consist of stretching, passive, active, and resistive movements applied to specific muscle groups or joints to maintain or increase range of motion, strength, or endurance.

Prognosis

The prognosis for the child with CP depends largely on the type and severity of the condition. Children with mild to moderate involvement (85%) have the capability of achieving ambulation between 2 and 7 years of age (Berker & Yalçin, 2008). If the child does not achieve independent ambulation by this time, chances are poor for later ambulation and independence. Approximately 30% to 50% of individuals with CP have significant cognitive impairments, and an even higher percentage have mild cognitive and learning deficits. However, many children with severe spastic tetraplegic CP have normal intelligence. Growth is affected in children with spastic tetraplegia, and many children remain below the fifth percentile for age and sex.

As children with CP become adults, about 30% remain in the home and are cared for by a parent or caregiver; 50% of individuals with spastic tetraplegia live in independent settings and function at appropriate social levels considering their disability (Green, Greenberg, & Hurwitz, 2003). Vocational rehabilitation and higher education are possible for adults with CP. Children with severe CP mobility impairment and feeding problems often succumb to respiratory tract infection in childhood. The few survival rate studies on children or adults with CP show that survival is influenced by existing comorbidities (Nehring, 2010).

Prevention of some cases of CP may become a reality in the near future. Studies indicate that early neuroprotection in term infants with moderate encephalopathy due to hypoxic-ischemic injury with the use of therapeutic hypothermia (head cooling or whole-body cooling to 33° to 35° C) within 6 hours of birth improved survival without CP by approximately 40% (Johnston, Fatemi, Wilson et al., 2011). A Cochrane Database Systematic Review of 11 randomized, controlled trials of therapeutic hypothermia in 1505 term and late preterm infants with intrapartum asphyxia showed significant reduction in mortality and neurodevelopmental disability at 18 months of age (Jacobs, Berg, Hunt et al., 2013). Erythropoietin, a hormone that increases red blood cells (RBCs) and oxygen in the blood, is being studied alone and in combination with therapeutic hypothermia treatment in preterm infants with the hope of improving outcomes when exposed to hypoxic ischemic encephalopathy (HIE).

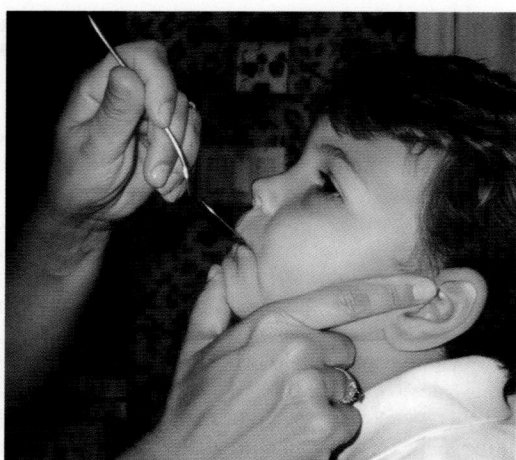

FIG 49.3 Manual jaw control provided anteriorly.

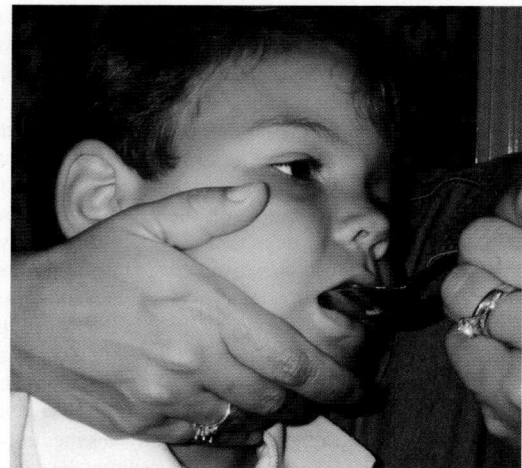

FIG 49.4 Manual jaw control provided from the side.

> **⚠ NURSING ALERT**
>
> The use of mobile infant walkers and door frame jumping seats should not be used; they pose a risk for injury to normal children and are especially hazardous for children with CP. Safer alternatives are available (e.g., stationary musical activity jumper).

Care Management

Because children with CP expend so much energy in their efforts to accomplish ADLs, more frequent rest periods should be arranged to avoid fatigue. Meeting the child's nutritional needs may be a challenge because of gastroesophageal reflux, feeding and swallowing difficulties, chronic constipation and subsequent anorexia, and absence or diminished ability to independently feed himself or herself. The diet should be tailored to the child's activity and metabolic needs. Gastrostomy feedings may be necessary to supplement regular feedings and ensure adequate weight gain, particularly in children at risk for growth failure and chronic malnutrition, those with severe CP and subsequent oral feeding difficulties, and children whose well-being is affected by illness and decreased fluid or medication intake (Rogers, 2004). Oral feedings may be continued to maintain oral motor skills as tolerated. Weight gain is perceived as an important measure of adequate oral feeding efficiency.

Parents may need assistance and advice with medication administration through a gastrostomy tube to prevent clogging. A skin-level gastrostomy is particularly suited for children with CP. Because jaw control is often compromised, more normal control can be achieved if the feeder provides stability of the oral mechanism from the side or front of the face. When directed from the front, the middle finger of the nonfeeding hand is placed posterior to the body portion of the chin, the thumb is placed below the bottom lip, and the index finger is placed parallel to the child's mandible (Fig. 49.3). Manual jaw control from the side assists with head control, correction of neck and trunk hyperextension, and jaw stabilization. The middle finger of the nonfeeding hand is placed posterior to the bony portion of the chin, the index finger is placed on the chin below the lower lip, and the thumb is placed obliquely across the cheek to provide lateral jaw stability (Fig. 49.4).

Safety precautions are implemented, such as having children wear protective helmets if they are subject to falls or capable of injuring their heads on hard objects. Because children with CP are at risk for altered proprioception and subsequent falls, the home and play environments should be adapted to their needs to prevent bodily harm. Appropriate immunizations should be administered to prevent childhood illnesses and protect against respiratory tract infections, such as influenza or pneumonia. Dental problems may be more common in children with CP, which creates a need for meticulous attention to all aspects of dental care. Transportation of the child with motor problems and restricted mobility may be especially challenging for the family and child. Attention must be given to the child's safety when riding in a motor vehicle; a federally-approved safety restraint should be used at all times. It is recommended that children with CP ride in a rear-facing position as long as possible because of their poor head, neck, and trunk control (Lovette, 2008). Car restraints especially designated for children with poor head and neck control are available and should be used.*

The involvement of physical therapy, speech therapy, and occupational therapy is particularly important in establishment and maintenance of muscle function, development of adequate speech and phonation, and identification of modifications necessary for the child's environment so that ADLs can be performed to the child's satisfaction.

As in all aspects of care, educational requirements are determined by the child's needs and potential. Children with mild to moderate cognitive involvement are generally able to participate in regular classes. Resource rooms are available in most schools to provide more individualized attention. Integration of children with CP into regular classrooms should be the initial goal. For those who are unable to benefit from formal education, a vocational training program may be appropriate. At adolescence, prevocational and vocational counseling and guidance are arranged. At any phase or in any setting, education is geared toward the child's assets.

Recreation and after-school activities should be considered for children who are unable to participate in regular athletic programs and other peer activities. Some children can compete in athletic and artistic endeavors, and many games and pastimes are suited to their capabilities. Competitive sports are also becoming increasingly available to children with disabilities and offer an added dimension to physical activities. Recreational activities serve to stimulate children's interest and curiosity, help them adjust to their disability, improve their functional abilities, and build self-esteem. Any accomplishment that helps children approach a normal way of life enhances their self-concept.

---

*For information on specially adapted molded-plastic chairs for children with CP, contact Snug Seat at 800-336-7684; http://www.snugseat.com/.

Support the Family

Probably the nursing interventions most valuable to the family are support and help in coping with the emotional aspects of the disorder, many of which are discussed in relation to the child with a disability (see Chapter 36). Initially, the parents need supportive counseling directed toward understanding the meaning of the diagnosis and all of the feelings that it engenders. Later, they need clarification regarding what they can expect from the child and from health care professionals. Educating families in the principles of family-centered care and parent/professional collaboration is essential. The family may require help in modifying the home environment for care of the child (see Chapter 36). Transportation to the practitioner's office and other health care agencies often requires special arrangements.

Care coordination for the child and family with CP is an important nursing role. In many cases, the family assumes complete care of the child and becomes quite adept at caring for his or her individual needs. The home health nurse or case manager has an important role in the support and encouragement for families/caregivers who assume the primary care of a child with CP. Having a child with CP implies numerous problems of daily management and changes in family life. The nurse can help with education, assessment, and mobilization of resources, and can stress principles of normalization.

The nurse can support the parents by acknowledging and addressing their concerns and frustrations; by noting and appreciating their problem-solving skills and their approaches to helping the child. Parents and other family members may need support and counseling. Siblings of a child with a disability are affected and may respond to the child's presence with overt or less evident behavioral problems. The family needs a relationship with nurses who can provide continued contact, support, and encouragement through the long process of habilitation.

Parents may find help and support from parent groups, where they can share experiences, accomplishments, problems, and concerns while deriving comfort and practical information. Parent support groups are most helpful through sharing experiences and accomplishments. For example, parents can learn from others what it is like to have a child with CP, which is generally not possible from professionals (see Family-Centered Care box: The Reality of Acceptance of Cerebral Palsy).

United Cerebral Palsy has branches in most communities and provides a variety of services for children and families.

A number of excellent books also are available to guide parents and nurses who work with children with CP. People with CP who have triumphed write many of the books.

Support the Hospitalized Child

CP is not a disorder that requires hospitalization; therefore, when children with CP are hospitalized, they are usually admitted for illness or corrective surgery. To facilitate the care and management of hospitalized children with CP, the therapy program should be continued (as their condition allows) while they are hospitalized. This should be incorporated into the multidisciplinary care plan, with every effort expended to make certain the ground that has been so laboriously gained is not lost. Nursing care of the child with CP is similar to that of any child with a disability, and children with CP should be approached as would any child in the hospital. Speech impairment is common in children with CP, but this may not correlate with their ability to understand. Therapy programs should be continued, when appropriate, during the time they are hospitalized. Encouraging the parent to room-in and actively participate in the child's care helps promote family-centered care. However, it is also important to remember that hospitalization may be the first time a parent can defer care to a nurse and not be the primary caregiver. This respite may be crucial to the parent's well-being. Respect the parent's preference in this regard.

NEURAL TUBE DEFECTS (MYELOMENINGOCELE)

Abnormalities that derive from the embryonic neural tube (neural tube defects [NTDs]) constitute the largest group of congenital anomalies that are consistent with multifactorial inheritance. Normally, the spinal cord and cauda equina are encased in a protective sheath of bone and meninges (Fig. 49.5, A). Failure of neural tube closure produces defects of varying degrees (Box 49.4). They may involve the entire length of the neural tube or may be restricted to a small area.

In the United States, rates of NTDs have declined from 1.3 per 1000 births in 1970 to 0.3 per 1000 births after the introduction of mandatory food fortification with folic acid in 1998. One concern is that NTD rates have not decreased in Hispanic and non-Hispanic white mothers since 1999 (CDC, 2009). In 2005, the CDC estimated the rates for spina bifida (SB) to be 17.96 per 100,000 live births, thus making this one of the most common birth defects in the United States (Matthews, 2009; Wolff, Witkop, Miller et al., 2009). Increased use of prenatal diagnostic

---

FAMILY-CENTERED CARE

The Reality of Acceptance of Cerebral Palsy

Acceptance is rarely achieved in the length of time implied in the literature.

In the first place, what is acceptance? To me, it is the end of comparing my son with every other child I see. I focus on his gains, not society's expectations.

It is also being able to laugh periodically at his "clumsiness." It is "gallows humor" as he achieves adulthood; jokes about CP can be funny now.

The bitterness is gone; I am now happy for people who have children without CP.

I no longer feel sorry for my son but rather for the people who cannot see him for the great person he is; the CP does not come first.

He is now a young man of 25 years, and I am learning to accept his independence.

It is a "never-ending story."

Elaine A. Dunham, RN
Shriners Hospitals for Children
Springfield, MA

BOX 49.4   Significant Neural Tube Defects

Cranioschisis: A congenital skull defect through which various tissues protrude

Exencephaly: Brain totally exposed or extruded through an associated skull defect; fetus usually aborted

Anencephaly: If fetus with exencephaly survives, degeneration of the brain to a spongiform mass with no bony covering; incompatible with life usually beyond a few days to weeks

Encephalocele: Herniation of brain and meninges through a defect in the skull, producing a fluid-filled sac; can be frontal or posterior

Rachischisis or spina bifida (SB): Fissure in the spinal column that leaves the meninges and spinal cord exposed

Meningocele: Hernial protrusion of a saclike cyst of meninges filled with spinal fluid (see Fig. 49.5, C)

Myelomeningocele (meningomyelocele): Hernial protrusion of a saclike cyst containing meninges, spinal fluid, and a portion of the spinal cord with its nerves (see Fig. 49.5, D)

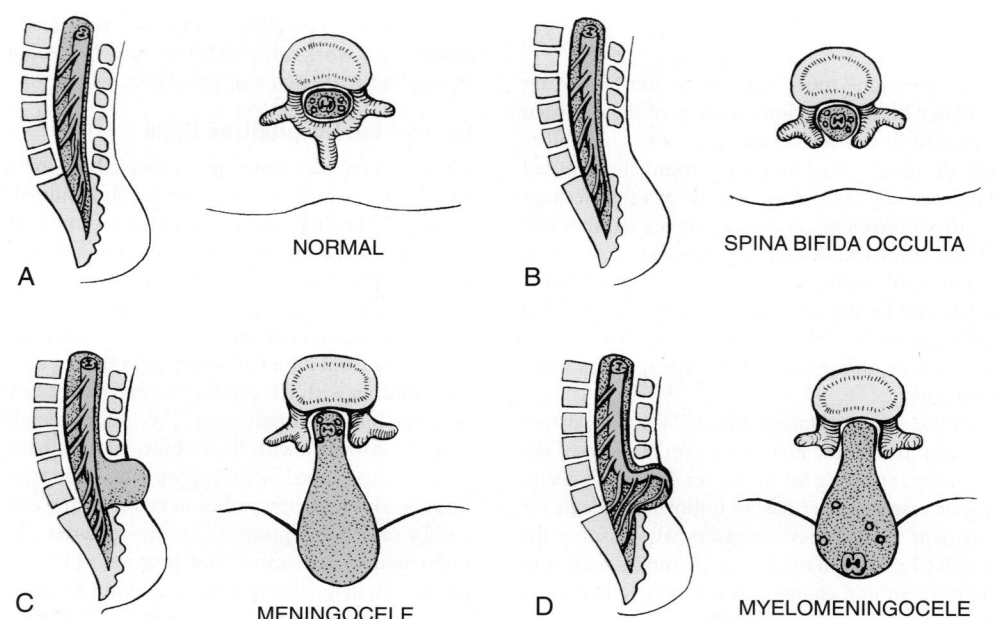

FIG 49.5 Midline defects of the osseous spine with varying degrees of neural herniations. **A,** Normal. **B,** Spina bifida occulta. **C,** Meningocele. **D,** Myelomeningocele

techniques and termination of pregnancies have also affected the overall incidence of NTDs (see the "Prevention" section later in this chapter).

Anencephaly, the most serious NTD, is a congenital malformation in which both cerebral hemispheres are absent. The condition is usually incompatible with life, and many affected infants are stillborn. For those who survive, no specific treatment is available. The infants have a functional portion of the brainstem and are able to maintain vital functions (e.g., temperature regulation and cardiac and respiratory function) for a few hours to several weeks but eventually die of respiratory failure.

Myelodysplasia refers broadly to any malformation of the spinal canal and cord. Midline defects involving failure of the osseous (bony) spine to close are called *spina bifida (SB),* the most common defect of the CNS. SB is categorized into two types—SB occulta and SB cystica.

Spina bifida occulta refers to a defect that is not visible externally. It occurs most frequently in the lumbosacral area (L5 and S1) (see Fig. 49.5, *B*). SB occulta may not be apparent unless there are associated cutaneous manifestations or neuromuscular disturbances.

Spina bifida cystica refers to a visible defect with an external saclike protrusion. The two major forms of SB cystica are *meningocele,* which encases meninges and spinal fluid but no neural elements (see Fig. 49.5, *C*), and *myelomeningocele* (or *meningomyelocele*), which contains meninges, spinal fluid, and nerves (see Fig. 49.5, *D*). Meningocele is not associated with neurologic deficit, which occurs in varying, often serious, degrees in myelomeningocele. Clinically, the term *spina bifida* is used to refer to myelomeningocele.

Pathophysiology

The pathophysiology of SB is best understood when related to the normal formative stages of the nervous system. At approximately 20 days of gestation, a decided depression, the neural groove, appears in the dorsal ectoderm of the embryo. During the fourth week of gestation, the groove deepens rapidly, and its elevated margins develop laterally and fuse dorsally to form the neural tube. Neural tube formation begins in the cervical region near the center of the embryo and advances in both directions—caudally and cephalically—until the end of the fourth week of gestation, when the ends of the neural tube, the anterior and posterior neuropores, close.

Most authorities believe the primary defect in neural tube malformations is a failure of neural tube closure. However, some evidence indicates that the defects are a result of splitting of the already closed neural tube as a result of an abnormal increase in cerebrospinal fluid (CSF) pressure during the first trimester.

Etiology

There is evidence of a multifactorial etiology, including drugs, radiation, maternal malnutrition, chemicals, and possibly a genetic mutation in folate pathways in some cases, which may result in abnormal development. There is also evidence of a genetic component in the development of SB; myelomeningocele may occur in association with syndromes, such as trisomy 18, PHAVER (limb **p**terygia, congenital **h**eart **a**nomalies, **v**ertebral defects, **e**ar anomalies, and **r**adial defects) syndrome, and Meckel-Gruber syndrome (Shaer, Chescheir, & Schulkin, 2007). Additional factors predisposing children to an increased risk for NTDs include prepregnancy maternal obesity, maternal diabetes mellitus, low maternal vitamin B_{12} status, maternal hyperthermia, and the use of AEDs in pregnancy. The genetic predisposition is supported by evidence of the risk for recurrence after one affected child (3% to 4%) and a 10% risk for recurrence with two previously affected children (Kinsman & Johnston, 2016).

The degree of neurologic dysfunction depends on where the sac protrudes through the vertebrae, the anatomic level of the defect, and the amount of nerve tissue involved. The majority of myelomeningoceles (75%) involve the lumbar or lumbosacral area (Fig. 49.6). Hydrocephalus is a frequently associated anomaly in 80% to 90% of patients. About 80% of patients with myelomeningocele have an associated type II Chiari malformation (Kinsman & Johnston, 2016). There is some evidence that prolonged exposure of the myelomeningocele sac to amniotic fluid predisposes to the development of hindbrain herniation and Chiari II malformation (Adzick, 2013).

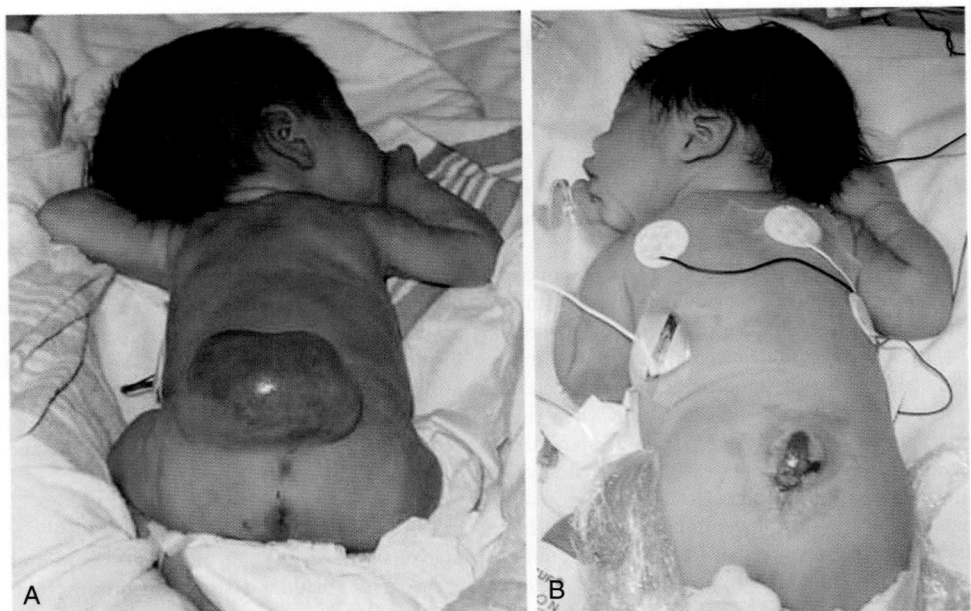

FIG 49.6 A, Myelomeningocele with an intact sac. **B,** Myelomeningocele with a ruptured sac. (Courtesy of Dr. Robert C. Dauser, Neurosurgery, Baylor College of Medicine, Houston, TX.)

BOX 49.5   Clinical Manifestations of Spina Bifida

Spina Bifida Cystica
Sensory disturbances usually parallel to motor dysfunction
- Below second lumbar vertebra:
  - Flaccid, partial paralysis of lower extremities
  - Varying degrees of sensory deficit
  - Overflow incontinence with constant dribbling of urine
  - Lack of bowel control
  - Rectal prolapse (sometimes)
- Below third sacral vertebra:
  - No motor impairment
  - May have saddle anesthesia with bladder and anal sphincter paralysis

Joint deformities (sometimes produced in utero):
- Talipes valgus or varus contractures
- Kyphosis
- Lumbosacral scoliosis
- Hip dislocation or subluxation

Spina Bifida Occulta
Frequently no observable manifestations
May be associated with one or more cutaneous manifestations:
- Skin depression or dimple
- Port-wine angiomatous nevi
- Dark tufts of hair
- Soft, subcutaneous lipomas

May have neuromuscular disturbances:
- Progressive disturbance of gait with foot weakness
- Bowel and bladder sphincter disturbances

Diagnostic Evaluation

The diagnosis of SB is made on the basis of clinical manifestations (Box 49.5) and examination of the meningeal sac. Diagnostic measures used to evaluate the brain and spinal cord include MRI, ultrasonography, and CT. A neurologic evaluation will determine the extent of involvement of bowel and bladder function as well as lower extremity neuromuscular involvement. Flaccid paralysis of the lower extremities is a common finding with absent deep tendon reflexes.

Prenatal Detection

It is possible to determine the presence of some major open NTDs prenatally. Ultrasonographic scanning of the uterus and elevated maternal concentrations of alpha-fetoprotein (AFP, or MS-AFP), a fetal-specific gamma-1-globulin, in amniotic fluid may indicate anencephaly or myelomeningocele. The optimum time for performing these diagnostic tests is between 16 and 18 weeks of gestation before AFP concentrations normally diminish and in sufficient time to permit a therapeutic abortion. It is recommended that such diagnostic procedures and genetic counseling be considered for all mothers who have borne an affected child, and testing is offered to all pregnant women (American College of Obstetrics and Gynecology Committee on Practice Bulletins, 2007). Chorionic villus sampling is also a method for prenatal diagnosis of NTDs; however, it carries certain risks (skeletal limb depletion) and is not recommended before 10 weeks of gestation (Simpson, Richards, & Otano, 2012).

Therapeutic Management

Management of the child who has a myelomeningocele requires a multidisciplinary team approach involving the specialties of neurology, neurosurgery, pediatrics, urology, orthopedics, rehabilitation, physical therapy, occupational therapy, and social services, as well as intensive nursing care in a variety of specialty areas. The collaborative efforts of these specialists focus on (1) the myelomeningocele and the problems associated with the defect—hydrocephalus, paralysis, orthopedic deformities (e.g., developmental dysplasia of the hip, clubfoot, scoliosis), and genitourinary abnormalities; (2) possible acquired problems that may or may not be associated, such as Chiari II malformation, meningitis, seizures, hypoxia, tethered cord, and hemorrhage; and (3) other abnormalities, such as cardiac or gastrointestinal (GI) malformations. Many hospitals have routine outpatient care by multidisciplinary teams to provide the complex follow-up care needed for children with myelodysplasia.

Many authorities believe that early closure, within the first 24 to 72 hours, offers the most favorable outcome. Surgical closure within the first 24 hours is recommended if the sac is leaking CSF (Kinsman & Johnston, 2016).

A variety of neurosurgical and plastic surgical procedures are used for skin closure without disturbing the neural elements or removing any portion of the sac. The objective is satisfactory skin coverage of the lesion and meticulous closure. Wide excision of the large membranous covering may damage functioning neural tissue.

Associated problems are assessed and managed by appropriate surgical and supportive measures. Shunt procedures provide relief from imminent or progressive hydrocephalus (see Chapter 46). When diagnosed, ventriculitis, meningitis, urinary tract infection, and pneumonia are treated with vigorous antibiotic therapy and supportive measures. Surgical intervention for Chiari II malformation is indicated only when the child is symptomatic (i.e., high-pitched crowing cry, stridor, respiratory difficulties, apnea, oral-motor difficulties, upper extremity spasticity).

Early surgical closure of the myelomeningocele sac through fetal surgery has been evaluated in relation to prevention of injury to the exposed spinal cord tissue and the improvement of neurologic and urologic outcomes in the affected child. The Management of Myelomeningocele Study, a clinical trial supported by the National Institutes of Health, found that prenatal surgery for myelomeningocele reduced the need for shunting (for hydrocephalus), evaluated at 12 months, and there was an improvement in mental and motor function scores at 30 months in children who had prenatal surgery (compared with children who had postnatal surgery) (Adzick, Thom, Spong et al., 2011). Outcome data for urologic and bowel function are not available at this time.

Infancy

Initial care of the newborn involves preventing infection; performing a neurologic assessment, including observing for associated anomalies; and dealing with the impact of the anomaly on the family. Although meningoceles are repaired early, especially if there is danger of rupture of the sac, the philosophy regarding skin closure of myelomeningocele varies. Most authorities believe that early closure, within the first 24 to 72 hours, offers the most favorable outcome. Early closure, preferably in the first 12 to 18 hours, not only prevents local infection and trauma to the exposed tissues but also avoids stretching of other nerve roots (which may occur as the meningeal sac expands during the first hours after birth), thus preventing further motor impairment. Broad-spectrum antibiotics are initiated, and neurotoxic substances, such as povidone/iodine are avoided at the malformation.

Improved surgical techniques do not alter the major physical disability and deformity or chronic urinary tract infections that affect the quality of life for these children. Superimposed on these physical problems are the disorder's effects on family life and finances and on school and hospital services.

Orthopedic Considerations

According to most orthopedists, musculoskeletal problems that will affect later locomotion should be evaluated early, and treatment, when indicated, should be instituted without delay. Neurologic assessment will determine the neurosegmental level of the lesion and enable recognition of spasticity and progressive paralysis, potential for deformity, and functional expectations. Orthopedic management includes prevention of joint contractures, correction of any existing deformities, prevention or minimization of the effects of motor and sensory deficits, prevention of skin breakdown, and obtaining the best possible function of affected lower extremities. Common orthopedic problems requiring attention in SB include deformities of the hips, knees, feet, and spine; fractures and insensate skin further complicate orthopedic care. Other problems

that may occur later include kyphosis and scoliosis (Lazzaretti & Pearson, 2010; Liptak & Dosa, 2010). Because children with this condition often have decreased sensitivity in their lower extremities, preventive skin care is important. A high percentage (60%) of children seen in a wound clinic for skin breakdown had myelomeningocele (Samaniego, 2003). The status of the neurologic deficit remains the most important factor in determining the child's ultimate functional abilities.

With technologic advances, a variety of lightweight orthoses, including braces, special "walking" devices, and custom-built wheelchairs, are available to provide mobility to children with spinal cord lesions (see Chapter 48). Early in infancy, intervention with passive range-of-motion exercises, positioning, and stretching exercises may help decrease the incidence of muscle contractures. Corrective surgical procedures, when indicated, are best initiated at an early age so the child will not lag significantly behind age mates in developmental progress. The degree of lower extremity function guides decisions about whether orthopedic surgery will be needed.

Management of Genitourinary Function

Myelomeningocele is one of the most common causes of neuropathic (neurogenic) bladder dysfunction among children. In infants, the goal of treatment is to preserve renal function. In older children, the goal is to preserve renal function and achieve optimal urinary continence. Urinary incontinence is a chronic, often debilitating problem for the child. In addition, the neuropathic bladder may produce urinary system distress, characterized by symptomatic urinary tract infections, ureterohydronephrosis, and vesicoureteral reflux or renal insufficiency. The characteristics of bladder dysfunction in children vary according to the level of the neurologic lesion and the influence of bony growth and development on the spine. Therefore, ongoing urologic monitoring is essential. Evidence is growing that early intervention, based on evaluation during the neonatal period and before complications occur, improves bladder function, reduces the risk for subsequent urinary system distress, and decreases the need for reconstructive surgery of the lower urinary tract (Snodgrass & Gargollo, 2010; Tarcan, Onol, Ilker et al., 2006).

Treatment of renal problems includes (1) regular urologic care with prompt and vigorous treatment of infections; (2) a method of regular emptying of the bladder, such as clean intermittent catheterization (CIC) taught to and performed by parents and self-catheterization taught to children; (3) medications to improve bladder storage and continence, such as oxybutynin chloride (Ditropan) and tolterodine (Detrol); and (4) surgical procedures such as vesicostomy (bladder surgically brought out to the abdominal wall, allowing continuous urinary drainage) and augmentation enterocystoplasty (using a segment of bowel or stomach to increase bladder capacity, thereby reducing high bladder pressures).

However, despite the combined efforts of CIC, medication, and surgical intervention, some children with myelodysplasia may continue to experience debilitating urinary incontinence. Many of these children are able to attain social continence with a continent urinary diversion commonly referred to as a *Mitrofanoff procedure*. In this procedure, a catheterizable channel is surgically created from appendix, ureter, or tapered bowel. The proximal end of the channel is connected to the bladder with the distal end brought out as a small stoma on the abdominal wall, usually near the umbilicus. The bladder neck may be sutured to prevent urinary leakage from the urethra. CIC through the easily accessible abdominal route fosters greater independence in children, especially in those unable to transfer from wheelchair to toilet to perform CIC.

Bowel Control

Some degree of fecal continence can be achieved in most children with myelomeningocele with diet modification, regular toilet habits, and prevention of constipation and impaction. It is frequently a lengthy process. Dietary fiber supplements (recommended 10 g/day), laxatives, suppositories, or enemas aid in producing regular evacuation. Older children and adolescents seeking more independence may attain bowel continence and higher quality of life after undergoing an antegrade continence enema (ACE) procedure (Doolin, 2006). In a procedure similar to the Mitrofanoff, the appendix or ileum is used to create a catheterizable channel with attachment of the proximal end to the colon. The distal end of the channel exits through a small abdominal stoma. Every 1 or 2 days, a catheter is passed through the stoma, allowing enema solution to be instilled directly into the colon. After administration of the enema solution, the child sits on the toilet for 30 to 60 minutes as stool is flushed out through the rectum. The frequency of enemas and volume of solution used to completely evacuate the bowel vary among individuals.

Prognosis

The early prognosis for the child with myelomeningocele depends on the neurologic deficit present at birth, including motor ability, bladder innervation, and associated neurologic anomalies. Early surgical repair of the spinal defect, antibiotic therapy to reduce the incidence of meningitis and ventriculitis, prevention of urinary system dysfunction, and early detection and correction of hydrocephalus have significantly increased the survival rate and quality of life in such children. *Children with SB have normal intelligence.* Many children with SB achieve partial independent living and gainful employment. Reports of survival rates vary, and many include adults who were born before medical advances and surgical techniques seen in the past 25 years. Coordinated care for adults with SB is essential; however, multidisciplinary adult care is often inadequate (Lazzaretti & Pearson, 2010). In children and adolescents with SB, the achievement of urinary continence is associated with improved self-concept and self-esteem, especially among girls (Moore, Kogans, & Parekh, 2004). This chronic condition has an array of associated complications, including hydrocephalus and shunt malfunctions, scoliosis, bowel and bladder management issues, latex allergy, and epilepsy. However, based on current medical knowledge and ethical considerations, aggressive, early management is favored for the child with myelomeningocele.

Prevention

The CDC (2009) continues to affirm that 50% to 70% of NTDs can be prevented by daily consumption of 0.4 mg of folic acid among women of childbearing age. The data indicate that serum folate concentrations among women of childbearing age decreased 16% from 2003 to 2004 in all ethnic groups studied. Lowest serum folate levels were seen in non-Hispanic whites in 2003 to 2004; however, overall serum folate levels remained below recommended levels in non-Hispanic African-Americans during all three periods studied (CDC, 2007). These results indicate that nurses and other health care professionals have an important task in disseminating information that may decrease the incidence of birth defects in children by promoting maternal consumption of folic acid.*

To ensure adequate daily intake of the recommended amount of folic acid, women must take a folic acid supplement, eat a fortified breakfast cereal containing 100% of the Recommended Dietary Allowance (RDA) of folic acid (e.g., Kellogg's Product 19, General Mills Total, Multigrain Cheerios Plus), or increase their consumption of fortified foods (cereal, bread, rice, grits, pasta) and foods naturally rich in folate (green, leafy vegetables and citrus fruits). For women who have had a previous pregnancy affected by NTDs, folic acid intake is increased to 4 mg under the supervision of a practitioner beginning 1 month before a planned pregnancy and continuing through the first trimester. Supplementation of 4 mg of folate should not be given solely in multivitamin preparations because of the risk for overdose of other vitamins. Drugs that affect folic acid metabolism and increase the risk for myelomeningocele should be avoided before pregnancy (if plans are to become pregnant in the near future) and during pregnancy; these include trimethoprim and the AEDs—carbamazepine, phenytoin, phenobarbital, valproic acid, and primidone (Kinsman & Johnston, 2016).

Care Management

At birth, an examination is performed to assess the integrity of the membranous cyst. During transport to the nursery, every effort is made to prevent trauma to this protective covering. In addition to the routine assessment of the newborn (see Chapter 23), assess the infant for the level of neurologic involvement. Note movement of extremities or skin response, especially an anal reflex that might provide clues to the degree of motor or sensory impairment. It is important to observe the infant's behavior in conjunction with the stimulus, because limb movements can be induced in response to spinal cord reflex activity that has no connection with the higher centers. Observation of urinary output, especially if a diaper remains dry, may indicate urinary retention. Abdominal assessment revealing bladder distention, even with a wet diaper, may indicate urinary overflow in a retentive bladder. The head circumference is measured daily (see Chapter 29), and the fontanels are examined for signs of tension or bulging.

Care of the Myelomeningocele Sac

The infant is usually placed in an incubator or warmer so temperature can be maintained without clothing or covers that might irritate the spinal lesion. When an overhead warmer is used, the dressings over the defect require more frequent moistening because of the dehydrating effect of the radiant heat.

Before surgical closure, the myelomeningocele is prevented from drying by the application of a sterile, moist, nonadherent dressing. The moistening solution is usually sterile normal saline. Dressings are changed frequently (every 2 to 4 hours), and the sac is closely inspected for leaks, abrasions, irritation, and any signs of infection. The sac must be carefully cleansed if it becomes soiled or contaminated. Sometimes the sac ruptures during delivery or transport, and any opening in the sac greatly increases the risk for infection to the CNS.

> **! NURSING ALERT**
>
> Observe for early signs of infection, such as temperature instability (axillary), irritability, and lethargy, and for signs of increased intracranial pressure, which might indicate developing hydrocephalus.

> **! NURSING ALERT**
>
> Avoid measuring rectal temperatures in infants with spina bifida (SB). Because bowel sphincter function is frequently affected, the thermometer can cause irritation and rectal prolapse.

---

*Information is available from the Centers for Disease Control and Prevention, National Center on Birth Defects and Developmental Disabilities, Division of Birth Defects and Developmental Disabilities, 1600 Clifton Road NE, MS E-86, Atlanta, GA 30333; 800-CDC-INFO; email: cdcinfo@cdc.gov; http://www.cdc.gov/ncbddd/folicacid and from the March of Dimes Resource Center, 1275 Mamaroneck Avenue, White Plains, NY 10605; http://www.marchofdimes.com.

One of the most important and challenging aspects in the early care of the infant with myelomeningocele is positioning. Before surgery, the infant is kept in the prone position to minimize tension on the sac and the risk for trauma. The prone position allows for optimal positioning of the legs, especially in cases of associated hip dysplasia. The infant is placed prone with the hips slightly flexed and supported to reduce tension on the defect. The legs are maintained in abduction with a pad between the knees to counteract hip subluxation, and a small roll is placed under the ankles to maintain a neutral foot position. A variety of aids, including diaper rolls, foam pads, or specially designed frames and appliances, can be used to maintain the desired position.

Prevent Complications

The prone position affects other aspects of the infant's care. For example, in this position, the infant is more difficult to keep clean, pressure areas are a constant threat, and feeding becomes a problem. The infant's head is turned to one side for feeding. Fortunately, most defects are repaired early, and the infant can be held for feeding soon after surgery. Special care must be taken to avoid pressure on the operative site.

Diapering the infant may be contraindicated until the defect has been repaired and healing is well advanced or epithelialization has taken place. The padding beneath the diaper area is changed as needed to keep the skin dry and free from irritation. When urinary retention is detected, CIC is used. Because the bowel sphincter is frequently affected, there is continual passage of stool, often misinterpreted as diarrhea, which is a constant irritant to the skin and a source of infection to the spinal lesion.

> **! NURSING ALERT**
>
> To prevent stool contamination of the spina bifida (SB) defect preoperatively, obtain a surgical drape (e.g., Steri-Drape). Cut a portion of the drape to fit the infant's sacrum, and secure the drape using nonlatex tape. Place the rest of the drape loosely over the dressing, covering the defect and thus preventing exposure to stool.

Areas of sensory and motor impairment are subject to skin breakdown and therefore require meticulous care. Placing the infant on a special mattress or mattress overlay reduces pressure on the knees and ankles. Periodic cleansing, application of lotion, and gentle massage aid circulation.

Gentle range-of-motion exercises are carried out to prevent contractures, and stretching of contractures is performed when indicated. However, these exercises may be restricted to the foot, ankle, and knee joint. When the hip joints are unstable, stretching against tight hip flexors or adductor muscles, which act much like bowstrings, may aggravate a tendency toward subluxation. Consultation with a physical therapist is an important aspect of the short- and long-term management of infants with myelomeningocele.

Cuddling infants with unrepaired myelomeningocele is contraindicated. Caressing, stroking, and other comfort measures meet their need for tactile stimulation. Individualized developmental care with age-appropriate stimulation is provided.

Provide Postoperative Care

Postoperative care of the infant with myelomeningocele involves the same basic care as that of any postsurgical infant and includes monitoring vital signs, monitoring intake and output, providing nourishment, observing for signs of infection, and managing pain. Care of the operative site is carried out under the direction of the surgeon and includes close observation for signs of leakage of CSF. General care is done as preoperatively.

The prone position is maintained after surgical closure, although many neurosurgeons allow a side-lying or partial side-lying position unless it aggravates a coexisting hip dysplasia or permits undesirable hip flexion. This offers an opportunity for position changes, which reduces the risk for pressure sores and facilitates feeding. If permitted, the infant can be held upright against the body, with care taken to avoid pressure on the operative site. After the effects of anesthesia have subsided and the infant is alert, feedings may be resumed unless there are other anomalies or associated complications.

Support the Family and Educate About Home Care

As soon as the parents are able to cope with the infant's condition, they are encouraged to become involved in care. They need to learn how to continue at home the care that has been initiated in the hospital, including positioning, feeding, skin care, and range-of-motion exercises when appropriate. They are taught CIC technique when it is prescribed. Parents also need to know the signs of complications (urinary, neurologic, orthopedic) and how to obtain assistance when needed.

The mother who wishes to breastfeed her infant is encouraged to do so, because this will be beneficial. Shortly after delivery, the mother is started on a program of pumping to initiate and maintain milk supply until the infant is stable enough to begin breastfeeding (Hurtekant & Spatz, 2007). This process may require considerable support from nurses, physicians, and family members because of separation from the infant for surgical care and recovery.

The long-range planning with and support of the parents and newborn begin in the hospital and continue throughout childhood and even into young adulthood. The life expectancy of children with SB extends well into adulthood; therefore, planning should involve long-term goals and plans for optimum function as an adult. Discussion about aspects of adulthood such as receiving educational or vocational training and education, living independently, having a mate, having sexual relationships, and bearing and rearing children is important and should not be overlooked (Rowe & Jadhav, 2008). The unique service needs of adolescents with SB as they attempt to gain independence from family and establish lives of their own have not been adequately addressed in the literature (Sawyer & Macnee, 2010). Betz, Linroth, Butler, and colleagues (2010) interviewed young people with SB making the transition to adulthood. Some common themes that emerged among these young people were as follows: (1) challenges in preparation for self-management; (2) limited social relationships; (3) awareness of their cognitive challenges; and (4) the cost of independence. Nurses assume an important role as central members of the health care team. As care managers and coordinators, nurses review information with the family, take responsibility for family teaching, and act as a liaison between inpatient and outpatient services. The child may require numerous hospitalizations over the years, and each one will be a source of stress to which the younger child is especially vulnerable (see Chapter 37 for a discussion of care of the child with a disability).

Habilitation involves not only solving problems of self-help and locomotion but also solving the most distressing problem of urinary or bowel incontinence, which threatens the child's social acceptability. Assistance in preparing the child and the school regarding the special needs of children with disabilities helps provide a better initial adjustment to this broader social experience.

A Life Course Model has been developed for patients, families, caregivers, teachers, and clinicians to facilitate, through a developmental approach, the care of the child and young person with SB; this program has been made into a Web-based tool that can be used to assist in the transition to adulthood (Dicianno, Fairman, Juengst et al., 2010). Additional information regarding this program is available through the Spina Bifida Association's website at http://www.spinabifidaassociation.org.

The Spina Bifida Association of America* is organized to provide services and support for families of children with spinal lesions.

Latex Allergy

Latex allergy, or latex hypersensitivity, was identified as being a serious health hazard when a report linked intraoperative anaphylaxis with latex in children with SB. Latex, a natural product derived from the rubber tree, is used in combination with other chemicals to give elasticity, strength, and durability to many products. Children with SB are at high risk for developing latex allergy because of repeated exposure to latex products during surgery and procedures. Therefore, such children should not be exposed to latex products from birth onward to minimize the occurrence of latex hypersensitivity. Allergic reactions range from urticaria, wheezing, watery eyes, and rashes to anaphylactic shock. More severe reactions tend to occur when latex comes in contact with mucous membranes, wet skin, the bloodstream, or an airway. There also can be cross-reactions to a number of foods (e.g., banana, avocado, kiwi, chestnut).

Allergic reactions to latex protein can also occur when the substance is transferred to food by food handlers wearing latex gloves, prompting several states to pass legislation that prohibits the use of latex gloves in food service. In addition to patients with SB, high-risk populations include patients with urogenital anomalies or multiple surgeries, as well as health care workers. Box 49.6 lists medical conditions associated with the risk for latex allergy.

The most important goals are prevention of latex sensitivity and identification of children with known hypersensitivity (see Guidelines box: Identifying Latex Allergy). High-risk and latex-allergic individuals must be managed in a latex-free environment. Take care that they do not come in direct or secondary contact with products or equipment containing latex at *any time* during medical treatment. Allergy testing can identify latex sensitivity with varying success. Skin prick testing and provocation testing carry the risk for allergic reaction or anaphylaxis. Several commercially available assays can be useful in confirming latex sensitivity. To date, none of these tests demonstrates complete diagnostic reliability, and they should not be the sole determinant of the presence or absence of an allergic response to latex.

Because children who have SB are prone to develop sensitivity to latex, reducing exposure from birth onward may decrease the chance of allergy development. Nonlatex product lists are available to parents and health care workers; these products may be substituted for those containing latex. In the health care arena, it is important to use products with the lowest potential risk for sensitizing patients and staff members.*

The identification of those sensitive to latex is best accomplished through careful screening of all patients. During the health interview with the parent or child, ask *all* patients, not only those at risk, about sensitivity to latex. Be certain this is a routine part of all preoperative and preprocedural histories. Stress the importance of the allergy history to all personnel (e.g., phlebotomists) (see the Guidelines box: Identifying Latex Allergy for questions related to latex allergy). Children with latex hypersensitivity should carry some form of allergy identification, such as a medical alert bracelet. Education programs regarding latex hypersensitivity are aimed at those who care for high-risk groups, such as children with SB, and may include relatives, school nurses, teachers, child care workers, and babysitters. In addition to educating caregivers about the child's exposure to medical products that contain latex, nurses need to inform them of common nonmedical latex objects, such as water toys, pacifiers, and plastic storage bags.[†] Items brought to the hospital, such as floral bouquets, should also be screened for latex toys and balloons. Parents should also receive literature explaining signs and symptoms of latex hypersensitivity and appropriate emergency treatment (see the "Anaphylaxis" section in Chapter 42).

BOX 49.6   Medical Conditions Associated With Risk for Latex Allergy

- Spina bifida (SB)
- Urogenital anomalies
- Imperforate anus
- Tracheoesophageal fistula
- VATER* association
- Preterm infants
- Ventriculoperitoneal shunt
- Cognitive impairment
- Cerebral palsy (CP)
- Spinal cord injuries (SCIs)
- Multiple surgeries
- Atopy

***V**ertebral defects, **A**nal atresia, **T**racheoesophageal fistula, **E**sophageal atresia, and **R**enal/radial defects.

 GUIDELINES

Identifying Latex Allergy

- Does your child have any symptoms, such as sneezing, coughing, rashes, or wheezing, when handling rubber products (e.g., balloons, tennis or Koosh balls, adhesive bandage strips) or when in contact with rubber hospital products (e.g., gloves, catheters)?
- Has your child ever had an allergic reaction during surgery?
- Does your child have a history of rashes; asthma; or allergic reactions to medication or foods, especially milk, kiwi, bananas, or chestnuts?
- How would you identify or recognize an allergic reaction in your child?
- What would you do if an allergic reaction occurred?
- Has anyone ever discussed latex or rubber allergy or sensitivity with you?
- Has your child had any allergy testing?
- When did your child last come in contact with any type of rubber product? Were you present?

Modified from Romanczuk, A. (1993). Latex use with infants and children: It can cause problems. *American Journal of Maternal/Child Nursing, 18*(4), 208–212.

SPINAL MUSCULAR ATROPHY, TYPE 1 (WERDNIG-HOFFMANN DISEASE)

Spinal muscular atrophy (SMA) type 1 (Werdnig-Hoffmann disease) is a disorder characterized by progressive weakness and wasting of skeletal muscles caused by degeneration of anterior horn cells. It is inherited as an autosomal recessive trait and is the most common paralytic form of the floppy infant syndrome (congenital hypotonia). The sites of the pathologic condition are the anterior horn cells of the spinal cord and the motor nuclei of the brainstem, but the primary effect is atrophy of skeletal muscles. The age of onset is variable, but the earlier the onset, the more disseminated and severe the motor weakness. The disorder may be manifested early—often at birth—and almost always before 2 years of age; death may occur as a result of respiratory failure by 2 years of age (Iannaccone & Burghes, 2002; Lunn & Wang, 2008). The manifestations (Box 49.7) and prognosis are categorized according to the age of onset, severity of weakness, and clinical course; some children may

---

*For a list of latex products and alternative products, visit the Spina Bifida Association's home page, http://www.spinabifidaassociation.org, and click the Learn tab for the Latex List.

†Latex-free product lists are available from the American Latex Allergy Association's online resource manual, available at http://latexallergyresources.org/latex-free-products. American Latex Allergy Association, PO Box 198, Slinger, WI 53086; 888-972-5378; http://www.latexallergyresources.org.

Type 1 (Werdnig-Hoffmann Disease)
Clinical manifestations within first few weeks or months of life
Onset within 6 months of life
Inactivity the most prominent feature
Infant lying in a frog-leg position with legs externally rotated, abducted, and flexed at knees
Generalized weakness
Absent deep tendon reflexes
Limited movements of shoulder and arm muscles
Active movement usually limited to fingers and toes
Diaphragmatic breathing with sternal retractions (diaphragmatic paralysis may occur)
Abnormal tongue movements (at rest)
Weak cry and cough
Poor suck reflex
Tiring quickly during feedings (if breastfed, may lose weight before noticeable)
Growth failure (nutritional)
Alert facies
Normal sensation and intellect
Affected infants not able to sit alone, roll over, or walk
Early death possible from respiratory failure or infection

Type 2 (Intermediate Spinal Muscular Atrophy)
Onset before 18 months of age
   Early: Weakness confined to arms and legs
   Later: Becomes generalized
Legs usually involved to greater extent than arms
Prominent pectus excavatum
Movements absent during complete relaxation or sleep
Some infants able to sit if placed in position, but few can ambulate
Life span from 7 months to 7 years, although many have normal life expectancy

Type 3 (Kugelberg-Welander Disease; Mild Spinal Muscular Atrophy)
Onset of symptoms after 18 months of age
Normal head control and ability to sit unassisted by 6 to 8 months of age
Thigh and hip muscles weak
Scoliosis common
Failure to walk a common presentation
In those who manage to walk:
   • Waddling gait
   • Genu recurvatum
   • Protuberant abdomen
   • Ambulation becoming increasingly difficult
   • Confinement to a wheelchair by second decade
   • Deep tendon reflexes possibly present early but disappear

*These classifications are general, but some research suggests there may be variations in life span and other characteristics (Iannaccone & Burghes, 2002; Russman, Buncher, White et al., 1996; Russman, Iannaccone, Buncher et al., 1992).

fluctuate between exhibiting symptoms of types 1 and 2 or types 2 and 3 in regard to clinical function (Sarnat, 2016a). Some experts also categorize SMA according to the highest level of motor function (Lunn & Wang); type 1 includes "nonsitters," type 2 includes "sitters," and type 3 includes "walkers" (Iannaccone, 2007). A severe rare fetal form of SMA, classified as type 0, is reported to be quite lethal in the perinatal period; motor neuron degeneration may be noted as early as midgestation

in type 0 (Sarnat, 2016a). Type 4 may present between 20 and 30 years of age and may be referred to as *proximal adult type SMA* (Sarnat, 2016a).

Diagnostic Evaluation and Therapeutic Management

The diagnosis is based on the molecular genetic marker for the *SMN* (survival motor neuron) gene, which is located on chromosome 5q13. Prenatal diagnosis may be made by genetic analysis of circulating fetal cells in maternal blood (Béroud, Karliova, Bonnefont et al., 2003) or circulating fetal cells in amniotic fluid. The risk for subsequent affected offspring in carriers of the mutant gene or in families with known cases of SMA may also be evaluated genetically. Further diagnostic studies include muscle electromyography (EMG), which demonstrates a denervation pattern, and muscle biopsy; however, the genetic analysis has become the gold standard for diagnosis of the condition (Sarnat, 2016a).

There is no cure for the disease, and treatment is symptomatic and preventive, primarily preventing joint contractures and treating orthopedic problems, the most serious of which is scoliosis. Hip subluxation and dislocation may also occur. Many children benefit from powered wheelchairs, lifts, special pressure-adjustable mattresses, and accessible environmental controls. Muscle and joint contractures require careful attention and care to prevent further complications. Nutritional growth failure may occur in infants and toddlers as a result of poor feeding; supplemental gastrostomy feedings may be required to maintain adequate nutritional status and maintain weight gain. The use of lower extremity orthoses may assist with ambulation, but eventually, the child may be confined to a wheelchair as muscle atrophy progresses. Restrictive lung disease is the most serious complication of SMA (Iannaccone, 2007). Upper respiratory tract infections often occur and are treated with antibiotic therapy; they are the cause of death in many children. Rapid eye movement (REM)–related sleep-disordered breathing is common in children with SMA type 1; this progresses to sleep-disordered breathing during REM and non-REM sleep followed by respiratory failure, which often requires nocturnal noninvasive mechanical ventilation (Schroth, 2009). Noninvasive ventilation methods such as bilevel positive airway pressure (BiPAP) have decreased the morbidity and increased the survival rate of children with SMA types 1 and 2. A decreased ability to cough and clear secretions may be managed with airway clearance therapies such as the cough-assist machine and manual cough assistance. Guidelines for the standardization of respiratory care for patients with SMA have been published elsewhere (Schroth).

Prognosis

Prognosis varies according to the age of onset or group as described in Box 49.7. Individuals with SMA type 1 may succumb to respiratory infections or failure between 1 and 24 months of age (Iannaccone & Burghes, 2002; Sarnat, 2016a); however, some may live into their third or fourth decade of life. A significant number of infants with SMA require a tracheotomy, and associated medical conditions in survivors include gastroesophageal reflux, scoliosis, early onset puberty, hip dysplasia, and recurrent oral candidiasis (Bach, 2007). Drug therapy with riluzole, valproic acid, gabapentin, and oral phenylbutyrate has been shown to slow the progression of the condition, but none has demonstrated significant overall benefits (Wadman, Bosboom, van der Pol et al., 2012; Sarnat, 2016a).

Care Management

An infant or small child with progressive muscle weakness requires nursing care similar to that of an immobilized patient (see Chapter 48). However, the underlying goal of treatment should be to assist the child and family in dealing with the illness while progressing toward a life of normalization within the child's capabilities. Special attention should be directed to preventing muscle and joint contractures, promoting independence in performance of ADLs, and becoming incorporated into the mainstream of school when possible. In addition, parents need support and resources to be able to provide for the child and remain an intact family. Because children with neuromuscular disease have abnormal breathing patterns that often contribute to early death, it is important to assess adequate oxygenation, especially during the sleep phase when shallow breathing occurs and hypoxemia may develop. Home pulse oximetry may be used to assess the child during sleep and provide noninvasive mechanical ventilation as necessary (Bush, Fraser, Jardine et al., 2005; Young, Lowe, Fitzgerald et al., 2007) (see the "Duchenne [Pseudohypertrophic] Muscular Dystrophy" section later in this chapter for respiratory management). Supportive care also includes management of orthoses and other orthopedic equipment as required. Because children with SMA are intellectually normal, verbal, tactile, and auditory stimulation are important aspects of developmental care. Supporting them so that they can see the activities around them and transporting them in appropriate conveyances (e.g., wagon, power wheelchair) for a change of environment provide stimulation and a broader scope of contacts.

Children who are able to sit require proper support and attention to alignment to prevent deformities and other complications. Children who survive beyond infancy need attention to educational needs and opportunities for social interaction with other children. The parents of a child who is chronically ill require much support and encouragement* (see Chapter 36). Parents who have not sought genetic counseling should be encouraged to do so to evaluate further risk potential.

Congenital muscular dystrophies have an onset at birth and clinical manifestations in the first 2 years of life. Although rare disorders, these are divided into three major groups: (1) collagenopathies, (2) merosinopathies, and (3) dystroglycanopathies. In addition to progressive skeletal muscle weakness and hypotonia, some are associated with joint hyperlaxity and eye or brain abnormalities. Genetic studies may help to correlate with specific phenotypes. Evidence-based guidelines for evaluation, diagnosis, and management of congenital muscular dystrophies have been published recently by the American Academy of Neurology (Kang, Morrison, Iannaccone et al., 2015).

SPINAL MUSCULAR ATROPHY, TYPE 3 (KUGELBERG-WELANDER DISEASE)

SMA type 3 (Kugelberg-Welander disease) is a result of anterior horn cell and motor nerve degeneration. The disease is characterized by a pattern of muscular weakness similar to that of type 1 SMA (see Box 49.7). Several modes of inheritance have been reported for the disease: autosomal recessive, autosomal dominant, and X-linked recessive.

The onset occurs from younger than 1 year of age into adulthood, with symptoms resembling type 3 SMA. Proximal muscle weakness (especially of the lower limbs) and muscular atrophy are the predominant features. The disease runs a slowly progressive course. Some children lose the ability to walk 8 to 9 years after the onset of symptoms, but many can still walk after 30 years or more. Many affected people have a normal life expectancy (Lunn & Wang, 2008).

*Family resources include Families of SMA, 925 Busse Road, Elk Grove Village, IL 60007; 800-886-1762; http://www.curesma.org. In Canada: Families of Spinal Muscular Atrophy Canada, 103–7134 Vedder Rd., Chilliwack, BC V2R 4G4; 855-824-1266; http://www.curesma.ca. Muscular Dystrophy Association—USA, 3300 E. Sunrise Drive, Tucson, AZ 85718; 800-572-1717; http://www.mda.org.

Therapeutic Management and Care Management

The management is primarily symptomatic and supportive and is related to maintaining mobility as long as possible, preventing complications such as skin breakdown, optimizing and maintaining respiratory function, and providing support to the child and family. The discussion of family support in the section for Duchenne muscular dystrophy (DMD) is also applicable to families of children with SMA.

MUSCULAR DYSTROPHIES

Muscular dystrophies (MDs) constitute the largest and most important single group of muscle diseases of childhood. The MDs have a genetic origin in which there is gradual degeneration of muscle fibers, and they are characterized by progressive weakness and wasting of symmetric groups of skeletal muscles, with increasing disability and deformity. In all forms of MD, there is an insidious loss of strength, but each type differs in regard to the muscle groups affected (Fig. 49.7), age of onset, rate of progression, and inheritance pattern. The most common form, Duchenne muscular dystrophy (DMD), is discussed separately in the next section.

Facioscapulohumeral (Landouzy-Dejerine) muscular dystrophy is inherited as an autosomal dominant disorder with onset in early adolescence. It is characterized by difficulty in raising the arms over the head, lack of facial mobility, and a forward slope of the shoulders. The progression is slow, and the life span is usually unaffected.

Limb-girdle muscular dystrophy (LGMD) is a heterogenous group of disorders with autosomal dominant and recessive inheritance whose clinical manifestations often appear in later childhood, adolescence, or early adulthood with variable but usually slow progression (Quan, 2011). All types of LGMD are characterized by weakness of proximal muscles of the pelvic and shoulder girdles. Other forms of MD include myotonic dystrophy, scapulohumeral MD (Emery-Dreifuss MD), fascioscapulohumeral MD (Landouzy-Dejerine disease), and congenital MD; these forms consist of subtypes of MD and are discussed at length elsewhere (Sarnat, 2016b).

Treatment of the MDs consists mainly of supportive measures, including physical therapy, orthopedic procedures to minimize deformity, ventilation support, and assistance for the affected child in meeting the demands of daily living.

DUCHENNE (PSEUDOHYPERTROPHIC) MUSCULAR DYSTROPHY

DMD is the most severe and the most common MD of childhood. It is inherited as an X-linked recessive trait, and the single-gene defect is located on the short arm of the X chromosome. DMD has a high mutation rate, with a positive family history in about 65% of cases. Genetic counseling is an important aspect of the care of the family. In about 30% of cases, it is a new mutation, and the mother is *not* the carrier (Sarnat, 2016b).

As in all X-linked disorders, males are affected almost exclusively. The female carrier may have an elevated serum creatine kinase, but muscle weakness is usually not a problem; however, about 10% of female carriers develop cardiomyopathy (Manzur, Kinali, & Muntoni, 2008). In rare instances, a female may be identified with DMD disease yet with muscular weakness that is milder than in boys (Sarnat, 2016b). At the genetic level, both DMD and Becker MD (a milder variant) result from mutations of the gene that encodes dystrophin, a protein product in skeletal muscle. Dystrophin is absent from the muscles of children with DMD and is reduced or abnormal in children with Becker MD. Children with Becker MD have a later onset of symptoms, which

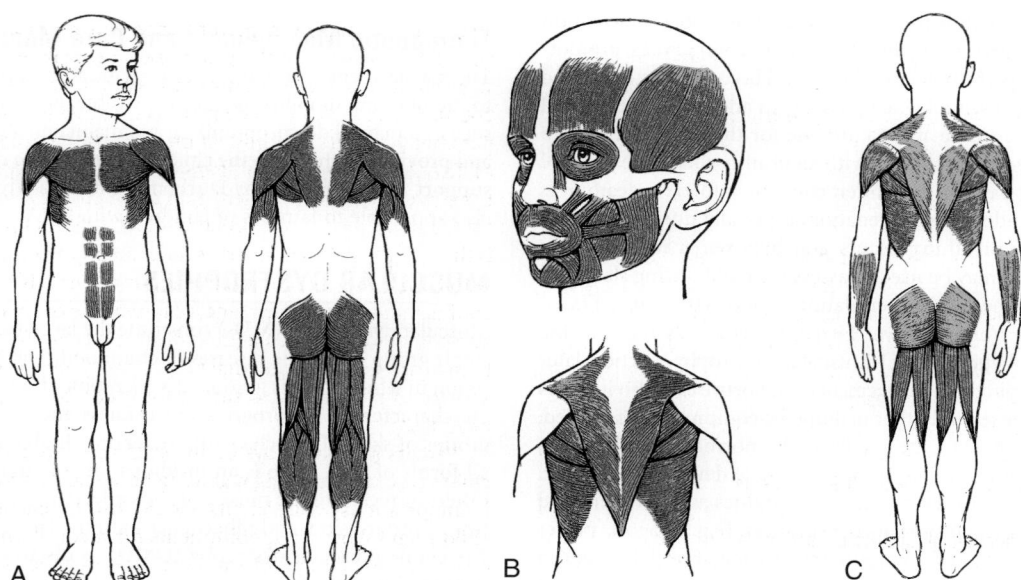

FIG 49.7 Initial muscle groups involved in muscular dystrophies (MDs). **A,** Pseudohypertrophic. **B,** Fascioscapulohumeral. **C,** Limb girdle.

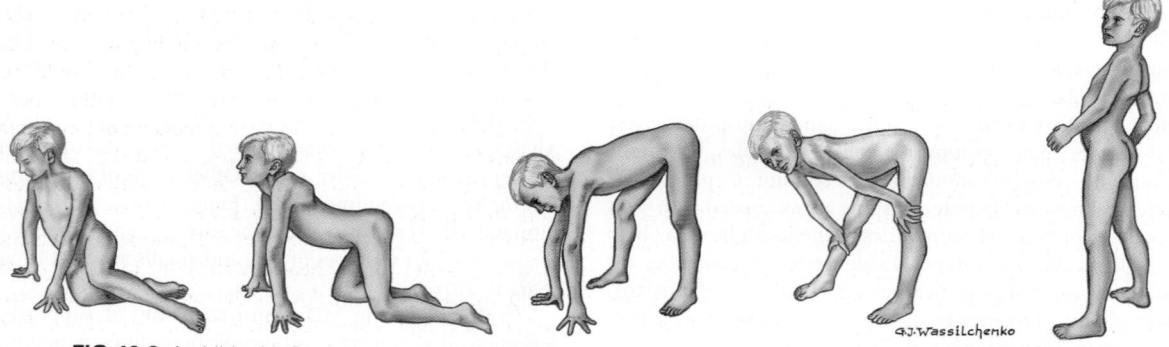

FIG 49.8 A child with Duchenne muscular dystrophy (DMD) attains standing posture by kneeling and then gradually pushing his torso upright (with knees straight) by "walking" his hands up his legs (Gower sign). Note the marked lordosis in an upright position.

BOX 49.8 Characteristics of Duchenne Muscular Dystrophy

- Early onset, usually between 3 and 7 years of age
- Progressive muscular weakness, wasting, and contractures
- Calf muscle pseudohypertrophy in most patients
- Loss of independent ambulation by 9 to 12 years of age
- Slowly progressive, generalized weakness during teenage years

---

are usually not as severe as those seen in DMD. The incidence is approximately 1 in 3600 male births for the Duchenne form and approximately 1 in 30,000 live births for the Becker type (Sarnat, 2016b). Box 49.8 describes the characteristics of DMD.

Most children with DMD reach the appropriate developmental milestones early in life, although they may have mild, subtle delays. Evidence of muscle weakness usually appears during the third to seventh year, although there may have been a history of delay in motor development, particularly walking. Difficulties in running, riding a bicycle, and climbing stairs are usually the first symptoms noted. Typically, affected boys have a waddling gait and lordosis, fall frequently, and develop a characteristic manner of rising from a squatting or sitting position on the floor (Gower sign) (Fig. 49.8). Lordosis occurs as a result of weakened pelvic muscles, and the waddling gait is a result of weakness in the gluteus medius and maximus muscles (Battista, 2010). In the early years, rapid developmental gains may mask the progression of the disease.

Muscles, especially in the calves, thighs, and upper arms, become enlarged from fatty infiltration and feel unusually firm or woody on palpation (Box 49.9). The term *pseudohypertrophy* is derived from this muscular enlargement. Profound muscular atrophy occurs in the later stages; contractures and deformities involving large and small joints are common complications as the disease progresses. Ambulation usually becomes impossible by 12 years of age. The loss of mobilization further increases the spectrum of complications, which may include osteoporosis, fractures, constipation, skin breakdown, and psychosocial and behavioral problems. Atrophy of facial, oropharyngeal, and respiratory muscles does not occur until the advanced stage of the disease. Ultimately, the disease process involves the diaphragm and auxiliary muscles of respiration, and cardiomyopathy is seen in approximately 50% to 80% of patients with DMD (Sarnat, 2016b).

BOX 49.9   Clinical Manifestations of Duchenne Muscular Dystrophy

Relentless progression of muscle weakness; possible death from respiratory or cardiac failure

Waddling gait

Lordosis

Frequent falls

Gower sign (child turns onto side or abdomen; flexes knees to assume a kneeling position; and then with knees extended, gradually pushes torso to an upright position by "walking" the hands up the legs)

Enlarged (hypertrophied) muscles (especially calves, thighs, and upper arms); feel unusually firm or woody on palpation

Later stages—profound muscular atrophy

Mental deficiency (common)

- Mild (≈20 IQ points below normal)
- Mental deficit present in 25% to 30% of patients

Complications:

- Contracture deformities of hips, knees, and ankles
- Disuse atrophy
- Cardiomyopathy
- Obesity and at times undernutrition
- Respiratory compromise and cardiac failure

IQ, Intelligence quotient.

Obesity is a common complication that contributes to premature loss of ambulation. Children who have restricted opportunities for physical activity and who are bored easily consume calories in excess of their needs. Overfeeding by well-meaning family and friends may compound this. Proper dietary intake and a diversified recreational program help reduce the likelihood of obesity and enable children to maintain ambulation and functional independence for a longer time.

Mild to moderate cognitive impairment is commonly associated with MD. A deficiency of dystrophin isoforms in brain tissue causes cognitive and intellectual impairment (Manzur, Kinali, & Muntoni, 2008). The mean intelligence quotient (IQ) is approximately 20 points below normal, and frank mental deficit is present in 20% to 30% of these children. Verbal IQ is markedly low in boys with DMD, and emotional disturbance is more common than in other children with disabilities; however, children with DMD should be involved in early learning programs and eventually moved into regular classrooms as much as possible. Patients with Becker MD present later in life than those with DMD, but they often do not survive past the middle of the second decade, with few patients living into their forties (Sarnat, 2016b).

Diagnostic Evaluation

The diagnosis of DMD is primarily established by blood polymerase chain reaction (PCR) for the dystrophin gene mutation (Sarnat, 2016b). Prenatal diagnosis is also possible as early as 12 weeks of gestation. Serum enzyme measurement, muscle biopsy, and EMG may also be used in establishing the diagnosis. Serum creatine kinase levels are extremely high in the first 2 years of life before the onset of clinical weakness. If the child demonstrates the usual characteristics, has a positive family history for DMD, and the PCR result is positive, the muscle biopsy may be deferred.

Therapeutic Management

No curative treatment exists for childhood MD. The use of the corticosteroids prednisone and deflazacort has been evaluated as a treatment for DMD. Several clinical trials demonstrated increased muscle strength and improved performance and pulmonary function, with significant decrease in the progression of weakness, when prednisone was administered for 6 months to 2 years (Manzur, Kuntzer, Pike et al., 2008). The American Academy of Neurology has published a practice parameter for the administration of corticosteroids in the treatment of DMD (Moxley, Ashwal, Pandya et al., 2005). Major side effects in these studies included weight gain and a cushingoid facial appearance.

Maintaining optimal function in all muscles for as long as possible is the primary goal; secondary is the prevention of contractures. Children with DMD who remain as active as possible are able to avoid wheelchair confinement for a longer time. Maintenance of function often involves stretching exercises, strength and muscle training, breathing exercises to increase and maintain vital lung capacity, range-of-motion exercises, surgery to release contracture deformities, bracing, and performance of ADLs.

Parents should always be involved in making decisions about the child's care, and teaching regarding home safety and prevention of falls is important as well. Parents should also be encouraged to have the child keep follow-up appointments for medical care and physical and occupational therapy. Because respiratory tract infections are most troublesome in these children, influenza and pneumococcal vaccines are encouraged, and contact with people with respiratory tract infections should be avoided. Action plans for prompt treatment of respiratory illness are important.

Eventually, respiratory and cardiac problems become the central focus of the debilitating illness. Children with neuromuscular disease develop abnormal breathing patterns, and hypoxia may occur as a result of inadequate oxygenation. Polysomnography should be performed once daytime symptoms of sleep-disordered breathing occur. The child and parents should be involved in a discussion of long-term ventilation options. Cardiac and respiratory assessment during wake/sleep cycles is imperative. Respiratory care for children with neuromuscular conditions such as SMA and DMD may involve the use of noninvasive ventilation with BiPAP on a temporary or full-time basis, mechanically assisted coughing (MAC), or tracheotomy and relief of airway obstruction with coughing and suctioning devices; the tracheotomy, however, is associated with more complications (Simonds, 2006; Young, Lowe, Fitzgerald et al., 2007). Home pulse oximetry may be used to monitor oxygenation during sleep or to aid in decision making regarding the use of MAC to clear the airways.

Several devices are available for children with neuromuscular disease to assist in clearing the airway when the cough reflex is ineffective or diminished. The mechanical in-exsufflator (MIE; also referred to as *cough assist*) has been found to be safe and effective in the daily management of respiratory function (Kravitz, 2009; Miske, Hickey, Kolb et al., 2004). The MIE delivers positive inspiratory pressures at a set rate followed by negative pressure exsufflation coordinated with the patient's own breathing rhythm. The exsufflation is designed to mimic a cough reflex so that mucus can be effectively cleared. Airway suctioning after exsufflation is accomplished as necessary to clear the airways. In children, the MIE device may be connected directly to a tracheostomy or used with a mouthpiece or face mask. Boitano's (2009) article provides a variety of equipment options, including various masks that can be used to deliver noninvasive positive pressure.

Manual cough-assisting techniques include glossopharyngeal breathing or air stacking (frog breathing); the abdominal thrust, which is similar to the Heimlich maneuver (Kravitz, 2009); and manual hyperinflation with a self-inflating resuscitation bag (without oxygen) and a mouthpiece. Hyperinflation may be used in conjunction with abdominal thrusts to improve peak cough flows (Boitano, 2009).

The use of routine chest physiotherapy (postural drainage) for DMD has not been adequately evaluated for its effectiveness in clearing the airway of mucus except when there is focal atelectasis and mucus plugging the airways (Kravitz, 2009).

Survival in individuals with DMD may be prolonged several years with the use of noninvasive ventilation and MAC as alternatives to tracheotomy and airway suctioning (Bach & Martinez, 2011; Simonds, 2006). The American Thoracic Society has published extensive guidelines for respiratory monitoring and care of children and adults with DMD (Finder, Birnkrant, Carl et al., 2004).

The American Academy of Pediatrics Section on Cardiology and Cardiac Surgery (2005) recommends an extensive cardiac evaluation of the child diagnosed with either DMD or Becker MD. Patients with neuromuscular conditions may not have the typical signs and symptoms of cardiac dysfunction. Therefore, symptoms such as weight loss, nausea and vomiting, cough, increased fatigue on performance of ADLs, and orthopnea should be carefully evaluated to detect early signs of cardiomyopathy.

Genetic counseling is recommended for parents, sisters, and maternal aunts and their daughters. Long-term care, end-of-life care, and palliative care options are issues that the health care team must discuss with the child and family affected by MD (Finder, 2009). Professional counseling is necessary in some cases to allow frank discussion of these issues, and referrals should be made as appropriate.

Care Management

The care and management of a child with MD involve the combined efforts of an interprofessional health care team. Nurses can help clarify the roles of these health care professionals to family and colleagues. The major emphasis of nursing care is to help the child and family cope with a chronic, progressive, incapacitating disease; to help design a program that will afford maximal independence and reduce the predictable and preventable disabilities associated with the disorder; and to help the child and family deal constructively with the limitations the disease imposes on their daily lives. Because of advances in technology, children with MD may live into early adulthood; therefore, the goals of care should also involve decisions regarding quality of life, achievement of independence, and transition to adulthood.

Working closely with other team members, nurses assist the family in developing the child's self-help skills to give the child the satisfaction of being as independent as possible for as long as possible. This requires continual evaluation of the child's capabilities, which are often difficult to assess. Fortunately, most children with MD instinctively recognize the need to become as independent as possible and strive to do so.

Practical difficulties faced by families are physical limitations of housing, transportation, and mobility. Some families live in houses or apartments that are unsuited to wheelchairs. Transportation may also be a barrier for families of children with MD. Assisting with these challenges requires team problem solving. Diet, nutritional needs, and nutrition modification are discussed according to the needs of the individual child and family.

Children with MD tend to become socially isolated as their physical condition deteriorates to the point that they can no longer keep up with their friends and classmates. Their physical capabilities diminish, and their dependency increases at the age at which most children are expanding their range of interests and relationships. To gain peer associations, they often learn and use behaviors that bring them the rewards of other children's company. These friends are often children who have been rejected by more able-bodied classmates.

The parents' social activities are also restricted, and the family's activities must be continually modified to accommodate the needs of the affected child. When the child becomes increasingly incapacitated, the family may consider home-based care, an assisted living facility, or respite care. Unless the child is severely incapacitated, he should also

be involved in the decisions regarding such care. Nurses can assist with decision making by exploring all available options and resources and support the child and family in the decision. Older boys with MD may also need psychiatric or psychologic counseling to deal with issues such as depression, anger, and quality of life. Parents need encouragement to become involved in support groups because there is evidence that adequate social support from family, community, and other parents is crucial to appropriate coping in families with children with chronic illness.

Regardless of how successful the program or how well the family adapts to the disorder, superimposed on the physical and emotional problems associated with a child with a long-term disability is the constant knowledge of the ultimate outcome of the disease. These families encounter all of the manifestations of the child with a chronic fatal illness (see Chapter 36).

Nurses are especially valuable health care professionals as they come to know the family and the family's challenges. Nurses can be alert to the problems and needs and make necessary referrals when supplementary services are indicated. The Muscular Dystrophy Association—USA* has branches in most communities to assist families that have a member with MD.

ACQUIRED NEUROMUSCULAR DISORDERS

GUILLAIN-BARRÉ SYNDROME (INFECTIOUS POLYNEURITIS)

Guillain-Barré syndrome (GBS), also known as *infectious polyneuritis,* is an uncommon acute demyelinating polyneuropathy with a progressive, usually ascending flaccid paralysis. The hallmark of GBS is acute peripheral motor weakness. The paralysis usually occurs approximately 10 days after a nonspecific viral infection; GBS has also been reported after administration of certain vaccines (rabies, influenza, polio, and meningococcal) (Sarnat, 2016c). Several subtypes of GBS include acute inflammatory demyelinating neuropathy, acute motor axonal neuropathy, acute motor sensory axonal neuropathy, and Miller Fisher syndrome. Children are less often affected than adults; among children, those between 4 and 10 years of age have higher susceptibility. The male-to-female ratio is reported to be 1.5 : 1. Two peak periods with an increased incidence of GBS have been identified: late adolescence and young adulthood.

Chronic inflammatory demyelinating polyradiculoneuropathies (CIDPs) are chronic types of GBS that recur intermittently or do not improve over a period of months to years (Sarnat, 2016c). The following discussion focuses on GBS.

Congenital GBS is rare yet may occur in the neonatal period and consists of hypotonia, weakness, and decreased or absent reflexes. Maternal neuromuscular disease may or may not be present. Diagnosis is established by the same criteria as in older children, but the symptoms gradually subside over the first few months of life and disappear by 12 months of age (Sarnat, 2016c).

Pathophysiology

GBS is an immune-mediated disease often associated with a number of viral or bacterial infections or the administration of certain vaccines.

---

*3300 E. Sunrise Drive, Tucson, AZ 85718; 800-572-1717; email: mda@mdausa.org; http://www.mda.org. In Canada: Muscular Dystrophy Canada, 2345 Yonge Street, Suite 900, Toronto, ON M4P 2E5; 866-MUSCLE-8; http://www.muscle.ca/national/home.html.

It has been associated with infectious mononucleosis, measles, mumps, *Campylobacter jejuni* (gastroenteritis), cytomegalovirus, *Borrelia burgdorferi* (Lyme disease), Epstein-Barr virus, *Helicobacter pylori,* and *Mycoplasma* and *Pneumocystis* infections. Onset of GBS symptoms usually occurs within 10 days of the primary infection. Pathologic changes in spinal and cranial nerves consist of inflammation and edema with rapid, segmented demyelination and compression of nerve roots within the dural sheath. Nerve conduction is impaired, producing ascending partial or complete paralysis of muscles innervated by the involved nerves. GBS has three phases:

1. **Acute:** Phase starts when symptoms begin and continues until new symptoms stop appearing or deterioration ceases; it may last as long as 4 weeks.
2. **Plateau:** Symptoms remain constant without further deterioration; it may last from days to weeks.
3. **Recovery:** Patient begins to improve and progress to optimal recovery; it usually lasts a few weeks to months depending on the deficits incurred by the illness.

Diagnostic Evaluation

The diagnosis of GBS is based on clinical manifestations (Box 49.10), CSF analysis, and EMG findings. CSF analysis reveals an abnormally elevated protein concentration, normal glucose, and fewer than 10 white blood cells (WBCs)/mm³ (Sarnat, 2016c). EMG shows evidence of acute muscle denervation, but other laboratory studies are usually noncontributory. The symmetric nature of the paralysis helps differentiate this disorder from spinal paralytic poliomyelitis, which usually affects sporadic muscles.

Therapeutic Management

Treatment of GBS is primarily supportive. In the acute phase, patients are hospitalized because respiratory and pharyngeal involvement may require assisted ventilation, sometimes with a temporary tracheostomy. Treatment modalities include aggressive ventilatory support in the event of respiratory compromise, intravenous immunoglobulin (IVIG), and sometimes steroids; plasmapheresis and immunosuppressive drugs may also be used. Plasmapheresis has been shown to decrease the length of recovery in patients with severe GBS yet is expensive, and the side effects

include hypotension, fever, bleeding disorders, chills, urticaria, and bradycardia. Some evidence reports equal benefits to treatment of GBS with IVIG administration or plasmapheresis; both sped up recovery time in studies reviewed (Hughes & Cornblath, 2005). There is evidence, however, of significant improvement in children with high-dose IVIG therapy (vs. supportive treatment alone) (Hughes, Swan, & van Doorn, 2012).

IVIG is now recommended as the primary treatment of GBS when administered within 2 weeks of disease onset (Hughes, 2008). Corticosteroids alone do not decrease the symptoms or shorten the duration of the disease.

Medications that may be administered during the acute phase include a low-molecular-weight heparin to prevent deep vein thrombosis (DVT), a mild laxative or stool softener to prevent constipation, pain medication such as acetaminophen, and a histamine antagonist to prevent stress ulcer formation. Chronic neuropathic pain after GBS may be treated with gabapentin, which is reported to be more effective than carbamazepine (Sarnat, 2016c).

Rehabilitation after the acute phase may involve physical therapy, occupational therapy, and speech therapy. Additional consideration should be given to problems of general weakness and retraining for toileting and feeding (Lyons, 2008).

Course and Prognosis

Better outcomes are associated with younger age, no requirement for mechanical respiratory assistance, slower progression of disease, normal peripheral nerve function on EMG, and treatment with either IVIG or plasmapheresis. Recovery usually begins within 2 to 3 weeks, and most patients regain full muscle strength. The recovery of muscle strength progresses in the reverse order of onset of paralysis, with lower extremity strength being the last to recover. Poor prognosis with subsequent residual effects in children is reportedly associated with cranial nerve involvement, extensive disability at time of presentation, and intubation.

Most deaths associated with GBS are caused by respiratory failure; therefore, early diagnosis and access to respiratory support are especially important. The rate of recovery is usually related to the degree of involvement and may extend from a few weeks to months. The greater the degree of paralysis, the longer the recovery phase.

Care Management

Nursing care is primarily supportive and is the same as that required for children with immobilization and respiratory compromise. The emphasis of care is on close observation to assess the extent of paralysis and on prevention of complications, including aspiration, ventilator-associated pneumonia (VAP), atelectasis, DVT, pressure ulcer, fear and anxiety, autonomic dysfunction, and pain.

During the acute phase of the disease, the nurse should carefully observe the child's condition for possible difficulty in swallowing and respiratory involvement. The child's respiratory function is closely monitored, and oxygen source, appropriate-sized insufflation bag and mask, endotracheal intubation and suctioning equipment, tracheotomy tray, and vasoconstrictor drugs are kept available. Vital signs are monitored frequently, as well as neurologic signs and level of consciousness. For children who develop respiratory impairment, the care is the same as that for any child with respiratory distress requiring mechanical ventilation.

Respiratory care, if intubation is required, requires close monitoring of oxygenation status (usually by pulse oximetry and sometimes arterial blood gases), maintenance of an open airway with suctioning, and postural changes to prevent pneumonia. Consideration should be given to preventing opportunistic infections such as VAP; meticulous oral care and hypopharynx suctioning, elevation of the head of bed 30

BOX 49.10   Clinical Manifestations of Guillain-Barré Syndrome

Initial Symptoms
Muscle tenderness
Paresthesia and cramps (sometimes)
Proximal symmetric muscle weakness
Ascending paralysis from lower extremities
Frequently involves muscles of trunk and upper extremities and those supplied by cranial nerves (especially facial)
Flaccid paralysis with loss of reflexes
May involve facial, extraocular, labial, lingual, pharyngeal, and laryngeal muscles
Intercostal and phrenic nerve involvement:
  • Breathlessness in vocalizations
  • Shallow, irregular respirations

Other Manifestations
Tendon reflexes depressed or absent
Variable degrees of sensory impairment
Muscle tenderness or sensitivity to slight pressure
Urinary incontinence or retention and constipation

degrees, and strict asepsis with suctioning equipment (including catheters, a Yankauer device, or both) should be implemented to prevent VAP. Children with oral and pharyngeal involvement may be fed via a nasogastric or gastrostomy tube to ensure adequate feeding. It is also important to consider the possibility of stress ulcers in such patients and administer a proton pump inhibitor. Immobilization, which occurs with GBS, decreases GI function; therefore, attention to problems such as decreased gastric emptying, constipation, and feeding residuals requires nursing assessment and appropriate collaborative interventions. Temporary urinary catheterization may be required; urinary retention is common, and appropriate assessment of urinary output is vital. Sensory impairment and paralysis in the lower extremities make the child susceptible to skin breakdown; therefore, attention should be given to meticulous skin care. Passive range-of-motion exercises and application of orthoses to prevent muscle contracture are important when paralysis is present. Prevention of DVT is accomplished with pneumatic compression (antiembolism) devices, administration of a low-molecular-weight heparin, and early mobilization and ambulation. Autonomic dysfunction may be life-threatening; thus, close monitoring of vital signs in the acute phase is essential.

A key to recovery in the child with GBS is the prevention of muscle and joint contractures, so passive range-of-motion exercises must be carried out routinely to maintain vital function. Although the child may have a generalized paralysis, cognitive function remains intact; therefore, it is important for nursing care to involve communication with the child or adolescent regarding procedures and treatments that may be frightening, especially if mechanical ventilation is required. Encourage parents to talk to the child and make eye and physical contact and to reassure the child during this phase of the illness.

Pain management is crucial in the care of children with GBS. Although neuromuscular impairment may make pain perception more difficult to accurately evaluate, objective pain scales should be used. Gabapentin and carbamazepine may be used to manage neuropathic pain in patients with GBS.

Physical therapy may be limited to passive range-of-motion exercises during the evolving phase of the disease. Later, as the disease stabilizes and recovery begins, an active physical therapy program is implemented to prevent contracture deformities and facilitate muscle recovery. This may include active exercise, gait training, and bracing.

Throughout the course of the illness, child and parent support is paramount. The usual rapidity of the paralysis and the long recovery period greatly tax the emotional reserves of all family members. The parents and child benefit from repeated reassurance by the interprofessional care team that recovery is occurring and from realistic information regarding the possibility of permanent disability. In the event of a residual disability, the family needs assistance in accepting and adjusting to the loss of function (see Chapter 38). The GBS/CIDP Foundation International* is a nonprofit organization devoted to support, education, and research. It provides families with support from recovered people, publishes informational literature and a newsletter, and maintains a list of practitioners experienced with the disease.

TETANUS

Tetanus, or lockjaw, is an acute, preventable, but often fatal disease caused by an exotoxin produced by the anaerobic spore-forming, gram-positive bacillus *Clostridium tetani*. It is characterized by painful muscular rigidity primarily involving the masseter and neck muscles. There are

---

*The Holly Building, 104½ Forrest Avenue, Narberth, PA 19072; 610-667-0131, 866-224-3301; http://www.gbs-cidp.org.

four requirements for the development of tetanus: (1) presence of tetanus spores or vegetative forms of the bacillus, (2) injury to the tissues, (3) wound conditions that encourage multiplication of the organism, and (4) a susceptible host.

Tetanus spores are found in soil; dust; and the intestinal tracts of humans and animals, especially herbivorous animals. The organisms are more prevalent in rural areas but are readily carried to urban areas by the wind. The organisms are not invasive but enter the body by way of wounds, particularly a puncture wound, burn, or crushed area. They may enter through a minor, unnoticed break in the skin, such as a thorn or needle prick, bee sting, or scratch. In newborns, infection may occur through the umbilical cord, usually in situations in which infants are delivered in contaminated surroundings, severing the umbilical cord with nonsterile instruments, or the mother is not adequately immunized. The disease has the greatest incidence in months when people are more involved in outdoor activities.

Pathophysiology

When prevention efforts are not effective and conditions are favorable, the organisms proliferate and form potent exotoxins, one of which is tetanospasmin. Tetanospasmin affects the CNS to produce the clinical manifestations of the disease. The ideal conditions for the organisms' growth are devitalized tissues without access to air, such as wounds that have not been washed or kept clean and those that have crusted over, trapping pus beneath. The exotoxin appears to reach the CNS by way of either the neuron axons or the vascular system. The toxin becomes fixed on nerve cells of the anterior horn of the spinal cord and the brainstem. The toxin acts at the myoneural junction to produce muscular stiffness and lower the threshold for reflex excitability.

The incubation period for tetanus varies from 3 days to 3 weeks and averages 8 days; most cases occur within 14 days. In neonates, it is usually 5 to 14 days. Shorter incubation periods have been associated with more heavily contaminated wounds, more severe disease, and a poorer prognosis (American Academy of Pediatrics, Committee on Infectious Diseases, & Pickering, 2012).

The manner of onset varies, but the initial symptoms are usually a progressive stiffness and tenderness of the muscles in the neck and jaw. Eventually, all voluntary muscles are affected (Box 49.11). As the child recovers from the disease, the paroxysms become less frequent and gradually subside. Survival beyond 4 days usually indicates recovery, but complete recovery may require weeks.

Therapeutic Management

Primary prevention is key and occurs through immunization and boosters (American Academy of Pediatrics, Committee on Infectious Diseases, & Pickering, 2012). Once an injury has occurred, further preventive measures are based on the child's immune status and the nature of the injury. Specific prophylactic therapy after trauma is administration of tetanus toxoid or tetanus antitoxin. A dose of tetanus toxoid is not necessary for clean, minor wounds in children who have completed the immunization series (see the "Immunizations" section in Chapter 31 for age-specific recommendations).

An unprotected or inadequately immunized child who sustains a "tetanus-prone" wound (including wounds contaminated with dirt, feces, soil, and saliva; puncture wounds; avulsions; and wounds resulting from missiles, crushing, burns, and frostbite) should receive tetanus immunoglobulin (TIG). Concurrent administration of both TIG and tetanus toxoid at separate sites is recommended both to provide protection and to initiate the active immune process (American Academy of Pediatrics, Committee on Infectious Diseases, & Pickering, 2012).

After the individual has received primary tetanus immunization, antitoxin is believed to provide protection for at least 10 years and for

BOX 49.11 Clinical Manifestations of Tetanus

Initial Symptoms

Progressive stiffness and tenderness of muscles in neck and jaw

Characteristic difficulty in opening the mouth (trismus)

Risus sardonicus (sardonic smile) caused by facial muscle spasm

Progressive Involvement

Opisthotonic positioning

Boardlike rigidity of abdominal and limb muscles

Difficulty swallowing

Extreme sensitivity to external stimuli (slight noise, gentle touch, or bright light):

- Trigger paroxysmal muscle contractions that last seconds to minutes
- Contractions recur with increased frequency until almost continuous (sustained, tetanic)

Laryngospasm and tetany of respiratory muscles:

- Accumulated secretions
- Respiratory arrest
- Atelectasis
- Pneumonia

Other Aspects

Mentation unaffected; patient alert

Pain, anxiety, and distress reflected in:

- Rapid pulse
- Sweating
- Anxious facial expression
- Fever usually absent or only mild

---

a longer period after booster immunization (American Academy of Pediatrics, Committee on Infectious Diseases, & Pickering, 2012). Recently, the Advisory Committee on Immunization Practices recommended no specific time intervals between the administration of a tetanus- or diphtheria-toxoid–containing vaccine and Tdap (tetanus, diphtheria, and pertussis) to provide protection against pertussis; other than a localized pain reaction, no other side effects were noted in people who received the Td and Tdap at intervals as short as 18 months (CDC, 2011). Completion of active immunization is carried out according to the usual pattern. Antibiotic treatment with penicillin G (or erythromycin or tetracycline in older children with allergy to penicillin) is important in the management of tetanus as an adjunct against clostridia; metronidazole is a viable alternative (Arnon, 2016a).

⚡ SAFETY ALERT

Tetanus immunoglobulin (TIG) and tetanus toxoid are always administered via the intramuscular (IM) route in separate syringes and at separate sites; they are never administered by the intravenous (IV) route.

Aggressive supportive care is necessary to treat tetanus in the acute phase. The acutely ill child is best treated in an intensive care facility where close and constant observation and equipment for monitoring and respiratory support are readily available.

General supportive care is indicated, including maintaining an adequate airway and fluid and electrolyte balance, managing pain, and ensuring adequate caloric intake. Indwelling oral or nasogastric feedings may be required to maintain adequate fluid and caloric intake; continued laryngospasm may necessitate total parenteral nutrition or gastrostomy feeding. Severe or recurrent laryngospasm or excessive secretions may require advanced airway management, such as endotracheal intubation or tracheotomy.

TIG therapy to neutralize toxins is the most specific therapy for tetanus. Local care of the wound by surgical debridement and cleansing helps reduce the numbers of proliferating organisms at the site of injury. The cleansing should be repeated several times during the first 48 hours, and deep, infected lacerations are usually exposed and debrided. Infiltration of the wound with TIG is no longer considered necessary (American Academy of Pediatrics, Committee on Infectious Diseases, & Pickering, 2012).

Diazepam is the drug of choice for seizure control and muscle relaxation (Arnon, 2016a), but lorazepam (Ativan) may be used in some cases. Intrathecal baclofen, IV magnesium sulfate, dantrolene sodium, and midazolam may also be used in the management of muscle spasticity associated with tetanus. Patients with severe tetanus and those who do not respond to other muscle relaxants may require the administration of a neuromuscular blocking agent, such as rocuronium or vecuronium; intrathecal baclofen may be used as a muscle relaxant but only in the intensive care unit, because it often induces apnea. Because of their paralytic effect on respiratory muscles, use of these drugs requires mechanical ventilation with endotracheal intubation or tracheotomy and constant cardiopulmonary monitoring. Endotracheal tube insertion or tracheotomy is often indicated and should be performed before severe respiratory distress develops. Despite the absence of pain manifestation with these drugs, it is important to administer adequate analgesia. The administration of corticosteroids has met with success in some cases.

Care Management

The care of the child with tetanus requires supportive management by the interprofessional team, with particular attention to airway and breathing. Respiratory status is carefully evaluated for any signs of distress, and appropriate emergency equipment is kept available at all times. The location, extent, and severity of muscle spasms are important nursing observations. Muscle relaxants, opioids, and sedatives that may be prescribed can also cause respiratory depression; therefore, the child should be assessed for excessive CNS depression. Attention to hydration and nutrition involves monitoring an IV infusion, monitoring nasogastric or gastrostomy feedings, and suctioning oropharyngeal secretions when indicated.

In caring for a child with tetanus during the acute phase, every effort should be made to control or eliminate stimulation from sound, light, and touch. Although a darkened room is ideal, sufficient light is essential so that the child can be carefully observed; light appears to be less irritating than vibratory or auditory stimuli. The infant or child is handled as little as possible, and extra effort is expended to avoid any sudden or loud noise to prevent seizures.

If a potent muscle relaxant such as vecuronium is used, the total paralysis makes oral communication impossible. The drug is not a sedative, however, and anxiety should be considered in children who are intubated. Therefore, all the child's needs must be anticipated and procedures carefully explained beforehand. Additional care is focused on preventing the complications associated with prolonged immobility, including decreased bowel and bladder tone and subsequent constipation, anorexia, DVT, pneumonia, and skin breakdown.

Because their mental status is clear, children are aware of what is happening to them and are often extremely anxious. They should not be left alone, and all efforts should be made to reduce anxiety, which can contribute to muscle spasms. Parents are encouraged to stay with the child to offer security and support. They also need support, information, and reassurance from the nurse.

BOTULISM

Botulism is an acute flaccid paralysis caused by the preformed toxin produced by the anaerobic bacillus *Clostridium botulinum*. In classic, or foodborne botulism, the most common source of the toxin is a contaminated food source. The disease has a wide variation in severity, from constipation to progressive sequential loss of neurologic function and respiratory failure. The most common source of the toxin is improperly sterilized home-canned foods. CNS symptoms appear abruptly approximately 12 to 36 hours after ingestion of contaminated food and may or may not be preceded by acute digestive disturbance (Box 49.12).

Human botulism is caused by neurotoxins A, B, E, and rarely F (American Academy of Pediatrics, Committee on Infectious Diseases, & Pickering, 2012). Types A and B are the most common causes of infant botulism. In addition to foodborne botulism, other forms include wound botulism; infant botulism; and artificial botulism, usually a result of bioterrorism.

Treatment consists of IV administration of botulism antitoxin and general supportive measures, primarily respiratory and nutritional. Toxins vary in protein-binding capacity. Some have a relatively short half-life and do not bind to tissues firmly; therefore, therapy is continued until paralysis subsides. Other toxins appear to bind irreversibly to nerve endings and are therefore not amenable to neutralization.

Infant Botulism

Infant botulism, unlike foodborne botulism in older people, is caused by ingestion of spores or vegetative cells of *C. botulinum* and the subsequent release of the toxin from organisms colonizing the GI tract. *C. botulinum* types A and B are the most common causative strains of infant botulism. This form of botulism has become more prevalent than any other form. Many cases of infant botulism occur in breastfed infants who are being introduced to nonhuman milk substances (American Academy of Pediatrics, Committee on Infectious Diseases, & Pickering, 2012). There appears to be no common food or drug source of the organisms; however, the *C. botulinum* organisms have been found in honey. Botulism may occur in infants as young as 1 week of age up to 12 months of age with a peak incidence between 2 and 4 months of age.

The severity of the disease varies widely, from mild constipation to progressive sequential loss of neurologic function and respiratory failure (see Box 49.12). The affected infant is usually well before the onset of symptoms. Constipation is a common presenting symptom, and almost all infants exhibit generalized weakness and a decrease in spontaneous movements. Deep tendon reflexes are usually diminished or absent. Cranial nerve deficits are common, as evidenced by loss of head control, difficulty in feeding, weak cry, and reduced gag reflex. SMA type 1 and metabolic disorders are often mistaken for infant botulism in the initial diagnostic phase because of the similarities in clinical manifestations of hypotonia, lethargy, and poor feeding (Arnon, 2016b). Presenting clinical signs also often mimic those of sepsis in young infants. Botulism toxin exerts its effect by inhibiting the release of acetylcholine at the myoneural junction, thereby impairing motor activity of muscles innervated by affected nerves.

Diagnosis is made on the basis of the clinical history, physical examination, and laboratory detection of the organism in the patient's stool and, less commonly, blood. However, isolation of the organism may take several days; therefore, suspicion of botulism by clinical presentation should require emergent treatment (Arnon, 2016b). EMG may be helpful in establishing the diagnosis; however, results may be normal early in the course of the illness.

Treatment consists of immediate administration of botulism immune globulin intravenously (BIG-IV) (Arnon, 2016b) without delaying for laboratory diagnosis. Early administration of BIG-IV neutralizes the toxin and stops the progression of the disease. The human-derived botulism antitoxin (BIG-IV) has been evaluated and is now available nationwide for use only in infant botulism. Infants treated with BIG-IV usually have a shortened hospital stay from approximately 6 weeks to 2 weeks, reportedly as a result of decreased requirements for mechanical ventilation and intensive care (Arnon, 2016b). Approximately 50% of affected infants require intubation and mechanical ventilation; therefore, respiratory support is crucial, as is nutritional support because theses infants are unable to feed. Trivalent equine botulinum antitoxin and bivalent antitoxin, used in adults and older children, are *not* administered to infants. Antibiotic therapy is not part of the management because the botulinum toxin is an intracellular molecule, and antibiotics would not be effective; aminoglycosides in particular should not be administered because they may potentiate the blocking effects of the neurotoxin (Arnon, 2016b).

The prognosis is generally good if the patient is adequately treated, although recovery may be slow, requiring a few weeks after severe illness. Untreated patients may require a longer hospitalization.

BOX 49.12 Clinical Manifestations of Botulism

General Signs	**Infant Botulism***
Weakness	Constipation (a common symptom)
Dizziness	Generalized weakness
Headache	Decrease in spontaneous movements
Difficulty talking and speaking	Diminished or absent deep tendon reflexes
Diplopia	Loss of head control
Vomiting	Poor feeding
Progressive, life-threatening respiratory paralysis	Weak cry
	Reduced gag reflex
	Progressive respiratory paralysis

*Most commonly diagnosed as "rule out sepsis" in the acute phase because of clinical presentation. Sometimes may be misdiagnosed as spinal muscular atrophy or metabolic disease.

> ## ! NURSING ALERT
>
> Although the precise source of *C. botulinum* spores has not been identified as originating from honey in many cases of infant botulism, it is still recommended that honey not be given to infants younger than 12 months of age because the spores have been found in honey (CDC, 2010).

Care Management

Nursing responsibilities include observing, recognizing, and reporting signs of poor feeding, constipation, and muscle impairment in the infant with botulism and providing intensive nursing care when an infant is hospitalized (see the "Care Management" section for the infant with SMA earlier in this chapter; also see Chapter 25). Parental support and reassurance are important. Most infants recover when the disorder is recognized and BIG-IV therapy is implemented. Nursing care of the infant on mechanical ventilation requires observation of oxygenation status and vigilance for any complications. Parents should be aware that during recovery, infants fatigue easily when muscular action is sustained. This has important implications for timing the resumption of feedings because of the risk for aspiration. Parents should also be advised that normal bowel activity may not return for several weeks. Therefore, a stool softener can be beneficial.

SPINAL CORD INJURIES

Spinal cord injuries (SCIs) with major neurologic involvement traditionally have not been a common cause of physical disability in children. However, many children with these injuries are admitted to major medical centers, and because of the increased survival rate as a result of improved management, nurses have an important role in the care and rehabilitation of children with SCI.

Mechanisms of Injury

The most common cause of serious spinal cord damage in children is trauma involving motor vehicle accidents (MVAs) (including automobile-bicycle, all-terrain vehicles, and snowmobiles), sports injuries (especially from diving, trampoline activities, gymnastics, and football), birth trauma, and nonaccidental trauma. MVAs accounted for 56% of SCIs in children, and adolescents and falls and firearm injury caused 14% and 9% of SCIs, respectively. The children injured (SCI) in MVAs were not properly restrained in 67.7% of the cases (Vitale, Goss, Matsumoto et al., 2006). The increased use of recreational activities involving motorized vehicles such as jet water skis, all-terrain vehicles, and motorcycles has also increased the incidence of SCIs in children. Congenital defects of the spine (e.g., myelomeningocele) also may in some cases produce the effects of SCI.

Transverse myelitis (inflammation of the spinal cord) may be caused by illness and has also been reported to develop from inadvertent intraarterial administration of long-acting penicillin injected into the buttocks. Damage can be extensive enough to result in paraplegia or even lower limb amputation.

In MVAs, most SCIs in children are a result of indirect trauma caused by sudden hyperflexion or hyperextension of the neck, often combined with a rotational force. Trauma to the spinal cord without evidence of vertebral fracture or dislocation (**spinal cord injury without radiographic abnormality [SCIWORA]**) is particularly likely to occur in an MVA when proper safety restraints are not used. An unrestrained child becomes a projectile during sudden deceleration and is subject to injury from contact with a variety of objects inside and outside the vehicle. Individuals who use only a lap seat belt restraint are at greater risk for SCI than those who use a combination lap and shoulder restraint. High cervical spine injuries have been reported in children younger than 2 years of age who are improperly restrained in forward-facing car seats. Infants who are improperly restrained in an infant car seat may experience cervical trauma in a car crash. Small children may also be severely injured by deploying front seat air bags.

Falling from heights occurs less often in children than in adults, but vertebral compression from blows to the head or buttocks can occur in water sports (diving and surfing), falls from horses, or other athletic activities. Birth injuries may occur in breech deliveries from traction force on the spinal cord during delivery of the head and shoulders. When shaken, infants commonly sustain cervical cord damage, as well as subdural hematoma and retinal hemorrhages; cognitive impairment and death may occur subsequent to the traumatic event. Infants have weak neck muscles, and during vigorous shaking, their large and heavy heads rapidly wobble back and forth. A significant number of adolescents receive SCIs secondary to gunshot wounds, stabbings, and other violent inflicted injury.

Because of the marked mobility of the neck, fracture or subluxation (partial dislocation) is the most common immediate cause of SCI, particularly in the lower cervical region. Although unusual in adults,

SCI without fracture is common in children, whose spines are suppler, weaker, and more mobile than those of adults. Therefore, the force is more easily dissipated over a larger number of segments. In infants and small children younger than 5 years of age, upper cervical spine fractures and spinal compression are more common, but adolescents tend to have lower cervical and thoracolumbar fracture dislocations (Pruitt & McMahon, 2016).

The severity of the force, the mechanisms of the injury, and the degree of the individual's muscular relaxation at the time of the injury greatly influence the extent of the trauma. SCIs are classified as either complete or incomplete. In a complete injury, there is no motor or sensory function more than three segments below the neurologic level of the injury (Mathison, Kadom, & Krug, 2008). Incomplete lesions have several typical characteristics (Mathison et al):

Central cord syndrome: Central gray matter destruction and preservation of peripheral tracts; tetraplegia with sacral sparing common; some motor recovery gained

Anterior cord syndrome: Complete motor and sensory loss with trunk and lower extremity proprioception and sensation of pressure

Posterior cord syndrome: Loss of sensation, pain, and proprioception with normal cord function, including motor function; able to move extremities but have difficulty controlling such movements

Brown-Séquard syndrome: Unilateral cord lesion with a motor deficit on the opposite side of the body from the primary insult; absence of pain and temperature sensation on the opposite side from the injury

Spinal cord concussion: Transient loss of neural function below the level of the acute spinal cord lesion, resulting in flaccid paralysis and loss of tendon, autonomic, and cutaneous reflex activity; may last hours to weeks

The ASIA Impairment Scale (Box 49.13) combines motor and sensory function and is used to determine the severity of impairment from the injury (complete or incomplete). It may also be used to measure neurologic changes and functional goals for rehabilitation (Mathison et al., 2008).

BOX 49.13 **American Spinal Injury Association Impairment Scale**

A—complete: No motor or sensory function is preserved in the sacral segments S4 to S5.

B—incomplete: Sensory but not motor function is preserved below the neurologic level and includes the sacral segments S4 to S5.

C—incomplete: Motor function is preserved below the neurologic level, and more than one-half of key muscles below the neurologic level have a muscle grade less than 3.

D—incomplete: Motor function is preserved below the neurologic level, and at least one-half of key muscles below the neurologic level have a muscle grade of 3 or more.

E—normal: Motor and sensory function are normal.

Clinical Syndromes (Optional)

Central cord
Brown-Séquard
Anterior cord
Conus medullaris
Cauda equina

Used with permission of American Spinal Injury Association. (2015). *Standard neurological classification of spinal cord injury.* Retrieved from www.asia-spinalinjury.org/wp-content/uploads/2016/02/International_Stds_Diagram_Worksheet.pdf.

The injury sustained can affect any of the spinal nerves, and the higher the injury, the more extensive the damage. The child can be left with complete or partial paralysis of the lower extremities (paraplegia) or with damage at a higher level and without functional use of any of the four extremities (tetraplegia). A high cervical cord injury that affects the phrenic nerve paralyzes the diaphragm and leaves the child dependent on mechanical ventilation.

A mild but equally frightening form of cord trauma is spinal cord compression, a temporary neural dysfunction without visible damage to the cord. Complete tetraplegia can result but initially may not be differentiated from serious cord injury.

Clinical Manifestations

It is often difficult to determine the extent and severity of damage at first. Immediate loss of function is caused by both anatomic and impaired physiologic function, and improved function may not be evident for weeks or even months. Manifestation of the initial response to acute SCI is flaccid paralysis below the level of the damage. This stage is often referred to as *spinal shock syndrome* and is caused by the sudden disruption of central and autonomic pathways. Local effects of cord edema and ischemia produce a physiologic transection with or without an anatomic severance. Most children with an SCI experience some spinal shock. Manifestations include the absence of reflexes at or below the cord lesion, with flaccidity or limpness of the involved muscles, loss of sensation and motor function, and autonomic dysfunction (symptoms of hypotension, low or high body temperature, loss of bladder and bowel control, and autonomic dysreflexia).

Autonomic paralysis also affects thermoregulatory functions. Afferent impulses from temperature receptors in the skin are not integrated; therefore, the patient is subject to temperature increases or decreases in response to alterations in environmental temperature. Hyperthermia can result from excessive ambient temperature, such as too many covers.

Except in the situations previously mentioned, flaccid paralysis is replaced by spinal reflex activity and increasing spasticity or, in incomplete lesions, greater or lesser degree of neurologic recovery.

The paralytic nature of autonomic function is replaced by autonomic dysreflexia, especially when the lesions are above the mid-thoracic level. This autonomic phenomenon is caused by visceral distention or irritation, particularly of the bowel or bladder. Sensory impulses are triggered and travel to the cord lesion, where they are blocked, which causes activation of sympathetic reflex action with disturbed central inhibitory control. Excessive sympathetic activity is manifested by a flushing face, sweating forehead, pupillary constriction, marked hypertension, headache, and bradycardia. The precipitating stimulus may be merely a full bladder or rectum or other internal or external sensory input. It can be a catastrophic event unless the irritation is relieved.

Additional clinical findings of SCI may include numbness, tingling, or burning; priapism; weakness; and loss of bowel and bladder control (Hayes & Arriola, 2005).

Neurogenic shock occurs as a result of a disruption in the descending sympathetic pathways with loss of vasomotor tone and sympathetic innervations to the cardiovascular system (Hayes & Arriola, 2005). Hypotension, bradycardia, and peripheral vasodilation occur as a result of neurogenic shock.

Children with suspected SCI may have suffered multiple injuries (e.g., head injury); therefore, multiple clinical manifestations may occur that may mask those of an SCI.

Therapeutic Management

Initial care begins at the scene of the accident with proper immobilization of the cervical, thoracic, and lumbar spine. Because of the complexity of these injuries, it is usually recommended that these patients be transported to a spinal injury center for care by specially trained health care professionals as soon as possible after the injury for appropriate diagnostic evaluation and intervention.

The initial management of the child with a suspected SCI should begin with an assessment of the ABCs—airway, breathing, and circulation. Guidelines for the child who is found unconscious with an unknown cause are discussed in Chapter 42. The airway should be opened using the jaw-thrust technique to minimize damage to the cervical spine. The child is monitored for cardiovascular instability, and measures are taken to support systemic blood pressure and maintain optimal cardiac output. Because MVA and other trauma in children may involve internal organ damage and potential bleeding, abdominal distention and other signs are acted on immediately to prevent further systemic shock. After the child is stabilized and transported to a regional trauma center, a thorough evaluation of neurologic status and any other associated trauma is carried out by the multidisciplinary team. In the emergency department, spinal immobilization should be maintained until a thorough neurologic assessment is completed; in children, this typically involves a CT scan and possibly an MRI. Additional interventions are discussed in the Care Management section.

The American Association of Neurological Surgeons and the Congress of Neurological Surgeons have published SCI management guidelines and standards of care for adult and pediatric patients with SCIs. Recently, evidence-based guidelines for the management of SCI in children were published (Rozelle, Aarabi, Dhall et al., 2013).

IV methylprednisone may be started within the first 12 hours after the injury to decrease inflammation and minimize further injury; however, its use in small children is controversial.

A number of progressive rehabilitation modalities have been developed in recent years that have the potential for increasing the quality of life for children with SCI. One treatment is functional electrical stimulation (FES), also referred to as *functional neuromuscular stimulation*, or *neuromuscular electrical stimulation (NMES)*. With this treatment, an electrical stimulator is surgically implanted under the skin in the abdomen, and electrode leads are tunneled to paralyzed leg muscles, enabling the child to sit, stand, and walk with the aid of crutches, a walker, or other orthoses. The stimulator can also be used to elicit a voluntary grasp and release with the hand. Before the latter can be accomplished, a number of surgical tendon transfers may be required for elbow extension, wrist extension, and finger and thumb flexion. In addition, FES has therapeutic benefits, which include increased muscle strength, improved gait function, and increased cardiovascular fitness (Thrasher & Popovic, 2008). Tendon transfers have been shown to be successful in enhancing hand and arm function, increasing pinch force, and facilitating independence in ADLs (Hosalkar, Pandya, Hsu et al., 2009). Restoration of hand and arm function enables children with SCI to perform self-catheterization and achieve greater independence in personal hygiene.

Exercise is considered an integral part of SCI rehabilitation; exercise may enhance neuroplasticity and decrease further muscle atrophy. Examples of exercise modalities in SCI patients include upper body strength training and hand cycling (Hosalkar et al., 2009).

Administration of pharmacologic agents such as clonidine hydrochloride may improve ambulation in patients with partial SCIs, and exercise therapy through interactive locomotor training has helped some individuals with SCI regain ambulatory function.

A number of orthoses or ambulation aids such as crutches may still be necessary to achieve upright mobility, yet as robotic technology advances, so do the chances for improved mobilization in children with SCI. Mechanical or robotic orthoses may be used in conjunction with FES to enable ambulation in patients with SCI (To, Kirsch, Kobetic et al., 2005). Gait training may be achieved with a number of different modalities, including a stationary cycle; however, no specific method has proved superior to the others. FES has also been effective in reducing complications from bladder and bowel incontinence and in assisting males in achieving penile erection.

Surgical interventions for SCI include early cord decompression (decompression laminectomy) and cervical or thoracic fusion. Crutchfield, Vinke, or Gardner-Wells tongs and skeletal traction may be used for early cervical vertebral stabilization. A halo vest may be suited for ambulation after the acute phase (see types of traction in Chapter 48). After cervical spinal fusion, a hard cervical collar or sterno-occipital-mandibular immobilizer brace may be worn until the fusion is solidified. When SCI occurs in young children and preteens, scoliosis develops over time and often requires surgical consideration (Parent, Mac-Thiong, Roy-Beaudry et al., 2011).

Care Management

The nursing care of the child affected by SCI is complex and challenging. An interprofessional care SCI team is equipped to manage the acute phase of the injury, and some members, including the nurse, may follow the patient to eventual recovery. Nursing management is concerned with ensuring adequate initial stabilization of the entire spinal column with a rigid cervical collar with supportive blocks on a rigid backboard. The traumatic event causing the injury may or may not be recalled if the child lost consciousness; such events are extremely frightening to the child. The immobilization process and the inability to move the extremities may also frighten the young child; therefore, it is important to reassure and comfort the child during this process.

During the acute phase of the injury, it is imperative that airway patency be ensured, complications prevented, and function maintained. Evaluate the extent of the neurologic damage early to establish a baseline for neurologic function. Continual assessment of sensory and motor function should occur to prevent further deterioration of neurologic status as a result of spinal cord edema. The ASIA Impairment Scale can be used to assess neurologic function on a routine basis during the patient's recovery. After the patient is admitted, further evaluation of his or her ability to perform ADLs and need for assistance during recovery can be made with the Functional Independence Measure Scale.

Nursing care during the acute phase should also focus on frequent monitoring of neurologic signs to determine any changes in neurologic function that require further intervention (e.g., level of consciousness using the Glasgow Coma Scale). In addition to airway maintenance, the nurse should monitor for changes in hemodynamic status that may require immediate medical attention. Neurogenic shock consists of hypotension, bradycardia, and vasodilation. Inotropic medications may be required to maintain adequate perfusion. Measuring urinary output and fluids administered closely monitors renal function. The child with a head injury may experience elevated intracranial pressure; therefore, changes in neurologic status are reported to the practitioner. Fluid restriction may be required if intracranial pressure is elevated, so fluid intake should be closely monitored.

The nursing care of the child with an SCI is, in most respects, the same as that of any immobilized child (see the "The Immobilized Child" section in Chapter 48). Additional aspects of care that should be addressed on an individual basis include hypercalcemia in adolescent boys, DVT, latex sensitization, pain, hypothermia and hyperthermia, spasticity, autonomic dysreflexia, and sleep-disordered breathing (Vogel, Betz, & Mulcahey, 2012).

Respiratory care often focuses on maintaining an adequate airway and effective ventilation. The child with a high-level cervical injury (C3 and above) requires continuous ventilatory assistance. In most instances, a tracheostomy is the method of choice for greater ease in clearing

secretions and for less trauma to tissues during long-term ventilatory dependence. In some children, breathing pacemaker devices (phrenic nerve stimulators) are implanted to stimulate the phrenic nerve and produce diaphragmatic contractions and lung expansion without assisted ventilation. In the child who does not require mechanical ventilation, special attention to clearance of secretions is vital because of decreased pulmonary function. In addition to percussion and postural drainage, the child may require a cough-assist device to clear secretions effectively (see the discussion of therapeutic management in the "Duchenne [Pseudohypertrophic] Muscular Dystrophy" section earlier in this chapter).

Temperature is often poorly regulated in children with SCI; therefore, body temperature must be monitored closely for fluctuations. Response to environmental temperature changes may be slow or absent, and the ability to dissipate heat through the process of shivering may be compromised.

Children with SCI have unique needs in relation to skin care. Because of decreased sensation and impaired mobility, they depend on others to assess and assist in the management of intact skin. Skin care practices are the same as those for any child who is immobilized. A skin score scale (e.g., the Braden Q Scale) should be used to objectively evaluate risks for skin breakdown and skin conditions (Noonan, Quigley & Curley, 2011). An alternating-pressure mattress or other pressure relief or reduction device is kept underneath the child, and the skin is thoroughly inspected at least once a day (or more often if there is increased risk) for signs of pressure and breakdown, especially over bony prominences.

Bowel and bladder function is often affected in the child with SCI. CIC may be required to regularly empty the neurogenic bladder and prevent urinary tract infections. A regular bowel management program is tailored to the child's needs.

Pain management is vital in children and adolescents with SCI. In children with upper motor neuron involvement, the spasticity that develops may require administration of an antispasmodic medication, such as diazepam. Baclofen is considered the drug of choice for reducing muscle spasticity. Gabapentin may be used to treat neuropathic pain. Botulinum toxin type A and α_2-adrenergic agonists may be used in older children with SCI to decrease muscle spasticity.

All adaptive devices help children increase their mobility, function, and endurance. Children with some lower extremity function progress to parallel bars and then to a walker; children with tetraplegia learn to

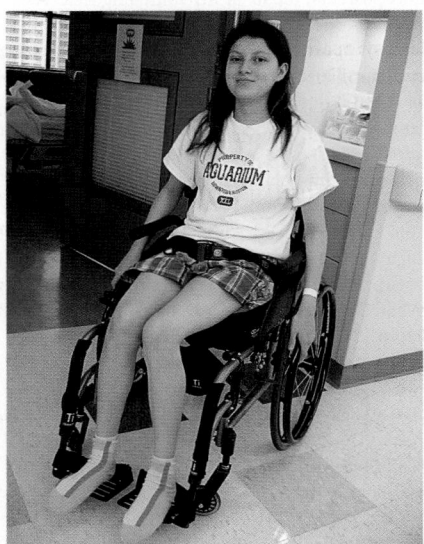

FIG 49.9 A wheelchair allows an adolescent mobility and independence. (Courtesy of Texas Children's Hospital, Houston, TX.)

use a wheelchair—among the most valuable aids available to children with SCIs (Fig. 49.9). The wheelchair should be selected carefully in relation to where it will be used, the architectural barriers, and the child's functional capacity. For children with severe upper extremity paralysis, a variety of motorized wheelchairs are used; however, the more complex they are, the greater their cost, weight, and tendency to break down. Wheelchair tolerance is gained over time and is accompanied by measures to prevent orthostatic hypotension and pressure ulcers.

A variety of orthoses and other appliances can be adapted for use by many children. The primary purpose of lower extremity bracing in children with SCIs is for ambulation.

During the recovery and rehabilitation phase, patients with SCI must be carefully monitored for complications of immobility such as DVT and pulmonary embolus. Children with high-level lesions are susceptible to the development of autonomic dysreflexia, which requires prompt action to prevent encephalopathy and shock. Clinical manifestations of autonomic dysreflexia include a drastic increase in systemic blood pressure, headache, bradycardia, profuse diaphoresis, cardiac arrhythmias, flushing, piloerection, blurred vision, nasal congestion, anxiety, spots on the visual field, or absent or minimum symptoms (Vogel, Hickey, Klaas et al., 2004).

The child and family with SCI are prepared by the interprofessional care team for the eventual discharge from the acute care facility to a rehabilitation center. The major aims of physical rehabilitation are to prepare the child and family to achieve normalization and resume life at home and in the community. Additional goals of rehabilitation in children with SCI are to promote independence in mobility and self-care skills, academic achievement, independent living, and employment.

The nurse is a crucial member of the health care team in relation to helping the family cope with the magnitude of the injury and disability, understand the extent of the disability, verbalize expected outcomes, and move toward eventual rehabilitation and normalization within the child's capabilities. The goals of rehabilitation include preparing the child and family to live at home and function as independently as possible.

REFERENCES

Adzick, N. S. (2013). Fetal surgery for spina bifida: Past, present, future. *Seminars in Pediatric Surgery, 22*(1), 10–17.

Adzick, N. S., Thom, E. A., Spong, C. Y., et al. (2011). A randomized trial of prenatal versus postnatal repair of myelomeningocele. *New England Journal of Medicine, 364*(11), 993–1104.

American Academy of Pediatrics, Committee on Infectious Diseases, & Pickering, L. (Eds.), (2012). *2012 red book: Report of the Committee on Infectious Diseases* (29th ed.). Elk Grove Village, IL: Author.

American Academy of Pediatrics Section on Cardiology and Cardiac Surgery. (2005). Cardiovascular health supervision for individuals affected by Duchenne or Becker muscular dystrophy. *Pediatrics, 116*(6), 1569–1573.

American College of Obstetrics and Gynecology Committee on Practice Bulletins. (2007). ACOG practice bulletin no. 77: Screening for fetal chromosomal abnormalities. *Obstetrics & Gynecology, 109*(1), 217–227.

Arnon, S. S. (2016a). Tetanus *(Clostridium tetani)*. In R. M. Kliegman, B. F. Stanton, J. W. St. Geme, et al. (Eds.), *Nelson textbook of pediatrics* (20th ed.). Philadelphia, PA: Saunders/Elsevier.

Arnon, S. S. (2016b). Anaerobic bacterial infections: botulism *(Clostridium botulinum)*. In R. M. Kliegman, B. F. Stanton, J. W. St. Geme, et al. (Eds.), *Nelson textbook of pediatrics* (20th ed.). Philadelphia, PA: Saunders/Elsevier.

Bach, J. R. (2007). Medical considerations of long-term survival of Werdnig-Hoffmann disease. *American Journal of Physical Medicine & Rehabilitation, 86*(5), 349–355.

Bach, J. R., & Martinez, D. (2011). Duchenne muscular dystrophy: Continuous noninvasive ventilatory support prolongs survival. *Respiratory Care, 56*(6), 744–750.

Battista, V. (2010). Muscular dystrophy, Duchenne. In P. L. Jackson, J. A. Vessey, & N. A. Schapiro (Eds.), *Primary care of the child with a chronic illness* (5th ed.). St. Louis, MO: Mosby/Elsevier.

Bax, M., Goldstein, M., Rosenbaum, P., et al. (2005). Proposed definition and classification of cerebral palsy. *Developmental Medicine & Child Neurology, 47*(8), 571–576.

Berker, A. N., & Yalçin, M. S. (2008). Cerebral palsy: Orthopedic aspects and rehabilitation. *Pediatric Clinics of North America, 55*(5), 1209–1225.

Béroud, C., Karliova, M., Bonnefont, J. P., et al. (2003). Prenatal diagnosis of spinal muscular atrophy by genetic analysis of circulating fetal cells. *Lancet, 361*(9362), 1013–1014.

Betz, C. L., Linroth, R., Butler, C., et al. (2010). Spina bifida: What we learned from consumers. *Pediatric Clinics of North America, 57*(4), 935–944.

Boitano, L. J. (2009). Equipment options for cough augmentation, ventilation, and noninvasive interfaces in neuromuscular respiratory management. *Pediatrics, 123*(4 suppl), S226–S230.

Bosanquet, M., Copeland, L., Ware, R., et al. (2013). A systematic review of tests to predict cerebral palsy in young children. *Developmental Medicine & Child Neurology, 55*(5), 418–426.

Bush, A., Fraser, J., Jardine, E., et al. (2005). Respiratory management of the infant with type 1 spinal muscular atrophy. *Archives of Disease in Childhood, 90*(7), 709–711.

Centers for Disease Control and Prevention. (2013). *Data and statistics for cerebral palsy: Prevalence and characteristics.* Retrieved from http://www.cdc.gov/NCBDDD/cp/data.html.

Centers for Disease Control and Prevention. (2011). Updated recommendation for use of tetanus toxoid, reduced diphtheria toxoid and acellular pertussis (Tdap) vaccine from the Advisory Committee on Immunization Practices, 2010. *Morbidity and Mortality Weekly Report, 60*(01), 13–15.

Centers for Disease Control and Prevention. (2010). *Botulism: General information: Frequently asked questions.* Retrieved from https://www.cdc.gov/botulism/prevention.html.

Centers for Disease Control and Prevention. (2009). Racial/ethnic differences in the birth prevalence of spina bifida—United States, 1995-2005. *Morbidity and Mortality Weekly Report, 57*(53), 1409–1413.

Centers for Disease Control and Prevention. (2007). Folate status in women of childbearing age, by race/ethnicity—United States, 1999-2000, 2001-2002, and 2003-2004. *Morbidity and Mortality Weekly Report, 55*(51-52), 1377–1380.

Dai, A. I., Wasay, M., & Awan, S. (2008). Botulinum toxin type A with oral baclofen versus oral tizanidine: A randomized pilot comparison in patients with cerebral palsy and equines foot deformity. *Journal of Child Neurology, 23*(12), 1464–1466.

Dicianno, B. E., Fairman, A. D., Juengst, S. B., et al. (2010). Using the spina bifida Life Course Model in clinical practice: An interdisciplinary approach. *Pediatric Clinics of North America, 57*(4), 945–957.

Doolin, E. (2006). Bowel management for patients with myelodysplasia. *Surgical Clinics of North America, 86*(2), 505–514.

Finder, J. D. (2009). A 2009 perspective on the 2004 American Thoracic Society statement, "respiratory care of the patient with Duchenne muscular dystrophy." *Pediatrics, 123*(4 suppl), S239–S241.

Finder, J. D., Birnkrant, D., Carl, J., et al. (2004). Respiratory care of the patient with Duchenne muscular dystrophy: ATS consensus statement. *American Journal of Respiratory and Critical Care Medicine, 170*(4), 456–465.

Golomb, M. R., Saha, C., Garg, B. P., et al. (2007). Association of cerebral palsy with other disabilities in children with perinatal arterial ischemic stroke. *Pediatric Neurology, 37*(4), 245–249.

Green, L., Greenberg, G. M., & Hurwitz, E. (2003). Primary care of children with cerebral palsy. *Clinics in Family Practice, 5*(2), 1–21.

Hack, M., & Costello, D. W. (2008). Trends in the rates of cerebral palsy associated with neonatal intensive care of preterm children. *Clinical Obstetrics and Gynecology, 51*(4), 763–774.

Hayes, J. S., & Arriola, T. (2005). Pediatric spinal injuries. *Pediatric Nursing, 31*(6), 464–467.

Hermansen, M. C., & Hermansen, M. G. (2006). Perinatal infections and cerebral palsy. *Clinics in Perinatology, 33*(2), 315–333.

Hirtz, D., Thurman, D. J., Gwinn-Hardy, K., et al. (2007). How common are the "common" neurological disorders? *Neurology, 68*(5), 326–337.

Hosalkar, H., Pandya, N. K., Hsu, J., et al. (2009). Specialty update: What's new in orthopaedic rehabilitation. *Journal of Bone and Joint Surgery (American), 91*(9), 2296–2310.

Hughes, R. (2008). The role of IVIG in autoimmune neuropathies: The latest evidence. *Journal of Neurology, 255*(3 suppl), 7–11.

Hughes, R. A., & Cornblath, D. R. (2005). Guillain-Barré syndrome. *Lancet, 366*(9497), 1653–1666.

Hughes, R. A., Swan, A. V., & van Doorn, P. A. (2012). Intravenous immunoglobulin for Guillain-Barré syndrome. *Cochrane Database of Systematic Reviews, 2012*(7), CD002063.

Hurtekant, K. M., & Spatz, D. L. (2007). Special considerations for breastfeeding the infant with spina bifida. *Journal of Perinatal & Neonatal Nursing, 21*(1), 69–75.

Iannaccone, S. T. (2007). Modern management of spinal muscular atrophy. *Journal of Child Neurology, 22*(8), 974–978.

Iannaccone, S. T., & Burghes, A. (2002). Spinal muscular atrophies. *Advances in Neurology, 88*, 83–98.

Jacobs, S. E., Berg, M., Hunt, R., et al. (2013). Cooling for newborns with hypoxic ischaemic encephalopathy. *Cochrane Database of Systematic Reviews, 2013*(1), CD003311.

Johnston, M. V. (2016). Cerebral palsy. In R. M. Kliegman, B. F. Stanton, J. W. St. Geme, et al. (Eds.), *Nelson textbook of pediatrics* (20th ed.). Philadelphia, PA: Saunders/Elsevier.

Johnston, M. V., Fatemi, A., Wilson, M. A., et al. (2011). Treatment advances in neonatal neuroprotection and neurointensive care. *Lancet Neurology, 10*(4), 372–382.

Kang, P. B., Morrison, L., Iannaccone, S. T., et al. (2015). Evidence-based guideline summary: Evaluation, diagnosis, and management of congenital muscular dystrophy. *Neurology, 84*(13), 1369–1378.

Kinsman, S. L., & Johnston, M. V. (2016). Myelomeningocele. In R. M. Kliegman, B. F. Stanton, J. W. St. Geme, et al. (Eds.), *Nelson textbook of pediatrics* (20th ed.). Philadelphia, PA: Saunders/Elsevier.

Krageloh-Mann, I., & Cans, C. (2009). Cerebral palsy update. *Brain & Development, 31*(7), 537–544.

Kravitz, R. M. (2009). Airway clearance in Duchenne muscular dystrophy. *Pediatrics, 123*(4 suppl), S231–S235.

Krigger, K. W. (2006). Cerebral palsy: An overview. *American Family Physician, 73*(1), 91–100, 101-102.

Lazzaretti, C. C., & Pearson, C. (2010). Myelodysplasia. In P. J. Allen & J. A. Vessey (Eds.), *Primary care of the child with a chronic condition* (5th ed.). St. Louis, MO: Mosby/Elsevier.

Liptak, G. S., & Dosa, N. P. (2010). Myelomeningocele. *Pediatrics in Review, 31*(11), 443–450.

Lovette, B. (2008). Safe transportation for children with special needs. *Journal of Pediatric Health Care, 22*(5), 323–328.

Lukban, M. B., Rosales, R. L., & Dressler, D. (2009). Effectiveness of botulinum toxin A for upper and lower limb spasticity in children with cerebral palsy: A summary of evidence. *Journal of Neural Transmission, 116*(3), 319–331.

Lundy, C., Lumsden, D., & Fairhurst, C. (2009). Treating complex movement disorders in children with cerebral palsy. *Ulster Medical Journal, 78*(3), 157–163.

Lunn, M. R., & Wang, C. H. (2008). Spinal muscular atrophy. *Lancet, 371*(9630), 2120–2133.

Lyons, R. (2008). Elusive belly pain and Guillain-Barré syndrome. *Journal of Pediatric Health Care, 22*(5), 310–314.

Manzur, A. Y., Kinali, M., & Muntoni, F. (2008). Update on the management of Duchenne muscular dystrophy. *Archives of Disease in Childhood, 93*(11), 986–990.

Manzur, A. Y., Kuntzer, T., Pike, M., et al. (2008). Glucocorticoid corticosteroids for Duchenne muscular dystrophy. *Cochrane Database of Systematic Reviews, 2008*(1), CD003725.

Mathison, D. J., Kadom, N., & Krug, S. E. (2008). Spinal cord injury in the pediatric patient. *Clinical Pediatric Emergency Medicine, 9*(2), 106–123.

Matthews, T. J. (2009). *Trends in spina bifida and anencephalus in the United States, 1991-2006.* Retrieved from http://www.cdc.gov/nchs/data/hestat/spine_anen/spine_anen.htm.

McKearnan, K. A., Kieckhefer, G. M., Engel, J. M., et al. (2004). Pain in children with cerebral palsy: A review. *Journal of Neuroscience Nursing, 36*(5), 252–259.

Miske, L. J., Hickey, E. M., Kolb, S. M., et al. (2004). Use of the mechanical in-exsufflator in pediatric patients with neuromuscular disease and impaired cough. *Chest, 125*(4), 1406–1412.

Moore, C., Kogan, B. A., & Parekh, A. (2004). Impact of urinary incontinence on self-concept in children with spina bifida. *Journal of Urology, 171*(4), 1659–1662.

Morton, R., Gray, N., & Vloeberghs, M. (2011). Controlled study of the effects of continuous intrathecal baclofen infusion in non-ambulant children with cerebral palsy. *Developmental Medicine & Child Neurology, 53*(8), 736–741.

Moster, D., Wilcox, A. J., Vollset, S. E., et al. (2010). Cerebral palsy among term and postterm births. *Journal of the American Medical Association, 304*(9), 976–982.

Motta, F., Antonello, C. E., & Stignani, C. (2011). Intrathecal baclofen and motor function in cerebral palsy. *Developmental Medicine & Child Neurology, 53*(5), 443–448.

Moxley, R. T., Ashwal, S., Pandya, S., et al. (2005). Practice parameter: Corticosteroid treatment of Duchenne dystrophy. *Neurology, 64*(1), 13–20.

National Institute of Neurologic Disorders and Stroke. (2015). *Cerebral palsy: Hope through research.* Retrieved from https://www.ninds.nih.gov/Disorders/Patient-Caregiver-Education/Hope-Through-Research/Cerebral-Palsy-Hope-Through-Research.

Nehring, W. M. (2010). Cerebral palsy. In P. L. Jackson, J. A. Vessey, & N. A. Schapiro (Eds.), *Primary care of the child with a chronic illness* (5th ed.). St. Louis, MO: Mosby/Elsevier.

Noonan, C., Quigley, S., & Curley, M. A. (2011). Using the Braden Q Scale to predict pressure ulcer risk in pediatric patients. *Journal of Pediatric Nursing, 26*(6), 566–575.

Nordmark, E., Josenby, A. L., Lagergren, J., et al. (2008). Long-term outcomes five years after selective dorsal rhizotomy. *BMC Pediatrics, 8*, 54.

Oskoui, M., Coutinho, F., Dykeman, J., et al. (2013). An update on the prevalence of cerebral palsy: A systematic review and meta-analysis. *Developmental Medicine & Child Neurology, 55*(6), 509–519.

Parent, S., Mac-Thiong, J. M., Roy-Beaudry, M., et al. (2011). Spinal cord in the pediatric population: A systematic review of the literature. *Journal of Neurotrauma, 28*(8), 1515–1524.

Quan, D. (2011). Muscular dystrophies and neurologic diseases that present as myopathy. *Rheumatic Disease Clinics of North America, 37*(2), 233–244.

Pruitt, D. W., & McMahon, M. A. (2016). Spinal cord injury and autonomic crisis management. In R. M. Kliegman, B. F. Stanton, J. W. St. Geme, et al. (Eds.), *Nelson textbook of pediatrics* (20th ed.). Philadelphia, PA: Saunders/Elsevier.

Rogers, B. (2004). Feeding method and health outcomes of children with cerebral palsy. *Journal of Pediatrics, 145*(2 suppl), S28–S32.

Rosenbaum, P., Paneth, N., Leviton, A., et al. (2007). A report: The definition and classification of cerebral palsy April 2006. *Developmental Medicine & Child Neurology Supplement, 109*, 8–14.

Rowe, D. E., & Jadhav, A. L. (2008). Care of the adolescent with spina bifida. *Pediatric Clinics of North America, 55*(6), 1359–1374.

Rozelle, C. J., Aarabi, B., Dhall, S. S., et al. (2013). Management of pediatric cervical spine and spinal cord injuries. *Neurosurgery, 72*(2 suppl), 205–226.

Russman, B. S., Buncher, C. R., White, M., et al. (1996). Function changes in spinal muscular atrophy II and III: The DCN/SMA Group. *Neurology, 47*(4), 973–976.

Russman, B. S., Iannaccone, S. T., Buncher, C. R., et al. (1992). Spinal muscular atrophy: New thoughts on the pathogenesis and classification schema. *Journal of Child Neurology, 7*(4), 347–353.

Samaniego, I. A. (2003). A sore spot in pediatrics: Risk factors for pressure ulcers. *Pediatric Nursing, 29*(4), 278–282.

Sarnat, H. B. (2016a). Spinal muscular atrophies. In R. M. Kliegman, B. F. Stanton, J. W. St. Geme, et al. (Eds.), *Nelson textbook of pediatrics* (20th ed.). Philadelphia, PA: Saunders/Elsevier.

Sarnat, H. B. (2016b). Muscular dystrophies. In R. M. Kliegman, B. F. Stanton, J. W. St. Geme, et al. (Eds.), *Nelson textbook of pediatrics* (20th ed.). Philadelphia, PA: Saunders/Elsevier.

Sarnat, H. B. (2016c). Guilain-Barre. In R. M. Kliegman, B. F. Stanton, J. W. St. Geme, et al. (Eds.), *Nelson textbook of pediatrics* (20th ed.). Philadelphia, PA: Saunders/Elsevier.

Sawyer, S. M., & Macnee, S. (2010). Transition to adult health care for adolescents with spina bifida: Research issues. *Developmental Disabilities Research Reviews, 16*(1), 60–65.

Schroth, M. K. (2009). Special considerations in the respiratory management of spinal muscular atrophy. *Pediatrics, 123*(4 suppl), S245–S249.

Shaer, C. M., Chescheir, N., & Schulkin, J. (2007). Myelomeningocele: A review of the epidemiology, genetics, risk factors for conception, prenatal diagnosis, and prognosis for affected individuals. *Obstetrical & Gynecological Survey, 62*(7), 471–479.

Shatrov, J. G., Birch, S. C., Lam, L. T., et al. (2010). Chorioamnionitis and cerebral palsy: A meta-analysis. *Obstetrics & Gynecology, 116*(2 pt 1), 387–392.

Simonds, A. K. (2006). Recent advances in respiratory care for neuromuscular disease. *Chest, 130*(6), 1879–1886.

Simpson, J. L., Richards, D. S., & Otano, L. (2012). Prenatal genetic diagnosis. In S. G. Gabbe, J. R. Niebyl, J. L. Simpson, et al. (Eds.), *Obstetrics: Normal and problem pregnancies* (6th ed.). Philadelphia, PA: Saunders/Elsevier.

Snodgrass, W. T., & Gargollo, P. C. (2010). Urologic care of the neurogenic bladder in children. *Urologic Clinics of North America, 37*(2), 207–214.

Tarcan, T., Onol, F. F., Ilker, Y., et al. (2006). The timing of primary neurosurgical repair significantly affects neurogenic bladder prognosis in children with myelomeningocele. *Journal of Urology, 176*(3), 1161–1165.

Thrasher, T. A., & Popovic, M. R. (2008). Functional electrical stimulation of walking: Function, exercise and rehabilitation. *Annales de Réadaptation et de Médecine Physique, 51*(6), 452–460.

To, C. S., Kirsch, R. F., Kobetic, R., et al. (2005). Simulation of a functional neuromuscular stimulation powered mechanical gait orthosis with coordinated joint locking. *IEEE Transactions on Neural Systems and Rehabilitation Engineering, 13*(2), 227–235.

Vitale, M. G., Goss, J. M., Matsumoto, H., et al. (2006). Epidemiology of pediatric spinal cord injury in the United States: Years 1997 and 2000. *Journal of Pediatric Orthopedics, 26*(6), 745–749.

Vogel, L. C., Betz, R. R., & Mulcahey, M. J. (2012). Spinal cord injuries in children and adolescents. *Handbook of Clinical Neurology, 109*(3), 131–148.

Vogel, L. C., Hickey, K. J., Klaas, S. J., et al. (2004). Unique issues in pediatric spinal cord injury. *Orthopaedic Nursing, 23*(5), 300–308.

Wadman, R. I., Bosboom, W. M., van der Pol, W. L., et al. (2012). Drug treatment for spinal muscular atrophy type I. *Cochrane Database of Systematic Reviews, 2004*(4), CD006281.

Wolff, T., Witkop, C. T., Miller, T., et al. (2009). Folic acid supplementation for the prevention of neural tube defects: An update of the evidence for the US Preventive Services Task Force. *Annals of Internal Medicine, 150*(9), 632–639.

Wright, P. A., Durham, S., Ewins, D. J., et al. (2012). Neuromuscular electrical stimulation for children with cerebral palsy: A review. *Archives of Disease in Childhood, 97*(4), 364–371.

Yeargin-Allsopp, M., Van Naarden Braun, K., Doernberg, N. S., et al. (2008). Prevalence of cerebral palsy in 8-year-old children in three areas of the United States in 2002: A multisite collaboration. *Pediatrics, 121*(3), 547–554.

Young, H. K., Lowe, A., Fitzgerald, D. A., et al. (2007). Outcome of noninvasive ventilation in children with neuromuscular disease. *Neurology, 68*(3), 198–201.

Pages followed by b, t, or f refer to boxes, tables, or figures, respectively.

Special Features

Special Features (cont'd)

FAMILY-CENTERED CARE

GUIDELINES

MEDICATION GUIDE